Chief Nurse: Anne Dabrow Woods, DNP, RN, CRNP, ANP-BC, AGACNP-BC, FAAN
Acquisitions Editor: Susan M. Hartman
Editor-in-Chief: Collette Bishop, RN, MS, MA, CIC
Clinical Project Manager: Janet Rader, RN, BSN
Clinical Editors: John Bodnar, RN, BSN, BS; Meghan Lynch, RN, BSN; Lisa Merenda, MSN, RN, CRRN;
Linda Lee Phelps, DNP, RN
Managing Editors: Carla A. Rudoy Vitale, PhD; Diane Labus; Ellen Sellers
Editors: Karen C. Comerford, Mary T. Durkin
Editorial Assistant: Linda K. Ruhf
Graphic Arts & Design Manager: Stephen Druding
Senior Production Associate: Bridgett Dougherty
Manufacturing Manager: Beth Welsh
Production Services: Aptara, Inc.

9 8 7 6 5 4 3 2 1
Printed in China

NDH44-010523
ISSN: 0273-320X
ISBN-13: 978-1-9751-9857-2
ISBN-10: 1-9751-9857-3

This work is provided "as is," and the publisher disclaims any and all warranties, express or implied, including any warranties as to accuracy, comprehensiveness, or currency of the content of this work.

This work is no substitute for individual patient assessment based upon health care professionals' examination of each patient and consideration of, among other things, age, weight, gender, current or prior medical conditions, medication history, laboratory data, and other factors unique to the patient. The publisher does not provide medical advice or guidance, and this work is merely a reference tool. Health care professionals, and not the publisher, are solely responsible for the use of this work, including all medical judgments and for any resulting diagnosis and treatments.

Given continuous, rapid advances in medical science and health information, independent professional verification of medical diagnoses, indications, appropriate pharmaceutical selections and dosages, and treatment options should be made and health care professionals should consult a variety of sources. When prescribing medication, health care professionals are advised to consult the product information sheet (the manufacturer's package insert) accompanying each drug to verify, among other things, conditions of use, warnings, and side effects and identify any changes in dosage schedule or contraindications, particularly if the medication to be administered is new, infrequently used, or has a narrow therapeutic range. To the maximum extent permitted under applicable law, no responsibility is assumed by the publisher for any injury and/or damage to persons or property, as a matter of products liability, negligence law or otherwise, or from any reference to or use by any person of this work.

shop.lww.com

CCS0323

S0-BSN-538

Includes only evidence-based off-label uses

Lists adverse reactions by body system

Indicates level of drug that can be reduced by dialysis

➤ **Acute ischemic stroke presenting 3 to 4.5 hours after symptom onset (Activase)** ◆
Adults: 0.9 mg/kg by IV infusion over 1 hour with 10% of total dose given as an initial IV bolus over 1 minute. Maximum total dose is 90 mg.

Route	Onset	Peak	Duration
PO	15 min	1 hr	6–12 hr
PO (extended-release)	15 min	6–12 hr	24 hr
IV	5 min	20 min	5–8 hr

Half-life: 3 to 10 hours.

CONTRAINDICATIONS & CAUTIONS
• Contraindicated in patients hypersensitive to drug or other beta blockers.
Dialyzable drug: Yes.
⚠ *Overdose S&S:* Bradycardia, nausea, hypotension, bronchospasm, HF, cardiac arrest, coma, AV block, vomiting.

Identifies known signs and symptoms of overdose

ADVERSE REACTIONS
CNS: fatigue, dizziness, depression, headache, insomnia, mental confusion, nightmares, short-term memory loss, hallucinations, vertigo, *stroke.* **CV:** hypotension, *bradycardia*, *HF*, edema, palpitations, Raynaud syndrome, cold extremity, first-degree AV block. **EENT:** blurred vision, tinnitus, rhinitis, dry mouth. **GI:** nausea, diarrhea, constipation, heartburn, flatulence, gastric pain, vomiting. **GU:** decreased libido, erectile dysfunction. **Respiratory:** dyspnea, wheezing, *bronchospasm.* **Skin:** rash, pruritus, gangrene (IV). **Other:** accidental injury.

PREGNANCY-LACTATION-REPRODUCTION
• There are no adequate studies during pregnancy. Drug crosses the placental barrier. Use during pregnancy only if clearly needed. Monitor fetal growth.
• Drug appears in human milk in very small quantities. Consider possible infant exposure with use during breastfeeding.

Highlights pregnancy, lactation, and reproduction concerns

NURSING CONSIDERATIONS
↻ *Alert:* Always check patient's apical pulse rate before giving drug. If it's slower than 60 beats/minute, withhold drug and contact prescriber immediately to verify dose.
• In patients with diabetes, monitor glucose level closely because drug masks common signs and symptoms of hypoglycemia.
• Monitor BP frequently; drug masks common signs and symptoms of shock.
• Beta blockers may mask tachycardia caused by hyperthyroidism. In patients with suspected thyrotoxicosis, taper off beta blocker to avoid thyroid storm.

Points out critical information that can't be overlooked

INTERACTIONS
Drug-drug. *Amiodarone:* May increase bradycardic effects. Monitor therapy.
Barbiturates: May reduce metoprolol effect. Monitor therapy.
Calcium channel blockers: May increase hypotensive effects. Monitor therapy.
Cardiac glycosides: May cause excessive bradycardia and increased depressant effect on myocardium. Use together cautiously.
Catecholamine-depleting drugs (MAO inhibitors): May have additive effect. Monitor patient for hypotension and bradycardia.
Clonidine: May increase risk of bradycardia. If clonidine and a beta blocker are coadministered, withdraw the beta blocker several days before the gradual withdrawal of clonidine.
CYP2D6 inhibitors (fluoxetine, paroxetine, propafenone, quinidine): May increase metoprolol level. Monitor vital signs carefully. Metoprolol dosage reduction may be needed.
Epinephrine: May blunt epinephrine effect during treatment of allergic reaction. Monitor therapy.
Hydralazine: May increase levels and effects of both drugs. Monitor patient closely.

Lists potential interactions with other drugs, herbs, and lifestyle factors

Boxed Warning When stopping long-term therapy, taper dosage over 1 to 2 weeks. Abrupt discontinuation may cause exacerbations of angina or MI. Don't discontinue therapy abruptly even in patients treated only for HTN. Restart metoprolol, at least temporarily, if angina markedly worsens or acute coronary insufficiency occurs. ■
• Beta selectivity is lost at higher doses. Watch for peripheral side effects.
• *Look alike–sound alike:* Don't confuse metoprolol succinate with metoprolol tartrate. Don't confuse metoprolol with metaproterenol, misoprostol, or metolazone. Don't confuse Toprol-XL with Topamax, Tegretol, or Tegretol-XR.

Easy-to-spot FDA boxed warnings

Identifies drugs with similar appearance or name

PATIENT TEACHING
• Instruct patient to take drug exactly as prescribed and with meals.
• Caution patient to avoid driving and other tasks requiring mental alertness until

Lists most important information patients should know

EFFECTS ON LAB TEST RESULTS
• May increase transaminase, ALP, and LDH levels.

Lists how results may be affected by taking drug

🍁Canada   ◇OTC   ◆Off-label use   ✐Photoguide   ⊜Do not crush   *Liquid contains alcohol   ▓Genetic

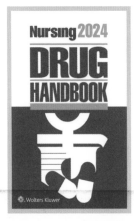

44TH EDITION

Nursing 2024

DRUG HANDBOOK®

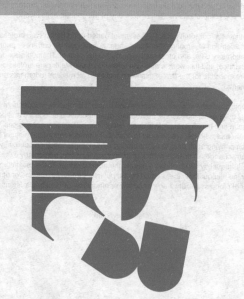

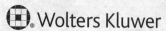 Wolters Kluwer

Philadelphia · Baltimore · New York · London
Buenos Aires · Hong Kong · Sydney · Tokyo

Contents

Contributors and consultants

Janine Barnaby, RPh, BCOP
Director, Outpatient Infusion Pharmacy
Lehigh Valley Health Network
Allentown, PA

David Bruch, BS, PharmD
Associate Lecturer
University of Wyoming–School of Pharmacy
Laramie, WY

Lawrence Carey, PharmD
Assistant Dean for Assessment,
    Accreditation, and Quality
Temple University School of Pharmacy
Philadelphia, PA

Jeffrey Cies, PharmD, MPH, BCPS-AQ ID, BCPPS,
    FCCP, FCCM, FPPA
Pharmacy Clinical Coordinator, Critical
    Care and Infectious Diseases
    Clinical Pharmacist
St. Christopher's Hospital for Children
Philadelphia, PA

Jason C. Cooper, PharmD
Clinical Specialist, MUSC Drug
    Information Center
Medical University of South Carolina
Charleston, SC

Lauren Falonk, PharmD
Pharmacist in Charge
Walgreens Pharmacy
Camden, NJ

Toshal Hallowell, PharmD
Pharmacist
Edward M. Kennedy Community
    Health Center
Worcester, MA

Rebecca Hoover, PharmD, MBA
Associate Professor
Idaho State University
Pocatello, ID

Jill Krabak, PharmD, BSPharm
Clinical Pharmacist
Justice Grown
Dickson City, PA

Chung-Shien Lee, PharmD, BCPS, BCOP
Associate Professor
St. John's University
Queens, NY

Celia Lu, PharmD, BCACP
Associate Professor–Industry Professional
St. John's University College of Pharmacy
    and Health Sciences
Queens, NY

Hannah McCaffery, PharmD
Manager, Pharmacy Regulations and
    Implementations
Health Partners Plans
Philadelphia, PA

Kimberly E. Ng, PharmD, BCPS
Associate Professor
St. John's University
Queens, NY

Michael N. Perza, PharmD, BCPS
Clinical Pharmacist
Christiana Care Health System
Newark, DE

Christine Price, PharmD
Clinical Coordinator/PGY1 Pharmacy
    Residency Director
Morton Plant Hospital
Clearwater, FL

Janet Rader, BSN, RN
Clinical Consultant
New Tripoli, PA

Melissa Rinaldi, PharmD
Clinical Pharmacist
Independence Blue Cross
Philadelphia, PA

Kerry Rinato, PharmD, BCPS
Clinical Pharmacist
Sunrise Hospital
Las Vegas, NV

Maha Saad, PharmD, BCGP, BCPS
Associate Clinical Professor
St. John's University College of Pharmacy
    and Health Sciences
Co-Director Drug Information Center
Long Island Jewish Medical Center—
    Northwell Health
Queens, NY

Michele F. Shepherd, PharmD, MS, BCPS, FASHP
Clinical Consultant
Jordan, MN

Michelle Smith, PharmD, BCPS
Clinical Consultant
Havre, MT

Maggie White-Jones, PharmD
Pharmacist
Walgreens Pharmacy
Berlin, MD

How to use *Nursing2024 Drug Handbook*®

The best-selling nursing drug guide for 44 years, *Nursing Drug Handbook* is meticulously reviewed and updated annually by pharmacists and nurses to include the most current, relevant information that practicing nurses and students need to know to administer medications safely in any health care setting. As in previous editions, *Nursing2024 Drug Handbook* emphasizes nursing and safety aspects of drug administration without attempting to replace detailed pharmacology texts. Only the most essential information is included, and helpful graphic symbols, logos, and highlighting draw special attention to critical details that can't be overlooked.

Outstanding features

The 44th edition provides a wealth of the latest drug information right at your fingertips:
• Tabbed "New Drugs" section–ensures quick access to 21 completely new drug monographs introduced in this edition
• Features the latest information on thousands of generic, brand, and combination drugs included in 690 comprehensive drug monographs and 27 appendices
• Drug safety always at the forefront–look for prominently displayed safety alerts, drug warnings, ISMP tall-man letters to help differentiate similarly spelled drug names, plus a special chapter on promoting safe drug administration—with updated guidelines on administering opioid analgesics, preventing and treating IV extravasation injury, safe handling of hazardous drugs, and best practices to ensure patient safety and reduce drug errors
• Special logos and symbols throughout to emphasize FDA boxed warnings, clinical alerts, new indications, necessary dosage adjustments, overdose signs and symptoms, off-label uses, drugs that shouldn't be crushed or chewed, over-the-counter drugs, biosimilar drugs, Canadian drugs, look alike–sound alike drugs, and the dialyzability status of each drug
• Genetic symbols pinpointing monographs and specific genetic-related information to help select and guide drug therapy
• Pregnancy-Lactation-Reproduction section in each monograph–captures all relevant information in one convenient place
• Key appendices reviewing prescription drug abuse, dangerous abbreviations to avoid, therapeutic monitoring guidelines, safe disposal of unused drugs, tumor lysis syndrome, serotonin syndrome, biosimilar drugs, and Canadian drug schedules and safe administration tools
• Thoroughly updated appendices containing indications and dosages of various classes and groupings of drugs–antidotes, antidiarrheals, ophthalmic drugs, laxatives, antacids, biologicals and blood derivatives, vaccines and toxoids, vitamins and minerals, common combination drugs, and less commonly used drugs
• Photoguide featuring 415 full-color, actual-sized tablets and capsules.

Introductory chapters

Chapter 1, "Drug actions, interactions, and reactions," explains how drugs work in the body. It provides a general overview of drug properties (absorption, distribution, metabolism, and excretion) and other significant factors affecting drug action (including protein binding, patient's age, underlying disease, dosage form, and route and timing of administration). Also discussed are drug interactions, adverse reactions, and toxic reactions. Chapter 2, "Drug therapy across the lifespan," discusses the danger associated with indiscriminate use of drugs during pregnancy and breastfeeding and the special precautions women should take when medications are necessary. This chapter also covers the unique challenges of giving drugs to children and older adults and offers practical suggestions on how to minimize problems with these special populations. Chapter 3, "Safe drug administration," explores the ongoing involvement of governmental and nongovernmental organizations weighing in on drug safety issues and the necessary measures nurses must take to prevent medication errors from occurring.

Chapter 4, "Selected therapeutic drug classifications," summarizes the indications, actions, and contraindications and cautions of more than 59 drug classes represented in *Nursing2024 Drug Handbook*. Generic drugs within each class are also listed, allowing nurses to quickly identify and compare similar drugs when patients can't tolerate or don't respond to a particular drug.

Drug monographs

Each generic drug monograph in *Nursing2024 Drug Handbook* includes the most pertinent clinical information nurses must know to administer medications safely, monitor for potential interactions and adverse effects, implement necessary care measures, and provide appropriate patient teaching. Entries are arranged alphabetically, with the generic drug name prominently displayed–along with its "tall man" lettering (if applicable), pronunciation, corresponding brand (or trade) names, therapeutic class, and pharmacologic class–on a shaded background for quick and easy identification. Banners or symbols to identify drugs that warrant a special safety alert, designate biosimilar drugs, or indicate drugs that appear in the color photoguide are also included in this highlighted area.

Specific information for each drug is then systematically organized under the headings below. Special icons and logos may be used throughout, as warranted, to point out the drug's safety concerns. For example, a clinical alert logo (🔔) provides important advice about life-threatening effects associated with the drug or its administration; a boxed warning (**Boxed Warning**) represents a specific warning issued by the FDA. A special icon (⬤) indicates oral drug forms that shouldn't be crushed or chewed. (See *Anatomy of a monograph*, on the inside book cover, for a visual guide to the various symbols that may appear within a drug entry.)

Available forms
This section lists the preparations available for each drug (for example, tablets, capsules, solutions for injection) and specifies available dosage forms and strengths. Dosage strengths specifically available in Canada are designated with a maple leaf (🍁). Preparations that may be obtained over the counter, without a prescription, are marked with an open diamond (◊). Liquid formulations that contain alcohol are indicated with an asterisk (*). Capsules or tablets that shouldn't be crushed are marked with a "Do Not Crush" symbol (⬤).

Indications & dosages
General dosage information for adults and children is found in this section. Dosage instructions reflect current trends in therapeutics and can't be considered absolute or universal. For individual patients, dosage instructions must be considered in light of the patient's condition.

Indications and dosages that aren't approved by the FDA are followed by a closed diamond (♦). It should be noted that only highly evidence-based off-label uses are included in this edition. An *Adjust-a-dose* logo appearing within this section indicates the need for a special dosage adjustment for certain patients, such as older adults or those with renal or hepatic impairment. In some cases, a dosage adjustment may apply to all patient populations for all of the indications listed; this is marked accordingly.

Administration
Here, readers will find guidelines for safely administering drugs by all applicable routes, including PO, IV, IM, subcut, ophthalmic, inhalational, topical, rectal, vaginal, transdermal, and buccal. A special screened background highlights IV administration guidelines (including specific instructions on how to reconstitute, mix, and store IV medications) and the major potential IV incompatibilities.

Action
This section succinctly describes the mechanism of action–that is, how the drug provides its therapeutic effect. For example, although all antihypertensives lower BP, they don't all do so by the same process. Also included, in table form, are the onset, peak (described in terms of effect or peak blood level), and duration of drug action for each route of administration, if data are available or applicable. Values listed are for patients with normal kidney function unless otherwise specified. The drug's half-life is also provided when known.

Adverse reactions
In this section, adverse reactions that are known to occur at a frequency of 1% or greater are listed according to body system. Life-threatening reactions appear in ***bold italic*** type.

Interactions
Within this section, readers can find each drug's confirmed, clinically significant interactions (additive effects, potentiated effects, and antagonistic effects) with other drugs, herbs, foods, beverages, and lifestyle behaviors (such as alcohol use, sun exposure, or smoking). Interactions with a rapid onset are highlighted in color; interactions with a delayed onset are in **bold** type.

Drug interactions are listed under the drug that's adversely affected. For example, because magnesium trisilicate, an antacid ingredient, interacts with tetracycline to decrease tetracycline's absorption, this interaction is listed under tetracycline. To check on the possible effects of using two or more drugs simultaneously, refer to the interactions section for each drug.

Effects on lab test results
This section lists increased and decreased levels, counts, and other values in lab test results that may be caused by the drug's systemic effects. It also indicates false-positive, false-negative, and otherwise altered results of lab tests a drug may cause.

Contraindications & cautions
This section outlines any conditions or special circumstances, such as diseases or conditions, in which use of the drug is undesirable or for which the drug should be given with caution. This section also contains information about whether or not the drug is dialyzable. When applicable, specific signs and symptoms of drug overdose are listed as the last bulleted item under this heading and highlighted by a special logo (⚠*Overdose S&S:*) for easy identification.

Pregnancy–lactation–reproduction
This section provides nurses with targeted, easy-to-understand safety information about each drug's use during pregnancy and breastfeeding. It also provides information about fertility effects, contraception recommendations, and enrollment information for registries that monitor drug safety during pregnancy.

Nursing considerations
Within this section, readers can find practical information on patient-monitoring techniques and suggestions for the prevention and treatment of adverse reactions as well as helpful tips on promoting patient comfort.

Patient teaching
Concise guidelines for explaining the drug's purpose, encouraging compliance, ensuring proper use and storage, and preventing or minimizing adverse reactions are included in this section.

Appendices and other helpful aids

Nursing2024 Drug Handbook includes 27 appendices that provide nurses and students with hands-on access to a wealth of supportive data and clinical information.

A handy visual "Quick guide to special symbols, logos, and highlighted terms" and "Guide to abbreviations" immediately follow this "How to use" piece.

Photoguide to tablets and capsules

To enhance patient safety and help make drug identification easier, *Nursing2024 Drug Handbook* offers a 32-page full-color photoguide to the most commonly prescribed tablets and capsules. Shown in actual size, the drugs are arranged alphabetically by generic name for quick reference followed by the brand names and their most common dosage strengths. Below the name of each drug is a cross-reference to where information on the drug can be found in the book. Brand names of drugs that appear in the photoguide are shown in text with a special capsule symbol (✔). Page references to the drug photos appear in boldface type in the index (for example, **C12**).

Photos for certain brands were provided by the following companies for use in this book: Novartis Pharmaceuticals (Enablex); Sepracor, Inc. (Lunesta); Teva Pharmaceuticals (Azilect); and Pfizer (Sutent). Additional photos were provided by Jeff Sigler of SFI Medical Publishing.

Lippincott NursingCenter®

Readers also have online access to a wealth of drug-related information at https://www.nursingcenter.com. Included are monthly FDA drug updates, drug warnings, and drug news abstracts. Also included are drug quizzes, best-practice medication safety guidelines, administration tips, real-life medication stories, CE tests, and so much more.

Quick guide to special symbols, logos, and highlighted terms

The following symbols or highlighted features appear throughout drug monographs and select appendices in this edition.

Special symbols and logos	Usage or meaning
SAFETY ALERT!	Drug that presents a heightened avoidable danger
BIOSIMILAR DRUG	FDA-approved biosimilar drug
buPROPion	"Tall man" lettering for FDA-designated generic drug names prone to mix-ups
▶	Indication for drug
✳ *NEW INDICATION:*	New indication for drug
Adjust-a-dose:	Dosage adjustment needed for certain populations
Adjust-a-dose (for all indications):	Dosage adjustment needed for all indications
⬲	Genetic considerations used to select and guide drug therapy
☾ *Alert:*	Clinical alert
✤	Available in Canada
◇	Over-the-counter (OTC)
◆	Off-label use
⬮	Appears in Photoguide
*	Liquid contains alcohol
DNC	Drugs that shouldn't be crushed or chewed
Look alike–sound alike:	Drugs with easily confused names
Boxed Warning	FDA boxed warning
⚠ *Overdose S&S:*	Overdose signs & symptoms
Highlighted reactions and interactions	
life-threatening	Life-threatening reaction
rapid onset	Causes interaction with rapid onset
delayed onset	Causes interaction with delayed onset

Guide to abbreviations

ACE	angiotensin-converting enzyme	CV	cardiovascular
		CVAD	central venous access device
ACS	acute coronary syndrome	D_5W	dextrose 5% in water
ADH	antidiuretic hormone	DEHP	di(2-ethylhexyl) phthalate
ADHD	attention deficit hyperactivity disorder	DIC	disseminated intravascular coagulation
ADLs	activities of daily living	dL	deciliter
ADP	adenosine 5′ diphosphate	DMARD	disease-modifying antirheumatic drug
AEDs	antiepileptic drugs		
AIDS	acquired immunodeficiency syndrome	DNA	deoxyribonucleic acid
		DPP-4	dipeptidyl peptidase-4
ALP	alkaline phosphatase	DRESS	drug reaction with eosinophilia and systemic symptoms
ALS	amyotrophic lateral sclerosis		
ALT	alanine transaminase		
ANA	antinuclear antibody	DVT	deep vein thrombosis
ANC	absolute neutrophil count	ECG	electrocardiogram
ARB	angiotensin receptor blocker	EEG	electroencephalogram
ARDS	acute respiratory distress syndrome	EENT	eyes, ears, nose, throat
		eGFR	estimated glomerular filtration rate
AST	aspartate transaminase		
AUC	area under the curve	ESRD	end-stage renal disease
AV	atrioventricular	ET	endotracheal
BCRP	breast cancer resistance protein	FDA	Food and Drug Administration
b.i.d.	twice daily	FSH	follicle-stimulating hormone
BMI	body mass index	5-FU	fluorouracil
BP	blood pressure	G	gauge
BPH	benign prostatic hypertrophy	g	gram
BSA	body surface area	G6PD	glucose-6-phosphate dehydrogenase
BUN	blood urea nitrogen		
CABG	coronary artery bypass graft	GABA	gamma-aminobutyric acid
CAD	coronary artery disease	G-CSF	granulocyte colony-stimulating factor
cAMP	cyclic 3′, 5′ adenosine monophosphate		
		GERD	gastroesophageal reflux disease
CBC	complete blood count		
CDAD	*Clostridioides difficile*–associated diarrhea	GFR	glomerular filtration rate
		GGT	gamma-glutamyltransferase
CDC	Centers for Disease Control and Prevention	GI	gastrointestinal
		GnRH	gonadotropin-releasing hormone
CK	creatine kinase		
CMV	cytomegalovirus	GU	genitourinary
CNS	central nervous system	GVHD	graft-versus-host disease
COPD	chronic obstructive pulmonary disease	H_1	histamine_1
		H_2	histamine_2
CrCl	creatinine clearance	Hb	hemoglobin
CSF	cerebrospinal fluid	HbA_1c	glycosylated hemoglobin
CT	computed tomography	HBsAg	hepatitis B virus surface antigen
CTCAE	Common Terminology Criteria for Adverse Events		
		HBV	hepatitis B virus

HCV	hepatitis C virus	MS	multiple sclerosis
HDL	high-density lipoprotein	msec	millisecond
HER2	human epidermal growth factor receptor 2	MUGA	multigated acquisition scan
HF	heart failure	NG	nasogastric
HIV	human immunodeficiency virus	NMS	neuroleptic malignant syndrome
HMG-CoA	3-hydroxy-3-methyl-glutaryl coenzyme A	NNRTI	non-nucleoside reverse transcriptase inhibitor
HPA	hypothalamic-pituitary-adrenal	NRTI	nucleoside reverse transcriptase inhibitor
HR	heart rate	NSAID	nonsteroidal anti-inflammatory drug
HTN	hypertension		
IBS	irritable bowel syndrome	NSCLC	non-small-cell lung cancer
ICP	intracranial pressure	NSS	normal (0.9%) saline solution
ICU	intensive care unit	NYHA	New York Heart Association
ID	intradermal	OCD	obsessive-compulsive disorder
Ig	immunoglobulin	ODT	orally disintegrating tablet
ILD	interstitial lung disease	OTC	over-the-counter
IM	intramuscular	oz	ounce
INR	International Normalized Ratio	PABA	para-aminobenzoic acid
		PAH	pulmonary arterial hypertension
IOP	intraocular pressure	PCA	patient-controlled analgesia
IPPB	intermittent positive-pressure breathing	PCI	percutaneous coronary intervention
ITP	immune thrombocytopenia	PDE5	phosphodiesterase type 5
IV	intravenous	PE	pulmonary embolus
kg	kilogram	P-gp	P-glycoprotein
L	liter	PML	progressive multifocal leukoencephalopathy
LABA	long-acting beta-agonist		
lb	pound	PO	by mouth
LDH	lactate dehydrogenase	PPI	proton pump inhibitor
LDL	low-density lipoprotein	PR	by rectum
LFTs	liver function tests	PRES	posterior reversible encephalopathy syndrome
LH	luteinizing hormone		
LVEF	left ventricular ejection fraction	PRN	as needed
		PSA	prostate-specific antigen
M	molar	PT	prothrombin time
m^2	square meter	PTCA	percutaneous transluminal coronary angioplasty
MAC	*Mycobacterium avium* complex		
		PTSD	posttraumatic stress disorder
MAO	monoamine oxidase	PTT	partial thromboplastin time
mcg	microgram	PVC	premature ventricular contraction
mEq	milliequivalent		
mg	milligram		
MI	myocardial infarction	PVD	peripheral vascular disease
min	minute	q.i.d.	four times daily
mL	milliliter	RA	rheumatoid arthritis
mm^3	cubic millimeter	RAAS	renin-angiotensin-aldosterone system
mo	month		
MRI	magnetic resonance imaging	RBC	red blood cell
MRSA	methicillin-resistant *Staphylococcus aureus*	RDA	recommended daily allowance
		REM	rapid eye movement

REMS	risk evaluation and mitigation strategy	T_4	thyroxine
		TB	tuberculosis
RNA	ribonucleic acid	TCA	tricyclic antidepressant
RSV	respiratory syncytial virus	TEN	toxic epidermal necrolysis
SA	sinoatrial	TIA	transient ischemic attack
SCAR	severe cutaneous adverse reaction	t.i.d.	three times daily
		TLS	tumor lysis syndrome
sec	second	TNF	tumor necrosis factor
SIADH	syndrome of inappropriate antidiuretic hormone	TPN	total parenteral nutrition
		TSH	thyroid-stimulating hormone
SJS	Stevens-Johnson syndrome	tsp	teaspoon
SL	sublingual	ULN	upper limit of normal
SLE	systemic lupus erythematosus	URI	upper respiratory infection
SSNRI	selective serotonin and norepinephrine reuptake inhibitor	USP	United States Pharmacopeia
		UTI	urinary tract infection
		UV	ultraviolet
SSRI	selective serotonin reuptake inhibitor	VLDL	very low density lipoprotein
		WBC	white blood cell
subcut	subcutaneous	WHO	World Health Organization
T_3	triiodothyronine	wk	week

1

Drug actions, interactions, and reactions

Any drug a patient takes causes a series of physical and chemical events in the body. The first event, when a drug combines with cellular drug receptors, is the *drug's mechanism of action*. What happens next is the *drug effect*. Depending on the type of cellular drug receptors affected by a given drug, an effect can be local, systemic, or both. A systemic drug effect can follow a local effect. For example, when you apply a drug to the skin, it causes a local effect. But transdermal absorption of that drug can also produce a systemic effect. A local effect can also follow systemic absorption. For example, the peptic ulcer drug cimetidine produces a local effect after it's swallowed by blocking histamine receptors in the stomach's parietal cells. Diphenhydramine, on the other hand, causes a systemic effect by blocking histamine receptors throughout the body.

Drug properties
Drug absorption, distribution, metabolism, and excretion make up a drug's pharmacokinetics. These processes determine a drug's onset of action, peak concentration, duration of action, and bioavailability.

Absorption
Before a drug can act in the body, it must be absorbed into the bloodstream—usually after oral administration, the most common route. Before an oral drug can be absorbed, it must disintegrate into particles small enough to dissolve in GI secretions. Only after dissolving can the drug be absorbed. Most absorption of orally given drugs occurs in the small intestine because the mucosal villi provide extensive surface area. Once absorbed and circulated in the bloodstream, the drug is *bioavailable*, or ready to exert its action and produce a drug effect. The speed of absorption and whether absorption is complete or partial depend on the drug's effects, dosage form, administration route, interactions with other substances in the GI tract such as other drugs and food, and various patient characteristics. Oral solutions and syrups bypass the need for disintegration and dissolution and are usually absorbed faster than solid dosage forms. Some tablets have enteric coatings to prevent disintegration in the acidic environment of the stomach; others have coatings of varying thicknesses that simply delay release of the drug.

Drugs given IM must first be absorbed through the muscle into the bloodstream. Rectal suppositories must dissolve to be absorbed through the rectal mucosa. Drugs given IV are injected directly into the bloodstream and are bioavailable completely and immediately.

Distribution
After absorption, a drug moves from the bloodstream into the fluids and tissues in the body, a movement known as *distribution*. The volume into which a drug is distributed throughout the body is known as the *volume of distribution*. Individual patient variations can change the amount of drug distributed throughout the body. For example, in a patient with edema, a given dose is distributed into a larger volume than in a patient without edema. Occasionally, a dose is increased to account for this difference. In this case, the dose should be decreased after the edema is corrected. Conversely, a dose given to a patient with dehydration may need to be decreased to allow for its distribution into a much smaller volume. Patients who are very obese may present another problem when considering drug distribution. Some drugs—such as digoxin, gentamicin, and tobramycin—aren't well-distributed into fatty tissue. Sometimes, doses based on actual body weight may lead to overdose and serious toxicity. In these cases, doses must be based on ideal body weight, or adjusted body weight, which may be estimated from mathematical formulas or actuarial tables that give an average weight range for height.

Metabolism
Most drugs are metabolized in the liver. Hepatic diseases may affect the liver's metabolic functions and may increase or decrease a drug's usual metabolism. Closely monitor all patients with hepatic disease for drug effect and toxicity.

The rate at which a drug is metabolized varies from person to person. Some patients metabolize drugs so quickly that the drug levels in their blood and tissues prove therapeutically inadequate. In other patients, the rate of metabolism is so slow that ordinary doses can produce toxicity or prolonged duration of action. Specific genetic tests can be performed to determine whether a patient metabolizes drugs slowly or quickly.

Excretion

The body eliminates drugs by metabolism (usually hepatic) and excretion (usually renal). *Drug excretion* is the movement of a drug or its metabolites from the tissues back into circulation and from the circulation into the organs of excretion, where they're removed from the body. Most drugs are excreted by the kidneys, but some can be eliminated through the lungs, exocrine (sweat, salivary, or mammary) glands, liver, skin, or intestinal tract. Drugs also may be removed artificially by direct mechanical intervention, such as peritoneal dialysis or hemodialysis.

Other modifying factors

One important factor influencing a drug's action and effect is its tendency to bind to plasma proteins, especially albumin, and other tissue components. Because only a free, unbound drug molecule can act in the body, protein binding greatly influences the degree and duration of a drug's effect. Malnutrition, renal failure, and the presence of other protein-bound drugs can influence protein binding. When protein-binding behavior changes, the drug dosage may need to be adjusted accordingly.

The patient's age is another important factor. Older adults usually have decreased hepatic function, less muscle mass, diminished renal function, and lower albumin levels. These patients may need lower doses and sometimes longer dosage intervals to avoid toxicity. Neonates have underdeveloped metabolic enzyme systems and inadequate renal function, so they need highly individualized dosages and careful monitoring.

Underlying disease also may affect drug action and effect. For example, acidosis may cause insulin resistance. Genetic diseases, such as G6PD deficiency and hepatic porphyria, may turn drugs into toxins, with serious consequences. Patients with G6PD deficiency may develop hemolytic anemia when given certain drugs, such as sulfonamides. A patient with genetic susceptibility can develop acute porphyria if given a barbiturate. A patient with a highly active hepatic enzyme system can develop hepatitis when treated with isoniazid because of the quick intrahepatic buildup of a toxic metabolite.

Drug administration issues

The dosage form of a drug is important because it can also influence the drug's action in the body. Some tablets and capsules are too large to be easily swallowed by patients who are sick. An oral solution may be substituted, but it may produce higher drug levels than a tablet because the liquid is more easily and completely absorbed. When a potentially toxic drug (such as digoxin) is given in the liquid form, its increased absorption can cause toxicity. Sometimes a change in dosage form also requires a change in dosage.

Routes of administration aren't always interchangeable. For example, diazepam is readily absorbed PO but is slowly and erratically absorbed IM. On the other hand, gentamicin must be given parenterally because oral administration results in drug levels too low to effectively treat systemic infections.

Improper storage can alter a drug's potency. Most drugs must be stored in tight containers protected from direct sunlight and extremes in temperature and humidity that can cause them to deteriorate. Some drugs require special storage conditions, such as refrigeration. Patients should be cautioned not to store drugs in a bathroom because of the constantly changing environment.

The timing of drug administration can be important. Sometimes, giving an oral drug during, shortly before, or after a meal changes the amount of drug absorbed. Sometimes, the presence of food in the GI tract may be desirable to increase absorption (such as with rivaroxaban) or to increase tolerability (such as with aspirin or other irritating drugs). But penicillins and tetracyclines shouldn't be taken at mealtimes because certain foods can inactivate them. If in doubt about the effect of food on a certain drug, the nurse should check with a pharmacist.

The nurse should always document the patient's age, actual height, and actual weight (in kg). Patient "stated" or "reported" weights aren't appropriate for dosing medications. The prescriber and pharmacist will need this information to be as accurate as possible when calculating the dosage for many drugs. It's especially important to record daily weights of patients who require intensive care, neonates, and infants because their weights can change frequently. Children and patients who are critically ill should always be weighed because most medications given to these patients are weight-based. The patient's medical record should also include all current lab data, especially results of renal and liver function studies, so the prescriber and pharmacist can adjust the dosage as needed.

The nurse should also watch for metabolic and physiologic changes (such as depressed respiratory function, acidosis, or alkalosis) that might alter drug effect.

The nurse should obtain a comprehensive family history from the patient or family, asking about past reactions to drugs, possible genetic traits that might affect drug response, and current use of other prescription and OTC drugs, illicit drugs, herbal supplements, and vitamin supplements. Multiple drug therapies can cause serious and fatal drug interactions and can dramatically change many drugs' effects.

Drug interactions

A *drug interaction* occurs when a drug given concomitantly with another drug alters the effect of either or both drugs. Usually the effect of one drug is increased or decreased. For instance, one drug may inhibit or stimulate the metabolism or excretion of the other or free it for further action by displacing the drug from protein-binding sites.

Combination therapy is based on drug interactions. One drug may be given to complement, enhance, or protect the effects of another. For example, imipenem and cilastatin are given together because cilastatin inhibits a renal enzyme that would degrade imipenem. In many cases, two drugs with similar actions are given together precisely because of the additive effect. For instance, acetaminophen and codeine are commonly given in combination because together they provide greater pain relief than if either is given alone.

Drug interactions are sometimes used to prevent or antagonize certain adverse reactions. The diuretics hydrochlorothiazide and spironolactone are often given together because the former is potassium-depleting and the latter potassium-sparing.

Not all drug interactions are beneficial. Many drugs interact to decrease efficacy or increase toxicity. An example of decreased efficacy occurs when a tetracycline is given with drugs or foods that contain calcium or magnesium (such as antacids or milk). These bind with tetracycline in the GI tract and cause inadequate drug absorption. An example of increased toxicity can be seen in a patient taking an NSAID and an anticoagulant such as warfarin. This combination of drugs increases the risk of GI bleeding. Avoid drug combinations that produce these effects, if possible.

Sometimes drug interactions occur after a drug that inhibits or increases the metabolism of another drug has been discontinued. After the drug is discontinued, the other drug's levels may increase or decrease, so the dosage may need adjustment.

Adverse reactions

Drugs cause adverse *effects;* patients have adverse *reactions.* An adverse reaction may be tolerated to obtain a therapeutic effect, or it may be hazardous and unacceptable. Some adverse reactions subside with continued use. For example, the drowsiness caused by paroxetine and the orthostatic hypotension caused by prazosin usually subside after several days, when the patient develops tolerance. But many adverse reactions are dose related and lessen or disappear only if the dosage is reduced. Most adverse reactions aren't therapeutically desirable, but a few can be put to clinical use. An example of this is the drowsiness caused by diphenhydramine, which makes it useful as a mild sedative.

Common Terminology Criteria for Adverse Events are standardized definitions that describe adverse events that may occur in the course of cancer therapy. An *adverse event* is considered any event that's unfavorable or that has an unfavorable outcome to a patient due to a medication and not to the underlying condition of the patient. (See *Common Terminology Criteria for Adverse Events*, page 4.)

Drug hypersensitivity, or drug allergy, is the result of an antigen–antibody immune reaction that occurs in the body when a drug is given to a patient who is susceptible. Signs and symptoms of a drug allergy may include rash, itching, angioedema, or shortness of breath. One of the most dangerous of all drug hypersensitivities is anaphylaxis. In its most severe form, anaphylaxis can rapidly become fatal. (See Appendix 15, *Anaphylaxis.*)

Rarely, idiosyncratic reactions occur. These reactions are highly unpredictable and unusual. One of the best known idiosyncratic adverse reactions is aspirin-induced asthma, which may be life-threatening. A more common idiosyncratic reaction is extreme sensitivity to very low doses of a drug or insensitivity to higher-than-normal doses.

To manage adverse reactions correctly, you need to be aware of changes in the patient's clinical condition, even subtle ones. Such changes may be an early warning of impending toxicity. Listen to the patient's complaints about reactions to a drug, and consider each objectively. You may be able to reduce adverse reactions in several ways. Dosage reduction can help. But, in many cases, so does a simple rescheduling of the dose. For example, the CNS stimulation that pseudoephedrine may produce may be managed if it's given early in the day rather than at bedtime. Similarly, drowsiness from antihistamines or tranquilizers can be less important if these drugs are given at bedtime. Most importantly, your patient needs to be told which adverse reactions to expect so that the patient won't become worried or even decide to stop taking the drug. Always advise the patient to report all adverse reactions to the prescriber, and teach the patient which adverse reactions must be reported immediately.

Your ability to recognize signs and symptoms of drug allergies or serious idiosyncratic reactions may save your patient's life. Ask each patient about the drugs currently being taken or those taken in the past and whether any unusual reactions occurred while taking them. If a patient claims to be allergic to a drug, ask for specific examples of what the patient experienced after taking the drug. The patient may be calling a harmless adverse reaction such as upset stomach an allergic reaction or may have a true history of anaphylaxis. In either case, you and the prescriber need to be aware of the reaction. Record and report clinical changes throughout the patient's course of treatment. If you suspect a severe adverse reaction, withhold the drug until you can check with a pharmacist and the prescriber.

Toxic reactions

Chronic drug toxicities are usually caused by the cumulative effect and resulting buildup of the drug in the body. These effects may be undesired extensions of the desired therapeutic effect. For example, standard doses of glyburide normalize the blood glucose level, but higher doses can produce hypoglycemia.

Drug toxicities may also occur when a drug level rises as a result of impaired metabolism or excretion. For example, hepatic dysfunction impairs the metabolism of amiodarone, raising its concentration in the blood. Similarly, renal dysfunction may cause digoxin toxicity because this drug is eliminated by the kidneys. Excessive dosage can also cause toxic levels. For instance, tinnitus is usually a sign that the safe dose of aspirin has been exceeded.

Many drug toxicities are predictable, dosage-related, and reversible upon dosage adjustment or discontinuation. Monitor patients carefully for physiologic changes that might alter drug effect. Watch especially for hepatic and renal impairment. Warn the patient about signs of impending toxicity and tell the patient what to do if a toxic reaction occurs. Also, make sure to emphasize the importance of taking a drug exactly as prescribed. Warn the patient that serious problems could arise if the patient changes the dose or schedule or stops taking the drug without the prescriber's knowledge.

Pharmacogenetics

Prescribers typically follow a standardized approach to prescribing drugs. Although decisions are made based on evidence-based approaches and with the best of intentions, some result in the development of adverse drug reactions. It would be helpful to be able to accurately predict which patients will (and which will not) respond and to what degree when prescribed a certain drug. Pharmacogenetics—the study of how varied responses to a drug can be caused by genetic differences between individuals—attempts to do just this.

The first pharmacogenetic detection occurred when Pythagoras recognized the dangers of ingesting fava beans in 510 B.C., which eventually led to the discovery of G6PD in 1956. Shortly after, the term *pharmacogenetics* was coined and later defined as the study of variability in drug response due to heredity. The goals of pharmacogenetics include identification of innovative drug targets, consideration of DNA sequence variation on drug effects, development of new agents, and optimization of drug efficacy while minimizing drug toxicity.

Pharmacogenetics considers the existence of *polymorphisms*, which are genetic variations that occur in 1% or more of the population. If clinicians are able to predict which patients express polymorphisms, they can provide targeted therapy. Researchers have learned that many polymorphisms involve cytochrome P450 (CYP450) isoenzymes.

Polymorphisms play a significant role in determining whether a drug will be predictably metabolized. Patients fall into one of four classes of metabolizers: extensive, ultrarapid, intermediate, and poor. Patients considered extensive metabolizers possess an overwhelming capacity to metabolize certain drugs and may exhibit therapeutic failure, whereas patients who are poor metabolizers, such as those with G6PD deficiency, exhibit toxicities due to their inability to metabolize certain drugs. Ethnicity may also play a role in determining how patients are classified in regard to metabolism.

It's vital to recognize the importance of the CYP450 system. Approximately 60 CYP enzymes are found in humans, and many genes that encode for these enzymes are polymorphic. Polymorphism associated with CYP enzymes may be expressed via amino acid substitution (thereby reducing enzymatic activity) or by amplification or duplication of activity (thereby increasing enzymatic activity). It's thought that approximately one-third of all medications prescribed today are metabolized by CYP450, including TCAs, antiarrhythmics, beta-receptor antagonists, codeine, warfarin, phenytoin, and nicotine.

In addition, enzymes that metabolize cancer chemotherapy drugs, such as thiopurine S-methyltransferase, dihydropyrimidine dehydrogenase, and UDP-glucuronosyl transferase, can have therapeutic implications; for example, polymorphisms affecting these enzymes can result in serious adverse reactions, such as anemia and neurotoxicity. Finally, miscellaneous polymorphisms affecting drug transport proteins such as P-gp may affect drug response. P-gp acts as a safety mechanism to remove toxins from cells and has a role in the distribution of cancer chemotherapy drugs, digoxin, cyclosporine, and protease inhibitors.

As a nurse, you need to be aware of the clinical ramifications of pharmacogenetics—having an effective knowledge of which drugs, diseases, or ethnic groups are affected by these variations can help you anticipate issues that may arise with patients under your care. For example, some patients of Asian descent have a significant reduction in enzyme activity secondary to amino acid substitution and therefore exhibit slower metabolism of certain drugs compared to patients from other ethnic groups. The effect of this on clinical practice is seen in the dosing of rosuvastatin; patients of Asian descent are typically started at 5 mg/day PO, whereas other patients are started at 10 mg/day. Giving a lower dose helps limit the development of serious adverse reactions in patients of Asian descent.

Another example of how drug metabolism is affected by genetic polymorphism involves the drug warfarin. Studies have shown that CYP2C9, which is the primary enzyme responsible for warfarin metabolism, has two genetic variants. These variants are associated with up to an 80% decrease in enzymatic activity that can affect approximately 7% to 11% of patients. Patients with these variant genotypes have 2.4 times an increase in the risk of serious or life-threatening bleeding after usual doses of warfarin. Consequently, patients with these variants retain warfarin longer and need significantly lower maintenance dosages.

Fortunately, genetic testing for polymorphisms is available when issues such as these arise. Although testing isn't done for every patient, it can be helpful for those who seem to be refractory or overly sensitive to the effects of certain drugs or who meet other criteria.

2

Drug therapy across the lifespan

Drug therapy is a fact of life for millions of people of all ages, and certain aspects of a patient's life, such as age, growth, and development, can affect drug therapy.

Drugs and pregnancy

Drug administration safety during pregnancy has been a source of serious medical concern and controversy since the thalidomide tragedy of the late 1950s, when thousands of malformed infants were born after their mothers were given this mild sedative-hypnotic while pregnant. To identify drugs that may cause such teratogenic effects, preclinical drug studies include tests on pregnant lab animals. These studies may reveal gross teratogenicity but don't establish absolute safety. This is because different animal species react to drugs in different ways. Consequently, animal studies can't reveal all possible teratogenic effects in humans. For example, the preliminary animal studies on thalidomide gave no warning of its teratogenic effects, and it was subsequently released for general use in Europe.

What about the placental barrier? Once thought to protect the fetus from drug effects, the placenta isn't much of a barrier at all. Almost every drug a patient takes during pregnancy crosses the placental barrier and enters fetal circulation, except for drugs with exceptionally large molecular structures, such as heparin, an injectable anticoagulant. By this standard, heparin could be used during pregnancy without fear of harming the fetus, but even heparin carries a warning for cautious use during pregnancy. Conversely, just because a drug crosses the placental barrier doesn't necessarily mean it's harmful to the fetus.

One factor—stage of fetal development—seems clearly related to greater risk during pregnancy. During the first and third trimesters of pregnancy, the fetus is especially vulnerable to damage from maternal use of drugs. During these times, give *all* drugs with extreme caution.

Organogenesis—when fetal organs differentiate—occurs in the first trimester. This is the most sensitive period for drug-induced fetal malformation. Strongly advise your patient not to take medications, including OTC drugs and supplements, without first discussing them with the health care provider.

Fetal sensitivity to drugs is also of special concern during the third trimester. At birth, after maternal separation, the neonate must rely on its own metabolism to eliminate any remaining drug. Because the neonate's detoxifying systems aren't fully developed, any residual drug may take a long time to be metabolized and thus may induce prolonged toxic reactions. For this reason, discourage patients from taking drugs except when absolutely necessary and advised by their prescribers during the last 3 months of pregnancy.

In many circumstances, patients must continue to take certain drugs during pregnancy. For example, a patient with a well-controlled seizure disorder may need to keep taking the anticonvulsant during pregnancy. Similarly, a patient with a bacterial infection must receive antibiotics during pregnancy. In such cases, the risk to the fetus is outweighed by the patient's medical needs, and drugs with lower teratogenic potential should be used whenever possible.

Complying with the following general guidelines can prevent indiscriminate and harmful use of drugs during pregnancy:
- Before a drug is prescribed for a patient of childbearing potential, ask the date of the patient's last menstrual period and whether the patient may be pregnant. If a drug is a known teratogen (for example, isotretinoin), some manufacturers may recommend special precautions to ensure that the drug isn't given to a patient of childbearing potential until pregnancy is ruled out and may require that contraceptives be used throughout the course of therapy.
- Caution a patient to avoid all drugs (including OTC drugs and herbs and supplements) except those essential to maintain the pregnancy and the patient's health—especially during the first and third trimesters.
- Topical drugs may be subject to the same warning against use during pregnancy. Many topically applied drugs can be absorbed in amounts large enough to be harmful to the fetus.
- When a patient needs to be prescribed a medication during pregnancy, use the safest drug in the lowest dose possible to minimize harm to the fetus.

• Instruct a patient to check with the prescriber before taking any drug during pregnancy.
• Encourage a patient to enroll in the pregnancy exposure registry for drugs that have one. Registries compile data on pregnancy outcomes to further define the risks of drug exposure in human pregnancies.
• During pregnancy, advise a patient to give the prescriber a list of all drugs, herbs, and supplements the patient is currently taking.
• Some drugs are part of a REMS drug safety program to ensure that benefits of the medication outweigh its risks through restricted access, education, and strict monitoring. Be sure to advise patients on the necessity to comply with these program requirements while taking such medications.

Drugs and breastfeeding
Many drugs a mother takes appear in human milk. Drug levels in human milk tend to be high when drug levels in maternal blood are high, especially after each dose. Many manufacturers' instructions advise the mother to breastfeed *before* taking each drug dose, not *after*. Also, in general, drugs with short half-lives are preferred because they peak quickly and are then eliminated and are less likely to be excreted in human milk.

A mother who wants to breastfeed usually may continue to do so with the prescriber's advice. However, breastfeeding should be temporarily interrupted and replaced with bottle-feeding when the mother must take certain drugs, such as a tetracycline, a sulfonamide (during the first 2 weeks postpartum), some oral anticoagulants, a drug that contains iodine, or an antineoplastic.

Caution the patient who is breastfeeding to protect the infant by not taking drugs indiscriminately. Instruct the mother to first check with the prescriber to be sure the patient is taking the safest drug at the lowest dose. Also instruct the patient to give the prescriber a list of all drugs, herbs, and supplements the patient is currently taking.

Drug therapy in children
Providing drug therapy to infants, children, and adolescents is challenging. Physiologic differences between children and adults, including those involving vital organ maturity and body composition, significantly influence a drug's effectiveness.

Physiologic changes affecting drug action
As a child develops, the processes of absorption, distribution (including drug binding to plasma proteins), metabolism, and excretion undergo profound changes that affect drug dosage. To ensure optimal drug effect and minimal toxicity, consider these factors when giving drugs to a child.

Absorption
Drug absorption in children depends on the form of the drug, its physical properties, simultaneous ingestion of other drugs or food, physiologic changes, and concurrent disease.

The pH of neonatal gastric fluid is neutral or slightly acidic; it becomes more acidic as the infant matures, which affects drug absorption. For example, ampicillin is better absorbed in an infant than in an adult because of the infant's low gastric acidity.

Various infant formulas or milk products may increase gastric pH and impede absorption of acidic drugs. If possible and so advised, give a child oral drugs on an empty stomach.

Gastric emptying time and transit time through the small intestine—which takes longer in children than in adults—can affect absorption. Also, intestinal hypermotility (as occurs in patients with diarrhea) can diminish a drug's absorption.

A child's comparatively thin epidermis allows increased absorption of topical drugs, increasing the risk of adverse systemic reactions.

Distribution
As with absorption, changes in body weight and physiology during childhood can significantly influence a drug's distribution and effects. In an infant born prematurely, body fluid makes up about 85% of total body weight; in an infant born at term, it makes up 55% to 70%; in an adult, 50% to 55%. Extracellular fluid (mostly blood) constitutes 40% of a neonate's body weight, compared with 20% in an adult. Intracellular fluid remains fairly constant throughout life and has little effect on drug dosage.

Extracellular fluid volume influences a water-soluble drug's concentration and effect because most drugs travel through extracellular fluid to reach their receptors. Compared with adults, distribution volume in children is proportionately greater because their fluid-to-solid body weight proportion is larger.

Because the proportion of fat to lean body mass increases with age, the distribution of fat-soluble drugs is more limited in children than in adults. As a result, a drug's fat or water solubility affects the dosage for a child.

Plasma protein binding

A decrease in albumin level or intermolecular attraction between drug and plasma protein causes many drugs to be less bound to plasma proteins in infants than in adults.

Highly protein-bound drugs may displace endogenous compounds, such as bilirubin or free fatty acids. Displacement of bound bilirubin can increase unbound (free) bilirubin, which can lead to increased risk of kernicterus at normal bilirubin levels. Conversely, an endogenous compound may displace a low protein-bound drug.

Because only an unbound drug molecule has a pharmacologic effect, a change in the ratio of a protein-bound to an unbound active drug can greatly influence the drug's effect.

Several diseases and disorders, such as nephrotic syndrome and malnutrition, can decrease plasma protein levels and increase the level of an unbound drug, which can either intensify the drug's effect or produce toxicity.

Metabolism

A neonate's ability to metabolize a drug depends on the integrity of the hepatic enzyme system, intrauterine exposure to the drug, and the properties of the drug itself.

Certain metabolic mechanisms are underdeveloped in neonates. Glucuronidation is a metabolic process occurring in the liver that renders most drugs more water soluble, facilitating renal excretion. This process isn't developed enough to permit larger doses of most drugs until the infant is 1 month old. The use of chloramphenicol sodium succinate in a neonate may cause gray baby syndrome because the infant's immature liver can't metabolize the drug; as a result, toxic levels accumulate in the blood. Reducing the dosage in a neonate and periodically monitoring drug levels are good ways to avoid toxicity. Conversely, intrauterine exposure to drugs may induce early development of hepatic enzyme mechanisms, thereby increasing the infant's capacity to metabolize potentially harmful substances.

Older children can metabolize some drugs (theophylline, for example) more rapidly than adults. This ability may arise from their increased hepatic metabolic activity. Doses larger than those recommended for adults may be required.

Also, more than one drug given simultaneously to a child may change hepatic metabolism and initiate production of hepatic enzymes.

Excretion

Renal excretion of a drug is the net result of glomerular filtration, active tubular secretion, and passive tubular reabsorption. Many drugs are excreted in the urine. The degree of renal development or presence of renal disease can greatly affect a child's dosage requirements because if a child can't excrete a drug renally, the drug may accumulate to toxic levels.

Physiologically, an infant's kidneys differ from an adult's in that infants have a high resistance to blood flow and their kidneys receive a smaller proportion of cardiac output. Infants have incomplete glomerular and tubular development and short, incomplete loops of Henle. (A child's GFR reaches an adult value between ages $2\frac{1}{2}$ and 5 months; the child's tubular secretion rate may reach an adult value between ages 7 and 12 months.) Infants also are less able to concentrate urine or reabsorb certain filtered compounds. The proximal tubules in infants also are less able to secrete organic acids.

Children and adults have diurnal variations in urine pH that correlate with sleep patterns. Changes in urine pH can affect the amount of drug excreted into the urine.

Special administration considerations

Biochemically, a drug displays the same mechanisms of action in all people. But the response to a drug can be affected by a child's age and size, as well as by the maturity of the target organ. To ensure optimal drug effect and minimal toxicity, consider the following factors when giving drugs to children.

Adjusting dosages for children

When calculating children's dosages, don't use formulas that modify adult dosages. A child isn't a scaled-down version of an adult. Base pediatric dosages on either body weight (mg/kg) or body surface area (mg/m^2).

Reevaluate dosages at regular intervals to ensure needed adjustments as the child develops. Although BSA provides a useful standard for adults and older children, use the body weight method in premature or full-term infants. Don't exceed the maximum adult dosage when calculating amounts per kilogram of body weight (except with certain drugs, such as theo-phylline, if indicated).

Obtain an accurate maternal drug history, including prescription and OTC drugs, vitamins, herbs, or supplements taken during pregnancy. Drugs passed into human milk can have adverse effects on the breastfeeding infant. Before giving a drug to a breastfeeding mother, investigate its potential effects on the infant.

For example, a sulfonamide given to a mother for a UTI appears in human milk and may cause kernicterus in an infant with low levels of unconjugated bilirubin.

Giving oral drugs

Remember the following when giving oral drugs to a child:

If the patient is an infant, give drugs in liquid form, if possible. For accurate administration, measure and give the preparation by oral syringe, never a parenteral syringe. It's very important to remove the syringe cap to keep the infant from swallowing or aspirating it. Be sure to instruct parents to do the same. Never use a vial or cup. Lift the patient's head to prevent aspiration of the drug, and press down on the chin to prevent choking. You may also place the drug in a nipple and allow the infant to suck the contents.

If the patient is a toddler, explain how you're going to give the drug. If possible, have the parents enlist the child's cooperation. Never call it "candy," even if it has a pleasant taste. Let the child take the liquid drug from a calibrated medication cup rather than a spoon. It's easier and more accurate. If the preparation is available only in tablet form, crush and mix it with an appropriate vehicle, such as applesauce. (First, verify with a pharmacist that the tablet can be crushed and mixed without compromising its effectiveness. For example, most long-acting or extended-release products shouldn't be crushed.)

If the patient is an older child who can swallow a tablet or capsule, have the child place the drug on the back of the tongue and swallow it with water or nonacidic fruit juice (such as apple juice), because milk and milk products may interfere with drug absorption.

Giving IV infusions

For IV infusions in infants, use a peripheral vein or a scalp vein in the temporal region. The scalp vein is safe because the needle isn't likely to dislodge. However, the hair must be clipped around the site, and the needle and infiltrated fluids may cause temporary disfigurement. For these reasons, scalp veins aren't used as commonly today as they were in the past.

The arms and legs are the most accessible insertion sites, but because children tend to move about, take these precautions:

● Protect the insertion site to keep the catheter or needle from being dislodged. Use a padded arm board to reduce the risk of dislodgment. Remove the arm board during range-of-motion exercises.

● Place the IV tubing clamp out of the child's reach. If extension tubing is used to allow the child greater mobility, securely tape the connection.

● Explain in simple terms to the child why restraints must be used while the child is asleep, to alleviate anxiety and maintain trust.

During an infusion, monitor flow rates and check the child's condition and the insertion site at least every hour. Titrate the flow rate only while the patient is composed; crying and emotional upset can constrict blood vessels. Flow rate may vary if a pump isn't used. Flow should be adequate because some drugs (calcium, for example) can be irritating at low flow rates. Infants, small children, and children with compromised cardiopulmonary status are especially vulnerable to fluid overload with IV drug administration. To prevent this problem and help ensure that a limited amount of fluid is infused in a controlled manner, use a volume-control device in the IV tubing and an infusion pump or a syringe. Don't place more than 2 hours of IV fluid in the volume-control set at a time.

Giving IM injections

IM injections are preferred when a drug can't be given by other parenteral routes and rapid absorption is needed.

The vastus lateralis muscle is the preferred injection site in children age 2 and younger. For children ages 3 to 18, the deltoid muscle is the preferred site. Though rarely used in children, the ventrogluteal site can be used in certain circumstances, such as when the child's condition prevents administration in other sites. To select the correct needle size, consider the patient's age, muscle mass, nutritional status, and drug viscosity.

Record and rotate injection sites. Explain to the patient that the injection will hurt but that the drug will help the patient feel better. Swaddle an infant or use an assistant during the injection, if needed, and comfort the infant afterward.

Giving topical drugs and inhalants

When giving a child a topical drug or inhalant, consider the following:

Use eardrops warmed to room temperature. Cold drops can cause pain and vertigo. To give drops, turn the patient on the side, with the affected ear up. If the patient is younger than age 3, pull the pinna down and back; if age 3 or older, pull the pinna up and back.

Avoid using inhalants in young children because it's difficult to get them to cooperate. Before you try to give a drug to an older child through a metered-dose inhaler, explain how to use the inhaler. Then have the child hold the inhaler and close the lips around the mouthpiece. Have the child exhale and pinch the nostrils shut. When the child starts to inhale, release one dose of the drug into the child's mouth. Tell the patient to continue inhaling until the lungs feel full; then the child can breathe normally and unpinch the nostrils. Most inhaled drugs aren't useful if the drug remains in the mouth or throat—if you doubt the patient's ability to use the inhaler correctly, don't use it. Devices such as spacers or assist devices may help. Check with a pharmacist, the prescriber, or a respiratory therapist for suggestions.

Use topical corticosteroids cautiously because prolonged use in children may delay growth. When you apply topical corticosteroids to the diaper area of infants, don't cover the area with plastic or rubber pants, which act as an occlusive dressing and may enhance systemic absorption.

Giving parenteral nutrition

Give IV nutrition to patients who can't or won't take adequate food orally and to patients with hypermetabolic conditions who need supplementation. The latter group includes infants born prematurely, children, and adolescents with burns or other major trauma, intractable diarrhea, malabsorption syndromes, GI abnormalities, emotional disorders (such as anorexia nervosa), and congenital abnormalities.

Before giving fat emulsions to infants and children, weigh the potential benefits against any possible risks. Fats—supplied as 10% or 20% lipid emulsions—are given both peripherally and centrally. Their use is limited by the child's ability to metabolize them. For example, an infant or child with a diseased liver can't efficiently metabolize fats.

Some fats, however, must be supplied both to prevent essential fatty acid deficiency and

to permit normal growth and development. A minimum of calories (2% to 4%) must be supplied as linoleic acid—an essential fatty acid found in lipids. Nevertheless, fat solutions may decrease oxygen perfusion and may adversely affect children with pulmonary disease. This risk can be minimized by supplying only the minimum fat needed for essential fatty acid requirements and not the usual intake of 40% to 50% of the child's total calories.

Fatty acids can also displace bilirubin bound to albumin, causing a rise in free, unconjugated bilirubin and an increased risk of kernicterus. Fat solutions may interfere with some bilirubin assays and cause falsely elevated bilirubin levels. To avoid this complication, draw a blood sample 4 hours after infusion of the lipid emulsion or, if the emulsion is infused over 24 hours, be sure the lab is aware so that the blood samples can be centrifuged before the assay is performed.

It isn't usually recommended to give other IV solutions or medications in the same line as parenteral nutrition because of the potential for precipitates to form. Refer to your facility's nutrition/pharmacy policy or contact a pharmacist for further information.

Drug therapy in older adults

If you're giving drugs to older adults, you'll need to understand the physiologic and pharmacokinetic changes in this population that may affect drug dosage, cause common adverse reactions, or create adherence problems.

Physiologic changes affecting drug action

As a person ages, gradual physiologic changes occur. Some of these age-related changes may alter the therapeutic and toxic effects of drugs.

Body composition

Proportions of fat, lean tissue, and water in the body change with age. Total body mass and lean body mass tend to decrease, but the proportion of body fat tends to increase.

Body composition varies from person to person, and these changes in body composition affect the relationship between a drug's concentration and distribution in the body.

For example, a water-soluble drug such as gentamicin isn't distributed to fat. Because there's relatively more fat tissue and less lean tissue in an older adult, more drug remains in the blood. Fat-soluble drugs tend to accumulate in older adults, resulting in prolonged half-lives and more pronounced effects.

Gastrointestinal function

In older adults, decreases in gastric acid secretion and GI motility slow the emptying of stomach contents and movement through the entire intestinal tract. Research suggests that older adults may not absorb drugs as easily as younger people. This is an especially significant problem with drugs that have a narrow therapeutic index such as digoxin, in which any change in absorption can be crucial.

Hepatic function

The liver's ability to metabolize certain drugs decreases with age. This decrease is caused by diminished blood flow to the liver, which results from an age-related decrease in cardiac output, and from the lessened activity of certain liver enzymes. When an older adult takes a sleep medication such as flurazepam, for example, the liver's reduced ability to metabolize the drug as well as the lipophilic property of the drug can produce residual effects the next morning.

Decreased hepatic function may result in more intense drug effects caused by higher levels, longer-lasting drug effects because of prolonged levels, and a greater risk of drug toxicity.

Renal function

An older adult's renal function is usually sufficient to eliminate excess body fluid and waste, but the ability to eliminate some drugs may be reduced by 50% or more.

Many drugs commonly used by older adults, such as digoxin, are excreted primarily through the kidneys. If the kidneys' ability to excrete the drug is decreased, high blood levels may result. Digoxin toxicity can occur in older adults who don't receive a reduced digoxin dosage to accommodate decreased renal function.

Drug dosages can be modified to compensate for age-related decreases in renal function. Aided by results of lab tests, such as BUN and creatinine levels, adjust drug dosages so the patient receives therapeutic benefits without the risk of toxicity. It's important to remember that serum creatinine is a function of muscle mass and that most older adults lose muscle mass as they age. An older adult can have significant renal impairment even with a serum creatinine level in the normal range. Observe the patient for signs and symptoms of toxicity.

Special administration considerations

Aging is usually accompanied by a decline in organ function that can affect drug distribution and clearance. This physiologic decline is likely to be worsened by a disease or a chronic disorder. Together, these factors can significantly increase the risk of adverse reactions and drug toxicity, as well as nonadherence.

Adverse reactions

Compared with younger people, older adults experience twice as many adverse drug reactions, mostly from increased use of concomitant medications, poor adherence, and physiologic changes.

Signs and symptoms of adverse drug reactions—including confusion, weakness, agitation, and lethargy—are often mistakenly attributed to senility or disease. If the adverse reaction isn't identified, the patient may continue to receive the drug and receive other, unnecessary drugs to treat the complications caused by the original drug. This prescribing cascade can sometimes result in a pattern of inappropriate and excessive drug prescribing, causing polypharmacy.

Any drug can cause adverse reactions, but most of the serious reactions in older adults are caused by relatively few drugs. Be particularly alert for toxicities resulting from diuretics, antihypertensives, digoxin, corticosteroids, anticoagulants, sleeping aids, and OTC drugs.

Diuretic toxicity

Because total body water content decreases with age, a normal dosage of a potassium-wasting diuretic, such as furosemide or hydrochlorothiazide, may result in fluid loss and even dehydration in an older adult.

These diuretics may deplete a patient's potassium level, making the patient feel weak, and they may raise blood uric acid and glucose levels, complicating gout and diabetes mellitus.

Antihypertensive toxicity

Many older adults experience light-headedness or fainting when taking antihypertensives, partly in response to atherosclerosis and decreased elasticity of the blood vessels. Antihypertensives can lower BP too rapidly, resulting in insufficient blood flow to the brain, which can cause dizziness, fainting, or even a stroke.

Consequently, dosages of antihypertensives must be carefully individualized. In older adults, aggressive treatment of high BP may be harmful. Treatment goals should be reasonable. Elevated BP needs to be reduced slowly in older adults. Tell the patient to change positions slowly and maintain adequate fluid intake to avoid orthostatic hypotension.

Digoxin toxicity

As the body's renal function and rate of excretion decline, the digoxin level in the blood of an older adult may increase to the point of causing nausea, vomiting, diarrhea and, most seriously, cardiac arrhythmias. Monitor the patient's digoxin level and observe for early signs and symptoms of toxicity, such as appetite loss, confusion, or depression.

Corticosteroid toxicity

Older adults taking a corticosteroid may experience short-term effects, including fluid retention and psychological effects ranging from mild euphoria to acute psychotic reactions. Long-term toxic effects, such as osteoporosis, can be especially severe in older adults who have been taking prednisone or related steroidal compounds for months or even years. To prevent serious toxicity, carefully monitor patients on long-term regimens. Observe them for subtle changes in appearance, mood, and mobility and for impaired healing and fluid and electrolyte disturbances.

Anticoagulant effects

Older adults taking an anticoagulant have an increased risk of bleeding, especially when they take NSAIDs or aspirin at the same time. Be sure to evaluate all drugs the patient is taking for increased risk of bleeding. Because older adults are more likely to fall, they're also at increased risk for bleeding as a result of a fall. If a patient is taking warfarin, monitor the INR carefully, if applicable, and monitor for bruising and other signs and symptoms of bleeding.

Sleeping aid toxicity

Sedatives and sleeping aids, such as zolpidem and diphenhydramine, may cause excessive sedation or drowsiness. Keep in mind that consumption of alcohol may increase CNS depressant effects, even if the sleeping aid was taken the previous evening. Use these drugs sparingly in older adults.

Over-the-counter drug toxicity

Prolonged ingestion of aspirin, aspirin-containing analgesics, and other OTC NSAIDs (such as ibuprofen and naproxen) may cause GI irritation—even ulcers—and gradual blood loss resulting in severe anemia. Prescription NSAIDs may cause similar problems. Both OTC and prescription NSAIDs can cause renal toxicity in older adults. Anemia from prolonged aspirin consumption can affect all age groups, but older adults may be less able to compensate because of their already reduced iron stores. These drugs should be used very carefully and at the lowest effective doses.

Acetaminophen is found in a variety of prescription and OTC products. Liver injury may occur from inadvertently taking excess acetaminophen from multiple sources.

Laxatives may cause diarrhea in older adults, who are extremely sensitive to drugs such as bisacodyl. Long-term oral use of mineral oil as a lubricating laxative may result in lipoid pneumonia from aspiration of small residual oil droplets in the patient's mouth.

Antihistamines such as diphenhydramine have anticholinergic effects and can cause confusion and mental status changes; they are also more likely to cause dizziness, sedation, and hypotension in older adults. OTC decongestants, including phenylephrine, can have systemic effects, such as hypertension, anxiety, insomnia, and agitation.

Nonadherence

Poor adherence can be a problem with patients of any age. Many hospitalizations result from nonadherence with a medical regimen. In older adults, factors linked to aging, such as diminished visual acuity, hearing loss, forgetfulness, the need for multiple drug therapy, and socioeconomic factors, can combine to make adherence a special problem. About one-third of older adults fail to adhere with their prescribed drug therapy. They may fail to take prescribed doses or to follow the correct schedule. They may take drugs prescribed for previous disorders, stop drugs prematurely, or indiscriminately use drugs that are to be taken as needed. Older adults may also have multiple prescriptions for the same drug and inadvertently take an overdose.

Review the patient's drug regimen with the patient. Make sure the patient understands the dose amount, the time and frequency of doses, and why the drug has been prescribed. Also, explain in detail if a drug is to be taken with food, with water, or separate from other drugs. To verify the patient's understanding, ask the patient to repeat the instructions back to you.

Help the patient avoid drug therapy problems by suggesting the use of drug calendars, pill sorters, or other aids to help with adherence. Refer the patient to the prescriber, a pharmacist, or social services if further information or assistance with drug therapy is needed.

3

Safe drug administration

Medication therapy is a primary intervention for many illnesses. It greatly benefits many patients and yet is involved in many instances of unintended harm to patients and health care workers from either unintended consequences of therapy (adverse drug reactions or exposure to hazardous drugs) or medication-related errors (preventable adverse drug events). (See *Preventing and treating IV vesicant extravasation injury*, page 14.) Medication errors are a significant cause of patient morbidity and mortality in the United States. In 1999, the Institute of Medicine (IOM) published its first Quality Chasm report, "To Err is Human: Building a Safer Health System," which reported that errors related to medications accounted for approximately 1 out of 131 outpatient deaths, 1 out of 854 inpatient deaths, and more than 7,000 deaths annually. Recent research indicates that the number of medication errors may actually be much higher. Of all sentinel events reviewed in 2020 (794) by The Joint Commission (a nonprofit organization that seeks to improve public health care through the voluntary accreditation of health care institutions), approximately 24 events were attributed to medication management. A sentinel event is a patient safety event that results in patient death or permanent harm or requires intervention to sustain life.

Many governmental and nongovernmental organizations are dedicated to improving the safety of drug administration. One mission of the FDA, for example, is to protect the public health by assuring the safety, effectiveness, and security of human drugs, vaccines, and medical devices. In 2007, the Food and Drug Administration Amendments Act expanded the FDA's authority regarding assessing and communicating risks associated with drugs. One of the new provisions of the law granted the FDA authority to require drug manufacturers to submit Risk Evaluation and Mitigation Strategies. (See *Risk Evaluation and Mitigation Strategies*, page 15.) The U.S. Pharmacopeia (USP), a nonprofit, nongovernmental public health organization, sets official public standards for drugs and other health care products manufactured or sold in the United States. It also sets standards for the quality, purity, and strength of food ingredients and dietary supplements.

In 2005, The Patient Safety and Quality Improvement Act authorized the creation of patient safety organizations (PSOs) to improve the quality and safety of U.S. health care delivery. One of these PSOs, the Institute for Safe Medication Practices (ISMP), is a nonprofit organization entirely dedicated to preventing medication errors and using medications safely. In addition, The Joint Commission has established National Patient Safety Goals and standards to improve the safe use of medications in its accredited facilities.

The CDC has a number of campaigns and initiatives to promote medication safety by developing evidence-based policies and using collaborative interventions.

One important initiative of the CDC, FDA, and other organizations is to address the use and misuse of opioids in treating chronic pain (pain not related to cancer or palliative care that lasts longer than 3 months or past the time of normal tissue healing). According to the CDC, in 2016 more than 11.5 million individuals in the United States reported misusing prescription opioids in the past year, and in 2017, the number of overdose deaths involving opioids was six times higher than in 1999. The death rate continues to increase. (See *Safe opioid administration*, page 16.)

The CDC has developed an evidence-based guideline, "CDC Guideline for Prescribing Opioids for Chronic Pain—United States, 2016" (https://www.cdc.gov/mmwr/volumes/65/rr/rr6501e1.htm), which addresses "1) when to initiate or continue opioids for chronic pain; 2) opioid selection, dosage, duration, follow-up, and discontinuation; and 3) assessing risk and addressing harms of opioid use." The CDC has also developed the "Checklist for Prescribing Opioids for Chronic Pain" (https://www.cdc.gov/drugoverdose/pdf/pdo_checklist-a.pdf), which provides guidance for primary care providers treating adults with chronic pain.

The FDA has developed a comprehensive action plan that focuses on policies to reduce the impact of the opioid abuse epidemic on families and communities while providing patients access to safe and effective pain relief. The FDA opioid medication action plan includes consulting expert advisory

Preventing and treating IV vesicant extravasation injury

Extravasation injuries occur when vesicant IV solutions or drugs—those with the potential to cause significant tissue injury (such as certain chemotherapy drugs, antibiotics, electrolyte solutions, vasopressors, and antiemetics)—escape from blood vessels into surrounding tissue (extravasate) during administration. Drugs or solutions that produce inflammation rather than serious or lasting tissue injury from extravasation are considered irritants. Extravasation injuries may occur when vesicants are given centrally or peripherally. Such injury can cause significant harm, including necrotic ulcers that may require surgical intervention, infection, loss of a limb or limb function, or complex regional pain syndrome.

Signs and symptoms of peripheral extravasation include:
- changes in IV site appearance (blanching, bruising) or temperature (coolness, erythema)
- pain, tightness, or itching at or surrounding the insertion site
- IV site fluid leakage
- numbness or tingling, diminished capillary refill, or decreased motor function in the extremity.

Signs and symptoms of CVAD extravasation include:
- discomfort at the insertion site or along the CVAD path
- fluid leakage from the insertion site
- increased resistance to solution injection
- shoulder, neck, or chest edema.

Preventing extravasation

Use the following measures to prevent extravasation injuries:
- Know facility policy for administering vesicant drugs and solutions. Make sure you've been properly trained in prevention measures and extravasation recognition and management.
- When administering vesicants, know the specific antidote for the drug being given, and make sure that the antidote and equipment needed to manage extravasation are on hand. Some antidotes for vesicants and solutions include sodium thiosulfate for alkylating agents, hyaluronidase for electrolytes and antibiotics (nafcillin, vancomycin [Vancocin]), and phentolamine for vasopressors (dopamine, norepinephrine).

- Ensure that the IV access site or CVAD is patent before giving the drug. Make sure the insertion site is visible, and use an appropriate catheter stabilization device.
- Make sure the drug is given by the proper route according to facility policy. Most vesicants administered by continuous infusion should be given utilizing a CVAD. Know when an IV infusion pump device should and shouldn't be used.
- Frequently monitor the patient for extravasation signs and symptoms, and teach the patient to immediately report them.

Treating extravasation

- Follow facility policy for treatment of extravasation injury. Stop the drug, and aspirate any residual drug and blood from the IV catheter or CVAD.
- Note the time the infusion started to provide an estimate of the amount of solution extravasated and notify the practitioner.
- If an antidote exists, prepare for administration through the existing IV catheter or CVAD. After antidote administration, remove the peripheral IV catheter, but avoid pressure to the site.
- For extravasation from a CVAD, prepare the patient for a CT scan to assess catheter placement and fluid collection, if appropriate.
- For peripheral extravasation, prepare for subcut injections of drug-specific antidote, if appropriate.
- Elevate the affected limb.
- Apply hot (for vasoconstrictors) or cold (for alkylating drugs) compresses, if ordered.
- Use a skin marker or photo for serial documentation of extravasation according to facility policy.
- Monitor the site for pain, erythema progression, induration, tissue necrosis, and possible compartment syndrome. Note that symptom development may be delayed for 48 hours.
- Document the date and time of the infusion, time when signs and symptoms were first noted, extravasation signs and symptoms, type and size of venous access device, estimated extravasation solution amount, treatment instituted, practitioner notification, and the patient's response to treatment. Patients with significant tissue damage may need surgery.

committees before new drug approvals for opioids without abuse-deterrent properties and for new labeling of appropriate opioid use in children, developing additional changes and warnings to immediate-release opioid labeling information to provide risk and safe prescribing guidance for physicians, strengthening the requirements for drug companies

to generate postmarket data on the long-term impact of using opioids to improve treatment of both addiction and pain, updating REMS requirements for opioids to increase pain management and safe prescribing training of prescribers and to decrease inappropriate opioid prescribing, supporting the development of and expanding the use of

Risk Evaluation and Mitigation Strategies

REMS is a risk management program that goes beyond the drug's package insert and is used when necessary to make certain that a drug's benefits outweigh its risks. REMS are designed to help reduce the occurrence or severity of certain serious risks by informing or supporting the execution of the safe use conditions described in the medication's FDA-approved prescribing information. The FDA can require a REMS at any stage of a drug's lifecycle (as part of a drug's New Drug Application or after approval as new safety information becomes available), and manufacturers who fail to comply with REMS requirements can face substantial monetary penalties. For a list of currently approved REMS, go to www.accessdata.fda.gov/scripts/cder/rems/index.cfm.

When evaluating the necessity of REMS, the FDA takes into consideration such factors as:
- the number of patients most likely to use the drug
- the seriousness of the patient's disease
- the drug's benefit
- the projected duration of treatment
- the severity of known or potential adverse events
- whether the drug is a new molecular entity.

The FDA has issued an outline of specific components that manufacturers should use to develop a REMS proposal. These include the development of specific REMS goals and elements to ensure a drug's safe and appropriate use. The REMS must also describe how the manufacturer plans to evaluate whether the REMS goal is being met and the timetable for periodic assessments and reassessments. The results of the evaluations must be reported to the FDA, and the FDA may require that the REMS be modified and will determine if additional actions must be taken.

REMS may contain one or all of the following components:
- **Medication guide:** Written safety information for patients that must be distributed by the pharmacist to each patient receiving the drug
- **Communication plan:** Plan that includes the tools to teach health care professionals how to use the drug safely and appropriately
- **Elements to Assure Safe Use (EASU):** Specific requirements and elements to ensure safe use of the drug, including requirements that each patient be enrolled in a registry, that essential lab monitoring be performed, that the drug may only be prescribed by a prescriber with a specific certification, and that the drug may only be distributed by a specialty pharmacy
- **Implementation plan:** Plan that describes how the EASUs will be put into action.

abuse-deterrent opioids, improving access to naloxone and other drug treatment options for opioid use disorders, and reexamining the risks and benefits of opioids and their effects on public health.

Causes of medication errors

The National Coordinating Council for Medication Error Reporting and Prevention (www.nccmerp.org) defines a *medication error* as "any preventable event that may cause or lead to inappropriate medication use or patient harm while the medication is in the control of the health care professional, patient, or consumer. Such events may be related to professional practice, health care products, procedures, and systems, including prescribing; order communication; product labeling, packaging, and nomenclature; compounding; dispensing; distribution; administration; education; monitoring; and use."

Medication errors were once thought to be caused by lapses in an individual's practice. Traditionally, teaching nurses to administer drugs safely focused on the individual nurse's practice and the application of the "rights" of safe medication administration. (See *The eight "rights" of medication administration*, page 17.)

Although individual nursing practice is still an extremely important part of safe drug administration, the focus of prevention efforts has widened. After medication errors had been systematically studied by numerous organizations who shared data, it became apparent that these errors are complex events with multiple factors and are most often caused by failures within systems. As a result of these findings, research has shifted to preventing medication errors by identifying their root causes and then developing and validating evidence-based prevention strategies. Organizational processes, management decisions, inadequate medication administration protocols, staffing shortages, environmental conditions, poor communication, inadequate drug knowledge and resources, and individual mistakes or protocol violations may all contribute to medication errors.

The medication administration process

Medication errors can occur from medication administration process problems or within any one or more than one of the five stages of medication administration. Because up to 40% of a

Safe opioid administration

Opioid analgesics are associated with adverse effects, most notably respiratory depression followed by sedation. Additional adverse effects include aspiration pneumonia, constipation, delirium, dizziness, falls, hallucinations, hypotension, and nausea and vomiting. Opioid analgesics are also linked with adverse drug events due to:

- lack of knowledge regarding differing potencies among opioids
- incorrect administration of multiple opioids, including their respective routes of administration
- inadequate monitoring of patients who take opioids.
  Nurses can help avoid opioid misuse by:
- identifying conditions that put patients at a higher risk for oversedation and respiratory depression (sleep disorders, morbid obesity, older age, habitual opioid use, major organ dysfunction or failure, respiratory disorders, smoking, polypharmacy)
- screening patients for respiratory depression risk factors using screening tools, such as the Pasero Opioid-induced Sedation Scale (POSS), Richmond Agitation-Sedation Scale (RASS), Screener and Opioid Assessment for Patients with Pain (SOAPP and SOAPP-R), the Opioid Risk Tool (ORT), and the Screening Instrument for Substance Abuse Potential (SISAP)
- assessing the patient's opioid history, including possible abuse, adverse effects, and intolerance
- assessing the patient's skin for an existing opioid patch, implanted drug delivery system, or infusion pump
- starting patients who are opioid-naive with a non-opioid pain regimen before moving on to opioids
- starting patients who are opioid-naive with the lowest dosage of opioid possible and titrating upwards
- consulting a pharmacist when changing opioid medications or their administration routes
- dosing opioids based on the individual patient's condition and needs
- being mindful of when opioids are administered; for instance, not administering opioids before a patient transfer to avoid possible injury to the patient if drug levels peak during the time of transfer
- using patient-controlled analgesia (PCA) devices
- educating patients and their caregivers about opioid misuse and the steps to take to prevent this occurrence.

Tips for safe opioid administration include the following:

- Double-check the medication order, appropriateness of the medication, the dose, line placement for infusions, and pump settings.
- Ensure standing orders are available for reversal agents.
- Label all IV and epidural lines to avoid confusion.
- Monitor the patient closely if identified as being at high risk for adverse outcomes related to opioid treatment. Frequently assess respiration quality and rate, and observe for signs and symptoms of oversedation.
- Use capnography and pulse oximetry readings to help detect opioid toxicity.
- Keep oxygen and naloxone in the area where opioids are administered.
- Utilize established pain guidelines and standardized formats that are consistent with the patient's age, condition, and ability to understand to monitor and document the patient's pain.
- In collaboration with the multidisciplinary team, involve the patient in the pain management planning process. Develop realistic expectations and measurable goals that the patient understands for the degree, duration, and reduction of pain. Discuss objectives used to evaluate treatment progress (for example, relief of pain and improved physical and psychosocial function).
- Educate patients and their caregivers about PCA use before surgical procedures and warn against dosing by proxy.
- Regularly observe and monitor patients who are using PCA.
- Provide education on pain management, treatment options, and safe use of the opioid.
- Teach the patient and family about pain management strategies during discharge planning. Include information about the patient's pain management plan and adverse effects of pain management treatment.
- Teach the patient and family about safe use, storage, and disposal of opioids. Instruct patients who use fentanyl patches to store them in a secure manner to prevent access by children, pets, and drug-seekers. Educate patients about how to properly apply patches and to protect them from heat.

nurse's time may be spent in medication administration and nursing practice intersects multiple stages, nurses may often be involved in medication errors. Here are some of the types of errors that have been reported in each stage.

Stage 1: Ordering and prescribing
- Prescriber orders are incomplete or illegible.
- Contraindicated drugs (such as drugs to which the patient is allergic) are prescribed.
- The prescriber specifies the wrong drug, dose, route, frequency, or duration, or fails to specify the indication.
- Drugs are prescribed using inappropriate or inadequate verbal orders.

The eight "rights" of medication administration

Traditionally, nurses have been taught the "five rights" of medication administration. These are broadly stated goals and practices to help individual nurses administer drugs safely and correctly.

1. The *right drug:* Check the drug label and verify that the drug and form to be given is the drug that was prescribed.
2. The *right patient:* Confirm the patient's identity by checking at least two patient identifiers.
3. The *right dose:* Verify that the dose and dosage form to be given are appropriate for the patient, and check the drug label with the prescriber's order.
4. The *right time:* Ensure that the drug is administered at the correct time and frequency.
5. The *right route:* Verify that the route by which the drug is to be given is specified by the prescriber and is appropriate for the patient.

In addition to the traditional "five rights" of individual practice, best-practice researchers have added three additional "rights":

6. The *right reason:* Verify that the drug prescribed is appropriate to treat the patient's condition.
7. The *right response:* Monitor the patient's response to the drug administered.
8. The *right documentation:* Completely and accurately document in the patient's medical record the drug administered; the monitoring of the patient, including the patient's response; and other nursing interventions.

Stage 2: Transcribing and verifying
• An incorrect drug, dose, route, time, or frequency is transcribed into the medication administration record (MAR) by the pharmacist or nurse.
• Drug verification and documentation in the MAR by the pharmacist or nurse are inadequate.

Stage 3: Dispensing and delivery
• The prescribed drug is filled incorrectly.
• Failure to deliver the right drug to the right place for the right patient occurs.

Stage 4: Administering
• The wrong drug is given to the wrong patient by the nurse or other licensed professional.
• The wrong dose is calculated and given or infused by the nurse or other licensed professional.
• The right drug is incorrectly prepared (such as crushing a drug that shouldn't be crushed) and is given by the nurse or other licensed professional.
• The correct drug is administered by the wrong route (such as an oral drug that is injected IV) by the nurse or other licensed professional.
• The correct drug is given at the wrong time or frequency by the nurse or other licensed professional.

Stage 5: Monitoring and reporting
• Monitoring of the patient by the nurse before and after medication administration is inadequate.
• Documentation and reporting of the patient's condition by the nurse before and after medication administration are inadequate.
• Hand-off communication between licensed professionals is inadequate.
• Reporting of medication errors is inadequate.

Elements contributing to safer drug administration

Ensuring the safe delivery of medication involves a system-wide, interdisciplinary approach, and research has shown that improvements in communication, education, and prevention of hazardous drug exposure can facilitate the safe delivery of medication.

Communication improvements

Communication issues have been implicated in approximately 60% of reported medication errors. Communication can be improved in many ways throughout the medication administration process. The traditional nursing process "rights" of safe drug administration are still important components of safe drug administration, but even when protocols are followed exactly, some medication errors still occur. For example, a nurse who's exactly following the eight "rights" might administer a drug to which a patient is allergic if the allergy information is incomplete or undocumented or hasn't been communicated effectively. Appropriate communication among all members of the health care team, including nurses, is vitally important.

Many health care facilities have instituted measures to help standardize and organize appropriate communication. One tool commonly used is SBAR (Situation, Background, Assessment, and Recommendation); its purpose is to logically organize information to optimize proper communication among health care providers.

Each institution must have tools and policies in place for the documentation of medication administration. Each prescribed medication order must be clearly written or entered into an electronic medical record system, and verbal orders must be used and documented according to facility policy. Each verbal order should be read back and verified with the prescriber before the drug is administered. The patient's condition must be monitored after each medication is given, and the patient's response and any nursing interventions must be documented appropriately. Clear communication through documentation is essential to safe practice.

The Joint Commission has developed goals and standards regarding medication reconciliation—the process of comparing a patient's medication regimen when medications are discontinued, dosages are changed, or new medications are added, and at every transition in care (for example, on admission, upon discharge, and between care settings and levels). Medication reconciliation helps ensure that essential information about the patient's medication regimen is communicated to the health care team. Medication reconciliation helps prevent the inadvertent omission of needed medications, prevents medication duplication, and helps identify medications with potentially harmful interactions.

Education improvements

Lack of knowledge has been implicated in many medication errors; therefore, education about medications is essential to their safe administration. All health care team members involved in the process of medication administration, including the prescriber, pharmacist, and nurse, must have access to accurate information about each drug's indications, appropriate dosing regimen, appropriate route, appropriate frequency, possible drug interactions, appropriate monitoring, any cautions, and possible adverse effects. Each facility should have processes in place to educate staff and communicate important drug information.

Governmental and nongovernmental agencies are doing their part toward educating facilities, prescribers, and nurses. The FDA established the boxed warning system to alert prescribers to drugs with increased risks to patients. These boxed warnings are the strongest labeling requirements for drugs that can have serious reactions. The Joint Commission requires accredited health care facilities to develop a list of abbreviations to avoid in all medication communications. The ISMP maintains a list of high-alert medications that may cause significant patient harm when given incorrectly. (Each facility should have protocols in place for administering high-alert medications with safeguards built into the process.) The FDA and ISMP have developed a list of drugs with similar names—look-alike, sound-alike (LASA) medications—that can be easily confused with each other. Dissimilarities in each drug's name are highlighted with uppercase letters (so each name has mixed-case letters, called *tall-man lettering*), making such mix-ups less likely to occur for each drug.

Patient education

Patients and their families should be active participants in the patient's care and should understand the patient's plan of care, including the purpose of newly prescribed medications. The patient and family need to be taught what to watch for, how the patient's condition will be monitored, what signs and symptoms to report, and to report anything that doesn't seem right, including unfamiliar medications. Before administering a medication, the nurse needs to verify with the patient medication allergies or unusual past reactions to medications.

The following general teaching guidelines will help ensure that the patient receives the maximum therapeutic benefit from the medication regimen and will help the patient avoid adverse reactions, accidental overdose, and harmful changes in effectiveness.

• Instruct the patient to learn the brand names, generic name, and dosages of all drugs and supplements (such as herbs and vitamins) being taken.

• Tell the patient to notify the pharmacist and prescriber about all medications the patient is taking, including prescription drugs, OTC drugs, and herbal or other supplements, and about any drug allergies or reactions.

• Advise the patient to always read the label and Medication Guide before taking a drug, to take it exactly as prescribed, and to never share prescription drugs with others.

• Warn the patient not to change manufacturers of a drug without consulting the prescriber, to avoid harmful changes in effectiveness.

• Tell the patient to check the expiration date before taking a drug.

• Teach the patient how to safely discard drugs that are outdated or no longer needed. (See Appendix 10: *Safe disposal of unused drugs: What patients need to know*.)

- Caution the patient to keep all drugs safely out of the reach of children and pets.
- Advise the patient to store drugs in their original containers, at the proper temperature, and in areas where they won't be exposed to sunlight or excessive heat or humidity. Sunlight, heat, and humidity can cause drug deterioration and reduce a drug's effectiveness.
- Encourage the patient to report all suspected adverse or unusual reactions to the prescriber, and teach proper techniques for self-monitoring the condition (for example, how to obtain a resting HR before taking digoxin).
- Suggest that the patient have all prescriptions filled at the same pharmacy or pharmacy system so that pharmacists can warn against potentially harmful drug interactions.
- Tell the patient to report the complete medication history to all health care providers involved in the patient's care, including the dentist.
- Instruct the patient to call the prescriber, poison control center, or pharmacist immediately and to seek immediate medical attention if the patient or someone else has taken an overdose. The National Poison Control Center emergency phone number is 1-800-222-1222. Tell the patient to keep this and other emergency numbers handy at all times.
- If the patient is taking an opioid, instruct the patient and caregiver on the signs and symptoms of an overdose and on the administration of naloxone as state law permits.
- Advise the patient to make sure a sufficient supply of drugs is on hand when traveling. The patient should personally carry the drugs in their original containers and not pack them in luggage. Also, recommend that the patient carry a letter from the prescriber authorizing the use of a drug, especially if the drug is a controlled substance.
- Encourage the patient to keep a wallet card or cell phone app that lists all medications the patient is taking, including dose, route, frequency, and indication.

Improvements in preventing hazardous drug exposure

The CDC estimates that 8 million U.S. health care workers are potentially exposed to hazardous drugs in the workplace. Hazardous drugs, as defined by the American Society of Health-System Pharmacists and the National Institute for Occupational Safety and Health (NIOSH), have one or more of the following characteristics:
- carcinogenicity (cause cancer)

- teratogenicity (cause defects in the developing fetus) or cause other developmental toxicities
- reproductive toxicity
- organ toxicity at low doses
- genotoxicity (cause damage to DNA)
- a structure and toxicity profile that mimics that of existing hazardous drugs.

The NIOSH list of antineoplastics and other hazardous drugs can be found at https://www.cdc.gov/niosh/docs/2016-161/pdfs/2016-161.pdf. Health care workers can be exposed to hazardous drugs through inhalation, ingestion, skin contact and absorption, or injection; exposure is most likely from skin contact and absorption or inhalation. Potential exposure can occur in many ways, such as:
- preparing drugs for administration (reconstituting powdered drugs, crushing tablets for oral liquids, compounding powders, or counting out oral doses from multidose bottles)
- administering hazardous drugs IM, IV, intrathecally, or subcut
- directly contacting drugs on the contaminated exteriors of drug vials, on drug-contaminated work surfaces, and on IV tubing and syringes
- handling body fluids that contain drugs or drug-contaminated dressings, linens, or waste
- transporting hazardous drugs
- removing and disposing of personal protective equipment (PPE)
- cleaning contaminated workspaces and spills.

Protecting workers and minimizing exposure

Protecting health care workers and minimizing their exposure to hazardous drugs can be achieved through engineering and administrative controls and use of appropriate PPE.

Engineering controls include:
- class II or III biological safety cabinets (also known as *vertical flow hoods* or *ventilated cabinets*) for hazardous drug preparation
- closed-system drug transfer devices
- needleless systems.

Administrative controls include:
- implementing training, retraining, and testing programs to educate and monitor staff about best practices to prevent hazardous drug exposure
- developing and implementing management policies and protocols to reduce staff risk
- using monitoring programs to identify hazardous drugs and staff exposure or development of early disease.

Appropriate use of PPE includes:
- making sure PPE fits and is used and disposed of properly, following facility policies and protocols
- selecting PPE based on assessment of the potential for hazardous drug exposure:
  – Gloves: Select gloves appropriate for the potential exposure. Double gloving may be necessary depending on the potential exposure. Polyvinyl chloride exam gloves offer little hazardous drug protection. Look for test information provided by the glove manufacturer showing resistance to specific hazardous drugs. If gloves are made with latex, make sure your patient doesn't have a latex allergy.
  – Gowns: These should be long-sleeved, with tight-fitting cuffs. Disposable gowns coated with laminate materials provide better protection than noncoated gowns. Refer to the manufacturer for permeation information. Don't reuse gowns; change gowns immediately after a spill or splash.
  – Respirators: A properly fit-tested certified N-95 respirator or surgical N-95 respirator provides protection from most airborne particles. Other types of respirators may be necessary to protect from airborne gases. Surgical masks don't provide adequate respiratory protection from drug exposure.
  – Face shields: Using face shields with goggles protects against splashes to the face and eyes. Full-face respirators also provide protection. Face shields or eye glasses with side shields don't provide full eye and face protection.
  – Sleeve, hair, and shoe covers: These covers help provide additional protection. They may be required in certain environments such as drug-compounding areas.

Strategies for reducing error rates
In addition to improvements in communication and education, other strategies that have helped reduce medication administration error rates include:
- providing adequate nurse-to-patient staffing ratios
- designing drug preparation areas as safety zones that promote making correct choices during the medication administration process according to drug importance, frequency of use, and sequence of use
- improving the medication administration environment (reduce noise to 50 dB, improve lighting to at least 100 foot-candles, obtain nonglare computer screens)
- developing and using protocols that reduce distractions for nursing staff directly involved in administering medications
- dispensing medications in unit-dose or unit-of-use packaging
- restricting high-alert drugs and administration routes (limiting their number, variety, and concentration in patient care areas). For example, remove all neuromuscular blockers from units where patients aren't normally intubated. Remove highly concentrated electrolytes from unit stock in patient care units. Remove concentrated oral opioids from unit stock and dispensing cabinets. Apply additional strong warnings to drug labels. Make sure emergency equipment is always available.
- switching from IV to oral or subcut forms as soon as possible
- dispensing IV and epidural infusions only from the pharmacy
- labeling all medications both on and off the sterile field
- posting drug information in patient care units and having drug information available for all health care providers at the point of care; using infusion rate and dosing charts in patient care areas
- avoiding unapproved abbreviations
- using leading zeros; for example, use "0.5 mg" rather than ".5 mg"
- avoiding trailing zeros; for example, use "5 mg" rather than "5.0 mg"
- requiring that medication orders be prescribed by metric weight, not by volume (for example, in mg/kg not mL). Never rely on a patient's stated or historical weight. Weigh patients as soon as possible, and measure and document actual weights only in metric units in all electronic and written formats.
- establishing protocols and checklists to double-check and document high-alert drugs or unusual drugs, dosages, or regimens
- always recalculating doses before giving drugs to children or neonates. Make sure that the dose formula is included for calculating the dose. Have a second clinician (preferably a pharmacist) double-check the calculations.
- making sure each patient is monitored appropriately before and after drug administration. Have appropriate monitoring equipment (cardiac monitors, capnography, pulse oximeters) available as needed.

Using technology to promote safety

Technology is becoming an increasingly important part of providing safer drug administration. The goal of medication administration technology is to enhance individual practice and help build safeguards into the medication administration process. Information about ISMP and safe medication practices can be found at http://ismp.org/.

Computerized provider order entry

In computerized provider order entry (CPOE), the prescriber enters the medication orders into a computerized record, thus eliminating errors due to illegible handwriting. Such safeguards as immediate order checking for errors (such as incorrect dosing or routes of administration) and drug interactions, allergy checks, and administration protocols can be built into the system. Orders can be immediately transmitted to the appropriate department and can also be linked to drug information databases. CPOE can be used to monitor how drugs are utilized and can provide data for quality improvement.

Bar codes

Bar-code technology is widely used and was initially developed to help control and track inventory for industry. The use of this technology for safer drug administration, dispensing, inventory control, and drug storage and preparation has been endorsed by the IOM, The Joint Commission, Agency for Healthcare Research and Quality, and ISMP. With this technology, the patient wears a bar-code identifier on a wristband; the medication also has a bar code that uses the medication's own unique National Drug Code to identify the name, dose, manufacturer, and type of packaging. The nurse scans the bar code using an optical scanner, verifying the patient's identity and medication. The system supports but does not replace the traditional "rights" of safe medication.

Bar-code systems have been shown to reduce medication errors, but they aren't without disadvantages. For example, they don't save time in the medication administration process. Problems with the technology can cause delays in treatment. Wristbands can become unreadable due to wear, and scanners can malfunction. These problems may tempt nurses to develop dangerous shortcuts, such as attaching patients' wristbands to clipboards or giving the patient the medication first and then scanning the wristband.

Automated dispensing cabinets

Automated dispensing cabinets (ADCs) are computer-controlled medication distribution systems in the patient care unit or ancillary department that are used to store, track, and dispense medications. ADCs can provide nurses with near-total access to medications needed in their patient care area and promote the control and security of medications. They electronically track the use of drugs such as controlled substances. They may have bar-code capabilities for restocking and correct medication selection, and can be programmed to provide safeguards such as drug safety alerts. ADCs can be linked with external databases and billing systems to increase the efficiency of drug dispensing and billing.

"Smart" pumps

From 2005 through 2009, the FDA received 56,000 reports of adverse events, including numerous injuries and deaths, linked to infusion pumps. Currently, there are initiatives to improve infusion systems and technology. "Smart" IV pumps can have such features as programmable drug libraries and dosage limits, can perform automatic calculations, have dose-error reduction software, and can be programmed to signal dosage alerts. ISMP recommends administering high-alert IV medications using programmable infusion pumps with dose error-reduction software. They can be integrated with bar-code and CPOE technologies and can be wireless. Smart pumps can help alert nurses when incorrect dosages have been selected or to dosages that may exceed recommended levels.

Smart pumps can't detect all problems with IV drug infusions, however. For example, an incorrect drug can be selected from the library database and, with some pumps, it's possible to override safety alerts. Other infusion pump problems include software defects and failure of built-in safety alarms. Some pumps have ambiguous on-screen directions that can lead to dosing errors. The FDA recommends reporting all infusion-related adverse events, planning ahead in case a pump fails, labeling the channels and tubing to prevent errors, checking all settings, and monitoring patients for signs and symptoms of infusion problems. Nurses should perform independent calculation of all doses and infusion rates and not rely solely on the pump. It's essential to double-check each dose calculation. Nurses shouldn't bypass pump alarms and must verify that the pump is functioning properly before beginning an infusion.

Other technologies

Using oral syringes that don't have luer-locks to administer oral or enteral medications helps prevent oral or enteral medications from being administered via the wrong route. (The ISMP has reported cases in which oral medications were drawn into parenteral syringes and inadvertently injected into IV lines, resulting in patient deaths.) Utilizing special tubing that doesn't have side ports for epidural medication administration prevents inadvertent injection of an incorrect drug into the epidural catheter. Certain drugs such as vincristine should always be dispensed in a minibag (25 to 50 mL) of solution and never in a syringe, to avoid accidental intrathecal instead of IV administration. Oral liquid dosing devices, such as syringes, cups, and droppers, should display the metric scale only.

Reporting medication errors

Clearly, medication errors are a major threat to patient safety. Only by sharing and analyzing data and performing more research can evidence-based quality improvements be developed and validated. Several agencies and organizations provide voluntary reporting systems to study the causes and prevalence of medication errors. The FDA has its Adverse Event Reporting System (FAERS), which is part of the MedWatch program. The National Coordinating Council for Medication Error Reporting and Prevention (NCC MERP) has 27 national organization members, including ISMP and United States Pharmacopeial Convention, cooperating to address the interdisciplinary issues. ISMP has reporting programs for practitioner-based medication errors, vaccine errors, and consumer medication errors. Nurses should be encouraged to report medication errors and "near misses" and to help identify problems within systems.

4

Selected therapeutic drug classifications

Alkylating drugs

bendamustine hydrochloride, busulfan, CARBOplatin, carmustine, chlorambucil, CISplatin, cyclophosphamide, dacarbazine, ifosfamide, lomustine, melphalan, oxaliplatin, temozolomide, thiotepa

INDICATIONS
➤ **Various tumors, especially those with large volume and slow cell-turnover rate**

ACTION
Alkylating drugs appear to act independently of a specific cell-cycle phase. Highly reactive, they primarily target nucleic acids and form links with the nuclei of different molecules. This allows the drugs to cross-link double-stranded DNA and to prevent strands from separating for replication, which may contribute to these drugs' ability to destroy cells. These polyfunctional compounds can be divided chemically into five groups: nitrogen mustards, ethyleneamines, alkyl sulfonates, triazines, and nitrosoureas.

ADVERSE REACTIONS
The most common adverse reactions are bone marrow depression (anemia, leukopenia, thrombocytopenia), chills, diarrhea, fever, flank pain, hair loss, nausea, vomiting, redness or pain at the injection site, sore throat, swelling of the feet or lower legs, secondary leukemia, and infertility.

CONTRAINDICATIONS & CAUTIONS
Boxed Warning Refer to individual drug monographs for boxed warnings. ■
• Contraindicated in patients hypersensitive to these drugs.
• Use cautiously in patients receiving other cell-destroying drugs or radiation.
• May cause fetal harm if administered during pregnancy. Females and males with female partners of childbearing potential should use effective contraception during therapy. Consult individual drug monographs for contraception recommendations after final dose of drug. Patients should stop breastfeeding during therapy because drugs appear in human milk. Safety and effectiveness of many alkylating drugs haven't been established in children. Older adults are at increased risk for adverse reactions; monitor closely.

Alpha blockers (peripherally acting)

alfuzosin hydrochloride, doxazosin mesylate, phentolamine mesylate, prazosin hydrochloride, silodosin, tamsulosin hydrochloride, terazosin hydrochloride

INDICATIONS
➤ **HTN, or mild to moderate urinary obstruction in men with BPH**

ACTION
Selective alpha blockers decrease vascular resistance and increase vein capacity, thereby lowering BP and causing nasal and scleroconjunctival congestion, ptosis, orthostatic and exercise hypotension, mild to moderate miosis, interference with ejaculation, and pink, warm skin. They also relax nonvascular smooth muscle, especially in the prostate capsule, which reduces urinary problems in men with BPH. Because alpha$_1$ blockers don't block alpha$_2$ receptors, they don't cause transmitter overflow.

Nonselective alpha blockers antagonize both alpha$_1$ and alpha$_2$ receptors. Generally, alpha blockade results in tachycardia, palpitations, and increased renin secretion because of abnormally large amounts of norepinephrine (from transmitter overflow) released from adrenergic nerve endings as a result of the blockade of alpha$_1$ and alpha$_2$ receptors. Norepinephrine's effects are counterproductive to the major uses of nonselective alpha blockers.

ADVERSE REACTIONS
Alpha blockers may cause severe orthostatic hypotension and syncope, especially with the first few doses. The most common adverse effects of alpha$_1$ blockade are dizziness, headache, drowsiness, somnolence, and malaise. These drugs also may cause tachycardia, palpitations, fluid retention (from excess renin secretion),

nasal and ocular congestion, weakness, and aggravation of respiratory tract infection.

CONTRAINDICATIONS & CAUTIONS
• Contraindicated in patients hypersensitive to these drugs or their components. Also contraindicated in combination therapy with PDE5 inhibitors (sildenafil, tadalafil, vardenafil) due to increased risk of hypotension. Discontinue if symptoms of angina or coronary insufficiency occur. May cause hypotension and increased risk of syncope. Use cautiously. Alfuzosin is contraindicated in patients with moderate or severe hepatic insufficiency and when given with strong CYP3A4 inhibitors. Silodosin is contraindicated in patients with severe renal or hepatic impairment and when given with strong CYP3A4 inhibitors.
• Use cautiously during pregnancy and breastfeeding. In children, safety and effectiveness of many alpha blockers haven't been established; use cautiously. In older adults, hypotensive effects may be more pronounced.
• Alpha-adrenergic blockers can cause marked hypotension and syncope, especially if the patient is in the upright position. Marked orthostatic effects are most common with the first dose but can also occur with a dosage increase or with therapy interruption of more than a few days. To decrease the likelihood of excessive hypotension and syncope, treatment must be initiated at a low dose; adjust dosage slowly.
• Patients undergoing dosage titration should avoid situations, both in the day and at night, in which injury could result if syncope occurs.

Alzheimer disease drugs
aducanumab-avwa, donepezil hydrochloride, galantamine hydrobromide, memantine hydrochloride, rivastigmine tartrate

INDICATIONS
➤ **Mild to moderate dementia of the Alzheimer type**

ACTION
Current theories attribute signs and symptoms of Alzheimer disease to a deficiency of cholinergic neurotransmission. It's suggested that these drugs improve cholinergic function by increasing acetylcholine levels through reversible inhibition of its hydrolysis by cholinesterase. Memantine is an N-methyl-D-aspartate (NMDA) receptor antagonist. Persistent activation of the NMDA receptors is thought to contribute to the symptoms of Alzheimer disease. No evidence indicates that these drugs alter the course of the underlying disease process. Aducanumab is an amyloid beta-directed antibody directed against amyloid plaques in the brain.

ADVERSE REACTIONS
Weight loss, diarrhea, anorexia, nausea, vomiting, dizziness, headache, bradyarrhythmias; HTN and constipation (memantine); cerebral microhemorrhage, superficial siderosis, falls (aducanumab).

CONTRAINDICATIONS & CAUTIONS
• Contraindicated in patients hypersensitive to these drugs or their components.
• May exaggerate neuromuscular blocking effects of succinylcholine-type and similar neuromuscular blockers used during anesthesia.
• Use cautiously with concomitant drugs that slow HR because of increased risk of heart block.
• Use cautiously with NSAIDs because the drugs increase gastric acid secretion. There is increased risk of developing ulcers and active or occult GI bleeding.
• Use cautiously in patients with moderate hepatic or renal impairment. Some drugs aren't recommended in severe hepatic impairment or severe renal impairment. Refer to manufacturer's instructions for use and dosage adjustments for patients with renal impairment.
• Use cautiously in patients with a history of asthma or COPD.
• Conditions that raise urine pH may decrease urinary elimination of memantine, resulting in increased memantine plasma level and increased incidence of adverse effects.

Aminoglycosides
amikacin sulfate, gentamicin sulfate, neomycin sulfate, tobramycin sulfate

INDICATIONS
➤ **Septicemia; postoperative, pulmonary, intra-abdominal, and urinary tract infections; skin, soft-tissue, bone, and joint infections; aerobic gram-negative bacillary meningitis not susceptible to other antibiotics; serious staphylococcal, *Pseudomonas***

aeruginosa, Klebsiella, and *Acinetobacter* infections; enterococcal infections; nosocomial pneumonia; TB; initial empirical therapy in patients who are febrile and leukopenic

ACTION

Aminoglycosides are bactericidal. They bind directly and irreversibly to 30S ribosomal subunits, inhibiting bacterial protein synthesis. They're active against many aerobic gramnegative and some aerobic gram-positive organisms and can be used with other antibiotics for short courses of therapy.

ADVERSE REACTIONS

Ototoxicity and nephrotoxicity are the most serious complications. Neuromuscular blockade also may occur. Oral forms (neomycin) most commonly cause diarrhea, nausea, and vomiting. Parenteral drugs may cause vein irritation, phlebitis, and sterile abscess.

CONTRAINDICATIONS & CAUTIONS

Boxed Warning Refer to individual drug monographs for boxed warnings. ▪
• Contraindicated in patients hypersensitive to these drugs.
Boxed Warning Aminoglycosides are associated with significant nephrotoxicity and ototoxicity. Toxicity may develop even with conventional doses, particularly in patients with prerenal azotemia or impaired renal function. Evidence of renal function impairment or ototoxicity requires drug discontinuation or appropriate dosage adjustments. When possible, monitor serum drug concentrations, renal function, and eighth nerve function. Avoid use with other ototoxic, neurotoxic, or nephrotoxic drugs. Aminoglycosides can cause fetal harm when given during pregnancy. Safety of treatment lasting longer than 14 days hasn't been established. ▪
• Use cautiously in patients with neuromuscular disorders and in those taking neuromuscular blockers.
• Use at lower dosages in patients with renal impairment.
• Use cautiously during pregnancy. Safety hasn't been established during breastfeeding. In neonates and infants born prematurely, the half-life of aminoglycosides is prolonged because of immature renal systems. In infants and children, dosage adjustment may be needed. Older adults have an increased risk of

nephrotoxicity and commonly need a lower dose and longer dosage intervals; they're also susceptible to ototoxicity and superinfection.

Angiotensin-converting enzyme inhibitors

benazepril hydrochloride, captopril, enalaprilat, enalapril maleate, fosinopril sodium, lisinopril, moexipril hydrochloride, perindopril erbumine, quinapril hydrochloride, ramipril, trandolapril

INDICATIONS
➤ HTN, HF, left ventricular dysfunction (LVD), MI, and diabetic nephropathy

ACTION

ACE inhibitors prevent conversion of angiotensin I to angiotensin II, a potent vasoconstrictor. Besides decreasing vasoconstriction and thus reducing peripheral arterial resistance, inhibiting angiotensin II decreases adrenocortical secretion of aldosterone. This reduces sodium and water retention and extracellular fluid volume. ACE inhibition also causes increased levels of bradykinin, which results in vasodilation. This decreases HR and systemic vascular resistance.

ADVERSE REACTIONS

The most common adverse effects of therapeutic doses are dry cough, dysgeusia, fatigue, headache, hyperkalemia, hypotension, proteinuria, rash, and tachycardia. Severe hypotension may occur at toxic drug levels. Angioedema of the face and limbs is a rare but serious complication.

CONTRAINDICATIONS & CAUTIONS
• Contraindicated in patients hypersensitive to these drugs.
• Angioedema of the face, extremities, lips, tongue, glottis, and larynx has been reported in patients treated with ACE inhibitors.
• Can cause serious anaphylactoid reactions, hypotension, neutropenia, and hepatic failure.
• Use cautiously in patients with impaired renal function or serious autoimmune disease and in those taking other drugs known to decrease WBC count or immune response.
Boxed Warning When pregnancy is detected, discontinue drug as soon as possible. Drugs that

DRUG CLASSES

act directly on the RAAS can cause fetal injury and death. ■

• High risks of fetal morbidity and mortality are linked to ACE inhibitors, especially in the second and third trimesters. Some ACE inhibitors appear in human milk; instruct patient to stop breastfeeding during therapy. Safety in children hasn't been established for all products; for use in children, refer to manufacturer's instructions for individual products. Older adults may need lower doses because of impaired drug clearance.

Antacids
aluminum hydroxide, calcium carbonate, magnesium hydroxide, magnesium oxide, sodium bicarbonate

INDICATIONS
➤ **Gastric hyperacidity; hyperphosphatemia (aluminum hydroxide); hypomagnesemia (magnesium oxide); postmenopausal hypocalcemia (calcium carbonate)**

ACTION
Antacids reduce the total acid load in the GI tract and elevate gastric pH to reduce pepsin activity. They also strengthen the gastric mucosal barrier and increase esophageal sphincter tone. Aluminum-containing antacids bind with phosphate ions in the intestine to form insoluble aluminum phosphate, which is excreted in feces. Calcium helps to prevent or treat negative calcium balance and bone loss in osteoporosis.

ADVERSE REACTIONS
Antacids containing aluminum may cause aluminum intoxication, constipation, hypophosphatemia, intestinal obstruction, and osteomalacia. Antacids containing magnesium may cause diarrhea or hypermagnesemia (in renal failure). Calcium carbonate, magnesium oxide, and sodium bicarbonate may cause constipation, milk-alkali syndrome, and rebound hyperacidity.

CONTRAINDICATIONS & CAUTIONS
• Potentially significant interactions may exist requiring dosage or frequency adjustment, additional monitoring, or selection of alternative therapy. Consult Drug Interactions in specific drug entries for more detailed information.

• Use calcium carbonate and magnesium oxide cautiously in patients with severe renal disease. Use sodium bicarbonate cautiously in patients with HTN, renal disease, or edema; in those who are vomiting; in those receiving diuretics or continuous GI suction; and in those on sodium-restricted diets.

• Give aluminum preparations and calcium carbonate cautiously in older adults; in patients receiving antidiarrheals, antispasmodics, or anticholinergics; and in those with dehydration, fluid restriction, chronic renal disease, or suspected intestinal absorption problems.

• Patients should consult prescriber before using antacids during pregnancy and breastfeeding. Serious adverse effects from changes in fluid and electrolyte balance are more likely in infants; monitor them closely. Older adults have an increased risk of adverse reactions; monitor them closely.

Antianginals
ranolazine

Beta blockers
atenolol, bisoprolol fumarate, metoprolol, nadolol, propranolol hydrochloride

Calcium channel blockers
amLODIPine besylate, dilTIAZem hydrochloride, niCARdipine hydrochloride, NIFEdipine, verapamil hydrochloride

Nitrates
isosorbide (dinitrate; mononitrate), nitroglycerin

INDICATIONS
➤ **Moderate to severe angina (beta blockers); classic, effort-induced angina and Prinzmetal angina (calcium channel blockers); recurrent angina (long-acting nitrates and topical, transdermal, transmucosal, and oral extended-release nitroglycerin); acute angina (SL nitroglycerin and SL or chewable isosorbide dinitrate); unstable angina (IV nitroglycerin); chronic angina (ranolazine)**

ACTION

The mechanism of action of ranolazine's antianginal effects hasn't been determined. Beta blockers decrease catecholamine-induced increases in HR, BP, and myocardial contraction. Calcium channel blockers inhibit the flow of calcium through muscle cells, which dilates coronary arteries and decreases systemic vascular resistance, known as *afterload*. Nitrates relax vascular smooth muscle, causing decreased afterload and left ventricular end-diastolic pressure, or *preload*, and increase blood flow through collateral coronary vessels.

ADVERSE REACTIONS

Ranolazine may cause QT-interval prolongation, dizziness, constipation, and nausea. Beta blockers may cause bradycardia, cough, diarrhea, disturbing dreams, dizziness, dyspnea, fatigue, fever, HF, hypotension, lethargy, nausea, peripheral edema, pruritus, rash, depression, shortness of breath, and wheezing. Calcium channel blockers may cause bradycardia, heart block, confusion, constipation, depression, diarrhea, dizziness, dyspepsia, edema, elevated liver enzyme levels (transient), fatigue, flushing, headache, hypotension, insomnia, nervousness, and rash. Nitrates may cause flushing, headache, orthostatic hypotension, reflex tachycardia, rash, syncope, and vomiting.

CONTRAINDICATIONS & CAUTIONS

• Contraindicated in patients hypersensitive to these drugs.

Boxed Warning Abrupt discontinuation of beta blocker therapy has been associated with angina exacerbation and, in some cases, MI and ventricular arrhythmias. When discontinuation of beta blockers is planned, gradually reduce dosage over at least a few weeks. ∎

• Ranolazine is contraindicated in patients taking strong inhibitors of CYP3A or inducers of CYP3A and in those with clinically significant hepatic impairment. Beta blockers are contraindicated in patients with cardiogenic shock, sinus bradycardia, sick sinus syndrome, heart block greater than first degree, decompensated heart failure, or bronchial asthma. Calcium channel blockers are contraindicated in patients with severe hypotension or heart block greater than first degree (except with functioning pacemaker). Nitrates are contraindicated in patients with pericardial tamponade, restrictive cardiomyopathy, constrictive pericarditis,

severe anemia, cerebral hemorrhage, head trauma, or glaucoma, and in patients using PDE5 inhibitors (sildenafil, tadalafil, vardenafil).

• Use beta blockers cautiously in patients with nonallergic bronchospastic disorders, diabetes, or impaired hepatic or renal function. Use calcium channel blockers cautiously in those with hepatic or renal impairment, bradycardia, HF, or cardiogenic shock. Use nitrates cautiously in those with hypotension or recent MI.

• Use beta blockers cautiously during pregnancy. Recommendations for breastfeeding vary by drug; use beta blockers and calcium channel blockers cautiously. Safety and effectiveness haven't been established in children. Check with the prescriber before giving these drugs to children. Older adults have an increased risk of adverse reactions; use cautiously.

Antiarrhythmics

adenosine

Class IA

disopyramide phosphate, procainamide hydrochloride, quiNIDine (gluconate; sulfate)

Class IB

lidocaine hydrochloride, mexiletine hydrochloride

Class IC

flecainide acetate, propafenone hydrochloride

Class II (beta blockers)

esmolol hydrochloride, propranolol hydrochloride

Class III

amiodarone hydrochloride, dofetilide, dronedarone, ibutilide fumarate, sotalol hydrochloride

Class IV (calcium channel blockers)

dilTIAZem hydrochloride, verapamil hydrochloride

INDICATIONS

➤ Atrial and ventricular arrhythmias

DRUG CLASSES

ACTION

Class I drugs reduce the inward current carried by sodium ions, which stabilizes neuronal cardiac membranes. Class IA drugs depress phase 0, prolong the action potential, and stabilize cardiac membranes. Class IB drugs depress phase 0, shorten the action potential, and stabilize cardiac membranes. Class IC drugs block the transport of sodium ions, which decreases conduction velocity but not repolarization rate. Class II drugs decrease HR, myocardial contractility, BP, and AV node conduction. Class III drugs prolong the repolarization phase. Class IV drugs decrease myocardial contractility and oxygen demand by inhibiting calcium ion influx; they also dilate coronary arteries and arterioles.

ADVERSE REACTIONS

Most antiarrhythmics can aggravate existing arrhythmias or cause new ones. They also may produce CNS disturbances, such as dizziness or fatigue; GI problems, such as nausea, vomiting, or altered bowel elimination; hypersensitivity reactions; and hypotension. Some antiarrhythmics may worsen HF. Class II drugs may cause bronchoconstriction. Amiodarone may cause hepatic injury, pulmonary toxicity, and thyroid abnormalities.

CONTRAINDICATIONS & CAUTIONS

Boxed Warning Refer to individual drug monographs for boxed warnings. ∎
• Contraindicated in patients hypersensitive to these drugs.
• Many antiarrhythmics are contraindicated or require cautious use in patients with cardiogenic shock, digitalis toxicity, and second- or third-degree heart block (unless patient has a pacemaker or implantable cardioverter defibrillator).
• Use during pregnancy only if potential benefits to the mother outweigh fetal risks. Use cautiously during breastfeeding; many antiarrhythmics appear in human milk. Monitor children closely because they have an increased risk of adverse reactions. Use cautiously in older adults, who may exhibit physiologic alterations in CV system.
• To minimize the risk of induced arrhythmia, patients initiated or reinitiated on sotalol should be placed for a minimum of 3 days (on their maintenance dose or until steady-state drug levels are achieved) in a facility that can provide cardiac resuscitation, continuous ECG monitoring, and CrCl calculations.

Antibiotic antineoplastics

bleomycin sulfate, DAUNOrubicin hydrochloride, DAUNOrubicin citrate (liposomal), DOXOrubicin hydrochloride, epiRUBicin hydrochloride, IDArubicin hydrochloride, mitoMYcin

INDICATIONS

➤ **Various solid tumors; leukemia**

ACTION

Although classified as antibiotics, these drugs destroy cells, thus ruling out their use as antimicrobials alone. They interfere with proliferation of malignant cells in several ways. Their action may be specific to cell-cycle phase, not specific to cell-cycle phase, or both. Some of these drugs act like alkylating drugs or antimetabolites. By binding to or creating complexes with DNA, antibiotic antineoplastics directly or indirectly inhibit DNA, RNA, and protein synthesis.

ADVERSE REACTIONS

The most common adverse reactions include anxiety, bone marrow depression, chills, confusion, diarrhea, ECG changes, extravasation, fever, flank or joint pain, hair loss, nausea, redness or pain at the injection site, sore throat, swelling of the feet or lower legs, vomiting, and cardiomyopathy.

CONTRAINDICATIONS & CAUTIONS

Boxed Warning Refer to individual drug monographs for boxed warnings. ∎
• Contraindicated in patients hypersensitive to these drugs.
• Avoid antineoplastics during pregnancy. Breastfeeding during therapy isn't recommended. Safety and effectiveness of some drugs haven't been established in children; use cautiously. Use cautiously in older adults because of their increased risk of adverse reactions.

Anticholinergics

atropine sulfate, benztropine mesylate, dicyclomine hydrochloride, scopolamine

INDICATIONS

➤ **Prevention of motion sickness, preoperative reduction of secretions and blockage of cardiac reflexes, adjunctive treatment of GI disorders, blockage of cholinomimetic** effects of cholinesterase inhibitors or other drugs, and (for benztropine) various spastic conditions, including acute dystonic reactions, muscle rigidity, parkinsonism, and extrapyramidal disorders

ACTION
Anticholinergics competitively antagonize the actions of acetylcholine and other cholinergic agonists at muscarinic receptors.

ADVERSE REACTIONS
Therapeutic doses commonly cause blurred vision, constipation, cycloplegia, decreased sweating or anhidrosis, dry mouth, headache, mydriasis, palpitations, tachycardia, urinary hesitancy, and urine retention. These reactions usually disappear when therapy stops. Toxicity can cause signs and symptoms resembling psychosis (disorientation, confusion, hallucinations, delusions, anxiety, agitation, and restlessness); dilated, nonreactive pupils; blurred vision; hot, dry, flushed skin; dry mucous membranes; dysphagia; decreased or absent bowel sounds; urine retention; hyperthermia; tachycardia; HTN; and increased respirations.

CONTRAINDICATIONS & CAUTIONS
• Contraindicated in patients hypersensitive to these drugs and in those with angle-closure glaucoma, renal or GI obstructive disease, reflux esophagitis, or myasthenia gravis.
• Use cautiously in patients with heart disease, GI infection, open-angle glaucoma, prostatic hypertrophy, HTN, hyperthyroidism, ulcerative colitis, autonomic neuropathy, or hiatal hernia with reflux esophagitis.
• Safety hasn't been established during pregnancy. During breastfeeding, avoid anticholinergics because they may decrease milk production; some may appear in human milk and cause infant toxicity. Safety and effectiveness in children haven't been established. Patients older than age 40 may be more sensitive to these drugs. In older adults, use cautiously and reduce dosage, as indicated.

Anticoagulants

Heparin derivative
heparin sodium

Low-molecular-weight heparins
dalteparin sodium, enoxaparin sodium

Selective factor Xa inhibitors
apixaban, betrixaban, edoxaban, fondaparinux sodium, rivaroxaban

Thrombin inhibitors
argatroban, bivalirudin, dabigatran etexilate mesylate

Vitamin K inhibitor
warfarin sodium

INDICATIONS
➤ PE, DVT, thrombus, DIC, unstable angina, MI, atrial fibrillation, heparin-induced thrombocytopenia, heparin-induced thrombosis–thrombocytopenia syndrome, PCI

ACTION
Heparin derivatives accelerate formation of an antithrombin–thrombin complex. They inactivate thrombin and prevent conversion of fibrinogen to fibrin. Thrombin inhibitors directly bind to thrombin and inhibit its action. Selective factor Xa inhibitors directly bind to factor Xa. Warfarin inhibits vitamin K–dependent activation of clotting factors II, VII, IX, and X, which are formed in the liver.

ADVERSE REACTIONS
Anticoagulants commonly cause bleeding and may cause hypersensitivity reactions or hemorrhage. Heparin derivatives may cause thrombocytopenia and may increase liver enzyme levels. Nonhemorrhagic adverse reactions associated with thrombin inhibitors may include back pain, bradycardia, and hypotension. Warfarin may cause agranulocytosis, alopecia (long-term use), anorexia, dermatitis, fever, nausea, tissue necrosis or gangrene, urticaria, and vomiting.

CONTRAINDICATIONS & CAUTIONS
Boxed Warning Refer to individual drug monographs for boxed warnings. ∎
• Contraindicated in patients hypersensitive to these drugs or their components; in patients with aneurysm, active bleeding, CV hemorrhage, hemorrhagic blood dyscrasias, hemophilia, severe HTN, pericardial effusions, or pericarditis; and in patients undergoing major surgery, neurosurgery, neuraxial anesthesia, spinal puncture, or ophthalmic surgery.
• Heparin formulations are contraindicated in patients with history of heparin-induced

DRUG CLASSES

thrombocytopenia or heparin-induced thrombosis–thrombocytopenia syndrome.
• Use cautiously in patients with severe diabetes, renal impairment, severe trauma, ulcerations, or vasculitis.
• Most anticoagulants (except warfarin) may be used in pregnancy only if potential benefit to the mother outweighs risk to the fetus. Warfarin is contraindicated during pregnancy and just after threatened or spontaneous abortion. Patients should avoid breastfeeding during therapy. Infants, especially neonates, may be more susceptible to anticoagulants because of vitamin K deficiency. Older adults are at greater risk for hemorrhage because of altered hemostatic mechanisms and age-related deterioration of hepatic and renal functions.
• Premature discontinuation leads to increased risk of thromboembolic events.

Anticonvulsants

brivaracetam, carBAMazepine, cloBAZam, clonazePAM, diazePAM, eslicarbazepine acetate, felbamate, fosphenytoin sodium, gabapentin, lacosamide, lamoTRIgine, levETIRAcetam, magnesium sulfate, OXcarbazepine, phenytoin sodium, primidone, rufinamide, tiaGABine hydrochloride, topiramate, valproic acid, vigabatrin, zonisamide

INDICATIONS
➤ **Seizure disorders; partial-onset seizures; acute, isolated seizures not caused by seizure disorders; status epilepticus; prevention of seizures after trauma or craniotomy; neuropathic pain; adjunctive therapy in treatment of seizures; adjunctive therapy for primary generalized tonic-clonic seizures**

ACTION
Anticonvulsants include six classes of drugs: selected hydantoin derivatives, barbiturates, benzodiazepines, succinimides, iminostilbene derivatives (carbamazepine), and valproic/carboxylic acid derivatives. Magnesium sulfate is a miscellaneous anticonvulsant. Some hydantoin derivatives and carbamazepine inhibit the spread of seizure activity in the motor cortex. Some barbiturates and succinimides limit seizure activity by increasing the threshold for motor cortex stimuli. Selected benzodiazepines and valproic/carboxylic acid derivatives may increase inhibition of GABA in brain neurons. Magnesium sulfate interferes with the release of acetylcholine at the myoneural junction.

ADVERSE REACTIONS
Anticonvulsants can cause adverse CNS effects, such as ataxia, confusion, somnolence, and tremor. Many anticonvulsants also cause CV disorders, such as arrhythmias and hypotension; GI effects, such as vomiting; and hematologic disorders, such as agranulocytosis, bone marrow depression, leukopenia, and thrombocytopenia. SJS, other severe rashes, and abnormal LFT results may also occur.

CONTRAINDICATIONS & CAUTIONS
Boxed Warning Refer to individual drug monographs for boxed warnings. ■
• Contraindicated in patients hypersensitive to these drugs.
• Carbamazepine is contraindicated within 14 days of MAO inhibitor use.
• Use cautiously in patients with blood dyscrasias. Also, use barbiturates cautiously in patients with suicidality.
• During pregnancy, therapy may continue despite the fetal risks caused by some anticonvulsants. Refer to manufacturer's instructions for each product for use during pregnancy and breastfeeding. Children, especially young ones, are sensitive to the CNS depression of some anticonvulsants; use cautiously. Older adults are sensitive to CNS effects and may need lower doses. Also, some anticonvulsants may take longer to be eliminated because of decreased renal function, and parenteral use is more likely to cause apnea, hypotension, bradycardia, and cardiac arrest.

Antidepressants, tricyclic

amitriptyline hydrochloride, amoxapine, clomiPRAMINE hydrochloride, desipramine hydrochloride, doxepin hydrochloride, imipramine (hydrochloride; pamoate), nortriptyline hydrochloride, protriptyline hydrochloride, trimipramine

INDICATIONS
➤ **Depression, anxiety (doxepin), OCD (clomipramine), enuresis in children older than age 6 (imipramine)**

ACTION
Unknown. TCAs may inhibit reuptake of nor-epinephrine and serotonin in CNS nerve termi-nals (presynaptic neurons), thus enhancing the concentration and activity of neurotransmitters in the synaptic cleft. TCAs also exert antihis-taminic, sedative, anticholinergic, vasodilatory, and quinidine-like effects.

ADVERSE REACTIONS
Adverse reactions include anticholinergic effects, orthostatic hypotension, and seda-tion. The tertiary amines (amitriptyline, dox-epin, imipramine, and trimipramine) exert the strongest sedative effects; tolerance usually de-velops in a few weeks. TCAs may cause CV ef-fects such as T-wave abnormalities, conduction disturbances, and arrhythmias.

CONTRAINDICATIONS & CAUTIONS
Boxed Warning Antidepressants can increase the risk of suicidality. Appropriately monitor patients of all ages who are started on antide-pressant therapy, and observe closely for clinical worsening, suicidality, or unusual changes in behavior. Advise families and caregivers of the need for close observation and communication with the prescriber. ■
• Contraindicated in patients hypersensitive to these drugs and in patients with urine retention or angle-closure glaucoma.
• TCAs are contraindicated within 2 weeks of MAO inhibitor therapy.
• Use cautiously in patients with suicidality, schizophrenia, paranoia, seizure disorders, CV disease, or impaired hepatic function.
• Use cautiously during pregnancy and breast-feeding; safety hasn't been established. In children younger than age 12, TCAs aren't recommended except for imipramine, which is used for enuresis in children age 6 and older. Older adults are more sensitive to therapeutic and adverse effects and need lower dosages.

Antidiabetics (type 2 diabetes)
acarbose, albiglutide, alogliptin benzoate, bromocriptine mesylate, canagliflozin, dapagliflozin propanediol, dulaglutide, empagliflozin, exenatide, glimepiride, glipiZIDE, glyBURIDE, linagliptin, liraglutide, lixisenatide, metFORMIN, miglitol, nateglinide, pioglitazone hydrochloride, pramlintide acetate, rosiglitazone maleate, sAXagliptin hydrochloride, semaglutide, SITagliptin phosphate

INDICATIONS
➤ As adjunct to diet and exercise in mild to moderately severe, stable, nonketotic, type 2 diabetes that can't be controlled by diet alone; as adjunct to diet and ex-ercise for long-term weight management in children with body weight above 60 kg and initial BMI corresponding to 30 kg/m² or greater for adults (obese) by interna-tional cut-offs (Refer to manufacturer's prescribing information for Cole Criteria [Saxenda].)

ACTION
Antidiabetics come in several types. Sulfonyl-ureas are sulfonamide derivatives that aren't an-tibacterial. They lower glucose levels by stimu-lating insulin release from the pancreas. These drugs work only in the presence of function-ing beta cells in the islet tissue of the pancreas. After prolonged administration, they produce hypoglycemia by acting outside of the pancreas, resulting in effects that include reduced glucose production by the liver and enhanced periph-eral sensitivity to insulin. The latter may result from an increased number of insulin receptors or from changes after insulin binding.

Meglitinides, such as nateglinide and repag-linide, are nonsulfonylurea antidiabetics that stimulate the release of insulin from the pancreas.

Metformin decreases hepatic glucose pro-duction, reduces intestinal glucose absorption, and improves insulin sensitivity by increasing peripheral glucose uptake and utilization. With metformin therapy, insulin secretion remains unchanged, and fasting insulin levels and all-day insulin response may decrease.

Alpha-glucosidase inhibitors, such as acar-bose and miglitol, delay digestion of carbo-hydrates, resulting in a smaller rise in glucose levels. Pramlintide, a human amylin analogue, slows the rate at which food leaves the stom-ach, decreasing postprandial increase in glucose level, and reduces appetite.

Rosiglitazone and pioglitazone are thiazol-idinediones, which lower glucose levels by im-proving insulin sensitivity. They are potent and highly selective agonists for receptors found in insulin-sensitive tissues, such as adipose tissue, skeletal muscle, and liver.

DRUG CLASSES

DPP-4 inhibitors, such as linagliptin and sitagliptin, increase insulin release by inhibiting the enzyme DPP-4. Sodium–glucose cotransporter 2 inhibitors, such as dapagliflozin and empagliflozin, reduce reabsorption of filtered glucose and lower plasma glucose concentration by increasing urinary excretion of glucose.

Glucagonlike peptide 1 receptor agonists (albiglutide, dulaglutide, and others) increase insulin secretion from pancreatic beta cells, suppress glucagon secretion, and slow gastric emptying. They may cause medullary thyroid cancer.

ADVERSE REACTIONS

⊙ *Alert:* Sulfonylureas and meglitinide have the potential to cause severe hypoglycemia. Metformin and glitazones rarely cause hypoglycemia unless taken with insulin stimulators or insulin injections. Acarbose and miglitol don't cause hypoglycemia.

Sulfonylureas cause dose-related reactions that usually respond to decreased dosage: anorexia, headache, heartburn, nausea, paresthesia, vomiting, and weakness.

The most serious adverse reaction linked to metformin is lactic acidosis. It's a rare effect and is most likely to occur in patients with renal dysfunction. Other reactions to metformin include dermatitis, GI upset, megaloblastic anemia, rash, and unpleasant or metallic taste.

Thiazolidinediones may cause fluid retention leading to or exacerbating HF. Alpha-glucosidase inhibitors can cause abdominal pain, diarrhea, and flatulence.

Sodium–glucose cotransporter 2 inhibitors may cause hypotension, abnormal renal function, and euglycemic diabetic ketoacidosis, and may increase risk of UTIs.

DPP-4 inhibitors may cause GI reactions, euglycemic diabetic ketoacidosis, and antibody formation.

CONTRAINDICATIONS & CAUTIONS

Boxed Warning Refer to individual drug monographs for boxed warnings. ∎
- Contraindicated in patients hypersensitive to these drugs, in patients with history of allergic reaction to sulfonamide derivatives (glimepiride), and in patients with diabetic ketoacidosis with or without coma. Metformin is also contraindicated in patients with metabolic acidosis; use cautiously in patients with renal or hepatic disease.

- Use sulfonylureas cautiously in patients with established atherosclerotic CV disease. These patients may have increased risk of mortality.
- Use sulfonylureas cautiously in patients with renal or hepatic disease or history of sulfonamide antibiotic hypersensitivity. Use metformin cautiously in patients with adrenal or pituitary insufficiency and in patients who are debilitated or malnourished. Alpha-glucosidase inhibitors should be used cautiously in patients with mild to moderate renal insufficiency. Thiazolidinediones aren't recommended in patients with edema, HF, or liver disease.
- DPP-4 inhibitors may increase the risk of pancreatitis and are contraindicated in patients with a personal or family history of medullary thyroid cancer and in patients with multiple endocrine neoplasia syndrome type 2.
- Use is contraindicated during pregnancy and breastfeeding. Oral antidiabetics appear in small amounts in human milk and may cause hypoglycemia in the infant. Older adults may be more sensitive to these drugs, usually need lower dosages, and are more likely to develop neurologic symptoms of hypoglycemia; monitor these patients closely.

Antidiarrheals
bismuth subsalicylate, diphenoxylate hydrochloride–atropine sulfate, loperamide, octreotide acetate

INDICATIONS
➤ **Mild, acute, or chronic diarrhea; carcinoid syndrome–related diarrhea (octreotide acetate)**

ACTION
Bismuth preparations may have a mild water-binding capacity, may absorb toxins, and provide a protective coating for the intestinal mucosa. Diphenoxylate and loperamide slow GI motility and excessive GI propulsion. Addition of atropine sulfate to diphenoxylate discourages abuse. Octreotide inhibits secretion of GI neurotransmitters and hormones to control diarrhea and has also been used to in treatment of acromegaly and carcinoid syndrome.

ADVERSE REACTIONS
Bismuth preparations may cause salicylism (with high doses), temporary darkening of tongue and stools, constipation, and abdominal cramps.

Octreotide may cause diarrhea, cholelithiasis, abdominal pain, flatulence, back pain, fatigue, headache, abdominal pain, nausea, and dizziness.

CONTRAINDICATIONS & CAUTIONS

• Contraindicated in patients hypersensitive to these drugs.
• Some antidiarrheals may appear in human milk; check individual drugs for specific recommendations.
• Use caution when giving antidiarrheals to older adults.
• For children or teenagers recovering from flu or chickenpox, consult prescriber before giving bismuth subsalicylate.
• Don't give bismuth to patients who are allergic to salicylates or aspirin or who are taking blood thinners. Don't give to children who have or are recovering from chickenpox or flu symptoms due to risk of Reye syndrome.
• Octreotide may cause changes in glucose metabolism and thyroid and cardiac function.
• Torsades de pointes, cardiac arrest, and death have been reported with higher than recommended loperamide doses.
• Loperamide and diphenoxylate-atropine are contraindicated in children younger than age 2.

Antiemetics

aprepitant, dimenhyDRINATE, dolasetron mesylate, dronabinol, fosaprepitant dimeglumine, granisetron hydrochloride, meclizine hydrochloride, metoclopramide hydrochloride, ondansetron hydrochloride, palonosetron hydrochloride, prochlorperazine, prochlorperazine maleate, promethazine hydrochloride, rolapitant hydrochloride, scopolamine, trimethobenzamide hydrochloride

INDICATIONS

➤ **Nausea, vomiting, motion sickness, and vertigo**

ACTION

For antihistamines (dimenhydrinate, meclizine hydrochloride, trimethobenzamide), the mechanism of action is unclear. Phenothiazines (prochlorperazine, promethazine hydrochloride) work by blocking the dopaminergic receptors in the chemoreceptor trigger zone of the brain. Serotonin receptor antagonists (dolasetron,

granisetron, ondansetron) block serotonin stimulation centrally in the chemoreceptor trigger zone and peripherally in vagal nerve terminals. Substance P/neurokinin 1 receptor (NK_1) antagonists (aprepitant, fosaprepitant, rolapitant) inhibit the NK_1 receptors in the brainstem.

ADVERSE REACTIONS

Antiemetics may cause asthenia, fatigue, dizziness, headache, insomnia, abdominal pain, anorexia, constipation, diarrhea, epigastric discomfort, gastritis, heartburn, nausea, vomiting, neutropenia, hiccups, tinnitus, dehydration, and fever. Metoclopramide and prochlorperazine may cause tardive dyskinesia. Rolapitant may cause neutropenia and anemia. Serotonin receptor antagonists may cause headache and increased QT interval. Promethazine administered IV can cause severe tissue injury.

CONTRAINDICATIONS & CAUTIONS

Boxed Warning Refer to individual drug monographs for boxed warnings. ∎
• Contraindicated in patients hypersensitive to these drugs or to any of their components.
• Contraindicated in severe vomiting until etiology of vomiting is established.
• Rolapitant is contraindicated in patients receiving CYP2D6 substrates with a narrow therapeutic index, such as thioridazine and pimozide, because of risk of QT-interval prolongation and torsades de pointes due to increased plasma levels of the substrates.
• Use cautiously in patients with tartrazine and sulfite sensitivities. Antiemetics may cause allergic-type reactions, including hives, itching, wheezing, asthma, and anaphylaxis.
Boxed Warning Don't use promethazine in children younger than age 2 due to risk of severe respiratory depression. ∎

Antifungals

amphotericin B (lipid complex; liposomal), anidulafungin, caspofungin acetate, clotrimazole, econazole nitrate, efinaconazole, fluconazole, flucytosine, griseofulvin, isavuconazonium sulfate, itraconazole, ketoconazole, luliconazole, micafungin sodium, miconazole nitrate, nystatin, posaconazole, sertaconazole nitrate, tavaborole, terbinafine hydrochloride, voriconazole

DRUG CLASSES

INDICATIONS
➤ **Various fungal infections**

ACTION
The amphotericin products bind to sterols in the fungal cell membrane, altering permeability and allowing intracellular components to leak out. These drugs usually inhibit fungal growth and multiplication, but if the level is high enough, the drugs can destroy fungi. Azole antifungals, nystatin, and terbinafine interfere with sterol synthesis in fungal cells, damaging cell membranes and increasing permeability. Caspofungin inhibits the synthesis of an integral component of fungal cell walls. Tavaborole inhibits fungal protein synthesis. Flucytosine penetrates into fungal cells and is converted to 5-FU, and then converted to several active metabolites, which inhibit protein synthesis. Griseofulvin inhibits cell mitosis at metaphase.

ADVERSE REACTIONS
Fluconazole may cause transient elevations of liver enzyme ALP and bilirubin levels; severe liver injury; and dizziness, nausea, vomiting, abdominal pain, diarrhea, rash, headache, and hypokalemia. Adverse reactions to itraconazole include headache and nausea. The most common adverse reactions to ketoconazole are nausea and vomiting. Efinaconazole, luliconazole, and tavaborole can cause local skin irritation. Adverse reactions to voriconazole are uncommon. However, the drug may alter renal function and cause vision changes. Common adverse reactions to caspofungin include paresthesia, tachycardia, anorexia, anemia, pain, myalgia, tachypnea, chills, and diaphoresis. Reactions to nystatin seldom occur, but may include diarrhea, nausea, vomiting, and abdominal pain. Terbinafine may cause abdominal pain, jaundice, diarrhea, flatulence, nausea, anaphylaxis, headache, rash, vision disturbances, and liver enzyme abnormalities. Flucytosine may cause headache, diarrhea, abdominal pain, and bone marrow depression. Griseofulvin may cause confusion, rash, diarrhea, nausea, vomiting, and decreased granulocyte count.

CONTRAINDICATIONS & CAUTIONS
Boxed Warning Refer to individual drug monographs for boxed warnings. ∎
• Contraindicated in patients hypersensitive to these drugs or to any of their components.

• Administer IV amphotericin under close clinical observation. Acute infusion reactions can occur, including fever, shaking chills, hypotension, anorexia, nausea, vomiting, and tachypnea.
• Use caution with concomitant use of caspofungin and cyclosporine because of the possibility of elevated liver enzymes.
• Amphotericin formulations aren't interchangeable and are each prescribed differently.
• Amphotericin, caspofungin, and micafungin can cause severe hypersensitivity reactions, including anaphylaxis.
• Fluconazole and caspofungin can cause severe liver injury.
• Terbinafine can cause hepatic failure and temporary or permanent loss of smell and taste.
↻ *Alert:* Anidulafungin is contraindicated in patients with known or suspected hereditary fructose intolerance (HFI). Drug contains fructose as an inactive ingredient, which may precipitate a metabolic crisis (life-threatening hypoglycemia, hypophosphatemia, lactic acidosis, and hepatic failure) in patients with HFI. Before administering, obtain careful history of HFI signs and symptoms (nausea, vomiting, abdominal pain) with fructose or sucrose ingestion.

Antihistamines
cetirizine hydrochloride, chlorpheniramine maleate, desloratadine, diphenhydrAMINE hydrochloride, fexofenadine hydrochloride, levocetirizine dihydrochloride, loratadine, promethazine hydrochloride

INDICATIONS
➤ **Allergic rhinitis, urticaria, pruritus, vertigo, motion sickness, nausea and vomiting, sedation, dyskinesia, parkinsonism**

ACTION
Antihistamines are structurally related chemicals that compete with histamine for H_1-receptor sites on smooth muscle of bronchi, GI tract, and large blood vessels, binding to cellular receptors and preventing access to and subsequent activity of histamine. They don't directly alter histamine or prevent its release.

ADVERSE REACTIONS
First-generation antihistamines cause drowsiness and impaired motor function early in

therapy. They also can cause blurred vision, constipation, and dry mouth and throat. Some antihistamines, such as promethazine, may cause cholestatic jaundice, which may be a hypersensitivity reaction, and may predispose patients to photosensitivity. Promethazine may also cause extrapyramidal reactions with high doses.

CONTRAINDICATIONS & CAUTIONS
Boxed Warning Refer to individual drug monographs for boxed warnings. ∎
• Contraindicated in patients hypersensitive to these drugs and in those with angle-closure glaucoma, stenosing peptic ulcer, pyloroduodenal obstruction, or bladder neck obstruction. Promethazine is contraindicated in those taking MAO inhibitors. Levocetirizine is contraindicated in patients with ESRD and in children younger than age 12 with renal impairment.
• Safe use hasn't been established during pregnancy. During breastfeeding, antihistamines shouldn't be used because many of these drugs appear in human milk and may cause unusual excitability in the infant. Neonates, especially those born prematurely, may experience seizures. Children, especially those younger than age 6, may experience paradoxical hyperexcitability with restlessness, insomnia, nervousness, euphoria, tremors, and seizures; give cautiously. Older adults usually are more sensitive to the adverse effects of antihistamines, especially dizziness, sedation, hypotension, and urine retention; use cautiously and monitor these patients closely.

Antihypertensives
ACE inhibitors
benazepril hydrochloride, captopril, enalaprilat, enalapril maleate, fosinopril sodium, lisinopril, moexipril hydrochloride, perindopril erbumine, quinapril hydrochloride, ramipril, trandolapril

Angiotensin II receptor blockers
azilsartan kamedoxomil, candesartan cilexetil, eprosartan mesylate, irbesartan, losartan potassium, olmesartan medoxomil, telmisartan, valsartan

Beta blockers
atenolol, bisoprolol fumarate, carvedilol, labetalol hydrochloride, metoprolol (succinate; tartrate), nadolol, propranolol hydrochloride

Calcium channel blockers
amLODIPine besylate, dilTIAZem hydrochloride, felodipine, niCARdipine hydrochloride, NIFEdipine, nisoldipine, verapamil hydrochloride

Centrally acting alpha blockers (sympatholytics)
cloNIDine hydrochloride, guanFACINE hydrochloride, methyldopa

Direct renin inhibitor
aliskiren hemifumarate

Peripherally acting alpha blockers
doxazosin mesylate, prazosin hydrochloride, terazosin hydrochloride

Vasodilators
hydrALAZINE hydrochloride, nitroglycerin, nitroprusside sodium

INDICATIONS
➤ Essential and secondary HTN

ACTION
For information on the action of ACE inhibitors, alpha blockers, ARBs, beta blockers, calcium channel blockers, and diuretics, see their individual drug class entries. Centrally acting sympatholytics stimulate central alpha-adrenergic receptors, reducing cerebral sympathetic outflow, thereby decreasing peripheral vascular resistance and BP. Vasodilators act directly on smooth muscle to reduce BP.

ADVERSE REACTIONS
Antihypertensives commonly cause orthostatic changes in HR, headache, hypotension, nausea, and vomiting. Other reactions vary greatly among different drug types. Centrally acting sympatholytics may cause constipation, depression, dizziness, drowsiness, dry mouth, headache, palpitations, severe rebound HTN, and sexual dysfunction; methyldopa also may cause aplastic anemia and thrombocytopenia. Vasodilators may cause ECG changes, diarrhea, dizziness, HF, palpitations, pruritus, and rash.

DRUG CLASSES

CONTRAINDICATIONS & CAUTIONS

Boxed Warning When pregnancy is detected in patients receiving ACE inhibitors, ARBs, or direct renin inhibitors, discontinue therapy as soon as possible. Drugs that act directly on the RAAS can cause fetal injury and death. ■

Boxed Warning Abrupt discontinuation of beta blocker therapy has been associated with angina exacerbation and, in some cases, MI and ventricular arrhythmias. When discontinuation of beta blockers is planned, gradually reduce dosage over at least a few weeks. ■

Boxed Warning Refer to individual drug monographs for additional boxed warnings. ■

• Contraindicated in patients hypersensitive to these drugs and in those with hypotension.

• Use cautiously in patients with hepatic or renal dysfunction.

• Refer to each manufacturer's instructions for use during pregnancy. During breastfeeding, refer to manufacturer's instructions for use because some antihypertensives appear in human milk. Safety and effectiveness of many antihypertensives haven't been established in children; refer to individual manufacturer's instructions. Older adults are more susceptible to adverse reactions and may need lower maintenance doses; monitor these patients closely.

• Alpha-adrenergic blockers can cause marked lowering of BP, especially postural hypotension, and syncope in association with the first dose or first few days of therapy. To decrease the likelihood of syncope or excessive hypotension, always initiate with a low dose, given at bedtime.

Antilipemics

alirocumab, atorvastatin calcium, cholestyramine, colesevelam hydrochloride, colestipol, evolocumab, ezetimibe, fenofibrate, fluvastatin sodium, gemfibrozil, lomitapide mesylate, lovastatin, mipomersen sodium, niacin, pitavastatin, pravastatin sodium, rosuvastatin calcium, simvastatin

INDICATIONS
➤ **Hyperlipidemia, hypercholesterolemia**

ACTION
Antilipemics lower elevated lipid levels. Bile-sequestering drugs (cholestyramine, colesevelam) lower LDL level by forming insoluble complexes with bile salts, triggering cholesterol to leave the bloodstream and other storage areas to make new bile acids. Fibric acid derivatives (gemfibrozil) reduce cholesterol formation, increase sterol excretion, and decrease lipoprotein and triglyceride synthesis. HMG-CoA reductase inhibitors (atorvastatin, fluvastatin, lovastatin, pitavastatin, pravastatin, rosuvastatin, simvastatin) interfere with the activity of enzymes that generate cholesterol in the liver. Selective cholesterol absorption inhibitors (ezetimibe, evolocumab) inhibit cholesterol absorption by the small intestine, reducing hepatic cholesterol stores and increasing cholesterol clearance from the blood.

ADVERSE REACTIONS
Antilipemics commonly cause GI upset. Bile-sequestering drugs may cause bloating, cholelithiasis, constipation, and steatorrhea. Fibric acid derivatives may cause cholelithiasis and have other GI or CNS effects. Use of gemfibrozil with HMG-CoA reductase inhibitors may affect liver function or cause rash, pruritus, increased CK levels, rhabdomyolysis, and myopathy. Alirocumab may cause hypersensitivity reactions. Evolocumab may cause rash and hypersensitivity.

CONTRAINDICATIONS & CAUTIONS
• Contraindicated in patients hypersensitive to these drugs. Also, bile-sequestering drugs are contraindicated in patients with complete biliary obstruction. Fibric acid derivatives are contraindicated in patients with primary biliary cirrhosis or significant hepatic or renal dysfunction. HMG-CoA reductase inhibitors and cholesterol absorption inhibitors are contraindicated in patients with active liver disease or persistently elevated transaminase levels.

• Use bile-sequestering drugs cautiously in patients who are constipated. Use fibric acid derivatives cautiously in patients with peptic ulcer. Use HMG-CoA inhibitors cautiously in patients who consume large amounts of alcohol or who have a history of liver or renal disease.

• Use bile-sequestering drugs and fibric acid derivatives cautiously and avoid using HMG-CoA inhibitors during pregnancy. Avoid using fibric acid derivatives and HMG-CoA inhibitors and give bile-sequestering drugs cautiously during breastfeeding. In children ages 10 to 17, certain antilipemics have been approved to treat heterozygous familial hypercholesterolemia.

Older adults have an increased risk of severe constipation; use bile-sequestering drugs cautiously and monitor patients closely.

Antimetabolite antineoplastics

azaCITIDine, capecitabine, cytarabine, decitabine, fludarabine phosphate, fluorouracil, gemcitabine hydrochloride, mercaptopurine, methotrexate, PEMEtrexed, PRALAtrexate, trifluridine–tipiracil hydrochloride

INDICATIONS
➤ **Various tumors and hematologic conditions**

ACTION
Antimetabolites are structurally similar to naturally occurring metabolites and can be divided into three subcategories: purine, pyrimidine, and folinic acid analogues. Most of these drugs interrupt cell reproduction at a specific phase of the cell cycle. Purine analogues are incorporated into DNA and RNA, interfering with nucleic acid synthesis (by miscoding) and replication. They also may inhibit synthesis of purine bases through pseudofeedback mechanisms. Pyrimidine analogues inhibit enzymes in metabolic pathways that interfere with biosynthesis of uridine and thymine. Folic acid antagonists prevent conversion of folic acid to tetrahydrofolate by inhibiting the enzyme dihydrofolic acid reductase.

ADVERSE REACTIONS
The most common adverse effects include anxiety, bone marrow depression (anemia, leukopenia, thrombocytopenia), chills, diarrhea, fever, flank or joint pain, hair loss, nausea, redness or pain at the injection site, stomatitis, swelling of the feet or lower legs, dose-dependent neurologic toxicity, and vomiting. Cytarabine may cause reversible corneal toxicity and hemorrhagic conjunctivitis, which may be prevented or diminished by prophylaxis with local corticosteroid eyedrops. Fludarabine may cause hemolytic anemia and ITP.

CONTRAINDICATIONS & CAUTIONS
Boxed Warning Refer to individual drug monographs for boxed warnings. ∎

• Contraindicated in patients hypersensitive to these drugs.
• Most drugs can cause fetal harm; patients exposed to them during pregnancy should be informed of fetal risk. Breastfeeding isn't recommended for patients taking these drugs. Safety and effectiveness of some drugs in children haven't been established. Older adults have an increased risk of adverse reactions; monitor them closely.

Antimigraine drugs
Calcitonin gene–related peptide (CGRP) receptor antagonists
atogepant, eptinezumab, rimegepant, ubrogepant

Serotonin 5-HT$_1$ receptor agonists
almotriptan malate, eletriptan hydrobromide, frovatriptan succinate, lasmiditan, naratriptan hydrochloride, rizatriptan benzoate, SUMAtriptan succinate, ZOLMitriptan

INDICATIONS
➤ **Migraines with or without aura; migraine prevention**

ACTION
CGRP receptor antagonists mediate trigeminovascular pain transmission. Serotonin 5-HT$_1$ receptor agonists constrict cranial vessels, inhibit neuropeptide release, and reduce transmission in the trigeminal nerve pathway.

ADVERSE REACTIONS
These drugs have a wide range of adverse reactions. These include weakness, drowsiness, tingling, warmth or hot sensations, flushing, nasal discomfort, hypersensitivity, visual disturbances, paresthesia, dizziness, fatigue, somnolence, chest pain, weakness, dry mouth, dyspepsia, nausea, diaphoresis, injection-site reactions, vertigo, malaise, and neck, throat, or jaw pain. Intranasal sumatriptan can cause nasal or throat discomfort and taste disturbances.

CONTRAINDICATIONS & CAUTIONS
• Contraindicated in patients hypersensitive to these drugs or their components.
• Serotonin 5-HT$_1$ receptor agonists are contraindicated in patients with ischemic heart disease, angina, CAD, Wolff-Parkinson-White

syndrome, previous MI, uncontrolled HTN or other significant underlying CV conditions, cerebrovascular disease, PVD, and ischemic bowel disease.

• Serotonin syndrome can occur, especially when used with other serotonergic drugs.

• Information regarding use of serotonin 5-HT$_1$ receptor agonists during pregnancy is limited; however, other drugs exist that are preferred for migraine therapy during pregnancy. CGRP receptor antagonists may cause fetal harm and appear in human milk. Sumatriptan and eletriptan appear in human milk; use cautiously during breastfeeding. Refer to manufacturer's instructions for each drug.

• Serotonin 5-HT$_1$ receptor agonists are contraindicated with recent use (within 24 hours) of another 5-HT$_1$ agonist (e.g., another triptan) or of an ergotamine-containing medication.

Antiparkinsonian drugs
amantadine hydrochloride, apomorphine hydrochloride, benztropine mesylate, bromocriptine mesylate, diphenhydrAMINE hydrochloride, entacapone, levodopa–carbidopa, levodopa–carbidopa–entacapone, pramipexole dihydrochloride, rasagiline mesylate, rOPINIRole hydrochloride, selegiline hydrochloride, tolcapone

INDICATIONS
➤ **Signs and symptoms of Parkinson disease and drug-induced extrapyramidal reactions**

ACTION
Unknown. Antiparkinsonians include synthetic anticholinergics, dopaminergics, and the antiviral amantadine. Anticholinergics probably prolong the action of dopamine by blocking its reuptake into presynaptic neurons and by suppressing central cholinergic activity. Dopaminergics act in the brain by increasing dopamine availability, thus improving motor function. Entacapone and tolcapone are reversible inhibitors of peripheral catechol-O-methyltransferase (commonly known as COMT), which is responsible for elimination of various catecholamines, including dopamine. Blocking this pathway when giving levodopa–carbidopa should result in higher levels of levodopa, thereby allowing greater dopaminergic stimulation in the CNS and leading to a greater effect in treating parkinsonian symptoms. Amantadine is thought to increase dopamine release in the substantia nigra. Apomorphine is thought to cause stimulation of postsynaptic dopamine D$_2$-type receptors.

ADVERSE REACTIONS
Anticholinergics may cause blurred vision, cycloplegia, constipation, decreased sweating or anhidrosis, dry mouth, headache, mydriasis, palpitations, tachycardia, urinary hesitancy, and urine retention. Dopaminergics may cause arrhythmias, confusion, disturbing dreams, dystonias, hallucinations, headache, muscle cramps, nausea, orthostatic hypotension, and vomiting. Amantadine also causes irritability, insomnia, and livedo reticularis (with prolonged use). Apomorphine causes yawning, drowsiness, somnolence, dyskinesia, dizziness/orthostatic hypotension, rhinorrhea, nausea, vomiting, hallucinations, confusion, and edema.

CONTRAINDICATIONS & CAUTIONS
Boxed Warning Refer to individual drug monographs for boxed warnings. ■

• Contraindicated in patients hypersensitive to these drugs.

• Use cautiously in patients with prostatic hyperplasia or tardive dyskinesia and in patients who are debilitated.

• NMS-like syndrome involving muscle rigidity, increased body temperature, and mental status changes may occur with abrupt withdrawal of antiparkinsonian agents.

• Safe use hasn't been established during pregnancy. Antiparkinsonians may appear in human milk; the patient should stop the drug or stop breastfeeding, taking into account the importance of the drug to the mother. Safety and effectiveness haven't been established in children. Older adults have an increased risk of adverse reactions; monitor closely.

• Nonselective MAO inhibitors are contraindicated for use with levodopa–carbidopa. Use caution with entacapone.

• Patients treated with ropinirole have reported falling asleep during ADLs.

• Selegiline is contraindicated for use with opioids.

Antiplatelet drugs

abciximab, aspirin, cangrelor tetrasodium, cilostazol, clopidogrel bisulfate, dipyridamole, eptifibatide, prasugrel, ticagrelor, ticlopidine hydrochloride, tirofiban hydrochloride, vorapaxar sulfate

INDICATIONS

➤ Reduction of thrombotic events by reducing platelet aggregation; adjunct to PCI, prevention of cardiac ischemic complications, or treatment of unstable angina not responding to conventional therapy when PCI is planned within 24 hours (abciximab); ACS and PCI (eptifibatide); ACS (tirofiban); non-ST-segment elevation ACS and ST-segment elevation MI, recent MI, recent stroke or PVD (clopidogrel, ticlopidine, vorapaxar); to reduce risk of stroke in patients with acute ischemic stroke (NIH Stroke Scale score of 5 or less) or high-risk TIA (ticagrelor)

ACTION

The IV drugs abciximab, eptifibatide, and tirofiban antagonize the glycoprotein (GP)IIb/IIIa receptors located on platelets, which are involved in platelet aggregation. Clopidogrel, cangrelor, prasugrel, and ticagrelor are inhibitors of platelet aggregation that inhibit the binding of ADP to its platelet receptor and the subsequent ADP-mediated activation of the GPIIb/IIIa complex. Ticlopidine inhibits the binding of fibrinogen to platelets. Vorapaxar inhibits thrombin-induced and thrombin receptor agonist peptide-induced platelet aggregation.

ADVERSE REACTIONS

The IV drugs can cause serious, sometimes fatal, bleeding, thrombocytopenia, and anaphylaxis. The most common adverse reactions to the oral agents include anaphylaxis, rash, stomach pain, nausea, and headache. Bleeding can also occur. Ticlopidine may cause neutropenia and elevated LFT values. Prasugrel can cause atrial fibrillation.

CONTRAINDICATIONS & CAUTIONS

Boxed Warning Refer to individual drug monographs for boxed warnings. ∎

• Can cause severe, sometimes fatal, bleeding.

• Contraindicated in patients hypersensitive to these drugs or their components.

• Contraindicated in active bleeding, bleeding disorders, intracranial neoplasm, AV malformation or aneurysm, cerebrovascular accident (within 2 years), recent major surgery or trauma, severe uncontrolled HTN, or thrombocytopenia.

• Avoid use of ticagrelor in patients with severe hepatic impairment.

• Because of its very long half-life, vorapaxar is effectively irreversible.

• Safe use during pregnancy hasn't been established. Refer to manufacturer's instructions. Drugs may appear in human milk. The patient should stop the drug or stop breastfeeding.

Antipsychotics

First generation (typical)

chlorproMAZINE hydrochloride, fluPHENAZine (decanoate; hydrochloride), haloperidol (decanoate; lactate), loxapine (hydrochloride; succinate), molindone hydrochloride, perphenazine, pimozide, prochlorperazine (edisylate; maleate), thioridazine hydrochloride, thiothixene hydrochloride, trifluoperazine hydrochloride

Second generation (atypical)

ARIPiprazole, ARIPiprazole lauroxil, asenapine maleate, brexpiprazole, cariprazine hydrochloride, cloZAPine, iloperidone, lurasidone hydrochloride, OLANZapine (pamoate), paliperidone (palmitate), QUEtiapine fumarate, risperiDONE, ziprasidone (hydrochloride; mesylate)

INDICATIONS

➤ Schizophrenia (all but pimozide); schizoaffective disorder (paliperidone); psychosis, acute agitation, depression, or mania in bipolar I disorder; depression (chlorpromazine); autism irritability (aripiprazole, risperidone); child hyperactivity and severe behavioral problems (chlorpromazine, haloperidol); acute intermittent porphyria (chlorpromazine); nausea, vomiting (chlorpromazine, prochlorperazine); anxiety, tetanus (chlorpromazine); hiccups

DRUG CLASSES

(chlorpromazine); Tourette syndrome (haloperidol, pimozide)

ACTION
Antipsychotics block several neurotransmitters, particularly dopamine. The exact mechanism of action and ideal combination of targeted neurotransmitters remain unknown.

ADVERSE REACTIONS
First-generation antipsychotics may cause cardiac arrhythmias, cardiac arrest, hypotension, tachycardia, agitation, akathisia, seizures, dizziness, sedation, dystonia, headache, insomnia, NMS, extrapyramidal symptoms, tardive dyskinesia, photosensitivity, pruritus, anorexia, constipation, dry mouth, nausea, weight gain, amenorrhea, galactorrhea, gynecomastia, impotence, urine retention, blurred vision, and hyperthermia/hyperpyrexia.

Second-generation antipsychotics may cause akathisia, dizziness, drowsiness, extrapyramidal symptoms, headache, constipation, nausea, QT-interval prolongation, weight gain, hyperprolactinemia, dyslipidemia, hyperglycemia, and hyperthermia/hyperpyrexia.

CONTRAINDICATIONS & CAUTIONS
Boxed Warning Older adults with dementia-related psychosis treated with antipsychotics are at increased risk for death. Antipsychotics aren't approved for treatment of patients with dementia-related psychosis. ■

Boxed Warning Increased risk of suicidality is seen in children, adolescents, and young adults taking antidepressants. Monitor these patients for worsening and emergence of suicidality. ■

Boxed Warning Refer to individual drug monographs for additional boxed warnings. ■

• Contraindicated in patients hypersensitive to these drugs.
• Use cautiously and observe for tardive dyskinesia, which may be irreversible.
• Use cautiously and watch for signs and symptoms of NMS (muscle rigidity, fever, delirium), especially with first-generation injectable antipsychotics.
• Use cautiously in patients who are depressed or agitated.
• Use cautiously with lithium because of risk of encephalopathic syndrome (weakness, lethargy, fever, confusion).
• Use cautiously in patients with MI, ischemic heart disease, HF, conduction abnormalities, or

cerebrovascular disease, and in those at risk for hypotension.
• Use cautiously in patients with dyslipidemia or diabetes, particularly with second-generation antipsychotics.
• Use cautiously in patients with respiratory infections or chronic disorders because of increased pneumonia risk.
• Use cautiously in patients with blood dyscrasias.
• Use cautiously in patients with history of seizures.
• Use cautiously in patients with Parkinson disease or dementia with Lewy bodies.
• Use cautiously in patients with renal impairment; lower dosage or discontinue drug if BUN level is abnormal.
• Risk during pregnancy is unknown; refer to manufacturer's instructions for use during pregnancy and breastfeeding. When used during the third trimester, there is an increased risk of extrapyramidal symptoms or withdrawal symptoms in the newborn that can be severe and require hospitalization.
• Patients taking antipsychotics should use caution when driving or performing hazardous work due to drowsiness.

Antirheumatics (disease-modifying, biologics, and Janus kinase [JAK] inhibitors)
abatacept, adalimumab, anakinra, baricitinib, canakinumab, certolizumab pegol, etanercept, golimumab, inFLIXimab, ixekizumab, leflunomide, sarilumab, secukinumab, tocilizumab, tofacitinib citrate, upadacitinib, ustekinumab

INDICATIONS
➤ **RA, ankylosing spondylitis, polyarticular juvenile idiopathic arthritis, systemic juvenile idiopathic arthritis**

ACTION
Activated T lymphocytes are found in the synovium of patients with RA. Some drugs bind to TNF so it can't bind to a receptor and exert an effect. TNF plays an important role in pathologic inflammation and joint destruction. Some drugs are antagonists of interleukin-6 receptor, interleukin-1 receptor, interleukin-12 receptor,

and interleukin-17 receptor, which leads to reduction of cytokine production. JAK inhibitors are intracellular enzymes that transmit signals arising from cytokine or growth factor–receptor interactions on the cellular membrane to influence cellular processes of hematopoiesis and immune cell function.

ADVERSE REACTIONS
The most serious adverse reactions include serious infections and malignancies. The most common adverse reactions include rash, pruritus, hair loss, urticaria, nausea, vomiting, anorexia, flatulence, dyspepsia, anemia, leukopenia, thrombocytopenia, elevated liver enzymes, stomatitis, HTN, headache, and hematuria. JAK inhibitors increase lipid levels and risk of thrombosis.

CONTRAINDICATIONS & CAUTIONS
Boxed Warning Refer to individual drug monographs for boxed warnings. ■
• May cause increased risk of serious infections leading to hospitalization or death, including TB, bacterial sepsis, invasive fungal infections (such as histoplasmosis), and infections due to other opportunistic pathogens. Perform tests for latent TB and start treatment for TB before starting therapy if indicated.
• Contraindicated in patients hypersensitive to these drugs or their components.
• Use cautiously in patients receiving two antirheumatics with similar mechanisms of action.
• Use cautiously in patients with a history of recurrent infections, COPD, CNS disorders, demyelinating disorders, HF, and immunosuppression.
• Safe use during pregnancy hasn't been established. Drugs may appear in human milk. Refer to manufacturer's instructions for use during pregnancy and breastfeeding.
• Due to immunosuppressive action, these drugs may also be indicated for Crohn disease, psoriatic arthritis, plaque psoriasis, ulcerative colitis, giant cell arteritis, cytokine release syndrome, moderate to severe hidradenitis suppurativa in patients age 12 and older, and uveitis and for GVHD prophylaxis. Refer to manufacturer's instructions for approved indications of individual drugs.

Antituberculotics
bedaquiline fumarate, cycloSERINE, ethambutol hydrochloride, isoniazid, pyrazinamide, rifabutin, rifAMPin, rifapentine

INDICATIONS
➤ **Acute pulmonary and extrapulmonary TB, acute UTIs**

ACTION
Cycloserine and isoniazid inhibit cell-wall synthesis in susceptible strains of gram-positive and gram-negative bacteria, including *Mycobacterium tuberculosis*. Rifampin, rifapentine, and rifabutin inhibit DNA-dependent RNA polymerase activity in susceptible *M. tuberculosis* organisms. Ethambutol causes impaired cell metabolism. Bedaquiline inhibits an enzyme essential to generate energy in *M. tuberculosis* organisms. The mechanism of action for pyrazinamide is unknown.

ADVERSE REACTIONS
Adverse reactions primarily affect the GI tract, peripheral nervous system, and hepatic system. Use cautiously in patients with hepatic impairment.

Isoniazid may precipitate seizures in patients with a seizure disorder, may produce optic or peripheral neuritis, and may cause fatal hepatitis.

Optic neuritis, blood dyscrasias, anaphylaxis, and hepatotoxicity may occur with ethambutol.

Rifampin may cause epigastric pain, nausea, vomiting, flatulence, abdominal cramps, anorexia, and diarrhea. It has been shown to produce liver dysfunction. Fatalities associated with jaundice have occurred in patients with liver disease and in patients taking rifampin with other hepatotoxic agents.

Cycloserine can cause seizures, confusion, dizziness, headache, and somnolence.

CONTRAINDICATIONS & CAUTIONS
Boxed Warning Severe, sometimes fatal, hepatitis associated with isoniazid has been reported and may develop even after many months of treatment. Carefully monitor patients given isoniazid and perform monthly interviews. Defer preventive treatment in persons with acute hepatic disease. ■
• Contraindicated in patients hypersensitive to these drugs or their components.

DRUG CLASSES

• Multidrug regimens should be used.
• Discontinue drugs or reduce dosage if patients develop signs of CNS toxicity, including seizures, psychosis, somnolence, depression, confusion, hyperreflexia, headache, tremor, vertigo, paresis, or dysarthria.
• May cause QT-interval prolongation. Use cautiously with other drugs that prolong QT interval.
• The use of medications for TB in patients who are pregnant may outweigh fetal risks. Refer to manufacturer's instructions for use during pregnancy and breastfeeding.

Benzodiazepines

ALPRAZolam, chlordiazePOXIDE hydrochloride, cloBAZam, clonazePAM, diazePAM, flurazepam, LORazepam, midazolam hydrochloride, oxazepam, temazepam, triazolam

INDICATIONS

➤ **Seizure disorders (clobazam, clonazepam, diazepam, midazolam, parenteral lorazepam); anxiety disorder (alprazolam, chlordiazepoxide, diazepam, lorazepam, oxazepam); insomnia (flurazepam, temazepam, triazolam); procedural/surgical sedation or amnesia (diazepam, lorazepam, midazolam); skeletal muscle spasm and tremor (diazepam); acute alcohol withdrawal (chlordiazepoxide, diazepam, oxazepam)**

ACTION

Benzodiazepines act selectively on polysynaptic neuronal pathways throughout the CNS. Precise sites and mechanisms of action aren't fully known. However, benzodiazepines enhance or facilitate the action of GABA, an inhibitory neurotransmitter in the CNS. These drugs appear to act at the limbic, thalamic, and hypothalamic levels of the CNS to produce anxiolytic, sedative, hypnotic, skeletal muscle relaxant, and anticonvulsant effects.

ADVERSE REACTIONS

Therapeutic doses may cause drowsiness, impaired motor function, constipation, diarrhea, vomiting, altered appetite, urinary changes, visual disturbances, and CV irregularities. Toxic doses may cause continuing problems with short-term memory, confusion, severe depression, shakiness, vertigo, slurred speech, staggering, bradycardia, respiratory depression, respiratory arrest, or severe weakness. Prolonged or frequent use can cause physical dependency and withdrawal syndrome when drug is stopped.

CONTRAINDICATIONS & CAUTIONS

Boxed Warning Refer to individual drug monographs for additional boxed warnings. ∎
Boxed Warning Benzodiazepine use exposes patient to risks of abuse, misuse, and addiction, which can lead to overdose or death. Assess each patient's risk for abuse, misuse, and addiction before prescribing and periodically during therapy. ∎
Boxed Warning Abrupt discontinuation or rapid dosage reduction of benzodiazepines after continued use may precipitate acute withdrawal reactions, which can be life-threatening. To reduce risk of withdrawal reactions, gradually taper drug to discontinue or reduce dosage. ∎
Boxed Warning Concomitant use of benzodiazepines and opioids may result in profound sedation, respiratory depression, coma, and death. Reserve concomitant prescribing of these drugs to patients for whom alternative treatment options are inadequate. Limit dosages and durations to the minimum required. Follow patients for signs and symptoms of respiratory depression and sedation. ∎
• Monitor patients for signs and symptoms of respiratory depression and sedation.
• Contraindicated in patients hypersensitive to these drugs, in those with acute angle-closure glaucoma, and in those with depressive neuroses or psychotic reactions in which anxiety isn't prominent.
• Avoid use in patients with suicidality and in patients with a history of drug abuse. If drug is necessary, monitor patient carefully.
• Use cautiously in patients with chronic pulmonary insufficiency or sleep apnea and in those with hepatic or renal insufficiency.
• Benzodiazepines increase risk of congenital malformation if taken in the first trimester. Use during labor may cause neonatal flaccidity. A neonate whose mother took a benzodiazepine during pregnancy may have withdrawal symptoms. Benzodiazepines appear in human milk; patients shouldn't breastfeed during therapy. In older adults, benzodiazepine elimination may be prolonged; consider a lower dosage.

Beta blockers

Beta₁-selective blockers
acebutolol hydrochloride, atenolol, betaxolol hydrochloride, bisoprolol fumarate, esmolol hydrochloride, metoprolol (succinate; tartrate), nebivolol hydrochloride

Beta₁ and beta₂ (nonselective) blockers
carvedilol phosphate (beta blocker and alpha₁ blocker), labetalol hydrochloride (beta blocker and alpha₁ blocker), nadolol, propranolol hydrochloride, sotalol hydrochloride, timolol maleate

INDICATIONS
➤ HTN (most drugs); angina pectoris (atenolol, metoprolol, nadolol, propranolol); arrhythmias (acebutolol, esmolol, propranolol, sotalol); glaucoma (betaxolol, timolol); prevention of MI (atenolol, metoprolol, propranolol); prevention of recurrent migraine and other vascular headaches (propranolol); pheochromocytomas or essential tremors (selected drugs); HF (atenolol, carvedilol, metoprolol)

ACTION
Beta blockers compete with beta agonists for available beta receptors; individual drugs differ in their ability to affect beta receptors. Some drugs are nonselective: they block beta₁ receptors in cardiac muscle and beta₂ receptors in bronchial and vascular smooth muscle. Several drugs are cardioselective and, in lower doses, inhibit mainly beta₁ receptors. Some beta blockers have intrinsic sympathomimetic activity and stimulate and block beta receptors, and thereby have less effect on slowing HR. Others stabilize cardiac membranes, which affects cardiac action potential.

ADVERSE REACTIONS
Therapeutic dose may cause bradycardia, dizziness, fatigue, and erectile dysfunction; some may cause other CNS disturbances, such as depression, hallucinations, memory loss, and nightmares. Toxic dose can produce severe hypotension, bradycardia, HF, or bronchospasm.

CONTRAINDICATIONS & CAUTIONS
Boxed Warning Abrupt discontinuation of beta blockers has been associated with angina exacerbation and, in some cases, MI and ventricular arrhythmias. When discontinuation of beta blockers is planned, gradually reduce dosage over at least a few weeks. ∎

Boxed Warning Refer to individual drug monographs for additional boxed warnings. ∎

• Contraindicated in patients hypersensitive to these drugs and in those with cardiogenic shock, sinus bradycardia, heart block greater than first degree, or bronchial asthma.

• Beta blockers may mask signs and symptoms of hypoglycemia (palpitations, tachycardia, tremor).

• Use cautiously in patients with nonallergic bronchospastic disorders, diabetes, impaired hepatic or renal function, and HF.

• Use cautiously during pregnancy. Drugs appear in human milk. Safety and effectiveness haven't been established in children; use only if the benefits outweigh the risks. Use cautiously in older adults; patients may need reduced maintenance doses because of increased bioavailability, delayed metabolism, and increased adverse effects.

Calcium channel blockers
amLODIPine besylate, clevidipine butyrate, dilTIAZem hydrochloride, felodipine, isradipine, niCARdipine hydrochloride, NIFEdipine, niMODipine, nisoldipine, verapamil hydrochloride

INDICATIONS & DOSAGES
➤ Prinzmetal variant angina; chronic stable angina; unstable angina; HTN; arrhythmias; subarachnoid hemorrhage (nimodipine)

ACTION
The main physiologic action of calcium channel blockers is to inhibit calcium influx across the slow channels of myocardial and vascular smooth muscle cells. By inhibiting calcium flow into these cells, calcium channel blockers reduce intracellular calcium levels. This, in turn, dilates coronary arteries, peripheral arteries, and arterioles and slows cardiac conduction.

When used to treat Prinzmetal variant angina, calcium channel blockers inhibit coronary spasm, which then increases oxygen delivery to the heart. Peripheral artery dilation reduces afterload, which decreases myocardial oxygen use. Inhibiting calcium flow into specialized cardiac conduction cells in the SA and AV nodes slows conduction through the heart. Verapamil and diltiazem have the greatest effect on the AV node, which slows the ventricular rate in atrial fibrillation or flutter and converts supraventricular tachycardia to a normal sinus rhythm.

ADVERSE REACTIONS

Symptomatic hypotension can occur. Verapamil may cause bradycardia, hypotension, various degrees of heart block, and worsening of HF after rapid IV delivery. Nifedipine may cause flushing, headache, heartburn, hypotension, light-headedness, and peripheral edema. The most common adverse reactions to diltiazem are headache and dizziness; it also may induce dyspepsia, bradycardia, HF, edema, and various degrees of heart block.

CONTRAINDICATIONS & CAUTIONS

Boxed Warning Refer to individual drug monographs for boxed warnings. ∎

• Contraindicated in patients hypersensitive to these drugs and in those with MI (nifedipine), second- or third-degree heart block (except those with a pacemaker), and cardiogenic shock. Use diltiazem and verapamil cautiously in patients with HF.

• Use cautiously during pregnancy and breastfeeding; refer to individual manufacturer's instructions. Calcium channel blockers may appear in human milk; some drugs may need to be stopped during breastfeeding. In older adults, the half-life of calcium channel blockers may be increased as a result of decreased clearance.

Cephalosporins

First generation
cefadroxil, ceFAZolin sodium, cephalexin

Second generation
cefaclor, cefOXitin sodium, cefprozil, cefuroxime (axetil; sodium)

Third generation
cefdinir, cefditoren pivoxil, cefotaxime sodium, cefpodoxime proxetil, cefTAZidime, cefTRIAXone sodium

Fourth generation
cefepime hydrochloride

Fifth generation
ceftaroline fosamil

INDICATIONS

➤ Infections of the lungs, skin, soft tissue, bones, joints, urinary and respiratory tracts, blood, abdomen, and heart; CNS infections caused by susceptible strains of *Neisseria meningitidis, Haemophilus influenzae,* and *Streptococcus pneumoniae;* meningitis caused by *Escherichia coli* or *Klebsiella;* infections that develop after surgical procedures classified as contaminated or potentially contaminated; perioperative prophylaxis; penicillinase-producing *Neisseria gonorrhoeae;* otitis media and ampicillin-resistant middle ear infections caused by *H. influenzae*

ACTION

Cephalosporins are chemically and pharmacologically similar to penicillin; they act by inhibiting bacterial cell-wall synthesis, causing rapid cell destruction. Their sites of action are enzymes known as *penicillin-binding proteins.* The affinity of certain cephalosporins for these proteins in various microorganisms helps explain the differing actions of these drugs. They are bactericidal: They act against many aerobic gram-positive and gram-negative bacteria and some anaerobic bacteria but don't kill fungi or viruses.

First-generation cephalosporins act against many gram-positive cocci, including penicillinase-producing *Staphylococcus aureus* and *S. epidermidis, S. pneumoniae,* group B streptococci, and group A beta-hemolytic streptococci. Susceptible gram-negative organisms include *Klebsiella pneumoniae, E. coli, Proteus mirabilis,* and *Shigella.*

Second-generation cephalosporins are effective against all organisms susceptible to first-generation drugs and have additional activity against *Moraxella catarrhalis, H. influenzae, Enterobacter, Citrobacter, Providencia, Acinetobacter, Serratia,* and *Neisseria. Bacteroides fragilis* are susceptible to cefoxitin.

Third-generation cephalosporins are less active than first- and second-generation drugs against gram-positive bacteria but are more active against gram-negative organisms, including those resistant to first- and second-generation drugs. They have the greatest stability against beta-lactamases produced by gram-negative bacteria. Susceptible gram-negative organisms include *E. coli, Klebsiella, Enterobacter, Providencia, Acinetobacter, Serratia, Proteus, Morganella,* and *Neisseria.* Some third-generation drugs are active against *B. fragilis* and *Pseudomonas.*

Cefepime shows activity against a wide range of gram-positive and gram-negative bacteria. Cefepime exhibits resistance to beta-lactamases. Susceptible gram-negative bacteria include *Enterobacter, E. coli, K. pneumoniae, P. mirabilis,* and *Pseudomonas aeruginosa.* Susceptible gram-positive bacteria include *S. aureus, S. pneumoniae,* and *Streptococcus pyogenes.*

Ceftaroline has antimicrobial activity against gram-negative bacteria similar to third-generation cephalosporins. It is also active against gram-positive bacteria such as MRSA and methicillin-resistant *S. pneumoniae.*

ADVERSE REACTIONS
Many cephalosporins have similar adverse effects. Hypersensitivity reactions range from mild rashes, fever, and eosinophilia to fatal anaphylaxis and are more common in patients with penicillin allergy. Adverse GI reactions include abdominal pain, diarrhea, dyspepsia, glossitis, nausea, tenesmus, and vomiting. CDAD ranging in severity from mild to fatal colitis can occur during treatment or after treatment ends. Hematologic reactions include positive direct and indirect antiglobulin on Coombs test, thrombocytopenia or thrombocythemia, transient neutropenia, and reversible leukopenia. Minimal elevation of LFT results occurs occasionally. Adverse renal effects may occur with any cephalosporin; they are most common in older adults, patients with decreased renal function, and those taking other nephrotoxic drugs. Some products increase risk of arrhythmia, chest pain, hypotension, and HTN.

Local reactions may occur after IV or IM administration; these reactions occur more often with higher doses and long-term therapy. Bacterial and fungal superinfections may result from suppression of normal flora.

CONTRAINDICATIONS & CAUTIONS
• Contraindicated in patients hypersensitive to cephalosporins and related antibiotics.
• Ceftriaxone is contraindicated in neonates if they require (or are expected to require) treatment with calcium-containing IV solutions, including continuous calcium-containing infusions such as parenteral nutrition, because of risk of precipitation of ceftriaxone-calcium.
• Use cautiously in patients with renal or hepatic impairment, history of GI disease, or allergy to penicillins.
• Use ceftriaxone cautiously in neonates with hyperbilirubinemia, especially if born prematurely.
• During pregnancy, use only when potential benefits outweigh potential fetal hazards; safety hasn't been definitively established. During breastfeeding, use cautiously because drugs appear in human milk. In neonates and infants, half-life is prolonged; use cautiously. Older adults are susceptible to superinfection and coagulopathies, commonly have renal impairment, and may need a lower dosage; use cautiously.

CNS stimulants
armodafinil, dexmethylphenidate hydrochloride, dextroamphetamine sulfate, doxapram hydrochloride, lisdexamfetamine dimesylate, methylphenidate hydrochloride, modafinil, phentermine hydrochloride

INDICATIONS
➤ **Stimulation of respiration in patients with drug-induced postanesthesia respiratory depression or CNS depression caused by overdose and as temporary measure in acute respiratory insufficiency (doxapram); obstructive sleep apnea (armodafinil, modafinil); narcolepsy (armodafinil, dextroamphetamine, methylphenidate, modafinil); shift-work sleep disorder (armodafinil, modafinil); obesity (phentermine); binge eating disorder (lisdexamfetamine); ADHD (dextroamphetamine, lisdexamfetamine, dexmethylphenidate, methylphenidate)**

ACTION
Doxapram produces respiratory stimulation through the peripheral carotid chemoreceptors. The exact mechanism of action of armodafinil and modafinil isn't known. Phentermine is a sympathomimetic amine. The exact mechanism of action in treating obesity hasn't been established. Dextroamphetamine, dexmethylphenidate, lisdexamfetamine, and methylphenidate promote nerve impulse transmission.

DRUG CLASSES

ADVERSE REACTIONS

The adverse effects of CNS stimulants are related to the stimulatory effect of these drugs and include HTN, palpitations, tachyarrhythmias, urticaria, constipation, decreased appetite, diarrhea, dizziness, excitement, insomnia, tremor, and restlessness. Armodafinil and modafinil may cause severe rash, including SJS, DRESS/multiorgan hypersensitivity, angioedema, and anaphylaxis. Lisdexamphetamine causes suppression of growth in children and serotonin syndrome in adults.

CONTRAINDICATIONS & CAUTIONS

Boxed Warning Refer to individual drug monographs for boxed warnings. ∎

• Contraindicated in patients hypersensitive to these drugs or their components.

• Use drugs cautiously in patients with psychiatric illness.

• Drugs have the potential for abuse and misuse.

• Doxapram is contraindicated in epilepsy, seizure disorders, mechanical disorders of ventilation such as muscle paresis, flail chest, pneumothorax, asthma, pulmonary fibrosis, head injury, stroke, cerebral edema, uncompensated HF, severe coronary disease, and severe HTN.

• Delay administration of doxapram in patients who have received general anesthesia utilizing a volatile agent until the volatile agent has been excreted. This will lessen the chance for arrhythmias, including ventricular tachycardia and ventricular fibrillation.

• Administer doxapram cautiously in patients taking MAO inhibitors or sympathomimetics because an added pressor effect may occur.

• Phentermine is contraindicated in agitated states, CV disease, history of drug abuse, severe HTN, hyperthyroidism, and glaucoma.

• Dextroamphetamine, phentermine, lisdexamfetamine, dexmethylphenidate, and methylphenidate are contraindicated during or within 14 days after use of MAO inhibitors.

• Drugs can cause arrhythmias, HTN, nervousness, and insomnia.

• Use lisdexamfetamine, dextroamphetamine, methylphenidate, dexmethylphenidate, and modafinil cautiously in patients with seizure disorder.

• Safety during pregnancy hasn't been established. Some amphetamines appear in human milk; breastfeeding isn't recommended.

• Serious CV reactions, including sudden death, have been reported in association with CNS stimulant treatment (such as lisdexamphetamine) at recommended doses in children with structural cardiac abnormalities or other serious heart problems. In adults, sudden death, stroke, and MI have been reported. Avoid use in patients with known structural cardiac abnormalities, cardiomyopathy, serious heart arrhythmia, or CAD.

Corticosteroids

beclomethasone dipropionate, betamethasone (dipropionate; valerate), budesonide, ciclesonide, cortisone acetate, deflazacort, dexamethasone (sodium phosphate), fludrocortisone acetate, flunisolide, fluticasone propionate, hydrocortisone (acetate; butyrate; cypionate; probutate; sodium succinate; valerate), methylPREDNISolone (acetate; sodium succinate), mometasone furoate, prednisoLONE (acetate; sodium phosphate), predniSONE, triamcinolone (acetonide; hexacetonide)

INDICATIONS

➤ **Duchenne muscular dystrophy; hypersensitivity; inflammation, particularly of eye, nose, and respiratory tract (asthma); to initiate immunosuppression; replacement therapy in adrenocortical insufficiency, dermatologic and GI diseases, and respiratory, endocrine, hematologic, and rheumatic disorders**

ACTION

Corticosteroids suppress cell-mediated and humoral immunity by reducing levels of leukocytes, monocytes, and eosinophils; by decreasing Ig binding to cell-surface receptors; and by inhibiting interleukin synthesis. They reduce inflammation by preventing hydrolytic enzyme release into the cells, preventing plasma exudation, suppressing polymorphonuclear leukocyte migration, and disrupting other inflammatory processes.

ADVERSE REACTIONS

Systemic corticosteroid therapy may suppress the HPA axis. Excessive use may cause cushingoid symptoms and various systemic disorders, such as diabetes and osteoporosis. Other effects may include dermatologic disorders, edema, mood changes, fluid and electrolyte imbalances, gastritis or GI irritation, HTN, ocular changes, immunosuppression, increased appetite, insomnia, psychosis, and weight gain.

CONTRAINDICATIONS & CAUTIONS

• Contraindicated in patients hypersensitive to these drugs or their components and in those with systemic fungal infection.
• Use cautiously in patients with GI ulceration, renal disease, HTN, osteoporosis, varicella, vaccinia, exanthem, diabetes, hypothyroidism, thromboembolic disorder, seizures, myasthenia gravis, HF, TB, ocular herpes simplex, hypoalbuminemia, emotional instability, or psychosis.
• Avoid use during pregnancy, if possible, because of risk to the fetus. If use during pregnancy is necessary, use the lowest effective dose for the shortest duration. Inhaled drugs are preferred for treating asthma during pregnancy. Patients should stop breastfeeding because these drugs appear in human milk and could cause serious adverse effects in infants. In children, long-term use should be avoided whenever possible because stunted growth may result. Older adults may have an increased risk of adverse reactions; monitor closely.

Diuretics, loop
bumetanide, ethacrynate sodium, ethacrynic acid, furosemide, torsemide

INDICATIONS
➤ **Edema from HF, hepatic cirrhosis, or nephrotic syndrome; mild to moderate HTN; adjunctive treatment in acute pulmonary edema or hypertensive crisis; short-term management of ascites due to malignancy, idiopathic edema, and lymphedema**

ACTION
Loop diuretics inhibit sodium and chloride reabsorption in the ascending loop of Henle, thus increasing excretion of sodium, chloride, and water. Like thiazide diuretics, loop diuretics increase excretion of potassium. Loop diuretics produce more diuresis and electrolyte loss than thiazide diuretics.

ADVERSE REACTIONS
Therapeutic doses commonly cause metabolic and electrolyte disturbances, particularly

potassium depletion, and also may cause hyperglycemia, hyperuricemia, hypochloremic alkalosis, and hypomagnesemia. Rapid parenteral administration may cause hearing loss (including deafness) and tinnitus. High doses can produce profound diuresis, leading to hypovolemia and CV collapse. Photosensitivity also may occur.

CONTRAINDICATIONS & CAUTIONS
Boxed Warning Refer to individual drug monographs for boxed warnings. ■
• Use of excessive amounts can lead to profound diuresis with water and electrolyte depletion; carefully individualize dosage and schedule.
• Use cautiously in patients with a sulfa allergy because of the potential for a cross-reaction.
• Contraindicated in patients hypersensitive to these drugs and in patients with anuria, hepatic coma, or severe electrolyte depletion.
• Use cautiously in patients with severe renal disease.
• Use cautiously during pregnancy. Don't use during breastfeeding. Use cautiously in neonates; the usual pediatric dose can be used, but dosage intervals should be extended. If needed in older adults, use a lower dose and monitor patient closely; these patients are more susceptible to drug-induced diuresis.

Diuretics, potassium-sparing
aMILoride hydrochloride, eplerenone, spironolactone, triamterene

INDICATIONS & DOSAGES
➤ **Edema from hepatic cirrhosis, nephrotic syndrome, and HF; mild or moderate HTN; diagnosis of primary hyperaldosteronism; aid in treatment of hypokalemia; prophylaxis of hypokalemia in patients taking cardiac glycosides; to improve survival of patients with left ventricular systolic dysfunction (LVEF less than or equal to 40%) who are stable and CHF after acute MI**

ACTION
Amiloride and triamterene act directly on the distal renal tubule of the nephron to inhibit sodium reabsorption and potassium and hydrogen excretion. Spironolactone and eplerenone competitively inhibit aldosterone at the distal renal tubules, also promoting sodium excretion and potassium retention.

DRUG CLASSES

ADVERSE REACTIONS

Hyperkalemia is the most serious adverse reaction; it could lead to arrhythmias. Other adverse reactions include nausea, vomiting, headache, weakness, fatigue, bowel disturbances, cough, and dyspnea.

CONTRAINDICATIONS & CAUTIONS

Boxed Warning Refer to individual drug monographs for boxed warnings. ■
• Contraindicated in patients hypersensitive to these drugs, in those taking other potassium-sparing diuretics or potassium supplements, and in those with anuria, acute or chronic renal insufficiency, severe hyperkalemia, or diabetic nephropathy.
• Use cautiously in patients with severe hepatic insufficiency because electrolyte imbalance may lead to hepatic encephalopathy and in patients with diabetes, who are at increased risk for hyperkalemia.
• No controlled studies of use during pregnancy exist. Refer to manufacturer's instructions for use during pregnancy and breastfeeding. Use cautiously in children, who are more susceptible to hyperkalemia. In older adults and in patients with debilitation, observe closely and reduce dosage, if needed; these patients are more susceptible to drug-induced diuresis and hyperkalemia.

Diuretics, thiazide and thiazide-like

Thiazide
hydroCHLOROthiazide

Thiazide-like
indapamide, metOLazone

INDICATIONS

➤ **Edema from right-sided HF, mild to moderate left-sided HF, corticosteroid or estrogen therapy, or nephrotic syndrome; edema and ascites caused by hepatic cirrhosis; HTN**

ACTION

Thiazide and thiazide-like diuretics interfere with sodium transport across the tubules of the cortical diluting segment in the nephron, thereby increasing renal excretion of sodium, chloride, water, and potassium and decreasing calcium excretion.

Thiazide diuretics also exert an antihypertensive effect. Although the exact mechanism is unknown, direct arteriolar dilation may be partially responsible. In diabetes insipidus, thiazides cause a paradoxical decrease in urine volume and an increase in renal concentration of urine, possibly because of sodium depletion and decreased plasma volume. This increases water and sodium reabsorption in the kidneys.

ADVERSE REACTIONS

Therapeutic doses cause electrolyte and metabolic disturbances, most commonly potassium depletion. Other abnormalities include hypotension, elevated cholesterol levels, hypercalcemia, hyperglycemia, hyperuricemia, hypochloremic alkalosis, hypomagnesemia, hyponatremia, and photosensitivity.

CONTRAINDICATIONS & CAUTIONS

Boxed Warning Refer to individual drug monographs for boxed warnings. ■
• Contraindicated in patients hypersensitive to these drugs and in those with anuria.
• Use cautiously in patients with severe renal disease, impaired hepatic function, or progressive liver disease.
• Use hydrochlorothiazide cautiously in patients with sulfonamide or penicillin allergy; use may increase risk of acute transient myopia and acute angle-closure glaucoma.
• Use cautiously during pregnancy. Drugs appear in human milk; patient should either discontinue breastfeeding or discontinue drug. Safety and effectiveness in children haven't been established. If needed in older adults, reduce dosage and monitor patient closely; these patients are more susceptible to drug-induced diuresis.

Estrogens

esterified estrogens, estradiol (cypionate; hemihydrate; valerate), estrogens (conjugated), estropipate

INDICATIONS

➤ **Prevention of moderate to severe vasomotor symptoms linked to menopause, such as hot flushes and dizziness; stimulation of vaginal tissue development, cornification, and secretory activity; inhibition of hormone-sensitive cancer growth; female hypogonadism; female castration; primary** ovulation failure; ovulation control; prevention of conception

ACTION

Estrogens promote the development and maintenance of the female reproductive system and secondary sexual characteristics. They inhibit the release of pituitary gonadotropins and have various metabolic effects, including retention of fluid and electrolytes, retention and deposition in bone of calcium and phosphorus, and mild anabolic activity.

Estrogens and estrogenic substances given as drugs have effects related to endogenous estrogen's mechanism of action. They can mimic the action of endogenous estrogen when used as replacement therapy and can inhibit ovulation or the growth of certain hormone-sensitive cancers.

ADVERSE REACTIONS

Acute adverse reactions include abdominal cramps; asthenia; back pain; bloating caused by fluid and electrolyte retention; breast swelling and tenderness; changes in menstrual bleeding patterns, such as spotting and prolongation or absence of bleeding; depression; endometrial hyperplasia; flatulence; headache; insomnia; leukorrhea; loss of appetite; loss of libido; nausea; photosensitivity; swollen feet or ankles; weight gain; vaginal hemorrhage, vaginitis.

Long-term effects include benign hepatomas, cholestatic jaundice, elevated BP (sometimes into the hypertensive range), endometrial carcinoma (rare), and thromboembolic disease (risk increases greatly with cigarette smoking, especially in women older than age 35).

CONTRAINDICATIONS & CAUTIONS

Boxed Warning Refer to individual drug monographs for boxed warnings. ■

Boxed Warning There is an increased risk of endometrial cancer in patients with a uterus who use unopposed estrogens. ■

Boxed Warning Estrogen-alone therapy shouldn't be used for the prevention of CV disease or dementia. ■

Boxed Warning Estrogen-alone therapy may increase risk of stroke and DVT. It also may increase probable dementia in patients age 65 and older who are postmenopausal. ■

• Contraindicated in women with thrombophlebitis or thromboembolic disorders,

unexplained abnormal genital bleeding, or estrogen-dependent neoplasia.

• Use cautiously in patients with HTN; metabolic bone disease; migraines; seizures; asthma; cardiac, renal, or hepatic impairment; blood dyscrasia; diabetes; family history of breast cancer; or fibrocystic disease.

• Contraindicated during pregnancy and breastfeeding. In adolescents whose bone growth isn't complete, use cautiously because of effects on epiphyseal closure. Women who are postmenopausal with a history of long-term estrogen use are at increased risk for endometrial cancer and stroke. Women who are postmenopausal also have increased risk of breast cancer, MI, stroke, and blood clots with long-term use of estrogen plus progestin.

Fluoroquinolones

ciprofloxacin, delafloxacin meglumine, gatifloxacin, gemifloxacin mesylate, levoFLOXacin, moxifloxacin hydrochloride, ofloxacin

INDICATIONS

➤ **Bone and joint infection; bacterial bronchitis; endocervical and urethral chlamydial infection; bacterial gastroenteritis; endocervical and urethral gonorrhea; intra-abdominal infection; empirical therapy for febrile neutropenia; pelvic inflammatory disease; bacterial pneumonia; bacterial prostatitis; acute sinusitis; skin and soft-tissue infection; typhoid fever; bacterial UTI (prevention and treatment); chancroid; meningococcal carriers; bacterial septicemia caused by susceptible organisms; bacterial conjunctivitis (gatifloxacin); infectious diarrhea; inhalational anthrax postexposure; plague**

ACTION

Fluoroquinolones produce a bactericidal effect by inhibiting intracellular DNA gyrase and topoisomerase IV. These enzymes are essential catalysts in the duplication, transcription, and repair of bacterial DNA.

Fluoroquinolones are broad-spectrum, systemic antibacterial drugs active against a wide range of aerobic gram-positive and gram-negative organisms. Gram-positive aerobic bacteria include *Staphylococcus aureus, S. epidermidis, S. hemolyticus, S. saprophyticus;*

penicillinase- and non–penicillinase-producing staphylococci and some methicillin-resistant strains; *Streptococcus pneumoniae;* group A (beta) hemolytic streptococci *(S. pyogenes);* group B streptococci *(S. agalactiae);* viridans streptococci; groups C, F, and G streptococci and nonenterococcal group D streptococci; and *Enterococcus faecalis* and *Bacillus anthracis.* Fluoroquinolones are also effective against gram-negative aerobic bacteria, including, but not limited to, *Escherichia coli, Neisseria meningitidis,* and most strains of penicillinase- and non–penicillinase-producing *Haemophilus ducreyi, H. influenzae, H. parainfluenzae, Moraxella catarrhalis, N. gonorrhoeae,* most clinically important *Enterobacteriaceae,* and *Vibrio parahaemolyticus.* Certain fluoroquinolones are active against *Chlamydia trachomatis, Legionella pneumophila, Mycobacterium avium-intracellulare, Mycoplasma hominis, M. pneumoniae,* and *Pseudomonas aeruginosa.*

ADVERSE REACTIONS
Adverse reactions that are rare but need medical attention include CNS stimulation (acute psychosis, agitation, hallucinations, tremors), hepatotoxicity, hypoglycemia or hyperglycemia, hypersensitivity reactions, interstitial nephritis, phlebitis, pseudomembranous colitis, and tendinitis or tendon rupture. Adverse reactions that need no medical attention unless they persist or become intolerable include CNS effects (dizziness, headache, nervousness, drowsiness, insomnia), GI reactions, and photosensitivity.

CONTRAINDICATIONS & CAUTIONS
Boxed Warning Fluoroquinolones are associated with increased risk of tendinitis and tendon rupture in all age-groups. The risk further increases in older adults (usually older than age 60), in patients taking corticosteroids, and in patients who have received kidney, heart, or lung transplants. For patients with sinusitis, bronchitis, and uncomplicated UTIs, use only if there are no alternative treatment options. ∎
Boxed Warning Fluoroquinolones may exacerbate muscle weakness in persons with myasthenia gravis. Avoid use in patients with known history of myasthenia gravis. ∎
🌢 *Alert:* Drug may increase risk of aortic dissection or rupture when used systemically. Avoid use in patients with known aortic aneurysm and patients at risk for an aortic aneurysm, including those with peripheral atherosclerotic vascular diseases, HTN, certain genetic conditions (Marfan syndrome, Ehlers-Danlos syndrome), and older adults. Drug should only be used in these patients if no other treatment options are available.
● Contraindicated in patients hypersensitive to fluoroquinolones because serious, possibly fatal, reactions can occur.
● Most systemic fluoroquinolones can cause QT-interval prolongations. Avoid in patients with a history of QTc-interval prolongation or uncorrected electrolyte disorders (hypokalemia, hypomagnesemia) and in patients taking class IA or class III antiarrhythmics and other drugs that prolong the QT interval.
● Hypoglycemia or hyperglycemia may occur in patients with or without diabetes.
● Use cautiously in patients with known or suspected CNS disorders that predispose them to seizures or lower the seizure threshold, cerebral ischemia, severe hepatic dysfunction, or renal insufficiency.
● CDAD ranging in severity from mild to fatal colitis can occur during treatment or even more than 2 months after therapy ends.
● If phototoxicity occurs, discontinue drug.
● Refer to manufacturer's instructions for use during pregnancy and breastfeeding. In children, fluoroquinolones aren't recommended because they can cause joint problems. If needed in older adults, reduce dosage; these patients are more likely to have reduced renal function.

Hematopoietic agents
darbepoetin alfa, epoetin alfa

INDICATIONS
➤ **Anemia associated with chronic renal failure, zidovudine therapy in patients with HIV, and cancer chemotherapy; to reduce need for allogeneic blood transfusions in patients undergoing elective, noncardiac, nonvascular surgical procedures**

ACTION
Epoetin alfa and darbepoetin alfa stimulate RBC production in the bone marrow.

ADVERSE REACTIONS
Hematopoietics may cause fatigue, headache, chest pain, HTN, nausea, vomiting, diarrhea, mucositis, stomatitis, myalgias, fever,

dyspnea, cough, sore throat, alopecia, rash, urticaria, seizures, stinging at injection site, peripheral edema, procedural hypotension, abdominal pain, thromboembolic events.

CONTRAINDICATIONS & CAUTIONS

Boxed Warning Refer to individual drug monographs for boxed warnings. ∎
- Contraindicated in patients hypersensitive to these drugs, their components, or human albumin.
- Contraindicated in uncontrolled HTN.
- Epoetin alfa isn't indicated for use in patients with cancer receiving hormonal agents, biologic products, or radiotherapy unless also receiving concomitant myelosuppressive chemotherapy; in patients with cancer receiving myelosuppressive chemotherapy when the anticipated outcome is cure or when chemotherapy-related anemia can be managed by transfusion; in patients scheduled for surgery who are willing to donate autologous blood; in patients undergoing cardiac or vascular surgery; or as a substitute for RBC transfusions in patients who require immediate correction of anemia.

Boxed Warning Don't use in patients with breast, non-small-cell lung, head and neck, or lymphoid cancers. Drug increases risk of tumor progression or recurrence or shortened overall survival. ∎
- Use cautiously in patients with cardiac disease, seizures, and porphyria.
- During pregnancy, consider the benefits and risks for the mother and possible risks to the fetus before starting therapy. It isn't known if drugs appear in human milk. Consider the benefits and risk of breastfeeding and potential adverse effects on infant; use cautiously during breastfeeding.

Histamine$_2$-receptor antagonists
cimetidine, famotidine, nizatidine

INDICATIONS
➤ **Duodenal or gastric ulcer; Zollinger-Ellison syndrome; GERD; heartburn**

ACTION
H$_2$-receptor antagonists inhibit the action of H$_2$ receptors in gastric parietal cells, reducing gastric acid output and concentration, regardless of stimulants, such as histamine, food, insulin, and caffeine, or basal conditions.

ADVERSE REACTIONS
H$_2$-receptor antagonists rarely cause adverse reactions. Cardiac arrhythmias, dizziness, fatigue, gynecomastia, headache, mild and transient diarrhea, and thrombocytopenia are possible.

CONTRAINDICATIONS & CAUTIONS
- Contraindicated in patients hypersensitive to these drugs.
- Use cautiously in patients with impaired renal or hepatic function.
- Use cautiously during pregnancy. Refer to manufacturer's instructions for use during breastfeeding as some drugs shouldn't be used. Older adults have increased risk of adverse reactions, particularly those affecting the CNS; use cautiously.

Immunosuppressants
anakinra, azaTHIOprine, basiliximab, belatacept, belimumab, cycloSPORINE, fingolimod, inFLIXimab, lymphocyte immune globulin, mycophenolate mofetil, siponimod, sirolimus, tacrolimus

INDICATIONS
➤ **Prevention of rejection in organ transplants; RA; MS (fingolimod, siponimod); SLE; Crohn disease; ulcerative colitis; cryopyrin-associated periodic syndromes; polyarticular juvenile idiopathic arthritis; psoriatic arthritis; ankylosing spondylitis; plaque psoriasis; moderate to severe aplastic anemia in patients unsuitable for bone marrow transplant (lymphocyte immune globulin); interleukin-1 receptor antagonist deficiency; active lupus nephritis; lymphangioleiomyomatosis (sirolimus)**

ACTION
Exact mechanism of action isn't fully known. Immunosuppressants act by suppressing cell-mediated hypersensitivity reactions and produce various alterations in antibody production, blocking the activity of interleukin, inhibiting helper T cells and suppressor T cells, and antagonizing the metabolism of purine, therefore inhibiting RNA and DNA structure and synthesis.

ADVERSE REACTIONS
Immunosuppressants may cause albuminuria, hematuria, proteinuria, renal failure, hepatotoxicity, oral *Candida* infections, gingival

DRUG CLASSES

hyperplasia, tremors, and headache. The most serious reactions include leukopenia, thrombocytopenia, risk of secondary infection, and severe (life-threatening) anaphylaxis.

CONTRAINDICATIONS & CAUTIONS

Boxed Warning Refer to individual drug monographs for boxed warnings. ∎

• Contraindicated in patients hypersensitive to these drugs or their components.
• Use cautiously in patients with severe renal disease or severe hepatic disease.
• Refer to manufacturer's instructions for use during pregnancy and breastfeeding.

Inotropes

digoxin, DOBUTamine hydrochloride, DOPamine hydrochloride, milrinone lactate

INDICATIONS

➤ HF and supraventricular arrhythmias, including supraventricular tachycardia, atrial fibrillation, and atrial flutter (digoxin); short-term HF (milrinone); low cardiac output (dopamine)

ACTION

Inotropics help move calcium into the cells, which increases cardiac output by strengthening contractility. Digoxin also acts on the CNS to slow HR. Dobutamine increases cardiac stroke volume and cardiac output without marked increases in HR. Milrinone relaxes vascular smooth muscle, decreasing peripheral vascular resistance (afterload) and the amount of blood returning to the heart (preload). Dopamine produces positive chronotropic and inotropic effects on the myocardium, resulting in increased HR and cardiac contractility.

ADVERSE REACTIONS

Inotropics may cause arrhythmias, nausea, vomiting, diarrhea, headache, fever, mental disturbances, visual changes, and chest pain. Milrinone may cause thrombocytopenia, hypotension, hypokalemia, and elevated liver enzymes.

CONTRAINDICATIONS & CAUTIONS

• Contraindicated in patients hypersensitive to these drugs or their components.
• Digoxin and dopamine are contraindicated in ventricular fibrillation.

• Use cautiously in patients with renal insufficiency because of the potential for toxicity.
• Use digoxin cautiously in patients with sinus node disease or AV block because of the potential for advanced heart block.
• Refer to manufacturer's instructions for use during pregnancy and breastfeeding.

Laxatives

Bulk-forming
calcium polycarbophil, psyllium

Emollient
mineral oil

Hyperosmolar
glycerin, lactulose, lubiprostone, polyethylene glycol

Saline
magnesium (citrate; hydroxide; sulfate), sodium phosphates

Stimulant
bisacodyl

Stool softener, stool surfactant
docusate (calcium; sodium)

INDICATIONS

➤ Constipation; IBS; diverticulosis; bowel cleansing; portal systemic encephalopathy (lactulose)

ACTION

Laxatives promote movement of intestinal contents through the colon and rectum in several ways: bulk-forming, emollient, hyperosmolar, and stimulant.

ADVERSE REACTIONS

All laxatives may cause flatulence, diarrhea, and abdominal disturbances. Bulk-forming laxatives may cause intestinal obstruction, impaction, or (rarely) esophageal obstruction. Emollient laxatives may irritate the throat. Hyperosmolar and saline laxatives may cause fluid and electrolyte imbalances. Stimulant laxatives may cause urine discoloration, malabsorption, and weight loss.

CONTRAINDICATIONS & CAUTIONS

• Contraindicated in patients with GI obstruction or perforation, toxic colitis, megacolon, nausea and vomiting, or acute surgical abdomen.

• Use cautiously in patients with rectal or anal conditions, such as rectal bleeding or large hemorrhoids.

• Refer to manufacturer's instructions for use during pregnancy and breastfeeding. Infants and children have an increased risk of fluid and electrolyte disturbances; use cautiously. In older adults, dependence is more likely to develop because of age-related changes in GI function. Monitor closely.

Macrolide anti-infectives

azithromycin, clarithromycin, erythromycin (ethylsuccinate; lactobionate; stearate), fidaxomicin

INDICATIONS

➤ **Various common infections; CDAD (fidaxomicin)**

ACTION

Inhibit RNA-dependent protein synthesis by acting on a small portion of the 50S ribosomal unit. They're active against *Staphylococcus aureus, Streptococcus pneumoniae, Streptococcus pyogenes, Streptococcus agalactiae, Moraxella catarrhalis, Chlamydia trachomatis, Mycoplasma pneumoniae, Haemophilus influenzae,* and *Neisseria gonorrhoeae.* Fidaxomicin is active against CDAD.

ADVERSE REACTIONS

These drugs may cause cardiac effects (prolonged QT interval, arrhythmias, torsades de pointes), nausea, vomiting, diarrhea, abdominal pain, palpitations, chest pain, vaginal candidiasis, nephritis, dizziness, headache, vertigo, somnolence, rash, and photosensitivity.

CONTRAINDICATIONS & CAUTIONS

• Contraindicated in patients hypersensitive to these drugs and their components.

• CDAD ranging in severity from mild to fatal colitis can occur during treatment or even more than 2 months after therapy ends (except fidaxomicin).

• Refer to manufacturer's instructions for use during pregnancy and breastfeeding.

Neuromuscular blockers

atracurium besylate, cisatracurium besylate, pancuronium bromide, rocuronium bromide, succinylcholine chloride, vecuronium bromide

INDICATIONS

➤ **To relax skeletal muscle during surgery; management of patients who are fighting mechanical ventilation; rapid sequence and routine tracheal intubation**

ACTION

Nondepolarizing blockers (atracurium, cisatracurium, pancuronium, rocuronium, vecuronium) compete with acetylcholine at cholinergic receptor sites on the skeletal muscle membrane. This action blocks acetylcholine's neurotransmitter actions, preventing muscle contraction. Succinylcholine is a depolarizing blocker. This drug isn't inactivated by cholinesterase, thereby preventing repolarization of the motor endplate and causing muscle paralysis.

ADVERSE REACTIONS

Neuromuscular blockers may cause apnea, hypotension, HTN, arrhythmias, tachycardia, bronchospasm, excessive bronchial or salivary secretions, and skin reactions.

CONTRAINDICATIONS & CAUTIONS

Boxed Warning Refer to individual drug monographs for boxed warnings. ∎

• Contraindicated in patients hypersensitive to these drugs or their components.

• The drugs should be used only by personnel skilled in airway management and respiratory support.

• Refer to manufacturer's instructions for use during pregnancy and breastfeeding.

Nonsteroidal anti-inflammatory drugs

aspirin, celecoxib, diclofenac, diflunisal, etodolac, fenoprofen, ibuprofen, indomethacin, ketoprofen, ketorolac tromethamine, meloxicam, nabumetone, naproxen, piroxicam, sulindac

DRUG CLASSES

INDICATIONS & DOSAGES
➤ **Mild to moderate pain, inflammation, stiffness, swelling, or tenderness caused by headache, arthralgia, myalgia, neuralgia, dysmenorrhea, RA, juvenile arthritis, osteoarthritis, dental or surgical procedures, or patent ductus arteriosus**

ACTION
The analgesic effect of NSAIDs may result from interference with the prostaglandins involved in pain. Prostaglandins appear to sensitize pain receptors to mechanical stimulation or to other chemical mediators. NSAIDs inhibit synthesis of prostaglandins peripherally and possibly centrally.

NSAIDs exert an anti-inflammatory effect that may result in part from inhibition of cyclooxygenase-1 and -2 enzymes and prostaglandin synthesis and release during inflammation. The exact mechanism isn't clear.

ADVERSE REACTIONS
Adverse reactions chiefly involve the GI tract, particularly erosion of the gastric mucosa. The most common symptoms are abdominal pain, dyspepsia, epigastric distress, heartburn, and nausea. CNS and skin reactions also may occur. Flank pain with other evidence of nephrotoxicity occurs occasionally. Fluid retention may aggravate HTN or HF.

CONTRAINDICATIONS & CAUTIONS
Boxed Warning Refer to individual drug monographs for additional boxed warnings. ■
Boxed Warning NSAIDs may increase risk of serious CV thrombotic events, MI, and stroke, which can be fatal, and are contraindicated after CABG surgery. ■
Boxed Warning NSAIDs increase risk of serious GI reactions, including inflammation, ulceration, and perforation of the stomach or intestines, which can be fatal. Older adults are at increased risk. ■
• Contraindicated in patients hypersensitive to these drugs.
🔵 *Alert:* MI or stroke can occur as early as the first week of using an NSAID (except aspirin). The risk appears higher with higher doses. Use the lowest effective dose for the shortest duration possible.
🔵 *Alert:* NSAIDs increase the risk of HF.
• Use cautiously in patients with HF, HTN, risk of MI (except low-dose aspirin), fluid retention, renal insufficiency, or coagulation defects.
• Safety during pregnancy hasn't been established. Use at 20 weeks or later during pregnancy may cause fetal renal impairment. Use during the third trimester increases risk of premature closure of the ductus arteriosus. Patients older than age 60 may be more susceptible to toxic effects of NSAIDs because of decreased renal function.

Nucleoside reverse transcriptase inhibitors
abacavir sulfate, emtricitabine, lamiVUDine, stavudine, zidovudine

INDICATIONS
➤ **HIV-1 infection; prevention of maternal-fetal HIV transmission; chronic HBV infection (lamivudine). HIV infection prophylaxis after occupational exposure (such as needle stick or mucous membrane or nonintact skin contact) or nonoccupational exposure to blood, genital secretions, or other potentially infectious body fluids of a person infected with HIV when there's substantial risk of transmission ◆**

ACTION
NRTIs inhibit DNA viral replication by chain termination, competitive inhibition of reverse transcriptase, or both.

ADVERSE REACTIONS
Because of the complexity of HIV infection, it's often difficult to distinguish between disease-related symptoms and adverse drug reactions. The most frequently reported adverse effects of NRTIs are anemia, leukopenia, and neutropenia. Thrombocytopenia is less common. Rare adverse effects of NRTIs are hepatotoxicity, myopathy, and neurotoxicity. Any of these adverse effects requires prompt medical attention.

Adverse effects that don't need medical attention unless they persist or are bothersome include headache, malaise, anorexia, vomiting, insomnia, myalgias, nausea, and hyperpigmentation of nails.

CONTRAINDICATIONS & CAUTIONS
Boxed Warning Refer to individual drug monographs for boxed warnings. ■

• Contraindicated in patients hypersensitive to these drugs and patients with moderate to severe hepatic impairment (abacavir) or pancreatitis (didanosine).

• Use cautiously in patients with mild hepatic impairment or risk factors for liver impairment, risk for pancreatitis (didanosine), or compromised bone marrow function (zidovudine).

• Use drug during pregnancy only if benefits outweigh risks. To reduce the risk of transmitting the virus, mothers infected with HIV shouldn't breastfeed. The pharmacokinetic and safety profiles of NRTIs are similar in children and adults. NRTIs may be used in children age 3 months and older, but the half-life may be prolonged in neonates. In older adults, elimination half-life may be prolonged.

Opioid analgesics

codeine, fentaNYL citrate, HYDROcodone, HYDROmorphone hydrochloride, meperidine hydrochloride, methadone hydrochloride, morphine sulfate, nalbuphine hydrochloride, oxyCODONE hydrochloride, oxyMORphone hydrochloride, tramadol

INDICATIONS

➤ **Moderate to severe pain from acute and some chronic disorders; management of pain severe enough to require daily, around-the-clock, long-term opioid treatment; management of opioid dependence (methadone); anesthesia support; sedation**

ACTION

Opioids act as agonists at specific opioid-receptor binding sites in the CNS and other tissues, altering perception of pain.

ADVERSE REACTIONS

Respiratory and circulatory depression (including orthostatic hypotension) are the major hazards of opioids. Other adverse CNS effects include agitation, coma, depression, dizziness, dysphoria, euphoria, faintness, mental clouding, nervousness, restlessness, sedation, seizures, visual disturbances, and weakness. Adverse GI effects include biliary colic, constipation, nausea, and vomiting. Urine retention or hypersensitivity also may occur. Drug tolerance and psychological or physical dependence may follow prolonged use.

CONTRAINDICATIONS & CAUTIONS

Boxed Warning Refer to individual drug monographs for additional boxed warnings. ∎

Boxed Warning Opioids should only be prescribed with benzodiazepines or other CNS depressants to patients for whom alternative treatment options are inadequate. ∎

• Take care when prescribing and administering to avoid dosing errors due to confusion among different concentrations and between mg and mL, which could result in accidental overdose and death.

• Contraindicated in patients hypersensitive to these drugs and in those who have recently taken an MAO inhibitor. Also contraindicated in those with acute or severe bronchial asthma or respiratory depression.

❸ *Alert:* When used concomitantly with serotonergic drugs, risk of serotonin syndrome increases.

❸ *Alert:* Use may lead to rare but serious decrease in adrenal gland cortisol production and, with long-term use, to decreased sex hormone levels.

• Use cautiously in patients with head injury, increased ICP or increased IOP, hepatic or renal dysfunction, mental illness, emotional disturbances, or drug-seeking behaviors.

❸ *Alert:* Don't stop drug abruptly; individualize the gradual taper plan to prevent withdrawal syndrome, worsening of pain, and psychological distress in patients who are physically dependent.

• Use cautiously during pregnancy and breastfeeding. Prolonged maternal use of opioids during pregnancy can cause neonatal withdrawal syndrome in the newborn, which may be life-threatening if not recognized and treated according to protocols developed by neonatology experts. Infants of patients who are breastfeeding and taking opioids may develop physical dependence. Safety and effectiveness of some opioids in children haven't been established. Older adults may be more sensitive to opioids, and lower doses are usually given.

Penicillins

Natural penicillins

penicillin G (benzathine; potassium; procaine; sodium), penicillin V potassium

DRUG CLASSES

Aminopenicillins
amoxicillin, amoxicillin–clavulanate potassium, ampicillin (trihydrate), ampicillin sodium–sulbactam sodium

Extended-spectrum penicillins
piperacillin sodium–tazobactam sodium

Penicillinase-resistant penicillins
dicloxacillin sodium, nafcillin sodium, oxacillin sodium

INDICATIONS
➤ Streptococcal pneumonia; enterococcal and nonenterococcal group D endocarditis; diphtheria; anthrax; meningitis; tetanus; botulism; actinomycosis; syphilis; relapsing fever; Lyme disease; pneumococcal infections; rheumatic fever; bacterial endocarditis; neonatal group B streptococcal disease; septicemia; gynecologic infections; infections of urinary, respiratory, and GI tracts; infections of skin, soft tissue, bones, and joints

ACTION
Generally bactericidal, penicillins inhibit synthesis of the bacterial cell wall, causing rapid cell destruction. They're most effective against fast-growing susceptible bacteria. Their sites of action are enzymes known as *penicillin-binding proteins* (PBPs). The affinity of certain penicillins for PBPs in various microorganisms helps explain the different activities of these drugs.

Susceptible aerobic gram-positive cocci include *Staphylococcus aureus;* nonenterococcal group D streptococci; groups A, B, D, G, H, K, L, and M streptococci; *Streptococcus viridans;* and *Enterococcus* (usually with an aminoglycoside). Susceptible aerobic gram-negative cocci include *Neisseria meningitidis* and non–penicillinase-producing *N. gonorrhoeae*.

Susceptible aerobic gram-positive bacilli include *Corynebacterium, Listeria,* and *Bacillus anthracis*. Susceptible anaerobes include *Peptococcus, Peptostreptococcus, Actinomyces, Clostridium, Fusobacterium, Veillonella,* and non–beta-lactamase–producing strains of *Streptococcus pneumoniae*. Susceptible spirochetes include *Treponema pallidum, T. pertenue, Leptospira, Borrelia recurrentis* and, possibly, *B. burgdorferi*.

Aminopenicillins have uses against more organisms, including many gram-negative organisms. Like natural penicillins, aminopenicillins are vulnerable to inactivation by penicillinase. Susceptible organisms include *Escherichia coli, Proteus mirabilis, Shigella, Salmonella, S. pneumoniae, N. gonorrhoeae, Haemophilus influenzae, S. aureus, S. epidermidis* (non–penicillinase-producing *Staphylococcus*), and *Listeria monocytogenes*.

Extended-spectrum penicillins offer a wider range of bactericidal action than the other three classes and usually are given in combination with aminoglycosides. Susceptible strains include *Enterobacter, Klebsiella, Citrobacter, Serratia, Bacteroides fragilis, Pseudomonas aeruginosa, Proteus vulgaris, Providencia rettgeri,* and *Morganella morganii*. These penicillins are also vulnerable to beta-lactamase and penicillinases.

Penicillinase-resistant penicillins are semisynthetic penicillins designed to remain stable against hydrolysis by most staphylococcal penicillinases and thus are the drugs of choice against susceptible penicillinase-producing staphylococci. They also act against most organisms susceptible to natural penicillins.

ADVERSE REACTIONS
With all penicillins, hypersensitivity reactions range from mild rash, fever, and eosinophilia to fatal anaphylaxis. Hematologic reactions include hemolytic anemia, leukopenia, thrombocytopenia, and transient neutropenia. Certain adverse reactions are more common with specific classes. For example, bleeding episodes are usually seen with high doses of extended-spectrum penicillins, whereas GI adverse effects are most common with ampicillin. In patients with renal disease, high doses (especially of penicillin G) irritate the CNS, causing confusion, twitching, lethargy, dysphagia, seizures, and coma. Hepatotoxicity may occur with penicillinase-resistant penicillins, and hypokalemia and hypernatremia have been reported with extended-spectrum penicillins. Local irritation from parenteral therapy may be severe enough to warrant administration by subclavian or centrally placed catheter or may warrant stopping therapy.

CONTRAINDICATIONS & CAUTIONS
Boxed Warning Refer to individual drug monographs for boxed warnings. ∎

• Contraindicated in patients hypersensitive to these drugs.
• Use cautiously in patients with history of asthma or drug allergy, mononucleosis, renal impairment, CV diseases, hemorrhagic condition, or electrolyte imbalance.
• May cause CDAD, requiring drug discontinuation and treatment with other drugs.
• Use cautiously during pregnancy. Recommendations during breastfeeding vary by drug. For children, dosage recommendations have been established for most penicillins. Older adults are susceptible to superinfection and renal impairment, which decreases excretion of penicillins; use cautiously and at a lower dosage.

Phenothiazines

chlorproMAZINE hydrochloride, fluPHENAZine decanoate, perphenazine, prochlorperazine maleate, promethazine hydrochloride, thioridazine hydrochloride, thiothixene, trifluoperazine hydrochloride

INDICATIONS
➤ **Agitated psychotic states; schizophrenia; hallucinations; manic-depressive illness; excessive motor and autonomic activity; nausea and vomiting; moderate anxiety; behavioral problems caused by chronic organic mental syndrome; tetanus; acute intermittent porphyria; intractable hiccups**

ACTION
Phenothiazines are believed to function as dopamine antagonists by blocking postsynaptic dopamine receptors in various parts of the CNS. Their antiemetic effects result from blockage of the chemoreceptor trigger zone. They also produce varying degrees of anticholinergic effects and alpha-adrenergic receptor blocking.

ADVERSE REACTIONS
Phenothiazines may produce extrapyramidal symptoms, such as dystonic movements, torticollis, oculogyric crises, and parkinsonian symptoms ranging from akathisia during early treatment to tardive dyskinesia after long-term use. An NMS resembling severe parkinsonism may occur, most often in young men taking fluphenazine.

Other adverse reactions include abdominal pain, agitation, anorexia, arrhythmias, confusion, constipation, dizziness, dry mouth, endocrine effects, fainting, hallucinations, hematologic disorders, local gastric irritation, nausea, orthostatic hypotension with reflex tachycardia, photosensitivity, seizures, skin eruptions, urine retention, visual disturbances, and vomiting. Promethazine injection can cause severe chemical irritation and tissue damage with such reactions as burning, pain, thrombophlebitis, tissue necrosis, and gangrene. Preferred route is IM.

CONTRAINDICATIONS & CAUTIONS
Boxed Warning Refer to individual drug monographs for boxed warnings. ■
• Contraindicated in patients with CNS depression, bone marrow suppression, HF, circulatory collapse, coronary artery or cerebrovascular disorders, subcortical damage, or coma. Also contraindicated in patients receiving spinal and epidural anesthetics and adrenergic blockers.
• Use cautiously in patients with debilitation and in those with hepatic, renal, or CV disease; respiratory disorders; hypocalcemia; seizure disorders; suspected brain tumor or intestinal obstruction; glaucoma; and prostatic hyperplasia.
• Use during pregnancy only if clearly needed; safety hasn't been established. Patients shouldn't breastfeed during therapy because most phenothiazines appear in human milk and directly affect prolactin levels. Phenothiazines aren't recommended for children younger than age 12 unless otherwise specified; use cautiously for nausea and vomiting. Children who are acutely ill, such as those with chickenpox, measles, CNS infections, or dehydration, have a greatly increased risk of dystonic reactions. Older adults are more sensitive to therapeutic and adverse effects, especially cardiotoxicity, tardive dyskinesia, and other extrapyramidal effects; use cautiously and reduce doses, adjusting dosage to patient response.

Progestins

HYDROXYprogesterone caproate, medroxyPROGESTERone acetate, norethindrone (acetate), ulipristal acetate

INDICATIONS
➤ **Amenorrhea; endometrial hyperplasia; advanced uterine adenocarcinoma;**

DRUG CLASSES

abnormal uterine bleeding; endometriosis; contraception; to reduce risk of preterm birth

ACTION
Unknown. Progestins transform proliferative endometrium into secretory endometrium.

ADVERSE REACTIONS
Progestins may cause amenorrhea, breakthrough bleeding, spotting, changes in menstrual flow, breast enlargement and tenderness, alterations in weight, and mood changes.

CONTRAINDICATIONS & CAUTIONS
Boxed Warning Refer to individual drug monographs for boxed warnings. ∎
• Contraindicated in patients with impaired liver function or liver disease; known or suspected breast cancer; active DVT, PE, or history of these conditions; active or recent arterial thromboembolic disease; and undiagnosed vaginal bleeding. Also contraindicated in patients hypersensitive to these drugs and their components.
• Use cautiously in patients with depression, epilepsy, migraine headaches, asthma, cardiac dysfunction, or renal dysfunction.
• Use is contraindicated during pregnancy. Use cautiously during breastfeeding because progestins have been detected in human milk. Progestins aren't indicated in children.

Protease inhibitors
atazanavir sulfate, darunavir ethanolate, fosamprenavir calcium, lopinavir, ritonavir, saquinavir mesylate, tipranavir

INDICATIONS
➤ HIV infection; postexposure prophylaxis (as off-label use)

ACTION
Protease inhibitors bind to the protease active site and inhibit HIV protease activity. This enzyme is required for the proteolysis of viral polyprotein precursors into the individual functional proteins found in infectious HIV. The net effect is formation of noninfectious, immature virus particles.

ADVERSE REACTIONS
The most common adverse effects that require immediate medical attention include kidney

stones, pancreatitis, diabetes or hyperglycemia, ketoacidosis, and paresthesia.
Common adverse effects that don't need medical attention unless they persist or are bothersome include generalized weakness, GI disturbances, headache, insomnia, and taste disturbance. Less common adverse effects include dizziness and somnolence, nausea, jaundice, scleral icterus, rash, abdominal pain, vomiting, peripheral neurologic symptoms, dizziness, myalgia, diarrhea, depression, and fever.

CONTRAINDICATIONS & CAUTIONS
Boxed Warning Refer to individual drug monographs for boxed warnings. ∎
• Contraindicated in patients hypersensitive to these drugs or their components and in patients taking a drug highly dependent on CYP3A4 for metabolism.
• Use cautiously in patients with impaired hepatic or renal function and those with diabetes or hemophilia.
• Use during pregnancy only if benefits outweigh risks. To reduce the risk of transmitting HIV to the infant, mothers infected with HIV shouldn't breastfeed.

Proton pump inhibitors
dexlansoprazole, esomeprazole (magnesium; sodium), lansoprazole, omeprazole (magnesium), pantoprazole sodium, RABEprazole

INDICATIONS
➤ Duodenal ulcers; gastric ulcers; erosive esophagitis; GERD; hypersecretory conditions (Zollinger-Ellison syndrome); NSAID-induced ulcer prophylaxis

ACTION
The drugs reduce stomach acid production by combining with hydrogen, potassium, and adenosine triphosphate in parietal cells of the stomach to block the last step in gastric acid secretion.

ADVERSE REACTIONS
PPIs may cause abdominal pain, diarrhea, constipation, flatulence, nausea, vomiting, dizziness, arthralgia, fever, rash, dry mouth, headache, asthenia, URI, abnormal LFT results, and hyperglycemia.

CONTRAINDICATIONS & CAUTIONS

• Contraindicated in patients hypersensitive to these drugs or their components.
• May increase risk of osteoporosis-related bone fractures and CDAD. Use lowest effective dose for the shortest duration.
• May increase risk of GI infections, hypomagnesemia and, with prolonged use, vitamin B_{12} deficiency.
• Studies are limited during pregnancy; consider the benefits and risks before starting therapy. Some drugs may appear in human milk. Refer to manufacturer's instructions for use during breastfeeding.

Selective serotonin reuptake inhibitors

citalopram hydrobromide, escitalopram oxalate, FLUoxetine hydrochloride, fluvoxaMINE maleate, PARoxetine hydrochloride, sertraline hydrochloride, vilazodone hydrochloride

INDICATIONS

➤ **Major depression; bipolar disorder (fluoxetine); OCD; bulimia nervosa (fluoxetine); premenstrual dysphoric disorders; panic disorders; PTSD (paroxetine, sertraline); vasomotor symptoms (paroxetine)**

ACTION

SSRIs selectively inhibit the reuptake of serotonin with little or no effects on other neurotransmitters in the CNS, such as norepinephrine and dopamine.

ADVERSE REACTIONS

Common adverse effects include headache, tremor, dizziness, sleep disturbances, abnormal dreams, anorexia, anxiety, asthenia, diarrhea, dry mouth, flulike symptoms, GI disturbances, and sexual dysfunction. Less common adverse effects include bleeding (ecchymoses, epistaxis), akathisia, breast tenderness or enlargement, extrapyramidal effects, dystonia, fever, hyponatremia, mania or hypomania, palpitations, serotonin syndrome, weight gain or loss, rash, urticaria, and pruritus.

CONTRAINDICATIONS & CAUTIONS

Boxed Warning Antidepressants can increase risk of suicidality, particularly in children, adolescents, and young adults. Appropriately monitor patients of all ages who are started on antidepressant therapy; observe closely for clinical worsening, suicidality, or unusual behavior changes. Advise families and caregivers of the need for close observation and communication with the prescriber. ∎
• Contraindicated in patients hypersensitive to these drugs or their components, within 14 days of MAO inhibitor therapy, and with concurrent use of linezolid or methylene blue.
• Use cautiously in patients with hepatic, renal, or cardiac disease.
• Use during pregnancy only if benefits outweigh risks; use of certain SSRIs in the first trimester may cause birth defects. Neonates born to patients who took an SSRI during the third trimester may develop complications that require prolonged hospitalization, respiratory support, and enteral feeding. Some SSRIs appear in human milk. Refer to manufacturer's instructions for use during breastfeeding. Older adults may be more sensitive to the insomniac effects of SSRIs.

Skeletal muscle relaxants

baclofen, carisoprodol, cyclobenzaprine hydrochloride, dantrolene sodium, methocarbamol, orphenadrine citrate, tiZANidine hydrochloride

INDICATIONS

➤ **Painful musculoskeletal disorders, muscle spasticity; prevention and treatment of malignant hyperthermia (dantrolene)**

ACTION

Baclofen may reduce impulse transmission from the spinal cord to skeletal muscle. Carisoprodol, cyclobenzaprine, methocarbamol, orphenadrine, and tizanidine's mechanisms of action are unclear. Dantrolene acts directly on skeletal muscle to decrease excitation and reduce muscle strength by interfering with intracellular calcium movement.

ADVERSE REACTIONS

Skeletal muscle relaxants may cause ataxia, confusion, depressed mood, dizziness, drowsiness, dry mouth, hallucinations, headache, hypotension, nervousness, tachycardia, tremor, and vertigo. Baclofen also may cause seizures with abrupt withdrawal.

DRUG CLASSES

CONTRAINDICATIONS & CAUTIONS
Boxed Warning Refer to individual drug monographs for boxed warnings. ∎
• Contraindicated in patients hypersensitive to these drugs.
• Use cautiously in patients with impaired renal or hepatic function.
• Refer to manufacturer's instructions for use during pregnancy and breastfeeding. In children, recommendations vary. Older adults have an increased risk of adverse reactions; monitor carefully.
• Due to sedative properties, may impair ability to perform hazardous tasks, such as driving or operating machinery.
• May have additive sedative effects when used with other CNS depressants, including alcohol.

Sulfonamides
sulfADIAZINE,
sulfamethoxazole–trimethoprim

INDICATIONS
➤ **Bacterial infections; nocardiosis; toxoplasmosis; chloroquine-resistant *Plasmodium falciparum* malaria; *Pneumocystis jiroveci* pneumonia; shigellosis; UTI; rheumatic fever prophylaxis**

ACTION
Sulfonamides are bacteriostatic. They inhibit biosynthesis of tetrahydrofolic acid, which is needed for bacterial cell growth. They're active against some strains of staphylococci, streptococci, *Nocardia asteroides* and *N. brasiliensis, Clostridium tetani* and *C. perfringens, Bacillus anthracis, Escherichia coli,* and *Neisseria gonorrhoeae* and *N. meningitidis, Haemophilus influenzae.* Sulfonamides are also active against organisms that cause UTIs, such as *E. coli, Proteus mirabilis* and *P. vulgaris, Klebsiella, Enterobacter,* and *Staphylococcus aureus.*

ADVERSE REACTIONS
Many adverse reactions stem from hypersensitivity, including bronchospasm, conjunctivitis, erythema multiforme, erythema nodosum, exfoliative dermatitis, fever, joint pain, pruritus, leukopenia, Lyell syndrome, photosensitivity, rash, SJS, and TEN. GI reactions include anorexia, diarrhea, folic acid malabsorption, nausea, pancreatitis, stomatitis, and vomiting.

Hematologic reactions include agranulocytosis, granulocytopenia, hypoprothrombinemia, thrombocytopenia and, in G6PD deficiency, hemolytic anemia. Renal effects usually result from crystalluria caused by precipitation of sulfonamide in the renal system.

CONTRAINDICATIONS & CAUTIONS
• Contraindicated in patients hypersensitive to these drugs.
• Use cautiously in patients with renal or hepatic impairment, bronchial asthma, severe allergy, or G6PD deficiency.
• During pregnancy, use is contraindicated in patients at term. Also contraindicated during breastfeeding; sulfonamides appear in human milk. Older adults are susceptible to bacterial and fungal superinfection and have an increased risk of folate deficiency anemia and adverse renal and hematologic effects.

Tetracyclines
doxycycline (hyclate; monohydrate),
minocycline hydrochloride, tetracycline hydrochloride

INDICATIONS & DOSAGES
➤ **Bacterial, protozoal, and rickettsial infections; acne**

ACTION
Tetracyclines are bacteriostatic but may be bactericidal against certain organisms. They bind reversibly to 30S and 50S ribosomal subunits, which inhibits bacterial protein synthesis.

Susceptible gram-positive organisms include *Bacillus anthracis, Actinomyces israelii, Clostridium perfringens* and *C. tetani, Listeria monocytogenes,* and *Nocardia.*

Susceptible gram-negative organisms include *Neisseria meningitidis, Pasteurella multocida, Legionella pneumophila, Brucella* species, *Vibrio cholerae, Yersinia enterocolitica, Y. pestis, Bordetella pertussis, Haemophilus influenzae, H. ducreyi, Campylobacter fetus, Shigella* species, and many other common pathogens.

Other susceptible organisms include *Rickettsia akari, R. typhi, R. prowazekii,* and *R. tsutsugamushi; Coxiella burnetii; Chlamydia trachomatis* and *C. psittaci; Mycoplasma pneumoniae* and *M. hominis; Leptospira* species;

Treponema pallidum and *T. pertenue;* and *Borrelia recurrentis.*

ADVERSE REACTIONS
The most common adverse effects involve the GI tract and may be dose related; they include abdominal discomfort; anorexia; bulky, loose stools; colitis; epigastric burning; flatulence; nausea; and vomiting. Superinfections and CDAD can occur.

Photosensitivity reactions may be severe. Permanent discoloration of teeth occurs if drug is given during tooth formation in children younger than age 8.

CONTRAINDICATIONS & CAUTIONS
• Contraindicated in patients hypersensitive to these drugs.
• Use cautiously in patients with renal or hepatic impairment.
• Tetracyclines can cause fetal harm; avoid use during pregnancy. Tetracyclines appear in human milk; the decision to continue or discontinue breastfeeding should take into account benefits to the mother and risks to the infant. Children younger than age 8 shouldn't take tetracyclines; these drugs can cause permanent tooth discoloration, enamel hypoplasia, and a reversible decrease in bone calcification. Older adults may have decreased esophageal motility; use these drugs cautiously, and monitor patients for local irritation from slow passage of oral forms.

Thrombolytics
alteplase, defibrotide sodium, reteplase, tenecteplase

INDICATIONS
➤ To lyse thrombi, often in acute or emergency situations; acute MI; acute ischemic stroke; PE; peripheral vascular occlusion; to restore patency to IV access devices (alteplase); hepatic sinusoidal obstruction syndrome after hematopoietic stem cell transplant (defibrotide)

ACTION
Thrombolytics convert plasminogen to plasmin, which lyses thrombi, and degrades fibrin, fibrinogen, and other plasma proteins.

ADVERSE REACTIONS
The most common adverse reactions are bleeding and allergic responses. Other common adverse reactions include nausea, vomiting, fever, and hypotension.

CONTRAINDICATIONS & CAUTIONS
• Contraindicated in patients hypersensitive to drugs and their components and in combination with other fibrinolytics.
• Contraindicated in active bleeding, history of stroke, recent intracranial or intraspinal surgery or trauma, intracranial neoplasm, arteriovenous malformation or aneurysm, bleeding diathesis, or severe uncontrolled HTN.
• Pregnancy is considered to be a relative contraindication, but drugs shouldn't be withheld in life-threatening situations. It isn't known if drugs appear in human milk; use cautiously during breastfeeding.

Vasopressors
DOBUTamine hydrochloride, DOPamine hydrochloride, ePHEDrine sulfate, EPINEPHrine hydrochloride, norepinephrine

INDICATIONS
➤ Correction of hemodynamic imbalances present in shock, trauma, septicemia, cardiac surgical procedures, spinal anesthesia, drug reactions, renal failure, HF; anaphylaxis, severe hypersensitivity reactions (epinephrine)

ACTION
Dobutamine is a direct-acting inotrope whose primary activity results from stimulation of the beta receptors of the heart while producing mild chronotropic, hypertensive, arrhythmogenic, and vasodilatory effects. Dobutamine increases cardiac output by decreasing peripheral vascular resistance, reducing ventricular filling pressure, and increasing AV node conduction. Dopamine is a natural catecholamine, a precursor to norepinephrine in noradrenergic nerves, and a neurotransmitter in certain areas of the CNS. It produces positive chronotropic and inotropic effects on the myocardium, resulting in increased HR and cardiac contractility, by directly exerting agonist action on beta-adrenergic receptors. Epinephrine and related medications (ephedrine, norepinephrine) act on receptors

DRUG CLASSES

in the heart to produce a positive chronotropic effect as well as constrict arteries in the skin, mucous membranes, and organs via action on alpha-adrenergic receptors.

ADVERSE REACTIONS

Adverse reactions to vasopressors may include ventricular arrhythmias, tachycardia, angina, palpitations, cardiac conduction abnormalities, widened QRS complex, bradycardia, hypotension, HTN, vasoconstriction, headache, anxiety, azotemia, dyspnea, phlebitis, peripheral cyanosis, and gangrene of the extremities. Difficult or painful urination can be seen with ephedrine. Less common are hypotension, thrombocytopenia, hypokalemia, and nausea.

CONTRAINDICATIONS & CAUTIONS

Boxed Warning Refer to individual drug monographs for boxed warnings. ■

• Contraindicated in patients hypersensitive to these drugs or their components.
• Contraindicated in patients with pheochromocytoma, uncorrected tachyarrhythmias, or ventricular fibrillation.
• Dobutamine is contraindicated in patients with idiopathic hypertrophic subaortic stenosis.
• Before treatment, correct hypovolemia.
• Some vasopressors must be used cautiously in patients with a sulfite allergy, particularly patients with asthma. Allergic-type reactions, including anaphylactic symptoms and severe asthmatic episodes, can occur.
• Administer infusion into a large vein to prevent extravasation into surrounding tissue, which can cause tissue necrosis.
• Use with extreme caution in patients taking MAO inhibitors or who have been treated with MAO inhibitors 2 to 3 weeks before infusion. Patients taking dopamine will require substantially reduced dosages.
• Dopamine, ephedrine, and norepinephrine shouldn't be used during cyclopropane and halothane anesthesia because of the risk of ventricular tachycardia or fibrillation.
• Use cautiously in patients with hyperthyroidism, bradycardia, partial heart block, myocardial disease, or severe arteriosclerosis.
• Give during pregnancy only if clearly indicated. Use cautiously during breastfeeding. Safety and effectiveness in children haven't been established.

abacavir sulfate ⌧
ah-BAK-ah-veer

Ziagen

Therapeutic class: Antiretrovirals
Pharmacologic class: Nucleoside reverse transcriptase inhibitors

AVAILABLE FORMS
Oral solution: 20 mg/mL
Tablets: 300 mg

INDICATIONS & DOSAGES
➤ **HIV-1 infection**
Adults: 300 mg PO b.i.d. or 600 mg PO daily with other antiretrovirals.
Children ages 3 months and older (oral solution): 8 mg/kg PO b.i.d. or 16 mg/kg PO once daily up to maximum of 600 mg PO daily, with other antiretrovirals.
Children weighing 25 kg or more (scored tablets): 300 mg PO b.i.d.
Children weighing 20 to less than 25 kg (scored tablets): 150 mg PO in the morning and 300 mg PO in the evening.
Children weighing 14 to less than 20 kg (scored tablets): 150 mg PO b.i.d.
Adjust-a-dose: In patients with mild hepatic impairment (Child-Pugh class A), give 200 mg (oral solution) PO b.i.d.

ADMINISTRATION
PO
⌧ **Boxed Warning** Screen for the HLA-B*5701 allele before start of therapy and before reinitiating therapy in patients with unknown status who previously tolerated drug. ▪
• Drug is considered hazardous; use safe handling and disposal precautions according to facility policy.
• Always give drug with other antiretrovirals, never alone.
• May give with or without food.
• Give missed dose as soon as possible; don't double dose.

ACTION
Converted intracellularly to the active metabolite carbovir triphosphate, which inhibits activity of HIV-1 reverse transcriptase, terminating viral DNA growth.

Route	Onset	Peak	Duration
PO	Unknown	0.7–1.7 hr	Unknown

Half-life: 1 to 2 hours.

ADVERSE REACTIONS
CNS: fever, headache, insomnia and sleep disorders, anxiety, depressive disorders, malaise, fatigue, dizziness. **EENT:** ear, nose, and throat infections. **GI:** diarrhea, nausea, vomiting, abdominal pain. **Hematologic:** *neutropenia, thrombocytopenia.* **Hepatic:** elevated transaminase levels. **Metabolic:** increased CK, amylase, triglyceride levels; hyperglycemia. **Musculoskeletal:** pain. **Respiratory:** bronchitis, pneumonia, viral infection. **Skin:** rash. **Other:** chills, *hypersensitivity reaction.*

INTERACTIONS
Drug-drug. *Methadone:* May slightly increase methadone elimination. Monitor effectiveness; increase methadone dosage if needed.
Riociguat: May increase riociguat serum concentration. Riociguat dosage decrease may be needed.
Drug-lifestyle. *Alcohol use:* May decrease elimination of drug, increasing overall exposure. Monitor alcohol consumption. Discourage use together.

EFFECTS ON LAB TEST RESULTS
• May increase ALT, AST, amylase, CK, and triglyceride levels.
• May decrease Hb level and platelet and neutrophil counts.

CONTRAINDICATIONS & CAUTIONS
⌧ **Boxed Warning** Contraindicated in patients who carry the HLA-B*5701 allele because they are at high risk for hypersensitivity reactions. ▪
Boxed Warning Drug can cause serious and sometimes fatal hypersensitivity reactions with multiple organ involvement. Contraindicated in patients with a prior hypersensitivity reaction to abacavir. ▪
• Contraindicated in patients with moderate to severe hepatic impairment.
🌓 *Alert:* Due to increased risk of hepatotoxicity, use cautiously when giving drug to patients at risk for liver disease. Lactic acidosis and severe hepatomegaly with steatosis, including fatal cases, have been reported with the use of nucleoside analogues alone or in

combination, including abacavir and other antiretrovirals. Stop treatment with drug and don't restart if events occur.

• Women are more likely than men to experience lactic acidosis and severe hepatomegaly with steatosis. Obesity and prolonged nucleoside exposure may be risk factors.

• Use cautiously in older adults.

Dialyzable drug: Unknown.

PREGNANCY-LACTATION-REPRODUCTION

• Use cautiously during pregnancy; drug crosses placental barrier. Use during pregnancy only if potential benefits outweigh risk.

• Register patients who are pregnant with the Antiretroviral Pregnancy Registry at 1-800-258-4263.

• Drug appears in human milk. To avoid postnatal HIV-1 infection transmission, viral resistance in infants who test positive for HIV, and possible adverse reactions, instruct patients not to breastfeed.

NURSING CONSIDERATIONS

Boxed Warning Monitor patient for signs or symptoms of hypersensitivity (such as fever, rash, fatigue, achiness, generalized malaise, nausea, vomiting, diarrhea, abdominal pain, cough, dyspnea, or pharyngitis); if present, stop drug and notify prescriber immediately. ∎

Boxed Warning Don't restart drug or any abacavir-containing product after a hypersensitivity reaction, regardless of HLA-B*5701 status, because severe signs and symptoms will recur within hours and may include life-threatening hypotension and death. ∎

• Because of a high rate of early virologic resistance, triple antiretroviral therapy with abacavir, lamivudine, and tenofovir shouldn't be used as a new treatment regimen for treatment-naive or pretreated patients. Monitor patients currently controlled with this combination in addition to other antiretrovirals, and consider modification of therapy.

• Monitor patient for immune reconstitution syndrome. Inflammatory response to indolent or residual opportunistic infection (MAC infection, CMV, *Pneumocystis jiroveci* pneumonia, or TB) may occur during initial treatment; autoimmune disorders (Graves disease, polymyositis, and Guillain-Barré syndrome) may occur at any time after start of therapy.

• Assess for CAD risk factors with antiretroviral use, and address modifiable risk factors

(such as HTN, hyperlipidemia, diabetes, and smoking).

• Drug may mildly elevate glucose level, especially in children.

PATIENT TEACHING

• Inform patient that drug can cause a life-threatening hypersensitivity reaction. Warn patient who develops signs or symptoms of hypersensitivity (such as fever, rash, severe tiredness, achiness, a generally ill feeling, nausea, vomiting, diarrhea, stomach pain, cough, shortness of breath, or sore throat) to stop taking drug and notify prescriber immediately.

• Encourage patient to review information leaflet about drug with each new prescription and refill and to carry a warning card summarizing the signs and symptoms of hypersensitivity.

• Inform patient that drug doesn't cure HIV infection. Tell patient that drug doesn't reduce the risk of HIV transmission to others through sexual contact or blood contamination and that its long-term effects are unknown.

• Caution patient not to stop anti-HIV medicines, even for a short time, because the virus may become harder to treat.

• Warn patient not to restart abacavir or other abacavir-containing drugs without being under medical care because of the risk of serious hypersensitivity reaction.

• Tell patient to take drug exactly as prescribed with or without food.

• Advise patient of childbearing potential to consult prescriber if pregnant or planning to become pregnant.

---

abatacept ⬚
ab-a-TA-sept

Orencia, Orencia ClickJect

Therapeutic class: Antirheumatics
Pharmacologic class: Selective costimulation modulators

AVAILABLE FORMS

Lyophilized powder for injection: 250 mg single-use vial (25 mg/mL when reconstituted)

Solution for subcut administration: 50 mg/ 0.4 mL, 87.5 mg/0.7 mL, 125 mg/mL single-dose prefilled syringe; 125 mg/mL prefilled autoinjector

---

INDICATIONS & DOSAGES
➤ **Moderate to severe RA, used alone or with other DMARDs (except biologic DMARDs, Janus kinase [JAK] inhibitors)**
Adults weighing more than 100 kg: 1 g IV over 30 minutes. Repeat 2 and 4 weeks after initial infusion and then every 4 weeks thereafter.
Adults weighing 60 to 100 kg: 750 mg IV over 30 minutes. Repeat 2 and 4 weeks after initial infusion and then every 4 weeks thereafter.
Adults weighing less than 60 kg: 500 mg IV over 30 minutes. Repeat 2 and 4 weeks after initial infusion and then every 4 weeks thereafter.
Adults (subcut): 125 mg subcut once weekly with or without IV loading dose. For patients receiving loading dose, give single IV dose based on weight. Then give 125 mg subcut within a day, followed by 125 mg subcut once weekly. Patients transferring from IV to subcut form should receive the first subcut dose instead of the next scheduled IV dose.
➤ **As monotherapy or with methotrexate to reduce signs and symptoms of moderately to severely active polyarticular juvenile idiopathic arthritis**
Children ages 6 and older weighing 75 kg or more: Use adult dosing regimen, not to exceed a maximum dose of 1,000 mg.
Children ages 6 and older weighing less than 75 kg: 10 mg/kg IV over 30 minutes. Repeat 2 and 4 weeks after initial infusion and then every 4 weeks thereafter. Calculate dosing based on body weight before each dose is administered.
Children ages 2 and older weighing 50 kg or more: 125 mg subcut once weekly without an IV loading dose.
Children ages 2 and older weighing 25 to less than 50 kg: 87.5 mg subcut once weekly without an IV loading dose.
Children ages 2 and older weighing 10 to less than 25 kg: 50 mg subcut once weekly without an IV loading dose.
➤ **Adult psoriatic arthritis**
Adults weighing more than 100 kg: 1 g IV over 30 minutes. Repeat 2 and 4 weeks after initial infusion, then every 4 weeks thereafter.
Adults weighing 60 to 100 kg: 750 mg IV over 30 minutes. Repeat 2 and 4 weeks after initial infusion, then every 4 weeks thereafter.
Adults weighing less than 60 kg: 500 mg IV over 30 minutes. Repeat 2 and 4 weeks after initial infusion, then every 4 weeks thereafter.
Adults (subcut): 125 mg subcut once weekly without IV loading dose. Patients transferring from IV to subcut form should receive first subcut dose instead of the next scheduled IV dose.
➤ **Prophylaxis of acute GVHD in combination with a calcineurin inhibitor and methotrexate in patients undergoing hematopoietic stem cell transplantation (HSCT) from a matched or 1 allele-mismatched unrelated donor** ▨
Adults and children age 6 and older: 10 mg/kg (maximum, 1,000 mg) IV over 60 minutes on day before transplantation; then a dose on days 5, 14, and 28 after transplantation.
Children ages 2 to younger than 6: 15 mg/kg IV over 60 minutes on day before transplantation; then 12 mg/kg on days 5, 14, and 28 after transplantation.

ADMINISTRATION
IV
▼ Reconstitute vial with 10 mL of sterile water for injection, using only the silicone-free disposable syringe provided, to yield 25 mg/mL. Use an 18G to 21G needle for preparation.
▼ Gently swirl contents until completely dissolved. Avoid vigorous shaking.
▼ Vent the vial with a needle to clear away foam.
▼ Solution should be clear and colorless to pale yellow. Don't use if opaque particles, discoloration, or other foreign particles are present.
▼ Further dilute solution to 100 mL total volume with NSS using silicone-free disposable syringe provided with each vial. Infuse using an infusion set and a sterile, nonpyrogenic, low–protein-binding 0.2- to 1.2-micron filter.
▼ Store diluted solution at room temperature or refrigerate at 36° to 46° F (2° to 8° C). Complete infusion within 24 hours of reconstituting.
▼ **Incompatibilities:** Don't infuse in the same line with other IV drugs.
Subcutaneous
● Prefilled syringes and autoinjectors aren't intended for IV administration.
● Remove prefilled syringe or autoinjector from refrigerator 30 to 60 minutes before administration so that it reaches room temperature.
● Abatacept should be clear and colorless to pale yellow; don't use if particulate matter or discoloration is present.

- Rotate injection sites. See product labeling for appropriate sites.
- Never inject into tender, bruised, red, or hard areas.
- The ability of children to self-inject with the autoinjector hasn't been tested.

ACTION

Inhibits T-cell activation, decreases T-cell proliferation, and inhibits production of TNF-alpha, interferon-gamma, and interleukin-2.

Route	Onset	Peak	Duration
IV, subcut	Unknown	Unknown	Unknown

Half-life: IV, 13 days; subcut, 14.3 days.

ADVERSE REACTIONS

CNS: headache, dizziness, fever. **CV:** HTN. **EENT:** epistaxis, nasopharyngitis, rhinitis, sinusitis. **GI:** nausea, diverticulitis, dyspepsia, diarrhea, abdominal pain. **GU:** acute pyelonephritis, UTI, acute kidney injury. **Hematologic:** anemia, decreased CD4 lymphocyte count. **Metabolic:** hypermagnesemia. **Musculoskeletal:** back pain, limb pain. **Respiratory:** URI, bronchitis, cough, pneumonia, rhonchi, dyspnea, hypoxia. **Skin:** cellulitis, rash, injection-site reaction. **Other:** infections, *malignancies,* herpes simplex, influenza, infusion reactions.

INTERACTIONS

Drug-drug. *Anakinra, TNF antagonists:* May increase risk of infection. Don't use together.
Biologic DMARDs, JAK inhibitors: Safety and effectiveness when used together haven't been determined. Concurrent use isn't recommended.
Live-virus vaccines: May decrease effectiveness of vaccine. Avoid giving vaccines during or for 3 months after abatacept therapy.
Non-live vaccines: May diminish therapeutic effect of vaccine. If given during treatment, consider revaccination at least 2 to 3 months after therapy is complete.
Drug-herb. *Echinacea:* May diminish the therapeutic effect of immunosuppressants. Avoid concurrent use.

EFFECTS ON LAB TEST RESULTS

- May increase magnesium level.
- May decrease CD4 lymphocyte count.
- GDH-PQQ (glucose dehydrogenase pyrroloquinoline quinone)–based glucose monitoring systems may react with maltose present in abatacept, causing falsely elevated blood glucose readings on the day of infusion (IV form only).

CONTRAINDICATIONS & CAUTIONS

- Contraindicated in patients hypersensitive to drug or its components.
- Rare cases of severe hypersensitivity reactions have been reported. Reactions may occur with the first dose or within 24 hours of infusion. Discontinue drug and treat emergently if hypersensitivity occurs.
- Use cautiously in patients with active infection, history of chronic infections, or underlying conditions that may predispose patient to infection; scheduled elective surgery; or COPD.
- Patients should be screened for viral hepatitis before starting therapy. Antirheumatic treatment may cause reactivation of HBV.
- Malignancies, including skin cancer, have been reported with abatacept use; periodic skin exams are recommended.
- Ensure patient's vaccination status is current with vaccination guidelines before starting abatacept.
- Safety and effectiveness in polyarticular juvenile idiopathic arthritis or acute GVHD in patients younger than age 2 haven't been established.
Dialyzable drug: Unknown.

PREGNANCY-LACTATION-REPRODUCTION

- Use cautiously during pregnancy and only if benefit to the mother justifies fetal risk.
- Register patients who are pregnant with the pregnancy registry (1-877-311-8972).
- It isn't known if drug appears in human milk. Patient should discontinue breastfeeding or discontinue drug, taking into account the importance of drug to the mother.

NURSING CONSIDERATIONS

- Make sure patient has been screened for TB and viral hepatitis before giving drug. Treat patients who test positive for TB before starting drug.
- Ensure patient receives antiviral prophylaxis for Epstein-Barr virus reactivation and continues for 6 months after HSCT. Consider prophylactic antivirals for CMV infection or reactivation during treatment and for 6 months after HSCT.
- Monitor patient, especially an older adult, carefully for infections and malignancies.

Reactions in bold italics are *life-threatening*. Interactions may have a *rapid onset* or a ***delayed onset***.

• If patient develops a severe infection, notify prescriber; therapy may need to be stopped.

⚠ *Alert:* If patient has COPD, watch for worsening respiratory status.

• Monitor patient for hypersensitivity reactions; ensure supportive measures are available to treat hypersensitivity reactions.

• Ensure that patients are up to date with all immunizations before start of therapy.

• *Look alike–sound alike:* Don't confuse Orencia with Oracea.

PATIENT TEACHING

• Instruct patient that TB and viral hepatitis screening is necessary before therapy.

• Tell patient with RA to continue taking prescribed arthritis drugs.

• Caution patient to avoid exposure to infections.

• Advise patient to immediately report signs and symptoms of infection, swollen face or tongue, and difficulty breathing.

• Instruct patient with COPD to report worsening signs and symptoms.

• Advise patient to avoid live-virus vaccines during and for 3 months after therapy.

• Caution patient to consult prescriber if pregnant or planning to breastfeed.

• Encourage patient who is pregnant to enroll in pregnancy registry at 1-877-311-8972.

• Advise patient to contact prescriber before taking any other drugs or herbal supplements.

• Remind patient to contact prescriber before scheduling surgery.

• Instruct patient or caregiver in subcut administration, drug storage, and syringe disposal.

SAFETY ALERT!

abemaciclib ☒
a-bem-a-SYE-klib

Verzenio

Therapeutic class: Antineoplastics
Pharmacologic class: Kinase inhibitors

AVAILABLE FORMS

Tablets ⓞ: 50 mg, 100 mg, 150 mg, 200 mg

INDICATIONS & DOSAGES

Adjust-a-dose (for all indications): For severe hepatic impairment (Child-Pugh class C), reduce abemaciclib dosing frequency to once daily. Refer to manufacturer's instructions for toxicity-related dosage adjustments. For concomitant use of strong CYP3A inhibitors (except ketoconazole), if recommended starting dose of abemaciclib is 150 or 200 mg b.i.d., reduce abemaciclib dose to 100 mg b.i.d. If a strong CYP3A inhibitor is begun and abemaciclib dose has been decreased to 100 mg b.i.d. due to adverse reactions, further reduce abemaciclib dose to 50 mg b.i.d. When a strong CYP3A inhibitor has been discontinued, increase abemaciclib dose (after three to five half-lives of the inhibitor) to the dose that was used before the strong CYP3A inhibitor was begun. With concomitant use of moderate CYP3A inhibitors, monitor patient for adverse reactions; consider reducing abemaciclib dose in 50-mg decrements.

➤ **Initial endocrine-based treatment of hormone receptor (HR)–positive, HER2–negative advanced or metastatic breast cancer, in combination with an aromatase inhibitor**

Men and women who are postmenopausal: 150 mg PO b.i.d. Treat men and women who are premenopausal and perimenopausal with a GnRH agonist per clinical practice standards. Continue treatment until disease progression or unacceptable toxicity occurs.

➤ **HR-positive, HER2-negative advanced or metastatic breast cancer with disease progression after endocrine therapy, in combination with fulvestrant**

Adults: 150 mg PO b.i.d. Coadminister fulvestrant. Treat women who are premenopausal and perimenopausal with a GnRH agonist per clinical practice standards. Continue treatment until disease progression or unacceptable toxicity occurs.

➤ **Monotherapy for the treatment of HR-positive, HER2-negative advanced or metastatic breast cancer with disease progression after endocrine therapy and prior chemotherapy in the metastatic setting** ☒

Adults: 200 mg PO b.i.d. Continue treatment until disease progression or unacceptable toxicity occurs.

✳ *NEW INDICATION:* Adjuvant treatment for HR-positive, HER2-negative, node-positive early breast cancer, in combination with endocrine therapy (tamoxifen or aromatase inhibitor), in patients at high risk for recurrence and with a Ki-67 score of 20% or more as determined by an FDA-approved test

Adults: 150 mg PO b.i.d. until completion of 2 years of treatment or disease recurrence or unacceptable toxicity occurs.

ADMINISTRATION

PO

- Give drug at approximately the same time every day.
- Patient must swallow tablets whole and not chew, crush, or split them. Only administer intact tablets.
- May give without regard for food.
- If patient vomits or misses a dose, give the next dose at its scheduled time.
- Store at 68° to 77° F (20° to 25° C).

ACTION

An inhibitor of cyclin-dependent kinases 4 and 6 (CDK4 and CDK6). In estrogen receptor–positive breast cancer cells, cyclin D1 and CDK4 and CDK6 promote cell-cycle progression and cell proliferation. Drug blocks progression from G1 into S phase of the cell cycle, resulting in cell aging and death.

Route	Onset	Peak	Duration
PO	Unknown	8 hr	Unknown

Half-life: 18.3 hours.

ADVERSE REACTIONS

CNS: fatigue, fever, headache, dysgeusia, dizziness. **CV:** peripheral edema, *venous thromboembolism.* **EENT:** dry mouth, increased tearing. **GI:** diarrhea, nausea, abdominal pain, vomiting, stomatitis, constipation, decreased appetite. **GU:** UTI, vaginal infection, increased creatinine level. **Hematologic:** *neutropenia,* anemia, *leukopenia, thrombocytopenia.* **Hepatic:** increased transaminase levels, *hepatotoxicity.* **Metabolic:** weight loss, dehydration, *hypokalemia.* **Musculoskeletal:** arthralgia. **Respiratory:** cough, dyspnea, ILD, pneumonitis. **Skin:** alopecia, pruritus, rash, nail disorder. **Other:** infections, flulike symptoms, *sepsis.*

INTERACTIONS

Drug-drug. *Ketoconazole:* May significantly increase abemaciclib level. Avoid concomitant use.
Moderate and strong CYP3A inducers (rifampin): May decrease abemaciclib plasma level and lead to reduced activity. Avoid concomitant use; consider alternative agents.
Moderate CYP3A inhibitors (diltiazem, verapamil): May increase abemaciclib level. Monitor patient for adverse reactions; consider reducing abemaciclib dose.

Strong CYP3A inhibitors (clarithromycin, itraconazole): May increase abemaciclib level and increase risk of toxicity. Decrease abemaciclib dosage.
Drug-food. *Grapefruit products:* May increase abemaciclib level. Avoid concomitant use.

EFFECTS ON LAB TEST RESULTS

- May increase ALT, AST, and creatinine levels.
- May decrease Hb level and hematocrit and WBC, RBC, neutrophil, and platelet counts.

CONTRAINDICATIONS & CAUTIONS

⚠ *Alert:* CDK4 or CDK6 inhibitors may cause rare but severe or fatal ILD and pneumonitis.
- Drug may cause GI toxicity (including diarrhea associated with dehydration and infection), bone marrow suppression, and hepatotoxicity.
- Venous thromboembolism has been reported in patients treated with abemaciclib with fulvestrant or with an aromatase inhibitor.
- Use in patients with severe renal impairment and ESRD hasn't been studied.
- Use cautiously in patients with severe hepatic impairment (Child-Pugh class C).
- Safety and effectiveness in children haven't been established.
Dialyzable drug: Unknown.

PREGNANCY-LACTATION-REPRODUCTION

- Drug may cause fetal harm. Advise patient of fetal risk.
- Pregnancy testing is recommended for patients of childbearing potential before treatment.
- Patients of childbearing potential should use effective contraception during treatment and for at least 3 weeks after final dose.
- Serious adverse reactions may occur in infants who are breastfed. Patient shouldn't breastfeed during treatment and for at least 3 weeks after final dose.
- Based on animal studies, drug may impair fertility in males of reproductive potential.

NURSING CONSIDERATIONS

⚠ *Alert:* Monitor patients for new or worsening pulmonary signs or symptoms (hypoxia, cough, dyspnea, interstitial infiltrates on radiologic images); if they occur, interrupt therapy immediately and evaluate patient. If infection, neoplasm, and other causes are

---

Reactions in bold italics are *life-threatening.* Interactions may have a *rapid onset* or a *delayed onset.*

excluded, permanently discontinue treatment in patients with severe ILD or pneumonitis.
• Monitor patients for loose stools and associated dehydration and infection. Initiate antidiarrheal therapy and increase oral fluids at first sign of diarrhea.
• Monitor CBC before therapy begins, every 2 weeks during therapy for the first 2 months, monthly for the next 2 months, then as clinically indicated.
• Monitor patients for signs and symptoms of hepatotoxicity (fatigue, right upper quadrant abdominal pain, loss of appetite) and bone marrow suppression (fatigue, unusual bleeding or bruising, fever, infection).
• Obtain LFTs before therapy begins, every 2 weeks during therapy for the first 2 months, monthly for the next 2 months, then as clinically indicated.
• Monitor patients for signs and symptoms of thrombosis (pain and swelling of the extremities) and PE (chest pain, dyspnea, tachycardia), and treat appropriately.

PATIENT TEACHING
🛈 *Alert:* Warn patient to immediately report breathing difficulty or discomfort, and shortness of breath while at rest or with low activity, which may indicate ILD or pneumonitis.
• Teach patient to take drug at the same time each day, to take only whole tablets, and not to take damaged tablets.
• Tell patient to report all adverse reactions and to immediately report signs and symptoms of hepatotoxicity or venous thromboembolism.
• Advise patient to immediately report fever, particularly in association with other signs and symptoms of infection (malaise, pain, cough, shortness of breath, drainage, changes in urine).
• Instruct patient to begin antidiarrheal therapy (such as loperamide) at first sign of loose stools, to increase fluid intake, and to notify prescriber for further instructions and follow-up.
• Warn patient of childbearing potential of fetal risk. Advise her that a pregnancy test will be done before therapy begins, to use effective contraception during therapy and for at least 3 weeks after final dose, and to report known or suspected pregnancy.
• Remind patient not to breastfeed during treatment and for at least 3 weeks after final dose.
• Advise male patient of reproductive potential that drug may impair fertility.

SAFETY ALERT!

abiraterone acetate
a-bir-A-ter-one

Yonsa, Zytiga

Therapeutic class: Antineoplastics
Pharmacologic class: Antiandrogen biosynthesis inhibitors

AVAILABLE FORMS
Tablets ⬛: 250 mg
Tablets (film-coated) ⬛: 500 mg
Tablets (micronized) ⬛: 125 mg

INDICATIONS & DOSAGES
Adjust-a-dose (for all indications): For patients with baseline moderate hepatic impairment (Child-Pugh class B), reduce starting dosage of Zytiga to 250 mg PO once daily or Yonsa starting dosage to 125 mg once daily. If hepatotoxicity develops during treatment, refer to manufacturer's instructions for dosage adjustments.
   For patients who must take a strong CYP3A4 inducer, increase dosing frequency to b.i.d. only during coadministration.
➤ **Metastatic, castration-resistant prostate cancer**
Adult men: 1,000 mg Zytiga PO once daily, in combination with 5 mg prednisone PO b.i.d. Or, 500 mg Yonsa PO once daily in combination with 4 mg methylprednisolone PO b.i.d.
➤ **Metastatic, high-risk castration-sensitive prostate cancer (Zytiga only)**
Adult men: 1,000 mg PO once daily in combination with 5 mg prednisone PO daily.

ADMINISTRATION
PO
• Patients receiving abiraterone should also receive a GnRH analogue concurrently (or have had a bilateral orchiectomy).
• Drug is hazardous: use safe handling and disposal precautions according to facility policy. Patients who are pregnant or may become pregnant should wear gloves when handling tablets.
• Zytiga and Yonsa tablets aren't interchangeable; don't substitute between formulations.
• Give Zytiga tablets on an empty stomach; patient shouldn't eat for 2 hours before or 1 hour after receiving drug. Give Yonsa tablets without regard to food.

- Patient should swallow tablets whole with water and not crush or chew them.
- Store tablets at room temperature.

ACTION

Inhibits biosynthesis of androgen production and increases mineralocorticoid production by the adrenal glands.

Route	Onset	Peak	Duration
PO	Rapid	2 hr	Unknown

Half-life: 7 to 17 hours.

ADVERSE REACTIONS

CNS: fatigue, fever, insomnia, headache. **CV:** edema, hot flushes, HTN, *arrhythmias,* chest pain, *cardiac failure.* **EENT:** nasopharyngitis. **GI:** diarrhea, dyspepsia, constipation, vomiting. **GU:** UTI, hematuria, urinary frequency, nocturia. **Hematologic:** anemia, bruising, *lymphopenia.* **Hepatic:** increased transaminase levels, bilirubinemia, *hepatotoxicity.* **Metabolic:** *hypokalemia, hypophosphatemia,* hyperglycemia, hyperlipidemia, hypernatremia. **Musculoskeletal:** joint swelling, joint discomfort, muscle discomfort, fractures, groin pain. **Respiratory:** URI, cough, dyspnea. **Skin:** rash. **Other:** falls.

INTERACTIONS

Drug-drug. *CYP2C8 substrates (pioglitazone):* May increase substrate level. Monitor patient closely.
Dextromethorphan, thioridazine, other CYP2D6 substrates: May inhibit metabolism of these drugs, causing higher levels. Avoid using together. If drugs must be used together, consider reducing dosage of substrate drug.
Strong CYP3A4 inducers (carbamazepine, phenobarbital, phenytoin, rifabutin, rifampin, rifapentine): May decrease abiraterone level. If drugs must be used together, increase abiraterone dosage during concomitant use; decrease back to the previous dose and frequency if the CYP3A4 inducer is discontinued.
Drug-food. *Any food:* May significantly increase drug absorption of Zytiga. Patient must take Zytiga on an empty stomach.

EFFECTS ON LAB TEST RESULTS

- May increase ALP, ALT, AST, bilirubin, glucose, sodium, cholesterol, and triglyceride levels.

- May decrease potassium, phosphate, and Hb levels.
- May decrease lymphocyte count.

CONTRAINDICATIONS & CAUTIONS

- Contraindicated in patients hypersensitive to drug or its components and in those with baseline severe hepatic impairment (Child-Pugh class C).
- Use cautiously in patients with a history of CV disease (HF, recent MI, ventricular arrhythmias), diabetes, or liver disease.
- Avoid use with radium Ra 223 dichloride; combined use increases mortality and fracture risk.
- Safety in patients with LVEF of less than 50% or NYHA Class III or IV HF hasn't been established.
Dialyzable drug: Unknown.

PREGNANCY-LACTATION-REPRODUCTION

- Drug isn't indicated for use in women and is contraindicated during pregnancy and breastfeeding.
- Patients who are pregnant or may become pregnant should use personal protective equipment (gloves) when handling drug.
- Based on animal studies, male patients with partners of childbearing potential should use effective contraception during treatment and for at least 3 weeks after final dose.

NURSING CONSIDERATIONS

- Monitor ALT, AST, and bilirubin levels in all patients at baseline, every 2 weeks for first 3 months, then monthly thereafter. For patients with moderate hepatic impairment, measure at baseline, every week during first month of treatment, every 2 weeks for next 2 months, and monthly thereafter. If AST or ALT level rises above 5 × ULN, or bilirubin level rises above 3 × ULN, interrupt treatment and closely monitor liver function.
- Monitor patient for signs and symptoms of hepatotoxicity (malaise, jaundice, abdominal pain, nausea, vomiting).
- Monitor patient with a history of CV disease at least monthly for HTN, hypokalemia, and fluid retention. Monitor serum potassium level before treatment and at least monthly. Control HTN and correct hypokalemia before and during treatment.
- Monitor blood glucose level in patient with diabetes during and after treatment with abiraterone. Adjust antidiabetic dosage, if

---

Reactions in bold italics are *life-threatening*. Interactions may have a *rapid onset* or a ***delayed onset***.

needed, to minimize risk of hypoglycemia. Severe hypoglycemia has been reported in patients receiving thiazolidinediones (including pioglitazone) or repaglinide.

• Monitor patient for signs and symptoms of adrenocortical insufficiency (chronic fatigue, loss of appetite, muscle weakness, weight loss, nausea, and vomiting). Patient may need an increased corticosteroid dosage before, during, and after stressful situations.

PATIENT TEACHING

• Teach patient safe drug administration.
• Instruct patient that abiraterone and either prednisone or methylprednisolone must be used together.
• Warn patient not to stop abiraterone, prednisone, methylprednisolone, or other chemotherapy drugs without consulting prescriber.
• Advise patient that if a single dose of abiraterone, methylprednisolone, or prednisone is missed, to take the regular dose the next day. If more than one dose is missed, advise patient to inform prescriber.
• Teach patient that periodic blood tests will be needed to monitor tolerance to therapy.
• Warn patient, female caregivers, and female sexual partners about risk of fetal harm from abiraterone therapy. Teach patient who is pregnant or may become pregnant to wear gloves while handling drug.
• Teach male patient and female sexual partners the importance of using condoms. If patient's partner is pregnant or of childbearing potential, patient should use a condom and another effective birth control method during treatment and for at least 3 weeks after final dose.

acamprosate calcium
a-kam-PROE-sate

Therapeutic class: Alcohol deterrents
Pharmacologic class: Synthetic amino acid neurotransmitter analogues

AVAILABLE FORMS
Tablets (delayed-release) ⬤: 333 mg

INDICATIONS & DOSAGES
➤ **Adjunct to management of alcohol abstinence**
Adults: 666 mg PO t.i.d.

Adjust-a-dose: In patients with CrCl of 30 to 50 mL/minute, give 333 mg t.i.d.

ADMINISTRATION
PO
• Don't crush or break tablets.
• Give drug without regard for food.

ACTION
Restores the balance of neuronal excitation and inhibition, probably by interacting with glutamate and GABA neurotransmitter systems, thus reducing alcohol dependence.

Route	Onset	Peak	Duration
PO	Unknown	3–8 hr	Unknown

Half-life: 20 to 33 hours.

ADVERSE REACTIONS
CNS: abnormal thinking, amnesia, anxiety, asthenia, depression, dizziness, headache, insomnia, migraine, paresthesia, somnolence, *suicidality,* syncope, tremor, pain. **CV:** chest pain, HTN, palpitations, peripheral edema, vasodilation. **EENT:** abnormal vision, dry mouth, pharyngitis, rhinitis. **GI:** abdominal pain, anorexia, constipation, diarrhea, dyspepsia, flatulence, increased appetite, nausea, taste disturbance, vomiting. **GU:** erectile dysfunction. **Metabolic:** weight gain. **Musculoskeletal:** arthralgia, back pain, myalgia. **Respiratory:** bronchitis, dyspnea, increased cough. **Skin:** increased sweating, pruritus, rash. **Other:** accidental injury, chills, decreased libido, flulike symptoms, infection.

INTERACTIONS
None significant.

EFFECTS ON LAB TEST RESULTS
• May increase ALT, AST, ALP, bilirubin, blood glucose, creatinine, LDH, and uric acid levels.
• May decrease sodium level.
• May decrease leukocyte count.

CONTRAINDICATIONS & CAUTIONS
• Contraindicated in patients hypersensitive to drug or its components and in those with CrCl of 30 mL/minute or less.
• Don't use it in patients with a history of sulfite sensitivity.
• Use cautiously in older adults, patients with moderate renal impairment, and patients with

a history of depression and suicidal thoughts or attempts.
• Safety and effectiveness in children haven't been established.
Dialyzable drug: Unknown.
⚠ *Overdose S&S:* Diarrhea, hypercalcemia in chronic overdose.

PREGNANCY-LACTATION-REPRODUCTION
• Use cautiously during pregnancy and only if potential benefit justifies fetal risk.
• It isn't known if drug appears in human milk. Use cautiously during breastfeeding.

NURSING CONSIDERATIONS
• Use only after patient successfully becomes abstinent from drinking.
• Drug doesn't eliminate or reduce withdrawal symptoms.
🖑 *Alert:* Monitor patient for development of depression or suicidality.
• Drug doesn't cause alcohol aversion or a disulfiram-like reaction if used with alcohol.

PATIENT TEACHING
• Tell patient to continue the alcohol abstinence program, including counseling and support.
🖑 *Alert:* Advise patient to notify prescriber if depression, anxiety, thoughts of suicide, or severe diarrhea develops.
• Caution patient's family or caregiver to watch for signs of depression or suicidality.
• Instruct patient in safe drug administration.
• Advise patient to use effective contraception during therapy. Tell patient to report pregnancy or plans to become pregnant.
• Explain that drug may impair judgment, thinking, or motor skills. Urge patient to use caution when driving or performing hazardous activities until drug's effects are known.
• Tell patient to continue taking acamprosate and to contact prescriber if patient resumes drinking alcohol.

acetaminophen (APAP, paracetamol) 📋
a-seet-a-MIN-a-fen

ACET✷ ◇, Arthritis Pain Relief ◇, Children's Silapap ◇, FeverAll ◇, Fortolin✷, Ofirmev, Pediatrix✷ ◇, Rapid Action✷ ◇, Taminol✷, Triaminic Fever Reducer ◇, Tylenol ◇

Therapeutic class: Analgesics
Pharmacologic class: Para-aminophenol derivatives

AVAILABLE FORMS
Caplets: 500 mg ◇
Caplets (extended-release) 🕓: 650 mg ◇
Capsules: 325 mg ◇, 500 mg ◇
Drops: 80 mg/mL✷ ◇
Elixir: 160 mg/5 mL✷ ◇*
Gelcaps: 350 mg, 500 mg ◇
Injection: 10 mg/mL
Oral liquid: 160 mg/5 mL✷ ◇, 500 mg/ 15 mL ◇
Oral solution: 80 mg/mL✷ ◇, 160 mg/ 5 mL✷ ◇, 167 mg/5 mL ◇
Oral suspension: 80 mg/0.8 mL ◇, 160 mg/ 5 mL✷ ◇
Oral syrup: 160 mg/5 mL ◇
Powder: 160 mg ◇, 500 mg ◇
Suppositories: 80 mg ◇, 120 mg ◇, 160 mg✷ ◇, 325 mg ◇, 650 mg ◇
Tablets: 325 mg ◇, 500 mg ◇, 650 mg ◇
Tablets (chewable): 80 mg ◇, 160 mg ◇
Tablets (dispersible): 80 mg ◇, 160 mg ◇
Tablets (extended-release) 🕓: 650 mg ◇

INDICATIONS & DOSAGES
Boxed Warning Maximum daily dose includes all routes of administration and all acetaminophen-containing products, including combination products. ∎
➤ **Mild pain or fever**
PO
Adults: 325 to 650 mg PO every 4 to 6 hours. Or, two extended-release caplets PO every 8 hours. Maximum, 3,250 mg daily unless under health care provider supervision, when 4 g daily (immediate-release) may be used. For long-term therapy, don't exceed 2.6 g daily unless prescribed and monitored closely by health care provider.
Children older than age 12: 325 to 650 mg PO every 4 to 6 hours or 1,300 mg PO

Reactions in bold italics are *life-threatening*. Interactions may have a *rapid onset* or a ***delayed onset***.

every 8 hours (extended-release) PRN. Maximum dose for immediate-release is 3,250 mg/24 hours unless under health care provider supervision, when up to 4 g/24 hours may be used. Maximum dose for extended-release is 3,900 mg/24 hours.

Children ages 6 to 11 (immediate-release): 325 mg PO every 4 to 6 hours. Maximum daily dose is 1,625 mg/day PO. Don't use for more than 5 days unless directed by health care provider.

Children age 11 weighing 32.7 to 43.2 kg: 480 to 500 mg PO (oral suspension or chewable tablets) every 4 hours PRN. Maximum, five doses/day.

Children ages 9 to 10 weighing 27.3 to 32.6 kg: 325 to 400 mg PO (oral suspension or chewable tablets) every 4 hours PRN. Maximum, five doses/day.

Children ages 6 to 8 weighing 21.8 to 27.2 kg: 320 to 325 mg PO (oral suspension or chewable tablets) every 4 hours PRN. Maximum, five doses/day.

Children ages 4 to 5 weighing 16.4 to 21.7 kg: 240 mg PO (oral suspension or chewable tablets) every 4 hours PRN. Maximum, five doses/day.

Children ages 2 to 3 weighing 10.9 to 16.3 kg: 160 mg PO (oral suspension or chewable tablets) every 4 hours PRN. Maximum, five doses/day.

Children ages 1 to 2 weighing 8.2 to 10.8 kg: 120 mg PO (oral suspension or chewable tablets) every 4 hours PRN. Maximum, five doses/day.

Children ages 4 to 11 months weighing 5.4 to 8.1 kg: 80 mg PO (oral suspension, drops, or liquid) every 4 hours PRN. Maximum, five doses/day.

Children ages 0 to 3 months weighing 2.7 to 5.3 kg: 40 mg PO (oral drops) every 4 hours PRN. Maximum, five doses/day.

Adjust-a-dose: For adults with GFR of 10 to 50 mL/minute/1.73 m^2, give every 6 hours; if GFR is less than 10 mL/minute/1.73 m^2, give every 8 hours. For patients receiving continuous renal replacement therapy, give every 6 hours. For infants, children, and adolescents with GFR less than 10 mL/minute/1.73 m^2, give every 8 hours. For infants, children, and adolescents receiving hemodialysis or peritoneal dialysis, give every 8 hours.

Rectal
Adults and children age 12 and older: 325 to 650 mg PR every 4 to 6 hours PRN.

Maximum, 3.9 g daily. For long-term therapy, don't exceed 2.6 g daily unless prescribed and monitored closely by health care provider.

Children ages 6 to 11: 325 mg PR every 4 to 6 hours PRN. Maximum, 1,625 mg in 24 hours.

Children ages 3 to 6: 120 mg PR every 4 to 6 hours PRN. Maximum, 600 mg in 24 hours.

Children ages 1 to 3: 80 mg PR every 4 to 6 hours PRN. Maximum, 400 mg in 24 hours.

Children ages 6 to 11 months: 80 mg PR every 6 hours PRN. Maximum, 320 mg in 24 hours.

➤ **Mild to moderate pain; mild to moderate pain with adjunctive opioid analgesics; fever**

Adults and children age 13 and older weighing 50 kg or more: 1,000 mg IV every 6 hours or 650 mg IV every 4 hours. Maximum dose is 1,000 mg as a single dose and 4,000 mg/day.

Adults and children age 13 and older weighing less than 50 kg: 15 mg/kg IV every 6 hours or 12.5 mg/kg IV every 4 hours. Maximum dose is 15 mg/kg (up to 750 mg) as a single dose and 75 mg/kg (up to 3,750 mg)/day.

Children ages 2 to 12: 15 mg/kg IV every 6 hours or 12.5 mg/kg IV every 4 hours. Maximum dose is 15 mg/kg as a single dose and 75 mg/kg (up to 3,750 mg)/day.

Infants age 29 days to 2 years for fever: 15 mg/kg IV every 6 hours. Maximum dose is 60 mg/kg/day, with minimum dosing interval of 6 hours.

Neonates (32 weeks' gestational age and greater) to age 28 days for fever: 12.5 mg/kg IV every 6 hours. Maximum dose is 50 mg/kg/day, with minimum dosing interval of 6 hours.

Adjust-a-dose: Longer dosing intervals and a reduced total daily dose may be warranted in patients with CrCl of 30 mL/minute or less.

ADMINISTRATION
PO
• Use liquid form for children and patients who have difficulty swallowing.
• Give drug without regard for food.
• Patient should allow dispersible tablet or powder to dissolve in the mouth.
• Shake liquid formulations well before using.
• Give extended-release forms whole; don't crush, dissolve, or allow patient to chew extended-release forms.

IV

▼ Examine vial; don't use if particulate matter or discoloration is observed.

▼ For 1,000-mg dose, give by inserting a vented IV set through the septum of a 100-mL vial.

▼ For doses less than 1,000 mg, withdraw appropriate dose and place into a separate container before administration.

▼ Place small-volume pediatric doses of up to 60 mL in a syringe and use a syringe-pump.

▼ May administer without further dilution.

▼ Don't add other medications to IV solution.

▼ Give over 15 minutes.

▼ Entire 100-mL vial isn't for use in patients weighing less than 50 kg.

▼ Monitor end of infusion to prevent possibility of air embolism.

▼ Use within 6 hours of penetrating vial seal.

▼ Vial is for single use only. Discard unused portion.

▼ **Incompatibilities:** Diazepam, chlorpromazine hydrochloride. Don't admix with other drugs.

Rectal

● If suppository is too soft, refrigerate for 15 minutes or run under cold water in wrapper.

ACTION

Thought to produce analgesia by inhibiting prostaglandin and other substances that sensitize pain receptors. Drug may relieve fever through central action in the hypothalamic heat-regulating center.

Route	Onset	Peak	Duration
PO	<1 hr	30–60 min	4–6 hr
IV	5–30 min	15 min	4–6 hr
PR	Unknown	1.5–5 hr	Unknown

Half-life: PO, 2 to 3 hours; IV, 2.4 hours (adults), 3 hours (children and adolescents), 4.2 hours (infants), 7 hours (neonates); PR, 2 to 3 hours.

ADVERSE REACTIONS

CNS: agitation (IV), anxiety, fatigue, headache, insomnia, fever. **CV:** HTN, hypotension, peripheral edema, periorbital edema, tachycardia (IV). **GI:** nausea, vomiting, abdominal pain, diarrhea, constipation (IV). **GU:** oliguria (IV). **Hematologic:** hemolytic anemia, *leukopenia, neutropenia, pancytopenia, anemia.* **Hepatic:** jaundice.

Metabolic: hypoalbuminemia (IV), *hypoglycemia, hypokalemia,* hypervolemia, *hypomagnesemia,* hypophosphatemia (IV). **Musculoskeletal:** muscle spasms, extremity pain (IV). **Respiratory:** abnormal breath sounds, dyspnea, *hypoxia,* atelectasis, pleural effusion, *pulmonary edema, stridor,* wheezing (IV). **Skin:** rash, urticaria; infusion-site pain (IV), pruritus.

INTERACTIONS

Drug-drug. *Barbiturates, carbamazepine, hydantoins, rifampin:* High doses or long-term use of these drugs may reduce therapeutic effects and enhance hepatotoxic effects of acetaminophen. Avoid using together.

Busulfan: May increase busulfan level. Monitor patient closely.

Cholestyramine resin: May decrease acetaminophen absorption. Give at least 1 hour after acetaminophen or consider therapy change.

Dasatinib: May enhance hepatotoxic effects of dasatinib and increase acetaminophen level. Avoid use together.

Imatinib, mipomersen: May increase hepatotoxic effects of these drugs. Monitor patient closely.

Isoniazid: May increase risk of acetaminophen adverse effects. Monitor patient closely.

Lamotrigine: Prolonged acetaminophen use may decrease lamotrigine level. Monitor patient for therapeutic effects; adjust lamotrigine dosage as needed.

Lomitapide: May increase risk of hepatotoxicity. Limit maximum adult dose of acetaminophen to 4 g or less daily for 3 or fewer days per week or consider therapy change.

Metyrapone, probenecid: May increase acetaminophen level and risk of hepatotoxicity. Avoid use together.

Warfarin: May increase anticoagulant effects with long-term use with high doses of acetaminophen. Monitor INR closely.

Drug-lifestyle. *Alcohol use:* May increase risk of hepatic damage. Discourage use together.

EFFECTS ON LAB TEST RESULTS

● May increase AST level. May decrease glucose, potassium, phosphorus, magnesium, albumin, and Hb level and hematocrit.

● May decrease neutrophil, WBC, RBC, and platelet counts.

● May cause false-positive test result for urinary 5-hydroxyindoleacetic acid. May falsely

---

Reactions in bold italics are *life-threatening.* Interactions may have a *rapid onset* or a ***delayed onset.***

decrease glucose level in home monitoring systems.

CONTRAINDICATIONS & CAUTIONS

Boxed Warning Drug can cause acute liver failure, which may require a liver transplant or cause death. Most cases of liver injury are associated with drug doses exceeding 4,000 mg/day and often involve more than one acetaminophen-containing product. ∎

🜊 *Alert:* May cause serious, potentially fatal skin reactions, including SJS, TEN, and acute generalized exanthematous pustulosis. Reaction may occur with first or subsequent use when acetaminophen is used as monotherapy or when it is one component of combination drug therapy. Monitor for reddening of the skin, rash, blisters, and detachment of the upper surface of the skin. Stop drug immediately if skin reaction is suspected.

• Contraindicated in patients hypersensitive to drug. IV form is contraindicated in patients with severe hepatic impairment or severe active liver disease.

• Use cautiously in patients with any type of liver disease, chronic malnutrition, severe hypovolemia (dehydration, blood loss), or severe renal impairment (CrCl of 30 mL/minute or less).

🜋 Use cautiously in patients with G6PD deficiency.

• Use cautiously in patients with long-term alcohol use because therapeutic doses cause hepatotoxicity in these patients. Patients with chronic alcoholism shouldn't take more than 2 g of acetaminophen every 24 hours.

Dialyzable drug: Unknown.

⚠ *Overdose S&S:* Stage 1 (up to 24 hours): abdominal pain, diaphoresis, nausea, vomiting, malaise, pallor; stage 2 (24 to 36 hours): right upper quadrant pain, elevated LFT results, prolonged PT; stage 3 (72 to 96 hours): hepatic failure, encephalopathy, coma.

PREGNANCY-LACTATION-REPRODUCTION

• Use cautiously during pregnancy. Embryo-fetal risk is very low.

• There are no studies of IV acetaminophen use during pregnancy; use only if clearly needed.

• Drug appears in human milk. Use cautiously during breastfeeding.

NURSING CONSIDERATIONS

Boxed Warning Many OTC and prescription products contain acetaminophen; be aware of this when calculating total daily dose. ∎

Boxed Warning Use caution when prescribing, preparing, and administering IV acetaminophen to avoid dosing errors leading to accidental overdose and death. Don't confuse dose in milliGRAMS and dose in milliLITERS. Be sure to base dose on weight for patients weighing less than 50 kg, to properly program infusion pump, and to ensure that total daily dose of acetaminophen from all sources doesn't exceed maximum daily limit. ∎

• Consider reducing total daily dose and increasing dosing intervals in patients with hepatic or renal impairment.

PATIENT TEACHING

• Tell parents and caregivers to consult prescriber before giving drug to children younger than age 2.

• Advise parents and caregivers that drug is only for short-term use; urge them to consult prescriber if giving to infants for longer than 3 days, children for longer than 5 days, or adults for longer than 10 days.

Boxed Warning Caution patient or caregiver that many OTC products contain acetaminophen and should be counted when calculating total daily dose. ∎

• Tell patient to consult prescriber for fever lasting longer than 3 days or recurrent fever.

🜊 *Alert:* Warn patient that high doses or unsupervised long-term use can cause liver damage. Excessive alcohol use may increase the risk of liver damage. Caution patient with long-term alcoholism to limit drug to 2 g/day or less.

• Caution patient to contact health care provider if signs and symptoms of liver damage (illogical thinking, severe dyspepsia, jaundice, inability to eat, weakness) occur.

🜊 *Alert:* Warn patient to stop drug and seek medical attention immediately if rash or other reactions occurs while using acetaminophen.

• Tell patient who is breastfeeding that drug appears in human milk in low levels. Drug may be used safely if therapy is short-term and doesn't exceed recommended doses.

🍁Canada   ◇OTC   ◆Off-label use   ⦕Photoguide   ⊜Do not crush   *Liquid contains alcohol   🜋Genetic

acetaZOLAMIDE
ah-set-a-ZOLE-ah-mide

acetaZOLAMIDE sodium
Therapeutic class: Diuretics
Pharmacologic class: Carbonic anhydrase inhibitors

AVAILABLE FORMS
acetazolamide
Capsules (extended-release) ⓄⓉⒸ: 500 mg
Tablets: 125 mg; 250 mg
acetazolamide sodium
Powder for injection: 500-mg vial

INDICATIONS & DOSAGES
➤ **Secondary glaucoma; preoperative treatment of acute angle-closure glaucoma**
Adults: 250 mg PO every 4 hours or 250 mg PO b.i.d. for short-term therapy. In acute cases, 500 mg PO; then 125 to 250 mg PO every 4 hours. Or, for extended-release capsules, 500 mg PO b.i.d. To rapidly lower IOP, initially, 500 mg IV; may repeat in 2 to 4 hours, if needed, followed by 125 to 250 mg PO or IV every 4 hours.
➤ **Chronic open-angle glaucoma**
Adults: 250 mg to 1 g PO daily in divided doses q.i.d., or 250 mg IV every 4 hours, or 500 mg extended-release PO b.i.d.
➤ **To prevent or treat acute mountain sickness (high-altitude sickness)**
Adults and children age 12 and older: 500 mg to 1 g (extended-release) PO daily in divided doses every 12 hours. Start 24 to 48 hours before ascent and continue for 48 hours while at high altitude. When rapid ascent is required, start with 1,000 mg PO daily.
➤ **Adjunct for epilepsy and myoclonic, refractory, generalized tonic-clonic, absence, or mixed seizures**
Adults: 8 to 30 mg/kg PO (immediate-release only) or IV daily in divided doses; optimum range is 375 mg to 1 g daily. If given with other anticonvulsants, start at 250 mg PO or IV once daily, and increase to 375 mg to 1 g daily.
➤ **Edema caused by HF; drug-induced edema**
Adults: 250 to 375 mg (5 mg/kg; immediate-release only) PO daily in the morning. For best results, use every other day or 2 days on followed by 1 to 2 days off. Or, 250 to 375 mg

IV once daily for 1 or 2 days, alternating with a day of rest.

ADMINISTRATION
PO
• Give oral drug with food to minimize GI upset.
• Don't crush or open extended-release capsules.
• If patient can't swallow oral form, pharmacist may make a suspension using crushed tablets.
• Refrigeration of suspension improves palatability but doesn't improve stability.
IV
▼ Reconstitute drug in 500-mg vial with at least 5 mL of sterile water for injection. Store reconstituted solution for 3 days under refrigeration or 12 hours at room temperature.
▼ Direct IV injection is the preferred route. Administer in divided doses for amounts more than 250 mg.
▼ IM administration isn't recommended.
▼ **Incompatibilities:** Multivitamins.

ACTION
Promotes renal excretion of sodium, potassium, bicarbonate, and water. As anticonvulsant, drug normalizes neuronal discharge. In mountain sickness, drug stimulates ventilation and increases cerebral blood flow. In glaucoma, drug reduces IOP.

Route	Onset	Peak	Duration
PO	60–90 min	1–4 hr	8–12 hr
PO (extended-release)	2 hr	3–6 hr	18–24 hr
IV	2–10 min	15 min	4–5 hr

Half-life: 3 to 6 hours.

ADVERSE REACTIONS
CNS: *seizures,* drowsiness, paresthesia, confusion, depression, ataxia, headache, malaise, fever, fatigue, excitement, dizziness, flaccid paralysis, taste alteration. **CV:** flushing. **EENT:** transient myopia, hearing dysfunction, tinnitus. **GI:** nausea, vomiting, anorexia, diarrhea, melena, constipation. **GU:** polyuria, hematuria, crystalluria, glycosuria, renal calculus. **Hematologic:** *aplastic anemia, leukopenia, thrombocytopenia purpura, hemolytic anemia, agranulocytosis, pancytopenia.* **Hepatic:** abnormal liver function, cholestatic jaundice, hepatic insufficiency, *fulminant hepatic necrosis.* **Metabolic:**

hypokalemia, hyponatremia, *hypoglycemia*, hyperglycemia, asymptomatic hyperuricemia, hyperchloremic acidosis. **Skin:** pain at injection site, photosensitivity, rash, urticaria. **Other:** growth retardation in children, *anaphylaxis*.

INTERACTIONS

Drug-drug. *Alpha blockers, beta blockers, antihypertensives:* May increase hypotensive effect. Monitor patient carefully.

Amphetamines, quinidine: May decrease renal clearance of these drugs, increasing toxicity. Monitor patient for toxicity.

Carbamazepine: May increase carbamazepine level. Monitor patient for toxicity.

Cyclosporine: May increase cyclosporine level, causing nephrotoxicity and neurotoxicity. Monitor patient for toxicity.

Flecainide: May increase flecainide concentration. Monitor patient for toxicity and cardiac rhythm disturbances.

Folic acid antagonists: May increase adverse effects of folic acid antagonists. Use cautiously together.

Lithium: May increase lithium excretion, decreasing its effect. Monitor lithium level.

Methenamine: May reduce methenamine effect. Avoid using together.

Phenytoin: May increase phenytoin level and risk of osteomalacia. Use together cautiously.

Primidone: May decrease serum and urine primidone levels and decrease anticonvulsant effect. Monitor patient closely.

◑ *Alert: Salicylates (aspirin):* May cause accumulation and toxicity of acetazolamide, resulting in CNS depression, metabolic acidosis, anorexia, and death. Administer with caution; monitor patient for toxicity.

Sodium bicarbonate: May increase risk of renal calculus. Monitor patient closely.

Drug-lifestyle. *Sun exposure:* May increase risk of photosensitivity reactions. Advise patient to avoid excessive sunlight exposure.

EFFECTS ON LAB TEST RESULTS

- May increase uric acid level. May decrease potassium, sodium, and Hb levels and hematocrit.
- May increase or decrease glucose level.
- May decrease WBC and platelet counts.
- May interfere with the HPLC method of assay for theophylline.

CONTRAINDICATIONS & CAUTIONS

◑ *Alert:* Cross-sensitivity between sulfonamides and sulfonamide-derivative diuretics such as acetazolamide has been reported.

◑ *Alert:* Fatalities have occurred due to severe reactions to sulfonamides, including SJS, TEN, fulminant hepatic necrosis, agranulocytosis, aplastic anemia, and other blood dyscrasias. Sensitizations may recur when a sulfonamide is readministered, irrespective of the route of administration. If signs and symptoms of hypersensitivity or other serious reactions occur, discontinue drug.

- Contraindicated in patients hypersensitive to drug and in those with hyponatremia or hypokalemia, marked renal or hepatic disease or dysfunction, suprarenal gland failure, hyperchloremic acidosis, or cirrhosis.
- Contraindicated in patients receiving long-term treatment for chronic noncongestive angle-closure glaucoma.
- Use cautiously in patients receiving other diuretics and in those with diabetes, renal impairment, respiratory acidosis, emphysema, or COPD.

Dialyzable drug: Unknown.

⚠ *Overdose S&S:* Electrolyte imbalance, acidotic state, CNS effects.

PREGNANCY-LACTATION-REPRODUCTION

- There are no well-controlled studies during pregnancy; use only if potential benefit justifies fetal risk.
- Enroll patients who are pregnant and taking acetazolamide for seizure disorders in the AED Pregnancy Registry (1-888-233-2334).
- Drug appears in human milk. Patient should discontinue drug or discontinue breastfeeding, taking into account the importance of the drug to the patient. Use during breastfeeding only when benefit to patient justifies risk to infant.

NURSING CONSIDERATIONS

- Monitor fluid intake and output, glucose, and electrolytes, especially potassium, bicarbonate, and chloride. When drug is used as diuretic therapy, consult prescriber and dietitian about providing a high-potassium diet.
- Monitor older adults closely because they are especially susceptible to excessive diuresis.
- Weigh patient daily. Rapid or excessive fluid loss may cause weight loss and hypotension.

- Diuretic effect decreases when acidosis occurs but can be reestablished by using intermittent administration schedules.
- Monitor patient for signs of hemolytic anemia (pallor, weakness, and palpitations).
- Monitor blood glucose level in patients with diabetes or impaired glucose tolerance.
- Monitor patient for hypersensitivity reactions.
- Monitor growth in children.
- *Look alike–sound alike:* Don't confuse acetazolamide with acetaminophen or acyclovir.

PATIENT TEACHING
- Teach patient safe drug administration.
- Caution patient not to perform hazardous activities if adverse CNS reactions occur.
- Instruct patient to avoid prolonged exposure to sunlight because drug may cause phototoxicity.
- Instruct patient to notify prescriber of unusual bleeding, bruising, tingling, tremors, rash, fever, kidney stones, or loss of appetite.

acetylcysteine
a-se-teel-SIS-tay-een

Acetadote

Therapeutic class: Mucolytics
Pharmacologic class: L-cysteine derivatives

AVAILABLE FORMS
Inhalation solution: 10%, 20%
IV injection: 200 mg/mL

INDICATIONS & DOSAGES
➤ **Adjunctive therapy for abnormal viscid or thickened mucous secretions in patients with pneumonia, bronchitis, bronchiectasis, primary amyloidosis of the lung, TB, cystic fibrosis, emphysema, atelectasis, pulmonary complications of thoracic surgery, or CV surgery**
Adults and children: 1 to 2 mL 10% or 20% solution by direct instillation into trachea as often as every hour. Or, 1 to 10 mL of 20% solution or 2 to 20 mL of 10% solution by nebulization every 2 to 6 hours PRN.
➤ **Diagnostic bronchial studies**
Adults and children: Two or three administrations of 1 to 2 mL of 20% solution or 2 to 4 mL of 10% solution by nebulization or intratracheal instillation before procedure.

➤ **Routine tracheostomy care**
Adults and children: 1 to 2 mL of 10% or 20% solution by direct instillation into tracheostomy every 1 to 4 hours.
➤ **Acetaminophen toxicity**
PO
Adults and children: Initially, 140 mg/kg PO; then 70 mg/kg PO 4 hours after initial dose, then every 4 hours for 17 doses (total).
IV
Adults and children weighing 41 to 100 kg or more: 150 mg/kg in 200 mL of diluent IV over 1 hour. Then, 50 mg/kg in 500 mL of diluent IV over 4 hours. Then, 100 mg/kg in 1,000 mL of diluent IV over 16 hours.
Adults and children weighing 21 to 40 kg: 150 mg/kg in 100 mL of diluent IV over 1 hour. Then, 50 mg/kg in 250 mL of diluent IV over 4 hours. Then, 100 mg/kg in 500 mL diluent IV over 16 hours.
Adults and children weighing 5 to 20 kg: 150 mg/kg in 3 mL/kg diluent IV over 1 hour. Then, 50 mg/kg in 7 mL/kg diluent IV over 4 hours. Then, 100 mg/kg in 14 mL/kg diluent IV over 16 hours.
Adjust-a-dose: Refer to manufacturer's instruction for dosing in patients weighing less than 40 kg and requiring fluid restriction.

ADMINISTRATION
PO
(inhalation formulation)
- Administer via the oral route. Dilute oral dose (used for acetaminophen overdose) with diet cola or other diet soft drinks or water. Dilute 20% solution to 5% (add 3 mL of diluent to each milliliter of drug). If patient vomits within 1 hour of receiving loading or maintenance dose, repeat dose. Use diluted solution within 1 hour.
- Drug smells strongly of sulfur. Mixing oral form with juice or cola improves its taste.
- Drug delivered through NG tube may be diluted with water.
- Store opened, undiluted oral solution in the refrigerator for up to 96 hours.
IV
▼ Drug may turn from a colorless liquid to a slight pink or purple color once the stopper is punctured. This color change doesn't affect the drug.
▼ Drug is hyperosmolar and is compatible with D_5W, half-NSS, and sterile water for injection.

▼ Adjust total volume given for patients who weigh less than 40 kg or who are fluid restricted.

▼ For patients who weigh 41 kg or more, dilute loading dose in 200 mL of D_5W, second dose in 500 mL, and third dose in 1,000 mL. Refer to manufacturer's instructions for dosage and dilution for patients weighing 40 kg or less.

▼ Reconstituted solution is stable for 24 hours at room temperature.

▼ Vials contain no preservatives; discard after opening.

▼ **Incompatibilities:** None listed by manufacturer. Consult a drug incompatibility reference for more information.

Inhalational

● Use plastic, glass, stainless steel, or another nonreactive metal when giving by nebulization. Hand-bulb nebulizers aren't recommended because output is too small and particle size too large.

● If only a portion of the solution in a vial is used for inhalation, store remainder in refrigerator and use within 96 hours.

● **Incompatibilities:** Physically or chemically incompatible with inhaled tetracyclines, erythromycin lactobionate, amphotericin B, and ampicillin sodium. If given by aerosol inhalation, nebulize these drugs separately. Iodized oil, trypsin, and hydrogen peroxide are physically incompatible with acetylcysteine; don't add to nebulizer.

ACTION

Reduces the viscosity of pulmonary secretions by splitting disulfide linkages between mucoprotein molecular complexes. Also restores liver stores of glutathione to treat acetaminophen toxicity.

Route	Onset	Peak	Duration
Inhalation	5–10 min	1–2 hr	1 hr
IV	Unknown	0.5–1 hr	Unknown

Half-life: Inhalation, 5.6 hours; IV, 5.6 hours.

ADVERSE REACTIONS

CNS: fever, drowsiness. **CV:** chest tightness, flushing, tachycardia, edema. **EENT:** rhinorrhea, pharyngitis, throat tightness. **GI:** nausea, stomatitis, vomiting. **Respiratory:** *bronchospasm,* cough, dyspnea, rhonchi. **Skin:** clamminess, pruritus, rash, urticaria. **Other:** *anaphylactoid reaction,* chills, hypersensitivity reaction.

INTERACTIONS

Drug-drug. *Activated charcoal:* May limit acetylcysteine's effectiveness. Avoid using activated charcoal before or with oral acetylcysteine.

EFFECTS ON LAB TEST RESULTS

None reported.

CONTRAINDICATIONS & CAUTIONS

● Contraindicated in patients hypersensitive to drug.

◑ **Alert:** Serious anaphylactoid reactions, including rash, hypotension, dyspnea, and wheezing, have been reported. Reactions usually occur 30 to 60 minutes after start of infusion and may require treatment and drug discontinuation.

● Use cautiously in older adults and patients with debilitation and severe respiratory insufficiency. Use IV form cautiously in patients with asthma or a history of bronchospasm, in those weighing less than 40 kg, and in patients requiring fluid restriction.

Dialyzable drug: Yes.

PREGNANCY-LACTATION-REPRODUCTION

● There are no adequate and well-controlled studies during pregnancy; use cautiously during pregnancy and only if clearly indicated.

● It's unknown if drug appears in human milk. Use cautiously during breastfeeding.

NURSING CONSIDERATIONS

● Monitor cough type and frequency.

◑ **Alert:** Monitor patient for bronchospasm, especially if patient has asthma.

● Ingestion of more than 150 mg/kg of acetaminophen may cause hepatotoxicity. Measure acetaminophen level 4 hours after ingestion to determine risk of hepatotoxicity. See manufacturer's information for nomogram for estimating potential for hepatotoxicity from acute acetaminophen ingestion and need for acetylcysteine therapy.

◑ **Alert:** Drug is used for acetaminophen overdose within 24 hours of ingestion. Start drug immediately; don't wait for results of acetaminophen level. Give within 10 hours of acetaminophen ingestion to minimize hepatic injury.

● For suspected acetaminophen overdose, obtain baseline INR and AST, ALT, bilirubin, BUN, creatinine, glucose, and electrolyte levels.

- In acetaminophen overdose, check acetaminophen, ALT, and AST levels and INR after the last maintenance dose. If acetaminophen level is still detectable, or if the ALT/AST level is still increasing or the INR remains elevated, the maintenance doses should be continued and the prescriber should contact a regional poison control center (1-800-222-1222) or a special health professional assistance line (1-800-525-6115) for assistance with dosing recommendations.
- Half-life elimination increases by 80% in patients with severe liver damage.

❶ *Alert:* Monitor patient receiving IV form for anaphylactoid reactions. Reactions involving more than simple skin flushing or erythema should be treated as anaphylactoid reactions. If anaphylactoid reaction occurs, stop infusion and treat reaction with antihistamines and epinephrine if needed. Once anaphylaxis treatment starts, carefully restart infusion. If anaphylactoid symptoms return, stop drug.
- Flushing and skin erythema may occur within 30 to 60 minutes of start of IV infusion and usually resolve without stopping infusion.
- When acetaminophen level is below toxic level according to nomogram, stop therapy.
- The vial stopper doesn't contain natural rubber latex, dry natural rubber, or blends of natural rubber.
- *Look alike–sound alike:* Don't confuse acetylcysteine with acetylcholine or acetazolamide.

PATIENT TEACHING
- Warn patient that drug may have a foul taste or smell that may be distressing.
- For maximum effect, instruct patient to cough to clear airway before aerosol administration.

acyclovir
ay-SYE-kloe-ver

Sitavig, Zovirax

acyclovir sodium

Therapeutic class: Antivirals
Pharmacologic class: Nucleosides and nucleotides

AVAILABLE FORMS
Capsules: 200 mg
Cream: 5%
Ointment: 5%
Solution (IV): 50 mg/mL
Suspension: 200 mg/5 mL
Tablets: 400 mg, 800 mg
Tablets (buccal) ⓞⓑⓒ: 50 mg

INDICATIONS & DOSAGES
Adjust-a-dose (for all indications): For patients receiving the IV form, if CrCl is 25 to 50 mL/minute/1.73 m^2, give 100% of dose every 12 hours; if CrCl is 10 to 25 mL/minute/1.73 m^2, give 100% of dose every 24 hours; if CrCl is less than 10 mL/minute/1.73 m^2, give 50% of dose every 24 hours.

For patients receiving the PO form, if normal dose is 200 mg every 4 hours five times daily and CrCl is less than 10 mL/minute/1.73 m^2, give 200 mg PO every 12 hours. If normal dose is 400 mg every 12 hours and CrCl is less than 10 mL/minute/1.73 m^2, give 200 mg every 12 hours. If normal dose is 800 mg every 4 hours five times daily and CrCl is 10 to 25 mL/minute/1.73 m^2, give 800 mg every 8 hours; if CrCl is less than 10 mL/minute/1.73 m^2, give 800 mg every 12 hours.

For patients who require hemodialysis, give additional dose after each dialysis.

➤ **First and recurrent episodes of mucocutaneous HSV (HSV-1 and HSV-2) infections in patients who are immunocompromised**
Adults and children age 12 and older: 5 mg/kg IV over 1 hour every 8 hours for 7 days.
Children ages 3 months to younger than 12 years: 10 mg/kg IV over 1 hour every 8 hours for 7 days.

➤ **Severe first episodes of genital herpes in patients who aren't immunocompromised**
Adults and children age 12 and older: 5 mg/kg IV over 1 hour every 8 hours for 5 days.

➤ **First genital herpes episode**
Adults: 200 mg PO every 4 hours while awake, five times daily. Continue for 10 days.

➤ **Initial genital herpes; limited, non-life-threatening mucocutaneous HSV infections in patients who are immunocompromised**
Adults and children age 12 and older: Adequately cover all lesions every 3 hours six times daily for 7 days. Although dosage varies depending on total lesion area, use about ½-inch (1.3-cm) ribbon of ointment on each 4-inch (10-cm) square of surface area.

➤ **Intermittent therapy for recurrent genital herpes**

Adults: 200 mg PO every 4 hours while awake, five times daily. Continue for 5 days. Begin therapy at first sign of recurrence.

➤ **Long-term suppressive therapy for recurrent genital herpes**

Adults: 400 mg PO b.i.d. for up to 12 months. Or, 200 mg PO t.i.d. to five times daily for up to 12 months.

➤ **Varicella zoster infections in patients who are immunocompromised**

Adults and children age 12 and older: 10 mg/kg IV over 1 hour every 8 hours for 7 days. Use ideal body weight for patients who are obese. Don't exceed maximum dosage equivalent of 20 mg/kg every 8 hours.

Children younger than age 12: 20 mg/kg IV over 1 hour every 8 hours for 7 days.

➤ **Varicella (chickenpox) infection in patients who are immunocompetent**

Adults and children weighing more than 40 kg: 800 mg PO q.i.d. for 5 days.

Children age 2 and older weighing less than 40 kg: 20 mg/kg (maximum, 80 mg/kg/day) PO q.i.d. for 5 days. Start therapy as soon as symptoms appear.

➤ **Acute herpes zoster infection in patients who are immunocompetent**

Adults and children age 12 and older: 800 mg PO every 4 hours five times daily for 7 to 10 days.

➤ **Herpes simplex encephalitis**

Adults and children age 12 and older: 10 mg/kg IV over 1 hour every 8 hours for 10 days.

Children ages 3 months to 12 years: 20 mg/kg IV over 1 hour every 8 hours for 10 days.

➤ **Neonatal HSV infections**

Neonates with postmenstrual age of at least 34 weeks: 20 mg/kg IV over 1 hour every 8 hours for 21 days.

Neonates with postmenstrual age of less than 34 weeks: 20 mg/kg IV over 1 hour every 12 hours for 21 days.

➤ **Recurrent herpes labialis in patients who are immunocompetent**

Topical

Adults and children age 12 and older: Apply cream five times daily for 4 days. Start therapy as early as possible after signs and symptoms occur. Or, apply ointment every 3 hours, six times daily for 7 days.

Oral/buccal

Adults: 50-mg buccal tablet as a single dose to upper gum region, on the same side as the symptoms, within 1 hour after onset of prodromal symptoms and before appearance of signs of cold sore.

ADMINISTRATION

PO
- Give drug without regard for meals, but give with food if stomach irritation occurs.
- Patient should take drug as prescribed, even after feeling better.

Buccal
- Patients shouldn't chew, suck, crush, or swallow tablets.
- Apply with dry finger immediately after taking tablet out of blister pack.
- Place tablet just above incisor tooth on upper gum on the same side of the mouth as prodromal symptoms appeared.
- Hold tablet in place with slight pressure over upper lip for 30 seconds to ensure adhesion. Place rounded side to gum for comfort, but either side can be applied.
- Tablet will stay in place and dissolve gradually.
- Food and drink can be taken normally with tablet in place.
- Patients should avoid chewing gum, touching or pressing tablet, wearing upper denture, brushing teeth, or other activity that may interfere with adhesion.
- Patients should drink plenty of liquids in case of dry mouth.
- If buccal tablet doesn't adhere or falls off within first 6 hours, reposition same tablet immediately. If tablet doesn't adhere, place a new tablet.
- If patient swallows buccal tablet within first 6 hours, have patient drink a glass of water; then apply a new tablet.
- If buccal tablet falls out or patient swallows it after first 6 hours, don't reapply.

IV
- ▼ Inspect solution for particulate matter and discoloration before administration.
- ▼ Once diluted, use each dose within 24 hours.
- ▼ Solutions concentrated at 7 mg/mL or more may cause a higher risk of phlebitis.
- ▼ Encourage fluid intake because patient must be adequately hydrated during infusion.
- ▼ Bolus injection, dehydration (decreased urine output), renal disease, and use with other nephrotoxic drugs increase the risk of renal toxicity. Don't give by bolus injection.
- ▼ Give IV infusion over at least 1 hour to prevent renal tubular damage.

▼ Monitor intake and output, especially during the first 2 hours after administration.

🌙 *Alert:* Don't give IM or subcut.

▼ **Incompatibilities:** None listed by manufacturer. Consult a drug incompatibility reference for more information.

Topical

• Apply with finger cot or rubber glove to prevent autoinoculation of other body sites and transmission of infection to others.

• Apply as early as possible after onset of prodromal symptoms or when lesions appear.

• Topical form is for cutaneous use only; don't apply to eyes.

ACTION

Interferes with DNA synthesis and inhibits viral multiplication.

Route	Onset	Peak	Duration
PO	Unknown	2.5 hr	Unknown
Buccal	Unknown	7 hr (in saliva)	Unknown
IV	Immediate	Immediate	Unknown
Topical	Unknown	Unknown	Unknown

Half-life: 2 to 3.5 hours with normal renal function; up to 19 hours with renal impairment.

ADVERSE REACTIONS

CNS: headache, malaise, *encephalopathic changes (including lethargy, obtundation, tremor, confusion, hallucinations, agitation, seizures, coma).* **EENT:** gum pain, canker sores (buccal tablets). **GI:** nausea, vomiting, diarrhea. **GU:** *acute renal failure,* hematuria. **Hematologic:** *leukopenia, neutropenia, thrombocytopenia,* thrombocytosis, anemia. **Hepatic:** bilirubinemia. **Skin:** inflammation or phlebitis at injection site, rash, urticaria, eczema, dryness, pruritus, contact dermatitis, application-site reaction; mild pain, burning, or stinging (topical or buccal form. **Other:** hypersensitivity reaction.

INTERACTIONS

Drug-drug. *Foscarnet:* May enhance nephrotoxicity. Don't use together.

Hydantoins: May decrease levels of these drugs. Monitor patient closely.

Probenecid: May increase acyclovir level. Monitor patient for possible toxicity.

Varicella vaccine: May diminish therapeutic effect of vaccine. Avoid use of acyclovir within 24 hours before vaccine administration and for 14 days after.

Zidovudine: May cause drowsiness or lethargy. Use together cautiously.

EFFECTS ON LAB TEST RESULTS

• May increase bilirubin, BUN, and creatinine levels.

• May increase Hb level.

• May decrease ANC and WBC count.

• May increase or decrease platelet count.

CONTRAINDICATIONS & CAUTIONS

• Contraindicated in patients hypersensitive to drug.

• Use cautiously in patients with neurologic problems, renal disease, hepatic disease, electrolyte abnormalities, significant hypoxia, or dehydration, and in those receiving other nephrotoxic drugs.

• Drug increases risk of thrombotic thrombocytopenic purpura and hemolytic-uremic syndrome in patients who are immunocompromised, which can be fatal.

Dialyzable drug: Yes.

⚠ *Overdose S&S:* Agitation, coma, seizures, lethargy, elevated BUN and creatinine levels, renal failure.

PREGNANCY-LACTATION-REPRODUCTION

• Use cautiously during pregnancy and only if potential benefit outweighs fetal risk.

• Drug appears in human milk. Use cautiously during breastfeeding and only when clearly indicated. Patients with active herpetic lesions near or on the breasts should avoid breastfeeding.

NURSING CONSIDERATIONS

• Start therapy as early as possible after signs or symptoms occur.

• Drug isn't a cure for herpes, but it helps improve signs and symptoms.

🌙 *Alert:* Long-term acyclovir use may result in nephrotoxicity. In patients with renal disease or dehydration and in those taking other nephrotoxic drugs, monitor renal function.

🌙 *Alert:* If signs and symptoms of extravasation occur, stop IV infusion immediately and notify prescriber. Hyaluronidase may need to be injected subcut at extravasation site as an antidote.

• Encephalopathic changes are more likely to occur in patients with neurologic disorders and in those who have had neurologic reactions to cytotoxic drugs.

- Monitor patient for hypersensitivity reactions, including SJS, TEN, anaphylaxis, and angioedema.
- *Look alike–sound alike:* Don't confuse acyclovir sodium with acetazolamide sodium vials. Don't confuse Zovirax with Zyvox.

PATIENT TEACHING
- Tell patient to take drug as prescribed, even after feeling better.
- Inform patient drug is effective in managing herpes infection but doesn't eliminate or cure it. Warn patient that drug won't prevent spread of infection to others.
- Avise patient to avoid sexual contact while visible lesions are present. Virus transmission can occur during treatment.
- Teach patient about early signs and symptoms of herpes infection (such as tingling, itching, or pain) and to notify prescriber and get a prescription for drug before the infection fully develops. Early treatment is most effective.

adalimumab
ay-da-LIM-yoo-mab

Humira

adalimumab-adaz
Hyrimoz

adalimumab-adbm
Cyltezo

adalimumab-afzb
Abrilada

adalimumab-aqvh
Yusimry

adalimumab-atto
Amjevita

adalimumab-bwwd
Hadlima

adalimumab-fkjp
Hulio

Therapeutic class: Antiarthritics
Pharmacologic class: TNF blockers

AVAILABLE FORMS
Injection: 10 mg/0.1 mL, 10 mg/0.2 mL, 20 mg/0.2 mL, 20 mg/0.4 mL, 40 mg/0.4 mL, 40 mg/0.8 mL, 80 mg/0.8 mL prefilled syringes or pens; 40 mg/0.8 mL single-use vial (institutional use only)

INDICATIONS & DOSAGES
➤ **RA; psoriatic arthritis; ankylosing spondylitis**
Adults: 40 mg subcut every other week. Patient may continue to take methotrexate, steroids, NSAIDs, salicylates, analgesics, or other DMARDs during therapy. Patients with RA who aren't also taking methotrexate may have the dose increased to 40 mg weekly, if needed.
➤ **Moderate to severe adult Crohn disease when response to conventional therapy is inadequate or when response to infliximab is lost or patient can't tolerate the drug; moderate to severe active ulcerative colitis when response to immunosuppressants (such as corticosteroids, azathioprine, or 6-mercaptopurine) is inadequate**
Adults: Initially, 160 mg subcut on day 1 given in 1 day or split over 2 consecutive days; then 80 mg 2 weeks later (day 15), followed by a maintenance dose of 40 mg every other week starting at week 4 (day 29). Patients not taking concomitant methotrexate may derive additional benefit from increasing dosage to 40 mg every week or 80 mg every other week. For ulcerative colitis, only continue in patients who have shown evidence of clinical remission by 8 weeks (day 57) of therapy.
➤ **Pediatric Crohn disease**
Children age 6 and older weighing 40 kg or more (Humira, Cyltezo, Yusimry only): Initially, 160 mg subcut on day 1 given in 1 day or split over 2 consecutive days; then 80 mg 2 weeks later (day 15), followed by a maintenance dose of 40 mg every other week starting at week 4 (day 29).
Children age 6 and older weighing from 17 to less than 40 kg (Humira, Cyltezo only): 80 mg subcut on day 1, followed by 40 mg 2 weeks later (day 15), followed by a maintenance dose of 20 mg every other week starting at week 4 (day 29).
➤ **Pediatric moderate to severe active ulcerative colitis (Humira only)**
Children age 5 and older weighing 40 kg or more: Initially, 160 mg subcut on day 1 given in 1 day or split over 2 consecutive days; then 80 mg on day 8 and 80 mg on day 15, followed by maintenance dose of 40 mg every

week or 80 mg every other week starting at week 4 (day 29).

Children age 5 and older weighing from 20 to less than 40 kg: 80 mg subcut on day 1; then 40 mg on day 8 and 40 mg on day 15, followed by maintenance dose of 20 mg every week or 40 mg every other week starting at week 4 (day 29).

➤ **To reduce signs and symptoms of moderately to severely active polyarticular juvenile idiopathic arthritis**

Children age 2 and older weighing 30 kg or more: 40 mg subcut every other week.

Children age 2 and older weighing between 15 and 30 kg: 20 mg subcut every other week.

Children age 2 and older weighing between 10 and 15 kg: 10 mg subcut every other week.

➤ **Moderate to severe chronic plaque psoriasis**

Adults: 80 mg subcut, followed by 40 mg subcut every other week starting 1 week after the initial dose. Treatment beyond 1 year has not been studied.

➤ **Noninfectious intermediate uveitis, posterior uveitis, and panuveitis (Humira only)**

Adults: 80 mg subcut, followed by 40 mg subcut every other week starting 1 week after initial dose.

Children age 2 and older weighing 30 kg or more: 40 mg subcut every other week.

Children age 2 and older weighing 15 to 30 kg: 20 mg subcut every other week.

Children age 2 and older weighing 15 kg or less: 10 mg subcut every other week.

➤ **Moderate to severe hidradenitis suppurativa (Humira only)**

Adults and adolescents age 12 and older weighing 60 kg or more: Initially, 160 mg subcut given in 1 day or split over 2 consecutive days; then 80 mg subcut on day 15, followed by 40 mg subcut weekly or 80 mg every other week (starting on day 29).

Adolescents age 12 and older weighing 30 to 60 kg: Initially, 80 mg subcut on day 1; then 40 mg subcut on day 8. Thereafter, give 40 mg subcut every other week.

ADMINISTRATION

Subcutaneous

- Inject subcut into lower abdomen or thigh at separate sites.
- Rotate injection sites.
- Don't give in an area that is bruised, tender, red, or hard.

- May leave drug (don't remove cap or cover) at room temperature for about 15 to 30 minutes before injecting.
- Don't use if particulates or discoloration is noted in autoinjector, pen, prefilled syringe, or single-use institutional-use vial.
- Refrigerate at 36° to 46° F (2° to 8° C); don't freeze. May store at room temperature (maximum, 77° F [25° C]) for up to 14 days if needed. Discard after 14 days. Protect from light.

⚠ *Alert:* Needle cap or cover of pen and prefilled syringe may contain latex. Check product packaging to confirm.

ACTION

A recombinant human IgG$_1$ monoclonal antibody that blocks human TNF-alpha. TNF-alpha participates in normal inflammatory and immune responses and in the inflammation and joint destruction of RA.

Route	Onset	Peak	Duration
Subcut	Variable	75–187 hr	Unknown

Half-life: 10 to 20 days.

ADVERSE REACTIONS

CNS: headache, syncope, hypertensive encephalopathy, confusion, paresthesia, subdural hematoma, tremor, myasthenia. **CV:** HTN, arrhythmia, atrial fibrillation, chest pain, CAD, *DVT, cardiac arrest, HF, MI,* palpitations, pericardial effusion, pericarditis. **EENT:** cataract, pharyngitis, caries. **GI:** abdominal pain, nausea, cholecystitis, cholelithiasis, esophagitis, gastroenteritis, *GI hemorrhage,* vomiting, diverticulitis. **GU:** hematuria, UTI, cystitis, pelvic pain, kidney stones, pyelonephritis, menstrual disorder. **Hematologic:** polycythemia, *agranulocytosis,* positive ANA titer, paraproteinemia. **Hepatic:** increased ALP level, *hepatic necrosis.* **Metabolic:** hypercholesterolemia, hyperlipidemia, dehydration, ketosis, increased CK level. **Musculoskeletal:** back pain, bone disorder, osteonecrosis, joint disorder, muscle cramps, synovitis, tendon disorder, septic arthritis, limb pain, bone fracture. **Respiratory:** URI, dyspnea, decreased lung function, pleural effusion, asthma, *bronchospasm,* pneumonia. **Skin:** rash, injection-site reactions (erythema, itching, pain, swelling), cellulitis, erysipelas. **Other:** accidental injury, *malignancy,* adenoma, hypersensitivity reactions, flulike

---

Reactions in bold italics are *life-threatening*. Interactions may have a *rapid onset* or a *delayed onset*.

syndrome, parathyroid disorder, infection, herpes simplex or zoster infection, *sepsis,* antibody development.

INTERACTIONS
Drug-drug. *Abatacept, anakinra, tocilizumab:* May increase risk of serious infections and neutropenia in patients with RA. Don't use together.

CYP450 substrates with narrow therapeutic index (cyclosporine, theophylline, warfarin): May affect CYP450 substrate level. Monitor levels closely when initiating or discontinuing adalimumab; adjust CYP450 substrate dosage as needed.

Live-virus vaccines: No data are available on secondary transmission of infection from live-virus vaccines. Avoid using together.

EFFECTS ON LAB TEST RESULTS
• May increase CK, ALP, and cholesterol levels.
• May decrease platelet and WBC counts.
• May cause positive ANA titer and development of antibodies.

CONTRAINDICATIONS & CAUTIONS
• Contraindicated in patients with immunosuppression or active chronic or localized infection.
🔵 *Alert:* Anaphylaxis and angioneurotic edema have been reported. If serious reaction occurs, discontinue drug immediately and treat appropriately.

Boxed Warning Patients taking TNF-alpha blockers are at increased risk for developing serious infections that can lead to hospitalization or death. Most patients were taking concomitant immunosuppressants, such as methotrexate or corticosteroids. Reported infections include *Legionella* and *Listeria* infections, active TB, and invasive fungal infections. Consider empirical antifungal therapy for patients at risk for invasive fungal infections who develop systemic illness. Carefully consider risk and benefits of therapy before starting drug in patients with chronic or recurrent infections. ∎

Boxed Warning Lymphoma and other malignancies, some fatal, have been reported in children and adolescents treated with TNF blockers, including adalimumab. ∎

Boxed Warning Hepatosplenic T-cell lymphoma, a rare type of T-cell lymphoma, has occurred in adolescents and young adults

with inflammatory bowel disease treated with TNF blockers, including adalimumab. ∎
• Use cautiously in patients with demyelinating disorders, a history of recurrent infection, those with underlying conditions that predispose them to infections, those who have lived in areas where TB and histoplasmosis are endemic, patients with HF, and older adults.
Dialyzable drug: Unknown.

PREGNANCY-LACTATION-REPRODUCTION
• Use during pregnancy only if clearly needed.
• Drug appears in human milk. Use cautiously during breastfeeding.

NURSING CONSIDERATIONS
• Give first dose under supervision of prescriber.
Boxed Warning Patient should be evaluated and treated, if necessary, for latent TB before start of adalimumab therapy. Closely monitor patient for possible development of TB even if patient has tested negative before start of therapy. ∎
Boxed Warning Serious infections and sepsis, including TB and invasive fungal infections, may occur. If patient develops new infection during treatment, monitor closely; if infection becomes serious, stop drug. ∎
🔵 *Alert:* Drug may increase the risk of malignancy. Patients with highly active RA may be at an increased risk for lymphoma.
🔵 *Alert:* If patient develops anaphylaxis, a severe infection, other serious allergic reaction, or evidence of a lupuslike syndrome, stop drug.
• Drug may cause reactivation of HBV in chronic carriers.
🔵 *Alert:* The needle covers or caps may contain latex and shouldn't be handled by those with latex sensitivity.
• Patients with arthritis may continue to take methotrexate as prescribed.
• *Look alike–sound alike:* Don't confuse Humira with Humulin or Humalog.

PATIENT TEACHING
• Tell patient to report all adverse reactions and any evidence of TB or other infection.
• Teach patient or caregiver how to safely give and store drug.
• Instruct patient not to place used needles and syringes in the household trash or recyclables but to dispose of them properly.

ⓘ *Alert:* Warn patient to seek immediate medical attention for symptoms of blood dyscrasias or infection, including fever, bruising, bleeding, and pallor.
• Inform patient of risk of malignancies.

adefovir dipivoxil
ah-DEF-oh-veer

Hepsera

Therapeutic class: Antivirals
Pharmacologic class: Nucleosides and nucleotides

AVAILABLE FORMS
Tablets: 10 mg

INDICATIONS & DOSAGES
➤ **Chronic HBV infection**
Adults and children age 12 and older: 10 mg PO once daily.
Adjust-a-dose: In adults with CrCl of 30 to 49 mL/minute, give 10 mg PO every 48 hours. In patients with CrCl of 10 to 29 mL/minute, give 10 mg PO every 72 hours. In patients receiving hemodialysis, give 10 mg PO every 7 days, after dialysis session. There are no dose recommendations for adolescents with renal impairment.

ADMINISTRATION
PO
• Give drug without regard for meals.
• Store at room temperature.

ACTION
An acyclic nucleotide analogue that inhibits HBV reverse transcription via viral DNA chain termination.

Route	Onset	Peak	Duration
PO	Unknown	0.5–4 hr	Unknown

Half-life: 7.5 hours.

ADVERSE REACTIONS
CNS: asthenia, headache. **GI:** abdominal pain, diarrhea, dyspepsia, flatulence, nausea, vomiting. **GU:** *renal failure, renal insufficiency.* **Hepatic:** *hepatic failure,* hepatomegaly with steatosis, *severe acute exacerbation of hepatitis.* **Metabolic:** *lactic acidosis.* **Skin:** pruritus, rash.

INTERACTIONS
Drug-drug. *Ibuprofen:* May increase adefovir bioavailability. Monitor patient for adverse effects.
Nephrotoxic drugs (aminoglycosides, cyclosporine, NSAIDs, tacrolimus, vancomycin): May increase risk of nephrotoxicity. Use together cautiously.
Tenofovir disoproxil fumarate–containing products (Atripla, Cimduo, Complera, Delstrigo, Stribild, Symfi, Temixys, Truvada, Viread): Use together increases risk for lactic acidosis and hepatotoxicity. Contraindicated for use together.

EFFECTS ON LAB TEST RESULTS
• May increase ALT, amylase, AST, CK, creatinine, and lactate levels.
• May decrease phosphorus level.

CONTRAINDICATIONS & CAUTIONS
Boxed Warning Offer patients HIV antibody testing; drug may promote resistance to antiretrovirals in those with chronic HBV infection who also have unrecognized or untreated HIV infection. ∎
• Contraindicated in patients hypersensitive to components of drug.
• Use cautiously in patients with renal dysfunction, in those receiving nephrotoxic drugs, and in those with known risk factors for hepatic disease.
• Use cautiously in older adults because they're more likely to have decreased renal and cardiac function.
• Safety and effectiveness in children younger than age 12 haven't been established.
Dialyzable drug: 35%.
⚠ *Overdose S&S:* GI adverse reactions.

PREGNANCY-LACTATION-REPRODUCTION
• Use cautiously during pregnancy and only if potential benefit justifies fetal risk.
• To monitor fetal outcomes of patients exposed to drug during pregnancy, prescribers should register patients in the antiretroviral pregnancy registry (1-800-258-4263).
• It isn't known if drug appears in human milk. Use cautiously during breastfeeding.

NURSING CONSIDERATIONS
Boxed Warning Due to increased risk of nephrotoxicity, monitor renal function, and adjust dosage if needed, especially in

patients with renal dysfunction or those taking nephrotoxic drugs. ∎

Boxed Warning Patients may develop lactic acidosis and severe hepatomegaly with steatosis during treatment. Women, patients who are obese, and patients taking antiretrovirals are at higher risk. Monitor hepatic function. Stop drug, if needed. ∎

Boxed Warning Stopping adefovir may cause severe worsening of hepatitis. Monitor hepatic function closely for at least several months in patients who stop anti-HBV therapy. ∎

• The ideal length of treatment hasn't been established.

PATIENT TEACHING

• Teach patient safe drug administration.
• Tell patient to immediately report weakness, muscle pain, trouble breathing, stomach pain with nausea and vomiting, dizziness, light-headedness, fast or irregular heartbeat, and feeling cold, especially in arms and legs.
• Warn patient not to stop taking this drug unless directed because it could cause hepatitis to become worse.
• Instruct patient to report pregnancy or breastfeeding.

SAFETY ALERT!

adenosine
a-DEN-oh-seen

Therapeutic class: Antiarrhythmics
Pharmacologic class: Nucleosides

AVAILABLE FORMS
Injection: 3 mg/mL

INDICATIONS & DOSAGES
➤ **To convert paroxysmal supraventricular tachycardia (PSVT) to sinus rhythm**
Adults and children weighing 50 kg or more: 6 mg IV by rapid bolus injection over 1 to 2 seconds, followed by a saline flush. If PSVT isn't eliminated in 1 to 2 minutes, give 12 mg by rapid IV push and repeat, if needed.
Children weighing less than 50 kg: Initially, 0.05 to 0.1 mg/kg IV by rapid bolus injection followed by a saline flush. If PSVT isn't eliminated in 1 to 2 minutes, give additional bolus injections, increasing the amount given in 0.05- to 0.1-mg/kg increments, followed by a saline flush. Continue, as needed, until

conversion of the PSVT or a maximum single dose of 0.3 mg/kg (up to 12 mg) is given.
Adjust-a-dose: Reduce initial adenosine dose to 3 mg IV bolus if patient is currently receiving carbamazepine or dipyridamole or has a transplanted heart, or if adenosine is given via central line.
➤ **Stress-testing diagnostic aid ◆**
Adults: 140 mcg/kg/minute infused over 6 minutes (total dose of 0.84 mg/kg).

ADMINISTRATION
IV
▼ Don't give single doses exceeding 12 mg.
▼ Crystals may form if solution is cold; gently warm solution to room temperature. Don't use solutions that aren't clear.
▼ In adults, avoid giving drug through a central line because central administration hasn't been studied.
▼ Give by rapid IV injection to ensure drug action.
▼ Give directly into a vein as proximal as possible to the trunk. When giving through an IV line, use the port closest to patient.
▼ Flush immediately and rapidly with NSS to ensure that drug quickly reaches the systemic circulation.
▼ Drug lacks preservatives. Discard unused portion. Don't refrigerate.
▼ **Incompatibilities:** Consult a drug incompatibility reference for information.

ACTION
Naturally occurring nucleoside that acts on the AV node to slow conduction and inhibit reentry pathways.

Route	Onset	Peak	Duration
IV	Immediate	Immediate	Unknown

Half-life: Less than 10 seconds.

ADVERSE REACTIONS
CNS: dizziness, light-headedness, numbness, tingling in arms, headache, nervousness.
CV: chest pressure, facial flushing, hypotension, arrhythmias, ST-segment depression, first- or second-degree AV block. **EENT:** throat, neck, or jaw discomfort. **GI:** nausea.
Respiratory: dyspnea.

INTERACTIONS
Drug-drug. *Carbamazepine:* May cause high-level heart block. Use together cautiously and consider using a lower initial adenosine dose.

✤Canada   ◇OTC   ◆Off-label use   ✔Photoguide   ⊜Do not crush   *Liquid contains alcohol   ▨Genetic

Digoxin, verapamil: May cause ventricular fibrillation. Monitor ECG closely.

Dipyridamole: May increase adenosine's effects. Adenosine dose may need to be reduced. Use together cautiously.

Methylxanthines (caffeine, theophylline): May decrease adenosine's effects. Adenosine dose may need to be increased, or patients may not respond to adenosine therapy.

EFFECTS ON LAB TEST RESULTS
None reported.

CONTRAINDICATIONS & CAUTIONS
• Contraindicated in patients hypersensitive to drug.
• Contraindicated in those with second- or third-degree heart block or sinus node disease (sick sinus syndrome and symptomatic bradycardia), except those with a pacemaker.
• Use cautiously in patients with obstructive lung disease not associated with bronchoconstriction (emphysema or bronchitis); avoid use in those with bronchoconstriction or bronchospasm (asthma).
• Drug may increase risk of seizures.
• Avoid use in patients with signs and symptoms of acute MI (unstable angina, CV instability). Drug may increase risk of serious CV reaction (fatal or nonfatal cardiac arrest, supraventricular tachycardia, MI). Make sure appropriate emergency equipment is readily available.
• Use cautiously in patients with autonomic dysfunction, stenotic valvular heart disease, pericarditis or pericardial effusions, stenotic carotid artery disease with cerebrovascular insufficiency, or uncorrected hypovolemia. Drug may increase risk of hypotensive complications.
Dialyzable drug: Unknown.

PREGNANCY-LACTATION-REPRODUCTION
• No studies have been performed during pregnancy. Use during pregnancy only if clearly indicated.
• There are no well-controlled studies during breastfeeding. Patient should discontinue breastfeeding or discontinue drug, taking into account importance of drug to the patient.

NURSING CONSIDERATIONS
🔆 *Alert:* By decreasing conduction through the AV node, drug may produce first-, second-, or third-degree heart block. Patients who develop high-level heart block after a single dose shouldn't receive additional doses.
🔆 *Alert:* New arrhythmias, including heart block and transient asystole, may develop; monitor cardiac rhythm and treat as indicated.
• Monitor BP closely. Discontinue drug in patients who develop persistent or symptomatic hypotension.
• Monitor patient for seizures during therapy.
🔆 *Alert:* Don't confuse adenosine with adenosine phosphate.

PATIENT TEACHING
• Instruct patient to report adverse reactions promptly.
• Teach patient to avoid products containing methylxanthines, including caffeinated coffee, tea, or other caffeinated beverages, caffeine-containing drug products, aminophylline, and theophylline before an imaging study.
• Tell patient to report discomfort at IV site.
• Inform patient that flushing or chest pain lasting 1 to 2 minutes may occur.

SAFETY ALERT!

ado-trastuzumab emtansine ⌧
ADD-oh tras-TOOZ-oo-mab em-TAN-seen

Kadcyla

Therapeutic class: Antineoplastics
Pharmacologic class: Antibody drug conjugates

AVAILABLE FORMS
Injection (lyophilized powder for solution): 100 mg, 160 mg in single-use vials

INDICATIONS & DOSAGES
Adjust-a-dose (for all indications): Refer to manufacturer's instructions for toxicity-related dosage adjustments.

➤ **HER2-positive, metastatic breast cancer in patients who previously received trastuzumab and a taxane, separately or in combination. Patients should have either received previous treatment for metastatic disease or developed recurrence during or within 6 months of completing adjuvant treatment**

Reactions in bold italics are *life-threatening*. Interactions may have a *rapid onset* or a **delayed onset**.

Adults: 3.6 mg/kg IV every 21 days until disease progression or unacceptable toxicity occurs. Maximum dose is 3.6 mg/kg.

➤ **Adjuvant treatment of HER2-positive early breast cancer with residual invasive disease after neoadjuvant taxane and trastuzumab-based treatment**
Adults: 3.6 mg/kg IV every 21 days for 14 cycles unless disease recurrence or unacceptable toxicity occurs.

ADMINISTRATION

IV

▼ Don't confuse or substitute this drug with trastuzumab (Herceptin). These drugs aren't interchangeable.

☉ *Alert:* The manufacturer recommends that the trade name be used and clearly recorded (with the batch number) in patient record to avoid confusion.

▼ Drug is considered hazardous; use safe handling and disposal precautions according to facility policy.

▼ To reconstitute, slowly inject 5 mL sterile water for injection into 100-mg vial or 8 mL sterile water for injection into 160-mg vial to yield concentration of 20 mg/mL.

▼ Swirl gently until dissolved. Don't shake. Solution should be colorless to pale brown.

▼ Add reconstituted dose to 250 mL of NSS in infusion bag and administer immediately through IV line containing 0.2- or 0.22-micron in-line nonprotein adsorptive polyethersulfone filter.

▼ Administer initial infusion over 90 minutes. Don't administer as IV push or bolus. Monitor patient for infusion-related reactions during administration and for 90 minutes after completion. Slow or interrupt infusion for infusion-related events. Discontinue drug if life-threatening infusion-related reactions occur.

▼ May administer subsequent infusions over 30 minutes if initial infusion was uneventful. Monitor patient during infusion and for 30 minutes after completion.

▼ Observe for subcut infiltration during infusion.

▼ Give at dosage and rate patient tolerated at most recent infusion.

▼ If dose is delayed or missed, give as soon as possible; don't wait for next planned cycle. Adjust schedule to maintain a 3-week interval between doses.

▼ Reconstituted vials can be stored in refrigerator for 24 hours at 36° to 46° F (2° to 8° C). Don't freeze.

▼ **Incompatibilities:** Dextrose solution, other drugs.

ACTION

Drug contains both trastuzumab and DM1 (a microtubule inhibitor), linked by a covalent bond, and targets the HER2 receptor by combined mechanisms of trastuzumab and DM1. The recombinant monoclonal antibody, trastuzumab, binds to the HER2 receptor and intracellular lysosomal degradation releases the cytotoxic component, DM1, resulting in microtubule disruption and cell death.

Route	Onset	Peak	Duration
IV	Unknown	End of infusion	Unknown

Half-life: 4 days.

ADVERSE REACTIONS

CNS: fatigue, headache, fever, asthenia, dizziness, peripheral neuropathy, taste perversion, insomnia. **CV: *left ventricular dysfunction, hemorrhage,*** edema, HTN. **EENT:** dry eye syndrome, blurred vision, conjunctivitis, increased lacrimation, epistaxis, dry mouth. **GI:** nausea, constipation, stomatitis, abdominal pain, vomiting, diarrhea, dyspepsia. **GU:** UTI. **Hematologic: *thrombocytopenia, neutropenia,*** anemia, hemorrhage. **Hepatic:** elevated transaminase levels, increased ALP level, bilirubinemia. **Metabolic: *hypokalemia.*** **Musculoskeletal:** pain, arthralgia, myalgia, weakness. **Respiratory:** pneumonitis, dyspnea, cough. **Skin:** pruritus, rash. **Other:** chills, hypersensitivity reactions, infusion reaction.

INTERACTIONS

Drug-drug. *Anthracyclines:* May enhance cardiotoxic effects of anthracyclines. When possible, avoid anthracycline-based therapy for up to 7 months after stopping ado-trastuzumab emtansine. Monitor patients who must receive this combination closely for cardiac dysfunction.
Anticoagulants (clopidogrel, heparin, warfarin), antiplatelet agents: May increase risk of hemorrhagic events. Monitor patient closely.
Strong CYP3A4 inhibitors (atazanavir, clarithromycin, ketoconazole, nefazodone, nelfinavir, ritonavir, telithromycin): May increase

ado-trastuzumab level and potential toxicity. Avoid use together. If use together is necessary, stop CYP3A4 inhibitor and delay treatment until inhibitor clears from patient's circulation, or monitor patient carefully for adverse effects.

EFFECTS ON LAB TEST RESULTS
• May increase bilirubin, AST, and ALT levels.
• May decrease potassium level.
• May decrease Hb level and platelet and neutrophil counts.

CONTRAINDICATIONS & CAUTIONS
Boxed Warning Severe liver injury (including fatal liver damage, liver failure, and death) has been reported. Monitor serum transaminase and bilirubin levels before starting drug and before each dose. Dosage modifications or discontinuation of therapy may be necessary. ∎

Boxed Warning Drug may significantly reduce LVEF. Assess LVEF before starting drug and every 3 months during treatment. Withhold or discontinue drug as clinically indicated. ∎

• Contraindicated in patients hypersensitive to drug or its components.
• Use cautiously in patients with liver failure, risk of hepatotoxicity, symptomatic HF, serious cardiac arrhythmia, history of MI, or unstable angina.
• Avoid use in patients with history of trastuzumab hypersensitivity or infusion-related events.
• Patients with shortness of breath at rest due to advanced malignancy and comorbidities may be at increased risk for pulmonary toxicity.
• Use cautiously in patients taking anticoagulants and antiplatelet agents and in those with preexisting thrombocytopenia.
▧ Patients of Asian ancestry may be at higher risk for thrombocytopenia.
Dialyzable drug: Unknown.
⚠ *Overdose S&S:* Thrombocytopenia, death.

PREGNANCY-LACTATION-REPRODUCTION
Boxed Warning Exposure to drug can result in embryo-fetal death or birth defects. ∎
• Verify pregnancy status before start of therapy.
Boxed Warning Patients of childbearing potential should use effective contraception during treatment and for 7 months after last dose.

Male patients with partners of childbearing potential should use effective contraception during treatment and for 4 months after last dose. ∎
• May impair fertility in females and males of reproductive potential. It isn't known if the effects are reversible.
🅘 *Alert:* Advise patient to immediately report suspected or confirmed pregnancy during therapy or within 7 months after last dose. Report drug exposure to manufacturer (1-888-835-2555).
• It isn't known if drug appears in human milk. Advise patients not to breastfeed during treatment and for 7 months after final dose.

NURSING CONSIDERATIONS
▧ Confirm HER2 testing with FDA-approved test by established lab. Only patients with HER2 protein overexpression should receive drug because those are the only patients studied for whom benefit has been shown.
• Infusion-related reactions, including hypersensitivity reactions, may occur. Closely monitor patient during and for 90 minutes after infusion for fever, chills, flushing, dyspnea, hypotension, wheezing, bronchospasm, or tachycardia. Slow or interrupt infusion as necessary. In most patients, these reactions resolve over the course of several hours to a day after the infusion is terminated.
• Monitor patient for extravasation, which may cause redness, tenderness, skin irritation, pain, or swelling at infusion site.
🅘 *Alert:* Permanently discontinue drug in patients diagnosed with ILD or pneumonitis.
• Monitor platelet count before treatment and before each dose.
• Discontinue drug in patients diagnosed with nodular regenerative hyperplasia of the liver.
• *Look alike–sound alike:* Don't confuse ado-trastuzumab emtansine with fam-trastuzumab deruxtecan, pertuzumab, trastuzumab, or trastuzumab–hyaluronidase.

PATIENT TEACHING
• Inform patient that drug may cause severe liver damage that may be life-threatening.
• Tell patient to report unexplained nausea, vomiting, abdominal pain, jaundice, dark urine, generalized itchiness, or anorexia.
• Caution patient that drug may cause heart problems, with or without symptoms. Instruct patient to report new-onset or worsening of

---

Reactions in bold italics are *life-threatening*. Interactions may have a *rapid onset* or a ***delayed onset***.

shortness of breath, cough, swelling of the ankles or legs, palpitations, weight gain of more than 5 lb in 24 hours, fatigue, dizziness, or loss of consciousness.
- Advise patient that drug may cause lung problems. Tell patient to report trouble breathing, cough, or tiredness.
- Alert patient that drug may cause low platelet count. Instruct patient to contact prescriber if excessive bleeding occurs.
- Warn patient that drug may cause nerve damage. Instruct patient to report numbness or tingling, burning or sharp pain, sensitivity to touch, lack of coordination, or muscle weakness or loss of muscle function.

Boxed Warning Inform patient that drug may cause birth defects and fetal death. Advise patient of childbearing potential to use effective contraception during treatment and for 7 months after last dose. Advise male patient with partner of childbearing potential to use effective contraception during treatment and for 4 months after last dose. ∎

🕒 *Alert:* Advise patient to immediately report suspected or confirmed pregnancy during therapy.
- Advise patient not to breastfeed during treatment and for 7 months after final dose.

albuterol sulfate
al-BYOO-ter-ole

Airomir♣, ProAir Digihaler, ProAir HFA, ProAir RespiClick, Proventil HFA, Ventolin HFA

Therapeutic class: Bronchodilators
Pharmacologic class: Adrenergics

AVAILABLE FORMS
Inhalation aerosol: 100 mcg/actuation ♣, 108 mcg/actuation
Inhalation powder: 108 mcg/actuation
Solution for inhalation: 0.021% (0.63 mg/3 mL), 0.042% (1.25 mg/3 mL), 0.083% (2.5 mg/3 mL), 0.5 mg/mL ♣, 1 mg/mL♣, 2 mg/mL ♣, 0.5% (5 mg/mL)
Syrup: 2 mg/5 mL
Tablets: 2 mg, 4 mg

INDICATIONS & DOSAGES
➤ **To prevent or treat bronchospasm in patients with reversible obstructive airway disease**

Adjust-a-dose (for oral forms): For older adults and patients sensitive to sympathomimetic amines, 2 mg PO t.i.d. or q.i.d. as oral tablets or syrup. Maximum, 32 mg daily.
Tablets
Adults and children older than age 12: 2 to 4 mg PO t.i.d. or q.i.d. Maximum, 32 mg daily.
Children ages 6 to 12: 2 mg PO t.i.d. or q.i.d. Maximum, 24 mg daily.
Syrup
Adults and children older than age 14: 2 to 4 mg PO t.i.d. or q.i.d. Maximum, 32 mg daily.
Children ages 6 to 14: 2 mg PO t.i.d. or q.i.d. Maximum, 24 mg daily.
Children ages 2 to 5: Initially, 0.1 mg/kg PO t.i.d. Starting dose shouldn't exceed 2 mg t.i.d. Maximum, 12 mg daily.
Solution for inhalation
Adults and children age 12 and older: 2.5 mg by nebulizer, given over 5 to 15 minutes, t.i.d. or q.i.d. To prepare solution, use 0.5 mL of 0.5% solution diluted with 2.5 mL of NSS. Or, use 3 mL of 0.083% solution.
Children ages 2 to 12 weighing more than 15 kg: 2.5 mg by nebulizer given over 5 to 15 minutes t.i.d. or q.i.d., with subsequent doses adjusted to response. Don't exceed 2.5 mg t.i.d. or q.i.d.
Children ages 2 to 12 weighing 15 kg or less: 0.63 mg or 1.25 mg by nebulizer given over 5 to 15 minutes t.i.d. or q.i.d., with subsequent doses adjusted to response. Don't exceed 2.5 mg t.i.d. or q.i.d.
Inhalation aerosol
Adults and children age 4 and older: 1 to 2 inhalations every 4 to 6 hours as needed. Regular use for maintenance therapy to control asthma symptoms isn't recommended.
Inhalational powder
Adults and children age 4 and older: 2 inhalations every 4 to 6 hours. In some patients, 1 inhalation every 4 hours may be sufficient.
➤ **To prevent exercise-induced bronchospasm**
Adults and children age 4 and older: 2 inhalations 15 to 30 minutes before exercise.
➤ **Adjuvant therapy for acute treatment of moderate to severe hyperkalemia ♦**
Adults: 10 to 20 mg via nebulization over 10 minutes, given in combination with other recommended therapy.

♣Canada ◇OTC ♦Off-label use ✐Photoguide ⊚Do not crush *Liquid contains alcohol ✄Genetic

ADMINISTRATION
PO
- May give without regard for food.
- Store at room temperature.

Inhalational
- If more than 1 inhalation is ordered, wait 1 minute, then shake the inhaler again if necessary, and repeat procedure.
- Inhalation powder inhaler device doesn't require priming. Use spacer device to improve drug delivery, if appropriate. Don't use ProAir RespiClick with a spacer or volume holding chamber.
- Shake the aerosol inhaler well before use and prime inhaler according to manufacturer's instructions before first use, when it has been dropped, or when it hasn't been used for more than 2 weeks.
- Keep cap on inhaler closed during storage.
- For nebulization, empty entire contents of one sterile unit-dose vial into nebulizer reservoir. Connect mouthpiece or face mask; then connect nebulizer to compressor and turn on compressor. Flow rate is regulated for the particular nebulizer to deliver albuterol inhalation solution over 5 to 15 minutes.
- Patient should breathe calmly, deeply, and evenly through the mouth until mist no longer appears in nebulizer chamber.
- Clean nebulizer according to manufacturer's instructions.

ACTION
Relaxes bronchial, uterine, and vascular smooth muscle by stimulating beta$_2$ receptors.

Route	Onset	Peak	Duration
PO	15–30 min	2–3 hr	4–8 hr
Inhalation (aerosol)	5–15 min	30–120 min	3–4 hr
Inhalation (powder)	Rapid	30 min	3–4 hr

Half-life: Oral, 5 to 6 hours; inhalation aerosol, 6 hours; inhalation powder, 5 hours.

ADVERSE REACTIONS
CNS: tremor, excitement, nervousness, anxiety, ataxia, depression, drowsiness, emotional lability, fatigue, headache, rigors, shakiness, headache, hyperactivity, insomnia, dizziness, weakness, CNS stimulation, malaise, altered taste, fever. **CV:** tachycardia, palpitations, HTN, chest pain, lymphadenopathy, edema, extrasystoles. **EENT:** conjunctivitis, otitis media, tinnitus, ear disorder, dry and irritated nose and throat (with inhaled form), nasal congestion, epistaxis, hoarseness, pharyngitis, rhinitis, glossitis. **GI:** nausea, vomiting, diarrhea, eructation, flatulence, gastroenteritis, heartburn, anorexia, increased appetite. **GU:** UTI. **Hematologic:** anemia, decreased WBC count, lymphadenopathy. **Hepatic:** increased transaminase levels. **Metabolic:** hyperglycemia, *hypokalemia.* **Musculoskeletal:** pain, hyperkinesia, muscle cramps, back pain. **Respiratory:** *bronchospasm,* exacerbation of asthma, URI, cough, wheezing, dyspnea, bronchitis, increased sputum, viral respiratory tract infection. **Skin:** diaphoresis, pallor, urticaria, rash. **Other:** hypersensitivity reactions, flulike syndrome, cold symptoms, infection.

INTERACTIONS
Drug-drug. *Antiarrhythmics (amiodarone, bretylium, disopyramide, dofetilide, procainamide, quinidine, sotalol), arsenic trioxide, chlorpromazine, dolasetron, droperidol, mefloquine, mesoridazine, moxifloxacin, pentamidine, pimozide, tacrolimus, thioridazine, ziprasidone:* May prolong QT interval and increase risk of life-threatening arrhythmias, including torsades de pointes. Monitor QT interval and patient.
Beta blockers (labetalol, propranolol): May block pulmonary effect and increase risk of severe bronchospasm in patients with asthma. Avoid use together. If unavoidable, cautiously use cardioselective beta blockers (atenolol, metoprolol).
CNS stimulants: May increase CNS stimulation. Avoid using together.
Digoxin: May decrease digoxin level. Monitor digoxin level closely.
Diuretics (furosemide, thiazides): May cause ECG changes and hypokalemia. Monitor potassium level. Use caution when administered with non-potassium-sparing diuretics.
Epinephrine, short-acting sympathomimetic bronchodilators (levalbuterol, pirbuterol): May increase risk of toxicity. Don't use together.
Linezolid, MAO inhibitors, TCAs: May increase adverse CV effects. Consider alternative therapy. Monitor patient closely if used together.
Propranolol, other beta blockers: May cause mutual antagonism. Monitor patient carefully.

EFFECTS ON LAB TEST RESULTS
- May increase glucose level.
- May decrease potassium level.

• May decrease Hb level, hematocrit, and WBC count.

CONTRAINDICATIONS & CAUTIONS
• Contraindicated in patients hypersensitive to drug or its ingredients and in those with severe hypersensitivity to milk proteins (dry powder inhalers).
• Use cautiously in patients with CV disorders (including coronary insufficiency and HTN), hyperthyroidism, or diabetes and in those who are unusually responsive to adrenergics.
Dialyzable drug: Unknown.
⚠ *Overdose S&S:* Exaggeration of adverse reactions, seizures, angina, hypotension, HTN, tachycardia, arrhythmias, nervousness, headache, tremor, dry mouth, palpitations, nausea, dizziness, fatigue, malaise, sleeplessness, hypokalemia, cardiac arrest.

PREGNANCY-LACTATION-REPRODUCTION
• There are no adequate and well-controlled studies during pregnancy. Use during pregnancy only if potential benefit justifies fetal risk.
• Data collection to monitor outcomes during pregnancy in patients with asthma and in infants and medications used to treat asthma in pregnancy is available at MotherToBaby Pregnancy Studies at 866-626-6847 or https://mothertobaby.org.
• It isn't known if drug appears in human milk. Use cautiously during breastfeeding.

NURSING CONSIDERATIONS
• Drug may decrease sensitivity of spirometry used for diagnosis of asthma.
• Syrup contains no alcohol or sugar and may be taken by children as young as age 2.
• Monitor patient for hypersensitivity reactions, including SJS.
• Monitor patient for effectiveness. Using drug alone may not be adequate to control asthma in some patients. Long-term control medications may be needed.
• In patients with COVID-19 who require a bronchodilator for asthma or COPD symptoms, use of pressurized metered-dose inhalers as opposed to nebulized delivery is preferred. Nebulized delivery may increase transmission of particles (SARS-CoV2) into the environment and potentially decrease the life of expiratory circuit filter.

🕓 *Alert:* Drug may cause paradoxical bronchospasm. Monitor patient closely; discontinue drug immediately and use alternative therapy if paradoxical bronchospasm occurs. Bronchospasm with inhaled formulations frequently occurs with first use of new canister or vial.
🕓 *Alert:* Patient may use tablets and aerosol together. Monitor these patients closely for signs and symptoms of toxicity.
• *Look alike–sound alike:* Don't confuse albuterol with atenolol or Albutein.

PATIENT TEACHING
• Warn patient about risk of paradoxical bronchospasm and advise patient to stop drug immediately if it occurs.
• Teach patient to perform oral inhalation correctly.
• If prescriber orders more than 1 inhalation, tell patient to wait 1 minute and shake the inhaler again before repeating procedure.
• Tell patient that use of a spacer device with appropriate inhaler may improve drug delivery to lungs.
• If patient is also using a corticosteroid inhaler, instruct patient to use the bronchodilator first and then to wait about 5 minutes before using the corticosteroid.
• Tell patient to remove canister and wash aerosol inhaler with warm, soapy water at least once a week.
• Warn patient not to wash or place any part of powder inhaler in water. If mouthpiece needs cleaning, advise patient to gently wipe it with dry cloth or tissue.
• Advise patient not to use more than prescribed and not to increase dose or frequency without consulting physician. Fatalities have been reported from excessive use.
• Instruct patient to report worsening symptoms.

SAFETY ALERT!

alectinib hydrochloride ※
al-EK-ti-nib

Alecensa

Therapeutic class: Antineoplastics
Pharmacologic class: Tyrosine kinase inhibitors

AVAILABLE FORMS
Capsules 🔵: 150 mg

INDICATIONS & DOSAGES

➤ **Anaplastic lymphoma kinase (ALK)-positive, metastatic NSCLC** ⚕
Adults: 600 mg PO b.i.d. until disease progression or unacceptable toxicity.
Adjust-a-dose: Recommended dosage in patients with severe hepatic impairment (Child-Pugh class C) is 450 mg PO b.i.d. Refer to manufacturer's instructions for toxicity-related dosage adjustments.

ADMINISTRATION

PO

• Hazardous drug; use safe handling and disposal precautions according to facility policy.
• Give with food.
• Don't open or dissolve contents of capsule; patient should swallow capsule whole.
• If a dose is missed or vomiting occurs after taking a dose, give next dose at the scheduled time.
• Don't store above 86° F (30° C). Store in the original container to protect from light and moisture.

ACTION

A tyrosine kinase inhibitor that targets *ALK* and *RET* gene abnormalities that alter signaling and expression and result in increased cellular proliferation and survival in tumors that express these fusion proteins. Inhibiting ALK signaling decreases tumor cell viability.

Route	Onset	Peak	Duration
PO	Unknown	4 hr	Unknown

Half-life: 33 hours (parent drug).

ADVERSE REACTIONS

CNS: fatigue, headache, dysgeusia. **CV:** *bradycardia,* edema. **EENT:** vision disorder. **GI:** vomiting, constipation, nausea, diarrhea. **GU:** renal impairment. **Hematologic:** anemia, hemolytic anemia, *lymphopenia, neutropenia.* **Hepatic:** hyperbilirubinemia, elevated ALP, AST, and ALT levels. **Metabolic:** increased weight, hypoalbuminemia, *hypocalcemia,* hyperglycemia, *hypokalemia, hyperkalemia,* hyponatremia, hypophosphatemia, increased CK and GGT levels. **Musculoskeletal:** myalgia, back pain. **Respiratory:** dyspnea, cough. **Skin:** rash, photosensitivity.

INTERACTIONS

Drug-drug. *Bradycardia-causing drugs:* May increase risk of bradycardia. Monitor patient closely.
Drug-lifestyle. *Sun exposure:* May increase risk of photosensitivity. Discourage sun exposure.

EFFECTS ON LAB TEST RESULTS

• May increase AST, ALT, ALP, CK, bilirubin, glucose, GGT, and creatinine levels.
• May decrease calcium, phosphorus, albumin, and sodium levels.
• May increase or decrease potassium level.
• May decrease WBC and RBC counts.

CONTRAINDICATIONS & CAUTIONS

⚕ Drug is only approved for use in patients with metastatic NSCLC who test positive for the abnormal *ALK* gene.
• Drug may increase risk of hepatotoxicity, pulmonary toxicity (ILD or pneumonitis), renal impairment, intestinal perforation, endocarditis, and hemorrhage.
• Safety and effectiveness in children haven't been determined.
Dialyzable drug: Unlikely.

PREGNANCY-LACTATION-REPRODUCTION

• Drug may cause fetal harm. Patients of childbearing potential should use effective contraception during treatment and for 1 week after therapy ends.
• Males with partners of childbearing potential should use effective contraception during treatment and for 3 months after final dose.
• It's unknown if drug appears in human milk. Due to the potential for serious adverse reactions in infants, breastfeeding isn't recommended during treatment and for 1 week after final dose.

NURSING CONSIDERATIONS

• Monitor LFTs (ALT, AST, and total bilirubin levels) every 2 weeks during first 3 months of treatment, then once a month and as clinically indicated during treatment. Monitor patients for signs and symptoms of hepatotoxicity and intestinal perforation.
• Monitor patients for signs and symptoms of ILD or pneumonitis (worsening of respiratory symptoms, cough, dyspnea, fever). Withhold drug if patients are diagnosed with ILD or pneumonitis and permanently discontinue drug if it's the causative factor.

Reactions in bold italics are *life-threatening*. Interactions may have a *rapid onset* or a *delayed onset*.

- Monitor patients for myalgia or musculoskeletal pain and assess CK level every 2 weeks for first month of treatment and as clinically indicated. Drug may need to be withheld or dosage reduced.
- Monitor patients for chest pain and monitor HR and BP regularly. Dosage modification isn't required in cases of asymptomatic bradycardia. Adjust dosage for non-life-threatening, symptomatic bradycardia and assess for concomitant bradycardia-contributing drugs. Treat life-threatening bradycardia appropriately.
- Monitor renal function.
- Monitor patients for abnormal bleeding.
- Monitor patients for signs and symptoms of photosensitivity.

PATIENT TEACHING
- Advise patient to report all drugs and supplements being taken before beginning therapy.
- Teach patient to report signs and symptoms of liver injury or intestinal perforation (tiredness, anorexia, jaundice, dark urine, pruritus, nausea, vomiting, right-sided stomach pain, sharp abdominal pain, fever, easy bleeding or bruising); explain the need for blood tests throughout treatment.
- Inform patient of the risks of severe ILD or pneumonitis. Advise patient to contact prescriber immediately for new or worsening respiratory symptoms.
- Educate patient about the possibility of muscle pain, tenderness, and weakness and to immediately report new, worsening, or persistent signs and symptoms of muscle pain or weakness.
- Counsel patient that drug may cause dizziness, light-headedness, syncope and, rarely, chest pain and to immediately report these symptoms to prescriber.
- Tell patient to report abnormal bleeding.
- Advise patient to avoid prolonged sun exposure while taking drug and for at least 7 days after last dose. Advise patient to use broad-spectrum sunscreen and lip balm (SPF 50 or higher) to protect from potential sunburn.
- Instruct patient in safe drug administration.
- Caution patient of childbearing potential of possible fetal harm if drug is taken during pregnancy. Advise patient to use effective contraception during treatment and for 1 week after final dose and to inform prescriber immediately of possible pregnancy.

- Explain to male patient with partners of childbearing potential the need to use effective contraception during and for 3 months after treatment ends.
- Warn patient not to breastfeed during treatment and for 1 week after treatment ends.

alendronate sodium
ah-LEN-dro-nate

Binosto, Fosamax✿

Therapeutic class: Antiosteoporotics
Pharmacologic class: Bisphosphonates

AVAILABLE FORMS
Oral solution: 70 mg/75 mL
Tablets: 5 mg, 10 mg, 35 mg, 70 mg
Tablets (effervescent): 70 mg

INDICATIONS & DOSAGES
➤ **Osteoporosis in men and women who are postmenopausal**
Adults: 10 mg PO daily or 70-mg tablet or solution PO once weekly.
➤ **Paget disease of bone (osteitis deformans) (excluding Binosto and oral solution)**
Adults: 40 mg PO daily for 6 months. May consider retreatment in 6 months.
➤ **To prevent osteoporosis in women who are postmenopausal (excluding Binosto and oral solution)**
Adults: 5 mg PO daily or 35-mg tablet PO once weekly.
➤ **Glucocorticoid-induced osteoporosis in patients receiving glucocorticoids in a daily dose equivalent to 7.5 mg or more of prednisone and who have low bone mineral density (excluding Binosto and oral solution)**
Adults: 5 mg PO daily. For women who are postmenopausal not receiving estrogen, recommended dose is 10 mg PO daily.
➤ **Prevention of androgen deprivation therapy–associated osteoporosis ◆**
Adults: 70 mg once weekly.

ADMINISTRATION
PO
- Give drug with 180 to 240 mL of plain water at least 30 minutes before patient's first food or drink of the day to facilitate delivery to the stomach and reduce esophageal irritation risk.

• Dissolve effervescent tablet in 120 mL of plain room-temperature water. Once effervescence stops, wait 5 minutes or more and stir solution for about 10 seconds before giving.
• Give at least 60 mL of water after oral solution.
• Don't allow patient to lie down for 30 minutes after taking drug and until after first food of the day.
• Don't give at bedtime or before patient arises for the day. Failure to follow these instructions may increase the risk of esophageal adverse effects.

ACTION
Suppresses osteoclast activity on newly formed resorption surfaces, which reduces bone turnover. Bone formation exceeds resorption at remodeling sites, leading to progressive gains in bone mass.

Route	Onset	Peak	Duration
PO	Unknown	Unknown	Unknown

Half-life: More than 10 years.

ADVERSE REACTIONS
CNS: headache, taste perversion. **GI:** abdominal pain, nausea, dyspepsia, constipation, diarrhea, flatulence, acid regurgitation, esophageal ulcer, vomiting, dysphagia, abdominal distention, gastritis, gastric ulcer, melena. **Musculoskeletal:** pain, muscle cramp.

INTERACTIONS
Drug-drug. *Antacids, calcium supplements, multivitamins and minerals, many oral drugs:* May interfere with absorption of alendronate. Instruct patient to wait at least 30 minutes after taking alendronate before taking other drug orally.
Aspirin, NSAIDs: May increase risk of upper GI adverse reactions. Monitor patient closely.
Levothyroxine: May decrease bioavailability of alendronate. Monitor patient.
PPIs: May diminish therapeutic effects of alendronate. Monitor therapy.
Drug-food. *Any food:* May decrease absorption of drug. Advise patient to take with full glass of plain water at least 30 minutes before food, beverages, or ingestion of other drugs.

EFFECTS ON LAB TEST RESULTS
• May decrease calcium and phosphate levels.

CONTRAINDICATIONS & CAUTIONS
• Contraindicated in patients hypersensitive to drug and in those with hypocalcemia or abnormalities of the esophagus that delay esophageal emptying.
• Contraindicated in patients unable to stand or sit upright for at least 30 minutes.
• Oral solution contraindicated in patients at increased risk for aspiration.
• Drug isn't recommended for patients with CrCl of less than 35 mL/minute.
◑ *Alert:* There may be an increased risk of atypical fractures of the thigh in patients treated with bisphosphonates.
• Use cautiously in patients with active upper GI problems (dysphagia, symptomatic esophageal diseases, gastritis, duodenitis, ulcers) or mild to moderate renal insufficiency.
• Use cautiously in patients with known risk factors for osteonecrosis of the jaw (diagnosis of cancer; concomitant treatment with chemotherapy, radiotherapy, corticosteroids), poor oral hygiene, and comorbid disorders, such as preexisting dental disease, anemia, coagulopathy, or infection.
• Use effervescent tablet cautiously in patients who must restrict sodium intake, including some patients with a history of HF, HTN, or other CV diseases. Each effervescent tablet contains 603 mg of sodium, equivalent to approximately 1,532 mg of salt (NaCl).
Dialyzable drug: No.
⚠ *Overdose S&S:* Hypocalcemia, hypophosphatemia, upset stomach, heartburn, esophagitis, gastritis, ulcer.

PREGNANCY-LACTATION-REPRODUCTION
• No data exist on fetal risk in humans, but there is a theoretical risk of fetal harm. Discontinue use during pregnancy.
• It isn't known if drug appears in human milk. Use cautiously during breastfeeding.

NURSING CONSIDERATIONS
• Correct hypocalcemia and other disturbances of mineral metabolism (such as vitamin D deficiency) before therapy begins.
• Patients at risk for vitamin D deficiency, such as those who are chronically ill, who are nursing home bound, who have a GI malabsorption syndrome, or who are older than age 70, may require vitamin D supplementation.

Reactions in bold italics are *life-threatening*. Interactions may have a *rapid onset* or a **delayed onset**.

• In Paget disease, drug is indicated for patients with ALP level at least 2 × ULN, for those who are symptomatic, and for those at risk for future complications from the disease.

• Monitor patient's calcium and phosphate levels throughout therapy.

• Severe musculoskeletal pain has been associated with bisphosphonate use and may occur within days, months, or years of start of therapy. When drug is stopped, symptoms may resolve partially or completely.

• Patients who develop osteonecrosis of the jaw should receive care by an oral surgeon.

• Optimal length of treatment hasn't been determined. Reevaluate need for continued therapy periodically. Patients at low risk for fracture should be considered for discontinuation after 3 to 5 years of treatment.

• *Look alike–sound alike:* Don't confuse Fosamax with Flomax.

PATIENT TEACHING

• Instruct patient in safe drug administration. Stress importance of taking drug as directed to avoid adverse effects.

• Warn patient not to lie down for at least 30 minutes after taking drug to facilitate delivery to stomach and to reduce risk of esophageal irritation.

• Tell patient who misses a once-weekly dose to take one dose on the morning after remembering and then return to weekly dosing on the chosen day as originally scheduled.

• Advise patient to report adverse reactions immediately, especially chest pain or difficulty swallowing.

• Advise patient to take supplemental calcium and vitamin D if dietary intake is inadequate.

• Advise patient to discuss usage and timing of OTC medications with prescriber.

• Tell patient about benefits of weight-bearing exercises in increasing bone mass. If applicable, explain importance of reducing or eliminating cigarette smoking and alcohol use.

• Warn patient of fetal risk and that drug will be discontinued during pregnancy.

aliskiren hemifumarate
a-lis-KYE-ren

Rasilez✤, Tekturna

Therapeutic class: Antihypertensives
Pharmacologic class: Renin inhibitors

AVAILABLE FORMS
Tablets: 150 mg, 300 mg

INDICATIONS & DOSAGES
➤ **HTN, alone or with other antihypertensives**
Adults and children age 6 and older weighing more than 50 kg: 150 mg PO daily; may increase to 300 mg PO daily.

ADMINISTRATION
PO
• Don't give drug with high-fat meal; may decrease drug's effectiveness.
• Give consistently at same time each day with or without meals. However, consistent administration with regard to meals is recommended.

ACTION
Decreases renin activity and inhibits conversion of angiotensin to angiotensin I, decreasing vasoconstriction and lowering BP.

Route	Onset	Peak	Duration
PO	Unknown	1–3 hr	Unknown

Half-life: 24 hours.

ADVERSE REACTIONS
CNS: headache, dizziness, fatigue. **CV:** hypotension. **GI:** abdominal pain, diarrhea, dyspepsia, gastroesophageal reflux. **GU:** increased creatinine and BUN levels. **Metabolic:** *hyperkalemia,* increased CK level. **Respiratory:** cough, URI. **Skin:** rash. **Other:** hypersensitivity reaction.

INTERACTIONS
Drug-drug. ✺ *Alert:* ACE inhibitors (benazepril, captopril, lisinopril, moexipril, quinapril), ARBs (azilsartan, candesartan, irbesartan, losartan, telmisartan, valsartan), other drugs that antagonize RAAS:* May increase risk of renal impairment, hypotension, and hyperkalemia. Concomitant use is contraindicated in patients with diabetes. Avoid

concomitant use in patients with moderate to severe renal impairment (GFR less than 60 mL/minute).

Atorvastatin: May increase aliskiren levels. Use cautiously together.

CYP3A4/P-gp inhibitors (cyclosporine, itraconazole, ketoconazole, verapamil): May increase aliskiren concentration and risk of adverse reactions. Use with caution. Avoid concurrent use with cyclosporine or itraconazole.

Furosemide: May reduce furosemide peak levels. Monitor patient for effectiveness.

NSAIDs: May increase risk of renal toxicity. Monitor renal function periodically.

Potassium-sparing diuretics, potassium supplements: May increase risk of hyperkalemia. Use cautiously together.

Rifampin: May decrease aliskiren plasma concentration. Larger aliskiren doses may be needed.

Drug-food. *Grapefruit juice:* May decrease aliskiren plasma level. Advise patient to avoid products containing fruit juice.

High-fat meals: May substantially decrease plasma levels of drug. Monitor patient for effectiveness.

EFFECTS ON LAB TEST RESULTS
• May increase potassium, CK, BUN, uric acid, and serum creatinine levels.
• May decrease Hb level and hematocrit.

CONTRAINDICATIONS & CAUTIONS
• Contraindicated in patients hypersensitive to drug or its components and in those with diabetes who are receiving ARBs or ACE inhibitors.
• Contraindicated in patients taking cyclosporine or itraconazole.
• Use cautiously in patients with history of angioedema, severe renal dysfunction (GFR of less than 30 mL/minute), HF, MI, volume depletion, history of dialysis, nephrotic syndrome, or renovascular HTN.
Dialyzable drug: No.
⚠ *Overdose S&S:* Hypotension.

PREGNANCY-LACTATION-REPRODUCTION
Boxed Warning Drug can cause fetal harm. Drugs that act on the RAAS can cause injury and death to the developing fetus. Discontinue drug as soon as possible once pregnancy is detected. ∎

• Patients of childbearing potential should avoid becoming pregnant while taking drug.
• It isn't known if drug appears in human milk. Patient should discontinue breastfeeding or discontinue drug.

NURSING CONSIDERATIONS
• Monitor BP for hypotension, especially if used in combination with other antihypertensives.
• Monitor potassium levels, especially in patients also taking ACE inhibitors.
🕒 *Alert:* Rarely, angioedema may occur at any time during treatment. Discontinue drug for angioedema or anaphylaxis and don't readminister. Early emergency treatment is critical and may include intubation, antihistamines, steroids, and epinephrine.
• Monitor renal function. It's unknown how patients with significant renal disorders will respond to the use of this drug.
• Correct volume or salt depletion before giving drug or start therapy under close monitoring.
• Effect of any dose is usually seen within 2 weeks.
• Monitor patient for serious skin reactions (SJS, TEN).
• *Look alike–sound alike:* Don't confuse Tekturna with Valturna.

PATIENT TEACHING
• Instruct patient not to take drug with a high-fat meal because this may decrease drug's effectiveness.
• Instruct patient to monitor BP daily, if possible, and to report low readings, dizziness, and headaches to prescriber.
• Tell patient to immediately report swelling of the face or neck or difficulty breathing.
• Advise patient of need for regular lab tests to monitor for adverse effects.
• Instruct patient to discontinue drug and notify prescriber if pregnancy is detected.

---

allopurinol ✖
al-oh-PURE-i-nole

Zyloprim✎

allopurinol sodium ✖
Aloprim

Therapeutic class: Antigout drugs
Pharmacologic class: Xanthine oxidase inhibitors

AVAILABLE FORMS
allopurinol
Tablets (scored): 100 mg, 200 mg✲, 300 mg
allopurinol sodium
Injection: 500-mg vial

INDICATIONS & DOSAGES
Adjust-a-dose (for all indications): If CrCl is 10 to 20 mL/minute, give 200 mg PO or IV daily; if CrCl is 3 to 10 mL/minute, give 100 mg PO or IV daily; if CrCl is less than 3 mL/minute, give a maximum of 100 mg PO or IV at extended intervals.
➤ **Gout or hyperuricemia**
Adults: Initially, 100 mg PO daily; then titrate in 100-mg increments weekly until serum urate concentration falls to 6 mg/dL or less. Maximum, 800 mg daily. Dosage varies with severity of disease; can be given as single dose or divided, but doses greater than 300 mg should be divided.
➤ **Hyperuricemia caused by malignancies**
Adults: 200 to 400 mg/m² daily IV as a single infusion or in equally divided doses every 6, 8, or 12 hours beginning 24 to 48 hours before initiation of chemotherapy. Maximum, 600 mg daily.
Children and adolescents: Initially, 200 mg/m² daily IV as single infusion or in equally divided doses every 6, 8, or 12 hours beginning 24 to 48 hours before initiation of chemotherapy. Then titrate according to uric acid levels. For children ages 6 to 10, give 300 mg PO daily or in three divided doses; for children younger than age 6, give 150 mg PO daily.
➤ **To prevent uric acid nephropathy (TLS) during cancer chemotherapy**
Adults: 600 to 800 mg PO daily for 2 to 3 days, with high fluid intake.

➤ **Recurrent calcium oxalate calculi**
Adults: 200 to 300 mg PO daily in single or divided doses.

ADMINISTRATION
PO
• Give drug with or immediately after meals to minimize GI upset.
• Store at room temperature; protect from light.
IV
▼ When possible, initiate therapy 24 to 48 hours before the start of chemotherapy known to cause tumor lysis.
▼ Dissolve contents of each 30-mL vial with 25 mL of sterile water for injection.
▼ Dilute solution to desired concentration (no greater than 6 mg/mL) with NSS for injection or D₅W. Can give as a single daily infusion or in equally divided infusions at 6-, 8-, or 12-hour intervals. Rate of infusion depends on volume of infusate.
▼ Store solution at 68° to 77° F (20° to 25° C) and use within 10 hours. Don't use solution if it contains particulates or is discolored.
▼ **Incompatibilities:** Amikacin, amphotericin B, carmustine, cefotaxime, chlorpromazine, cimetidine, clindamycin, cytarabine, dacarbazine, daunorubicin, diphenhydramine, doxorubicin, doxycycline, droperidol, floxuridine, gentamicin, haloperidol, hydroxyzine, idarubicin, imipenem–cilastatin, mechlorethamine, meperidine, methylprednisolone, metoclopramide, minocycline, nalbuphine, netilmicin, ondansetron, prochlorperazine, promethazine, sodium bicarbonate (or solutions containing sodium bicarbonate), streptozocin, tobramycin, vinorelbine.

ACTION
Reduces uric acid production by inhibiting xanthine oxidase.

Route	Onset	Peak	Duration
PO	Unknown	1.5 hr (allopurinol); 4.5 hr (oxypurinol)	1–2 wk
IV	Unknown	30 min	Unknown

Half-life: Allopurinol, 1 to 2 hours; oxypurinol, 15 hours.

ADVERSE REACTIONS
GI: nausea, vomiting, abdominal pain, diarrhea. **GU:** *renal failure.* **Hepatic:** increased ALP and transaminase levels.

Musculoskeletal: acute gout attack.
Skin: rash, maculopapular rash.

INTERACTIONS

Drug-drug. *Amoxicillin, ampicillin:* May increase possibility of rash. Avoid using together.

Antineoplastics: May increase potential for bone marrow suppression. Monitor patient carefully.

Azathioprine, mercaptopurine: May increase levels of these drugs. Concomitant administration of 300 to 600 mg of oral allopurinol per day requires dosage reduction to ⅓ to ¼ of usual dose of azathioprine or mercaptopurine. Make subsequent dosage adjustments based on therapeutic response and appearance of toxic effects.

Chlorpropamide: May increase hypoglycemic effect. Avoid using together.

Cyclosporine: May increase cyclosporine level. Monitor cyclosporine level and adjust dosage as necessary.

Ethacrynic acid, thiazide diuretics: May increase risk of allopurinol toxicity. Reduce allopurinol dosage, and monitor renal function closely.

Theophylline: May increase theophylline level. Adjust theophylline dosage as needed.

Uricosurics (colchicine, probenecid): May have additive effect. May be used to therapeutic advantage.

Warfarin: May increase anticoagulant effect. Adjust warfarin dosage, if needed.

EFFECTS ON LAB TEST RESULTS

• May increase creatinine, uric acid, glucose, phosphorus, ALP, ALT, and AST levels.
• May decrease magnesium level.
• May increase or decrease calcium, potassium, and sodium levels.
• May increase eosinophil count.
• May decrease Hb level, hematocrit, and granulocyte and platelet counts.
• May increase or decrease WBC count.

CONTRAINDICATIONS & CAUTIONS

• Contraindicated in patients hypersensitive to drug.
⚕ ❶ *Alert:* To avoid risk of SCAR, avoid use of allopurinol in patients who are HLA-B*5801-positive. The American College of Rheumatology recommends HLA-B*5801 screening in patients at elevated risk for SCAR, including patients of Korean descent who have chronic kidney disease stage 3 or greater as well as patients of Han Chinese or Thai descent regardless of kidney function. Some experts suggest screening in all patients of Korean ethnicity regardless of renal function.
• Use cautiously in patients with renal impairment.
Dialyzable drug: Yes.

PREGNANCY-LACTATION-REPRODUCTION

• Use in pregnancy only if clearly needed.
• Drug appears in human milk. Use cautiously during breastfeeding.

NURSING CONSIDERATIONS

❶ *Alert:* Rash can be followed by more severe hypersensitivity reactions (SJS, vasculitis, irreversible hepatotoxicity), which can be fatal. Discontinue drug at first sign of rash.
• Monitor uric acid level to evaluate drug's effectiveness.
• Monitor fluid intake and output; daily urine output of at least 2 L and maintenance of neutral or slightly alkaline urine are desirable.
• Periodically monitor CBC and hepatic and renal function, especially at start of therapy.
• Optimal benefits when used for gout may need 2 to 6 weeks of therapy. Because acute gout attacks may occur during this time, concurrent use of colchicine may be prescribed prophylactically.
• Don't restart drug in patients who have a severe reaction.
• *Look alike–sound alike:* Don't confuse Zyloprim with ZORprin or zolpidem.

PATIENT TEACHING

• To minimize GI adverse reactions, tell patient to take drug with or immediately after meals.
⚕ ❶ *Alert:* Advise patient who is known to be HLA-B*5801-positive to avoid allopurinol.
• Encourage patient to drink plenty of fluids while taking drug unless otherwise contraindicated.
• Drug may cause drowsiness; tell patient not to drive or perform hazardous tasks requiring mental alertness until CNS effects of drug are known.
• If patient is taking drug for recurrent calcium oxalate stones, advise patient also to reduce dietary intake of animal protein, sodium, refined sugars, oxalate-rich foods, and calcium.
• Tell patient to stop drug at first sign of rash, which may precede severe hypersensitivity or

---

Reactions in bold italics are *life-threatening*. Interactions may have a *rapid onset* or a ***delayed onset***.

other adverse reactions. Rash is more common in patients taking diuretics and in those with renal disorders. Tell patient to report all adverse reactions.

• Teach patient importance of continuing drug even if asymptomatic.

---

almotriptan malate
al-moh-TRIP-tan

Therapeutic class: Antimigraine drugs
Pharmacologic class: Serotonin 5-HT$_1$ receptor agonists

AVAILABLE FORMS
Tablets: 6.25 mg, 12.5 mg

INDICATIONS & DOSAGES
➤ **Acute migraine with or without aura**
Adults and adolescents age 12 and older: 6.25 mg or 12.5 mg PO, with one additional dose after 2 hours if headache is unresolved or recurs. The 12.5-mg dose tends to be more effective in adults. Maximum, two doses (total of 25 mg) within 24 hours.
Adjust-a-dose: For patients with hepatic or renal impairment, initially 6.25 mg, with maximum daily dose of 12.5 mg.

ADMINISTRATION
PO
• Give drug without regard for food.
• Give only one repeat dose within 24 hours, no sooner than 2 hours after first dose.

ACTION
May act as an agonist at serotonin receptors on extracerebral intracranial blood vessels, which constricts the affected vessels, inhibits neuropeptide release, and reduces pain transmission in the trigeminal pathways.

Route	Onset	Peak	Duration
PO	1–3 hr	1–3 hr	Unknown

Half-life: 3 to 4 hours.

ADVERSE REACTIONS
CNS: paresthesia, headache, dizziness, somnolence. **GI:** nausea, vomiting, dry mouth.

INTERACTIONS
Drug-drug. *Antiemetics (5-HT$_3$ antagonists), antipsychotics, metolazone, methylene blue, metoclopramide, opioid analgesics,*
tramadol: May increase serotonergic effects and serotonin syndrome. Monitor therapy.
CYP3A4 inhibitors (such as ketoconazole): May increase almotriptan level. Monitor patient for potential adverse reaction. May need to reduce dosage. Avoid concomitant use in patients with renal or hepatic impairment.
Ergot-containing drugs, serotonin 5-HT$_{1B/1D}$ agonists: May cause additive effects. Contraindicated for use within 24 hours of almotriptan.
MAO inhibitors, verapamil: May increase almotriptan level. No dose adjustment is necessary.
SSNRIs, SSRIs: May cause additive serotonin effects, resulting in weakness, hyperreflexia, or incoordination. Monitor patient closely if given together.

EFFECTS ON LAB TEST RESULTS
None reported.

CONTRAINDICATIONS & CAUTIONS
• Contraindicated in patients hypersensitive to drug.
• Contraindicated in patients with angina pectoris, history of MI, silent ischemia, coronary artery vasospasm, Prinzmetal variant angina, or other CV disease; uncontrolled HTN; PVD, including ischemic bowel disease; cerebrovascular disease (history of stroke or TIA); and hemiplegic or basilar migraine.
• Use cautiously in patients with renal or hepatic impairment, known hypersensitivity to sulfonamide, and in those with cataracts because of the potential for corneal opacities.
• Use cautiously in patients with risk factors for CAD, such as obesity, diabetes, smoking, hypercholesterolemia, HTN, females after menopause or males older than age 40, and family history of CAD. CV evaluation to exclude CV disease is recommended.
• Drug isn't intended for migraine prophylaxis or treatment of cluster headaches.
Dialyzable drug: Unknown.
⚠ *Overdose S&S:* HTN, more serious CV symptoms.

PREGNANCY-LACTATION-REPRODUCTION
• Use during pregnancy only if potential benefit justifies fetal risk.
• It isn't known if drug appears in human milk. Use cautiously during breastfeeding.

NURSING CONSIDERATIONS

• Overuse of acute migraine drugs for 10 or more days per month may lead to migraine-like daily headaches or a marked increase in frequency of migraine attacks (medication overuse headache). Withdrawal of the overused drugs may be necessary.
• Consider obtaining ECG with first dose of drug in patients with positive CAD risk factors.
• Assess patients with signs and symptoms of angina after almotriptan dose for CAD and Prinzmetal or variant angina, including ECG monitoring.
• Monitor patient for vasospastic events, such as peripheral ischemia (Raynaud syndrome), blindness, partial vision loss, or GI ischemia (abdominal pain, bloody diarrhea). Consider further evaluation for signs or symptoms suggesting decreased arterial flow after triptan use.
⚠ *Alert:* Combining triptans with SSRIs or SSNRIs may cause serotonin syndrome. Signs and symptoms include restlessness, hallucinations, loss of coordination, rapid heartbeat, rapid changes in BP, increased body temperature, overactive reflexes, nausea, vomiting, and diarrhea. Serotonin syndrome occurs more often when starting or increasing the dose of a triptan, SSRI, or SSNRI.

PATIENT TEACHING

• Tell patient that drug can be taken with or without food.
• Advise patient to take drug only when having a migraine; explain that drug isn't taken on a regular schedule.
• Advise patient to use only one repeat dose within 24 hours, no sooner than 2 hours after first dose.
• Advise patient that other commonly prescribed migraine drugs can interact with almotriptan.
• Advise patient to report chest or throat tightness, pain, or heaviness.

SAFETY ALERT!

alogliptin benzoate
AL-oh-GLIP-tin

Nesina

Therapeutic class: Antidiabetics
Pharmacologic class: DPP-4 inhibitors

AVAILABLE FORMS
Tablets: 6.25 mg, 12.5 mg, 25 mg

INDICATIONS & DOSAGES
➤ **Adjunct to diet and exercise to improve glycemic control in adults with type 2 diabetes**
Adults: 25 mg PO daily.
Adjust-a-dose: For patients with moderate renal impairment (CrCl of 30 to less than 60 mL/minute), give 12.5 mg PO daily. For patients with severe renal impairment (CrCl of 15 to less than 30 mL/minute) and for those with ESRD (CrCl of less than 15 mL/minute) or requiring hemodialysis, give 6.25 mg PO daily.

ADMINISTRATION
PO
• Give without regard for food.
• Store at room temperature.

ACTION
Slows inactivation of incretin, which increases blood concentrations of incretin and reduces fasting or postprandial glucose in patients with type 2 diabetes.

Route	Onset	Peak	Duration
PO	Unknown	1–2 hr	Unknown

Half-life: 21 hours.

ADVERSE REACTIONS
CNS: headache. **CV:** *HF.* **EENT:** nasopharyngitis. **GU:** decreased CrCl, decreased GFR. **Metabolic:** *hypoglycemia.* **Respiratory:** URI.

INTERACTIONS
Drug-drug. *ACE inhibitors:* May enhance the adverse effects of ACE inhibitor, especially angioedema. Monitor therapy.
Androgens (except danazol), pegvisomant: May enhance hypoglycemic effect. Monitor therapy.
Danazol, fluoroquinolones, thiazide diuretics: May diminish hypoglycemic effect. Monitor therapy.
Insulin, sulfonylureas: May enhance hypoglycemic activity. Adjust dosage of insulin or sulfonylurea.
MAO inhibitors, salicylates, SSRIs: May increase hypoglycemic effect. Monitor therapy.

EFFECTS ON LAB TEST RESULTS
• May increase ALT level.
• May decrease GFR and CrCl.

Reactions in bold italics are *life-threatening*. Interactions may have a *rapid onset* or a **delayed onset**.

CONTRAINDICATIONS & CAUTIONS
• Contraindicated in patients hypersensitive to drug or its components and in those with type 1 diabetes or ketoacidosis.
• Use cautiously in patients with liver disease or injury, history of pancreatitis, gallstones, history of alcoholism, renal disease, or history of angioedema with another DPP-4 inhibitor.
🕖 *Alert:* Use cautiously in patients with a history of HF or renal disease. Drug may increase risk of HF in these patients.
• Safety and effectiveness in children haven't been established.
Dialyzable drug: No.

PREGNANCY-LACTATION-REPRODUCTION
• Use cautiously during pregnancy and only if clearly needed.
• It isn't known if drug appears in human milk. Use cautiously during breastfeeding.

NURSING CONSIDERATIONS
🕖 *Alert:* Monitor patient for signs and symptoms of HF (shortness of breath, orthopnea, tiredness, weakness, fatigue, weight gain, peripheral or abdominal edema). Drug may need to be discontinued and other antidiabetics may be needed.
• Assess renal function at baseline and periodically during treatment.
• Monitor patient for hypersensitivity reactions, including SJS. Stop drug immediately if hypersensitivity is suspected.
• Monitor patients for development of blisters or skin erosions; consider dermatologist referral for diagnosis and treatment if present.
• Monitor patient for signs and symptoms (rare) of acute pancreatitis (severe abdominal pain that may radiate to the back, with or without vomiting).
• Assess LFTs before treatment. If liver injury is suspected during treatment (fatigue, anorexia, abdominal discomfort, dark urine, jaundice), obtain LFTs. If elevated LFT values are present, persist, or worsen, withhold drug and determine probable cause. Restart drug only if cause isn't alogliptin-related.
• Monitor blood glucose level if patient is receiving concurrent antidiabetics; adjust dosages of these medications if needed.
🕖 *Alert:* May cause joint pain that can be severe and disabling. Report severe and persistent joint pain to prescriber; drug may need to be discontinued.

PATIENT TEACHING
🕖 *Alert:* Instruct patient to immediately report signs and symptoms of HF. Patient shouldn't stop drug without first discussing with prescriber.
• Instruct patient to monitor blood glucose level carefully.
• Advise patient to seek medical attention for hypersensitivity symptoms.
• Caution patient to seek medical attention for signs and symptoms of pancreatitis (severe abdominal pain that may radiate to the back, with or without vomiting) or liver injury (fatigue, anorexia, abdominal discomfort, dark urine, or jaundice).

SAFETY ALERT!

alpelisib 🗵
al-pe-LIS-ib

Piqray, Vijoice

Therapeutic class: Antineoplastics
Pharmacologic class: Kinase inhibitors

AVAILABLE FORMS
Tablets: 50 mg, 125 mg, 200 mg
Tablets 🕖: 50 mg, 150 mg, 200 mg

INDICATIONS & DOSAGES
➤ **Hormone receptor (HR)–positive, HER2-negative, *PIK3CA*-mutated, advanced, or metastatic breast cancer as detected by an FDA-approved test following progression on or after an endocrine-based regimen** 🗵
Women who are postmenopausal and men:
300 mg PO once daily. Continue treatment until disease progression or unacceptable toxicity occurs. When fulvestrant is given with alpelisib, recommended fulvestrant dosage is 500 mg IM on days 1, 15, and 29, and once monthly thereafter.
Adjust-a-dose: Refer to manufacturer's instructions for toxicity-related dosage adjustments of alpelisib and fulvestrant.
✳ *NEW INDICATION:* **Severe manifestations of PIK3CA-related overgrowth spectrum requiring systemic therapy (Vijoice)** 🗵
Adults: 250 mg PO once daily until disease progression or unacceptable toxicity occurs.
Children ages 6 to younger than 18: Initially, 50 mg PO once daily. May increase after 24 weeks to 125 mg for response

---

optimization. Continue until disease progression or unacceptable toxicity occurs.
Children ages 2 to younger than 6: 50 mg PO once daily until disease progression or unacceptable toxicity occurs.
Adjust-a-dose: Refer to manufacturer's instructions for toxicity-related dosage adjustments.

ADMINISTRATION

PO
• Drug may be considered hazardous; use safe handling precautions.
• Give at approximately the same time each day with food.
• Patient should swallow tablets whole and not chew, crush, or split them. Don't give tablets that are broken, cracked, or otherwise not intact.
• For patients unable to swallow Vijoice tablets, place tablets in glass with 60 to 120 mL of water and let stand for 5 minutes then crush tablets with a spoon and stir until an oral suspension is obtained. Give immediately or discard if not given within 60 minutes. After giving, place 30 to 45 mL in same glass, stir with the same spoon to re-suspend any remaining particle and give to patient. Repeat rinse step if particles remain to ensure full dose is given.
• If a dose is missed, give within 9 hours after the usual time. If it has been more than 9 hours, skip the dose for that day. The next day, give drug at the usual time.
• If patient vomits after taking the dose, don't give an additional dose on that day, and resume the dosing schedule the next day at the usual time.
• Store at 68° to 77° F (20° to 25° C).

ACTION
A phosphatidylinositol-3-kinase inhibitor that increases estrogen receptor transcription in breast cancer cells. The combination of alpelisib and fulvestrant provided greater antitumor activity compared with either treatment alone.

Route	Onset	Peak	Duration
PO	Unknown	2–4 hr	Unknown

Half-life: 8 to 9 hours.

ADVERSE REACTIONS
CNS: fatigue, fever, dysgeusia, headache.
CV: peripheral edema. **GI:** diarrhea, stomatitis, vomiting, nausea, abdominal pain, dyspepsia, decreased appetite. **GU:** UTI, *acute kidney injury.* **Hematologic:** *lymphocytopenia,* anemia, prolonged PTT, *thrombocytopenia.* **Hepatic:** increased lipase and transaminase levels, hypoalbuminemia, increased bilirubin. **Metabolic:** weight loss, hyperglycemia, hypophosphatemia, hyponatremia, increased GGT level, *hypocalcemia, hypoglycemia, hypokalemia, hyperkalemia, hypomagnesemia,* hyperlipidemia. **Musculoskeletal:** osteonecrosis of the jaw. **Respiratory:** pneumonitis. **Skin:** rash, alopecia, pruritus, eczema, dry skin, cellulitis, *SCAR (SJS, TEN, erythema multiforme).* **Other:** mucosal dryness, mucosal inflammation, hypersensitivity reaction.

INTERACTIONS
Drug-drug. *BCRP inhibitors (estrone, omeprazole, saquinavir, verapamil):* May increase alpelisib level and risk of toxicity. Avoid use together. If use together can't be avoided, closely monitor patient for adverse reactions.
CYP2C9 substrates (bosentan, candesartan, celecoxib, diclofenac, glipizide, indomethacin, losartan, phenobarbital, phenytoin, rosuvastatin, warfarin): May decrease substrate plasma concentration and therapeutic effects. Monitor patient closely.
CYP3A4 inducers (carbamazepine, efavirenz, phenytoin, rifampin): May decrease alpelisib level and therapeutic effect. Avoid use together.

EFFECTS ON LAB TEST RESULTS
• May increase creatinine, GGT, ALT, AST, cholesterol, triglyceride, HbA$_{1c}$, and lipase levels.
• May decrease calcium, sodium, albumin, phosphate, and magnesium levels.
• May increase or decrease glucose and potassium levels.
• May prolong PTT.
• May increase eosinophil count.
• May decrease Hb level and lymphocyte and platelet counts.

CONTRAINDICATIONS & CAUTIONS
• Contraindicated in patients with severe hypersensitivity to drug or its components; severe reactions, including anaphylaxis and anaphylactic shock, have been reported.

- Severe cutaneous reactions have been reported, including SJS, erythema multiforme (EM), TEN, and DRESS syndrome.
- Severe hyperglycemia, including ketoacidosis, has been reported.
- Use cautiously in patients with diabetes. The safety of drug in patients with type 1 and uncontrolled type 2 diabetes hasn't been established. Patients with a history of diabetes may require intensified diabetic treatment.
- Drug may increase risk of severe pneumonitis, including acute interstitial pneumonitis and ILD. Consider a diagnosis of noninfectious pneumonitis in patients with nonspecific respiratory signs and symptoms (hypoxia, cough, dyspnea, or interstitial infiltrates on radiologic exams) and in whom infectious, neoplastic, and other causes have been excluded by means of appropriate investigations.
- Safety and effectiveness in children haven't been established.

Dialyzable drug: Unknown.

⚠ *Overdose S&S:* Hyperglycemia, nausea, asthenia, rash.

PREGNANCY-LACTATION-REPRODUCTION
- Drug can cause fetal harm. Advise patient of potential fetal risk if used during pregnancy.
- Advise patients of childbearing potential to use effective contraception during therapy and for 1 week after final dose.
- Advise males with partners of childbearing potential to use condoms and effective contraception during treatment and for 1 week after final dose.
- Drug may impair fertility in males and females of reproductive potential.
- It isn't known if drug appears in human milk. Because of the potential for serious adverse reactions in the infant, patients shouldn't breastfeed during treatment and for 1 week after final dose.

NURSING CONSIDERATIONS
- Verify pregnancy status before starting therapy.
- Monitor patient for hypersensitivity reactions, such as dyspnea, flushing, rash, fever, or tachycardia. Permanently discontinue drug for severe hypersensitivity reactions.
- Monitor patient for severe cutaneous reaction (SCAR), including SJS, EM, TEN, and DRESS syndrome. If signs or symptoms of SCAR occur (severe rash, worsening rash,

reddened skin, peeling skin; blistering of the lips, eyes, mouth, or skin; flulike symptoms, fever), interrupt therapy and consult a dermatologist. If SCAR is confirmed, permanently discontinue drug. If SCAR isn't confirmed, dosage modifications and management of rash may be required per the manufacturer's instructions.
- Monitor patient for hyperglycemia, including ketoacidosis. If hyperglycemia occurs, therapy interruption, dosage reduction, or drug discontinuation may be required per the manufacturer's instructions.
- Before starting drug, obtain fasting plasma glucose (FPG) and HbA$_{1c}$ levels and optimize blood glucose level. After initiating drug, monitor blood glucose level, FPG, or both, at least once every week for the first 2 weeks, then at least once every 4 weeks, and as clinically indicated. Monitor HbA$_{1c}$ every 3 months and as clinically indicated.
- If hyperglycemia occurs during therapy, monitor blood glucose or FPG level as clinically indicated, and at least twice weekly until blood glucose or FPG level decreases to normal. During treatment with an antidiabetic, continue monitoring blood glucose or FPG level at least once a week for 8 weeks, then once every 2 weeks and as clinically indicated.
- Monitor patient for new or worsening respiratory signs and symptoms or for development of pneumonitis. If signs or symptoms occur, immediately interrupt therapy and evaluate for pneumonitis. Permanently discontinue drug in patients with confirmed pneumonitis.
- Monitor patient for severe diarrhea, including dehydration and acute kidney injury. If diarrhea occurs, therapy interruption, dosage reduction, or drug discontinuation may be required. Treat diarrhea as clinically indicated.

PATIENT TEACHING
- Instruct patient in safe drug administration.
- Teach patient to report all adverse reactions.
- Inform patient to immediately report signs and symptoms of hypersensitivity.
- Caution patient that severe skin reactions can occur and to immediately report signs and symptoms of severe cutaneous reactions (flulike symptoms; severe rash or rash that worsens; reddened skin; blistering of the lips, eyes, or mouth; blisters on the skin or peeling skin, with or without fever).

• Warn patient that hyperglycemia may develop. Advise patient to closely monitor blood glucose level during therapy and to report signs and symptoms of hyperglycemia (increased thirst, dry mouth, frequent urination, and increased appetite with weight loss).

• Inform patient to immediately report respiratory problems, as drug can increase risk of pneumonitis.

• Advise patient that drug may cause diarrhea, which may be severe. Inform patient to start antidiarrheal treatment, increase fluid intake, and notify prescriber if diarrhea occurs.

• Warn patient of childbearing potential that drug can cause fetal harm and that pregnancy testing will be performed before therapy begins. Advise patient to immediately report a known or suspected pregnancy.

• Advise patient of childbearing potential and male patient with partners of childbearing potential to use effective contraception during therapy and for 1 week after final dose.

• Advise patient not to breastfeed during treatment and for 1 week after final dose.

• Advise male or female patient of reproductive potential that drug may impair fertility.

SAFETY ALERT!

ALPRAZolam
al-PRAH-zoe-lam

Apo-Alpraz✳, Xanax✦, Xanax TS✳, Xanax XR

Therapeutic class: Anxiolytics
Pharmacologic class: Benzodiazepines
Controlled substance schedule: IV

AVAILABLE FORMS
Oral solution: 1 mg/mL (concentrate)
Tablets: 0.25 mg, 0.5 mg, 1 mg, 2 mg
Tablets (extended-release) ⓞⓝⓒ: 0.5 mg, 1 mg, 2 mg, 3 mg
Tablets (ODTs): 0.25 mg, 0.5 mg, 1 mg, 2 mg

INDICATIONS & DOSAGES
Adjust-a-dose (for all indications): For older adults and patients with debilitation or advanced hepatic disease, usual first dose is 0.25 mg PO b.i.d. or t.i.d. For extended-release tablets, 0.5 mg PO once daily.

To discontinue drug or reduce dosage, decrease by no more than 0.5 mg every 3 days.

Some patients may benefit from more gradual discontinuation.

Boxed Warning To reduce risk of withdrawal reactions, use a gradual taper to discontinue or reduce dosage. If withdrawal reactions develop, consider pausing the taper or increasing the dosage to the previous tapered dosage level. Subsequently decrease the dosage more slowly. ∎

➤ **Anxiety**
Adults: Usual first dose, 0.25 to 0.5 mg (immediate-release) PO t.i.d. Maximum, 4 mg daily in divided doses.

➤ **Panic disorders with or without agoraphobia**
Adults: 0.5 mg PO t.i.d., increased at intervals of 3 to 4 days in increments of no more than 1 mg/day. Maximum, 10 mg daily in divided doses. For extended-release tablets, start with 0.5 to 1 mg PO once daily. Increase by no more than 1 mg/day every 3 to 4 days. Maximum daily dose, 10 mg.

ADMINISTRATION
PO
• Don't break or crush extended-release tablets.

• Mix oral solution with liquids or semisolid food, such as water, juices, carbonated beverages, applesauce, and puddings. Use only calibrated dropper provided with this product. Give drug immediately after mixing.

• Use dry hands to remove ODTs from bottle. Place tablet on top of the tongue and allow to disintegrate; water isn't necessary. Discard cotton from inside bottle.

• Discard unused portion if breaking scored ODT.

• Patients treated with divided doses of immediate-release tablets can be switched to extended-release tablets at same total daily dose. Patients should take extended-release tablets in the morning.

ACTION
Unknown. Probably potentiates the effects of GABA, depresses the CNS, and suppresses the spread of seizure activity.

Route	Onset	Peak	Duration
PO	Unknown	1–2 hr	Unknown
PO (extended-release)	Unknown	10 hr	Unknown

Half-life: Immediate-release, 6.3 to 26.9 hours; extended-release, 10.7 to 15.8 hours.

Reactions in bold italics are *life-threatening*. Interactions may have a *rapid onset* or a **delayed onset**.

ADVERSE REACTIONS

CNS: insomnia, irritability, dizziness, headache, anxiety, confusion, drowsiness, sedation, somnolence, difficulty speaking, impaired coordination, memory impairment, fatigue, depression, mental impairment, ataxia, dyskinesia, hypoesthesia, lethargy, vertigo, malaise, tremor, nervousness, restlessness, agitation, nightmare, akathisia, disorientation, derealization, depersonalization, talkativeness, disinhibition, disturbance in attention, equilibrium disturbance. **CV:** palpitations, chest pain, hypotension. **EENT:** blurred vision, dry mouth, allergic rhinitis, nasal congestion. **GI:** diarrhea, constipation, nausea, increased appetite, anorexia, vomiting, dyspepsia, abdominal pain, increased or decreased salivation. **GU:** dysmenorrhea, sexual dysfunction, difficulty urinating, incontinence. **Metabolic:** increased or decreased weight. **Musculoskeletal:** arthralgia, myalgia, limb pain, back pain, muscle cramps, muscle twitch. **Respiratory:** dyspnea, hyperventilation. **Skin:** rash, pruritus, increased sweating, dermatitis, allergic reaction. **Other:** injury, dependence, feeling warm, increased or decreased libido.

INTERACTIONS

Drug-drug. *Anticonvulsants, antidepressants, antihistamines, barbiturates, benzodiazepines, general anesthetics, narcotics, phenothiazines, protease inhibitors:* May increase CNS depressant effects. Avoid using together.
CYP3A inducers (carbamazepine): May induce alprazolam metabolism and may reduce therapeutic effects. May need to increase dosage.
Delavirdine, strong CYP3A inhibitors (atazanavir, clarithromycin, itraconazole, ketoconazole, miconazole, saquinavir, telithromycin): May increase alprazolam level, CNS depression, and psychomotor impairment. Use together is contraindicated.
Digoxin: May increase digoxin level, especially in older adults. Monitor level and adjust digoxin dosage if necessary.
Hydantoins (phenytoin): May decrease effects of alprazolam and increase hydantoin levels. Monitor patient closely.
Methadone: May significantly increase risk of CNS depression. Avoid use if possible or monitor patient closely.

Moderate or weak CYP3A inhibitors (cimetidine, fluoxetine, fluvoxamine, hormonal contraceptives): May increase alprazolam level. Use cautiously together; consider alprazolam dosage reduction.
Boxed Warning *Opioids:* May cause slow or difficult breathing, sedation, and death. Avoid use together. If use together is necessary, limit dosage and duration of each drug to the minimum necessary for desired effect. ∎
Rifamycins (rifampin): May decrease effects of alprazolam. Alprazolam dosage increase may be needed.
Ritonavir: May increase alprazolam level with short-term use; after 10 days, alprazolam exposure isn't affected. Reduce alprazolam dosage when initiating ritonavir. May increase dosage after 10 to 14 days of concomitant ritonavir dosing.
TCAs (amitriptyline, doxepin, imipramine, nortriptyline): May increase adverse effects. Monitor patient closely.
Drug-herb. *Kava, valerian root:* May increase sedation. Discourage use together.
St. John's wort: May decrease drug level. Discourage use together.
Drug-food. *Grapefruit juice:* May increase drug level. Discourage use together.
Drug-lifestyle. *Alcohol and cannabis use:* May cause additive CNS effects. Discourage use together.
Smoking: May decrease effectiveness of drug. Monitor patient closely.

EFFECTS ON LAB TEST RESULTS
• May increase liver enzyme levels.

CONTRAINDICATIONS & CAUTIONS
Boxed Warning Benzodiazepine use exposes patient to risks of abuse, misuse, and addiction, which can lead to overdose or death. Assess each patient's risk of abuse, misuse, and addiction before prescribing and periodically during therapy. ∎
Boxed Warning Abrupt discontinuation or rapid dosage reduction of benzodiazepines after continued use may precipitate acute withdrawal reactions, which can be life-threatening. To reduce risk of withdrawal reactions, gradually taper drug to discontinue or reduce dosage. ∎
• Contraindicated in patients hypersensitive to drug or other benzodiazepines and in those with acute angle-closure glaucoma.

Boxed Warning Opioids should only be prescribed with benzodiazepines or other CNS depressants to patients for whom alternative treatment options are inadequate. ■
- Use cautiously in patients with hepatic, renal, or pulmonary disease or history of substance abuse.
- Use cautiously in older adults.
- Safety and effectiveness in children haven't been established.

Dialyzable drug: No.

⚠ *Overdose S&S:* Somnolence, confusion, impaired coordination, diminished reflexes, coma.

PREGNANCY-LACTATION-REPRODUCTION
- Drug may cause fetal harm. Neonates exposed during late pregnancy may experience sedation, respiratory depression, and neonatal withdrawal. Use isn't recommended during pregnancy.
- The National Pregnancy Registry for Psychiatric Medications is available at 866-961-2388 or https://womensmentalhealth.org/research/pregnancyregistry/
- Drug appears in human milk. Use isn't recommended during breastfeeding.

NURSING CONSIDERATIONS
Boxed Warning Monitor patient also taking an opioid for signs and symptoms of respiratory depression and sedation. ■
- The optimum duration of therapy is unknown.
- Give smallest effective dose to prevent ataxia or oversedation, especially in older adults or patients who are debilitated.
- Monitor hepatic, renal, and hematopoietic function periodically in patients receiving repeated or prolonged therapy.
- ⏹ *Alert:* Panic disorder is associated with major depressive disorders and increased reports of suicide among patients who are untreated. Monitor patients with depression for suicidality or plans for suicide.
- Consider giving same total daily dose of immediate-release formulation in divided doses more frequently in patients being treated for panic disorder who experience early-morning anxiety or anxiety symptoms between doses.
- *Look alike–sound alike:* Don't confuse alprazolam with alprostadil or lorazepam. Don't confuse Xanax with Fanapt, Zantac, Xopenex, or Tenex.

PATIENT TEACHING
Boxed Warning Caution patient or caregiver of patient taking an opioid with a benzodiazepine, CNS depressant, or alcohol to seek immediate medical attention if patient experiences dizziness, light-headedness, extreme sleepiness, slowed or difficult breathing, or unresponsiveness. ■

Boxed Warning Caution patient that benzodiazepines, even at recommended doses, increase risk of abuse, misuse, and addiction, which can lead to overdose and death, especially when used in combination with other drugs (opioid analgesics), alcohol, or illicit substances. ■

Boxed Warning Instruct patient to seek emergency medical help for signs and symptoms of benzodiazepine abuse, misuse, and addiction (abdominal pain, amnesia, anorexia, anxiety, aggression, ataxia, blurred vision, confusion, depression, disinhibition, disorientation, dizziness, euphoria, impaired concentration and memory, indigestion, irritability, muscle pain, slurred speech, tremors, vertigo, delirium, paranoia, suicidal thoughts or actions, seizures, difficulty breathing, coma). Teach patient proper disposal of unused drug. Advise patient not to take drug at a higher dose, more frequently, or for longer than prescribed. ■

Boxed Warning Tell patient that continued use of drug for several days to weeks may lead to physical dependence and that abrupt discontinuation or rapid dosage reduction may precipitate acute withdrawal reactions (unusual movements, responses, or expressions; seizures; sudden and severe mental or nervous system changes; depression; seeing or hearing things that others don't; homicidal thoughts; extreme increase in activity or talking; losing touch with reality; suicidal thoughts or actions), which can be life-threatening. Instruct patient that discontinuation or dosage reduction may require a slow taper. ■

Boxed Warning Stress the possibility of developing protracted withdrawal syndrome (anxiety; trouble remembering, learning, or concentrating; depression; problems sleeping; feeling like insects are crawling under the skin; weakness; shaking; muscle twitching; burning or prickling feeling in the hands, arms, legs, or feet; ringing in the ears), with symptoms lasting weeks to more than 12 months. ■

Reactions in bold italics are *life-threatening*. Interactions may have a *rapid onset* or a **delayed onset**.

- Warn patient not to stop drug abruptly because withdrawal symptoms or seizures may occur.
- Warn patient to avoid hazardous activities that require alertness and good coordination until effects of drug are known.
- Tell patient to avoid use of alcohol while taking drug.
- Advise patient that smoking may decrease drug's effectiveness.
- Tell patient to swallow extended-release tablets whole.
- Instruct patient in safe drug administration and storage.
- Warn patient not to use drug during pregnancy or breastfeeding and to report pregnancy to prescriber.

alteplase
al-ti-PLAZE

Activase, Cathflo Activase

Therapeutic class: Thrombolytics
Pharmacologic class: Enzymes

AVAILABLE FORMS
Cathflo Activase injection: 2-mg single-patient vials
Injection: 50-mg, 100-mg vials

INDICATIONS & DOSAGES
➤ **Lysis of thrombi obstructing coronary arteries in acute MI (Activase)**
3-hour infusion
Adults weighing 65 kg or more: 6 to 10 mg IV bolus over first 1 to 2 minutes, then 50 to 54 mg IV infusion for remainder of first hour (for a total of 60 mg the first hour). Then 20 mg/hour infused for 2 hours. Don't exceed total dose of 100 mg.
Adults weighing less than 65 kg: 0.075 mg/kg IV bolus over 1 to 2 minutes, followed by 0.675 mg/kg in rest of first hour. Then 0.25 mg/kg/hour infused for 2 hours. Don't exceed total dose of 100 mg.
Accelerated infusion
Adults weighing more than 67 kg: 100 mg maximum total dose. Give 15 mg IV bolus over 1 to 2 minutes, followed by 50 mg infused over the next 30 minutes; then 35 mg infused over the next hour. Don't exceed total dose of 100 mg.
Adults weighing 67 kg or less: 15 mg IV bolus over 1 to 2 minutes, followed by 0.75 mg/kg (not to exceed 50 mg) infused over the next 30 minutes; then 0.5 mg/kg (not to exceed 35 mg) infused over the next hour. Don't exceed total dose of 100 mg.
➤ **To manage acute massive PE (Activase)**
Adults: 100 mg by IV infusion over 2 hours. Begin parenteral anticoagulation at end of infusion when PTT or thrombin time returns to twice normal or less. Don't exceed 100-mg dose. Higher doses may increase risk of intracranial bleeding.
➤ **Acute ischemic stroke (Activase)**
Adults: 0.9 mg/kg by IV infusion over 1 hour with 10% of total dose given as an initial IV bolus over 1 minute. Maximum total dose is 90 mg.
➤ **To restore function to CVADs (Cathflo Activase)**
Adults and children older than age 2: For patients weighing more than 30 kg, instill 2 mg in 2 mL sterile water into catheter. For patients weighing less than 30 kg, instill 110% of the internal lumen volume of the catheter, not to exceed 2 mg in 2 mL sterile water. After 30 minutes of dwell time, assess catheter function by aspirating blood. If function is restored, aspirate 4 to 5 mL of blood in patients weighing 10 kg or more or 3 mL in patients weighing less than 10 kg to remove drug and residual clot, and gently irrigate the catheter with NSS. If catheter function isn't restored after 120 minutes, instill a second dose.
➤ **Acute ischemic stroke presenting 3 to 4.5 hours after symptom onset (Activase)** ♦
Adults: 0.9 mg/kg by IV infusion over 1 hour with 10% of total dose given as an initial IV bolus over 1 minute. Maximum total dose is 90 mg.

ADMINISTRATION
IV
▼ Immediately before use, reconstitute solution with unpreserved sterile water for injection. Check manufacturer's labeling for specific information.
▼ Don't use 50-mg vial if vacuum isn't present; 100-mg vials don't have a vacuum.
▼ Using an 18G needle, direct stream of sterile water at lyophilized cake. Don't shake.
▼ Slight foaming is common. Let it settle before giving drug. Solution should be colorless or pale yellow.

▼ Drug may be given reconstituted (at 1 mg/mL) or diluted with an equal volume of NSS or D_5W to yield 0.5 mg/mL.

▼ Give drug using a controlled infusion device.

▼ Discard any unused drug after 8 hours.

Cathflo Activase

▼ Assess the cause of catheter dysfunction before using drug. Possible causes of occlusion include catheter malposition, mechanical failure, constriction by a suture, and lipid deposits or drug precipitates in the catheter lumen. Don't try to suction the catheter because you risk damaging the vessel wall or collapsing a soft-walled catheter.

▼ Reconstitute Cathflo Activase with 2.2 mL sterile water to yield 1 mg/mL. Dissolve completely to produce a colorless to pale yellow solution. Don't shake.

▼ Don't use excessive pressure while instilling drug into catheter; doing so could rupture the catheter or expel a clot into circulation.

▼ Solution is stable for up to 8 hours at room temperature.

▼ **Incompatibilities:** Bivalirudin, dobutamine, dopamine, heparin, morphine, nitroglycerin. Consult detailed reference for other specific incompatibilities.

ACTION

Converts plasminogen to plasmin by directly cleaving peptide bonds at two sites, causing fibrinolysis.

Route	Onset	Peak	Duration
IV	Unknown	Unknown	Unknown

Half-life: Less than 5 minutes.

ADVERSE REACTIONS

CNS: *cerebral hemorrhage,* fever. **CV:** *arrhythmias,* hypotension, edema, *cholesterol embolization, venous thrombosis.* **GI:** *bleeding,* nausea, vomiting. **GU:** *bleeding.* **Hematologic:** *spontaneous bleeding.* **Skin:** ecchymosis. **Other:** *anaphylaxis, sepsis (Cathflo Activase),* bleeding at puncture sites, hypersensitivity reactions.

INTERACTIONS

Drug-drug. *Aspirin, clopidogrel, dipyridamole, drugs affecting platelet activity (abciximab), heparin, warfarin, anticoagulants:* May increase risk of bleeding. Monitor patient carefully.

Nitroglycerin: May decrease alteplase serum concentration. Monitor therapy.
Tranexamic acid: May diminish therapeutic effect of alteplase. Avoid combination.

EFFECTS ON LAB TEST RESULTS

● May alter coagulation and fibrinolytic test results.

CONTRAINDICATIONS & CAUTIONS

● Contraindicated in patients hypersensitive to drug or its components.

● Activase therapy for acute MI or PE is contraindicated in patients with active internal bleeding; history of stroke; recent intracranial or intraspinal surgery or trauma; intracranial neoplasm, AV malformation, or aneurysm; known bleeding diathesis; or severe uncontrolled HTN.

● Activase therapy for acute ischemic stroke is contraindicated in patients with evidence of intracranial hemorrhage; suspected subarachnoid hemorrhage; recent (within 3 months) intracranial or intraspinal surgery; serious head trauma or previous stroke; history of intracranial hemorrhage; uncontrolled HTN at time of treatment; seizure at onset of stroke; active internal bleeding; intracranial neoplasm, AV malformation, or aneurysm; bleeding diathesis (which may include current use of oral anticoagulants, INR greater than 1.7, PT longer than 15 seconds, platelet count less than $100,000/mm^3$, current use of direct thrombin inhibitors or direct factor Xa inhibitors with elevated sensitive lab tests, or patients who have received heparin within the previous 48 hours and who at presentation have a prolonged PTT).

● In patients with acute ischemic stroke without recent use of oral anticoagulants or heparin, may initiate Activase before available coagulation study results. Discontinue infusion if either a pretreatment INR is greater than 1.7 or a prolonged PTT is identified.

● Patients with severe neurologic deficits (National Institutes of Health Stroke Scale greater than 22) or who have major early infarct signs on a CT scan may have increased risk of bleeding.

● Use cautiously in patients who have had a recent major surgery or procedure or who have other conditions in which bleeding constitutes a significant hazard or would be difficult to control because of its location.

Reactions in bold italics are *life-threatening*. Interactions may have a *rapid onset* or a *delayed onset*.

• Use cautiously in patients with previous puncture of a noncompressible vessel; concomitant oral anticoagulant therapy; organ biopsy; trauma (including cardiopulmonary resuscitation); GI or GU bleeding; cerebrovascular disease; systolic pressure of 175 mm Hg or higher or diastolic pressure of 110 mm Hg or higher; mitral stenosis, atrial fibrillation, or other conditions that may lead to left heart thrombus; acute pericarditis or subacute bacterial endocarditis; hemostatic defects caused by hepatic or renal impairment; septic thrombophlebitis; or diabetic hemorrhagic retinopathy.

• Use cautiously in patients receiving anticoagulants and in patients age 75 and older.

• Use of thrombolytics can increase risk of thromboembolic events in patients at risk for left heart thrombus, such as patients with mitral stenosis or atrial fibrillation. Drug hasn't been shown to adequately treat underlying DVT in patients with PE. Consider the possible risk of reembolization due to lysis of underlying deep venous thrombi in these patients.

• Safety and effectiveness in children haven't been established.

Dialyzable drug: Unknown.

PREGNANCY-LACTATION-REPRODUCTION
• Information related to use during pregnancy is limited; most guidelines consider pregnancy a relative contraindication. Drug shouldn't be withheld during pregnancy in life-threatening situations but should be avoided if safer alternatives are available.

• It isn't known if drug appears in human milk. Use cautiously during breastfeeding.

NURSING CONSIDERATIONS
🖐 *Alert:* When used for acute ischemic stroke, give drug within 3 hours after symptoms occur and only when intracranial bleeding has been ruled out.

• Drug may be given to menstruating patients.

• To recannulize occluded coronary arteries and improve heart function, begin treatment as soon as possible after symptoms start.

• Anticoagulant and antiplatelet therapy is commonly started during or after treatment, to decrease risk of another thrombosis.

• Monitor vital signs and neurologic status carefully. Keep patient on strict bed rest.

• Coronary thrombolysis is linked with arrhythmias caused by reperfusion of ischemic myocardium. Such arrhythmias don't differ from those commonly linked with MI. Have antiarrhythmics readily available, and carefully monitor ECG.

• Avoid invasive procedures, IM injections, and nonessential handling of patient during thrombolytic therapy. Perform essential venipunctures carefully. Closely monitor patient for signs of internal bleeding, and frequently check all puncture sites. Bleeding is the most common adverse effect and may occur internally and at external puncture sites.

• If an arterial puncture is necessary during Activase infusion, use an arm vessel that can be manually compressed. Apply pressure for at least 30 minutes followed by a pressure dressing. Check the site regularly for bleeding.

• If uncontrollable bleeding occurs, stop infusion (and parenteral anticoagulant) and notify prescriber.

• Don't use the "tPA" abbreviation when ordering this drug. "tPA" has been mistaken for TNKase (tenecteplase), TPN, or TXA (errorprone).

• *Look alike–sound alike:* Don't confuse alteplase with Altace. Don't confuse Activase with Cathflo Activase or TNKase.

PATIENT TEACHING
• Explain use and administration of drug to patient and family.

• Tell patient to report adverse reactions promptly and to immediately report signs and symptoms of bleeding, urinary problems, abdominal pain, nausea, vomiting, confusion, severe headache, one-sided weakness, trouble speaking or thinking, visual disturbances, dizziness, passing out, chest pain, or cathetersite pain.

amantadine hydrochloride
a-MAN-ta-deen

Gocovri, Osmolex ER

Therapeutic class: Antivirals
Pharmacologic class: Synthetic cyclic primary amines

AVAILABLE FORMS
Capsules: 100 mg

Capsules (extended-release) ⓄⓃⒸ*: 68.5 mg, 137 mg*
Oral syrup: 50 mg/5 mL
Tablets: 100 mg
Tablets (extended-release) ⓄⓃⒸ*: 129 mg, 193 mg*

INDICATIONS & DOSAGES

Adjust-a-dose (for all indications): Lower dosages are recommended for patients with renal impairment. Refer to the manufacturer's product information.

➤ **Parkinson disease**
Adults: Initially, if used as monotherapy, 100 mg PO b.i.d. In patients with serious illness or in those already receiving high doses of other antiparkinsonian drugs, begin dose at 100 mg PO once daily. Increase to 100 mg b.i.d. if needed after at least 1 week. Some patients may benefit from 400 mg daily in divided doses. For extended-release tablet (Osmolex ER), 129 mg PO once daily; increase weekly to maximum daily dose of 322 mg. For extended-release capsule (Gocovri), 137 mg PO once daily; increase in 1 week to maximum daily dose of 274 mg.

➤ **Adjunct to levodopa–carbidopa in patients with Parkinson disease experiencing "off" episodes (Gocovri)**
Adults: 137 mg PO once daily. Increase in 1 week to maximum daily dose of 274 mg.

➤ **Drug-induced extrapyramidal reactions**
Adults: 100 mg PO b.i.d. May increase to 300 mg daily in divided doses. Extended-release (Osmolex ER), 129 mg PO once daily. Maximum daily dose, 322 mg.

ADMINISTRATION
PO
- Give without regard for food.
- Give extended-release tablets in the morning; extended-release capsules at bedtime.
- Don't crush or break extended-release forms. May sprinkle entire contents of capsule on a small amount (tsp) of soft food such as applesauce and administer immediately. Patient shouldn't chew extended-release forms.

ACTION
May exert its antiparkinsonian effect by causing the release of dopamine in the substantia nigra.

Route	Onset	Peak	Duration
PO	Unknown	2–4 hr	Unknown
PO (extended-release)	Unknown	5–12 hr	Unknown

Half-life: About 10 to 25 hours; with renal dysfunction, as long as 10 days.

ADVERSE REACTIONS
CNS: dizziness, delusions, illusion, paranoia, insomnia, irritability, light-headedness, depression, fatigue, confusion, hallucinations, anxiety, ataxia, headache, nervousness, dream abnormalities, agitation, somnolence, dystonia, syncope, apathy, *suicidality.* **CV:** *HF,* peripheral edema, orthostatic hypotension. **EENT:** blurred vision, cataract, dry eye, dry nose, dry mouth. **GI:** nausea, anorexia, constipation, vomiting, diarrhea. **GU:** UTI, BPH. **Musculoskeletal:** joint swelling, muscle spasms. **Respiratory:** cough. **Skin:** livedo reticularis, contusion, dyschromia. **Other:** falls.

INTERACTIONS
Drug-drug. *Alkalinizing agents, quinidine, sulfamethoxazole–trimethoprim, thiazide diuretics, triamterene:* May increase amantadine level, increasing the risk of toxicity. Use together cautiously.
Anticholinergics: May increase anticholinergic effects. Use together cautiously; reduce dosage of anticholinergic before starting amantadine.
Antipsychotics (clozapine, quetiapine): May decrease therapeutic effect of both drugs. Avoid use together. If use is unavoidable, decrease antipsychotic dose or consider a non-dopamine antagonist (pimavanserin).
CNS stimulants (amphetamines, modafinil): May increase CNS stimulation. Use together cautiously.
Live attenuated influenza vaccines: May interfere with efficacy of live attenuated influenza vaccines. Use together cautiously.
Drug-lifestyle. *Alcohol use:* May increase CNS effects, including dizziness, confusion, and orthostatic hypotension. Discourage use together.

EFFECTS ON LAB TEST RESULTS
- May increase CK, BUN, creatinine, ALP, LDH, bilirubin, GGT, AST, and ALT levels.

Reactions in bold italics are *life-threatening*. Interactions may have a *rapid onset* or a ***delayed onset***.

CONTRAINDICATIONS & CAUTIONS
• Contraindicated in patients hypersensitive to drug and in those with ESRD.
• Use cautiously in older adults and in patients with seizure disorders, psychosis, impulse control disorders, HF, peripheral edema, hepatic disease, mental illness, eczematoid rash, renal impairment, orthostatic hypotension, and CV disease.
• Avoid use in patients with untreated angle-closure glaucoma.
• Don't use drug for prophylaxis or treatment of influenza A due to high resistance rates.
Dialyzable drug: No.
⚠ *Overdose S&S:* Arrhythmia, HTN, tachycardia, pulmonary edema, respiratory distress, increased BUN level, decreased CrCl, renal insufficiency, insomnia, anxiety, aggressive behavior, hypertonia, hyperkinesia, tremor, confusion, disorientation, depersonalization, fear, delirium, hallucinations, psychotic reactions, lethargy, somnolence, coma, seizures, hyperthermia.

PREGNANCY-LACTATION-REPRODUCTION
• Drug may cause fetal harm. Use during pregnancy isn't recommended.
• Drug appears in human milk. Use isn't recommended during breastfeeding.

NURSING CONSIDERATIONS
• Patients with Parkinson disease who don't respond to anticholinergics may respond to this drug.
• Older adults are more susceptible to adverse neurologic effects. Monitor patient for mental status changes.
🕒 *Alert:* Monitor all patients for suicidality. Suicidal ideation and attempts may occur in any patient, regardless of psychiatric history.
🕒 *Alert:* Sporadic cases of NMS have been reported with dosage reduction or drug withdrawal. Observe patient carefully when dosage is abruptly reduced or drug is discontinued.
• Drug must be discontinued gradually. Abrupt discontinuation may cause an increase in signs and symptoms of Parkinson disease or cause delirium, agitation, delusions, hallucinations, paranoid reaction, stupor, anxiety, depression, or slurred speech.
• Drug can worsen mental health conditions in patients with a history of psychiatric disorders or substance abuse.
• Monitor liver and renal function tests.

• *Look alike–sound alike:* Don't confuse amantadine with amiodarone or rimantadine.

PATIENT TEACHING
🕒 *Alert:* Tell patient to take drug exactly as prescribed because not doing so may result in serious adverse reactions or death.
• Advise patient that drug must be stopped gradually and not to stop taking drug or change the dose before consulting prescriber.
• Caution patient to report increases in Parkinson disease signs or symptoms or adverse effects.
• Stress importance of taking extended-release capsules at bedtime or extended release tablets in the morning.
• If insomnia occurs, tell patient to take drug several hours before bedtime.
• Tell patient that if dizziness occurs when standing up, not to stand or change positions too quickly.
• Instruct patient to notify prescriber of adverse reactions, especially dizziness, depression, anxiety, nausea, and urine retention.
• Caution patient to avoid activities that require mental alertness until effects of drug are known.
• Encourage patient with Parkinson disease to gradually increase physical activity as symptoms improve.
• Advise patient to avoid alcohol while taking drug.

SAFETY ALERT!

ambrisentan
am-bree-SEN-tan

Letairis, Volibris✤

Therapeutic class: Vasodilators
Pharmacologic class: Endothelin-receptor antagonists

AVAILABLE FORMS
Tablets ⓓⓝ: 5 mg, 10 mg

INDICATIONS & DOSAGES
➤ **PAH (WHO Group 1) to improve exercise tolerance and decrease rate of clinical worsening; in combination with tadalafil to reduce risks of disease progression and hospitalization for worsening PAH, and to improve exercise ability**

Adults: 5 mg PO once daily with or without tadalafil 20 mg once daily; at 4-week intervals, may increase ambrisentan to 10 mg PO once daily or tadalafil to 40 mg once daily if tolerated.

ADMINISTRATION
PO
- Drug is considered hazardous: use safe handling and disposal precautions according to facility policy.
- Give without regard for food.
- Give whole; don't crush or split tablets.

ACTION
Blocks endothelin-1 receptors on vascular endothelin and smooth muscle. Stimulation of these receptors in smooth muscle cells is associated with vasoconstriction and PAH.

Route	Onset	Peak	Duration
PO	Rapid	2 hr	Unknown

Half-life: 9 hours.

ADVERSE REACTIONS
CNS: headache. **CV:** peripheral edema, flushing. **EENT:** nasal congestion, sinusitis. **GI:** dyspepsia. **Hematologic:** anemia. **Hepatic:** hepatic impairment. **Respiratory:** cough, bronchitis.

INTERACTIONS
Drug-drug. *Cyclosporine:* May increase ambrisentan level. Use together cautiously. Limit ambrisentan dosage to 5 mg daily.

EFFECTS ON LAB TEST RESULTS
- May increase AST, ALT, and bilirubin levels.
- May decrease Hb level and hematocrit.

CONTRAINDICATIONS & CAUTIONS
- Contraindicated in patients hypersensitive to drug or its components and in those with idiopathic pulmonary fibrosis, including patients with pulmonary HTN.
- Use cautiously in patients with mild hepatic impairment. Not recommended in patients with moderate or severe hepatic impairment.
- Use cautiously in those with renal impairment; drug hasn't been studied in those with severe renal impairment.
- **Alert:** Patients who develop acute pulmonary edema during initial treatment may have pulmonary veno-occlusive disease.

Discontinue drug if pulmonary veno-occlusive disease is confirmed.
Dialyzable drug: Unknown.
⚠ *Overdose S&S:* Headache, flushing, dizziness, nausea, nasal congestion, hypotension.

PREGNANCY-LACTATION-REPRODUCTION
Boxed Warning Contraindicated during pregnancy. May cause birth defects ■
Boxed Warning Must exclude pregnancy before starting therapy. Obtain monthly pregnancy tests during treatment and for 1 month after final dose. ■
Boxed Warning Patients of childbearing potential must use one highly effective form of contraception (intrauterine device, contraceptive implant, or tubal sterilization) or a combination of methods (hormonal method with a barrier method or two barrier methods) during treatment and for 1 month after treatment ends. If a partner's vasectomy is the chosen method of contraception, a hormonal or barrier method must also be used. ■
Boxed Warning Because of risk of embryo-fetal toxicity, ambrisentan is available to females only through the Ambrisentan REMS Program. Only registered prescribers and pharmacies may prescribe and dispense ambrisentan and only to patients enrolled in and meeting all the conditions of REMS at www.ambrisentanrems.us.com or 1-888-417-3172. ■
- It isn't known if drug appears in human milk. Patient should discontinue breastfeeding or discontinue drug.
- Drug may adversely affect spermatogenesis.

NURSING CONSIDERATIONS
- Treat patients of childbearing potential only after negative pregnancy tests.
- Assess Hb level at initiation, at 1 month, and periodically thereafter. Use isn't recommended in patients with significant anemia.
- Monitor patient for fluid retention; diuretic or fluid management may be needed.

PATIENT TEACHING
Boxed Warning Inform patient that monthly pregnancy testing is required during therapy and to immediately report suspected pregnancy to prescriber. ■
- **Alert:** Counsel patient of childbearing potential on contraceptive use.

Reactions in bold italics are *life-threatening*. Interactions may have a *rapid onset* or a *delayed onset*.

• Tell patient that monthly blood tests will be done to monitor for adverse effects.
• Instruct patient in safe drug administration.
• **🛈 Alert:** Teach patient to notify prescriber immediately of signs or symptoms of liver injury, including anorexia, nausea, vomiting, fever, malaise, fatigue, right upper quadrant abdominal discomfort, itching, and jaundice.
• Tell patient to report edema and weight gain.
• Inform male patient of potential for decreased sperm count.

amikacin sulfate
am-i-KAY-sin

Therapeutic class: Antibiotics
Pharmacologic class: Aminoglycosides

AVAILABLE FORMS
Injection: 250 mg/mL vial

INDICATIONS & DOSAGES
Adjust-a-dose (for all indications): Adjust dosage to avoid peak drug level above 35 mcg/mL and trough drug level above 10 mcg/mL. For adults with impaired renal function, initially, 7.5 mg/kg IM or IV. Subsequent doses and frequency determined by amikacin levels and renal function studies. For adults receiving hemodialysis, monitor drug levels and adjust dosage accordingly.
➤ **Serious infections caused by sensitive strains of** *Pseudomonas aeruginosa,* *Escherichia coli, Proteus, Klebsiella,* *Staphylococcus, Providencia, Enterobacter,* *Serratia,* **or** *Acinetobacter*
Adults and children: Maximum dosage is 15 mg/kg/day IM or IV infusion, in divided doses every 8 to 12 hours, for 7 to 10 days. Don't exceed 1.5 g/day.
Neonates: Initially, loading dose of 10 mg/kg IV; then 7.5 mg/kg every 12 hours for 7 to 10 days.
➤ **Uncomplicated UTI caused by organisms not susceptible to less toxic drugs**
Adults: 250 mg IM or IV b.i.d.

ADMINISTRATION
IV
▼ Obtain specimen for culture and sensitivity tests before giving first dose. Begin therapy while awaiting results.

▼ For adults, dilute IV drug in 100 to 200 mL of D₅W or NSS. For children, the amount of fluid will depend on the ordered dose.
▼ In adults and children, infuse over 30 to 60 minutes. In infants, infuse over 1 to 2 hours.
▼ Don't premix with other drugs.
▼ Inspect solution for particulate matter and discoloration before administration.
▼ After infusion, flush line with NSS or D₅W.
▼ Refer to manufacturer's instructions for stability and storage after dilution in D₅W, NSS, and other solutions.
▼ May store vials at room temperature.
▼ **Incompatibilities:** None listed by manufacturer. Consult a drug incompatibility reference for more information.
IM
• Obtain specimen for culture and sensitivity tests before giving first dose. Begin therapy while awaiting results.

ACTION
Inhibits protein synthesis by binding directly to the 30S ribosomal subunit; bactericidal.

Route	Onset	Peak	Duration
IV	Immediate	30 min	8–12 hr
IM	Unknown	1 hr	8–12 hr

Half-life: Adults, 2 hours; patients with severe renal damage, 17 to 150 hours.

ADVERSE REACTIONS
CNS: *neuromuscular blockade.* **EENT:** ototoxicity. **GU:** azotemia, *nephrotoxicity,* increase in urinary excretion of casts. **Respiratory:** *apnea.*

INTERACTIONS
Drug-drug. **Boxed Warning** *Acyclovir,* *amphotericin B, bacitracin, cisplatin, colistin,* *paromomycin, polymyxin B, vancomycin,* *other aminoglycosides:* May increase nephrotoxicity. Avoid use together and monitor renal function test results. ∎
Cephalosporins, penicillins: May inactivate each other in vitro. Don't mix.
Dimenhydrinate: May mask ototoxicity symptoms. Monitor patient's hearing.
Boxed Warning *General anesthetics:* May increase neuromuscular blockade. Monitor patient for increased effects. ∎
Boxed Warning *IV loop diuretics* *(ethacrynic acid, furosemide):* May increase

ototoxicity. Avoid use together and monitor patient's hearing. ∎

Boxed Warning *Neuromuscular blockers:* May increase effects of nondepolarizing muscle relaxants, including prolonged respiratory depression. Use together only when necessary, and expect to reduce dosage of nondepolarizing muscle relaxant. ∎

NSAIDs (indomethacin): May increase amikacin level in premature infants. Avoid administering together or monitor amikacin level if unavoidable.

EFFECTS ON LAB TEST RESULTS
• May increase BUN and creatinine levels.

CONTRAINDICATIONS & CAUTIONS
• Contraindicated in patients hypersensitive to drug or other aminoglycosides.
• Use cautiously in patients with sulfite sensitivity.
• Use cautiously in patients with impaired renal function, hypocalcemia, neuromuscular disorders (myasthenia gravis, parkinsonism), or hearing impairment; neonates and infants; and older adults.
• Drug can cause superinfection such as CDAD, which can be severe and can occur more than 2 months after therapy ends.
Dialyzable drug: Yes.
⚠ *Overdose S&S:* Nephrotoxicity, ototoxicity, neurotoxicity.

PREGNANCY-LACTATION-REPRODUCTION
• There are no well-controlled studies during pregnancy. Other aminoglycosides can cause fetal harm. Not recommended for use during pregnancy. If used during pregnancy, or if patient becomes pregnant while taking drug, apprise patient of potential fetal hazard.
• It isn't known if drug appears in human milk. Patient should discontinue breastfeeding or discontinue drug.

NURSING CONSIDERATIONS
• Obtain blood for peak level 1 hour after IM injection and 30 minutes to 1 hour after IV infusion ends; for trough level, draw blood just before next dose. Don't collect blood in a heparinized tube; heparin is incompatible with aminoglycosides.
Boxed Warning Due to increased risk of ototoxicity, evaluate patient's hearing before and during therapy if patient will be receiving the drug for longer than 2 weeks. Notify

prescriber if patient has tinnitus, vertigo, or hearing loss. ∎

Boxed Warning Weigh patient and review renal function studies before and periodically during therapy.
• Correct dehydration before therapy because of increased risk of toxicity.

Boxed Warning Monitor serum amikacin peak and trough concentrations periodically during therapy. Peak drug levels greater than 35 mcg/mL and trough levels greater than 10 mcg/mL may be linked to a higher risk of toxicity. ∎

Boxed Warning Due to increased risk of nephrotoxicity, monitor renal function: urine output, specific gravity, urinalysis, BUN and creatinine levels, and CrCl. Report evidence of declining renal function to prescriber. Safe use for longer than 14 days hasn't been established. ∎
• Watch for signs and symptoms of superinfection (especially of upper respiratory tract), such as continued fever, chills, and increased pulse rate.

Boxed Warning Neuromuscular blockade and respiratory paralysis have been reported after aminoglycoside administration, especially in patients receiving anesthetics, neuromuscular blockers, or massive transfusions of citrate-anticoagulated blood. If blockade occurs, calcium salts may reverse these phenomena, but mechanical ventilation may be necessary. Monitor patient closely. ∎
• Therapy usually continues for 7 to 10 days. If no response occurs after 3 to 5 days, stop therapy and obtain new specimens for culture and sensitivity testing.
• *Look alike–sound alike:* Don't confuse amikacin with anakinra.

PATIENT TEACHING
• Instruct patient to promptly report all adverse reactions, especially changes in urine, weight gain, edema, hearing impairment, fever, diarrhea, and abdominal pain.
• Inform patient that CDAD may occur a few months after taking antibiotics and to immediately report abdominal pain, cramps, or very loose, watery, or bloody stools.
• Warn patient about risks to fetus if drug is taken during pregnancy and to immediately report possible pregnancy to prescriber.
• Encourage patient to maintain adequate fluid intake.

aMILoride hydrochloride
a-MILL-oh-ride

Midamor✦

Therapeutic class: Diuretics
Pharmacologic class: Potassium-sparing diuretics

AVAILABLE FORMS
Tablets: 5 mg

INDICATIONS & DOSAGES
➤ **To counteract hypokalemia induced by thiazide or other potassium-wasting diuretics in patients with HTN or HF**
Adults: 5 mg PO daily in addition to patient's antihypertensive or diuretic. May increase to 10 mg daily if needed. If hypokalemia persists with 10 mg, may increase to 15 mg, then 20 mg with careful monitoring of electrolyte levels.

ADMINISTRATION
PO
• Give with food to minimize GI upset.
• Store at room temperature.

ACTION
Inhibits sodium reabsorption and potassium excretion in the distal tubules.

Route	Onset	Peak	Duration
PO	2 hr	3–4 hr	24 hr

Half-life: 6 to 9 hours.

ADVERSE REACTIONS
CNS: dizziness, fatigue, headache, weakness, *encephalopathy.* **GI:** abdominal pain, anorexia, appetite changes, constipation, diarrhea, nausea, vomiting, flatulence. **GU:** erectile dysfunction. **Metabolic:** *hyperkalemia.* **Musculoskeletal:** muscle cramps. **Respiratory:** cough, dyspnea.

INTERACTIONS
Drug-drug. *ACE inhibitors, ARBs, canagliflozin, cyclosporine, eplerenone, indomethacin, other potassium-sparing diuretics, potassium supplements, tacrolimus, tolvaptan:* May cause hyperkalemia. Use cautiously together. Monitor potassium level closely.
Digoxin: May affect digoxin clearance and decrease inotropic effects. Monitor digoxin level.
Lithium: May decrease lithium clearance, increasing risk of lithium toxicity. Avoid use together.
NSAIDs: May decrease diuretic effectiveness and cause severe hyperkalemia. Avoid use together.
Drug-food. *Foods high in potassium (such as bananas, oranges), salt substitutes containing potassium:* May cause hyperkalemia. Advise patient to choose diet carefully and to use low-potassium salt substitutes.

EFFECTS ON LAB TEST RESULTS
• May increase BUN and potassium levels.
• May decrease pH and liver enzyme, chloride, and sodium levels.
• May decrease Hb level and neutrophil count.

CONTRAINDICATIONS & CAUTIONS
• Contraindicated in patients hypersensitive to drug, in those with potassium level greater than 5.5 mEq/L, and in those with anuria, acute or chronic renal insufficiency, or diabetic nephropathy.
• Use cautiously in patients with diabetes, cardiopulmonary disease, or severe hepatic insufficiency.
• Use cautiously in older adults or patients who are debilitated.
• Safety and effectiveness in children haven't been established.
Dialyzable drug: Unknown.
⚠ *Overdose S&S:* Dehydration, electrolyte imbalance.

PREGNANCY-LACTATION-REPRODUCTION
• Use during pregnancy only if clearly needed.
• It isn't known if drug appears in human milk. Patient should discontinue breastfeeding or discontinue drug.

NURSING CONSIDERATIONS
Boxed Warning Carefully monitor potassium level because of the risk of hyperkalemia, especially in patients with renal impairment or diabetes and in older adults. Monitor potassium level when drug is initiated, when diuretic dosages are adjusted, and during an illness that could affect renal function. Alert prescriber immediately if potassium level exceeds 5.5 mEq/L; expect to stop drug. ■

• Drug may cause severe hyperkalemia after glucose tolerance testing in patients with diabetes; stop drug at least 3 days before testing.
• Monitor serum electrolyte levels and renal function.
• Monitor acid-base balance in patients who are severely ill and at risk for respiratory or metabolic acidosis.
• *Look alike–sound alike:* Don't confuse amiloride with amiodarone, amlodipine, or inamrinone.

PATIENT TEACHING
• Instruct patient to take drug with food to minimize GI upset.
• Advise patient to avoid sudden posture changes and to rise slowly to avoid dizziness.
• Caution patient not to perform hazardous activities if adverse CNS reactions occur.
• To prevent serious hyperkalemia, warn patient to avoid eating potassium-rich foods, potassium-containing salt substitutes, and potassium supplements.
• Advise patient to report signs of hyperkalemia, such as tingling, muscle weakness, muscle cramps, fatigue, and limb paralysis.
• Instruct patient to check with prescriber before taking new prescriptions or OTC drugs.

SAFETY ALERT!

amiodarone hydrochloride
am-ee-OH-dah-rohn

Nexterone, Pacerone

Therapeutic class: Antiarrhythmics
Pharmacologic class: Benzofuran derivatives

AVAILABLE FORMS
Injection: 50 mg/mL vial; 150 mg/100 mL, 360 mg/200 mL, 450 mg/200 mL, 900 mg/500 mL premixed bag
Tablets: 100 mg, 200 mg, 300 mg, 400 mg

INDICATIONS & DOSAGES
Boxed Warning Amiodarone is intended for use only in patients with life-threatening arrhythmias unresponsive to adequate doses of other antiarrhythmics or when alternative drugs can't be tolerated. ∎
➤ **Prevention of recurrent life-threatening ventricular arrhythmias, such as ventricular fibrillation or hemodynamically unstable ventricular tachycardia**
Adults: Give loading dose of 800 to 1,600 mg PO daily or divided into two equal doses daily for 1 to 3 weeks until first therapeutic response occurs; then 600 to 800 mg PO daily for 1 month, followed by maintenance dose of 400 mg PO daily or, for patients with severe GI intolerance, 200 mg PO b.i.d. Determine long-term maintenance dose according to antiarrhythmic effect.

Or, give loading dose of 150 mg IV over 10 minutes (15 mg/minute); then 360 mg IV over next 6 hours (1 mg/minute), followed by 540 mg IV over next 18 hours (0.5 mg/minute). After first 24 hours, continue with maintenance IV infusion of 720 mg/24 hours (0.5 mg/minute).

Maintenance infusion can continue cautiously for 2 to 3 weeks. To convert to oral form from IV (based on a 720-mg/day infusion): If IV infusion has been for less than 1 week, initial dose is 800 to 1,600 mg PO daily; if IV infusion has been from 1 to 3 weeks, initial dose is 600 to 800 mg PO daily; if IV infusion has been more than 3 weeks, initial dose is 400 mg PO daily.

If breakthrough episodes of ventricular fibrillation or hemodynamically unstable ventricular tachycardia occur, may give supplemental infusions of 150 mg IV over 10 minutes.

ADMINISTRATION
Boxed Warning Drug can exacerbate arrhythmias and should be initiated in a clinical setting where continuous ECG monitoring and cardiac resuscitation are available. ∎
PO
• Divide oral loading dose into two or three equal doses and give with meals to decrease GI intolerance. Give maintenance dose once daily or divide into two doses with meals to decrease GI intolerance.
IV
▼ Give drug IV only if continuous ECG and electrophysiologic monitoring are available.
▼ Mix first dose of 150 mg in 100 mL of D_5W solution followed by 360 mg in 200 mL of D_5W solution for maintenance infusion.
▼ If infusion will last 2 hours or longer, mix solution in glass or polyolefin bottles.

▼ If concentration is 2 mg/mL or more, give drug through a central line. If possible, use a dedicated line.

▼ Drug may be a vesicant; ensure proper needle or catheter placement before and during IV infusion and avoid extravasation.

▼ Use an in-line filter.

▼ Continuously monitor patient's cardiac status. If hypotension occurs, reduce infusion rate.

▼ IV amiodarone leaches out plasticizers from IV tubing and adsorbs to polyvinyl chloride (PVC) tubing, which can adversely affect male reproductive tract development in fetuses, infants, and toddlers when used at concentrations or flow rates outside of recommendations.

▼ **Incompatibilities:** Aminophylline, ampicillin sodium–sulbactam sodium, bivalirudin, cefazolin sodium, ceftazidime, digoxin, furosemide, heparin sodium, imipenem–cilastatin sodium, magnesium sulfate, micafungin, nitroprusside sodium, NSS, piperacillin sodium, piperacillin–tazobactam sodium, quinidine gluconate, sodium bicarbonate, sodium phosphates, potassium phosphates. Refer to a compatibility reference for other drugs.

ACTION
Inhibits adrenergic stimulation and blocks sodium and potassium channels, leading to a prolongation of action potential duration.

Route	Onset	Peak	Duration
PO	Variable	3–7 hr	Variable
IV	Unknown	Unknown	Variable

Half-life: Oral, 15 to 142 days; IV single dose mean range, 9 to 36 days.

ADVERSE REACTIONS
CNS: fatigue, malaise, tremor, peripheral neuropathy, ataxia, paresthesia, insomnia, sleep disturbances, headache, dizziness, lack of coordination, abnormal taste, abnormal smell. **CV:** hypotension, *asystole,* atrial fibrillation, *bradycardia, arrhythmias, HF, heart block, sinus arrest,* edema, flushing. **EENT:** asymptomatic corneal microdeposits, visual disturbances, optic neuropathy or neuritis resulting in visual impairment, abnormal salivation. **GI:** nausea, vomiting, anorexia, constipation, abdominal pain, diarrhea. **Hematologic:** *coagulation abnormalities.* **Hepatic:** *hepatic failure,* hepatic

dysfunction. **Metabolic:** hypothyroidism, hyperthyroidism. **Respiratory:** *ARDS, severe pulmonary toxicity, pulmonary edema, eosinophilic pneumonitis.* **Skin:** photosensitivity, blue-gray skin. **Other:** decreased libido.

INTERACTIONS
Drug-drug. *Antiarrhythmics:* May reduce hepatic or renal clearance of certain antiarrhythmics, especially flecainide, procainamide, and quinidine. Use of amiodarone with other antiarrhythmics, especially mexiletine, propafenone, disopyramide, and procainamide, may induce torsades de pointes. Avoid using together.

Azole antifungals, disopyramide, pimozide: May increase the risk of arrhythmias, including torsades de pointes. Avoid using together.

Beta blockers, calcium channel blockers: May potentiate bradycardia, sinus arrest, and AV block; may increase hypotensive effect. Use together cautiously.

Cimetidine: May increase amiodarone level. Use together cautiously.

Cyclosporine: May increase cyclosporine level, resulting in an increase in serum creatinine level and renal toxicity. Monitor cyclosporine levels and renal function tests.

Dabigatran: May increase bleeding risk. Monitor patient closely.

Digoxin: May increase digoxin level 70% to 100%. Monitor digoxin level closely, and reduce digoxin dosage by half or stop drug completely when starting amiodarone therapy.

Fentanyl: May cause hypotension, bradycardia, and decreased cardiac output. Monitor patient closely.

Fluoroquinolones: May increase risk of arrhythmias, including torsades de pointes. Avoid using together.

HMG-CoA reductase inhibitors (lovastatin, simvastatin): May cause myopathy or rhabdomyolysis. Lovastatin dosage shouldn't exceed 40 mg daily. Simvastatin dosage shouldn't exceed 20 mg daily. Lower the dosages of other drugs in this class. Monitor patient carefully.

Loratadine, trazodone: May cause prolonged QT interval and torsades de pointes. Monitor closely.

Macrolide antibiotics (azithromycin, clarithromycin, erythromycin): May cause additive prolongation of the QT interval. Use with caution.

Phenytoin: May decrease phenytoin metabolism and increase phenytoin level. May decrease amiodarone level. Monitor phenytoin level and adjust dosages of drugs if needed.

Protease inhibitors (amprenavir, atazanavir, lopinavir–ritonavir, nelfinavir, ritonavir, saquinavir): May increase the risk of amiodarone toxicity. Use of ritonavir or nelfinavir with amiodarone is contraindicated. Use other protease inhibitors cautiously.

Quinidine: May increase quinidine level, causing life-threatening cardiac arrhythmias. Avoid using together, or monitor patient closely if use together can't be avoided. Adjust quinidine dosage as needed.

Rifamycins: May decrease amiodarone level. Monitor patient closely.

Theophylline: May increase theophylline level and cause toxicity. Monitor theophylline level.

Warfarin: May increase anticoagulant response, with the potential for serious or fatal bleeding. Decrease warfarin dosage 33% to 50% when starting amiodarone. Monitor patient closely.

Drug-herb. *St. John's wort:* May decrease amiodarone levels. Discourage use together.

Drug-food. *Grapefruit juice:* May inhibit CYP3A4 metabolism of drug in the intestinal mucosa, causing increased levels and risk of toxicity. Discourage use together.

Drug-lifestyle. *Sun exposure:* May cause photosensitivity reaction. Advise patient to take precautions.

EFFECTS ON LAB TEST RESULTS
- May increase ALP, ALT, AST, GGT, inactive reverse T_3, and T_4 levels.
- May decrease T_3 level.
- May prolong PT and increase INR.

CONTRAINDICATIONS & CAUTIONS
- Contraindicated in patients hypersensitive to drug or to iodine.
- Contraindicated in those with cardiogenic shock, second- or third-degree AV block, severe SA node disease resulting in bradycardia unless an artificial pacemaker is present, and in those for whom bradycardia has caused syncope.
- Use cautiously in patients receiving other antiarrhythmics. Upon starting amiodarone,

attempt to gradually discontinue prior antiarrhythmics.
- Use cautiously in patients with pulmonary, hepatic, or thyroid disease.

Boxed Warning Drug may cause pulmonary and liver toxicity, which can be fatal. ▐

🕒 *Alert:* Avoid use in patients with Wolff-Parkinson-White syndrome and preexcited atrial fibrillation or flutter.
- Safety and effectiveness in children haven't been established. Life-threatening gasping syndrome may occur in neonates given IV solutions containing benzyl alcohol.

Dialyzable drug: No.

⚠ *Overdose S&S:* AV block, bradycardia, hypotension, cardiogenic shock, hepatotoxicity.

PREGNANCY-LACTATION-REPRODUCTION
- Drug may cause fetal harm. Use during pregnancy only to treat life-threatening or refractory arrhythmias.
- Drug appears in human milk. Contraindicated during breastfeeding.

NURSING CONSIDERATIONS
- Be aware of the high risk of adverse reactions.
- Obtain baseline thyroid function tests.

🕒 *Alert:* Drug may cause hyperthyroidism or hypothyroidism. Hyperthyroidism can result in fatal thyrotoxicosis or arrhythmia. If hyperthyroidism or hypothyroidism occurs, reduce dosage or discontinue drug. Thyroid nodules and thyroid cancer have been reported. Use cautiously in patients with thyroid disease. Monitor thyroid function during treatment, particularly in older adults and patients with underlying thyroid dysfunction.

Boxed Warning Drug may pose life-threatening management problems in patients at risk for sudden death. Use only in patients with life-threatening, recurrent ventricular arrhythmias unresponsive to or intolerant of other antiarrhythmics or alternative drugs. ▐

Boxed Warning Drug is highly toxic. Watch carefully for pulmonary toxicity. Obtain baseline chest X-ray and pulmonary function tests. Reassess history, physical exam, and chest X-ray every 3 to 6 months and as clinically indicated. ▐
- Watch for evidence of pneumonitis, exertional dyspnea, nonproductive cough, and pleuritic chest pain.

Boxed Warning Monitor patient for hepatotoxicity. Obtain baseline and periodic LFTs.

Reactions in bold italics are *life-threatening*. Interactions may have a *rapid onset* or a *delayed onset*.

Discontinue or reduce dosage if LFT values exceed 3 × ULN or double in a patient with elevated baseline LFT values. Discontinue for signs or symptoms of liver injury. Liver injury is common and is usually mild but has been fatal in a few cases. ■

- Correct electrolyte imbalances before start of therapy and throughout treatment.
- Monitor electrolyte levels, particularly potassium and magnesium.
- Monitor PT and INR if patient takes warfarin and digoxin level if patient takes digoxin.
- Regular ophthalmic exams are advised to monitor patient for optic neuropathy, optic neuritis, and corneal microdeposits.
- Monitor BP and HR and rhythm frequently. Perform continuous ECG monitoring when starting or changing dosage. Notify prescriber of significant change in assessment results.

◑ *Alert:* Patients may continue to be at risk for drug-related adverse reactions or drug interactions after discontinuation of amiodarone.

◑ *Alert:* May cause life-threatening or fatal reactions, including SJS and TEN. Discontinue drug immediately if such signs or symptoms as progressive rash with blisters or mucosal lesions occur.

- During or after treatment with IV form, patient may be transferred to oral therapy.
- *Look alike–sound alike:* Don't confuse amiodarone with amiloride.

PATIENT TEACHING

- Advise patient to wear sunscreen or protective clothing to prevent sensitivity reaction to the sun. Monitor patient for skin burning or tingling, followed by redness and blistering. Exposed skin may turn blue-gray.
- Advise patient to keep follow-up appointments, including eye exams and blood tests.
- Tell patient to report vision changes, weakness, "pins and needles" or numbness, poor coordination, weight change, heat or cold intolerance, neck swelling, progressive rash, or mucosal lesions.
- Tell patient to take oral drug with food if GI reactions occur.
- Inform patient that adverse effects of drug are more common at high doses and become more frequent with treatment lasting longer than 6 months, but are generally reversible when drug is stopped. Resolution of adverse reactions may take up to 4 months.

- Tell patient not to stop taking drug without consulting prescriber.
- Inform patient of potential hazard to the fetus if drug is used during pregnancy.

amitriptyline hydrochloride
a-mih-TRIP-ti-leen

Elavil✤

Therapeutic class: Antidepressants
Pharmacologic class: TCAs

AVAILABLE FORMS
Tablets: 10 mg, 25 mg, 50 mg, 75 mg, 100 mg, 150 mg

INDICATIONS & DOSAGES
➤ **Depression (outpatients)**
Adults: 75 mg PO daily in divided doses. Or, 50 to 100 mg PO daily as single dose at bedtime or in divided doses. May increase by 25 to 50 mg, as needed, to a total of 150 mg/day. Make increases preferably in late afternoon or at bedtime. Titrate maintenance dosage to lowest dose that will maintain relief of symptoms, usually 40 to 100 mg daily. Continue maintenance therapy for at least 3 months.
Older adults and adolescents: 10 mg PO t.i.d. plus 20 mg at bedtime daily.
➤ **Depression (patients who are hospitalized)**
Adults: Initially, 100 mg PO daily. If necessary, gradually increase to 200 to 300 mg daily.

ADMINISTRATION
PO
- Give drug without regard for food.
- Give higher doses in late afternoon or at bedtime to minimize daytime sedation.
- May give maintenance dose as a single dose at bedtime.

ACTION
Unknown. May increase amount of norepinephrine, serotonin, or both in the CNS by blocking their reuptake by the presynaptic neurons.

Route	Onset	Peak	Duration
PO	Unknown	2–5 hr	Unknown

Half-life: 13 to 36 hours.

ADVERSE REACTIONS

CNS: *stroke, seizures, coma,* ataxia, tremor, peripheral neuropathy, anxiety, insomnia, nightmares, restlessness, drowsiness, dizziness, syncope, weakness, fatigue, headache, extrapyramidal reactions, hallucinations, delusions, confusion, incoordination, numbness, tingling, paresthesia, dysarthria, disturbed concentration, excitement, disorientation, fever, peculiar taste. **CV:** orthostatic hypotension, tachycardia, *heart block, arrhythmias, MI,* ECG changes, HTN, edema, palpitations. **EENT:** blurred vision, mydriasis, increased IOP, tinnitus, dry mouth, black tongue, parotid swelling. **GI:** nausea, vomiting, anorexia, epigastric pain, diarrhea, constipation, paralytic ileus, stomatitis. **GU:** urine retention, urinary frequency, erectile dysfunction, testicular swelling. **Hematologic:** *agranulocytosis, thrombocytopenia, leukopenia,* purpura, eosinophilia. **Metabolic:** *hypoglycemia,* hyperglycemia, SIADH, weight gain or loss. **Skin:** rash, urticaria, alopecia, photosensitivity reactions, diaphoresis. **Other:** hypersensitivity reactions, gynecomastia, female galactorrhea, altered libido.

INTERACTIONS

Drug-drug. *Antiemetics (5HT₃), antipsychotics, linezolid, methylene blue:* May cause serotonin syndrome. Avoid combination.
Barbiturates: May increase amitriptyline metabolism. Consider therapy modification.
Cimetidine: May decrease TCA metabolism. Monitor therapy.
CNS depressants: May enhance CNS depression. Avoid using together.
Disulfiram: May increase amitriptyline level and risk of CNS toxicity. Monitor patient closely.
Drugs that prolong QT interval (antiarrhythmics, chlorpromazine, clarithromycin, haloperidol, levofloxacin, quinolones, thioridazine): May increase risk of life-threatening arrhythmia, including torsades de pointes. Use together cautiously.
Epinephrine, norepinephrine: May increase hypertensive effect. Use together cautiously.
Fluoxetine, fluvoxamine, hormonal contraceptives, paroxetine, sertraline: May increase TCA level. Consider therapy modification.
MAO inhibitors: May cause severe excitation, hyperpyrexia, or seizures, usually with high doses. Avoid using within 14 days of MAO inhibitor therapy.
Topiramate: May increase amitriptyline level. Adjust amitriptyline dosage.
Drug-herb. *SAM-e, St. John's wort, yohimbe:* May cause serotonin syndrome and decrease amitriptyline level. Discourage use together.
Drug-lifestyle. *Alcohol use:* May enhance CNS depression. Discourage use together.
Smoking: May lower drug level. Watch for lack of effect.
Sun exposure: May increase risk of photosensitivity reactions. Advise patient to take precautions.

EFFECTS ON LAB TEST RESULTS

- May increase LFT values.
- May increase or decrease glucose level.
- May increase eosinophil count.
- May decrease granulocyte, platelet, and WBC counts.

CONTRAINDICATIONS & CAUTIONS

- Contraindicated in patients hypersensitive to drug, in those who have received an MAO inhibitor within the past 14 days, and in the acute MI recovery phase.
- ⚠ *Alert:* Concomitant use with linezolid or methylene blue can cause serotonin syndrome (fever, mental status changes, muscle twitching, excessive sweating, shivering or shaking, diarrhea, loss of coordination). Use drug with linezolid or methylene blue only for life-threatening or urgent conditions when the potential benefits outweigh the risks of toxicity.
- Drug isn't approved for use in children younger than age 12.
- Use cautiously in patients with history of seizures, urine retention, angle-closure glaucoma, or increased IOP; in those with hyperthyroidism, CV disease, diabetes, or impaired liver function; and in those receiving thyroid drugs.
- Use cautiously in older adults and in patients with suicidality.
- Use cautiously in those receiving electroconvulsive therapy.
- Avoid use in patients with bipolar disorder; drug may precipitate a shift to mania or hypomania.
Dialyzable drug: No.
- ⚠ *Overdose S&S:* Cardiac arrhythmias, severe hypotension, seizures, CNS depression, coma, impaired myocardial contractility, confusion, disturbed concentration, transient

---

visual hallucinations, dilated pupils, disorders of ocular motility, agitation, hyperactive reflexes, polyradiculoneuropathy, stupor, drowsiness, muscle rigidity, vomiting, hypothermia, hyperpyrexia.

PREGNANCY-LACTATION-REPRODUCTION

• There are no adequate and well-controlled studies during pregnancy. Use during pregnancy only if potential benefit outweighs fetal risk.
• Drug appears in human milk. Patient should discontinue breastfeeding or discontinue drug.

NURSING CONSIDERATIONS

Boxed Warning Drug may increase the risk of suicidal thinking and behavior in children, adolescents, and young adults with major depressive disorder or other psychiatric disorder. Monitor all patients closely for clinical worsening, suicidality, or unusual changes in behavior, especially at start of therapy. ■
◐ *Alert:* If linezolid or methylene blue must be given, amitriptyline must be stopped and patient should be monitored for serotonin toxicity for 2 weeks, or until 24 hours after the last dose of methylene blue or linezolid, whichever comes first. Treatment with amitriptyline may be resumed 24 hours after last dose of methylene blue or linezolid.
• Amitriptyline has strong anticholinergic effects and is one of the most sedating TCAs. Anticholinergic effects have rapid onset even though therapeutic effect is delayed for weeks.
• Older adults may have an increased sensitivity to anticholinergic effects of drug; sedating effects of drug may increase the risk of falls in this population.
• If signs or symptoms of psychosis occur or increase, expect prescriber to reduce dosage. Record mood changes. Monitor patient for suicidal tendencies and allow only minimum supply of drug.
• Because patients using TCAs may suffer hypertensive episodes and arrhythmias during surgery, stop drug gradually several days before surgery.
• Monitor glucose level.
• Watch for nausea, headache, and malaise after abrupt withdrawal of long-term therapy; these symptoms don't indicate addiction.
• Don't withdraw drug abruptly.

• *Look alike–sound alike:* Don't confuse amitriptyline with nortriptyline or aminophylline. Don't confuse Elavil with Eldepryl or enalapril.

PATIENT TEACHING

Boxed Warning Advise family and caregivers to closely observe patient for increased suicidal thinking and behavior. ■
◐ *Alert:* Teach patient to recognize and immediately report symptoms of serotonin toxicity (fever, mental status changes, muscle twitching, excessive sweating, shivering or shaking, diarrhea, loss of coordination).
• Advise patient to take full dose at bedtime when possible; however, caution patient that morning orthostatic hypotension may occur.
• Tell patient to avoid alcohol during drug therapy.
• Advise patient to consult prescriber before taking other drugs.
• Warn patient to avoid activities that require alertness and psychomotor coordination until CNS effects of drug are known. Drowsiness and dizziness usually subside after a few weeks.
• Inform patient that dry mouth may be relieved with sugarless hard candy or gum. Saliva substitutes may be useful.
• Advise patient to use a sunblock, wear protective clothing, and avoid prolonged exposure to strong sunlight.
• Warn patient not to stop drug abruptly.
• Advise patient that it may take as long as 30 days to achieve full therapeutic effect.

amLODIPine besylate
am-LOE-di-peen

Katerzia, Norvasc🖉

Therapeutic class: Antihypertensives
Pharmacologic class: Calcium channel blockers

AVAILABLE FORMS
Suspension: 1 mg/mL
Tablets: 2.5 mg, 5 mg, 10 mg

INDICATIONS & DOSAGES
Adjust-a-dose (for all indications): For older adults, patients who are small or frail or have hepatic insufficiency, and those taking other antihypertensives, initially 2.5 mg PO daily.

➤ **Chronic stable angina, vasospastic angina (Prinzmetal or variant angina); to reduce risk of hospitalization because of angina; to reduce risk of coronary revascularization procedure in patients with recently documented CAD by angiography and without HF or with LVEF less than 40%**

Adults: Initially, 5 to 10 mg PO daily. Titrate over 7 to 14 days according to response and tolerance. Most patients need 10 mg daily.

➤ **HTN**

Adults: Initially, 5 mg PO daily. Titrate over 7 to 14 days according to response and tolerance. Maximum daily dose, 10 mg.

Children ages 6 to 17: 2.5 to 5 mg PO once daily. Maximum dose, 5 mg daily.

ADMINISTRATION

PO
- Give without regard for food.
- Shake suspension before using.
- Refrigerate oral suspension; don't freeze.

ACTION

Inhibits calcium ion influx across cardiac and smooth-muscle cells, dilates coronary arteries and arterioles, and decreases BP and myocardial oxygen demand.

Route	Onset	Peak	Duration
PO	Unknown	6–12 hr	24 hr

Half-life: 30 to 50 hours.

ADVERSE REACTIONS

CNS: headache, somnolence, fatigue, dizziness, asthenia. **CV:** edema, flushing, palpitations. **GI:** nausea, abdominal pain. **GU:** sexual dysfunction. **Musculoskeletal:** cramps. **Respiratory:** dyspnea. **Skin:** pruritus, rash.

INTERACTIONS

Drug-drug. *Conivaptan, moderate and strong CYP3A4 inhibitors (clarithromycin, itraconazole, ketoconazole, ritonavir):* May increase amlodipine plasma concentration. Monitor patient for hypotension and edema.
Cyclosporine (systemic), tacrolimus: May increase cyclosporine or tacrolimus level. Monitor levels and patient.
Sildenafil: May increase risk of hypotension. Monitor BP closely.
Simvastatin: May increase risk of myopathy, including rhabdomyolysis. Simvastatin dosage shouldn't exceed 20 mg daily.

EFFECTS ON LAB TEST RESULTS

None reported.

CONTRAINDICATIONS & CAUTIONS

- Contraindicated in patients hypersensitive to drug.
- Use cautiously in patients receiving other peripheral vasodilators, especially those with severe aortic stenosis or hypertrophic cardiomyopathy with outflow tract obstruction, and in patients with HF with reduced LVEF. Because drug is metabolized by the liver, use cautiously and in reduced dosage in patients with severe hepatic disease.
- Safety and effectiveness in children younger than age 6 haven't been established.
Dialyzable drug: No.
⚠ *Overdose S&S:* Marked peripheral vasodilation with hypotension and possibly reflex tachycardia.

PREGNANCY-LACTATION-REPRODUCTION

- Use in pregnancy only if potential benefit justifies the risk to the fetus. Other antihypertensives are preferred during pregnancy.
- Drug appears in human milk. Use cautiously during breastfeeding.

NURSING CONSIDERATIONS

⚠ *Alert:* Monitor patient carefully. Some patients, especially those with severe obstructive CAD, have developed increased frequency, duration, or severity of angina or acute MI after initiation of calcium channel blocker therapy or at time of dosage increase.
- Monitor BP frequently during initiation of therapy. Because drug-induced vasodilation has a gradual onset, acute hypotension is rare.
- Notify prescriber if signs of HF occur, such as swelling of hands and feet or shortness of breath.
⚠ *Alert:* Abrupt withdrawal of drug may increase frequency and duration of chest pain. Taper dose gradually under medical supervision.
- *Look alike–sound alike:* Don't confuse amlodipine with amiloride.

PATIENT TEACHING

- Caution patient to report all adverse reactions and to continue taking drug, even when feeling better.
- Tell patient SL nitroglycerin may be taken as needed when angina symptoms are acute. If patient continues nitrate therapy during

---

Reactions in bold italics are *life-threatening*. Interactions may have a *rapid onset* or a *delayed onset*.

adjustment of amlodipine dosage, urge continued adherence.
• Advise patient to shake suspension before using.

amoxicillin
a-moks-i-SIL-in

Amoxil, Apo-Amoxi ✦, Auro-Amoxicillin ✦, Novamoxin ✦

Therapeutic class: Antibiotics
Pharmacologic class: Aminopenicillins

AVAILABLE FORMS
Capsules: 250 mg, 500 mg
Oral suspension: 50 mg/mL (pediatric drops); 125 mg/5 mL, 200 mg/5 mL, 250 mg/5 mL, 400 mg/5 mL (after reconstitution)
Tablets: 500 mg, 875 mg
Tablets (chewable): 125 mg, 250 mg

INDICATIONS & DOSAGES
Adjust-a-dose (for all indications): Adults with GFR of less than 30 mL/minute shouldn't receive the 875-mg tablet. Adults with GFR of 10 to 30 mL/minute should receive 250 or 500 mg every 12 hours depending on the infection. Adults with GFR of less than 10 mL/minute should receive 250 or 500 mg every 24 hours depending on the severity of the infection. Adults on hemodialysis should receive 250 or 500 mg every 24 hours with an extra dose both during and at the end of dialysis.
➤ **Mild to moderate infections of the ear, nose, and throat; skin and skin structure; or GU tract**
Adults and children weighing 40 kg or more: 500 mg PO every 12 hours or 250 mg PO every 8 hours.
Children older than age 3 months weighing less than 40 kg: 25 mg/kg/day PO divided every 12 hours or 20 mg/kg/day PO divided every 8 hours.
Neonates and infants up to age 3 months: Up to 30 mg/kg/day PO divided every 12 hours.
➤ **Mild to severe infections of the lower respiratory tract and severe infections of the ear, nose, and throat; skin and skin structure; or GU tract**
Adults and children weighing 40 kg or more: 875 mg PO every 12 hours or 500 mg PO every 8 hours.

Children older than age 3 months weighing less than 40 kg: 45 mg/kg/day PO divided every 12 hours or 40 mg/kg/day PO divided every 8 hours.
Neonates and infants up to age 3 months: Up to 30 mg/kg/day PO divided every 12 hours.
➤ **Pharyngitis, tonsillitis, or both secondary to *Streptococcus pyogenes* infection**
Adults and children weighing 40 kg or more: 875 mg every 12 hours or 500 mg every 8 hours for at least 10 days.
Children older than age 3 months weighing less than 40 kg: 45 mg/kg/day PO divided every 12 hours or 40 mg/kg/day PO divided every 8 hours for at least 10 days.
Neonates and infants up to age 3 months: Up to 30 mg/kg/day PO divided every 12 hours for at least 10 days.
➤ ***Helicobacter pylori* eradication to reduce risk of duodenal ulcer recurrence**
Adults: Amoxicillin 1 g with lansoprazole 30 mg PO every 8 hours for 14 days (dual therapy). Or, amoxicillin 1 g, clarithromycin 500 mg, and lansoprazole 30 mg, all given PO every 12 hours for 14 days (triple therapy). Consult latest guidelines for recommendations due to increasing macrolide resistance.

ADMINISTRATION
PO
• Before giving, ask patient about allergic reactions to penicillin. A negative history of penicillin allergy is no guarantee against allergic reaction.
• Obtain specimen for culture and sensitivity tests before giving first dose. Begin therapy while awaiting results.
• Give drug with or without food.
• Shake oral suspension vigorously after reconstitution and before giving.
• For a child, place drops directly on child's tongue for swallowing or add to formula, milk, fruit juice, water, ginger ale, or other cold drink for immediate and complete consumption.
• Store reconstituted oral suspension in refrigerator, if possible. Be sure to check individual product labels for storage information.

ACTION
Inhibits cell-wall synthesis during bacterial multiplication.

Route	Onset	Peak	Duration
PO	Unknown	1–2 hr	6–8 hr

Half-life: 1 to 1.5 hours (7.5 hours in severe renal impairment).

ADVERSE REACTIONS

GI: diarrhea, nausea, *pseudomembranous colitis,* vomiting. **GU:** interstitial nephritis, nephropathy. **Skin:** rash. **Other:** *anaphylaxis,* hypersensitivity reactions, overgrowth of nonsusceptible organisms.

INTERACTIONS

Drug-drug. *Allopurinol:* Increases incidence of rashes from both drugs as compared to amoxicillin alone. Monitor patient closely for rashes.

Chloramphenicol, macrolides, sulfonamides, tetracycline: May reduce therapeutic action of penicillins. Monitor therapy.

Hormonal contraceptives: May decrease oral contraceptive effectiveness. Advise use of additional form of contraception during penicillin therapy.

Live-virus vaccines: May decrease effectiveness of live-virus vaccines. Concurrent use isn't recommended.

Methotrexate: May increase methotrexate serum concentration. Monitor patient closely for toxicity.

Probenecid: May increase levels of amoxicillin and other penicillins. Probenecid may be used for this purpose.

Warfarin: May enhance anticoagulant effect. Use together cautiously.

EFFECTS ON LAB TEST RESULTS

- May increase AST and ALT levels.
- May decrease aminoglycoside level.
- May increase eosinophil count.
- May decrease Hb level and granulocyte, platelet, and WBC counts.
- May alter results of urine glucose tests that use cupric sulfate, such as Benedict reagent and Clinitest.
- May cause transient decrease in total conjugated estriol, estriol glucuronide, conjugated estrone, and estradiol during pregnancy.

CONTRAINDICATIONS & CAUTIONS

- Contraindicated in patients hypersensitive to drug or other penicillins.
- Use cautiously in patients with other drug allergies (especially to cephalosporins) because of possible cross-sensitivity.
- Use cautiously in those with mononucleosis because of high risk of maculopapular rash.
- Use cautiously in older adults.

Dializable drug: Yes.

⚠ *Overdose S&S:* Oliguric renal failure.

PREGNANCY-LACTATION-REPRODUCTION

- Use during pregnancy only if clearly needed.
- Drug appears in human milk. Use cautiously during breastfeeding.

NURSING CONSIDERATIONS

- If large doses are given or if therapy is prolonged, bacterial or fungal superinfection may occur, especially in older adults and patients with immunosuppression or debilitation.
- CDAD, ranging from mild diarrhea to fatal colitis, has been reported with nearly all antibacterial agents, including amoxicillin. Evaluate patient if diarrhea occurs.
- Amoxicillin usually causes fewer cases of diarrhea than ampicillin.
- Monitor patient for hypersensitivity reactions, including anaphylaxis and SJS.
- *Look alike–sound alike:* Don't confuse amoxicillin with ampicillin, amoxapine.

PATIENT TEACHING

- Tell patient to take entire quantity of drug exactly as prescribed, even after feeling better.
- Instruct patient in proper drug administration and storage.
- Tell patient to report rash, fever, or chills. Rash is the most common allergic reaction, especially if patient is also taking allopurinol.

amoxicillin–clavulanate potassium

a-mox-i-SILL-in/KLAV-yu-lah-nate

Augmentin, Augmentin ES-600, Clavulin ✦

Therapeutic class: Antibiotics
Pharmacologic class: Aminopenicillins–beta-lactamase inhibitors

AVAILABLE FORMS

Oral suspension (after reconstitution): 125 mg amoxicillin trihydrate, 31.25 mg clavulanic acid/5 mL; 200 mg amoxicillin trihydrate, 28.5 mg clavulanic acid/5 mL; 250 mg amoxicillin trihydrate, 62.5 mg clavulanic acid/5 mL; 400 mg amoxicillin

---

Reactions in bold italics are *life-threatening.* Interactions may have a *rapid onset* or a *delayed onset.*

trihydrate, 57 mg clavulanic acid/5 mL;
600 mg amoxicillin trihydrate, 42.9 mg clavulanic acid/5 mL
Tablets: 875 mg amoxicillin trihydrate,
125 mg clavulanic acid
Tablets (chewable): 200 mg amoxicillin trihydrate, 28.5 mg clavulanic acid; 400 mg amoxicillin trihydrate, 57 mg clavulanic acid
Tablets (extended-release): 1 g amoxicillin trihydrate, 62.5 mg clavulanic acid
Tablets (film-coated): 250 mg amoxicillin trihydrate, 125 mg clavulanic acid; 500 mg amoxicillin trihydrate, 125 mg clavulanic acid

INDICATIONS & DOSAGES

➤ **Lower respiratory tract infections, otitis media, sinusitis, skin and skin-structure infections, and UTIs caused by susceptible strains of gram-positive and gram-negative organisms**
Adults and children weighing 40 kg or more:
250 mg PO, based on amoxicillin component, every 8 hours; or 500 mg every 12 hours. For more severe infections, 500 mg every 8 hours or 875 mg every 12 hours.
Children age 3 months and older weighing less than 40 kg: 20 to 45 mg/kg/day PO, based on amoxicillin component and severity of infection, daily in divided doses every 8 to 12 hours.
Children younger than age 3 months: 30 mg/kg/day PO, based on amoxicillin component of the 125 mg/5 mL oral suspension, in divided doses every 12 hours.
Adjust-a-dose: Don't give the 875-mg tablet to patients with CrCl of less than 30 mL/minute. If CrCl is 10 to 30 mL/minute, give 250 to 500 mg PO every 12 hours. If CrCl is less than 10 mL/minute, give 250 to 500 mg PO every 24 hours. Give patients on hemodialysis 250 to 500 mg PO every 24 hours with an additional dose both during and after dialysis.
➤ **Otitis media caused by *Streptococcus pneumoniae, Haemophilius influenzae*, or *Moraxella catarrhalis* after antibiotic exposure for otitis media within the preceding 3 months in child age 2 or younger or attending day-care center**
Children age 3 months to younger than 2 years: 90 mg/kg/day PO based on amoxicillin component of 600 mg/5 mL oral suspension in divided doses every 12 hours.
➤ **Acute bacterial sinusitis or community-acquired pneumonia caused by**

Haemophilus influenzae, M. catarrhalis, H. parainfluenzae, Klebsiella pneumoniae, methicillin-susceptible *Staphylococcus aureus,* or *S. pneumoniae*
Adults and children weighing more than 40 kg: 2 g amoxicillin/125 mg clavulanic acid (two extended-release tablets) PO every 12 hours for 10 days (sinusitis) or 7 to 10 days (pneumonia).

ADMINISTRATION
PO
• Before giving drug, ask patient about allergic reactions to penicillin. A negative history of penicillin allergy is no guarantee against an allergic reaction.
• Obtain specimen for culture and sensitivity tests before giving first dose. Begin therapy while awaiting results.
• Give drug at the start of a meal to enhance absorption and decrease GI intolerance.
• Give drug at least 1 hour before a bacteriostatic antibiotic.
• Avoid use of 250-mg tablet in children weighing less than 40 kg. Use chewable form instead.
• After reconstitution, refrigerate the oral suspension; discard after 10 days.

ACTION
Amoxicillin prevents bacterial cell-wall synthesis during replication. Clavulanic acid increases amoxicillin's effectiveness by inactivating beta-lactamases, which destroy amoxicillin.

Route	Onset	Peak	Duration
PO	Unknown	1–2.5 hr	Unknown

Half-life: 1 to 1.5 hours. For patients with severe renal impairment, 7.5 hours for amoxicillin and 4.5 hours for clavulanate.

ADVERSE REACTIONS
GI: nausea, vomiting, diarrhea. **GU:** vaginal candidiasis, vaginitis. **Skin:** rash, candidal diaper rash, diaper rash, urticaria. **Other:** hypersensitivity reactions.

INTERACTIONS
Drug-drug. *Allopurinol:* May increase risk of rash. Monitor patient for rash.
Hormonal contraceptives: May decrease hormonal contraceptive effectiveness. Advise use of additional form of contraception during penicillin therapy.

Live-virus vaccines: May decrease effectiveness of live-virus vaccines. Concurrent use isn't recommended.

Methotrexate: May increase risk of methotrexate toxicity. Monitor methotrexate levels.

Oral anticoagulants (warfarin): May prolong PT. Monitor PT closely during coadministration.

Probenecid: May increase levels of amoxicillin and other penicillins. Use together isn't recommended.

Tetracyclines: May reduce therapeutic action of penicillins. Avoid administering together.

EFFECTS ON LAB TEST RESULTS
• May decrease aminoglycoside level.
• May decrease platelet, leukocyte, and granulocyte counts.
• May increase or decrease eosinophil count.
• May alter results of urine glucose tests that use cupric sulfate, such as Benedict reagent and Clinitest.

CONTRAINDICATIONS & CAUTIONS
• Contraindicated in patients hypersensitive to drug or other penicillins and in those with a history of amoxicillin-related cholestatic jaundice or hepatic dysfunction.
• Use cautiously in patients with other drug allergies (especially to cephalosporins) because of possible cross-sensitivity.
• Use cautiously in older adults and patients with hepatic dysfunction.
• Drug may increase risk of hepatic dysfunction (hepatitis, cholestatic jaundice), especially in older adults, males, and patients on prolonged treatment.
• Don't give ampicillin-class antibiotics to patients with mononucleosis due to high incidence of erythematous rash.
Dialyzable drug: Yes.
⚠ *Overdose S&S:* Crystalluria, oliguric renal failure, GI symptoms, rash, hyperactivity or drowsiness.

PREGNANCY-LACTATION-REPRODUCTION
• Use during pregnancy only if clearly needed.
• Drug appears in human milk. Use cautiously during breastfeeding.

NURSING CONSIDERATIONS
🕒 *Alert:* Ratios of amoxicillin and clavulanic acid aren't consistent from product

to product. Therefore, formulations aren't equivalent. For example, don't substitute two 250-mg tablets for one 500-mg tablet or substitute one 250-mg film-coated tablet for one 250-mg chewable tablet.
• If large doses are given or therapy is prolonged, bacterial or fungal superinfection may occur, especially in older adults and patients with debilitation or immunosuppression.
• CDAD, ranging from mild diarrhea to fatal colitis, has been reported with nearly all antibacterial agents, including amoxicillin–clavulanate. Evaluate patient if diarrhea occurs.
• Chewable tablets and powder for oral solution contain phenylalanine.
• Monitor LFTs periodically in patients with hepatic impairment. Discontinue drug if signs of hepatitis occur.
• This drug combination is useful in settings with a high prevalence of amoxicillin-resistant organisms.
• *Look alike–sound alike:* Don't confuse amoxicillin with ampicillin, amoxapine, or Azulfidine.

PATIENT TEACHING
• Tell patient to take entire quantity of drug exactly as prescribed, even after feeling better.
• Instruct patient to take drug with food to prevent GI upset. Advise patient taking the oral suspension to keep drug refrigerated, to shake it well before taking it, and to discard remaining drug after 10 days.
• Tell patient to report all adverse reactions and to call prescriber if a rash occurs because rash may indicate an allergic reaction.

SAFETY ALERT!

amphotericin B lipid complex
am-foe-TER-i-sin

Abelcet

Therapeutic class: Antifungals
Pharmacologic class: Polyene antibiotics

AVAILABLE FORMS
Suspension for injection: 100 mg/20 mL vial

INDICATIONS & DOSAGES
➤ **Invasive fungal infections, including** *Aspergillus* **and** *Candida* **species, in patients**

---

refractory to or intolerant of conventional amphotericin B therapy

Adults and children: 5 mg/kg daily IV as a single infusion given at rate of 2.5 mg/kg/hour.

Adjust-a-dose: Determine dosage based on overall clinical condition of individual patient.

ADMINISTRATION

IV

▼ To prepare, shake vial gently until there's no yellow sediment. Withdraw calculated dose into one or more 20-mL syringes using an 18G needle. More than one vial will be needed.

▼ Attach a 5-micron filter needle to syringe and inject dose into IV bag of D_5W. Volume of D_5W should be sufficient to yield 1 mg/mL (2 mg/mL for children and those with CV disorders). One filter needle can be used for up to four vials of amphotericin B lipid complex.

▼ Don't use an in-line filter.

▼ If infusing through an existing IV line, flush first with D_5W.

▼ If infusion time exceeds 2 hours, mix contents by shaking infusion bag every 2 hours.

▼ Monitor vital signs closely. Fever, shaking chills, and hypotension may appear within 2 hours of starting infusion. Slowing infusion rate may decrease risk of infusion-related reactions.

▼ If severe respiratory distress occurs, stop infusion, provide supportive therapy for anaphylaxis, and notify prescriber. Don't restart drug.

▼ Reconstituted drug is stable up to 48 hours if refrigerated (36° to 46° F [2° to 8° C]) and up to 6 hours at room temperature.

▼ Discard any unused drug because it contains no preservative.

▼ **Incompatibilities:** Electrolytes, other IV drugs, saline solutions.

ACTION

Binds to sterols of fungal cell membranes, altering cell permeability and causing cell death.

Route	Onset	Peak	Duration
IV	Unknown	Unknown	Unknown

Half-life: About 1 week.

ADVERSE REACTIONS

CNS: fever, headache, pain. **CV:** *cardiac arrest,* chest pain, HTN, hypotension. **GI:** *GI hemorrhage,* abdominal pain, diarrhea, nausea, vomiting. **GU:** increased creatinine level, *renal failure.* **Hematologic:** *leukopenia, thrombocytopenia,* anemia. **Hepatic:** hyperbilirubinemia. **Metabolic:** *hypokalemia.* **Respiratory:** *respiratory failure,* dyspnea, respiratory disorder. **Skin:** rash. **Other:** *multiple organ failure,* chills, *sepsis,* infection.

INTERACTIONS

Drug-drug. *Antineoplastics:* May increase risk of renal toxicity, bronchospasm, and hypotension. Use together cautiously.

Cardiac glycosides: May increase risk of digitalis toxicity from amphotericin B–induced hypokalemia. Monitor potassium level closely.

Clotrimazole, fluconazole, itraconazole, ketoconazole, miconazole: May counteract effects of amphotericin B by inducing fungal resistance. Monitor patient closely.

Corticosteroids, corticotropin: May enhance hypokalemia, which could lead to cardiac toxicity. Monitor electrolyte levels and cardiac function.

Cyclosporine: May increase renal toxicity. Monitor renal function test results closely.

Flucytosine: May increase risk of flucytosine toxicity from increased cellular uptake or impaired renal excretion. Use together cautiously.

Leukocyte transfusions: May increase risk of pulmonary reactions, such as acute dyspnea, tachypnea, hypoxemia, hemoptysis, and interstitial infiltrates. Don't coadminister.

Nephrotoxic drugs (such as aminoglycosides, pentamidine): May increase risk of renal toxicity. Use together cautiously and monitor renal function closely.

Skeletal muscle relaxants (tubocurarine): May enhance skeletal muscle relaxant effects of amphotericin B–induced hypokalemia. Monitor potassium level closely.

Zidovudine: May increase myelotoxicity and nephrotoxicity. Monitor renal and hematologic function.

EFFECTS ON LAB TEST RESULTS

• May increase ALP, ALT, AST, bilirubin, BUN, creatinine, GGT, and LDH levels.
• May decrease magnesium and potassium levels.
• May decrease Hb level and platelet and WBC counts.

CONTRAINDICATIONS & CAUTIONS

• Contraindicated in patients hypersensitive to amphotericin B or its components.
• Anaphylaxis can occur. If patient develops severe respiratory distress, discontinue infusion, treat appropriately, and don't restart drug.
• Use cautiously in patients with renal impairment. Adjust dosage based on patient's overall condition. Renal toxicity is more common at higher dosages.
Dialyzable drug: No.
⚠ *Overdose S&S:* Cardiorespiratory arrest.

PREGNANCY-LACTATION-REPRODUCTION

• Use cautiously during pregnancy, taking into account importance of drug to the mother.
• It isn't known if drug appears in human milk. Patient should discontinue breastfeeding or discontinue drug.

NURSING CONSIDERATIONS

🖢 *Alert:* Different amphotericin B preparations aren't interchangeable, so dosages will vary. Confusing the preparations may cause permanent damage or death.
• Hydrate before infusion to reduce risk of nephrotoxicity.
• Frequently monitor creatinine and electrolyte levels (especially magnesium and potassium), LFT values, and CBC during therapy.
• Acute infusion reactions, including fever and chills, may occur 1 to 2 hours after start of infusion and are more common with first few doses. Infusion has rarely been associated with arrhythmias, hypotension, and shock.
🖢 *Alert:* Immediately stop infusion if severe respiratory distress occurs. Patient shouldn't receive further infusions.
• *Look alike–sound alike:* Don't confuse Abelcet with AmBisome or amphotericin B lipid complex with conventional amphotericin B.

PATIENT TEACHING

• Inform patient that fever, chills, nausea, and vomiting may develop during infusion, but that these symptoms usually subside with subsequent doses.
• Instruct patient to report any redness or pain at infusion site.
• Teach patient to recognize and report to prescriber signs and symptoms of acute hypersensitivity, such as respiratory distress.
• Warn patient that therapy may take several months.

• Tell patient to expect frequent lab testing to monitor kidney and liver function.

SAFETY ALERT!

amphotericin B liposomal
am-foe-TER-i-sin

AmBisome

Therapeutic class: Antifungals
Pharmacologic class: Polyene antibiotics

AVAILABLE FORMS

Powder for injection: 50-mg vial

INDICATIONS & DOSAGES

➤ **Empirical therapy for presumed fungal infection in patients who are febrile and neutropenic**
Adults and children: 3 mg/kg IV infusion over 2 hours daily.
➤ **Systemic fungal infections caused by *Aspergillus* species, *Candida* species, or *Cryptococcus* species refractory to conventional amphotericin B therapy; patients for whom renal impairment or unacceptable toxicity precludes use of conventional amphotericin B therapy**
Adults and children: 3 to 5 mg/kg IV infusion over 2 hours daily.
➤ **Visceral leishmaniasis in patients who are immunocompetent**
Adults and children: 3 mg/kg IV infusion over 2 hours daily on days 1 to 5, day 14, and day 21. A repeat course of therapy may be beneficial if initial treatment fails to clear parasites.
➤ **Visceral leishmaniasis in patients who are immunocompromised**
Adults and children: 4 mg/kg IV infusion over 2 hours daily on days 1 to 5, day 10, day 17, day 24, day 31, and day 38.
➤ **Cryptococcal meningitis in patients with HIV infection**
Adults and children: 6 mg/kg/day IV infusion over 2 hours.

ADMINISTRATION
IV
▼ Don't reconstitute with bacteriostatic water for injection, and don't allow bacteriostatic product in solution.

Reactions in bold italics are *life-threatening*. Interactions may have a *rapid onset* or a *delayed onset*.

▼ Don't reconstitute with saline solutions, add saline solutions to reconstituted concentration, or mix with other drugs.

▼ Reconstitute each 50-mg vial with 12 mL of sterile water for injection to yield 4 mg/mL. A yellow, translucent suspension will form.

▼ After reconstitution, shake vial vigorously for 30 seconds or until particulate matter disperses.

▼ Dilute to 1 to 2 mg/mL by withdrawing calculated amount of reconstituted solution into a sterile syringe and injecting it through a 5-micron filter into an appropriate amount of D_5W. Use only one filter needle per vial. Concentrations of 0.2 to 0.5 mg/mL may provide sufficient volume of infusion for children.

▼ Flush existing IV line with D_5W before infusing drug. If this isn't possible, give drug through a separate line.

▼ Use a controlled infusion device and an in-line filter with a mean pore diameter of 1 micron or larger.

▼ Initially, infuse drug over at least 2 hours. If drug is tolerated well, reduce infusion time to 1 hour. If discomfort occurs, increase infusion time.

▼ Store unopened vial at 36° to 46° F (2° to 8° C). Store reconstituted drug for up to 24 hours at 36° to 46° F. Use within 6 hours of dilution with D_5W. Don't freeze.

▼ **Incompatibilities:** Other IV drugs, saline solutions.

ACTION
Binds to sterols of fungal cell membranes, altering cell permeability and causing cell death.

Route	Onset	Peak	Duration
IV	Unknown	Unknown	Unknown

Half-life: About 4 to 6 days.

ADVERSE REACTIONS
CNS: fever, anxiety, confusion, headache, insomnia, asthenia, pain. **CV:** chest pain, hypotension, tachycardia, HTN, edema, phlebitis, flushing. **EENT:** epistaxis, rhinitis. **GI:** anorexia, constipation, nausea, vomiting, abdominal pain, diarrhea, *GI hemorrhage.* **GU:** hematuria, increased BUN and creatinine levels. **Hematologic:** anemia, *thrombocytopenia, leukopenia.* **Hepatic:** increased ALP and transaminase levels, bilirubinemia, *hepatotoxicity.* **Metabolic:** hyperglycemia,

hypernatremia, hyponatremia, *hypocalcemia, hypokalemia,* hypovolemia, *hypomagnesemia.* **Musculoskeletal:** back pain. **Respiratory:** increased cough, dyspnea, hypoxia, pleural effusion, lung disorder. **Skin:** pruritus, rash, diaphoresis. **Other:** chills, infection, hypersensitivity reaction, *sepsis,* blood product infusion reaction, procedural complication.

INTERACTIONS
Drug-drug. *Antineoplastics:* May enhance potential for renal toxicity, bronchospasm, and hypotension. Use together cautiously.
Cardiac glycosides: May increase risk of digitalis toxicity caused by amphotericin B–induced hypokalemia. Monitor potassium level closely.
Clotrimazole, fluconazole, ketoconazole, miconazole: May induce fungal resistance to amphotericin B. Use together cautiously.
Corticosteroids, corticotropin: May increase potassium depletion, which could cause cardiac dysfunction. Monitor electrolyte levels and cardiac function.
Cyclosporine: May increase renal toxicity. Monitor renal function test results closely.
Flucytosine: May increase flucytosine toxicity by increasing cellular reuptake or impairing renal excretion of flucytosine. Use together cautiously.
Leukocyte transfusions: Increases risk of pulmonary toxicity. Don't use together.
Other nephrotoxic drugs, such as antibiotics and antineoplastics: May cause additive nephrotoxicity. Use together cautiously; monitor renal function closely.
Skeletal muscle relaxants: May enhance effects of skeletal muscle relaxants resulting from amphotericin B–induced hypokalemia. Monitor potassium level.

EFFECTS ON LAB TEST RESULTS
• May increase ALP, ALT, AST, bilirubin, BUN, creatinine, GGT, glucose, and LDH levels.
• May decrease calcium, magnesium, and potassium levels.
• May increase or decrease sodium level.
• May decrease Hb level and leukocyte and platelet counts.

CONTRAINDICATIONS & CAUTIONS
• Contraindicated in patients hypersensitive to drug or its components.

• Use cautiously in older adults and patients with impaired renal function.
Dialyzable drug: No.
⚠ *Overdose S&S:* Cardiorespiratory arrest.

PREGNANCY-LACTATION-REPRODUCTION
• Use during pregnancy only if potential benefits outweigh fetal risk.
• It isn't known if drug appears in human milk. Patient should discontinue breastfeeding or discontinue drug.

NURSING CONSIDERATIONS
• Patients also receiving chemotherapy or bone marrow transplantation and those with HIV disease are at greater risk for additional adverse reactions, such as cardiac arrest, hallucinations, seizures, arrhythmias, and thrombocytopenia. Refer to manufacturer's instructions for a complete list of reactions.
🔔 *Alert:* Different amphotericin B preparations aren't interchangeable, so dosages will vary. Confusing the preparations may cause permanent damage or death.
• Hydrate before infusion to reduce the risk of nephrotoxicity.
• Monitor BUN, creatinine, and electrolyte levels (particularly magnesium and potassium), LFT, and CBC.
• Watch for signs and symptoms of hypokalemia (ECG changes, muscle weakness, cramping, drowsiness).
• Patients treated with this drug have a lower risk of chills, elevated BUN level, hypokalemia, HTN, and vomiting than patients treated with conventional amphotericin B.
• Therapy may take several weeks or months.
• Observe patient closely for adverse reactions during infusion. If anaphylaxis occurs, stop infusion immediately, provide supportive therapy, and notify prescriber.
• Consider premedication to prevent infusion-related reactions.
• *Look alike–sound alike:* Don't confuse amphotericin B liposomal with AmBisome or amphotericin B liposomal lipid complex with conventional amphotericin B.

PATIENT TEACHING
• Teach patient signs and symptoms of hypersensitivity, and stress importance of reporting them immediately.
• Warn patient that therapy may take several months; teach personal hygiene and other

measures to prevent spread and recurrence of lesions.
• Instruct patient to report any adverse reactions that occur while receiving drug.
• Tell patient to watch for and report signs and symptoms of low blood potassium levels (muscle weakness, cramping, drowsiness).
• Advise patient that frequent lab testing will be needed.

ampicillin
am-pi-SIL-in

ampicillin sodium

Therapeutic class: Antibiotics
Pharmacologic class: Aminopenicillins

AVAILABLE FORMS
Capsules: 250 mg, 500 mg
Injection: 125 mg, 250 mg✳, 500 mg, 1 g, 2 g, 10 g

INDICATIONS & DOSAGES
➤ **Respiratory tract infections**
Adults and children weighing more than 20 kg: 250 mg PO every 6 hours.
Children weighing 20 kg or less: 50 mg/kg/day PO in equally divided doses every 6 to 8 hours. Maximum dose is 250 mg q.i.d.
➤ **Respiratory tract and soft-tissue infections**
Adults and children weighing 40 kg or more: 250 to 500 mg IV or IM every 6 hours.
Adults and children weighing less than 40 kg: 25 to 50 mg/kg/day IV or IM in equally divided doses every 6 to 8 hours.
➤ **GI or GU infections (excluding gonorrhea)**
Adults and children weighing 20 kg or more: 500 mg PO every 6 hours. For severe infections, larger doses may be needed.
Children weighing less than 20 kg: 100 mg/kg/day PO in equally divided doses every 6 hours. Maximum dose is 500 mg q.i.d.
➤ **GI and GU tract infections (including gonorrhea in females)**
Adults and children weighing 40 kg or more: 500 mg IV or IM every 6 hours.
Adults and children weighing less than 40 kg: 50 mg/kg/day IV or IM in equally divided doses every 6 to 8 hours.

> **Uncomplicated gonorrhea**

Adults and children weighing more than 20 kg: 3.5 g PO with 1 g probenecid given as a single dose.

> **Urethritis in males due to gonorrhea**

Adult men: Two doses of 500 mg each IV or IM at 8- to 12-hour intervals. May repeat or extend treatment if necessary.

> **Bacterial meningitis or septicemia**

Adults and children: 150 to 200 mg/kg/day IM or IV in divided doses every 3 to 4 hours. May start with IV therapy, then continue with IM injections. For sepsis, give IV at least 3 days before switching to IM.

Neonates gestational age greater than 34 weeks and postnatal 28 days or less: 150 mg/kg/day in divided doses every 8 hours.

Neonates gestational age 34 weeks or less and postnatal 8 to less than 28 days: 150 mg/kg/day in divided doses every 12 hours.

Neonates gestational age 34 weeks or less and postnatal 7 days or less: 100 mg/kg/day in divided doses every 12 hours.

ADMINISTRATION

PO

• Before giving drug, ask patient about allergic reactions to penicillin. A negative history of penicillin allergy is no guarantee against a future allergic reaction.

• Obtain specimen for culture and sensitivity tests before giving. Begin therapy while awaiting results.

• When given orally, drug may cause GI disturbances. Food may interfere with absorption. Give drug with 8 oz of water ½ hour before or 2 hours after meals.

• Give drug IM or IV if infection is severe or if patient can't take oral dose.

IV

▼ Before giving drug, ask patient about allergic reactions to penicillin. A negative history of penicillin allergy is no guarantee against a future allergic reaction.

▼ Obtain specimen for culture and sensitivity tests before giving. Begin therapy while awaiting results.

▼ Give drug IV only if infection is severe or if patient can't take oral dose.

▼ Give drug intermittently to prevent vein irritation. Change site every 48 hours.

▼ For direct injection, reconstitute with bacteriostatic water for injection. Use 5 mL

for 250-mg or 500-mg vials, 7.4 mL for 1-g vials, and 14.8 mL for 2-g vials. Give drug over 10 to 15 minutes to avoid seizures. Don't exceed 100 mg/minute.

▼ For intermittent infusion, dilute in 50 to 100 mL of NSS for injection. Give drug over 15 to 30 minutes.

▼ Use first dilution within 1 hour. Follow manufacturer's directions for stability data when drug is further diluted for IV infusion.

▼ **Incompatibilities:** None listed by manufacturer. Consult a drug incompatibility reference for more information.

IM

• Before giving drug, ask patient about allergic reactions to penicillin. A negative history of penicillin allergy is no guarantee against a future allergic reaction.

• Obtain specimen for culture and sensitivity tests before giving. Begin therapy while awaiting results.

• Give drug IM only if infection is severe or patient can't take oral dose.

• Dissolve contents of vial with sterile water or bacteriostatic water for injection. Final concentration is 125 mg or 250 mg/mL.

• Use solution for IM injection within 1 hour of preparation.

ACTION

Inhibits cell-wall synthesis during bacterial multiplication.

Route	Onset	Peak	Duration
PO	Unknown	2 hr	6–8 hr
IV	Immediate	Immediate	Unknown
IM	Unknown	1 hr	Unknown

Half-life: 1 to 1.8 hours (10 to 24 hours in severe renal impairment).

ADVERSE REACTIONS

CNS: *seizures.* **EENT:** glossitis. **GI:** diarrhea, nausea, *pseudomembranous colitis,* abdominal pain, black hairy tongue, enterocolitis, gastritis, stomatitis, vomiting. **Hematologic:** *leukopenia, thrombocytopenia, thrombocytopenic purpura,* anemia, eosinophilia, hemolytic anemia, *agranulocytosis.* **Skin:** rash, urticaria. **Other:** hypersensitivity reactions, overgrowth of nonsusceptible organisms.

INTERACTIONS

Drug-drug. *Allopurinol:* May increase risk of rash. Monitor patient for rash.

H_2 antagonists, PPIs: May decrease ampicillin absorption and level. Separate administration times. Monitor patient for continued antibiotic effectiveness.

Hormonal contraceptives: May decrease hormonal contraceptive effectiveness. Advise use of another form of contraception during therapy.

Live-virus vaccines: May decrease effectiveness of live-virus vaccines. Concurrent use isn't recommended.

Methotrexate: May increase methotrexate level, increasing risk of toxicity. Monitor methotrexate level.

Probenecid: May increase levels of ampicillin and other penicillins. Probenecid may be used for this purpose.

Warfarin: May increase bleeding risk. Monitor PT and INR.

EFFECTS ON LAB TEST RESULTS
• May decrease Hb level.
• May increase eosinophil count. May decrease granulocyte, platelet, and WBC counts.
• May decrease aminoglycoside level.
• May alter results of urine glucose tests that use cupric sulfate, such as Benedict reagent and Clinitest.

CONTRAINDICATIONS & CAUTIONS
• Contraindicated in patients hypersensitive to drug or other penicillins and in those with infections caused by penicillinase-producing organisms.
• Use cautiously in patients with other drug allergies (especially to cephalosporins) because of possible cross-sensitivity, and in those with mononucleosis because of high risk of maculopapular rash.
• Use cautiously in patients with renal impairment.
Dialyzable drug: Yes.

PREGNANCY-LACTATION-REPRODUCTION
• Ampicillin crosses the placental barrier. Use during pregnancy only if clearly needed.
• Drug appears in human milk. Use cautiously during breastfeeding.

NURSING CONSIDERATIONS
• Monitor sodium levels frequently because each gram of ampicillin sodium injection contains 2.9 mEq of sodium.
• If large doses are given or if therapy is prolonged, bacterial or fungal superinfection may

occur, especially in older adults and patients with immunosuppression or debilitation.
• Watch for signs and symptoms of hypersensitivity, such as erythematous maculopapular rash, urticaria, and anaphylaxis.
• Use lowest dosage compatible with effective treatment in neonates and infants because of incompletely developed renal function in these patients.
• Monitor patients for CDAD, which can be fatal and can occur even more than 2 months after therapy ends. Antibiotic may need to be stopped and other treatment begun.

PATIENT TEACHING
• Tell patient to take entire quantity of drug exactly as prescribed, even after feeling better.
• Instruct patient in safe drug administration.
• Inform patient to report all adverse reactions and to notify prescriber if rash, fever, or chills develop. A rash is the most common allergic reaction, especially if allopurinol is also being taken.
• Instruct patient to report diarrhea.

ampicillin sodium–sulbactam sodium
am-pi-SIL-in/sul-BAK-tam

Unasyn

Therapeutic class: Antibiotics
Pharmacologic class: Aminopenicillins–beta-lactamase inhibitors

AVAILABLE FORMS
Injection: Vials and piggyback vials containing 1.5 g (1 g ampicillin sodium and 0.5 g sulbactam sodium), 3 g (2 g ampicillin sodium and 1 g sulbactam sodium); vial containing 15 g (10 g ampicillin sodium and 5 g sulbactam sodium)

INDICATIONS & DOSAGES
Adjust-a-dose (for all indications): If CrCl in adults is 15 to 29 mL/minute/1.73 m², give 1.5 to 3 g every 12 hours; if CrCl is 5 to 14 mL/minute/1.73 m², give 1.5 to 3 g every 24 hours. Give dose after hemodialysis.
➤ **Intra-abdominal, gynecologic, and skin-structure infections caused by susceptible strains**
Adults: 1.5 to 3 g IM or IV every 6 hours. Don't exceed 4 g/day of sulbactam.

Children age 1 or older weighing 40 kg or more (skin and skin-structure infections only): 1.5 to 3 g IV or IM every 6 hours for no longer than 14 days. Don't exceed 4 g/day sulbactam.

Children age 1 or older weighing less than 40 kg (skin and skin-structure infections only): 300 mg/kg/day (200 mg ampicillin/ 100 mg sulbactam) IV in divided doses every 6 hours for no longer than 14 days. Continue therapy with an appropriate oral anti-infective agent if necessary.

ADMINISTRATION

• Before giving, ask patient about allergic reactions to penicillin. A negative history of penicillin allergy is no guarantee against future allergic reaction.
• Obtain specimen for culture and sensitivity tests. Begin therapy while awaiting results.

IV

▼ Reconstitute powder with NSS, sterile water for injection, D_5W, lactated Ringer injection, M/6 sodium lactate, dextrose 5% in half-NSS for injection, or 10% invert sugar.

▼ After reconstitution, let vials stand for a few minutes so foam can dissipate. Inspect solution for particles.

▼ Give drug at least 1 hour before giving a bacteriostatic antibiotic.

▼ For infusion, can give dose by slow IV injection over at least 10 to 15 minutes or can dilute in 50 to 100 mL of compatible diluent and infuse over 15 to 30 minutes.

▼ Stability varies with diluent, temperature, and concentration of solution.

▼ **Incompatibilities:** Acyclovir, aminoglycosides, amiodarone, amphotericin B cholesteryl, amphotericin B lipid complex, amphotericin B liposomal, caspofungin, chlorpromazine, ciprofloxacin, daunorubicin, dobutamine, ganciclovir, ondansetron, phenytoin, prochlorperazine, verapamil. Refer to a drug compatibility reference for full listing.

IM

• For IM injection, reconstitute with sterile water for injection or 0.5% or 2% lidocaine hydrochloride injection. Add 3.2 mL to a 1.5-g vial (or 6.4 mL to a 3-g vial) to yield 375 mg/mL. Give deep into muscle within 1 hour after preparation.
• IM injection may cause pain at injection site.
• In children, don't use IM route.

ACTION

Inhibits cell-wall synthesis during bacterial multiplication.

Route	Onset	Peak	Duration
IV	Immediate	15 min	Unknown
IM	Unknown	30–52 min	Unknown

Half-life: 1 to 1.5 hours (10 to 24 hours in severe renal impairment).

ADVERSE REACTIONS

CV: thrombophlebitis, phlebitis. **GI:** diarrhea. **Skin:** pain at injection site, rash, urticaria. **Other:** hypersensitivity reactions.

INTERACTIONS

Drug-drug. *Allopurinol:* May increase risk of rash. Monitor patient for rash.

Hormonal contraceptives: May decrease hormonal contraceptive effectiveness. Strongly advise use of another contraceptive during therapy.

Live-virus vaccines: May decrease effectiveness of live-virus vaccines. Use together isn't recommended.

Methotrexate: May increase methotrexate level, increasing risk of toxicity. Monitor methotrexate level.

Oral anticoagulants: May increase risk of bleeding. Monitor PT and INR.

Probenecid: May increase ampicillin level. Probenecid may be used for this purpose.

Tetracycline: May decrease effectiveness of ampicillin–sulbactam. Avoid coadministration if possible.

Drug-herb. *Khat:* May decrease antimicrobial effect of certain penicillins. Discourage khat chewing, or tell patient to take drug 2 hours after khat chewing.

EFFECTS ON LAB TEST RESULTS

• May increase ALP, ALT, AST, bilirubin, BUN, CK, creatinine, and LDH levels.
• May decrease albumin and protein levels.
• May increase eosinophil, lymphocyte, monocyte, and basophil counts.
• May decrease Hb level, hematocrit, and granulocyte, RBC, and WBC counts.
• May increase or decrease platelet count.
• May increase urine RBC and hyaline casts.
• May transiently decrease conjugated estriol, conjugated estrone, estradiol, and estriol glucuronide levels during pregnancy.

• May alter results of urine glucose tests that use cupric sulfate, such as Benedict reagent and Clinitest.

CONTRAINDICATIONS & CAUTIONS
• Contraindicated in patients hypersensitive to drug or other penicillins, in those with other drug allergies (especially to cephalosporins) because of possible cross-sensitivity, and in those with mononucleosis because of high risk of maculopapular rash.
• Contraindicated in patients with a history of cholestatic jaundice or hepatitis.
• Use cautiously in patients with renal impairment.
Dialyzable drug: Yes.
⚠ *Overdose S&S:* Neuromuscular hyperexcitability, seizures.

PREGNANCY-LACTATION-REPRODUCTION
• There are no adequate and well-controlled studies during pregnancy. Use cautiously during pregnancy and only if clearly needed.
• Drug appears in human milk. Use cautiously during breastfeeding.

NURSING CONSIDERATIONS
• Dosage is expressed as total drug. Each vial contains a 2:1 ratio of ampicillin sodium to sulbactam sodium.
• Monitor LFT results during therapy, especially in patients with impaired liver function.
• If large doses are given or if therapy is prolonged, bacterial or fungal superinfection may occur, especially in older adults and patients with debilitation or immunosuppression.
• Watch for signs and symptoms of hypersensitivity, such as erythematous maculopapular rash, urticaria, and anaphylaxis.
• Monitor for CDAD, which can be fatal. Antibiotic may need to be stopped and other treatment begun.

PATIENT TEACHING
• Tell patient to report all adverse reactions, including rash, fever, or chills. A rash is the most common allergic reaction.
• Warn patient that IM injection may cause pain at injection site.

anastrozole
an-AS-troe-zole

Arimidex♦

Therapeutic class: Antineoplastics
Pharmacologic class: Aromatase inhibitors

AVAILABLE FORMS
Tablets: 1 mg

INDICATIONS & DOSAGES
➤ **First-line treatment of women who are postmenopausal with hormone receptor (HR)–positive or HR–unknown locally advanced or metastatic breast cancer; advanced breast cancer in women who are postmenopausal with disease progression after tamoxifen therapy; adjunctive treatment of women who are postmenopausal with HR–positive early breast cancer**
Adults: 1 mg PO daily.
➤ **Risk reduction for breast cancer in women who are postmenopausal ♦**
Adults: 1 mg PO daily for 5 years.

ADMINISTRATION
PO
• Drug is considered a hazardous agent and is a potential teratogen. Follow safe handling procedures when preparing, administering, or dispensing.
• Give drug without regard for meals.

ACTION
A selective nonsteroidal aromatase inhibitor that significantly lowers estradiol levels, which inhibits breast cancer cell growth in women who are postmenopausal.

Route	Onset	Peak	Duration
PO	<24 hr	2–5 hr	<7 days

Half-life: 50 hours.

ADVERSE REACTIONS
CNS: headache, fatigue, asthenia, pain, dizziness, fatigue, depression, mood disturbance, paresthesia, anxiety, insomnia, *stroke.* **CV:** hot flashes, *thromboembolic disease,* chest pain, peripheral edema, HTN, vasodilation, *cardiac ischemia.* **EENT:** cataracts, dry mouth, pharyngitis, sinusitis. **GI:** nausea, vomiting, diarrhea, constipation, abdominal pain, anorexia, dyspepsia. **GU:** vaginal

---

dryness, leukorrhea, vaginitis, vulvovaginitis, *vaginal hemorrhage,* pelvic pain, UTI. **Hematologic:** anemia. **Metabolic:** weight gain, increased cholesterol level. **Musculoskeletal:** bone pain, back pain, arthritis, arthralgia, osteoporosis, fractures, arthrosis, joint disorder, myalgia. **Respiratory:** dyspnea, bronchitis, cough. **Skin:** alopecia, rash, diaphoresis. **Other:** infection, accidental injury, *neoplasm,* lymphedema, flulike symptoms, breast pain.

INTERACTIONS
Drug-drug. *Estrogen:* May decrease pharmacologic action of anastrozole. Use together isn't recommended.
Tamoxifen: May reduce anastrozole plasma level. Don't use together.

EFFECTS ON LAB TEST RESULTS
• May increase liver enzyme and cholesterol levels.

CONTRAINDICATIONS & CAUTIONS
• Contraindicated in patients hypersensitive to drug or its components.
• Use cautiously in patients with preexisting ischemic heart disease.
Dialyzable drug: Unknown.

PREGNANCY-LACTATION-REPRODUCTION
• Drug can cause fetal harm. Contraindicated during pregnancy and in patients who plan to become pregnant.
• Patients of childbearing potential should use effective contraception during therapy and for at least 3 weeks after final dose.
• It isn't known if drug appears in human milk. Patient shouldn't breastfeed during therapy and for 2 weeks after final dose.
• May impair fertility in patients of childbearing potential.

NURSING CONSIDERATIONS
• Give drug under supervision of a prescriber experienced in use of antineoplastics.
• Patients with hormone receptor–negative disease and patients who didn't respond to previous tamoxifen therapy rarely respond to anastrozole.
• For patients with advanced breast cancer, continue anastrozole until tumor progresses.
• Monitor bone mineral density because drug can decrease bone mineral density.

• Use drug only in women who are postmenopausal.
• Rule out pregnancy before starting drug.

PATIENT TEACHING
• Instruct patient to report adverse reactions, especially difficulty breathing, chest pain, or skin lesions or blisters.
• Tell patient to take medication at the same time each day.
• Stress need for follow-up care.
• Counsel patient about risks of pregnancy during therapy. Advise use of effective contraception during therapy and for at least 3 weeks after final dose.
• Advise patient not to breastfeed during treatment and for 2 weeks after final dose.
• Inform patient that cholesterol level may increase.
• Tell patient that drug lowers estrogen level, which may lead to decreased bone strength and increased risk of fractures.
• Tell patient of childbearing potential that drug may impair fertility.

SAFETY ALERT!

apalutamide
a-pa-LOO-ta-mide

Erleada

Therapeutic class: Antineoplastics
Pharmacologic class: Androgen receptor inhibitors

AVAILABLE FORMS
Tablets ⬤: 60 mg

INDICATIONS & DOSAGES
Adjust-a-dose (for all indications): If grade 3 or greater toxicity occurs, withhold drug until symptoms improve to grade 1 or less or to original grade; then resume at same dosage or a reduced dosage (180 or 120 mg), if warranted.
➤ **Castration-resistant prostate cancer**
Adult males: 240 mg (four 60-mg tablets) PO once daily.

ADMINISTRATION
PO
• May give with or without food.

- Make sure patient swallows tablets whole. Don't break, crush, or allow patient to chew tablets.
- If patient can't swallow tablets, mix whole tablets in 4 oz (120 mL) of applesauce by stirring. Don't crush tablets. Wait 15 minutes, then stir mixture. Wait another 15 minutes, then stir mixture until tablets are well mixed, with no chunks remaining. Using a spoon, have patient swallow mixture right away. Rinse container with 2 oz (60 mL) of water and have patient immediately drink contents. Repeat the rinse with 2 oz of water to ensure entire dose is taken. Give mixture within 1 hour of preparation.
- Give a missed dose as soon as possible on the same day; then return to the normal schedule on the following day. Don't give extra tablets to make up for a missed dose.
- Store in original container; don't discard desiccant. Protect from light and moisture.

ACTION

Binds to androgen receptors to decrease tumor cell proliferation and increase apoptosis, leading to decreased tumor volume.

Route	Onset	Peak	Duration
PO	Unknown	2 hr	Unknown

Half-life: 3 days.

ADVERSE REACTIONS

CNS: fatigue, asthenia. **CV:** peripheral edema, HTN, hot flushes, *ischemic heart disease, HF.* **GI:** decreased appetite, diarrhea, nausea, stomatitis. **GU:** hematuria. **Hematologic:** anemia, *leukopenia, lymphopenia.* **Metabolic:** weight loss, hypothyroidism, hypercholesterolemia, hyperglycemia, hypertriglyceridemia, *hyperkalemia.* **Musculoskeletal:** arthralgia, fracture. **Skin:** rash, pruritus. **Other:** fall.

INTERACTIONS

Drug-drug. *Strong CYP3A4/CYP2C8 inducers (rifampin):* May decrease apalutamide level. Monitor patient for loss of apalutamide activity.
Strong CYP3A4 (itraconazole, ketoconazole) or CYP2C8 (gemfibrozil) inhibitors: May increase apalutamide level. Monitor patient and reduce apalutamide dosage if necessary.
Substrates of CYP2C9 (warfarin), CYP2C19 (omeprazole), CYP3A4 (midazolam), and uridine diphosphate glycosyltransferase: May

reduce levels of these drugs. Use other drugs as substitutes for these drugs if possible, or if use with apalutamide is necessary, monitor patient for loss of activity of these drugs.
Substrates of P-gp (fexofenadine), BCRP, and organic anion transporting polypeptide 1B1 (rosuvastatin): May reduce levels of these drugs. Use cautiously together if necessary. If use with apalutamide is necessary, monitor patient for loss of activity of these drugs.

EFFECTS ON LAB TEST RESULTS

- May increase TSH, potassium, cholesterol, glucose, and triglyceride levels.
- May decrease RBC, WBC, and lymphocyte counts.

CONTRAINDICATIONS & CAUTIONS

- Drug isn't indicated for use in females.
- Use cautiously in patients with a risk of falls and fractures.
- Drug may increase risk of seizures. Avoid use in patients with a history of seizures or with predisposing factors for seizures and in those receiving drugs known to decrease seizure threshold or to induce seizures.
- Drug may increase risk of hypothyroidism and CV disease.
- Drug may increase risk of cerebrovascular and ischemic CV events, including events leading to death.
- Safety and effectiveness in children haven't been established.

Dialyzable drug: Unknown.

PREGNANCY-LACTATION-REPRODUCTION

⚠️ *Alert:* Contraindicated during pregnancy. May cause fetal harm and loss of pregnancy.
- Patients with partners of childbearing potential should use effective contraception (condom) during treatment and for 3 months after final dose
- Drug may impair fertility in males of reproductive potential.

NURSING CONSIDERATIONS

- Administer a GnRH analogue concurrently unless patient has had a bilateral orchiectomy.
- Use appropriate precautions (such as wearing single gloves) when receiving, handling, administering, and disposing of drug.
- Evaluate patient for risk of falls and fractures. Consider use of bone-targeted agents, if appropriate.

Reactions in bold italics are *life-threatening*. Interactions may have a *rapid onset* or a ***delayed onset***.

• Monitor patient for seizures. If seizure occurs, permanently discontinue drug.
• Monitor patient for signs and symptoms of cerebrovascular disorders and ischemic heart disease. Optimize management of CV risk factors.
• Monitor patient for rash, including generalized urticaria, conjunctivitis, erythema multiforme, skin exfoliation, stomatitis, mouth ulcers, blisters, dermatitis, and SJS.
• *Look alike–sound alike:* Don't confuse apalutamide with bicalutamide, flutamide, or nilutamide.

PATIENT TEACHING
• Instruct patient in safe drug administration and handling.
• Inform patient receiving a GnRH analogue that he will need to continue this drug while taking apalutamide.
• Warn patient that drug isn't indicated for use in females.
• Tell patient that drug may increase risk of falls and fractures.
• Tell patient that drug may increase risk of heart disease, stroke, and ministroke and to seek help immediately if experiencing chest pain or discomfort; numbness or weakness of the face, arm, or leg; trouble speaking; or loss of balance.
• Caution patient that drug may increase the risk of seizures and to use care when involved in activities in which loss of consciousness could cause harm to himself or others.
• Tell patient to report all adverse reactions and to immediately report seizure, falls, or rash.
• *Alert:* Advise patient of reproductive potential to use effective contraception during treatment and for 3 months after final dose.
• Caution patient to use condoms while having sex. Drug may cause fetal harm.
• Educate patient of reproductive potential about the risk of impaired fertility. Advise patient not to donate sperm during treatment and for 3 months after final dose.

apixaban
a-PIX-a-ban

Eliquis⚭

Therapeutic class: Anticoagulants
Pharmacologic class: Factor Xa inhibitors

AVAILABLE FORMS
Tablets: 2.5 mg, 5 mg

INDICATIONS & DOSAGES
➤ **Reduction of risk of stroke and systemic embolism in patients with nonvalvular atrial fibrillation**
Adults: 5 mg PO b.i.d.
Adjust-a-dose: Reduce dosage to 2.5 mg b.i.d. in patients with any two of the following characteristics: age 80 or older, body weight 60 kg or less, or serum creatinine 1.5 mg/dL or greater.
➤ **DVT prophylaxis after hip or knee replacement surgery**
Adults: 2.5 mg PO b.i.d. beginning 12 to 24 hours after surgery. Continue for 35 days after hip replacement surgery or for 12 days after knee replacement surgery.
➤ **DVT and PE**
Adults: 10 mg PO b.i.d. for 7 days followed by 5 mg PO b.i.d.; then, to reduce risk of recurrence after at least 6 months of treatment, 2.5 mg PO b.i.d.

ADMINISTRATION
PO
• May give without regard for food.
• Give a missed dose as soon as possible on the same day, then resume twice-daily administration. Patient shouldn't double the dose to make up for a missed dose.
• If patient can't swallow tablets, crush and suspend in water, D_5W, or apple juice or mix with applesauce and give promptly PO, or crush and suspend in 60 mL of water or D_5W and give promptly through NG tube. Crushed tablets are stable in water, D_5W, apple juice, or applesauce for up to 4 hours.
• Store at room temperature.

ACTION
Selectively inhibits factor Xa, decreasing thrombin generation and thrombus development.

Route	Onset	Peak	Duration
PO	Unknown	3–4 hr	Unknown

Half-life: 12 hours.

ADVERSE REACTIONS
EENT: epistaxis, bleeding gums. **GI:** nausea, rectal hemorrhage. **GU:** hematuria, menorrhagia. **Hematologic:** *major bleeding,* anemia, hematoma, bruising. **Respiratory:** hemoptysis.

INTERACTIONS
Drug-drug. *Aspirin and other antiplatelet agents/anticoagulants, heparin, NSAIDs, SSNRIs, SSRIs, thrombolytics:* May increase bleeding risk. Avoid use together.
Combined strong dual inducers of CYP3A4 and P-gp (carbamazepine, phenytoin, rifampin): May decrease apixaban concentration. Avoid use together.
Combined strong dual inhibitors of CYP3A4 and P-gp (clarithromycin, itraconazole, ketoconazole, ritonavir): May increase apixaban concentration. Decrease dosage by 50% in patients taking 5 or 10 mg b.i.d.; avoid use together in patients already taking 2.5 mg b.i.d.
Drug-herb. *Alfalfa, anise, bilberry:* May increase bleeding risk. Consider therapy modification.
St. John's wort: May decrease apixaban concentration. Avoid use together.
Drug-food. *Grapefruit juice:* May increase drug level and risk of bleeding. Use cautiously and monitor patient for bleeding.

EFFECTS ON LAB TEST RESULTS
• May increase LFT values.
• May prolong PT, INR, and PTT.

CONTRAINDICATIONS & CAUTIONS
• Contraindicated in patients hypersensitive to drug or its components and in those with active pathological bleeding.
• Use cautiously in patients at risk for severe bleeding (especially those concomitantly taking drugs that affect hemostasis).
• Use of apixaban isn't recommended in patients with acute PE who are hemodynamically unstable, patients who require thrombolysis or pulmonary embolectomy, or patients with antiphospholipid syndrome.
• Use isn't recommended in patients with triple positive antiphospholipid syndrome.

Boxed Warning Discontinuing drug prematurely increases risk of thrombotic events. If anticoagulation with apixaban must be discontinued for a reason other than pathological bleeding, strongly consider coverage with another anticoagulant. ∎

Boxed Warning Consider potential risk of epidural or spinal hematoma versus benefit in patients scheduled for spinal procedures, such as spinal or epidural anesthesia or spinal puncture. Hematomas may result in long-term or permanent paralysis. Risk may increase with use of indwelling epidural catheters, concomitant use of drugs that affect hemostasis (NSAIDs, platelet inhibitors, anticoagulants), history of traumatic or repeated epidural or spinal punctures, or history of spinal deformity or surgery. ∎

◔ *Alert:* Discontinue apixaban at least 48 hours before elective surgery or invasive procedures with a moderate or high risk of unacceptable or clinically significant bleeding.

◔ *Alert:* Discontinue apixaban at least 24 hours before elective surgery or invasive procedures with a low risk of bleeding or when the bleeding would be noncritical in location and easily controlled.

• Bridging anticoagulation before the intervention isn't generally required. Restart apixaban as soon as adequate hemostasis has returned.

• Drug isn't recommended for patients with severe hepatic impairment or prosthetic heart valves.

• Bleeding risk is increased in patients with severe renal impairment.

• Safety and effectiveness in children haven't been established.

Dialyzable drug: 14%.

⚠ *Overdose S&S:* Increased risk of bleeding.

PREGNANCY-LACTATION-REPRODUCTION
• Drug may cross the placental barrier. Not recommended during pregnancy.
• It isn't known if drug appears in human milk. Not recommended during breastfeeding.

NURSING CONSIDERATIONS
• Monitor patient for bleeding. Discontinue drug if acute pathologic bleeding occurs.
◔ *Alert:* Promptly evaluate signs and symptom of blood loss. Drug can cause serious, potentially fatal bleeding.

Reactions in bold italics are *life-threatening*. Interactions may have a *rapid onset* or a *delayed onset*.

Boxed Warning Monitor patients receiving neuraxial anesthesia or undergoing spinal puncture for neurologic impairment (midline back pain, sensory or motor deficits, such as numbness or weakness in lower limbs, bowel or bladder dysfunction). Treat impairment urgently. ■

❸ *Alert:* Removal of indwelling epidural or intrathecal catheters should be delayed for at least 24 hours after last dose of apixaban. Next dose of apixaban should be given no earlier than 5 hours after catheter removal. Don't give drug for at least 48 hours after traumatic or repeated epidural or spinal punctures.

• Administration of activated charcoal may be useful in the management of apixaban overdose or accidental ingestion. Andexanet alfa is available for reversal of the anti-factor Xa activity of apixaban.

• When switching from warfarin to apixaban, discontinue warfarin and start apixaban when INR is below 2.0.

• If switching from apixaban to warfarin, discontinue apixaban and begin both a parenteral anticoagulant and warfarin at the time the next dose of apixaban would have been taken. Discontinue the parenteral anticoagulant when INR reaches an acceptable range. Initial INR measurements during the transition to warfarin may not be useful because apixaban affects the INR.

• If switching between apixaban and anticoagulants other than warfarin, discontinue drug being taken and begin other drug at next scheduled dose.

PATIENT TEACHING

• Warn patient not to discontinue drug without first talking to prescriber, because of risk of clot formation and stroke.

• Tell patient to report all adverse reactions; caution patient that bruising or bleeding may occur more easily.

• Advise patient to report unusual bleeding.

• Instruct patient to inform all health care providers (including dentists) about taking this drug as well as other products known to affect bleeding (including nonprescription products, such as aspirin or NSAIDs) before scheduling surgery or medical or dental procedure and before taking any new drug.

• Tell patient to report pregnancy or plans to become pregnant or breastfeed during treatment.

apremilast
a-PRE-mil-ast

Otezla

Therapeutic class: Antiarthritics
Pharmacologic class: Phosphodiesterase-4 inhibitors

AVAILABLE FORMS
Tablets ⬛: 10 mg, 20 mg, 30 mg

INDICATIONS & DOSAGES
➤ **Active psoriatic arthritis; moderate to severe plaque psoriasis in patients who are candidates for phototherapy or systemic therapy; oral ulcers associated with Behçet disease**
Adults: Initially, 10 mg PO in a.m. on day 1; 10 mg PO b.i.d. (a.m. and p.m.) on day 2; 10 mg PO in a.m. and 20 mg PO in p.m. on day 3; 20 mg PO b.i.d. (a.m. and p.m.) on day 4; 20 mg PO in a.m. and 30 mg PO in p.m. on day 5; then 30 mg PO b.i.d. (a.m. and p.m.) on day 6 and thereafter.
Adjust-a-dose: In patients with severe renal impairment (CrCl less than 30 mL/minute), give doses according to a.m. schedule only (omit p.m. doses) from days 1 through 5. For day 6 and onward, give 30 mg once daily.

ADMINISTRATION
PO
• Give without regard to meals.
• Don't crush, split, or allow patient to chew tablets.
• Store tablets below 86° F (30° C).

ACTION
Increases intracellular cAMP level. Its action in the treatment of psoriatic arthritis and psoriasis isn't well defined.

Route	Onset	Peak	Duration
PO	Unknown	2.5 hr	Unknown

Half-life: 6 to 9 hours.

ADVERSE REACTIONS
CNS: headache, depression, fatigue, insomnia, migraine. **EENT:** nasopharyngitis, tooth abscess. **GI:** diarrhea, frequent bowel movements, nausea, vomiting, upper abdominal pain, decreased appetite, dyspepsia, GERD. **Metabolic:** weight loss. **Musculoskeletal:**

back pain, arthralgia. **Respiratory:** URI, bronchitis. **Skin:** folliculitis.

INTERACTIONS

Drug-drug. *Strong CYP450 inducers (carbamazepine, phenobarbital, phenytoin, rifampin):* May decrease apremilast level, causing loss of effectiveness. Use together isn't recommended.
Drug-herb. *St. John's wort:* May decrease apremilast level. Consider therapy modification.

EFFECTS ON LAB TEST RESULTS

None reported.

CONTRAINDICATIONS & CAUTIONS

- Contraindicated in patients hypersensitive to drug or its components.

Alert: Use cautiously in patients with history of depression or suicidality. Weigh risks and benefits of using drug in these patients.
- Use cautiously in patients with severe renal impairment.
- Use cautiously in older adults and patients taking medications that can lead to volume depletion or hypotension; they are at increased risk of complications from severe diarrhea, nausea, or vomiting.
- Safety and effectiveness in children haven't been established.

Dialyzable drug: Unknown.

PREGNANCY-LACTATION-REPRODUCTION

- Use cautiously during pregnancy and only if benefits outweigh fetal risk. Enroll patients who are pregnant in pregnancy exposure registry (1-877-311-8972 or https://mothertobaby.org/ongoing-study/otezla-apremilast/) to monitor pregnancy outcomes.
- It isn't known if drug appears in human milk. Use cautiously during breastfeeding.

NURSING CONSIDERATIONS

- Titration to maintenance dose is intended to reduce GI symptoms with initial therapy.
- Monitor patient for complications of diarrhea or vomiting. Severe symptoms may require dosage reductions or drug suspension.
- Monitor patient for depression or suicidality.
- Monitor patient regularly for unexplained or significant weight loss. Evaluate cause and consider discontinuing drug.

PATIENT TEACHING

- Explain to patient that drug may cause weight loss.

Alert: Warn patient and caregivers to immediately report signs and symptoms of depression or suicidality.
- Instruct patient to titrate drug as directed to reduce GI symptoms.
- Advise patient that drug may be taken without regard to food and not to crush, chew, or split tablets.

aprepitant

ah-PRE-pit-ant

Cinvanti, Emend

fosaprepitant dimeglumine

Emend

Therapeutic class: Antiemetics
Pharmacologic class: Substance P and neurokinin-1 receptor antagonists

AVAILABLE FORMS

aprepitant
Capsules: 40 mg, 80 mg, 125 mg
Injection (emulsion): 130 mg/18 mL single-dose vial
Powder for oral suspension (kit): 125 mg
fosaprepitant dimeglumine
Injection: 150-mg single-dose vial

INDICATIONS & DOSAGES

➤ **To prevent nausea and vomiting after highly emetogenic chemotherapy (HEC) (including cisplatin) and moderately emetogenic chemotherapy (MEC), with a 5-HT_3 antagonist and a corticosteroid**
Adults and children age 12 and older (capsules): On day 1 of chemotherapy, 125 mg PO 1 hour before treatment; on days 2 and 3, give 80 mg PO 1 hour before chemotherapy or if no chemotherapy is scheduled, give in the morning.
Adults unable to swallow capsules and children age 6 months to younger than 12 years weighing 6 kg or more (oral suspension): On day 1 of chemotherapy, 3 mg/kg PO 1 hour before treatment; maximum dose, 125 mg. On days 2 and 3, 2 mg/kg PO 1 hour before chemotherapy or, if no chemotherapy is scheduled, give in the morning; maximum dose, 80 mg.

Fosaprepitant single-day regimen
Adults: 150 mg IV over 20 to 30 minutes 30 minutes before chemotherapy.
Children age 12 and older: 150 mg IV over 30 minutes 30 minutes before chemotherapy.
Children ages 2 to younger than 12 weighing at least 6 kg: 4 mg/kg (maximum dose, 150 mg) IV over 60 minutes 30 minutes before chemotherapy.
Children ages 6 months to younger than 2 years weighing at least 6 kg: 5 mg/kg (maximum dose, 150 mg) IV over 60 minutes 30 minutes before chemotherapy.
Fosaprepitant and aprepitant 3-day regimen
Children ages 12 to 17: On day 1, 115 mg IV over 30 minutes 30 minutes before chemotherapy; on days 2 and 3, give 80 mg capsule PO 1 hour before treatment or, if no chemotherapy is scheduled, give in the morning.
Children ages 6 months to younger than 12 years weighing at least 6 kg: On day 1, 3 mg/kg (maximum dose, 115 mg) IV over 60 minutes 30 minutes before chemotherapy; on days 2 and 3, give 2 mg/kg (maximum dose, 80 mg) oral suspension PO 1 hour before chemotherapy or, if no chemotherapy is scheduled, give in the morning.
Aprepitant (Cinvanti)
Adults: Single-dose regimen for HEC: On day 1, 130 mg IV over 30 minutes 30 minutes before chemotherapy. Single-dose regimen for MEC: On day 1, 130 mg IV over 30 minutes 30 minutes before chemotherapy.
➤ **Prevention of nausea and vomiting associated with initial and repeat courses of MEC chemotherapy as a 3-day regimen with dexamethasone and a 5-HT$_3$ antagonist (Cinvanti)**
Adults: On day 1 of chemotherapy, give 100 mg IV emulsion and complete 30 minutes before treatment. On days 2 and 3, give 80 mg PO once daily.
➤ **To prevent postoperative nausea and vomiting**
Adults: 40 mg PO within 3 hours before induction of anesthesia.

ADMINISTRATION
PO
• Give drug without regard for food.
• Drug may be given with other antiemetics.
• Oral suspension should be prepared by a health care provider according to manufacturer's instructions, but once prepared may be administered by a health care provider, patient, or caregiver.
• Refer to manufacturer's instructions and instructions for dexamethasone and 5-HT$_3$ antagonist for concomitant administration.
• Refrigerate prepared oral suspension until administered. May store at room temperature for up to 3 hours before use. Discard any dose remaining after 72 hours.
IV
Fosaprepitant (Emend)
▼ Reconstitute with 5 mL of NSS. Add the NSS along the vial wall to prevent foaming. Swirl gently and avoid shaking.
▼ Add entire reconstituted volume to infusion bag containing 145 mL of NSS. Total volume will be 150 mL and concentration will be 1 mg/mL.
▼ Gently invert the bag two to three times.
▼ Final fosaprepitant (Emend) solution is stable for 24 hours at room temperature.
Aprepitant (Cinvanti)
▼ For 130-mg dose, aseptically prepare an infusion bag filled with 130 mL NSS or D$_5$W; then withdraw 18 mL from the vial and transfer it into infusion bag to yield a total volume of 148 mL.
▼ For 100-mg dose, aseptically prepare an infusion bag filled with 100 mL NSS or D$_5$W; then withdraw 14 mL from the vial and transfer it into infusion bag to yield a total volume of 114 mL.
▼ Gently invert the prepared bag four to five times. Avoid shaking.
▼ Before administering either drug, inspect bag for particulate matter and discoloration. Discard if particulates or discoloration is observed.
▼ Cinvanti is stable for 6 hours in NSS or 12 hours in D$_5$W.
▼ **Incompatibilities:** Solutions containing divalent cations (e.g., Ca^{2+}, Mg^{2+}), including lactated Ringer solution and Hartmann solution.

ACTION
Inhibits emesis by selectively antagonizing substance P and neurokinin-1 receptors in the brain; appears to be synergistic with 5-HT$_3$ antagonists and corticosteroids.

Route	Onset	Peak	Duration
PO	Unknown	3–4 hr	Unknown
IV	Unknown	<30 min	Unknown

Half-life: 9 to 13 hours.

ADVERSE REACTIONS
CNS: asthenia, fatigue, dizziness, fever, headache, peripheral neuropathy, syncope, anxiety, hypoesthesia. **CV:** *bradycardia,* HTN, hypotension. **EENT:** dry mouth, mucous membrane disorder, tinnitus. **GI:** anorexia, constipation, diarrhea, nausea, abdominal pain, eructation, flatulence, gastritis, heartburn, vomiting, dyspepsia. **GU:** UTI. **Hematologic:** *neutropenia, leukopenia, thrombocytopenia,* anemia. **Hepatic:** increased ALT level. **Metabolic:** dehydration. **Musculoskeletal:** extremity pain. **Skin:** pruritus, alopecia, infusion-site reaction. **Other:** candidiasis, hiccups.

INTERACTIONS
Drug-drug. *Alprazolam, midazolam, triazolam:* May increase levels of these drugs. Watch for CNS effects, such as increased sedation. Decrease benzodiazepine dose.
Atazanavir, clarithromycin, diltiazem, erythromycin, itraconazole, ketoconazole, nefazodone, nelfinavir, ritonavir, troleandomycin, other CYP3A4 inhibitors: May increase aprepitant level and risk of toxicity. Use together cautiously.
Carbamazepine, phenytoin, rifampin, other CYP3A4 inducers: May decrease aprepitant level. Watch for decreased antiemetic effect.
Dexamethasone, methylprednisolone: May increase levels of these drugs and risk of toxicity. Decrease PO corticosteroid dose by 50%; decrease IV methylprednisolone dose by 25%.
Diltiazem: May increase diltiazem level. Monitor HR and BP. Avoid using together.
Docetaxel, etoposide, ifosfamide, imatinib, irinotecan, paclitaxel, vinorelbine, vinblastine, vincristine: May increase levels and risk of toxicity of these drugs. Use together cautiously.
Hormonal contraceptives: May decrease contraceptive effectiveness. Female patients should use additional birth control method during therapy and for 1 month after last dose.
Paroxetine: May decrease paroxetine and aprepitant effects. Monitor patient for effectiveness.
Phenytoin: May decrease effectiveness of aprepitant. Avoid use together.
Pimozide: May increase pimozide level. Use together is contraindicated.

Warfarin: May decrease warfarin effectiveness. Monitor INR carefully for 2 weeks after each aprepitant treatment.
Drug-herb. *St. John's wort:* May decrease antiemetic effects by inducing CYP3A4. Discourage use together.
Drug-food. *Grapefruit juice:* May increase drug level and risk of toxicity. Discourage use together.

EFFECTS ON LAB TEST RESULTS
• May increase ALP, AST, ALT, BUN, creatinine, glucose, and urine protein levels.
• May decrease sodium levels.
• May decrease Hb level and WBC, platelet, and neutrophil counts.

CONTRAINDICATIONS & CAUTIONS
• Contraindicated in patients hypersensitive to fosaprepitant, aprepitant, or their components. Hypersensitivity reactions have been reported.
• Use cautiously in patients receiving chemotherapy drugs metabolized mainly via CYP3A4 and in those with severe hepatic disease.
• Drug isn't approved for use in children.
Dialyzable drug: No.
⚠ *Overdose S&S:* Drowsiness, headache.

PREGNANCY-LACTATION-REPRODUCTION
• Use during pregnancy only if clearly needed.
• Cinvanti contains alcohol and shouldn't be used during pregnancy.
• Patients taking hormonal contraceptives should use an additional form of contraception during therapy and for 1 month after final dose.
• It isn't known if drug appears in human milk. Use cautiously during breastfeeding.

NURSING CONSIDERATIONS
• Avoid giving drug for more than 3 days per chemotherapy cycle.
🕐 *Alert:* IV form is only given on day 1 of a 3-day antiemetic regimen.
🕐 *Alert:* Before giving drug, screen patient carefully for possible drug and herb interactions.
• Monitor patients for hypersensitivity reactions (dyspnea, flushing, eye swelling, pruritus and wheezing) directly after administration.

Reactions in bold italics are *life-threatening*. Interactions may have a *rapid onset* or a *delayed onset*.

• Don't give drug for established nausea or vomiting.

• Expect to give drug with other antiemetics to treat breakthrough emesis.

• Monitor CBC, LFT results, and creatinine level periodically during therapy.

• *Look alike–sound alike:* Don't confuse aprepitant (oral and IV form) with fosaprepitant (IV form). Don't confuse Emend with Vfend.

PATIENT TEACHING

• Advise patient to report all adverse reactions to prescriber.

• Tell patient that severe hypersensitivity reactions have occurred and that patient will be monitored after therapy.

• If nausea or vomiting occurs, instruct patient to take breakthrough antiemetics rather than more aprepitant.

• Urge patient to report use of any other drugs or herbs.

• Instruct patient in safe oral drug administration.

• Advise patient who takes a hormonal contraceptive to use an additional form of birth control during therapy and for 1 month after last dose.

• Tell patient who takes warfarin that PT and INR will be monitored closely for 2 weeks after therapy starts.

SAFETY ALERT!

argatroban
ahr-GAH-troh-ban

Therapeutic class: Anticoagulants
Pharmacologic class: Direct thrombin inhibitors

AVAILABLE FORMS

Injection: 1 mg/mL in 50-mL, 125-mL vial; 100 mg/mL in 2.5-mL vial

INDICATIONS & DOSAGES

➤ **To prevent or treat thrombosis in patients with heparin-induced thrombocytopenia**

Adults without hepatic impairment: 2 mcg/kg/minute, given as a continuous IV infusion; adjust dose until the steady-state PTT is 1½ to 3 times the initial baseline value, not to exceed 100 seconds; maximum dose, 10 mcg/kg/minute. See current manufacturer's label for recommended doses and infusion rates.

Adjust-a-dose: For adults with moderate or severe hepatic impairment, reduce first dose to 0.5 mcg/kg/minute, given as a continuous infusion. Monitor PTT closely and adjust dosage as needed.

➤ **Anticoagulation in patients with or at risk for heparin-induced thrombocytopenia during PCI**

Adults: Start a continuous IV infusion at 25 mcg/kg/minute and give a 350 mcg/kg IV bolus over 3 to 5 minutes. Check activated clotting time (ACT) 5 to 10 minutes after bolus dose is completed. Proceed with procedure if ACT is more than 300 seconds.

Adjust-a-dose: Use the following table to adjust dosage.

Activated clotting time (ACT)	Additional IV bolus	Continuous IV infusion
<300 sec	150 mcg/kg	30 mcg/kg/min*
>450 sec	None needed	15 mcg/kg/min*

*Check ACT again after 5 to 10 minutes.

Once a therapeutic ACT (300 to 450 sec) has been achieved, continue this dose for the duration of the procedure. In case of dissection, impending abrupt closure, thrombus formation during the procedure, or inability to achieve or maintain an ACT exceeding 300 seconds, give an additional bolus of 150 mcg/kg and increase infusion rate to 40 mcg/kg/minute. Check ACT again after 5 to 10 minutes.

ADMINISTRATION

IV

▼ Before starting therapy, obtain a complete list of patient's prescription and OTC drugs and supplements, including herbs.

▼ Stop all parenteral anticoagulants before giving drug. Giving with antiplatelets, thrombolytics, and other anticoagulants may increase risk of bleeding.

▼ Before starting drug, get results of baseline coagulation tests, platelet count, Hb level, and hematocrit, and report any abnormalities to prescriber.

▼ Dilute each 2.5-mL vial with 250 mL of NSS, D_5W, or lactated Ringer injection to a final concentration of 1 mg/mL. Dilution isn't required for the 50-mL or 125-mL vial.

▼ Mix the solution by repeated inversion of the diluent bag for 1 minute.

▼ Don't expose solution to direct sunlight.

▼ See manufacturer's instructions for storage.

▼ **Incompatibilities:** Other IV drugs.

ACTION

Reversibly binds to the thrombin-active site and inhibits thrombin-catalyzed or -induced reactions: fibrin formation; coagulation factor V, VIII, and XIII activation; protein C activation; and platelet aggregation. Inhibits the action of free and clot-associated thrombin.

Route	Onset	Peak	Duration
IV	Rapid	1–3 hr	Duration of infusion

Half-life: 39 to 51 minutes.

ADVERSE REACTIONS

CNS: *cerebrovascular disorder, intracranial bleeding,* fever, pain, headache. **CV:** *hemorrhage,* atrial fibrillation, *cardiac arrest,* hypotension, *ventricular tachycardia,* chest pain, angina, *bradycardia, MI,* groin or brachial bleeding. **GI:** abdominal pain, diarrhea, *GI bleeding,* nausea, vomiting. **GU:** abnormal renal function, hematuria, UTI. **Hematologic:** anemia. **Respiratory:** cough, dyspnea, pneumonia, hemoptysis. **Skin:** *injection-site hemorrhage.* **Other:** allergic reactions, infection, *sepsis.*

INTERACTIONS

Drug-drug. *Glycoprotein IIb/IIIa inhibitors (abciximab, eptifibatide, tirofiban), thrombolytics:* May increase risk of bleeding, including intracranial bleeding. Avoid using together. Safety and effectiveness of concurrent use haven't been established.
Heparin: May increase risk of bleeding. Allow sufficient time for heparin's effect on PTT to decrease before starting argatroban.
Warfarin: May prolong PT and INR and may increase risk of bleeding. Monitor patient closely.

Drug-herb. *Herbs with anticoagulant or antiplatelet properties (alfalfa, anise, bilberry, others):* May increase risk of bleeding. Discourage use together.

EFFECTS ON LAB TEST RESULTS

- May decrease Hb level and hematocrit.
- May prolong PTT and ACT.

CONTRAINDICATIONS & CAUTIONS

- Contraindicated in patients who have overt major bleeding or who are hypersensitive to drug or any of its components.
- Use cautiously in patients with hepatic disease or conditions that increase the risk of hemorrhage, such as severe HTN.
- Use cautiously in patients who have just had lumbar puncture, spinal anesthesia, or major surgery, especially of the brain, spinal cord, or eye; patients with hematologic conditions causing increased bleeding tendencies, such as congenital or acquired bleeding disorders; and patients with GI ulcers or other lesions.
- Use cautiously in patients who are critically ill; reduced dosages may be needed.
- Safety and effectiveness in children haven't been established.

Dialyzable drug: 20% during 4-hour hemodialysis session.

⚠ *Overdose S&S:* Excessive anticoagulation, with or without bleeding.

PREGNANCY-LACTATION-REPRODUCTION

- There are no adequate well-controlled studies during pregnancy. Use during pregnancy only if clearly needed.
- It isn't known if drug appears in human milk. Patient should discontinue breastfeeding or discontinue drug.

NURSING CONSIDERATIONS

- Check PTT 2 hours after giving drug; dose adjustments may be required to get a targeted PTT of 1½ to 3 times the baseline, no longer than 100 seconds. Steady state is achieved 1 to 3 hours after starting drug.
- Draw blood for ACT every 20 to 30 minutes during prolonged PCI.

🔆 *Alert:* Patients can hemorrhage from any site in body. Unexplained decreases in hematocrit or BP or other unexplained symptoms may signify a hemorrhagic event.

- To convert to warfarin therapy, give expected daily dose of warfarin PO with argatroban at up to 2 mcg/kg/minute until INR exceeds 4 on combined therapy. If argatroban infusion rate is greater than 2 mcg/kg/minute, decrease rate to 2 mcg/kg/minute before administering warfarin. After argatroban is stopped, repeat INR in 4 to 6 hours. If the repeat INR is less than desired therapeutic range, resume IV argatroban infusion. Repeat procedure daily until desired therapeutic range on warfarin alone is reached.

Reactions in bold italics are *life-threatening*. Interactions may have a *rapid onset* or a ***delayed onset***.

- *Look alike–sound alike:* Don't confuse argatroban with Aggrastat.

PATIENT TEACHING
- Instruct patient who is pregnant, has recently delivered, or is breastfeeding to notify prescriber.
- Advise patient to report bleeding, tarry stools, bruising, rash, or difficulty breathing immediately.

ARIPiprazole ☒
ar-i-PIP-ra-zole

Abilify✔, Abilify Maintena, Abilify MyCite

ARIPiprazole lauroxil ☒
Aristada, Aristada Initio

Therapeutic class: Antipsychotics
Pharmacologic class: Quinolinone derivatives

AVAILABLE FORMS
Oral solution: 1 mg/mL
Suspension for IM use (extended-release): 300-mg, 400-mg vial or prefilled syringe (Abilify Maintena); 441 mg/1.6 mL, 662 mg/2.4 mL, 882 mg/3.2 mL, 1,064 mg/3.9 mL in prefilled syringes (Aristada); 675 mg/2.4 mL in prefilled syringe (Aristada Initio)
Tablets: 2 mg, 5 mg, 10 mg, 15 mg, 20 mg, 30 mg
Tablets (ODTs): 10 mg, 15 mg
Tablets (with sensor [Abilify MyCite]) ⓒ: 2 mg, 5 mg, 10 mg, 15 mg, 20 mg, 30 mg

INDICATIONS & DOSAGES
Adjust-a-dose (for all indications except adjunctive treatment of major depressive disorder): Refer to manufacturer's instructions for drug interactions, CYP2D6 poor metabolizers, and missed dose dosage adjustments.
➤ **Schizophrenia (oral, IM [Abilify Maintena])**
Adults: Initially, 10 to 15 mg PO daily; increase to maximum daily dose of 30 mg, if needed, after at least 2 weeks. Continue patients who respond on the lowest dosage needed to maintain remission. Periodically reassess patients to determine the need for maintenance treatment.

Or, 400 mg IM monthly. For patients who have never taken aripiprazole, establish

tolerability with aripiprazole PO before initiating treatment with Abilify Maintena. It may take up to 2 weeks to fully assess tolerability. After the first IM injection, administer 10 to 20 mg aripiprazole PO for 14 days. For patients already stable on another oral antipsychotic and known to tolerate aripiprazole, after the first IM injection, continue treatment with the other antipsychotic for 14 days.

Maintenance dosage is 400 mg IM monthly, no sooner than 26 days after previous injection.
Adjust-a-dose: If adverse reactions occur with 400-mg dose or if patient is a poor metabolizer of CYP2D6, consider reducing dosage to 300 mg IM monthly. ☒
Adolescents ages 13 to 17: Initially, 2 mg PO daily; increase to 5 mg after 2 days, then to recommended dose of 10 mg in 2 more days. May titrate to maximum daily dose of 30 mg in 5-mg increments. Continue patients who respond on the lowest dosage needed to maintain remission. Periodically reassess patients to determine need for maintenance treatment.
➤ **Schizophrenia (Aristada, Aristada Initio)**
Adults: Establish tolerability with oral aripiprazole before initiating treatment with aripiprazole lauroxil, which may take up to 2 weeks. Base initial monthly dose of Aristada on current oral daily aripiprazole dose. If current oral aripiprazole dose is 10 mg/day, give 441 mg IM in the deltoid or gluteal muscle once per month. If current oral aripiprazole dose is 15 mg/day, give 662 mg once per month, 882 mg once every 6 weeks, or 1,064 mg once every 2 months IM in the gluteal muscle. If current oral aripiprazole dose is 20 mg/day or more, give 882 mg IM in the gluteal muscle once every month. Continue oral aripiprazole for 21 consecutive days after initiation of the first monthly dose or give a single injection of 675 mg Aristada Initio in the deltoid or gluteal muscle and one dose of oral aripiprazole 30 mg. Avoid injecting both preparations into the same deltoid or gluteal muscle.

The first Aristada injection may be administered on the same day as Aristada Initio or up to 10 days after.
Adjust-a-dose: Adjust dosage as needed; if a dose is required earlier than the recommended interval, don't administer earlier than 14 days after the previous injection.
➤ **Bipolar mania, including manic and mixed episodes, with or without psychotic**

---

features; adjunctive therapy with either lithium or valproate for treatment of manic and mixed episodes associated with bipolar I disorder with or without psychotic features

Adults: Initially, 15 mg PO once daily as monotherapy or 10 to 15 mg PO once daily as adjunctive therapy with lithium or valproate. Target dose is 15 mg/day as monotherapy or adjunctive therapy. May increase dose to maximum of 30 mg/day based on clinical response. For maintenance, continue patients who respond on monotherapy on the lowest dosage needed to maintain remission. Periodically reassess patients to determine the long-term usefulness of maintenance treatment.

Children ages 10 to 17: Initially, 2 mg PO daily; increase to 5 mg PO daily after 2 days, then to recommended dose of 10 mg after 2 additional days. May titrate to maximum daily dose of 30 mg in 5-mg increments every 5 days. Give as monotherapy or as adjunct to lithium or valproate. For maintenance, continue patients who respond on monotherapy on the lowest dosage needed to maintain remission. Periodically reassess patients to determine the need for maintenance treatment.

➤ **Bipolar I disorder maintenance monotherapy**

Adults: For patients who have never taken aripiprazole, establish tolerability with oral aripiprazole before initiating treatment with extended-release IM suspension. Once tolerability is established, give 400 mg (extended-release suspension) IM monthly. After first injection, continue oral aripiprazole for 14 consecutive days to achieve therapeutic aripiprazole concentrations during initiation of therapy. Maintenance dosage is 400 mg IM monthly, given no sooner than 26 days after previous injection.

Adjust-a-dose: If adverse reactions occur with 400-mg dose or if patient is a poor metabolizer of CYP2D6, consider reducing dosage to 300 mg IM monthly. ▧

➤ **Adjunctive treatment of major depressive disorder**

Adults: Initially, 2 to 5 mg PO daily. Dose range is 2 to 15 mg/day. Dosage adjustments of up to 5 mg/day should occur gradually, at intervals of no less than 1 week.

➤ **Irritability associated with autistic disorder**

Children ages 6 to 17: Initially, 2 mg PO daily for 7 days. Increase dosage to 5 mg/day, with subsequent increases to 10 or 15 mg/day if needed. Gradually adjust dosage up to 5 mg/day at intervals of no less than 1 week.

➤ **Tourette disorder**

Children ages 6 to 18 weighing 50 kg or more: Initially, 2 mg/day PO for 2 days; then increase to 5 mg/day with a target dose of 10 mg/day on day 8. If optimal control of tics isn't achieved, increase by 5 mg/day at intervals of no less than 1 week to maximum of 20 mg/day.

Children ages 6 to 18 weighing less than 50 kg: Initially, 2 mg/day PO, increasing to target dose of 5 mg/day after 2 days. If optimal control of tics isn't achieved, increase to 10 mg/day. Adjust dosage at intervals of no less than 1 week.

➤ **Agitation associated with schizophrenia or bipolar mania**

Adults: 9.75 mg IM (range, 5.25 to 15 mg). No additional benefit was demonstrated for 15 mg compared to 9.75 mg. May repeat every 2 hours to a total of 30 mg/day. If ongoing therapy is indicated, switch to oral therapy as soon as possible.

ADMINISTRATION
PO

• Give drug without regard for food.

• Substitute the oral solution on a mg-per-mg basis up to 25 mg. Give patients taking 30-mg tablets 25 mg of solution.

• Keep ODTs in blister package until ready to use. Don't split tablet. Place tablet on the tongue and allow to dissolve; no liquid is needed.

• Abilify MyCite drug-device combination system consists of tablets with an embedded ingestible event marker (IEM) to track drug ingestion, a wearable patch containing a sensor that detects the signal from the IEM after ingestion and transmits data to a smartphone, a smartphone application (app) to display patient information, and a Web-based portal for health care professionals and caregivers. Refer to manufacturer's detailed instructions for use.

• Apply the MyCite patch when instructed by the app to the left side of the body just above the lower edge of the rib cage. Don't place patch over skin that is irritated, inflamed, or not intact, or is overlapping the area where the last patch was located.

• Patient must swallow tablets with sensor whole; don't divide, crush, or allow patient to chew these tablets.

- Don't repeat dose if tablet with sensor isn't detected after ingestion.
- Store oral solution at room temperature; it can be used up to 6 months after opening.

IM
- Inject slowly into the deltoid or gluteal muscle according to manufacturer's instructions; rotate injection sites.

⚠ *Alert:* Don't confuse IM dosage forms (Abilify Maintena, Aristada, Aristada Initio).

ACTION
Thought to exert partial agonist activity at dopamine 2 and 5-HT_{1A} receptors and antagonist activity at 5-HT_{2A} receptors.

Route	Onset	Peak	Duration
PO	Unknown	3–5 hr	Unknown
IM	Unknown	1–3 hr	Unknown
		4–7 days (Abilify Maintena)	

Half-life: About 75 hours in patients with normal metabolism. Abilify Maintena, 30 to 45 days; Aristada, 54 to 57 days; Aristada Initio, 15 to 18 days.

ADVERSE REACTIONS
CNS: headache, anxiety, insomnia, somnolence, sedation, akathisia, extrapyramidal disorder, tremor, asthenia, fatigue, lethargy, pain, dizziness, irritability, fever, restlessness, agitation, impaired concentration. **CV:** tachycardia, orthostatic hypotension. **EENT:** blurred vision, epistaxis, toothache, increased salivation, drooling, nasopharyngitis, dry mouth, pharyngolaryngeal pain. **GI:** nausea, vomiting, constipation, anorexia, dyspepsia, diarrhea, abdominal pain, increased appetite. **GU:** urinary incontinence. **Hematologic: neutropenia. Metabolic:** weight gain, weight loss, hyperglycemia, hypercholesterolemia. **Musculoskeletal:** stiffness, muscle spasms, muscle rigidity, dystonia, myalgia, arthralgia, extremity pain. **Respiratory:** cough, URI. **Skin:** rash, application-site rash (patch), injection-site reaction.

INTERACTIONS
Drug-drug. *Antihypertensives:* May enhance antihypertensive effects. Monitor BP.
Benzodiazepines (lorazepam): May cause excessive sedation and orthostatic hypotension. Monitor patient closely.
Carbamazepine and other CYP3A4 inducers: May decrease aripiprazole level and effectiveness. See manufacturer's

instructions for dosage adjustments. Monitor patient closely.
CNS depressants: May lead to enhanced CNS depression. Use together with caution.
Ketoconazole and other CYP3A4 inhibitors: May increase risk of serious toxic effects. Start treatment with reduced dose of aripiprazole, and monitor patient closely.
Metoclopramide: May increase risk of extrapyramidal reactions. Use together is contraindicated.
Opioid class warning: May cause slow or difficult breathing, sedation, and death. Avoid use together. If use together is necessary, limit dosage and duration of each drug to the minimum necessary for desired effect.
Strong CYP2D6 inhibitors (fluoxetine, paroxetine, quinidine): May increase aripiprazole level and toxicity. See manufacturer's instructions for dosage adjustments.
Drug-food. *Grapefruit juice:* May increase drug level. Tell patient not to take drug with grapefruit juice.
Drug-lifestyle. *Alcohol use:* May increase CNS effects. Discourage use together.

EFFECTS ON LAB TEST RESULTS
- May increase CK, LDL cholesterol, triglyceride, and glucose levels.
- May decrease HDL cholesterol level.
- May decrease WBC count and ANC.

CONTRAINDICATIONS & CAUTIONS
- Contraindicated in patients hypersensitive to drug.
- Safety and effectiveness in children with major depressive disorder, agitation associated with schizophrenia, and bipolar mania haven't been established.

Boxed Warning Older adults with dementia-related psychosis treated with atypical antipsychotics are at an increased risk for death. Drug isn't approved for treatment of patients with dementia-related psychosis. ■
- Use cautiously in patients with CV disease, cerebrovascular disease, or conditions that could predispose patient to hypotension, such as dehydration or hypovolemia.
- Life-threatening arrhythmias have occurred with therapeutic doses of antipsychotics.
- Use cautiously in patients with history of seizures or with conditions that lower the seizure threshold.
- Use cautiously in patients who engage in strenuous exercise, are exposed to extreme

heat, take anticholinergics, or are susceptible to dehydration.

- Use cautiously in patients with Lewy body dementia or Parkinson disease; drug may aggravate motor disturbances.
- Use cautiously in patients at risk for aspiration pneumonia, such as those with Alzheimer disease.
- Use cautiously in patients at risk for falls, including those who have diseases or conditions or are taking medications that may cause somnolence, orthostatic hypotension, or motor or sensory instability.
- Discontinue drug at first sign of blood dyscrasia or if ANC is less than $1,000/mm^3$.
- Abilify MyCite drug-device product is only approved for use in adults.

Dialyzable drug: Unlikely.

⚠ *Overdose S&S:* Somnolence, tremor, vomiting, acidosis, aggression, atrial fibrillation, bradycardia, coma, confusion, seizures, depressed level of consciousness, HTN, hypokalemia, hypotension, increased AST and blood CK levels, lethargy, loss of consciousness, aspiration pneumonia, prolonged QRS complex, prolonged QT interval, respiratory arrest, status epilepticus, tachycardia.

PREGNANCY-LACTATION-REPRODUCTION

- Safety of atypical antipsychotic use during pregnancy hasn't been well studied; routine use isn't recommended. Use during pregnancy only if potential benefit justifies fetal risk.
- 🛈 *Alert:* Neonates exposed to antipsychotics during the third trimester are at risk for developing extrapyramidal signs and symptoms (repetitive muscle movements of the face and body) and withdrawal signs and symptoms (agitation, abnormally increased or decreased muscle tone, tremors, sleepiness, severe difficulty breathing, difficulty feeding) after delivery.
- Enroll patients exposed to aripiprazole during pregnancy in the National Pregnancy Registry for Atypical Antipsychotics (1-866-961-2388 or http://womensmentalhealth.org/clinical-and-research-programs/pregnancyregistry/).
- Drug appears in human milk. Use isn't recommended during breastfeeding.

NURSING CONSIDERATIONS

- 🛈 *Alert:* NMS may occur. Monitor patient for hyperpyrexia, muscle rigidity, altered mental status, irregular pulse or BP, tachycardia, diaphoresis, and cardiac arrhythmias.

- If signs and symptoms of NMS occur, immediately stop drug and notify prescriber.
- Monitor patient for signs and symptoms of tardive dyskinesia. Older adults, especially women, are at highest risk of developing this adverse effect.
- 🛈 *Alert:* Fatal cerebrovascular adverse events (stroke, TIA) may occur in older adults with dementia. Drug isn't safe or effective in these patients.

Boxed Warning Drug may increase the risk of suicidal thinking and behavior in children, adolescents, and young adults ages 18 to 24 during the first 2 months of treatment, especially in those with major depressive or other psychiatric disorder. Monitor all patients for worsening or emergence of suicidal thoughts and behaviors. ■

- 🛈 *Alert:* Hyperglycemia may occur. Monitor patient with diabetes regularly. Patient with risk factors for diabetes should undergo fasting blood glucose testing at baseline and periodically. Monitor all patients for symptoms of hyperglycemia, including increased hunger, thirst, frequent urination, and weakness. Hyperglycemia may resolve when patient stops taking drug.
- Monitor patient for symptoms of metabolic syndrome (significant weight gain and increased BMI, HTN, hyperglycemia, hypercholesterolemia, and hypertriglyceridemia).
- Monitor patient for new or increasing compulsive or uncontrollable urges to gamble, binge eat, shop, and have sex. Dosage may need to be reduced or drug discontinued if urges occur.
- Monitor patients with clinically significant neutropenia for fever or other signs and symptoms of infection; treat promptly if they occur. Discontinue drug if ANC is less than $1,000/mm^3$ and monitor WBC count until recovery.
- Assess fall risk at start of treatment then periodically for patients who have diseases or conditions or are taking drugs that may cause somnolence, orthostatic hypotension, or motor or sensory instability.
- Monitor patient for abnormal body temperature regulation, especially if patient exercises, is exposed to extreme heat, takes anticholinergics, or is dehydrated.
- 🗝 Dosage adjustments may be indicated in patients who are known CYP2D6 poor metabolizers.

Reactions in bold italics are *life-threatening*. Interactions may have a *rapid onset* or a ***delayed onset***.

• Treat patient with the smallest dose for the shortest time, and periodically reevaluate for need to continue.

• Give prescriptions only for small quantities of drug, to reduce risk of overdose.

• Change Abilify MyCite patch weekly or sooner, as needed. Patient should keep patch on while showering, swimming, or exercising.

• Remove Abilify MyCite patch before an MRI or if patch causes skin irritation.

• Detection of tablet by the MyCite sensor takes 30 minutes to 2 hours and may not occur in some cases.

• Tracking drug ingestion in "real time" or during an emergency isn't recommended because detection of MyCite sensor may be delayed or not occur, causing a false-negative reading.

• *Look alike–sound alike:* Don't confuse aripiprazole with rabeprazole, omeprazole, or pantoprazole. Don't confuse IM dosage forms (Abilify Maintena, Aristada, Aristada Initio).

PATIENT TEACHING

Boxed Warning Advise families and caregivers to closely observe patient for clinical worsening, suicidality, or unusual changes in behavior. ■

• Caution patient or caregiver of patient taking an opioid with a benzodiazepine, CNS depressant, or alcohol to seek immediate medical attention if patient experiences dizziness, light-headedness, extreme sleepiness, slowed or difficult breathing, or unresponsiveness.

• Advise patient and caregiver to notify prescriber if compulsive or uncontrollable urges occur.

◑ *Alert:* Caution patient not to stop drug without first discussing with prescriber.

• Tell patient to use caution while driving or operating hazardous machinery because psychoactive drugs may impair judgment, thinking, or motor skills.

• Advise patient that grapefruit juice may interact with aripiprazole and to avoid its use.

• Advise patient that gradual improvement in symptoms should occur over several weeks rather than immediately.

◑ *Alert:* Warn patient with phenylketonuria that ODTs contain phenylalanine.

• Advise patient that each milliliter of oral solution contains 400 mg of sucrose and 200 mg of fructose.

• Tell patient to avoid alcohol use while taking drug.

• Advise patient to limit strenuous activity while taking drug to avoid dehydration.

• Instruct patient in safe drug administration and storage.

• Teach patient that the Abilify MyCite drug-device combination product is used to track drug ingestion. Ensure that patient is capable and willing to use a smartphone and app, and that the app is compatible with the specific phone. Assist patient to download app and encourage patient to follow instructions for use.

• Instruct patient to verify that the Abilify MyCite app is paired with the sensor patch before use.

• Teach patient that the Abilify MyCite app will direct patient to apply and remove the patch correctly. Tell patient to change the patch weekly and to keep it on while showering, swimming, or exercising.

• Tell patient that the Abilify MyCite patch will need to be removed before an MRI, then replaced with a new patch as soon as possible afterwards.

• Instruct patient to remove the patch if skin irritation occurs and to report this to prescriber.

• Instruct patient to take Abilify MyCite tablets whole.

• Teach patient that the Abilify MyCite tablets are usually detected within 30 minutes but there may be a delay of more than 2 hours for the smartphone app/Web portal to detect it. Inform patient that sometimes the tablet may not be detected at all. If tablet isn't detected, instruct patient not to repeat dose.

• Advise patient not to become pregnant or breastfeed without first discussing with prescriber.

asenapine
a-SEN-a-peen

Saphris, Secuado

Therapeutic class: Antipsychotics
Pharmacologic class: Dopamine–serotonin antagonists

AVAILABLE FORMS

Tablets (SL) ⊛*:* 2.5 mg, 5 mg, 10 mg
Transdermal system: 3.8 mg/24 hour, 5.7 mg/24 hour, 7.6 mg/24 hour

INDICATIONS & DOSAGES
➤ **Schizophrenia (acute and maintenance therapy)**
Adults: 5 mg SL b.i.d. May increase up to 10 mg b.i.d. after 1 week based on tolerability. For maintenance therapy, give 5 to 10 mg SL b.i.d. Or, 3.8 mg/24 hours (transdermal system). May increase to 5.7 mg/24 hours or 7.6 mg/24 hours after a week.
➤ **Acute manic or mixed episodes associated with bipolar I disorder as adjunctive therapy with either lithium or valproate**
Adults: 5 mg SL b.i.d. Dosage may be increased to a maximum of 10 mg SL b.i.d. as tolerated.
➤ **Acute manic or mixed episodes associated with bipolar I disorder as monotherapy**
Adults: 5 to 10 mg SL b.i.d.
Children ages 10 to 17: Initially, 2.5 mg SL b.i.d. May increase after 3 days to 5 mg SL b.i.d., then to 10 mg SL b.i.d. after 3 additional days based on tolerability.
➤ **Maintenance treatment of bipolar I disorder as monotherapy**
Adults: Continue dosage that patient received during stabilization (5 or 10 mg SL b.i.d.). Based on clinical response and tolerability, can decrease a dose of 10 mg SL b.i.d. to 5 mg SL b.i.d.

ADMINISTRATION
Sublingual
• Make sure patient doesn't split, crush, chew, or swallow tablet.
• Peel back colored tab on tablet pack, gently remove tablet, place under patient's tongue, and allow to dissolve completely.
• Patient shouldn't eat or drink for 10 minutes after taking drug.
Transdermal
• Don't open pouch until ready to apply a patch.
• Apply 1 patch daily to clean, dry, intact skin of the upper arm, upper back, abdomen, or hip, and leave on for only 24 hours.
• Patient should wear only 1 patch at a time and not use the same application site two times in a row.
• Don't cut patches.
• If patch comes completely off, apply a new one.
• Patient may shower while wearing patch; swimming and bathing haven't been evaluated.
• Don't apply heat over patch; prolonged heat application increases drug's plasma concentration.

ACTION
Unknown. May block dopamine and 5-HT receptors.

Route	Onset	Peak	Duration
SL	Immediate	0.5–1.5 hr	Unknown
Transdermal	Rapid	12–24 hr	Unknown

Half-life: SL, 24 hours; transdermal, 30 hours.

ADVERSE REACTIONS
CNS: akathisia, agitation, anxiety, depression, dizziness, extrapyramidal symptoms, fatigue, headache, insomnia, irritability, somnolence, manic symptoms, anger, taste perversion. **CV:** HTN, peripheral edema, tachycardia. **EENT:** dry mouth, oral hypoesthesia, salivary hypersecretion, toothache, glossitis, nasopharyngitis, oropharyngeal pain, nasal congestion. **GI:** constipation, dyspepsia, increased appetite, stomach discomfort, abdominal pain, nausea, vomiting. **GU:** dysmenorrhea. **Hematologic:** anemia. **Hepatic:** increased transaminase levels. **Metabolic:** weight gain, hyperinsulinemia, increased prolactin level, dehydration. **Musculoskeletal:** arthralgia, muscle strain, extremity pain. **Respiratory:** dyspnea, URI. **Skin:** rash, application-site reaction. **Other:** *suicidality.*

INTERACTIONS
Drug-drug. *Alpha₁ blockers (doxazosin, terazosin):* May increase risk of hypotension. Use together cautiously.
Antiarrhythmics, class IA (procainamide, quinidine) and class III (amiodarone, sotalol); antibiotics (gatifloxacin, moxifloxacin); antipsychotics (chlorpromazine, thioridazine, ziprasidone); citalopram: May prolong QTc interval, leading to lethal arrhythmias such as torsades de pointes. Avoid use together.
Antidepressants (fluvoxamine, imipramine, paroxetine): May increase asenapine level. Use together cautiously. Reduce paroxetine dosage by half if using with asenapine.
CNS agents: May enhance CNS depression. Use with caution.
CYP2D2 substrates and inhibitors (paroxetine): May increase substrate and inhibitor level. Reduce dosage of these drugs.

Reactions in bold italics are *life-threatening*. Interactions may have a *rapid onset* or a **delayed onset**.

Dextromethorphan: May increase dextromethorphan level. Use together cautiously.
Metoclopramide: May increase risk of extrapyramidal reactions. Avoid administering together.
Opioid class warning: May cause slow or difficult breathing, sedation, and death. Avoid use together. If use together is necessary, limit dosage and duration of each drug to the minimum necessary for desired effect.
Strong CYP1A2 inhibitors (fluvoxamine): May increase asenapine level. Monitor therapy; adjust asenapine dose as needed.
Drug-lifestyle. *Alcohol use:* May increase CNS effects. Discourage use together.

EFFECTS ON LAB TEST RESULTS

• May increase glucose, total cholesterol, LDL, ALT, AST, serum triglyceride, CK, and prolactin levels.
• May decrease sodium and HDL cholesterol level.
• May decrease Hb level and platelet, WBC, and neutrophil counts.

CONTRAINDICATIONS & CAUTIONS

Boxed Warning Older adults with dementia-related psychosis treated with atypical or conventional antipsychotics are at increased risk for death. Antipsychotics aren't approved for the treatment of dementia-related psychosis. ▪
• *Opioid class warning:* Opioids should only be prescribed with benzodiazepines or other CNS depressants to patients for whom alternative treatment options are inadequate.
• Contraindicated in patients with a known hypersensitivity and in patients with severe hepatic failure (Child-Pugh class C). Hypersensitivity reactions may occur as early as the first dose.
• *Alert:* Avoid use in patients with conditions that may increase risk of torsades de pointes and in those taking other drugs that prolong QTc interval.
• Use cautiously in patients with or at risk for diabetes; in those with known CV or cerebrovascular disease, preexisting low WBC count, difficulty swallowing, history of leukopenia or neutropenia, Parkinson disease, or history of seizures or conditions that lower the seizure threshold; and in patients who are antipsychotic-naive.
• Don't use in patients at risk for aspiration pneumonia.

• Use cautiously in patients at risk for falls, including those who have diseases or conditions or are taking medications that may cause somnolence, orthostatic hypotension, or motor or sensory instability.
• Safe and effective use for bipolar I disorder in children younger than age 10 or for schizophrenia in children younger than age 12 hasn't been established.
Dializable drug: Unknown.
⚠ *Overdose S&S:* Agitation, confusion, hypotension, circulatory collapse.

PREGNANCY-LACTATION-REPRODUCTION

• Drug may cause fetal harm. Safety of atypical antipsychotic use during pregnancy hasn't been well studied; routine use isn't recommended. Use during pregnancy only if potential benefit justifies fetal risk.
• *Alert:* Neonates exposed to antipsychotics during the third trimester are at risk for developing extrapyramidal signs and symptoms (repetitive muscle movements of the face and body) and withdrawal signs and symptoms (agitation, abnormally increased or decreased muscle tone, tremors, sleepiness, severe difficulty breathing, difficulty feeding) after delivery.
• Patients exposed to asenapine during pregnancy should be enrolled in National Pregnancy Registry for Atypical Antipsychotics (1-866-961-2388 or https://womensmentalhealth.org/research/pregnancyregistry/).
• It isn't known if drug appears in human milk. Use cautiously during breastfeeding weighing benefits of treatment and risk to the infant.

NURSING CONSIDERATIONS

• Monitor ECG before and regularly during treatment for prolongation of QTc interval.
• Obtain BP before starting drug, and monitor BP regularly. Watch for orthostatic hypotension.
• Monitor waist circumference and BMI.
• Monitor patient for tardive dyskinesia, which may occur after prolonged use. It may disappear spontaneously or persist for life, despite stopping drug.
• Monitor patient for suicidality, especially at start of therapy.
• *Alert:* Watch for signs and symptoms of NMS (extrapyramidal effects, hyperthermia, autonomic disturbance), which are rare but

can be fatal. Discontinue drug immediately if they occur, and monitor patient closely.

• Monitor patient for serious allergic reactions (anaphylaxis, angioedema, hypotension, difficulty breathing, wheezing, swollen tongue, rash).

• Drug may alter glucose control in patients with diabetes. Monitor glucose levels closely.

• Monitor CBC frequently during first few months of therapy in those with history of leukopenia or neutropenia. If WBC count decreases, monitor patient for signs and symptoms of infection; if infection occurs, discontinue drug in the absence of another cause.

• Monitor patient for dysphagia, which can lead to aspiration and aspiration pneumonia.

• Dispense lowest appropriate quantity of drug, to reduce risk of overdose.

• Monitor patient for abnormal body temperature regulation, especially if patient exercises, is exposed to extreme heat, takes anticholinergics, or is dehydrated.

• Complete fall risk assessments at start of treatment then periodically for patients on long-term therapy who have diseases or conditions or are taking medications that may cause somnolence, orthostatic hypotension, or motor or sensory instability.

• Reduce dosage gradually to avoid withdrawal symptoms when discontinuing antipsychotic therapy.

PATIENT TEACHING

• *Opioid class warning:* Caution patient or caregiver of patient taking an opioid with a benzodiazepine, CNS depressant, or alcohol to seek immediate medical attention if patient experiences dizziness, light-headedness, extreme sleepiness, slowed or difficult breathing, or unresponsiveness.

• Instruct patient in safe drug administration.

• Warn patient to avoid activities that require mental alertness, such as operating hazardous machinery or operating a motor vehicle, until drug's effects are known.

• Advise patient to contact prescriber if palpitations or rapid heartbeat occurs.

• Advise patient not to stand up quickly but to get up slowly from a sitting position to avoid dizziness.

• Inform patient that weight gain may occur.

• Warn patient against exposure to extreme heat because drug may impair body's ability to reduce temperature.

• Advise patient to avoid alcohol.

aspirin (acetylsalicylic acid, ASA) 💉
AS-pir-in

Asaphen✽ ◇, Asatab✽ ◇, Bayer Aspirin ◇, Durlaza, Ecotrin ◇, Entrophen✽ ◇, Rivasa✽ ◇, St. Joseph ◇, Vazalore ◇

Therapeutic class: Anti-inflammatory drugs
Pharmacologic class: Salicylates

AVAILABLE FORMS
Capsules (immediate-release)) 💊 81 mg ◇, 325 mg ◇
Capsules (extended-release) 💊 162.5 mg
Suppositories: 60 mg ◇, 160 mg✽ ◇, 300 mg ◇, 600 mg ◇
Tablets: 80 mg ◇, 325 mg ◇, 500 mg ◇
Tablets (chewable): 80 mg✽ ◇, 81 mg ◇
Tablets (delayed-release): 81 mg ◇, 325 mg ◇, 500 mg ◇
Tablets (enteric-coated) 💊 80 mg✽ ◇, 81 mg ◇, 162 mg✽ ◇, 325 mg ◇, 500 mg ◇

INDICATIONS & DOSAGES
➤ **RA, osteoarthritis, or other polyarthritic or inflammatory conditions**
Adults: Initially, 3 g PO daily in divided doses. Increase as needed, with target plasma salicylate levels of 150 to 300 mcg/mL.
➤ **Juvenile RA**
Children: 90 to 130 mg/kg/day PO in divided doses. Increase as needed, with target plasma salicylate levels of 150 to 300 mcg/mL.
➤ **Mild pain or fever; spondyloarthropathies**
Adults and children age 12 and older weighing 50 kg or more: 325 to 650 mg PO or PR every 4 hours PRN. Or, for delayed-release products, 1,300 mg PO followed by 650 to 1,300 mg PO every 8 hours. Maximum dose is 4,000 mg in 24 hours.
Children ages 2 to 11 weighing less than 50 kg: 10 to 15 mg/kg/dose PO or PR every 4 hours up to 90 mg/kg daily.
➤ **Suspected acute MI**
Adults: Initially, 160 to 325 mg PO (nonenteric-coated) chewed or crushed; or 160 to 162.5 mg immediate-release capsule (Vazalore) as soon as MI is suspected. Continue maintenance dose of 160 to 325 mg PO daily for 30 days after infarction. After 30 days, consider further therapy for prevention of MI.

➤ **To reduce risk of MI in patients with previous MI, unstable angina, and chronic stable angina pectoris**
Adults: 75 to 325 mg PO daily. Or, 162.5 mg extended-release capsule PO daily.

➤ **To reduce risk of recurrent TIAs and stroke or death in patients at risk**
Adults: 50 to 325 mg PO daily. Or, 162.5 mg extended-release capsule PO daily.

➤ **Acute ischemic stroke**
Adults: 50 to 325 mg PO daily, started within 48 hours of stroke onset; continue indefinitely.

➤ **CABG**
Adults: 325 mg PO daily starting 6 hours postprocedure. Continue for up to 1 year.

➤ **Venous thromboembolism extended therapy to prevent recurrence (in patients who have completed anticoagulation treatment and have decided to stop oral anticoagulation)** ◆
Adults: 100 mg PO once daily.

➤ **Venous thromboembolism prophylaxis for total hip arthroplasty (THA) or total knee arthroplasty (TKA) (immediate-release)** ◆
Adults: After 5-day course of postoperative rivaroxaban prophylaxis, initiate aspirin 81 mg once daily starting on postoperative day 6 and continue for 9 days for TKA (total duration: 14 days) or 30 days for THA (total duration: 35 days).

ADMINISTRATION
PO
• For patient with swallowing difficulties, crush non-enteric-coated aspirin and dissolve in soft food or liquid. Give liquid immediately after mixing because drug will break down rapidly.
• Give capsules with full glass of water.
• Give tablets with food, milk, antacid, or large glass of water to reduce GI effects.
• Give enteric-coated, immediate-release capsules, or extended-release forms whole; don't crush or break.
• For acute MI, have patient chew non-enteric-coated tablet.
Rectal
• Refrigerate suppositories.

ACTION
Thought to produce analgesia and exert its anti-inflammatory effect by inhibiting prostaglandin and other substances that sensitize pain receptors. Drug may relieve fever through central action in the hypothalamic heat-regulating center. In low doses, drug also appears to interfere with clotting by keeping a platelet-aggregating substance from forming.

Route	Onset	Peak	Duration
PO (buffered)	5–30 min	1–2 hr	1–4 hr
PO (enteric-coated)	5–30 min	Variable	1–4 hr
PO (tablet)	5–30 min	25–40 min	1–4 hr
PO (extended-release)	Unknown	2 hr	4–8 hr
PR	Unknown	3–4 hr	Unknown

Half-life: 15 minutes to 6 hours (dose dependent).

ADVERSE REACTIONS
CNS: agitation, *cerebral edema, coma,* confusion, dizziness, headache, lethargy, hyperthermia, nervousness, *seizures, subdural or intracranial hemorrhage.* **CV:** *arrhythmias,* edema, hypotension, tachycardia, *hemorrhage.* **EENT:** tinnitus, hearing loss. **GI:** nausea, *GI bleeding,* dyspepsia, GI distress, gastritis, GI erosion, heartburn, occult bleeding, *pancreatitis,* vomiting, ulcer. **GU:** *antepartum and postpartum bleeding,* interstitial nephritis, papillary necrosis, prolonged pregnancy and labor, proteinuria, renal insufficiency, renal failure. **Hematologic:** anemia, prolonged bleeding time, *leukopenia, thrombocytopenia,* coagulopathy, *DIC.* **Hepatic:** *hepatitis, hepatotoxicity,* increased transaminase levels. **Metabolic:** dehydration, *hyperkalemia,* hyponatremia, hyperglycemia, *hypoglycemia* (children), *metabolic acidosis,* respiratory alkalosis. **Musculoskeletal:** acetabular bone destruction, rhabdomyolysis, weakness. **Respiratory:** *asthma, bronchospasm,* dyspnea, hyperventilation, *laryngeal edema, noncardiogenic pulmonary edema,* tachypnea. **Skin:** rash, bruising, urticaria, hives. **Other:** *angioedema, Reye syndrome,* hypersensitivity reactions, low birth weight, *stillbirth.*

INTERACTIONS
Drug-drug. *ACE inhibitors:* May decrease antihypertensive effects. Monitor BP closely. *Acetazolamide:* May cause accumulation and toxicity of acetazolamide, resulting in CNS depression, metabolic acidosis, anorexia, and death. Administer together with caution and monitor patient for toxicity.

Ammonium chloride and other urine acidifiers: May increase levels of aspirin products. Watch for aspirin toxicity.

Antacids in high doses and other urine alkalinizers: May decrease levels of aspirin products. Watch for decreased aspirin effect.

Anticoagulants, antiplatelet agents: May increase risk of bleeding. Use with extreme caution if these drugs must be used together.

Beta blockers: May decrease antihypertensive effect. Avoid long-term aspirin use if patient is taking antihypertensives.

Corticosteroids: May enhance salicylate elimination and decrease drug level. Watch for decreased aspirin effect. May increase risk of GI ulceration and bleeding. Monitor therapy.

Diuretics: May decrease effectiveness of diuretics in patients with underlying renal or CV disease. Monitor therapy.

Heparin: May increase risk of bleeding. Monitor coagulation studies and patient closely if used together.

Ibuprofen, other NSAIDs: May negate antiplatelet effect of low-dose aspirin therapy and decrease renal function. Patients using immediate-release aspirin (not enteric-coated) should take ibuprofen at least 30 minutes after or more than 8 hours before aspirin. Patients using extended-release aspirin should take ibuprofen at least 2 to 4 hours after or more than 8 hours before aspirin. Occasional use of ibuprofen is unlikely to have a negative effect.

Influenza virus vaccine, live; varicella virus vaccine, live: Increased risk of Reye syndrome. Use together is contraindicated in children and adolescents.

Methotrexate: May increase risk of methotrexate toxicity. Avoid using together.

Oral antidiabetics: May increase hypoglycemic effect. Monitor patient closely.

Phenytoin, valproic acid: May increase valproic acid level. Avoid using together.

Probenecid: May decrease uricosuric effect. Avoid using together.

Vitamin E: May enhance antiplatelet effect of agents with antiplatelet properties. Monitor patient closely.

Drug-herb. *White willow:* Contains salicylates and may increase risk of adverse effects. Discourage use together.

Drug-food. *Caffeine:* May increase drug absorption. Watch for increased effects.

Drug-lifestyle. *Alcohol use:* May increase risk of GI bleeding. Discourage use together.

EFFECTS ON LAB TEST RESULTS

• May increase LFT values and BUN, creatinine, sodium, and potassium levels.
• May decrease platelet and WBC counts.
• May falsely decrease protein-bound iodine level.
• May interfere with urine glucose analysis with Diastix, Chemstrip uG, Clinitest, and Benedict solution; with urinary 5-hydroxyindoleacetic acid and vanillylmandelic acid tests; and with Gerhardt test for urine acetoacetic acid.

CONTRAINDICATIONS & CAUTIONS

• Contraindicated in patients hypersensitive to drug and in those with NSAID-induced sensitivity reactions or bleeding disorders, such as hemophilia, von Willebrand disease, telangiectasia, bleeding ulcers, and hemorrhagic states.
• Use cautiously in patients with GI lesions, impaired renal function, hypoprothrombinemia, vitamin K deficiency, thrombocytopenia, or thrombotic thrombocytopenic purpura.
▨ Avoid use in patients with severe hepatic or renal impairment, G6PD deficiency, or history of active peptic ulcer disease.
◔ *Alert:* Oral and rectal OTC products containing aspirin and nonaspirin salicylates shouldn't be given to children or teenagers who have or are recovering from chickenpox or flulike symptoms with or without fever because of the risk of Reye syndrome.
• Safe use of extended-release capsules in children hasn't been established.
Dialyzable drug: Yes.
⚠ *Overdose S&S:* Severe acid-base and electrolyte disturbance, hyperthermia, dehydration, tinnitus, vertigo, headache, confusion, drowsiness, diaphoresis, hyperventilation, vomiting, diarrhea.

PREGNANCY-LACTATION-REPRODUCTION

• Use in pregnancy only if clearly needed and specifically directed to do so by a physician. Avoid use during third trimester.
• Drug appears in human milk. Patients who are breastfeeding should avoid aspirin if possible.
• Use of NSAIDs (including aspirin) at 20 weeks or later in pregnancy may cause fetal renal dysfunction leading to oligohydramnios and potential neonatal renal impairment; use at 30 weeks or later in pregnancy may

---

Reactions in bold italics are *life-threatening*. Interactions may have a *rapid onset* or a ***delayed onset***.

increase risk of premature closure of the ductus arteriosus.

• Avoid NSAID use during pregnancy starting at 20 weeks' gestation. If potential benefit justifies fetal risk, use lowest effective dose for shortest duration. Consider ultrasound monitoring of amniotic fluid if NSAID use is longer than 48 hours.

• Use of 81 mg of low-dose aspirin for certain pregnancy-related conditions under prescriber direction is acceptable.

NURSING CONSIDERATIONS

• For inflammatory conditions, rheumatic fever, and thrombosis, give aspirin on a schedule rather than as needed.

• Because enteric-coated tablets are slowly absorbed, they aren't suitable for rapid relief of acute pain, fever, or inflammation. They cause less GI bleeding and may be better suited for long-term therapy, such as for arthritis.

• For patients who can't tolerate oral drugs, ask prescriber about using aspirin rectal suppositories. Watch for rectal mucosal irritation or bleeding.

• Febrile, dehydrated children can develop toxicity rapidly.

• Monitor older adults closely because they may be more susceptible to aspirin's toxic effects.

• Monitor salicylate level. Therapeutic salicylate level for arthritis is 150 to 300 mcg/mL. Tinnitus may occur at levels above 200 mcg/mL, but this isn't a reliable indicator of toxicity, especially in very young patients and those older than age 60. With long-term therapy, severe toxic effects may occur with levels exceeding 400 mcg/mL.

• During prolonged therapy, assess hematocrit, Hb level, PT, INR, and renal function periodically.

• Drug irreversibly inhibits platelet aggregation. Stop drug 5 to 7 days before elective surgery to allow time for production and release of new platelets.

• Monitor patient for hypersensitivity reactions, such as anaphylaxis and asthma.

• **Look alike–sound alike:** Don't confuse aspirin with Asendin or Afrin.

PATIENT TEACHING

• Tell patient who's allergic to tartrazine to avoid aspirin.

• Advise patient on a low-salt diet that 1 tablet of buffered aspirin contains 553 mg of sodium.

• Instruct patient in safe drug administration.

• Warn patient not to drink alcohol 2 hours before or 1 hour after taking extended-release capsule and not to take extra capsule to make up for a missed dose.

• Remind patient taking drug for a chronic condition not to stop drug without first discussing with prescriber.

• Instruct patient to discard aspirin tablets that have a strong vinegar-like odor.

• Tell patient to consult prescriber if giving drug to children for longer than 5 days or adults for longer than 10 days.

• Advise patient receiving prolonged treatment with large doses of aspirin to watch for small, round, red pinprick spots; bleeding gums; and signs of GI bleeding; advise patient to drink plenty of fluids. Encourage use of a soft-bristled toothbrush.

• Because of the many drug interactions with aspirin, warn patient taking prescription drugs to check with prescriber or pharmacist before taking aspirin or OTC products containing aspirin.

• Warn patient who is pregnant not to take NSAIDs at 20 weeks' gestation or later unless instructed to do so by prescriber due to potential fetal risk. Advise patient to consult pharmacist or health care provider about taking OTC medications during pregnancy.

• Drug is a leading cause of poisoning in children. Caution parents to keep drug out of reach of children. Encourage use of child-resistant containers.

atazanavir sulfate
at-a-za-NA-veer

Reyataz✐

Therapeutic class: Antiretrovirals
Pharmacologic class: Protease inhibitors

AVAILABLE FORMS
Capsules ⓤ: 150 mg, 200 mg, 300 mg
Oral powder: 50 mg

INDICATIONS & DOSAGES
Adjust-a-dose (for all indications): In patients with Child-Pugh class B hepatic insufficiency who haven't experienced prior

virologic failure, reduce dosage to 300 mg PO once daily. Patients with ESRD who are treatment-naive and on hemodialysis should receive atazanavir 300 mg with ritonavir 100 mg. Don't give to patients who are treatment-experienced and on hemodialysis.

Significant drug interactions exist requiring dosage adjustment or drug avoidance. Refer to manufacturer's instructions or interactions reference for dosage adjustments.

➤ **HIV-1 infection, with other antiretrovirals in patients who are treatment-experienced**

Adults: Give 300 mg once daily, plus 100 mg ritonavir once daily with food. In patients also taking an H_2-receptor antagonist (H2RA) and tenofovir, give 400 mg PO once daily, plus 100 mg ritonavir.

Children and adolescents ages 6 to younger than 18 who are treatment-experienced and receiving ritonavir: For patients weighing 35 kg or more, give 300 mg with ritonavir 100 mg PO once daily. For patients weighing 15 to 34 kg, give 200 mg with ritonavir 100 mg PO once daily. For patients weighing 5 to 15 kg, capsules aren't recommended. Use oral powder.

Children at least age 3 months and weighing at least 5 kg and less than 25 kg: For patients weighing 15 to less than 25 kg, give 250 mg oral powder PO immediately followed by 80 mg ritonavir daily. For patients weighing 5 to less than 15 kg, give 200 mg oral powder PO immediately followed by 80 mg ritonavir daily.

➤ **HIV-1 infection, with other antiretrovirals, in patients who are treatment-naive**

Adults: Recommended regimen is 300 mg PO once daily with ritonavir 100 mg. When drug is given with efavirenz, give atazanavir 400 mg and ritonavir 100 mg as a single daily dose with food and efavirenz on an empty stomach, preferably at bedtime. For adults unable to tolerate ritonavir, give 400 mg PO once daily.

Adolescents at least age 13 and weighing at least 40 kg who can't tolerate ritonavir: 400 mg PO once daily with food.

Children and adolescents ages 6 to younger than 18: For patients weighing 35 kg or more, give 300 mg with ritonavir 100 mg PO once daily. For patients weighing 15 to less than 34 kg, give 200 mg with ritonavir 100 mg PO once daily. For patients weighing 5 to 15 kg,

capsules aren't recommended. Use oral powder.

Children at least age 3 months and weighing at least 5 kg and less than 25 kg: For patients weighing 15 to less than 25 kg, give 250 mg oral powder PO immediately followed by 80 mg ritonavir daily. For patients weighing 5 to less than 15 kg, give 200 mg oral powder PO immediately followed by 80 mg ritonavir daily.

Adjust-a-dose: Administration with ritonavir in patients with any degree of hepatic impairment isn't recommended. In adults with mild hepatic impairment (Child-Pugh class A), give 400 mg PO daily; for moderate hepatic impairment (Child-Pugh class B), give 300 mg daily; for severe hepatic impairment (Child-Pugh class C), atazanavir isn't recommended.

➤ **HIV-1 infection, with other antiretrovirals, in patients who are treatment-experienced and pregnant**

Women: Give 300 mg PO daily with 100 mg ritonavir. For patients who are treatment-experienced during second or third trimester when given with either H2RA or tenofovir, give 400 mg PO daily with 100 mg ritonavir.

ADMINISTRATION
PO
• Give drug with food.
• Don't open capsules.
• Mix oral powder with food (such as applesauce or yogurt) or beverage (such as milk, infant formula, or water).
• When mixing with food, mix powder with a minimum of 1 tablespoon of food in small container and feed to child. Add additional tablespoon of food to container, mix, and feed residual mixture to child.
• When mixing with beverage, mix powder with minimum of 30 mL of beverage and give to child to drink. Add additional 15 mL of beverage to the drinking cup, mix, and give to child to drink residual mixture. If water is used, also give food at same time.
• For young infants who can't eat solid food or drink from a cup, mix powder with 10 mL of infant formula in a medicine cup and draw up into oral syringe. Give to infant into either inner cheek. Pour additional 10 mL of formula into medicine cup and mix. Give residual mixture to infant in the same manner. Don't give in an infant bottle.

• Give entire dose of powder after mixing within 1 hour of preparation. Additional food may be given after dose is given.

ACTION

Inhibits viral maturation in HIV-1–infected cells, resulting in the formation of immature noninfectious viral particles.

Route	Onset	Peak	Duration
PO	Unknown	2–3 hr	Unknown

Half-life: Unboosted, 7 to 8 hours; boosted with ritonavir, 9 to 18 hours.

ADVERSE REACTIONS

CNS: headache, depression, dizziness, fatigue, fever, insomnia, pain, peripheral neuropathy. **CV:** prolonged PR interval, first- and second-degree heart block, peripheral edema. **EENT:** nasal congestion, rhinorrhea, oropharyngeal pain. **GI:** abdominal pain, diarrhea, nausea, vomiting. **Hematologic:** anemia, *neutropenia.* **Hepatic:** hyperbilirubinemia, increased LFT values, jaundice. **Metabolic:** increased CK level, hyperlipidemia, *hypoglycemia.* **Musculoskeletal:** arthralgia, myalgia, limb pain. **Respiratory:** increased cough, wheezing. **Skin:** rash.

INTERACTIONS

Refer to a drug interactions resource for both atazanavir and ritonavir for complete information.

Drug-drug. *Alfuzosin:* May increase alfuzosin plasma concentration, increasing risk of hypotension. Use together is contraindicated.

Antacids, buffered medications (didanosine buffered preparation): May reduce atazanavir plasma concentration. Administer atazanavir 2 hours before or 1 hour after these medications.

Antiarrhythmics (amiodarone, bepridil, systemic lidocaine, quinidine): May produce serious or life-threatening adverse reactions. Use cautiously. Monitor antiarrhythmic therapeutic concentration.

Anticoagulants (apixaban, rivaroxaban, warfarin): May cause serious or life-threatening bleeding. Monitor INR.

Antifungals (itraconazole, ketoconazole, posaconazole, voriconazole): May increase risk of toxicity of both antifungal and atazanavir. Use cautiously when high doses of ketoconazole or itraconazole are administered with atazanavir and ritonavir. Administration

of voriconazole with atazanavir and ritonavir isn't recommended.

Aprepitant: May increase aprepitant serum concentration. Avoid combination.

Aripiprazole: May increase aripiprazole plasma concentration. Monitor patient and adjust aripiprazole dosage as needed when atazanavir is started or stopped.

Benzodiazepines (midazolam, triazolam): May increase plasma concentrations of these drugs. Oral midazolam and triazolam are contraindicated because of the potential for serious or life-threatening events, such as prolonged or increased sedation or respiratory depression. Use IV midazolam with caution and close monitoring. Consider reducing the IV midazolam dosage.

Bosentan: May decrease atazanavir plasma concentration when administered without ritonavir; coadministration of atazanavir and bosentan without ritonavir isn't recommended. May increase bosentan plasma concentration. Adjust bosentan dose when used with atazanavir–ritonavir. Consider therapy modification.

Calcium channel blockers (amlodipine, diltiazem, felodipine, nicardipine, nifedipine, verapamil): May prolong PR interval in some patients; use caution. Consider reducing diltiazem dosage by 50% and titrating dosages of other calcium channel blockers. Monitor ECG.

Carbamazepine: May increase carbamazepine level. May decrease atazanavir level, resulting in antiretroviral treatment failure. If coadministration can't be avoided, monitor patient closely. Consider alternative therapy for carbamazepine.

Clarithromycin: May prolong QTc interval; reduce clarithromycin dosage by 50%. Significantly reduces concentration of active metabolite (14-OH clarithromycin); consider alternative therapy for indications other than MAC.

Colchicine: May increase plasma concentrations of colchicine. Don't give colchicine and atazanavir together to patients with hepatic or renal impairment. In those with normal renal and hepatic function, reduce colchicine dose. Consider therapy modification.

Corticosteroids (fluticasone, prednisone): May increase corticosteroid plasma concentration. Monitor patient for signs and symptoms of adrenal insufficiency. Consider alternatives to fluticasone for long-term use.

Delavirdine: May increase atazanavir plasma concentration and decrease delavirdine plasma concentration. Closely monitor patient and adjust therapy as needed.

Didanosine (buffered): May decrease atazanavir concentration. Give atazanavir 2 hours before or 1 hour after buffered formulation of didanosine. Coadministration of enteric-coated didanosine capsules and atazanavir decreases didanosine exposure. Separate atazanavir and didanosine administration times.

Digoxin: May prolong PR interval. Use with caution.

Eplerenone: May increase eplerenone plasma concentration. Avoid combination.

Ergot derivatives (dihydroergotamine, ergonovine, ergotamine, methylergonovine): May cause serious or life-threatening events such as acute ergot toxicity (peripheral vasospasm, ischemia of the extremities). Use together is contraindicated.

Fluoxetine: May increase plasma concentrations of both drugs. Closely monitor patient for adverse reactions, including serotonin syndrome. Fluoxetine or atazanavir dosage reduction may be needed.

Hepatitis C antivirals (elbasvir/grazoprevir, glecaprevir/pibrentasvir): May increase serum concentrations of these drugs, which can lead to increased liver toxicity. Coadministration is contraindicated.

HMG-CoA reductase inhibitors (atorvastatin, lovastatin, rosuvastatin, simvastatin): May increase serum concentrations of these drugs, possibly increasing their toxicity, including rhabdomyolysis. Administration with simvastatin or lovastatin is contraindicated. If using atorvastatin or rosuvastatin, start with lowest possible dosage with careful monitoring. Consider pravastatin or fluvastatin in combination with atazanavir.

Hormonal contraceptives (ethinyl estradiol, norethindrone, norgestimate): See manufacturer's instructions. Alternative methods of nonhormonal contraception are recommended.

H2RAs (famotidine): May decrease atazanavir plasma concentration, possibly causing development of resistance. See manufacturer's instructions for H2RA administration recommendations.

Immunosuppressants (cyclosporine, sirolimus, tacrolimus): May increase levels of these drugs. Monitor immunosuppressant concentrations.

Irinotecan: May interfere with irinotecan metabolism, resulting in increased toxicity. Use together is contraindicated.

Lurasidone: May increase lurasidone plasma concentration. Use together is contraindicated if administered with ritonavir.

mTOR inhibitors (everolimus, temsirolimus): May increase plasma concentrations of these drugs. If coadministration can't be avoided, monitor clinical response and adjust mTOR inhibitor dosage as needed.

NNRTIs (efavirenz, nevirapine): May decrease atazanavir plasma level. In patients who are treatment-naive, give atazanavir 400 mg with food and ritonavir 100 mg with efavirenz 600 mg on an empty stomach. Don't administer atazanavir with efavirenz in patients who are treatment-experienced. Nevirapine may decrease atazanavir exposure; administering them together may increase nevirapine exposure. Use together is contraindicated.

Opioid analgesics (buprenorphine, fentanyl, oxycodone, sufentanil): May increase plasma concentration and half-life of opioid; reduced opioid dosage may be needed. Closely monitor respiratory function during opioid administration and for a longer period than usual after stopping opioid. Atazanavir without ritonavir shouldn't be administered with buprenorphine.

PDE5 inhibitors (sildenafil, tadalafil, vardenafil): Coadministration of atazanavir and sildenafil for PAH is contraindicated. When used for erectile dysfunction, see manufacturer's instructions for dosage adjustments. Monitor patient closely.

Pimozide: May cause serious or life-threatening reactions (cardiac arrhythmias). Use is contraindicated.

Protease inhibitors (amprenavir, darunavir, fosamprenavir, nelfinavir, ritonavir, saquinavir, tipranavir): Drug may increase concentration of other protease inhibitors. Atazanavir–ritonavir isn't recommended with other protease inhibitors. Other combinations may require dosage changes. Consider therapy modification.

PPIs (omeprazole): Substantially decrease atazanavir plasma concentration, possibly causing development of resistance. In patients who are treatment-naive, give PPI 12 hours before atazanavir dose. PPI shouldn't exceed dose equivalent to omeprazole 20 mg. Don't use PPIs in patients

---

Reactions in bold italics are ***life-threatening***. Interactions may have a *rapid onset* or a ***delayed onset***.

who are treatment-experienced receiving atazanavir.

Quetiapine: May increase quetiapine plasma concentration. Administer cautiously; closely monitor clinical response. Adjust quetiapine dosage to one-sixth of current dose.

Ranolazine: Increases risk of dose-related QTc-interval prolongation, torsades de pointes–type arrhythmias, and sudden death. Avoid use together. Contraindicated with cobicistat-boosted atazanavir.

Rifabutin: May increase rifabutin blood level. Rifabutin dosage reduction of up to 75% (150 mg every other day or three times/week) is recommended.

Rifampin: May decrease atazanavir plasma concentration, possibly causing development of resistance. Use together is contraindicated.

Salmeterol: May increase salmeterol concentration, increasing risk of CV events, including QT-interval prolongation, palpitations, and sinus tachycardia. Use together isn't recommended.

Saxagliptin: May increase saxagliptin plasma concentration. Limit saxagliptin dosage to 2.5 mg daily.

Strong CYP3A4 inhibitors (brentuximab, cabazitaxel, cilostazol, eletriptan, eplerenone, maraviroc, risperidone, romidepsin, trazodone): May increase inhibitor level. Refer to interactions resource for complete information.

TCAs (amitriptyline): May cause serious or life-threatening adverse reactions. Monitor TCA concentration.

Tenofovir: May decrease atazanavir level. Don't administer atazanavir with tenofovir unless also administering ritonavir; administer as atazanavir 300 mg, ritonavir 100 mg, and tenofovir 300 mg. Atazanavir increases tenofovir concentration; watch for tenofovir-associated adverse reactions.

Tetracyclines (minocycline): May reduce atazanavir plasma concentration. Closely monitor atazanavir concentration and clinical response. Adjust atazanavir dosage as needed.

Tyrosine kinase inhibitors (dasatinib, lapatinib, nilotinib, pazopanib, sorafenib, sunitinib): May increase tyrosine kinase inhibitor plasma concentrations. If use together can't be avoided, closely monitor clinical response and adjust tyrosine kinase inhibitor dosage as needed.

Vasopressin receptor antagonists (conivaptan, tolvaptan): May increase plasma concentration of these drugs. Avoid coadministration.

Vemurafenib: May increase vemurafenib plasma concentration. Avoid combination.

Vilazodone: May increase vilazodone plasma concentration. Reduce vilazodone dosage to 20 mg in patients receiving atazanavir.

Vinca alkaloids (vinblastine, vincristine): May increase pharmacologic effects of these drugs and risk of toxicity (characterized by profound neutropenia or severe neuropathy). Consider temporarily suspending atazanavir in patients experiencing hematologic or GI toxicity during administration of atazanavir and vinca alkaloids. Or, reducing vinca alkaloid dosage may decrease toxicity.

Drug-herb. *St. John's wort:* May decrease drug level, reducing therapeutic effect and causing drug resistance. Use together is contraindicated.

Drug-food. *Any food:* May increase bioavailability of drug. Tell patient to take drug with food.

EFFECTS ON LAB TEST RESULTS

• May increase ALT, AST, amylase, bilirubin, lipase, CK, glucose, triglyceride, and total cholesterol levels.
• May decrease glucose level.
• May decrease Hb level and neutrophil and platelet counts.

CONTRAINDICATIONS & CAUTIONS

• Contraindicated in patients hypersensitive to drug or its ingredients.
• Contraindicated in patients taking drugs cleared mainly by CYP3A4 or drugs that can cause serious or life-threatening reactions at high levels (alfuzosin, amiodarone [with ritonavir], dihydroergotamine, elbasvir–grazoprevir, ergonovine, ergotamine, glecaprevir–pibrentasvir, irinotecan, lovastatin, lurasidone [with ritonavir], methylergonovine, midazolam [PO], nevirapine, pimozide, quinidine [with ritonavir], rifampin, sildenafil [Revatio], St. John's wort, simvastatin, triazolam).
• Don't use in patients with Child-Pugh class C hepatic insufficiency or ESRD managed with hemodialysis.
• Use cautiously in patients with cardiac conduction system disease, hepatic impairment, diabetes, or hemophilia types A and B.
• Use cautiously in older adults because of the increased likelihood of other disease,

additional drug therapy, and decreased hepatic, renal, or cardiac function.
• Use isn't recommended in children younger than age 3 months due to risk of kernicterus.
Dialyzable drug: No.
⚠ *Overdose S&S:* Asymptomatic bifascicular block, PR-interval prolongation, jaundice.

PREGNANCY-LACTATION-REPRODUCTION
• Use during pregnancy only if potential benefit justifies fetal risk. The U.S. Department of Health and Human Services Perinatal HIV Guidelines recommend atazanavir as a preferred protease inhibitor for patients who are pregnant and antiretroviral-naive when combined with low-dose ritonavir boosting. Enroll patients who are pregnant in the Antiretroviral Pregnancy Registry (1-800-258-4263).
• Drug appears in human milk. Breastfeeding is contraindicated in patients infected with HIV because of risk of postnatal transmission of HIV.

NURSING CONSIDERATIONS
⚠ *Alert:* Drug may prolong the PR interval. Monitor ECG, especially in patients with pre-existing conduction system disease.
• Monitor patient for hyperglycemia and new-onset diabetes or worsened diabetes. Insulin and oral antidiabetic dosages may need adjustment.
• Monitor patient with HBV or HCV infection for elevated liver enzyme levels or hepatic decompensation.
• Monitor patient for immune reconstitution syndrome. Evaluate and treat indolent or residual opportunistic infections, such as MAC, CMV, *Pneumocystis jiroveci* pneumonia, or TB. Some autoimmune disorders, such as Graves disease, polymyositis, and Guillain-Barré syndrome, have also occurred, even after many months of treatment.
• Watch for life-threatening lactic acidosis syndrome and symptomatic hyperlactatemia, especially in women and patients who are obese.
• If patient has hemophilia, watch for bleeding.
• Drug may cause nephrolithiasis or cholelithiasis. Evaluate patient for signs or symptoms of nephrolithiasis (flank pain) or cholelithiasis (abdominal pain, nausea, vomiting, jaundice); interrupt or discontinue drug

as clinically indicated should signs or symptoms occur.
• Monitor patient for rash. Discontinue drug if rash occurs.
• Most patients have an asymptomatic increase in indirect bilirubin, possibly with yellowed skin or sclerae. This hyperbilirubinemia will resolve when therapy stops.
• Monitor liver enzyme levels and renal function before and periodically during treatment.
• Although cross-resistance occurs among protease inhibitors, resistance to drug doesn't preclude use of other protease inhibitors.
⚠ *Alert:* For patients with phenylketonuria, be aware that oral powder contains 35 mg of phenylalanine; capsules don't.

PATIENT TEACHING
• Urge patient to take drug with food every day and to take other antiretrovirals as prescribed.
• Advise patient to maintain adequate hydration to decrease risk of chronic kidney disease.
• Explain that drug doesn't cure HIV infection and that patient may develop opportunistic infections and other complications of HIV disease.
• Caution patient that drug doesn't reduce the risk of transmitting HIV to others.
• Tell patient that drug may cause altered or increased body fat, central obesity, buffalo hump, peripheral wasting, facial wasting, breast enlargement, and a cushingoid appearance.
• Advise patient to report all adverse drug reactions.
• Caution patient not to take other prescriptions or OTC or herbal medicines without first consulting prescriber.
• Advise patient to discuss pregnancy with prescriber.

SAFETY ALERT!

atenolol
a-TEN-o-loll

Tenormin♦

Therapeutic class: Antihypertensives
Pharmacologic class: Beta blockers

AVAILABLE FORMS
Tablets: 25 mg, 50 mg, 100 mg

INDICATIONS & DOSAGES

Adjust-a-dose (for all indications): If CrCl is 15 to 35 mL/minute/1.73 m², maximum dose is 50 mg daily; if CrCl is below 15 mL/minute/1.73 m², maximum dose is 25 mg daily. Patients on hemodialysis need 25 to 50 mg after each dialysis session. For older adults, consider starting initial dose at 25 mg PO daily.

➤ **HTN**

Adults: Initially, 50 mg PO daily alone or in combination with a diuretic as a single dose, increased to 100 mg once daily after 7 to 14 days. Dosages of more than 100 mg daily are unlikely to produce further benefit.

➤ **Angina pectoris**

Adults: 50 mg PO once daily, increased as needed to 100 mg daily after 7 days for optimal effect. Maximum, 200 mg daily.

➤ **Acute MI**

Adults: 100 mg PO daily or 50 mg b.i.d. for at least 7 days; may continue for 1 to 3 years if no contraindications.

ADMINISTRATION
PO

- May give without regard for meals.
- Give drug exactly as prescribed, at the same time each day.

ACTION

Selectively blocks beta₁-adrenergic receptors, decreases cardiac output and cardiac oxygen consumption, and depresses renin secretion.

Route	Onset	Peak	Duration
PO	1 hr	2–4 hr	24 hr

Half-life: 6 to 7 hours.

ADVERSE REACTIONS

CNS: depression, dizziness, fatigue, lethargy, vertigo, drowsiness, fever, light-headedness, dreaming. **CV:** orthostatic hypotension, ***bradycardia, HF, heart block,*** bundle-branch block, intermittent claudication, atrial fibrillation, atrial flutter, ***supraventricular tachycardia, cardiac arrest, cardiogenic shock, ventricular tachycardia, MI.*** **GI:** nausea, diarrhea. **Musculoskeletal:** leg pain. **Respiratory:** *bronchospasm,* dyspnea, *PE,* wheezing. **Skin:** rash. **Other:** cold extremities, ***death.***

INTERACTIONS

Drug-drug. *Amiodarone:* May increase risk of bradycardia, AV block, and myocardial depression. Monitor ECG and vital signs.
Antihypertensives: May increase hypotensive effect. Use together cautiously.
Calcium carbonate, calcium citrate: May decrease atenolol level. Separate doses by at least 2 hours. Monitor patient and adjust atenolol dosage as needed.
Calcium channel blockers, hydralazine, methyldopa: May cause additive hypotension and bradycardia. Adjust dosage as needed.
Cardiac glycosides, diltiazem, verapamil: May cause excessive bradycardia and increased depressant effect on myocardium. Use together cautiously.
Catecholamine-depleting drugs (reserpine): May increase risk of hypotension and bradycardia. Use together cautiously.
Clonidine: May exacerbate rebound HTN if clonidine is withdrawn. Atenolol should be withdrawn before clonidine by several days or added several days after clonidine is stopped.
Dolasetron: May increase risk of irregular heart rhythm. Monitor patient.
Insulin, oral antidiabetics: May alter dosage requirements in patient with diabetes who has been previously stabilized. Observe patient carefully.
IV lidocaine: May reduce hepatic metabolism of lidocaine, increasing risk of toxicity. Give bolus doses of lidocaine at a slower rate and monitor therapy.
NSAIDs: May decrease antihypertensive effects. Monitor BP.
Prazosin: May increase the risk of orthostatic hypotension in the early phases of use together.
Rivastigmine: May enhance bradycardic effect of atenolol. Avoid combination.

EFFECTS ON LAB TEST RESULTS

- May increase bilirubin and liver enzyme levels.
- May decrease glucose level.
- May increase platelet count.

CONTRAINDICATIONS & CAUTIONS

- Contraindicated in patients hypersensitive to drug or its components.
- Contraindicated in patients with sinus bradycardia, heart block greater than first degree, overt cardiac failure, untreated pheochromocytoma, and cardiogenic shock.

• Contraindicated in patients with acute MI and HF who don't promptly respond to IV furosemide or equivalent therapy.
• Use cautiously in older adults, patients at risk for HF, and in those with diabetes, hyperthyroidism, myasthenia gravis, and impaired renal or hepatic function.
• Beta blockers shouldn't be routinely used in patients with bronchospastic disease. Atenolol may be used cautiously in patients who don't respond to or can't tolerate other antihypertensive treatment. Use lowest possible dosage and have bronchodilator available. Consider divided doses if atenolol dosage must be increased.
• Drug may precipitate or aggravate signs and symptoms of PVD and Raynaud disease and worsen anginal symptoms in patients with vasospastic angina.
• Don't routinely stop long-term beta blocker therapy before major surgery; however, risks associated with general anesthesia and surgery may be increased due to the heart's impaired ability to respond to reflex adrenergic stimuli.
• Safe use in children hasn't been established.
Dialyzable drug: Yes.
⚠ *Overdose S&S:* Lethargy, decreased respiratory drive, wheezing, sinus pause, bradycardia.

PREGNANCY-LACTATION-REPRODUCTION
• Drug can cause fetal harm. Use cautiously during pregnancy; inform patient of the potential fetal hazard.
• Drug appears in human milk. Use cautiously during breastfeeding.
• Neonates born to patients receiving atenolol at parturition and infants being breastfed by patients receiving atenolol may be at risk for hypoglycemia and significant bradycardia.

NURSING CONSIDERATIONS
• Monitor HR and BP, preferably just before next dose, to evaluate effectiveness.
• Monitor patients on hemodialysis closely because of hypotension risk.
• Beta blockers may mask tachycardia caused by hyperthyroidism. In patients with suspected thyrotoxicosis, withdraw beta blocker gradually to avoid thyroid storm.
• Drug may mask signs and symptoms of hypoglycemia in patients with diabetes.
• Drug may cause changes in exercise tolerance and ECG.

• Monitor patient for cardiac failure. Discontinue drug in patients who develop cardiac failure that doesn't respond to standard treatment.
Boxed Warning Avoid abrupt discontinuation of therapy. Withdraw drug gradually to avoid serious adverse reactions, such as severe exacerbations of angina, MI, and ventricular arrhythmias. Because CAD is common and may be unrecognized, avoid abrupt discontinuation even in patients treated only for HTN. ∎
• *Look alike–sound alike:* Don't confuse atenolol with timolol or albuterol.

PATIENT TEACHING
• Instruct patient to take drug exactly as prescribed, at the same time every day.
Boxed Warning Caution patient not to stop drug suddenly. ∎
• Advise patient to report all adverse reactions to prescriber.
• Teach patient how to take pulse, when to withhold drug, and when to report HR according to prescriber's instructions.
• Tell patient of childbearing potential to notify prescriber about planned, suspected, or known pregnancy.
• Advise patient who is breastfeeding to contact prescriber; drug may cause hypoglycemia or significant bradycardia in the infant.

---

atomoxetine hydrochloride ⚠
AT-oh-mox-e-teen

Strattera✐

Therapeutic class: ADHD drugs
Pharmacologic class: Selective norepinephrine reuptake inhibitors

---

AVAILABLE FORMS
Capsules ⒹⓃⒼ: 10 mg, 18 mg, 25 mg, 40 mg, 60 mg, 80 mg, 100 mg

INDICATIONS & DOSAGES
➤ **ADHD**
Adults and children older than age 6 and adolescents weighing more than 70 kg: Initially, 40 mg PO daily; increase after at least 3 days to a total of 80 mg/day PO, as a single dose in the morning or two evenly divided doses in the morning and late afternoon or early evening. After 2 to 4 weeks, increase total dose to a maximum of 100 mg, if needed.

Children age 6 and older and adolescents weighing 70 kg or less: Initially, 0.5 mg/kg PO daily; increase after a minimum of 3 days to a target total daily dose of 1.2 mg/kg PO as a single dose in the morning or two evenly divided doses in the morning and late afternoon or early evening. Don't exceed 1.4 mg/kg or 100 mg daily, whichever is less.

Adjust-a-dose: In patients with moderate hepatic impairment (Child-Pugh class B), reduce to 50% of the normal dose; in those with severe hepatic impairment (Child-Pugh class C), reduce to 25% of the normal dose.

☒ In children and adults weighing more than 70 kg who are also receiving strong CYP2D6 inhibitors or are known CYP2D6 poor metabolizers, start at 40 mg daily and increase to 80 mg daily only if symptoms don't improve after 4 weeks and if first dose is tolerated.

☒ In children weighing less than 70 kg who are also receiving strong CYP2D6 inhibitors or are known CYP2D6 poor metabolizers, adjust dosage to 0.5 mg/kg daily and increase to 1.2 mg/kg daily only if symptoms don't improve after 4 weeks and if first dose is tolerated.

ADMINISTRATION
PO
• Give drug without regard for meals.
• Capsules should be swallowed whole and not opened.
• Give missed dose as soon as possible but give no more than prescribed total daily amount in a 23-hour period.
• May discontinue drug without tapering.
• Store tablets at controlled room temperature of 59° to 86° F (15° to 30° C).

ACTION
May be related to selective inhibition of the presynaptic norepinephrine transporter.

Route	Onset	Peak	Duration
PO	Rapid	1–2 hr	Unknown

Half-life: 5 hours; 24 hours in poor metabolizers.

ADVERSE REACTIONS
CNS: headache, insomnia, dizziness, somnolence, irritability, mood swings, fatigue, sedation, depression, tremor, early-morning awakening, paresthesia, abnormal dreams, sleep disorder, syncope, anxiety. **CV:** orthostatic hypotension, tachycardia, HTN, palpitations,

hot flush. **EENT:** mydriasis, conjunctivitis, dry mouth, oropharyngeal pain, pharyngolaryngeal pain, sinus headache. **GI:** abdominal pain, constipation, dyspepsia, nausea, anorexia, vomiting, decreased appetite. **GU:** urine retention, urinary hesitation, ejaculatory problems, difficulty in micturition, dysmenorrhea, erectile dysfunction, menstrual disorder, prostatitis. **Metabolic:** weight loss, thirst. **Skin:** pruritus, excoriation, increased sweating, rash. **Other:** decreased libido, chills.

INTERACTIONS
Drug-drug. *Albuterol:* May increase CV effects. Use together cautiously.
MAO inhibitors: May cause hyperthermia, rigidity, myoclonus, autonomic instability with possible rapid fluctuations of vital signs, and mental status changes. Avoid use within 2 weeks of MAO inhibitor.
Pressor agents: May increase BP. Use together cautiously.
Strong CYP2D6 inhibitors (fluoxetine, paroxetine, quinidine): May increase atomoxetine level. Adjust atomoxetine dosage based on effect and tolerance.

EFFECTS ON LAB TEST RESULTS
None reported.

CONTRAINDICATIONS & CAUTIONS
• Contraindicated in patients hypersensitive to drug or its components; in those with current or history of pheochromocytoma, or narrow-angle glaucoma; in those with serious CV disorders who are intolerant of increased BP or HR; and in those who have taken an MAO inhibitor within the past 2 weeks.
• Drug may increase risk of sudden death, stroke, and MI in patients with preexisting structural cardiac disorders or other serious heart problems, including cardiomyopathy, CAD, and arrhythmias.
☒ Use cautiously in patients with HTN, tachycardia, hypotension, urine retention, cerebrovascular disease or poor CYP2D6 metabolizers.

Boxed Warning Drug may increase risk of suicidality in children and adolescents. ■
• Safety and effectiveness in children younger than age 6 haven't been established.
Dialyzable drug: No.
⚠ **Overdose S&S:** Somnolence, agitation, hyperactivity, abnormal behavior, GI symptoms, mydriasis, tachycardia, dry mouth, prolonged

QT interval, disorientation, hallucinations, seizures.

PREGNANCY-LACTATION-REPRODUCTION
• Don't use during pregnancy unless potential benefit justifies fetal risk. Patients of child-bearing potential should be advised to use effective contraception.
• It isn't known if drug appears in human milk. Use cautiously during breastfeeding.
• Health care providers are encouraged to register patients in the National Pregnancy Registry for ADHD Medications, which monitors pregnancy outcomes in patients exposed to ADHD medications during pregnancy (1-866-961-2388 or https://womensmentalhealth.org/adhd-medications/).

NURSING CONSIDERATIONS
• Use drug as part of a total treatment program for ADHD, including psychological, educational, and social intervention. Drug may be discontinued without tapering.
Boxed Warning Monitor children and adolescents closely for worsening of condition, agitation, irritability, suicidal thinking or behaviors, and unusual changes in behavior, especially the first few months of therapy or when dosage is increased or decreased. ■
• Periodically monitor patients for changes in HR or BP.
• Assess patients carefully for cardiac disease, including family history of sudden death or ventricular arrhythmia. Evaluate patients with new cardiac symptoms promptly.
• Screen patients for bipolar disorder or risk factors for bipolar disorder before treatment, including family history of mania or depression. Drug may increase risk of emergence or worsening of disorder.
• Patients taking drug for extended periods must be reevaluated periodically to determine drug's usefulness.
• Monitor growth during treatment. If growth or weight gain is unsatisfactory, consider interrupting therapy.
۞ **Alert:** Severe liver injury may occur and progress to liver failure. Notify prescriber of any sign of liver injury: yellowing of the skin or the sclera of the eyes, pruritus, dark urine, upper right-sided tenderness, or unexplained flulike syndrome.

• Monitor BP and pulse rate at baseline, after each dosage increase, and periodically during treatment.
• Monitor patient for urinary hesitancy, urine retention, or priapism.
• Monitor patient for appearance or worsening of psychotic or manic symptoms, aggressive behavior, or hostility.
• Monitor patient for hypersensitivity reactions, including anaphylaxis.

PATIENT TEACHING
Boxed Warning Advise patient or caregivers to immediately report unusual behavior or suicidality. ■
• Instruct patient to immediately report chest pain, shortness of breath, or fainting.
• Tell patient to use caution when operating a vehicle or machinery until the effects of drug are known.
• Warn male patient to seek prompt medical attention for an erection that lasts more than 4 hours.
• Inform patient that therapy may be interrupted periodically to check ADHD symptoms.
• Tell patient who is pregnant, planning to become pregnant, or breastfeeding to consult prescriber before taking atomoxetine.

---

atorvastatin calcium ۞
a-TORE-va-sta-tin

Lipitor✦

Therapeutic class: Antilipemics
Pharmacologic class: HMG-CoA reductase inhibitors

AVAILABLE FORMS
Tablets ⓄⓃⒸ: 10 mg, 20 mg, 40 mg, 80 mg

INDICATIONS & DOSAGES
Adjust-a-dose (for all indications): Significant drug interactions exist requiring dosage or frequency adjustment or drug avoidance. Refer to manufacturer's instructions for dosage adjustments.
➤ **In patients with clinically evident CAD, to reduce risk of nonfatal MI, fatal and nonfatal strokes, angina, HF, and revascularization procedures**
Adults: Initially, 10 to 20 mg PO daily. May increase based on patient response and tolerance; usual dosage, 10 to 80 mg PO daily.

➤ **To reduce risk of MI, stroke, angina, or revascularization procedures in patients with multiple risk factors for CAD but who don't yet have the disease**
Adults: Initially, 10 to 20 mg PO daily. May increase based on patient response and tolerance; usual dosage, 10 to 80 mg PO daily.

➤ **To reduce risk of MI or stroke in patients with type 2 diabetes and multiple risk factors for CAD but who don't yet have the disease**
Adults: Initially, 10 to 20 mg PO daily. May increase based on patient response and tolerance; usual dosage, 10 to 80 mg PO daily.

➤ **Adjunct to diet to reduce LDL, total cholesterol, apolipoprotein B, and triglyceride levels and to increase HDL levels in patients with primary hypercholesterolemia (heterozygous familial and nonfamilial) and mixed dyslipidemia (Fredrickson types IIa and IIb); adjunct to diet to reduce triglyceride level (Fredrickson type IV); primary dysbetalipoproteinemia (Fredrickson type III) in patients who don't respond adequately to diet** ☒
Adults: Initially, 10 or 20 mg PO once daily. Patient who requires a reduction of more than 45% in LDL level may be started at 40 mg once daily. Increase dose, as needed, to maximum of 80 mg daily as single dose. Dosage based on lipid levels drawn within 2 to 4 weeks of starting therapy and after dosage adjustment.

➤ **Alone or as an adjunct to lipid-lowering treatments, such as LDL apheresis, to reduce total and LDL cholesterol in patients with homozygous familial hypercholesterolemia** ☒
Adults: 10 to 80 mg PO once daily.

➤ **Heterozygous familial hypercholesterolemia in children who don't respond adequately to dietary treatment** ☒
Children ages 10 to 17 (girls should be 1 year postmenarche): Initially, 10 mg PO once daily. Adjustment intervals should be at least 4 weeks. Maximum daily dose is 20 mg.

ADMINISTRATION
PO
• Give drug without regard for meals at any time of the day.

ACTION
Inhibits HMG-CoA reductase, an early (and rate-limiting) step in cholesterol biosynthesis.

Route	Onset	Peak	Duration
PO	Unknown	1–2 hr	Unknown

Half-life: 14 hours.

ADVERSE REACTIONS
CNS: insomnia. **EENT:** nasopharyngitis, pharyngolaryngeal pain. **GI:** abdominal pain, diarrhea, dyspepsia, flatulence, nausea. **GU:** UTI. **Hepatic:** increased LFT values. **Metabolic:** *diabetes.* **Musculoskeletal:** *rhabdomyolysis,* arthralgia, myalgia, extremity pain, muscle spasms, musculoskeletal pain. **Skin:** rash.

INTERACTIONS
Drug-drug. *Amiodarone:* May increase risk of severe myopathy or rhabdomyolysis. Avoid use together or decrease atorvastatin dose.
Antacids, cholestyramine, colestipol: May decrease atorvastatin level. Separate administration times.
Colchicine, **diltiazem,** *fibric acid derivatives,* **nefazodone,** *niacin, protease inhibitors,* **verapamil:** May decrease metabolism of HMG-CoA reductase inhibitors, increasing toxicity. Monitor patient for adverse effects and report unexplained muscle pain.
Cyclosporine, *tacrolimus, telaprevir, tipranavir plus ritonavir:* May increase statin level and risk of myopathy and rhabdomyolysis. Avoid use together.
Darunavir and ritonavir, fosamprenavir, fosamprenavir and ritonavir, saquinavir and ritonavir: May increase atorvastatin level and risk of myopathy and rhabdomyolysis. Atorvastatin dosage shouldn't exceed 20 mg daily.
Digoxin: May increase digoxin level. Monitor digoxin level and patient for evidence of toxicity.
Fluconazole, itraconazole, ketoconazole, voriconazole: May increase atorvastatin level and adverse effects. Avoid using together or, if unavoidable, atorvastatin dosage shouldn't exceed 20 mg daily.
Gemfibrozil: May increase risk of myopathy/rhabdomyolysis. Avoid combination.
Hormonal contraceptives: May increase norethindrone and ethinyl estradiol levels. Consider increased drug effect when selecting an oral contraceptive.
Lopinavir and ritonavir: May increase statin level and risk of myopathy and rhabdomyolysis. Use together cautiously and at lowest atorvastatin dosage necessary.

Macrolides (azithromycin, clarithromycin, erythromycin, telithromycin): May increase atorvastatin level and risk of myopathy and rhabdomyolysis. Atorvastatin dosage shouldn't exceed 20 mg daily or withhold atorvastatin during macrolide therapy.
Nelfinavir: May increase statin level and risk of myopathy and rhabdomyolysis. Atorvastatin dosage shouldn't exceed 40 mg daily.
Drug-herb. *Jin bu huan, kava:* May increase risk of hepatotoxicity. Discourage use together.
Drug-food. *Grapefruit juice:* May increase drug levels when consumed in large quantities, increasing risk of adverse reactions. Discourage use together.
Drug-lifestyle. *Alcohol use:* May increase hepatotoxic effects. Monitor patient closely.

EFFECTS ON LAB TEST RESULTS
• May increase LFT values and CK levels.

CONTRAINDICATIONS & CAUTIONS
• Contraindicated in patients hypersensitive to drug and in those with active liver disease or unexplained persistent elevations of transaminase levels.
• There is increased risk of myopathy and rhabdomyolysis with drug use, especially in patients age 65 and older; in those with uncontrolled hypothyroidism or renal impairment; and in patients taking certain other drugs.
• Some dosage forms contain polysorbate 80, which can cause delayed hypersensitivity reactions.
• Use cautiously in patients with hepatic impairment or heavy alcohol use.
• Withhold or stop drug in patients at risk for renal failure caused by rhabdomyolysis resulting from trauma; in serious, acute conditions that suggest myopathy; and in major surgery, severe acute infection, hypotension, uncontrolled seizures, or severe metabolic, endocrine, or electrolyte disorders.
⚕ Limit use in children to those older than age 10 with homozygous familial hypercholesterolemia.
Dialyzable drug: No.

PREGNANCY-LACTATION-REPRODUCTION
• Drug may cause fetal harm. Contraindicated in most patients who are pregnant or may become pregnant. Consider use in patients at high risk for CV events during pregnancy (homozygous familial

hypercholesterolemia, established CV disease) on an individual basis.
• Patients of childbearing potential should use effective contraception during treatment and be apprised of potential hazards to the fetus.
• It isn't known if drug appears in human milk. Use is contraindicated during breastfeeding.

NURSING CONSIDERATIONS
• Patient should follow a standard cholesterol-lowering diet before and during therapy.
• Before treatment, assess patient for underlying causes for hypercholesterolemia and obtain a baseline lipid profile. Obtain periodic LFT results and lipid levels before starting treatment and at 4 and 12 weeks after initiation, or after an increase in dosage and periodically thereafter.
• Watch for signs of myositis and myopathy (unexplained muscle pain, tenderness, weakness, malaise, dark urine, fever). Drug may need to be discontinued.
• *Look alike–sound alike:* Don't confuse atorvastatin with atomoxetine or other statins.

PATIENT TEACHING
• Teach patient about proper dietary management, weight control, and exercise. Explain their importance in controlling high fat levels.
• Warn patient to avoid alcohol.
• Tell patient to inform prescriber of all adverse reactions. Stress the risk of myopathy (unexplained muscle pain, tenderness or weakness, particularly if accompanied by malaise, and fever).
• Advise patient that drug can be taken at any time of day, without regard for meals.
⊘ *Alert:* Tell patient to stop drug and notify prescriber immediately if pregnant or breastfeeding.

atovaquone
a-TOE-va-kwone

Mepron

Therapeutic class: Antiprotozoals
Pharmacologic class: Ubiquinone analogues

AVAILABLE FORMS
Oral suspension: 750 mg/5 mL

INDICATIONS & DOSAGES

➤ **Acute, mild to moderate *Pneumocystis jiroveci* pneumonia in patients who can't tolerate sulfamethoxazole–trimethoprim**
Adults and adolescents age 13 and older: 750 mg (5 mL) PO b.i.d. for 21 days.

➤ **To prevent *P. jiroveci* pneumonia in patients who are unable to tolerate sulfamethoxazole–trimethoprim**
Adults and adolescents age 13 and older: 1,500 mg (10 mL) PO daily.

ADMINISTRATION

PO
- Give with food; taking with meals enhances absorption.
- Shake bottle gently before using.
- Give entire contents of foil pouch, which can be poured into a dosing spoon or cup or be taken directly into the mouth.

ACTION

May interfere with electron transport in protozoal mitochondria, inhibiting enzymes needed to synthesize nucleic acids and adenosine triphosphate.

Route	Onset	Peak	Duration
PO	Unknown	Unknown	Unknown

Half-life: 2 to 4 days.

ADVERSE REACTIONS

CNS: headache, insomnia, fever, pain, asthenia, anxiety, dizziness, taste perversion, depression. **CV:** hypotension. **EENT:** sinusitis, rhinitis, oral candidiasis. **GI:** abdominal pain, nausea, diarrhea, vomiting, constipation, anorexia, dyspepsia. **Hematologic:** *neutropenia,* anemia. **Hepatic:** elevated transaminase levels, increased ALP level. **Metabolic:** *hypoglycemia,* hyponatremia, increased amylase level. **Musculoskeletal:** myalgia. **Respiratory:** cough, dyspnea. **Skin:** rash, diaphoresis, pruritus. **Other:** flulike syndrome.

INTERACTIONS

Drug-drug. *Metoclopramide:* May decrease atovaquone bioavailability. Use another antiemetic.
Rifabutin, rifampin: May decrease atovaquone's steady-state level. Avoid using together.
Tetracycline: May decrease atovaquone level. Monitor patient for continued or reactivated infection.

Zidovudine: May elevate zidovudine level and lead to toxicity. Monitor closely.

EFFECTS ON LAB TEST RESULTS

- May increase glucose, amylase, ALP, ALT, and AST levels. May decrease Hb and sodium levels.
- May decrease neutrophil count.

CONTRAINDICATIONS & CAUTIONS

- Contraindicated in patients hypersensitive to drug.
- Serious hypersensitivity reactions have been reported.
- Use cautiously in patients with severe hepatic impairment.
- Use cautiously with other highly protein-bound drugs; if used together, assess patient for toxicity.
- **⚕ *Alert:*** Patients with GI disorders may not absorb drug well and may not achieve adequate plasma levels. Consider parenteral therapy with alternative drugs.
- Safety and effectiveness in children age 12 and younger haven't been established.
Dialyzable drug: Unknown.
⚠ ***Overdose S&S:*** Methemoglobinemia, rash.

PREGNANCY-LACTATION-REPRODUCTION

- Use cautiously during pregnancy and only if potential benefit justifies fetal risk.
- It isn't known if drug appears in human milk. Use cautiously during breastfeeding.

NURSING CONSIDERATIONS

- **⚕ *Alert:*** Monitor patient closely during therapy because of risk of pulmonary infection.
- Monitor patients with hepatic impairment closely.
- Monitor patient for GI disorders (nausea, vomiting, diarrhea) that might affect patient's ability to absorb drug.

PATIENT TEACHING

- Instruct patient to take drug with meals; food significantly enhances absorption.
- Stress importance of taking atovaquone as prescribed.
- Advise patient to report all adverse reactions and to immediately report nausea, vomiting, diarrhea, white mouth patches, flulike symptoms, dark urine, tiredness, lack of appetite, yellow skin, and light stools.

atovaquone–proguanil hydrochloride
a-TOE-va-kwon/pro-GWA-nil

Malarone

Therapeutic class: Antimalarials
Pharmacologic class: Hydroxynaphtho-
quinone and biguanide derivatives

AVAILABLE FORMS
Tablets (adult-strength): 250 mg atovaquone
and 100 mg proguanil hydrochloride
Tablets (pediatric-strength): 62.5 mg atovaquone and 25 mg proguanil hydrochloride

INDICATIONS & DOSAGES
➤ **To prevent *Plasmodium falciparum*
malaria, including in areas where chloroquine resistance has been reported, beginning 1 or 2 days before entering a malaria-
endemic area and continuing during stay
and for 7 days after return**
*Adults and children weighing more than
40 kg:* 1 adult-strength tablet PO once daily.
Children weighing 31 to 40 kg: 3 pediatric-
strength tablets PO once daily.
Children weighing 21 to 30 kg: 2 pediatric-
strength tablets PO once daily.
Children weighing 11 to 20 kg: 1 pediatric-
strength tablet PO daily.
Adjust-a-dose: Don't use for malaria prophylaxis in patients with severe renal impairment
(CrCl less than 30 mL/minute).
➤ **Acute, uncomplicated *P. falciparum*
malaria**
*Adults and children weighing more than
40 kg:* 4 adult-strength tablets PO once daily
for 3 consecutive days.
Children weighing 31 to 40 kg: 3 adult-
strength tablets PO once daily for 3 consecutive days.
Children weighing 21 to 30 kg: 2 adult-
strength tablets PO once daily for 3 consecutive days.
Children weighing 11 to 20 kg: 1 adult-
strength tablet PO once daily for 3 consecutive days.
Children weighing 9 to 10 kg: 3 pediatric-
strength tablets PO once daily for 3 consecutive days.
Children weighing 5 to 8 kg: 2 pediatric-
strength tablets PO once daily for 3 consecutive days.

ADMINISTRATION
PO
• Give dose at same time each day, with food
or milk.
• If patient has difficulty swallowing tablets,
crush tablets and mix in condensed milk.
• If vomiting occurs within 1 hour of drug
administration, repeat dose.
• Store tablets at controlled room temperature
of 59° to 86° F (15° to 30° C).

ACTION
Thought to interfere with nucleic acid replication in the malarial parasite. Atovaquone
selectively inhibits mitochondrial electron
transport in the parasite. Cycloguanil, an active metabolite of proguanil hydrochloride,
inhibits dihydrofolate reductase. Atovaquone
and cycloguanil are active against the erythro-
cytic and exoerythrocytic stages of *Plasmodium* species.

Route	Onset	Peak	Duration
PO	Unknown	Unknown	Unknown

Half-life: Atovaquone: 2 to 3 days in adults, 1 to
2 days in children; proguanil: 12 to 21 hours in
adults and children.

ADVERSE REACTIONS
CNS: headache, asthenia, dizziness, dreams,
insomnia. **EENT:** vision changes, oral ulcers.
GI: abdominal pain, nausea, vomiting, diarrhea, anorexia, dyspepsia, gastritis. **Respiratory:** cough. **Skin:** pruritus.

INTERACTIONS
Drug-drug. *Metoclopramide:* May decrease
atovaquone bioavailability. Use another
antiemetic.
Rifabutin, rifampin: May significantly decrease atovaquone level. Avoid using together.
Tetracycline: May decrease atovaquone level.
Monitor patient closely for continued or reactivated infection.
Warfarin: May increase anticoagulation effect. Monitor INR.

EFFECTS ON LAB TEST RESULTS
• May increase LFT values.
• May decrease Hb level, hematocrit, and
neutrophil count.

CONTRAINDICATIONS & CAUTIONS
• Contraindicated in patients hypersensitive
to atovaquone, proguanil hydrochloride, or

Reactions in bold italics are ***life-threatening***. Interactions may have a *rapid onset* or a ***delayed onset***.

components of drug and in those with severe renal impairment or severe or complicated malaria.
• Use cautiously in patients with vomiting or diarrhea; drug absorption may be decreased.
• Use cautiously in older adults because they have a greater frequency of decreased renal, hepatic, and cardiac function.
• Safety and effectiveness haven't been established for prevention in children who weigh less than 11 kg or for treatment in children who weigh less than 5 kg.
Dialyzable drug: Unknown.
⚠ *Overdose S&S:* Rash, methemoglobinemia (atovaquone); epigastric discomfort, vomiting, reversible hair loss, scaling of the skin on the palms or soles, reversible aphthous ulceration, hematologic adverse effects (proguanil).

PREGNANCY-LACTATION-REPRODUCTION
• Use during pregnancy only if potential benefit justifies fetal risk.
• It isn't known if atovaquone appears in human milk, but proguanil does appear in small amounts. Use cautiously during breastfeeding.

NURSING CONSIDERATIONS
• Monitor patient for persistent diarrhea or vomiting. Patients with these symptoms may need a different antimalarial.
• Monitor patients on prophylactic therapy for elevated liver enzyme levels, hepatitis, and hepatic failure.

PATIENT TEACHING
• Teach patient safe drug administration.
• Advise patient to notify prescriber if patient can't complete the course of therapy as prescribed.
• Instruct patient to supplement preventive antimalarial with use of protective clothing, bed nets, and insect repellents.
• Caution patient that prophylaxis isn't assured and to seek medical attention for any febrile illness during or after return from malaria-endemic area.

SAFETY ALERT!

atropine sulfate ⓧ
AT-troe-peen

AtroPen

Therapeutic class: Antiarrhythmics
Pharmacologic class: Anticholinergics–belladonna alkaloids

AVAILABLE FORMS
Injection: 0.4 mg/mL, 1 mg/mL vials
Prefilled autoinjectors: 0.25 mg, 0.5 mg, 1 mg, 2 mg
Prefilled syringe: 0.05 mg/mL in 5-mL syringe, 0.1 mg/mL in 5- and 10-mL syringe

INDICATIONS & DOSAGES
➤ **Bradyasystolic cardiac arrest**
Adults: 1 mg IV (preferred) every 3 to 5 minutes; maximum total dose is 3 mg.
➤ **Symptomatic bradycardia**
Adults: 0.5 mg IV push or IM, repeated every 3 to 5 minutes, not to exceed a total of 3 mg or 0.04 mg/kg.
Children and adolescents: 0.02 mg/kg IV. May repeat once in 3 to 5 minutes; maximum dose is 1 mg.
➤ **Organophosphorus or muscarinic mushroom poisoning**
Adults: 2 to 3 mg IV (preferred), IM, or subcut; may repeat every 20 to 30 minutes.
➤ **Initial treatment of muscarinic symptoms of insecticide (organophosphorus or carbamate) poisoning or organophosphorus nerve agent poisoning**
Adults and children weighing more than 41 kg: For severe symptoms, immediately give three AtroPen 2 mg IM injections in rapid succession. For mild symptoms, give one AtroPen 2 mg IM injection. If patient then develops severe symptoms, give two additional 2 mg IM injections in rapid succession 10 minutes after first injection.
Children weighing 18 to 41 kg: For severe symptoms, immediately give three AtroPen 1 mg IM injections in rapid succession. For mild symptoms, give one AtroPen 1 mg IM injection. If patient then develops severe symptoms, give two additional 1 mg IM injections in rapid succession 10 minutes after first injection.
Children weighing 7 to 18 kg: For severe symptoms, immediately give three AtroPen

0.5 mg IM injections in rapid succession. For mild symptoms, give one AtroPen 0.5 mg IM injection. If patient then develops severe symptoms, give two additional 0.5 mg IM injections in rapid succession 10 minutes after first injection.

Infants weighing less than 7 kg: For severe symptoms, immediately give three AtroPen 0.25 mg IM injections in rapid succession. For mild symptoms, give one AtroPen 0.25 mg IM injection. If patient then develops severe symptoms, give two additional 0.25 mg IM injections in rapid succession 10 minutes after first injection.

➤ **Preoperatively to diminish secretions and block cardiac vagal reflexes**
Adults: 0.5 to 1 mg IV (preferred), IM, or subcut 30 to 60 minutes before anesthesia. May repeat in 1 to 2 hours PRN. Maximum total dose, 3 mg.

➤ **Stress echocardiography (adjunct chronotropic agent)** ♦
Adults: 0.25 to 0.5 mg IV up to a total dose of 1 to 2 mg until 85% of target HR is achieved.

ADMINISTRATION
IV
▼ Give into a large vein or into IV tubing by rapid injection.
▼ Slow delivery may cause paradoxical bradycardia.
▼ **Incompatibilities:** None listed by manufacturer. Consult a drug incompatibility reference for more information.
Subcutaneous
• Document administration site.
IM
• Autoinjection may be given through clothing.
• Firmly jab autoinjector needle tip into midlateral thigh at 90-degree angle.
• Hold autoinjector in place for at least 10 seconds to allow time for complete administration.
• Make sure needle is visible after removing autoinjector. If needle didn't engage, repeat injection, jabbing more firmly.
• Massage injection site for several seconds after removing autoinjector.
• In patients who are young or very thin, pinch the skin on the thigh together before injection.

ACTION
Inhibits muscarinic actions of acetylcholine at parasympathetic neuroeffector junction,

blocking vagal effects on SA and AV nodes, enhancing conduction through AV node and increasing HR.

Route	Onset	Peak	Duration
IV	Immediate	Unknown	Unknown
IM	Rapid	3–60 min	4 hr
Subcut	Unknown	Unknown	Unknown

Half-life: IM: adults, 2 to 4 hours; children older than age 2, 1.5 to 3.5 hours; children younger than age 2, 4 to 10 hours.

ADVERSE REACTIONS
Severity and frequency of adverse reactions are dose-related.
CNS: headache, restlessness, insomnia, dizziness, ataxia, disorientation, hallucinations, delirium, excitement, agitation, anxiety, amnesia, decreased deep tendon reflex, drowsiness, dysarthria, hyperreflexia, *seizure,* vertigo, confusion, fever, weakness. **CV:** *bradycardia,* palpitations, tachycardia, chest pain, hypotension, *prolonged QT interval, atrial and ventricular arrhythmias.* **EENT:** blurred vision, mydriasis, photophobia, cycloplegia, increased IOP, dry mouth. **GI:** constipation, nausea, vomiting, abdominal distention, abdominal pain, delayed gastric emptying, diminished bowel sounds. **GU:** urine retention, urinary hesitancy or urgency, erectile dysfunction. **Hematologic:** leukocytosis, anemia, petechiae, increased Hb level. **Metabolic:** hyperglycemia, *hypoglycemia,* hyponatremia, *hypokalemia,* thirst, dehydration. **Musculoskeletal:** muscle twitching. **Respiratory:** *bradypnea,* dyspnea, *pulmonary edema.* **Skin:** rash, anhidrosis, hyperhidrosis, dermatitis, injection-site reaction, cyanosis. **Other:** hypersensitivity reaction, *anaphylaxis.*

INTERACTIONS
Drug-drug. *Anticholinergics, drugs with anticholinergic effects (amantadine, antiarrhythmics, antiparkinsonian drugs, meperidine, phenothiazines, TCAs):* May increase anticholinergic effects. Use together cautiously.
Potassium chloride, potassium citrate: May increase risk of mucosal lesions. Avoid combination.

EFFECTS ON LAB TEST RESULTS
• May increase BUN level.
• May decrease sodium and potassium levels.

Reactions in bold italics are *life-threatening*. Interactions may have a *rapid onset* or a *delayed onset*.

- May increase or decrease glucose level.
- May increase or decrease Hb level. May increase RBC and WBC counts.

CONTRAINDICATIONS & CAUTIONS
- Contraindicated in patients hypersensitive to drug and in patients with hyperthermia.
- Drug may increase risk of acute angle-closure glaucoma, obstructive uropathy, obstructive disease of GI tract, and paralytic ileus, toxic megacolon, and intestinal atony.
- Use cautiously in patients with hyperthyroidism, CAD, HTN, HF, tachycardia, hiatal hernia with reflux esophagitis, prostatic hypertrophy, myasthenia gravis, or renal or hepatic impairment, and in older adults.
- Use cautiously in patients with Down syndrome because they may be more sensitive to drug.
- Drug will be ineffective treatment of bradycardia in patients with heart transplants due to lack of vagal nerve innervation.
Dialyzable drug: No.
⚠ *Overdose S&S:* Delirium, seizures, coma, tachycardia, fever, mydriasis, decreased salivation and sweating, urine retention, HTN, vasodilation, hyperthermia.

PREGNANCY-LACTATION-REPRODUCTION
- Use during pregnancy only if clearly needed.
- Safe use during breastfeeding hasn't been established. Atropine has been reported in human milk. Use cautiously during breastfeeding.

NURSING CONSIDERATIONS
- Doses less than 0.5 mg in adults and less than 0.1 mg in children may increase risk of paradoxical bradycardia.
- Monitor pulse rate, BP, and mental status.
- IV administration requires cardiac monitoring.
- ⓘ *Alert:* Watch for tachycardia in patients with cardiac conditions because it may lead to ventricular fibrillation.
- Monitor fluid intake and urine output. Drug causes urine retention and urinary hesitancy.

PATIENT TEACHING
- Instruct patient to report all adverse reactions and to immediately report urine retention, abnormal heartbeat, dizziness, passing out, difficulty breathing, weakness, tremors, and abdominal edema.

- Teach patient signs and symptoms of insecticide poisoning (nausea, diarrhea, muscle spasms).
- Explain to patient how to use, store, and dispose of the AtroPen.

SAFETY ALERT!

axitinib
ax-i-TI-nib

Inlyta

Therapeutic class: Antineoplastics
Pharmacologic class: Kinase inhibitors

AVAILABLE FORMS
Tablets ⓓⓝⓒ: 1 mg, 5 mg

INDICATIONS & DOSAGES
➤ **Advanced renal cell carcinoma after failure of one prior systemic therapy**
Adults: 5 mg PO b.i.d. If patient tolerates drug for at least 2 consecutive weeks with adverse reactions no greater than grade 2 CT-CAE guidelines, is normotensive, and isn't receiving antihypertensives, may increase dosage to 7 mg b.i.d., then 10 mg b.i.d.
Adjust-a-dose: Base dosage adjustment on individual safety and tolerability. Management of adverse reactions may require temporary interruption or permanent discontinuation. If dosage reduction from 5 mg b.i.d. is needed, recommended dosage is 3 mg b.i.d. If a strong CYP3A4/5 inhibitor must be coadministered, decrease axitinib dosage by approximately half; may increase or decrease subsequent doses based on individual safety and tolerability. If strong CYP3A4/5 inhibitor is discontinued, return axitinib dosage to that used before initiation after inhibitor is out of system (3 to 5 half-life periods of the strong inhibitor). Reduce axitinib starting dose by approximately half in patients with baseline moderate hepatic impairment (Child-Pugh class B); may increase or decrease subsequent doses based on individual safety and tolerability.
➤ **First-line treatment of advanced renal cell carcinoma in combination with avelumab**
Adults: 5 mg PO b.i.d. in combination with avelumab 800-mg IV infusion every 2 weeks. If patient tolerates drug for at least 2 consecutive weeks with adverse reactions no greater

than grade 2 CTCAE guidelines, is normotensive, and isn't receiving antihypertensives, may increase dosage to 7 mg b.i.d., then 10 mg b.i.d. Continue until disease progression or unacceptable toxicity occurs. Refer to manufacturer's instructions for avelumab prescribing information.

Adjust-a-dose: See manufacturer's labeling for hepatotoxicity-related dosage adjustments in patients receiving axitinib in combination with avelumab.

➤ **First-line treatment of advanced renal cell carcinoma in combination with pembrolizumab**

Adults: 5 mg PO b.i.d. in combination with pembrolizumab 200-mg IV infusion every 3 weeks or 400-mg IV infusion every 6 weeks. If patient tolerates drug for at least 6 consecutive weeks with adverse reactions no greater than grade 2 CTCAE guidelines, is normotensive, and isn't receiving antihypertensives, may increase dosage to 7 mg b.i.d., then 10 mg b.i.d. Continue until disease progression or unacceptable toxicity occurs. Refer to manufacturer's instructions for pembrolizumab prescribing information.

Adjust-a-dose: See manufacturer's labeling for hepatotoxicity-related dosage adjustments in patients receiving axitinib in combination with pembrolizumab.

ADMINISTRATION
PO
- Drug is considered hazardous: use safe handling and disposal precautions according to facility policy.
- May give without regard for food.
- Give tablets approximately 12 hours apart.
- Have patient swallow tablets whole with a glass of water.
- If a dose is missed or patient vomits, don't give an additional dose; give next prescribed dose at usual time.
- Store at 68° to 77° F (20° to 25° C).

ACTION
Inhibits receptor tyrosine kinase, which decreases cell proliferation, tumor growth, angiogenesis, and cancer progression.

Route	Onset	Peak	Duration
PO	Unknown	2.5–4.1 hr	Unknown

Half-life: 2.5 to 6.1 hours.

ADVERSE REACTIONS
CNS: asthenia, fatigue, headache, dizziness, dysgeusia, TIA. **CV:** *HF, thromboembolism, hemorrhage,* HTN, *DVT.* **EENT:** dysphonia, mucosal inflammation, stomatitis, epistaxis, tinnitus, retinal vein occlusion thrombosis, glossodynia. **GI:** diarrhea, nausea, vomiting, constipation, mucositis, stomatitis, abdominal pain, dyspepsia, hemorrhoids, *GI perforation,* fistula formation, *rectal hemorrhage.* **GU:** hematuria, increased creatinine level, proteinuria. **Hematologic:** anemia, *thrombocytopenia, polycythemia.* **Hepatic:** increased transaminase levels, bilirubinemia, increased lipase level, *hepatotoxicity.* **Metabolic:** decreased appetite, decreased weight, hypothyroidism, hyponatremia, *hyperkalemia,* dehydration, hypertriglyceridemia, hypercholesterolemia. **Musculoskeletal:** arthralgia, musculoskeletal pain, extremity pain, myalgia. **Respiratory:** cough, *hemoptysis,* dyspnea, *PE.* **Skin:** alopecia, hand-foot syndrome, rash, dry skin, pruritus, erythema.

INTERACTIONS
Drug-drug. *Moderate CYP3A4/5 inducers (bosentan, efavirenz, etravirine, modafinil, nafcillin), strong CYP3A4/5 inducers (carbamazepine, dexamethasone, phenobarbital, phenytoin, rifabutin, rifampin, rifapentine):* May reduce axitinib level. Avoid concurrent use.

Strong CYP3A4/5 inhibitors (atazanavir, clarithromycin, itraconazole, ketoconazole, nefazodone, nelfinavir, ritonavir, saquinavir, telithromycin, voriconazole): May increase axitinib level. Avoid concurrent use; if strong CYP3A4/5 inhibitor is absolutely necessary, reduce axitinib dosage.

Drug-herb. *St. John's wort:* May decrease axitinib plasma concentration. Discourage concurrent use.

Drug-food. *Grapefruit, grapefruit juice:* May increase axitinib plasma concentration. Discourage concurrent use.

EFFECTS ON LAB TEST RESULTS
- May increase potassium, amylase, lipase, ALP, ALT, AST, bilirubin, cholesterol, triglyceride, and creatinine levels.
- May decrease bicarbonate, calcium, albumin, phosphate, and thyroid hormone levels.
- May increase or decrease glucose, sodium, and TSH levels.

Reactions in bold italics are *life-threatening*. Interactions may have a *rapid onset* or a *delayed onset*.

• May decrease Hb level and lymphocyte, neutrophil, and platelet counts.

CONTRAINDICATIONS & CAUTIONS
• Use isn't recommended in patients with recent GI bleeding or untreated brain metastases.
• Combination use with avelumab can cause severe and fatal CV events. Optimize management of CV risk factors (HTN, diabetes, dyslipidemia) before use.
• Drug may be associated with impaired wound healing.
• Use cautiously in patients with HTN; in those at risk for GI perforation, HF, fistula formation, thyroid dysfunction, or arterial or venous thromboembolic events; and in patients with moderate hepatic impairment (Child-Pugh class B) or ESRD (CrCl less than 15 mL/minute). Drug hasn't been studied in patients with Child-Pugh class C hepatic impairment.
• Cases of reversible posterior leukoencephalopathy syndrome (RPLS) have been reported.
• Safety and effectiveness in children haven't been established.
Dialyzable drug: Unknown.
⚠ *Overdose S&S:* Dizziness, HTN, seizures, possible fatal hemoptysis.

PREGNANCY-LACTATION-REPRODUCTION
• Drug can cause fetal harm. Patients of childbearing potential should be advised of fetal risk and to avoid becoming pregnant during therapy.
• Patients of childbearing potential should have a pregnancy test before starting drug.
• Patients of childbearing potential and men with partners of childbearing potential should use effective contraception during therapy and for 1 week after final dose.
• It isn't known if drug appears in human milk. Patient should discontinue drug or discontinue breastfeeding during treatment and for 2 weeks after final dose.
• Drug may impair both female and male fertility.

NURSING CONSIDERATIONS
• HTN should be well controlled before start of therapy. Monitor patient for increased BP; treat as indicated. If HTN persists despite antihypertensive use, decrease axitinib dosage, as ordered.

• Watch for hypotension if drug is withheld for any reason and patient continues antihypertensive use.
• Monitor patient for signs and symptoms of hematologic or neurologic disease, thromboembolic events, and GI disorders.
• Monitor patient for bleeding or hemorrhagic event. Temporarily interrupt treatment if bleeding occurs.
• Monitor patient for CV events; obtain baseline and periodic evaluations of LVEF.
• Monitor use of all prescription drugs, OTC medications, grapefruit or grapefruit juice, and supplements.
• Obtain LFTs and renal and thyroid function tests before and periodically during therapy. Consider more frequent monitoring of liver enzymes when therapy is combined with avelumab and pembrolizumab.
• Stop drug at least 2 days before elective surgery; resume at least 2 weeks after major surgery and adequate wound healing. Monitor wound healing carefully.
• Monitor patient for signs and symptoms of RPLS (headache, seizures, lethargy, confusion, blindness, and other visual disturbances) and other neurologic signs and symptoms. Discontinue drug if these occur.
• Monitor patient for proteinuria before and during therapy. For moderate or severe proteinuria, reduce dosage or withhold drug.

PATIENT TEACHING
• Advise female patient and male patient with partner of childbearing potential to use effective birth control during treatment and for 1 week after final dose.
• Instruct patient in safe drug administration.
• Advise patient to report all adverse reactions.
• Caution patient to tell prescriber of planned surgeries.
• Teach patient to consult prescriber before starting new drugs or supplements.
• Instruct patient to keep lab test appointments as requested by prescriber to monitor drug's safety and effectiveness.

azaTHIOprine ⚕
ay-za-THYE-oh-preen

Azasan, Imuran

azaTHIOprine sodium ⚕
Imuran✦

Therapeutic class: Immunosuppressants
Pharmacologic class: Purine antagonists

AVAILABLE FORMS
Powder for injection: 50-mg vial✦, 100-mg vial
Tablets: 25 mg, 50 mg, 75 mg, 100 mg

INDICATIONS & DOSAGES
⚕ *Adjust-a-dose (for all indications):* Reduce dosage in patients with thiopurine S-methyltransferase (TPMT) or NUDT15 deficiency. In patients receiving allopurinol or febuxostat, decrease azathioprine dosage to one-third to one-fourth of usual dose.
➤ **Immunosuppression in kidney transplantation**
Adults: Initially, 3 to 5 mg/kg PO or IV daily, usually beginning on day of transplantation but may begin 1 to 3 days prior. Maintained at 1 to 3 mg/kg daily based on patient response and tolerance.
Adjust-a-dose: Give drug in lower doses to patients with oliguria in the posttransplant period and in those with impaired renal function.
➤ **RA**
Adults: Initially, 1 mg/kg PO or IV as single dose or divided into two doses. Usual dose is 50 to 100 mg. If patient response isn't satisfactory after 6 to 8 weeks, dosage may be increased by 0.5 mg/kg daily to maximum of 2.5 mg/kg daily at 4-week intervals. Maintenance therapy should be at lowest effective dose. Attempt gradual dose reduction once patient is stable. Reduce dosage by 0.5 mg/kg (about 25 mg daily) every 4 weeks.

ADMINISTRATION
PO
• Give drug after meals to minimize adverse GI effects.
• Drug is a potential teratogen and mutagen. Use safe-handling procedures.

IV
▼ Drug is a potential teratogen and mutagen. Use safe handling procedures.
▼ Use only in patients who can't tolerate oral drugs.
▼ Reconstitute drug in 50-mg vial with 5 mL of sterile water for injection. Give by direct IV injection, or further dilute in NSS or D_5W solution.
▼ Reconstitute drug in 100-mg vial with 10 mL of sterile water for injection. Dilute further in NSS or D_5W solution.
▼ When drug is diluted further, the final volume depends on desired infusion time, usually 30 to 60 minutes, but may be as short as 5 minutes and as long as 8 hours for the daily dose.
▼ Inspect for particles before use.
▼ **Incompatibilities:** None listed by manufacturer. Consult a drug incompatibility reference for more information.

ACTION
May alter antibody production and suppress T-cell effects.

Route	Onset	Peak	Duration
PO, IV	Unknown	1–2 hr	Unknown

Half-life: About 5 hours.

ADVERSE REACTIONS
CNS: fever. **GI:** nausea, vomiting, diarrhea. **Hematologic:** anemia, *leukopenia, myelosuppression, pancytopenia, thrombocytopenia, immunosuppression.* **Hepatic:** *hepatotoxicity.* **Musculoskeletal:** myalgia. **Other:** infections, *increased risk of neoplasia.*

INTERACTIONS
Drug-drug. *ACE inhibitors:* May cause severe leukopenia and increase risk of anemia. Monitor patient closely.
Aminosalicylate derivatives (mesalazine, olsalazine, sulfasalazine): Inhibits TPMT. Use together cautiously.
⚕ *Allopurinol:* May impair inactivation of azathioprine. Avoid using if possible; decrease azathioprine to one third to one fourth usual dose. Consider further dosage reduction or alternative therapy for patients with low or absent TPMT activity.
Cyclosporine: May decrease cyclosporine level. Monitor cyclosporine level closely.
DMARDs (abatacept, adalimumab, etanercept, hydroxychloroquine, leflunomide,

---

Reactions in bold italics are *life-threatening*. Interactions may have a *rapid onset* or a ***delayed onset***.

methotrexate, minocycline, sulfasalazine, tocilizumab): Concomitant use hasn't been studied. Use together isn't recommended.
Febuxostat: May increase risk of toxicity. Concomitant use is contraindicated.
Live-virus vaccines: May reduce effectiveness of live-virus vaccines. Patients who are immunocompromised may be at increased risk for vaccine-induced infection. Defer live-virus vaccines until immune function improves.
Mercaptopurine: May increase risk of myelosuppression, including pancytopenia. Avoid concomitant use.
Ribavirin: May increase risk of severe pancytopenia and azathioprine-related myelotoxicity. Monitor CBC, including platelet count.
Sulfamethoxazole–trimethoprim and other drugs that interfere with myelopoiesis: May cause severe leukopenia, especially in patients with renal transplants. Use together cautiously.
Tacrolimus (topical): May increase risk of adverse effects of tacrolimus. Avoid use together.
Warfarin: May inhibit warfarin's anticoagulant effect. Monitor patient. Adjust warfarin dosage as needed.
Drug-herb. *Cat's claw, echinacea:* May increase immune function and reduce drug's therapeutic effects. Avoid using together.

EFFECTS ON LAB TEST RESULTS
• May increase ALP, ALT, AST, and bilirubin levels.
• May decrease Hb level and platelet, RBC, and WBC counts.

CONTRAINDICATIONS & CAUTIONS
• Contraindicated in patients hypersensitive to drug or its components.
Boxed Warning Long-term immunosuppression with this drug increases risk of neoplasia, including posttransplant lymphoma and hepatosplenic T-cell lymphoma in patients with inflammatory bowel disease. Prescribers using this drug should be very familiar with its risks, the mutagenic potential to both men and women, and possible hematologic toxicities. ■
▧ Patients with intermediate TPMT activity may be at increased risk for myelotoxicity if receiving conventional doses of drug. Patients with low or absent TPMT or NUDT15 activity are at increased risk for developing severe, life-threatening myelotoxicity if receiving

conventional doses of azathioprine. TPMT genotyping or phenotyping and NUDT15 genotyping can help identify patients who are at increased risk for developing azathioprine toxicity.
• Use cautiously in patients with hepatic or renal dysfunction.
• Benefits must be weighed against risk when giving to patient with systemic viral infection, such as chickenpox or herpes zoster.
• Rare but life-threatening hepatic veno-occlusive disease has been reported in patients with transplants. If this is suspected, permanently discontinue drug.
• Patients with RA previously treated with alkylating drugs, such as cyclophosphamide, chlorambucil, or melphalan, may be at increased risk for tumor development if treated with this drug. Use together is contraindicated.
Dialyzable drug: 45% in an 8-hour dialysis session.
▲ *Overdose S&S:* Nausea, vomiting, diarrhea, abnormal liver function, leukopenia.

PREGNANCY-LACTATION-REPRODUCTION
• There are no adequate and well-controlled studies during pregnancy Drug can cause fetal harm. Avoid use during pregnancy when possible. Don't use to treat RA during pregnancy. Patients of childbearing potential should avoid becoming pregnant.
• Drug appears in human milk. Avoid use during breastfeeding.

NURSING CONSIDERATIONS
• Use appropriate precautions for receiving, handling, storing, preparing, dispensing, transporting, administering, and disposing of drug. Follow NIOSH and USP 800 recommendations and facility policies and procedures for containment strategy.
▧ Consider genotype or phenotype testing for TPMT and genotype testing for NUDT15. Patients with low or absent levels are at greater risk for the hematologic effects of and severe bone marrow toxicity from azathioprine therapy.
• To prevent bleeding, avoid all IM injections when platelet count falls below 100,000/mm³.
• Monitor CBC and platelet counts weekly for 1 month, twice monthly for 2 months, then monthly unless more frequent monitoring is clinically indicated. Also monitor counts at dosage changes. Notify prescriber if counts drop suddenly or become dangerously low. Drug may need to be temporarily withheld.

• Watch for early signs and symptoms of hepatotoxicity (such as clay-colored stools, dark urine, pruritus, and yellow skin and sclera) and monitor patient periodically for increased ALP, bilirubin, AST, and ALT levels.

• Monitor patient for bacterial, viral, fungal, protozoal, and opportunistic infections, including reactivation of latent infections such as TB.

• Watch for new-onset neurologic symptoms. Patients on immunosuppressive therapy may be at increased risk for JC virus–associated infection resulting in multifocal leukoencephalopathy.

• Aspirin, NSAIDs, and low-dose glucocorticoids may be continued during azathioprine therapy for RA.

• Therapeutic response for RA usually occurs within 8 weeks. Consider patients not improved after 12 weeks refractory to treatment.

• *Look alike–sound alike:* Don't confuse azathioprine with Azulfidine. Don't confuse Imuran with Inderal.

PATIENT TEACHING

Boxed Warning Warn patient of the risk of malignancy. ▮

• Warn patient to report even mild infections (colds, fever, sore throat, malaise), because drug is a potent immunosuppressant.

• Warn patient that some hair thinning is possible.

• Tell patient taking drug for refractory RA that it may take up to 12 weeks to be effective.

• Advise patient to report unusual bleeding or bruising.

• Instruct patient in safe drug administration and handling.

• Advise patient to use soft toothbrush and perform oral care cautiously.

azelastine hydrochloride
a-ZEL-as-teen

Astepro Allergy ◇

Therapeutic class: Antihistamines
Pharmacologic class: H$_1$-receptor antagonists

AVAILABLE FORMS
Intranasal: 0.1%, 0.15% ◇
Ophthalmic solution: 0.05%

INDICATIONS & DOSAGES
➤ **Pruritus from allergic conjunctivitis**
Adults and children age 3 and older: Instill 1 drop into affected eye b.i.d.
➤ **Perennial allergic rhinitis**
Adults and children age 12 and older: Instill 2 sprays (0.15%) per nostril b.i.d.
Children ages 6 to 11: Instill 1 spray (0.1% or 0.15%) per nostril b.i.d.
Children age 6 months to 5 years: Instill 1 spray (0.1%) per nostril b.i.d.
➤ **Seasonal allergic rhinitis**
Adults and children age 12 and older: Instill 1 to 2 sprays (0.1% or 0.15%) per nostril b.i.d. or 2 sprays (0.15%) per nostril once daily.
Children ages 6 to 11: Instill 1 spray (0.15%) per nostril b.i.d.
Children ages 5 to 11: Instill 1 spray (0.1%) per nostril b.i.d.
➤ **Vasomotor rhinitis**
Adults and adolescents age 12 and older: Instill 2 sprays (0.1%) per nostril b.i.d.

ADMINISTRATION
Ophthalmic
• Keep bottle tightly closed when not in use.
• Don't touch tip of dropper to any surface.
Intranasal
• Before initial use of nasal spray, prime the delivery system with 4 sprays (0.1%) or 6 sprays (0.15%), or until a fine mist appears.
• Tilting head downward while spraying will help avoid bitter taste.
• If 3 or more days have elapsed since last use, reprime the delivery system with 2 sprays or until a fine mist appears.
• After each use, wipe spray tip with a clean tissue or cloth.
🔊 *Alert:* Be aware of different concentrations of nasal spray as some aren't indicated for use in all indications or certain age-groups.

ACTION
Inhibits the release of histamine and other mediators from cells involved in the allergic response.

Route	Onset	Peak	Duration
Ophthalmic	3 min	Unknown	8 hr
Intranasal	Unknown	2–4 hr	Unknown

Half-life: 22 to 25 hours.

ADVERSE REACTIONS
CNS: anxiety, depression, dizziness, drowsiness, headache, fatigue, malaise, nervousness,

---

sleep disorder, vertigo, dysesthesia, fever. **CV:** flushing, HTN, tachycardia. **EENT:** transient eye burning or stinging, conjunctivitis, eye pain, temporary blurring, otitis media, epistaxis, nasal discomfort, nasal congestion, nasal mucosa ulcer, postnasal drip, rhinitis, pharyngitis, pharyngolaryngeal pain, sinusitis, dry mouth, sneezing, bitter taste. **GI:** abdominal pain, constipation, diarrhea, nausea, vomiting, gastroenteritis, increased appetite. **GU:** hematuria, increased urinary frequency. **Metabolic:** weight gain. **Musculoskeletal:** myalgia. **Respiratory:** *asthma, bronchospasm,* dyspnea, cough, URI. **Skin:** pruritus, contact dermatitis. **Other:** flulike syndrome, cold symptoms.

INTERACTIONS
Drug-drug. *Cimetidine:* May increase azelastine plasma concentration. Avoid use together. *CNS depressants:* May enhance CNS depressant effect of azelastine. Avoid combination. **Drug-lifestyle.** *Alcohol use:* May increase CNS depressant effect of azelastine. Avoid use together.

EFFECTS ON LAB TEST RESULTS
None reported.

CONTRAINDICATIONS & CAUTIONS
• Contraindicated in patients hypersensitive to drug or its components.
Dialyzable drug: Unknown.

PREGNANCY-LACTATION-REPRODUCTION
• Use cautiously during pregnancy and only if potential benefit justifies fetal risk.
• It isn't known if drug appears in human milk. Use cautiously during breastfeeding.

NURSING CONSIDERATIONS
• Drug is for ophthalmic or intranasal use only. Don't inject or give orally.
• Don't use ophthalmic form for irritation caused by contact lenses.

PATIENT TEACHING
• Instruct patient not to touch any surface, eyelid, or surrounding areas with tip of eye dropper.
• Tell patient to keep bottle tightly closed when not in use.
• Advise patient not to wear contact lens if eye is red.

• Warn patient that soft contact lenses may absorb the preservative benzalkonium.
• Instruct patient who wears soft contact lenses and whose eyes aren't red to wait at least 10 minutes after instilling drug before inserting contact lenses.
• Tell patient to report all adverse reactions and to immediately report shortness of breath or severe nose irritation if taking intranasal form.
• Because drug may cause CNS depression, advise patient using intranasal form to avoid hazardous activities requiring complete mental alertness, such as driving or operating machinery.
• Advise patient and caregivers that different concentrations of nasal spray exist and may not be indicated for use in certain conditions or age-groups.

azelastine hydrochloride–fluticasone propionate
a-ZEL-as-teen/floo-TIK-a-sone

Dymista

Therapeutic class: Antihistamines–corticosteroids
Pharmacologic class: H_1-receptor antagonists–corticosteroids

AVAILABLE FORMS
Nasal spray: 137 mcg azelastine hydrochloride and 50 mcg fluticasone propionate/spray

INDICATIONS & DOSAGES
➤ **Symptoms of seasonal allergic rhinitis**
Adults and children age 6 and older: 1 spray/nostril b.i.d.

ADMINISTRATION
Intranasal
• Shake gently before each use.
• Prime the spray before initial use; spray six times or until a fine mist appears. If the spray hasn't been used within the past 14 days, prime the spray again with 1 spray or until a fine mist appears.
• Store upright at room temperature with dust cap in place. Don't freeze or refrigerate.
• Protect from light.

ACTION

Azelastine inhibits release of histamine and other mediators from cells involved in the allergic response. Fluticasone may decrease inflammation by inhibiting mast cells, macrophages, and mediators such as leukotrienes.

Route	Onset	Peak	Duration
Intranasal	Rapid	0.5 hr (azelastine), 1 hr (fluticasone)	Unknown

Half-life: Azelastine, 25 hours; fluticasone, 7.8 hours.

ADVERSE REACTIONS

CNS: headache, fever, dysgeusia, pain.
EENT: epistaxis, nasal congestion, rhinitis, pharyngitis, oropharyngeal pain, otitis media, otitis externa. **GI:** diarrhea, nausea, vomiting, upper abdominal pain. **Respiratory:** cough, URI. **Skin:** urticaria. **Other:** viral infection.

INTERACTIONS

Drug-drug. *CNS depressants:* May increase risk of drowsiness. Use together cautiously.
CYP3A4 inhibitors (fluconazole, ketoconazole): May increase fluticasone plasma level. Use together cautiously.
Desmopressin: Fluticasone may enhance hyponatremic effect of desmopressin. Avoid concurrent use.
Ritonavir: May increase fluticasone plasma level and risk of systemic corticosteroid effects, including Cushing syndrome and adrenal suppression. Avoid use together.
Drug-lifestyle. *Alcohol use:* May increase risk of somnolence and CNS impairment. Discourage use together.

EFFECTS ON LAB TEST RESULTS

None reported.

CONTRAINDICATIONS & CAUTIONS

• Contraindicated in patients hypersensitive to either drug or its components.
• Avoid use in patients with current nasal ulcers, nasal trauma, or nasal surgery until healing occurs.
• Use cautiously in patients with glaucoma, cataracts, ongoing infection, immunosuppression, or history of adrenal suppression.
• Safety and effectiveness in children younger than age 6 haven't been established.
Dialyzable drug: Unknown.

PREGNANCY-LACTATION-REPRODUCTION

• Use cautiously during pregnancy or breast-feeding and only if benefits outweigh risks to the fetus or infant.

NURSING CONSIDERATIONS

• Monitor patient for fungal, bacterial, or viral infections.
• Monitor patient for localized nasopharyngeal *Candida albicans* infection with prolonged use.
• Ensure that patient receives regular eye exams to screen for cataracts and glaucoma with long-term use.
• Monitor growth rate in children using the spray long-term.
• Monitor patient for adrenal insufficiency (tiredness, weakness, nausea, vomiting, hypotension).

PATIENT TEACHING

• Instruct patient to follow full package directions for use.
• Caution patient to avoid spraying into eyes and, if exposure occurs, to flush eyes with water for 10 minutes.
• Warn patient to watch for changes in vision, which can indicate serious eye problems, such as glaucoma or cataracts. Advise patient to have regular eye exams while taking drug.
• Tell patient to watch for nasal problems, such as nosebleeds and nasal septal perforation.
• Advise patient that drug can decrease the body's ability to heal or fight infection. Tell patient to report fever, aches or pains, chills, fatigue, or exposure to chickenpox or measles. Caution patient to avoid exposure to communicable diseases.
• Warn patient that drug can cause drowsiness. Instruct patient to avoid alcohol and other drugs that cause drowsiness while taking this medication.
• Advise patient to avoid driving or tasks that require alertness until drug's effects are known.
• Instruct patient to report pregnancy, plans to become pregnant, or breastfeeding.

Reactions in bold italics are *life-threatening*. Interactions may have a *rapid onset* or a **delayed onset**.

azithromycin
ay-zi-thro-MY-sin

AzaSite, Zithromax🕮

Therapeutic class: Antibiotics
Pharmacologic class: Macrolides

AVAILABLE FORMS
Injection: 500 mg
Ophthalmic solution: 1%
Powder for oral suspension: 100 mg/5 mL,
200 mg/5 mL; 1,000 mg/single-dose packet
Tablets: 250 mg, 500 mg, 600 mg

INDICATIONS & DOSAGES
➤ **Acute bacterial worsening of COPD
caused by *Haemophilus influenzae,
Moraxella catarrhalis,* or *Streptococcus
pneumoniae;* uncomplicated skin and skin-
structure infections caused by *Staphylococcus aureus, Streptococcus pyogenes,* or
Streptococcus agalactiae; second-line therapy for pharyngitis or tonsillitis caused by
*S. pyogenes***
Adults and adolescents age 16 and older: Initially, 500 mg PO as a single dose on day 1,
followed by 250 mg daily on days 2 through
5. Total cumulative dose is 1.5 g. Or, for
worsening COPD, 500 mg PO daily for
3 days.
➤ **Community-acquired pneumonia
caused by *Chlamydophila pneumoniae,
H. influenzae, Mycoplasma pneumoniae,
S. pneumoniae, Legionella pneumophila,
M. catarrhalis,* or *S. aureus***
Adults and adolescents age 16 and older: For
mild infections, give 500 mg PO as a single
dose on day 1; then 250 mg PO daily on days
2 through 5. Total dose is 1.5 g. For more severe infections or those caused by *S. aureus,*
give 500 mg IV as a single daily dose for at
least 2 days; then 500 mg PO as a single daily
dose to complete a 7- to 10-day course of
therapy. Switch from IV to oral therapy based
on patient response.
➤ **Community-acquired pneumonia
caused by *C. pneumoniae, H. influenzae,
M. pneumoniae,* or *S. pneumoniae***
Children age 6 months and older: 10 mg/kg
oral suspension PO (maximum of 500 mg) as
a single dose on day 1, followed by 5 mg/kg
(maximum, 250 mg) daily on days 2 through 5.

➤ **Acute bacterial sinusitis caused by
H. influenzae, M. catarrhalis, or
*S. pneumoniae***
Adults: 500 mg PO daily for 3 days.
Children age 6 months and older: 10 mg/kg
oral suspension PO once daily for 3 days.
Maximum daily dose, 500 mg.
➤ **Chancroid**
Adults: 1 g PO as a single dose.
➤ **Nongonococcal urethritis or cervicitis
caused by *Chlamydia trachomatis***
Adults and adolescents age 16 and older: 1 g
PO as a single dose.
➤ **To prevent disseminated MAC in pa-
tients with advanced HIV infection**
Adults: 1.2 g PO once weekly.
➤ ***MAC* in patients with advanced HIV in-
fection**
Adults: 600 mg PO daily with ethambutol
15 mg/kg daily.
➤ **Urethritis and cervicitis caused by
*Neisseria gonorrhoeae***
Adults: 2 g PO as a single dose.
➤ **Pelvic inflammatory disease caused by
C. trachomatis, N. gonorrhoeae, or *My-
coplasma hominis* in patients who need initial IV therapy**
Adults and adolescents age 16 and older:
500 mg IV as a single daily dose for at least
2 days; then 250 mg PO daily to complete a
7-day course of therapy. Switch from IV to
oral therapy based on patient response.
➤ **Otitis media**
Children older than age 6 months: 30 mg/kg
oral suspension PO as a single dose (maximum dose, 1,500 mg); or 10 mg/kg PO
once daily for 3 days (maximum daily dose,
500 mg); or 10 mg/kg PO on day 1 (maximum dose, 500 mg), then 5 mg/kg once
daily on days 2 to 5 (maximum daily dose,
250 mg).
➤ **Pharyngitis, tonsillitis**
Children age 2 and older: 12 mg/kg oral suspension (maximum, 500 mg) PO daily for
5 days.
➤ **Bacterial conjunctivitis caused by
coryneform group G, *H. influenzae,
Staphylococcus aureus, Streptococcus mitis* group, and *S. pneumoniae***
Adults and children age 1 and older: Instill
1 drop in affected eye(s) b.i.d., 8 to 12 hours
apart for first 2 days; then instill 1 drop in affected eye(s) once daily for next 5 days.
➤ **Cat scratch disease (*Bartonella henselae*
infection) ♦**

Adults and children weighing 45.5 kg or more: 500 mg PO on day 1, then 250 mg PO daily on days 2 to 5.

Children weighing less than 45.5 kg: 10 mg/kg on day 1, then 5 mg/kg PO daily on days 2 to 5.

➤ **Severe cholera ♦**
Adults: 1 g PO as a single dose.

➤ **COPD, prevention of exacerbations ♦**
Adults: 250 to 500 mg PO three times/week or 250 mg PO once daily.

➤ **Cystic fibrosis to improve lung function and reduce exacerbations ♦**
Adults and children age 6 and older: 500 mg PO for patients weighing 40 kg or more or 250 mg PO for patients weighing less than 40 kg three times/week or 250 mg PO once daily. Screen patients before treatment; don't give to those who test positive for nontuberculous mycobacterial infection.

ADMINISTRATION
PO
• Obtain specimen for culture and sensitivity tests before giving first dose. Begin therapy while awaiting results.
• Reconstitute suspension packet with 2 oz (60 mL) of water. After patient has taken dose, rinse glass with additional 2 oz of water and have patient drink it to ensure entire dose has been taken. Packets aren't for children.
• Reconstitute oral suspension by adding 9 mL of water to the 300-mg and 600-mg bottles, 12 mL of water to the 900-mg bottle, and 15 mL to the 1,200-mg bottle. Shake well after each use. Store at 41° to 86° F (5° to 30° C) for up to 10 days.

IV
▼ Reconstitute drug in 500-mg vial with 4.8 mL of sterile water for injection to yield 100 mg/mL.
▼ Shake well until all drug is dissolved.
▼ Further dilute in 250- or 500-mL NSS solution, half-NSS, D_5W, or lactated Ringer solution to yield a final concentration of 1 or 2 mg/mL, respectively.
▼ Infuse a 250-mL infusion (2-mg/mL dose) over 1 hour or 500-mL infusion (1-mg/mL dose) over 3 hours. Never give it as a bolus or IM injection.
▼ Reconstituted solution and diluted solution are stable for 24 hours when stored below 86° F (30° C). Diluted solution is stable for 7 days when refrigerated at 41° F (5° C).

▼ **Incompatibilities:** Amikacin sulfate, aztreonam, cefotaxime, ceftazidime, ceftriaxone sodium, cefuroxime, ciprofloxacin, clindamycin phosphate, famotidine, fentanyl citrate, furosemide, gentamicin sulfate, imipenem–cilastatin sodium, ketorolac tromethamine, levofloxacin, morphine sulfate, piperacillin–tazobactam sodium, potassium chloride, tobramycin sulfate. Consult a compatibility reference for additional information.

Ophthalmic
• Avoid contaminating applicator tip. Don't allow it to touch eye, fingers, or other surfaces.
• Invert closed bottle and shake once before each use. Remove cap with bottle still in the inverted position. Tilt head back, and with bottle inverted, gently squeeze bottle to instill 1 drop into affected eye(s).
• Store unopened bottle under refrigeration at 36° to 46° F (2° to 8° C). Once bottle has been opened, store at 36° to 77° F (2° to 25° C) for up to 14 days. Discard after 14 days.

ACTION
Binds to the 50S subunit of bacterial ribosomes, blocking protein synthesis; bacteriostatic or bactericidal, depending on concentration.

Route	Onset	Peak	Duration
PO	Unknown	2–5 hr	Unknown
IV, ophthalmic	Unknown	Unknown	Unknown

Half-life: About 3 days.

ADVERSE REACTIONS
CNS: fatigue, headache, somnolence, dizziness, dysgeusia, fever. **CV:** chest pain, palpitations, edema. **EENT:** eye irritation (ophthalmic), oral candidiasis. **GI:** abdominal pain, anorexia, diarrhea, constipation, nausea, vomiting, stomatitis, dyspepsia, enteritis, gastritis, flatulence, melena. **GU:** candidiasis, nephritis, vaginitis. **Hepatic:** cholestatic jaundice. **Metabolic:** increased LDH level. **Respiratory:** *bronchospasm,* cough, pleural effusion. **Skin:** photosensitivity reactions, rash, injection-site reaction, diaphoresis, eczema, dermatitis, pruritus. **Other:** *angioedema,* fungal infection.

Reactions in bold italics are *life-threatening.* Interactions may have a *rapid onset* or a ***delayed onset.***

INTERACTIONS

Drug-drug. *Antacids containing aluminum and magnesium:* May lower peak azithromycin level (immediate-release form). Separate doses by at least 2 hours.

Antiarrhythmics (amiodarone, quinidine): May increase risk of life-threatening arrhythmias, including torsades de pointes. Monitor ECG rhythm carefully.

Carbamazepine, phenytoin: May increase levels of these drugs. Monitor drug levels.

Cyclosporine: May elevate cyclosporine concentrations, with increased risk of nephrotoxicity and neurotoxicity. Monitor cyclosporine levels and renal function.

Digoxin: May increase digoxin level. Monitor digoxin level.

Drugs that prolong QT interval (fluoroquinolones, lithium, methadone, paliperidone, perflutren): May prolong QT interval. Use together with caution and monitor patient.

Ergotamine: May cause acute ergotamine toxicity. Monitor patient closely.

HMG-CoA reductase inhibitors (atorvastatin, lovastatin): May increase HMG-CoA reductase inhibitor levels, resulting in severe myopathy or rhabdomyolysis. Consider alternative therapy.

Nelfinavir: May increase azithromycin level. Monitor for liver enzyme abnormalities and hearing impairment.

Pimozide: May prolong QT interval and cause ventricular tachycardia. Concurrent use is contraindicated.

Warfarin: May increase INR. Monitor INR carefully.

Drug-lifestyle. *Sun exposure:* May cause photosensitivity reactions. Advise patient to avoid excessive sunlight exposure.

EFFECTS ON LAB TEST RESULTS

• May increase ALT, AST, creatinine, LDH, CK, and bilirubin levels.

CONTRAINDICATIONS & CAUTIONS

• Contraindicated in patients hypersensitive to azithromycin, erythromycin, or other macrolide or ketolide antibiotics and in those with history of cholestatic jaundice or hepatic dysfunction from prior use of azithromycin.

• Serious cases of allergic reactions, including angioedema, anaphylaxis, SJS, TEN, and DRESS syndrome have been reported, some with fatalities. Prolonged observation and symptomatic treatment may be necessary.

• Infantile hypertrophic pyloric stenosis has been reported after the use of azithromycin in neonates (treatment up to 42 days of life).

• Use cautiously in patients with impaired hepatic function or myasthenia gravis.

• The National Institutes of Health (NIH) and Infectious Diseases Society of America COVID-19 guidelines recommend against the use of azithromycin (in combination with hydroxychloroquine or chloroquine) for the treatment of COVID-19, except in the setting of a clinical trial.

🔷 *Alert:* Use cautiously in patients at increased risk for torsades de pointes and fatal arrhythmias, including those with known prolonged QT interval, history of torsades de pointes, congenital long QT syndrome, bradyarrhythmias, uncompensated HF, uncorrected hypokalemia or hypomagnesemia, clinically significant bradycardia, or concomitant use of drugs known to prolong the QT interval or class IA (procainamide, quinidine) or class III (amiodarone, dofetilide, sotalol) antiarrhythmics.

🔷 *Alert:* Older adults may be at increased risk for drug-associated QT-interval effects.

• Drug may cause CDAD ranging in severity from mild diarrhea to fatal colitis, which may occur more than 2 months after administration. If CDAD is suspected or confirmed, drug may need to be discontinued and appropriate treatment begun.

• Prolonged use of ophthalmic solution may result in overgrowth of nonsusceptible organisms, including fungi. If superinfection occurs, discontinue drug and institute alternative therapy.

Dialyzable drug: Unknown.

PREGNANCY-LACTATION-REPRODUCTION

• There are no adequate and well-controlled studies during pregnancy. Use during pregnancy only if clearly needed.

• Drug appears in human milk. Use cautiously during breastfeeding.

NURSING CONSIDERATIONS

• Monitor patient for superinfection. Drug may cause overgrowth of nonsusceptible bacteria or fungi.

🔷 *Alert:* Monitor patient for CDAD, which may range in severity from mild diarrhea to fatal colitis.

۞ *Alert:* Consider full risk profile when choosing appropriate antibiotic therapy. Alternative macrolide or fluoroquinolone class drugs also have the potential to cause QT-interval prolongation and other significant adverse effects.

• Monitor patient for allergic and skin reactions. Discontinue drug if reactions occur. Be aware that allergic symptoms may recur when symptomatic therapy is discontinued; patient may require prolonged monitoring and treatment.

• Monitor patient for jaundice, hepatotoxicity, and hepatitis. Discontinue drug immediately if signs and symptoms (yellowing of skin or sclera, abdominal pain, nausea, vomiting, dark urine) occur.

• Exacerbation and new onset of myasthenia gravis have occurred with azithromycin use. Monitor patient for neurologic changes.

PATIENT TEACHING
• Tell patient to take drug as prescribed, even after feeling better.

• Advise patient to avoid excessive sunlight and to wear protective clothing and use sunscreen when outside.

• Tell patient to report adverse reactions promptly.

• Instruct parents and caregivers to contact prescriber if vomiting or irritability with feeding occurs during or after azithromycin use in neonates (treatment up to 42 days of life).

۞ *Alert:* Warn patient to seek immediate medical care for irregular heartbeat, shortness of breath, dizziness, or fainting.

• Tell patient that tablets and suspension can be taken with or without food. Food may reduce GI upset.

• Instruct patient to thoroughly wash hands before instilling ophthalmic solution.

• Tell patient to avoid contaminating ophthalmic applicator tip and not to let tip touch eye, fingers, or other surfaces.

• Instruct patient how to instill ophthalmic solution.

• Advise patient to avoid contact lenses when diagnosed with bacterial conjunctivitis.

aztreonam
AZ-tree-oh-nam

Azactam, Cayston

Therapeutic class: Antibiotics
Pharmacologic class: Monobactams

AVAILABLE FORMS
Inhalation (Cayston): 75-mg ampule
Injection: 500-mg, 1-g, 2-g vials

INDICATIONS & DOSAGES
➤ **UTI; septicemia; infections of lower respiratory tract, skin, and skin structures; intra-abdominal infections, surgical infections, and gynecologic infections caused by susceptible** *Escherichia coli, Klebsiella pneumoniae, Proteus mirabilis, Pseudomonas aeruginosa, Enterobacter cloacae, Klebsiella oxytoca, Citrobacter* **species, and** *Serratia marcescens;* **respiratory infections caused by** *Haemophilus influenzae*
Adults: 500 mg, 1 g, or 2 g IV or IM every 8 to 12 hours. For severe systemic or life-threatening infections, 2 g every 6 to 8 hours. Maximum dose is 8 g daily.
Children ages 9 months and older: 30 mg/kg IV every 6 to 8 hours. Maximum dose is 120 mg/kg/day.
Adjust-a-dose: For adults with CrCl of 10 to 30 mL/minute/1.73 m^2, give 1 to 2 g; then give 50% of the usual dose at usual interval. If CrCl is less than 10 mL/minute/1.73 m^2, give 500 mg to 2 g; then give 25% of the usual dose at usual interval. For serious infections, add ⅛ of the initial dose to maintenance doses after each hemodialysis session.
➤ **To improve respiratory symptoms in patients with** *P. aeruginosa* **infection (Cayston) who have cystic fibrosis**
Adults and children age 7 and older: 75 mg inhalation t.i.d. at least 4 hours apart for 28 days, followed by 28 days off.

ADMINISTRATION
Inhalational
• Patient should use bronchodilator before Cayston administration.

• Give short-acting bronchodilators 15 minutes to 4 hours before each dose of aztreonam or long-acting bronchodilators 30 minutes to 12 hours before each dose.

Reactions in bold italics are *life-threatening*. Interactions may have a *rapid onset* or a **delayed onset**.

- Space doses at least 4 hours apart.
- Treatment order for patients on multiple therapies is bronchodilator, mucolytics, then aztreonam.
- Don't reconstitute until ready to give dose.
- Add one ampule of diluent to one amber glass vial of aztreonam. Replace rubber stopper on vial and gently swirl until contents have completely dissolved. Administer immediately.
- Don't use diluent or reconstituted drug if it's cloudy or if there are particles in the solution.
- Use only Altera Nebulizer System to administer drug.
- Never mix with other drugs in nebulizer.
- Administration usually takes 2 to 3 minutes.

IV

▼ Obtain specimen for culture and sensitivity tests before giving first dose. Begin therapy while awaiting results.

▼ For direct injection, reconstitute with 6 to 10 mL of sterile water for injection and immediately shake vial vigorously. Constituted solutions aren't for multiple-dose use. Discard unused solution.

▼ To give a bolus, inject drug over 3 to 5 minutes, directly into IV tubing.

▼ For infusion, reconstitute with a compatible IV solution to yield 20 mg/mL or less.

▼ Give infusions over 20 minutes to 1 hour.

▼ Give thawed solutions only by IV infusion.

▼ **Incompatibilities:** Acyclovir, amphotericin B, ampicillin sodium, azithromycin, chlorpromazine, daunorubicin hydrochloride, ganciclovir, lorazepam, metronidazole, mitomycin, mitoxantrone, nafcillin, prochlorperazine, streptozocin, vancomycin. Consult a compatibility reference for additional information.

IM

- To prepare IM injection, add at least 3 mL of one of the following solutions per gram of aztreonam: sterile water for injection, bacteriostatic water for injection, NSS, or bacteriostatic NSS.
- Give IM injections deep into a large muscle, such as the upper outer quadrant of the gluteus maximus or the side of the thigh.
- Give doses larger than 1 g by IV route.

③ *Alert:* Don't give IM injection to children.
- Pain and swelling may occur at injection site.

ACTION

Inhibits bacterial cell-wall synthesis, ultimately causing cell-wall destruction; bactericidal.

Route	Onset	Peak	Duration
IV	Unknown	Immediate	Unknown
IM	Unknown	<1 hr	Unknown
Inhalation	Unknown	1 hr	Unknown

Half-life: 1.5 to 2.1 hours.

ADVERSE REACTIONS

CNS: *seizures,* confusion, headache, insomnia, fever. **CV:** hypotension, phlebitis, thrombophlebitis, chest discomfort. **EENT:** nasal congestion, sore throat. **GI:** *pseudomembranous colitis,* diarrhea, abdominal pain, nausea, vomiting. **GU:** increased creatinine level. **Hematologic:** *neutropenia, pancytopenia, thrombocytopenia,* eosinophilia, anemia, leukocytosis, thrombocytosis. **Hepatic:** increased transaminase levels. **Respiratory:** bronchospasm, cough, wheezing. **Skin:** discomfort and swelling at IM injection site, rash, erythema multiforme. **Other:** hypersensitivity reactions.

INTERACTIONS

Drug-drug. *Aminoglycosides:* May have synergistic nephrotoxic effects. Monitor renal function.
Cefoxitin, imipenem: May have antagonistic effect. Avoid using together.

EFFECTS ON LAB TEST RESULTS

- May increase ALT, AST, BUN, creatinine, and LDH levels.
- May decrease Hb level and neutrophil and RBC counts.
- May increase or decrease platelet and WBC counts.
- May prolong PT and PTT and increase INR.
- May cause false-positive Coombs test result. May alter urine glucose determinations using cupric sulfate (Clinitest or Benedict reagent).

CONTRAINDICATIONS & CAUTIONS
• Contraindicated in patients hypersensitive to drug or its components.
⊘ Alert: Use cautiously in patients with hypersensitivity to other beta-lactam antibiotics (penicillins, cephalosporins, carbapenems).
• Use cautiously in older adults and in patients with impaired renal or hepatic function. Dosage adjustment may be needed. Monitor renal function test results.
• Drug may cause CDAD ranging in severity from mild diarrhea to fatal colitis occurring up to 2 months after administration. If CDAD is suspected or confirmed, drug may need to be discontinued and appropriate treatment begun.
• Rare cases of TEN have been reported in patients undergoing bone marrow transplant with multiple risk factors, including sepsis, radiation therapy, and concomitantly administered drugs associated with TEN.
Dialyzable drug: Yes.

PREGNANCY-LACTATION-REPRODUCTION
• Drug crosses the placental barrier. There are no adequate and well-controlled studies during pregnancy. Use during pregnancy only if clearly needed.
• Drug appears in human milk. Patient should temporarily discontinue breastfeeding.

NURSING CONSIDERATIONS
• Observe patient for signs and symptoms of superinfection.
⊘ Alert: Because drug is ineffective against gram-positive and anaerobic organisms, combine it with other antibiotics for immediate treatment of life-threatening illnesses.
• Monitor patient for hypersensitivity reactions
• Antibiotics may promote overgrowth of nonsusceptible organisms. Monitor patient for signs of superinfection.

PATIENT TEACHING
• Warn patient receiving IM drug that pain and swelling may occur at injection site.
• Tell patient to report discomfort at IV insertion site.
• Instruct patient to report adverse reactions and signs and symptoms of superinfection promptly.
• Instruct patient or caregiver in proper administration of drug by nebulizer.
• Teach patient or caregiver to use bronchodilator before using Cayston.

baclofen
BAK-loe-fen

Fleqsuvy, Gablofen, Lioresal
Intrathecal, Lyvispah, Ozobax

Therapeutic class: Skeletal muscle relaxants
Pharmacologic class: Gamma-aminobutyric acid derivatives

AVAILABLE FORMS
Intrathecal injection: 50 mcg/mL, 500 mcg/mL, 1,000 mcg/mL, 2,000 mcg/mL
Oral granules: 5-mg, 10-mg, 20-mg packets
Oral solution: 5 mg/5 mL, 25 mg/5 mL
Tablets: 5 mg, 10 mg, 20 mg

INDICATIONS & DOSAGES
Adjust-a-dose (for all indications): For patients with impaired renal function, decrease oral and intrathecal doses.
➤ **Spasticity in MS; spinal cord injury**
Adults and children age 12 and older: Initially, 5 mg PO t.i.d. for 3 days; then 10 mg t.i.d. for 3 days, 15 mg t.i.d. for 3 days, 20 mg t.i.d. for 3 days. Increase daily dosage, based on response, to maximum of 80 mg (given as 20 mg q.i.d.).
Adjust-a-dose: For older adults and patients with psychiatric or brain disorders, increase dose gradually.
➤ **To manage severe spasticity in patients who don't respond to or can't tolerate oral baclofen therapy**
Adults: For screening phase, after test dose to check responsiveness, give drug via implantable infusion pump. Give test dose of 1 mL of 50 mcg/mL dilution into intrathecal space by barbotage over 1 minute or longer. Significantly decreased severity or frequency of muscle spasm or reduced muscle tone should appear within 4 to 8 hours. If response is inadequate, give second test dose of 75 mcg/1.5 mL 24 hours after the first. If response is still inadequate, give final test dose of 100 mcg/2 mL after 24 hours. Patients unresponsive to the 100-mcg dose shouldn't be considered candidates for implantable pump.
Children age 4 and older: Initial test dose is the same as that for adults (50 mcg); for very small children, initial dose is 25 mcg.
For maintenance therapy: Adjust first dose based on screening dose that elicited an adequate response. Double this effective dose

and give over 24 hours. However, if screening dose effectiveness was maintained for 8 hours or longer, don't double dose. After first 24 hours, increase dose slowly as needed and tolerated by 10% to 30% increments at 24-hour intervals in spasticity of spinal cord origin. In children with spasticity of spinal cord origin and adults and children with spasticity of cerebral origin, increase by 5% to 15% increments at 24-hour intervals. During prolonged maintenance therapy, increase daily dose by 10% to 40% in spasticity of spinal cord origin, or increase daily dose by 5% to 20% in spasticity of cerebral origin, if needed; if patient experiences adverse effects, decrease dose by 10% to 20%. Maintenance dosages range from 12 to 2,003 mcg daily based on diagnosis, but experience with dosages of more than 1,000 mcg daily is limited. Most patients need 300 to 800 mcg daily for spasticity of spinal cord origin and 90 to 703 mcg daily for spasticity of cerebral origin.

ADMINISTRATION
PO
• Give drug with meals or milk to prevent GI distress.
• May give granules without water by emptying packet into the mouth and allowing to dissolve. Or, mix with 15 mL of liquid or soft food (applesauce, yogurt, pudding) and give within 2 hours. If giving multiple packets, mix each packet with a separate volume of liquid or soft food.
• May give granules through an 8F or larger feeding tube after mixing well with 15 mL of liquid; flush tube before and after giving. Give within 2 hours of mixing suspension and remix if suspension left standing for more than 15 minutes.
• Shake oral suspensions well.
• Discard unused oral solution 2 months after first opening bottle.
• Use calibrated measuring device to deliver prescribed dose of solution.
Intrathecal
Boxed Warning Don't discontinue abruptly. This can result in high fever, altered mental status, exaggerated rebound spasticity, and muscle rigidity, which in rare cases, has led to rhabdomyolysis, multiple organ-system failure, and death. ∎
• Don't give intrathecal injection by IV, IM, subcut, or epidural route.

• Maintenance infusions that require dilution must be diluted with sterile preservative-free sodium chloride for injection.
• If patient suddenly requires a large intrathecal dose increase, check for a catheter complication, such as kinking or dislodgment.
• With long-term intrathecal use, about 5% of patients may develop tolerance to drug. In some cases, this may be treated by hospitalizing patient and slowly withdrawing drug over a 2- to 4-week period. After the "drug holiday," drug may be restarted at the initial continuous infusion dose.

ACTION
Hyperpolarizes fibers to reduce impulse transmission. Appears to reduce transmission of impulses from the spinal cord to skeletal muscle, thus decreasing the frequency and amplitude of muscle spasms in patients with spinal cord lesions.

Route	Onset	Peak	Duration
PO	Unknown	30 min– 4 hr	Unknown
Intrathecal	30 min–1 hr	4 hr	4–8 hr

Half-life: Oral, children with cerebral palsy, 4.5 hours; adults, 2.75 to 5.7 hours. Intrathecal, 1.5 hours over first 4 hours.

ADVERSE REACTIONS
CNS: agitation, drowsiness, dizziness, headache, weakness, fatigue, hypotonia, tremor, confusion, insomnia, *seizures with intrathecal use,* paresthesia, asthenia, pain, speech disorder, depression, *coma.* **CV:** hypotension, peripheral edema. **EENT:** amblyopia, nasal congestion, dry mouth, excessive salivation. **GI:** nausea, constipation, diarrhea, vomiting. **GU:** urinary frequency, urine retention, erectile dysfunction, incontinence. **Metabolic:** hyperglycemia, weight gain. **Musculoskeletal:** muscle rigidity or spasticity, muscle weakness, back pain. **Respiratory:** dyspnea, hypoventilation, pneumonia. **Skin:** rash, pruritus, urticaria, diaphoresis. **Other:** chills, accidental injury.

INTERACTIONS
Drug-drug. *CNS depressants:* May increase CNS depression. Avoid using together.
Boxed Warning *Opioid class warning:* May cause slow or difficult breathing, sedation, and death. Avoid use together. If use together is necessary, limit dosage and duration of

each drug to minimum necessary for desired effect. ∎

Drug-lifestyle. *Alcohol use:* May increase CNS depression. Discourage use together.

EFFECTS ON LAB TEST RESULTS

• May increase ALP, AST, CK, and glucose levels.
• May increase leukocyte count.

CONTRAINDICATIONS & CAUTIONS

• Contraindicated in patients hypersensitive to drug.
• Use cautiously in patients with impaired renal function, respiratory disease, or seizure disorder or when spasticity is used to maintain motor function.
• Use cautiously in patients with psychotic disorders, schizophrenia, confusional states, or autonomic dysreflexia. Exacerbations of these conditions have occurred.
• Use cautiously in patients who have had a stroke; drug is poorly tolerated and not significantly beneficial.

Boxed Warning Opioids should only be prescribed with benzodiazepines or other CNS depressants to patients for whom alternative treatment options are inadequate. ∎

• Safety and effectiveness in children younger than age 4 (intrathecal use) and age 12 (oral use) haven't been established.

Dialyzable drug: Yes.

⚠ **Overdose S&S:** Coma, dizziness, light-headedness, diminished reflexes, vomiting, hypotonia, increased salivation, drowsiness, vision changes, respiratory depression, seizures.

PREGNANCY-LACTATION-REPRODUCTION

• Use during pregnancy only when potential benefits justify fetal risk.
• Drug may increase risk of late-onset neonatal withdrawal symptoms.
• Oral drug appears in human milk. It isn't known if drug appears in human milk after intrathecal administration. Patient should avoid breastfeeding during therapy unless potential benefit justifies risk to the infant. Withdrawal symptoms can occur in infants when breastfeeding is stopped.

NURSING CONSIDERATIONS

🕒 **Alert:** Don't use oral drug to treat muscle spasm caused by rheumatic disorders, cerebral palsy, Parkinson disease, or stroke

because drug's effectiveness for these indications hasn't been established.
• Life-threatening CNS depression, CV collapse, and respiratory failure may occur with intrathecal use. Have trained staff and resuscitation equipment available during screening, dosage titration, and pump refill.
• Avoid contamination of sterile surfaces through contact with the nonsterile exterior of the Gablofen prefilled syringe while refilling implantable intrathecal pumps. Use of the prefilled syringe in an aseptic setting (e.g., operating room) to fill sterile intrathecal pumps before implantation in patients isn't recommended unless external surface of syringe is treated to ensure sterility.
• Reservoir refilling must be performed by fully trained and qualified personnel following directions provided by the pump manufacturer.

🕒 **Alert:** Use extreme caution when filling an FDA-approved implantable pump equipped with an injection port that allows direct access to the intrathecal catheter. Direct injection into the catheter through the catheter access port may cause a life-threatening overdose.

Boxed Warning Consult the infusion system's technical manual for postimplant information. ∎

• Watch for sensitivity reactions, such as fever, skin eruptions, and respiratory distress.
• Expect an increased risk of seizures in patients with seizure disorder.
• The amount of relief determines whether dosage (and drowsiness) can be reduced.
• Some degree of muscle tone and spasticity may be necessary to sustain upright posture and balance with movement or to obtain optimal function, help support circulatory function, and prevent formation of DVT.
• When switching to intrathecal baclofen, attempt to discontinue concomitant oral antispasmodics to avoid overdose or increased adverse effects. Reduce oral antispasmodic dosage slowly while monitoring patient closely.

Boxed Warning Don't withdraw intrathecal drug abruptly after long-term use unless severe adverse reactions demand it; doing so may precipitate seizures, high fever, hallucinations, or rebound spasticity. ∎

• **Look alike–sound alike:** Don't confuse baclofen with Bactroban.

PATIENT TEACHING

Boxed Warning Advise patient and caregivers, especially patients with spinal cord injuries at T6 or above, communication difficulties, or history of withdrawal symptoms from oral or intrathecal baclofen, of risks associated with abrupt discontinuation of intrathecal form. Tell them to keep scheduled refill visits and teach them the signs and symptoms of baclofen withdrawal. ■

• Instruct patient and caregivers in safe oral drug administration and storage.

Boxed Warning Opioid class warning: Caution patient or caregiver of patient taking an opioid with a benzodiazepine, CNS depressant, or alcohol to seek immediate medical attention for dizziness, light-headedness, extreme sleepiness, slowed or difficult breathing, or unresponsiveness. ■

• Tell patient to avoid activities that require alertness until CNS effects of drug are known. Drowsiness usually is transient.

• Caution patient to avoid alcohol and OTC antihistamines while taking drug.

• Advise patient to follow prescriber's orders regarding rest and physical therapy.

• Instruct patient and caregivers about the signs and symptoms of overdose and what to do if an overdose occurs.

• Teach patient and caregivers proper home care of pump and insertion site.

---

baloxavir marboxil
bal-OX-a-vir mar-BOX-il

Xofluza

Therapeutic class: Antivirals
Pharmacologic class: Endonuclease inhibitors

AVAILABLE FORMS
Oral suspension (granules): 40 mg/20 mL
Tablets: 40 mg, 80 mg

INDICATIONS & DOSAGES
➤ **Acute, uncomplicated influenza in patients who have been symptomatic for no more than 48 hours who are otherwise healthy or at high risk for developing influenza-related complications; postexposure influenza prophylaxis**
Adults and children age 12 and older weighing 80 kg or more: 80 mg PO as a single dose.

Adults and children age 12 and older weighing 40 to less than 80 kg: 40 mg PO as a single dose.

ADMINISTRATION
PO
• Give drug with or without food. Avoid giving with dairy products and calcium-fortified beverages.

• Give drug as soon as possible within 48 hours of symptom onset or after contact with an individual with influenza.

• Oral suspension may be used for oral or enteral administration.

• Oral suspension contains no preservative and must be given within 10 hours after constitution.

• Prepare oral suspension by gently tapping bottom of the bottle to loosen the granules. Add 20 mL of drinking water or sterile water and gently swirl to ensure that the granules are evenly suspended. Don't shake. Write expiration time and date on the bottle label in the space provided.

• Use a measuring device (oral syringe, measuring cup) to deliver the suspension dose.

• For enteral administration (e.g., feeding tube), draw up suspension with an enteral syringe. Flush with 1 mL of water before and after enteral administration.

• The total prescribed oral suspension dose requires two bottles for adults and adolescents weighing at least 80 kg.

• Store drug in original blister card or bottle at 68° to 77° F (20° to 25° C).

ACTION
Inhibits the activity of polymerase acidic protein to halt viral gene transcription.

Route	Onset	Peak	Duration
PO	Unknown	4 hr	Unknown

Half-life: 79.1 hours.

ADVERSE REACTIONS
CNS: headache. **EENT:** sinusitis. **GI:** diarrhea, nausea. **Respiratory:** bronchitis.

INTERACTIONS
Drug-drug. *Live attenuated influenza vaccine:* May decrease effectiveness of the vaccine. Avoid concurrent use.
Polyvalent cation–containing antacids, laxatives, or oral supplements (calcium, iron, magnesium, selenium, zinc): May decrease

---

baloxavir level and effectiveness. Avoid concurrent use.
Drug-food. *Calcium-fortified beverages, dairy products, milk:* May decrease baloxavir concentration and effectiveness. Avoid use together.

EFFECTS ON LAB TEST RESULTS
None reported.

CONTRAINDICATIONS & CAUTIONS
• Contraindicated in patients hypersensitive to drug or its components.
• Serious bacterial infections may begin with influenza-like symptoms or may coexist with or occur as a complication of influenza.
• Safety and effectiveness in children younger than age 12 or weighing less than 40 kg haven't been established.
Dialyzable drug: Unlikely.

PREGNANCY-LACTATION-REPRODUCTION
• No data exist on the use of drug during pregnancy or on developmental risk to a fetus. Due to lack of data, the CDC doesn't recommend use of drug during pregnancy.
• Pregnancy may increase risk of severe complications from influenza, including maternal death, stillbirth, birth defects, preterm delivery, and low-birth-weight and small-for-gestational-age infants.
• It isn't known if drug appears in human milk. Consider the benefits of breastfeeding and the potential adverse effects on the infant before using drug.

NURSING CONSIDERATIONS
• Monitor patient for secondary bacterial infection, which may begin with influenza-like symptoms or coexist with or occur as a complication of influenza, and treat appropriately.

PATIENT TEACHING
• Instruct patient that drug should be taken as soon as possible within 48 hours of onset of symptoms or after contact with an individual with influenza.
• Counsel patient on safe drug administration.
• Inform patient that a pharmacist will mix oral suspension before it's dispensed and to take drug before the expiration time and date written on the bottle label. Caution patient not to take suspension if the expiration time and date have passed.

• Alert patient that the total prescribed dose of oral suspension may require two bottles.
• Tell patient to report all adverse reactions.
• Advise patient to consider postponing receiving live attenuated influenza vaccine while taking drug.

beclomethasone dipropionate (inhalation)
be-kloe-METH-a-sone

QVAR RediHaler

Therapeutic class: Antiasthmatics
Pharmacologic class: Corticosteroids

AVAILABLE FORMS
Oral inhalation aerosol: 40 mcg/metered spray, 80 mcg/metered spray

INDICATIONS & DOSAGES
➤ **Chronic asthma**
Adults and children age 12 and older: Starting dose, 40 to 80 mcg b.i.d. when patient previously used bronchodilators alone, or 40 to 320 mcg b.i.d. when patient previously used inhaled corticosteroids. If patient doesn't respond adequately to initial dosage after 2 weeks, increasing dosage may provide additional asthma control. Maximum, 320 mcg b.i.d.
Children ages 4 to 11: 40 mcg b.i.d. May increase to 80 mcg b.i.d. after 2 weeks if needed. Maximum, 80 mcg b.i.d.

ADMINISTRATION
Inhalational
• No need to prime or shake RediHaler.
• Close the white cap to prepare the inhaler with medicine before each inhalation.
• Instruct patient to hold breath for 5 to 10 seconds to enhance drug action.
• Have patient rinse mouth and spit after use.
• Space doses 12 hours apart.
• Don't shake inhaler with cap open to avoid possible actuation.
• Don't wash or put any part of the inhaler in water; gently wipe mouthpiece with a dry cloth or tissue as needed.
• Don't use with a spacer or volume holding chamber.
• Discard the inhaler when the dose counter displays "0."
• Store drug at room temperature.

Reactions in bold italics are **life-threatening**. Interactions may have a *rapid onset* or a **delayed onset**.

ACTION
May decrease inflammation by decreasing the number and activity of inflammatory cells, inhibiting bronchoconstrictor mechanisms, producing direct smooth-muscle relaxation, and decreasing airway hyperresponsiveness.

Route	Onset	Peak	Duration
Inhalation	1–4 wk	0.5 hr	Unknown

Half-life: 4 hours.

ADVERSE REACTIONS
CNS: headache, pain, fever. **EENT:** ear infection, nasopharyngitis, pharyngitis, allergic rhinitis, sinusitis, oral candidiasis, oropharyngeal pain, dry mouth. **GI:** nausea, vomiting, diarrhea, viral gastroenteritis. **Musculoskeletal:** back pain, myalgia. **Respiratory:** cough, URI, viral URI, exacerbation of asthma, wheezing. **Other:** flulike symptoms, hypersensitivity reactions.

INTERACTIONS
None reported by manufacturer.

EFFECTS ON LAB TEST RESULTS
None reported.

CONTRAINDICATIONS & CAUTIONS
• Contraindicated in patients hypersensitive to drug or its ingredients and in those with status asthmaticus, nonasthmatic bronchial diseases, or asthma controlled by bronchodilators or other noncorticosteroids alone.
• Use cautiously, if at all, in patients with TB, ocular HSV, or untreated systemic fungal, bacterial, parasitic, or viral infections.
• Use cautiously in patients receiving systemic corticosteroid therapy.
• Safety and effectiveness in children younger than age 4 haven't been established.
Dialyzable drug: No.

PREGNANCY-LACTATION-REPRODUCTION
• Use during pregnancy only when potential benefits justify fetal risk.
• After delivery, evaluate neonates for adrenal suppression if mother received substantial doses during pregnancy.
• Serious adverse reactions may occur in breastfeeding infants. A decision should be made to discontinue breastfeeding or discontinue drug, taking into account importance of drug to the mother.

NURSING CONSIDERATIONS
• Check oral mucous membranes frequently for signs and symptoms of fungal infection.
• During times of stress (trauma, surgery, infection), systemic corticosteroids may be needed to prevent adrenal insufficiency in patients who have been corticosteroid-dependent.
• Periodic measurement of growth and development may be needed during high-dose or prolonged therapy in children.
• Cataracts and decreases in bone mineral density can occur with long-term use. Closely monitor patients for vision changes and for decreased bone mineral content, especially patients with major risk factors.
⚠ *Alert:* Taper oral corticosteroid therapy slowly. Acute adrenal insufficiency and death may occur in patients with asthma who change abruptly from oral corticosteroids to beclomethasone.
⚠ *Alert:* Bronchospasm may occur after dosing; discontinue drug and treat immediately with a short-acting inhaled bronchodilator.
• Monitor patient for hypersensitivity reactions (urticaria, angioedema, rash, bronchospasm) and infections.

PATIENT TEACHING
• Teach patient or caregiver safe drug administration and care of inhaler.
• Inform patient that drug doesn't relieve acute asthma attacks.
• Tell patient who needs a bronchodilator to use it several minutes before beclomethasone.
• Instruct patient who hasn't had chickenpox or measles or been properly immunized to use particular care to avoid exposure.
• Instruct patient to carry or wear medical identification indicating patient's need for supplemental systemic corticosteroids during stress.
• Tell patient it may take up to 4 weeks to feel the full benefit of the drug.
• Advise patient to prevent oral fungal infections by gargling or rinsing mouth with water after each use. Caution patient not to swallow the water.
• Tell patient to report evidence of corticosteroid withdrawal, including fatigue, weakness, arthralgia, orthostatic hypotension, and dyspnea.

---

beclomethasone dipropionate (intranasal)
be-kloe-METH-a-sone

Beconase AQ, Qnasl, Rivanase AQ✤

Therapeutic class: Corticosteroids
Pharmacologic class: Corticosteroids

AVAILABLE FORMS
Nasal aerosol solution (Qnasl): 40 mcg/actuation, 80 mcg/actuation
Nasal spray (Beconase AQ): 42 mcg/metered spray

INDICATIONS & DOSAGES
➤ **To relieve symptoms of seasonal or perennial allergic and nonallergic (vaso-motor) rhinitis; to prevent nasal polyp recurrence after surgical removal (Beconase AQ)**
Adults and children age 12 and older: 1 or 2 sprays (42 to 84 mcg Beconase AQ) in each nostril b.i.d.
Children ages 6 to 12: Initially, 1 spray (42 mcg) in each nostril b.i.d. May increase to 2 sprays in each nostril b.i.d. Once adequate control is achieved, decrease to 1 spray in each nostril b.i.d. Maximum, 336 mcg daily.
➤ **To relieve symptoms of seasonal or perennial allergic rhinitis (Qnasl)**
Adults and children age 12 and older: 2 sprays (160 mcg total) in each nostril once daily. Maximum, 320 mcg/day.
Children ages 4 to 11: 1 spray (40 mcg) in each nostril once daily. Maximum, 80 mcg/day.

ADMINISTRATION
Intranasal
• Pump nasal spray six times or until a fine mist is produced before first use; repeat priming if nasal spray hasn't been used for 7 days (Beconase AQ). Qnasl doesn't need to be primed.
• Shake Beconase AQ well before use.
• Instruct patient to blow nose to clear nasal passages before use.
• Insert nozzle into nostril, pointing away from septum; patient's head should tilt forward slightly for Beconase AQ. Hold other nostril closed while spraying; patient should hold breath for a few seconds, then exhale through the mouth. Repeat in other nostril.
• After administering, remove Beconase AQ nasal applicator, wash with cold water, dry, and replace protective cap. Wipe Qnasl nasal tip with clean dry tissue or cloth and replace protective cap; keep dry at all times.

ACTION
May reduce nasal inflammation by inhibiting mediators of inflammation.

Route	Onset	Peak	Duration
Intranasal	5–7 days	3 wk	Unknown

Half-life: About 2.8 hours (major active metabolite).

ADVERSE REACTIONS
CNS: headache, light-headedness, fever. **EENT:** mild, transient nasal burning and stinging; dryness, epistaxis, nasal congestion, nasopharyngeal fungal infections, rhinorrhea, sneezing, watery eyes. **GI:** nausea. **Metabolic:** growth velocity reduction in children and adolescents. **Respiratory:** URI.

INTERACTIONS
None reported by manufacturer.

EFFECTS ON LAB TEST RESULTS
None reported.

CONTRAINDICATIONS & CAUTIONS
• Contraindicated in patients hypersensitive to drug or its components.
• Use cautiously, if at all, in patients with active or quiescent respiratory tract tuberculous infections, untreated local or systemic fungal or bacterial infections, systemic viral or parasitic infections, or ocular HSV infections.
• Avoid use in patients who have recently had nasal septal ulcers, nasal surgery, or trauma until wound healing occurs.
• Use cautiously in patients receiving systemic corticosteroid therapy.
• Safety and effectiveness in children younger than age 6 (Beconase AQ) or age 4 (Qnasl) haven't been established.
Dialyzable drug: No.
⚠ *Overdose S&S:* Hypercorticism, adrenal suppression.

PREGNANCY-LACTATION-REPRODUCTION
• Use during pregnancy only when potential benefits justify fetal risk.

Reactions in bold italics are *life-threatening*. Interactions may have a *rapid onset* or a ***delayed onset***.

• After delivery, evaluate neonates for adrenal suppression if mother received substantial doses during pregnancy.
• It isn't known if drug appears in human milk. Use cautiously during breastfeeding.

NURSING CONSIDERATIONS
• Observe patient for infections.
• Drug isn't effective for acute exacerbations of rhinitis. Decongestants or antihistamines may be needed.
• Stop drug if no significant symptom improvement occurs after 3 weeks.
• Monitor growth routinely in children; reduced growth rate may occur.
• Glaucoma and cataracts can occur. Closely monitor patients for vision changes and increased IOP.
• Watch for hypercorticism and adrenal suppression with very high doses, or with standard doses in patients who are susceptible. If signs and symptoms occur, taper and discontinue drug.
• Monitor patient for hypersensitivity reactions (anaphylaxis, angioedema, urticaria, rash).

PATIENT TEACHING
• Advise patient or parent to read package insert for instructions on drug use and canister and applicator care.
• Tell patient not to blow nose for 15 minutes after using Qnasl.
• Advise patient to use drug as prescribed, because its effectiveness depends on regular use.
• Explain that unlike decongestants, drug doesn't work right away. Most patients notice improvement within a few days, but some may need 2 to 3 weeks.
• Warn patient not to exceed recommended dosage because of risk of HPA axis suppression.
• Instruct patient who hasn't had chickenpox or measles or been properly immunized to use particular care to avoid exposure.
• Tell patient to notify prescriber if signs and symptoms don't improve within 3 weeks or if nasal irritation persists.
• Teach patient good nasal and oral hygiene.

belimumab ☒
beh-LIM-oo-mab

Benlysta

Therapeutic class: Immunosuppressants
Pharmacologic class: Human monoclonal antibodies

AVAILABLE FORMS
IV injection: 120 mg, 400 mg in single-use vials
Subcut injection: 200 mg/mL single-dose prefilled autoinjector or prefilled syringe

INDICATIONS & DOSAGES
➤ **Active, autoantibody-positive SLE**
Adults and children age 5 and older:
10 mg/kg IV infusion every 2 weeks for first three doses, then every 4 weeks thereafter.
Adults older than age 18: 200 mg subcut once weekly.
➤ **Active lupus nephritis in patients who are receiving standard therapy**
Adults: 10 mg/kg IV infusion every 2 weeks for first three doses, then every 4 weeks thereafter. Or, 400 mg subcut (two 200-mg injections) once weekly for four doses, then 200 mg once weekly thereafter.

ADMINISTRATION
IV
▼ Consider premedicating with an antihistamine and antipyretic for prophylaxis against infusion or hypersensitivity reactions.
▼ Store unopened vials in refrigerator.
▼ Once vial has been at room temperature for 10 to 15 minutes, reconstitute with sterile water: 1.5 mL for 120-mg vial and 4.8 mL for 400-mg vial.
▼ Direct stream of sterile water toward side of vial to minimize foaming. Gently swirl for 60 seconds every 5 minutes until dissolved. Don't shake. Protect solution from light while dissolving. Usual reconstitution time is 10 to 15 minutes but may take up to 30 minutes.
▼ Solution should be opalescent and colorless to pale yellow. Small air bubbles are expected and acceptable.
▼ Dilute only in NSS, half-NSS, or lactated Ringer solution to a volume of 250 mL.

▼ To dilute, withdraw a volume of fluid equal to amount of medication to be added from a 250-mL infusion bag, so total volume will remain at 250 mL when the medication is added. Add the medication to the 250-mL infusion bag and gently invert to mix the solution. Discard any unused drug solution.

▼ Protect unused reconstituted solution from light and store in refrigerator. Solutions in NSS, half-NSS, or lactated Ringer solution may be stored in refrigerator or at room temperature.

▼ Administer as an IV infusion over 1 hour. Don't give as an IV push or bolus.

▼ Complete infusion within 8 hours of reconstitution.

▼ **Incompatibilities:** Dextrose solution, other IV drugs.

Subcutaneous

• If changing from IV therapy to subcut administration for SLE, give first subcut dose 1 to 4 weeks after last IV dose. If changing from IV therapy for lupus nephritis, give first subcut dose any time after first two IV doses and 1 to 2 weeks after last IV dose.

• Administer by subcut injection in abdomen or thigh.

• Allow at least 5 cm between injections when giving more than one injection at the same site.

• Rotate injection sites weekly; never inject into areas where skin is tender, bruised, red, or hard.

• Remove from refrigerator and allow to sit at room temperature for 30 minutes before use.

• Inspect visually for particulate matter and discoloration before administration; use only if solution appears clear to opalescent and colorless to pale yellow.

• Administer once a week, preferably on the same day each week.

• If a dose is missed, administer injection as soon as possible; then resume schedule or start a new weekly schedule from the day that the missed dose was administered. Don't administer two doses on the same day.

ACTION

B-lymphocyte stimulator-specific inhibitor that inhibits survival of B cells, including autoreactive B cells, and reduces their differentiation into Ig-producing plasma cells.

Route	Onset	Peak	Duration
IV, subcut	Unknown	Unknown	Unknown

Half-life: IV, 19.4 days; subcut, 18.3 days.

ADVERSE REACTIONS

CNS: anxiety, headache, insomnia, migraine, depression, fever. **EENT:** nasopharyngitis, pharyngitis. **GI:** nausea, diarrhea, viral gastroenteritis. **GU:** cystitis, UTI. **Hematologic:** *leukopenia.* **Musculoskeletal:** extremity pain. **Respiratory:** bronchitis, URI. **Skin:** injection-site reactions. **Other:** infection, antibody detection, hypersensitivity reactions, infusion reactions.

INTERACTIONS

Drug-drug. *Biologic agents (including B-cell targeted therapies):* Use together hasn't been studied. Don't use together.

Live-virus vaccines: May impair response to vaccines. Don't give live-virus vaccines for 30 days before or concurrently with belimumab.

Drug-herb. *Echinacea:* May decrease drug's therapeutic effects. Consider therapy modification.

EFFECTS ON LAB TEST RESULTS

• May decrease leukocyte count.

CONTRAINDICATIONS & CAUTIONS

• Contraindicated in patients with a history of anaphylaxis to belimumab.

• Use cautiously in patients with a history of chronic infection, hypersensitivity reactions, infusion reactions, depression, or malignancies.

▧ Use cautiously in patients who are Black because response rate may be lower.

• More deaths occurred with belimumab than with placebo during the controlled period of the main clinical trials. No single cause of death predominated, but possible causes included infection, CV disease, and suicide.

• Use isn't recommended for patients with severe active lupus nephritis or severe active CNS lupus.

• IV administration in children younger than age 5 with SLE isn't indicated.

• Safety and effectiveness of IV administration in patients younger than age 18 with active lupus nephritis haven't been established.

• Safety and effectiveness of subcut administration in patients younger than age 18 haven't been established.
Dialyzable drug: Unknown.

PREGNANCY-LACTATION-REPRODUCTION

• There are no adequate well-controlled studies during pregnancy. Use cautiously during pregnancy and only if potential benefit outweighs risk to the fetus.
• Patients who are pregnant should enroll in a pregnancy registry that monitors maternal-fetal outcomes of exposure to belimumab by calling 1-877-681-6296.
• Patients of childbearing potential should use adequate contraception during treatment and for at least 4 months after final dose.
• Monitor the infant of a treated mother for B-cell reduction and other immune dysfunction; consider risks and benefits before giving live or live-attenuated vaccines to the infant.
• It isn't known if drug appears in human milk. A decision should be made to discontinue breastfeeding or discontinue drug, taking into account the importance of the drug to the mother.

NURSING CONSIDERATIONS

• IV drug should be administered only by a health care professional prepared to manage anaphylaxis.
• Patient or caregiver may administer subcut after proper training and if prescriber determines it's appropriate.
• Watch for hypersensitivity reactions, even in patients who previously tolerated infusions.
• Monitor patient for infection. Serious and sometimes fatal infections have occurred in patients receiving immunosuppressants.
• Monitor patient for depression, suicidality, malignancies, allergic reactions, and infusion reactions.
• Assess patients with new-onset or deteriorating neurologic signs and symptoms for JC virus–associated progressive multifocal leukoencephalopathy (PML). If PML is confirmed, therapy may have to be discontinued.

PATIENT TEACHING

• Warn patient not to skip appointments to ensure that drug is given on schedule to improve effectiveness of treatment.
• Tell patient to immediately report signs and symptoms of an allergic reaction (itching, hives, shortness of breath, swelling of

the face, and throat closure) and new or worsening depression, suicidality, or other mood changes.
• Teach patient infection-prevention measures.
• Instruct patient to immediately report signs and symptoms of infection (fever, body aches, cough, and sore throat).
• Tell patient to report history of cancer to health care provider.
• Instruct patient not to receive live-virus vaccines while taking drug.
• If patient or caregiver will be administering subcut at home, provide training and instruct patient or caregiver to follow directions for administration provided in the "Instructions for Use."
• Counsel patient of childbearing potential to use adequate contraception during treatment and for at least 4 months after final dose.
• Advise patient to tell prescriber if pregnant or breastfeeding.

---

benazepril hydrochloride ⚥
ben-A-za-pril

Lotensin✒

Therapeutic class: Antihypertensives
Pharmacologic class: ACE inhibitors

AVAILABLE FORMS

Tablets: 5 mg, 10 mg, 20 mg, 40 mg

INDICATIONS & DOSAGES

➤ **HTN**
Adults: For patients not receiving a diuretic, 10 mg PO daily initially. Adjust dosage as needed and tolerated; usually 20 to 40 mg daily in one or two divided doses. For patients receiving a diuretic, 5 mg PO daily initially.
Children age 6 and older: 0.2 mg/kg (between 0.1 and 0.6 mg/kg) PO daily. Adjust as needed up to 0.6 mg/kg (maximum 40 mg) PO daily.
Adjust-a-dose: In adults, if CrCl is below 30 mL/minute/1.73 m^2 or serum creatinine level is greater than 3 mg/dL, give 5 mg PO daily. May adjust daily dose up to 40 mg.

ADMINISTRATION

PO
• Protect tablets from moisture.
• Suspension may be prepared by a pharmacist.

• Refrigerate suspension at 36° to 46° F (2° to 8° C); shake before each use. Discard unused portion after 30 days.

ACTION
Inhibits ACE, preventing conversion of angiotensin I to angiotensin II, a potent vasoconstrictor. Less angiotensin II decreases peripheral arterial resistance, decreasing aldosterone secretion, which reduces sodium and water retention and lowers BP. Drug also acts as antihypertensive in patients with low-renin HTN.

Route	Onset	Peak	Duration
PO	1 hr	1–2 hr	24 hr

Half-life: 10 to 11 hours.

ADVERSE REACTIONS
CNS: headache, fatigue, postural dizziness, somnolence. **CV:** symptomatic hypotension. **Respiratory:** cough.

INTERACTIONS
Drug-drug. *Aliskiren:* May increase risk of renal impairment, hypotension, and hyperkalemia in patients with diabetes and those with moderate to severe renal impairment (GFR less than 60 mL/minute). Concomitant use is contraindicated in patients with diabetes. Avoid concomitant use in those with moderate to severe renal impairment.
Angiotensin II receptor antagonists (telmisartan): May increase risk of renal dysfunction. Avoid concurrent use.
Antidiabetics, insulin: May increase risk of hypoglycemia. Monitor patient carefully.
Azathioprine: May increase risk of anemia or leukopenia. Monitor hematologic study results if used together.
Diuretics, other antihypertensives: May cause excessive hypotension. Stop diuretic or lower dosage of benazepril, as needed.
Everolimus, neprilysin inhibitors (sacubitril), sirolimus, temsirolimus: May increase risk of angioedema. Discontinue one or both agents if an interaction is suspected.
Gold salts: May increase risk of nitritoid reaction. Carefully monitor patient.
Iron salts (parenteral): May increase risk of adverse reactions to iron salts. Monitor patient closely.
Lithium: May increase lithium level and toxicity. Use together cautiously; monitor lithium level.

Nesiritide: May increase risk of hypotension. Monitor BP.
NSAIDs (including selective cyclooxygenase-2 inhibitors): May decrease antihypertensive effects. Monitor BP. May also increase risk of renal dysfunction. Monitor renal function periodically.
Potassium-sparing diuretics, potassium supplements: May cause hyperkalemia. Monitor potassium level and renal function.
Salicylates: May decrease hypotensive effects of benazepril and increase risk of nephrotoxicity. Use cautiously together. Consider increasing benazepril dosage or decreasing or stopping salicylate.
Thiazide diuretics: May attenuate potassium loss. Also may increase risk of renal failure. Monitor serum potassium level and renal function.
Trimethoprim: May increase risk of hyperkalemia. Monitor serum potassium level and clinical response.
Drug-herb. *Ma huang, yohimbe:* May decrease antihypertensive effects. Discourage use together.
Drug-food. *Salt substitutes containing potassium:* May cause hyperkalemia. Monitor potassium level and renal function.

EFFECTS ON LAB TEST RESULTS
• May increase BUN, creatinine, potassium, uric acid, glucose, bilirubin, urine protein, and liver enzyme levels.
• May decrease sodium level.
• May increase eosinophil count.
• May lead to false-negative aldosterone/renin ratio.

CONTRAINDICATIONS & CAUTIONS
• Contraindicated in patients hypersensitive to ACE inhibitors and in those with a history of angioedema regardless of prior ACE inhibitor use.
• Use cautiously in patients with impaired hepatic or renal function. If jaundice develops or liver enzyme levels are markedly elevated, discontinue drug.
• Use cautiously in patients with history of airway surgery or other risk factors for airway obstruction.
• Use cautiously in older adults.
• Use cautiously in patients post-MI and in those with renal artery stenosis, chronic kidney disease, severe HF, or volume depletion (increased risk of acute kidney injury).

Reactions in bold italics are *life-threatening*. Interactions may have a *rapid onset* or a *delayed onset*.

• Safety and effectiveness in children younger than age 6 or in children with GFR less than 30 mL/minute/1.73 m² haven't been established.
Dialyzable drug: Slightly.

PREGNANCY-LACTATION-REPRODUCTION

Boxed Warning Drugs that act on the RAAS can cause injury and death to a developing fetus. Discontinue drug if pregnancy detected. ■

• Small amounts of drug appear in human milk. Patient should either discontinue drug or discontinue breastfeeding.

NURSING CONSIDERATIONS

• Monitor patient for hypotension. Excessive hypotension can occur when drug is given with diuretics. If possible, diuretic therapy should be stopped 2 to 3 days before starting benazepril to decrease potential for excessive hypotensive response. If drug doesn't adequately control BP, diuretic may be cautiously reinstituted.

☒ Although ACE inhibitors reduce BP in patients of all races, they reduce it less in patients who are Black and are taking ACE inhibitors alone. These patients should take drug with a thiazide diuretic for a more favorable response.

• Monitor patient for angioedema and anaphylactoid reactions, including intestinal angioedema (abdominal pain with or without nausea or vomiting).

☒ Drug may increase risk of angioedema in patients who are Black.

• Measure BP when drug level is at peak (2 to 6 hours after administration) and at trough (just before a dose) to verify adequate BP control.

• Assess renal and hepatic function before and periodically during therapy. Monitor potassium level.

• Monitor patient for excessive cough. Therapy may need to be changed if cough is intolerable.

• *Look alike–sound alike:* Don't confuse benazepril with Benadryl. Don't confuse Lotensin with lovastatin.

PATIENT TEACHING

• Instruct patient to avoid salt substitutes because they may contain potassium, which can cause high potassium level in patients taking drug.

• Inform patient that light-headedness can occur, especially during first few days of therapy. Tell patient to rise slowly to minimize this effect, to report dizziness to prescriber and, if fainting occurs, to stop drug and call prescriber immediately.

• Warn patient to use caution in hot weather and during exercise. Inadequate fluid intake, vomiting, diarrhea, and excessive perspiration can lead to light-headedness and fainting.

• Advise patient to report signs and symptoms of infection (such as fever and sore throat), easy bruising or bleeding; swelling of tongue, lips, face, eyes, mucous membranes, or extremities; difficulty swallowing or breathing; or hoarseness.

• Caution patient with diabetes to monitor blood glucose level closely.

⊙ *Alert:* Tell patient of childbearing potential to notify prescriber if pregnancy occurs. Drug will need to be stopped.

• Tell patient to contact prescriber if intolerable cough develops.

benztropine mesylate
BENZ-troe-peen

Therapeutic class: Antiparkinsonian drugs
Pharmacologic class: Anticholinergics

AVAILABLE FORMS
Injection: 1 mg/mL
Tablets: 0.5 mg, 1 mg, 2 mg

INDICATIONS & DOSAGES
➤ **Drug-induced extrapyramidal disorders (except tardive dyskinesia)**
Adults: 1 to 4 mg PO, IV, or IM once daily or b.i.d.
➤ **Transient extrapyramidal disorders**
Adults: 1 to 2 mg PO, IV, or IM b.i.d. or t.i.d. After 1 or 2 weeks, withdraw drug to determine continued need.
➤ **Acute dystonic reaction**
Adults: 1 to 2 mg PO, IV, or IM; then 1 to 2 mg PO once daily or b.i.d. to prevent recurrence. IV or IM route is preferred for severe acute reactions.
➤ **Parkinsonism**
Adults: 0.5 to 6 mg PO, IV, or IM daily in a single dose at bedtime or divided in two to four doses. First dose is 0.5 to 1 mg, increased by 0.5 mg every 5 to 6 days. Adjust dosage

to meet individual requirements. Maximum, 6 mg daily.

➤ **Postencephalitic parkinsonism**
Adults: 2 mg PO, IV, or IM daily in one or more doses. For patients who are highly sensitive, may initiate at 0.5 mg PO or IM at bedtime, and increase as needed. Maximum, 6 mg daily.

ADMINISTRATION
PO
• May give before or after meals, depending on patient reaction. If patient is prone to excessive salivation, give drug after meals. If patient's mouth dries excessively, give drug before meals unless it causes nausea.
• Store at room temperature.
IV
▼ Reserve IV delivery for emergencies, such as acute dystonic reactions.
▼ The IV form is seldom used because no significant difference in onset exists between it and the IM form.
▼ Use filtered needle to draw up solution from ampule.
▼ Visually inspect solution for particulate matter and discoloration before administration.
▼ Discard unused portion.
▼ Store at room temperature.
▼ **Incompatibilities:** Haloperidol lactate.
IM
• Use filtered needle to draw up solution from ampule.
• Visually inspect solution for particulate matter and discoloration before giving.
• Discard unused portion.
• Store at room temperature.

ACTION
Unknown. May block central cholinergic receptors, helping to balance cholinergic activity in the basal ganglia.

Route	Onset	Peak	Duration
PO	1 hr	7 hr	24 hr
IV, IM	15 min	Unknown	24 hr

Half-life: Unknown.

ADVERSE REACTIONS
CNS: confusion, memory impairment, nervousness, depression, disorientation, hallucinations, toxic psychosis, fever, finger numbness. **CV:** tachycardia. **EENT:** dilated pupils, blurred vision, dry mouth. **GI:** constipation, nausea, vomiting, paralytic ileus. **GU:** urine retention, dysuria. **Musculoskeletal:** muscle weakness. **Skin:** decreased sweating. **Other:** hypersensitivity reaction, hyperthermia, *heat stroke.*

INTERACTIONS
Drug-drug. *Amantadine, phenothiazines, TCAs:* May cause additive anticholinergic adverse reactions, such as confusion, hallucinations, GI effects, fever, or heat intolerance. Reduce dosage before giving.
Cholinergics (donepezil, galantamine, rivastigmine, tacrine): May antagonize the therapeutic effects of these drugs. If used together, monitor patient for therapeutic effect.

EFFECTS ON LAB TEST RESULTS
None reported.

CONTRAINDICATIONS & CAUTIONS
• Contraindicated in patients hypersensitive to drug or its components, in those with angle-closure glaucoma, and in children younger than age 3.
• Drug isn't recommended for use in patients with tardive dyskinesia.
• Drug may produce anhidrosis. Use cautiously in hot weather, in patients with mental disorders, in older adults, and in children age 3 and older.
• Use cautiously in patients with prostatic hyperplasia, arrhythmias, or seizure disorders.
Dializable drug: Unknown.
⚠ *Overdose S&S:* CNS depression preceded or followed by stimulation; confusion, nervousness, listlessness, intensification of mental symptoms or toxic psychosis (in patients with mental illness being treated with neuroleptic drugs), hallucinations, dizziness, muscle weakness, ataxia, dry mouth, mydriasis, blurred vision, palpitations, tachycardia, HTN, nausea, vomiting, dysuria, numbness of fingers, dysphagia, allergic reactions, headache, delirium, coma, shock, seizures, respiratory arrest, anhidrosis, hyperthermia, glaucoma, constipation; hot, dry, flushed skin.

PREGNANCY-LACTATION-REPRODUCTION
• Safe use during pregnancy hasn't been established.
• It isn't known if drug appears in human milk. Anticholinergic agents may suppress lactation.

Reactions in bold italics are *life-threatening*. Interactions may have a *rapid onset* or a ***delayed onset***.

NURSING CONSIDERATIONS
- Monitor vital signs carefully.
- Watch closely for adverse reactions, especially in older adults and patients who are debilitated. Report adverse reactions promptly.
- At certain doses, drug produces atropine-like toxicity, which may aggravate tardive dyskinesia.
- Watch for intermittent constipation and abdominal distention and pain, which may indicate onset of paralytic ileus.
- **❶ Alert:** Never stop drug abruptly. Reduce dosage gradually.
- **Look alike–sound alike:** Don't confuse benztropine with bromocriptine.

PATIENT TEACHING
- Warn patient to avoid activities that require alertness until CNS effects of drug are known.
- Advise patient who takes a single daily dose to do so at bedtime.
- Caution patient to report signs and symptoms of urinary hesitancy or urine retention.
- Tell patient to relieve dry mouth with cool drinks, ice chips, sugarless gum, or hard candy.
- Advise patient to limit hot weather activities because drug-induced lack of sweating may cause overheating.

betamethasone dipropionate
bay-ta-METH-a-sone

Diprolene, Sernivo

betamethasone valerate
Luxiq

Therapeutic class: Corticosteroids
Pharmacologic class: Corticosteroids

AVAILABLE FORMS
betamethasone dipropionate
Cream: 0.05%
Gel: 0.05%
Lotion: 0.05%
Ointment: 0.05%
Spray: 0.05%
betamethasone valerate
Cream: 0.1%
Foam: 0.12%
Lotion: 0.1%
Ointment: 0.1%

INDICATIONS & DOSAGES
➤ **Inflammation and pruritus from corticosteroid-responsive dermatoses**
Adults and children older than age 12: Clean area; apply cream, ointment, lotion, or gel sparingly. Give dipropionate products once daily to b.i.d.; give valerate 0.1% lotion b.i.d., or valerate 0.1% cream or ointment once daily to t.i.d. Maximum dosage of augmented betamethasone dipropionate 0.05% ointment, cream, gel, or lotion is 45 g, 45 g, 50 g, or 50 mL per week, respectively. Therapy with augmented formulations shouldn't exceed 2 weeks.
➤ **Inflammation and pruritus from corticosteroid-responsive dermatoses of scalp (valerate foam only)**
Adults: Gently massage small amounts of foam into affected scalp areas b.i.d., morning and evening, until control is achieved. If no improvement is seen in 2 weeks, reassess diagnosis.
➤ **Mild to moderate plaque psoriasis**
Adults: Apply spray to affected skin areas b.i.d. for up to 4 weeks; rub in gently. Discontinue when control is achieved.

ADMINISTRATION
Topical
- Apply sparingly to affected areas. To prevent skin damage, rub in gently, leaving a thin coat.
- May decrease dosing frequency of cream or ointment to once daily as directed by prescriber, if clinical improvement is seen.
- Avoid applying near eyes or mucous membranes or in ear canal, groin area, or armpit.
- Don't dispense foam directly into warm hands because foam will begin to melt on contact; dispense onto a plate or other cool surface and pick up small amounts of foam with fingers to apply immediately.
- **❶ Alert:** Foam product is flammable. Avoid fire, flame, or smoking during use. Don't expose to heat.
- For patients with eczematous dermatitis whose skin may be irritated by adhesive material, hold dressing in place with gauze, elastic bandages, stockings, or stockinette.
- **❶ Alert:** Don't use occlusive dressings unless directed by prescriber.
- Shake spray well before use. Avoid use on face, scalp, axilla, groin, or other intertriginous areas.
- Store at room temperature.

ACTION

Unclear. Is diffused across cell membranes to form complexes with receptors. Has anti-inflammatory, antipruritic, vasoconstrictive, and antiproliferative activity. Considered a medium-potency to very-high-potency drug (depending on product), according to vasoconstrictive properties.

Route	Onset	Peak	Duration
Topical	Unknown	Unknown	Unknown

Half-life: Unknown.

ADVERSE REACTIONS

GU: glucosuria (with dipropionate).
Metabolic: hyperglycemia. **Skin:** burning, pruritus, irritation, dryness, erythema, folliculitis, striae, acneiform eruptions, scaling, perioral dermatitis, hypopigmentation, hypertrichosis, allergic contact dermatitis, secondary infection, maceration, atrophy, alopecia, miliaria with occlusive dressings, application-site pain. **Other:** *HPA axis suppression,* Cushing syndrome.

INTERACTIONS

None significant.

EFFECTS ON LAB TEST RESULTS

- May increase glucose level.
- May suppress the wheal and flare reactions to skin test antigens.

CONTRAINDICATIONS & CAUTIONS

- Contraindicated in patients hypersensitive to corticosteroids.
- Don't use as monotherapy in primary bacterial infections (impetigo, paronychia, erysipelas, cellulitis, angular cheilitis), rosacea, perioral dermatitis, or acne.
- Don't use augmented betamethasone dipropionate 0.05% ointment; betamethasone dipropionate 0.05% gel, cream, and ointment; betamethasone 0.05% spray; or betamethasone valerate 0.1% ointment on the face, groin, or axilla.
Dialyzable drug: No.
⚠ *Overdose S&S:* Systemic effects.

PREGNANCY-LACTATION-REPRODUCTION

- There are no adequate and well-controlled studies during pregnancy. Use during pregnancy only if potential benefit justifies fetal risk.
- Use cautiously during breastfeeding.

NURSING CONSIDERATIONS

- Drug isn't for ophthalmic use.
- Because of alcohol content of vehicle, gel products may cause mild, transient stinging, especially when used on or near excoriated skin.
- If antifungal or antibiotic combined with corticosteroid fails to provide prompt improvement, stop corticosteroid until infection is controlled.
- Monitor patient for allergic contact dermatitis, often identified as failure to heal.
- Systemic absorption is likely with prolonged or extensive body surface treatment. Watch for symptoms of HPA axis suppression, manifestations of Cushing syndrome, hyperglycemia, and glucosuria. If HPA axis suppression occurs, attempt to withdraw drug or substitute a less potent steroid. Withdraw gradually.
- Evaluate patient for HPA axis suppression by using the urinary free cortisol and corticotropin stimulation tests.
- Drug may increase risk of posterior subcapsular cataracts and glaucoma. Consider referral to an ophthalmologist for evaluation if symptoms develop.
- ⚠ *Alert:* Children may demonstrate greater susceptibility to HPA axis suppression and Cushing syndrome.
- Avoid using plastic pants or tight-fitting diapers on treated areas in young children. Children may absorb larger amounts of drug and be more susceptible to systemic toxicity.
- ⚠ *Alert:* Don't replace Diprolene with generics because other products have different potencies.

PATIENT TEACHING

- Teach patient how to apply drug.
- Emphasize that drug is for external use only.
- Tell patient to wash hands after application.
- Advise patient to stop drug and report signs of systemic absorption, skin irritation or ulceration, hypersensitivity, visual changes, or infection.
- Instruct patient not to use occlusive dressings unless directed by prescriber.
- Discuss personal hygiene measures to reduce chance of infection.

Reactions in bold italics are *life-threatening*. Interactions may have a *rapid onset* or a *delayed onset*.

bethanechol chloride
be-THAN-e-kole

Duvoid

Therapeutic class: Urinary stimulants
Pharmacologic class: Cholinergic agonists

AVAILABLE FORMS
Tablets: 5 mg, 10 mg, 25 mg, 50 mg

INDICATIONS & DOSAGES
➤ **Acute postoperative and postpartum nonobstructive (functional) urine retention, neurogenic atony of urinary bladder with urine retention**
Adults: 10 to 50 mg PO t.i.d. to q.i.d. Determine minimum effective dose by giving 5 or 10 mg and repeating same amount at hourly intervals until satisfactory response or maximum of 50 mg has been given.

ADMINISTRATION
PO
• Give drug 1 hour before or 2 hours after meals because drug may cause nausea and vomiting if taken soon after eating.
• Store at room temperature.

ACTION
Directly stimulates muscarinic cholinergic receptors, mimicking acetylcholine action, increasing GI tract tone and peristalsis and contraction of the detrusor muscle of the urinary bladder.

Route	Onset	Peak	Duration
PO	30 min	60–90 min	1 hr

Half-life: Unknown.

ADVERSE REACTIONS
CNS: headache, malaise, *seizures.* **CV:** *bradycardia,* profound hypotension with reflexive tachycardia, flushing. **EENT:** lacrimation, miosis. **GI:** abdominal cramps, diarrhea, excessive salivation, nausea, belching, borborygmus. **GU:** urinary urgency. **Respiratory:** *bronchoconstriction, asthma attack.* **Skin:** diaphoresis.

INTERACTIONS
Drug-drug. *Anticholinergics, atropine, belladonna alkaloids, procainamide, quinidine:*
May reverse cholinergic effects. Observe patient for lack of drug effect.
Cholinesterase inhibitors (donepezil), cholinergic agonists: May cause additive effects or increase toxicity. Avoid using together.
Ganglionic blockers (pentolinium, trimethaphan): May cause critical drop in BP, usually preceded by severe abdominal pain. Avoid using together.

EFFECTS ON LAB TEST RESULTS
• None reported.

CONTRAINDICATIONS & CAUTIONS
• Contraindicated in patients hypersensitive to drug or its components and in those with uncertain strength or integrity of bladder wall, mechanical obstruction of GI or urinary tract, hyperthyroidism, peptic ulceration, latent or active bronchial asthma, obstructive pulmonary disease, pronounced bradycardia or hypotension, vasomotor instability, cardiac disease or CAD, AV conduction defects, HTN, seizure disorder, Parkinson disease, spastic GI disturbances, acute inflammatory lesions of the GI tract, peritonitis, or marked vagotonia.
• Safe use in children hasn't been established.
Dialyzable drug: Unknown.
⚠ **Overdose S&S:** Abdominal discomfort, excessive salivation, flushing, hot feeling, diaphoresis, nausea, vomiting.

PREGNANCY-LACTATION-REPRODUCTION
• It isn't known if drug affects reproduction. Use during pregnancy only if clearly needed.
• It isn't known if drug appears in human milk. Patient should discontinue breastfeeding or discontinue drug.

NURSING CONSIDERATIONS
• Monitor patient for orthostatic hypotension.
• Watch closely for adverse reactions that may indicate drug toxicity.

PATIENT TEACHING
• Tell patient to take drug on an empty stomach and at regular intervals.
• Inform patient that drug is usually effective 30 to 90 minutes after use.

♣Canada   ◇OTC   ◆Off-label use   ✐Photoguide   ⊜Do not crush   *Liquid contains alcohol   ▓Genetic

bevacizumab
be-vuh-SIZ-uh-mab

Avastin

bevacizumab-awwb
Mvasi

bevacizumab-bvzr
Zirabev

Therapeutic class: Antineoplastics
Pharmacologic class: Monoclonal antibodies

AVAILABLE FORMS
Solution: 25 mg/mL in 4-mL, 16-mL vials

INDICATIONS & DOSAGES
Adjust-a-dose (for all indications): Although there are no recommended dosage reductions, temporarily suspend or stop drug in patients with severe infusion reactions (GI perforations and fistulae, wound healing complications, hemorrhage, thromboembolic events, PRES, renal injury and proteinuria, HF), severe HTN that isn't controlled with medical management, or moderate to severe proteinuria.

➤ **Platinum-resistant recurrent epithelial ovarian, fallopian tube, or primary peritoneal cancer**
Adults: 10 mg/kg IV every 2 weeks in combination with paclitaxel, pegylated liposomal doxorubicin, or weekly topotecan; or 15 mg/kg IV every 3 weeks in combination with topotecan.

➤ **Platinum-sensitive recurrent epithelial ovarian, fallopian tube, or primary peritoneal cancer**
Adults: Initially, 15 mg/kg IV every 3 weeks in combination with carboplatin and paclitaxel for six cycles up to eight cycles, followed by continued use of bevacizumab 15 mg/kg IV every 3 weeks as a single agent until disease progression. Or, give 15 mg/kg IV every 3 weeks in combination with carboplatin and gemcitabine for six cycles up to 10 cycles, followed by continued use of bevacizumab 15 mg/kg IV every 3 weeks as a single agent until disease progression.

➤ **Stage III or IV epithelial ovarian, fallopian tube, or primary peritoneal cancer after initial surgical resection**
Adults: 15 mg/kg every 3 weeks with carboplatin and paclitaxel for up to six cycles, followed by 15 mg/kg every 3 weeks as a single agent, for a total of up to 22 cycles.

➤ **Metastatic colorectal cancer with fluoropyrimidine-irinotecan–based or fluoropyrimidine-oxaliplatin–based chemotherapy for second-line treatment after progression on a first-line bevacizumab-containing regimen**
Adults: 5 mg/kg IV every 2 weeks or 7.5 mg/kg IV every 3 weeks.

➤ **Persistent, recurrent, or metastatic cervical cancer with paclitaxel and cisplatin or paclitaxel and topotecan**
Adults: 15 mg/kg IV infusion once every 3 weeks.

➤ **First- or second-line treatment, with 5-FU–based chemotherapy, for metastatic colon or rectal cancer**
Adults: If used with bolus irinotecan, 5-FU, and leucovorin (IFL) regimen, give 5 mg/kg IV every 14 days. If used with oxaliplatin, 5-FU, and leucovorin (FOLFOX 4) regimen, give 10 mg/kg IV every 14 days. Infusion rate varies by patient tolerance and number of infusions.

➤ **With carboplatin and paclitaxel as first-line treatment of unresectable, locally advanced, recurrent, or metastatic nonsquamous NSCLC**
Adults: 15 mg/kg IV infusion once every 3 weeks.

➤ **With interferon alfa for metastatic renal cell carcinoma; as single agent for progressive glioblastoma following prior therapy**
Adults: 10 mg/kg IV every 14 days.

➤ **Unresectable or metastatic hepatocellular carcinoma in combination with atezolizumab in patients who haven't received prior systemic therapy (Avastin only)**
Adults: 15 mg/kg IV infusion after 1,200-mg IV infusion of atezolizumab on the same day, every 3 weeks until disease progression or unacceptable toxicity occurs. Refer to manufacturer's instructions for atezolizumab prescribing information.

➤ **Unresectable malignant pleural mesothelioma** ◆
Adults: 15 mg/kg IV every 3 weeks in combination with pemetrexed and cisplatin for up to six cycles, followed by bevacizumab maintenance therapy at 15 mg/kg once every 3 weeks until disease progression or unacceptable toxicity.

Reactions in bold italics are *life-threatening*. Interactions may have a *rapid onset* or a ***delayed onset***.

➤ **Age-related macular degeneration ♦**
Adults: Intravitreal bevacizumab 1.25 mg
(0.05 mL) monthly for 3 months; then may
give scheduled (monthly) or as needed based
on monthly ophthalmologic assessment.
➤ **Diabetic macular edema ♦**
Adults: Initially, intravitreal bevacizumab
1.25 mg (0.05 mL); repeat every 4 weeks depending on ophthalmologic response.

ADMINISTRATION
IV
▼ Don't freeze or shake vials.
▼ Dilute drug using aseptic technique. With-
draw proper dose and mix in a total volume
of 100 mL NSS in an IV bag.
▼ Don't give by IV push or bolus.
▼ Give first infusion over 90 minutes and, if
tolerated, second infusion over 60 minutes.
Later infusions can be given over 30 minutes
if previous infusions were tolerated.
▼ Discard unused portion; drug is
preservative-free.
▼ Diluted drug is stable 8 hours if refriger-
ated at 36° to 46° F (2° to 8° C).
▼ Protect from light.
▼ **Incompatibilities:** Dextrose solutions.

ACTION
A recombinant humanized vascular endothelial growth factor inhibitor.

Route	Onset	Peak	Duration
IV	Unknown	Unknown	Unknown

Half-life: About 20 days.

ADVERSE REACTIONS
Includes adverse reactions as part of
chemotherapy regimens.
CNS: asthenia, dysarthria, dizziness,
headache, taste disorder, anxiety, pain, syncope, fatigue, insomnia, myasthenia, fever.
CV: *intra-abdominal thrombosis,* HTN, *arterial thrombosis, thromboembolism, DVT,
hemorrhage,* edema, chest pain, left ventricular dysfunction, *PE.* **EENT:** excess lacrimation, blurred vision, tinnitus, deafness, epistaxis, rhinitis, rhinorrhea, nasal congestion,
sinusitis, gum bleeding, voice alteration,
oropharyngeal pain, oral ulceration, tooth
abscess. **GI:** anorexia, constipation, diarrhea, stomatitis, vomiting, *GI hemorrhage,*
abdominal pain, gastritis, nausea, bile duct
fistula, rectal fistula, rectal pain, tracheoesophageal fistula. **GU:** *vaginal hemorrhage,*

increased creatinine level, proteinuria, UTI,
ovarian failure, pelvic pain, bladder fistula,
vaginal fistula, renal fistula. **Hematologic:**
*leukopenia, neutropenia, thrombocytope-
nia.* **Hepatic:** bilirubinemia, increased liver
enzyme levels. **Metabolic:** *hypokalemia,
hyperkalemia,* weight loss, hyperglycemia,
hypomagnesemia, hyponatremia, hypoalbuminemia, *hypocalcemia,* dehydration. **Musculoskeletal:** back pain, limb pain, myalgia,
arthralgia, muscle weakness. **Respiratory:**
hemoptysis, pulmonary hemorrhage, dyspnea, cough, bronchopleural fistula. **Skin:**
dry skin, bruise, acne, cellulitis, exfoliative
dermatitis, nail disorder, palmar-plantar erythrodysesthesia. **Other:** postoperative wound
complication, infection, infusion-related reaction.

INTERACTIONS
Drug-drug. *Bisphosphonate derivatives:*
May increase risk of osteonecrosis of the jaw.
Monitor therapy.
Live-virus vaccines: May reduce immune re-
sponse. Avoid use together.
Sunitinib: May increase bevacizumab toxic-
ities, including microangiopathic hemolytic
anemia and HTN. Avoid combination.

EFFECTS ON LAB TEST RESULTS
● May increase bilirubin, glucose, and urine
protein levels.
● May decrease albumin, magnesium, cal-
cium, and sodium levels.
● May increase or decrease potassium level.
● May decrease neutrophil, platelet, and
WBC counts.

CONTRAINDICATIONS & CAUTIONS
● Use cautiously in patients hypersensitive to
drug or its components and in those who need
surgery, have a bowel obstruction or fistulae,
are at increased risk for kidney failure, are
taking anticoagulants, or have significant CV
disease (HTN, HF, thromboembolism).
● Use cautiously in patients with prior
anthracycline-based chemotherapy as the incidence of HF and decreased LVEF may increase with use of bevacizumab. Discontinue
drug in patients who develop HF.
● Use cautiously in older adults; adverse reactions occur more often in these patients.
● Drug increases risk of severe or fatal hemorrhage, hemoptysis, GI bleeding, CNS hemorrhage, and vaginal bleeding. Don't give to

patients with serious hemorrhage or recent hemoptysis.
• Safety and effectiveness in children haven't been established.
Dialyzable drug: Unknown.
⚠ *Overdose S&S:* Headache.

PREGNANCY-LACTATION-REPRODUCTION
• Drug has shown teratogenic effects in animal studies. Avoid use during pregnancy.
• Because of bevacizumab's long half-life, females should use adequate contraception during therapy and for 6 months after final dose.
◑ *Alert:* May increase risk of ovarian failure and may impair fertility. Long-term effects on fertility are unknown.
• It isn't known if drug appears in human milk. Patients should avoid breastfeeding during therapy and for 6 months after final dose.

NURSING CONSIDERATIONS
◑ *Alert:* PRES-associated symptoms (HTN, headache, visual disturbances, altered mental function, seizures) may occur 16 hours to 1 year after starting drug. PRES can be confirmed only by MRI. Monitor patient closely. If syndrome occurs, stop drug and provide supportive care.
◑ *Alert:* Monitor patient for arterial thromboembolic events and venous thromboembolic events (VTEs). Patients treated for cervical cancer may be at increased risk for VTEs. Permanently discontinue drug for grade 4 VTE, including PE.
◑ *Alert:* Drug may increase risk of developing fistula, including non-GI fistulae (tracheoesophageal, bronchopleural, biliary, vaginal, renal, or bladder), which can be fatal.
• Permanently stop drug if patient develops any fistula of an internal organ.
• Hypersensitivity reactions can occur during infusion. Monitor patient closely for hypertensive crisis with neurologic changes, wheezing, oxygen desaturation, chest pain, headache, rigors, and diaphoresis.
• If patient develops severe HTN, hypertensive crisis, serious hemorrhage, or GI perforation that needs intervention, stop drug.
◑ *Alert:* Drug may increase risk of serious arterial thromboembolic events, including MI, TIAs, stroke, HF, and angina. Patients at highest risk are age 65 or older, have a history of arterial thromboembolism, and have taken

drug before. If patient has an arterial thrombotic event, permanently stop drug.
• Drug may cause fatal GI perforation. Monitor patient closely.
• Bevacizumab can result in life-threatening wound dehiscence. Permanently discontinue bevacizumab therapy in patients who experience wound dehiscence that requires medical intervention. Discontinue drug at least 28 days before elective surgery and don't restart drug for at least 28 days after surgery and until the surgical wound is fully healed.
• Monitor urinalysis for worsening proteinuria. Patients with 2+ or greater urine dipstick test should undergo 24-hour urine collection. Discontinue use in patients with nephrotic syndrome.
• Monitor patient's BP every 2 to 3 weeks.

PATIENT TEACHING
• Inform patient about potential adverse reactions. Tell patient to report adverse reactions immediately, especially abdominal pain, constipation, and vomiting.
• Advise patient that BP and urinalysis will be monitored during treatment.
• Caution patient of childbearing potential to avoid pregnancy during treatment and for 6 months after final dose.
• Tell patient not to breastfeed during therapy and for 6 months after final dose.
◑ *Alert:* Inform patient of the potential for ovarian failure and impaired fertility before starting treatment.
• Urge patient to alert other health care providers about bevacizumab therapy and to avoid elective surgery during treatment.

bisoprolol fumarate
bis-OH-proe-lol

Therapeutic class: Antihypertensives
Pharmacologic class: Selective beta blockers

AVAILABLE FORMS
Tablets: 5 mg, 10 mg

INDICATIONS & DOSAGES
Adjust-a-dose (for all indications): In patients with bronchospastic disease or hepatic or renal insufficiency (CrCl less than 40 mL/minute), initially give 2.5 mg; then titrate with caution.

Reactions in bold italics are *life-threatening*. Interactions may have a *rapid onset* or a *delayed onset*.

B

➤ **HTN**
Adults: Initially, 2.5 to 5 mg PO daily alone or with other antihypertensives. May increase to 10 mg daily, then to 20 mg once daily if needed.

➤ **HF with reduced ejection fraction** ♦
Adults: 1.25 mg PO once daily. Titrate gradually up to 10 mg/day.

➤ **Angina** ♦
Adults: 10 mg PO once daily; may increase to maximum dose of 20 mg once daily after at least 1 week if needed.

ADMINISTRATION
PO
• May give without regard to meals.
• Store at room temperature. Protect from moisture.

ACTION
Selectively blocks cardiac adrenoceptors, reducing resting and exercise HR, decreasing cardiac output, depressing renin secretion, and decreasing tonic sympathetic outflow from the vasomotor centers in the brain.

Route	Onset	Peak	Duration
PO	1–2 hr	2–4 hr	Unknown

Half-life: 9 to 12 hours.

ADVERSE REACTIONS
CNS: headache, dizziness, hypoesthesia, insomnia, asthenia, fatigue. **CV:** chest pain, peripheral edema, *bradycardia.* **EENT:** dry mouth, pharyngitis, rhinitis, sinusitis. **GI:** diarrhea, nausea, vomiting. **Musculoskeletal:** arthralgia. **Respiratory:** cough, dyspnea, URI. **Skin:** diaphoresis.

INTERACTIONS
Drug-drug. *Antiarrhythmics (disopyramide), calcium channel blockers (diltiazem, verapamil):* May increase myocardial depression or conduction delay. Use cautiously together.
Beta blockers: May increase beta blocker effects to unsafe level. Use together is contraindicated.
Catecholamine-depleting drugs (guanethidine, reserpine): May cause hypotension or bradycardia. Monitor patient closely.
Clonidine: May cause rebound HTN if clonidine is discontinued. Stop bisoprolol for several days before discontinuing clonidine.
Digoxin: May increase risk of slow AV conduction and bradycardia. Use together cautiously.

Insulin, oral antidiabetics: May mask signs and symptoms of hypoglycemia, particularly tachycardia. Use together cautiously.
Rifampin: May increase bisoprolol metabolism. Monitor patient for decreased bisoprolol effects.

EFFECTS ON LAB TEST RESULTS
• May increase serum triglyceride, AST, ALT, uric acid, creatinine, BUN, potassium, glucose, and phosphorus levels.
• May decrease WBC and platelet counts.
• May cause ANA conversion.

CONTRAINDICATIONS & CAUTIONS
• Contraindicated in patients hypersensitive to drug and in those with cardiogenic shock, overt cardiac failure, second- or third-degree AV block, or marked sinus bradycardia.
• Use cautiously in patients with hepatic or renal insufficiency, hyperthyroidism, HF, arterial insufficiency, PVD, or diabetes.
• Use cautiously in patients with a history of severe anaphylactic reaction to a variety of allergens. Patients may be more sensitive if allergen is reintroduced; usual epinephrine doses may not be effective.
• Use cautiously in patients with bronchospastic disease who don't tolerate or respond to other antihypertensive treatment. Patients should have a bronchodilator on hand in the event of an episode.
• Safety and effectiveness in children haven't been established.
Dialyzable drug: No.

PREGNANCY-LACTATION-REPRODUCTION
• There are no adequate and well-controlled studies during pregnancy. Use during pregnancy only if potential benefit justifies fetal risk.
• It isn't known if drug appears in human milk. Use cautiously during breastfeeding.

NURSING CONSIDERATIONS
• Monitor BP closely.
• Avoid use in patients with acute HF because of worsening of disease. If bisoprolol administration is necessary, monitor patient closely.
• Use cautiously in patients with known compensated HF. In patients without a history of HF, drug may precipitate signs and symptoms of new HF. Consider stopping drug at first indication of new HF. Drug may be continued while HF is being treated with other drugs.

• Drug interruption or abrupt discontinuation may exacerbate angina pectoris, MI, or ventricular arrhythmia and may exacerbate the signs and symptoms of hyperthyroidism, possibly leading to thyroid storm. If drug is to be discontinued, taper over approximately 1 week while monitoring patient. If withdrawal signs and symptoms occur, restart drug at least temporarily.

• A long-term bisoprolol regimen shouldn't be discontinued before major surgery. However, the impaired ability of the heart to respond to reflex adrenergic stimuli may increase risks of general anesthesia and surgical procedures.

• Drug may mask tachycardia caused by hyperthyroidism. In patients with suspected thyrotoxicosis, withdraw drug gradually to avoid thyroid storm.

• Drug may mask signs and symptoms of hypoglycemia in patients with diabetes.

• Drug may cause or aggravate signs and symptoms of arterial insufficiency in patients with PVD.

PATIENT TEACHING

• Tell patient to report slowed heartbeat, difficulty breathing, or other signs of HF.

• Caution patient not to discontinue bisoprolol without first consulting health care provider.

• Warn patient with diabetes that bisoprolol may mask signs and symptoms of hypoglycemia (such as tachycardia, dizziness, and weakness).

• Urge patient to use caution when operating automobiles and machinery or performing activities requiring alertness.

SAFETY ALERT!

bivalirudin
bye-VAL-ih-roo-din

Angiomax

Therapeutic class: Anticoagulants
Pharmacologic class: Direct thrombin inhibitors

AVAILABLE FORMS

Injection: 250-mg vial; 5 mg/mL in 50-mL and 100-mL single-dose container

INDICATIONS & DOSAGES

➤ **Anticoagulation in patients undergoing PCI, including patients with heparin-induced thrombocytopenia and heparin-induced thrombocytopenia and thrombosis syndrome**

Adults: 0.75 mg/kg IV bolus followed by a continuous infusion of 1.75 mg/kg/hour during the procedure. Check activated clotting time 5 minutes after bolus dose is given. May give additional 0.3 mg/kg bolus dose if needed. Infusion may continue for up to 4 hours after procedure in patients with ST-segment elevation MI.

Adjust-a-dose: For patients with CrCl of 30 mL/minute or less, decrease maintenance infusion rate to 1 mg/kg/hour; for patients on hemodialysis, reduce infusion rate to 0.25 mg/kg/hour. No reduction of bolus dose is needed.

ADMINISTRATION
IV

▼ Lyophilized powder must be reconstituted and diluted. Reconstitute each 250-mg vial with 5 mL of sterile water for injection. Gently swirl until all material is dissolved.

▼ Reconstituted material will be a clear to slightly opalescent, colorless to slightly yellow solution.

▼ Withdraw and discard 5 mL from a 50-mL infusion bag containing D_5W or NSS. Then add contents of reconstituted vial to infusion bag to yield a final concentration of 5 mg/mL.

▼ Store unopened vials at room temperature. Refrigerate reconstituted vials for up to 24 hours; don't freeze.

▼ Store premixed solution at or below -4° F (-20° C). Thaw at room temperature or under refrigeration; don't thaw in microwave or by bath immersion. May store thawed solution for 14 days under refrigeration; don't refreeze.

▼ Solutions are stable at room temperature for 24 hours. Discard remaining unused solution.

▼ **Incompatibilities:** Alteplase, amiodarone, amphotericin B, chlorpromazine, diazepam, dobutamine, prochlorperazine, reteplase, streptokinase, vancomycin.

ACTION

Binds specifically and rapidly to thrombin, inhibiting its effects, thereby producing an anticoagulant effect.

Route	Onset	Peak	Duration
IV	Rapid	Immediate	1–2 hr

Half-life: 25 minutes in patients with normal renal function.

ADVERSE REACTIONS

CNS: anxiety, headache, insomnia, nervousness, fever, pain. **CV:** *bradycardia,* HTN, hypotension, angina pectoris, *thrombosis.* **GI:** abdominal pain, dyspepsia, nausea, vomiting. **GU:** urine retention, pelvic pain. **Hematologic:** *severe, spontaneous bleeding (cerebral, retroperitoneal, GU, GI).* **Musculoskeletal:** back pain. **Skin:** pain at injection site.

INTERACTIONS

Drug-drug. *GPIIa/IIIb inhibitors (abciximab, eptifibatide, tirofiban), heparin, thrombolytics, warfarin:* May increase risk of hemorrhage. Use together cautiously.
Drug-herb. *Herbs with anticoagulant or antiplatelet properties (alfalfa, anise, bilberry, ginseng):* May increase risk of bleeding. Discourage use together.

EFFECTS ON LAB TEST RESULTS

- May decrease Hb level, hematocrit, and platelet count.
- May increase INR.

CONTRAINDICATIONS & CAUTIONS

- Contraindicated in patients hypersensitive to drug or its components and in patients with significant active bleeding.
- Use cautiously in patients undergoing brachytherapy due to an increased risk of thrombus formation, and in those with diseases linked to increased bleeding risk.
- Use cautiously in older adults; bleeding events occur more frequently in these patients.
- Safety and effectiveness in children haven't been established.
Dialyzable drug: 25%.
⚠ *Overdose S&S:* Bleeding, death due to hemorrhage.

PREGNANCY-LACTATION-REPRODUCTION

- Use cautiously during pregnancy and only if clearly indicated.
- It's unknown if drug appears in human milk. Use cautiously during breastfeeding.

NURSING CONSIDERATIONS

- There is no antidote for drug.
- Monitor coagulation test results, Hb level, and hematocrit before starting therapy and periodically thereafter.
- Obtain a complete list of patient's prescription and OTC drugs and supplements, including herbs.
- 🔔 *Alert:* Hemorrhage can occur at any site in the body. If patient has unexplained decrease in hematocrit, decrease in BP, or other unexplained symptoms, suspect hemorrhage.
- Monitor venipuncture sites for bleeding, hematoma, or inflammation.
- Don't give drug IM.

PATIENT TEACHING

- Advise patient that drug can cause bleeding and to immediately report unusual bruising or bleeding (nosebleeds, bleeding gums) or melena.
- Counsel patient that drug is given with aspirin. Caution patient to avoid other aspirin-containing drugs or NSAIDs while receiving this drug.
- Advise patient to consult with prescriber before initiating any herbal therapy; many herbs have anticoagulant, antiplatelet, and fibrinolytic properties.
- Caution patient to avoid activities that carry a risk of injury and to use a soft toothbrush and electric razor while taking drug.

SAFETY ALERT!

bleomycin sulfate
blee-oh-MYE-sin

Therapeutic class: Antineoplastics
Pharmacologic class: Cytotoxic glycopeptide antibiotics

AVAILABLE FORMS

Injection: 15-unit vials, 30-unit vials

INDICATIONS & DOSAGES

Adjust-a-dose (for all indications): For patients with CrCl of 40 to 50 mL/minute, give 70% of dose; for CrCl of 30 to 39 mL/minute, give

60% of dose; for CrCl of 20 to 29 mL/minute, give 55% of dose; for CrCl of 10 to 19 mL/minute, give 45% of dose; and for CrCl of 5 to 9 mL/minute, give 40% of dose.

➤ **Squamous cell carcinoma (head, neck, skin, penis, cervix, and vulva), non-Hodgkin lymphoma, testicular carcinoma**
Adults: Because an anaphylactoid reaction is possible, treat patients with lymphoma with 2 units or less for first two doses. If no acute reaction occurs, then may follow regular dosage schedule: 0.25 to 0.5 units/kg (10 to 20 units/m^2) IV, IM, or subcut once or twice weekly to total of 400 units.

➤ **Hodgkin lymphoma**
Adults: Because an anaphylactoid reaction is possible, treat patients with lymphoma with 2 units or less for first two doses. If no acute reaction occurs, then may follow regular dosage schedule: 0.25 to 0.5 units/kg (10 to 20 units/m^2) IV, IM, or subcut one or two times weekly. After 50% response, maintenance dose is 1 unit IV or IM daily or 5 units IV or IM weekly. Total cumulative dose is 400 units.

➤ **Malignant pleural effusion**
Adults: 60 units given as single-dose bolus intrapleural injection.

ADMINISTRATION

IV
▼ Preparing and giving parenteral form of drug may be mutagenic, teratogenic, and carcinogenic. Use safe handling and disposal precautions according to facility policy.
▼ Reconstitute 15-unit or 30-unit vial with 5 or 10 mL, respectively, of NSS for injection to equal 3 units/mL solution.
▼ Administer slowly over 10 minutes.
▼ Use reconstituted solution within 24 hours.
▼ Refrigerate unopened vials containing dry powder.
▼ Drug is an irritant and may cause phlebitis. It isn't known to cause tissue damage with extravasation. If signs or symptoms of extravasation occur, stop infusion immediately and institute appropriate care according to facility policy.
▼ **Incompatibilities:** Amino acids; aminophylline; amphotericin B conventional/lipid complex/liposome; ascorbic acid injection; cefazolin; dantrolene; diazepam; drugs containing sulfhydryl groups; fluids containing dextrose; furosemide; hydrocortisone; methotrexate; mitomycin; nafcillin; penicillin G; phenytoin; riboflavin; solutions containing divalent and trivalent cations, especially calcium salts and copper; terbutaline sulfate.

IM
• Dilute 15-unit vial in 1 to 5 mL or 30-unit vial in 2 to 10 mL of sterile water for injection, bacteriostatic water for injection, or NSS for injection.
• Monitor injection site for irritation.

Subcutaneous
• Dilute 15-unit vial in 1 to 5 mL or 30-unit vial in 2 to 10 mL of sterile water for injection, bacteriostatic water for injection, or NSS for injection.
• Monitor injection site for irritation.

Intrapleural
• For intrapleural use, dilute 60 units of drug in 50 to 100 mL NSS for injection; give drug through a thoracotomy tube.
• If patient's condition requires sclerosis, instill drug when chest tube drainage is 100 to 300 mL/24 hours; ideally, drainage should be less than 100 mL/24 hours. After instillation, clamp thoracotomy tube and move patient from the back to the left then right side several times for the next 4 hours. Remove clamp and reestablish suction. Length of time chest tube is left in place after sclerosis depends on patient's condition.

ACTION
May inhibit DNA synthesis and cause scission of single- and double-stranded DNA; also inhibits RNA and protein synthesis.

Route	Onset	Peak	Duration
IV, IM, subcut	Unknown	30–60 min	Unknown

Half-life: 2 hours.

ADVERSE REACTIONS
CNS: fever. **GI:** stomatitis, anorexia, nausea, vomiting, diarrhea. **Metabolic:** weight loss, hyperuricemia. **Respiratory:** *pneumonitis, pulmonary fibrosis.* **Skin:** erythema, hyperpigmentation, acne, rash, striae, skin tenderness, pruritus, reversible alopecia, hyperkeratosis, nail changes. **Other:** chills, *anaphylactoid reactions.*

Reactions in bold italics are *life-threatening*. Interactions may have a *rapid onset* or a *delayed onset*.

INTERACTIONS
Drug-drug. *Anesthesia:* May increase oxygen requirements. Monitor patient closely.
Brentuximab: May increase risk of pulmonary toxicity. Avoid use together.
Cisplatin: May decrease bleomycin elimination. Monitor renal function and adjust bleomycin dosage as needed.
Fosphenytoin, phenytoin: May decrease phenytoin and fosphenytoin levels. Monitor drug levels closely.
Live-virus vaccines: May increase risk of vaccine-induced adverse reactions. Avoid concomitant use.
Nephrotoxic drugs: May decrease bleomycin elimination and increase risk of pulmonary toxicity. Monitor patient closely.
Other antineoplastics: May increase risk of pulmonary toxicities at lower doses. Monitor patient closely.
Oxygen: May increase risk of pulmonary toxicity during surgery due to increased sensitization of lung tissue from bleomycin. Use together cautiously.

EFFECTS ON LAB TEST RESULTS
• May increase uric acid level.

CONTRAINDICATIONS & CAUTIONS
• Contraindicated in patients hypersensitive to drug.
• Use cautiously in patients with renal or pulmonary impairment.
🕭 **Alert:** Adverse pulmonary reactions are more common in patients older than age 70. Pulmonary toxic adverse effects may be increased in patients receiving radiation therapy, patients with lung disease, and patients who need oxygen therapy.
Dialyzable drug: Unknown.

PREGNANCY-LACTATION-REPRODUCTION
• Drug can cause fetal harm when administered during pregnancy. Inform patient of the fetal risk.
• Patients of childbearing potential should avoid becoming pregnant during therapy.
• It isn't known if drug appears in human milk. Patient should discontinue breastfeeding during therapy.

NURSING CONSIDERATIONS
Boxed Warning Drug should be administered under the supervision of a physician experienced in the use of cancer chemotherapeutic agents. ∎
• Pulmonary toxicities are common. Obtain pulmonary function tests before start of treatment and at regular intervals during treatment. If tests show a marked decline, stop drug.
Boxed Warning Fatal pulmonary fibrosis may occur, especially when cumulative dose exceeds 400 units. ∎
• Monitor chest X-ray every 1 to 2 weeks and listen to lungs regularly.
Boxed Warning Monitor patient with lymphoma for idiosyncratic reactions (hypotension, confusion, fever, chills, wheezing) after receiving drug. ∎
• Severe idiosyncratic reactions can occur, usually after first or second dose. Monitor patient carefully.
• Monitor liver and kidney function.
• Watch for fever, which may be treated with antipyretics. Fever usually occurs within 3 to 6 hours of administration.
• Hodgkin disease and testicular tumor improvement is prompt and noted within 2 weeks. If no improvement is seen by this time, improvement is unlikely. Squamous cell cancers sometimes require as long as 3 weeks before improvement is noted.
🕭 **Alert:** Watch for hypersensitivity reactions, which may be delayed for several hours, especially in patients with lymphoma. (Give test dose of 1 to 2 units before first two doses in patients with lymphoma. If no reaction occurs, follow regular dosage schedule.)

PATIENT TEACHING
• Warn patient that hair loss may occur but is usually reversible.
• Tell patient to report adverse reactions promptly and to take infection-control and bleeding precautions.
• Advise patient who is to receive anesthesia to inform anesthesiologist about taking this drug. High oxygen levels inhaled during surgery may enhance pulmonary toxicity of drug.

bortezomib
bore-TEZ-oh-mib

Velcade

Therapeutic class: Antineoplastics
Pharmacologic class: Proteasome inhibitors

AVAILABLE FORMS
Powder for injection: 3.5 mg

INDICATIONS & DOSAGES
Adjust-a-dose (for all indications): Refer to manufacturer's instructions for toxicity-related dosage adjustments in patients with hepatic impairment or peripheral neuropathy and in those on combination therapies.

➤ **Previously untreated multiple myeloma**
Adults: 1.3 mg/m^2 IV bolus over 3 to 5 seconds or subcut in combination with oral melphalan and oral prednisone for nine 6-week treatment cycles. In cycles 1 to 4, bortezomib is given twice weekly (days 1, 4, 8, 11, 22, 25, 29, and 32). In cycles 5 to 9, bortezomib is given once weekly (days 1, 8, 22, and 29). Separate consecutive doses of drug by at least 72 hours. Prior to initiating any cycle, platelet count should be 70 × 10^9/L or greater, ANC should be 1 × 10^9/L or greater, and non-hematologic toxicities should have resolved to grade 1 or baseline.

➤ **Previously untreated mantle cell lymphoma**
Adults: 1.3 mg/m^2 IV bolus over 3 to 5 seconds in combination with IV rituximab, cyclophosphamide, doxorubicin, and oral prednisone for six 3-week treatment cycles. Bortezomib is administered first followed by rituximab. Bortezomib is given twice weekly for 2 weeks (days 1, 4, 8, and 11) followed by 10-day rest period on days 12 to 21. Patients who respond at cycle 6 should receive two additional cycles for a total of 8 cycles. Separate consecutive doses of drug by at least 72 hours. Before initiating any cycle other than cycle 1, platelet count should be 100 × 10^9/L or greater, ANC should be 1.5 × 10^9/L or greater, Hb level should be at least 8 g/dL or greater, and nonhematologic toxicities should have resolved to grade 1 or baseline.

➤ **Multiple myeloma or mantle cell lymphoma that still progresses after at least one therapy**

Adults: 1.3 mg/m^2 by IV bolus over 3 to 5 seconds or subcut twice weekly for 2 weeks (days 1, 4, 8, and 11), followed by a 10-day rest period (days 12 through 21). This 3-week period is a treatment cycle. For therapy longer than eight cycles, may adjust dosage schedule to once weekly for 4 weeks (days 1, 8, 15, and 22) followed by a 13-day rest period (days 23 through 35). Separate consecutive doses of drug by at least 72 hours.

ADMINISTRATION
● Drug is hazardous. Use appropriate precautions for handling and disposal.
● Use caution and aseptic technique when preparing and handling drug. Wear gloves and protective clothing to prevent skin contact.
● Inspect solution before administration. Don't give if solution is discolored or contains particles.

IV
▼ Reconstitute with 3.5 mL of NSS to a final concentration of 1 mg/mL and give by IV bolus over 3 to 5 seconds within 8 hours of preparation.
▼ Reconstituted drug may be stored in original vial or a syringe at 77° F (25° C); total storage time must not exceed 8 hours.
▼ Store unopened vial at a controlled room temperature, in original packaging, protected from light.
▼ **Incompatibilities:** None listed by manufacturer. Consult a drug incompatibility reference for more information.

Subcutaneous
● Reconstitute with 1.4 mL of NSS to a final concentration of 2.5 mg/mL and give within 8 hours of preparation.
● Reconstituted drug may be stored in original vial or a syringe at 77° F (25° C); total storage time must not exceed 8 hours.
● Rotate injection sites. New injections should be given at least 1 inch (2.54 cm) from an old site and never in areas that are tender, bruised, reddened, or hard.
● If injection-site reactions occur, a less concentrated solution (1 mg/mL) may be used.

ACTION
Disrupts intracellular homeostatic mechanisms by inhibiting the 26S proteasome, which regulates intracellular levels of certain proteins, causing cells to die.

Route	Onset	Peak	Duration
IV, subcut	Unknown	Unknown	Unknown

Half-life: 40 to 193 hours (1-mg/m^2 dose); 76 to 108 hours (1.3-mg/m^2 dose).

ADVERSE REACTIONS

CNS: anxiety, asthenia, dizziness, dysesthesia, fatigue, fever, headache, insomnia, paresthesia, peripheral neuropathy, neuralgia, rigors, weakness. **CV:** edema, HTN, hypotension, cardiac disease, **hemorrhage. EENT:** blurred vision. **GI:** abdominal pain, constipation, decreased appetite, diarrhea, dysgeusia, dyspepsia, nausea, vomiting. **Hematologic:** *neutropenia, thrombocytopenia,* anemia, *leukopenia, lymphopenia.* **Hepatic:** *acute liver failure, hepatitis,* hyperbilirubinemia, increased liver enzyme levels. **Metabolic:** dehydration, anorexia, hyperglycemia. **Musculoskeletal:** arthralgia, back pain, bone pain, limb pain, muscle cramps, myalgia. **Respiratory:** cough, dyspnea, pneumonia, URI. **Skin:** alopecia, pruritus, rash, injection-site reaction. **Other:** infection, herpes zoster, herpes simplex.

INTERACTIONS

Drug-drug. *Antihypertensives:* May cause hypotension. Monitor patient's BP closely.
Drugs linked to peripheral neuropathy (amiodarone, antivirals, isoniazid, nitrofurantoin, statins): May worsen neuropathy. Use together cautiously.
Drugs that prolong QT interval (antiarrhythmics [bretylium, disopyramide, dofetilide, procainamide, quinidine, sotalol], chlorpromazine, dolasetron, droperidol, mefloquine, mesoridazine, moxifloxacin, pentamidine, pimozide, tacrolimus, thioridazine, ziprasidone): May prolong QT interval and increase risk of life-threatening ventricular arrhythmias. Use together with caution.
Oral antidiabetics: May cause hypoglycemia or hyperglycemia. Monitor glucose level closely.
Strong CYP3A4 inducers (rifampin): May reduce drug's effects. Avoid use together.
Strong CYP3A4 inhibitors (ketoconazole): May increase risk of toxicity. Monitor patient closely; consider bortezomib dosage reduction.
Drug-herb. *St. John's wort:* May decrease bortezomib exposure. Avoid concomitant use.

Drug-food. *Grapefruit:* May increase risk of toxicity. Discourage use together.
Green tea: May decrease therapeutic effect of drug. Avoid use together.

EFFECTS ON LAB TEST RESULTS
• May increase liver enzyme, bilirubin, and uric acid levels.
• May decrease calcium level.
• May increase or decrease potassium, sodium, and glucose levels.
• May decrease Hb level and neutrophil and platelet counts.

CONTRAINDICATIONS & CAUTIONS
• Contraindicated in patients hypersensitive to bortezomib, boron, or mannitol.
• Intrathecal administration is contraindicated.
• Use cautiously in patients with hepatic or renal impairment or with a history of syncope and in those who are dehydrated or receiving other drugs known to cause hypotension.
• Use cautiously in patients with risk factors for, or existing, heart disease. Closely monitor patients for acute development or exacerbation of HF and new-onset decreased LVEF.
• Use cautiously in older adults, who may be at greater risk for adverse effects.
Dialyzable drug: Yes.
⚠ **Overdose S&S:** Symptomatic hypotension, thrombocytopenia.

PREGNANCY-LACTATION-REPRODUCTION
• There are no adequate and well-controlled studies during pregnancy. Drug may cause fetal harm. Use during pregnancy isn't recommended.
• Patients of childbearing potential should avoid becoming pregnant and should use effective contraception during treatment and for 7 months after final dose.
• Males with partners of childbearing potential should use effective contraception during treatment and for at least 4 months after final dose.
• It isn't known if drug appears in human milk. Patients shouldn't breastfeed during treatment and for 2 months after final dose.

NURSING CONSIDERATIONS
• Monitor patient for evidence of neuropathy, such as a burning sensation, hyperesthesia, hypoesthesia, paresthesia, discomfort, or neuropathic pain.

- Consider subcut administration for patients at high risk for or with preexisting peripheral neuropathy.
- Be aware that the IV and subcut concentrations are different. Be sure to check that patient is receiving appropriate concentration of drug before administration.
- Monitor patient closely for PRES-associated symptoms (HTN, headache, visual disturbances, altered mental function, seizures), which may occur after starting drug. PRES can be confirmed only by MRI. If syndrome occurs, stop drug and provide supportive care.
- Monitor patient for signs and symptoms of TLS (hyperuricemia, hyperkalemia, hyperphosphatemia, hypocalcemia, acute renal failure).
- Monitor patient for pulmonary and cardiac toxicity (HF, pneumonitis, lung infiltrates).
- Monitor patient for thrombotic microangiopathy (anemia, thrombocytopenia, confusion, HTN, decreased urine output, edema, fever).
- Monitor glucose levels in patients with diabetes who are taking oral hypoglycemics.
- Watch carefully for adverse effects, especially in older adults.
- Be sure patient has an order for an antiemetic, antidiarrheal, or both to treat drug-induced nausea, vomiting, or diarrhea.
- Provide fluid and electrolyte replacement to prevent dehydration.
- To manage orthostatic hypotension, adjust antihypertensive dosage, maintain hydration status, and give mineralocorticoids or sympathomimetics.
- Dialysis may reduce drug level; give after dialysis.
- **❸ Alert:** Because thrombocytopenia is common, monitor patient's CBC and platelet counts carefully during treatment, before each dose, and especially on day 11.

PATIENT TEACHING
- Instruct patient to report all adverse effects.
- Tell patient to notify prescriber about new or worsening peripheral neuropathy.
- Urge patient to use effective contraception during treatment and for 7 months after final dose and not to breastfeed during treatment and for 2 months after final dose.
- Teach patient how to avoid dehydration, and stress the need to tell prescriber about dizziness, light-headedness, or fainting spells.

- Tell patient to use caution when driving or performing other hazardous activities because drug may cause fatigue, dizziness, faintness, light-headedness, and doubled or blurred vision.
- Advise patient with diabetes to check blood glucose level frequently if using an oral antidiabetic and to report changes in blood glucose level.
- Caution patient to report bleeding or signs or symptoms of infection immediately.

bosentan ⚕
bow-SEN-tan

Tracleer

Therapeutic class: Vasodilators
Pharmacologic class: Endothelin-receptor antagonists

AVAILABLE FORMS
Tablets: 62.5 mg, 125 mg
Tablets (for suspension): 32 mg

INDICATIONS & DOSAGES
Adjust-a-dose (for all indications): Refer to manufacturer's instructions for toxicity-related dosage adjustments. Discontinue bosentan at least 36 hours before start of ritonavir; at least 10 days after ritonavir start, resume bosentan at recommended initial dose once daily or every other day based on tolerability.
➤ **PAH (WHO Group 1) in patients with WHO/NYHA Class II to IV symptoms to improve exercise ability and decrease rate of clinical worsening** ⚕
Adults: 62.5 mg PO b.i.d., in the morning and evening, for 4 weeks. If patient weighs 40 kg or more, increase to maintenance dosage of 125 mg PO b.i.d., in the morning and evening. If patient weighs less than 40 kg, maintenance dosage is 62.5 mg PO b.i.d.
➤ **To improve pulmonary vascular resistance in PAH (idiopathic or congenital) in children** ⚕
Children older than age 12 weighing more than 40 kg: Initially, 62.5 mg PO b.i.d. After 4 weeks, increase to 125 mg PO b.i.d.
Children older than age 12 weighing less than 40 kg: Initial and maintenance dosage is 62.5 mg PO b.i.d.

Children age 12 and younger weighing more than 24 to 40 kg: Initial and maintenance dosage is 64 mg PO b.i.d.
Children age 12 and younger weighing more than 16 to 24 kg: Initial and maintenance dosage is 48 mg PO b.i.d.
Children age 12 and younger weighing more than 8 to 16 kg: Initial and maintenance dosage is 32 mg PO b.i.d.
Children age 12 and younger weighing 4 to 8 kg: Initial and maintenance dosage is 16 mg PO b.i.d.

ADMINISTRATION
PO
• Give drug in morning and evening without regard for meals.
• Disperse tablets for oral suspension, or dispersible tablet half, in a minimal amount of water immediately before administration.
• Store divided dispersible tablet pieces at 68° to 77° F (20° to 25° C) in opened blister for up to 7 days.

ACTION
Specific and competitive antagonist for endothelin-1 (ET-1). ET-1 levels are elevated in patients with PAH, suggesting a pathogenic role for ET-1 in this disease.

Route	Onset	Peak	Duration
PO	Unknown	3–5 hr	Unknown

Half-life: About 5 hours.

ADVERSE REACTIONS
CNS: headache, fatigue, syncope. **CV:** edema, flushing, hypotension, palpitations, chest pain. **EENT:** sinusitis. **GU:** decreased sperm count. **Hematologic:** anemia. **Hepatic:** abnormal transaminase levels, *hepatotoxicity.* **Musculoskeletal:** arthralgia. **Respiratory:** respiratory tract infection.

INTERACTIONS
Drug-drug. *Clarithromycin:* May increase risk of bosentan hepatotoxicity and increase active metabolite of clarithromycin. Monitor patient closely. Stop one or both drugs if an interaction is suspected.
Cyclosporine: May increase bosentan level and decrease cyclosporine level. Use together is contraindicated.
CYP2C9 inhibitor (amiodarone, fluconazole) plus moderate CYP3A inhibitor (amprenavir, diltiazem, erythromycin, flucona-

zole) or strong CYP3A inhibitor (ketoconazole, itraconazole): May cause large increase in bosentan plasma concentration. Administration of bosentan with a CYP2C9 inhibitor plus a strong or moderate CYP3A inhibitor isn't recommended.
Glyburide: May increase risk of elevated LFT values and decrease levels of both drugs. Use together is contraindicated.
Hormonal contraceptives: May cause contraceptive failure. Patient should use two reliable methods of birth control during treatment and for 1 month after stopping drug.
Ketoconazole: May increase bosentan effect. Watch for adverse effects.
PDE5 inhibitors (sildenafil): May increase bosentan level and decrease sildenafil level. Use together with caution.
Rifampin: May alter bosentan level. Monitor hepatic function weekly for 4 weeks followed by routine monitoring.
Ritonavir: May increase risk of bosentan toxicity. Dosage adjustment may be needed.
Simvastatin, other statins: May decrease levels of these drugs. Monitor cholesterol levels to assess need to adjust statin dose.
Tacrolimus: May decrease tacrolimus level. Use together cautiously.
Warfarin: May decrease warfarin level. Monitor coagulation tests and adjust warfarin dosage as needed.

EFFECTS ON LAB TEST RESULTS
Boxed Warning May increase AST, ALT, and bilirubin levels. ∎
• May decrease Hb level and hematocrit.

CONTRAINDICATIONS & CAUTIONS
Boxed Warning Only prescribers and pharmacies registered with the Bosentan REMS Program (1-866-359-2612 or www.BosentanREMSProgram.com) may prescribe and distribute bosentan. ∎
• Contraindicated in patients hypersensitive to drug; reactions may include DRESS syndrome, anaphylaxis, rash, and angioedema.
Boxed Warning Generally avoid using in patients with moderate to severe hepatic impairment or in those with elevated aminotransferase levels greater than 3 × ULN. ∎
• Use cautiously in patients with mild hepatic impairment.
Dialyzable drug: Unlikely.
⚠ *Overdose S&S:* Headache, nausea, vomiting, hypotension, dizziness, blurred vision.

PREGNANCY-LACTATION-REPRODUCTION

Boxed Warning Drug is likely to cause major birth defects. Contraindicated in pregnancy. Verify pregnancy status of patients of childbearing potential before starting drug, monthly during treatment, and 1 month after final dose. ■

Boxed Warning Patients of childbearing potential must use one highly effective form of contraception (intrauterine device [IUD] or tubal sterilization) or a combination of methods (hormone method with a barrier method or two barrier methods). If a partner's vasectomy is the chosen method of contraception, a hormone or barrier method must be also used along with this method. Ensure contraception is continued until 1 month after completion of bosentan therapy. ■

Boxed Warning There is a possibility of contraception failure when bosentan is administered with hormonal contraceptives; patient shouldn't use hormonal contraceptives alone when taking bosentan. ■

• Decreased sperm counts have been observed in patients receiving drug.
• It isn't known if drug appears in human milk. Use isn't recommended during breastfeeding.

NURSING CONSIDERATIONS

Boxed Warning Use of this drug can cause serious liver injury. AST and ALT level elevations may be dose dependent and reversible, so measure these levels before treatment and monthly thereafter, adjusting dosage accordingly. If elevations are accompanied by symptoms of liver injury (nausea, vomiting, fever, abdominal pain, jaundice, or unusual lethargy or fatigue) or if bilirubin level increases by $2 \times$ ULN or greater, discontinue drug and notify prescriber immediately. ■

• Fluid retention and HF may occur. Patient may require diuretics, fluid management, or hospitalization for decompensating HF.
• Monitor patient for pulmonary edema.
• Monitor Hb level after 1 and 3 months of therapy; then every 3 months.
• Gradually reduce dosage before stopping drug.

PATIENT TEACHING

• Advise patient to take doses in the morning and evening, with or without food.

Boxed Warning Warn patient to avoid becoming pregnant while taking this drug and for 1 month after final dose. Hormonal contraceptives, including oral, implantable, and injectable methods, may not be effective when used with this drug. Advise patient to use two acceptable methods of contraception during and for 1 month after treatment with bosentan. A monthly pregnancy test must be performed. ■

• Inform patient of risk of low sperm count.
• Advise patient to have LFTs and blood counts performed regularly.

SAFETY ALERT!

brentuximab vedotin ☒
bren-TUK-see-mab ve-DOE-tin

Adcetris

Therapeutic class: Antineoplastics
Pharmacologic class: CD30-directed antibodies

AVAILABLE FORMS

Powder for injection: 50 mg single-use vial

INDICATIONS & DOSAGES

Adjust-a-dose (for all indications): Refer to manufacturer's instructions for toxicity-related dosage adjustments and dosage adjustments for patients with hepatic and renal impairment.

➤ **Classic Hodgkin lymphoma (cHL) in patients at high risk for relapse or progression after autologous hematopoietic stem cell transplantation (auto-HSCT) consolidation**
Adult: 1.8 mg/kg IV every 3 weeks in 4 to 6 weeks after auto-HSCT or upon recovery from auto-HSCT for a maximum of 16 cycles or until disease progression or toxicities occur. Maximum dose is 180 mg.

➤ **Hodgkin lymphoma after failure of auto-HSCT or after failure of at least two multiagent chemotherapy regimens in patients who aren't auto-HSCT candidates; systemic anaplastic large cell lymphoma (ALCL) after failure of at least one multiagent chemotherapy regimen**
Adults: 1.8 mg/kg IV infusion every 3 weeks, or until disease progression or toxicities occur. Maximum dose is 180 mg.

➤ **Relapsed primary cutaneous ALCL or CD30-expressing mycosis fungoides**

Adults: 1.8 mg/kg IV infusion every 3 weeks for a maximum of 16 cycles or until disease progression or toxicities occur. Maximum dose is 180 mg.

➤ **Previously untreated stage III or IV cHL, in combination with chemotherapy**
Adults: 1.2 mg/kg IV infusion every 2 weeks until a maximum of 12 doses are given, or until disease progression or unacceptable toxicity occurs. Maximum dose is 120 mg.

➤ **Previously untreated systemic ALCL or other CD30-expressing peripheral T-cell lymphomas (PTCL), including angioimmunoblastic T-cell lymphoma and PTCL not otherwise specified, in combination with cyclophosphamide, doxorubicin, and prednisone** ⊠
Adults: 1.8 mg/kg IV infusion every 3 weeks, with each cycle of chemotherapy for six to eight doses. Maximum dose is 180 mg.

ADMINISTRATION

IV

▼ Drug is considered hazardous; use safe handling and disposal precautions.

▼ Reconstitute each 50-mg vial with 10.5 mL sterile water for injection to yield a single-use solution containing 5 mg/mL.

▼ Gently swirl contents; don't shake vial. Inspect for particulates and discoloration.

▼ Dilute further to yield 0.4 to 1.8 mg/mL in infusion bag of NSS injection, 5% dextrose injection, or lactated Ringer injection. Gently mix by inverting bag.

▼ After reconstitution, infuse immediately or store at 36° to 46° F (2° to 8° C) and use within 24 hours of reconstitution. Don't freeze. Discard unused portion left in vial.

▼ Administer drug only by IV infusion over 30 minutes; don't give by IV push or bolus.

▼ **Incompatibilities:** Don't mix or administer drug with other medications or fluids.

ACTION

Disrupts microtubule network of the cancer cell, which induces cell-cycle arrest and apoptotic death of the cells.

Route	Onset	Peak	Duration
IV	Rapid	1–3 days	Unknown

Half-life: 4 to 6 days.

ADVERSE REACTIONS

CNS: peripheral neuropathy (sensory, motor), headache, dizziness, fatigue, chills, insomnia, anxiety, pain, fever. **CV:** peripheral edema, *PE, supraventricular arrhythmia,* lymphadenopathy. **EENT:** oropharyngeal pain. **GI:** nausea, diarrhea, abdominal pain, vomiting, constipation, decreased appetite. **GU:** pyelonephritis, UTI. **Hematologic:** *neutropenia,* anemia, *thrombocytopenia.* **Metabolic:** decreased weight, hyperglycemia. **Musculoskeletal:** arthralgia, myalgia, back pain, extremity pain, muscle spasms. **Respiratory:** URI, cough, dyspnea, pneumonitis, pneumothorax. **Skin:** rash, pruritus, alopecia, night sweats, dry skin, cellulitis. **Other:** *septic shock, anaphylaxis,* immunogenicity, infusion-related reactions.

INTERACTIONS

Drug-drug. *Bleomycin:* Increases risk of pulmonary toxicity. Concomitant use is contraindicated.
Strong CYP3A4 inducers (rifampin): May decrease brentuximab level. Monitor patient for brentuximab effectiveness.
Strong CYP3A4 inhibitors (ketoconazole): May increase brentuximab level. Monitor patient for increased adverse effects.

EFFECTS ON LAB TEST RESULTS

● May increase glucose, transaminase, and bilirubin levels.
● May decrease RBC, WBC, platelet, and neutrophil counts.

CONTRAINDICATIONS & CAUTIONS

● Contraindicated in patients hypersensitive to drug.

Boxed Warning John Cunningham virus infection resulting in progressive multifocal leukoencephalopathy (PML) and death can occur in patients receiving brentuximab. ▮

☕ *Alert:* Infusion-related reactions, including anaphylaxis, have occurred. If anaphylaxis occurs, discontinue drug immediately and permanently and initiate appropriate therapy. Interrupt infusion for other infusion-related reactions and treat appropriately. Patients with prior infusion-related reactions should be premedicated (acetaminophen, antihistamine, corticosteroid) for subsequent infusions.

● Avoid use in patients with severe renal impairment or moderate or severe hepatic impairment due to increased risk of grade 3 or greater adverse events.

• Serious infections (pneumonia, bacteremia, sepsis, fatal septic shock) have been reported.
• Safety and effectiveness in children haven't been established.
Dialyzable drug: Unknown.

PREGNANCY-LACTATION-REPRODUCTION

• Drug may cause fetal harm. Patients of childbearing potential should avoid pregnancy during and for 6 months after therapy ends.
• Drug may damage spermatozoa and testicular tissue, resulting in possible genetic abnormalities. Males with partners of childbearing potential should use effective contraception during therapy and for 6 months after therapy ends.
• Drug may compromise male fertility.
• It isn't known if drug appears in human milk. Breastfeeding isn't recommended during treatment.

NURSING CONSIDERATIONS

• Drug may cause severe peripheral neuropathy. Monitor patient for new or worsening signs and symptoms.
• Drug may cause hepatotoxicity, which can be fatal, especially in patients with preexisting liver disease or elevated baseline liver enzymes and in those taking concomitant medications. Monitor liver enzymes and bilirubin. Delay or reduce dose, or discontinue drug as clinically indicated for new, worsening, or recurrent hepatotoxicity.
• Monitor patient closely for infusion-related adverse effects; interrupt therapy and treat as necessary.
• Monitor patient for signs and symptoms of neutropenia and anemia. Monitor CBC before each dose, and more frequently if patient exhibits grade 3 or 4 neutropenia. Delay or reduce dose, or discontinue drug as required. May give G-CSF prophylaxis.
• Monitor patient for TLS, characterized by changes in electrolytes and kidney damage.
• Monitor patient for skin reactions, especially SJS. Discontinue drug if reactions occur.
Boxed Warning Monitor patient for vision loss, impaired speech, muscle weakness or paralysis, and cognitive deterioration, which may indicate PML. Hold drug for suspected PML and discontinue if diagnosis is confirmed. ∎

• Monitor patient for noninfectious pulmonary toxicity (pneumonitis, ILD, ARDS). Hold drug during evaluation of new or worsening pulmonary symptoms and until symptoms improve.
• Monitor patient for infection (bacterial, fungal, or viral) during treatment.
• Monitor patient for new or worsening GI signs and symptoms of perforation, hemorrhage, erosion, ulcer, intestinal obstruction, enterocolitis, neutropenic colitis, and ileus.
• Monitor patient for hyperglycemia, exacerbation of preexisting diabetes, and ketoacidosis. Give antihyperglycemic agent as clinically indicated.
• Verify pregnancy status before therapy.

PATIENT TEACHING

• Tell patient to report muscle weakness or numbness or tingling of the hands or feet.
• Advise patient to report signs or symptoms of possible infection, including temperature of 100.5° F (38° C) or greater, chills, cough, or pain on urination.
• Warn patient to report signs or symptoms of possible infusion-related reactions, including fever, chills, rash, or breathing problems (wheezing, cough, chest tightness), blue skin color, and swelling of the face, lips, tongue, or throat.
• Instruct patient to immediately report signs or symptoms of PML (changes in mood or unusual behavior, confusion, thinking problems, memory loss, vision changes, altered speech, gait abnormalities, decreased strength on one side of the body).
• Tell patient to report all adverse effects.
• Caution patient to avoid becoming pregnant during and for 6 months after therapy ends and to report possible pregnancy immediately.
• Breastfeeding isn't recommended during therapy.
• Caution patient with partner of childbearing potential to use effective contraception during and for 6 months after therapy ends.

Reactions in bold italics are *life-threatening*. Interactions may have a *rapid onset* or a *delayed onset*.

brexpiprazole ⚕
brex-PIP-ra-zole

Rexulti⬧

Therapeutic class: Antipsychotics
Pharmacologic class: Atypical antipsychotics

AVAILABLE FORMS
Tablets: 0.25 mg, 0.5 mg, 1 mg, 2 mg, 3 mg, 4 mg

INDICATIONS & DOSAGES
Adjust-a-dose (for all indications): Refer to manufacturer's instructions for drug-interaction dosage adjustments. Reduce dosage by half in patients who are CYP2D6 poor metabolizers.

➤ **Adjunctive treatment of major depressive disorder (MDD)**
Adults: Initially, 0.5 or 1 mg PO once daily. If starting at 0.5 mg, increase to 1 mg PO once daily after 1 week based on patient's response and tolerability. Then, increase to target dose of 2 mg PO once daily after 1 week. Maximum daily dose is 3 mg.
Adjust-a-dose: If Child-Pugh score is 7 or more or CrCl is less than 60 mL/minute, maximum daily dose is 2 mg.

➤ **Schizophrenia**
Adults: Initially, 1 mg PO once daily on days 1 through 4; then titrate to 2 mg PO once daily on days 5 through 7; then increase to 4 mg PO once daily on day 8 based on patient's response and tolerability. Recommended target dose is 2 to 4 mg daily. Maximum daily dose is 4 mg.
Children age 13 and older: Initially, 0.5 mg PO once daily on days 1 through 4; then titrate to 1 mg PO once daily on days 5 through 7; then increase to 2 mg PO once daily on day 8 based on response and tolerability. Increase by 1 mg weekly, if indicated. Recommended target dose, 2 to 4 mg daily. Maximum dose, 4 mg.
Adjust-a-dose: If Child-Pugh score is 7 or more or CrCl is less than 60 mL/minute, maximum daily dose is 3 mg.

ADMINISTRATION
PO
• Give without regard for food.

• If a dose is missed, give as soon as possible. If it's close to the time for next dose, skip missed dose and give next dose at the regular time. Don't double-dose.
• Store at 68° to 77° F (20° to 25° C).

ACTION
Exact mechanism unknown. Its effect may occur through partial agonist activity at serotonin 5-HT_{1A} and dopamine D_2 receptors, as well as antagonist activity at serotonin 5-HT_{2A} receptors.

Route	Onset	Peak	Duration
PO	Unknown	4 hr	Unknown

Half-life: 91 hours.

ADVERSE REACTIONS
CNS: fatigue, drowsiness, akathisia, headache, tremor, dizziness, anxiety, restlessness, somnolence, sedation, abnormal dreams, insomnia, extrapyramidal reactions. **EENT:** blurred vision, nasopharyngitis, dry mouth, sialorrhea. **GI:** constipation, dyspepsia, increased appetite, diarrhea, nausea, abdominal pain, flatulence. **GU:** UTI. **Metabolic:** weight gain, increased CK level, increased prolactin level, decreased cortisol level. **Musculoskeletal:** myalgia. **Skin:** hyperhidrosis.

INTERACTIONS
Drug-drug. *Anticholinergics (diphenhydramine, meclizine, scopolamine):* May increase risk of body temperature dysregulation. Use together cautiously.
CNS depressants: May increase CNS depressant effects. Monitor therapy.
Strong CYP2D6 inhibitors (bupropion, fluoxetine, paroxetine, quinidine), strong CYP3A4 inhibitors (clarithromycin, itraconazole, ketoconazole, ritonavir): May increase brexpiprazole concentration. Reduce brexpiprazole dosage.
Strong CYP3A4 inducers (carbamazepine, phenytoin, rifampin): May decrease brexpiprazole concentration. Increase brexpiprazole dosage.
Drug-herb. *St. John's wort:* May decrease brexpiprazole concentration. Increase brexpiprazole dosage.

EFFECTS ON LAB TEST RESULTS
• May increase CK, glucose, triglyceride, and prolactin levels.

- May decrease cortisol level.
- May decrease WBC count.

CONTRAINDICATIONS & CAUTIONS

- Contraindicated in patients hypersensitive to drug or its components.

Boxed Warning Older adults with dementia-related psychosis treated with antipsychotics are at increased risk for death. Drug isn't approved for treatment of patients with dementia-related psychosis. ∎

Boxed Warning Antidepressants have increased the risk of suicidality in patients younger than age 24. Safety and effectiveness in children with MDD haven't been established. ∎

- Antipsychotics can cause NMS, which can be fatal.
- Antipsychotics can cause tardive dyskinesia, especially in older adults, most notably older women, and may be irreversible.
- Atypical antipsychotics are associated with metabolic changes, such as weight gain, dyslipidemia, hyperglycemia, and diabetes.
- Antipsychotics may increase the risk of seizures. Use cautiously in patients with a history of seizures or conditions that could lower the seizure threshold.
- Drug may alter the body's ability to lower the core temperature.
- ⚕ Use cautiously in patients who are poor metabolizers of CYP2D6, in patients with moderate to severe hepatic impairment (Child-Pugh score of 7 or more), and in those with moderate, severe, or end-stage renal impairment (CrCl less than 60 mL/minute); adjust dosage appropriately.
- Use cautiously in patients with preexisting hypotension or who are taking other antihypertensives; drug can cause orthostatic hypotension or syncope.
- Use cautiously in patients at risk for aspiration pneumonia. Esophageal dysmotility and aspiration have been associated with antipsychotic use.
- Antipsychotics can impair thinking, judgment, and motor skills.
- Drug may cause intense impulsive or compulsive behavior urges, particularly for gambling, and the inability to control these urges. Other compulsive urges reported less frequently include sexual urges, shopping, and eating or binge eating.
- Drug may cause somnolence, orthostatic hypotension, and motor and sensory

instability, which may lead to falls and, consequently, fractures or other injuries.
- Tablets may contain lactose; avoid use in patients with lactose-intolerant conditions.
- Use cautiously in older adults because of the increased risk of adverse events.

Dialyzable drug: Unlikely.

PREGNANCY-LACTATION-REPRODUCTION

- There are no adequate studies in pregnancy. Neonates exposed to antipsychotics during the third trimester are at risk for extrapyramidal or withdrawal signs and symptoms, which can vary in severity but may require prolonged hospitalization. Routine use during pregnancy isn't recommended; risks and benefits should be considered.
- Enroll patients exposed to drug during pregnancy in the National Pregnancy Registry for Atypical Antipsychotics (1-866-961-2388 or https://womensmentalhealth.org/research/pregnancyregistry/).
- It's unknown if drug appears in human milk. Consider risks and benefits before using during breastfeeding.

NURSING CONSIDERATIONS

Boxed Warning Monitor patients for suicidality, especially during the first few months of treatment and after dosage changes. Consider discontinuing drug in patients whose depression worsens or who experience suicidality. ∎

- Monitor patients for signs and symptoms of NMS (hyperpyrexia, muscle rigidity, change in mental status, tachycardia, change in BP or pulse, diaphoresis, arrhythmias, elevated CK level, rhabdomyolysis, acute renal failure). Discontinue drug if reactions appear, and treat appropriately.
- Monitor blood glucose, triglyceride, and lipid levels; observe for weight changes.
- Monitor patients for seizures, difficulty swallowing, and aspiration.
- Monitor patients with diabetes regularly for worsening of glucose control.
- Monitor patients at risk for diabetes (obesity, family history) before and periodically during treatment.
- Avoid exposing patients to extreme heat; make sure they are well hydrated.
- Monitor patients for tardive dyskinesia (involuntary, dyskinetic movements). Reassess need for continued treatment periodically. If

---

tardive dyskinesia develops, consider discontinuing drug.
- Monitor patients with a history of significantly low WBC count or ANC or drug-induced neutropenia frequently during first few months of therapy. Consider discontinuing drug at first sign of significant decline in WBC count; monitor patients for fever or other signs or symptoms of infection. Discontinue drug in patients with severe neutropenia (ANC less than 1,000/mm^3).
- Monitor patients for orthostatic hypotension and syncope. Patients at increased risk include those with dehydration, hypovolemia, history of CV disease (HF, MI, ischemia, conduction abnormalities), or history of cerebrovascular disease; those taking antihypertensives; and patients who are antipsychotic-naive. Lower starting dose and slower titration may be needed in these patients.
- Complete fall risk assessments when initiating antipsychotic treatment and periodically for patients on long-term therapy, especially for patients who have diseases or conditions or are taking other medications that could exacerbate their fall risk.
- Monitor patients for impulsive or compulsive behavior urges; consider reducing dosage or stopping drug if they develop.
- Check with pharmacist regarding potential interactions with other drugs that are metabolized via the CYP450 enzyme system in the liver.
- *Look alike–sound alike:* Don't confuse Rexulti with Maxalt.

PATIENT TEACHING
- ⚠ *Alert:* Counsel family members or caregivers to monitor for changes in behavior and to immediately report suicidality to prescriber.
- Advise patient or caregivers to watch for and report new or intense gambling urges, compulsive sexual urges, compulsive shopping, binge or compulsive eating, or other urges.
- Explain the potential for dystonic or extrapyramidal symptoms (involuntary, abnormal movements). Instruct patient to immediately report symptoms to prescriber.
- Teach patient with diabetes to monitor blood glucose level closely and to report changes in glucose level.
- Advise patient to report lactose intolerance before starting therapy.

- Educate patient about the risk of metabolic changes, how to recognize hyperglycemia, and the need for blood tests for glucose and lipid levels. Encourage patient to report weight gain.
- Caution patient about risk of orthostatic hypotension and syncope, especially at start of therapy and with dosage changes.
- Advise patient to contact prescriber immediately if patient is or plans to become pregnant or is breastfeeding.
- Remind patient to avoid strenuous exercise, dehydration, or exposure to extreme heat. Encourage patient to drink plenty of water while taking drug.
- Instruct patient to report muscle rigidity, diaphoresis, changes in BP, or irregular heartbeats.
- Warn patient about potential for drug interactions and advise patient to report to prescriber all OTC drugs, prescription medications, and supplements being taken before start of therapy.
- Caution patient about risk of impaired judgment, thinking, or motor skills. Advise patient not to perform activities that require mental alertness, such as operating hazardous machinery, including motor vehicles, until drug's effects are known.

brimonidine tartrate
bri-MOE-ni-deen

Alphagan P, Lumify ◇, Mirvaso, Onreltea ✤

Therapeutic class: Antiglaucoma drugs–dermatologic agents
Pharmacologic class: Selective alpha$_2$ agonists

AVAILABLE FORMS
Ophthalmic solution: 0.025% ◇, 0.1%, 0.15%, 0.2%
Topical gel: 0.33%

INDICATIONS & DOSAGES
➤ **To reduce IOP in open-angle glaucoma or ocular HTN**
Adults and children age 2 and older: 1 drop in affected eye t.i.d., about 8 hours apart.
➤ **Relief of redness of the eye due to minor irritations (OTC only)**

Adults and children age 5 and older: Instill 1 drop in affected eye every 6 to 8 hours. Don't use more often than q.i.d.

➤ **Persistent erythema of rosacea (Mirvaso)**

Adults: Apply a pea-size amount to five areas of the face (central forehead, chin, nose, and each cheek) once daily.

ADMINISTRATION
Ophthalmic
• Don't touch tip of dropper to eye or surrounding tissue.
• If more than one ophthalmic product is being used, give them at least 5 minutes apart.
• Patient should remove contact lenses before administration and wait 10 minutes before reinserting or, if using products that contain benzalkonium chloride, wait 15 minutes.

Topical
• Apply a thin layer across the entire face, avoiding the lips and eyes.
• Don't apply to open wounds or irritated skin.
• Wash hands immediately after applying.
• Store at room temperature.

ACTION
Ophthalmic form reduces aqueous humor production and increases uveoscleral outflow. Topical form may reduce erythema through direct vasoconstriction.

Route	Onset	Peak	Duration
Ophthalmic	Unknown	30 min–2.5 hr	Unknown
Topical	Unknown	15 days	Unknown

Half-life: Ophthalmic, 2 hours; topical, unknown.

ADVERSE REACTIONS
CNS: asthenia, dizziness, headache, fatigue, somnolence, paresthesia, abnormal taste. **CV:** HTN, hypotension, flushing, chest pain. **EENT:** increased IOP, allergic conjunctivitis, ocular hyperemia, pruritus, abnormal vision, allergic reaction, blepharitis, burning; conjunctival edema, hemorrhage, or inflammation; dryness, eyelid edema or erythema, foreign body sensation, increased tearing, pain, photophobia, stinging (ophthalmic only); nasal congestion, nasopharyngitis, rhinitis, sinusitis, dry mouth. **GI:** dyspepsia. **Metabolic:** hypercholesterolemia. **Musculoskeletal:** pain. **Respiratory:** bronchitis, cough, dyspnea. **Skin:** rash; acne rosacea, acne vulgaris, allergic contact dermatitis, dermatitis, erythema, burning sensation, pain (topical only). **Other:** infection, flulike symptoms.

INTERACTIONS
Drug-drug. *Antihypertensives, beta blockers, cardiac glycosides:* May further decrease BP or pulse rate. Monitor vital signs.
Apraclonidine, dorzolamide, pilocarpine, timolol: May have additive IOP-lowering effects. Use cautiously together.
CNS depressants: May increase effects of depressant. Use cautiously together.
Linezolid, MAO inhibitors: May increase effects of brimonidine. Use cautiously together.
TCAs: May interfere with brimonidine's effect. Use cautiously together.
Drug-lifestyle. *Alcohol use:* May increase CNS depressant effect. Discourage use together.

EFFECTS ON LAB TEST RESULTS
• May increase cholesterol level.

CONTRAINDICATIONS & CAUTIONS
• Ophthalmic form is contraindicated in patients hypersensitive to drug or its components and in neonates, infants, and children younger than age 2.
• Topical gel is contraindicated in patients hypersensitive to drug or its components; reactions have included angioedema, urticaria, and contact dermatitis.
• Use cautiously in patients with CV disease, cerebral or coronary insufficiency, hepatic or renal impairment, depression, Raynaud phenomenon, Sjögren syndrome, orthostatic hypotension, or thromboangiitis obliterans.
Dialyzable drug: Unknown.
⚠ **Overdose S&S:** Hypotension.

PREGNANCY-LACTATION-REPRODUCTION
• Use during pregnancy only if potential benefit justifies fetal risk.
• It isn't known if drug appears in human milk. Consider discontinuing breastfeeding or discontinuing drug.

NURSING CONSIDERATIONS
• Monitor IOP because drug effect may reverse after first month of therapy.
• Erythema, intermittent flushing, or pallor or excessive whitening may occur after topical application and may resolve when therapy is discontinued.

PATIENT TEACHING
• Instruct patient in safe drug administration.
• Caution patient to avoid hazardous activities because of risk of decreased mental alertness, fatigue, or drowsiness.
• Advise patient to avoid alcohol.

brodalumab
broe-DAL-ue-mab

Siliq

Therapeutic class: Immunomodulators
Pharmacologic class: Interleukin receptor antagonists

AVAILABLE FORMS
Injection: 210 mg/1.5 mL in single-dose, prefilled syringe

INDICATIONS & DOSAGES
➤ **Moderate to severe plaque psoriasis in patients who are candidates for systemic therapy or phototherapy and have failed to respond or have lost response to other systemic therapies**
Adults: 210 mg subcut at weeks 0, 1, and 2, then every 2 weeks. If adequate response hasn't been achieved after 12 to 16 weeks of treatment, consider discontinuing therapy as success is less likely.

ADMINISTRATION
Subcutaneous
• Allow syringe to reach room temperature (approximately 30 minutes) before injecting. Don't warm in any other way. Don't remove gray needle cap until ready to inject.
• Once syringe has reached room temperature, don't rerefrigerate.
• Don't use drug if cloudy or discolored or if foreign matter is present. A few translucent to white particles may be present.
• Inject full amount of 1.5 mL to administer a 210-mg dose.
• Inject subcut into thigh, abdomen, or upper outer arm.
• Don't inject into areas where skin is tender, bruised, red, hard, thick, scaly, or affected by psoriasis.
• Store drug refrigerated at 36° to 46° F (2° to 8° C) in original carton to protect from light and damage during storage. When necessary, may store drug at room temperature

up to a maximum of 77° F (25° C) for a maximum single period of 14 days. Discard after 14 days at room temperature.
• Don't freeze or shake syringe or carton filled with syringes.

ACTION
A monoclonal antibody that binds to interleukin-17RA and inhibits proinflammatory cytokines and other inflammatory mediators, leading to decreased inflammation.

Route	Onset	Peak	Duration
Subcut	Unknown	3 days	Unknown

Half-life: Unknown.

ADVERSE REACTIONS
CNS: headache, fatigue. **EENT:** oropharyngeal pain. **GI:** diarrhea, nausea. **Hematologic:** *neutropenia.* **Musculoskeletal:** arthralgia, myalgia. **Skin:** injection-site reactions, tinea infections. **Other:** flulike symptoms, infections.

INTERACTIONS
Drug-drug. *Cyclosporine:* May decrease effect of cytokines on cyclosporine, a CYP450 substrate. Monitor cyclosporine level; adjust cyclosporine dosage as clinically indicated.
CYP450 substrates: May decrease effect of cytokines on CYP450 substrates. Adjust CYP450 substrate dosage as clinically indicated by drug concentration or therapeutic effect.
Live-virus vaccines: May affect ability to elicit immune response. Avoid use together.
Warfarin: May decrease effect of cytokines on warfarin, a CYP450 substrate. Monitor INR; adjust warfarin dosage as clinically indicated.

EFFECTS ON LAB TEST RESULTS
• May decrease ANC.

CONTRAINDICATIONS & CAUTIONS
• Contraindicated in patients with Crohn disease; drug may worsen disease.
Boxed Warning Suicidality, including completed suicides, have occurred in patients treated with this drug. ■
Boxed Warning Because of suicide risk, drug is available only through the restricted SILIQ REMS Program. ■
• Drug increases risk of infections, including serious infections.

• Drug increases risk of latent TB reactivation.

• Use cautiously in patients with chronic infection or history of recurrent infection.

• Safety and effectiveness in children haven't been evaluated.

Dialyzable drug: Unknown.

PREGNANCY-LACTATION-REPRODUCTION

• There are no human data concerning use during pregnancy. Because human IgG antibodies cross the placental barrier, drug may be transmitted from patient to developing fetus.

• It isn't known if drug appears in human milk. Drug's effect on infants who are breast-fed or on milk production is also unknown. Use only if benefit clearly outweighs risk to infant.

NURSING CONSIDERATIONS

• Discontinue drug if patient develops Crohn disease during therapy.

Boxed Warning Suicidality, including completed suicides, have occurred in patients treated with this drug. Before therapy, consider risks and benefits in patients with a history of depression or suicidality. ∎

Boxed Warning Assess for new or worsening suicidality, new-onset or worsening depression, anxiety, or other mood changes; refer patient to mental health professional, as appropriate. Reevaluate continued use of drug if changes occur. ∎

• Evaluate patients for TB before therapy begins. Consider anti-TB therapy before starting drug in patients with a history of latent TB or active TB when an adequate course of TB treatment can't be confirmed.

• Closely monitor patient for signs and symptoms of active TB during and after treatment.

• Monitor patient for signs and symptoms of infection (fever, malaise, cough, pain, skin changes, wound or rash with drainage). If a serious infection develops or patient isn't responding to standard treatment for the infection, discontinue drug until infection resolves.

• *Look alike–sound alike:* Don't confuse Siliq with Actiq.

PATIENT TEACHING

Boxed Warning Instruct patient and caregivers to watch for suicidality, new or worsening depression, anxiety, or other mood changes. Tell patient to carry provided Siliq patient wallet card and to call the National Suicide Prevention Lifeline (1-800-273-8255) if suicidality occurs. ∎

• Explain that drug may lower the ability to fight infection. Tell patient to report signs and symptoms of infection.

• Teach patient to report signs and symptoms of Crohn's disease (diarrhea, bloody stools, stomach pain or cramping, sudden or uncontrollable bowel movements, constipation, loss of appetite, weight loss, fever, fatigue).

• Show patient who plans to self-administer drug the injection technique. Explain need to follow manufacturer's instructions for use.

• Tell patient not to use the syringe if it has been dropped on a hard surface because a break in the syringe (which may or may not be obvious) may have occurred. Instruct patient to use a new syringe and to call 1-800-321-4576.

budesonide (inhalation, intranasal)
byoo-DES-oh-nide

Pulmicort Flexhaler, Pulmicort Respules, Pulmicort Nebuamp ✽, Pulmicort Turbuhaler ✽, Rhinocort Allergy ◇

Therapeutic class: Corticosteroids
Pharmacologic class: Corticosteroids

AVAILABLE FORMS

Dry powder inhaler: 90 mcg/dose, 100 mcg/dose ✽, 180 mcg/dose, 200 mcg/dose ✽, 400 mcg/dose ✽
Inhalation suspension (Respules): 0.25 mg/2 mL, 0.5 mg/2 mL, 1 mg/2 mL
Nasal spray: 32 mcg/metered spray

INDICATIONS & DOSAGES

➤ **As a preventative in maintenance of asthma**

All patients: Use lowest effective dose after stabilizing asthma.

Respules

Children ages 1 to 8 previously taking bronchodilator alone: 0.5 mg daily or 0.25 mg b.i.d. suspension via jet nebulizer. Maximum dose is 0.5 mg/day.

Children ages 1 to 8 previously taking inhaled corticosteroid: 0.5 mg daily or 0.25 mg b.i.d.

suspension via jet nebulizer to maximum dose of 1 mg/day.

Children ages 1 to 8 previously taking oral corticosteroid: 1 mg daily or 0.5 mg b.i.d. via jet nebulizer. Maximum dose is 1 mg/day.

Adjust-a-dose: Symptomatic children not responding to nonsteroidal therapy may require starting dose of 0.25 mg daily.

Flexhaler

Adults: Initially, inhaled dose of 360 mcg b.i.d. to maximum of 720 mcg b.i.d. Starting dose of 180 mcg b.i.d. may be adequate in some adults.

Children ages 6 to 17: Initially, inhaled dose of 180 mcg b.i.d. to maximum of 360 mcg b.i.d. Starting dose of 360 mcg b.i.d. may be appropriate in some children.

Turbuhaler

Adults and children age 12 and older when treatment with inhaled glucocorticoids is started, during periods of severe asthma, and while oral glucocorticoids are being reduced or discontinued: Initially, inhaled dose of 400 to 2,400 mcg daily divided into two to four administrations. Maintenance dose is usually 200 to 400 mcg b.i.d. Individualize dose to the lowest possible to meet therapeutic objective.

Children ages 6 to 12 when beginning budesonide, during periods of severe asthma, and while oral corticosteroids are being reduced or discontinued: Initially, inhaled dose of 100 to 200 mcg b.i.d. For maintenance, use lowest dose necessary to control symptoms.

➤ **Symptoms of seasonal or perennial allergic rhinitis**

Adults and children age 12 and older: 1 to 2 sprays in each nostril once daily. Once allergy symptoms improve, reduce to 1 spray in each nostril daily. Maximum dose, 4 sprays (256 mcg) per nostril once daily.

Children ages 6 to younger than 12: 1 spray per nostril daily. If allergy symptoms don't improve, may increase to 2 sprays per nostril daily. Once allergy symptoms improve, reduce to 1 spray in each nostril daily. Maximum dose, 2 sprays (128 mcg) per nostril daily.

ADMINISTRATION

Inhalational

• Give inhalation suspension at regular intervals daily or b.i.d., as directed.

• Give suspension with a jet nebulizer connected to a compressor with adequate airflow.

Make sure that it's equipped with a mouthpiece or suitable face mask.

• Total daily dose may be increased or given as a divided dose to improve control if needed. Titrate dosage downward again after asthma is stabilized.

• When aluminum foil envelope has been opened, the shelf-life of unused ampules is 2 weeks when protected from light.

• Refer to manufacturer's instructions before use. Prime inhaler before first use. Have patient inhale deeply and forcefully each time unit is used. Remind patient to rinse mouth with water after inhalation.

• Discard inhaler after 60 (90-mcg dose) or 120 (180-mcg dose) actuations.

Intranasal

• Prime pump by actuating eight times before first use. Reprime pump if not used for 2 or more days. Discard bottle after 120 sprays.

• If applicator hasn't been used for 14 days or more, rinse it and reprime with one spray or until a fine mist appears.

• Shake before each actuation.

• To instill intranasal drug, have patient blow nose to clear nasal passages and tilt head slightly forward. Insert nozzle into nostril, pointing away from septum. Patient should hold other nostril closed and inhale gently during spraying. Next, shake container and repeat in other nostril. Patient should avoid blowing nose for 15 minutes after administration.

• Wipe spray tip clean with a tissue.

• Store nasal canister with valve upward and away from extreme heat or cold.

ACTION

Exhibits potent glucocorticoid activity and weak mineralocorticoid activity. Drug inhibits mast cells, macrophages, and mediators (such as leukotrienes) involved in inflammation.

Route	Onset	Peak	Duration
Inhalation, powder	24 hr	1–2 wk	Unknown
Inhalation, Respules	2–8 days	4–6 wk	Unknown
Intranasal	10 hr	2 wk	Unknown

Half-life: Inhalation and intranasal, 2 to 3 hours.

ADVERSE REACTIONS

CNS: headache, asthenia, fever, hypertonia, insomnia, pain, syncope, taste perversion, fatigue, emotional lability. **CV:** chest pain.

EENT: conjunctivitis, otitis media, otitis externa, sinusitis, pharyngitis, rhinitis, voice alteration, dry mouth; epistaxis and nasal irritation (intranasal). **GI:** abdominal pain, dyspepsia, diarrhea, gastroenteritis, nausea, oral candidiasis, vomiting, anorexia. **Metabolic:** weight gain. **Musculoskeletal:** back pain, fractures, myalgia. **Respiratory:** respiratory tract infection, *bronchospasm,* increased cough, stridor. **Skin:** ecchymoses, rash, dermatitis, pruritus, eczema. **Other:** flulike symptoms, hypersensitivity reactions, viral infection, cervical lymphadenopathy.

INTERACTIONS

Drug-drug. *Strong CYP3A4 inhibitors (atazanavir, clarithromycin, itraconazole, ketoconazole, nefazodone, nelfinavir, ritonavir, saquinavir, telithromycin):* May inhibit metabolism and increase level of budesonide. Monitor patient for adverse reactions and adjust dosage as needed.

EFFECTS ON LAB TEST RESULTS
None reported.

CONTRAINDICATIONS & CAUTIONS
• Contraindicated in patients hypersensitive to drug, in those with severe hypersensitivity to milk proteins (powder for inhalation), and in those with status asthmaticus or other acute asthma episodes.
• Use nasal formulation cautiously in patients with septal ulcers, nasal surgery, nasal trauma, or untreated localized nasal mucosa infections.
• Use cautiously, if at all, in patients with active or inactive TB, ocular HSV infections, or untreated systemic fungal, bacterial, viral, or parasitic infections.
Dialyzable drug: Unlikely.
⚠ *Overdose S&S:* Hyperadrenocorticism.

PREGNANCY-LACTATION-REPRODUCTION
• Hypoadrenalism may occur in infants of patients who received corticosteroids during pregnancy. Monitor these infants carefully.
• Studies during pregnancy of patients using inhaled or intranasal form haven't demonstrated an increased risk of abnormalities. Inhaled corticosteroids are recommended for the treatment of asthma during pregnancy.
• Drug appears in human milk. Patient should use lowest possible dose immediately after breastfeeding to maximize time between dose and breastfeeding.

NURSING CONSIDERATIONS
⚠ *Alert:* When transferring from systemic corticosteroid to inhalation drug, use caution and gradually decrease corticosteroid dose to prevent adrenal insufficiency.
• Inhalation drug doesn't remove the need for systemic corticosteroid therapy in some situations.
• Systemic effects of corticosteroid therapy may occur if recommended daily dosage is exceeded.
• If bronchospasm occurs after inhalation use, stop therapy and treat with a bronchodilator.
• Lung function may improve within 24 hours of starting therapy, but maximum benefit may not be achieved for 1 to 2 weeks or longer.
• For Pulmicort Respules, lung function improves in 2 to 8 days, but maximum benefit may not be seen for 4 to 6 weeks.
• Watch for *Candida* infections of the mouth or pharynx.
⚠ *Alert:* Corticosteroids may increase risk of developing serious or fatal infections in patients exposed to viral illnesses, such as chickenpox or measles.
• In rare cases, inhaled corticosteroids have been linked to increased IOP and cataract development. Stop drug if local irritation occurs.
• Monitor bone mineral density in patients at risk for decreased bone mineral content (prolonged immobilization, family history of osteoporosis, postmenopausal status).
• Monitor children for reduction in growth velocity. Use lowest effective dose.
• Monitor patients for hypercorticism and adrenal suppression and if they occur, reduce dosage slowly.
• Rare cases of vasculitis (eosinophilic granulomatosis with polyangiitis) and other eosinophilic conditions have occurred when systemic corticosteroids have been reduced or withdrawn. Monitor patients for eosinophilia, vasculitic rash, worsening pulmonary symptoms, cardiac symptoms, and neuropathy.

PATIENT TEACHING
• Tell patient that budesonide inhaler isn't a bronchodilator and isn't intended to treat acute episodes of asthma.

Reactions in bold italics are *life-threatening*. Interactions may have a *rapid onset* or a ***delayed onset***.

• Instruct patient to use the inhaler according to manufacturer's instructions at regular intervals because effectiveness depends on twice-daily use on a regular basis.
• Tell patient that improvement in asthma control may be seen within 24 hours, although maximum benefit may not appear for 1 to 2 weeks. If signs or symptoms worsen during this time, instruct patient to contact prescriber.
• Advise patient to avoid exposure to chickenpox or measles and to contact prescriber if exposure occurs.
• Instruct patient using inhaler to carry or wear medical identification indicating need for supplementary corticosteroids during periods of stress or an asthma attack.
• Tell patient to read and follow patient information leaflet contained in package.
• Advise patient using nasal formula to notify prescriber if signs or symptoms don't improve or if they worsen in 3 weeks.
• Teach patient good nasal and oral hygiene and not to share drug because this could spread infection.

budesonide (oral, rectal)
byoo-DES-oh-nide

Entocort EC, Ortikos, Tarpeyo, Uceris

Therapeutic class: Corticosteroids
Pharmacologic class: Glucocorticoids

AVAILABLE FORMS
Capsules (delayed-release 🌕*):* 3 mg, 4 mg
Capsules (extended-release 🌕*):* 6 mg, 9 mg
Foam: 2 mg/actuation
Tablets (extended-release 🌕*):* 9 mg

INDICATIONS & DOSAGES
Adjust-a-dose (for all indications): In patients with moderate to severe liver disease who have increased signs or symptoms of hypercorticism, reduce dosage or avoid use
➤ **Mild to moderate active Crohn disease involving the ileum, ascending colon, or both (capsules)**
Adults: 9 mg PO once daily in morning for up to 8 weeks. For recurrent episodes of active Crohn disease, may give a repeat 8-week course.

Children ages 8 to 17 weighing more than 25 kg: 9 mg PO once daily in the morning for up to 8 weeks, followed by 6 mg once daily in the morning for 2 weeks.
➤ **To maintain remission in mild to moderate Crohn disease that involves the ileum or ascending colon (capsules)**
Adults: 6 mg PO daily in the morning for up to 3 months. Taper dosage to complete cessation after 3 months. Therapy for longer than 3 months doesn't have added benefit.
➤ **Induction of remission in active mild to moderate ulcerative colitis (tablets)**
Adults: 9 mg PO once daily in the morning for up to 8 weeks.
➤ **Induction of remission in mild to moderate distal ulcerative colitis (rectal foam)**
Adults: 2 mg (1 metered dose) PR b.i.d. for 2 weeks then 2 mg PR once daily for 4 weeks.
✳ *NEW INDICATION:* **Proteinuria in patients with primary IgA neuropathy at risk for rapid disease progression**
Adults: 16 mg PO daily in the morning at least 1 hour before a meal.
Adjust-a-dose: Reduce dosage to 8 mg daily for 2 weeks before discontinuing drug.

ADMINISTRATION
PO
• Give drug whole; don't break or crush capsule or tablet.
• For patients unable to swallow an intact capsule: open capsule (Entocort EC), mix contents with 1 tablespoon of applesauce; have patient consume within 30 minutes of mixing. Follow with a full glass of water. For other formulations (Ortikos, Uceris, Tarpeyo): patient should swallow whole and not chew, crush, or open.
Rectal
• Attach applicator to canister nozzle. Warm canister in the hands while shaking it for 10 to 15 seconds.
• Unlock canister top; then turn it upside down and insert applicator tip into rectum.
• Push down on pump dome for 2 seconds and hold applicator in place for 10 to 15 seconds.
• Withdraw and discard used applicator.

ACTION
Significant glucocorticoid effects caused by drug's high affinity for glucocorticoid receptors.

🍁Canada ◇OTC ◆Off-label use ✐Photoguide 🌕Do not crush *Liquid contains alcohol ⚚Genetic

Route	Onset	Peak	Duration
PO	Unknown	0.5–10 hr	Unknown
PO (extended-release)	Unknown	7.4–19.2 hr	Unknown
Rectal	Unknown	Unknown	Unknown

Half-life: 2 to 8 hours.

ADVERSE REACTIONS

CNS: headache, dizziness, asthenia, hyperkinesia, paresthesia, tremor, weakness, vertigo, fatigue, malaise, agitation, confusion, drowsiness, insomnia, nervousness, somnolence, pain, sleep disorder, fever. **CV:** chest pain, HTN, edema, palpitations, tachycardia, flushing. **EENT:** facial edema, eye abnormality, abnormal vision, ear infection, sinusitis, rhinitis, pharyngeal disorder, glossitis, tooth disorder. **GI:** nausea, diarrhea, dyspepsia, abdominal pain, flatulence, vomiting, anal disorder, aggravated Crohn disease, enteritis, epigastric pain, fistula, glossitis, hemorrhoids, intestinal obstruction, increased appetite, abdominal distention, constipation. **GU:** dysuria, micturition frequency, nocturia, intermenstrual bleeding, menstrual disorder, hematuria, pyuria, UTI. **Hematologic:** leukocytosis, anemia. **Metabolic:** hypercorticism, adrenocortical insufficiency, *hypokalemia*, increased weight. **Musculoskeletal:** back pain, aggravated arthritis, cramps, arthralgia, myalgia. **Respiratory:** respiratory tract infection, bronchitis, dyspnea. **Skin:** acne, alopecia, dermatitis, eczema, skin disorder, diaphoresis, purpura, hirsutism, bruising. **Other:** flulike disorder, candidiasis, viral infection.

INTERACTIONS

Drug-drug. *CYP3A4 inhibitors (cyclosporine, erythromycin, itraconazole, ketoconazole, ritonavir, saquinavir):* May increase effects of budesonide. If use together is unavailable, reduce budesonide dosage.
Gastric acid secretion inhibitors (antacids, H_2 blockers, PPIs): May affect dissolution of extended-release budesonide. Avoid use together or separate administration times by as much as possible and monitor clinical response to budesonide.
Quinolones (levofloxacin): May increase risk of tendon rupture when taken concomitantly with corticosteroids. Avoid use together.
Salicylates (aspirin): May decrease salicylate level and effectiveness and increase risk of GI bleeding. Monitor patient response and adjust salicylate dosage as needed.
Drug-food. *Grapefruit juice:* May increase drug effects. Discourage use together.

EFFECTS ON LAB TEST RESULTS
• May increase ALP and C-reactive protein levels. May decrease potassium, cortisol, and Hb levels.
• May increase erythrocyte sedimentation rate and WBC count.

CONTRAINDICATIONS & CAUTIONS
• Contraindicated in patients hypersensitive to drug.
• Use cautiously in patients with TB, HTN, diabetes, osteoporosis, hepatic impairment, peptic ulcer disease, glaucoma, or cataracts; those with a family history of diabetes or glaucoma; and those with any other condition in which glucocorticoids may have unwanted effects.
Dialyzable drug: Unlikely.
⚠ *Overdose S&S:* Hypercorticism, adrenal suppression.

PREGNANCY-LACTATION-REPRODUCTION
• May use drug cautiously during pregnancy for the induction of remission in patients with inflammatory bowel disease. Use only if potential benefit justifies fetal risk.
• Monitor infants born of patients receiving corticosteroids during pregnancy for signs and symptoms of hypoadrenalism, such as poor feeding, irritability, weakness, and vomiting.
• Glucocorticoids appear in human milk, and infants may have adverse reactions. Use cautiously during breastfeeding and only if benefits outweigh risks.

NURSING CONSIDERATIONS
• Reduced liver function affects elimination of this drug; systemic availability of drug may increase in patients with liver cirrhosis. Consider dosage reduction or discontinue drug with severe liver dysfunction.
• Patients undergoing surgery or other stressful situations may need systemic glucocorticoid supplementation in addition to budesonide therapy.
• Carefully monitor patients transferred from systemic glucocorticoid therapy to budesonide for signs and symptoms of corticosteroid withdrawal. Watch for

---

immunosuppression, especially in patients who haven't had diseases such as chickenpox or measles; these can be fatal in patients who are immunosuppressed or receiving glucocorticoids.
• Replacement of systemic glucocorticoids with this drug may unmask allergies, such as eczema and rhinitis, which were previously controlled by systemic drug.
• Long-term use of drug may cause hypercorticism and adrenal suppression.

PATIENT TEACHING
• Tell patient to swallow capsules and tablets whole and not to chew, crush, or break them. Inform patient that Entocort EC capsules can be opened and the contents sprinkled on applesauce.
• Advise patient to avoid grapefruit juice while taking drug.
• Tell patient to notify prescriber immediately if patient is exposed to or develops chickenpox or measles or develops signs and symptoms of infection during treatment.
• Tell patient to keep container tightly closed.
• Teach patient how to administer rectal formulation and to keep it away from flame.

bumetanide
byoo-MET-a-nide

Bumex◆, Burinex✤

Therapeutic class: Diuretics
Pharmacologic class: Loop diuretics

AVAILABLE FORMS
Injection: 0.25 mg/mL
Tablets: 0.5 mg, 1 mg, 2 mg, 5 mg✤

INDICATIONS & DOSAGES
➤ **Edema caused by HF or hepatic or renal disease**
Adults: 0.5 to 2 mg PO once daily. If diuretic response isn't adequate, a second or third dose may be given at 4- to 5-hour intervals. Or (recommended as the safest and most effective method for the continued control of edema) give on an intermittent-dose schedule on alternate days or for 3 to 4 days with rest periods of 1 to 2 days in between. Maximum, 10 mg daily.

May give parenterally if oral route isn't possible or if risk of impaired GI absorption

exists. Usual first dose is 0.5 to 1 mg IV or IM. If response isn't adequate, may give a second or third dose at 2- to 3-hour intervals. Maximum, 10 mg daily.

ADMINISTRATION
PO
• To prevent nocturia, give drug in morning. If second dose is needed, give in early afternoon.
IV
▼ For direct injection, give drug over 1 to 2 minutes.
▼ For intermittent infusion, give diluted drug through an intermittent infusion device or piggyback into an IV line containing a free-flowing, compatible solution.
▼ Solutions should be freshly prepared and used within 24 hours. Protect from light.
▼ **Incompatibilities:** None listed by manufacturer. Consult a drug incompatibility reference for more information.
IM
• Document injection site.

ACTION
Inhibits sodium and chloride reabsorption in the ascending loop of Henle.

Route	Onset	Peak	Duration
PO	30–60 min	1–2 hr	4–6 hr
IV	Within min	15–30 min	2–3 hr
IM	40 min	Unknown	5–6 hr

Half-life: 1 to 1.5 hours.

ADVERSE REACTIONS
CNS: dizziness, headache. **CV:** hypotension. **EENT:** impaired hearing. **GU:** increased creatinine level, azotemia. **Hepatic:** increased LDH level. **Metabolic:** volume depletion, dehydration, *hypokalemia,* hypochloremia, *hypomagnesemia,* hyperuricemia, hyponatremia, hyperglycemia. **Musculoskeletal:** muscle cramps.

INTERACTIONS
Drug-drug. *Aminoglycoside antibiotics:* May increase ototoxicity. Avoid using together if possible.
Antidiabetics: May decrease hypoglycemic effects. Monitor glucose level.
Antihypertensives: May increase hypotensive effects. Consider dosage adjustment.
Cardiac glycosides: May increase risk of digoxin toxicity from bumetanide-induced

hypokalemia. Monitor potassium and digoxin levels.

Chlorothiazide, chlorthalidone, furosemide, hydrochlorothiazide, indapamide, metolazone: May cause excessive diuretic response, causing serious electrolyte abnormalities or dehydration. Adjust doses carefully, and monitor patient closely for signs and symptoms of excessive diuretic response.

Cisplatin: May increase risk of ototoxicity and nephrotoxicity. Monitor patient closely.

Lithium: May decrease lithium clearance, increasing risk of lithium toxicity. Monitor lithium level.

Neuromuscular blockers: May prolong neuromuscular blockade. Monitor patient closely.

NSAIDs, probenecid: May inhibit diuretic response. Use together cautiously.

Other potassium-wasting drugs (amphotericin B, corticosteroids): May increase risk of hypokalemia. Use together cautiously.

Drug-herb. *Dandelion:* May increase diuresis. Discourage use together.

Licorice: May cause unexpected, rapid potassium loss. Discourage use together.

EFFECTS ON LAB TEST RESULTS
• May increase ALP, ALT, AST, bilirubin, protein, cholesterol, creatinine, glucose, LDH, BUN, and urine urea levels.
• May decrease calcium, magnesium, potassium, sodium, and chloride levels.
• May decrease platelet count.

CONTRAINDICATIONS & CAUTIONS
• Contraindicated in patients hypersensitive to drug and in patients with anuria, hepatic coma, or severe electrolyte depletion.
• Patients allergic to sulfonamides may show hypersensitivity to bumetanide.
• Use cautiously in patients with hepatic cirrhosis and ascites or decreased renal function and in older adults.

Dialyzable drug: Unknown.

⚠ *Overdose S&S:* Electrolyte depletion, weakness, dizziness, confusion, anorexia, lethargy, vomiting, cramps, dehydration, circulatory collapse, vascular thrombosis, and embolism.

PREGNANCY-LACTATION-REPRODUCTION
• There are no adequate well-controlled studies during pregnancy. Use during pregnancy only if potential benefits justify fetal risk.

• Use isn't recommended during breast-feeding.

NURSING CONSIDERATIONS
Boxed Warning Profound diuresis with electrolyte depletion can occur. Adjust dosage and dosing schedule to individual patient's needs; careful medical supervision is required. ∎
• Monitor fluid intake and output, weight, and electrolyte, BUN, creatinine, and carbon dioxide levels frequently, especially in older adults.
• Watch for evidence of hypokalemia, such as muscle weakness and cramps. Instruct patient to report these symptoms.
• Consult prescriber and dietitian about a high-potassium diet. Foods rich in potassium include citrus fruits, tomatoes, bananas, dates, and apricots.
• Monitor glucose level in patients with diabetes.
• Monitor uric acid level, especially in patients with history of gout.
• If oliguria or azotemia develops or increases, prescriber may stop drug.
• Drug can be safely used in patients allergic to furosemide; 1 mg of bumetanide equals about 40 mg of furosemide.
• Monitor patient for ototoxicity, especially when drug is given IV, at high doses, and in combination with other ototoxins.

PATIENT TEACHING
• Instruct patient to weigh self daily to monitor fluid status.
• Advise patient to take drug in morning to avoid need to urinate at night. Tell patient who needs second dose to take it in early afternoon.
• Advise patient to avoid sudden posture changes and to rise slowly to avoid dizziness upon standing quickly.
• Instruct patient to notify prescriber about extreme thirst, muscle weakness, cramps, nausea, or dizziness.

Reactions in bold italics are *life-threatening*. Interactions may have a *rapid onset* or a ***delayed onset***.

B

buprenorphine
byoo-pre-NOR-feen

Butrans, Sublocade

buprenorphine hydrochloride
Belbuca, Buprenex

Therapeutic class: Opioid analgesics
Pharmacologic class: Opioid agonist-antagonists–opioid partial agonists
Controlled substance schedule: III

AVAILABLE FORMS
Buccal film: 75 mcg, 150 mcg, 300 mcg, 450 mcg, 600 mcg, 750 mcg, 900 mcg
Injection: 0.324 mg (equivalent to 0.3 mg base/mL)
Injection (extended-release): 100 mg/0.5 mL, 300 mg/1.5 mL prefilled syringes
Sublingual tablets ⊖*:* 2 mg, 8 mg (as base)
Transdermal patch: 5 mcg/hour, 7.5 mcg/hour, 10 mcg/hour, 15 mcg/hour, 20 mcg/hour

INDICATIONS & DOSAGES
➤ **Moderate to severe pain**
Adults and children age 13 and older: 0.3 mg IM or slow IV (over at least 2 minutes) every 6 hours PRN, or around the clock; repeat dose once (up to 0.3 mg), as needed, 30 to 60 minutes after first dose. May increase IM dosing to 0.6 mg/dose.
Children ages 2 to 12: 2 to 6 mcg/kg IM or slow IV (over at least 2 minutes) every 4 to 6 hours.
Adjust-a-dose: In patients at high risk, such as older adults and patients who are debilitated, use minimum dose required.
➤ **Moderate to severe chronic pain in patients requiring continuous opioid analgesia for an extended period of time and alternative treatment options are inadequate**
Adults (opioid-naive): 5 mcg/hour transdermal patch once every 7 days. May titrate dosage to maximum of 20 mcg/hour. Allow minimum of 72 hours between dosage increases. Or, 75 mcg buccal film once daily or, if tolerated, every 12 hours for at least 4 days; then increase to 150 mcg every 12 hours. May titrate dosage as needed in increments of 150 mcg every 12 hours, no more frequently than every 4 days. Maximum, 450 mcg every 12 hours.

Adults (non-opioid-naive): Buprenorphine may precipitate withdrawal in patients already on opioids. For conversion from other opioids to transdermal buprenorphine, taper patient's current around-the-clock opioids for up to 7 days to no more than morphine 30 mg or equivalent per day before beginning treatment with buprenorphine. Patients may use short-acting analgesics as needed until analgesic efficacy with buprenorphine is attained. For patients whose daily dose was less than morphine 30 mg PO or equivalent, initiate treatment with buprenorphine transdermal patch 5 mcg/hour. For patients whose daily dose was between 30 and 80 mg of morphine equivalents, initiate treatment with buprenorphine transdermal patch 10 mcg/hour.

For patients whose daily dose was greater than 80 mg of morphine equivalents, buprenorphine transdermal system 20 mcg/hour may not provide adequate analgesia. Consider the use of an alternative analgesic.

May titrate dosage to maximum of 20 mcg/hour transdermal patch once every 7 days. Allow minimum of 72 hours between dosage increases. If patch must be discontinued, taper dosage gradually every 7 days to prevent withdrawal in patient who is physically dependent; consider initiating immediate-release opioids, if needed.

Or, for conversion from other opioids to buccal buprenorphine, taper dosage to no more than 30 mg PO morphine sulfate equivalents (MSE) per day. For patients taking less than 30 mg PO MSE per day, start treatment with 75 mcg buccal film once daily or every 12 hours. For patients taking between 30 and 89 mg PO MSE, start treatment with 150 mcg every 12 hours. For patients taking between 90 and 160 mg PO MSE, start treatment with 300 mcg every 12 hours. Buccal buprenorphine may not provide adequate analgesia for patients requiring greater than 160 mg PO MSE per day. Consider using an alternative analgesic. Titrate dosage in increments of 150 mcg every 12 hours, no more frequently than every 4 days to a maximum dose of 900 mcg every 12 hours.

To discontinue buccal therapy, taper dosage gradually while monitoring patient carefully for signs and symptoms of withdrawal. If patient develops withdrawal signs or symptoms, increase dosage to previous level and taper more slowly by increasing the interval between decreases, decreasing the amount of change in dose, or both.

Adjust-a-dose: Transdermal buprenorphine hasn't been evaluated in patients with severe hepatic impairment. Consider use of an alternative analgesic that may permit more dosing flexibility in these patients.

In patients with severe hepatic impairment, reduce the buccal starting dose and reduce the buccal titration dose by half that of patients with normal liver function, from 150 to 75 mcg. In patients with known or suspected mucositis, reduce starting dosage and titration incremental dosage by half compared to patients without mucositis.

➤ **Opioid use disorder**

Adults: 8 mg SL on day 1 and 16 mg SL on day 2. Titrate buprenorphine dosage in increments or decrements of 2 or 4 mg to a level that holds patient in treatment and suppresses opioid withdrawal signs and symptoms. Maintenance dose is generally in the range of 4 to 24 mg SL per day. Recommended target dosage is 16 mg as a single daily dose. Continue treatment for as long as patient is benefiting and the drug contributes to intended treatment goals.

➤ **Moderate to severe opioid use disorder in patients who have initiated treatment with a transmucosal buprenorphine-containing product, followed by dosage adjustment for a minimum of 7 days (Sublocade)**

Adults: 300 mg (extended-release) subcut monthly for first 2 months, followed by 100 mg (extended-release) subcut maintenance dose monthly. May increase maintenance dose to 300 mg monthly for patients who tolerate 100-mg dose but don't demonstrate a satisfactory clinical response. Administer drug with a minimum of 26 days between doses.

ADMINISTRATION

IV

▼ For direct injection, give slowly over at least 2 minutes into a vein or through tubing of a free-flowing, compatible IV solution.

▼ **Incompatibilities:** None listed by manufacturer. Consult a drug incompatibility reference for more information.

IM

• Inspect for particulate matter and discoloration.

• Give drug as deep IM injection.

Subcutaneous

Boxed Warning Sublocade may cause serious harm or death if given IV. Don't administer Sublocade IV or IM. ∎

• Only health care providers should prepare and administer Sublocade.

• Use only syringe and safety needle supplied.

• Remove drug from refrigerator at least 15 minutes before use. Don't open foil pack until ready for use. Discard drug if left at room temperature for longer than 7 days.

• Don't use if particles or discoloration is present.

• Remove excess air from syringe and inject drug subcut in abdomen only. Select a site between the transpyloric and transtubercular planes, avoiding areas where skin is irritated, red, bruised, infected, or scarred.

• Don't rub skin after injection. A lump may be felt for several weeks that will shrink over time.

• Rotate injection sites.

• Give a missed dose as soon as possible, with the next dose no sooner than 26 days later. Occasional dosing delays up to 2 weeks aren't expected to significantly impact treatment.

Sublingual

• Place all tablets of the dose under the tongue until dissolved. Must give tablets whole.

• Patient shouldn't eat or drink anything until the tablets are completely dissolved.

• After transmucosal medicine has completely dissolved, assist patient with gently rinsing teeth and gums with water then swallowing the water. Have patient wait at least 1 hour before brushing teeth.

Transdermal

⟳ *Alert:* Avoid exposing patch or surrounding area to direct external heat source or direct sunlight. Such exposure may increase amount of drug released, which can result in overdose and death.

• Each patch is intended to be worn for 7 days. If patch falls off during 7-day dosing interval, apply new patch to different site.

• Don't use if pouch seal is broken or patch is cut, damaged, or altered. Apply patch to intact skin immediately after opening.

• Appropriate application sites are upper outer arm, upper chest, upper back, or side of the chest (eight total available sites).

Reactions in bold italics are *life-threatening*. Interactions may have a *rapid onset* or a ***delayed onset***.

• Application site should be hairless; clip hair if needed but don't shave site. If needed, clean selected site with water only and allow to dry completely before applying patch.

• Edges of patch may be taped to the skin if needed.

• After removing patch, fold it in half, seal it in patch-disposal unit, and place it in trash.

• Wait minimum of 3 weeks before applying new patch to same application site.

• Exposure of patch to water, such as while bathing or showering, is acceptable.

Buccal

• Don't use film if package seal is broken or film is cut, damaged, or altered.

• To administer, first have patient moisten inside of cheek with tongue or water.

• Apply film immediately after removal from sealed package. Place yellow side of film against inside of cheek and hold in place with dry fingers for 5 seconds; then leave in place until film fully dissolves (about 30 minutes).

• Make sure patient doesn't chew or swallow film and doesn't eat or drink until film has dissolved.

🔵 *Alert:* After medication completely dissolves, assist patient with gently rinsing teeth and gums with water then swallowing the water. Have patient wait at least 1 hour before brushing teeth.

ACTION

Unknown. Binds with opioid receptors in the CNS, altering perception of and emotional response to pain.

Route	Onset	Peak	Duration
IV	Immediate	2 min	6 hr
IM	15 min	1 hr	6 hr
Subcut	Unknown	24 hr	Unknown
SL	Unknown	30–60 min	Unknown
Transdermal	17 hr	3–6 days	7 days
Buccal	Unknown	0.5–4 hr	Unknown

Half-life: 1 to 7 hours; subcut, 43 to 60 days; transdermal, 26 hours; buccal, 16 to 39 hours.

ADVERSE REACTIONS

CNS: dizziness, sedation, vertigo, depression, dreaming, fatigue, headache, insomnia, anxiety, pain, paresthesia, weakness, somnolence, fever. **CV:** HTN, hypotension, tachycardia, peripheral edema. **EENT:** conjunctivitis, diplopia, miosis, nasopharyngitis, sinus congestion, sinusitis, dry mouth, oropharyngeal pain. **GI:** nausea, abdominal pain, constipation, diarrhea, vomiting, anorexia, dyspepsia, gastroenteritis. **GU:** urine retention, UTI. **Hematologic:** anemia. **Hepatic:** increased AST and ALT levels. **Metabolic:** increased GGT and CK levels. **Musculoskeletal:** arthralgia, back pain, muscle spasm, joint swelling, extremity pain. **Respiratory:** *respiratory depression*, dyspnea, hypoventilation, URI, bronchitis. **Skin:** application-site rash or erythema (patch), diaphoresis, injection-site reactions, pruritus, rash, bruising. **Other:** chills, hot flashes, infection, withdrawal syndrome, flulike symptoms.

INTERACTIONS

Drug-drug. *Anticholinergics:* May increase risk of constipation and urine retention. Monitor therapy.

Boxed Warning *Benzodiazepines, CNS depressants:* May cause slow or difficult breathing, sedation, and death. Avoid use together. If use together is necessary, limit dosage and duration of each drug to the minimum necessary for desired effect. ■

Class IA or III antiarrhythmics: May increase risk of prolonged QT syndrome. Monitor patient closely.

CYP3A4 inducers (carbamazepine, phenobarbital, phenytoin, rifampin): May increase clearance of buprenorphine. Monitor patient for clinical effects of drug. If patient is taking Sublocade, patient may need to be transitioned back to a formulation that permits dosage adjustments.

CYP3A4 inhibitors (erythromycin, ketoconazole, ritonavir, saquinavir): May decrease clearance of buprenorphine. Monitor patient for increased adverse effects.

Diuretics: May decrease therapeutic effects of diuretics. Monitor therapy.

MAO inhibitors: May cause additive effects. Avoid use together.

NNRTIs (delavirdine, efavirenz, etravirine, nevirapine): May increase or decrease therapeutic effects of Sublocade. Monitor therapy closely.

🔵 *Alert: Serotonergic drugs (amoxapine, antiemetics [dolasetron, granisetron, ondansetron, palonosetron], antimigraine drugs, buspirone, cyclobenzaprine, dextromethorphan, linezolid, lithium, MAO inhibitors, maprotiline, methylene blue, mirtazapine, nefazodone, SSNRIs, SSRIs, TCAs, trazodone, tryptophan, vilazodone):* Can increase risk of serotonin syndrome. Use together cautiously; monitor patient for serotonin syndrome.

Skeletal muscle relaxants: May enhance neuromuscular blocking action and increase respiratory depression. Use together cautiously.

Drug-lifestyle. *Alcohol or illicit drug use:* May cause additive effects. Discourage use together.

EFFECTS ON LAB TEST RESULTS

• May increase amylase, ALT, AST, GGT, and CK levels.

CONTRAINDICATIONS & CAUTIONS

• Contraindicated in patients hypersensitive to drug and in those with paralytic ileus or GI obstruction.

Boxed Warning Serious, life-threatening, or fatal respiratory depression may occur, especially during drug initiation or after a dosage increase. Misuse or abuse of drug by chewing, swallowing, snorting, or injecting buprenorphine extracted from the transdermal system will result in the uncontrolled delivery of buprenorphine and will pose a significant risk of overdose and death. ■

Boxed Warning *Opioid class warning:* Opioids should only be prescribed with benzodiazepines or other CNS depressants to patients for whom alternative treatment options are inadequate. ■

Boxed Warning Buprenorphine is only available through REMS Program. Health care settings and pharmacies that order and dispense this drug must be certified in this program and comply with the REMS requirements. ■

Boxed Warning Never inject Sublocade IV. Serious harm or death can occur as drug forms a solid mass upon contact with body fluids. If given IV, local tissue damage and thromboembolic events can occur. ■

• To achieve adequate analgesia and minimize adverse effects, consider patient's tolerance, condition, and other medications.

◐ *Alert:* Don't exceed dose of one 20-mcg/hour transdermal patch every 7 days or 900 mcg every 12 hours for buccal film due to risk of prolonging QTc interval.

◐ *Alert:* Patients are at increased risk for oversedation and respiratory depression if they snore or have a history of sleep apnea, haven't used opioids recently or are first-time opioid users, have increased opioid dosage requirements or opioid habituation, received general anesthesia for longer lengths of time, received other sedating drugs, have thoracic or other surgical incisions that may impair breathing, or have preexisting pulmonary or cardiac disease. Monitor these patients carefully.

◐ *Alert:* Drug may lead to rare but serious decrease in adrenal gland cortisol production.

◐ *Alert:* Combined use of medication-assisted treatment (MAT) drugs methadone or buprenorphine with benzodiazepines or other CNS depressants increases risk of serious adverse effects; however, the harm caused by untreated opioid addiction may outweigh these risks. Patients may require MAT for opioid addiction indefinitely, and the use of these drugs should continue for as long as patients are benefiting and their use contributes to the intended treatment goals.

• Use cautiously in older adults and patients who are debilitated or morbidly obese; patients who are opioid dependent; in those undergoing biliary tract surgery and those with biliary tract disease or pancreatitis; in those with head injury, intracranial lesions, and increased ICP; severe respiratory, liver, or kidney impairment; CNS depression or coma; those at risk for hypotension and circulatory shock; and in those with thyroid irregularities, adrenal insufficiency, prostatic hypertrophy, urethral stricture, acute alcoholism, delirium tremens, or kyphoscoliosis.

• Don't use Sublocade in patients with preexisting moderate to severe hepatic impairment as buprenorphine levels can't be rapidly adjusted. If patient develops moderate to severe hepatic impairment during treatment, and buprenorphine toxicity or overdose occurs within 2 weeks of drug administration, surgical removal of the depot may be needed.

Dialyzable drug: Unknown.

⚠ *Overdose S&S:* Respiratory depression, pinpoint pupils, sedation, hypotension, death, snoring, bradycardia, cool and clammy skin, partial or complete airway obstruction, skeletal muscle flaccidity, somnolence.

PREGNANCY-LACTATION-REPRODUCTION

• There are no adequate and controlled studies during pregnancy. Use during pregnancy only if potential benefits justify fetal risk.

Boxed Warning Prolonged use during pregnancy can result in neonatal opioid withdrawal syndrome, which may be

---

Reactions in bold italics are *life-threatening*. Interactions may have a *rapid onset* or a ***delayed onset***.

life-threatening if not recognized and treated and requires management according to protocols developed by neonatology experts. If prolonged opioid use is required during pregnancy, advise patient of the risk of neonatal opioid withdrawal syndrome and ensure patient that appropriate treatment will be available. ▉

• Drug appears in human milk. Use during breastfeeding isn't recommended.

• Monitor infants exposed to large doses of opioids during breastfeeding for apnea and sedation. Withdrawal symptoms can occur in infants when drug or breastfeeding is stopped.

NURSING CONSIDERATIONS

Boxed Warning Buprenorphine has potential for abuse similar to other opioids and is a controlled substance. Patients at risk for opioid abuse include those with personal or family history of substance abuse or mental illness. Assess for risk of abuse before prescribing, and monitor patients regularly. ▉

Boxed Warning Accidental exposure to drug, especially in children, can cause a fatal overdose. ▉

• Don't stop drug abruptly; withdraw slowly and individualize the gradual taper plan to prevent signs and symptoms of withdrawal, worsening pain, and psychological distress in patients who are physically dependent. Refer to manufacturer's label for specific tapering instructions.

• When tapering opioids, watch closely for signs and symptoms of opioid withdrawal. Such symptoms may indicate a need to taper more slowly. Also monitor patient for suicidality, use of other substances, and mood changes.

🜂 *Alert:* Carefully monitor vital signs, pain level, respiratory status, and sedation level in patients receiving opioids, especially those receiving IV opioids postoperatively.

🜂 *Alert:* If patient is taking opioids with serotonergic drugs, watch for signs and symptoms of serotonin syndrome (agitation, hallucinations, rapid HR, fever, diaphoresis, shivering or shaking, muscle twitching or stiffness, trouble with coordination, nausea, vomiting, diarrhea), especially when starting treatment or increasing dosages. Signs and symptoms may occur within several hours of coadministration but may also occur later, especially after dosage increase. Discontinue the opioid,

serotonergic drug, or both if serotonin syndrome is suspected.

• Monitor patient for signs and symptoms of adrenal insufficiency (nausea, vomiting, loss of appetite, fatigue, weakness, dizziness, low BP). Perform diagnostic testing if adrenal insufficiency is suspected. If adrenal insufficiency is confirmed, treat with corticosteroids and wean patient off opioids if appropriate. Discontinue corticosteroids when clinically appropriate.

• Monitor patient for signs and symptoms of decreased sex hormone levels (low libido, erectile dysfunction, amenorrhea, infertility); drug may cause decreased sex hormone levels with long-term use. If signs or symptoms occur, evaluate patient and obtain lab testing.

• Work with patient to develop strategies to manage the use of prescribed or illicit benzodiazepines or other CNS depressants when starting MAT. Taper benzodiazepine or CNS depressant to discontinuation, if possible.

🜂 *Alert:* If patient is receiving prescribed benzodiazepines or other CNS depressants for anxiety or insomnia, verify diagnosis and consider other treatment options for these conditions, if possible.

🜂 *Alert:* Coordinate care to ensure other prescribers are aware of patient's MAT.

• Monitor patient for illicit drug use, including urine or blood screening.

• Assess patient's oral health history before transmucosal use. Tooth decay, cavities, oral infections, and loss of teeth have been reported in patients taking transmucosal buprenorphine. These problems can be serious and can occur in patients with no history of dental issues.

• Drug may prolong QT interval and increase risk of ventricular arrhythmias. Avoid use in patients with a personal or family history of long QT syndrome. Use caution and periodically monitor ECGs in patients with hypokalemia, hypomagnesemia, unstable cardiac disease including atrial fibrillation, unstable HF, or active myocardial ischemia.

• For patients at risk for hepatotoxicity, monitor LFTs before and during treatment.

• Drug should be used as part of a complete treatment program that includes counseling and psychosocial support.

• Drug may worsen increased ICP and mask its signs and symptoms. Carefully monitor patient's pupillary reflexes and level of consciousness.

- Monitor patients with history of seizure disorders for worsening of condition.
- Monitor patients for signs and symptoms of hypotension after initiating therapy or increasing dosage.
- Monitor patients with fever or increased core body temperature after exertion; adjust dosage if signs or symptoms of respiratory or CNS depression occur.
- Watch for worsening of symptoms in patients with biliary tract disease, including acute pancreatitis; drug may cause spasm of sphincter of Oddi.
- Reassess patient's level of pain 15 and 30 minutes after parenteral administration.
- **Alert:** Naloxone won't completely reverse the respiratory depression caused by buprenorphine overdose; an overdose may require mechanical ventilation. Larger-than-usual doses of naloxone (more than 0.4 mg) and doxapram also may be indicated.
- Treat accidental skin exposure by removing exposed clothing and rinsing skin with water.
- Drug may cause constipation. Assess bowel function and need for stool softeners and stimulant laxatives.
- **Alert:** Drug's opioid antagonist properties may cause withdrawal syndrome in patients who are opioid dependent.
- If dependence occurs, withdrawal symptoms may appear up to 14 days after drug is stopped.
- If Sublocade depot must be surgically removed, or treatment discontinued, monitor patient for signs and symptoms of withdrawal and treat appropriately.
- Regularly monitor Sublocade subcut injection site for evidence of tampering or attempted removal of the drug depot.
- In patients with oral mucositis using the buccal film, consider reducing dose; oral mucositis may lead to faster absorption and higher blood concentration of drug.
- *Look alike–sound alike:* Don't confuse Buprenex with Bumex. Don't confuse buprenorphine with bupropion.

PATIENT TEACHING

- **Alert:** Encourage patient to report all medications being taken, including prescription and OTC drugs and supplements.
- **Boxed Warning** *Opioid class warning:* Caution patient or caregiver of patient taking an opioid with a benzodiazepine, CNS depressant, or alcohol to seek immediate medical attention for dizziness, light-headedness, extreme sleepiness, slowed or difficult breathing, or unresponsiveness. ■
- **Alert:** Caution patient to immediately report signs and symptoms of hypersensitivity reaction (rash, hives, itching, facial swelling, wheezing, dizziness), serotonin syndrome, adrenal insufficiency, decreased sex hormone levels, or liver impairment (yellowing of skin or eyes, dark urine, light-colored stools, abdominal pain, nausea).
- **Alert:** Teach patient to avoid nonprescribed benzodiazepines, sedatives, or alcohol when taking MAT due to increased risk of overdose and death.
- Stress to patient taking transmucosal formulations the importance of oral care and potential for dental problems. Instruct patient in proper oral care after transmucosal dose.
- Tell patient to obtain a dental evaluation before starting drug and to establish a dental caries prevention plan with regular dental checkups.
- Advise patient to notify all prescribers of MAT and not to stop MAT or other prescribed drugs without first consulting prescriber to determine need for gradual tapering regimen.
- Tell patient and family to immediately report adverse reactions to prescriber.
- Caution patient who is ambulatory about getting out of bed or chair quickly or walking, as hypotension can occur.
- Warn patient that drug can cause dependence, and withdrawal can occur when drug is discontinued.
- Teach patient not to drive, operate heavy machinery, or perform dangerous activities until drug's effects are known.
- When drug is used after surgery, encourage patient to turn, cough, and breathe deeply to prevent breathing problems.
- Explain assessment and monitoring process to patient and family. Instruct them to immediately report difficulty breathing or other signs or symptoms of potential adverse opioid-related reaction.
- Instruct patient in proper drug administration, storage, and disposal.
- Warn patient not to apply heat to patch application site or to cut patch.
- Warn patient not to take other long-acting opioids while using transdermal system or buccal film.
- Teach patient that naloxone is prescribed in conjunction with the opioid when beginning

and renewing treatment as a preventive measure to reduce opioid overdose and death.

buPROPion hydrobromide
byoo-PROE-pee-on

Aplenzin

buPROPion hydrochloride
Forfivo XL, Wellbutrin SR♦, Wellbutrin XL

Therapeutic class: Antidepressants
Pharmacologic class: Aminoketones

AVAILABLE FORMS
bupropion hydrobromide
Tablets (extended-release) ⓓ: 174 mg, 348 mg, 522 mg
bupropion hydrochloride
Tablets (extended-release 12-hour) ⓓ: 100 mg, 150 mg, 200 mg
Tablets (extended-release 24-hour) ⓓ: 150 mg, 300 mg, 450 mg
Tablets (immediate-release) ⓓ: 75 mg, 100 mg

INDICATIONS & DOSAGES
Adjust-a-dose (for all indications): In patients with renal impairment (GFR less than 90 mL/minute) or mild hepatic impairment (Child-Pugh score 5 to 6), consider reduced frequency or dosage. In patients with moderate to severe hepatic impairment (Child-Pugh score 7 to 15), don't exceed 174 mg every other day (Aplenzin); 100 mg per day or 150 mg every other day (sustained-release tablets); 150 mg every other day (extended-release tablets); 75 mg per day (immediate-release tablets). Forfivo XL isn't recommended in patients with renal or hepatic impairment.
➤ **Major depressive disorder (Aplenzin only)**
Adults: Initially, 174 mg PO (equivalent to 150 mg/day bupropion HCl) given as a single daily dose in the morning. If the 174-mg dose is adequately tolerated, increase to target dose of 348 mg once daily in the morning as early as day 4 of dosing. The full antidepressant effect may not be evident for several months of treatment or longer. When switching patients from Wellbutrin SR or Wellbutrin XL to Aplenzin, give the equivalent total

daily dose when possible (522 mg bupropion HBr is equivalent to 450 mg bupropion HCl; 348 mg bupropion HBr is equivalent to 300 mg bupropion HCl; 174 mg bupropion HBr is equivalent to 150 mg bupropion HCl).
➤ **Major depressive disorder (except Aplenzin)**
Adults: For immediate-release, initially, 100 mg PO b.i.d.; increase after 3 days to 100 mg PO t.i.d., if needed. If patient doesn't improve after several weeks of therapy, increase dosage to 150 mg t.i.d. No single dose should exceed 150 mg. Allow at least 6 hours between successive doses. Maximum dose is 450 mg daily. For sustained-release, initially, 150 mg PO every morning; increase to target dose of 150 mg PO b.i.d., as tolerated, as early as day 4 of dosing. Allow at least 8 hours between successive doses. Maximum dose is 400 mg daily. For extended-release, initially, 150 mg PO every morning; increase to target dosage of 300 mg PO daily, as tolerated, as early as day 4 of dosing. Allow at least 24 hours between successive doses. Maximum is 450 mg daily. Don't initiate treatment with Forfivo XL.
➤ **Seasonal affective disorder**
Adults: Start treatment in autumn before depressive symptoms appear. Wellbutrin XL: Initially, 150 mg extended-release PO once daily in the morning. After 1 week, may increase to 300 mg once daily, if tolerated. Continue 300 mg daily during autumn and winter and taper to 150 mg daily for 2 weeks before stopping drug in early spring. Aplenzin: 174 mg PO daily in the morning. May increase to 348 mg PO once daily after 7 days. Taper and discontinue drug in early spring.
➤ **Aid to smoking-cessation treatment (extended-release tablets 12-hour)**
Adults: 150 mg PO daily for 3 days; increased to maximum of 300 mg daily in two divided doses at least 8 hours apart. Begin therapy at least 1 week before target cessation date; continue therapy for at least 12 weeks. Some patients may need continued treatment.

ADMINISTRATION
PO
• Don't crush, split, or allow patients to chew tablets.
• Give without regard to meals.
• When switching patients from immediate-release or sustained-release tablets to extended-release tablets, give the same total

daily dose (when possible) as the once-daily dosage provided.

ACTION
Unknown. Drug doesn't inhibit MAO, but it weakly inhibits norepinephrine, dopamine, and serotonin reuptake. Noradrenergic or dopaminergic mechanisms, or both, may cause drug's effect.

Route	Onset	Peak	Duration
PO (extended-release)	Unknown	5 hr	Unknown
PO (immediate-release)	Unknown	2 hr	Unknown
PO (sustained-release)	Unknown	3 hr	Unknown

Half-life: 8 to 24 hours.

ADVERSE REACTIONS
CNS: abnormal dreams, insomnia, headache, sedation, tremor, agitation, dizziness, *seizures, suicidality,* anxiety, confusion, delusions, euphoria, fever, hostility, impaired concentration, impaired sleep quality, akinesia, akathisia, paresthesia, abnormal thinking, depression, fatigue, syncope, taste disturbance, somnolence. **CV:** tachycardia, *arrhythmias,* HTN, hypotension, palpitations, chest pain, flushing. **EENT:** blurred vision, tinnitus, auditory disturbances, epistaxis, rhinitis, pharyngitis, nasopharyngitis, sinusitis, dry mouth. **GI:** constipation, nausea, vomiting, anorexia, dyspepsia, diarrhea, abdominal pain, flatulence. **GU:** erectile dysfunction, decreased libido, menstrual complaints, urinary frequency, urine retention. **Metabolic:** increased appetite, weight loss, weight gain. **Musculoskeletal:** arthritis, myalgia, arthralgia, muscle spasm or twitch. **Respiratory:** URI, bronchitis, cough, increased coughing. **Skin:** diaphoresis, pruritus, rash, dry skin, cutaneous temperature disturbance, urticaria. **Other:** chills, accidental injury, hot flashes.

INTERACTIONS
Drug-drug. *Amantadine, levodopa:* May increase risk of adverse reactions. If used together, give small first doses of bupropion and increase dosage gradually.
Antidepressants (desipramine, fluoxetine, imipramine, nortriptyline, sertraline), antipsychotics (haloperidol, risperidone, thioridazine), systemic corticosteroids, theophylline: May lower seizure threshold. Use cautiously together.

Beta blockers, class IC antiarrhythmics: May increase levels of these drugs and adverse reactions. Use a reduced dose if used with bupropion.
Carbamazepine, phenobarbital, phenytoin: May enhance metabolism of bupropion and decrease its effect. Monitor patient closely.
CYP2B6 substrates or inhibitors (cyclophosphamide, orphenadrine, thiotepa), efavirenz, fluvoxamine, nelfinavir, norfluoxetine, paroxetine, ritonavir, sertraline: May increase bupropion activity. Monitor patient for expected therapeutic effects and adverse effects.
Linezolid, methylene blue: May increase hypertensive effect of bupropion. Use together is contraindicated.
MAO inhibitors: May increase hypertensive effect of bupropion. Don't use these drugs within 14 days of each other.
Nicotine replacement agents: May increase risk of HTN. Monitor BP.
SSRIs: May increase risk of suicidality in children, adolescents, and young adults with major depressive disorder. Use together cautiously.
Drug-lifestyle. *Alcohol use:* May alter seizure threshold. Discourage use together.
Sun exposure: May increase risk of photosensitivity reactions. Advise patient to avoid excessive sunlight exposure.

EFFECTS ON LAB TEST RESULTS
• May increase LFT values.
• May cause false-positive results for urine detection of amphetamines.

CONTRAINDICATIONS & CAUTIONS
• Contraindicated in patients hypersensitive to drug and in those with seizure disorders or history of bulimia or anorexia nervosa because of a higher risk of seizures.
• **Alert:** Concomitant use with SSRIs, linezolid, or methylene blue can cause serotonin syndrome (fever, mental status changes, muscle twitching, diaphoresis, shivering or shaking, diarrhea, loss of coordination). Use drug with SSRIs, linezolid, or methylene blue only for life-threatening or urgent conditions when the potential benefits outweigh the risks of toxicity.
• Hypersensitivity reactions, including anaphylaxis, pruritus, urticaria, angioedema, dyspnea, erythema multiforme, and SJS, have occurred.

Reactions in bold italics are *life-threatening.* Interactions may have a *rapid onset* or a **delayed onset**.

- Contraindicated in patients abruptly stopping use of alcohol, sedatives (including benzodiazepines), or antiepileptics.
- Don't use with other drugs containing bupropion.
- Don't initiate therapy with Forfivo XL or taper Forfivo XL dosage; use another bupropion formulation for initial dosage titration and for tapering dosage before discontinuation.
- 🔵 *Alert:* Bupropion isn't approved for use in children.
- Use cautiously in patients with recent history of MI; unstable heart disease; renal or hepatic impairment; a history of seizures, head trauma, or other predisposition to seizures; and in those being treated with drugs that lower seizure threshold.
- *Dialyzable drug:* Unknown.
- ⚠ *Overdose S&S:* Seizures, ECG changes, hallucinations, loss of consciousness, sinus tachycardia, coma, fever, hypotension, muscle rigidity, rhabdomyolysis, respiratory failure, stupor.

PREGNANCY-LACTATION-REPRODUCTION
- Use during pregnancy only when potential benefits justify fetal risk.
- Notify prescriber if patient plans to or becomes pregnant.
- Health care providers are encouraged to register patients who are pregnant in the National Pregnancy Registry for Antidepressants (1-866-961-2388 or https://womensmentalhealth.org/clinical-and-research-programs/pregnancyregistry/antidepressants/).
- Drug and its metabolites appear in human milk. Recommendations for breastfeeding vary by individual product; refer to manufacturer's labeling for recommendations.

NURSING CONSIDERATIONS
- Many patients experience a period of increased restlessness, including agitation, insomnia, and anxiety, especially at start of therapy.
- 🔵 *Alert:* To minimize the risk of seizures, don't exceed maximum recommended dose.
- 🔵 *Alert:* Patient with major depressive disorder may experience a worsening of depression and suicidality. Carefully monitor patient for worsening depression or suicidality, especially at the beginning of therapy and during dosage changes.

Boxed Warning Drug may increase the risk of suicidality in children, adolescents, and young adults with major depressive disorder or other psychiatric disorder. ∎
🔵 *Alert:* If SSRIs, linezolid, or methylene blue must be given, bupropion must be stopped and patient monitored for serotonin toxicity for 2 weeks or until 24 hours after the last dose of SSRIs, methylene blue, or linezolid, whichever comes first. Treatment with bupropion may be resumed 24 hours after last dose of SSRIs, methylene blue, or linezolid.
- Closely monitor patient with history of bipolar disorder. Antidepressants can cause manic episodes during the depressed phase of bipolar disorder. This may be less likely to occur with bupropion than with other antidepressants.
- Begin smoking-cessation treatment while patient is still smoking; about 1 week is needed to achieve steady-state drug levels.
- Stop smoking-cessation treatment if patient hasn't progressed toward abstinence by week 7. Treatment usually lasts up to 12 weeks. Patient can stop taking drug without tapering off.
- Monitor patients without iridectomy for narrow-angle glaucoma.
- Monitor BP for HTN before and periodically during treatment.
- *Look alike–sound alike:* Don't confuse bupropion with buspirone. Don't confuse Wellbutrin SR with Wellbutrin XL.

PATIENT TEACHING
Boxed Warning Advise families and caregivers to closely observe patient for increased suicidality, as well as hostility, agitation, and depressed mood, and to contact health care provider immediately should these occur. ∎
🔵 *Alert:* Explain that excessive use of alcohol, abrupt withdrawal from alcohol or other sedatives, and addiction to cocaine, opiates, or stimulants during therapy may increase risk of seizures. Seizure risk also increases in those using OTC stimulants, in anorectics, and in patients with diabetes using oral antidiabetics or insulin.
🔵 *Alert:* Teach patient to recognize and immediately report symptoms of serotonin toxicity (fever, mental status changes, muscle twitching, diaphoresis, shivering or shaking, diarrhea, loss of coordination).
- Tell patient not to chew, crush, or divide tablets.

• Advise patient to consult prescriber before taking other prescription or OTC drugs.
• Advise patient to avoid hazardous activities that require alertness and good psychomotor coordination until effects of drug are known.
• Tell patient that it may take 4 weeks or longer to reach full antidepressant effect.
• Inform patient that tablets may have an odor.
• Tell patient taking extended-release form that the empty shell may appear in stool.

busPIRone hydrochloride
byoo-SPYE-rone

Therapeutic class: Anxiolytics
Pharmacologic class: Azaspirodecane-dione derivatives

AVAILABLE FORMS
Tablets: 5 mg, 7.5 mg, 10 mg, 15 mg, 30 mg

INDICATIONS & DOSAGES
➤ **Generalized anxiety disorder**
Adults: Initially, 7.5 mg PO b.i.d. Increase dosage by 5 mg daily at 2- to 3-day intervals. Usual maintenance dosage is 20 to 30 mg daily in divided doses. Don't exceed 60 mg daily.

ADMINISTRATION
PO
• Give drug at the same times each day, and always with or always without food.

ACTION
May inhibit neuronal firing and reduce serotonin turnover in cortical, amygdaloid, and septohippocampal tissue.

Route	Onset	Peak	Duration
PO	Unknown	40–90 min	Unknown

Half-life: 2 to 3 hours.

ADVERSE REACTIONS
CNS: dizziness, drowsiness, headache, nervousness, insomnia, light-headedness, fatigue, numbness, excitement, confusion, depression, anger, decreased concentration, paresthesia, incoordination, tremor, hostility. **CV:** tachycardia, nonspecific chest pain. **EENT:** blurred vision, dry mouth. **GI:** nausea, diarrhea, abdominal distress, constipation,

vomiting. **Musculoskeletal:** aches and pains. **Skin:** rash, diaphoresis, clamminess.

INTERACTIONS
Drug-drug. *Azole antifungals:* May inhibit first-pass metabolism of buspirone. Monitor patient closely for adverse effects; adjust dosage as needed.
CNS depressants: May increase CNS depression. Use together cautiously.
CYP3A4 inducers (carbamazepine, dexamethasone, phenobarbital, phenytoin, rifabutin, rifampin): May decrease buspirone level. Adjust dosage as needed.
Drugs metabolized by CYP3A4 (clarithromycin, diltiazem, erythromycin, fluvoxamine, itraconazole, ketoconazole, nefazodone, ritonavir, verapamil): May increase buspirone level. Monitor patient; decrease buspirone dosage and adjust carefully.
Linezolid, methylene blue: May cause serotonin syndrome. Use extreme caution and monitor closely.
MAO inhibitors: May elevate BP and increase risk of serotonin syndrome. Avoid use together; don't use MAO inhibitors within 14 days of stopping or starting buspirone.
Nefazodone: May increase levels of both drugs. Use lower buspirone dosage if used together.
Sodium oxybate: May increase sleep duration and CNS depression. Use together is contraindicated.
Drug-food. *Grapefruit juice:* May increase drug level, increasing adverse effects. Discourage use together.
Drug-lifestyle. *Alcohol use:* May increase CNS depression. Discourage use together.

EFFECTS ON LAB TEST RESULTS
• May interfere with urinary metanephrine/catecholamine assay testing for pheochromocytoma, resulting in a false-positive result.

CONTRAINDICATIONS & CAUTIONS
• Contraindicated in patients hypersensitive to drug and within 14 days of MAO inhibitor therapy.
🕔 *Alert:* Concomitant use with linezolid or methylene blue can cause serotonin syndrome (fever, mental status changes, muscle twitching, diaphoresis, shivering or shaking, diarrhea, loss of coordination). Use drug with linezolid or methylene blue only for

life-threatening or urgent conditions when the potential benefits outweigh the risks of toxicity.

• Drug isn't recommended for patients with severe hepatic or renal impairment.

Dialyzable drug: No.

⚠ *Overdose S&S:* Nausea, vomiting, dizziness, drowsiness, miosis, gastric distress.

PREGNANCY-LACTATION-REPRODUCTION
• Use during pregnancy and breastfeeding isn't recommended. Use during pregnancy only if clearly needed.

NURSING CONSIDERATIONS
• Monitor patient closely for adverse CNS reactions. Drug is less sedating than other anxiolytics, but CNS effects may be unpredictable.

⊙ *Alert:* Before starting therapy, don't stop a previous benzodiazepine regimen abruptly because a withdrawal reaction may occur.

⊙ *Alert:* If linezolid or methylene blue must be given, buspirone must be stopped and patient should be monitored for serotonin toxicity for 2 weeks or until 24 hours after the last dose of methylene blue or linezolid, whichever comes first. Treatment with buspirone may be resumed 24 hours after last dose of methylene blue or linezolid.

• Drug shows no potential for abuse and isn't classified as a controlled substance.

• *Look alike–sound alike:* Don't confuse buspirone with bupropion or risperidone.

PATIENT TEACHING
⊙ *Alert:* Teach patient to recognize and immediately report symptoms of serotonin toxicity (fever, mental status changes, muscle twitching, diaphoresis, shivering or shaking, diarrhea, loss of coordination).

• Warn patient to avoid hazardous activities that require alertness and good coordination until effects of drug are known.

• Remind patient that drug effects may not be noticeable for several weeks.

• Warn patient not to abruptly stop a benzodiazepine because of risk of withdrawal symptoms.

• Tell patient to avoid use of alcohol and grapefruit juice during therapy.

• Advise patient to take consistently; that is, always with or always without food.

butorphanol tartrate
byoo-TOR-fa-nole

B

Therapeutic class: Opioid analgesics
Pharmacologic class: Opioid agonist-antagonists–opioid partial agonists

AVAILABLE FORMS
Injection: 1 mg/mL, 2 mg/mL
Nasal spray: 10 mg/mL (1 mg/spray)

INDICATIONS & DOSAGES
➤ **Moderate to severe pain**
Adults: Initially, 2 mg IM every 3 to 4 hours PRN, or around the clock; then individualize dose to 1 to 4 mg, not to exceed 4 mg per dose. Or initially, 1 mg IV every 3 to 4 hours PRN; then individualize dose to 0.5 to 2 mg. Or, 1 mg by nasal spray every 3 to 4 hours (1 spray in one nostril); repeat in 60 to 90 minutes if pain relief is inadequate. For severe pain, 2 mg (1 spray in each nostril) every 3 to 4 hours.

Adjust-a-dose: For patients with renal or hepatic impairment, increase dosage interval to 6 to 8 hours and give 50% of the normal dose. For older adults, give 1 mg IM or 0.5 mg IV; wait 6 hours before repeating dose. For nasal use, 1 mg (1 spray in one nostril). May give another 1 mg in 1.5 to 2 hours. Wait 6 hours before repeating sequence.

➤ **Labor for patients at full term; early labor (without signs of fetal distress)**
Adults: 1 or 2 mg IV or IM; repeat after 4 hours as needed. Don't give dose less than 4 hours before anticipated delivery.

➤ **Preoperative anesthesia or preanesthesia**
Adults: 2 mg IM 60 to 90 minutes before surgery.

➤ **Adjunct to balanced anesthesia**
Adults: 2 mg IV shortly before induction, or 0.5 to 1 mg IV in increments during anesthesia.

Older adults: One-half usual dose, with repeat doses determined by patient's response.

ADMINISTRATION
IV
▼ Compatible solutions include D_5W and NSS.
▼ Give by direct injection into a vein or into the tubing of a free-flowing IV solution.

▼ **Incompatibilities:** None listed by manufacturer. Consult a drug incompatibility reference for more information.

IM
• Give drug IM; don't give subcut.

Intranasal
• Prime pump before initial use; if not used for 2 days or more, reprime with one or two strokes.
• Have patient blow nose gently to clear both nostrils.
• Insert spray tip into one nostril, pointing toward back of the nose; close other nostril with fingertip and tilt head slightly forward.
• Have patient sniff gently with mouth closed during spray, then tilt head backwards and sniff gently a few more seconds. Repeat with other nostril if prescribed.
• Store at room temperature.

ACTION
May bind with opioid receptors in the CNS, altering perception of and emotional response to pain.

Route	Onset	Peak	Duration
IV	1 min	30–60 min	3–4 hr
IM	10–30 min	30–60 min	3–4 hr
Nasal	15 min	1–2 hr	2.5–5 hr

Half-life: About 3 to 5 hours.

ADVERSE REACTIONS
CNS: dizziness, insomnia, somnolence, anxiety, asthenia, confusion, euphoria, floating feeling, headache, lethargy, nervousness, paresthesia, tremor, weakness, sensation of heat, unpleasant taste. **CV:** flushing, palpitations, vasodilation. **EENT:** blurred vision, tinnitus, earache, nasal congestion, nasal irritation, epistaxis, pharyngitis, sinus congestion, sinusitis, rhinitis, dry mouth. **GI:** nausea, vomiting, anorexia, constipation, stomach pain. **Respiratory:** bronchitis, cough, dyspnea, URI. **Skin:** clamminess, diaphoresis, pruritus.

INTERACTIONS
Drug-drug. **Boxed Warning** *Benzodiazepines, CNS depressants:* May cause slow or difficult breathing, sedation, and death. Avoid use together. If use together is necessary, limit dosage and duration of each drug to the minimum necessary for desired effect. ∎

CNS depressants: May cause additive effects. Use together cautiously.
Boxed Warning *CYP3A4 inducers (carbamazepine, phenytoin, rifampin):* May decrease level of intranasally administered drug, causing decreased effectiveness or drug withdrawal syndrome. Monitor patient closely. ∎
Boxed Warning *CYP3A4 inhibitors (azole antifungals, macrolide antibiotics, protease inhibitors):* May increase level of intranasally administered drug, resulting in increased or prolonged adverse reactions; may cause potentially fatal respiratory depression. Avoid use together. ∎
🔵 *Alert: Serotonergic drugs:* May increase risk of serotonin syndrome. Use together cautiously; monitor patient for serotonin syndrome.
Drug-herb. 🔵 *Alert: St. John's wort:* May increase risk of serotonin syndrome. Use together cautiously; monitor patient for serotonin syndrome.
Drug-lifestyle. *Alcohol use:* May cause additive effects. Discourage use together.

EFFECTS ON LAB TEST RESULTS
None reported.

CONTRAINDICATIONS & CAUTIONS
• Contraindicated in patients hypersensitive to drug or to preservative, benzethonium chloride, and in those with opioid addiction; may cause withdrawal syndrome.
Boxed Warning Drug is available through a REMS program for opioid analgesics. ∎
Boxed Warning Drug exposes patients and other users to risks of opioid addiction, abuse, and misuse, which can lead to overdose and death. Assess each patient's risk before prescribing butorphanol tartrate, and monitor all patients regularly for development of these behaviors or conditions. ∎
Boxed Warning Serious, life-threatening, or fatal respiratory depression may occur with use of butorphanol tartrate. Monitor patients for respiratory depression, especially during drug initiation and after dosage increase. ∎
Boxed Warning *Opioid class warning:* Opioids should only be prescribed with benzodiazepines or other CNS depressants to patients for whom alternative treatment options are inadequate. ∎
🔵 *Alert:* Drug may lead to rare but serious decrease in adrenal gland cortisol production.

Reactions in bold italics are *life-threatening*. Interactions may have a *rapid onset* or a ***delayed onset***.

◐ *Alert:* Drug may cause decreased sex hormone levels with long-term use.

• Use cautiously in patients with head injury, increased ICP, acute MI, ventricular dysfunction, coronary insufficiency, respiratory disease or depression, and renal or hepatic dysfunction.

• Use cautiously in patients who have recently received repeated doses of opioid analgesic.

• For patients who have been taking drug regularly, gradually taper dosage to prevent signs and symptoms of withdrawal.

• Safety and efficacy in patients younger than age 18 haven't been established.

• Older adults may have increased sensitivity to drug. Use caution when selecting a dosage for such patients, and usually start at low end of dosing range.

Dialyzable drug: Unknown.

⚠ *Overdose S&S:* Respiratory depression, CNS depression, CV insufficiency, coma, death.

PREGNANCY-LACTATION-REPRODUCTION

• There are no adequate and well-controlled studies in pregnancy before 37 weeks' gestation. Use during pregnancy only if potential benefit justifies fetal risk.

• There have been rare reports of infant respiratory distress and apnea after butorphanol administration during labor. These reports have been associated with administration of a dose within 2 hours of delivery, use of multiple doses, use with additional analgesics or sedatives, or use in preterm pregnancies.

• If fetal HR pattern is abnormal, use butorphanol cautiously.

• The decision to continue therapy or discontinue breastfeeding should take into account risks versus benefits to mother and infant.

◐ *Alert:* Monitor patients who are breastfeeding and infants for psychomimetic reactions. Monitor infants exposed to drug during breastfeeding for apnea and sedation. Withdrawal symptoms can occur in infants when drug or breastfeeding is stopped.

Boxed Warning Closely monitor neonates with prolonged opioid exposure during pregnancy for signs and symptoms of withdrawal, which may be life-threatening and may require management according to protocols developed by neonatology experts. ∎

NURSING CONSIDERATIONS

◐ *Alert:* If patient is taking opioids with serotonergic drugs, monitor for signs and symptoms of serotonin syndrome, especially when starting treatment or increasing dosages. Signs and symptoms may occur within several hours of coadministration but may also occur later, especially after dosage increase. Discontinue the opioid, serotonergic drug, or both if serotonin syndrome is suspected.

Boxed Warning Use of any coadministered CYP3A4 inhibitors or inducers can cause an increase or decrease in drug levels, leading to fatal adverse effects. ∎

• Don't stop drug abruptly; withdraw slowly and individualize the gradual taper plan to prevent signs and symptoms of withdrawal, worsening pain, and psychological distress in patients who are physically dependent. Refer to manufacturer's label for specific tapering instructions.

• When tapering opioids, watch closely for signs and symptoms of opioid withdrawal. Such symptoms may indicate a need to taper more slowly. Monitor patient for suicidality, use of other substances, and mood changes.

◐ *Alert:* Monitor patient for signs and symptoms of adrenal insufficiency. Perform diagnostic testing if adrenal insufficiency is suspected. If adrenal insufficiency is confirmed, treat with corticosteroids and wean patient off opioids if appropriate. Discontinue corticosteroids when clinically appropriate.

◐ *Alert:* Monitor patient for signs and symptoms of decreased sex hormone levels. If signs and symptoms occur, evaluate patient and obtain lab testing.

• Drug may cause constipation. Assess bowel function and need for stool softener and stimulant laxatives.

Boxed Warning Psychological and physical addiction may occur. ∎

• Periodically monitor postoperative vital signs and bladder function. Because drug decreases both rate and depth of respirations, monitor arterial oxygen saturation to help assess respiratory depression.

PATIENT TEACHING

◐ *Alert:* Encourage patient to report all medications being taken, including prescription and OTC drugs and supplements.

• Caution patient to avoid alcohol during therapy.

♣Canada ◇OTC ◆Off-label use 𝒫Photoguide ⊕Do not crush *Liquid contains alcohol ☒Genetic

Boxed Warning Caution patient or caregiver of patient taking an opioid with a benzodiazepine, CNS depressant, or alcohol to seek immediate medical attention for dizziness, light-headedness, extreme sleepiness, slowed or difficult breathing, or unresponsiveness. ■

• Counsel patient not to discontinue opioids without first discussing with prescriber the need for a gradual tapering regimen.

🜂 *Alert:* Caution patient to immediately report signs and symptoms of serotonin syndrome, adrenal insufficiency, and decreased sex hormone levels.

• Caution patient who is ambulatory about getting out of bed or walking. Warn outpatient to avoid driving and other hazardous activities that require mental alertness until it's clear how the drug affects the CNS.

Boxed Warning Accidental ingestion of even one dose of nasal solution, especially by children, can result in a fatal overdose. ■

• Teach patient how to take nasal spray and how to store in child-resistant container.

• Inform patient that naloxone is prescribed in conjunction with the opioid at start and renewal of treatment as a preventive measure to reduce opioid overdose and death.

cabotegravir–rilpivirine
ka-boe-TEG-ra-vir/ril-pi-VIR-een

Cabenuva

Therapeutic class: Antiretrovirals
Pharmacologic class: HIV-1 integrase strand transfer inhibitors/HIV-1 NNRTIs

AVAILABLE FORMS
Injection (extended-release suspension): 400 mg cabotegravir and 600 mg rilpivirine single-dose vials (kit); 600 mg cabotegravir and 900 mg rilpivirine single-dose vials (kit)

INDICATIONS & DOSAGES
➤ **HIV-1 infection to replace current antiretroviral regimen in patients who are virologically suppressed on a stable antiretroviral regimen with no history of treatment failure and no known or suspected resistance to cabotegravir or rilpivirine**
Adults and adolescents age 12 and older weighing at least 35 kg: Initially, cabotegravir

30 mg PO daily and rilpivirine 25 mg PO daily for at least 28 days to assess tolerability. On the last day of oral dosing, initiate injections with cabotegravir 600 mg IM and rilpivirine 900 mg IM as separate gluteal injections. Starting 1 month after initial injections, give cabotegravir 400 mg IM and rilpivirine 600 mg IM as separate gluteal injections once monthly.

Alternatively, on last day of oral dosing or current antiretroviral therapy, initiate injections with cabotegravir 600 mg IM and rilpivirine 900 mg IM as separate gluteal injections and repeat in 1 month. May give the next doses of cabotegravir 600 mg IM and rilpivirine 900 mg IM in 2 months, then every 2 months thereafter.

Adjust-a-dose: If switching from monthly to every-2-month regimen, give cabotegravir 600 mg IM and rilpivirine 900 mg IM 1 month after last monthly injection, then ever 2 months thereafter. If switching from every-2-month to monthly regimen, give cabotegravir 400 mg IM and rilpivirine 600 mg IM 2 months after last every-2-month injection, then every month thereafter.

ADMINISTRATION
IM
• Complete dose requires an injection of cabotegravir and an injection of rilpivirine given during the same visit.

• Don't further dilute or reconstitute vials. Don't mix with other products or diluents.

• Before use, remove vials from refrigerator; allow products to reach room temperature (not to exceed 77° F [25° C]) for 15 minutes.

• Inspect vials for particulate matter and discoloration. Don't use if present. Cabotegravir vial has a brown tint, which may limit inspection.

• Shake vials vigorously until suspension looks uniform before withdrawing into syringes. Small air bubbles are expected and acceptable.

• Give as soon as possible; suspension may remain in syringe for up to 2 hours. After 2 hours, discard drug and syringe.

• Order of giving both injections isn't important.

• Give each injection at separate gluteal sites on opposite sides or at least 2 cm apart using the Z-track technique. The ventrogluteal site is preferred. Don't give by other routes or anatomic sites. May need longer needle

---

Reactions in bold italics are *life-threatening*. Interactions may have a *rapid onset* or a *delayed onset*.

C

lengths sufficient to reach the gluteus muscle for patients with higher BMI.

• May give dose up to 7 days before or after the date patient is scheduled to receive maintenance injections.

• If patient plans to miss a scheduled injection by more than 7 days, give oral therapy to replace up to two consecutive months. Recommended dose is cabotegravir 30 mg PO daily and rilpivirine 25 mg PO daily with the first dose starting when the next injection is due and continued until the day injection dosing is restarted. If oral therapy lasts for more than 2 months, an alternative regimen is recommended.

• Refer to manufacturer's instructions for unplanned missed injections.

• Store vials at 36° to 46° F (2° to 8° C) in original carton. Don't freeze. Vials may remain in original carton at room temperature for up to 6 hours; discard vials after 6 hours.

ACTION

Cabotegravir inhibits the integrase strand transfer step of retroviral DNA integration essential for HIV-1 replication. Rilpivirine inhibits HIV-1 replication by noncompetitive inhibition of HIV-1 reverse transcriptase.

Route	Onset	Peak	Duration
IM (cabotegravir)	Unknown	7 days	Unknown
IM (rilpivirine)	Unknown	3–4 days	Unknown

Half-life: Cabotegravir, 5.6 to 11.5 weeks; rilpivirine, 13 to 28 weeks.

ADVERSE REACTIONS

CNS: abnormal dreams, anxiety, depressive disorders, dizziness, fatigue, fever, headache, sleep disorder. **GI:** abdominal pain, diarrhea, dyspepsia, flatulence, gastritis, nausea, vomiting. **Hepatic:** *hepatotoxicity.* **Metabolic:** weight gain, increased CK and lipase levels. **Musculoskeletal:** bone and muscle pain. **Skin:** rash, injection-site reaction. **Other:** hypersensitivity reaction.

INTERACTIONS

Drug-drug. *Anticonvulsants (carbamazepine, oxcarbazepine, phenobarbital, phenytoin):* May decrease cabotegravir and rilpivirine levels and decrease antiviral effect. Avoid use together.

Antimycobacterials (rifabutin, rifampin, rifapentine): May decrease cabotegravir and rilpivirine levels and decrease antiviral effect. Avoid use together.

Drugs that increase risk of torsades de pointes (amiodarone, ciprofloxacin, haloperidol, SSRIs): May increase risk of prolonged QTc interval. Use together cautiously.

Macrolide or ketolide antibiotics (azithromycin, clarithromycin, erythromycin): May increase rilpivirine level and risk of torsades de pointes. Consider alternatives or use other macrolides with less effect on rilpivirine level (azithromycin).

Methadone: May decrease methadone level. Monitor patient closely and adjust methadone maintenance dosage as needed.

Other anti-HIV-1 medications: May increase risk of adverse effects. Avoid use together.

Systemic glucocorticoids (dexamethasone): May decrease rilpivirine level and decrease antiviral effect if more than a single dose is given. Avoid use together.

Drug-herb. *St. John's wort:* May decrease rilpivirine level and decrease antiviral effect. Discourage use together.

EFFECTS ON LAB TEST RESULTS

• May increase ALT, AST, CK, and lipase levels.

• May affect response to corticotropin stimulation tests.

CONTRAINDICATIONS & CAUTIONS

• Contraindicated in patients with previous hypersensitivity reaction to cabotegravir or rilpivirine.

• Hypersensitivity reactions to rilpivirine, including DRESS syndrome, have been reported. Skin reactions may be accompanied by constitutional symptoms such as fever or organ dysfunction.

• Drug may increase risk of hepatotoxicity in patients with preexisting hepatic disease or identifiable risk factors.

• Use in patients with severe renal impairment (CrCl of 15 to less than 30 mL/minute), ESRD (CrCl less than 15 mL/minute), or severe hepatic impairment (Child-Pugh class C) hasn't been studied. Use cautiously and monitor patients for adverse effects.

• Residual levels of cabotegravir and rilpivirine may remain in systemic circulation for 12 months or longer.

• Use only in patients who agree to required injections because nonadherence to injections or missed doses could lead to loss of virologic response and viral resistance. To minimize risk of viral resistance, initiate an alternative, suppressive antiretroviral regimen no later than when injection is due. If virologic failure is suspected, switch patient to an alternative regimen as soon as possible.

• Safety and effectiveness in children younger than age 12 or weighing less than 35 kg haven't been established.

• Use cautiously in older adults.

Dialyzable drug: No.

PREGNANCY-LACTATION-REPRODUCTION

• It isn't known if drug increases risk of birth defects and miscarriage. Consider benefits and risks when using in patients of childbearing potential or during pregnancy.

• Enroll patients exposed to drug during pregnancy in the Antiretroviral Pregnancy Registry (1-800-258-4263).

• It isn't known if drug appears in human milk or how drug affects milk production or infants who are breastfed. Patients with HIV-1 infection shouldn't breastfeed to avoid transmission to infant.

NURSING CONSIDERATIONS

• Follow injection instructions carefully to avoid accidental IV administration.

• Monitor patient for approximately 10 minutes after injection. If patient experiences postinjection reaction (dyspnea, agitation, abdominal cramping, flushing, sweating, oral numbness, and changes in BP), treat as indicated.

• Monitor patient for signs or symptoms of hypersensitivity (severe rash or rash accompanied by fever, general malaise, fatigue, muscle or joint aches, blisters, mucosal involvement [oral blisters or lesions], conjunctivitis, facial edema, hepatitis, eosinophilia, angioedema, difficulty breathing, dark or tea-colored urine). Discontinue drug immediately if they occur and treat patient as appropriate.

• Monitor LFT values routinely and discontinue drug if hepatotoxicity is suspected.

• Monitor patient with depressive symptoms to assess whether symptoms are related to drug and to determine risk of continued therapy.

PATIENT TEACHING

🜂 *Alert:* Stress importance of maintaining viral suppression by adhering to medication regimen and scheduled visits. Tell patient to contact prescriber if patient plans to or misses

a scheduled injection and that oral therapy may be used to replace up to two consecutive monthly injections.

• Inform patient that injection-site reactions (pain, erythema, tenderness, pruritus, and local swelling) or systemic reactions (fever, musculoskeletal pain, and sciatica pain) may occur.

• Teach patient to immediately report signs and symptoms of hypersensitivity reaction.

• Advise patient of the need for lab tests to monitor liver function.

• Tell patient to immediately report depressive symptoms (depressed mood, depression, major depression, altered mood, mood swings, feeling tense, negative thoughts, suicidal ideation or attempt).

• Advise patient that if drug is stopped, other medicine will be given to treat HIV-1 infection.

• Warn patient of reproductive potential about the long duration of drug exposure and that drug's effect in pregnancy is still under study.

SAFETY ALERT!

calaspargase pegol-mknl
kal-AS-par-jase PEG-ol

Asparlas

Therapeutic class: Antineoplastics
Pharmacologic class: Amino acid enzymes

AVAILABLE FORMS
Injection: 3,750 units/5 mL (750 units/mL) single-dose vial

INDICATIONS & DOSAGES
➤ **Acute lymphoblastic leukemia as part of a multiagent regimen**
Adults ages 18 to 21 and children age 1 month and older: 2,500 units/m^2 IV infusion no more frequently than once every 21 days.
Adjust-a-dose: Refer to manufacturer's instructions for toxicity-related and infusion reaction adjustments.

ADMINISTRATION
IV
▼ Premedicate with acetaminophen, an H$_1$ blocker (diphenhydramine), and an H$_2$ blocker (famotidine) 30 to 60 minutes before infusion.

Reactions in bold italics are *life-threatening*. Interactions may have a *rapid onset* or a ***delayed onset***.

▼ Visually inspect vial for particulate matter, cloudiness, or discoloration before administration. If present, discard.

▼ Dilute in 100 mL NSS or D₅W. Discard any drug remaining in vial.

▼ After dilution, administer immediately into an infusion of the same type of solution as used for vial dilution.

▼ Infuse over 1 hour.

▼ May store diluted solution for up to 4 hours at room temperature (59° to 77° F [15° to 25° C]) or refrigerated at 36° to 46° F (2° to 8° C) for up to 24 hours.

▼ Refrigerate vials and protect from light. Don't use if vial has been shaken or vigorously agitated, frozen, or stored at room temperature for more than 48 hours.

▼ **Incompatibilities:** Don't infuse other drugs or solutions through the same IV line during administration.

ACTION

An enzyme that converts L-asparagine into aspartic acid and ammonia and depletes plasma L-asparagine levels. This decreases the amount of L-asparagine available to leukemia cells and leads to cell death.

Route	Onset	Peak	Duration
IV	Unknown	1 hr	Unknown

Half-life: 16 days.

ADVERSE REACTIONS

CV: *HF,* arrhythmia, *embolic and thrombotic events.* **GI:** *pancreatitis,* diarrhea. **Hematologic:** *hemorrhage,* abnormal clotting studies. **Hepatic:** *hepatotoxicity,* elevated transaminase levels, hyperbilirubinemia. **Respiratory:** dyspnea, pneumonia. **Other:** hypersensitivity, *anaphylaxis, sepsis,* fungal infection.

INTERACTIONS

Drug-drug. *Oral contraceptives:* May decrease efficacy of contraceptive. Patient should use a nonhormonal contraceptive method.

EFFECTS ON LAB TEST RESULTS

• May increase ALT, AST, bilirubin, amylase, and lipase levels.
• May decrease fibrinogen and albumin ss levels.
• May prolong PT and PTT.

CONTRAINDICATIONS & CAUTIONS

• Contraindicated in patients with a history of serious hypersensitivity reactions, including anaphylaxis, to pegylated L-asparaginase therapy.
• Contraindicated in patients with a history of serious pancreatitis, thrombosis, or hemorrhage during previous L-asparaginase therapy.
• Contraindicated in patients with severe hepatic impairment.
• Use isn't indicated in adults older than age 21.
Dialyzable drug: Unknown.

PREGNANCY-LACTATION-REPRODUCTION

• Drug may cause fetal harm. Advise patients who are pregnant of fetal risk before use.
• It isn't known if drug appears in human milk. Patient should avoid breastfeeding during therapy and for 3 months after final dose.
• Patients of childbearing potential should use effective nonhormonal contraception, including a barrier method, during treatment and for at least 3 months after final dose.

NURSING CONSIDERATIONS

• Monitor bilirubin and transaminase levels at least weekly during treatment and for at least 6 weeks after final dose. Provide supportive care and discontinue drug for serious liver toxicity.
• *Alert:* Administer drug in a setting with available resuscitation equipment and agents to treat anaphylaxis (epinephrine, oxygen, IV steroids, antihistamines).
• Observe patients for 1 hour after administration. Watch for hypersensitivity reactions (angioedema, lip or eye swelling, erythema, decreased BP, bronchospasm, dyspnea, pruritus, rash). Discontinue drug in patients with serious hypersensitivity reactions.
• Monitor patients for signs and symptoms of pancreatitis (upper abdominal pain, fever, rapid HR, nausea, vomiting, steatorrhea). Assess amylase and lipase levels to confirm signs and symptoms. Withhold drug if pancreatitis is suspected and discontinue if confirmed.
• Monitor glucose level at least weekly until recovery therapy cycle.
• Monitor patients for hyperglycemia and glucose intolerance related to pancreatitis (excessive thirst, increase in urine volume or frequency of urination).

• Monitor patients for thrombotic events (severe headache, arm or leg swelling, dyspnea, chest pain); discontinue drug if serious event occurs.

• Monitor PT, PTT, and fibrinogen level and watch for signs and symptoms of hemorrhage (unusual bleeding or bruising). Consider replacement therapy in patients with severe or symptomatic coagulopathy.

• Monitor patients for signs and symptoms of hepatotoxicity (jaundice, severe nausea, vomiting, bruising, bleeding).

• Obtain pregnancy test in patients of childbearing potential before starting drug.

• *Look alike–sound alike:* Don't confuse calaspargase with L-asparaginase.

PATIENT TEACHING

• Advise patient to report all adverse reactions.
• Teach patient to recognize and immediately report signs or symptoms of hypersensitivity, pancreatitis, thrombosis, hemorrhage, and hepatotoxicity.
• Advise patient of childbearing potential to use effective nonhormonal contraception, including a barrier method, during treatment and for at least 3 months after final dose.
• Caution patient to immediately report pregnancy or suspected pregnancy during therapy.
• Instruct patient not to breastfeed during treatment and for at least 3 months after final dose.

calcitonin salmon
kal-si-TOE-nin

Miacalcin

Therapeutic class: Antiosteoporotics
Pharmacologic class: Polypeptide hormones

AVAILABLE FORMS
Injection: 200 units/mL in 2-mL vials
Nasal spray: 200 units/activation

INDICATIONS & DOSAGES
➤ **Paget disease of bone (osteitis deformans)**
Adults: 100 units daily IM or subcut.
➤ **Hypercalcemia**
Adults: 4 units/kg every 12 hours IM or subcut. If response is inadequate after 1 or 2 days, increase dosage to 8 units/kg every 12 hours.

If response remains unsatisfactory after 2 additional days, increase dosage to maximum of 8 units/kg every 6 hours.
➤ **Postmenopausal osteoporosis in patients more than 5 years after menopause**
Adults: 200 units (one activation) daily intranasally, alternating nostrils daily. Or, 100 units IM or subcut daily. Patient should receive adequate vitamin D and calcium supplements (at least 1,000 mg elemental calcium and 400 units of vitamin D) daily.

ADMINISTRATION
IM
• IM route is preferred if volume of dose exceeds 2 mL; use multiple injection sites.
• Visually inspect solution for particles, cloudiness, or discoloration. If present, discard.
• Store in refrigerator between 36° and 46° F (2° and 8° C).
Intranasal
• Alternate nostrils daily.
• Allow bottle to reach room temperature and prime pump before first use by releasing until a full spray is produced. Don't prime pump every day. Don't shake bottle.
• Carefully insert nozzle into the nostril while patient's head is upright and firmly depress pump toward bottle.
• Wipe nozzle with a clean, damp cloth and dry.
• Discard spray container after 30 doses.
• Keep bottle refrigerated between 36° and 46° F (2° and 8° C) while unopened; store in an upright position at room temperature after opening.
Subcutaneous
• Visually inspect solution for particles, cloudiness, or discoloration. If present, discard.
• Alternate injection sites.
• Store in refrigerator between 36° and 46° F (2° and 8° C).

ACTION
Decreases osteoclastic activity by inhibiting osteocytic osteolysis; decreases mineral release and matrix or collagen breakdown in bone.

Route	Onset	Peak	Duration
IM, subcut	2 hr	23 min	6–8 hr
Intranasal	Rapid	10–13 min	Unknown

Half-life: IM and subcut, 58 to 64 minutes. intranasal, 18 minutes.

ADVERSE REACTIONS

CNS: depression, headache, dizziness, paresthesia, fatigue. **CV:** flushing, pedal edema. **EENT:** eye pain, abnormal tearing, conjunctivitis, epistaxis, nasal congestion, rhinitis, sinusitis, facial edema. **GI:** transient nausea, salty taste, anorexia, nausea, abdominal pain. **GU:** increased urinary frequency, nocturia. **Hematologic:** infection, lymphadenopathy. **Musculoskeletal:** arthrosis, myalgia, back pain, osteoarthritis. **Respiratory:** *bronchospasm,* URI, shortness of breath, sinusitis. **Skin:** rash, pruritus of ear lobes, injection-site reaction. **Other:** hypersensitivity reactions, flulike symptoms, *malignancy.*

INTERACTIONS

Drug-drug. *Lithium:* May reduce plasma lithium concentration due to increased urinary clearance of lithium. Monitor level and adjust lithium dosage as needed.
Zoledronic acid: May enhance hypocalcemic effect of zoledronic acid. Monitor therapy.

EFFECTS ON LAB TEST RESULTS
• May reduce calcium level.

CONTRAINDICATIONS & CAUTIONS
• Contraindicated in patients hypersensitive to drug.
• For osteoporosis, reserve for patients with contraindications to alternative agents.
• Safety and effectiveness in children haven't been established.
Dialyzable drug: Unknown.
⚠ *Overdose S&S:* Hypocalcemic tetany (increased neuromuscular irritability, repetitive neuromuscular movements after a single stimulus).

PREGNANCY-LACTATION-REPRODUCTION
• Use during pregnancy only if potential benefits justify fetal risk.
• Nasal spray isn't indicated for use in patients of childbearing potential.
• It isn't known if drug appears in human milk, but it has been shown to decrease milk production in animals. Before use during breastfeeding, consider risk of infant exposure, benefits of breastfeeding to the infant, and benefits of treatment to the patient.

NURSING CONSIDERATIONS
• Skin test is usually done in patients with suspected drug sensitivity before therapy.

• Calcium and vitamin D supplements are recommended in patients with osteoporosis or Paget disease who have inadequate dietary intake.
⚠ *Alert:* Systemic allergic reactions are possible because the hormone is a protein. Monitor patient for hypersensitivity reactions, including anaphylaxis, and prepare for emergency treatment if needed.
⚠ *Alert:* Observe patient for signs of hypocalcemic tetany during therapy (muscle twitching, tetanic spasms, and seizures when hypocalcemia is severe).
⚠ *Alert:* Periodically reevaluate need for continued therapy because of the possible association between malignancy and long-term calcitonin salmon use.
• Monitor calcium level closely. Watch for symptoms of hypercalcemia relapse: bone pain, renal calculi, polyuria, anorexia, nausea, vomiting, thirst, constipation, lethargy, bradycardia, muscle hypotonicity, pathologic fracture, psychosis, and coma.
• Periodic exams of urine sediment are recommended.
• Periodic nasal exam with visualization of nasal mucosa, turbinates, septum, and mucosal blood vessel status is recommended to assess for ulceration in patients using intranasal form.
• Nasal reactions occur more commonly in older adults.
• Monitor periodic ALP and 24-hour urine hydroxyproline levels to evaluate drug effect.
• In Paget disease, maximum reductions of ALP and urinary hydroxyproline excretion may take 6 to 24 months of continuous treatment.
• In patients with good first response to drug who have a relapse, expect to evaluate antibody response to the hormone protein.
• If symptoms have been relieved after 6 months, treatment may be stopped until symptoms or radiologic signs recur.
• *Look alike–sound alike:* Don't confuse calcitonin with calcifediol or calcitriol.

PATIENT TEACHING
• When drug is given for Paget disease or postmenopausal osteoporosis, remind patient to take adequate calcium and vitamin D supplements.
• Inform patient that local inflammatory reactions at subcut or IM injection sites and facial

flushing and warmth may occur within minutes of injection and usually last about 1 hour.
• Tell patient that nausea may occur at the onset of therapy.
• Instruct patient to promptly report signs and symptoms of hypercalcemia.
• Advise patient who is breastfeeding that drug may inhibit lactation.
• Instruct patient in proper nasal spray administration and storage.

calcitriol (1,25-dihydroxycholecalciferol)
kal-SIH-trye-ol

Rocaltrol, Vectical

Therapeutic class: Antihypocalcemics
Pharmacologic class: Vitamin D analogues

AVAILABLE FORMS
Capsules: 0.25 mcg, 0.5 mcg
Injection: 1 mcg/mL
Oral solution: 1 mcg/mL
Topical ointment: 3 mcg/g

INDICATIONS & DOSAGES
➤ **Hypocalcemia in patients undergoing long-term dialysis (PO)**
Adults: Initially, 0.25 mcg PO daily. Increase by 0.25 mcg daily at 4- to 8-week intervals. Maintenance oral dosage is 0.25 mcg every other day up to 1 mcg daily (most patients undergoing hemodialysis respond to doses between 0.5 and 1 mcg/day).
➤ **Hypocalcemia in patients undergoing long-term dialysis (IV)**
Adults and children age 13 and older: Usual IV dosage is 1 to 2 mcg IV three times weekly (approximately every other day). Increase dose by 0.5 to 1 mcg at 2- to 4-week intervals.
➤ **Hypoparathyroidism, pseudohypoparathyroidism**
Adults and children age 6 and older: Initially, 0.25 mcg PO daily in the morning. Dosage may be increased at 2- to 4-week intervals. Maintenance dosage is 0.5 to 2 mcg PO daily.
➤ **Hypoparathyroidism**
Children ages 1 to 5: 0.25 to 0.75 mcg PO daily.
➤ **To manage secondary hyperparathyroidism and resulting metabolic bone disease in patients in predialysis (with CrCl of 15 to 55 mL/minute)**

Adults and children age 3 and older: Initially, 0.25 mcg PO daily. Dosage may be increased to 0.5 mcg/day if needed.
Children younger than age 3: Initially, 0.01 to 0.015 mcg/kg PO daily.
➤ **Mild to moderate plaque psoriasis**
Adults and children age 7 and older: Apply ointment topically to affected area b.i.d., morning and evening. Maximum weekly dose is 200 g.
Children age 2 to 6: Apply ointment topically to affected area b.i.d., morning and evening. Maximum weekly dose is 100 g.

ADMINISTRATION
PO
• Give drug without regard for food.
• Don't give with magnesium-containing antacids.
IV
▼ For hypocalcemia in patient undergoing hemodialysis, give drug by rapid injection through catheter at end of hemodialysis session.
▼ Discard unused portion.
▼ Store at room temperature.
▼ **Incompatibilities:** None listed by manufacturer. Consult a drug incompatibility reference for more information.
Topical
• Topical form isn't for oral, ophthalmic, or intravaginal use. Don't use on facial skin.
• Gently rub into skin until no longer visible.
• Don't apply an occlusive dressing.

ACTION
Stimulates calcium absorption from the GI tract and promotes movement of calcium from bone to blood.

Route	Onset	Peak	Duration
PO	2–6 hr	3–6 hr	3–5 days
IV	Immediate	Unknown	3–5 days
Topical	Unknown	Unknown	Unknown

Half-life: 5 to 8 hours.

ADVERSE REACTIONS
CNS: headache, somnolence, weakness, irritability. **CV:** HTN, *arrhythmias.* **EENT:** conjunctivitis, photophobia, dry mouth, rhinorrhea. **GI:** nausea, vomiting, constipation, polydipsia, *pancreatitis,* metallic taste, anorexia. **GU:** polyuria, nocturia, nephrocalcinosis, hypercalciuria, decreased libido. **Metabolic:** weight loss. **Musculoskeletal:**

C

bone and muscle pain. **Skin:** pruritus, skin discomfort at application area or injection site. **Other:** hyperthermia.

INTERACTIONS
Drug-drug. *Aluminum hydroxide:* May increase aluminum concentration. Don't use together.
Calcium supplements: May increase risk of hypercalcemia. Avoid unmonitored calcium use.
Cardiac glycosides: May increase risk of arrhythmias. Monitor therapy.
Cholestyramine, colestipol, excessive use of mineral oil: May decrease absorption of oral vitamin D analogues. Avoid using together.
Corticosteroids: May diminish vitamin D analogue effects. Monitor therapy.
Magnesium-containing antacids: May cause hypermagnesemia, especially in patients with chronic renal failure. Avoid using together.
Phenobarbital, phenytoin: May inhibit calcitriol synthesis. Dose may need to be increased.
Phosphate binders (lanthanum carbonate, sevelamer): May alter phosphate level. Monitor phosphate level and adjust binder dosage, as needed.
Sucralfate: May increase serum concentrations of sucralfate and aluminum concentrations. Avoid using together.
Thiazide, thiazide-like diuretics: May cause hypercalcemia. Use together cautiously.

EFFECTS ON LAB TEST RESULTS
• May increase AST, ALT, BUN, creatinine, cholesterol, urine albumin, and calcium levels.

CONTRAINDICATIONS & CAUTIONS
• Contraindicated in patients with hypercalcemia or vitamin D toxicity. Withhold all preparations containing vitamin D.
• Contraindicated in patients hypersensitive to drug or its components or to drugs in the same class.
• Use cautiously in patients receiving cardiac glycosides or in those with sarcoidosis or hyperparathyroidism.
Dialyzable drug: Unknown.
⚠ *Overdose S&S:* Hypercalcemia, hyperphosphatemia, hypercalciuria.

PREGNANCY-LACTATION-REPRODUCTION
• Use in pregnancy only if potential benefits justify fetal risk.

• Ingested calcitriol may appear in human milk. Patient shouldn't breastfeed during therapy.
• Use topical calcitriol cautiously in patients who are breastfeeding. If maternal use of a topical vitamin D analogue is needed, patient should ensure infant doesn't come in contact with treated area.

NURSING CONSIDERATIONS
• Effective therapy is dependent on adequate calcium intake.
• Monitor calcium level; this level multiplied by the phosphate level shouldn't exceed 70. After dosage adjustment, determine calcium level daily until level returns to normal. Once level is within normal limits, determine calcium level at least twice weekly. If hypercalcemia occurs, stop drug and notify prescriber but resume after calcium level returns to normal. Patient should receive adequate daily intake of calcium. Observe for hypocalcemia, bone pain, and weakness before and during therapy.
• Monitor phosphate level, especially in patients with hypoparathyroidism and patients on dialysis.
• Reduce dose as parathyroid hormone levels decrease in response to therapy.
• Make sure patient taking calcitriol maintains adequate fluid status.
• The symptoms of vitamin D intoxication include headache, somnolence, weakness, irritability, HTN, arrhythmias, conjunctivitis, photophobia, rhinorrhea, nausea, vomiting, constipation, polydipsia, pancreatitis, metallic taste, dry mouth, anorexia, nephrocalcinosis, polyuria, nocturia, weight loss, bone and muscle pain, pruritus, hyperthermia, and decreased libido.
• *Look alike–sound alike:* Don't confuse calcitriol with calcifediol or calcitonin.

PATIENT TEACHING
• Tell patient to report all adverse reactions and to immediately report early signs and symptoms of vitamin D intoxication: weakness, nausea, vomiting, dry mouth, constipation, muscle or bone pain, or metallic taste.
• Instruct patient to adhere to diet and calcium supplementation and to avoid OTC drugs and antacids that contain magnesium.
🔆 *Alert:* Tell patient that drug is the most potent form of vitamin D available and shouldn't be taken by anyone else.

calcium acetate
Calphron ◇, Phoslyra

calcium chloride

calcium citrate ◇
Cal-Citrate ◇, Cal-C-Cap ◇, Citracal ◇

calcium gluconate

calcium lactate

Therapeutic class: Calcium supplements
Pharmacologic class: Calcium salts

AVAILABLE FORMS
1 mEq of elemental calcium equals 20 mg
calcium acetate
Contains 169 mg or 8.45 mEq of elemental calcium/g
Capsules: 667 mg
Gelcaps: 667 mg
Solution: 667 mg/5 mL
Tablets ⓞⓝⓒ: 667 mg, 668 mg ◇
calcium chloride
Contains 273 mg or 13.6 mEq of elemental calcium/g
Injection: 10% solution in 10-mL ampules, vials, and syringes
calcium citrate
Contains 211 mg or 10.6 mEq of elemental calcium/g
Capsules: 180 mg ◇, 225 mg ◇
Granules for oral solution: 760 mg/3.5 g
Tablets: 200 mg ◇, 250 mg ◇, 950 mg ◇
calcium gluconate
Contains 93 mg or 4.5 mEq of elemental calcium/g
Capsules: 500 mg ◇
Injection: 10 mg/mL, 20 mg/mL, 100 mg/mL
Tablets: 50 mg ◇, 500 mg ◇
calcium lactate
Contains 130 mg or 6.5 mEq of elemental calcium/g
Capsules: 100 mg ◇, 500 mg ◇
Tablets: 100 mg ◇, 325 mg ◇, 648 mg ◇

INDICATIONS & DOSAGES
➤ **Hypocalcemia**
Adults: 7 to 14 mEq elemental calcium IV. May give as a 10% calcium chloride solution. Or, initially, 1 to 2 g calcium gluconate IV.
Children: 0.136 to 0.252 mEq elemental calcium/kg IV. Or, initially, 29 to 200 mg/kg

calcium gluconate IV based on age and serum calcium level.
➤ **Adjunctive treatment of magnesium intoxication**
Adults: Initially, 7 mEq IV. Base subsequent doses on patient's response.
➤ **During exchange transfusions**
Adults: 1.35 mEq IV with each 100 mL citrated blood.
Neonates: 0.45 mEq IV after each 100 mL citrated blood.
➤ **Hyperphosphatemia**
Adults: Initially, 2 capsules or tablets or 10 mL oral solution PO t.i.d. with meals. Titrate dose every 2 to 3 weeks until an acceptable serum phosphorus level is reached; watch for hypercalcemia. Most patients on dialysis need 3 to 4 capsules or tablets or 15 to 20 mL oral solution with each meal.
➤ **Dietary supplement**
Adults: 500 mg to 2 g PO daily.

ADMINISTRATION
PO
• Give drug with a full glass of water.
• Give 1 to 1.5 hours after meals if GI upset occurs.
IV
▼ Give calcium chloride and gluconate only by IV route.
▼ Dilute calcium gluconate before use in 5% dextrose or NSS per manufacturer's instructions and assess for potential drug or IV fluid incompatibilities, especially with concurrent phosphate administration.
▼ Monitor ECG when giving calcium IV. Stop drug and notify prescriber if patient complains of discomfort.
🛇 *Alert:* Extravasation may cause severe necrosis and tissue sloughing. Calcium gluconate is less irritating to veins and tissues than calcium chloride.
Direct injection
▼ Don't use scalp veins in children.
▼ Warm solution to body temperature before giving it.
▼ For calcium chloride, give at 0.5 to 1 mL/minute (1.36 mEq/minute). For calcium gluconate bolus injection, don't exceed an infusion rate of 200 mg/minute in adults or 100 mg/minute in children, including neonates.
▼ Give slowly through a small needle into a large vein or through an IV line containing a free-flowing, compatible solution.

Reactions in bold italics are *life-threatening*. Interactions may have a *rapid onset* or a ***delayed onset***.

▼ After injection, keep patient recumbent for 15 minutes.

Intermittent infusion

▼ Infuse diluted solution through an IV line containing a compatible solution.

▼ **Incompatibilities:** Calcium chloride: None listed by manufacturer. Consult a drug incompatibility reference for more information. Calcium gluconate: ceftriaxone, fluids containing bicarbonate or phosphate, lipid products, methylprednisolone, minocycline.

ACTION

Replaces calcium and maintains calcium level.

Route	Onset	Peak	Duration
PO	Unknown	Unknown	Unknown
IV	Immediate	Immediate	30 min–2 hr

Half-life: Unknown.

ADVERSE REACTIONS

CNS: anxiety, tingling sensations, sense of oppression or heat waves with IV use, syncope with rapid IV use. **CV:** *bradycardia, arrhythmias, cardiac arrest with rapid IV use,* decreased BP, vasodilation. **GI:** constipation, irritation, chalky taste, *hemorrhage,* nausea, vomiting, thirst, abdominal pain. **GU:** polyuria, renal calculi. **Metabolic:** hypercalcemia. **Skin:** infusion-site reactions.

INTERACTIONS

Drug-drug. *Bisphosphonates:* May reduce absorption of bisphosphonate from GI tract. Give calcium salts at least 30 minutes after alendronate or risedronate, at least 60 minutes after ibandronate, and not within 2 hours of tiludronate or etidronate.

Calcium channel blockers: May diminish therapeutic effects of calcium channel blockers. Monitor therapy.

Cardiac glycosides: May increase digoxin toxicity. Give calcium cautiously, if at all, to patients taking cardiac glycosides.

Deferiprone: May decrease deferiprone serum concentration. Separate administration of deferiprone and oral calcium medications or supplements by at least 4 hours.

Fluoroquinolones: Oral calcium may decrease absorption of oral quinolones. Consider therapy modification. Give at least 2 hours before or 6 hours after Phoslyra.

Iron supplements: May reduce iron absorption. Separate drug administration by 2 hours.

Levothyroxine: May decrease effects of thyroid products. Separate by at least 4 hours.

Raltegravir: May decrease raltegravir serum concentration. Give raltegravir 2 hours before or 6 hours after calcium or avoid concurrent use.

Sodium polystyrene sulfonate: May cause metabolic acidosis in patients with renal disease and a reduction of the resin's binding of potassium. Separate drugs by several hours.

Tetracyclines: May decrease serum concentration of tetracyclines. Avoid use together or, if concurrent use is absolutely necessary, consider separating administration of each agent by several hours.

Thiazide diuretics: May cause hypercalcemia. Avoid using together.

Drug-food. *Foods containing oxalic acid (rhubarb, spinach), phytic acid (bran, whole-grain cereals), or phosphorus (dairy products, milk):* May interfere with calcium absorption. Discourage use together.

EFFECTS ON LAB TEST RESULTS

• May increase calcium level.
• May decrease phosphorus level.

CONTRAINDICATIONS & CAUTIONS

• Contraindicated in patients with cancer who have bone metastases and in those with ventricular fibrillation, hypercalcemia, hypophosphatemia, or renal calculi.

• Use calcium products with extreme caution in patients taking cardiac glycosides and in those with sarcoidosis, renal or cardiac disease, and electrolyte disturbances.

• Use calcium chloride cautiously in patients with cor pulmonale, respiratory acidosis, or respiratory failure.

Dialyzable drug: Yes.

⚠ *Overdose S&S:* Hypercalcemia, confusion, delirium, stupor, coma.

PREGNANCY-LACTATION-REPRODUCTION

• It isn't known if drug can cause fetal harm when used during pregnancy or if it can affect reproductive capacity. Use during pregnancy only if clearly needed; monitor maternal serum calcium level.

• Calcium appears in human milk, but is thought to be compatible with breastfeeding. Monitor maternal serum calcium level.

NURSING CONSIDERATIONS

🔔 *Alert:* Double-check that you're giving the correct form of calcium; resuscitation cart may contain both calcium gluconate and calcium chloride.

• Monitor calcium levels frequently. Hypercalcemia may result after large doses in chronic renal failure. Report abnormalities.

• Signs and symptoms of severe hypercalcemia may include stupor, confusion, delirium, and coma. Signs and symptoms of mild hypercalcemia may include anorexia, nausea, and vomiting.

• *Look alike–sound alike:* Don't confuse calcium with calcitriol, or calcium chloride with calcium gluconate.

PATIENT TEACHING

• Tell patient to take oral calcium 1 to 1½ hours after meals if GI upset occurs.

• Tell patient to take oral calcium with a full glass of water.

• Tell patient to report anorexia, nausea, vomiting, constipation, abdominal pain, dry mouth, thirst, or polyuria.

• Advise patient to notify prescriber if taking OTC products such as iron.

• Warn patient not to eat rhubarb, spinach, bran and whole-grain cereals, or dairy products in the meal before taking calcium; these foods may interfere with calcium absorption.

• Inform patient that some products may contain phenylalanine or tartrazine.

SAFETY ALERT!

canagliflozin
kan-a-gli-FLOE-zin

Invokana

Therapeutic class: Antidiabetics
Pharmacologic class: Sodium-glucose cotransporter 2 inhibitors

AVAILABLE FORMS

Tablets: 100 mg, 300 mg

INDICATIONS & DOSAGES

Adjust-a-dose (for all indications): Refer to manufacturer's instructions for renal impairment and drug interaction dosage adjustments.

➤ **Adjunct to diet and exercise to improve glycemic control in patients with type 2 diabetes; to reduce risk of major adverse CV events in patients with type 2 diabetes and established CV disease**

Adults: 100 mg PO once daily before first meal of the day. May increase to 300 mg/day.

➤ **To reduce risk of ESRD, doubling of serum creatinine level, CV death, and hospitalization for HF in patients with type 2 diabetes and diabetic nephropathy with albuminuria greater than 300 mg/day**

Adults: 100 mg PO once daily. May increase to 300 mg/day.

ADMINISTRATION

PO

• Give before first meal of the day.

• Give missed dose as soon as possible unless it's close to time of next regularly scheduled dose. Don't give two doses at the same time.

• Store tablets at room temperature.

ACTION

Inhibits SGLT2, which reabsorbs glucose filtered by the kidneys, increasing amount of urinary glucose that is excreted.

Route	Onset	Peak	Duration
PO	Unknown	1–2 hr	Unknown

Half-life: 10.6 hours for 100-mg dose; 13.1 hours for 300-mg dose.

ADVERSE REACTIONS

CNS: fatigue, asthenia, syncope, postural dizziness. **CV:** hypotension, orthostatic hypotension. **GI:** thirst, constipation, nausea, abdominal pain, dehydration, *pancreatitis.* **GU:** genital fungal infection, UTI, increased urination, vulvovaginal pruritus, renal impairment. **Hematologic:** increased Hb level. **Metabolic:** *hypoglycemia, hyperkalemia,* hypercholesterolemia, hypermagnesemia, hyperphosphatemia. **Musculoskeletal:** bone fracture, increased risk of lower limb amputation. **Other:** hypersensitivity reactions, falls.

INTERACTIONS

Drug-drug. *ACE inhibitors (enalapril, lisinopril, moexipril, quinapril), ARBs (candesartan, losartan, olmesartan, valsartan), eplerenone, potassium-sparing diuretics (amiloride, spironolactone):* May increase risk of hyperkalemia. Monitor potassium level closely.

Antihypertensives: May increase hypotension. Monitor patient closely.

Reactions in bold italics are *life-threatening*. Interactions may have a *rapid onset* or a *delayed onset*.

Carbamazepine, efavirenz: May decrease canagliflozin serum concentration. Consider increasing canagliflozin dosage based on GFR.

Digoxin: May increase digoxin level. Monitor digoxin level periodically.

Fosphenytoin, phenytoin: May decrease canagliflozin concentration. Consider increasing canagliflozin to 200 mg/day in patients tolerating 100 mg/day and to 300 mg/day in patients with eGFR of 60 mL/minute/1.73 m^2 or greater.

Insulin and insulin secretagogues (glipizide, repaglinide): May increase risk of hypoglycemia. Consider lower dosage of insulin or insulin secretagogue.

Lomitapide: May increase lomitapide level. Limit maximum adult dosage of lomitapide to 30 mg daily.

Loop diuretics: May cause hypotension and intravascular volume depletion. Consider alternative therapy.

Salicylates: May increase hypoglycemic effects. Monitor patient closely.

SSRIs (citalopram, fluoxetine, sertraline): May increase canagliflozin level. Monitor patient closely. Canagliflozin dosage may need adjustment if SSRI is discontinued.

UGT inducers (phenobarbital, rifampin, ritonavir): May decrease canagliflozin level. Adjust canagliflozin dosage based on estimated GFR.

Drug-herb. *St. John's wort:* May decrease canagliflozin serum concentration. Consider increasing canagliflozin dosage based on GFR.

EFFECTS ON LAB TEST RESULTS

• May increase serum creatinine, potassium, magnesium, phosphate, Hb, LDL cholesterol, non-HDL cholesterol, and urine glucose levels.

• May decrease GFR and serum glucose level.

• May cause positive test for glycosuria and interfere with 1,5-anhydroglucitol assay. Use other methods to monitor glycemic control.

CONTRAINDICATIONS & CAUTIONS

• Contraindicated in patients hypersensitive to drug or its components, in those with severe renal impairment (eGFR of less than 30 mL/minute/1.73 m^2) or ESRD, and in patients on dialysis.

• Drug isn't recommended for patients with severe hepatic disease (Child-Pugh class C), type 1 diabetes, or diabetic ketoacidosis.

• For patients who will undergo scheduled surgery, consider temporarily stopping drug for at least 3 days before surgery; temporarily stop drug and resolve ketoacidosis before restarting drug.

⚠ *Alert:* Drug may cause acidosis, which may require emergency department care or hospitalization.

⚠ *Alert:* Drug may cause hyperkalemia, especially in patients with renal impairment or who are taking potassium-sparing diuretics, ACE inhibitors, or ARBs.

• Drug may increase risk of bone fracture as early as 12 weeks after start of treatment and has been linked to decreased bone mineral density. Consider factors that may contribute to bone fracture risk prior to prescribing.

⚠ *Alert:* Drug may increase risk of severe UTI, including urosepsis and pyelonephritis. Monitor patient and treat promptly if indicated.

⚠ *Alert:* SGLT2 inhibitors such as canagliflozin increase the risk of a rare but serious necrotizing fasciitis of the perineum (Fournier gangrene). If necrotizing fasciitis is suspected, immediately discontinue SGL2 drug and begin broad-spectrum antibiotics. Surgical debridement may be necessary. Monitor blood glucose level and start alternative therapy for glycemic control. Serious outcomes have included hospitalization, multiple surgeries, and death.

• Drug increases serum creatinine level and decreases eGFR; patients with hypovolemia may be more susceptible to these changes. Renal function abnormalities can occur after drug initiation. More frequent renal function monitoring is recommended in patients with an eGFR of less than 60 mL/minute/1.73 m^2.

• Use cautiously in older adults; in patients with volume depletion, impaired renal function, chronic low systolic BP, or hypotension; and in those on concurrent diuretics.

• Safety and effectiveness in children haven't been established.

Dialyzable drug: No.

PREGNANCY-LACTATION-REPRODUCTION

• There are no adequate well-controlled studies in patients who are pregnant. Use during pregnancy only if potential benefit justifies fetal risk.

• Due to adverse effects on renal development observed in animal studies, the manufacturer doesn't recommend use of canagliflozin during the second and third trimesters.

• It isn't known if drug appears in human milk. Patient should discontinue breastfeeding or discontinue drug, taking into account importance of drug to the patient.

NURSING CONSIDERATIONS

• Monitor patient for infections, new pain or tenderness, and sores or ulcers of the lower limbs. Discontinue drug if these complications occur.

⚠ *Alert:* Drug can increase risk of acute kidney injury. Before start of therapy, assess patient for factors that may predispose patient to acute kidney injury (decreased blood volume, chronic renal insufficiency, HF, or concurrent use of other medications, such as diuretics, ACE inhibitors, ARBs, metformin, NSAIDs). Assess renal function before starting drug and monitor patient periodically. If acute kidney injury occurs, drug should be discontinued and the kidney impairment treated.

• Correct volume depletion before initiating drug. Observe for hypotension during therapy.

⚠ *Alert:* Monitor patients for ketoacidosis, especially those with major illness, reduced food or fluid intake, or reduced insulin dose. Elevated urine or serum ketone levels without associated very high glucose levels have occurred with SGLT2 inhibitor use.

⚠ *Alert:* Immediately report signs and symptoms of necrotizing fasciitis of the perineum (temperature above 100.4° F [38° C]); general feeling of being unwell; tenderness, redness, or swelling of the genitals back to the rectum); signs and symptoms can worsen quickly. Immediately stop drug and prepare to administer broad-spectrum antibiotics; surgical debridement may be necessary. Monitor blood glucose levels and start alternative therapy for glycemic control.

• Monitor blood glucose level. Assess for signs and symptoms of hypoglycemia.

• Be aware that because of the drug's mechanism of action, urine test will be positive for glucose.

• Monitor electrolytes, such as potassium and magnesium. Correct levels as clinically indicated.

• Drug may increase lipid levels. Assess levels periodically and treat as clinically indicated.

• Assess for genital mycotic (fungal) infections, especially in patients with a history of infection and in uncircumcised males. Treat appropriately.

• Monitor patient for hypersensitivity reaction (urticaria); reaction may occur hours to days after start of therapy. Discontinue drug and treat appropriately if hypersensitivity reaction occurs.

PATIENT TEACHING

• Counsel patient about the increased risk of lower limb amputations. Instruct patient about the importance of routine preventive foot care and to immediately report infections, new pain or tenderness, and sores or ulcers involving the lower limbs.

• Advise patient to discontinue drug and immediately report hypersensitivity reaction (generalized urticarial rash).

⚠ *Alert:* Teach patient the signs and symptoms of necrotizing fasciitis (temperature above 100.4° F [38° C], general feeling of being unwell, and tenderness, redness, or swelling of the genitals back to the rectum) and to seek immediate medical attention if any occur.

⚠ *Alert:* Instruct patient to seek medical attention immediately for signs and symptoms of ketoacidosis (difficulty breathing, hyperventilation, anorexia, nausea, vomiting, abdominal pain, confusion, unusual fatigue or sleepiness).

⚠ *Alert:* Instruct patient to seek medical attention for signs and symptoms of UTI (dysuria, frequency, pelvic pain, hematuria, urgency, fever, back pain, nausea, vomiting).

⚠ *Alert:* Advise patient to seek immediate medical attention for signs and symptoms of acute kidney injury (decreased urine output, swelling in legs or feet). Warn patient not to stop drug without first discussing with prescriber.

• Warn patient of possible risks to fetus and infant during pregnancy or breastfeeding. Instruct patient who is breastfeeding to discontinue drug or discontinue breastfeeding.

• Caution patient to avoid dehydration, which can cause hypotension. Instruct patient regarding adequate fluid intake and to report signs and symptoms of hypotension (postural dizziness, weakness, syncope).

- Advise patient to use care during first few weeks of therapy because of an increased risk of falls.
- Instruct patient on general diabetes care, including importance of diet and exercise and monitoring blood glucose and HbA_{1c} levels; signs and symptoms and management of hypoglycemia and hyperglycemia; and assessing for diabetes complications.
- Advise patient to seek medical advice promptly during periods of stress (such as fever, trauma, infection, or surgery) because medication requirements may change.
- Instruct patient in safe drug administration.

candesartan cilexetil
kan-de-SAR-tan

Atacand🔊

Therapeutic class: Antihypertensives
Pharmacologic class: ARBs

AVAILABLE FORMS
Tablets: 4 mg, 8 mg, 16 mg, 32 mg

INDICATIONS & DOSAGES
Adjust-a-dose (for all indications): If patient, especially patient with impaired renal function, is taking a diuretic, administer under close medical supervision and consider a lower starting dose.
➤ **HTN (used alone or with other antihypertensives)**
Adults: Initially, 16 mg PO once daily when used alone in patients who aren't volume-depleted; usual dosage range, 8 to 32 mg PO daily as a single dose or in two divided doses. Adjust dosage about every 2 weeks, as tolerated, to target effect.
Adjust-a-dose: In patients with moderate hepatic impairment, initially give 8 mg PO once daily.
➤ **Pediatric HTN (used alone or with other antihypertensives)**
⚠ *Alert:* Don't use in children with GFR less than 30 mL/minute/1.73 m^2.
Children ages 6 to younger than 17: Initially for patients weighing more than 50 kg, 8 to 16 mg PO once daily. May adjust dosage to between 4 and 32 mg PO as single dose or divided doses as indicated.

Initially for patients weighing less than 50 kg, 4 to 8 mg PO once daily. May adjust dosage to between 2 and 16 mg PO as single dose or divided doses as needed.
Children ages 1 to younger than 6: Initially, 0.2 mg/kg PO once daily. Dosage range, 0.05 to 0.4 mg/kg/day PO as single dose or divided doses.
➤ **HF with reduced ejection fraction (NYHA Class II to IV)**
Adults: Initially, 4 mg PO once daily. Double the dose about every 2 weeks as tolerated to a target dose of 32 mg once daily.

ADMINISTRATION
PO
- Give drug without regard for food.
- Pharmacist may make tablets into suspension for patients unable to swallow pills.
- Shake suspension well before each use.
- Suspension may be stored unopened at room temperature for 100 days.
- Use suspension within 30 days of opening bottle.

ACTION
Inhibits vasoconstrictive action of angiotensin II by blocking angiotensin II receptor on the surface of vascular smooth muscle and other tissue cells.

Route	Onset	Peak	Duration
PO	Unknown	3–4 hr	24 hr

Half-life: 9 hours.

ADVERSE REACTIONS
CNS: dizziness, headache. **CV:** hypotension. **EENT:** pharyngitis, rhinitis, sinusitis. **GU:** renal function abnormality. **Metabolic:** *hyperkalemia.* **Musculoskeletal:** back pain. **Respiratory:** URI.

INTERACTIONS
Drug-drug. *ACE inhibitors, other ARBs:* May increase risk of hypotension, hyperkalemia, and changes in renal function (including acute renal failure) when used with other drugs that cause blockade of the RAAS. Consider therapy modification.
Aliskiren: May increase risk of renal impairment, hypotension, and hyperkalemia in patients with diabetes and those with moderate to severe renal impairment (GFR less than 60 mL/minute). Concomitant use is contraindicated in patients with diabetes. Avoid concomitant use in those with moderate to severe renal impairment.

🍁Canada ◇OTC ◆Off-label use 🔊Photoguide ⊕Do not crush *Liquid contains alcohol ▦Genetic

Canagliflozin: May enhance hyperkalemic and hypotensive effects. Monitor closely.
Lithium: May increase lithium concentration. Monitor lithium levels closely.
NSAIDs (celecoxib, ibuprofen): May decrease antihypertensive effect of candesartan. Coadministration in patients who are volume-depleted (including those taking diuretics) or with decreased renal function and in older adults may result in deteriorating renal function. Monitor BP and renal function.
Potassium-sparing diuretics, potassium supplements: May cause hyperkalemia. Monitor patient closely.
Drug-food. *Salt substitutes containing potassium:* May cause hyperkalemia. Monitor patient closely.

EFFECTS ON LAB TEST RESULTS

• May increase potassium, BUN, and serum creatinine levels.
• May cause false-negative aldosterone-to-renin ratio.

CONTRAINDICATIONS & CAUTIONS

• Contraindicated in patients hypersensitive to drug or its components, in children with GFR of less than 30 mL/min/1.73 m^2, and in children younger than age 1.
• Use cautiously in patients whose renal function depends on the RAAS (such as patients with HF) because of risk of oliguria and progressive azotemia with acute renal failure or death.
• Use cautiously in patients who are volume or salt depleted; may cause symptoms of hypotension. Start therapy with a lower dosage range, and monitor BP carefully.
• Don't use for HTN in children younger than age 1 because of potential effects on the developing immature kidneys.
Dialyzable drug: No.
⚠ *Overdose S&S:* Hypotension, dizziness, tachycardia; possible bradycardia from parasympathetic stimulation.

PREGNANCY-LACTATION-REPRODUCTION

Boxed Warning Drugs such as candesartan that act directly on the RAAS can cause injury and death to the developing fetus. Discontinue candesartan as soon as possible if pregnancy occurs. ▮
• It isn't known if drug appears in human milk. Consider discontinuing breastfeeding or

drug, taking into account importance of drug to the patient.

NURSING CONSIDERATIONS

• Most of drug's antihypertensive effect occurs within 2 weeks. Maximal effect may take 4 to 6 weeks. Diuretic may be added if BP isn't controlled by drug alone.
• Monitor BP during dosage escalation and periodically thereafter.
• If hypotension occurs after a candesartan dose, position patient supine and treat appropriately.
• Monitor renal function and serum potassium level periodically.

PATIENT TEACHING

Boxed Warning Inform patient of childbearing potential of the consequences of exposure to drug during pregnancy and to immediately report suspected pregnancy. ▮
• Advise patient who is breastfeeding of the risk of adverse effects on the infant and the need to stop either breastfeeding or drug.
• Instruct patient or caregiver in safe drug administration and storage.
• Inform patient to report all adverse reactions without delay.

SAFETY ALERT!

cangrelor
KAN-grel-or

Kengreal

Therapeutic class: Antiplatelet drugs
Pharmacologic class: Platelet aggregation inhibitors

AVAILABLE FORMS

Lyophilized powder for injection: 50 mg

INDICATIONS & DOSAGES

➤ **As an adjunct to PCI for reducing risk of periprocedural MI, repeat coronary revascularization, and stent thrombosis in patients who haven't been treated with a P2Y$_{12}$ platelet inhibitor and aren't receiving a glycoprotein IIb/IIIa inhibitor**
Adults: 30 mcg/kg IV bolus before PCI followed immediately by a 4 mcg/kg/minute IV infusion continued for at least 2 hours or for duration of PCI, whichever is longer. Transition patient to oral P2Y$_{12}$ platelet inhibitor to

maintain platelet inhibition. Recommended inhibitors include ticagrelor 180 mg PO at any time during infusion or immediately after discontinuation, or prasugrel 60 mg or clopidogrel 600 mg immediately after discontinuation of infusion.

ADMINISTRATION

IV

▼ For each 50-mg vial, reconstitute by adding 5 mL sterile water for injection. Swirl gently until dissolved; avoid vigorous mixing. Ensure contents are fully dissolved, clear, colorless to pale yellow, and free from particulate matter.

▼ Dilute reconstituted drug immediately. Don't use without dilution.

▼ Further dilute each reconstituted vial by withdrawing contents from one reconstituted vial and adding to one 250-mL NSS or dextrose 5% bag. Mix bag thoroughly. This dilution will result in a concentration of 200 mcg/mL and should be sufficient for at least 2 hours of dosing. Patients weighing 100 kg or more will require a minimum of two bags.

▼ Discard any unused portion of reconstituted solution remaining in vial.

▼ Administer via a dedicated IV line.

▼ Administer bolus volume rapidly (over less than 1 minute) from the diluted bag via manual IV push or pump. Ensure bolus is completely administered before start of PCI. Start infusion immediately after administration of bolus.

▼ Diluted drug remains stable for up to 12 hours in 5% dextrose injection and 24 hours in NSS at room temperature.

▼ **Incompatibilities:** None listed by manufacturer. Consult a drug incompatibility reference for more information.

ACTION

A direct P2Y$_{12}$ platelet receptor inhibitor that blocks ADP-induced platelet activation and aggregation. Binds selectively and reversibly to the P2Y$_{12}$ platelet receptor to prevent further signaling and platelet activation.

Route	Onset	Peak	Duration
IV	2 min	2 min	1 hr after discontinuation of infusion

Half-life: 3 to 6 minutes.

ADVERSE REACTIONS

CNS: *intracranial hemorrhage.* **CV:** *hemorrhage.* **GU:** worsening renal function in patients with severe renal impairment (CrCl less than 30 mL/minute). **Respiratory:** dyspnea.

INTERACTIONS

Drug-drug. *Agents with antiplatelet properties (NSAIDs, P2Y$_{12}$ platelet inhibitors, SSRIs):* May enhance antiplatelet effects. Monitor therapy.
Anticoagulants: May increase anticoagulant effects. Monitor therapy.
Glucosamine: May enhance antiplatelet effects. Monitor therapy.
Thienopyridines (clopidogrel, prasugrel): Negate antiplatelet effect. Don't give clopidogrel or prasugrel until the cangrelor infusion has been discontinued.

EFFECTS ON LAB TEST RESULTS

• May inhibit platelet aggregation.

CONTRAINDICATIONS & CAUTIONS

• Contraindicated in patients hypersensitive to drug or its components and in those with significant active bleeding.
• Drug can cause serious hypersensitivity reactions, including anaphylaxis, bronchospasm, angioedema, and stridor.
• Safety and effectiveness in children haven't been established.
Dialyzable drug: Unlikely.

PREGNANCY-LACTATION-REPRODUCTION

• There are no adequate studies during pregnancy. Untreated MI can be fatal.
• When possible, discontinue cangrelor 1 hour before labor, delivery, or neuraxial blockade.
• It isn't known if drug appears in human milk.

NURSING CONSIDERATIONS

• Monitor patients for hypersensitivity reactions, including anaphylactic reactions, anaphylactic shock, bronchospasm, angioedema, and stridor. Discontinue drug immediately and treat emergently.
• Monitor patients for signs of overt bleeding and symptoms of active bleeding.
• Platelet function will normalize 1 hour after discontinuation of infusion.

PATIENT TEACHING

• Explain to patient that drug is used to inhibit platelet function during PCI and that platelet function and ability for clot formation will normalize 1 hour after infusion.

• Warn patient of the risk of bleeding; advise patient to immediately report signs and symptoms of bleeding (mental status changes, light-headedness, low BP, blood in stool or urine, bleeding from gums, joint pain and swelling, abnormal bruising, abdominal or chest pain).

• Caution patient that hypersensitivity reactions may occur and to immediately report difficulty breathing, swelling of throat and lips, feeling faint, hives, or rash.

SAFETY ALERT!

capecitabine ☒
kap-ah-SEAT-ah-been

Xeloda

Therapeutic class: Antineoplastics
Pharmacologic class: Pyrimidine analogues

AVAILABLE FORMS

Tablets ⬤*:* 150 mg, 500 mg

INDICATIONS & DOSAGES

Adjust-a-dose (for all indications): Round to nearest dose that gives a whole tablet; don't cut tablets in half. Reduce dosage by 25% in patients with moderate renal impairment (30 to 50 mL/minute). Refer to manufacturer's instructions for toxicity-related dosage adjustments.

➤ **With docetaxel or alone, metastatic breast cancer resistant to both paclitaxel and an anthracycline-containing chemotherapy regimen or resistant to paclitaxel in patients for whom further anthracycline therapy isn't indicated; first-line treatment of metastatic colorectal cancer when fluoropyrimidine therapy alone is preferred; Dukes stage C colon cancer after complete resection of primary tumor when fluoropyrimidine alone is preferred**
Adults: 1,250 mg/m² PO b.i.d. for 2 weeks, followed by a 1-week rest period; repeat every 3 weeks. Adjuvant treatment in patients with Dukes C colon cancer is recommended for a total of eight cycles (24 weeks). Maximum

dose is 5,600 mg/day with BSA of 2.18 m² or more for both breast and colon cancers.

➤ **Breast cancer (adjuvant therapy) in patients with HER2-negative primary breast cancer who had residual invasive disease after neoadjuvant therapy (containing an anthracycline, taxane, or both) and surgery** ◆
Adults: 1,250 mg/m² PO b.i.d. on days 1 to 14 of a 21-day treatment cycle for six to eight cycles.

➤ **Pancreatic cancer (adjuvant therapy) after complete resection of pancreatic adenocarcinoma** ◆
Adults: 830 mg/m² PO b.i.d. on days 1 to 21 every 28 days (in combination with gemcitabine) for six cycles beginning within 12 weeks of resection.

➤ **Pancreatic cancer (locally advanced or metastatic)** ◆
Adults: 1,250 mg/m² PO b.i.d. on days 1 to 14 of a 3-week cycle or 830 mg/m² b.i.d. (in combination with gemcitabine) on days 1 to 21 of a 4-week cycle until disease progression or unacceptable toxicity.

ADMINISTRATION

PO

• Give drug whole with water within 30 minutes after a meal.

• Don't cut or crush tablets.

• Use gloves and safety glasses to avoid exposure if tablets break.

• Pharmacist may compound drug into a suspension if patient can't swallow tablets.

• Give missed dose as soon as possible unless it's close to next regularly scheduled dose. Don't give two doses at the same time.

ACTION

Converts to active 5-FU, which causes cellular injury by interfering with DNA synthesis to inhibit cell division and with RNA processing and protein synthesis.

Route	Onset	Peak	Duration
PO	Unknown	90–120 min	Unknown

Half-life: About 45 minutes.

ADVERSE REACTIONS

CNS: dizziness, fatigue, weakness, headache, insomnia, pain, paresthesia, fever, lethargy, peripheral neuropathy, mood alteration, depression, hypoesthesia, encephalopathy, asthenia, taste perversion. **CV:** edema, *venous*

Reactions in bold italics are *life-threatening*. Interactions may have a *rapid onset* or a *delayed onset*.

thrombosis, flushing, lymphedema. **EENT:** eye irritation, increased lacrimation, abnormal vision, conjunctivitis, epistaxis, rhinorrhea, oral discomfort, pharyngeal disorder, sore throat, dry mouth, oral candidiasis. **GI:** diarrhea, nausea, vomiting, stomatitis, abdominal pain, constipation, anorexia, dyspepsia, GI motility disorder, upper GI inflammatory disorder, *GI hemorrhage,* ileus. **GU:** UTI. **Hematologic:** *neutropenia, febrile neutropenia, thrombocytopenia,* anemia, *lymphopenia.* **Hepatic:** increased ALT level, hyperbilirubinemia. **Metabolic:** dehydration, weight loss, hypercalcemia, *hypocalcemia.* **Musculoskeletal:** myalgia, arthralgia, bone pain, limb pain, back pain, chest pain. **Respiratory:** dyspnea, cough, hemoptysis, pneumonia, pleural effusion, URI. **Skin:** hand-foot syndrome, dermatitis, skin discoloration, nail disorder, alopecia, rash, erythema, pruritus. **Other:** flulike illness.

INTERACTIONS

Drug-drug. *Antacids containing aluminum hydroxide or magnesium hydroxide:* May increase exposure to capecitabine and its metabolites. Monitor patient.

Allopurinol: May decrease capecitabine metabolite concentration. Avoid concurrent use.

Clozapine: May enhance neutropenia. Monitor concurrent use.

Fosphenytoin, phenytoin: May increase toxicity or fosphenytoin/phenytoin effect. Consider therapy modification or monitor phenytoin level.

Leucovorin: May increase cytotoxic effects of 5-FU with enhanced toxicity. Monitor patient carefully.

Boxed Warning *Warfarin:* May decrease clearance of warfarin and increase risk of bleeding. Monitor PT and INR frequently. ∎

Drug-herb. *Echinacea:* May diminish therapeutic effects of 5-FU. Avoid concurrent use.

Drug-food. *Any food:* Reduces rate and extent of capecitabine absorption. Patient should take consistently within 30 minutes after a meal.

EFFECTS ON LAB TEST RESULTS

• May increase triglyceride, ALT, and bilirubin levels.

• May decrease potassium and magnesium levels.

• May increase or decrease calcium level.

• May decrease Hb level and neutrophil, platelet, and WBC counts.

Boxed Warning May prolong PT and increase INR (in patients taking warfarin concomitantly). ∎

CONTRAINDICATIONS & CAUTIONS

⊠ Contraindicated in patients hypersensitive to capecitabine or 5-FU, in patients with known dihydropyrimidine dehydrogenase deficiency or absence, and in those with severe renal impairment (CrCl less than 30 mL/minute).

• Severe bone marrow suppression can occur and occurs more commonly when drug used in combination therapy. Dosage adjustment may be needed.

• Cardiotoxicity may occur, including MI, angina, arrhythmias, cardiac arrest, HF, ECG changes, and cardiomyopathy.

• Use cautiously in older adults and patients with history of CAD, mild to moderate hepatic dysfunction from liver metastases, hyperbilirubinemia, and renal insufficiency.

• Use cautiously in patients also taking warfarin, especially if older than age 60, due to higher risk of coagulopathy.

Dialyzable drug: Unknown.

⚠ *Overdose S&S:* Nausea, vomiting, diarrhea, GI irritation and bleeding, bone marrow depression.

PREGNANCY-LACTATION-REPRODUCTION

• Fetal harm may occur if drug is used during pregnancy. Patients of childbearing potential should use effective contraception during treatment and for 6 months after final dose.

• Male patients with partners of childbearing potential should use effective contraception during treatment and for 3 months after final dose.

• It isn't known if drug appears in human milk. Patient should discontinue breastfeeding during treatment and for 2 weeks after final dose.

NURSING CONSIDERATIONS

• Older adults may have a greater risk of adverse GI effects.

• Assess patient for severe diarrhea, and notify prescriber if it occurs. Give fluid and electrolyte replacement if patient becomes dehydrated. Drug may need to be immediately interrupted until diarrhea resolves or becomes less intense.

• Monitor patients for renal failure, especially patients with preexisting renal compromise or dehydration due to anorexia, asthenia, nausea, vomiting, or diarrhea.

• Discontinue drug for severe mucocutaneous reactions, such as SJS and TEN.

• Monitor patient for hand-foot syndrome (numbness, paresthesia, painless or painful swelling, erythema, desquamation, blistering, and severe pain of hands or feet), hyperbilirubinemia, and severe nausea. Drug therapy must be immediately adjusted. Hand-foot syndrome is staged from 1 to 4; drug may be stopped if severe or recurrent episodes occur.

Boxed Warning Frequently monitor INR and PT of patients taking capecitabine and oral coumarin-derivative anticoagulant therapy; adjust anticoagulant dose accordingly. Altered coagulation studies and bleeding may occur within several days to several months after start of therapy and within a month after therapy ends. ■

Boxed Warning Patients older than age 60 and those with a diagnosis of cancer are at increased risk of coagulopathy. ■

☉ Alert: Monitor patient carefully for toxicity, which may be managed by symptomatic treatment, dose interruptions, and dosage adjustments.

• **Look alike–sound alike:** Don't confuse Xeloda with Xenical.

PATIENT TEACHING

• Teach patient safe drug administration, handling, and storage.

• If a combination of tablets is prescribed, teach patient importance of correctly identifying the tablets to avoid possible dosing error.

☉ Alert: Tell patient also taking warfarin to report significant bleeding or bruising.

• Inform patient and caregiver about expected adverse effects of drug (especially nausea, vomiting, diarrhea, and hand-foot syndrome [pain, swelling, or redness of hands or feet]) and that patient-specific dosage adaptations during therapy are expected and needed.

☉ Alert: Instruct patient to stop taking drug and immediately report diarrhea (more than four bowel movements daily or diarrhea at night), vomiting (two to five episodes in 24 hours), nausea, appetite loss or decreased daily food intake, stomatitis (pain, redness, swelling, or sores in mouth), hand-foot syndrome, temperature of 100.5° F (38° C) or higher, or other evidence of infection.

• Tell patient that most adverse effects improve within 2 to 3 days after stopping drug. Advise patient who doesn't improve to contact prescriber.

• Advise patient of childbearing potential to avoid becoming pregnant during therapy.

• Advise patient who is breastfeeding to stop breastfeeding during therapy.

captopril ▨
KAP-toe-pril

Therapeutic class: Antihypertensives
Pharmacologic class: ACE inhibitors

AVAILABLE FORMS
Tablets: 12.5 mg, 25 mg, 50 mg, 100 mg

INDICATIONS & DOSAGES
Adjust-a-dose (for all indications): Patients with impaired renal function may respond to smaller or less frequent doses. In patients with significant renal impairment, reduce initial daily dosage, and use smaller increments for a slow titration (1- to 2-week intervals). Slowly back-titrate dosage after desired therapeutic effect has been achieved to determine the minimal effective dose. A loop diuretic such as furosemide, rather than a thiazide diuretic, is preferred in patients with severe renal impairment when concomitant diuretic therapy is required.

➤ **HTN (alone or in combination with other antihypertensives)**
Adults: Initially, 25 mg PO b.i.d. or t.i.d. If dosage doesn't control BP satisfactorily in 1 or 2 weeks, increase it to 50 mg b.i.d. or t.i.d. If that dosage doesn't control BP satisfactorily after another 1 or 2 weeks, expect to add a diuretic. If patient needs further BP reduction, may increase dosage to 100 mg b.i.d. or t.i.d., then if necessary, to 150 mg b.i.d. or t.i.d. while continuing diuretic. Usual dosage range is 25 to 150 mg b.i.d. or t.i.d. Maximum daily dosage is 450 mg.

➤ **Diabetic nephropathy**
Adults: 25 mg PO t.i.d.

➤ **HF**
Adults: Initially, 25 mg PO t.i.d. Patients with normal or low BP who have been vigorously treated with diuretics and who may be hyponatremic or hypovolemic may start with 6.25 or 12.5 mg PO t.i.d.; starting dosage may be adjusted over several days. Gradually

increase dosage to 50 mg PO t.i.d.; once patient reaches this dosage, delay further dosage increases for at least 2 weeks to assess satisfactory response. Usual dosage is 50 to 100 mg PO t.i.d.; maximum dosage is 450 mg daily. Generally used in conjunction with a diuretic; may also add a cardiac glycoside in select patients.

➤ **Left ventricular dysfunction after acute MI**

Adults: Start therapy as early as 3 days after MI with 6.25 mg PO for one dose, followed by 12.5 mg PO t.i.d. Increase over several days to 25 mg PO t.i.d.; then increase to 50 mg PO t.i.d. over several weeks.

ADMINISTRATION
PO
• Give 1 hour before meals to enhance drug absorption.
• Pharmacist may compound drug into a suspension if patient can't swallow tablets.
• Refrigerate suspension and shake well before use. Suspension is stable for 56 days if refrigerated.

ACTION
Inhibits ACE, preventing conversion of angiotensin I to angiotensin II, a potent vasoconstrictor. Less angiotensin II decreases peripheral arterial resistance, decreasing aldosterone secretion, which reduces sodium and water retention and lowers BP.

Route	Onset	Peak	Duration
PO	Within 15 min	60–90 min	Unknown

Half-life: Less than 2 hours.

ADVERSE REACTIONS
CNS: dizziness, headache, malaise, fatigue, fever, insomnia, dysgeusia, paresthesia. **CV:** tachycardia, hypotension, chest pain, palpitations. **EENT:** oral ulceration. **GI:** gastritis, abdominal pain, anorexia, constipation, diarrhea, dry mouth, nausea, vomiting, peptic ulcer. **GU:** proteinuria. **Hematologic:** *leukopenia, agranulocytosis, thrombocytopenia, pancytopenia,* anemia. **Metabolic:** hyperkalemia. **Respiratory:** dry, persistent, nonproductive cough; dyspnea. **Skin:** urticarial rash, maculopapular rash, pruritus, alopecia. **Other:** *angioedema.*

INTERACTIONS
Drug-drug. *Aliskiren:* May increase risk of renal impairment, hypotension, and hyperkalemia in patients with diabetes and those with moderate to severe renal impairment (GFR less than 60 mL/minute). Concomitant use is contraindicated in patients with diabetes. Avoid concomitant use in those with moderate to severe renal impairment.
Antacids: May decrease captopril effect. Separate dosage times.
ARBs (candesartan, valsartan), other ACE inhibitors: May increase toxic effects of captopril. Consider alternative therapy.
Canagliflozin: May enhance hyperkalemic and hypotensive effects. Monitor potassium level and BP.
Diuretics, other antihypertensives: May cause excessive hypotension. May need to stop diuretic or reduce captopril dosage.
Gold: May cause nitritoid reactions (facial flushing, nausea, vomiting, hypotension). Monitor therapy.
Insulin, oral antidiabetics: May cause hypoglycemia when captopril therapy is started. Monitor patient closely.
Lithium: May increase lithium level; symptoms of toxicity possible. Monitor lithium level and patient closely.
Neprilysin inhibitors (sacubitril): May increase risk of angioedema. Use together is contraindicated. Don't give within 36 hours of switching to or from sacubitril.
NSAIDs: May reduce antihypertensive effect. Monitor BP.
Potassium-sparing diuretics, potassium supplements: May cause hyperkalemia. Avoid using together unless hypokalemia is confirmed.
Drug-food. *Salt substitutes containing potassium:* May cause hyperkalemia. Monitor patient closely.

EFFECTS ON LAB TEST RESULTS
• May increase ALP, bilirubin, liver transaminase, BUN, serum creatinine, and potassium levels.
• May decrease serum sodium and glucose levels.
• May decrease Hb level, hematocrit, and granulocyte, platelet, RBC, and WBC counts.
• May cause positive ANA titer.
• May cause false-positive urine acetone test results.

CONTRAINDICATIONS & CAUTIONS
• Contraindicated in patients hypersensitive to drug or other ACE inhibitors and in patients who had angioedema related to previous treatment with an ACE inhibitor.
• Use cautiously in patients with impaired renal function or serious autoimmune disease, especially SLE, and in those who have been exposed to other drugs that affect WBC counts or immune response.
Dialyzable drug: Yes (hemodialysis in adults only).
⚠ *Overdose S&S:* Hypotension.

PREGNANCY-LACTATION-REPRODUCTION
Boxed Warning Use during pregnancy can cause injury and death to the developing fetus. When pregnancy is detected, stop drug as soon as possible. ■
• Drug appears in human milk. Patient should discontinue breastfeeding or discontinue drug, taking into account importance of drug to the patient.

NURSING CONSIDERATIONS
⚝ Patients who are Black and taking ACE inhibitors as monotherapy for HTN have a smaller reduction in BP than patients of other ethnicities.
⚝ Patients who are Black and taking ACE inhibitors have a higher incidence of angioedema than patients of other ethnicities.
• Monitor patient's BP and pulse rate frequently.
🌑 *Alert:* Older adults may be more sensitive to drug's hypotensive effects.
• Assess patient for signs of angioedema.
• Drug causes cough, most frequently of all ACE inhibitors.
• In patients with impaired renal function or collagen vascular disease, monitor WBC and differential counts before starting treatment, every 2 weeks for the first 3 months of therapy, and periodically thereafter.
• *Look alike–sound alike:* Don't confuse captopril with carvedilol.

PATIENT TEACHING
• Instruct patient in proper drug administration and storage.
• Inform patient that light-headedness is possible, especially during first few days of therapy, and to rise slowly to minimize this effect and to report occurrence to prescriber. If fainting occurs, tell patient to stop drug and call prescriber immediately.
• Tell patient to use caution in hot weather and during exercise. Lack of fluids, vomiting, diarrhea, and excessive perspiration can lead to light-headedness and syncope.
• Advise patient to report signs and symptoms of infection, such as fever and sore throat.
Boxed Warning Tell patient to notify prescriber if pregnancy occurs. Drug will need to be stopped. ■
• Urge patient to promptly report swelling of the face, lips, or mouth or difficulty breathing.
• Advise patient not to use potassium-sparing diuretics, ARBs, potassium supplements, or potassium-containing salt substitutes without first consulting prescriber.

---

carBAMazepine ⚝
kar-ba-MAZ-e-peen

Carbatrol, Epitol, Equetro, TEGretol, TEGretol-XR

Therapeutic class: Anticonvulsants
Pharmacologic class: Iminostilbene derivatives

AVAILABLE FORMS
Capsules (extended-release) ⓝ: 100 mg, 200 mg, 300 mg
Oral suspension: 100 mg/5 mL
Tablets ⓝ: 100 mg, 200 mg, 300 mg, 400 mg
Tablets (chewable): 100 mg, 200 mg
Tablets (extended-release) ⓝ: 100 mg, 200 mg, 400 mg

INDICATIONS & DOSAGES
➤ **Generalized tonic-clonic and complex partial seizures, mixed seizure patterns**
Adults and children older than age 12: Initially, 200 mg PO b.i.d. (conventional or extended-release tablets or capsules), or 100 mg suspension PO q.i.d. with meals. May be increased every 7 days by 200 mg daily in divided doses at 12-hour intervals for extended-release tablets or capsules or 6- to 8-hour intervals for conventional tablets or suspension, adjusted to minimum effective level.
    After 2 to 3 months of treatment, serum concentrations may decrease due to hepatic enzyme autoinduction and dosage may need

---

C

to be further increased to 15 to 20 mg/kg/day; doses up to approximately 2 g/day may be needed in some patients for optimal effect.

Maximum, 1,000 mg daily in children ages 12 to 15 and 1,200 mg daily in patients older than age 15. Doses up to 1,600 mg daily have been used in adults in rare instances. Usual maintenance dosage is 800 to 1,200 mg daily.
Children younger than age 12 (extended-release capsules): Children taking total daily dosages of immediate-release carbamazepine of 400 mg or greater may be converted to the same total daily dosage of extended-release capsules, using a twice-daily regimen. Usually, optimal clinical response is achieved at daily doses below 35 mg/kg.
Children ages 6 to 12: Initially, 100 mg PO b.i.d. (conventional or extended-release tablets) or 50 mg suspension PO q.i.d. with meals, increased at weekly intervals by up to 100 mg PO in three to four divided doses daily (in two divided doses for extended-release form). Maximum, 1,000 mg daily. Usual maintenance dosage is 400 to 800 mg daily.
Children younger than age 6: 10 to 20 mg/kg/day in two to three divided doses (conventional tablets) or four divided doses (suspension). Maximum dosage is 35 mg/kg in 24 hours.
➤ **Acute manic and mixed episodes associated with bipolar I disorder**
Adults: Initially, 100 to 400 mg PO daily in divided doses. Increase by 200 mg every 1 to 4 days to achieve therapeutic response. Doses up to 1,800 mg daily may be needed in some patients.
Equetro
Adults: Initially, 200 mg Equetro PO b.i.d. Increase by 200 mg daily to achieve therapeutic response. Doses higher than 1,600 mg daily haven't been studied.
➤ **Trigeminal neuralgia**
Adults: Initially, 100 mg PO b.i.d. (conventional or extended-release tablets) or 50 mg suspension PO q.i.d. with meals, increased by 100 mg every 12 hours for tablets or 50 mg q.i.d. for suspension until pain is relieved. Maximum, 1,200 mg daily. Maintenance dosage is usually 200 to 400 mg PO b.i.d.

Or, initially, 200-mg extended release capsule PO daily. May increase daily dosage by up to 200 mg/day every 12 hours, only as needed to achieve freedom from pain. Don't exceed 1,200 mg daily.

ADMINISTRATION
PO
• Shake oral suspension well before measuring dose.
• When converting from tablets to suspension, administer the same number of milligrams per day in smaller, more frequent doses.
• When converting from immediate-release to extended-release tablets, administer same total daily dosage.
• Give chewable, immediate-release, and extended-release tablets with meals.
• Contents of extended-release capsules may be sprinkled over applesauce if patient has difficulty swallowing capsules. Extended-release capsules may be administered with or without food. Capsules and tablets shouldn't be crushed or chewed, unless labeled as chewable form.
• When giving by NG tube, mix dose with an equal volume of water, NSS, or D_5W. Flush tube with 100 mL of diluent after giving dose.
• Don't crush or split extended-release form or give broken or chipped tablets.

ACTION
Thought to stabilize neuronal membranes and limit seizure activity by either increasing efflux or decreasing influx of sodium ions across cell membranes in the motor cortex during generation of nerve impulses.

Route	Onset	Peak	Duration
PO	Unknown	1.5–12 hr	Unknown
PO (extended-release)	Unknown	4–8 hr	Unknown

Half-life: 25 to 65 hours with single dose; 8 to 29 hours with long-term use.

ADVERSE REACTIONS
CNS: ataxia, dizziness, drowsiness, somnolence, vertigo, ***worsening of seizures,*** confusion, fatigue, fever, headache, syncope, pain, depression including ***suicidality,*** speech disorder, asthenia, abnormal thinking, paresthesia, twitching, tremor, weakness, disturbances of coordination, hallucinations. **CV:** ***arrhythmias, AV block, HF,*** edema, aggravation of CAD, HTN, hypotension, thrombophlebitis, embolism, lymphadenopathy. **EENT:** blurred vision, cortical lens opacities, increased IOP, conjunctivitis, diplopia, nystagmus, tinnitus, hyperacusis, dry pharynx, dry mouth.

GI: nausea, vomiting, constipation, abdominal pain, anorexia, diarrhea, dyspepsia, glossitis, stomatitis, *pancreatitis*. **GU:** albuminuria, glycosuria, erectile dysfunction, urinary frequency, urine retention. **Hematologic:** *agranulocytosis, aplastic anemia, thrombocytopenia, pancytopenia,* eosinophilia, leukocytosis, porphyria. **Hepatic:** abnormal LFT values, jaundice, *hepatitis*. **Metabolic:** hyponatremia, *hypocalcemia*. **Musculoskeletal:** leg cramps, arthralgia, myalgia. **Respiratory:** pulmonary hypersensitivity. **Skin:** *erythema multiforme, SJS, TEN,* diaphoresis, rash, urticaria, pruritus, photosensitivity reactions, skin disorder, alopecia, nail disorder. **Other:** SIADH, chills.

INTERACTIONS
Drug-drug. *Aprepitant, other CYP3A4 inhibitors:* Increases plasma carbamazepine level. Monitor carbamazepine level; adjust carbamazepine dosage as necessary.
Aripiprazole: May decrease aripiprazole serum concentration. Double aripiprazole dose when carbamazepine is added, then base additional dosage increases on clinical evaluation. If carbamazepine is later withdrawn, reduce aripiprazole dose.
Atracurium, cisatracurium, pancuronium, rocuronium, vecuronium: May decrease the effects of nondepolarizing muscle relaxant, causing it to be less effective. May need to increase the dose of the nondepolarizing muscle relaxant.
Azole antifungals (itraconazole, ketoconazole): May increase carbamazepine level and decrease antifungal level. Monitor levels and effectiveness of drugs.
Cimetidine, danazol, diltiazem, fluoxetine, fluvoxamine, isoniazid, loratadine, olanzapine, valproic acid, verapamil: May increase carbamazepine level. Use with isoniazid may increase risk of hepatotoxicity. Use together cautiously.
Clarithromycin, erythromycin: May inhibit metabolism of carbamazepine, increasing carbamazepine level and risk of toxicity. Avoid using together.
CNS depressants (antihistamines, benzodiazepines, hypnotics, opioids): May increase risk of respiratory depression, sedation, hypotension, and syncope. Consider reducing dosage of either drug if used together.

Cyclophosphamide: May increase risk of cyclophosphamide-related toxicities. Monitor carefully.
CYP1A2 and CYP3A4 substrates (acetaminophen, alprazolam, doxycycline, felbamate, haloperidol, hormonal contraceptives, phenytoin, sirolimus, theophylline, tiagabine, topiramate, valproate): May decrease levels of these drugs. Watch for decreased effect.
Lamotrigine: May decrease lamotrigine level and increase carbamazepine level. Monitor patient for clinical effects and toxicity.
Lapatinib: May decrease lapatinib serum concentration; lapatinib dosage may need to be increased. Avoid use together when possible.
Lithium: May increase CNS toxicity of lithium. Avoid using together.
MAO inhibitors: May increase depressant and anticholinergic effects. Avoid using together. Discontinue MAO inhibitors at least 14 days before starting carbamazepine.
Nefazodone: May increase carbamazepine levels and toxicity while reducing nefazodone levels and therapeutic benefits. Use together is contraindicated.
Oral and other hormonal contraceptives: May cause breakthrough bleeding and reduced contraceptive effectiveness. Consider back-up method of birth control.
Phenobarbital, phenytoin, primidone: May decrease carbamazepine level. Watch for decreased effect.
SSRIs, TCAs: May increase carbamazepine level and decrease levels of antidepressant. Closely monitor patient and adjust dosage as needed.
Warfarin: May reduce anticoagulant effect. Monitor PT when starting or stopping carbamazepine.
Drug-herb. *Plantains (psyllium seed):* May inhibit GI absorption of drug. Discourage use together.
Drug-food. *Grapefruit juice:* May increase carbamazepine level. Don't use together.

EFFECTS ON LAB TEST RESULTS
• May increase BUN level and LFT values. May decrease sodium levels and thyroid function test values.
• May increase eosinophil and WBC counts. May decrease granulocyte and platelet counts.
• May interact with some pregnancy tests.

CONTRAINDICATIONS & CAUTIONS

• Contraindicated in patients hypersensitive to this drug or TCAs and in those with a history of bone marrow suppression; also contraindicated in those who have taken an MAO inhibitor within 14 days.

• Use cautiously in patients with mixed seizure disorders because they may experience an increased risk of seizures. Also, use cautiously in patients with myasthenia gravis, renal and hepatic dysfunction. Avoid use in patients with porphyria.

• Serious and sometimes fatal DRESS syndrome can occur; drug may need to be stopped and patient converted to another therapy.

Boxed Warning Serious, sometimes fatal, dermatologic reactions, including TEN and SJS, have been reported. Patients of Asian ancestry with the HLA-B*1502 allele are at increased risk. Screen patients with ancestry in genetically at-risk populations for HLA-B*1502 before carbamazepine treatment. Don't use carbamazepine in patients testing positive unless benefit clearly outweighs risk. ▪

• Drug may cause AV heart block conduction abnormalities. Use cautiously in patients at risk for conduction abnormalities, in those with abnormal ECGs, and in patients with preexisting heart damage.

• Drug can cause hyponatremia. Risk appears dose-related and may be increased in older adults or patients taking diuretics. For symptomatic hyponatremia, drug may need to be discontinued.

▧ Oral suspension may contain sorbitol; avoid use in patients with hereditary fructose intolerance.

• Safety and effectiveness of Equetro in children and adolescents haven't been established for indications other than epilepsy.

Dialyzable drug: Yes.

⚠ *Overdose S&S:* Conduction disorders, hypotension or HTN, impairment of consciousness, irregular breathing, respiratory depression, tachycardia, shock, seizures, adiadochokinesia, ataxia, athetoid movements, ballism, dizziness, drowsiness, dysmetria, motor restlessness, muscular twitching, mydriasis, nystagmus, opisthotonos, psychomotor disturbances, tremor; hyperreflexia followed by anuria or oliguria, hyporeflexia, nausea and vomiting, urine retention.

PREGNANCY-LACTATION-REPRODUCTION

• Drug can cause fetal harm, including major congenital malformations, when administered during pregnancy. Weigh benefits against the risks. If used during pregnancy, monotherapy, rather than use in combination with other anticonvulsants, is recommended to possibly reduce risk of teratogenic effects.

• Consider tests to detect fetal defects as part of routine prenatal care in patients receiving drug during pregnancy.

• Patients taking carbamazepine during pregnancy should enroll in the North American Antiepileptic Drug Pregnancy Registry (1-888-233-2334 or www.aedpregnancyregistry.org).

• Drug and its metabolite appear in human milk. Patient should discontinue breastfeeding or discontinue drug, taking into account importance of drug to the patient.

NURSING CONSIDERATIONS

• Watch for worsening of seizures, especially in patients with mixed seizure disorders, including atypical absence seizures.

❶ *Alert:* Closely monitor all patients taking or starting AEDs for changes in behavior indicating worsening of suicidality or depression. Symptoms such as anxiety, agitation, hostility, mania, and hypomania may be precursors to emerging suicidality.

• Obtain baseline determinations of urinalysis, renal function, iron levels, electrolyte levels, liver function, CBC, and platelet and reticulocyte counts. Monitor these values periodically thereafter.

Boxed Warning Aplastic anemia and agranulocytosis have been reported in association with carbamazepine therapy. Obtain complete pretreatment hematologic testing as a baseline. If patient in the course of treatment exhibits low or decreased WBC or platelet counts, monitor patient closely. Consider discontinuing drug if significant bone marrow depression develops. ▪

• Never stop drug suddenly when treating seizures. Notify prescriber immediately if adverse reactions occur.

• Adverse reactions may be minimized by increasing dosages gradually.

• Therapeutic level is 4 to 12 mcg/mL. Monitor level and effects closely. Ask patient when last dose was taken to better evaluate drug level.

• When managing seizures, take appropriate precautions.

🌓 *Alert:* Watch for signs of anorexia or subtle appetite changes, which may indicate excessive drug level.

• *Look alike–sound alike:* Don't confuse carbamazepine with oxcarbazepine. Don't confuse Tegretol or Tegretol-XR with Topamax or Toprol-XL. Don't confuse Carbatrol with carvedilol.

PATIENT TEACHING

• Tell patient that genetic testing may be needed before start of therapy.

• Instruct patient in safe drug administration and storage.

• Tell patient that TEGretol-XR tablet coating may appear in stool because it isn't absorbed.

• Inform patient using drug for trigeminal neuralgia that an attempt should be made to decrease dosage or withdraw drug every 3 months.

• Advise patient to report adverse reactions and to immediately report fever, sore throat, mouth ulcers, or easy bruising or bleeding.

• Tell patient that drug may cause mild to moderate dizziness and drowsiness when first taken and to avoid hazardous activities until effects disappear, usually within 3 to 4 days.

• Advise patient that periodic eye exams are recommended.

• Inform patient of risks to fetus if pregnancy occurs while taking carbamazepine; advise patient to enroll in the North American Antiepileptic Drug Pregnancy Registry.

• Advise patient that breastfeeding isn't recommended during therapy.

SAFETY ALERT!

CARBOplatin
KAR-boe-pla-tin

Paraplatin

Therapeutic class: Antineoplastics
Pharmacologic class: Platinum-containing compounds

AVAILABLE FORMS

Aqueous solution for injection: 10 mg/mL in 5-mL, 15-mL, 45-mL, 60-mL,100-mL vials

INDICATIONS & DOSAGES

➤ **Advanced ovarian cancer**

Adults: 360 mg/m² IV on day 1 every 4 weeks as a single agent. Or, 300 mg/m² on day 1 every 4 weeks for six cycles when used with other chemotherapy drugs such as cyclophosphamide. Or, use the Calvert formula to calculate initial dosage:

$$\text{Total dose (mg)} = \text{(target AUC in mg/mL/minute)} \times \text{(GFR in mL/minute} + 25)$$

where *target AUC* is usually 4 to 6 mg/mL/minute and *GFR* is measured in mL/minute.

Doses shouldn't be repeated until platelet count exceeds 100,000/mm³ and neutrophil count exceeds 2,000/mm³. Subsequent doses are based on blood counts: If platelet count is greater than 100,000/mm³ and neutrophil count is greater than 2,000/mm³, give 125% of prior dose. If platelet count is 50,000/mm³ to 100,000/mm³ and neutrophil count is 500/mm³ to 2,000/mm³, keep same dose. If platelet count is less than 50,000/mm³ and neutrophil count is less than 500/mm³, give 75% of dose.

Adjust-a-dose: If CrCl is 41 to 59 mL/minute, first dose is 250 mg/m². If CrCl is 16 to 40 mL/minute, first dose is 200 mg/m². Drug isn't recommended for patients with CrCl of 15 mL/minute or less.

➤ **Neuroblastoma, localized and unresectable ◆**

Children weighing 10 kg or more: 200 mg/m²/day IV on days 1, 2, and 3 every 21 days for two cycles (in combination with etoposide for two cycles, then followed by cyclophosphamide, doxorubicin, and vincristine).

Children younger than age 1: 6.6 mg/kg/day IV on days 1, 2, and 3 (in combination with etoposide for two cycles, then followed by cyclophosphamide, doxorubicin, and vincristine).

➤ **Glioma ◆**

Children and adolescents age 3 months and older: For induction, 175 mg/m² IV weekly for 4 weeks every 6 weeks for two cycles, with a 2-week recovery period between courses (in combination with vincristine).

For maintenance, 175 mg/m² IV weekly for 4 weeks (in combination with vincristine) for up to 12 cycles, with a 3-week recovery period between cycles.

Reactions in bold italics are *life-threatening*. Interactions may have a *rapid onset* or a *delayed onset*.

ADMINISTRATION

IV

> **Boxed Warning** Anaphylaxis may occur within minutes of administration. Keep epinephrine, corticosteroids, and antihistamines available when giving carboplatin. ▮

▼ Hazardous agent; use facility's safe handling and disposal precautions.

▼ Don't use aluminum needles or IV administration sets because drug may precipitate or lose potency.

▼ For premixed aqueous solution of 10 mg/mL, dilute for infusion with NSS or D$_5$W to a concentration as low as 0.5 mg/mL; however, most clinicians generally dilute dose in either 100 or 250 mL of NSS or D$_5$W.

▼ Give drug by continuous or intermittent infusion over at least 15 minutes.

▼ Store unopened vials at room temperature. Protect from light.

▼ Once diluted as directed, drug is stable at room temperature for 8 hours.

▼ Because drug contains no preservatives, discard after 8 hours.

▼ **Incompatibilities:** None listed by manufacturer. Consult a drug incompatibility reference for more information.

ACTION

May cross-link strands of cellular DNA and interfere with RNA transcription, causing an imbalance of growth that leads to cell death. Not specific to cell cycle.

Route	Onset	Peak	Duration
IV	Unknown	Unknown	Unknown

Half-life: Carboplatin, about 2.5 to 6 hours; platinum, 5 or more days.

ADVERSE REACTIONS

CNS: dizziness, confusion, *stroke,* peripheral neuropathy, *central neurotoxicity,* pain, asthenia, taste perversion, fever. **CV:** *HF, embolism, bleeding.* **EENT:** ototoxicity. **GI:** abdominal pain, constipation, diarrhea, nausea, vomiting, mucositis, stomatitis. **GU:** renal toxicity. **Hematologic:** *thrombocytopenia, leukopenia, neutropenia,* anemia, *bone marrow suppression.* **Hepatic:** hyperbilirubinemia, elevated LFT values. **Metabolic:** hyponatremia, *hypokalemia, hypocalcemia, hypomagnesemia.* **Skin:** alopecia, injection-site reactions. **Other:** hypersensitivity reactions, infection.

INTERACTIONS

Drug-drug. *Bone marrow suppressants, including radiation therapy:* May increase hematologic toxicity. Monitor CBC with differential closely.

Live-virus vaccines: May diminish vaccine's effect. Don't give live-virus vaccines for 3 months after carboplatin.

Nephrotoxic drugs, especially aminoglycosides and amphotericin B: May enhance nephrotoxicity of carboplatin. Use together cautiously.

Phenytoin: May decrease phenytoin level. Monitor serum level and patient for decreased effectiveness.

Drug-herb. *Echinacea:* May diminish therapeutic effects of carboplatin. Avoid concurrent use.

EFFECTS ON LAB TEST RESULTS

• May increase ALP, AST, BUN, and creatinine levels.

• May decrease calcium, sodium, magnesium, and potassium levels.

• May decrease Hb level, hematocrit, and neutrophil, platelet, RBC, and WBC counts.

CONTRAINDICATIONS & CAUTIONS

• Contraindicated in patients with severe bone marrow suppression or bleeding and in patients with history of hypersensitivity to cisplatin or platinum-containing compounds

• Patients older than age 65 and those previously treated with cisplatin are at greater risk for neurotoxicity.

• Safety and effectiveness in children haven't been established.

Dialyzable drug: Yes.

⚠ **Overdose S&S:** Bone marrow suppression, hepatotoxicity.

PREGNANCY-LACTATION-REPRODUCTION

• There are no adequate well-controlled studies during pregnancy. Drug may cause fetal harm when administered during pregnancy. Avoid use in patients of childbearing potential. Patients shouldn't become pregnant during therapy.

• It's unknown if drug appears in human milk. Patient should discontinue breastfeeding during therapy.

NURSING CONSIDERATIONS

> **Boxed Warning** Carboplatin should be administered under the supervision of a

physician experienced in the use of chemotherapeutic agents. Appropriate management of therapy and complications is possible only when adequate treatment facilities are readily available. ■

• Determine electrolyte, creatinine, and BUN levels; CBC with differential; platelet count; and CrCl before first infusion and before each course of treatment.

🕭 *Alert:* When using the Calvert formula, the total dose is calculated in mg, not mg/m^2.

• Monitor CBC with differential and platelet count frequently during therapy and, when indicated, until recovery. Lowest WBC and platelet counts usually occur by day 21. Levels usually return to baseline by day 28. Don't repeat unless platelet count exceeds 100,000/mm^3.

Boxed Warning Anaphylactic-like reactions to carboplatin injection have been reported and may occur within minutes of administration. Epinephrine, corticosteroids, and antihistamines have been employed to alleviate symptoms. ■

Boxed Warning Bone marrow suppression is dose related and may be severe, resulting in infection or bleeding. Anemia may be cumulative and require transfusion support. ■

Boxed Warning Vomiting is another frequent drug-related adverse effect. ■

• Antiemetics are recommended to prevent nausea and vomiting.

• Bone marrow suppression may be more severe in patients with CrCl below 60 mL/minute; adjust dosage.

🕭 *Alert:* Carefully check ordered dose against lab test results. Only one increase in dosage is recommended. Subsequent doses shouldn't exceed 125% of starting dose.

• Therapeutic effects are commonly accompanied by toxicity.

• Drug has less nephrotoxicity and neurotoxicity than cisplatin, but it causes more severe myelosuppression.

• To prevent bleeding, avoid all IM injections when platelet count is below 50,000/mm^3.

• Monitor vital signs during infusion.

• Monitor patient for hearing and vision changes.

• *Look alike–sound alike:* Don't confuse carboplatin with cisplatin.

PATIENT TEACHING

• Advise patient of most common adverse reactions: nausea, vomiting, bone marrow suppression, anemia, and reduction in blood platelets.

• Advise patient to watch for signs of infection (fever, sore throat, fatigue) and bleeding (easy bruising, nosebleeds, bleeding gums, melena). Tell patient to take temperature daily.

• Because of risk of sterility and menstruation cessation, counsel both men and women of reproductive potential before starting therapy. Also recommend that patient consult prescriber before becoming pregnant.

• Advise patient to stop breastfeeding during therapy because of risk of toxicity to infant.

cariprazine hydrochloride
kar-IP-ra-zeen

Vraylar

Therapeutic class: Antipsychotics
Pharmacologic class: Atypical antipsychotics

AVAILABLE FORMS
Capsules: 1.5 mg, 3 mg, 4.5 mg, 6 mg

INDICATIONS & DOSAGES
Adjust-a-dose (for all indications): If a strong CYP3A4 inhibitor is initiated while patient is on a stable dose of cariprazine, reduce cariprazine dosage by half; if patient is taking 4.5 mg daily, reduce to 1.5 or 3 mg daily; if patient is taking 1.5 mg daily, give every other day. Adjust cariprazine dosage when CYP3A4 inhibitor is discontinued. If initiating cariprazine while patient is on a strong CYP3A4 inhibitor, give 1.5 mg on days 1 and 3 (with no dose on day 2); from day 4 onward, give 1.5 mg daily, and increase to a maximum dose of 3 mg daily. Adjust cariprazine dosage when CYP3A4 inhibitor is discontinued. Concomitant use of cariprazine and CYP3A4 inducers hasn't been studied and isn't recommended.

➤ **Schizophrenia; manic or mixed episodes associated with bipolar I disorder**
Adults: Initially, 1.5 mg PO once daily on day 1. May increase to 3 mg PO once daily on day 2. Based on patient's response and tolerability, may make further dosage adjustments in 1.5- or 3-mg increments. Recommended dosage range for schizophrenia is 1.5 to 6 mg once daily. Recommended dosage for bipolar I

disorder is 3 to 6 mg once daily. Maximum, 6 mg daily.

➤ **Depressive episodes associated with bipolar I disorder (bipolar depression)**
Adults: Initially, 1.5 mg PO once daily. May increase to 3 mg PO once daily on day 15 based on response and tolerability. Maximum dosage, 3 mg daily.

ADMINISTRATION
PO
• May give with or without food.
• Store at room temperature.
• Protect 3- and 4.5-mg capsules from light to prevent potential color fading.

ACTION
Exact mechanism unknown. Action thought to occur through partial agonist activity at central dopamine D_2 and serotonin 5-HT$_{1A}$ receptors as well as antagonist activity at serotonin 5-HT$_{2A}$ receptors.

Route	Onset	Peak	Duration
PO	Unknown	3–6 hr	Unknown

Half-life: 48 to 96 hours (parent compound); 1 day to 3 weeks (major metabolites).

ADVERSE REACTIONS
CNS: fatigue, fever, extrapyramidal symptoms, akathisia, headache, somnolence, dizziness, agitation, insomnia, restlessness, anxiety. **CV:** tachycardia, HTN. **EENT:** blurred vision, nasopharyngitis, toothache, oropharyngeal pain, dry mouth. **GI:** abdominal pain, constipation, diarrhea, dyspepsia, nausea, vomiting, decreased appetite. **GU:** UTI. **Hepatic:** increased hepatic enzyme levels. **Metabolic:** weight gain, increased CK level. **Musculoskeletal:** arthralgia, back pain, extremity pain. **Respiratory:** cough. **Skin:** rash.

INTERACTIONS
Drug-drug. *Antiparkinsonian drugs (dopamine agonists):* May diminish therapeutic effect of dopamine agonists; when possible in patients with Parkinson disease, consider using an alternative antipsychotic, such as clozapine or quetiapine, which may convey the lowest interaction risk.
CNS depressants: May increase CNS depression. Monitor therapy.
CYP3A4 inducers (carbamazepine, rifampin): May increase or decrease

cariprazine concentration. Use together isn't recommended.
Opioid class warning: May cause slow or difficult breathing, sedation, and death. Avoid use together. If use together is necessary, limit dosage and duration of each drug to the minimum necessary for desired effect.
Strong CYP3A4 inhibitors (itraconazole, ketoconazole): May increase cariprazine concentration. Reduce cariprazine dosage.
Drug-herb. *Kava kava:* May enhance adverse or toxic effects of cariprazine. Monitor concurrent use.
St. John's wort: May decrease cariprazine concentration. Discourage use together.
Drug-food. *Grapefruit juice (CYP3A4 inhibitor):* May increase cariprazine concentration. Discourage use together.

EFFECTS ON LAB TEST RESULTS
• May increase CK and liver enzyme levels.
• May decrease WBC count.

CONTRAINDICATIONS & CAUTIONS
• Contraindicated in patients hypersensitive to drug or its components.
Boxed Warning Antipsychotics increase the risk of death in older adults with dementia-related psychosis. Drug isn't approved to treat patients with dementia-related psychosis. ∎
• *Opioid class warning:* Opioids should only be prescribed with benzodiazepines or other CNS depressants to patients for whom alternative treatment options are inadequate.
Boxed Warning Antidepressants increase the risk of suicidality in children and young adults. Closely monitor all patients treated with antidepressants for clinical worsening and emergence of suicidality. ∎
🔾 *Alert:* Antipsychotics can cause leukopenia and neutropenia, which can be fatal. Use cautiously in patients with preexisting low WBC count or ANC or history of drug-induced leukopenia or neutropenia.
• Antipsychotics can cause orthostatic hypotension and syncope. Drug hasn't been evaluated in patients with a recent history of MI or unstable CV disease.
• Antipsychotics can cause NMS, which can be fatal.
• Drug may cause irreversible tardive dyskinesia, especially in older adults, most notably older women.
• Antipsychotics can disrupt the body's ability to reduce core body temperature; impair

judgment, thinking, or motor skills; and increase risk of metabolic changes (hyperglycemia, diabetes, dyslipidemia, weight gain), esophageal dysmotility, aspiration, aspiration pneumonia, and falls.

• Antipsychotics increase risk of seizures, especially in patients with a history of seizures or with conditions that lower the seizure threshold.

• Drug is associated with dystonia, especially in males and younger age-groups, most commonly during first few days of treatment.

• Use isn't recommended in patients with severe hepatic or renal impairment.

Boxed Warning Safety and effectiveness in children haven't been established. ∎

Dialyzable drug: Unlikely.

⚠ *Overdose S&S:* Orthostasis, sedation.

PREGNANCY-LACTATION-REPRODUCTION

• Drug may cause fetal harm. Neonates exposed to antipsychotics during the third trimester are at risk for extrapyramidal and withdrawal signs and symptoms, which can vary in severity and require prolonged hospitalization.

• Encourage patients exposed to drug during pregnancy to enroll in the National Pregnancy Registry for Atypical Antipsychotics (1-866-961-2388 or http://womensmentalhealth.org/research/pregnancyregistry/atypicalantipsychotic/).

• It isn't known if drug appears in human milk. Consider risks and benefits before using during breastfeeding.

NURSING CONSIDERATIONS

• Monitor patients for hypersensitivity reactions (rash, pruritus, urticaria, swollen tongue or lips, facial edema, pharyngeal edema).

• Monitor patients for signs and symptoms of NMS (hyperpyrexia, muscle rigidity, delirium, autonomic instability, elevated CK level, rhabdomyolysis, acute kidney injury); discontinue drug immediately if reactions appear. Provide intensive symptomatic treatment and monitoring.

• Monitor patients for signs and symptoms of tardive dyskinesia (potentially irreversible, involuntary, dyskinetic movements). Drug may need to be discontinued.

• Monitor patients for signs and symptoms of dystonia (throat tightness, difficulty swallowing or breathing, tongue protrusion).

• Monitor blood glucose, triglyceride, and lipid levels and for changes in weight, waist circumference, and BMI.

• Monitor patients for clinically significant leukopenia, neutropenia, fever, or other signs and symptoms of infection; treat promptly. Agranulocytosis (sometimes fatal) has been reported with antipsychotic use. Discontinue drug for ANC less than 1,000/mm^3 and monitor WBC count until abnormalities resolve.

• Monitor patients for orthostatic hypotension, especially in older adults and patients with dehydration, hypovolemia, concomitant treatment with antihypertensives, and known CV or cerebrovascular disease. Complete fall risk assessments at baseline and periodically during treatment.

• Ask patients about a history of seizures and review patients' medications for those that might lower the seizure threshold, as drug may increase the risk of seizures.

• Monitor patients who are exposed to strenuous exercise or extreme heat, are dehydrated, or are taking anticholinergics for elevated core body temperature.

• Monitor patients for clinical worsening and emergence of suicidality.

• *Look alike–sound alike:* Don't confuse Vraylar with Valchlor.

PATIENT TEACHING

• *Opioid class warning:* Caution patient or caregiver of patient taking an opioid with a benzodiazepine, CNS depressant, or alcohol to seek immediate medical attention for dizziness, light-headedness, extreme sleepiness, slowed or difficult breathing, or unresponsiveness.

• Counsel patient on importance of following dosage escalation instructions.

• Explain potential for dystonic or extrapyramidal signs and symptoms (involuntary, abnormal movements). Advise patient to immediately report signs and symptoms to prescriber, as drug may need to be discontinued.

• Instruct patient to report signs and symptoms of NMS.

• Educate patient about risk of metabolic changes and how to recognize signs and symptoms of hyperglycemia and diabetes. Instruct patient that lab monitoring of blood glucose and lipid levels and monitoring weight for changes may be necessary.

Reactions in bold italics are *life-threatening*. Interactions may have a *rapid onset* or a ***delayed onset***.

- Advise patient to report fever or other signs or symptoms of infection, which may indicate blood dyscrasias.
- Remind patient to avoid strenuous exercise or exposure to extreme heat and to drink plenty of water, as drug may impair body temperature–regulating ability.
- Counsel patient on risk of orthostatic hypotension and syncope, especially during treatment initiation and dosage increases.
- Warn patient about potential for drug interactions and advise patient to report to prescriber all OTC and prescription drugs and natural supplements being taken.
- Caution patient about operating hazardous machinery, including motor vehicles, until drug's effects on cognitive and motor skills are known.
- Advise patient who is pregnant, considering pregnancy, or is breastfeeding to discuss risks and benefits with prescriber.

SAFETY ALERT!

carmustine (BCNU)
kar-MUS-teen

BiCNU, Gliadel Wafer

Therapeutic class: Antineoplastics
Pharmacologic class: Nitrosoureas

AVAILABLE FORMS
Injection: 100-mg vial (lyophilized), with a 3-mL vial of dehydrated alcohol supplied as a diluent
Wafer: 7.7 mg, for intracavitary use

INDICATIONS & DOSAGES
➤ **Brain tumor, Hodgkin lymphoma, non-Hodgkin lymphoma, multiple myeloma**
Adults: 150 to 200 mg/m^2 IV by slow infusion every 6 weeks; may be divided into daily injections of 75 to 100 mg/m^2 on 2 successive days; repeat dose every 6 weeks if platelet count is greater than 75,000/mm^3 and WBC count is greater than 3,000/mm^3.
Adjust-a-dose: Dosage is reduced by 30% when WBC nadir is 2,000 to 2,999/mm^3 and platelet nadir is 25,000 to 74,999/mm^3. Dosage is reduced by 50% when WBC nadir is less than 2,000/mm^3 and platelet nadir is less than 25,000/mm^3.
➤ **Adjunct to surgery in patients with recurrent glioblastoma for whom surgical resection is indicated; adjunct to surgery and radiation in patients with newly diagnosed high-grade malignant glioma**
Adults: 8 wafers placed in the resection cavity if size and shape of cavity allow. If 8 wafers can't be accommodated, use maximum number of wafers allowed.

ADMINISTRATION
IV
▼ Preparing and giving parenteral form of drug may be mutagenic, teratogenic, or carcinogenic. Follow facility policy to reduce risks. Wear gloves when handling any form of drug.
▼ Prepare drug only in glass or polypropylene containers. Ensure the containers used are polyvinyl chloride (PVC) free and DEHP free. Solution is unstable in PVC IV bags.
▼ If powder liquefies or appears oily, discard because decomposition has occurred.
▼ To reconstitute, dissolve 100 mg of drug in 3 mL of dehydrated alcohol provided by manufacturer.
▼ Dilute solution with 27 mL of sterile water for injection. Resulting solution should be clear and colorless to yellowish and contains 3.3 mg of carmustine/mL in 10% alcohol.
▼ For infusion, further dilute in 500 mL D$_5$W or NSS in glass or polypropylene container to a concentration of 0.2 mg/mL.
▼ Don't use PVC IV tubing. May use polyethylene IV tubing.
▼ Don't mix with other drugs during administration.
▼ Give over at least 2 hours; don't exceed a rate of 1.66 mg/m^2/minute.
▼ To reduce pain on infusion, dilute further, slow infusion rate, or administer via a central catheter.
▼ Reconstituted solution may be stored in refrigerator for 24 hours. Once further diluted in D$_5$W or NSS, store at room temperature and give within 8 hours. It may decompose at temperatures above 80° F (27° C). Solution is also stable for 24 hours refrigerated followed by 6 additional hours at room temperature. Protect from light.
▼ **Incompatibilities:** Sodium bicarbonate.
Intracavitary
• Unopened foil pouches of wafers may be kept at room temperature for a maximum of 6 hours. Open only in the operating room immediately before implantation.

• Wafers broken in half may be used; however, discard wafers as hazardous waste if broken into more than two pieces.
• Use double gloves when handling wafers. Discard outer gloves into a biohazard waste container after use.

ACTION

Inhibits enzymatic reactions involved with DNA synthesis, cross-links strands of cellular DNA, and interferes with RNA transcription, causing an imbalance of growth that leads to cell death. Not specific to cell cycle.

Route	Onset	Peak	Duration
IV, intracavitary	Unknown	Unknown	Unknown

Half-life: IV, 15 to 75 minutes.

ADVERSE REACTIONS

IV only
CNS: headache, encephalopathy, *seizures.*
CV: tachycardia, chest pain, veno-occlusive disease. **EENT:** conjunctival edema, conjunctival hemorrhage, visual disturbances. **GI:** nausea, vomiting, anorexia, diarrhea. **GU:** *nephrotoxicity,* renal impairment. **Hematologic:** *leukopenia, thrombocytopenia, acute leukemia or bone marrow dysplasia,* anemia. **Hepatic:** increased transaminase levels, increased ALP level, hyperbilirubinemia, *hepatotoxicity.* **Metabolic:** hyperglycemia, *hypokalemia,* hyponatremia. **Respiratory:** pneumonitis, ILD, pulmonary fibrosis. **Skin:** alopecia, hyperpigmentation, erythema, burning sensation; injection-site pain, burning, erythema, swelling, tissue necrosis. **Other:** hypersensitivity reaction, opportunistic infection, gynecomastia.
Intracavitary wafer only
CNS: fever, depression, *intracranial HTN,* pain, asthenia, *seizures, cerebral edema, cerebral hemorrhage,* brain abscess, brain cyst, hydrocephalus, meningitis. **CV:** chest pain, *PE.* **GI:** nausea, vomiting, constipation, abdominal pain. **GU:** UTI. **Musculoskeletal:** back pain. **Other:** abnormal healing.

INTERACTIONS

Drug-drug. *Cimetidine:* May increase carmustine's bone marrow toxicity. Avoid using together.
Clozapine: May increase risk of neutropenia. Monitor concurrent use.

Live-virus vaccines: May increase risk of infection in patients who are immunocompromised. Don't use together; don't give for at least 3 months after carmustine.
Myelosuppressants: May increase myelosuppression. Monitor patient.
Phenobarbital: Induces carmustine metabolism, reducing exposure and possibly leading to reduced efficacy. Consider alternative to phenobarbital.
Phenytoin: May decrease levels of these drugs. Monitor patient. Consider alternative to phenytoin.
Drug-herb. *Echinacea:* May diminish therapeutic effect of immunosuppressants. Consider therapy modification.

EFFECTS ON LAB TEST RESULTS

• May increase ALP, AST, bilirubin, Hb, and urine urea levels.
• May decrease platelet and WBC counts.

CONTRAINDICATIONS & CAUTIONS

• Contraindicated in patients hypersensitive to drug.
Boxed Warning Bone marrow suppression (thrombocytopenia and leukopenia), the most common and severe toxic effect, may cause bleeding and overwhelming infections in patients who are already immunocompromised. ∎
Boxed Warning Pulmonary toxicity appears to be dose related. Patients receiving greater than 1,400 mg/m^2 cumulative dose are at higher risk. Pulmonary toxicity can occur years after treatment and can result in death, particularly in patients treated in childhood. ∎
• Drug may increase risk of secondary malignancies.
• Injection-site reactions may occur, especially during rapid IV infusion. Intense skin and flushing suffusion of the conjunctiva may occur within 2 hours, lasting about 4 hours.
• Use cautiously in older adults.
Dialyzable drug: No.

PREGNANCY-LACTATION-REPRODUCTION

• Drug may cause fetal harm. Patients of childbearing potential should use effective contraception during treatment and for at least 6 months after final dose.
• Males of reproductive potential should use effective contraception during treatment and for 3 months after final dose.
• Drug may impair male fertility.

Reactions in bold italics are *life-threatening*. Interactions may have a *rapid onset* or a *delayed onset*.

• It isn't known if drug appears in human milk. Patient should discontinue breastfeeding during treatment.

NURSING CONSIDERATIONS

❂ *Alert:* Carmustine for injection should be administered under the supervision of a physician experienced in the use of cancer chemotherapeutic agents.

• Obtain pulmonary function tests before and during therapy.

Boxed Warning Bone marrow suppression is delayed with carmustine. Blood counts should be monitored weekly for at least 6 weeks after a dose and drug shouldn't be given more often than every 6 weeks. ■

Boxed Warning Bone marrow toxicity of carmustine for injection is cumulative; dosage adjustment must be considered on the basis of nadir blood cell counts from prior dose. Don't administer a repeat course of drug until blood counts recover. ■

• Drug is associated with a moderate to high emetic potential (dose-related); give antiemetic before drug to reduce nausea.

• If drug touches skin, wash off thoroughly. Avoid contact with skin because drug will stain skin brown and skin contact may increase extravasation risk.

• Monitor infusion site for possible infiltration during drug administration.

• Obtain liver and renal function tests periodically.

• Monitor CBC with differential. May use ANC to assess patient's immunosuppressive state.

• Monitor uric acid level. To prevent hyperuricemia with resulting uric acid nephropathy, allopurinol may be used with adequate hydration.

• Therapeutic levels are commonly toxic.

• Acute leukemia or bone marrow dysplasia may occur after long-term use.

• Anticipate blood transfusions during treatment because of cumulative anemia.

• Monitor patient for secondary malignancies.

PATIENT TEACHING

• Advise patient about common adverse reactions to drug.

• Tell patient to watch for signs and symptoms of infection (fever, sore throat, fatigue), stiff neck, and bleeding (easy bruising, nosebleeds, bleeding gums, melena) and to take temperature daily.

• Instruct patient to avoid OTC products containing aspirin and NSAIDs unless prescribed by health care provider.

• Advise patient to stop breastfeeding during therapy because of possible risk of toxicity to infant.

• Caution patient of childbearing potential to avoid becoming pregnant during therapy and to consult prescriber before becoming pregnant.

• Instruct male patient of reproductive potential to use effective contraception during treatment and for 3 months after final dose.

carvedilol
kar-VAH-da-lol

Coreg✿

carvedilol phosphate
Coreg CR✿

Therapeutic class: Antihypertensives
Pharmacologic class: Alpha-nonselective beta blockers

AVAILABLE FORMS

Capsules (extended-release) ⏣: 10 mg, 20 mg, 40 mg, 80 mg
Tablets: 3.125 mg, 6.25 mg, 12.5 mg, 25 mg

INDICATIONS & DOSAGES

Adjust-a-dose (for all indications): In patients with pulse rate below 55 beats/minute, reduce dosage.

➤ **HTN**

Adults: Dosage highly individualized. For immediate-release tablets, initially, 6.25 mg PO b.i.d. Measure standing BP 1 hour after first dose. If tolerated, continue dosage for 7 to 14 days. May increase to 12.5 mg PO b.i.d. for 7 to 14 days, following same BP monitoring protocol as before. Maximum dose is 25 mg PO b.i.d. as tolerated. May be switched to extended-release capsule after controlled on immediate-release tablets. Or, for extended-release capsule, initially 20 mg PO once daily. Measure standing BP 1 hour after dose. May increase by 20 mg every 7 to 14 days to maximum of 80 mg PO once daily if needed and tolerated, using standing systolic pressure 1 hour after dosing as a guide for tolerance.

> **Left ventricular dysfunction after MI**

Adults: Dosage individualized. Start therapy after patient is hemodynamically stable and fluid retention has been minimized. For immediate-release tablets, initially, 3.125 to 6.25 mg PO b.i.d. Increase after 3 to 10 days to 12.5 mg b.i.d. as tolerated, then again after 3 to 10 days to a target dose of 25 mg b.i.d. May be switched to extended-release capsule after controlled on immediate-release tablets. Or, 10 to 20 mg extended-release capsules PO once daily. May increase after 3 to 10 days to 20 to 40 mg PO once daily; continue increasing dose every 3 to 10 days until target dose of 80 mg PO once daily based on tolerability is reached.

> **Mild to severe HF**

Adults: Dosage highly individualized. For immediate-release tablets, initially, 3.125 mg PO b.i.d. for 2 weeks; if tolerated, may increase to 6.25 mg PO b.i.d. Dosage may be doubled every 2 weeks, as tolerated. Maximum dose for patients in severe HF or who weigh less than 85 kg is 25 mg PO b.i.d.; for those weighing more than 85 kg, dose is 50 mg PO b.i.d. May be switched to extended-release capsule after controlled on immediate-release tablets. Or, 10-mg extended-release capsule PO once daily for 2 weeks. May increase to 20, 40, and 80 mg over successive intervals of at least 2 weeks to maximum tolerated dose.

ADMINISTRATION
PO

- Give drug with food.
- Make sure patient doesn't crush, chew, or take capsules in divided doses.
- Capsules may be opened, contents sprinkled on cool applesauce, and taken immediately; don't store.
- Give capsules in the morning.
- Extended-release equivalent of 3.125 mg immediate-release b.i.d. is 10 mg once daily, 6.25 mg immediate-release b.i.d. is 20 mg once daily, 12.5 mg immediate-release b.i.d. is 40 mg once daily, and 25 mg immediate-release b.i.d. is 80 mg once daily.
- Administer extended-release form and drugs that contain alcohol 2 hours apart.

ACTION

Nonselective beta blocker with alpha-blocking activity.

Route	Onset	Peak	Duration
PO	Rapid	1–2 hr	7–10 hr
PO (extended-release)	30 min	5 hr	Unknown

Half-life: Immediate-release, 7 to 10 hours; extended-release, unknown.

ADVERSE REACTIONS

CNS: asthenia, dizziness, fatigue, *stroke,* headache, malaise, fever, hypoesthesia, hypotonia, vertigo, somnolence, depression, insomnia, syncope, paresthesia, abnormal thinking, nervousness, sleep disorder. **CV:** hypotension, orthostatic hypotension, *AV block, bradycardia,* edema, angina pectoris, HTN, palpitations, PVD, peripheral ischemia, tachycardia. **EENT:** abnormal vision, blurred vision, tinnitus, periodontitis, dry mouth, nasopharyngitis, nasal congestion, sinus congestion. **GI:** diarrhea, vomiting, nausea, melena, GI pain. **GU:** erectile dysfunction, renal insufficiency, increased BUN level, increased creatinine level, albuminuria, glycosuria, hematuria, UTI. **Hematologic:** *thrombocytopenia,* purpura, hypoprothrombinemia. **Hepatic:** increased transaminase levels, increase ALP level, hyperbilirubinemia, increased liver enzyme levels. **Metabolic:** hyperglycemia, weight gain or loss, *hyperkalemia, hypoglycemia,* hypercholesterolemia, hyperuricemia, hypovolemia, fluid overload, hyponatremia, diabetes, gout. **Musculoskeletal:** arthralgia, muscle cramps. **Respiratory:** *lung edema,* cough, dyspnea, rales. **Skin:** diaphoresis, rash, pruritus, photosensitivity. **Other:** hypersensitivity reactions, decreased libido, flulike symptoms.

INTERACTIONS

Drug-drug. *Amiodarone:* May increase risk of bradycardia, AV block, and myocardial depression. Monitor patient's ECG and vital signs.

Catecholamine-depleting drugs (MAO inhibitors): May cause bradycardia or severe hypotension. Monitor patient closely.

Cimetidine: May increase bioavailability of carvedilol. Monitor vital signs closely.

Clonidine: May increase BP-lowering and HR-lowering effects. Monitor vital signs closely.

Cyclosporine: May increase cyclosporine level. Monitor cyclosporine level.

Reactions in bold italics are *life-threatening*. Interactions may have a *rapid onset* or a ***delayed onset***.

CYP2D6 inhibitors (fluoxetine, paroxetine, propafenone, quinidine): May increase level of carvedilol. Monitor patient for hypotension and dizziness.

Digoxin: May increase digoxin level by about 15% when given together. Monitor digoxin level.

Diltiazem, verapamil: May cause isolated conduction disturbances. Monitor patient's heart rhythm and BP.

Insulin, oral antidiabetics: May enhance hypoglycemic properties. Monitor glucose level.

NSAIDs, salicylates: May decrease antihypertensive effects. Monitor BP.

Rifamycin (except rifabutin): May significantly reduce carvedilol level. Monitor vital signs closely.

EFFECTS ON LAB TEST RESULTS
• May increase ALP, ALT, AST, BUN, bilirubin, cholesterol, creatinine, GGT, nonprotein nitrogen, potassium, triglyceride, sodium, and uric acid levels.
• May increase or decrease glucose level.
• May shorten PT and decrease platelet and leukocyte counts.

CONTRAINDICATIONS & CAUTIONS
• Contraindicated in patients hypersensitive to drug and in those with NYHA Class IV decompensated cardiac failure requiring IV inotropic therapy.
• Contraindicated in patients with bronchial asthma or related bronchospastic conditions, second- or third-degree AV block, sick sinus syndrome (unless a pacemaker is in place), cardiogenic shock, severe bradycardia, or severe hepatic impairment.
• Use cautiously in patients with left-sided HF who are hypertensive, perioperative patients who receive anesthetics that depress myocardial function, patients with diabetes receiving insulin or oral antidiabetics, and those subject to spontaneous hypoglycemia.
• Use cautiously in patients with thyroid disease (may mask hyperthyroidism; withdrawal may precipitate thyroid storm or exacerbation of hyperthyroidism), myasthenia gravis, untreated pheochromocytoma, Prinzmetal or variant angina, bronchospastic disease (in those who can't tolerate other antihypertensives), or PVD (may precipitate or aggravate symptoms of arterial insufficiency).
• Safety and effectiveness in children younger than age 18 haven't been established.

Dialyzable drug: No.

⚠ *Overdose S&S:* Hypotension, bradycardia, cardiac insufficiency, cardiogenic shock, cardiac arrest, respiratory problems, bronchospasm, vomiting, lapses of consciousness, generalized seizures.

PREGNANCY-LACTATION-REPRODUCTION
• There are no adequate well-controlled studies during pregnancy. Use during pregnancy only if potential benefit outweighs potential risk to the fetus.
• Beta blocker use in the third trimester may increase risk of hypotension, bradycardia, hypoglycemia, and respiratory depression in the neonate.
• It's unknown if drug appears in human milk. Patient should discontinue breastfeeding or discontinue drug, taking into account importance of drug to the patient.

NURSING CONSIDERATIONS
🕔 *Alert:* Patients who have a history of severe anaphylactic reaction to several allergens may be more reactive to repeated challenge (accidental, diagnostic, or therapeutic). They may be unresponsive to dosages of epinephrine typically used to treat allergic reactions.
• Mild hepatocellular injury may occur during therapy. At first sign of hepatic dysfunction, perform tests for hepatic injury or jaundice; if present, stop drug.
• If drug must be stopped, do so gradually over 1 to 2 weeks, if possible.
• Monitor patient with HF for worsened condition, renal dysfunction, or fluid retention; diuretics may need to be increased.
• Monitor patient with diabetes closely; drug may mask signs of hypoglycemia, or hyperglycemia may be worsened.
• Hypotension can occur. Observe patient for dizziness or light-headedness for 1 hour after giving each new dose. Reduce dose in patient with HR less than 55 beats/minute.
• Monitor older adults carefully; drug levels are about 50% higher in older adults than in patients who are younger.
• *Look alike–sound alike:* Don't confuse carvedilol with carteolol or captopril.

PATIENT TEACHING
• Tell patient not to interrupt or stop drug without medical approval.

- Inform patient that improvement of HF symptoms might take several weeks of drug therapy.
- Advise patient with HF to call prescriber if weight gain or shortness of breath occurs.
- Inform patient that low BP when standing may occur. If patient feels dizzy or faint (rare), advise sitting or lying down and tell patient to notify prescriber if symptoms persist.
- Caution patient against performing hazardous tasks during start of therapy.
- Advise patient with diabetes to promptly report changes in glucose level.
- Inform patient who wears contact lenses that eyes may feel dry.
- Teach patient safe drug administration and storage.
- Instruct patient considering cataract surgery to inform ophthalmologist of carvedilol use due to risk of intraoperative floppy iris syndrome.

caspofungin acetate
KAS-po-fun-gin

Cancidas

Therapeutic class: Antifungals
Pharmacologic class: Echinocandins

AVAILABLE FORMS
Lyophilized powder for injection: 50 mg, 70 mg in single-dose vials

INDICATIONS & DOSAGES
Adjust-a-dose (for all indications): For adults receiving rifampin, give 70 mg IV once daily. Adults receiving nevirapine, efavirenz, carbamazepine, dexamethasone, or phenytoin may also require 70 mg IV once daily. For children receiving rifampin, give 70 mg/m² IV once daily (not to exceed 70 mg). Also consider giving 70 mg/m² IV once daily (not to exceed 70 mg) for children receiving nevirapine, efavirenz, carbamazepine, dexamethasone, or phenytoin. For patients with Child-Pugh class B (score of 7 to 9), after initial 70-mg loading dose (when indicated), give 35 mg/day. There's no clinical experience in adults with Child-Pugh score of more than 9 or in children with any degree of hepatic impairment.

➤ **Invasive aspergillosis in patients who are refractory to or intolerant of other therapies (amphotericin B, lipid forms of amphotericin B, itraconazole); candidemia and *Candida*-caused intra-abdominal abscesses, peritonitis, and pleural space infections**
Adults: 70-mg IV loading dose on day 1, followed by 50 mg IV once daily. Base treatment duration on severity of patient's underlying disease, recovery from immunosuppression, and clinical response. Patients with invasive aspergillosis may need 6 to 12 weeks of therapy.
Children age 3 months to 17 years: 70-mg/m² IV loading dose on day 1, followed by 50 mg/m² daily thereafter. May increase daily maintenance dose to 70 mg/m². Maximum loading dose and daily maintenance dose shouldn't exceed 70 mg.

➤ **Empirical treatment of presumed fungal infections in patients who are febrile and neutropenic**
Adults: 70-mg IV loading dose on day 1, followed by 50 mg IV once daily thereafter. Continue empirical therapy until neutropenia resolves. If fungal infection is confirmed, treat for a minimum of 14 days and continue therapy for at least 7 days after neutropenia and symptoms resolve. May increase daily dose to 70 mg if the 50-mg dose is well tolerated but clinical response is suboptimal.
Children age 3 months to 17 years: 70-mg/m² IV loading dose on day 1, followed by 50 mg/m² daily thereafter. May increase daily maintenance dose to 70 mg/m². Maximum loading dose and daily maintenance dose shouldn't exceed 70 mg.

➤ **Esophageal candidiasis**
Adults: 70-mg loading dose on day 1, followed by 50 mg IV daily for 7 to 14 days after symptoms resolve. May transition to oral fluconazole once oral intake tolerable. In patients with fluconazole-refractory disease, continue caspofungin for 14 to 21 days.
Children age 3 months to 17 years: 70-mg/m² IV loading dose on day 1, followed by 50 mg/m² daily thereafter. May increase daily maintenance dose to 70 mg/m². Maximum loading dose and daily maintenance dose shouldn't exceed 70 mg.
Adjust-a-dose: Consider suppressive oral therapy in adults with HIV infection due to the risk of oropharyngeal candidiasis relapse.

Reactions in bold italics are *life-threatening*. Interactions may have a *rapid onset* or a ***delayed onset***.

ADMINISTRATION
IV
▼ Let refrigerated vial warm to room temperature.
▼ Reconstitute drug by adding 10.8 mL of NSS, sterile water for injection, bacteriostatic water for injection with methylparaben and propylparaben, or bacteriostatic water for injection with benzyl alcohol 0.9% to the vial. Resulting solution will be clear.
▼ Reconstitution will lead to a concentration of 5 mg/mL for 50-mg vial and 7 mg/mL for 70-mg vial.
▼ Use reconstituted vials within 1 hour of reconstitution or discard. Vials are for single dose only. Discard unused portion.
▼ Transfer appropriate volume (mL) of reconstituted drug to an IV bag containing 250 mL of NSS, 0.45% or 0.225% sodium chloride, or lactated Ringer solution. Or, for patients on fluid restrictions, may add reconstituted volume of drug to a reduced volume of solution, not to exceed a final concentration of 0.5 mg/mL.
▼ Give drug by slow infusion over about 1 hour. Don't administer as an IV bolus.
▼ Monitor site carefully for phlebitis.
▼ The final product for infusion (solution in IV bag or bottle) can be stored at room temperature for 24 hours or at 36° to 46° F (2° to 8° C) for 48 hours.
▼ **Incompatibilities:** Don't mix or infuse with other drugs or dextrose solutions.

ACTION
Inhibits synthesis of 1,3-β-D-glucan, an essential component of the cell wall, in susceptible *Aspergillus* and *Candida* species. Drug is extensively distributed and has a prolonged half-life.

Route	Onset	Peak	Duration
IV	Unknown	Unknown	Unknown

Half-life: 9 to 11 hours; terminal, 40 to 50 hours.

ADVERSE REACTIONS
CNS: fever, headache, asthenia, fatigue, *seizure,* dizziness, somnolence, tremor, anxiety, confusion, depression, insomnia. **CV:** edema, tachycardia, phlebitis, infused vein complications, hypotension, HTN, flushing, arrythmia, *bradycardia.* **EENT:** epistaxis. **GI:** anorexia, nausea, vomiting, diarrhea, abdominal pain, abdominal distention, constipation, dyspepsia, mucosal inflammation.

GU: proteinuria, increased creatinine level, increased BUN level, hematuria, UTI, *renal failure.* **Hematologic:** anemia, eosinophilia, coagulopathy, *neutropenia, thrombocytopenia.* **Hepatic:** increased transaminase levels, hyperbilirubinemia, *hepatotoxicity.* **Metabolic:** *hypokalemia, hypomagnesemia,* hyperglycemia, hypercalcemia, fluid overload. **Musculoskeletal:** arthralgia, back pain, extremity pain. **Respiratory:** dyspnea, *hypoxia,* crackles, cough, pneumonia, tachypnea. **Skin:** rash. **Other:** chills, hypersensitivity reaction. infusion reaction, *sepsis.*

INTERACTIONS
Drug-drug. *Cyclosporine:* May increase caspofungin level. May increase risk of elevated ALT level; avoid using together unless benefit outweighs risk.
CYP inducers (carbamazepine, dexamethasone, efavirenz, nevirapine, phenytoin, rifampin): May reduce caspofungin level. May need to adjust dosage upward to 70 mg in patients who are clinically unresponsive.
Tacrolimus: May reduce tacrolimus level. Monitor tacrolimus level; expect to adjust dosage.

EFFECTS ON LAB TEST RESULTS
• May increase glucose, calcium, BUN, creatinine, bilirubin, ALP, and liver enzyme levels.
• May decrease albumin, potassium, magnesium, and protein levels.
• May increase eosinophil count.
• May decrease Hb level, hematocrit, and neutrophil and platelet counts.

CONTRAINDICATIONS & CAUTIONS
• Contraindicated in patients hypersensitive to drug or its components.
• Anaphylaxis, other hypersensitivity reactions, and possible histamine-mediated adverse reactions, including rash, facial swelling, angioedema, pruritus, sensation of warmth, and bronchospasm, have been reported during administration.
• Cases of SJS and TEN, some with a fatal outcome, have been reported.
• Safety and effectiveness in neonates and infants younger than age 3 months aren't known.
Dialyzable drug: No.

PREGNANCY-LACTATION-REPRODUCTION

• Based on animal data, drug may cause fetal harm. Use during pregnancy only if potential benefit justifies fetal risk. Other antifungals are recommended for *Aspergillus* or *Candida* infections during pregnancy.
• It's unknown if drug appears in human milk. Drug was found in study of animal milk. Use cautiously during breastfeeding; use of other antifungals is recommended. Monitor infants for signs and symptoms of histamine release, such as facial swelling, rash, and GI symptoms.

NURSING CONSIDERATIONS

• Safety information is limited, but drug is well tolerated for therapy lasting longer than 2 weeks.
• Observe patients for histamine-mediated reactions, including rash, facial swelling, pruritus, and a sensation of warmth.
• Discontinue drug at first sign or symptom of a hypersensitivity reaction and administer appropriate treatment.
• Monitor patients who develop abnormal LFT values during therapy for evidence of worsening hepatic function and evaluate for the risks and benefits of continuing therapy.

PATIENT TEACHING

• Instruct patient to report signs and symptoms of phlebitis.
• Instruct patient to immediately report signs or symptoms of a hypersensitivity reaction, rash, or other skin reactions.

cefadroxil
sef-a-DROX-ill

Therapeutic class: Antibiotics
Pharmacologic class: First-generation cephalosporins

AVAILABLE FORMS

Capsules: 500 mg
Oral suspension: 250 mg/5 mL, 500 mg/5 mL
Tablets: 1 g

INDICATIONS & DOSAGES

➤ UTIs caused by *Escherichia coli, Proteus mirabilis,* and *Klebsiella* species; skin and soft-tissue infections caused by staphylococci and streptococci; pharyngitis or tonsillitis caused by group A beta-hemolytic streptococci *(Streptococcus pyogenes)*

Adults: 1 to 2 g PO daily, depending on infection being treated. Usually given once daily or in two divided doses. For pharyngitis and tonsillitis, treat for 10 days.
Children: 30 mg/kg PO daily in a single dose or in two divided doses every 12 hours for tonsillitis, pharyngitis, and impetigo, and in two divided doses every 12 hours for other skin infections and UTIs. For beta-hemolytic strep infection, treat for at least 10 days.
Adjust-a-dose: In adults with renal impairment, give first dose of 1 g. Reduce additional doses based on CrCl. If CrCl is 25 to 50 mL/minute, give 500 mg PO every 12 hours. If CrCl is 10 to 25 mL/minute, give 500 mg PO every 24 hours; if CrCl is less than 10 mL/minute, give 500 mg PO every 36 hours.

ADMINISTRATION

PO

• Before administration, ensure patient isn't allergic to penicillins or cephalosporins.
• Obtain specimen for culture and sensitivity tests before giving first dose. Begin therapy while awaiting results.
• Administer without regard to meals but can give drug with food or milk to lessen GI discomfort.
• Keep oral suspension refrigerated and discard unused portion after 14 days. Shake well before using.

ACTION

Inhibits cell-wall synthesis, promoting osmotic instability; usually bactericidal.

Route	Onset	Peak	Duration
PO	Unknown	70–90 min	Unknown

Half-life: About 1 to 2 hours.

ADVERSE REACTIONS

CNS: *seizures,* fever. **GI:** diarrhea, glossitis, abdominal cramps. **GU:** genital pruritus, candidiasis, vaginitis, renal dysfunction. **Hematologic:** *transient neutropenia, leukopenia, agranulocytosis, thrombocytopenia,* anemia, eosinophilia. **Hepatic:** hepatic dysfunction, cholestasis. **Musculoskeletal:** arthralgia. **Skin:** rash, urticaria, pruritus. **Other:** hypersensitivity reactions, including *anaphylaxis* and *angioedema*.

Reactions in bold italics are *life-threatening*. Interactions may have a *rapid onset* or a *delayed onset*.

INTERACTIONS

Drug-drug. *Aminoglycosides:* May increase risk of nephrotoxicity. Avoid using together.
Estrogen-based contraceptives: May decrease contraceptive absorption and effectiveness. Patient should avoid use together or use non-hormonal contraception during antibiotic therapy and for 7 days after completion of antibiotic.
Live-virus vaccines: May decrease vaccine effectiveness. Don't give together.
Probenecid: May inhibit excretion and increase cefadroxil level. Use together cautiously.
Warfarin: May enhance anticoagulant effects. Monitor therapy.

EFFECTS ON LAB TEST RESULTS

• May increase ALP, ALT, AST, bilirubin, GGT, and LDH levels.
• May increase eosinophil count.
• May decrease Hb level and granulocyte, neutrophil, platelet, and WBC counts.
• May prolong PT.
• May falsely increase serum or urine creatinine level in tests using Jaffé reaction. May cause false-positive results of Coombs test and urine glucose tests that use cupric sulfate, such as Benedict reagent and Clinitest.

CONTRAINDICATIONS & CAUTIONS

• Contraindicated in patients hypersensitive to drug or other cephalosporins.
• To reduce development of drug-resistant bacteria and maintain effectiveness of antibacterial drugs, use drug only to treat or prevent infections proven or strongly suspected to be caused by bacteria.
• Use cautiously in patients with a history of sensitivity to penicillin or GI diseases (colitis).
• Use cautiously in patients with impaired renal function; adjust dosage as needed.
🕔 *Alert:* Seizures have occurred, particularly in patients with renal impairment when the dosage wasn't reduced. If seizures occur, discontinue drug and treat if clinically indicated.
🕔 *Alert:* Drug can cause CDAD and pseudomembranous colitis ranging from mild to life-threatening that can occur more than 2 months after treatment.
Dialyzable drug: Yes.

PREGNANCY-LACTATION-REPRODUCTION

• There are no adequate studies during pregnancy. Use during pregnancy only if potential benefit justifies fetal risk.
• It isn't known if drug appears in human milk. Use cautiously during breastfeeding.

NURSING CONSIDERATIONS

• If CrCl is less than 50 mL/minute, lengthen dosage interval so drug doesn't accumulate. Monitor renal function in patients with renal dysfunction.
• If large doses are given, therapy is prolonged, or patient is high risk, monitor patient for superinfection.
• Monitor patient for diarrhea and treat appropriately.
• *Look alike–sound alike:* Don't confuse drug with other cephalosporins that sound alike.

PATIENT TEACHING

• Instruct patient in safe drug administration and storage.
• Tell patient to take entire amount of drug exactly as prescribed, even if feeling better.
• Advise patient to notify prescriber if rash develops or if signs and symptoms of superinfection appear, such as recurring fever, chills, and malaise.

ceFAZolin sodium
sef-AH-zoe-lin

Therapeutic class: Antibiotics
Pharmacologic class: First-generation cephalosporins

AVAILABLE FORMS

Infusion: 1 g/50 mL, 2 g/50 mL in 50-mL bag; 2 g/100 mL, 3 g/100 mL in 100-mL bag
Injection (parenteral): 500 mg, 1 g, 2 g
Injection (prefilled syringe): 1 g/10 mL, 2 g/10 mL, 2 g/20 mL

INDICATIONS & DOSAGES

Adjust-a-dose (for all indications): For adults with CrCl of 55 mL/minute or greater, give full dose every 6 to 8 hours; if CrCl is 35 to 54 mL/minute, give full dose every 8 hours or longer; if CrCl is 11 to 34 mL/minute, give 50% of usual dose every 12 hours; if CrCl is below 10 mL/minute, give 50% of usual dose every 18 to 24 hours.

For children with CrCl of 40 to 70 mL/minute, give 60% of normal daily dose divided every 12 hours; if CrCl is 20 to 40 mL/minute, give 25% of usual daily dose divided every 12 hours; if CrCl is 5 to 20 mL/minute, give 10% of usual dose every 24 hours.

➤ **Perioperative prevention in contaminated surgery**

Adults: 1 to 2 g IM or IV 30 to 60 minutes before surgery; then 0.5 to 1 g IM or IV every 6 to 8 hours for 24 hours. In operations lasting longer than 2 hours, give another 0.5- to 1-g dose IM or IV intraoperatively. Continue treatment for 3 to 5 days if life-threatening infection is likely.

Children ages 10 to 17 with CrCl of 70 mL/minute or more: 2 g if weight is 50 kg or more or 1 g if weight is less than 50 kg IM or IV 30 to 60 minutes before surgery; then 0.5 to 1 g IM or IV every 6 to 8 hours for 24 hours. In operations lasting longer than 2 hours, give another 0.5- to 1-g dose IM or IV intraoperatively. Continue treatment for 3 to 5 days if life-threatening infection is likely.

➤ **Infections of respiratory, biliary, and GU tracts; skin, soft-tissue, bone, and joint infections; septicemia; endocarditis caused by *Escherichia coli*, Enterobacteriaceae, gonococci, *Haemophilus influenzae*, *Klebsiella* species, *Proteus mirabilis*, *Staphylococcus aureus*, *Streptococcus pneumoniae*, and group A beta-hemolytic streptococci (*Streptococcus pyogenes*)**

Adults: 250 to 500 mg IM or IV every 8 hours for mild infections or 500 mg to 1.5 g IM or IV every 6 to 8 hours for moderate to severe or life-threatening infections. Maximum, 12 g/day in life-threatening situations.

Children older than age 1 month: 25 to 50 mg/kg/day IM or IV in three or four divided doses. In severe infections, dose may be increased to 100 mg/kg/day.

ADMINISTRATION

IV

▼ Before giving first dose, obtain specimen for culture and sensitivity tests. Begin therapy while awaiting results.

▼ Before giving drug, ensure patient isn't allergic to penicillins or cephalosporins.

▼ Give commercially available frozen solutions in D₅W only by intermittent or continuous IV infusion.

▼ Reconstitute drug with sterile water, bacteriostatic water, or NSS as follows: Add 2 mL to 500-mg vial or 2.5 mL to 1-g vial, yielding 225 mg/mL or 330 mg/mL, respectively.

▼ Shake well until dissolved.

▼ For direct injection, further dilute with 5 mL of sterile water for injection.

▼ Inject into a large vein or into the tubing of a free-flowing IV solution over 3 to 5 minutes or as an intermittent infusion over 30 to 60 minutes.

▼ For intermittent infusion, add reconstituted drug to 50 to 100 mL of compatible solution or use premixed solution.

▼ If IV therapy lasts longer than 3 days, alternate injection sites. Use of small IV needles in larger available veins may be preferable.

▼ Reconstituted drug is stable 24 hours at room temperature or 10 days refrigerated.

▼ **Incompatibilities:** None listed by manufacturer. Consult a drug incompatibility reference for more information.

IM

● Before giving first dose, obtain specimen for culture and sensitivity tests. Begin therapy while awaiting results.

● After reconstitution, inject drug IM without further dilution. This drug isn't as painful as other cephalosporins. Give injection deep into a large muscle.

ACTION

Inhibits cell-wall synthesis, promoting osmotic instability; usually bactericidal.

Route	Onset	Peak	Duration
IV	Immediate	Immediate	Unknown
IM	Unknown	0.5–2 hr	Unknown

Half-life: About 2 hours.

ADVERSE REACTIONS

CNS: dizziness, syncope, confusion, weakness, fatigue, headache, somnolence. **CV:** hypotension, phlebitis, thrombophlebitis with IV injection. **EENT:** oral candidiasis, oral ulcers. **GI:** diarrhea, *pseudomembranous colitis,* anorexia, glossitis, dyspepsia, abdominal cramps, anal pruritus, vomiting, nausea, epigastric pain, flatus. **GU:** genital pruritus, candidiasis, vaginitis. **Hematologic:** *neutropenia, leukopenia, thrombocytopenia,* eosinophilia. **Skin:** maculopapular and erythematous rashes, urticaria, pruritus, pain,

---

Reactions in bold italics are *life-threatening*. Interactions may have a *rapid onset* or a *delayed onset*.

induration, sterile abscesses, tissue sloughing at injection site, *SJS.* **Other:** *anaphylaxis,* hypersensitivity reactions, drug fever.

INTERACTIONS

Drug-drug. *Aminoglycosides:* May increase risk of nephrotoxicity. Avoid using together.
Anticoagulants: May increase anticoagulant effects. Monitor PT and INR.
Estrogen-based contraceptives: May decrease contraceptive absorption and effectiveness. Patient should avoid use together or use non-hormonal contraception for duration of antibiotic (or 14 days, whichever is longer) and for 7 days after completion of antibiotic.
Live-virus vaccines: May decrease effectiveness of live-virus vaccines. Concurrent use isn't recommended.
Phenytoin: May decrease protein binding of phenytoin. Monitor phenytoin level.
Probenecid: May inhibit excretion and increase cefazolin level. Use together isn't recommended.
Warfarin: May enhance anticoagulant effects. Monitor therapy.

EFFECTS ON LAB TEST RESULTS

- May increase ALP, ALT, AST, bilirubin, GGT, and LDH levels.
- May increase eosinophil count.
- May decrease neutrophil, platelet, and WBC counts.
- May prolong INR.
- May falsely increase serum or urine creatinine level in tests using Jaffé reaction.
- May cause false-positive results of Coombs test and urine glucose tests that use cupric sulfate, such as Benedict reagent and Clinitest.

CONTRAINDICATIONS & CAUTIONS

- Contraindicated in patients hypersensitive to drug or other cephalosporins and in those with immediate hypersensitivity reactions (anaphylaxis or serious skin reactions) to penicillins or other beta-lactams.
- Use cautiously in patients hypersensitive to penicillin because of the possibility of cross-sensitivity with other beta-lactam antibiotics.
- Solutions containing dextrose may be contraindicated in patients with corn product hypersensitivity.
- Use cautiously in patients with a history of colitis, seizure disorders, or renal insufficiency.

- To reduce development of drug-resistant bacteria and maintain effectiveness of antibacterial drugs, use drug only to treat or prevent infections proven or strongly suspected to be caused by bacteria.
- Prolonged use may result in fungal or bacterial superinfection, including CDAD and pseudomembranous colitis, which can occur more than 2 months after treatment ends.
Dialyzable drug: Yes.
⚠ *Overdose S&S:* Pain, inflammation, and phlebitis at injection site; dizziness, paresthesia, headache, seizures; elevated creatinine, BUN, liver enzymes, and bilirubin levels; positive Coombs test; thrombocytosis, thrombocytopenia, eosinophilia, leukopenia; prolonged PT.

PREGNANCY-LACTATION-REPRODUCTION

- There are no adequate studies during pregnancy. Use during pregnancy only if clearly needed and potential benefit justifies fetal risk.
- Drug appears in very low concentrations in human milk. Use cautiously during breast-feeding.

NURSING CONSIDERATIONS

- If CrCl falls below 55 mL/minute in adults or 70 mL/minute in children, adjust dosage.
- If large doses are given, therapy is prolonged, or patient is at high risk, monitor patient for signs and symptoms of superinfection.
- Monitor patient for diarrhea and treat appropriately.
- Monitor patient for hypersensitivity reactions.
- *Look alike–sound alike:* Don't confuse drug with other cephalosporins that sound alike.

PATIENT TEACHING

- Instruct patient to report adverse reactions promptly.
- Tell patient to report discomfort at IV injection site.
- Advise patient to notify prescriber if a rash develops or if signs and symptoms of superinfection, such as recurring fever, chills, and malaise, appear.

---

cefdinir
sef-DIN-er

Therapeutic class: Antibiotics
Pharmacologic class: Third-generation cephalosporins

AVAILABLE FORMS
Capsules: 300 mg
Oral suspension: 125 mg/5 mL, 250 mg/5 mL

INDICATIONS & DOSAGES
Adjust-a-dose (for all indications): If CrCl is less than 30 mL/minute, reduce dosage to 300 mg PO once daily for adults and 7 mg/kg (up to 300 mg) PO once daily for children ages 6 months to 12 years. In patients receiving long-term hemodialysis, give 300 mg or 7 mg/kg PO at end of each dialysis session and then every other day.
➤ **Mild to moderate infections caused by susceptible strains of microorganisms in community-acquired pneumonia, acute worsening of chronic bronchitis, acute maxillary sinusitis, acute bacterial otitis media, and uncomplicated skin and skin-structure infections**
Adults and children age 13 and older: 300 mg PO every 12 hours or 600 mg PO every 24 hours for 10 days. Give every 12 hours for pneumonia and skin infections.
Children ages 6 months to 12 years: 7 mg/kg PO every 12 hours or 14 mg/kg PO every 24 hours for 10 days, up to maximum dose of 600 mg daily. Give every 12 hours for skin infections.
➤ **Pharyngitis, tonsillitis**
Adults and children age 13 and older: 300 mg PO every 12 hours for 5 to 10 days or 600 mg PO every 24 hours for 10 days.
Children ages 6 months to 12 years: 7 mg/kg PO every 12 hours for 5 to 10 days; or 14 mg/kg PO every 24 hours for 10 days.

ADMINISTRATION
PO
• Before administration, ensure patient isn't allergic to penicillins or cephalosporins.
• Give drug without regard for meals.
• Give twice-daily doses every 12 hours.
• Shake suspension well before use.
• Suspension can be stored at room temperature (68° to 77° F [20° to 25° C]) for 10 days.

ACTION
Inhibits cell-wall synthesis, promoting osmotic instability; usually bactericidal.

Route	Onset	Peak	Duration
PO	Unknown	2–4 hr	Unknown

Half-life: 1.75 hours.

ADVERSE REACTIONS
CNS: headache. **GI:** diarrhea, abdominal pain, nausea. **GU:** vaginal moniliasis, vaginitis, increased urine proteins. **Hematologic:** increased WBC and RBC counts. **Other:** hypersensitivity reactions, ***anaphylaxis.***

INTERACTIONS
Drug-drug. *Aminoglycosides:* May increase risk of nephrotoxicity. Avoid using together.
Antacids containing aluminum and magnesium, iron supplements, multivitamins containing iron: May decrease rate of absorption and bioavailability of cefdinir. Give such preparations 2 hours before or after cefdinir.
Estrogen-based contraceptives: May decrease contraceptive absorption and effectiveness. Patient should avoid use together or use nonhormonal contraception for duration of antibiotic (or 14 days, whichever is longer) and for 7 days after completion of antibiotic.
Live-virus vaccines: May decrease effectiveness of live-virus vaccines. Concurrent use isn't recommended.
Probenecid: May inhibit renal excretion of cefdinir. Monitor patient for adverse reactions.
Warfarin: May enhance anticoagulant effects. Monitor therapy.

EFFECTS ON LAB TEST RESULTS
• May increase ALP, GGT, bilirubin, potassium, and LDH levels.
• May decrease bicarbonate level.
• May increase WBC, RBC, eosinophil, lymphocyte, and platelet counts.
• May decrease Hb level.
• May falsely increase serum or urine creatinine level in tests using Jaffé reaction.
• May cause false-positive results of Coombs test and urine glucose tests that use cupric sulfate, such as Benedict reagent and Clinitest.

CONTRAINDICATIONS & CAUTIONS
• Contraindicated in patients hypersensitive to drug or other cephalosporins.

- To reduce development of drug-resistant bacteria and maintain effectiveness of antibacterial drugs, use drug only to treat or prevent infections proven or strongly suspected to be caused by bacteria.
- Use cautiously in patients hypersensitive to penicillin because of the possibility of cross-sensitivity with other beta-lactam antibiotics.
- Use cautiously in patients with history of colitis or renal insufficiency.
Dialyzable drug: 63%.

PREGNANCY-LACTATION-REPRODUCTION
- There are no adequate studies during pregnancy. Use during pregnancy only if clearly needed.
- It isn't known if drug appears in human milk. Use cautiously during breastfeeding.

NURSING CONSIDERATIONS
- Prolonged drug treatment may result in emergence and overgrowth of resistant organisms. Monitor patient for signs and symptoms of superinfection.
- Pseudomembranous colitis and CDAD have been reported with cefdinir and can occur more than 2 months after therapy ends. Monitor for diarrhea in patients after antibiotic therapy and in those with history of colitis.
- Monitor patient for hypersensitivity reactions.
- *Look alike–sound alike:* Don't confuse drug with other cephalosporins that sound alike.

PATIENT TEACHING
- Instruct patient or caregiver in safe drug administration and storage.
- Inform patient with diabetes that suspension contains sucrose.
- Tell patient that drug may be taken without regard to meals.
- Instruct patient to take drug as prescribed, even if feeling better.
- Advise patient to report severe diarrhea or diarrhea with abdominal pain.
- Tell patient to report all adverse reactions or signs and symptoms of superinfection promptly.

cefepime hydrochloride
SEF-e-pim

Maxipime

Therapeutic class: Antibiotics
Pharmacologic class: Fourth-generation cephalosporins

AVAILABLE FORMS
Injection: 500-mg, 1-g, 2-g vials; 2 g/100 mL; 1-g, 2-g ADD-Vantage vials; 1 g/50 mL, 2 g/50 mL

INDICATIONS & DOSAGES
Adjust-a-dose (for all indications): Adjust adult dosage based on CrCl, as shown in the table below. For patients receiving hemodialysis, about 68% of drug is removed after a 3-hour dialysis session. Cefepime dosage for patients receiving hemodialysis is 1 g on day 1, followed by 500 mg every 24 hours for treatment of all infections except febrile neutropenia. For patients with febrile neutropenia, give 1 g every 24 hours. Give cefepime after hemodialysis and at the same time each day. For patients receiving continuous ambulatory peritoneal dialysis, give normal dose every 48 hours. Because pediatric and adult cefepime pharmacokinetics are similar, change the pediatric dosing regimen proportional to the adult regimen.
➤ **Mild to moderate UTI caused by *Escherichia coli*, *Klebsiella pneumoniae*, or *Proteus mirabilis*, including concurrent bacteremia with these microorganisms**
Adults and children age 16 and older: 0.5 to 1 g IM or IV over 30 minutes every 12 hours for 7 to 10 days. Use IM only for *E. coli* infection when IM route is considered more appropriate route of administration.
➤ **Severe UTI, including pyelonephritis, caused by *E. coli*, *P. mirabilis*, or *K. pneumoniae***
Adults and children age 16 and older: 2 g IV over 30 minutes every 12 hours for 10 days.

CrCl (mL/min)	Recommended maintenance dosing schedule			
>60	500 mg every 12 hr	1 g every 12 hr	2 g every 12 hr	2 g every 8 hr
30–60	500 mg every 24 hr	1 g every 24 hr	2 g every 24 hr	2 g every 12 hr
11–29	500 mg every 24 hr	500 mg every 24 hr	1 g every 24 hr	2 g every 24 hr
<11	250 mg every 24 hr	250 mg every 24 hr	500 mg every 24 hr	1 g every 24 hr

Adult dosage adjustments for renal impairment (cefepime hydrochloride)

✤Canada ◊OTC ◆Off-label use ✐Photoguide ⊛Do not crush *Liquid contains alcohol ✄Genetic

➤ **Moderate to severe pneumonia caused by *Streptococcus pneumoniae*, *Pseudomonas aeruginosa*, *K. pneumoniae*, or *Enterobacter* species**
Adults and children age 16 and older: 1 to 2 g IV over 30 minutes every 8 to 12 hours for 10 days. For *P. aeruginosa*, 2 g IV every 8 hours for 10 days.

➤ **Moderate to severe skin infection, uncomplicated skin infection, and skin-structure infection caused by *Streptococcus pyogenes* or methicillin-susceptible strains of *Staphylococcus aureus***
Adults and children age 16 and older: 2 g IV over 30 minutes every 12 hours for 10 days.

➤ **Complicated intra-abdominal infection caused by *E. coli*, viridans group streptococci, *P. aeruginosa*, *K. pneumoniae*, *Enterobacter* species, or *Bacteroides fragilis***
Adults and children age 16 and older: 2 g IV over 30 minutes every 8 to 12 hours for 7 to 10 days. Give with metronidazole. For *P. aeruginosa*, 2 g IV every 8 hours.

➤ **Empirical therapy for febrile neutropenia**
Adults and children age 16 and older: 2 g IV every 8 hours for 7 days or until neutropenia resolves. If fever resolves but patient remains neutropenic for more than 7 days, frequently reevaluate the need for continued antimicrobial therapy.

➤ **Uncomplicated and complicated UTI (including pyelonephritis), uncomplicated skin and skin-structure infection, pneumonia, empirical therapy for febrile neutropenic children**
Children ages 2 months to 16 years weighing up to 40 kg: 50 mg/kg/dose IV over 30 minutes every 12 hours for 7 to 10 days. For febrile neutropenia or moderate to severe pseudomonal pneumonia, 50 mg/kg IV every 8 hours for 7 days or until neutropenia resolves (10 days for pseudomonal pneumonia). For UTI, treat for 7 to 10 days. Don't exceed 2 g/dose. May consider IM route only for mild to moderate, uncomplicated or complicated UTIs due to *E. coli*.

ADMINISTRATION
• Before giving, ensure patient isn't allergic to penicillins or cephalosporins.
• Obtain specimen for culture and sensitivity tests before giving. Start therapy while awaiting results.

IV
▼ Follow manufacturer's guidelines closely when reconstituting drug. They vary with concentration of drug ordered and how drug is packaged.
▼ The type of diluent varies with the product used. Use only solutions recommended by the manufacturer.
▼ Give intermittent IV infusion with a Y-type administration set and compatible solutions over 30 minutes.
▼ Interrupt flow of primary IV solution while drug is infusing.
▼ May also give by direct IV injection after vial reconstitution over 5 minutes.
▼ **Incompatibilities:** Aminophylline, ciprofloxacin, netilmicin sulfate, gentamicin, metronidazole, tobramycin, vancomycin.

IM
• Reconstitute drug using sterile water for injection, NSS for injection, D_5W injection, 0.5% or 1% lidocaine hydrochloride, or bacteriostatic water for injection with parabens or benzyl alcohol. Follow manufacturer's guidelines for quantity of diluent to use.
• Inspect solution for particulate matter before use. The powder and its solutions tend to darken, depending on storage conditions. If stored as recommended, potency isn't adversely affected.
• Pain may occur at injection site. Give deep IM into large muscle mass.

ACTION
Inhibits bacterial cell-wall synthesis, promotes osmotic instability, and destroys bacteria.

Route	Onset	Peak	Duration
IV	Unknown	30 min	Unknown
IM	Unknown	1–2 hr	Unknown

Half-life: Adults, 2 to 2.5 hours.

ADVERSE REACTIONS
CNS: fever, headache. **CV:** injection-site phlebitis. **GI:** diarrhea, nausea, vomiting. **Hepatic:** increased transaminase levels. **Metabolic:** hypophosphatemia. **Skin:** rash, pruritus. **Other:** injection-site reaction (pain, inflammation), hypersensitivity reactions.

INTERACTIONS
Drug-drug. *Aminoglycosides, potent diuretics:* May increase risk of nephrotoxicity. Monitor renal function closely.

Reactions in bold italics are *life-threatening*. Interactions may have a *rapid onset* or a *delayed onset*.

Estrogen-based contraceptives: May decrease contraceptive absorption and effectiveness. Patient should avoid use together or use nonhormonal contraception for duration of antibiotic (or 14 days, whichever is longer) and for 7 days after completion of antibiotic.
Live-virus vaccines: May decrease effectiveness of live-virus vaccines. Concurrent use isn't recommended.
Probenecid: May inhibit renal excretion of cefepime. Monitor patient for adverse reactions.
Warfarin: May enhance anticoagulant effects. Monitor therapy.

EFFECTS ON LAB TEST RESULTS
• May increase BUN, creatinine, potassium, bilirubin, ALK, ALT, and AST levels.
• May increase or decrease phosphorus and calcium levels.
• May increase eosinophil count.
• May decrease hematocrit and neutrophil, platelet, and WBC counts.
• May alter PT and PTT.
• May falsely increase serum or urine creatinine level in tests using Jaffé reaction. May cause false-positive results of Coombs test and urine glucose tests that use cupric sulfate, such as Benedict reagent and Clinitest.

CONTRAINDICATIONS & CAUTIONS
• Contraindicated in patients hypersensitive to drug or other cephalosporins and in patients with immediate hypersensitivity reactions to beta-lactam antibiotics or penicillins.
• Use cautiously in patients sensitive to penicillin.
• Dextrose solutions may be contraindicated in patients with corn product hypersensitivity.
• To reduce development of drug-resistant bacteria and maintain effectiveness of antibacterial drugs, use drug only to treat or prevent infections proven or strongly suspected to be caused by bacteria.
🔊 *Alert:* Drug may increase risk of nonconvulsive status epilepticus (altered mental status, confusion, decreased responsiveness), especially in patients with renal impairment. To decrease risk, follow dosage adjustment guidelines for patients with CrCl of 60 mL/minute or less. Discontinue drug in patients with seizures associated with drug.
• Use cautiously in patients with history of colitis or renal insufficiency.
Dializable drug: 68%.

⚠ *Overdose S&S:* Encephalopathy, myoclonus, seizures, neuromuscular excitability, nonconvulsive status epilepticus.

PREGNANCY-LACTATION-REPRODUCTION
• There are no adequate studies during pregnancy. Use during pregnancy only if clearly needed and potential benefit justifies fetal risk.
• Drug appears in human milk in very low concentrations (0.5 mcg/mL). Use cautiously during breastfeeding.

NURSING CONSIDERATIONS
• Monitor patient for superinfection, including CDAD and pseudomembranous colitis, which can occur more than 2 months after final dose. Drug may cause overgrowth of nonsusceptible bacteria or fungi.
• Drug may alter PT and increase bleeding risk. Patients at risk include those with renal or hepatic impairment or poor nutrition and those receiving prolonged therapy. Monitor PT and INR in these patients. Give vitamin K, as indicated.
• Monitor patient for neurologic changes.
• Monitor patient for hypersensitivity reactions.
• *Look alike–sound alike:* Don't confuse drug with other cephalosporins that sound alike.

PATIENT TEACHING
• Warn patient receiving drug IM that pain may occur at injection site.
• Advise patient to promptly report all adverse reactions, including rash, and signs and symptoms of superinfection (such as recurring fever, chills, malaise, and diarrhea).

cefotaxime sodium
sef-oh-TAKS-eem

Therapeutic class: Antibiotics
Pharmacologic class: Third-generation cephalosporins

AVAILABLE FORMS
Injection: 500 mg, 1 g, 2 g

INDICATIONS & DOSAGES
Adjust-a-dose (for all indications): For patients with CrCl less than 20 mL/minute/1.73 m^2, give half of usual dose at regular time interval.

♣ Canada ◇ OTC ◆ Off-label use 🖉 Photoguide ⊜ Do not crush *Liquid contains alcohol ▓ Genetic

➤ **Perioperative prophylaxis in contaminated surgery**

Adults: 1 g IM or IV 30 to 90 minutes before surgery. In patients undergoing bowel surgery, provide preoperative mechanical bowel cleansing and give a nonabsorbable anti-infective, such as neomycin. In patients undergoing cesarean delivery, give 1 g IM or IV as soon as the umbilical cord is clamped; then 1 g IM or IV 6 and 12 hours later.

Adjust-a-dose: For patients who are obese weighing at least 120 kg (or defined as BMI greater than 30 kg/m^2), administer 2 g within 60 minutes before surgical incision.

➤ **Uncomplicated gonorrhea caused by penicillinase-producing strains or non–penicillinase-producing strains of *Neisseria gonorrhoeae***

Adults and adolescents: 500 mg IM as a single dose.

➤ **Rectal gonorrhea**

Men: 1 g IM as a single dose.
Women: 500 mg IM as a single dose.

➤ **Serious infection of the lower respiratory and urinary tract, CNS, skin, bone, and joints; gynecologic and intra-abdominal infection; bacteremia; septicemia caused by susceptible microorganisms, such as streptococci (including *Streptococcus pneumoniae* and *Streptococcus pyogenes*, *Staphylococcus aureus* [penicillinase- and non–penicillinase-producing], and *Staphylococcus epidermidis*), *Escherichia coli*, *Klebsiella*, *Haemophilus influenzae*, *Serratia marcescens*, and species of *Pseudomonas* (including *P. aeruginosa*), *Enterobacter*, *Proteus*, and *Peptostreptococcus***

Adults and children weighing 50 kg or more: 1 to 2 g IV or IM every 6 to 8 hours. Up to 12 g IV daily can be given for life-threatening infections.

Children ages 1 month to 12 years weighing less than 50 kg: 50 to 180 mg/kg/day IM or IV in four to six divided doses.

Neonates ages 1 to 4 weeks: 50 mg/kg IV every 8 hours.

Neonates to age 1 week: 50 mg/kg IV every 12 hours.

ADMINISTRATION

• Before giving, ensure patient isn't allergic to penicillins or cephalosporins.

• Obtain specimen for culture and sensitivity tests before giving. Begin therapy while awaiting results.

IV

▼ For direct injection, reconstitute drug in 500-mg, 1-g, or 2-g vials with 10 mL of sterile water for injection. Solutions containing 1 g/14 mL are isotonic.

▼ Inject drug over 3 to 5 minutes into a large vein or into the tubing of a free-flowing IV solution. Potentially life-threatening arrhythmias have been reported with more rapid administration.

▼ For infusion, reconstitute drug in infusion vials with 50 to 100 mL of D$_5$W or NSS.

▼ Interrupt flow of primary IV solution, and infuse this drug over 15 to 30 minutes.

▼ **Incompatibilities:** Allopurinol, azithromycin, doxapram, filgrastim, fluconazole, pentamidine, sodium bicarbonate injection, vancomycin.

IM

• Reconstitute 500-mg vial with 2 mL, 1-g vial with 3 mL, and 2-g vial with 5 mL sterile water for injection.

• For doses of 2 g, divide the dose and give at different sites.

• Inject deep into a large muscle, such as the gluteus maximus or the side of the thigh.

ACTION

Inhibits cell-wall synthesis, promoting osmotic instability; usually bactericidal.

Route	Onset	Peak	Duration
IV	Immediate	Immediate	Unknown
IM	Unknown	30 min	Unknown

Half-life: 1 to 2 hours.

ADVERSE REACTIONS

CNS: fever, headache. **CV:** IV-site phlebitis and thrombophlebitis. **GI:** diarrhea, nausea, vomiting. **Hematologic:** *agranulocytosis, thrombocytopenia, transient neutropenia,* eosinophilia. **Skin:** rash, pruritus, IM-site pain and induration, IV-site inflammation. **Other:** hypersensitivity reactions, including *anaphylaxis*.

INTERACTIONS

Drug-drug. *Aminoglycosides:* May increase risk of nephrotoxicity. Monitor patient's renal function tests.

Estrogen-based contraceptives: May decrease contraceptive absorption and effectiveness.

Reactions in bold italics are *life-threatening*. Interactions may have a *rapid onset* or a *delayed onset*.

Patient should avoid use together or use non-hormonal contraception for duration of antibiotic (or 14 days, whichever is longer) and for 7 days after completion of antibiotic.
Live-virus vaccines: May decrease effectiveness of live-virus vaccines. Concurrent use isn't recommended.
Probenecid: May inhibit excretion and increase cefotaxime level. Use together cautiously.
Warfarin: May enhance anticoagulant effects. Monitor therapy.

EFFECTS ON LAB TEST RESULTS
• May increase ALP, ALT, AST, bilirubin, GGT, and LDH levels. May decrease Hb level.
• May increase eosinophil count. May decrease granulocyte, neutrophil, and platelet counts.
• May falsely increase serum or urine creatinine level in tests using Jaffé reaction. May cause false-positive results of Coombs test and urine glucose tests that use cupric sulfate, such as Benedict reagent and Clinitest.

CONTRAINDICATIONS & CAUTIONS
• Contraindicated in patients hypersensitive to drug or other cephalosporins.
• Use cautiously in patients hypersensitive to penicillin because of possibility of cross-sensitivity with other beta-lactam antibiotics.
• CDC guidelines for sexually transmitted diseases don't recommend cefotaxime as a treatment option for uncomplicated or rectal gonorrhea; ceftriaxone plus azithromycin is preferred.
• Prolonged use may result in fungal or bacterial superinfection, including CDAD and pseudomembranous colitis, which can occur more than 2 months after treatment ends.
• To reduce development of drug-resistant bacteria and maintain effectiveness of antibacterial drugs, use drug only to treat or prevent infections proven or strongly suspected to be caused by bacteria.
• Use cautiously in patients with history of colitis or renal insufficiency.
Dialyzable drug: Yes.
⚠ *Overdose S&S:* Elevated BUN and creatinine levels.

PREGNANCY-LACTATION-REPRODUCTION
• There are no adequate studies during pregnancy. Use during pregnancy only if clearly needed.

• Low concentrations of drug appear in human milk. Use cautiously during breastfeeding.

NURSING CONSIDERATIONS
• If large doses are given, therapy is prolonged, or patient is at high risk, monitor patient for superinfection.
• Monitor patient for diarrhea and treat appropriately.
• Monitor patient for signs and symptoms of allergic reaction.
• *Look alike–sound alike:* Don't confuse drug with other cephalosporins that sound alike.

PATIENT TEACHING
• Tell patient to promptly report adverse reactions and signs and symptoms of superinfection, including diarrhea.
• Instruct patient to report discomfort at IV insertion site.

cefpodoxime proxetil
SEF-pode-OKS-eem

Therapeutic class: Antibiotics
Pharmacologic class: Third-generation cephalosporins

AVAILABLE FORMS
Granules for oral suspension: 50 mg/5 mL or 100 mg/5 mL when reconstituted
Tablets (film-coated): 100 mg, 200 mg

INDICATIONS & DOSAGES
Adjust-a-dose (for all indications): For patients with CrCl less than 30 mL/minute, increase dosage interval to every 24 hours. Give to patients receiving hemodialysis three times weekly after hemodialysis.
➤ **Acute community-acquired pneumonia caused by strains of *Haemophilus influenzae* or *Streptococcus pneumoniae***
Adults and children age 12 and older: 200 mg PO every 12 hours for 14 days.
➤ **Acute bacterial worsening of chronic bronchitis caused by *S. pneumoniae* or *H. influenzae* (strains that don't produce beta-lactamase only), or *Moraxella catarrhalis* (tablets only)**
Adults and children age 12 and older: 200 mg PO every 12 hours for 10 days.
➤ **Uncomplicated gonorrhea in men and women; rectal gonococcal infections in women**

Adults and children age 12 and older: 200 mg PO as a single dose.

➤ **Uncomplicated skin and skin-structure infections caused by *Staphylococcus aureus* or *Streptococcus pyogenes***

Adults and children age 12 and older: 400 mg PO every 12 hours for 7 to 14 days.

➤ **Acute otitis media caused by *S. pneumoniae* (penicillin-susceptible strains only), *S. pyogenes*, *H. influenzae*, or *M. catarrhalis***

Children ages 2 months to 12 years: 5 mg/kg oral suspension PO every 12 hours for 5 days. Don't exceed 200 mg per dose.

➤ **Pharyngitis or tonsillitis caused by *S. pyogenes***

Adults: 100 mg PO every 12 hours for 5 to 10 days.

Children ages 2 months to 12 years: 5 mg/kg PO every 12 hours for 5 to 10 days. Don't exceed 100 mg per dose.

➤ **Uncomplicated UTIs caused by *Escherichia coli*, *Klebsiella pneumoniae*, *Proteus mirabilis*, or *Staphylococcus saprophyticus***

Adults and adolescents age 12 and older: 100 mg PO every 12 hours for 7 days.

➤ **Mild to moderate acute maxillary sinusitis caused by *H. influenzae*, *S. pneumoniae*, or *M. catarrhalis***

Adults and adolescents age 12 and older: 200 mg PO every 12 hours for 10 days.

Children ages 2 months to 12 years: 5 mg/kg PO every 12 hours for 10 days; maximum, 200 mg/dose.

ADMINISTRATION
PO
• Before administration, ensure patient isn't allergic to penicillins or cephalosporins.
• Obtain specimen for culture and sensitivity tests before giving. Begin therapy while awaiting results.
• Give tablets with food to enhance absorption. May give oral suspension without regard to food. Shake suspension well before using.
• Store suspension in the refrigerator (36° to 46° F [2° to 8° C]). Discard unused portion after 14 days.

ACTION
Inhibits cell-wall synthesis, promoting osmotic instability; usually bactericidal.

Route	Onset	Peak	Duration
PO	Unknown	2–3 hr	Unknown

Half-life: 2 to 3 hours.

ADVERSE REACTIONS
CNS: headache. **GI:** diarrhea, *CDAD,* nausea, abdominal pain. **GU:** vaginal fungal infections. **Skin:** rash. **Other:** hypersensitivity reactions, including *anaphylaxis.*

INTERACTIONS
Drug-drug. *Aminoglycosides:* May increase risk of nephrotoxicity. Monitor renal function tests closely.

Antacids, H2-receptor antagonists: May decrease absorption of cefpodoxime. Separate H2-receptor antagonist and cefpodoxime doses by at least 2 hours. Monitor therapy.

Estrogen-based contraceptives: May decrease contraceptive absorption and effectiveness. Patient should avoid use together or use nonhormonal contraception for duration of antibiotic (or 14 days, whichever is longer) and for 7 days after completion of antibiotic.

Live-virus vaccines: May decrease effectiveness of live-virus vaccines. Concurrent use isn't recommended.

Probenecid: May decrease excretion of cefpodoxime. Monitor patient for toxicity.

Warfarin: May prolong PT and increase INR. Monitor levels closely, and adjust warfarin dosage.

EFFECTS ON LAB TEST RESULTS
• May increase AST, ALT, GGT, ALP, bilirubin, potassium, and LDH levels.
• May decrease albumin and sodium levels.
• May increase or decrease glucose level.
• May decrease Hb level, hematocrit, ANC, and WBC, platelet, and lymphocyte counts.
• May falsely increase serum or urine creatinine level in tests using Jaffé reaction.
• May cause false-positive results of Coombs test and urine glucose tests that use cupric sulfate, such as Benedict reagent and Clinitest.

CONTRAINDICATIONS & CAUTIONS
• Contraindicated in patients hypersensitive to drug or other cephalosporins.
⚠ *Alert:* Drug can cause CDAD and pseudomembranous colitis ranging from mild to life-threatening due to overgrowth of nonsusceptible bacteria or fungi.

Reactions in bold italics are *life-threatening*. Interactions may have a *rapid onset* or a *delayed onset*.

- To reduce development of drug-resistant bacteria and maintain effectiveness of antibacterial drugs, use drug only to treat or prevent infections proven or strongly suspected to be caused by bacteria.
- Use cautiously in patients with a history of penicillin hypersensitivity because of risk of cross-sensitivity.
- Use cautiously in patients receiving nephrotoxic drugs because other cephalosporins have been shown to have nephrotoxic potential.
- For children with otitis media, American Academy of Pediatrics guidelines recommend basing duration on patient age: For patients younger than age 2 or with severe symptoms (any age), 10-day course; for patients age 2 to 5 with mild to moderate symptoms, 7-day course; for patients age 6 and older with mild to moderate symptoms, 5-day course.
- ☺ *Alert:* Some dosage forms may contain benzoate, which is a metabolite of benzyl alcohol. Benzyl alcohol in large amounts has been linked to potentially fatal gasping syndrome in neonates. Avoid dosage forms with benzyl alcohol derivatives in neonates. Refer to manufacturer's labeling.
- Safety and effectiveness in children younger than age 2 months haven't been established.
Dialyzable drug: 23%.

PREGNANCY-LACTATION-REPRODUCTION

- There are no adequate studies during pregnancy. Use during pregnancy only if clearly needed.
- Drug appears in human milk. Patient should discontinue breastfeeding or discontinue drug, taking into account importance of drug to the patient.

NURSING CONSIDERATIONS

- Monitor renal function closely.
- Monitor patient for superinfection and diarrhea and treat appropriately. Use extreme caution when using drug in patients at increased risk for antibiotic-induced pseudomembranous colitis due to exposure to institutional settings (such as nursing homes or hospitals) with endemic *Clostridioides difficile* infection.
- Monitor patient for hypersensitivity reactions.
- *Look alike–sound alike:* Don't confuse drug with other cephalosporins that sound alike.

PATIENT TEACHING

- Tell patient to take drug as prescribed, even if feeling better.
- Instruct patient in safe drug administration and storage.
- Tell patient to report all adverse reactions, especially rash or signs and symptoms of superinfection.
- Advise patient to promptly report loose stools or diarrhea.

---

cefprozil
sef-PRO-zil

Therapeutic class: Antibiotics
Pharmacologic class: Second-generation cephalosporins

AVAILABLE FORMS

Powder for oral suspension: 125 mg/5 mL, 250 mg/5 mL when reconstituted
Tablets: 250 mg, 500 mg

INDICATIONS & DOSAGES

Adjust-a-dose (for all indications): If CrCl is less than 30 mL/minute, give 50% of standard dose at standard intervals. If patient is receiving dialysis, give dose after hemodialysis is completed; drug is removed by hemodialysis.
➤ **Pharyngitis or tonsillitis caused by** *Streptococcus pyogenes*
Adults and children age 13 and older: 500 mg PO daily for at least 10 days.
Children ages 2 to 12: 7.5 mg/kg PO every 12 hours for 10 days. Don't exceed 500 mg/day.
➤ **Otitis media caused by** *Streptococcus pneumoniae, Haemophilus influenzae,* **or** *Moraxella catarrhalis*
Infants and children ages 6 months to 12 years: 15 mg/kg PO every 12 hours for 10 days. Don't exceed 500 mg/dose.
American Academy of Pediatrics guidelines don't routinely recommend cefprozil use.
➤ **Secondary bacterial infections of acute bronchitis and acute bacterial worsening of chronic bronchitis caused by** *S. pneumoniae, H. influenzae,* **or** *M. catarrhalis*
Adults and children age 13 and older: 500 mg PO every 12 hours for 10 days.
➤ **Uncomplicated skin and skin-structure infections caused by** *Staphylococcus aureus* **or** *S. pyogenes*

Adults and children age 13 and older: 250 or 500 mg PO every 12 hours or 500 mg PO daily for 10 days.

Children ages 2 to 12: 20 mg/kg PO every 24 hours for 10 days. Don't exceed adult dose.

ADMINISTRATION

PO

- Obtain specimen for culture and sensitivity tests before giving first dose. Start therapy while awaiting results.
- Before giving, ensure patient isn't allergic to penicillins or cephalosporins.
- Give without regard to meals.
- Give around the clock to limit variation in peak and trough serum levels.
- Shake suspension well before using.
- Refrigerate suspension and discard after 14 days.

ACTION

Inhibits cell-wall synthesis, promoting osmotic instability; usually bactericidal.

Route	Onset	Peak	Duration
PO	Unknown	1.5 hr	Unknown

Half-life: 1.25 hours in adults with normal renal function; 1.5 hours in children; 2 hours in patients with impaired hepatic function; 5 to 6 hours in patients with renal impairment or ESRD.

ADVERSE REACTIONS

CNS: dizziness. **GI:** diarrhea, nausea, vomiting, abdominal pain. **GU:** genital pruritus, vaginitis. **Hematologic:** eosinophilia. **Hepatic:** increased transaminase levels. **Skin:** rash. **Other:** superinfection, hypersensitivity reaction, including *anaphylaxis*.

INTERACTIONS

Drug-drug. *Aminoglycosides:* May increase risk of nephrotoxicity. Monitor renal function tests closely.

Estrogen-based contraceptives: May decrease contraceptive absorption and effectiveness. Patient should avoid use together or use nonhormonal contraception for duration of antibiotic (or 14 days, whichever is longer) and for 7 days after completion of antibiotic.

Live-virus vaccines: May decrease effectiveness of live-virus vaccines. Concurrent use isn't recommended.

Probenecid: May inhibit excretion and increase cefprozil level. Use together cautiously.

Warfarin: May enhance anticoagulant effects. Monitor therapy.

EFFECTS ON LAB TEST RESULTS

- May increase ALP, ALT, AST, bilirubin, BUN, creatinine, and LDH levels.
- May increase eosinophil count. May decrease platelet and WBC counts.
- May prolong PT and PTT.
- May provide false-negative reaction in the ferricyanide test for blood glucose.
- May falsely increase serum or urine creatinine level in tests using Jaffé reaction. May cause false-positive results of Coombs test and urine glucose tests that use cupric sulfate, such as Benedict reagent and Clinitest.

CONTRAINDICATIONS & CAUTIONS

- Contraindicated in patients hypersensitive to drug or other cephalosporins.
- To reduce development of drug-resistant bacteria and maintain effectiveness of antibacterial drugs, use drug only to treat or prevent infections proven or strongly suspected to be caused by bacteria.
- Use cautiously in patients hypersensitive to penicillin because of possibility of cross-sensitivity with other beta-lactam antibiotics.

⚠ Alert: May cause mild to life-threatening CDAD and pseudomembranous colitis, which can occur even more than 2 months after therapy; drug may need to be discontinued and other treatment initiated. Use cautiously in patients with a history of GI disease, especially colitis.

- Use cautiously in patients with history of colitis and renal insufficiency.

Dialyzable drug: Yes.

PREGNANCY-LACTATION-REPRODUCTION

- There are no adequate studies during pregnancy. Use during pregnancy only if clearly needed.
- Small amounts of drug appear in human milk. Use cautiously during breastfeeding.

NURSING CONSIDERATIONS

- Monitor renal function test and LFT results.
- Drug may cause overgrowth of nonsusceptible bacteria or fungi. Monitor patient for superinfection.

Reactions in bold italics are *life-threatening*. Interactions may have a *rapid onset* or a ***delayed onset***.

- Monitor patient for diarrhea and treat accordingly.
- Monitor patient for hypersensitivity reactions.
- *Look alike–sound alike:* Don't confuse drug with other cephalosporins that sound alike.

PATIENT TEACHING

- Advise patient to take drug as prescribed, even if feeling better.
- Inform patient with phenylketonuria that product may contain phenylalanine.
- Teach proper drug administration and storage.
- Instruct patient to report all adverse reactions and to immediately report rash or signs and symptoms of superinfection, including diarrhea.

---

cefTAZidime
sef-TAZ-i-deem

Fortaz, Tazicef

Therapeutic class: Antibiotics
Pharmacologic class: Third-generation cephalosporins

AVAILABLE FORMS

Infusion: 1 g, 2 g in 50-mL premixed solution
Injection (with sodium carbonate): 500 mg, 1 g, 2 g

INDICATIONS & DOSAGES

Adjust-a-dose (for all indications): If CrCl is 31 to 50 mL/minute, give 1 g every 12 hours; if CrCl is 16 to 30 mL/minute, give 1 g every 24 hours; if CrCl is 6 to 15 mL/minute, give 500 mg every 24 hours; if CrCl is less than 5 mL/minute, give 500 mg every 48 hours. Ceftazidime is removed by hemodialysis; give a loading dose of 1 g, followed by 1 g after each hemodialysis period. If patient is receiving continuous ambulatory peritoneal dialysis, give a loading dose of 1 g, followed by 500 mg every 24 hours. Or, add 250 mg per 2 L of dialysis fluid.

➤ **Serious lower respiratory tract infection; skin, gynecologic, intra-abdominal, bone and joint, and CNS infection; bacteremia; and septicemia caused by susceptible microorganisms, such as streptococci (including *Streptococcus pneumoniae* and *Streptococcus pyogenes*), penicillinase- and** non–penicillinase-producing *Staphylococcus aureus, Escherichia coli, Klebsiella, Proteus, Enterobacter, Haemophilus influenzae, Pseudomonas,* **and some strains of *Bacteroides***
Adults and children age 12 and older: 1 to 2 g IV or IM every 8 to 12 hours. Route and dosage are determined by susceptibility of the organism, severity of infection, and condition of patient. Give up to 6 g daily in life-threatening infections.
Children ages 1 month to 12 years: 30 to 50 mg/kg IV every 8 hours. Maximum dose is 6 g/day.
Neonates up to age 4 weeks: 30 mg/kg IV every 12 hours.
➤ **Uncomplicated UTI**
Adults: 250 mg IV or IM every 12 hours.
➤ **Complicated UTI**
Adults and children age 12 and older: 500 mg to 1 g IV or IM every 8 to 12 hours.
➤ **Uncomplicated pneumonia; mild skin and skin-structure infections**
Adults and children age 12 and older: 500 mg to 1 g IV or IM every 8 hours.
➤ **Lung infections caused by *Pseudomonas* in patients with cystic fibrosis with normal renal function**
Adults and children age 12 and older: 30 to 50 mg/kg IV every 8 hours. Maximum dose is 6 g/day.
➤ **Very severe life-threatening infections, especially in patients who are immunocompromised**
Adults and children older than age 12: 2 g IV every 8 hours.

ADMINISTRATION
IV

▼ Before administration, ensure patient isn't allergic to penicillins or cephalosporins.
▼ Obtain specimen for culture and sensitivity tests before giving. Begin therapy while awaiting results.
▼ Each brand of drug includes specific instructions for reconstitution. Read and follow them carefully.
▼ To reconstitute solution that contains sodium carbonate, add 5.3 mL sterile water for injection to a 500-mg vial, or add 10 mL to a 1-g or 2-g vial. Shake well to dissolve drug. Because carbon dioxide is released during dissolution, positive pressure will develop in vial.

▼ Inspect solution for particulate matter and discoloration before giving. Use only if solution is clear.

▼ Infuse drug over 15 to 30 minutes.

▼ **Incompatibilities:** Aminophylline, amiodarone, azithromycin, clarithromycin, fluconazole, idarubicin, midazolam, pentamidine, ranitidine, sargramostim, vancomycin.

IM

• Before administration, ensure patient isn't allergic to penicillins or cephalosporins.

• Obtain specimen for culture and sensitivity tests before giving. Begin therapy while awaiting results.

• Inject deep into a large muscle, such as the gluteus maximus or the side of the thigh.

ACTION

Inhibits cell-wall synthesis, promoting osmotic instability; usually bactericidal.

Route	Onset	Peak	Duration
IV	Immediate	Immediate	Unknown
IM	Unknown	1 hr	Unknown

Half-life: 2 hours.

ADVERSE REACTIONS

CNS: headache, dizziness, paresthesia, fever. **CV:** injection-site phlebitis and thrombophlebitis. **GI:** *CDAD,* nausea, vomiting, diarrhea, abdominal cramps. **GU:** vaginitis. **Hematologic:** *agranulocytosis, leukopenia, thrombocytopenia,* eosinophilia, thrombocytosis. **Skin:** rash, pruritus, pain, injection-site inflammation. **Other:** hypersensitivity reactions, including *anaphylaxis,* candidiasis.

INTERACTIONS

Drug-drug. *Aminoglycosides:* May cause additive or synergistic effect against some strains of *Pseudomonas aeruginosa* and *Enterobacteriaceae;* may increase risk of nephrotoxicity. Monitor patient for effects and monitor renal function.
Chloramphenicol: May cause antagonistic effect. Avoid using together.
Estrogen-based contraceptives: May decrease contraceptive absorption and effectiveness. Patient should avoid use together or use non-hormonal contraception for duration of antibiotic (or 14 days, whichever is longer) and for 7 days after completion of antibiotic.
Live-virus vaccines: May decrease effectiveness of live-virus vaccines. Concurrent use isn't recommended.

Probenecid: May increase serum concentrations of cephalosporins. Monitor therapy.
Warfarin: May increase anticoagulation effect. Monitor PT and INR closely.

EFFECTS ON LAB TEST RESULTS

• May increase ALP, ALT, AST, bilirubin, and LDH levels. May decrease Hb level.

• May increase eosinophil count. May decrease granulocyte and WBC counts. May increase or decrease platelet count.

• May prolong PTT and PT, and increase INR.

• May falsely increase serum or urine creatinine level in tests using Jaffé reaction. May cause false-positive results of Coombs test and urine glucose tests that use cupric sulfate, such as Benedict reagent and Clinitest.

CONTRAINDICATIONS & CAUTIONS

• Contraindicated in patients hypersensitive to drug or other cephalosporins.

• To reduce development of drug-resistant bacteria and maintain effectiveness of antibacterial drugs, use drug only to treat or prevent infections proven or strongly suspected to be caused by bacteria.

• Use cautiously in patients hypersensitive to penicillin; may cause cross-sensitivity with other beta-lactam antibiotics.

• Prolonged use can result in superinfection, including CDAD and pseudomembranous colitis, which can occur even more than 2 months after treatment ends.

• Use cautiously in patients with history of colitis, renal insufficiency, or seizures.
Dialyzable drug: Yes.

⚠ *Overdose S&S:* Seizures, encephalopathy, asterixis, neuromuscular excitability, coma (in patients with renal failure).

PREGNANCY-LACTATION-REPRODUCTION

• There are no adequate studies during pregnancy. Use during pregnancy only if clearly needed.

• Drug appears in human milk in low concentrations. Use caution during breastfeeding.

NURSING CONSIDERATIONS

• If large doses are given, therapy is prolonged, or patient is at high risk, monitor patient for superinfection.

• Monitor patient for diarrhea and treat appropriately.

Reactions in bold italics are *life-threatening*. Interactions may have a *rapid onset* or a ***delayed onset***.

- Monitor patient for hypersensitivity reactions.
- *Look alike–sound alike:* Don't confuse drug with other cephalosporins that sound alike.

PATIENT TEACHING
- Tell patient to report adverse reactions or signs of superinfection promptly.
- Instruct patient to report discomfort at IV insertion site.
- Advise patient to notify prescriber about loose stools or diarrhea.

---

cefTAZidime–avibactam sodium

sef-TAZ-i-deem/A-vi-BAK-tam sodium

Avycaz

Therapeutic class: Antibiotics
Pharmacologic class: Cephalosporins–beta-lactamase inhibitors

AVAILABLE FORMS
Injection (single-use vials): 2 g ceftazidime and 0.5 g avibactam per vial

INDICATIONS & DOSAGES
⚠ *Alert:* Dosage recommendations are expressed as total grams of the ceftazidime–avibactam combination.
Adjust-a-dose (for all indications): For adults: If CrCl is 31 to 50 mL/minute, give 1.25 g every 8 hours; if CrCl is 16 to 30 mL/minute, give 0.94 g every 12 hours; if CrCl is 6 to 15 mL/minute, give 0.94 g every 24 hours; if CrCl is 5 mL/minute or less, give 0.94 g every 48 hours. If patient is on hemodialysis, administer after hemodialysis on hemodialysis days.
➤ **Complicated intra-abdominal infections caused by susceptible microorganisms** (*Escherichia coli, Klebsiella pneumoniae, Proteus mirabilis, Providencia stuartii, Enterobacter cloacae, Klebsiella oxytoca,* or *Pseudomonas aeruginosa*) in combination with metronidazole
Adults: 2.5 g IV every 8 hours for 5 to 14 days.
Children ages 2 to 18: 62.5 mg/kg IV every 8 hours for 5 to 14 days. Maximum dose, 2.5 g.
Children ages 6 months to 2 years: 62.5 mg/kg IV every 8 hours for 5 to 14 days.

Children ages 3 to 6 months: 50 mg/kg IV every 8 hours for 5 to 14 days.
Adjust-a-dose: In children ages 2 and older with eGFR of 31 to 50 mL/minute/1.73 m^2, give 31.25 mg/kg to maximum of 1.2 g every 8 hours; with eGFR of 16 to 30 mL/minute/1.73 m^2, give 23.75 mg/kg to maximum of 0.94 g every 12 hours; with eGFR of 6 to 15 mL/minute/1.73 m^2, give 23.75 mg/kg to maximum of 0.94 g every 24 hours; with eGFR of 5 mL/minute/1.73 m^2 or less, give 23.75 mg/kg to maximum of 0.94 g every 48 hours.
➤ **Complicated UTI, including pyelonephritis, caused by susceptible microorganisms** (*E. coli, K. pneumoniae, Citrobacter koseri, Enterobacter aerogenes, E. cloacae, Citrobacter freundii, Proteus* spp., or *P. aeruginosa*)
Adults: 2.5 g IV every 8 hours for 7 to 14 days.
Children ages 2 to 18: 62.5 mg/kg IV every 8 hours for 7 to 14 days. Maximum dose, 2.5 g.
Children ages 6 months to 2 years: 62.5 mg/kg IV every 8 hours for 7 to 14 days.
Children ages 3 to 6 months: 50 mg/kg IV every 8 hours for 7 to 14 days.
Adjust-a-dose: In children age 2 and older with eGFR of 31 to 50 mL/minute/1.73 m^2, give 31.25 mg/kg to maximum of 1.2 g every 8 hours; with eGFR of 16 to 30 mL/minute/1.73 m^2, give 23.75 mg/kg to maximum of 0.94 g every 12 hours; with eGFR of 6 to 15 mL/minute/1.73 m^2, give 23.75 mg/kg to maximum of 0.94 g every 24 hours; with eGFR of 5 mL/minute/1.73 m^2 or less, give 23.75 mg/kg to maximum of 0.94 g every 48 hours.
➤ **Hospital-acquired bacterial pneumonia and ventilator-associated bacterial pneumonia caused by susceptible microorganisms** (*K. pneumoniae, E. cloacae, E. coli, Serratia marcescens, P. mirabilis, P. aeruginosa,* or *Haemophilus influenzae*)
Adults: 2.5 g IV every 8 hours for 7 to 14 days.

ADMINISTRATION
IV
▼ Store unconstituted vials at 77° F (25° C). Protect from light.
▼ Reconstitute vial with 10 mL sterile water for injection, NSS, 5% dextrose, lactated

Ringer solution, or all combinations of dextrose injection and sodium chloride injection containing up to 2.5% dextrose and 0.45% sodium chloride. Mix gently.

▼ Refer to package insert for specific information regarding volume to withdraw from vial to dilute further to 50 or 250 mL to administer renal doses of drug.

▼ After reconstitution, transfer contents of vial within 30 minutes to an infusion bag for further dilution.

▼ Further dilute constituted solution with the same diluent used for constitution to achieve a total volume between 50 and 250 mL. Mix gently. Inspect for particulate matter and discoloration (the color of solution ranges from clear to light yellow).

▼ Final admixed solution is stable for 12 hours at room temperature and for 24 hours if refrigerated at 36° to 46° F (2° to 8° C). Use final solution within 12 hours of subsequent storage at room temperature.

▼ Infuse final solution over 2 hours.

▼ **Incompatibilities:** Solutions other than those listed above. Refer to manufacturer's instructions for a list of compatible drugs or consult a drug incompatibility reference for more information.

ACTION

Ceftazidime is a bactericidal agent that inhibits cell-wall synthesis, promoting osmotic instability. Avibactam increases ceftazidime's effectiveness by inactivating certain beta-lactamases, which destroy ceftazidime.

Route	Onset	Peak	Duration
IV	Rapid	Unknown	Unknown

Half-life: Ceftazidime, about 3 hours; avibactam, about 2.5 hours.

ADVERSE REACTIONS

CV: injection-site phlebitis. **GI:** nausea, diarrhea, vomiting, constipation, abdominal pain. **Hematologic:** eosinophilia, *thrombocytopenia.* **Hepatic:** increased ALP, ALT, and GGT levels. **Metabolic:** *hypokalemia.* **Skin:** rash, pruritus. **Other:** hypersensitivity reaction.

INTERACTIONS

Drug-drug. *Aminoglycosides:* May increase risk of nephrotoxicity. Monitor closely.
Estrogen-based contraceptives: May decrease contraceptive absorption and effectiveness. Patient should avoid use together or use

nonhormonal contraception for duration of antibiotic (or 14 days, whichever is longer) and for 7 days after completion of antibiotic.
Live-virus vaccines: May decrease effectiveness of live-virus vaccines. Concurrent use isn't recommended.
Probenecid: May decrease ceftazidime–avibactam excretion. Avoid use together.
Vitamin K antagonists (warfarin): May enhance anticoagulation effects. Monitor therapy.

EFFECTS ON LAB TEST RESULTS

● May increase ALP, GGT, and ALT levels. May decrease potassium level.
● May prolong PT.
● May cause false-positive reaction for glucose in the urine with certain methods.
● May result in seroconversion from a negative to a positive direct Coombs test.

CONTRAINDICATIONS & CAUTIONS

● Contraindicated in patients hypersensitive to cephalosporins or avibactam.
● To reduce development of drug-resistant bacteria and maintain effectiveness of antibacterial drugs, use drug only to treat or prevent infections proven or strongly suspected to be caused by susceptible bacteria.
● Use cautiously in patients with penicillin or other beta-lactam allergy because of cross-sensitivity.
🕭 *Alert:* Drug may cause severe neurologic reactions, including encephalopathy, myoclonus, seizures, and nonconvulsive status epilepticus. Risk may increase in patients with renal impairment; ensure dosage adjustment for renal function. Discontinue drug if neurotoxicity occurs.
🕭 *Alert:* Serious and fatal hypersensitivity reactions and anaphylaxis can occur.
● Use cautiously in patients with renal impairment.
● CDAD has been reported with the use of nearly all systemic antibacterial drugs, and may range in severity from mild diarrhea to fatal colitis. CDAD may occur more than 2 months after use of antibacterial drugs.
● Safety and effectiveness in children younger than age18 with hospital-acquired or ventilated-associated bacterial pneumonia haven't been established.
● Safety and effectiveness in children younger than age 3 for treatment of UTI and

---

Reactions in bold italics are *life-threatening*. Interactions may have a *rapid onset* or a *delayed onset*.

intra-abdominal infection haven't been established.

• Use cautiously in older adults, who are more likely to have renal dysfunction.
Dialyzable drug: Yes.

PREGNANCY-LACTATION-REPRODUCTION

• There are no adequate studies during pregnancy. Use during pregnancy only if clearly needed.

• Ceftazidime appears in human milk in low concentrations; it isn't known if avibactam appears in human milk. Use cautiously during breastfeeding.

NURSING CONSIDERATIONS

• To reduce the development of drug-resistant bacteria and maintain the effectiveness of antibacterial drugs, ceftazidime–avibactam should be used only to treat infections that are proven or strongly suspected to be caused by susceptible bacteria.

🜂 *Alert:* Monitor renal function at baseline and at least daily in patients with renal impairment.

🜂 *Alert:* Monitor patients for CNS reactions (including seizures, nonconvulsive status epilepticus, encephalopathy, coma, asterixis, neuromuscular excitability, and myoclonia), particularly in those with renal impairment. Adjust dosage based on CrCl level or discontinue therapy as clinically indicated.

• Watch for CDAD in patients who develop diarrhea. If CDAD is suspected or confirmed, antibacterial drugs not directed against CDAD may need to be discontinued.

• Assess carefully for previous hypersensitivity reactions to cephalosporins, penicillins, or carbapenems.

• Monitor patient closely for hypersensitivity reaction. Discontinue drug if allergic reactions occur.

• Urine glucose tests based on enzymatic glucose oxidase reactions are recommended. False-positive reactions may occur with other methods.

• *Look alike–sound alike:* Don't confuse Avycaz with Fortaz or Avelox. Don't confuse avibactam with aztreonam.

PATIENT TEACHING

• Instruct patient to immediately report changes in CNS status (disturbance of consciousness, including confusion, hallucinations, stupor, and coma; myoclonus, seizures).

• Advise patient that diarrhea, including frequent watery or bloody diarrhea, may occur even months after antibacterial treatment ends and to consult health care provider for evaluation.

• Teach patient to report signs and symptoms of hypersensitivity reactions.

• Inform patient that blood tests to assess renal function will be needed during treatment.

• Counsel patient, family, or caregivers that antibacterial drugs should be used to treat bacterial infections only and aren't effective in treating viral infections (such as the common cold).

• Advise patient that it's common to feel better early in the course of therapy but to take the full course of the drug as prescribed. Skipping doses or not completing the full course of therapy may decrease the effectiveness of treatment and increase the likelihood that bacteria will develop resistance and won't be treatable in the future.

• Instruct patient to report pregnancy, plans to become pregnant, or breastfeeding.

ceftolozane sulfate–tazobactam sodium
sef-TOL-oh-zane/TAZ-oh-BAK-tam

Zerbaxa

Therapeutic class: Antibiotics
Pharmacologic class: Cephalosporins–beta-lactamase inhibitors

AVAILABLE FORMS
Powder for injection: 1 g ceftolozane and 0.5 g tazobactam in single-dose vial

INDICATIONS & DOSAGES

🜂 *Alert:* Dosage recommendations are expressed as total grams of the ceftolozane–tazobactam combination.

Adjust-a-dose (for all indications): On hemodialysis days, give maintenance dose immediately after completion of dialysis. For patients with changing renal function, monitor CrCl at least daily and adjust dosage accordingly.

➤ **Complicated intra-abdominal infections caused by *Enterobacter cloacae, Escherichia coli, Klebsiella oxytoca, Klebsiella pneumoniae, Proteus mirabilis,***

Pseudomonas aeruginosa, Bacteroides fragilis, Streptococcus anginosus, Streptococcus constellatus, **or** *Streptococcus salivarius*
Adults: 1.5 g IV every 8 hours for 4 to 14 days based on infection severity and clinical response. Give with metronidazole 500 mg IV every 8 hours.
Children from birth to younger than age 18: 30 mg/kg (to maximum 1.5 g) IV every 8 hours for 5 to 14 days.
Adjust-a-dose: If CrCl is 30 to 50 mL/minute, give 750 mg IV every 8 hours; if CrCl is 15 to 29 mL/minute, give 375 mg IV every 8 hours; if on hemodialysis or with ESRD, give single loading dose of 750 mg IV followed by maintenance dose of 150 mg IV every 8 hours for remainder of treatment period. Use isn't recommended in children with eGFR of 50 mL/minute/1.73 m^2 or less.
➤ **Complicated UTIs, including pyelonephritis, caused by** *E. coli, K. pneumoniae, P. mirabilis,* **or** *P. aeruginosa*
Adults: 1.5 g IV every 8 hours for 7 days.
Children from birth to younger than age 18: 30 mg/kg (to maximum 1.5 g) IV every 8 hours for 7 to 14 days.
Adjust-a-dose: If CrCl is 30 to 50 mL/minute, give 750 mg IV every 8 hours; if CrCl is 15 to 29 mL/minute, give 375 mg IV every 8 hours; if on hemodialysis or with ESRD, give single loading dose of 750 mg IV followed by maintenance dose of 150 mg IV every 8 hours for remainder of treatment period. Use isn't recommended in children with eGFR of 50 mL/minute/1.73 m^2 or less.
➤ **Hospital-acquired bacterial pneumonia and ventilator-associated bacterial pneumonia caused by susceptible gram-negative bacteria** *(E. cloacae, E. coli, Haemophilus influenzae, K. oxytoca, K. pneumoniae, P. mirabilis, P. aeruginosa, Serratia marcescens)*
Adults: 3 g IV infusion every 8 hours for 8 to 14 days (may need longer duration) based on infection severity and clinical response.
Adjust-a-dose: If CrCl is 30 to 50 mL/minute, give 1.5 g IV every 8 hours; if CrCl is 15 to 29 mL/minute, give 750 mg IV every 8 hours; for patients with ESRD on hemodialysis, give a single loading dose of 2.25 g followed by 450 mg maintenance dose IV every 8 hours for remainder of treatment.

ADMINISTRATION

IV

▼ Reconstitute vial with 10 mL sterile water for injection or NSS; gently shake to dissolve. The final volume is approximately 11.4 mL and must be added to a larger volume for infusion.
▼ To prepare required dose, withdraw appropriate volume from vial and add withdrawn volume to infusion bag containing 100 mL NSS or D_5W.
▼ Administer by infusion over 60 minutes.
▼ Once reconstituted, vials are stable for 1 hour; once placed in infusion bag, drug is stable for 24 hours at room temperature or 7 days under refrigeration. Don't freeze vials or infusion bags that contain drug.
▼ Infusions range from clear, colorless solutions to solutions that are clear and slightly yellow. Variations in color within this range don't affect product's potency.
▼ Vial doesn't contain a bacteriostatic preservative. Discard unused portion.
▼ **Incompatibilities:** Don't mix with other drugs or solutions except D_5W or NSS.

ACTION

Ceftolozane inhibits cell-wall synthesis by binding to penicillin-binding proteins. Tazobactam is an irreversible inhibitor of some beta-lactamases.

Route	Onset	Peak	Duration
IV	Unknown	1 hr	Unknown

Half-life: Ceftolozane, 3 to 4 hours; tazobactam, 2 to 3 hours.

ADVERSE REACTIONS

CNS: headache, insomnia, anxiety, dizziness, fever, *intracranial hemorrhage.* **CV:** hypotension, atrial fibrillation. **GI:** nausea, diarrhea, CDAD, constipation, vomiting, abdominal pain. **GU:** renal impairment. **Hematologic:** anemia, *thrombocytosis.* **Hepatic:** increased AST and ALT levels. **Metabolic:** *hypokalemia.* **Skin:** rash.

INTERACTIONS

Drug-drug. *Aminoglycosides:* May increase risk of nephrotoxicity. Monitor patient closely.
Estrogen-based contraceptives: May decrease contraceptive absorption and effectiveness. Patient should avoid use together or use nonhormonal contraception for duration of

antibiotic (or 14 days, whichever is longer) and for 7 days after completion of antibiotic.
Live-virus vaccines: May decrease effectiveness of live-virus vaccines. Concurrent use isn't recommended.
Probenecid: May increase ceftolozane–tazobactam serum concentration. Monitor therapy.
Vitamin K antagonists (warfarin): May enhance anticoagulant effects. Monitor PT and INR.

EFFECTS ON LAB TEST RESULTS
• May increase ALT and AST levels.
• May decrease potassium, magnesium, and phosphate levels.
• May increase platelet count.
• May decrease Hb level, hematocrit, and RBC count.
• May cause positive Coombs test.

CONTRAINDICATIONS & CAUTIONS
• Contraindicated in patients with serious hypersensitivity to ceftolozane–tazobactam, piperacillin–tazobactam, or other members of the beta-lactam class.
• Use cautiously in patients hypersensitive to cephalosporins, penicillin, or tazobactam.
• To reduce development of drug-resistant bacteria and maintain effectiveness of antibacterial drugs, use drug only to treat or prevent infections proven or strongly suspected to be caused by bacteria.
• May cause fungal or bacterial superinfection, including CDAD and pseudomembranous colitis. Stop drug and take appropriate measures if diarrhea develops. CDAD has occurred more than 2 months after antibacterial treatment.
• Use cautiously in older adults.
• Safety and effectiveness in children with pneumonia haven't been established.
• Use isn't recommended in children with eGFR of 50 mL/minute/1.73 m^2 or less. Infants may not have sufficient eGFR in the first few months of life.
Dialyzable drug: Ceftolozane, 66%; tazobactam, 56%.

PREGNANCY-LACTATION-REPRODUCTION
• Use during pregnancy hasn't been studied. Use cautiously and only if benefits outweigh fetal risk.
• It isn't known if drug appears in human milk. Use cautiously during breastfeeding.

NURSING CONSIDERATIONS
• Obtain daily renal function tests in patients with changing renal function. Adjust dosage as necessary based on CrCl.
• Monitor patient for signs and symptoms of hypersensitivity; institute appropriate therapy if needed.
• Monitor patient for development of superinfection, including diarrhea.
• *Look alike–sound alike:* Don't confuse Zerbaxa with Pradaxa.

PATIENT TEACHING
• Teach patient that drug is given IV and to immediately report signs or symptoms of allergic reactions (wheezing, chest tightness, itching, or swelling of the face, lips, tongue, or throat).
• Advise patient not to skip doses even if feeling better, as this may decrease effectiveness of treatment.
• Counsel patient to report GI adverse effects such as severe watery or bloody diarrhea.

cefTRIAXone sodium
sef-try-AX-ohn

Therapeutic class: Antibiotics
Pharmacologic class: Third-generation cephalosporins

AVAILABLE FORMS
Infusion: 1 g/50 mL, 2 g/50 mL premixed
Injection: 250 mg, 500 mg, 1 g, 2 g

INDICATIONS & DOSAGES
Adjust-a-dose (for all indications): In patients with significant renal disease and hepatic dysfunction, maximum dose is 2 g/day. In patients receiving intermittent hemodialysis, no dosage adjustment is necessary as drug is poorly dialyzed.
➤ **Uncomplicated gonorrhea**
Adults: 250 mg IM as a single dose, plus azithromycin 1 g PO as a single dose or doxycycline 100 mg PO b.i.d. for 7 days.
➤ **UTI; lower respiratory tract, gynecologic, bone or joint, intra-abdominal, skin, or skin-structure infection; septicemia caused by susceptible microorganisms, including *Streptococcus pneumoniae, Staphylococcus aureus, Haemophilus influenzae, Klebsiella pneumoniae, Klebsiella oxytoca, Escherichia coli, Enterobacter aerogenes,***

Proteus mirabilis, Serratia marcescens, Morganella morganii, Bacteroides fragilis, Acinetobacter calcoaceticus, **and** *Neisseria gonorrhoeae*

Adults and children older than age 12: 1 to 2 g IM or IV daily or in equally divided doses every 12 hours. Total daily dose shouldn't exceed 4 g. Treat for 4 to 14 days. Complicated infections may require longer treatment.

Children age 12 and younger: 50 to 75 mg/kg IM or IV daily or in divided doses every 12 hours. Total daily dose not to exceed 2 g.

➤ **Meningitis caused by** *Haemophilus influenzae, Neisseria meningitidis,* **or** *S. pneumoniae*

Adults: 2 g IV b.i.d. Usual duration of therapy is 7 to 21 days depending on clinical response.

Children: Initially, 100 mg/kg IM or IV; then 100 mg/kg/day as a single dose or in divided doses every 12 hours for 7 to 14 days. Maximum dose is 4 g/day.

➤ **Perioperative prophylaxis**

Adults: 1 g IV as a single dose 30 minutes to 2 hours before surgery.

➤ **Acute bacterial otitis media caused by** *S. pneumoniae, H. influenzae,* **or** *Moraxella catarrhalis*

Adults: 1 to 2 g IM or IV once daily or in two equally divided doses daily for 3 days.

Children: 50 mg/kg IM as a single dose. Don't exceed 1 g.

➤ **Acute otitis media ♦**

Children: 50 mg/kg/day IV or IM for 1 to 3 consecutive days in patients unresponsive to initial antibiotic therapy and in patients with penicillin allergy.

ADMINISTRATION

• Before giving drug, ensure patient isn't allergic to penicillins or cephalosporins.
• Obtain specimen for culture and sensitivity testing before giving first dose. Begin therapy while awaiting results.

IV

▼ Reconstitute drug with sterile water for injection, NSS for injection, D₅W, or a combination of NSS and dextrose injection and other compatible solutions.

▼ Add 2.4 mL of diluent to the 250-mg vial, 4.8 mL to the 500-mg vial, 9.6 mL to the 1-g vial, and 19.2 mL to the 2-g vial. All reconstituted solutions average 100 mg/mL. For intermittent infusion, dilute further to

achieve desired concentration, and give over 30 minutes.

▼ Diluted IV preparation is stable for 48 hours at room temperature or 10 days if refrigerated.

⊕ *Alert:* Don't mix or administer ceftriaxone with calcium-containing IV solutions, including parenteral nutrition.

▼ **Incompatibilities:** Aminoglycosides, aminophylline, azithromycin, calcium-containing solutions, clindamycin phosphate, filgrastim, fluconazole, gentamicin, labetalol, linezolid, pentamidine, theophylline, vancomycin, vinorelbine tartrate. Consult a drug compatibility reference for more information.

IM

• Inject deep into a large muscle, such as the gluteus maximus or the lateral aspect of the thigh.
• Can dilute with 1% lidocaine to decrease discomfort.

ACTION

Inhibits cell-wall synthesis, promoting osmotic instability; usually bactericidal.

Route	Onset	Peak	Duration
IV	Immediate	Immediate	Unknown
IM	Unknown	2–3 hr	Unknown

Half-life: Adults with normal renal and hepatic function, 5 to 9 hours.

ADVERSE REACTIONS

GI: diarrhea. **GU:** increased BUN level. **Hematologic:** eosinophilia, *thrombocytosis, leukopenia.* **Hepatic:** increased transaminase levels. **Skin:** pain, induration, tenderness at injection site; rash. **Other:** hypersensitivity reactions, serum sickness, *anaphylaxis.*

INTERACTIONS

Drug-drug. *Aminoglycosides:* May increase nephrotoxicity and cause synergistic effect against some strains of *Enterobacteriaceae* species. Monitor patient.

Estrogen-based contraceptives: May decrease contraceptive absorption and effectiveness. Patient should avoid use together or use nonhormonal contraception for duration of antibiotic (or 14 days, whichever is longer) and for 7 days after completion of antibiotic.

Live-virus vaccines: May decrease effectiveness of live-virus vaccines. Concurrent use isn't recommended.

Reactions in bold italics are *life-threatening*. Interactions may have a *rapid onset* or a *delayed onset*.

Probenecid: May increase ceftriaxone concentration. Monitor therapy.

Warfarin: May increase anticoagulation effect. Monitor PT and INR closely.

EFFECTS ON LAB TEST RESULTS
• May increase ALP, ALT, AST, bilirubin, BUN, and LDH levels.
• May increase eosinophil and platelet counts.
• May decrease WBC count.
• May prolong PTT and PT, and increase INR.
• May falsely increase serum or urine creatinine level in tests using Jaffé reaction. May cause false-positive results of Coombs test and urine glucose tests that use cupric sulfate, such as Benedict reagent and Clinitest.

CONTRAINDICATIONS & CAUTIONS
• Contraindicated in patients hypersensitive to drug or other cephalosporins.
• Contraindicated in premature neonates up to postmenstrual age of 41 weeks, hyperbilirubinemic neonates, and neonates requiring calcium-containing IV solutions.
• Use cautiously in patients hypersensitive to penicillin because of possibility of cross-sensitivity with other beta-lactam antibiotics.
• To reduce development of drug-resistant bacteria and maintain effectiveness of antibacterial drugs, use drug only to treat or prevent infections proven or strongly suspected to be caused by bacteria.
🔶 *Alert:* May cause superinfection and mild to fatal CDAD. If suspected, manage appropriately; discontinue drug if needed.
🔶 *Alert:* May cause hemolytic anemia, which can be fatal. If anemia develops during therapy, stop drug until cause is determined.
• Use cautiously in patients with history of colitis, renal insufficiency, or GI or gallbladder disease.
Dialyzable drug: No.

PREGNANCY-LACTATION-REPRODUCTION
• There are no adequate studies during pregnancy. Use during pregnancy only if clearly needed.
• Drug appears in human milk in low concentrations. Use cautiously during breastfeeding.

NURSING CONSIDERATIONS
• If large doses are given, therapy is prolonged, or patient is at high risk, monitor patient for signs and symptoms of superinfection.
• Monitor PT and INR in patients with impaired vitamin K synthesis or low vitamin K stores. Vitamin K therapy may be needed.
• Monitor patients for diarrhea and anemia and treat appropriately.
• Monitor patient for hypersensitivity reactions.
• *Look alike–sound alike:* Don't confuse drug with other cephalosporins that sound alike.

PATIENT TEACHING
• Tell patient to report adverse reactions promptly.
• Instruct patient to report discomfort at IV insertion site.
• If patient with diabetes is receiving home care and is testing urine for glucose, tell patient drug may affect results of cupric sulfate tests and to use an enzymatic test instead.
• Tell patient to notify prescriber about loose stools or diarrhea.

---

cefuroxime axetil
se-fyoor-OX-eem

cefuroxime sodium
Zinacef

Therapeutic class: Antibiotics
Pharmacologic class: Second-generation cephalosporins

AVAILABLE FORMS
cefuroxime axetil
Tablets: 125 mg, 250 mg, 500 mg
cefuroxime sodium
Infusion: 750 mg, 1.5 g
Injection: 750 mg, 1.5 g

INDICATIONS & DOSAGES
Adjust-a-dose (for all indications): For injectable form in adults with CrCl of 10 to 20 mL/minute, give 750 mg IV or IM every 12 hours; if CrCl is less than 10 mL/minute, give 750 mg IV or IM every 24 hours. Give patients on hemodialysis an additional dose after hemodialysis.
➤ **Serious lower respiratory tract infection, UTI, skin or skin-structure infection, bone or joint infection, septicemia, meningitis, and gonorrhea**

Adults and children age 13 and older: 750 mg to 1.5 g cefuroxime sodium IV or IM every 8 hours for 5 to 10 days. For life-threatening infections and infections caused by less susceptible organisms, 1.5 g IV or IM every 6 hours; for bacterial meningitis, up to 3 g IV every 8 hours.

Children ages 3 months to 12 years: 50 to 100 mg/kg/day cefuroxime sodium IV or IM in equally divided doses every 6 to 8 hours. Use higher dosage of 100 mg/kg/day, not to exceed maximum adult dosage, for more severe or serious infections. For bacterial meningitis, 200 to 240 mg/kg/day cefuroxime sodium IV in divided doses every 6 to 8 hours.

➤ **Perioperative prophylaxis**
Adults: 1.5 g IV 30 to 60 minutes before initial incision; in lengthy operations, 750 mg IV or IM every 8 hours. For open-heart surgery, 1.5 g IV at induction of anesthesia and then every 12 hours for a total dose of 6 g.

➤ **Mild to moderate acute bacterial exacerbations of chronic bronchitis**
Adults and children age 13 and older: 250 or 500 mg PO every 12 hours for 10 days.

➤ **Acute bacterial maxillary sinusitis**
Adults and children age 13 and older: 250 mg PO every 12 hours for 10 days.
Children age 12 and younger able to swallow pills: 250 mg every 12 hours for 10 days.

➤ **Pharyngitis and tonsillitis**
Adults and children age 13 and older: 250 mg PO every 12 hours for 10 days.

➤ **Otitis media**
Children age 12 and younger able to swallow pills: 250 mg PO every 12 hours for 10 days.

➤ **Uncomplicated skin and skin-structure infection**
Adults and children age 13 and older: 250 or 500 mg PO every 12 hours for 10 days.

➤ **Uncomplicated UTI**
Adults: 250 mg PO every 12 hours for 7 to 10 days.

➤ **Uncomplicated gonorrhea**
Adults: 1,000 mg PO as a single dose. Or, 1.5 g IM with 1 g probenecid PO for one dose.

➤ **Early Lyme disease**
Adults and children age 13 and older: 500 mg PO every 12 hours for 20 days.

ADMINISTRATION
● Obtain specimen for culture and sensitivity tests before giving first dose. May start therapy while awaiting results.
● Before giving drug, ensure patient isn't allergic to penicillins or cephalosporins.
PO
● Give tablets without regard for meals; give oral suspension with food.
● Some products may contain phenylalanine or sodium.
● Don't crush tablets due to bitter taste.
IV
▼ Reconstitute each 750-mg vial with 8.3 mL and each 1.5-g vial with 16 mL of sterile water for injection.
▼ Withdraw entire contents of vial for a dose.
▼ For direct injection, inject over 3 to 5 minutes into a large vein or into the tubing of a free-flowing IV solution.
▼ For intermittent infusion, add reconstituted drug to 100 mL D$_5$W, NSS for injection, or other compatible IV solution.
▼ Infuse over 15 to 30 minutes.
▼ **Incompatibilities:** Azithromycin, ciprofloxacin, cisatracurium, clarithromycin, doxapram, filgrastim, fluconazole, gentamicin, midazolam, ranitidine, sodium bicarbonate injection, vancomycin, vinorelbine tartrate.
IM
● Reconstitute 750-mg vial with 3 mL sterile water for injection.
● Inject deep into a large muscle, such as the gluteus maximus or the side of the thigh.

ACTION
Inhibits cell-wall synthesis, promoting osmotic instability; usually bactericidal.

Route	Onset	Peak	Duration
PO	Unknown	2–4 hr	Unknown
IV	Immediate	2–3 min	Unknown
IM	Unknown	15–60 min	Unknown

Half-life: 1 to 2 hours.

ADVERSE REACTIONS
CV: phlebitis, local thrombophlebitis. **GI:** diarrhea, nausea, vomiting. **GU:** vaginitis. **Hematologic:** anemia, *thrombocytopenia, transient neutropenia,* eosinophilia. **Metabolic:** increased LDH level. **Skin:** rash. **Other:** hypersensitivity reactions, including *anaphylaxis.*.

Reactions in bold italics are *life-threatening*. Interactions may have a *rapid onset* or a *delayed onset*.

INTERACTIONS

Drug-drug. *Aminoglycosides:* May cause synergistic activity against some organisms; may increase nephrotoxicity. Monitor patient's renal function closely.

Antacids: May decrease cefuroxime serum concentration. Give oral drug at least 1 hour before or 2 hours after short-acting antacids.

Estrogen-based contraceptives: May decrease contraceptive absorption and effectiveness. Patient should avoid use together or use nonhormonal contraception for duration of antibiotic (or 14 days, whichever is longer) and for 7 days after completion of antibiotic.

Live-virus vaccines: May decrease effectiveness of live-virus vaccines. Concurrent use isn't recommended.

Loop diuretics: May increase risk of adverse renal reactions. Monitor renal function.

Probenecid: May inhibit excretion and increase cefuroxime level. Probenecid may be used for this effect.

Warfarin: May increase anticoagulation effects. Monitor PT and INR closely.

EFFECTS ON LAB TEST RESULTS

• May increase ALP, ALT, AST, bilirubin, and LDH levels.
• May decrease Hb level and hematocrit.
• May increase INR and eosinophil count.
• May decrease neutrophil and platelet counts.
• May prolong PT.
• May falsely increase serum or urine creatinine level in tests using Jaffé reaction. May cause false-positive results of Coombs test and urine glucose tests that use cupric sulfate, such as Benedict reagent and Clinitest.

CONTRAINDICATIONS & CAUTIONS

• Contraindicated in patients hypersensitive to drug or other cephalosporins.
• Use cautiously in patients hypersensitive to penicillin because of possibility of cross-sensitivity with other beta-lactam antibiotics.
• Solutions containing dextrose may be contraindicated in patients with hypersensitivity to corn.
• According to the CDC, oral cephalosporins aren't recommended to treat gonococcal infections.
• Use cautiously in patients with history of colitis and in those with renal insufficiency.
• Some products may contain phenylalanine or sodium.

⚠ *Alert:* Drug may cause CDAD and pseudomembranous colitis ranging from mild to life-threatening, which can occur even 2 months after therapy.
• Some cephalosporins have been associated with seizures in patients with renal impairment when the dosage wasn't reduced. If drug-associated seizures occur, discontinue drug and treat with anticonvulsant therapy if indicated.
Dialyzable drug: Yes.

PREGNANCY-LACTATION-REPRODUCTION

• There are no adequate studies during pregnancy. Use during pregnancy only if clearly needed.
• Drug appears in human milk. Patient should consider temporarily discontinuing breastfeeding during treatment.

NURSING CONSIDERATIONS

• Monitor patient for signs and symptoms of superinfection and diarrhea and treat appropriately.
• Drug may increase INR and risk of bleeding. Monitor patient.
• Monitor patient for hypersensitivity reactions.
• *Look alike–sound alike:* Don't confuse drug with other cephalosporins that sound alike.

PATIENT TEACHING

• Tell patient to take drug as prescribed, even if feeling better.
• Instruct patient to notify prescriber about rash, loose stools, diarrhea, or evidence of superinfection.
• Caution patient to report hypersensitivity reactions.
• Advise patient receiving drug IV to report discomfort at IV insertion site.

---

celecoxib ⚜
sell-ah-COCKS-ib

CeleBREX🔗, Elyxyb

Therapeutic class: NSAIDs
Pharmacologic class: Cyclooxygenase-2 inhibitors

AVAILABLE FORMS

Capsules: 50 mg, 100 mg, 200 mg, 400 mg
Solution: 120 mg/4.8 mL (25 mg/mL)

INDICATIONS & DOSAGES

⚮ *Adjust-a-dose (for all indications):* For older adults and patients weighing less than 50 kg, start at lowest dosage. For patients with Child-Pugh class B hepatic impairment, reduce dosage by about 50%. For patients who are poor metabolizers of CYP2C9, start treatment at half the lowest recommended dose.

➤ **To relieve signs and symptoms of osteoarthritis**
Adults: 200 mg PO daily as a single dose or in two equally divided doses.
➤ **To relieve signs and symptoms of RA**
Adults: 100 to 200 mg PO b.i.d.
➤ **To relieve signs and symptoms of ankylosing spondylitis**
Adults: 200 mg PO once daily or in two divided doses. If no response after 6 weeks, may increase dose to 400 mg daily. If no response after 6 more weeks, consider other treatment.
➤ **To relieve signs and symptoms of juvenile RA**
Children age 2 and older weighing 10 to 25 kg: 50 mg PO b.i.d.
Children age 2 and older weighing more than 25 kg: 100 mg PO b.i.d.
➤ **Acute pain and primary dysmenorrhea**
Adults: 400 mg PO, initially, followed by another 200-mg dose if needed on the first day. On subsequent days, 200 mg PO b.i.d. as needed.
✳ *NEW INDICATION:* **Acute migraine (Elyxyb only)**
Adults: 120 mg PO, as needed. Maximum dosage, 120 mg/day. Use for fewest number of days per month.
Adjust-a-dose: For patients with moderate hepatic impairment (Child-Pugh class B) or patients who are poor CYP2C9 metabolizers, give 60-mg dose.

ADMINISTRATION
PO
• May give without regard to meals.
• For patients with difficulty swallowing capsules, may add capsule contents to applesauce. Carefully empty entire contents of capsule onto a level teaspoon of cool or room-temperature applesauce and give immediately with water. The capsule contents sprinkled on applesauce are stable for up to 6 hours under refrigeration.
• Use calibrated medication measuring device to measure and deliver solution.
• Store at room temperature.

ACTION
Thought to inhibit prostaglandin synthesis, impeding cyclooxygenase-2, to produce anti-inflammatory, analgesic, and antipyretic effects.

Route	Onset	Peak	Duration
PO	Unknown	3 hr	Unknown
PO (solution)	Unknown	1 hr	Unknown

Half-life: 11 hours; solution, 6 hours.

ADVERSE REACTIONS
CNS: headache, dizziness, insomnia, dysgeusia, fever. **CV:** HTN, peripheral edema. **EENT:** eye disorder, pharyngitis, rhinitis, sinusitis. **GI:** abdominal pain, diarrhea, dyspepsia, flatulence, GERD, nausea. **GU:** nephrolithiasis. **Metabolic:** hyperchloremia. **Musculoskeletal:** back pain, arthralgia. **Respiratory:** dyspnea, URI, cough. **Skin:** rash. **Other:** accidental injury, hypersensitivity reaction.

INTERACTIONS
Drug-drug. *ACE inhibitors, ARBs, beta blockers (propranolol):* May decrease antihypertensive effects. Monitor BP.
Antacids containing aluminum or magnesium: May decrease celecoxib level. Separate doses.
Anticoagulants, antiplatelets (clopidogrel, prasugrel): May increase bleeding risk. Use cautiously.
Aspirin: May increase risk of ulcers; low aspirin dosages can be used safely to reduce the risk of CV events. Monitor patient for signs and symptoms of GI bleeding.
Corticosteroids: May increase risk of GI bleeding. Use together cautiously.
Cyclosporine: May increase risk of nephrotoxicity. Monitor renal function.
CYP2C9 inducers (rifampin): May decrease effect of celecoxib. Monitor therapy.
CYP2C9 inhibitors (amiodarone, fluconazole, metronidazole, ritonavir, zafirlukast): May increase celecoxib level and risk of toxicity. Use together cautiously.
CYP2D6 substrates (atomoxetine): May increase exposure and toxicity of substrates. Monitor therapy.
Digoxin: May increase digoxin serum concentration. Monitor concurrent therapy.
Lithium: May increase lithium level. Monitor patient for lithium toxicity.

Reactions in bold italics are *life-threatening*. Interactions may have a *rapid onset* or a **delayed onset**.

Loop and thiazide diuretics: May increase nephrotoxicity; may decrease antihypertensive effects. Monitor therapeutic effects and renal function.

Methotrexate: May increase risk of methotrexate toxicity (neutropenia, thrombocytopenia, renal dysfunction). Monitor patient.

Boxed Warning *NSAIDs:* Can increase risk of serious CV thrombotic events, including MI or stroke, which can be fatal. Risk may occur early in treatment and may increase with duration of use in patients with or without heart disease or risk factors for heart disease. Risk appears greater at higher doses. Use lowest effective dose for shortest duration possible. ■

Pemetrexed: May increase risk of myelosuppression and renal and GI toxicity. Monitor patient closely, especially patients with renal impairment.

SSNRIs, SSRIs: May increase bleeding risk. Monitor closely.

Vancomycin: May increase vancomycin serum concentration. Monitor concurrent use.

Warfarin: May prolong PT and risk of bleeding complications. Monitor PT and INR, and check for signs and symptoms of bleeding.

Drug-herb. *Alfalfa, anise, bilberry:* May increase risk of bleeding. Discourage use together.

White willow: Herb and drug contain similar components. Discourage use together.

Drug-lifestyle. *Long-term alcohol use, smoking:* May cause GI irritation or bleeding. Check for signs and symptoms of bleeding.

EFFECTS ON LAB TEST RESULTS
• May increase ALT, AST, BUN, creatinine, CK, glucose, uric acid, and potassium levels.
• May decrease Hb level and hematocrit.
• May prolong PTT.

CONTRAINDICATIONS & CAUTIONS
Boxed Warning Contraindicated for the treatment of perioperative pain after CABG. ■
• Contraindicated in patients hypersensitive to drug, sulfonamides, aspirin, or other NSAIDs.
• Contraindicated in patients who experienced asthma, urticaria, or allergic-type reactions after taking aspirin or other NSAIDs and in those who have demonstrated allergic-type reactions to sulfonamides.
• Avoid use in patients with recent MI.

• Use in patients with severe renal or severe hepatic impairment isn't recommended.
• Use may lead to new-onset HTN or worsening of preexisting HTN.
• Drug may increase risk of DIC in children with juvenile RA.
🔆 *Alert:* NSAIDs increase risk of HF.
🜊 Use cautiously in patients with history of ulcers or GI bleeding, advanced renal disease, dehydration, anemia, symptomatic liver disease, HTN, edema, HF, or asthma and in poor CYP2C9 metabolizers.
🜊 Consider alternative therapies for treatment of juvenile RA in patients identified to be poor CYP2C9 metabolizers.
• Use cautiously in older adults and patients who are debilitated.
Boxed Warning Older adults and patients with a prior history of peptic ulcer disease or GI bleeding are at greater risk for serious GI events, which can be fatal. ■
Dialyzable drug: Unlikely.
⚠ *Overdose S&S:* Lethargy, drowsiness, nausea, vomiting, epigastric pain, GI bleeding, HTN, acute renal failure, respiratory depression, coma, anaphylaxis.

PREGNANCY-LACTATION-REPRODUCTION
🔆 *Alert:* Use of NSAIDs at 20 weeks or later in pregnancy may cause fetal renal dysfunction leading to oligohydramnios and potential neonatal renal impairment. NSAID use at 30 weeks or later in pregnancy may increase risk of premature closure of the ductus arteriosus. Avoid use during pregnancy starting at 20 weeks' gestation. If potential benefit justifies fetal risk, use lowest effective dose for shortest duration. Consider ultrasound monitoring of amniotic fluid if NSAID use is longer than 48 hours. Use of low-dose aspirin (81 mg) for certain pregnancy-related conditions under the direction of a prescriber is acceptable.
• Drug appears in human milk. Use cautiously during breastfeeding. Patient should consider temporarily discontinuing breastfeeding during treatment.
• Long-term use of NSAIDs in patients of childbearing potential may be associated with infertility that's reversible on discontinuation of NSAID.

NURSING CONSIDERATIONS
Boxed Warning NSAIDs cause an increased risk of serious GI adverse events, including

bleeding, ulceration, and perforation of the stomach or intestines, which can be fatal. ∎
- Additional risk factors for GI bleeding include treatment with corticosteroids or anticoagulants, longer duration of NSAID treatment, smoking, alcoholism, older age, and poor overall health.
- Although drug may be used with low aspirin dosages, the combination may increase risk of GI bleeding.
- Watch for signs and symptoms of overt and occult bleeding and abnormal clotting.
- ○ *Alert:* Watch for and immediately evaluate signs and symptoms of heart attack (chest pain, shortness of breath, trouble breathing) or stroke (weakness in one part or side of the body, slurred speech).
- Drug can cause fluid retention; monitor patient with HTN, edema, or HF.
- Drug may impair response of antihypertensives. Monitor BP.
- Drug may mask signs and symptoms of infection and fever due to anti-inflammatory effect.
- Assess patient for CV risk factors before therapy.
- Drug may be hepatotoxic; watch for signs and symptoms of liver toxicity.
- Before starting drug therapy, rehydrate patient who is dehydrated.
- Monitor patient's renal function; renal insufficiency is possible in patients with preexisting renal disease. Long-term administration may cause renal papillary necrosis and other renal injury.
- Monitor patient for hypersensitivity reactions, including serious skin reactions (SJS, exfoliative dermatitis, DRESS syndrome). Discontinue at first appearance of rash.
- *Look alike–sound alike:* Don't confuse Celebrex with Cerebyx or Celexa.

PATIENT TEACHING
- Tell patient to report history of allergic reactions to sulfonamides, aspirin, or other NSAIDs before therapy.
- Instruct patient to promptly report signs of GI bleeding, such as melena or blood in vomit, urine, or stool.
- Tell patient to report pregnancy or plans to become pregnant during therapy.
- ○ *Alert:* Warn patient who is pregnant not to take NSAIDs at 20 weeks' gestation or later unless instructed to do so by prescriber, due to

potential fetal risk. Advise patient to discuss taking OTC medications with a pharmacist or health care provider during pregnancy.
- ○ *Alert:* Advise patient to immediately report rash, unexplained weight gain, or swelling.
- ○ *Alert:* Advise patient to seek medical attention immediately if chest pain, shortness of breath or trouble breathing, weakness in one part or side of the body, or slurred speech occurs.
- Instruct patient in proper drug administration and storage.
- Tell patient that drug may harm the liver. Advise patient to stop therapy and notify prescriber immediately if experiencing signs and symptoms of hepatotoxicity, including nausea, fatigue, lethargy, itching, yellowing of skin or eyes, right upper quadrant tenderness, and flulike syndrome.
- Inform patient that it may take several days before consistent pain relief occurs.
- Advise patient that using OTC NSAIDs with celecoxib may increase the risk of GI toxicity.

SAFETY ALERT!

cemiplimab-rwlc
se-MIP-li-mab

Libtayo

Therapeutic class: Antineoplastics
Pharmacologic class: Programmed death receptor-1 blocking antibodies

AVAILABLE FORMS
Injection: 350 mg/7 mL (50 mg/mL) single-dose vial

INDICATIONS & DOSAGES
Adjust-a-dose (for all indications): Refer to manufacturer's instructions for toxicity-related dosage adjustments.
➤ **Metastatic cutaneous squamous cell carcinoma (CSCC) or locally advanced CSCC in patients who aren't candidates for curative surgery or curative radiation**
Adults: 350 mg IV infusion over 30 minutes every 3 weeks until disease progression or unacceptable toxicity occurs.
➤ **Locally advanced or metastatic basal cell carcinoma previously treated with a hedgehog pathway inhibitor or when a**

hedgehog pathway inhibitor isn't appropriate

Adults: 350 mg IV infusion over 30 minutes every 3 weeks until disease progression or unacceptable toxicity occurs.

➤ **First-line treatment of patients with advanced NSCLC (locally advanced, in which patients aren't candidates for surgical resection or definitive chemoradiation or who are metastatic) whose tumors have high PD-L1 expression as determined by FDA-approved test, with no *EGFR, ALK,* or *ROS1* alterations**

Adults: 350 mg IV infusion over 30 minutes every 3 weeks until disease progression or unacceptable toxicity occurs.

ADMINISTRATION

IV

▼ Store unopened vials in refrigerator at 36° to 46° F (2° to 8° C) in original carton and protected from light; don't freeze or shake.

▼ Inspect vial for particulate matter and discoloration. Drug should appear clear to slightly opalescent, colorless to pale yellow, and may contain trace amounts of translucent to white particles. Discard vial if solution is cloudy, discolored, or contains other particulate matter.

▼ Withdraw 7 mL from vial and dilute with NSS or D_5W to a final concentration between 1 and 20 mg/mL; mix diluted solution by gentle inversion but don't shake; discard any unused drug.

▼ Infuse over 30 minutes through an IV line containing an in-line filter or add-on 0.2- to 5-micron filter.

▼ Store at room temperature up to 77° F (25° C) for no more than 8 hours or refrigerate at 36° to 46° F (2° to 8° C) for no more than 24 hours from the time of preparation to the end of infusion. Diluted solution should come to room temperature before administration; don't freeze.

▼ Store unopened vials at 36° to 46° F (2° to 8° C) in original carton and protected from light; don't freeze or shake.

▼ **Incompatibilities:** Don't give with solutions other than NSS or D_5W.

ACTION

IgG4 monoclonal antibody that binds to programmed death-receptor (PD) antibodies, thereby blocking PD-1 activity and decreasing tumor growth.

Route	Onset	Peak	Duration
IV	Unknown	Unknown	Unknown

Half-life: 20.3 days.

ADVERSE REACTIONS

CNS: *aseptic meningitis,* complex regional pain syndrome, fatigue, headache. **CV:** HTN. **GI:** diarrhea, nausea, constipation, vomiting, decreased appetite, immune-mediated colitis. **GU:** UTI, increased creatinine level. **Hematologic:** anemia, *lymphocytopenia, prolonged bleeding time.* **Hepatic:** increased transaminase levels, hyperbilirubinemia, *hepatitis.* **Metabolic:** decreased appetite, *endocrinopathies,* hyponatremia, *hypokalemia, hyperkalemia,* hypophosphatemia, hypercalcemia, *hypocalcemia,* hypoalbuminemia, hypermagnesemia, hypothyroidism. **Musculoskeletal:** pain, arthralgia, muscular weakness. **Respiratory:** URI, dyspnea, pneumonia, *pneumonitis,* cough. **Skin:** rash, pruritus, cellulitis, skin infection, immune-mediated dermatologic reactions (rash, dermatitis). **Other:** *sepsis,* antibody development.

INTERACTIONS

None reported.

EFFECTS ON LAB TEST RESULTS

● May increase AST and magnesium levels.
● May decrease albumin, phosphate, and sodium levels.
● May increase or decrease calcium and potassium levels.
● May increase INR.
● May decrease Hb level and hematocrit and lymphocyte and RBC counts.

CONTRAINDICATIONS & CAUTIONS

🖐 *Alert:* Immune-mediated adverse reactions, which may be severe or fatal, can occur in any organ system or tissue and include pneumonitis, GI toxicities (colitis, hepatitis, pancreatitis), endocrinopathies (adrenal insufficiency, hypophysitis, hypothyroidism, hyperthyroidism, type 1 diabetes), nephritis with renal dysfunction, dermatologic toxicities (erythema multiforme, SJS, pemphigoid, TEN), myocarditis, neurologic toxicities (meningitis, encephalitis, myelitis and demyelination, myasthenic syndrome, myasthenia gravis, Guillain-Barré syndrome, nerve paresis, autoimmune neuropathy), ocular inflammatory toxicities (uveitis, iritis, retinal detachment, vision loss), musculoskeletal toxicities (myositis, rhabdomyolysis, arthritis, polymyalgia rheumatica), and hematologic and immunologic toxicities (hemolytic anemia, aplastic anemia, hemophagocytic lymphohistiocytosis, systemic inflammatory response syndrome, histiocytic necrotizing lymphadenitis, Kikuchi lymphadenitis, sarcoidosis, and immune thrombocytopenic purpura [solid]). Monitor patient closely.

🕚 *Alert:* Fatal and other serious complications can occur in patients who receive allogeneic hematopoietic stem cell transplantation (HSCT) despite intervening therapy between drug administration and allogeneic HSCT. Consider risk versus benefit.

• Drug may cause rejection of a transplanted organ. Monitor patient closely.

• Safety and effectiveness in children haven't been established.

Dialyzable drug: Unknown.

PREGNANCY-LACTATION-REPRODUCTION

• Drug can cause fetal harm based on mechanism of action. Advise patients of childbearing potential about fetal risk and the need to use effective contraception during treatment and for at least 4 months after final dose.

• It isn't known if drug appears in human milk. Patient shouldn't breastfeed during treatment and for at least 4 months after final dose.

NURSING CONSIDERATIONS

• Monitor patient for infusion-related reactions (chills, rash, pruritus, flushing, shortness of breath, dizziness, fever, syncope, back or neck pain, facial swelling). Interrupt or slow rate of infusion, or permanently discontinue infusion based on severity of the reaction.

• Monitor patient for development of immune-mediated adverse reactions.

• When immune-mediated adverse reactions occur, withhold or discontinue drug as needed and administer corticosteroids until resolved, followed by a corticosteroid taper over 1 month.

• Consider use of other systemic immunosuppressants when immune-mediated adverse reactions aren't controlled with corticosteroids and begin hormone replacement therapy for endocrinopathies as warranted.

• Evaluate LFTs, creatinine and thyroid function tests at baseline and periodically during treatment.

• Assess pregnancy status before start of treatment.

PATIENT TEACHING

• Teach patient to report all adverse reactions.

• Counsel patient to immediately report immune-mediated adverse reactions or infusion-related reactions.

• Advise patient of childbearing potential that drug can cause harm to a fetus and to inform prescriber of a known or suspected pregnancy.

• Warn patient of childbearing potential to use effective contraception during treatment and for at least 4 months after final dose.

• Instruct patient not to breastfeed while taking drug and for at least 4 months after final dose.

cephalexin
sef-a-LEX-in

Apo-Cephalex ✤

Therapeutic class: Antibiotics
Pharmacologic class: First-generation cephalosporins

AVAILABLE FORMS
Capsules: 250 mg, 330 mg, 500 mg, 750 mg
Oral suspension: 125 mg/5 mL, 250 mg/5 mL
Tablets: 250 mg, 500 mg

INDICATIONS & DOSAGES
➤ **Respiratory tract infections caused by susceptible isolates of *Streptococcus pneumoniae* and *Streptococcus pyogenes;* GU tract infections caused by susceptible isolates of *Escherichia coli, Proteus mirabilis,* and *Klebsiella pneumoniae;* skin and skin-structure infections caused by susceptible isolates of *Staphylococcus aureus* or *S. pyogenes;* bone infections caused by susceptible isolates of *S. aureus* and *P. mirabilis;* and otitis media caused by susceptible isolates of *S. pneumoniae, Haemophilus influenzae, S. aureus, S. pyogenes,* and *Moraxella catarrhalis***

Adults and children age 15 and older: 250 mg to 1 g PO every 6 hours or 500 mg every 12 hours for 7 to 14 days. Maximum, 4 g daily.

Children older than age 1: 25 to 50 mg/kg/day PO in two to four equally divided doses for 7 to 14 days. For otitis media, 75 to

---

Reactions in bold italics are *life-threatening*. Interactions may have a *rapid onset* or a *delayed onset*.

100 mg/kg PO in equally divided doses every 6 hours. For severe infections, 50 to 100 mg/kg PO in equally divided doses. Don't exceed recommended adult dosage.

Adjust-a-dose: For adults and children age 15 and older with CrCl of 30 to 59 mL/minute, no dosage adjustment is needed but maximum daily dose shouldn't exceed 1 g; for CrCl of 15 to 29 mL/minute, reduce dosage to 250 mg every 8 or 12 hours; for CrCl of 5 to 14 mL/minute in patients not yet on dialysis, reduce dosage to 250 mg every 24 hours; for CrCl of 1 to 4 mL/minute in patients not yet on dialysis, reduce dosage to 250 mg every 48 or 60 hours.

ADMINISTRATION
PO
• Before giving, ensure patient isn't allergic to penicillins or cephalosporins.
• Obtain specimen for culture and sensitivity tests before giving. Begin therapy while awaiting results.
• To prepare oral suspension, add required amount of water to powder in two portions. Shake well after each addition. After mixing, store in refrigerator. Mixture will remain stable for 14 days. Keep tightly closed and shake well before using.
• May give without regard to meals but give drug with food or milk to lessen GI discomfort.

ACTION
Inhibits cell-wall synthesis, promoting osmotic instability; usually bactericidal.

Route	Onset	Peak	Duration
PO	Unknown	1 hr	Unknown

Half-life: Adults, 30 minutes to 1.25 hours; children ages 3 to 12 months, 2.5 hours; neonates, 5 hours.

ADVERSE REACTIONS
CNS: dizziness, headache, fatigue, agitation, confusion, hallucinations. **GI:** anorexia, nausea, vomiting, diarrhea, *CDAD,* gastritis, glossitis, dyspepsia, abdominal pain, anal pruritus. **GU:** genital pruritus, candidiasis, vaginitis, vaginal discharge, interstitial nephritis. **Hematologic:** *neutropenia, thrombocytopenia,* eosinophilia, anemia. **Musculoskeletal:** arthritis, arthralgia, joint pain. **Skin:** rash, urticaria. **Other:** *anaphylaxis,* hypersensitivity reactions, including *anaphylaxis.*

INTERACTIONS
Drug-drug. *Aminoglycosides:* May increase risk of nephrotoxicity. Avoid using together.
Estrogen-based contraceptives: May decrease contraceptive absorption and effectiveness. Patient should avoid use together or use non-hormonal contraception for duration of antibiotic (or 14 days, whichever is longer) and for 7 days after completion of antibiotic.
Live-virus vaccines: May decrease effectiveness of live-virus vaccines. Concurrent use isn't recommended.
Metformin: May increase metformin level. Monitor blood glucose level closely.
Multivitamins containing zinc: May decrease cephalexin absorption. Consider administering at least 3 hours after cephalexin. Consider therapy modification.
Probenecid: May increase cephalosporin level. Use together isn't recommended.
Warfarin: May enhance anticoagulant effects. Monitor therapy.

EFFECTS ON LAB TEST RESULTS
• May increase ALP, ALT, AST, bilirubin, and LDH levels.
• May increase eosinophil count.
• May decrease Hb level and neutrophil and platelet counts and prolong PT.
• May falsely increase serum or urine creatinine level in tests using Jaffé reaction. May cause false-positive results of Coombs test and urine glucose tests that use cupric sulfate, such as Benedict reagent and Clinitest.

CONTRAINDICATIONS & CAUTIONS
• Contraindicated in patients hypersensitive to cephalosporins.
• Use cautiously in patients hypersensitive to penicillin because of possibility of cross-sensitivity with other beta-lactam antibiotics.
• Severe hypersensitivity reactions, including anaphylactic severe skin reactions (SJS, erythema multiforme), can occur. If an allergic reaction occurs, discontinue drug immediately and treat appropriately.
• Drug may increase risk of seizures. Use cautiously in patients with history of seizures.
• Use cautiously in older adults, patients with history of colitis, and in those with renal or hepatic impairment.
⏺ *Alert:* Drug can cause superinfection and CDAD and pseudomembranous colitis ranging from mild to life-threatening, which can occur even 2 months after therapy.

Dialyzable drug: Unknown.

⚠ *Overdose S&S:* Nausea, vomiting, epigastric distress, diarrhea, hematuria.

PREGNANCY-LACTATION-REPRODUCTION
• There are no adequate studies during pregnancy. Use during pregnancy only if clearly needed and potential benefit justifies fetal risk.
• Drug appears in human milk. Use cautiously during breastfeeding.

NURSING CONSIDERATIONS
• If large doses are given or if therapy is prolonged, monitor patient for superinfection and diarrhea, especially if patient is high risk.
• Treat group A beta-hemolytic streptococcal infections for a minimum of 10 days.
• If anemia develops during or after cephalexin therapy, obtain a diagnostic work-up for drug-induced hemolytic anemia, discontinue drug, and institute appropriate therapy.
• Monitor PT in patients with renal or hepatic impairment or poor nutritional state, in those on prolonged therapy, and in patients taking anticoagulants.
• Monitor patients for hypersensitivity reactions.
• *Look alike–sound alike:* Don't confuse drug with other cephalosporins that sound alike.

PATIENT TEACHING
• Tell patient to take drug exactly as prescribed, even if feeling better.
• Instruct patient in safe drug administration and storage.
• Tell patient to report all adverse reactions and to immediately report rash and signs and symptoms of superinfection or diarrhea.

---

certolizumab pegol
SERT-oh-LIZ-u-mahb PEGH-ol

Cimzia

Therapeutic class: Immunomodulators
Pharmacologic class: TNF blockers

AVAILABLE FORMS
Lyophilized powder for injection: 200 mg
Prefilled syringe: 200 mg/mL

INDICATIONS & DOSAGES
➤ **Crohn disease when response to conventional therapy is inadequate**
Adults: Initially and at weeks 2 and 4, 400 mg subcut (given as two injections of 200 mg), followed by a maintenance dose of 400 mg every 4 weeks, if adequate response.
➤ **RA**
Adults: Initially and at weeks 2 and 4, 400 mg subcut (given as two injections of 200 mg), followed by maintenance dose of 200 mg every other week, or may consider 400 mg every 4 weeks.
➤ **Psoriatic arthritis; active ankylosing spondylitis; nonradiographic axial spondyloarthritis, with objective signs of inflammation**
Adults: 400 mg subcut (given as two injections of 200 mg) initially; repeat dose at week 2 and then again at week 4. Maintenance dosage is 200 mg every other week, or may consider 400 mg every 4 weeks.
➤ **Moderate to severe plaque psoriasis in patients who are candidates for systemic therapy or phototherapy**
Adults: 400 mg (given as 2 subcut injections of 200 mg) every other week.
Adults weighing 90 kg or less: Consider initial dose of 400 mg (given as 2 subcut injections of 200 mg) at weeks 0, 2 and 4, then 200 mg every other week.

ADMINISTRATION
Subcutaneous
• Bring drug to room temperature for 30 minutes before reconstituting.
• Each 400-mg dose requires two vials. Reconstitute each vial with 1 mL of sterile water for injection, using provided 20G needle. Gently swirl the vial without shaking. May take up to 30 minutes to fully reconstitute. Inspect vial for particulate matter and discoloration, and discard if present.
• Draw up each vial in its own syringe, switching each 20G needle to a 23G needle. Inject prepared or prefilled syringes into separate sites in the abdomen or thigh. Don't inject in areas where skin is tender, bruised, red, or hard. Discard unused portion of vial or syringe.
• Reconstituted drug is stable for 2 hours at room temperature or for up to 24 hours if refrigerated. Don't freeze.
• May store prefilled syringes at room temperature for up to 7 days; write date removed

---

Reactions in bold italics are *life-threatening*. Interactions may have a *rapid onset* or a ***delayed onset***.

from refrigerator and discard if not used within 7 days. Store in original carton (to protect from light) and don't return to refrigerator.
• Give prefilled syringe at room temperature.
• The needle shield inside removable cap of prefilled syringe contains natural rubber latex, which may cause an allergic reaction in latex-sensitive individuals.

ACTION

Selectively neutralizes TNFα, a proinflammatory cytokine responsible for stimulating the production of inflammatory mediators.

Route	Onset	Peak	Duration
Subcut	Unknown	54–171 hr	Unknown

Half-life: 14 days.

ADVERSE REACTIONS

CNS: anxiety, bipolar disorder, *suicidality,* fever, headache, *stroke,* TIA. **CV:** angina pectoris, *arrhythmias, HF,* HTN, *MI,* pericardial effusion, pericarditis, vasculitis, thrombophlebitis, *hemorrhage.* **EENT:** optic neuritis, retinal hemorrhage, uveitis, nasopharyngitis. **GI:** abdominal pain. **GU:** UTI, nephrotic syndrome, menstrual disorder. **Hematologic:** anemia, *leukopenia,* lymphadenopathy, *pancytopenia, thrombophilia.* **Hepatic:** elevated liver enzyme levels, *hepatitis.* **Musculoskeletal:** arthralgia, extremity pain. **Respiratory:** URI, TB, cough, bronchitis. **Skin:** alopecia, dermatitis, peripheral edema, erythema nodosum, urticaria, injection-site reactions. **Other:** viral infection (herpes), bacterial infection.

INTERACTIONS

Drug-drug. *Abatacept, anakinra, natalizumab, rilonacept, rituximab:* May increase risk of serious infection and neutropenia. Avoid using together.
Live-virus vaccines: May cause infection. Avoid using together.
Immunosuppressants (pimecrolimus, tacrolimus [topical], tocilizumab, tofacitinib, vedolizumab): May enhance adverse or toxic effects of immunosuppressants. Avoid using together.
Drug-herb. *Echinacea:* May diminish therapeutic effects. Consider therapy modification.

EFFECTS ON LAB TEST RESULTS

• May falsely prolong PTT.

CONTRAINDICATIONS & CAUTIONS

• Contraindicated in patients with a history of hypersensitivity reaction to drug or its components, including angioedema, anaphylactoid reaction, serum sickness, and urticaria.
• Use cautiously in patients with known hypersensitivity to other TNF blockers and those with underlying conditions that may increase the risk of infections.
• Use cautiously in patients with underlying hematologic disorders because significant hematologic abnormalities have occurred.
• Don't use in combination with biological DMARDs or other TNF-blocker therapy.
Boxed Warning Patients treated with certolizumab are at increased risk for serious infections that may lead to hospitalization or death. Most patients who developed these infections were taking concomitant immunosuppressants, such as methotrexate or corticosteroids. ■
Boxed Warning Consider empirical antifungal therapy for patients at risk for invasive fungal infections who develop severe systemic illness. ■
• Use cautiously in patients with a history of recurrent infections or concomitant immunosuppressive therapy and in those who have resided in regions where TB and histoplasmosis are endemic. Don't begin drug in patients with active infections.
• Use cautiously in patients with a history of CNS demyelinating disorder, hematologic disorders, or HF.
• Drug may increase risk of malignancies. Periodic skin exams are recommended in patients with risk factors for skin cancer.
• Rare reactivation of HBV infection can occur, usually in chronic carriers who are also receiving immunosuppressants. Evaluate patient for HBV infection before initiating treatment. Monitor HBV carriers for clinical signs and symptoms of active infection and altered lab values during and for several months after therapy ends.
Boxed Warning Certolizumab isn't indicated for use in children or adolescents because of the risk of lymphoma and other malignancies reported with the use of TNF blockers. ■
• Use cautiously in older adults because of increased risk of infection.
Dialyzable drug: Unknown.

PREGNANCY-LACTATION-REPRODUCTION

• Use during pregnancy only when clearly needed and benefits outweigh risks to the fetus. Enroll patients exposed to certolizumab pegol during pregnancy in the Autoimmune Diseases in Pregnancy Study (1-877-311-8972 or https://mothertobaby.org/pregnancy-studies/).

• Drug may affect immune response in in utero–exposed newborn and infant.

• It isn't known if drug appears in human milk. For use during breastfeeding, prescriber should take into account importance of drug to the patient and potential adverse effects on the infant.

NURSING CONSIDERATIONS

Boxed Warning Carefully consider risks and benefits of treatment before initiating therapy in patients with chronic or recurrent infection. ∎

Boxed Warning Monitor patient for signs and symptoms of invasive fungal infection and other opportunistic infections during and after treatment. Discontinue treatment if serious infection or sepsis develops. Fatal infections have occurred. ∎

Boxed Warning Invasive fungal infections, including histoplasmosis, coccidioidomycosis, candidiasis, aspergillosis, blastomycosis, and pneumocystosis, may present with disseminated, rather than localized disease. Antigen and antibody testing for histoplasmosis may be negative in some patients with active infection. Consider empirical antifungal therapy in patients at risk for invasive fungal infections who develop severe systemic illness. ∎

Boxed Warning Bacterial, viral, and other infections due to opportunistic pathogens, including *Legionella* and *Listeria*, have occurred. ∎

Boxed Warning Test patient for latent TB before and during therapy; active TB, including reactivation of latent TB, has occurred. Initiate treatment for latent infection before starting therapy. ∎

Boxed Warning Closely monitor patient for signs and symptoms of infection during and after treatment, including the possible development of TB in patients who tested negative for latent TB before starting therapy. ∎

• Before therapy, evaluate patients at risk for HBV infection and test for previous HBV infection.

• Monitor patient for hypersensitivity reactions, including severe skin reactions.

• Monitor patient for new or worsening neurologic disorders, including seizures, optic neuritis, and peripheral neuropathy.

• Monitor patient for signs and symptoms of blood dyscrasias (bruising, bleeding, pallor).

PATIENT TEACHING

Boxed Warning Teach patient to seek prompt medical attention for signs and symptoms of infection, such as persistent fever, cough, shortness of breath, or fatigue. ∎

• Advise patient to seek immediate medical attention for unusual bruising or bleeding.

• Instruct patient to seek immediate medical attention if symptoms of allergic reaction develop.

• Tell patient to report signs and symptoms of HF or neurologic changes.

• Advise patient of the risk of lymphoma and other malignancies.

• Instruct patient or caregiver capable of drug administration in safe technique, storage, and syringe disposal.

SAFETY ALERT!

cetuximab ⬦
seh-TUX-eh-mab

Erbitux

Therapeutic class: Antineoplastics
Pharmacologic class: Monoclonal antibodies

AVAILABLE FORMS

Injection: 2 mg/mL

INDICATIONS & DOSAGES

Adjust-a-dose (for all indications): If patient develops a grade 1 or 2 CTCAE infusion reaction, permanently reduce infusion rate by 50%. If patient develops a grade 3 or 4 CTCAE infusion reaction, stop drug immediately and permanently. Refer to manufacturer's instructions for dosage modifications for other toxicities.

➤ **Squamous cell carcinoma of the head and neck, in combination with radiation therapy**
Adults: Loading dose of 400 mg/m² IV infusion over 120 minutes followed by weekly maintenance dose of 250 mg/m² IV infusion

---

over 60 minutes. If used with radiation therapy, begin drug 1 week before radiation course. Complete administration 1 hour before radiation. Continue for the duration (6 or 7 weeks) of radiation therapy or until disease progression or unacceptable toxicity occurs.

➤ **Squamous cell carcinoma of the head and neck, as single-agent or in combination with platinum-based therapy and 5-FU**
Adults: 500 mg/m^2 IV infusion over 2 hours every 2 weeks. Or, initially, 400 mg/m^2 IV infusion over 120 minutes followed by weekly maintenance dose of 250 mg/m^2 IV infusion over 60 minutes. Complete infusion 1 hour before platinum-based therapy with 5-FU. Continue therapy until disease progression or unacceptable toxicity occurs.

➤ *KRAS* **mutation-negative (wild type), epidermal growth factor receptor (EGFR)–expressing, metastatic colorectal cancer as determined by FDA-approved tests in combination with FOLFIRI (irinotecan, 5-FU, leucovorin) chemotherapy regimen for first-line treatment, or in combination with irinotecan in patients refractory to irinotecan-based chemotherapy, or as a single agent in patients who have failed oxaliplatin- and irinotecan-based chemotherapy or who are intolerant to irinotecan** ▨
Adults: 500 mg/m^2 IV infusion over 2 hours every 2 weeks. Or, initially, 400 mg/m^2 IV infusion over 120 minutes followed by weekly maintenance dose of 250 mg/m^2 IV infusion over 60 minutes. Complete infusion 1 hour before irinotecan or FOLFIRI regimen. Continue therapy until disease progression or unacceptable toxicity occurs.

✳ *NEW INDICATION:* **Metastatic colorectal cancer with** *BRAF* **V600E mutation, as detected by FDA-approved test, after prior therapy, in combination with encorafenib** ▨
Adults: Initially, 400 mg/m^2 IV infusion over 120 minutes, then 250 mg/m^2 infusion over 60 minutes weekly with encorafenib 300 mg PO daily until disease progression or unacceptable toxicity occurs. Refer to encorafenib prescribing information.

ADMINISTRATION
IV

▼ Drug is a potential teratogen. Follow safe handling procedures when preparing or administering.

▼ Premedicate with an H$_1$-antagonist such as diphenhydramine 50 mg IV 30 to 60 minutes before first dose. Premedication before subsequent doses should be based on clinical judgment and severity of prior infusion reactions.

▼ Solution should be clear and colorless and may contain a small amount of particulates.

▼ Don't shake or dilute.

▼ Drug can be given by infusion pump or syringe pump, piggybacked into patient's infusion line. Don't give drug by IV push or bolus.

▼ Give initial loading dose over 120 minutes and subsequent infusions over 60 minutes. Don't exceed infusion rate of 10 mg/minute.

▼ Give drug through a low–protein-binding 0.22-micron in-line filter.

▼ Flush line with NSS at the end of the infusion.

▼ Observe patient for 1 hour after administration.

▼ Store vials at 36° to 46° F (2° to 8° C). Don't freeze.

▼ Solution in infusion container is stable up to 12 hours at 36° to 46° F (2° to 8° C) and up to 8 hours at 68° to 77° F (20° to 25° C).

▼ **Incompatibilities:** Don't dilute with other solutions.

ACTION
An EGFR antagonist that binds to the EGFR on normal and tumor cells.

Route	Onset	Peak	Duration
IV	Unknown	Unknown	Unknown

Half-life: 3 to 10 days.

ADVERSE REACTIONS
CNS: asthenia, depression, fever, headache, fatigue, insomnia, anxiety, confusion, pain, peripheral neuropathy, taste disturbance. **CV:** edema, *cardiopulmonary arrest, PE.* **EENT:** conjunctivitis, pharyngitis. **GI:** abdominal pain, anorexia, constipation, diarrhea, dyspepsia, dysphagia, mucositis, nausea, stomatitis, vomiting, xerostomia. **GU:** *acute renal failure.* **Hematologic:** anemia, *neutropenia, leukopenia.* **Hepatic:** increased transaminase levels, increased ALP level. **Metabolic:** dehydration, *hypomagnesemia, hypocalcemia, hypokalemia,* weight loss. **Musculoskeletal:** back pain, bone pain, arthralgia. **Respiratory:** cough, dyspnea. **Skin:** alopecia, rash, pruritus, radiation dermatitis, nail changes,

hand-foot syndrome, skin fissures. **Other:** antibody development, chills, infection, infusion reaction, *sepsis.*

INTERACTIONS
Drug-lifestyle. *Sun exposure:* May worsen skin reactions. Advise patient to avoid excessive sun exposure.

EFFECTS ON LAB TEST RESULTS
• May increase LFT values.
• May decrease magnesium, calcium, and potassium levels.
• May decrease Hb level and lymphocyte and neutrophil counts.

CONTRAINDICATIONS & CAUTIONS
• Use cautiously in patients hypersensitive to drug, its components, or murine proteins. If used with radiation, use cautiously in patients with a history of CAD, arrhythmias, and HF.
• Risk of anaphylactic reactions may be increased in patients with a history of tick bites or red meat allergy, or in the presence of IgE antibodies directed against galactose-α-1,3-galactose (alpha-gal).
▨ Determine *RAS* mutation and EGFR-negative expression status using FDA-approved tests before initiating treatment for colorectal cancer. Drug isn't indicated for treatment of *RAS*-mutant colorectal cancer or when results of *RAS* mutation tests are unknown; increased tumor progression, increased mortality, or lack of benefit may occur in patients with *RAS*-mutant metastatic colorectal cancer.
• ILD has been reported in patients using drug.
• Dermatologic toxicity has been reported in the majority of patients. Acneiform rash usually develops in first 2 weeks of therapy and may require dosage modification and treatment with topical or oral antibiotics.
• Adverse reactions may occur more frequently when drug is given with cisplatin and radiation.
• Electrolyte abnormalities are common, especially hypomagnesemia.
• Life-threatening and fatal bullous mucocutaneous disease with blisters, erosions, and skin sloughing has been observed in patients treated with cetuximab. It couldn't be determined if these mucocutaneous adverse reactions were directly related to EGFR inhibition

or to idiosyncratic immune-related effects (such as SJS or TEN).
Dialyzable drug: No.

PREGNANCY-LACTATION-REPRODUCTION
• There are no adequate studies during pregnancy. Drug may cause fetal harm and isn't recommended for use during pregnancy. Inform patient of fetal risk.
• Patients of childbearing potential should use effective contraception during treatment and for 2 months after final dose.
• Patients shouldn't breastfeed during therapy and for at least 2 months after final dose.
• Drug may impair female fertility.

NURSING CONSIDERATIONS
Boxed Warning Severe and fatal infusion reactions, including acute airway obstruction, urticaria, and hypotension, may occur, usually with the first infusion. If a severe infusion reaction occurs, stop drug immediately and permanently and provide symptomatic treatment. ■
• Keep epinephrine, corticosteroids, IV antihistamines, bronchodilators, and oxygen available for severe infusion reactions.
• Manage mild to moderate infusion reactions by decreasing infusion rate and premedicating with an antihistamine for subsequent infusions.
• Monitor patient for infusion reactions for 1 hour after infusion ends.
• Verify pregnancy status in patients of childbearing potential before starting drug.
• ILD can occur. Assess patient for acute onset or worsening of pulmonary symptoms. If ILD is confirmed, interrupt therapy or stop drug.
• Monitor patient for skin toxicity, which starts most often during first 2 weeks of therapy. Treat with topical and oral antibiotics.
• Monitor magnesium, calcium, and potassium levels weekly during treatment and for at least 8 weeks after therapy ends.
Boxed Warning In patients also receiving radiation therapy or platinum-based therapy with 5-FU, closely monitor electrolytes, especially magnesium, potassium, and calcium, during and after therapy. Cardiopulmonary arrest or sudden death has occurred. ■

PATIENT TEACHING
• Tell patient to promptly report adverse reactions, including dyspnea, chills, or fever.

Reactions in bold italics are *life-threatening*. Interactions may have a *rapid onset* or a *delayed onset*.

• Inform patient that skin reactions may occur, typically during the first 2 weeks of treatment.

• Advise patient to avoid prolonged or unprotected sun exposure during and 2 months after treatment.

• Instruct patient not to breastfeed during therapy and for at least 2 months after final dose.

• Advise patient of childbearing potential to use adequate contraception during therapy and for 2 months after final dose.

chloroquine phosphate
KLO-ro-kwin

Therapeutic class: Antimalarials
Pharmacologic class: Aminoquinolines

AVAILABLE FORMS
Tablets: 250 mg (equivalent to 150 mg base), 500 mg (equivalent to 300 mg base)

INDICATIONS & DOSAGES
⚠️ *Alert:* Prescribers should be completely familiar with this drug before prescribing.

➤ **Acute malarial attacks caused by** *Plasmodium vivax, Plasmodium malariae, Plasmodium ovale,* **and susceptible strains of** *Plasmodium falciparum*
Adults: Initially, 1 g (600 mg base) PO; then 500 mg (300 mg base) at 6, 24, and 48 hours.
Adults of low body weight and children: Initially, 16.6 mg/kg (10 mg/kg base) PO; then 8.3 mg/kg (5 mg/kg base) at 6, 24, and 36 hours. Don't exceed adult dose of 1,000 mg (600 mg base) for initial dosage and 500 mg (300 mg base) for subsequent doses.
Adjust-a-dose: For adults and children, for treatment of chloroquine-sensitive *P. vivax* and *P. malariae,* concomitant therapy with an 8-aminoquinoline (e.g., primaquine) is necessary.

➤ **To prevent malaria**
Adults: 500 mg (300 mg base) PO once weekly on the same day each week, for 1 to 2 weeks before entering a malaria-endemic area and continued for 4 weeks after leaving the area. If beginning after entering a malaria-endemic area, give 1 g (600 mg base) PO initially, in two divided doses 6 hours apart. Continue for 8 weeks after leaving the endemic area.

Adults of low body weight and children: Initially, 8.3 mg/kg (5 mg/kg base) PO once weekly on the same day each week, for 1 to 2 weeks before entering a malaria-endemic area and continued for 4 weeks after leaving the area. Don't exceed 500 mg (300 mg base). If beginning after entering a malaria-endemic area, give 16.7 mg/kg (10 mg/kg base) PO initially, in two divided doses 6 hours apart, followed by the usual dosing regimen.

➤ **Extraintestinal amebiasis**
Adults: 1 g (600 mg base) PO once daily for 2 days; then 500 mg (300 mg base) daily for 2 to 3 weeks. Treatment is usually combined with an intestinal amebicide.

ADMINISTRATION
PO
⚠️ *Alert:* Drug dosage may be discussed in "mg" or "mg base"; be aware of the difference.

• To improve adherence when drug is used for prevention, advise patient to take drug immediately before or after a meal on the same day each week.

• Pharmacist can prepare an oral suspension if patient can't swallow pills.

• Shake suspension before use.

ACTION
May bind to and alter the properties of DNA in susceptible parasites.

Route	Onset	Peak	Duration
PO	Unknown	1–2 hr	Unknown

Half-life: 3 to 5 days.

ADVERSE REACTIONS
CNS: *seizures,* agitation, anxiety, confusion, mild and transient headache, psychic stimulation, neuropathy, acute extrapyramidal reactions, hallucinations. **CV:** hypotension, ECG changes, *cardiomyopathy.* **EENT:** blurred vision, difficulty in focusing, reversible corneal changes; typically irreversible, sometimes progressive or delayed retinal changes (such as narrowing of arterioles, macular lesions, pallor of optic disk, optic atrophy, and patchy retinal pigmentation, typically leading to blindness); ototoxicity, nerve deafness, vertigo, tinnitus. **GI:** anorexia, abdominal cramps, diarrhea, nausea, vomiting. **Hematologic:** *agranulocytosis, aplastic anemia, thrombocytopenia.* **Hepatic:** *hepatitis.* **Musculoskeletal:** myopathy or neuromyopathy

---

♣Canada   ◇OTC   ♦Off-label use   ✐Photoguide   ⊘Do not crush   *Liquid contains alcohol   ▩Genetic

leading to progressive weakness and atrophy of proximal muscle groups. **Skin:** pruritus, lichen planus eruptions, skin and mucosal pigmentary changes, pleomorphic skin eruptions, *erythema multiforme, SJS, TEN,* exfoliative dermatitis, urticaria, DRESS syndrome, hair loss and bleaching of hair pigment. **Other:** *anaphylaxis, angioedema.*

INTERACTIONS

Drug-drug. *Aluminum salts (kaolin), antacids, magnesium:* May decrease GI absorption. Separate dose times by 4 hours.
Ampicillin: May significantly reduce bioavailability of ampicillin. Separate dose times by 2 hours.
Cimetidine: May decrease hepatic metabolism of chloroquine. Avoid use together.
Cyclosporine: May increase serum cyclosporine level. Monitor patient closely. If necessary, discontinue chloroquine.
Drugs that prolong QT interval: May have additive effects on QT interval and increase risk of life-threatening arrhythmias. Avoid concurrent use if possible.
Insulin, other antidiabetics: May increase hypoglycemic effect. Adjust antidiabetic dosage.
Lumefantrine: May enhance adverse/toxic effects of lumefantrine. Don't use artemether–lumefantrine combination concurrently with chloroquine unless no option exists.
Mefloquine: May increase seizure risk. Avoid concurrent use, and delay administration of mefloquine until at least 12 hours after the last dose of chloroquine when possible.
Praziquantel: May reduce praziquantel bioavailability. Monitor patient.
Tamoxifen: May increase risk of retinal toxicity. Monitor patient.
Drug-lifestyle. *Sun exposure:* May cause drug-induced dermatoses. Advise patient to avoid sun exposure.

EFFECTS ON LAB TEST RESULTS
• May increase liver enzyme levels.
• May decrease Hb level and granulocyte and platelet counts.

CONTRAINDICATIONS & CAUTIONS
• Contraindicated in patients hypersensitive to drug and in those with retinal or visual field changes or porphyria.
⌧ Use cautiously in patients with severe GI, neurologic, or blood disorders; hepatic disease or alcoholism; or G6PD deficiency or psoriasis.
• Don't use to treat *Plasmodium* species acquired in an area of known chloroquine resistance or when chloroquine prophylaxis has failed. Use other antimalarials if patient has a resistant strain of plasmodia.
• Risk of toxic reactions may be greater in older adults and in patients with impaired renal function because drug is substantially excreted by the kidneys. Monitor renal function closely.
Dialyzable drug: Unknown.
⚠ **Overdose S&S:** Headache, drowsiness, visual disturbances, nausea, vomiting, CV collapse, seizures, sudden and early respiratory and cardiac arrest; atrial standstill, nodal rhythm, prolonged intraventricular conduction time, progressive bradycardia leading to ventricular fibrillation or arrest.

PREGNANCY-LACTATION-REPRODUCTION
• Safety and effectiveness of chloroquine in during pregnancy aren't known. Avoid use during pregnancy except in the suppression or treatment of malaria when benefit outweighs fetal risk.
• Serious adverse reactions may occur in breastfed infants. Patient should discontinue breastfeeding or discontinue drug, taking into account importance of drug to the patient.

NURSING CONSIDERATIONS
• Ensure that baseline and periodic ophthalmic exams are performed. Check periodically for ocular muscle weakness after long-term use. Risk factors for development of retinopathy during treatment include advanced age, subnormal glomerular filtration, concomitant use of tamoxifen citrate or concurrent macular disease, duration of treatment, and high daily or accumulated dosage.
• Make sure patient is tested with an audiometer before, during, and after therapy, especially if therapy is long-term.
• Monitor CBC and LFTs periodically during long-term therapy. If a severe blood disorder—not caused by the disease—develops, drug may need to be stopped.
• Monitor all patients for hypoglycemia.
• For malaria prevention, the CDC recommends that patient take drug for 4 weeks after leaving the area.
⚡ *Alert:* Monitor patient for overdose, which can quickly lead to toxic symptoms. Children

---

are extremely susceptible to toxicity; avoid long-term treatment.

PATIENT TEACHING

• To improve adherence when using drug for prevention, advise patient to take drug immediately before or after a meal on the same day each week.

• Instruct patient to avoid excessive sun exposure to prevent worsening of drug-induced dermatoses.

• Tell patient to report adverse reactions promptly, especially blurred vision, increased sensitivity to light, tinnitus, hearing loss, or muscle weakness.

• Instruct patient to keep drug out of reach of children. Overdose may be fatal.

• Caution patient that hypoglycemia may occur with or without antidiabetics and to immediately report hypoglycemia signs and symptoms (dizziness, headache, weakness, shaking, fast heartbeat, confusion, hunger, sweating).

• Advise patient of childbearing potential to discuss pregnancy or breastfeeding with provider.

---

ciclesonide (inhalation, intranasal)
sik-le-SON-ide

Alvesco, Omnaris, Zetonna

Therapeutic class: Corticosteroids
Pharmacologic class: Corticosteroids

AVAILABLE FORMS

Nasal aerosol solution: 37 mcg/metered spray
Nasal suspension: 50 mcg/metered spray
Oral inhalation aerosol: 80 mcg, 160 mcg

INDICATIONS & DOSAGES

➤ **Preventative during asthma maintenance (Alvesco)**

Adults and children age 12 and older who were previously taking bronchodilators alone: Initially, inhaled dose of 80 mcg b.i.d.; increase to maximum of 160 mcg b.i.d. after 4 weeks if not controlled.

Adults and children age 12 and older who were previously taking inhaled corticosteroids: Initially, 80 mcg b.i.d.; increase to maximum of 320 mcg b.i.d. after 4 weeks if not controlled.

Adults and children age 12 and older who were previously taking oral corticosteroids: 320 mcg b.i.d.

➤ **Signs and symptoms of perennial allergic rhinitis**

Adults and children age 12 and older: 2 sprays of Omnaris in each nostril once daily (200 mcg/day). Or, 1 actuation of Zetonna per nostril once daily.

➤ **Signs and symptoms of seasonal allergic rhinitis**

Adults and children age 12 and older: 1 actuation of Zetonna per nostril once daily.
Adults and children age 6 and older: 2 sprays of Omnaris in each nostril once daily (200 mcg/day).

ADMINISTRATION

Inhalational

• Before first use or when inhaler hasn't be used for more than 10 days, prime by actuating three times.

• Patient should rinse mouth after inhalation.

Intranasal

• Before first use of Omnaris, gently shake container, then prime by spraying eight times. If not used for 4 consecutive days, gently shake and reprime with 1 spray or until a fine mist appears.

• Before first use of Zetonna, prime by actuating three times. If not used for 10 consecutive days, prime by actuating three times. If the product is dropped, the canister and actuator may become separated; if this happens, instruct patient to reassemble product and test spray once into the air before using.

ACTION

May decrease inflammation by inhibiting macrophages, eosinophils, and mediators such as leukotrienes involved in the asthmatic response.

Route	Onset	Peak	Duration
Inhalation	>4 wk	1 hr	Unknown
Intranasal	1–2 days	1–5 wk	Unknown

Half-life: Inhalation drug, less than 1 hour; inhalation drug's active metabolite, 6 to 7 hours; intranasal drug, unknown.

ADVERSE REACTIONS

CNS: headache. **EENT:** ear pain, nasopharyngitis, sinusitis, pharyngolaryngeal pain, nasal congestion or discomfort, epistaxis, nasal mucosal or septum disorders. **GI:** nausea.

GU: UTI. **Metabolic:** growth retardation. **Musculoskeletal:** arthralgia, pain in the extremities or back. **Respiratory:** URI, cough, bronchitis. **Other:** flulike symptoms.

INTERACTIONS

Drug-drug. *Desmopressin:* May enhance hyponatremic effect of desmopressin. Avoid concurrent use.

Esketamine: Nasal corticosteroids may diminish therapeutic effect of esketamine. Give ciclesonide at least 1 hour before esketamine.

Ketoconazole, other inhibitors of CYP450: May increase ciclesonide level and adverse effects. Use together cautiously; adjust ciclesonide dosage as needed.

EFFECTS ON LAB TEST RESULTS

None reported.

CONTRAINDICATIONS & CAUTIONS

• Contraindicated as primary treatment of status asthmaticus or other acute asthmatic episodes, and in patients hypersensitive to drug or its components.

• Intranasal form is contraindicated in patients who have had recent nasal septal ulcers, nasal surgery, or nasal trauma until healing has occurred.

• Use cautiously in patients who have changed from systemic to inhaled corticosteroids because renal insufficiency, steroid withdrawal (pain, lassitude, depression), or acute worsening of symptoms may occur.

• Use cautiously in patients who are immunosuppressed and in those with wounds; corticosteroids suppress the immune system.

• Use cautiously in children; may cause a decline in growth rate.

• Use cautiously, if at all, in patients with active or quiescent respiratory TB infection; untreated systemic fungal, bacterial, viral, or parasitic infections; or ocular HSV infection.

Dialyzable drug: Unknown.

⚠ *Overdose S&S:* Hyperadrenocorticism.

PREGNANCY-LACTATION-REPRODUCTION

• There are no adequate well-controlled studies during pregnancy. Use during pregnancy only if potential benefit justifies fetal risk.

• If patient takes a corticosteroid during pregnancy, monitor neonate for hypoadrenalism.

• It isn't known if drug appears in human milk. Use cautiously during breastfeeding.

NURSING CONSIDERATIONS

⚠ *Alert:* Don't use inhaler for acute bronchospasm or acute asthma.

• Assess patient for bone loss during long-term use.

• Watch for evidence of localized mouth infections, glaucoma, cataracts, and immunosuppression.

• Monitor infants born to mothers using drug during pregnancy for hypoadrenalism.

• Monitor patients who are switched from systemic to inhaled corticosteroids for worsening of signs and symptoms and other adverse effects of withdrawal. Wean patient off oral corticosteroids slowly.

• Monitor children for decline in growth rate; the potential to regain growth after drug is stopped hasn't been studied.

• Monitor patients for nasal adverse effects.

• For patients who don't respond adequately to starting dose after 4 weeks of therapy, higher doses may provide additional asthma control.

• After asthma stability has been achieved, titrate to lowest effective dosage to minimize systemic effects.

PATIENT TEACHING

• Teach patient how to use drug properly. Refer patient to manufacturer's instructions.

• Inform patient that drug isn't indicated for the relief of acute bronchospasm.

• Instruct patient to rinse mouth with water and spit out after oral inhalation.

• Advise patient to use drug at regular intervals or about the same time every day, as directed.

• Instruct patient using intranasal form to contact prescriber if there is no relief from symptoms after 1 week.

• Warn patient to avoid exposure to chickenpox, measles, or other infections and, if exposed, to consult prescriber immediately.

• Inform patient that asthma-related therapeutic results may take several weeks and to contact prescriber if symptoms don't improve after 4 weeks of treatment or if condition worsens.

• Advise parents of child receiving long-term therapy that child should have periodic growth measurements.

cilostazol
sill-AHS-tah-zoll

Therapeutic class: Antiplatelet drugs
Pharmacologic class: cAMP phosphodiesterase inhibitors

AVAILABLE FORMS
Tablets: 50 mg, 100 mg

INDICATIONS & DOSAGES
➤ **To reduce symptoms of intermittent claudication**
Adults: 100 mg PO b.i.d.
Adjust-a-dose: Decrease dosage to 50 mg PO b.i.d. when giving with CYP3A4 or CYP2C19 inhibitors.

ADMINISTRATION
PO
• Give drug at least 30 minutes before or 2 hours after breakfast and dinner.

ACTION
Thought to inhibit the enzyme phosphodiesterase III, thus inhibiting platelet aggregation and causing vasodilation.

Route	Onset	Peak	Duration
PO	2–4 wk	Unknown	Unknown

Half-life: 11 to 13 hours.

ADVERSE REACTIONS
CNS: dizziness, headache, vertigo. **CV:** palpitations, peripheral edema, tachycardia. **EENT:** pharyngitis, rhinitis. **GI:** abnormal stools, diarrhea, abdominal pain, dyspepsia, flatulence, nausea. **Musculoskeletal:** back pain, myalgia. **Respiratory:** cough. **Other:** infection.

INTERACTIONS
Drug-drug. *Anticoagulants, antiplatelet agents:* May increase bleeding risk. Use together cautiously.
CYP2C19 inhibitors (fluconazole, omeprazole, ticlopidine), strong or moderate CYP3A4 inhibitors (diltiazem, erythromycin, itraconazole, ketoconazole): May increase level of cilostazol and its metabolites. Reduce cilostazol dosage to 50 mg b.i.d.
Drug-herb. *Herbs with anticoagulant properties (alfalfa, anise, bilberry):* May prolong bleeding time. Discourage use together.

Drug-food. *Grapefruit juice:* May increase drug level. Discourage use together.
Drug-lifestyle. *Smoking:* May decrease drug exposure. Discourage smoking.

EFFECTS ON LAB TEST RESULTS
• May reduce triglyceride levels. May increase HDL level.

CONTRAINDICATIONS & CAUTIONS
• Contraindicated in patients hypersensitive to drug or its components.
• Drug hasn't been studied in patients with hemostatic disorders or active bleeding. Avoid use in these patients.
Boxed Warning Contraindicated in patients with HF of any severity. Cilostazol and similar drugs that inhibit the enzyme phosphodiesterase decrease likelihood of survival compared with placebo in patients with class III and IV HF. ∎
⚠ *Alert:* CV risk is unknown in patients using drug long-term and in those with severe underlying heart disease.
• Use cautiously in patients with severe underlying heart disease.
• Use cautiously in patients with severe renal impairment (CrCl less than 25 mL/minute) and in those with moderate to severe hepatic impairment.
• Left ventricular outflow tract obstruction has been reported in patients with sigmoid-shaped interventricular septum.
Dialyzable drug: No.
⚠ *Overdose S&S:* Severe headache, diarrhea, hypotension, tachycardia, cardiac arrhythmias.

PREGNANCY-LACTATION-REPRODUCTION
• There are no adequate studies during pregnancy. Fetal risk is unknown.
• Drug may appear in human milk. Patient should discontinue breastfeeding or discontinue drug, taking into account importance of drug to the patient.

NURSING CONSIDERATIONS
• Beneficial effects may not be seen for up to 12 weeks after therapy starts. If symptoms haven't improved after 3 months, discontinue drug.
• Monitor patients for development of a new systolic murmur or cardiac signs or symptoms after drug initiation.

✤Canada ◇OTC ◆Off-label use ✐Photoguide ⊛Do not crush *Liquid contains alcohol ▨Genetic

- Dosage can be reduced or stopped without such rebound effects as platelet hyperaggregation.
- Monitor platelet and WBC counts periodically.

PATIENT TEACHING

- Instruct patient in safe drug administration.
- Tell patient that beneficial effect of drug on cramping pain isn't likely to be noticed for 2 to 4 weeks and that it may take as long as 12 weeks.
- Inform patient that CV risk is unknown in patients who use drug on a long-term basis and in those with severe underlying heart disease.
- Tell patient that drug may cause dizziness. Caution patient not to drive or perform other activities that require alertness until response to drug is known.

---

cinacalcet hydrochloride
sin-ah-KAL-set

Sensipar

Therapeutic class: Hyperparathyroidism drugs
Pharmacologic class: Calcimimetics

AVAILABLE FORMS

Tablets ⓄⒾⒸ: 30 mg, 60 mg, 90 mg

INDICATIONS & DOSAGES

Adjust-a-dose (for all indications): Patients with moderate to severe hepatic impairment (Child-Pugh class B or C) may experience increased exposure to cinacalcet and increased half-life. Dosage adjustments may be necessary based on serum calcium, serum phosphorus, or intact parathyroid hormone (iPTH) level.

➤ **Primary hyperparathyroidism**
Adults: Initially, 30 mg PO b.i.d. Titrate every 2 to 4 weeks through sequential doses of 30 mg, 60 mg, and 90 mg PO b.i.d., and 90 mg PO t.i.d. or q.i.d. to normalize calcium levels.
➤ **Secondary hyperparathyroidism in patients with chronic kidney disease undergoing dialysis**
Adults: Initially, 30 mg PO once daily; adjust no more than every 2 to 4 weeks through sequential doses of 30 mg, 60 mg, 90 mg, 120 mg, and 180 mg PO once daily to reach

target range of 150 to 300 picograms (pg)/mL for iPTH level.
➤ **Hypercalcemia in patients with parathyroid carcinoma**
Adults: Initially, 30 mg PO b.i.d.; adjust every 2 to 4 weeks through sequential doses of 30 mg, 60 mg, and 90 mg PO b.i.d., and 90 mg PO t.i.d. or q.i.d. daily if needed to normalize calcium level. Measure serum calcium level within 1 week after drug initiation or dosage adjustment.

ADMINISTRATION
PO
- Don't break or crush tablets; give them whole, with food or shortly after a meal.
- Stop etelcalcetide at least 4 weeks before starting cinacalcet. Ensure corrected serum calcium level is at or above lower limit of normal (LLN) before cinacalcet use.

ACTION
Increases sensitivity of calcium-sensing receptor on the parathyroid gland to extracellular calcium, which lowers PTH level and subsequently lowers serum calcium level.

Route	Onset	Peak	Duration
PO	Unknown	2–6 hr	Unknown

Half-life: Terminal half-life, 30 to 40 hours.

ADVERSE REACTIONS
CNS: dizziness, asthenia, *seizures,* depression, fatigue, headache, paresthesia. **CV:** hypotension, HTN. **GI:** diarrhea, nausea, vomiting, anorexia, constipation, abdominal pain, dyspepsia. **Hematologic:** anemia. **Metabolic:** *hypocalcemia,* hypercalcemia, dehydration, *hyperkalemia,* hypoparathyroidism. **Musculoskeletal:** myalgia, arthralgia, fracture, limb pain, noncardiac chest pain, muscle spasms. **Respiratory:** URI, cough, dyspnea. **Skin:** rash. **Other:** hypersensitivity reaction, dialysis access infection.

INTERACTIONS
Drug-drug. *CYP2D6 substrates (carvedilol, desipramine, metoprolol), especially with a narrow therapeutic index (flecainide, thioridazine, most TCAs, vinblastine):* May increase levels of these drugs. Adjust dosage of substrate, as needed.
Etelcalcetide: May enhance hypocalcemic effect of etelcalcetide. Avoid concurrent use.
Strong CYP3A4 inhibitors (erythromycin,

---

itraconazole, ketoconazole): May increase cinacalcet level. Use together cautiously, monitoring PTH and calcium level closely and adjusting cinacalcet dosage, as needed.
Drug-lifestyle. *Smoking:* May increase cinacalcet clearance. Discourage smoking. Adjust dosage if smoking stops or starts.

EFFECTS ON LAB TEST RESULTS
• May decrease calcium and phosphorus levels.

CONTRAINDICATIONS & CAUTIONS
• Contraindicated in patients hypersensitive to drug or its components and in patients with calcium level less than LLN range.
• Use cautiously in patients with history of seizures and in those with moderate to severe hepatic impairment.
• Isolated, idiosyncratic cases of hypotension, worsening HF, or arrhythmia have been reported in patients with impaired cardiac function.
• Safety and effectiveness in children haven't been established.
Dialyzable drug: No.
⚠ *Overdose S&S:* Hypocalcemia.

PREGNANCY-LACTATION-REPRODUCTION
• There are no adequate studies during pregnancy. Use during pregnancy only if potential benefit justifies fetal risk.
• It isn't known if drug appears in human milk. Patient should discontinue breastfeeding or discontinue drug, taking into account importance of drug to the patient.

NURSING CONSIDERATIONS
🔵 *Alert:* Monitor calcium level closely. Hypocalcemia can prolong QT interval, potentially resulting in ventricular arrhythmia, and lower the seizure threshold.
• Monitor patients for worsening of common GI adverse reactions (nausea and vomiting) and for signs and symptoms of GI bleeding and ulcerations. Patients with risk factors for upper GI bleeding (known gastritis, esophagitis, ulcers, severe vomiting) may be at increased risk. Promptly evaluate and treat suspected GI bleeding.
• Patients with moderate to severe hepatic impairment may need dosage adjustment based on PTH and calcium levels. Monitor these patients closely.

• Give drug alone or with vitamin D sterols, phosphate binders, or both.
• Measure calcium level within 1 week after starting therapy or adjusting dosage. After maintenance dose is established, measure calcium level monthly for patients with chronic kidney disease receiving dialysis and every 2 months for those with primary hyperparathyroidism or parathyroid carcinoma.
• Watch carefully for evidence of hypocalcemia: paresthesia, myalgias, cramping, tetany, and seizures.
• For patients with secondary hyperparathyroidism: If calcium level is 7.5 to 8.4 mg/dL or patient develops symptoms of hypocalcemia, give calcium-containing phosphate binders, vitamin D sterols, or both, to raise calcium level. If calcium level is below 7.5 mg/dL or hypocalcemia symptoms persist and the vitamin D dose can't be increased, withhold drug until calcium level reaches 8.0 mg/dL, hypocalcemia symptoms resolve, or both. Resume therapy with the next lowest dose.
• Measure iPTH level 1 to 4 weeks after therapy starts or with dosage changes (wait at least 12 hours after dose before measuring iPTH level). After the maintenance dose is established, monitor PTH level every 1 to 3 months. Levels in patients with chronic kidney disease receiving dialysis should be 150 to 300 pg/mL.
• If iPTH level is less than 150 pg/mL, reduce cinacalcet or vitamin D sterols dosage or discontinue therapy.
• Adynamic bone disease may develop if iPTH levels are suppressed below 100 pg/mL. If this occurs, notify prescriber.
🔵 *Alert:* Don't use drug in patients with chronic kidney disease who aren't receiving dialysis because they have an increased risk of hypocalcemia.

PATIENT TEACHING
• Teach patient safe drug administration.
• Advise patient to report to prescriber adverse reactions and signs of hypocalcemia, which include paresthesia, muscle weakness, muscle cramping, and muscle spasm.
• Advise patient to immediately report signs or symptoms of GI bleeding, such as black or tarry stool, bright red blood in vomit, dark or bright red blood mixed with stool, and abdominal cramps.

• Emphasize importance of regular blood tests to monitor safety and efficacy.

ciprofloxacin
si-proe-FLOX-a-sin

Cipro◆

Therapeutic class: Antibiotics
Pharmacologic class: Fluoroquinolones

AVAILABLE FORMS
Infusion (premixed): 200 mg in 100 mL, 400 mg in 200 mL
Injection: 200 mg/20 mL, 400 mg/40 mL
Suspension (oral): 250 mg/5 mL, 500 mg/ 5 mL
Tablets (extended-release, film-coated) **ONE***:* 500 mg, 1,000 mg
Tablets (film-coated): 100 mg, 250 mg, 500 mg, 750 mg

INDICATIONS & DOSAGES
Boxed Warning Use in patients with acute sinusitis, acute exacerbations of chronic bronchitis, and acute uncomplicated cystitis isn't recommended because of risk of serious adverse effects. Use in these patients only when there are no other treatment options. ∎
Adjust-a-dose (for all indications): For patients with a CrCl of 30 to 50 mL/minute, give 250 to 500 mg PO every 12 hours or the usual IV dose; if CrCl is 5 to 29 mL/minute, give 250 to 500 mg PO every 18 hours or 200 to 400 mg IV every 18 to 24 hours. If patient is receiving hemodialysis or peritoneal dialysis, give 250 to 500 mg PO every 24 hours.
➤ **Complicated intra-abdominal infection**
Adults: 500 mg PO or 400 mg IV every 12 hours for 7 to 14 days. Give with metronidazole.
➤ **Severe or complicated bone or joint infection, severe respiratory tract infection, severe skin or skin-structure infection**
Adults: 500 to 750 mg PO every 12 hours (if treating *Pseudomonas aeruginosa* osteomyelitis, give 750 mg) or 400 mg IV every 8 hours.
➤ **Severe or complicated UTI; mild to moderate bone or joint infection; mild to moderate respiratory infection; mild to moderate skin or skin-structure infection; infectious diarrhea; typhoid fever**
Adults: 500 mg PO or 400 mg IV every 12 hours. Or, 1,000 mg extended-release tablets PO every 24 hours.
➤ **Complicated UTI or pyelonephritis**
Adults: 500 mg PO every 12 hours for 5 to 7 days. Or 1,000 mg extended-release tablets PO every 24 hours for 5 to 7 days. If prevalence of fluoroquinolone resistance is more than 10%, an initial dose of a long-acting parenteral antimicrobial (ceftriaxone, ertapenem, or a consolidated 24-hour dose of an aminoglycoside) is recommended for outpatients.
Children ages 1 to 17: 6 to 10 mg/kg IV every 8 hours for 10 to 21 days. Maximum IV dose, 400 mg. Or, 10 to 20 mg/kg PO every 12 hours. Maximum PO dose, 750 mg. Treat for 10 to 21 days. Don't exceed maximum dose, even in patients who weigh more than 51 kg.
Adjust-a-dose: If CrCl is less than 30 mL/ minute, reduce dosage of extended-release form from 1,000 to 500 mg daily. Give 500 mg extended-release form after hemodialysis or peritoneal dialysis is completed.
➤ **Nosocomial pneumonia**
Adults: 400 mg IV every 8 hours for 10 to 14 days.
➤ **Mild to moderate UTI**
Adults: 250 mg PO or 200 mg IV every 12 hours for 7 to 14 days.
➤ **Uncomplicated UTI**
Adults: 500 mg extended-release tablet PO once daily for 3 days, or 250 mg PO every 12 hours for 3 days.
➤ **Chronic bacterial prostatitis**
Adults: 500 mg PO every 12 hours or 400 mg IV every 12 hours for 28 days.
➤ **Lower respiratory tract infections**
Adults: 500 to 750 mg PO every 12 hours or 400 mg IV every 8 to 12 hours for 7 to 14 days.
➤ **Mild to moderate acute sinusitis**
Adults: 500 mg PO or 400 mg IV every 12 hours for 10 days.
➤ **Empirical therapy in patients who are febrile and neutropenic**
Adults: 400 mg IV every 8 hours used with piperacillin 50 mg/kg IV every 4 hours (not to exceed 24 g/day of piperacillin) for 7 to 14 days.
➤ **Inhalation anthrax (postexposure)**
Adults: 400 mg IV every 12 hours initially until susceptibility test results are known; then 500 mg PO every 12 hours. Give drug

---

Reactions in bold italics are *life-threatening*. Interactions may have a *rapid onset* or a **delayed onset**.

with one or two additional antimicrobials. Switch to oral therapy when appropriate. Treat for 60 days (IV and PO combined). *Children:* 10 mg/kg IV every 12 hours; then 15 mg/kg PO every 12 hours. Don't exceed 800 mg/day IV or 1,000 mg/day PO. Give drug with one or two additional antimicrobials. Switch to oral therapy when appropriate. Treat for 60 days (IV and PO combined).

➤ **Plague due to *Yersinia pestis*; plague prophylaxis as soon as possible after suspected or confirmed exposure**
Adults: 400 mg IV every 8 to 12 hours or 500 to 750 mg PO every 12 hours for 14 days.
Children ages 1 to 17: 10 mg/kg IV or 15 mg/kg PO every 8 to 12 hours for 10 to 21 days. Maximum dosage, 500 mg/dose PO and 400 mg/dose IV.

ADMINISTRATION
PO
• Extended- and immediate-release oral forms aren't interchangeable.
• Obtain specimen for culture and sensitivity tests before giving first dose. Begin therapy while awaiting results.
• To avoid decreasing the effects of ciprofloxacin, give at least 2 hours before or 6 hours after certain drugs and vitamins. Food doesn't affect absorption but may delay peak levels.
• Give drug with plenty of fluids to reduce risk of urine crystals.
• Don't crush or split extended-release tablets.
• Shake oral suspension vigorously each time before use for approximately 15 seconds; don't give through feeding tube.
• Give dose post dialysis.
IV
▼ Obtain specimen for culture and sensitivity tests before giving first dose. Begin therapy while awaiting results.
▼ Dilute drug to 1 to 2 mg/mL using D_5W or NSS for injection.
▼ If giving drug through a Y-type set, stop the other IV solution while infusing.
▼ Infuse over 1 hour into a large vein to minimize discomfort and vein irritation.
▼ **Incompatibilities:** Aminophylline, ampicillin–sulbactam, azithromycin, cefepime, clindamycin phosphate, dexamethasone sodium phosphate, furosemide, heparin sodium, methylprednisolone sodium succinate, phenytoin sodium. Consult a drug compatibility reference for complete listing.

ACTION
Inhibits bacterial DNA synthesis, mainly by blocking DNA gyrase; bactericidal.

Route	Onset	Peak	Duration
PO	Unknown	30–120 min	Unknown
PO (extended-release)	Unknown	1–4 hr	Unknown
IV	Unknown	Immediate	Unknown

Half-life: 4 hours; extended-release, 6 hours in adults with normal renal function.

ADVERSE REACTIONS
CNS: dizziness, drowsiness, insomnia, nervousness, neurologic changes, confusion, headache, restlessness, fever. **GI:** abdominal pain, dyspepsia, diarrhea, nausea, vomiting. **GU:** vulvovaginal candidiasis. **Hematologic:** *leukopenia, neutropenia, thrombocytopenia, thrombocytosis,* eosinophilia. **Hepatic:** abnormal LFT values. **Musculoskeletal:** musculoskeletal symptoms. **Respiratory:** asthma. **Skin:** rash, injection-site reaction. **Other:** hypersensitivity reactions.

INTERACTIONS
Drug-drug. *Aluminum hydroxide, aluminum-magnesium hydroxide, calcium carbonate, didanosine (chewable tablets, buffered tablets, or pediatric powder for oral solution), magnesium hydroxide, products containing zinc:* May decrease ciprofloxacin absorption and effects. Give ciprofloxacin 2 hours before or 6 hours after these drugs.
Cyclosporine: May increase risk of cyclosporine toxicity. Monitor renal function and cyclosporine level.
Drugs primarily metabolized by CYP1A2 (clozapine, methylxanthines, olanzapine, ropinirole, zolpidem): May increase plasma level of coadministered drug, leading to clinically significant adverse reactions of coadministered drug. Monitor patient for adverse reactions.
Drugs that prolong QT interval (amiodarone, procainamide, TCAs): May additionally increase QT interval and risk of life-threatening cardiac arrhythmias. Use together cautiously.
Duloxetine: May significantly increase duloxetine level. Avoid concurrent use.
Iron salts: May decrease absorption of ciprofloxacin, reducing anti-infective response. Give at least 2 hours apart.
NSAIDs: May increase risk of CNS stimulation. Monitor patient closely.

Oral antidiabetics (glimepiride, glyburide): May increase risk of hypoglycemia. Monitor glucose level closely if used together.

Phenytoin: May increase or decrease phenytoin level. Monitor phenytoin level during and after use together.

Probenecid: May elevate level of ciprofloxacin. Monitor patient for toxicity.

Boxed Warning *Steroids:* May increase risk of tendinitis and tendon rupture. ∎

Sildenafil: May increase sildenafil level. Use together cautiously and monitor patient for sildenafil toxicity.

Sucralfate: May decrease ciprofloxacin absorption, reducing anti-infective response. If use together can't be avoided, give at least 6 hours apart.

Theophylline: May increase theophylline level and prolong theophylline half-life. If concomitant use can't be avoided, monitor theophylline level and watch for adverse effects.

Tizanidine: Increases tizanidine levels, causing low BP, somnolence, dizziness, and slowed psychomotor skills. Use together is contraindicated.

Warfarin: May increase anticoagulant effects. Monitor PT and INR closely.

Drug-food. *Caffeine:* May increase effect of caffeine. Discourage use together.

Dairy products, other foods: May delay peak drug levels. Advise patient to take drug on an empty stomach.

Orange juice fortified with calcium: May decrease GI absorption of drug, reducing its effects. Discourage use together.

Drug-lifestyle. *Sun, UV light exposure:* May cause photosensitivity reactions. Advise patient to avoid excessive sunlight or UV light exposure.

EFFECTS ON LAB TEST RESULTS
• May increase ALP, ALT, AST, bilirubin, BUN, creatinine, LDH, and GGT levels.
• May increase eosinophil count.
• May decrease WBC, neutrophil, and platelet counts.
• May increase crystals in urine.

CONTRAINDICATIONS & CAUTIONS
• Contraindicated in patients sensitive to fluoroquinolones.
🕃 *Alert:* Serious and occasionally fatal hypersensitivity reactions, some after first dose, have been reported. Emergency treatment for anaphylaxis may be necessary. Immediately discontinue drug at first appearance of rash, jaundice, or other signs and symptoms of hypersensitivity.

🕃 *Alert:* Cases of severe hepatotoxicity, including fatal events, have been reported. Acute liver injury can be rapid and is frequently associated with hypersensitivity. If signs and symptoms of hepatitis occur, discontinue drug immediately.

🕃 *Alert:* Patients receiving systemic drug have an increased risk of hyperglycemia and hypoglycemia, which can result in coma. Hypoglycemia has been reported more frequently in the older adults and in patients with diabetes.

🕃 *Alert:* Drug may increase risk of aortic dissection or rupture when used systemically. Avoid use in patients with known aortic aneurysm, patients at risk for aortic aneurysm, including those with peripheral atherosclerotic vascular diseases, HTN, certain genetic conditions (Marfan syndrome, Ehlers-Danlos syndrome), and older adults. Use drug in these patients only if no other treatment options are available.

• Use cautiously in patients with CNS disorders, such as severe cerebral arteriosclerosis or seizure disorders, and in those at risk for seizures. Drug may cause CNS stimulation.

Boxed Warning Drug is associated with increased risk of tendinitis and tendon rupture, especially in patients older than age 60 and those with heart, kidney, or lung transplants. ∎

Boxed Warning Drug may exacerbate muscle weakness in patients with myasthenia gravis. Avoid use of fluoroquinolones in patients with a known history of myasthenia gravis. ∎

• Oral or parenteral fluoroquinolones may increase the risk of peripheral neuropathy of the arms or legs. Symptoms can occur anytime during treatment and can last for months to years or be permanent. Stop drug immediately if patient develops symptoms and switch to a nonfluoroquinolone antibacterial drug unless the benefits of continued treatment outweigh the risks.

Boxed Warning Fluoroquinolones have been associated with disabling and potentially irreversible serious adverse reactions that have occurred together, including tendinitis and tendon rupture, peripheral neuropathy, and CNS effects. Drug is associated with increased risk of serious adverse CNS reactions

C

(seizures, toxic psychoses, increased ICP, pseudotumor cerebri, tremors, restlessness, anxiety, light-headedness, confusion, hallucinations, paranoia, depression, nightmares, insomnia, disturbances in attention, disorientation, agitation, memory impairment, delirium and, rarely, suicidality). If any of these serious adverse reactions occur, discontinue drug immediately. ∎

Boxed Warning Reserve drug for use in patients who have no alternative treatment options for acute exacerbation of chronic bronchitis, acute sinusitis, and acute uncomplicated cystitis. ∎

• Drug may cause CDAD ranging in severity from mild diarrhea to fatal colitis and possibly occurring more than 2 months after therapy ends. Drug may need to be discontinued if CDAD develops during therapy.

Dialyzable drug: Less than 10%.

PREGNANCY-LACTATION-REPRODUCTION

• There are no adequate studies during pregnancy. Use during pregnancy only if potential benefit justifies fetal risk.

• Patients should receive the usual doses and regimens for anthrax postexposure prophylaxis during pregnancy.

• Drug appears in human milk, and the amount absorbed by an infant is unknown. Because of the risk of serious adverse reactions (including articular damage), a decision should be made to discontinue breastfeeding or discontinue drug, taking into account importance of drug to the patient.

• Patients who are breastfeeding may pump and discard human milk during and for 2 days after treatment.

NURSING CONSIDERATIONS

• Patients who are immunocompromised should receive the usual doses and regimens for anthrax postexposure prophylaxis.

• Monitor patient's intake and output, and observe patient for signs of crystalluria.

Boxed Warning Monitor patients receiving systemic drug for CNS (seizures, increased ICP, pseudotumor cerebri, dizziness, tremors) and psychiatric (disturbances in attention, disorientation, agitation, nervousness, memory impairment, delirium) adverse reactions. Discontinue drug for CNS adverse effects, including psychiatric adverse reactions. ∎

Boxed Warning Tendon rupture may occur in patients receiving quinolones. If pain or

inflammation occurs or if patient ruptures a tendon, stop drug. ∎

⚠ *Alert:* Monitor patients for signs and symptoms of aortic aneurysm, dissection, and rupture (sudden, severe, and constant pain in the stomach, chest, or back; throbbing in the stomach area, deep pain in the back or the side of the stomach; steady, gnawing pain in the stomach that lasts for hours or days; pain in the jaw, neck, back, or chest; coughing or hoarseness; shortness of breath, trouble swallowing). Discontinue drug immediately if any of these aortic disorders are suspected.

• Monitor patient for symptoms of peripheral neuropathy (pain, burning, tingling, numbness, weakness, or a change in sensation to light touch, pain, temperature, or sense of body position), and report them immediately to the practitioner.

⚠ *Alert:* Immediately report signs and symptoms of hepatitis (anorexia, jaundice, dark urine, pruritus, abdominal tenderness) and discontinue drug.

• Long-term therapy may result in overgrowth of drug-resistant organisms.

• Patients with cutaneous anthrax and signs and symptoms of systemic involvement, extensive edema, or lesions on the head or neck need IV therapy and a multidrug approach.

⚠ *Alert:* Monitor patients receiving systemic drug for symptoms of hypoglycemia (confusion, pounding or rapid heartbeat, dizziness, pale skin, shakiness, diaphoresis, unusual hunger, trembling, headache, weakness, irritability, unusual anxiety). Immediately discontinue drug for blood glucose disturbances, and switch to a nonfluoroquinolone antibiotic if possible.

PATIENT TEACHING

• Tell patient to take drug as prescribed, even after feeling better.

• Advise patient to drink plenty of fluids to reduce risk of urine crystals.

• Instruct patient in safe drug administration.

⚠ *Alert:* Warn patient to seek immediate medical attention for signs or symptoms of aortic aneurysm.

⚠ *Alert:* Warn patient to immediately notify prescriber for signs and symptoms of serious adverse reactions, including unusual joint or tendon pain, muscle weakness, "pins and needles" tingling or pricking sensation, numbness in the arms or legs, confusion or hallucinations.

♣Canada   ◇OTC   ◆Off-label use   ✐Photoguide   ⬤Do not crush   *Liquid contains alcohol   ▨Genetic

🜀 *Alert:* Caution patients that significantly low blood sugar levels can occur. Instruct patients how to manage symptoms and to immediately report any occurrence to the prescriber.

🜀 *Alert:* Advise patients with diabetes that they may need to monitor blood glucose levels more frequently during therapy.

🜀 *Alert:* Inform patients to immediately report psychiatric adverse reactions and that these can occur after just one dose.

• Warn patient to avoid hazardous tasks that require alertness, such as driving, until effects of drug are known.

• Advise patient that hypersensitivity reactions may occur even after first dose. If a rash or other allergic reaction occurs, tell patient to stop drug immediately and notify prescriber.

• Tell patient that tendon rupture can occur with drug and to notify prescriber if pain or inflammation occurs.

• Tell patient to avoid excessive sunlight or artificial UV light during therapy.

SAFETY ALERT!

cisatracurium besylate
sis-ah-trah-KYOO-ee-hum

Nimbex

Therapeutic class: Skeletal muscle relaxants
Pharmacologic class: Nondepolarizing neuromuscular blockers

AVAILABLE FORMS
Injection: 2 mg/mL, 10 mg/mL*

INDICATIONS & DOSAGES
Adjust-a-dose (for all indications): In patients with neuromuscular disease, such as myasthenia gravis or carcinomatosis, don't exceed 0.02 mg/kg. Patients with burns may need increased amount.

➤ **Adjunct to general anesthesia to facilitate ET intubation and relax skeletal muscles during surgery**
Adults: First dose of 0.15 to 0.2 mg/kg IV; then maintenance dose of 0.03 mg/kg IV 40 to 50 minutes after initial 0.15 mg/kg dose or 50 to 60 minutes after 0.2 mg/kg dose PRN. Adjust maintenance dose based on clinical criteria, including response to peripheral nerve stimulation.

Or, as a continuous infusion in operating room, after an initial bolus dose, give a maintenance infusion at 3 mcg/kg/minute and reduce to 1 to 2 mcg/kg/minute as needed. Initiate infusion only after early evidence of spontaneous recovery from initial bolus dose.

Children ages 2 to 12: 0.1 to 0.15 mg/kg IV over 5 to 10 seconds. After first dose, give a maintenance infusion of 3 mcg/kg/minute, then reduce to 1 to 2 mcg/kg/minute as needed.

Children ages 1 to 23 months: 0.15 mg/kg over 5 to 10 seconds. No information is available for continuous infusion.

Adjust-a-dose: During CABG surgery (adults) with induced hypothermia, reduce infusion rate by 50%.

➤ **To maintain neuromuscular blockade during mechanical ventilation in ICU**
Adults: Principles for infusion in operating room apply to use in ICU. After first dose, give 3 mcg/kg/minute by IV infusion. Range, 0.5 to 10.2 mcg/kg/minute.

ADMINISTRATION
IV

🜀 *Alert:* Accidental administration of neuromuscular blockers may be fatal. Store drug with the cap and wrapper around the cap intact and in a manner that minimizes the possibility of selecting the wrong product.

▼ Drug is colorless to slightly yellow or green-yellow. Inspect vials for particulates and discoloration before use. Don't use unclear solutions or those with visible particulates.

🜀 *Alert:* The 20-mL vial is only intended for use as an infusion for a single patient in the ICU.

▼ Use only under direct supervision of medical staff skilled in using neuromuscular blockers and maintaining airway patency. Don't give drug unless resources for intubation, mechanical ventilation, and oxygen therapy are within reach.

▼ Keep refrigerated; don't freeze. After removal from refrigeration to room temperature (77° F [25° C]), use within 21 days, even if rerefrigerated.

▼ Use drug within 24 hours when diluted to a concentration of 0.1 mg/mL in D_5W, NSS, or 5% dextrose and NSS.

▼ **Incompatibilities:** Alkaline solutions with pH higher than 8.5, propofol, ketorolac.

Reactions in bold italics are *life-threatening*. Interactions may have a *rapid onset* or a ***delayed onset***.

ACTION

Binds to cholinergic receptors on the motor end plate, antagonizing acetylcholine and blocking neuromuscular transmission.

Route	Onset	Peak	Duration
IV	2–3 min	3–5 min	35–45 min

Half-life: 22 to 29 minutes; about 3 hours for laudanosine metabolite.

ADVERSE REACTIONS

CV: *bradycardia,* hypotension, flushing. **Respiratory:** *bronchospasm.* **Skin:** rash.

INTERACTIONS

Drug-drug. *Aminoglycosides, bacitracin, calcium channel blockers, clindamycin, colistimethate sodium, colistin, lincomycin, lithium, local anesthetics, magnesium salts, polymyxins, procainamide, quinidine, quinine, tetracyclines, vancomycin:* May enhance neuromuscular blocking action of cisatracurium. Use together cautiously.
Carbamazepine, phenytoin: May decrease the effects of cisatracurium. May need to increase cisatracurium dose.
Enflurane or isoflurane given with nitrous oxide or oxygen: May prolong cisatracurium duration of action. Patient may need less frequent maintenance doses, lower maintenance doses, or reduced infusion rate of cisatracurium. Effects are dependent on duration of volatile agent administration.
Succinylcholine: May shorten time to onset of maximal neuromuscular block. Monitor patient.

EFFECTS ON LAB TEST RESULTS

None reported.

CONTRAINDICATIONS & CAUTIONS

• Contraindicated in patients who are hypersensitive to drug, to other bisbenzylisoquinolinium drugs, or to benzyl alcohol (found in 10-mg/mL vial). Don't use 10-mL vials with benzyl alcohol in neonates and premature infants.
• Severe hypersensitivity reactions, including fatal and life-threatening anaphylactic reactions, have been reported. Wheezing, laryngospasm, bronchospasm, rash, and itching have been reported in children.
• Patients with renal or hepatic impairment receiving extended administration may be at higher risk for seizures.

Dialyzable drug: Unknown.
⚠ **Overdose S&S:** Prolonged neuromuscular blockade.

PREGNANCY-LACTATION-REPRODUCTION

• There are no adequate studies during pregnancy. Use during pregnancy only if clearly needed and potential benefit justifies fetal risk.
• It isn't known if drug appears in human milk. Use cautiously during breastfeeding.

NURSING CONSIDERATIONS

• Drug isn't recommended for rapid-sequence ET intubation because of its intermediate onset.
• Consider extending interval between administering drug and attempting intubation by at least 1 minute to achieve adequate intubation conditions in older adults and patients with ESRD.
• Dosage requirements vary widely among patients. Base subsequent dosage on patient's response to initial doses.
• Drug has been associated with residual paralysis. To prevent complications resulting from drug-associated residual paralysis, extubation is recommended only after patient has recovered sufficiently from neuromuscular blockade. Consider using a reversal agent, especially in cases in which residual paralysis is more likely to occur.
• To reduce the risk of respiratory arrest and death, confirm proper selection and dose of intended product and avoid confusion with other injectable solutions present in critical care and other clinical settings.
🕙 *Alert:* Drug has no known effect on consciousness, pain threshold, or cerebration. To avoid patient distress, don't induce neuromuscular block before unconsciousness.
🕙 *Alert:* Never give by IM injection. Administer undiluted as bolus injection over 5 to 10 seconds. Continuous infusion requires use of an infusion pump.
• Monitor neuromuscular function with nerve stimulator during drug administration. If stimulation doesn't elicit a response, stop infusion until response returns.
🕙 *Alert:* Drug should only be given by clinicians experienced in its use. Don't give drug unless personnel and facilities for resuscitation, life-support, and drug antagonist are immediately available.

• To avoid inaccurate dosing, perform neuromuscular monitoring on a nonparetic arm or leg in patients with hemiparesis or paraparesis.
• Monitor acid-base balance and electrolyte levels. Abnormalities may potentiate or antagonize the action of cisatracurium.
• Monitor patient for malignant hyperthermia.
• Give analgesics, if indicated. Patient can feel pain but can't indicate its presence.
◐ *Alert:* Careful dosage calculation is essential. Always verify dosage with another health care professional.

PATIENT TEACHING
• Explain purpose of drug.
• Assure patient that monitoring will be continuous.
• Explain all procedures and events because patient can still hear.

SAFETY ALERT!

CISplatin
SIS-pla-tin

Therapeutic class: Antineoplastics
Pharmacologic class: Platinum-containing compounds

AVAILABLE FORMS
Injection: 1 mg/mL
Lyophilized powder for injection: 50 mg

INDICATIONS & DOSAGES
◐ *Alert:* Dosages greater than 100 mg/m²/cycle are rarely used and should be confirmed with prescriber.
Adjust-a-dose (for all indications): Other dosage regimens may be used. Consider alternative treatment or dosage reductions for impaired CrCl, myelosuppression, or neuropathy. Consider permanent discontinuation for grade 3 or 4 neuropathy.

Don't give repeat course of cisplatin until serum creatinine level is below 1.5 mg/dL or BUN level is below 25 mg/dL, platelets are 100,000/mm³ or higher, WBCs are 4,000/mm³ or higher, and audiometric analysis indicates that auditory acuity is within normal limits.
➤ **Adjunctive therapy in advanced testicular cancer**
Adults: 20 mg/m² IV daily for 5 days. Repeat every 3 weeks for three cycles.

➤ **Adjunctive therapy in advanced ovarian cancer**
Adults: 75 to 100 mg/m² IV once every 3 to 4 weeks on day 1.
➤ **Advanced bladder cancer**
Adults: 50 to 70 mg/m² IV every 3 to 4 weeks. Give 50 mg/m² every 4 weeks in patients who have received other antineoplastics or radiation therapy.

ADMINISTRATION
IV
▼ Drug may be mutagenic, teratogenic, or carcinogenic. Follow facility policy on preparing and giving drug to reduce risks.
▼ Hydrate with 1 to 2 L of fluid for 8 to 12 hours before giving drug, with continued hydration for 24 hours after administration.
◐ *Alert:* Don't use needles or IV sets containing aluminum parts for preparation or administration.
▼ Infusions are most stable in solutions containing chloride (such as NSS or half-NSS and 0.22% sodium chloride). Don't use D₅W alone.
▼ Reconstitute 50-mg powder vial with 50 mL sterile water for injection to produce a 1-mg/1 mL clear or colorless to slightly yellow solution. Don't refrigerate reconstituted solution.
▼ Visually inspect solution for particulate matter and discoloration before administration, whenever solution and container permit.
▼ Further dilute reconstituted solution in 1 to 2 L of a compatible infusion solution with or without 37.5 g of mannitol. Refer to detailed references for specific infusion solution stability and compatibility information.
▼ Reconstituted solution is stable for 20 hours at controlled room temperature; don't refrigerate. Protect solution removed from amber vial from light if not used within 6 hours.
▼ Administer over 6 to 8 hours
Boxed Warning Premedicate with highly effective antiemetic. Drug can cause severe nausea and vomiting. Posttreatment antiemetics may be necessary. ■
▼ Solutions in vials that have been entered are stable for 7 days at room temperature under fluorescent light; if protected from light, stability is 28 days. Don't refrigerate.
▼ **Incompatibilities:** None listed by manufacturer. Consult a drug compatibility reference for more information.

Reactions in bold italics are *life-threatening*. Interactions may have a *rapid onset* or a *delayed onset*.

ACTION
May cross-link strands of cellular DNA and interfere with RNA transcription, causing an imbalance of growth that leads to cell death. Not specific to cell cycle.

Route	Onset	Peak	Duration
IV	Rapid	Unknown	Several days

Half-life: Initial phase, 14 to 49 minutes; beta, 0.7 to 4.6 hours; gamma, 24 to 127 hours.

ADVERSE REACTIONS
CNS: peripheral neuropathy. **EENT:** tinnitus, hearing loss. **GI:** anorexia, diarrhea, loss of taste, nausea, vomiting. **GU:** *nephrotoxicity.* **Hematologic:** *myelosuppression, leukopenia, thrombocytopenia,* anemia. **Hepatic:** increased liver enzyme levels. **Metabolic:** *hypomagnesemia, hypokalemia, hypocalcemia.* **Skin:** local irritation. **Other:** hypersensitivity reactions.

INTERACTIONS
Drug-drug. *Aminoglycosides (gentamicin, tobramycin):* May increase nephrotoxicity. Avoid use together.
Aminoglycosides, bumetanide, ethacrynic acid, furosemide, torsemide: May increase ototoxicity. Avoid using together, if possible.
Aspirin, NSAIDs: May increase risk of nephrotoxicity. Avoid using together.
Clozapine: May increase neutropenic risk. Monitor concurrent use.
Fosphenytoin, phenytoin: May decrease phenytoin and fosphenytoin levels. Monitor levels.
Live-virus vaccines: May increase vaccine-associated infection and decrease effectiveness of chemotherapy. Concurrent use isn't recommended.
Myelosuppressants (chemotherapy, radiation therapy): May increase myelosuppression. Monitor patient.
Drug-herb. *Echinacea:* May diminish drug's therapeutic effect. Monitor patient.

EFFECTS ON LAB TEST RESULTS
• May increase uric acid level. May decrease calcium, Hb, magnesium, phosphate, potassium, and sodium levels.
• May decrease platelet and WBC counts.

CONTRAINDICATIONS & CAUTIONS
• Hypersensitivity reactions, including anaphylaxis, requiring emergency treatment have been reported. Facial edema, bronchoconstriction, tachycardia, and hypotension may occur within minutes of administration. Epinephrine, corticosteroids, and antihistamines have been used effectively to alleviate symptoms.
• Contraindicated in patients hypersensitive to drug or other platinum-containing compounds and in those with preexisting renal impairment, hearing impairment, or myelosuppression.
• Use cautiously in patients previously treated with radiation or cytotoxic drugs and in those with peripheral neuropathies; also use cautiously with other ototoxic and nephrotoxic drugs.
Boxed Warning Drug can cause severe renal toxicity, including acute renal failure, which is dose-related and cumulative. Ensure adequate hydration and monitor renal function and electrolyte levels. Consider dosage reductions or alternative treatment in patients with renal impairment. ∎
Boxed Warning Drug can cause dose-related peripheral neuropathy that becomes more severe with repeated courses of drug. ∎
• Secondary malignancies have been reported.
• Drug can cause hyperuricemia and TLS requiring antihyperuricemia therapy to reduce uric acid levels, especially with dosages higher than 50 mg/m^2.
• Use cautiously in older adults.
• Safe use in children hasn't been established.
Dialyzable drug: No.
⚠ **Overdose S&S:** Renal failure, liver failure, deafness, ocular toxicity, significant myelosuppression, intractable nausea and vomiting, neuritis, death.

PREGNANCY-LACTATION-REPRODUCTION
• Drug can cause fetal harm when used during pregnancy. Patients of childbearing potential should use effective contraception during and for 14 months after treatment. Males with partners of childbearing potential should use effective contraception during and for 11 months after treatment.
• Drug may cause ovarian failure, premature menopause, impaired spermatogenesis, and decreased fertility.
• Drug appears in human milk. Patients shouldn't breastfeed during therapy.

NURSING CONSIDERATIONS

- Drug should be administered under the supervision of a physician experienced in the use of cancer chemotherapeutic agents.

Boxed Warning Severe myelosuppression with fatalities due to infection can occur. Monitor blood counts accordingly. Therapy interruption may be required. ∎

⚠ *Alert:* Cisplatin is considered a vesicant if more than 20 mL is administered or if it's given at a concentration of 0.5 mg/mL or more. Monitor infusion site; stop infusion immediately and notify prescriber if extravasation occurs. Don't flush the line.

- Monitor CBC, electrolyte levels (especially potassium and magnesium), platelet count, and renal function studies before initial and subsequent doses.
- Ototoxicity, which may be more pronounced in children, is manifested by tinnitus or loss of high-frequency hearing and, occasionally, deafness.
- To detect hearing loss, obtain audiometry tests before initial and subsequent doses.
- Prehydration and mannitol diuresis may significantly reduce renal toxicity and ototoxicity. Maintain adequate hydration and urine output for 24 hours after drug administration.
- Therapeutic effects are frequently accompanied by toxicity.
- Drug is highly emetogenic. Nausea and vomiting may occur immediately or may be delayed. Antiemetics are recommended. Monitor intake and output. Continue IV hydration until patient can tolerate adequate oral intake.

Boxed Warning Renal toxicity is cumulative; don't give next dose until renal function returns to normal. ∎

- To prevent bleeding, avoid all IM injections when platelet count is less than 50,000/mm^3.
- Anticipate need for blood transfusions during treatment because of cumulative anemia.
- Monitor patient for hypersensitivity reactions; treat as clinically indicated.
- Verify pregnancy status before treatment.
- *Look alike–sound alike:* Don't confuse cisplatin with carboplatin; they aren't interchangeable.

PATIENT TEACHING

- Teach patient to report all adverse reactions, including nausea and vomiting and infusion-site discomfort.
- Advise patient to watch for signs and symptoms of infection (fever, sore throat, fatigue)

and bleeding (easy bruising, nosebleeds, bleeding gums, tarry stools). Tell patient to take temperature daily.
- Tell patient to immediately report ringing in the ears or numbness in hands or feet.
- Instruct patient to avoid OTC products containing aspirin or other NSAIDs.
- Advise patient to stop breastfeeding during therapy because of risk of toxicity to infant.
- Warn patient of childbearing potential about need for contraception due to risk of fetal harm.

---

citalopram hydrobromide ☒
si-TAL-oh-pram

CeleXA✒

Therapeutic class: Antidepressants
Pharmacologic class: SSRIs

AVAILABLE FORMS

Capsules: 30 mg
Solution: 10 mg/5 mL
Tablets: 10 mg, 20 mg, 40 mg

INDICATIONS & DOSAGES

☒ *Adjust-a-dose (for all indications):* For patients with significant hepatic impairment and for those who are CYP2C19 poor metabolizers, are taking cimetidine or another CYP2C19 inhibitor, or are older than age 60, maximum dosage is 20 mg/day.

➤ **Depression**
Adults: Initially, 20 mg PO once daily, increasing to maximum of 40 mg daily after no less than 1 week.
Patients older than age 60: 20 mg PO daily.

ADMINISTRATION

PO
- Give without regard for food.
- Capsules are only available in 30-mg strength. Use of tablets or solution is necessary for initial dosage and titration.

ACTION

Probably linked to potentiation of serotonergic activity in the CNS resulting from inhibition of neuronal reuptake of serotonin.

Route	Onset	Peak	Duration
PO	1–4 wk	4 hr	1–2 days

Half-life: 35 hours.

Reactions in bold italics are *life-threatening*. Interactions may have a *rapid onset* or a *delayed onset*.

ADVERSE REACTIONS
CNS: somnolence, insomnia, *suicidality,* anxiety, agitation, dizziness, paresthesia, migraine, impaired concentration, amnesia, depression, apathy, tremor, confusion, fatigue, fever, asthenia, taste perversion, yawning. **CV:** tachycardia, orthostatic hypotension, hypotension, *prolonged QT interval.* **EENT:** rhinitis, sinusitis, dry mouth, abnormal accommodation. **GI:** nausea, diarrhea, anorexia, dyspepsia, vomiting, abdominal pain, increased saliva, flatulence, increased appetite. **GU:** dysmenorrhea, amenorrhea, ejaculation disorder, erectile dysfunction, anorgasmia, polyuria, decreased libido. **Metabolic:** decreased or increased weight. **Musculoskeletal:** arthralgia, myalgia. **Respiratory:** URI, coughing. **Skin:** rash, pruritus, diaphoresis.

INTERACTIONS
Drug-drug. *Amphetamines, antiemetics, antipsychotics, buspirone, dextromethorphan, dihydroergotamine, opioids, other SSRIs or SSNRIs (duloxetine, venlafaxine), TCAs,* **tramadol,** *trazodone, tryptophan:* May increase risk of serotonin syndrome. Avoid other drugs that increase the availability of serotonin in the CNS; monitor patient closely if used together.

Antiarrhythmics (Class IA [procainamide, quinidine], Class III [amiodarone, sotalol]), antibiotics (clarithromycin, erythromycin, levofloxacin, moxifloxacin), antipsychotics (chlorpromazine, thioridazine), drugs that prolong QTc interval (dolasetron, methadone, ondansetron, pentamidine): May cause QTc prolongation and increase risk of torsades de pointes. Use together isn't recommended.

Anticoagulants, antiplatelet agents: May increase bleeding risk. Monitor therapy.

Carbamazepine: May increase citalopram clearance. Monitor patient for effects.

CNS drugs: May cause additive effects. Use together cautiously.

CYP2C19 inhibitors: May increase risk of QT-interval prolongation or ventricular arrhythmias. Limit citalopram dosage to 20 mg daily.

Drugs that affect coagulation (aspirin, NSAIDs): May increase bleeding risk. Monitor patient closely.

Drugs that inhibit CYP3A4 and CYP2C19: May cause decreased clearance of citalopram. Monitor patient for increased adverse effects.

Linezolid, methylene blue: May cause serotonin syndrome. Use together is contraindicated.

Lithium: May enhance serotonergic effect of citalopram. Use together cautiously, and monitor lithium level.

MAO inhibitors (phenelzine, selegiline, tranylcypromine): May cause serotonin syndrome or signs and symptoms resembling NMS. Use together is contraindicated. Avoid using within 14 days of MAO inhibitor therapy.

Pimozide: May increase risk of QT-interval prolongation or ventricular arrhythmias. Use together is contraindicated.

Sumatriptan: May cause weakness, hyperreflexia, and incoordination. Monitor patient closely.

Drug-lifestyle. *Alcohol use:* May increase CNS effects. Discourage use together.

EFFECTS ON LAB TEST RESULTS
None reported.

CONTRAINDICATIONS & CAUTIONS
• Contraindicated in patients hypersensitive to drug or its inactive components.

🜨 ☙ *Alert:* Drug isn't recommended for patients with congenital long QT syndrome, bradycardia, hypokalemia, hypomagnesemia, recent acute MI, or uncompensated HF.

🜨 ☙ *Alert:* High doses can prolong the QT interval and cause torsades de pointes, a potentially fatal heart rhythm. Maximum dose is 40 mg/day in patients age 60 and younger. Maximum dose is 20 mg/day in patients older than age 60, patients with hepatic impairment, and CYP2C19 poor metabolizers or patients taking cimetidine or another CYP2C19 inhibitor.

☙ *Alert:* Discontinue drug in patients with persistent QTc interval measurement longer than 500 msec.

☙ *Alert:* Concomitant use with linezolid or methylene blue can cause serotonin syndrome (fever, mental status changes, muscle twitching, diaphoresis, shivering or shaking, diarrhea, loss of coordination). Use together is contraindicated.

• Use cautiously in patients with history of mania, seizures, suicidality, or significant hepatic or renal impairment.

Dialyzable drug: No.

⚠ *Overdose S&S:* Dizziness, diaphoresis, nausea, vomiting, tremor, somnolence, sinus tachycardia, amnesia, confusion, coma, seizures, hyperventilation, cyanosis, rhab-domyolysis, ECG changes.

PREGNANCY-LACTATION-REPRODUCTION

• There are no adequate well-controlled studies during pregnancy. Use during pregnancy only if potential benefit justifies fetal risk
• Encourage patients to register in National Pregnancy Registry for Antidepressants at 1-844-405-6185 or https://womensmentalhealth.org/research/pregnancyregistry/antidepressants.
• Use in third trimester may be linked to neonatal complications at birth requiring respiratory support and tube feeding. Consider risk versus benefit of treatment during this time.
• Drug appears in human milk. Infants exposed in utero may have irritability, restlessness, excessive somnolence, decreased feeding, and weight loss. Consider patient's clinical need and risk to infant before use.

NURSING CONSIDERATIONS

• Correct electrolyte disturbances before starting drug; monitor patients at high risk for electrolyte disturbances periodically during therapy.
• Although drug hasn't been shown to impair psychomotor performance, any psychoactive drug has the potential to impair judgment, thinking, or motor skills.
Boxed Warning The possibility of a suicide attempt is inherent in depression and may persist until significant remission occurs. Closely supervise all patients for clinical worsening, suicidality, or unusual changes in behavior at start of drug therapy. ■
• Reduce risk of overdose by limiting amount of drug available per refill.
Boxed Warning Drug may increase the risk of suicidality in children, adolescents, and young adults with major depressive disorder or other psychiatric disorders. Drug isn't approved for use in children. ■
🕒 *Alert:* Monitor patient for serotonin syndrome. Signs and symptoms of serotonin syndrome may include restlessness, hallucinations, loss of coordination, fast heartbeat, rapid changes in BP, increased body temperature, overactive reflexes, nausea, vomiting, and diarrhea. Serotonin syndrome may be more likely to occur when starting or increasing the dose of the triptan, SSRI, or SSNRI.
🕒 *Alert:* If linezolid or methylene blue must be given, stop drug and monitor patient for serotonin toxicity for 2 weeks, or until

24 hours after the last dose of methylene blue or linezolid, whichever comes first. Treatment may be resumed 24 hours after last dose of methylene blue or linezolid.
• Don't discontinue drug abruptly because a discontinuation syndrome can develop, with varying symptoms.
• *Look alike–sound alike:* Don't confuse CeleXA with Zyprexa, CelebREX, or Cerebyx.

PATIENT TEACHING
Boxed Warning Advise families and caregivers to closely observe patient for increased suicidality. ■
🕒 *Alert:* Teach patient to recognize and immediately report symptoms of serotonin toxicity (fever, mental status changes, muscle twitching, excessive sweating, shivering or shaking, diarrhea, loss of coordination).
• Caution patient against use of MAO inhibitors while taking citalopram.
• Although improvement may take 1 to 4 weeks, inform patient to continue therapy as prescribed.
• Advise patient not to stop drug abruptly.
• Tell patient that drug may be taken in the morning or evening without regard to meals. If drowsiness occurs, patient should take drug in evening.
• Instruct patient to exercise caution when driving or operating hazardous machinery; drug may impair judgment, thinking, and motor skills.
• Advise patient to consult prescriber before taking other prescription or OTC drugs.
• Warn patient to avoid alcohol during therapy.
• Advise patient of childbearing potential to consult prescriber before breastfeeding.
• Instruct patient of childbearing potential to notify prescriber immediately if pregnancy is planned or suspected.

clarithromycin
kla-RITH-roe-mye-sin

Therapeutic class: Antibiotics
Pharmacologic class: Macrolides

AVAILABLE FORMS
Suspension: 125 mg/5 mL, 250 mg/5 mL
Tablets (extended-release) ⓄⓉⒸ: 500 mg
Tablets (film-coated): 250 mg, 500 mg

INDICATIONS & DOSAGES

Adjust-a-dose (for all indications): In patients with CrCl of less than 30 mL/minute, reduce dosage by 50%. For concomitant use with atazanavir or ritonavir in patients with CrCl of 30 to 60 mL/minute, reduce dosage by 50%; if CrCl is less than 30 mL/minute, reduce dosage by 75%. In patients with normal renal function, decrease clarithromycin dose by 50% when administered with atazanavir.

➤ **Pharyngitis or tonsillitis caused by *Streptococcus pyogenes***
Adults: 250 mg PO every 12 hours for 10 days.
Children age 6 months and older: 7.5 mg/kg PO every 12 hours for 10 days.

➤ **Acute maxillary sinusitis caused by *Streptococcus pneumoniae, Haemophilus influenzae,* or *Moraxella catarrhalis***
Adults: 500 mg PO every 12 hours for 14 days. Or, if using extended-release form, give two 500-mg tablets PO daily for 14 days.
Children age 6 months and older: 7.5 mg/kg PO every 12 hours for 10 days.

➤ **Acute worsening of chronic bronchitis caused by *M. catarrhalis* or *S. pneumoniae***
Adults: 250 mg PO every 12 hours for 7 to 14 days.

➤ **Acute worsening of chronic bronchitis caused by *H. influenzae* or *Haemophilus parainfluenzae***
Adults: 500 mg PO every 12 hours for 7 days *(H. parainfluenzae)* or 7 to 14 days *(H. influenzae)*.

➤ **Acute worsening of chronic bronchitis caused by *M. catarrhalis, S. pneumoniae, H. parainfluenzae,* or *H. influenzae***
Adults: Two 500-mg extended-release tablets PO daily for 7 days.

➤ **Mild to moderate community-acquired pneumonia caused by *H. influenzae, S. pneumoniae, Chlamydophila pneumoniae,* or *Mycoplasma pneumoniae***
Adults: 250 mg PO every 12 hours for 7 days *(H. influenzae)* or 7 to 14 days (other bacteria).

➤ **Mild to moderate community-acquired pneumonia caused by *H. influenzae, H. parainfluenzae, M. catarrhalis, S. pneumoniae, C. pneumoniae,* or *M. pneumoniae***
Adults: Two 500-mg extended-release tablets PO once daily for 7 days.

➤ **Mild to moderate community-acquired pneumonia caused by *S. pneumoniae, C. pneumoniae,* or *M. pneumoniae***
Children age 6 months and older: 7.5 mg/kg PO every 12 hours for 10 days.

➤ **Uncomplicated skin and skin-structure infections caused by *Staphylococcus aureus* or *S. pyogenes***
Adults: 250 mg PO every 12 hours for 7 to 14 days.
Children age 6 months and older: 7.5 mg/kg PO every 12 hours for 10 days.

➤ **Acute otitis media**
Children age 6 months and older: 7.5 mg/kg PO every 12 hours for 10 days.

➤ **To prevent and treat disseminated infection caused by MAC in patients with advanced HIV infection**
Adults: 500 mg PO b.i.d. Therapy should continue if clinical response is observed; can be discontinued when patient is considered at low risk for disseminated infection.
Children age 20 months and older: 7.5 mg/kg PO b.i.d., up to 500 mg b.i.d.

➤ **To reduce risk of duodenal ulcer recurrence in *Helicobacter pylori* infection**
Adults: 500 mg clarithromycin with 30 mg lansoprazole and 1 g amoxicillin, all given PO every 12 hours for 10 to 14 days. Or, 500 mg clarithromycin with 20 mg omeprazole and 1 g amoxicillin, all given PO every 12 hours for 10 days. Or, two-drug regimen with 500 mg clarithromycin PO every 8 hours and 40 mg omeprazole PO once daily for 14 days. Continue omeprazole for 14 additional days for symptom relief and ulcer healing. *Note:* Avoid use of clarithromycin triple therapy in patients with risk factors for macrolide resistance (e.g., prior macrolide exposure, local clarithromycin resistance rates of 15% or more).

ADMINISTRATION
PO

• There is resistance to macrolides in certain bacterial infections caused by *S. pneumoniae* and *S. aureus.* Obtain specimen for culture and sensitivity tests before giving. Begin therapy while awaiting results.
• Give immediate-release form with or without food; give extended-release tablets with food. Extended-release tablets should not be crushed.
• Don't refrigerate the suspension form; discard unused portion after 14 days.

ACTION

Binds to the 50S subunit of bacterial ribosomes, blocking protein synthesis; bacteriostatic or bactericidal, depending on concentration.

Route	Onset	Peak	Duration
PO	Unknown	2–3 hr	Unknown
PO (extended-release)	Unknown	5–8 hr	Unknown

Half-life: 3 to 7 hours; 5 to 9 hours (extended-release).

ADVERSE REACTIONS

CNS: headache, insomnia, taste perversion. **GI:** abdominal pain or discomfort, diarrhea, nausea, dyspepsia, flatulence, vomiting. **GU:** increased BUN level. **Hematologic:** coagulation abnormalities. **Hepatic:** abnormal LFT values. **Skin:** rash. **Other:** hypersensitivity reaction, including *anaphylaxis;* candidiasis.

INTERACTIONS

Drug-drug. *Alfuzosin, alprazolam, midazolam, triazolam:* May decrease clearance of these drugs, causing adverse reactions. Use together cautiously.

Almotriptan: May increase almotriptan serum concentration. Limit initial almotriptan adult dose to 6.25 mg and maximum adult dose to 12.5 mg/24 hours; avoid concurrent use in patients with impaired hepatic or renal function. Consider therapy modification.

Apixaban, dabigatran, edoxaban, rivaroxaban: May increase concentrations of these drugs. Apixaban, dabigatran, rivaroxaban, or edoxaban dosage reductions or avoidance of combination may be necessary. Consider therapy modification.

Atazanavir, ritonavir: May increase clarithromycin level. Reduce clarithromycin dosage in patients with renal impairment and in all patients taking atazanavir.

Carbamazepine, phenytoin: May inhibit metabolism of these drugs, increasing serum levels and risk of toxicity. Use together cautiously.

Colchicine: May increase colchicine level. Concomitant use is contraindicated in patients with renal or hepatic impairment. In those with normal renal and hepatic function, reduce colchicine dose.

Cyclosporine: May increase cyclosporine levels. Monitor cyclosporine level.

CYP3A4 inducers (efavirenz, nevirapine, rifabutin, rifampin): May decrease clarithromycin level. Consider alternative antibacterial treatment.

CYP3A4 substrates (amlodipine, diltiazem, nifedipine, verapamil): May increase substrate concentration. Avoid use together or reduce substrate dosage.

Digoxin, other P-gp substrates: May increase digoxin and substrate levels. Monitor patient for toxicity.

Dihydroergotamine, ergotamine: May cause acute ergot toxicity. Use together is contraindicated.

Fluconazole: May increase clarithromycin level. Monitor patient closely.

HMG-CoA reductase inhibitors: Lovastatin and simvastatin are contraindicated. Use with other statins may increase levels of these drugs and may rarely cause rhabdomyolysis. Use together cautiously. For adults, limit atorvastatin to a maximum dose of 20 mg/day and pravastatin to 40 mg/day.

Itraconazole: May increase itraconazole and clarithromycin concentrations. Use together cautiously.

Oral hypoglycemic agents (nateglinide, pioglitazone, repaglinide, rosiglitazone)/ insulin: May result in significant hypoglycemia. Monitor patient.

Other drugs that prolong QTc interval (amiodarone, antipsychotics, disopyramide, dofetilide, fluoroquinolones, fluoxetine, procainamide, quinidine, sotalol, TCAs): May have additive effects. Monitor ECG for QTc interval prolongation. Avoid using together if possible.

PDE5 inhibitors (sildenafil, tadalafil, vardenafil): May increase level of PDE5 inhibitor. Coadministration not recommended. Consider reduced PDE5 inhibitor dosage.

Pimozide: May cause torsades de pointes. Use together is contraindicated.

Theophylline: May increase theophylline level. Monitor drug level.

Warfarin: May prolong PT and increase INR. Monitor PT and INR carefully.

Zidovudine: May alter zidovudine level. Separate doses by at least 2 hours.

Drug-herb. *St. John's wort:* May decrease clarithromycin level. Avoid use.

EFFECTS ON LAB TEST RESULTS

- May increase BUN level and LFT values.
- May decrease WBC count.
- May prolong PT and increase INR.

Reactions in bold italics are *life-threatening*. Interactions may have a *rapid onset* or a *delayed onset*.

CONTRAINDICATIONS & CAUTIONS

⚠️ *Alert:* Use in patients with CAD has shown an increased risk of all-cause mortality 1 year or more after the end of treatment. Consider potential risk versus benefits before using in patients with suspected or confirmed heart disease. Use of an alternative antibiotic is recommended.

• Severe acute hypersensitivity reactions, including anaphylaxis, SJS, TEN, drug rash with eosinophilia, and Henoch-Schönlein purpura, have been reported. Discontinue drug and begin immediate treatment if these occur.

• Contraindicated in patients hypersensitive to clarithromycin, erythromycin, or other macrolides and in those receiving pimozide or other drugs that prolong QT interval or cause cardiac arrhythmias.

• Contraindicated in patients with a history of cholestatic jaundice or hepatic impairment associated with prior use of clarithromycin.

• Avoid use in patients with ongoing proarrhythmic conditions, such as uncorrected hypokalemia or hypomagnesemia or clinically significant bradycardia, and in patients receiving Class IA or Class III antiarrhythmics. Older adults may be more susceptible to drug-associated effects on the QT interval.

• Use cautiously in patients with hepatic or renal impairment.

• May cause exacerbation of or new signs and symptoms in patients with myasthenia gravis. Use cautiously in these patients.

• Drug may cause CDAD and pseudomembranous colitis, which can occur more than 2 months after therapy ends.

• Safety in patients with MAC infection younger than age 20 months hasn't been studied. Safety and effectiveness for pharyngitis, tonsillitis, community-acquired pneumonia, sinusitis, otitis media, and skin and skin-structure infections in children younger than age 6 months haven't been established. Safety and effectiveness of extended-release tablets in children haven't been established.
Dialyzable drug: No.

PREGNANCY-LACTATION-REPRODUCTION

• There are no adequate well-controlled studies during pregnancy; animal studies show adverse pregnancy outcome and embryo-fetal risk. Use during pregnancy only in clinical circumstances in which no alternative therapy is appropriate. Inform patient of fetal risk.

• Drug appears in human milk. Use cautiously during breastfeeding and weigh benefits against risks.

NURSING CONSIDERATIONS

⚠️ *Alert:* Be sure to use extended-release form to only treat infections for which it is approved.

• Monitor patient for superinfection. Drug may cause overgrowth of nonsusceptible bacteria or fungi.

• Monitor patient for hypersensitivity reactions and diarrhea.

• For MAC treatment, use drug in combination with other antimycobacterial drugs.

PATIENT TEACHING

• Tell patient to take drug as prescribed, even after feeling better.

• Caution patient to report all adverse reactions.

• Advise patient of the importance of taking immediate-release product every 12 hours.

• Instruct patient in safe drug administration and storage.

• Advise patient to inform prescriber of concurrent drugs patient may be taking, because of risk of significant drug interactions.

---

clascoterone
klas-KOE-ter-one

Winlevi

Therapeutic class: Antiacne drugs
Pharmacologic class: Androgen receptor inhibitors

AVAILABLE FORMS
Cream: 1%

INDICATIONS & DOSAGES
➤ **Acne vulgaris**
Adults and children age 12 and older: Apply thin uniform layer to affected area b.i.d., in morning and evening.

ADMINISTRATION
Topical
• Gently wash and dry affected area before applying drug.

• For topical use only; not for ophthalmic, oral, or vaginal use.

• Avoid getting drug in eyes, mouth, and mucous membranes; if contact occurs, rinse thoroughly with water.
• Avoid applying to cuts, abrasions, or eczematous or sunburned skin.
• Wash hands after applying drug.
• Store at room temperature. Discard drug 180 days after date prescription was filled or 1 month after first opening, whichever is sooner.

ACTION
Inhibits androgen receptors and decreases sebum production and inflammation.

Route	Onset	Peak	Duration
Topical	Unknown	Unknown	Unknown

Half-life: Unknown.

ADVERSE REACTIONS
CV: edema. **GU:** amenorrhea, polycystic ovaries. **Metabolic:** *hyperkalemia,* HPA axis suppression. **Skin:** dryness, erythema, pruritus, scaling, skin atrophy, stinging or burning, striae rubrae, telangiectasia.

INTERACTIONS
Drug-drug. *Astringents, medicated soaps and cleansers:* May increase skin irritation. Avoid use together.

EFFECTS ON LAB TEST RESULTS
• May increase potassium level.
• May decrease cortisol level.

CONTRAINDICATIONS & CAUTIONS
• HPA axis suppression may occur with prolonged use on large surface areas or use of occlusive dressings over drug.
• Avoid concomitant use of other potentially irritating topical products (medicated or abrasive soaps and cleansers, soaps and cosmetics with strong drying effect, products with high alcohol concentrations, astringents, spices, or lime).
• Safety and effectiveness in children younger than age 12 haven't been established. Use cautiously in children as they are more prone to systemic toxicity.
• Use cautiously in older adults.
Dialyzable drug: Unknown.

PREGNANCY-LACTATION-REPRODUCTION
• There are no studies during pregnancy. It's unknown if drug increases risk of major birth defects, miscarriage, or adverse maternal or fetal outcomes.
• It isn't known if drug appears in human milk or how drug affects milk production or infants who are breastfed. Consider benefit to the mother against possible risk to the infant.

NURSING CONSIDERATIONS
• Monitor patient for local skin reactions and avoid concomitant use of other potentially irritating topical products.
• Monitor patient for HPA axis suppression (decreased cortisol level, fatigue, muscle and joint pain, hypotension, irregular menstruation); if HPA suppression occurs, attempt to withdraw drug.

PATIENT TEACHING
• Instruct patient to gently wash and dry affected area before applying drug and to wash hands well after application.
• Advise patient to keep drug away from eyes, mouth, and mucous membranes. If contact occurs, tell patient to rinse areas thoroughly with water.
• Warn patient to avoid applying drug to cuts and abrasions, eczematous areas, and sunburned skin.
• Tell patient to avoid concomitant use of other potentially irritating topical products.

clevidipine
cle-VIH-deh-peen

Cleviprex

Therapeutic class: Antihypertensives
Pharmacologic class: Dihydropyridine calcium channel blockers

AVAILABLE FORMS
Injection: 0.5 mg/mL in 50- and 100-mL single-use vials

INDICATIONS & DOSAGES
➤ **To lower BP when oral therapy isn't feasible or desirable**
Adults: Begin infusion at 1 to 2 mg/hour and titrate by doubling the dose every 90 seconds. When BP approaches goal, titrate every 5 to 10 minutes at less than double the dose. Maintenance dose is usually 4 to 6 mg/hour. Maximum dose is 1,000 mL (average of

21 mg/hour) per 24-hour period. Drug isn't recommended for use beyond 72 hours.

ADMINISTRATION
IV

▼ Store vials in cartons in refrigerator because drug is photosensitive. May store unopened vials at controlled room temperature (77° F [25° C]) for up to 2 months.

▼ Upon transfer to room temperature, mark vials in cartons with date. Don't return to refrigerated storage after beginning room temperature storage.

▼ Maintain aseptic technique when handling solution. Drug can support growth of microorganisms.

▼ Invert vial several times to mix emulsion before use.

▼ Inspect solution and discard if particulate matter or discoloration is present before use. Don't dilute.

▼ Use a continuous infusion pump to regulate flow.

▼ Discard unused portion within 12 hours after stopper puncture.

▼ **Incompatibilities:** Don't administer drug in same IV line with other medications.

ACTION
Inhibits calcium ion influx across cardiac and smooth-muscle cells, decreasing contractility and oxygen demand. Dilates coronary arteries and arterioles, decreasing systemic vascular resistance.

Route	Onset	Peak	Duration
IV	2–4 min	Unknown	5–15 min

Half-life: 15 minutes; metabolite, 9 hours.

ADVERSE REACTIONS
CNS: headache. **CV:** atrial fibrillation, hypotension, reflex tachycardia. **GI:** nausea, vomiting. **GU:** *acute renal failure.*

INTERACTIONS
None reported.

EFFECTS ON LAB TEST RESULTS
None reported.

CONTRAINDICATIONS & CAUTIONS
• Contraindicated in patients hypersensitive to soybeans, soy products, eggs, or egg products and in those with defective lipid metabolism (pathologic hyperlipidemia, lipoid nephrosis, acute pancreatitis) or severe aortic stenosis.

• Use cautiously in patients with HF, and monitor for exacerbations.

• Safety and effectiveness in children younger than age 18 haven't been established.
Dialyzable drug: Unknown.

⚠ *Overdose S&S:* Hypotension, reflex tachycardia.

PREGNANCY-LACTATION-REPRODUCTION
• There are no adequate well-controlled studies during pregnancy. Use during pregnancy only if potential benefit justifies fetal risk.

• It isn't known if drug appears in human milk. Consider the possibility of infant exposure during breastfeeding; monitor infant for adverse effects.

NURSING CONSIDERATIONS
• Monitor BP and HR continuously, especially when starting drug and during dosage adjustments.

• Drug may exacerbate HF; monitor patient closely.

• Titrate dose slowly; rapid titration may cause hypotension and reflex tachycardia. If either occurs, decrease clevidipine dosage.

• Monitor patient who received prolonged infusion for rebound HTN for at least 8 hours after infusion is stopped if no other antihypertensive is prescribed.

• To convert to oral therapy, discontinue or titrate drug downward while appropriate oral therapy is established. When an oral antihypertensive is started, consider the lag time of onset of the oral agent's effect and continue BP monitoring until desired effect is achieved.

• Drug isn't a beta-adrenergic blocker; if given with beta-adrenergic blocker, gradually reduce beta-adrenergic blocker dosage to avoid withdrawal symptoms.

PATIENT TEACHING
• Tell patient to report adverse reactions promptly.

• Advise patient to seek medical attention immediately if signs and symptoms of hypertensive emergency occur (visual changes, neurologic symptoms, HF).

clindamycin hydrochloride
klin-da-MYE-sin

Cleocin Hydrochloride, Dalacin C ✽

clindamycin palmitate hydrochloride
Cleocin Pediatric, Dalacin C Flavored Granules ✽

clindamycin phosphate (injection)
Cleocin Phosphate, Dalacin C Phosphate ✽

Therapeutic class: Antibiotics
Pharmacologic class: Lincomycin derivatives

AVAILABLE FORMS
clindamycin hydrochloride
Capsules: 75 mg, 150 mg, 300 mg
clindamycin palmitate hydrochloride
Granules for oral solution: 75 mg/5 mL
clindamycin phosphate (injection)
Infusion (premixed): 300 mg (50 mL), 600 mg (50 mL), 900 mg (50 mL)
Injection: 150 mg/mL

INDICATIONS & DOSAGES
➤ **Infections caused by sensitive staphylococci, streptococci, pneumococci, *Bacteroides, Fusobacterium, Clostridium perfringens*, or other sensitive aerobic and anaerobic organisms**
Adults: 150 to 450 mg PO every 6 hours; or 300 to 600 mg IM or IV every 6, 8, or 12 hours. In more severe infections, dosage may be increased to 1,200 to 2,700 mg/day IM or IV in two, three, or four divided doses. In life-threatening infections, dosages as high as 4,800 mg daily can be given.
Children able to swallow capsules: 8 to 20 mg/kg/day PO divided in three or four equal doses.
Children ages 1 month to 16 years: 20 to 40 mg/kg/day or 350 to 450 mg/m^2/day IM or IV in three or four equal doses. In beta-hemolytic streptococcal infections, treatment should continue for at least 10 days.
Neonates younger than age 1 month: 15 to 20 mg/kg/day IM or IV in three or four equal doses. Consider 15 mg/kg/day for small premature infants.

ADMINISTRATION
PO
• Obtain specimen for culture and sensitivity tests before giving first dose. Begin therapy while awaiting results.
• Give capsule form with a full glass of water to prevent esophageal irritation.
• Don't refrigerate reconstituted oral solution because it will thicken. Drug is stable for 2 weeks at room temperature.
IV
▼ Obtain specimen for culture and sensitivity tests before giving first dose. Begin therapy while awaiting results.
▼ Never give undiluted as a bolus.
▼ For infusion, dilute each 300 mg in 50-mL solution and give over 10 to 60 minutes at no more than 30 mg/minute.
▼ Check site daily for phlebitis and irritation.
▼ Drug may contain benzyl alcohol. Benzyl alcohol has been associated with a fatal gasping syndrome in premature infants.
▼ **Incompatibilities:** Aminophylline, ampicillin, barbiturates, calcium gluconate, magnesium sulfate, phenytoin.
IM
• Obtain specimen for culture and sensitivity tests before giving first dose. Begin therapy while awaiting results.
• IM administration uses undiluted solution.
• Inject deep into muscle. Rotate sites. Don't exceed 600 mg per injection.

ACTION
Inhibits bacterial protein synthesis by binding to the 50S subunit of the ribosome.

Route	Onset	Peak	Duration
PO	Unknown	45–60 min	Unknown
IV	Immediate	Immediate	Unknown
IM	Unknown	1–3 hr	Unknown

Half-life: 2.5 to 3 hours.

ADVERSE REACTIONS
CNS: metallic taste. **CV:** thrombophlebitis. **GI:** nausea, *CDAD,* abdominal pain, diarrhea, vomiting, esophageal ulcer, esophagitis. **Hematologic:** *thrombocytopenia, transient leukopenia,* eosinophilia. **Hepatic:** jaundice, elevated LFT values. **Skin:** rash, urticaria, pruritus, dermatitis. **Other:** hypersensitivity reactions.

Reactions in bold italics are *life-threatening*. Interactions may have a *rapid onset* or a ***delayed onset***.

INTERACTIONS

Drug-drug. *CYP3A4 inducers (phenytoin, rifampin):* May decrease clindamycin concentration. Monitor patient for loss of efficacy.
CYP3A4 and CYP3A5 inhibitors (diltiazem, erythromycin, itraconazole, ritonavir, saquinavir, verapamil): May increase clindamycin concentration. Monitor patient for adverse effects.
Live-virus vaccines: May decrease vaccine effectiveness. Don't give together.
Neuromuscular blockers: May increase neuromuscular blockade. Monitor patient closely.

EFFECTS ON LAB TEST RESULTS

• May increase ALP, AST, and bilirubin levels.
• May increase eosinophil count. May decrease platelet and WBC counts.

CONTRAINDICATIONS & CAUTIONS

• Contraindicated in patients hypersensitive to drug or lincomycin. Severe hypersensitivity reactions requiring emergency treatment have been reported. Severe skin reactions and DRESS syndrome have been reported. Discontinue drug if these occur.
• Use only to treat or prevent infections proven or strongly suspected to be caused by bacteria to reduce development of drug-resistant bacteria.
• Clindamycin use may result in overgrowth of nonsusceptible organisms, particularly yeasts. Monitor patient for sign of superinfection.
• Use cautiously in neonates and patients with renal or hepatic disease, asthma, history of GI disease, or significant allergies.
• Severe or fatal reactions, such as TEN, DRESS syndrome, and SJS, have been reported. Discontinue drug if severe skin reaction occurs.
Boxed Warning Clindamycin has been associated with development of CDAD, which may evolve into severe, possibly fatal, colitis; its use should be reserved for serious infections. Don't use drug in nonbacterial infections. ■
Dialyzable drug: No.

PREGNANCY-LACTATION-REPRODUCTION

• There are no adequate studies during pregnancy. Use during pregnancy only if clearly needed and potential benefit justifies fetal risk.
• Drug appears in human milk. Use during breastfeeding isn't recommended. Monitor infant who is breastfed for diarrhea and candidiasis.

NURSING CONSIDERATIONS

• IM injection may raise CK level in response to muscle irritation.
• Monitor renal, hepatic, and hematopoietic functions during prolonged therapy.
• Observe patient for signs and symptoms of superinfection.
• *Alert:* Don't give opioid antidiarrheals to treat drug-induced diarrhea; they may prolong and worsen this condition.
Boxed Warning Diarrhea, colitis, and pseudomembranous colitis have developed up to 2 months after cessation of drug therapy. If CDAD is suspected or confirmed, the antibiotic not directed against *C. difficile* may need to be discontinued. Initiate fluid and electrolyte management, protein supplementation, antibiotic treatment of *C. difficile*, and surgical evaluation as clinically indicated. ■
• Drug doesn't penetrate blood-brain barrier.

PATIENT TEACHING

• Advise patient to take capsule form with a full glass of water to prevent esophageal irritation.
• Warn patient that IM injection may be painful.
• Tell patient to report discomfort at IV insertion site.
• Instruct patient to report all adverse reactions (especially diarrhea and hypersensitivity reactions). Warn patient not to self-treat diarrhea because drug may cause life-threatening colitis.

clindamycin phosphate (intravaginal, topical)

klin-da-MYE-sin

Cleocin, Cleocin T, Clinda-Derm, Clindagel, Clinda-T✚, Clindesse, Clindets, Dalacin✚, Evoclin, Xaciato

Therapeutic class: Antibiotics
Pharmacologic class: Lincomycin derivatives

AVAILABLE FORMS

Foam: 1%
Gel: 1%, 2%
Lotion: 1%
Pledget: 1%*

Topical cream: 2%
Topical solution: 1%*
Vaginal cream: 2%
Vaginal suppositories: 100 mg

INDICATIONS & DOSAGES

➤ **Inflammatory acne vulgaris**
Adults and children age 12 and older: Apply to skin b.i.d., morning and evening, or once daily if using Clindagel or Evoclin.

➤ **Bacterial vaginosis**
Adults: 1 applicatorful vaginally at bedtime for 3 to 7 days in patients who aren't pregnant or 7 days in patients who are pregnant, or 1 suppository vaginally at bedtime for 3 days, or 1 applicatorful of Clindesse vaginally as a single dose.
Adults and children age 12 and older: 1 applicatorful 2% gel vaginally as a single dose.

ADMINISTRATION

Topical
• Wash area with warm water and soap, rinse, pat dry, and wait 30 minutes after washing or shaving to apply.
• Avoid excessive washing of affected area.
• Apply to entire area, but avoid contact with eyes, nose, mouth, and other mucous membranes.
• Remove pledgets from foil just before use.
• Use pledgets only once and then discard; more than 1 pledget may be used per application.
• If using foam or Clindagel, discontinue use if there has been no improvement after 6 to 8 weeks, or if condition worsens.

Vaginal
• Make sure patient knows how to use applicators that come with drug.

ACTION

Bacteriostatic or bactericidal based on drug level and susceptibility of organism; suppresses growth of susceptible organisms in sebaceous glands by blocking protein synthesis.

Route	Onset	Peak	Duration
Topical, vaginal	Unknown	Unknown	Unknown
Vaginal (2% gel)	Unknown	6 hr	Unknown

Half-life: Topical and vaginal cream, 1.5 to 2.5 hours; vaginal suppositories, 11 hours.

ADVERSE REACTIONS

CNS: headache. **EENT:** pharyngitis. **GI:** constipation. **GU:** vulvovaginal disease, vulvovaginitis, vulvar irritation, vaginal discomfort, vaginal candidiasis. **Musculoskeletal:** back pain. **Skin:** dryness, redness, burning, irritation, pruritus, swelling, oily skin, exfoliation.

INTERACTIONS

Drug-drug. *Erythromycin (topical or systemic):* May diminish clindamycin's effect. Avoid combination.
Isotretinoin: May cause cumulative dryness, resulting in excessive skin irritation. Use together cautiously.
Neuromuscular blockers: May increase action of neuromuscular blocker. Use together cautiously.
Drug-lifestyle. *Abrasive or medicated soaps or cleansers, acne products, or other preparations containing peeling drugs (benzoyl peroxide, resorcinol, salicylic acid, sulfur, tretinoin), alcohol-containing products (aftershave, cosmetics, perfumed toiletries, shaving creams or lotions), astringent soaps or cosmetics, medicated cosmetics or cover-ups:* May cause cumulative dryness, resulting in excessive skin irritation. Urge caution.

EFFECTS ON LAB TEST RESULTS

• May increase liver enzyme levels.

CONTRAINDICATIONS & CAUTIONS

• Contraindicated in patients hypersensitive to clindamycin or lincomycin and in those with history of ulcerative colitis, regional enteritis, or antibiotic-related colitis.
• Intravaginal form can be absorbed systemically and cause CDAD even 2 months after therapy ends.
Dialyzable drug: No.
⚠ *Overdose S&S:* Systemic effects.

PREGNANCY-LACTATION-REPRODUCTION

• There are no adequate studies during pregnancy. Use during pregnancy only if clearly needed and potential benefit justifies fetal risk.
• Drug appears in human milk. Use cautiously during breastfeeding. If topical drug is applied to the chest, patient should avoid accidental ingestion by the infant.

Reactions in bold italics are *life-threatening*. Interactions may have a *rapid onset* or a *delayed onset*.

C

NURSING CONSIDERATIONS
• For treating acne, drug may be used with tretinoin or benzoyl peroxide, as well as systemic antibiotics.
• Drug can cause excessive dryness.
• Topical solution and pledgets contain alcohol base, which may irritate eyes.
• Monitor older adults for systemic effects.
• Monitor patients for diarrhea.
• Monitor patient for vulvovaginal candidiasis, which may require antifungal treatment in patients receiving vaginal form.

PATIENT TEACHING
• Instruct patient in proper drug administration.
• Tell patient to wash area with warm water and soap, rinse, pat dry, and wait 30 minutes after washing or shaving before applying topically.
• Warn patient to avoid excessive washing of area. Tell patient to cover entire affected area but to avoid contact with eyes, nose, mouth, and other mucous membranes.
• Instruct patient to use other prescribed acne medicines at a different time.
• Tell patient to use only as prescribed.
• Instruct patient to dab, not roll, applicator-tipped bottle. If tip becomes dry, patient should invert bottle and depress tip several times to moisten.
• Warn patient not to smoke while applying topical solution or foam.
• Advise patient that some vaginal forms contain mineral oil, which can weaken latex or rubber products, such as condoms and diaphragms, and that patient should use another form of birth control during and within 3 days of therapy (Cleocin) or 5 days (Clindesse). Polyurethane condoms aren't recommended during or for 7 days after treatment with Xaciato; patient may use latex or polyisoprene condoms.
• Advise patient to avoid sexual intercourse and use of tampons or douches during vaginal treatment.
• Instruct patient to notify prescriber immediately if abdominal pain or diarrhea occurs. Inform patient that an antidiarrheal may worsen condition and should only be used as directed by prescriber.
• Advise patient to complete entire course of therapy.

clobetasol propionate
kloe-BAY-ta-sol

Clobex, Clodan, Impeklo, Impoyz, Olux, Olux-E, Tasoprol, Tovet

Therapeutic class: Corticosteroids
Pharmacologic class: Corticosteroids

AVAILABLE FORMS
Cream: 0.025%, 0.05%
Cream (emollient): 0.05%
Foam: 0.05%*
Gel: 0.05%
Lotion: 0.05%
Ointment: 0.05%
Scalp application: 0.05%*
Shampoo: 0.05%*
Solution: 0.05%*
Spray: 0.05%*

INDICATIONS & DOSAGES
➤ **Short-term topical treatment for moderate to severe plaque-type psoriasis of nonscalp regions, excluding the face and intertriginous areas**
Adults: Apply thin layer of lotion or cream to affected areas b.i.d., morning and evening, for up to 14 days. Or, apply spray directly onto affected areas b.i.d. and rub in gently and completely. For localized lesions (less than 10% of BSA) that haven't improved sufficiently, continue treatment for up to 2 more weeks. Total dose shouldn't exceed 50 g (50 mL) weekly.
Adolescents age 16 and older: Apply thin layer of emollient cream to affected areas b.i.d. and rub in gently and completely. If applied to 5% to 10% of BSA, can be used for up to 4 consecutive weeks. Total dosage shouldn't exceed 50 g (50 mL) weekly.
➤ **Inflammation and pruritus from corticosteroid-responsive dermatoses**
Adults: Apply thin layer of cream, emollient cream, foam, gel, lotion, solution, or ointment to affected areas b.i.d., morning and evening, for maximum of 14 days. Total dose shouldn't exceed 50 g (50 mL) weekly.
Children age 12 and older: Apply thin layer of cream, emollient cream, foam, gel, solution, or ointment to affected areas b.i.d., morning and evening, for maximum of 14 days. Total dose shouldn't exceed 50 g (50 mL) weekly.

➤ **Short-term topical treatment of mild to moderate plaque-type psoriasis of non-scalp regions, excluding the face and intertriginous areas**

Adults and children age 12 and older: Apply thin layer of foam to affected areas b.i.d., morning and evening, for maximum of 14 days. Total dose shouldn't exceed 50 g (21 capfuls) weekly.

➤ **Inflammation and pruritus of moderate to severe corticosteroid-responsive dermatoses of the scalp**

Adults and children age 12 and older: Apply thin layer of solution to the affected scalp area b.i.d., morning and evening. Massage into affected scalp area gently and completely. Limit treatment to 14 days, with no more than 50 g (50 mL) weekly.

➤ **Moderate to severe scalp psoriasis**

Adults: Apply thin film of shampoo to affected areas of dry scalp once daily. Leave in place for 15 minutes before lathering and rinsing. Limit treatment to 4 consecutive weeks. If complete disease control isn't achieved after 4 weeks, substitute treatment with a less potent topical steroid. Maximum dose is 50 g (50 mL) weekly. Or, apply thin layer of foam to scalp b.i.d. for up to 2 weeks. Maximum dose is 50 g (21 capfuls) weekly.

Children age 12 and older: Apply thin layer of foam to scalp b.i.d. for up to 2 weeks. Maximum dose is 50 g (21 capfuls) weekly.

ADMINISTRATION
Topical
- Apply the smallest amount that will cover affected area.
- Apply shampoo to dry scalp.
- Gently wash skin before applying. To prevent skin damage, rub medication in gently and completely. When treating hairy sites, part hair and apply directly to lesions.
- To dispense foam, hold the can upside down and depress the actuator.
- Avoid applying near eyes or mucous membranes or in ear canal.
- � *Alert:* Don't use occlusive dressings or bandages. Don't cover or wrap treated areas unless directed by prescriber.

ACTION
Unclear. Diffuses across cell membranes to form complexes with receptors, showing antiinflammatory, antipruritic, vasoconstrictive, and antiproliferative activity. Considered a very-high-potency to high-potency drug, according to vasoconstrictive properties.

Route	Onset	Peak	Duration
Topical	Unknown	Unknown	Unknown

Half-life: Unknown.

ADVERSE REACTIONS
CNS: headache. **EENT:** nasopharyngitis, streptococcal pharyngitis (spray). **GU:** glycosuria. **Metabolic:** hyperglycemia. **Skin:** burning, pruritus, irritation, dryness, erythema, folliculitis, skin fissure, stinging, perioral dermatitis, allergic contact dermatitis, hypopigmentation, hypertrichosis, acneiform eruptions, eczema, skin atrophy, telangiectasia. **Respiratory:** URI (spray). **Other:** *HPA axis suppression,* Cushing syndrome, finger numbness.

INTERACTIONS
None significant.

EFFECTS ON LAB TEST RESULTS
- May increase glucose level.

CONTRAINDICATIONS & CAUTIONS
- Contraindicated in patients hypersensitive to corticosteroids and in those with primary scalp infections (scalp solution only).
- Topical corticosteroids may be absorbed and cause hyperadrenocorticism (Cushing syndrome), hyperglycemia, glycosuria, or suppression of the HPA axis, particularly in younger children and in patients receiving high doses for prolonged periods.
- Rarely, prolonged treatment with corticosteroids is associated with development of Kaposi sarcoma.
- Don't use as monotherapy for primary bacterial infections (impetigo, paronychia, erysipelas, cellulitis, angular cheilitis, erythrasma), rosacea, perioral dermatitis, or acne.
- Don't use very-high-potency or high-potency agents on the face, groin, or axilla areas.
- Drug isn't for ophthalmic use. Avoid contact with eyes as drug may increase risk of posterior subcapsular cataracts and glaucoma.
- Use cautiously in children. Use in children younger than age 12 isn't recommended.

Reactions in bold italics are *life-threatening*. Interactions may have a *rapid onset* or a ***delayed onset***.

Lotion, shampoo, and spray formulations aren't recommended for use in children age 17 and younger.
Dialyzable drug: Unknown.
⚠ *Overdose S&S:* Systemic effects.

PREGNANCY-LACTATION-REPRODUCTION
• There are no adequate studies during pregnancy. Use during pregnancy only if potential benefit justifies fetal risk. Extensive use during pregnancy isn't recommended.
• It isn't known if drug appears in human milk. Use cautiously during breastfeeding.

NURSING CONSIDERATIONS
• If antifungal or antibiotic combined with corticosteroid fails to provide prompt improvement, stop corticosteroid until infection is controlled.
• Stop drug and notify prescriber if skin infection, striae, or atrophy occurs.
• HPA axis suppression occurs at doses as low as 2 g daily. Monitor children closely.

PATIENT TEACHING
• Teach patient how to apply drug, to avoid contact with eyes, and to wash hands after application.
• Tell patient to stop drug and report signs of systemic absorption, skin irritation or ulceration, hypersensitivity, or infection.
• Warn patient to use drug for no longer than 14 consecutive days, except shampoo, which can be used for 4 consecutive weeks.
• Tell patient using the foam to invert can and dispense a small amount of Olux foam (up to a golf ball-size dollop) into the cap of the can, onto a saucer or other cool surface, or directly on the lesion, taking care to avoid contact with the eyes. Dispensing directly onto hands isn't recommended because foam will melt immediately on contact with warm skin. Tell patient to move hair away from affected area of scalp so that foam can be applied to each affected area.
• Tell patient using foam that contents are flammable and under pressure, and to avoid smoking during and immediately after application and to keep can away from flames. Also tell patient not to puncture or incinerate container.

clonazePAM
kloe-NAZ-e-pam

KlonoPIN⌀

Therapeutic class: Anticonvulsants
Pharmacologic class: Benzodiazepines
Controlled substance schedule: IV

AVAILABLE FORMS
Tablets: 0.5 mg, 1 mg, 2 mg
Tablets (ODTs): 0.125 mg, 0.25 mg, 0.5 mg, 1 mg, 2 mg

INDICATIONS & DOSAGES
➤ **Lennox-Gastaut syndrome, atypical absence seizures, akinetic and myoclonic seizures**
Adults and children older than age 10 or weighing more than 30 kg: Initially, no more than 1.5 mg/day PO in three divided doses. May be increased by 0.5 to 1 mg every 3 days until seizures are controlled or adverse effects prevent further increases. If given in unequal doses, give largest dose at bedtime. Maximum recommended daily dose is 20 mg.
Children age 10 and younger or weighing 30 kg or less: Initially, 0.01 to 0.03 mg/kg PO daily (not to exceed 0.05 mg/kg daily) in two or three divided doses. Increase by 0.25 to 0.5 mg every third day to maximum maintenance dose of 0.1 to 0.2 mg/kg PO daily divided into three equal doses, as needed.
➤ **Panic disorder**
Adults: Initially, 0.25 mg PO b.i.d.; increase in increments of 0.125 to 0.25 mg b.i.d. every 3 days until panic disorder is controlled, or adverse reactions are seen, to target dose of 1 mg daily. Some patients may benefit from dosages up to maximum of 4 mg daily. To achieve 4 mg daily, increase dosage in increments of 0.125 to 0.25 mg b.i.d. every 3 days, as tolerated, until panic disorder is controlled or adverse effects make further increases undesired. Taper drug with decrease of 0.125 mg b.i.d. every 3 days until drug is stopped.

ADMINISTRATION
PO
• Have patient swallow tablets whole with water. Give ODT to patient with or without water.

• Peel back the foil of the ODT pouch carefully. Don't push ODT through foil.
• Pharmacist can prepare oral suspension from tablets if necessary for younger patients.

ACTION

Unknown. Probably acts by facilitating the effects of the inhibitory neurotransmitter GABA.

Route	Onset	Peak	Duration
PO	20–40 min	1–4 hr	6–12 hr

Half-life: Adults, 17 to 60 hours; children, 22 to 33 hours; neonates, 22 to 81 hours.

ADVERSE REACTIONS

CNS: amnesia, aphonia, choreiform movements, confusion, depression, emotional lability, drowsiness, memory impairment, dysarthria, dysdiadochokinesis, "glassy-eyed" appearance, headache, hemiparesis, hypotonia, hysteria, insomnia, psychosis, slurred speech, tremor, vertigo, paradoxical reactions (aggressive behavior, agitation, anxiety, excitability, hostility, irritability, nervousness, nightmares and vivid dreams, sleep disturbances), fever, ataxia, abnormal coordination, somnolence, dizziness, reduced intellectual ability. **CV:** palpitations, edema.
EENT: abnormal eye movements, diplopia, nystagmus, blurred vision, pharyngitis, rhinitis, rhinorrhea, sinusitis, coated tongue, dry mouth, sore gums. **GI:** constipation, diarrhea, encopresis, gastritis, increased or decreased appetite, nausea, abdominal pain.
GU: dysuria, enuresis, nocturia, urine retention, dysmenorrhea, vaginitis, delayed ejaculation, erectile dysfunction, increased libido, urinary frequency, UTI. **Hematologic:** anemia, eosinophilia, *leukopenia, thrombocytopenia.* **Hepatic:** hepatomegaly, transient elevations of serum transaminases and ALP.
Metabolic: dehydration, weight loss or gain.
Musculoskeletal: muscle weakness, myalgia. **Respiratory:** chest congestion, hypersecretion in upper respiratory tract passages, respiratory depression, shortness of breath, bronchitis, URI, cough. **Skin:** hair loss, hirsutism, rash. **Other:** hypersensitivity reaction, general deterioration, lymphadenopathy, flulike symptoms.

INTERACTIONS

Drug-drug. *Carbamazepine, phenobarbital:* May lower clonazepam levels. Monitor patient closely.

Clozapine: May increase clozapine-related toxicities. Consider therapy modification.
CNS depressants: May increase CNS depression. Avoid using together.
Digoxin: May increase digoxin level and toxicity. Monitor digoxin level.
Fluconazole, itraconazole, ketoconazole, miconazole: May increase and prolong clonazepam level, CNS depression, and psychomotor impairment. Avoid using together.
Methadone: May increase potential for fatal respiratory depression. Use cautiously.
Olanzapine: May enhance clonazepam-related toxicity. Avoid concomitant use with IM olanzapine due to risks of additive adverse events.
Boxed Warning *Opioids:* May cause slow or difficult breathing, sedation, coma, and death. Avoid use together. If use together is necessary, limit dosage and duration of each drug to the minimum necessary for desired effect. ∎
Phenytoin: May lower clonazepam level or increase phenytoin level. Monitor serum concentrations of both drugs.
Protease inhibitors (nelfinavir, ritonavir): May cause severe respiratory depression. Monitor patient carefully.
SSRIs: May enhance adverse/toxic effects of SSRIs and increase risk of psychomotor impairment. Monitor patient closely.
Thalidomide: May enhance CNS depressant effect of thalidomide. Avoid concurrent use.
Theophylline: May decrease clonazepam effects. Monitor patient closely.
Valproic acid: May increase clonazepam toxicity and absence status and increase seizure risk and teratogenic effects of both drugs in first trimester. Use cautiously.
Drug-herb. *Kava kava:* May enhance adverse or toxic effects of drug. Use cautiously.
St. John's wort: May decrease clonazepam serum concentration, resulting in decreased drug effects. Consider therapy modification.
Drug-lifestyle. *Alcohol use:* May cause additive CNS effects. Discourage use together.

EFFECTS ON LAB TEST RESULTS
• May increase LFT values.
• May increase eosinophil count.
• May decrease Hb level and platelet and WBC counts.

CONTRAINDICATIONS & CAUTIONS

Boxed Warning *Opioid class warning:* Opioids should only be prescribed with benzodiazepines or other CNS depressants to patients for whom alternative treatment options are inadequate. ■

Boxed Warning Benzodiazepine use exposes patient to risks of abuse, misuse, and addiction, which can lead to overdose or death. Assess each patient's risk of abuse, misuse, and addiction before prescribing and periodically during therapy. ■

Boxed Warning Continued use of benzodiazepines, including clonazepam, may lead to clinically significant physical dependence. Risk increases with longer treatment duration and higher daily dose. ■

Boxed Warning Abrupt discontinuation or rapid dosage reduction of benzodiazepines after continued use may precipitate acute withdrawal reactions, which can be life-threatening. To reduce risk of withdrawal reactions, gradually taper drug to discontinue or reduce dosage. ■

• Contraindicated in patients hypersensitive to benzodiazepines and in those with significant hepatic disease or acute angle-closure glaucoma.

• Use cautiously in patients with mixed-type seizures because drug may cause generalized tonic-clonic seizures.

• Use cautiously in children; in patients with chronic respiratory disease, open-angle glaucoma, porphyria, or a history of drug or alcohol addiction; in patients who are debilitated, and in those at risk for falls.

• Use cautiously in older adults. Drug may accumulate due to potential decrease in hepatic and renal function.

Dialyzable drug: No.

⚠ *Overdose S&S:* Somnolence, confusion, coma, diminished reflexes.

PREGNANCY-LACTATION-REPRODUCTION

• Drug may cause fetal harm. Use during pregnancy only if clearly needed and potential benefit justifies fetal risk.

• Drug may cause neonatal flaccidity, respiratory and feeding difficulties, and hypothermia in infants born to patients who received benzodiazepines late in pregnancy. In addition, neonates born to patients who received benzodiazepines late in pregnancy may be at some risk for experiencing withdrawal symptoms during the postnatal period.

• Encourage patients who are taking drug during pregnancy to register in the North American AED Pregnancy Registry (1-888-233-2334 or www.aedpregnancyregistry.org); registration must be done by patients themselves.

• Drug appears in human milk. Patient should discontinue breastfeeding or discontinue drug, taking into account importance of drug to the patient.

NURSING CONSIDERATIONS

⊕ *Alert:* Closely monitor all patients for changes in behavior that may indicate worsening of suicidality or depression.

• Don't stop drug abruptly because this may worsen seizures. Notify prescriber at once if adverse reactions develop.

• Closely assess response of older adults, who are more sensitive to drug's CNS effects.

• Monitor patient for oversedation.

• Monitor CBC and LFTs.

• Withdrawal symptoms are similar to those of barbiturates.

• To reduce inconvenience of somnolence when drug is used for panic disorder, giving one dose at bedtime may be desirable.

Boxed Warning Monitor patient taking an opioid concomitantly with clonazepam for signs and symptoms of respiratory depression and sedation. ■

• *Look alike–sound alike:* Don't confuse clonazepam with clonidine, clozapine, or lorazepam. Don't confuse Klonopin with clonidine.

PATIENT TEACHING

Boxed Warning Caution patient that benzodiazepines, even at recommended doses, increase risk of abuse, misuse, and addiction, which can lead to overdose and death, especially when used with other drugs (opioid analgesics), alcohol, or illicit substances. Warn patient or caregiver of patient taking an opioid with a benzodiazepine, CNS depressant, or alcohol to seek immediate medical attention for dizziness, light-headedness, extreme sleepiness, slowed or difficult breathing, or unresponsiveness. ■

Boxed Warning Teach patient signs and symptoms of benzodiazepine abuse, misuse, and addiction (abdominal pain, amnesia, anorexia, anxiety, aggression, ataxia, blurred vision, confusion, depression, disinhibition, disorientation, dizziness, euphoria, impaired concentration and memory, indigestion, irritability, muscle pain, slurred speech, tremors, vertigo, delirium, paranoia, suicidality, seizures, difficulty breathing, coma) and to seek emergency medical help if they occur. Demonstrate proper disposal of unused drug. Advise patient not to take drug at a higher dose, more frequently, or for longer than prescribed. ▪

Boxed Warning Tell patient that continued use of drug for several days to weeks may lead to physical dependence and that abrupt discontinuation or rapid dosage reduction may precipitate acute withdrawal reactions (unusual movements, responses, or expressions; seizures; sudden and severe mental or nervous system changes; depression; seeing or hearing things that others don't; homicidal thoughts; extreme increase in activity or talking; losing touch with reality; suicidality), which can be life-threatening. Instruct patient that drug discontinuation or dosage reduction may require a slow taper. ▪

Boxed Warning Stress the possibility of development of protracted withdrawal syndrome (anxiety; trouble remembering, learning, or concentrating; depression; problems sleeping; feeling like insects are crawling under the skin; weakness; shaking; muscle twitching; burning or prickling feeling in the hands, arms, legs, or feet; ringing in the ears), with symptoms lasting weeks to more than 12 months. ▪

• Advise patient to avoid driving and other hazardous activities that require mental alertness until drug's CNS effects are known.
• Instruct parent to monitor child's school performance because drug may interfere with attentiveness.
• Warn patient and parents not to stop drug abruptly because seizures may occur.
• Advise patient that drug isn't for use during pregnancy or breastfeeding.
• Teach patient proper drug administration and storage.

cloNIDine
KLOE-ni-deen

cloNIDine hydrochloride
Catapres, Catapres-TTS, Duraclon, Kapvay, Nexiclon XR

Therapeutic class: Antihypertensives
Pharmacologic class: Centrally acting alpha agonists

AVAILABLE FORMS
Injection for epidural use: 100 mcg/mL
Injection for epidural use, concentrate: 500 mcg/mL
Tablets: 0.1 mg, 0.2 mg, 0.3 mg
Tablets (extended-release) ⓞⓃⓒ: 0.1 mg, 0.2 mg
Tablets (scored extended-release): 0.17 mg, 0.26 mg
Transdermal: 0.1 mg/24 hours, 0.2 mg/ 24 hours, 0.3 mg/24 hours

INDICATIONS & DOSAGES
➤ **Essential and renal HTN**
Adults: Initially, 0.1 mg PO b.i.d.; then increase by 0.1 mg daily on a weekly basis. Or, 0.17 mg Nexiclon XR PO daily; then increase by 0.09 mg daily on a weekly basis. Usual range is 0.2 to 0.6 mg daily in divided doses; infrequently, dosages as high as 2.4 mg daily are used.

Or, apply transdermal patch once every 7 days, starting with 0.1-mg system and adjusted with another 0.1-mg or larger system after 1 or 2 weeks if desired BP reduction isn't achieved. Don't exceed concurrent use of two clonidine 0.3-mg systems.
Adjust-a-dose: In patients with ESRD on dialysis, initially 0.09 mg Nexiclon XR PO daily; then titrate as tolerated.
➤ **Severe cancer pain that is unresponsive to epidural or spinal opiate analgesia or other more conventional methods of analgesia**
Adults: Initially, 30 mcg/hour by continuous epidural infusion. Experience with rates greater than 40 mcg/hour is limited.
Children old enough to tolerate placement and management of an epidural catheter: Initially, 0.5 mcg/kg/hour by epidural infusion. Dosage should be cautiously adjusted, based on response.
➤ **ADHD as monotherapy or as adjunctive therapy to stimulant medications**

Children ages 6 to 17: Initially, 0.1 mg extended-release tablet (Kapvay) PO at bedtime. Adjust by 0.1 mg/day at weekly intervals to desired response. With first dosage increase, give tablets b.i.d., with equal or higher dose given at bedtime. Maximum dose is 0.4 mg/day.

ADMINISTRATION
PO
- Don't crush, break, or allow patient to chew extended-release tablets except Nexiclon XR tablets, which are scored to be broken.
- Immediate-release and extended-release forms can't be substituted on a milligram-per-milligram basis.
- Give initial extended-release dose at bedtime.
- Give last dose immediately before bedtime.
- Reduce dosage gradually over 2 to 4 days before discontinuing. Decrease dosage of extended-release form by no more than 0.1 mg every 3 to 7 days.

Transdermal
- Apply patch to nonhairy area of intact skin on upper arm or torso.
- When converting from oral to patch form, place patch on patient and gradually decrease oral dose over several days. Antihypertensive effect of patch takes 2 to 3 days to appear.

Epidural
Boxed Warning The injection form concentrate, containing 500 mcg/mL, must be diluted in NSS injection before use to yield 100 mcg/mL. ∎

☉ *Alert:* The injection form must not be used with a preservative.

ACTION
Unknown. Thought to stimulate alpha$_2$ receptors and inhibit the central vasomotor centers, decreasing sympathetic outflow to the heart, kidneys, and peripheral vasculature and lowering peripheral vascular resistance, BP, and HR.

Route	Onset	Peak	Duration
PO (immediate-release)	30–60 min	1–3 hr	6–10 hr
PO (extended-release)	1–2 wk	7–8 hr	Unknown
Transdermal	2–3 days	3 days	7 days
Epidural	Unknown	30–60 min	Unknown

Half-life: Immediate- and extended-release, 12 to 16 hours; transdermal, 20 hours; epidural, 1 to 2 hours.

ADVERSE REACTIONS
CNS: drowsiness, dizziness, confusion, sedation, fatigue, irritability, malaise, hallucinations, agitation, depression, nightmares, night terrors, restless sleep, emotional disorder, aggression, tearfulness, headache, insomnia, tremor, somnolence, nervousness. **CV:** *bradycardia,* chest pain, edema, hypotension, orthostatic hypotension, tachycardia. **EENT:** otitis media, tinnitus, nasal congestion, sore throat, dry mouth. **GI:** constipation, nausea, vomiting, anorexia, abdominal pain, viral GI infection. **GU:** enuresis, nocturia, urine retention, erectile dysfunction, loss of libido. **Metabolic:** weight gain. **Musculoskeletal:** myalgia, arthralgia, weakness. **Skin:** pruritus; dermatitis; burning sensation, contact allergy, or localized blanching with transdermal patch; hyperpigmentation, diaphoresis, rash. **Other:** withdrawal syndrome, gynecomastia.

INTERACTIONS
Drug-drug. *Amitriptyline, amoxapine, clomipramine, desipramine, doxepin, imipramine, mirtazapine, nortriptyline, protriptyline, trimipramine:* May cause loss of BP control with life-threatening elevations in BP. Avoid using together.
Beta blockers: May increase risk of sinus node dysfunction. May increase rebound HTN if clonidine is withdrawn abruptly. Use cautiously together and closely monitor BP.
Calcium channel blockers (verapamil), digoxin: May cause AV block and severe hypotension. Monitor BP and ECG.
CNS depressants (barbiturates, cannabinoid-containing products, opioids): May increase CNS depression. Use together cautiously.
Diuretics, other antihypertensives: May increase hypotensive effect. Monitor patient closely.
Levodopa: May increase hypotensive effects. Monitor patient.
Drug-herb. *Capsicum:* May reduce antihypertensive effectiveness. Discourage use together.
Ma huang: May decrease antihypertensive effects. Discourage use together.
Drug-lifestyle. *Alcohol use:* May increase CNS depression and clonidine level. Discourage use together.

EFFECTS ON LAB TEST RESULTS
- None.

CONTRAINDICATIONS & CAUTIONS

• Contraindicated in patients hypersensitive to drug.

• Transdermal form is contraindicated in patients hypersensitive to any component of the adhesive layer of transdermal system.

• Epidural form is contraindicated in patients receiving anticoagulant therapy, in those with bleeding diathesis, in those with an injection-site infection, and in those who are hemodynamically unstable or have severe CV disease.

• Use cautiously in patients with severe coronary insufficiency, conduction disturbances, recent MI, cerebrovascular disease, chronic renal failure, or impaired liver function.

• Safety and effectiveness in children for essential and renal HTN haven't been established in adequate and well-controlled trials.
Dialyzable drug: No.

⚠ *Overdose S&S:* Early HTN, then hypotension; bradycardia; respiratory and CNS depression; hypothermia; drowsiness; decreased or absent reflexes; weakness; irritability; miosis. With large overdoses: Reversible cardiac conduction defects or arrhythmias, apnea, coma, seizures.

PREGNANCY-LACTATION-REPRODUCTION

• There are no adequate well-controlled studies during pregnancy. Drug crosses the placental barrier. Use during pregnancy only if clearly needed.

Boxed Warning Epidural clonidine isn't recommended for obstetric, postpartum, or perioperative pain management due to the risk of hemodynamic instability, especially hypotension and bradycardia, except in rare cases in which the potential benefits outweigh the risks. ∎

• Register patient exposed to ADHD medications during pregnancy in the National Pregnancy Registry for ADHD Medications (1-866-961-2388 or https://womensmentalhealth.org/adhd-medications/).

• Drug appears in human milk. Use cautiously during breastfeeding; monitor infant for sedation, lethargy, tachypnea, and poor feeding.

NURSING CONSIDERATIONS

• Drug may be given to lower BP rapidly in some hypertensive emergencies.

• Monitor BP and pulse rate frequently. Dosage is usually adjusted to patient's BP and tolerance.

• Older adults may be more sensitive to drug's hypotensive effects than patients who are younger.

• Observe patient for tolerance to drug's therapeutic effects, which may require increased dosage.

• Noticeable antihypertensive effects of transdermal clonidine may take 2 to 3 days. Oral antihypertensive therapy may have to be continued in the interim; wean patient from oral dose over 1 to 3 days after first patch is applied.

🛈 *Alert:* Remove transdermal patch before defibrillation or cardioversion to prevent arcing.

• Stop drug gradually by reducing dosage over 2 to 4 days to avoid rapid rebound in BP, agitation, headache, and tremor. When stopping therapy in patients receiving both clonidine and a beta blocker, gradually withdraw the beta blocker several days before gradually stopping clonidine to minimize adverse reactions.

• Don't stop drug before surgery because of risk of rebound HTN from abrupt withdrawal. Withhold immediate-release forms within 4 hours of surgery and restart as soon as possible afterward. May give Nexiclon XR up to 28 hours before surgery and resume the following day. Consider transitioning to transdermal patch at least 3 days before surgery if patients aren't expected to resume PO medications within 12 hours of surgery.

• When drug is given epidurally, carefully monitor infusion pump, and inspect catheter tubing for obstruction or dislodgment.

• *Look alike–sound alike:* Don't confuse clonidine with clonazepam, clozapine, Klonopin, quinidine, or clomiphene.

PATIENT TEACHING

• Instruct patient to take drug exactly as prescribed and to report adverse reactions.

• Advise patient that stopping drug abruptly may cause severe rebound HTN; dosage must be reduced gradually over 2 to 4 days, as instructed by prescriber.

• Tell patient to take the last dose immediately before bedtime.

• Reassure patient that the transdermal patch usually remains attached despite showering and other routine daily activities. Instruct patient on the use of the adhesive overlay to provide additional skin adherence, if needed. Also tell patient to place patch at a different site each week.

Reactions in bold italics are *life-threatening*. Interactions may have a *rapid onset* or a *delayed onset*.

- Caution patient that drug may cause drowsiness but that this adverse effect usually diminishes over 4 to 6 weeks.
- Inform patient that dizziness upon standing can be minimized by rising slowly from a sitting or lying position and avoiding sudden position changes.
- Advise patient that, if an MRI is scheduled, to alert the facility about wearing a transdermal patch.

clopidogrel bisulfate ⓧ
cloe-PID-oh-grel

Plavix✔

Therapeutic class: Antiplatelet drugs
Pharmacologic class: Platelet aggregation inhibitors

AVAILABLE FORMS
Tablets: 75 mg, 300 mg

INDICATIONS & DOSAGES
➤ **To reduce rate of MI and stroke in patients with established peripheral arterial disease or history of recent MI or stroke**
Adults: 75 mg PO daily.
➤ **To reduce rate of MI and stroke in patients with unstable angina/non-ST-elevation MI (NSTEMI), including those managed medically and those managed with coronary revascularization; to reduce rate of MI and stroke in patients with acute ST-elevation MI (STEMI) who are to be managed medically**
Adults: Initially, a single 300-mg PO loading dose; then 75 mg PO once daily. Start and continue aspirin with clopidogrel; also use a parenteral anticoagulant initially. Initiating clopidogrel without a loading dose will delay (by several days) establishing antiplatelet effects.

ADMINISTRATION
PO
- Give drug without regard to meals.

ACTION
Inhibits the binding of the P2Y$_{12}$ component of ADP to its platelet receptor, impeding ADP-mediated activation and subsequent platelet aggregation, and irreversibly modifies the platelet ADP receptor.

Route	Onset	Peak	Duration
PO	2 hr	45 min	5 days

Half-life: 6 hours.

ADVERSE REACTIONS
CV: hematoma, *hemorrhage.* **EENT:** epistaxis.
Other: hypersensitivity reactions.

INTERACTIONS
Drug-drug. *Apixaban, dabigatran, edoxaban, rivaroxaban:* May increase risk of bleeding. Use together cautiously.
Aspirin, NSAIDs: May increase risk of GI bleeding. Monitor patient.
CYP2C19 inducers (rifamycins): May increase antiplatelet effect. Carefully monitor platelet function when starting, stopping, or changing rifamycin dosage. Adjust clopidogrel dosage as needed.
CYP2C8 substrates (repaglinide): May increase substrate level. Avoid use together or adjust substrate dosage and monitor patient closely.
Opioids: May delay and reduce clopidogrel absorption. Consider parenteral antiplatelet agents in patients with ACS requiring opioids.
Salicylates: May increase the risk of serious bleeding in patients with TIA or ischemic stroke. Avoid use together.
SNRIs, SSRIs: May increase bleeding risk. Use together cautiously.
Strong or moderate CYP2C19 inhibitors (cimetidine, esomeprazole, etravirine, felbamate, fluconazole, ketoconazole, omeprazole, ticlopidine, voriconazole), PPIs: May decrease effects of clopidogrel. Avoid use together.
Warfarin: May increase risk of bleeding. Use together cautiously.
Drug-herb. *Herbs with antiplatelet activity (capsicum, fenugreek, garlic, ginkgo biloba, turmeric, many others):* May increase risk of bleeding. Discourage use together.
Drug-food. *Grapefruit, grapefruit juice:* May reduce drug's antiplatelet effects. Avoid use together.

EFFECTS ON LAB TEST RESULTS
- May decrease platelet count.

CONTRAINDICATIONS & CAUTIONS
- Contraindicated in patients hypersensitive to drug or its components, in those with a history of hypersensitivity or hematologic

reaction to other thienopyridines, and in those with pathologic bleeding (such as peptic ulcer or intracranial hemorrhage).

• Hypersensitivity reactions, including rash, angioedema, and hematologic reactions, have been reported.

• Consider discontinuing drug 5 days before elective surgery, including elective CABG, except in patients with cardiac stents who haven't completed the full course of dual antiplatelet therapy; discuss patient-specific situations with cardiologist. Platelet aggregation won't return to normal for at least 5 days after drug has been stopped.

• Premature interruption of therapy may result in stent thrombosis with subsequent fatal or nonfatal MI. Duration of therapy, in general, is determined by type of stent placed (bare metal or drug eluting) and whether an ACS event was ongoing at the time of placement.

• Use cautiously in patients at risk for increased bleeding from trauma, surgery, or other pathologic conditions and in those with renal or hepatic impairment.

Dialyzable drug: Unknown.

⚠ *Overdose S&S:* Prolonged bleeding time, bleeding complications.

PREGNANCY-LACTATION-REPRODUCTION

• Information related to use during pregnancy is limited. Use cautiously during pregnancy and only if clearly needed.

• It isn't known if drug appears in human milk. Patient should discontinue breastfeeding or discontinue drug, taking into account importance of drug to the patient.

NURSING CONSIDERATIONS

■ **Boxed Warning** Drug effectiveness depends on the drug's activation to an active metabolite by the cytochrome P450 system, principally CYP2C19. Patients who are poor metabolizers form less of the active metabolite and the effects of the drug on platelet activity are reduced. Tests are available to assess a patient's CYP2C19 genotype. Consider alternative treatment for patients identified as poor metabolizers. ■

※ Approximately 2% of white patients and 4% of Black patients are poor metabolizers of CYP2C19, and the prevalence is higher in patients of Asian descent (14% of patients of Chinese descent).

● *Alert:* Drug may cause fatal thrombotic thrombocytopenic purpura (thrombocytopenia, hemolytic anemia, neurologic findings, renal dysfunction, and fever) that requires urgent treatment, including plasmapheresis.

• *Look alike–sound alike:* Don't confuse Plavix with Paxil.

PATIENT TEACHING

• Advise patient that it may take longer than usual to stop bleeding and to refrain from activities in which trauma and bleeding may occur. Encourage patient to wear a seat belt when in a car.

• Instruct patient to notify prescriber if unusual bleeding or bruising occurs.

• Tell patient to inform all health care providers, including dentists, before undergoing procedures or starting new drug therapy, about taking drug.

• Caution patient not to stop drug without first discussing with prescriber.

clotrimazole
kloe-TRIM-a-zole

Canesten❋, Clotrimaderm❋, Cruex ◇, Desenex ◇, Lotrimin AF ◇, Trivagizole 3 ◇

Therapeutic class: Antifungals
Pharmacologic class: Imidazole derivatives

AVAILABLE FORMS

Topical cream: 1%
Topical lotion: 1%
Topical ointment: 1%
Topical solution: 1%
Troches (lozenges) Ⓞ: 10 mg
Vaginal cream: 1% ◇, 2% ◇
Vaginal tablets: 200 mg❋ ◇, 500 mg❋ ◇

INDICATIONS & DOSAGES

➤ **Superficial fungal infections (tinea corporis, tinea cruris, tinea pedis, tinea versicolor, candidiasis)**

Adults and children age 2 and older: Apply thin film and massage into affected and surrounding area b.i.d., morning and evening, for 2 to 4 weeks. Continue treatment of tinea pedis until 1 week after clinical resolution. If improvement doesn't occur after 2 to 4 weeks, reevaluate patient.

➤ **Vulvovaginal candidiasis**
Adults and children age 12 and older: 1 applicatorful of vaginal cream daily at bedtime for 3 days (2%) or 7 days (1%).

➤ **Oropharyngeal candidiasis**
Adults and children age 3 and older: 1 lozenge dissolved in mouth over 15 to 30 minutes five times daily for 14 consecutive days. When drug is used for initial treatment in patients with HIV-1 infection, duration of therapy is 7 to 14 days.

➤ **To prevent oropharyngeal candidiasis in patients immunocompromised by chemotherapy, radiotherapy, or corticosteroid therapy in the treatment of leukemia, solid tumors, or renal transplantation**
Adults: 1 lozenge dissolved in mouth over 15 to 30 minutes t.i.d. for duration of chemotherapy or until corticosteroid is reduced to maintenance levels.

ADMINISTRATION
PO
• Lozenges should dissolve in mouth and not be chewed, for full benefit.
Topical
• Clean and dry area before applying drug.
• Don't use occlusive wrappings or dressings.
Vaginal
• If applicator for cream isn't disposable, wash applicator with soap and warm water immediately after use. Rinse thoroughly and dry.

ACTION
Fungistatic or fungicidal, depending on drug level. Alters fungal cell-wall permeability and produces osmotic instability.

Route	Onset	Peak	Duration
PO	Unknown	Unknown	3 hr
Topical, vaginal	Unknown	Unknown	Unknown

Half-life: Unknown.

ADVERSE REACTIONS
GI: lower abdominal cramps, nausea and vomiting with lozenges. **GU:** mild vaginal burning or irritation, urinary frequency. **Hepatic:** elevated AST level (lozenges). **Skin:** erythema, blistering, burning, edema, general irritation, peeling, pruritus, skin fissures, stinging, urticaria.

INTERACTIONS
None significant.

EFFECTS ON LAB TEST RESULTS
• May increase liver enzyme levels.

CONTRAINDICATIONS & CAUTIONS
• Contraindicated in patients hypersensitive to drug.
• Contraindicated for ophthalmic use.
Dialyzable drug: Unknown.

PREGNANCY-LACTATION-REPRODUCTION
• There are no adequate studies during pregnancy. Use lozenges during pregnancy only if potential benefit justifies fetal risk.
• Use topical clotrimazole during first trimester only if clearly indicated.
• Manual insertion may be preferred over use of vaginal applicator. Use only on advice of physician.
• It's unknown if drug appears in human milk. Use cautiously during breastfeeding. Patient should consider discontinuing breastfeeding.

NURSING CONSIDERATIONS
• Consult prescriber before using topical preparations in children younger than age 2. Don't use troches in children younger than age 3; don't use vaginal preparations in children younger than age 12.
• Watch for irritation or sensitivity; stop if irritation occurs, and notify prescriber.
• Improvement usually occurs within 1 week; if no improvement is seen within 2 to 4 weeks, review diagnosis.

PATIENT TEACHING
• Reassure patient that hypopigmentation from tinea versicolor will resolve gradually.
• Warn patient not to use occlusive wrappings or dressings.
• Warn patient to avoid contact with eyes.
• Caution patient that frequent or persistent yeast infections may suggest a more serious medical problem.
• Tell patient to refrain from sexual intercourse during vaginal treatment.
• Warn patient that topical preparation may stain clothing.
• Tell patient that using a sanitary napkin protects clothing when using vaginal preparation.
• Stress need to continue use of vaginal preparations, as prescribed, even if menstruation begins.

• Tell patient with athlete's foot to change shoes and cotton socks daily and to dry between the toes after bathing.
• Tell patient to allow lozenges to dissolve in mouth and not to chew, for full benefit.
• Stress need to continue treatment for full course and to notify prescriber if no improvement occurs after 2 to 4 weeks.

SAFETY ALERT!

cloZAPine ⚕
KLOE-za-peen

Clozaril♦, Versacloz

Therapeutic class: Antipsychotics
Pharmacologic class: Dibenzapine derivatives

AVAILABLE FORMS
Oral suspension: 50 mg/mL
Tablets: 25 mg, 50 mg, 100 mg, 200 mg
Tablets (ODTs): 12.5 mg, 25 mg, 100 mg, 150 mg, 200 mg

INDICATIONS & DOSAGES
➤ **Schizophrenia in patients who are severely ill and unresponsive to other therapies; to reduce risk of recurrent suicidality in schizophrenia or schizoaffective disorders**
Adults: Initially, 12.5 mg PO once daily or b.i.d. Adjust dose upward by 25 to 50 mg daily (if tolerated) to 300 to 450 mg daily in one to three doses by end of 2 weeks. Individual dosage is based on clinical response, patient tolerance, and adverse reactions. Subsequent dosage shouldn't be increased more than once or twice weekly and shouldn't exceed 100-mg increments. Don't exceed 900 mg daily.
⚕ **Boxed Warning** For the general population, if ANC is $1,500/mm^3$ or greater (normal baseline range), treatment may be initiated. Confirm all initial reports of ANC less than $1,500/mm^3$ with a repeat ANC within 24 hours. For patients with benign ethnic neutropenia (BEN), obtain two baseline ANC levels before initiating treatment (normal ANC range for those with BEN is $1,000/mm^3$ or greater). For patients with BEN, if ANC is $1,000/mm^3$ or greater, treatment may be initiated. ∎

⚕ *Adjust-a-dose:* Refer to manufacturer's instructions for ANC monitoring and dosage interruption for neutropenia, and for concurrent use with CYP1A2, CYP2D6, or CYP3A4 inhibitors or CYP1A2 or CYP3A4 inducers. Reduce dosages in those with significant renal or hepatic impairment and in those who are poor metabolizers of CYP2D6.

In older adults, start with 12.5 mg once daily for 3 days; then increase to 25 mg once daily for 3 days as tolerated. May further increase, as tolerated, in increments of 12.5 to 25 mg daily every 3 days to desired response, up to 700 mg/day (mean dose is 300 mg/day).

Discontinue drug in patients with QT interval greater than 500 msec, those with symptoms of ventricular arrhythmias, or those with cardiomyopathy/myocarditis or NMS.

When restarting drug in patients who have discontinued clozapine for 2 days or more, reinitiate at 12.5 mg once daily or b.i.d. to minimize risk of hypotension, bradycardia, and syncope. If that dose is well tolerated, may increase dose to the previously therapeutic dose more quickly than recommended for initial treatment.

ADMINISTRATION
PO
• Give with or without food.
• May divide total daily dose into uneven doses, with larger dose given at bedtime.
• Peel the foil from the ODT blister and gently remove the tablet immediately before giving. Don't push tablet through foil.
• Give ODT with or without water.
• Shake bottle for 10 seconds before withdrawing suspension using provided oral syringe and syringe adaptor.
• If patient has missed more than 2 days of treatment, restart drug at 12.5 mg once daily or b.i.d. and retitrate. May titrate more quickly than initial treatment, if tolerated.

ACTION
Unknown. Binds selectively to dopaminergic receptors in the CNS and may interfere with adrenergic, cholinergic, histaminergic, and serotonergic receptors.

Route	Onset	Peak	Duration
PO	Unknown	1–6 hr	4–12 hr

Half-life: Proportional to dose; may range from 4 to 66 hours.

ADVERSE REACTIONS

CNS: drowsiness, sedation, dizziness, vertigo, headache, *seizures,* syncope, tremor, disturbed sleep or nightmares, restlessness, hypokinesia or akinesia, agitation, rigidity, akathisia, confusion, fatigue, insomnia, lethargy, ataxia, slurred speech, depression, myoclonus, anxiety, fever. **CV:** tachycardia, hypotension, HTN, chest pain, ECG changes, orthostatic hypotension. **EENT:** visual disturbances, increased salivation, dry mouth. **GI:** constipation, nausea, vomiting, heartburn, diarrhea. **GU:** urinary frequency or urgency, urine retention, incontinence, abnormal ejaculation. **Hematologic:** *leukopenia, neutropenia,* eosinophilia. **Metabolic:** hyperglycemia, weight gain, hypercholesterolemia, hypertriglyceridemia. **Musculoskeletal:** hypokinesia, muscle rigidity, muscle weakness. **Skin:** rash, diaphoresis.

INTERACTIONS

Drug-drug. *Anticholinergics:* May potentiate anticholinergic effects of clozapine. Use together cautiously.

Antihypertensives: May potentiate hypotensive effects. Monitor BP.

۞ Alert: *Benzodiazepines other psychotropic drugs:* May increase risk of sedation and CV and respiratory arrest. Use together cautiously.

Bone marrow suppressants: May increase bone marrow toxicity. Avoid using together.

CYP2D6 or CYP3A4 inhibitors (bupropion, cimetidine, duloxetine, erythromycin, escitalopram, fluoxetine, paroxetine, quinidine, sertraline, terbinafine); moderate or weak CYP1A2 inhibitors (caffeine, oral contraceptives): Monitor patient for adverse reactions. Reduce clozapine oral dosage if necessary.

CYP2D6 substrates (carbamazepine, flecainide, phenothiazines, propafenone): May increase substrate levels. Use cautiously together.

Digoxin, other highly protein-bound drugs, warfarin: May increase levels of these drugs. Monitor patient closely for adverse reactions.

Drugs that prolong the QT interval (antiarrhythmics, citalopram, ziprasidone): May increase risk of prolonged QT interval and ventricular arrhythmias. Avoid use together.

Opioid class warning: May cause slow or difficult breathing, sedation, and death. Avoid use together. If use together is necessary, limit dosage and duration of each drug to the minimum necessary for desired effect.

Psychoactive drugs: May cause additive effects. Use together cautiously.

Ritonavir: May increase clozapine levels and toxicity. Avoid using together.

Strong CYP3A4 inducers (carbamazepine, phenytoin, rifampin): May decrease clozapine effectiveness. Use together isn't recommended. If coadministration is necessary, consider increasing clozapine dosage.

Strong CYP1A2 inhibitors (ciprofloxacin, fluvoxamine): May increase clozapine level. Reduce clozapine dosage to one third during coadministration.

Drug-herb. *St. John's wort:* May decrease drug level. Discourage use together.

Drug-lifestyle. *Alcohol use:* May increase CNS depression. Discourage use together.

Smoking: May decrease drug level. Urge patient to quit smoking. Monitor patient for effectiveness and adjust dosage.

EFFECTS ON LAB TEST RESULTS

• May increase glucose, cholesterol, and triglyceride levels.

• May increase eosinophil count. May decrease granulocyte, WBC counts, and ANC.

CONTRAINDICATIONS & CAUTIONS

Boxed Warning Because of risk of severe neutropenia, which can lead to fatal infections, drug is available only through the Clozapine REMS Program. ∎

• *Opioid class warning*: Opioids should only be prescribed with benzodiazepines or other CNS depressants to patients for whom alternative treatment options are inadequate.

• Contraindicated in patients with a history of serious hypersensitivity to drug or its components, in patients who experienced clozapine-induced agranulocytosis or severe granulocytopenia, and in patients with uncontrolled epilepsy.

• Closely monitor patients taking other drugs that suppress bone marrow function.

• Use cautiously in patients with prostatic hyperplasia or angle-closure glaucoma because drug has potent anticholinergic effects. Severe GI reactions (constipation, intestinal obstruction, fecal impaction, paralytic ileus) can also occur.

Boxed Warning Fatal myocarditis and cardiomyopathy may occur at any time during treatment. If signs or symptoms (chest

---

🍁Canada   ◇OTC   ◆Off-label use   🖉Photoguide   💊Do not crush   *Liquid contains alcohol   ▨Genetic

pain, tachycardia, palpitations, dyspnea, fever, flulike symptoms, hypotension, ECG changes) occur, obtain a cardiac evaluation, and discontinue drug. Generally, patients with clozapine-related myocarditis or cardiomyopathy shouldn't be re-challenged with the drug. ∎

• Eosinophilia associated with organ involvement (myocarditis, pancreatitis, hepatitis, colitis, nephritis) frequently develops during first month of treatment. If eosinophilia develops, evaluate for systemic reactions and, if clozapine-related disease is suspected, discontinue drug immediately. If clonidine isn't the cause, treat underlying cause before continuing clozapine.

• Drug may cause QT-interval prolongation and life-threatening ventricular arrhythmias. Use caution in those with risk factors for QT-interval prolongation or serious CV reactions and in those taking drugs known to prolong the QT interval. Consider obtaining a baseline ECG and serum chemistry panel, and correct electrolyte abnormalities before starting treatment. Discontinue clozapine if QTc interval is greater than 500 msec. Obtain a cardiac evaluation and discontinue drug if patient has symptoms of torsades de pointes or other arrhythmias (syncope, presyncope, dizziness, palpitations).

• Drug can cause NMS, which can be fatal. If signs and symptoms of NMS (*hyperpyrexia, muscle rigidity, altered mental status, irregular pulse, fluctuating BP, tachycardia, diaphoresis, cardiac arrhythmias, elevated CK level, myoglobinuria, rhabdomyolysis, acute renal failure*) occur, discontinue drug and begin appropriate treatment and monitoring.

• Tardive dyskinesia (TD), a syndrome of potentially irreversible, involuntary dyskinetic movements, has occurred in patients taking antipsychotics. Use the lowest effective dosage for the shortest duration possible. Consider discontinuing drug if TD occurs. (*Note:* Some patients may require treatment despite TD.)

• Somnolence, orthostatic hypotension, and motor and sensory instability have been reported, which may lead to falls and, consequently, fractures or other fall-related injuries.

• Older adults may have an increased sensitivity to anticholinergic effects of drug; sedating effects of drug may increase the risk of falls in this population.

Boxed Warning Drug isn't indicated for use in older adults with dementia-related psychoses because of an increased risk of death from CV disease or infection. ∎

• Safe and effective use in children hasn't been established.

Dialyzable drug: No.

⚠ *Overdose S&S:* Altered state of consciousness, drowsiness, delirium, coma, tachycardia, hypotension, respiratory depression or failure, hypersalivation, aspiration pneumonia, cardiac arrhythmias, seizures.

PREGNANCY-LACTATION-REPRODUCTION

• There are no adequate studies during pregnancy. Use during pregnancy only if clearly needed and potential benefit justifies fetal risk.

⚠ *Alert:* Neonates exposed to antipsychotics during the third trimester are at risk for developing extrapyramidal signs and symptoms (repetitive muscle movements of the face and body) and withdrawal symptoms (agitation, abnormally increased or decreased muscle tone, tremors, sleepiness, severe difficulty breathing, and difficulty feeding) after delivery.

• Drug appears in human milk. Patient shouldn't breastfeed during therapy.

NURSING CONSIDERATIONS

⚠ *Alert:* Drug may cause hyperglycemia. Monitor patients with diabetes regularly. In patients with risk factors for diabetes, obtain fasting blood glucose test results at baseline and periodically.

⚠ *Alert:* Monitor patient for metabolic syndrome, including significant weight gain and increased BMI, HTN, hyperglycemia, hypercholesterolemia, and hypertriglyceridemia.

• Monitor patient for signs and symptoms of myocarditis and cardiomyopathy.

• Monitor patient for anticholinergic effects, including constipation and urine retention.

Boxed Warning Monitor patient for neutropenia. Obtain ANC before and regularly during treatment. ∎

Boxed Warning Orthostatic hypotension, syncope, bradycardia, and cardiac arrest can occur. Orthostatic hypotension is more likely to occur during initial titration with rapid dose escalation and can occur with the first dose and with doses as low as 12.5 mg. Start treatment with 12.5 mg once daily or b.i.d. and titrate slowly using divided dosages. Use

---

cautiously in patients with CV or cerebrovascular disease or conditions that may cause hypotension. ∎

Boxed Warning Seizures may occur, especially in patients receiving high doses. Begin treatment at 12.5 mg, titrate gradually, and use divided dosing. Use caution with patients with a history of seizures or risk factors for seizures (CNS pathology, drugs that lower the seizure threshold, alcohol abuse). ∎

• Some patients experience transient fever with temperature higher than 100.4° F (38° C), especially in the first 3 weeks of therapy. Monitor these patients closely.

⚠ *Alert:* Fever may be the first sign of neutropenic infection. Interrupt therapy and obtain ANC level in patients who develop fever (temperature of 101.3° F [38.5° C]). If fever occurs in patient with ANC less than 1,000/mm³, initiate appropriate workup and treatment and monitor and manage patient appropriately.

🔲 If drug is to be discontinued and patient doesn't have moderate to severe neutropenia, reduce dose gradually over 1 to 2 weeks. To discontinue the drug abruptly for a reason unrelated to neutropenia, continue to monitor ANC until it is 1,500/mm³ or greater (for the general population), or until ANC is 1,000/mm³ or greater or above patient's baseline (for those with BEN).

• If patient reports onset of fever (temperature 101.3° F or greater) while discontinuing drug, continue to monitor ANC for an additional 2 weeks after drug is discontinued.

• When discontinuing drug, monitor patients carefully for recurrence of psychotic symptoms and symptoms related to cholinergic rebound (diaphoresis, headache, nausea, vomiting, diarrhea).

• PE and DVT have occurred in patients taking clozapine. It isn't known whether these can be attributed to the drug or to some other patient characteristic. Monitor for PE if patient develops DVT, acute dyspnea, chest pain, or other respiratory signs and symptoms.

• Drug can cause sedation and impair cognitive and motor performance. Monitor patient carefully for CNS changes.

• Assess fall risk when initiating therapy and recurrently for patients on long-term therapy, especially older adults and patients with diseases or conditions or who are taking other medications that could exacerbate fall risk.

• *Look alike–sound alike:* Don't confuse clozapine with clonidine, clonazepam, or Klonopin. Don't confuse Clozaril with Colazal.

PATIENT TEACHING

Boxed Warning Tell patient about need for regular blood tests to check for low ANC. Advise patient to report flulike symptoms, fever, sore throat, lethargy, weakness, malaise, or other signs of neutropenia or infection. ∎

Boxed Warning Warn patient taking drug to avoid hazardous activities that require alertness and good coordination and where sudden loss of consciousness and falls could cause serious risk to patient or others. ∎

• Tell patient to check with prescriber before taking alcohol or OTC drugs.

• Advise patient that smoking may decrease drug effectiveness.

• Caution patient to rise slowly to avoid dizziness and to immediately report feeling faint, loss of consciousness, or irregular or slow heartbeat.

• Inform patient that drug may cause somnolence, orthostatic hypotension, and motor and sensory instability, which may lead to falls and, consequently, fractures or other injuries.

• Teach patient safe drug administration.

• Inform patient about risk of metabolic changes, seizures, and TD.

SAFETY ALERT!

codeine phosphate–acetaminophen 🗓
koe-DEEN/a-seet-a-MIN-a-fen

Therapeutic class: Opioid analgesics
Pharmacologic class: Opioids–para-aminophenol derivatives
Controlled substance schedule: III (tablets); V (liquid)

AVAILABLE FORMS
Oral solution or suspension: 12 mg codeine and 120 mg acetaminophen/5 mL*
Tablets: 15 mg codeine and 300 mg acetaminophen, 30 mg codeine and 300 mg acetaminophen, 60 mg codeine and 300 mg acetaminophen

INDICATIONS & DOSAGES
➤ **Mild to moderately severe pain**
Adults: Codeine 15 to 60 mg and acetaminophen 300 to 1,000 mg PO every 4 hours as

needed for pain; adjust dosage based on pain severity and patient response. Maximum total daily dosage: acetaminophen 4,000 mg and codeine 360 mg.

Adjust-a-dose: Initiate dosing regimen for each patient individually, taking into consideration pain severity, patient response, prior analgesic treatment experience, and risk factors for addiction, abuse, and misuse. Consider decreased dosage in patients with renal impairment, older adults, and patients overly sensitive to effects of opioids. For patients with hepatic impairment, maximum total daily acetaminophen dose is 2,000 mg.

ADMINISTRATION
PO

- Store tablets at room temperature.
- Give with milk or meals to avoid GI upset.
- For oral solution or suspension, be sure to use a calibrated measuring device.

ACTION
Codeine may bind with opioid receptors in the CNS, altering perception and emotional response to pain. Acetaminophen is thought to produce analgesia by inhibiting prostaglandin and other substances that sensitize pain receptors.

Route	Onset	Peak	Duration
PO (codeine)	30–45 min	1–2 hr	4–6 hr
PO (acetaminophen)	Rapid	0.5–2 hr	3–4 hr

Half-life: Codeine, 2.9 hours; acetaminophen, 1.25 to 3 hours.

ADVERSE REACTIONS
CNS: drowsiness, light-headedness, dizziness, sedation, euphoria, dysphoria. **GI:** nausea, vomiting, constipation, abdominal pain. **Hematologic:** *thrombocytopenia, agranulocytosis.* **Respiratory:** shortness of breath, *respiratory depression.* **Skin:** pruritus, rash, diaphoresis. **Other:** hypersensitivity reactions.

INTERACTIONS
Drug-drug. *Antipsychotics, general anesthetics, opioid analgesics, sedative-hypnotics, tranquilizers, other CNS depressants:* May increase CNS depression. Use together cautiously.

Boxed Warning *Benzodiazepines, CNS depressants:* May cause slow or difficult breathing, sedation, and death. Avoid use together.

If use together is necessary, limit dosage and duration of each drug to the minimum necessary for desired effect.

Boxed Warning *CYP2D6 inducers:* May decrease analgesic effects or result in opioid withdrawal. Use cautiously.

Boxed Warning *CYP3A4 inducers and inhibitors, CYP2D6 inhibitors:* Effects of concomitant use or discontinuation of these drugs with codeine are complex. Their use with codeine requires careful consideration of the effects on the parent drug, codeine, and the active metabolite, morphine.

Boxed Warning *CYP3A4 inhibitors:* May increase codeine concentration and increase adverse reactions, including fatal respiratory depression. Use cautiously.

Diuretics: May decrease effect of diuretic. Monitor patient for diminished diuresis or effects on BP.

MAO inhibitors: May cause serotonin syndrome or opioid toxicity (respiratory depression, coma). Use together or within 14 days is contraindicated. If urgent use of an opioid is necessary, use test doses and frequent titration of small doses of other opioids (such as oxycodone, hydrocodone, oxymorphone, or buprenorphine) to treat pain while closely monitoring BP and signs and symptoms of CNS and respiratory depression.

Muscle relaxants (baclofen, methocarbamol): May increase neuromuscular blocking effect and risk of respiratory depression. Monitor patient closely.

Serotonergic drugs (amoxapine, antiemetics [dolasetron, granisetron, ondansetron, palonosetron], antimigraine drugs, buspirone, cyclobenzaprine, dextromethorphan, lithium, maprotiline, methylene blue, mirtazapine, nefazodone, SSNRIs, SSRIs, TCAs, trazodone, tryptophan, vilazodone): May increase risk of serotonin syndrome. Use together cautiously and monitor patient for serotonin syndrome.

Drug-herb. *St. John's wort:* May increase risk of serotonin syndrome. Use together cautiously.

Drug-lifestyle. **Boxed Warning** *Alcohol use:* May cause slow or difficult breathing, sedation, and death. Avoid use together.

EFFECTS ON LAB TEST RESULTS
- May increase serum amylase level.
- May cause false-positive results for urinary 5-hydroxyindoleacetic acid.

Reactions in bold italics are *life-threatening*. Interactions may have a *rapid onset* or a *delayed onset*.

• May cause urine drug screen to be positive for morphine.

CONTRAINDICATIONS & CAUTIONS

• Contraindicated in patients hypersensitive to codeine or acetaminophen and in patients with significant respiratory depression, acute or severe bronchial asthma in an unmonitored setting or in the absence of resuscitative equipment, and in those with known or suspected GI obstruction, including paralytic ileus.

Boxed Warning Use exposes patient and others to the risk of opioid addiction, abuse, and misuse. To ensure that the benefits of opioid analgesics outweigh the risks of addiction, abuse, and misuse, the FDA has required a REMS program for these products. Assess each patient's risk before prescribing; monitor all patients for these behaviors. ∎

Boxed Warning *Opioid class warning:* Opioids should only be prescribed with benzodiazepines or other CNS depressants to patients for whom alternative treatment options are inadequate. ∎

Boxed Warning *Opioid class warning:* Life-threatening respiratory depression and death have occurred in children who received codeine. Most of the reported cases occurred after tonsillectomy or adenoidectomy, and many of the children had evidence of being an ultrarapid metabolizer of codeine due to a CYP2D6 polymorphism. Codeine phosphate–acetaminophen is contraindicated in children younger than age 12 and in children younger than age 18 after tonsillectomy or adenoidectomy. Avoid using drug in adolescents ages 12 to 18 who have other risk factors that may increase their sensitivity to the respiratory depressant effects of codeine unless benefits outweigh risks. Risk factors include conditions associated with hypoventilation, such as postoperative status, obstructive sleep apnea, obesity, severe pulmonary disease, neuromuscular disease, and concomitant use of other drugs that cause respiratory depression. ∎

Boxed Warning Accidental ingestion of even one dose of codeine–acetaminophen, especially by children, can result in a fatal overdose. ∎

Boxed Warning May cause life-threatening or fatal respiratory depression. Monitor carefully when starting or increasing dosages. ∎

⚕ *Alert:* For managing pain (not associated with tonsillectomy or adenoidectomy),

codeine should be used in children only if benefits outweigh risks.

• Safety and effectiveness in children younger than age 18 haven't been established.

• Drug may lead to a rare but serious decrease in adrenal gland cortisol production.

• Drug may decrease sex hormone levels with long-term use.

⚕ *Alert:* Patients are at increased risk for oversedation and respiratory depression if they snore or have a history of sleep apnea, no recent history of opioid use or are first-time opioid users, have increased opioid dose requirements or opioid habituation, received general anesthesia for longer lengths of time, received other sedating drugs, have preexisting pulmonary or cardiac disease, or have thoracic or other surgical incisions that may impair breathing. Monitor patients carefully.

• Use cautiously in patients with head injury, intracranial lesions, increased ICP, or acute abdominal conditions.

Boxed Warning Acetaminophen has been associated with acute liver failure, usually at doses greater than 4,000 mg/day and often when more than one acetaminophen-containing product is used. Liver failure may result in liver transplant or death. ∎

⚕ *Alert:* May cause SCAR, including SJS, TEN, and acute generalized exanthematous pustulosis. Reaction may occur with first or subsequent use when acetaminophen is used as monotherapy or when it is one component of combination drug therapy. Monitor for reddening of the skin, rash, blisters, and detachment of the upper surface of the skin. Stop drug immediately if skin reaction is suspected.

• Use cautiously in patients with asthma or sulfite sensitivity because allergy-type reactions, anaphylaxis, and asthmatic episodes may occur.

▨ Use cautiously in older adults and patients who are debilitated; in those with severe renal or hepatic impairment, hypothyroidism, urethral stricture, Addison disease, or prostatic hypertrophy; in patients identified as ultrarapid metabolizers of codeine; and in those with identified polymorphism of CYP2D6 genotype.

Dialyzable drug: Unknown.

⚠ *Overdose S&S:* Extreme sleepiness, confusion, shallow breathing. Codeine: Pinpoint pupils, respiratory depression, loss of consciousness, seizures. Acetaminophen:

Hepatic necrosis, nausea, vomiting, diaphoresis, malaise, renal tubular necrosis, hypoglycemia, coma, coagulation defects.

PREGNANCY-LACTATION-REPRODUCTION

Boxed Warning Prolonged use during pregnancy can result in neonatal opioid withdrawal syndrome, which may be life-threatening and requires management according to expert neonatology protocols. If prolonged use is needed, advise patient of the risks and ensure appropriate treatment will be available. ∎

◑ *Alert:* There are no adequate studies during pregnancy. Use during pregnancy only if potential benefit justifies fetal risk; dependence and withdrawal in newborns may occur.

• Don't administer drug during labor when delivery of a premature infant is anticipated.

◑ *Alert:* Codeine and its metabolites and acetaminophen appear in human milk. Breastfeeding isn't recommended for patients taking codeine due to risk of serious adverse reactions in infants, such as excess sleepiness, difficulty breastfeeding, or serious breathing problems that could result in death.

NURSING CONSIDERATIONS

Boxed Warning Serious, life-threatening, or fatal respiratory depression may occur with use of codeine–acetaminophen. Monitor patients for respiratory depression, especially during initiation or after a dosage increase. ∎

Boxed Warning Monitor all patients regularly for development of opioid addiction, abuse, and misuse, which can lead to overdose and death. ∎

• Prescribe lowest effective dosage for shortest period of time and inform patients of risks and signs and symptoms of acetaminophen and codeine toxicity.

• Ensure accuracy when prescribing, dispensing, and administering codeine 12 mg–acetaminophen 120 mg/5 mL. Dosing errors due to confusion between mg and mL and other codeine–acetaminophen oral suspensions of different concentrations can result in accidental overdose and death.

◑ *Alert:* If patient is taking opioids with serotonergic drugs, watch for signs and symptoms of serotonin syndrome (agitation, hallucinations, rapid HR, fever, diaphoresis, shivering or shaking, muscle twitching or stiffness, trouble with coordination, nausea, vomiting,

diarrhea), especially when at start of treatment or after dosage increases. Signs and symptoms may occur within several hours of coadministration but may occur later, especially after dosage increase. Discontinue opioid, serotonergic drug, or both for suspected serotonin syndrome.

◑ *Alert:* Monitor patient for signs and symptoms of adrenal insufficiency (nausea, vomiting, loss of appetite, fatigue, weakness, dizziness, low BP). Perform diagnostic testing for suspected adrenal insufficiency. For confirmed adrenal insufficiency, treat with corticosteroids and wean patient off opioids if appropriate. Discontinue corticosteroids when clinically appropriate.

• Monitor patient for signs and symptoms of decreased sex hormone levels (low libido, erectile dysfunction, amenorrhea, infertility). If signs and symptoms occur, evaluate patient and obtain lab testing.

◑ *Alert:* Carefully monitor vital signs, pain level, respiratory status, and sedation level in all patients receiving opioids, especially those receiving IV drugs, even those given postoperatively.

⚕ Carefully monitor patients identified as ultrarapid metabolizers of codeine and those with identified polymorphism of CYP2D6 genotype. Overdose signs and symptoms and exaggerated adverse effects may occur at normal doses in these patients.

• Monitor serial renal function tests or LFTs in patients with severe hepatic or renal disease.

◑ *Alert:* Don't stop drug abruptly; withdraw slowly and individualize the gradual taper plan to prevent signs and symptoms of withdrawal, worsening pain, and psychological distress in patients who are physically dependent. Refer to manufacturer's label for specific tapering instructions.

◑ *Alert:* When tapering opioids, monitor patient closely for signs and symptoms of opioid withdrawal (restlessness, lacrimation, rhinorrhea, yawning, perspiration, chills, myalgia, mydriasis, irritability, anxiety, insomnia, backache, joint pain, weakness, abdominal cramps, anorexia, nausea, vomiting, diarrhea, increased BP or HR, increased respiratory rate). Such symptoms may indicate a need to taper more slowly. Also monitor patient for suicidality, use of other substances, and mood changes.

Reactions in bold italics are *life-threatening*. Interactions may have a *rapid onset* or a ***delayed onset***.

PATIENT TEACHING

Boxed Warning Caution patient or caregiver of patient taking an opioid with a benzodiazepine, CNS depressant, or alcohol to seek immediate medical attention for dizziness, light-headedness, extreme sleepiness, slowed or difficult breathing, or unresponsiveness. ■

• **Alert:** Warn patient and caregiver of patient taking codeine to watch for slow or shallow breathing, difficult or noisy breathing, confusion, excessive sleepiness, or trouble breastfeeding or limpness (in infant). If any of these signs occur, tell patient to stop drug and immediately seek emergency medical attention.

• Warn patient to stop drug and seek medical attention immediately if skin rash or reaction occurs while using acetaminophen.

• Encourage patient to report all medications being taken, including prescriptions and OTC medications and supplements.

• Caution patient to immediately report signs and symptoms of serotonin syndrome, adrenal insufficiency, and decreased sex hormone levels.

• **Alert:** Counsel patient not to discontinue opioids without first discussing the need for gradual tapering of the regimen with prescriber.

• Teach patients that naloxone may be prescribed in conjunction with the opioid when beginning and renewing treatment as a preventive measure to reduce opioid overdose and death.

• Inform patient with severe hepatic or renal disease that serial renal function tests or LFTs will be needed.

• Caution patient not to drive a car or operate heavy machinery while taking this drug.

• Warn patient about alcohol use during therapy.

• Warn patient that codeine may be habit-forming and to take only as long as it's prescribed and in the amounts prescribed.

⬚ Advise patient who is breastfeeding and is an ultrarapid metabolizer to obtain emergency treatment if the infant shows signs and symptoms of codeine toxicity (sleepiness, difficulty breastfeeding or breathing, limpness).

codeine sulfate ⬚

Therapeutic class: Opioid analgesics
Pharmacologic class: Opioids
Controlled substance schedule: II

AVAILABLE FORMS

Tablets: 15 mg, 30 mg, 60 mg

INDICATIONS & DOSAGES

➤ **Mild to moderately severe pain**

Adults: 15 to 60 mg PO up to every 4 hours PRN for pain. Adjust dosage to obtain appropriate balance between pain management and opioid-related adverse reactions. Maximum is 360 mg/24 hours.

Adjust-a-dose: For older adults or patients with renal or hepatic impairment, begin with lower-than-normal dosages or with longer dosing intervals and titrate slowly while monitoring for respiratory depression, sedation, and hypotension. Initiate individual dosing regimen for each patient, taking into account pain severity, patient response, prior analgesic treatment experience, and risk factors for addiction, abuse, and misuse.

ADMINISTRATION

PO

• Give drug with milk or meals to avoid GI upset.

• Pharmacist may compound drug into an oral suspension if patient can't swallow tablets.

• Store at room temperature.

ACTION

May bind with opioid receptors in the CNS, altering perception of and emotional response to pain. Also suppresses the cough reflex by direct action on the cough center in the medulla.

Route	Onset	Peak	Duration
PO	30–60 min	1–2 hr	4–6 hr

Half-life: 2.5 to 3.5 hours.

ADVERSE REACTIONS

CNS: drowsiness, sedation, dizziness, euphoria, dysphoria, light-headedness. **CV:** *bradycardia,* flushing, hypotension. **EENT:** dry mouth. **GI:** constipation, nausea, vomiting, abdominal pain. **GU:** urine retention.

Respiratory: shortness of breath, *respiratory depression.* **Skin:** diaphoresis, pruritus. **Other:** hypersensitivity reaction.

INTERACTIONS

Drug-drug. `Boxed Warning`
Benzodiazepines, CNS depressants: May cause respiratory depression, sedation, coma, and death. Avoid use together. If use together is necessary, limit dosage and duration of each drug to the minimum necessary for desired effect. ▪

CNS depressants, general anesthetics, hypnotics, other opioid analgesics, sedatives, TCAs, tranquilizers: May cause additive effects. Use together cautiously; monitor patient response.

`Boxed Warning` *CYP3A4 inducers and inhibitors, CYP2D6 inhibitors:* Effects of concomitant use or discontinuation of these drugs with codeine are complex. Their use with codeine sulfate requires careful consideration of the effects on the parent drug, codeine, and the active metabolite, morphine. ▪

CYP2D6 inhibitors (bupropion, paroxetine), CYP3A4 inducers (carbamazepine, phenytoin, rifampin): May decrease analgesic effect or increase risk of opioid withdrawal. Avoid use if possible. If concomitant use is necessary, monitor patient closely.

CYP3A4 inhibitors (azole antifungals, macrolide antibiotics, protease inhibitors): May increase codeine effects and risk of adverse reactions, including respiratory depression. Consider reducing codeine dosage; monitor patient closely.

Diuretics: May decrease effect of diuretic. Monitor patient for diminished diuresis or effects on BP.

MAO inhibitors (linezolid, phenelzine): May cause serotonin syndrome or opioid toxicity (respiratory depression, coma). Use together or within 14 days is contraindicated. If urgent use of an opioid is necessary, use test doses and frequent titration of small doses of other opioids (such as oxycodone, hydrocodone, oxymorphone, or buprenorphine) to treat pain while closely monitoring BP and signs and symptoms of CNS and respiratory depression.

Muscle relaxants (baclofen, methocarbamol): May increase neuromuscular blocking effect and risk of respiratory depression. Monitor patient closely.

Opioid antagonists (nalbuphine, pentazocine): May reduce analgesic effect or precipitate withdrawal symptoms. Avoid use together.

🕓 *Alert:* Serotonergic drugs (amoxapine, antiemetics [dolasetron, granisetron, ondansetron, palonosetron], antimigraine drugs, buspirone, cyclobenzaprine, dextromethorphan, lithium, maprotiline, methylene blue, mirtazapine, nefazodone, SSNRIs, SSRIs, TCAs, trazodone, tryptophan, vilazodone): May increase risk of serotonin syndrome. Use together cautiously and monitor patient for serotonin syndrome.

Drug-herb. *St. John's wort:* May increase risk of serotonin syndrome. Use together cautiously.

Drug-lifestyle. `Boxed Warning` *Alcohol use:* May cause slow or difficult breathing, sedation, and death. Avoid use together. ▪

EFFECTS ON LAB TEST RESULTS

• May increase amylase and lipase levels.
• May cause urine drug screen to be positive for morphine.

CONTRAINDICATIONS & CAUTIONS

• Contraindicated in patients hypersensitive to drug and in patients with significant respiratory depression, acute or severe bronchial asthma in an unmonitored setting or in the absence of resuscitative equipment, and in those with known or suspected GI obstruction, including paralytic ileus.

`Boxed Warning` Opioids should only be prescribed with benzodiazepines or other CNS depressants to patients for whom alternative treatment options are inadequate. ▪

`Boxed Warning` Drug exposes users to the risks of opioid addiction, abuse, and misuse, which can lead to overdose and death. To ensure that the benefits of opioid analgesics outweigh the risks of addiction, abuse, and misuse, the FDA has required a REMS program for these products. Assess each patient's risk (previous substance use disorder, younger age, major depression, psychotropic drug use) before prescribing drug. ▪

🕓 *Alert:* Safety and effectiveness and pharmacokinetics of codeine in children younger than age 18 haven't been established.

`Boxed Warning` Children who receive codeine for pain relief after a tonsillectomy or adenoidectomy and are ultrarapid metabolizers due to a CYP2D6 polymorphism have

---

Reactions in bold italics are *life-threatening*. Interactions may have a *rapid onset* or a *delayed onset*.

an increased risk of death. Codeine is contraindicated for pain management after these surgeries. ∎

• Drug may lead to a rare but serious decrease in adrenal gland cortisol production.

• Drug may decrease sex hormone levels with long-term use.

Alert: Patients are at increased risk of oversedation and respiratory depression if they have snoring or history of sleep apnea, no recent opioid use or are first-time opioid users, have increased opioid dose requirements or opioid habituation, received general anesthesia for longer lengths of time, received other sedating drugs, have preexisting pulmonary or cardiac disease, or have thoracic or other surgical incisions that may impair breathing. Monitor patients carefully.

Boxed Warning Accidental ingestion of even one dose of codeine sulfate tablets, especially by children, can result in a fatal overdose. ∎

• Use cautiously in older adults, patients who are debilitated, and in those with head injury, increased ICP, increased CSF pressure, hepatic or renal disease, hypothyroidism, Addison disease, acute alcoholism, seizures, severe CNS depression, bronchial asthma, COPD, respiratory depression, and shock.
Dialyzable drug: Unknown.

Overdose S&S: CNS depression, respiratory depression, apnea, flaccid skeletal muscles, bradycardia, hypotension, circulatory collapse, death.

PREGNANCY-LACTATION-REPRODUCTION

Alert: There are no adequate well-controlled studies during pregnancy. Use during pregnancy only if potential benefit justifies fetal risk.

Boxed Warning Prolonged use during pregnancy can cause neonatal withdrawal syndrome, which can be life-threatening and requires management by neonatology experts. If used during pregnancy, advise patient of risks and ensure appropriate treatment is available. ∎

• Don't administer drug during labor when delivery of a premature infant is anticipated.

Alert: Breastfeeding isn't recommended for patients taking codeine because of the risk of serious adverse reactions in breastfed infants, such as excess sleepiness, difficulty breastfeeding, or serious breathing problems that could result in death.

NURSING CONSIDERATIONS

Boxed Warning Serious, life-threatening, or fatal respiratory depression may occur with use of codeine sulfate tablets. Monitor patients for respiratory depression, especially during initiation or after a dosage increase. ∎

Boxed Warning Monitor all patients regularly for development of opioid addiction, abuse, and misuse, which can lead to overdose and death. ∎

• If patient is taking opioids with serotonergic drugs, watch for signs and symptoms of serotonin syndrome (agitation, hallucinations, rapid HR, fever, diaphoresis, shivering or shaking, muscle twitching or stiffness, trouble with coordination, nausea, vomiting, diarrhea), especially at start of treatment or after dosage increases. Signs and symptoms may occur within several hours of coadministration but may occur later, especially after dosage increase. Discontinue opioid, serotonergic drug, or both if serotonin syndrome is suspected.

• Monitor patient for signs and symptoms of adrenal insufficiency (nausea, vomiting, loss of appetite, fatigue, weakness, dizziness, low BP). Perform diagnostic testing if adrenal insufficiency is suspected. If adrenal insufficiency is confirmed, treat with corticosteroids and wean patient off opioids if appropriate. Discontinue corticosteroids when clinically appropriate.

• Monitor patient for signs and symptoms of decreased sex hormone levels (low libido, erectile dysfunction, amenorrhea, infertility). If signs and symptoms occur, evaluate patient and obtain lab testing.

Alert: Don't stop drug abruptly; withdraw slowly and individualize the gradual taper plan to prevent signs and symptoms of withdrawal, worsening pain, and psychological distress in patients who are physically dependent. Refer to manufacturer's label for specific tapering instructions.

Alert: When tapering opioids, monitor patient closely for signs and symptoms of opioid withdrawal (restlessness, lacrimation, rhinorrhea, yawning, perspiration, chills, myalgia, mydriasis, irritability, anxiety, insomnia, backache, joint pain, weakness, abdominal cramps, anorexia, nausea, vomiting, diarrhea, increased BP or HR, increased respiratory rate). Such symptoms may indicate a need to taper more slowly. Also monitor patient for

suicidality, use of other substances, and mood changes.
- Reassess patient's level of pain at least 15 and 30 minutes after use.
- For full analgesic effect, give drug before patient has intense pain.
- Drug is an antitussive; don't use when cough is a valuable diagnostic sign or is beneficial (as after thoracic surgery). Monitor cough type and frequency.
- Monitor respiratory and circulatory status.
- Opioids may cause constipation. Assess bowel function and need for stool softeners and stimulant laxatives.
- Codeine may delay gastric emptying, increase biliary tract pressure from contraction of the sphincter of Oddi, and interfere with hepatobiliary imaging studies.
- *Look alike–sound alike:* Don't confuse codeine with Cardene or Cordran.

PATIENT TEACHING
Boxed Warning Caution patient or caregiver of patient taking an opioid with a benzodiazepine, CNS depressant, or alcohol to seek immediate medical attention for dizziness, light-headedness, extreme sleepiness, slowed or difficult breathing, or unresponsiveness. ∎
🕓 *Alert:* Warn patient and caregiver of patient taking codeine to watch for slow or shallow breathing, difficult or noisy breathing, confusion, excessive sleepiness, or trouble breastfeeding or limpness (in infant). If any of these signs occur, tell patient or caregiver to stop drug and immediately seek emergency medical attention.
🕓 *Alert:* Encourage patient to report all medications being taken, including prescriptions and OTC medications and supplements.
- Caution patient to immediately report signs and symptoms of serotonin syndrome, adrenal insufficiency, and or decreased sex hormone levels.
🕓 *Alert:* Counsel patient not to discontinue opioids without first discussing the need for a gradual tapering regimen with prescriber.
- Teach patients that naloxone may be prescribed in conjunction with the opioid when beginning and renewing treatment as a preventive measure to reduce opioid overdose and death.
- Advise patient that GI distress caused by taking drug orally can be eased by taking drug with milk or meals.

- Instruct patient to ask for or to take drug before pain is intense.
- Caution patient who is ambulatory about getting out of bed or walking. Warn outpatient to avoid driving and other hazardous activities that require mental alertness until drug's effects on the CNS are known.
- Advise patient to avoid alcohol during therapy.
Boxed Warning Warn patient that accidental ingestion of even one dose of codeine sulfate, especially by children, can result in a fatal overdose of codeine. ∎
- Warn patient who is breastfeeding to watch for increased sleepiness, difficulty breastfeeding or breathing, or limpness (in infant). Tell patient to immediately seek medical attention if this occurs.

---

colchicine ⬚
KOL-chi-seen

Colcrys🗸, Gloperba, Mitigare

Therapeutic class: Antigout drugs
Pharmacologic class: Colchicum autumnale alkaloids

AVAILABLE FORMS
Capsules: 0.6 mg
Oral solution: 0.6 mg/5 mL
Tablets: 0.6 mg

INDICATIONS & DOSAGES
Adjust-a-dose (for all indications): Administration of CYP3A4 or P-gp inhibitors or inhibitors of both CYP3A4 and P-gp with colchicine in patients who are on or have recently completed treatment (within the past 14 days) has been reported to lead to colchicine toxicity and fatal drug interactions, particularly in patients with hepatic or renal impairment. If coadministration is required, colchicine dose may need to be reduced or therapy interrupted; monitor patient carefully for colchicine toxicity. Refer to Colcrys manufacturer's instructions for dosage adjustments by drug and indication for CYP3A4, P-gp, and protease inhibitors.
➤ **Prevention of gout flares**
Adults: 0.6 mg PO once daily or b.i.d. Maximum daily dose is 1.2 mg.

Reactions in bold italics are *life-threatening*. Interactions may have a *rapid onset* or a **delayed onset**.

Children older than age 16 (Colcrys): 0.6 mg PO once daily or b.i.d. Maximum daily dose, 1.2 mg.

Adjust-a-dose: For patients taking Colcrys with CrCl of less than 30 mL/minute, give 0.3 mg/day. Closely monitor patient after dosage increases. For patients on dialysis, starting doses should be 0.3 mg twice a week with close monitoring. Closely monitor patients with mild to moderate hepatic impairment; no dosage adjustment is required. Consider dosage reduction in patients with severe hepatic impairment.

For patients taking Mitigare or Gloperba, consider dosage reduction or alternative drug in patients with severe renal impairment; closely monitor patients undergoing hemodialysis for toxicity. Consider dosage reduction or alternative drug in patients with severe hepatic impairment.

➤ **Gout flares (Colcrys)**
Adults and adolescents older than age 16: 1.2 mg PO at first sign of a flare, followed by 0.6 mg 1 hour later; maximum dosage is 1.8 mg over a 1-hour period. Wait 12 hours before resuming gout prophylaxis.

Adjust-a-dose: For patients with CrCl of less than 30 mL/minute or severe hepatic impairment, no dosage adjustment is needed but treatment course should be repeated no more than once every 2 weeks. For patients with severe renal or hepatic impairment requiring repeated courses for the treatment of gout flares, consider alternative therapy. For patients on dialysis, reduce total recommended dose for treatment of gout flares to a single dose of 0.6 mg (one tablet) no more than once every 2 weeks.

➤ **Familial Mediterranean fever (Colcrys)** 🧬
Adults: 1.2 to 2.4 mg PO daily; may increase by 0.3 mg/day to maximum daily dose given once daily or in two divided doses.
Adolescents age 13 and older: 1.2 to 2.4 mg PO once daily or in two divided doses.
Children ages 6 to 12: 0.9 to 1.8 mg PO once daily or in two divided doses.
Children ages 4 to 6: 0.3 to 1.8 mg PO once daily or in two divided doses.

Adjust-a-dose: For patients with CrCl of less than 30 mL/minute or ESRD requiring dialysis, initially 0.3 mg/day, carefully increasing dosage as needed. For patients with severe hepatic disease, consider dosage reduction with careful monitoring. Decrease

dosage by 0.3 mg/day, if intolerable adverse effects.

➤ **Behçet syndrome with arthritis, cutaneous lesions, or mucocutaneous ulcers** ◆
Adults: 1.2 to 1.8 mg/day in two to three divided doses.

➤ **Pericarditis, acute and recurrent, in combination with aspirin or NSAIDs** ◆
Adults: For maintenance, with or without loading dose: In patients weighing 70 kg or more, give 0.6 mg b.i.d.; for those weighing less than 70 kg or unable to tolerate higher dosing regimen, give 0.6 mg once daily.

ADMINISTRATION
PO
• Hazardous drug; use safe handling and disposal precautions.
• Give drug with or without food.
• Give missed dose as soon as possible; then return to normal dosing schedule. Don't double dose.

ACTION
Exact mechanism of action is not fully known; thought to involve a reduction in lactic acid produced by leukocytes, reducing uric acid deposits and phagocytosis, thereby decreasing the inflammatory process.

Route	Onset	Peak	Duration
PO	Unknown	30–180 min	Unknown

Half-life: 27 to 31 hours.

ADVERSE REACTIONS
CNS: fatigue, headache. **EENT:** pharyngolaryngeal pain. **GI:** diarrhea, nausea, vomiting, abdominal discomfort. **Hematologic:** *aplastic anemia, granulocytopenia, leukopenia, pancytopenia, thrombocytopenia.* **Metabolic:** gout.

INTERACTIONS
Drug-drug. *Acidifying agents:* May inhibit action of colchicine. Avoid use together.
Alkalinizing agents: May increase action of colchicine. Avoid use together.
CNS depressants, sympathomimetics (such as phenylephrine): May increase sensitivity to these drugs. Monitor patient closely and adjust dosage as needed.
Digoxin, HMG-CoA reductase inhibitors (atorvastatin, simvastatin): May increase risk of myopathy or rhabdomyolysis. Avoid use together. If coadministration can't be

avoided, monitor patient carefully. Discontinue colchicine if signs or symptoms occur. *Moderate CYP3A4 inhibitors (amprenavir, aprepitant, diltiazem, erythromycin, fluconazole, fosamprenavir, verapamil), P-gp inhibitors (cyclosporine, ranolazine), strong CYP3A4 inhibitors (atazanavir, clarithromycin, itraconazole, ketoconazole, nefazodone, nelfinavir, ritonavir, saquinavir; fixed combination of elvitegravir–cobicistat–emtricitabine–tenofovir):* May increase colchicine level, increasing the risk of toxic effects. Reduce colchicine dosage if alternative treatment isn't available. Concurrent use in patients with renal or hepatic impairment is contraindicated.

Drug-food. *Grapefruit, grapefruit juice:* May increase drug level. Discourage use together.

EFFECTS ON LAB TEST RESULTS
• May increase AST, ALT, and CK levels.
• May decrease Hb level, hematocrit, and leukocyte, granulocyte, and platelet counts.
• May cause false-positive results when testing urine for RBCs or Hb.

CONTRAINDICATIONS & CAUTIONS
• Contraindicated in patients with serious CV, renal, hepatic, or GI impairment and in those taking P-gp inhibitors or strong CYP3A4 inhibitors.
• Don't give Mitigare or Gloperba to patients with both renal and hepatic impairment.
• Myelosuppression has been reported. Use cautiously in patients with hematologic disorders.
◑ *Alert:* Fatal overdoses, both accidental and intentional, have been reported in adults and children who have ingested colchicine.
Dialyzable drug: No.
⚠ *Overdose S&S:* Abdominal pain, nausea, vomiting, diarrhea, hypovolemia, multiorgan failure, death.

PREGNANCY-LACTATION-REPRODUCTION
• There are no adequate studies during pregnancy. Use during pregnancy only if potential benefit justifies fetal risk.
• Drug isn't expected to appear in human milk. Use cautiously during breastfeeding and observe infants for adverse effects related to vitamin absorption.

NURSING CONSIDERATIONS
• Safety and effectiveness of repeat treatment for gout flares haven't been established.
◑ *Alert:* Colcrys, Gloperba, and Mitigare are the only FDA-approved single-ingredient colchicine products.
• Drug isn't an analgesic and shouldn't be used to treat pain from other causes.
• Obtain baseline lab studies, including CBC, before starting therapy and periodically thereafter; watch for myelosuppression, leukopenia, granulocytopenia, thrombocytopenia, pancytopenia, and aplastic anemia.
• Monitor patient who has used drug for a prolonged period for neuromuscular toxicity and rhabdomyolysis.
• If nausea, vomiting, or diarrhea occurs, discontinue drug.
• Drug may increase risk of malignancy.
• When used for gout prophylaxis, colchicine must be given with allopurinol or a uricosuric drug (such as probenecid) to decrease serum uric acid level. However, colchicine should be started before the other agent because a sudden change in uric acid level may cause a gout attack.
• *Look alike–sound alike:* Don't confuse colchicine with Cortrosyn.

PATIENT TEACHING
• Teach patient proper drug administration.
• Advise patient to take drug as prescribed even if feeling better and not to alter dosage or discontinue drug without first discussing with prescriber.
• Caution patient that many drugs and other substances may interact with colchicine and to tell prescriber and pharmacist all prescription and OTC medications and supplements used. Patient should check with prescriber before starting new medications, especially antibiotics.
• Tell patient to keep drug out of the reach of children due to risk of fatal overdose.
• Advise patient to report all adverse reactions, including muscle pain or weakness, tingling or numbness in fingers or toes, unusual bleeding or bruising, increased infections, weakness, tiredness, cyanosis, nausea, vomiting, or diarrhea; advise patient to discontinue drug.

Reactions in bold italics are *life-threatening*. Interactions may have a *rapid onset* or a ***delayed onset***.

crisaborole
kris-a-BOR-ole

Eucrisa

Therapeutic class: Dermatologic agents
Pharmacologic class: Phosphodiesterase 4 inhibitors

AVAILABLE FORMS
Topical ointment: 2%

INDICATIONS & DOSAGES
➤ **Mild to moderate atopic dermatitis**
Adults and children age 3 months and older:
Apply a thin film to affected areas b.i.d.

ADMINISTRATION
Topical
• Drug is for external use only; not for ophthalmic, oral, or intravaginal use.
• Store at room temperature.
• Keep tube tightly closed.

ACTION
Exact mechanism unknown. Drug is a phosphodiesterase 4 inhibitor that increases intracellular cAMP levels.

Route	Onset	Peak	Duration
Topical	Unknown	Unknown	Unknown

Half-life: Unknown.

ADVERSE REACTIONS
Skin: application-site pain, burning, or stinging.

INTERACTIONS
None reported.

EFFECTS ON LAB TEST RESULTS
None reported.

CONTRAINDICATIONS & CAUTIONS
• Contraindicated in patients hypersensitive to drug or its components.
• Hypersensitivity reactions have been reported, including contact urticaria.
• Safety and effectiveness in children younger than age 3 months haven't been established.
Dialyzable drug: Unlikely.

PREGNANCY-LACTATION-REPRODUCTION
• Drug hasn't been studied during pregnancy. In animal studies, there were no adverse developmental effects.
• Drug is systemically absorbed; risk of harm in infants who are breastfed is unknown. Consider benefits to patient and risks to infant before using.

NURSING CONSIDERATIONS
• Monitor patient for severe pruritus, swelling, and erythema, which may indicate hypersensitivity. If these occur, discontinue drug.

PATIENT TEACHING
• Advise patient to discontinue drug and immediately report signs or symptoms of hypersensitivity reactions, such as hives, itching, swelling, and redness.
• Warn patient that effects of drug in patient who is pregnant or breastfeeding are unknown.
• Remind patient or caregivers to wash hands after applying drug unless patient's hands are being treated.

cyclobenzaprine hydrochloride
sye-kloe-BEN-za-preen

Amrix, Fexmid

Therapeutic class: Skeletal muscle relaxants
Pharmacologic class: TCA derivatives

AVAILABLE FORMS
Capsules (extended-release) 🚫: 15 mg, 30 mg
Tablets: 5 mg, 7.5 mg, 10 mg

INDICATIONS & DOSAGES
➤ **Adjunct to rest and physical therapy to relieve muscle spasm from acute, painful musculoskeletal conditions**
Adults and children age 15 and older: 5 mg PO t.i.d. Based on response, may increase to 7.5 or 10 mg t.i.d. Don't exceed 30 mg/day. Or, initially, 15 mg extended-release capsule PO once daily; may increase to 30 mg daily (adults only). Use for longer than 2 or 3 weeks isn't recommended.
Adjust-a-dose: In older adults and patients with mild hepatic impairment, start with

5-mg conventional tablets and adjust slowly upward; consider less frequent dosing. Don't use extended-release capsules in children, older adults, or patients with impaired hepatic function.

ADMINISTRATION
PO
• Don't split the generic 10-mg tablets because of the high risk of inconsistent doses.
• Give extended-release capsules whole; don't crush or break.
• In patients able to reliably swallow applesauce without chewing, sprinkle capsule contents onto a tablespoon of applesauce; have patient consume immediately without chewing then rinse the mouth to ensure all of the contents have been swallowed.

ACTION
Unknown. Relieves skeletal muscle spasm of local origin without disrupting muscle function.

Route	Onset	Peak	Duration
PO	1 hr	4 hr	12–24 hr
PO (extended-release)	1.5 hr	7–8 hr	Unknown

Half-life: Tablets, 18 hours; extended-release capsules, 32 hours.

ADVERSE REACTIONS
CNS: dizziness, irritability, somnolence, drowsiness, *seizures*, headache, tremor, insomnia, fatigue, asthenia, nervousness, decreased mental acuity, attention disturbances, dysgeusia. **CV:** palpitations. **EENT:** visual disturbances, blurred vision, pharyngitis, dry mouth. **GI:** dyspepsia, constipation, nausea, diarrhea, abdominal pain. **Respiratory:** URI. **Skin:** acne.

INTERACTIONS
Drug-drug. *CNS depressants:* May increase CNS depression. Avoid using together.
MAO inhibitors: May cause hyperpyretic crisis, seizures, and death when MAO inhibitors are used with TCAs; may also occur with cyclobenzaprine. Avoid using within 2 weeks of MAO inhibitor therapy.
Boxed Warning *Opioid class warning:* Use with opioids may cause slow or difficult breathing, sedation, and death. Avoid use together. If use together is necessary, limit dosage and duration of each drug to the minimum necessary for desired effect. ∎

Naproxen: May increase drowsiness. Make patient aware of this interaction.
Tramadol: May increase risk of seizures. Use together cautiously.
Drug-lifestyle. *Alcohol use:* May increase CNS depression. Discourage use together.

EFFECTS ON LAB TEST RESULTS
• May cause false-positive serum TCA screen.

CONTRAINDICATIONS & CAUTIONS
• Contraindicated in patients hypersensitive to drug; in those with hyperthyroidism, heart block, arrhythmias, conduction disturbances, or HF; and in those in the acute recovery phase of an MI.
• Drug isn't recommended in patients with moderate to severe hepatic impairment.
• There is increased risk of potentially life-threatening serotonin syndrome when drug is used in combination with SSRIs, SSNRIs, other TCAs, tramadol, bupropion, meperidine, or verapamil.
• Use cautiously in older adults, patients who are debilitated, and patients with a history of urine retention, acute angle-closure glaucoma, or increased IOP.
• Safety and effectiveness of immediate-release form in children younger than age 15 or of extended-release in all children haven't been established.
Dialyzable drug: Unknown.
⚠ **Overdose S&S:** Drowsiness, tachycardia, tremor, agitation, coma, ataxia, HTN, slurred speech, confusion, dizziness, nausea, vomiting, hallucinations, cardiac arrest, chest pain, cardiac arrhythmias, ECG changes (changes in QRS axis or width).

PREGNANCY-LACTATION-REPRODUCTION
• There are no adequate well-controlled studies during pregnancy. Use during pregnancy only if clearly needed.
• It isn't known if drug appears in human milk. Use cautiously during breastfeeding.

NURSING CONSIDERATIONS
• Drug may cause toxic reactions similar to those caused by TCAs, including arrhythmias and prolonged conduction time leading to MI and stroke. Observe same precautions as when giving TCAs.
• Monitor patient for nausea, headache, and malaise, which may occur if drug is stopped abruptly after long-term use.

Reactions in bold italics are *life-threatening*. Interactions may have a *rapid onset* or a **delayed onset**.

• Monitor patient for serotonin syndrome (mental status changes, diaphoresis, tachycardia, labile BP, hyperthermia, neuromuscular abnormalities, GI symptoms).

🌙 *Alert:* Notify prescriber immediately of signs and symptoms of overdose, including cardiac toxicity.

PATIENT TEACHING

Boxed Warning Caution patient or caregiver of patient taking an opioid with a benzodiazepine, CNS depressant, or alcohol to seek immediate medical attention for dizziness, light-headedness, extreme sleepiness, slowed or difficult breathing, or unresponsiveness. ■

• Advise patient to report urinary hesitancy or urine retention. If constipation is a problem, suggest that patient increase fluid intake and use a stool softener.

• Warn patient to avoid activities that require alertness until CNS effects of drug are known.

• Warn patient not to combine with alcohol or other CNS depressants, including OTC cold or allergy remedies.

• Instruct patient in proper drug administration.

• Advise patient that using drug for longer than 2 to 3 weeks isn't recommended.

SAFETY ALERT!

cyclophosphamide
sye-kloe-FOSS-fa-mide

Procytox ❦

Therapeutic class: Antineoplastics
Pharmacologic class: Nitrogen mustards

AVAILABLE FORMS
Capsules 🔘: 25 mg, 50 mg
Injection: 200-mg❦, 500-mg, 1-g, 2-g vials

INDICATIONS & DOSAGES
Adjust-a-dose (for all indications): Consider dosage reduction to 75% of usual dosage in patients with severe renal failure (CrCl of 0 to 10 mL/minute). Adjust dosage for patients with hepatic dysfunction: If bilirubin level is 3.1 to 5 mg/dL or transaminase levels are greater than 3 × ULN, give 75% of dose. Don't give if bilirubin level is greater than 5 mg/dL.

➤ **Breast or ovarian cancer, Hodgkin lymphoma, chronic lymphocytic leukemia, chronic myelocytic leukemia, acute lymphoblastic leukemia, acute myelocytic and monocytic leukemia, neuroblastoma, retinoblastoma, malignant lymphoma, multiple myeloma, mycosis fungoides**
Adults and children: Initially for induction, 40 to 50 mg/kg IV in divided doses over 2 to 5 days. Or, 10 to 15 mg/kg IV every 7 to 10 days, 3 to 5 mg/kg IV twice weekly, or 1 to 5 mg/kg PO daily, based on patient tolerance. Adjust subsequent doses according to evidence of antitumor activity or leukopenia.
➤ **Minimal-change nephrotic syndrome in patients who failed to adequately respond to or are unable to tolerate adrenocorticosteroid therapy**
Children: 2 mg/kg PO daily for 8 to 12 weeks. Maximum cumulative dose, 168 mg/kg.

ADMINISTRATION
• Preparing and administering drug may be mutagenic, teratogenic, or carcinogenic. Follow facility protocol to reduce risks. Always wear gloves.

PO
• Give oral form in the morning; infrequent urination during the night may increase possibility of cystitis.

• Drug is associated with moderate to high emetic potential. Consider antiemetics to prevent nausea and vomiting.

• Make sure patient receives adequate fluids or is infused to force diuresis to reduce risk of urinary tract toxicity.

• Don't open, cut, crush, or allow patient to chew capsules.

• Pharmacist can prepare solution for oral administration. Must refrigerate solution for up to 14 days. Shake before use.
IV
▼ For direct IV injection, reconstitute powder with NSS for injection only.

▼ For IV infusion, first reconstitute powder using NSS for injection or sterile water for injection.

▼ Add 25 mL to 500-mg vial, 50 mL to 1-g vial, or 100 mL to 2-g vial to produce a solution containing 20 mg/mL. Shake vigorously to dissolve. If powder doesn't dissolve completely, let vial stand for a few minutes.

▼ Check reconstituted solution for small particles. Filter solution, if needed.

❦Canada   ◊OTC   ◆Off-label use   ✐Photoguide   🔘Do not crush   *Liquid contains alcohol   ▨Genetic

▼ For infusion, further dilute with D_5W, dextrose 5% in NSS for injection, or half-NSS for injection to minimum concentration of 2 mg/mL.

▼ Give by direct IV injection slowly or IV infusion over 1 to 2 hours.

▼ Without further dilution, solution reconstituted in NSS for injection is stable for 6 days if refrigerated or 24 hours at room temperature. Solution reconstituted in sterile water for injection must be used immediately.

▼ Reconstituted solutions further diluted in half-NSS for injection are stable for 24 hours at room temperature or 6 days if refrigerated; those diluted in D_5W or dextrose 5% in NSS for injection are stable for 24 hours at room temperature or 36 hours if refrigerated.

▼ Use stored solutions cautiously because drug contains no preservatives.

▼ **Incompatibilities:** None listed by manufacturer. Consult a drug incompatibility reference for more information.

ACTION

Cross-links strands of cellular DNA and interferes with RNA transcription, causing an imbalance of growth that leads to cell death. Not specific to cell cycle.

Route	Onset	Peak	Duration
PO	Unknown	Unknown	Unknown
IV	Unknown	2–3 hr	Unknown

Half-life: 3 to 12 hours.

ADVERSE REACTIONS

GI: nausea, vomiting, anorexia, abdominal discomfort, stomatitis. **Hematologic:** *leukopenia, neutropenia, thrombocytopenia,* anemia. **Hepatic:** *hepatotoxicity.* **Metabolic:** hyperuricemia, hyponatremia. **Skin:** alopecia. **Other:** hypersensitivity reactions.

INTERACTIONS

Drug-drug. *ACE inhibitors, allopurinol, clozapine, natalizumab, paclitaxel, thiazide diuretics, zidovudine:* May increase hematotoxicity and immunosuppression. Monitor therapy.
Amiodarone, G-CSF drugs: May increase risk of pulmonary toxicity. Monitor therapy.

Amphotericin B, indomethacin: May increase risk of nephrotoxicity. Monitor patient closely.
Azathioprine: May increase risk of hepatotoxicity (liver necrosis). Monitor patient closely.
Busulfan: May increase risk of hepatic venoocclusive disease. Monitor patient closely.
Cardiotoxic drugs (anthracycline), cytarabine, pentostatin, trastuzumab): May increase adverse cardiac effects. Monitor patient for toxicity.
Cyclosporine: May decrease cyclosporine concentration and increase risk of GVHD. Monitor patient closely.
Etanercept: May increase risk of malignant solid tumors in patients with Wegener granulomatosis. Use cautiously.
Leflunomide: May increase risk of hematologic toxicity, such as pancytopenia, agranulocytosis, or thrombocytopenia. Don't use a leflunomide loading dose and monitor patient for bone marrow suppression at least monthly.
Live-virus vaccines: May increase vaccine-induced adverse reactions. Don't give together.
Metronidazole: May increase risk of acute encephalopathy. Monitor patient response.
Protease inhibitors: May increase cyclophosphamide-related toxicities and mucositis. Monitor therapy.
Succinylcholine: May prolong neuromuscular blockade and cause apnea. Avoid using together and alert anesthesiologist if drug has been given within 10 days of general anesthesia.
Tamoxifen: May increase risk of thromboembolism. Monitor patient closely.
Warfarin: May increase or decrease warfarin effects. Monitor patient closely.
Drug-herb. *Echinacea:* May decrease effect of cyclophosphamide. Consider alternative agents.

EFFECTS ON LAB TEST RESULTS

• May increase uric acid level. May decrease Hb and pseudocholinesterase levels.
• May decrease platelet, RBC, and WBC counts.
• May suppress positive reaction to *Candida,* mumps, *Trichophyton,* and tuberculin skin test results. May cause a false-positive Papanicolaou test result.

Reactions in bold italics are *life-threatening.* Interactions may have a *rapid onset* or a *delayed onset.*

C

CONTRAINDICATIONS & CAUTIONS

• Contraindicated in patients hypersensitive to drug and in those with severe bone marrow suppression or urinary outflow obstruction.
• Use cautiously in patients with hypersensitivity to other alkylating agents; cross-sensitivity can occur.
• Use cautiously in patients with leukopenia, thrombocytopenia, malignant cell infiltration of bone marrow, or hepatic, cardiac, or renal disease and in those who have recently undergone radiation therapy or chemotherapy; radiation therapy of the cardiac region may increase risk of cardiotoxicity.
• Combined effect of cyclophosphamide and past or concomitant radiation treatment may increase risk of hemorrhagic cystitis.
• Drug may increase risk of secondary malignancies and veno-occlusive liver disease.
Dialyzable drug: Yes.
⚠ ***Overdose S&S:*** Infection, myelosuppression, cardiotoxicity.

PREGNANCY-LACTATION-REPRODUCTION

• Drug may cause fetal harm if used during pregnancy. Patients of childbearing potential should avoid pregnancy while receiving cyclophosphamide and for up to 1 year after completion of treatment. Male patients who are sexually active with partners of childbearing potential should use a condom during and for at least 4 months after treatment.
• Amenorrhea, transient or permanent, develops in a proportion of patients treated with drug. The risk of premature menopause increases with age.
• Men treated with drug may develop oligospermia or azoospermia. Development of sterility appears to depend on dose, duration of therapy, and state of gonadal function at time of treatment. Sterility may be irreversible in some patients. Treatment for nephrotic syndrome beyond 90 days in boys increases the probability of sterility.
• Drug appears in human milk. Patient should discontinue breastfeeding or discontinue drug, taking into account importance of drug to the patient.

NURSING CONSIDERATIONS

• If cystitis occurs, stop drug and notify prescriber. Cystitis can occur months after therapy ends. Mesna may be given to reduce frequency and severity of bladder toxicity. Test urine for blood.
• Adequately hydrate patients before and after dose to decrease risk of cystitis.
• Use caution to ensure correct dose to decrease risk of cardiac toxicity.
• Monitor CBC and renal function tests and LFT results.
• Monitor patient closely for leukopenia (nadir between days 8 and 15, recovery in 17 to 28 days). Withhold drug for ANC less than $1,500/\text{mm}^3$.
• Monitor uric acid level. To prevent hyperuricemia with resulting uric acid nephropathy, allopurinol may be used with adequate hydration.
• To prevent bleeding, avoid all IM injections when platelet count is less than $50,000/\text{mm}^3$. *
• Monitor patients for renal, pulmonary, and cardiac toxicities, veno-occlusive liver disease, secondary malignancies, impaired wound healing, and hyponatremia.
• Anticipate blood transfusions because of cumulative anemia.
• Therapeutic effects are often accompanied by toxicity.
• Drug is associated with a moderate to high emetic potential (depending on dose, regimen, or administration route); antiemetics are recommended to prevent nausea and vomiting.

PATIENT TEACHING

• Warn patient that hair loss is likely to occur but is reversible.
• Advise patient to report all adverse reactions, especially signs and symptoms of infection (fever, sore throat, fatigue) and bleeding (easy bruising, nosebleeds, bleeding gums, tarry stools, bloody urine), dyspnea, cough, edema, and dizziness. Tell patient to take temperature daily.
• Instruct patient to avoid OTC products that contain aspirin.
• To minimize risk of hemorrhagic cystitis, encourage patient to urinate every 1 to 2 hours while awake and to drink at least 3 L of fluid daily.
• Tell patient taking capsules to take them in the morning because infrequent urination during night increases risk of cystitis.
• Advise patient that drug is associated with a moderate to high emetic potential and that antiemetics are recommended.
• Advise both male and female patients to practice contraception during therapy and for 4 months afterward for men and 12 months for women; drug may cause birth defects.

• Advise patient to stop breastfeeding during therapy because of risk of toxicity to infant.
• Drug can cause irreversible sterility in both males and females. Before therapy, counsel patient who is considering parenthood. Also recommend that patient consult prescriber before becoming pregnant.

cycloSPORINE
sye-kloe-SPOR-een

Sandimmune

cycloSPORINE (modified)
Gengraf, Neoral

Therapeutic class: Immunosuppressants
Pharmacologic class: Immunosuppressants

AVAILABLE FORMS
Capsules for microemulsion (modified):*
25 mg, 100 mg
Capsules (nonmodified): 25 mg, 50 mg, 100 mg
Injection: 50 mg/mL
Oral solution (modified and nonmodified):
100 mg/mL*

INDICATIONS & DOSAGES
➤ **To prevent organ rejection in renal, hepatic, or cardiac transplantation**
Adults and children: 15 mg/kg PO 4 to 12 hours before transplantation, continued daily for 1 or 2 weeks postoperatively. Then reduce dosage by 5% each week to maintenance level of 5 to 10 mg/kg daily. Or, 5 to 6 mg/kg IV concentrate 4 to 12 hours before transplantation as a slow IV infusion over 2 to 6 hours. Postoperatively, repeat dose daily until patient can tolerate oral forms.

For conversion from Sandimmune to Gengraf or Neoral, use same daily dose as previously used for Sandimmune. Monitor blood levels every 4 to 7 days after conversion, and monitor BP and creatinine level every 2 weeks during the first 2 months.
➤ **Severe, active RA that hasn't adequately responded to methotrexate (Gengraf or Neoral)**
Adults: 1.25 mg/kg PO b.i.d. Onset of action generally occurs between 4 and 8 weeks. Dosage may be increased by 0.5 to 0.75 mg/kg daily after 8 weeks and again after 12 weeks

to a maximum of 4 mg/kg daily. If no response is seen after 16 weeks, stop therapy.
Adjust-a-dose: Decrease dosage by 25% to 50% to control adverse reactions (such as HTN, serum creatinine elevations [30% above patient's pretreatment level], or clinically significant lab abnormalities). If dosage reduction doesn't control abnormalities, or if adverse reaction or abnormality is severe, discontinue drug.
➤ **Psoriasis (Gengraf or Neoral)**
Adults: 1.25 mg/kg daily PO b.i.d. for at least 4 weeks. Increase dosage by 0.5 mg/kg daily once every 2 weeks as needed to a maximum of 4 mg/kg daily.
Adjust-a-dose: Decrease dosage by 25% to 50% to control adverse reactions (such as HTN, serum creatinine elevations [25% above patient's pretreatment level], or clinically significant lab abnormalities). If dosage reduction doesn't control abnormalities, or if adverse reaction or abnormality is severe, discontinue drug.

ADMINISTRATION
• Hazardous drug; follow safe handling procedures when preparing, administering, or dispensing.
PO
• Give Neoral or Gengraf on an empty stomach in two divided doses.
• Measure oral solution doses carefully in an oral syringe. Don't rinse dosing syringe with water. If syringe is cleaned, it must be completely dry before reuse.
• To improve the taste of Sandimmune oral solution, mix it with milk, chocolate milk, or orange juice. Gengraf or Neoral oral solution may be mixed with orange or apple juice (not grapefruit juice); it's less palatable when mixed with milk.
• Use a glass container to mix, and have patient drink at once.
IV
▼ This form is usually reserved for patients who can't tolerate oral drugs.
▼ Immediately before use, dilute each milliliter of concentrate in 20 to 100 mL of D_5W or NSS for injection. Give at one-third the oral dose.
▼ Infuse over 2 to 6 hours.
▼ Protect diluted drug from light.
▼ **Incompatibilities:** Amphotericin B cholesteryl sulfate complex, magnesium sulfate.

Reactions in bold italics are *life-threatening*. Interactions may have a *rapid onset* or a ***delayed onset***.

ACTION
May inhibit proliferation and function of T lymphocytes and inhibit production and release of lymphokines.

Route	Onset	Peak	Duration
PO	Unknown	90 min–3 hr	Unknown
IV	Unknown	Unknown	Unknown

Half-life: Initial phase, about 1 hour; terminal phase, 8.5 to 27 hours.

ADVERSE REACTIONS
CNS: tremor, headache, confusion, dizziness, pain, insomnia, depression, migraine, paresthesia, *seizures.* **CV:** HTN, flushing, edema, chest pain, arrhythmias. **EENT:** rhinitis, sinusitis, gum hyperplasia, gingivitis. **GI:** nausea, vomiting, diarrhea, abdominal discomfort, dyspepsia, flatulence. **GU:** increased creatinine level, UTI, menstrual disorder, *renal insufficiency.* **Hematologic:** anemia, *leukopenia, thrombocytopenia, lymphoma.* **Hepatic:** *hepatotoxicity.* **Metabolic:** hyperglycemia, hypertriglyceridemia. **Musculoskeletal:** leg cramps, arthralgia. **Respiratory:** URI, pneumonia, cough, dyspnea, bronchospasm. **Skin:** hirsutism, acne. **Other:** infections, *sepsis,* gynecomastia, flulike symptoms, *anaphylaxis.*

INTERACTIONS
Drug-drug. *Acyclovir, aminoglycosides, amphotericin B, cimetidine, diclofenac, gentamicin, ketoconazole, melphalan, NSAIDs, ranitidine, sulfamethoxazole–trimethoprim, tacrolimus, tobramycin, vancomycin:* May increase risk of nephrotoxicity. Avoid using together.
Allopurinol, azathioprine, **azole antifungals,** *bromocriptine, calcium channel blockers,* **caspofungin,** *cimetidine, clarithromycin, corticosteroids, cyclophosphamide, danazol, erythromycin, imipenem–cilastatin, metoclopramide,* **micafungin:** May increase cyclosporine level and immunosuppression. Monitor patient closely.
Carbamazepine, isoniazid, nafcillin, octreotide, **orlistat,** *phenobarbital,* **phenytoin, rifabutin, rifampin,** *ticlopidine:* May decrease immunosuppressant effect from low cyclosporine level. Cyclosporine dosage may need to be increased.
Digoxin, HMG-CoA reductase inhibitors (lovastatin, other statins), prednisolone: May decrease clearance of these drugs. Use together cautiously.
Mycophenolate mofetil: May decrease mycophenolate level. Monitor patient closely when cyclosporine is added to or removed from therapy.
Potassium-sparing diuretics: May induce hyperkalemia. Avoid concurrent use.
Pravastatin: May increase concentrations of both drugs. Limit pravastatin to 20 mg/day.
Protease inhibitors (indinavir, ritonavir): May increase cyclosporine level. Use together cautiously.
Rosuvastatin: May decrease clearance of statin. Limit rosuvastatin dose to 5 mg/day.
Sirolimus: May increase sirolimus level. Take sirolimus at least 4 hours after cyclosporine dose. If separating doses isn't possible, monitor patient for increased adverse effects.
Vaccines: May decrease immune response. Delay routine immunization.
Drug-herb. *Astragalus, echinacea, licorice:* May interfere with drug's effect. Discourage use together.
St. John's wort: May reduce drug level, resulting in transplant failure. Discourage use together.
Drug-food. *Alfalfa sprouts:* May interfere with drug's effect. Discourage use together.
Grapefruit and grapefruit juice: May increase drug level and cause toxicity. Advise patient to avoid use together.
Drug-lifestyle. *Sun exposure:* May increase risk of sensitivity to sunlight. Advise patient to avoid excessive sun exposure.

EFFECTS ON LAB TEST RESULTS
• May increase ALT, AST, bilirubin, BUN, creatinine, glucose, and LDL levels.
• May decrease Hb and magnesium levels.
• May decrease platelet and WBC counts.

CONTRAINDICATIONS & CAUTIONS
• Contraindicated in patients hypersensitive to drug or polyoxyethylated castor oil (found in injectable form).
• Contraindicated in patients with RA or psoriasis with abnormal renal function, uncontrolled HTN, or malignancies (Neoral or Gengraf).
• Contraindicated with psoralen and UVA light (PUVA), methotrexate or other immunosuppressive agents, UVB light, coal tar, or radiation therapy in patients with psoriasis (Neoral or Gengraf).

- Obtain biopsy of skin lesions not typical for psoriasis before starting drug. Use in patients with malignant or premalignant skin changes only after appropriate treatment of such lesions and if no other treatment option exists.

Boxed Warning Manage patients receiving drug in facilities equipped and staffed with adequate lab and supportive medical resources. ∎

Dialyzable drug: No.

PREGNANCY-LACTATION-REPRODUCTION
- There are no adequate studies during pregnancy; use during pregnancy isn't recommended. If drug is needed during pregnancy, use only if potential benefit justifies fetal risk.
- Alcohol is present in cyclosporine preparations; consider this fact when using drug during pregnancy.
- Drug and ethanol present in cyclosporine preparations appear in human milk. Patient should discontinue breastfeeding or discontinue drug, taking into account importance of drug to the patient.

NURSING CONSIDERATIONS
Boxed Warning Only experienced physicians should prescribe this drug. ∎

Boxed Warning Patients with psoriasis previously treated with PUVA, methotrexate or other immunosuppressive agents, UVB, coal tar, or radiation therapy are at an increased risk for skin malignancies when taking Neoral or Gengraf. ∎

- Drug can cause hepatotoxicity.

Boxed Warning Neoral and Gengraf may increase the patient's susceptibility to infection and the development of neoplasia. ∎

🕙 *Alert:* Drugs causing immunosuppression increase the risk of opportunistic infections, including activation of latent viral infections such as BK virus–associated neuropathy, which may lead to serious outcomes, including kidney graft loss.

Boxed Warning Monitor patient's renal function. ∎

Boxed Warning Monitor cyclosporine level at regular intervals with prolonged Sandimmune use. Absorption of capsules and oral solution can be erratic during long-term use. ∎

Boxed Warning Neoral and Gengraf have greater bioavailability than Sandimmune. A lower dose of Neoral or Gengraf may be needed to provide blood level similar to that achieved with Sandimmune. Monitor blood level when switching patients between these two brands. ∎

Boxed Warning Gengraf is bioequivalent to and interchangeable with Neoral capsules, but neither is interchangeable with Sandimmune. ∎

Boxed Warning Always give Sandimmune with corticosteroids; however, don't give Sandimmune with other immunosuppressants. ∎

Boxed Warning Drug can cause systemic HTN and nephrotoxicity; risk increases with increasing dosage and duration of therapy. ∎

- Use Neoral or Gengraf to treat RA or psoriasis.

RA
- Before starting treatment, measure BP at least twice and obtain two creatinine levels to estimate baseline.
- Evaluate BP and creatinine level every 2 weeks during first 3 months and then monthly if patient is stable.
- Monitor BP and creatinine level after an increase in NSAID dosage or introduction of a new NSAID. Monitor CBC and LFTs monthly if patient also receives methotrexate.

Psoriasis
- Measure BP at least twice to determine a baseline. Monitor BP after dosage changes.
- Evaluate patient for occult infection and tumors initially and throughout treatment.
- Obtain baseline creatinine level (on two occasions), CBC, and BUN, magnesium, uric acid, potassium, and lipid levels.
- Evaluate BP, CBC, and uric acid, potassium, lipid, magnesium, creatinine, and BUN levels every 2 weeks during first 3 months and then monthly thereafter if patient is stable.
- Monitor creatinine level after increasing NSAID dose or starting a new NSAID.
- Improvement in psoriasis takes 12 to 16 weeks of therapy.
- *Look alike–sound alike:* Don't confuse cyclosporine with cyclophosphamide or cycloserine. Don't confuse Sandimmune with Sandostatin.

PATIENT TEACHING
- Encourage patient to take drug at same time each day and to be consistent with relation to meals.
- Teach patient how to measure dosage and mask taste of oral solution. Tell patient not to take drug with grapefruit juice.

Reactions in bold italics are *life-threatening*. Interactions may have a *rapid onset* or a ***delayed onset***.

• Instruct patient to fill glass with water after dose and drink it to make sure all of drug has been consumed.
• Advise patient to take drug with meals if nausea occurs.
• Advise patient to take Neoral or Gengraf on an empty stomach.
• Tell patient being treated for psoriasis that improvement may not occur until after 12 to 16 weeks of therapy.
• Stress that drug shouldn't be stopped without prescriber's approval.
• Explain to patient the importance of frequent lab monitoring while receiving therapy.
• Tell patient to avoid people with infections because drug lowers resistance to infection.
• Advise patient to perform careful oral care and to see a dentist regularly because drug can cause gum disease.
• Advise patient of childbearing potential to use barrier contraception, not hormonal contraceptives, during therapy. Advise patient of the potential risk during pregnancy and the increased risk of tumors, high BP, and renal problems.
• Warn patient to wear protection in the sun and to avoid excessive sun exposure.

SAFETY ALERT!

cytarabine (ara-C, cytosine arabinoside)
sye-TARE-a-been

Cytosar ✤

Therapeutic class: Antineoplastics
Pharmacologic class: Pyrimidine analogues

AVAILABLE FORMS
Injection: 20 mg/mL, 100 mg/mL

INDICATIONS & DOSAGES
Adjust-a-dose (for all indications): Consider dosage reduction in patients with poor renal function.
➤ **Acute nonlymphocytic leukemia**
Adults and children: 100 mg/m^2 IV daily by continuous IV infusion or 100 mg/m^2 IV every 12 hours by rapid IV injection or IV infusion on days 1 to 7 in a course of therapy or daily until remission is attained.
➤ **Acute lymphocytic leukemia**
Consult literature for current recommendations.

➤ **Meningeal leukemia**
Adults and children: Varies from 5 to 75 mg/m^2 intrathecally. Frequency varies from once daily for 4 days to once every 4 days. The most frequently used dose is 30 mg/m^2 every 4 days until CSF is normal; then one additional dose.
➤ **Acute promyelocytic leukemia (induction)** ◆
Adults: 200 mg/m^2 IV daily by continuous IV infusion for 7 days beginning on day 3 of treatment (in combination with tretinoin and daunorubicin).

ADMINISTRATION
• Hazardous drug; use safe handling and disposal precautions.
IV
▼ To reduce nausea, give antiemetic before drug. Nausea and vomiting are more likely with large doses given by IV push. Dizziness may occur with rapid infusion.
▼ For IV infusion, dilute solution in vial using NSS for injection or D$_5$W and administer as a continuous infusion.
▼ **Incompatibilities:** None listed by manufacturer. Consult a drug incompatibility reference for more information.
Intrathecal
• The single-use vial doesn't contain any preservative; drug should be used as soon as possible after preparation. Discard unused portions of each vial properly.
• After drug administration by lumbar puncture, instruct patient to lie flat for 1 hour.
• Patients should be observed by physician for immediate toxic reactions.

ACTION
Inhibits DNA synthesis.

Route	Onset	Peak	Duration
IV, intrathecal	Unknown	Unknown	Unknown

Half-life: Initial, 8 minutes; terminal, 1 to 3 hours; in CSF, 2 hours.

ADVERSE REACTIONS
CNS: *neurotoxicity,* malaise, dizziness, headache, cerebellar syndrome, fever. **CV:** thrombophlebitis, edema, *hemorrhage.* **EENT:** conjunctivitis, oral ulcers. **GI:** nausea, vomiting, diarrhea, anorexia, anal ulceration, abdominal pain, projectile vomiting, *bowel necrosis with high doses given by rapid IV.* **GU:** urine retention, renal

dysfunction. **Hematologic:** *leukopenia,* anemia, reticulocytopenia, *thrombocytopenia,* megaloblastosis. **Hepatic:** *hepatotoxicity,* jaundice. **Metabolic:** hyperuricemia. **Musculoskeletal:** myalgia, bone pain. **Respiratory:** shortness of breath. **Skin:** rash, pruritus, alopecia, freckling. **Other:** infection, hypersensitivity reactions.

INTERACTIONS
Drug-drug. *Digoxin, except oral liquid:* May decrease oral digoxin absorption. Monitor digoxin level closely.
Flucytosine: May decrease flucytosine activity. Avoid using together.

EFFECTS ON LAB TEST RESULTS
- May increase BUN, creatinine, and uric acid levels.
- May increase megaloblast count.
- May decrease Hb level and platelet, RBC, reticulocyte, and WBC counts.

CONTRAINDICATIONS & CAUTIONS
- Contraindicated in patients hypersensitive to drug. Anaphylaxis has been reported (rare).
- Use cautiously in patients with hepatic or renal impairment, gout, or myelosuppression.
- TLS may occur. Consider antihyperuricemic therapy and ensure adequate hydration.
- Patients receiving continuous infusion or patients receiving cytarabine who were previously treated with L-asparaginase may be at increased risk for pancreatitis.
- **Alert:** With high-dose therapy, drug is associated with sudden respiratory distress syndrome, which can be fatal.
Dialyzable drug: Yes.
Overdose S&S: Irreversible CNS toxicity, death.

PREGNANCY-LACTATION-REPRODUCTION
- Drug can cause fetal harm if patient is exposed to drug systemically during pregnancy. Patients of childbearing potential should avoid becoming pregnant during therapy. If drug is used during pregnancy or if patient becomes pregnant while taking drug, advise patient of fetal risk.
- It isn't known if drug appears in human milk. Patient should discontinue breastfeeding or discontinue drug, taking into account importance of drug to the patient.

NURSING CONSIDERATIONS
Boxed Warning Cytarabine should be administered by physicians experienced in cancer chemotherapy. For induction therapy, patients should be treated in a facility with lab and supportive resources sufficient to monitor drug tolerance and protect and maintain a patient compromised by drug toxicity. Prescriber must judge possible benefit to patient against known toxic effects of cytarabine. ■
- Drug is an irritant. If extravasation occurs, stop the infusion immediately and follow facility policy for monitoring and treatment.
- Monitor fluid intake and output carefully. Maintain high fluid intake and give allopurinol to avoid urate nephropathy in leukemia-induction therapy. Monitor uric acid level.
- Anticipate the need for antiemetics, as IV doses of more than 1,000 mg/m^2 in adults are associated with a moderate emetic potential; in children, a 75-mg/m^2 IV dose is associated with a moderate emetic potential and IV doses of 3,000 mg/m^2 or more are associated with a high emetic potential.
- Monitor renal function studies, LFTs, and CBC with differential.
- Therapy may be modified or stopped if granulocyte count is below 1,000/mm^3 or platelet count is below 50,000/mm^3.
- Corticosteroid eye drops help prevent drug-induced conjunctivitis.
- Provide diligent mouth care to help minimize stomatitis.
- **Alert:** Assess patient receiving high doses for neurotoxicity, which may first appear as nystagmus but can progress to ataxia and cerebellar dysfunction.
- To prevent bleeding, avoid all IM injections when platelet count is below 50,000/mm^3.
- Anticipate blood transfusions because of cumulative anemia. Patient may receive RBC colony-stimulating factors to promote RBC production and decrease need for blood transfusions.
Boxed Warning Monitor patient for toxic effects, including bone marrow suppression, nausea, vomiting, diarrhea, oral ulceration, and hepatic dysfunction. ■
- In leukopenia, initial WBC count nadir occurs 7 to 9 days after drug is stopped. A second, more severe nadir occurs 15 to 24 days after drug is stopped. In thrombocytopenia, platelet count nadir occurs on days 12 to 15.

Reactions in bold italics are *life-threatening*. Interactions may have a *rapid onset* or a **delayed onset**.

D

🖐 *Alert:* A cytarabine syndrome has been described and is characterized by fever, myalgia, bone pain, occasionally chest pain, maculopapular rash, conjunctivitis, and malaise. It usually occurs 6 to 12 hours after drug administration. Corticosteroids have been shown to be beneficial in the treatment or prevention of this syndrome.

• *Look alike–sound alike:* Don't confuse cytarabine with clofarabine or vidarabine.

PATIENT TEACHING
• Instruct patient to watch for signs and symptoms of infection (fever, sore throat, fatigue) and bleeding (easy bruising, nosebleeds, bleeding gums, tarry stools). Tell patient to take temperature daily.
• Advise patient to report vision changes, blurred vision, or eye pain to prescriber.
• Advise breastfeeding patient to stop breastfeeding during therapy because of risk of toxicity in infant.
• Caution patient of childbearing potential to consult prescriber before becoming pregnant because drug may harm fetus.

SAFETY ALERT!

dabigatran etexilate mesylate
da-BIG-a-tran e-TEX-i-late

Pradaxa🍃

Therapeutic class: Anticoagulants
Pharmacologic class: Direct thrombin inhibitors

AVAILABLE FORMS
Capsules 🆗*:* 75 mg, 110 mg, 150 mg
Oral pellets: 20 mg, 30 mg, 40 mg, 50 mg, 110 mg, 150 mg

INDICATIONS & DOSAGES
➤ **To reduce risk of stroke and systemic embolism in patients with nonvalvular atrial fibrillation**
Adults: 150 mg PO b.i.d. if CrCl is greater than 30 mL/minute. Refer to manufacturer's instructions when converting to and from warfarin or parenteral anticoagulants.
Adjust-a-dose: For patients with CrCl of 15 to 30 mL/minute or for those with CrCl of 30 to 50 mL/minute who are taking dronedarone or oral ketoconazole

concurrently, give 75 mg PO b.i.d. Avoid use in patients with CrCl of less than 30 mL/minute also taking P-gp inhibitors. Don't use in patients on dialysis or in those with CrCl of less than 15 mL/minute.
➤ **To treat DVT and PE in patients with CrCl greater than 30 mL/minute who have been treated with a parenteral anticoagulant for 5 to 10 days; to reduce risk of recurrence of DVT and PE in patients with CrCl greater than 30 mL/minute who have been previously treated**
Adults: 150 mg PO b.i.d.
Adjust-a-dose: There are no dosing recommendations for patients with CrCl of 30 mL/minute or less or for those on dialysis. Avoid use in patients with CrCl of less than 50 mL/minute also taking P-gp inhibitors.
➤ **Prophylaxis of DVT and PE after hip replacement surgery**
Adults: 110 mg PO 1 to 4 hours after surgery and after hemostasis has been achieved, then 220 mg once daily for 28 to 35 days. If drug isn't started on day of surgery, after hemostasis has been achieved, start treatment with 220 mg once daily.
Adjust-a-dose: There are no dosing recommendations for patients with CrCl of less than 30 mL/minute or for those on dialysis. Avoid use in patients with CrCl of less than 50 mL/minute also taking P-gp inhibitors.
✳ *NEW INDICATION:* **Venous thromboembolism (VTE) in children previously treated with parenteral anticoagulant for at least 5 days**
Children ages 8 to younger than 18 (capsules): If 81 kg or more, 260 mg PO b.i.d.; if 61 to less than 81 kg, 220 mg PO b.i.d.; if 41 to less than 61 kg, 185 mg PO b.i.d.; if 26 to less than 41 kg, 150 mg PO b.i.d.; if 16 to less than 26 kg, 110 mg PO b.i.d.; if 11 to less than 16 kg, 75 mg PO b.i.d.
Children ages 3 months to younger than 12 years (pellets): Weight-based dose PO b.i.d. according to manufacturer's instructions.
Adjust-a-dose: Avoid use in children with eGFR less than 50 mL/minute/1.73 m².
✳ *NEW INDICATION:* **To reduce risk of VTE recurrence in previously treated children**
Children ages 8 to younger than 18 (capsules): If 81 kg or more, 260 mg PO b.i.d.; if 61 to less than 81 kg, 220 mg PO b.i.d.; if 41 to less than 61 kg, 185 mg PO b.i.d.; if 26 to less than 41 kg, 150 mg PO b.i.d.; if 16 to

less than 26 kg, 110 mg PO b.i.d.; if 11 to less than 16 kg, 75 mg PO b.i.d.

Children ages 3 months to younger than 12 years (pellets): Weight-based dose PO b.i.d. after previous treatment according to manufacturer's instructions.

Adjust-a-dose: Avoid use in children with eGFR less than 50 mL/minute/1.73 m^2.

ADMINISTRATION
PO
- Give without regard to food as close to 12 hours apart as possible. Give with food if GI distress occurs with capsules.
- Don't crush capsule, empty its contents, or allow patient to chew capsule. Patient must swallow capsule whole with full glass of water.
- Give pellets before a meal to ensure patient takes full dose.
- Mix pellets in 2 tsp (10 mL) of mashed carrots or bananas, or apple sauce. Or, may spoon pellets directly into patient's mouth and have patient swallow with apple juice, or add to approximately 1 to 2 oz (30 to 60 mL) of apple juice for drinking.
- Don't mix pellets with milk, milk products, or soft foods containing milk.
- Don't give pellets via syringe or feeding tube.
- Give pellets within 30 minutes of mixing; discard dose after 30 minutes if not given.
- Give missed dose as soon as possible on same day; if it's less than 6 hours before next scheduled dose, skip missed dose.
- If a partial dose of pellets is ingested, don't give additional dose; give next dose as scheduled.
- Temporarily discontinue drug before invasive or surgical procedures. Restart drug as soon as medically appropriate.

ACTION
Reversible, direct thrombin inhibitor that prevents development of a thrombus.

Route	Onset	Peak	Duration
PO	Unknown	1–2 hr	Unknown

Half-life: Adults, 12 to 17 hours; children, 12 to 14 hours; children (pellets), 9 to 11 hours.

ADVERSE REACTIONS
EENT: epistaxis. **GI:** abdominal pain or discomfort, gastritis-like symptoms, GERD, esophagitis, erosive gastritis, *gastric*

hemorrhage, hemorrhagic erosive gastritis, GI ulcer, diarrhea, nausea, vomiting, *GI bleeding.* **GU:** menorrhagia. **Hematologic:** *major bleeding event,* minor bleeding.

INTERACTIONS
Drug-drug. *Antiplatelet drugs, aspirin, fibrinolytic therapy, heparin, NSAIDs:* May increase risk of bleeding. Carefully consider risks and benefits of using together, monitor closely, and consider therapy modification.
P-gp inducers (rifampin): May reduce dabigatran level. Avoid use together.
P-gp inhibitors (dronedarone, systemic ketoconazole): May increase effectiveness of dabigatran; dosage reductions may be needed. Refer to indication-specific dosage adjustments above and manufacturer's instructions for additional information.
Drug-herb. *Herbs with anticoagulant/ antiplatelet properties (alfalfa, anise, bilberry):* May increase risk of bleeding. Consider therapy modification.

EFFECTS ON LAB TEST RESULTS
- May increase PTT, ecarin clotting time (ECT), and thrombin time.

CONTRAINDICATIONS & CAUTIONS
Boxed Warning Consider risk of epidural or spinal hematoma versus potential benefit in patients scheduled for spinal procedures, such as spinal or epidural anesthesia or spinal puncture. Hematomas may result in long-term or permanent paralysis. Increased risk may occur with use of indwelling epidural catheters, concomitant use of drugs that affect hemostasis (NSAIDs, platelet inhibitors, anticoagulants), history of traumatic or repeated epidural or spinal punctures, or history of spinal deformity or surgery. Optimal timing between administration of drug and spinal or epidural procedure isn't known. ■
- Contraindicated in patients hypersensitive to drug and in those with active pathologic bleeding.
- Contraindicated in patients with mechanical prosthetic valves. Use in patients with atrial fibrillation in the setting of other forms of valvular heart disease, including the presence of a bioprosthetic heart valve, isn't recommended.
- Use cautiously in older adults, in patients with a history of bleeding, and when used

---

with other drugs that increase the risk of bleeding.

• Because of risk of clot formation and stroke, avoid lapses in therapy when possible. Restart therapy as soon as possible.

Boxed Warning Discontinuing drug prematurely increases risk of thrombotic events. If drug must be discontinued for a reason other than pathologic bleeding or completion of a course of therapy, consider coverage with another anticoagulant. ∎

• Use in children with an eGFR less than 50 mL/minute/1.73 m² hasn't been studied; avoid use in these patients.

Dialyzable drug: Approximately 49% to 57%.

⚠ *Overdose S&S:* Hemorrhagic complications.

PREGNANCY-LACTATION-REPRODUCTION

• There are no adequate well-controlled studies during pregnancy. Consider risks of bleeding and stroke if drug is used during pregnancy.

• Drug may increase bleeding risk in the fetus and neonate. Monitor neonates for bleeding.

• It isn't known if drug appears in human milk. Breastfeeding isn't recommended during treatment. Patient should discontinue breastfeeding or discontinue drug, taking into account importance of drug to the patient.

NURSING CONSIDERATIONS

• Monitor patient for signs of bleeding. If bleeding occurs, stop drug, investigate cause, and provide supportive measures.

• A specific reversal agent (idarucizumab) is available. Refer to the idarucizumab prescribing information for additional information.

• Monitor ECT or PPT to assess treatment effectiveness.

Boxed Warning After spinal procedure, monitor patient for neurologic impairment (midline back pain, sensory or motor deficits such as numbness or weakness in lower limbs, bowel or bladder dysfunction). Treat impairment urgently. ∎

• Discontinue dabigatran 1 to 2 days before invasive or surgical procedures in patients with CrCl of 50 mL/minute or more and 3 to 5 days in patients with CrCl of less than 50 mL/minute. Consider longer times for patients undergoing major surgery, spinal puncture, or placement of a spinal or epidural catheter or port, in whom complete hemostasis may be required.

• For children, discontinue drug 24 hours before elective surgery if GFR greater than 80 mL/minute/1.73 m² or 2 days before elective surgery if eGFR 50 to 80 mL/minute/1.73 m².

PATIENT TEACHING

🕭 *Alert:* Advise patient to keep drug in original bottle to protect from moisture, to remove only one capsule from the opened bottle at the time of use, to tightly close the bottle immediately after removing drug, and not to put drug in pill boxes or pill organizers.

• Teach patient safe drug administration and storage.

• Caution patient to take drug as prescribed and not to stop or change dosage without first consulting prescriber.

• Advise patient to tell all health care providers about taking drug.

• Tell patient to inform prescriber about use of other drugs, including OTCs, vitamins, and herbs.

• Warn patient that bruising may occur more easily and bleeding may last longer during therapy.

• Instruct patient to report bleeding when brushing teeth or shaving; blood in vomit, urine, or stool; heavier menstrual bleeding; or nosebleeds.

• Tell patient regular blood tests to monitor drug's effects will be needed.

• Instruct patient to inform health care provider of scheduled invasive procedures, including dental work. Drug may need to be stopped temporarily.

SAFETY ALERT!

dacarbazine (DTIC)
da-KAR-ba-zeen

Therapeutic class: Antineoplastics
Pharmacologic class: Triazenes

AVAILABLE FORMS
Injection: 100 mg, 200 mg, 500 mg

INDICATIONS & DOSAGES
➤ **Metastatic malignant melanoma**
Adults: 2 to 4.5 mg/kg IV daily for 10 days; repeat every 4 weeks as tolerated. Or, 250 mg/m² IV daily for 5 days; repeat every 3 weeks.

➤ **Hodgkin lymphoma as second-line therapy**

Adults: 150 mg/m^2 IV daily (with other drugs) for 5 days; repeat every 4 weeks. Or, 375 mg/m^2 on first day of combination regimen; repeat every 15 days.

➤ **Advanced soft-tissue sarcomas ◆**

Adults: 250 mg/m^2 daily by continuous IV infusion for 4 days every 3 weeks (total dacarbazine dose is 1,000 mg/m^2 over 96 hours) (MAID regimen; in combination with mesna, doxorubicin, and ifosfamide).

ADMINISTRATION

IV

▼ Preparing and giving parenteral drug may be mutagenic, teratogenic, or carcinogenic. Follow facility policy to reduce risks.

▼ Reconstitute drug using sterile water for injection. Add 9.9 mL to 100-mg vial, 19.7 mL to 200-mg vial, and 49.25 mL to 500-mg vial to yield a concentration of 10 mg/mL.

▼ For infusion, dilute further with NSS or D$_5$W.

▼ Infuse over 15 to 60 minutes. To decrease pain at insertion site, dilute drug further or decrease infusion rate.

▼ Watch for irritation and infiltration during infusion; extravasation can cause severe pain, tissue damage, and necrosis. If solution infiltrates, notify prescriber and follow facility protocol.

▼ Reconstituted solutions in the vial are stable 8 hours at room temperature and with normal lighting conditions, or up to 3 days if refrigerated.

▼ Solution should be colorless to clear yellow. If solution turns pink, it has decomposed. Discard it.

▼ Diluted solutions are stable 8 hours at room temperature and with normal lighting, or up to 24 hours if refrigerated.

▼ Protect from light.

▼ **Incompatibilities:** Allopurinol sodium, cefepime, piperacillin–tazobactam. Consult a drug incompatibility reference for more information.

ACTION

Alkylating agent that binds to DNA, breaking the strands and interfering with protein synthesis.

Route	Onset	Peak	Duration
IV	Unknown	Unknown	Unknown

Half-life: Initial phase, 19 minutes; terminal phase, 5 hours. Renal and hepatic dysfunction: initial phase, 55 minutes; terminal phase, 7.2 hours.

ADVERSE REACTIONS

GI: anorexia, severe nausea and vomiting, stomatitis. **Hematologic:** *leukopenia, thrombocytopenia.* **Skin:** alopecia. **Other:** hypersensitivity reaction, local pain, burning and irritation at injection site.

INTERACTIONS

Drug-lifestyle. *Sun exposure:* May cause photosensitivity reaction. Advise patient to avoid excessive sunlight exposure.

EFFECTS ON LAB TEST RESULTS

● May increase BUN and liver enzyme levels.
● May decrease platelet, RBC, and WBC counts.

CONTRAINDICATIONS & CAUTIONS

● Contraindicated in hypersensitivity to drug.
● Use cautiously in patients with impaired bone marrow function and those with severe renal or hepatic dysfunction.
Dialyzable drug: Unknown.

PREGNANCY-LACTATION-REPRODUCTION

■ **Boxed Warning** Studies have demonstrated this agent to have a carcinogenic and teratogenic effect when used in animals. ■

● There are no adequate well-controlled studies during pregnancy. Use during pregnancy only if potential benefit justifies potential risk to the fetus.

● Drug is contraindicated in first trimester.

● It isn't known if drug appears in human milk. Patient should discontinue breastfeeding or discontinue drug, taking into account importance of drug to the patient.

NURSING CONSIDERATIONS

■ **Boxed Warning** Dacarbazine should be administered under the supervision of a prescriber experienced in the use of cancer chemotherapeutic agents. Prescriber must carefully weigh the possibility of therapeutic benefit against the risk of toxicity for each patient. ■

● Give antiemetics before giving this drug. Nausea and vomiting may subside after several doses.

Reactions in bold italics are *life-threatening*. Interactions may have a *rapid onset* or a *delayed onset*.

• To prevent bleeding, avoid all IM injections when platelet count falls below 50,000/mm³.
Boxed Warning Hematopoietic depression is the most common toxicity. ■

• Anticipate need for blood transfusions to combat anemia.

• Therapeutic effects commonly occur with toxicity. Monitor CBC and platelet count.
Boxed Warning Hepatic necrosis may occur. Monitor LFTs. ■

• For Hodgkin lymphoma, drug is usually given in combination with other antineoplastics.

• Monitor patient for extravasation during administration.

• Locally applied hot packs may relieve local pain, burning sensation, and irritation at injection site.

• *Look alike–sound alike:* Don't confuse dacarbazine with procarbazine.

PATIENT TEACHING

• Tell patient to watch for signs of infection (fever, sore throat, fatigue) and bleeding (easy bruising, nosebleeds, bleeding gums, melena) and to take temperature daily.

• Tell patient to avoid people with URIs.

• Advise patient to avoid sunlight.

• Reassure patient that fever, malaise, and muscle pain, beginning 7 days after treatment ends and possibly lasting 7 to 21 days, may be treated with mild fever reducers such as acetaminophen.

• Tell patient that restricting food intake for 4 to 6 hours before dose may help to decrease adverse GI effects.

• Reassure patient that hair loss is reversible.

• Advise patient to avoid pregnancy and breastfeeding during therapy.

dalbavancin hydrochloride
dal-ba-VAN-sin

Dalvance

Therapeutic class: Antibiotics
Pharmacologic class: Lipoglycopeptides

AVAILABLE FORMS
Injection: 500-mg single-use vial

INDICATIONS & DOSAGES
➤ **Acute bacterial skin and skin-structure infections caused by susceptible strains of**
gram-positive microorganisms (*Staphylococcus aureus* [including MRSA], *Streptococcus pyogenes, Streptococcus agalactiae, Streptococcus dysgalactiae, Streptococcus anginosus* group [*S. anginosus, S. intermedius, S. constellatus*]), *Enterococcus faecalis* (vancomycin-susceptible strains)
Adults: 1,500 mg IV infusion as a single dose, or 1,000 mg IV infusion followed by a second dose of 500 mg IV infusion 1 week later.
Children ages 6 to younger than 18: 18 mg/kg IV infusion as a single dose, up to maximum of 1,500 mg.
Children from birth to younger than age 6: 22.5 mg/kg IV infusion as a single dose, up to maximum of 1,500 mg.
Adjust-a-dose: For patients with CrCl of less than 30 mL/minute who aren't receiving hemodialysis, give 1,125 mg IV infusion as a single dose, or 750 mg IV infusion followed by a second dose of 375 mg IV infusion 1 week later. No dosage adjustment is necessary for patients on regularly scheduled hemodialysis; give without regard to hemodialysis timing. Dosage adjustment for children with CrCl less than 30 mL/minute hasn't been established.

ADMINISTRATION
IV

▼ Reconstitute each vial with 25 mL sterile water for injection or 5% dextrose injection. Swirl gently, and invert vial until vial contents are completely dissolved. Don't shake. Reconstituted vial contains a concentration of 20 mg/mL. Dilute further with dextrose 5% to a final concentration of 1 to 5 mg/mL.

▼ Inspect for particulate matter before infusion. Don't infuse if particulate matter is identified. Solution should be clear and colorless to yellow.

▼ To reduce risk of infusion-related reactions, infuse drug over 30 minutes.

▼ Flush IV line before and after each dalbavancin infusion with 5% dextrose injection if line is used to administer other drugs in addition to dalbavancin.

▼ Store reconstituted vials or final IV bags or bottles in refrigerator or at room temperature. Use within 48 hours.

▼ **Incompatibilities:** Other medications, electrolytes, saline-based solutions.

ACTION

Bactericidal; interferes with cell-wall peptidoglycan, preventing cross-linking in bacterial cell-wall synthesis.

Route	Onset	Peak	Duration
IV	Unknown	Unknown	7 days

Half-life: About 8.5 days (204 hours).

ADVERSE REACTIONS

CNS: headache, dizziness. **CV:** flushing, phlebitis, spontaneous hematoma. **EENT:** oral candidiasis. **GI:** nausea, vomiting, diarrhea, *GI hemorrhage,* melena, hematochezia, abdominal pain, *C. difficile colitis.* **GU:** vulvovaginal mycotic infection. **Hematologic:** anemia, *hemorrhagic anemia, leukopenia, neutropenia, thrombocytopenia,* eosinophilia, *thrombocytosis.* **Hepatic:** *hepatotoxicity.* **Metabolic:** *hypoglycemia.* **Respiratory:** *bronchospasm.* **Skin:** rash, pruritus, urticaria, petechiae. **Other:** infusion-site reactions, *anaphylactoid reaction, wound hemorrhage.*

INTERACTIONS

None reported.

EFFECTS ON LAB TEST RESULTS

• May increase INR and LDH, GGT, ALT, AST, and ALP levels.
• May decrease Hb level and platelet and WBC counts.

CONTRAINDICATIONS & CAUTIONS

• Contraindicated in patients hypersensitive to drug or its components.
• Don't use unless proven or strongly suspected bacterial infection exists.
• Use cautiously in patients with known hypersensitivity to glycopeptides.
• Use cautiously in patients with moderate to severe hepatic impairment (Child-Pugh class B or C).
• Use cautiously in older adults. Drug is substantially excreted by the kidneys.
Dialyzable drug: No.

PREGNANCY-LACTATION-REPRODUCTION

• There are no adequate well-controlled studies during pregnancy. Use during pregnancy only if clearly needed and potential benefit justifies fetal risk.
• It isn't known if drug appears in human milk. Use cautiously during breastfeeding.

NURSING CONSIDERATIONS

🛈 *Alert:* Monitor patient for development of CDAD, which can range from mild to fatal colitis and can occur more than 2 months after treatment ends.
• Ensure a suspected or confirmed serious bacterial infection exists before administering drug.
• Monitor patient for infusion reactions or hypersensitivity. Discontinue drug if reaction occurs.
• Rapid infusion (less than 30 minutes) may result in "red man syndrome" (upper body flushing, urticaria, pruritus, rash, back pain). Stopping or slowing infusion may stop this reaction.

PATIENT TEACHING

• Instruct patient to notify prescriber of allergy or hypersensitivity to other glycopeptides such as vancomycin before treatment.
• Explain to patient that drug is used only for presumed or confirmed serious bacterial infections.
• Teach patient that drug will be given intravenously, and to immediately report signs or symptoms of reactions.
• Advise patient not to skip any doses of antibacterial drugs as this may decrease effectiveness of treatment.
• Tell patient to report GI adverse effects such as diarrhea, which is common and may be serious.
• Warn patient to alert prescriber if pregnant or breastfeeding.

SAFETY ALERT!

dalteparin sodium
DAHL-tep-ah-rin

Fragmin

Therapeutic class: Anticoagulants
Pharmacologic class: Low-molecular-weight heparins

AVAILABLE FORMS

Injection: 2,500 antifactor Xa international units/0.2-mL syringe, 5,000 antifactor Xa international units/0.2-mL syringe, 7,500 antifactor Xa international units/0.3-mL syringe, 10,000 antifactor Xa international units/1-mL syringe, 12,500 antifactor Xa international units/0.5-mL syringe, 15,000 antifactor Xa international units/0.6-mL syringe, 18,000 antifactor Xa international units/0.72-mL syringe, 95,000 antifactor Xa international units/3.8-mL vial*

INDICATIONS & DOSAGES

➤ **To prevent DVT in patients undergoing abdominal surgery who are at moderate to high risk for thromboembolic complications**

Adults: 2,500 international units subcut daily, starting 1 to 2 hours before surgery and repeated once daily for 5 to 10 days postoperatively. Or, for patients at high risk, give 5,000 international units subcut the evening before surgery, then once daily postoperatively for 5 to 10 days. Or, in patients with malignancy, give 2,500 international units subcut 1 to 2 hours before surgery followed by 2,500 international units subcut 12 hours later, then 5,000 international units subcut once daily for 5 to 10 days postoperatively.

➤ **To prevent DVT in patients undergoing hip replacement surgery**

Adults: 2,500 international units subcut within 2 hours before surgery and second dose of 2,500 international units subcut in the evening after surgery (4 to 8 hours after surgery or later if hemostasis hasn't been achieved). Starting on first postoperative day, allowing a minimum of 6 hours after postoperative dose, give 5,000 international units subcut once daily for 5 to 10 days. Or, give 5,000 international units subcut 10 to 14 hours before surgery; then 5,000 international units subcut once daily starting 4 to 8 hours after surgery for 5 to 10 days postoperatively. Allow approximately 24 hours between preoperative and first postoperative doses.

If starting postoperatively, give 2,500 international units subcut in the evening after surgery (4 to 8 hours after surgery, or later if hemostasis hasn't been achieved). Starting on first postoperative day, allowing a minimum of 6 hours after postoperative dose, give 5,000 international units subcut once daily for 5 to 10 days.

➤ **Prophylaxis of ischemic complications in patients with unstable angina; non-Q-wave MI**

Adults: 120 international units/kg subcut every 12 hours with aspirin (75 to 165 mg daily) PO, unless contraindicated. Maximum dose,

10,000 international units. Treatment usually lasts 5 to 8 days.

➤ **To prevent DVT in patients at risk for thromboembolic complications because of severely restricted mobility during acute illness**

Adults: 5,000 international units subcut once daily for 12 to 14 days.

➤ **Symptomatic venous thromboembolism (VTE) in patients with cancer**

Adults: Initially, 200 international units/kg (maximum, 18,000 international units) subcut daily for 30 days; then 150 international units/kg (maximum, 18,000 international units) subcut daily months 2 through 6.

Adjust-a-dose: In patients with platelet count 50,000 to 100,000/mm^3, reduce dose by 2,500 international units until platelet count exceeds 100,000/mm^3. In patients with platelet count less than 50,000/mm^3, stop drug until platelet count exceeds 50,000/mm^3. In patients with CrCl of 30 mL/minute or less, monitor anti-Xa levels to determine appropriate dose. Target anti-Xa range is 0.5 to 1.5 international units/mL. Draw anti-Xa 4 to 6 hours after dose and only after patient has received three to four doses.

➤ **Symptomatic VTE in children**

Children ages 8 to younger than 17: 100 international units/kg b.i.d. for three doses; then assess anti-Xa level.

Children ages 2 to younger than 8: 125 international units/kg b.i.d. for three doses; then assess anti-Xa level.

Children ages 4 weeks to younger than 2 years: 150 international units/kg b.i.d. for three doses; then assess anti-Xa level.

Adjust-a-dose: Adjust dosage in increments of 25 international units/kg to achieve target anti-Xa level between 0.5 and 1 international unit/mL. If platelet count is 50,000 to 100,000/mm^3, reduce dosage by 50% until platelet count exceeds 100,000/mm^3. If platelet count is less than 50,000/mm^3, stop drug until platelet count exceeds 50,000/mm^3.

➤ **Acute symptomatic superficial lower extremity vein thrombosis 5 cm or greater in length** ♦

Adults: 5,000 units subcut every 12 hours for 45 days.

Adjust-a-dose: Recurrence risk is high if anticoagulation is discontinued earlier than 45 days. Monitor D-dimer at baseline and again at 45 days; if D-dimer remains elevated, a longer course may be necessary.

ADMINISTRATION
Subcutaneous
• Injection sites include a U-shaped area around the navel, upper outer side of thigh, and upper outer quadrangle of buttock. Rotate sites daily.
• Give subcut injection deeply, inserting entire length of needle at a 45- to 90-degree angle.
• After first penetration of rubber stopper, store multidose vial at room temperature for up to 2 weeks. Discard any unused solution after 2 weeks.
• Whenever possible, use benzyl alcohol–free formulations (prefilled syringes) in children.
• The needle shield of the prefilled syringe may contain natural rubber latex. Use cautiously in patients with latex allergies.
• Don't mix with other injections or infusions unless specific compatibility data support such mixing.
• Store at room temperature.

ACTION
Inhibition of factor Xa and thrombin by antithrombin.

Route	Onset	Peak	Duration
Subcut	1–2 hr	4 hr	>12 hr

Half-life: 2 to 5 hours.

ADVERSE REACTIONS
CNS: fever. **EENT:** epistaxis. **GU:** hematuria. **Hematologic:** *thrombocytopenia, hemorrhage,* ecchymoses, bleeding complications. **Hepatic:** elevated transaminase levels. **Skin:** pruritus, rash, hematoma at injection site, wound hematoma, injection-site pain. **Other:** hypersensitivity reaction.

INTERACTIONS
Drug-drug. *Antiplatelet drugs (aspirin, NSAIDs, clopidogrel, dipyridamole, ticlopidine), oral anticoagulants, SSRIs (fluoxetine), thrombolytics:* May increase risk of bleeding. Use together cautiously.
Drug-herb. *Herbs with anticoagulant/antiplatelet properties (alfalfa, anise, bilberry, willow):* May increase risk of bleeding. Discourage use together.

EFFECTS ON LAB TEST RESULTS
• May increase ALT and AST levels.
• May decrease Hb level and platelet count.

CONTRAINDICATIONS & CAUTIONS
• Contraindicated in patients hypersensitive to drug, heparin, or pork products; in those with active major bleeding; and in those with a history of heparin-induced thrombocytopenia or heparin-induced thrombocytopenia with thrombosis.
• Contraindicated in patients with unstable angina or non-Q-wave MI or prolonged VTE prophylaxis who are undergoing epidural/neuraxial anesthesia.
• Use cautiously in patients at increased risk for hemorrhage, such as those with severe uncontrolled HTN, bacterial endocarditis, congenital or acquired bleeding disorders, active ulceration, angiodysplastic GI disease, or hemorrhagic stroke; also use with caution shortly after brain, spinal, or ophthalmic surgery. Monitor vital signs.
• Use cautiously in patients with bleeding diathesis, thrombocytopenia, platelet defects, severe hepatic or renal insufficiency, hypertensive or diabetic retinopathy, or recent GI bleeding.
• Use preservative-free dalteparin in neonates and infants because serious and fatal adverse reactions, including gasping syndrome, can occur in neonates and low-birth-weight infants treated with medications containing benzyl alcohol.
Dialyzable drug: Unknown.
⚠ *Overdose S&S:* Hemorrhagic complications.

PREGNANCY-LACTATION-REPRODUCTION
• There are no adequate well-controlled studies during pregnancy. Use during pregnancy only if clearly needed.
• Use preservative-free formulations without benzyl alcohol (not multidose vial) when possible during pregnancy and only if clearly needed. Benzyl alcohol may cross the placental barrier.
• Small amounts of anti-Xa activity have been detected in human milk; clinical implications, if any, for a breastfeeding infant are unknown. Use cautiously during breastfeeding.

NURSING CONSIDERATIONS
Boxed Warning Patients who have received epidural or spinal anesthesia or spinal

---

Reactions in bold italics are *life-threatening*. Interactions may have a *rapid onset* or a *delayed onset*.

puncture are at increased risk for developing an epidural or spinal hematoma, which may result in long-term or permanent paralysis. Increased risk may occur with use of indwelling epidural catheters, concomitant use of drugs that affect hemostasis (NSAIDs, platelet inhibitors, anticoagulants), history of traumatic or repeated epidural or spinal punctures, or history of spinal deformity or surgery. Monitor these patients closely for neurologic impairment and treat urgently. ∎

Boxed Warning Monitor patients for neurologic impairment (midline back pain, sensory or motor deficits such as numbness or weakness in lower limbs, bowel or bladder dysfunction). Treat impairment urgently. ∎

Boxed Warning Optimal timing between administration of drug and neuraxial procedures isn't known. Consider benefits and risks before neuraxial intervention in patients anticoagulated or to be anticoagulated for thromboprophylaxis. ∎

• DVT is a risk factor in patients who are candidates for therapy, including those older than age 40, those who are obese, those undergoing surgery under general anesthesia lasting longer than 30 minutes, and those who have additional risk factors (such as malignancy or history of DVT or PE).
• Never give drug IM.
☺ *Alert:* Drug isn't interchangeable (unit for unit) with unfractionated heparin or other low–molecular-weight heparin.
• Periodic, routine CBC and fecal occult blood tests are recommended during therapy. Patients don't need regular monitoring of PT or PTT.
• Monitor patient closely for thrombocytopenia.
• Stop drug if a thromboembolic event occurs despite dalteparin prophylaxis.

PATIENT TEACHING
• Instruct patient and family to watch for and report signs and symptoms of bleeding (bruising and blood in stools) and to report all adverse reactions promptly.
• Inform patient it may take longer than usual to stop bleeding.
• Tell patient to avoid OTC drugs containing aspirin or other salicylates unless ordered by prescriber.
• Advise patient to consult with prescriber before initiating any herbal therapy; many

herbs have anticoagulant, antiplatelet, and fibrinolytic properties.
• Tell patient to use a soft toothbrush and electric razor during treatment.
• Instruct patient or caregiver in drug administration if appropriate.
• Urge patient to tell prescriber and care givers if patient is allergic to natural rubber latex.

SAFETY ALERT!

dapagliflozin
dap-a-gli-FLOE-zin

Farxiga

Therapeutic class: Antidiabetics
Pharmacologic class: Sodium-glucose cotransporter 2 inhibitors

AVAILABLE FORMS
Tablets: 5 mg, 10 mg

INDICATIONS & DOSAGES
➤ **Adjunct to diet and exercise to improve glycemic control in patients with type 2 diabetes**
*Adults with eGFR of 45 mL/minute/1.73 m²
or greater:* Initially, 5 mg PO once daily; may increase to 10 mg daily for patients who require additional glycemic control.
➤ **To reduce risk of CV death and hospitalization for HF in patients with NYHA Class II, III, or IV HF with reduced ejection fraction**
*Adults with eGFR of 25 mL/minute/1.73 m²
or greater:* 10 mg PO once daily.
➤ **To reduce risk of hospitalization for HF in patients with type 2 diabetes and established CV disease or multiple CV risk factors**
*Adults with eGFR of 45 mL/minute/1.73 m²
or greater:* 10 mg PO once daily.
➤ **To reduce risk of sustained eGFR decline, ESRD, CV death, and hospitalization for HF in patients with chronic kidney disease at risk of progression**
Adults: 10 mg PO once daily.
Adjust-a-dose: Drug isn't recommended for initiation when eGFR is less than 25 mL/minute/1.73 m²; however, patient may continue 10 mg PO once daily to reduce risk of eGFR decline, ESRD, CV death, and hospitalization for HF.

ADMINISTRATION
PO
- Give dose in the morning.
- May give without regard for food.
- Give missed dose as soon as possible unless it's almost time for next dose; don't double dose.
- Store at room temperature.

ACTION
Inhibitor of sodium-glucose cotransporter 2 (SGLT2). This reduces reabsorption of filtered glucose from the proximal renal tubule and lowers the renal threshold for glucose, resulting in increased urinary glucose excretion.

Route	Onset	Peak	Duration
PO	Unknown	2 hr	Unknown

Half-life: About 12.9 hours.

ADVERSE REACTIONS
CV: volume depletion (dehydration, hypovolemia, orthostatic hypotension, hypotension). **EENT:** nasopharyngitis. **GI:** nausea, constipation. **GU:** genital mycotic infection, UTI, increased urination, dysuria. **Metabolic:** dyslipidemia. **Musculoskeletal:** back pain, extremity pain. **Other:** influenza.

INTERACTIONS
Drug-drug. *Insulin, insulin secretagogues (glimepiride, glipizide, glyburide, nateglinide, repaglinide):* May increase risk of hypoglycemia. Monitor patient closely and adjust insulin and secretagogue dosages as necessary.
Loop diuretics: May increase risk of hypotension. Monitor patient closely.

EFFECTS ON LAB TEST RESULTS
- May increase creatinine and LDL cholesterol levels.
- May decrease eGFR level.
- May increase hematocrit.
- May cause positive urine glucose test.
- May interfere with 1,5-AG assay. Use alternative methods to monitor glycemic control.

CONTRAINDICATIONS & CAUTIONS
- Contraindicated in patients with ESRD or who are on dialysis and in patients with history of serious hypersensitivity reactions (anaphylaxis, angioedema, SCAR) to dapagliflozin-containing products.
- Use isn't recommended in patients with an eGFR less than 45 mL/minute/1.73 m² in patients without CV disease or risk factors.
- Not recommended for use in patients with type 1 diabetes or for treatment of diabetic ketoacidosis.
- Not recommended for treatment of chronic kidney disease in patients with polycystic kidney disease or those with current or recent immunosuppressive therapy for kidney disease.
- Use cautiously in older adults because of increased risk of adverse events.
- Drug increases serum creatinine level and decreases eGFR; older adults and patients with hypovolemia may be more susceptible to these changes.
- Don't use in patients with active bladder cancer; use cautiously in patients with history of bladder cancer. Drug may increase risk of cancer reactivation.
- *Alert:* SGLT2 inhibitors such as dapagliflozin increase the risk of necrotizing fasciitis of the perineum (Fournier gangrene), a rare but serious and life-threatening infection requiring urgent surgical intervention, that has been reported in both females and males. Serious outcomes have included hospitalization, multiple surgeries, and death.
- *Alert:* Drug may cause ketoacidosis, which may require emergency department care or hospitalization. Monitor patients for ketoacidosis, especially those with major illness, reduced food or fluid intake, or reduced insulin dosage. Elevated urine or serum ketone levels without associated very high glucose levels have occurred with SGLT2 inhibitor use.
Dialyzable drug: Unknown.

PREGNANCY-LACTATION-REPRODUCTION
- There are no adequate studies during pregnancy. Use during pregnancy, especially during the second and third trimesters, isn't recommended. If needed during pregnancy, use only if potential benefit justifies fetal risk.
- It isn't known if drug appears in human milk. Use while breastfeeding isn't recommended. Patient should discontinue breastfeeding or discontinue drug.

NURSING CONSIDERATIONS
- *Alert:* Drug can increase risk of acute kidney injury. Before starting therapy, assess patient for factors that may predispose to acute kidney injury (decreased blood volume,

---

Reactions in bold italics are *life-threatening*. Interactions may have a *rapid onset* or a **delayed onset**.

chronic renal insufficiency, HF, concurrent use of other medications such as diuretics, ACE inhibitors, ARBs, and NSAIDs). Assess renal function before start of therapy and monitor periodically. Correct volume depletion before starting drug. If acute kidney injury occurs, drug should be discontinued and the kidney impairment treated.

• Drug may increase risk of severe UTI, including urosepsis and pyelonephritis. Monitor patient and treat promptly if indicated.

🔔 *Alert:* Monitor and immediately report signs and symptoms of necrotizing fasciitis of the perineum (temperature above 100.4° F [38° C], general feeling of being unwell; tenderness, redness, or swelling of the genitals back to the rectum). Signs and symptoms can worsen quickly. Immediately discontinue drug and prepare to administer broad-spectrum antibiotics. Surgical debridement may be necessary. Monitor blood glucose level and start alternative therapy for glycemic control.

• Monitor glucose level closely, especially if patient is taking antidiabetics concurrently. Adjust hypoglycemic dosages if needed.

• Monitor patient for genital mycotic infections.

• Stop drug immediately if hypersensitivity, or reduced renal function, or bladder cancer is suspected.

• Monitor volume status and watch for signs and symptoms of hypotension, particularly in patients with impaired renal function (eGFR less than 60 mL/minute/1.73 m^2), older adults, and patients taking loop diuretics. Increased urinary glucose excretion also results in increased urine volume.

• Consider temporarily discontinuing drug for at least 3 days before scheduled surgery or other clinical situations known to predispose patient to ketoacidosis (prolonged fasting due to acute illness, postsurgery). Ensure risk factors are resolved before resuming therapy.

PATIENT TEACHING
• Warn patient to use drug only as directed.

🔔 *Alert:* Advise patient to seek immediate medical attention for signs and symptoms of acute kidney injury (decreased urine output, swelling in legs or feet). Warn patient not to stop taking drug without first discussing with prescriber.

🔔 *Alert:* Teach patient signs and symptoms of necrotizing fasciitis (temperature above 100.4° F [38° C], general feeling of being

unwell, and tenderness, redness, or swelling of the genitals back to the rectum) and to seek immediate medical attention if any occur.

• Instruct patient to report signs and symptoms of yeast infections (itching, burning, discharge) promptly.

• Counsel patient on importance of diet and exercise in addition to medication for diabetes control.

• Teach patient to obtain periodic blood testing as requested by prescriber.

🔔 *Alert:* Instruct patient to seek medical attention immediately for signs and symptoms of ketoacidosis (difficulty breathing, hyperventilation, anorexia, nausea, vomiting, abdominal pain, confusion, unusual fatigue or sleepiness).

• Inform patient of increased UTI risk. Instruct patient to seek medical attention for signs and symptoms of UTI (painful urination, urinary frequency, blood in urine, urgency, pelvic pain, fever, back pain, nausea, vomiting).

• Advise patient to watch for signs and symptoms of hypoglycemia (fatigue, weakness, confusion, headache, pallor, or profuse sweating) when taking with insulin or insulin secretagogues.

• Caution patient to maintain adequate fluid intake to decrease risk of hypotension.

• Warn patient to contact prescriber for signs and symptoms of hypotension, such as lightheadedness (especially with position change) and weakness.

• Advise patient to seek medical attention promptly for fever, trauma, infection, or when surgery is needed; dosage adjustment may be needed owing to stress.

DAPTOmycin
dap-toe-MYE-sin

Cubicin, Cubicin RF

Therapeutic class: Antibiotics
Pharmacologic class: Cyclic lipopeptides

AVAILABLE FORMS
Powder for injection: 350-mg, 500-mg vial
Powder for infusion: 350-mg, 500-mg vial

INDICATIONS & DOSAGES
➤ **Bacteremia caused by *Staphylococcus aureus* (including right-sided endocarditis**

caused by methicillin-susceptible and methicillin-resistant strains)

Adults: 6 mg/kg IV infusion over 30 minutes or IV injection over 2 minutes every 24 hours for at least 2 to 6 weeks based on patient response.

Adjust-a-dose: For patients with bacteremia and CrCl of less than 30 mL/minute, including those on hemodialysis or continuous ambulatory peritoneal dialysis, give 6 mg/kg IV every 48 hours. When possible, give drug after hemodialysis on hemodialysis days.

➤ **Bacteremia caused by *S. aureus* in children with normal renal function**

Children ages 12 to 17: 7 mg/kg IV infusion over 30 minutes once every 24 hours for up to 42 days.

Children ages 7 to 11: 9 mg/kg IV infusion over 30 minutes once every 24 hours for up to 42 days.

Children ages 1 to 6: 12 mg/kg IV infusion over 60 minutes once every 24 hours for up to 42 days.

➤ **Complicated skin or skin-structure infection (cSSSI) caused by susceptible strains of *S. aureus* (including MRSA), *Streptococcus pyogenes*, *Streptococcus agalactiae*, *Streptococcus dysgalactiae*, and *Enterococcus faecalis* (vancomycin-susceptible strains only)**

Adults: 4 mg/kg IV infusion over 30 minutes or IV injection over 2 minutes every 24 hours for 7 to 14 days.

Children ages 12 to 17: 5 mg/kg IV infusion over 30 minutes once every 24 hours for up to 14 days.

Children ages 7 to 11: 7 mg/kg IV infusion over 30 minutes once every 24 hours for up to 14 days.

Children ages 2 to 6: 9 mg/kg IV infusion over 60 minutes once every 24 hours for up to 14 days.

Children ages 1 to younger than 2: 10 mg/kg IV infusion over 60 minutes once every 24 hours for up to 14 days.

Adjust-a-dose: In adults with cSSSI and CrCl of less than 30 mL/minute, including those on hemodialysis or continuous ambulatory peritoneal dialysis, give 4 mg/kg IV every 48 hours. When possible, give drug after hemodialysis on hemodialysis days. Dosage adjustment for children with renal impairment hasn't been established.

ADMINISTRATION

IV

▼ Obtain specimen for culture and sensitivity tests before giving first dose. Begin therapy while awaiting results.

⚠ *Alert:* The two formulations of daptomycin, Cubicin and Cubicin RF, differ concerning storage and reconstitution. Refer to, and carefully follow, the manufacturer's instructions for reconstituting and storing each drug when preparing these drugs for administration.

▼ Infuse over 30 minutes in adults and children age 7 and older. For children ages 1 to 6, infuse over 60 minutes.

▼ For IV injection over 2 minutes, give at a concentration of 50 mg/mL (adults only).

▼ Vials are for single use; discard excess.

▼ Don't use drug with ReadyMED elastomeric infusion pumps (Cardinal Health); an impurity may leach from the pump into the solution.

▼ **Incompatibilities:** Dextrose-containing solutions and other IV drugs. If an IV line is used for several drugs, flush the line with NSS or lactated Ringer solution injection between drugs.

ACTION

Bactericidal; binds to and depolarizes susceptible bacterial membranes to inhibit protein, DNA, and RNA synthesis.

Route	Onset	Peak	Duration
IV	Rapid	<1 hr	Unknown

Half-life: About 3.7 to 9 hours.

ADVERSE REACTIONS

CNS: confusion, dizziness, fever, headache, insomnia. **CV:** chest pain, edema, HTN, hypotension. **EENT:** sore throat. **GI:** abdominal pain, diarrhea, nausea, vomiting. **GU:** UTI. **Hepatic:** abnormal LFT values. **Metabolic:** increase CK level. **Respiratory:** cough, dyspnea. **Skin:** injection-site reactions, pruritus, rash, diaphoresis. **Other:** infection, bacteremia, *sepsis.*

INTERACTIONS

Drug-drug. *HMG-CoA reductase inhibitors (simvastatin):* May increase risk of myopathy. Consider stopping these drugs while giving daptomycin.

Reactions in bold italics are **life-threatening**. Interactions may have a *rapid onset* or a **delayed onset**.

Warfarin: May alter anticoagulant activity. Monitor PT and INR for the first several days of daptomycin therapy.

EFFECTS ON LAB TEST RESULTS
• May increase ALP and CK levels and LFT values.
• May decrease Hb level, platelet count, and hematocrit.
• May cause false elevation of INR and false prolongation of PT.

CONTRAINDICATIONS & CAUTIONS
• Contraindicated in patients hypersensitive to drug.
• Use cautiously in patients with renal insufficiency and in older adults.
• Safety and effectiveness haven't been established in children younger than age 12 months. Avoid use in children with renal impairment and those younger than age 12 months because of risk of potential effects on muscular, neuromuscular, or nervous systems (peripheral or central).
Dialyzable drug: Yes.

PREGNANCY-LACTATION-REPRODUCTION
• There are no adequate well-controlled studies during pregnancy. Use during pregnancy only if potential benefit justifies fetal risk.
• Drug appears in human milk in low amounts. Use cautiously during breastfeeding.

NURSING CONSIDERATIONS
• Monitor CBC, renal function tests, and LFTs periodically.
• Monitor patient for muscle pain or weakness, particularly of the distal extremities.
⚠ *Alert:* Because drug may increase the risk of myopathy, monitor CK level weekly or more frequently with renal impairment. If CK level rises, monitor it more often. In patients with unexplained signs and symptoms of myopathy with CK level greater than 1,000 units/L (approximately 5 × ULN) and in patients without reported signs and symptoms with CK level greater than 2,000 units/L (10 × ULN or greater), stop drug. Consider stopping all other drugs linked with myopathy (such as HMG-CoA reductase inhibitors) during therapy.
• Monitor patient for superinfection because drug may cause overgrowth of nonsusceptible organisms.

⚠ *Alert:* Drug may cause eosinophilic pneumonia, a rare type of pneumonia in which eosinophil-type WBCs fill the lungs, causing fever, cough, shortness of breath, and difficulty breathing. Monitor patient closely.
• DRESS syndrome has been reported. Monitor patient for rash, fever, peripheral eosinophilia, and systemic organ impairment. If DRESS syndrome is suspected, discontinue drug and start appropriate treatment.
• Tubulointerstitial nephritis (TIN) has been reported. Monitor patient for new or worsening renal impairment. If TIN is suspected, discontinue drug and start appropriate treatment.
• Monitor patient for signs and symptoms of neuropathy; consider stopping drug if neuropathy occurs.
• Watch for evidence of CDAD, which can occur more than 2 months after therapy.
• *Look alike–sound alike:* Don't confuse daptomycin with dactinomycin.

PATIENT TEACHING
• Advise patient to immediately report muscle weakness and infusion-site irritation.
• Tell patient to report all adverse reactions, especially severe diarrhea, rash, fever, and infection.
• Inform patient about possible adverse reactions.

daratumumab
dar-a-TOOM-ue-mab

Darzalex

Therapeutic class: Antineoplastics
Pharmacologic class: Monoclonal antibodies

AVAILABLE FORMS
Injection: 100 mg/5 mL, 400 mg/20 mL in single-dose vials

INDICATIONS & DOSAGES
Adjust-a-dose (for all indications): Refer to manufacturer's instructions for toxicity-related and infusion reaction adjustments. No dosage reductions of daratumumab are recommended.
➤ **Multiple myeloma monotherapy in patients who received at least three prior**

lines of therapy, including a proteasome inhibitor (PI) and an immunomodulatory agent or who are double refractory to a PI and an immunomodulatory agent; multiple myeloma in combination with lenalidomide and low-dose dexamethasone in patients who have received at least one prior therapy

Adults: Initially, 16 mg/kg (actual body weight) IV infusion once weekly for weeks 1 through 8 (total of eight doses); then for weeks 9 through 24, give 16 mg/kg IV infusion every 2 weeks (total of eight doses). Then, beginning week 25 onwards, give 16 mg/kg IV infusion every 4 weeks until disease progression. Refer to manufacturer's instructions for dosing instructions for combination agents.

➤ **Multiple myeloma in combination with bortezomib and dexamethasone in patients who have received at least one prior therapy**

Adults: Initially, 16 mg/kg (actual body weight) IV infusion once weekly for weeks 1 through 9 (total of nine doses); then give 16 mg/kg IV infusion every 3 weeks beginning week 10 through week 24 (total of five doses); then give 16 mg/kg IV infusion every 4 weeks beginning week 25 onwards until disease progression. Refer to manufacturer's instructions for dosing instructions for combination agents.

➤ **Multiple myeloma in combination with pomalidomide and low-dose dexamethasone for patients who have received at least two prior therapies, including lenalidomide and a PI**

Adults: Initially, 16 mg/kg (actual body weight) IV infusion once weekly for weeks 1 through 8 (total of eight doses); then for weeks 9 through 24, give 16 mg/kg IV infusion every 2 weeks (total of eight doses). Then, beginning week 25 onward, give 16 mg/kg IV infusion every 4 weeks until disease progresses. Refer to manufacturer's dosing instructions for combination agents.

➤ **Newly diagnosed multiple myeloma in patients ineligible for autologous stem cell transplant (ASCT), in combination with bortezomib, melphalan, and prednisone**

Adults: Initially, 16 mg/kg (actual body weight) IV infusion once weekly for weeks 1 through 6 (total of six doses); then, for weeks 7 through 54, give 16 mg/kg IV infusion every 3 weeks (total of 16 doses). Then, beginning on week 55 and onward, give 16 mg/kg IV infusion every 4 weeks until disease

progresses. Refer to manufacturer's dosing instructions for bortezomib, melphalan, and prednisone.

➤ **Newly diagnosed multiple myeloma in patients eligible for ASCT, in combination with bortezomib, thalidomide, and dexamethasone**

Adults: Induction treatment phase: initially, 16 mg/kg (actual body weight) IV infusion once weekly for weeks 1 through 8 (total of eight doses); then for weeks 9 through 16, give 16 mg/kg IV infusion every 2 weeks (total of four doses). Consolidation treatment phase: for weeks 1 through 8 upon reinitiation of treatment after ASCT, give 16 mg/kg IV infusion every 2 weeks (total of four doses). Refer to manufacturer's dosing instructions for combination agents.

➤ **Newly diagnosed multiple myeloma in patients ineligible for ASCT, in combination with lenalidomide and low-dose dexamethasone**

Adults: Initially, 16 mg/kg (actual body weight) IV infusion once weekly for weeks 1 through 8 (total of eight doses); then, for weeks 9 through 24, 16 mg/kg IV infusion every 2 weeks (total of eight doses). Then, beginning on week 25 and onward, 16 mg/kg IV infusion every 4 weeks until disease progression. Refer to manufacturer's dosing instructions for combination agents.

➤ **Multiple myeloma in combination with carfilzomib and dexamethasone for patients who have received one to three prior lines of therapies**

Adults: Initially, 8 mg/kg (actual body weight) IV infusion once daily on days 1 and 2 (total of two doses); then, for weeks 2 through 8, 16 mg/kg IV infusion once weekly (total of seven doses); then, for weeks 9 to 24, 16 mg/kg IV infusion every 2 weeks (total of eight doses). Then, beginning on week 25 and onward, 16 mg/kg IV infusion every 4 weeks until disease progression. Refer to manufacturer's dosing instructions for combination agents.

ADMINISTRATION

IV

▼ One to three hours before each infusion, premedicate with IV corticosteroid (methylprednisolone 100 mg or equivalent dose of an intermediate- or long-acting corticosteroid for monotherapy or 20 mg dexamethasone or equivalent dose for combination therapy), an oral antipyretic (acetaminophen 650 to 1,000 mg), and an oral or IV antihistamine (diphenhydramine 25 to 50 mg or equivalent). After second monotherapy infusion, may reduce methylprednisolone dose to 60 mg PO or IV.

▼ When dexamethasone is the background regimen-specific corticosteroid, the dexamethasone dose will serve as the premedication on daratumumab infusion days. Don't give additional background regimen-specific corticosteroids (e.g., prednisone) on daratumumab infusion days when patient receives dexamethasone (or equivalent) as premedication.

▼ On first and second day after monotherapy infusions, administer an oral corticosteroid (20 mg methylprednisolone or equivalent dose of an intermediate- or long-acting corticosteroid). For combination therapy, may consider methylprednisolone 20 mg or less PO or equivalent the day after infusion. If a background regimen-specific corticosteroid (e.g., dexamethasone, prednisone) is given the day after the infusion, additional corticosteroids may not be needed.

▼ For patients with a history of obstructive pulmonary disorder, postinfusion medications, such as short- and long-acting bronchodilators and inhaled corticosteroids, may be indicated. After first four infusions, if patient has no major infusion reactions, the additional postinfusion drugs may be discontinued.

▼ Solution should be colorless to pale yellow; don't use if vials contain opaque particles, discoloration, or other foreign particles.

▼ Remove volume of NSS from infusion bag that's equal to the volume of drug. Infusion bags should be made of polyvinyl chloride (PVC), polypropylene (PP), polyethylene (PE), or polyolefin blend.

▼ Withdraw medication from vial and add to infusion bag. Discard unused solution.

▼ Gently invert bag; don't shake.

▼ May keep diluted solution at room temperature for a maximum of 15 hours (including infusion time). May store infusion bag up to 24 hours in refrigerator at 36° to 46° F (2° to 8° C). Protect from light; don't freeze.

▼ Allow infusion bag to come to room temperature; then use immediately, as the solution doesn't contain a preservative.

▼ Administer with infusion set with flow regulator and in-line, sterile, nonpyrogenic,

low-protein-binding polyethersulfone filter (pore size 0.22 or 0.2 micron). Polyurethane, polybutadiene, PVC, PP, or PE administration sets must be used.

▼ For the week-1 infusion (500 mL on days 1 and 2 or 1,000 mL on day 1), give initially at 50 mL/hour for the first hour. May increase by 50 mL/hour every hour to maximum rate of 200 mL/hour if no infusion reactions occur. For week-2 infusion, if there are no infusion reactions during the previous week's infusion, may decrease second infusion dilution volume to 500 mL and begin infusion at 50 mL/hour for the first hour and increase by 50 mL/hour to a maximum of 200 mL/hour if no infusion reactions occur. Otherwise, continue the dilution volume of 1,000 mL. For subsequent infusions week 3 onwards, if there are no infusion reactions during the previous infusion, may give infusions in 500 mL at an initial rate of 100 mL/hour; may increase by 50 mL/hour every hour to maximum rate of 200 mL/hour if no infusion reactions occur. Otherwise, continue to use instructions for week-2 infusion.

▼ Complete infusion within 15 hours.

▼ Give missed dose as soon as possible and adjust dosing schedule accordingly to maintain treatment interval.

▼ **Incompatibilities:** Don't infuse in same IV line with other agents.

ACTION

An IgG1kappa human monoclonal antibody that binds to CD38 and inhibits growth of CD38-expressing tumor cells by inducing apoptosis.

Route	Onset	Peak	Duration
IV	Unknown	Unknown	Unknown

Half-life: 9 to 27 days.

ADVERSE REACTIONS

CNS: fatigue, fever, headache, asthenia, peripheral sensory neuropathy, paresthesia. **CV:** HTN, peripheral edema, atrial fibrillation. **EENT:** nasal congestion, nasopharyngitis. **GI:** nausea, vomiting, diarrhea, constipation, decreased appetite. **GU:** UTI. **Hematologic:** anemia, *thrombocytopenia, neutropenia, leukopenia, lymphopenia.* **Metabolic:** dehydration, hyperglycemia, *hypocalcemia.* **Musculoskeletal:** back pain, arthralgia, muscle spasms, extremity pain, musculoskeletal chest pain. **Respiratory:** cough, dyspnea, URI, bronchitis, pneumonia. **Skin:** rash, pruritus. **Other:** infusion reactions, chills, herpes zoster reactivation, infection, *sepsis.*

INTERACTIONS
None reported.

EFFECTS ON LAB TEST RESULTS
• May increase glucose level.
• May decrease calcium level.
• May decrease RBC, platelet, neutrophil, and lymphocyte counts.
• May cause positive indirect antiglobulin tests (Coombs test), interfering with cross-matching and RBC antibody screening that may persist for up to 6 months after last daratumumab infusion.
• May cause false-positive serum protein electrophoresis and immunofixation assay results in patients with IgG1kappa myeloma protein affecting assessment of complete response by International Myeloma Working Group criteria.

CONTRAINDICATIONS & CAUTIONS
• Contraindicated in patients with a history of severe hypersensitivity (anaphylaxis) to daratumumab or its components.
❸ *Alert:* Drug should only be given by health care professional with immediate access to emergency equipment and medical support to manage severe infusion reactions. Approximately half of all patients may experience an infusion reaction, and most occur during the first infusion. Infusion reactions can occur with subsequent infusions and within 4 hours of completing an infusion.
• Drug may increase risk of herpes zoster reactivation. Initiate antiviral prophylaxis within 1 week of starting treatment and continue for 3 months after treatment ends.
• Safety and effectiveness in children haven't been established.
Dialyzable drug: Unknown.

PREGNANCY-LACTATION-REPRODUCTION
• Risk during pregnancy is unknown. Patient should use contraception during therapy and for up to 3 months after therapy ends.
• Based on the mechanism of action, drug may cause fetal myeloid- or lymphoid-cell depletion and decrease bone density with in utero exposure. Delay administering live-virus vaccines to neonates and infants exposed to drug in utero until hematology evaluation is completed.
• It isn't known if drug appears in human milk. Discuss risk and benefits with patient who plans to breastfeed. However, if drug is given with lenalidomide, pomalidomide, or thalidomide, patient shouldn't breastfeed.

NURSING CONSIDERATIONS
❸ *Alert:* Be sure to premedicate patient and frequently monitor for signs and symptoms of infusion reaction (bronchospasm, hypoxia, dyspnea, HTN or hypotension, cough, wheezing, larynx and throat tightness or irritation, laryngeal edema, pulmonary edema, nasal congestion, allergic rhinitis, headache, rash, urticaria, pruritus, nausea, vomiting, chills). Emergency treatment may be needed for severe infusion reactions.
• Monitor patient for ocular signs and symptoms (acute myopia, increased IOP). Interrupt treatment and seek ophthalmologic evaluation.
• Risk of neutropenia and thrombocytopenia is increased, especially when drug is used in combination with other chemotherapy agents. Monitor CBC periodically. Growth factors or platelet transfusion may be needed.
• Patients should be typed and screened for blood transfusions before start of therapy because drug can interfere with cross-matching and antibody screening. Inform blood bank that patient is taking drug if typed and screened after initiating therapy.

PATIENT TEACHING
• Advise patient to immediately report signs and symptoms of infusion reaction.
• Caution patient to report all adverse reactions and to immediately report fever or signs and symptoms of bruising or bleeding.
• Explain to patient that blood test results to match blood type for transfusions may be affected for up to 6 months after last dose. Advise patient to inform all health care providers about taking daratumumab in the event of a planned transfusion.
• Inform patient that drug may occasionally affect results of some tests used to determine complete response and additional tests may be needed.

Reactions in bold italics are *life-threatening*. Interactions may have a *rapid onset* or a ***delayed onset***.

• Instruct patient to avoid pregnancy and to use effective contraception during therapy and for up to 3 months after last dose.
• Warn patient who wants to breastfeed that it isn't known if drug appears in human milk.
• Caution patient to take postinfusion medications and antiviral prophylaxis, as prescribed.
• Advise patient to inform prescriber about a previous or existing hepatitis B infection and that drug may cause virus to become active again.

SAFETY ALERT!

darbepoetin alfa
dar-bah-poe-E-tin

Aranesp

Therapeutic class: Colony stimulating factors
Pharmacologic class: Recombinant human erythropoietins

AVAILABLE FORMS
Injection: 25 mcg/mL, 40 mcg/mL, 60 mcg/mL, 100 mcg/mL, 200 mcg/mL, 300 mcg/mL in single-dose vials
Injection (prefilled syringe): 10 mcg/0.4 mL, 25 mcg/0.42 mL, 40 mcg/0.4 mL, 60 mcg/0.3 mL, 100 mcg/0.5 mL, 150 mcg/0.3 mL, 200 mcg/0.4 mL, 300 mcg/0.6 mL, 500 mcg/mL

INDICATIONS & DOSAGES
➤ **Anemia due to chronic kidney disease (CKD)**
Adults: Initiate drug only if Hb level is less than 10 g/dL. The IV route is preferred for patients on dialysis. For patients on dialysis, give 0.45 mcg/kg IV or subcut once weekly. Or, give 0.75 mcg/kg IV or subcut once every 2 weeks. For patients not on dialysis, give 0.45 mcg/kg IV or subcut at 4-week intervals. Give the lowest effective dose to gradually increase Hb to a level at which blood transfusion isn't necessary. Refer to manufacturer's instructions for specific dosing. Don't increase dose more often than once every 4 weeks.
Children younger than age 18: Initiate drug only if Hb level is less than 10 g/dL. For patients on dialysis, give 0.45 mcg/kg IV or subcut once weekly. For patients not on dialysis,

give 0.75 mcg/kg IV or subcut once every 2 weeks.
Adults and children older than age 1 who are on dialysis and converting from epoetin alfa: Refer to manufacturer's instructions.
Adjust-a-dose: For patients with chronic renal disease who aren't on dialysis, if the Hb level exceeds 10 g/dL, reduce dosage or interrupt therapy; use the lowest dosage sufficient to reduce the need for RBC transfusions. For patients with chronic renal disease who are on dialysis, if Hb level approaches or exceeds 11 g/dL, reduce dosage or interrupt therapy.
➤ **Anemia due to chemotherapy in patients with nonmyeloid malignancies**
Adults: Initiate drug only if Hb level is less than 10 g/dL and if there is a minimum of 2 additional months of planned chemotherapy; 2.25 mcg/kg subcut once weekly or 500 mcg subcut once every 3 weeks until completion of chemotherapy course.
Adjust-a-dose: For either dosing schedule, adjust dose to maintain a target Hb level necessary to avoid RBC transfusions. Give the lowest effective dose to gradually increase Hb to a level at which blood transfusion isn't necessary. Refer to manufacturer's instructions for dosing adjustment.

If after 8 weeks of therapy there is no response as measured by Hb levels or if transfusions are still required, discontinue drug. Discontinue drug after completion of chemotherapy course.

ADMINISTRATION
IV
⚠ *Alert:* The needle cover of the prefilled syringe contains dry natural rubber (a derivative of latex). Assess patient for a history of latex allergy.
▼ Don't shake. Shaking can denature drug.
▼ If drug contains particles or is discolored, don't use.
▼ Give undiluted by IV injection.
▼ Single-dose vials contain no preservatives; don't pool unused portions.
▼ Store drug in refrigerator; don't freeze. Don't use if drug has been frozen. Protect drug from light.
▼ **Incompatibilities:** Other IV drugs or solutions.
Subcutaneous
⚠ *Alert:* The needle cover of the prefilled syringe contains dry natural rubber (a derivative

of latex). Assess patient for a history of latex allergy.
- Don't shake. Shaking can denature drug.
- Store drug in refrigerator; don't freeze. Protect drug from light.

ACTION
Induces erythropoiesis. Stimulates erythropoiesis by same mechanism as endogenous erythropoietin.

Route	Onset	Peak	Duration
IV	Unknown	Unknown	Unknown
Subcut	Slow	48 hr (CKD); 71 hr (cancer)	Unknown

Half-life: IV: 21 hours. Subcut: patients with CKD on dialysis, 46 hours; patients with CKD not on dialysis, 70 hours.

ADVERSE REACTIONS
CNS: *stroke.* **CV:** edema, HTN, hypotension, peripheral edema, *PE, acute MI, HF, thrombosis,* angina, vascular access thrombosis. **GI:** abdominal pain. **Metabolic:** fluid overload. **Respiratory:** cough, dyspnea. **Skin:** pruritus, rash, erythema. **Other:** injection-site pain, hypersensitivity reactions.

INTERACTIONS
Drug-drug. *Lenalidomide, pomalidomide, thalidomide:* May increase thrombogenic effects. Monitor therapy.

EFFECTS ON LAB TEST RESULTS
- May increase Hb level.

CONTRAINDICATIONS & CAUTIONS
- Contraindicated in patients hypersensitive to drug or its components, in those with uncontrolled HTN, and in patients with pure red cell aplasia that begins after treatment with Aranesp or other erythropoietin protein drugs.
- Some forms contain polysorbate 80, which may cause hypersensitivity reactions.
- Not indicated for use in patients with cancer receiving hormonal agents, biologic products, or radiotherapy unless patients are also receiving concomitant myelosuppressive chemotherapy; in those receiving myelosuppressive chemotherapy when the anemia can be managed by transfusion; or as a substitute for RBC transfusions in patients who require immediate correction of anemia.

Boxed Warning Drug isn't indicated for patients receiving myelosuppressive therapy when the anticipated outcome is cure. ∎
- Blistering and skin exfoliation reactions, including erythema multiforme, SJS, and TEN, have been reported. Discontinue therapy immediately if SCAR is suspected.
- Safety and effectiveness in children with cancer haven't been established.
Dialyzable drug: No.
⚠ *Overdose S&S:* CV and thrombotic reactions, polycythemia.

PREGNANCY-LACTATION-REPRODUCTION
- There are no adequate well-controlled studies during pregnancy; animal studies show that drug may cause fetal harm. Use during pregnancy only if potential benefit justifies fetal risk.
- It isn't known if drug appears in human milk. Use cautiously during breastfeeding.

NURSING CONSIDERATIONS
Boxed Warning Erythropoiesis-stimulating agents increase risk of death, MI, stroke, venous thromboembolism, vascular access thrombosis, and tumor progression or recurrence. No trial has identified an Hb target level, drug dose, or dosing strategy that doesn't increase these risks. ∎
Boxed Warning Patients with chronic renal disease have an increased risk of death and serious CV events, including stroke, when erythropoiesis-stimulating agents are used to increase Hb level to greater than 11 g/dL. Therapy should be individualized for each patient; the lowest possible dose sufficient to reduce the need for RBC transfusions should be used. ∎
Boxed Warning In patients with NSCLC and breast, head and neck, lymphoid, and cervical cancers, there is a risk of tumor growth and shortened survival when Hb levels exceed the lowest dose needed to avoid RBC transfusion. Target for the lowest dosage needed to avoid RBC transfusions. Use only for treatment of anemia due to concomitant myelosuppressive chemotherapy, and discontinue drug after chemotherapy course. ∎
- Evaluate iron status in all patients before and during treatment. Administer supplemental iron when serum ferritin level is less than 100 mcg/L or when serum transferrin saturation is less than 20%. The majority of patients

---

with CKD will require supplemental iron during the course of erythropoietin-stimulating agent therapy.

• When initiating therapy or adjusting dosage, monitor Hb level at least weekly until stable; then, at least monthly.

• Hb level may not increase until 2 to 6 weeks after starting therapy.

• If patient has a minimal response or lack of response at recommended dose, check for deficiencies in folic acid, iron, or vitamin B_{12}. Other contributing factors include infection, malignancy, and occult blood loss.

🕓 *Alert:* If patient develops a sudden loss of response with severe anemia and low reticulocyte count, withhold drug and test patient for antierythropoietin antibodies. If antibodies are present, stop treatment. Don't switch to another erythropoietic protein because a cross-reaction is possible.

• Control BP and monitor it carefully.

• Monitor renal function and electrolytes in patients in predialysis.

• Monitor patency of vascular and dialysis access and report problems immediately.

• Patients who are marginally dialyzed may need adjustments in dialysis prescriptions.

• Serious allergic reactions, including skin rash and urticaria, may occur. If an anaphylactic reaction occurs, stop the drug and give appropriate therapy.

• Drug increases risk of seizures in patients with CKD. Monitor patients closely for premonitory neurologic signs and symptoms during first few months of therapy.

PATIENT TEACHING

• Instruct patient on proper administration and use and disposal of needles.

• Advise patient of possible side effects and allergic reactions.

• Inform patient of the need for frequent monitoring of BP and Hb level; stress adherence with treatment for high BP.

• Instruct patient how to take drug correctly at home, including how to store drug and dispose of supplies properly.

• Advise patient to report new-onset seizures or symptoms, or change in seizure frequency.

darifenacin hydrobromide
dar-i-FEN-a-sin

Therapeutic class: Antispasmodics
Pharmacologic class: Anticholinergics

D

AVAILABLE FORMS
Tablets (extended-release) ⓝ: 7.5 mg, 15 mg

INDICATIONS & DOSAGES
➤ **Urge incontinence, urgency, and frequency from an overactive bladder**
Adults: Initially, 7.5 mg PO once daily. After 2 weeks, may increase to 15 mg PO once daily if needed.
Adjust-a-dose: If patient has moderate hepatic impairment (Child-Pugh class B) or when drug is administered with strong CYP3A4 inhibitors, don't exceed 7.5 mg PO once daily. Drug isn't recommended for use in patients with severe hepatic impairment (Child-Pugh class C).

ADMINISTRATION
PO
• Don't crush, divide, or allow patient to chew tablet; patient should swallow tablet whole with water.
• Give drug without regard for food.

ACTION
Relaxes smooth muscle of bladder by selectively antagonizing M3 muscarinic receptors.

Route	Onset	Peak	Duration
PO	Unknown	7 hr	Unknown

Half-life: 13 to 19 hours.

ADVERSE REACTIONS
CNS: asthenia, dizziness, pain, headache. **CV:** HTN, peripheral edema. **EENT:** abnormal vision, dry eyes, rhinitis, sinusitis, pharyngitis, dry mouth. **GI:** constipation, abdominal pain, diarrhea, dyspepsia, nausea, vomiting. **GU:** urinary tract disorder, UTI, vaginitis, urine retention. **Metabolic:** weight gain. **Musculoskeletal:** arthralgia, back pain. **Respiratory:** bronchitis. **Skin:** dry skin, pruritus, rash. **Other:** accidental injury, flulike syndrome.

INTERACTIONS
Drug-drug. *Anticholinergics:* May increase anticholinergic effects, such as dry mouth,

blurred vision, and constipation. Monitor patient closely.

Digoxin: May increase digoxin level. Monitor digoxin level.

Drugs metabolized by CYP2D6 (flecainide, TCAs, thioridazine): May increase levels of these drugs. Use together cautiously.

Strong CYP3A4 inhibitors (clarithromycin, itraconazole, ketoconazole, nefazodone, nelfinavir, ritonavir): May increase darifenacin level. Maintain dosage no higher than 7.5 mg PO daily.

Drug-lifestyle. *Hot weather:* May cause heat exhaustion or heat stroke from decreased sweating. Urge caution.

EFFECTS ON LAB TEST RESULTS
None reported.

CONTRAINDICATIONS & CAUTIONS
• Contraindicated in patients hypersensitive to drug or its components. Angioedema can be life-threatening and has been reported after the first dose. If angioedema occurs, discontinue drug, start appropriate therapy, and ensure patent airway.
• Contraindicated in those with or at risk for urine retention, gastric retention, or uncontrolled angle-closure glaucoma.
• Use cautiously in patients with bladder outflow or GI obstruction, ulcerative colitis, myasthenia gravis, severe constipation, controlled angle-closure glaucoma, decreased GI motility, or Child-Pugh class B hepatic impairment.

Dialyzable drug: Unknown.

⚠ *Overdose S&S:* Severe antimuscarinic effects (mydriasis, decreased secretions, ileus, urine retention, tachycardia, altered mental status).

PREGNANCY-LACTATION-REPRODUCTION
• There are no studies during pregnancy. Use only if potential benefit justifies fetal risk.
• It isn't known if drug appears in human milk. Use cautiously during breastfeeding.

NURSING CONSIDERATIONS
• Assess bladder function, and monitor drug effects.
• If patient has bladder outlet obstruction, watch for urine retention.
• Assess patient for decreased gastric motility and constipation.

• Monitor patient for CNS anticholinergic effects (headache, confusion, hallucinations, somnolence), particularly after starting treatment or increasing dosage.
• Monitor patient for hypersensitivity reactions, including angioedema.

PATIENT TEACHING
• Teach patient safe drug administration.
• Tell patient to use caution, especially when performing hazardous tasks, until drug effects are known.
• Tell patient to report blurred vision, constipation, and urine retention and to immediately report swelling of the face, lips, or tongue or difficulty speaking.
• Discourage use of other drugs that may cause dry mouth, constipation, urine retention, or blurred vision.
• Tell patient that drug increases risk of heat exhaustion or heat stroke (decreased sweating, dizziness, fatigue, nausea, fever). Advise cautious use in hot environments and during strenuous activity.

dasiglucagon
das-i-GLOO-ka-gon

Zegalogue

Therapeutic class: Antihypoglycemics
Pharmacologic class: Glucagon receptor agonists

AVAILABLE FORMS
Injection: 0.6 mg/0.6 mL single-dose autoinjector; 0.6 mg/0.6 mL single-dose prefilled syringe

INDICATIONS & DOSAGES
➤ **Severe hypoglycemia in patients with diabetes**
Adults and children age 6 and older: 0.6 mg subcut. If no response after 15 minutes, may repeat with an additional 0.6 mg subcut.

ADMINISTRATION
Subcutaneous
🕐 *Alert:* The needle shield of the autoinjector and the needle cap of the syringe contain dry natural rubber (a derivative of latex) and may cause allergic reactions in patients sensitive to latex.

• Inspect drug for particulate matter or discoloration before administration.
• Inject into lower abdomen, buttock, thigh, or outer upper arm.
• Store in protected case refrigerated at 36° to 46° F (2° to 8° C) until expiration date. Don't freeze.
• May store at room temperature for up to 12 months. Discard after 12 months.
• Protect from light.
• Don't refrigerate drug after storing at room temperature.

ACTION
Increases blood glucose concentration by activating hepatic glucagon receptors and stimulating glycogen breakdown and hepatic glucose release.

Route	Onset	Peak	Duration
Subcut	Unknown	35 min	Unknown

Half-life: 30 minutes.

ADVERSE REACTIONS
CNS: headache. **CV:** *bradycardia,* HTN, hypotension, palpitations, presyncope, *bradycardia,* orthostatic intolerance. **GI:** diarrhea, nausea, vomiting. **Skin:** injection-site pain. **Other:** hypersensitivity reactions.

INTERACTIONS
Drug-drug. *Beta blockers:* May transiently increase pulse rate and BP. Monitor vital signs.
Indomethacin: May decrease antihypoglycemic effect of dasiglucagon or may produce hypoglycemia. Use together cautiously.
Warfarin: May increase anticoagulant effect of warfarin. Monitor patient closely.

EFFECTS ON LAB TEST RESULTS
• May increase or decrease blood glucose level.

CONTRAINDICATIONS & CAUTIONS
• Contraindicated in patients with pheochromocytoma. In patients with suspected undiagnosed pheochromocytoma who have substantial increase in BP, consider giving 5 to 10 mg of IV phentolamine mesylate.
• Contraindicated in patient with insulinoma. Drug may stimulate exaggerated insulin release from an insulinoma and cause hypoglycemia. If patient develops signs or symptoms of hypoglycemia after a dose, give PO or IV glucose.
• Allergic reactions have been reported with glucagon products.
• Drug is effective in treating hypoglycemia only if sufficient hepatic glycogen stores are present. Patients in a starvation state or with adrenal insufficiency or chronic hypoglycemia may not have adequate levels of hepatic glycogen for drug to be effective. Treat these patients with glucose.
• Safety and effectiveness in children younger than age 6 haven't been established.
Dialyzable drug: Unknown.
⚠ *Overdose S&S:* Nausea, vomiting, inhibition of GI tract motility, increased BP and HR, decreased serum potassium level.

PREGNANCY-LACTATION-REPRODUCTION
• There are no studies during pregnancy. Hypoglycemia during pregnancy can cause complications and may be fatal.
• It isn't known if drug appears in human milk or how drug affects milk production or infants who are breastfed.

NURSING CONSIDERATIONS
• Once patient responds to treatment, give carbohydrates PO to prevent recurrence of hypoglycemia and restore liver glycogen level.
• Monitor patient for allergic reactions (generalized rash, anaphylactic shock with breathing difficulties, hypotension).
• *Look alike–sound alike:* Don't confuse dasiglucagon with glucagon.

PATIENT TEACHING
🛈 *Alert:* Educate patient and family members or caregivers about signs and symptoms of severe hypoglycemia (confusion, sleepiness, slurred speech, blurred vision, seizures) and risks of prolonged hypoglycemia.
• Tell patient about allergic reactions and to seek immediate medical attention if signs or symptoms of serious hypersensitivity reactions occur.
• Advise patient and caregiver to read the information and instructions for use before drug is needed.
• Teach patient and caregiver how to store and dispose of injectors and syringes.
• Instruct patient and caregiver to seek emergency medical help or call health care provider immediately after injection, even if patient awakens.

• Educate patient and caregiver that if no response occurs within 15 minutes, another dose of drug may be given.

• Instruct patient and caregiver, that when safely able, patient should ingest a fast-acting source of sugar (fruit juice) and a long-acting source of sugar (crackers with cheese or peanut butter).

degarelix acetate
deg-a-REL-ix

Firmagon

Therapeutic class: Antineoplastics
Pharmacologic class: GnRH receptor antagonists

AVAILABLE FORMS
Injection: 80-mg, 120-mg vial

INDICATIONS & DOSAGES
➤ **Advanced prostate cancer**
Adult men: Initially, 240 mg subcut, administered as two 120-mg injections at a concentration of 40 mg/mL. Maintenance dose is 80 mg subcut given as one injection at a concentration of 20 mg/mL every 28 days starting 28 days after first dose.

ADMINISTRATION
Subcutaneous
• Drug is considered hazardous; use safe handling and disposal precautions.

• Give drug within 1 hour of reconstitution.

• Attach vial adaptor and reconstitute with provided prefilled syringe containing preservative-free sterile water for injection (reconstitute each 120-mg vial with 3 mL; reconstitute 80-mg vial with 4.2 mL). Leave syringe in place.

• Keeping vial in an upright position, swirl it very gently until liquid looks clear and has no undissolved powder or particles. If powder adheres to vial over the liquid surface, vial can be tilted slightly to dissolve powder. Avoid shaking, to prevent foam formation. A ring of small air bubbles on surface of liquid is acceptable. The reconstitution procedure may take up to 15 minutes.

• To withdraw for administration, turn vial completely upside down and pull down on the plunger to withdraw all of the reconstituted solution from vial to the syringe; expel all air bubbles. Detach the syringe by unscrewing it from vial adaptor.

• While holding the syringe with the tip pointing up, screw the injection needle clockwise onto the syringe.

• Inject drug only in areas of the abdomen that won't be exposed to pressure, for example, not close to waistband or belt nor close to the ribs.

• Inject degarelix subcut immediately after reconstitution. Pinch skin of abdomen, and elevate subcutaneous tissue. Insert needle deeply (all the way to the hub) at angle of not less than 45 degrees. Gently pull back plunger to check if blood is aspirated. If blood appears in syringe, reconstituted product can no longer be used. Discontinue procedure and discard syringe and needle. Reconstitute new dose. Slowly inject over 30 seconds.

• Remove the needle; then release the skin.

• Repeat reconstitution procedure for second 120-mg initial dose. Choose different injection site and inject.

ACTION
Binds to and antagonizes GnRH receptors, which reduces the release of gonadotropins and, consequently, testosterone.

Route	Onset	Peak	Duration
Subcut	Unknown	2 days	Unknown

Half-life: Loading dose, about 53 days; maintenance dose, about 31 days.

ADVERSE REACTIONS
CNS: asthenia, dizziness, fatigue, fever, headache, insomnia. **CV:** HTN, hot flashes. **GI:** constipation, diarrhea, nausea. **GU:** erectile dysfunction, UTI, testicular atrophy. **Hepatic:** increased transaminase levels. **Metabolic:** weight gain, weight loss, increased GGT. **Musculoskeletal:** arthralgia, back pain. **Skin:** injection-site reactions (including pain, erythema, swelling, induration, and nodule formation), night sweats, hyperhidrosis. **Other:** chills, gynecomastia.

INTERACTIONS
Drug-drug. *Class IA, Class III antiarrhythmics (amiodarone, procainamide, quinidine, sotalol), other drugs known to prolong QT interval:* May prolong QT interval. Avoid use together.

Reactions in bold italics are *life-threatening*. Interactions may have a *rapid onset* or a ***delayed onset***.

EFFECTS ON LAB TEST RESULTS
• May increase PSA, AST, ALT, and GGT levels.

CONTRAINDICATIONS & CAUTIONS
• Contraindicated in patients hypersensitive to drug or its components. Discontinue drug for serious hypersensitivity reactions and don't rechallenge.
• Androgen deprivation therapy may increase risk of CV disease, anemia, decreased bone density, and diabetes.
• Androgen deprivation therapy may prolong the QT interval. Prescribers should consider whether benefits of therapy outweigh potential risks. Use cautiously in patients with congenital long QT syndrome, electrolyte abnormalities, or HF and in those taking drugs known to prolong the QT interval.
• Use cautiously in patients with CrCl of less than 50 mL/minute or severe hepatic impairment.
Dialyzable drug: Unknown.

PREGNANCY-LACTATION-REPRODUCTION
• Drug isn't indicated for use in women and is contraindicated in patients who are or may become pregnant or are breastfeeding.
• Drug may impair fertility in males and females of reproductive potential.

NURSING CONSIDERATIONS
• Drug is only to be administered by a health care professional.
• Monitor QT interval and electrolyte levels in patients with congenital long QT syndrome, electrolyte abnormalities, or HF, and in those taking drugs known to prolong the QT interval.
• Monitor PSA level; if level is elevated, monitor testosterone level.
• Monitor bone density tests periodically.
• Monitor LFT values, CBC, and glucose level.
• Monitor patient for mental status changes.

PATIENT TEACHING
• Advise patient about possible adverse effects, including hot flashes, flushing of the skin, weight gain, decreased sex drive, and difficulties with erectile function. Injection-site reactions are usually mild, self-limiting, and decrease within 3 days.
• Stress importance of reporting heart problems, such as HF, irregular heart rhythm, or salt imbalance, before taking drug.

• Advise patient to inform all health care providers about taking drug.

delafloxacin meglumine
del-a-FLOKS-a-sin

Baxdela

Therapeutic class: Antibiotics
Pharmacologic class: Fluoroquinolones

AVAILABLE FORMS
Injection: 300 mg in single-dose vial
Tablets: 450 mg

INDICATIONS & DOSAGES
Adjust-a-dose (for all indications): If eGFR is between 15 and 29 mL/minute/1.73 m², no dosage adjustment is needed for tablets but decrease IV dosage to 200 mg every 12 hours, or give 200 mg IV every 12 hours, then switch to 450 mg PO every 12 hours at prescriber's discretion.

➤ Acute bacterial skin and skin-structure infections caused by susceptible bacteria, including gram-positive organisms (*Staphylococcus aureus* [including MRSA and methicillin-susceptible isolates], *Staphylococcus haemolyticus, Staphylococcus lugdunensis, Streptococcus agalactiae, Streptococcus anginosus* group [including *S. anginosus, Streptococcus intermedius,* and *Streptococcus constellatus*], *Streptococcus pyogenes,* and *Enterococcus faecalis*) and gram-negative organisms (*Escherichia coli, Enterobacter cloacae, Klebsiella pneumoniae,* and *Pseudomonas aeruginosa*)
Adults: 300 mg IV infusion or 450 mg PO every 12 hours for 5 to 14 days. May switch from IV to PO dosing at prescriber's discretion.

➤ Community-acquired bacterial pneumonia caused by susceptible microorganisms (*Streptococcus pneumoniae, S. aureus* [methicillin-susceptible [MSSA] isolates only]), *K. pneumoniae, E. coli, P. aeruginosa, Haemophilus influenzae, Haemophilus parainfluenzae, Chlamydia pneumoniae, Legionella pneumophila,* and *Mycoplasma pneumoniae*)
Adults: 300 mg IV infusion or 450 mg PO every 12 hours for 5 to 10 days. May switch from IV to PO dosing at prescriber's discretion.

ADMINISTRATION

PO

• May give with or without food.

• Administer at least 2 hours before or 6 hours after antacids containing magnesium or aluminum, sucralfate, metal cations such as iron, multivitamin preparations containing zinc or iron, or didanosine buffered tablets for oral suspension or didanosine pediatric powder for oral solution.

• May give missed dose any time up to 8 hours before next scheduled dose. If less than 8 hours remain before next dose, wait until next scheduled dose.

IV

▼ Reconstitute vial using 10.5 mL of D_5W or NSS for each 300-mg vial.

▼ Shake vial vigorously until contents are completely dissolved. Final concentration is 300 mg/12 mL (25 mg/mL) as a clear yellow to amber solution.

▼ Withdraw 12 mL from reconstituted vial for a 300-mg dose and 8 mL for a 200-mg dose. Add volume withdrawn to a total volume of 250 mL using either NSS or D_5W to achieve a final concentration of 1.2 mg/mL before administration.

▼ Infuse over 60 minutes. If a common IV line is used to administer other drugs, flush line before and after infusion with NSS or D_5W.

▼ Inspect for particulate matter and discoloration before administration.

▼ Store unopened vials at room temperature (68° to 77° F [20° to 25° C]).

▼ Reconstituted vials or diluted IV bag may be stored either refrigerated at 36° to 46° F (2° to 8° C) or at room temperature (68° to 77° F [20° to 25° C]) for up to 24 hours; don't freeze.

▼ **Incompatibilities:** Magnesium, other multivalent cations given through same IV line, and other drugs.

ACTION

Inhibits bacterial topoisomerase IV and DNA gyrase enzymes.

Route	Onset	Peak	Duration
PO	Unknown	0.75–1 hr	Unknown
IV	Unknown	1 hr	Unknown

Half-life: Oral, 4.2 to 8.5 hours; IV, 3.7 hours.

ADVERSE REACTIONS

CNS: headache, dizziness, hypoesthesia, paresthesia, presyncope, syncope, anxiety, dysgeusia, insomnia, abnormal dreams. **CV:** sinus tachycardia, palpitations, bradycardia, hypotension, HTN, flushing. **EENT:** blurred vision, tinnitus, vertigo, oral candidiasis. **GI:** nausea, diarrhea, vomiting, abdominal pain, dyspepsia, *CDAD.* **GU:** vulvovaginal candidiasis, renal impairment, *renal failure.* **Hepatic:** elevated transaminase levels. **Metabolic:** *hypoglycemia,* hyperglycemia. **Musculoskeletal:** myalgia. **Skin:** infusion-site extravasation, infusion-site reactions (bruising, discomfort, edema, erythema, irritation, pain, phlebitis, swelling, thrombosis), pruritus, urticaria, dermatitis, rash. **Other:** hypersensitivity reaction, fungal infection.

INTERACTIONS

Drug-drug. *Antacids containing aluminum or magnesium, didanosine, iron, multivitamins containing iron or zinc, sucralfate:* May lower delafloxacin level when taken with PO formulation. Separate delafloxacin dose by at least 2 hours before or 6 hours after these drugs.

Corticosteroids: May increase risk of tendon injury. Avoid concurrent use.

Insulin, oral hypoglycemics (glyburide): May increase risk of hypoglycemia. Monitor glucose level closely.

EFFECTS ON LAB TEST RESULTS

• May increase liver transaminase, ALP, creatinine, and CK levels.

• May increase or decrease blood glucose level.

CONTRAINDICATIONS & CAUTIONS

• Contraindicated in patients hypersensitive to drug, its components, or other fluoroquinolones.

⚠ *Alert:* Patients receiving systemic drug have an increased risk of hyperglycemia and hypoglycemia, which can result in coma. Hypoglycemia has been reported more frequently in older adults and in patients with diabetes.

⚠ *Alert:* Drug may increase risk of aortic dissection or rupture when used systemically. Avoid use in patients with known aortic aneurysm, in patients at risk for an aortic aneurysm, including those with peripheral atherosclerotic vascular diseases, HTN, or certain genetic conditions (Marfan syndrome, Ehlers-Danlos syndrome), and in older adults. Drug should only be used in these patients if no other treatment options are available.

• Use should be limited to infections that are proven or strongly suspected to be caused by susceptible bacteria to reduce risk of drug-resistant bacteria and to maintain drug's effectiveness.

Boxed Warning Fluoroquinolones have been associated with disabling and potentially irreversible serious adverse reactions that have occurred together, including tendinitis and tendon rupture, peripheral neuropathy, and CNS effects. Discontinue immediately if signs and symptoms occur; avoid using fluoroquinolones in patients who experience any of these serious adverse reactions. ■

Boxed Warning Fluoroquinolones may exacerbate muscle weakness in patients with myasthenia gravis. Avoid using fluoroquinolones in patients with known history of myasthenia gravis. ■

Boxed Warning Oral or parenteral fluoroquinolones may increase risk of peripheral neuropathy of the arms or legs. Signs or symptoms can occur anytime during treatment and can last for months to years or be permanent. Stop drug immediately if patient develops signs or symptoms. Avoid use in patients who have previously experienced peripheral neuropathy. ■

Boxed Warning Use cautiously in patients with a history of known or suspected CNS disorders (severe cerebral arteriosclerosis, epilepsy) or other risk factors that increase the risk of seizures or lower the seizure threshold. Drug may increase risk of CNS reactions, including seizures, increased ICP (including pseudotumor cerebri), dizziness, and tremors. If these reactions occur, discontinue drug immediately and institute appropriate measures. ■

Boxed Warning Fluoroquinolones have been associated with an increased risk of psychiatric adverse reactions, including toxic psychosis; hallucinations or paranoia; depression or suicidality; delirium, disorientation, confusion, or disturbances in attention; anxiety, agitation, or nervousness; insomnia or nightmares; and memory impairment. These adverse reactions may occur after first dose. Stop drug immediately and institute appropriate measures if patient develops any of these reactions. ■

• Drug isn't indicated for patients with eGFR of less than 15 mL/minute/1.73 m^2, including patients receiving hemodialysis.

• Drug may cause CDAD ranging in severity from mild diarrhea to fatal colitis and possibly occurring more than 2 months after therapy ends. Drug may need to be discontinued if CDAD develops during therapy.

• Use cautiously in older adults; patients taking corticosteroids; patients with kidney, heart, or lung transplant; patients with renal impairment; patients with previous tendon disorders, including RA; and those participating in strenuous physical activity as risk of tendinitis or tendon rupture may be increased.

• Drug isn't approved for children younger than age 18.

Dialyzable drug: Yes.

PREGNANCY-LACTATION-REPRODUCTION

• Data are limited on the safety of delafloxacin during pregnancy. Use cautiously and only if benefits outweigh risk to the fetus.

• It isn't known if drug appears in human milk. Consider benefits of therapy and risks of breastfeeding in the infant.

NURSING CONSIDERATIONS

• Whenever possible, obtain specimen for culture and sensitivity testing before first dose. Begin therapy while awaiting results.

🖐 *Alert:* Monitor patients for signs and symptoms of aortic aneurysm, dissection, or rupture (sudden, severe, and constant pain in the stomach, chest, or back; throbbing in the stomach area; deep pain in the back or the side of the stomach; steady, gnawing pain in the stomach that lasts for hours or days; pain in the jaw, neck, back, or chest; coughing or hoarseness; shortness of breath or trouble swallowing). Discontinue drug immediately if any of these aortic disorders are suspected.

• Monitor patient for tendinitis (pain, swelling, inflammation), tendon rupture, arthralgia, and myalgia. Symptoms may occur from hours after starting drug to several months after therapy ends. Discontinue drug immediately if symptoms occur.

• Monitor patient for peripheral neuropathy (pain; burning; tingling; numbness; weakness; alterations in light touch, pain, temperature, position sense, and vibratory sensation; and motor strength) and CNS effects (seizures, increased ICP, pseudotumor cerebri, severe headaches, dizziness, tremors).

Signs and symptoms may occur hours or weeks after initial dose. Discontinue drug if these reactions occur.

• Monitor patients with myasthenia gravis for exacerbation of muscle weakness; discontinue drug immediately if symptoms occur.

• Monitor patients for rash or other signs and symptoms of hypersensitivity. Discontinue drug at first appearance of reaction.

• Monitor patients for CDAD, which has been reported in users of nearly all systemic antibacterial drugs. Stop drug and provide appropriate therapy if CDAD occurs.

◑ *Alert:* Monitor patients receiving systemic drug for symptoms of hypoglycemia (confusion, pounding or rapid heartbeat, dizziness, pale skin, shakiness, diaphoresis, unusual hunger, trembling, headache, weakness, irritability, unusual anxiety). Immediately discontinue drug for blood glucose disturbances, and switch to a nonfluoroquinolone antibiotic if possible.

◑ *Alert:* Monitor patients receiving systemic drug for psychiatric adverse reactions (toxic psychosis, hallucinations, paranoia, depression, suicidality, confusion, insomnia or nightmares, disturbances in attention, disorientation, agitation, nervousness, memory impairment, delirium). Discontinue drug if these reactions occur.

PATIENT TEACHING

• Discuss importance of taking every dose and of completing a full treatment course to prevent antibacterial resistance and to avoid decreasing drug's effectiveness. If drug is stopped because of adverse effects, patient should discuss with prescriber completing treatment with another antibacterial drug.

◑ *Alert:* Warn patient to seek immediate medical attention for signs or symptoms of aortic aneurysm, dissection, or rupture.

Boxed Warning Tell patient that tendon rupture can occur during therapy and to notify prescriber if pain, swelling, or inflammation of tendon or weakness or inability to use a joint occurs. Advise patient to stop drug and to rest and refrain from exercise. ∎

Boxed Warning Inform patient with myasthenia gravis that drug may exacerbate signs and symptoms of muscle weakness, including respiratory difficulties, and to immediately report worsening. ∎

Boxed Warning Caution patient to immediately report signs and symptoms of peripheral neuropathy (pain, tingling, burning, numbness, weakness) to prescriber and to stop drug. ∎

Boxed Warning Explain risk of CNS adverse effects (seizures, dizziness, lightheadedness, increased ICP, headache with or without blurred vision) with use of drug and advise patient to notify prescriber immediately if these occur. ∎

• Warn patient to avoid hazardous tasks that require alertness such as driving until drug's effects are known.

• Advise patient to report all adverse reactions and to immediately report hypersensitivity reactions (rash, hives, other skin reactions, tachycardia, difficulty swallowing or breathing, tightness of the throat, hoarseness, and swelling of the lips, tongue, or face), which can occur even after a single dose.

◑ *Alert:* Caution patients that significantly low blood sugar levels can occur. Instruct patients how to manage symptoms and to immediately report any occurrence to the prescriber.

◑ *Alert:* Advise patients with diabetes that they may need to monitor blood glucose levels more frequently during therapy.

Boxed Warning Inform patients to immediately report psychiatric adverse reactions and that these can occur after just one dose. ∎

• Caution patient to immediately report watery or bloody stools with or without abdominal cramping and fever. Diarrhea may occur during therapy or 2 months or more after last dose.

---

denosumab
deh-KNOW-sue-mab

Prolia, Xgeva

Therapeutic class: Antiosteoporotics–antiresorptives
Pharmacologic class: Monoclonal antibodies

AVAILABLE FORMS
Injection: 60 mg/mL in prefilled syringe (Prolia); 120 mg/1.7 mL (70 mg/mL) in single-use vial (Xgeva)

INDICATIONS & DOSAGES
➤ **Osteoporosis in men and women who are postmenopausal at risk for fracture (Prolia only)**

Reactions in bold italics are *life-threatening*. Interactions may have a *rapid onset* or a ***delayed onset***.

Adults: 60 mg subcut every 6 months. All patients should receive 1,000 mg of calcium daily and at least 400 international units of vitamin D daily.

➤ **To increase bone mass in men at high risk for fracture who are receiving androgen deprivation therapy for nonmetastatic prostate cancer and in women who are receiving adjuvant aromatase inhibitor therapy for breast cancer (Prolia only)**
Adults: 60 mg subcut once every 6 months. All patients should receive calcium 1,000 mg daily and at least 400 international units of vitamin D daily.

➤ **Glucocorticoid-induced osteoporosis in men and women at high risk for fracture who are either initiating or continuing systemic glucocorticoids in a daily dosage equivalent to 7.5 mg or greater of prednisone and expected to remain on glucocorticoids for at least 6 months (Prolia only)**
Adults: 60 mg subcut once every 6 months. All patients should receive calcium 1,000 mg daily and at least 400 international units of vitamin D daily.

➤ **Giant cell tumor of bone (Xgeva only)**
Adults and skeletally mature adolescents age 13 and older: 120 mg subcut every 4 weeks with additional 120-mg doses on days 8 and 15 of first month of therapy. Administer calcium and vitamin D as necessary to prevent or treat hypocalcemia.

➤ **Hypercalcemia of malignancy refractory to bisphosphonate therapy (Xgeva only)**
Adults: 120 mg subcut every 4 weeks with additional 120-mg doses on days 8 and 15 of first month of therapy.

➤ **Bone metastases from solid tumors; prevention of skeletal-related events in patients with multiple myeloma (Xgeva only)**
Adults: 120 mg subcut every 4 weeks, with calcium and vitamin D as necessary to prevent or treat hypocalcemia.

ADMINISTRATION
Subcutaneous
• Don't use if solution is discolored or cloudy or contains many particles or foreign particulate matter.
• Before administration, drug may be removed from refrigerator and brought to room temperature (up to 77° F [25° C]) by letting stand in original container. This generally takes 15 to 30 minutes. Don't warm drug in any other way. Avoid vigorous shaking of drug. Once removed from refrigerator, maintain at 77° F or lower and use within 14 days. Discard after 14 days if not used.
• Protect from direct light and heat.
• Use 27G needle to withdraw drug from single-use vial, and inject entire contents of vial. Don't reenter vial.
• Administer via subcut injection in upper arm, upper thigh, or abdomen.
• Drug is intended for subcut route only and shouldn't be administered IV, IM, or intradermally.
🛈 *Alert:* Needle cap on single-use syringe contains latex; keep away from patients with latex allergy.
• If a Prolia dose is missed, give as soon as convenient. Schedule injections every 6 months from date of last injection.

ACTION
Inhibits osteoclast activity, thereby decreasing bone resorption and increasing bone mass and strength.

Route	Onset	Peak	Duration
Subcut	Unknown	10 days	4–5 mo

Half-life: About 25 to 28 days.

ADVERSE REACTIONS
CNS: asthenia, insomnia, sciatica, headache, fatigue. **CV:** angina, atrial fibrillation, peripheral edema. **EENT:** vertigo, pharyngitis. **GI:** flatulence, GERD, upper abdominal pain, nausea, decreased appetite, vomiting, constipation, diarrhea. **GU:** cystitis. **Hematologic:** anemia, *thrombocytopenia.* **Metabolic:** hypercholesterolemia, *hypocalcemia,* hypophosphatemia. **Musculoskeletal:** osteonecrosis of jaw, back pain, bone pain, extremity pain, musculoskeletal pain, myalgia, spinal osteoarthritis. **Respiratory:** pneumonia, URI, dyspnea, cough, bronchitis. **Skin:** pruritus, rash, dermatitis. **Other:** *anaphylaxis,* facial swelling, herpes zoster.

INTERACTIONS
Drug-drug. *Calcimimetic drugs, calcium-lowering drugs:* May worsen hypocalcemia risk. Monitor serum calcium level closely.
Immunosuppressants (except cytarabine [liposomal]): May enhance adverse effects of immunosuppressants and increase risk of serious infections. Monitor patient closely.

Drug-lifestyle. *Alcohol use:* May increase risk of osteoporosis. Avoid use together.

EFFECTS ON LAB TEST RESULTS
• May increase cholesterol level.
• May decrease calcium, magnesium, and phosphate levels.
• May decrease Hb level and platelet count.

CONTRAINDICATIONS & CAUTIONS
• Contraindicated in patients with a history of systemic hypersensitivity to components of the product. Reactions have included anaphylaxis, facial swelling, and urticaria.
• Contraindicated in patients with hypocalcemia.
• Discontinue use if severe bone, joint, or muscle pain occurs.
• Use cautiously in patients with history of hypoparathyroidism, thyroid surgery, parathyroid surgery, malabsorption syndromes, excision of small intestine, or severe renal impairment.
• Clinically significant hypercalcemia requiring hospitalization and complicated by acute renal injury has been reported within the first year after treatment discontinuation in patients with giant cell tumor of bone being treated with Xgeva and in patients with growing skeletons.
• Use cautiously in older adults and patients with an impaired immune system.
• Safety and effectiveness in children haven't been established except for Xgeva in skeletally mature adolescents (ages 12 to 16) with giant cell tumor of bone.
Dialyzable drug: Unknown.

PREGNANCY-LACTATION-REPRODUCTION
• Drug may cause fetal harm; use is contraindicated during pregnancy. Inform patient of fetal risk.
• Caution patients of childbearing potential to use highly effective contraception during therapy and for at least 5 months after last dose.
• It isn't known if drug appears in human milk. Patient should discontinue breastfeeding or discontinue drug, taking into account importance of drug to the patient.

NURSING CONSIDERATIONS
• Drug should only be administered by a health care professional.

• Verify pregnancy status of patients of childbearing potential before starting drug.
• Make sure patient has adequate intake of calcium and vitamin D.
• Monitor calcium (especially in first weeks of therapy), vitamin D, magnesium, and phosphorus levels before and during therapy. Administer calcium, magnesium, and vitamin D as needed.
• Drug can cause severe symptomatic hypocalcemia; fatal cases have been reported. Correct hypocalcemia before starting drug.
• Multiple vertebral fractures have been reported after treatment ends. Evaluate patient's individual risk of vertebral fractures and consider transitioning to an alternative antiresorptive therapy.
• Drug may cause osteonecrosis of the jaw, which can occur spontaneously and is commonly associated with tooth extraction, local infection with delayed healing, or both. Monitor patients for signs and symptoms and perform an oral exam and ensure appropriate preventive dentistry before starting drug and periodically during therapy.
• Consider stopping drug if severe skin reactions occur.
• When treatment is discontinued, monitor patients for signs and symptoms of hypercalcemia (nausea, vomiting, headache, decreased alertness), assess serum calcium level periodically, reevaluate patient's calcium and vitamin D supplementation requirements, and treat appropriately.
🛑 *Alert:* Prolia and Xgeva contain the same active ingredient, denosumab. Patients receiving Prolia should not receive Xgeva.

PATIENT TEACHING
• Warn patient to immediately report signs and symptoms of low calcium (spasms, twitching or muscle cramps, and numbness or tingling of fingers or toes or around mouth); emphasize the importance of maintaining normal calcium levels.
• Advise patient to have a dental exam before treatment and to follow good oral hygiene practices during therapy.
• Instruct patient to tell dentist before dental procedures about taking drug, and to inform dentist or prescriber if persistent pain or slow healing of mouth or jaw occurs after dental surgery.
• Tell patient to report jaw pain, swelling, or numbness; loose teeth; or dramatic gum loss.

• Advise patient to seek prompt medical care if signs and symptoms of severe infection occur, including cellulitis or skin reactions (such as dermatitis, rash, or eczema).

• Advise patient to contact health care provider if severe bone, joint, or muscle pain occurs.

• Instruct patient with severe renal impairment about signs and symptoms of hypocalcemia and the importance of maintaining normal calcium levels.

• Tell patient to take calcium and vitamin D supplement, as directed by prescriber.

• Advise patient of childbearing potential to use highly effective contraception during therapy and for at least 5 months after final dose.

---

desmopressin acetate ░
des-moe-PRESS-in

DDAVP, Nocdurna, Stimate

Therapeutic class: Hemostatics
Pharmacologic class: Posterior pituitary hormones

AVAILABLE FORMS
Injection: 4 mcg/mL
Metered nasal spray: 10 mcg/spray, 150 mcg/spray
Nasal solution: 0.1 mg/mL
Tablets: 0.1 mg, 0.2 mg
Tablets (SL): 27.7 mcg, 55.3 mcg

INDICATIONS & DOSAGES
➤ **Nonnephrogenic diabetes insipidus, temporary polyuria, and polydipsia related to pituitary trauma**
IV, subcutaneous
Adults and children older than age 12: 2 to 4 mcg (0.5 to 1 mL) IV or subcut daily, usually in two divided doses.
PO
Adults and children older than age 4: Initially, 0.05 mg (half of the 0.1-mg tablet) PO b.i.d.; adjust dosage to patient response. If patient previously received the drug intranasally, begin oral therapy 12 hours after last intranasal dose. Maximum dose is 1.2 mg/day (divided into two or three doses) for patients with diabetes insipidus.
Intranasal
Adults and children older than age 12: 10 to 40 mcg (0.1 to 0.4 mL) intranasally daily in

one to three doses. Most adults need 0.2 mL (20 mcg) daily in two divided doses.
Children ages 4 to 12: 10 to 30 mcg (0.1 to 0.3 mL) intranasally daily in one or two doses.
➤ **Hemophilia A and von Willebrand disease** ░
Adults and children age 3 months and older: 0.3 mcg/kg diluted in NSS and infused IV over 15 to 30 minutes. Repeat dose, if needed, as indicated by lab response and patient's condition. If used preoperatively, give 30 minutes before the scheduled procedure.
Adults and children age 11 months and older: A total dose of 300 mcg (one spray [150 mcg] of solution containing 1.5 mg/mL in each nostril. Dose of 150 mcg (one spray of solution containing 1.5 mg/mL into a single nostril) may be adequate for patients weighing less than 50 kg. If used preoperatively, give drug 2 hours before surgery.
➤ **Primary nocturnal enuresis**
Adults and children age 6 and older: Initially, 0.2 mg PO at bedtime; adjust dose up to 0.6 mg to achieve desired response.
➤ **Nocturnal polyuria in adults who awaken at least two times per night to void (Nocdurna)**
Women: 27.7 mcg SL daily without water, 1 hour before bedtime.
Men: 55.3 mcg SL daily without water, 1 hour before bedtime.

ADMINISTRATION
PO
• Discontinue in patient with acute illness that may result in fluid or electrolyte imbalance.
• Store at controlled room temperature.
IV
▼ When given IV push for diabetes insipidus, dilution isn't required.
▼ Don't give injection to patients with hemophilia A with factor VIII activity of up to 5% or with severe von Willebrand disease.
▼ For adults and children weighing more than 10 kg, dilute with 50 mL sterile physiologic saline solution. For children weighing 10 kg or less, 10 mL of diluent is recommended. Infuse over 15 to 30 minutes.
▼ Inspect drug for particulates and discoloration before infusing.
▼ Monitor BP and pulse rate during infusion.
▼ The comparable antidiuretic dose of the injection is about one-tenth of the intranasal dose.

▼ Solution and injection must be refrigerated.

▼ **Incompatibilities:** None listed by manufacturer. Consult a drug incompatibility reference for more information.

Intranasal

• Ensure nasal passages are intact, clean, and free of obstruction before giving intranasally.

• Nasal spray pump delivers only doses of 10 mcg DDAVP (per 0.1-mL dose) or 150 mcg Stimate (per 0.1-mL dose). If doses other than these are required, use injection.

• Spray pump must be primed before first use. To prime pump, press down four times. If pump isn't used for 1 week, reprime by pressing down on pump once. Discard bottle after 25 doses (150 mcg/spray) or 50 doses (10 mcg/spray), depending on the strength, since the amount delivered thereafter per spray may be substantially less than the required dose.

• Nasal spray may be stored at room temperature.

Subcutaneous

• Dilution isn't required before injection.

• Teach patient to rotate injection sites to prevent tissue damage.

Sublingual

• Patient should empty bladder immediately before bedtime and limit fluid intake to a minimum from 1 hour before until 8 hours after administration.

• Patient should keep tablet under tongue until it has fully dissolved.

ACTION

Synthetic analogue of ADH that increases the permeability of renal tubular epithelium to adenosine monophosphate and water, enabling the epithelium to promote reabsorption of water and produce a concentrated urine. Also increases factor VIII activity by releasing endogenous factor VIII from plasma storage sites.

Route	Onset	Peak	Duration
PO	1 hr	0.9–1.5 hr	12 hr
IV	30 min	1.5–2 hr	6–14 hr
Intranasal	15–30 min	0.25–1.5 hr	6–14 hr
Subcut	Unknown	Unknown	Unknown
SL	30 min	Unknown	6 hr

Half-life: PO, 1.5 to 2.5 hours; IV, 3 hours; intranasal (DDAVP), 7.8 minutes (initial phase) and 75.5 minutes (terminal phase); intranasal (Stimate), 3.3 to 3.5 hours; SL (Nocdurna), 2.8 hours.

ADVERSE REACTIONS

CNS: headache, *seizures,* dizziness, asthenia. **CV:** flushing, HTN, fluid retention. **EENT:** conjunctivitis, edema around eyes, abnormal lacrimation, nasal discomfort or congestion, epistaxis, rhinitis, sore throat, nasopharyngitis, dry mouth. **GI:** nausea, abdominal cramps. **GU:** vulvar pain. **Metabolic:** *hyponatremia.* **Musculoskeletal:** back pain. **Respiratory:** cough, bronchitis. **Skin:** local erythema, swelling, or burning after injection. **Other:** chills.

INTERACTIONS

Drug-drug. *Carbamazepine, chlorpropamide:* May increase ADH; may increase desmopressin effect. Avoid using together. *Chlorpromazine, lamotrigine, NSAIDs, opioid analgesics, oxybutynin, SSRIs, TCAs:* May increase risk of water intoxication with hyponatremia. Monitor patient closely. *Clofibrate:* May enhance and prolong effects of desmopressin. Monitor patient closely. *Demeclocycline, lithium, tolvaptan:* May decrease effect of desmopressin. Use together cautiously. Avoid use with tolvaptan.

Boxed Warning *Loop diuretics, systemic or inhaled glucocorticoids:* May increase risk of hyponatremia. Use with Nocdurna is contraindicated. Drug can be started or resumed 3 days or 5 half-lives after the glucocorticoid is discontinued, whichever is longer. ∎

Pressor agents: May enhance pressor effects with large doses of desmopressin. Monitor patient closely.

Drug-lifestyle. *Alcohol use:* May increase risk of adverse effects. Discourage use together.

EFFECTS ON LAB TEST RESULTS

• May decrease sodium level.

CONTRAINDICATIONS & CAUTIONS

▩ Contraindicated in patients hypersensitive to drug and in those with type IIB von Willebrand disease, moderate to severe renal impairment, hyponatremia, or a history of hyponatremia.

Boxed Warning Nocdurna is contraindicated in patients at increased risk for severe hyponatremia, such as patients with excessive fluid intake or illnesses that can cause fluid or electrolyte imbalances (e.g., gastroenteritis, salt-wasting nephropathies, systemic

---

infection) and in those using loop diuretics or systemic or inhaled glucocorticoids. ■

• Nocdurna is contraindicated in patients with HF (NYHA Class II to IV), uncontrolled HTN, hyponatremia or a history of hyponatremia, polydipsia, primary nocturnal enuresis, renal impairment with an eGFR less than 50 mL/minute/1.73 m², and known or suspected SIADH secretion due to an increased risk of severe hyponatremia.

Boxed Warning Nocdurna can cause hyponatremia. Severe hyponatremia can be lifethreatening, leading to seizures, coma, respiratory arrest, or death. ■

• Use cautiously in patients with coronary artery insufficiency, hypertensive CV disease, and conditions linked to fluid and electrolyte imbalances, such as cystic fibrosis, because these patients are susceptible to hyponatremia.

• Use cautiously in patients at risk for water intoxication with hyponatremia.

Dialyzable drug: Unknown.

⚠ *Overdose S&S:* Confusion, drowsiness, continuing headache, problems passing urine, rapid weight gain due to fluid retention.

PREGNANCY-LACTATION-REPRODUCTION

• There are no adequate well-controlled studies during pregnancy. Use during pregnancy only if clearly needed.

• Drug appears in small amounts in human milk, and is poorly absorbed orally by infants. Use cautiously during breastfeeding.

• Drug isn't recommended for nocturia caused by normal physiologic changes that occur during pregnancy.

NURSING CONSIDERATIONS

• Before starting Nocdurna, evaluate patient for possible causes of nocturia, including excessive fluid intake before bedtime, and optimize the treatment of underlying conditions that may be contributing to nocturia. Confirm the diagnosis of nocturnal polyuria with a 24-hour urine collection, if one hasn't been obtained previously.

Boxed Warning Ensure serum sodium concentrations are normal before starting or resuming Nocdurna or increasing the dosage. Measure serum sodium level within 7 days and approximately 1 month after initiating therapy or increasing the dosage, and periodically during treatment. Monitor serum sodium level more frequently in patients age

65 and older and in patients at increased risk for hyponatremia. ■

Boxed Warning If hyponatremia occurs, Nocdurna may need to be temporarily or permanently discontinued. ■

• Morning and evening doses are adjusted separately for adequate diurnal rhythm of water turnover.

• Intranasal use can cause changes in the nasal mucosa, resulting in erratic, unreliable absorption. Report worsening condition to prescriber, who may recommend injectable DDAVP.

• Restrict fluid intake to reduce risk of water intoxication and sodium depletion, especially in children or older adults.

🕓 *Alert:* Overdose may cause oxytocic or vasopressor activity. Withhold drug and notify prescriber. If fluid retention is excessive, give furosemide.

• *Look alike–sound alike:* Don't confuse desmopressin with vasopressin.

PATIENT TEACHING

• Advise patient taking Nocdurna to moderate fluid intake in the evening and nighttime hours to decrease risk of hyponatremia and to avoid caffeine and alcohol before bedtime.

• Teach patient to immediately report signs or symptoms associated with hyponatremia (headache, nausea, vomiting, weight gain, restlessness, fatigue, lethargy, disorientation, depressed reflexes, loss of appetite, irritability, muscle weakness, muscle spasms or cramps, abnormal mental status, such as hallucinations, decreased consciousness, and confusion). Severe symptoms may include one or a combination of the following: seizure, coma, or respiratory arrest.

• Some patients may have trouble measuring and inhaling drug into nostrils. Teach patient and caregivers correct administration method.

• Instruct patient to clear nasal passages before giving drug.

• Instruct patient in safe drug administration.

• Advise patient to report nasal congestion, allergic rhinitis, or URI to prescriber; dosage adjustment may be needed.

• Warn patient to drink only enough water to satisfy thirst.

🖹 Inform patient with hemophilia A or von Willebrand disease that taking desmopressin may prevent hazards of using blood products.

• Advise patient to carry medical identification indicating use of drug.

desoximetasone
de-soks-i-MET-a-sone

Topicort

Therapeutic class: Corticosteroids
Pharmacologic class: Corticosteroids

AVAILABLE FORMS
Cream: 0.05%, 0.25%
Gel: 0.05%*
Ointment: 0.05%, 0.25%
Spray: 0.25%

INDICATIONS & DOSAGES
➤ **Inflammation and pruritus from corticosteroid-responsive dermatoses (except spray)**
Adults and children: Clean area; apply a thin film and rub in gently b.i.d. Don't use 0.25% ointment on children younger than age 10. If no improvement within 4 weeks, contact prescriber.
➤ **Plaque psoriasis (spray only)**
Adults: Apply a thin film to affected areas and rub in gently b.i.d. Treatment beyond 4 weeks isn't recommended.

ADMINISTRATION
Topical
• Gently wash skin before applying. To prevent skin damage, rub in gently, leaving thin coat. When treating hairy sites, part hair and apply directly to lesions.
• Avoid applying near eyes, mucous membranes, or in ear canal.
• Don't bandage, cover, or wrap treated skin area unless ordered; adverse reactions may occur more frequently.
• Stop drug and notify prescriber if skin infection, striae, or atrophy occurs.
• Discontinue therapy when control is achieved.
• Avoid using spray on face, axilla, or groin or if atrophy is present.
• Discard unused portion of the spray after 30 days.

ACTION
Diffuses across cell membranes to form complexes with receptors, showing anti-inflammatory, antipruritic, vasoconstrictive, and antiproliferative activity.

Route	Onset	Peak	Duration
Topical	Unknown	Unknown	Unknown

Half-life: 13 to 17 hours (urine).

ADVERSE REACTIONS
Skin: burning, pruritus, irritation, dryness, erythema, folliculitis, hypertrichosis, acneiform eruptions, perioral dermatitis, hypopigmentation, allergic contact dermatitis, maceration, secondary infection, atrophy, striae, miliaria. **Other:** *HPA axis suppression,* Cushing syndrome.

INTERACTIONS
None significant.

EFFECTS ON LAB TEST RESULTS
• May increase glucose level.

CONTRAINDICATIONS & CAUTIONS
• Contraindicated in patients hypersensitive to drug or its components.
• Don't use as monotherapy in primary bacterial infections (impetigo, paronychia, erysipelas, cellulitis, angular cheilitis), treatment of rosacea, perioral dermatitis, or acne.
• Don't use very-high-potency or high-potency agents on the face, groin, or axillae.
• Don't use spray if atrophy is present at treatment site.
• Drug isn't for ophthalmic use.
• Use cautiously in children. Spray isn't recommended for use in children.
Dialyzable drug: Unknown.
⚠ *Overdose S&S:* Systemic effects.

PREGNANCY-LACTATION-REPRODUCTION
• There are no adequate well-controlled studies during pregnancy. Use during pregnancy only if potential benefit justifies fetal risk.
• Don't use extensively, in large amounts, or for prolonged periods during pregnancy.
• It isn't known if topical corticosteroids are sufficiently absorbed systemically to produce detectable quantities in human milk. Use cautiously during breastfeeding. If used during breastfeeding, don't apply on the chest, to avoid accidental ingestion by the infant.

NURSING CONSIDERATIONS
• If fever develops and occlusive dressing is in place, notify prescriber and remove occlusive dressing.

Reactions in bold italics are *life-threatening*. Interactions may have a *rapid onset* or a ***delayed onset***.

D

- If antifungal or antibiotic combined with corticosteroid fails to provide prompt improvement, stop corticosteroid until infection is controlled.
- Systemic absorption is likely with use of occlusive dressings, prolonged treatment, or extensive body surface treatment. Watch for symptoms of HPA axis suppression, Cushing syndrome, hyperglycemia, and glycosuria.
- Avoid using plastic pants or tight-fitting diapers on treated areas in young children. Children may absorb larger amounts of drug and be more susceptible to systemic toxicity.
- Gel contains alcohol and may cause burning or irritation in open lesions.
- *Look alike–sound alike:* Don't confuse desoximetasone with dexamethasone.

PATIENT TEACHING
- Teach patient how to apply drug and to report all adverse reactions.
- Tell patient this drug is for external use only and to avoid contact with the eyes.
- If an occlusive dressing is ordered, advise patient to leave it in place for no longer than 12 hours each day and not to use the dressing on infected or weeping lesions.
- Tell patient to stop drug and report signs of systemic absorption, skin irritation or ulceration, hypersensitivity, or infection.
- Inform patient that spray is flammable and to keep away from heat, flame, or smoke while applying.

desvenlafaxine succinate
des-ven-la-FAX-in

Pristiq✐

Therapeutic class: Antidepressants
Pharmacologic class: SSNRIs

AVAILABLE FORMS
Tablets (extended-release) ⓄⓃⒸ: 25 mg, 50 mg, 100 mg

INDICATIONS & DOSAGES
Adjust-a-dose (for all indications): For patients with CrCl of 30 to 50 mL/minute, give maximum of 50 mg PO once daily. For patients with CrCl of less than 30 mL/minute or ESRD, give 25 mg PO daily or 50 mg PO every other day. Don't give supplemental doses after dialysis. For patients with moderate to severe hepatic impairment, give 50 mg PO daily; dosage escalation above 100 mg/day isn't recommended. Use 25-mg/day dose for gradual reduction when discontinuing treatment, to minimize discontinuation symptoms.

➤ **Major depressive disorder**
Adults: 50 mg PO once daily.

➤ **Vasomotor symptoms associated with menopause** ◆
Adults: Initially, 50 mg once daily. Titrate to 100 mg once daily; 150 mg once daily has also been studied and has been shown to be effective.

ADMINISTRATION
PO
- Administer at approximately the same time each day with or without food.
- Patient must swallow tablets whole with fluid and not divide, crush, chew, or dissolve them.

ACTION
Thought to potentiate serotonin and norepinephrine in the CNS through inhibition of their reuptake.

Route	Onset	Peak	Duration
PO	Unknown	Unknown	Unknown

Half-life: About 10 to 11 hours.

ADVERSE REACTIONS
CNS: abnormal dreams, anxiety, asthenia, dizziness, fatigue, jittery feeling, headache, insomnia, paresthesia, somnolence, tremor, disturbance in attention, nervousness. **CV:** increased BP, hot flashes, HTN, palpitations, tachycardia. **EENT:** blurred vision, mydriasis, tinnitus, vertigo, dry mouth. **GI:** constipation, diarrhea, dysgeusia, nausea, vomiting. **GU:** proteinuria, sexual dysfunction. **Metabolic:** decreased appetite, weight loss, hyperlipidemia. **Skin:** hyperhidrosis, rash. **Other:** chills, yawning.

INTERACTIONS
Drug-drug. *Amphetamines, buspirone, fentanyl, lithium, SSNRIs, SSRIs, TCAs, tramadol, triptans, tryptophan:* May increase risk of serotonin syndrome. Monitor patient closely if used together.
Aspirin, NSAIDs, warfarin, other drugs that affect coagulation: May increase risk of bleeding. Use together cautiously.

🍁Canada ◇OTC ◆Off-label use ✐Photoguide ⓄⓃⒸDo not crush *Liquid contains alcohol ▧Genetic

CNS drugs: Drug may cause additive CNS effects. Avoid using together.

CYP3A4 inhibitors (ketoconazole): May increase desvenlafaxine levels. Use together cautiously.

Desipramine, metoprolol, other drugs metabolized by CYP2D6: May increase levels of these drugs. Use together cautiously.

Linezolid, methylene blue: Increases risk of serotonin syndrome. Use together is contraindicated. If urgent treatment with either of these drugs is needed, stop desvenlafaxine immediately; then administer linezolid or methylene blue. Watch for signs and symptoms of serotonin syndrome for 7 days or until 24 hours after last dose of linezolid or methylene blue. Restart desvenlafaxine 24 hours after last dose of linezolid or methylene blue.

MAO inhibitors: May cause serotonin syndrome or signs and symptoms resembling NMS. Allow at least 14 days between discontinuation of an MAO inhibitor and starting desvenlafaxine, and 7 days after stopping desvenlafaxine before starting an MAO inhibitor.

Venlafaxine: Drug is a major active metabolite of venlafaxine. Avoid using together.

Drug-lifestyle. *Alcohol use:* May enhance CNS depression. Discourage use together.

EFFECTS ON LAB TEST RESULTS

• May increase total cholesterol, LDL, and triglyceride levels.
• May decrease sodium level.
• May cause false-positive test for phencyclidine and amphetamines.

CONTRAINDICATIONS & CAUTIONS

• Contraindicated in patients hypersensitive to drug.

🖐 *Alert:* Concomitant use with linezolid or methylene blue can cause serotonin syndrome (fever, mental status changes, muscle twitching, diaphoresis, shivering or shaking, diarrhea, loss of coordination). Use with linezolid or methylene blue is contraindicated.

• Potentially life-threatening serotonin syndrome has been reported with desvenlafaxine alone, but particularly with concomitant use of other serotonergic drugs and with drugs that impair serotonin metabolism.

• Use cautiously in older adults and in patients with renal impairment, diseases or conditions that could affect hemodynamic responses or metabolism, and in those with a history of mania or seizures.

• Drug may increase risk of bleeding events ranging from bruising, hematoma, epistaxis, and petechiae to life-threatening hemorrhage.

• Angle-closure glaucoma has occurred in patients with untreated anatomically narrow angles who have taken antidepressants.

Boxed Warning Desvenlafaxine isn't approved for use in children. ∎

Dialyzable drug: No.

⚠ *Overdose S&S:* Headache, vomiting, agitation, dizziness, nausea, constipation, diarrhea, dry mouth, paresthesia, tachycardia, change in level of consciousness, mydriasis, seizures, ECG changes.

PREGNANCY-LACTATION-REPRODUCTION

• There are no adequate well-controlled studies during pregnancy. Use during pregnancy only if clearly needed and potential benefit justifies fetal risk.

• Drug appears in human milk. Patient should discontinue breastfeeding or discontinue drug, taking into account importance of drug to the patient.

• Health care providers are encouraged to register patients in the National Pregnancy Registry for Antidepressants, which monitors pregnancy outcomes in patients exposed to antidepressants during pregnancy (1-844-405-6185).

NURSING CONSIDERATIONS

Boxed Warning Closely monitor all patients being treated for depression for signs and symptoms of clinical worsening and suicidality, especially at the beginning of therapy and with dosage adjustments. Symptoms may include agitation, insomnia, anxiety, aggressiveness, or panic attacks. ∎

• Carefully monitor BP. Drug may cause dose-related increases in BP.

• Monitor IOP in patients at risk for angle-closure glaucoma.

• Record mood changes. Monitor patient for suicidality and allow patient only a minimal supply of the drug.

• Monitor patient for signs and symptoms of bleeding.

• Monitor lipid and sodium levels before and during therapy.

- Hyponatremia can occur with desvenlafaxine use. Consider stopping drug in patients with symptomatic hyponatremia; institute appropriate medical intervention.
- ⓘ *Alert:* Don't stop drug abruptly. Withdrawal or discontinuation syndrome may occur if drug is stopped abruptly. Signs and symptoms of withdrawal syndrome include dizziness, nausea, headache, irritability, insomnia, diarrhea, anxiety, fatigue, abnormal dreams, and hyperhidrosis. Taper drug slowly.
- Monitor respiratory status. Drug may cause ILD or eosinophilic pneumonia. If patient develops dyspnea, cough, or chest discomfort, discontinue drug.
- Monitor patient for signs and symptoms of serotonin syndrome, including mental status changes, autonomic instability, neuromuscular symptoms, seizures, and GI symptoms.

PATIENT TEACHING

Boxed Warning Warn family members to closely monitor patient for signs and symptoms of worsening condition or suicidality. ∎

ⓘ *Alert:* Teach patient to recognize and immediately report symptoms of serotonin toxicity (fever, mental status changes, muscle twitching, diaphoresis, shivering or shaking, diarrhea, loss of coordination).

- Instruct patient in safe drug administration.
- Tell patient to avoid alcohol and to consult prescriber before taking other prescription or OTC drugs.
- If drug is to be stopped, tell patient to stop drug gradually by tapering dosage as instructed by prescriber and not to abruptly stop taking drug.
- Teach patient to report all adverse reactions, including abnormal bleeding.
- Warn patient to avoid hazardous activities that require alertness and good coordination until effects of drug are known.
- Advise patient of childbearing potential to inform prescriber if pregnant or breastfeeding or if planning to become pregnant.

dexamethasone (oral)
dex-a-METH-a-sone

Dexamethasone Intensol*, Hemady

dexamethasone sodium phosphate injection

Therapeutic class: Corticosteroids
Pharmacologic class: Glucocorticoids

AVAILABLE FORMS
dexamethasone
Elixir: 0.5 mg/5 mL*
Oral concentrate: 1 mg/mL*
Oral solution: 0.5 mg/5 mL
Tablets: 0.5 mg, 0.75 mg, 1 mg, 1.5 mg, 2 mg, 4 mg, 6 mg, 20 mg
dexamethasone sodium phosphate
Injection: 4-mg/mL, 10-mg/mL vials and prefilled syringes

INDICATIONS & DOSAGES
➤ **Cerebral edema**
Adults: Initially, 10 mg phosphate IV; then 4 mg IM every 6 hours until symptoms subside (usually 2 to 4 days); then taper over 5 to 7 days. Oral therapy (1 to 3 mg t.i.d.) should replace IM dosing as soon as possible.
➤ **Palliative management of recurrent or inoperable brain tumors**
Adults: 2 mg PO, IM, or IV b.i.d. to t.i.d. for maintenance therapy.
➤ **Inflammatory conditions, neoplasias**
Adults: 0.75 to 9 mg/day PO or 0.5 to 9 mg/day phosphate IM or IV, depending on size and location of affected area.
➤ **Acute, self-limited allergic disorders; acute exacerbations of chronic allergic disorders**
Adults: On day one, give 4 or 8 mg IM (using 4 mg/mL preparation). On days two and three, give four 0.75-mg tablets PO in two divided doses. On day four, give two 0.75-mg tablets PO in two divided doses. On days five and six, give one 0.75-mg tablet PO. A follow-up visit should take place on day eight.
➤ **Shock**
Adults: 1 to 6 mg/kg phosphate IV as single dose. Or, 40 mg phosphate IV every 2 to 6 hours, as needed, while shock persists.
➤ **Dexamethasone suppression test for Cushing syndrome**

Adults: Determine baseline 24-hour urine levels of 17-hydroxycorticosteroids; then, give 0.5 mg PO every 6 hours for 48 hours. Repeat 24-hour urine collection to determine 17-hydroxycorticosteroid excretion during second 24 hours of dexamethasone administration. Or, 1 mg PO as single dose at 11:00 p.m. with determination of plasma cortisol at 8 a.m. the next morning.

➤ **Adrenocortical insufficiency**
Children: 0.02 to 0.3 mg/kg/day or 0.6 to 9 mg/m²/day PO in three or four divided doses.

➤ **Acute exacerbation of MS**
Adults: 30 mg PO daily for 1 week, followed by 4 to 12 mg every other day for 1 month.

➤ **Adjunctive therapy for short-term administration in synovitis of osteoarthritis, RA, bursitis, acute gouty arthritis, epicondylitis, acute nonspecific tenosynovitis, posttraumatic osteoarthritis; lesions (keloids; localized, hypertrophic, infiltrated, inflammatory lesions of lichen planus, psoriatic plaques, granuloma annulare, or lichen simplex chronicus; discoid lupus erythematosus; necrobiosis lipoidica diabeticorum; alopecia areata; cystic tumors of an aponeurosis or tendon [ganglia])**
Adults: 0.2 to 6 mg intra-articular or intralesional injection ranging from one single injection to injection every 3 to 5 days to once every 2 to 3 weeks. Dosage and frequency of injection vary depending on condition and site of injection.

➤ **Multiple myeloma, in combination with other antimyeloma products (Hemady only)**
Adults: 20 or 40 mg PO once daily on specific days depending on treatment regimen. Refer to prescribing information of the other antimyeloma products used in combination for specific dosing.
Adjust-a-dose: Reduce dosage in older adults because of increased toxicity.

ADMINISTRATION
PO
• Give oral dose with food when possible. Patient may need measures to prevent GI irritation.
• Only give concentrated oral solution using calibrated dropper supplied with product. Discard opened bottle after 90 days.

• Mix concentrated oral solution with liquid or semisolid food, such as water, juices, soda or sodalike beverages, applesauce, and puddings. Have patient consume immediately.

IV
▼ For direct injection, inject undiluted over at least 1 minute (doses 10 mg or less).
▼ For intermittent or continuous infusion, dilute solution according to manufacturer's instructions and give over prescribed duration.
▼ During continuous infusion, change solution every 24 hours.
▼ **Incompatibilities:** Ciprofloxacin, diphenhydramine, doxapram, glycopyrrolate, idarubicin, midazolam, vancomycin.

IM
• Give IM injection deep into gluteal muscle. Rotate injection sites to prevent muscle atrophy. Avoid subcut injection because atrophy and sterile abscesses may occur.

Intra-articular, intralesional
• Frequent intra-articular injection may damage joint tissues.
• Use when affected joints or areas are limited to one or two sites.

ACTION
Decreases inflammation, mainly by stabilizing leukocyte lysosomal membranes; suppresses immune response; stimulates bone marrow; and influences protein, fat, and carbohydrate metabolism.

Route	Onset	Peak	Duration
PO	1–2 hr	1–2 hr	2.5 days
IV	1 hr	1 hr	Variable
IM	1 hr	1 hr	6 days
Intra-articular, intralesional	Unknown	Unknown	Unknown

Half-life: PO, 3 to 5 hours; IV, 1 to 5 hours (adults), 2 to 9.5 hours (children).

ADVERSE REACTIONS
CNS: euphoria, insomnia, psychotic behavior, *pseudotumor cerebri,* vertigo, headache, paresthesia, *seizures,* depression. **CV:** *HF,* HTN, edema, *arrhythmias,* thrombophlebitis, *thromboembolism.* **EENT:** cataracts, glaucoma, increase IOP. **GI:** peptic ulceration, abdominal distention, GI irritation, increased appetite, *pancreatitis,* nausea, vomiting. **GU:** menstrual irregularities, increased urine glucose and calcium levels. **Metabolic:**

---

hypokalemia, alkalosis, hyperglycemia, carbohydrate intolerance, hypercholesterolemia, *hypocalcemia,* sodium retention, fluid retention, weight gain. **Musculoskeletal:** growth suppression in children, muscle weakness, loss of muscle mass, osteoporosis, vertebral compression fracture, aseptic necrosis of femoral and humeral heads, pathologic long bone fracture, tendon rupture, myopathy. **Skin:** hirsutism, delayed wound healing, acne, various skin eruptions, atrophy at IM injection site, thin fragile skin, increased or decreased pigmentation, facial erythema, diaphoresis, petechiae, ecchymosis. **Other:** cushingoid state, susceptibility to infections, acute adrenal insufficiency after increased stress or abrupt withdrawal after long-term therapy, *angioedema.* **After abrupt withdrawal:** rebound inflammation, fatigue, weakness, arthralgia, fever, dizziness, lethargy, fainting, orthostatic hypotension, dyspnea, anorexia, *hypoglycemia. After prolonged use, sudden withdrawal may be fatal.*

INTERACTIONS

Drug-drug. *Antidiabetics, including insulin:* May decrease response. May need dosage adjustment.

Aspirin, indomethacin, other NSAIDs: May increase risk of GI distress and bleeding. Use together cautiously.

Cardiac glycosides: May increase risk of arrhythmia resulting from hypokalemia. May need dosage adjustment.

Cyclosporine: May increase toxicity. Monitor patient closely.

CYP3A4 inducers (barbiturates, carbamazepine, phenytoin, rifampin): May decrease corticosteroid effect. Increase corticosteroid dosage.

CYP3A4 inhibitors (clarithromycin, ketoconazole, itraconazole): May decrease metabolism of dexamethasone and increase risk of corticosteroid-related adverse effects. Consider therapy modification.

Oral anticoagulants: May alter dosage requirements. Monitor PT and INR closely.

Potassium-depleting drugs such as thiazide diuretics: May enhance potassium-wasting effects of dexamethasone. Monitor potassium level.

Salicylates: May decrease salicylate level. Monitor patient for lack of salicylate effectiveness.

Skin-test antigens: May decrease response. Postpone skin testing until therapy is completed.

Toxoids, vaccines: May decrease antibody response and may increase risk of neurologic complications. Avoid using together.

Drug-herb. *Echinacea:* May reduce drug's therapeutic effects. Don't use together.

Drug-lifestyle. *Alcohol use:* May increase risk of gastric irritation and GI ulceration. Discourage use together.

EFFECTS ON LAB TEST RESULTS

• May increase cholesterol and glucose levels. May decrease calcium, potassium, T_3, and T_4 levels.

• May decrease ^{131}I uptake and protein-bound iodine levels in thyroid function tests.

• May cause false-negative results in nitro blue tetrazolium test for systemic bacterial infections. May alter reactions to skin tests.

CONTRAINDICATIONS & CAUTIONS

• Contraindicated in patients hypersensitive to drug or its ingredients, in those with systemic fungal infections, and in those receiving immunosuppressive doses together with live-virus vaccines. IM administration is contraindicated in patients with ITP.

• Use cautiously in patients with recent MI.

• Use cautiously in patients with GI ulcer, renal disease, HTN, osteoporosis, diabetes, hypothyroidism, cirrhosis, diverticulitis, nonspecific ulcerative colitis, recent intestinal anastomoses, thromboembolic disorders, seizures, myasthenia gravis, HF, TB, active hepatitis, ocular HSV infection, emotional instability, or psychotic tendencies.

• Because some forms contain sulfite preservatives, also use cautiously in patients sensitive to sulfites.

Dialyzable drug: No.

PREGNANCY-LACTATION-REPRODUCTION

• Dexamethasone crosses the placental barrier. Use during pregnancy only if potential benefit justifies fetal risk. When systemic corticosteroids are needed during pregnancy, it's generally recommended to use lowest effective dose for shortest duration of time, avoiding high doses during first trimester.

• When giving in combination for multiple myeloma (20-mg tablet), use is contraindicated. Obtain pregnancy test before start of therapy. Patients of reproductive potential

should use effective contraception during treatment and for 1 month after final dose.
• Drug appears in human milk. Patients shouldn't breastfeed during treatment and for 2 weeks after final dose or should discontinue drug, taking into account importance of drug to the patient.
• Steroids can increase or decrease motility and number of spermatozoa in some males.

NURSING CONSIDERATIONS
⚠ *Alert:* Epidural corticosteroid injections to treat neck and back pain and radiating pain in the arms and legs may result in rare but serious adverse events (vision loss, stroke, paralysis, death). The use of epidural corticosteroid injections isn't approved by the FDA.
• Most adverse reactions to corticosteroids are dose- or duration-dependent.
• For better results and less toxicity, give once-daily dose in morning.
• Always adjust to lowest effective dose.
• Monitor patient's weight, BP, and electrolyte levels.
• Monitor patient for cushingoid effects, including moon face, buffalo hump, central obesity, thinning hair, HTN, and increased susceptibility to infection.
• Watch for depression or psychotic episodes, especially in high-dose therapy.
• Patient with diabetes may need increased insulin; monitor glucose levels.
• Drug may mask or worsen infections, including latent amebiasis.
• Older adults may be more susceptible to osteoporosis with long-term use.
• Inspect patient's skin for petechiae.
• Gradually reduce dosage after long-term therapy.
• *Look alike–sound alike:* Don't confuse dexamethasone with desoximetasone.

PATIENT TEACHING
• Instruct patient to take drug with food or milk.
⚠ *Alert:* Counsel patient to discuss benefits, risks, and other possible treatments with provider before undergoing epidural corticosteroid injection and to seek immediate medical attention for loss of vision or vision changes; tingling in the arms or legs; sudden weakness or numbness of the face, arm, or leg on one or both sides of the body; dizziness; severe headache; or seizures.

• Tell patient not to stop drug abruptly or without prescriber's consent.
• Teach patient signs and symptoms of early adrenal insufficiency: fatigue, muscle weakness, joint pain, fever, anorexia, nausea, shortness of breath, dizziness, and fainting.
• Instruct patient to carry medical identification indicating the need for supplemental systemic glucocorticoids during stress, especially when dosage is decreased. This card should contain prescriber's name, drug name, and drug dosage.
• Warn patient on long-term therapy about cushingoid effects (moon face, buffalo hump) and the need to notify prescriber about sudden weight gain or swelling.
• Warn patient about easy bruising.
• Advise patient receiving long-term therapy to consider exercise or physical therapy. Tell patient to ask prescriber about vitamin D or calcium supplement.
• Instruct patient receiving long-term therapy to have periodic eye exams.
• Advise patient to avoid exposure to infections (such as measles and chickenpox) and to notify prescriber if such exposure occurs.
• Tell patient to avoid alcohol.
• Advise patient of reproductive potential who is taking Hemady to use effective contraception during treatment and for at least 1 month after final dose.

dexmethylphenidate hydrochloride
dex-meth-il-FEN-i-date

Focalin, Focalin XR✒

Therapeutic class: CNS stimulants
Pharmacologic class: Methylphenidate derivatives
Controlled substance schedule: II

AVAILABLE FORMS
Capsules (extended-release) ⓘ: 5 mg, 10 mg, 15 mg, 20 mg, 25 mg, 30 mg, 35 mg, 40 mg
Tablets: 2.5 mg, 5 mg, 10 mg

INDICATIONS & DOSAGES
➤ **ADHD**
Immediate-release tablets
Adults and children age 6 and older:
For patients who aren't currently taking

methylphenidate, initially, 2.5 mg PO b.i.d., given at least 4 hours apart. Increase weekly by 2.5 to 5 mg daily, up to a maximum of 20 mg daily in divided doses.

For patients who are currently taking methylphenidate, initially give half the current methylphenidate dosage, up to a maximum of 20 mg PO daily in divided doses at least 4 hours apart.

Extended-release capsules
Adults: For patients who aren't currently taking dexmethylphenidate or methylphenidate, or who are on stimulants other than methylphenidate, give 10 mg PO once daily in the morning. May adjust in weekly increments of 10 mg to a maximum dose of 40 mg daily.

For patients who are currently taking methylphenidate, initially give half the total daily dose of methylphenidate. Patients who are currently taking the immediate-release form of dexmethylphenidate may be switched to the same daily dose of extended-release form. Maximum daily dose is 40 mg.
Children age 6 and older: For patients who aren't currently taking dexmethylphenidate or methylphenidate, or who are on stimulants other than methylphenidate, give 5 mg PO daily in the morning. May adjust in weekly increments of 5 mg to a maximum daily dose of 30 mg.

For patients who are currently taking methylphenidate, initially give half the total daily dose of methylphenidate. Patients who are currently taking the immediate-release form of dexmethylphenidate may be switched to the same daily dose of extended-release form. Maximum daily dose is 30 mg.

ADMINISTRATION
PO
• Patient may swallow capsules whole with or without food or may sprinkle contents on a small amount of applesauce and eat immediately without chewing.
• Don't crush or divide the capsule or its contents.
• Separate tablet twice-daily dosing by at least 4 hours.

ACTION
Blocks presynaptic reuptake of norepinephrine and dopamine and increases their release, increasing concentration in the synapse.

Route	Onset	Peak	Duration
PO (immediate-release)	Unknown	1–1.5 hr	Unknown
PO (extended-release)	Unknown	1–4 hr; 4.5–7 hr	Unknown

Half-life: Extended-release, about 3 hours (adults), 2 to 3 hours (children); immediate-release, 2.2 hours.

ADVERSE REACTIONS
CNS: headache, anxiety, feeling jittery, insomnia, fever, dizziness, mood swings, depression, irritability. **CV:** tachycardia. **EENT:** nasal congestion, pharyngolaryngeal pain, dry mouth. **GI:** anorexia, abdominal pain, nausea, dyspepsia, vomiting. **Musculoskeletal:** twitching (motor or vocal tics). **Skin:** pruritus. **Other:** hypersensitivity reactions.

INTERACTIONS
Drug-drug. *Antacids, acid suppressants:* May alter the release of extended-release form. Avoid using together.
Anticoagulants, phenobarbital, phenytoin, primidone, TCAs: May inhibit metabolism of these drugs. May need to decrease dosage of these drugs; monitor drug levels.
Antihypertensives (ACE inhibitors, ARBs, beta blockers, calcium channel blockers, centrally acting alpha-2 receptor agonists, potassium-sparing and thiazide diuretics): May decrease effectiveness of these drugs. Use together cautiously; monitor BP.
Halogenated anesthetics (halothane, isoflurane): May increase risk of sudden BP and HR increase during surgery. Avoid dexmethylphenidate in patients being treated with anesthetics on day of surgery.
MAO inhibitors (isocarboxazid, linezolid, methylene blue, selegiline): May increase risk of hypertensive crisis. Using together within 14 days of MAO inhibitor therapy is contraindicated.
Risperidone: May increase risk of extrapyramidal symptoms with dosage change of either agent. Monitor patient closely.

EFFECTS ON LAB TEST RESULTS
None reported.

CONTRAINDICATIONS & CAUTIONS
• Contraindicated in patients hypersensitive to methylphenidate or other components.
⚠ *Alert:* Avoid use in patients with known serious structural cardiac abnormalities,

---

♣Canada ◇OTC ♦Off-label use ✐Photoguide ⬤Do not crush *Liquid contains alcohol ⬚Genetic cardiomyopathy, serious heart rhythm abnormalities, CAD, and other serious heart problems. Sudden death, stroke, and MI have been reported.

Boxed Warning Use cautiously in patients with a history of substance abuse, including alcoholism. Chronic abuse can lead to marked tolerance and psychological dependence. Psychotic episodes can occur. Withdraw patient carefully from abusive use because severe depression can occur. Withdrawal after long-term use may unmask signs and symptoms of an underlying disorder that may require follow-up. ∎

- Use cautiously in patients with a psychiatric illness, bipolar disorder, depression, or family history of suicide, and in patients with seizures, HTN, hyperthyroidism, HF, stroke, or recent MI.
- Rare cases of priapism have been reported.
Dialyzable drug: Unknown.

⚠ *Overdose S&S:* Agitation, cardiac arrhythmias, confusion, seizures, delirium, dryness of mucous membranes, euphoria, flushing, hallucinations, headache, hyperpyrexia, hyperreflexia, HTN, muscle twitching, mydriasis, palpitations, diaphoresis, tachycardia, tremors, vomiting.

PREGNANCY-LACTATION-REPRODUCTION
- There are no adequate well-controlled studies during pregnancy. Use during pregnancy only if clearly needed and potential benefit justifies potential risk to the fetus.
- It isn't known if drug appears in human milk. Use cautiously during breastfeeding.

NURSING CONSIDERATIONS
- Diagnosis of ADHD must be based on complete history and evaluation of patient by psychological and educational experts.
- Obtain a detailed patient history, including a family history for mental disorders, family suicide, ventricular arrhythmias, or sudden death.
- Refer patient for psychological, educational, and social support.
- Periodically reevaluate the long-term usefulness of the drug.
- Monitor CBC and differential and platelet counts during prolonged therapy.
- Don't use for severe depression or normal fatigue states.
- Stop treatment or reduce dosage if symptoms worsen or adverse reactions occur.

- Long-term stimulant use may temporarily suppress growth. Monitor children for growth and weight gain. If growth slows or weight gain is lower than expected, stop drug.
- ⊕ *Alert:* Periodically monitor patient for changes in HR or BP. Promptly evaluate patients with chest pain, unexplained syncope, or other signs or symptoms of cardiac disease.
- Monitor patient for signs of drug dependence or abuse.
- If seizures occur, stop drug.
- Monitor patient for digital changes during therapy. Drug is associated with peripheral vasculopathy, including Raynaud phenomenon.
- *Look alike–sound alike:* Don't confuse dexmethylphenidate with methadone, methylphenidate, or dextroamphetamine.

PATIENT TEACHING
- Stress the importance of taking the correct dose of drug at the same time every day. Report accidental overdose immediately.
- ⊕ *Alert:* Warn patient that misuse of amphetamines can have serious effects, including sudden death.
- Instruct patient in safe drug administration.
- Advise parents to monitor child for medication abuse or sharing. Also inform parents to watch for increased aggression or hostility and to report worsening behavior.
- ⊕ *Alert:* Instruct patient to immediately report chest pain, shortness of breath, or fainting.
- Warn patient to seek immediate medical attention for prolonged or painful erections.
- Instruct parents to monitor child's height and weight and to tell prescriber if they suspect growth is slowing.
- Advise patient or caregivers to report new numbness, pain, skin color change, or sensitivity to temperature in fingers or toes, because of the risk of peripheral vasculopathy, including Raynaud phenomenon.
- Caution patient that blurred vision or difficulty with accommodation may occur and to exercise caution while performing activities that require a clear visual field. Advise patient to report blurred vision to prescriber.

Reactions in bold italics are *life-threatening*. Interactions may have a *rapid onset* or a *delayed onset*.

dextroamphetamine
dex-troe-am-FET-a-meen

Xelstrym

dextroamphetamine sulfate
Dexedrine, ProCentra, Zenzedi

Therapeutic class: CNS stimulants
Pharmacologic class: Amphetamines
Controlled substance schedule: II

AVAILABLE FORMS
Capsules (extended-release) ⓓⓝⓖ: 5 mg,
10 mg, 15 mg
Oral solution: 5 mg/5 mL
Tablets: 2.5 mg, 5 mg, 7.5 mg, 10 mg, 15 mg,
20 mg, 30 mg
Transdermal system: 4.5 mg/9 hours, 9 mg/
9 hours, 13.5 mg/9 hours, 18 mg/9 hours

INDICATIONS & DOSAGES
➤ **Narcolepsy**
Adults: 5 to 60 mg PO daily in divided doses.
Children age 12 and older: 10 mg PO daily.
Increase by 10 mg at weekly intervals until
optimal response is obtained. Give first dose
on awakening; give additional doses (one or
two) at intervals of 4 to 6 hours.
Children ages 6 to 12: 5 mg PO daily. Increase by 5 mg at weekly intervals as needed
until optimal response is obtained. Give first
dose on awakening; give additional doses
(one or two) at intervals of 4 to 6 hours.
➤ **ADHD**
Adults: Initially, 9 mg/9 hours transdermal
system daily. May titrate to maximum dose of
18 mg/9 hours.
Children age 6 and older: 5 mg PO once daily
or b.i.d. Increase by 5 mg at weekly intervals
until optimal response is obtained. It's rarely
necessary to exceed 40 mg/day. Or, initially,
4.5 mg/9 hours transdermal system daily.
Titrate weekly by 4.5 mg up to maximum recommended dose of 18 mg/9 hours.
Children ages 3 to 5: Initially, 2.5 mg
immediate-release tablets or solution PO
daily. May increase daily dosage in increments of 2.5 mg at weekly intervals until optimal response is obtained.
Adjust-a-dose: If severe renal impairment
(GFR of 15 to less than 30 mL/minute/
1.73 m^2), maximum transdermal dose is

13.5 mg/9 hours. If ESRD, maximum transdermal dose is 9 mg/9 hours.

ADMINISTRATION
PO
• Avoid late-evening doses, particularly with
extended-release capsules, due to resulting
insomnia. Give initial dose upon awakening.
• Some formulations may contain tartrazine
(immediate-release tablets) or benzoic acid,
which is a derivative of benzyl alcohol (oral
solution). Derivatives of benzyl alcohol are
associated with potentially fatal gasping syndrome in neonates.
• Make sure patient doesn't chew or crush
extended-release capsules.
Transdermal
• Apply to clean, dry, intact skin of hip, upper
arm, chest, upper back, or flank.
• Select different application site each time a
new system is applied.
• Apply system 2 hours before an effect is
needed; remove within 9 hours after application.
• Don't touch adhesive side of system to
avoid absorption of drug.
• If adhesive is touched, wash hands with
soap and water immediately. If system comes
off, apply new system; don't reapply with
dressing, tape, or other common adhesive.
• Avoid exposing application site to direct external heat source, such as hair dryer, heating
pad, electric blanket, or heated water bed; heat
increases both rate and extent of absorption.
• After removing system, fold so that adhesive adheres to itself and place in a lidded
container. Don't flush down the toilet.
• Don't substitute for other amphetamine
products on a mg-per-mg basis because of
differing pharmacokinetics.

ACTION
Promotes release of dopamine and norepinephrine from nerve terminals in the brain
and, to a lesser extent, the reuptake of catecholamines.

Route	Onset	Peak	Duration
PO	Unknown	3 hr	4–6 hr
PO (extended-release)	Unknown	8 hr	8 hr
Transdermal	Unknown	9 hr	Unknown

Half-life: PO, 10 to 12 hours; transdermal, 6.4 to
11.5 hours.

ADVERSE REACTIONS

CNS: insomnia, nervousness, restlessness, tremor, dizziness, headache, chills, overstimulation, dysphoria, euphoria, dyskinesia, aggressive behavior, taste perversion, fatigue, irritability, labile affect. **CV:** tachycardia, palpitations, *arrhythmias,* elevated BP. **EENT:** blurred vision, dry mouth. **GI:** diarrhea, constipation, anorexia, other GI disturbances, abdominal pain, nausea, vomiting. **GU:** erectile dysfunction. **Hematologic:** *neutropenia, leukopenia.* **Metabolic:** weight loss. **Musculoskeletal:** exacerbation of motor and phonic tics, *rhabdomyolysis.* **Skin:** urticaria, alopecia, application-site reaction (pain, pruritus, burning, erythema, edema). **Other:** changes in libido, slowed growth rate.

INTERACTIONS

Drug-drug. *Acetazolamide, alkalizing drugs, antacids, sodium bicarbonate:* May increase renal reabsorption. Monitor patient for enhanced amphetamine effects.

Acidifying drugs, ammonium chloride, ascorbic acid: May decrease level and increase renal clearance of dextroamphetamine. Monitor patient for decreased amphetamine effects.

Adrenergic blockers: May inhibit adrenergic blocking effects. Avoid using together.

Antihypertensives: May diminish antihypertensive effects. Monitor BP.

Lithium: May inhibit central stimulant effects of amphetamines. Monitor therapy.

MAO inhibitors: May cause severe HTN or hypertensive crisis. Avoid using within 14 days of MAO inhibitor therapy.

Meperidine: May potentiate analgesic effect. Use together cautiously.

Methenamine: May increase urinary excretion of amphetamines and reduce effectiveness. Monitor drug effects.

Norepinephrine: May enhance adrenergic effect of norepinephrine. Monitor patient.

Phenobarbital, phenytoin: May delay absorption of these drugs. Monitor patient closely.

Serotonergic drugs (SSNRIs, SSRIs, TCAs, triptans): Increases risk of serotonin syndrome. Start dextroamphetamine at lower doses and monitor patient for signs and symptoms of serotonin syndrome, especially during initiation or dosage increases.

TCAs: May increase adverse amphetamine effects and potentiate CV effects. Monitor patient closely; adjust dosage or use alternative therapy.

Drug-food. *Acidic foods, fruit juice:* Decreases amphetamine absorption. May decrease effectiveness of oral solution. Avoid giving together.

EFFECTS ON LAB TEST RESULTS

• May increase corticosteroid levels.
• May interfere with urinary steroid determinations.

CONTRAINDICATIONS & CAUTIONS

• Contraindicated in patients hypersensitive to or with idiosyncratic reactions to sympathomimetic amines, in those hypersensitive to amphetamine, and in those with hyperthyroidism, moderate to severe HTN, symptomatic CV disease, glaucoma, advanced arteriosclerosis, and history of drug abuse.

🔵 *Alert:* Use cautiously in patients who are agitated and patients with motor tics, phonic tics, or Tourette syndrome. Also use cautiously in patients whose underlying condition may be worsened by an increase in BP or HR (preexisting HTN, HF, recent MI); patients with a psychiatric illness, bipolar disorder, depression, or family history of suicide; and those with a seizure disorder.

• Don't use in children or adolescents with structural cardiac abnormalities or other serious heart problems.

Dialyzable drug: Unknown.

⚠ *Overdose S&S:* Assaultiveness, confusion, hallucinations, hyperreflexia, rapid respiration, restlessness, rhabdomyolysis, tremor, hyperpyrexia, panic states, fatigue, depression, arrhythmias, HTN, hypotension, circulatory collapse, nausea, vomiting, diarrhea, abdominal cramps, seizures, coma.

PREGNANCY-LACTATION-REPRODUCTION

• There are no adequate well-controlled studies during pregnancy. Use during pregnancy only if potential benefit justifies fetal risk.

• Enroll patients in the National Pregnancy Registry for Psychiatric Medications (866-961-2388 or https://womensmentalhealth. org/research/pregnancyregistry/adhd-medications/).

• Infants born to patients dependent on amphetamines have an increased risk of premature delivery and low birth weight, and may experience signs and symptoms of

---

Reactions in bold italics are *life-threatening*. Interactions may have a *rapid onset* or a ***delayed onset***.

withdrawal, as demonstrated by dysphoria, including agitation and significant drowsiness.
• Drug appears in human milk. Use during breastfeeding isn't recommended.

NURSING CONSIDERATIONS
• Obtain a detailed patient history, including a family history for mental disorders, family suicide, ventricular arrhythmias, or sudden death.
• Monitor patients beginning treatment for ADHD for aggressive behavior or hostility.
• Drug shouldn't be used to prevent fatigue.

Boxed Warning Drug has a high abuse potential and may cause dependence. Monitor patient closely. Pay particular attention to the possibility of patients obtaining amphetamines for nontherapeutic use or distribution to others. ■
• Periodically monitor patient for changes in HR or BP.
• Monitor for growth retardation in children.
• *Look alike–sound alike:* Don't confuse Dexedrine with dextran or Excedrin.

PATIENT TEACHING
Boxed Warning Warn patient that the misuse of amphetamines can cause serious CV adverse events, including sudden death. ■
• Instruct patient in safe drug administration and disposal.
• ⚠ *Alert:* Instruct patient to immediately report chest pain, shortness of breath, or fainting.
• Warn patient to avoid activities that require alertness, a clear visual field, or good coordination until CNS effects of drug are known.
• Tell patient fatigue may occur as drug effects wear off.
• Ask patient to report signs and symptoms of excessive stimulation.
• Inform parents that children may show increased aggression or hostility and to report worsening of behavior.
• Warn patient with a seizure disorder that drug may decrease seizure threshold and to notify prescriber if seizures occur.

---

dextroamphetamine sulfate–dextroamphetamine saccharate–amphetamine aspartate–amphetamine sulfate
dex-tro-am-PHET-ta-meen/
am-PHET-ta-meen

Adderall, Adderall XR, Mydayis

Therapeutic class: CNS stimulants
Pharmacologic class: Amphetamines
Controlled substance schedule: II

AVAILABLE FORMS
Capsules (extended-release) ⓓⓝⓒ: 5 mg, 10 mg, 12.5 mg, 15 mg, 20 mg 25 mg, 30 mg, 37.5 mg, 50 mg
Tablets: 5 mg, 7.5 mg, 10 mg, 12.5 mg, 15 mg, 20 mg, 30 mg

INDICATIONS & DOSAGES
➤ **Narcolepsy**
Adults and children age 12 and older: Initially, 10 mg (immediate-release) tablet PO daily. May increase daily dose by 10 mg at weekly intervals to maximum of 60 mg/day. Give in one to three divided doses per day.
Children ages 6 to younger than 12: Initially, 5 mg (immediate-release) tablet PO daily. May increase daily dose by 5 mg at weekly intervals until optimal response is achieved. Give in one to three divided doses per day.
Adjust-a-dose: For adverse reactions (insomnia or anorexia), reduce dosage.

➤ **ADHD**
Adults: Initially, 5 mg (immediate-release) tablet PO once daily or b.i.d. May increase daily dose by 5 mg at weekly intervals until optimal response achieved; maximum dose, 40 mg/day. Or, 20-mg extended-release capsule PO once daily in morning. Maximum dose, 30 mg/day. Or, in adults ages 18 to 55, 12.5 to 25 mg Mydayis PO once daily in the morning. May increase daily dose by 12.5 mg at weekly intervals until optimal response achieved; maximum dose, 50 mg/day.
Adolescents ages 13 to 17 (extended-release): Initially, 10 mg PO daily in morning. May increase to 20 mg/day after 1 week if symptoms aren't controlled. Or, 12.5 mg Mydayis PO daily in the morning. May increase to maximum of 25 mg/day after 1 week if symptoms aren't controlled.

Children age 6 and older (immediate-release): Initially, 5 mg PO once daily or b.i.d. May increase daily dose by 5 mg at weekly intervals until optimal response is achieved. Give in one to three divided doses per day. Rarely necessary to exceed a total of 40 mg/day.

Children ages 6 to 12 (extended-release): Initially, 5 to 10 mg PO once daily in morning. May increase daily dose by 5 or 10 mg at weekly intervals. Maximum dose, 30 mg/day.

Children ages 3 to 5 (immediate-release): Initially, 2.5 mg PO daily. May increase daily dose by 2.5 mg at weekly intervals until optimal response is achieved. Give in one to three divided doses per day.

Adjust-a-dose: In patients with severe renal impairment, dosage reduction may be needed. Refer to manufacturer's instructions.

ADMINISTRATION
PO
• May give with or without food. Give My-dayis consistently either with or without food.
• Give extended-release dose upon awakening; don't give immediate-release dose in late evening to avoid insomnia.
• Make sure patient takes extended-release capsules whole, or open the capsules and sprinkle entire contents on applesauce and have patient consume immediately without chewing.
• Don't give missed Mydayis dose later in the day because the effects may last up to 16 hours.

ACTION
Promotes release of dopamine and norepinephrine from nerve terminals in the brain and, to a lesser extent, the reuptake of catecholamines.

Route	Onset	Peak	Duration
PO (immediate-release)	Unknown	3 hr	4–6 hr
PO (extended-release)	Unknown	7–8 hr	Unknown

Half-life: Immediate-release, 9 to 14 hours; extended-release, 10 to 14 hours.

ADVERSE REACTIONS
CNS: headache, insomnia, agitation, anxiety, dizziness, drowsiness, emotional lability, nervousness, irritability, jitteriness, fatigue, speech disturbance, twitching, fever, depression. **CV:** systolic HTN, palpitations, tachycardia, Raynaud phenomenon. **EENT:** dry mouth, teeth clenching, tooth infection. **GI:** abdominal pain, decreased appetite, anorexia, constipation, diarrhea, dyspepsia, nausea, vomiting. **GU:** erectile dysfunction, UTI, dysmenorrhea. **Metabolic:** weight loss. **Respiratory:** dyspnea. **Skin:** diaphoresis, skin photosensitivity. **Other:** decreased libido, infection, accidental injury, hypersensitivity reaction.

INTERACTIONS
Drug-drug. *Acetazolamide, sodium bicarbonate, thiazides:* May increase amphetamine concentration through decreased urine excretion. Monitor patient response.
Adrenergic blockers, antihistamines, antihypertensives, ethosuximide, phenobarbital, phenytoin: Amphetamines may reduce therapeutic effects of these drugs. Monitor patient response.
Ammonium chloride, ascorbic acid, glutamic acid, guanethidine, methenamine, reserpine, sodium acid phosphate: May lower amphetamine blood level and absorption. Don't use together.
CYP2D6 inhibitors (fluoxetine, paroxetine, ritonavir): May increase amphetamine level and risk of serotonin syndrome. Monitor patient, especially during amphetamine initiation and dosage increase.
MAO inhibitors (isocarboxazid, linezolid, methylene blue, selegiline): May increase risk of hypertensive crisis. Concurrent use or use within 14 days of MAO inhibitors is contraindicated.
Lithium carbonate: May reduce therapeutic effects of amphetamines. Monitor patient response.
PPIs (omeprazole): May increase amphetamine absorption rate. Monitor therapy.
Serotonergic agents (buspirone, fentanyl, lithium, SSNRIs, SSRIs, TCAs, tramadol, triptans): May increase risk of serotonin syndrome. Monitor patient. Discontinue both drugs if syndrome occurs and provide supportive care.
TCAs (desipramine, protriptyline): May increase amphetamine level and risk of CV effects. Monitor patient closely.
Drug-herb. *Ephedra:* May cause HTN or arrhythmias. Don't use together.

Reactions in bold italics are *life-threatening*. Interactions may have a *rapid onset* or a *delayed onset*.

St. John's wort: May increase risk of serotonin syndrome. Use together cautiously.
Drug-lifestyle. *Alcohol use:* May increase risk of drug dependency. Concurrent use is contraindicated in patients with a history of ethanol or drug dependency.

EFFECTS ON LAB TEST RESULTS
- May increase plasma corticosteroid level.
- May interfere with urinary steroid testing.

CONTRAINDICATIONS & CAUTIONS
Boxed Warning Amphetamines have a high potential for abuse. Administration of amphetamines for prolonged periods of time may lead to drug dependence and must be avoided. Particular attention should be paid to the possibility of persons obtaining amphetamines for nontherapeutic use or distribution to others, and the drugs should be prescribed or dispensed sparingly. ∎
Boxed Warning Misuse of amphetamines may cause sudden death and serious CV adverse events. ∎
- Contraindicated in patients with advanced arteriosclerosis, symptomatic CV disease, moderate to severe HTN, hyperthyroidism, known hypersensitivity or idiosyncrasy to sympathomimetic amines, glaucoma, agitated states, or history of drug abuse.
- **Alert:** Sudden death has been reported at usual doses in patients with structural cardiac abnormalities and other serious heart problems. Stimulants generally should not be used in adults, children, or adolescents with structural cardiac abnormalities, cardiomyopathy, serious heart rhythm abnormalities, or other serious cardiac problems.
- Drug can increase BP. Use cautiously in patients with underlying medical conditions (preexisting HTN, HF, recent MI, ventricular arrhythmia) that might be compromised by increases in BP or HR.
- Use cautiously in patients with a history of seizures, tics or Tourette syndrome, or mental problems, including psychosis, bipolar illness, mania, or depression.
- Drug may cause peripheral vasculopathy, including Raynaud phenomenon, which may improve after dosage reduction or drug discontinuation.
- Drug hasn't been studied in older adults.
- Immediate-release tablets aren't recommended for children with ADHD younger than age 3 or for children with narcolepsy younger than age 6. Use of extended-release capsules in children younger than age 6 hasn't been studied.
- Safety and effectiveness of Mydayis in children age 12 and younger haven't been established.
Dialyzable drug: Unknown.
⚠ *Overdose S&S:* Restlessness, tremor, hyperreflexia, rapid respiration, confusion, assaultiveness, hallucinations, panic states, hyperpyrexia, rhabdomyolysis; fatigue, depression (usually follow central stimulation); arrhythmias, HTN or hypotension, circulatory collapse; nausea, vomiting, diarrhea, abdominal cramps; seizures, coma (usually precede fatal poisoning).

PREGNANCY-LACTATION-REPRODUCTION
- There are no adequate well-controlled studies during pregnancy. Use during pregnancy only if potential benefit justifies fetal risk.
- Infants born to patients dependent on amphetamines have an increased risk of premature delivery and low birth weight. These infants may also experience signs and symptoms of withdrawal, such as dysphoria, including agitation, and excessive drowsiness.
- Register patients in the National Pregnancy Registry for Psychostimulants (1-866-961-2388 or https://womensmentalhealth.org/clinical-and-research-programs/pregnancyregistry/othermedications/).
- Drug appears in human milk. Don't use during breastfeeding.

NURSING CONSIDERATIONS
- Interrupt therapy occasionally to assess if behavioral symptoms warrant continued therapy, if possible.
- Perform a careful history and physical exam in all patients to assess for the presence of cardiac disease. Further cardiac evaluation may be needed. All patients who develop cardiac signs and symptoms (chest pain, syncope) during therapy should have a prompt cardiac evaluation.
- Evaluate patient for dependence on other prescription drugs, illicit drugs, or alcohol before start of therapy.
- Monitor HR and BP during therapy.
- Screen patient for a family history of suicide, bipolar disorder, and depression before

use. Monitor patient for increased aggression, worsening of existing psychiatric signs and symptoms, or psychosis.

• When used long term, drug may slow growth rate in children. Monitor growth rate; interrupt treatment for children not growing or gaining weight as expected.

• Monitor patient for risk of vasculopathies, including Raynaud phenomenon, and evaluate unexplained wounds on fingers and toes.

• Single doses of 20 mg extended-release capsules and 10 mg immediate-release tablets given b.i.d. (4 hours apart) have been shown to produce comparable plasma amphetamine concentrations.

• When switching from other dextroamphetamine–amphetamine preparations to Mydayis, discontinue previous formation and titrate per package labeling. Don't substitute on a milligram-per-milligram basis.

• *Look alike–sound alike:* Don't confuse Adderall XR with Inderal.

PATIENT TEACHING

• Tell patient to report all drugs and supplements being taken before start of therapy, especially if patient has taken an MAO inhibitor within the past 2 weeks.

• Explain that serious cardiac effects are possible during therapy. Advise patient to immediately report chest pain, shortness of breath, or fainting.

• Advise patient to report development of such conditions as glaucoma, high BP, or hyperthyroidism.

• Instruct patient to keep regular follow-up appointments for monitoring of HR and BP, and for growth checks in children. Patient who isn't growing or gaining weight as expected may need treatment interruption.

• Advise patient to report worsening of psychiatric signs and symptoms or behavioral changes during therapy.

• Explain that drug may cause circulatory problems. Advise patient to immediately report unexplained wounds on fingers or toes.

• Instruct patient or caregiver in safe drug administration.

• Caution patient that abruptly stopping drug may cause withdrawal signs and symptoms (extreme fatigue, depression, increased appetite, agitation, abnormal dreams).

SAFETY ALERT!

diazePAM ⚠

dye-AZ-e-pam

Diastat*, Diastat AcuDial*, Diazepam Intensol*, Valium♥, Valtoco

Therapeutic class: Anxiolytics
Pharmacologic class: Benzodiazepines
Controlled substance schedule: IV

AVAILABLE FORMS

Injection: 5 mg/mL
Nasal spray: 5 mg/0.1 mL, 7.5 mg/0.1 mL, 10 mg/0.1 mL
Oral solution: 5 mg/5 mL, 5 mg/mL*
Rectal gel twin packs: 2.5 mg (pediatric); 10 mg, 20 mg (adult)
Tablets: 2 mg, 5 mg, 10 mg

INDICATIONS & DOSAGES

Adjust-a-dose (for all indications): For older adults or patients who are debilitated, give 2 to 2.5 mg PO daily or b.i.d. initially; increase gradually as needed and tolerated. Or, when using injection, use lower doses (2 to 5 mg) and increase dosage more gradually. Or, when using nasal spray, consider reducing dosage due to increased half-life in older adults.

➤ **Anxiety**
Adults: Depending on severity, 2 to 10 mg PO b.i.d. to q.i.d. Or, 2 to 10 mg IM or IV. May repeat in 3 to 4 hours if needed.
Children age 6 months and older: 1 to 2.5 mg PO t.i.d. or q.i.d., increased gradually, as needed and tolerated.

➤ **Acute alcohol withdrawal**
Adults: 10 mg PO t.i.d. or q.i.d. during first 24 hours; reduce to 5 mg PO t.i.d. or q.i.d., PRN. Or, 10 mg IV or IM initially; then 5 to 10 mg IV or IM again in 3 to 4 hours if needed.

➤ **Before endoscopic procedures**
Adults: Adjust IV dose to desired sedative response (up to 20 mg). If IV can't be used, give 5 to 10 mg IM 30 minutes before procedure.

➤ **Muscle spasm**
Adults: 2 to 10 mg PO b.i.d. to q.i.d. as an adjunct. Or, 5 to 10 mg IV or IM initially; then 5 to 10 mg IV or IM again in 3 to 4 hours if needed.

➤ **Preoperative sedation**
Adults: 10 mg IM or IV before surgery.

➤ **Adjunctive treatment for seizure disorders**
Adults: 2 to 10 mg PO b.i.d. to q.i.d.
Children age 6 months and older: 1 to 2.5 mg PO t.i.d. or q.i.d. initially; increase as needed and as tolerated.

➤ **Status epilepticus, severe recurrent seizures**
Adults: 5 to 10 mg IV or IM initially. Use IM route only if IV access is unavailable. Repeat every 10 to 15 minutes PRN, up to maximum dose of 30 mg. Repeat every 2 to 4 hours PRN.
Children age 5 and older: 1 mg IV slowly every 2 to 5 minutes to a maximum of 10 mg (IV preferred). Repeat in 2 to 4 hours PRN.
Children ages 30 days to younger than 5 years: 0.2 to 0.5 mg IV slowly every 2 to 5 minutes up to a maximum of 5 mg (IV preferred). Repeat in 2 to 4 hours PRN.

➤ **Patients on stable regimens of antiepileptic drugs who need diazepam intermittently to control bouts of increased seizure activity**
Adults and children age 12 and older: 0.2 mg/kg PR, rounding up to the nearest available dose form. A second dose may be given 4 to 12 hours later.
Children ages 6 to 11: 0.3 mg/kg PR, rounding up to the nearest available dose form. A second dose may be given 4 to 12 hours later.
Children ages 2 to 5: 0.5 mg/kg PR, rounding up to the nearest available dose form. A second dose may be given 4 to 12 hours later.

➤ **Tetanus**
Adults: Initially, 5 to 10 mg IV or IM then 5 to 10 mg in 3 to 4 hours if needed. Larger doses may be required.
Children age 5 and older: 5 to 10 mg IM or IV repeated every 3 to 4 hours PRN.
Children ages 30 days to younger than 5 years: 1 to 2 mg IM or IV slowly repeated every 3 to 4 hours PRN.

➤ **Acute treatment of intermittent, stereotypic episodes of frequent seizure activity (i.e., seizure clusters, acute repetitive seizures) that are distinct from usual seizure pattern in patients with epilepsy**
Rectal
Adults and children age 12 and older: 0.2 mg/kg PR, rounding up to nearest available dose form. May give second dose 4 to 12 hours later.
Children ages 6 to 11: 0.3 mg/kg PR, rounding up to nearest available dose form. May give second dose 4 to 12 hours later.

Children ages 2 to 5: 0.5 mg/kg PR, rounding up to nearest available dose form. May give second dose 4 to 12 hours later.
Intranasal
Adults and children age 12 and older weighing 76 kg or more: 10 mg intranasally in both nostrils (20 mg total).
Adults and children age 12 and older weighing 51 to 75 kg: 7.5 mg intranasally in both nostrils (15 mg total).
Adults and children age 12 and older weighing 28 to 50 kg: 10 mg intranasally in one nostril (10 mg total).
Adults and children age 12 and older weighing 14 to 27 kg: 5 mg intranasally in one nostril (5 mg total).
Children ages 6 to 11 weighing 56 to 74 kg: 10 mg intranasally in both nostrils (20 mg total).
Children ages 6 to 11 weighing 38 to 55 kg: 7.5 mg intranasally in both nostrils (15 mg total).
Children ages 6 to 11 weighing 19 to 37 kg: 10 mg intranasally in one nostril (10 mg total).
Children ages 6 to 11 weighing 10 to 18 kg: 5 mg intranasally in one nostril (5 mg total).
Adjust-a-dose: If a second dose is needed, give at least 4 hours after initial dose. Don't use more than two doses to treat a single episode. Nasal spray shouldn't be used to treat more than one episode every 5 days or five episodes per month.

ADMINISTRATION
PO
● When using oral solution, dilute dose just before giving with liquid or semisolid food, such as water, juices, soda or sodalike beverages, applesauce, or pudding.
● Discard opened bottle of concentrated solution after 90 days.
IV
▼ Keep emergency resuscitation equipment and oxygen at bedside.
▼ For adults, give at no more than 5 mg/minute.
▼ For children, administer slowly over 3 minutes. Don't exceed 0.25 mg/kg.
▼ Avoid infusion sets or containers made from polyvinyl chloride.
▼ If possible, inject directly into a large vein. If not, inject slowly through infusion tubing as near to the insertion site as possible. Watch closely for phlebitis at injection site.

▼ Monitor respirations every 5 to 15 minutes and before each dose.
▼ Don't store parenteral solution in plastic syringes.
▼ **Incompatibilities:** All other IV drugs, most IV solutions.

IM
• Use the IM route if IV administration is impossible.

Rectal
• Use Diastat rectal gel to treat no more than five episodes per month and no more than one episode every 5 days.

🔔 *Alert:* Only caregivers who can distinguish the distinct cluster of seizures or events from patient's ordinary seizure activity, who have been instructed and can give the treatment competently, who understand which seizures may be treated with Diastat, and who can monitor the clinical response and recognize when immediate professional medical evaluation is needed should give Diastat rectal gel.

Intranasal
• Use nasal spray to treat no more than five episodes per month and no more than one episode every 5 days.
• Each single-use nasal spray device delivers 1 spray and cannot be reused. Do not prime or attempt to use for more than one administration per device.
• Don't open blister packs or test devices before use.
• Store at 20° C to 25° C (68° F to 77° F). Don't freeze; protect from light.

ACTION
Potentiates the effects of GABA, depresses the CNS, and suppresses the spread of seizure activity.

Route	Onset	Peak	Duration
PO	30 min	0.25–2.5 hr	20–80 hr
IV	1–5 min	1–5 min	15–60 min
IM	Unknown	1 hr	Unknown
PR, intranasal	Unknown	90 min	Unknown

Half-life: About 1 to 12 days. Varies with route and patient age.

ADVERSE REACTIONS
CNS: drowsiness, abnormal thinking, agitation, emotional lability, euphoria, nervousness, asthenia, dysarthria, slurred speech, tremor, transient amnesia, fatigue, ataxia, headache, insomnia, paradoxical anxiety, disinhibition, hallucinations, minor changes in EEG patterns, pain, vertigo, confusion, depression, dysgeusia (nasal form). **CV:** hypotension, vasodilation. **EENT:** diplopia, blurred vision, nystagmus; with nasal form: nasal discomfort, nasal congestion, epistaxis, dry mouth. **GI:** nausea, abdominal pain, constipation, diarrhea with rectal form. **GU:** incontinence, urine retention. **Hematologic:** *neutropenia.* **Hepatic:** jaundice. **Respiratory:** hiccups. **Skin:** rash, phlebitis at injection site. **Other:** altered libido, physical or psychological dependence.

INTERACTIONS
Drug-drug. *Cimetidine, disulfiram, fluoxetine, fluvoxamine, hormonal contraceptives, isoniazid, metoprolol, propranolol, valproic acid:* May decrease clearance of diazepam and increase risk of adverse effects. Monitor patient for excessive sedation and impaired psychomotor function.
CNS depressants: May increase CNS and respiratory depression. Use together cautiously.
Digoxin: May increase digoxin level and risk of toxicity. Monitor patient and digoxin level closely.
Diltiazem: May increase CNS depression and prolong effects of diazepam. Reduce dose of diazepam.
Fluconazole, itraconazole, ketoconazole, miconazole: May increase and prolong diazepam level, CNS depression, and psychomotor impairment. Avoid using together.
Levodopa: May decrease levodopa effectiveness. Monitor patient.
Boxed Warning *Opioids:* May cause slow or difficult breathing, sedation, and death. Avoid use together. If use together is necessary, limit dosage and duration of each drug to the minimum necessary for desired effect. ∎
Phenobarbital: May increase effects of both drugs. Use together cautiously.
Drug-herb. *Kava kava:* May increase sedation. Discourage use together.
Drug-lifestyle. **Boxed Warning** *Alcohol use:* May cause additive CNS effects. Don't use together. ∎
Smoking: May decrease effectiveness of drug. Monitor patient closely.

EFFECTS ON LAB TEST RESULTS
• May increase LFT values.
• May decrease neutrophil count.

Reactions in bold italics are *life-threatening*. Interactions may have a *rapid onset* or a ***delayed onset***.

CONTRAINDICATIONS & CAUTIONS

Boxed Warning Opioids should only be prescribed with benzodiazepines or other CNS depressants to patients for whom alternative treatment options are inadequate. Limit doses and durations to the minimum required. ■

Boxed Warning Benzodiazepine use exposes patient to risks of abuse, misuse, and addiction, which can lead to overdose or death. Assess each patient's risk of abuse, misuse, and addiction before prescribing and periodically during therapy. ■

Boxed Warning Abrupt discontinuation or rapid dosage reduction of benzodiazepines after continued use may precipitate acute withdrawal reactions, which can be life-threatening. To reduce risk of withdrawal reactions, gradually taper drug to discontinue or reduce dosage. ■

• Contraindicated in patients hypersensitive to drug, patients with acute angle-closure glaucoma, and children younger than age 6 months (oral form).

• Diazepam (oral form) is contraindicated in patients with myasthenia gravis, severe respiratory insufficiency, severe hepatic insufficiency, or sleep apnea syndrome.

• Use cautiously in patients experiencing shock, coma, or acute alcohol intoxication (parenteral form).

• Use cautiously in older adults; patients who are debilitated; patients with hepatic or renal impairment, depression, history of substance abuse, impaired gag reflex, or chronic open-angle glaucoma (who are receiving appropriate therapy); and in those at risk for falls.

• Some injectable forms may contain propylene glycol; large amounts are potentially toxic and have been associated with hyperosmolality, lactic acidosis, seizures, and respiratory depression.

▨ Use cautiously in patients with renal or hepatic dysfunction, impaired alcohol dehydrogenase enzymes, or history of alcoholism.

• Safety and effectiveness and approval for drug's use in children vary by formulation. Use only for ages indicated.

Dialyzable drug: No.

⚠ *Overdose S&S:* Somnolence, confusion, coma, diminished reflexes.

PREGNANCY-LACTATION-REPRODUCTION

• Use during pregnancy isn't recommended, especially during first and third trimesters. If drug is needed during pregnancy, use only if potential benefit justifies fetal risk.

• Neonatal flaccidity, respiratory and feeding difficulties, hypothermia, and withdrawal symptoms have been reported in infants born to patients who received benzodiazepines late in pregnancy.

• Drug appears in human milk. Don't use during breastfeeding.

NURSING CONSIDERATIONS

• Periodically monitor LFTs, CBC, and renal function in patients receiving repeated or prolonged therapy.

• Monitor HR, BP, and mental status changes. Patients are at an increased risk for falls.

🕭 *Alert:* Use of drug may lead to abuse, misuse, and addiction, which can lead to overdose or death. Abuse and misuse of benzodiazepines frequently involves concomitant use of other medications, alcohol, or illicit substances, which increase frequency of serious adverse outcomes. Assess each patient's risk of abuse, misuse, and addiction before prescribing and throughout treatment.

Boxed Warning Continued use of benzodiazepines may lead to physical dependence. Abrupt discontinuation or rapid dosage reduction may precipitate acute withdrawal reactions, which can be life-threatening; taper gradually. ■

• *Look alike–sound alike:* Don't confuse diazepam with diazoxide or Ditropan. Don't confuse Valium with Valcyte.

PATIENT TEACHING

Boxed Warning Caution patient or caregiver of a patient taking an opioid with a benzodiazepine, CNS depressant, or alcohol to seek immediate medical attention for dizziness, light-headedness, extreme sleepiness, slowed or difficult breathing, or unresponsiveness. ■

Boxed Warning Caution patient that benzodiazepines, even at recommended doses, increase risk of abuse, misuse, and addiction, which can lead to overdose and death, especially when used with other drugs (opioid analgesics), alcohol, or illicit substances. ■

Boxed Warning Teach patient signs and symptoms of benzodiazepine abuse, misuse, and addiction (abdominal pain, amnesia, anorexia, anxiety, aggression, ataxia, blurred vision, confusion, depression, disin-hibition, disorientation, dizziness, euphoria, impaired concentration and memory, indigestion, irritability, muscle pain, slurred speech, tremors, vertigo, delirium, paranoia, suicidality, seizures, difficulty breathing, coma) and to seek emergency help if they occur, proper disposal of unused drug, and not to take drug at a higher dose, more frequently, or for longer than prescribed. ∎

Boxed Warning Tell patient that continued use of drug for several days to weeks may lead to physical dependence and that abrupt discontinuation or rapid dosage reduction may precipitate acute withdrawal reactions (unusual movements, responses, or expressions; seizures; sudden and severe mental or nervous system changes; depression; seeing or hearing things that others don't; homicidal thoughts; extreme increase in activity or talking; losing touch with reality; suicidality), which can be life-threatening. Instruct patient that discontinuation or dosage reduction may require a slow taper. ∎

Boxed Warning Stress the possibility of development of protracted withdrawal syndrome (anxiety; trouble remembering, learning or concentrating; depression; problems sleeping; feeling like insects are crawling under the skin; weakness, shaking, muscle twitching; burning or prickling feeling in the hands, arms, legs, or feet; ringing in the ears), with symptoms lasting weeks to more than 12 months. ∎

• Warn patient to report all adverse reactions and to avoid activities that require alertness and good coordination until effects of drug are known.

• Tell patient to avoid alcohol while taking drug.

• Warn patient not to abruptly stop drug because withdrawal symptoms may occur.

• Instruct caregiver on proper use of Diastat rectal gel and Valtoco nasal spray.

• Advise patient to avoid use during pregnancy due to fetal risk; instruct patient to notify prescriber of pregnancy or intention to become pregnant.

---

diclofenac (oral)
dye-KLOE-fen-ak

Zorvolex

diclofenac potassium
Cambia, Cataflam, Voltaren Rapide✦, Zipsor

diclofenac sodium (oral)
Voltaren✦

Therapeutic class: NSAIDs
Pharmacologic class: NSAIDs

AVAILABLE FORMS
diclofenac (oral)
Capsules: 18 mg, 35 mg
diclofenac potassium
Capsules: 25 mg*
Powder for solution: 50 mg/packet
Tablets: 25 mg, 50 mg
diclofenac sodium (oral)
Tablets (delayed-release) ⓒ: 25 mg, 50 mg, 75 mg
Tablets (extended-release) ⓒ: 100 mg

INDICATIONS & DOSAGES
Adjust-a-dose (for all indications): Patients with hepatic impairment may require lower initial dosages. Initiate treatment with Zorvolex or Zipsor at the lowest dosage; if efficacy isn't achieved with the lowest dosage, discontinue drug.

➤ **Ankylosing spondylitis**
Adults: 25 mg delayed-release diclofenac sodium PO q.i.d.; may add another 25-mg dose at bedtime if needed.

➤ **Osteoarthritis**
Adults: 50 mg diclofenac potassium or delayed-release diclofenac sodium PO b.i.d. or t.i.d., or 75 mg delayed-release diclofenac sodium PO b.i.d. Or, 35 mg Zorvolex PO t.i.d. Or, 100 mg extended-release diclofenac sodium PO daily.

➤ **RA**
Adults: 50 mg diclofenac potassium or delayed-release diclofenac sodium PO t.i.d. or q.i.d., or 75 mg delayed-release diclofenac sodium PO b.i.d. Or, 100 mg extended-release diclofenac sodium PO daily or b.i.d.

➤ **Analgesia**
Adults: 50 mg diclofenac potassium PO t.i.d. For some patients, the first dose on the first

---

day may be 100 mg, followed by 50 mg for the second and third doses; maximum dose for first day is 200 mg. Don't exceed 150 mg daily after the first day. Or, 25 mg Zipsor PO q.i.d. or 18 or 35 mg Zorvolex PO t.i.d.
Children age 12 and older (Zipsor): 25 mg PO q.i.d.

➤ **Primary dysmenorrhea**
Adults: 50 mg diclofenac potassium PO t.i.d. For some patients, the first dose on the first day may be 100 mg, followed by 50 mg for the second and third doses; maximum dose for first day is 200 mg. Don't exceed 150 mg daily after the first day.

➤ **Migraine**
Adults: 50 mg (1 packet) PO as a single dose.

ADMINISTRATION
PO
• Give drug (except Cambia) with milk, meals, or antacids.
• Don't crush or break delayed- or extended-release tablets.
• Mix powder (Cambia) in 30 to 60 mL water only. Use no other liquid.
• Mix solution well and have patient drink immediately.
• Powder (Cambia) and Zorvolex may be less effective if taken with food.
• Cambia, Zorvolex, and Zipsor aren't interchangeable with other formulations of oral diclofenac even if the milligram strength is the same.

ACTION
Reversibly inhibits cyclooxygenase 1 and 2 enzymes, which decreases proinflammatory processes. Has analgesic, anti-inflammatory, and antipyretic properties.

Route	Onset	Peak	Duration
PO (delayed-release)	30 min	2–3 hr	8 hr
PO (extended-release)	Unknown	5–6 hr	Unknown
PO	10 min	1 hr	8 hr

Half-life: 1 to 2.3 hours.

ADVERSE REACTIONS
CNS: dizziness, drowsiness, headache. **CV:** edema, fluid retention, HTN. **EENT:** tinnitus, nasopharyngitis, sinusitis. **GI:** abdominal pain, *bleeding or perforation,* constipation, diarrhea, flatulence, heartburn, nausea, peptic ulceration, vomiting, dyspepsia. **GU:** UTI,

increased creatinine level, renal function abnormality. **Hepatic:** increased transaminase levels. **Hematologic:** increased bleeding time. **Musculoskeletal:** osteoarthritis, arthralgia, back or limb pain. **Respiratory:** URI, cough, bronchitis. **Skin:** bruising, pruritus, rash, diaphoresis. **Other:** falls, flulike symptoms, hypersensitivity reactions.

INTERACTIONS
Drug-drug. *ACE inhibitors, ARBs:* May enhance adverse or toxic effect of NSAIDs and result in a significant decrease in renal function. May diminish antihypertensive effect of ACE inhibitors and ARBs. Monitor therapy.
Anticoagulants, antiplatelet agents, SSNRIs, SSRIs, warfarin: May cause bleeding. Monitor patient closely.
Aspirin: May decrease effectiveness of diclofenac and increase GI toxicity. Avoid using together.
Beta blockers: May decrease antihypertensive effects. Monitor patient closely.
Cyclosporine, digoxin, lithium, methotrexate: May reduce renal clearance of these drugs and increase risk of toxicity. Monitor patient closely.
CYP2C9 inducers (rifampin): May decrease diclofenac effect. Monitor therapy; adjust dosage as needed.
CYP2C9 inhibitors (voriconazole): May increase diclofenac level and risk of toxicity. Monitor therapy; adjust dosage as needed.
Diuretics: May decrease effectiveness of diuretics and risk of nephrotoxicity. Avoid using together.
NSAIDs, salicylates: May increase risk of GI toxicity. Avoid use together.
Pemetrexed: May increase risk of pemetrexed-associated myelosuppression and renal and GI toxicity. Monitor patient closely.
Potassium-sparing diuretics: May enhance retention and increase level of potassium. Monitor potassium level.
Drug-herb. *Alfalfa, anise, bilberry, willow:* May cause bleeding. Don't use together.
Drug-lifestyle. *Sun exposure:* May cause photosensitivity reactions. Advise patient to avoid excessive sunlight exposure.

EFFECTS ON LAB TEST RESULTS
• May increase ALT, AST, bilirubin, BUN, potassium, glucose, and creatinine levels.

CONTRAINDICATIONS & CAUTIONS

Boxed Warning Contraindicated for the treatment of pain after CABG surgery. ■

• Contraindicated in patients hypersensitive to drug and in those with hepatic porphyria or history of asthma, urticaria, or other allergic reactions after taking aspirin or other NSAIDs. Zipsor is contraindicated in patients hypersensitive to bovine protein.

Boxed Warning NSAID use increases risk of serious CV thrombotic events, including MI and stroke, which can be fatal. This risk may occur early in treatment and increase with duration of use. Risk appears greater at higher doses. Risk may be greater in patients with CV disease or risk factors for CV disease. Use lowest effective dose for shortest duration possible. ■

⚠ *Alert:* NSAIDs increase the risk of HF. Don't use in patients with severe HF unless the benefits are expected to outweigh risks.

• Use cautiously in patients with history of peptic ulcer disease, hepatic dysfunction, cardiac disease, HTN, fluid retention, or impaired renal function.

• Drug may cause photosensitivity as well as SCAR, including exfoliative dermatitis, SJS, and TEN, which can be fatal. Discontinue at first sign of rash or hypersensitivity.

Dialyzable drug: Unknown.

⚠ *Overdose S&S:* Drowsiness, confusion, GI bleeding, hypotonia, loss of consciousness, vomiting, aspiration, pneumonitis, increased ICP.

PREGNANCY-LACTATION-REPRODUCTION

⚠ *Alert:* Drug can cause fetal harm when administered at 30 weeks' gestation or later. Use during pregnancy before 30 weeks' gestation only if potential benefit justifies potential risk to the fetus.

⚠ *Alert:* Use of NSAIDs at 20 weeks or later in pregnancy may cause fetal renal dysfunction leading to oligohydramnios and potential neonatal renal impairment. Use at 30 weeks or later in pregnancy may increase risk of premature closure of the ductus arteriosus. Avoid use starting at 20 weeks' gestation. If potential benefit justifies fetal risk, use lowest effective dose for shortest duration. Consider ultrasound monitoring of amniotic fluid if NSAID use is longer than 48 hours. Use of low-dose aspirin (81 mg) for certain pregnancy-related conditions under direction of prescriber is acceptable.

• Drug may appear in human milk. Patient should discontinue breastfeeding or discontinue drug.

• May increase risk of reversible infertility in females.

NURSING CONSIDERATIONS

⚠ *Alert:* Monitor patient and immediately evaluate signs and symptoms of heart attack (chest pain, shortness of breath, trouble breathing) or stroke (weakness in one part or side of the body, slurred speech).

• Because NSAIDs impair the synthesis of renal prostaglandins, they can decrease renal blood flow and lead to reversible renal impairment, especially in patients with renal failure, HF, or liver dysfunction; in older adults; and in patients taking diuretics. Monitor these patients closely.

• LFT values may increase during therapy. Monitor transaminase, especially ALT, levels periodically in patients undergoing long-term therapy. Make first transaminase measurement no later than 8 weeks after therapy begins.

• Discontinue drug immediately if hepatic impairment occurs, including persistent or worsening abnormal LFT values, clinical signs or symptoms consistent with liver disease, or systemic manifestations of liver disease.

Boxed Warning NSAIDs cause an increased risk of serious GI adverse events, including bleeding, ulceration, and perforation of the stomach or intestines, which can be fatal. Older adults are at greater risk. ■

⚠ *Alert:* Different formulations of oral diclofenac are not bioequivalent even if the milligram strength is the same.

• Because of their antipyretic and anti-inflammatory actions, NSAIDs may mask the signs and symptoms of infection.

• Consider periodic CBC and chemistry profile monitoring with long-term NSAID treatment because serious GI bleeding, hepatotoxicity, and renal injury can occur without warning.

• Older adults are at greater risk for NSAID-associated serious CV, GI, or renal adverse reactions. Monitor patient closely for adverse effects.

• *Look alike–sound alike:* Don't confuse diclofenac with Diflucan.

PATIENT TEACHING
• Teach patient safe drug administration.
🕒 *Alert:* Advise patient to seek medical attention immediately if chest pain, shortness of breath or trouble breathing, weakness in one part or side of the body, or slurred speech occurs.
🕒 *Alert:* Warn patient who is pregnant not to take NSAIDs at 20 weeks' gestation or later unless instructed to do so by prescriber due to potential fetal risk. Advise patient to discuss taking OTC medications with pharmacist or health care provider during pregnancy.
• Advise patient not to take drug with other diclofenac-containing products (such as Arthrotec), other NSAIDs, or salicylates (salsalate, diflunisal).
• Teach patient signs and symptoms of GI bleeding (blood in vomit, urine, or stool; coffee-ground vomit; black, tarry stools) and to notify prescriber immediately if any of these occur.
• Teach patient the signs and symptoms of damage to the liver, including nausea, fatigue, lethargy, itching, yellowed skin or eyes, right upper quadrant tenderness, and flulike symptoms. Tell patient to contact prescriber immediately if these symptoms occur.
• Advise patient to avoid drinking alcohol or taking aspirin during drug therapy.
• Tell patient to wear sunscreen or protective clothing because drug may cause sensitivity to sunlight.
• Warn patient to avoid hazardous activities that require alertness until it is known whether the drug causes CNS symptoms.
• Advise patient that use of OTC NSAIDs (which may be present in OTC medications for treatment of colds, fever, or insomnia) and diclofenac may increase risk of GI toxicity.

---

diclofenac epolamine
dye-KLOE-fen-ak

Flector, Licart

diclofenac sodium (topical)
Pennsaid, Voltaren ◊

Therapeutic class: NSAIDs
Pharmacologic class: NSAIDs

AVAILABLE FORMS
Topical gel: 1% ◊, 3%
Topical solution: 1.5%, 2%
Transdermal patch: 1.3%

INDICATIONS & DOSAGES
➤ **Actinic keratosis (3% gel only)**
Adults: Apply gel to lesion b.i.d. for 60 to 90 days.
➤ **Osteoarthritis**
Adults: Apply 4 g of 1% gel to affected foot, knee, or ankle q.i.d. Maximum dose of 16 g to any single joint of the lower extremities. Or apply 2 g of 1% gel to affected hand, elbow, or wrist q.i.d. Maximum dose of 8 g to any single joint of the upper extremities. Total dose shouldn't exceed 32 g daily for all affected joints.
➤ **Acute pain due to minor strains, sprains, and contusions**
Adults: Apply 1 patch to most painful area b.i.d.
Children age 6 and older (Flector only): Apply 1 patch to most painful area b.i.d.
➤ **Osteoarthritis of the knee**
Adults: Count 10 drops at a time of 1.5% topical solution onto hand or directly onto knee. Apply to each side, front and back, spreading evenly, using a total of 40 drops q.i.d. Or, 2 pump actuations (40 mg) of 2% topical solution on each painful knee b.i.d. Dispense solution directly onto the knee or first into the hand and then onto the knee. Spread evenly around front, back, and sides of the knee.

ADMINISTRATION
Topical
• Apply to clean, dry skin.
• Don't apply on open wounds or broken skin.
• Avoid contact with eyes.
• Use enough gel to cover the lesion; for example, use 0.5 g of gel on a 5 × 5-cm lesion.
• Don't apply Flector or Licart patch to non-intact or damaged skin, including from exudative dermatitis, eczema, infected lesions, burns, or wounds.
• Patient shouldn't wear patch while bathing or showering.
• Measure gel using supplied dosing cards in package.
• Wash hands after applying. If treatment area is the hands, patient should wait at least 1 hour before washing hands.
• Don't cover treated area with an occlusive dressing or apply moist heat.
• Pump for 2% topical solution must be primed before first use. Depress pump four times while holding bottle upright; discard solution obtained during priming.

ACTION

Reversibly inhibits cyclooxygenase 1 and 2 enzymes, which decreases proinflammatory processes. Has analgesic, anti-inflammatory, and antipyretic properties.

Route	Onset	Peak	Duration
Topical	Unknown	4–12 hr	Unknown
Transdermal	Unknown	10–20 hr	Unknown

Half-life: 1 to 3 hours; 12 hours for patch.

ADVERSE REACTIONS

CNS: paresthesia, headache, hyperesthesia, pain, asthenia, migraine, hypokinesia, dysgeusia, somnolence. **CV:** chest pain, HTN. **EENT:** conjunctivitis, eye pain, sinusitis, pharyngitis, rhinitis. **GI:** diarrhea, dyspepsia, abdominal pain, flatulence, nausea. **GU:** hematuria, renal impairment. **Hepatic:** increased transaminase levels. **Metabolic:** hypercholesterolemia, hyperglycemia, increased CK level. **Musculoskeletal:** arthralgia, arthrosis, back pain, myalgia, neck pain. **Respiratory:** *asthma,* dyspnea, pneumonia. **Skin:** application-site reaction, contact dermatitis, dry skin, localized pain, pruritus, rash, vesicles, erythema, localized edema, acne, alopecia, photosensitivity reactions, skin ulcer. **Other:** *anaphylaxis,* flulike syndrome, infection, hypersensitivity reaction.

INTERACTIONS

Drug-drug. *ACE inhibitors, ARBs:* May enhance adverse or toxic effect of NSAIDs and result in a significant decrease in renal function. May diminish antihypertensive effect of ACE inhibitors and ARBs. Monitor therapy.
Anticoagulants, antiplatelet agents, SSNRIs, SSRIs, warfarin: May cause bleeding. Monitor patient closely.
Aspirin: May decrease effectiveness of diclofenac and increase GI toxicity. Avoid using together.
Beta blockers: May decrease antihypertensive effects. Monitor patient closely.
Cyclosporine, digoxin, lithium, methotrexate: May reduce renal clearance of these drugs and increase risk of toxicity. Monitor patient closely.
Diuretics: May decrease effectiveness of diuretics. Avoid using together.
Insulin, oral antidiabetics: May alter requirements for antidiabetics. Monitor patient closely.

Oral NSAIDs: May increase diclofenac effects. Minimize use together.
Pemetrexed: May increase risk of pemetrexed-associated myelosuppression and renal and GI toxicity. Avoid topical NSAID use 2 days before, day of, and 2 days after pemetrexed.
Potassium-sparing diuretics: May enhance retention and increase potassium level. Monitor potassium level.
Herb-drug. *Alfalfa, anise, bilberry, willow:* May cause bleeding. Don't use together.
Drug-lifestyle. *Sun exposure:* May increase risk of photosensitivity reactions. Advise patient to avoid excessive sun exposure.

EFFECTS ON LAB TEST RESULTS

• May increase ALT, AST, cholesterol, creatinine, glucose, and transaminase levels.

CONTRAINDICATIONS & CAUTIONS

• Contraindicated in patients hypersensitive to diclofenac. Diclofenac 3% sodium gel is also contraindicated in patients with a known hypersensitivity to benzyl alcohol, polyethylene glycol monomethyl ether 350, or hyaluronate sodium.
• Contraindicated in patients with a history of asthma, urticaria, or other allergic reactions after taking aspirin or other NSAIDs.
• Flector and Licart patches are contraindicated for use on nonintact or damaged skin, including from exudative dermatitis, eczema, infected lesions, burns, or wounds.
Boxed Warning Contraindicated for perioperative pain for CABG surgery. ■
Boxed Warning NSAIDs can increase risk of MI or stroke in patients with or without heart disease or risk factors for heart disease. Risk of MI or stroke can occur as early as the first weeks of NSAID use and can be fatal. ■
• Risk of MI or stroke appears greater at higher doses. Use lowest effective dose for shortest duration possible.
◆ *Alert:* NSAIDs increase risk of HF. Don't use in patients with severe HF unless benefits are expected to outweigh risks.
• Use cautiously in patients with the aspirin triad; these patients are usually asthmatics who develop rhinitis, with or without nasal polyps, after taking aspirin or other NSAIDs.

Reactions in bold italics are *life-threatening*. Interactions may have a *rapid onset* or a *delayed onset*.

- Use cautiously in patients with active GI bleeding or ulceration and in those with severe renal or hepatic impairment.
- May cause SCAR, including exfoliative dermatitis, SJS, and TEN, which can be fatal. Discontinue use at first sign of rash or hypersensitivity.

Dialyzable drug: Unknown.

PREGNANCY-LACTATION-REPRODUCTION

🕛 *Alert:* Drug can cause fetal harm when administered at 30 weeks' gestation or later. Use during pregnancy before 30 weeks' gestation only if potential benefit justifies fetal risk.
- Drug may cause constriction of ductus arteriosus. Avoid use in late pregnancy.
- Drug may appear in human milk. Patient should discontinue breastfeeding or discontinue drug, taking into account importance of drug to the patient.
- Drug may increase risk of reversible female infertility.

NURSING CONSIDERATIONS

Boxed Warning NSAIDs may increase the risk of serious CV thrombotic events. The risk may increase with duration of use. Patients with CV disease or risk factors for CV disease may be at greater risk. ∎

Boxed Warning NSAIDs increase the risk of serious GI adverse reactions, including bleeding, ulceration, and perforation of the stomach or intestines, which can be fatal. These reactions can occur at any time and without warning. Older adults are at greater risk. ∎

🕛 *Alert:* Monitor patient and immediately evaluate signs and symptoms of MI (chest pain, shortness of breath, trouble breathing) or stroke (weakness in one part or side of the body, slurred speech).
- Avoid use in patients with recent MI unless benefits are expected to outweigh risk of recurrent CV thrombotic events. If used in patients with recent MI, watch for signs and symptoms of cardiac ischemia.
- Avoid use in patients with severe HF unless benefits are expected to outweigh risk of worsening HF. If used in patients with severe HF, watch for signs and symptoms of worsening HF.
- Evaluate patient with signs or symptoms of liver dysfunction or with abnormal LFT

results for development of more severe hepatic reaction while taking drug.
- If clinical signs or symptoms of liver disease develop, or if systemic manifestation (eosinophilia, rash) occurs, discontinue drug.
- Safety and effectiveness of sunscreens, cosmetics, or other topical medications used with drug are unknown.
- Complete healing or optimal therapeutic effect may not be seen until 30 days after therapy is complete.
- Reevaluate treatment if signs or symptoms worsen or don't respond to therapy.

PATIENT TEACHING

- Inform patient about risk of skin reactions (rash, itchiness, pain, irritation) at the application site. Urge patient to seek medical attention if adverse reactions occur.

🕛 *Alert:* Advise patient to seek medical attention immediately if chest pain, shortness of breath or trouble breathing, weakness in one part or side of the body, or slurred speech occurs.
- Instruct patient in safe drug administration
- Encourage patient to minimize sun exposure during therapy. Explain that sunscreen may be helpful but that the safety of using sunscreen with drug is unknown.
- Advise patient needing an MRI to inform the facility about wearing a transdermal patch.
- Tell patient using diclofenac 3% sodium gel that complete healing or optimal therapeutic effect may not occur for up to 30 days after stopping therapy.
- Instruct patient not to apply other topical drugs or cosmetics to affected area while using drug, unless directed.
- Inform patient that if Flector or Licart patch begins to peel off, the edges may be taped down. Instruct patient not to wear Flector patch during bathing or showering. Bathing should take place in between scheduled patch removal and application.
- Instruct patient not to cover area with clothing for at least 10 minutes after applying gel and to wait at least 1 hour before showering or bathing.
- Tell patient to notify prescriber if pregnant or breastfeeding.

♣Canada ◇OTC ♦Off-label use ✐Photoguide ⬤Do not crush *Liquid contains alcohol ⁛Genetic

dicyclomine hydrochloride
dye-SYE-kloe-meen

Bentyl

Therapeutic class: Antispasmodics
Pharmacologic class: Anticholinergics–antimuscarinics

AVAILABLE FORMS
Capsules: 10 mg
Injection: 10 mg/mL
Syrup: 10 mg/5 mL
Tablets: 10 mg✹, 20 mg

INDICATIONS & DOSAGES
➤ **IBS, other functional GI disorders**
Adults: Initially, 20 mg PO q.i.d.; may increase to 40 mg PO q.i.d. after 1 week unless adverse effects limit dosage escalation. If efficacy isn't achieved within 2 weeks or adverse effects require doses below 80 mg per day, discontinue drug.

Or, 10 to 20 mg IM q.i.d. Don't use IM form for longer than 1 to 2 days.

ADMINISTRATION
PO
• May give without regard for food.
• Protect from excessive heat. Store in light-resistant container.

IM
� *Alert:* Don't give subcut or IV.
• Thrombosis and injection-site reaction may occur if drug is inadvertently injected IV.
☺ *Alert:* Injection concentration is 10 mg/mL. Carefully calculate appropriate amount of solution for administering correct dose.

ACTION
Inhibits action of acetylcholine on postganglionic, parasympathetic muscarinic receptors, decreasing GI motility. Drug possesses local anesthetic properties that may be partly responsible for spasmolysis.

Route	Onset	Peak	Duration
PO, IM	Unknown	1–1.5 hr	Unknown

Half-life: Initially, about 1.8 hours.

ADVERSE REACTIONS
CNS: asthenia, dizziness, somnolence, nervousness. **EENT:** blurred vision, dry mouth. **GI:** nausea.

INTERACTIONS
Drug-drug. *Amantadine, antihistamines, antiparkinsonian drugs, disopyramide, glutethimide, meperidine, phenothiazines, procainamide, quinidine, TCAs:* May have additive adverse effects. Avoid using together.
Antacids: May interfere with dicyclomine absorption. Give dicyclomine at least 1 hour before antacid.
Antiglaucoma drugs: May decrease therapeutic effect of these drugs. Use together is contraindicated.
GI motility agents (metoclopramide): May decrease effectiveness of motility agents. Monitor therapy.

EFFECTS ON LAB TEST RESULTS
None reported.

CONTRAINDICATIONS & CAUTIONS
• Contraindicated in patients hypersensitive to anticholinergics, in children younger than age 6 months, and in those with obstructive uropathy, obstructive disease of the GI tract, reflux esophagitis, severe ulcerative colitis, toxic megacolon, myasthenia gravis, unstable CV status in acute hemorrhage, or glaucoma.
• Use cautiously in patients with tachycardia secondary to cardiac insufficiency or thyrotoxicosis.
• Don't use in patients with myasthenia gravis except to reduce adverse muscarinic effects of an anticholinesterase.
• Use cautiously in patients with autonomic neuropathy, hyperthyroidism, CAD, arrhythmias, HF, HTN, hiatal hernia, hepatic or renal disease, prostatic hyperplasia, known or suspected GI infection, and ulcerative colitis.
• Use cautiously in patients in hot or humid environments; drug can cause heatstroke.
• May affect GI absorption of various drugs (such as slowly dissolving dosage forms of digoxin) by affecting GI motility, which may increase serum concentrations.
• Drug may increase risk of intestinal dilation and perforation when given to patients with *Salmonella* dysentery.
☺ *Alert:* Use cautiously in patients sensitive to anticholinergic drugs, especially older adults and patients with mental illness, because of the risk of psychosis and delirium. When present, these signs and symptoms usually resolve within 12 to 24 hours after discontinuation of drug.

Reactions in bold italics are **life-threatening**. Interactions may have a *rapid onset* or a **delayed onset**.

• Safety and effectiveness in children haven't been established.

Dialyzable drug: Unknown.

⚠ *Overdose S&S:* Headache; nausea; vomiting; blurred vision; dilated pupils; hot, dry skin; dry mouth; dysphagia; CNS stimulation; muscle weakness; paralysis.

PREGNANCY-LACTATION-REPRODUCTION
• Use during pregnancy only if clearly needed. Epidemiologic studies didn't show an increased risk of structural malformations among infants exposed to products containing dicyclomine at doses up to 40 mg/day during first trimester.
• Drug appears in human milk. Contraindicated during breastfeeding.

NURSING CONSIDERATIONS
• Adjust dosage based on patient's needs and response. Safety and effectiveness for longer than 2 weeks haven't been established.
• IM injection is about twice as bioavailable as oral form.
• Dicyclomine may have atropine-like adverse reactions.
❸ *Alert:* Overdose may cause curare-like effects, such as respiratory paralysis. Keep emergency equipment available.
• Monitor patient's vital signs and urine output carefully.
• *Look alike–sound alike:* Don't confuse dicyclomine with dyclonine or doxycycline. Don't confuse Bentyl with Benadryl.

PATIENT TEACHING
• Tell patient when to take drug, and stress importance of doing so on time and at evenly spaced intervals and to report all adverse reactions.
• Advise patient to avoid driving and other hazardous activities if drowsiness, dizziness, or blurred vision occurs; to drink plenty of fluids to help prevent constipation; and to report hypersensitivity reactions, including rash or other skin eruption.
• Warn patient that heat prostration may occur during therapy when environmental temperatures are high. If signs and symptoms (fever, decreased sweating) occur, instruct patient to stop drug and contact prescriber.
• Caution patient not to breastfeed during therapy.

SAFETY ALERT!

digoxin
di-JOX-in

Digitek, Lanoxin✔*, Lanoxin Pediatric, Toloxin✦

Therapeutic class: Inotropes
Pharmacologic class: Cardiac glycosides

AVAILABLE FORMS
Injection*: 0.1 mg/mL (pediatric), 0.25 mg/mL
Oral elixir: 0.05 mg/mL (pediatric)
Tablets: 0.0625 mg, 0.125 mg, 0.25 mg

INDICATIONS & DOSAGES
❸ *Alert:* Factors to consider when a digoxin dosing regimen is selected include body weight, age, renal function, concomitant drugs, and disease. Toxic levels of digoxin are only slightly higher than therapeutic levels.
Adjust-a-dose (for all indications): Refer to manufacturer's information for recommended dosage adjustments based on renal function and weight.
➤ **HF, rapid digitalization**
Tablets
Adults and children older than age 10: Total loading dose is 10 to 15 mcg/kg PO. Initially, give half the total loading dose followed by one-quarter of the loading dose every 6 to 8 hours twice. Carefully assess clinical response and toxicity before each dose. Recommended starting maintenance dose for patients with normal renal function is 3.4 to 5.1 mcg/kg/day PO once daily. May increase every 2 weeks based on clinical response, serum drug levels, and toxicity. Refer to manufacturer's instructions for once-daily maintenance dose recommendations based on renal function and lean body weight.
Children ages 5 to 10: Total loading dose is 20 to 45 mcg/kg PO. Initially, give half the total loading dose followed by one-quarter of the loading dose every 6 to 8 hours twice. Carefully assess clinical response and toxicity before each dose. Recommended starting maintenance dosage for patients with normal renal function is 3.2 to 6.4 mcg/kg PO b.i.d. Refer to manufacturer's instructions for daily maintenance dose recommendations based on renal function and lean body weight.

✦Canada ◇OTC ◆Off-label use ✔Photoguide ⊕Do not crush *Liquid contains alcohol ▓Genetic

Oral elixir

In children, if a loading dose is needed, it can be administered with roughly half the total given as the first dose. Additional fractions of this planned total dose may be given at 4- to 8-hour intervals, with careful assessment of clinical response before each additional dose. If patient's clinical response necessitates a change from the calculated loading dose of digoxin, base the calculation of the maintenance dose on the amount actually given as the loading dose.

Children older than age 10: Loading dose is 10 to 15 mcg/kg PO given in divided doses, followed by maintenance dose of 3 to 4.5 mcg/kg PO once daily.

Children ages 5 to 10: Loading dose is 20 to 35 mcg/kg PO given in divided doses, followed by maintenance dose of 2.8 to 5.6 mcg/kg/dose PO b.i.d.

Children ages 2 to 5: Loading dose is 30 to 45 mcg/kg PO given in divided doses, followed by maintenance dose of 4.7 to 6.6 mcg/kg/dose PO b.i.d.

Infants ages 1 to 24 months: Loading dose is 35 to 60 mcg/kg PO given in divided doses, followed by maintenance dose of 5.6 to 9.4 mcg/kg/dose PO b.i.d.

Full-term infants: Loading dose is 25 to 35 mcg/kg PO in divided doses, followed by maintenance dose of 3.8 to 5.6 mcg/kg/dose PO b.i.d.

Preterm infants: Loading dose is 20 to 30 mcg/kg PO given in divided doses, followed by maintenance dose of 2.3 to 3.9 mcg/kg/dose PO b.i.d.

IV

Initially for all patients, give half the total loading dose followed by one-quarter of the loading dose every 6 to 8 hours twice. Carefully assess clinical response and toxicity before each dose. Recommended starting maintenance doses assume the presence of normal renal function. May increase every 2 weeks based on clinical response, serum drug levels, and toxicity. Refer to manufacturer's instructions for maintenance dose recommendations based on renal function and lean body weight.

Adults and children older than age 10: Total loading dose is 8 to 12 mcg/kg IV in divided doses, followed by a starting maintenance dose of 2.4 to 3.6 mcg/kg IV once daily.

Children ages 5 to 10: Total loading dose is 15 to 30 mcg/kg IV in divided doses, followed by a starting maintenance dose of 2.3 to 4.5 mcg/kg/dose IV b.i.d.

Children ages 2 to 5: Total loading dose is 25 to 35 mcg/kg IV in divided doses, followed by a starting maintenance dose of 3.8 to 5.3 mcg/kg/dose IV b.i.d.

Infants ages 1 to 24 months: Total loading dose is 30 to 50 mcg/kg IV in divided doses, followed by a starting maintenance dose of 4.5 to 7.5 mcg/kg/dose IV b.i.d.

Full-term infants: Total loading dose is 20 to 30 mcg/kg IV in divided doses, followed by a starting maintenance dose of 3 to 4.5 mcg/kg/dose IV b.i.d.

Preterm infants: Total loading dose is 15 to 25 mcg/kg IV in divided doses, followed by a starting maintenance dose of 1.9 to 3.1 mcg/kg/dose IV b.i.d.

➤ HF, gradual digitalization

Tablets

More gradual attainment of digoxin levels can also be accomplished by beginning an appropriate maintenance dosage without a loading dose in patients with normal renal function.

Adults and children older than age 10: Give starting maintenance dose of 3.4 to 5.1 mcg/kg PO once daily.

Children ages 5 to 10: Give starting maintenance dose of 3.2 to 6.4 mcg/kg/dose PO b.i.d.

Adjust-a-dose: Refer to manufacturer's instructions for dosage adjustment based on renal function and lean body weight.

Oral elixir

More gradual attainment of digoxin levels can also be accomplished by beginning an appropriate maintenance dosage without a loading dose in patients with normal renal function. In general, divided daily dosing is recommended for infants and children younger than age 10. In newborns, renal clearance of digoxin is diminished and suitable dosage adjustments must be observed, especially in preterm infants. Beyond the immediate newborn period, children generally require proportionally larger doses than adults on the basis of body weight or surface area. Children older than age 10 require adult dosages in proportion to their body weight.

Adults and children older than age 10: 3 to 4.5 mcg/kg PO once daily.

Children ages 5 to 10: 2.8 to 5.6 mcg/kg/dose PO b.i.d.

Children ages 2 to 5: 4.7 to 6.6 mcg/kg/dose PO b.i.d.

Infants ages 1 to 24 months: 5.6 to 9.4 mcg/kg/dose PO b.i.d.

Full-term infants: 3.8 to 5.6 mcg/kg/dose PO b.i.d.

Preterm infants: 2.3 to 3.9 mcg/kg/dose PO b.i.d.

Adjust-a-dose: Refer to manufacturer's instructions for dosage adjustment based on renal function and lean body weight.

IV

Gradual digitalization can be accomplished by beginning an appropriate maintenance dose. Recommended starting doses assume the presence of normal renal function. May increase every 2 weeks based on clinical response, serum drug levels, and toxicity. Refer to manufacturer's instructions for dose recommendations based on renal function and lean body weight.

Adults and children older than age 10: Give a starting dose of 2.4 to 3.6 mcg/kg IV once daily.

Children ages 5 to 10: Give a starting dose of 2.3 to 4.5 mcg/kg/dose IV b.i.d.

Children ages 2 to 5: Give a starting dose of 3.8 to 5.3 mcg/kg/dose IV b.i.d.

Infants ages 1 to 24 months: Give a starting dose of 4.5 to 7.5 mcg/kg/dose IV b.i.d.

Full-term infants: Give a starting dose of 3 to 4.5 mcg/kg/dose IV b.i.d.

Preterm infants: Give a starting dose of 1.9 to 3.1 mcg/kg/dose IV b.i.d.

➤ **Atrial fibrillation (chronic)**

PO, IV

Adults: If a loading dose is used, total loading dose is 10 to 15 mcg/kg PO (tablets, elixir). Initially, give half the total loading dose followed by one-quarter of the loading dose every 6 to 8 hours twice. Carefully assess clinical response and toxicity before each dose. Recommended starting maintenance dosage for patients with normal renal function is 3.4 to 5.1 mcg/kg (tablets) PO once daily or 3 to 4.5 mcg/kg (elixir) PO once daily.

Or, for more gradual PO digitalization in patients with normal renal function, begin with the starting maintenance dosage of 3.4 to 5.1 mcg/kg (tablets) PO once daily or 3 to 4.5 mcg/kg (oral elixir) PO once daily. May increase every 2 weeks based on clinical response, serum drug levels, and toxicity. Refer to manufacturer's instructions for once-daily maintenance dose recommendations based on renal function and lean body weight.

Or, if using an IV loading dose, give a total loading dose of 8 to 12 mcg/kg IV by initially giving half the total loading dose followed by one-quarter of the loading dose every 6 to 8 hours twice. Carefully assess clinical response and toxicity before each dose. Recommended starting maintenance dosage for patients with normal renal function is 2.4 to 3.6 mcg/kg IV once daily.

Or, for more gradual IV digitalization in patients with normal renal function, begin with the starting maintenance dosage of 2.4 to 3.6 mcg/kg IV once daily. Increase every 2 weeks according to clinical response, serum drug levels, and toxicity. Refer to manufacturer's instructions for dosage recommendations based on renal function and lean body weight.

ADMINISTRATION
PO
- Before giving loading dose, obtain baseline data (HR and rhythm, BP, and electrolyte levels) and ask patient about use of cardiac glycosides within the previous 2 to 3 weeks.
- Before giving drug, take apical-radial pulse for 1 minute. Record and notify prescriber of significant changes (sudden increase or decrease in pulse rate, pulse deficit, irregular beats and, particularly, regularization of a previously irregular rhythm). If these occur, check BP and obtain a 12-lead ECG.

IV

▼ Before giving loading dose, obtain baseline data (HR and rhythm, BP, and electrolyte levels) and ask patient about use of cardiac glycosides within the previous 2 to 3 weeks.

▼ Before giving drug, take apical-radial pulse for 1 minute. Record and notify prescriber of significant changes (sudden increase or decrease in pulse rate, pulse deficit, irregular beats and, particularly, regularization of a previously irregular rhythm). If these occur, check BP and obtain a 12-lead ECG.

▼ May administer undiluted or diluted with a fourfold or greater volume of D_5W, NSS, or sterile water for injection; use immediately. Using less than a fourfold volume of diluent could lead to precipitation of the digoxin.

▼ Infuse drug slowly over at least 5 minutes or longer.

▼ Protect solution from light.

▼ **Incompatibilities:** Other IV drugs.

ACTION
Inhibits sodium-potassium–activated adenosine triphosphatase, promoting movement of calcium from extracellular to intracellular cytoplasm and strengthening myocardial contraction. Also acts on CNS to enhance vagal tone, slowing conduction through the SA and AV nodes.

Route	Onset	Peak	Duration
PO	30–120 min	2–6 hr	3–4 days
IV	5–30 min	1–4 hr	3–4 days

Half-life: With normal renal function: adults, 36 to 48 hours; children, 18 to 36 hours.

ADVERSE REACTIONS
CNS: confusion, weakness, mental disturbances (anxiety, hallucinations, depression, delirium), dizziness, headache. **CV:** *arrhythmias, heart block.* **EENT:** blurred vision, diplopia, light flashes, photophobia, yellow-green color disturbance, halos around visual images. **GI:** anorexia, nausea, diarrhea, vomiting.

INTERACTIONS
Drug-drug. *ACE inhibitors, ARBs, COX-2 inhibitors, NSAIDs, other drugs that affect renal function:* May increase digoxin level. Monitor therapy.
Amiloride: May decrease digoxin effect and increase renal clearance of digoxin. Monitor patient for altered digoxin effect.
Amiodarone, diltiazem, **dronedarone,** *indomethacin, nifedipine,* **protease inhibitors, quinidine, verapamil:** May increase digoxin level. Monitor patient for toxicity.
Amphotericin B, carbenicillin, corticosteroids, **diuretics (chlorthalidone, loop diuretics, metolazone),** *ticarcillin:* May cause hypokalemia and hypomagnesemia, predisposing patient to cardiac glycoside toxicity. Monitor electrolyte levels.
Antacids: May decrease absorption of oral digoxin. Separate doses as much as possible.
Antibiotics (azole antifungals, macrolides, telithromycin, tetracyclines), propafenone, ritonavir: May increase risk of cardiac glycoside toxicity. Monitor patient for toxicity.
Beta blockers, calcium channel blockers: May have additive effects on AV node conduction, causing advanced or complete heart block. Use cautiously.
Cholestyramine, colestipol, metoclopramide: May decrease absorption of oral digoxin.

Monitor patient for decreased digoxin level and effect. Give digoxin 1.5 hours before or 2 hours after other drugs.
Dronedarone: May increase risk of sudden death. Monitor patient closely or consider therapy modification.
Parenteral calcium, thiazides: May cause hypercalcemia and hypomagnesemia, predisposing patient to digitalis toxicity. Monitor calcium and magnesium levels.
P-gp inducers or inhibitors: May alter digoxin level and effect. Consult interactions resource for specific drug.
Sotalol: May increase proarrhythmic effect. Use together cautiously.
Sympathomimetics (dopamine, epinephrine, norepinephrine): May increase risk of arrhythmias. Use together cautiously.
Drug-herb. *Foxglove, fumitory, goldenseal, hawthorn:* May increase cardiac effects. Discourage use together.
Licorice, Siberian ginseng: May increase toxicity. Monitor patient closely.
St. John's wort: May decrease digoxin serum concentration. Monitor therapy.

EFFECTS ON LAB TEST RESULTS
• May prolong PR interval or depress ST segment on ECG.

CONTRAINDICATIONS & CAUTIONS
• Contraindicated in patients hypersensitive to drug and in those with digitalis-induced toxicity, ventricular fibrillation, or ventricular tachycardia unless caused by HF.
• Don't use in patients with Wolff-Parkinson-White syndrome unless the conduction accessory pathway has been pharmacologically or surgically disabled.
• Use with extreme caution in older adults and in patients with acute MI, incomplete AV block, sinus bradycardia, PVCs, chronic constrictive pericarditis, hypertrophic cardiomyopathy, renal insufficiency, severe pulmonary disease, or hypothyroidism.
• Loading doses to initiate digoxin therapy in patients with HF aren't recommended by the American College of Cardiology Foundation/American Heart Association for management of HF. If patient is older than age 70, has impaired renal function, or has a low lean body mass, initially use low doses (0.125 mg daily or every other day).

Reactions in bold italics are *life-threatening*. Interactions may have a *rapid onset* or a ***delayed onset***.

D

• Safety and effectiveness in control of ventricular rate in children with atrial fibrillation haven't been established.

Dialyzable drug: No.

⚠ *Overdose S&S:* Ventricular tachycardia, ventricular fibrillation, bradycardia, heart block, cardiac arrest, hyperkalemia.

PREGNANCY-LACTATION-REPRODUCTION

• It isn't known if drug can cause fetal harm when used during pregnancy or if drug can affect reproductive capacity. Use during pregnancy only if clearly needed.

• If given during pregnancy, monitor neonate for signs and symptoms of digoxin toxicity, including vomiting and cardiac arrhythmias.

• Drug appears in human milk; however, an infant who is breastfed is exposed to an amount estimated to be far below the usual infant maintenance dose. Use cautiously, but the amount should have no pharmacologic effect on the infant.

NURSING CONSIDERATIONS

• Drug-induced arrhythmias may increase the severity of HF and hypotension.

• In children, cardiac arrhythmias, including sinus bradycardia, are usually early signs of toxicity.

• Patients with hypothyroidism are extremely sensitive to cardiac glycosides and may need lower doses.

• Monitor patient for toxicity. Toxic effects on the heart may be life-threatening and require immediate attention. Signs and symptoms of toxicity include anorexia, nausea, vomiting, visual changes, and cardiac arrhythmias. Patients with low body weight, advanced age, renal impairment, and electrolyte disturbances are at increased risk.

• Monitor digoxin level. Therapeutic level ranges from 0.5 to 2 nanograms/mL. Obtain blood for digoxin level at least 6 to 8 hours after last oral dose, preferably just before next scheduled dose.

🕚 *Alert:* Excessively slow pulse rate (60 beats/minute [bpm] or less) may be a sign of digitalis toxicity. Withhold drug and notify prescriber.

• Monitor potassium level carefully. Take corrective action before hypokalemia occurs. Hyperkalemia may result from digoxin toxicity.

• Reduce dose or discontinue drug for 1 or 2 days before elective cardioversion. Adjust dosage after cardioversion.

• *Look alike–sound alike:* Don't confuse digoxin with doxepin.

PATIENT TEACHING

• Teach patient and a responsible family member about drug action, dosage regimen, how to take pulse, reportable signs, and follow-up care.

• Tell patient to report pulse rate less than 60 bpm or more than 110 bpm or skipped beats or other rhythm changes.

• Instruct patient to report all adverse reactions promptly. Nausea, vomiting, diarrhea, appetite loss, and visual disturbances may indicate toxicity.

• Encourage patient to eat a consistent amount of potassium-rich foods.

• Tell patient not to substitute one brand for another without discussing with prescriber.

• Advise patient to avoid using herbal supplements and to consult prescriber before taking one.

---

dilTIAZem hydrochloride
dil-TYE-a-zem

Cardizem✐, Cardizem CD✐, Cardizem LA✐, Cartia XT, Dilt XR, Taztia XT, Tiazac, Tiazac XC ✲

Therapeutic class: Antihypertensives
Pharmacologic class: Calcium channel blockers

AVAILABLE FORMS

Capsules (extended-release) 🚫: 60 mg, 90 mg, 120 mg, 180 mg, 240 mg, 300 mg, 360 mg, 420 mg
Injection: 5 mg/mL in 5-, 10-, and 25-mL vials
Powder for injection: 100 mg
Tablets: 30 mg, 60 mg, 90 mg, 120 mg
Tablets (extended-release) 🚫: 120 mg, 180 mg, 240 mg, 300 mg, 360 mg, 420 mg

INDICATIONS & DOSAGES

➤ **To manage Prinzmetal or variant angina or chronic stable angina pectoris**
Adults: 30 mg PO q.i.d. (immediate-release tablets) before meals and at bedtime. Increase dose gradually to maximum of 360 mg/day

---

divided into three or four doses, as indicated. Or, give 120- or 180-mg extended-release capsule or 180-mg extended-release tablet PO once daily. Adjust over a 7- to 14-day period as needed and tolerated up to a maximum dose of 360 mg/day (Cardizem LA), 480 mg/day (Cardizem CD, Cartia XT), or 540 mg/day (Tiazac, Taztia XT).

➤ **HTN, alone or as combination therapy**
Adults: Initially 180 to 240 mg extended-release capsules PO once daily. Adjust dosage based on patient response to a maximum dose of 480 mg/day (Cardizem CD, Cartia XT). Or, 120 to 240 mg extended-release capsules PO once daily. Adjust dosage based on patient response to a maximum dose of 540 mg/day (Tiazac, Taztia XT). Or, 180 to 240 mg extended-release tablet PO once daily. Dosage can be adjusted approximately every 14 days to a maximum of 540 mg daily.

➤ **To control rapid ventricular rate in atrial fibrillation or atrial flutter; to rapidly convert paroxysmal supraventricular tachycardia (PSVT) to sinus rhythm**
Adults: 0.25 mg/kg IV bolus. If after 15 minutes rate control is insufficient, repeat with dose of 0.35 mg/kg IV bolus. If patient with atrial fibrillation or flutter responds after one to two bolus doses, begin continuous infusion of 5 to 10 mg/hour. May increase infusion rate in 5-mg/hour increments according to ventricular response up to maximum of 15 mg/hour. If patient with PSVT fails to respond, consider alternative therapy.

ADMINISTRATION
PO
• Don't crush or allow patient to chew extended-release tablets or capsules; they should be swallowed whole.
• Tiazac and Taztia extended-release capsules can be opened and the contents sprinkled onto a spoonful of applesauce. The applesauce must be eaten immediately and without chewing, followed by a glass of cool water.
IV
▼ For direct injection, no need to dilute 5-mg/mL injection. Give over 2 minutes.
▼ For continuous infusion, refer to manufacturer's instructions for dilution and administration. Compatible solutions include NSS, D_5W, or 5% dextrose and half-NSS.
▼ Continuous infusion rate ranges from 5 to 15 mg/hour.

▼ For direct injection or continuous infusion, give slowly while monitoring ECG and BP continuously.
▼ Don't infuse for longer than 24 hours.
▼ **Incompatibilities:** Acetazolamide, acyclovir, aminophylline, ampicillin, ampicillin sodium–sulbactam sodium, diazepam, furosemide, heparin, hydrocortisone, insulin, methylprednisolone, nafcillin, phenytoin, rifampin, sodium bicarbonate, thiopental.

ACTION
Inhibits calcium ion influx across cardiac and smooth-muscle cells, decreasing myocardial contractility and oxygen demand. Drug also dilates coronary arteries and arterioles.

Route	Onset	Peak	Duration
PO	30–60 min	2–4 hr	6–8 hr
PO (extended-release capsule)	2–3 hr	10–14 hr	12–24 hr
PO (LA)	3–4 hr	11–18 hr	6–9 hr
IV	<3 min	2–7 min	1–10 hr

Half-life: 3 to 9 hours.

ADVERSE REACTIONS
CNS: headache, dizziness, asthenia. **CV:** edema, *arrhythmias, AV block, bradycardia, HF,* flushing, hypotension, conduction abnormalities, abnormal ECG, palpitations, vasodilation. **EENT:** conjunctivitis, sinus congestion, pharyngitis, rhinitis. **GI:** nausea, vomiting, constipation, diarrhea, dyspepsia, abdominal discomfort. **GU:** erectile dysfunction. **Metabolic:** gout. **Respiratory:** bronchitis, cough, dyspnea. **Skin:** rash, injection-site reaction. **Other:** infection, flulike symptoms.

INTERACTIONS
Drug-drug. *Anesthetics:* May increase effects of anesthetics. Monitor patient.
Atazanavir, cimetidine: May inhibit diltiazem metabolism, increasing additive AV node conduction slowing. Monitor patient for toxicity.
Beta blockers (propranolol): May increase risk of bradycardia, AV block, and depressed contractility. Use together cautiously.
Buspirone, quinidine, sirolimus, tacrolimus: May increase level of these drugs. Monitor drug levels and patient for toxicity.

Carbamazepine: May increase level of carbamazepine. Monitor carbamazepine level, and watch for signs and symptoms of toxicity.

Cyclosporine: May increase cyclosporine level. Monitor cyclosporine level with each dosage change.

Diazepam, midazolam, triazolam: May increase CNS depression and prolong effects of these drugs. Use lower dose of these benzodiazepines.

Digoxin: May have additive effect that slows AV node conduction and increases digoxin level. Monitor patient for digoxin toxicity.

HMG-CoA reductase inhibitors (lovastatin, simvastatin): May increase risk of myopathy, rhabdomyolysis, and kidney failure. Use lower starting and maintenance doses of diltiazem and statins.

Ivabradine: May increase ivabradine level, which may exacerbate bradycardia and conduction disturbances. Avoid use together.

Lithium: May reduce lithium level, causing loss of mania control. May also enhance lithium's neurotoxic effects. Monitor therapy.

Rifampin: May lower diltiazem level significantly. Avoid use together.

Theophylline: May enhance action of theophylline, causing intoxication. Monitor theophylline levels.

EFFECTS ON LAB TEST RESULTS
• May increase CK, glucose, ALT, AST, LDH, bilirubin, and ALP levels.
• May decrease Hb level and leukocyte and platelet counts.
• May increase urine crystals and uric acid level.

CONTRAINDICATIONS & CAUTIONS
• Contraindicated in patients hypersensitive to drug and in those with sick sinus syndrome or second- or third-degree AV block in the absence of an artificial pacemaker, hypotension (systolic less than 90 mm Hg), acute MI, and pulmonary congestion.
• Additional contraindications for IV form include patients who have atrial fibrillation or flutter with an accessory bypass tract, as in Wolff-Parkinson-White syndrome or short PR interval syndrome, cardiogenic shock, and ventricular tachycardia, and within a few hours of IV beta-blocker therapy.
• Use cautiously in older adults and patients with HF, hypertrophic obstructive cardiomyopathy, or impaired hepatic or renal function.

• Safety and effectiveness in children haven't been established.

Dialyzable drug: No.

⚠ *Overdose S&S:* Bradycardia, hypotension, heart block, cardiac failure.

PREGNANCY-LACTATION-REPRODUCTION
• There are no adequate well-controlled studies during pregnancy. Use during pregnancy only if clearly needed.
• Drug appears in human milk. Patient should discontinue breastfeeding or discontinue drug.

NURSING CONSIDERATIONS
• Monitor BP and HR when starting therapy and during dosage adjustments.
• Maximal antihypertensive effect may not be seen for 14 days.
• If systolic BP is below 90 mm Hg or HR is below 60 beats/minute, withhold dose and notify prescriber.
• Monitor ECG and hepatic and renal function.
• *Look alike–sound alike:* Don't confuse Tiazac with Ziac.

PATIENT TEACHING
• Instruct patient in safe drug administration, to take drug as prescribed, even when feeling better, and to report all adverse reactions.
• Advise patient to avoid hazardous activities during start of therapy.
• If nitrate therapy is prescribed during dosage adjustment, stress patient adherence. Tell patient that SL nitroglycerin may be taken with drug, as needed, when angina symptoms are acute.

diphenhydrAMINE hydrochloride
dye-fen-HYE-drah-meen

Banophen ◇, Benadryl ◇, Children's Benadryl Allergy ◇, Sominex ◇, Unisom SleepMelts ◇, ZzzQuil ◇

Therapeutic class: Antihistamines
Pharmacologic class: Ethanolamines

AVAILABLE FORMS
Capsules: 25 mg ◇, 50 mg ◇
Elixir: 12.5 mg/5 mL ◇*
Injection: 50 mg/mL
Liquid: 12.5 mg/5 mL ◇*, 50 mg/30 mL*

Tablets: 25 mg ◇, 50 mg ◇
Tablets (chewable): 12.5 mg ◇
Tablets (ODTs): 25 mg ◇

INDICATIONS & DOSAGES

➤ **Rhinitis, allergy symptoms, motion sickness, Parkinson disease**
Adults and children age 12 and older: 25 to 50 mg PO every 4 to 6 hours. Maximum, 300 mg PO daily. Or, 10 to 50 mg IV or deep IM. Maximum IV or IM dosage, 400 mg daily. Don't exceed 25 mg/minute when giving IV.
Children ages 6 to 11: 12.5 to 25 mg PO every 4 to 6 hours. Maximum dose is 150 mg daily.
Children other than premature infants and neonates: 5 mg/kg/24 hours deep IM or IV divided into four doses. Don't exceed 25 mg/minute when giving IV. Maximum dose is 300 mg daily.

➤ **Nighttime sleep aid**
Adults and children age 12 and older: 25 to 50 mg PO at bedtime.

➤ **Nonproductive cough**
Adults and children age 12 and older: 25 to 50 mg (liquid) PO every 4 hours. Don't exceed 300 mg daily.
Children ages 6 to 11: 12.5 to 25 mg (liquid) PO every 4 to 6 hours or as directed. Don't exceed six doses in 24 hours.

ADMINISTRATION
PO
• Give drug with food or milk to reduce GI distress.
• Give 30 minutes before bedtime when given for insomnia, or 30 minutes before exposure when given for motion sickness.
IV
▼ For injection, don't exceed 25 mg/minute.
▼ May further dilute and give as an intermittent infusion over 10 to 15 minutes for children.
▼ **Incompatibilities:** Allopurinol, amobarbital, amphotericin B, cefepime, dexamethasone, foscarnet, haloperidol, pentobarbital, phenobarbital, phenytoin, thiopental.
IM
• Give IM injection deep into large muscle; alternate injection sites to prevent irritation.

ACTION
Competes with histamine for H_1-receptor sites. Prevents, but doesn't reverse, histamine-mediated responses, particularly those of the bronchial tubes, GI tract, uterus, and blood vessels.

Route	Onset	Peak	Duration
PO	15 min	1–4 hr	3–6 hr
IV	Immediate	1–4 hr	3–6 hr
IM	Unknown	1–4 hr	3–6 hr

Half-life: About 4 to 18 hours.

ADVERSE REACTIONS
CNS: ataxia, drowsiness, euphoria, sedation, sleepiness, dizziness, incoordination, *seizures*, confusion, insomnia, headache, vertigo, fatigue, restlessness, tremor, nervousness, irritability, paradoxical excitation, paresthesia. **CV:** palpitations, hypotension, tachycardia, chest tightness. **EENT:** diplopia, blurred vision, tinnitus, dry mouth, nasal congestion, pharyngeal edema. **GI:** nausea, epigastric distress, vomiting, diarrhea, constipation, anorexia. **GU:** dysuria, urine retention, urinary frequency, early menses. **Hematologic:** *thrombocytopenia, agranulocytosis,* hemolytic anemia. **Respiratory:** thickening of bronchial secretions, wheezing. **Skin:** urticaria, photosensitivity, diaphoresis, rash. **Other:** chills, dry mucous membranes, *anaphylactic shock.*

INTERACTIONS
Drug-drug. *CNS depressants:* May increase sedation. Use together cautiously.
MAO inhibitors: May increase anticholinergic effects. Avoid using together.
Other products that contain diphenhydramine (including topical therapy): May increase risk of adverse reactions. Avoid using together.
Drug-lifestyle. *Alcohol use:* May increase CNS depression. Discourage use together.
Sun exposure: May cause photosensitivity reactions. Advise patient to avoid extensive sunlight exposure.

EFFECTS ON LAB TEST RESULTS
• May decrease Hb level and hematocrit.
• May decrease granulocyte and platelet counts.
• May prevent, reduce, or mask positive result in diagnostic skin test.
• May produce false-positives in urine detection of methadone and phencyclidine and in serum TCA screens.

Reactions in bold italics are *life-threatening*. Interactions may have a *rapid onset* or a *delayed onset*.

CONTRAINDICATIONS & CAUTIONS

• Contraindicated in patients hypersensitive to drug and other similar antihistamines, in newborns, and in premature neonates.
• Don't use parenteral form as a local anesthetic due to risk of local necrosis.
• Use cautiously in patients with angle-closure glaucoma, stenosing peptic ulcer, symptomatic prostatic hyperplasia, bladder neck obstruction, pyloroduodenal obstruction, or asthma.
• Use with caution in patients with prostatic hyperplasia, asthma, COPD, increased IOP, hyperthyroidism, CV disease, and HTN.
• Children younger than age 6 should use drug only as directed by prescriber.
Dialyzable drug: Unlikely.
⚠ *Overdose S&S:* Dry mouth, fixed or dilated pupils, flushing, GI symptoms.

PREGNANCY-LACTATION-REPRODUCTION

• There are no adequate well-controlled studies during pregnancy. Use during pregnancy only if clearly needed.
• Drug appears in human milk. Contraindicated during breastfeeding.

NURSING CONSIDERATIONS

• Stop drug 4 days before diagnostic skin testing.
• Dizziness, excessive sedation, syncope, toxicity, paradoxical stimulation, and hypotension are more likely to occur in older adults.
• *Look alike–sound alike:* Don't confuse diphenhydramine with dimenhydrinate. Don't confuse Benadryl with Bentyl or benazepril.

PATIENT TEACHING

• Drug is in many OTC sleep and cold products. Advise patient to consult prescriber before using these products.
• Warn patient not to take this drug with any other products that contain diphenhydramine (including topical therapy) because of increased adverse reactions.
• Instruct patient in safe drug administration.
• Warn patient to avoid alcohol and hazardous activities that require alertness until CNS effects of drug are known.
• Tell patient to notify prescriber if tolerance develops because a different antihistamine may need to be prescribed.
• Warn patient of possible photosensitivity reactions. Advise use of a sunblock.

dipyridamole
dye-peer-IH-duh-mohl

Therapeutic class: Antiplatelet drugs
Pharmacologic class: Pyrimidine analogues

D

AVAILABLE FORMS

Injection: 5 mg/mL
Tablets: 25 mg, 50 mg, 75 mg

INDICATIONS & DOSAGES

➤ **To inhibit platelet adhesion in prosthetic heart valves (given together with warfarin)**
Adults and children age 12 and older: 75 to 100 mg PO q.i.d.
➤ **Alternative to exercise in evaluation of CAD during thallium myocardial perfusion scintigraphy**
Adults: 0.57 mg/kg (total dose) as an IV infusion at a constant rate over 4 minutes (0.142 mg/kg/minute).

ADMINISTRATION
PO
• Give 1 hour before or 2 hours after meals. If GI distress develops, may give with meals.
• Pharmacist can prepare oral suspension for patients unable to swallow tablets. Shake well before use.
IV
▼ For use as a diagnostic drug, dilute in half-NSS, NSS, or D_5W in at least a 1:2 ratio for a total volume of 20 to 50 mL.
▼ Inject thallium-201 within 5 minutes after completing the 4-minute dipyridamole infusion.
▼ Don't mix in same syringe or infusion container with other drugs.
▼ **Incompatibilities:** Other drugs.

ACTION

Inhibits adenosine deaminase and phosphodiesterase, which increases adenosine, a coronary vasodilator and platelet aggregation inhibitor.

Route	Onset	Peak	Duration
PO	Unknown	75 min	Unknown
IV	Unknown	2 min	Unknown

Half-life: 1 to 12 hours; alpha half-life of oral form, 40 minutes; beta half-life of oral form, 10 hours.

ADVERSE REACTIONS

CNS: dizziness, headache, fatigue, pain, paresthesia. **CV:** angina pectoris, chest pain, *ECG abnormalities*, flushing, hypotension, HTN, labile BP. **GI:** nausea, abdominal distress, diarrhea, vomiting. **Skin:** rash, pruritus.

INTERACTIONS

Drug-drug. *Adenosine:* May increase levels and cardiac effects of adenosine. Adjust adenosine dose as needed.

Anticoagulants, apixaban, dabigatran, drugs with antiplatelet properties (NSAIDs, P2Y$_{12}$ inhibitors, SSRIs), edoxaban, heparin, rivaroxaban, salicylates, thrombolytics: May increase bleeding risks. Monitor therapy.

Cholinesterase inhibitors: May counteract anticholinesterase effects and aggravate myasthenia gravis. Monitor patient.

Theophylline, other xanthine derivatives: May prevent coronary vasodilation by IV dipyridamole, causing a false-negative thallium-imaging result. Avoid using together.

EFFECTS ON LAB TEST RESULTS

• May increase liver enzyme levels.

CONTRAINDICATIONS & CAUTIONS

• Contraindicated in patients hypersensitive to drug.

• Use cautiously in patients with hypotension, hepatic impairment, or severe CAD.

🕭 *Alert:* IV drug is associated with cardiac death, fatal and nonfatal MI, ventricular fibrillation, symptomatic ventricular tachycardia, stroke, transient cerebral ischemia, seizures, anaphylactoid reaction, and bronchospasm.

• Safety and effectiveness in children younger than age 12 haven't been established.

Dialyzable drug: Unlikely.

⚠ *Overdose S&S:* Hypotension, warm feeling, flushes, diaphoresis, restlessness, weakness, dizziness, tachycardia.

PREGNANCY-LACTATION-REPRODUCTION

• There are no adequate well-controlled studies during pregnancy. Use during pregnancy only if clearly needed.

• Drug appears in human milk. Use cautiously during breastfeeding.

NURSING CONSIDERATIONS

• Observe for adverse reactions, especially with large doses. Monitor BP.

• Observe for signs and symptoms of bleeding.

• Dipyridamole injection may contain tartrazine, which may cause allergic reactions in some patients.

• *Look alike–sound alike:* Don't confuse dipyridamole with disopyramide.

PATIENT TEACHING

• Instruct patient to take drug exactly as prescribed.

• Advise patient to report adverse reactions promptly.

• Tell patient receiving drug IV to report discomfort at IV insertion site.

SAFETY ALERT!

DOBUTamine hydrochloride
doe-BYOO-ta-meen

Therapeutic class: Inotropes
Pharmacologic class: Adrenergics–beta$_1$ agonists

AVAILABLE FORMS

Dobutamine in 5% dextrose: 1 mg/mL (250 or 500 mg); 2 mg/mL (500 mg); 4 mg/mL (1,000 mg)
Injection: 12.5 mg/mL

INDICATIONS & DOSAGES

➤ **To increase cardiac output during short-term treatment of cardiac decompensation caused by depressed contractility from heart disease; adjunctive therapy in cardiac surgery**

Adults: Initially, 0.5 to 1 mcg/kg/minute IV infusion, titrating to optimum dosage of 2 to 20 mcg/kg/minute. Usual effective range to increase cardiac output is 2.5 to 15 mcg/kg/minute. Usual maximum dosage is 20 mcg/minute and, rarely, rates up to 40 mcg/kg/minute may be needed.

ADMINISTRATION

IV

▼ Before starting therapy, give a plasma volume expander to correct hypovolemia and, in patients who have atrial fibrillation with rapid ventricular response, a cardiac glycoside.

▼ Dilute concentrate before injecting. Compatible solutions include D$_5$W, D$_{10}$W, D$_5$W

---

and NSS injection, D_5W and half-NSS injection, D_5W in lactated Ringer injection, NSS for injection, lactated Ringer solution for injection, Isolyte-M with D_5W, Normosol-M in D_5W, 20% mannitol in water for injection, and sodium lactate injection.

▼ Oxidation may slightly discolor admixture. This doesn't indicate a significant loss of potency, provided drug is used within 24 hours of reconstitution.

▼ Don't administer unless solution is clear and container is undamaged.

▼ Give through a CVAD or large peripheral vein using an infusion pump.

▼ Titrate rate according to patient's condition.

▼ Infusions lasting up to 72 hours produce no more adverse effects than shorter infusions.

▼ Watch for irritation and infiltration; extravasation can cause tissue damage and necrosis. Change IV sites regularly to avoid phlebitis.

▼ Solution remains stable for 24 hours. Don't freeze.

▼ **Incompatibilities:** Diluents containing both sodium bisulfite and ethanol and other drugs; 5% sodium bicarbonate injection and other strongly alkaline solutions. Consult a drug incompatibility reference for more information.

ACTION

Stimulates heart's $beta_1$ receptors to increase myocardial contractility and stroke volume. At therapeutic dosages, drug increases cardiac output by decreasing peripheral vascular resistance, reducing ventricular filling pressure, and facilitating AV node conduction.

Route	Onset	Peak	Duration
IV	1–2 min	10 min	<5 min after infusion

Half-life: 2 minutes.

ADVERSE REACTIONS

CNS: headache. **CV:** increased BP, increased HR, angina, PVCs, phlebitis, nonspecific chest pain, palpitations, ventricular ectopy, hypotension. **GI:** nausea, vomiting. **Respiratory:** *asthma attack,* shortness of breath. **Other:** hypersensitivity reactions.

INTERACTIONS

Drug-drug. *Beta blockers:* May antagonize dobutamine effects. Avoid using together.

Guanethidine, oxytocic drugs: May increase pressor response, causing severe HTN. Monitor BP closely.

Linezolid: May increase hypertensive effect of sympathomimetics. May need to decrease initial doses of dobutamine and titrate to effect.

EFFECTS ON LAB TEST RESULTS

- May decrease potassium level.
- May decrease platelet count.

CONTRAINDICATIONS & CAUTIONS

- Contraindicated in patients hypersensitive to drug or its components and in those with idiopathic hypertrophic subaortic stenosis.
- Solutions containing dextrose may be contraindicated in patients with known allergy to corn or corn products.
- Use cautiously in patients with history of HTN because drug may increase pressor response.
- Use cautiously after acute MI.
- Use cautiously in patients with history of sulfite sensitivity. Anaphylaxis or asthmatic episodes can occur.
- May precipitate or exacerbate ventricular ectopic activity, but rarely has caused ventricular tachycardia.

Dialyzable drug: Unknown.

⚠ *Overdose S&S:* Anorexia, nausea, vomiting, tremor, anxiety, palpitations, headache, shortness of breath, anginal and nonspecific chest pain, HTN, tachyarrhythmias, myocardial ischemia, ventricular fibrillation, hypotension.

PREGNANCY-LACTATION-REPRODUCTION

- There are no adequate well-controlled studies during pregnancy. Use during pregnancy only if clearly needed and potential benefit justifies fetal risk.
- It isn't known if drug appears in human milk. Use cautiously during breastfeeding.

NURSING CONSIDERATIONS

🔔 *Alert:* Because drug increases AV node conduction, patients with atrial fibrillation may develop a rapid ventricular rate.
- Continuously monitor ECG, BP, pulmonary artery wedge pressure, cardiac output, and urine output during therapy.
- Correct hypovolemia before therapy.
- Monitor electrolyte levels. Drug may lower potassium level.

• *Look alike–sound alike:* Don't confuse dobutamine with dopamine.

PATIENT TEACHING
• Tell patient to report all adverse reactions promptly, especially labored breathing, angina, palpitations, dizziness, and drug-induced headache.
• Instruct patient to report discomfort at IV insertion site.

SAFETY ALERT!

DOCEtaxel
dohs-eh-TAX-ell

Taxotere*

Therapeutic class: Antineoplastics
Pharmacologic class: Taxoids

AVAILABLE FORMS
*Injection concentrate**: 20 mg/0.5 mL, 20 mg/mL, 80 mg/2 mL, 80 mg/4 mL, 160 mg/8 mL, 200 mg/10 mL
Injection solution: 20 mg/2 mL*, 80 mg/8 mL*, 160 mg/16 mL*

INDICATIONS & DOSAGES
Adjust-a-dose (for all indications): Refer to manufacturer's instructions for toxicity-related dosage adjustments and treatment.
➤ **Locally advanced or metastatic breast cancer after failure of previous chemotherapy**
Adults: 60 to 100 mg/m^2 IV over 1 hour every 3 weeks.
➤ **Adjuvant postsurgery treatment of operable, node-positive breast cancer**
Adults: 75 mg/m^2 IV as a 1-hour infusion given 1 hour after doxorubicin 50 mg/m^2 and cyclophosphamide 500 mg/m^2 every 3 weeks for six cycles. May use prophylactic G-CSF therapy to decrease risk of hematologic toxicities.
➤ **Locally advanced or metastatic NSCLC after failure of previous cisplatin-based chemotherapy**
Adults: 75 mg/m^2 IV over 1 hour every 3 weeks.
➤ **With cisplatin, unresectable, locally advanced, or metastatic NSCLC not previously treated with chemotherapy**
Adults: 75 mg/m^2 docetaxel IV over 1 hour, immediately followed by cisplatin 75 mg/m^2 IV over 30 to 60 minutes every 3 weeks.

➤ **Metastatic castration-resistant prostate cancer, with prednisone**
Adults: 75 mg/m^2 IV, as a 1-hour infusion every 3 weeks, given with 5 mg prednisone PO b.i.d. continuously. Premedicate with dexamethasone 8 mg PO at 12 hours, 3 hours, and 1 hour before docetaxel infusion.
➤ **Advanced gastric adenocarcinoma, in combination with cisplatin and 5-FU**
Adults: Premedicate with antiemetics and hydration per cisplatin recommendations. Give 75 mg/m^2 docetaxel IV over 1 hour, followed by cisplatin 75 mg/m^2 IV over 1 to 3 hours both on day 1 only, then 5-FU 750 mg/m^2 IV daily as a 24-hour continuous infusion for 5 days beginning at the end of cisplatin infusion. Repeat cycle every 3 weeks.
➤ **Induction treatment of inoperable locally advanced squamous cell cancer of the head and neck (SCCHN), with cisplatin and 5-FU**
Adults: Premedicate with antiemetics and hydration per cisplatin recommendations. Use prophylaxis for neutropenic infections. Give 75 mg/m^2 IV infusion over 1 hour, followed by cisplatin 75 mg/m^2 IV infusion over 1 hour, on day 1, followed by 5-FU 750 mg/m^2 daily as a continuous IV infusion for 5 days. Repeat this regimen every 3 weeks for four cycles. After chemotherapy, patients should receive radiotherapy.
➤ **Induction treatment for locally advanced (unresectable, low surgical cure, or organ preservation) SCCHN with cisplatin and 5-FU before chemoradiotherapy**
Adults: Premedicate with antiemetics and hydration per cisplatin recommendations. Give 75 mg/m^2 IV infusion over 1 hour, followed by cisplatin 100 mg/m^2 IV infusion over 30 minutes to 3 hours on day 1, followed by 5-FU 1,000 mg/m^2 daily as a continuous IV infusion from day 1 to day 4. Repeat this regimen every 3 weeks for three cycles. After chemotherapy, patients should receive chemoradiotherapy.

ADMINISTRATION
IV
▼ Give oral corticosteroid such as dexamethasone 16 mg PO (8 mg b.i.d.) daily for 3 days, starting 1 day before docetaxel administration, to reduce risk or severity of fluid retention and hypersensitivity reactions.

Reactions in bold italics are *life-threatening*. Interactions may have a *rapid onset* or a **delayed onset**.

▼ Drug is a hazardous agent; use safe handling precautions according to facility protocol.

⚠ *Alert:* Carefully read package instructions and confirm concentration being used; admixture errors have occurred due to the availability of various concentrations.

▼ If using the 2-vial formulation, dilute using supplied diluent. Let drug and diluent stand at room temperature for 5 minutes before mixing. After adding all the diluent to drug vial, gently rotate vial for about 45 seconds. Let solution stand for a few minutes so foam dissipates. All foam need not dissipate before preparing infusion solution.

▼ If using the 1-vial formulation, no dilution is needed. The product comes ready to add to the infusion solution.

▼ Prepare infusion solution by withdrawing needed amount of premixed solution from vial and injecting it into 250 mL NSS or D_5W to yield 0.3 to 0.74 mg/mL. Doses of more than 200 mg need a larger volume to stay below 0.74 mg/mL of drug. Mix infusion thoroughly by manual rotation.

▼ Prepare and store infusion solution in bottles (glass, polyolefin, or polypropylene) or plastic bags, and give through polyethylene-lined administration sets.

▼ Contact between undiluted concentrate and polyvinyl chloride equipment or devices isn't recommended.

▼ If solution isn't clear or if it contains precipitate, discard.

▼ Infuse over 1 hour.

▼ Store unopened vials between 36° and 77° F (2° and 25° C).

⚠ *Alert:* Mark all waste materials with CHEMOTHERAPY HAZARD labels.

▼ **Incompatibilities:** None listed by manufacturer. Consult a drug incompatibility reference for more information.

ACTION

Promotes formation and stabilization of nonfunctional microtubules. This prevents mitosis and leads to cell death.

Route	Onset	Peak	Duration
IV	Rapid	Unknown	Unknown

Half-life: Terminal phase, 11 hours.

ADVERSE REACTIONS

CNS: asthenia, paresthesia, dysesthesia, fatigue, dizziness, peripheral neuropathy, weakness, dysgeusia, drug fever, syncope. **CV:** peripheral edema, *arrhythmias,* chest tightness, flushing, vasodilation, hypotension, lymphedema, phlebitis, left ventricular dysfunction. **EENT:** tearing, conjunctivitis, altered hearing. **GI:** anorexia, diarrhea, dysphagia, esophagitis, nausea, stomatitis, abdominal pain, vomiting. **GU:** amenorrhea. **Hematologic:** *febrile neutropenia, leukopenia, myelosuppression, neutropenia, thrombocytopenia,* anemia. **Hepatic:** *hepatotoxicity.* **Metabolic:** fluid retention. **Musculoskeletal:** myalgia, arthralgia. **Respiratory:** dyspnea, cough, *pulmonary edema.* **Skin:** alopecia, skin toxicity, nail disorder, rash, reaction at injection site. **Other:** infection, chills, hypersensitivity reactions, *death.*

INTERACTIONS

Drug-drug. *Compounds that induce, inhibit, or are metabolized by CYP3A4 (cyclosporine, erythromycin, ketoconazole, troleandomycin):* May modify metabolism of docetaxel. Use together cautiously.

Ketoconazole or other CYP3A4 inhibitors: May increase docetaxel level and toxicity, including neutropenia. Monitor patient closely. Consider docetaxel dosage reduction if administration with strong CYP3A4 inhibitors can't be avoided.

EFFECTS ON LAB TEST RESULTS

• May increase ALP, ALT, AST, and bilirubin levels. May decrease Hb level.
• May decrease platelet and WBC counts.

CONTRAINDICATIONS & CAUTIONS

Boxed Warning Contraindicated in patients with neutrophil counts less than $1,500/mm^3$. Perform frequent blood cell counts during therapy. ∎

Boxed Warning Treatment-related mortality increases in patients with abnormal liver function, those receiving higher doses, and patients with NSCLC and a history of prior treatment with platinum-based chemotherapy who receive docetaxel as a single agent at a dose of $100 mg/m^2$. ∎

Boxed Warning Patients with severe hepatic impairment shouldn't receive this drug. Don't give drug to patients with bilirubin levels exceeding the ULN, or those with ALT or AST levels above $1.5 \times$ ULN and ALP levels above $2.5 \times$ ULN. Obtain bilirubin, AST or ALT, and ALP levels before each therapy cycle. ∎

Boxed Warning Contraindicated in patients severely hypersensitive to drug or with a history of hypersensitivity to polysorbate 80. Some dosage forms may contain polysorbate 80. ∎

• SCAR, such as SJS, TEN, and acute generalized exanthematous pustulosis, has occurred.

• Safety and effectiveness in children haven't been established.

• Discontinue treatment if cystoid macular edema develops.

⚫ *Alert:* Some drug formulations may contain alcohol. Use cautiously in patients with hepatic impairment and in those in whom ethanol intake should be avoided or minimized. Some medications, such as pain relievers and sleep aids, may interact with the alcohol in the docetaxel infusion and worsen the intoxicating effects. A generic, nonalcoholic form of docetaxel is available.

Dialyzable drug: No.

⚠ *Overdose S&S:* Severe neutropenia, mild asthenia, cutaneous reactions, mild paresthesia, bone marrow suppression, peripheral neurotoxicity, mucositis.

PREGNANCY-LACTATION-REPRODUCTION

• Drug can cause fetal harm when used during pregnancy. Advise patients of childbearing potential to avoid becoming pregnant during therapy.

• Patients of childbearing potential should use effective contraception during treatment and for 6 months after final dose. Males with partners of childbearing potential should use effective contraception during treatment and for 3 months after final dose.

• It isn't known if drug appears in human milk. Patient should discontinue breastfeeding or discontinue drug, taking into account importance of drug to the patient.

NURSING CONSIDERATIONS

⚫ *Alert:* Drug should be administered only under the supervision of a physician experienced with antineoplastics and in a facility equipped to handle anaphylaxis.

• Verify pregnancy status before starting therapy.

• Bone marrow toxicity is the most frequent and dose-limiting toxicity. Frequent blood count monitoring is needed during therapy.

Boxed Warning Monitor patient closely for hypersensitivity reactions, especially during first and second infusions. Severe and even fatal reactions have occurred in patients who have received recommended 3-day dexamethasone premedication. For severe reactions, discontinue docetaxel immediately and administer appropriate therapy. ∎

• Patients who have previously experienced a hypersensitivity reaction to paclitaxel may develop a hypersensitivity reaction to docetaxel that may include severe or fatal reactions such as anaphylaxis. Monitor patients with a previous history of hypersensitivity to paclitaxel closely during initiation of therapy. Hypersensitivity reactions may occur within a few minutes after infusion is started. If minor reactions, such as flushing or localized skin reactions, occur, therapy interruption isn't required.

Boxed Warning Fluid retention is dose related and may be severe. Monitor patient closely. ∎

• Enterocolitis and neutropenic colitis (typhlitis) have occurred in patients treated with docetaxel alone and in combination with other chemotherapeutic agents, despite the coadministration of G-CSF. Use cautiously in patients with neutropenia, particularly those at risk for developing GI complications. Enterocolitis and neutropenic colitis may develop at any time, and could lead to death as early as the first day of symptom onset. Monitor patients closely from onset of signs and symptoms of GI toxicity.

⚫ *Alert:* Evaluate patients for history of problems with alcohol or drinking, liver disease, or other conditions that may be affected by alcohol intake.

⚫ *Alert:* Monitor patients for signs and symptoms of alcohol intoxication during and after treatment (appearance of being drunk, confusion, stumbling, somnolence). Consider using formulation with lowest alcohol content for patients who experience adverse reactions. Slowing infusion rate during administration may help resolve signs and symptoms of alcohol intoxication.

⚫ *Alert:* When indicated, cisplatin dose should follow docetaxel dose.

• Monitor patient for vision changes. If they occur, patient should have a prompt, comprehensive eye exam.

Reactions in bold italics are *life-threatening*. Interactions may have a *rapid onset* or a ***delayed onset***.

D

- Monitor patient who received docetaxel, doxorubicin, and cyclophosphamide for delayed myelodysplasia or myeloid leukemia.
- Monitor patient closely for signs and symptoms of SJS and TEN (fever, blistering and peeling of the skin, eye irritation and redness) and acute generalized exanthematous pustulosis (sudden high fever and rash). Consider permanently discontinuing drug in patients who experience these types of reactions.
- *Look alike–sound alike:* Don't confuse docetaxel with paclitaxel. Don't confuse Taxotere with Taxol.

PATIENT TEACHING

🕒 *Alert:* Caution patient to avoid driving, operating machinery, or performing other hazardous activities for 1 to 2 hours after treatment.

🕒 *Alert:* Instruct patient to immediately report signs and symptoms of alcohol intoxication that may occur during or 1 to 2 hours after treatment.

- Caution patient of childbearing potential to avoid pregnancy or breastfeeding during therapy.
- Inform patient of potential hazard to the fetus if drug is used during pregnancy.
- Advise patient to report any pain or burning at injection site during or after administration.
- Warn patient that hair loss occurs in almost 80% of patients and usually reverses when treatment stops; cases of permanent hair loss have been reported.
- Tell patient to report all adverse reactions and to promptly report sore throat, fever, skin reactions, or unusual bruising or bleeding, as well as signs and symptoms of fluid retention, such as swelling or shortness of breath.
- Tell patient to report new or worsening signs or symptoms of GI toxicity.

---

dofetilide
doe-FE-ti-lyed

Tikosyn

Therapeutic class: Antiarrhythmics
Pharmacologic class: Antiarrhythmics

AVAILABLE FORMS
Capsules: 125 mcg, 250 mcg, 500 mcg

INDICATIONS & DOSAGES

➤ **To maintain normal sinus rhythm in patients with symptomatic atrial fibrillation or atrial flutter lasting longer than 1 week who have been converted to normal sinus rhythm; to convert atrial fibrillation and atrial flutter to normal sinus rhythm**

Adults: Individualized dosage based on CrCl and baseline QTc interval (or QT interval if HR is below 60 beats/minute), determined before first dose; usually 500 mcg PO b.i.d.

Adjust-a-dose: If CrCl is 40 to 60 mL/minute, starting dose is 250 mcg PO b.i.d.; if CrCl is 20 to 39 mL/minute, starting dose is 125 mcg PO b.i.d. Don't use drug at all if CrCl is less than 20 mL/minute.

Determine QTc interval 2 to 3 hours after first dose. If QTc interval has increased by more than 15% above baseline or if it's more than 500 msec (550 msec in patients with ventricular conduction abnormalities), adjust dosage as follows: If starting dose based on CrCl was 500 mcg PO b.i.d., give 250 mcg PO b.i.d. If starting dose based on CrCl was 250 mcg b.i.d., give 125 mcg b.i.d. If starting dose based on CrCl was 125 mcg b.i.d., give 125 mcg once a day.

Determine QTc interval 2 to 3 hours after each subsequent dose while patient is in hospital. If at any time after second dose the QTc interval exceeds 500 msec (550 msec in patients with ventricular conduction abnormalities), stop drug.

ADMINISTRATION
PO
- Give drug without regard for food or antacid administration.
- Protect from moisture and humidity.
- If a dose is missed, don't double the dose. Give next dose at the usual time.

ACTION
Prolongs repolarization without affecting conduction velocity (Vaughan-Williams Class III antiarrhythmic). Drug doesn't affect sodium channels, alpha-adrenergic receptors, or beta-adrenergic receptors.

Route	Onset	Peak	Duration
PO	Unknown	2–3 hr	Unknown

Half-life: 10 hours.

ADVERSE REACTIONS

CNS: headache, *stroke*, dizziness, insomnia, anxiety, migraine, *cerebral ischemia*, asthenia, paresthesia, syncope, pain. **CV:** chest pain, *ventricular fibrillation, ventricular tachycardia, torsades de pointes, AV block, heart block, bradycardia, cardiac arrest, MI,* bundle-branch block, angina, atrial fibrillation, supraventricular tachycardia, HTN, palpitations, peripheral edema. **GI:** nausea, diarrhea, abdominal pain. **GU:** UTI. **Hepatic:** liver damage. **Musculoskeletal:** back pain, arthralgia, facial paralysis. **Respiratory:** respiratory tract infection, dyspnea, increased cough. **Skin:** rash, diaphoresis. **Other:** *angioedema,* flulike syndrome, accidental injury.

INTERACTIONS

Drug-drug. *Antiarrhythmics (Class I and III):* May increase dofetilide level. Withhold other antiarrhythmics for at least three plasma half-lives before giving dofetilide.
CYP3A4 inhibitors (amiodarone, **azole antifungals,** *cannabinoids, diltiazem,* **macrolides,** *nefazodone, norfloxacin, protease inhibitors, quinine, SSRIs, zafirlukast):* May decrease metabolism and increase dofetilide level. Use together cautiously.
Drugs secreted by renal tubular cationic transport (amiloride, metformin, triamterene): May increase dofetilide level. Use together cautiously; monitor patient for adverse effects.
Drugs that prolong QT interval: May increase risk of QT interval prolongation. Avoid using together.
Inhibitors of renal cationic secretion (cimetidine, ketoconazole, megestrol, prochlorperazine, sulfamethoxazole–trimethoprim), trimethoprim, verapamil: May increase dofetilide level. Use together is contraindicated.
Potassium-depleting diuretics: May increase risk of hypokalemia or hypomagnesemia. Monitor potassium and magnesium levels.
Thiazide diuretics: May cause hypokalemia and arrhythmias. Use together is contraindicated.
Drug-food. *Grapefruit juice:* May decrease hepatic metabolism and increase drug level. Discourage use together.

EFFECTS ON LAB TEST RESULTS

None reported.

CONTRAINDICATIONS & CAUTIONS

- Contraindicated in patients hypersensitive to drug, in those with congenital or acquired long QT interval syndromes or with baseline QTc interval greater than 440 msec (500 msec in patients with ventricular conduction abnormalities), and in those with CrCl less than 20 mL/minute.
- Use cautiously in patients with severe hepatic impairment.
- Safety and effectiveness in children haven't been studied.
Dialyzable drug: Unknown.
⚠ *Overdose S&S:* Prolonged QT interval, ventricular fibrillation, torsades de pointes, cardiac arrest.

PREGNANCY-LACTATION-REPRODUCTION

- There are no adequate well-controlled studies during pregnancy. Use during pregnancy only if clearly needed and potential benefit justifies fetal risk.
- It isn't known if drug appears in human milk. Patients shouldn't breastfeed during therapy.

NURSING CONSIDERATIONS

Boxed Warning When dofetilide is initiated or reinitiated, patients should be hospitalized for a minimum of 3 days in a facility that can provide calculations of CrCl, continuous ECG monitoring, and cardiac resuscitation. ■
- Don't discharge patient within 12 hours of conversion to normal sinus rhythm.
- Before discharge, ensure patient has an adequate supply of medication to allow uninterrupted dosing until patient can fill a prescription as an outpatient.
- Monitor patient for prolonged diarrhea, diaphoresis, and vomiting. Report these signs to prescriber because electrolyte imbalance may increase potential for arrhythmia development.
- Monitor renal function and QTc interval every 3 months. Drug can cause torsades de pointes ventricular arrhythmia.
- Use of potassium-depleting diuretics may cause hypokalemia and hypomagnesemia, increasing the risk of torsades de pointes. Give dofetilide after potassium level reaches and stays in normal range.
- Before starting dofetilide, stop previous antiarrhythmics while carefully monitoring patient for a minimum of three plasma half-lives. Don't give drug after amiodarone

---

Reactions in bold italics are *life-threatening*. Interactions may have a *rapid onset* or a *delayed onset*.

therapy until amiodarone level falls below 0.3 mcg/mL or until amiodarone has been stopped for at least 3 months.
• If dofetilide must be stopped to allow dosing with interacting drugs, allow at least 2 days before starting other drug therapy.

PATIENT TEACHING
• Tell patient to report any change in OTC drug, prescription drug, supplement, or herb use.
• If antiulcer therapy is needed, tell patient that omeprazole, ranitidine, or antacids (aluminum and magnesium hydroxide) will be prescribed.
• Instruct patient in safe drug administration.
• Tell patient to immediately report chest pain, dyspnea, palpitations, excessive or prolonged diarrhea, diaphoresis, vomiting, or loss of appetite or thirst.
• Instruct patient to notify prescriber of pregnancy.
• Advise patient not to breastfeed while taking dofetilide.

dolutegravir–rilpivirine
doe-loo-TEG-ra-vir/ril-pi-VIR-een

Juluca

Therapeutic class: Antiretrovirals
Pharmacologic class: Integrase strand transfer inhibitors–NNRTIs

AVAILABLE FORMS
Tablets: 50 mg dolutegravir base/25 mg rilpivirine base

INDICATIONS & DOSAGES
➤ **HIV-1 infection in patients who are virologically suppressed (HIV-1 RNA less than 50 copies/mL) on a stable antiretroviral regimen for at least 6 months with no history of treatment failure and no known substitutions associated with resistance to the individual components of the drug**
Adults: 50 mg dolutegravir/25 mg rilpivirine (1 tablet) PO once daily.
Adjust-a-dose: If administered with rifabutin, give an additional 25-mg rilpivirine tablet once daily for the duration of rifabutin coadministration.

ADMINISTRATION
PO
• Give with a meal.
• If a dose is missed, give it as soon as possible. Don't double the next dose.
• Store in original bottle; don't remove desiccant. Protect from moisture.
• Store at 68° to 77° F (20° to 25° C).

ACTION
Dolutegravir inhibits HIV integrase by binding to the integrase active site and blocking retroviral DNA integration essential for HIV replication. Rilpivirine inhibits HIV-1 replication by noncompetitive inhibition of HIV-1 reverse transcriptase.

Route	Onset	Peak	Duration
PO (dolutegravir)	Unknown	3 hr	Unknown
PO (rilpivirine)	Unknown	4 hr	Unknown

Half-life: Dolutegravir, 14 hours; rilpivirine, 50 hours.

ADVERSE REACTIONS
CNS: headache, depressive disorders (including *suicidality*), fatigue, dizziness, somnolence, anxiety, insomnia, sleep disorders, abnormal dreams. **GI:** diarrhea, abdominal pain or discomfort, flatulence, nausea, vomiting, decreased appetite. **GU:** membranous glomerulonephritis, mesangioproliferative glomerulonephritis, nephrolithiasis, renal impairment. **Hepatic:** *hepatotoxicity,* cholecystitis, cholelithiasis, *hepatitis.* **Metabolic:** hyperglycemia. **Musculoskeletal:** myositis, decreased bone mineral density. **Skin:** rash, pruritus. **Other:** immune reconstitution syndrome.

INTERACTIONS
Drug-drug. *Antacids (aluminum hydroxide, magnesium hydroxide, calcium carbonate):* May decrease rilpivirine level. Administer drug 4 hours before or 6 hours after antacids.
Anticonvulsants (carbamazepine, oxcarbazepine, phenobarbital, phenytoin): May decrease dolutegravir and rilpivirine levels, resulting in loss of virologic response. Use together is contraindicated.
Calcium and iron supplements (oral), multivitamins containing calcium or iron: May decrease dolutegravir level. Administer supplements and dolutegravir–rilpivirine together with a meal or give supplements 4 hours before or 6 hours after dolutegravir–rilpivirine.

Clarithromycin, erythromycin: May increase rilpivirine level. Consider alternative antibiotics such as azithromycin.

Dalfampridine: May increase dalfampridine level and risk of seizures. Consider benefits of concomitant therapy against the seizure risk. Consider alternative treatments.

Dexamethasone (systemic): May decrease rilpivirine level when dexamethasone is given as more than a single-dose treatment, resulting in loss of virologic response. Use together is contraindicated except for a single dose of dexamethasone.

Dofetilide: May increase dofetilide level, causing serious or life-threatening events. Use together is contraindicated.

Drugs containing polyvalent cations (aluminum, magnesium), such as buffered drugs, cation-containing products or laxatives, sucralfate: May decrease dolutegravir level. Administer dolutegravir–rilpivirine 4 hours before or 6 hours after drugs containing polyvalent cations.

Drugs known to prolong QTc interval and increase risk of torsades de pointes (amiodarone, erythromycin, haloperidol, oxycodone): May increase risk of QT-interval prolongation and torsades de pointes. Avoid use together.

H_2-receptor antagonists (cimetidine, famotidine, nizatidine): May decrease rilpivirine level. Give dolutegravir–rilpivirine at least 4 hours before or 12 hours after H_2-receptor antagonist.

Metformin: May increase metformin level. When used together, limit metformin to 1,000 mg daily when starting metformin or dolutegravir–rilpivirine. When starting or stopping dolutegravir–rilpivirine, monitor glucose level and adjust metformin dosage. Monitor glucose level when initiating concomitant use and after withdrawal of dolutegravir–rilpivirine.

Methadone: May decrease methadone level. No dosage adjustments are required when starting administration of methadone with dolutegravir–rilpivirine. Monitor patients on methadone maintenance therapy, as dosage adjustments may be needed.

Other antiretrovirals to treat HIV-1: Dolutegravir–rilpivirine is a complete regimen. Use with other antiretrovirals isn't recommended.

PPIs (esomeprazole, lansoprazole, omeprazole, pantoprazole, rabeprazole): May decrease rilpivirine level due to gastric pH increase, which may result in loss of virologic response. Use together is contraindicated.

Rifabutin: May decrease rilpivirine level. Give an additional 25-mg tablet of rilpivirine once daily for duration of the rifabutin coadministration.

Rifampin, rifapentine: May decrease dolutegravir and rilpivirine levels, resulting in loss of virologic response. Use together is contraindicated.

Drug-herb. *St. John's wort:* May decrease dolutegravir and rilpivirine levels, resulting in loss of virologic response. Use together is contraindicated.

EFFECTS ON LAB TEST RESULTS
• May increase ALT, AST, total bilirubin, CK, lipase, and glucose levels.
• May decrease cortisol level.

CONTRAINDICATIONS & CAUTIONS
• Contraindicated in patients hypersensitive to dolutegravir, rilpivirine, or other components of the tablet.
• Use cautiously in patients with underlying HBV or HCV infection or marked elevations in transaminase levels before treatment. Drug may increase risk of worsening or development of transaminase elevations, immune reconstitution syndrome, or HBV reactivation.
• Use cautiously in older adults and in patients with severe ESRD or severe hepatic impairment (Child-Pugh class C).
• Safety and effectiveness in children haven't been established.
Dialyzable drug: Unlikely.

PREGNANCY-LACTATION-REPRODUCTION
⚠ *Alert:* Dolutegravir may increase risk of neural tube birth defects, especially when taken at the time of conception and during the first trimester. Prescribers should weigh risks and benefits of drug and consider the use of alternative antiretrovirals before prescribing dolutegravir–rilpivirine to patients of childbearing potential.
⚠ *Alert:* Obtain pregnancy test to exclude pregnancy before start of therapy. Don't start drug in patients actively trying to become pregnant unless there's no suitable alternative.
⚠ *Alert:* Patients of childbearing potential using drug should use consistent, effective contraception.

Reactions in bold italics are *life-threatening*. Interactions may have a *rapid onset* or a *delayed onset*.

D

🌢 *Alert:* Enroll patients exposed to drug during pregnancy in the Antiretroviral Pregnancy Registry (1-800-258-4263).

• The CDC recommends that patients infected with HIV-1 shouldn't breastfeed due to the potential risk of HIV-1 transmission to the infant.

NURSING CONSIDERATIONS

• Verify pregnancy status before starting therapy.

🌢 *Alert:* Drug may cause severe skin reactions and severe hypersensitivity reactions such as DRESS syndrome with organ dysfunction, including liver injury. Monitor LFT values and initiate appropriate therapy.

🌢 *Alert:* Monitor patient for severe rash (or rash accompanied by fever, general malaise, skin blisters or skin peeling, oral blisters or lesions, conjunctivitis, facial edema, hepatitis, eosinophilia, angioedema, or difficulty breathing). Discontinue drug immediately if these signs or symptoms occur; delay in stopping drug may result in a life-threatening reaction.

• Monitor patient for severe depressive symptoms (depressed mood, depression, dysphoria, major depression, altered mood, negative thoughts, suicidality). Promptly evaluate depressive symptoms to assess whether the symptoms are related to the drug and to determine whether the risks of continued therapy outweigh the benefits.

• Monitor patient for signs and symptoms of hepatotoxicity (elevated LFT values, yellowing of the skin or whites of the eyes, dark urine, pale-colored stools, nausea, vomiting, loss of appetite, right-sided abdominal pain or tenderness), especially in patients with HBV or HCV infection, who may be at increased risk. Hepatotoxicity has also occurred in patients without preexisting hepatic disease or identifiable risk factors.

• *Look alike–sound alike:* Don't confuse rilpivirine with ritonavir. Don't confuse Juluca with Jublia or Januvia.

PATIENT TEACHING

• Teach patient to report all adverse reactions and to stop drug and immediately report a rash with signs or symptoms of hypersensitivity, DRESS syndrome, or hepatotoxicity.

• Tell patient to report all drugs and supplements being taken before start of therapy, as drug interactions may lead to loss of therapeutic effect, development of resistance, and an increase in adverse reactions.

• Advise patient that drug isn't a cure for HIV or AIDS. Stress the importance of taking drug as directed and staying on continuous antiretroviral therapy to control HIV infection and prevent resistance to therapy.

• Instruct patient on safe drug administration.

• Caution patient and caregiver to immediately report depressive symptoms (depressed mood, depression, dysphoria, major depression, altered mood, negative thoughts, suicidality).

• Instruct patient to immediately report pregnancy. Inform patient that there is an antiretroviral registry to monitor fetal outcomes if exposed to drug during pregnancy.

• Caution patient not to breastfeed during therapy.

donepezil hydrochloride
doe-NEP-eh-zill

Adlarity, Aricept🍁, Aricept ODT

Therapeutic class: Anti-Alzheimer drugs
Pharmacologic class: Acetylcholinesterase inhibitors

AVAILABLE FORMS

Tablets 🚫*:* 5 mg, 10 mg, 23 mg
Tablets (ODTs) 🚫*:* 5 mg, 10 mg
Transdermal patch: 5 mg/day, 10 mg/day

INDICATIONS & DOSAGES

➤ **Mild to moderate dementia of Alzheimer type**
Adults: 5 mg PO once daily for 4 to 6 weeks; may then increase dosage to 10 mg PO once daily.

➤ **Moderate to severe dementia of Alzheimer type**
Adults: Initially, 5 mg PO once daily for 4 to 6 weeks; dose may then be increased to 10 mg PO once daily. The dose may be increased to 23 mg PO once daily after patient has been taking 10 mg daily for 3 months.

✱ *NEW INDICATION:* **Mild, moderate, or severe Alzheimer dementia**
Adults: 5 mg/day transdermal patch applied once weekly. After 4 to 6 weeks, may increase to maximum dose of 10 mg/day. May switch patients taking 5 or 10 mg of PO donepezil to once weekly transdermal patch at the same

dose. May switch patients taking 5 mg PO donepezil for at least 4 weeks immediately to once weekly 10 mg/day transdermal system.

ADMINISTRATION
PO
- Allow ODT to dissolve on tongue; then follow with water.
- Give drug at bedtime, without regard for food.
- Don't split or crush tablets.

Transdermal
- At the end of 7 days, remove patch and apply a new one; apply only one patch at a time.
- When switching from PO, apply first patch with the last oral dose.
- Remove from refrigerator and allow pouch to reach room temperature before opening. Don't use heat source to warm patch. Don't apply a cold patch.
- Use within 24 hours of warming.
- Apply to back (avoid spine) or, if needed, may apply to upper buttocks or upper outer thigh on skin that won't be rubbed by tight clothing.
- Don't apply to same location for at least 2 weeks.
- Don't apply where medication, cream, lotion, or powder has recently been applied, or to reddened, irritated, or cut skin. Don't shave the site.
- Apply patch immediately after removing from pouch to clean, dry, intact skin with minimal hair.
- Press down firmly for 30 seconds to ensure good contact at edges of patch.
- Patch may remain on for bathing.
- Avoid prolonged exposure of patch to external heat sources (sunlight, saunas, heating pads).
- If patch falls off or a dose is missed, apply new patch immediately, then replace 7 days later.
- Store in refrigerator at 36° to 46° F (2° to 8° C).

ACTION
Inhibits acetylcholinesterase, the enzyme that causes acetylcholine hydrolysis, resulting in increased acetylcholine available for synaptic transmission in the CNS.

Route	Onset	Peak	Duration
PO	Unknown	3–8 hr	Unknown

Half-life: 70 hours.

ADVERSE REACTIONS
CNS: headache, insomnia, *seizures,* dizziness, fatigue, depression, somnolence, syncope, pain, hallucinations, abnormal dreams, hostility, nervousness, fever, confusion, emotional lability, personality disorder. **CV:** chest pain, HTN, hypotension, *hemorrhage.* **GI:** nausea, diarrhea, vomiting, anorexia, abdominal pain, *GI bleeding.* **GU:** urinary incontinence, urinary frequency, UTI. **Metabolic:** weight loss, dehydration, increased CK level, hyperlipidemia. **Musculoskeletal:** muscle cramps, arthritis, back pain. **Respiratory:** dyspnea, bronchitis. **Skin:** eczema, diaphoresis, ecchymosis, laceration; application-site pruritus, dermatitis, or pain. **Other:** accidental injury, infection.

INTERACTIONS
Drug-drug. *Anesthesia:* May exaggerate succinylcholine-type muscle relaxation during anesthesia. Use together cautiously.
Anticholinergics: May decrease donepezil effects. Avoid using together.
Anticholinesterases, bethanechol, cholinomimetics, succinylcholine: May have synergistic effect. Monitor patient closely.
Carbamazepine, dexamethasone, phenobarbital, phenytoin, rifampin: May increase rate of donepezil elimination. Monitor patient.
Drugs that prolong QT interval: May increase risk of QT-interval prolongation. Monitor patient; consider therapy modification.
NSAIDs: May increase gastric acid secretions. Monitor for active or occult GI bleeding.

EFFECTS ON LAB TEST RESULTS
- May increase CK and lipid levels.

CONTRAINDICATIONS & CAUTIONS
- Contraindicated in patients hypersensitive to drug or piperidine derivatives.
- Patches are contraindicated in patients with a history of allergic contact dermatitis with transdermal donepezil. Suspect contact dermatitis if reaction spreads beyond size of patch, if there's an intense reaction (increasing erythema, edema, papules, vesicles), or if symptoms don't improve within 48 hours of patch removal.
- Use cautiously in patients who take NSAIDs or have CV disease, are at risk for rhabdomyolysis and renal failure, or have asthma, obstructive pulmonary disease,

---

Reactions in bold italics are *life-threatening*. Interactions may have a *rapid onset* or a *delayed onset*.

seizure disorders, or urinary outflow impairment.
• Drug may increase gastric acid secretion. Use cautiously in patients with a history of GI bleeding or ulcer disease.
• Drug may prolong QT interval and increase risk of torsades de pointes and may cause vagotonic bradycardia, heart block, or syncope. Use cautiously in patients with sick sinus syndrome, bradycardia, or conduction abnormalities.
• Some products contain aspartame; avoid use or use cautiously in patients with phenylketonuria.
Dialyzable drug: Unknown.
⚠ *Overdose S&S:* Severe nausea, vomiting, salivation, diaphoresis, bradycardia, hypotension, respiratory depression, collapse, seizures, increasing muscle weakness.

PREGNANCY-LACTATION-REPRODUCTION
• There are no adequate well-controlled studies during pregnancy. Use during pregnancy only if clearly needed and potential benefit justifies fetal risk.
• It isn't known if drug appears in human milk. Use cautiously during breastfeeding.

NURSING CONSIDERATIONS
• Monitor patient for evidence of active or occult GI bleeding.
• Monitor patient for bradycardia because of potential for vagotonic effects.
• Monitor patient for signs and symptoms of GI intolerance (nausea, vomiting, diarrhea) at start of therapy and after dosage increases.
• Patients weighing less than 55 kg may experience increased nausea, vomiting, and weight loss.
• *Look alike–sound alike:* Don't confuse Aricept with Ascriptin, Aciphex, or Azilect.

PATIENT TEACHING
• Stress that drug doesn't alter underlying degenerative disease but can temporarily stabilize or relieve symptoms. Effectiveness depends on taking drug at regular intervals.
• Teach patient and caregiver safe drug administration.
• Advise patient and caregiver to report significant adverse effects or changes in overall health status immediately and to inform health care team that patient is taking drug before patient receives anesthesia.

• Tell patient to avoid OTC cold or sleep remedies because of risk of increased anticholinergic effects.

SAFETY ALERT!

DOPamine hydrochloride
DOE-pa-meen

D

Therapeutic class: Vasopressors
Pharmacologic class: Adrenergics

AVAILABLE FORMS
Injection: 40 mg/mL concentrate for IV infusion
Injection (premixed in D_5W): 0.8 mg/mL, 1.6 mg/mL, 3.2 mg/mL

INDICATIONS & DOSAGES
➤ **To treat shock and correct hemodynamic imbalances; to improve perfusion to vital organs; to increase cardiac output; to correct hypotension**
Adults: Initially, 2 to 5 mcg/kg/minute by IV infusion. Titrate dosage to desired hemodynamic or renal response. In patients who are seriously ill, start with 5 mcg/kg/minute and increase gradually in increments of 5 to 10 mcg/kg/minute to a rate of 20 to 50 mcg/kg/minute, as needed.
Adjust-a-dose: In patients with occlusive vascular disease, consider decreasing dosage for changes in extremity skin color or temperature. Initial dopamine dosages shouldn't exceed one-tenth of the usual dosage in patients who have received MAO inhibitors within the prior 2 to 3 weeks.

ADMINISTRATION
IV
▼ Dilute vials (concentrated solution) before administration. Dilute with D_5W, NSS, D_5W in NSS or half-NSS, lactated Ringer solution, D_5W in lactated Ringer solution, or sodium lactate injection. Mix just before use.
▼ Use a central line or large vein, as in the antecubital fossa, to minimize risk of extravasation.
▼ Use a continuous infusion pump to regulate flow rate. Avoid inadvertent administration of a bolus of the drug.
Boxed Warning Watch infusion site carefully for extravasation; if it occurs, stop

---

♣ Canada   ◇ OTC   ◆ Off-label use   🖉 Photoguide   ⓒ Do not crush   *Liquid contains alcohol   ▓ Genetic infusion immediately and call prescriber. To prevent sloughing and necrosis in ischemic areas, infiltrate the area with 5 to 10 mg phentolamine in 10 to 15 mL NSS as soon as possible. ▮

▼ Because solution will deteriorate rapidly, discard after 24 hours or earlier if it's discolored.

▼ Don't use product if it's darker than slightly yellow or discolored in another way.

▼ **Incompatibilities:** Alkalies (including sodium bicarbonate), oxidizing agents, iron salts.

ACTION
Stimulates dopaminergic, alpha and beta receptors of the sympathetic nervous system, resulting in a positive inotropic effect and increased cardiac output. Action is dose-related; large doses cause mainly alpha stimulation.

Route	Onset	Peak	Duration
IV	5 min	Unknown	<10 min after infusion

Half-life: 2 minutes.

ADVERSE REACTIONS
CNS: headache, anxiety. **CV:** hypotension, HTN, *ventricular arrhythmias,* atrial fibrillation, ectopic beats, tachycardia, angina, palpitations, conduction abnormalities, *bradycardia,* vasoconstriction. **GI:** nausea, vomiting. **Metabolic:** azotemia, hyperglycemia. **Respiratory:** dyspnea. **Skin:** necrosis and tissue sloughing with extravasation, piloerection.

INTERACTIONS
Drug-drug. *Alpha and beta blockers:* May antagonize dopamine effects. Monitor patient closely.
Diuretics (furosemide): May potentiate diuresis. Use together cautiously and monitor fluid volume closely.
Ergot alkaloids: May cause extremely high BP. Avoid using together.
Haloperidol: May suppress renal and mesenteric vasodilation. Monitor therapy.
Inhaled anesthetics: May increase risk of arrhythmias or HTN. Monitor patient closely.
⊕ *Alert: MAO inhibitors (phenelzine, tranylcypromine):* May cause fever, hypertensive crisis, or severe headache. Avoid using together; if patient received an MAO inhibitor in the past 2 to 3 weeks, initial dopamine dose is less than or equal to 10% of the usual dose.

Oxytocics, vasopressors: May cause severe, persistent HTN. Use together cautiously.
Phenytoin: May cause severe hypotension, bradycardia, and cardiac arrest. Monitor patient carefully.
TCAs: May increase pressor response. Monitor patient closely.

EFFECTS ON LAB TEST RESULTS
• May increase catecholamine, glucose, creatinine, and BUN levels.

CONTRAINDICATIONS & CAUTIONS
• Contraindicated in patients with uncorrected tachyarrhythmias, pheochromocytoma, or ventricular fibrillation.
• Use cautiously in patients with sulfite sensitivity. Hypersensitivity reactions, including anaphylaxis and asthmatic episodes, may occur.
• Use cautiously in patients with occlusive vascular disease, cold injuries, diabetic endarteritis, and arterial embolism, and in those taking MAO inhibitors.
Dialyzable drug: Unlikely.
⚠ *Overdose S&S:* Excessive BP elevation.

PREGNANCY-LACTATION-REPRODUCTION
• There are no adequate well-controlled studies during pregnancy. Use during pregnancy only if potential benefit justifies fetal risk.
• If vasopressors are used to correct hypotension or are added to a local anesthetic solution during labor or delivery, the interaction with some oxytocics may cause severe persistent HTN. Monitor patient closely.
• It isn't known if drug appears in human milk. Use cautiously during breastfeeding.

NURSING CONSIDERATIONS
• Most patients receive less than 20 mcg/kg/minute. Doses of 0.5 to 2 mcg/kg/minute mainly stimulate dopamine receptors and dilate the renal vasculature. Doses of 2 to 10 mcg/kg/minute stimulate beta receptors for a positive inotropic effect. Higher doses also stimulate alpha receptors, constricting blood vessels and increasing BP.
• Drug isn't a substitute for blood or fluid volume deficit. If deficit exists, replace fluid before giving vasopressors.
• During infusion, frequently monitor ECG, BP, cardiac output, central venous pressure, pulmonary artery wedge pressure, pulse rate,

---

urine output, and color and temperature of limbs.

• If diastolic pressure rises disproportionately with a significant decrease in pulse pressure, decrease infusion rate and watch carefully for further evidence of predominant vasoconstrictor activity, unless such an effect is desired.

• Observe patient closely for adverse reactions; dosage may need to be adjusted or drug stopped.

• Check urine output often. If urine flow decreases without hypotension, notify prescriber because dosage may need to be reduced.

🖱 *Alert:* After stopping drug, watch closely for sudden drop in BP. Taper dosage slowly to evaluate stability of BP, and provide IV fluids as clinically indicated to expand blood volume.

• Acidosis decreases effectiveness of drug. Correct before or during dopamine infusion.

• *Look alike–sound alike:* Don't confuse dopamine with dobutamine.

PATIENT TEACHING
• Tell patient to report adverse reactions promptly.
• Instruct patient to immediately report discomfort at IV insertion site.

doxazosin mesylate
dox-AY-zo-sin

Cardura🖊, Cardura XL

Therapeutic class: Antihypertensives
Pharmacologic class: Alpha blockers

AVAILABLE FORMS
Tablets (immediate-release): 1 mg, 2 mg, 4 mg, 8 mg
Tablets (extended-release) 🌀: 4 mg, 8 mg

INDICATIONS & DOSAGES
➤ **Essential HTN**
Adults: Initially, 1 mg immediate-release tablet PO daily. After the initial dose and with each dosage increase, monitor BP for at least 6 hours. May increase to 2 mg and thereafter 4 mg and 8 mg once daily, if needed. Maximum daily dose is 16 mg, but doses over 4 mg daily increase the risk of adverse reactions. Don't use extended-release formulation to treat HTN.

➤ **BPH**
Adults: Initially, 1 mg immediate-release tablet PO once daily in the morning or evening; may increase at 1- or 2-week intervals to 2 mg and, thereafter, 4 mg and 8 mg once daily, if needed. Or, one 4-mg extended-release tablet once daily with breakfast. May increase to 8 mg in 3 to 4 weeks.

ADMINISTRATION
PO
• Patient should swallow extended-release tablets whole and not chew, divide, cut, or crush them.
• Give extended-release tablet with breakfast.
• Don't give evening dose the night before switching to extended-release tablets from immediate-release formula. Start extended-release tablets at lowest dose (4 mg once daily) the next morning.
• If therapy is interrupted for several days, restart drug at initial dosing regimen.

ACTION
An alpha$_1$ blocker that acts on the peripheral vasculature to reduce peripheral vascular resistance and produce vasodilation. Drug also decreases smooth muscle tone in the prostate and bladder neck.

Route	Onset	Peak	Duration
PO	1–2 hr	2–13.5 hr	24 hr

Half-life: Extended-release, 15 to 19 hours; immediate-release, 22 hours.

ADVERSE REACTIONS
CNS: dizziness, asthenia, headache, vertigo, somnolence, malaise, drowsiness, pain, fatigue. **CV:** orthostatic hypotension, *arrhythmias,* hypotension, edema. **EENT:** rhinitis, dry mouth. **GI:** abdominal pain, nausea, dyspepsia. **GU:** polyuria, UTI. **Hematologic:** *leukopenia, neutropenia.* **Musculoskeletal:** myalgia. **Respiratory:** dyspnea, respiratory tract infection.

INTERACTIONS
Drug-drug. *Antihypertensives, diuretics:* May increase hypotensive effects. Adjust dosages as necessary.
PDE5 inhibitors (sildenafil, tadalafil, vardenafil): May cause additive hypotensive effects and symptomatic hypotension. Initiate PDE5 therapy at lowest possible dosage.

Strong CYP3A4 inhibitors (atazanavir, clarithromycin, ketoconazole, ritonavir): May increase doxazosin level. Use together with caution; monitor BP and watch for hypotension signs and symptoms.

Drug-herb. *Ma huang:* May decrease antihypertensive effects. Discourage use together.

EFFECTS ON LAB TEST RESULTS
• May decrease WBC and neutrophil counts.

CONTRAINDICATIONS & CAUTIONS
• Contraindicated in patients hypersensitive to drug and quinazoline derivatives (including prazosin and terazosin).
• Use cautiously in patients with impaired hepatic function. Monitor BP and observe for signs and symptoms of hypotension. Drug isn't recommended for use in patients with severe hepatic impairment.
• Intraoperative floppy iris syndrome has been observed during cataract surgery in some patients on or previously treated with alpha₁ blockers.
• Rarely, drug has been associated with priapism (painful penile erection, sustained for hours and unrelieved by sexual intercourse or masturbation), which can lead to permanent erectile dysfunction if not promptly treated.
• Safety and effectiveness in children haven't been established.

Dialyzable drug: No.

⚠ *Overdose S&S:* Hypotension.

PREGNANCY-LACTATION-REPRODUCTION
• There are no adequate well-controlled studies during pregnancy. Use immediate-release form during pregnancy only if clearly needed; extended-release form isn't indicated for use in females.
• Drug may appear in human milk. Use immediate-release form cautiously.

NURSING CONSIDERATIONS
• Monitor BP closely.
• If syncope occurs, place patient in a recumbent position and treat supportively. A transient hypotensive response isn't considered a contraindication to continued therapy.
• Rule out prostate cancer before starting treatment for BPH.
• Watch for new or worsening angina, especially in patients with acute MI within the last 6 months or HF.

• *Look alike–sound alike:* Don't confuse doxazosin with doxapram, doxorubicin, or doxepin. Don't confuse Cardura with Coumadin, K-Dur, Cardene, or Cordarone.

PATIENT TEACHING
• Instruct patient to take drug exactly as prescribed.
🌓 *Alert:* Advise patient that a first-dose effect (marked low BP on standing up, with dizziness or fainting) may occur. This is most common after first dose but also can occur during dosage adjustment or interruption of therapy.
• Instruct patient to consult prescriber if dizziness or palpitations are bothersome.
• Caution patient to rise slowly from sitting or lying position.
• Advise patient to avoid driving and other hazardous activities until drug's effects are known.
• Instruct patient to inform surgeon of alpha₁-blocker therapy before having cataract surgery.
• Inform patient that drug has been associated with rare, but serious, priapism and to seek immediate medical treatment for a painful penile erection lasting longer than 4 hours.
• Advise patient not to be concerned if a tablet occasionally appears in the stool. Explain that the medication in the extended-release tablet is contained within a nonabsorbable shell designed to release the drug at a controlled rate. When this process is completed, the empty tablet is eliminated from the body through the stool.

doxepin hydrochloride
DOKS-eh-pin

Silenor

Therapeutic class: Antidepressants
Pharmacologic class: TCAs

AVAILABLE FORMS
Capsules: 10 mg, 25 mg, 50 mg, 75 mg, 100 mg, 150 mg
Oral concentrate: 10 mg/mL
Tablets: 3 mg, 6 mg

INDICATIONS & DOSAGES
➤ **Depression; anxiety**
Adults: Initially, 75 mg PO daily. Usual dosage range is 75 to 150 mg daily to maximum of 300 mg daily in divided doses. Mild symptoms may require only 25 to 50 mg/day. Or, may give entire maintenance dose once daily to a maximum dose of 150 mg/day at bedtime.
➤ **Insomnia (Silenor only)**
Adults: 6 mg PO once daily within 30 minutes of bedtime.
Adjust-a-dose: For older adults, give 3 mg PO once daily within 30 minutes of bedtime. May increase daily dose to 6 mg if indicated. For patients with hepatic impairment, initial dose is 3 mg PO once daily. For administration with cimetidine, give maximum dose of 3 mg once daily.

ADMINISTRATION
PO
• Dilute oral concentrate with 4 oz (120 mL) of water, milk, or juice (orange, grapefruit, tomato, prune, or pineapple, but not grape); don't mix preparation with carbonated beverages.
• Give at bedtime, if possible, because it may cause drowsiness and dizziness.
• Don't give Silenor within 3 hours of a meal to minimize potential for next-day effect.

ACTION
Increases amount of norepinephrine, serotonin, or both in the CNS by blocking their reuptake by the presynaptic neurons.

Route	Onset	Peak	Duration
PO	Unknown	3.5 hr	Unknown

Half-life: About 15 hours.

ADVERSE REACTIONS
CNS: drowsiness, dizziness, *seizures*, confusion, numbness, hallucinations, paresthesia, ataxia, weakness, headache, extrapyramidal reactions, tardive dyskinesia, tremor, taste disturbance, fatigue. **CV:** orthostatic hypotension, HTN, tachycardia, ECG changes, flushing. **EENT:** blurred vision, closed-angle glaucoma, mydriasis, tinnitus, dry mouth, aphthous stomatitis. **GI:** constipation, nausea, vomiting, indigestion, diarrhea, anorexia. **GU:** urine retention, change in libido, testicular swelling. **Hepatic:** jaundice. **Metabolic:** *hypoglycemia,* hyperglycemia, weight gain.

Respiratory: asthma exacerbation. **Skin:** diaphoresis, rash, urticaria, photosensitivity reactions, alopecia. **Other:** hypersensitivity reactions, breast enlargement, galactorrhea, chills.

INTERACTIONS
Drug-drug. *Barbiturates, CNS depressants:* May enhance CNS depression. Avoid using together.
Cimetidine: May increase doxepin level. If Silenor is used with cimetidine, maximum Silenor dose of 3 mg is recommended in adults and patients who are older.
Clonidine: May cause life-threatening HTN. Avoid using together.
Drugs metabolized by CYP2D6 (cimetidine, flecainide, phenothiazines, propafenone, quinidine, SSRIs [fluoxetine, fluvoxamine, paroxetine, sertraline]): May increase doxepin level. Monitor drug levels and watch for signs and symptoms of toxicity.
Epinephrine, norepinephrine: May increase hypertensive effect. Use together cautiously.
Linezolid, methylene blue: May cause serotonin syndrome. Use with extreme caution and monitor patient closely.
MAO inhibitors: May increase risk of serotonin syndrome. Contraindicated within 14 days of MAO inhibitor therapy.
Quinolones: May increase risk of life-threatening arrhythmias. Avoid use together.
Tolazamide: May increase risk of severe hypoglycemia. Monitor patient closely.
Drug-herb. *Evening primrose oil:* May cause additive or synergistic effect, resulting in lower seizure threshold and increasing the risk of seizure. Discourage use together.
St. John's wort, SAM-e, yohimbe: May cause serotonin syndrome. Discourage use together.
Drug-lifestyle. *Alcohol use:* May enhance CNS depression. Discourage use together.
Sun exposure: May increase risk of photosensitivity reactions. Advise patient to avoid excessive sunlight exposure.

EFFECTS ON LAB TEST RESULTS
• May increase or decrease glucose level.
• May increase LFT values.

CONTRAINDICATIONS & CAUTIONS
• Contraindicated in patients hypersensitive to drug and in those with glaucoma or tendency toward urine retention and during acute recovery phase of an MI.

Boxed Warning Doxepin isn't approved for use in children. Clinicians considering the use of doxepin in a child, adolescent, or young adult must balance risk with clinical need. ∎

🕄 *Alert:* Concomitant use with linezolid or methylene blue can cause serotonin syndrome (fever, mental status changes, muscle twitching, diaphoresis, shivering or shaking, diarrhea, loss of coordination). Use with linezolid or methylene blue only for life-threatening or urgent conditions when the potential benefits outweigh the risks of toxicity.

• Avoid use in patients with bipolar disorder. Drug isn't approved to treat bipolar depression.

• Drug may increase risk of SIADH and hyponatremia, especially in females, older adults, and patients who are volume depleted; in those with concurrent diuretic use; and in patients with low body weight or debilitation.
Dialyzable drug: No.

⚠ *Overdose S&S:* Cardiac arrhythmias, severe hypotension, seizures, CNS depression, coma, confusion, disturbed concentration, transient visual hallucinations, dilated pupils, agitation, hyperactive reflexes, stupor, drowsiness, muscle rigidity, vomiting, hypothermia, hyperpyrexia.

PREGNANCY-LACTATION-REPRODUCTION

• There are no adequate well-controlled studies during pregnancy. Use during pregnancy only if clearly needed and potential benefit justifies fetal risk.

• Drug appears in human milk. Patients shouldn't breastfeed due to risk of excess sedation and respiratory depression.

NURSING CONSIDERATIONS

• Don't withdraw drug abruptly; gradually taper dosage to minimize withdrawal symptoms.

• Monitor patient for nausea, headache, and malaise after abrupt withdrawal of long-term therapy; these symptoms don't indicate addiction.

🕄 *Alert:* If linezolid or methylene blue must be given, stop drug and monitor patient for serotonin toxicity for 2 weeks, or until 24 hours after the last dose of methylene blue or linezolid, whichever comes first. Treatment may be resumed 24 hours after last dose of methylene blue or linezolid.

• If signs or symptoms of psychosis occur or increase, expect prescriber to reduce dosage.

Record mood changes. Monitor patient for suicidality, and allow only a minimum supply of drug.

• If using drug for insomnia and symptoms don't resolve after 10 days, evaluate for primary psychiatric or medical illness.

Boxed Warning Drug may increase risk of suicidality in children, adolescents, and young adults ages 18 to 24, especially during the first few months of treatment, especially in those with major depressive disorder or other psychiatric disorder. ∎

Boxed Warning Monitor all patients for clinical worsening, suicidality, or unusual changes in behavior. ∎

• Drug has strong anticholinergic effects and is one of the most sedating TCAs. Adverse anticholinergic effects can occur rapidly.

• *Look alike–sound alike:* Don't confuse doxepin with doxazosin, digoxin, doxapram, or Doxidan.

PATIENT TEACHING

🕄 *Alert:* Teach patient to recognize and immediately report symptoms of serotonin toxicity (fever, mental status changes, muscle twitching, diaphoresis, shivering or shaking, diarrhea, loss of coordination).

• Instruct patient in safe drug administration.

• Warn patient not to stop drug suddenly.

Boxed Warning Advise families and caregivers to closely observe patient for increased suicidality. ∎

• Tell patient to take full dose at bedtime whenever possible but to watch for possible morning dizziness on standing up quickly.

• Advise patient to consult prescriber before taking other prescription or OTC drugs.

• Warn patient to avoid hazardous activities that require alertness and good psychomotor coordination until effects of drug are known. Drowsiness and dizziness usually subside after a few weeks.

• Advise patient to report episodes of complex sleep behaviors (driving, preparing and eating food, making phone calls, or having sex while not fully awake, with amnesia of the event).

• Caution patient to avoid alcohol during drug therapy.

• Tell patient that antianxiety effect is apparent before antidepressant effect; maximal effect may not be evident for 2 to 3 weeks.

• To prevent sensitivity to the sun, advise patient to use sunblock, wear protective

---

clothing, and avoid prolonged exposure to strong sunlight.

• Recommend use of sugarless hard candy or gum to relieve dry mouth.

SAFETY ALERT!

DOXOrubicin hydrochloride
dox-oh-ROO-bi-sin

Adriamycin

Therapeutic class: Antineoplastics
Pharmacologic class: Anthracycline glycoside antibiotics

AVAILABLE FORMS
Injection (preservative-free): 2 mg/mL
Powder for injection: 10 mg, 20 mg, 50 mg

INDICATIONS & DOSAGES
Adjust-a-dose (for all indications): Refer to manufacturer's instructions for toxicity-related dosage adjustments.

➤ **Bladder, breast, lung, ovarian, stomach, and thyroid cancers; non-Hodgkin lymphoma; Hodgkin lymphoma; acute lymphoblastic and myeloblastic leukemia; Wilms tumor; neuroblastoma; lymphoma; soft-tissue and bone sarcomas**
Adults and children: 60 to 75 mg/m^2 IV as single dose every 21 days, or when used in combination with other chemotherapy drugs, 40 to 75 mg/m^2 IV every 21 to 28 days.

➤ **Adjuvant treatment as a component of multiagent chemotherapy in women with evidence of axillary lymph node involvement after resection of primary breast cancer**
Women: 60 mg/m^2 IV bolus on day 1 of each 21-day treatment cycle in combination with cyclophosphamide for a total of four cycles.

➤ **Endometrial carcinoma** ◆
Women: 60 mg/m^2 IV on day 1 of each 21-day treatment cycle for eight cycles in combination with cisplatin.

➤ **Multiple myeloma** ◆
Adults: In combination with other chemotherapy drugs, 9 mg/m^2/day IV on days 1 to 4 for three cycles or 10 mg/m^2/day IV as a continuous infusion on days 1 to 4 of each cycle.

➤ **Uterine sarcoma** ◆
Women: 60 mg/m^2 IV on day 1 every 21 days; maximum cumulative dose, 480 mg/m^2. Or, 50 mg/m^2 IV (over 15 minutes) on day 1

every 21 days in combination with ifosfamide/mesna; maximum cumulative dose, 450 mg/m^2.

➤ **Waldenström macroglobulinemia** ◆
Adults: 50 mg/m^2 IV on day 1 of each 21-day treatment cycle for four to eight cycles in combination with other drugs (cyclophosphamide, vincristine, prednisone, and rituximab).

ADMINISTRATION
IV
▼ Never give drug IM or subcut.

Boxed Warning If extravasation occurs, stop infusion immediately, apply ice to affected area, and notify prescriber. Extravasation can result in severe local tissue injury and necrosis requiring wide excision and skin grafting. ∎

▼ Preparing and giving parenteral drug may be mutagenic, teratogenic, or carcinogenic. Follow facility policy to reduce risks.

▼ Reconstitute with preservative-free NSS for injection to yield 2 mg/mL; add 5 mL to 10-mg vial, 10 mL to 20-mg vial, or 25 mL to 50-mg vial. Shake vial to dissolve drug.

▼ Don't place IV catheter over joints or in limbs with poor venous or lymphatic drainage.

▼ Give by direct injection over 3 to 10 minutes into the tubing of a free-flowing IV solution containing D$_5$W or NSS for injection.

▼ Some protocols give doxorubicin as a prolonged infusion, which requires central venous access.

▼ If vein streaking proximal to the site of infusion or facial flushing occurs, slow administration rate. If welts appear, stop drug and notify prescriber.

▼ Refrigerated, reconstituted solution is stable for 15 days; at room temperature, it's stable for 7 days.

▼ Protect from light.

▼ **Incompatibilities:** Other drugs and alkaline solutions.

ACTION
Interferes with DNA-dependent RNA synthesis by intercalation.

Route	Onset	Peak	Duration
IV	Unknown	Unknown	Unknown

Half-life: Initial, 5 minutes; terminal, 20 to 48 hours.

ADVERSE REACTIONS

CNS: malaise. **CV:** cardiac depression, *arrhythmias, HF, acute left ventricular failure, irreversible cardiomyopathy, shock, myocarditis, pericarditis.* **GI:** nausea, vomiting, diarrhea, abdominal pain, stomatitis, esophagitis, anorexia, ulcer, mucositis. **GU:** transient red urine. **Hematologic:** anemia, *myelosuppression.* **Metabolic:** hyperuricemia, weight loss, weight gain. **Skin:** alopecia, severe cellulitis and tissue sloughing (extravasation), discolored sweat, pruritus, urticaria, rash, photosensitivity, facial flushing, radiation recall effect. **Other:** chills, systemic infection, *sepsis, anaphylaxis, secondary malignancy (acute myelogenous leukemia [AML], myelodysplastic syndrome).*

INTERACTIONS

Drug-drug. *Calcium channel blockers:* May increase cardiotoxic effects. Monitor patient's ECG closely.

CYP2D6, CYP3A4, or P-gp inhibitors (cyclosporine, erythromycin, ketoconazole, ritonavir, verapamil): May increase doxorubicin level. Avoid use together.

CYP3A4 or P-gp inducers (carbamazepine, phenobarbital, phenytoin, rifampin): May decrease doxorubicin level. Avoid use together.

Dexrazoxane: May decrease tumor response and time to progression. Don't give dexrazoxane as a cardioprotectant at start of doxorubicin therapy. May consider use as a cardioprotectant in patients who have received a cumulative doxorubicin dose of 300 mg/m^2 and who will continue to receive doxorubicin.

Digoxin: May decrease digoxin level. Monitor digoxin level closely.

Fosphenytoin, phenytoin: May decrease level of phenytoin or fosphenytoin. Monitor drug level.

Paclitaxel: May decrease doxorubicin clearance. Give doxorubicin before paclitaxel if used together.

Progesterone: May enhance myelosuppression. Monitor patient and lab values closely.

Streptozocin: May increase risk of adverse effects. Use cautiously together.

Trastuzumab: May increase risk of cardiac dysfunction. Consider therapy modification.

Vaccines (inactivated): May diminish therapeutic effect of vaccines. If patient is vaccinated during therapy, revaccinate 3 months after stopping immunosuppressant.

Vaccines (live-virus): May increase vaccine-related toxicities and decrease vaccine's therapeutic effects. Avoid use of live-virus vaccines with immunosuppressants.

Drug-herb. *St. John's wort:* May decrease doxorubicin serum concentration. Avoid combination.

EFFECTS ON LAB TEST RESULTS

- May increase transaminase, bilirubin, and uric acid levels.
- May decrease platelet and WBC counts.

CONTRAINDICATIONS & CAUTIONS

- Contraindicated in patients with a history of sensitivity reactions to drug or its components.
- Contraindicated in patients with severe myocardial insufficiency, recent (past 4 to 6 weeks) MI, severe persistent drug-induced myelosuppression, baseline neutrophil count less than 1,500 cells/mm^3, or severe hepatic impairment (Child-Pugh class C or serum bilirubin level above 5 mg/dL).
- Don't use in patients who had previous treatment with complete cumulative doses of doxorubicin, daunorubicin, idarubicin, or other anthracyclines or anthracenediones.
Dialyzable drug: No.

PREGNANCY-LACTATION-REPRODUCTION

- May cause fetal harm if used during pregnancy. Advise patients of the risk. Patients of childbearing potential and male patients with partners of childbearing potential should avoid pregnancy.
- Advise patients of childbearing potential to use effective nonhormonal contraception during and for 6 months after therapy ends. Advise male patients with partners of childbearing potential to use effective contraception during and for 3 months after therapy ends.
- Drug appears in human milk. Patient shouldn't breastfeed during therapy.
- Drug may cause oligospermia, azoospermia, and permanent loss of fertility in males. Sperm counts have returned to normal levels in some men, which may occur several years after stopping treatment.
- Drug may cause amenorrhea, infertility, and premature menopause in females. Recovery of menses and ovulation is related to age at time of treatment.

NURSING CONSIDERATIONS

Boxed Warning Drug should be administered under the supervision of a physician experienced with cancer chemotherapeutic agents. ∎

• Verify pregnancy status before starting treatment.

• Perform cardiac function studies, including a MUGA or echocardiogram, ECG, and LVEF, before treatment, periodically throughout therapy, and after therapy is completed.

• Take preventive measures, including adequate hydration of patient, before starting treatment. Rapid lysis of leukemic cells may cause hyperuricemia and TLS. Allopurinol may be ordered.

• Premedicate with antiemetic to reduce nausea.

• If skin or mucosal contact occurs, immediately wash with soap and water.

Boxed Warning Reduce dosage in patients with hepatic impairment. ∎

Boxed Warning Severe myelosuppression may occur, possibly resulting in hospitalization or death. ∎

Boxed Warning Risk of secondary AML or myelodysplastic syndrome increases with doxorubicin use, especially when given with DNA-damaging antineoplastics or radiotherapy, when patients have been heavily pretreated with cytotoxic drugs, when doses have been escalated, or when patients age 50 and older had an existing increased risk of secondary AML or myelodysplastic syndrome. Children are also at risk for developing secondary AML. ∎

• Monitor CBC with differential, electrolyte levels, renal function, and LFT values; monitor ECG during therapy.

• Leukopenia may occur during days 10 to 14, with recovery by day 21.

• Monitor ECG for changes, such as sinus tachycardia, T-wave flattening, ST-segment depression, and voltage reduction.

Boxed Warning Cardiomyopathy risk is proportional to the cumulative exposure, with incidence rates of 1% to 20% for cumulative doses ranging from 300 to 500 mg/m^2 when drug is given every 3 weeks. Cardiomyopathy risk is further increased with concomitant cardiotoxic therapy. Assess LVEF before, regularly during, and after doxorubicin treatment. ∎

• If tachycardia develops, stop drug or slow rate of infusion, and notify prescriber.

Boxed Warning Myocardial toxicity, including acute left ventricular failure, may occur during therapy or months to years after termination of therapy. Assess LVEF regularly, during, and after treatment with doxorubicin. Children are at increased risk for developing delayed cardiotoxicity. ∎

⊕ *Alert:* If signs of HF develop, stop drug and notify prescriber. HF can often be prevented by increasing frequency of ECG assessments or multigated radionuclide angiography as the cumulative dose exceeds 300 mg/m^2 when patient is also receiving or has received cyclophosphamide, trastuzumab, or radiation therapy to cardiac area.

⊕ *Alert:* Reddish color of drug is similar to that of daunorubicin; don't confuse the two drugs.

• Esophagitis is common in patients who also have received radiation therapy.

⊕ *Alert:* Patient who has previously received radiation therapy is susceptible to radiation recall effect.

• *Look alike–sound alike:* Don't confuse doxorubicin with doxorubicin liposomal, daunorubicin, or idarubicin.

PATIENT TEACHING

⊕ *Alert:* Advise patient to immediately report pain or burning at injection site during or after administration.

• Tell patient to report all adverse effects.

• Inform patient of the increased risk of treatment-related leukemia.

• Instruct patient to watch for signs and symptoms of infection (fever, sore throat, fatigue) and bleeding (easy bruising, nosebleeds, bleeding gums, tarry stools) and to take temperature daily.

• Advise patient that orange to red urine for 1 to 2 days is normal and doesn't indicate presence of blood.

• Inform patient that hair loss may occur but that it's usually reversible. Hair may regrow 2 to 5 months after drug is stopped.

• Counsel patient to take antiemetics on a regular basis to avoid nausea and vomiting.

• Advise patient of fetal risk and to use effective contraception during and after treatment.

• Inform patient of changes to fertility and risk to infant with breastfeeding.

• Warn patient that drug can cause heart muscle damage that may lead to HF and serious heart rhythm problems that may lead to death.

DOXOrubicin hydrochloride liposomal

dox-oh-ROO-bi-sin

Doxil

Therapeutic class: Antineoplastics
Pharmacologic class: Anthracycline glycoside antibiotics

AVAILABLE FORMS

Injection: 2 mg/mL

INDICATIONS & DOSAGES

Adjust-a-dose (for all indications): Refer to manufacturer's instructions for toxicity-related dosage adjustments.

➤ **Ovarian cancer that has progressed or recurred after platinum-based chemotherapy**
Women: 50 mg/m^2 IV. Repeat treatment once every 28 days until disease progression or unacceptable toxicity.

➤ **AIDS-related Kaposi sarcoma after failure of prior systemic chemotherapy or intolerance to such therapy**
Adults: 20 mg/m^2 IV every 21 days until disease progression or unacceptable toxicity.

➤ **Multiple myeloma in patients who haven't previously received bortezomib and have received at least one prior therapy**
Adults: 30 mg/m^2 IV on day 4 of every 21-day cycle (administer after bortezomib) for eight cycles or until disease progression or unacceptable toxicity.

➤ **Refractory metastatic breast cancer ♦**
Adults: 50 mg/m^2 IV every 4 weeks.

ADMINISTRATION

IV

▼ Drug is cytotoxic. Follow applicable special handling and disposal procedures. Immediately wash thoroughly with soap and water if drug contacts skin or mucosa.

▼ Don't give as an undiluted suspension or as an IV bolus. Don't give IM or subcut.

▼ Dilute doses up to 90 mg in 250 mL D$_5$W using aseptic technique. Dilute doses exceeding 90 mg in 500 mL D$_5$W.

🔵 *Alert:* Carefully check label on IV bag before giving drug. Accidentally substituting doxorubicin hydrochloride liposomal for conventional doxorubicin hydrochloride may cause severe adverse reactions. The two products can't be substituted on a milligram-per-milligram basis.

▼ Don't use an in-line filter.

▼ Inspect product visually for particulate matter and discoloration before administration; don't use if a precipitate or foreign matter is present.

▼ Initiate infusion at 1 mg/minute and if no infusion-related reactions occur, increase rate to complete administration over 60 minutes. Monitor patient carefully during infusion. Never give as bolus injection.

Boxed Warning Serious, sometimes fatal, allergic infusion reactions can occur. Make sure emergency equipment and medications are available. Acute infusion-related reactions include flushing, shortness of breath, facial swelling, headache, chills, back pain, tightness in chest or throat, and hypotension. ■

▼ If extravasation occurs, stop infusion immediately and attempt to aspirate extravasated fluid before removing needle. Don't flush line or apply pressure to the site. Apply ice to the site intermittently for 15 minutes four times a day for 3 days. If extravasation is in an extremity, elevate the extremity. Restart infusion in another vein.

▼ Refrigerate diluted solution at 36° to 46° F (2° to 8° C) and give within 24 hours.

▼ **Incompatibilities:** Other IV drugs.

ACTION

Consists of doxorubicin hydrochloride encapsulated in liposomes. Inhibits DNA and RNA synthesis through intercalation.

Route	Onset	Peak	Duration
IV	Unknown	Unknown	Unknown

Half-life: 3.6 to 6.6 hours in first phase; 46.7 to 59.8 hours in second phase with doses of 10 to 20 mg/m^2.

ADVERSE REACTIONS

CNS: asthenia, paresthesia, headache, somnolence, dizziness, depression, insomnia, anxiety, malaise, emotional lability, fatigue, neuralgia, peripheral neuropathy, taste perversion, fever. **CV:** vasodilation, *DVT,* chest pain, hypotension, tachycardia, flushing, peripheral edema, *cardiomyopathy, HF, arrhythmias,* pericardial effusion, *cardiac*

---

arrest. **EENT:** conjunctivitis, dry eyes, optic neuritis, retinitis, epistaxis, rhinitis, pharyngitis, sinusitis, oral moniliasis, oral ulcers, secondary oral cancers, glossitis. **GI:** nausea, vomiting, constipation, anorexia, diarrhea, abdominal pain, dyspepsia, enlarged abdomen, esophagitis, dysphagia, stomatitis, rectal bleeding, ileus. **GU:** UTI, hematuria, vaginal candidiasis. **Hematologic:** *leukopenia, neutropenia, thrombocytopenia,* anemia. **Hepatic:** hyperbilirubinemia, increased ALP level, increased transaminase levels. **Metabolic:** dehydration, weight loss, hypercalcemia, *hypokalemia,* hyponatremia. **Musculoskeletal:** myalgia, back pain. **Respiratory:** dyspnea, increased cough, pneumonia. **Skin:** rash, alopecia, dry skin, pruritus, ecchymosis, skin discoloration, skin disorder, exfoliative dermatitis, fungal dermatitis, acne, diaphoresis, palmar–plantar erythrodysesthesia. **Other:** allergic reaction, chills, herpes zoster, herpes simplex, infection, *infusion-related reactions.*

INTERACTIONS

No formal drug interaction studies have been conducted. However, doxorubicin hydrochloride liposomal may interact with drugs that interact with the conventional form of doxorubicin hydrochloride.

Drug-drug. *Other antineoplastics:* May increase toxicity of other antineoplastics. Use together cautiously.

EFFECTS ON LAB TEST RESULTS

• May increase bilirubin, calcium, ALT, and ALP levels.
• May decrease potassium and sodium levels.
• May decrease Hb level and neutrophil, platelet, and WBC counts.
• May prolong PT and increase INR.

CONTRAINDICATIONS & CAUTIONS

• Contraindicated in patients hypersensitive to conventional formulation of doxorubicin hydrochloride or any component of the liposomal form.
Boxed Warning May cause myocardial damage, including acute left ventricular failure, as the total cumulative doxorubicin dose approaches 550 mg/m^2. Risk of cardiomyopathy may be increased at lower cumulative doses in patients with prior mediastinal irradiation. Prior use of other anthracyclines or anthracenediones should be

included in calculations of total cumulative dosage. ■
• Risk of cardiomyopathy with doxorubicin is generally proportional to the cumulative exposure, although the relationship between cumulative doxorubicin liposomal dose and risk of cardiotoxicity isn't known. Anthracycline-induced cardiotoxicity may be delayed (after discontinuation of anthracycline treatment).
• Give drug to patient with history of CV disease only when benefit outweighs risk to patient.
• Safety and effectiveness in children haven't been established.
Dialyzable drug: Unknown.
⚠ *Overdose S&S:* Leukopenia, mucositis, thrombocytopenia.

PREGNANCY-LACTATION-REPRODUCTION

• Drug may cause fetal harm if used during pregnancy. Advise patient of fetal risk.
• Patients of childbearing potential and male patients with partners of childbearing potential should use effective contraception during therapy and for 6 months after final dose.
• It isn't known if drug appears in human milk. Patient should discontinue breastfeeding during treatment.
• Drug may damage spermatozoa and testicular tissue in males and may result in oligospermia, azoospermia, and permanent loss of fertility.
• Drug may cause amenorrhea, infertility, and premature menopause in females. Recovery of menses and ovulation is related to age at time of treatment.

NURSING CONSIDERATIONS

• Verify pregnancy status before starting treatment.
• Consider previous or current therapy with related compounds such as daunorubicin when calculating total dose of drug to be given. HF and cardiomyopathy may occur after therapy ends.
Boxed Warning Assess left ventricular cardiac function (multigated radionuclide angiogram scan or echocardiogram) before drug initiation, during treatment to detect acute changes, and after treatment to detect delayed cardiotoxicity. ■
• Monitor patient for infusion reactions (flushing, dyspnea, facial swelling, headache, chills, chest pain, back pain, chest and throat tightness, fever, tachycardia, pruritus, rash,

cyanosis, syncope, bronchospasm, asthma, apnea, hypotension). Most reactions occur with first infusion. Ensure emergency equipment is readily available.

• Monitor patient for signs and symptoms of hand-foot syndrome, hematologic toxicity, and stomatitis. These adverse reactions may be managed with dosage delays and adjustments.

Boxed Warning If an infusion-related reaction occurs, temporarily stop drug until resolution, then resume at a reduced infusion rate. Discontinue infusion for serious or life-threatening reactions. ▪

• Evaluate patient's hepatic function before therapy, and reduce dosage for serum bilirubin level of 1.2 mg/dL or higher.

• Monitor CBC, including platelets, before each dose and frequently throughout therapy. Leukopenia is usually transient. Persistent severe myelosuppression may result in superinfection or hemorrhage. Patient may need G-CSF to support blood counts.

• Secondary oral cancers, primarily squamous cell carcinoma, have been reported during treatment and for up to 6 years after last dose in patients with long-term exposure to drug. Assess patients at regular intervals for the presence of oral ulceration or any oral discomfort that may indicate secondary oral cancer.

• *Look alike–sound alike:* Don't confuse doxorubicin with daunorubicin. Don't confuse Doxil with Paxil. Don't confuse regular formulation of doxorubicin with liposomal formulation.

PATIENT TEACHING

• Tell patient to notify prescriber of all adverse reactions, including signs and symptoms of hand-foot syndrome (such as tingling or burning, redness, flaking, bothersome swelling, small blisters, or small sores on palms of hands or soles of feet).

• Advise patient to report signs and symptoms of stomatitis (such as painful redness, swelling, or sores in mouth).

• Inform patient of risk of secondary oral cancers.

• Warn patient to avoid exposure to people with infections. Tell patient to report temperature of 100.5° F (38° C) or higher.

• Tell patient to report nausea, vomiting, tiredness, weakness, rash, or mild hair loss.

• Advise patient of childbearing potential to avoid pregnancy and to use effective contraception during treatment and for 6 months after final dose. Discontinue breastfeeding during therapy.

• Advise male patient with partner of childbearing potential to use effective contraception during treatment and for 6 months after final dose.

doxycycline calcium
dox-i-SYE-kleen

Vibramycin

doxycycline hyclate
Acticlate, Acticlate Cap, Doryx, Doryx MPC, Doxy 100, Morgidox, Vibramycin

doxycycline monohydrate
Apprilon ✦, Oracea, Vibramycin

Therapeutic class: Antibiotics
Pharmacologic class: Tetracyclines

AVAILABLE FORMS
doxycycline calcium
Syrup: 50 mg/5 mL
doxycycline hyclate
Capsules: 50 mg, 100 mg
Injection: 100 mg, 200 mg
Tablets: 20 mg, 50 mg, 75 mg, 100 mg, 150 mg
Tablets (delayed-release) ⦿: 50 mg, 75 mg, 80 mg, 100 mg, 120 mg, 150 mg, 200 mg
doxycycline monohydrate
Capsules: 50 mg, 75 mg, 100 mg, 150 mg
Capsules (Oracea): 40 mg (30 mg immediate-release and 10 mg delayed release)
Oral suspension: 25 mg/5 mL
Tablets: 50 mg, 75 mg, 100 mg, 150 mg

INDICATIONS & DOSAGES
➤ **Infections caused by susceptible gram-positive and gram-negative organisms (including *Haemophilus ducreyi*, *Yersinia pestis*, *Francisella tularensis*, and *Campylobacter fetus*), *Rickettsiae* species, *Mycoplasma pneumoniae*, *Chlamydia trachomatis*, or *Borrelia burgdorferi* (Lyme disease); *Chlamydophila* psittacosis; granuloma inguinale; adjunctive therapy in acute intestinal amebiasis or severe acne (PO)**

Adults and children older than age 8 weighing 45 kg or more: 100 mg PO or 120 mg (Doryx MPC) PO every 12 hours on first day; then 100 mg PO or 120 mg Doryx MPC daily as a single dose or in two divided doses. Or, 200 mg IV on first day in one or two infusions; then 100 to 200 mg IV daily. Daily doses of 200 mg IV can be given as a single dose or in two divided doses.

Children older than age 8 weighing less than 45 kg for severe or life-threatening infections: 2.2 mg/kg PO or IV or 2.6 mg/kg Doryx MPC PO every 12 hours.

Children older than age 8 weighing less than 45 kg for less severe infections: 4.4 mg/kg PO or IV divided into two doses on first day of treatment, followed by maintenance dose of 2.2 mg/kg PO given as a single daily dose or divided into twice-daily doses or 2.2 to 4.4 mg/kg/day IV given as one or two infusions, depending on the severity of the infection. Or, 5.3 mg/kg Doryx MPC PO divided into two doses on first day of treatment, followed by maintenance dose of 2.6 mg/kg given as a single daily dose or divided into twice-daily doses.

Give IV infusion slowly (minimum 1 hour). Refer to manufacturer's instructions for duration of therapy.

➤ **Gonorrhea in patients allergic to penicillin**
Adults: 100 mg PO b.i.d. for 7 days. Or, 300 mg PO once, followed in 1 hour with a second 300-mg PO dose.

➤ **Uncomplicated gonococcal infections (except anorectal infections in men)**
Adults: 120 mg Doryx MPC PO b.i.d. for 7 days. Or, 360 mg Doryx MPC PO followed by 360 mg PO in 1 hour.

➤ **Acute epididymo-orchitis caused by *Neisseria gonorrhoeae* or *C. trachomatis* (Doryx MPC)**
Adults: 120 mg PO b.i.d. for at least 10 days.

➤ **Syphilis in patients allergic to penicillin**
Adults: 100 mg PO or 120 mg Doryx MPC PO b.i.d. for 14 days (early). If more than 1-year duration, 100 mg PO or 120 mg Doryx MPC PO b.i.d. for 4 weeks.

➤ **Primary or secondary syphilis in patients allergic to penicillin**
Adults: 300 mg PO daily in divided doses for 14 days.

➤ **Uncomplicated urethral, endocervical, or rectal infections caused by *C. trachomatis* or *Ureaplasma urealyticum***

Adults: 100 mg PO or 120 mg Doryx MPC b.i.d. for at least 7 days.

➤ **To prevent malaria**
Adults: 100 mg PO or 120 mg Doryx MPC PO daily beginning 1 to 2 days before travel to endemic area and continued for 4 weeks after travel.

Children older than age 8: Give 2 mg/kg (2.4 mg/kg for Doryx MPC) PO once daily beginning 1 to 2 days before travel to endemic area and continued for 4 weeks after travel. Don't exceed daily dose of 100 mg (excluding Doryx MPC).

➤ **Adjunct to other antibiotics for inhalation, GI, and oropharyngeal anthrax**
Adults: 100 mg every 12 hours IV initially until susceptibility test results are known. Switch to 100 mg PO or 120 mg Doryx MPC PO b.i.d. when appropriate. Treat for 60 days total.

Children older than age 8 weighing more than 45 kg: 100 mg every 12 hours IV; then switch to 100 mg PO b.i.d. when appropriate. Treat for 60 days total.

Children older than age 8 weighing 45 kg or less: 2.2 mg/kg every 12 hours IV; then switch to 2.2 mg/kg (up to 100 mg) PO b.i.d. when appropriate. Treat for 60 days total.

Children age 8 and younger: 2.2 mg/kg IV every 12 hours; then switch to 2.2 mg/kg (up to 100 mg) PO b.i.d. when appropriate. Treat for 60 days total.

➤ **Inhalational anthrax (postexposure) (Doryx MPC)**
Adults and children weighing 45 kg or more: 120 mg PO b.i.d. for 60 days.
Children weighing less than 45 kg: 2.6 mg/kg PO b.i.d. for 60 days.

➤ **Cutaneous anthrax**
Adults: 100 mg PO every 12 hours for 60 days.
Children older than age 8 weighing more than 45 kg: 100 mg PO every 12 hours for 60 days.
Children older than age 8 weighing 45 kg or less: 2.2 mg/kg (up to 100 mg) PO every 12 hours for 60 days.
Children age 8 and younger: 2.2 mg/kg (up to 100 mg) PO every 12 hours for 60 days.

➤ **Inflammatory lesions of rosacea (Oracea)**
Adults: 40 mg PO once daily in the morning, 1 hour before or 2 hours after a meal. Give with a full glass of water. Reevaluate treatment after 16 weeks.

D

◆Canada   ◇OTC   ◆Off-label use   ✔Photoguide   ⊚Do not crush   *Liquid contains alcohol   ▓Genetic

ADMINISTRATION

PO

• Obtain specimen for culture and sensitivity tests before giving. Begin therapy while awaiting results.

• Doryx MPC can't be substituted on a milligram-per-milligram basis with other oral doxycyclines.

⚠️ *Alert:* Check expiration date. Outdated or deteriorated tetracyclines may cause reversible nephrotoxicity (Fanconi syndrome).

• Give drug with food or milk if stomach upset occurs.

• Increase fluid intake and don't administer tablets or capsules within 1 hour of bedtime because of possible esophageal irritation or ulceration.

• Give Oracea with a full glass of water.

• Don't crush delayed-release tablets or capsules. Delayed-released tablets and capsules can be carefully broken apart and their contents sprinkled onto a spoonful of applesauce and swallowed without chewing.

IV

▼ Obtain specimen for culture and sensitivity tests before giving. Begin therapy while awaiting results.

▼ Reconstitute powder for injection with sterile water for injection. Use 10 mL in 100-mg vial and 20 mL in 200-mg vial. Further dilute solution to a concentration of 0.1 mg/mL to 1 mg/mL; don't infuse solution that contains more than 1 mg/mL. Refer to manufacturer's instructions for compatible solutions.

▼ Don't expose drug to light or heat. Protect it from sunlight during infusion.

▼ Infusion time varies with dose but usually ranges from 1 to 4 hours. Infusion must be completed within 12 hours or within 6 hours in lactated Ringer solution or dextrose 5% in lactated Ringer solution.

▼ Monitor infusion site for evidence of thrombophlebitis.

▼ Reconstituted injectable solution is stable 72 hours if refrigerated and protected from light.

▼ **Incompatibilities:** Allopurinol, drugs that are unstable in acidic solutions (such as barbiturates), erythromycin lactobionate, heparin, meropenem, nafcillin, penicillin G potassium, piperacillin–tazobactam, riboflavin, sulfonamides. Refer to an IV drug compatibilities reference for full listing.

ACTION

Exerts bacteriostatic effect by binding to the 30S and possibly 50S ribosomal subunits of microorganisms and inhibiting protein synthesis.

Route	Onset	Peak	Duration
PO	Unknown	1.5–4 hr	Unknown
PO (delayed-release)	Unknown	2–4 hr	Unknown
IV	Immediate	Unknown	Unknown

Half-life: About 1 day after multiple dosing.

ADVERSE REACTIONS

CNS: *intracranial HTN,* headache, anxiety, pain. **CV:** HTN, pericarditis, thrombophlebitis. **EENT:** nasopharyngitis, sinusitis, nasal congestion, dry mouth, permanent tooth discoloration, enamel defects. **GI:** diarrhea, epigastric distress, nausea, anorexia, glossitis, dysphagia, vomiting, oral candidiasis, enterocolitis, anogenital inflammatory lesions, esophagitis, abdominal distention, *pancreatitis.* **GU:** vaginitis, vulvovaginal mycotic infection. **Hematologic:** *neutropenia, thrombocytopenia,* eosinophilia, hemolytic anemia. **Hepatic:** increased transaminase levels. **Metabolic:** hyperglycemia, increased LDH level. **Musculoskeletal:** back pain, bone growth retardation in children younger than age 8. **Skin:** rash, photosensitivity reactions, increased pigmentation, urticaria. **Other:** superinfection, flulike symptoms, hypersensitivity reactions, including *anaphylaxis.*

INTERACTIONS

Drug-drug. *Antacids and laxatives containing aluminum, magnesium, or calcium; antidiarrheals:* May decrease antibiotic absorption. Give antibiotic 1 hour before or 2 hours after these drugs.

Barbiturates, carbamazepine, phenobarbital, phenytoin, rifamycins: May decrease antibiotic effect. Consider therapy modification.

Ferrous sulfate and other iron products, zinc: May decrease antibiotic absorption. Give drug 2 hours before or 3 hours after iron.

Hormonal contraceptives: May decrease contraceptive effectiveness and increase risk of breakthrough bleeding. Advise use of a nonhormonal contraceptive.

Isotretinoin: May increase risk of pseudotumor cerebri. Avoid using together.

Methoxyflurane: May cause nephrotoxicity with tetracyclines. Avoid using together.

Reactions in bold italics are *life-threatening*. Interactions may have a *rapid onset* or a *delayed onset*.

Penicillins: May interfere with bactericidal action of penicillins. Avoid using together.
Warfarin: May increase anticoagulant effect. Monitor PT and INR; adjust dosage.
Drug-lifestyle. *Alcohol use:* May decrease drug's effect. Discourage use together.
Sun exposure: May cause photosensitivity reactions. Advise patient to avoid excessive sunlight exposure.

EFFECTS ON LAB TEST RESULTS

• May increase BUN and liver enzyme levels. May decrease Hb level.
• May increase eosinophil count. May decrease platelet, neutrophil, and WBC counts.
• May falsely elevate fluorometric tests for urine catecholamines. May cause false-negative results in urine glucose tests using glucose oxidase reagent (Diastix or Chemstrip uG). Parenteral form may cause false-positive Clinitest results.

CONTRAINDICATIONS & CAUTIONS

• Contraindicated in patients hypersensitive to drug or other tetracyclines.
• Use cautiously in patients with impaired renal or hepatic function.
• CDAD has been reported and may range in severity from mild diarrhea to fatal colitis. If CDAD is suspected or confirmed, ongoing antibiotic use not directed against *Clostridioides difficile* may need to be discontinued. Institute appropriate treatment.
• In a fetus in the last half of gestation or in a child younger than age 8, drug may cause permanently discolored teeth, enamel defects, and bone growth retardation. Drug shouldn't be used in this age-group unless other drugs aren't likely to be effective or are contraindicated.
• Use in patients age 8 and younger only when potential benefits are expected to outweigh risks in severe or life-threatening conditions, such as anthrax or Rocky Mountain spotted fever, particularly when there are no alternative therapies.
• Drug doesn't completely suppress malaria of *Plasmodium* strains. Patients may still transmit infection to mosquitoes outside endemic areas.
• Don't use Oracea for treatment or prevention of infections. Oracea should only be used as indicated for rosacea.
Dialyzable drug: No.
⚠ **Overdose S&S:** Dizziness, nausea, vomiting.

PREGNANCY-LACTATION-REPRODUCTION

• Tetracyclines cross the placental barrier. Drug is generally considered a second-line antibiotic during pregnancy and use should be avoided. Use during pregnancy only when other drugs are contraindicated or ineffective.
• During pregnancy, use the usual dosage schedule for anthrax.
• Drug appears in human milk. Patient should take into account benefits of breastfeeding versus risk of exposure to the infant.

NURSING CONSIDERATIONS

• If patient receives large doses or prolonged therapy or if patient is at high risk, watch for signs and symptoms of superinfection. If superinfection occurs, drug should be discontinued and appropriate therapy instituted.
• Use usual dosage schedule for anthrax in patients who are immunocompromised.
• Cutaneous anthrax with signs of systemic involvement, extensive edema, or lesions on the head or neck requires IV therapy and a multidrug approach.
• Ciprofloxacin and doxycycline are first-line therapies for anthrax. If patient with anthrax also has meningitis, ciprofloxacin is preferred because of better distribution to the CNS.
• Drug may increase risk of intracranial HTN (IH) and pseudotumor cerebri, especially in women who are overweight or have a history of IH. Monitor patient for headache, blurred vision, diplopia, and vision loss. If visual changes occur, prompt ophthalmic evaluation is needed.
• Monitor patient for superinfection.
• Check patient's tongue for signs of fungal infection. Emphasize good oral hygiene.
• Photosensitivity reactions may occur within a few minutes to several hours after exposure and may last after therapy ends. Discontinue drug at first evidence of skin erythema.
• *Look alike–sound alike:* Don't confuse doxycycline with doxylamine or dicyclomine. Don't confuse Oracea with Orencia.

PATIENT TEACHING

• Tell patient to take entire amount of drug exactly as prescribed, even if feeling better.
• Instruct patient to report adverse reactions promptly, especially signs or symptoms of hypersensitivity or IH. If drug is being given IV, tell patient to report discomfort at IV site.
• Instruct patient in safe drug administration.

• Warn patient to avoid direct sunlight and UV light, wear protective clothing, and use sunscreen.
• Tell patient to report signs and symptoms of superinfection to prescriber.

doxylamine succinate–pyridoxine hydrochloride
docks-ILL-ah-meen/peer-reh-DOCK-seen

Bonjesta, Diclectin✶, Diclegis

Therapeutic class: Antiemetics
Pharmacologic class: Antihistamines–vitamin B_6 analogues

AVAILABLE FORMS
Tablets (delayed-release) ⓄⓉⒸ: doxylamine succinate 10 mg/pyridoxine hydrochloride 10 mg
Tablets (extended-release) ⓄⓉⒸ: doxylamine succinate 20 mg/pyridoxine hydrochloride 20 mg

INDICATIONS & DOSAGES
➤ **Nausea and vomiting of pregnancy in patients who don't respond to conservative management**
Adults (delayed-release): 2 tablets at bedtime on day 1. If that dosage adequately controls symptoms the next day, patient should continue taking 2 tablets at bedtime. If symptoms persist into the afternoon of day 2, patients should take 2 tablets at bedtime that night, then take 1 tablet in the morning and 2 tablets at bedtime on day 3. If that dosage adequately controls symptoms on day 4, patients should continue taking 1 tablet in the morning and 2 tablets at bedtime. Otherwise, they should take 1 tablet in the morning, 1 tablet in the midafternoon, 2 tablets at bedtime on day 4. Maximum dose, 4 tablets/day.
Adults (extended-release): Initially, 1 tablet at bedtime on day 1. If symptoms aren't adequately controlled on day 2, increase dose to 1 tablet in the morning and 1 tablet at bedtime. Maximum dose is 1 tablet b.i.d.

ADMINISTRATION
PO
• Give tablets whole on an empty stomach with a glass of water. Don't crush, split, or allow patient to chew tablets.
• Patient should take tablets daily and not PRN.

• Store bottle at room temperature. Keep bottle tightly closed and protect from moisture. Don't remove desiccant canister from bottle.

ACTION
Unknown. The combination of antihistamine and vitamin B_6 may cause anticholinergic effects, decreasing nausea.

Route	Onset	Peak	Duration
PO (doxylamine)	Unknown	1.7–8.5 hr	Unknown
PO (pyridoxine)	Unknown	0.5–4.7 hr	Unknown

Half-life: Doxylamine, 11.9 to 12.6 hours; pyridoxine, 0.4 hour.

ADVERSE REACTIONS
CNS: somnolence.

INTERACTIONS
Drug-drug. *CNS depressants (sedative-hypnotics and tranquilizers):* May have additive effects. Don't use together.
MAO inhibitors (selegiline, tranylcypromine): May prolong and intensify CNS anticholinergic effects. Use together is contraindicated.
Other ethanolamine derivative antihistamines (diphenhydramine): May have additive effects. Avoid use together.
Drug-food. *Any food:* May delay onset and reduce absorption if taken with food. Patient should take drug on an empty stomach.
Drug-lifestyle. *Alcohol use:* May cause additive CNS depression. Alcohol isn't recommended during pregnancy.

EFFECTS ON LAB TEST RESULTS
• May cause false-positive urine screening tests for methadone, opiates, and phencyclidine.

CONTRAINDICATIONS & CAUTIONS
• Contraindicated in patients hypersensitive to drug, its components, and other ethanolamine-derivative antihistamines.
• Use cautiously in patients with asthma, increased IOP, angle-closure glaucoma, stenosing peptic ulcer, or pyloroduodenal or urinary bladder neck obstruction because of anticholinergic effects.
• Safety and effectiveness in children haven't been established.
Dializable drug: Unknown.

Reactions in bold italics are **life-threatening**. Interactions may have a *rapid onset* or a **delayed onset**.

PREGNANCY-LACTATION-REPRODUCTION
• Drug is intended for use during pregnancy. Drug hasn't been studied in patients with hyperemesis gravidarum.
• Drug appears in human milk and shouldn't be used during breastfeeding.

NURSING CONSIDERATIONS
• Reassess for continued need for drug as the pregnancy progresses.
• Monitor patient for anticholinergic effects (dry mouth, tachycardia, urine retention, constipation, ataxia).
• Monitor patient for somnolence, increased falls, and other CNS depressant effects.

PATIENT TEACHING
• Warn patient about adverse reactions, including somnolence, increased falls, other CNS depressant effects, dry mouth, dilated pupils, dizziness, confusion, fast heartbeat, and fluid retention.
• Teach patient to take drug as prescribed and that drug isn't to be used on an as-needed basis.
• Advise patient to avoid alcohol and sedating medications, including antihistamine cough and cold products, opioids, and sleep aids, while taking this drug because of increased risk of additive effects.
• Caution patient to avoid driving and operating heavy equipment or other activities that require complete mental alertness.

---

dronabinol (delta-9-tetrahydrocannabinol) ☒
droe-NAB-i-nol

Marinol, Syndros

Therapeutic class: Antiemetics
Pharmacologic class: Cannabinoids
Controlled substance schedule: III (Marinol); II (Syndros)

AVAILABLE FORMS
Capsules: 2.5 mg, 5 mg, 10 mg
Oral solution: 5 mg/mL*

INDICATIONS & DOSAGES
➤ **Nausea and vomiting from cancer chemotherapy after failure of conventional antiemetics**

Adults and children: 5 mg/m^2 (capsules) PO 1 to 3 hours before chemotherapy session. Then, 5 mg/m^2 (capsules) PO every 2 to 4 hours after chemotherapy, for total of four to six doses per day. If needed, increase dosage in 2.5-mg/m^2 increments to maximum of 15 mg/m^2 (capsules) per dose.
Adults: 4.2 mg/m^2 (oral solution) 1 to 3 hours before chemotherapy, then every 2 to 4 hours after chemotherapy for a total of four to six doses per day. If needed, increase oral solution dosage as tolerated in increments of 2.1 mg/m^2. Maximum dosage is 12.6 mg/m^2 (oral solution)/dose.
Adjust-a-dose: For older adults: Initiate capsules at low end of dosing range; may initiate oral solution at 2.1 mg/m^2 once daily before chemotherapy to reduce risk of CNS symptoms.
➤ **Anorexia and weight loss in patients with AIDS**
Adults: 2.5 mg (capsules) PO b.i.d. 1 hour before lunch and dinner. If patient can't tolerate twice-daily dosing, decrease to 2.5 mg (capsules) PO given as a single dose daily before dinner or at bedtime. May gradually increase to maximum of 20 mg (capsules) daily given in divided doses. Or, 2.1 mg (oral solution) PO b.i.d. 1 hour before lunch and dinner. If needed, may increase dosage gradually to 2.1 mg (oral solution) PO 1 hour before lunch and 4.2 mg 1 hour before dinner. If needed, may further increase dosage to 4.2 mg (oral solution) PO 1 hour before lunch and 4.2 mg 1 hour before dinner. Maximum dosage is 8.4 mg b.i.d.
Adjust-a-dose: For older adults, initiate capsules at low end of dosing range; may initiate at 2.1 mg (oral solution) PO once daily 1 hour before dinner or at bedtime to reduce risk of CNS symptoms. For patients with severe or persistent CNS symptoms, may reduce dosage to 2.5 mg (capsules) PO or 2.1 mg (oral solution) PO once daily 1 hour before dinner or at bedtime.

ADMINISTRATION
PO
• Give 1 to 3 hours before chemotherapy.
• For nausea and vomiting, give first dose on an empty stomach at least 30 minutes before patient eats; can give subsequent doses without regard to meals.
• When giving for nausea and vomiting, keep timing of dosing in relation to meal times

---

consistent for each chemotherapy cycle, once dosage has been determined from the titration process.
- Dosing later in the day may reduce frequency of CNS adverse reactions.
- Always use the calibrated oral dosing syringe when administering oral solution. Patient should take each dose with 180 to 240 mL of water.
- Can give Syndros via a silicone enteral feeding tube, #14 French or greater. Don't use tubes made of polyurethane. If prescribed dose is greater than 5 mg, divide total dose and draw up in two or more portions using the oral syringe. Flush the feeding tube with 30 mL of water after administration.
- Store capsules in cool environment, but protect from freezing. May store opened bottle of oral solution at 77° F (25° C); discard unused oral solution 42 days after opening.

ACTION

Cannabinoid that potentiates the activity of CB-1 and CB-2 receptors.

Route	Onset	Peak	Duration
PO	30–60 min	0.5–4 hr	4–6 hr (psychoactive effect); >24 hr (appetite stimulation)

Half-life: 4 to 36 hours.

ADVERSE REACTIONS

CNS: ataxia, dizziness, euphoria, paranoia, amnesia, asthenia, confusion, depersonalization, hallucinations, abnormal thinking, somnolence, anxiety, nervousness. **CV:** orthostatic hypotension, palpitations, tachycardia, vasodilation, facial flushing. **GI:** abdominal pain, dry mouth, nausea, vomiting.

INTERACTIONS

Drug-drug. *CNS depressants, psychomimetic substances, sedatives, TCAs:* May cause additive CNS depression. Avoid using together.
CYP2C9 inhibitors (amiodarone, fluconazole), CYP3A4 inhibitors (clarithromycin, erythromycin, itraconazole, ketoconazole, ritonavir): May increase dronabinol-related adverse reactions. Monitor carefully.
Disulfiram, metronidazole (Syndros only): May cause disulfiram-like reaction. Discontinue products containing disulfiram or metronidazole at least 14 days before starting treatment and don't give them within 7 days of completing treatment.

Drugs with cardiac effects (anticholinergics, TCAs): May have additive effects. Use cautiously together.
Drug-food. *Grapefruit juice:* May increase dronabinol-related adverse reactions. Discourage use together.
Drug-lifestyle. *Alcohol use:* May cause additive CNS depression. Discourage use together.

EFFECTS ON LAB TEST RESULTS
- May increase LFT values.

CONTRAINDICATIONS & CAUTIONS
- Contraindicated in patients hypersensitive to drug.
- Capsules are contraindicated in patients hypersensitive to sesame oil.
- Oral solution is contraindicated in patients hypersensitive to alcohol and within 14 days of products containing disulfiram or metronidazole.
- Oral solution contains propylene glycol; large amounts are toxic and are associated with hyperosmolarity, lactic acidosis, renal toxicity, CNS depression, seizures, cardiac arrhythmias, ECG changes, and hemolysis. Use caution.
- Use cautiously in children, older adults, and patients with heart disease, seizure disorders, or history of substance abuse.
- Safety and effectiveness of oral solution in children haven't been established.
Dialyzable drug: Unknown.
⚠ **Overdose S&S:** Drowsiness, euphoria, heightened sensory awareness, altered time perception, reddened conjunctiva, dry mouth, tachycardia, memory impairment, depersonalization, mood alteration, panic reactions, urine retention, decreased bowel motility, decreased motor coordination, lethargy, slurred speech, orthostatic hypotension; lactic acidosis, hypoglycemia, CNS depression, coma, seizures (oral solution).

PREGNANCY-LACTATION-REPRODUCTION
- Drug may cause fetal harm. Avoid use during pregnancy.
- Data are limited on the presence of dronabinol in human milk and its effects on infant who is breastfed or on milk production. Patients with HIV shouldn't breastfeed due to the risk of postnatal HIV transmission. Because of the possible adverse effects on the

---

Reactions in bold italics are ***life-threatening***. Interactions may have a *rapid onset* or a ***delayed onset***.

infant, patient shouldn't breastfeed during therapy and for 9 days after final dose.

NURSING CONSIDERATIONS
• Expect drug to be prescribed only for patients who haven't responded satisfactorily to other antiemetics.

🜲 *Alert:* Drug is the principal active substance in *Cannabis sativa* (marijuana), which can produce both physiologic and psychological dependence and has a high risk of abuse. Use cautiously in patients receiving sedatives, hypnotics, or other psychoactive drugs.

• Assess patient's risk of abuse or misuse before drug is prescribed. Monitor patients with a history of substance abuse for abuse or misuse behaviors during treatment.

▨ Patients who are known to carry genetic variants associated with CYP2C9 function (CYP2C9 polymorphism) have increased risk of adverse drug-related effects.

• Monitor patient for hypotension, HTN, syncope, and tachycardia.

• Drug can exacerbate mania, depression, and schizophrenia. Screen patients for these illnesses before giving drug. If drug must be used, monitor patient for worsening signs and symptoms of psychiatric illness. Older adults may be more sensitive to drug's effects.

• CNS effects are intensified at higher dosages.

• Drug effects may persist for days after treatment ends.

• New or worsening nausea, vomiting, or abdominal pain can occur during treatment. Ask patients about these symptoms as they may not recognize them as abnormal.

• *Look alike–sound alike:* Don't confuse dronabinol with droperidol.

PATIENT TEACHING
• Tell patient to report all adverse reactions; tell patient that drug may induce unusual changes in mood or other adverse behavioral effects.

• Advise patient to report new or worsening nausea, vomiting, or abdominal pain.

• Caution patient that oral solution can't be taken within 14 days of disulfiram or metronidazole.

• Advise patient against performing activities that require alertness until CNS effects of drug are known.

• Warn caregivers to supervise patient during and immediately after treatment.

• Advise patient to store drug securely.
• Advise patient not to breastfeed during therapy and for 9 days after final dose.

---

dronedarone
dro-neh-DAR-rone

Multaq

Therapeutic class: Antiarrhythmics
Pharmacologic class: Benzofuran derivatives

AVAILABLE FORMS
Tablets: 400 mg

INDICATIONS & DOSAGES
➤ **To reduce risk of hospitalization for atrial fibrillation in patients in sinus rhythm with a history of paroxysmal or persistent atrial fibrillation**
Adults: 400 mg PO b.i.d.

ADMINISTRATION
PO
• Give drug with morning and evening meals.
• Omit a missed dose and give next regularly scheduled dose.
• Store at room temperature.

ACTION
Blocks sodium and potassium channels and decreases atrial ventricular node and sinus node conduction by blocking calcium and beta$_1$ channels.

Route	Onset	Peak	Duration
PO	Unknown	3–6 hr	Unknown

Half-life: 13 to 19 hours.

ADVERSE REACTIONS
CNS: asthenia. **CV:** *bradycardia, HF, QT-interval prolongation.* **GI:** abdominal pain, diarrhea, dyspepsia, nausea, vomiting. **GU:** prerenal azotemia, *acute renal failure,* elevated creatinine level. **Metabolic:** hypovolemia. **Skin:** allergic dermatitis, dermatitis, eczema, pruritus, rash.

INTERACTIONS
Drug-drug. *Beta blockers:* May increase risk of bradycardia. Initially, give low dose of beta blocker and increase dosage only after monitoring ECG for tolerance.

Calcium channel blockers: May cause additive AV-blocking effects. Reduce initial dosage of calcium channel blocker; increase dosage only after monitoring ECG for tolerance.

CYP2C9 substrates (losartan, warfarin): May increase metabolite levels. Monitor patient closely; monitor INR in patient taking warfarin.

CYP3A inducers (carbamazepine, phenobarbital, phenytoin, rifampin): May decrease dronedarone level. Avoid use together.

CYP3A inhibitors (clarithromycin, erythromycin, itraconazole, ketoconazole, ritonavir, voriconazole): May increase dronedarone level. Use together is contraindicated.

CYP3A substrates (sirolimus, tacrolimus): May increase levels of these drugs. Monitor drug levels.

Dabigatran: May increase dabigatran level. Reduce dabigatran dose. Avoid use together in patients with severe renal impairment.

Digoxin: May increase digoxin level and electrophysiologic effects of dronedarone. Avoid use together; if necessary to use together, decrease digoxin dosage, monitor levels, and observe for toxicity.

Drugs that prolong QT interval (Class I and III antiarrhythmics, macrolide antibiotics, phenothiazines, TCAs): May further increase QT interval, leading to torsades de pointes. Use together is contraindicated.

Statins: May increase statin level. Use together cautiously. Limit simvastatin dosage to 10 mg once daily.

Drug-herb. *St John's wort:* May decrease drug level. Discourage use together.

Drug-lifestyle. *Grapefruit juice:* May increase drug level. Don't use together.

EFFECTS ON LAB TEST RESULTS
- May increase serum creatinine level.
- May decrease potassium and magnesium levels (in patients taking potassium-depleting diuretics).

CONTRAINDICATIONS & CAUTIONS
Boxed Warning Contraindicated in patients with NYHA Class IV HF or Class II to III HF with recent decompensation requiring hospitalization or referral to an HF clinic. Drug doubles risk of death in these patients. ∎

Boxed Warning Contraindicated in patients with atrial fibrillation who won't or can't be restored to normal sinus rhythm. Drug doubles risk of death, stroke, and hospitalization for HF in patients with permanent atrial fibrillation. ∎

- Contraindicated in patients hypersensitive to drug or its components.
- Contraindicated in patients with second- or third-degree AV block or sick sinus syndrome (unless a functioning pacemaker is in place), bradycardia (less than 50 beats/minute), severe hepatic impairment, QTc interval of 500 msec or greater, or PR interval greater than 280 msec.
- Contraindicated in patients with previous hepatic or pulmonary toxicity with amiodarone use.
- **⚠ Alert:** Drug may increase risk of severe hepatic injury or failure.
- Use cautiously in patients with new or worsening HF.
- ILD has been reported. Discontinue drug if pulmonary toxicity is confirmed.
- Marked increase in serum creatinine level, prerenal azotemia, and acute renal failure, frequently in the setting of HF or hypovolemia, have been reported. Effects appear to be reversible upon drug discontinuation and with appropriate medical treatment. Monitor renal function periodically.
- Safety and effectiveness in children haven't been established.

Dialyzable drug: Unknown.

⚠ Overdose S&S: QTc-interval prolongation.

PREGNANCY-LACTATION-REPRODUCTION
- Drug may cause fetal harm, and use during pregnancy is contraindicated. Patients of childbearing potential should use effective contraception during therapy.
- It isn't known if drug appears in human milk. Drug is contraindicated during breastfeeding.

NURSING CONSIDERATIONS
- Potassium-depleting diuretics may cause hypokalemia and hypomagnesemia, increasing the risk of torsades de pointes. Initiate dronedarone therapy after potassium and magnesium levels reach and stay within normal range.
- Ensure that patients discontinue Class I or III antiarrhythmics or drugs that are strong inhibitors of CYP3A before starting drug.
- Monitor CV status, ECG, electrolyte levels, and QTc interval routinely.

• Monitor renal function regularly. Renal impairment can occur.
• Monitor hepatic serum enzyme levels, especially during the first 6 months of therapy. Discontinue drug if hepatic injury is suspected.

PATIENT TEACHING
• Instruct patient in safe drug administration.
• Advise patient to report weight gain, dyspnea, fatigue, and peripheral edema, which may indicate worsening HF.
• Tell patient to report changes in OTC or prescription drug use, or in supplement or herb use.
• Instruct patient to report slowed heartbeat, diarrhea, nausea, vomiting, abdominal pain, indigestion, fatigue, or rash.
• Advise patient of childbearing potential to use an effective method of birth control while taking drug and to notify prescriber if becoming pregnant or thinking of becoming pregnant.
• Advise patient not to breastfeed while taking dronedarone because drug may appear in human milk.

drospirenone–estetrol
droh-SPYE-re-none/ES-te-trol

Nextstellis

Therapeutic class: Contraceptives
Pharmacologic class: Estrogen-progestin combinations

AVAILABLE FORMS
Tablets: 3 mg drospirenone/14.2 mg estetrol as 24 active tablets and 4 inert tablets per pack

INDICATIONS & DOSAGES
➤ **Prevention of pregnancy in women of childbearing potential**
Women with no current use of hormonal contraceptives: 1 active tablet PO daily for 24 days beginning on day 1 of menstrual cycle. Then, 1 inert tablet PO daily on days 25 through 28. Begin each subsequent 28-day pack on same day of week on which first regimen began, following same schedule. Restart active tablets on next day after last inert tablet.
Adjust-a-dose: Refer to manufacturer's instructions for patients switching from another

contraceptive method or starting after delivery, abortion, or miscarriage.

ADMINISTRATION
PO
• Give 1 tablet at same time each day without regard to food.
• If 1 active tablet is missed, give missed tablet as soon as possible and next tablet at scheduled time, even if 2 active tablets are taken on same day; then continue 1 tablet a day until pack is finished.
• If 2 or more active tablets are missed in weeks 1 or 2, give 1 missed tablet as soon as possible with tablet for current day and discard other missed tablet(s). Continue 1 tablet a day until pack is finished. Give additional nonhormonal contraceptive until active tablets are taken for 7 consecutive days.
• If 2 active tablets are missed in week 3, give 1 missed tablet as soon as possible with tablet for current day and discard other missed tablets. Finish active tablets and discard inert tablets in pack. Start new pack of tablets on next day. Give additional nonhormonal contraceptive until active tablets are taken for 7 consecutive days.
• If 1 or more inert tablets are missed, skip missed tablet days and continue taking 1 tablet a day until pack is finished.
• If patient vomits or acute diarrhea occurs within 3 to 4 hours after giving an active tablet, give active tablet scheduled for next day as soon as possible and within 12 hours of usual time of tablet-taking if possible. If more than 2 tablets are missed, follow above information on missed tablets, including use of additional nonhormonal contraceptives.
• Store tablets at 68° to 77° F (20° to 25° C).

ACTION
Prevents pregnancy primarily by suppressing ovulation.

Route	Onset	Peak	Duration
PO (drospirenone)	Unknown	1–3 hr	Unknown
PO (estetrol)	Unknown	30 min–2 hr	Unknown

Half-life: 34 hours (drospirenone); 27 hours (estetrol).

ADVERSE REACTIONS
CNS: headache, mood disturbance. **CV:** **thromboembolism.** **GU:** dysmenorrhea, decreased libido. **Hematologic:** bleeding

irregularities. **Metabolic:** weight gain. **Skin:** acne. **Other:** breast symptoms.

INTERACTIONS

Drug-drug. *Antibiotics:* May decrease contraceptive effect. Advise patient on additional contraception during concomitant use.

Antidiabetics: May decrease blood glucose–lowering effect of antidiabetic. Increase frequency of glucose monitoring and increase antidiabetic dose, as needed, based on glucose levels.

Bile acid sequestrants (cholestyramine, colesevelam, colestipol): May cause contraceptive failure or increase breakthrough bleeding. Separate administration times. Refer to sequestrant prescribing information for additional information.

Drugs that may increase serum potassium level (ACE inhibitors, ARBs, NSAIDs, potassium supplements, spironolactone): May increase serum potassium level. Monitor serum potassium level.

Hepatitis C drug combinations containing ombitasvir/paritaprevir/ritonavir with or without dasabuvir: May increase liver enzyme levels. Avoid use together. May initiate drospirenone–estetrol 2 weeks after completion of hepatitis C combination drug regimen.

Lamotrigine: May decrease effect of lamotrigine. Adjust lamotrigine dosage according to prescribing information based on hormonal contraceptive initiation or discontinuation.

Moderate and weak CYP3A4 inducers (dabrafenib, dexamethasone, modafinil, nafcillin): May cause contraceptive failure. Advise use of additional contraceptive method during concomitant use and for 28 days after discontinuing CYP3A inducer, unless prescribing information of inducer indicates no clinically significant interaction.

Strong CYP3A inducers (dexamethasone, phenobarbital, phenytoin, rifampin, rifamycin): May lead to contraceptive failure. Avoid concomitant use. If concomitant use is unavoidable, advise use of alternative contraceptive method or additional nonhormonal contraceptive during concomitant use and for 28 days after discontinuing inducer.

Strong CYP3A inhibitors (diltiazem, ketoconazole, loperamide, saquinavir): May increase risk of adverse drug reactions. Monitor serum potassium level in patients taking concomitantly long term.

Systemic corticosteroids: May increase risk of corticosteroid-related adverse reactions. Monitor patient closely. Follow recommendation for corticosteroid according to its prescribing information.

Thyroid hormone replacement therapy: May increase thyroid-binding globulin level. Monitor TSH level and follow recommendation for thyroid hormone replacement according to its prescribing information.

Drug-herb. *St. John's wort:* May decrease contraceptive effect or increase breakthrough bleeding. Discourage use together or recommend alternative contraceptive method.

Drug-lifestyle. **Boxed Warning** *Smoking:* May increase risk of CV events. Use is contraindicated in women older than age 35 who smoke. ∎

Sunlight, UV light: May increase risk of chloasma. Encourage patient to limit exposure and wear sunscreen while taking drug.

EFFECTS ON LAB TEST RESULTS
• May increase potassium, liver enzyme, blood glucose, triglyceride, corticosteroid-binding globulin, aldosterone, and total T_3 and total T_4 levels.
• May decrease LDL level.
• May increase platelet count.
• May decrease PT, PTT, and platelet aggregation time.

CONTRAINDICATIONS & CAUTIONS
• Contraindicated in patients at risk for arterial or venous thrombotic events. Evaluate patient for personal or family history of thrombotic or thromboembolic disorders and consider whether history suggests inherited or acquired hypercoagulopathy before starting drug.
• Contraindicated in patients with current or history of hormonally sensitive malignancy (breast cancer), hepatic adenoma, hepatocellular carcinoma, acute hepatitis, or decompensated cirrhosis.
• Contraindicated in patients with uterine bleeding of undiagnosed etiology.
• Contraindicated in patients at risk for hyperkalemia (renal impairment, hepatic impairment, adrenal insufficiency).
• Contraindicated in patients with uncontrolled HTN or HTN with vascular disease.
• Contraindicated in patients with migraine headaches with aura. Discontinue drug in patients who develop new migraines that are

recurrent, persistent, or severe, or who experience increased frequency or severity of migraines while taking drug.
• Avoid use in patients with hereditary angioedema; drug may induce or exacerbate symptoms.
• Avoid use in patients with history of chloasma gravidarum or increased sensitivity to sun or UV exposure.
• Drug may be ineffective in patients with BMI of 30 kg/m^2 or greater. Safety and effectiveness in patients with BMI of 35 kg/m^2 or greater haven't been established.
• Drug may increase risk of CV events, especially in patients older than age 40; those with HTN, dyslipidemia, diabetes, or obesity; and those who use nicotine-containing products.
• Drug may decrease glucose tolerance. Use cautiously in patients who are prediabetic or diabetic.
• Drug may increase triglyceride levels and risk of pancreatitis. Consider alternative contraceptive method in patients with history of hypertriglyceridemia.
• Drug may increase risk of development or worsening of gallbladder disease. Consider discontinuing drug in patients with symptomatic gallbladder or cholestatic disease.
Dialyzable drug: Unknown.
⚠ **Overdose S&S:** Nausea, vomiting, severe headache, thromboembolic complications, vaginal bleeding.

PREGNANCY-LACTATION-REPRODUCTION
• Use during pregnancy isn't indicated. Discontinue if pregnancy is confirmed.
• Drug appears in human milk and may decrease milk production. Patient should use other forms of contraception while breastfeeding. Evaluate benefits of breastfeeding, keeping in mind the patient's clinical need and potential adverse effects on the infant.

NURSING CONSIDERATIONS
• Monitor patient for thrombotic and thromboembolic events; discontinue drug if an event occurs.
• Monitor patient for unexplained vision changes. Stop drug and immediately evaluate patient for retinal vein thrombosis.
• Stop drug during prolonged periods of immobilization.
• Monitor patient with history of depression; stop drug if depression recurs to a serious degree.

• In patient at high risk for hyperkalemia and patient in whom taking drug may increase potassium level, check serum potassium level during first treatment cycle.
• Monitor BP periodically. Stop drug if BP rises significantly.
• Monitor liver enzyme levels. Withhold or permanently discontinue drug for significant liver enzyme elevations.
• Monitor glucose level in patients who are prediabetic or diabetic.
• Evaluate patient for other causes if irregular bleeding or amenorrhea persists.

PATIENT TEACHING
Boxed Warning Inform patient that smoking increases risk of a serious CV event when combined with drug and that hormonal contraceptives are contraindicated in females older than age 35 who smoke. ■
• Instruct patient in proper administration (including managing missed doses) and storage.
• Warn patient about increased risk of arterial or venous thrombotic or thromboembolic events while taking drug, especially patient with HTN, dyslipidemia, diabetes, or obesity.
• Instruct patient to immediately report limb pain or swelling, sudden shortness of breath, sudden change in vision, chest pain, sudden severe headache, weakness or numbness in arm or leg, or trouble speaking.
• Tell patient to contact prescriber if prolonged immobilization occurs.
• Teach patient to report signs or symptoms of hyperkalemia (weakness, palpitations or irregular heartbeat, nausea, vomiting, severe chest pain, dyspnea).
• Instruct patient about regular BP checks and to report BP increases to prescriber.
• Alert patient that drug may cause elevated liver enzyme levels and can increase risk of liver tumors. Instruct patient to report signs or symptoms of liver disease (jaundice).
• Instruct patient who is prediabetic or diabetic to contact prescriber for signs or symptoms of hyperglycemia (increased thirst, dry mouth, frequent urination, increased appetite with weight loss).
• Advise patient about risk of development or worsening of gallbladder disease and to report signs or symptoms of gallbladder disease (rapidly intensifying pain in the upper portion of the abdomen or in the center of the abdomen just below the breastbone, back pain

between the shoulder blades, pain in the right shoulder, nausea, vomiting).
• Inform patient that drug may cause unscheduled bleeding and spotting.
• Tell patient to contact prescriber if amenorrhea occurs in two or more consecutive cycles or signs and symptoms of pregnancy occur (morning sickness, unusual breast tenderness). Inform patient to stop drug if pregnancy is confirmed.
• Inform patient that drug may cause chloasma (dark patches of facial skin), especially in patient with history of chloasma gravidarum.
• Instruct patient to avoid exposure to UV light or prolonged exposure to sunlight and to wear sunscreen while taking drug.

---

drospirenone–ethinyl estradiol

droh-SPYE-re-none/ETH-i-nill es-tra-DYE-ole

Jasmiel, Loryna, Lo-Zumandimine, Mya✹, Nikki, Ocella, Quismette 21✹, Quismette 28✹, Syeda, Yasmin, Yaz, Zamine 21✹, Zamine 28✹, Zumandimine

Therapeutic class: Contraceptives
Pharmacologic class: Estrogen–progestin combinations

AVAILABLE FORMS
Tablets: 3 mg drospirenone and 0.03 mg ethinyl estradiol as 21 active tablets (Quismette 21, Zamine 21) and 7 inert tablets (Ocella, Quismette 28, Syeda, Yasmin, Zamine 28, Zumandimine); 3 mg drospirenone and 0.02 mg ethinyl estradiol as 24 active tablets and 4 inert tablets (Jasmiel, Loryna, Lo-Zumandimine, Mya, Nikki, Yaz)

INDICATIONS & DOSAGES
➤ **Contraception**
Women: 1 active tablet PO daily for 21 days beginning on day 1 of menstrual cycle or first Sunday after onset of menstruation. Then 1 inert tablet PO daily on days 22 through 28. Or 1 active tablet PO daily for 24 days beginning on day 1 of menstrual cycle or first Sunday after onset of menstruation. Then 1 inert tablet PO daily on days 25 through 28. Begin next and all subsequent 28-day

regimens on same day of week that first regimen began, following same schedule. Restart active tablets on next day after last inert tablet.
➤ **Premenstrual dysphoric disorder (Yaz)**
Women: 1 active tablet PO daily for 24 days beginning on day 1 of menstrual cycle or first Sunday after menstruation begins. Then 1 inert tablet PO daily on days 25 through 28. Begin next and all subsequent 28-day regimens on same day of week that first regimen began, following same schedule. Restart active tablets on next day after last inert tablet.
➤ **Acne in women at least age 14 and only if patient desires an oral contraceptive for birth control (Loryna, Nikki, Yaz)**
Women: Follow guidelines of use for contraception. The 28-day dosing regimen consists of 1 active tablet PO for 24 consecutive days followed by 1 inert tablet PO daily for 4 days. After 28 tablets are taken, new course is started next day.

ADMINISTRATION
PO
• Give at same time each day.
• Give tablets in order directed on blister pack.

ACTION
Reduces chance of conception by inhibiting ovulation, inhibiting sperm progression, and reducing chance of implantation.

Route	Onset	Peak	Duration
PO	Unknown	1–2 hr	Unknown

Half-life: Drospirenone, 30 hours; ethinyl estradiol, 24 hours.

ADVERSE REACTIONS
CNS: depression, dizziness, emotional lability, headache, migraine, irritability, nervousness, mood changes. **CV: *arterial or venous thromboembolism,*** HTN, fluid retention. **EENT:** cataracts, steepening of corneal curvature, intolerance to contact lenses, retinal thrombosis. **GI:** abdominal pain, abdominal cramping, bloating, changes in appetite, colitis, diarrhea, nausea, vomiting, gallbladder disease. **GU:** amenorrhea, breakthrough bleeding, change in cervical erosion and secretion, change in menstrual flow, cystitis, cystitis-like syndrome, dysmenorrhea, impaired renal function, leukorrhea, menstrual

---

Reactions in bold italics are ***life-threatening***. Interactions may have a *rapid onset* or a ***delayed onset***.

disorder, premenstrual syndrome, spotting, temporary infertility after discontinuing treatment, vaginal candidiasis, vaginitis. **Hepatic:** *Budd-Chiari syndrome, hepatic adenomas,* cholestatic jaundice, benign liver tumors. **Metabolic:** reduced glucose tolerance, porphyria, weight change, *hyperkalemia.* **Musculoskeletal:** back pain. **Skin:** *erythema multiforme,* acne, erythema nodosum, hemorrhagic eruption, hirsutism, loss of scalp hair, melasma, pruritus, rash. **Other:** hypersensitivity reaction, changes in libido, breast tenderness.

INTERACTIONS

Drug-drug. *ACE inhibitors, aldosterone antagonists, ARBs, NSAIDs, potassium-sparing diuretics:* May increase risk of hyperkalemia. Monitor potassium level.

Acetaminophen: May increase level of contraceptive and decrease effectiveness of acetaminophen. Monitor patient for adverse effects. Adjust acetaminophen dose as needed.

Antibiotics, griseofulvin, penicillins, tetracycline: May decrease contraceptive effect. Advise patient to use additional method of birth control while taking the antibiotic.

Ascorbic acid, atorvastatin: May increase level of contraceptive. Monitor patient for adverse effects.

Carbamazepine, modafinil, oxcarbazepine, phenobarbital, phenytoin, protease inhibitors: May increase metabolism of ethinyl estradiol and decrease contraceptive effectiveness. Advise patient to use another method of birth control.

Cyclosporine, prednisolone, theophylline: May increase levels of these drugs. Monitor patient for adverse effects and toxicity.

Hepatitis C drug combinations containing ombitasvir, paritaprevir, ritonavir, dasabuvir: May increase ALT level. Use together is contraindicated. Discontinue drospirenone–ethinyl estradiol before starting therapy due to risk of significant liver enzyme level increases. May restart approximately 2 weeks after completion of the combination drug regimen.

Lamotrigine: May decrease lamotrigine level and reduce seizure control. Dosage adjustment may be necessary.

Rifampin: May decrease contraceptive effectiveness and increase menstrual irregularities. Advise patient to use another method of birth control.

Warfarin, other anticoagulants: May increase or decrease anticoagulation effect. Monitor INR or consider therapy modification.

Drug-herb. *St. John's wort:* May decrease contraceptive effectiveness and increase breakthrough bleeding. Discourage use together, or advise use of additional method of birth control.

Drug-lifestyle. *Smoking:* May increase risk of adverse CV effects. Advise patient to avoid smoking.

EFFECTS ON LAB TEST RESULTS

• May increase potassium, corticoid, prothrombin, thyroid-binding globulin, total circulating sex steroid, total thyroid hormone, triglyceride, amylase, GGT, transferrin, prolactin, renin activity, vitamin A, and factor VII, VIII, IX, and X levels, as well as iron-binding capacity.

• May decrease antithrombin III level, folate, albumin, zinc, and vitamin B_{12}.

• May increase norepinephrine-induced platelet aggregation. May decrease glucose tolerance and free T_3 resin uptake.

CONTRAINDICATIONS & CAUTIONS

• Contraindicated in females with hepatic dysfunction, tumor, or disease; renal or adrenal insufficiency; thrombophlebitis, thromboembolic disorders, or history of DVT or thromboembolic disorders, inherited hypercoagulopathies; cerebrovascular disease or CAD; uncontrolled HTN; diabetes with vascular disease; thrombogenic valvular or thrombogenic rhythm diseases of the heart; headaches with focal neurologic symptoms or migraine headaches with or without aura if older than age 35; known, suspected, or history of breast cancer, endometrial cancer, or other estrogen-dependent neoplasia; undiagnosed abnormal uterine bleeding; or cholestatic jaundice of pregnancy or jaundice with other hormonal contraceptive use; and in patients older than age 35 who smoke.

• Contraindicated in patients hypersensitive to components of formulation and in women age 65 or older.

• Contraindicated after major surgery with prolonged immobilization.

• Use cautiously in patients with CV risk factors such as HTN, hyperlipidemias, obesity, and diabetes.

• Don't use in patients predisposed to hyperkalemia; drug may increase potassium level.

• Use cautiously in patients with conditions aggravated by fluid retention.

Dialyzable drug: Unknown.

⚠ *Overdose S&S:* Nausea, withdrawal uterine bleeding.

PREGNANCY-LACTATION-REPRODUCTION

• Contraindicated in patients who are or may become pregnant. There is little or no increased risk of birth defects with inadvertent use of combined oral contraceptives during early pregnancy.

• Small amounts of hormonal contraceptives appear in human milk. Use of drug during breastfeeding isn't recommended; may reduce milk production.

NURSING CONSIDERATIONS

❂ *Alert:* The use of contraceptives causes increased risk of MI, thromboembolism, stroke, hepatic neoplasia, gallbladder disease, and HTN. Risk increases in patients with HTN, diabetes, hyperlipidemia, and obesity.

Boxed Warning Smoking increases risk of serious CV adverse effects. Risk increases with age, especially in women older than age 35, and with the number of cigarettes smoked. ■

• Relationship between use of hormonal contraceptives and breast and cervical cancers is unclear. Encourage patients to schedule a complete gynecologic exam at least yearly and to perform breast self-exams monthly.

• In patients scheduled to have elective surgery that may increase the risk of thromboembolism, stop contraceptive use from at least 4 weeks before until 2 weeks after surgery. Also stop use during and after prolonged immobilization.

• Because of increased risk of thromboembolism in the postpartum period, don't start contraceptive earlier than 4 to 6 weeks after delivery.

• Stop use and evaluate patient if loss of vision, proptosis, diplopia, papilledema, or retinal vascular lesions occur. Recommend that contact lens wearers be evaluated by an ophthalmologist if visual changes or lens intolerance occurs.

• If patient misses two consecutive periods, she should obtain a negative pregnancy test result before continuing use of contraceptive.

• Immediately stop use if pregnancy is confirmed.

• Closely monitor patient with diabetes. Glucose intolerance may occur.

• Closely monitor patient with HTN or a history of depression. Stop drug if these events occur.

• In patient at high risk for hyperkalemia and patient taking medications that may increase potassium, check potassium level during the first treatment cycle.

• Stop drug and evaluate patient if persistent, severe headaches occur or if migraines occur or are worsened.

• Evaluate patient for malignancy or pregnancy if she experiences breakthrough bleeding or spotting.

• Closely monitor patient with hyperlipidemias.

• Stop use if jaundice occurs.

• Monitor patient on thyroid replacement therapy as estrogens may lead to decreased total thyroid hormone levels. Thyroid medication dosage may need to be increased while patient is taking estrogens.

• *Look alike–sound alike:* Don't confuse Yaz with Yasmin.

PATIENT TEACHING

• Advise patient to use additional method of birth control during the first 7 days of the first cycle of hormonal contraceptive.

• Inform patient that pills don't protect against sexually transmitted diseases such as HIV.

• Advise patient of the dangers of smoking while taking hormonal contraceptives. Suggest smokers choose a different form of birth control.

• Tell patient to schedule gynecologic exams yearly and to perform breast self-exam monthly.

• Inform patient that spotting, light bleeding, or stomach upset may occur while she is taking the first one to three packs of pills. Tell her to continue taking the pills and to notify health care provider if these symptoms persist.

• Teach patient safe drug administration.

• Tell patient to immediately report sharp chest pain, coughing of blood or sudden shortness of breath, calf pain, crushing chest pain or chest heaviness, sudden severe headache or vomiting, dizziness or fainting, visual or speech disturbances, weakness or numbness in an arm or leg, vision loss, breast lumps, severe stomach pain or tenderness,

---

Reactions in bold italics are *life-threatening*. Interactions may have a *rapid* onset or a *delayed onset*.

difficulty sleeping, lack of energy, fatigue, change in mood, or jaundice with fever, fatigue, loss of appetite, dark urine, or light-colored bowel movements.

• Tell patient to notify health care provider if she wears contact lenses and notices a change in vision or has trouble wearing the lenses.
• Tell patient that risk of pregnancy increases with each active tablet she forgets to take. Inform patient what to do if she misses pills.
• Tell patient to use an additional method of birth control and to notify health care provider if she isn't sure what to do about missed pills.
• Advise patient that amenorrhea may occur. Rule out pregnancy if amenorrhea occurs in two or more consecutive cycles.
• Advise patient who is breastfeeding to use an alternative method of birth control until infant is completely weaned. Quality and quantity of human milk may be decreased. Yellowing of skin and eyes (jaundice) and breast enlargement may occur in breastfed neonates.

SAFETY ALERT!

dulaglutide
doo-la-GLOO-tide

Trulicity

Therapeutic class: Antidiabetics
Pharmacologic class: Glucagon-like peptide-1 receptor agonists

AVAILABLE FORMS
Injection: 0.75 mg/0.5 mL, 1.5 mg/0.5 mL, 3 mg/0.5 mL, 4.5 mg/0.5 mL in single-dose pens

INDICATIONS & DOSAGES
➤ **Adjunct to diet and exercise to improve glycemic control in patients with type 2 diabetes; to reduce risk of major adverse CV events in patients with type 2 diabetes who have established CV disease or multiple CV risk factors**
Adults: 0.75 mg subcut once weekly. Increase dosage to 1.5 mg once weekly for additional glycemic control. If additional glycemic control is needed, increase dosage to 3 mg once weekly after at least 4 weeks on the 1.5-mg dose. If further glycemic control is needed, increase dosage to the maximum dose of

4.5 mg once weekly after at least 4 weeks on the 3-mg dose.

ADMINISTRATION
Subcutaneous
• Inject into abdomen, thigh, or upper arm once weekly any time of day. Use a different injection site each week.
• May give without regard to meals.
• ⚠ *Alert:* Don't mix dulaglutide with insulin. Give as separate injections in nonadjacent areas.
• Don't give IM or IV.
• Inspect for particulate matter and discoloration before administration. Don't give if present.
• Refrigerate at 36° to 46° F (2° to 8° C). May store at room temperature for a total of 14 days if temperature doesn't exceed 86° F (30° C).
• Don't freeze. Don't use drug if it has been frozen.
• Protect from light by storing in original carton until time of administration.
• Discard injection device after each use in puncture-resistant container.
• If a dose is missed, give within 3 days of missed dose; then resume prior schedule. If less than 3 days remain until next scheduled dose, skip the missed dose and give the next dose on schedule.
• The day of weekly administration may be changed if necessary as long as the last dose was 3 or more days before the new day.

ACTION
A human glucagon-like peptide-1 (GLP-1) receptor agonist that, like endogenous GLP-1, binds to and activates the GLP-1 receptor in the pancreatic beta cells, leading to glucose-dependent insulin release. Also decreases glucagon secretion and slows gastric emptying.

Route	Onset	Peak	Duration
Subcut	Unknown	24–72 hr	Unknown

Half-life: About 5 days.

ADVERSE REACTIONS
CNS: fatigue. **CV:** tachycardia, increased PR interval, first-degree AV block. **GI:** nausea, diarrhea, vomiting, decreased appetite, dyspepsia, constipation, flatulence, GERD, eructation; abdominal pain, tenderness, or distention. **GU:** renal impairment.

Hepatic: elevated lipase and amylase levels.
Metabolic: *hypoglycemia.* **Other:** antidrug
antibody formation.

INTERACTIONS

Drug-drug. *Insulin, insulin secretagogues
(meglitinides, sulfonylureas):* May increase
risk of hypoglycemia. Consider reducing insulin or insulin secretagogue dosage; monitor
blood glucose level closely.
Oral medications: May affect absorption of
oral medications since dulaglutide delays gastric emptying. Monitor effects, especially
when given with other drugs with a narrow
therapeutic index such as warfarin.

EFFECTS ON LAB TEST RESULTS

• May increase lipase and amylase levels.
May decrease glucose level.

CONTRAINDICATIONS & CAUTIONS

Boxed Warning Contraindicated in patients
with a personal or family history of medullary
thyroid carcinoma (MTC) and in patients
with multiple endocrine neoplasia syndrome
type 2. ∎
Boxed Warning Thyroid C-cell adenomas
and carcinomas occurred in animal studies.
It isn't known if dulaglutide causes thyroid
C-cell tumors, including MTC, in humans. ∎
• Contraindicated in patients with a serious
hypersensitivity reaction to drug or its components.
• Hypersensitivity reactions (including anaphylaxis and angioedema) have been reported
with other GLP-1 receptor agonists. Use
cautiously in patients with a history of angioedema or anaphylaxis with another GLP-1
receptor agonist.
• Drug hasn't been studied in patients with a
history of pancreatitis. Consider alternative
antidiabetic therapy.
• Drug shouldn't be used in patients with
type 1 diabetes or for treatment of diabetic ketoacidosis. Drug isn't a substitute for insulin.
• To reduce risk of hypoglycemia, consider
dosage reduction of concomitantly administered secretagogues or insulin when initiating
dulaglutide.
• Avoid use in patients with severe GI disease, including severe gastroparesis; drug
slows gastric emptying and hasn't been studied in this population.
• Use cautiously in patients with hepatic or
renal insufficiency.

• Drug may cause diabetic retinopathy complications, especially in patients with a history of diabetic retinopathy.
• Safety and effectiveness in children haven't
been established.
Dialyzable drug: Unknown.
⚠ *Overdose S&S:* Mild or moderate GI symptoms, nonsevere hypoglycemia.

PREGNANCY-LACTATION-REPRODUCTION

• There are no adequate studies during pregnancy. Use cautiously during pregnancy
and only if potential benefit justifies fetal
risk.
• It isn't known if drug appears in human
milk. Use cautiously during breastfeeding
after considering risks.

NURSING CONSIDERATIONS

• Use caution when initiating dulaglutide
therapy or escalating dosage in patients with
renal insufficiency. Monitor renal function,
especially in patients who report severe GI
adverse reactions (nausea, vomiting, diarrhea,
dehydration).
• Monitor patients for hypoglycemia; patients
with concomitant use of insulin secretagogues
or insulin are at increased risk.
• Monitor patients for signs and symptoms
of pancreatitis (including persistent severe
abdominal pain, sometimes radiating to the
back, which may or may not be accompanied
by vomiting). Discontinue drug if pancreatitis
is suspected. Don't restart drug if pancreatitis
is confirmed.
• Monitor patient for tachycardia; monitor
ECG for PR-interval prolongation.
• Refer patients with elevated serum calcitonin level or thyroid nodules on exam or
neck imaging to an endocrinologist.
• Monitor patients with a history of diabetic
retinopathy for disease progression.
• *Look alike–sound alike:* Don't confuse dulaglutide with duloxetine or dutasteride.

PATIENT TEACHING

• Explain to patient that dulaglutide isn't a
substitute for insulin. Educate patient on general diabetes care, including the need to monitor glucose and HbA$_{1c}$ levels, how to recognize the signs and symptoms of hypoglycemia
or hyperglycemia, the importance of diet and
exercise, and the impact stress or trauma may
have on glucose levels.

Reactions in bold italics are *life-threatening*. Interactions may have a *rapid onset* or a ***delayed onset***.

- Warn patient to immediately discontinue drug and inform prescriber if hypersensitivity reactions occur.
- Advise patient to report heart palpitations or feelings of a racing heartbeat while at rest.
- Teach patient of risk of dehydration due to GI adverse reactions, including the associated risk of worsening renal function. Counsel patient to take precautions to avoid fluid depletion.
- Teach patient signs and symptoms of acute pancreatitis (persistent severe abdominal pain, sometimes radiating to the back, which may or may not be accompanied by vomiting) and to discontinue drug promptly and contact prescriber if any of these signs and symptoms occur.
- **Boxed Warning** Inform patient of risk of MTC. Teach the signs and symptoms of thyroid tumors (a mass in the neck, dysphagia, dyspnea, persistent hoarseness). ■
- Instruct patient on the proper use of drug (rotating sites, inspecting solution for particles, discarding needles, storing pens and syringes, handling a missed dose).
- Caution patient never to mix insulin and dulaglutide but to give as separate injections. Although dulaglutide and insulin may be injected in the same body area, they shouldn't be injected adjacent to each other.
- Instruct patient to report pregnancy or plans to become pregnant or to breastfeed.

DULoxetine hydrochloride
doo-LOX-ah-teen

Cymbalta✇, Drizalma Sprinkle

Therapeutic class: Antidepressants
Pharmacologic class: SSNRIs

AVAILABLE FORMS
Capsules (delayed-release) ⓞⓣⓒ: 20 mg, 30 mg, 40 mg, 60 mg

INDICATIONS & DOSAGES
Adjust-a-dose (for all indications): If possible, gradually taper dosage when discontinuing drug to avoid adverse reactions.
➤ **Major depressive disorder**
Adults: Initially, 20 mg PO b.i.d. to 60 mg PO once daily or divided in two equal doses. May also start at 30 mg/day for 1 week to allow patients to adjust to medication. Maximum, 120 mg daily.

➤ **Generalized anxiety disorder**
Adults: 60 mg PO daily. Or, 30 mg PO daily for 1 week; then increase to 60 mg PO daily. May increase in increments of 30 mg daily to 120 mg PO once daily.
Children ages 7 to 17: 30 mg PO once daily for 2 weeks; may increase to 60 mg once daily. For doses greater than 60 mg/day, increase dosage in increments of 30 mg/day. Maximum, 120 mg daily.
Adjust-a-dose: In older adults, initially, 30 mg PO once daily for 2 weeks before considering an increase to target dose of 60 mg once daily. If needed, increase dosage further in increments of 30 mg once daily. Maximum, 120 mg daily.
➤ **Fibromyalgia**
Adults: Initially, 30 mg PO once daily for 1 week; increase to 60 mg PO once daily after a week. Some patients may respond to the starting dose. Maximum dose is 60 mg/day. Base continued treatment on individual patient response.
Children age 13 to 17: 30 mg PO once daily. May increase to 60 mg PO once daily based on response and tolerability.
➤ **Neuropathic pain related to diabetic peripheral neuropathy**
Adults: 60 mg PO once daily.
Adjust-a-dose: Consider a lower starting dose and a gradual increase in dose for patients with renal impairment.
➤ **Chronic musculoskeletal pain**
Adults: Initially, 30 mg PO once daily for 1 week; then increase to 60 mg PO once daily.

ADMINISTRATION
PO
- Give without regard to meals.
- Give capsule whole; don't crush or allow patient to chew capsules.
- Drizalma only: For patients with difficulty swallowing, may open capsule, sprinkle contents over applesauce, and have patient swallow immediately along with tablespoon of applesauce.
- Drizalma only: For patients unable to take medication by mouth, may open capsule and add contents to an all-plastic catheter tip syringe containing 50 mL water. Shake syringe gently for 10 seconds. Deliver immediately through a 12 French or larger NG tube. Ensure no pellets are left in syringe; rinse with additional 15 mL water if needed.

ACTION
Inhibits serotonin and norepinephrine reuptake and is a weak inhibitor of dopamine reuptake in the CNS.

Route	Onset	Peak	Duration
PO	Unknown	5–6 hr (fasting)	Unknown

Half-life: 7.8 to 22.2 hours.

ADVERSE REACTIONS
CNS: dizziness, fatigue, headache, insomnia, somnolence, *suicidality,* fever, hypoesthesia, paresthesia, irritability, lethargy, nervousness, abnormal dreams, insomnia, restlessness, sleep disorder, anxiety, asthenia, tremor, agitation, dysgeusia. **CV:** flushing, increased BP, palpitations. **EENT:** blurred vision, nasopharyngitis, pharyngolaryngeal pain, dry mouth. **GI:** constipation, diarrhea, nausea, dyspepsia, gastritis, vomiting, flatulence, abdominal pain, increased or decreased appetite, viral gastroenteritis. **GU:** abnormal orgasm, urinary frequency, ejaculatory disorder, dysuria, erectile dysfunction, urinary hesitation. **Hepatic:** increased ALT level. **Metabolic:** weight gain or loss, hyponatremia. **Musculoskeletal:** myalgia. **Respiratory:** cough, URI. **Skin:** diaphoresis, night sweats, pruritus, rash. **Other:** decreased libido, hot flash, chills, rigors, yawning.

INTERACTIONS
Drug-drug. *Anticoagulants (aspirin, NSAIDs, warfarin):* May increase bleeding risk. Monitor patient closely.
Class IC antiarrhythmics (flecainide, propafenone), phenothiazines: May increase levels of these drugs. Use together cautiously.
CNS drugs: May increase adverse effects. Use together cautiously.
CYP1A2 inhibitors (cimetidine, fluvoxamine, certain quinolones): May increase duloxetine level. Avoid use together.
CYP1A2 substrates (caffeine, theophylline): May increase substrate level. Use together cautiously.
CYP2D6 inhibitors (fluoxetine, paroxetine, quinidine): May increase duloxetine level. Use together cautiously.
Drugs that reduce gastric acidity: May cause premature breakdown of duloxetine's protective coating and early release of the drug. Monitor patient for effects.
Linezolid, methylene blue: May cause serotonin syndrome. Don't use together.

Lithium, SSNRIs, SSRIs, tramadol: May increase risk of serotonin syndrome. Avoid use together.
⚠ *Alert: MAO inhibitors (phenelzine, rasagiline, selegiline):* May cause hyperthermia, rigidity, myoclonus, autonomic instability, rapid fluctuations of vital signs, agitation, delirium, and coma. Avoid use within 2 weeks after MAO inhibitor therapy; wait at least 5 days after stopping duloxetine before starting MAO inhibitor.
TCAs (amitriptyline, imipramine, nortriptyline): May increase levels of these drugs. Reduce TCA dose, and monitor drug levels closely.
Thioridazine: May prolong the QT interval and increase risk of serious ventricular arrhythmias and sudden death. Avoid using together.
Triptans: May cause serotonin syndrome (restlessness, hallucinations, loss of coordination, fast heartbeat, rapid changes in BP, increased body temperature, hyperreflexia, nausea, vomiting, and diarrhea) or NMS. Use cautiously and with increased monitoring, especially when starting or increasing dosages.
Drug-herb. *St. John's wort:* May increase risk of serotonin syndrome. Discourage use together.
Drug-lifestyle. *Alcohol use:* May increase risk of liver damage. Discourage use together.

EFFECTS ON LAB TEST RESULTS
• May increase ALP, ALT, AST, bilirubin, glucose, and CK levels.
• May decrease sodium level.

CONTRAINDICATIONS & CAUTIONS
• Contraindicated in patients hypersensitive to drug or its ingredients and in patients taking MAO inhibitors. Drug isn't recommended for patients with hepatic dysfunction, severe renal impairment, or ESRD.
⚠ *Alert:* Before using duloxetine in a child or adolescent, balance potential risks with clinical need.
• Safety and effectiveness in children younger than age 7 for generalized anxiety disorder or younger than age 13 for fibromyalgia haven't been established. Use for other indications hasn't been studied.
• Don't begin duloxetine in patients receiving linezolid or methylene blue. If urgent treatment with linezolid or methylene blue is needed in patient already receiving

---

Reactions in bold italics are *life-threatening*. Interactions may have a *rapid onset* or a *delayed onset*.

duloxetine, discontinue duloxetine; then administer linezolid or methylene blue.
• Use cautiously in patients with a history of mania or seizures, patients who drink substantial amounts of alcohol, patients with HTN, patients with controlled angle-closure glaucoma, and those with conditions that slow gastric emptying.
• Pupil dilation that occurs after duloxetine use may trigger an angle-closure attack in a patient with anatomically narrow angles who doesn't have a patent iridectomy.
• Drug may increase risk of bleeding events.
• Orthostatic hypotension, falls, and syncope have been reported with therapeutic doses and tend to occur within first week of therapy but can occur at any time during treatment, particularly after dosage increases. Fall risk appears to increase steadily with age and be related to degree of orthostatic decrease in BP as well as other factors that may increase the underlying risk of falls. Consider dosage reduction or discontinuing drug if falls occur.
Dialyzable drug: Unlikely.

⚠ Overdose S&S: Coma, hypotension, HTN, seizures, serotonin syndrome, somnolence, syncope, tachycardia, vomiting.

PREGNANCY-LACTATION-REPRODUCTION
• There are no adequate well-controlled studies during pregnancy. Use during pregnancy only if potential benefit justifies fetal risk.
• To monitor pregnancy outcomes, enroll patients exposed to drug during pregnancy in the Cymbalta Pregnancy Registry (1-866-814-6975) or www.cymbaltapregnancyregistry.com).
• Use during the third trimester may cause neonatal complications, including respiratory distress, cyanosis, apnea, seizures, vomiting, hypoglycemia, hypotonia, and hyperreflexia, which may require prolonged hospitalization, respiratory support, and tube feeding.
• Drug appears in human milk. Use cautiously during breastfeeding and only when benefits outweigh risks.

NURSING CONSIDERATIONS
Boxed Warning Drug may increase risk of suicidality in children, adolescents, and young adults ages 18 to 24, especially during the first few months of treatment, and in those with major depressive disorder or other psychiatric disorder. ▪

Boxed Warning Monitor all patients for worsening of depression or emergence of suicidality, especially when therapy starts or dosage changes. ▪
🔋 Alert: Concomitant use with linezolid or methylene blue can cause serotonin syndrome (fever, mental status changes, muscle twitching, diaphoresis, shivering or shaking, diarrhea, loss of coordination). If linezolid or methylene blue must be given, stop drug and monitor patient for serotonin toxicity for 5 days or until 24 hours after last dose of methylene blue or linezolid, whichever comes first. May resume treatment 24 hours after last dose of methylene blue or linezolid.
• If taken with TCAs, duloxetine metabolism will be prolonged, and patient will need extended monitoring.
• Severe skin reactions, including erythema multiforme and SJS, can occur. Discontinue at first sign of blisters, peeling rash, mucosal erosions, or other signs or symptoms of hypersensitivity if no other etiology can be identified.
• Periodically reassess patient to determine the need for continued therapy.
• Don't stop drug abruptly. Decrease dosage gradually, and watch for symptoms that may arise when drug is stopped, such as dizziness, nausea, headache, paresthesia, vomiting, irritability, and nightmares.
• If intolerable symptoms arise when decreasing or stopping drug, restart at previous dose and decrease even more gradually.
• Monitor BP periodically during treatment.
• Older adults may be more sensitive to drug effects than younger adults.
🔋 Alert: Combining triptans with an SSRI or an SSNRI may cause serotonin syndrome or NMS-like reactions. Signs and symptoms of serotonin syndrome may include restlessness, hallucinations, loss of coordination, fast heartbeat, rapid changes in BP, increased body temperature, overactive reflexes, nausea, vomiting, and diarrhea. Serotonin syndrome may be more likely to occur when starting or increasing the dose of triptan, SSRI, or SSNRI.
• May worsen glycemic control in patients with diabetes. Monitor blood glucose levels.
• *Look alike–sound alike:* Don't confuse duloxetine with fluoxetine or paroxetine. Don't confuse Cymbalta with Symbyax.

♣Canada   ◇OTC   ◆Off-label use   ✐Photoguide   ⊜Do not crush   *Liquid contains alcohol   ▓Genetic

PATIENT TEACHING

Boxed Warning Warn families or caregivers to report signs of worsening depression (such as agitation, irritability, insomnia, hostility, impulsivity) and signs of suicidality to prescriber immediately. ■

⚠ Alert: Teach patient to recognize and immediately report signs and symptoms of serotonin toxicity (fever, mental status changes, muscle twitching, diaphoresis, shivering or shaking, diarrhea, loss of coordination).

• Tell patient to contact prescriber immediately and to discontinue drug at first sign of hypersensitivity (including blisters, peeling rash, or mucosal erosions).

• Tell patient to not stop drug abruptly; dosage must be gradually reduced to avoid adverse effects.

• Tell patient to consult prescriber or pharmacist before taking other prescription or OTC drugs or herbal or other dietary supplements.

• Urge patient to avoid activities that are hazardous or require mental alertness until drug's effects are known.

• Warn against drinking alcohol during therapy.

• If patient takes drug for depression, explain that it may take 1 to 4 weeks to notice an effect.

• Advise patients with diabetes to closely monitor blood glucose level.

dutasteride
doo-TAS-teh-ride

Avodart*

Therapeutic class: BPH drugs
Pharmacologic class: 5-alpha-reductase enzyme inhibitors

AVAILABLE FORMS
Capsules ⊙: 0.5 mg

INDICATIONS & DOSAGES

➤ **To treat and improve the symptoms of BPH, reduce the risk of acute urine retention, and reduce the need for BPH-related surgery**

Men: 0.5 mg PO once daily as monotherapy. May be given with tamsulosin 0.4 mg PO once daily as combination therapy.

ADMINISTRATION
PO
• Drug is considered a teratogen. Follow safe handling and disposal procedures.
• Don't crush, break, or allow patient to chew capsules; contact with contents may cause oropharyngeal irritation.
• Give drug without regard for food.

ACTION
Inhibits conversion of testosterone to dihydrotestosterone, the androgen primarily responsible for the initial development and subsequent enlargement of the prostate gland.

Route	Onset	Peak	Duration
PO	Unknown	2–3 hr	Unknown

Half-life: About 5 weeks.

ADVERSE REACTIONS
GU: impotence, erectile dysfunction, decreased libido, ejaculation disorder. **Other:** gynecomastia, breast tenderness.

INTERACTIONS
Drug-drug. *CYP3A4 inhibitors (cimetidine, ciprofloxacin, diltiazem, ketoconazole, ritonavir, verapamil):* May increase dutasteride level. Use together cautiously and monitor therapy.

EFFECTS ON LAB TEST RESULTS
• May increase total testosterone and TSH levels.
• May lower PSA level.

CONTRAINDICATIONS & CAUTIONS
• Contraindicated in patients hypersensitive to dutasteride or its ingredients or to other 5-alpha-reductase inhibitors.
• Drug isn't indicated for use in females or children.
⚠ Alert: 5-Alpha-reductase inhibitors may increase the risk of high-grade prostate cancer. Before start of therapy, evaluate patients to rule out other urologic conditions, including prostate cancer that might mimic BPH. Any increase in PSA level in patient receiving dutasteride should be considered significant; evaluate patient for prostate cancer.
• Use cautiously in patients with hepatic disease.
Dialyzable drug: Unknown.

PREGNANCY-LACTATION-REPRODUCTION

• Drug isn't indicated for use in females. Contraindicated during pregnancy.

☙ *Alert:* Because drug may be absorbed through the skin, patients who are or may become pregnant shouldn't handle drug, especially avoiding contact with crushed or broken tablets. If contact occurs, wash contact area immediately with soap and water.

• It isn't known if drug appears in human milk. Contraindicated for use during breast-feeding.

• Drug appears in semen. Effects on male fertility are unknown.

NURSING CONSIDERATIONS

• Carefully monitor patients with a large residual urine volume or severely diminished urine flow, or both, for obstructive uropathy.

• Patients should wait at least 6 months after their last dose before donating blood.

• Establish a new baseline PSA level at least 3 months after start of treatment, and use it to assess potentially cancer-related changes in PSA level.

• To interpret PSA values in men treated for 3 months or more, double the PSA value for comparison with normal values in untreated men.

• Evaluate patients for prostate cancer and other urologic conditions that may cause similar signs and symptoms before initiating therapy and periodically thereafter.

PATIENT TEACHING

• Instruct patient in safe drug administration and handling.

• Inform patient that ejaculate volume may decrease but that sexual function should remain normal.

• Caution patient who is pregnant or may become pregnant not to handle drug. A male fetus exposed to drug by the mother's swallowing or absorbing the drug through the skin may be born with abnormal sex organs.

☙ *Alert:* Tell patient not to donate blood for at least 6 months after final dose to prevent drug administration to a transfusion recipient who is pregnant.

• Advise patient that drug is present in semen.

• Tell patient periodic blood tests will be needed to monitor therapeutic effects.

SAFETY ALERT!

edoxaban tosylate
e-DOX-a-ban

Savaysa

Therapeutic class: Factor Xa inhibitors
Pharmacologic class: Anticoagulants

E

AVAILABLE FORMS
Tablets: 15 mg, 30 mg, 60 mg

INDICATIONS & DOSAGES

Adjust-a-dose (for all indications): If CrCl is 15 to 50 mL/minute, decrease dosage to 30 mg PO once daily.

➤ **To reduce risk of stroke and systemic embolism in patients with nonvalvular atrial fibrillation (NVAF)**

Adults: 60 mg PO once daily. Refer to manufacturer's instructions for transitioning to or from other anticoagulants.

Boxed Warning Don't use for treatment of NVAF in patients with CrCl greater than 95 mL/minute because of increased risk of ischemic stroke ∎

➤ **DVT and PE**

Adults weighing more than 60 kg: 60 mg PO once daily after 5 to 10 days of therapy with a parenteral anticoagulant. Refer to manufacturer's instructions for transitioning to or from other anticoagulants.

Adjust-a-dose: If patient weighs 60 kg or less or is taking certain concomitant P-gp inhibitors, decrease dosage to 30 mg PO once daily.

ADMINISTRATION
PO

• Give without regard to meals.

• For patients who can't swallow whole tablets, crush tablets and mix with applesauce or 60 to 90 mL water; give immediately. For patients with a gastric tube, mix crushed tablets with 60 to 90 mL water and give immediately.

• If a dose is missed, give as soon as possible on the same day. Resume normal schedule the following day. Don't double the dose to make up for missed dose.

ACTION

Inhibits free factor Xa, prothrombinase activity, and thrombin-induced platelet

---

♣Canada   ◇OTC   ◆Off-label use   ✐Photoguide   ⊜Do not crush   *Liquid contains alcohol   ▩Genetic aggregation. Inhibition of factor Xa in the coagulation cascade reduces thrombin generation and thrombus formation.

Route	Onset	Peak	Duration
PO	Unknown	1–2 hr	Unknown

Half-life: 10 to 14 hours.

ADVERSE REACTIONS
CNS: *intracranial hemorrhage, hemorrhagic stroke, epidural or spinal hematoma.* **CV:** *hemorrhage.* **EENT:** epistaxis, *oral hemorrhage.* **GI:** *GI hemorrhage.* **GU:** *vaginal hemorrhage,* hematuria. **Hematologic:** anemia, bruising. **Hepatic:** abnormal LFT values. **Skin:** rash, puncture-site bleeding.

INTERACTIONS
Drug-drug. *Anticoagulants, antiplatelet drugs (aspirin, P2Y12 inhibitors), NSAIDs, omega-3-fatty acids, SSNRIs, SSRIs, thrombolytics, vitamin E, vorapaxar:* May increase risk of bleeding. Monitor patient for bleeding during therapy.
Aspirin: May cause bleeding. Monitor patients on long-term low-dose aspirin therapy for bleeding.
Digoxin: May increase digoxin level. Monitor digoxin level closely.
P-gp inducers (rifampin): May increase P-gp inducer exposure and decrease edoxaban serum concentration. Avoid concomitant use.
P-gp inhibitors (itraconazole[oral], ketoconazole [oral],macrolide antibiotics, quinidine, verapamil): May increase edoxaban level when edoxaban is used for DVT or PE; reduce edoxaban dosage to 30 mg if patient is receiving these medications. Edoxaban dosage adjustment isn't recommended when edoxaban is used to treat NVAF.
Drug-herb. *Alfalfa, anise, bilberry:* May increase bleeding risk. Don't use together.

EFFECTS ON LAB TEST RESULTS
• May increase LFT values.
• May increase PT, PTT, and INR.
• May decrease thrombocyte and RBC counts.

CONTRAINDICATIONS & CAUTIONS
• Contraindicated in patients hypersensitive to drug or its components and in those with active pathological bleeding.
Boxed Warning Contraindicated in patients with CrCl greater than 95 mL/minute.

Efficacy is reduced in patients with NVAF with CrCl greater than 95 mL/minute, increasing the risk of stroke. There is an increased risk of ischemic stroke in patients with NVAF if their renal function improves and edoxaban blood level decreases. ∎
• Drug isn't recommended in patients with triple positive antiphospholipid syndrome due to increased risk of thrombotic events.
• Drug hasn't been studied in patients with mechanical heart valves or moderate to severe mitral stenosis or when CrCl is less than 15 mL/minute. Use isn't recommended in these patients.
• Use isn't recommended in patients with moderate to severe hepatic impairment (Child-Pugh classes B and C) because of possible intrinsic coagulation abnormalities.
Boxed Warning Epidural or spinal hematomas may occur in patients treated with edoxaban who are receiving neuraxial anesthesia or undergoing spinal puncture. Risk increases with indwelling epidural catheters, concomitant drugs that affect hemostasis (NSAIDs, platelet inhibitors, anticoagulants), spinal surgery or deformity, or a history of traumatic or repeated epidural or spinal punctures. The optimal timing between edoxaban administration and neuraxial procedures isn't known. Weigh risks and benefits before neuraxial intervention in patients who are or will be anticoagulated. ∎
• Safety and effectiveness in children haven't been established.
Dialyzable drug: Less than 7%.
⚠ *Overdose S&S:* Bleeding.

PREGNANCY-LACTATION-REPRODUCTION
• There are no adequate studies during pregnancy. Use during pregnancy only if benefit outweighs fetal risk.
• It isn't known if drug appears in human milk. Patient should discontinue breastfeeding or discontinue drug.

NURSING CONSIDERATIONS
Boxed Warning Premature discontinuation of drug increases risk of ischemic events. If drug is stopped for a reason other than pathological bleeding or completion of treatment, consider transitioning to an alternative anticoagulant. ∎
• Monitor patient for bleeding. Immediately evaluate signs or symptoms of blood loss; discontinue drug if acute pathological bleeding

---

Reactions in bold italics are *life-threatening*. Interactions may have a *rapid onset* or a ***delayed onset***.

occurs. Drug can cause serious and potentially fatal bleeding.

• A reversal agent for edoxaban isn't available.

• Discontinue edoxaban at least 24 hours before invasive or surgical procedures. If surgery can't be delayed, weigh risk of bleeding against urgency of intervention.

• After surgery or other procedure, may restart edoxaban as soon as hemostasis has been achieved and patient can take oral medication.

⚠️ *Alert:* Don't remove indwelling epidural or intrathecal catheters earlier than 12 hours after last dose of edoxaban. Don't give next dose earlier than 2 hours after removal of the catheter.

Boxed Warning Monitor patients frequently after spinal or epidural anesthesia or puncture for signs and symptoms of neurologic impairment (numbness or weakness of the legs, bowel or bladder dysfunction). Evaluate impairment urgently. ∎

• Be aware that vitamin K, protamine, tranexamic acid, and dialysis aren't expected to reverse the effects of edoxaban.

PATIENT TEACHING

• Warn patient that bruising and bleeding may occur more easily and that bleeding may last longer during therapy.

• Instruct patient to immediately report unusual bleeding to prescriber.

• Teach patient to take drug exactly as prescribed.

• Advise patient not to discontinue drug without first consulting prescriber.

• Caution patient to inform health care providers about taking edoxaban before scheduling surgery or medical or dental procedures.

• Instruct patient to inform health care providers and dentists about prescription medications, OTC drugs, or herbal products currently being taken or that may be taken.

• Advise patient to immediately report pregnancy, plans to become pregnant, or intent to breastfeed during treatment.

• Warn patient having neuraxial anesthesia or spinal puncture to watch for signs and symptoms of spinal or epidural hematoma, such as back pain, tingling, numbness (especially in the lower limbs), muscle weakness, and stool or urine incontinence. If any of these

symptoms occur, advise patient to immediately contact health care provider.

• Warn patient to immediately report signs and symptoms of hemorrhage or adverse reactions, such as one-sided weakness, problems thinking or speaking, dizziness, balance changes, blurred vision, severe headache, and pale skin.

efavirenz
eff-ah-VYE-renz

Sustiva

Therapeutic class: Antiretrovirals
Pharmacologic class: NNRTIs

AVAILABLE FORMS
Capsules ⓘ: 50 mg, 100 mg, 200 mg
Tablets ⓘ: 600 mg

INDICATIONS & DOSAGES
➤ **HIV-1 infection, with other antiretrovirals**

Adults and children age 3 months and older weighing 40 kg or more: 600 mg (three 200-mg capsules or one 600-mg tablet) PO once daily on an empty stomach, preferably at bedtime.

Children age 3 months and older weighing 32.5 to less than 40 kg: 400 mg PO once daily, preferably at bedtime.

Children age 3 months and older weighing 25 to less than 32.5 kg: 350 mg PO once daily, preferably at bedtime.

Children age 3 months and older weighing 20 to less than 25 kg: 300 mg PO once daily, preferably at bedtime.

Children age 3 months and older weighing 15 to less than 20 kg: 250 mg PO once daily, preferably at bedtime.

Children age 3 months and older weighing 7.5 to less than 15 kg: 200 mg PO once daily, preferably at bedtime.

Children age 3 months and older weighing 5 to less than 7.5 kg: 150 mg PO once daily, preferably at bedtime.

Children age 3 months and older weighing 3.5 to less than 5 kg: 100 mg PO once daily, preferably at bedtime.

Adjust-a-dose: For adults also taking voriconazole, increase voriconazole maintenance dose to 400 mg every 12 hours and decrease efavirenz dose to 300 mg once daily using capsule formulation. For adults and children weighing 50 kg or more who are also taking rifampin, recommended efavirenz dosage is 800 mg once daily.

ADMINISTRATION
PO
• Drug must be given in combination with other antiretrovirals.
• Give drug at bedtime to decrease CNS adverse effects.
• In children, consider prophylaxis with antihistamines before initiating therapy, to prevent rash.
• Don't break or crush tablets. Don't crush capsules.
• Give once daily on an empty stomach.
• For patients who can't swallow capsules or tablets, capsule contents may be sprinkled over a small amount (1 or 2 tsp) of food and mixed gently. For patients who can tolerate solid foods, mix with soft food, such as applesauce, grape jelly, or yogurt.
• For young infants, dose from capsules can be gently mixed into 10 mL of reconstituted room-temperature infant formula in a 30-mL medicine cup. If more than 1 capsule is needed for a dose, add contents of all capsules needed to 10 mL of formula; don't add more formula. Draw up dose mixture into a 10-mL dosing syringe to administer; then add an additional 10 mL to mixing cup and stir to disperse any remaining residue. Administer to infant.
• Give efavirenz mixture within 30 minutes of mixing. Patient shouldn't consume any additional food or additional formula for 2 hours after administration.

ACTION
Inhibits nonnucleoside reverse transcriptase, which inhibits the transcription of HIV-1 RNA to DNA, a critical step in the viral replication process, suppressing viral replication.

Route	Onset	Peak	Duration
PO	Unknown	3–5 hr	Unknown

Half-life: Single dose, 52 to 76 hours; multiple doses, 40 to 55 hours.

ADVERSE REACTIONS
CNS: dizziness, abnormal dreams or thinking, anxiety, agitation, amnesia, confusion, depersonalization, depression, euphoria, fever, fatigue, pain, hallucinations, headache, hypoesthesia, impaired concentration, insomnia, nervousness, somnolence. **GI:** diarrhea, nausea, abdominal pain, anorexia, dyspepsia, vomiting. **Hematologic:** neutropenia. **Hepatic:** increased transaminase levels, increased GGT level. **Metabolic:** increased amylase level, hyperglycemia, hypertriglyceridemia. **Skin:** rash, *erythema multiforme,* pruritus.

INTERACTIONS
Efavirenz can interact significantly with many drugs. Consult a drug interaction resource or pharmacist for additional information.
Drug-drug. *Amprenavir, clarithromycin, lopinavir:* May decrease levels of these drugs. Consider alternative therapy or dosage adjustment.
Atorvastatin, calcium channel blockers, itraconazole, pravastatin, simvastatin: May decrease levels of these drugs. Dosage adjustments may be necessary.
Bepridil, ergot derivatives, midazolam, pimozide: May inhibit metabolism of these drugs and cause serious or life-threatening adverse events (such as arrhythmias, prolonged sedation, or respiratory depression). Avoid using together.
Bupropion: May decrease plasma concentrations and clinical effects of bupropion. Guide bupropion dosage by clinical response.
Carbamazepine: May decrease both carbamazepine and efavirenz levels. Avoid using together.
CYP2B6 inducers (strong): May increase metabolism of CYP2B6 substrates. Consider an alternative for one of the interacting drugs. Some combinations may be specifically contraindicated. Consult appropriate manufacturer labeling. Consider therapy modification.
CYP2B6 inhibitors: May decrease metabolism of CYP2B6 substrates. Consider therapy modification.
CYP2C19 substrates: CYP2C19 moderate inhibitors may decrease metabolism of CYP2C19 substrates. Monitor therapy.
CYP3A4 inducers (strong): May increase metabolism of CYP3A4 substrates. Consider an alternative for one of the interacting drugs. Some combinations may be specifically contraindicated. Consult appropriate manufacturer labeling. Consider therapy modification.
CYP3A4 substrates: CYP3A4 moderate inhibitors may decrease metabolism of CYP3A4 substrates. Monitor therapy.

Reactions in bold italics are *life-threatening*. Interactions may have a *rapid onset* or a *delayed onset*.

Drugs that induce the CYP3A enzyme system (phenobarbital, phenytoin, rifampin): May decrease efavirenz level. Avoid using together. Refer to manufacturer's instructions for contraindications.

Drugs that prolong QT interval (amiodarone, haloperidol, lithium, procainamide, thioridazine): May increase risk of torsades de pointes. Consider alternative to efavirenz.

Estrogens, ritonavir: May increase drug levels. Monitor patient.

Hormonal contraceptives (ethinyl estradiol–norgestimate, etonogestrel): May decrease norgestimate and etonogestrel levels. Advise use of a reliable method of barrier contraception in addition to use of hormonal contraceptives.

Nevirapine: May decrease efavirenz clinical effectiveness and increase risk of adverse reactions. Avoid using together.

Psychoactive drugs: May cause additive CNS effects. Avoid using together.

Ranolazine: May decrease ranolazine concentration. Don't use together.

Rifabutin: May decrease rifabutin level. Increase daily rifabutin dosage by 50%. Consider doubling rifabutin dosage when rifabutin is given two to three times per week.

Rifampin: May decrease efavirenz concentration. Monitor therapy.

Ritonavir: May increase levels of both drugs. Monitor patient and liver function closely.

Saquinavir: May decrease saquinavir level and efavirenz exposure to the body. Don't use with saquinavir as sole protease inhibitor.

Voriconazole (in standard doses): Decreases voriconazole level significantly, while efavirenz level significantly increases. Avoid using together unless doses of each are adjusted.

Warfarin: May increase or decrease level and effects of warfarin. Monitor INR.

Drug-herb. *St. John's wort:* May decrease response and lead to possible resistance to efavirenz or all same-class drugs. Don't use together.

Ginkgo biloba: May decrease efavirenz concentration. Monitor concurrent use.

Kava kava: May enhance adverse or toxic effect of CNS depressants. Monitor therapy.

Drug-food. *High-fat meals:* May increase absorption of drug. Instruct patient to maintain a proper low-fat diet.

Drug-lifestyle. *Alcohol use:* May enhance CNS effects. Discourage use together.

EFFECTS ON LAB TEST RESULTS
- May increase ALT, AST, GGT, triglyceride, glucose, amylase, and cholesterol levels.
- May decrease neutrophil count.
- May cause false-positive urine cannabinoid and benzodiazepine test results.

CONTRAINDICATIONS & CAUTIONS
- Contraindicated in patients hypersensitive to drug or its components and when used concomitantly with elbasvir or grazoprevir.
- Use in patients with moderate or severe hepatic impairment (Child-Pugh class B or C) isn't recommended.
- Use cautiously in patients with mild hepatic impairment (Child-Pugh class A) and in those receiving hepatotoxic drugs. Monitor LFT values in patients with history of hepatitis B or C and in those taking ritonavir.
- Administration with Atripla (efavirenz 600 mg/emtricitabine 200 mg/tenofovir disoproxil fumarate 300 mg) isn't recommended unless needed for dosage adjustment (e.g., with rifampin), because efavirenz is one of its active ingredients.
- Serious psychiatric adverse reactions have been reported, including aggressive behavior, severe depression, suicidality, nonfatal suicide attempts, paranoia, and mania. Use cautiously in patients with a history of mental illness or substance abuse.
- Drug may prolong QT interval. Avoid use in patients at increased risk for or with other drugs with known risk of torsades de pointes. Consider an alternative to efavirenz.
- Use cautiously in patients with a history of seizures.
- Immune reconstitution syndrome has been reported in patients treated with combination antiretroviral therapy.
- Drug frequently affects the nervous system. Signs and symptoms usually begin 1 to 2 days after start of therapy and resolve in 2 to 4 weeks but don't indicate onset of psychiatric signs and symptoms. Giving dose at bedtime may improve tolerability.
- Late-onset neurotoxicity, including ataxia and encephalopathy (impaired consciousness, confusion, psychomotor slowing, psychosis, delirium), may occur months to years after therapy.
- Rash usually begins within 1 to 2 weeks after start of therapy and resolves within 4 weeks. Discontinue drug if severe rash (SJS) develops.

Dialyzable drug: No.

⚠ *Overdose S&S:* Increased nervous system symptoms, involuntary muscle contractions.

PREGNANCY-LACTATION-REPRODUCTION

• Because of the risk of neural tube defects, don't use drug in first trimester. Advise patients who are pregnant of the risk to a fetus. Strongly consider other antiretrovirals.

• Register patients who are pregnant in the Antiretroviral Pregnancy Registry at 1-800-258-4263 or www.apregistry.com.

• Patients should avoid breastfeeding because of the risk of HIV transmission.

• Patients of childbearing potential should use barrier contraception in combination with other (hormonal) contraception methods during therapy and for 12 weeks after therapy ends.

NURSING CONSIDERATIONS

🖑 *Alert:* Drug shouldn't be used as monotherapy or added on as a single drug to a regimen failing because of viral resistance.

• Verify pregnancy status before treatment

• Using drug with ritonavir may increase liver enzyme levels and adverse effects (such as dizziness, nausea, and paresthesia).

• Monitor LFT values before and during treatment in all patients. Consider discontinuing drug in patients with persistent elevations of serum transaminase levels greater than $5 \times$ ULN. Discontinue drug if elevation is accompanied by clinical signs or symptoms of hepatitis or hepatic decompensation.

• Children may be more prone to adverse reactions, especially diarrhea, nausea, vomiting, and rash. Consider prophylaxis with antihistamines before initiating therapy, to prevent rash in this population.

• Discontinue drug if patient develops severe rash associated with blistering, desquamation, mucosal involvement, or fever.

• Monitor patients for elevated triglyceride and cholesterol levels before therapy and periodically during treatment.

• Monitor patients for nervous system and psychiatric symptoms.

PATIENT TEACHING

• Tell patient to take drug exactly as prescribed and not to stop drug without medical approval. Also instruct patient to report adverse reactions.

• Tell patient to immediately report signs and symptoms of serious psychiatric adverse effects.

• Inform patient about need for blood tests to monitor LFT values and triglyceride levels.

• Tell patient to use a barrier contraceptive with a hormonal contraceptive during therapy and for 12 weeks after therapy ends and to notify prescriber immediately if pregnancy is suspected; drug is a known risk to the fetus. Hormonal methods that contain progesterone may have decreased effectiveness.

• Inform patient that drug doesn't cure HIV infection, that opportunistic infections and other complications of HIV infection may continue to occur, and that transmission of HIV to others through sexual contact or blood contamination is still possible.

• Inform patient that rash is a common adverse effect. Tell patient to report rash immediately because it may be serious in rare cases.

• Instruct patient to report use of other drugs, including OTC drugs and herbal supplements.

• Advise patient that dizziness, difficulty sleeping or concentrating, drowsiness, or unusual dreams may occur during the first few days of therapy. Reassure patient that these symptoms typically resolve after 2 to 4 weeks and may be less problematic if drug is taken at bedtime.

• Tell patient to avoid alcohol, driving, or operating machinery until the drug's effects are known.

elagolix
el-a-GOE-lix

Orilissa

Therapeutic class: Endocrine drugs
Pharmacologic class: GnRH receptor antagonists

AVAILABLE FORMS
Tablets: 150 mg, 200 mg

INDICATIONS & DOSAGES

Adjust-a-dose (for all indications): For patients with moderate hepatic impairment (Child-Pugh class B), give 150 mg PO once daily for up to 6 months. Use of 200 mg b.i.d. isn't recommended.

Reactions in bold italics are *life-threatening*. Interactions may have a *rapid onset* or a ***delayed onset***.

➤ **Management of moderate to severe pain associated with endometriosis**
Women age 18 and older: 150 mg PO once daily for up to 24 months.
➤ **Management of moderate to severe pain associated with endometriosis with dyspareunia**
Women age 18 and older: 200 mg PO b.i.d. for up to 6 months.

ADMINISTRATION
PO
• Exclude pregnancy before starting drug or start drug within 7 days from the onset of menses.
• Give at approximately the same time each day, with or without food.
• Give missed dose on the same day as soon as possible; then resume regular dosing schedule.
• Store at 36° to 86° F (2° to 30° C).

ACTION
A GnRH receptor antagonist that suppresses the pituitary gland and decreases concentrations of the ovarian sex hormones, estradiol and progesterone.

Route	Onset	Peak	Duration
PO	Unknown	1 hr	Unknown

Half-life: 4 to 6 hours.

ADVERSE REACTIONS
CNS: headache, insomnia, anxiety, depression, mood changes, exacerbation of mood disorders, dizziness, irritability. **GI:** nausea, diarrhea, abdominal pain, constipation. **GU:** changes in menstrual bleeding pattern, amenorrhea, decreased libido. **Metabolic:** night sweats, weight gain. **Musculoskeletal:** arthralgia, bone loss. **Skin:** rash. **Other:** hot flushes, hypersensitivity reactions.

INTERACTIONS
Drug-drug. *CYP3A inducers (carbamazepine, phenytoin):* May decrease elagolix level. Monitor therapy.
Hormonal contraceptives: May reduce efficacy of elagolix if contraceptive contains estrogen. Use of nonhormonal contraception is recommended during treatment and for at least 28 days after final dose.
Midazolam: May decrease midazolam level. Monitor patient for effectiveness; adjust midazolam dosage as clinically indicated.

Rifampin: May increase elagolix level. Limit elagolix dosage to 150 mg once daily and concomitant use to 6 months.
Rosuvastatin: May decrease rosuvastatin level. Consider increasing rosuvastatin dosage.
Strong CYP3A inhibitors (cobicistat, conivaptan, danoprevir, elvitegravir, itraconazole, ketoconazole, lopinavir, posaconazole, ritonavir, saquinavir, tipranavir, voriconazole): May increase elagolix concentration. Limit 200-mg b.i.d. regimen to 1 month and limit concomitant use of 150-mg once-daily regimen to 6 months.
Strong OATP1B1 inhibitors (cyclosporine, gemfibrozil): May decrease elagolix concentration. Use together is contraindicated.
Substrates of CYP3A (alprazolam, atorvastatin, buspirone, colchicine, darunavir, rivaroxaban, saquinavir, simvastatin, tipranavir, triazolam): May decrease concentrations of these drugs. Monitor patient for therapeutic effect; adjust substrate dosage as clinically indicated.
Substrates of P-gp (digoxin): May increase digoxin concentration. Monitor digoxin level; adjust dosage as indicated.

EFFECTS ON LAB TEST RESULTS
• May increase hepatic transaminase, total cholesterol, LDL-C, HDL-C, and triglyceride levels.

CONTRAINDICATIONS & CAUTIONS
• Contraindicated in patients hypersensitive to drug and in those with severe hepatic impairment (Child-Pugh class C) or known osteoporosis.
• **Alert:** Use cautiously in patients with a history of suicidality or depression. Drug may increase risk of suicidality and mood disorders.
• Drug can cause liver impairment and should be used at the lowest effective dose.
• Drug may cause bone loss, which may not be completely reversible. Assess bone mineral density in patients with additional risk factors for osteoporosis. Limit duration of use in all patients.
• Safety and effectiveness in patients younger than age 18 haven't been studied.
Dialyzable drug: No.

PREGNANCY-LACTATION-REPRODUCTION

• Contraindicated during pregnancy. Drug may increase risk of early pregnancy loss. Discontinue drug if pregnancy occurs during treatment.

• Patients who become pregnant during treatment should enroll in the pregnancy registry (1-833-782-7241).

• Exclude pregnancy before start of treatment and obtain pregnancy test if pregnancy is suspected during treatment.

• Patients should use nonhormonal contraception during treatment and for 28 days after final dose.

• There are no data on the presence of drug or its metabolites in human milk or on the effects on the breastfed infant or on milk production. Consider benefits of treatment and risks to the breastfed infant before use.

NURSING CONSIDERATIONS

🕒 *Alert:* Monitor patient for suicidality and exacerbation of existing mood disorders.

🕒 *Alert:* Promptly evaluate patient with depressive symptoms to determine whether risks of continued therapy outweigh benefits.

🕒 *Alert:* Refer patients with new or worsening depression, anxiety, or other mood changes to a mental health professional for assessment.

• Monitor bone mineral density in patients with a history of low-trauma fracture or other risk factors for osteoporosis or bone loss.

• Consider supplementation with calcium and vitamin D. The benefit of patients taking these supplements during treatment with elagolix hasn't been studied, but supplements may be beneficial for all patients.

• Monitor patient for changes in menstrual bleeding (reduction in amount, intensity, or duration). These changes can make it difficult to recognize pregnancy. Perform pregnancy testing if pregnancy is suspected; discontinue treatment if confirmed.

• Monitor patient for signs and symptoms of liver injury (jaundice, abdominal pain, dark amber–colored urine, fatigue, nausea, vomiting, generalized swelling, easy bruising). Obtain LFT values if signs and symptoms occur.

PATIENT TEACHING

🕒 *Alert:* Advise patient to seek immediate medical attention for suicidality, new-onset or worsening depression, anxiety, or other mood changes.

🕒 *Alert:* Counsel family member or caregivers to watch for changes in behavior and to immediately report suicidality to prescriber.

• Advise patient that drug may cause menstrual changes, which can make it difficult to detect an early pregnancy. Counsel patient to obtain a pregnancy test if pregnancy is suspected and to discontinue drug if pregnancy is confirmed.

• Caution patient to avoid pregnancy while using drug and to use nonhormonal contraceptives during and for 28 days after treatment, even if taking oral contraceptives.

• Inform patient that estrogen-containing contraceptives are expected to reduce drug's efficacy.

• Inform patient about the risk of bone loss. Advise adequate intake of calcium and vitamin D and supplementation if prescribed.

• Counsel patient to immediately report signs and symptoms of liver injury.

• Instruct patient in safe drug administration.

---

elbasvir–grazoprevir ▨
ELB-as-vir/graz-OH-pre-vir

Zepatier

Therapeutic class: Antivirals
Pharmacologic class: HCV NS5A inhibitors/HCV NS3/4A protease inhibitors

AVAILABLE FORMS
Tablets: elbasvir 50 mg/grazoprevir 100 mg

INDICATIONS & DOSAGES
➤ **Chronic HCV genotypes 1 or 4 infection, with or without ribavirin** ▨
Adults and children age 12 and older or weighing at least 30 kg: 1 tablet PO once daily. See manufacturer's instructions for recommended dosing regimens and durations for treatment of HCV genotype 1 or 4 in patients with or without cirrhosis.
Adjust-a-dose: If ALT level is greater than $10 \times$ ULN, consider discontinuing drug. If ALT level is elevated and accompanied by signs or symptoms of liver inflammation, increased conjugated bilirubin or ALP level, or increased INR, discontinue drug. If CrCl is 50 mL/minute or less and ribavirin is used, refer to ribavirin prescribing information for ribavirin dosage adjustment.

ADMINISTRATION
PO
- May give without regard for food.
- Store at 68° to 77° F (20° to 25° C).
- Store in original container. Protect from moisture.

ACTION
Elbasvir inhibits HCV NS5A, which is an enzyme needed for viral RNA replication and assembly of virions. Grazoprevir inhibits HCV NS3/4A protease, which is an enzyme that is essential for viral replication and is responsible for HCV protein cleavage.

Route	Onset	Peak	Duration
PO (elbasvir)	Unknown	3 hr	Unknown
PO (grazoprevir)	Unknown	2 hr	Unknown

Half-life: Elbasvir, 24 hours; grazoprevir, 31 hours.

ADVERSE REACTIONS
CNS: headache, fatigue, insomnia, irritability, depression. **GI:** nausea; diarrhea, abdominal pain (with ribavirin). **Hematologic:** anemia. **Hepatic:** ALT elevations, bilirubin elevations. **Musculoskeletal:** arthralgia (with ribavirin). **Respiratory:** dyspnea (with ribavirin). **Skin:** rash, pruritus (with ribavirin).

INTERACTIONS
Drug-drug. *Antibiotics (nafcillin):* May decrease concentrations of elbasvir and grazoprevir and therapeutic effects. Use together isn't recommended.
Asunaprevir: May increase asunaprevir concentration. Avoid concurrent use.
HIV medications (cobicistat, elvitegravir, emtricitabine, etravirine, tenofovir): May increase elbasvir–grazoprevir concentrations. Use together isn't recommended. Etravirine may decrease elbasvir–grazoprevir concentrations and lead to decreased effectiveness. Use together isn't recommended.
HMG-CoA reductase inhibitors (atorvastatin, rosuvastatin): May increase atorvastatin and rosuvastatin concentrations. Maximum recommended doses are atorvastatin 20 mg/day and rosuvastatin 10 mg/day.
HMG-CoA reductase inhibitors (fluvastatin, lovastatin, simvastatin): May increase concentrations of HMG-CoA reductase inhibitors. Use lowest necessary statin dosage and monitor patient closely for statin-associated adverse effects such as myopathy.

Immunosuppressants (tacrolimus): May increase tacrolimus concentration. Frequently monitor renal function and tacrolimus level, and watch for tacrolimus-associated adverse effects.
Moderate CYP3A inducers (bosentan, modafinil): May decrease elbasvir–grazoprevir plasma concentrations. Use together isn't recommended.
OATP1B1/3 inhibitors (atazanavir, cyclosporine, darunavir, lopinavir, saquinavir, tipranavir): May increase risk of ALT elevation. Use together is contraindicated.
Strong CYP3A inducers (carbamazepine, efavirenz, phenytoin, rifampin): May cause loss of virologic response. Use together is contraindicated.
Strong CYP3A inhibitors (clarithromycin, itraconazole, ketoconazole, nefazodone, nelfinavir, ritonavir, telithromycin): May increase elbasvir or grazoprevir concentrations. Use together isn't recommended.
Drug-herb. *St. John's wort:* May decrease elbasvir–grazoprevir concentrations and cause loss of virologic response. Use together is contraindicated.

EFFECTS ON LAB TEST RESULTS
- May increase ALT and bilirubin levels.
- May decrease Hb level.

CONTRAINDICATIONS & CAUTIONS
⚕ Patients with HCV genotype 1a infection should undergo testing for NS5A resistance-associated polymorphisms before starting treatment, to determine the need for ribavirin and treatment duration.
- If elbasvir–grazoprevir is administered with ribavirin, the contraindications with ribavirin also apply.

Boxed Warning Reactivation of HBV may occur in patients who are coinfected with HCV, and result in fulminant hepatitis, hepatic failure, and death. Screen all patients for current or prior HBV infection before treatment and if positive for HBV infection, assess baseline HBV DNA. ∎

- Contraindicated in patients with moderate or severe hepatic impairment (Child-Pugh class B or C).

⚠ *Alert:* Use cautiously in patients with risk factors for liver failure (hepatocellular carcinoma, alcohol abuse).

Female patients, patients of Asian descent, and patients age 65 and older are at increased risk for elevated ALT level.
• Safe use in children younger than age 12 or weighing less than 35 kg, recipients of liver transplants, and patients with HBV and HCV coinfection hasn't been established.
Dialyzable drug: No.

PREGNANCY-LACTATION-REPRODUCTION
• There are no human data regarding use during pregnancy. If drug is used with ribavirin, the combination regimen is contraindicated in patients who are pregnant and in men whose partners are pregnant.
• If drug is given with ribavirin, a negative pregnancy test is required immediately before initiation, monthly during therapy, and for 6 months after treatment ends.
• It isn't known if elbasvir or grazoprevir appears in human milk. Use cautiously during breastfeeding.

NURSING CONSIDERATIONS
Boxed Warning Monitor patient with current or prior HBV infection for hepatitis flare or HBV reactivation with lab testing and watch for signs and symptoms of liver injury during active and posttreatment follow-up. ∎
• Obtain LFT values before start of therapy, at treatment week 8, at week 12 in patients receiving 16 weeks of treatment, and as clinically indicated.
• Drug is approved for patients with or without cirrhosis.
⚕ *Alert:* Monitor patients closely for liver failure; discontinue drug if signs and symptoms of decompensation develop or as clinically indicated.
• Monitor patients for signs and symptoms of liver inflammation (fatigue, weakness, lack of appetite, abdominal pain, nausea, vomiting, jaundice, and discolored feces).

PATIENT TEACHING
⚕ *Alert:* Warn patient to immediately report signs and symptoms of liver injury (fatigue, weakness, loss of appetite, nausea, vomiting, yellowing of skin or eyes, light-colored stool).
• Instruct patient to report current or new prescription or OTC medications or supplements being taken before starting therapy because of possible interactions.
• Explain importance of taking drug around the same time every day, without missing or skipping doses. Advise patient to contact prescriber if a dose is missed and not to double a dose.
• Teach patient importance of adherence and regular follow-up with prescriber during therapy.
• Advise patient to avoid pregnancy during and for 6 months after final dose when drug is used concomitantly with ribavirin.

eletriptan hydrobromide
ell-ah-TRIP-tan

Relpax✦

Therapeutic class: Antimigraine drugs
Pharmacologic class: Serotonin 5-HT$_1$ receptor agonists

AVAILABLE FORMS
Tablets ⊙*:* 20 mg, 40 mg

INDICATIONS & DOSAGES
➤ **Acute migraine with or without aura**
Adults: 20 to 40 mg PO at first migraine symptom. If headache recurs, dose may be repeated at least 2 hours later to a maximum of 80 mg in any 24-hour period.

ADMINISTRATION
PO
• Give drug without regard for food.
• Give drug whole; don't crush or break tablet.
• Give drug with a full glass of water.

ACTION
Binds to 5-HT$_{1B/1D/1F}$ receptors and may constrict intracranial blood vessels and inhibit proinflammatory neuropeptide release.

Route	Onset	Peak	Duration
PO	0.5 hr	1.5–2 hr	Unknown

Half-life: About 4 hours.

ADVERSE REACTIONS
CNS: asthenia, dizziness, drowsiness, headache, paresthesia, somnolence. **CV:** chest tightness, pain, and pressure; flushing. **EENT:** dry mouth, pharyngitis. **GI:** abdominal pain, discomfort, or cramps; dyspepsia, dysphagia, nausea.

Reactions in bold italics are *life-threatening*. Interactions may have a *rapid onset* or a **delayed onset**.

INTERACTIONS

Drug-drug. *CYP3A4 inhibitors (clarithromycin, itraconazole, ketoconazole, nefazodone, nelfinavir, ritonavir):* May increase eletriptan metabolism. Avoid use within 72 hours of these drugs.

Ergotamine-containing or ergot-type drugs (dihydroergotamine, methysergide), other triptans: May prolong vasospastic reactions. Avoid use within 24 hours of these drugs.

Linezolid: May enhance serotonergic effect of eletriptan, possibly resulting in serotonin syndrome. If urgent initiation of linezolid is needed, discontinue eletriptan immediately and monitor patient.

MAO inhibitors: May increase risk of serotonin syndrome. Avoid use together.

Methylene blue: May increase risk of serotonin syndrome. Avoid concurrent use.

Other 5-HT$_1$ antagonists: Concomitant use is contraindicated. Avoid concurrent use.

SSNRIs, SSRIs, TCAs: May increase risk of serotonin syndrome. Monitor patient closely.

EFFECTS ON LAB TEST RESULTS
• None known.

CONTRAINDICATIONS & CAUTIONS

• Contraindicated in patients hypersensitive to drug or its components. Hypersensitivity reactions, including anaphylaxis, have been reported. Anaphylactic reactions are more likely in patients with a history of sensitivity to multiple allergens.

• Contraindicated in patients with severe hepatic impairment, ischemic heart disease, history of MI, or silent ischemia; coronary artery vasospasm, including Prinzmetal variant angina; Wolff-Parkinson-White syndrome or arrhythmias associated with other cardiac accessory conduction pathway disorders; and other significant CV conditions.

• Contraindicated in patients with cerebrovascular syndromes, such as stroke or TIA; PVD, including ischemic bowel disease; uncontrolled HTN; or hemiplegic or basilar migraine.

• Contraindicated in patients with risk factors for CAD, such as uncontrolled HTN, hypercholesterolemia, smoking, obesity, diabetes, strong family history of CAD, patients who are postmenopausal, or men older than age 40, unless patient is free from cardiac disease. Monitor patient closely after first dose.

• Use cautiously in older adults.

• Safety of treating more than three migraine headaches in 30 days hasn't been established.

• Safety and effectiveness in children haven't been established.

Dialyzable drug: Unknown.

⚠ **Overdose S&S:** HTN, serious CV reactions.

PREGNANCY-LACTATION-REPRODUCTION

• Data related to eletriptan use in pregnancy is limited. Use of other agents for migraine management is preferred.

• Drug appears in human milk. Use cautiously during breastfeeding.

NURSING CONSIDERATIONS

• Drug isn't intended for migraine prevention.

🔵 **Alert:** Combining a triptan with an SSRI or SSNRI, TCAs, linezolid, methylene blue, or MAO inhibitors may cause serotonin syndrome. Signs and symptoms, which may include restlessness, hallucinations, loss of coordination, fast heartbeat, rapid changes in BP, increased body temperature, hyperreflexia, nausea, vomiting, and diarrhea, occur within minutes to hours of patient receiving a new or increased dosage of the serotonergic drug; signs and symptoms may be more likely to occur at start of therapy or when serotonergic drug dosage is increased.

• Use drug only when patient has a clear diagnosis of migraine. If the first use produces no response, reconsider the migraine diagnosis.

🔵 **Alert:** Serious cardiac events, including acute MI, arrhythmias, and death, occur rarely within a few hours after use of 5-HT$_1$ agonists. Don't use in patients with a history of CV disease.

• Significant HTN can occur even in patients with no history of HTN. Monitor BP closely.

PATIENT TEACHING

• Instruct patient in safe drug administration.

• Warn patient to avoid driving and operating machinery if dizziness or fatigue occurs.

• Tell patient to immediately report signs or symptoms of MI (pain, tightness, heaviness, or pressure in the chest, throat, neck, or jaw); stroke (trouble speaking, change in balance, one-sided weakness); or vasospasm (changes in color or sensation of fingers or toes, GI cramps or pain, bloody diarrhea, leg cramps or pain, burning or aching pain in feet while resting, numbness or tingling in legs).

SAFETY ALERT!

elotuzumab
el-oh-TOOZ-ue-mab

Empliciti

Therapeutic class: Antineoplastics
Pharmacologic class: Monoclonal antibodies

AVAILABLE FORMS
Injection: 300-mg, 400-mg single-dose vials

INDICATIONS & DOSAGES
➤ **Multiple myeloma in combination with lenalidomide and dexamethasone in patients who have received one to three prior therapies**
Adults: 10 mg/kg IV every week for first two 28-day cycles, then every 2 weeks thereafter in combination with lenalidomide 25 mg PO on days 1 through 21 of every cycle until disease progression or unacceptable toxicity. Between 3 and 24 hours before elotuzumab is given, administer dexamethasone 28 mg PO. Additionally, give dexamethasone 8 mg IV between 45 and 90 minutes before elotuzumab is administered. On days that elotuzumab isn't administered (days 8 and 22 of cycle 3 and all subsequent cycles), give dexamethasone 40 mg PO. Elotuzumab must be given with premedications.
➤ **Multiple myeloma in combination with pomalidomide and dexamethasone in patients who have received at least two prior therapies including lenalidomide and a proteasome inhibitor**
Adults age 75 and older: 10 mg/kg IV once every week for the first two 28-day cycles; then starting at cycle 3, give 20 mg/kg every 4 weeks thereafter. Use in combination with pomalidomide 4 mg PO on days 1 through 21 of every cycle. Between 3 and 24 hours before elotuzumab is given, administer dexamethasone 8 mg PO. Additionally, give dexamethasone 8 mg IV between 45 and 90 minutes before elotuzumab is administered. On days that elotuzumab isn't administered (days 8, 15, and 22 of cycle 3 and all subsequent cycles), give dexamethasone 20 mg PO. Continue treatment until disease progression or unacceptable toxicity.
Adults age 75 and younger: 10 mg/kg IV once every week for the first two 28-day cycles;

then starting at cycle 3, give 20 mg/kg every 4 weeks thereafter. Use in combination with pomalidomide 4 mg PO on days 1 through 21 of every cycle. Between 3 and 24 hours before elotuzumab is given, administer dexamethasone 28 mg PO. Additionally, give dexamethasone 8 mg IV between 45 and 90 minutes before elotuzumab is administered. On days that elotuzumab isn't administered (days 8, 15, and 22 of cycle 3 and all subsequent cycles), give dexamethasone 40 mg PO. Continue treatment until disease progression or unacceptable toxicity.
Adjust-a-dose: If the dose of one drug in the regimen is delayed or interrupted or the drug is discontinued, treatment with the other drugs may continue as scheduled. However, if dexamethasone is delayed or discontinued, base the decision whether to administer drug on clinical judgment for the risk of hypersensitivity. For grade 2 or higher infusion reaction, interrupt infusion and institute appropriate medical and supportive measures; upon resolution to grade 1 or lower, restart drug at 0.5 mL/minute and gradually increase at a rate of 0.5 mL/minute every 30 minutes as tolerated to rate at which the infusion reaction occurred. Resume the escalation regimen if there's no recurrence of the infusion reaction. If an infusion reaction recurs, stop infusion and don't restart on that day; monitor vital signs every 30 minutes for 2 hours after infusion. Severe infusion reactions may require permanent discontinuation of drug and emergency treatment.

Delay and modify dosage of dexamethasone and lenalidomide as recommended in their prescribing information. Delay and modify dosage of dexamethasone and pomalidomide as recommended in their prescribing information.

ADMINISTRATION
IV
▼ Premedicate patient 45 to 90 minutes before infusion with diphenhydramine 25 to 50 mg PO or IV, or equivalent H_1 blocker; ranitidine 50 mg IV or 150 mg PO, or equivalent H_2 blocker; and acetaminophen 650 to 1,000 mg PO.
▼ Reconstitute each vial with sterile water for injection; 13 mL for 300-mg vial and 17 mL for 400-mg vial for a final concentration in either vial of 25 mg/mL.

Reactions in bold italics are *life-threatening*. Interactions may have a *rapid onset* or a ***delayed onset***.

▼ Hold vial upright and swirl solution by rotating vial to dissolve the lyophilized cake. Invert vial a few times to dissolve any powder that may be present on top of vial or stopper; don't shake. Powder should dissolve in less than 10 minutes. After dissolution, allow reconstituted solution to stand for 5 to 10 minutes.

▼ Solution should be colorless to slightly yellow, clear to slightly opalescent. Discard solution if particulate matter or discoloration is observed.

▼ After reconstitution, withdraw necessary volume for the calculated dose from each vial, up to a maximum of 16 mL from 400-mg vial and 12 mL from 300-mg vial and further dilute with either NSS or D_5W into an infusion bag made of polyvinyl chloride or polyolefin. Final infusion concentration should range between 1 and 6 mg/mL. Volume of NSS or D_5W can be adjusted so as not to exceed 5 mL/kg of patient weight at any given dose of drug.

▼ Complete infusion within 24 hours of reconstitution. If not used immediately, store under refrigeration at 36° to 46° F (2° to 8° C) and protected from light for up to 24 hours. A maximum of 8 hours of the total 24 hours can be at room temperature and room light.

▼ Administer infusion through a nonpyrogenic low-protein-binding filter (with a pore size of 0.2 to 1.2 microns) using an automated infusion pump.

▼ Initiate infusion at a rate of 0.5 mL/minute and increase in stepwise fashion as follows if no infusion reactions develop: For cycle 1/dose 1, infuse at 0.5 mL/minute for first 30 minutes, then increase to 1 mL/minute for next 30 minutes, then increase to 2 mL/minute until infusion is completed. For cycle 1/dose 2, for first 30 minutes, infuse at 3 mL/minute, then 4 mL/minute from 30 minutes until finished; all infusions after this may be infused at 5 mL/minute. Maximum infusion rate shouldn't exceed 5 mL/minute. Adjust infusion rate after any grade 2 or higher infusion reaction.

▼ Keep unopened vials under refrigeration.

▼ **Incompatibilities:** Administer alone; don't mix or infuse in same line with other drugs.

ACTION
A humanized IgG1 monoclonal antibody that specifically targets the SLAMF7 signaling protein, activating natural killer cells and targeting the SLAMF7 protein on myeloma cells to kill the cells.

Route	Onset	Peak	Duration
IV	Unknown	Unknown	Unknown

Half-life: Unknown.

ADVERSE REACTIONS
CNS: peripheral neuropathy, headache, hypoesthesia, fatigue, fever, altered mood. **CV:** chest pain, HTN, hypotension, edema, tachycardia, *bradycardia.* **EENT:** cataracts, nasopharyngitis, oropharyngeal pain. **GI:** diarrhea, constipation, vomiting, decreased appetite. **GU:** *acute renal failure.* **Hematologic:** anemia, *leukopenia, thrombocytopenia.* **Hepatic:** elevated ALP level, *hepatotoxicity.* **Metabolic:** weight loss, hyperglycemia, *hyperkalemia,* hypoalbuminemia, *hypocalcemia.* **Musculoskeletal:** pain in extremities, bone pain, muscle spasms. **Respiratory:** cough, URI, pneumonia, *PE.* **Skin:** night sweats. **Other:** hypersensitivity, infusion reactions.

INTERACTIONS
Drug-drug. *Immunosuppressants (natalizumab, ocrelizumab, pidotimod, pimecrolimus, tacrolimus [topical], upadacitinib):* May enhance infection risk or toxic effects. Avoid combination.
Live-virus vaccines: May enhance adverse or toxic effect of vaccines. Don't give live-virus vaccines for at least 3 months after elotuzumab.

Drug-herb. *Echinacea:* May diminish therapeutic effect of elotuzumab. Avoid concurrent use.

EFFECTS ON LAB TEST RESULTS
• May increase transaminase, bilirubin, ALP, glucose, and potassium levels.
• May decrease albumin, calcium, and bicarbonate levels.
• May decrease lymphocyte, leukocyte, and platelet counts.
• May interfere with gamma region serum protein electrophoresis and immunofixation assay results.

CONTRAINDICATIONS & CAUTIONS

• May cause hypersensitivity reactions. Patient must be premedicated with dexamethasone, diphenhydramine, ranitidine, and acetaminophen.
• Infections can occur. Monitor patients for fever and other signs and symptoms of infection; treat promptly.
• Second primary malignancies can occur.
• Drug can interfere with assays used to monitor M-protein, which can impact the determination of complete response.
• Safety and effectiveness in children haven't been established.
Dialyzable drug: No.

PREGNANCY-LACTATION-REPRODUCTION

• There are no studies of elotuzumab use during pregnancy. Drug may cause fetal harm. Lenalidomide and pomalidomide are contraindicated for use during pregnancy.
• Males and females of reproductive potential must use effective contraception during treatment and for a significant amount of time after final dose. Follow lenalidomide and pomalidomide prescribing information for specific details on pregnancy testing, contraception, and blood and sperm donation.
• It isn't known if drug appears in human milk. Breastfeeding isn't recommended.

NURSING CONSIDERATIONS

• Monitor patients for development of infusion reactions (fever, chills, HTN or hypotension, bradycardia). Interrupt infusion for grade 2 or higher infusion reactions and treat appropriately.
• In patients who experience an infusion reaction, monitor vital signs every 30 minutes for 2 hours after end of infusion.
• Ensure patient has taken premedications before infusion.
• Monitor patients for development of infection, which can be fatal, and treat promptly.
• Monitor patients for second primary malignancies.
• Obtain baseline liver enzyme levels and monitor periodically during treatment. Stop drug for grade 3 or higher liver enzyme elevations. May consider continuing treatment after results return to baseline.

PATIENT TEACHING

• Advise patient that lenalidomide and pomalidomide used in combination with elotuzumab can cause fetal harm and have specific requirements regarding contraception, pregnancy testing, blood and sperm donation, and transmission in sperm.
• Inform patient of risk of liver toxicity during treatment; tell patient to report signs and symptoms of toxicity (tiredness, weakness, loss of appetite, confusion, jaundice, change in stool color, abdominal pain, swelling of stomach area).
• Advise patient to immediately report signs and symptoms of infusion reactions (fever, chills, rash, breathing problems, dizziness, light-headedness) that could occur within 24 hours of infusion.
• Instruct patient that oral dexamethasone, an H_1 blocker, an H_2 blocker, and acetaminophen will be required before infusions to reduce risk of infusion reactions.
• Caution patient about risk of developing infections during treatment; teach patient to report signs and symptoms of infection (fever, flulike symptoms, cough, shortness of breath, burning with urination, painful rash).
• Warn patient of risk of developing second primary malignancies during treatment.
• Advise patient that lab testing will be needed to monitor treatment.

SAFETY ALERT!

eluxadoline
el-ux-AD-oh-leen

Viberzi

Therapeutic class: Anti–IBS drugs
Pharmacologic class: Mu-opioid receptor agonists, delta-opioid receptor antagonists, kappa-opioid receptor agonists
Controlled substance schedule: IV

AVAILABLE FORMS
Tablets: 75 mg, 100 mg

INDICATIONS & DOSAGES
➤ **IBS with diarrhea (IBS-D)**
Adults: 100 mg PO b.i.d.
Adjust-a-dose: Reduce dosage to 75 mg b.i.d. in patients who can't tolerate 100-mg dose, are receiving concomitant OATP1B1 inhibitors, or have mild to moderate (Child-Pugh class A or B) hepatic impairment.

Reactions in bold italics are ***life-threatening***. Interactions may have a *rapid onset* or a ***delayed onset***.

E

ADMINISTRATION
PO
- Give with food.
- If a dose is missed, give next dose at the regular time. Don't give two doses at the same time to make up for a missed dose.
- Store at room temperature.

ACTION
Mu-opioid receptor agonist, delta-opioid receptor antagonist, and kappa-opioid receptor agonist that decreases peristaltic action of the intestines. Acts locally to reduce abdominal pain and IBS-D without constipating adverse effects.

Route	Onset	Peak	Duration
PO (with food)	Unknown	1.5 hr (range, 1–8 hr)	Unknown

Half-life: 3.7 to 6 hours.

ADVERSE REACTIONS
CNS: dizziness, fatigue, drowsiness, euphoria, intoxicated feeling, sedation. **EENT:** nasopharyngitis. **GI:** constipation, nausea, vomiting, abdominal pain, abdominal distention, flatulence, viral gastroenteritis, gastroesophageal reflux. **Hepatic:** elevated ALT and AST levels. **Respiratory:** URI, bronchitis, *asthma, bronchospasm, respiratory failure,* increased bronchial secretions. **Skin:** rash. **Other:** hypersensitivity reactions.

INTERACTIONS
Drug-drug. *Drugs that cause constipation (alosetron, anticholinergics, opioids):* May increase risk of constipation-related adverse reactions. Avoid use together.
OATP1B1 inhibitors (atazanavir, cyclosporine, eltrombopag, gemfibrozil, lopinavir, rifampin, ritonavir, saquinavir, tipranavir): May increase eluxadoline concentration. Give eluxadoline at a dose of 75 mg b.i.d.; monitor patient for eluxadoline-related adverse reactions.
Rosuvastatin: May increase rosuvastatin concentration and risk of myopathy/rhabdomyolysis. Use lowest effective rosuvastatin dose.
Drug-lifestyle. *Alcohol use:* May increase risk of acute pancreatitis. Patient should avoid prolonged or acute excessive alcohol use while taking drug. Monitor patient closely.

EFFECTS ON LAB TEST RESULTS
- May increase ALT and AST levels.

CONTRAINDICATIONS & CAUTIONS
- Contraindicated in patients hypersensitive to drug or its components.
- Contraindicated in patients without a gallbladder, with known or suspected biliary duct obstruction, or sphincter of Oddi disease or dysfunction. Permanently discontinue drug in patients who develop biliary duct obstruction or sphincter of Oddi spasm while taking eluxadoline.
- Contraindicated in patients with alcohol abuse, alcohol addiction, alcoholism, or consumption of more than three alcoholic beverages each day; history of pancreatitis or structural diseases of the pancreas or suspected pancreatic duct obstruction with severe hepatic impairment (Child-Pugh class C); history of chronic or severe constipation or sequelae from constipation; or known or suspected mechanical GI obstruction.
- Drug has potential for abuse and psychological dependence. Consider naloxone in the event of overdose.
- Safety and effectiveness in children haven't been established.
- Use cautiously in older adults, for whom the same effectiveness was observed but with a higher incidence of adverse reactions.
Dialyzable drug: Unlikely.

PREGNANCY-LACTATION-REPRODUCTION
- Use cautiously during pregnancy. Risk to fetus is unknown.
- It isn't known if drug appears in human milk. Use cautiously during breastfeeding, taking into account maternal benefits and fetal risk.

NURSING CONSIDERATIONS
- Monitor patients with hepatic impairment for impaired mental or physical abilities needed to perform potentially hazardous activities, such as driving or operating machinery.
- Monitor patients for sphincter of Oddi spasm (unusual or severe epigastric or upper right quadrant abdominal pain that may radiate to the back or shoulder, with or without nausea and vomiting, and with liver or pancreatic enzyme elevations). Discontinue drug if signs or symptoms develop.

- Monitor patients, especially those with excessive alcohol intake, for pancreatitis (new or worsening abdominal or epigastric pain that may radiate to the back, associated with elevated pancreatic enzyme levels). Discontinue drug if signs and symptoms occur.
- Monitor patients for constipation. Discontinue drug immediately if severe constipation develops.
- Watch for signs and symptoms of abuse of drug, including psychological dependence.

PATIENT TEACHING
- Advise patient to read the FDA-approved medication guide.
- Instruct patient in safe drug administration.
- Warn patient to stop drug and seek medical attention for new or worsening upper right quadrant abdominal pain that radiates to the shoulder or back or if nausea or vomiting occurs.
- Advise patient to avoid prolonged and acute excessive alcohol use while taking drug.
- Counsel patient to discontinue drug and contact prescriber immediately for severe constipation.
- Instruct patient to avoid taking drug with other medications that may cause constipation and to ask prescriber for a list of these medications.
- Inform patient that loperamide may occasionally be used with eluxadoline but must be stopped if constipation develops.
- Caution patient with hepatic impairment not to drive, operate machinery, or perform other dangerous activities until effects of drug are known.
- Advise patient that if a dose is missed to take the next dose at the regular time and not to take two doses at the same time to make up for the missed dose.

elvitegravir–cobicistat–emtricitabine–tenofovir disoproxil fumarate
el-vye-TEG-ra-veer/koe-BIK-i-stat/em-tra-SYE-tah-ben/te-NOE-fo-veer

Stribild

Therapeutic class: Antiretrovirals
Pharmacologic class: Antivirals

AVAILABLE FORMS
Tablet: Each tablet contains 150 mg elvitegravir, 150 mg cobicistat, 200 mg emtricitabine, and 300 mg tenofovir disoproxil fumarate

INDICATIONS & DOSAGES
➤ **HIV-1 infection in patients who are antiretroviral treatment–naive; to replace current antiretroviral regimen in patients who are virologically suppressed (HIV-1 RNA fewer than 50 copies/mL) on a stable regimen for at least 6 months with no history of treatment failure and no known substitutions associated with resistance to individual components**
Adults and children age 12 and older weighing at least 35 kg: 1 tablet PO once daily.
Adjust-a-dose: Initiation of drug in patients with estimated CrCl below 70 mL/minute or in patients with Child-Pugh class C hepatic impairment isn't recommended. Discontinue drug in patients whose estimated CrCl declines to less than 50 mL/minute.

ADMINISTRATION
PO
- Give with food.
- Drug is used as a complete treatment; don't give with other antiretrovirals.

ACTION
Combination of agents with differing mechanisms of action (integrase strand transfer inhibition, pharmacokinetic enhancement, nucleoside and nucleotide analogue HIV-1 reverse transcriptase inhibition) working together to inhibit HIV replication.

Reactions in bold italics are *life-threatening*. Interactions may have a *rapid onset* or a ***delayed onset***.

Route	Onset	Peak	Duration
PO (elvitegravir)	Unknown	4 hr	Unknown
PO (cobicistat, emtricitabine)	Unknown	3 hr	Unknown
PO (tenofovir)	Unknown	2 hr	Unknown

Half-life: Elvitegravir, 12.9 hours; cobicistat, 3.5 hours; emtricitabine, 10 hours; tenofovir, 12 to 18 hours.

ADVERSE REACTIONS

CNS: anxiety, headache, dizziness, insomnia, abnormal dreams, fatigue, somnolence, depression, fever, pain. **GI:** diarrhea, nausea, flatulence. **GU:** increased creatinine level, proteinuria, hematuria. **Hepatic:** increased transaminase levels. **Metabolic:** increased amylase, lipase, CK, lipid levels. **Musculoskeletal:** arthralgia, back pain, bone fracture, myalgia. **Respiratory:** cough, pneumonia. **Skin:** rash.

INTERACTIONS

⚠ *Alert:* Drug can interact with many drugs. Consult a drug interaction resource or pharmacist for additional information.
Drug-drug. *Acyclovir, cidofovir, ganciclovir, valacyclovir, valganciclovir:* May increase concentrations of these drugs, emtricitabine, and tenofovir due to competition for renal excretion. Use together carefully.
Additional antiretrovirals: May increase risk of drug interactions and altered pharmacokinetics of drug components. Use together is contraindicated.
Alfuzosin: May increase alfuzosin level and risk of severe hypotension. Use together is contraindicated.
Antacids, calcium or iron supplements, cation-containing laxatives, buffered medications: May decrease elvitegravir concentration. Separate administration times by 2 hours.
Antiarrhythmics, digoxin: May increase levels of these drugs. Use together cautiously and monitor drug levels if possible.
Antidepressants (SSRIs, TCAs, trazodone): May increase levels of these drugs. Use together cautiously and titrate antidepressant according to response.
Antifungals (itraconazole, ketoconazole, voriconazole): May increase levels of these drugs, elvitegravir, and cobicistat. Use together cautiously. Don't exceed 200 mg/day of ketoconazole or itraconazole.

Antiplatelet drugs (clopidogrel, ticagrelor): May increase ticagrelor level or decrease clopidogrel level. Use together isn't recommended.
Beta blockers (metoprolol, timolol): May increase beta blocker concentration. Monitor patient carefully and decrease beta blocker dosage as necessary.
Bosentan: May increase bosentan level. Give bosentan dose based on manufacturer's instructions and adjust according to patient tolerance.
Calcium channel blockers (amlodipine, diltiazem, felodipine, nicardipine, nifedipine, verapamil): May increase level of calcium channel blocker. Use together cautiously and monitor patient closely.
Carbamazepine, oxcarbazepine, phenobarbital, phenytoin: May significantly decrease elvitegravir and cobicistat levels; may increase carbamazepine level. Use together is contraindicated.
Clarithromycin: May increase clarithromycin and cobicistat levels. Use together cautiously. Decrease clarithromycin dosage by 50% if CrCl falls between 50 and 60 mL/minute.
Clonazepam, ethosuximide: May increase levels of these drugs. Use together cautiously.
Colchicine: May increase colchicine concentration. Adjust dosage according to manufacturer's instructions. Use together is contraindicated in patients with renal or hepatic impairment.
CYP2D6, CYP3A, P-gp substrates: May alter plasma concentrations of the four drug components (elvitegravir, cobicistat, emtricitabine, and tenofovir). Use together cautiously.
Dexamethasone: May significantly decrease cobicistat and elvitegravir levels. Monitor patient carefully for loss of therapeutic effect (elvitegravir, cobicistat) and development of resistance.
Direct oral anticoagulants (apixaban, dabigatran, edoxaban, rivaroxaban): May increase bleeding risk. Adjust anticoagulant dosage.
Ergot derivatives (dihydroergotamine, ergotamine, methylergonovine): May increase levels of these drugs. Use together is contraindicated.
Fluticasone: May increase fluticasone level. Choose an alternative corticosteroid.
HMG-CoA reductase inhibitors (atorvastatin): May increase statin drug level and risk of

E

myopathy. Start statin at lowest dosage and titrate carefully.

Hormonal contraceptives: May alter levels of these drugs. Consider nonhormonal forms of birth control.

Immunosuppressants (cyclosporine, sirolimus, tacrolimus): May increase immunosuppressant level. Use together cautiously.

Lovastatin, simvastatin: May increase statin level and risk of myopathy. Use together is contraindicated.

Lurasidone, pimozide: May increase risk of cardiac adverse effects. Use together is contraindicated.

Midazolam: May increase midazolam level. Use with oral midazolam is contraindicated. Use parenteral form cautiously and monitor patient closely.

Neuroleptics (perphenazine, quetiapine, risperidone, thioridazine): May increase neuroleptic drug level. Decrease neuroleptic dosage as needed.

PDE5 inhibitors (sildenafil, tadalafil, vardenafil): May increase effects of PDE5 inhibitors. Adjust dosage according to manufacturer's instructions. Use with sildenafil for PAH is contraindicated.

Rifabutin, rifapentine: May decrease cobicistat and elvitegravir levels. Avoid use together.

Rifampin: May decrease elvitegravir and cobicistat concentrations, decreasing therapeutic effect. Use together is contraindicated.

Salmeterol: May increase risk of CV effects of salmeterol, including QT-interval prolongation, palpitations, and tachycardia. Avoid use together.

Sedative/hypnotics (buspirone, clorazepate, diazepam, estazolam, flurazepam, zolpidem): May increase concentrations of sedative/ hypnotics. Use cautiously together and monitor patient carefully.

Triazolam: May increase triazolam concentration. Use together is contraindicated.

Warfarin: Effect on warfarin concentration isn't known. Monitor INR carefully.

Drug-herb. *St. John's wort:* May reduce concentrations of drug components and decrease therapeutic effect. Use together is contraindicated.

EFFECTS ON LAB TEST RESULTS

• May increase AST, ALT, GGT, amylase, creatinine, CK, total cholesterol, HDL, LDL, and triglyceride levels.

• May decrease potassium and phosphate levels.

• May increase urine RBC count.

CONTRAINDICATIONS & CAUTIONS

• Contraindicated in patients hypersensitive to drugs or their components and in those with CrCl of less than 70 mL/minute or severe hepatic impairment (Child-Pugh class C).

• Contraindicated with drugs that are highly dependent on CYP3A for clearance or strongly induce CYP3A.

• Use cautiously in new-onset or worsening renal impairment, including acute renal failure and Fanconi syndrome. Avoid administering with other nephrotoxic agents.

• Use cautiously in patients with a history of pathologic fracture or other risk factors for osteoporosis or bone loss. Consider calcium and vitamin D supplementation.

Boxed Warning Drug isn't approved for the treatment of chronic HBV infection; safety and effectiveness of drug haven't been established in patients infected with both HBV and HIV-1. Severe acute exacerbations of hepatitis B have been reported in patients who are infected with both HBV and HIV-1 and who have discontinued emtricitabine (Emtriva) or tenofovir (Viread), which are components of this drug. Monitor hepatic function closely with both clinical and lab follow-up for at least several months in patients who are infected with both HBV and HIV-1 and who discontinue this drug. If appropriate, initiation of anti–hepatitis B therapy may be warranted. ∎

• Lactic acidosis and severe hepatomegaly with steatosis, including fatal cases, have been reported with use of nucleoside analogues, including tenofovir and emtricitabine, in combination with other antiretrovirals.

• Drug may cause immune reconstitution syndrome.

• Safety and effectiveness in children younger than age 12 or weighing less than 35 kg haven't been established.

Dialyzable drug: Elvitegravir, unlikely; cobicistat, unlikely; emtricitabine, 30% hemodialysis; tenofovir, 10% hemodialysis.

PREGNANCY-LACTATION-REPRODUCTION

• Register patients who are pregnant in the Antiretroviral Pregnancy Registry at 1-800-258-4263.

Reactions in bold italics are *life-threatening*. Interactions may have a *rapid onset* or a *delayed onset*.

• Not recommended for use during pregnancy.
• Drug (emtricitabine, tenofovir) appears in human milk. Because of risk of HIV transmission, patient shouldn't breastfeed.

NURSING CONSIDERATIONS
• Monitor LFT values.
• Suspend treatment in patients who develop signs and symptoms or lab findings suggestive of lactic acidosis or pronounced hepatotoxicity (including nausea, vomiting, unusual or unexpected stomach discomfort, and weakness).
• Test for HBV before starting therapy; severe acute exacerbations of hepatitis B have been reported in patients infected with both HBV and HIV-1.
• Avoid concurrent or recent use of a nephrotoxic agent because renal impairment is possible.
• Assess CrCl, urine glucose, and urine protein before initiating and periodically during treatment.
• Monitor serum phosphorus level in patients at risk for renal impairment.
• Closely monitor patients with a confirmed increase in serum creatinine level of greater than 0.4 mg/dL from baseline for renal safety.
• Consider assessing bone mineral density (BMD) in patients with a history of pathologic bone fracture or other risk factors for osteoporosis or bone loss because of risk of drug-related decreased BMD.
• Monitor patients for infection and development of immune reconstitution syndrome (inflammatory response to indolent or residual opportunistic infections, such as MAC infection, CMV, *Pneumocystis jiroveci* pneumonia, or TB), which may necessitate further evaluation and treatment.
• Autoimmune disorders (such as Graves disease, polymyositis, and Guillain-Barré syndrome) have also been reported in the setting of immune reconstitution; however, the time to onset is more variable, and the disorder can occur many months after initiation of treatment.

PATIENT TEACHING
• Caution patient to remain under the care of a health care provider and to comply with routine monitoring to decrease risk of adverse events.

• Inform patient that this drug isn't a cure for HIV-1 infection; patient must stay on continuous HIV therapy to control HIV-1 infection and decrease HIV-related illnesses.
• Instruct patient to avoid behaviors that can spread HIV-1 infection to others (such as sharing needles or other injection equipment; sharing personal items that may have blood or body fluids on them, such as toothbrushes and razor blades; or having sex without the protection of a latex or polyurethane condom).
• Warn patient not to breastfeed because HIV-1 can be passed to the infant in human milk.
• Teach patient to take drug on a regular dosing schedule with food and not to miss doses.
• Instruct patient not to change dose or stop drug without first consulting health care provider.
• Advise patient to immediately report nausea, vomiting, unusual or unexpected stomach discomfort, and weakness.
• Caution patient to report signs and symptoms of infection.
• Teach patient to report yellowing of skin or sclera, dark urine, light-colored stools, loss of appetite, or nausea.

SAFETY ALERT!

empagliflozin
em-pa-gli-FLOE-zin

Jardiance

Therapeutic class: Antidiabetics
Pharmacologic class: Sodium-glucose cotransporter 2 inhibitors

AVAILABLE FORMS
Tablets: 10 mg, 25 mg

INDICATIONS & DOSAGES
Adjust-a-dose (for all indications): Discontinue drug if GFR is less than 45 mL/minute/1.73 m^2.
➤ **As adjunct to diet and exercise to improve glycemic control in patients with type 2 diabetes**
Adults: 10 mg PO daily in the morning. May increase to 25 mg daily after 4 to 12 weeks if needed for additional glycemic control.
➤ **To reduce risk of CV death in patients with type 2 diabetes and established CV disease.**

Adults: 10 mg PO daily in the morning.

✳ *NEW INDICATION:* **To reduce risk of CV death and hospitalization for HF in patients with HF**

Adults: 10 mg PO daily in the morning.

ADMINISTRATION
PO
- May give without regard for food.
- Store at room temperature.

ACTION
Inhibits renal reabsorption of glucose and lowers renal threshold for glucose, resulting in increased urinary excretion of glucose.

Route	Onset	Peak	Duration
PO	Unknown	1.5 hr	Unknown

Half-life: 12.4 hours.

ADVERSE REACTIONS
GI: nausea. **GU:** genital mycotic infections, UTI, renal impairment, increased urination. **Hematologic:** increased hematocrit. **Metabolic:** dyslipidemia, increased thirst. **Musculoskeletal:** arthralgia. **Respiratory:** URI.

INTERACTIONS
Drug-drug. *Diuretics:* May enhance diuretic effect. Closely monitor patient for volume depletion.

Insulin, insulin secretagogues, sulfonylureas, other antidiabetics: May increase hypoglycemic risk. Monitor patient closely.

EFFECTS ON LAB TEST RESULTS
- May increase serum creatinine level.
- May increase hematocrit.
- May decrease GFR.
- May cause false-positive urine glucose tests.
- Interferes with 1,5-anhydroglucitol assay.

CONTRAINDICATIONS & CAUTIONS
- Contraindicated in patients with history of serious hypersensitivity reaction to drug or its components.
- Contraindicated in patients with severe renal impairment or ESRD and in those on dialysis.
- Don't start or use in patients with GFR of less than 45 mL/minute.
- Drug isn't recommended for glycemic control in patients with eGFR of less than 30 mL/minute/1.73 m^2.

- Dosing recommendations haven't been determined for patients with type 2 diabetes and established CV disease with eGFR of less than 30 mL/minute/1.73 m^2, or for patients who have HF with reduced ejection fraction with eGFR of less than 20 mL/minute/1.73 m^2.
- Drug isn't recommended for type 1 diabetes or for treatment of diabetic ketoacidosis.
- Serious hypersensitivity reactions, including angioedema, have been reported in patients treated with empagliflozin. Discontinue drug if a hypersensitivity reaction occurs, treat promptly per standard of care, and monitor patients until signs and symptoms resolve.

❸ *Alert:* Sodium-glucose cotransporter 2 (SGLT2) inhibitors increase risk of a rare but serious necrotizing fasciitis of the perineum, also known as Fournier gangrene. If necrotizing fasciitis is suspected, immediately discontinue SGLT2 drug and begin broad-spectrum antibiotics. Surgical debridement may be necessary. Monitor blood glucose levels and start alternative therapy for glycemic control.

❸ *Alert:* Drug may cause ketoacidosis, which may require emergency department care or hospitalization for treatment. Monitor for ketoacidosis, especially in patients with major illness, reduced food or fluid intake, or reduced insulin dose. Elevated urine or serum ketone level without associated very high glucose levels has occurred with SGLT2 inhibitor use.

- Consider temporarily discontinuing drug at least 3 days before scheduled surgery to reduce risk of ketoacidosis.
- Use cautiously in patients with low BP or moderate renal impairment and in those taking diuretics; drug may increase risk of hypotension.
- Drug may increase risk of adverse events related to volume depletion and reduced renal function, especially in older adults and patients with renal impairment.
- Drug may increase incidence of bone fractures. Per American Diabetes Association guidelines, SGLT2 inhibitors should be avoided in patients with fracture risk factors.
- Use cautiously in patients with elevated hematocrit at baseline, as value may increase.
- Safety and effectiveness in children haven't been established.

Dialyzable drug: Unknown.

Reactions in bold italics are *life-threatening*. Interactions may have a *rapid onset* or a *delayed onset*.

PREGNANCY-LACTATION-REPRODUCTION

- Drug hasn't been studied in patients who are pregnant. Drug isn't recommended during second and third trimesters. Use during pregnancy only if benefit justifies fetal risk.
- It isn't known if drug appears in human milk. Patient should discontinue breastfeeding or discontinue drug.

NURSING CONSIDERATIONS

- Assess renal function before initiating therapy and periodically during treatment. Don't start therapy if GFR is less than 30 mL/minute. Closely monitor patients with GFR of less than 60 mL/minute.
- Assess fluid status. Correct volume depletion before starting therapy and monitor during therapy.
- Monitor patients for signs and symptoms of hypotension (fatigue, dizziness, blurred vision, clammy skin) during therapy. Drug may increase risk of hypotension due to intravascular volume contraction.
- Monitor glucose level closely during drug initiation. Concomitant use of insulin and other antidiabetics may increase risk of hypoglycemia.
- Watch for genital mycotic infections and treat appropriately.
- ☻ *Alert:* Monitor patient and immediately report signs and symptoms of necrotizing fasciitis of the perineum (temperature above 100.4° F [38° C], malaise along with genital or perianal pain, tenderness, erythema, or swelling). Symptoms can worsen quickly. Immediately discontinue drug and prepare to administer broad-spectrum antibiotics.
- ☻ *Alert:* Drug may increase risk of severe UTI, including urosepsis and pyelonephritis. Monitor patient and treat promptly if indicated.
- Monitor LDL cholesterol periodically; treat appropriately.
- Drug causes positive urine glucose tests. Avoid urine glucose testing for glycemic control monitoring.
- *Look alike–sound alike:* Don't confuse empagliflozin with canagliflozin or dapagliflozin. Don't confuse Jardiance with Januvia, Jantoven, or Janumet.

PATIENT TEACHING

- Instruct patient in safe drug administration.
- Stress importance of adhering to diet, weight reduction, exercise, personal hygiene, and blood glucose monitoring while on therapy.
- Teach patient to report all adverse reactions and how to identify and manage signs and symptoms of hypoglycemia (dizziness, weakness, shaking, fast heartbeat).
- Teach patient how to identify and manage signs and symptoms of hypotension (fatigue, dizziness, blurred vision, clammy skin). Encourage patient to maintain adequate fluid intake.
- ☻ *Alert:* Teach patient signs and symptoms of necrotizing fasciitis and to seek immediate medical attention if they occur.
- ☻ *Alert:* Instruct patient to seek medical attention immediately for signs and symptoms of ketoacidosis (difficulty breathing, hyperventilation, anorexia, nausea, vomiting, abdominal pain, confusion, unusual fatigue or sleepiness) or necrotizing fasciitis (fever or malaise along with genital or perianal pain, tenderness, erythema, swelling).
- Instruct patient to seek medical advice during periods of stress or illness because medication requirements may change.
- ☻ *Alert:* Instruct patient to seek medical attention for signs and symptoms of UTI (difficulty urinating, frequency, urgency, pelvic pain, blood in urine, fever, back pain, nausea, vomiting).
- Inform patient that periodic monitoring of blood glucose and HbA_{1c} levels and renal function will be needed.
- Advise patient that urine glucose tests will be falsely positive because drug increases glucose excretion, and recommend alternative methods to monitor glycemic control.
- Counsel patient to consult prescriber before starting new prescription or OTC medications or supplements.
- Tell patient to report pregnancy or plans to become pregnant or breastfeed during treatment.

emtricitabine
em-tra-SYE-tah-ben

Emtriva

Therapeutic class: Antiretrovirals
Pharmacologic class: NRTIs

AVAILABLE FORMS
Capsules: 200 mg
Oral solution: 10 mg/mL

INDICATIONS & DOSAGES
➤ **HIV-1 infection, with other antiretrovirals**

Adults: One 200-mg capsule or 240 mg (24 mL) oral solution PO once daily.
Children ages 3 months to 17 years: For children weighing more than 33 kg who can swallow intact capsules, one 200-mg capsule PO once daily. Otherwise, 6 mg/kg, up to a maximum dose of 240 mg (24 mL) oral solution PO once daily.
Children younger than age 3 months: 3 mg/kg oral solution PO once daily.
Adjust-a-dose: In adults with CrCl of 30 to 49 mL/minute, give one 200-mg capsule every 48 hours or 120 mg oral solution every 24 hours; if CrCl is 15 to 29 mL/minute, give one 200-mg capsule every 72 hours or 80 mg oral solution every 24 hours; if CrCl is less than 15 mL/minute or patient is receiving hemodialysis, give one 200-mg capsule every 96 hours or 60 mg oral solution every 24 hours. Give dose after hemodialysis session. In children with renal insufficiency, consider a dose reduction or increased dosing interval.

ADMINISTRATION
PO
• Give drug with or without food.
• Refrigerate oral solution; if stored at room temperature, use within 3 months.
• Dispense in original containers; keep containers tightly closed.

ACTION
Inhibits replication of HIV by blocking viral DNA synthesis and inhibits reverse transcriptase by acting as an alternative for the enzyme's substrate, deoxycytidine triphosphate.

Route	Onset	Peak	Duration
PO	Unknown	1–2 hr	Unknown

Half-life: About 10 hours.

ADVERSE REACTIONS
CNS: abnormal dreams, asthenia, dizziness, headache, insomnia, depression, fatigue, neuritis, paresthesia, peripheral neuropathy, fever. **EENT:** rhinitis, otitis media. **GI:** abdominal pain, diarrhea, nausea, dyspepsia, vomiting, gastroenteritis. **Hematologic:** anemia. **Hepatic:** increased transaminase levels, hyperbilirubinemia, *hepatotoxicity.*

Metabolic: hyperglycemia, *hypoglycemia,* increased amylase level, hypertriglyceridemia. **Musculoskeletal:** arthralgia, myalgia. **Respiratory:** increased cough, pneumonia. **Skin:** allergic skin reaction, discoloration, rash, pruritus, urticarial and purpuric lesions. **Other:** infection.

INTERACTIONS
Drug-drug. *Cladribine:* May decrease effects of cladribine. Don't use together.
Orlistat: May decrease serum concentration of antiretrovirals. Monitor concurrent use.

EFFECTS ON LAB TEST RESULTS
• May increase ALT, amylase, AST, bilirubin, CK, lipase, and triglyceride levels.
• May increase or decrease glucose level.
• May decrease Hb level and neutrophil count.
• May increase urine glucose level.

CONTRAINDICATIONS & CAUTIONS
• Contraindicated in patients hypersensitive to drug or its ingredients.
• In older adults, use cautiously because of the potential for other diseases and drug therapies and for decreased hepatic, renal, or cardiac function.
• Use cautiously in patients with impaired renal function.
Boxed Warning Severe acute exacerbations of HBV infection have been reported in patients infected with both HBV and HIV-1 who have discontinued emtricitabine. Monitor hepatic function closely with both clinical and lab follow-up for at least several months in patients infected with both HIV-1 and HBV who discontinue this drug. If appropriate, initiation of anti–HBV therapy may be warranted. ■
• Lactic acidosis and severe hepatomegaly with steatosis, including fatal cases, have been reported with use of nucleoside analogues, alone or in combination with other antiretrovirals.
Dialyzable drug: 30% over 3-hour hemodialysis period.

PREGNANCY-LACTATION-REPRODUCTION
• Use drug during pregnancy only if clearly needed.
• Register patients who are pregnant in the Antiretroviral Pregnancy Registry at 1-800-258-4263.

Reactions in bold italics are *life-threatening.* Interactions may have a *rapid onset* or a ***delayed onset.***

- Patients should avoid breastfeeding because of potential for HIV-1 transmission and serious adverse reactions in breastfed infants.

NURSING CONSIDERATIONS
- Test all patients for HBV before starting drug.
- Suspend treatment in patients who develop signs and symptoms or lab findings suggestive of lactic acidosis or pronounced hepatotoxicity (including nausea, vomiting, unusual or unexpected stomach discomfort, and weakness).

Boxed Warning Monitor hepatic function closely with both clinical and lab follow-up for at least several months in patients infected with both HIV-1 and HBV who discontinue this drug. Severe acute exacerbations of hepatitis B have been reported. ∎

- Monitor patients for infection and development of immune reconstitution syndrome (inflammatory response to opportunistic infections, such as MAC infection, CMV, *Pneumocystis jiroveci* pneumonia, or TB), which may necessitate further evaluation and treatment.
- Hyperpigmentation occurs more frequently in children.

PATIENT TEACHING
- Instruct patient in safe drug administration.
- Remind patient that anti-HIV medicine must be taken for life.
- Inform patient that drug doesn't cure HIV infection, that opportunistic infections and other complications of HIV infection may continue to occur, and that transmission of HIV to others through sexual contact or blood contamination is still possible.
- Explain possible adverse reactions, including lactic acidosis and hepatotoxicity; advise patient to report all adverse reactions.
- Tell patient to notify prescriber immediately of known or suspected pregnancy.
- Warn patient against breastfeeding.

emtricitabine–rilpivirine–tenofovir alafenamide fumarate
em-tra-SYE-ta-ben/ril-pi-VIR-een/
te-NOE-fo-veer

Odefsey

Therapeutic class: Antiretrovirals
Pharmacologic class: NRTIs–NNRTIs

AVAILABLE FORMS
Tablets: 200 mg emtricitabine, 25 mg rilpivirine, and 25 mg tenofovir alafenamide fumarate

INDICATIONS & DOSAGES
➤ **HIV-1 infection as initial therapy in patients with no antiretroviral treatment history and HIV-1 RNA 100,000 copies/mL or less; or to replace a stable antiretroviral regimen in patients who are virologically suppressed (HIV-1 RNA less than 50 copies/mL) for at least 6 months with no history of treatment failure and no known substitutions associated with resistance to the individual components**
Adults and children age 12 and older weighing at least 35 kg: 1 tablet PO once daily with a meal.
Adjust-a-dose: For patients on hemodialysis, give 1 tablet once daily; give after hemodialysis on dialysis days. Drug isn't recommended for patients with CrCl of less than 30 mL/minute who aren't receiving long-term dialysis.

ADMINISTRATION
PO
- Give drug once daily with a meal.
- Store below 86° F (30° C).
- Keep only in tightly closed, original container.

ACTION
Nucleoside, nonnucleoside, and nucleotide inhibitor combination of reverse transcriptase that inhibits viral replication.

Route	Onset	Peak	Duration
PO (emtricitabine)	Unknown	1–2 hr	Unknown
PO (rilpivirine)	Unknown	4–5 hr	Unknown
PO (tenofovir)	Unknown	0.48 hr	Unknown

Half-life: Emtricitabine, 10 hours; rilpivirine, 50 hours; tenofovir, 0.51 hour.

ADVERSE REACTIONS

CNS: headache, insomnia, sleep disturbances, depression, somnolence, dizziness. **GI:** flatulence, diarrhea, nausea, vomiting, abdominal pain. **Metabolic:** hypophosphatemia, increased lipid levels. **Musculoskeletal:** decreased bone mineral density. **Skin:** rash. **Other:** hypersensitivity reaction.

INTERACTIONS

☙ *Alert:* Drug combination can interact significantly with many drugs. Consult a drug interaction resource or pharmacist for additional information.

Drug-drug. *Acyclovir, aminoglycosides, cidofovir, ganciclovir, valacyclovir, valganciclovir:* May increase Odefsey (specifically tenofovir) concentration. Monitor patient for Odefsey-related increased adverse effects. Tenofovir products may increase ganciclovir or valganciclovir serum concentration. Monitor therapy.

Antacids (aluminum, magnesium hydroxide, calcium carbonate): May decrease rilpivirine level. Give antacids at least 2 hours before or at least 4 hours after Odefsey.

Anticonvulsants (carbamazepine, oxcarbazepine, phenobarbital, phenytoin): May decrease rilpivirine level, resulting in loss of virologic response and possible drug resistance. Use together is contraindicated.

Antimycobacterial drugs (rifabutin, rifampin, rifapentine): May decrease rilpivirine and tenofovir levels, resulting in loss of virologic response and possible drug resistance. Use together is contraindicated.

Azole antifungals (fluconazole, itraconazole, ketoconazole): May decrease azole level. Monitor patient for breakthrough fungal infections.

CYP3A inducers: May decrease rilpivirine level, resulting in loss of virologic response and possible drug resistance. Use together is contraindicated.

CYP3A inhibitors: May increase rilpivirine level and risk of adverse events. Monitor therapy.

Dexamethasone (systemic): May decrease rilpivirine level, resulting in loss of virologic response and possible drug resistance. Use of more than a single dose of dexamethasone is contraindicated.

Didanosine: May decrease didanosine serum concentration. Give didanosine on an empty stomach at least 2 hours before or 4 hours after Odefsey due to the requirement that rilpivirine be administered with food.

H_2-receptor antagonists (cimetidine, famotidine, nizatidine): May decrease rilpivirine level. Administer H_2-receptor antagonist at least 12 hours before or 4 hours after Odefsey. Consider therapy modification.

Ketolide or macrolide antibiotics (clarithromycin, erythromycin): May increase rilpivirine level. Consider using an alternative antibiotic.

Methadone: May increase methadone metabolism. Adjust methadone dosage as clinically indicated.

NSAIDs: May increase risk of nephrotoxicity and adverse effects, especially at high doses. Use alternatives to these combinations if possible.

P-gp inducers: May decrease tenofovir level, which may lead to loss of therapeutic effect and resistance. Monitor patient closely.

P-gp inhibitors: May increase tenofovir level. Monitor patient for increased Odefsey-related adverse effects.

PPIs (dexlansoprazole, esomeprazole, lansoprazole, omeprazole, pantoprazole, rabeprazole): May decrease rilpivirine level, resulting in loss of virologic response and possible drug resistance. Use together is contraindicated.

QTc interval–prolonging agents: May enhance QTc interval–prolonging effect. Consider alternative medications to Odefsey in patients with known risk of torsades de pointes.

Drug-herb. *St. John's wort:* May decrease Odefsey serum concentration, resulting in loss of virologic response and possible resistance to drug combination. Discourage use together.

EFFECTS ON LAB TEST RESULTS

• May increase phosphorus, triglyceride, lipid and serum lactate levels.

CONTRAINDICATIONS & CAUTIONS

Boxed Warning Odefsey isn't approved for treatment of chronic HBV infection, and safety and effectiveness haven't been established in patients coinfected with HIV-1 and HBV. Severe acute exacerbations of HBV infection have been reported in patients coinfected with HIV-1 and HBV after discontinuation of antiretroviral therapy. Monitor hepatic function during and for several months

after discontinuation of treatment. If appropriate, initiate anti-HBV therapy. ■
- Contraindicated in patients hypersensitive to drug or its components.
- Consider alternative therapy in patients at high risk for torsades de pointes or when administered with medications known to increase risk of torsades de pointes. Supratherapeutic dosages of Odefsey have been shown to prolong QTc interval and may increase risk of ventricular arrhythmias.
- Use isn't recommended in patients with CrCl of less than 30 mL/minute unless they are receiving long-term hemodialysis.
- Use cautiously in patients at risk for renal dysfunction. Hypophosphatemia has been reported secondary to proximal renal tubulopathy.
- Use cautiously in patients at risk for liver disease. Hepatic adverse events have been reported.
- Use in patients with severe hepatic impairment hasn't been studied..
- Drug may cause lactic acidosis and hepatomegaly with steatosis, including fatal cases. These effects may occur without elevated transaminase levels and in patients with no known risk factors. Risk factors include long-term antiretroviral use, obesity, and being female. Monitor all patients closely.
- May increase risk of immune reconstitution syndrome, resulting in an inflammatory response to an indolent or opportunistic infection or activation of autoimmune disorders (MAC infection, CMV, *Pneumocystis jiroveci* pneumonia, TB, Graves disease, polymyositis, Guillain-Barré syndrome).
- Safety and effectiveness in children younger than age 12 or weighing less than 35 kg haven't been established.
Dialyzable drug: Emtricitabine, 30%; rilpivirine, unlikely; tenofovir, 54%.

PREGNANCY-LACTATION-REPRODUCTION
- There are no well-controlled studies during pregnancy. Use cautiously during pregnancy.
- Patients who become pregnant during therapy and who are virologically suppressed (HIV-1 RNA less than 50 copies per mL) may continue drug. Monitor viral load closely.
- To monitor pregnancy outcomes, health care providers are encouraged to register patients in the Antiretroviral Pregnancy Registry (1-800-258-4263).
- Some components of drug appear in human milk. It isn't known if Odefsey affects

lactation effects on an infant. The CDC recommends that patients with HIV infection not breastfeed to avoid HIV transmission to the infant.

NURSING CONSIDERATIONS
- Discontinue Odefsey if clinical or lab findings suggestive of lactic acidosis or hepatotoxicity develop.
- Test for HBV before initiation of antiretroviral therapy in all patients.
- Assess CD4 count, HIV-1 RNA plasma levels, LFT values, serum creatinine, urine glucose, and urine protein before initiation and during therapy.
- In patients who are virologically suppressed, additional monitoring of HIV-1 RNA and regimen tolerability is recommended after replacing therapy to assess for potential virologic failure or rebound.
- Monitor patient for hypersensitivity, rash, and severe skin reactions, including DRESS syndrome (severe rash or rash accompanied by fever, blisters, mucosal involvement, conjunctivitis, facial edema, angioedema, hepatitis, eosinophilia). Most rashes occur within first 4 to 6 weeks of therapy. Monitor lab parameters and clinical status. Stop drug immediately if hypersensitivity or rash develops.
- Monitor serum phosphorus level in patients with chronic kidney disease. Odefsey may increase risk of Fanconi syndrome. Discontinue drug for significantly decreased renal function or evidence of Fanconi syndrome.
- Calcium and vitamin D supplementation may be beneficial for all patients.
- Monitor patient for depression, dysphoria, mood changes, negative thoughts, suicidality, or suicide attempts. Patients who develop these symptoms should be promptly evaluated; consider risks versus benefits of continued treatment.
- Monitor patient for infection.

PATIENT TEACHING
- **Alert:** Counsel patient, family members, or caregivers to watch for signs and symptoms of depression and to immediately report depression, negative thoughts, dysphoria, or suicidality to prescriber.
- Advise patient that Odefsey can cause buildup of lactic acid in the blood. Instruct patient to seek immediate medical attention for weakness, fatigue, muscle pain, trouble breathing, stomachache with nausea and

vomiting, dizziness, chills, or fast or irregular heartbeat.

• Caution patient that Odefsey may cause liver problems. Instruct patient to seek immediate medical attention for yellowing of the skin or eyes, dark-colored urine, loss of appetite, light-colored stool, nausea, or pain or tenderness on right side of the stomach.

🌙 *Alert:* Warn patient to stop taking drug and immediately seek medical attention for allergic reactions (rash, fever, blisters, mucosal involvement, eye inflammation; swelling of the face, eyes, lips, mouth, tongue, or throat, which may lead to difficulty swallowing or breathing).

• Caution patient not to discontinue drug combination without first discussing with prescriber. Advise patient of the importance of not running out of the medications and of not missing doses.

Boxed Warning Inform patient that severe acute exacerbations of hepatitis B have been reported in patients who are coinfected and who discontinue drug. ∎

• Remind patient to notify prescriber about other prescription or OTC drugs, including herbal and vitamin supplements, patient is taking or plans to take.

• Inform patient that blood tests will be needed to check for effectiveness and adverse effects of therapy.

• Advise patient to immediately report signs and symptoms of infection.

• Tell patient of childbearing potential to notify prescriber about planned, suspected, or known pregnancy and that there is a pregnancy registry for use of antivirals during pregnancy.

• Advise patient not to breastfeed during therapy.

emtricitabine–tenofovir alafenamide

em-tra-SYE-tah-ben/te-NOE-fo-veer

Descovy

Therapeutic class: Antiretrovirals
Pharmacologic class: NNRTIs

AVAILABLE FORMS

Tablets: 120 mg emtricitabine and 15 mg tenofovir alafenamide, 200 mg emtricitabine and 25 mg tenofovir alafenamide

INDICATIONS & DOSAGES

Adjust-a-dose (for all indications): In adults with CrCl below 15 mL/minute who are receiving long-term hemodialysis, give daily dose on days of hemodialysis after completion of hemodialysis treatment. Use isn't recommended in patients with CrCl of 15 to less than 30 mL/minute or in those with ESRD not receiving hemodialysis.

➤ **HIV-1 infection in combination with other antiretrovirals**
Adults and children weighing 35 kg or more: One 200 mg/25 mg tablet PO once daily.

➤ **HIV-1 infection in combination with other antiretrovirals other than protease inhibitors that require a CYP3A inhibitor**
Children weighing at least 25 to less than 35 kg: One 200 mg/25 mg tablet PO once daily.
Children weighing at least 14 to less than 25 kg: One 120 mg/15 mg tablet PO once daily.

➤ **Preexposure prophylaxis (PrEP) in patients who are at risk with a negative HIV-1 test immediately before treatment, to reduce risk of HIV-1 infection from sexual acquisition, excluding those at risk from receptive vaginal sex**
Adults and adolescents weighing at least 35 kg: One 200 mg/25 mg tablet PO once daily.

ADMINISTRATION
PO
• May give with or without food.
• Give missed dose as soon possible. If it's close to time for next dose, skip missed dose. Don't give two doses at the same time or extra doses.
• Don't remove drug from original container; keep container tightly closed.

ACTION
Interferes with HIV viral RNA-dependent DNA polymerase activities, resulting in inhibition of viral replication.

Route	Onset	Peak	Duration
PO (emtricitabine)	Unknown	1–2 hr	Unknown
PO (tenofovir)	Unknown	0.48 hr	Unknown

Half-life: Emtricitabine, 10 hours; tenofovir, 0.51 hour.

Reactions in bold italics are *life-threatening*. Interactions may have a *rapid onset* or a ***delayed onset***.

ADVERSE REACTIONS
CNS: headache, fatigue. **GI:** nausea, diarrhea, vomiting, abdominal pain. **Metabolic:** increased triglyceride levels. **Musculoskeletal:** decreased bone mineral density.

INTERACTIONS
⚠ *Alert:* Drug combination can interact significantly with many drugs. Consult a drug interaction resource or pharmacist for additional information.

Drug-drug. *Acyclovir, valacyclovir:* May increase serum concentration of tenofovir products. Tenofovir products may increase serum concentration of acyclovir or valacyclovir. Monitor therapy.

Adefovir: May diminish therapeutic effect of tenofovir products. Tenofovir products may increase adefovir serum concentration. Avoid use together.

Aminoglycosides: May increase serum concentration of tenofovir products and aminoglycosides. Monitor therapy.

Anticonvulsants (carbamazepine, oxcarbazepine, phenobarbital, phenytoin, primidone): May decrease tenofovir serum concentration. Consider alternative anticonvulsant.

Antimycobacterial drugs (rifabutin, rifampin, rifapentine): May decrease tenofovir level. Use together isn't recommended.

Cidofovir: May increase serum concentrations of tenofovir products and cidofovir. Monitor therapy.

Cobicistat: May increase risk of adverse effects of tenofovir. Monitor therapy.

Ganciclovir, valganciclovir: May increase serum level of tenofovir, ganciclovir, or valganciclovir concentration. Monitor patient closely for increased adverse effects.

Lamivudine: May increase risk of adverse effects of emtricitabine. Avoid use together.

NSAIDs: May enhance nephrotoxic effect of tenofovir. Seek alternatives to this combination whenever possible. Avoid use of tenofovir with multiple NSAIDs or with any NSAID given at a high dose.

P-gp inducers: May decrease tenofovir absorption, causing loss of therapeutic effect and development of resistance. Monitor therapy closely or consider therapy modification.

P-gp inhibitors: May increase tenofovir level. Use cautiously together.

Protease inhibitors (ritonavir, tipranavir): May decrease tenofovir serum concentration. Use together isn't recommended.

Ribavirin (oral inhalation, systemic): May increase risk of hepatotoxicity. Use together cautiously.

Drug-herb. *St. John's wort:* May decrease tenofovir serum concentration. Discourage use together.

EFFECTS ON LAB TEST RESULTS
- May increase total cholesterol, LDL, HDL, triglyceride, ALT, amylase, AST, bilirubin, CK, lipase, serum creatinine, and glucose levels.
- May decrease phosphate level.
- May decrease neutrophil count.

CONTRAINDICATIONS & CAUTIONS
- Contraindicated for use in PrEP in individuals with unknown or positive HIV-1 status.

Boxed Warning Drug isn't approved for treatment of chronic HBV infection. Safety and effectiveness haven't been established for patients coinfected with HIV and HBV; acute, severe exacerbations of HBV infection (liver decompensation and liver failure) have been reported after discontinuation of antiretroviral therapy. ■

Boxed Warning When used for HIV-1 PrEP, drug must only be prescribed to individuals confirmed to be HIV-negative immediately before drug initiation and at least every 3 months during use. Drug-resistant HIV-1 variants have been identified with use of emtricitabine–tenofovir for HIV-1 PrEP after undetected acute HIV-1 infection. Don't use for HIV-1 PrEP in patients with signs or symptoms of acute HIV-1 infection unless HIV-1 negative infection status is confirmed. ■

- Descovy isn't recommended for patient with CrCl of less than 30 mL/minute unless patient is on hemodialysis.
- Drug may increase risk of acute renal failure and Fanconi syndrome. Patients with pre-existing renal impairment and those taking nephrotoxic agents (including NSAIDs) are at increased risk.
- Use in patients with severe hepatic impairment (Child-Pugh class C) hasn't been studied.
- Immune reconstitution syndrome may occur, resulting in an inflammatory response to an opportunistic infection (MAC infection, CMV, *Pneumocystis jiroveci* pneumonia, TB) or an autoimmune disorder (Graves

disease, polymyositis, Guillain-Barré syndrome); evaluate and treat appropriately.

🔄 *Alert:* Lactic acidosis and severe hepatomegaly with steatosis, including fatal cases, have been reported with nucleoside analogues (tenofovir) in combination with other antiretrovirals. Interrupt treatment in patients who develop clinical or lab findings suggestive of lactic acidosis or hepatotoxicity (hepatomegaly and steatosis with or without transaminase elevations). Some cases of hepatotoxicity have occurred in patients with no hepatic disease before treatment.

• Safety and effectiveness when administered with an HIV-1 protease inhibitor that's given with either ritonavir or cobicistat haven't been established in children weighing less than 35 kg or adults with CrCl below 15 mL/minute, with or without hemodialysis.

• Safety and effectiveness in children with HIV infection weighing less than 14 kg or in children weighing less than 35 kg treated for HIV-1 PrEP haven't been established.

Dialyzable drug: Emtricitabine, 30%; tenofovir alafenamide, 54%.

PREGNANCY-LACTATION-REPRODUCTION

• If indicated, drug shouldn't be withheld because of pregnancy.

• Emtricitabine and tenofovir appear in human milk. Both drugs are contraindicated during breastfeeding.

• The CDC recommends that HIV-infected patients not breastfeed to avoid postnatal transmission of HIV.

• To monitor pregnancy outcomes, health care providers are encouraged to register patients in the Antiretroviral Pregnancy Registry (1-800-258-4263).

NURSING CONSIDERATIONS

• Test for HBV before initiation of antiretroviral therapy. Drug isn't approved for the treatment of chronic HBV infection.

• Descovy must be given as part of a regimen with other antiretrovirals unless used for PrEP.

• Screen all individuals for HIV-1 infection immediately before initiating drug for HIV-1 PrEP, at least once every 3 months during treatment, and upon diagnosis of other sexually transmitted infections (STIs).

• If recent (less than 1 month) exposure to HIV-1 is suspected or clinical symptoms are consistent with acute HIV-1 infection, use a test approved or cleared by the FDA to help diagnose acute or primary HIV-1 infection.

• Use drug for HIV-1 PrEP to reduce risk of HIV-1 infection as part of a comprehensive prevention strategy, including adherence to daily administration and safer sex practices, including condoms, to reduce risk of STIs.

• Monitor CD4 counts and HIV RNA plasma levels to evaluate effectiveness of treatment.

• Assess serum creatinine level, estimated CrCl, urine protein, and urine glucose before initiation and during therapy. Monitor serum phosphorus level in patients with chronic kidney disease due to increased risk of developing Fanconi syndrome. Discontinue drug in patients who develop clinically significant decreases in renal function or evidence of Fanconi syndrome.

• Evaluate patients with persistent or worsening bone or muscle signs or symptoms for renal dysfunction (including Fanconi syndrome), hypophosphatemia, and osteomalacia.

• Monitor lipid levels periodically.

Boxed Warning Monitor patients with HIV and HBV coinfection for several months after therapy discontinuation for acute exacerbations of HBV infection. Monitor hepatic function by clinical assessment and lab testing. Start anti–hepatitis B therapy as clinically indicated, especially in patients with advanced liver disease or cirrhosis. ∎

• Calcium and vitamin D supplements may benefit all patients.

PATIENT TEACHING

• Advise patient that hepatitis B sometimes worsens after therapy; closely monitor patient for a few months after therapy.

• Caution patient not to stop drug without first discussing with prescriber.

• Advise patient of importance of taking drug without missing doses, to avoid loss of treatment effectiveness.

• Warn patient to report signs and symptoms of kidney problems (inability to pass urine, change in how much urine is passed, blood in the urine, weight gain).

Boxed Warning Instruct patient to report signs and symptoms of liver problems (dark urine, loss of appetite, nausea, right upper quadrant abdominal pain, achiness or tenderness, light-colored stools, vomiting, yellowing of skin or eyes). ∎

Reactions in bold italics are *life-threatening*. Interactions may have a *rapid onset* or a ***delayed onset***.

• Advise patient to report signs and symptoms of lactic acidosis (trouble breathing, fast or irregular heartbeat, stomach pain with nausea or vomiting, fatigue, shortness of breath, weakness, dizziness or light-headedness, feeling cold, muscle pain or cramps).

• Instruct patient to report signs and symptoms of infection (fever, sore throat, weakness, cough, shortness of breath).

• Teach patient to avoid behaviors that can spread HIV-1 infection to others, including sharing or reusing needles, sharing razors or toothbrushes, or having sex without using a latex or polyurethane condom.

• Teach patient about the use of other prevention measures (consistent and correct condom use, knowledge of partners' HIV-1 status [including viral suppression status], regular testing for STIs that can facilitate HIV-1 transmission). Inform uninfected individuals about potential for HIV-1 infection and support their efforts in reducing sexual risk behavior.

• Caution patient not to breastfeed, to avoid transmitting HIV-1 to infant.

• Inform patient that there is an antiretroviral pregnancy registry to monitor fetal outcomes in patients exposed to Descovy during pregnancy.

enalaprilat ✂
eh-NAH-leh-prel-at

enalapril maleate ✂
Epaned, Vasotec♥

Therapeutic class: Antihypertensives
Pharmacologic class: ACE inhibitors

AVAILABLE FORMS
enalaprilat
Injection: 1.25 mg/mL
enalapril maleate
Oral solution: 1 mg/mL
Tablets: 2.5 mg, 5 mg, 10 mg, 20 mg

INDICATIONS & DOSAGES
➤ **HTN**
Adults: In patients not taking diuretics, initially, 5 mg PO once daily; then adjusted based on response. Usual dosage ranges from 10 to 40 mg daily as a single dose or two divided doses. Or, 1.25 mg IV infusion over 5 minutes every 6 hours.

Children ages 1 month to 16 years: 0.08 mg/kg (up to 5 mg) PO once daily; dosage should be adjusted as needed up to 0.58 mg/kg (maximum 40 mg). Don't use if CrCl is less than 30 mL/minute/1.73 m².
Adjust-a-dose: If adult patient is taking diuretics or CrCl is 30 mL/minute or less, initially, 2.5 mg PO once daily and titrate to a maximum dose of 40 mg daily. Or, 0.625 mg IV over 5 minutes, and repeat in 1 hour, if needed; then 1.25 mg IV every 6 hours. For adult patients on dialysis, give 2.5 mg PO on dialysis days; adjust dosage on dialysis days based on BP response.
➤ **To convert from IV therapy to oral therapy in patients receiving diuretics**
Adults: Initially, 2.5 mg PO once daily; if patient was receiving 0.625 mg IV every 6 hours, then 2.5 mg PO once daily. Adjust dosage based on response.
➤ **To convert from oral therapy to IV therapy**
Adults: 1.25 mg IV over 5 minutes every 6 hours.
➤ **To convert from IV therapy to oral therapy**
Adults: 5 mg PO once daily.
Adjust-a-dose: For patients with CrCl of 30 mL/minute or less, give 2.5 mg PO once daily.
➤ **To manage symptomatic HF**
Adults: Initially, 2.5 mg PO b.i.d., increased gradually as tolerated over a few days or weeks. Maintenance is 5 to 40 mg daily in two divided doses. Maximum daily dose is 40 mg in two divided doses.
Adjust-a-dose: For patients with hyponatremia (serum sodium level of less than 130 mEq/L) or serum creatinine level greater than 1.6 mg/dL, recommended initial dose is 2.5 mg once daily.
➤ **Asymptomatic left ventricular dysfunction**
Adults: Initially, 2.5 mg PO b.i.d. Increase as tolerated to target daily dose of 20 mg PO in divided doses.

ADMINISTRATION
PO
• Give drug without regard for food.
• Request oral suspension for patient who has difficulty swallowing.

IV

▼ Inspect solution for particulate matter and discoloration before administration.

▼ Compatible solutions include D₅W, NSS for injection, dextrose 5% in lactated Ringer injection, and dextrose 5% in NSS for injection.

▼ Inject drug slowly over at least 5 minutes, or dilute in 50 mL of a compatible solution and infuse over 15 minutes.

▼ **Incompatibilities:** Amphotericin B, cefepime, phenytoin.

ACTION

Inhibits ACE, preventing conversion of angiotensin I to angiotensin II, a potent vasoconstrictor. Less angiotensin II decreases peripheral arterial resistance, decreasing aldosterone secretion, reducing sodium and water retention, and lowering BP.

Route	Onset	Peak	Duration
PO	1 hr	3–4 hr	12–24 hr
IV	15 min	1–4 hr	6 hr

Half-life: 11 hours, but varies by age and comorbidities.

ADVERSE REACTIONS

CNS: asthenia, headache, dizziness, fatigue, vertigo, syncope, weakness. **CV:** hypotension, orthostatic hypotension, chest pain, angina, *MI.* **GI:** anorexia, diarrhea, nausea, abdominal pain, vomiting. **GU:** UTI. **Hematologic:** bone marrow depression. **Respiratory:** bronchitis; dry, persistent, tickling, nonproductive cough; dyspnea, pneumonia. **Skin:** rash. **Other:** hypersensitivity reactions.

INTERACTIONS

Drug-drug. *ACE inhibitors, ARBs (candesartan, telmisartan):* May increase risk of hypotension, hyperkalemia, and renal failure. Avoid use together; if use together is unavoidable, closely monitor BP, renal function, and electrolyte levels.

Aldosterone blockers (eplerenone): May increase risk of hyperkalemia. Monitor therapy.

Aliskiren: May increase risk of hypotension, hyperkalemia, and renal failure. Use together is contraindicated in patients with diabetes.

Azathioprine: May increase risk of anemia or leukopenia. Monitor hematologic study results if used together.

Diuretics: May excessively reduce BP. Use together cautiously.

Gold sodium thiomalate: May increase risk of nitritoid reactions. Use cautiously together.

Insulin, oral antidiabetics: May cause hypoglycemia, especially at start of enalapril therapy. Monitor patient closely.

Lithium: May cause lithium toxicity. Monitor lithium level.

mTOR inhibitors (sirolimus, temsirolimus): May increase risk of angioedema. Monitor patient closely.

Neprilysin inhibitors (sacubitril): May increase risk of angioedema. Use together is contraindicated. Don't give within 36 hours of switching to or from sacubitril–valsartan, a neprilysin inhibitor.

NSAIDs: May increase risk of renal failure in older adults or patients with volume depletion or impaired renal function. Monitor renal function.

Potassium-sparing diuretics, potassium supplements: May cause hyperkalemia. Avoid using together unless hypokalemia is confirmed.

Drug-herb. *Capsaicin:* May cause cough. Discourage use together.

Ma huang: May decrease antihypertensive effects. Discourage use together.

Drug-food. *Salt substitutes containing potassium:* May cause hyperkalemia. Monitor patient closely.

EFFECTS ON LAB TEST RESULTS

• May increase bilirubin, BUN, creatinine, and potassium levels and LFT values.

• May decrease sodium and Hb levels and hematocrit.

CONTRAINDICATIONS & CAUTIONS

▧ Contraindicated in patients hypersensitive to drug, in those with a history of angioedema related to previous treatment with an ACE inhibitor, and in patients with hereditary or idiopathic angioedema.

• Safety and effectiveness of IV use in children haven't been established.

• Oral drug isn't recommended in neonates (younger than age 1 month), preterm infants who haven't reached a corrected postconceptual age of 44 weeks, and in children with GFR of less than 30 mL/minute/1.73 m².

• Use cautiously in patients with renal impairment or those with aortic stenosis or hypertrophic cardiomyopathy.

Dialyzable drug: Yes.

⚠ *Overdose S&S:* Hypotension.

PREGNANCY-LACTATION-REPRODUCTION
Boxed Warning Use during pregnancy can cause injury and death to the developing fetus. If pregnancy is detected, stop drug as soon as possible. ■

- Drug appears in human milk. Breastfeeding isn't recommended.

NURSING CONSIDERATIONS
- Closely monitor BP response to drug.
- Monitor CBC with differential counts before and during therapy.
- Patients with diabetes, those with impaired renal function or HF, and those receiving drugs that can increase potassium level may develop hyperkalemia. Monitor potassium intake and potassium level.
- Monitor renal function, especially in patients who are post-MI and in those with bilateral renal artery stenosis, chronic kidney disease, volume depletion, or HF.
- Monitor patients for angioedema and anaphylactoid reactions (airway obstruction; edema of the face, extremities, lips, tongue; abdominal pain with or without nausea or vomiting).
- Monitor patients for hepatotoxicity (jaundice, increased LFT values).
- ▧ Patients who are Black taking ACE inhibitors as monotherapy for HTN have a smaller reduction in BP than those who are non-Black. Patients who are Black taking ACE inhibitors have a higher incidence of angioedema than those who are non-Black.
- *Look alike–sound alike:* Don't confuse enalapril with Anafranil or Eldepryl.

PATIENT TEACHING
- Instruct patient to report breathing difficulty or swelling of face, eyes, lips, or tongue. Swelling of the face and throat (including swelling of the larynx) may occur, especially after first dose.
- Advise patient to report signs and symptoms of infection, such as fever and sore throat.
- Instruct patient to report persistent nonproductive cough.
- Inform patient that light-headedness can occur, especially during first few days of therapy. Tell patient to rise slowly to minimize this effect and to notify prescriber if symptoms develop. If fainting occurs, advise patient to stop drug and call prescriber immediately.

- Tell patient to use caution in hot weather and during exercise. Inadequate fluid intake, vomiting, diarrhea, and excessive perspiration can lead to light-headedness and fainting.
- Advise patient to avoid salt substitutes; these products may contain potassium, which can cause high potassium levels in patients taking this drug.
- **Boxed Warning** Tell patient of childbearing potential to notify prescriber if pregnancy occurs. Drug will need to be stopped. ■

SAFETY ALERT!

enfuvirtide
en-foo-VEER-tide

Fuzeon

Therapeutic class: Antiretrovirals
Pharmacologic class: Fusion inhibitors

AVAILABLE FORMS
Powder for injection: 108-mg single-use vials (90 mg/mL after reconstitution)

INDICATIONS & DOSAGES
➤ **HIV-1 infection, with other antiretrovirals, in patients who have continued HIV-1 replication despite antiretroviral therapy**
Adults: 90 mg subcut b.i.d.
Children weighing at least 11 kg: 2 mg/kg subcut b.i.d. Maximum, 90 mg/dose.

ADMINISTRATION
Subcutaneous
- Reconstitute vial with 1 mL sterile water for injection. Tap vial with fingertip for 10 seconds, then gently roll, making sure powder doesn't adhere to vial wall. Let drug stand for up to 45 minutes to ensure reconstitution but allow more time if solution is foamy or jelled. When completely mixed, solution should be clear, colorless, and without bubbles or particulate matter. If solution appears foamy or jelled, allow more time for it to dissolve. Then draw up correct dose and inject drug.
- If drug isn't used immediately after reconstitution, refrigerate in original vial and use within 24 hours. Don't inject drug until it's at room temperature.
- Vial is for single use; discard unused portion.
- Inject into upper arm, anterior thigh, or abdomen. Rotate injection sites. Don't inject

into same site for two consecutive doses, and don't inject into moles, scar tissue, bruises, tattoos, or the navel, where large nerves course close to the skin.

• Store unreconstituted vials at room temperature.

ACTION

Interferes with entry of HIV-1 into cells by inhibiting fusion of HIV-1 to CD4 cell membranes.

Route	Onset	Peak	Duration
Subcut	Unknown	4–8 hr	Unknown

Half-life: 3.8 hours.

ADVERSE REACTIONS

CNS: fatigue, insomnia, anxiety, asthenia. **EENT:** conjunctivitis, sinusitis, dry mouth. **GI:** diarrhea, nausea, *pancreatitis*, abdominal pain, anorexia, constipation. **Hematologic:** eosinophilia. **Hepatic:** increased transaminase levels. **Metabolic:** weight loss, increased CK level. **Musculoskeletal:** myalgia, limb pain. **Respiratory:** pneumonia, cough. **Skin:** injection-site reactions, folliculitis. **Other:** herpes simplex, flulike illness.

INTERACTIONS

Drug-drug. *Orlistat:* May decrease enfuvirtide serum concentration. Monitor therapeutic response.

EFFECTS ON LAB TEST RESULTS

• May increase CK, ALT, AST, GGT, lipase, amylase, and triglyceride levels.
• May increase eosinophil count.
• May decrease Hb level.

CONTRAINDICATIONS & CAUTIONS

• Contraindicated in patients hypersensitive to drug and in those not infected with HIV.
• Safety and effectiveness in children weighing less than 11 kg haven't been determined. *Dialyzable drug:* Unlikely.

PREGNANCY-LACTATION-REPRODUCTION

• There are no well-controlled studies during pregnancy. Use during pregnancy only if clearly needed.
• Register patients who are pregnant in the Antiretroviral Pregnancy Registry at 1-800-258-4263.
• Because of the potential for HIV transmission, patients shouldn't breastfeed.

NURSING CONSIDERATIONS

• Injection-site reactions (pain, discomfort, induration, erythema, pruritus, nodules, cysts, ecchymosis), which are common, may require analgesics or rest.
• Monitor patients for infection and development of immune reconstitution syndrome (inflammatory response to opportunistic infections, such as MAC infection, CMV, *Pneumocystis jiroveci* pneumonia, or TB), which may necessitate further evaluation and treatment. Autoimmune disorders (such as Graves disease, polymyositis, and Guillain-Barré syndrome) have also been reported in the setting of immune reconstitution; however, time to onset varies, and can occur months after initiation of treatment.
• Nerve pain (neuralgia or paresthesia) lasting up to 6 months and associated with administration at sites where large nerves course close to the skin, bruising, and hematomas have occurred. Patients receiving anticoagulants and those with hemophilia or other coagulation disorders may have a higher risk of postinjection bleeding.
⚠ *Alert:* Monitor patient closely for evidence of bacterial pneumonia. Patients at high risk include those with a low initial CD4 count or high initial viral load, those who use IV drugs or smoke, and those with history of lung disease.
• Hypersensitivity may occur with first dose or later doses. If systemic symptoms occur, stop drug and don't rechallenge.

PATIENT TEACHING

• Teach patient how to prepare and give drug and how to safely dispose of used needles and syringes.
• Tell patient to rotate injection sites and to watch for cellulitis or local infection.
• Urge patient to immediately report evidence of pneumonia, such as cough with fever, rapid breathing, or shortness of breath.
• Tell patient to stop taking drug and seek medical attention if evidence of hypersensitivity develops, such as rash, fever, nausea, vomiting, chills, rigors, and hypotension.
• Teach patient that drug doesn't cure HIV infection and that it must be taken with other antiretrovirals.
• Tell patient to inform prescriber of pregnancy or plans to become pregnant or to breastfeed while taking drug. Because HIV

Reactions in bold italics are *life-threatening*. Interactions may have a *rapid onset* or a **delayed onset**.

could be transmitted to the infant, patients infected with HIV shouldn't breastfeed.
- Tell patient that drug may affect the ability to drive or operate machinery.
- Tell patient that information on self-administration is available (1-877-4FUZEON [1-877-438-9366]).

SAFETY ALERT!

enoxaparin sodium
en-OCKS-a-par-in

Lovenox

Therapeutic class: Anticoagulants
Pharmacologic class: Low-molecular-weight heparins

AVAILABLE FORMS
Multidose vial: 300 mg/3 mL*
Syringes (graduated prefilled): 60 mg/0.6 mL, 80 mg/0.8 mL, 100 mg/mL, 120 mg/0.8 mL, 150 mg/mL
Syringes (prefilled): 30 mg/0.3 mL, 40 mg/0.4 mL

INDICATIONS & DOSAGES
➤ **To prevent PE and DVT after hip or knee replacement surgery**
Adults: 30 mg subcut every 12 hours for 7 to 10 days. Treatment for up to 14 days has been well tolerated. Give initial dose between 12 and 24 hours postoperatively, as long as hemostasis has been established. Continue treatment during postoperative period until risk of DVT has diminished. Before hip replacement surgery, patients may receive 40 mg subcut given 12 hours (range, 9 to 15 hours) preoperatively. After initial phase of therapy, patients should continue with 40 mg subcut daily for 3 weeks.
Adjust-a-dose: In patients with CrCl of less than 30 mL/minute, give 30 mg subcut once daily.
➤ **To prevent PE and DVT after abdominal surgery**
Adults: 40 mg subcut daily with initial dose 2 hours before surgery. Give subsequent dose, as long as hemostasis has been established, 24 hours after initial preoperative dose, and continue once daily for 7 to 10 days. Treatment for up to 12 days has been well tolerated. Continue treatment during postoperative period until risk of DVT has diminished.

Adjust-a-dose: In patients with CrCl of less than 30 mL/minute, give 30 mg subcut once daily.
➤ **To prevent PE and DVT in patients with acute illness who are at increased risk because of decreased mobility**
Adults: 40 mg subcut once daily for 6 to 11 days. Treatment for up to 14 days has been well tolerated.
Adjust-a-dose: In patients with CrCl of less than 30 mL/minute, give 30 mg subcut once daily.
➤ **To prevent ischemic complications of unstable angina and non–Q-wave MI with oral aspirin therapy**
Adults: 1 mg/kg subcut every 12 hours until clinical stabilization (minimum 2 days) with aspirin 100 to 325 mg PO once daily. Usual duration of treatment is 2 to 8 days.
Adjust-a-dose: In patients with CrCl of less than 30 mL/minute, give 1 mg/kg subcut once daily.
➤ **Acute ST-segment elevation MI**
Adults younger than age 75: 30 mg single IV bolus plus 1 mg/kg subcut followed by 1 mg/kg subcut every 12 hours (maximum of 100 mg for the first two doses only) with aspirin 75 to 325 mg PO once daily. When given with a thrombolytic, give enoxaparin from 15 minutes before to 30 minutes after the start of fibrinolytic therapy. For patients undergoing PCI, if the last subcut dose was given less than 8 hours before balloon inflation, no additional dose is needed. If the last dose was given more than 8 hours before balloon inflation, give 0.3 mg/kg IV bolus.
Adults age 75 and older: Don't use an initial IV bolus. Give 0.75 mg/kg subcut every 12 hours (maximum 75 mg for the first two doses only).
Adjust-a-dose: In adults younger than age 75 with severe renal impairment (CrCl less than 30 mL/minute), 30 mg single IV bolus plus 1 mg/kg subcut followed by 1 mg/kg subcut once daily. In adults age 75 and older with severe renal impairment, 1 mg/kg subcut once daily with no initial bolus. Give with aspirin.
➤ **Inpatient treatment of acute DVT with and without PE when given with warfarin sodium**
Adults: 1 mg/kg subcut every 12 hours. Or, 1.5 mg/kg subcut once daily (at same time daily) for 5 to 7 days until therapeutic oral anticoagulant effect (INR 2 to 3) is achieved.

E

Warfarin sodium therapy is usually started within 72 hours of enoxaparin injection.
Adjust-a-dose: In patients with CrCl of less than 30 mL/minute, give 1 mg/kg subcut once daily.

➤ **Outpatient treatment of acute DVT without PE when given with warfarin sodium**

Adults: 1 mg/kg subcut every 12 hours for 5 to 7 days until therapeutic oral anticoagulant effect (INR 2 to 3) is achieved. Warfarin sodium therapy usually is started within 72 hours of enoxaparin injection.
Adjust-a-dose: In patients with CrCl of less than 30 mL/minute, give 1 mg/kg subcut once daily.

ADMINISTRATION

• Solution appears clear and colorless to pale yellow; discard if discolored or if it contains particulate matter.

IV

▼ Use multidose vial for IV injections.

▼ Flush IV access with sufficient amount of saline or dextrose solution before and after IV bolus administration.

▼ **Incompatibilities:** Don't mix or administer with other IV drugs.

Subcutaneous

• With patient lying down, give by deep subcut injection, alternating doses between left and right anterolateral and posterolateral abdominal walls. Don't expel air bubble from prefilled syringe before injecting to prevent drug loss and an incorrect dose. Hold skinfold between thumb and forefinger and insert entire length of needle. Push plunger to bottom of syringe.

• Don't massage after subcut injection. Watch for signs of bleeding at site. Rotate sites and keep record.

ACTION

Accelerates formation of antithrombin III–thrombin complex and deactivates thrombin, preventing conversion of fibrinogen to fibrin. Drug has a higher antifactor-Xa-to-antifactor-IIa activity ratio than heparin.

Route	Onset	Peak	Duration
IV	Unknown	Unknown	Unknown
Subcut	Unknown	4 hr	Unknown

Half-life: 4.5 hours after a single dose; 7 hours after repeated dosing.

ADVERSE REACTIONS

CNS: confusion, fever, pain. **CV:** edema, peripheral edema. **GI:** nausea, diarrhea. **GU:** hematuria. **Hematologic:** *thrombocytopenia, hemorrhage,* ecchymoses, bleeding complications, anemia. **Hepatic:** increased transaminase levels. **Respiratory:** dyspnea. **Skin:** irritation, pain, hematoma, ecchymosis, and erythema at injection site.

INTERACTIONS

Drug-drug. *Anticoagulants, antiplatelet drugs, NSAIDs:* May increase risk of bleeding. Use together cautiously and monitor patient for bleeding.
SSRIs: May increase risk of severe bleeding. Monitor patient for bleeding. Adjust therapy as needed.
Drug-herb. *Alfalfa, anise, bilberry:* May increase risk of bleeding. Discourage use together.

EFFECTS ON LAB TEST RESULTS

• May increase potassium, ALT, and AST levels.
• May decrease Hb level and platelet count.

CONTRAINDICATIONS & CAUTIONS

• Contraindicated in patients hypersensitive to drug, heparin, pork products, or benzyl alcohol (multidose vial only); in those with active major bleeding; and in those with history of immune-mediated heparin-induced thrombocytopenia (HIT) within the past 100 days or in the presence of circulating antibodies.

• Use drug in patients with a history of HIT only if more than 100 days have elapsed since the prior HIT episode and no circulating antibodies are present. Because HIT may still occur in these circumstances, the decision to use enoxaparin in such a case must be made only after a careful benefit-risk assessment and after nonheparin alternative treatments have been considered.

• Use cautiously in patients with history of aneurysms, cerebrovascular hemorrhage, spinal or epidural punctures (as with anesthesia), uncontrolled HTN, or threatened abortion.

• Use cautiously in older adults and in patients with conditions that place them at increased risk for hemorrhage, such as bacterial endocarditis, congenital or acquired bleeding disorders, ulcer disease, angiodysplastic GI disease, hemorrhagic stroke, or recent spinal, eye, or brain surgery.

Reactions in bold italics are *life-threatening*. Interactions may have a *rapid onset* or a *delayed onset*.

Boxed Warning Consider risks and benefits before neuraxial intervention (neuraxial anesthesia or spinal puncture) in patients who are or will be anticoagulated for thrombus prevention. Monitor patient frequently for signs and symptoms of neurologic impairment; if present, treat urgently. ■

• Use cautiously in patients with prosthetic heart valves, with regional or lumbar block anesthesia, blood dyscrasias, recent childbirth, pericarditis or pericardial effusion, renal insufficiency, or severe CNS trauma.

Dialyzable drug: No.

⚠ *Overdose S&S:* Hemorrhagic complications.

PREGNANCY-LACTATION-REPRODUCTION

• There are no well-controlled studies in during pregnancy. Monitor patients who are pregnant closely for evidence of bleeding or excessive coagulation. Warn patients about risk of therapy during pregnancy.

• Consider using a shorter-acting anticoagulant as delivery approaches.

• It isn't known if drug appears in human milk. Consider the developmental and health benefits of breastfeeding, patient's need for the drug, and potential adverse effects on the infant from the drug or the patient's underlying condition.

NURSING CONSIDERATIONS

• It's important to achieve hemostasis at the puncture site after PCI. The vascular access sheath for instrumentation should remain in place for 6 hours after enoxaparin dose if manual compression method is used; give next dose no sooner than 6 to 8 hours after sheath removal. Monitor vital signs and site for hematoma and bleeding.

• Obtain baseline coagulation studies before therapy.

• Monitor anti-Xa levels if abnormal coagulation parameters or bleeding occurs. PT and PTT aren't adequate for monitoring drug's anticoagulant effects.

• Monitor anti-Xa levels during pregnancy in patients with mechanical heart valves and in patients with significant renal impairment.

Boxed Warning Patients who receive epidural or spinal anesthesia or spinal puncture during therapy are at increased risk for developing an epidural or spinal hematoma, which may result in long-term or permanent paralysis. Factors that can increase these risks

include use of indwelling epidural catheters, concurrent use of other drugs that affect hemostasis, history of traumatic or repeated epidural or spinal puncture, and history of spinal deformity or spinal surgery. Monitor these patients closely for neurologic impairment, as urgent treatment is necessary. ■

Boxed Warning Optimal timing between administration of enoxaparin and spinal procedures isn't known. ■

⊙ *Alert:* For spinal procedures, consider both dose and elimination half-life of drug. Delay placement or removal of a spinal catheter for at least 12 hours after prophylactic doses or for 24 hours for higher therapeutic doses of 1 mg/kg b.i.d. or 1.5 mg/kg daily. Give postprocedure doses no sooner than 4 hours after catheter removal.

• Never give drug IM.

• Avoid IM injections of other drugs to prevent or minimize hematoma.

• Monitor platelet counts regularly. Patients with normal coagulation won't need close monitoring of PT or PTT.

• Regularly inspect patient for bleeding gums, bruises on arms or legs, petechiae, nosebleeds, melena, hematuria, and hematemesis.

• To treat severe overdose, give protamine sulfate (a heparin antagonist) by slow IV injection. Refer to manufacturer's instructions for protamine use.

⊙ *Alert:* Drug isn't interchangeable with heparin or other low-molecular-weight heparins.

PATIENT TEACHING

• Instruct patient and family to watch for signs of bleeding or abnormal bruising and to notify prescriber immediately.

Boxed Warning Tell patient to immediately report signs and symptoms of spinal or epidural hematoma, such as numbness (especially of the lower limbs) and muscle weakness. ■

• Advise patient to consult prescriber before initiating herbal therapy; many herbs have anticoagulant, antiplatelet, or fibrinolytic properties.

• Show patient how to properly administer subcut injection and dispose of syringe.

• Inform patient that a longer-than-usual time may be needed to stop bleeding and that bruising or bleeding may occur more easily.

• Instruct patient to inform health care providers and dentists of all medications being taken, including OTC products.

- Tell patient to avoid OTC drugs containing aspirin or other salicylates unless ordered by prescriber.
- Tell patient to inform prescriber of pregnancy or plans to become pregnant or to breastfeed during therapy.

entecavir
en-TEK-ah-veer

Baraclude

Therapeutic class: Antivirals
Pharmacologic class: Nucleosides–nucleotides

AVAILABLE FORMS
Oral solution: 0.05 mg/mL
Tablets: 0.5 mg, 1 mg

INDICATIONS & DOSAGES
➤ **Chronic HBV infection in patients with active viral replication and either persistently increased aminotransferase levels or histologically active disease**
Adults and adolescents age 16 and older with no previous nucleoside treatment and with compensated liver disease: 0.5 mg PO once daily.
Adjust-a-dose: If CrCl is 30 to less than 50 mL/minute, give 0.25 mg PO once daily or 0.5 mg PO every 48 hours. If CrCl is 10 to less than 30 mL/minute, give 0.15 mg PO once daily or 0.5 mg PO every 72 hours. If CrCl is less than 10 mL/minute or patient is undergoing hemodialysis or continuous ambulatory peritoneal dialysis (CAPD), give 0.05 mg PO once daily or 0.5 mg PO every 7 days.
Children age 2 to younger than age 16 and weighing at least 10 kg who have had no previous nucleoside treatment: For children weighing more than 30 kg, 10 mL (0.5 mg) oral solution or one 0.5-mg tablet PO once daily. For children weighing more than 26 to 30 kg, 9 mL (0.45 mg) oral solution PO once daily. For children weighing more than 23 to 26 kg, 8 mL (0.4 mg) oral solution PO once daily. For children weighing more than 20 to 23 kg, 7 mL (0.35 mg) oral solution PO once daily. For children weighing more than 17 to 20 kg, 6 mL (0.3 mg) oral solution PO once daily. For children weighing more than 14 to 17 kg, 5 mL (0.25 mg) oral solution PO once daily. For children weighing more than 11 to 14 kg, 4 mL (0.2 mg) oral solution PO once daily. For children weighing more than 10 to 11 kg, 3 mL (0.15 mg) oral solution PO once daily.
Adjust-a-dose: Insufficient data are available for specific dosage adjustments in children with renal impairment. Consider reducing dosage or increasing dosing interval similar to adjustments for adults.
⚠ **Alert:** While an FDA-approved indication, treatment of lamivudine-refractory or -resistant HBV infection isn't recommended by The American Association for the Study of Liver Disease. If needed, refer to manufacturer's instructions for dosing.

ADMINISTRATION
PO
- Hazardous drug; use safe handling and disposal procedures.
- Give on an empty stomach at least 2 hours after a meal and 2 hours before next meal to increase absorption.
- Store tablets at room temperature in tightly closed container.
- Use oral solution for patients weighing up to 30 kg and for doses less than 0.5 mg.
- Only give oral solution with provided dosing spoon.
- Don't mix oral solution with other liquids.
- Protect oral solution from light by storing in the outer carton.
- After oral solution has been opened, it can be used up to expiration date on the bottle.
- Give missed dose as soon as possible unless it's almost time for the next dose.

ACTION
Reduces viral DNA levels by inhibiting HBV viral polymerase, which blocks reverse transcriptase activity.

Route	Onset	Peak	Duration
PO	Unknown	0.5–1.5 hr	Unknown

Half-life: About 5 to 6 days.

ADVERSE REACTIONS
CNS: dizziness, fatigue, headache, fever, hepatic encephalopathy. **CV:** edema. **GI:** abdominal pain, diarrhea, dyspepsia, nausea, vomiting. **GU:** glycosuria, hematuria, increased creatinine level. **Hepatic:** increased transaminase levels, hyperbilirubinemia, ascites, hepatomegaly. **Metabolic:** increased lipase level,

---

hyperglycemia, *lactic acidosis.* **Respiratory:** URI. **Skin:** rash.

INTERACTIONS

Drug-drug. *Drugs that reduce renal function or compete for active tubular secretion:* May increase level of either drug. Monitor renal function, and watch for adverse effects.
Orlistat: May increase entecavir serum concentration. Monitor therapy.

Drug-food. *All foods:* Delays absorption and decreases drug level. Give drug on an empty stomach.

EFFECTS ON LAB TEST RESULTS

• May increase ALT, amylase, AST, blood glucose, creatinine, lipase, and total bilirubin levels.
• May decrease platelet count.

CONTRAINDICATIONS & CAUTIONS

• Contraindicated in patients hypersensitive to drug or its components.
Boxed Warning Don't use in patients infected with both HIV and HBV who aren't also receiving highly active antiretroviral therapy (HAART) due to risk of resistance. ∎
• Use cautiously in patients with renal impairment and in patients who have had a liver transplant.
• Safety and effectiveness in children younger than age 2 haven't been established.
Dialyzable drug: 13% after 4-hour hemodialysis.

PREGNANCY-LACTATION-REPRODUCTION

• Use cautiously during pregnancy and only if benefit outweighs fetal risk.
• Register patients who are pregnant in the Antiretroviral Pregnancy Registry at 1-800-258-4263.
• It isn't known if drug appears in human milk. Use cautiously during breastfeeding.

NURSING CONSIDERATIONS

Boxed Warning Drug may cause life-threatening lactic acidosis and severe hepatomegaly with steatosis when used alone or in combination with antiretrovirals. ∎
Boxed Warning HBV infection may worsen severely after therapy stops. Monitor hepatic function for several months in patients who stop therapy. If appropriate, start therapy for HBV infection. ∎

• Closely monitor patients with renal impairment and patients who have had a liver transplant.
• In older adults, adjust dosage for age-related decrease in renal function.

PATIENT TEACHING

• Instruct patient in safe drug administration and handling.
• Tell patient to report all adverse effects of this drug and any new drugs being taken.
• Explain that drug doesn't reduce the risk of HBV transmission to others.
• Teach patient the signs and symptoms of lactic acidosis, such as muscle pain, weakness, dyspnea, GI distress, cold hands and feet, dizziness, or fast or irregular heartbeat.
• Teach patient the signs and symptoms of hepatotoxicity, such as jaundice, dark urine, light-colored stool, loss of appetite, nausea, and stomach pain.
• Warn patient that missed doses increase risk of resistance and to be sure to refill drug before it runs out.

SAFETY ALERT!

EPINEPHrine (adrenaline)
ep-i-NEF-rin

EPINEPHrine hydrochloride
Adrenaclick, Adrenalin, Auvi-Q, EpiPen, EpiPen Jr, Symjepi

Therapeutic class: Vasopressors
Pharmacologic class: Adrenergics

AVAILABLE FORMS

Injection: 0.1 mg/mL, 1 mg/mL
Injection device: 0.1 mg/0.1 mL, 0.15 mg/0.15 mL, 0.15 mg/0.3 mL, 0.3 mg/0.3 mL

INDICATIONS & DOSAGES
➤ **Anaphylaxis**

Adults and children weighing 30 kg or more: 0.3 to 0.5 mg IM or subcut, repeated every 5 to 10 minutes as needed. Maximum single dose is 0.5 mg. Or, 0.3 mg IM or subcut with autoinjector to maximum of 0.5 mg per injection; repeat every 5 to 10 minutes as needed.
Children weighing 15 to less than 30 kg: 0.01 to 0.15 mg/kg IM or subcut to maximum of 0.3 mg per injection; repeat every 5 to 10 minutes as needed.

Children weighing 7.5 to less than 15 kg: 0.01 mg/kg IM or subcut to maximum of 0.3 mg per injection; repeat every 5 to 10 minutes as needed.

➤ **Hypotension associated with septic shock**

Adults: 0.05 to 2 mcg/kg/minute IV infusion titrated to achieve desired mean arterial pressure. May adjust dosage every 10 to 15 minutes in increments of 0.05 to 0.2 mcg/kg/minute to achieve desired BP goal. Titrate to patient response. After hemodynamic stabilization, wean incrementally over time, such as by decreasing epinephrine dosages every 10 minutes, to determine patient tolerance.

➤ **Cardiac resuscitation**

Adults: 1 mg IV or intraosseously every 3 to 5 minutes until return of spontaneous circulation.

Children: 0.01 mg/kg IV or intraosseously, up to 1 mg, repeated every 3 to 5 minutes until return of spontaneous circulation.

➤ **Asthma ◆**

Adults and children older than age 12: 0.01 mg/kg divided into three doses of approximately 0.3 to 0.5 mg IM (preferred) or subcut every 20 minutes as needed. Start with small dose and increase if needed. Use product with 1 mg/mL concentration.

ADMINISTRATION

IV

▼ Keep solution in light-resistant container, and don't remove before use.

▼ For IV infusion, just before use, mix with D_5W, combinations of dextrose in saline solution, or NSS

▼ Monitor BP, HR, and ECG when therapy starts and frequently thereafter.

▼ Discard solution if it's discolored or contains precipitate or after 24 hours.

▼ When giving as a continuous infusion, use a central line with an infusion pump. Extravasation can cause tissue necrosis.

▼ Don't give autoinjectors IV.

▼ **Incompatibilities:** Don't mix with alkaline solutions (such as sodium bicarbonate). Consult a drug incompatibility reference for more information.

IM

• Give into the anterolateral aspect of the thigh through clothing if necessary. May repeat injection every 5 to 15 minutes if necessary.

• Massage site after IM injection to counteract vasoconstriction. Repeated local injection can cause necrosis at injection site.

• Don't give if solution is discolored or contains precipitate.

Subcutaneous

• Don't give if solution is discolored or contains precipitate.

• Protect from light and freezing; store between 68° and 77° F (20° and 25° C).

ACTION

Potentiates alpha and beta receptors. Relaxes bronchial smooth muscle by stimulating $beta_2$ receptors. Stimulates alpha and beta receptors in the sympathetic nervous system.

Route	Onset	Peak	Duration
IV	Immediate	5 min	Short
IM	Rapid	Unknown	1–4 hr
Subcut	5–15 min	30 min	1–4 hr

Half-life: IV injection, less than 5 minutes. IM and subcut, unknown.

ADVERSE REACTIONS

CNS: drowsiness, headache, nervousness, tremor, *cerebral hemorrhage, stroke,* vertigo, pain, disorientation, agitation, asthenia, tremor, anxiety, apprehensiveness, fear, restlessness, dizziness, weakness, paresthesia, *subarachnoid hemorrhage.* **CV:** palpitations, *ventricular fibrillation, shock,* widened pulse pressure, HTN, tachycardia, anginal pain, cardiac arrhythmias, altered ECG (including decreased T-wave amplitude). **GI:** nausea, vomiting. **GU:** renal insufficiency. **Metabolic:** hyperglycemia, *hypoglycemia, hypokalemia, lactic acidosis,* insulin resistance. **Respiratory:** dyspnea, pulmonary edema, respiratory difficulties. **Skin:** urticaria, hemorrhage at injection site, pallor, diaphoresis. **Other:** tissue necrosis at injection site.

INTERACTIONS

Drug-drug. *Alpha blockers (phentolamine):* May cause hypotension from unopposed beta-adrenergic effects. Avoid using together.

Antihistamines, thyroid hormones: When given with sympathomimetics, may cause severe adverse cardiac effects. Avoid using together.

Beta-adrenergic blockers (propranolol): May increase BP and decrease HR. Use together cautiously.

Reactions in bold italics are *life-threatening*. Interactions may have a *rapid onset* or a *delayed onset*.

Cardiac glycosides, diuretics, general anesthetics (halogenated hydrocarbons): May increase risk of ventricular arrhythmias. Monitor ECG closely.

Carteolol, nadolol, penbutolol, pindolol, propranolol, timolol: May cause HTN followed by bradycardia. Stop beta blocker 3 days before starting epinephrine.

Doxapram, methylphenidate: May enhance CNS stimulation or pressor effects. Monitor patient closely.

Ergot alkaloids: May decrease vasoconstrictor activity. Monitor patient closely.

Levodopa: May enhance risk of arrhythmias. Monitor ECG closely.

MAO inhibitors: May increase risk of hypertensive crisis. Monitor BP closely.

TCAs: May potentiate the pressor response and cause arrhythmias. Use together cautiously.

EFFECTS ON LAB TEST RESULTS

- May increase BUN, glucose, and lactic acid levels.
- Interferes with tests for urinary catecholamines.

CONTRAINDICATIONS & CAUTIONS

- Contraindicated in patients with angle-closure glaucoma, shock (other than anaphylactic shock), organic brain damage, HF, cardiac dilation, arrhythmias, coronary insufficiency, or cerebral arteriosclerosis.
- Contraindicated in patients receiving general anesthesia with halogenated hydrocarbons or cyclopropane and in patients in labor (may delay second stage).
- Commercial products containing sulfites (including epinephrine) are contraindicated in patients with sulfite allergies, except when epinephrine is used to treat serious allergic reactions or other emergency situations.
- Don't use epinephrine with local anesthetic in fingers, toes, ears, nose, or genitalia.
- Use cautiously in patients with longstanding bronchial asthma or emphysema who have developed degenerative heart disease.
- Use cautiously in older adults and in patients with hyperthyroidism, CV disease, HTN, psychoneurosis, and diabetes.

Dialyzable drug: Unknown.

⚠ *Overdose S&S:* Precordial distress, vomiting, headache, dyspnea, HTN, peripheral vascular constriction, pulmonary edema, cerebral hemorrhage, arrhythmias, extreme pallor and coldness of the skin, metabolic acidosis, kidney failure.

PREGNANCY-LACTATION-REPRODUCTION

- Use during pregnancy only if potential benefit justifies fetal risk.
- Parenteral administration of epinephrine, if used to support BP during low or other spinal anesthesia for delivery, can cause accelerated fetal HR and shouldn't be used in obstetrics when maternal BP exceeds 130/80 mm Hg.
- It isn't known if drug appears in human milk. Use cautiously during breastfeeding.

NURSING CONSIDERATIONS

- Use phentolamine to prevent tissue sloughing and necrosis if epinephrine extravasation occurs.
- In patients with Parkinson disease, drug increases rigidity and tremor.
- Epinephrine is drug of choice in emergency treatment of acute anaphylactic reactions.
- Observe patient closely for adverse reactions. Notify prescriber if adverse reactions develop; adjusting dosage or stopping drug may be necessary.
- If BP increases sharply, give rapid-acting vasodilators, such as nitrates and alpha blockers, to counteract the marked pressor effect of large doses.
- Oxidizing products, such as iodine, chromates, nitrites, oxygen, and salts of easily reducible metals (such as iron), rapidly destroy drug.
- When treating patient with reactions caused by other drugs given IM or subcut, inject this drug into the site where the other drug was given to minimize further absorption.
- *Look alike–sound alike:* Don't confuse epinephrine with ephedrine or norepinephrine.

PATIENT TEACHING

- If patient has acute hypersensitivity reactions (such as to bee stings), it may be necessary to teach patient how to self-inject.
- Instruct patient in autoinjector use and disposal. Tell patient to give autoinjector in outer thigh and not into buttock.
- Caution patient or caregiver to only give two sequential doses unless under direct medical supervision. Patient should seek immediate medical care for acute hypersensitivity reactions.

• Tell patient to promptly report all adverse reactions.

epiRUBicin hydrochloride
ep-i-ROO-bi-sin

Ellence

Therapeutic class: Antineoplastics
Pharmacologic class: Anthracycline glycoside antibiotics

AVAILABLE FORMS
Injection: 50 mg/25 mL, 200 mg/100 mL single-dose vials

INDICATIONS & DOSAGES
➤ **Adjuvant therapy in patients with evidence of axillary node tumor involvement after resection of primary breast cancer**
Adults: 100 to 120 mg/m^2 IV infusion on day 1 of each cycle, or divided equally in two doses on days 1 and 8 of each cycle; cycle repeated every 3 to 4 weeks for six cycles; used with regimens containing cyclophosphamide and 5-FU.

Dosage modification after first cycle is based on toxicity. For patients with platelet count nadir below 50,000/mm^3, ANC below 250/mm^3, neutropenic fever, or grade 3 or 4 nonhematologic toxicity, reduce day 1 dose in subsequent cycles to 75% of day 1 dose given in current cycle. Delay day 1 therapy in subsequent cycles until platelet count is at least 100,000/mm^3, ANC is at least 1,500/mm^3, and nonhematologic toxicities recover to grade 1 or less.

For patients receiving divided doses (days 1 and 8), day 8 dose should be 75% of day 1 dose if platelet count is 75,000 to 100,000/mm^3 and ANC is 1,000 to 1,499/mm^3. If day 8 platelet count is below 75,000/mm^3, ANC is below 1,000/mm^3, or grade 3 or 4 nonhematologic toxicity has occurred, omit day 8 dose.

Adjust-a-dose: For patients with bone marrow dysfunction (patients heavily pretreated, patients with bone marrow depression, or those with neoplastic bone marrow infiltration), start at lower doses of 75 to 90 mg/m^2.

For patients with hepatic dysfunction, if bilirubin is 1.2 to 3 mg/dL or AST is 2 to 4 × ULN, give half recommended starting dose.

If bilirubin level is above 3 mg/dL or AST is more than 4 × ULN, give one-quarter the recommended starting dose.

For patients with severe renal dysfunction (creatinine level over 5 mg/dL), consider lower doses.

➤ **Esophageal cancer; gastric cancer** ♦
Adults: 50 mg/m^2 IV on day 1 every 21 days for up to eight cycles, in combination with cisplatin, oxaliplatin, 5-FU, or capecitabine.

ADMINISTRATION
IV

▼ Wear protective clothing (goggles, gown, disposable gloves) when handling drug, which is a vesicant.

Boxed Warning Extravasation can result in severe local tissue injury and necrosis requiring wide excision and skin grafting. Immediately terminate drug and apply ice to affected area. ∎

Boxed Warning If burning or stinging occurs indicating perivenous infiltration, stop infusion immediately and restart in another vein. ∎

▼ Never give drug IM or subcut; severe tissue necrosis may result.

▼ Always give IV in free-flowing NSS or D$_5$W over 3 to 20 minutes depending on dosage and volume of infusion solution. Infuse doses of 100 to 120 mg/m^2 over 15 to 20 minutes.

▼ Avoid veins over joints or in limbs with compromised venous or lymphatic drainage.

▼ Avoid repeated injection into the same vein.

▼ Facial flushing and erythematous streaking along vein may indicate overly rapid delivery.

▼ After vial has been penetrated, discard unused solution after 24 hours.

▼ Store refrigerated solution between 36° and 46° F (2° and 8° C). Don't freeze. Protect from light.

▼ **Incompatibilities:** 5-FU, heparin, any alkaline pH solutions, other IV drugs.

ACTION
Known to form a complex with DNA by getting between nucleotide base pairs, inhibiting DNA, RNA, and protein synthesis; DNA cleavage occurs, resulting in cytocidal activity. Drug may also interfere with replication and transcription of DNA and may generate cytotoxic free radicals.

Route	Onset	Peak	Duration
IV	Unknown	Unknown	Unknown

Half-life: 33 hours.

ADVERSE REACTIONS

CNS: lethargy, fever. **CV:** *cardiomyopathy, HF.* **EENT:** conjunctivitis, keratitis. **GI:** nausea, vomiting, diarrhea, anorexia, mucositis. **GU:** amenorrhea, red urine. **Hematologic:** *leukopenia, neutropenia, febrile neutropenia, thrombocytopenia,* anemia. **Skin:** alopecia, rash, pruritus, skin changes, local toxicity. **Other:** hot flashes, infection.

INTERACTIONS

Drug-drug. *Calcium channel blockers, other cardioactive compounds:* May increase risk of HF. Monitor cardiac function closely.
Cimetidine: May significantly increase epirubicin level. Don't use together.
Cytotoxic drugs (anthracyclines, trastuzumab): May cause additive toxicities (especially hematologic and GI). Monitor patient closely.
Live-virus vaccines: May increase risk of vaccine-induced adverse reactions. Avoid concomitant use; don't give for at least 3 months after drug.
Pimecrolimus, tacrolimus (topical): May enhance adverse and toxic effects of epirubicin. Don't use together.
Taxanes (doxorubicin, paclitaxel): May increase level of epirubicin metabolites and risk of toxicity. Monitor patient closely for CV toxicity and separate administration times as much as possible.

EFFECTS ON LAB TEST RESULTS

• May decrease Hb level and neutrophil, platelet, and WBC counts.

CONTRAINDICATIONS & CAUTIONS

• Contraindicated in patients hypersensitive to drug, other anthracyclines, or anthracenediones and in those with persistent myelosuppression, severe myocardial insufficiency, recent MI, cardiomyopathy or HF, serious arrhythmias, previous treatment with anthracyclines up to the maximum cumulative dose, or severe hepatic dysfunction.
• Use cautiously in patients with active or dormant cardiac disease, previous or current radiotherapy to mediastinal and pericardial areas, or previous therapy with other anthracyclines or anthracenediones.
• Use cautiously in patients receiving other cardiotoxic drugs.
Boxed Warning Secondary acute myeloid leukemia and myelodysplastic syndromes have been reported in patients with breast cancer treated with anthracyclines, including epirubicin. ■
🕒 *Alert:* Drug may increase risk of thrombophlebitis and thromboembolic events, including fatal PE. Venous sclerosis may result from injection into a small vessel or repeated injections into the same vein.
• Safety and effectiveness in children haven't been established.
Dialyzable drug: Unknown.
⚠ *Overdose S&S:* Bone marrow aplasia, grade 4 mucositis, GI bleeding, hyperthermia, multiple organ failure, lactic acidosis, increased LDH level, anuria, death.

PREGNANCY-LACTATION-REPRODUCTION

• Drug can cause fetal harm. If drug is used during pregnancy, or if patient becomes pregnant during therapy, apprise patient of fetal risk.
• Patients of childbearing potential should use effective contraception during treatment and for 6 months after final dose.
• Men with partners of childbearing potential should use effective contraception during treatment and for 3 months after final dose. Men with partners who are pregnant should use condoms during treatment and for at least 7 days after final dose.
• It isn't known if drug appears in human milk. Patient shouldn't breastfeed during treatment and for at least 7 days after final dose.
• Drug may impair female fertility and induce premature menopause.

NURSING CONSIDERATIONS

• Verify pregnancy status before starting drug.
• Don't handle drug if you are pregnant.
• For patients taking 120 mg/m² regimen, give prophylactic antibiotic therapy.
• Drug is moderately to highly emetogenic; give antiemetic before drug to reduce nausea and vomiting.
Boxed Warning Myocardial damage, including acute left ventricular failure, can occur. Cardiomyopathy risk is proportional

to the cumulative exposure, with incidence rates from 0.9% at a cumulative dose of 550 mg/m^2, 1.6% at 700 mg/m^2, and 3.3% at 900 mg/m^2. Risk of cardiomyopathy increases with concomitant cardiotoxic therapy. Assess LVEF before and regularly during and after treatment. ∎

• Monitor LVEF regularly during therapy. Stop drug at first sign of impaired cardiac function. Early signs of cardiac toxicity include sinus tachycardia, ECG abnormalities, tachyarrhythmias, bradycardia, AV block, and bundle-branch block.

Boxed Warning Severe myelosuppression resulting in serious infection, septic shock, requirement for transfusions, hospitalization, and death may occur. ∎

• Obtain total and differential WBC, CBC, and platelet count, and LFTs before and during each cycle of therapy.

• WBC nadir is usually reached 10 to 14 days after drug administration, and WBC count returns to normal by day 21.

• Monitor uric acid, potassium, calcium, phosphate, and creatinine levels immediately after initial chemotherapy administration in patients susceptible to TLS. Hydration, urine alkalinization, and prophylaxis with allopurinol may prevent hyperuricemia and minimize potential complications of TLS.

• Drug may enhance the effects of radiation therapy or cause an inflammatory cell reaction at irradiation site. Monitor patient closely.

PATIENT TEACHING

• Advise patient to report any pain or burning at injection site during or after administration.

• Instruct patient to report nausea, vomiting, mouth inflammation, dehydration, fever, evidence of infection, or symptoms of HF (rapid heartbeat, labored breathing, swelling).

• Tell patient that urine will be reddish pink for 1 to 2 days after treatment.

• Inform patient of risk of heart damage and treatment-related leukemia with use of drug.

• Advise patient of fetal and fertility risk. Provide contraception and breastfeeding recommendations.

• Tell patient that hair usually regrows within 2 to 3 months after final dose.

eplerenone
ep-LER-eh-nown

Inspra

Therapeutic class: Antihypertensives
Pharmacologic class: Selective aldosterone receptor antagonists

AVAILABLE FORMS
Tablets: 25 mg, 50 mg

INDICATIONS & DOSAGES
➤ **HTN**
Adults: 50 mg PO once daily. If response is inadequate after 4 weeks, increase dosage to 50 mg PO b.i.d. Maximum daily dose, 100 mg/day.
Adjust-a-dose: In patients taking moderate CYP3A4 inhibitors, reduce eplerenone starting dose to 25 mg PO once daily. If BP response is inadequate, may increase dosage to a maximum of 25 mg b.i.d.
➤ **HF with reduced ejection fraction after an MI**
Adults: Initially, 25 mg PO once daily. Increase within 4 weeks, as tolerated and according to potassium level, to 50 mg PO once daily.
Adjust-a-dose: Once treatment begins, if potassium level is less than 5 mEq/L, increase dosage from 25 mg every other day to 25 mg daily; or increase dosage from 25 mg daily to 50 mg daily. If potassium level is 5 to 5.4 mEq/L, don't adjust dosage. If potassium level is 5.5 to 5.9 mEq/L, decrease dosage from 50 mg daily to 25 mg daily; or decrease dosage from 25 mg daily to 25 mg every other day; or if dosage was 25 mg every other day, withhold drug. If potassium level is 6 mEq/L or greater, withhold drug. May restart drug at 25 mg every other day when potassium level is less than 5.5 mEq/L. In patients receiving a moderate CYP3A inhibitor, don't exceed 25 mg once daily.
➤ **HF (NYHA Class II to IV) with reduced LVEF of 35% or less in patients already taking optimal doses of other HF medications** ◆
Adults: Initially, 25 mg once daily. May double the dose after 4 weeks, if serum potassium level remains less than 5 mEq/L and renal function is stable, to a maximum target dose of 50 mg once daily.

ADMINISTRATION
PO
- Give drug without regard for meals.

ACTION
Binds to mineralocorticoid receptors and blocks aldosterone, which increases BP through induction of sodium reabsorption and possibly other mechanisms.

Route	Onset	Peak	Duration
PO	Unknown	1.5–2 hr	Unknown

Half-life: 3 to 6 hours.

ADVERSE REACTIONS
CNS: headache, dizziness. **CV:** angina, *MI.* **GU:** increased creatinine level, abnormal vaginal bleeding. **Metabolic:** *hyperkalemia.* **Other:** gynecomastia.

INTERACTIONS
Drug-drug. *ACE inhibitors, ARBs:* May increase risk of hyperkalemia. Use together cautiously.
Canagliflozin: May increase risk of hyperkalemia. Monitor therapy.
Lithium: May increase risk of lithium toxicity. Monitor lithium level.
Moderate CYP3A4 inhibitors (erythromycin, fluconazole, saquinavir, verapamil): May increase eplerenone level. Reduce eplerenone starting dose to 25 mg PO once daily.
NSAIDs: May reduce the antihypertensive effect and cause severe hyperkalemia in patients with impaired renal function. Monitor BP and potassium level.
Potassium supplements, potassium-sparing diuretics (amiloride, spironolactone, triamterene): May increase risk of hyperkalemia and sometimes-fatal arrhythmias. Use together is contraindicated.
Strong CYP3A inhibitors (azole antifungals [fluconazole, itraconazole, ketoconazole], macrolides [clarithromycin], nefazodone, protease inhibitors [nelfinavir, ritonavir]): Inhibits CYP3A4 metabolism of eplerenone. Use together is contraindicated.
Drug-herb. *St. John's wort:* May decrease eplerenone level over time. Discourage use together.
Drug-food. *Grapefruit juice:* May increase eplerenone level. Discourage use together.

EFFECTS ON LAB TEST RESULTS
- May increase BUN, creatinine, GGT, and potassium levels.
- May decrease sodium level.

CONTRAINDICATIONS & CAUTIONS
- When used for HTN, contraindicated in patients with type 2 diabetes with microalbuminuria, creatinine level greater than 2 mg/dL in males or greater than 1.8 mg/dL in females, or CrCl of less than 50 mL/minute.
- Contraindicated in all patients with potassium level greater than 5.5 mEq/mL at initiation or CrCl of 30 mL/minute.
- Use cautiously in patients with mild to moderate hepatic impairment.
Dialyzable drug: No.
⚠ *Overdose S&S:* Hypotension, hyperkalemia.

PREGNANCY-LACTATION-REPRODUCTION
- Use during pregnancy only if potential benefits justify fetal risk.
- It isn't known if drug appears in human milk. Patient should discontinue breastfeeding or discontinue drug.
- Drug may impair male fertility.

NURSING CONSIDERATIONS
- Drug may be used alone or with other antihypertensives.
- Full therapeutic effect of the drug occurs in 4 weeks.
- Measure potassium level at baseline, within first week or after dosage adjustment, at 1 month after starting therapy, and periodically thereafter.
- Monitor patient for signs and symptoms of hyperkalemia.
- *Look alike–sound alike:* Don't confuse Inspra with Spiriva.

PATIENT TEACHING
- Instruct patient in safe drug administration.
- Advise patient to avoid potassium supplements and salt substitutes during treatment.
- Inform male patient that drug may compromise fertility.
- Tell patient to report adverse reactions.

🍁Canada   ◇OTC   ♦Off-label use   ✏Photoguide   ⊕Do not crush   *Liquid contains alcohol   ▨Genetic

epoetin alfa (erythropoietin)
i-POE-i-tin

Epogen, Eprex✦, Procrit

epoetin alfa-epbx
Retacrit

Therapeutic class: Colony-stimulating factors
Pharmacologic class: Recombinant human erythropoietins

AVAILABLE FORMS
Injection (single-use vial): 1,000 units/ 0.5 mL✦, 2,000 units/0.5 mL✦, 2,000 units/ mL, 3,000 units/0.3 mL, 3,000 units/mL, 4,000 units/ 0.4 mL✦, 4,000 units/mL, 5,000 units/0.5 mL✦, 6,000 units/0.5 mL✦, 8,000 units/0.8 mL✦, 10,000 units/mL, 20,000 units/0.5 mL✦, 20,000 units/mL, 30,000 units/0.75 mL✦, 40,000 units/mL
Injection (multidose vial)* (Epogen, Procrit): 20,000 units/mL, 20,000 units/2 mL

INDICATIONS & DOSAGES
➤ **Anemia caused by chronic renal disease**
Adults: Dosage is individualized. For patients on hemodialysis, start treatment only if Hb level is less than 10 g/dL. For patients not on hemodialysis, start treatment only if Hb level is less than 10 g/dL, the rate of decline of Hb level indicates that patient will require an RBC transfusion, and reducing the risk of alloimmunization and other RBC transfusion–related risks is a treatment goal. Starting dose is 50 to 100 units/kg subcut or IV three times weekly. IV route is preferred for patients receiving hemodialysis.

Maintenance dosage is highly individualized. Give the lowest effective dose to gradually increase Hb to a level at which blood transfusion isn't necessary.
Children age 1 month and older: Initially, 50 units/kg IV or subcut three times weekly. Start treatment only if Hb level is less than 10 g/dL. IV route is preferred for patients receiving hemodialysis.

Maintenance dosage is highly individualized to keep Hb level within target range. Give the lowest effective dose to gradually increase Hb to a level at which blood transfusion isn't necessary.

Adjust-a-dose: For all patients, don't increase dosage more frequently than every 4 weeks. Reduce dosage by 25% or more as needed to reduce rapid responses if Hb level rises more than 1 g/dL in any 2-week period. Increase dosage by 25% for Hb level less than 10 g/dL that hasn't increased by 1 g/dL after 4 weeks or falls below 10 g/dL. For adults on dialysis, if Hb level approaches or exceeds 11 g/dL, reduce dosage or interrupt therapy. For adults not on dialysis, if Hb level exceeds 10 g/dL, reduce dosage or interrupt therapy. For children, if Hb level approaches or exceeds 12 g/dL, reduce dosage or interrupt therapy.
➤ **Anemia from zidovudine therapy (4,200 mg/week or less) in patients infected with HIV**
Adults: Initially, 100 units/kg IV or subcut three times weekly for 8 weeks or until Hb level reaches target level. If response isn't satisfactory after 8 weeks, increase dosage by 50 to 100 units/kg IV or subcut three times weekly. Evaluate response every 4 to 8 weeks thereafter; further increase dosage in increments of 50 to 100 units/kg three times weekly, up to maximum of 300 units/kg IV or subcut. Give the lowest effective dose to gradually increase Hb to a level where blood transfusion isn't necessary.
Adjust-a-dose: Withhold drug if Hb level exceeds 12 g/dL. Restart drug at 25% below the previous dosage if Hb level declines to less than 11 g/dL. Discontinue if an increase in Hb isn't achieved at 300 units/kg for 8 weeks.
➤ **Anemia from chemotherapy**
Adults: Start therapy if Hb level is less than 10 g/dL and a minimum of 2 additional months of chemotherapy is planned. Initially, 150 units/kg subcut three times weekly or 40,000 units subcut weekly until completion of a chemotherapy course. If Hb level hasn't increased by at least 1 g/dL (in the absence of RBC transfusion) and remains below 10 g/dL after initial 4 weeks of therapy, increase dosage up to 300 units/kg subcut three times weekly or 60,000 units weekly. Give the lowest effective dose to gradually increase Hb to a level at which blood transfusion isn't necessary. Discontinue drug after 8 weeks if no response, as measured by Hb level or if transfusions are still required.
Children ages 5 to 18: 600 units/kg IV once weekly until completion of a chemotherapy course. If Hb level hasn't increased by at least 1 g/dL (in the absence of RBC

transfusion) and remains below 10 g/dL after initial 4 weeks of therapy, increase dosage to 900 units/kg IV (maximum, 60,000 units). Discontinue drug after 8 weeks if no response, as measured by Hb level or if transfusions are still required.

Adjust-a-dose: Withhold drug if Hb level exceeds level needed to avoid an RBC transfusion. Restart drug at dosage 25% below previous dosage when Hb level approaches a level at which an RBC transfusion may be required. Reduce dosage by 25% if Hb level increases more than 1 g/dL in a 2-week period or reaches a level needed to avoid an RBC transfusion.

➤ **To reduce need for allogenic blood transfusion in patients with anemia scheduled to have elective, noncardiac, nonvascular surgery**

Adults: 300 units/kg subcut daily for 10 days before surgery, on day of surgery, and for 4 days after surgery. Or, 600 units/kg subcut in once-weekly doses (21, 14, and 7 days before surgery), plus a fourth dose on day of surgery. DVT prophylaxis is recommended for patients undergoing surgery during epoetin therapy.

➤ **Symptomatic anemia in myelodysplastic syndromes ♦**

Adults: 150 to 300 units/kg subcut once daily or 450 to 1,000 units/kg/week in divided doses, three to seven times a week or 60,000 units once weekly.

ADMINISTRATION

IV

▼ Store solution in refrigerator; don't freeze.

▼ Protect from light. Don't shake.

▼ Give by direct injection without dilution.

▼ If patient is having dialysis, drug may be given into venous return line after dialysis session. To keep drug from adhering to tubing, inject drug with blood still in the line. Then flush with NSS.

▼ Single-dose vials contain no preservatives. Discard unused portion. Don't reenter preservative-free vials.

▼ Store unused portions of multidose vials at 36° to 46° F (2° to 8° C). Discard 21 days after initial entry.

🕒 *Alert:* Multidose vials contain benzyl alcohol, which has been associated with sometimes fatal neurologic and other complications in premature infants.

▼ **Incompatibilities:** Other IV drugs.

Subcutaneous

• Store solution in refrigerator; don't freeze.

• Protect from light. Don't shake.

• Don't use if solution is discolored or has particulate matter.

• Give in upper arm, abdomen, mid-thigh, or outer buttocks.

• Single-use vial without preservative may be admixed in a syringe with bacteriostatic NSS for injection with benzyl alcohol 0.9% (bacteriostatic saline) at a 1:1 ratio to provide local anesthetic.

• Rotate injection sites and document.

ACTION

Functions as a growth factor and as a differentiating factor, enhancing RBC production.

Route	Onset	Peak	Duration
IV	Immediate	Immediate	Unknown
Subcut	Unknown	5–24 hr	Unknown

Half-life: 4 to 13 hours.

ADVERSE REACTIONS

CNS: asthenia, dizziness, depression, fatigue, headache, insomnia, paresthesia, fever, chills, *seizures.* **CV:** edema, HTN, vascular occlusion by clot of arteriovenous graft, *DVT, thrombosis.* **EENT:** pharyngitis. **GI:** diarrhea, nausea, vomiting, stomatitis. **Hematologic:** *leukopenia.* **Metabolic:** hyperglycemia, *hypokalemia,* hyperuricemia, weight loss. **Musculoskeletal:** arthralgia, myalgia, bone pain, muscle spasm. **Respiratory:** cough, congestion, *PE,* shortness of breath, URI. **Skin:** injection-site reactions, rash, urticaria, pruritus. **Other:** medical device malfunction (clotting), chills.

INTERACTIONS

Drug-drug. *Lenalidomide, pomalidomide, thalidomide:* May enhance thrombogenic effects of these drugs. Monitor therapeutic response.

EFFECTS ON LAB TEST RESULTS

• May increase BUN, creatinine, potassium, Hb, and uric acid levels.

• May decrease leukocyte count.

CONTRAINDICATIONS & CAUTIONS

• Contraindicated in patients hypersensitive to products derived from mammal cells or albumin (human) and in those with uncontrolled HTN or pure RBC aplasia that begins after treatment with epoetin.

Boxed Warning In patients with NSCLC or breast, head and neck, lymphoid, or cervical cancers, there is a risk of tumor growth or recurrence and shortened survival. Use lowest dosage needed to avoid RBC transfusions. Use only for treatment of anemia due to concomitant myelosuppressive chemotherapy and discontinue drug after chemotherapy course. Erythropoiesis-stimulating agents aren't indicated for patients receiving myelosuppressive therapy when the anticipated outcome is cure. ■

Boxed Warning Patients with chronic renal disease have an increased risk of death, serious adverse CV events, and stroke when erythropoiesis-stimulating agents are used to increase Hb level to more than 11 g/dL. Individualize therapy and use lowest dosage needed to reduce the need for RBC transfusion. ■

• SCAR, including erythema multiforme, SJS, and TEN, may occur with use of erythropoiesis-stimulating agents; discontinue drug if SCAR is suspected.

Dialyzable drug: Unknown.

⚠ *Overdose S&S:* Severe HTN.

PREGNANCY-LACTATION-REPRODUCTION

• Use single-dose formulations during pregnancy only if potential benefit justifies fetal risk.

• Multidose vials contain benzyl alcohol and are contraindicated during pregnancy and breastfeeding, and in neonates and infants. Patients shouldn't breastfeed for at least 2 weeks after final dose.

• It isn't known if drug appears in human milk. Use single-dose vials cautiously during breastfeeding.

NURSING CONSIDERATIONS

• Before starting therapy, evaluate patient's iron status. Patient should receive adequate iron supplementation beginning no later than when epoetin alfa treatment starts and continuing throughout therapy. Patient also may need vitamin B_{12} and folic acid.

• Monitor BP before therapy. Most patients with chronic renal failure have HTN. BP may increase, especially when hematocrit increases in the early part of therapy.

• Institute diet restrictions or drug therapy to control BP.

• Monitor Hb level twice weekly until it stabilizes in the target range and maintenance dose is established, then continue to monitor at least monthly. Resume twice-weekly testing after any dosage adjustments.

• When used in HIV-infected adults, dosage recommendations are for those with endogenous erythropoietin levels of 500 milliunits/mL or less and cumulative zidovudine doses of 4.2 g/week or less.

• Monitor blood counts; elevated hematocrit may cause excessive clotting. For patients with chronic renal disease, monitor Hb level weekly until stable and then at least monthly.

• Monitor patient for hypersensitivity reactions and SCAR.

• For patients who don't respond adequately over a 12-week escalation period, increasing dosage further may increase risks and not improve response. Evaluate other causes of anemia and discontinue drug if responsiveness doesn't improve.

• Patient may need additional heparin to prevent clotting during dialysis treatments.

• Drug increases risk of seizures in patients with chronic kidney disease. Monitor patients closely for neurologic signs and symptoms.

Boxed Warning Due to increased risk of DVT, prophylaxis is recommended. ■

🔵 *Alert:* Evaluate patient who experiences a lack or loss of effect for pure red cell aplasia.

• *Look alike–sound alike:* Don't confuse Epogen with Neupogen.

PATIENT TEACHING

• Instruct patient or caregiver in safe drug administration, storage, and disposal, if appropriate,

• Inform patient that pain or discomfort in limbs (long bones) and pelvis, feelings of cold, and diaphoresis may occur after injection (usually within 2 hours). Symptoms may last for 12 hours and then disappear.

• Counsel patient on the increased risks of mortality, CV reactions, thromboembolic events, stroke, and tumor progression.

• Teach patient that routine blood tests will be needed to monitor drug effect.

• Advise patient to avoid driving or operating heavy machinery at start of therapy. There may be a relationship between too-rapid increase in hematocrit and seizures.

• Tell patient to monitor BP at home and to adhere to dietary restrictions.

Reactions in bold italics are *life-threatening*. Interactions may have a *rapid onset* or a *delayed onset*.

• Advise patient that menstruation may resume after therapy and to consider need for contraception.

SAFETY ALERT!

eptifibatide
ep-tiff-IB-ah-tide

Therapeutic class: Antiplatelet drugs
Pharmacologic class: Glycoprotein IIb/IIIa inhibitors

AVAILABLE FORMS
Injection (bolus): 20 mg/10 mL (2 mg/mL) vial
Injection (premixed for infusion): 75 mg/ 100 mL (0.75 mg/mL), 200 mg/100 mL (2 mg/mL)

INDICATIONS & DOSAGES
➤ **ACS (unstable angina or non–ST-segment elevation MI) in patients receiving drug therapy and in those undergoing PCI**
Adults: 180 mcg/kg IV bolus as soon as possible after diagnosis, followed by a continuous IV infusion at a rate of 2 mcg/kg/minute until hospital discharge or start of CABG surgery, for up to 72 hours. Give aspirin (160 to 325 mg) daily and heparin (target PTT, 50 to 70 sec) unless PCI is scheduled.
Adjust-a-dose: If CrCl is less than 50 mL/ minute, give 180 mcg/kg IV bolus as soon as possible after diagnosis, followed by a continuous IV infusion at 1 mcg/kg/minute.
➤ **PCI**
Adults: 180 mcg/kg IV bolus given just before the procedure, immediately followed by an infusion of 2 mcg/kg/minute and a second IV bolus of 180 mcg/kg given 10 minutes after the first bolus. Continue infusion until hospital discharge or for 18 to 24 hours, whichever comes first. Minimum duration of infusion is 12 hours; maximum duration is 96 hours. Give aspirin 160 to 325 mg PO 1 to 24 hours before PCI and daily thereafter; give heparin to maintain ACT target of 200 to 300 seconds before PCI (but not after).
Adjust-a-dose: If CrCl is less than 50 mL/minute, give 180 mcg/kg IV bolus just before the procedure, immediately followed by a continuous IV infusion at 1 mcg/kg/minute and a second bolus of 180 mcg/kg given 10 minutes after the first bolus.

ADMINISTRATION
IV
▼ Inspect solution for particles before use; if they appear, drug may not be sterile. Discard it.
▼ Protect drug from light before giving.
▼ May give drug in same line with NSS, D₅NSS, alteplase, atropine, dobutamine, heparin, lidocaine, meperidine, metoprolol, midazolam, morphine, nitroglycerin, or verapamil. Main infusion may also contain up to 60 mEq/L of potassium chloride.
▼ For IV push, withdraw bolus dose from 10-mL vial into a syringe and give over 1 or 2 minutes. Discard unused drug left in vial.
▼ For infusion, give undiluted drug directly from 100-mL vial or container using an infusion pump. Vials require a vented infusion set.
▼ Administer drug with heparin titrated to dosing parameters.
▼ If patient needs thrombolytics, stop infusion.
▼ Refrigerate vials at 36° to 46° F (2° to 8° C). Store vials at room temperature for no longer than 2 months; afterward, discard them.
▼ **Incompatibilities:** Furosemide.

ACTION
Reversibly binds to the glycoprotein IIb/IIIa (GPIIb/IIIa) receptor on human platelets and inhibits platelet aggregation.

Route	Onset	Peak	Duration
IV	Immediate	Immediate	4–8 hr

Half-life: 2.5 hours.

ADVERSE REACTIONS
CV: hypotension. **GU:** hematuria. **Hematologic:** *thrombocytopenia, major bleeding,* minor bleeding. **Other:** bleeding at femoral artery access site.

INTERACTIONS
Drug-drug. *Apixaban, clopidogrel, dabigatran, dipyridamole, edoxaban, NSAIDs, oral anticoagulants (warfarin), rivaroxaban, SSRIs, thrombolytics, ticlopidine:* May increase risk of bleeding. Monitor patient closely for signs of bleeding.
Other inhibitors of GPIIb/IIIa: May cause serious bleeding. Avoid using together.

EFFECTS ON LAB TEST RESULTS
• May decrease platelet count.

CONTRAINDICATIONS & CAUTIONS
• Contraindicated in patients hypersensitive to drug or its components and in those with history of bleeding diathesis or evidence of active abnormal bleeding within previous 30 days; severe HTN (systolic BP higher than 200 mm Hg or diastolic BP higher than 110 mm Hg) not adequately controlled with antihypertensives; major surgery within previous 6 weeks; history of stroke within 30 days or history of hemorrhagic stroke; current or planned use of another parenteral GPIIb/IIIa inhibitor; or dependency on dialysis.
• There is no clinical experience with drug use in patients with a baseline platelet count less than 100,000/mm^3.
• Safety and effectiveness in children haven't been established.
Dialyzable drug: Yes.

PREGNANCY-LACTATION-REPRODUCTION
• Use during pregnancy only if clearly needed.
• It isn't known if drug appears in human milk. Use cautiously during breastfeeding.

NURSING CONSIDERATIONS
• Drug is intended for use with heparin and aspirin.
• At least 4 hours before hospital discharge, stop this drug and heparin and achieve sheath hemostasis by standard compressive techniques.
• Remove sheath during infusion only after heparin has been stopped and its effects largely reversed.
• Stop infusion at least 2 to 4 hours before CABG surgery.
• Minimize use of arterial and venous punctures, IM injections, urinary catheters, and nasotracheal and NG tubes.
• When obtaining IV access, avoid use of noncompressible sites (such as subclavian or jugular veins).
• Monitor patient for bleeding.
• **Alert:** If platelet count falls below 100,000/mm^3, stop this drug and heparin. Monitor patient closely.
• Obtain baseline lab tests before start of drug therapy; also determine Hb level, hematocrit, PT, INR, PTT, platelet count, and creatinine level.
• Obtain platelet count 2 to 4 hours after initiation and at 24 hours or before discharge, whichever comes first.

PATIENT TEACHING
• Advise patient to inform health care provider of all drugs and supplements being taken.
• Counsel patient that benefits of drug outweigh risk of serious bleeding.
• Tell patient to report chest discomfort or other adverse effects to prescriber immediately.
• Instruct patient to report unusual bleeding, bruising, or blood in stools.

---

erenumab-aooe
e-REN-ue-mab

Aimovig

Therapeutic class: Antimigraine drugs
Pharmacologic class: Monoclonal antibodies

AVAILABLE FORMS
Injection: 70 mg/mL, 140 mg/mL prefilled autoinjectors or syringes

INDICATIONS & DOSAGES
➤ **Migraine prevention**
Adults: 70 mg subcut once monthly. If ineffective, 140 mg subcut monthly.

ADMINISTRATION
Subcutaneous
• **Alert:** The needle shield of the autoinjector and the needle cap of the syringe contain dry natural rubber (a derivative of latex) and may cause allergic reactions in patients sensitive to latex.
• Before administration, allow product to sit at room temperature for at least 30 minutes protected from direct sunlight. Don't warm by using a heat source, such as hot water or microwave.
• Don't shake product.
• Visually inspect solution for discoloration or particulate matter. Don't use if solution is cloudy, discolored, or contains flakes or particles.

• Products are for single use; give entire contents.

• Administer subcut in the abdomen, thigh, or upper arm. Don't inject into areas where skin is tender, bruised, red, or hard.

• Give missed dose as soon as possible; then schedule monthly from the date of the last dose.

• Store product refrigerated at 36° to 46° F (2° to 8° C) in original carton to protect from light until time of use. Don't freeze.

• If removed from the refrigerator, store at room temperature (up to 77° F [25° C]) in original carton and use within 7 days. Don't return product to the refrigerator after it has been warmed. Discard product if left at room temperature for more than 7 days.

ACTION

Human monoclonal antibody that binds to the calcitonin gene-related peptide (CGRP) receptor and antagonizes CGRP receptor function.

Route	Onset	Peak	Duration
Subcut	Unknown	6 days	Unknown

Half-life: 28 days.

ADVERSE REACTIONS

CV: HTN. **GI:** constipation. **Musculoskeletal:** muscle spasms, cramps. **Skin:** injection-site reaction (pain, erythema, pruritus). **Other:** antibody development.

EFFECTS ON LAB TEST RESULTS

None reported.

CONTRAINDICATIONS & CAUTIONS

• Hypersensitivity reactions (rash, angioedema, anaphylaxis) have been reported; discontinue use if serious reaction occurs.

• Safety and effectiveness in children haven't been established.

• Use cautiously in patients age 65 and older. Begin at lowest dosage and consider how hepatic, renal, and cardiac function; other disease states; or other drug therapy may affect drug effectiveness.

Dialyzable drug: Unknown.

PREGNANCY-LACTATION-REPRODUCTION

• There are no data regarding drug's use during pregnancy. Data suggest that patients with migraine may be at increased risk for preeclampsia during pregnancy.

• It isn't known if drug appears in human milk or how drug affects an infant who is breastfed. Before use in breastfeeding, consider patient's need for the drug and potential adverse effects on the infant.

NURSING CONSIDERATIONS

• Monitor patients for injection-site and other adverse reactions.

• Monitor BP.

PATIENT TEACHING

• Advise patient to read the Patient Information leaflet enclosed with drug.

⚠ *Alert:* Warn patient who is latex-sensitive about the risk of allergic reaction since the needle shield of the autoinjector and the needle cap of the syringe contain dry natural rubber.

• Teach patient how to properly administer and store drug according to manufacturer's instructions and to dispose of syringes safely.

• Advise patient to report injection-site reactions, allergic reactions, or other adverse effects.

• Advise patient that development of HTN and worsening of preexisting HTN can occur and to contact prescriber if experiencing elevated BP.

• Warn patient not to use an autoinjector or syringe that has been dropped on a hard surface as it may have broken, even if no visible damage is seen. Tell patient to use a new autoinjector or syringe and to call 1-800-77-AMGEN (1-800-772-6436).

SAFETY ALERT!

eriBULin mesylate
er-ih-BYOO-lin

Halaven

Therapeutic class: Antineoplastics
Pharmacologic class: Microtubule inhibitors

AVAILABLE FORMS

Injection: 1 mg/2 mL vial

INDICATIONS & DOSAGES

➤ **Metastatic breast cancer in patients who have received at least two chemotherapeutic regimens for the treatment of metastatic disease, and whose treatments have included an anthracycline and a taxane**

---

in either the adjuvant or metastatic setting; unresectable or metastatic liposarcoma in patients who have received a prior anthracycline-containing regimen

Adults: 1.4 mg/m^2 IV on days 1 and 8 of a 21-day cycle. Assess for peripheral neuropathy and obtain CBC before each dose. Don't administer drug on day 1 or 8 if ANC falls below 1,000/mm^3, platelet count falls below 75,000/mm^3, or grade 3 or 4 nonhematologic toxicities exist. May delay day-8 dose for a maximum of 1 week.

If toxicities don't resolve or improve to grade 2 or less by day 15, omit dose. If toxicities resolve or improve to grade 2 or less by day 15, give eribulin at a reduced dose and initiate next cycle no sooner than 2 weeks later. Don't reescalate eribulin dose after it has been reduced.

Adjust-a-dose: In mild hepatic impairment (Child-Pugh class A) and in patients with moderate or severe renal impairment (CrCl of 15 to 49 mL/minute), give 1.1 mg/m^2 IV on days 1 and 8 of a 21-day cycle. In moderate hepatic impairment (Child-Pugh class B), give 0.7 mg/m^2 IV on days 1 and 8 of a 21-day cycle. If toxicities occur, refer to manufacturer's instructions for dosage adjustments. Don't reescalate dosage after it has been reduced. Discontinue drug for any event requiring permanent dosage reduction while patient receives 0.7 mg/m^2.

ADMINISTRATION

IV

▼ Hazardous drug; use safe handling and disposal precautions.

▼ Draw up required amount from vial and administer undiluted, or dilute in 100 mL NSS. Don't use dextrose.

▼ Administer IV over 2 to 5 minutes.

▼ May store undiluted drug in a syringe or diluted solutions for 4 hours at room temperature or 24 hours if refrigerated.

▼ Discard unused portion of vial.

▼ **Incompatibilities:** Dextrose, other IV drugs.

ACTION

Inhibits growth phase of cells by blocking mitotic spindles and stopping the cell cycle.

Route	Onset	Peak	Duration
IV	Unknown	Unknown	Unknown

Half-life: About 40 hours.

ADVERSE REACTIONS

CNS: dizziness, depression, peripheral neuropathy, headache, insomnia, asthenia, fatigue, dysgeusia, fever. **CV:** *QT-interval prolongation,* peripheral edema, hypotension. **EENT:** increased lacrimation, oropharyngeal pain. **GI:** anorexia, dyspepsia, abdominal pain, stomatitis, dry mouth, constipation, diarrhea, nausea, vomiting. **GU:** UTI. **Hematologic:** *neutropenia,* anemia, *thrombocytopenia.* **Metabolic:** weight loss, *hypokalemia, hypocalcemia,* hypophosphatemia, hyperglycemia. **Musculoskeletal:** muscle spasms, muscle weakness, arthralgia, myalgia, back pain, bone pain, pain in extremity. **Respiratory:** URI, cough, dyspnea. **Skin:** rash, alopecia. **Other:** mucosal inflammation.

INTERACTIONS

Drug-drug. *Class IA and III antiarrhythmics, other drugs known to prolong QT interval:* May further prolong QT interval. Use together cautiously and monitor patient carefully.

EFFECTS ON LAB TEST RESULTS

• May increase ALT, AST and bilirubin levels.

• May decrease potassium, calcium, magnesium, and phosphorus levels.

• May decrease Hb level and neutrophil and platelet counts.

CONTRAINDICATIONS & CAUTIONS

• Contraindicated in patients hypersensitive to drug or its components.

• Avoid use in patients with existing congenital long QT syndrome.

• Use cautiously in patients with liver or renal insufficiency and in those at risk for neutropenia or peripheral motor or sensory neuropathy.

• Use cautiously in patients with HF, bradyarrhythmias, or electrolyte imbalance and in those taking drugs known to prolong QT interval or with a history of prolonged QT interval.

• Safety and effectiveness in children haven't been established.

Dializable drug: Unknown.

⚠ *Overdose S&S:* Neutropenia, hypersensitivity reaction.

Reactions in bold italics are *life-threatening*. Interactions may have a *rapid onset* or a *delayed onset*.

PREGNANCY-LACTATION-REPRODUCTION
• There are no well-controlled studies during pregnancy, but drug is expected to cause fetal harm. Patients should use effective contraception during treatment and for at least 2 weeks after final dose.
• Males with partners of childbearing potential should use effective contraception during treatment and for 3½ months after final dose.
• It isn't known if drug appears in human milk. Patient shouldn't breastfeed during treatment and for 2 weeks after final dose.
• Animal data show drug may damage male reproductive tissues, leading to impaired fertility of unknown duration.

NURSING CONSIDERATIONS
• Assess patient for peripheral neuropathy before each dose.
• Monitor patient for hypokalemia, hypomagnesemia, hypocalcemia, and hypophosphatemia before and periodically during therapy. Correct potassium or magnesium level before treatment.
• Monitor ECG for changes, especially QT-interval prolongation.
• Monitor patient for signs and symptoms of infection.
• Monitor blood counts and obtain CBC before each dose.
• Monitor LFTs and renal function tests during therapy.
• Consider prophylactic antiemetics for nausea and vomiting.

PATIENT TEACHING
• Tell patient to report a temperature of 100.4° F (38° C) or greater and other signs or symptoms of infection, such as chills, cough, or burning or pain on urination.
• Advise patient that drug may cause nerve damage and to contact prescriber if burning, tingling, or radiating pain occurs in any extremity.
• Caution patient to immediately report irregular heartbeat.
• Warn patient to avoid pregnancy and to use effective contraception during treatment and for 2 weeks after final dose.
• Advise male patient with partners of childbearing potential to use effective contraception during treatment and for 3½ months after final dose.
• Tell patient not to breastfeed during treatment and for 2 weeks after final dose.

• Advise male patient that drug may damage reproductive tissues, leading to impaired fertility of unknown duration.

SAFETY ALERT!

erlotinib ⌷
er-LOE-tye-nib

Tarceva

Therapeutic class: Antineoplastics
Pharmacologic class: Epidermal growth factor receptor inhibitors

AVAILABLE FORMS
Tablets ⓪: 25 mg, 100 mg, 150 mg

INDICATIONS & DOSAGES
Adjust-a-dose (for all indications): Refer to manufacturer's instructions for toxicity-related dosage adjustments.
➤ **With gemcitabine, first-line treatment of locally advanced, unresectable, or metastatic pancreatic cancer**
Adults: 100 mg PO once daily taken at least 1 hour before or 2 hours after meals. Continue until disease progresses or intolerable toxicity occurs.
➤ **Metastatic NSCLC in patients with tumors with epidermal growth factor receptor (*EGFR*) exon 19 deletions or exon 21 (L858R) substitution mutations as detected by an FDA-approved test receiving first-line, maintenance, or second or greater line treatment after progression following at least one prior chemotherapy regimen ⌷**
Adults: 150 mg PO once daily at least 1 hour before or 2 hours after a meal. Continue until disease progresses or intolerable toxicity occurs.

ADMINISTRATION
PO
• Hazardous drug; use appropriate precautions for handling and disposal.
• Give drug on an empty stomach 1 hour before or 2 hours after a meal.
• For patients unable to swallow tablets whole, tablets may be dissolved in 100 mL water and given orally or via feeding tube (silicone-based). To ensure patient receives full dose, rinse container with 40 mL water, administer residue, and repeat rinse.

ACTION

Inhibits tyrosine kinase activity in EGFRs, which are expressed on the surface of normal and cancer cells.

Route	Onset	Peak	Duration
PO	Unknown	4 hr	Unknown

Half-life: 36.2 hours.

ADVERSE REACTIONS

CNS: fatigue, syncope, *stroke,* anxiety, depression, dizziness, headache, insomnia, neuropathies, fever, voice disorder, taste disorder. **CV:** chest pain, arrhythmias, edema, *MI, DVT.* **EENT:** conjunctivitis, keratoconjunctivitis sicca, decreased tear production, abnormal eyelash growth, tinnitus, dry mouth. **GI:** abdominal pain, anorexia, diarrhea, decreased appetite, nausea, stomatitis, vomiting, constipation, dyspepsia, flatulence, *pancreatitis.* **GU:** UTI, renal insufficiency. **Hematologic:** anemia, *thrombocytopenia, leukopenia, lymphocytopenia.* **Hepatic:** increased ALT level, hyperbilirubinemia, increased GGT level, *hepatic failure.* **Metabolic:** weight loss. **Musculoskeletal:** pain, weakness, back pain, arthralgia, myalgia. **Respiratory:** cough, dyspnea. **Skin:** acne, dry skin, pruritus, rash, alopecia, paronychia. **Other:** infection, mucosal inflammation.

INTERACTIONS

Drug-drug. *Antacids:* May reduce bioavailability of drug. Separate doses by several hours if an antacid is necessary.
Anticoagulants, such as warfarin: May increase risk of bleeding. Monitor PT and INR.
Ciprofloxacin: May increase erlotinib plasma concentration. Consider reducing erlotinib dosage if severe adverse reactions occur; avoid use together if possible.
CYP3A4 inducers (carbamazepine, phenobarbital, phenytoin, rifabutin, rifampin): May increase erlotinib metabolism. Avoid use if possible or increase erlotinib dosage by 50-mg increments at 2-week intervals to a maximum of 450 mg as tolerated.
H₂-receptor antagonists (cimetidine, famotidine): May reduce bioavailability of drug. Give erlotinib 10 hours after and at least 2 hours before H₂-antagonist dosing.
PPIs (esomeprazole, omeprazole): May reduce bioavailability of drug. Dose separation may not eliminate interaction; avoid use together if possible.

Strong CYP3A4 inhibitors (atazanavir, clarithromycin, itraconazole, ketoconazole, nefazodone, nelfinavir, ritonavir, saquinavir, voriconazole): May decrease erlotinib metabolism. Avoid use together if possible or reduce erlotinib dosage by 50-mg decrements.
Drug-herb. *St. John's wort:* May increase drug metabolism. Drug dosage may need to be increased. Discourage use together.
Drug-food. *Any food:* May increase bioavailability of drug. Give drug 1 hour before or 2 hours after meals.
Grapefruit or grapefruit juice: May increase drug level. Avoid use together.
Drug-lifestyle. *Cigarette smoking:* May decrease drug level. Increase drug dosage by 50-mg increments at 2-week intervals to a maximum of 300 mg. Immediately reduce dosage to recommended dose (100 or 150 mg daily) upon smoking cessation.
Sun exposure: May cause photosensitivity reactions. Patient should use alcohol-free emollient cream and sunscreen and avoid sun exposure.

EFFECTS ON LAB TEST RESULTS

- May increase ALT, AST, GGT, bilirubin, BUN, and creatinine levels.
- May decrease Hb level and platelet and WBC counts.
- May increase INR and prolong PT.

CONTRAINDICATIONS & CAUTIONS

- Use cautiously in patients with pulmonary disease or liver impairment. Also use cautiously in patients who have received or are receiving chemotherapy because it may worsen adverse pulmonary effects.
- Withhold drug for acute onset of new or progressive unexplained pulmonary signs and symptoms, such as dyspnea, cough, and fever (pending diagnostic evaluation), and for grade 3 or 4 keratitis lasting more than 2 weeks. Withhold drug for acute or worsening ocular disorders such as eye pain, and consider discontinuation.
- Use cautiously in patients receiving other antiangiogenic agents, corticosteroids, NSAIDs, or taxane-based chemotherapy, and in those with a history of peptic ulcer disease because of increased risk of GI perforation.
- Interrupt therapy or discontinue drug in patients with hepatic impairment or dehydration, which increases risk of renal failure.

Reactions in bold italics are *life-threatening*. Interactions may have a *rapid onset* or a ***delayed onset***.

- SCAR, including SJS, TEN, and exfoliative dermatitis, can occur.
- Safety and effectiveness in children haven't been established.

Dialyzable drug: Unknown.

⚠ *Overdose S&S:* Severe adverse reactions (diarrhea, ALT or AST elevation, rash).

PREGNANCY-LACTATION-REPRODUCTION

- Drug may cause fetal harm. If used during pregnancy, or if patient becomes pregnant during therapy, apprise patient of fetal risk.
- Patients of childbearing potential should use effective contraception during therapy and for 1 month after final dose.
- It isn't known if drug appears in human milk. Patients shouldn't breastfeed during treatment and for 2 weeks after final dose.

NURSING CONSIDERATIONS

- Monitor renal function tests and LFTs periodically during therapy.
- ☙ *Alert:* GI perforation with fatalities has been reported. Permanently discontinue drug if GI perforation occurs.
- ☙ *Alert:* Rarely, serious ILD may occur. If patient develops dyspnea, cough, and fever, notify prescriber. Therapy may need to be interrupted or stopped.
- Monitor patient for severe diarrhea, and give loperamide if needed.
- Monitor patient for eye ulcers, bullous blistering, and exfoliative skin conditions.

PATIENT TEACHING

- ☙ *Alert:* Tell patient to immediately report new or worsened cough, shortness of breath, eye irritation or pain, or severe or persistent diarrhea, nausea, anorexia, or vomiting.
- Instruct patient in safe drug administration.
- Explain the likelihood of serious interactions with other drugs and herbal supplements and the need to tell prescriber about any change in drugs and supplements taken.
- Counsel patient about smoking cessation, as smoking may decrease drug level and effectiveness.

ertapenem sodium
er-tah-PEN-em

INVanz

Therapeutic class: Antibiotics
Pharmacologic class: Carbapenems

AVAILABLE FORMS
Injection: 1 g

INDICATIONS & DOSAGES

Adjust-a-dose (for all indications): In adults with CrCl of 30 mL/minute/1.73 m² or less, give 500 mg/day. In patients on hemodialysis receiving daily 500-mg dose less than 6 hours before hemodialysis, give supplementary 150-mg dose afterward. In patients on hemodialysis receiving dose 6 hours or more before hemodialysis, no supplementary dose is needed.

➤ **Complicated intra-abdominal infection caused by** *Escherichia coli, Clostridium clostridioforme, Eubacterium lentum, Peptostreptococcus* **species,** *Bacteroides fragilis, Bacteroides distasonis, Bacteroides ovatus, Bacteroides thetaiotaomicron,* **or** *Bacteroides uniformis*
Adults and children age 13 and older: 1 g IV or IM once daily for 5 to 14 days.
Infants and children ages 3 months to 12 years: 15 mg/kg IV or IM every 12 hours for 5 to 14 days. Don't exceed 1 g daily.

➤ **Complicated skin or skin-structure infection, including diabetic foot infections without osteomyelitis, caused by** *Staphylococcus aureus* **(methicillin-susceptible strains),** *Streptococcus agalactiae, Streptococcus pyogenes, E. coli, Klebsiella pneumoniae, Proteus mirabilis, B. fragilis, Peptostreptococcus* **species,** *Porphyromonas asaccharolytica,* **or** *Prevotella bivia*
Adults and children age 13 and older: 1 g IV or IM once daily for 7 to 14 days. Diabetic foot infections may need up to 28 days of treatment.
Infants and children ages 3 months to 12 years: 15 mg/kg IV or IM every 12 hours for 7 to 14 days. Don't exceed 1 g daily.

➤ **Community-acquired pneumonia from** *S. pneumoniae* **(penicillin-susceptible strains),** *Haemophilus influenzae* **(beta-lactamase–negative strains), or** *Moraxella catarrhalis;* **complicated UTI, including**

pyelonephritis caused by *E. coli* or *K. pneumoniae*

Adults and children age 13 and older: 1 g IV or IM once daily for 10 to 14 days. If patient improves after at least 3 days of treatment, use appropriate oral therapy to complete the full course of therapy.

Infants and children ages 3 months to 12 years: 15 mg/kg IV or IM every 12 hours for 10 to 14 days. Don't exceed 1 g daily. If patient improves after at least 3 days of treatment, use appropriate oral therapy to complete the full course of therapy.

➤ **Acute pelvic infection, including post-partum endomyometritis, septic abortion, and postsurgical gynecologic infection caused by *S. agalactiae*, *E. coli*, *B. fragilis*, *P. asaccharolytica*, *Peptostreptococcus* species, or *P. bivia***

Adults and children age 13 and older: 1 g IV or IM once daily for 3 to 10 days.

Infants and children ages 3 months to 12 years: 15 mg/kg IV or IM every 12 hours for 3 to 10 days. Don't exceed 1 g daily.

➤ **Prevention of surgical site infection after elective colorectal surgery**

Adults: 1 g IV 1 hour before surgical incision.

➤ **Complicated urinary tract infections, including pyelonephritis**

Adults and children age 13 and older: 1 g IV or IM once daily for 10 to 14 days.

Infants and children ages 3 months to 12 years: 15 mg/kg IV or IM every 12 hours for 10 to 14 days. Don't exceed 1 g daily.

ADMINISTRATION

IV

▼ Obtain specimens for culture and sensitivity testing before giving. Begin therapy while awaiting results.

▼ Before giving first dose, check for previous hypersensitivity to penicillin, cephalosporin, beta-lactam, or local amide-type anesthetics.

▼ May give IV infusions for up to 14 days.

▼ Reconstitute 1-g vial with 10 mL of sterile water for injection, NSS for injection, or bacteriostatic water for injection.

▼ Shake well to dissolve, and then immediately transfer contents to 50 mL of NSS.

▼ For children ages 3 months to 12 years, immediately withdraw a volume equal to 15 mg/kg (not to exceed 1 g/day); dilute in NSS to a final concentration of 20 mg/mL or less.

▼ Infuse over 30 minutes.

▼ Complete the infusion within 6 hours of reconstitution or refrigerate for up to 24 hours. Infuse within 4 hours once removed from refrigeration. Don't freeze.

▼ **Incompatibilities:** Diluents containing dextrose, other IV drugs.

IM

● Obtain specimens for culture and sensitivity testing before giving. Begin therapy while awaiting results.

● Before giving first dose, check for previous hypersensitivity to penicillin, cephalosporin, beta-lactam, or local amide-type anesthetics.

● May give IM injections for up to 7 days.

● Reconstitute 1-g vial with 3.2 mL of 1% lidocaine hydrochloride injection (without epinephrine). Shake vial thoroughly to form solution. Immediately withdraw volume equal to 15 mg/kg of body weight (not to exceed 1 g/day) and give by deep IM injection into a large muscle, such as the gluteal muscles or lateral part of the thigh. Use the reconstituted IM solution within 1 hour after preparation. Don't give reconstituted solution IV.

ACTION

Inhibits cell-wall synthesis through binding to penicillin-binding proteins.

Route	Onset	Peak	Duration
IV	Immediate	30 min	24 hr
IM	Unknown	2.3 hr	24 hr

Half-life: 4 hours.

ADVERSE REACTIONS

CNS: altered mental status, anxiety, asthenia, dizziness, fatigue, fever, headache, insomnia. **CV:** chest pain, edema, HTN, hypotension, phlebitis, swelling, tachycardia, thrombophlebitis. **EENT:** pharyngitis, oral candidiasis. **GI:** diarrhea, abdominal pain, acid regurgitation, constipation, dyspepsia, nausea, vomiting. **GU:** renal dysfunction, vaginitis. **Hematologic:** *leukopenia, neutropenia, thrombocytopenia,* anemia, coagulation abnormalities, eosinophilia, *thrombocytosis.* **Hepatic:** jaundice, increased transaminase levels, increased ALP level. **Metabolic:** *hyperkalemia, hypokalemia,* hyperglycemia. **Musculoskeletal:** leg pain. **Respiratory:** cough, dyspnea, URI, crackles, *respiratory distress,* rhonchi. **Skin:** erythema, extravasation, infusion-site pain and redness, pruritus, rash, diaper dermatitis.

Reactions in **bold italics** are *life-threatening*. Interactions may have a *rapid onset* or a *delayed onset*.

Other: hypersensitivity reactions, infused vein complications, **death.**

INTERACTIONS

Drug-drug. *Probenecid:* May reduce renal clearance; may increase half-life. Use together isn't recommended to extend half-life.
Valproic acid: May decrease valproic acid level, leading to loss of seizure control. Monitor valproic acid level, and observe patient for signs of seizure activity. Use of carbapenems with valproic acid or divalproex sodium isn't recommended.

EFFECTS ON LAB TEST RESULTS
- May increase albumin, ALT, ALP, AST, bilirubin, creatinine, glucose, and potassium levels.
- May increase eosinophil count, urine RBC count, or urine WBC count.
- May decrease Hb level, hematocrit, and segmented neutrophil and serum WBC counts.
- May increase or decrease platelet count.
- May prolong PT.

CONTRAINDICATIONS & CAUTIONS
- Contraindicated in patients hypersensitive to components of the drug or to other drugs in the same class and in patients who have had anaphylactic reactions to beta-lactams.
- IM use is contraindicated in patients hypersensitive to local anesthetics of the amide type because of the use of lidocaine as the diluent.
- Drug may cause CDAD, ranging in severity from mild to fatal colitis, which may occur during treatment or more than 2 months after treatment. Drug may need to be discontinued for suspected CDAD.
- Use cautiously in patients with CNS disorders and compromised renal function, as CNS reactions, including seizures, may occur in these patients.
- Use cautiously in older adults.
Dialyzable drug: Yes.
⚠ *Overdose S&S:* Nausea, diarrhea, dizziness.

PREGNANCY-LACTATION-REPRODUCTION
- There are no well-controlled studies during pregnancy. Use during pregnancy only if clearly needed.
- Drug appears in human milk. Use cautiously and only when expected benefit outweighs risk.

NURSING CONSIDERATIONS
- If patient has diarrhea during therapy, notify prescriber and collect stool specimen for culture to rule out CDAD.
- Vomiting occurs more frequently in children than adults. Monitor children closely for signs and symptoms of dehydration and electrolyte imbalance.
- If allergic reaction occurs, stop drug immediately.
- Anaphylactic reactions require immediate emergency treatment with epinephrine, oxygen, IV steroids, and airway management.
- Anticonvulsants may continue in patients with seizure disorders. If focal tremors, myoclonus, or seizures occur, notify prescriber. Dosage may need to be decreased or drug stopped.
- Monitor renal, hepatic, and hematopoietic function during prolonged therapy.
- MRSA and *Enterococcus* species are resistant to drug.
- *Look alike–sound alike:* Don't confuse IN-Vanz with AVINza.

PATIENT TEACHING
- Tell patient to report all adverse reactions.
- Instruct patient to report discomfort at injection site.
- Advise patient to report diarrhea as soon as possible.

SAFETY ALERT!

ertugliflozin
er-too-gli-FLOE-zin

Steglatro

Therapeutic class: Antidiabetics
Pharmacologic class: Sodium-glucose cotransporter 2 inhibitors

AVAILABLE FORMS
Tablets: 5 mg, 15 mg

INDICATIONS & DOSAGES
➤ **Adjunct to diet and exercise to improve glycemic control in patients with type 2 diabetes**
Adults: 5 mg PO once daily in the morning. May increase to 15 mg once daily.

ADMINISTRATION
PO
- May give with or without food.
- Give a missed dose as soon as possible. If it's almost time for the next dose, skip the missed dose and give at the next regularly scheduled time. Don't give two doses at the same time.
- Store in a dry place at controlled room temperature (68° to 77° F [20° to 25° C]).

ACTION
Increases the amount of urinary glucose excreted by inhibiting sodium-glucose cotransporter 2 (SGLT2), which reabsorbs glucose through the kidneys.

Route	Onset	Peak	Duration
PO	Unknown	1–2 hr	Unknown

Half-life: 16.6 hours.

ADVERSE REACTIONS
CNS: headache. **EENT:** nasopharyngitis. **GI:** thirst. **GU:** genital fungal infections, UTI, vaginal pruritus, increased urination, renal impairment. **Metabolic:** volume depletion, weight loss, hyperphosphatemia, increased LDL level, *hypoglycemia*. **Musculoskeletal:** back pain.

INTERACTIONS
Drug-drug. *ACE inhibitors (enalapril, lisinopril), ARBs (candesartan, losartan, valsartan), diuretics, NSAIDs:* May increase risk of acute kidney injury. Monitor patient closely and use together cautiously.
Insulin, insulin secretagogues (glipizide, repaglinide): May increase risk of hypoglycemia. Consider lower dosage of insulin or insulin secretagogue.

EFFECTS ON LAB TEST RESULTS
- May increase serum creatinine, LDL cholesterol, phosphate, and Hb levels.
- Causes false-positive urine glucose tests. Use alternative methods to monitor glycemic control.
- May cause unreliable 1,5-AG assay results. Use alternative methods to monitor glycemic control.

CONTRAINDICATIONS & CAUTIONS
- Contraindicated in patients hypersensitive to drug or its components and in patients with severe renal impairment (eGFR less than 30 mL/minute/1.73 m^2) or ESRD, or on dialysis.
- Drug isn't indicated in patients with type 1 diabetes or for the treatment of ketoacidosis.
- Use in patients with severe hepatic impairment isn't recommended.
- Use cautiously in patients with an eGFR less than 60 mL/minute/1.73 m^2, in patients with low systolic BP, and in patients on diuretics as these patients are at increased risk for hypotension due to the intravascular volume contraction effect of drug.
- Drug isn't recommended in patients with eGFR less than 45 mL/minute/1.73 m^2. Drug hasn't shown improved glycemic control in patients whose eGFR is persistently 30 to 60 mL/minute/1.73 m^2.
- Use cautiously in patients with pancreatic insulin deficiency, individuals on calorie restrictions, and patients with a history of alcohol abuse as ketoacidosis is more likely to occur in these individuals.
- Consider temporarily discontinuing drug for at least 4 days before scheduled surgery, to reduce risk of ketoacidosis.
- Use cautiously in patients with hypovolemia, chronic renal insufficiency, or HF as renal impairment and acute kidney injury can occur.
- Drug may increase risk of serious UTIs, including urosepsis and pyelonephritis.
- Use cautiously in patients with a history of prior amputation, peripheral vascular disease, neuropathy, and diabetic foot ulcers as studies have shown an increased risk of lower limb amputation with another SGLT2 inhibitor.
- Safety and effectiveness in children haven't been established.
- Use cautiously in older adults, who may be more at risk for hypovolemia and hypotension.
- **Alert:** SGLT2 inhibitors increase risk of a rare but serious necrotizing fasciitis of the perineum, also known as Fournier gangrene. If necrotizing fasciitis is suspected, immediately discontinue the SGLT2 inhibitor and begin broad-spectrum antibiotics. Surgical debridement may be necessary. Monitor blood glucose levels and start alternative therapy for glycemic control.
Dialyzable drug: Unknown.

PREGNANCY-LACTATION-REPRODUCTION
- Drug may cause adverse renal effects; use isn't recommended during second and third trimesters.

Reactions in bold italics are *life-threatening*. Interactions may have a *rapid onset* or a *delayed onset*.

• There are no data regarding the presence of drug in human milk, the effects on the breastfed infant, or the effects on milk production. Because of the potential for serious adverse reactions in breastfed infants, patients shouldn't breastfeed during therapy.

NURSING CONSIDERATIONS

• Correct fluid volume depletion before starting drug, if clinically indicated.
• Monitor patients for hypovolemia (dehydration, dizziness, orthostatic hypotension, presyncope, syncope, hypotension, acute renal injury).
• Monitor patients for signs and symptoms of acute kidney injury. Assess renal function at baseline and periodically throughout therapy.
• Monitor patients for signs and symptoms of UTI and treat promptly if indicated.
• Monitor patients for signs and symptoms of genital mycotic infections, especially uncircumcised males and patients with a history of genital mycotic infections. Treat promptly.
🕭 *Alert:* Watch for and immediately report signs and symptoms of necrotizing fasciitis of the perineum (temperature above 100.4° F [38° C], general feeling of being unwell, and tenderness, redness, or swelling of the genitals back to the rectum). Signs and symptoms can worsen quickly. Immediately discontinue drug and prepare to administer broad-spectrum antibiotics.
• Monitor blood glucose level. Assess for signs and symptoms of hypoglycemia.
• Monitor patients for ketoacidosis (dehydration, severe metabolic acidosis, nausea, vomiting, abdominal pain, generalized malaise, shortness of breath), even patients with glucose levels less than 250 mg/dL. Discontinue drug for suspected ketoacidosis and treat appropriately.
• Consider temporarily discontinuing therapy in patients with reduced oral intake (such as acute illness or prolonged fasting for surgery) or fluid losses (such as GI illness or excessive heat exposure), as renal impairment and acute kidney injury can occur.
• Drug may increase LDL cholesterol levels. Assess periodically and treat if clinically indicated.
• Monitor patients for signs and symptoms of infection, new pain or tenderness, and sores or ulcers of the lower limbs. Treat as indicated; discontinue drug if these complications occur.

• *Look alike–sound alike:* Don't confuse ertugliflozin with canagliflozin, dapagliflozin, or empagliflozin. Don't confuse Steglatro with Segluromet or Steglujan.

PATIENT TEACHING
• Instruct patient in safe drug administration.
• Stress importance of adherence to dietary instructions, regular physical activity, periodic blood glucose monitoring, and HbA$_{1c}$ testing.
• Advise patient to report all adverse reactions.
• Teach patient how to recognize and manage hypoglycemia and hyperglycemia, and to watch for diabetic complications.
• Advise patient to seek medical advice promptly during periods of stress, such as fever, trauma, infection, or surgery, as drug requirements may change.
• Caution patient to avoid dehydration, which can cause hypotension. Instruct patient to maintain adequate fluid intake and to report signs and symptoms of hypotension (postural dizziness, weakness, syncope).
• Instruct patient to stop drug and seek medical attention immediately if signs and symptoms of ketoacidosis (nausea, vomiting, abdominal pain, tiredness, and labored breathing) occur.
• Inform patient that acute kidney injury has been reported and to immediately report reduced oral intake (due to acute illness or fasting) or increased fluid losses (due to vomiting, diarrhea, or excessive heat exposure), as ertugliflozin may need to be temporarily discontinued.
• Advise patient that lab monitoring of renal function will be needed.
• Teach patient signs and symptoms of UTIs (changes in urination, frequent urination, burning with urination) and to seek medical attention if they occur.
• Inform patient of the increased risk of amputation. Counsel patient about the importance of routine preventive foot care.
• Instruct patient to watch for and immediately report new pain or tenderness, sores or ulcers, or infections involving the leg or foot.
• Teach patient to recognize and report signs and symptoms of genital yeast infections (redness or rash of the glans or foreskin of the penis or vulva, burning with urination, discharge).

---

❸ *Alert:* Teach patient signs and symptoms of necrotizing fasciitis and to seek immediate medical attention if any of these signs and symptoms occur.

• Advise patient of the risk to a fetus and to immediately report pregnancy or plans to become pregnant.

• Advise patient not to breastfeed during therapy.

• Inform patient that urine will test positive for glucose during therapy.

SAFETY ALERT!

ertugliflozin–metformin hydrochloride
er-too-gli-FLOE-zin/met-FORE-min

Segluromet

Therapeutic class: Antidiabetics
Pharmacologic class: Sodium-glucose cotransporter 2 inhibitors–biguanides

AVAILABLE FORMS
Tablets: 2.5 mg ertugliflozin/500 mg metformin hydrochloride; 2.5 mg ertugliflozin/1,000 mg metformin hydrochloride; 7.5 mg ertugliflozin/500 mg metformin hydrochloride; 7.5 mg ertugliflozin/1,000 mg metformin hydrochloride

INDICATIONS & DOSAGES
➤ **Adjunct to diet and exercise to improve glycemic control in patients with type 2 diabetes**
Adults: In patients taking metformin, switch to tablets containing 2.5 mg ertugliflozin with a similar total daily dose of current metformin regimen and give PO in divided doses b.i.d. In patients taking ertugliflozin, switch to tablets containing 500 mg metformin with a similar total daily dose of current ertugliflozin regimen and give PO in divided doses b.i.d. In patients taking ertugliflozin and metformin, switch to tablets containing the same total daily dose of current ertugliflozin regimen and a similar daily dose of current metformin regimen and give PO in divided doses b.i.d. Gradually escalate dose based on effectiveness and tolerability to a maximum daily dose of 15 mg ertugliflozin and 2,000 mg metformin.

ADMINISTRATION
PO
• Give with meals.
• Give missed dose as soon as it's remembered. If it's almost time for the next dose, skip the missed dose and give drug at the next regularly scheduled time. Don't give two doses at the same time.
• Store at controlled room temperature (68° to 77° F [20° to 25° C]).
• Protect from moisture; store in a dry place.

ACTION
Ertugliflozin increases the amount of urinary glucose excreted by inhibiting sodium-glucose cotransporter 2 (SGLT2), which reabsorbs glucose through the kidneys. Metformin decreases hepatic glucose production and intestinal absorption of glucose and improves insulin sensitivity by increasing peripheral glucose uptake and utilization.

Route	Onset	Peak	Duration
PO (ertugliflozin)	Unknown	1–2 hr	Unknown
PO (metformin hydrochloride)	Unknown	2–3 hr	Unknown

Half-life: Ertugliflozin, 16.6 hours; metformin hydrochloride, 6.2 hours.

ADVERSE REACTIONS
CNS: headache, asthenia. **CV:** hypotension. **EENT:** nasopharyngitis. **GI:** diarrhea, nausea, vomiting, flatulence, abdominal discomfort, indigestion. **GU:** genital fungal infections, UTI, vaginal pruritus, increased urination, renal impairment. **Metabolic:** volume depletion, weight loss, increased LDL level, decreased vitamin B_{12} level, hyperphosphatemia, *hypoglycemia, lactic acidosis.* **Musculoskeletal:** back pain.

INTERACTIONS
Drug-drug. *Calcium channel blockers, corticosteroids, estrogens, isoniazid, nicotinic acid, oral contraceptives, phenothiazines, phenytoin, sympathomimetics, thiazides and other diuretics, thyroid products:* May increase risk of hyperglycemia and lead to loss of glycemic control. Closely monitor glycemic control.
Boxed Warning *Carbonic anhydrase inhibitors (acetazolamide, dichlorphenamide, topiramate, zonisamide):* May increase risk of lactic acidosis. Consider more frequent monitoring of patient. ∎

Reactions in bold italics are *life-threatening*. Interactions may have a *rapid onset* or a *delayed onset*.

Drugs that reduce metformin clearance (cimetidine, dolutegravir, ranolazine, vandetanib): May increase systemic exposure to metformin and risk of lactic acidosis. Consider benefits and risks of concomitant use.

Insulin, insulin secretagogues (sulfonylureas): May increase risk of hypoglycemia. Lower insulin or insulin secretagogue dosages may be needed.

Boxed Warning *Radiologic contrast dye:* May cause acute decrease in renal function and increase risk of lactic acidosis. Stop drug at the time of, or before, an iodinated contrast imaging procedure in patients with an eGFR of less than 60 mL/minute/1.73 m². Reevaluate eGFR 48 hours after imaging procedure. May restart drug if renal function stabilizes. ∎

Drug-lifestyle. **Boxed Warning** *Alcohol use (excessive):* May increase risk of lactic acidosis. Discourage use together. ∎

EFFECTS ON LAB TEST RESULTS

- May increase serum creatinine, LDL cholesterol, phosphate, and Hb levels.
- May decrease vitamin B_{12} level and eGFR.
- May cause unreliable 1,5-AG assay results and false-positive urine glucose test results.

CONTRAINDICATIONS & CAUTIONS

Boxed Warning Metformin-containing drugs increase the risk of lactic acidosis and can result in hypothermia, hypotension, resistant bradyarrhythmias, and death. For suspected metformin-associated lactic acidosis, immediately discontinue drug. Prompt hemodialysis is recommended. ∎

Boxed Warning Risk factors for metformin-associated lactic acidosis include renal impairment, use of carbonic anhydrase inhibitors, age 65 and older, radiologic study with contrast, surgery or other procedures, and hypoxic states (HF, MI, sepsis, shock). ∎

Boxed Warning Patients with hepatic impairment are at increased risk for developing metformin-associated lactic acidosis. Avoid use in patients with hepatic disease. ∎

- Contraindicated in patients hypersensitive to ertugliflozin or metformin or its components, in those with severe renal impairment or ESRD, and in patients on dialysis.
- Contraindicated in patients with an eGFR less than 30 mL/minute/1.73 m². Use isn't recommended in patients with an eGFR less than 45 mL/minute/1.73 m².

- Contraindicated in patients with acute or chronic metabolic acidosis, including diabetic ketoacidosis, with or without coma.
- Consider temporarily discontinuing drug for at least 4 days before scheduled surgery, to reduce risk of ketoacidosis.
- Drug isn't indicated for patients with type 1 diabetes or for treatment of diabetic ketoacidosis.
- Use cautiously in patients with an eGFR of less than 60 mL/minute/1.73 m², in patients age 65 or older, in patients with low systolic BP, and in patients on diuretics, as intravascular volume contraction and hypotension can occur.
- Use cautiously in patients with pancreatic insulin deficiency, patients with calorie restrictions, and patients with a history of excessive alcohol intake, as ketoacidosis is more likely to occur.
- Use cautiously in patients with hypovolemia, chronic renal insufficiency, or HF and in those receiving concomitant diuretic, ACE inhibitor, ARB, or NSAID therapy, as renal impairment and acute kidney injury can occur.
- If acute kidney injury occurs, discontinue drug and begin treatment.
- Use cautiously in patients with a history of prior amputation, peripheral vascular disease, neuropathy, and diabetic foot ulcers, as an increased risk of lower limb amputation (primarily of the toe) was observed in clinical studies with another SGLT2 inhibitor.
- Use cautiously in patients with a history of genital mycotic infections and in patients who aren't circumcised, as they are more likely to develop genital mycotic infections.
- **Alert:** SGLT2 inhibitors increase risk of a rare but serious necrotizing fasciitis of the perineum, also known as Fournier gangrene. If necrotizing fasciitis is suspected, immediately discontinue the SGLT2 inhibitor and begin broad-spectrum antibiotics. Surgical debridement may be necessary. Monitor blood glucose levels and start alternative therapy for glycemic control.
- Use cautiously in patients with inadequate vitamin B_{12} or calcium intake or absorption. Drug may decrease vitamin B_{12} level. Monitor vitamin B_{12} levels every 2 to 3 years in patients at high risk; monitor hematologic parameters annually in all patients to assess for anemia.
- Safety and effectiveness in children haven't been established.

Dialyzable drug: Ertugliflozin, unknown; metformin hydrochloride, yes.

⚠ *Overdose S&S:* Hypoglycemia, lactic acidosis.

PREGNANCY-LACTATION-REPRODUCTION

• Drug isn't recommended during the second and third trimesters, as animal studies suggest increased risk of adverse renal effects from ertugliflozin.

• It isn't known if ertugliflozin appears in human milk or how drug affects the infant who is breastfed or milk production. Metformin is present in human milk. Because of the potential for serious adverse reactions in infants, patients shouldn't breastfeed.

• Metformin may cause ovulation in some patients who are premenopausal and anovulatory. Advise patients of the potential for unintended pregnancy.

NURSING CONSIDERATIONS

• Correct volume depletion before start of treatment. Monitor patients for signs and symptoms of hypovolemia (hypotension, dizziness, syncope, thirst) after initiating therapy.

• Monitor patients for signs and symptoms of acute kidney injury, and assess renal function, including eGFR, at baseline and periodically throughout therapy.

• Monitor patients for signs and symptoms of genital mycotic infections; treat promptly if indicated.

↻ *Alert:* Watch for and immediately report signs and symptoms of necrotizing fasciitis of the perineum (temperature above 100.4° F [38° C], general feeling of being unwell, tenderness, redness, or swelling of the genitals back to the rectum). Signs and symptoms can worsen quickly. Immediately discontinue drug and prepare to administer broad-spectrum antibiotics.

• Monitor blood glucose level. Assess for signs and symptoms of hypoglycemia.

• Drug may increase LDL cholesterol level. Assess periodically and treat if clinically indicated.

• Monitor B_{12} level.

• Monitor patients for signs and symptoms of infection, osteomyelitis, new pain, and ulcers of the lower limbs. Discontinue drug if these occur.

• Monitor patients for peripheral vascular disease, neuropathy, and diabetic foot ulcers. Treat as indicated.

• Monitor patients for signs and symptoms of UTIs and treat promptly.

Boxed Warning Monitor patients for signs and symptoms of metformin-associated lactic acidosis (hypothermia, hypotension, resistant bradyarrhythmias), including subtle, nonspecific signs and symptoms (dehydration, nausea, vomiting, malaise, myalgia, abdominal pain, respiratory distress, increased somnolence) and lab abnormalities (elevated blood lactate levels, anion gap acidosis, increased lactate/pyruvate ratios, metformin level greater than 5 mcg/mL). Treat suspected lactic acidosis as clinically indicated and immediately discontinue drug. Hemodialysis may reverse symptoms and lead to recovery. ∎

↻ *Alert:* Drug may need to be temporarily discontinued during times of reduced oral intake of food and fluids (such as surgery, acute illness or fasting, fluid losses from GI illness or excessive heat exposure). Renal impairment and acute kidney injury can occur.

• Don't use urine tests to monitor glycemic control.

• *Look alike–sound alike:* Don't confuse ertugliflozin with canagliflozin, dapagliflozin, or empagliflozin. Don't confuse Segluromet with Steglatro or Steglujan.

PATIENT TEACHING

Boxed Warning Inform patient of the risks of lactic acidosis due to the metformin component. Teach patient the signs and symptoms of lactic acidosis and conditions that predispose to lactic acidosis. Advise patient to discontinue drug immediately and report unexplained hyperventilation, malaise, myalgia, unusual somnolence, slow or irregular heartbeat, sensation of feeling cold (especially in the extremities), or other nonspecific symptoms. Stress importance of adhering to dietary instructions, regular physical activity, periodic blood glucose and HbA_{1c} monitoring, and renal function testing. ∎

• Teach patient to report all adverse reactions.

• Instruct patient how to recognize and manage hypoglycemia and hyperglycemia, and to watch for diabetic complications.

Reactions in bold italics are *life-threatening*. Interactions may have a *rapid onset* or a *delayed onset*.

- Advise patient to promptly seek medical advice during periods of stress (such as fever, trauma, infection, or surgery), as drug requirements may change.
- Caution patient to avoid dehydration, which can cause hypotension. Instruct patient to maintain adequate fluid intake and to immediately report signs and symptoms of hypotension (postural dizziness, weakness, temporary loss of consciousness).
- Instruct patient to seek immediate medical advice if signs and symptoms of ketoacidosis (nausea, vomiting, abdominal pain, tiredness, labored breathing) occur.
- Inform patient that acute kidney injury has been reported and to seek medical advice immediately if reduced oral intake (due to acute illness or fasting) or increased fluid losses (due to vomiting, diarrhea, or excessive heat exposure) occur, as drug may need to be temporarily discontinued.
- Instruct patient to recognize and immediately report signs and symptoms of UTIs (abdominal, pelvic, or back pain; frequent urination; burning with urination; fever; nausea; vomiting).
- Inform patient that drug may increase the risk of amputations. Stress importance of routine preventive foot care. Instruct patient to watch for and immediately report new pain or tenderness, sores or ulcers, or infections involving the leg or foot.
- Tell patient to report signs and symptoms of genital yeast infections (itching, redness, rash, discharge, genital pain).
- 🕲 *Alert:* Teach patient signs and symptoms of necrotizing fasciitis and to seek immediate medical attention if any of these signs and symptoms occur.
- Inform patient that urine glucose tests shouldn't be used for monitoring glycemic control during therapy because patient's urine will test positive for glucose.
- Advise patient of the risk to a fetus and to immediately report pregnancy or plans to become pregnant.
- Advise patient not to breastfeed during therapy.
- Inform patient who is premenopausal and anovulatory that metformin therapy may result in ovulation.

SAFETY ALERT!

ertugliflozin–sitagliptin
er-TOO-gli-FLOE-zin/sit-a-GLIP-tin

Steglujan

Therapeutic class: Antidiabetics
Pharmacologic class: Sodium-glucose cotransporter 2 inhibitors–DPP-4 enzyme inhibitors

AVAILABLE FORMS
Tablets: 5 mg ertugliflozin/100 mg sitagliptin; 15 mg ertugliflozin/100 mg sitagliptin

INDICATIONS & DOSAGES
➤ **Adjunct to diet and exercise to improve glycemic control in adults with type 2 diabetes**
Adults: Initially, 5 mg ertugliflozin/100 mg sitagliptin PO once daily in the morning. May increase to a maximum dose of 15 mg/100 mg PO once daily if tolerated and additional glycemic control is needed. For patients already treated with ertugliflozin, maintain current ertugliflozin dose when switching to combination product.

ADMINISTRATION
PO
- May give with or without food.
- If a dose is missed, give it as soon as it's remembered. If it's almost time for the next dose, skip the missed dose and give drug at the next regularly scheduled time. Don't give two doses at the same time.
- Store at room temperature 68° to 77° F (20° to 25° C).

ACTION
Ertugliflozin increases the amount of urinary glucose excreted by inhibiting sodium-glucose cotransporter 2 (SGLT2), which reabsorbs glucose through the kidneys. Sitagliptin inhibits DPP-4. By increasing and prolonging active incretin levels, sitagliptin helps increase insulin release and decrease circulating glucose.

Route	Onset	Peak	Duration
PO (ertugliflozin)	Unknown	1–2 hr	Unknown
PO (sitagliptin)	Rapid	1–4 hr	Unknown

Half-life: Ertugliflozin, 16.6 hours; sitagliptin, 12.4 hours.

ADVERSE REACTIONS

CNS: headache. **CV:** peripheral edema. **EENT:** nasopharyngitis. **GI:** thirst, abdominal pain, nausea, diarrhea. **GU:** genital fungal infections, UTI, vaginal pruritus, increased urination, renal impairment. **Hematologic:** volume depletion, increased Hb level. **Metabolic:** weight loss, increased LDL cholesterol level, *hypoglycemia*, hyperphosphatemia. **Musculoskeletal:** back pain. **Respiratory:** URI.

INTERACTIONS

Drug-drug. *ACE inhibitors, ARBs, diuretics, NSAIDs:* May increase risk of renal impairment and acute kidney injury. Use cautiously together.
Digoxin: May increase digoxin concentration. Monitor digoxin level.
Insulin, insulin secretagogues: May increase risk of hypoglycemia. Consider lower insulin or insulin secretagogue dosage.

EFFECTS ON LAB TEST RESULTS

- May increase serum creatinine, LDL cholesterol, phosphate, and digoxin levels.
- May increase Hb level.
- May decrease eGFR.
- May cause false-positive urine glucose tests and unreliable 1,5-AG assay results.

CONTRAINDICATIONS & CAUTIONS

- Contraindicated in patients hypersensitive to sitagliptin, ertugliflozin, or components of product, in patients with severe renal impairment (eGFR less than 30 mL/minute/1.73 m^2) or ESRD, and in patients on dialysis.
- Rare but serious allergic and hypersensitivity reactions, such as anaphylaxis, angioedema, and exfoliative skin conditions including SJS, have been reported with sitagliptin and other DPP-4 inhibitors. If reactions occur, discontinue drug and begin appropriate monitoring and treatment.
- Drug isn't for treatment of patients with type 1 diabetes or diabetic ketoacidosis.
- Drug hasn't been studied in patients with a history of pancreatitis. There are postmarketing reports of acute pancreatitis, including fatal and nonfatal hemorrhagic or necrotizing pancreatitis, in patients taking sitagliptin. It's unknown if a history of pancreatitis increases risk of sitagliptin-related pancreatitis.
- Drug may increase risk of symptomatic hypotension from intravascular volume contraction. Use cautiously in patients with impaired renal function (eGFR less than 60 mL/minute/1.73 m^2) or preexisting hypotension and in those age 65 and older.
- Drug isn't recommended in patients with eGFR less than 45 mL/minute/1.73 m^2. Drug increases serum creatinine level and decreases eGFR. Monitor these patients more frequently.
- Consider temporarily discontinuing drug for at least 4 days before scheduled surgery, to reduce risk of ketoacidosis.
- HF has occurred with other DPP-4 inhibitors. Before starting drug, consider risks and benefits of therapy in patients with known risk factors for HF.
- Serious and life-threatening ketoacidosis has been reported in patients taking SGLT2 inhibitors and in patients taking ertugliflozin. For suspected ketoacidosis, discontinue drug, evaluate patient, and treat promptly. In some cases, risk factors for ketoacidosis (insulin dosage reduction, acute febrile illness, reduced calorie intake due to illness or surgery, pancreatic insulin deficiency, or alcohol abuse) were identified.
- Use cautiously in patients with hypovolemia, chronic renal insufficiency, and HF as drug may increase risk of renal impairment and acute kidney injury.
- Use cautiously in patients with a history of prior amputation, peripheral vascular disease, neuropathy, and diabetic foot ulcers as an increased risk of lower limb amputation (primarily of the toe) was observed in clinical studies with another SGLT2 inhibitor.
- Use cautiously in patients with a history of genital mycotic infections and in patients who aren't circumcised as they are more likely to develop genital mycotic infections.
- **Alert:** SGLT2 inhibitors increase risk of a rare but serious necrotizing fasciitis of the perineum, also known as Fournier gangrene. For suspected necrotizing fasciitis, immediately discontinue the SGLT2 inhibitor and begin broad-spectrum antibiotics. Surgical debridement may be necessary. Monitor blood glucose levels and start alternative therapy for glycemic control.
- Drug may increase risk of severe and disabling arthralgia, which may occur soon after therapy begins or years later. If disabling joint pain occurs, discontinue drug if appropriate.
- Postmarketing cases of bullous pemphigoid requiring hospitalization have been reported.

Reactions in bold italics are *life-threatening*. Interactions may have a *rapid onset* or a **delayed onset**.

• Safety and effectiveness in children haven't been determined.

Dialyzable drug: Ertugliflozin, unknown; sitagliptin, 13.5%.

PREGNANCY-LACTATION-REPRODUCTION

• Drug isn't recommended during the second and third trimesters, as animal studies suggest increased risk of adverse renal effects from ertugliflozin.

• Report prenatal exposure to drug to the Merck Pregnancy Registry (1-800-986-8999).

• It isn't known if drug appears in human milk or how drug affects milk production or an infant who is breastfed. Because of the potential for serious adverse reactions in infants who are breastfed, patient shouldn't breastfeed during therapy.

NURSING CONSIDERATIONS

• Assess for volume depletion at baseline and correct fluid balance before initiating therapy. Monitor patient for hypovolemia (dehydration, dizziness, presyncope, syncope, hypotension, orthostatic hypotension) during therapy.

• Monitor patients for signs and symptoms of acute kidney injury. Assess renal function at baseline and periodically during therapy.

🕓 *Alert:* Drug may need to be temporarily discontinued during times of reduced oral intake of food or fluids (such as acute illness or fasting, fluid losses due to GI illness or excessive heat exposure), as renal impairment and acute kidney injury can occur.

• Monitor patients for signs and symptoms of UTIs, urosepsis, and pyelonephritis; treat promptly if indicated.

• Monitor patients for signs and symptoms of genital mycotic infections; treat promptly if indicated.

🕓 *Alert:* Watch for and immediately report signs and symptoms of necrotizing fasciitis of the perineum (temperature above 100.4° F [38° C], general feeling of being unwell, and tenderness, redness, or swelling of the genitals back to the rectum). Signs and symptoms can worsen quickly. Immediately discontinue drug and prepare to administer broad-spectrum antibiotics.

• Monitor blood glucose level. Assess for signs and symptoms of hypoglycemia.

• Drug may increase LDL cholesterol level. Assess periodically and treat if clinically indicated.

• Monitor patients for signs and symptoms of infection, osteomyelitis, new pain, and ulcers of the lower limbs. Discontinue drug if these occur.

• Monitor patients for PVD, neuropathy, and diabetic foot ulcers. Treat as indicated.

• Monitor patients for acute pancreatitis; if suspected, promptly discontinue drug and treat appropriately.

• Monitor patients for signs and symptoms of HF. If HF develops, treat as clinically indicated; drug may need to be discontinued.

• Monitor patients for serious allergic and hypersensitivity reactions. If reactions occur, discontinue drug and institute appropriate monitoring and treatment.

• Monitor patients for arthralgia. If severe joint pain occurs, drug may need to be discontinued.

• Monitor patients for blisters or erosions, as this may indicate bullous pemphigoid. For suspected bullous pemphigoid, discontinue drug and refer patient to a dermatologist for diagnosis and treatment.

• Urine tests shouldn't be used to monitor glycemic control.

• *Look alike–sound alike:* Don't confuse ertugliflozin with canagliflozin, dapagliflozin, or empagliflozin. Don't confuse sitagliptin with saxagliptin, linagliptin, or alogliptin. Don't confuse Steglujan with Steglatro or Segluromet.

PATIENT TEACHING

• Advise patient to report all adverse reactions.

• Stress importance of adhering to dietary instructions, regular physical activity, periodic blood glucose and HbA$_{1c}$ monitoring, and renal function testing.

• Teach patient how to recognize and manage hypoglycemia and hyperglycemia, and to watch for diabetic complications. Caution patient that use with insulin and insulin secretagogues may increase the risk of hypoglycemia.

• Advise patient to discontinue drug and seek immediate medical attention for allergic reactions (rash; hives; swelling of the face, lips, tongue, and throat; difficulty swallowing or breathing).

• Caution patient to promptly seek medical advice during periods of stress (such as fever, trauma, infection, or surgery), as drug requirements may change.

• Teach patient to avoid dehydration, which can cause hypotension. Instruct patient regarding adequate fluid intake and to report signs and symptoms of hypotension (postural dizziness, weakness, temporary loss of consciousness).

• Instruct patient to immediately seek medical advice if signs and symptoms of ketoacidosis (nausea, vomiting, abdominal pain, tiredness, and labored breathing) occur.

• Inform patient that acute kidney injury has been reported and to immediately seek medical advice if reduced oral intake (due to acute illness or fasting) or increased fluid losses (due to vomiting, diarrhea, or excessive heat exposure) occur, as drug may need to be temporarily discontinued.

• Caution patient to immediately report symptoms of HF (increasing shortness of breath, rapid increase in weight, or swelling of the feet).

• Advise patient that acute pancreatitis can occur. Tell patient to discontinue drug and immediately report severe, persistent abdominal pain that may radiate to the back, with or without vomiting.

• Instruct patient to recognize and immediately report signs and symptoms of UTIs (abdominal, pelvic, or back pain; frequent urination; burning with urination; fever; nausea; vomiting).

• Inform patient of the increased risk of amputations. Counsel patient about the importance of routine preventive foot care.

• Instruct patient to watch for and immediately report new pain or tenderness, sores or ulcers, or infections involving the leg or foot.

• Advise patient that arthralgia can occur at any time during treatment and to report severe joint pain to prescriber.

• Advise patient that bullous pemphigoid requiring hospitalization can occur and to immediately report blisters or skin erosions.

• Tell patient to report signs and symptoms of genital yeast infections (itching, redness, rash, discharge, genital pain).

🙂 *Alert:* Teach patient signs and symptoms of necrotizing fasciitis and to seek immediate medical attention if any of these signs and symptoms occur.

• Inform patient that urine glucose tests shouldn't be used for monitoring glycemic control during therapy because patient's urine will test positive for glucose.

• Advise patient of the risk to a fetus and to immediately report pregnancy or plans to become pregnant.

• Caution patient not to breastfeed during therapy.

erythromycin (ophthalmic, topical)
er-ith-roe-MYE-sin

Erygel, Ery 2% Pads

Therapeutic class: Antibiotics
Pharmacologic class: Macrolides

AVAILABLE FORMS
Ophthalmic ointment: 0.5%
Topical gel: 2%
Topical pad: 2%
Topical solution: 2%*

INDICATIONS & DOSAGES
➤ **Superficial ocular infections involving the conjunctiva or cornea caused by organisms susceptible to erythromycin (ophthalmic ointment)**
Adults and children: Apply a ribbon of ointment about 1 cm long directly to infected eye up to six times daily, depending on severity of infection.

➤ **To prevent ophthalmia neonatorum caused by *Neisseria gonorrhoeae* or *Chlamydia trachomatis* (ophthalmic ointment)**
Neonates: Apply a ribbon of ointment about 1 cm long in lower conjunctival sac of each eye shortly after birth.

➤ **Inflammatory acne vulgaris (topical gel, topical pads, topical solution)**
Adults and children: Apply pads and solution to affected areas b.i.d., morning and evening. Apply gel once daily or b.i.d. If no improvement in 6 to 8 weeks, discontinue drug; prescriber should reevaluate treatment.

ADMINISTRATION
Ophthalmic
• Don't use for infection unless causative organism has been identified.

• Clean eye area of excessive discharge before application.

• To prevent ophthalmia neonatorum, apply ointment no later than 1 hour after birth. Use drug in neonates born either vaginally or by

---

Reactions in bold italics are *life-threatening*. Interactions may have a *rapid onset* or a ***delayed onset***.

cesarean birth. Gently massage eyelids for 1 minute to spread ointment.
• Use new tube for each neonate.
• Store ophthalmic ointment at room temperature in tightly closed, light-resistant container.
Topical
• Wash, rinse, and pat affected areas dry before application.
• Wash hands after each application.
• Avoid contact with eyes, nose, mouth, other mucous membranes, and broken skin.

ACTION

Inhibits RNA-dependent protein synthesis by binding to bacterial 50s ribosomal subunits.

Route	Onset	Peak	Duration
Ophthalmic, topical	Unknown	Unknown	Unknown

Half-life: Unknown.

ADVERSE REACTIONS

EENT: minor ocular irritations, redness.
Skin: burning, dryness, pruritus, erythema, irritation, oily skin, peeling, sensitivity reactions, leather appearance, tenderness. **Other:** hypersensitivity reactions.

INTERACTIONS

Drug-drug. *Clindamycin (topical):* Topical form may antagonize clindamycin's effect. Avoid using together.
Isotretinoin (topical): May increase adverse effects of erythromycin. Use together cautiously.
Drug-lifestyle. *Abrasive or medicated soaps or cleansers, acne products or other preparations containing peeling drugs (benzoyl peroxide, resorcinol, salicylic acid, sulfur, tretinoin), alcohol-containing products (aftershave, cosmetics, perfumed toiletries, shaving creams or lotions), astringent soaps or cosmetics, medicated cosmetics or cover-ups:* May cause cumulative dryness, resulting in excessive skin irritation. Urge caution.

EFFECTS ON LAB TEST RESULTS

None reported.

CONTRAINDICATIONS & CAUTIONS

• Contraindicated in patients hypersensitive to drug.
• Safety and effectiveness of topical drug in children haven't been established.
Dialyzable drug: Unknown.

PREGNANCY-LACTATION-REPRODUCTION

• Use during pregnancy only if clearly needed. Topical drug may be used to treat acne during pregnancy.
• It isn't known if drug appears in human milk after topical application. Use cautiously during breastfeeding.

NURSING CONSIDERATIONS

• Ointment and pads are intended only for treatment of inflammatory acne and not for treatment of superficial skin infections.
⚠ *Alert:* Prolonged topical use may result in fungal or bacterial superinfection, including pseudomembranous colitis and CDAD, during and even 2 months after treatment. Consider these diagnoses in patients who present with diarrhea; stop drug for significant diarrhea, abdominal cramps, or passage of blood or mucus.

PATIENT TEACHING

• Teach patient how to apply drug and to wash hands before and after applying ointment. Warn patient not to touch tip of applicator to eye or surrounding tissue.
• Tell patient that vision may be blurred for a few minutes after applying ophthalmic ointment. Instruct patient to keep eyes closed for 1 to 2 minutes after applying drug.
• Advise patient to watch for and report signs and symptoms of sensitivity (itching lids, redness, swelling, or constant burning of eyes or skin).
• Tell patient not to share drug, washcloths, or towels with family members and to notify prescriber if anyone develops same signs or symptoms.
• Instruct patient to wash hands after each application.
• Stress importance of adherence with recommended therapy.
• Teach patient to wash, rinse, and dry face thoroughly before each topical use.
• Advise patient to avoid topical use near eyes, nose, mouth, or other mucous membranes.
• Tell patient to stop using drug and notify prescriber if condition worsens or if there is no improvement.
• Caution patient to keep topical drug away from heat and open flame.
• Advise patient to report diarrhea immediately.

erythromycin base
er-ith-roe-MYE-sin

Eryc✐, Ery-Tab✐

erythromycin ethylsuccinate
E.E.S. Granules, EryPed

erythromycin lactobionate
Erythrocin

erythromycin stearate
Erythrocin Stearate

Therapeutic class: Antibiotics
Pharmacologic class: Macrolides

AVAILABLE FORMS
erythromycin base
Capsules (delayed-release): 250 mg
Tablets (delayed-release): 250 mg, 333 mg, 500 mg
erythromycin ethylsuccinate
Oral suspension: 200 mg/5 mL, 400 mg/5 mL
Powder for oral suspension: 200 mg/5 mL, 400 mg/5 mL
Tablets: 400 mg
erythromycin lactobionate
Injection: 500 mg*
erythromycin stearate
Tablets (film-coated): 250 mg

INDICATIONS & DOSAGES
➤ **Acute pelvic inflammatory disease caused by *Neisseria gonorrhoeae* in females with a history of penicillin sensitivity**
Adults: 500 mg IV every 6 hours for 3 days; then 500 mg (base) PO every 12 hours, or 333 mg (base) PO every 8 hours for 7 days.
➤ **Intestinal amebiasis caused by *Entamoeba histolytica***
Adults: 500 mg (base or stearate) PO every 12 hours, or 333 mg (base) PO every 8 hours, or 250 mg (base or stearate) PO every 6 hours, or 400 mg (ethylsuccinate) q.i.d. for 10 to 14 days.
Children: 30 to 50 mg/kg PO daily in divided doses for 10 to 14 days. Don't exceed 4 g/day.
➤ **To prevent rheumatic fever recurrence in patients allergic to penicillin and sulfonamides**
Adults: 250 mg (base or stearate) PO b.i.d., or 400 mg (ethylsuccinate) PO b.i.d.
➤ **Mild to moderately severe respiratory tract, skin, or soft-tissue infection from**
sensitive group A beta-hemolytic streptococci, *Streptococcus pneumoniae, Mycoplasma pneumoniae, Corynebacterium diphtheriae,* or *Bordetella pertussis; Listeria monocytogenes* **infection**
Adults: 250 mg PO every 6 hours, 333 mg PO every 8 hours, or 500 mg PO every 12 hours. Maximum dose is 4 g daily. Or 15 to 20 mg/kg IV daily, as continuous infusion or in divided doses every 6 hours for 10 days (3 weeks for *Mycoplasma* species infection). Maximum dosage is 4 g/day.
Children: 30 to 50 mg/kg PO daily, in divided doses every 6 hours; or 15 to 20 mg/kg IV daily, in divided doses every 4 to 6 hours for 10 days (3 weeks for *Mycoplasma* species infection).
➤ **Nongonococcal urethritis caused by *Ureaplasma urealyticum* when tetracycline is contraindicated or not tolerated**
Adults: 500 mg (base or stearate) PO every 6 hours, or 666 mg (base) PO every 8 hours, or 800 mg (ethylsuccinate) PO every 8 hours for at least 7 days.
➤ **Legionnaires disease**
Adults: 1 to 4 g (base or stearate) or 1.6 to 4 g (ethylsuccinate) PO daily in divided doses for 10 to 14 days alone or with rifampin. IV route may be used initially in severe cases.
➤ **Uncomplicated urethral, endocervical, or rectal infection caused by *Chlamydia trachomatis,* when tetracyclines are contraindicated**
Adults: 500 mg base PO q.i.d. for at least 7 days, or 666 mg PO every 8 hours for at least 7 days, or 250 mg PO q.i.d. for 14 days if patient can't tolerate higher doses.
➤ **Urogenital *C. trachomatis* infection during pregnancy**
Women: 500 mg (base or stearate) PO q.i.d. or 666 mg (base) PO every 8 hours for at least 7 days. Patients who can't tolerate this regimen may receive 500 mg (base or stearate) PO every 12 hours, or 333 mg (base) PO every 8 hours, or 250 mg (base or stearate) PO q.i.d. for at least 14 days.
➤ **Conjunctivitis of the newborn caused by *C. trachomatis***
Neonates: 50 mg/kg/day PO in 4 divided doses for at least 2 weeks.
➤ **Pneumonia in infants caused by *C. trachomatis***
Infants: 50 mg/kg/day (base or stearate) PO in four divided doses for 21 days.

Reactions in bold italics are *life-threatening*. Interactions may have a *rapid onset* or a **delayed onset**.

➤ **Pertussis**
Adults: 40 to 50 mg/kg/day PO in divided doses for 5 to 14 days.

➤ **Preoperative prophylaxis for elective colorectal surgery**
Adults: Two 500-mg tablets, three 333-mg tablets, or four 250-mg tablets PO at 1 p.m., 2 p.m., and 11 p.m. on preoperative day 1 before 8 a.m. surgery.

➤ **Primary syphilis**
Adults: 30 to 40 g (base or stearate) PO or 48 to 64 g (ethylsuccinate) PO in divided doses for 10 to 15 days. (CDC guidelines don't recommend erythromycin for this indication.)

ADMINISTRATION
PO
• Obtain specimen for culture and sensitivity tests before giving. Begin therapy while awaiting results.
• When giving suspension, note the concentration.
• Give base or stearate with full glass of water 2 hours before or 2 hours after meals for best absorption; may give ethylsuccinate or delayed release without regard to meals.
• Give drug with food if GI upset occurs. Don't give drug with milk, soda, or fruit juice.
• Coated tablets or encapsulated pellets cause less GI upset, so they may be better tolerated by patients who have trouble tolerating drug.
• Protect capsules from moisture and excessive heat.
IV
▼ Obtain specimen for culture and sensitivity tests before giving. Begin therapy while awaiting results.
▼ Reconstitute drug according to manufacturer's directions.
▼ Dilute each 250 mg in at least 100 mL of NSS. Don't give IV push.
▼ Infuse each dose over 20 to 60 minutes.
▼ **Incompatibilities:** None listed by manufacturer. Consult a drug incompatibility reference for more information.

ACTION

Inhibits bacterial protein synthesis by binding to the 50S subunit of the ribosome. Bacteriostatic or bactericidal, depending on concentration.

Route	Onset	Peak	Duration
PO	Unknown	0.5–4 hr	Unknown
IV	Immediate	2.5 hr	Unknown

Half-life: 1.5 to 2 hours.

ADVERSE REACTIONS
CNS: fever. **CV:** vein irritation or thrombophlebitis after IV injection, *ventricular arrhythmias, prolonged QT interval.* **GI:** *pseudomembranous colitis,* abdominal pain and cramping, diarrhea, nausea, vomiting, anorexia. **Hepatic:** hepatic dysfunction. **Skin:** eczema, rash, urticaria. **Other:** hypersensitivity reactions, including *anaphylaxis,* overgrowth of nonsusceptible bacteria or fungi.

INTERACTIONS
Drug-drug. *Azole antifungals (ketoconazole):* May increase erythromycin and antifungal concentrations, leading to increased risk of adverse reactions, including sudden death from cardiac causes. Avoid use together.
Benzodiazepines (midazolam, triazolam): May increase effects of these drugs. Monitor patient closely.
Carbamazepine: May inhibit metabolism of carbamazepine, increasing blood level and risk of toxicity. Avoid using together.
Clarithromycin: May increase QTc interval and risk of arrhythmias. Avoid use together.
Clindamycin, lincomycin: May be antagonistic. Avoid using together.
Clopidogrel: May inhibit antiplatelet effect of clopidogrel. Monitor platelet function when starting or stopping erythromycin. Adjust clopidogrel dosage as needed.
Colchicine: May increase colchicine level and risk of colchicine-related adverse reactions. Use cautiously and monitor patient for colchicine-related toxicity.
Cyclosporine: May increase cyclosporine level. Monitor drug level.
Digoxin: May increase digoxin level. Monitor patient for digoxin toxicity.
Dihydroergotamine, ergotamine: May increase ergot toxicity. Use together is contraindicated.
Disopyramide: May increase disopyramide level, which may cause arrhythmias and prolonged QT intervals. Monitor ECG.
Fluoroquinolones, other drugs that prolong the QTc interval (amiodarone, antipsychotics, procainamide, quinidine, sotalol, TCAs): May have additive effects. Monitor ECG for QTc interval prolongation. Avoid using together, if possible.
HMG-CoA reductase inhibitors (lovastatin, simvastatin): May increase concentrations of HMG-CoA reductase inhibitors;

rhabdomyolysis has occurred rarely. Monitor CK and serum transaminase levels.

Oral anticoagulants: May increase anticoagulant effect. Monitor PT and INR closely.

Pimozide: May increase QTc interval and risk of ventricular arrhythmias. Use together is contraindicated.

Rifamycins (rifabutin, rifampin, rifapentine): May decrease therapeutic effects of erythromycin while increasing adverse effects of rifamycin. Monitor patient.

Sildenafil: May increase sildenafil systemic exposure (AUC). Consider reducing sildenafil dosage.

Strong CYP3A inhibitors (diltiazem, verapamil): May increase the risk of sudden death from cardiac causes. Don't use together.

Theophylline: May decrease erythromycin level and increase theophylline toxicity. Use together cautiously.

Drug-food. Grapefruit juice: May inhibit drug's metabolism; caution patient to avoid grapefruit juice during therapy.

EFFECTS ON LAB TEST RESULTS

• May increase ALP, ALT, AST, and bilirubin levels.
• May interfere with fluorometric determination of urine catecholamines and with colorimetric assays.

CONTRAINDICATIONS & CAUTIONS

• Contraindicated in patients hypersensitive to drug or other macrolides.
• **Alert:** Drug has been associated with prolonged QT interval and infrequent cases of arrhythmia, including torsades de pointes. Avoid drug in patients with known prolonged QT interval, proarrhythmic conditions, or clinically significant bradycardia, and in those receiving class IA (quinidine, procainamide) or class III (dofetilide, amiodarone, sotalol) antiarrhythmics.
• Use erythromycin salts cautiously in patients with impaired hepatic function.
• May cause infantile hypertrophic pyloric stenosis (IHPS) requiring surgery. Benefit of therapy needs to be weighed against risk of developing IHPS.
• Prolonged or repeated use may result in superinfection. If superinfection occurs, discontinue drug.
• Drug may cause CDAD, ranging in severity from mild to life-threatening colitis, during treatment and for up to 2 months after

treatment. Drug may need to be discontinued for suspected or confirmed CDAD.
• Use cautiously in older adults, who are at increased risk for developing drug-induced hearing loss, fluid retention, and QT prolongation.
• Don't use drug to treat neurosyphilis.
Dialyzable drug: No.

PREGNANCY-LACTATION-REPRODUCTION

• Use drug during pregnancy only if clearly needed.
• Drug may not reach the fetus adequately to prevent congenital syphilis; a penicillin regimen is recommended.
• **Alert:** Some IV formulations contain benzyl alcohol, which is associated with neonatal gasping syndrome, a sometimes fatal condition.
• Drug appears in human milk. Use cautiously during breastfeeding.

NURSING CONSIDERATIONS

• Monitor patient for superinfection and diarrhea. Drug may cause overgrowth of nonsusceptible bacteria or fungi.
• Monitor hepatic function. Drug may cause hepatotoxicity.
• Monitor patients for new hearing loss.
• Monitor patient for fluid retention.

PATIENT TEACHING

• Instruct patient in safe drug administration.
• Tell patient to take drug as prescribed, even after feeling better.
• Caution patient to report all adverse reactions, especially diarrhea, nausea, abdominal pain, vomiting, and fever.
• Instruct parents or caregivers of infants to immediately report signs and symptoms of IHPS (vomiting or irritability with feeding).
• Advise patient to use cautiously if breastfeeding.

---

escitalopram oxalate
ess-si-TAL-oh-pram

Lexapro⬧

Therapeutic class: Antidepressants
Pharmacologic class: SSRIs

AVAILABLE FORMS

Oral solution: 5 mg/5 mL
Tablets: 5 mg, 10 mg, 20 mg

Reactions in bold italics are *life-threatening*. Interactions may have a *rapid onset* or a *delayed onset*.

INDICATIONS & DOSAGES
Adjust-a-dose (for all indications): For older adults and patients with hepatic impairment, 10 mg PO daily, initially and as maintenance dosages.

➤ **Acute and maintenance therapy for patients with major depressive disorder**
Adults and adolescents age 12 and older: Initially, 10 mg PO once daily, increasing to 20 mg if needed after at least 1 week in adults and 3 weeks in adolescents.

➤ **Generalized anxiety disorder**
Adults: Initially, 10 mg PO once daily, increasing to 20 mg if needed after at least 1 week.

➤ **Obsessive-compulsive disorder** ♦
Adults and adolescents age 12 and older: Initially, 10 mg PO once daily. May increase dose in 10-mg increments at 1-week or greater intervals up to 40 mg once daily.

➤ **Premenstrual dysphoric disorder** ♦
Adult women: Continuous daily dosing regimen: Initially, 5 to 10 mg PO once daily. Over the first month, may increase dose, based on response and tolerability, to 20 mg once daily.
Luteal phase dosing regimen: 5 to 10 mg PO once daily, starting 14 days before anticipated onset of menstruation and continuing to the onset of menses. Over the first month, may increase dose to 20 mg once daily during the luteal phase.
Symptom-onset dosing regimen: 5 to 10 mg PO once daily from the day of symptom onset until a few days after start of menses. Over the first month, may increase dose, based on response and tolerability, to 20 mg once daily.

ADMINISTRATION
PO
• Give without regard for food.
• Give in the morning or evening.

ACTION
Selectively inhibits reuptake of serotonin.

Route	Onset	Peak	Duration
PO	Unknown	5 hr	Unknown

Half-life: 27 to 32 hours.

ADVERSE REACTIONS
CNS: fever, insomnia, dizziness, somnolence, paresthesia, headache, light-headedness, migraine, tremor, vertigo, abnormal dreams, irritability, impaired concentration, fatigue, lethargy. **CV:** palpitations, HTN, flushing, chest pain. **EENT:** blurred vision, tinnitus, earache, rhinitis, sinusitis, dry mouth, toothache. **GI:** nausea, diarrhea, constipation, indigestion, abdominal pain, vomiting, increased or decreased appetite, flatulence, heartburn, cramps, gastroesophageal reflux. **GU:** ejaculation disorder, erectile dysfunction, anorgasmia, menstrual cramps, UTI, urinary frequency. **Metabolic:** weight gain or loss, hyponatremia. **Musculoskeletal:** arthralgia, myalgia, muscle cramps, pain in neck, shoulder, arms, or legs. **Respiratory:** bronchitis, cough. **Skin:** rash, diaphoresis. **Other:** decreased libido, yawning, flulike symptoms.

INTERACTIONS
Drug-drug. *Antiparkinsonians (rasagiline, selegiline):* May cause serotonin syndrome. Avoid use together.
Aspirin, NSAIDs, other drugs known to affect coagulation: May increase the risk of bleeding. Use together cautiously.
Beta blockers: May cause bradycardia and increase risk of CNS toxicity. Monitor patient closely.
Buspirone, methylphenidate: May increase risk of serotonin syndrome. Monitor patient closely.
Carbamazepine: May increase escitalopram clearance. Monitor patient for expected antidepressant effect and adjust dose as needed.
Cimetidine: May increase escitalopram level. Monitor patient for increased adverse reactions to escitalopram.
Citalopram: May cause additive effects. Using together is contraindicated.
CNS drugs: May cause additive effects. Use together cautiously.
Desipramine, other drugs metabolized by CYP2D6 substrates: May increase levels of these drugs. Use together cautiously.
Linezolid, methylene blue: May cause serotonin syndrome. Avoid use together.
MAO inhibitors: May cause fatal serotonin syndrome or signs and symptoms resembling NMS. Avoid using within 14 days of MAO inhibitor therapy.
Pimozide: May increase risk of QTc-interval prolongation. Use together is contraindicated.
Serotonergic drugs (amphetamines, buspirone, fentanyl, lithium, SSRIs, TCAs, tramadol, triptans): May increase risk of serotonin syndrome. Use together cautiously, especially at the start of therapy or at dosage increases.

♣Canada ◇OTC ♦Off-label use ✐Photoguide ⊕Do not crush *Liquid contains alcohol ▨Genetic

Drug-herb. *St. John's wort:* May cause serotonin syndrome. Use with caution.
Drug-lifestyle. *Alcohol use:* May increase CNS effects. Discourage use together.

EFFECTS ON LAB TEST RESULTS
• May increase bilirubin and cholesterol levels and LFT values.
• May decrease serum potassium and sodium levels.
• May increase or decrease glucose level.
• May decrease serum prothrombin level.
• May increase INR.

CONTRAINDICATIONS & CAUTIONS
• Contraindicated in patients taking pimozide, MAO inhibitors, or within 14 days of MAO inhibitor therapy and in those hypersensitive to escitalopram, citalopram, or any of its inactive ingredients.
�ことり **Alert:** Concomitant use with methylene blue or linezolid can cause serotonin syndrome (fever, mental status changes, muscle twitching, diaphoresis, shivering, shaking, diarrhea, loss of coordination). Don't start drug in patients receiving methylene blue or linezolid.
🌜 **Alert:** If linezolid or methylene blue must be given, stop escitalopram and monitor patient for serotonin toxicity for 2 weeks or until 24 hours after last dose of methylene blue or linezolid, whichever comes first. May resume escitalopram 24 hours after last dose of methylene blue or linezolid.
• Use cautiously in patients with a history of mania, seizure disorders, suicidality, or renal or hepatic impairment.
• Use cautiously in patients with diseases that produce altered metabolism or hemodynamic responses.
• Use cautiously in older adults as they may have greater sensitivity to drug.
Boxed Warning Escitalopram isn't approved for use in children younger than age 12. ∎
• Safety and effectiveness in children younger than age 18 with generalized anxiety disorder haven't been established.
Dialyzable drug: Unknown.
⚠ **Overdose S&S:** Seizures, coma, dizziness, ECG changes, hypotension, insomnia, nausea, sinus tachycardia, somnolence, vomiting, acute renal failure.

PREGNANCY-LACTATION-REPRODUCTION
• Use during pregnancy only if potential benefit justifies fetal risk.

• Prescriber should consider tapering dosage in the third trimester by carefully weighing established benefit of treating depression with an antidepressant against risks; decision can only be made on a case-by-case basis.
• Health care providers are encouraged to register patients in the National Pregnancy Registry for Antidepressants at 1-866-961-2388 or https://womensmentalhealth.org/research/pregnancyregistry/antidepressants/.
• Drug appears in human milk. Use cautiously during breastfeeding; monitor infants for adverse reactions.

NURSING CONSIDERATIONS
Boxed Warning Drug may increase risk of suicidality in children, adolescents, and young adults ages 18 to 24, especially during the first few months of treatment, especially in patients with major depressive disorder or other psychiatric disorder. ∎
Boxed Warning Closely monitor all patients for clinical worsening and for emergence of suicidality. ∎
• Evaluate patient for history of drug abuse, and observe for signs of misuse or abuse.
• When discontinuing drug, taper gradually and monitor patient for reemerging signs and symptoms.
• Periodically reassess patient to determine need for maintenance treatment and appropriate dosing.
🌜 **Alert:** Combining triptans with an SSRI or an SSNRI may cause serotonin syndrome or NMS-like reactions. Serotonin syndrome may be more likely to occur when starting or increasing the dose of triptan, SSRI, or SSNRI.
• *Look alike–sound alike:* Don't confuse escitalopram with estazolam.

PATIENT TEACHING
• Instruct patient in safe drug administration.
• Inform patient that symptoms should improve gradually over several weeks, rather than immediately.
• Tell patient that although improvement may occur within 1 to 4 weeks, to continue drug as prescribed.
Boxed Warning Caution patient and patient's family to report signs of worsening depression (such as agitation, irritability, insomnia, hostility, impulsivity) and suicidality to prescriber immediately. ∎

E

❸ *Alert:* Teach patient to recognize and immediately report symptoms of serotonin toxicity (fever, mental status changes, muscle twitching, diaphoresis, shivering or shaking, diarrhea, loss of coordination).

• Tell patient to use caution while driving or operating hazardous machinery because of drug's potential to impair judgment, thinking, and motor skills.

• Advise patient to consult health care provider before taking other prescription or OTC drugs.

• Encourage patient to avoid alcohol while taking drug.

• Advise patient to report pregnancy or breastfeeding before starting therapy.

esketamine
es-KET-a-meen

Spravato

Therapeutic class: Antidepressants
Pharmacologic class: Noncompetitive N-methyl-D-aspartate receptor antagonists
Controlled substance schedule: III

AVAILABLE FORMS
Nasal spray: 28 mg (2 sprays)/device

INDICATIONS & DOSAGES
➤ **Treatment-resistant depression in conjunction with an oral antidepressant**
Adults: Induction phase (weeks 1 to 4): On day 1, starting dose is 56 mg intranasal with a subsequent dose that week of 56 or 84 mg based on efficacy and tolerability. For weeks 2 to 4, give 56 or 84 mg intranasal twice per week. For maintenance phase weeks 5 to 8, give 56 or 84 mg intranasal once weekly. For maintenance phase week 9 and after, give 56 or 84 mg intranasal once weekly or once every 2 weeks. Individualize to the least frequent dosing to maintain response.
Adjust-a-dose: If patient misses treatment sessions and depression symptoms worsen, consider returning patient to previous dosing schedule.
➤ **Depressive symptoms in patients with major depressive disorder with acute suicidality**
Adults: 84 mg intranasal twice per week for 4 weeks. May reduce dosage to 56 mg twice per week, based on tolerability. After 4 weeks,

assess for therapeutic benefit to determine need for continued treatment. Concomitant use with an oral antidepressant beyond 4 weeks hasn't been systematically evaluated.

ADMINISTRATION
Intranasal
• Drug must be administered under direct supervision of a health care provider.
• A treatment session consists of nasal administration and postadministration observation under supervision.
• Patients should avoid food for at least 2 hours and liquids for at least 30 minutes before administration.
• Patients should blow their nose before first dose only to clear the nasal passages. Patients shouldn't blow their nose between doses.
• Patients who require a nasal corticosteroid or nasal decongestant on dosing day should use these medications at least 1 hour before administration of esketamine.
• Don't prime device before use.
• Use two devices for a 56-mg dose or three devices for an 84-mg dose, with a 5-minute rest period between use of each device.
• Ensure indicator shows two green dots. If it doesn't, dispose of device and obtain a new one.
• Recline patient's head to about 45 degrees during administration.
• Insert tip straight into the nostril until the nose rest touches the skin between the nostrils; close the opposite nostril. Have patient inhale while pushing the plunger in until it stops. Repeat to deliver dose to the other nostril. Instruct patient to sniff gently to keep drug inside nose.
• Ensure administration by confirming that the indicator shows no green dots when the device is empty. When one dose is delivered, one green dot will indicate that a dose remains in the device.
• Dab patient's nose with a tissue if liquid drops out. Patient shouldn't blow nose.
• If patient misses treatment sessions and there is no worsening of depressive symptoms, continue current dosing schedule. If patient misses maintenance-phase treatment sessions and depression symptoms worsen, consider returning to previous dosing schedule.
• Store at room temperature (68° to 77° F [20° to 25° C]).

ACTION
Mechanism for antidepressant effect is unknown.

Route	Onset	Peak	Duration
Intranasal	Unknown	20–40 min	Unknown

Half-life: 7 to 12 hours.

ADVERSE REACTIONS
CNS: dissociation, dizziness, sedation, vertigo, hypoesthesia, anxiety, depression, lethargy, feeling drunk, feeling abnormal, dysarthria, headache, tremor, euphoric mood, insomnia, mental impairment, intentional self-injury, dysphoria. **CV:** increased BP, tachycardia. **EENT:** nasal discomfort, oropharyngeal pain, throat irritation, dry mouth, toothache. **GI:** dysgeusia, nausea, vomiting, constipation, diarrhea. **GU:** urinary frequency. **Musculoskeletal:** myalgia. **Skin:** hyperhidrosis.

INTERACTIONS
Drug-drug. *CNS depressants (benzodiazepines, opioids):* May increase sedation. Use cautiously together and monitor patient closely for additive sedative effects.
MAO inhibitors (rasagiline, selegiline), psychostimulants (amphetamines, armodafinil, methylphenidate, modafinil): May increase BP. Use cautiously together and monitor patient closely.
Drug-lifestyle. *Alcohol use:* May increase sedation. Avoid use together.

EFFECTS ON LAB TEST RESULTS
None reported.

CONTRAINDICATIONS & CAUTIONS
• Contraindicated in patients hypersensitive to esketamine or ketamine or its components and in those with aneurysmal vascular disease (including thoracic and abdominal aorta and intracranial and peripheral arterial vessels), AV malformation, or history of intracerebral hemorrhage.
• Use cautiously in patients with history of hypertensive encephalopathy.
Boxed Warning Drug can cause delayed or prolonged sedation. Closely monitor patients for sedation with concomitant use of CNS depressants. ∎
Boxed Warning Dissociative or perceptual changes (including distortion of time and space and illusions), derealization, and

depersonalization may occur. Because of drug's potential to induce dissociative effects, carefully assess patients with psychosis before giving drug. Initiate treatment only if benefit outweighs risk. ∎
Boxed Warning Because of risks of sedation and dissociation, patients must be monitored by a health care provider for at least 2 hours at each treatment session and assessed to determine whether they are clinically stable and ready to leave the health care setting. ∎
Boxed Warning Drug is a controlled substance with potential for abuse, misuse, and diversion. Assess patient's risk of abuse or misuse before prescribing and monitor all patients for development of these behaviors or conditions, including drug-seeking behavior, during therapy. Individuals with a history of drug abuse or dependence are at greater risk. ∎
Boxed Warning Drug is only available through a REMS program because of the risks of serious adverse outcomes from sedation, dissociation, and abuse and misuse. ∎
Boxed Warning There is increased risk of suicidality in children and young adults taking antidepressants. Closely monitor all patients treated with antidepressants for clinical worsening and emergence of suicidality. Drug isn't approved for use in children. ∎
• Drug may increase risk of short- or long-term cognitive or memory impairment.
• Use cautiously in patients with moderate hepatic impairment because of increased risk of adverse reactions.
• Drug hasn't been studied in patients on dialysis or in those with severe hepatic impairment (Child-Pugh class C).
• Drug's effectiveness in preventing suicide or reducing suicidality hasn't been proven. Patient may still require in-patient treatment.
• Drug hasn't been studied or approved for use as an anesthetic.
Dialyzable drug: Unknown.

PREGNANCY-LACTATION-REPRODUCTION
• Drug may cause fetal harm and isn't recommended for use during pregnancy.
• If pregnancy occurs during treatment, discontinue drug and counsel patient about fetal risk.
• Patients of childbearing potential should consider pregnancy planning and prevention during treatment.

Reactions in bold italics are *life-threatening*. Interactions may have a *rapid onset* or a *delayed onset*.

E

• Prescribers should register patients in the antidepressant exposure registry by contacting the National Pregnancy Registry for Antidepressants (1-866-961-2388 or https://womensmentalhealth.org/research/pregnancyregistry/antidepressants).

• Drug appears in human milk. Breastfeeding isn't recommended during treatment.

NURSING CONSIDERATIONS

• Assess BP before administration. If baseline BP is greater than 140 mm Hg systolic or 90 mm Hg diastolic, consider risks of short-term increases in BP and benefit of treatment.

• Don't give if an increase in BP or ICP poses a serious risk.

• After administration, reassess BP for at least 2 hours, beginning at approximately 40 minutes. If BP drops and patient appears clinically stable for at least 2 hours, may discharge patient at end of postdose monitoring period; if not, continue to monitor.

• Assess for hypertensive crisis (chest pain, shortness of breath) or hypertensive encephalopathy (sudden severe headache, visual disturbances, seizures, diminished consciousness, or focal neurologic deficits) and provide emergency care as indicated.

Boxed Warning Monitor patient for sedation and dissociation for at least 2 hours after administration. ∎

Boxed Warning Monitor all patients for signs and symptoms of abuse, misuse, dependence, and tolerance. ∎

Boxed Warning Closely monitor all patients for clinical worsening and emergence of suicidality. Consider changing the therapeutic regimen, including possibly discontinuing drug or the concomitant oral antidepressant, in patients whose depression is persistently worse, or who are experiencing emergent suicidality. ∎

• Drug may increase risk of ulcerative or interstitial cystitis. Monitor patients for urinary tract and bladder signs and symptoms (urinary frequency, dysuria, urinary urgency, nocturia, cystitis) and refer for appropriate follow-up as clinically indicated.

• **Look alike–sound alike:** Don't confuse esketamine with ketamine or escitalopram.

PATIENT TEACHING

• Advise patient to report all adverse reactions.

Boxed Warning Inform patient that sedation, dissociative symptoms, perception disturbances, dizziness, vertigo, anxiety, and increased BP may occur and that monitoring by a health care provider will be needed until these effects resolve. ∎

Boxed Warning Advise patient that drug is a federally controlled substance because it can be abused, misused, or lead to dependence. ∎

Boxed Warning Tell patient that drug is available only through a REMS program. Inform patient that enrollment in the REMS program is necessary before drug administration, that drug must be administered under the direct observation of a health care provider, and that patient will need to be monitored by a health care provider for at least 2 hours after administration. ∎

Boxed Warning Advise patient and caregivers to look for emergence of suicidality, especially early during treatment and when dosage is adjusted, and to immediately contact prescriber if changes occur. ∎

• Because drug may impair the ability to drive or operate machinery, caution patient to avoid potentially hazardous activities requiring complete mental alertness and motor coordination (driving, operating machinery) until the next day after a restful sleep.

• Warn patient that someone must be available to drive patient home after each treatment session.

• Caution patient of childbearing potential about risk to a fetus. Advise patient to report pregnancy or plan to become pregnant during treatment.

• Advise patient not to breastfeed during treatment.

SAFETY ALERT!

esmolol hydrochloride
ES-moe-lol

Brevibloc

Therapeutic class: Antiarrhythmics
Pharmacologic class: Selective beta blockers

AVAILABLE FORMS

Injection: 10 mg/mL vial
Premixed IV bags in sodium chloride: 10 mg/mL in 250-mL bags; 20 mg/mL in 100-mL bags

INDICATIONS & DOSAGES

➤ **Supraventricular tachycardia; noncompensatory sinus tachycardia**

Adults: 500 mcg/kg as loading dose by IV infusion over 1 minute; then 4-minute maintenance infusion of 50 mcg/kg/minute. If adequate response doesn't occur within 5 minutes, may repeat loading dose and follow with maintenance infusion of 100 mcg/kg/minute for 4 minutes. May repeat loading dose and increase maintenance infusion by increments of 50 mcg/kg/minute. Maintenance dose general range, 50 to 200 mcg/kg/minute. Maximum maintenance infusion for tachycardia is 200 mcg/kg/minute. May continue maintenance infusions for up to 48 hours.

➤ **Intraoperative and postoperative tachycardia or HTN**

Adults: For immediate control: 1,000 mcg/kg as a bolus dose over 30 seconds, followed by 150 mcg/kg/minute IV infusion, if needed. For gradual control (stepwise dosing): Loading dose is 500 mcg/kg over 1 minute, then 50 mcg/kg/minute for 4 minutes. Optional loading dose if needed, then 100 mcg/kg/minute for 4 minutes. Optional loading dose if needed, then 150 mcg/kg/minute for 4 minutes. If necessary, may increase to 200 mcg/kg/minute. Maximum doses are 200 mcg/kg/minute for tachycardia and 300 mcg/kg/minute for HTN.

ADMINISTRATION

IV

▼ Don't dilute single-dose vials or premixed containers.

▼ Give with an infusion-control device rather than by IV push. Administer by continuous IV infusion with or without a loading dose and titrate based on ventricular rate or BP at 4-minute or more intervals. Avoid infusing into small veins or through a butterfly catheter.

▼ If concentration exceeds 10 mg/mL, give drug through a central line.

▼ Don't use for longer than 48 hours. Watch infusion site carefully for signs of extravasation; if they occur, stop infusion immediately and call prescriber.

▼ **Incompatibilities:** Amphotericin B cholesteryl sulfate complex, diazepam, furosemide, procainamide, sodium bicarbonate 5%.

ACTION

A class II antiarrhythmic and ultra-short-acting selective beta-1 blocker that decreases HR, contractility, and BP.

Route	Onset	Peak	Duration
IV	Immediate	5 min (with loading dose); 30 min (without loading dose)	30 min after discontinuation of infusion

Half-life: About 9 minutes.

ADVERSE REACTIONS

CNS: dizziness, somnolence, headache, agitation, confusion. **CV:** hypotension, peripheral ischemia. **GI:** nausea, vomiting. **Skin:** inflammation or induration at infusion site, hyperhidrosis.

INTERACTIONS

Drug-drug. *Antidiabetic agents:* May increase blood glucose-lowering effect of antidiabetic. Closely monitor blood glucose concentration.

Calcium channel blockers (diltiazem, nicardipine, nifedipine, verapamil), flecainide: May potentiate pharmacologic effects of both drugs. IV administration in close proximity is contraindicated. Monitor cardiac function closely and adjust therapy as needed.

Clonidine: May cause life-threatening BP increases. Closely monitor BP. Discontinue either agent gradually, preferably esmolol first.

Digoxin: May increase digoxin level and bradycardia. Monitor digoxin level.

Lidocaine: May increase lidocaine concentration. Monitor patient closely and adjust dosage as needed.

MAO inhibitors: May worsen bradycardia or HTN. Discontinue esmolol or reduce esmolol dosage if needed.

Morphine: May increase esmolol level. Adjust esmolol dosage carefully.

NSAIDs: May impair antihypertensive effect of esmolol. Monitor BP and adjust esmolol dosage as needed.

Prazosin: May increase risk of orthostatic HTN. Help patient to stand slowly until effects are known.

Salicylates (aspirin): May impair antihypertensive effect of esmolol. Monitor patient and consider alternative therapy as needed.

Succinylcholine: May prolong neuromuscular blockade. Monitor patient closely.

Reactions in bold italics are *life-threatening*. Interactions may have a *rapid onset* or a ***delayed onset***.

Vasoconstrictive and positive inotropic agents (dopamine, epinephrine, norepinephrine): May increase risk of reduced cardiac contractility in presence of high systemic vascular resistance. Don't use together.

EFFECTS ON LAB TEST RESULTS
• May increase serum potassium level.

CONTRAINDICATIONS & CAUTIONS
• Contraindicated in patients hypersensitive to drug or its components, in those with severe sinus bradycardia, second- or third-degree heart block, sick sinus syndrome, cardiogenic shock, decompensated HF, and pulmonary HTN, and in patients taking calcium channel blockers.
• Use cautiously in patients with renal impairment, hypovolemia, peripheral circulatory disorders, diabetes, or bronchospasm.
• May cause myocardial ischemia when abruptly discontinued in patients with CAD.
⚠ *Alert:* Don't withdraw drug abruptly, as angina, MI, and ventricular arrhythmias can occur.
• Use in combination with an alpha blocker (after starting the alpha blocker) in patients with pheochromocytoma to avoid paradoxical BP increases.
• Safety and effectiveness in children haven't been established.
Dialyzable drug: Unknown.
⚠ *Overdose S&S:* Bradycardia, hypotension, loss of consciousness, cardiac arrest, pulseless electrical activity.

PREGNANCY-LACTATION-REPRODUCTION
• Use during third trimester can cause fetal bradycardia. Use during pregnancy only if potential benefit justifies fetal risk.
• It isn't known if drug appears in human milk. Patient should discontinue breastfeeding or discontinue drug.

NURSING CONSIDERATIONS
⚠ *Alert:* Monitor ECG and BP continuously during infusion. Nearly half of patients will develop hypotension. Diaphoresis and dizziness may accompany hypotension. Monitor patient closely, especially if patient had low BP before treatment.
• Hypotension can usually be reversed within 30 minutes by decreasing the dose or, if

needed, by stopping the infusion. Notify prescriber if this becomes necessary.
• If a local reaction develops at infusion site, change to another site. If extravasation occurs, stop infusion immediately and disconnect tubing from cannula. Gently aspirate extravasated solution without flushing the catheter; then remove the IV catheter and elevate the extremity.
• When HR stabilizes, replace IV drug with an alternative antiarrhythmic. Reduce esmolol infusion rate by 50% 30 minutes after first dose of the new drug. Monitor patient response and, if HR is controlled for 1 hour after administration of second dose of the replacement drug, stop esmolol infusion.
• Monitor serum electrolyte levels, as hyperkalemia can occur, especially in patients with renal impairment.
• Drug can mask signs and symptoms of hyperthyroidism. Monitor patient for thyrotoxicosis when withdrawing drug.
• Monitor patient for and correct hypovolemia.

PATIENT TEACHING
• Instruct patient to report all adverse reactions promptly.
• Tell patient to report discomfort at IV site.

esomeprazole magnesium
ess-oh-ME-pray-zol

Nexium✐, Nexium 24 HR ◊

esomeprazole sodium
Nexium IV

Therapeutic class: Antiulcer drugs
Pharmacologic class: PPIs

AVAILABLE FORMS
esomeprazole magnesium
Capsules (delayed-release) ⓓⓒ: 20 mg ◊, 40 mg
Powder for suspension (delayed-release): 2.5 mg, 5 mg, 10 mg, 20 mg, 40 mg
Tablets (delayed-release): 20 mg ◊
esomeprazole sodium
Powder for injection: 20-mg, 40-mg single-use vials

INDICATIONS & DOSAGES

Adjust-a-dose (for all indications): For patients with severe hepatic failure (Child-Pugh class C), maximum daily dose is 20 mg.

➤ **GERD; to heal erosive esophagitis**
Adults: 20 or 40 mg PO daily for 4 to 8 weeks. Maintenance dose for healing erosive esophagitis is 20 mg PO daily for up to 6 months.
Children ages 1 to 11 weighing 20 kg or more: 10 or 20 mg PO once daily for up to 8 weeks.
Children ages 1 to 11 weighing less than 20 kg: 10 mg PO once daily for up to 8 weeks.

➤ **Symptomatic GERD**
Adults: 20 mg PO daily for 4 weeks. If symptoms are unresolved, may continue treatment for 4 more weeks.
Children and adolescents ages 12 to 17: 20 mg PO once daily for up to 4 weeks.
Children ages 1 to 11: 10 mg PO once daily for up to 8 weeks.

➤ **Erosive esophagitis due to acid-mediated GERD only**
Infants ages 1 to 11 months weighing more than 7.5 to 12 kg: 10 mg PO once daily for up to 6 weeks.
Infants ages 1 to 11 months weighing more than 5 to 7.5 kg: 5 mg PO once daily for up to 6 weeks.
Infants ages 1 to 11 months weighing 3 to 5 kg: 2.5 mg PO once daily for up to 6 weeks.

➤ **Short-term treatment (up to 10 days) of GERD in patients with a history of erosive esophagitis who can't take drug orally**
Adults: 20 or 40 mg IV bolus over at least 3 minutes. Or, dilute to a total volume of 50 mL and give by IV infusion over 10 to 30 minutes. Switch patient to oral therapy as soon as tolerated.
Children ages 1 to 17 weighing 55 kg or more: 20 mg IV infusion once daily over 10 to 30 minutes.
Children ages 1 to 17 weighing less than 55 kg: 10 mg IV infusion once daily over 10 to 30 minutes.
Children ages 1 month to younger than 1 year: 0.5 mg/kg IV infusion once daily over 10 to 30 minutes.

➤ **To reduce the risk of gastric ulcers in patients receiving continuous NSAID therapy**
Adults: 20 or 40 mg PO once daily for up to 6 months.

➤ **Long-term treatment of pathologic hypersecretory conditions, including Zollinger-Ellison syndrome**
Adults: 40 mg PO b.i.d. Adjust dosage based on patient response.

➤ **To eliminate *Helicobacter pylori***
Adults: 40 mg (magnesium) PO daily, 1,000 mg amoxicillin PO b.i.d., and 500 mg clarithromycin PO b.i.d., given together for 10 days to reduce duodenal ulcer recurrence.

➤ **Reduction of risk of rebleeding of gastric or duodenal ulcers after therapeutic endoscopy**
Adults: 80 mg IV infusion over 30 minutes, followed by continuous infusion of 8 mg/hour for a total IV treatment duration of 72 hours, followed by oral acid-suppressive therapy.
Adjust-a-dose: In patients with mild to moderate hepatic impairment (Child-Pugh classes A and B), maximum continuous infusion rate is 6 mg/hour. In patients with severe hepatic impairment (Child-Pugh class C), maximum continuous infusion rate is 4 mg/hour.

ADMINISTRATION

PO

• Give drug at least 1 hour before meals. If patient has difficulty swallowing the capsule, contents of the capsule can be emptied and mixed with 1 tablespoon of applesauce and swallowed (without chewing the enteric-coated pellets).

• If giving capsule via NG tube, open capsule and empty the granules into a 60-mL syringe. Mix with 50 mL of water. Replace the plunger and shake vigorously for 15 seconds. Flush NG tube with additional water after use. Don't give if pellets have dissolved or disintegrated.

• For oral suspension, mix contents of a 2.5- or 5-mg packet with 5 mL of water; mix contents of a 10-, 20-, or 40-mg packet with 15 mL of water. Then let it sit for 2 to 3 minutes to thicken. Stir the suspension and drink within 30 minutes.

• To give oral suspension via NG tube, add 5 mL of water to a syringe, then add contents of 2.5- or 5-mg packet; or add 15 mL of water to a syringe, then add contents of 10-, 20-, or 40-mg packet. Shake syringe and leave for 2 to 3 minutes to thicken. Shake syringe again and inject through NG or gastric tube within 30 minutes. Flush any remaining contents into the stomach with additional water.

Reactions in bold italics are *life-threatening*. Interactions may have a *rapid onset* or a ***delayed onset***.

IV

▼ For IV bolus, reconstitute powder with 5 mL of NSS and inject over at least 3 minutes.

▼ For IV infusion, reconstitute powder with 5 mL of NSS, lactated Ringer injection, or D_5W. Further dilute with 45 mL of NSS, lactated Ringer injection, or D_5W. Infuse over 10 to 30 minutes.

▼ For continuous IV infusion, add two 40-mg vials reconstituted with NSS to 100 mL NSS. Infuse at 8 mg/hour for 71.5 hours.

▼ Flush IV line with D_5W, NSS, or lactated Ringer injection before and after administration.

▼ Use reconstituted powder within 12 hours.

▼ Use admixture diluted with D_5W within 6 hours.

▼ If diluted with NSS or lactated Ringer injection, use within 12 hours.

▼ Store reconstituted solution and admixture at room temperature.

▼ **Incompatibilities:** Other IV drugs.

ACTION

Reduces gastric acid secretion and decreases gastric acidity.

Route	Onset	Peak	Duration
PO	Unknown	1.5 hr	13–17 hr
IV	Unknown	Unknown	Unknown

Half-life: 1 to 1.5 hours.

ADVERSE REACTIONS

CNS: headache, dizziness, fever. **EENT:** dry mouth. **GI:** abdominal pain, constipation, diarrhea, flatulence, nausea, vomiting. **Respiratory:** cough. **Skin:** pruritus, injection-site reaction.

INTERACTIONS

Drug-drug. *Calcium salts (calcium carbonate):* May interfere with GI absorption of calcium salts. Closely monitor clinical response to calcium; larger dosages of calcium may be needed.

Cilostazol: May increase concentrations of cilostazol and its active metabolite. Consider a cilostazol dose reduction when giving concurrently with esomeprazole.

Clopidogrel: May decrease antiplatelet activity. Use esomeprazole magnesium or esomeprazole sodium cautiously with clopidogrel.

Dabigatran: May decrease concentration of active metabolite of dabigatran. Monitor patient closely.

Diazepam: May decrease clearance of diazepam. Monitor patient for diazepam toxicity.

Digoxin: May increase serum digoxin level. Monitor digoxin concentration and clinical response. For suspected interaction, adjust digoxin dosage as needed.

Drugs metabolized by CYP2C19: May alter clearance of esomeprazole, especially in older adults or patients with hepatic insufficiency. Monitor patient for toxicity.

Fluvoxamine: May increase risk of adverse reactions. Use cautiously.

Iron salts (ferrous sulfate): May interfere with absorption of iron salts. Temporary cessation of esomeprazole may be required to achieve appropriate clinical response to oral iron. If stopping esomeprazole isn't an option, parenteral iron may be a suitable alternative.

Ketoconazole, voriconazole: May increase esomeprazole concentration. Monitor therapy.

Methotrexate: May increase methotrexate concentration and risk of toxicity. Monitor patient closely.

Mycophenolate: May decrease mycophenolate plasma concentration and pharmacologic effects. Monitor clinical response and adjust mycophenolate dosage as needed.

Protease inhibitors (atazanavir, nelfinavir, saquinavir): May reduce atazanavir or nelfinavir plasma level. Use together isn't recommended. May increase saquinavir level. Monitor patient carefully. Refer to protease inhibitor prescribing information.

Rifampin: May decrease esomeprazole levels. Avoid using together.

Rilpivirine: May cause loss of virologic response or resistance. Use together is contraindicated.

Tacrolimus: May increase pharmacologic effects of tacrolimus and risk of adverse reactions. Closely monitor tacrolimus trough concentration when starting or stopping esomeprazole. Adjust tacrolimus dosage as needed.

Warfarin: May prolong PT and increase INR, causing abnormal bleeding. Monitor patient and PT and INR.

Drug-herb. *St. John's wort:* May decrease esomeprazole level. Avoid use together.

Drug-food. *Any food:* May reduce drug level. Advise patient to take drug 1 hour before food.

EFFECTS ON LAB TEST RESULTS

• May decrease magnesium and vitamin B_{12} levels.
• May cause false-positive results in diagnostic investigations for neuroendocrine tumors (CgA level).
• May cause false-positive results for urine screening for tetrahydrocannabinol (THC).
• May cause a hyperresponse in gastrin secretion in response to secretin stimulation test, falsely suggesting gastrinoma.

CONTRAINDICATIONS & CAUTIONS

• Contraindicated in patients hypersensitive to drug or components of esomeprazole or omeprazole (a drug similar to this one).
• **Alert:** There may be an increased risk of osteoporosis-related hip, wrist, and spine fractures associated with PPIs. Risk is increased in patients who received high-dose and long-term (longer than 1 year) therapy. The lowest dosage for the shortest duration should be used. Consider vitamin D and calcium supplementation.
• Use cautiously in patients receiving continuous NSAID therapy who are at increased risk for gastric ulcers (those age 60 and older and those with a history of gastric ulcers).
• Symptomatic response to drug doesn't preclude the presence of gastric malignancy. Consider reevaluating patient with suboptimal response or early relapse.
• Drug-induced decreases in gastric acidity may increase serum chromogranin A (CgA) level, possibly causing false-positive results in diagnostic investigations for neuroendocrine tumors. Temporarily stop esomeprazole at least 14 days before assessing CgA level; consider repeating the test if initial CgA level is high.
• If cutaneous lupus or SLE occurs, discontinue drug.
• American College of Gastroenterology Clinical Guideline 2017 recommends avoiding use of clarithromycin triple therapy (a PPI, clarithromycin, and amoxicillin or metronidazole) to eliminate *H. pylori* in patients with risk factors for macrolide resistance (prior macrolide exposure, local clarithromycin resistance rates of 15% or higher,

eradication rates with clarithromycin-based regimens of 85% or lower).
Dialyzable drug: Unlikely.
⚠ **Overdose S&S:** Blurred vision, confusion, tremor, ataxia, intermittent clonic seizures, diaphoresis, drowsiness, flushing, headache, nausea, tachycardia.

PREGNANCY-LACTATION-REPRODUCTION

• Use during pregnancy only if potential benefit justifies fetal risk.
• It isn't known if drug appears in human milk, but omeprazole does. Use cautiously during breastfeeding.

NURSING CONSIDERATIONS

• Antacids can be used while taking drug, unless otherwise directed by prescriber.
• Monitor patient for rash or signs and symptoms of hypersensitivity. Monitor GI symptoms for improvement or worsening. Monitor LFTs, especially in patients with preexisting hepatic disease.
• **Alert:** Prolonged use may cause low magnesium levels that require magnesium supplementation and possibly discontinuation of drug. Monitor magnesium level before treatment and periodically during treatment. Monitor patient for signs and symptoms of low magnesium level, such as abnormal HR or heart rhythm, palpitations, muscle spasms, tremor, and seizures. In children, abnormal HR may present as fatigue, upset stomach, dizziness, and light-headedness.
• **Alert:** May increase risk of CDAD. Evaluate for CDAD in patients who develop diarrhea that doesn't improve.
• **Alert:** Prolonged treatment (at least 3 years or more) may lead to vitamin B_{12} malabsorption and subsequent vitamin B_{12} deficiency, which is dose-related and more severe in women and those younger than age 30; prevalence decreases after discontinuation of therapy.
• Monitor patient for acute tubulointerstitial nephritis (rash, fever, arthralgia, decreased renal function, malaise, nausea, anorexia).
• **Look alike–sound alike:** Don't confuse Nexium with Nexavar.

PATIENT TEACHING

• Instruct patient to take drug exactly as prescribed.
• Teach patient safe drug administration.

- Tell patient to inform prescriber of worsening signs and symptoms, pain, or diarrhea that doesn't improve.
- Instruct patient to alert prescriber if rash or other signs and symptoms of allergy occur.
- Warn patient to immediately report symptoms of low magnesium level, such as involuntary muscle movements or seizures.

esterified estrogens
es-TER-i-fied ES-troe-jenz

Menest

Therapeutic class: Estrogens
Pharmacologic class: Estrogens

AVAILABLE FORMS
Tablets (film-coated): 0.3 mg, 0.625 mg, 1.25 mg, 2.5 mg

INDICATIONS & DOSAGES
➤ **Inoperable progressing prostate cancer**
Men: 1.25 to 2.5 mg PO t.i.d.
➤ **Palliative treatment for metastatic breast cancer**
Men and women who are postmenopausal: 10 mg PO t.i.d. for 3 or more months.
➤ **Hypoestrogenism due to hypogonadism**
Women: 2.5 to 7.5 mg PO daily in divided doses in cycles of 20 days on, 10 days off.
➤ **Hyperestrogenism due to castration, primary ovarian failure**
Women: 1.25 mg PO daily in cycles of 3 weeks on, 1 week off. Adjust for symptoms. Can be given continuously.
➤ **Vasomotor menopausal symptoms**
Women: 1.25 mg PO daily in cycles of 3 weeks on, 1 week off. If patient is menstruating, cyclic administration is started on day 5 of bleeding.
➤ **Moderate to severe menopausal vulvar and vaginal atrophy**
Women: 0.3 to 1.25 mg or more PO daily, depending on tissue response of individual patient, in cycles of 3 weeks on, 1 week off.

ADMINISTRATION
PO
- Use lowest effective dose needed for specific indication.
- Give without regard to food.

ACTION
Mimics the actions of endogenous estrogens; increases synthesis of DNA, RNA, and protein in responsive tissues; reduces release of FSH and LH from pituitary gland.

Route	Onset	Peak	Duration
PO	Unknown	Unknown	Unknown

Half-life: Unknown.

ADVERSE REACTIONS
CNS: headache, migraine, dizziness, chorea, depression, nervousness, mood disturbance, irritability, exacerbation of epilepsy, dementia exacerbation, *stroke, seizure exacerbation.* **CV:** thrombophlebitis, *thromboembolism,* HTN, edema, *PE, MI.* **EENT:** worsening myopia or astigmatism, intolerance of contact lenses, retinal thrombosis. **GI:** nausea, vomiting, abdominal cramps, bloating, anorexia, increased appetite, *pancreatitis,* gallbladder disease. **GU:** breakthrough bleeding, altered menstrual flow, dysmenorrhea, amenorrhea, premenstrual-like syndrome, *endometrial cancer, ovarian cancer,* endometrial hyperplasia, cervical erosion, altered cervical secretions, enlargement of uterine fibromas, vaginal candidiasis, testicular atrophy, impotence, cystitis-like syndrome. **Hepatic:** cholestatic jaundice, benign hepatic adenoma. **Metabolic:** hypercalcemia, weight gain or loss, hypertriglyceridemia, carbohydrate intolerance. **Respiratory:** asthma exacerbation. **Skin:** melasma, rash, pruritus, urticaria, hirsutism or hair loss, erythema nodosum, *erythema multiforme,* dermatitis. **Other:** change in libido; breast tenderness, enlargement, or secretion; gynecomastia; *breast cancer;* hypersensitivity reaction, including *anaphylaxis.*

INTERACTIONS
Drug-drug. *Anastrozole:* May interfere with anastrozole effectiveness. Avoid use together. *Carbamazepine, fosphenytoin, phenobarbital, phenytoin, rifampin:* May decrease effectiveness of estrogen therapy. Monitor patient closely.
Clarithromycin, erythromycin, itraconazole, ketoconazole, ritonavir: May increase estrogen plasma levels and side effects. Monitor patient.
Corticosteroids: May increase corticosteroid effects. Monitor patient closely.

Dantrolene, hepatotoxic drugs: May increase risk of hepatotoxicity. Monitor liver function closely.

Exemestane: May interfere with exemestane effectiveness. Avoid use together.

Oral anticoagulants: May decrease anticoagulant effects. Adjust dosage if needed. Monitor PT and INR.

Ospemifene: May enhance adverse or toxic effect of and interfere with effectiveness of ospemifene. Avoid use together.

Thyroid replacement therapy: May decrease thyroid hormone levels. Higher doses of thyroid hormone may be required.

Tranexamic acid: May enhance thrombogenic effect. Avoid if possible.

Drug-herb. *Red clover:* May increase estrogen effects. Discourage use together.

St. John's wort: May decrease effects of drug. Discourage use together.

Drug-food. *Folic acid:* May decrease absorption of folic acid. Monitor levels.

Grapefruit, grapefruit juice: May increase risk of adverse effects. Discourage use together.

Drug-lifestyle. *Alcohol use:* May increase estrogen level and risk of breast cancer and osteoporosis. Avoid concurrent use.

Smoking: May increase risk of CV effects. If smoking continues, may need another form of therapy.

EFFECTS ON LAB TEST RESULTS

• May increase calcium, thyroid-binding globulin, circulating thyroid hormone, serum triglyceride, HDL, and serum phospholipid levels.
• May decrease LDL level.
• May increase platelet count.
• May alter clotting factors.
• May accelerate PT, PTT, and platelet aggregation times.
• May reduce response to metyrapone test. May cause impaired glucose tolerance.

CONTRAINDICATIONS & CAUTIONS

• Contraindicated in patients hypersensitive to drug and in patients with breast cancer (except metastatic disease), estrogen-dependent neoplasia, active thrombophlebitis, thromboembolic disorders, undiagnosed abnormal genital bleeding, liver dysfunction or disease, or history of thromboembolic disease.
• Use cautiously in patients with history of HTN, mental depression, cardiac or renal

dysfunction, gallbladder disease, bone disease, migraine, seizures, SLE, porphyria, asthma, or diabetes.

Boxed Warning Don't use drug for prevention of CV disease. Drug is associated with development of dementia in patients age 65 and older who are postmenopausal. Estrogens with or without progestins should be prescribed at the lowest effective doses for the shortest duration consistent with treatment goals. ■

Dialyzable drug: Unknown.

⚠ *Overdose S&S:* Nausea, withdrawal bleeding in females.

PREGNANCY-LACTATION-REPRODUCTION

• Estrogens shouldn't be used during pregnancy.
• There is no indication for use in pregnancy. There appears to be little or no increased risk of birth defects in infants born to patients who have used estrogens and progestins from oral contraceptives inadvertently during early pregnancy.
• Estrogens appear in human milk and have been shown to decrease quantity and quality of human milk. Use only if clearly needed; closely monitor infant's growth.

NURSING CONSIDERATIONS

🕒 *Alert:* Drug is considered a high-risk medication for older adults.

Boxed Warning Close clinical surveillance of all patients taking estrogens is important because estrogens have been reported to increase risk of endometrial cancer. Adequate diagnostic measures, including endometrial sampling when indicated, should be undertaken to rule out malignancy in all cases of undiagnosed persistent or recurring abnormal vaginal bleeding. ■

• Reevaluate therapy as clinically appropriate to determine treatment necessity.
• When given cyclically for short-term use, administration should be cyclic and attempts to discontinue or taper the medication should be made at 3- to 6-month intervals.
• Make sure patient has thorough physical exams before starting estrogen therapy. Patients receiving long-term therapy should have annual exams. Periodically monitor body weight, BP, lipid levels, and hepatic function.
• Notify pathologist about patient's estrogen therapy when sending specimens to the lab for evaluation.

⟲ Alert: Because of risk of thromboembolism, stop therapy at least 4 to 6 weeks before procedures that cause prolonged immobilization or increased risk of thromboembolism, such as knee or hip surgery.

• May impair glucose tolerance. Monitor glucose level closely in patients with diabetes.

PATIENT TEACHING

• Advise patient to report all adverse reactions promptly.

Boxed Warning Emphasize importance of regular physical exams. Patients who are postmenopausal and use estrogen replacement for longer than 5 years to treat menopausal symptoms may be at increased risk for endometrial cancer. Risk is reduced by using cyclic rather than continuous therapy and the lowest possible estrogen dosage. Adding progestins to the regimen decreases risk of endometrial hyperplasia, but it's unknown whether progestins affect risk of endometrial cancer. ∎

⟲ Alert: Warn patient to immediately report abdominal pain; pain, numbness, or stiffness in legs or buttocks; pressure or pain in chest or shortness of breath; severe headaches; visual disturbances, such as blind spots, flashing lights, or blurriness; vaginal bleeding or discharge; breast lumps; swelling of hands or feet; yellow skin or sclera; dark urine; or light-colored stools.

• Tell patient with diabetes to report elevated glucose level so that antidiabetic dosage can be adjusted.

• Explain to patient receiving cyclic therapy for postmenopausal symptoms that withdrawal bleeding may occur during week off drug. Tell patient to report unusual vaginal bleeding.

• Teach patient to perform routine breast self-exam.

• Advise patient of childbearing potential to consult prescriber before taking drug and to inform prescriber of pregnancy immediately.

• Teach patient methods to decrease risk of blood clots.

• Encourage patient to stop smoking or reduce number of cigarettes smoked because of the risk of CV complications.

estradiol ⚛
es-tra-DYE-ole

Alora, Climara, Dotti, Estrace, Estrace Vaginal Cream, Estring Vaginal Ring, Evamist, Menostar, Minivelle, Vagifem, Vivelle, Vivelle-Dot, Yuvafem

estradiol acetate
Femring

estradiol cypionate
Depo-Estradiol

estradiol gel
Divigel, Elestrin, EstroGel

estradiol valerate
Delestrogen

Therapeutic class: Estrogens
Pharmacologic class: Estrogens

AVAILABLE FORMS
estradiol
Spray, topical solution: 1.53 mg/spray
Tablets (micronized): 0.5 mg, 1 mg, 2 mg
Transdermal: 0.014 mg/24 hours, 0.025 mg/24 hours, 0.0375 mg/24 hours, 0.05 mg/24 hours, 0.06 mg/24 hours, 0.075 mg/24 hours, 0.1 mg/24 hours
Vaginal cream (in nonliquefying base): 0.1 mg/g
Vaginal ring (extended-release): 2 mg (0.0075 mg/24 hours)
Vaginal tablets: 4 mcg, 10 mcg
estradiol acetate
Vaginal ring: 0.05 mg/24 hours; 0.1 mg/24 hours
estradiol cypionate
Injection (in oil): 5 mg/mL
estradiol gel
Transdermal gel: 0.06% (1.25 g/metered dose), 0.06% (0.87 g/activation), 0.1% (in 0.25 mg, 0.5 mg, 0.75 mg, 1 mg, and 1.25 mg single-dose packets)
estradiol valerate
Injection (in oil): 10 mg/mL, 20 mg/mL, 40 mg/mL

INDICATIONS & DOSAGES
➤ **Vasomotor menopausal symptoms, female hypogonadism, female castration, primary ovarian failure**

Women: 1 to 2 mg PO estradiol daily. Or, for vasomotor symptoms, 1 to 5 mg cypionate IM once every 3 to 4 weeks; for female hypogonadism, 1.5 to 2 mg cypionate IM once every month.

Transdermal patch

Women: Apply patch according to manufacturer's instructions. Apply to clean, dry area of the trunk. Adjust dose, if necessary, after the first 2 or 3 weeks of therapy; then every 3 to 6 months as needed. Rotate application sites weekly with an interval of at least 1 week between particular sites used. Adjust dosage as needed.

➤ **Postmenopausal urogenital symptoms**

Women: One ring inserted into the upper third of the vagina. Ring is kept in place for 3 months.

➤ **Vulvar and vaginal atrophy**

Women: 0.05 mg/24 hours applied twice weekly in a cyclic regimen. Or, 0.05 mg/24 hours Climara applied weekly in a cyclic regimen. Or, 2 to 4 g vaginal applications of cream daily for 1 to 2 weeks; then gradually reduce to one-half initial dosage for 1 to 2 weeks. When vaginal mucosa is restored, maintenance dose is 1 g one to three times weekly in a cyclic regimen. Attempt to taper or discontinue at 3- to 6-month intervals. If using Vagifem or Yuvafem for atrophic vaginitis, give 1 tablet vaginally once daily for 2 weeks. Maintenance dose is 1 tablet inserted vaginally twice weekly. Or, 10 to 20 mg valerate IM every 4 weeks as needed. Or, 1 to 5 mg cypionate IM once every 3 to 4 weeks. Or, 0.05 to 0.1 mg daily by vaginal ring. Replace vaginal ring every 3 months. Or, 1.25 g EstroGel applied once daily to skin.

➤ **Palliative treatment of advanced, inoperable breast cancer**

Men and women who are postmenopausal: 10 mg PO estradiol t.i.d. for 3 months.

➤ **Palliative treatment of advanced, inoperable prostate cancer**

Men: 30 mg valerate IM every 1 to 2 weeks, or 1 to 2 mg estradiol PO t.i.d.

➤ **To prevent postmenopausal osteoporosis**

Women: Place a 6.5-cm² (0.025 mg/24 hours) Climara patch once weekly on clean, dry skin of lower abdomen or upper quadrant of buttock. Or, place a 3.25-cm² (0.014 mg/24 hours) Menostar patch once weekly to clean, dry area of the lower abdomen. Or, place a 0.025 mg/24 hours patch twice weekly in a cyclic regimen in patients with an intact uterus. In patients with a hysterectomy,

apply one patch twice weekly in a continuous regimen. For each system, press firmly in place for about 10 seconds; ensure complete contact, especially around edges. Or, 0.025-mg/24 hours Vivelle, Vivelle-Dot, or Alora system applied to a clean, dry area of the trunk twice weekly. Or, 0.5 mg PO daily for 23 days, followed by 5 days without drug.

➤ **Moderate to severe vasomotor symptoms from menopause**

Women: Start with Divigel 0.25 g daily and adjust dosage based on patient response (range, up to 1.25 g/day). Or, 1 pump per day of Elestrin applied to the upper arm. Or, Evamist 1 spray per day initially; may adjust dose based on clinical response (1 to 3 sprays/day). Or, 0.05 to 0.1 mg daily by vaginal ring. Replace vaginal ring every 3 months. Or, 1.25 g EstroGel applied once daily to arm.

ADMINISTRATION

PO

- Give without regard for food. If stomach upset occurs, give with food.
- Store at controlled room temperature.

IM

- To give IM injection, make sure drug is well dispersed by rolling vial between palms.
- Visually inspect solution to ensure that it's clear and colorless to pale yellow. If solution is stored at low temperature, some crystals may form that redissolve readily with warming.
- Inject deep into upper outer quadrant of the gluteal muscle. Rotate injection sites to prevent muscle atrophy. Never give IV.

Transdermal

- Apply Elestrin once daily to the upper arm.
- Apply EstroGel over the entire area of one arm on the inside and outside from wrist to shoulder. Don't massage or rub EstroGel. Patient should allow gel to dry for 5 minutes before getting dressed.
- Apply Evamist each morning to adjacent, nonoverlapping areas on the inner surface of the forearm, starting near the elbow. Allow to dry for 2 minutes and do not wash the site for 30 minutes.
- Apply Divigel once daily on skin of either right or left upper thigh. Application surface area should be about 5 by 7 inches (about 12.5 by 18 cm; about the size of two palm prints). Apply entire contents of a unit-dose packet each day. To avoid potential skin irritation, apply

Divigel to right or left upper thigh on alternating days. Don't apply Divigel on face, breasts, or irritated skin, or in or around the vagina. After application, allow gel to dry before dressing. Don't wash application site within 1 hour after applying Divigel. Avoid contact of gel with eyes. Wash hands after application.
• Apply transdermal patch to clean, dry, hairless, intact skin on abdomen or buttock. Don't apply to breasts, waistline, or other areas where clothing can loosen patch. When applying, ensure thorough contact between patch and skin, especially around edges, and hold in place for about 10 seconds. Apply patch immediately after opening and removing protective cover. Rotate application sites.
• Dispose of patches by folding adhesive ends together and discarding properly in trash away from children and pets.

Vaginal
• Using the applicator, insert vaginal tablet as far into vagina as it can comfortably go, without using force.
• Remove vaginal ring from its pouch. Squeeze sides together and insert ring into vagina where comfortable.
• Rinse vaginal ring in lukewarm water and reinsert if ring falls out or is removed before end of treatment.
• Attach applicator to vaginal cream tube and squeeze tube from the bottom to expel prescribed amount of cream into applicator. Remove applicator from tube and insert deeply into the vagina. Press plunger downward to its original position.
• Cleanse vaginal cream applicator by washing in mild soap and water; allow it to dry thoroughly.

ACTION

Increases synthesis of DNA, RNA, and protein in responsive tissues; reduces release of FSH and LH from the pituitary gland.

Route	Onset	Peak	Duration
PO, IM, vaginal	Unknown	Unknown	Unknown
Transdermal gel (EstroGel)	Immediate	1 hr	24–36 hr

Half-life: Alora transdermal patch, 1.75 ± 2.87 hours; Vivelle transdermal patch, 4.4 ± 2.3 hours; Vivelle-Dot transdermal patch, 5.9 to 7.7 hours; other forms, unknown. Estradiol apparent elimination half-life, 21 to 26 hours. Estradiol apparent terminal half-life, about 10 hours after Divigel administration.

ADVERSE REACTIONS

CNS: *stroke,* headache, migraine, pain, asthenia, dizziness, fatigue, anxiety, nervousness, mood disturbance, irritability, dementia, chorea, depression, *seizure exacerbation.* **CV:** thrombophlebitis, *thromboembolism,* HTN, edema, *DVT, PE, MI.* **EENT:** worsening myopia or astigmatism, intolerance of contact lenses, retinal thrombosis, sinusitis, nasopharyngitis. **GI:** nausea, vomiting, abdominal pain or cramps, bloating, constipation, flatulence, gastroenteritis, *pancreatitis,* gallbladder disease, dyspepsia. **GU:** UTI, breakthrough bleeding, altered menstrual flow, dysmenorrhea, *endometrial cancer,* cervical erosion (ring), altered cervical secretions, uterine pain, enlargement of uterine fibromas, vaginal candidiasis, genital pruritus, vaginal discomfort, vaginal discharge, vaginitis. **Hepatic:** cholestatic jaundice. **Metabolic:** weight gain, hypothyroidism, hypercalcemia (in patients with breast cancer and bone metastases). **Musculoskeletal:** arthralgia, back pain, myalgia, neck pain, limb pain, fractures. **Respiratory:** URI, asthma exacerbation, bronchitis. **Skin:** application-site reaction, acne, rash, melasma, erythema nodosum, dermatitis, hair loss, hirsutism, pruritus. **Other:** gynecomastia, *breast cancer,* hot flashes, breast tenderness or enlargement, nipple pain or discharge, flulike syndrome, accidental injury.

INTERACTIONS

Drug-drug. *Anastrozole:* May interfere with anastrozole effectiveness. Avoid use together.
Carbamazepine, fosphenytoin, phenobarbital, phenytoin, rifampin: May decrease effectiveness of estrogen therapy. Monitor patient closely.
Clarithromycin, erythromycin, itraconazole, ketoconazole, ritonavir: May increase estrogen plasma levels and side effects. Monitor patient.
Corticosteroids: May enhance effects of corticosteroids. Monitor patient closely.
Cyclosporine: May increase risk of toxicity. Use together with caution, and monitor cyclosporine level frequently.
Dantrolene, other hepatotoxic drugs: May increase risk of hepatotoxicity. Monitor liver function closely.
Exemestane: May interfere with exemestane effectiveness. Avoid use together.

Oral anticoagulants: May decrease anticoagulant effect. Dosage adjustments may be needed. Monitor PT and INR.

Ospemifene: May enhance adverse or toxic effects of ospemifene and interfere with its effectiveness. Avoid use together.

Thyroid hormones: May decrease therapeutic effect. Monitor therapy.

Drug-herb. *Red clover:* May increase estrogen effects. Discourage use together.

Saw palmetto: May negate drug's effects. Discourage use together.

St. John's wort: May decrease effects of drug. Discourage use together.

Drug-food. *Caffeine:* May increase caffeine level. Advise patient to avoid or minimize use of caffeine.

Folic acid: May decrease absorption of folic acid. Monitor levels.

Grapefruit juice: May elevate drug level. Tell patient to take drug with liquid other than grapefruit juice.

Drug-lifestyle. *Alcohol use:* May increase estrogen level and risk of breast cancer and osteoporosis. Avoid concurrent use.

Smoking: May increase risk of adverse CV effects. If smoking continues, may need another therapy.

EFFECTS ON LAB TEST RESULTS

- May increase LFT values and total T_4, thyroid-binding globulin, HDL, and triglyceride levels.
- May decrease LDL level.
- May increase platelet count.
- May alter clotting factors.
- May accelerate PT, PTT, and platelet aggregation times.
- May decrease metyrapone test results. May impair glucose tolerance.

CONTRAINDICATIONS & CAUTIONS

- Contraindicated in patients with active or history of thrombophlebitis or thromboembolic disorders, estrogen-dependent neoplasia, breast or reproductive organ cancer, or undiagnosed abnormal genital bleeding.
- Contraindicated in patients with protein C, protein S, or antithrombin deficiency or other known thrombophilic disorders.
- Contraindicated in patients with liver dysfunction or disease.
- Contraindicated in patients with known anaphylactic reaction or angioedema caused by drug. Exogenous estrogens may exacerbate signs and symptoms of angioedema in women with hereditary angioedema.
- Use cautiously in patients with cerebrovascular disease or CAD, asthma, bone disease, diabetes, gallbladder disease, hypothyroidism, porphyria, SLE, migraine, seizures, or cardiac or renal dysfunction.
- Use cautiously in patients with a strong family history (grandmother, mother, sister) of breast cancer, breast nodules, fibrocystic breasts, or abnormal mammogram findings.

Boxed Warning Patients ages 50 to 79 who are postmenopausal and are taking estrogen and progestin have an increased risk of MI, stroke, invasive breast cancer, PE, and thrombosis. Patients age 65 or older who are postmenopausal also have an increased risk of dementia. ▪

Dialyzable drug: Unknown.

⚠ *Overdose S&S:* Nausea, vomiting, withdrawal uterine bleeding.

PREGNANCY-LACTATION-REPRODUCTION

- Drug is contraindicated in pregnancy.
- Use of estrogen and progestin as in combination hormonal contraceptives hasn't been associated with teratogenic effects when inadvertently taken early in pregnancy.
- Estrogens have been shown to decrease quantity and quality of human milk. Estrogens can appear in human milk. Use only if clearly needed; closely monitor infant's growth.

NURSING CONSIDERATIONS

- Ensure that patient has physical exam before starting therapy. Patients receiving long-term therapy should have yearly exams. Monitor lipid levels, BP, body weight, and hepatic function.

Boxed Warning Estrogen increases the risk of endometrial cancer. Use adequate diagnostic measures, including endometrial sampling when indicated, to rule out malignancy in all cases of undiagnosed persistent or recurring abnormal vaginal bleeding. ▪

Boxed Warning Don't use estrogens with or without progestins to prevent CV disease or dementia. Use the lowest effective doses and for the shortest duration consistent with treatment goals. ▪

- When estrogen is prescribed for a patient with a uterus who is postmenopausal, also initiate a progestin to reduce risk of endometrial cancer.

• *Alert:* EstroGel contains alcohol. Avoid fire, flame, or smoking until area dries in 2 to 5 minutes.

• In patients also taking oral estrogen, treatment with the transdermal patch can begin 1 week after withdrawal of oral therapy, or sooner if menopausal symptoms appear before the end of the week.

• Transdermal systems may be used continually rather than cyclically in patients without an intact uterus. Other alternative regimens are 1 to 5 mg cypionate IM every 3 to 4 weeks and 10 to 20 mg valerate IM every 4 weeks, as needed.

• Prescriber should assess patient's need to continue estradiol therapy. Make attempts to stop or taper at 3- to 6-month intervals.

• Because of risk of thromboembolism, stop therapy at least 1 month before high-risk procedures or those that cause prolonged immobilization, such as knee or hip surgery.

• Glucose tolerance may be impaired. Monitor glucose level closely in patients with diabetes.

• Notify pathologist about estrogen therapy when sending specimens to the lab for evaluation.

PATIENT TEACHING

• Tell patient to read package insert describing estrogen's adverse effects and give her a verbal explanation of those effects.

• Emphasize importance of regular physical exams. Patients who are postmenopausal and use estrogen replacement for longer than 5 years may be at increased risk for endometrial cancer. Risk is reduced by using cyclic rather than continuous therapy and the lowest possible dosages of estrogen. Adding progestins to the regimen decreases risk of endometrial hyperplasia; however, it isn't known whether progestins affect risk of endometrial cancer. No increased risk of breast cancer has been reported.

Boxed Warning Advise patient not to allow contact between children and Evamist application site. Accidental exposure may cause breast budding and breast masses in prepubertal females and gynecomastia and breast masses in prepubertal males. Ensure children don't come in contact with application site. ∎

• Teach patient safe drug administration and to follow package insert for specific prescribed product.

• Instruct patient or caregiver how to inject estradiol valerate if able to administer.

• Caution patient using Vagifem who has severely atrophic vaginal mucosa to be careful when inserting applicator.

• After gynecologic surgery, tell patient to use any vaginal applicator cautiously and only if clearly indicated.

• *Alert:* Warn patient to immediately report abdominal pain, pressure or pain in chest, shortness of breath, severe headaches, visual disturbances, vaginal bleeding or discharge, breast lumps, swelling of hands or feet, yellow skin or sclera, dark urine, light-colored stools, and pain, numbness, or stiffness in legs or buttocks.

• Explain to patient receiving cyclic therapy for postmenopausal symptoms that withdrawal bleeding may occur during week off drug. Tell her to report unusual vaginal bleeding.

• Tell patient with diabetes to report elevated glucose level so that antidiabetic dosage can be adjusted.

• Teach patient how to perform routine breast self-exam.

• Teach patient methods to decrease risk of blood clots.

• Advise patient not to become pregnant during estrogen therapy.

• Encourage patient to stop or reduce smoking because of the risk of CV complications.

• Advise patient not to allow pets to lick or touch Evamist application site. If signs of illness occur, patient should contact pet's veterinarian.

estradiol–norethindrone acetate transdermal system

ess-tra-DYE-ole/nor-ETH-in-drone

CombiPatch

Therapeutic class: Estrogens
Pharmacologic class: Estrogen–progestin combinations

AVAILABLE FORMS

Transdermal: 9-cm^2 system releasing 0.05 mg estradiol and 0.14 mg norethindrone acetate daily; 16-cm^2 system releasing 0.05 mg estradiol and 0.25 mg norethindrone acetate daily

INDICATIONS & DOSAGES

➤ **Moderate to severe vasomotor symptoms from menopause; vulval and vaginal atrophy; hypoestrogenemia from hypogonadism, castration, or primary ovarian failure in patient with intact uterus**

Continuous combined regimen

Women: Wear 9-cm^2 patch system continuously on lower abdomen. Replace system twice weekly during 28-day cycle. May increase to 16-cm^2 patch.

Continuous sequential regimen

Women: For use in sequential regimen with an estradiol transdermal system (such as Alora, Vivelle), wear 0.05-mg estradiol transdermal patch for first 14 days of 28-day cycle; replace system twice weekly. Wear 9-cm^2 patch system on lower abdomen for rest of 28-day cycle; replace system according to product directions. May increase to 16-cm^2 patch.

ADMINISTRATION

Transdermal

• Apply patch system to a smooth (fold-free), clean, dry, nonirritated area of skin on lower abdomen, avoiding the waistline. Rotate application sites, with an interval of at least 1 week between applications to same site.

• Don't apply patch on or near breasts.

• Avoid applying to areas that may get prolonged sun exposure.

• Reapply patch, if needed, to another area of lower abdomen. If patch fails to adhere, replace with a new one in a different area.

• Remove patch slowly to avoid skin irritation and fold patch so that it sticks to itself. Discard in trash out of reach of children or pets. Don't flush down the toilet.

• Keep patch sealed until ready to apply.

ACTION

Estrogen replacement therapy can reduce menopausal symptoms and release of FSH and LH by binding to nuclear receptors in estrogen-responsive tissues in patients who are postmenopausal. Norethindrone blocks gonadotropin, which inhibits ovulation.

Route	Onset	Peak	Duration
Transdermal	12–24 hr	Unknown	Unknown

Half-life: Estradiol, 2 to 3 hours; norethindrone, 6 to 8 hours.

ADVERSE REACTIONS

CNS: asthenia, *stroke,* depression, insomnia, nervousness, dizziness, headache, weakness, pain. **CV:** *thromboembolism,* thrombophlebitis, HTN, edema, *DVT, PE, MI.* **EENT:** pharyngitis, rhinitis, sinusitis, tooth disorder, retinal vascular thrombosis, intolerance to contact lenses. **GI:** abdominal pain, diarrhea, dyspepsia, flatulence, nausea, constipation, gallbladder disease. **GU:** dysmenorrhea, leukorrhea, menstrual disorder, suspicious Papanicolaou smears, vaginitis, menorrhagia, *vaginal hemorrhage.* **Hepatic:** cholestatic jaundice. **Metabolic:** weight gain, hypercalcemia (in patients with breast cancer and bone metastases), hypertriglyceridemia. **Musculoskeletal:** arthralgia, back pain. **Respiratory:** respiratory disorder, bronchitis. **Skin:** application-site reactions, acne, rash, melasma, chloasma. **Other:** accidental injury, flulike syndrome, breast pain, breast enlargement, infection, changes in libido.

INTERACTIONS

Drug-drug. *Anastrozole:* May interfere with anastrozole effectiveness. Avoid using together.

Carbamazepine, fosphenytoin, phenobarbital, phenytoin, rifampin: May decrease estrogen therapy effectiveness. Monitor patient closely.

Clarithromycin, erythromycin, itraconazole, ketoconazole, ritonavir: May increase estrogen plasma levels and side effects. Monitor patient.

Corticosteroids: May enhance effects of corticosteroids. Monitor patient closely.

Cyclosporine: May increase risk of toxicity. Use together with caution; monitor cyclosporine level frequently.

Dantrolene, hepatotoxic drugs: May increase risk of hepatotoxicity. Monitor liver function closely.

Exemestane: May interfere with exemestane effectiveness. Avoid use together.

Oral anticoagulants: May decrease effect of anticoagulant. May need to adjust dose. Monitor PT and INR.

Ospemifene: May enhance adverse or toxic effects of ospemifene and interfere with its effectiveness. Avoid use together.

Drug-herb. *Red clover:* May increase estrogen effects. Discourage together use.

Saw palmetto: May cause antiestrogenic effects. Discourage use together.

Reactions in bold italics are *life-threatening*. Interactions may have a *rapid onset* or a ***delayed onset***.

St. John's wort: May decrease effects of drug. Discourage use together.

Drug-food. *Caffeine:* May increase caffeine level. Advise patient to avoid or minimize use of caffeine.

Folic acid: May decrease absorption of folic acid. Monitor levels.

Grapefruit juice: May elevate estrogen level. Advise patient to take with liquid other than grapefruit juice.

Drug-lifestyle. *Alcohol use:* May increase estrogen level and risk of breast cancer and osteoporosis. Avoid concurrent use.

Smoking: May increase risk of adverse CV effects. If smoking continues, may need alternative therapy.

Sun exposure: May cause photosensitivity reactions. Don't expose patch to the sun for long periods of time.

EFFECTS ON LAB TEST RESULTS

• May increase T_3 and T_4, HDL, and triglyceride and transaminase levels.
• May decrease LDL level.
• May increase fibrinogen activity and platelet count.
• May decrease T_3 resin uptake.
• May accelerate PT, PTT, and platelet aggregation times.
• May reduce response to metyrapone test. May alter glucose tolerance test results.

CONTRAINDICATIONS & CAUTIONS

• Contraindicated in patients hypersensitive to estrogen, progestin, or any component of the patch and in patients with known or suspected breast cancer, known or suspected estrogen-dependent neoplasia, known anaphylactic reaction or angioedema, known hepatic impairment or disease, undiagnosed abnormal genital bleeding, active thrombophlebitis, or thromboembolic disorders, including MI, DVT, PE, or stroke.
▧ Contraindicated in patients with known protein C, protein S, or antithrombin deficiency, or other known thrombophilic disorders.
Boxed Warning Don't use estrogens, with or without progestins, to prevent CV disease or dementia. Use drug with or without progestins at the lowest effective doses and for the shortest duration consistent with treatment goals. ∎
Boxed Warning Patients ages 50 to 79 who are postmenopausal and taking estrogen and progestin have an increased risk of MI, stroke,

invasive breast cancer, PE, and DVT. Patients age 65 and older who are postmenopausal also have an increased risk of dementia. ∎
▧ Exogenous estrogens may exacerbate signs and symptoms of angioedema in patients with hereditary angioedema.
• Use cautiously in patients with asthma, epilepsy, migraine, SLE, porphyria, diabetes, hepatic hemangiomas, or cardiac or renal dysfunction.
Dialyzable drug: Unknown.
⚠ *Overdose S&S:* Nausea, withdrawal bleeding.

PREGNANCY-LACTATION-REPRODUCTION

• Contraindicated during pregnancy.
• Estrogen has been shown to appear in and decrease quantity and quality of human milk. Use cautiously during breastfeeding.

NURSING CONSIDERATIONS

• Treatment of postmenopausal symptoms usually starts during menopausal stage when vasomotor symptoms occur.
• A combined estrogen–progestin regimen is indicated for a patient with an intact uterus. Progestins taken with estrogen significantly reduce, but don't eliminate, risk of endometrial cancer linked to use of estrogen alone.
Boxed Warning Estrogen increases risk of endometrial cancer. Adding a progestin to estrogen therapy reduces risk of endometrial hyperplasia. For patient who is postmenopausal, use adequate diagnostic measures, including endometrial sampling when indicated, to rule out malignancy if undiagnosed persistent or recurring abnormal vaginal bleeding occurs. ∎
• Patients not receiving continuous estrogen or combined estrogen–progestin therapy may start therapy at any time.
• Patients receiving continuous hormone replacement therapy should complete the current cycle before starting therapy. Patients commonly have withdrawal bleeding at completion of cycle; first day of withdrawal bleeding is an appropriate time to start therapy.
• Reevaluate therapy at 3- to 6-month intervals.
• Because of risk of thromboembolism, stop therapy at least 4 to 6 weeks before surgery associated with an increased risk of thromboembolism, or during periods of prolonged immobilization.
• BP increases have been linked to estrogen use. Monitor patient's BP regularly.
• Monitor glucose level closely in patients with diabetes.

⟲ *Alert:* Don't interchange CombiPatch with other estrogen patches. Verify therapy before application.

PATIENT TEACHING

• Teach patient how to properly apply, remove, and dispose of patch.
• Tell patient that an oil-based cream or lotion may help remove adhesive from the skin after patch has been removed and the area allowed to dry for 15 minutes.
• Advise patient not to use patch if pregnant or planning to become pregnant.
• Instruct patient that the continuous combined regimen may lead to irregular bleeding, particularly in the first 6 months, but that it usually decreases with time and often stops completely.
• Tell patient that, for the continuous sequential regimen, monthly withdrawal bleeding is common.
• Advise patient to alert prescriber and remove patch at first sign of clotting disorders (thrombophlebitis, cerebrovascular disorders, PE).
• Instruct patient to stop using patch and call prescriber about any loss of vision, sudden onset of protrusion of the eyeball (proptosis), double vision, or migraine.
• Encourage patient to stop or reduce smoking because of the risk of CV complications.
• Tell patient to perform monthly breast self-exams and to have annual gynecologic and breast exams by a health care provider.
• Tell patient undergoing an MRI to alert facility that she's using a transdermal patch.

---

estradiol–progesterone ⚕

ES-tra-dye-ole/proe-JES-te-rone

Bijuva

Therapeutic class: Menopause drugs
Pharmacologic class: Estrogen–progestin combinations

AVAILABLE FORMS

Capsules: 1 mg estradiol/100 mg progesterone

INDICATIONS & DOSAGES

➤ **Moderate to severe vasomotor symptoms due to menopause**

Patients with intact uterus: 1 capsule PO once daily.

ADMINISTRATION
PO

• Give with food in the evening.
• Give a missed dose as soon as possible unless it's within 2 hours of the next dose.
• Store at 68° to 77° F (20° to 25° C).

ACTION

Circulating estrogens modulate the pituitary secretion of the gonadotropins LH and FSH through a negative feedback mechanism. Estrogens reduce the elevated levels of these hormones seen in patients who are postmenopausal. Progesterone opposes the action of estrogen by decreasing estrogen receptor levels, increasing the metabolism of estrogen to less active metabolites, or blunting the response to estrogen at the cellular level.

Route	Onset	Peak	Duration
PO	Unknown	Estradiol, 5 hr; progesterone, 3 hr	Unknown

Half-life: Estradiol, 26 hours; progesterone, 10 hours.

ADVERSE REACTIONS

CNS: headache. **GU:** vaginal bleeding, vaginal discharge, pelvic pain. **Other:** breast tenderness.

INTERACTIONS

Drug-drug. *CYP3A4 inducers (carbamazepine, phenobarbital, rifampin):* May decrease estrogen and progestin levels, decreasing therapeutic effect and causing changes in uterine bleeding. Monitor patient closely.
CYP3A4 inhibitors (clarithromycin, erythromycin, itraconazole, ketoconazole, ritonavir): May increase estrogen and progestin levels and increase adverse effects. Monitor patient closely.
Drug-herb. *St. John's wort:* May decrease estrogen and progestin levels, decreasing therapeutic effect and causing changes in uterine bleeding. Monitor patient closely.
Drug-food. *Grapefruit juice:* May increase plasma concentrations of estrogens and progestins. Discourage use together.
Drug-lifestyle. *Smoking:* May increase risk of adverse CV effects. Discourage use

---

Reactions in bold italics are *life-threatening*. Interactions may have a *rapid onset* or a ***delayed onset***.

together. If smoking continues, consider alternative therapy.

EFFECTS ON LAB TEST RESULTS
• May increase HDL and triglyceride levels.
• May decrease LDL level.
• May increase or decrease calcium level.
• May accelerate PT, PTT, and platelet aggregation time.
• May increase platelet count and clotting factors.
• May decrease antifactor Xa and antithrombin III levels.
• May increase fibrinogen and plasminogen levels and activity.
• May increase circulating total thyroid hormone levels, corticosteroid binding globulin levels, sex hormone-binding globulin levels, free testosterone levels, free estradiol levels, and other plasma protein tests.
• May impair glucose tolerance.

CONTRAINDICATIONS & CAUTIONS
• Contraindicated in patients with undiagnosed abnormal genital bleeding; known, suspected, or history of breast cancer; known or suspected estrogen-dependent neoplasia; active DVT, PE, arterial thromboembolic disease, or history of these conditions; known anaphylactic reaction, angioedema, or hypersensitivity to estrogen or progesterone or capsule ingredients; or known liver impairment or disease.
▧ Contraindicated in patients with known protein C, protein S, or antithrombin deficiency, or other known thrombophilic disorders.
Boxed Warning Patients ages 50 to 79 who are postmenopausal and are taking estrogen and progestin have an increased risk of DVT, PE, stroke, MI, and invasive breast cancer. Patients age 65 and older who are postmenopausal also have an increased risk of developing probable dementia. ∎
Boxed Warning There is an increased risk of endometrial cancer in patients with a uterus who use unopposed estrogen. Adding a progestin to estrogen therapy has been shown to reduce the risk of endometrial hyperplasia, which may be a precursor to endometrial cancer. ∎
Boxed Warning Estrogen plus progestin therapy should not be used for the prevention of CV disease or dementia. ∎

Boxed Warning Use the lowest effective dose and for the shortest duration consistent with treatment goals and individual risks. Reevaluate patients periodically as clinically appropriate to determine if treatment is still necessary. ∎
• Estrogen therapy may cause retinal vascular thrombosis.
• Drug may increase risk of gallbladder disease after menopause.
• Drug may increase risk of pancreatitis in patients with preexisting hypertriglyceridemia. If pancreatitis occurs, consider discontinuing drug.
• Drug may be poorly metabolized by patients with impaired liver function. Use cautiously in patients with a history of cholestatic jaundice associated with estrogen use or with pregnancy. If cholestatic jaundice recurs, discontinue drug.
• Use cautiously in patients with a history of asthma, diabetes, cardiac or renal dysfunction, epilepsy, migraine headaches, porphyria, SLE, hepatic hemangiomas, or hereditary angioedema, as estrogen therapy may exacerbate these conditions.
• Drug isn't indicated for use in children.
Dialyzable drug: Unknown.
⚠ *Overdose S&S:* Nausea, vomiting, breast tenderness, abdominal pain, drowsiness, fatigue, withdrawal bleeding.

PREGNANCY-LACTATION-REPRODUCTION
• Drug isn't indicated for use in pregnancy or in patients of childbearing potential.
• Estrogens appear in human milk and can decrease milk production in patients who are breastfeeding.

NURSING CONSIDERATIONS
Boxed Warning Assess patients who are postmenopausal with undiagnosed persistent or recurring abnormal genital bleeding to rule out malignancy. ∎
• Assess baseline risk of breast cancer and CV disease before starting drug.
• Monitor BP, fluid status, lipid levels, LFT values, and thyroid function during therapy as clinically indicated. Patients on thyroid replacement therapy may require a higher dose of thyroid hormone.
• Monitor calcium level in patients with breast cancer and bone metastases. Discontinue drug for hypercalcemia and treat calcium level as appropriate.

E

- Ensure that patient receives age-appropriate breast and pelvic exams.
- Monitor patient for vision abnormalities. If sudden partial or complete loss of vision, or a sudden onset of proptosis, diplopia, or migraine occurs, discontinue drug and obtain eye exam. If eye exam reveals papilledema or retinal vascular lesions, permanently discontinue drug.
- Discontinue estrogen therapy at least 4 to 6 weeks before surgery when there is an increased risk of thromboembolism, or during periods of prolonged immobilization.
- *Look alike–sound alike:* Don't confuse this product with other estrogen or progesterone products.

PATIENT TEACHING
- Teach patient safe drug administration and to report all adverse reactions.

Boxed Warning Warn patient of possible serious adverse reactions related to drug, including CV disorders, malignant neoplasms, and age-related probable dementia. ■

- Instruct patient to immediately report abnormal vaginal bleeding; new breast lumps; changes in vision or speech; sudden, new headaches; severe chest or leg pain with or without shortness of breath; weakness and fatigue; or vomiting.
- Instruct patient that drug may need to be stopped before surgery or if patient will be on bed rest.
- Tell patient that prescriber will evaluate continued need for treatment every 3 to 6 months.
- Teach patient that she should have yearly pelvic and breast exams and mammograms unless otherwise directed by prescriber.

---

estradiol valerate–estradiol valerate with dienogest ▧
ess-tra-DYE-ole VAL-er-ate/ dye-EN-oh-jest

Natazia

Therapeutic class: Estrogens
Pharmacologic class: Estrogen–progestin combinations

AVAILABLE FORMS
Tablets: 28-day blister pack containing two 3-mg estradiol valerate, five 2-mg estradiol valerate with 2-mg dienogest, seventeen 2-mg estradiol valerate with 3-mg dienogest, two 1-mg estradiol valerate, and two inert tablets

INDICATIONS & DOSAGES
➤ **Contraception; treatment of heavy menstrual bleeding in patients without organic pathology who choose to use an oral contraceptive as their method of contraception**
Women: 1 tablet PO daily beginning on first day of menstrual cycle (first day of menstrual bleeding) in order directed on blister pack at same time each day. When changing from another combination hormonal contraceptive, begin on first day of withdrawal bleeding. When changing from combination hormonal vaginal ring or transdermal patch, begin on day vaginal ring or transdermal patch is removed. When changing from progestin-only contraceptive, begin on day patient would have taken the next progestin-only pill. When changing from implant contraceptive or intrauterine system, begin day of implant or intrauterine system removal. When changing from injection contraceptive, begin day next injection is due.

ADMINISTRATION
PO
- Give at same time each day; don't skip or delay intake by more than 12 hours.
- Follow manufacturer's detailed instructions if 1 or 2 tablets are missed; patient should use additional backup nonhormonal forms of contraception if necessary.
- If patient experiences severe vomiting or diarrhea within 3 to 4 hours after taking a colored tablet, treat as a missed tablet.
- Must give tablets in order indicated on blister pack.

ACTION
Prevents pregnancy by suppressing ovulation. May also cause changes in endometrium and cervical mucus, inhibiting sperm penetration and reducing likelihood of implantation.

Route	Onset	Peak	Duration
PO	Unknown	3 hr (estradiol); 1.5 hr (dienogest)	Unknown

Half-life: Estradiol, 14 hours; dienogest, 11 hours.

ADVERSE REACTIONS
CNS: mood changes (depression, mood swings, dysthymic disorder, crying),

---

Reactions in bold italics are *life-threatening*. Interactions may have a *rapid onset* or a ***delayed onset***.

headache, migraine, dizziness. **CV: *venous and arterial thromboembolic events (MI, DVT, PE, stroke, cerebral thrombosis),*** HTN, fluid retention. **GI:** nausea, vomiting, gallbladder disease, GI symptoms (abdominal pain). **GU:** menstrual disorder, amenorrhea, irregular uterine bleeding, metrorrhagia, oligomenorrhea, uterine leiomyoma, vulvovaginal candidiasis, *ruptured ovarian cyst.* **Hepatic:** *hepatitis.* **Metabolic:** hypertriglyceridemia, weight gain, hyperglycemia. **Skin:** acne, chloasma, erythema nodosum, erythema multiforme. **Other:** breast pain, tenderness, or discomfort; hypersensitivity reaction.

INTERACTIONS
Drug-drug. *Antibiotics:* May reduce contraceptive effectiveness. Advise use of backup contraception during therapy.
HIV protease inhibitors, NNRTIs: May either increase or decrease estrogen and progesterone levels. Use together cautiously and monitor patient for effectiveness of hormone treatment.
Lamotrigine: May decrease lamotrigine serum level, reducing seizure control. Adjust lamotrigine dosage as necessary.
Strong CYP3A4 inducers (barbiturates, carbamazepine, felbamate, griseofulvin, oxcarbazepine, phenytoin, rifampin, topiramate): May reduce contraceptive effectiveness or increase breakthrough bleeding. An alternative method of birth control should be used.
Strong and moderate inhibitors of CYP3A4 (cimetidine, clarithromycin, diltiazem, erythromycin, fluconazole, itraconazole, ketoconazole, SSRIs, verapamil, voriconazole): May increase levels of hormones. Avoid use together. If drugs must be used together, monitor patient for adverse effects.
Thyroid hormone: May increase serum concentration of thyroid-binding globulin, leading to decreased effectiveness of thyroid replacement therapy. Monitor patient; thyroid hormone dosage may need adjustment.
Drug-herb. *Red clover:* May increase estrogen effects. Discourage use together.
St. John's wort: May reduce contraceptive effectiveness or increase breakthrough bleeding. Recommend alternative method of birth control.
Drug-food. *Grapefruit juice:* May increase levels of hormones. Avoid use together.
Drug-lifestyle. **Boxed Warning** *Smoking:* Increases risk of serious CV events, such as

stroke, emboli, or heart disease. Recommend smoking cessation. ∎

EFFECTS ON LAB TEST RESULTS
• May increase thyroid-binding globulin, glucose, cholesterol, and lipid levels.
• May alter clotting factors.
• May affect glucose tolerance test results.

CONTRAINDICATIONS & CAUTIONS
• Contraindicated in patients with benign or malignant liver tumors; liver disease; current or history of breast cancer or other estrogen- or progestin-sensitive cancer; undiagnosed abnormal uterine bleeding; headaches with focal neurologic symptoms or migraine headaches with or without aura if older than age 35; diabetes with vascular disease; uncontrolled HTN; HTN with vascular disease; thrombogenic valvular or thrombogenic rhythm disease of heart, such as endocarditis or atrial fibrillation; CAD; cerebrovascular disease; and current or past DVT or PE.
▨ Contraindicated in patients with inherited or acquired hypercoagulopathies.
Boxed Warning Contraindicated in patients who smoke and who are older than age 35. ∎
• Use cautiously in females with CV disease risk factors, history of cholestasis, history of well-controlled HTN, prediabetes or well-controlled diabetes, history of hyperlipidemia, new-onset headaches, history of bleeding irregularities, history of emotional disorders, angioedema, or chloasma.
▨ Exogenous estrogens may exacerbate signs and symptoms of angioedema in patients with hereditary angioedema.
• Use isn't recommended in patients with complicated solid organ transplant or SLE.
• Safety and effectiveness in women with BMI greater than 30 kg/m² haven't been evaluated.
• Drug hasn't been studied in patients who are postmenopausal and isn't indicated in this population.
Dialyzable drug: Unknown.
⚠ **Overdose S&S:** Nausea, withdrawal bleeding.

PREGNANCY-LACTATION-REPRODUCTION
• Contraindicated during pregnancy.
• There is little or no increased risk of birth defects in patients who inadvertently use combined oral contraceptives during early pregnancy.

• Estrogen has been shown to decrease quantity and quality of human milk. Drug shouldn't be used during breastfeeding.
• Use before menarche isn't indicated.

NURSING CONSIDERATIONS

• Start drug no earlier than 4 weeks after delivery in patients who aren't breast-feeding. Risk of postpartum venous thromboembolic event (VTE) decreases and ovulation risk increases after third postpartum week.
• Monitor BP; elevations are possible in women who are nonhypertensive.
• Monitor coagulation factors as appropriate.
• Monitor glucose and cholesterol levels regularly, especially in women who are prediabetic and in those with history of elevated lipid levels.
• Monitor patients for headache. New-onset headaches may require discontinuing oral contraceptives.
• Carefully monitor patients with a history of depression for recurrence or exacerbation.
• Stop drug if arterial or deep VTE occurs. Highest risk of VTE occurs during first year of contraceptive use. If feasible, stop tablets at least 4 weeks before and for 2 weeks after major surgery.
• Oral contraceptives are associated with increased risk of thrombotic and hemorrhagic strokes, especially in females older than age 35, in those with HTN, and in smokers. Stop drug if unexplained vision loss, proptosis, diplopia, papilledema, or retinal vascular changes occur. Evaluate retinal vein thrombosis immediately.
• Risk of drug causing breast, cervical, or endometrial cancer remains controversial and uncertain. As a precaution, patients should have regular Papanicolaou tests, breast exams, and mammograms.
• Discontinue drug if jaundice develops. Patients who take oral contraceptives are at slightly higher risk for developing liver tumors and gallstones. Monitor patient for skin color changes and pain in right upper quadrant.
• Ensure that patient uses a nonhormonal contraceptive method, such as a condom or spermicide, for the first 9 days.

PATIENT TEACHING

• Teach patient safe drug administration and to read the patient guide for information on missed tablets and when to contact pharmacist or prescriber; tell patient that backup contraception must be used.
• Tell patient starting drug for first time to begin taking tablets on day 1 of menses and to use backup contraceptive method for first 9 days.
• Inform patient that spotting or light bleeding may occur at first.
• Advise patient that nausea is possible, especially during first few months, but that this symptom usually disappears and that patient shouldn't stop taking tablets. Tell patient to report to prescriber if nausea doesn't resolve.
• Warn patient to start drug no earlier than 4 weeks after giving birth.
• Advise patient to notify prescriber if pregnant before taking drug.
• Tell patient that breastfeeding while taking tablets isn't recommended because milk production may be reduced and small amounts of drug appear in human milk.
• Inform patient taking tablets that blood tests may be needed to assess blood clotting and blood glucose and cholesterol levels, and that BP monitoring may be needed.
• Tell patient to inform prescriber if taking prescription or OTC medications or herbal supplements.
• Advise patient, if appropriate, to quit smoking before taking drug.

Boxed Warning Advise patient who smokes of the increased risk of serious CV events from combination oral contraceptive use. Risk increases with age, especially after age 35, and with number of cigarettes smoked. ■

• Warn patient that contraceptive use doesn't protect against HIV infection or other sexually transmitted diseases.
• Tell patient that a missed period may occur but that pregnancy should be ruled out for two or more consecutive missed menstrual cycles.
• Advise patient to immediately report persistent leg pain; sudden shortness of breath; sudden blindness (partial or complete); severe chest pain; sudden, severe headache; weakness or numbness in an arm or leg; trouble speaking; or yellowing of skin or eyes.
• Inform patient with tendency to chloasma to avoid sun exposure and UV radiation.

Reactions in bold italics are *life-threatening*. Interactions may have a *rapid onset* or a *delayed onset*.

estrogens (conjugated) (estrogenic substances, conjugated; oestrogens, conjugated) ▨
Premarin♦

Therapeutic class: Estrogens
Pharmacologic class: Estrogens

AVAILABLE FORMS
Injection: 25-mg vial
Tablets: 0.3 mg, 0.45 mg, 0.625 mg, 0.9 mg, 1.25 mg
Vaginal cream: 0.625 mg/g

INDICATIONS & DOSAGES
➤ **Abnormal uterine bleeding (hormonal imbalance)**
Women: 25 mg slow IV (preferred) or IM. Repeat dose in 6 to 12 hours, if necessary.
➤ **Vulvar or vaginal atrophy; kraurosis vulvae**
Women: 0.5 to 2 g cream intravaginally once daily in cycles of 21 days on, 7 days off.
➤ **Moderate to severe dyspareunia due to menopause-related vulvar and vaginal atrophy**
Women: 0.5 g cream intravaginally twice weekly as a continuous regimen. Or, 0.5 g intravaginally once daily for 21 days followed by 7 days off.
➤ **Hypoestrogenism due to castration or primary ovarian failure**
Women: Initially, 1.25 mg PO daily in cycles of 3 weeks on, 1 week off. Adjust dose as needed.
➤ **Hypoestrogenism due to female hypogonadism**
Women: 0.3 to 0.625 mg PO daily, given cyclically 3 weeks on, 1 week off. Adjust dose depending on symptom severity and responsiveness of the endometrium.
➤ **Moderate to severe vasomotor symptoms with or without moderate to severe symptoms of vulvar and vaginal atrophy associated with menopause**
Women: Initially, 0.3 mg PO daily. May also give cyclically 25 days on, 5 days off. Adjust dosage based on patient response.
➤ **To prevent osteoporosis**
Women: 0.3 mg PO daily, or cyclically 25 days on, 5 days off. Adjust dose based on response of bone mineral density testing.
➤ **Palliative treatment of inoperable prostatic cancer**
Men: 1.25 to 2.5 mg PO t.i.d. Judge effectiveness based on phosphatase determinations and symptomatic improvement.
➤ **Palliative treatment of breast cancer**
Adults (men and women): 10 mg PO t.i.d. for at least 3 months.

ADMINISTRATION
PO
- Give drug at same time each day.
- May give with or without food.
- Store tablets at controlled room temperature.

IV
▼ IV use is preferred over IM because a more rapid response can be expected.
▼ Refrigerate before reconstituting.
▼ Store injection in refrigerator (36° to 46° F [2° to 8° C]).
▼ Reconstitute slowly with 5 mL sterile water for injection. Gently agitate; don't shake.
▼ Drug is compatible with NSS and dextrose and invert sugar solutions.
▼ Use solutions immediately after reconstitution.
▼ Give direct injection slowly to avoid flushing reaction.
▼ **Incompatibilities:** Acidic solutions, ascorbic acid, protein hydrolysate.

IM
- Reconstitute with sterile water for injection. Agitate gently after adding diluent.
- Inject deep into large muscle. Rotate injection sites to prevent muscle atrophy.

Vaginal
- Wash the vaginal area with soap and water, insert about two-thirds the length of the applicator into the vagina, and release drug.
- Give drug at bedtime or when patient will lie flat for 30 minutes after use to minimize drug loss.
- Store cream at controlled room temperature.

ACTION
Increases synthesis of DNA, RNA, and protein in responsive tissues. Also reduces release of FSH and LH from the pituitary gland.

Route	Onset	Peak	Duration
PO, IV, IM, vaginal	Unknown	7 hr	Unknown

Half-life: 27 hours.

ADVERSE REACTIONS
CNS: headache, pain, dizziness, chorea, migraine, depression, nervousness, *stroke,*

exacerbation of seizures. **CV:** flushing with rapid IV administration; vasodilation, thrombophlebitis, *thromboembolism,* HTN, edema, *PE, MI.* **EENT:** worsening myopia or astigmatism, intolerance of contact lenses. **GI:** nausea, vomiting, abdominal pain or cramps, bloating, flatulence, diarrhea, *pancreatitis,* gallbladder disease. **GU:** *vaginal hemorrhage,* breakthrough bleeding, altered menstrual flow, dysmenorrhea, amenorrhea, leukorrhea, *endometrial cancer,* altered cervical secretions, enlargement of uterine fibromas, vaginal candidiasis, vaginitis, vulvovaginal disorder, dysuria, urinary frequency, impotence. **Hepatic:** cholestatic jaundice. **Metabolic:** weight gain, hypercalcemia, hypertriglyceridemia. **Musculoskeletal:** arthralgia, back pain, muscle cramps, myalgia. **Respiratory:** *asthma exacerbation.* **Skin:** chloasma, acne, erythema, pruritus, rash, urticaria, hirsutism or hair loss, erythema nodosum, *erythema multiforme.* **Other:** breast tenderness or secretion; gynecomastia; *breast cancer;* changes in libido.

INTERACTIONS

Drug-drug. *Anastrozole:* May interfere with anastrozole effectiveness. Avoid use together.
Corticosteroids: May enhance corticosteroid effects. Monitor patient closely.
Cyclosporine: May increase risk of toxicity. Use together with caution, and monitor cyclosporine level frequently.
CYP3A4 inducers (carbamazepine, fosphenytoin, phenobarbital, phenytoin, rifampin): May decrease effectiveness of estrogen therapy. Monitor patient closely.
CYP3A4 inhibitors (itraconazole, ketoconazole, macrolide antibiotics, ritonavir): May increase estrogen plasma levels and risk of adverse effects. Monitor patient.
Dantrolene, other hepatotoxic drugs: May increase risk of hepatotoxicity. Monitor liver function closely.
Exemestane: May interfere with exemestane effectiveness. Avoid use together.
Oral anticoagulants: May decrease anticoagulant effects. May need to adjust dosage. Monitor PT and INR.
Ospemifene: May enhance adverse or toxic effects of ospemifene and interfere with its effectiveness. Avoid use together.
Thyroid hormones: May increase serum thyroxine-binding globulin levels, which may increase thyroid hormone requirements.

Drug-herb. *Red clover:* May increase estrogen effects. Discourage use together.
Saw palmetto: May have antiestrogenic effects. Discourage use together.
St. John's wort: May decrease effects of drug. Discourage use together.
Drug-food. *Caffeine:* May increase caffeine level. Advise caution.
Grapefruit juice: May increase concentration of estrogen. Avoid using together.
Drug-lifestyle. *Smoking:* May increase risk of adverse CV effects. Recommend smoking cessation. If smoking continues, recommend nonhormonal contraception.

EFFECTS ON LAB TEST RESULTS

• May increase T_3 and total T_4, phospholipid, thyroid-binding globulin, HDL, and triglyceride levels.
• May decrease LDL level.
• May increase platelet count.
• May alter clotting factors.
• May accelerate PT, PTT, and platelet aggregation.
• May cause a false-positive metyrapone test result.
• May interfere with glucose tolerance test.

CONTRAINDICATIONS & CAUTIONS

• Contraindicated in patients with liver dysfunction; known or suspected pregnancy; thrombophlebitis, thromboembolic disorders; active or history of DVT or PE; estrogen-dependent neoplasia; breast or reproductive cancer (except for palliative treatment); undiagnosed abnormal genital bleeding; and known anaphylactic reaction or angioedema to conjugated estrogens.
⚕ Contraindicated in patients with known protein C, protein S, or antithrombin deficiency or other thrombophilic disorders.
• Use cautiously in patients with cerebrovascular disease or CAD, asthma, bone disease, migraine, seizures, SLE, porphyria, hepatic hemangioma, gallbladder disease, diabetes, hypoparathyroidism, or renal dysfunction.
⚕ Use cautiously in patients who have a strong family history (mother, grandmother, sister) of breast or reproductive tract cancer, breast nodules, fibrocystic breasts, or abnormal mammogram findings.
⚕ Exogenous estrogens may exacerbate signs and symptoms of angioedema in women with hereditary angioedema.
Dialyzable drug: Unknown.

Reactions in bold italics are *life-threatening.* Interactions may have a *rapid onset* or a *delayed onset.*

⚠ **Overdose S&S:** Nausea, vomiting, breast tenderness, abdominal pain, drowsiness or fatigue, withdrawal uterine bleeding.

PREGNANCY-LACTATION-REPRODUCTION
• Contraindicated during pregnancy.
• Drug shouldn't be used during breastfeeding. Estrogen has been shown to decrease the quantity and quality of human milk.

NURSING CONSIDERATIONS
• Make sure patient has thorough physical exam before starting therapy; patients receiving long-term therapy should have yearly exams. Periodically monitor lipid levels, BP, body weight, and hepatic function.
• Rapid treatment of dysfunctional uterine bleeding or reduction of surgical bleeding usually requires delivery by IV or IM route.
Boxed Warning Don't use to prevent CV disease. In patients who are postmenopausal receiving therapy for more than 5 years, drug may increase risks of MI, stroke, invasive breast cancer, PE, and DVT. Use the lowest effective doses for the shortest time, considering the benefits and risks. ■
Boxed Warning In patients who are postmenopausal receiving therapy for more than 5 years, drug may increase risk of endometrial cancer. Cyclic therapy and the lowest possible dose reduce risk. Adding progestins decreases risk of endometrial hyperplasia, but it's unknown whether they affect risk of endometrial cancer. ■
Boxed Warning Drug may increase risk of dementia in patients after menopause who are age 65 and older and receiving conjugated estrogens plus medroxyprogesterone acetate for 4 years. ■
• Periodically reevaluate need for therapy.
• When used solely for the treatment of vulval and vaginal atrophy, consider topical products.
• Ensure adequate calcium and vitamin D intake when using drug to prevent osteoporosis.
• Because of thromboembolism risk, stop therapy at least 4 to 6 weeks before procedures that prolong immobilization or raise risk of thromboembolism, such as knee or hip surgery.
• Notify pathologist about estrogen therapy when sending specimens for lab evaluation.
• Glucose tolerance may be impaired. Monitor glucose level closely in patients with diabetes.

• **Look alike–sound alike:** Don't confuse Premarin with Primaxin, Provera, or Remeron.

PATIENT TEACHING
• Teach patient safe drug administration.
• Teach patient about adverse effects and to promptly report them.
• Emphasize importance of regular physical exams.
• Explain to patient that cyclic therapy for postmenopausal symptoms may cause withdrawal bleeding during week off drug. Tell patient to report unusual vaginal bleeding.
🛈 **Alert:** Warn patient to immediately report abdominal pain; pain, numbness, or stiffness in legs or buttocks; pressure or pain in chest; shortness of breath; severe headaches; visual disturbances, such as blind spots, flashing lights, or blurriness; vaginal bleeding or discharge; breast lumps; swelling of hands or feet; yellow skin or sclera; dark urine; and light-colored stools.
• Tell patient with diabetes to report elevated glucose level so that antidiabetic dosage can be adjusted.
• Teach patient how to perform routine breast self-exam.
• Advise patient not to become pregnant during estrogen therapy.
• Encourage patient to stop smoking or reduce number of cigarettes smoked because of the risk of CV complications.
• Tell patient using drug for osteoporosis prevention to ensure adequate intake of calcium and vitamin D.
• Inform patient that vaginal cream has been reported to weaken latex condoms and to use an alternative method of contraception.

SAFETY ALERT!

eszopiclone
es-zoe-PIK-lone

Lunesta✏

Therapeutic class: Hypnotics
Pharmacologic class: Pyrrolopyrazine derivatives
Controlled substance schedule: IV

AVAILABLE FORMS
Tablets: 1 mg, 2 mg, 3 mg

E

INDICATIONS & DOSAGES
➤ **Insomnia**
Adults: 1 mg PO immediately before bedtime. Increase to 2 or 3 mg as needed.
Older adults and patients who are debilitated: 1 mg PO immediately before bedtime. Increase to 2 mg as needed. Maximum dose is 2 mg.
Adjust-a-dose: In patients with severe hepatic impairment and in those also taking a potent CYP3A4 inhibitor, don't exceed 2-mg dose.

ADMINISTRATION
PO
• Don't give with or immediately after a meal.
• Give drug immediately before bedtime because drug may cause dizziness or lightheadedness.

ACTION
Probably interacts with GABA receptors at allosteric binding sites close to or connected to benzodiazepine receptors.

Route	Onset	Peak	Duration
PO	Rapid	1 hr	Unknown

Half-life: 6 hours.

ADVERSE REACTIONS
CNS: abnormal dreams, anxiety, complex sleep-related behavior, confusion, depression, dizziness, hallucinations, headache, migraine, nervousness, pain, somnolence, neuralgia, unpleasant taste. **CV:** chest pain, edema. **EENT:** dry mouth. **GI:** diarrhea, dyspepsia, nausea, vomiting. **GU:** dysmenorrhea, UTI, decreased libido. **Respiratory:** URI. **Skin:** pruritus, rash. **Other:** accidental injury, viral infection, gynecomastia.

INTERACTIONS
Drug-drug. *CNS depressants:* May have additive CNS effects. Adjust dosage of either drug as needed.
CYP3A4 inducers (rifampin): May decrease level and effects of eszopiclone. Monitor therapy.
Olanzapine: May impair cognitive function or memory. Use together cautiously.
Boxed Warning *Opioid class warning:* May cause slow or difficult breathing, sedation, and death. Avoid use together. If use together is necessary, limit dosage and duration of each drug to minimum necessary for desired effect. ■
Strong CYP3A4 inhibitors (clarithromycin, itraconazole, ketoconazole, nefazodone, nelfinavir, ritonavir): May decrease eszopiclone elimination, increasing toxicity risk. Use together cautiously. Limit eszopiclone dose.
Drug-herb. *St. John's wort:* May decrease eszopiclone serum concentration. Discourage concurrent use.
Drug-food. *High-fat meals:* May delay drug's effects. Discourage high-fat meals with or just before taking drug.
Drug-lifestyle. *Alcohol use:* May decrease psychomotor ability. Discourage taking drug if patient drank alcohol that evening or before bed.

EFFECTS ON LAB TEST RESULTS
None reported.

CONTRAINDICATIONS & CAUTIONS
• Contraindicated in patients with known hypersensitivity to eszopiclone.
Boxed Warning Drug may cause rare but serious injury, including death, due to complex sleep behaviors, such as sleepwalking, sleep driving, and engaging in other activities while not fully awake. These behaviors can occur at the lowest recommended dosages and after just one dose. Drug is contraindicated in patients with a history of complex sleep behavior after taking eszopiclone. ■
• Rarely, drug may cause angioedema and anaphylaxis that require emergency treatment and can be fatal. Don't rechallenge patients who develop angioedema after treatment with drug.
Boxed Warning *Opioid class warning:* Opioids should only be prescribed with benzodiazepines or other CNS depressants when alternative treatment options are inadequate. ■
• Use cautiously in older adults and patients who are debilitated, in patients with diseases or conditions that could affect metabolism or hemodynamic responses, and in patients with compromised respiratory function or severe hepatic impairment. Also use cautiously in patients with signs and symptoms of depression because of the increased risk of suicide.
• The 2019 Updated Beers Criteria suggest avoiding use in older adults.
• Dosage adjustments may be needed when drug is combined with other CNS depressants because of potentially additive effects.

Reactions in bold italics are **life-threatening**. Interactions may have a *rapid onset* or a **delayed onset**.

- Safety and effectiveness in children haven't been established.

⚠ **Overdose S&S:** CNS depression.

PREGNANCY-LACTATION-REPRODUCTION
- Use during pregnancy only if potential benefit justifies fetal risk.
- It isn't known if drug appears in human milk. Breastfeeding isn't recommended.

NURSING CONSIDERATIONS
🛈 **Alert:** Anaphylaxis and angioedema may occur as early as the first dose; monitor patient closely.

🛈 **Alert:** Drug may increase risk of next-day impairment of driving and other activities that require full alertness. Risk increases with dosage and if drug is taken with less than 7 or 8 hours of sleep. Patient taking 3-mg dose shouldn't drive or perform activities requiring complete mental alertness during the morning after use.

- Evaluate patient for physical and psychiatric disorders before treatment.
- Use the lowest effective dose.

🛈 **Alert:** Give drug immediately before patient goes to bed or after patient has gone to bed and has trouble falling asleep.

- Use only for short periods (for example, 7 to 10 days). If patient still has trouble sleeping, check for other psychological disorders.
- Risk of abuse and dependence increases with the dose and duration of treatment and the concurrent use of other psychoactive drugs. Abrupt discontinuation may cause withdrawal symptoms.
- Monitor patient for changes in behavior, such as decreased inhibition, aggression, and agitation, and including those that suggest depression or suicidality. Amnesia and other neuropsychiatric symptoms may occur unpredictably.

PATIENT TEACHING
Boxed Warning *Opioid class warning:* Caution patient or caregiver of patient taking an opioid with a benzodiazepine, CNS depressant, or alcohol to seek immediate medical attention for dizziness, light-headedness, extreme sleepiness, slowed or difficult breathing, or unresponsiveness. ∎

Boxed Warning Warn patient of the risk of injury or death related to complex sleep behaviors. Direct patient to stop drug and immediately inform prescriber if an episode of complex sleep behavior occurs or if patient doesn't remember activities performed while taking drug. ∎

🛈 **Alert:** Warn patient that drug may cause allergic reactions, facial swelling, and complex sleep-related behaviors, such as driving, eating, and making phone calls while asleep. Advise patient to report these adverse effects.

🛈 **Alert:** Caution patient taking 3 mg of eszopiclone not to drive or engage in activities that are hazardous or require complete mental alertness the day after use.

- Urge patient to take drug immediately before going to bed because drug may cause dizziness or light-headedness.
- Caution patient not to take drug unless a full night's sleep is possible.
- Advise patient to avoid taking drug after a high-fat meal and to avoid alcohol.
- Tell patient to avoid activities that require mental alertness until the drug's effects are known.
- Urge patient to immediately report changes in behavior and thinking.
- Warn patient not to stop drug abruptly or change dose without consulting the prescriber.
- Inform patient that tolerance or dependence may develop if drug is taken for a prolonged period.

etanercept
ee-TAN-er-sept

Enbrel, Enbrel SureClick

etanercept-szzs
Erelzi

etanercept-ykro
Eticovo

Therapeutic class: Antiarthritics
Pharmacologic class: TNF blockers

AVAILABLE FORMS
Injection (powder): 25 mg multidose vial
Injection (solution): 25 mg/0.5 mL single-dose vial
Prefilled autoinjector: 50 mg/mL
Prefilled single-dose Sensoready pen: 50 mg/mL
Prefilled single-dose syringe: 25 mg/0.5 mL, 50 mg/mL

INDICATIONS & DOSAGES

➤ **To reduce signs and symptoms of moderately to severely active polyarticular juvenile idiopathic arthritis in patients whose response to one or more DMARDs has been inadequate**

Children ages 2 to 17: For children weighing 63 kg or more, 50 mg subcut once weekly. For children weighing less than 63 kg (Enbrel only), 0.8 mg/kg subcut once weekly as two injections, either on the same day or 3 or 4 days apart using the multiuse vial. Maximum dosage is 50 mg/week. Glucocorticoids, NSAIDs, or analgesics may be continued during treatment. Use with methotrexate hasn't been studied in children.

➤ **RA, ankylosing spondylitis**

Adults: 50 mg subcut once weekly. Methotrexate, glucocorticoids, salicylates, NSAIDs, and analgesics may be continued during treatment.

➤ **Psoriatic arthritis**

Adults: 50 mg subcut once weekly. May continue methotrexate, glucocorticoids, salicylates, NSAIDs, and analgesics during treatment.

➤ **Chronic moderate to severe plaque psoriasis in patients who are candidates for systemic therapy or phototherapy**

Adults: 50 mg subcut twice weekly for 3 months. Then, reduce dosage to 50 mg subcut once weekly.

Children age 4 and older: For patients weighing 63 kg or more, 50 mg (Enbrel or Eticovo) subcut once weekly. For patients weighing less than 63 kg, 0.8 mg/kg (Enbrel) subcut once weekly. Maximum dosage is 50 mg/week.

ADMINISTRATION

Subcutaneous

● Give 50-mg dose as one subcut injection using a 50-mg/mL single-use prefilled syringe or prefilled autoinjector or pen or as two 25-mg subcut injections using prefilled syringe or multidose vial. May give the two 25-mg injections on the same day or 3 to 4 days apart.

● No dosage form for Erelzi or Eticovo allows weight-based dosing for children weighing less than 63 kg.

● To achieve pediatric doses other than 25 or 50 mg, use reconstituted Enbrel.

● Store prefilled syringe or pen refrigerated at 36° to 46° F (2° to 8° C), but let it reach room temperature (15 to 30 minutes) before use.

Don't remove needle cover while allowing syringe to reach room temperature.

● Store prefilled autoinjector refrigerated at 36° to 46° F (2° to 8° C), but let it reach room temperature before use. Don't remove the needle cover while allowing syringe to reach room temperature.

● Don't return an autoinjector, prefilled syringe, dose tray, or prefilled pen to the refrigerator after it has reached room temperature. Protect from light and heat and discard after 14 days (Enbrel, Eticovo) or 28 days (Erelzi).

● Reconstitute multiple-use vial aseptically with 1 mL of supplied sterile bacteriostatic water for injection (0.9% benzyl alcohol). Use a 25G needle rather than the supplied vial adapter if the vial will be used for multiple doses, but use a 27G needle for injection. Don't filter reconstituted solution when preparing or giving drug. Inject diluent slowly into vial. Refrigerate reconstituted vial for up to 14 days at 36° to 46° F (2° to 8° C) and discard 14 days after reconstitution.

● Minimize foaming by gently swirling during dissolution rather than shaking. Dissolution takes less than 10 minutes.

● Don't use solution if it's discolored or cloudy, or if it contains particulate matter.

● Separate injection sites by at least 1 inch (2.5 cm), rotate regularly, and never use areas where skin is tender, bruised, red, or hard. Use sites on the thigh, abdomen, and upper arm.

⊙ *Alert:* Needle covers of diluent syringe and prefilled syringe and internal needle cover within cap of the pen contain latex and shouldn't be handled by persons sensitive to latex.

ACTION

Binds specifically to TNF and blocks its action with cell-surface TNF receptors, reducing inflammatory and immune responses found in RA.

Route	Onset	Peak	Duration
Subcut	Unknown	72 hr	Unknown

Half-life: About 5 days.

ADVERSE REACTIONS

CNS: headache, asthenia, dizziness, fever. **CV:** peripheral edema. **EENT:** rhinitis, pharyngitis, sinusitis, mouth ulcers. **GI:** abdominal pain, dyspepsia, nausea, vomiting, diarrhea. **Respiratory:** URI, cough, respiratory disorder, lower respiratory infection.

Reactions in bold italics are *life-threatening*. Interactions may have a *rapid onset* or a ***delayed onset***.

Skin: injection-site reaction, rash, alopecia, urticaria, pruritus. **Other:** infection, antibody development, hypersensitivity, *malignancies.*

INTERACTIONS
Drug-drug. *Antidiabetics:* Increase risk of hypoglycemia. Antidiabetic dosage reduction may be needed.

Cyclophosphamide: May increase risk of solid malignancies. Concurrent use not recommended.

Immunomodulators (abatacept, anakinra, belimumab, canakinumab, certolizumab pegol, infliximab, natalizumab, vedolizumab): Increases risk of serious infection. Use together isn't recommended.

Sulfasalazine: May cause decreased neutrophil count. Monitor patient carefully.

Vaccines (inactivated): May reduce vaccine effectiveness. Complete all age-appropriate vaccinations at least 2 weeks before start of immunosuppressive therapy.

Vaccines (live-virus): May affect normal immune response. Postpone live-virus vaccination until 3 months after etanercept discontinuation.

Drug-herb. *Echinacea:* May diminish drug's therapeutic effect. Discourage use together. If used together, monitor patient for decreased effect of etanercept.

EFFECTS ON LAB TEST RESULTS
None reported.

CONTRAINDICATIONS & CAUTIONS
• Contraindicated in patients hypersensitive to drug or its components and in those with sepsis.

• Use cautiously in patients age 65 and older and in patients with underlying diseases that predispose them to infection, such as diabetes, HF, or history of active or chronic infections.

• Rare cases of new-onset or exacerbations of CNS and peripheral nervous system demyelinating disorders (transverse myelitis, optic neuritis, MS, Guillain-Barré syndrome) and seizure disorders have occurred.

• Use cautiously in patients with a history of HF and moderate to severe alcoholic hepatitis.

• Don't start drug in patients with an active infection, patients who have been exposed to TB, or patients with a history of an opportunistic infection, including clinically important localized infections, because of the increased risk of the development of serious infections that may lead to hospitalizations or death.

• Use cautiously in patients who have resided or traveled in areas of endemic TB or endemic mycoses, such as histoplasmosis, coccidioidomycosis, or blastomycosis.

• Use cautiously in patients previously infected with HBV. Evaluate patients at increased risk for HBV infection before treatment and monitor patients for reactivation during and for several months after therapy ends. If reactivation occurs, drug may need to be stopped and antiviral therapy begun.

• Avoid use in patients with Wegener granulomatosis who are receiving immunosuppressants; drug may increase risk of malignancy.

• Temporarily interrupt treatment in patients with varicella virus exposure; consider prophylactic treatment with varicella zoster immune globulin.

• Children should be up to date with all immunizations before start of therapy.

Dialyzable drug: Unknown.

PREGNANCY-LACTATION-REPRODUCTION
• Use during pregnancy only if clearly needed.

• Drug is present in low levels in human milk and is minimally absorbed by an infant who is breastfed. Use cautiously during breastfeeding.

NURSING CONSIDERATIONS
• Etanercept-szzs (Erelzi) and etanercept-ykro (Eticovo) are biosimilar to the FDA-approved reference product etanercept (Enbrel). There are no clinically meaningful differences between the biosimilar product and the reference product based on the conditions of their use. However, they aren't considered to be interchangeable.

• Methotrexate, glucocorticoids, salicylates, NSAIDs, or analgesics may be continued during treatment in adults.

Boxed Warning Patients treated with anti-TNF therapies are at increased risk for developing serious, sometimes fatal, infections (TB; invasive fungal infections; bacterial, viral, and other infections). Most patients who developed serious infections were also receiving immunosuppressants, such as methotrexate or corticosteroids. Monitor patient carefully; if serious infection or sepsis occurs, stop therapy and notify prescriber. ∎

Boxed Warning Infections, including bacterial sepsis and TB, have been reported. Evaluate patient's risk factors and test for latent TB. Begin treatment for latent TB before therapy with etanercept and monitor patient for active TB during treatment, even if initial latent TB test is negative. ■

🜂 *Alert:* Don't give live-virus vaccines during therapy.

Boxed Warning Histoplasmosis, coccidioidomycosis, blastomycosis, and other opportunistic infections may develop with use of this drug. Consider empirical antifungal therapy in patients at risk for invasive fungal infections who develop severe systemic illness. ■

Boxed Warning Lymphoma and other malignancies, sometimes fatal, have been reported in children and adolescents. ■

• Monitor patient for hypersensitivity reactions and new or worsening HF.

• *Look alike–sound alike:* Don't confuse etanercept-szzs (Erelzi) or etanercept-ykro (Eticovo) with the reference drug etanercept (Enbrel).

PATIENT TEACHING

• Teach patient who is self-administering drug about mixing and injection techniques, including rotating injection sites.

• Tell patient that injection-site reactions usually disappear in 3 to 5 days but to contact prescriber if they persist beyond that.

• Inform patient about avoiding live-virus vaccine administration during therapy.

• Advise patient to report signs or symptoms of pancytopenia, such as bruising, bleeding, persistent fever, or pallor.

• Instruct patient to report signs or symptoms of new or worsening medical conditions, such as CNS demyelinating disorders (numbness, tingling, vision changes, weakness of arms and legs, dizziness), seizures, or HF.

• Stress importance of alerting other health care providers about this therapy.

• Instruct patient to promptly report signs of infection, including persistent fever, cough, shortness of breath, or fatigue.

• Advise patient to discuss pregnancy, plans to become pregnant, and breastfeeding with prescriber.

ethacrynate sodium
eth-a-KRIH-nayt

Edecrin

ethacrynic acid
Edecrin

Therapeutic class: Diuretics
Pharmacologic class: Loop diuretics

AVAILABLE FORMS
ethacrynate sodium
Injection: 50 mg/vial
ethacrynic acid
Tablets: 25 mg

INDICATIONS & DOSAGES
➤ **Edema (rapid diuresis)**
Adults: 50 mg or 0.5 to 1 mg/kg IV. Usually only one dose is needed, although may give a second dose PRN.
➤ **Edema**
Adults: 50 to 200 mg PO daily. May increase to 200 mg b.i.d. if needed for desired effect in 25- to 50-mg increments.
Children age 13 months and older: First dose is 25 mg PO, increased cautiously by 25 mg daily until desired effect is achieved.
Adjust-a-dose: If added to an existing diuretic regimen, first dose is 25 mg and dosage adjustments are made in 25-mg increments.

ADMINISTRATION
PO
• Give in morning to prevent nocturia.
• Give after meals.
IV
▼ Add 50 mL of D_5W or NSS to vial.
▼ Don't use cloudy or opalescent solution.
▼ Give over several minutes through tubing of running infusion.
▼ If more than one IV dose is needed, use a new injection site to avoid thrombophlebitis.
▼ Discard unused solution after 24 hours.
▼ **Incompatibilities:** Hydralazine, Normosol-M, procainamide, ranitidine, solutions or drugs with pH below 5, whole blood and its derivatives.

ACTION
Potent loop diuretic; inhibits sodium and chloride reabsorption at the proximal and distal tubules and the ascending loop of Henle.

Route	Onset	Peak	Duration
PO	30 min	2 hr	6–8 hr
IV	5 min	15–30 min	2 hr

Half-life: 2 to 4 hours.

ADVERSE REACTIONS

CNS: malaise, confusion, fatigue, apprehension, vertigo, headache, fever. **CV:** orthostatic hypotension, thrombophlebitis (IV). **EENT:** transient or permanent deafness with overrapid IV injection, blurred vision, tinnitus. **GI:** cramping, diarrhea, anorexia, nausea, vomiting, abdominal discomfort, dysphagia, *GI bleeding.* **GU:** oliguria, hematuria, nocturia, polyuria, frequent urination, azotemia. **Hematologic:** *agranulocytosis, neutropenia, thrombocytopenia.* **Metabolic:** hyperuricemia; gout; *hypokalemia*; hypochloremic alkalosis; fluid and electrolyte imbalances, including dilutional *hyponatremia, hypocalcemia, and hypomagnesemia*; hyperglycemia and impaired glucose tolerance; volume depletion, dehydration. **Skin:** rash. **Other:** chills.

INTERACTIONS

Drug-drug. *Aminoglycoside antibiotics:* May increase ototoxicity and nephrotoxicity. Use together cautiously.
Antidiabetics: May decrease hypoglycemic effects. Monitor glucose level.
Antihypertensives: May increase risk of hypotension. Use together cautiously.
Cardiac glycosides: May increase risk of digoxin toxicity from ethacrynate-induced hypokalemia. Monitor potassium and digoxin levels.
Chlorothiazide, chlorthalidone, hydrochlorothiazide, indapamide, metolazone: May cause excessive diuretic response, causing serious electrolyte abnormalities or dehydration. Adjust doses carefully, and monitor patient closely for signs and symptoms of excessive diuretic response.
Cisplatin: May increase risk of ototoxicity and nephrotoxicity. Avoid using together.
Furosemide: May increase risk of ototoxicity. Avoid use together.
Lithium: May decrease lithium clearance, increasing risk of lithium toxicity. Monitor lithium level.
Neuromuscular blockers: May alter neuromuscular blockade. Monitor patient closely.
NSAIDs: May decrease diuretic effect. Use together cautiously.

Other potassium-wasting drugs (amphotericin B, corticosteroids): May increase risk of hypokalemia and hypocalcemia. Use cautiously.
Probenecid: May decrease diuretic effect. Avoid using together.
Risperidone: May enhance adverse or toxic effect of risperidone. Consider therapy modification and maintain adequate hydration.
Warfarin: May increase anticoagulant effect. Use together cautiously.
Drug-herb. *Dandelion:* May increase diuresis. Discourage use together.
Licorice: May cause unexpected rapid potassium loss. Discourage use together.

EFFECTS ON LAB TEST RESULTS
• May increase glucose and uric acid levels.
• May decrease calcium, magnesium, potassium, and sodium levels.
• May decrease granulocyte, neutrophil, and platelet counts.

CONTRAINDICATIONS & CAUTIONS
• Contraindicated in infants, patients hypersensitive to drug, and patients with anuria.
⚠ *Alert:* Drug is potent diuretic and can cause severe diuresis with water and electrolyte depletion. Monitor patient closely.
• Use cautiously in patients with electrolyte abnormalities or hepatic impairment.
• Ototoxicity has been reported, most often with IV use and with excessive doses.
• Rarely, pancreatitis has been reported.
Dialyzable drug: Unknown.
⚠ *Overdose S&S:* Dehydration, electrolyte depletion.

PREGNANCY-LACTATION-REPRODUCTION
• Use in pregnancy only if clearly needed.
• It isn't known if drug appears in human milk. Patient should discontinue breastfeeding or discontinue drug.

NURSING CONSIDERATIONS
• Monitor fluid intake and output, weight, BP, and electrolyte levels.
• Watch for signs and symptoms of orthostatic hypotension (dizziness, vertigo, syncope) and hypokalemia (muscle weakness and cramps).
• Monitor glucose level in patients with diabetes.
• Consult prescriber and dietitian about providing a high-potassium diet. Potassium chloride and sodium supplements may be needed.

• Dosage may be on an alternate-day schedule, or more prolonged periods of diuretic therapy may be interspersed with rest periods. Intermittent dosage schedule allows time to correct electrolyte imbalance and may provide a more efficient diuretic response.

• Drug may increase risk of gastric hemorrhage caused by steroid treatment.

• Monitor older adults, who are especially susceptible to hypotension and other effects of excessive diuresis.

• Monitor uric acid level, especially in patients with history of gout.

⚠️ *Alert:* If patient develops severe diarrhea, stop drug. Patient shouldn't receive drug again after diarrhea has resolved.

PATIENT TEACHING

• Instruct patient to take drug with food to minimize GI upset.

• Advise patient to take drug in morning to avoid need to urinate at night. If a second dose is needed, tell patient to take it in early afternoon.

• Advise patient to avoid sudden posture changes and to rise slowly to avoid dizziness upon standing quickly.

• Tell patient to notify prescriber about muscle weakness, cramps, nausea, diarrhea, or dizziness.

• Caution patient not to perform hazardous activities if drug causes drowsiness.

• Advise patient with diabetes to closely monitor glucose level.

ethambutol hydrochloride
e-THAM-byoo-tole

Etibi✣, Myambutol

Therapeutic class: Antituberculotics
Pharmacologic class: Synthetic antituberculotics

AVAILABLE FORMS
Tablets: 100 mg, 400 mg

INDICATIONS & DOSAGES
➤ **Adjunctive treatment for pulmonary TB**
Adults and children age 13 and older: In patients who haven't received prior antituberculotics, 15 mg/kg PO daily as a single dose once every 24 hours, combined with other antituberculous therapy. For retreatment, 25 mg/kg PO every 24 hours as a single dose

for 60 days (or until bacteriologic smears and cultures become negative) with at least one other antituberculotic; after 60 days, decrease to 15 mg/kg/day as a single dose every 24 hours.

ADMINISTRATION
PO
• Always give with other antituberculotics to prevent development of resistant organisms.

• Give without regard to food; if GI upset occurs, give with food.

• Give on a once-every-24-hour basis only.

ACTION
May inhibit synthesis of one or more metabolites of susceptible bacteria, changing cell metabolism during cell division; bacteriostatic.

Route	Onset	Peak	Duration
PO	Unknown	2–4 hr	Unknown

Half-life: About 2.5 to 3.6 hours.

ADVERSE REACTIONS
CNS: dizziness, fever, disorientation, hallucinations, headache, malaise, mental confusion, peripheral neuritis. **EENT:** optic neuritis, irreversible blindness, decreased visual acuity. **GI:** abdominal pain, anorexia, GI upset, nausea, vomiting. **Hematologic:** *thrombocytopenia, leukopenia, neutropenia,* lymphadenopathy. **Hepatic:** abnormal LFT values. **Metabolic:** hyperuricemia, precipitation of acute gout. **Musculoskeletal:** joint pain. **Skin:** *erythema multiforme,* dermatitis, pruritus. **Other:** *anaphylactoid reactions,* hypersensitivity reactions.

INTERACTIONS
Drug-drug. *Aluminum salts:* May delay and reduce ethambutol absorption. Separate doses by at least 4 hours.

EFFECTS ON LAB TEST RESULTS
• May increase ALT, AST, bilirubin, and uric acid levels.

• May decrease WBC and platelet counts.

CONTRAINDICATIONS & CAUTIONS
• Contraindicated in children younger than age 13, patients hypersensitive to drug, and patients with optic neuritis.

• Use cautiously in patients with impaired renal function, cataracts, recurrent eye

---

Reactions in bold italics are *life-threatening*. Interactions may have a *rapid onset* or a ***delayed onset***.

inflammation, gout, or diabetic retinopathy. Irreversible blindness has occurred.
• Liver toxicities, including fatalities, have been reported. Obtain baseline and periodic assessment of hepatic function.
Dialyzable drug: Unknown.

PREGNANCY-LACTATION-REPRODUCTION
• Drug crosses the placental barrier. Ophthalmic abnormalities have occurred in infants exposed to antituberculotics in utero. Use during pregnancy only if benefit justifies fetal risk.
• Use of effective contraception during treatment for multidrug-resistant TB is recommended for patients of childbearing potential.
• Drug appears in human milk. Use only if expected benefit to the patient outweighs risk to the infant. Monitor infant for jaundice.
• Patients with multidrug-resistant TB and positive sputum smear shouldn't breastfeeding.

NURSING CONSIDERATIONS
• Perform visual acuity and color discrimination tests before and during therapy. Patients taking more than 15 mg/kg/day should have monthly eye exams.
• Ensure that any changes in vision don't result from an underlying condition.
• Obtain AST and ALT levels before therapy, and monitor these levels every 3 to 4 weeks.
• In patients with impaired renal function, base dosage on drug level.
• Monitor uric acid level; observe patient for signs and symptoms of gout.

PATIENT TEACHING
• Tell patient to report all vision changes immediately; explain that eye exams will be necessary. Advise patient that visual disturbances usually disappear several weeks to months after drug is stopped. Inflammation of the optic nerve is related to dosage and duration of treatment.
• Inform patient that drug is given with other antituberculotics.
• Stress importance of adherence with drug therapy.
• Instruct patient to report adverse reactions to prescriber.
• Advise patient of childbearing potential to use effective contraception during treatment of multidrug-resistant TB.

ethinyl estradiol–desogestrel
ETH-in-il/DAY-so-jest-rul

Monophasic
Emoquette, Isibloom, Kalliga

Biphasic
Kariva, Pimtrea, Simliya, Viorele, Volnea

Triphasic
Cyclessa, Velivet

ethinyl estradiol–ethynodiol diacetate
Monophasic
Kelnor 1/35, Kelnor 1/50, Zovia 1/35-28

ethinyl estradiol–levonorgestrel
Monophasic
Afirmelle, Altavera, Ashlyna, Aviane-28, Ayuna, Balcoltra, Falmina, Iclevia, Introvale, Kurvelo, Lessina-28, Levora 0.15/30-28, Marlissa, Orsythia, Portia-28, Seasonale, Setlakin, Tyblume, Vienva

Biphasic
Daysee, Jaimiess, LoSeasonique, Lo Simpesse, Seasonique, Simpesse

Triphasic
Enpresse-28, Levonest, Quartette, Trivora-28

ethinyl estradiol–norethindrone
Monophasic
Alyacen 1/35, Balziva-28, Brevicon 28-Day, Briellyn, Cyclafem 1/35, Cyonanz, Dasetta 1/35, Kaitlib Fe, Nexesta Fe, Nortrel 0.5/35, Nortrel 1/35, Nylia 1/35, Philith, Vyfemla, Wera

Biphasic
Aranelle

Triphasic
Alyacen 7/7/7, Aranelle, Dasetta 7/7/7, Nortrel 7/7/7, Nylia 7/7/7, Pirmella 7/7/7

E

---

ethinyl estradiol–norethindrone acetate

Monophasic
Activella, Fyavolv, Junel 1/20, Junel 1.5/30, Larin 1/20, Larin 1.5/30, Loestrin 21 1/20, Loestrin 21 1.5/30, Microgestin 1/20, Microgestin 1.5/30, Taytulla

ethinyl estradiol–norgestimate

Monophasic
Estarylla, Mili, Mono-Linyah, Previfem, Sprintec

Triphasic
Tri-Estarylla, Tri-Linyah, Tri-Lo-Estarylla, Tri-Lo-Mili, Tri-Lo-Sprintec, Tri-Mili, Tri-Previfem, Tri-Sprintec

ethinyl estradiol–norgestrel

Monophasic
Cryselle, Elinest, Low-Ogestrel

ethinyl estradiol–norethindrone acetate–ferrous fumarate

Monophasic
Blisovi 24 Fe, Blisovi Fe 1.5/30, Blisovi Fe 1/20, Gemmily, Junel Fe 1/20, Junel Fe 1.5/30, Larin 24 Fe, Larin Fe 1/20, Larin Fe 1.5/30, Loestrin 24 Fe, Loestrin Fe 1/20, Loestrin Fe 1.5/30, Lo Loestrin Fe, Merzee, Microgestin Fe 1/20, Microgestin Fe 1.5/30, Minastrin 24 Fe

Triphasic
Estrostep Fe, Tri-Legest Fe

Therapeutic class: Contraceptives
Pharmacologic class: Estrogen–progestin combinations

AVAILABLE FORMS
Monophasic hormonal contraceptives
ethinyl estradiol–desogestrel
Tablets: ethinyl estradiol 30 mcg and desogestrel 0.15 mg (Emoquette, Isibloom, Kalliga)
ethinyl estradiol–ethynodiol diacetate
Tablets: ethinyl estradiol 35 mcg and ethynodiol diacetate 1 mg (Kelnor 1/35, Zovia 1/35-28); ethinyl estradiol 50 mcg and ethynodiol diacetate 1 mg (Kelnor 1/50)

ethinyl estradiol–levonorgestrel
Tablets: ethinyl estradiol 20 mcg and levonorgestrel 0.1 mg (Afirmelle, Aviane-28, Balcoltra, Falmina, Lessina-28, Orsythia, Tyblume, Vienva); ethinyl estradiol 30 mcg and levonorgestrel 0.15 mg (Altavera, Ayuna, Kurvelo, Levora 0.15/30-28, Marlissa, Portia-28); ethinyl estradiol 30 mcg and 0.15 mg levonorgestrel (84 tablets) (Ashlyna, Iclevia, Introvale, Seasonale, Setlakin)
ethinyl estradiol–norethindrone
Tablets: ethinyl estradiol 20 mcg and norethindrone 1 mg (Taytulla), ethinyl estradiol 35 mcg and norethindrone 0.4 mg (Balziva-28, Briellyn, Nexesta Fe, Philith, Vyfemla); ethinyl estradiol 25 mcg and norethindrone 0.8 mg (Kaitlib Fe); ethinyl estradiol 35 mcg and norethindrone 0.5 mg (Aranelle, Brevicon 28-Day, Cyonanz, Nortrel 0.5/35, Wera); ethinyl estradiol 35 mcg and norethindrone 0.75 mg; ethinyl estradiol 35 mcg and norethindrone 1 mg (Alyacen 1/35, Cyclafem 1/35, Dasetta l/35, Nortrel 1/35, Nylia 1/35, Pirmella 1/35)
ethinyl estradiol–norethindrone acetate
Tablets: ethinyl estradiol 2.5 mcg and norethindrone acetate 1 mg; ethinyl estradiol 5 mcg and norethindrone acetate 1 mg; ethinyl estradiol 20 mcg and norethindrone acetate 1 mg (Junel 1/20, Larin 1/20, Loestrin 21 1/20, Microgestin 1/20, Taytulla); ethinyl estradiol 30 mcg and norethindrone acetate 1.5 mg (Junel 1.5/30, Larin 1.5/30, Loestrin 21 1.5/30, Microgestin 1.5/30)
Tablets for menopausal symptoms or osteoporosis: ethinyl estradiol 0.0025 mg and norethindrone acetate 0.5 mg (Fyavolv); ethinyl estradiol 0.005 mg and norethindrone acetate 1 mg (Fyavolv); ethinyl estradiol 0.5 mg and norethindrone acetate 0.1 mg (Activella), ethinyl estradiol 1 mg and norethindrone acetate 0.5 mg (Activella)
ethinyl estradiol–norgestimate
Tablets: ethinyl estradiol 35 mcg and norgestimate 0.25 mg (Estarylla, Mili, Mono-Linyah, Previfem, Sprintec)
ethinyl estradiol–norgestrel
Tablets: ethinyl estradiol 30 mcg and norgestrel 0.3 mg (Cryselle, Elinest, Low-Ogestrel)
ethinyl estradiol–norethindrone acetate–ferrous fumarate
Chewable tablets: norethindrone 0.4 mg and ethinyl estradiol 35 mcg; inactive tablets contain ferrous fumarate 75 mg

Tablets: ethinyl estradiol 10 mcg, norethindrone acetate 1 mg, and ferrous fumarate 75 mg (Lo Loestrin Fe); ethinyl estradiol 20 mcg, norethindrone acetate 1 mg, and ferrous fumarate 75 mg (Blisovi 24 Fe, Blisovi Fe 1/20, Gemmily, Junel Fe 1/20, Larin 24 Fe, Larin Fe 1/20, Loestrin Fe 1/20, Loestrin 24 Fe, Merzee, Microgestin Fe 1/20, Minastrin 24 Fe); ethinyl estradiol 30 mcg, norethindrone acetate 1.5 mg, and ferrous fumarate 75 mg(Blisovi Fe 1.5/30, Junel Fe 1.5/30, Larin Fe 1.5/30, Loestrin Fe 1.5/30, Microgestin Fe 1.5/30)

Biphasic hormonal contraceptives
ethinyl estradiol–desogestrel
Tablets: ethinyl estradiol 20 mcg and desogestrel 0.15 mg (21 days), then inert tablets (2 days), then ethinyl estradiol 10 mcg (5 days) (Kariva, Pimtrea, Simliya, Viorele, Volnea)
ethinyl estradiol–levonorgestrel
Tablets: ethinyl estradiol 0.02 mg and levonorgestrel 0.1 mg (84 days), then ethinyl estradiol 0.01 mg (7 days) (LoSeasonique, Lo Simpesse); ethinyl estradiol 30 mcg and levonorgestrel 0.15 mg (84 days), then ethinyl estradiol 10 mcg (7 days) (Daysee, Jaimiess, Seasonique, Simpesse)
ethinyl estradiol–norethindrone
Tablets: ethinyl estradiol 35 mcg and norethindrone 0.5 mg (12 tablets), then ethinyl estradiol 35 mcg and norethindrone 1 mg (9 tablets) (Aranelle)

Triphasic hormonal contraceptives
ethinyl estradiol–desogestrel
Tablets: 0.1 mg desogestrel and 25 mcg ethinyl estradiol (7 tablets), 0.125 mg desogestrel and 25 mcg ethinyl estradiol (7 tablets), 0.15 mg desogestrel and 25 mcg ethinyl estradiol (7 tablets) (Cyclessa, Velivet)
ethinyl estradiol–levonorgestrel
Tablets: ethinyl estradiol 30 mcg and levonorgestrel 0.05 mg (6 days), ethinyl estradiol 40 mcg and levonorgestrel 0.075 mg (5 days), ethinyl estradiol 30 mcg and levonorgestrel 0.125 mg (10 days) (Enpresse-28, Levonest, Myzilra, Trivora-28); ethinyl estradiol 20 mcg and 0.15 mg levonorgestrel (42 days), ethinyl estradiol 25 mcg and 0.15 mg levonorgestrel (21 days), ethinyl estradiol 30 mcg and 0.15 mg levonorgestrel (21 days), ethinyl estradiol 10 mcg (7 days) (Quartette)
ethinyl estradiol–norethindrone
Tablets: ethinyl estradiol 30 mcg and norethindrone 0.5 mg (7 days), ethinyl estradiol 35 mcg and norethindrone 1 mg (9 days),

ethinyl estradiol 35 mcg and norethindrone 0.5 mg (5 days) (Aranelle); ethinyl estradiol 35 mcg and norethindrone 0.5 mg (7 days), ethinyl estradiol 35 mcg and norethindrone 0.75 mg (7 days) ethinyl estradiol 35 mcg and norethindrone 1 mg (7 days) (Alyacen 7/7/7, Dasetta 7/7/7, Nortrel 7/7/7, Nylia, 7/7/7, Pirmella 7/7/7)
ethinyl estradiol–norgestimate
Tablets: ethinyl estradiol 25 mcg and norgestimate 0.18 mg (7 days), ethinyl estradiol 25 mcg and norgestimate 0.215 mg (7 days), ethinyl estradiol 25 mcg and norgestimate 0.25 mg (7 days) (Tri-Lo-Estarylla, Tri-Lo-Mili, Tri-Lo-Sprintec); ethinyl estradiol 35 mcg and norgestimate 0.18 mg (7 days), ethinyl estradiol 35 mcg and norgestimate 0.215 mg (7 days), ethinyl estradiol 35 mcg and norgestimate 0.25 mg (7 days) (Tri-Estarylla, Tri-Linyah, Tri-Mili, Tri-Previfem, Tri-Sprintec)
ethinyl estradiol–norethindrone acetate–ferrous fumarate
Tablets: ethinyl estradiol 20 mcg and norethindrone acetate 1 mg (5 days), ethinyl estradiol 30 mcg and norethindrone acetate 1 mg (7 days), ethinyl estradiol 35 mcg and norethindrone acetate 1 mg (9 days), 75-mg ferrous fumarate tablets (7 days) (Estrostep Fe, Tri-Legest Fe)

INDICATIONS & DOSAGES
➤ **Contraception**
Monophasic hormonal contraceptives
Women: 1 tablet PO daily beginning on first day of menstrual cycle or first Sunday after menstrual cycle begins. With 20- and 21-tablet package, new cycle begins 7 days after last tablet taken. With 28-tablet package, dosage is 1 tablet daily without interruption; extra tablets taken on days 22 to 28 are placebos or contain iron. Or, for Seasonale, 1 pink tablet PO daily beginning on first menstrual cycle begins, for 84 consecutive days, followed by 7 days of white (inert) tablets. Or, for Taytulla, capsule pack has 24 active pink capsules (with hormones) to be taken one daily for 24 days, followed by 4 reminder maroon capsules (without hormones) to be taken one daily for the next 4 days.

When changing from 21-day or 28-day combination oral contraceptive, begin on first day of withdrawal bleeding, at the latest 7 days after last active tablet. When changing from progestin-only pill, begin the next day. When changing from implant contraceptive, begin the day of implant removal. When changing from injection contraceptive, begin the day when next injection is due.

Biphasic hormonal contraceptives
Women: 1 color tablet PO daily for 10 days; then next color tablet for 11 days. With 21-tablet packages, new cycle begins 7 days after last tablet taken. With 28-tablet packages, dosage is 1 tablet daily without interruption. Or, for Seasonique, 1 light blue-green tablet PO once daily for 84 consecutive days followed by 1 yellow tablet for 7 consecutive days; then repeat cycle.

Triphasic hormonal contraceptives
Women: 1 tablet PO daily in the sequence specified by the brand. With 21-tablet packages, new dosing cycle begins 7 days after last tablet taken. With 28-tablet packages, dosage is 1 tablet daily without interruption.

➤ **Moderate acne vulgaris in women age 14 and older who have no known contraindications to hormonal contraceptive therapy, who want oral contraception for at least 6 months, who have reached menarche, and who are unresponsive to topical antiacne drugs (ethinyl estradiol–norgestimate, ethinyl estradiol–norethindrone acetate–ferrous fumarate)**
Women age 15 and older: 1 tablet PO daily.

➤ **Menopausal signs and symptoms; to prevent osteoporosis (Activella, Fyavolv)**
Women with intact uterus: 1 tablet PO daily.

ADMINISTRATION
PO
• Give drug at the same time each day; give at night to reduce nausea and headaches.
• Patient may swallow chewable tablet whole and follow with a full glass of liquid.

ACTION
Inhibits ovulation and may prevent transport of the ovum (if ovulation should occur) through the fallopian tubes.

Estrogen suppresses FSH, blocking follicular development and ovulation.

Progestin suppresses LH so that ovulation can't occur even if the follicle develops; it also thickens cervical mucus, interfering with sperm migration, and prevents implantation of the fertilized ovum.

Route	Onset	Peak	Duration
PO	Unknown	2 hr (ethinyl estradiol), 0.5–4 hr (varies by progestin)	Unknown

Half-life: 6 to 20 hours (ethinyl estradiol); 5 to 45 hours (varies by progestin).

ADVERSE REACTIONS
CNS: headache, dizziness, depression, lethargy, migraine, *stroke, cerebral hemorrhage.* **CV:** *thromboembolism,* HTN, edema, *PE, MI.* **EENT:** worsening myopia or astigmatism, intolerance of contact lenses, exophthalmos, diplopia. **GI:** nausea, vomiting, abdominal cramps, bloating, anorexia, changes in appetite, gallbladder disease, *pancreatitis.* **GU:** breakthrough bleeding, spotting, granulomatous colitis, dysmenorrhea, amenorrhea, cervical erosion or abnormal secretions, enlargement of uterine fibromas, vaginal candidiasis. **Hepatic:** cholestatic jaundice, *liver tumors,* gallbladder disease. **Metabolic:** weight change, additive insulin resistance in those with diabetes. **Skin:** rash, acne, *erythema multiforme,* melasma, hirsutism. **Other:** breast tenderness, enlargement, secretion.

INTERACTIONS
Drug-drug. *Anastrozole:* May inhibit anastrozole effect. Avoid use together.
Anti-infectives (chloramphenicol, fluconazole, griseofulvin, neomycin, nitrofurantoin, penicillins, sulfonamides, tetracyclines): May decrease contraceptive effect. Advise patient to use another method of contraception.
Atorvastatin: May increase norethindrone and ethinyl estradiol levels. Monitor patient for adverse effects.
Benzodiazepines: May decrease or increase benzodiazepine levels. Adjust dosage, if necessary.
Beta blockers: May increase beta blocker level. Dosage adjustment may be necessary.
Carbamazepine, fosphenytoin, phenobarbital, phenytoin, rifampin: May decrease estrogen effect. Use together cautiously.
Corticosteroids: May enhance corticosteroid effect. Monitor patient closely.
Exemestane: May interfere with exemestane effectiveness. Avoid use together.
Insulin, sulfonylureas: Glucose intolerance may decrease antidiabetic effects. Monitor these effects.

Reactions in bold italics are *life-threatening*. Interactions may have a *rapid onset* or a *delayed onset*.

Iron supplements: Increase risk of iron-related toxicity if blister card contains iron. Don't use together.

NNRTIs, protease inhibitors: May decrease hormonal contraceptive effect. Avoid using together, if possible.

Oral anticoagulants: May decrease anticoagulant effect. Dosage adjustments may be needed. Monitor PT and INR.

Ospemifene: May enhance adverse or toxic effects of ospemifene and interfere with its effectiveness. Avoid use together.

Drug-herb. *Red clover:* May interfere with drug. Discourage use together.

St. John's wort: May decrease drug effect because of increased hepatic metabolism. Discourage use together, or advise patient to use an additional method of contraception.

Drug-food. *Caffeine:* May increase caffeine level. Urge caution.

Grapefruit juice: May increase estrogen level. Advise patient to take with liquid other than grapefruit juice.

Drug-lifestyle. *Smoking:* May increase risk of adverse CV effects. If smoking continues, may need alternative therapy.

EFFECTS ON LAB TEST RESULTS
• May increase thyroid-binding globulin, total T_4, lipid, and triglyceride levels.
• May alter clotting factors.
• May increase norepinephrine-induced platelet aggregation and prolong PT.
• May reduce response to metyrapone test.
• May cause false-positive result in nitroblue tetrazolium test.

CONTRAINDICATIONS & CAUTIONS
• Contraindicated in patients with thromboembolic disorders, cerebrovascular disease or CAD, diplopia or ocular lesions arising from ophthalmic vascular disease, classic migraine, MI, known or suspected breast cancer, known or suspected estrogen-dependent neoplasia, benign or malignant liver tumors, active liver disease or history of cholestatic jaundice with pregnancy or previous use of hormonal contraceptives, or undiagnosed abnormal vaginal bleeding. Also contraindicated in patients receiving hepatitis C drug combinations containing ombitasvir–paritaprevir–ritonavir, with or without dasabuvir.
• Use cautiously in patients with hyperlipidemia, HTN, migraines, seizure disorders,

asthma, bleeding irregularities, gallbladder disease, ocular disease, diabetes, emotional disorders, and cardiac, renal, or hepatic insufficiency.

Dialyzable drug: Unknown.

⚠ **Overdose S&S:** Nausea, withdrawal uterine bleeding.

PREGNANCY-LACTATION-REPRODUCTION
• Use during pregnancy isn't indicated. Discontinue if pregnancy is confirmed. There is little or no increased risk of birth defects in patients who accidently use drug during early pregnancy.
• Estrogens can reduce quantity and quality of human milk. Patient should use other forms of contraception during breastfeeding.

NURSING CONSIDERATIONS
Boxed Warning Cigarette smoking increases the risk of serious CV adverse effects from oral contraceptives. Women who use oral contraceptives shouldn't smoke. ∎
• Triphasic hormonal contraceptives may cause fewer adverse reactions, such as breakthrough bleeding and spotting.
• The CDC reports that use of hormonal contraceptives may decrease risk of ovarian and endometrial cancers and doesn't seem to increase risk of breast cancer. However, the FDA reports that some studies suggest that hormonal contraceptives may be linked to an increase in cervical cancer.
• Monitor lipid levels, BP, body weight, and hepatic function.
• **Alert:** Many hormonal contraceptives share similar names. Make sure to check the hormone strength for verification.
• Estrogens and progestins may alter glucose tolerance, thus changing dosage requirements for antidiabetics. Monitor glucose level.
• Stop hormonal contraceptives for a few weeks before adrenal function tests.
• Stop hormonal contraceptive and notify prescriber if patient develops granulomatous colitis.
• Stop drug at least 1 week before surgery to decrease risk of thromboembolism. Tell patient to use an alternative method of birth control.
• Patients who are nonlactating or those who have had second-trimester abortion must wait 28 days before starting oral contraception.

PATIENT TEACHING

• Tell patient to take tablets or capsules at same time each day; nighttime doses may reduce nausea and headaches.

• Advise patient to use additional method of birth control, such as condom or diaphragm with spermicide, for first week of first cycle.

• Inform patient that missing doses in midcycle greatly increases likelihood of pregnancy.

• Teach patient that missing a dose may cause spotting or light bleeding.

• Counsel patient that hormonal contraceptives don't protect against HIV or other sexually transmitted diseases.

• Tell patient using 91-day method that there will be four planned menses per year, but spotting or bleeding between menses may occur.

• If 1 pill or capsule is missed, tell patient to take it as soon as possible (2 pills or capsules if remembered on the next day) and then to continue regular schedule. Advise an additional method of contraception for remainder of cycle. If 2 consecutive pills or capsules are missed, tell patient to take 2 pills or capsules a day for next 2 days and then resume regular schedule. Advise an additional method of contraception for the next 7 days or preferably for the remainder of cycle. If 2 consecutive pills or capsules are missed in the 3rd or 4th week or if patient misses 3 consecutive pills or capsules, tell patient to contact prescriber for instructions.

• Warn patient of common adverse effects, such as headache, nausea, dizziness, breast tenderness, spotting, and breakthrough bleeding, which usually diminish after 3 to 6 months.

• Instruct patient to weigh herself at least twice a week and to report any sudden weight gain or swelling to prescriber.

• Caution patient to avoid exposure to UV light or prolonged exposure to sunlight.

• **Alert:** Warn patient to immediately report abdominal pain; numbness, stiffness, or pain in legs or buttocks; pressure or pain in chest; shortness of breath; severe headache; visual disturbances, such as blind spots, blurriness, or flashing lights; undiagnosed vaginal bleeding or discharge; two consecutive missed menstrual periods; lumps in the breast; swelling of hands or feet; or severe pain in the abdomen (tumor rupture in liver).

• Advise patient of increased risks created by simultaneous use of cigarettes and hormonal contraceptives.

• If one menstrual period is missed and tablets or capsules have been taken on schedule, tell patient to continue taking them. If two consecutive menstrual periods are missed, tell patient to stop drug and have pregnancy test. Progestins may cause birth defects if taken early in pregnancy.

• Tell patient to chew chewable tablet and follow with a full glass of liquid or swallow whole.

• Caution patient not to take same drug for longer than 12 months without consulting prescriber. Stress importance of Papanicolaou tests and annual gynecologic exams.

• Advise patient to check with prescriber about how soon pregnancy may be attempted after hormonal therapy is stopped. Many prescribers recommend that patients not become pregnant within 2 months after stopping drug.

• Warn patient of possible delay in achieving pregnancy when drug is stopped.

• Teach patient methods to decrease risk of thromboembolism.

• Advise patient taking hormonal contraceptives to use additional form of birth control during concurrent treatment with certain antibiotics.

• Inform patient that hormonal contraceptives may change the fit of contact lenses.

etonogestrel–ethinyl estradiol vaginal ring
et-oh-noe-JES-trel/ETH-in-il

EluRyng, NuvaRing

Therapeutic class: Contraceptives
Pharmacologic class: Progestin–estrogen combinations

AVAILABLE FORMS
Vaginal ring: Delivers 0.12 mg/day etonogestrel and 0.015 mg/day ethinyl estradiol

INDICATIONS & DOSAGES
➤ **Contraception**
Women: Insert 1 ring into the vagina and leave in place for 3 weeks. Insert new ring 1 week after the previous ring is removed.

ADMINISTRATION
Vaginal
• In women who didn't use hormonal contraception during the previous month, initiate

---

Reactions in bold italics are *life-threatening*. Interactions may have a *rapid onset* or a *delayed onset*.

therapy on the first day of the menstrual cycle; may also insert on days 2 to 5, even if bleeding isn't complete, but a barrier method, such as male condoms or spermicide, should be used for the following 7 days. Women using a combination oral contraceptive may switch to a vaginal ring on any day, but at the latest on the day after the usual hormone-free interval. See manufacturer's instructions for use after progestin-only methods, abortion, miscarriage, or childbirth.

• Leave ring in place continuously for a full 3 weeks to maintain effect. It's then removed for 1 week. During this time, withdrawal bleeding occurs (usually starting 2 or 3 days after removal). Insert a new ring 1 week after removal of the previous one, at approximately the same time of day, regardless of whether patient is still menstruating.

• Before dispensing to user, store refrigerated (36° to 46° F [2° to 8° C]). After dispensing, can be stored for up to 4 months at 77° F (25° C).

ACTION

Suppresses gonadotropins, which inhibits ovulation, increases the viscosity of cervical mucus (decreasing the ability of sperm to enter the uterus), and alters the endometrial lining (reducing potential for implantation).

Route	Onset	Peak	Duration
Vaginal	Rapid	200 hr (etonogestrel); 59 hr (ethinyl estradiol)	Unknown

Half-life: Etonogestrel, 29 hours; ethinyl estradiol, 45 hours.

ADVERSE REACTIONS

CNS: headache, emotional lability, mood changes, depression, migraine. **CV:** HTN, edema, *thromboembolic events, MI.* **EENT:** changes in corneal curvature, intolerance to contact lenses, sinusitis. **GI:** nausea, vomiting, abdominal pain. **GU:** vaginitis, leukorrhea, device-related events (for example, foreign body sensation, coital difficulties, device expulsion), vaginal discomfort, breakthrough bleeding, vaginal discharge, dysmenorrhea. **Hepatic:** cholestatic jaundice. **Metabolic:** weight gain. **Respiratory:** URI. **Skin:** chloasma, acne. **Other:** breast pain or tenderness, decreased libido.

INTERACTIONS

Drug-drug. *Acetaminophen:* May decrease acetaminophen level and increase ethinyl estradiol level. Monitor patient for effects.
Ampicillin, barbiturates, carbamazepine, felbamate, griseofulvin, oxcarbazepine, phenytoin, rifampin, tetracyclines, topiramate: May decrease contraceptive effect and increase risk of pregnancy, breakthrough bleeding, or both. Tell patient to use an additional form of contraception while taking these drugs.
Anastrozole: May diminish therapeutic effect of anastrozole. Avoid use together.
Ascorbic acid, atorvastatin, itraconazole: May increase ethinyl estradiol level. Monitor patient for adverse effects.
Clofibrate, morphine, salicylic acid, temazepam: May increase clearance of these drugs. Monitor patient for effectiveness.
Cyclosporine, prednisolone, theophylline: May increase levels of these drugs. Monitor levels if appropriate and adjust dosage.
Exemestane: May interfere with exemestane effectiveness. Avoid use together.
HCV combination products (ombitasvir–paritaprevir–ritonavir with or without dasabuvir): May elevate liver enzyme levels. Use together is contraindicated.
HIV protease inhibitors (lopinavir, ritonavir), NNRTIs (efavirenz, nevirapine): May affect contraceptive effect. Refer to the specific protease inhibitor drug literature. May need to use a backup method of contraception.
Miconazole (oil-based vaginal capsule): May increase serum concentrations of etonogestrel and ethinyl estradiol. Monitor patient for adverse effects.
Ospemifene: May enhance adverse or toxic effects of ospemifene and interfere with its effectiveness. Avoid use together.
Drug-herb. *St. John's wort:* May reduce drug effectiveness and increase the risk of breakthrough bleeding and pregnancy. Discourage use together.
Drug-lifestyle. **Boxed Warning** *Smoking:* May increase risk of serious CV adverse effects, especially in patients older than age 35 who smoke. Drug shouldn't be used in those older than age 35 who smoke. Urge patient to avoid smoking. ∎

EFFECTS ON LAB TEST RESULTS

• May increase coagulation factors, thyroid-binding globulin (leading to increased circulating total thyroid hormone levels), sex hormone-binding globulin (and other binding proteins), and lipid levels.

• May decrease T_3 resin uptake and glucose tolerance.

CONTRAINDICATIONS & CAUTIONS

• Contraindicated in patients hypersensitive to components of drug and in patients older than age 35 who smoke 15 or more cigarettes daily.

• Contraindicated in patients with thrombophlebitis, thromboembolic disorder, history of DVT, cerebrovascular disease or CAD (current or previous), valvular heart disease with complications, severe HTN, diabetes with vascular complications, headache with focal neurologic symptoms or migraine headaches with aura, known or suspected cancer of the endometrium or breast, estrogen-dependent neoplasia, abnormal undiagnosed genital bleeding, jaundice related to pregnancy or previous use of hormonal contraceptives, active liver disease, or benign or malignant hepatic tumors.

• Contraindicated in women older than age 35 with migraine headaches or headaches with focal neurologic symptoms, and in those undergoing major surgery with prolonged immobilization.

• Use cautiously in patients with HTN, hyperlipidemias, obesity, or diabetes.

• Use cautiously in patients with conditions that could be aggravated by fluid retention, and in patients with a history of depression.

• Ring may not be suitable for patients with conditions that make the vagina more susceptible to vaginal irritation or ulceration. Vaginal/cervical erosion or ulceration has been reported.

• Ring may interfere with the correct placement and position of barrier contraceptive methods, such as a diaphragm, cervical cap, or female condom. These methods aren't recommended as backup methods with ring use.
Dialyzable drug: Unknown.

PREGNANCY-LACTATION-REPRODUCTION

• Not indicated for use in pregnancy; drug is contraindicated. Discontinue drug if pregnancy is confirmed.

• There is little or no increased risk of birth defects in patients who accidently use combined hormonal contraceptives during early pregnancy.

• Drug may appear in human milk and may decrease quantity and quality of milk. Patients who are breastfeeding should use other forms of contraception.

• Drug isn't indicated before menarche.

NURSING CONSIDERATIONS

🛇 *Alert:* Drug may increase the risk of MI, thromboembolism, stroke, hepatic neoplasia, and gallbladder disease.

Boxed Warning Cigarette smoking increases the risk of serious adverse cardiac effects. The risk increases with age and in patients who smoke 15 or more cigarettes daily. ■

• Stop drug at least 4 weeks before and for 2 weeks after procedures that may increase the risk of thromboembolism, and during and after prolonged immobilization.

• Stop drug and notify prescriber if patient develops unexplained partial or complete loss of vision, proptosis, diplopia, papilledema, retinal vascular lesions, migraines, depression, or jaundice.

• Monitor BP closely if patient has HTN or renal disease.

• Rule out pregnancy if patient hasn't adhered to the prescribed regimen and a period is missed, if prescribed regimen has been adhered to and two periods are missed, or if patient has retained the ring for longer than 4 weeks.

PATIENT TEACHING

• Stress importance of having regular annual physical exams to check for adverse effects or developing contraindications.

• Tell patient that drug doesn't protect against HIV and other sexually transmitted diseases.

• Advise patient not to smoke while using contraceptive.

• Caution patient to use backup method of contraception until ring has been used continuously for 7 days. Tell patient not to use diaphragm, cervical cap, or female condom if backup method is needed.

• Inform patient who wears contact lenses to contact an ophthalmologist if vision or lens tolerance changes.

• Advise patient to follow manufacturer's instructions for use if switching from different form of hormonal contraceptive.

• Teach patient to insert ring into vagina (using fingers) and keep it in place continuously for 3 weeks to maintain effect, saving foil

---

Reactions in bold italics are *life-threatening*. Interactions may have a *rapid onset* or a *delayed onset*.

package for later disposal. Explain that it is then removed for 1 full week and that, during this time, withdrawal bleeding occurs (usually starting 2 or 3 days after removal). Tell patient to insert new ring 1 week after removing previous one at approximately the same time of day, regardless of menstrual bleeding. Tell patient to reseal ring in the package after removing it from vagina.

• Advise patient to regularly check for presence of ring in the vagina and not to deviate from the recommended regimen.

• Inform patient that, if the ring is removed or expelled (such as while removing a tampon, straining, or moving bowels), it should be washed with cool to lukewarm (not hot) water and reinserted immediately. Stress that contraceptive effect may be compromised if the ring stays out for longer than 3 hours and that she should use a backup method of contraception until the newly reinserted ring has been used continuously for 7 days.

• Tell patient that there's no danger of the vaginal ring being pushed too far up in the vagina or getting lost.

SAFETY ALERT!

etoposide
e-toe-POE-side

etoposide phosphate
Etopophos

Therapeutic class: Antineoplastics
Pharmacologic class: Podophyllotoxin derivatives

AVAILABLE FORMS
etoposide
Capsules: 50 mg
Injection: 20 mg/mL in 5-mL, 25-mL, 50-mL vials
etoposide phosphate
Injection: 114-mg vials equivalent to 100 mg etoposide

INDICATIONS & DOSAGES
Adjust-a-dose (for all indications): For patients with CrCl of 15 to 50 mL/minute, reduce dose by 25%. For patients with CrCl of less than 15 mL/minute, consider further dosage reduction. Adjust dosage to account for myelosuppressive effects of coadministered

drugs or effects of prior radiation therapy or chemotherapy.

➤ **Refractory testicular cancer in combination with other chemotherapeutic agents**
Adults: 50 to 100 mg/m^2 daily IV on 5 consecutive days every 21- to 28-day cycle. Or, 100 mg/m^2 daily IV on days 1, 3, and 5 every 21- to 28-day cycle.

➤ **Small-cell carcinoma of the lung in combination with other chemotherapeutic agents**
Adults: 35 mg/m^2 daily IV for 4 days. Or, 50 mg/m^2 daily IV for 5 days. Repeat cycles every 3 to 4 weeks. Oral dose is two times IV dose (70 mg/m^2 for 4 days to 100 mg/m^2 for 5 days), rounded to nearest 50 mg.

ADMINISTRATION
PO
• Hazardous drug; use appropriate handling and disposal precautions.
• Consider antiemetics because oral etoposide is associated with mild to moderate emetic potential.
• Give drug without regard for food.
• Refrigerate capsules at 36° to 46° F (2° to 8° C). Don't freeze. Capsules are stable for 36 months under refrigeration.
IV
▼ Preparing and giving parenteral drug may be mutagenic, teratogenic, or carcinogenic. Follow facility policy to reduce risks. Use gloves.
▼ Plastic devices made of acrylic or ABS (acrylonitrile butadiene styrene) have been reported to crack and leak when used with undiluted etoposide injection.
▼ Drug is an irritant; monitor IV site to avoid extravasation.
▼ For etoposide infusion, dilute to 0.2 or 0.4 mg/mL in either D$_5$W or NSS. Higher concentrations may crystallize.
▼ Give etoposide by slow infusion over at least 30 to 60 minutes to prevent severe hypotension. Never give by rapid injection.
▼ For etoposide phosphate, reconstitute each vial with sterile water for injection, D$_5$W, NSS, bacteriostatic water for injection with benzyl alcohol, or bacteriostatic sodium chloride for injection with benzyl alcohol to a concentration of 20 mg/mL or 10 mg/mL. After reconstitution, give without further dilution or dilute to as low as 0.1 mg/mL in either D$_5$W or NSS.

⬥Canada ◇OTC ◆Off-label use ✐Photoguide ⬚Do not crush *Liquid contains alcohol ▨Genetic

▼ Give etoposide phosphate over 5 minutes to 3.5 hours.

▼ Check BP every 15 minutes during infusion. Hypotension may occur if infusion is too rapid. If systolic pressure falls below 90 mm Hg, stop infusion and notify prescriber.

▼ Etoposide diluted to 0.2 mg/mL is stable for 96 hours at room temperature in plastic or glass, unprotected from light; at 0.4 mg/mL, it's stable for 24 hours under same conditions. Diluted etoposide phosphate solution stored in glass or plastic containers is stable under refrigeration for 7 days or for 24 to 48 hours at room temperature, depending on diluent. Further diluted solutions are stable under refrigeration or at room temperature for 24 hours.

▼ **Incompatibilities:** Cefepime, diazepam, filgrastim, gallium nitrate, idarubicin.

ACTION
Inhibits topoisomerase II enzyme, causing inability to repair DNA strand breaks, which leads to cell death. Cell-cycle specific to G_2 portion of cell cycle.

Route	Onset	Peak	Duration
PO, IV	Unknown	Unknown	Unknown

Half-life: Terminal phase, 4 to 11 hours.

ADVERSE REACTIONS
CNS: peripheral neuropathy, fatigue, aftertaste, fever, *seizures.* **CV:** hypotension. **EENT:** transient cortical blindness, optic neuritis. **GI:** anorexia, diarrhea, nausea, vomiting, abdominal pain, stomatitis, mucositis, constipation, dysphagia, esophagitis. **Hematologic:** *leukopenia, neutropenia, thrombocytopenia, secondary leukemia,* anemia, *myelosuppression.* **Hepatic:** *hepatotoxicity.* **Respiratory:** interstitial pneumonitis, pulmonary fibrosis. **Skin:** reversible alopecia, rash, radiation recall dermatitis, pigmentation, *SJS.* **Other:** hypersensitivity reactions, including *anaphylaxis-like reaction.*

INTERACTIONS
Drug-drug. *Cyclosporine:* May increase etoposide level and toxicity. Monitor CBC and adjust etoposide dose.
CYP3A4 inducers (carbamazepine, fosphenytoin, rifampin): May decrease etoposide phosphate concentration. Use alternative when possible.

Live-virus vaccines: May increase risk of adverse reactions to live-virus vaccine. Concurrent use isn't recommended.
Phosphatase inhibitors: May decrease etoposide effectiveness. Monitor drug effects.
Warfarin: May further prolong PT. Monitor PT and INR closely.
Drug-food. *Grapefruit juice:* May reduce etoposide concentrations. Avoid using together.

EFFECTS ON LAB TEST RESULTS
• May decrease Hb level and neutrophil, platelet, RBC, and WBC counts.

CONTRAINDICATIONS & CAUTIONS
• Contraindicated in patients hypersensitive to drug.
• Use cautiously in patients with hepatic impairment.
• Secondary leukemias have occurred with long-term use.
• Safety and effectiveness in children haven't been established.
Dialyzable drug: No.

PREGNANCY-LACTATION-REPRODUCTION
• Drug can cause fetal harm if used during pregnancy. Advise patient of childbearing potential to use effective contraception during treatment and for at least 6 months after final dose. If drug is used during pregnancy, or if patient becomes pregnant during therapy, apprise patient of fetal hazard.
• Males with partners of childbearing potential should use effective contraception during treatment and for 4 months after final dose.
• Drug appears in human milk. Patient should discontinue breastfeeding or discontinue drug.
• In females, drug may cause infertility and result in amenorrhea. Recovery of menses and ovulation is related to age at treatment. In males, drug may result in oligospermia, azoospermia, and permanent loss of fertility. Sperm counts have been reported to return to normal levels in some men; in some cases, normal levels have occurred several years after therapy ends.

NURSING CONSIDERATIONS
Boxed Warning Give drug under the supervision of a physician experienced in the use of cancer chemotherapy. Severe myelosuppression with infection or bleeding may occur. ∎

Reactions in bold italics are *life-threatening*. Interactions may have a *rapid onset* or a *delayed onset*.

- Obtain baseline BP before starting therapy.
- Anticipate need for antiemetics.
- Have diphenhydramine, hydrocortisone, epinephrine, and emergency equipment available to establish an airway in case anaphylaxis occurs.

Boxed Warning Monitor CBC. Watch for evidence of bone marrow suppression, which could lead to infection or bleeding. ∎

- Patients with low serum albumin level may be at increased risk for toxicities.
- Observe patient's mouth for signs of ulceration.
- To prevent bleeding, avoid all IM injections when platelet count is below 50,000/mm³.

PATIENT TEACHING

- Tell patient to report all adverse reactions and to watch for signs and symptoms of infection (fever, sore throat, fatigue) and bleeding (easy bruising, nosebleeds, bleeding gums, melena). Tell patient to take temperature daily.
- Inform patient of need for frequent BP readings during IV administration.
- Inform patient of the risk of secondary cancers with long-term use.
- Caution patient of childbearing potential to avoid pregnancy and breastfeeding during therapy and to use effective contraception during treatment and for 6 months after final dose.
- Advise male patient to use effective contraception for 4 months after final dose.

---

etravirine
eh-trah-VIGH-reen

Intelence

Therapeutic class: Antiretrovirals
Pharmacologic class: NNRTIs

AVAILABLE FORMS
Tablets ⊙: 25 mg, 100 mg, 200 mg

INDICATIONS & DOSAGES
➤ **HIV-1 in patients who are treatment-experienced, in combination with other antiretrovirals**
Adults: 200 mg PO b.i.d.
Children age 2 and older weighing 30 kg or more: 200 mg PO b.i.d.
Children age 2 and older weighing 25 to less than 30 kg: 150 mg PO b.i.d.

Children age 2 and older weighing 20 to less than 25 kg: 125 mg PO b.i.d.
Children age 2 and older weighing 10 to less than 20 kg: 100 mg PO b.i.d.

ADMINISTRATION
PO
- Give drug after meals.
- Have patient swallow tablets whole with a liquid such as water.
- If patient can't swallow whole tablets, place tablets in a glass with 5 mL of water. Stir water well until it looks milky. May add 15 mL more water, orange juice, or milk to glass (avoid grapefruit juice, fluids warmer than 104° F [40° C], or carbonated beverages) and have patient drink immediately. Rinse glass with water several times and have patient swallow each rinse completely.

ACTION
Binds to reverse transcriptase, an enzyme that replicates HIV.

Route	Onset	Peak	Duration
PO	Unknown	2.5–4 hr	Unknown

Half-life: About 41 ± 20 hours.

ADVERSE REACTIONS
CNS: abnormal dreams, amnesia, anxiety, confusion, disorientation, fatigue, headache, hypoesthesia, insomnia, paresthesia, peripheral neuropathy, *seizures,* sluggishness, syncope, tremors. **CV:** angina, *atrial fibrillation,* HTN, **MI. EENT:** blurred vision, vertigo, dry mouth. **GI:** abdominal distension, abdominal pain, anorexia, constipation, diarrhea, flatulence, gastritis, GERD, *hematemesis,* nausea, *pancreatitis,* retching, stomatitis, vomiting. **GU:** *renal failure.* **Hematologic:** anemia, hemolytic anemia. **Hepatic:** *hepatitis,* hepatomegaly, increased liver enzyme levels. **Metabolic:** hyperglycemia, hypercholesterolemia, *diabetes,* dyslipidemia. **Respiratory:** *bronchospasm,* dyspnea. **Skin:** rash, night sweats, hyperhidrosis, dry skin, lipohypertrophy, itchy lesions. **Other:** hypersensitivity reactions, immune reconstitution syndrome, gynecomastia.

INTERACTIONS
Etravirine can interact significantly with many drugs. Consult a drug interaction resource or pharmacist for additional information.

Drug-drug. *Antiarrhythmics (amiodarone, bepridil, disopyramide, flecainide, lidocaine, mexiletine, propafenone, quinidine):* May decrease levels of these drugs. Use caution, and monitor patient closely.

Atazanavir: May decrease atazanavir level and increase etravirine level. Avoid use unless atazanavir is boosted with ritonavir.

Atorvastatin, lovastatin, simvastatin: May decrease levels of these drugs. Adjust dosage, if needed.

Clarithromycin: May decrease clarithromycin level and increase etravirine level. Consider using azithromycin for treating MAC.

CYP3A4 inhibitors (itraconazole, ketoconazole): May decrease levels of these drugs. May increase etravirine level. Adjust dosage, if needed.

CYP450 inducers (carbamazepine, phenobarbital, phenytoin): May decrease etravirine level. Avoid use together.

Delavirdine: May increase etravirine level. Avoid use together.

Dexamethasone: May decrease etravirine level. Avoid use together.

Diazepam: May increase diazepam level. Reduce diazepam dose, as needed.

Dolutegravir: May decrease dolutegravir level. Use only when administered with atazanavir–ritonavir, darunavir–ritonavir, or lopinavir–ritonavir.

Efavirenz, nevirapine: May decrease etravirine level. Avoid use together.

Fluconazole, posaconazole: May increase etravirine level. Use together cautiously.

Fluvastatin: May increase fluvastatin level. Adjust dosage, if needed.

Immunosuppressants (cyclosporine, sirolimus, tacrolimus): May decrease levels of these drugs. Use together cautiously, and monitor patient closely.

Lopinavir–ritonavir: May decrease etravirine level. Use together cautiously.

Methadone: May cause withdrawal symptoms. Monitor patient, and consider increasing methadone dosage.

NNRTIs (delavirdine, efavirenz, nevirapine, rilpivirine): May alter etravirine level and hasn't been shown to be beneficial. Administration with other NNRTIs isn't recommended.

PDE5 inhibitors (sildenafil, tadalafil, vardenafil): May decrease effectiveness of these drugs. Adjust dosage, as needed.

Protease inhibitors (atazanavir, fosamprenavir, nelfinavir): May alter protease inhibitor level if given without ritonavir. Avoid use together unless given with low-dose ritonavir.

Rifabutin: May decrease etravirine and rifabutin levels. If etravirine isn't given with a protease inhibitor and ritonavir, give rifabutin 300 mg daily. If etravirine is given with darunavir and ritonavir or with saquinavir and ritonavir, avoid rifabutin.

Rifampin, rifapentine: May decrease etravirine level. Avoid use together.

Ritonavir: May decrease etravirine level. Avoid use together.

Ritonavir and tipranavir: May decrease etravirine level. Avoid use together.

Warfarin: May increase warfarin level. Monitor INR closely, and adjust warfarin dosage if needed.

Drug-herb. *St. John's wort:* May decrease etravirine level. Avoid use together.

EFFECTS ON LAB TEST RESULTS
• May increase amylase, lipase, creatinine, total cholesterol, LDL, triglyceride, AST, ALT, and glucose levels.
• May decrease Hb level and WBC, neutrophil, and platelet counts.

CONTRAINDICATIONS & CAUTIONS
• Contraindicated in patients hypersensitive to etravirine or its components.
• Hypersensitivity reactions, including DRESS syndrome (ranging from rash to organ dysfunction), and severe, potentially life-threatening and fatal skin reactions (SJS, TEN, erythema multiforme) have been reported. Discontinue drug immediately if signs or symptoms of hypersensitivity reactions or severe skin reactions develop.
• Concomitant use with other drugs may result in potentially significant drug interactions, some of which may lead to loss of therapeutic effect and possible resistance. See manufacturer's recommendations for dosage adjustments.
• Use cautiously in older adults and patients with hepatic impairment or HBV or HCV infection.
• For children, don't exceed adult dosage or give to children younger than age 2.
Dialyzable drug: Unlikely.

Reactions in bold italics are *life-threatening*. Interactions may have a *rapid onset* or a ***delayed onset***.

PREGNANCY-LACTATION-REPRODUCTION

- Use only if potential benefit outweighs fetal risk.
- Register patients who are pregnant in the Antiretroviral Pregnancy Registry at 1-800-258-4263.
- It isn't known if drug appears in human milk. Patients with HIV infection shouldn't breastfeed.

NURSING CONSIDERATIONS

⚠ *Alert:* Etravirine may interact with many drugs. Review patient's complete drug regimen.
⚠ *Alert:* Monitor patient closely for skin reactions. Fatalities have occurred due to TEN, SJS, or erythema multiforme, and hypersensitivity reactions that may be accompanied by hepatic failure. Discontinue drug if severe skin or hypersensitivity reactions develop.
- Monitor patient for signs of fat redistribution (central obesity, buffalo hump, peripheral wasting, breast enlargement, cushingoid appearance).
- Immune reconstitution syndrome can occur. Monitor patient for inflammatory response to indolent or residual infections or autoimmune disorders.
- Notify prescriber if signs, symptoms, or lab abnormalities suggest pancreatitis. Monitor amylase and lipase levels.
- Monitor patient's CBC, platelet count, LFTs, and renal function studies. Report abnormalities.

PATIENT TEACHING

- Instruct patient in safe drug administration.
- Warn patient to tell prescriber about any other prescription drugs, OTC drugs, and herbal supplements being taken.
- Advise patient to report adverse effects to prescriber.
- Inform patient that drug doesn't cure HIV infection, that opportunistic infections and other complications of HIV infection may still occur, and that HIV may still be transmitted to others through sexual contact or blood contamination.
- Advise patient to take drug as prescribed and not to alter dose or stop drug without medical approval.
- Stress importance of taking every dose; missed doses can result in development of resistance.
- Tell patient that routine blood tests will be needed to assess tolerance of drug therapy.

SAFETY ALERT!

everolimus ▨
eh-ver-OH-lih-mus

Afinitor, Afinitor Disperz, Zortress

Therapeutic class: Antineoplastics
Pharmacologic class: Kinase inhibitors

AVAILABLE FORMS

Tablets (Afinitor) ⦺: 2.5 mg, 5 mg, 7.5 mg, 10 mg
Tablets (Zortress) ⦺: 0.25 mg, 0.5 mg, 0.75 mg, 1 mg
Tablets for oral suspension (Afinitor Disperz) ⦺: 2 mg, 3 mg, 5 mg

INDICATIONS & DOSAGES

➤ **Advanced renal cell carcinoma after treatment with sunitinib or sorafenib fails; renal angiomyolipoma with tuberous sclerosis complex; advanced hormone-receptor positive, HER2-negative breast cancer in patients who are postmenopausal in combination with exemestane for recurrence or progression after treatment with letrozole or anastrozole; progressive neuroendocrine tumors of pancreatic origin (unresectable, locally advanced, or metastatic); progressive, well-differentiated, nonfunctional neuroendocrine tumors of GI or lung origin (locally advanced or metastatic) (Afinitor)**
Adults: 10 mg PO once daily. Continue until disease progression or unacceptable toxicity occurs.
Adjust-a-dose: Refer to manufacturer's instructions for dosage modifications for adverse effects, for patients with hepatic impairment, and for those taking drugs that inhibit or induce P-gp and CYP3A4.
➤ **Prevention of organ rejection in liver transplantation (Zortress only)**
Adults: 1 mg PO b.i.d. starting at least 30 days after transplant in combination with reduced-dose tacrolimus and corticosteroids. Adjust dosage based on trough concentrations obtained 4 to 5 days after previous dosing.
Adjust-a-dose: In patients with mild hepatic impairment, reduce initial dose by a third. In patients with moderate to severe hepatic impairment, reduce initial dose by half and monitor blood concentrations.

➤ **Prevention of kidney transplant rejection in patients at low to moderate immunologic risk (Zortress only)**

Adults: Initially, 0.75 mg PO b.i.d. in combination with basiliximab induction and a reduced dose of cyclosporine and corticosteroids as soon as possible after transplantation. Dosage adjustments may be made at 4- to 5-day intervals based on patient response and clinical situation.

Adjust-a-dose: In patients with mild hepatic impairment (Child-Pugh class A), reduce initial dose by a third. In patients with moderate to severe hepatic impairment (Child-Pugh class B or C), reduce initial dose by half and monitor blood concentrations.

➤ **Subependymal giant cell astrocytoma with tuberous sclerosis in patients who aren't surgical candidates (Afinitor or Afinitor Disperz)**

Adults and children age 1 and older: Initially, 4.5 mg/m² PO once daily until disease progression or unacceptable toxicity; round dose to nearest strength. Adjust dosage per manufacturer's instructions in 1- to 2-week intervals to trough concentration of 5 to 15 ng/mL. Maximum dose increment at any titration must not exceed 5 mg. Don't combine the two dosage forms (Afinitor tablets and Afinitor Disperz tablets) to achieve the desired dose. Use one dosage form or the other. Once a stable dose is attained, monitor trough concentrations every 3 to 6 months in patients with changing BSA or every 6 to 12 months in patients with stable BSA for duration of treatment.

Adjust-a-dose: Refer to manufacturer's instructions for dosage modifications for adverse effects, for patients with hepatic impairment, and for those taking drugs that inhibit or induce P-gp and CYP3A4.

➤ **Adjunctive treatment of patients with tuberous sclerosis complex (TSC)–associated partial-onset seizures (Afinitor Disperz)** ▨

Adults and children age 2 and older: Initially, 5 mg/m² PO once daily. Titrate dosage to attain trough concentration of 5 to 15 ng/mL. Maximum dose increase is 5 mg every 1 to 2 weeks. Once a stable dose is attained, monitor trough concentrations every 3 to 6 months in patients with changing BSA or every 6 to 12 months in patients with stable BSA for duration of treatment.

Adjust-a-dose: For patients with severe hepatic impairment (Child-Pugh class C), initially, 2.5 mg/m² once daily; adjust dosage based on trough concentrations as recommended. Refer to manufacturer's instructions for toxicity-related dosage adjustments and for dosage adjustments when drug is used concurrently with P-gp and CYP3A4 inhibitors and P-gp and CYP3A4 inducers.

ADMINISTRATION
PO
Afinitor, Zortress
• Give drug at same time(s) each day, consistently with or without food.
• Have patient swallow tablets whole with a glass of water. Tablets shouldn't be chewed or crushed.
Afinitor Disperz
• Wear gloves to avoid possible contact with everolimus when preparing suspension.
• Give as a suspension only.
• Give drug orally once daily at the same time every day, either consistently with or without food.
• Administer suspension immediately after preparation. Discard suspension if not administered within 60 minutes after preparation. Prepare suspension in water only.
• To administer drug using an oral syringe, place the prescribed dose into a 10-mL syringe. Don't exceed a total of 10 mg per syringe. If higher doses are required, prepare an additional syringe. Don't break or crush tablets. Draw approximately 5 mL of water and 4 mL of air into the syringe. Place the filled syringe into a container (tip up) for 3 minutes, until the tablets are in suspension. Gently invert the syringe five times immediately before administration. After administration of prepared suspension, draw approximately 5 mL of water and 4 mL of air into the same syringe, and swirl contents to suspend remaining particles. Administer the entire contents of the syringe.
• To administer using a small drinking glass, place the prescribed dose into a small drinking glass (maximum size 100 mL) containing approximately 25 mL of water. Don't exceed a total of 10 mg per glass. If higher doses are required, prepare an additional glass. Don't break or crush tablets. Allow 3 minutes for suspension to occur. Stir the contents gently with a spoon, immediately prior to drinking. After administration of the prepared

suspension, add 25 mL of water and stir with the same spoon to re-suspend remaining particles. Administer the entire contents of the glass.

• May give a missed Afinitor dose up to 6 hours after the normally scheduled dose. If more than 6 hours have elapsed, omit that day's dose and give it at the usual time the next day.

ACTION
Binds to an intracellular protein, thereby inhibiting mammalian target rapamycin (mTOR), a kinase. Inhibiting mTOR reduces cancer cell proliferation, angiogenesis, and glucose uptake.

Route	Onset	Peak	Duration
PO	Unknown	1–2 hr	Unknown

Half-life: 30 hours.

ADVERSE REACTIONS
CNS: asthenia, dizziness, headache, insomnia, paresthesia, fever, fatigue, dysgeusia, *seizures.* **CV:** chest pain, peripheral edema, *HF,* HTN, tachycardia, edema, hot flush, *hemorrhage.* **EENT:** conjunctivitis, eyelid edema, epistaxis, nasopharyngitis, oropharyngeal pain, rhinitis, dry mouth. **GI:** abdominal pain, anorexia, diarrhea, dysphagia, hemorrhoids, nausea, stomatitis, vomiting, constipation. **GU:** increased creatinine level, renal failure, UTI, menstrual irregularities. **Hematologic:** anemia, *leukopenia, neutropenia, thrombocytopenia.* **Hepatic:** elevated ALP, AST, ALT levels. **Metabolic:** diabetes exacerbation, weight loss, *hypokalemia,* hyperglycemia, hypercholesterolemia, hypertriglyceridemia, hypophosphatemia. **Musculoskeletal:** extremity pain, jaw pain, arthralgia, back pain. **Respiratory:** cough, dyspnea, pleural effusion, URI, *pneumonitis.* **Skin:** acneiform dermatitis, dry skin, erythema, hand-foot syndrome, nail disorder, pruritus, onychoclasis, rash, alopecia, skin lesion. **Other:** chills, infection, hypersensitivity reactions, *angioedema.*

INTERACTIONS
Drug-drug. *Clozapine:* May enhance risk of neutropenia. Monitor patient response.
Boxed Warning *Cyclosporine:* Increased nephrotoxicity can occur with standard cyclosporine dosing in combination with Zortress. Decrease cyclosporine dosage, and monitor serum cyclosporine and everolimus levels. ■

Strong CYP3A4 inducers (carbamazepine, dexamethasone, phenobarbital, phenytoin, rifabutin, rifampin): May decrease everolimus level. Avoid using together; if drugs must be used together, increase everolimus dosage per manufacturer's instructions.

Strong or moderate CYP3A4 inhibitors (amprenavir, aprepitant, atazanavir, clarithromycin, delavirdine, diltiazem, erythromycin, fluconazole, fosamprenavir, itraconazole, ketoconazole, nefazodone, nelfinavir, ritonavir, saquinavir, telithromycin, verapamil, voriconazole) and P-gp inhibitors (amiodarone, spironolactone): May increase everolimus level. Avoid using together; if drugs must be used together, reduce everolimus dosage per manufacturer's instructions.

Vaccines (live-virus): Toxic effects of vaccines may increase and drug's therapeutic effects diminish. Avoid use together.
Drug-herb. *St. John's wort:* May alter drug level. Don't use together.
Drug-food. *Grapefruit, grapefruit juice:* May increase drug level. Don't use together.

EFFECTS ON LAB TEST RESULTS
• May increase AST, ALT, urinary protein and creatinine, cholesterol, triglyceride, and glucose levels.
• May decrease phosphate level.
• May decrease Hb level and lymphocyte, neutrophil, and platelet counts.
• May increase PT.

CONTRAINDICATIONS & CAUTIONS
Boxed Warning Use of Zortress has been shown to increase mortality in a heart transplant clinical trial. Use in patients after heart transplantation isn't recommended. ■
• Contraindicated in patients hypersensitive to drug, its components, or other rapamycin derivatives.
• Afinitor isn't indicated to treat functional carcinoid tumors.
• Avoid use in patients with severe hepatic impairment or severe infection.
Dialyzable drug: No.

PREGNANCY-LACTATION-REPRODUCTION
• Avoid use during pregnancy because of fetal risk.

• Patients of childbearing potential should avoid pregnancy and use highly effective contraception during treatment and for 8 weeks after last dose.

• Males with partners of childbearing potential should use effective contraception during treatment and for 4 weeks after final dose.

• The National Transplantation Pregnancy Registry (NTPR) follows patients who are pregnant and taking immunosuppressants after any solid organ transplant. The NTPR encourages reporting all immunosuppressant exposures during pregnancy in patients who have undergone organ transplantation (1-877-955-6877 or https://www.transplantpregnancyregistry.org/).

• Drug may cause male and female infertility.

• It isn't known if drug appears in human milk.

NURSING CONSIDERATIONS

Boxed Warning Zortress should only be prescribed by providers experienced in immunosuppressive therapy and management of patients who have undergone organ transplantation. ■

• Don't crush tablets. Avoid direct contact with skin or mucous membranes. If contact occurs, wash area thoroughly.

• Drug can adversely affect wound healing. Withhold drug for at least 1 week before elective surgery. Don't give for at least 2 weeks after major surgery and until adequate wound healing.

Boxed Warning Zortress increases risk of infection and malignancies, such as lymphoma and skin cancer, due to immunosuppression. ■

◑ *Alert:* Drug may cause immunosuppression, predisposing patients to bacterial, fungal, viral, or protozoal infections, including reactivation of hepatitis B virus. Infections may be severe or even fatal. Complete treatment of preexisting invasive fungal infections before starting therapy. Consider holding or stopping everolimus if infection occurs. Discontinue drug if invasive systemic fungal infection is diagnosed, and treat infection appropriately. Incidence of serious infections was reported at a higher frequency in patients younger than age 6.

• Monitor patient for signs of infection (fever, chills, sore throat, fatigue).

Boxed Warning There is an increased risk of arterial and venous renal thrombosis leading to graft loss in patients taking Zortress, mostly in first 30 days after transplant. ■

Boxed Warning When drug is used with cyclosporine, increased nephrotoxicity can occur and reduced dosages of everolimus are needed. Monitor cyclosporine and everolimus whole blood trough concentrations. ■

• Hyperglycemia, hypercholesterolemia, and hypertriglyceridemia have been reported. Withhold or permanently discontinue drug based on severity.

• Monitor renal function studies, glucose and lipid levels, and CBC before and during therapy.

• Monitor respiratory status for signs and symptoms of noninfectious pneumonitis (hypoxia, pleural effusion, cough, dyspnea). For severe cases, discontinue therapy and administer corticosteroids.

PATIENT TEACHING

• Advise patient of need for contraception.

• Inform male and female patient that use may impair fertility.

• Teach patient safe drug administration and handling.

• Advise patient to limit sun exposure.

• Advise patient to report mouth ulcers, fever, shortness of breath, cough, rash, headache, loss of appetite, nausea, vomiting, diarrhea, swelling of the extremities or face, weakness, tiredness, or nosebleeds.

• Tell patient not to receive live-virus vaccines and to avoid close contact with anyone who has received a live-virus vaccine.

SAFETY ALERT!

exenatide ☒
eks-EHN-uh-tyde

Bydureon BCise, Byetta

Therapeutic class: Antidiabetics
Pharmacologic class: Incretin mimetics

AVAILABLE FORMS

Injection: 5 mcg/dose in 1.2-mL; 10 mcg/dose in 2.4-mL prefilled multidose pen
Injection (extended-release): 2 mg/dose in single-dose pen

INDICATIONS & DOSAGES
➤ **Adjunct to diet and exercise to improve glycemic control in patients with type 2 diabetes**

Adults: 5 mcg (immediate-release) subcut b.i.d. within 60 minutes before morning and evening meals. Give doses at least 6 hours apart. If needed, increase to 10 mcg b.i.d. after 1 month. Or, 2 mg (extended-release) subcut once every 7 days any time of day, with or without a meal.

Adjust-a-dose: Use caution when escalating doses of Byetta (injection) from 5 to 10 mcg in patients with moderate renal impairment (CrCl of 30 to 50 mL/minute).

When converting from Byetta immediate-release to Bydureon BCise extended-release formulation, initiate weekly administration of extended-release exenatide the day after discontinuing exenatide immediate-release. Patient may experience increased blood glucose levels for approximately 2 to 4 weeks after conversion. Pretreatment with exenatide immediate-release isn't required before initiating extended-release exenatide.

ADMINISTRATION
Subcutaneous
🖑 *Alert:* Multidose pens are for single patient use only. Pens should never be shared even if the needle is changed. Clearly label with patient identifying information where it will not obstruct the dosing window, warning, or other product information.

Bydureon BCise
• Give Bydureon BCise at any time during the day and without regard to meals.
• Remove autoinjector from refrigerator 15 minutes before mixing the injection, to reach room temperature.
• Mix by shaking vigorously for at least 15 seconds. After mixing, Bydureon BCise should appear as an opaque, white to off-white suspension, evenly mixed with no residual medicine along the side, bottom, or top of the inspection window.
• Inspect visually for particulate matter and discoloration before administration; drug contains microspheres that appear as white to off-white particles. Don't use if foreign particulate matter or discoloration is observed.
• Give immediately as a subcut injection in thigh, abdomen, or back of upper arm. Rotate injection sites each week.

• Hold autoinjector straight up with the orange cap toward the ceiling. Turn the knob on bottom from the lock to unlock position until you hear a click; then unscrew and discard the orange cap.
• Push autoinjector against the skin. You will hear a click when the injection begins.
• Keep holding autoinjector against the skin for 15 seconds and until an orange rod appears in the window, to make sure the full dose is delivered.
• Give missed dose of extended-release form as soon as noticed, provided next regularly scheduled dose is due 3 or more days later. Then, resume usual dosing schedule of once every 7 days (weekly). If a dose is missed and the next regularly scheduled dose is due 1 or 2 days later, don't give the missed dose; instead, resume treatment with the next regularly scheduled dose.
• Store flat in the refrigerator between 36° and 46° F (2° and 8° C). Can keep at room temperature not to exceed 86° F (30° C) for no more than a total of 4 weeks, if needed.

Byetta
• Drug comes in two strengths; check cartridge carefully before use.
• Don't give after a meal.
• Give as a subcut injection in the thigh, abdomen, or upper arm.
• Inject subcut within 60 minutes before morning and evening meals or before the two main meals of the day approximately 6 hours or more apart.
• If a dose is missed, resume treatment with the next scheduled dose.
• Before first use, store drug in refrigerator at 36° to 46° F (2° to 8° C). After first use, drug can be kept at room temperature up to 77° F (25° C). Don't freeze, and don't use drug if it has been frozen. Protect drug from light. Discard pen 30 days after first use, even if some drug remains.
• Don't mix with insulin.

ACTION
Reduces fasting and postprandial glucose levels in type 2 diabetes, as an incretin analogue (glucagon-like peptide 1), by stimulating insulin production in response to elevated glucose levels, inhibiting glucagon release after meals, and slowing gastric emptying.

Route	Onset	Peak	Duration
Subcut	Unknown	2.1 hr	Unknown
Subcut (extended-release)	Unknown	2 wk, 6–7 wk	10 wk

Half-life: 2.4 hours; extended-release, about 2 weeks.

ADVERSE REACTIONS

CNS: dizziness, headache, fatigue, jittery feeling, nervousness, asthenia. **GI:** anorexia, constipation, decreased appetite, diarrhea, dyspepsia, nausea, vomiting, GERD, abdominal distention, flatulence. **Metabolic:** *hypoglycemia.* **Skin:** diaphoresis.

INTERACTIONS

Drug-drug. *Digoxin, lovastatin:* May decrease concentrations of these drugs. Monitor patient.

Oral drugs that need to maintain a threshold concentration to maintain effectiveness (antibiotics, hormonal contraceptives): May reduce rate and extent of absorption of these drugs. Give these drugs at least 1 hour before giving exenatide.

Other antidiabetics (insulin, meglitinides [repaglinide], sulfonylureas): May increase risk of hypoglycemia. Closely monitor blood glucose concentrations when exenatide is started or stopped, and reinforce patient instructions for hypoglycemia management, especially in patients receiving insulin. Reduce insulin or sulfonylurea dose as needed, and monitor patient closely.

Warfarin: May increase INR and increase bleeding risk when administered together. Monitor INR frequently, especially when starting drug or changing dosage.

EFFECTS ON LAB TEST RESULTS

• Decreases glucose level.
• May increase INR.

CONTRAINDICATIONS & CAUTIONS

Boxed Warning Extended-release form is contraindicated in patients with personal or family history of medullary thyroid carcinoma (MTC) and in patients with multiple endocrine neoplasia syndrome type 2. ▮

• Contraindicated in patients hypersensitive to drug or its components. Serious reactions (anaphylaxis, angioedema) have been reported. If hypersensitivity occurs, discontinue drug.

• Contraindicated in patients with a history of drug-induced immune-mediated thrombocytopenia from exenatide products.

• Possibly fatal serious bleeding from drug-induced immune-mediated thrombocytopenia has been reported with exenatide use.

Boxed Warning Exenatide extended-release causes an increased incidence in thyroid C-cell tumors at clinically relevant exposures in rats compared to controls. It's unknown whether it causes thyroid C-cell tumors, including MTC, in humans, as the human relevance of exenatide extended-release–induced rodent thyroid C-cell tumors hasn't been determined. ▮

• Exenatide extended-release isn't recommended as first-line therapy for patients with inadequate glycemic control on diet and exercise because of the uncertain relevance of the rat thyroid C-cell tumor findings to humans.

• Drug isn't recommended for patients with ESRD or severe renal impairment (CrCl of less than 30 mL/minute). Use cautiously in patients with kidney transplantation or moderate renal impairment.

• Drug has been associated with acute pancreatitis, including fatal and nonfatal hemorrhagic or necrotizing pancreatitis. Discontinue immediately if pancreatitis is suspected. Don't restart if pancreatitis is confirmed.

• Don't use in patients with type 1 diabetes or diabetic ketoacidosis.

• Don't use in patients with severe GI disease (including gastroparesis).

• Risk of hypoglycemia increases when drug is used in combination with other drugs that can lower blood glucose level (eg, insulin, insulin secretagogues). Dosage reductions may be necessary.

• Safety and effectiveness in children younger than age 10 haven't been established.

Dialyzable drug: Unknown.

⚠ *Overdose S&S:* Severe nausea, severe vomiting, hypoglycemia.

PREGNANCY-LACTATION-REPRODUCTION

• Use only if potential benefit justifies fetal risk.

• It isn't known if drug appears in human milk. Patient should discontinue breastfeeding or discontinue drug.

Reactions in bold italics are *life-threatening*. Interactions may have a *rapid onset* or a ***delayed onset***.

NURSING CONSIDERATIONS
• Assess GI and renal function before and during treatment.

Boxed Warning Routine monitoring of serum calcitonin level or the use of thyroid ultrasound is of uncertain value for detection of MTC in patients treated with exenatide extended-release. ∎

⊖ *Alert:* Drug-related nausea, vomiting, and diarrhea resulting in dehydration have led to increased serum creatinine levels and acute renal failure.

• Monitor patient receiving extended-release form for serious injection-site reactions, such as abscess, cellulitis, and necrosis, with or without subcutaneous nodules.

• Monitor glucose level regularly and HbA_{1c} level periodically.

⊖ *Alert:* Stop drug if pancreatitis is suspected. Initiate appropriate treatment, and monitor patient carefully. Drug shouldn't be readministered.

• *Look alike–sound alike:* Don't confuse exenatide with ezetimibe.

PATIENT TEACHING
Boxed Warning Explain to patient taking extended-release exenatide the risk and signs and symptoms of thyroid tumors (mass in the neck, dysphagia, dyspnea, persistent hoarseness). ∎

• Explain the risks of drug.

• Review proper use and storage of medication, particularly the one-time setup for each new pen or reconstitution procedure for powder.

• Instruct patient in the proper use of autoinjector.

⊖ *Alert:* Warn patient not to share the multidose pen device with other people, even if the needle is changed due to the risk of transmission of blood-borne pathogens, including HIV and hepatitis viruses.

• Advise patient that drug may decrease appetite, food intake, and body weight, and that these changes don't warrant a change in dosage.

• Advise patient to seek immediate medical care if unexplained, persistent, severe abdominal pain, with or without vomiting, occurs.

• Inform patient receiving extended-release form about risk of serious injection-site reactions and to report signs and symptoms (erythema, pain, drainage, skin color changes) immediately.

• Review steps for managing hypoglycemia, especially if patient takes a sulfonylurea or insulin.

• Inform patient of risk of worsening renal function and signs and symptoms of renal dysfunction.

• Tell patient changing from immediate-release to extended-release form that transient blood glucose elevations are possible during the first 2 to 4 weeks of therapy.

• Stress importance of proper storage (refrigeration), infection prevention, and timing of exenatide dose in relation to other oral drugs.

---

ezetimibe ⚲
ee-ZET-ah-mibe

Zetia⬦

Therapeutic class: Antilipemics
Pharmacologic class: Selective cholesterol absorption inhibitors

AVAILABLE FORMS
Tablets: 10 mg

INDICATIONS & DOSAGES
➤ **Adjunct to diet to reduce total cholesterol, LDL cholesterol (LDL-C), and apolipoprotein B (apo B) levels in patients with primary hypercholesterolemia, alone or combined with HMG-CoA reductase inhibitors (statins); adjunct to other lipid-lowering drugs (combined with atorvastatin or simvastatin) to reduce total cholesterol and LDL-C levels in patients with homozygous familial hypercholesterolemia; adjunct to diet in patients with homozygous sitosterolemia to reduce sitosterol and campesterol levels; adjunct to fenofibrate and diet to reduce total cholesterol, LDL-C, apo B, and non-HDL-C levels in patients with mixed hyperlipidemia** ⚲
Adults and children age 10 and older: 10 mg PO daily.

ADMINISTRATION
PO
• Give drug without regard for meals.
• May give dose at same time as an HMG-CoA reductase inhibitor or fenofibrate.
• Give at least 2 hours before or at least 4 hours after administration of a bile acid sequestrant.

ACTION

Inhibits absorption of cholesterol by the small intestine, unlike other drugs used for cholesterol reduction; causes reduced hepatic cholesterol stores and increased cholesterol clearance from the blood.

Route	Onset	Peak	Duration
PO	Within 1 wk; max effect in 2–4 wk	4–12 hr	Unknown

Half-life: 22 hours.

ADVERSE REACTIONS

CNS: dizziness, fatigue. **EENT:** nasopharyngitis, sinusitis. **GI:** diarrhea. **Musculoskeletal:** arthralgia, back pain, pain in extremity, myalgia. **Respiratory:** URI. **Other:** viral infection, flulike symptoms.

INTERACTIONS

Drug-drug. *Bile acid sequestrant (cholestyramine):* May decrease ezetimibe level. Give ezetimibe at least 2 hours before or 4 hours after cholestyramine.
Coumarin anticoagulants (warfarin): May alter anticoagulant effects. Monitor INR.
Cyclosporine: May increase levels of both drugs. Monitor cyclosporine level and patient for adverse reactions.
Fenofibrate: May increase risk of cholelithiasis. Monitor patient; consider alternative therapy if cholelithiasis occurs.
Fibrates: May increase excretion of cholesterol into the gallbladder bile. Avoid using together.
Gemfibrozil: May increase risk of myopathy and cholelithiasis. Avoid use together.

EFFECTS ON LAB TEST RESULTS

• May increase LFT values and CK level.

CONTRAINDICATIONS & CAUTIONS

• Contraindicated in patients hypersensitive to components of drug.
• Contraindicated in combination with HMG-CoA reductase inhibitors in patients with active liver disease or unexplained increased transaminase levels.
• Rarely, myopathy, including rhabdomyolysis, has been reported. Risk may increase with concurrent use of fibrate drugs or high-dose statins, age greater than 65, hypothyroidism, or renal impairment. Discontinue ezetimibe and statin or fibrate immediately if myopathy is suspected or confirmed.

• Administration with fibrates other than fenofibrate isn't recommended until use in patients is adequately studied.
Dialyzable drug: Unknown.

PREGNANCY-LACTATION-REPRODUCTION

• Use only if potential benefit justifies fetal risk.
• When drug is used with a statin in a patient of childbearing potential, refer to pregnancy information and product labeling for the statin. Statins are contraindicated during breastfeeding.
• It isn't known if drug appears in human milk. Use drug only if potential benefit justifies risk to the infant.

NURSING CONSIDERATIONS

• Before starting treatment, assess patient for underlying causes of dyslipidemia.
• Obtain baseline triglyceride and total cholesterol, LDL-C, and HDL-C levels.
• Using drug with an HMG-CoA reductase inhibitor significantly decreases total cholesterol and LDL-C, apo B, and triglyceride levels and (except with pravastatin) increases HDL-C level more than use of an HMG-CoA reductase inhibitor alone. Check LFT values when therapy starts and thereafter according to the HMG-CoA reductase inhibitor manufacturer's recommendations.
• Patient should maintain a cholesterol-lowering diet during treatment.
• Monitor patient for muscle pain, weakness, or tenderness. Discontinue drug if signs or symptoms of myopathy occur with CK more than 10 × ULN.

PATIENT TEACHING

• Emphasize importance of following a cholesterol-lowering diet during drug therapy.
• Instruct patient in safe drug administration.
• Advise patient to report unexplained muscle pain, weakness, or tenderness.
• Urge patient to tell prescriber about any herbal or dietary supplements being taken.
• Advise patient to visit prescriber for routine follow-ups and to obtain monitoring blood tests.
• Tell patient to report pregnancy.

Reactions in bold italics are *life-threatening*. Interactions may have a *rapid onset* or a *delayed onset*.

famciclovir 🐾
fam-SYE-kloe-vir

Therapeutic class: Antivirals
Pharmacologic class: Nucleosides–nucleotides

AVAILABLE FORMS
Tablets: 125 mg, 250 mg, 500 mg

INDICATIONS & DOSAGES
➤ **Acute herpes zoster infection (shingles)**
Adults: 500 mg PO every 8 hours for 7 days.
Adjust-a-dose: For patients with CrCl of 40 to 59 mL/minute, give 500 mg PO every 12 hours; if CrCl is 20 to 39 mL/minute, give 500 mg PO every 24 hours; if CrCl is less than 20 mL/minute, give 250 mg PO every 24 hours. For patients on hemodialysis, give 250 mg PO after each hemodialysis session.
➤ **Recurrent genital herpes**
Adults: 1,000 mg PO b.i.d. for a single day. Begin therapy at the first sign or symptom.
Adjust-a-dose: For patients with CrCl of 40 to 59 mL/minute, give 500 mg every 12 hours for 1 day; for CrCl of 20 to 39 mL/minute, give 500 mg PO as a single dose; if CrCl is less than 20 mL/minute, give 250 mg as a single dose. For patient on hemodialysis, give 250 mg single dose after hemodialysis session.
➤ **Suppression of recurrent genital herpes**
Adults: 250 mg PO b.i.d. for up to 1 year.
Adjust-a-dose: For patients with CrCl of 20 to 39 mL/minute, give 125 mg PO every 12 hours; if CrCl is less than 20 mL/minute, give 125 mg PO every 24 hours. For patients on hemodialysis, give 125 mg PO after each hemodialysis session.
➤ **Recurrent mucocutaneous (orolabial/genital) herpes simplex infections in patients infected with HIV**
Adults: 500 mg PO b.i.d. for 7 days.
Adjust-a-dose: For patients with CrCl of 20 to 39 mL/minute, give 500 mg PO every 24 hours; if CrCl is less than 20 mL/minute, give 250 mg PO every 24 hours. For patients on hemodialysis, give 250 mg PO after each hemodialysis session.
➤ **Recurrent herpes labialis (cold sores)**
Adults: 1,500 mg PO for one dose. Give at the first sign or symptom of cold sore.
Adjust-a-dose: For patients with CrCl of 40 to 59 mL/minute, give 750 mg as a single dose;

for CrCl of 20 to 39 mL/minute, give 500 mg PO as a single dose; if CrCl is less than 20 mL/minute, give 250 mg as a single dose. For patient on hemodialysis, give 250 mg single dose after hemodialysis session.

ADMINISTRATION
PO
• Give drug without regard for meals.
• Store at 68° to 77° F (20° to 25° C).

ACTION
A guanosine nucleoside that is converted to penciclovir, which enters viral cells and inhibits DNA polymerase and viral DNA synthesis.

Route	Onset	Peak	Duration
PO	Unknown	1 hr	Unknown

Half-life: Penciclovir, 2 to 4 hours.

ADVERSE REACTIONS
CNS: headache, migraine, fatigue, dizziness, paresthesia, somnolence. **GI:** nausea, abdominal pain, diarrhea, vomiting, flatulence. **GU:** dysmenorrhea. **Hematologic:** *leukopenia, neutropenia.* **Hepatic:** elevated AST and ALT levels, bilirubinemia. **Metabolic:** increased amylase and lipase levels. **Skin:** pruritus, rash.

INTERACTIONS
Drug-drug. *Varicella virus vaccine, zoster vaccine (live, attenuated):* May diminish effect of vaccines. When possible, discontinue famciclovir for at least 24 hours before and 14 days after vaccinations.

EFFECTS ON LAB TEST RESULTS
• May increase AST, ALT, amylase, lipase, and bilirubin levels.
• May decrease Hb level and leukocyte and neutrophil counts.

CONTRAINDICATIONS & CAUTIONS
• Contraindicated in patients hypersensitive to drug, its components, or penciclovir cream.
• Use cautiously in patients with renal or hepatic impairment and in older adults.
🔲 Efficacy and safety haven't been established for patients with first episode of genital herpes or ophthalmic zoster; patients who are immunocompromised, other than for treatment of recurrent episodes of orolabial or genital herpes in patients infected with HIV;

and patients who are Black or African American with recurrent genital herpes.
• Efficacy in children hasn't been established.
Dialyzable drug: Yes.

PREGNANCY-LACTATION-REPRODUCTION
• Use drug during pregnancy only if benefit clearly outweighs fetal risk.
• It isn't known if drug appears in human milk. Use only if benefits outweigh risk to the infant.

NURSING CONSIDERATIONS
• Monitor LFTs and renal function tests.
• Periodically monitor CBC during long-term therapy.

PATIENT TEACHING
• Inform patient that drug doesn't cure herpes but can decrease the duration and severity of symptoms.
• Teach patient how to avoid spreading infection to others.
• Urge patient to recognize the early signs and symptoms of herpes infection, such as tingling, itching, burning, pain, or lesion and to report them. Therapy is more effective if started within 48 hours of rash onset.
• Drug may contain lactose. If patient is lactose-intolerant, advise patient to notify prescriber before taking drug.
• Advise patient who experiences dizziness, somnolence, confusion or other CNS disturbance to refrain from driving or operating machinery.

famotidine
fa-MOE-ti-deen

Pepcid◆, Pepcid AC ◇,
Zantac 360° ◇

Therapeutic class: Antiulcer drugs
Pharmacologic class: H$_2$-receptor antagonists

AVAILABLE FORMS
Injection: 0.4 mg/mL in NSS (premixed), 10 mg/mL
Powder for oral suspension: 40 mg/5 mL after reconstitution
Tablets: 10 mg ◇, 20 mg ◇, 40 mg

INDICATIONS & DOSAGES
Adjust-a-dose (for all indications): For patients with CrCl below 60 mL/minute, refer to manufacturer's product information because dosage varies based on form being administered, indication, and CrCl value.
➤ **Short-term treatment for duodenal ulcer**
Adults, children, and adolescents weighing more than 40 kg: For acute therapy, 40 mg PO once daily at bedtime or 20 mg PO b.i.d. for up to 4 to 8 weeks. Healing usually occurs within 4 weeks.

For maintenance therapy (adults), 20 mg PO once daily at bedtime for 1 year or as clinically indicated.
Children ages 1 to 16: 0.5 mg/kg/day oral suspension PO at bedtime or divided b.i.d. (maximum dose, 40 mg/day); doses up to 1 mg/kg/day have been used.
➤ **Short-term treatment for benign gastric ulcer**
Adults, children, and adolescents weighing more than 40 kg: 40 mg PO daily at bedtime for up to 8 weeks.
Children ages 1 to 16: 0.5 mg/kg/day PO at bedtime or in two divided doses, up to 40 mg daily; doses up to 1 mg/kg/day have been used.
➤ **Pathologic hypersecretory conditions (such as Zollinger-Ellison syndrome)**
Adults: 20 mg PO every 6 hours, up to 160 mg every 6 hours. Maximum, 640 mg/day.
➤ **Patients who are hospitalized who can't take oral drug or who have intractable ulcers or hypersecretory conditions**
Adults: 20 mg IV every 12 hours.
Children ages 1 to 16: 0.25 mg/kg IV every 12 hours (maximum dose, 40 mg/day); doses up to 0.5 mg/kg every 12 hours have been used.
➤ **GERD**
Adults, children, and adolescents weighing more than 40 kg: Short-term therapy: 20 mg PO b.i.d. for up to 6 weeks. For esophagitis caused by GERD, 20 to 40 mg b.i.d. for up to 12 weeks.
Children ages 1 to 16: Short-term therapy: 0.5 mg/kg/dose PO b.i.d. (maximum dose, 40 mg b.i.d.). Up to 1 mg/kg/dose b.i.d. has been used.
Children ages 3 months to younger than 1 year: Short-term therapy: 0.5 mg/kg/dose oral suspension PO b.i.d. for up to 8 weeks.

Reactions in bold italics are *life-threatening*. Interactions may have a *rapid onset* or a **delayed onset**.

Children younger than age 3 months: Short-term therapy: 0.5 mg/kg/dose oral suspension once daily for up to 8 weeks.

➤ **To prevent or treat heartburn (only indication for OTC)**
Adults and children older than age 12: 10 to 20 mg up to b.i.d. for maximum of 40 mg/day.

ADMINISTRATION
PO
• Give without regard to meals.
• May give OTC tablets 10 to 60 minutes before patient eats food or drinks beverages that cause heartburn. Patient shouldn't chew regular tablets.
• May give with antacids.
• Shake oral suspension before use.
• Store reconstituted oral suspension below 77° F (25° C). Discard after 30 days. Don't freeze.
• Store tablets at 68° to 77° F (20° to 25° C). Protect from light.
IV
▼ Compatible solutions include sterile water for injection, NSS for injection, D₅W or dextrose 10% in water for injection, 5% sodium bicarbonate injection, and lactated Ringer injection. Drug also can be added to TPN solutions.
▼ Before use, store at 36° to 46° F (2° to 8° C). If solution freezes, allow to solubilize at room temperature. Protect from light.
▼ For direct injection, dilute 2 mL (20 mg) with compatible solution to a total volume of either 5 or 10 mL. Inject over at least 2 minutes.
▼ For intermittent infusion, dilute 20 mg (2 mL) in 100-mL compatible solution. The premixed 50-mL solution doesn't need further dilution. Infuse over 15 or 30 minutes.
▼ After dilution, solution is stable for 7 days at room temperature.
▼ **Incompatibilities:** Amphotericin B cholesteryl sulfate complex, azathioprine, cefepime, chloramphenicol, dantrolene, diazepam, ganciclovir, gemtuzumab, lansoprazole, mitomycin, pantoprazole, piperacillin–tazobactam, trimethoprim–sulfamethoxazole.

ACTION
Competitively inhibits action of histamine on the H₂-receptor sites of parietal cells, decreasing gastric acid secretion.

Route	Onset	Peak	Duration
PO	1 hr	1–3 hr	10–20 hr
IV	1 hr	1–4 hr	10–20 hr

Half-life: 2.5 to 3.5 hours.

ADVERSE REACTIONS
CNS: headache, dizziness; irritability, agitation (younger than age 1). **GI:** constipation, diarrhea; vomiting (younger than age 1).

INTERACTIONS
Drug-drug. *Cefditoren, dasatinib, delavirdine, fosamprenavir:* May decrease absorption of these drugs due to reduced gastric acidity. Avoid use together.
Drugs dependent on gastric pH for absorption (atazanavir, cefuroxime, erlotinib, ketoconazole, itraconazole, nilotinib, rilpivirine): May decrease absorption of these drugs. Refer to prescribing information of the individual drug.
Drugs that prolong QT interval (antiarrhythmics, chlorpromazine, citalopram, clarithromycin, fluoxetine, levofloxacin): May increase risk of cardiac arrhythmias, including torsades de pointes. Use together cautiously unless specifically contraindicated. Refer to prescribing information of the individual drug.
Risedronate (delayed-release): May increase risedronate serum concentration. Avoid combination.

EFFECTS ON LAB TEST RESULTS
• May increase liver enzyme levels.
• May cause false-negative results in skin tests using allergen extracts. May antagonize pentagastrin in gastric acid secretion tests.

CONTRAINDICATIONS & CAUTIONS
• Contraindicated in patients with a history of serious hypersensitivity to drug and other H₂-receptor antagonists.
• Use for OTC self-medication is contraindicated in patients with trouble or pain when swallowing, vomiting with blood, bloody or black stools, allergic reactions to other acid reducers, or renal impairment and in those using other acid reducers unless directed by health care provider.
• Drug may cause reversible confusional states that clear within 3 to 4 days after discontinuation. Patients older than age 50 and

those with renal or hepatic impairment may be more at risk.

🌑 *Alert:* Symptomatic response doesn't preclude the presence of gastric malignancy. Consider further evaluation in patients with suboptimal response or an early symptomatic relapse after treatment with drug.

🌑 *Alert:* QT-interval prolongation and torsades de pointes have been reported rarely in patients with renal dysfunction.

• Treatment lasting 2 years can cause vitamin B$_{12}$ deficiency, which is dose-related and more likely to occur in women and those younger than age 30.

🌑 *Alert:* Some forms may contain benzyl alcohol, which is linked to gasping syndrome (metabolic acidosis, respiratory distress, CNS dysfunction, hypotension, CV collapse) in neonates.

Dialyzable drug: No.

⚠ *Overdose S&S:* Similar to adverse reactions with use at recommended dosages.

PREGNANCY-LACTATION-REPRODUCTION

• Drug crosses placental barrier and appears in human milk. Use cautiously during pregnancy and breastfeeding.

NURSING CONSIDERATIONS

• Assess patient for abdominal pain.
• Look for blood in emesis, stool, or gastric aspirate.
• Monitor patients with renal dysfunction for QT-interval prolongation.

PATIENT TEACHING

• Instruct patient in proper use of OTC product, if appropriate.
• Tell patient to take prescription drug with a snack, if desired.
• Advise patient to limit use of prescription drug to no longer than 8 weeks, unless ordered by prescriber, and OTC drug to no longer than 2 weeks.
• With prescriber's knowledge, let patient take antacids together, especially at beginning of therapy when pain is severe.
• Urge patient to avoid cigarette smoking because it may increase gastric acid secretion and worsen disease.
• Advise patient to report abdominal pain, blood in stools or vomit, melena, or coffee-ground emesis.

febuxostat
feb-UX-oh-stat

Uloric

Therapeutic class: Antigout drugs
Pharmacologic class: Xanthine oxidase inhibitors

AVAILABLE FORMS
Tablets: 40 mg, 80 mg

INDICATIONS & DOSAGES

Boxed Warning Only use drug in patients who have an inadequate response to a maximally titrated dose of allopurinol, who are intolerant to allopurinol, or for whom treatment with allopurinol isn't advisable. ∎

➤ **Chronic management of hyperuricemia associated with gout**
Adults: 40 mg PO daily. May increase dosage to 80 mg after 2 weeks if uric acid level remains above 6 mg/dL.

Adjust-a-dose: Maximum dose in patients with severe renal impairment (CrCl of less than 30 mL/minute) is 40 mg/day.

ADMINISTRATION
PO
• Give drug without regard to food or antacid use.
• Store at 77° F (25° C). Protect from light.

ACTION
Reduces uric acid production by inhibiting xanthine oxidase.

Route	Onset	Peak	Duration
PO	Rapid	1–1.5 hr	Unknown

Half-life: 5 to 8 hours.

ADVERSE REACTIONS
CNS: dizziness. **GI:** nausea. **Hepatic:** liver function abnormalities. **Musculoskeletal:** arthralgia. **Skin:** rash.

INTERACTIONS
Drug-drug. *Azathioprine, mercaptopurine:* May increase levels of these drugs, leading to toxicity. Use together is contraindicated.
Pegloticase: May increase toxic effects of pegloticase. Avoid use together.
Theophylline: May increase theophylline level. Use cautiously together.

Reactions in bold italics are *life-threatening*. Interactions may have a *rapid onset* or a ***delayed onset***.

EFFECTS ON LAB TEST RESULTS
• May increase ALP, AST, and ALT levels.

CONTRAINDICATIONS & CAUTIONS
• Contraindicated in patients hypersensitive to drug or its components.

Boxed Warning Drug may increase risk of CV death in patients with CV disease compared to those treated with allopurinol, based on a CV outcomes study. Consider the risks and benefits of drug when deciding to prescribe or continue patients on febuxostat. Consider use of prophylactic low-dose aspirin in patients with a history of CV disease. ■

• Use in patients with secondary hyperuricemia (including organ transplant recipients and patients with malignancy) hasn't been studied; use isn't recommended.
• Use cautiously in patients with severe hepatic impairment (Child-Pugh class C) or renal impairment (CrCl of less than 30 mL/minute).
• Serious skin and hypersensitivity reactions, including SJS, DRESS syndrome, and TEN, have been reported; if suspected, discontinue drug.
• Use cautiously in patients reporting serious skin reactions to allopurinol.
• Not recommended for the treatment of asymptomatic hyperuricemia.
• Safety and effectiveness in children haven't been established.
Dialyzable drug: Unlikely.

PREGNANCY-LACTATION-REPRODUCTION
• It isn't known if drug crosses the placental barrier. Use during pregnancy only if potential benefit justifies fetal risk.
• It isn't known if drug appears in human milk. Use cautiously during breastfeeding.

NURSING CONSIDERATIONS
Boxed Warning Monitor all patients for signs and symptoms of CV events. ■
• Acute gout flares may occur during first 6 weeks of therapy; colchicine or another anti-inflammatory may be added prophylactically, and drug should be continued.
• Monitor hepatic function at baseline, 2 months and 4 months after starting therapy, and periodically thereafter.
• Monitor patients for signs and symptoms of hypersensitivity or severe skin reactions.
🖢 *Alert:* Patients with unexplained serum ALT level greater than 3 × ULN with total bilirubin level greater than 2 × ULN

are at risk for severe drug-induced liver injury. Stop drug in these patients and don't restart.
• Monitor uric acid level.

PATIENT TEACHING
Boxed Warning Advise patient of the risk of CV events. Teach patient to seek immediate emergency medical care for chest pain, shortness of breath, dizziness, fainting, lightheadedness, fast or irregular heartbeat, numbness or weakness on one side of the body, slurred speech, blurred vision, or sudden severe headache. ■

• Warn patient about the risk of gout flares and the importance of taking an NSAID or colchicine during the first 6 weeks of treatment.
• Advise patient to report all adverse reactions, including abnormal bleeding, nausea, malaise, light-colored stools, yellowing of eyes or skin, rash, chest pain, dyspnea, or neurologic symptoms of a stroke.
• Instruct patient to report signs or symptoms of severe skin reactions immediately.

felodipine
fe-LOE-di-peen

Plendil🍁

Therapeutic class: Antihypertensives
Pharmacologic class: Calcium channel blockers

AVAILABLE FORMS
Tablets (extended-release) 🕳 : 2.5 mg, 5 mg, 10 mg

INDICATIONS & DOSAGES
➤ **HTN**
Adults: Initially, 2.5 to 5 mg PO daily. Adjust dosage based on patient response, usually at intervals of not less than 2 weeks. Maximum dosage, 10 mg daily.
Older adults: 2.5 mg PO daily; adjust dosage as for adults. Maximum dosage, 10 mg daily.
Adjust-a-dose: Patients with impaired hepatic function may respond to lower doses.
➤ **Chronic stable angina (alternative agent)** ◆
Adults: Initially, 5 to 10 mg PO once daily; if initiated at 5 mg, increase to 10 mg once daily as tolerated after 2 to 4 weeks.

ADMINISTRATION
PO
• Give drug whole; don't crush or cut tablets.
• Give drug without food or with a light meal low in fat and carbohydrates.
• Store at 68° to 77° F (20° to 25° C). Protect from light.

ACTION
A dihydropyridine-derivative calcium channel blocker that prevents entry of calcium ions into vascular smooth muscle and cardiac cells; shows some selectivity for smooth muscle compared with cardiac muscle.

Route	Onset	Peak	Duration
PO	2–5 hr	2.5–5 hr	24 hr

Half-life: 11 to 16 hours.

ADVERSE REACTIONS
CNS: headache, dizziness, paresthesia, asthenia, warm sensation. **CV:** peripheral edema, tachycardia, palpitations, flushing. **EENT:** rhinorrhea, pharyngitis. **GI:** abdominal pain, nausea, constipation, diarrhea, dyspepsia. **Musculoskeletal:** arthralgia, muscle cramps, back or limb pain. **Respiratory:** URI, cough, sneezing. **Skin:** rash.

INTERACTIONS
Drug-drug. *Anticonvulsants (long term):* May decrease felodipine level. Avoid using together.
Antipsychotics (atypical second-generation): May enhance hypotensive effects. Monitor therapy.
CYP3A4 inhibitors (azole antifungals, cimetidine, erythromycin): May decrease clearance of felodipine. Reduce doses of felodipine; monitor patient for toxicity.
Metoprolol: May alter pharmacokinetics of metoprolol. Monitor patient for adverse reactions.
Tacrolimus: May increase tacrolimus level. Monitor patient closely.
Drug-herb. *Herbs with hypertensive or hypotensive properties:* May increase or decrease antihypertensive effects. Discourage use together.
Drug-food. *Grapefruit:* May increase drug level and adverse effects. Discourage use together.
Drug-lifestyle. *Alcohol use:* May increase felodipine absorption. Monitor patient for increased hypotensive effect.

EFFECTS ON LAB TEST RESULTS
• May lead to false-negative aldosterone/renin ratio.

CONTRAINDICATIONS & CAUTIONS
• Contraindicated in patients hypersensitive to drug.
• Drug may cause significant hypotension and rarely syncope.
• Safe use in patients with HF hasn't been established. Use cautiously in patients with HF or decreased ventricular function.
• Use cautiously and in lower doses in older adults and in patients with hepatic impairment.
• Drug may contain lactose. If necessary, consider alternative agent in patients who are lactose-intolerant.
• Safety and effectiveness in children haven't been established.
Dialyzable drug: Unlikely.
⚠ *Overdose S&S:* Peripheral vasodilation, hypotension, bradycardia.

PREGNANCY-LACTATION-REPRODUCTION
• There are no well-controlled studies during pregnancy, but animal studies show potential fetal hazards. If treatment for HTN during pregnancy is needed, other agents are preferred.
• It isn't known if drug appears in human milk. Patient should discontinue breastfeeding or discontinue drug.

NURSING CONSIDERATIONS
• Monitor BP and HR for response.
• Monitor patient for peripheral edema, which appears to be both dose- and age-related. It's more common in patients taking higher doses, especially those older than age 60.

PATIENT TEACHING
• Teach patient safe drug administration.
• Advise patient to continue taking drug even when feeling better, to watch diet, and to check with prescriber or pharmacist before taking other drugs, including OTC drugs, nutritional supplements, or herbal remedies.
• Teach patient to report all adverse reactions.
• Advise patient to observe good oral hygiene and to see a dentist regularly; use of drug may cause mild gum problems.

Reactions in bold italics are *life-threatening*. Interactions may have a *rapid onset* or a *delayed onset*.

fenofibrate
fee-no-FYE-brate

Antara, Fenoglide, Lipofen, TriCor🖋

fenofibrate (choline)
Trilipix

fenofibric acid
Fibricor

Therapeutic class: Antilipemics
Pharmacologic class: Fibric acid derivatives

AVAILABLE FORMS
fenofibrate
Capsules 🔴*:* 50 mg, 150 mg
Capsules (micronized) 🔴*:* 30 mg, 43 mg, 67 mg, 90 mg, 130 mg, 134 mg, 200 mg
Tablets 🔴*:* 40 mg, 48 mg, 54 mg, 120 mg, 145 mg, 160 mg
fenofibrate (choline)
Capsules (delayed-release) 🔴*:* 45 mg, 135 mg
fenofibric acid
Tablets: 35 mg, 105 mg

INDICATIONS & DOSAGES
Adjust-a-dose (for all indications): Refer to specific product information for guidelines regarding dosing for patients with renal impairment.

➤ **Hypertriglyceridemia (Fredrickson types IV and V hyperlipidemia) in patients who don't respond adequately to diet alone**
Adults: For Antara and generics, initial dose is 30 to 90 mg PO daily, with maximum dose of 90 mg daily. For Fibricor and generics, initial dose is 35 to 105 mg daily, with maximum dose of 105 mg daily. For fenofibrate (micronized), initial dose is 43 to 130 mg once daily, with maximum dose of 130 mg daily. For Fenoglide and generics, initial dose is 40 to 120 mg/day, with maximum dose of 120 mg daily. For Lipofen and generics, initial dose is 50 to 150 mg daily, with maximum dose of 150 mg daily. For TriCor and generics, initial dose is 48 to 145 mg daily, with maximum dose of 145 mg daily. For Trilipix and generics, initial dose is 45 to 135 mg once daily, with maximum dose of 135 mg once daily. For all forms, adjust dose based on patient response and repeat lipid determinations every 4 to 8 weeks.

➤ **Primary hypercholesterolemia or mixed dyslipidemia (Fredrickson types IIa and IIb) in patients who don't respond adequately to diet alone**
Adults: For Antara and generics, initial dose is 90 mg PO daily. For Fenoglide, initial dose is 120 mg/day. For fenofibrate (micronized), initial dose is 130 mg once daily. For Fibricor and generics, the dose is 105 mg PO daily. For Lipofen and generics, initial dose is 150 mg daily. For TriCor and generics, initial dose is 145 mg daily. For Trilipix and generics, initial dose is 135 once daily. May reduce dose if lipid levels fall significantly below the target range.

ADMINISTRATION
PO
• Administer Fenoglide and Lipofen with meals.
• Administer Antara, Fibricor, TriCor, and Trilipix with or without food.
• Ensure patient swallows capsules and tablets whole. Don't open capsules or crush, dissolve, or allow patient to chew capsules or tablets.
• Store at room temperature.

ACTION
May lower triglyceride levels by inhibiting triglyceride synthesis with less VLDL released into circulation. Drug may also stimulate breakdown of triglyceride-rich protein.

Route	Onset	Peak	Duration
PO	Unknown	2–8 hr	Unknown

Half-life: 20 hours.

ADVERSE REACTIONS
CNS: dizziness, headache, localized pain. **CV:** *PE,* thrombophlebitis. **EENT:** rhinitis, sinusitis, nasopharyngitis. **GI:** abdominal pain, constipation, diarrhea, dyspepsia, nausea. **Hepatic:** elevated AST and ALT levels. **Metabolic:** increased CK level. **Musculoskeletal:** arthralgia, back pain, limb pain, myalgia. **Respiratory:** URI. **Skin:** urticaria, rash.

INTERACTIONS
Drug-drug. *Bile acid sequestrants:* May bind and inhibit absorption of fenofibrate. Give drug 1 hour before or 4 to 6 hours after bile acid sequestrants.

Coumarin-type anticoagulants: May potentiate anticoagulant effect, prolonging PT and INR. Monitor PT and INR closely.

Cyclosporine, immunosuppressants, nephrotoxic drugs: May induce renal dysfunction that may affect fenofibrate elimination. Use together cautiously.

HMG-CoA reductase inhibitors: May increase risk of adverse musculoskeletal effects. Avoid using together, unless potential benefit outweighs risk.

Drug-food. *Any food:* May increase capsule absorption. Advise patient to take Fenoglide and Lipofen with meals. Refer to specific product for more information.

Drug-lifestyle. *Alcohol use:* May increase triglyceride levels. Discourage use together.

EFFECTS ON LAB TEST RESULTS
• May increase ALT, AST, BUN, CK, and creatinine levels.
• May decrease uric acid and Hb levels, hematocrit, and platelet and WBC counts.

CONTRAINDICATIONS & CAUTIONS
• Contraindicated in patients hypersensitive to drug and in those with gallbladder disease, hepatic dysfunction, primary biliary cirrhosis, severe renal dysfunction or ESRD (including those receiving hemodialysis), or unexplained persistent liver function abnormalities.
• Some formulations may contain peanut oil or soya lecithin and are contraindicated in patients with these allergies. Refer to individual products.
• Use cautiously in older adults and patients with a history of pancreatitis and renal impairment.
• Anaphylaxis and angioedema have been reported with fenofibrate. In some cases, reactions were life-threatening and required emergency treatment.
• Safety and effectiveness in children haven't been established.
Dialyzable drug: No.

PREGNANCY-LACTATION-REPRODUCTION
• Triglyceride and lipid concentrations increase during pregnancy. May consider using fenofibrate beginning in second trimester to treat severe hypertriglyceridemia. Use other agents for hypercholesterolemia, if necessary. Refer to individual manufacturer's instructions for use during pregnancy.
• Contraindicated during breastfeeding.

NURSING CONSIDERATIONS
• Obtain baseline lipid levels and LFT results before therapy, and monitor liver function periodically during therapy. Stop drug if enzyme levels persist above 3 × ULN.
• Monitor renal function in patients with current or risk of renal impairment
◖ **Alert:** Watch for signs and symptoms of pancreatitis, myositis, rhabdomyolysis, hepatic impairment, cholelithiasis, and renal failure. Monitor patient for muscle pain, tenderness, or weakness, especially with malaise or fever.
• SCARs, including SJS, TEN, and DRESS syndrome, have been reported, occurring days to weeks after drug initiation. Discontinue drug and treat appropriately.
• If an adequate response isn't obtained after 2 to 3 months of treatment with maximum daily dose, stop therapy.
• Drug lowers uric acid level by increasing uric acid excretion in patients with or without hyperuricemia.
• Beta blockers, estrogens, and thiazide diuretics may increase triglyceride levels; evaluate need for continued use of these drugs.
• Hb level, hematocrit, and WBC count may decrease when therapy starts but will stabilize with long-term administration.
• Discontinue if gallstones are found upon gallbladder studies.
• Discontinue if patient develops markedly elevated CK concentration or if myopathy or myositis is suspected or diagnosed.
• Permanently discontinue if high-density lipoprotein cholesterol (HDL-C) becomes severely depressed; monitor HDL-C level.

PATIENT TEACHING
• Teach patient safe drug administration.
• Inform patient that drug therapy doesn't reduce need for following a triglyceride-lowering diet.
• Advise patient to promptly report all adverse reactions, especially unexplained muscle weakness, pain, or tenderness, abdominal pain, and yellowing of skin or eyes, particularly with malaise or fever.
• Warn patient to immediately report development of skin reactions, such as a rash or exfoliative dermatitis.
• Advise patient to continue weight control measures, including diet and exercise, and to limit alcohol before therapy.

Reactions in bold italics are *life-threatening*. Interactions may have a *rapid onset* or a *delayed onset*.

SAFETY ALERT!

fentaNYL citrate
FEN-ta-nil

fentaNYL nasal spray
Lazanda

fentaNYL sublingual spray
Subsys

fentaNYL transdermal system
Duragesic-12, Duragesic-25,
Duragesic-50, Duragesic-75,
Duragesic-100

fentaNYL transmucosal
Actiq, Fentora

Therapeutic class: Opioid analgesics
Pharmacologic class: Opioid agonists
Controlled substance schedule: II

AVAILABLE FORMS
Injection: 50 mcg/mL
Nasal spray: 100 mcg, 300 mcg, 400 mcg
Transdermal system: Patches that release
12.5 mcg, 25 mcg, 37.5 mcg, 50 mcg,
62.5 mcg, 75 mcg, 87.5 mcg, or 100 mcg of
drug per hour
Transmucosal (buccal tablet): 100 mcg,
200 mcg, 400 mcg, 600 mcg, 800 mcg
Transmucosal (lozenge): 200 mcg, 400 mcg,
600 mcg, 800 mcg, 1,200 mcg, 1,600 mcg
Transmucosal (SL spray): 100 mcg, 200 mcg,
400 mcg, 600 mcg, 800 mcg, 1,200 mcg,
1,600 mcg

INDICATIONS & DOSAGES
➤ **Adjunct to general anesthetic**
Adults: For low-dose therapy, 1 to 2 mcg/kg
IV. For moderate-dose therapy, 2 to 20 mcg/kg
IV; then 25 to 100 mcg IV or IM PRN. For
high-dose therapy, 20 to 50 mcg/kg IV; then
25 mcg to one-half initial loading dose IV PRN.
➤ **Adjunct to regional anesthesia**
Adults: 50 to 100 mcg IM or slowly IV over 1
to 2 minutes PRN.
➤ **To induce and maintain anesthesia**
Children ages 2 and older: 2 to 3 mcg/kg IV
every 1 to 2 hours as needed.
➤ **Postoperative pain, restlessness, tachyp-
nea, and emergence delirium**
Adults: 50 to 100 mcg IM every 1 to 2 hours
PRN.

➤ **Preoperative medication**
Adults: 50 to 100 mcg IM 30 to 60 minutes
before surgery.
➤ **To manage persistent, moderate to
severe chronic pain in patients who are
opioid-tolerant and require around-the-
clock opioid analgesics for an extended
time**
Adults and children age 2 and older: When
converting to transdermal system, base the
first dose on the daily dose, potency, and characteristics of the current opioid therapy; the
reliability of the relative potency estimates
used to calculate the needed dose; the degree
of opioid tolerance; and patient's condition.
Each patch may be worn for 72 hours, although some adult patients may need a patch
to be applied every 48 hours during the first
dosage period. May increase dose 3 days after
the first dose, then every 6 days thereafter.
Adjust-a-dose: For older adults and patients who are cachectic or debilitated, start
transdermal system doses at no higher than
25 mcg/hr unless these patients are already
tolerating around-the-clock opioid at a
dose and potency comparable to fentanyl
25 mcg/hr transdermal system.
➤ **To manage breakthrough cancer pain
in patients already receiving and tolerating
an opioid**
Adults: 200 mcg Actiq initially; may give second dose 15 minutes after completing the
first (30 minutes after first lozenge is placed
in mouth). Maximum dose is 2 lozenges per
breakthrough episode. If several episodes of
breakthrough pain requiring 2 lozenges occur,
dose may be increased to the next available
strength. After a successful dosage has been
reached, patient should limit use to no more
than 4 lozenges daily.

Or, initially 100 mcg buccal tablet between
the upper cheek and gum. May repeat same
dose once per breakthrough episode after at
least 30 minutes. Adjust in 100-mcg increments. Doses above 400 mcg can be increased
by 200 mcg. Generally, dosage should be increased when patient requires more than one
dose per breakthrough episode. Once a successful maintenance dose has been established, reevaluate if patient experiences more
than four breakthrough episodes per day.

Or, initially 100 mcg nasal spray. Titrate
as needed to an effective dosage (from 100
to 200, to 300, to 400, to 600 mcg, up to
maximum of 800 mcg) that gives adequate

analgesia with tolerable adverse effects. Dose is a single spray into one nostril or single spray into each nostril per episode. Don't give more than four doses per 24 hours. Wait at least 2 hours before treating another episode. During an episode, if analgesia isn't achieved within 30 minutes, patient may use a rescue medication as directed by the health care provider.

Or, initially 100 mcg SL spray. If pain isn't relieved after 30 minutes during each breakthrough pain episode treated, one additional dose of the same strength may be given for that episode. May use a maximum of two doses for any breakthrough pain episode, and 4 hours must elapse before treating another episode of breakthrough pain with a higher dose. Titrate dosage level as needed to an effective dosage (from 100 to 200, to 400, to 600, to 800, to 1,200, to 1,600 mcg) that gives adequate analgesia with tolerable adverse effects using a single dose per breakthrough cancer pain episode. When drug has been titrated to an effective dosage, patients should generally use only one dose of the appropriate strength per breakthrough pain episode.

➤ **Switching from Actiq to Fentora or Subsys to manage breakthrough cancer pain in patients who are opioid-tolerant**

Adults: If current Actiq dose is 200 to 400 mcg, start with 100 mcg Fentora or Subsys; if current Actiq dose is 600 to 800 mcg, use 200 mcg Fentora or Subsys; if current Actiq dose is 1,200 to 1,600 mcg, use 400 mcg Fentora or Subsys. Refer to manufacturer's information for titration instructions if needed. Actiq, Fentora, and Subsys aren't bioequivalent.

Adjust-a-dose: For patients with renal or hepatic impairment, use lowest possible dose.

ADMINISTRATION

Boxed Warning Substantial differences exist in the pharmacokinetic profile of fentanyl buccal, intranasal, and SL compared with other fentanyl products that result in clinically important differences in the extent of absorption of fentanyl, which could result in fatal overdose. When prescribing, don't convert patients on a mcg-per-mcg basis from other fentanyl products to fentanyl buccal. When dispensing, don't substitute a fentanyl buccal prescription for other fentanyl products. ∎

IV

▼ Only those trained to give IV anesthetics and manage adverse effects should give this form.

▼ Keep opioid antagonist (naloxone) and resuscitation equipment available.

▼ IV form often used with droperidol to produce neuroleptanalgesia.

▼ Inject slowly over 1 to 2 minutes.

▼ **Incompatibilities:** Azithromycin, dantrolene, gemtuzumab ozogamicin, pantoprazole, phenytoin, sulfamethoxazole–trimethoprim. Compatibility of many other drugs is undetermined.

IM

• Document administration site.

Intranasal

• Prime device by spraying into the pouch (4 sprays in total). Reprime if product hasn't been used for 5 days.

• Insert the nozzle about ½ inch (1 cm) into the nose and point toward the bridge of the nose, tilting the bottle slightly.

• Press down firmly until a click is heard and the number in the counting window advances by one.

Transdermal

• Dosage equivalent charts are available to calculate the fentanyl transdermal dose based on the daily morphine intake; for example, for every 60 mg of oral morphine or 15 mg of IM morphine per 24 hours, 25 mcg/hour of transdermal fentanyl is needed.

• Clip hair at application site but don't use a razor, which may irritate skin. Wash area with clear water, if needed, but not with soaps, oils, lotions, alcohol, or other substances that may irritate skin or prevent adhesion. Dry area completely before application.

• Remove transdermal system from package just before applying, hold in place for 30 seconds, and be sure edges of patch stick to skin.

• Don't cut or otherwise alter transdermal patch before applying.

• Place transdermal patch on the upper back for a child or patient who's cognitively impaired to reduce the chance the patch will be removed and placed in the mouth.

• If another patch is needed after 48 to 72 hours, apply it to a different skin site.

Boxed Warning Heat from fever or heating pads, electric blankets, heat lamps, hot tubs, or water beds may increase transdermal delivery and cause toxicity. ∎

Reactions in bold italics are *life-threatening*. Interactions may have a *rapid onset* or a *delayed onset*.

- Always wear gloves when handling transdermal system.

Transmucosal

- Remove foil just before giving.
- For Actiq: Place lozenge between patient's cheek and gum and allow to dissolve over about 15 to 20 minutes; it must not be bitten, sucked, or chewed. May move lozenge from one side to the other using stick. Discard stick in the trash after use or, if any drug matrix remains on the stick, place under low running tap water until dissolved. Or, place in child-resistant container provided and discard as for Schedule II drugs.
- For buccal tablet: Place tablet between patient's cheek and gum and leave there until disintegrated, usually 14 to 25 minutes. Patient shouldn't suck, chew, or swallow tablet; doing so results in lower plasma concentrations. After 30 minutes, if remnants from tablet remain, they may be swallowed with a glass of water.
- For SL spray: Open blister package with scissors immediately before use. Carefully spray contents of unit into the mouth under the tongue. Patient should hold medicine under the tongue for 30 to 60 seconds; patient shouldn't spit or rinse mouth.

ACTION

Binds with opioid receptors in the CNS, altering perception of and emotional response to pain.

Route	Onset	Peak	Duration
IV	1–2 min	3–5 min	30–60 min
IM	7–15 min	20–30 min	1–2 hr
Intranasal	15–21 min	25–35 min	Unknown
Transdermal	12–24 hr	1–3 days	Variable
Transmucosal	5–15 min	20–90 min	Unknown

Half-life: Parenteral, 3.5 hours; intranasal, 15 to 24.9 hours; transmucosal, 5 to 15 hours; transdermal, 18 hours.

ADVERSE REACTIONS

CNS: asthenia, clouded sensorium, confusion, euphoria, lethargy, sedation, somnolence, *seizures,* anxiety, depression, dizziness, fatigue, hallucinations, headache, migraine, hypoesthesia, insomnia, agitation, nervousness, dysgeusia, fever, tremor. **CV:** edema, *bradycardia, arrhythmias, cardiorespiratory arrest,* tachycardia, vasodilation, chest pain, HTN, hypotension, *DVT, PE.* **EENT:** dry eyes, dry mouth, abnormal vision,

eye swelling, strabismus, ptosis, epistaxis, pharyngitis, oral ulcer, nasal discomfort, rhinorrhea, nasal congestion, postnasal drip, rhinitis (intranasal). **GI:** constipation, abdominal pain, anorexia, diarrhea, dyspepsia, flatulence, ileus, nausea, vomiting, stomatitis. **GU:** urine retention. **Hematologic:** anemia, *neutropenia.* **Hepatic:** jaundice, increased ALP level. **Metabolic:** *hypokalemia,* dehydration, weight loss, hypercalcemia, hyperglycemia, hypoalbuminemia, *hypocalcemia, hypomagnesemia,* hyponatremia, *lactic acidosis.* **Musculoskeletal:** back pain, abnormal gait. **Respiratory:** *apnea, hypoventilation, respiratory depression,* dyspnea, cough, URI, bronchitis. **Skin:** diaphoresis, pruritus, rash, pressure injury, erythema at application site (transdermal). **Other:** accidental injury, hypersensitivity reactions, chills, infection, physical dependence.

INTERACTIONS

Drug-drug. *Amiodarone:* May cause hypotension, bradycardia, and decreased cardiac output. Monitor patient closely.

Anticholinergics (benztropine, cyclopentolate, dicyclomine, fesoterodine): May increase risk of urine retention, severe constipation, and paralytic ileus. Monitor patient closely.

Boxed Warning *Benzodiazepines, CNS depressants:* May cause slow or difficult breathing, sedation, and death. Avoid use together. If use together is necessary, limit dosage and duration of each drug to the minimum necessary for desired effect. ∎

Buprenorphine, butorphanol, nalbuphine, pentazocine: May reduce analgesic effect of fentanyl or precipitate withdrawal signs and symptoms. Avoid use together.

Boxed Warning *CYP3A4 inducers (carbamazepine, phenytoin, rifampin):* May decrease fentanyl level and result in decreased efficacy or precipitate a withdrawal syndrome in patients with a physical dependence on fentanyl. If CYP3A4 inducer is discontinued, fentanyl level may increase and cause fentanyl-related adverse reactions. Taper CYP3A4 inducers cautiously and adjust fentanyl dosage as needed. ∎

Boxed Warning *CYP3A4 inhibitors (erythromycin, ketoconazole, ritonavir):* May increase fentanyl level and increase risk of potentially fatal respiratory depression. Use together cautiously and monitor patient closely. ∎

✤Canada ◇OTC ◆Off-label use ✐Photoguide ⊕Do not crush *Liquid contains alcohol ▨Genetic

Diuretics: Opioids may decrease diuresis or BP effects. Monitor therapy.

Droperidol: May cause hypotension and decrease pulmonary arterial pressure. Use together cautiously.

General anesthetics, hypnotics, other opioid analgesics, sedatives, TCAs: May cause additive effects. Use together cautiously. Consider dosage reduction of one or both drugs if adverse effects occur.

Muscle relaxants (cyclobenzaprine, metaxalone): May enhance neuromuscular blocking effect of relaxant and risk of respiratory depression. Use cautiously together.

Protease inhibitors: May increase fentanyl levels and adverse effects. Monitor patient closely for respiratory depression.

🌢 *Alert:* Serotonergic drugs (antiemetics [dolasetron, granisetron, ondansetron, palonosetron], amoxapine, antimigraine drugs, buspirone, cyclobenzaprine, dextromethorphan, linezolid, lithium, MAO inhibitors, maprotiline, methylene blue, mirtazapine, nefazodone, SSNRIs, SSRIs, TCAs, trazodone, tryptophan, vilazodone): May increase risk of serotonin syndrome. Use together cautiously; monitor for serotonin syndrome. Don't use fentanyl while patient is taking an MAO inhibitor or within 14 days of stopping one.

Drug-herb. 🌢 *Alert:* St. John's wort May increase risk of serotonin syndrome. Use together cautiously; monitor for serotonin syndrome.

Drug-lifestyle. *Alcohol use:* May cause additive effects. Discourage use together.

EFFECTS ON LAB TEST RESULTS
• May increase amylase and lipase levels.

CONTRAINDICATIONS & CAUTIONS
• Contraindicated in patients hypersensitive to drug or its components and in those with acute or severe bronchial asthma in an unmonitored setting or in the absence of resuscitative equipment, or known or suspected GI obstruction, including paralytic ileus.

Boxed Warning Opioids should only be prescribed with benzodiazepines or other CNS depressants to patients for whom alternative treatment options are inadequate. ∎

Boxed Warning Transdermal form contraindicated in patients hypersensitive to adhesives, those who are opioid-naive, those who need postoperative pain management, and those with acute, mild, or intermittent pain that can be managed with nonopioids. Don't use in patients with increased intracranial pressure, head injury, impaired consciousness, or coma. ∎

Boxed Warning Transmucosal forms contraindicated in those who need acute or postoperative pain management. ∎

Boxed Warning Nasal spray is contraindicated in patients who are opioid-nontolerant and in those who need acute or postoperative pain management. ∎

Boxed Warning Drug may increase risks of opioid addiction, abuse, and misuse, which can lead to overdose and death. Risks increase in patients with a personal or family history of substance abuse or mental illness. Assess risks before drug is prescribed. ∎

Boxed Warning Refer to manufacturer's instructions for REMS requirements. ∎

🌢 *Alert:* Drug may lead to rare but serious decrease in adrenal gland cortisol production.

🌢 *Alert:* Drug may cause decreased sex hormone levels with long-term use.

• Fentora contraindicated in patients with mucositis more severe than grade 1.

• Use with caution in patients with brain tumors, COPD, decreased respiratory reserve, potentially compromised respirations, hepatic or renal disease, or cardiac bradyarrhythmias.

• Use with caution in older adults and patients who are debilitated.

• Opioids can cause sleep-related breathing disorders, including central sleep apnea (CSA) and sleep-related hypoxemia. Opioid use increases risk of CSA in a dose-dependent fashion. In patients who present with CSA, consider decreasing opioid dosage using best practices for opioid taper.

Dialyzable drug: Unknown.

⚠ *Overdose S&S:* CNS depression, respiratory depression, apnea, flaccid skeletal muscles, bradycardia, hypotension, circulatory collapse.

PREGNANCY-LACTATION-REPRODUCTION
• There are no well-controlled studies during pregnancy. Use during pregnancy only if potential benefit justifies fetal risk.

Boxed Warning Prolonged maternal use of opioids during pregnancy can cause neonatal withdrawal syndrome, which may be life-threatening and requires management by

---

neonatology experts. Advise patient of the risk of neonatal withdrawal syndrome. ■

• Drug appears in human milk. Refer to individual manufacturer's instructions for use during breastfeeding.

NURSING CONSIDERATIONS

Boxed Warning Respiratory depression or death can occur even when transdermal drug has been used as recommended and has not been misused or abused. Drug should only be prescribed by health care providers knowledgeable in the use of potent opioids for management of long-term pain. Drug is contraindicated for use in conditions in which the risk of life-threatening respiratory depression is significantly increased. Transdermal patch is for hospital use only. ■

Boxed Warning Regularly monitor patients for development of opioid addiction, abuse, and misuse. ■

Boxed Warning Serious, life-threatening or fatal respiratory depression can occur. Monitor patient closely, especially within first 24 to 72 hours of drug initiation and after dosage increase. ■

❸ *Alert:* If patient is taking opioids with serotonergic drugs, monitor for signs and symptoms of serotonin syndrome (agitation, hallucinations, rapid HR, fever, diaphoresis, shivering or shaking, muscle twitching or stiffness, trouble with coordination, nausea, vomiting, diarrhea), especially when starting treatment or increasing dosage. Symptoms may occur within several hours of coadministration but may also occur later, especially after dosage increase. Discontinue the opioid, serotonergic drug, or both if serotonin syndrome is suspected.

❸ *Alert:* Monitor patient for signs and symptoms of adrenal insufficiency (nausea, vomiting, loss of appetite, fatigue, weakness, dizziness, low BP). Perform diagnostic testing if adrenal insufficiency is suspected. If adrenal insufficiency is confirmed, treat with corticosteroids and wean patient off opioids if appropriate. Discontinue corticosteroids when clinically appropriate.

❸ *Alert:* Don't stop drug abruptly; withdraw slowly and individualize the gradual taper plan to prevent signs and symptoms of withdrawal, worsening pain, and psychological distress in patients who are physically dependent. Refer to manufacturer's label for specific tapering instructions.

❸ *Alert:* When tapering opioids, monitor patient closely for signs and symptoms of opioid withdrawal (restlessness, lacrimation, rhinorrhea, yawning, perspiration, chills, myalgia, mydriasis, irritability, anxiety, insomnia, backache, joint pain, weakness, abdominal cramps, anorexia, nausea, vomiting, diarrhea, increased BP or HR, increased respiratory rate). Such symptoms may indicate a need to taper more slowly. Also watch for suicidality, use of other substances, and mood changes.

❸ *Alert:* Monitor patient for signs and symptoms of decreased sex hormone levels (low libido, erectile dysfunction, amenorrhea, infertility). If signs and symptoms occur, evaluate patient and obtain lab testing.

• For better analgesic effect, give drug before patient has intense pain.

❸ *Alert:* High doses can produce muscle rigidity, which can be reversed with neuromuscular blockers; however, patient must be artificially ventilated.

❸ *Alert:* Watch for sedation and respiratory depression in patients with increased ICP, brain tumors, head injury, or impaired consciousness. Avoid use in patients with impaired consciousness or coma.

• Monitor circulatory and respiratory status and urinary function carefully. Drug may cause respiratory depression, hypotension, urine retention, nausea, vomiting, ileus, or altered level of consciousness, no matter how it's given.

• Periodically monitor postoperative vital signs and bladder function. Because drug decreases both rate and depth of respirations, monitoring of arterial oxygen saturation (SaO_2) may help assess respiratory depression. Immediately report respiratory rate below 12 breaths/minute, decreased respiratory volume, or decreased SaO_2.

• Drug may cause constipation. Assess bowel function and need for stool softeners and stimulant laxatives.

Boxed Warning Fentanyl is an opioid agonist and schedule II controlled substance with potential for abuse. Be alert for signs of misuse, abuse, or diversion. ■

Transdermal form

• Transdermal drug levels peak between 24 and 72 hours after initial application and dose increases. Monitor patients for life-threatening hypoventilation, especially during these times.

- Fentanyl patches should be used only in patients age 2 or older who are opioid tolerant, who have chronic moderate to severe pain poorly controlled by other drugs, and who need a total daily opioid dose at least equivalent to the 25-mcg/hour fentanyl patch.
- When converting patient from another opioid, determine the initial fentanyl dosage with great care; overestimating the dosage could be dangerous or fatal.
- Identify all daily drugs, particularly CYP3A4 inhibitors, which may increase fentanyl levels.
- Monitor patients closely, and provide immediate care for evidence of overdose, such as slow or shallow breathing, a slow heartbeat, severe sleepiness, cold and clammy skin, trouble walking and talking, and feeling faint, dizzy, or confused.
- Give patients detailed instructions for using fentanyl patches correctly and safely.
- Make dosage adjustments gradually in patient using the transdermal system. Reaching steady-state level of a new dosage may take up to 6 days; delay dosage adjustment until after at least two applications.
- Monitor patient who develops adverse reactions to the transdermal system for at least 12 hours after removal. Drug level drops gradually; it may take as long as 17 hours to decline by 50%.
- Most patients experience good control of pain for 3 days while wearing the transdermal system, but a few may need a new application after 48 hours.
- Because the drug level rises for the first 24 hours after application, analgesic effect can't be evaluated on the first day. Make sure patient has adequate supplemental analgesic to prevent breakthrough pain.
- When reducing opioid therapy or switching to a different analgesic, withdraw the transdermal system gradually. Because the drug level drops gradually after removal, give half the equianalgesic dose of the new analgesic 12 to 18 hours after removal.
- **Alert:** Transdermal patches must be stored, used, and disposed of properly to prevent poisonings or other harm, especially to children and pets. A patch that has been worn for 3 days may still contain enough fentanyl to cause harm, or be fatal to a child or pet. Patches should only be handled by patient or patient's caregivers.

Intranasal and transmucosal forms
Boxed Warning Intranasal and transmucosal forms are used only to manage breakthrough cancer pain in patients who are already receiving and tolerating opioids. ■
Boxed Warning Intranasal and transmucosal forms aren't bioequivalent and can't be substituted on a microgram-per-microgram basis. ■
- *Look alike–sound alike:* Don't confuse fentanyl with alfentanil.

PATIENT TEACHING
Boxed Warning Caution patient or caregiver of patient taking an opioid with a benzodiazepine, CNS depressant, or alcohol to seek immediate medical attention for dizziness, light-headedness, extreme sleepiness, slowed or difficult breathing, or unresponsiveness. ■
Boxed Warning Advise patient that drug increases risk of opioid addiction, abuse, and misuse, which can lead to overdose and death. Teach patient proper use of drug. ■
- When drug is used for pain control, instruct patient to request drug before pain becomes intense.
- **Alert:** Encourage patient to report all medications being taken, including prescription and OTC medications and supplements.
- **Alert:** Caution patient to immediately report signs and symptoms of serotonin syndrome, adrenal insufficiency, and decreased sex hormone levels to health care provider.
- **Alert:** Counsel patient not to discontinue opioids without first discussing need for a gradual tapering regimen with prescriber.
- Teach patients that naloxone is prescribed in conjunction with the opioid when beginning and renewing treatment as a preventive measure to reduce opioid overdose and death.
- Tell patient to avoid drinking alcohol or taking other CNS-type drugs, unless specifically prescribed by practitioner, because additive effects can occur.
- Teach patient about proper application and disposal of transdermal patch.
- **Alert:** Teach patient not to alter the transdermal patch (such as by cutting it) before applying.
- Advise parent or caregiver to place transdermal patch on the upper back for child or patient who's cognitively impaired, to reduce chance the patch will be removed and placed in the mouth.

Reactions in bold italics are *life-threatening*. Interactions may have a *rapid onset* or a ***delayed onset***.

• Teach patient to dispose of the transdermal patch by folding it so the adhesive side adheres to itself and then flushing it down the toilet.

• Tell patient that pain relief with the patch may not occur for several hours after the patch is applied. Oral, immediate-release opioids may be needed for initial pain relief.

Boxed Warning Inform patient that heat from fever or environment, such as from heating pads, electric blankets, heat lamps, hot tubs, or water beds, may increase transdermal delivery and cause toxicity requiring dosage adjustment. Instruct patient to notify prescriber if fever occurs or if patient will be spending time in a hot climate. ■

◔ *Alert:* Instruct patient that if an MRI is required, to inform the facility that patient is wearing a transdermal patch.

• Teach patient proper administration of transmucosal forms.

• Advise patient that transmucosal lozenge contains 2 g sugar per unit.

• Teach patient proper administration of the nasal spray, and explain that a fine mist isn't always felt and to rely on the audible click and advancement of the dose counter.

Boxed Warning Warn patient and patient's family that the amount of drug in transmucosal and intranasal forms can be fatal to a child. Advise patient to keep medicine well secured and out of children's reach. ■

ferric carboxymaltose
FER-ik car-box-ee-MAL-tose

Injectafer

Therapeutic class: Iron supplements
Pharmacologic class: Hematinics

AVAILABLE FORMS
Injection: 750 mg of elemental iron in 15-mL single-dose vial; 1,000 mg of elemental iron in 20-mL single-dose vial

INDICATIONS & DOSAGES
➤ **Iron deficiency anemia in patients with non-dialysis-dependent chronic kidney disease**
Adults: For patients weighing at least 50 kg, 750 mg IV on day 1; repeat dose after at least 7 days. May repeat course of therapy if anemia recurs. For patients weighing less than 50 kg, give 15 mg/kg body weight on day 1; repeat dose after at least 7 days. May repeat course of therapy if anemia recurs. Maximum cumulative dose is 1,500 mg per treatment course.

➤ **Iron deficiency anemia in patients intolerant to or who have had unsatisfactory response to oral iron**
Adults: For patients weighing at least 50 kg, 750 mg IV on day 1; repeat dose after at least 7 days. May repeat course of therapy if anemia recurs. For patients weighing less than 50 kg, give 15 mg/kg body weight on day 1; repeat dose after at least 7 days. May repeat course of therapy if anemia recurs. Maximum cumulative dose is 1,500 mg per treatment course.

Children age 1 and older weighing 50 kg or more: 750 mg IV on day 1; repeat dose after at least 7 days. May repeat course of therapy if anemia recurs. Maximum cumulative dose is 1,500 mg per course.

Children age 1 and older weighing less than 50 kg: 15 mg/kg IV on day; repeat dose after at least 7 days. May repeat course of therapy if anemia recurs.

ADMINISTRATION
IV

▼ Inspect vial for particulate matter and discoloration before administration.

▼ Give either as an undiluted slow IV push (at 100 mg [2 mL]/minute) or as an infusion. To administer by infusion, dilute up to 1,000 mg iron in maximum of 250 mL sterile NSS injection. Infusion concentration must be not less than 2 mg iron/mL.

▼ Give infusion over at least 15 minutes.

▼ Infusion is stable for 72 hours at room temperature at 2- to 4-mg/mL concentrations.

▼ Store vials at 68° to 77° F (20° to 25° C). Don't freeze vials.

▼ Vials are single-use and have no preservative. Discard any excess drug remaining in vial.

▼ **Incompatibilities:** None listed by manufacturer. Consult a drug incompatibility reference for more information.

ACTION
Colloidal iron (III) hydroxide acts in complex with carboxymaltose, a carbohydrate polymer that releases iron, an essential component in the formulation of Hb.

Route	Onset	Peak	Duration
IV	Unknown	15 min–1.21 hr	Unknown

Half-life: 7 to 12 hours.

ADVERSE REACTIONS

CNS: dizziness, headache, fever, chills, dysgeusia, syncope. **CV:** HTN, hypotension, flushing, tachycardia, chest discomfort. **EENT:** nasopharyngitis. **GI:** nausea, vomiting, constipation, GI infection. **Hepatic:** increased hepatic enzyme levels. **Hematologic:** decreased platelet and WBC counts. **Metabolic:** hypophosphatemia. **Skin:** rash, injection-site reaction, including discomfort, discoloration, pruritus, extravasation.

INTERACTIONS

Drug-drug. *Dimercaprol:* May enhance nephrotoxic effect of iron salts. Avoid combination.

EFFECTS ON LAB TEST RESULTS

- May increase ALT and GGT levels.
- May decrease phosphorus level.
- May decrease platelet and WBC counts.
- May falsely elevate serum iron and transferrin-bound iron levels in the 24 hours after administration.

CONTRAINDICATIONS & CAUTIONS

- Contraindicated in patients hypersensitive to drug or its components, in patients with evidence of iron overload, and in those with anemia not caused by iron deficiency.
- Symptomatic hypophosphatemia has been reported in patients at risk for low serum phosphate levels, mostly after repeated exposure to ferric carboxymaltose in patients with no reported history of renal impairment.
- Transient HTN has been reported immediately after administration.
- Serious hypersensitivity reactions, including anaphylaxis, have been reported.
- Safety and effectiveness in children younger than age 1 haven't been established.
Dialyzable drug: No.
⚠ *Overdose S&S:* Hemosiderosis, hypophosphatemic osteomalacia.

PREGNANCY-LACTATION-REPRODUCTION

- Hypersensitivity reaction to infusion may have serious consequences such as fetal bradycardia. Use during pregnancy only if potential benefit justifies fetal risk.
- Drug appears in human milk. Use cautiously during breastfeeding.

NURSING CONSIDERATIONS

- Before administering, assess patient for prior history of reactions to parenteral iron products.
- Monitor serum phosphate level in patients at risk for low serum phosphate who require a repeat course of treatment.
- Monitor patient for extravasation during administration. Extravasation may cause persistent discoloration. If extravasation occurs, discontinue infusion at that site.
- Monitor vital signs before and after each dose. Monitor patient for HTN after each dose.
- Monitor patient for hypersensitivity reactions during infusion and for at least 30 minutes after infusion or until patient is clinically stable. Only administer drug when personnel and therapies are immediately available for treatment of serious hypersensitivity reactions.
- Monitor iron status (Hb level and hematocrit, serum ferritin level, iron saturation) frequently during therapy.

PATIENT TEACHING

- Advise patient to report signs and symptoms of hypersensitivity reactions, such as rash, itching, dizziness, light-headedness, swelling, and breathing problems.
- Caution patient not to take oral iron supplements while receiving iron by infusion.
- Advise patient to report pregnancy or plans to become pregnant.

fidaxomicin
fye-DAX-oh-MYE sin

Dificid

Therapeutic class: Antibiotics
Pharmacologic class: Macrolides

AVAILABLE FORMS

Granules for oral suspension: 40 mg/mL
Tablets: 200 mg

Reactions in bold italics are *life-threatening*. Interactions may have a *rapid onset* or a **delayed onset**.

INDICATIONS & DOSAGES
➤ **CDAD**

Adults and children weighing 12.5 kg or more and able to swallow tablets: 200 mg PO b.i.d. for 10 days.

Children ages 6 months to younger than 18 years: For those weighing 9 to less than 12.5 kg, 160 mg (4 mL) oral solution PO b.i.d. for 10 days; for 7 to less than 9 kg, 120 mg (3 mL) oral solution PO b.i.d. for 10 days; for 4 to less than 7 kg, 80 mg (2 mL) oral solution PO b.i.d. for 10 days.

ADMINISTRATION
PO
- May give without regard for food.
- Remove reconstituted oral solution from refrigerator 15 minutes before administration. Shake vigorously; then give using an oral dosing syringe.
- Store tablets at room temperature. Store reconstituted oral suspension in refrigerator; discard after 12 days.

ACTION
Acts on *Clostridioides difficile* locally in the GI tract by inhibiting RNA synthesis through RNA polymerases.

Route	Onset	Peak	Duration
PO	<1 hr	1–5 hr	Unknown

Half-life: About 12 hours.

ADVERSE REACTIONS
GI: nausea, vomiting, abdominal pain or discomfort, abdominal distention, *GI bleeding*, dyspepsia, dysphagia, flatulence, intestinal obstruction, megacolon. **Hematologic:** anemia, *neutropenia.* **Hepatic:** increased ALP and hepatic enzyme levels. **Metabolic:** hyperglycemia, *metabolic acidosis.* **Skin:** drug eruption, rash, pruritus.

INTERACTIONS
None reported.

EFFECTS ON LAB TEST RESULTS
- May increase ALP, liver enzyme, and blood glucose levels.
- May decrease serum bicarbonate level.
- May decrease WBC, RBC, and platelet counts.

CONTRAINDICATIONS & CAUTIONS
- Contraindicated in patients hypersensitive to drug.
- Acute hypersensitivity reactions have been reported. Discontinue drug and treat appropriately. Patients with known macrolide allergies may have increased risk.
- Drug isn't an effective treatment for systemic *Clostridium* infections. Don't prescribe fidaxomicin unless a *C. difficile* infection has been proven or is strongly suspected because this may lead to the development of drug-resistant bacteria.
- Safety and effectiveness in children younger than age 6 months haven't been determined.

Dialyzable drug: Unknown.

PREGNANCY-LACTATION-REPRODUCTION
- Use drug in pregnancy only if clearly needed.
- It isn't known if drug appears in human milk. Use cautiously if breastfeeding.

NURSING CONSIDERATIONS
- Obtain specimen for culture before start of treatment.
- Monitor response to treatment.
- Monitor glucose level, especially in patients with diabetes.
- Monitor patient for abdominal pain or bleeding.
- Monitor patient for acute hypersensitivity.

PATIENT TEACHING
- Instruct patient or caregiver in safe drug administration.
- Advise patient that drug is used to treat CDAD only and shouldn't be used to treat other infections.
- Counsel patient to take the drug exactly as directed. Missing or skipping doses, or not completing the full course of therapy, may lead to reinfection, continued infection, or bacterial resistance.

filgrastim (G-CSF)
fill-GRASS-tim

Grastofil ✤, Neupogen

filgrastim-aafi
Nivestym

filgrastim-ayow
Releuko

filgrastim-sndz
Zarxio

tbo-filgrastim
Granix

Therapeutic class: Colony-stimulating factors
Pharmacologic class: Hematopoietics

AVAILABLE FORMS
Injection: 300 mcg/mL, 480 mcg/1.6 mL vials; 300 mcg/0.5 mL, 480 mcg/0.8 mL prefilled syringes

INDICATIONS & DOSAGES
➤ **Acute exposure to myelosuppressive doses of radiation (hematopoietic syndrome of acute radiation syndrome) (Neupogen)**
Adults and children: 10 mcg/kg subcut as soon as possible after suspected or confirmed exposure to radiation doses greater than 2 gray (Gy). Continue daily administration until ANC remains greater than 1,000/mm³ for three consecutive CBCs or exceeds 10,000/mm³ after a radiation-induced nadir.
➤ **To decrease incidence of infection in patients with nonmyeloid malignancies receiving myelosuppressive chemotherapy associated with risk of severe febrile neutropenia; to reduce time to neutrophil recovery and duration of fever after induction or consolidation chemotherapy for acute myeloid leukemia (Neupogen, Nivestym, Releuko, Zarxio)**
Adults and children: 5 mcg/kg by a single subcut injection or short IV infusion (15 to 30 minutes), or continuous IV infusion once daily at least 24 hours after chemotherapy. Give daily for up to 2 weeks, until ANC reaches 10,000/mm³.

Adjust-a-dose: May increase dosage by increments of 5 mcg/kg for each chemotherapy cycle, depending on duration and severity of ANC nadir.
➤ **To decrease incidence of infection in patients with nonmyeloid malignancies receiving myelosuppressive chemotherapy associated with risk of severe febrile neutropenia (Granix)**
Adults and children age 1 month and older: 5 mcg/kg/day subcut. Continue until anticipated nadir has passed and neutrophil count has recovered to normal range.
➤ **To decrease risk of infection in patients with nonmyeloid malignant disease receiving myelosuppressive antineoplastics followed by bone marrow transplantation (Neupogen, Nivestym, Releuko, Zarxio)**
Adults and children: 10 mcg/kg daily IV infusion for no longer than 24 hours or as continuous 24-hour subcut infusion at least 24 hours after cytotoxic chemotherapy and bone marrow infusion. Adjust subsequent dosages based on neutrophil response.
Adjust-a-dose: For patients with ANC above 1,000/mm³ for 3 consecutive days, reduce dosage to 5 mcg/kg/day. If ANC decreases to less than 1,000/mm³ with 5-mcg/kg/day dose, increase dosage to 10 mcg/kg/day. If ANC remains above 1,000/mm³ for 3 more consecutive days, stop drug. If ANC decreases to below 1,000/mm³, resume therapy at 5 mcg/kg daily.
➤ **Chronic severe neutropenia (Neupogen, Nivestym, Releuko, Zarxio)**
Adults and children: For patients with congenital neutropenia, starting dose is 6 mcg/kg subcut b.i.d. For patients with idiopathic or cyclic neutropenia, starting dose is 5 mcg/kg as a single daily subcut injection. Adjust dosage based on patient response.
➤ **Peripheral blood progenitor cell collection and therapy in patients with cancer (Neupogen, Nivestym, Zarxio)**
Adults and children: 10 mcg/kg/day subcut (as bolus or continuous infusion). Begin treatment at least 4 days before leukapheresis and continue until last leukapheresis.
Adjust-a-dose: Monitor daily neutrophil count after 4 days of treatment; discontinue drug for WBC count above 100,000/mm³.
➤ **Hematopoietic stem cell mobilization in autologous transplantation in patients with non-Hodgkin lymphoma or multiple**

Reactions in bold italics are *life-threatening*. Interactions may have a *rapid onset* or a ***delayed onset***.

myeloma (in combination with plerixafor) (Neupogen) ◆

Adults: 10 mcg/kg subcut daily; begin 4 days before plerixafor initiation and continue on each day before apheresis for up to 8 days.

ADMINISTRATION

• Give at least 24 hours after cytotoxic chemotherapy.

🕓 **Alert:** Direct administration of less than 0.3 mL isn't recommended because of potential for dosing errors.

🕓 **Alert:** Removable needle cap in prefilled syringes contains natural rubber latex. Don't use in patients with latex allergies.

• Store in refrigerator at 36° to 46° F (2° to 8° C) in original pack to protect from light. Don't shake.

• Before use, allow drug to reach room temperature for at least 30 minutes to a maximum of 24 hours. (If beyond 24 hours, discard drug.)

• Solution should be clear and colorless to slightly yellow. Discard if solution is discolored or contains particulate matter.

• Avoid freezing; if frozen, thaw in refrigerator before administering. Discard drug if frozen more than once.

• Discard unused portion of prefilled syringes.

• Refer to manufacturer's instructions for further administration details.

IV

▼ Dilute in 50 to 100 mL of D_5W. Dilution to less than 5 mcg/mL isn't recommended.

▼ Don't dilute with NSS; product may precipitate.

▼ If drug yield is 5 to 15 mcg/mL, add albumin at 2 mg/mL (0.2%) to minimize binding of drug to plastic containers or tubing.

▼ Give by intermittent infusion over 15 to 30 minutes or by continuous infusion over 24 hours.

▼ Once a dose is withdrawn, don't reuse vial. Discard unused portion. Vials are for single-dose use only.

▼ **Incompatibilities:** Sodium solutions. No other incompatibilities are listed by manufacturer. Consult a drug incompatibility reference for more information.

Subcutaneous

• Rotate administration sites and record.

• Administer in outer upper arms, abdomen, thighs, or upper outer areas of the buttock.

• Don't inject into areas that are tender, red, bruised, hardened, or scarred or into sites with stretch marks.

ACTION

Binds cell receptors to stimulate proliferation, differentiation, commitment, and end-cell function of neutrophils.

Route	Onset	Peak	Duration
IV	1–2 days	Unknown	4 days
Subcut	1–2 days	2–8 hr	4 days
Subcut (tbo-filgrastim)	3–5 days to max ANC	4–6 hr	21 days to baseline ANC return after chemotherapy completion

Half-life: 3 to 3.5 hours.

ADVERSE REACTIONS

CNS: fever, headache, weakness, fatigue, dizziness, insomnia, pain, hypoesthesia. **CV:** chest pain, HTN, peripheral edema. **EENT:** epistaxis, sore throat, oral pain. **GI:** nausea, vomiting, diarrhea, decreased appetite, constipation. **GU:** UTI. **Hematologic:** *thrombocytopenia,* anemia, leukocytosis, splenomegaly, *neutropenic fever.* **Hepatic:** increased ALP level. **Metabolic:** increased LDH level. **Musculoskeletal:** bone pain, back pain, extremity pain, arthralgia, muscle spasms. **Respiratory:** dyspnea, cough, bronchitis, URI. **Skin:** alopecia, rash, erythema, cutaneous vasculitis. **Other:** hypersensitivity reactions, transfusion reaction, *sepsis,* antibody development.

INTERACTIONS

Drug-drug. *Bleomycin, cyclophosphamide:* May increase pulmonary toxicity. Monitor therapy.

Chemotherapeutic drugs: Rapidly dividing myeloid cells may be sensitive to cytotoxic drugs. Don't use within 24 hours before or after a dose of one of these drugs.

EFFECTS ON LAB TEST RESULTS

• May increase ALP, creatinine, LDH, and uric acid levels.

• May increase WBC count.

• May decrease Hb level and platelet count.

CONTRAINDICATIONS & CAUTIONS

• Contraindicated in patients hypersensitive to drug or its components or to proteins derived from *Escherichia coli.*

🍁Canada   ◇OTC   ◆Off-label use   ✔Photoguide   ⊕Do not crush   *Liquid contains alcohol   ▩Genetic

• Severe allergic reactions, including anaphylaxis, can occur. Permanently discontinue drug for serious allergic reactions.

• Splenic rupture (including fatal cases), sickle cell crisis (including fatal cases), ARDS, cutaneous vasculitis, glomerulonephritis, and capillary leak syndrome, which may be life-threatening, have been reported.

• Use cautiously in severe chronic neutropenia; confirm diagnosis before initiating drug. Drug may increase risk of myelodysplastic syndrome and acute myelogenous leukemia.

• G-CSF drugs may act as a growth factor on any type of tumor. Transmission of tumor cells by peripheral blood progenitor cell therapy infusion may occur and hasn't been well studied.

• Use cautiously in children as studies regarding safety and effectiveness in children are limited.

Dializable drug: Unknown.

⚠ *Overdose S&S:* Excessive leukocytosis.

PREGNANCY-LACTATION-REPRODUCTION

• Adverse effects have been seen in animal studies. Use during pregnancy only if potential benefit justifies fetal risk.

• It isn't known if drug appears in human milk. Use with extreme caution during breast-feeding.

NURSING CONSIDERATIONS

🛈 *Alert:* Obtain baseline CBC after exposure to myelosuppressive doses of radiation; don't delay administration if CBC isn't readily available. Monitor CBC every third day until ANC remains greater than $1,000/mm^3$ for three consecutive CBCs.

• Obtain baseline CBC and platelet count before therapy.

• Obtain CBC and platelet count two to three times weekly during therapy. Patients who receive drug also receive high doses of chemotherapy, which may increase risk of toxicities.

• A transiently increased neutrophil count is common 1 or 2 days after therapy starts. Give daily for up to 2 weeks or until ANC has returned to $10,000/mm^3$ after the expected chemotherapy-induced neutrophil nadir.

• For severe chronic neutropenia, monitor CBC with differential and platelet count during initial 4 weeks of treatment and during the 2 weeks after dosage adjustments. Once patient is clinically stable, monitor monthly during first year of treatment, then as

clinically indicated. Consider risks and benefits of continued treatment if abnormal cytogenetics or myelodysplasia occurs.

• Glomerulonephritis can occur; dosage reduction or drug discontinuation may be necessary.

• Monitor patients with left upper abdominal or shoulder pain for enlarged spleen or splenic rupture.

• Monitor patients for capillary leak syndrome (hypotension, hypoalbuminemia, edema, hemoconcentration), which can be life-threatening. Monitor patients closely; intensive care may be needed.

• Assess patients with fever, lung infiltrates, or respiratory distress for ARDS. Discontinue drug if ARDS is confirmed.

• Watch for sickle cell crisis in patients with sickle cell trait or sickle cell disease.

• Monitor patients for signs and symptoms of cutaneous vasculitis (purpura, erythema), especially patients on long-term therapy. Withhold drug if cutaneous vasculitis develops. Consider restarting drug at a reduced dosage when signs and symptoms have resolved and ANC has decreased.

• *Look alike–sound alike:* Don't confuse Neupogen with Epogen or Neumega. Don't confuse filgrastim-sndz with filgrastim.

PATIENT TEACHING

• Instruct patient and caregivers on proper timing, administration, and disposal of subcut self-administered drug.

• Patient with latex allergy shouldn't administer or receive drug in prefilled syringes.

• Instruct patient to report all adverse reactions promptly.

• Teach patient signs and symptoms of allergic reaction (rash, facial edema, wheezing, dyspnea, hypotension, rapid HR); advise patient to seek immediate medical attention if they occur.

• Advise patient to immediately report purpura or erythema.

• Warn patient to seek immediate medical attention if swelling, decreased urination, shortness of breath, abdominal swelling or feeling of fullness, dizziness, or fatigue occurs.

🛈 *Alert:* Rarely, splenic rupture may occur. Advise patient to immediately report left upper abdominal or shoulder tip pain.

• Tell patient that routine blood tests will be needed before and during treatment to monitor for effectiveness and safe use.

Reactions in bold italics are *life-threatening*. Interactions may have a *rapid onset* or a ***delayed onset***.

• Warn patient who is pregnant or breastfeeding about drug's risks.

finasteride
fin-AS-teh-ride

Propecia✐, Proscar✐

Therapeutic class: BPH drugs
Pharmacologic class: 5-alpha reductase inhibitors

AVAILABLE FORMS
Tablets: 1 mg, 5 mg

INDICATIONS & DOSAGES
➤ **To improve symptoms of BPH and reduce risk of acute urine retention and need for surgery, including transurethral resection of prostate and prostatectomy; to reduce risk of BPH, with or without doxazosin (Proscar)**
Men: 5 mg PO daily.
➤ **Male pattern hair loss (androgenetic alopecia) in men only (Propecia)**
Men: 1 mg PO daily.

ADMINISTRATION
PO
• Give drug without regard for food.
• Store at room temperature. Protect from moisture and light.
⚠ *Alert:* Drug is a potential teratogen. Follow safe handling procedures.

ACTION
Inhibits 5-alpha reductase, resulting in inhibition of the conversion of testosterone to dihydrotestosterone (DHT), the androgen primarily responsible for the initial development and subsequent enlargement of the prostate gland. In male pattern baldness, the scalp contains miniaturized hair follicles and increased DHT level; drug decreases scalp DHT level in such cases.

Route	Onset	Peak	Duration
PO	Unknown	1–2 hr	24 hr

Half-life: 6 hours; 8 hours in older adults.

ADVERSE REACTIONS
CNS: dizziness, drowsiness, asthenia, headache. **CV:** hypotension, orthostatic hypotension, peripheral edema. **EENT:** rhinitis.

GU: erectile dysfunction, decreased volume of ejaculate, decreased libido, breast tenderness. **Respiratory:** dyspnea. **Other:** gynecomastia, rash.

INTERACTIONS
None reported.

EFFECTS ON LAB TEST RESULTS
• May decrease PSA level.

CONTRAINDICATIONS & CAUTIONS
• Contraindicated in patients hypersensitive to drug or to other 5-alpha reductase inhibitors, such as dutasteride.
⚠ *Alert:* Drug may increase the risk of high-grade prostate cancer. Before starting drug, patient should be evaluated to rule out other urologic conditions, including prostate cancer, that might mimic BPH. An increase in PSA level during therapy should be considered significant and patient should be evaluated for prostate cancer.
• Use cautiously in patients with liver dysfunction.
• Drug isn't indicated for use in children or females.
Dialyzable drug: Unknown.

PREGNANCY-LACTATION-REPRODUCTION
• Contraindicated in pregnancy and in patients of childbearing potential.
• Patients who are pregnant should avoid contact with drug and with semen from a male partner taking drug.
• It isn't known if drug appears in human milk.

NURSING CONSIDERATIONS
• Before therapy, evaluate patient for conditions that mimic BPH, including hypotonic bladder, prostate cancer, infection, or stricture.
• Carefully monitor patients who have a large residual urine volume or severely diminished urine flow.
• Sustained increase in PSA level could indicate nonadherence with therapy.
• A minimum of 6 months of therapy may be needed for treatment of BPH.

PATIENT TEACHING
• Teach patient safe drug administration and handling.

♣Canada   ◇OTC   ◆Off-label use   ✐Photoguide   ⊜Do not crush   *Liquid contains alcohol   ▒Genetic

• Warn patient who is or may become pregnant not to handle crushed or broken tablets because of risk of adverse effects on male fetus and to avoid contact with semen from a male partner exposed to finasteride.
• Inform patient that signs of improvement may require at least 3 months of daily use when drug is used to treat hair loss or at least 6 months when taken for BPH.
• Reassure patient that drug may decrease volume of ejaculate without impairing normal sexual function.
• Instruct patient to report breast changes, such as lumps, pain, or nipple discharge.

finerenone
fin-ER-e-none

Kerendia

Therapeutic class: Miscellaneous renal drugs
Pharmacologic class: Mineralocorticoid receptor antagonists

AVAILABLE FORMS
Tablets: 10 mg, 20 mg

INDICATIONS & DOSAGES
➤ **To reduce risk of sustained eGFR decline, ESRD, CV death, nonfatal MI, and hospitalization for HF in patients with chronic kidney disease associated with type 2 diabetes**
Adults: Initially, 10 or 20 mg PO once daily based on eGFR and serum potassium thresholds. Don't initiate drug if serum potassium level is more than 5.0 mEq/L. If eGFR is 60 mL/minute/1.73 m^2 or more, start at 20 mg once daily; if eGFR is 25 to less than 60 mL/minute/1.73 m^2, start at 10 mg once daily. If starting with 10 mg, increase dosage after 4 weeks to target dosage of 20 mg once daily, based on eGFR and serum potassium thresholds.
Adjust-a-dose: Adjust dosage as needed based on every-4-week eGFR and potassium level. If current serum potassium level is 4.8 mEq/L or less and patient is taking 10 mg, increase to 20 mg daily except if eGFR has decreased by more than 30% compared to previous measurement; if so, maintain 10-mg dose. If patient is already taking 20-mg dose, maintain 20 mg daily.

If current serum potassium level is more than 4.8 to 5.5 mEq/L and patient is taking 10 mg daily, stay at 10 mg daily. If patient is already taking 20-mg dose, stay at 20 mg daily.

If current serum potassium level is more than 5.5 mEq/L and patient is taking 10 mg, withhold drug and consider restarting at 10 mg once daily when serum potassium level is 5.0 mEq/L or less. If patient is already taking 20-mg dose, withhold drug and restart at 10 mg once daily when serum potassium level is 5.0 mEq/L or less.

ADMINISTRATION
PO
• Give without regard to food.
• If patient can't swallow, crush tablet and mix with applesauce or water; give immediately.
• Give a missed dose as soon as possible but only on same day; if not on same day, skip dose and continue with regular dosing schedule next day.
• Store tablets at 68° to 77° F (20° to 25° C).

ACTION
Blocks mineralocorticoid-mediated sodium reabsorption and mineralocorticoid activation in renal, cardiac, and vascular tissue, reducing fibrosis and inflammation.

Route	Onset	Peak	Duration
PO	Unknown	0.5–1.25 hr	Unknown

Half-life: 2 to 3 hours.

ADVERSE REACTIONS
CV: hypotension. **Metabolic:** *hyperkalemia,* hyponatremia.

INTERACTIONS
Drug-drug. *Drugs that may increase potassium level (ACE inhibitors, ARBs, potassium-sparing diuretics):* May increase potassium retention. Monitor potassium level frequently.
Moderate (erythromycin) and weak (amiodarone) CYP3A inhibitors: May increase finerenone level and risk of adverse reactions. Use together cautiously and monitor potassium level.
Strong (rifampin) or moderate (efavirenz) CYP3A inducers: May decrease finerenone level. Avoid use together.
Strong CYP3A inhibitors (itraconazole): May significantly increase finerenone level. Use together is contraindicated.

Reactions in bold italics are *life-threatening*. Interactions may have a *rapid onset* or a *delayed onset*.

Drug-herb. *St. John's wort:* May decrease finerenone level. Discourage use together.
Drug-food. *Grapefruit, grapefruit juice:* May increase finerenone level. Discourage use together.

EFFECTS ON LAB TEST RESULTS
• May increase potassium level.
• May decrease sodium level and eGFR.

CONTRAINDICATIONS & CAUTIONS
• Contraindicated in patients with adrenal insufficiency.
• Drug isn't recommended if eGFR is less than 25 mL/minute/1.73 m^2.
• Drug increases risk of hyperkalemia in patients who have higher baseline potassium levels, risk factors for hyperkalemia (concomitant drugs that increase serum potassium level or impair its excretion), or decreased kidney function. If serum potassium levels are more than 4.8 to 5.0 mEq/L, consider initiation with additional serum potassium monitoring within the first 4 weeks based on clinical judgment and serum potassium levels.
• Avoid use in patients with severe hepatic impairment (Child-Pugh class C). Consider additional potassium monitoring in patients with moderate hepatic impairment (Child-Pugh class B).
• Safety and effectiveness in children haven't been established.
• Use cautiously in older adults.
Dialyzable drug: Unlikely.

PREGNANCY-LACTATION-REPRODUCTION
• There are no studies during pregnancy.
• It isn't known if drug appears in human milk or how drug affects milk production or infants who are breastfed.
• Patient shouldn't breastfeed during therapy and for 1 day after final dose.

NURSING CONSIDERATIONS
• Monitor serum potassium level and eGFR at baseline, at 4 weeks, after dosage adjustment, and periodically during therapy.

PATIENT TEACHING
• Advise patient of the need for periodic monitoring of serum potassium level.
• Caution patient to consult prescriber before using potassium supplements or salt substitutes containing potassium.

• Instruct patient to inform prescriber if taking other prescription and OTC medications, herbs, and supplements.
• Tell patient to avoid grapefruit or grapefruit juice while taking drug.
• Warn patient not to breastfeed during therapy and for 1 day after final dose.

fingolimod
fin-GOL-ih-mod

Gilenya, Tascenso ODT

Therapeutic class: Immunomodulators
Pharmacologic class: Sphingosine 1-phosphate receptor modulators

AVAILABLE FORMS
Capsules: 0.25 mg, 0.5 mg
ODTs: 0.25 mg

INDICATIONS & DOSAGES
➤ **To reduce frequency of clinical exacerbations and to delay accumulation of physical disability in relapsing forms of MS**
Adults and children age 10 and older weighing more than 40 kg: 0.5 mg PO once daily.
Children age 10 and older weighing 40 kg or less: 0.25 mg PO once daily.

ADMINISTRATION
PO
• Hazardous drug; use appropriate handling and disposal precautions.
• May give without regard for food.
• May give ODT with or without water.
• Place ODT directly on the tongue and allow it to dissolve before patient swallows it.
• Give ODT as soon as it's removed from blister pack; don't store outside of blister pack.
• Store at room temperature. Protect from moisture.

ACTION
Blocks activity of lymphocytes leaving lymph nodes, which reduces number of lymphocytes in the peripheral blood.

Route	Onset	Peak	Duration
PO	Unknown	12–16 hr	Unknown

Half-life: 6 to 9 days.

ADVERSE REACTIONS

CNS: asthenia, depression, dizziness, paresthesia, headache, migraine. **CV:** *bradycardia,* HTN. **EENT:** sinusitis, blurred vision, eye pain. **GI:** abdominal pain, gastroenteritis, diarrhea, nausea. **Hematologic:** *lymphopenia, leukopenia.* **Hepatic:** increased transaminase levels, *hepatotoxicity.* **Metabolic:** hypertriglyceridemia, weight loss. **Musculoskeletal:** back pain, extremity pain. **Respiratory:** bronchitis, cough, dyspnea. **Skin:** tinea infections, alopecia, actinic keratosis, basal cell carcinoma, skin papilloma. **Other:** flulike symptoms, herpes viral infections.

INTERACTIONS

Drug-drug. *Antineoplastics, immunomodulators, immunosuppressants:* May increase risk of immunosuppression. Use cautiously together.

❂ *Alert: Beta blockers HR-lowering calcium channel blockers (diltiazem, verapamil), digoxin:* May increase risk of severe bradycardia or heart block. If possible, switch patient to cardiac drug that doesn't cause bradycardia before starting fingolimod. If change isn't possible, monitor patient with continuous ECG overnight after first dose to determine effects.

Drugs that prolong QT interval (Class IA or III antiarrhythmics [amiodarone, procainamide, quinidine, sotalol], citalopram, chlorpromazine, erythromycin, haloperidol, methadone): May increase risk of QT-interval prolongation and torsades de pointes. Contraindicated together.

Ketoconazole: May increase fingolimod level and risk of adverse effects. Use cautiously and monitor patient closely.

Live attenuated virus vaccines: May decrease vaccination effects or increase infection risk. Don't use together or give vaccine within 60 days of prior fingolimod use.

Drug-lifestyle. *Sun exposure:* May cause photosensitivity reactions. Advise patient to wear protective clothing and use a sunscreen with a high protection factor.

EFFECTS ON LAB TEST RESULTS

• May increase ALT, AST, GGT, and triglyceride levels.
• May decrease lymphocyte and neutrophil counts.

CONTRAINDICATIONS & CAUTIONS

• Contraindicated in patients hypersensitive to drug and in those with active acute or chronic infection.

❂ *Alert:* Contraindicated in patients with MI, unstable angina, stroke, TIA, decompensated HF requiring hospitalization, or class III/IV HF within the past 6 months; in those with history or presence of Mobitz Type II second- or third-degree AV block or sick sinus syndrome unless patient has a functioning pacemaker; in those with cardiac arrhythmias requiring treatment with Class IA or Class III antiarrhythmics; and in those with baseline QTc interval of 500 msec or greater.

❂ *Alert:* Use cautiously after cardiac evaluation in patients with ischemic heart disease, history of MI, HF, history of cardiac arrest, cerebrovascular disease, history of symptomatic bradycardia, recurrent syncope, severe untreated sleep apnea, AV block, or SA heart block. Monitor patient in a setting with resources and personnel capable of managing symptomatic bradycardia.

• Use cautiously in patients with sick sinus syndrome and in those taking beta blockers or calcium channel blockers.

• Use cautiously in patients with history of infection, macular edema, decreased pulmonary function test results, or liver disease.

• Use cautiously in patients older than age 65 who have concomitant disease or are taking other drugs.

• Safety and effectiveness in children younger than age 10 haven't been established.
Dialyzable drug: No.

⚠ *Overdose S&S:* Chest tightness or discomfort.

PREGNANCY-LACTATION-REPRODUCTION

• Drug may cause fetal harm. Use during pregnancy only if benefit justifies fetal risk.
• Patients who are pregnant should enroll in the Gilenya Pregnancy Registry (1-877-598-7237 or https://www.gilenyapregnancyregistry.com).
• Patients of childbearing potential should use effective contraception during therapy and for 2 months after final dose.
• Patients planning to become pregnant should stop drug 2 months before planned conception.
• It isn't known if drug appears in human milk. Use cautiously during breastfeeding.

Reactions in bold italics are *life-threatening*. Interactions may have a *rapid onset* or a *delayed onset*.

NURSING CONSIDERATIONS

• Verify pregnancy status before treatment.

⚠ *Alert:* Monitor HR and BP hourly for at least 6 hours after first dose in all patients. Obtain ECG before first dose and at the end of the observation period. Monitor BP routinely during treatment.

⚠ *Alert:* Monitor patients at high risk and those who may not tolerate bradycardia with continuous ECG overnight. Patients at high risk include those who develop severe bradycardia after receiving the first dose, those with preexisting conditions who may not tolerate bradycardia, those receiving other drugs that slow the HR or AV conduction, those with QT-interval prolongation before taking fingolimod or prolonged QT interval that occurs during monitoring period, those receiving other drugs that prolong QT interval, and those at risk for QT-interval prolongation due to hypokalemia, hypomagnesemia, or congenital long-QT syndrome.

⚠ *Alert:* If CV symptoms occur (HR less than 45 beats/minute [bpm] in adults, less than 55 bpm in children age 12 and older, or less than 60 bpm in children age 10 or 11; at its lowest value 6 hours after dose; or new-onset second-degree or higher AV block 6 hours after dose), continue monitoring until symptoms resolve.

⚠ *Alert:* Repeat first-dose monitoring guidelines after second dose in patients who required pharmacologic intervention for symptomatic bradycardia after first dose.

• Obtain baseline ECG if one wasn't done within 6 months before start of therapy, especially in patients receiving antiarrhythmics, beta blockers, or calcium channel blockers and in those with cardiac risk factors or slow or irregular HR on physical exam.

⚠ *Alert:* Drug may cause PML, which can cause severe disability or death. Monitor patient for progressive and diverse symptoms of PML (progressive weakness on one side of the body, clumsiness, vision problems, confusion, and changes in thinking, personality, memory, and orientation). Stop drug and perform diagnostic evaluation, including MRI, if PML is suspected.

• Test for varicella antibodies before treatment initiation, especially if patient has no history of chickenpox or immunization; consider vaccination against varicella zoster 1 month before start of fingolimod therapy.

• Obtain baseline ophthalmic exam and monitor patient for macular edema at 3 to 4 months after treatment initiation and if patient complains of visual disturbances. Although macular edema is a rare adverse reaction, patients with uveitis and diabetes are at increased risk.

• Drug may increase risk of infections. Monitor patient for signs and symptoms of infection during treatment and for 2 months after therapy ends. Obtain baseline CBC with differential within 6 months of beginning therapy. Stop treatment if patient has active infection.

• Human papilloma virus (HPV) infections, including papilloma, dysplasia, warts, and HPV-related cancer, have been reported in patients treated with fingolimod. Consider vaccination against HPV before treatment initiation, taking into account vaccination recommendations. Cancer screening, including Papanicolaou test, is recommended as per standard of care for patients receiving an immunosuppressive therapy.

• Monitor patient for hepatic impairment (unexplained nausea, vomiting, abdominal pain, fatigue, anorexia, jaundice, dark urine). Obtain LFTs within 6 months before start of treatment, promptly in patients who report symptoms that may indicate liver injury, and periodically until 2 months after therapy ends. Most enzyme elevations occur within 3 to 4 months of treatment initiation. Drug may need to be discontinued if severe liver injury occurs.

• Monitor patient for respiratory changes. Obtain spirometry and diffusion lung capacity tests if clinically indicated.

• Drug is associated with basal cell carcinoma and melanoma. Monitor patient for suspicious skin lesions and evaluate promptly.

• Restart therapy as at initiation if patient discontinues treatment for more than 2 weeks.

PATIENT TEACHING

⚠ *Alert:* Teach patient to immediately contact the health care provider if signs and symptoms of a slowing HR, such as dizziness, tiredness, irregular heartbeat, or palpitations, occur.

⚠ *Alert:* Advise patient to immediately report symptoms of PML (new or worsening weakness; trouble using arms or legs; changes in thinking, eyesight, strength, or balance).

F

Tell patient not to stop drug without first discussing with prescriber.

• Instruct patient to report visual disturbances, trouble breathing, changes in HR (low HR, dizziness, fatigue, chest pain) or rhythm (palpitations), infection (pain, fever, malaise), or suspicious skin lesions.

• Tell patient to immediately report unexplained nausea, vomiting, abdominal pain, fatigue, anorexia, jaundice, or dark urine.

• Advise patient to notify prescriber of any medication changes.

• Warn patient of childbearing potential about fetal risk; advise patient to use effective contraception during treatment and for 2 months after treatment ends.

• Advise patient to immediately report pregnancy or plans to become pregnant.

• Advise patient to promptly report suspicious skin lesions and to limit exposure to sun and UV light by wearing protective clothing and using a sunscreen with a high protection factor.

flecainide acetate
FLEH-kay-nide

Therapeutic class: Antiarrhythmics
Pharmacologic class: Benzamide derivatives

AVAILABLE FORMS
Tablets: 50 mg, 100 mg, 150 mg

INDICATIONS & DOSAGES
➤ **Prevention of paroxysmal supraventricular tachycardia, including AV nodal reentrant tachycardia and AV reentrant tachycardia or paroxysmal atrial fibrillation or flutter in patients without structural heart disease; life-threatening ventricular arrhythmias such as sustained ventricular tachycardia**

Adults: For paroxysmal supraventricular tachycardia or paroxysmal atrial fibrillation or flutter, 50 mg PO every 12 hours. Increase in increments of 50 mg b.i.d. every 4 days. Maximum dose is 300 mg/day. For life-threatening ventricular arrhythmias, 50 to 100 mg PO every 12 hours. Increase in increments of 50 mg b.i.d. every 4 days until desired effect occurs. Maximum dose for most patients is 400 mg/day.

Children older than age 6 months: Initially, 100 mg/m^2/day in divided doses every 8 to 12 hours. May titrate dosage at 4-day intervals. Maximum dosage is 200 mg/m^2/day.
Children age 6 months and younger: 50 mg/m^2/day in divided doses every 8 to 12 hours. May titrate dosage at 4-day intervals. Maximum dosage is 200 mg/m^2/day.
Adjust-a-dose: For adults, if CrCl is 35 mL/minute or less, first dose is 100 mg PO once daily or 50 mg PO b.i.d.

ADMINISTRATION
PO
• Give drug without regard for food.
• Oral suspension can be prepared by a pharmacist. Shake well before use. May refrigerate or keep at room temperature, protected from light, for 60 days.

ACTION
A Class IC antiarrhythmic that decreases excitability, conduction velocity, and automaticity by slowing atrial, AV node, His-Purkinje system, and intraventricular conduction; prolongs refractory periods in these tissues.

Route	Onset	Peak	Duration
PO	Unknown	1–6 hr	Unknown

Half-life: 12 to 27 hours (adults); 11 to 12 hours (adolescents age 12 to 15); 8 hours (children); 6 hours (12 months [infants]); 11 to 12 hours (3 months [infants]); 29 hours or less (newborns).

ADVERSE REACTIONS
CNS: dizziness, headache, light-headedness, syncope, fatigue, fever, tremor, anxiety, insomnia, hypoesthesia, depression, malaise, paresis, paresthesia, ataxia, vertigo, asthenia, somnolence. **CV:** *new or worsened arrhythmias, bradycardia, HF, cardiac arrest,* chest pain, palpitations, edema, flushing. **EENT:** blurred vision and other visual disturbances, eye pain, eye irritation, dry mouth. **GI:** nausea, constipation, abdominal pain, dyspepsia, vomiting, diarrhea, anorexia. **Respiratory:** dyspnea. **Skin:** diaphoresis, rash.

INTERACTIONS
Drug-drug. *Amiodarone, cimetidine, CYP2D6 inhibitors (clozapine, quinidine):* May increase level of flecainide. Watch for toxicity. In the presence of amiodarone, reduce usual flecainide dose by 50% and monitor patient for adverse effects.

Reactions in bold italics are *life-threatening*. Interactions may have a *rapid onset* or a ***delayed onset***.

Digoxin: May increase digoxin level. Monitor digoxin level.

Disopyramide, verapamil: May increase negative inotropic properties. Avoid using together.

Propranolol, other beta blockers: May increase flecainide and propranolol levels. Watch for propranolol and flecainide toxicity (negative inotropic effects).

QTc interval–prolonging drugs (fluoroquinolones, ondansetron, posaconazole): May increase risk of cardiotoxicity and arrhythmias. Consider therapy modification.

Ritonavir: May significantly increase flecainide levels and toxicity. Use together is contraindicated.

Drug-food. *Milk:* May interfere with drug absorption. Monitor trough drug levels during major changes in dietary milk intake.

EFFECTS ON LAB TEST RESULTS
None reported.

CONTRAINDICATIONS & CAUTIONS
• Contraindicated in hypersensitivity to drug and in those with second- or third-degree AV block or right bundle-branch block with left hemiblock (in the absence of an artificial pacemaker), recent MI, structural heart disease, or cardiogenic shock.

Boxed Warning Patients who received flecainide for atrial fibrillation or flutter were at increased risk for ventricular tachycardia and ventricular fibrillation. Its use in patients with chronic atrial fibrillation isn't recommended. ■

• Use cautiously in patients with severe renal disease, prolonged QT interval, sick sinus syndrome, or blood dyscrasia. Avoid use in HF.

• In patients with hepatic disease, use drug only if potential benefits outweigh risk, and use frequent and early drug-level monitoring to guide dosage.

• When transferring patient from another antiarrhythmic to flecainide, allow two to four plasma half-lives to elapse for the drug being discontinued before starting flecainide at the usual dosage. Consider hospitalizing patients in whom withdrawal of a previous antiarrhythmic produced life-threatening arrhythmias.

• Safety and effectiveness in children haven't been determined.

Dialyzable drug: No.

PREGNANCY-LACTATION-REPRODUCTION
• Use during pregnancy only if potential benefit justifies risk to the fetus.

• Drug appears in human milk. Consider discontinuing breastfeeding or drug.

NURSING CONSIDERATIONS
Boxed Warning When used to prevent ventricular arrhythmias, reserve drug for patients with documented life-threatening arrhythmias. For patients with sustained ventricular tachycardia, initiate therapy in the hospital and monitor rhythm. ■

Boxed Warning Patients treated with flecainide for atrial flutter have a 1:1 AV conduction due to slowing of the atrial rate. A paradoxical increase in the ventricular rate may occur. Concomitant negative chronotropic therapy with digoxin or beta blockers may lower the risk of this complication. ■

• Due to safety risks, flecainide should be reserved for symptomatic supraventricular tachycardia in patients without structural or ischemic heart disease who aren't candidates for, or prefer not to undergo, catheter ablation and in whom other therapies have failed or are contraindicated.

• Flecainide is an appropriate adjunctive therapy in patients with type 3 long QT syndrome or catecholaminergic polymorphic ventricular tachycardia who are already taking a maximally tolerated beta blocker but are still experiencing symptoms.

• Check that pacing threshold was determined 1 week before and after starting therapy in patient with a pacemaker; flecainide can alter endocardial pacing thresholds.

• Correct hypokalemia or hyperkalemia before giving flecainide; these electrolyte disturbances may alter drug's effect.

• Monitor ECG for proarrhythmic effects.

• Most patients can be maintained on an every-12-hours dosing schedule; some need to receive flecainide every 8 hours.

• Monitor flecainide level, especially if patient has renal failure or HF. Therapeutic flecainide levels range from 0.2 to 1 mcg/mL. Risk of adverse effects increases when trough blood level exceeds 1 mcg/mL.

PATIENT TEACHING
• Stress importance of taking drug exactly as prescribed.

• Instruct patient to report adverse reactions promptly and to limit fluid and sodium intake to minimize fluid retention.
• Advise patient to immediately report pregnancy, plans to become pregnant, breastfeeding, or plans to breastfeed during treatment.

---

fluconazole ☒
floo-KON-a-zole

Diflucan✸

Therapeutic class: Antifungals
Pharmacologic class: Triazoles

AVAILABLE FORMS
Injection: 100 mg/50 mL, 200 mg/100 mL, 400 mg/200 mL
Powder for oral suspension: 50 mg/5 mL, 200 mg/5 mL
Tablets: 50 mg, 100 mg, 150 mg, 200 mg

INDICATIONS & DOSAGES
Adjust-a-dose (for all indications except vulvovaginal candidiasis): If CrCl is less than 50 mL/minute and patient isn't receiving dialysis, give initial loading dose of 50 to 400 mg for patients about to receive multiple doses; then reduce dosage by 50%. Patients receiving regular hemodialysis treatment should receive usual dose after each dialysis session.

➤ **Oropharyngeal candidiasis**
Adults: 200 mg PO or IV on first day, then 100 mg once daily for at least 2 weeks.
Children: 6 mg/kg PO or IV on first day, then 3 mg/kg daily for 2 weeks.
Adjust-a-dose (for premature neonates [gestational age, 26 to 29 weeks]): For first 2 weeks of life, give same dosage as for older children every 72 hours. After first 2 weeks, give dose once daily. Maximum daily dose 600 mg.

➤ **Esophageal candidiasis**
Adults: 200 mg PO or IV on first day, then 100 mg once daily. Up to 400 mg daily has been used, depending on patient's condition and tolerance of treatment. Patients should receive drug for at least 3 weeks and for 2 weeks after symptoms resolve.
Children: 6 mg/kg PO or IV on first day, then 3 to 12 mg/kg daily for at least 3 weeks and for at least 2 weeks after symptoms resolve. Maximum daily dose, 12 mg/kg (or 600 mg).

Adjust-a-dose (for premature neonates [gestational age, 26 to 29 weeks]): For first 2 weeks of life, give same dosage as for older children every 72 hours. After first 2 weeks, give dose once daily.

➤ **Vulvovaginal candidiasis**
Adults: 150 mg PO for one dose only.

➤ **Systemic candidiasis**
Adults: Optimal therapeutic dosage and duration of therapy haven't been established; doses of up to 400 mg PO or IV daily have been used.
Children: 6 to 12 mg/kg/day PO or IV. Maximum daily dose, 600 mg.
Adjust-a-dose (for premature neonates [gestational age, 26 to 29 weeks]): For first 2 weeks of life, give same dosage as for older children every 72 hours. After first 2 weeks, give dose once daily.

➤ **Cryptococcal meningitis**
Adults: 400 mg PO or IV on first day, then 200 mg once daily for 10 to 12 weeks after CSF culture result is negative. Doses up to 400 mg/day may be used.
Children: 12 mg/kg/day PO or IV on first day, then 6 to 12 mg/kg/day for 10 to 12 weeks after CSF culture result is negative. Maximum daily dose, 600 mg.
Adjust-a-dose (for premature neonates [gestational age, 26 to 29 weeks]): For the first 2 weeks of life, administer the same dosage as for older children every 72 hours. After the first 2 weeks, administer dose once daily.

➤ **To prevent candidiasis in patients receiving bone marrow transplant and patients with cancer**
Adults: 400 mg PO or IV once daily. Start treatment several days before anticipated agranulocytosis, and continue for 7 days after neutrophil count exceeds 1,000/mm³.

➤ **To suppress relapse of cryptococcal meningitis in patients with AIDS**
Adults: 200 mg PO or IV daily.
Children: 6 mg/kg/day PO or IV once daily.
Adjust-a-dose (for premature neonates [gestational age, 26 to 29 weeks]): For first 2 weeks of life, give same dosage as for older children every 72 hours. After first 2 weeks, give dose once daily.

➤ ***Candida*-related peritonitis; UTI**
Adults: 50 to 200 mg PO or IV once daily.

ADMINISTRATION
PO
- Drug is considered hazardous; use safe handling and disposal precautions.
- Give drug without regard for food.
- Add 24 mL of distilled or purified water to the bottle and shake oral suspension well before giving.
- Store tablets and powder for oral suspension below 86° F (30° C). Store reconstituted suspension between 41° and 86° F (5° and 30° C). Discard unused portion after 2 weeks.
- Protect from freezing.
IV
▼ Drug is considered hazardous; use safe handling and disposal precautions.
▼ To ensure product sterility, don't remove protective wrap from IV bag until just before use.
▼ The plastic container may show some opacity from moisture absorbed during sterilization. This doesn't affect drug and diminishes over time.
▼ To prevent air embolism, don't connect in series with other infusions.
▼ Use an infusion pump.
▼ Give by continuous infusion at no more than 200 mg/hour.
▼ Don't use if solution is cloudy or precipitated.
▼ **Incompatibilities:** Many other IV drugs are incompatible. Consult a drug incompatibility reference for more information. Don't add other drugs to IV bag.

ACTION
Inhibits fungal CYP450 (responsible for fungal sterol synthesis); weakens fungal cell walls.

Route	Onset	Peak	Duration
PO	Rapid	1–2 hr	30 hr
IV	Immediate	Immediate	Unknown

Half-life: 20 to 50 hours.

ADVERSE REACTIONS
CNS: headache, dizziness, taste perversion. **GI:** nausea, vomiting, abdominal pain, diarrhea, dyspepsia. **Skin:** rash.

INTERACTIONS
Fluconazole can significantly interact with many drugs. Consult a drug interaction resource or pharmacist for additional information.

Drug-drug. *Alprazolam, chlordiazepoxide, clonazepam, clorazepate, diazepam, estazolam, flurazepam, midazolam, quazepam, triazolam:* Fluconazole may increase levels of these drugs and may cause increased CNS depression and psychomotor impairment. Avoid using together.
Carbamazepine, celecoxib, cyclosporine, phenytoin, theophylline: May increase levels of these drugs. Monitor carbamazepine, cyclosporine, phenytoin, and theophylline levels. Consider reducing celecoxib dosage by half when using with fluconazole.
Cimetidine: May decrease fluconazole level. Monitor patient's response to fluconazole.
CYP3A4 substrates that may lead to QT-interval prolongation (erythromycin, pimozide, quinidine): May cause prolonged QT interval and sudden death. Use together is contraindicated.
HMG-CoA reductase inhibitors (atorvastatin, fluvastatin, lovastatin, pravastatin, simvastatin): May increase levels and adverse effects of these drugs. Avoid using together or reduce dosage of HMG-CoA reductase inhibitor.
Hydrochlorothiazide: May increase fluconazole level. Monitor patient for fluconazole toxicity.
Isoniazid, oral sulfonylureas, phenytoin, rifampin, valproic acid: May increase hepatic transaminase level. Monitor LFT results closely.
Oral sulfonylureas (glipizide, glyburide): May increase levels of these drugs. Monitor patient for enhanced hypoglycemic effect.
Rifampin: May enhance fluconazole metabolism. Monitor patient for lack of response to fluconazole.
Tacrolimus: May increase tacrolimus level and nephrotoxicity. Monitor patient carefully.
Warfarin: May increase risk of bleeding. Monitor PT and INR.
Zidovudine: May increase zidovudine-related toxicities. Monitor patient closely; zidovudine dosage decrease may be needed.
Zolpidem: May increase therapeutic effects of zolpidem. Monitor patient closely. A decrease in dosage may be needed.

EFFECTS ON LAB TEST RESULTS
- May increase ALP, ALT, AST, GGT, cholesterol, and triglyceride levels.
- May decrease potassium level.
- May decrease platelet and WBC counts.

✚Canada   ◇OTC   ◆Off-label use   ✐Photoguide   ⊕Do not crush   *Liquid contains alcohol   ▧Genetic

CONTRAINDICATIONS & CAUTIONS

- Rarely, anaphylaxis has been reported.
- Contraindicated in patients hypersensitive to drug.
- Use dosage forms containing benzyl alcohol derivatives cautiously in neonates or avoid use.
- Use cautiously in patients hypersensitive to other antifungal azole compounds.
- Use cautiously in patients with renal dysfunction or proarrhythmic conditions.
- Reversible adrenal insufficiency has been reported in patients receiving fluconazole.
- ▧ Oral suspension contains sucrose and shouldn't be used in patients with hereditary fructose, glucose, or galactose malabsorption or sucrase-isomaltase deficiency.

Dialyzable drug: 50%.

⚠ *Overdose S&S:* Hallucinations, paranoid behavior.

PREGNANCY-LACTATION-REPRODUCTION

- Contraindicated for most indications during pregnancy. Long-term treatment with high doses (400 to 800 mg/day) during first trimester may be associated with birth defects.
- Patients of childbearing potential should use effective contraception during treatment and for 1 week after final dose.
- Drug appears in human milk. Use cautiously during breastfeeding.

NURSING CONSIDERATIONS

- 🜂 *Alert:* Serious hepatotoxicity has occurred in patients with underlying medical conditions. Monitor LFTs and discontinue drug if hepatic dysfunction develops.
- Rare cases of exfoliative skin disorders have been reported. Closely monitor patients who develop mild rash. Stop drug if lesions progress.
- Monitor renal function during treatment; dosage adjustment may be necessary.
- Monitor potassium level.
- Monitor patient for adrenal insufficiency (fatigue, weakness, anorexia, weight loss, abdominal pain).
- Likelihood of adverse reactions may be greater in patients with HIV infection.

PATIENT TEACHING

- Tell patient to take drug as directed, even after feeling better.
- Instruct patient to report all adverse reactions promptly.

flumazenil
FLOO-ma-zeh-nil

Therapeutic class: Antidotes
Pharmacologic class: Benzodiazepine antagonists

AVAILABLE FORMS
Injection: 0.1 mg/mL in 5-mL and 10-mL multiple-dose vials

INDICATIONS & DOSAGES

➤ **Complete or partial reversal of sedative effects of benzodiazepines after anesthesia (adults) or conscious sedation (adults and children)**

Adults: Initially, 0.2 mg IV over 15 seconds. If patient doesn't reach desired level of consciousness after 45 seconds, repeat dose. Repeat at 1-minute intervals, if needed, until cumulative dose of 1 mg has been given (first dose plus four more doses). Most patients respond after 0.6 to 1 mg of drug. In case of resedation, dosage may be repeated after 20 minutes, but never give more than 1 mg at any one time or exceed 3 mg in any 1 hour.

Children age 1 year and older: 0.01 mg/kg (up to 0.2 mg) IV over 15 seconds. If patient doesn't reach desired level of consciousness after 45 seconds, repeat dose. Repeat at 1-minute intervals, if needed, until cumulative dose of 0.05 mg/kg or 1 mg, whichever is lower, has been given (first dose plus four more doses).

➤ **Suspected benzodiazepine overdose**

Adults: Initially, 0.2 mg IV over 30 seconds. If patient doesn't reach desired level of consciousness after 30 seconds, give 0.3 mg over 30 seconds. If patient still doesn't respond adequately, give 0.5 mg over 30 seconds. Repeat 0.5-mg doses, as needed, at 1-minute intervals until cumulative dose of 3 mg has been given. Most patients with benzodiazepine overdose respond to cumulative doses between 1 and 3 mg; rarely, patients who respond partially after 3 mg may need additional doses, up to 5 mg total. If patient doesn't respond in 5 minutes after receiving 5 mg, sedation is unlikely to be caused by benzodiazepines. In case of resedation, may repeat dose after 20 minutes, but never give more than 1 mg (give as 0.5 mg/minute) at any one time or exceed 3 mg in any 1 hour.

Reactions in bold italics are *life-threatening*. Interactions may have a *rapid onset* or a **delayed onset**.

ADMINISTRATION

IV

▼ Make sure airway is secure and patent.

▼ Compatible solutions include D$_5$W, lactated Ringer injection, and NSS.

▼ To minimize pain at injection site, inject drug over 15 to 30 seconds into large vein through free-flowing solution.

▼ Monitor patient for signs and symptoms of extravasation.

▼ Drug is stable in a syringe for 24 hours.

▼ Store drug in vial at 68° to 77° F (20° to 25° C) until use; protect from light.

▼ **Incompatibilities:** None listed by manufacturer. Consult a drug incompatibility reference for more information.

ACTION

Competitively inhibits the actions of benzodiazepines on the GABA–benzodiazepine receptor complex.

Route	Onset	Peak	Duration
IV	1–2 min	6–10 min	1 hr (variable range: 19–50 min)

Half-life: Adults: 40 to 80 minutes (terminal); children: 20 to 75 minutes (terminal).

ADVERSE REACTIONS

CNS: dizziness, headache, *seizures,* agitation, emotional lability, anxiety, nervousness, tremor, insomnia, vertigo, fatigue, malaise, paresthesia, ataxia, depersonalization, depression, dysphoria, euphoria, paranoia. **CV:** cutaneous vasodilation, thrombophlebitis, palpitations, flushing. **EENT:** abnormal or blurred vision, lacrimation, dry mouth. **GI:** nausea, vomiting. **Respiratory:** dyspnea, hyperventilation. **Skin:** diaphoresis, rash. **Other:** pain at injection site, injection-site reaction.

INTERACTIONS

None significant.

EFFECTS ON LAB TEST RESULTS

None reported.

CONTRAINDICATIONS & CAUTIONS

• Contraindicated in patients hypersensitive to flumazenil or benzodiazepines, in those with evidence of serious TCA overdose, and in those who have received benzodiazepines to treat a potentially life-threatening condition, such as status epilepticus or increased ICP.

• *Alert:* Don't use in patients with mixed-overdose who are seriously ill when seizures from any cause are likely.

• Use cautiously in patients with head injury, psychiatric disorders, or alcohol dependence.

• Use cautiously in patients at high risk for developing seizures and in those who have recently received multiple doses of a parenteral benzodiazepine, who display signs of seizure activity, or who may be at risk for benzodiazepine dependence, such as patients in the ICU.

Dialyzable drug: No.

⚠ *Overdose S&S:* Anxiety, agitation, increased muscle tone, hyperesthesia, seizures.

PREGNANCY-LACTATION-REPRODUCTION

• There are no adequate and well-controlled studies during pregnancy. Use during pregnancy only if benefit outweighs fetal risk.

• It isn't known if drug appears in human milk. Use cautiously during breastfeeding.

NURSING CONSIDERATIONS

• Monitor patient closely for resedation, respiratory depression, or other residual effects that may occur after reversal of benzodiazepine effects; drug's duration of action is the shortest of all benzodiazepines. Length of monitoring depends on specific drug being reversed. Monitor patient closely after doses of long-acting benzodiazepines such as diazepam, or after high doses of short-acting benzodiazepines such as 10 mg of midazolam. In most cases, severe resedation and respiratory depression are unlikely in patients who fail to show signs of resedation 2 hours after a 1-mg dose.

• Repeat doses of flumazenil in patients with liver disease should be reduced in size or frequency; dose of flumazenil used for initial reversal of benzodiazepine effects isn't affected.

Boxed Warning Monitor patients for seizures, especially those who have been on benzodiazepines for long-term sedation or in overdose cases in which patients are showing signs of serious TCA overdose. Practitioners should individualize flumazenil dosage and be prepared to manage seizures. ■

PATIENT TEACHING

• Warn patient not to perform hazardous activities within 24 hours of procedure because of the risk of residual sedative effects of the benzodiazepine.

• Tell patient to avoid alcohol, CNS depressants, and OTC drugs for 24 hours and to report all adverse reactions.

• Give family necessary instructions and provide patient with written instructions. Patient may not be able to recall information given after the procedure; drug doesn't reverse amnesic effects of benzodiazepines.

fluocinolone acetonide
floo-oh-SIN-oh-lone

Capex, Derma-Smoothe/FS, DermOtic, Flac, Synalar, Synalar TS

Therapeutic class: Corticosteroids
Pharmacologic class: Corticosteroids

AVAILABLE FORMS
Cream: 0.01%, 0.025%
Oil: 0.01%
Oil/drops (otic): 0.01%
Ointment: 0.025%
Shampoo: 0.01%
Topical solution: 0.01%

INDICATIONS & DOSAGES
➤ **Inflammation from corticosteroid-responsive dermatoses (cream, ointment, solution)**
Adults and children: Clean area; apply product sparingly b.i.d. to q.i.d.
➤ **Atopic dermatitis**
Adults: Apply thin film of body oil t.i.d.
Children age 3 months and older: Moisten skin then apply thin film of body oil b.i.d. for maximum of 4 weeks. Avoid face and diaper area.
➤ **Scalp psoriasis**
Adults: Wet or dampen hair and scalp thoroughly. Apply a thin film of scalp oil and massage into scalp. Cover with supplied shower cap overnight or for a minimum of 4 hours before washing thoroughly with regular shampoo and then rinsing thoroughly with water.
➤ **Seborrheic dermatitis of the scalp**
Adults: Apply no more than 30 mL of 0.01% shampoo to the scalp once daily, lather, and rinse thoroughly with water after 5 minutes.

➤ **Eczematous external otitis**
Adults and children age 2 and older: Apply 5 drops of oil (otic) into affected ear b.i.d. for 7 to 14 days.

ADMINISTRATION
Otic
• Tilt head to one side so the affected ear is facing up. Gently pull earlobe backward and upward and apply 5 drops of oil into the ear. Keep head tilted for at least 1 minute.
• Gently pat excess material dripping out of ear using a clean cotton ball.
• Otic formulation isn't for ophthalmic use.
Topical
• Gently wash skin before applying. To prevent skin damage, rub in gently, leaving a thin coat. When treating hairy sites, part hair and apply directly to lesions.
• Avoid application near eyes or mucous membranes; in armpits, groin, or rectal area; or in ear canal if eardrum is perforated.
• Do not use occlusive dressing unless ordered.
• For patients with eczematous dermatitis whose skin may be irritated by adhesive material, hold dressing in place with gauze, elastic bandages, stockings, or stockinette.
• Change dressing as prescribed. Stop drug and notify prescriber if skin infection, striae, or atrophy occur.
• Shake shampoo well before use. Discard shampoo after 2 months.

ACTION
Unclear. Is diffused across cell membranes to form complexes with receptors, resulting in decreased formation, release, and activity of inflammatory mediators.

Route	Onset	Peak	Duration
Otic, topical	Unknown	Unknown	Unknown

Half-life: Unknown.

ADVERSE REACTIONS
EENT: ear infection (otic). **Skin:** burning, pruritus, irritation, dryness, erythema, folliculitis, hypertrichosis, hypopigmentation, hyperpigmentation, acneiform eruptions, perioral dermatitis, keratosis pilaris, papules, pustules, skin atrophy, allergic contact dermatitis, maceration, secondary infection, atrophy, striae, miliaria with occlusive dressings, abscess. **Other:** herpes simplex, secondary infection.

Reactions in bold italics are **life-threatening**. Interactions may have a *rapid onset* or a **delayed onset**.

INTERACTIONS
None significant.

EFFECTS ON LAB TEST RESULTS
• May increase glucose level.

CONTRAINDICATIONS & CAUTIONS
• Contraindicated in patients hypersensitive to drug or its components.
• Don't use as monotherapy in primary bacterial infections (impetigo, paronychia, erysipelas, cellulitis, angular cheilitis), treatment of rosacea, perioral dermatitis, or acne.
• Children are at higher risk for HPA-axis suppression and Cushing syndrome than adults when treated with topical corticosteroids. Linear growth retardation, delayed weight gain, and intracranial HTN have been reported.
• Drug isn't indicated for use in children younger than age 3 months.
Dialyzable drug: Unknown.
⚠ *Overdose S&S:* Systemic effects.

PREGNANCY-LACTATION-REPRODUCTION
• Use lowest effective dose during pregnancy and breastfeeding.

NURSING CONSIDERATIONS
• If an occlusive dressing has been applied and a fever develops, notify prescriber and remove dressing.
• If antifungal or antibiotic combined with corticosteroid fails to provide prompt improvement, stop corticosteroid until infection is controlled.
• Systemic absorption is likely with use of occlusive dressings, prolonged treatment, or extensive body surface treatment. Watch for symptoms, such as hyperglycemia, glycosuria, HPA axis suppression, or Cushing syndrome.
• Avoid using plastic pants or tight-fitting diapers on treated areas in young children. Children may absorb larger amounts of drug and be more susceptible to systemic toxicity.
• *Alert:* Body oil and scalp oil formulations contain peanut oil.
• *Look alike–sound alike:* Don't confuse fluocinolone with fluocinonide or fluticasone.

PATIENT TEACHING
• Teach patient or family how to apply drug using gloves or sterile applicator.
• Tell patient to wash hands after application.

• Caution patient to use an occlusive dressing only if directed by prescriber. If an occlusive dressing is used, advise patient to leave it in place for no longer than 12 hours each day and not to use dressing on infected or weeping lesions.
• Tell patient to stop using solution and notify prescriber if signs of systemic absorption, skin irritation or ulceration, hypersensitivity, or infection develop.
• Advise patient using the shampoo not to bandage, cover, or wrap the treated scalp area unless directed.

fluocinonide
floo-oh-SIN-oh-nide

Lidex✥, Vanos

Therapeutic class: Corticosteroids
Pharmacologic class: Corticosteroids

AVAILABLE FORMS
Cream: 0.05%, 0.1%
Gel: 0.05%
Ointment: 0.05%
Topical solution: 0.05%

INDICATIONS & DOSAGES
➤ **Inflammation from corticosteroid-responsive dermatoses**
Adults and children age 12 and older: Clean area; apply cream, gel, ointment, or topical solution sparingly b.i.d. to q.i.d. In children, use lowest dosage that promotes healing. If using Vanos 0.1% cream in adults and children age 12 and older, apply a thin layer once daily or b.i.d. for up to 2 weeks. Maximum, 60 g/week.

ADMINISTRATION
Topical
• Gently wash skin before applying. To prevent skin damage, rub in gently, leaving a thin coat. When treating hairy sites, part hair and apply directly to lesion.
• Avoid applying near eyes or mucous membranes, in ear canal, or on groin or axilla.
• Occlusive dressings may be used in severe or resistant dermatoses.
• For patients with eczematous dermatitis whose skin may be irritated by adhesive material, hold dressing in place with gauze, elastic bandages, stockings, or stockinette.

F

- Change dressing as prescribed. Stop drug and notify prescriber if skin infection, striae, or atrophy occur.
- Continue treatment for a few days after lesions clear.

ACTION
Diffuses across cell membranes to form complexes with cytoplasmic receptors.

Route	Onset	Peak	Duration
Topical	Unknown	Unknown	Unknown

Half-life: Unknown.

ADVERSE REACTIONS
CNS: headache. **CV:** telangiectasia. **EENT:** nasopharyngitis, nasal congestion. **Skin:** burning, pruritus, irritation, dryness, erythema, folliculitis, hypertrichosis, hypopigmentation, acneiform eruptions, perioral dermatitis, allergic contact dermatitis, maceration, secondary infection, atrophy, striae, miliaria with occlusive dressings.

INTERACTIONS
None significant.

EFFECTS ON LAB TEST RESULTS
- May increase glucose level.

CONTRAINDICATIONS & CAUTIONS
- Contraindicated in patients hypersensitive to drug or its components.
- Don't use as monotherapy in primary bacterial infections (impetigo, paronychia, erysipelas, cellulitis, angular cheilitis), treatment of rosacea, perioral dermatitis, or acne.
- Don't use very-high-potency or high-potency agents on the face, groin, or armpits.
- Children are at higher risk for HPA-axis suppression and Cushing syndrome than adults when treated with topical corticosteroids. Linear growth retardation, delayed weight gain, and intracranial HTN have been reported.
- Safety and effectiveness in children younger than age 12 haven't been established.
Dialyzable drug: Unknown.
⚠ *Overdose S&S:* Systemic effects.

PREGNANCY-LACTATION-REPRODUCTION
- Use lowest effective dose in pregnancy and breastfeeding.

NURSING CONSIDERATIONS
- If an occlusive dressing has been applied and a fever develops, notify prescriber and remove dressing.
- If antifungal or antibiotic combined with corticosteroid fails to provide prompt improvement, stop corticosteroid until infection is controlled.
- Systemic absorption is likely with use of occlusive dressings, prolonged treatment, or extensive body surface treatment. Watch for such symptoms as hyperglycemia, glycosuria, and HPA axis suppression.
- Avoid using plastic pants or tight-fitting diapers on treated areas in young children. Children may absorb larger amounts of drug and be more susceptible to systemic toxicity.
- *Look alike–sound alike:* Don't confuse fluocinonide with fluocinolone or fluticasone.

PATIENT TEACHING
- Teach patient and family how to apply drug using careful hand washing and gloves or sterile applicator.
- If an occlusive dressing is ordered, advise patient to leave it in place no more than 12 hours each day and not to use the dressing on infected or weeping lesions.
- Tell patient to stop drug and report signs of systemic absorption, skin irritation or ulceration, hypersensitivity, or infection.

SAFETY ALERT!

fluorouracil (5-FU)
flure-oh-YOOR-a-sill

Carac, Efudex, Fluoroplex, Tolak

Therapeutic class: Antineoplastics
Pharmacologic class: Pyrimidine analogues

AVAILABLE FORMS
Cream: 0.5%, 1%, 4%, 5%
Injection: 50 mg/mL
Topical solution: 2%, 5%

INDICATIONS & DOSAGES
Adjust-a-dose (for all indications): Individualize 5-FU dosage and dosing schedule based on tumor type, specific regimen administered, disease state, response to treatment, and patient risk factors. Refer to manufacturer's instructions for toxicity-related dosage adjustments.

Reactions in bold italics are *life-threatening*. Interactions may have a *rapid onset* or a *delayed onset*.

➤ **Colon and rectal adenocarcinoma**
Adults (infusional regimen in combination with leucovorin alone, or in combination with leucovorin and oxaliplatin or irinotecan): 400 mg/m^2 by IV bolus on day 1, followed by 2,400 to 3,000 mg/m^2 IV as a continuous infusion over 46 hours every 2 weeks.
Adults (bolus dosing regimen in combination with leucovorin): 500 mg/m^2 by IV bolus on days 1, 8, 15, 22, 29, and 36 in 8-week cycles for four cycles.

➤ **Breast adenocarcinoma as part of a cyclophosphamide-based multidrug regimen**
Adults: 500 or 600 mg/m^2 IV on days 1 and 8 every 28 days for six cycles.

➤ **Gastric adenocarcinoma as part of a platinum-containing multidrug chemotherapy regimen**
Adults: 200 to 1,000 mg/m^2 IV as a continuous infusion over 24 hours. Frequency of dosing in each cycle and length of each cycle will depend on the dose of 5-FU injection and the specific regimen administered.

➤ **Pancreatic adenocarcinoma in combination with leucovorin or as a component of a multidrug chemotherapy regimen that includes leucovorin**
Adults: 400 mg/m^2 IV bolus on day 1, followed by 2,400 mg/m^2 IV as a continuous infusion over 46 hours every 2 weeks.

➤ **Multiple actinic (solar) keratoses**
Adults: Apply Carac cream (0.5%) once daily for up to 4 weeks. Apply Tolak cream (4%) once daily for 4 weeks. Or, apply Efudex (5%) cream or topical solution or Fluoroplex cream (1%) b.i.d. for 2 to 6 weeks.

➤ **Superficial basal cell carcinoma**
Adults: Apply 5% Efudex cream or topical solution b.i.d. usually for 3 to 6 weeks; maximum, 12 weeks.

➤ **Anal carcinoma, in combination with mitomycin and radiation ◆**
Adults: 1,000 mg/m^2/day continuous IV infusion days 1 to 4 and days 29 to 32.

➤ **Muscle-invasive bladder cancer, in combination with mitomycin and radiation ◆**
Adults: 500 mg/m^2/day continuous IV infusion during radiation therapy fractions 1 to 5 and 16 to 20.

➤ **Cervical cancer, in combination with cisplatin and radiation ◆**
Adults: 1,000 mg/m^2/day continuous IV infusion days 1 to 4 every 3 weeks for three cycles.

➤ **Advanced esophageal cancer, in combination with mitomycin and cisplatin ◆**
Adults: 300 mg/m^2/day continuous IV infusion for up to 6 months.

➤ **Preoperatively and postoperatively for management of adenocarcinoma of the stomach, esophagogastric junction, or lower esophagus, in combination with epirubicin and cisplatin ◆**
Adults: 200 mg/m^2/day continuous IV infusion days 1 to 21 every 3 weeks for six cycles (three cycles preoperatively and three cycles postoperatively).

➤ **Gastric and gastroesophageal cancer, in combination with cisplatin and docetaxel ◆**
Adults: 750 mg/m^2/day continuous IV infusion days 1 to 5 every 3 weeks until disease progression or unacceptable toxicity occurs.

➤ **Advanced esophagogastric cancer, in combination with epirubicin and either cisplatin or oxaliplatin ◆**
Adults: 200 mg/m^2/day continuous IV infusion days 1 to 21 every 3 weeks for a planned duration of 24 weeks.

➤ **Preoperative esophageal cancer, in combination with cisplatin and radiation ◆**
Adults: 1,000 mg/m^2/day continuous IV infusion days 1 to 4 and days 29 to 32 of a 35-day treatment cycle.

➤ **Head and neck cancer ◆**
Adults: 1,000 mg/m^2/day continuous IV infusion days 1 to 4 every 3 weeks (in combination with cisplatin) for at least six cycles, or 1,000 mg/m^2/day continuous IV infusion days 1 to 4 every 4 weeks (in combination with carboplatin), or 600 mg/m^2/day continuous IV infusion days 1 to 4, 22 to 25, and 43 to 46 (in combination with carboplatin and radiation).

Or, 1,000 mg/m^2/day continuous IV infusion days 1 to 4 every 3 weeks (in combination with docetaxel and cisplatin) for three cycles, followed by chemoradiotherapy, or 750 mg/m^2/day continuous IV infusion days 1 to 5 every 3 weeks (in combination with docetaxel and cisplatin) for up to four cycles, followed by radiation in patients without progressive disease.

Or, 1,000 mg/m^2/day continuous IV infusion days 1 to 4 every 3 weeks (in combination with cetuximab and either cisplatin or carboplatin) for a total of up to six cycles.

ADMINISTRATION

IV

▼ Preparing and giving parenteral drug may be mutagenic, teratogenic, or carcinogenic. Follow facility policy to reduce risks.

▼ To reduce nausea, give antiemetic before 5-FU.

▼ Don't use cloudy solution. If crystals form, redissolve by warming and shaking vigorously. Allow solution to cool to body temperature before administration.

▼ May give drug by direct injection without dilution or as a continuous infusion. IV administration rates vary by protocol. Refer to specific reference for protocol.

▼ For infusion, dilute drug with D_5W, sterile water for injection, or NSS for injection.

▼ For continuous infusion, use plastic IV containers. Solution is more stable in plastic than in glass bottles.

▼ For IV infusion regimens, administer through CVAD using an infusion pump.

🕙 *Alert:* Serious dosing errors involving continuous ambulatory infusion pumps have occurred. Carefully select the device and double-check flow rate. Drug should be prescribed in single daily doses (not course doses) and include instructions to infuse over a specific time period. Utilize independent double-checks during administration.

▼ Don't refrigerate. Protect drug from sunlight.

▼ Can store diluted solutions and syringes (nondiluted) at room temperature for up to 4 hours.

▼ **Incompatibilities:** Don't administer in same IV line concomitantly with other medicinal products.

Topical

• Use appropriate precautions for receiving, handling, administering, and disposing of drug. Wear gloves (single) during receiving, unpacking, and placing in storage.

• Apply topical form cautiously near patient's eyes, nose, and mouth.

• Not for vaginal use.

• Apply 10 minutes after washing, rinsing, and drying affected area.

• Avoid occlusive dressings with topical form because they increase risk of inflammatory reactions in adjacent normal skin.

• Apply topical form with nonmetal applicator or suitable gloves. Wash hands immediately after handling topical form.

• The 1% topical strength is used on patient's face. Higher strengths, such as 5%, are used for thicker skinned areas or resistant lesions, such as superficial basal cell carcinoma.

ACTION

Nucleoside metabolic inhibitor that interferes with DNA and RNA synthesis, which affects rapidly growing cells and may lead to cell death.

Route	Onset	Peak	Duration
IV, topical	Unknown	Unknown	Unknown

Half-life: 8 to 20 minutes (IV).

ADVERSE REACTIONS

CNS: malaise, acute cerebellar syndrome, headache, disorientation, confusion, ataxia, euphoria. **CV:** *cardiotoxicity.* **EENT:** visual changes, nystagmus, lacrimal duct stenosis, photophobia. **GI:** stomatitis, GI ulcer, nausea, vomiting, diarrhea, anorexia, *GI bleeding.* **Hematologic:** *leukopenia, thrombocytopenia, agranulocytosis,* anemia. **Skin:** dermatitis, erythema, scaling, pruritus, nail changes, pigmented palmar creases, erythematous contact dermatitis, desquamative rash of hands and feet, hand-foot syndrome, photosensitivity reactions, reversible alopecia, pain, burning, soreness, suppuration, swelling, dryness, erosion with topical use, fissuring (IV). **Other:** hypersensitivity reactions, including *anaphylaxis.*

INTERACTIONS

Drug-drug. *Leucovorin calcium:* May increase cytotoxicity and toxicity of fluorouracil. Monitor patient closely.

Live-virus vaccines: May increase risk of vaccine-induced adverse reactions. Concomitant use isn't recommended.

Warfarin: May prolong PT and increase INR. Monitor PT and INR closely; adjust warfarin dosage accordingly.

Drug-lifestyle. *Sun exposure:* May cause photosensitivity reactions. Advise patient to avoid excessive sunlight exposure.

EFFECTS ON LAB TEST RESULTS

• May increase ALP, AST, ALT, bilirubin, 5-hydroxyindoleacetic acid (in urine), and LDH levels.

• May decrease plasma albumin level.

• May decrease Hb level and granulocyte, platelet, RBC, and WBC counts.

Reactions in bold italics are *life-threatening*. Interactions may have a *rapid onset* or a *delayed onset*.

CONTRAINDICATIONS & CAUTIONS
• Contraindicated in patients hypersensitive to drug. Some topical dosage forms contain peanut oil.

⌧ Patients with dihydropyrimidine dehydrogenase gene mutations have increased risk of acute early-onset of toxicity and severe, life-threatening, or fatal adverse reactions. Drug may need to be withheld or permanently discontinued based on clinical assessment of toxicities.

⟳ *Alert:* Withhold IV drug for cardiotoxicity, hyperammonemic encephalopathy, neurologic toxicity, GI toxicity, hand-foot syndrome, severe mucositis, and severe hematologic toxicity. Bone marrow suppression can be fatal.

• Use cautiously in patients who have received high-dose pelvic radiation or alkylating drugs and in those with impaired hepatic or renal function or widespread neoplastic infiltration of bone marrow.

• Safety and effectiveness in children haven't been established.

Dialyzable drug: Yes.

⚠ *Overdose S&S:* Nausea, vomiting, diarrhea, GI ulceration and bleeding, bone marrow depression (thrombocytopenia, leukopenia, agranulocytosis).

PREGNANCY-LACTATION-REPRODUCTION
• There are no well-controlled studies during pregnancy. Drug may cause fetal harm. Use during pregnancy only if potential benefit justifies fetal risk. Inform patient about potential fetal hazard.

• Topical formulations contraindicated in patients who are or may become pregnant during therapy.

• Patients of childbearing potential and males with partners of childbearing potential should use effective contraception during therapy and for 3 months after final dose.

• Contraindicated during breastfeeding.

NURSING CONSIDERATIONS
⟳ *Alert:* IV drug should be administered under the supervision of a physician experienced in cancer chemotherapy. Patient should be hospitalized at least during the initial course of IV therapy.

• Ingestion and systemic absorption of topical form may cause leukopenia, thrombocytopenia, stomatitis, diarrhea, or GI ulceration, bleeding, and hemorrhage. Application to large ulcerated areas may cause systemic toxicity.

• Monitor patient and withhold drug and notify prescriber for signs and symptoms of cardiotoxicity (angina, MI, ischemia, arrhythmia, HF), neurologic toxicity (confusion, disorientation, ataxia, visual disturbances), GI toxicities (severe diarrhea, mucositis, stomatitis, or esophagopharyngitis with mucosal sloughing or ulceration), hyperammonemic encephalopathy (altered mental status, confusion, disorientation, coma, or ataxia, with elevated serum ammonia level), hand-foot syndrome (tingling pain, edema, erythema with tenderness, skin desquamation), and severe hematologic toxicity (neutropenia, thrombocytopenia, anemia).

• Encourage diligent oral hygiene to prevent superinfection of denuded mucosa.

• Monitor CBC with differential and platelet count before each treatment cycle and as clinically indicated.

• Watch for ecchymoses, petechiae, easy bruising, and anemia, especially in patients taking warfarin.

• Monitor fluid intake and output, LFT values, and renal function test results.

• Long-term use may cause erythematous, desquamative rash of the hands and feet (hand-foot syndrome). Syndrome gradually resolves over 5 to 7 days after therapy interruption.

• Dermatologic adverse effects are reversible when drug is stopped.

• To prevent bleeding, avoid IM injections when platelet count is below $50,000/mm^3$.

• Anticipate blood transfusions because of cumulative anemia.

• For overdose, give uridine triacetate within 96 hours of 5-FU infusion.

⟳ *Alert:* Toxicity may be delayed for 1 to 3 weeks.

• The WBC count nadir occurs 9 to 14 days after first dose; the platelet count nadir occurs in 7 to 14 days.

⟳ *Alert:* Drug may be ordered as "5-fluorouracil" or "5-FU." The numeral "5" is part of the drug name and shouldn't be confused with dosage units.

• *Look alike–sound alike:* Don't confuse fluorouracil with floxuridine, fludarabine, or flucytosine.

PATIENT TEACHING
• Advise patient to immediately report all adverse reactions, especially infection, bleeding, chest pain, palpitations, swelling,

dyspnea, severe nausea, vomiting, diarrhea, dark urine, yellowing of skin or eyes, malaise, confusion, visual or gait disturbances, or redness of hands or feet.

• Instruct patient to take temperature daily and to immediately report signs or symptoms of infection.

• Warn patient that hair loss may occur but usually is reversible after drug is stopped.

• Caution patient to avoid prolonged exposure to sunlight or UV light when topical form is used.

• Tell patient to use highly protective sunblock to avoid inflammatory skin irritation.

• Warn patient that topically treated area may be unsightly during therapy and for several weeks afterward. Complete healing may take 1 or 2 months.

• Advise patient of childbearing potential and male patient with partner of childbearing potential to use effective contraception during therapy and for 3 months after final dose.

• Counsel patient not to breastfeed.

FLUoxetine hydrochloride

floo-OX-e-teen

Prozac

Therapeutic class: Antidepressants
Pharmacologic class: SSRIs

AVAILABLE FORMS

Capsules (delayed-release) ⒹⓇ: 90 mg
Capsules: 10 mg, 20 mg, 40 mg
Oral solution: 20 mg/5 mL
Tablets: 10 mg, 20 mg, 60 mg

INDICATIONS & DOSAGES

Adjust-a-dose (for all indications): For patients with renal or hepatic impairment and those taking several drugs at the same time, reduce dose or increase dosing interval.

➤ **Major depressive disorder (MDD), OCD**

Adults: Initially, 20 mg PO in the morning; increase dosage after several weeks based on patient response. Doses over 20 mg/day can be given once daily in the morning or divided into b.i.d. dosing (morning and noon). Maximum daily dose is 80 mg.

Children ages 7 to 17 (OCD): 10 mg PO daily. After 2 weeks, increase to 20 mg daily. Dosage range is 20 to 60 mg daily.

In lower weight children, initially 10 mg/day. Consider additional dosage increases after several more weeks if insufficient clinical improvement is observed. Dosage range of 20 to 30 mg/day is recommended.

Children ages 8 to 18 (MDD): 10 mg PO once daily for 1 week; then increase to 20 mg daily. Due to higher plasma levels in lower weight children, the starting and target dose in this group may be 10 mg/day. Consider a dosage increase to 20 mg/day after several weeks if insufficient clinical improvement is observed.

➤ **Maintenance therapy for depression in patients who are stabilized (not for newly diagnosed depression)**

Adults: 90 mg fluoxetine delayed-release capsules PO once weekly. Start once-weekly doses 7 days after the last daily dose of fluoxetine 20 mg.

➤ **Short-term and long-term treatment of bulimia nervosa**

Adults: 60 mg PO daily in the morning. For some patients, it may be advisable to titrate up to this target dose over several days.

➤ **Short-term treatment of panic disorder with or without agoraphobia**

Adults: 10 mg PO once daily for 1 week, then increase dose as needed to 20 mg daily. Maximum daily dose is 60 mg.

➤ **Depressive episodes associated with bipolar I disorder (with olanzapine)**

Adults: 20 mg PO with 5 mg PO olanzapine once daily in the evening. Dosage adjustments can be made based on efficacy and tolerability within ranges of fluoxetine 20 to 50 mg and olanzapine 5 to 12.5 mg.

Children ages 10 to 17: Initially, 20 mg PO with 2.5 mg olanzapine PO once daily in evening. Dosage adjustments can be made based on efficacy and tolerability. Safety of doses above 12 mg olanzapine with 50 mg fluoxetine hasn't been evaluated in pediatric clinical studies.

➤ **Treatment-resistant depression**

Adults: 20 mg PO with 5 mg PO olanzapine once daily in the evening. Dosage adjustments can be made based on efficacy and tolerability within ranges of fluoxetine 20 to 50 mg and olanzapine 5 to 20 mg.

ADMINISTRATION

PO

• Give drug without regard for food.

Reactions in bold italics are *life-threatening*. Interactions may have a *rapid onset* or a *delayed onset*.

• Avoid giving drug in the afternoon, whenever possible, because doing so commonly causes nervousness and insomnia.

• Delayed-release capsules must be swallowed whole; don't crush or open.

ACTION

Thought to be linked to drug's inhibition of CNS neuronal uptake of serotonin.

Route	Onset	Peak	Duration
PO	Unknown	6–8 hr	Unknown

Half-life: Acute administration, 1 to 3 days; long-term administration, 4 to 6 days.

ADVERSE REACTIONS

CNS: nervousness, somnolence, anxiety, insomnia, headache, drowsiness, tremor, dizziness, asthenia, abnormal thinking, abnormal dreams, sleep disorder, amnesia, personality disorder, fatigue, fever, emotional lability, taste perversion, yawning. **CV:** chest pain, HTN, palpitations, vasodilation, hot flashes, *prolonged QT interval.* **EENT:** epistaxis, dry mouth, pharyngitis, sinusitis. **GI:** nausea, diarrhea, anorexia, dyspepsia, constipation, abdominal pain, vomiting, flatulence, increased appetite. **GU:** sexual dysfunction, decreased libido, micturition disorder, urinary frequency. **Metabolic:** weight loss, increased thirst, hyponatremia. **Musculoskeletal:** muscle pain, hyperkinetic muscle activity. **Skin:** rash, pruritus, diaphoresis. **Other:** flulike syndrome, chills, hypersensitivity reaction.

INTERACTIONS

Drug-drug. *Amphetamines, antiemetics, antipsychotics, buspirone, dextromethorphan, dihydroergotamine, lithium salts, meperidine, opioids, other SSRIs or SSNRIs (duloxetine, venlafaxine), TCAs,* **tramadol,** *trazodone, triptans:* May increase the risk of serotonin syndrome. Avoid combinations of drugs that increase the availability of serotonin in the CNS; monitor patient closely if used together.
Antiplatelet agents, aspirin, NSAIDs: May increase risk of bleeding. Use together cautiously.
Benzodiazepines, lithium, TCAs: May increase levels of these drugs, resulting in additional CNS effects. Monitor patient closely.
Beta blockers, carbamazepine, flecainide, vinblastine: May increase levels of these drugs. Monitor drug levels and monitor patient for adverse reactions.

Cyproheptadine: May reverse or decrease fluoxetine effect. Monitor patient closely.
Dextromethorphan: May cause unusual side effects such as visual hallucinations. Advise use of cough suppressant that doesn't contain dextromethorphan while taking fluoxetine.
Highly protein-bound drugs: May increase level of fluoxetine or other highly protein-bound drugs. Monitor patient closely.
Insulin, oral antidiabetics: May alter glucose level and antidiabetic requirements. Adjust dosage.
Linezolid, methylene blue: May cause serotonin syndrome. Use extreme caution and monitor closely.
MAO inhibitors (phenelzine, selegiline, tranylcypromine): May cause serotonin syndrome and signs and symptoms resembling NMS. Avoid using at the same time and for at least 5 weeks after stopping fluoxetine.
Phenytoin: May increase phenytoin level and risk of toxicity. Monitor phenytoin level and adjust dosage.
Pimozide, thioridazine: May increase levels of these drugs, increasing risk of serious ventricular arrhythmias and sudden death. Don't use together and don't use thioridazine for at least 5 weeks after stopping fluoxetine.
Tamoxifen: May decrease tamoxifen plasma level, leading to breast cancer recurrence. Monitor patient carefully.
Warfarin: May increase risk for bleeding. Monitor PT and INR.
Drug-herb. *Kava kava, St. John's wort, tryptophan, valerian:* May increase sedative and hypnotic effects; may cause serotonin syndrome. Discourage use together.
Drug-lifestyle. *Alcohol use:* May increase CNS depression. Discourage use together.

EFFECTS ON LAB TEST RESULTS

• May decrease sodium level.

CONTRAINDICATIONS & CAUTIONS

• Contraindicated in patients hypersensitive to drug, with pimozide, and within 14 days of stopping an MAO inhibitor intended to treat psychiatric disorders. MAO inhibitors shouldn't be started within 5 weeks of stopping fluoxetine. Avoid using thioridazine with fluoxetine or within 5 weeks after stopping fluoxetine.

Boxed Warning Drug may increase the risk of suicidality in children, adolescents, and young adults with MDD or other psychiatric disorder. ■

Boxed Warning Fluoxetine is approved for use in children with MDD and OCD. Fluoxetine isn't approved for use in children younger than age 7. ■

🕓 *Alert:* Concomitant use with linezolid or methylene blue can cause serotonin syndrome (fever, mental status changes, muscle twitching, diaphoresis, shivering or shaking, diarrhea, loss of coordination). Use drug with linezolid or methylene blue only for life-threatening or urgent conditions when the potential benefits outweigh the risks of toxicity.

• Use cautiously in patients at high risk for suicide and in those with history of diabetes, glaucoma, seizures, mania, or hepatic, renal, or CV disease.

Dialyzable drug: No.

⚠ *Overdose S&S:* Nausea, seizures, somnolence, tachycardia, HTN, vomiting, coma, delirium, ECG abnormalities, hypotension, mania, NMS-like reactions, fever, stupor, syncope.

PREGNANCY-LACTATION-REPRODUCTION

• Use cautiously during pregnancy and only if benefit justifies fetal risk.

• Enroll patients in the National Pregnancy Registry for Antidepressants at 1-866-961-2388 or https://womensmentalhealth.org/research/pregnancyregistry/antidepressants/.

• Drug appears in human milk. Use during breastfeeding isn't recommended.

NURSING CONSIDERATIONS

Boxed Warning Monitor all patients for worsening or emergence of suicidality. ■

🕓 *Alert:* If linezolid or methylene blue must be given, fluoxetine must be stopped and patient monitored for serotonin toxicity for 5 weeks or until 24 hours after final dose of linezolid or methylene blue, whichever comes first. Treatment with fluoxetine may be resumed 24 hours after final dose of linezolid or methylene blue.

• Use antihistamines or topical corticosteroids to treat rashes or pruritus.

• Watch for weight change during therapy, particularly in patients who are underweight or bulimic.

• Record mood changes. Watch for suicidality.

• Drug has a long half-life; monitor patient for adverse effects for up to 2 weeks after drug is stopped.

• Monitor patient for serotonin syndrome, particularly when drug is used in combination with other serotonergic agents.

🕓 *Alert:* Combining triptans with an SSRI or an SSNRI may cause serotonin syndrome or NMS-like reactions. Serotonin syndrome may be more likely to occur when starting or increasing the dose of triptan, SSRI, or SSNRI.

• Monitor blood glucose level (in patients with diabetes) and liver and renal function (baseline and as clinically indicated).

• Obtain ECG and monitor periodically in patients with risk factors for QT-interval prolongation and ventricular arrhythmia.

• Monitor mental status for depression, suicidality (especially at beginning of therapy and with dosage changes), anxiety, social functioning, mania, or panic attacks.

• Observe patient for signs or symptoms of abnormal bleeding, akathisia, or sleep disturbances.

• When discontinuing drug, taper dosage over 2 weeks to 1 month to avoid withdrawal syndrome.

• Evaluate patient for sexual dysfunction before and periodically during treatment.

• *Look alike–sound alike:* Don't confuse fluoxetine with fluvoxamine or fluvastatin. Don't confuse Prozac with Proscar or Prilosec.

PATIENT TEACHING

Boxed Warning Advise family and caregivers to carefully observe patient for worsening suicidality. ■

🕓 *Alert:* Teach patient to recognize and immediately report symptoms of serotonin toxicity (fever, mental status changes, muscle twitching, diaphoresis, shivering or shaking, diarrhea, loss of coordination).

• Tell patient to avoid taking drug in the afternoon whenever possible because doing so commonly causes nervousness and insomnia.

• Drug may cause dizziness or drowsiness. Warn patient to avoid driving and other hazardous activities that require alertness and good psychomotor coordination until effects of drug are known.

• Instruct patient to report adverse effects and to not stop drug suddenly without first discussing with prescriber due to risk of discontinuation reactions.

• Tell patient to consult prescriber before taking other prescription or OTC drugs.

• Advise patient that full therapeutic effect may not be seen for 4 weeks or longer.

Reactions in bold italics are *life-threatening*. Interactions may have a *rapid onset* or a ***delayed onset***.

fluticasone furoate
floo-TIK-a-sone

Arnuity Ellipta, Flonase Sensimist
Allergy Relief ◇

fluticasone propionate
ArmonAir Digihaler, Flonase Allergy
Relief ◇, Flovent Diskus, Flovent HFA,
Xhance

Therapeutic class: Corticosteroids
Pharmacologic class: Corticosteroids

AVAILABLE FORMS
Nasal spray (furoate): 27.5 mcg/spray
Nasal spray (propionate): 50 mcg/metered
spray, 93 mcg/metered spray
Oral inhalation aerosol: 44 mcg, 110 mcg,
220 mcg
Oral inhalation powder: 50 mcg, 100 mcg,
200 mcg, 250 mcg
Oral inhalation powder (ArmonAir): 30 mcg,
55 mcg, 113 mcg, 232 mcg

INDICATIONS & DOSAGES
➤ **As preventive in maintenance of chronic
asthma in patients requiring oral corticosteroid**
Flovent Diskus
*Adults and children age 12 and older not
on an inhaled corticosteroid:* Initially, inhaled dose of 100 mcg b.i.d. approximately
12 hours apart. For patients who don't respond adequately to starting dosage after
2 weeks of therapy, may increase dosage to
maximum of 1,000 mcg b.i.d.
*Adults and children age 12 and older previ-
ously taking inhaled corticosteroids:* Base
dosage on strength of previously inhaled corticosteroid product and disease severity, including consideration of patient's current control of asthma symptoms and risk of future
exacerbation, to maximum of 1,000 mcg b.i.d.
Children ages 4 to 11: For patients not on an
inhaled corticosteroid, recommended starting dosage is 50 mcg b.i.d. approximately
12 hours apart. For other patients, and for patients who don't respond adequately to starting dosage after 2 weeks of therapy, may increase dosage to maximum 100 mcg b.i.d.
Flovent HFA
*Adults and children age 12 and older not on
an inhaled corticosteroid:* Initially, inhaled

dose of 88 mcg b.i.d. approximately 12 hours
apart. For patients who don't respond adequately to starting dosage after 2 weeks of
therapy, may increase dosage to maximum
of 880 mcg b.i.d.
*Adults and children age 12 and older previ-
ously taking inhaled corticosteroids:* Base
dosage on strength of previously inhaled corticosteroid product and disease severity, including consideration of patient's current control of asthma symptoms and risk of future
exacerbation, to maximum of 880 mcg b.i.d.
Children ages 4 to 11: 88 mcg inhaled b.i.d.
approximately 12 hours apart, regardless of
prior therapy.
Arnuity Ellipta
Adults and children age 12 and older: Base
starting dosage on patient's asthma severity.
Usual recommended starting dose for patients
not on an inhaled corticosteroid is 100 mcg
given as 1 inhalation at the same time every
day. For other patients, base starting dose on
previous asthma drug therapy and disease
severity. For patients who don't respond to
100 mcg after 2 weeks of therapy, replacement with 200-mcg formulation may provide
additional control. Don't use more than once
every 24 hours.
Children ages 5 to 11: 50 mcg given as 1 inhalation daily.
ArmonAir Digihaler
*Adults and children age 12 and older not on
an inhaled corticosteroid:* 55 mcg by oral inhalation b.i.d. Patients with greater asthma
severity may use 113 mcg or 232 mcg by oral
inhalation b.i.d. Maximum dose is 232 mcg
b.i.d.
*Adults and children age 12 and older previ-
ously taking inhaled corticosteroids:* 55 mcg,
113 mcg, or 232 mcg by oral inhalation b.i.d.
based on asthma severity and strength of prior
therapy. Maximum dose is 232 mcg b.i.d.
*Children ages 4 to 11 not on an inhaled cor-
ticosteroid:* 30 mcg by oral inhalation b.i.d.
After 2 weeks, may increase to 55 mcg b.i.d.
*Children ages 4 to 11 previously taking in-
haled corticosteroids:* 30 mcg or 55 mcg by
oral inhalation b.i.d. based on asthma severity and strength of prior therapy. Doses above
55 mcg b.i.d. haven't been established in children ages 4 to 11.
Adjust-a-dose: For patients who don't respond
adequately to starting dose after 2 weeks
of therapy, an increased dose may improve
control.

F

➤ **Nasal symptoms of seasonal and perennial allergic and nonallergic rhinitis**
Flonase

Adults: Initially, 2 sprays (100 mcg) in each nostril daily or 1 spray b.i.d. Once symptoms are controlled, decrease to 1 spray in each nostril daily. Or, for seasonal allergic rhinitis, 2 sprays in each nostril once daily, as needed, for symptom control.

Adolescents and children age 4 and older: Initially, 1 spray (50 mcg) in each nostril daily. If not responding, increase to 2 sprays in each nostril daily. Once symptoms are controlled, decrease to 1 spray in each nostril daily. Maximum dose is 2 sprays in each nostril daily.

Flonase Sensimist Allergy Relief (OTC)

Adults and children age 12 and older: 110 mcg once daily administered as 2 sprays (27.5 mcg/spray) in each nostril for 1 week. For week 2 through 6 months, 1 or 2 sprays in each nostril once daily, as needed. Reevaluate treatment after 6 months of daily use.

Children ages 2 to 11: 55 mcg once daily administered as 1 spray (27.5 mcg/spray) in each nostril. Use for the shortest amount of time necessary to achieve symptom relief. Reevaluate treatment if child needs to use spray for longer than 2 months a year.

➤ **Nasal polyps (*Xhance*)**
Adults: 1 spray (93 mcg/spray) in each nostril b.i.d. May increase to 2 sprays in each nostril b.i.d. (maximum dose).

ADMINISTRATION

Inhalational
• For best results, aerosol canister should be at room temperature.
• Prime and shake well before each use.
• Patients should rinse mouth after inhalation.
• Refer to specific manufacturer's guideline for discard date and storage.

Intranasal
• Prime and shake well before use.

ACTION
Anti-inflammatory and vasoconstrictor that may decrease inflammation by inhibiting mast cells, macrophages, and mediators such as leukotrienes.

Route	Onset	Peak	Duration
Inhalation (nasal)	12 hr	Several days	1–2 wk
Inhalation (oral)	24 hr	0.5-1 hr	1–2 wk

Half-life: 7.8 to 24 hours, depending on formulation.

ADVERSE REACTIONS
CNS: headache, dizziness, fever, migraine, nervousness, fatigue, malaise, pain, voice disorder. **CV:** HTN. **EENT:** cataracts, conjunctivitis, dry eye, eye irritation, nasal burning or irritation, nasal discharge, blood in nasal mucus, epistaxis, nasal congestion, rhinitis, oral candidiasis, sinusitis, sinus infection, pharyngitis, hoarseness, laryngitis, mouth irritation, tooth ache. **GI:** abdominal discomfort, abdominal pain, diarrhea, nausea, viral gastroenteritis, vomiting. **GU:** UTI. **Hematologic:** eosinophilia. **Metabolic:** weight gain. **Musculoskeletal:** arthralgia, symptoms of neck sprain or strain, joint pain, muscular soreness or spasm, muscle injury, osteoporosis. **Respiratory:** URI, ***bronchospasm,*** asthma symptoms, bronchitis, chest congestion, cough, dyspnea. **Skin:** dermatitis, urticaria, rash, pruritus. **Other:** *angioedema,* influenza, viral infections.

INTERACTIONS
Drug-drug. *Cobicistat:* May increase serum concentration of oral inhalation drug. Avoid use together.
Ketoconazole, other CYP3A4 inhibitors: May increase mean fluticasone level and systemic corticosteroid adverse effects. Use together cautiously.
Ritonavir: May cause systemic corticosteroid effects, such as Cushing syndrome and adrenal suppression. Avoid using together.

EFFECTS ON LAB TEST RESULTS
• May cause abnormal response to the 6-hour cosyntropin stimulation test in patients taking high fluticasone doses.

CONTRAINDICATIONS & CAUTIONS
• Contraindicated in patients hypersensitive to components in these preparations. Immediate hypersensitivity reactions, including anaphylaxis, can occur.

Reactions in bold italics are *life-threatening*. Interactions may have a *rapid onset* or a ***delayed onset***.

• Contraindicated as primary treatment of patients with status asthmaticus or other acute, intense episodes of asthma.

• Use cautiously in patients at risk for decreased bone mineralization.

• Drug can increase risk of infections, vasculitis, Kaposi sarcoma, psychiatric disturbances, HTN, fluid retention, GI perforation, hyperglycemia, and IOP.

• Avoid intranasal use in patients with recent nasal septal ulcers, nasal surgery, or nasal trauma until healing has occurred.

Dialyzable drug: Unknown.

⚠ *Overdose S&S:* Hypercorticism.

PREGNANCY-LACTATION-REPRODUCTION

• Use during pregnancy only if potential benefit justifies risk to the fetus.

• Use cautiously in breastfeeding.

NURSING CONSIDERATIONS

• Because of risk of systemic absorption of inhaled corticosteroids, observe patient carefully for evidence of systemic corticosteroid effects.

⚠ *Alert:* Monitor patient, especially postoperatively, during periods of stress or severe asthma attack for evidence of inadequate adrenal response.

⚠ *Alert:* During withdrawal from oral corticosteroids, some patients may experience signs and symptoms of systemically active corticosteroid withdrawal, such as joint or muscle pain, lassitude, and depression, despite maintenance or even improvement of respiratory function. Deaths due to adrenal insufficiency have occurred with transfer from active corticosteroids to fluticasone propionate inhaler.

• For patients starting therapy who are currently receiving oral corticosteroid therapy, reduce dose of prednisone to no more than 2.5 mg/day on a weekly basis, beginning after at least 1 week of therapy with fluticasone.

⚠ *Alert:* As with other inhaled asthma drugs, bronchospasm may occur, with an immediate increase in wheezing after a dose. If bronchospasm occurs after a dose of inhalation aerosol, treat immediately with a fast-acting inhaled bronchodilator.

• Drug may increase risk of glaucoma and cataracts. Monitor patient.

• Inhaled corticosteroids can reduce growth trajectory in children. Monitor growth.

• If a dosage regimen fails to provide adequate control of asthma, reevaluate the therapeutic regimen and consider additional therapeutic options, such as replacing the current strength with a higher strength, initiating an inhaled corticosteroid and long-acting beta$_2$-agonist combination product, or initiating oral corticosteroids.

• After asthma stability has been achieved, titrate to the lowest effective dosage to reduce the possibility of adverse effects.

PATIENT TEACHING

• Teach patient how to safely administer and store drug.

• Advise patient to report all adverse reactions.

• Tell patient that inhalation drug isn't indicated for the relief of acute bronchospasm.

• Instruct patient to use drug at regular intervals, as directed.

• Advise patient that maximum inhalation benefit may not be achieved for 1 to 2 weeks or longer after starting treatment.

• Instruct patient to contact prescriber if nasal spray doesn't improve condition after 4 days of treatment.

• Caution patient to immediately contact prescriber if asthma episodes unresponsive to bronchodilators occur during treatment with fluticasone. During such episodes, patient may need therapy with oral corticosteroids.

• Warn patient to avoid exposure to chickenpox or measles and, if exposed, to consult prescriber immediately.

• Tell patient to carry or wear medical identification indicating that patient may need supplementary corticosteroids during stress or a severe asthma attack.

⚠ *Alert:* During periods of stress or a severe asthma attack, instruct patient who has been withdrawn from systemic corticosteroids to resume prescribed oral corticosteroids immediately and to contact prescriber for further instruction.

• Advise patient to rinse mouth without swallowing after oral inhalation to reduce risk of oral thrush.

fluticasone furoate–vilanterol trifenatate
floo-TIK-a-sone/vye-LAN-ter-ol

Breo Ellipta

Therapeutic class: Corticosteroids–bronchodilators
Pharmacologic class: Corticosteroids–beta$_2$-adrenergic agonists

AVAILABLE FORMS
Powder for inhalation: Inhaler containing two double-foil blister strips of powder formulation: One strip contains fluticasone furoate 100 mcg/blister or 200 mcg/blister; the other contains vilanterol 25 mcg/blister

INDICATIONS & DOSAGES
➤ **Asthma**
Adults: 1 inhalation of 100 mcg fluticasone furoate–25 mcg vilanterol trifenatate or 200 mcg fluticasone furoate–25 mcg vilanterol trifenatate once daily.
➤ **Maintenance treatment of COPD**
Adults: 1 inhalation of 100 mcg fluticasone furoate–25 mcg vilanterol trifenatate once daily.

ADMINISTRATION
Inhalational
- Patient shouldn't use more than 1 inhalation in 24 hours; may cause adverse effects.
- Have patient exhale fully before taking one long, steady, deep breath through the mouthpiece (patient shouldn't breathe through the nose), hold breath for 3 to 4 seconds, and exhale slowly and gently.
- After use, have patient rinse mouth with water without swallowing to help reduce the risk of oropharyngeal candidiasis.
- Give at the same time every day and not more than one time every 24 hours.
- Store at room temperature between 68° and 77° F (20° and 25° C) in a dry place away from heat and sunlight.
- Keep drug stored inside the unopened moisture-protective foil tray; remove from tray immediately before initial use.
- Discard drug 6 weeks after opening foil tray or when the counter reads "0" (after all blisters have been used).
- Inhaler isn't reusable.
- Don't attempt to take the inhaler apart.

ACTION
Fluticasone is an anti-inflammatory and vasoconstrictor that may decrease inflammation by inhibiting mast cells, macrophages, and mediators such as leukotrienes. Vilanterol trifenatate relaxes bronchial smooth muscle and inhibits inflammatory mediators, especially mast cells.

Route	Onset	Peak	Duration
Inhalation (fluticasone)	Unknown	30–60 min	Unknown
Inhalation (vilanterol)	Unknown	10 min	Unknown

Half-life: Fluticasone, 24 hours; vilanterol, 21 hours.

ADVERSE REACTIONS
CNS: headache, fever. **CV:** HTN, peripheral edema, extrasystoles. **EENT:** nasopharyngitis, oropharyngeal candidiasis, oropharyngeal pain, pharyngitis, rhinitis, sinusitis. **GI:** diarrhea, upper abdominal pain. **Musculoskeletal:** back pain, arthralgia. **Respiratory:** URI, pneumonia, bronchitis, cough. **Other:** flulike symptoms.

INTERACTIONS
Drug-drug. *CYP3A4 inhibitors (clarithromycin, conivaptan, itraconazole, ketoconazole, lopinavir, nefazodone, nelfinavir, ritonavir, saquinavir, voriconazole):* May increase systemic effects of corticosteroids, and increased CV adverse effects may occur. Use together cautiously.
Loop or thiazide diuretics (furosemide, hydrochlorothiazide, torsemide): May increase risk of hypokalemia or ECG changes. Monitor patient closely with concurrent use.
MAO inhibitors, TCAs, other drugs known to prolong QTc interval: May increase adrenergic effects or risk of ventricular arrhythmias. Don't use together.
Nonselective beta blockers (carvedilol, propranolol, sotalol): May increase risk of bronchospasm. Use cardioselective agents only if absolutely needed.
Other LABAs (arformoterol tartrate, formoterol fumarate, indacaterol, salmeterol): May increase risk of overdose. Don't use together.

EFFECTS ON LAB TEST RESULTS
- May increase glucose level.
- May decrease potassium level.

Reactions in bold italics are *life-threatening*. Interactions may have a *rapid onset* or a ***delayed onset***.

CONTRAINDICATIONS & CAUTIONS

• Contraindicated in patients with severe hypersensitivity to milk proteins and in those who have demonstrated hypersensitivity to fluticasone furoate, vilanterol, or their components.

🔔 **Alert:** Contraindicated as primary treatment of status asthmaticus or other acute episodes of COPD or asthma when other intensive measures are required.

• Use of LABAs as monotherapy (without inhaled corticosteroids [ICS]) for asthma is associated with an increased risk of asthma-related death. Available data from controlled clinical trials also suggest that use of LABAs as monotherapy increases the risk of asthma-related hospitalization in children and adolescents. These findings are considered a class effect of LABA monotherapy. When LABAs are used in fixed-dose combination with ICS, data from large clinical trials don't show a significant increase in the risk of serious asthma-related events (hospitalizations, intubations, death) compared with ICS alone.

🔔 **Alert:** Don't exceed recommended dosage; serious adverse events, including fatalities, have been associated with excessive use of inhaled sympathomimetics.

• Use cautiously in patients with existing TB; fungal, bacterial, viral, or parasitic infections; or ocular herpes simplex. Drug may suppress the immune system and infection may worsen.

• Use cautiously in patients with thyrotoxicosis, diabetes, ketoacidosis, or CV disorders (coronary insufficiency, arrhythmias, HTN).

• Use cautiously in patients with increased IOP, cataracts, or glaucoma. Increased IOP, glaucoma, and cataracts have occurred with prolonged use.

• Use cautiously in patients with seizure disorders; beta agonists may cause CNS stimulation.

Dialyzable drug: Unknown.

PREGNANCY-LACTATION-REPRODUCTION

• Use cautiously during pregnancy and breastfeeding.

• Avoid use during labor as drug may interfere with uterine contractility.

NURSING CONSIDERATIONS

• If not already prescribed, initiate an inhaled, short-acting beta$_2$ agonist in patients taking this drug.

• Patients who have been taking oral or inhaled short-acting beta$_2$ agonists on a regular basis (q.i.d.) should discontinue regular use of these drugs and use them only for relief of acute respiratory symptoms.

• Determine if patient has an allergy or intolerance to lactose; anaphylactic reactions have occurred in patients with severe milk protein allergies.

• Monitor short-acting beta$_2$ agonist rescue use. Increased use signals disease deterioration.

• Slowly wean patients requiring oral corticosteroids from systemic corticosteroid use after switch to an inhaler. Reduce daily prednisone dosage by 2.5 mg on a weekly basis during therapy with inhaled drug.

• Patients may require supplemental corticosteroid during times of stress when weaning from systemic corticosteroids.

• Monitor lung function and watch for COPD signs and symptoms and adrenal insufficiency (fatigue, lassitude, weakness, nausea, vomiting, hypotension).

• Discontinue drug slowly if hypercortisolism or adrenal suppression is suspected.

• Monitor patient periodically for candidal infections of the mouth. Have patient rinse mouth after inhalation without swallowing to help reduce the risk.

• Monitor patient for signs and symptoms of pneumonia.

• If paradoxical bronchospasm occurs, discontinue drug and institute alternative therapy.

• Monitor patient for increased IOP and for development or worsening of glaucoma or cataracts.

• Monitor patient for hypokalemia and hyperglycemia.

• Serious or even fatal courses of chickenpox or measles can occur in patients who are susceptible.

• Monitor patient for CV effects (tachycardia, HTN, supraventricular tachycardia, extrasystoles).

• Monitor patient for reduction in bone mineral density (BMD) initially and periodically with long-term use. Patients who use tobacco and those with prolonged immobilization, family history of osteoporosis, postmenopausal status, advanced age, poor nutrition, or long-term use of other drugs that can reduce BMD (anticonvulsants, oral corticosteroids) are at increased risk.

◑ *Alert:* Orally inhaled corticosteroids may slow growth rate when given to children and adolescents.

PATIENT TEACHING
• Teach patient to rinse mouth without swallowing after inhalation to help reduce the risk of candidal infections.
• Caution patient not to use drug for acute symptoms or asthma.
• Warn patient not to use drug with other LABAs.
• Instruct patient to immediately notify health care provider if adverse reactions occur, symptoms worsen, more inhalations than usual of rescue medication are needed, or a significant decrease in lung function occurs.
• Instruct patient not to discontinue drug without the guidance of health care provider.
• Advise patient to obtain regular eye exams.
• Caution patient to report pregnancy to health care provider as soon as possible.

fluticasone propionate (topical)
floo-TIK-a-sone

Therapeutic class: Corticosteroids
Pharmacologic class: Corticosteroids

AVAILABLE FORMS
Cream: 0.05%
Lotion: 0.05%
Ointment: 0.005%

INDICATIONS & DOSAGES
➤ **Inflammation and pruritus from dermatoses responsive to corticosteroids**
Adults: Apply a thin film of cream or ointment to affected area b.i.d.; rub in gently and completely.
Children age 3 months and older: Apply a thin film of cream to affected areas b.i.d. Rub in gently. Don't use for longer than 4 weeks.
➤ **Inflammation and pruritus from atopic dermatitis**
Adults and children age 3 months and older: Apply thin film of cream to affected areas once daily or b.i.d. Or, apply a thin film of lotion to affected areas once daily. Rub in gently. Don't use for longer than 4 weeks.

ADMINISTRATION
Topical
• Don't use drug with an occlusive dressing or in diaper area.
• Not for ophthalmic, oral, or intravaginal use.

ACTION
Is diffused across cell membranes to form complexes with cytoplasmic receptors. Shows anti-inflammatory, antipruritic, vasoconstrictive, and antiproliferative activity. Considered a medium-potency drug, according to vasoconstrictive properties.

Route	Onset	Peak	Duration
Topical	Rapid	Unknown	10 hr

Half-life: About 7.5 hours.

ADVERSE REACTIONS
CNS: finger numbness, light-headedness. **GI:** diarrhea, vomiting. **GU:** glycosuria. **Metabolic:** hyperglycemia. **Skin:** urticaria, burning, eczema, hypertrichosis, pruritus, irritation, erythema, hives, dryness, rash, stinging, telangiectasia. **Other:** *HPA-axis suppression,* Cushing syndrome.

INTERACTIONS
None significant.

EFFECTS ON LAB TEST RESULTS
• May increase glucose level.

CONTRAINDICATIONS & CAUTIONS
• Contraindicated in patients hypersensitive to drug or its components.
• Don't use as monotherapy in primary bacterial, viral, fungal, herpetic, or tubercular skin infections or for treatment of rosacea, perioral dermatitis, or acne.
• Drug isn't for ophthalmic use.
• Safety and effectiveness of ointment haven't been established in children. Safety and effectiveness of lotion and cream haven't been established in children younger than age 3 months.
Dialyzable drug: Unknown.
⚠ *Overdose S&S:* Systemic effects (including reversible HPA axis suppression, Cushing syndrome, hyperglycemia, glycosuria).

PREGNANCY-LACTATION-REPRODUCTION
• Use during pregnancy only if potential benefit justifies fetal risk.
• Use cautiously during breastfeeding.

Reactions in bold italics are *life-threatening*. Interactions may have a *rapid onset* or a *delayed onset*.

NURSING CONSIDERATIONS
- Don't mix drug with other bases or vehicles because doing so may affect potency.
- If adverse reactions occur, prescriber may order less potent drug.
- Stop drug if local irritation or systemic infection, absorption, or hypersensitivity occurs.
- May cause suppression of HPA axis in patients receiving high doses for prolonged periods, particularly in children.
- Absorption of corticosteroid is increased when drug is applied to inflamed or damaged skin, eyelids, or scrotal area; it's lowest when applied to intact normal skin, palms of hands, or soles of feet.
- *Look alike–sound alike:* Don't confuse fluticasone with fluconazole, fluocinolone, or fluocinonide.

PATIENT TEACHING
- Teach patient or family member how to apply drug using gloves, sterile applicator, or after careful hand washing.
- Tell patient to wash hands after application.
- Caution patient to avoid prolonged use and contact with eyes. Warn patient not to apply to face, in skin creases, or around eyes, genitals, underarms, or rectum.
- Instruct patient to notify prescriber of all adverse reactions, if condition persists or worsens, or if burning or irritation develops.

---

fluticasone propionate-salmeterol (inhalation)
floo-TIK-a-sone/sal-MEE-ter-ol

Advair Diskus 100/50, Advair Diskus 250/50, Advair Diskus 500/50, Advair HFA 45/21, Advair HFA 115/21, Advair HFA 230/21, Airduo RespiClick, Wixela Inhub

Therapeutic class: Antiasthmatics
Pharmacologic class: Corticosteroids–LABAs

AVAILABLE FORMS
Inhalation powder: 55 mcg fluticasone propionate and 14 mcg salmeterol, 100 mcg fluticasone propionate and 50 mcg salmeterol, 113 mcg fluticasone propionate and 14 mcg salmeterol, 232 mcg fluticasone propionate and 14 mcg salmeterol, 250 mcg fluticasone propionate and 50 mcg salmeterol, 500 mcg fluticasone propionate and 50 mcg salmeterol
Aerosol spray: 45 mcg fluticasone propionate and 21 mcg salmeterol, 115 mcg fluticasone propionate and 21 mcg salmeterol, 230 mcg fluticasone propionate and 21 mcg salmeterol

INDICATIONS & DOSAGES
➤ **Asthma in patients not adequately controlled on a long-term asthma control medication such as inhaled corticosteroid (ICS) or whose disease warrants initiation of treatment with both ICS and LABA**
Adults and children age 12 and older:
1 inhalation of Advair Diskus, Airduo RespiClick, or Wixela Inhub b.i.d., about 12 hours apart, or 2 inhalations of Advair HFA b.i.d. about 12 hours apart. Starting doses are dependent on patient's disease severity, based on previous asthma therapy (including ICS dosage), current control of asthma symptoms, and risk of future exacerbation. May increase dose after 2 weeks in patients who aren't adequately controlled. Maximum dose of Advair Diskus or Wixela Inhub is 1 inhalation of fluticasone 500 mcg and salmeterol 50 mcg b.i.d. Maximum dose of Advair HFA is 2 inhalations of fluticasone 230 mcg and salmeterol 21 mcg b.i.d.

Or, for patients not adequately controlled on a long-term asthma control medication such as ICS or whose disease warrants initiation of treatment with both ICS and LABA, base starting dose on patient's asthma severity; usual recommended starting dose for patients not on ICS is 55 mcg fluticasone/ 14 mcg salmeterol b.i.d. approximately 12 hours apart. For other patients, base starting dose on previous asthma drug therapy and disease severity.

For patients switching from another inhaled corticosteroid, base initial Airduo RespiClick dose strength on strength of previous ICS and disease severity. Highest recommended Airduo RespiClick dose is 232 mcg fluticasone/14 mcg salmeterol b.i.d.
Children ages 4 to 11 not controlled on ICS:
1 inhalation of Advair Diskus or Wixela Inhub fluticasone 100 mcg and salmeterol 50 mcg b.i.d. about 12 hours apart.
➤ **Maintenance therapy for airflow obstruction in patients with COPD; to reduce exacerbations of COPD in patients with a history of exacerbations**

Adults: 1 inhalation of Advair Diskus or Wixela Inhub 250/50 only b.i.d. about 12 hours apart.

ADMINISTRATION
Inhalational
• Prime Advair HFA before first use by releasing 4 test sprays into the air, away from the face, shaking well for 5 seconds before each spray. If inhaler hasn't been used for 4 weeks or has been dropped, prime inhaler again by shaking well before each spray and releasing 2 test sprays into the air.
• Discard Advair HFA canister when counter reads "000."
• Airduo RespiClick doesn't require priming. Never place inhaler in water; clean mouthpiece with dry cloth or tissue as needed.
• Must discard Advair Diskus and Wixela Inhub 1 month after removal from the foil pouch or when the counter reads "0."
• After administration, have patient rinse mouth without swallowing.

ACTION
Fluticasone is a synthetic corticosteroid with potent anti-inflammatory activity. Salmeterol, an LABA, relaxes bronchial smooth muscle and inhibits release of mediators.

Route	Onset	Peak	Duration
Inhalation (fluticasone)	Unknown	1–2 hr	Unknown
Inhalation (salmeterol)	Unknown	5 min	Unknown

Half-life: Fluticasone, 8 hours; salmeterol, 5.5 to 12.6 hours.

ADVERSE REACTIONS
CNS: headache, dizziness, migraine, sleep disorders, pain. **CV:** *arrhythmia, MI,* tachycardia, palpitations. **EENT:** eye redness, keratitis, congestion, nasal irritation, rhinorrhea, rhinitis, sinusitis, pharyngitis, dental discomfort and pain, decreased salivation, hoarseness or dysphonia, oral candidiasis, oral discomfort and pain, oral erythema and rashes, oral ulcerations, EENT infections. **GI:** abdominal pain and discomfort, diarrhea, gastroenteritis, nausea, unusual taste, vomiting. **Metabolic:** weight gain. **Musculoskeletal:** arthralgia, bone and cartilage disorders, musculoskeletal pain, muscle stiffness, rigidity, tightness. **Respiratory:** URI, bronchitis, cough, lower respiratory tract infection, pneumonia. **Skin:** dermatologic disorders (dermatosis, disorders of sweat and sebum),

dermatitis, eczema, contact dermatitis, pruritus, infection, skin flakiness. **Other:** allergic reactions, fluid retention, viral or bacterial infections.

INTERACTIONS
Drug-drug. *Beta blockers:* Blocked pulmonary effect of salmeterol may produce severe bronchospasm in patients with asthma. Avoid using together. If necessary, use a cardioselective beta blocker cautiously.
Ketoconazole, other inhibitors of CYP450: May increase fluticasone level and adverse effects. Use together cautiously.
Loop diuretics, thiazide diuretics: Potassium-wasting diuretics may cause or worsen ECG changes or hypokalemia. Use together cautiously.
MAO inhibitors, TCAs: May potentiate the action of salmeterol on the vascular system. Separate doses by 2 weeks.

EFFECTS ON LAB TEST RESULTS
• May increase liver enzyme levels.

CONTRAINDICATIONS & CAUTIONS
• Contraindicated in patients hypersensitive to drug or its components, as primary treatment of status asthmaticus or other acute episodes of asthma or COPD in which intensive measures are required, and in those with severe hypersensitivity to milk proteins.
• Use of LABA as monotherapy (without ICS) for asthma is associated with an increased risk of asthma-related death. Available data from controlled clinical trials also suggest that use of LABA as monotherapy increases the risk of asthma-related hospitalization in children and adolescents. These findings are considered a class effect of LABA monotherapy. When LABAs are used in fixed-dose combination with ICS, data from large clinical trials don't show a significant increase in the risk of serious asthma-related events (hospitalizations, intubations, death) compared with ICS alone.
🌓 *Alert:* Don't use drug for transferring patients from systemic corticosteroid therapy. Deaths from adrenal insufficiency have occurred in patients with asthma during and after transfer from systemic corticosteroids to less systemically available inhaled corticosteroids.
• Use cautiously, if at all, in patients with active or quiescent respiratory TB infection;

Reactions in bold italics are *life-threatening*. Interactions may have a *rapid onset* or a *delayed onset*.

untreated systemic fungal, bacterial, viral, or parasitic infection; or ocular herpes simplex.
• Use cautiously in patients with CV disorders, seizure disorders, diabetes, or thyrotoxicosis; in patients unusually responsive to sympathomimetic amines; and in patients with hepatic impairment.
• Glaucoma, increased IOP, and cataracts have been reported in patients with asthma and COPD after long-term ICS use. Consider referral to an ophthalmologist in patients who develop ocular symptoms or use drug long term.
Dialyzable drug: Unknown.
⚠ *Overdose S&S:* Hypercorticism, angina, arrhythmias, dizziness, dry mouth, fatigue, headache, HTN, hypotension, insomnia, malaise, muscle cramps, nausea, nervousness, palpitations, seizures, tachycardia, prolonged QTc interval, hypokalemia, hyperglycemia, cardiac arrest, death.

PREGNANCY-LACTATION-REPRODUCTION
• Use during pregnancy only if potential benefit justifies fetal risk.
• Avoid use during labor as drug can interfere with uterine contractility.
• Use cautiously during breastfeeding.

NURSING CONSIDERATIONS
🕒 *Alert:* Patient shouldn't be switched from systemic corticosteroids to Advair Diskus or Advair HFA because of HPA axis suppression. Death from adrenal insufficiency can occur. Several months are required for recovery of HPA function after withdrawal of systemic corticosteroids.
• Don't start therapy during rapidly deteriorating or potentially life-threatening episodes of asthma. Serious acute respiratory events, including fatality, can occur.
• Periodically reevaluate patient with COPD to assess for benefits or risks of therapy.
• Monitor patient for urticaria, angioedema, rash, bronchospasm, or other signs of hypersensitivity.
• Don't use this drug to stop an asthma attack. Patients should carry an inhaled, short-acting beta$_2$ agonist (such as albuterol) for acute symptoms.
• If drug causes paradoxical bronchospasm, treat immediately with a short-acting inhaled bronchodilator (such as albuterol), and notify prescriber.
• Monitor patient for increased use of inhaled short-acting beta$_2$ agonist. Dose of

fluticasone and salmeterol may need to be increased.
• Closely monitor children for growth suppression.

PATIENT TEACHING
• Instruct patient on proper use of the prescribed inhaler to provide effective treatment and on handling and storage. Remind patient to read and follow instructions for use.
• Tell patient to avoid exhaling into the dry-powder multidose inhaler; to activate and use the dry-powder multidose inhaler in a level, horizontal position; and not to use Advair Diskus or Wixela Inhub with a spacer device.
• Instruct patient to rinse mouth after inhalation to prevent oral candidiasis.
• Instruct patient to discard Airduo RespiClick inhaler 30 days after opening the foil pouch or when the counter reads "0," whichever comes first (device isn't reusable).
• Inform patient that improvement may occur within 30 minutes after dose, but the full benefit may not occur for 1 week or more.
• Advise patient not to exceed recommended prescribed dose.
• Warn patient not to relieve acute symptoms with drug. Treat acute symptoms with an inhaled short-acting beta$_2$ agonist.
• Instruct patient to report decreasing effects or use of increasing doses of the inhaled short-acting beta$_2$ agonist.
• Tell patient to report all adverse reactions, especially palpitations, chest pain, rapid HR, tremor, or nervousness.
• Instruct patient to call prescriber immediately if exposed to chickenpox or measles.

fluvastatin sodium 🅇
flue-va-STA-tin

Lescol XL

Therapeutic class: Antilipemics
Pharmacologic class: HMG-CoA reductase inhibitors

AVAILABLE FORMS
Capsules 🆗: 20 mg, 40 mg
Tablets (extended-release) 🆗: 80 mg

INDICATIONS & DOSAGES
➤ **To reduce LDL cholesterol (LDL-C) and total cholesterol levels in patients with**

primary hypercholesterolemia (types IIa and IIb); to slow progression of coronary atherosclerosis in patients with CAD; to reduce elevated triglyceride and apolipoprotein B (apo B) levels in patients with primary hypercholesterolemia and mixed dyslipidemia whose response to dietary restriction and other nonpharmacologic measures has been inadequate

Adults: Initially, 20 to 40 mg PO at bedtime, increasing if needed to maximum of 80 mg daily in divided doses or 80 mg extended-release tablet PO at bedtime for patients requiring LDL-C reduction to a goal of at least 25%, or 20 mg daily for patients requiring LDL-C reduction to a goal of less than 25%.

➤ **Adjunct to diet to reduce LDL-C, total cholesterol, and apo B levels in children with heterozygous familial hypercholesterolemia whose response to dietary restriction hasn't been adequate and for whom the following findings are present: LDL-C remains at 190 mg/dL or more, or LDL-C remains at 160 mg/dL or more and there's a positive family history of premature CV disease or two or more other CV disease risk factors are present** 🔲

Adolescent boys and girls (who are at least 1 year postmenarche) ages 10 to 16: 20 mg PO once daily at bedtime. Dosage adjustments may be made at 6-week intervals up to maximum of 40 mg (capsule) PO b.i.d. or 80 mg extended-release tablet PO once daily.

➤ **To reduce risk of undergoing coronary revascularization procedures and slow progression of coronary atherosclerosis**

Adults: In patients who must reduce LDL-C level by at least 25%, initially 40 mg PO once daily or b.i.d.; or one 80-mg extended-release tablet as a single dose at any time of the day. In patients who must reduce LDL-C level by less than 25%, initially 20 mg PO daily. Dosages range from 20 to 80 mg daily.

ADMINISTRATION
PO
- Give drug without regard for meals.
- For once-daily dosage, give immediate-release capsules in the evening.
- Don't crush or break tablets; don't open or crush capsules.
- Administer extended-release tablet as a single dose at any time of the day.
- Don't give two 40-mg capsules at one time.

ACTION
Inhibits HMG-CoA reductase, an early (and rate-limiting) step in the cholesterol synthesis pathway.

Route	Onset	Peak	Duration
PO	Unknown	1 hr	Unknown

Half-life: About 3 hours.

ADVERSE REACTIONS
CNS: dizziness, fatigue, headache, insomnia. **CV:** HTN, edema. **EENT:** pharyngitis, rhinitis, sinusitis, tooth disorder. **GI:** abdominal pain, constipation, diarrhea, dyspepsia, flatulence, nausea, vomiting. **GU:** UTI. **Hematologic:** *leukopenia, thrombocytopenia,* hemolytic anemia. **Musculoskeletal:** *rhabdomyolysis,* arthralgia, back pain, myalgia, arthropathy, extremity pain. **Respiratory:** URI, bronchitis, cough. **Other:** hypersensitivity reactions, accidental trauma, flulike illness.

INTERACTIONS
Drug-drug. *Cholestyramine, colestipol:* May bind with fluvastatin in the GI tract and decrease absorption. Separate doses by at least 4 hours.

Cimetidine, omeprazole, ranitidine: May decrease fluvastatin metabolism. Monitor patient for enhanced effects.

Cyclosporine and other immunosuppressants, colchicine, erythromycin, niacin: May increase risk of polymyositis and rhabdomyolysis. Avoid using together. Don't exceed 20 mg b.i.d. in patients taking cyclosporine.

Digoxin: May alter digoxin pharmacokinetics. Monitor digoxin level carefully.

Erythromycin, nicotinic acid: May increase risk of myopathy and rhabdomyolysis. Don't use together.

Fibric acids (fenofibrate, gemfibrozil): May cause severe myopathy or rhabdomyolysis. If coadministration can't be avoided, monitor CK closely.

Fluconazole, itraconazole, ketoconazole: May increase fluvastatin level and adverse effects. Use cautiously together or, if given together, reduce dose of fluvastatin. Don't exceed 20 mg b.i.d. in patients taking fluconazole.

Glyburide: May increase levels of both drugs. Monitor serum glucose and signs and symptoms of toxicity.

Phenytoin: May increase phenytoin levels. Monitor phenytoin levels.

Reactions in bold italics are *life-threatening*. Interactions may have a *rapid onset* or a ***delayed onset***.

Protease inhibitors (atazanavir, darunavir, fosamprenavir, nelfinavir, ritonavir, saquinavir, tipranavir): May increase fluvastatin level and risk of myopathy and rhabdomyolysis. Use together cautiously.

Rifampin: May enhance fluvastatin metabolism and decrease levels. Monitor patient for lack of effect.

Warfarin: May increase anticoagulant effect with bleeding. Monitor PT and INR.

Drug-herb. *Eucalyptus, jin bu huan, kava:* May increase risk of hepatotoxicity. Discourage use together.

Red yeast rice: May increase risk of adverse reactions because herb contains compounds similar to those in drug. Discourage use together.

Drug-lifestyle. *Alcohol use:* May increase risk of hepatotoxicity. Discourage use together.

EFFECTS ON LAB TEST RESULTS
- May increase ALT, AST, HbA_{1c}, fasting glucose, and CK levels.
- May decrease Hb level, hematocrit, and platelet and WBC counts.

CONTRAINDICATIONS & CAUTIONS
- Contraindicated in patients hypersensitive to drug and in those with active liver disease or unexplained persistent elevations of transaminase levels.
- Drug may cause rhabdomyolysis in patients with renal function impairment.
- Temporarily withhold drug in patient experiencing an acute or serious condition predisposing to development of renal failure secondary to rhabdomyolysis (sepsis; hypotension; major surgery; trauma; severe metabolic, endocrine, or electrolyte disorder; uncontrolled epilepsy).
- Use cautiously in patients with severe renal impairment or history of liver disease or heavy alcohol use, in those with inadequately treated hypothyroidism, and in patients age 65 or older.

Dialyzable drug: Unknown.

⚠ *Overdose S&S:* GI complaints, elevated AST and ALT levels.

PREGNANCY-LACTATION-REPRODUCTION
- Use contraindicated in pregnancy for most patients and during breastfeeding.
- The FDA has determined that statin use in patients at high risk for CV events during pregnancy (such as established CV disease) may be considered on an individual basis.

NURSING CONSIDERATIONS
- Patient should follow a diet restricted in saturated fat and cholesterol during therapy.
- Exercise caution when giving to patients with a history of liver disease or heavy alcohol ingestion. Closely monitor these patients.
- Perform LFTs before initiating therapy and if signs and symptoms of liver injury occur.
- Monitor lipid levels before starting therapy, at 4 weeks, at times of dosage changes, and periodically thereafter.
- Watch for signs and symptoms of myopathy. Monitor patient for muscle pain or weakness with malaise and fever. Discontinue drug for markedly elevated CK levels or if myopathy is suspected or confirmed.
- *Look alike–sound alike:* Don't confuse fluvastatin with fluoxetine.

PATIENT TEACHING
- Teach patient safe drug administration.
- Advise patient who is also taking a bile acid sequestrant such as cholestyramine to take fluvastatin at bedtime, at least 4 hours after taking the sequestrant.
- Teach patient about proper dietary management, weight control, and exercise. Explain their importance in controlling elevated cholesterol and triglyceride levels.
- Warn patient to avoid alcohol.
- Tell patient to notify prescriber of adverse reactions, especially muscle aches and pains.
- Advise patient that it may take up to 4 weeks for the drug to be completely effective.
- ⚠ *Alert:* Tell patient of childbearing potential to stop drug and immediately report pregnancy.

fluvoxaMINE maleate
floo-VOX-a-meen

Therapeutic class: Antidepressants
Pharmacologic class: SSRIs

AVAILABLE FORMS
Capsules (extended-release) ⓝ: 100 mg, 150 mg
Tablets: 25 mg, 50 mg, 100 mg

INDICATIONS & DOSAGES

Adjust-a-dose (for all indications): In older adults and patients with hepatic impairment, give lower first dose and adjust dose more slowly. When using extended-release capsules, titrate dosage more slowly after initial 100-mg dose.

➤ **OCD**

Adults: Initially, 50 mg (tablet) PO daily at bedtime; increase by 50 mg every 4 to 7 days. Maximum, 300 mg daily. Give total daily amounts above 100 mg in two divided doses. Or, 100-mg extended-release capsule PO once per day as a single daily dose at bedtime. Increase in 50-mg increments every week, as tolerated, until maximum therapeutic benefit is achieved. Maximum dose is 300 mg/day.

Children ages 8 to 17: Initially, 25 mg PO daily at bedtime; increase by 25 mg every 4 to 7 days. Maximum, 200 mg daily for children ages 8 to 11 and 300 mg daily for children ages 12 to 17. Give total daily amounts over 50 mg in two divided doses.

ADMINISTRATION

PO

- Give drug without regard for food.
- Capsules shouldn't be crushed or chewed.
- Give extended-release capsules at bedtime.
- Store at 77° F (25° C). Avoid exposure to temperatures above 86° F (30° C); protect from high humidity and light.

ACTION

Unknown. Selectively inhibits the presynaptic neuronal uptake of serotonin, which may improve OCD.

Route	Onset	Peak	Duration
PO (capsules)	Unknown	Unknown	Unknown
PO (tablets)	Unknown	3–8 hr	Unknown

Half-life: 14 to 16 hours.

ADVERSE REACTIONS

CNS: agitation, apathy, headache, malaise, asthenia, somnolence, insomnia, nervousness, pain, dizziness, tremor, anxiety, hypertonia, depression, psychoneurosis, twitching, amnesia, CNS stimulation, hyperkinesia, hypokinesia, abnormal dreams, abnormal thinking, paresthesia, yawning, taste perversion, manic reaction, myoclonus, syncope, weakness. **CV:** palpitations, chest pain, HTN, edema, hypotension, vasodilation. **EENT:** amblyopia, epistaxis, pharyngitis, laryngitis, tooth disorder, dry mouth. **GI:** nausea, diarrhea, constipation, dyspepsia, vomiting, anorexia, flatulence, dysphagia. **GU:** abnormal ejaculation, urinary frequency, polyuria, erectile dysfunction, anorgasmia, UTI, urine retention, dysmenorrhea, decreased libido. **Hepatic:** abnormal LFT values. **Metabolic:** weight gain or loss. **Musculoskeletal:** myalgia. **Respiratory:** URI, dyspnea, cough, bronchitis. **Skin:** diaphoresis, acne, ecchymoses. **Other:** flulike syndrome, viral infection, chills.

INTERACTIONS

⊕ *Alert:* Fluvoxamine can significantly interact with many drugs. Consult a drug interaction resource or pharmacist for additional information.

Drug-drug. *Alosetron (other 5-HT$_3$ inhibitors), pimozide, thioridazine:* May prolong QTc interval. Use together is contraindicated.

Benzodiazepines (alprazolam, diazepam, midazolam, triazolam): May reduce clearance of these drugs. Use together cautiously (except for diazepam, which shouldn't be used with fluvoxamine). Adjust benzodiazepine dosage as needed. Initial alprazolam dosage should be at least halved; titration to the lowest effective dosage is recommended.

Carbamazepine, clozapine, methadone, metoprolol, propranolol, tacrine, TCAs, theophylline: May increase levels of these drugs. Use together cautiously, and monitor patient closely for adverse reactions. Dosage adjustments may be needed.

Diltiazem: May cause bradycardia. Monitor HR.

Linezolid, methylene blue: May cause serotonin syndrome. Don't start drug in patients receiving linezolid or methylene blue.

MAO inhibitors (phenelzine, selegiline, tranylcypromine): May increase risk of serotonin syndrome. Concomitant use is contraindicated. Avoid using within 2 weeks of MAO inhibitor.

Mexiletine: May increase mexiletine level. Monitor level.

Ramelteon: May increase ramelteon concentration. Avoid concomitant use.

Serotonergic drugs (amphetamines, buspirone, fentanyl, lithium, TCAs, tramadol, triptans, tryptophan): May increase risk of serotonin syndrome. Avoid use together.

Reactions in bold italics are *life-threatening*. Interactions may have a *rapid onset* or a ***delayed onset***.

Monitor patient closely if use can't be avoided.

Tizanidine: May significantly increase drowsiness and impair psychomotor skills. Use together is contraindicated.

Warfarin, other drugs that interfere with hemostasis (aspirin, NSAIDs): May increase levels of these drugs and the risk of bleeding and prolong PT. Monitor INR and adjust anticoagulant dosage accordingly.

Drug-herb. *Alfalfa, anise, bilberry:* May increase antiplatelet activity. Avoid use together.

Kava kava, SAM-e, St. John's wort, tryptophan, valerian: May increase sedative-hypnotic effects and risk of serotonin syndrome. Avoid use together.

Melatonin: May increase melatonin bioavailability. Avoid use together.

Drug-lifestyle. *Alcohol use:* May increase CNS effects. Discourage use together.

Smoking: May decrease drug's effectiveness. Urge patient to stop smoking.

EFFECTS ON LAB TEST RESULTS
None reported.

CONTRAINDICATIONS & CAUTIONS
• Contraindicated in patients hypersensitive to drug or to other phenyl piperazine antidepressants; in those receiving pimozide, alosetron, tizanidine, ramelteon, or thioridazine therapy; and within 2 weeks of MAO inhibitor.

⚠ *Alert:* Concomitant use with linezolid or methylene blue can cause serotonin syndrome (fever, mental status changes, muscle twitching, diaphoresis, shivering or shaking, diarrhea, loss of coordination). Use drug with linezolid or methylene blue only for life-threatening or urgent conditions when the potential benefits outweigh the risks of toxicity.

• Use cautiously in patients with hepatic dysfunction, other conditions that may affect hemodynamic responses or metabolism, or history of mania or seizures.

Boxed Warning Fluvoxamine tablets aren't approved for use in children, except for those with OCD. Fluvoxamine extended-release capsules shouldn't be used in children. ∎

• Use cautiously in patients with CV disease. Fluvoxamine hasn't been systemically evaluated in patients with a recent history of MI or unstable heart disease.

• Bone fractures have been associated with antidepressant use. Consider the possibility of a fragility fracture if patient treated with an antidepressant presents with unexplained bone pain, point tenderness, swelling, or bruising.

Dialyzable drug: Unlikely.

⚠ *Overdose S&S:* Nausea, vomiting, diarrhea, coma, hypokalemia, hypotension, respiratory difficulties, somnolence, tachycardia, ECG abnormalities, seizures, dizziness, liver function disturbances, tremor, increased reflexes, unsteady gait, hypoxic encephalopathy.

PREGNANCY-LACTATION-REPRODUCTION
• Neonates exposed to drug late in third trimester have developed complications requiring prolonged hospitalization, respiratory support, and tube feeding. Neonates exposed to SSRIs in late pregnancy may have an increased risk of persistent pulmonary HTN of the newborn, which is associated with substantial neonatal morbidity and mortality. Carefully consider risks and benefits of treatment on a case-by-case basis.

• Register patients in the National Pregnancy Registry for Antidepressants at 1-866-961-2388 or https://womensmentalhealth.org/research/pregnancyregistry/antidepressants/.

• Drug appears in human milk. Patient should discontinue breastfeeding or discontinue drug.

NURSING CONSIDERATIONS
Boxed Warning Drug may increase risk of suicidality in young adults ages 18 to 24, especially during first few months of treatment. Monitor all patients closely for clinical worsening. ∎

• Record mood changes. Monitor patient for suicidality.

⚠ *Alert:* Combining an SSRI with a triptan may cause serotonin syndrome or NMS-like reactions. Serotonin syndrome is more likely to occur when starting or increasing the triptan dose.

⚠ *Alert:* If linezolid or methylene blue must be given, fluvoxamine must be stopped and patient should be monitored for serotonin toxicity for 2 weeks or until 24 hours after final dose of linezolid or methylene blue, whichever comes first. Treatment with fluvoxamine may be resumed 24 hours after final dose of linezolid or methylene blue.

• Patients shouldn't stop drug without first consulting prescriber; abruptly stopping drug may cause withdrawal syndrome, including headache, muscle ache, and flulike symptoms.

• Consider age and gender differences when determining dosages in children and women; therapeutic effect in women may be achieved with lower doses.

• *Look alike–sound alike:* Don't confuse fluvoxamine with fluoxetine.

PATIENT TEACHING
Boxed Warning Advise families and caregivers to closely observe patient for increased suicidality. ■

• Teach patient safe drug administration and handling.

• Caution patient to avoid alcohol.

🌙 *Alert:* Teach patient to recognize and immediately report signs and symptoms of serotonin toxicity (fever, mental status changes, muscle twitching, rigidity, hyperflexes, labile BP, increased HR, diaphoresis, shivering or shaking, nausea, vomiting, diarrhea, loss of coordination).

• Warn patient to avoid hazardous activities until CNS effects of drug are known.

• Advise patient to notify prescriber about planned, suspected, or known pregnancy.

• Tell patient who develops a rash, hives, or a related allergic reaction to notify prescriber.

• Inform patient that drug may cause sexual dysfunction and to discuss changes and management with health care provider.

• Inform patient that several weeks of therapy may be needed to obtain full therapeutic effect. Once improvement occurs, advise patient not to stop drug until directed by prescriber.

• Suggest that patient keep a diary of changes in mood or behavior. Tell patient to report suicidality immediately.

• Advise patient to check with prescriber before taking OTC medications, supplements, or other prescription drugs; drug interactions can occur.

fondaparinux sodium
fon-da-PAR-i-nuks

Arixtra

Therapeutic class: Anticoagulants
Pharmacologic class: Activated factor X inhibitors

AVAILABLE FORMS
Injection: 2.5 mg/0.5 mL, 5 mg/0.4 mL, 7.5 mg/0.6 mL, 10 mg/0.8 mL in single-dose, prefilled syringe

INDICATIONS & DOSAGES
➤ **To prevent DVT, which may lead to PE, in patients undergoing surgery for hip fracture, hip replacement, knee replacement, or abdominal surgery**
Adults weighing 50 kg or more: 2.5 mg subcut once daily for 5 to 9 days. Give first dose after hemostasis is established, 6 to 8 hours after surgery. Giving the dose earlier than 6 hours after surgery increases the risk of major bleeding. Patients undergoing hip fracture surgery should receive an extended prophylaxis course of up to 24 additional days.
➤ **Acute DVT (with warfarin); acute PE (with warfarin) when treatment is started in the hospital**
Adults weighing more than 100 kg: 10 mg subcut daily for 5 to 9 days and until INR is 2 to 3. Begin warfarin therapy as soon as possible, usually within 72 hours.
Adults weighing 50 to 100 kg: 7.5 mg subcut daily for 5 to 9 days and until INR is 2 to 3. Begin warfarin therapy as soon as possible, usually within 72 hours.
Adults weighing less than 50 kg: 5 mg subcut daily for 5 to 9 days and until INR is 2 to 3. Begin warfarin therapy as soon as possible, usually within 72 hours.
➤ **Acute symptomatic superficial vein thrombosis (at least 5 cm in length) of the legs ♦**
Adults: 2.5 mg subcut once daily for 45 days.
➤ **ACS (non-ST-elevation ACS [NSTE-ACS] or ST-elevation MI [STEMI]) ♦**
Adults: For NSTE-ACS, 2.5 mg subcut once daily for duration of hospitalization or until PCI is done. For STEMI, 2.5 mg IV once, then 2.5 mg subcut once daily starting the following day; treat for duration of

---

hospitalization, up to 8 days, or until revascularization.

ADMINISTRATION
Subcutaneous
• Give subcut only, never IM. Inspect the single-dose, prefilled syringe for particulate matter and discoloration before giving.
⚠ *Alert:* To avoid loss of drug, don't expel air bubble from the syringe.
• Give drug in fatty tissue of the lower abdomen, rotating injection sites. If drug has been properly injected, the needle will pull back into the syringe security sleeve and the white safety indicator will appear above the blue upper body. A soft click may be heard or felt when the syringe plunger is fully released. After injection of the syringe contents, the plunger automatically rises while the needle withdraws from the skin and retracts into the security sleeve. Don't recap the needle.

ACTION
Binds to antithrombin III (AT-III) and potentiates the neutralization of factor Xa by AT-III, which interrupts coagulation and inhibits formation of thrombin and blood clots.

Route	Onset	Peak	Duration
Subcut	Unknown	2–3 hr	Unknown

Half-life: 17 to 21 hours.

ADVERSE REACTIONS
CNS: insomnia, dizziness, confusion. **CV:** hypotension. **EENT:** epistaxis. **Hematologic: hemorrhage,** anemia, hematoma, *postoperative hemorrhage, thrombocytopenia.* **Hepatic:** increased AST and ALT levels. **Metabolic:** *hypokalemia.* **Skin:** mild local irritation (injection-site bleeding, rash, pruritus), bullous eruption, purpura, rash, increased wound drainage and infection.

INTERACTIONS
Drug-drug. *Drugs that increase risk of bleeding (anticoagulants, NSAIDs, platelet inhibitors):* May increase risk of hemorrhage. Stop these drugs before starting fondaparinux. If use together is unavoidable, monitor patient closely.
Drug-herb. *Angelica (dong quai), ginkgo, ginseng, willow:* May increase risk of bleeding. Discourage use together.

EFFECTS ON LAB TEST RESULTS
• May increase AST, ALT, and bilirubin levels.
• May decrease potassium level.
• May decrease Hb level, hematocrit, and platelet count.

CONTRAINDICATIONS & CAUTIONS
• Contraindicated in patients with CrCl of less than 30 mL/minute and for venous thromboembolism prophylaxis in patients weighing less than 50 kg who are undergoing hip fracture, hip replacement, knee replacement, or abdominal surgery.
• Contraindicated in patients with history of serious hypersensitivity reaction (angioedema, anaphylactoid, or anaphylactic reactions) to fondaparinux.
• Contraindicated in patients with active major bleeding, bacterial endocarditis, or thrombocytopenia with a positive test result for antiplatelet antibody after taking fondaparinux.
• Use cautiously in patients being treated with platelet inhibitors; in those at increased risk for bleeding, such as those with congenital or acquired bleeding disorders; in those with active ulcerative and angiodysplastic GI disease; in those with hemorrhagic stroke; and in patients shortly after brain, spinal, or ophthalmologic surgery.
• Use cautiously in older adults, in patients with CrCl of 30 to 50 mL/minute, and in those with a history of heparin-induced thrombocytopenia, a bleeding diathesis, uncontrolled arterial HTN, or a history of recent GI ulceration, diabetic retinopathy, or hemorrhage.
⚠ *Alert:* Use cautiously in patients who are latex-sensitive; the packaging (needle guard) contains dry natural rubber.
• Safety and effectiveness in children haven't been established.
Dializable drug: Yes.
⚠ *Overdose S&S:* Hemorrhagic complications.

PREGNANCY-LACTATION-REPRODUCTION
• Use cautiously during pregnancy and only if benefit justifies fetal risk.
• It isn't known if drug appears in human milk. Use cautiously during breastfeeding.

NURSING CONSIDERATIONS

• Don't use interchangeably with heparin, low–molecular-weight heparins, or heparinoids.

Boxed Warning Patients who receive epidural or spinal anesthesia, epidural catheters, or spinal puncture or have a history of spine deformity or surgery are at increased risk for developing an epidural or spinal hematoma, which may result in long-term or permanent paralysis. Other factors that increase risk include concurrent use of NSAIDs, platelet inhibitors, and other anticoagulants; use of indwelling epidural catheters; and history of traumatic or repeated epidural or spinal surgery. Monitor these patients closely for neurologic impairment, and treat urgently. Consider the risk before neuraxial intervention in patients anticoagulated or to be anticoagulated for thromboprophylaxis. ■

• Monitor renal function periodically, and stop drug in patients who develop unstable renal function or severe renal impairment while receiving therapy.

• Routinely assess patient for signs and symptoms of bleeding, and regularly monitor CBC, platelet count, creatinine level, and stool occult blood test results. Stop use if platelet count is less than $100,000/mm^3$.

• Anticoagulant effects may last for 2 to 4 days after stopping drug in patients with normal renal function.

• PT and PTT aren't suitable monitoring tests to measure drug activity. If coagulation parameters change unexpectedly or patient develops major bleeding, stop drug.

• Drug has been given safely for up to 26 days in clinical trials of DVT and PE treatment.

• Refer to label and local protocol for additional details for transitioning between anticoagulants.

PATIENT TEACHING

• Tell patient to report all adverse reactions, especially signs and symptoms of bleeding or neurologic impairment.

• Instruct patient to avoid OTC products that contain aspirin or other salicylates.

• Advise patient to consult with prescriber before starting herbal therapy; many herbs have anticoagulant, antiplatelet, or fibrinolytic properties.

• Teach patient the correct technique for subcut use, if needed.

formoterol fumarate
for-MOH-te-rol

Perforomist

Therapeutic class: Bronchodilators
Pharmacologic class: Selective beta$_2$-adrenergic agonists

AVAILABLE FORMS
Inhalation solution: 20 mcg/2 mL vial

INDICATIONS & DOSAGES
➤ **Maintenance treatment of bronchoconstriction in patients with COPD (chronic bronchitis, emphysema)**
Adults: 20 mcg by oral inhalation through a jet nebulizer every 12 hours. Maximum dose, 40 mcg/day.

ADMINISTRATION
Inhalational
• Give inhalational solution through a standard jet nebulizer connected to an air compressor.

• Solution doesn't require dilution before giving; don't mix other medications with formoterol solution.

• Patient should breathe deeply and evenly until all medication has been inhaled, about 9 minutes.

• Store in foil pouch and remove immediately before use. Drug is colorless; discard drug if solution isn't colorless.

• Clean nebulizer after use.

ACTION
Long-acting selective beta$_2$ agonist that causes bronchodilation. It ultimately increases cAMP, leading to relaxation of bronchial smooth muscle and inhibition of mediator release from mast cells.

Route	Onset	Peak	Duration
Inhalation solution	12 min	1–3 hr	12 hr

Half-life: 7 hours.

ADVERSE REACTIONS
CNS: tremor, dizziness, insomnia, nervousness, headache, fatigue, malaise, anxiety. **CV:** *arrhythmias*, chest pain, angina, HTN, hypotension, tachycardia, palpitations. **EENT:** nasopharyngitis, sinusitis, dysphonia, dry mouth, tonsillitis. **GI:** nausea, vomiting,

---

Reactions in bold italics are *life-threatening*. Interactions may have a *rapid onset* or a *delayed onset*.

diarrhea. **Metabolic:** *metabolic acidosis, hypokalemia,* hyperglycemia. **Musculoskeletal:** muscle cramps. **Respiratory:** bronchitis, respiratory tract infection, dyspnea. **Skin:** rash, pruritus. **Other:** viral infection.

INTERACTIONS

Drug-drug. *Adrenergics:* May potentiate sympathetic effects of formoterol. Use together cautiously.

Beta blockers: May antagonize effects of each other, causing bronchospasm in patients with COPD. Avoid use except when benefit outweighs risks. Use cardioselective beta blockers with caution to minimize risk of bronchospasm.

Diuretics, steroids, xanthine derivatives: May increase hypokalemic effect of formoterol. Use together cautiously.

MAO inhibitors, TCAs, other drugs that prolong QT interval: May increase risk of ventricular arrhythmias. Use together cautiously.

Non–potassium-sparing diuretics, such as loop or thiazide diuretics: May worsen ECG changes or hypokalemia. Use together cautiously, and monitor patient for toxicity.

EFFECTS ON LAB TEST RESULTS

- May increase glucose level.
- May decrease potassium level.

CONTRAINDICATIONS & CAUTIONS

- Contraindicated in patients hypersensitive to drug or its components, or with other LABAs.
- Use of a LABA without an inhaled corticosteroid is contraindicated in patients with asthma. Drug isn't indicated for the treatment of asthma.
- Use of a LABA as monotherapy for asthma is associated with an increased risk of asthma-related hospitalizations and death.
- Don't begin drug in patients with acutely deteriorating COPD, which may be life-threatening.
- Don't use drug to relieve acute symptoms (such as rescue therapy for acute episodes of bronchospasm). Treat acute symptoms with an inhaled short-acting beta$_2$ agonist.
- Use cautiously in patients with CV disease, especially coronary insufficiency, cardiac arrhythmias, and HTN, and in those who are unusually responsive to sympathomimetic amines.

- Use cautiously in patients with diabetes because hyperglycemia and ketoacidosis have occurred rarely with the use of beta agonists.
- Use cautiously in patients with seizure disorders or thyrotoxicosis.
- Safety and effectiveness in children haven't been established.

Dialyzable drug: Unknown.

⚠ *Overdose S&S:* Exaggeration of adverse reactions, hypotension, cardiac arrest.

PREGNANCY-LACTATION-REPRODUCTION

- Use cautiously during pregnancy and only if benefit outweighs fetal risk.
- Drug may interfere with uterine contractility if used during labor; use only if clearly needed.
- Use cautiously during breastfeeding.

NURSING CONSIDERATIONS

⚡ *Alert:* If maintenance regimen fails to provide usual response, contact prescriber immediately, as this indicates COPD destabilization.

⚡ *Alert:* As with all beta$_2$ agonists, drug may produce life-threatening paradoxical bronchospasm. If bronchospasm occurs, treat immediately and notify prescriber promptly.

⚡ *Alert:* If patient develops tachycardia, HTN, or other adverse CV effects, drug may need to be stopped.

- Watch for immediate hypersensitivity reactions, such as anaphylaxis, urticaria, angioedema, rash, and bronchospasm.

PATIENT TEACHING

- Tell patient not to increase dosage or frequency of use without medical advice and to only use drug with a nebulizer.
- Show patient how to use nebulizer according to manufacturer's instructions.
- Advise patient who misses a dose to skip that dose and take the next dose at the usual time.
- Caution patient that drug isn't to be used for acute asthmatic episodes. Prescriber should give a short-acting beta$_2$ agonist for this use.
- Advise patient to immediately report worsening symptoms, treatment that becomes less effective, or increased use of short-acting beta$_2$ agonists.
- Tell patient to report nausea, vomiting, shakiness, headache, fast or irregular heartbeat, or sleeplessness.
- Advise patient to notify prescriber of pregnancy or breastfeeding.

foscarnet sodium (PFA, phosphonoformic acid)
foss-CAR-net

Foscavir

Therapeutic class: Antivirals
Pharmacologic class: Pyrophosphate analogues

AVAILABLE FORMS
Injection: 24 mg/mL

INDICATIONS & DOSAGES
Adjust-a-dose (for all indications): Adjust dosage when CrCl is less than 1.4 mL/minute/kg. If CrCl falls below 0.4 mL/minute/kg, stop drug. Consult manufacturer's package insert for specific dosage adjustments.

Boxed Warning Drug is only indicated for use in patients who are immunocompromised with CMV retinitis and mucocutaneous acyclovir-resistant HSV infections. ■

➤ **CMV retinitis in patients with AIDS**
Adults: Initially, for induction, 60 mg/kg IV over a minimum of 1 hour every 8 hours or 90 mg/kg IV over 1½ to 2 hours every 12 hours for 2 to 3 weeks, depending on patient response. Follow with a maintenance infusion of 90 to 120 mg/kg over 2 hours daily. Maximum dosage, 180 mg/kg/day (initial dosage) and 120 mg/kg/day (maintenance dosage).

➤ **Acyclovir-resistant HSV infections**
Adults: 40 mg/kg IV over 1 hour every 8 to 12 hours for 2 to 3 weeks or until healed. Maximum dosage, 120 mg/kg/day.

ADMINISTRATION
IV

Boxed Warning To minimize renal toxicity, make sure patient is adequately hydrated before and during infusion. ■

▼ Don't exceed the recommended dosage, rate, or frequency of infusion. Doses must be individualized according to patient's renal function.

▼ Drug may be infused via a central or peripheral vein with enough blood flow for rapid distribution and dilution. If infusing into a central vein, don't dilute the commercially available form (24 mg/mL). If infusing into a peripheral vein, dilute to 12 mg/mL with D_5W or NSS to decrease risk of local irritation. Use an infusion pump. Use diluted solutions within 24 hours.

▼ Give induction treatment over 1 to 2 hours, depending on dose, and maintenance infusions over 2 hours and at no more than 1 mg/kg/minute.

▼ **Incompatibilities:** Acyclovir, amphotericin B, dextrose 30%, diazepam, digoxin, ganciclovir, lactated Ringer solution, leucovorin, midazolam, pentamidine, phenytoin, prochlorperazine, promethazine, solutions containing calcium (such as TPN), sulfamethoxazole–trimethoprim, vancomycin. Other drugs may also be incompatible. Consult a drug incompatibility reference for more information.

ACTION
Inhibits herpes virus replication in vitro by blocking the pyrophosphate-binding site on DNA polymerases and reverse transcriptases.

Route	Onset	Peak	Duration
IV	Unknown	Immediate	Unknown

Half-life: 3 to 4 hours.

ADVERSE REACTIONS
CNS: asthenia, dizziness, fatigue, fever, headache, hypoesthesia, malaise, neuropathy, paresthesia, *seizures,* abnormal coordination, agitation, aggression, amnesia, anxiety, aphasia, ataxia, cerebrovascular disorder, confusion, dementia, depression, EEG abnormalities, generalized spasms, hallucinations, insomnia, meningitis, peripheral neuropathy, nervousness, pain, sensory disturbances, somnolence, stupor, taste perversion, tremor. **CV:** ECG abnormalities, first-degree AV block, flushing, HTN, hypotension, palpitations, sinus tachycardia, chest pain, edema, *thrombosis.* **EENT:** conjunctivitis, eye pain, visual disturbances, pharyngitis, rhinitis, sinusitis, dry mouth. **GI:** abdominal pain, anorexia, diarrhea, nausea, vomiting, *pancreatitis,* constipation, dysphagia, dyspepsia, flatulence, melena, rectal hemorrhage, ulcerative stomatitis. **GU:** *acute renal failure,* abnormal renal function, albuminuria, candidiasis, dysuria, polyuria, nocturia, urethral disorder, urine retention, UTI. **Hematologic:** anemia, *bone marrow suppression, granulocytopenia, leukopenia, thrombocytopenia,* thrombocytosis. **Hepatic:** abnormal hepatic function. **Metabolic:** hyperphosphatemia,

---

Reactions in bold italics are *life-threatening*. Interactions may have a *rapid onset* or a *delayed onset*.

hypocalcemia, hypokalemia, hypomagnesemia, hypophosphatemia, hyponatremia, *acidosis,* thirst, cachexia, weight loss.
Musculoskeletal: arthralgia, back pain, leg cramps, myalgia. **Respiratory:** *bronchospasm,* cough, dyspnea, hemoptysis, pneumonia, pneumonitis, *pneumothorax,* pulmonary infiltration, *respiratory insufficiency, stridor.* **Skin:** diaphoresis, rash, erythematous rash, facial edema, pruritus, seborrhea, skin discoloration, skin ulceration.
Other: *sarcoma, sepsis,* abscess, bacterial or fungal infections, flulike symptoms, inflammation and pain at infusion site, lymphadenopathy, lymphoma-like disorder, rigors.

INTERACTIONS
Drug-drug. *Calcium:* May decrease serum level of ionized calcium. Avoid concurrent use.
Nephrotoxic drugs (acyclovir, aminoglycosides, amphotericin B, cyclosporine): May increase risk of nephrotoxicity. Avoid using together.
Pentamidine: May increase risk of nephrotoxicity; severe hypocalcemia also has been reported. Monitor renal function tests and electrolytes.
🜂 *Alert: QT-interval prolonging drugs (amiodarone, dofetilide, fluoroquinolones, phenothiazines, procainamide, quinidine, some macrolides, sotalol, TCAs):* May increase risk of prolonged QT interval and torsades de pointes. Avoid use together.

EFFECTS ON LAB TEST RESULTS
• May increase ALP, ALT, AST, bilirubin, creatinine, and phosphate levels.
• May decrease calcium, magnesium, phosphate, potassium, and sodium levels.
• May decrease Hb level and granulocyte and WBC counts.
• May increase or decrease platelet count.

CONTRAINDICATIONS & CAUTIONS
• Contraindicated in patients hypersensitive to drug.
Boxed Warning In patients with abnormal renal function, use cautiously, maintain adequate hydration, and reduce dosage. Drug is nephrotoxic and can worsen renal impairment. Some degree of nephrotoxicity occurs in most patients. ∎
• Drug may cause QT-interval prolongation and increase risk of ventricular arrhythmias.

Use cautiously in patients with a history of or at risk for QT-interval prolongation.
Dialyzable drug: Yes.
⚠ *Overdose S&S:* Seizures, renal impairment, paresthesia (limb or perioral), calcium and phosphate electrolyte disturbances.

PREGNANCY-LACTATION-REPRODUCTION
• Use cautiously in pregnancy and only if clearly needed. Monitoring of amniotic fluid volumes by ultrasound is recommended weekly after 20 weeks' gestation to detect oligohydramnios.
• Patient should discontinue breastfeeding or discontinue drug.

NURSING CONSIDERATIONS
🜂 *Alert:* Because drug is highly toxic, which is probably dose-related, always use the lowest effective maintenance dose.
Boxed Warning Frequent monitoring of serum creatinine, with dosage adjustment for changes in renal function, is imperative. ∎
• Monitor CrCl frequently during therapy because of drug's adverse effects on renal function. Obtain a baseline 24-hour CrCl. Monitor level two to three times weekly during induction and at least once every 1 to 2 weeks during maintenance.
Boxed Warning Drug can cause seizures related to altered mineral and electrolyte levels; monitor levels using a schedule similar to that established for monitoring of CrCl. Assess patient for tetany and seizures, and treat with supplementation if necessary. ∎
• Monitor patient's Hb level and hematocrit. Anemia occurs in about one-third of patients and may be severe enough to require transfusions.
• Drug may cause a dose-related transient decrease in ionized calcium, which may not always show up in patient's lab values.

PATIENT TEACHING
• Explain the importance of adequate hydration throughout therapy.
• Advise patient to report all adverse reactions, including tingling around the mouth, numbness in the arms and legs, pins-and-needles sensations, chest pain, palpitations, dyspnea, and changes in urine volume or color.
• Tell patient to report discomfort at IV insertion site.

- Advise patient to notify prescriber if pregnant or breastfeeding.

---

fosinopril sodium ▩
foe-SIN-oh-pril

Therapeutic class: Antihypertensives
Pharmacologic class: ACE inhibitors

AVAILABLE FORMS
Tablets: 10 mg, 20 mg, 40 mg

INDICATIONS & DOSAGES
➤ **HTN**
Adults: Initially, 10 mg PO daily; adjust dosage based on BP response at peak and trough levels. Usual dosage is 10 to 40 mg daily; maximum is 80 mg daily. Dosage may be divided.
Children age 6 and older weighing more than 50 kg: Initially, 5 to 10 mg PO once daily. Maximum dosage is 40 mg/day.
➤ **Adjunctive therapy for HF with diuretics or digoxin**
Adults: Initially, 10 mg PO once daily. Increase dosage over several weeks to a maximum of 40 mg PO daily, if needed.

ADMINISTRATION
PO
- Give drug without regard for meals.

ACTION
Inhibits ACE, preventing conversion of angiotensin I to angiotensin II, a potent vasoconstrictor. Less angiotensin II decreases peripheral arterial resistance, thus decreasing aldosterone secretion, which reduces sodium and water retention and lowers BP.

Route	Onset	Peak	Duration
PO	1 hr	3 hr	24 hr

Half-life: 11.5 to 14 hours.

ADVERSE REACTIONS
CNS: dizziness, headache, fatigue, syncope, somnolence, depression, paresthesia, weakness, fever. **CV:** chest pain, rhythm disturbances, hypotension, orthostatic hypotension, edema, flushing. **EENT:** tinnitus, pharyngitis, sinusitis. **GI:** *pancreatitis,* nausea, vomiting, diarrhea, abdominal pain, gastritis. **GU:** sexual dysfunction, UTI, dysuria, renal insufficiency, urinary frequency. **Musculoskeletal:** musculoskeletal pain, myalgia. **Respiratory:** URI; dry, persistent, tickling, nonproductive cough. **Skin:** rash, photosensitivity reactions, pruritus. **Other:** *angioedema,* change in libido, breast mass, viral infection.

INTERACTIONS
Drug-drug. *Aliskiren:* Increases risk of hypotension, hyperkalemia, and renal dysfunction. Don't use together in patients with GFR less than 60 mL/minute. Contraindicated in patients with diabetes.
Antacids: May impair absorption. Separate dosage times by at least 2 hours.
ARBs: May increase toxic effects of ACE inhibitors. Avoid use together when possible.
Azathioprine: May increase risk of anemia or leukopenia. Monitor hematologic studies if used together.
Diuretics, other antihypertensives: May cause excessive hypotension. Stop diuretic or lower fosinopril dosage.
Everolimus: May increase risk of angioedema. Use extreme caution.
Insulin: May alter insulin requirements in patients with diabetes. Monitor patient closely.
Lithium: May increase lithium level and lithium toxicity. Monitor lithium level.
NSAIDs: May decrease antihypertensive effects and increase potential for renal dysfunction. Monitor BP.
Potassium-sparing diuretics, potassium supplements: May cause hyperkalemia. Use cautiously and monitor patient closely.
Drug-herb. *Capsaicin:* May cause cough. Discourage use together.
Ma huang: May decrease antihypertensive effects. Discourage use together.
Drug-food. *Salt substitutes containing potassium:* May increase risk of hyperkalemia. Discourage use together.

EFFECTS ON LAB TEST RESULTS
- May increase BUN, creatinine, and potassium levels and LFT values.
- May decrease sodium level.
- May increase Hb level and hematocrit.
- May cause falsely low digoxin level with the Digi-Tab radioimmunoassay kit for digoxin.

CONTRAINDICATIONS & CAUTIONS
- Contraindicated in patients hypersensitive to drug or other ACE inhibitors.

Reactions in bold italics are *life-threatening*. Interactions may have a *rapid onset* or a ***delayed onset***.

• Use cautiously in patients with impaired renal or hepatic function.
Dialyzable drug: 2% to 7%.
⚠ *Overdose S&S:* Hypotension.

PREGNANCY-LACTATION-REPRODUCTION
• Use in pregnancy and during breastfeeding isn't recommended.
Boxed Warning Use during pregnancy can cause injury and death to the developing fetus. When pregnancy is detected, stop drug as soon as possible. ∎

NURSING CONSIDERATIONS
• Monitor BP for drug effect.
• Drug can increase risk of angioedema, including intestinal angioedema. Monitor patient for facial swelling, airway obstruction, and abdominal pain.
⚛ Patients who are Black and who take ACE inhibitors as monotherapy for HTN have a smaller reduction in BP and a higher incidence of angioedema than patients who are non-Black.
• Monitor potassium intake and potassium level. Patients with diabetes, those with impaired renal function, and those receiving drugs that can increase potassium level may develop hyperkalemia.
• ACE inhibitors may cause agranulocytosis and neutropenia. Monitor CBC with differential counts before therapy and periodically thereafter.
• Assess renal and hepatic function before and periodically throughout therapy.
• *Look alike–sound alike:* Don't confuse fosinopril with lisinopril.

PATIENT TEACHING
• Tell patient to avoid potassium-containing salt substitutes, which may increase risk of hyperkalemia when taken with fosinopril.
• Instruct patient to contact prescriber if light-headedness or fainting occurs.
• Advise patient to report evidence of infection, such as fever and sore throat.
• Instruct patient to report easy bruising or bleeding; swelling of tongue, lips, face, eyes, mucous membranes, arms, or legs; difficulty swallowing or breathing; cough; or hoarseness.
• Urge patient to use caution in hot weather and during exercise. Inadequate fluid intake, vomiting, diarrhea, and excessive perspiration can lead to light-headedness and fainting.

• Tell patient with diabetes using oral antidiabetics or insulin who is starting an ACE inhibitor to closely watch for hypoglycemia, especially during first month of combined use.
• Tell patient of childbearing potential to notify prescriber if pregnancy occurs. Drug will need to be stopped.

fosphenytoin sodium ⚛
FOS-fen-i-toyn

Cerebyx

Therapeutic class: Anticonvulsants
Pharmacologic class: Hydantoin derivatives

AVAILABLE FORMS
Injection: 100 mg phenytoin sodium equivalents/2 mL, 500 mg phenytoin sodium equivalents/10 mL vials

INDICATIONS & DOSAGES
Adjust-a-dose (for all indications): Phenytoin clearance is decreased slightly in older adults; lower or less frequent dosing may be required.
➤ **Status epilepticus**
Adults: Loading dose, 15 to 20 mg phenytoin sodium equivalent (PE)/kg IV at infusion rate of 100 to 150 mg PE/minute; then 4 to 6 mg PE/kg/day IV or IM in divided doses as maintenance dose. Don't exceed maximum rate of 150 mg PE/minute.
Children from birth to younger than age 17: Loading dose, 15 to 20 mg PE/kg IV at 2 mg PE/minute or 150 mg PE/minute, whichever is slower; then initial maintenance dose of 2 to 4 mg PE/kg IV 12 hours after loading dose, then continue 2 to 4 mg PE/kg once every 12 hours at 1 to 2 mg PE/kg/minute or 100 mg PE/minute, whichever is slower.
➤ **To prevent and treat seizures during neurosurgery (nonemergent loading or maintenance dosing)**
Adults: Loading dose, 10 to 20 mg PE/kg IM or IV at infusion rate not exceeding 150 mg PE/minute. Maintenance dose is 4 to 6 mg PE/kg/day IV or IM in divided doses.
Children from birth to younger than age 17: Loading dose, 10 to 15 mg PE/kg IV at 1 to 2 mg PE/minute or 150 mg PE/minute, whichever is slower; then initial maintenance dose of 2 to 4 mg PE/kg IV 12 hours after loading dose, then continue 2 to 4 mg PE/kg once every 12 hours at 1 to 2 mg

PE/kg/minute or 100 mg PE/minute, whichever is slower.

➤ **Traumatic brain injury; prevention of early posttraumatic seizure (alternative agent)** ◆

Adults: Loading dose, 17 to 20 mg PE/kg IV at 100 to 150 mg PE/minute; usual maximum dose, 2 g PE. Begin maintenance dose 8 to 12 hours after loading dose. Maintenance dose, 100 mg PE IV every 8 hours or 5 mg PE/kg/day (round to the nearest 100 mg PE) IV in divided doses every 8 hours. Duration of prophylaxis varies, but is generally short term.

ADMINISTRATION

IV

▼ If rapid phenytoin loading is a main goal, this form is preferred.

▼ For status epilepticus, give IV rather than IM because therapeutic phenytoin level occurs more rapidly.

▼ For infusion, dilute in D_5W or NSS for injection to yield 1.5 to 25 mg PE/mL.

Boxed Warning Don't give more than 150 mg PE/minute in adults and 2 mg PE/kg/minute (or 150 mg PE/minute) in children because of risk of severe hypotension and cardiac arrhythmias. Careful cardiac monitoring is needed during and after administering IV drug. Although risk of CV toxicity increases with infusion rates above the recommended infusion rate, these events have also been reported at or below the recommended infusion rate. Reducing rate of administration or discontinuing drug may be needed. ■

▼ Maintenance infusion rates in children shouldn't exceed 1 to 2 mg PE/kg/minute (or 100 mg PE/minute, whichever is slower).

▼ Patients receiving 20 mg PE/kg at 150 mg PE/minute typically feel discomfort, usually in the groin. To reduce discomfort, slow or temporarily stop infusion.

▼ Monitor patient's ECG, BP, and respirations continuously during maximum phenytoin level—about 10 to 20 minutes after end of fosphenytoin infusion. Severe CV complications are most common in older adults and patients who are gravely ill. If needed, decrease rate or stop infusion.

▼ Store drug under refrigeration. Don't store at room temperature longer than 48 hours. Discard vials that develop particulate matter.

▼ **Incompatibilities:** Other IV drugs.

IM

• Depending on dose ordered, may require two separate IM injections.

• IM administration generates systemic phenytoin levels similar enough to oral phenytoin sodium to allow essentially interchangeable use.

• Don't use IM route in children unless IV access is unavailable.

• Store drug under refrigeration. Don't store at room temperature longer than 48 hours. Discard vials that develop particulate matter.

ACTION

May stabilize neuronal membranes and limit seizure activity either by increasing efflux or decreasing influx of sodium ions across cell membranes in the motor cortex during generation of nerve impulses.

Route	Onset	Peak	Duration
IV	Unknown	End of infusion	Unknown
IM	Unknown	30 min	Unknown

Half-life: Fosphenytoin, 15 minutes; phenytoin, 12 to 29 hours.

ADVERSE REACTIONS

CNS: ataxia, dizziness, somnolence, *brain edema, intracranial HTN,* agitation, asthenia, dysarthria, extrapyramidal syndrome, fever, headache, hypesthesia, incoordination, increased or decreased reflexes, nervousness, paresthesia, speech disorders, stupor, thinking abnormalities, tremor, taste perversion, vertigo. **CV:** HTN, hypotension, tachycardia, vasodilation. **EENT:** nystagmus, amblyopia, diplopia, deafness, tinnitus, tongue disorder, dry mouth. **GI:** constipation, nausea, vomiting. **Metabolic:** *hypokalemia.* **Musculoskeletal:** back pain, myasthenia. **Respiratory:** pneumonia. **Skin:** pruritus, ecchymoses, injection-site reaction and pain, rash. **Other:** chills, facial edema, infection, pelvic pain.

INTERACTIONS

Drug-drug. *Amiodarone, capecitabine, chloramphenicol, chlordiazepoxide, cimetidine, disulfiram, estrogens, ethosuximide, felbamate, 5-FU, fluconazole, fluoxetine, fluvastatin, fluvoxamine, H_2-receptor antagonists, isoniazid, itraconazole, ketoconazole, methylphenidate, miconazole, omeprazole, oxcarbazepine, phenothiazines, salicylates,*

---

sertraline, succinimides, sulfonamides, ticlopidine, tolbutamide, topiramate, trazodone, voriconazole, warfarin: May increase phenytoin level and effect. Use together cautiously.

Bleomycin, carbamazepine, carboplatin, cisplatin, diazepam, diazoxide, doxorubicin, folic acid, fosamprenavir, methotrexate, nelfinavir, reserpine, rifampin, ritonavir, theophylline, vigabatrin: May decrease phenytoin level. Monitor patient.

Cisatracurium, corticosteroids, delavirdine, doxycycline, estrogens, fluconazole, furosemide, hormonal contraceptives, irinotecan, itraconazole, ketoconazole, paclitaxel, pancuronium, paroxetine, posaconazole, quinidine, rifampin, rocuronium, sertraline, teniposide, theophylline, vecuronium, vitamin D, voriconazole, warfarin: May decrease effects of these drugs because of increased hepatic metabolism. Monitor patient closely.

Lithium: May increase lithium toxicity. Monitor patient's neurologic status closely. Marked neurologic symptoms have been reported despite normal lithium level.

Phenobarbital, valproate sodium, valproic acid: May increase or decrease phenytoin level. May increase or decrease levels of these drugs. Monitor patient.

TCAs: May lower seizure threshold and require adjustments in phenytoin dosage. Use together cautiously.

Drug-herb. *St. John's wort:* May decrease phenytoin level. Monitor patient.

Drug-lifestyle. *Alcohol use:* Acute intoxication may increase phenytoin level and effect. Discourage use together.

Long-term alcohol use: May decrease phenytoin level. Monitor patient and strongly discourage use together.

EFFECTS ON LAB TEST RESULTS
• May increase ALP, GGT, and glucose levels.
• May decrease folate, potassium, and T_4 levels.
• May cause falsely low dexamethasone and metyrapone test results.

CONTRAINDICATIONS & CAUTIONS
• Contraindicated in patients hypersensitive to drug or its components, phenytoin, or other hydantoins.
• Contraindicated in patients with a history of prior acute hepatotoxicity attributable to fosphenytoin or phenytoin.

• Contraindicated in patients with sinus bradycardia, SA block, second- or third-degree AV block, or Adams-Stokes syndrome.
• Contraindicated in patients taking delavirdine because of potential loss of virologic response and possible resistance to delavirdine or to NNRTIs.
• Use cautiously in patients with porphyria and in those with history of hypersensitivity to similarly structured drugs, such as barbiturates, oxazolidinediones, and succinimide.
• Use cautiously in patients with low albumin level.
🔵 *Alert:* If patient develops acute hepatotoxicity, discontinue drug and don't readminister.
🔵 *Alert:* Serious and sometimes fatal TEN and SJS have been reported; usually onset of symptoms occurs within 28 days but sometimes later. Discontinue drug at first sign of rash unless rash is clearly not drug related. If rash occurs, evaluate patient for signs and symptoms of DRESS syndrome.
Dialyzable drug: Unknown.
⚠ *Overdose S&S:* Asystole, bradycardia, cardiac arrest, hypocalcemia, hypotension, lethargy, metabolic acidosis, nausea, syncope, tachycardia, vomiting, death.

PREGNANCY-LACTATION-REPRODUCTION
• Prenatal exposure to phenytoin may increase risk of congenital malformations and other adverse developmental outcomes. Use with extreme caution in pregnancy after assessing maternal benefits and fetal risk.
• A potentially life-threatening bleeding disorder related to decreased levels of vitamin K–dependent clotting factors may occur in newborns exposed to phenytoin in utero. This drug-induced condition can be prevented with vitamin K administration to the mother before delivery and to the neonate after birth.
• Encourage patients to enroll in the North American Antiepileptic Drug Pregnancy Registry.
• It isn't known if fosphenytoin appears in human milk but phenytoin does appear in human milk. Weigh benefits of breastfeeding along with patient's need for drug and potential adverse effects on the infant.

NURSING CONSIDERATIONS

⚠️ *Alert:* Because of risk of cardiac and local toxicity with IV fosphenytoin administration, use oral phenytoin whenever possible.

• Angioedema has been reported in patients treated with phenytoin and fosphenytoin. Discontinue immediately if symptoms of angioedema, such as facial, perioral, or upper airway swelling, occur.

• Most significant drug interactions are those commonly seen with phenytoin.

⚠️ *Alert:* Drug should always be prescribed and dispensed in phenytoin sodium equivalent units. Don't make adjustments in the recommended doses when substituting fosphenytoin for phenytoin, and vice versa.

• In status epilepticus, phenytoin may be used as maintenance instead of fosphenytoin, using the appropriate dose.

• Phosphate load provided by fosphenytoin (0.0037 millimole phosphate/mg PE) must be taken into consideration when treating patients who need phosphate restriction, such as those with severe renal impairment. Monitor lab values.

▧ Patients with Chinese ancestry who have tested positive for the allele HLA-B*1502 have a potentially increased risk of SCAR, including SJS and TEN. Monitor these patients carefully.

▧ Some patients treated with phenytoin have been shown to metabolize the drug slowly, which appears to be genetically determined. If early signs and symptoms of dose-related CNS toxicity develop, check serum levels immediately.

• If patient develops exfoliative, purpuric, or bullous rash or signs and symptoms of SLE, SJS, or TEN, stop drug and notify prescriber. If rash is mild (measles-like or scarlatiniform), therapy may resume after rash disappears. If rash recurs when therapy is resumed, further fosphenytoin or phenytoin administration is contraindicated. Document that patient is allergic to drug.

• Stop drug in patients with acute hepatotoxicity.

• Doses are usually selected to attain therapeutic serum total phenytoin concentrations of 10 to 20 mcg/mL (unbound phenytoin concentrations of 1 to 2 mcg/mL). Trough levels provide information about clinically effective serum level range and are obtained just before patient's next scheduled dose.

• After administration, phenytoin levels shouldn't be monitored until conversion to phenytoin is essentially complete—about 2 hours after the end of an IV infusion or 4 hours after IM administration.

• Interpret total phenytoin levels cautiously in patients with renal or hepatic disease or hypoalbuminemia caused by an increased fraction of unbound phenytoin. It may be more useful to monitor unbound phenytoin levels in these patients. When giving drug IV, monitor patients with renal and hepatic disease because they are at increased risk for more frequent and severe adverse reactions.

• Monitor glucose level closely in patients with diabetes; drug may cause hyperglycemia.

⚠️ *Alert:* Abrupt withdrawal of drug may precipitate status epilepticus.

• *Look alike–sound alike:* Don't confuse Cerebyx with Cerezyme, Celexa, or Celebrex.

PATIENT TEACHING

• Warn patient that sensory disturbances may occur with IV administration.

• Instruct patient to immediately report adverse reactions, especially rash, palpitations, dyspnea, chest pain, and dizziness.

• Instruct patient to discuss drug therapy with prescriber if considering pregnancy.

• Advise patient that the benefits of breastfeeding should be weighed along with patient's need for drug and potential adverse effects on the breastfed infant.

• Recommend that patient taking drug during pregnancy enroll in the North American AED Pregnancy Registry (www.aedpregnancyregistry.org or 1-888-233-2334).

---

frovatriptan succinate
frow-vah-TRIP-tan

Frova♦

Therapeutic class: Antimigraine drugs
Pharmacologic class: Serotonin 5-HT$_1$ receptor agonists

AVAILABLE FORMS
Tablets: 2.5 mg

Reactions in bold italics are *life-threatening*. Interactions may have a *rapid onset* or a *delayed onset*.

INDICATIONS & DOSAGES
➤ **Acute treatment of migraine attacks with or without aura**
Adults: 2.5 mg PO taken at the first sign of migraine attack. If the headache recurs, a second tablet may be taken at least 2 hours after the first dose. The total daily dose (per 24 hours) shouldn't exceed 7.5 mg.

ADMINISTRATION
PO
• Give drug without regard for food.
• Give drug with fluids as soon as signs or symptoms appear.

ACTION
May cause vasoconstriction in response to excessive dilation of extracerebral and intracranial arteries during migraine headaches.

Route	Onset	Peak	Duration
PO	Unknown	2–4 hr	Unknown

Half-life: 26 hours.

ADVERSE REACTIONS
CNS: dizziness, headache, fatigue, paresthesia, insomnia, anxiety, somnolence, dysesthesia, hypoesthesia, hot or cold sensation, pain, drowsiness. **CV:** chest pain, palpitations, flushing. **EENT:** abnormal vision, tinnitus, sinusitis, rhinitis, dry mouth. **GI:** dyspepsia, vomiting, abdominal pain, diarrhea, nausea. **Musculoskeletal:** skeletal pain. **Skin:** diaphoresis.

INTERACTIONS
Drug-drug. *Ergotamine-containing or ergot-type drugs (dihydroergotamine):* May cause prolonged vasospastic reactions. Separate doses by 24 hours.
5-HT$_1$ agonists (such as triptans): May cause additive effects. Separate doses by 24 hours.
MAO inhibitors, SNRIs, SSRIs (citalopram, fluoxetine, fluvoxamine, paroxetine, sertraline), TCAs: May cause serotonin syndrome. Discontinue drug if serotonin syndrome is suspected.

EFFECTS ON LAB TEST RESULTS
None reported.

CONTRAINDICATIONS & CAUTIONS
• Contraindicated in patients hypersensitive to drug or its components.

• Contraindicated in patients with history or symptoms of ischemic heart disease or coronary artery vasospasm, including Prinzmetal variant angina, Wolff-Parkinson-White syndrome, or other cardiac accessory conduction pathway disorders; in those with history of stroke, TIA, or PVD, including ischemic bowel disease; in those with uncontrolled HTN; and in those with hemiplegic or basilar migraine.
• Contraindicated within 24 hours of another triptan, drug containing ergotamine, or ergot-type drug.
• Before use in patients with risk factors for CAD, such as HTN, hypercholesterolemia, smoking, obesity, diabetes, or strong family history of CAD; patients after menopause; or men older than age 40, obtain a CV evaluation and show patient is free from cardiac disease. If drug is used in such a patient, monitor patient closely and consider obtaining an ECG after the first dose. Intermittent, long-term users of triptans or those with risk factors should undergo periodic cardiac evaluation while using drug.
• Safety of treating an average of more than four migraine headaches in a 30-day period hasn't been established.
• Safety and effectiveness in patients younger than age 18 haven't been established.
Dialyzable drug: Unknown.

PREGNANCY-LACTATION-REPRODUCTION
• It isn't known if drug affects fetal development. Use during pregnancy only if potential benefit justifies risk to the fetus.
• It isn't known if drug appears in human milk. Patient should discontinue breastfeeding or discontinue drug.

NURSING CONSIDERATIONS
⚠ *Alert:* Rare but serious cardiac events, including acute MI, life-threatening cardiac arrhythmias, and death, may occur within a few hours of a triptan dose.
• Use drug only when patient has a clear diagnosis of migraine. If patient has no response for the first migraine attack treated with frovatriptan, reconsider the diagnosis of migraine.
⚠ *Alert:* Combining a triptan with an SSRI or SSNRI, a TCA, MAO inhibitors, or agents that reduce frovatriptan's metabolism may cause serotonin syndrome. Signs and symptoms may include restlessness, hallucinations,

loss of coordination, fast heartbeat, rapid changes in BP, increased body temperature, hyperreflexia, nausea, vomiting, and diarrhea. Serotonin syndrome is more likely to occur when starting or increasing dosage of a serotonergic drug and usually occurs within minutes to hours.

• Monitor BP in patients taking 5-HT$_1$ agonists.

PATIENT TEACHING

• Instruct patient in safe drug administration and to take with a full glass of fluid.
• Caution patient to take extra care or avoid driving and operating machinery if dizziness or fatigue develops after taking drug.
• Stress importance of reporting all adverse reactions. Advise patient to immediately report pain, tightness, heaviness, or pressure in chest, throat, neck, or jaw; or rash or itching after taking drug.
• Instruct patient not to take drug within 24 hours of taking another serotonin-receptor agonist or ergot-type drug.

SAFETY ALERT!

fulvestrant ▧
full-VES-trant

Faslodex

Therapeutic class: Antineoplastics
Pharmacologic class: Estrogen antagonists

AVAILABLE FORMS

Injection: 50 mg/mL in 5-mL prefilled syringes*

INDICATIONS & DOSAGES

Adjust-a-dose (for all indications): For patients with moderate hepatic impairment (Child-Pugh class B), give 250 mg IM slowly as one 5-mL injection on days 1, 15, and 29, then monthly thereafter.

➤ **Hormone receptor (HR)–positive metastatic breast cancer with disease progression after antiestrogen therapy**
Women after menopause: 500 mg IM slowly into buttocks (over 1 to 2 minutes per injection) as two 5-mL injections, one in each buttock on days 1, 15, and 29, then once monthly thereafter.

➤ **HR-positive, HER2-negative advanced or metastatic breast cancer in combination with palbociclib or abemaciclib in women with disease progression after endocrine therapy** ▧
Adults: 500 mg IM slowly into buttocks (1 to 2 minutes per injection) as two 5-mL injections, one in each buttock, on days 1, 15, 29, and then once monthly thereafter. Recommended palbociclib dose is a 125-mg capsule PO once daily for 21 consecutive days followed by 7 days off each 28-day cycle. Recommended abemaciclib dosage is one 150-mg tablet PO b.i.d. Patients who are premenopausal and perimenopausal treated with this combination should be treated with luteinizing hormone-releasing hormone (LHRH) agonists according to current clinical practice standards.
Adjust-a-dose: Refer to palbociclib or abemaciclib prescribing information for dosage adjustments and management of toxicity, use with concomitant medications, and other relevant safety information related to palbociclib and abemaciclib.

➤ **HR-positive, HER2-negative advanced breast cancer in women not previously treated with endocrine therapy** ▧
Patients who are postmenopausal: 500 mg IM slowly into buttocks (over 1 to 2 minutes per injection) as two 5-mL injections, one in each buttock on days 1, 15, and 29, then once monthly thereafter.

➤ **HR-positive, HER2-negative advanced or metastatic breast cancer in women who are postmenopausal in combination with ribociclib, as initial endocrine-based therapy or after disease progression on endocrine therapy** ▧
Adults: 500 mg IM slowly into buttocks (over 1 to 2 minutes per injection) as two 5-mL injections, one in each buttock on days 1, 15, and 29, then once monthly thereafter. Recommended ribociclib dose is 600 mg PO once daily for 21 consecutive days followed by 7 days off treatment for each 28-day cycle.
Adjust-a-dose: Refer to ribociclib prescribing information for dosage adjustments and management of ribociclib-related toxicities.

ADMINISTRATION
IM

• Drug is a potential teratogen. Follow safe handling procedures.
• Drug may be warmed before use by storing at room temperature for 1 hour or rolling injection gently in hands.

- Expel gas bubble from syringe before giving.
- Give slowly into buttocks.

ACTION

Competitively binds estrogen receptors and downregulates estrogen-receptor protein in human breast cancer cells. It's effective in treating estrogen receptor–positive breast tumors.

Route	Onset	Peak	Duration
IM	Unknown	7 days	1 mo

Half-life: About 40 days.

ADVERSE REACTIONS

CNS: asthenia, headache, pain, dizziness, insomnia, fever, paresthesia, depression, anxiety, fatigue. **CV:** hot flashes, chest pain, peripheral edema, vasodilation. **EENT:** pharyngitis. **GI:** nausea, vomiting, constipation, abdominal pain, diarrhea, anorexia. **GU:** UTI. **Hematologic:** anemia. **Hepatic:** elevated AST and ALT levels. **Musculoskeletal:** bone pain, back pain, extremity pain, arthralgia, musculoskeletal pain, myalgia, pelvic pain, arthritis. **Respiratory:** dyspnea, cough. **Skin:** injection-site pain, rash, diaphoresis. **Other:** accidental injury, flulike syndrome.

INTERACTIONS

None reported.

EFFECTS ON LAB TEST RESULTS

- May increase ALT and AST levels.
- May decrease Hb level and hematocrit.
- May interfere with estradiol measurement by immunoassay, resulting in falsely elevated estradiol levels.

CONTRAINDICATIONS & CAUTIONS

- Contraindicated in patients allergic to drug or its components.
- Use cautiously in patients with moderate or severe hepatic impairment.
- When drug is used with palbociclib or abemaciclib, leukopenia, thrombocytopenia, neutropenia, and febrile neutropenia may occur. *Dialyzable drug:* Unknown.

PREGNANCY-LACTATION-REPRODUCTION

- Drug can cause fetal harm. Patients shouldn't become pregnant during therapy. If drug is used during pregnancy, or if patient becomes pregnant during therapy, apprise patient of potential fetal hazard. Patients should use effective contraception during therapy and for 1 year after final dose.
- It isn't known if drug appears in human milk. Patients shouldn't breastfeed during therapy and for 1 year after final dose.
- Drug may impair male and female fertility.

NURSING CONSIDERATIONS

- Because drug is given IM, use cautiously in patients with bleeding diatheses or thrombocytopenia, and in those taking anticoagulants.
- Pregnancy testing is recommended within 7 days before initiating drug.

PATIENT TEACHING

- Caution patient to avoid pregnancy and breastfeeding during therapy and for 1 year after final dose and to report suspected pregnancy immediately.
- Inform patient of the most common adverse effects, including pain at injection site, headache, GI symptoms, back pain, hot flashes, and sore throat. Advise patient to report all adverse reactions.

furosemide
fur-OH-se-mide

Lasix🖉, Lasix Special🍁

Therapeutic class: Antihypertensives
Pharmacologic class: Loop diuretics

AVAILABLE FORMS

Injection: 10 mg/mL
Oral solution: 8 mg/mL, 10 mg/mL
Tablets: 20 mg, 40 mg, 80 mg, 500 mg🍁

INDICATIONS & DOSAGES

➤ **Acute pulmonary edema**
Adults: 40 mg IV injected slowly over 1 to 2 minutes; then 80 mg IV over 1 to 2 minutes after 1 hour if needed.
➤ **Edema**
Adults: 20 to 80 mg PO daily in the morning. If response is inadequate, give a second dose, and each succeeding dose, every 6 to 8 hours. Carefully increase dose in 20- to 40-mg increments up to 600 mg daily. Once effective dose is attained, may give once daily or b.i.d. Or, 20 to 40 mg IV or IM, increased by 20 mg 2 hours after previous dose until desired effect achieved.

Infants and children: 2 mg/kg PO daily, increased by 1 to 2 mg/kg in 6 to 8 hours if needed; carefully adjusted up to maximum of 6 mg/kg if needed. Or, 1 mg/kg slowly IV or IM. May increase dosage by 1 mg/kg 2 hours after previous dose if needed up to 6 mg/kg. Maximum dose is 1 mg/kg/day for premature infants.

➤ **HTN**

Adults: 20 to 40 mg PO b.i.d. Dosage adjusted based on response. Usual dose is 40 to 80 mg/day in two divided doses. May be used as adjunct to other antihypertensives if needed.

ADMINISTRATION
PO
• To prevent nocturia, give in the morning. Give second dose if ordered in early afternoon, 6 to 8 hours after morning dose.
• Store tablets in light-resistant container to prevent discoloration (doesn't affect potency).

IV
▼ If discolored yellow, don't use.
▼ For direct injection, give over 1 to 2 minutes.
◐ *Alert:* For high-dose (160 mg or more), intermittent infusion in adults, dilute with D₅W, NSS, or lactated Ringer solution. To avoid ototoxicity, infuse at a rate no greater than 4 mg/minute.
▼ Use prepared infusion solution within 24 hours.
▼ **Incompatibilities:** Acidic solutions, amrinone, ciprofloxacin, milrinone, and various others. Consult a drug incompatibility reference for more information.

IM
• To prevent nocturia, give in the morning. Give second dose if ordered in early afternoon, 6 to 8 hours after morning dose.
• Give solution undiluted.
• Record administration site.
• IV administration is preferred over IM.

ACTION
Inhibits sodium and chloride reabsorption at the proximal and distal tubules and the ascending loop of Henle.

Route	Onset	Peak	Duration
PO	20–60 min	1–2 hr	6–8 hr
IV	Within 5 min	30 min	2 hr
IM	Unknown	30 min	2 hr

Half-life: 2 hours.

ADVERSE REACTIONS
CNS: vertigo, headache, dizziness, paresthesia, weakness, restlessness, fever. **CV:** orthostatic hypotension, thrombophlebitis with IV administration. **EENT:** blurred or yellowed vision, transient deafness, tinnitus. **GI:** abdominal discomfort and pain, GI irritation, diarrhea, anorexia, nausea, vomiting, constipation, *pancreatitis.* **GU:** azotemia, nocturia, polyuria, frequent urination, bladder spasm, oliguria, interstitial nephritis. **Hematologic:** *agranulocytosis, aplastic anemia, leukopenia, thrombocytopenia,* anemia. **Hepatic:** hepatic dysfunction, jaundice, increased liver enzyme levels. **Metabolic:** volume depletion and dehydration, asymptomatic hyperuricemia, increased cholesterol and triglyceride levels, impaired glucose tolerance, *hypokalemia,* hypochloremic alkalosis, hyperglycemia, dilutional hyponatremia, *hypocalcemia, hypomagnesemia.* **Musculoskeletal:** muscle spasm. **Skin:** dermatitis, purpura, rash, pruritus, photosensitivity reactions, transient pain at IM injection site, *TEN, SJS, erythema multiforme, DRESS syndrome.* **Other:** hypersensitivity reaction, including *anaphylaxis,* gout.

INTERACTIONS
Drug-drug. *Aminoglycoside antibiotics, cisplatin:* May increase ototoxicity. Use together cautiously.
Amphotericin B, corticosteroids, corticotropin, metolazone: May increase risk of hypokalemia. Monitor potassium level closely.
Antidiabetics: May decrease hypoglycemic effects. Monitor glucose level.
Antihypertensives: May increase risk of hypotension. Use together cautiously. Decrease antihypertensive dose if needed.
Cardiac glycosides, neuromuscular blockers: May increase toxicity of these drugs from furosemide-induced hypokalemia. Monitor potassium level.
Chlorothiazide, chlorthalidone, hydrochlorothiazide, indapamide, metolazone: May cause excessive diuretic response, causing serious electrolyte abnormalities or dehydration. Adjust doses carefully, and monitor patient closely for signs and symptoms of excessive diuretic response.
Ethacrynic acid: May increase risk of ototoxicity. Avoid using together.

Reactions in bold italics are *life-threatening*. Interactions may have a *rapid onset* or a *delayed onset*.

Lithium: May decrease lithium excretion, resulting in lithium toxicity. Monitor lithium level.

NSAIDs: May inhibit diuretic response. Use together cautiously.

Phenytoin: May decrease diuretic effects of furosemide. Use together cautiously.

Propranolol: May increase propranolol level. Monitor patient closely.

Salicylates: May cause salicylate toxicity, including ototoxicity. Use together cautiously.

Sucralfate: May reduce diuretic and antihypertensive effect. Separate doses by 2 hours.

Drug-herb. *Aloe:* May increase drug effect. Discourage use together.

Bayberry, blue cohosh, cayenne, ephedra, ginger, ginseng (American), kola, licorice: May worsen HTN. Discourage use together.

Licorice: May cause unexpected rapid potassium loss. Discourage use together.

Drug-food. *Any food:* May decrease furosemide serum level. Don't give with food.

Drug-lifestyle. *Sun exposure:* May increase risk of photosensitivity reactions. Advise patient to avoid excessive sunlight exposure.

EFFECTS ON LAB TEST RESULTS

• May increase cholesterol, triglyceride, glucose, BUN, creatinine, liver enzyme, and uric acid levels.

• May decrease calcium, magnesium, potassium, and sodium levels.

• May decrease Hb level and granulocyte, platelet, and WBC counts.

CONTRAINDICATIONS & CAUTIONS

• Contraindicated in patients hypersensitive to drug and in those with anuria.

• Use cautiously in patients with hepatic cirrhosis and in those allergic to sulfonamides.

⊕ Alert: Drug may cause tinnitus and reversible or irreversible hearing loss. Ototoxicity is associated with rapid injection, severe renal impairment, use of higher-than-recommended doses, hypoproteinemia, or use with other ototoxic drugs.

• Drug may exacerbate or activate SLE.

• Premature infants may be at increased risk for persistent patent ductus arteriosus with furosemide treatment during first weeks of life.

Dialyzable drug: No.

⚠ Overdose S&S: Dehydration, blood volume reduction, hypotension, electrolyte imbalance.

PREGNANCY-LACTATION-REPRODUCTION

• There are no well-controlled studies during pregnancy. Drug crosses the placental barrier. Use during pregnancy only if potential benefit justifies fetal risk.

• Drug may increase birth weight; monitor fetal growth.

• Drug appears in human milk. Avoid use during breastfeeding.

NURSING CONSIDERATIONS

⊕ Alert: Monitor weight, BP, and pulse rate routinely with long-term use.

Boxed Warning Drug is potent diuretic and can cause severe diuresis with water and electrolyte depletion. Monitor patient closely and adjust dose carefully. ▇

• If oliguria or azotemia develops or increases, drug may need to be stopped.

• Monitor fluid intake and output and electrolyte, BUN, and carbon dioxide levels frequently.

• Watch for signs of hypokalemia, such as muscle weakness and cramps.

• Consult prescriber and dietitian about a high-potassium diet or potassium supplements.

• Monitor glucose level in patients with diabetes.

• Drug may not be well absorbed orally in patient with severe HF. Drug may need to be given IV even if patient is taking other oral drugs.

• Monitor uric acid level, especially in patients with a history of gout.

• Monitor older adults, who are especially susceptible to excessive diuresis, because circulatory collapse and thromboembolic complications are possible.

• Monitor patients with severe symptoms of urine retention due to bladder emptying disorders, prostate enlargement, or urethral narrowing or worsening of symptoms, especially during initial treatment.

• Nephrocalcinosis and nephrolithiasis have occurred in infants born prematurely and in children younger than age 4 on long-term furosemide therapy. Monitor renal function and renal ultrasounds.

• *Look alike–sound alike:* Don't confuse furosemide with torsemide.

PATIENT TEACHING

• Advise patient to take drug in morning to prevent need to urinate at night. If a second dose is needed, tell patient to take it in early afternoon, 6 to 8 hours after morning dose.
• Inform patient of possible need for potassium or magnesium supplements.
• Instruct patient to stand slowly to prevent dizziness and to limit alcohol intake and strenuous exercise in hot weather to avoid worsening dizziness upon standing quickly.
• Advise patient to report all adverse reactions and to immediately report ringing in ears, severe abdominal pain, or sore throat and fever; these symptoms may indicate toxicity.
◑ *Alert:* Discourage patient from storing different types of drugs in the same container, increasing risk of drug errors. (The most popular strengths of furosemide and digoxin are white tablets that are about equal in size.)
• Tell patient to consult prescriber or pharmacist before taking OTC drugs.
• Teach patient to avoid direct sunlight and to use protective clothing and sunblock because of risk of photosensitivity reactions.

gabapentin
gab-ah-PEN-tin

Gralise, Neurontin●

gabapentin enacarbil
Horizant

Therapeutic class: Anticonvulsants
Pharmacologic class: GABA structural analogues

AVAILABLE FORMS

Capsules: 100 mg, 300 mg, 400 mg
Oral solution: 250 mg/5 mL
Tablets ⓄⓉⒸ: 100 mg, 300 mg, 400 mg, 600 mg, 800 mg
Tablets (extended-release) ⓄⓉⒸ: 300 mg, 600 mg

INDICATIONS & DOSAGES

Adjust-a-dose (for all indications): For immediate-release formulation in patients age 12 and older with CrCl of 30 to 59 mL/minute, give 400 to 1,400 mg daily divided into two doses. For CrCl of 15 to 29 mL/minute, give 200 to 700 mg daily in a single dose. For CrCl of less than 15 mL/minute, give 100 to 300 mg daily in a single dose. Reduce daily dosage in proportion to CrCl (patients with a CrCl of 7.5 mL/minute should receive half the daily dosage of those with a CrCl of 15 mL/minute). For patients receiving hemodialysis, maintenance dosage is based on estimates of CrCl. Give supplemental dose of 125 to 350 mg after each 4 hours of hemodialysis.

➤ **Adjunctive treatment of partial seizures with or without secondary generalization in patients with epilepsy (excluding Gralise and Horizant)**
Adults and children age 12 and older: Initially, 300 mg PO t.i.d. Increase dosage as needed and tolerated to 1,800 mg daily in three divided doses. Dosages up to 3,600 mg daily have been well tolerated.
Starting dosage, children ages 3 to 11: 10 to 15 mg/kg daily PO in three divided doses, adjusting over 3 days to reach effective dosage.
Effective dosage, children ages 5 to 11: 25 to 35 mg/kg daily PO in three divided doses.
Effective dosage, children ages 3 to 4: 40 mg/kg daily PO in three divided doses.

➤ **Moderate to severe primary restless legs syndrome (Horizant)**
Adults: 600 mg extended-release tablet PO daily at about 5 p.m. If dose isn't taken at the recommended time, the next dose should be taken the following day as prescribed.
Adjust-a-dose: If CrCl is 30 to 59 mL/minute, give 300 mg daily (may increase to 600 mg if needed). If CrCl is 15 to 29 mL/minute, give 300 mg daily. If CrCl is less than 15 mL/minute, give 300 mg every other day. Don't give to patients receiving hemodialysis.

➤ **Postherpetic neuralgia (immediate-release)**
Adults: 300 mg PO once daily on first day, 300 mg b.i.d. on day 2, and 300 mg t.i.d. on day 3. Adjust as needed for pain to a maximum daily dose of 1,800 mg in three divided doses.

➤ **Postherpetic neuralgia (Gralise)**
Adults: Titrate dosage to 1,800 mg PO once daily with the evening meal. On day 1, give 300 mg; on day 2, 600 mg; on days 3 to 6, 900 mg; on days 7 to 10, 1,200 mg; on days 11 to 14, 1,500 mg; and on day 15 and thereafter, 1,800 mg.
Adjust-a-dose: For patients with reduced renal function, initiate Gralise at a daily dose of 300 mg. For patients with CrCl of 30 to

60 mL/minute, titrate dosage to 600 to 1,800 mg daily as tolerated. Don't give Gralise to patients with CrCl of less than 30 mL/minute or to those receiving hemodialysis. Decrease dosage over 1 week or longer to reduce dosage, discontinue drug, or substitute with alternative medication.

➤ **Postherpetic neuralgia (Horizant)**
Adults: 600 mg PO in morning for 3 days; increase to 600 mg b.i.d. on day 4. If dose isn't taken at recommended time, skip dose, and take next dose at time of next scheduled dose.

Adjust-a-dose: If CrCl is 30 to 59 mL/minute, give 300 mg in the morning for 3 days; then increase to 300 mg b.i.d. (may increase to 600 mg b.i.d. as needed). If CrCl is 15 to 29 mL/minute, give 300 mg in the morning on days 1 and 3, then 300 mg daily in the morning (increase to 300 mg b.i.d. if needed). If CrCl is less than 15 mL/minute, give 300 mg in the morning every other day (increase to 300 mg daily in the morning if needed). If CrCl is less than 15 mL/minute and patient is on hemodialysis, give 300 mg after each dialysis treatment (increase to 600 mg after every dialysis treatment if needed).

➤ **Neuropathic pain (immediate-release)** ♦
Adults: 100 to 300 mg daily to t.i.d. For patients who are critically ill, initially 100 mg t.i.d. in combination with IV opioids. Maintenance dose, 300 to 1,200 mg t.i.d.; maximum dose, 3,600 mg daily.

ADMINISTRATION
PO
- Give immediate-release forms without regard for food.
- Give extended-release tablets with food.
- Give Gralise tablets with the evening meal.
- When giving drug t.i.d., maximum interval between doses should be no more than 12 hours.
- Refrigerate oral solution.
- Patient should swallow extended-release tablets whole and shouldn't cut, crush, or chew them.
- May divide scored 600- or 800-mg Neurontin tablets and give as a half-tablet. Use half-tablets within 28 days of dividing or discard.
- Gralise, Horizant, and other gabapentin products aren't interchangeable.

ACTION
Unknown. Structurally related to GABA but doesn't interact with GABA receptors, isn't converted into GABA or GABA agonist, doesn't inhibit GABA reuptake, and doesn't prevent degradation.

Route	Onset	Peak	Duration
PO (immediate-release)	Unknown	2–4 hr	Unknown
PO (extended-release)	Unknown	8 hr	Unknown
PO (enacarbil)	Unknown	5–7 hr	Unknown

Half-life: Gabapentin, 5 to 7 hours; gabapentin enacarbil, 5.1 to 6 hours.

ADVERSE REACTIONS
CNS: asthenia, ataxia, dizziness, fatigue, somnolence, abnormal thinking, amnesia, depression, fever, dysarthria, incoordination, tremor, headache, drowsiness, irritability, hostility, emotional lability, abnormal or drunken feeling, insomnia, hyperkinesia. **CV:** peripheral edema, vasodilation. **EENT:** amblyopia, diplopia, nystagmus, vertigo, otitis media, pharyngitis, nasopharyngitis. dental abnormalities, dry throat, dry mouth. **GI:** constipation, dyspepsia, increased appetite, flatulence, nausea, vomiting, diarrhea. **GU:** decreased libido, erectile dysfunction; UTI (Gralise). **Hematologic:** *leukopenia.* **Metabolic:** weight gain, hyperglycemia. **Musculoskeletal:** back pain, fractures, myalgia, limb pain. **Respiratory:** coughing, bronchitis, URI. **Skin:** abrasion, pruritus. **Other:** viral infections, infection, accidental injury.

INTERACTIONS
Drug-drug. *Antacids:* May decrease absorption of gabapentin. Separate dosage times by at least 2 hours.
CNS depressants: May increase risk of CNS depressant–related adverse effects. Monitor therapy.
Opioid analgesics (hydrocodone): May enhance CNS depressant effect of opioid analgesics. Consider therapy modification or limit dosages and duration of each drug.
Drug-herb. *Kava kava:* May enhance adverse or toxic CNS effects. Monitor therapy.
Drug-lifestyle. ◐ *Alert: Alcohol use:* May increase risk of CNS depression and respiratory difficulties. Discourage use together.

G

EFFECTS ON LAB TEST RESULTS
• May decrease WBC count.
• May increase glucose level.
• May cause false-positive results with the Ames N-Multistix SG dipstick test for urine protein when used with other anticonvulsants.

CONTRAINDICATIONS & CAUTIONS
• Contraindicated in patients hypersensitive to drug or its components.
• In older adults, adjust dosage based on CrCl values due to potentially decreased renal function.
• Gabapentin enacarbil isn't recommended for patients who must sleep during the day and remain awake at night.
• Anaphylaxis and angioedema can occur any time during therapy and require emergency treatment and discontinuation of drug.
⊖ *Alert:* May cause life-threatening and fatal respiratory depression in older adults and in patients with respiratory risk factors (CNS depressant or opioid use, COPD). Begin treatment at lowest dose and monitor patient closely.
• DRESS syndrome (with such symptoms as fever, rash, lymphadenopathy, and other organ system involvement), which can be life-threatening, can occur. Evaluate patient immediately if symptoms occur and discontinue drug.
Dialyzable drug: Yes.
⚠ *Overdose S&S:* Double vision, slurred speech, drowsiness, lethargy, diarrhea.

PREGNANCY-LACTATION-REPRODUCTION
• Use during pregnancy only if potential benefit justifies fetal risk.
• Use during breastfeeding only if benefit to patient outweighs risk to the infant.
• Encourage patients who are pregnant to enroll in the North American Antiepileptic Drug Pregnancy Registry at 1-888-233-2334 or www.aedpregnancyregistry.org.

NURSING CONSIDERATIONS
⊖ *Alert:* Closely monitor all patients taking or starting AEDs for changes in behavior indicating worsening of suicidality or depression. Such symptoms as anxiety, agitation, hostility, mania, and hypomania may be precursors to emerging suicidality.
⊖ *Alert:* Don't suddenly withdraw AEDs because of the risk of increased seizure frequency.

• Routine monitoring of drug levels isn't necessary. Drug doesn't appear to alter levels of other anticonvulsants.
• Monitor patient for hypersensitivity reactions, including anaphylaxis, angioedema, and SCAR.
• Monitor patient for CNS depression.

PATIENT TEACHING
• Instruct patient in safe drug administration and storage.
• Advise patient to take first dose at bedtime to minimize adverse reactions.
• Warn patient that extended-release formulas can cause significant dizziness and sleepiness.
• Warn patient to report all adverse reactions and to avoid driving and operating heavy machinery until drug's CNS effects are known.
⊖ *Alert:* Caution patient or caregiver to seek immediate medical attention for confusion or disorientation; unusual dizziness or lightheadedness; lethargy; extreme sleepiness; slow, shallow or difficult breathing; unresponsiveness; or cyanosis of the lips, fingers, or toes.
• Advise patient not to take gabapentin with alcohol or other drugs that may cause sleepiness or dizziness.
• Warn patient not to stop drug abruptly.
• Instruct patient to discuss drug therapy with prescriber if considering pregnancy.

ganciclovir (DHPG)
gan-SYE-kloe-vir

Zirgan

Therapeutic class: Antivirals
Pharmacologic class: Nucleosides–nucleotides

AVAILABLE FORMS
Injection: 500 mg/vial; 500 mg/250 mL single-dose bag
Ophthalmic gel: 0.15%

INDICATIONS & DOSAGES
⊖ *Alert:* IV ganciclovir is indicated only for the treatment of CMV retinitis in patients who are immunocompromised and for the prevention of CMV disease in patients who have received a transplant and are at risk for CMV disease.

Reactions in bold italics are *life-threatening*. Interactions may have a *rapid onset* or a **delayed onset**.

Adjust-a-dose (for all indications): Adjust IV dosage in patient with renal impairment according to the table. If patient is receiving hemodialysis, give dose shortly after session is complete.

Initial IV therapy

CrCl (mL/min)	Dose (mg/kg)	Interval
50–69	2.5	12 hr
25–49	2.5	24 hr
10–24	1.25	24 hr
<10	1.25	3 times weekly after hemodialysis

Maintenance IV therapy

CrCl (mL/min)	Dose (mg/kg)	Interval
50–69	2.5	24 hr
25–49	1.25	24 hr
10–24	0.625	24 hr
<10	0.625	3 times weekly after hemodialysis

➤ **CMV retinitis in patients who are immunocompromised, including those with AIDS**
Adults: Induction treatment is 5 mg/kg IV every 12 hours for 14 to 21 days. Maintenance treatment is 5 mg/kg IV daily 7 days per week or 6 mg/kg IV once daily five times weekly.

➤ **To prevent CMV disease in transplant recipients**
Adults: 5 mg/kg IV every 12 hours for 7 to 14 days; then 5 mg/kg daily 7 days per week or 6 mg/kg once daily five times weekly. Duration of therapy is 100 to 120 days post-transplantation.

➤ **Acute herpetic keratitis (Zirgan)**
Adults and children age 2 and older: 1 drop in affected eye five times daily (approximately every 3 hours while awake) until the corneal ulcer heals; then 1 drop t.i.d. for 7 days.

ADMINISTRATION

IV

▼ Drug is hazardous. Use safe handling precautions. IV solutions are alkaline; avoid direct contact with skin or mucous membranes. If contact occurs, wash area thoroughly with soap and water; thoroughly rinse eyes with plain water.

▼ Inspect vial; discard if particulate matter or discoloration is observed.

▼ To reconstitute, add 10 mL sterile water for injection to 500-mg vial. Gently swirl vial until solution appears clear. Don't use bacteriostatic water containing parabens, as precipitation can result.

▼ Further dilute in 50 to 250 mL (usually 100 mL) of compatible IV solution.

▼ If fluids are being restricted, dilute to no more than 10 mg/mL.

▼ Don't give as rapid or bolus injection.

▼ Use an infusion pump.

▼ Infuse slowly over at least 1 hour at a constant rate. Infusing drug too rapidly has toxic effects.

▼ Redissolve any crystals that formed in premixed bag by gently shaking. Solution must be clear at time of use.

⊘ *Alert:* Don't give subcut or IM.

▼ Flush IV line with NSS before and after administration.

▼ Reconstituted solution in the vial is stable at room temperature for 12 hours. Don't refrigerate or freeze. Use solution within 24 hours of dilution to reduce risk of bacterial contamination.

▼ Diluted solutions for infusion should be refrigerated and used within 24 hours of preparation; don't freeze.

▼ Store commercially premixed solution at room temperature.

▼ **Incompatibilities:** None listed by manufacturer. Consult a drug incompatibility reference for more information.

Ophthalmic

● Store at 59° to 77° F (15° to 20° C). Don't freeze.

ACTION

Inhibits binding of deoxyguanosine triphosphate to DNA polymerase, resulting in inhibition of DNA synthesis.

Route	Onset	Peak	Duration
IV	Unknown	Immediate	Unknown
Ophthalmic	Unknown	Unknown	Unknown

Half-life: IV, about 2.4 to 4.4 hours; ophthalmic, unknown.

ADVERSE REACTIONS

CNS: fever, asthenia, headache, peripheral neuropathy. **EENT:** retinal detachment in patients with CMV retinitis; blurred vision, eye irritation, punctate keratitis, conjunctival hyperemia (ophthalmic). **GI:** abdominal pain, anorexia, diarrhea, nausea, vomiting. **GU:** increased serum creatinine level. **Hematologic:** anemia, *agranulocytosis, leukopenia, thrombocytopenia.* **Respiratory:** cough, dyspnea, pneumonia. **Skin:** diaphoresis, pruritus, pain and phlebitis at injection site. **Other:** *sepsis*, chills, infection.

INTERACTIONS

Drug-drug. *Amphotericin B, cyclosporine, other nephrotoxic drugs:* May increase risk of nephrotoxicity. Monitor renal function.
Cytotoxic drugs: May increase toxic effects, especially hematologic effects and stomatitis. Use together only if benefits outweigh risks; monitor patient closely.
Imipenem–cilastatin: May increase seizure activity. Use together only if potential benefits outweigh risks.
Immunosuppressants (azathioprine, corticosteroids, cyclosporine, mycophenolate mofetil): May enhance immune and bone marrow suppression. Use together cautiously.
Probenecid: May increase ganciclovir level. Monitor patient closely.
Tenofovir products: May increase serum concentration of both drugs. Monitor therapy.
Zidovudine: May increase risk of agranulocytosis. Use together cautiously; monitor hematologic function closely.

EFFECTS ON LAB TEST RESULTS
• May increase ALP, ALT, AST, creatinine, and GGT levels.
• May decrease Hb level and granulocyte, neutrophil, platelet, and WBC counts.

CONTRAINDICATIONS & CAUTIONS
Boxed Warning Clinical toxicity of IV ganciclovir includes granulocytopenia, anemia, thrombocytopenia, and pancytopenia. Animal studies indicate that drug is carcinogenic and teratogenic. ■
• Contraindicated in patients hypersensitive to ganciclovir, valganciclovir, acyclovir, or components of the formulation.
• Drug isn't recommended in patients with ANC below 500/mm³, Hb below 8 g/dL, or platelet count below 25,000/mm³.
• Use cautiously and reduce dosage in patients with renal dysfunction. Monitor renal function test results.
Dialyzable drug: About 50%.
⚠ **Overdose S&S:** Persistent bone marrow suppression, reversible neutropenia or granulocytopenia, hepatitis, renal toxicity, seizures (all with IV form).

PREGNANCY-LACTATION-REPRODUCTION
Boxed Warning Based on animal studies, IV ganciclovir may be teratogenic or embryotoxic at recommended doses. ■
• Use during pregnancy only if potential benefits justify fetal risk.
• Patients of childbearing potential should use effective contraception during treatment and for 30 days after final dose. Men should practice barrier contraception during treatment and for at least 90 days after final dose.
• Breastfeeding isn't recommended during treatment or by patient who tests positive for HIV. It isn't known when breastfeeding can be safely resumed after final dose.
Boxed Warning Based on animal data, IV drug at recommended doses may cause temporary or permanent aspermatogenesis in males and may cause suppression of fertility in females. ■

NURSING CONSIDERATIONS
• Verify pregnancy status before start of treatment.
• Monitor CBC and platelet count frequently, especially in patients with renal impairment, prior drug-induced leukopenia, or baseline ANC below 1,000/mm³.
• Carefully monitor renal function, particularly in older adults and in patients taking other nephrotoxic drugs, at least weekly; adjust dosages in patients with renal impairment.
• Monitor ophthalmologic disease status during treatment.

PATIENT TEACHING
• Explain importance of drinking plenty of fluids during therapy.
• Instruct patient to report adverse reactions promptly.
• Tell patient to report discomfort at IV insertion site.
Boxed Warning Advise patient that IV use may impair fertility. ■
• Advise patient of childbearing potential to use effective contraception during IV treatment and for at least 30 days after final dose. Caution male patient to practice barrier contraception during and for at least 90 days after treatment.
• Advise patient to use soft toothbrush and electric razor because of increased bleeding risk with IV use.

- Emphasize importance of adhering to blood work as requested by prescriber.
- Instruct patient not to let sterile eye dropper touch any surface.
- Caution patient not to wear contact lenses while undergoing ophthalmic treatment.
- Advise patient undergoing ophthalmic treatment to notify prescriber if eye pain, redness, itching, or inflammation becomes aggravated.

SAFETY ALERT!

gemcitabine hydrochloride
jem-SITE-ah-been

Infugem

Therapeutic class: Antineoplastics
Pharmacologic class: Pyrimidine analogues

AVAILABLE FORMS
Injection: 10 mg/mL premixed infusion bag
Powder for injection: 200-mg, 1-g vials
Solution for injection: 200-mg, 1-g, 1.5-g, 2-g vials

INDICATIONS & DOSAGES
Adjust-a-dose (for all indications): If patient is on hemodialysis, begin hemodialysis 6 to 12 hours after drug infusion. If serum bilirubin level is greater than 1.6 mg/dL, use initial dose of 800 mg/m^2 and escalate if tolerated. Refer to manufacturer's instructions for toxicity-related dosage adjustments.

Permanently discontinue drug for any of the following nonhematologic adverse reactions: unexplained dyspnea or other evidence of severe pulmonary toxicity, severe hepatotoxicity, hemolytic-uremic syndrome, capillary leak syndrome, or PRES. Withhold drug or reduce dosage by 50% for other severe (grade 3 or 4) nonhematologic toxicity until resolved.

➤ **Locally advanced (nonresectable stage II or III) or metastatic (stage IV) adenocarcinoma of pancreas in patients previously treated with 5-FU**
Adults: 1,000 mg/m^2 IV over 30 minutes once weekly for 7 weeks followed by 1 week rest, unless toxicity occurs. Subsequent cycles should consist of infusions once weekly on days 1, 8, and 15 of each 28-day cycle. Monitor CBC with differential and platelet count before giving each dose.

➤ **With cisplatin, first-line treatment of inoperable, locally advanced (stage IIIA or IIIB), or metastatic (stage IV) NSCLC**
Adults: For 4-week schedule, 1,000 mg/m^2 IV over 30 minutes on days 1, 8, and 15 of each 28-day cycle. Administer cisplatin IV at 100 mg/m^2 on day 1 after gemcitabine infusion. For 3-week schedule, 1,250 mg/m^2 IV over 30 minutes on days 1 and 8 of each 21-day cycle. Administer cisplatin IV at 100 mg/m^2 on day 1 after gemcitabine infusion. Monitor CBC with differential and platelet count before each dose. During combination therapy with cisplatin, monitor serum creatinine, serum potassium, serum calcium, and serum magnesium levels.

➤ **With carboplatin, for treatment of advanced ovarian cancer that relapsed at least 6 months after platinum-based therapy**
Adults: 1,000 mg/m^2 IV over 30 minutes on days 1 and 8 of each 21-day cycle. Give carboplatin IV on day 1 after gemcitabine infusion. Check CBC with differential and platelet count before each dose.
Adjust-a-dose: Adjust dosage based on total ANC and platelet counts taken on days 1 and 8 of the cycle.

➤ **With paclitaxel, metastatic breast cancer (first-line treatment after failure of adjuvant anthracycline chemotherapy)**
Adults: 1,250 mg/m^2 IV over 30 minutes on days 1 and 8 of each 21-day cycle. Give paclitaxel as a 3-hour IV infusion on day 1 before gemcitabine. Check CBC with differential before each dose.
Adjust-a-dose: Adjust dosage based on total ANC and platelet counts taken on days 1 and 8 of the cycle.

➤ **Pancreatic cancer (adjuvant therapy)** ◆
Adults: 1,000 mg/m^2 IV on days 1, 8, and 15 every 28 days (combination with capecitabine) for six cycles beginning within 12 weeks of resection.

➤ **Bladder cancer (advanced or metastatic)** ◆
Adults: 1,000 mg/m^2 IV over 30 to 60 minutes days 1, 8, and 15; repeat cycle every 28 days (in combination with cisplatin), or 1,000 mg/m^2 IV over 30 minutes days 1 and 8; repeat cycle every 21 days (in combination with carboplatin) until disease progression or unacceptable toxicity.

G

➤ **Hepatobiliary cancer (advanced or metastatic)** ◆

Adults: 1,000 mg/m^2 IV over 30 minutes days 1 and 8; repeat cycle every 21 days (in combination with cisplatin), or 1,000 mg/m^2 IV over 30 minutes days 1 and 8; repeat cycle every 21 days (in combination with capecitabine), or 1,000 mg/m^2 IV infused at 10 mg/m^2/minute every 2 weeks (in combination with oxaliplatin).

ADMINISTRATION

IV

▼ Preparing and giving parenteral drug may be mutagenic, teratogenic, or carcinogenic. Follow safe handling precautions and use gloves.

▼ To prepare solution, add 5 mL of unpreserved NSS for injection to 200-mg vial, 25 mL to 1-g vial, or 50 mL to 2-g vial. Shake to dissolve.

▼ Resulting concentration is 38 mg/mL (accounting for the volume displaced by the powder); reconstitution at concentrations higher than 40 mg/mL isn't recommended.

▼ If needed, dilute to as little as 0.1 mg/mL by adding NSS for injection.

▼ Make sure solution is clear to light straw-colored and free of particles.

▼ Don't extend infusion time beyond 60 minutes or give drug more often than once weekly; doing so may increase toxicity.

▼ Drug is stable for 24 hours at room temperature.

▼ Don't refrigerate reconstituted drug because it may crystallize.

▼ Premixed bags remain stable until package expiration date when stored at 68° to 77° F (20° to 25° C). Don't freeze premixed bags as crystallization can occur.

▼ **Incompatibilities:** None listed by manufacturer. Consult a drug incompatibility reference for more information.

ACTION

Cytotoxic and specific to cell cycle; inhibits DNA synthesis and blocks progression of cells.

Route	Onset	Peak	Duration
IV	Unknown	30 min	Unknown

Half-life: About 1.7 to 19.4 hours (influenced by length of the infusion, age, and gender).

ADVERSE REACTIONS

CNS: drowsiness, paresthesia, pain, fever. **CV:** edema, peripheral edema. **GI:** stomatitis, nausea, vomiting, diarrhea. **GU:** proteinuria, hematuria. **Hematologic:** anemia, *leukopenia, neutropenia, thrombocytopenia, hemorrhage.* **Hepatic:** *hepatotoxicity.* **Respiratory:** dyspnea, *bronchospasm.* **Skin:** alopecia, rash, pain at injection site. **Other:** flulike syndrome, infection, injection-site reactions.

INTERACTIONS

Drug-drug: *Bleomycin:* May increase risk of pulmonary toxicity. Consider therapy modification.

Clozapine: May increase risk of neutropenia. Avoid combination.

Inactivated vaccines: May decrease effectiveness of vaccines. Give inactivated vaccine at least 2 weeks before gemcitabine therapy or revaccinate at least 3 months after therapy completion.

Live-virus vaccines: May increase risk of vaccine-induced adverse reactions. Defer use of live-virus vaccines.

Warfarin: May increase the anticoagulant effect of warfarin. Monitor patient and INR.

EFFECTS ON LAB TEST RESULTS

• May increase ALP, ALT, AST, BUN, creatinine, and urine protein levels.

• May decrease Hb level and neutrophil, platelet, and WBC counts.

CONTRAINDICATIONS & CAUTIONS

• Contraindicated in patients hypersensitive to drug.

• Use cautiously in patients with renal or hepatic impairment.

• Use cautiously when given within 7 days of radiation therapy.

• Prolonging infusion duration beyond 60 minutes or administering more frequently than weekly has resulted in an increased incidence of toxicities, including clinically significant hypotension, severe flulike symptoms, myelosuppression, and asthenia.

• Capillary leak syndrome with severe consequences has been reported when drug has been used alone or in combination with other chemotherapeutic agents. Discontinue if syndrome develops.

• Hemolytic-uremic syndrome that may lead to renal failure has been reported. Watch for evidence of anemia with microangiopathic

---

Reactions in bold italics are *life-threatening*. Interactions may have a *rapid onset* or a *delayed onset*.

hemolysis (elevated bilirubin or LDH level, reticulocytosis, severe thrombocytopenia, or renal failure), and monitor renal function at baseline and periodically during treatment. Permanently discontinue if hemolytic-uremic syndrome or severe renal impairment occurs; renal failure may not be reversible despite discontinuation.

• Myelosuppression, manifested by neutropenia, thrombocytopenia, and anemia, occurs with gemcitabine used alone; risk increases when combined with other cytotoxic drugs.

• Pulmonary toxicity, including interstitial pneumonitis, pulmonary fibrosis, pulmonary edema, and ARDS, has been reported; it may lead to respiratory failure (some fatal) despite discontinuation of therapy. Onset of pulmonary symptoms may occur up to 2 weeks after last dose of gemcitabine. Discontinue for unexplained dyspnea, with or without bronchospasm, or other evidence of pulmonary toxicity.

• Serious hepatotoxicity, including liver failure and death, has been reported with gemcitabine alone or in combination with other potentially hepatotoxic drugs. Administration in patients with concurrent liver metastases or preexisting medical history of hepatitis, alcoholism, or liver cirrhosis can lead to exacerbation of the underlying hepatic insufficiency. Assess hepatic function before initiating gemcitabine and periodically during treatment. Discontinue if severe liver injury develops.

• PRES has been reported in patients receiving gemcitabine alone or in combination with other chemotherapeutic agents. PRES can present with headache, seizure, lethargy, HTN, confusion, blindness, and other visual and neurologic disturbances. Confirm PRES diagnosis with MRI; discontinue gemcitabine if PRES develops during therapy.

• Safety and effectiveness in children haven't been determined.

Dialyzable drug: Unknown.

⚠ *Overdose S&S:* Myelosuppression, paresthesia, severe rash.

PREGNANCY-LACTATION-REPRODUCTION

• There are no adequate studies during pregnancy. Based on drug's mechanism of action, its use is expected to result in adverse reproductive effects. If drug is used during pregnancy or if patient becomes pregnant during therapy, apprise patient of potential fetal hazard.

• Patient should discontinue breastfeeding during treatment and for at least 1 week after final dose.

• Advise patient of childbearing potential to use effective contraception during treatment and for 6 months after final dose.

• Advise males with partners of childbearing potential to use effective contraception during treatment and for 3 months after final dose.

• May impair fertility in males of reproductive potential.

NURSING CONSIDERATIONS

• Verify pregnancy status before start of treatment.

• Monitor patient closely. Expect dosage modification according to toxicity and degree of myelosuppression. Age, gender, and presence of renal impairment may predispose patient to toxicity.

• Monitor hematologic values carefully, especially neutrophil and platelet counts.

• Obtain baseline and periodic renal and hepatic lab tests.

• *Look alike–sound alike:* Don't confuse gemcitabine with gemtuzumab.

PATIENT TEACHING

• Advise patient to report all adverse reactions and to immediately report evidence of infection (fever, sore throat, fatigue) and bleeding (easy bruising, nosebleeds, bleeding gums, melena). Tell patient to take temperature daily.

• Caution patient to immediately report changes in color or volume of urine output.

• Instruct patient to promptly report flulike symptoms, breathing problems, abdominal pain, or yellowing of skin.

• Tell patient that adverse effects may continue after treatment ends.

gemfibrozil
jem-FI-broe-zil

Lopid🔗

Therapeutic class: Antilipemics
Pharmacologic class: Fibric acid derivatives

AVAILABLE FORMS
Tablets: 600 mg

INDICATIONS & DOSAGES

➤ **As adjunct to diet in adults with hypertriglyceridemia (types IV and V hyperlipidemia) unresponsive to diet and who are at risk for pancreatitis; to reduce risk of CAD in patients without CAD symptoms and with type IIb hyperlipidemia who are refractory to treatment with diet, exercise, and other drugs, and who have decreased HDL levels and increased LDL and triglyceride levels**

Adults: 1,200 mg PO daily in two divided doses.

ADMINISTRATION

PO
- Give drug 30 minutes before breakfast and dinner.
- Store at room temperature.

ACTION

Inhibits peripheral lipolysis and reduces triglyceride synthesis in the liver; lowers triglyceride and VLDL levels and increases HDL levels.

Route	Onset	Peak	Duration
PO	2–5 days	1–2 hr	Unknown

Half-life: 1.5 hours.

ADVERSE REACTIONS

CNS: fatigue, headache, vertigo. **GI:** abdominal and epigastric pain, dyspepsia, acute appendicitis, constipation, diarrhea, nausea, vomiting. **Hematologic:** *leukopenia, thrombocytopenia,* anemia, eosinophilia. **Hepatic:** bile duct obstruction. **Metabolic:** *hypokalemia.* **Skin:** dermatitis, eczema, pruritus, rash.

INTERACTIONS

Drug-drug. *Bile acid sequestrants (colestipol):* May decrease absorption of fibric acid derivatives. Separate doses by at least 2 hours to minimize interaction; fenofibric acid labeling recommends giving drug 1 hour before or 4 to 6 hours after a bile acid sequestrant.

Colchicine: May increase risk of myopathy, especially in patients with renal dysfunction and in older adults. Use cautiously.

Cyclosporine: May decrease cyclosporine level and increase risk of nephrotoxicity. Monitor renal function and cyclosporine level, and adjust dose as needed.

CYP2C8, CYP2C9, CYP2C19, OATP1B1 substrates (bosentan, dabrafenib, glyburide, loperamide, montelukast, olmesartan, paclitaxel, rosiglitazone, rifampin): May increase levels of substrates metabolized through these enzymes. Consider therapy modification or decrease substrate dose.

Dasabuvir: May prolong QT interval and increase risk of ventricular arrhythmias. Use together is contraindicated.

Enzalutamide: May increase enzalutamide exposure and risk of seizures. If use together is unavoidable, reduce enzalutamide dose.

Ezetimibe: May enhance adverse or toxic effect of ezetimibe; may increase risk of myopathy and cholelithiasis. Avoid combination.

Glyburide, pioglitazone: May increase hypoglycemic effects. Monitor glucose level, and watch for signs of hypoglycemia.

HMG-CoA reductase inhibitors: May cause myopathy with rhabdomyolysis. Avoid using together. Use with simvastatin is contraindicated.

Repaglinide: May increase risk of severe hypoglycemia. Concurrent use is contraindicated.

Selexipag: May increase selexipag exposure. Concomitant use is contraindicated.

Warfarin: May prolong PT and increase bleeding risk. Reduce warfarin dosage and monitor PT and INR.

EFFECTS ON LAB TEST RESULTS

- May increase ALT, AST, ALP, bilirubin, and CK levels.
- May decrease potassium level.
- May decrease Hb level, hematocrit, and eosinophil, WBC, and platelet counts.

CONTRAINDICATIONS & CAUTIONS

- Contraindicated in patients hypersensitive to drug and in those with hepatic or severe renal dysfunction (including primary biliary cirrhosis) or gallbladder disease.
- The 2018 American College of Cardiology/American Heart Association Multisociety guidelines on cholesterol recommend avoiding use of gemfibrozil with all statins.
- Evaluate patient for secondary causes of hyperlipidemia before use.
- May increase risk of malignancy, gall stones, and myositis.
- Safety and effectiveness in children haven't been established.

Dialyzable drug: Unknown.

Reactions in bold italics are *life-threatening*. Interactions may have a *rapid onset* or a ***delayed onset***.

⚠ *Overdose S&S:* Abdominal cramps, abnormal LFT values, diarrhea, increased CK level, joint and muscle pain, nausea and vomiting.

PREGNANCY-LACTATION-REPRODUCTION
• Use in pregnancy only if potential benefit justifies fetal risk.
• Patient should discontinue breastfeeding or discontinue drug.

NURSING CONSIDERATIONS
• Check CBC and LFTs periodically during the first 12 months of therapy.
• If drug has shown no benefit after 3 months of therapy, stop drug.

PATIENT TEACHING
• Instruct patient to take drug 30 minutes before breakfast and dinner.
• Teach patient about proper dietary management of cholesterol and triglycerides. When appropriate, recommend weight control, exercise, and smoking cessation programs.
• Because of possible dizziness and blurred vision, advise patient to avoid driving and other hazardous activities until effects of drug are known.
• Tell patient to observe bowel movements and to report evidence of excess fat in feces or other signs of bile duct obstruction.
• Advise patient to report all adverse reactions and muscle pain to prescriber.

gentamicin sulfate (injection)
jen-ta-MYE-sin

Therapeutic class: Antibiotics
Pharmacologic class: Aminoglycosides

AVAILABLE FORMS
Injection: 10 mg/mL, 40 mg/mL
IV infusion (premixed): 60 mg, 80 mg, 100 mg in 50 mL NSS; 80 mg, 100 mg, 120 mg in 100 mL NSS

INDICATIONS & DOSAGES
➤ **Serious infections caused by sensitive strains of *Pseudomonas aeruginosa, Escherichia coli, Proteus, Klebsiella, Enterobacter, Serratia, Citrobacter,* or *Staphylococcus***
Adults: 3 mg/kg IM or IV infusion daily in three divided doses every 8 hours. For life-threatening infections, may give up to 5 mg/kg daily in divided doses every 8 hours; reduce dosage to 3 mg/kg daily as soon as patient improves.
Children: 2 to 2.5 mg/kg IM or IV infusion every 8 hours.
Neonates older than 1 week and infants: 2.5 mg/kg IM or IV infusion every 8 hours.
Neonates younger than 1 week and preterm infants: 2.5 mg/kg IM or IV infusion every 12 hours.
Adjust-a-dose: For adults with impaired renal function, dosages and frequency are determined by drug level and renal function. Refer to manufacturer's instructions for renal function dosage adjustments. To maintain therapeutic levels, adults should receive 1 to 1.7 mg/kg IM or IV infusion after each dialysis session, and children should receive 2 to 2.5 mg/kg IM or IV infusion after each dialysis session.

ADMINISTRATION
IV
▼ Obtain specimen for culture and sensitivity tests before giving. Begin therapy while awaiting results.
▼ For intermittent infusion, dilute vial with 50 to 200 mL of D_5W or NSS for injection. For infants and children, the diluent volume should be less, but allow for accurate measurement and administration. Maximum concentration isn't addressed by the manufacturer; the concentration of the pediatric-specific product is 10 mg/mL.
▼ Infuse over 30 minutes to 2 hours.
▼ After completing infusion, flush the line with NSS or D_5W.
▼ Premixed, single-dose, flexible containers should be administered IV only.
▼ **Incompatibilities:** Don't physically premix gentamicin with other drugs; administer separately according to the recommended route of administration and dosage schedule.
IM
• Obtain specimen for culture and sensitivity tests before giving. Begin therapy while awaiting results.
• Obtain blood for peak level 1 hour after IM injection or 30 minutes after IV infusion finishes; for trough levels, draw blood just before next dose. Don't collect blood in a heparinized tube; heparin is incompatible with aminoglycosides.

• Give undiluted. Gentamicin in NSS isn't intended for IM administration.

ACTION
Inhibits protein synthesis by binding directly to the 30S ribosomal subunit; bactericidal.

Route	Onset	Peak	Duration
IV	Immediate	30–60 min	Unknown
IM	Unknown	30–90 min	Unknown

Half-life: 2 to 3 hours; longer in patients with renal impairment and in infants.

ADVERSE REACTIONS
CNS: *encephalopathy, seizures,* fever, headache, lethargy, confusion, dizziness, numbness, depression, peripheral neuropathy, tingling. **CV:** hypotension, HTN. **EENT:** vision disturbance, tinnitus, vertigo, ototoxicity, increased salivation. **GI:** vomiting, nausea, decreased appetite, stomatitis. **GU:** increased BUN and creatinine levels, oliguria, *nephrotoxicity*; increased urine protein, cells or casts. **Hematologic:** *granulocytopenia, transient agranulocytosis, leukopenia, thrombocytopenia,* anemia, eosinophilia. **Metabolic:** weight loss. **Musculoskeletal:** muscle twitching, myasthenia gravis–like syndrome, joint pain. **Respiratory:** *respiratory depression,* laryngeal edema, pulmonary fibrosis. **Skin:** rash, urticaria, pruritus, burning sensation, alopecia, pseudotumor cerebri, purpura, injection-site pain. **Other:** *anaphylactoid reaction.*

INTERACTIONS
Drug-drug. **Boxed Warning** *Amikacin, carboplatin, cephaloridine, cidofovir, cisplatin, colistin, neomycin, paramycin, polymyxin B, streptomycin, tobramycin, vancomycin, viomycin, other aminoglycosides:* May increase ototoxicity and nephrotoxicity. Monitor hearing and renal function test results. Avoid concurrent or sequential use. ■
Atracurium, pancuronium, rocuronium, vecuronium: May increase effects of nondepolarizing muscle relaxants, including prolonged respiratory depression. Use together only when necessary, and expect to reduce dosage of nondepolarizing muscle relaxant.
Bisphosphonate derivatives: May enhance hypocalcemic effect of bisphosphonate derivatives. Monitor therapy.
General anesthetics: May increase neuromuscular blockade. Monitor patient closely.

Indomethacin: May increase peak and trough levels of gentamicin. Monitor gentamicin level.
Boxed Warning *IV loop diuretics (ethacrynic acid, furosemide):* May increase risk of ototoxicity. Avoid use together. ■
Parenteral penicillins (ampicillin): May inactivate gentamicin in vitro. Don't mix together. ■

EFFECTS ON LAB TEST RESULTS
• May increase ALT, AST, bilirubin, BUN, creatinine, LDH, and nonprotein nitrogen levels.
• May decrease serum calcium, magnesium, sodium, and potassium levels.
• May increase eosinophil count.
• May decrease Hb level and platelet and WBC counts.

CONTRAINDICATIONS & CAUTIONS
• Contraindicated in patients hypersensitive to drug or other aminoglycosides.
• Use cautiously in neonates, infants, older adults, and patients with impaired renal function or neuromuscular disorders.
• Use drug for short-term treatment if possible. Prolonged use may result in fungal or bacterial superinfection, including CDAD.
Dialyzable drug: 50%.
⚠ *Overdose S&S:* Nephrotoxicity, neurotoxicity, ototoxicity.

PREGNANCY-LACTATION-REPRODUCTION
Boxed Warning Aminoglycosides can cause fetal harm when used during pregnancy. ■
• If drug is used during pregnancy or if patient becomes pregnant during therapy, apprise patient of potential fetal hazard (deafness).
• Drug appears in human milk.

NURSING CONSIDERATIONS
Boxed Warning Evaluate patient's hearing before and during therapy. Notify prescriber if patient complains of tinnitus, vertigo, or hearing loss. Anticipate dosage adjustment or drug discontinuation. ■
• Weigh patient and review renal function studies before therapy begins.
⚡ *Alert:* Use preservative-free form when intrathecal or intraventricular route is used adjunctively for serious CNS infections, such as meningitis and ventriculitis.
Boxed Warning Maintain peak levels at 4 to 12 mcg/mL and trough levels at 1 to

---

Reactions in bold italics are *life-threatening*. Interactions may have a *rapid onset* or a *delayed onset*.

2 mcg/mL. Prolonged peak levels above 12 mcg/mL or prolonged trough levels greater than 2 mcg/mL may increase risk of toxicity. Hemodialysis may help remove gentamicin, especially with compromised renal function. Peritoneal dialysis is considerably less effective than hemodialysis. ■

Boxed Warning Nephrotoxicity risk is greater in patients with renal impairment and in those who receive high-dosage or prolonged therapy. Monitor renal function: urine output, specific gravity, urinalysis, BUN and creatinine levels, and CrCl. Report to prescriber evidence of declining renal function. ■

Boxed Warning Older adults and patients with dehydration are at increased risk for toxicity. ■

• Watch for signs and symptoms of superinfection (especially of upper respiratory tract), such as continued fever, chills, and increased pulse rate.

• Therapy usually continues for 7 to 10 days. If no response occurs in 3 to 5 days, stop therapy and obtain new specimens for culture and sensitivity testing.

PATIENT TEACHING

• Instruct patient to promptly report adverse reactions, such as vision changes, dizziness, vertigo, unsteady gait, ringing in the ears, hearing loss, numbness, tingling, muscle twitching, seizures, changes in urine amount, edema.

• Encourage patient to drink plenty of fluids to avoid dehydration.

• Warn patient to avoid hazardous activities if adverse CNS reactions occur.

SAFETY ALERT!

glatiramer acetate
gla-TIR-a-mer

Copaxone, Glatopa

Therapeutic class: MS drugs
Pharmacologic class: Biological response modifiers

AVAILABLE FORMS

Injection: 20 mg glatiramer acetate and 40 mg mannitol (20 mg/mL); 40 mg glatiramer acetate and 40 mg mannitol (40 mg/mL) single-use prefilled syringe

INDICATIONS & DOSAGES

➤ **Relapsing forms of MS, including clinically isolated syndrome, relapsing-remitting disease, and active secondary progressive disease**

Adults: 20 mg subcut daily, or 40 mg subcut three times per week given at least 48 hours apart.

ADMINISTRATION
Subcutaneous

⚠ *Alert:* 20 mg/mL and 40 mg/mL formulations of glatiramer aren't interchangeable.

• Give drug only subcut in arms, abdomen, hips, or thighs; rotate injection sites to prevent lipoatrophy. Don't give IV.

• Administer 40-mg dose on same 3 days each week (eg, Monday, Wednesday, Friday) at least 48 hours apart.

• Drug doesn't contain preservatives; discard if solution is cloudy or contains particulate matter.

• Don't try to expel the air bubble from the prefilled syringe. This may lead to loss of drug and an incorrect dose.

• An optional autoinjector is available by separate prescription for use with Copaxone. Ensure autoinjector is compatible before use to avoid administering a partial dose or other medication error.

• Store drug in refrigerator (36° to 46° F [2° to 8° C]); allow drug to warm to room temperature for 20 minutes before use.

• If refrigeration isn't available, may store at room temperature for up to 1 month.

• Avoid exposure to higher temperatures; protect from intense light. Don't freeze; discard if syringe freezes.

ACTION

May modify immune processes responsible for the pathogenesis of MS.

Route	Onset	Peak	Duration
Subcut	Unknown	Unknown	Unknown

Half-life: Unknown.

ADVERSE REACTIONS

CNS: anxiety, asthenia, abnormal dreams, emotional lability, fever, migraine, nervousness, pain, speech disorder, stupor, syncope, tremor. **CV:** chest pain, palpitations, vasodilation, HTN, tachycardia, edema. **EENT:** eye disorder, diplopia, visual field deficit, rhinitis, oral candidiasis, salivary gland enlargement, dental caries, *laryngospasm,* nasopharyngitis. **GI:** nausea, dysphagia, bowel urgency, gastroenteritis, ulcerative stomatitis, vomiting. **GU:** urinary urgency, *vaginal hemorrhage,* abnormal Papanicolaou smear, amenorrhea, hematuria, erectile dysfunction, menorrhagia, vaginal candidiasis. **Hematologic:** lymphadenopathy. **Metabolic:** weight gain. **Musculoskeletal:** arthralgia, back pain. **Respiratory:** dyspnea, cough, bronchitis, hyperventilation. **Skin:** diaphoresis, injection-site reaction, pruritus, rash, eczema, erythema, residual mass at injection site, benign neoplasm (cyst, polyp), skin atrophy, urticaria, warts. **Other:** hypersensitivity, flu-like syndrome, infection, abscess, chills, hay fever, herpes simplex and zoster.

INTERACTIONS

Drug-drug. *Denosumab, natalizumab, roflumilast:* May increase risk of serious infection. Consider therapy modification.
Leflunomide: May increase risk of hematologic toxicity, such as pancytopenia, agranulocytosis, or thrombocytopenia. Consider therapy modification.
Live-virus vaccines: Immunosuppressants may enhance adverse or toxic effect of live-virus vaccines. Avoid use for at least 3 months after immunosuppressive therapy.
Pimecrolimus, tacrolimus (topical): May enhance adverse or toxic effect of immunosuppressants. Avoid this combination.
Tofacitinib: May enhance immunosuppressive effect of tofacitinib. Avoid combination.
Trastuzumab: May enhance neutropenic effect of immunosuppressants. Monitor therapy.
Drug-herb. *Echinacea:* May diminish therapeutic effect of immunosuppressants. Consider therapy modification.

EFFECTS ON LAB TEST RESULTS

- May increase cholesterol level and LFT values.
- May diminish diagnostic effect of coccidioidin skin test.

CONTRAINDICATIONS & CAUTIONS

- Contraindicated in patients hypersensitive to drug or mannitol.
- Drug may increase risk of infection and hepatic injury.
- Safety and effectiveness in children haven't been established.
Dialyzable drug: Unknown.

PREGNANCY-LACTATION-REPRODUCTION

- There are no well-controlled studies during pregnancy. Use in pregnancy only if clearly needed.
- Use cautiously during breastfeeding.

NURSING CONSIDERATIONS

- Immediate postinjection reactions may occur; symptoms include flushing, chest pain, palpitations, anxiety, dyspnea, constriction of the throat, and urticaria. They typically are transient and self-limiting and don't need specific treatment. Onset of postinjection reaction may occur several months after treatment starts, and patients may have more than one episode.
- Patient may experience at least one episode of transient chest pain, which usually begins at least 1 month after treatment starts; it isn't accompanied by other signs or symptoms.
- Monitor patient for injection-site reactions.
- Monitor patient for signs or symptoms of liver dysfunction (nausea, anorexia, fatigue, jaundice, dark-colored urine, pale stools, increased bleeding or bruising).

PATIENT TEACHING

- Instruct patient how to self-inject drug. Supervise first injection. Injection sites include arms, abdomen, hips, and thighs.
- Tell patient to rotate injection sites daily.
- Explain need for aseptic self-injection techniques, and warn patient against reuse of needles and syringes. Periodically review proper disposal of needles, syringes, drug containers, and unused drug.
- Instruct patient to notify prescriber about planned, suspected, or known pregnancy.
- Tell patient to notify prescriber if breastfeeding.
- Advise patient not to change drug or dosage schedule or to stop drug without medical approval.
- Tell patient to notify prescriber of all adverse reactions and to immediately report if dizziness, flushing, fast heartbeat, anxiety, breathing problems or tightness in throat, swelling, rash, itching, hives, diaphoresis, chest pain, or severe pain occurs after drug injection.
- Warn patient to seek medical attention for chest pain of unusual duration or intensity.
- Inform patient that an autoinjector may be prescribed for Copaxone and to ensure syringe compatibility before use.

Reactions in bold italics are *life-threatening*. Interactions may have a *rapid onset* or a **delayed onset**.

glecaprevir–pibrentasvir ⌘
glek-A-pre-vir/pi-BRENT-as-vir

Mavyret

Therapeutic class: Antivirals
Pharmacologic class: HCV NS3/4A
protease inhibitors–HCV NS5A inhibitors

AVAILABLE FORMS
Oral pellets ⓄTC: 50 mg glecaprevir/20 mg
pibrentasvir
Tablets: 100 mg glecaprevir/40 mg
pibrentasvir

INDICATIONS & DOSAGES
Adjust-a-dose (for all indications): In patients
age 3 and older who have received a liver or
kidney transplant, a 12-week treatment duration is recommended. In patients with a genotype 1 infection who are NS5A inhibitor–
experienced without prior treatment with an
NS3/4A protease inhibitor or patients with
genotype 3 infection, a 16-week treatment duration is recommended.

➤ **Chronic HCV genotype 1, 2, 3, 4, 5, or
6 infection in patients who are treatment-
naive without cirrhosis or with compensated cirrhosis (Child-Pugh class A)** ⌘
*Adults and children age 12 and older or
weighing at least 45 kg:* 3 tablets (total daily
dose of 300 mg glecaprevir/120 mg pibrentasvir) PO once daily for 8 weeks.
*Children age 3 and older or weighing at
least 45 kg:* 300 mg glecaprevir/120 mg pibrentasvir PO once daily for 8 weeks.
*Children age 3 and older or weighing 30 to
less than 45 kg:* 250 mg glecaprevir/100 mg
pibrentasvir PO once daily for 8 weeks.
*Children age 3 and older weighing 20 to less
than 30 kg:* 200 mg glecaprevir/80 mg pibrentasvir PO once daily for 8 weeks.
*Children age 3 and older weighing less than
20 kg:* 150 mg glecaprevir/60 mg pibrentasvir
PO once daily for 8 weeks.

➤ **HCV genotype 1 infection with or without compensated cirrhosis (Child-Pugh
class A) in patients previously treated with
a regimen containing an HCV NS5A inhibitor but without an NS3/4A protease inhibitor (PI)** ⌘
*Adults and children age 12 and older or
weighing at least 45 kg:* 3 tablets (total daily

dose of 300 mg glecaprevir/120 mg pibrentasvir) PO once daily for 16 weeks.
*Children age 3 and older or weighing at
least 45 kg:* 300 mg glecaprevir/120 mg pibrentasvir PO once daily for 16 weeks.
*Children age 3 and older or weighing 30 to
less than 45 kg:* 250 mg glecaprevir/100 mg
pibrentasvir PO once daily for 16 weeks.
*Children age 3 and older weighing 20 to less
than 30 kg:* 200 mg glecaprevir/80 mg pibrentasvir PO once daily for 16 weeks.
*Children age 3 and older weighing less than
20 kg:* 150 mg glecaprevir/60 mg pibrentasvir
PO once daily for 16 weeks.

➤ **HCV genotype 1 infection with or without compensated cirrhosis (Child-Pugh
class A) in patients who previously received
an NS3/4A PI without prior treatment with
an NS5A inhibitor** ⌘
*Adults and children age 12 and older or
weighing at least 45 kg:* 3 tablets (total daily
dose of 300 mg glecaprevir/120 mg pibrentasvir) PO once daily for 12 weeks.
*Children age 3 and older or weighing at
least 45 kg:* 300 mg glecaprevir/120 mg pibrentasvir PO once daily for 12 weeks.
*Children age 3 and older or weighing 30 to
less than 45 kg:* 250 mg glecaprevir/100 mg
pibrentasvir PO once daily for 12 weeks.
*Children age 3 and older weighing 20 to less
than 30 kg:* 200 mg glecaprevir/80 mg pibrentasvir PO once daily for 12 weeks.
*Children age 3 and older weighing less than
20 kg:* 150 mg glecaprevir/60 mg pibrentasvir
PO once daily for 12 weeks.

➤ **HCV genotype 1, 2, 4, 5, or 6 infection
without cirrhosis in patients who previously received regimens containing interferon, pegylated interferon, ribavirin, or
sofosbuvir but have no prior treatment experience with an HCV NS3/4A PI or NS5A
inhibitor** ⌘
*Adults and children age 12 and older or
weighing at least 45 kg:* 3 tablets (total daily
dose of 300 mg glecaprevir/120 mg pibrentasvir) PO once daily for 8 weeks.
*Children age 3 and older or weighing at
least 45 kg:* 300 mg glecaprevir/120 mg pibrentasvir PO once daily for 8 weeks.
*Children age 3 and older or weighing 30 to
less than 45 kg:* 250 mg glecaprevir/100 mg
pibrentasvir PO once daily for 8 weeks.
*Children age 3 and older weighing 20 to less
than 30 kg:* 200 mg glecaprevir/80 mg pibrentasvir PO once daily for 8 weeks.

G

Children age 3 and older weighing less than 20 kg: 150 mg glecaprevir/60 mg pibrentasvir PO once daily for 8 weeks.

▶ **HCV genotype 1, 2, 4, 5, or 6 infection and compensated cirrhosis (Child-Pugh class A) in patients who previously received regimens containing interferon, pegylated interferon, ribavirin, or sofosbuvir but have no prior treatment experience with an HCV NS3/4A PI or NS5A inhibitor**

Adults and children age 12 and older or weighing at least 45 kg: 3 tablets (total daily dose of 300 mg glecaprevir/120 mg pibrentasvir) PO once daily for 12 weeks.

Children age 3 and older or weighing at least 45 kg: 300 mg glecaprevir/120 mg pibrentasvir PO once daily for 12 weeks.

Children age 3 and older or weighing 30 to less than 45 kg: 250 mg glecaprevir/100 mg pibrentasvir PO once daily for 12 weeks.

Children age 3 and older weighing 20 to less than 30 kg: 200 mg glecaprevir/80 mg pibrentasvir PO once daily for 12 weeks.

Children age 3 and older weighing less than 20 kg: 150 mg glecaprevir/60 mg pibrentasvir PO once daily for 12 weeks.

▶ **HCV genotype 3 infection with or without cirrhosis (Child-Pugh class A) in patients who previously received regimens containing interferon, pegylated interferon, ribavirin, or sofosbuvir but have no prior treatment experience with an HCV NS3/4A PI or NS5A inhibitor**

Adults and children age 12 and older or weighing at least 45 kg: 3 tablets (total daily dose of 300 mg glecaprevir/120 mg pibrentasvir) PO once daily for 16 weeks.

Children age 3 and older or weighing at least 45 kg: 300 mg glecaprevir/120 mg pibrentasvir PO once daily for 16 weeks.

Children age 3 and older or weighing 30 to less than 45 kg: 250 mg glecaprevir/100 mg pibrentasvir PO once daily for 16 weeks.

Children age 3 and older weighing 20 to less than 30 kg: 200 mg glecaprevir/80 mg pibrentasvir PO once daily for 16 weeks.

Children age 3 and older weighing less than 20 kg: 150 mg glecaprevir/60 mg pibrentasvir PO once daily for 16 weeks.

ADMINISTRATION
PO
• Give with food.
• Sprinkle pellets on a small amount of soft food low in water content that sticks to a spoon (peanut butter, chocolate hazelnut spread, cream cheese, thick jam, Greek yogurt); pellets mixed in liquid or food that would slide off a spoon may dissolve and become less effective.

• Give pellets with food within 15 minutes of preparation and have patient swallow dose without chewing.

• Give a missed dose as soon as possible if it's less than 18 hours from the scheduled time; then resume normal schedule. If it has been more than 18 hours from the scheduled time, skip missed dose; then resume normal schedule.

• Store at or below 86° F (30° C).

ACTION
Glecaprevir is an HCV NS3/4A protease inhibitor; pibrentasvir is an HCV NS5A inhibitor. Both are direct-acting antivirals that prevent viral replication of HCV.

Route	Onset	Peak	Duration
PO	Unknown	5 hr	Unknown

Half-life: Glecaprevir, 6 hours; pibrentasvir, 13 hours.

ADVERSE REACTIONS
CNS: headache, fatigue, asthenia. **GI:** nausea, diarrhea. **Metabolic:** hyperbilirubinemia. **Skin:** pruritus.

INTERACTIONS
Drug-drug. *Atazanavir:* May increase glecaprevir and pibrentasvir levels and ALT level. Use together is contraindicated.

Atorvastatin, lovastatin, simvastatin: May increase statin level, increasing risk of myopathy and rhabdomyolysis. Use together isn't recommended.

Carbamazepine, efavirenz: May decrease glecaprevir and pibrentasvir levels. Use together isn't recommended.

Cyclosporine: May increase glecaprevir and pibrentasvir levels. Coadministration isn't recommended in patients requiring more than 100 mg cyclosporine/day.

Dabigatran: May increase dabigatran level. Refer to dabigatran prescribing information for dosage modifications in combination with P-gp inhibitors in patients with renal impairment.

Darunavir, lopinavir, ritonavir: May increase glecaprevir and pibrentasvir levels. Use together isn't recommended.

Reactions in bold italics are *life-threatening*. Interactions may have a *rapid onset* or a *delayed onset*.

Digoxin: May increase digoxin level. Measure digoxin level before therapy with glecaprevir and pibrentasvir. Decrease digoxin dosage by 50% or by modifying dosing and frequency; continue monitoring.

Ethinyl estradiol: May increase ALT level. Use together isn't recommended.

Fluvastatin, pitavastatin: May increase fluvastatin and pitavastatin levels, increasing risk of myopathy and rhabdomyolysis. Use lowest approved dosage of fluvastatin and pitavastatin. If higher doses are needed, use lowest dosage necessary based on risk and benefit analysis.

Pravastatin: May increase pravastatin level, increasing risk of myopathy and rhabdomyolysis. Reduce pravastatin dosage by 50%.

Rifampin: May decrease glecaprevir and pibrentasvir levels and their therapeutic effect. Use together is contraindicated.

Rosuvastatin: May increase rosuvastatin level, increasing risk of myopathy and rhabdomyolysis. Don't exceed 10 mg of rosuvastatin.

Warfarin: May alter INR. Monitor INR closely.

Drug-herb. *St. John's wort:* May decrease glecaprevir and pibrentasvir levels and reduce their therapeutic effect. Discourage use together.

EFFECTS ON LAB TEST RESULTS
• May increase total bilirubin level.

CONTRAINDICATIONS & CAUTIONS
• Contraindicated in patients with moderate or severe hepatic impairment (Child-Pugh class B or C) and in those with history of prior hepatic decompensation.

🔆 *Alert:* Use cautiously in patients with risk factors for liver failure (hepatocellular carcinoma, alcohol abuse, portal hypertension).

Boxed Warning HBV reactivation may occur and can result in fulminant hepatitis, hepatic failure, and death. ∎

• Safety and effectiveness in children younger than age 3 haven't been studied.

Dialyzable drug: No.

PREGNANCY-LACTATION-REPRODUCTION
• There are no studies during pregnancy. Patients should postpone pregnancy until therapy completion.

• It isn't known if drug appears in human milk. Consider benefit to patient against possible risk to the infant.

NURSING CONSIDERATIONS
Boxed Warning Before initiating treatment, test all patients for evidence of current or prior HBV infection by measuring HBsAg and hepatitis B core antigen (anti-HBc). ∎

Boxed Warning Monitor patients coinfected with HCV and HBV for hepatitis flare or HBV reactivation during HCV treatment and posttreatment follow-up. Initiate appropriate management for HBV infection as clinically indicated. ∎

🔆 *Alert:* Monitor patients closely for liver failure; discontinue drug in patients who develop signs and symptoms of decompensation or as clinically indicated.

• Monitor LFT values at baseline and periodically when clinically indicated.

• Monitor patients for changes in glucose tolerance. Modification of antidiabetic therapy may be necessary.

• *Look alike–sound alike:* Don't confuse Mavyret with Mavik.

PATIENT TEACHING
Boxed Warning Teach patient about risk of HBV reactivation in patients coinfected with HBV during or after treatment of HCV infection. Advise patient to tell prescriber about a history of HBV infection. ∎

• Advise patient to report all medications being taken, including OTC and herbal agents, because of the risk of drug interactions.

• Inform patient of the risk of hypoglycemia, particularly within first 3 months of therapy, and that antidiabetic dosage modification may be necessary.

• Tell patient to report all adverse reactions and to immediately report signs and symptoms of hepatic impairment (fatigue, abdominal pain, nausea, vomiting, dark urine, light-colored stools, yellowing of the skin or eyes).

• Instruct patient not to skip doses and to take drug for entire treatment duration.

glimepiride
glye-MEH-per-ide

Amaryl

Therapeutic class: Antidiabetics
Pharmacologic class: Sulfonylureas

AVAILABLE FORMS
Tablets: 1 mg, 2 mg, 3 mg, 4 mg

INDICATIONS & DOSAGES
➤ **Adjunct to diet and exercise to lower glucose level in patients with type 2 diabetes**
Adults: Initially, 1 or 2 mg PO once daily; usual maintenance dose is 1 to 4 mg PO once daily. After reaching 2 mg, dosage is increased in increments not exceeding 2 mg every 1 to 2 weeks, based on patient's glucose level response. Maximum dose is 8 mg daily.
Adjust-a-dose: For patients with renal impairment, those at risk for hypoglycemia, and older adults, initially, 1 mg PO once daily; then adjust cautiously to appropriate dosage, if needed. If transferring to glimepiride from longer half-life sulfonylureas (e.g., chlorpropamide), overlapping drug effect may occur for 1 to 2 weeks; monitor patient closely for hypoglycemia.

ADMINISTRATION
PO
- Give drug with breakfast or first main meal of the day.
- Patients on nothing-by-mouth status or those requiring decreased caloric intake may need doses withheld to avoid hypoglycemia.

ACTION
Lowers glucose level by stimulating release of insulin from functioning pancreatic beta cells, and may lead to increased sensitivity of peripheral tissues to insulin.

Route	Onset	Peak	Duration
PO	1 hr	2–3 hr	>24 hr

Half-life: 5 to 9 hours.

ADVERSE REACTIONS
CNS: dizziness, asthenia, headache. **GI:** nausea. **Hepatic:** increased ALT level. **Metabolic:** *hypoglycemia,* dilutional hyponatremia, weight gain. **Other:** accidental injury, flulike symptoms.

INTERACTIONS
Many drugs affect glucose metabolism, which may require glimepiride dosage adjustment. Monitor glycemic control closely. Consult manufacturer's product information for additional information.
Drug-drug. *Beta blockers, clonidine:* May mask symptoms of hypoglycemia. Monitor glucose level.
Colesevelam: May decrease glimepiride serum concentration. Give glimepiride at least 4 hours before colesevelam. Consider therapy modification.
CYP2C9 inducers (rifampin)/inhibitors (fluconazole): Inducers may increase glimepiride metabolism, leading to worsening glycemic control; inhibitors may decrease glimepiride metabolism, leading to hypoglycemia. Monitor therapy.
Drugs that tend to produce hyperglycemia (corticosteroids, estrogens, fosphenytoin, hormonal contraceptives, isoniazid, nicotinic acid, phenothiazines, phenytoin, thyroid products): May lead to loss of glucose control. Adjust dosage.
Insulin: May increase risk of hypoglycemia. Use together cautiously.
Miconazole (oral): May increase serum concentration and enhance hypoglycemic effect of glimepiride. Monitor therapy.
NSAIDs, other drugs that are highly protein-bound (beta blockers, chloramphenicol, coumarin, MAO inhibitors, probenecid, sulfonamides): May increase hypoglycemic action of sulfonylureas such as glimepiride. Monitor glucose level carefully.
Rifamycins, thiazide diuretics: May increase risk of hyperglycemia. Monitor glucose level.
Salicylates: May increase hypoglycemic effects of sulfonylurea. Monitor glucose level.
Warfarin: Sulfonylureas may enhance anticoagulant effect of vitamin K antagonists; vitamin K antagonists may enhance hypoglycemic effect of sulfonylureas. Monitor therapy.
Drug-herb. *Herbs with hypoglycemic properties:* May enhance hypoglycemic effect of glimepiride. Monitor therapy.
Drug-lifestyle. *Alcohol use:* May alter glycemic control, most commonly causing hypoglycemia. May also cause disulfiram-like reaction. Discourage use together.

Reactions in bold italics are *life-threatening*. Interactions may have a *rapid onset* or a *delayed onset*.

EFFECTS ON LAB TEST RESULTS
• May increase ALT, AST, BUN, and creatinine levels.
• May decrease glucose and sodium levels.
• May decrease Hb level and granulocyte, platelet, RBC, and WBC counts.

CONTRAINDICATIONS & CAUTIONS
• Contraindicated in patients hypersensitive to drug or sulfonamides.
• Contraindicated as therapy for type 1 diabetes or diabetic ketoacidosis as drug wouldn't be effective.
◐ **Alert:** Use of oral antidiabetics may carry higher risk of CV mortality than use of diet alone or of diet and insulin therapy.
• Use cautiously in patients who are debilitated or malnourished and in those with adrenal, pituitary, or renal insufficiency; these patients are more susceptible to the hypoglycemic action of glucose-lowering drugs.
• Use cautiously with drugs that can cause hypoglycemia.
• Use cautiously in older adults.
▨ Patients with G6PD deficiency may be at increased risk for sulfonylurea-induced hemolytic anemia. Use cautiously and consider therapy modification.
• Safety and effectiveness in children haven't been established.
Dialyzable drug: Unknown.
⚠ **Overdose S&S:** Hypoglycemia.

PREGNANCY-LACTATION-REPRODUCTION
• Use in pregnancy only if potential benefit justifies fetal risk.
◐ **Alert:** Prolonged severe hypoglycemia (4 to 10 days) has been reported in neonates born to patients receiving a sulfonylurea at time of delivery. Discontinue drug at least 2 weeks before expected delivery.
• May cause hypoglycemia in infants who are breastfed. Consider risk of exposure to the infant, benefits of breastfeeding, and benefits of treatment for the patient. Monitor infant who is breastfeeding for signs and symptoms of hypoglycemia (jitters, cyanosis, apnea, hypothermia, excessive sleepiness, poor feeding, seizures).

NURSING CONSIDERATIONS
• Glimepiride and insulin may be used together in patients who lose glucose control after first responding to therapy.

• Monitor fasting glucose level periodically to determine therapeutic response. Also monitor HbA$_{1c}$ level, usually every 3 to 6 months, to precisely assess long-term glycemic control.
• When changing patient from other sulfonylureas to glimepiryide, a transition period isn't needed. Monitor patient carefully for 1 to 2 weeks when changing from longer half-life sulfonylureas, such as chlorpropamide.
• *Look alike–sound alike:* Don't confuse glimepiride with glyburide or glipizide. Don't confuse Amaryl with Altace.

PATIENT TEACHING
• Instruct patient in safe drug administration.
• Make sure patient understands that therapy relieves symptoms but doesn't cure the disease. Patient should also understand risks and advantages of taking drug and of other treatment methods.
• Stress importance of adhering to diet, weight reduction, exercise, and personal hygiene programs. Explain to patient and family how and when to monitor glucose level, and teach recognition of and intervention for signs and symptoms of high and low glucose levels.
• Advise patient to wear or carry medical identification at all times.
• Instruct patient to consult prescriber before taking OTC products or supplements.
• Teach patient to carry candy or other simple sugars to treat mild episodes of low glucose level. Patient experiencing severe episode may need hospital treatment.
• Advise patient to avoid alcohol, which lowers glucose level.

SAFETY ALERT!

glipiZIDE ▨
GLIP-i-zide

Glucotrol XL◢

Therapeutic class: Antidiabetics
Pharmacologic class: Sulfonylureas

AVAILABLE FORMS
Tablets (extended-release) ⬤**:** 2.5 mg, 5 mg, 10 mg
Tablets (immediate-release): 5 mg, 10 mg

INDICATIONS & DOSAGES
➤ **Adjunct to diet and exercise to lower glucose level in patients with type 2 diabetes**
Immediate-release tablets
Adults: Initially, 5 mg PO daily 30 minutes before breakfast. Titrate by 2.5- to 5-mg increments no less than every few days based on blood glucose levels. Maximum once-daily dose is 15 mg. Divide doses of more than 15 mg. Maximum total daily dose is 40 mg.
Adjust-a-dose: For patients with hepatic or renal insufficiency, patients older than age 65, or patients who are debilitated or malnourished, initially give 2.5 mg PO daily.
Extended-release tablets
Adults: Initially, 2.5 to 5 mg PO with breakfast daily. Increase by 5 mg every 3 months, depending on level of glycemic control. Maximum daily dose is 20 mg.
➤ **To replace insulin therapy (immediate-release)**
Adults: If insulin dosage is 20 units or less daily, insulin may be stopped when glipizide starts. If insulin dosage is more than 20 units daily, start patient at usual dosage in addition to 50% of insulin dose. In some cases, especially if insulin dose is more than 40 units daily, it may be advisable to transition to glipizide in a hospital setting.

ADMINISTRATION
PO
- Give immediate-release tablet about 30 minutes before meals.
- Give extended-release tablet with breakfast.
- Don't split or crush extended-release tablets.
- Patients on nothing-by-mouth status or those requiring decreased caloric intake may need doses withheld to avoid hypoglycemia.

ACTION
Stimulates insulin release from pancreatic beta cells, reduces glucose output by the liver, and increases peripheral sensitivity to insulin.

Route	Onset	Peak	Duration
PO (immediate-release)	15–30 min	1–3 hr	12–24 hr
PO (extended-release)	2–3 hr	6–12 hr	12–24 hr

Half-life: 2 to 5 hours.

ADVERSE REACTIONS
CNS: dizziness, drowsiness, headache, nervousness, tremor. **GI:** nausea, dyspepsia, flatulence, constipation, diarrhea, vomiting. **Hematologic:** *leukopenia,* hemolytic anemia, *agranulocytosis, thrombocytopenia.* **Metabolic:** *hypoglycemia.* **Skin:** rash, pruritus, urticaria, photosensitivity reactions.

INTERACTIONS
Many drugs affect glucose metabolism, which may require glimepiride dosage adjustment. Monitor glycemic control closely. Consult manufacturer's product information for additional information.
Drug-drug. *Amantadine, anabolic steroids, antifungals, chloramphenicol, MAO inhibitors, NSAIDs, probenecid, quinolones, ranitidine,* **salicylates,** *sulfonamides:* May increase hypoglycemic activity. Monitor glucose level.
Beta blockers, clonidine: May prolong hypoglycemic effect and mask symptoms of hypoglycemia. Use together cautiously.
Colesevelam: May decrease glipizide serum concentration. Give glipizide at least 4 hours before colesevelam. Consider therapy modification.
Corticosteroids, glucagon, phenytoin, **rifamycins, thiazide diuretics:** May decrease hypoglycemic response. Monitor glucose level.
Fluconazole: May increase glipizide serum concentration, leading to hypoglycemia. Monitor patient closely.
Miconazole (oral): May increase serum concentration and enhance hypoglycemic effect of glipizide. Monitor therapy.
Oral anticoagulants: May increase hypoglycemic activity or enhance anticoagulant effect. Monitor glucose level, PT, and INR.
Drug-herb. *Herbs with hypoglycemic properties:* May enhance hypoglycemic effect of glipizide. Monitor therapy.
Drug-lifestyle. *Alcohol use:* May alter glycemic control, most commonly causing hypoglycemia. May cause disulfiram-like reaction. Discourage use together.

EFFECTS ON LAB TEST RESULTS
- May increase ALP, AST, LDH, BUN, cholesterol, and creatinine levels.
- May decrease glucose level.
- May decrease Hb level and granulocyte, platelet, and WBC counts.

Reactions in bold italics are *life-threatening*. Interactions may have a *rapid onset* or a ***delayed onset***.

CONTRAINDICATIONS & CAUTIONS
• Contraindicated in patients hypersensitive to drug or sulfonamides and in those with diabetic ketoacidosis with or without coma.

⚠ *Alert:* Use of oral antidiabetics may carry a higher risk of CV mortality than use of diet alone or of diet and insulin therapy.

☒ Patients with G6PD deficiency may be at increased risk for sulfonylurea-induced hemolytic anemia. Use cautiously and consider therapy modification.

• Use cautiously in patients with severe GI disease or renal or hepatic disease, in older adults, and in patients who are debilitated or malnourished.

Dialyzable drug: Unknown.

⚠ *Overdose S&S:* Hypoglycemia.

PREGNANCY-LACTATION-REPRODUCTION
• Insulin is drug of choice to control diabetes during pregnancy. If glipizide is used during pregnancy, discontinue at least 1 month before expected delivery date because prolonged severe hypoglycemia (4 to 10 days) has been reported in neonates born to mothers receiving a sulfonylurea at the time of delivery.

• Drug may cause hypoglycemia in infants who are breastfed. Consider risk of exposure to infant, benefits of breastfeeding, and benefits of treatment for patient. Monitor infant who is breastfeeding for signs and symptoms of hypoglycemia (jitters, cyanosis, apnea, hypothermia, excessive sleepiness, poor feeding, seizures).

NURSING CONSIDERATIONS
• Some patients may attain effective control on a once-daily regimen, whereas others respond better with divided dosing.

• Patient may switch from immediate-release to extended-release tablets at the nearest equivalent total daily dose.

• Glipizide is a second-generation sulfonylurea. The frequency of adverse reactions appears to be lower than with first-generation drugs such as chlorpropamide.

• During periods of increased stress, patient may need insulin therapy. Monitor patient closely for hyperglycemia in these situations.

• Patient switching from insulin therapy to an oral antidiabetic should check glucose level at least three times a day before meals. Patient may need hospitalization during transition.

• *Look alike–sound alike:* Don't confuse glipizide with glyburide or glimepiride.

PATIENT TEACHING
• Instruct patient about disease and importance of following therapeutic regimen, adhering to diet, losing weight, getting exercise, and avoiding infection. Explain how and when to monitor glucose level, and teach recognition of episodes of low and high glucose levels.

• Tell patient to carry candy or other simple sugars to treat mild low-glucose episodes. Patient experiencing severe episode may need hospital treatment.

• Caution patient not to change drug dosage without prescriber's consent and to report abnormal blood or urine glucose test results.

• Tell patient not to take other drugs, including OTC drugs, without first checking with prescriber.

• Advise patient to wear or carry medical identification at all times.

• Warn patient to avoid alcohol, which lowers glucose level.

• Inform patient that something resembling a tablet may appear in the stool; assure patient that it's the nonabsorbable shell of the extended-release tablet.

SAFETY ALERT!

glyBURIDE (glibenclamide) ☒
GLYE-byoor-ide

Glynase

Therapeutic class: Antidiabetics
Pharmacologic class: Sulfonylureas

AVAILABLE FORMS
Tablets: 1.25 mg, 2.5 mg, 5 mg
Tablets (micronized): 1.5 mg, 3 mg, 6 mg

INDICATIONS & DOSAGES
➤ **Adjunct to diet to lower glucose level in patients with type 2 diabetes**
Nonmicronized form
Adults: Initially, 2.5 to 5 mg PO once daily with breakfast or first main meal. Adjust to maintenance dose at no more than 2.5-mg increments at weekly intervals. Usual maintenance dose is 1.25 to 20 mg, in single dose or divided doses. For dosages exceeding

10 mg daily, b.i.d. dosing may achieve better response. Maximum daily dose is 20 mg PO.

Micronized form

Adults: Initially, 1.5 to 3 mg PO daily with breakfast or first main meal. Adjust to maintenance dose at no more than 1.5-mg increments at weekly intervals. Usual daily maintenance dose is 0.75 to 12 mg as a single dose or in divided doses. Dosages exceeding 6 mg daily may have better response with b.i.d. dosing. Maximum dose is 12 mg PO daily.

Adjust-a-dose: For older adults, patients who are more sensitive to antidiabetics, and those with renal, hepatic, adrenal, or pituitary insufficiency, start with 1.25 mg (nonmicronized) or 0.75 mg (micronized) daily.

➤ **To replace insulin therapy**

Adults: If insulin dose is less than 40 units/day, may switch patient directly to glyburide when insulin is stopped. If insulin dose is less than 20 units/day, initial dose is 2.5 to 5 mg (1.5 to 3 mg micronized) PO daily. If insulin dose is 20 to 40 units/day, initial dose is 5 mg (3 mg micronized) PO daily. If insulin dose is 40 or more units/day, initially, 5 mg (3 mg micronized) PO once daily in addition to 50% of insulin dose. Gradually taper off insulin as the glyburide dose is increased.

ADMINISTRATION
PO

• Give drug with breakfast or first main meal.
• Twice-daily dosing may be beneficial if conventional glyburide doses are greater than 10 mg or micronized glyburide doses are greater than 6 mg.
• Patients on nothing-by-mouth status or those requiring decreased caloric intake may need doses withheld to avoid hypoglycemia.

ACTION
Unknown. Probably stimulates insulin release from pancreatic beta cells, reduces glucose output by the liver, and increases peripheral sensitivity to insulin.

Route	Onset	Peak	Duration
PO (micronized)	1 hr	2–3 hr	<24 hr
PO (nonmicronized)	1 hr	2–4 hr	<24 hr

Half-life: 4 to 10 hours.

ADVERSE REACTIONS
GI: nausea, epigastric fullness, heartburn.
Hematologic: *leukopenia,* hemolytic anemia, *agranulocytosis, thrombocytopenia, aplastic anemia.* **Metabolic:** *hypoglycemia, hyponatremia.* **Musculoskeletal:** arthralgia, myalgia. **Skin:** rash, pruritus, other allergic reactions. **Other:** *angioedema.*

INTERACTIONS
Many drugs affect glucose metabolism, which may require glimepiride dosage adjustment. Monitor glycemic control closely. Consult manufacturer's product information for additional information.

Drug-drug. *Anabolic steroids, azole antifungals, chloramphenicol, fluoroquinolones, MAO inhibitors, NSAIDs, probenecid, ranitidine,* **salicylates,** *sulfonamides:* May increase hypoglycemic activity. Monitor glucose level.

Beta blockers: May prolong hypoglycemic effect and mask symptoms of hypoglycemia. Use together cautiously.

Bosentan: Increases risk of elevated LFT values. Use together is contraindicated.

Carbamazepine, corticosteroids, glucagon, **rifamycins, thiazide diuretics:** May decrease hypoglycemic response. Monitor glucose level.

Colesevelam: May decrease glyburide serum concentration. Give glyburide at least 4 hours before colesevelam.

CYP2C9 inducers (rifampin): May increase glimepiride metabolism, leading to worsening glycemic control; Monitor therapy.

CYP2C9 inhibitors (fluconazole): May decrease glimepiride metabolism, leading to hypoglycemia. Monitor therapy.

Miconazole (oral): May increase serum concentration and enhance hypoglycemic effect of glyburide. Monitor therapy.

Oral anticoagulants: May increase hypoglycemic activity or enhance anticoagulant effect. Monitor glucose level, PT, and INR.

Drug-herb. *Herbs with hypoglycemic properties:* May enhance hypoglycemic effect of glimepiride. Monitor therapy.

Drug-lifestyle. *Alcohol use:* May alter glycemic control, most commonly causing hypoglycemia. May cause disulfiram-like reaction. Discourage use together.

EFFECTS ON LAB TEST RESULTS
• May increase ALP, AST, ALT, bilirubin, BUN, and cholesterol levels.
• May decrease glucose and sodium levels.
• May decrease Hb level and granulocyte, platelet, and WBC counts.

Reactions in bold italics are *life-threatening*. Interactions may have a *rapid onset* or a ***delayed onset***.

CONTRAINDICATIONS & CAUTIONS
• Contraindicated in patients hypersensitive to drug and in those with type 1 diabetes or diabetic ketoacidosis with or without coma.

⚠ *Alert:* Oral antidiabetics may have a higher risk of CV mortality than use of diet alone or of diet and insulin therapy.

• Use cautiously in patients with hepatic or renal impairment (eGFR less than 60 mL/minute); in older adults and patients who are debilitated or malnourished; and in patients allergic to sulfonamides.

⚕ Patients with G6PD deficiency may be at increased risk for sulfonylurea-induced hemolytic anemia. Use cautiously and consider therapy modification.

• Safety and effectiveness in children haven't been established.

Dialyzable drug: Unknown.

⚠ *Overdose S&S:* Hypoglycemia.

PREGNANCY-LACTATION-REPRODUCTION
• Insulin is drug of choice to control diabetes during pregnancy. If glyburide is used during pregnancy, discontinue at least 2 weeks before expected delivery date.

⚠ *Alert:* Prolonged severe hypoglycemia (4 to 10 days) has been reported in neonates born to mothers receiving a sulfonylurea at the time of delivery.

• Drug may cause hypoglycemia in infants who are breastfed. Patient should discontinue breastfeeding or discontinue drug.

NURSING CONSIDERATIONS
⚠ *Alert:* Micronized glyburide (Glynase) contains drug in a smaller particle size and isn't bioequivalent to regular glyburide tablets. In patients who have been taking nonmicronized form, adjust dosage.

• Drug is a second-generation sulfonylurea. Adverse effects are less common with second-generation drugs than with first-generation drugs such as chlorpropamide.

• During periods of increased stress, such as infection, fever, surgery, or trauma, patient may need insulin therapy. Monitor patient closely for hyperglycemia in these situations.

• Patient switching from insulin therapy to an oral antidiabetic should check glucose level at least three times a day before meals. Patient may need hospitalization during transition.

• *Look alike–sound alike:* Don't confuse glyburide with glimepiride or glipizide.

PATIENT TEACHING
• Teach patient about diabetes and the importance of following therapeutic regimen, adhering to specific diet, losing weight, getting exercise, following personal hygiene programs, and avoiding infection. Explain how and when to monitor glucose level, and teach recognition of and intervention for low and high glucose levels.

• Tell patient not to change drug dosage without prescriber's consent and to report abnormal blood or urine glucose test results.

• Teach patient to carry candy or other simple sugars for mild low glucose level. Patient experiencing severe episode may need hospital treatment.

• Advise patient not to take supplements or other drugs, including OTC drugs, without first checking with prescriber.

• Caution patient to wear or carry medical identification at all times.

⚠ *Alert:* Instruct patient to report episodes of low glucose to prescriber immediately; a severely low glucose level is sometimes fatal in patients receiving as little as 2.5 to 5 mg daily.

• Advise patient to avoid alcohol, which may lower glucose level.

golimumab
go-LIM-ue-mab

Simponi, Simponi Aria

Therapeutic class: Antiarthritics
Pharmacologic class: TNF blockers

AVAILABLE FORMS
Injection (IV): 50 mg/4 mL single-dose vial
Injection (subcut): 50 mg/0.5 mL, 100 mg/mL prefilled syringe or prefilled autoinjector

INDICATIONS & DOSAGES
➤ **Moderate to severe active RA in combination with methotrexate; active psoriatic arthritis or active ankylosing spondylitis alone or in combination with methotrexate or other nonbiologic DMARDs**

Adults: 50 mg subcut monthly. Or 2 mg/kg IV infusion over 30 minutes at weeks 0 and 4, then every 8 weeks thereafter.

➤ **Moderate to severe ulcerative colitis in patients who have demonstrated an inadequate response or intolerance to**

prior treatment or who require continuous steroid therapy

Adults: Initially, 200 mg subcut, followed by 100 mg subcut at week 2, then 100 mg subcut every 4 weeks.

➤ **Active polyarticular juvenile idiopathic arthritis; active psoriatic arthritis**

Children age 2 and older: 80 mg/m^2 IV infusion over 30 minutes at weeks 0 and 4, and every 8 weeks thereafter.

ADMINISTRATION

● The efficacy and safety of switching between IV and subcut formulations and routes of administration haven't been established.

IV

▼ Dilute with NSS or half-NSS to a final volume of 100 mL.

▼ Administer over 30 minutes. Use a 0.22-micron low protein-binding filter.

▼ Don't infuse with other drugs in the same IV line.

▼ Solutions diluted for infusion may be stored at room temperature for 4 hours.

▼ **Incompatibilities:** Don't infuse concomitantly in same IV line with other agents; compatibility studies haven't been conducted.

Subcutaneous

● Remove drug from refrigerator 30 minutes before administration and allow it to reach room temperature.

● Inspect solution before administration. Don't use solution if discolored or cloudy or if foreign particles are present. Drug is normally colorless to slightly opalescent to light yellow.

● Prefilled syringe and prefilled autoinjector contain latex. Don't handle if sensitive to latex.

● To administer, hold autoinjector firmly against skin and inject subcut into thigh, lower abdomen (below navel), or upper arm. A loud click is heard when injection begins. Continue to hold autoinjector against skin until second click is heard (may take 3 to 15 seconds). After second click, lift autoinjector from injection site.

● Don't use any leftover product remaining in prefilled syringe or prefilled autoinjector.

● Rotate injection sites. Don't inject drug into areas where skin is tender, bruised, red, or hard.

● If multiple injections are required, administer injections at different sites on the body.

ACTION

Binds to human TNF-alpha to neutralize its activity and inhibit its binding with receptors, thereby reducing the infiltration of inflammatory cells.

Route	Onset	Peak	Duration
IV	Unknown	12 weeks	Unknown
Subcut	Unknown	2–6 days	Unknown

Half-life: 2 weeks.

ADVERSE REACTIONS

CNS: fever. **CV:** HTN. **EENT:** nasopharyngitis, oral herpes, pharyngitis, laryngitis, rhinitis. **Hematologic:** *leukopenia.* **Hepatic:** increase ALT level. **Respiratory:** bronchitis, URI. **Skin:** injection-site reactions, rash. **Other:** flulike syndrome, infection, antibody development.

INTERACTIONS

Drug-drug. *Abatacept, anakinra, other immunosuppressants:* May increase risk of serious infection. Avoid using together. *CYP450 substrates (cyclosporine, theophylline, warfarin):* May alter levels of these drugs. Monitor patient closely and adjust dosages as needed.

Live-virus vaccines: May increase risk of infection. Postpone live-virus vaccine until 3 months after therapy has ended.

EFFECTS ON LAB TEST RESULTS

● May increase LFT values.

● May decrease platelet, WBC, and neutrophil counts.

● May diminish diagnostic effect of coccidioidin skin test.

● May cause positive ANA titer.

CONTRAINDICATIONS & CAUTIONS

Boxed Warning Consider risks and benefits of treatment before start of therapy in patients with chronic or recurrent infection. ■

● Use cautiously in patients with malignancies; invasive fungal infection; hematologic abnormalities, or HF.

● Drug may increase risk of malignancies, especially when patient is receiving concomitant immunosuppressants.

● Drug may increase risk of or worsening demyelinating disorders, including multiple sclerosis and Guillain-Barré syndrome. Use cautiously in patients with preexisting or

---

recent onset of CNS or peripheral demyelination disorders.
Dialyzable drug: Unknown.

PREGNANCY-LACTATION-REPRODUCTION
• Use during pregnancy only if benefit justifies fetal risk and only if clearly needed.
• Administration of live-virus vaccines to infants exposed to golimumab in utero isn't recommended for 6 months after mother's last dose during pregnancy.
• It isn't known if drug appears in human milk. Patient should discontinue breastfeeding or discontinue drug.

NURSING CONSIDERATIONS
Boxed Warning Monitor patient closely for signs and symptoms of infection before and after treatment. TB, invasive fungal infection, and other bacterial and viral opportunistic infections, which are sometimes fatal, may occur in patients receiving golimumab. Stop drug if serious infection or sepsis develops during treatment. ▮
Boxed Warning Evaluate patient for latent TB with tuberculin skin test before initiating treatment. Treat latent TB before therapy with golimumab. Monitor all patients for active TB during treatment even if initial latent TB test is negative. ▮
• Drug increases risk of reactivation of HBV infection, which can be fatal, in patients who are HBV carriers. Before starting therapy, patient should be tested for HBV infection.
• Monitor patient for new or worsening HF; stop drug if signs and symptoms occur.
Boxed Warning Lymphoma and other malignancies, some fatal, have been reported in children and adolescents treated with TNF blockers, including golimumab. ▮
• Monitor patient for lymphomas and other malignancies.
• Pancytopenia and other significant cytopenias, including aplastic anemia, can occur. Monitor CBC regularly during therapy. May discontinue drug if hematologic abnormalities develop.

PATIENT TEACHING
• Teach patient how to give subcut injection. First self-injection should be under supervision of qualified health care practitioner.
• Advise patient that prefilled syringes and prefilled autoinjectors contain latex or a latex derivative.

• Instruct patient to report all adverse reactions, especially signs and symptoms of infection, new or worsening HF, or liver or nervous system problems.
• Tell patient to avoid live-virus vaccines while taking drug.

---

granisetron
gran-IZ-e-tron

Sancuso, Sustol

granisetron hydrochloride

Therapeutic class: Antiemetics
Pharmacologic class: 5-HT$_3$ receptor antagonists

AVAILABLE FORMS
Injection: 0.1 mg/mL, 1 mg/mL single-dose, preservative-free vials and 4-mL multidose vials containing benzyl alcohol
Injection (extended-release): 10 mg/0.4 mL prefilled syringe
Tablets: 1 mg
Transdermal patch: 3.1 mg per 24 hours

INDICATIONS & DOSAGES
➤ **Prevention of nausea and vomiting from emetogenic cancer chemotherapy**
Adults and children ages 2 to 16: 10 mcg/kg IV undiluted and given by direct injection over 30 seconds, or diluted and infused over 5 minutes. Start giving at least 30 minutes before chemotherapy. Or, for adults, 1 mg PO up to 1 hour before chemotherapy and repeated 12 hours later. Or, for adults, 2 mg PO daily given up to 1 hour before chemotherapy. Or, for adults, apply a single patch to the upper outer arm 24 to 48 hours before chemotherapy. Remove the patch a minimum of 24 hours after completion of chemotherapy or a maximum of 7 days.

Or, for adults, 10 mg extended-release form subcut with dexamethasone at least 30 minutes before chemotherapy on day 1. Don't give extended-release form more frequently than once every 7 days. Refer to manufacturer's instructions for dexamethasone dosages.
Adjust-a-dose: In patients with moderate renal impairment (CrCl of 30 to 59 mL/minute), don't give extended-release form more frequently than once every 14 days. Don't give

extended-release form to patients with severe renal impairment (CrCl of less than 30 mL/minute).

➤ **Prevention of nausea and vomiting from radiation, including total body irradiation and fractionated abdominal radiation**
Adults: 2 mg PO once daily within 1 hour of radiation.

➤ **Prevention of postoperative nausea and vomiting**
Adults: 1 mg IV over 30 seconds before anesthetic induction or immediately before reversal of anesthesia.

➤ **Postoperative nausea and vomiting**
Adults: 1 mg IV over 30 seconds after surgery.

ADMINISTRATION
PO
• Oral suspension may be compounded by a pharmacist for patients who can't swallow tablets.
• Store tablets between 68° and 77° F (20° and 25° C). Protect from light.
IV
▼ For direct injection, give drug undiluted over 30 seconds.
▼ For intermittent infusion, dilute with NSS for injection or D_5W to a volume of 20 to 50 mL.
▼ Infuse over 5 minutes, starting within 30 minutes before chemotherapy and only on days chemotherapy is given.
▼ Diluted solutions are stable for 24 hours at room temperature. Protect from light.
▼ Don't freeze vials.
▼ Once the multiuse vial is penetrated, use contents within 30 days.
▼ **Incompatibilities:** Other IV drugs.
Subcutaneous
• Extended-release form is for subcut injection only.
• Drug should only be administered by a health care provider.
• Remove extended-release form kit from refrigerator 1 hour before administration.
• Refer to manufacturer's syringe preparation instructions for warming syringe to body temperature using syringe warming pouches included in kit.
• Don't give drug if discoloration or particulate matter is noted in syringe; be aware that syringe is amber-colored glass.
• Give drug by subcut injection in the skin of the back of the upper arm or in the skin of the

abdomen at least 1 inch (2.54 cm) from the umbilicus.
• Topical anesthetic may be used at injection site before giving drug.
• Avoid injecting into skin that's burned, hardened, inflamed, swollen, or otherwise compromised.
• Give drug as a slow, sustained subcut injection over 20 to 30 seconds.
• Store in refrigerator at 36° to 46° F (2° to 8° C). Protect from light; don't freeze.
• Once drug has been removed from refrigerator, it can remain at room temperature for up to 7 days.
Transdermal
• Apply patch to clean, intact, healthy skin on the upper outer arm.
• Each patch is packed in a pouch and should be applied directly after the pouch has been opened.
• Don't cut patch into pieces.
• Don't apply heating pad or heat lamp over or in vicinity of transdermal system; avoid extended exposure to heat.
• Cover transdermal system application site with clothing if there's a risk of exposure to direct natural or artificial sunlight while patch is applied and for 10 days after its removal.
• Fold removed patch in half with sticky side together; discard to avoid accidental contact or ingestion by others.

ACTION
May block 5-HT_3 in the CNS in the chemoreceptor trigger zone and in the peripheral nervous system on nerve terminals of the vagus nerve.

Route	Onset	Peak	Duration
PO	Unknown	Unknown	24 hr
IV	1–3 min	Unknown	24 hr
Subcut (extended-release)	Unknown	11–12 hr	7 days
Transdermal	Unknown	48 hr	Unknown

Half-life: PO, IV, transdermal, 5 to 9 hours; extended-release, 24 hours.

ADVERSE REACTIONS
CNS: asthenia, headache, fever, agitation, anxiety, CNS stimulation, dizziness, insomnia, somnolence, pain, weakness, drowsiness, taste disorder, syncope. **CV:** HTN, hypotension, prolonged QT interval; flushing, atrial fibrillation (extended-release form).

Reactions in bold italics are *life-threatening*. Interactions may have a *rapid onset* or a ***delayed onset***.

GI: constipation, nausea, vomiting, abdominal pain, decreased appetite, diarrhea, dyspepsia, flatulence, GERD. **Hematologic:** anemia, *leukocytosis, leukopenia, thrombocytopenia.* **Hepatic:** increased ALT and AST levels. **Skin:** alopecia, rash, dermatitis, injection-site reactions, application-site reactions. **Other:** *hypersensitivity reactions.*

INTERACTIONS

Drug-drug. *Apomorphine:* May increase risk of profound hypotension and loss of consciousness. Avoid use together.
Drugs that prolong QT interval: May increase risk of life-threatening cardiac arrhythmias, including torsades de pointes. Use together cautiously and monitor patient.
Serotonin modulators (fentanyl, lithium, MAO inhibitors, methylene blue IV, mirtazapine, SSNRIs, SSRIs, tramadol): May increase risk of serotonin syndrome. Monitor therapy.

EFFECTS ON LAB TEST RESULTS

• May increase ALT and AST levels.
• May alter fluid and electrolyte levels with prolonged use.
• May decrease Hb level and hematocrit and platelet and WBC counts.

CONTRAINDICATIONS & CAUTIONS

• Contraindicated in patients hypersensitive to drug or other 5-HT₃ receptor antagonists.
• Hypersensitivity reactions, including anaphylaxis, may occur up to 7 days or longer after administration of extended-release form.
• **Alert:** QT-interval prolongation has been reported, and drug may increase risk of ventricular arrhythmias. Use caution in patients with preexisting arrhythmias, cardiac conduction disorders, cardiac disease, or electrolyte abnormalities; in patients receiving cardiotoxic chemotherapy; and in those receiving medications that prolong QT interval.
• May increase risk of serotonin syndrome, which can be fatal, especially if drug is used with other serotonergic drugs.
• Use of extended-release form with successive emetogenic chemotherapy cycles for more than 6 months isn't recommended.
• Injection-site bruising and hematoma, which can be severe, may occur more than 5 days after administration of extended-release form. Patients receiving

anticoagulants or antiplatelet drugs may be at greater risk.
• Safety and effectiveness in children haven't been established.
Dialyzable drug: Unknown.
⚠ *Overdose S&S:* Headache.

PREGNANCY-LACTATION-REPRODUCTION

• Use in pregnancy only if clearly needed.
• Use cautiously in breastfeeding.

NURSING CONSIDERATIONS

• Drug regimen is given only on days when chemotherapy is given. Treatment at other times isn't useful.
• Monitor patient for signs and symptoms of serotonin syndrome (mental status changes, neuromuscular signs and symptoms, autonomic instability, seizures, GI symptoms). If signs or symptoms of serotonin syndrome occur, discontinue drug and initiate treatment.
• Monitor patients receiving extended-release form for injection-site infections, bruising, and hematoma.
• Monitor patients receiving extended-release form for signs and symptoms of hypersensitivity reactions (dyspnea, wheezing, rash, hives, fever, swelling).
• Monitor patients for constipation and decreased bowel activity, especially patients at risk for GI obstruction.

PATIENT TEACHING

• Stress importance of taking second dose of oral drug 12 hours after the first for maximum effectiveness.
• Instruct patient in safe patch administration and disposal.
• Tell patient to report adverse reactions immediately.
• Inform patient receiving extended-release form that hypersensitivity reactions can occur up to 7 days or later after subcut administration and to immediately report signs and symptoms.
• Teach patient signs and symptoms of serotonin syndrome and advise patient to report them immediately.
• Tell patient to report injection-site reactions (infection, bruising, hematoma, pain, warmth, bleeding) to prescriber.

haloperidol
ha-loe-PER-i-dole

haloperidol decanoate
Haldol Decanoate

haloperidol lactate
Haldol

Therapeutic class: Antipsychotics
Pharmacologic class: Butyrophenone derivatives

AVAILABLE FORMS
haloperidol
Tablets: 0.5 mg, 1 mg, 2 mg, 5 mg, 10 mg, 20 mg
haloperidol decanoate
Injection: 50 mg/mL*, 100 mg/mL*
haloperidol lactate
Injection: 5 mg/mL
Oral solution (concentrate): 2 mg/mL

INDICATIONS & DOSAGES
Adjust-a-dose (for all indications): For oral dosing in older adults and patients who are debilitated, initially, 0.5 to 2 mg PO b.i.d. or t.i.d.; increase gradually, as needed.
➤ **Schizophrenia**
Adults and children older than age 12: Dosage varies for each patient. Initially, 0.5 to 2 mg PO b.i.d. or t.i.d. For severe symptoms, initially, 3 to 5 mg PO b.i.d. or t.i.d. Maximum, 100 mg PO daily. Or, 2 to 5 mg lactate IM every 4 to 8 hours, although hourly administration may be needed until control is obtained. Maximum dose, 20 mg/day.
Children ages 3 to 12 weighing 15 to 40 kg: Initially, 0.5 mg PO in two or three divided doses daily. May increase dose by 0.5 mg at 5- to 7-day intervals, depending on therapeutic response and patient tolerance. Maintenance dose, 0.05 to 0.15 mg/kg PO daily given in two or three divided doses. Children who are severely disturbed may need higher doses. Maximum dose, 6 mg/day.
➤ **Chronic schizophrenia requiring prolonged therapy (haloperidol decanoate)**
Adults stable on low daily oral dose, older adults, or patients who are debilitated: Initial and maintenance dose, 10 to 15 times daily oral dose, given IM every 4 weeks.

Adults on high oral dose, at risk for relapse, or tolerant to oral haloperidol: Initial dose, 10 to 20 times daily oral dose; maintenance dose, 10 to 15 times daily oral dose, given IM every 4 weeks.
➤ **Nonpsychotic behavior disorders**
Children ages 3 to 12 weighing 15 to 40 kg: 0.05 to 0.075 mg/kg PO daily, in two or three divided doses. Maximum, 6 mg daily. Children with severe mental illness who don't have psychosis or who are hyperactive with conduct disorders may only require short-term use.
➤ **Tourette syndrome**
Adults: Initially, 0.5 to 5 mg PO b.i.d., t.i.d., or as needed. Maximum, 100 mg/day.
Children ages 3 to 12 weighing 15 to 40 kg: 0.05 to 0.075 mg/kg PO daily, in two or three divided doses.

ADMINISTRATION
⚠ *Alert:* Haloperidol isn't approved for IV use. Never administer haloperidol decanoate IV.
PO
• Give with food or milk to decrease GI distress.
• Avoid skin contact with oral solution; may cause contact dermatitis.
IM
• Protect drug from light. Slight yellowing of solution is common and doesn't affect potency. Discard very discolored solutions.
• Use a 21G needle. Maximum volume per injection site shouldn't exceed 3 mL. Give in gluteal muscle by deep IM injection; Z-track techniques are recommended (haloperidol decanoate).
• When switching from tablets to IM decanoate injection, if initial dose conversion requires more than 100 mg, give in two injections (100 mg maximum) separated by 3 to 7 days.

ACTION
A butyrophenone that probably exerts antipsychotic effects by blocking postsynaptic dopamine receptors in the brain.

Route	Onset	Peak	Duration
PO	Unknown	2–6 hr	Unknown
IM (decanoate)	Unknown	6 days	Unknown
IM (lactate)	Unknown	10–20 min	Unknown

Half-life: PO, 14 to 37 hours; IM decanoate, 3 weeks; IM lactate, 20 hours.

Reactions in bold italics are *life-threatening*. Interactions may have a *rapid onset* or a ***delayed onset***.

ADVERSE REACTIONS

CNS: extrapyramidal reactions, dystonia, drowsiness, headache, agitation, restlessness, hallucinations, parkinsonian-like syndrome, tremor, hypertonia, dystonia, bradykinesia, hyperkinesia. **EENT:** oculogyric crisis, dry mouth, salivary hypersecretion. **GI:** constipation, abdominal pain. **Metabolic:** hyperglycemia, hyponatremia.

INTERACTIONS

Drug-drug. *Anticholinergics:* May increase anticholinergic effects and glaucoma. Use together cautiously.

Antiparkinsonian drugs (dopamine agonist): May diminish therapeutic effect of both haloperidol and antiparkinsonian drug (dopamine agonist). Avoid using together. If use together can't be avoided, monitor patient for decreased effects of both agents.

Buspirone, CYP2D6 inhibitors (chlorpromazine, paroxetine, quinidine, sertraline), CYP3A4 inhibitors (alprazolam, itraconazole, nefazodone, ritonavir): May increase haloperidol level and risk of adverse effects. Monitor QTc interval and adverse reactions. Dosage reduction may be needed.

Carbamazepine: May decrease haloperidol level. Monitor patient.

CNS depressants: May increase CNS depression. Use together cautiously.

Corticosteroids, diuretics: May cause electrolyte imbalance and increase risk of QT-interval prolongation. Monitor electrolyte levels.

CYP3A4 inducers (carbamazepine, phenytoin, rifampin): May decrease haloperidol level and effectiveness. Monitor patient for clinical effect.

Lithium: May enhance neurotoxic effects and cause lethargy and confusion after high doses. Monitor patient.

Opioids: May cause slow or difficult breathing, sedation, and death. Avoid use together. If use together is necessary, limit dosage and duration of each drug to minimum necessary for desired effect.

QT-interval-prolonging drugs (amiodarone, ondansetron): May prolong QT interval. Monitor ECG. Consider therapy modification.

Drug-herb. *St. John's wort:* May decrease haloperidol level. Discourage use together.

Drug-lifestyle. *Alcohol use, cannabidiol:* May increase CNS depression. Discourage use together.

Smoking: May decrease haloperidol serum concentration. Monitor therapy.

EFFECTS ON LAB TEST RESULTS

- May increase LFT values.
- May decrease sodium level and platelet count.
- May increase or decrease glucose level and WBC count.

CONTRAINDICATIONS & CAUTIONS

- Contraindicated in patients hypersensitive to drug and in those with dementia with Lewy bodies, Parkinson disease, coma, or CNS depression.

Boxed Warning Older adults with dementia-related psychosis treated with atypical or conventional antipsychotics are at increased risk for death. Antipsychotics aren't approved for the treatment of dementia-related psychosis. ∎

- Use cautiously in older adults and patients who are debilitated; in patients with history of seizures or EEG abnormalities, prolonged QT interval and other severe CV disorders, allergies, glaucoma, myasthenia gravis, or urine retention.
- Use cautiously in patients at risk for falls, including those with diseases or conditions or who are taking drugs that may cause somnolence, orthostatic hypotension, or motor or sensory instability.
- *Opioid class warning:* Use opioids with benzodiazepines or other CNS depressants only when alternative treatment options are inadequate.
- Decanoate form contains benzyl alcohol.
- Off-label IV administration of lactate form requires ECG monitoring for arrhythmias and prolonged QT interval.
- Blood dyscrasias have been reported. Discontinue drug for ANC less than $1,000/mm^3$ or for leukopenia or agranulocytosis.

Dialyzable drug: Unknown.

⚠ *Overdose S&S:* Severe extrapyramidal reactions, hypotension, sedation, EEG abnormalities including torsades de pointes.

PREGNANCY-LACTATION-REPRODUCTION

⊕ *Alert:* Antipsychotic use during third trimester may result in extrapyramidal and withdrawal symptoms in newborns. May cause limb malformation if used during first trimester. Alternative agents are recommended. Use during pregnancy only if

benefits outweigh fetal risk and at minimum effective maternal dose.
- Drug appears in human milk. Breastfeeding isn't recommended.

NURSING CONSIDERATIONS
- Monitor patient for tardive dyskinesia, which may occur after prolonged use. It may not appear until months or years later and may disappear spontaneously or persist for life, despite ending drug.
- **Alert:** Watch for signs and symptoms of NMS (mental status changes, muscle rigidity, hyperthermia, autonomic disturbance [arrhythmias, labile BP, tachycardia, diaphoresis], elevated CK level, rhabdomyolysis, acute kidney injury), which are rare but commonly fatal.
- **Alert:** Monitor ECG when drug is given in high doses or when patient is taking other QT interval–prolonging drugs because of the increased risk of QT-interval prolongation and torsades de pointes.
- Don't withdraw drug abruptly unless required by severe adverse reactions.
- Complete fall risk assessments at start of antipsychotic treatment and recurrently for patients on long-term therapy, especially those at increased risk for falls.
- Esophageal dysmotility and aspiration can occur. Use cautiously in patients at risk for aspiration (those with pneumonia, Alzheimer disease).
- **Look alike–sound alike:** Don't confuse Haldol with Halcion or Halog.

PATIENT TEACHING
- Caution patient or caregiver of patient taking an opioid with a benzodiazepine, CNS depressant, or alcohol to seek immediate medical attention for dizziness, lightheadedness, extreme sleepiness, slowed or difficult breathing, or unresponsiveness.
- Advise patient to report all adverse reactions.
- Although drug is the least sedating of the antipsychotics, warn patient to avoid activities that require alertness and good coordination until effects of drug are known. Drowsiness and dizziness usually subside after a few weeks.
- Advise patient that drug may cause somnolence, orthostatic hypotension, and motor and sensory instability, which may lead to falls.
- Warn patient to avoid alcohol during therapy.

- Tell patient to relieve dry mouth with sugarless gum or hard candy.
- Tell patient to report changes in medications to physicians and pharmacist.

heparin sodium
HEP-a-rin

Therapeutic class: Anticoagulants
Pharmacologic class: Anticoagulants

AVAILABLE FORMS
Products are derived from beef lung or pork intestinal mucosa.
Injection: 1,000 units/mL, 5,000 units/mL, 10,000 units/mL, 20,000 units/mL
Premixed IV solutions: Units of heparin and type of solution vary by manufacturer.
Syringes: 1,000 units/mL, 5,000 units/0.5 mL, 5,000 units/mL

INDICATIONS & DOSAGES
➤ **Thromboprophylaxis**
Adults: 5,000 units subcut every 8 to 12 hours for a minimum of 7 days or for 10 to 14 days for patients undergoing total hip arthroplasty, total knee arthroplasty, or hip fracture surgery according to American College of Chest Physicians guidelines.
➤ **Full-dose continuous IV infusion therapy for DVT or PE**
Adults: 80 units/kg by IV bolus; then 18 units/kg/hour by IV infusion with pump. Titrate hourly rate based on PTT results (every 4 to 6 hours in the early stages of treatment).
Children: Initially, 75 to 100 units/kg IV over 10 minutes; then, for infants, maintenance dose of 25 to 30 units/kg/hour IV. For children older than age 1 year, maintenance dose is 18 to 20 units/kg/hour IV. Titrate dosage based on PTT.
➤ **Full-dose subcut therapy for DVT or PE**
Adults: Initially, 5,000 units IV bolus and 10,000 to 20,000 units in a concentrated solution subcut; then 8,000 to 10,000 units subcut every 8 hours or 15,000 to 20,000 units in a concentrated solution subcut every 12 hours.
➤ **Full-dose intermittent anticoagulation IV therapy for DVT or PE**
Adults: Initially, 10,000 units by IV bolus; then 5,000 to 10,000 units (or 50 to 70 units/kg) IV every 4 to 6 hours titrated according to PTT.

Reactions in bold italics are *life-threatening*. Interactions may have a *rapid onset* or a **delayed onset**.

➤ **Fixed low-dose therapy for prevention of venous thrombosis, PE, embolism associated with atrial fibrillation, and postoperative DVT**

Adults: 5,000 units subcut every 12 hours. For patients after surgery, give first dose 2 hours before procedure; then 5,000 units subcut every 8 to 12 hours for 5 to 7 days or until patient can walk.

ADMINISTRATION
IV

▼ Confirm selection of the correct formulation and strength before administration.

▼ Establish baseline coagulation parameters before therapy.

▼ For continuous infusion, use an infusion pump to provide maximum safety. Check infusions regularly, even when pumps are in good working order, to ensure correct dosing. Place notice above patient's bed to caution IV team or lab personnel to apply pressure dressings after venipuncture.

▼ When adding heparin to infusion solution, invert IV container at least six times to adequately mix solution.

▼ During intermittent administration, always draw blood 30 minutes before next scheduled dose to avoid falsely prolonged PTT. Blood for PTT may be drawn 4 hours after continuous IV heparin therapy starts. Never draw blood for PTT from the tubing of the heparin infusion or from the infused vein, because falsely prolonged PTT will result. Always draw blood from the opposite arm.

▼ Don't skip a dose or try to "catch up" with a solution containing heparin. If solution runs out, restart it as soon as possible, and reschedule bolus dose immediately. Monitor PTT.

▼ Concentrated heparin solutions (more than 100 units/mL) can irritate blood vessels.

▼ Never piggyback other drugs into an infusion line while heparin infusion is running. Never mix another drug and heparin in same syringe when giving a bolus.

▼ **Incompatibilities:** Alteplase, amiodarone, ciprofloxacin, diazepam, doxycycline hyclate, droperidol, ergotamine, erythromycin, filgrastim, gentamicin, haloperidol, idarubicin, levofloxacin, nesiritide, phenytoin sodium, reteplase. For additional information, consult detailed drug reference.

Subcutaneous

• Give low-dose injections sequentially between iliac crests in lower abdomen deep into subcutaneous fat. Inject drug subcut slowly into fat pad.

• Don't massage injection site; watch for signs of bleeding there.

• Alternate sites. Record location.

ACTION
Accelerates formation of antithrombin III–thrombin complex and deactivates thrombin, preventing conversion of fibrinogen to fibrin.

Route	Onset	Peak	Duration
IV	Immediate	Immediate	Variable
Subcut	20–30 min	2–4 hr	Variable

Half-life: 0.5 to 2 hours. Half-life is dose-dependent and nonlinear and may be disproportionately prolonged at higher doses.

ADVERSE REACTIONS
CNS: fever. **EENT:** rhinitis. **Hematologic: hemorrhage, heparin-induced thrombocytopenia, thrombocytopenia. Metabolic: hyperkalemia,** hypoaldosteronism. **Musculoskeletal:** osteoporosis. **Skin:** irritation, mild pain, hematoma, ulceration, cutaneous or subcutaneous necrosis, pruritus, urticaria, transient alopecia. **Other:** hypersensitivity reactions, including chills; *anaphylactoid reactions.*

INTERACTIONS
Drug-drug. *Antihistamines, digoxin, nicotine, nitrates, nitroglycerin, tetracyclines:* May decrease heparin effect. Monitor coagulation tests.

Antiplatelet drugs, salicylates: May increase anticoagulant effect. Use together cautiously. Monitor coagulation studies and patient closely.

Oral anticoagulants: May increase additive anticoagulation. Monitor PT, INR, and PTT. Avoid combination use unless bridging for long-term warfarin use.

Oritavancin, telavancin: May diminish therapeutic effect of heparin; may artificially increase results of lab tests commonly used to monitor IV heparin. Avoid combination.

Thrombolytics: May increase risk of hemorrhage. Monitor patient closely.

Drug-lifestyle. *Smoking:* May interfere with anticoagulant effect of heparin. Discourage smoking.

H

♣Canada ◇OTC ◆Off-label use ✒Photoguide ⊜Do not crush *Liquid contains alcohol ▨Genetic

EFFECTS ON LAB TEST RESULTS

• May increase ALT, AST, and potassium levels.
• May increase INR and prolong PT and PTT.
• May decrease platelet count.
• Drug may cause false elevations in some tests for thyroxine level.

CONTRAINDICATIONS & CAUTIONS

• Contraindicated in patients hypersensitive to heparin except in life-threatening situations when alternative anticoagulation isn't possible.
• Contraindicated in patients with a history of heparin-induced thrombocytopenia (HIT) and heparin-induced thrombocytopenia and thrombosis (HITT), in those with an uncontrolled bleeding state (except DIC), and when blood coagulation tests can't be performed at appropriate intervals (for full-dose heparin).
• Some products are derived from animal tissues and may be contraindicated in patients with pork allergy; consult manufacturer's instructions.
• Use cautiously in patients at increased risk for hemorrhage, such as those with hemophilia, thrombocytopenia, vascular purpuras, subacute bacterial endocarditis, severe HTN, hereditary antithrombin III deficiency receiving concurrent antithrombin III therapy, ulcerative lesions and continuous tube drainage of stomach or small intestine, liver disease with impaired hemostasis, and during and immediately after spinal tap or spinal anesthesia or major surgery (especially involving the brain, spinal cord, or eye).
• May reduce bone mineral density with prolonged use (longer than 6 months).
• Drug may increase risk of bleeding in women older than age 60.
Dialyzable drug: Unknown.
⚠ *Overdose S&S:* Bleeding, nosebleeds, hematuria, melena, easy bruising, petechial formations.

PREGNANCY-LACTATION-REPRODUCTION

• Drug doesn't cross placental barrier. Use during pregnancy only if potential benefit justifies fetal risk.
• Heparin doesn't appear in human milk.
• Use preservative-free formulations (without benzyl alcohol) in patients who are pregnant and breastfeeding and in neonates. Benzyl alcohol may cause gasping syndrome in neonates.

NURSING CONSIDERATIONS

🌢 *Alert:* Some commercially available heparin injections contain benzyl alcohol.
• Drug requirements are higher in early phases of thrombogenic diseases and febrile states; they are lower when patient's condition stabilizes.
• Older adults should usually start at lower dosage.
• Monitor patients for hyperkalemia during therapy.
🌢 *Alert:* Check order and vial carefully; heparin comes in various concentrations. Label must clearly state the strength of the entire container followed by how much medication is in 1 mL.
🌢 *Alert:* USP and international units are equivalent for heparin.
🌢 *Alert:* Heparin and low-molecular-weight heparins aren't interchangeable.
🌢 *Alert:* Don't change concentrations of infusions unless absolutely necessary. This is a common source of dosage errors.
🌢 *Alert:* There is the potential for delayed onset of HIT, a serious antibody-mediated reaction resulting from irreversible aggregation of platelets. HIT may progress to the development of venous and arterial thromboses, a condition referred to as heparin-induced thrombocytopenia and thrombosis (HITT). Thrombotic events may be the initial presentation for HITT, which can occur up to several weeks after stopping heparin therapy. Evaluate patients presenting with thrombocytopenia or thrombosis after stopping heparin for HIT and HITT.
• Draw blood for PTT 4 to 6 hours after subcut dose or after starting infusion.
• Avoid IM injections of other drugs to prevent or minimize hematoma.
• Monitor PTT regularly. Anticoagulation is present when PTT values are 1½ to 2 times the normal control values.
• Monitor platelet count regularly. When new thrombosis accompanies thrombocytopenia (white clot syndrome), stop heparin.
• Regularly inspect patient for bleeding gums, bruises on arms or legs, petechiae, nosebleeds, melena, hematuria, and hematemesis.
• Monitor vital signs.
🌢 *Alert:* To treat severe overdose, use protamine sulfate, a heparin antagonist. Base dosage on the dose of heparin, its route of administration, and the time since it was given.

Reactions in bold italics are *life-threatening*. Interactions may have a *rapid onset* or a *delayed onset*.

Generally, 1 mg of protamine neutralizes 100 USP units of heparin. Don't give more than 50 mg protamine in a 10-minute period. Protamine can cause severe hypotension and anaphylactoid reactions. Ensure emergency treatment is available.

• Abrupt withdrawal may cause increased coagulability; warfarin therapy usually overlaps heparin therapy for continuation of prophylaxis or treatment.

• *Look alike–sound alike:* Don't confuse heparin with Hespan or low-molecular-weight heparin.

PATIENT TEACHING

• Instruct patient to report all drug and food allergies.

• Caution patient and family to report all adverse reactions.

• Advise patient and family to watch for and immediately report signs and symptoms of bleeding (abnormal bleeding or bruising, red or black vomit or feces, abdominal pain, change in mental status, headache).

• Tell patient to avoid OTC drugs containing aspirin, other salicylates, or drugs that may interact with heparin unless ordered by prescriber.

• Advise patient to consult prescriber before starting herbal therapy; many herbs have anticoagulant, antiplatelet, or fibrinolytic properties.

• Counsel patient to inform practitioners and dentists about receiving heparin before scheduling surgical procedures.

hydrALAZINE hydrochloride
hye-DRAL-a-zeen

Apresoline ✤

Therapeutic class: Antihypertensives
Pharmacologic class: Peripheral vasodilators

AVAILABLE FORMS
Injection: 20 mg/mL
Tablets: 10 mg, 25 mg, 50 mg, 100 mg

INDICATIONS & DOSAGES
➤ **HTN**
Adults: Initially, 10 mg PO q.i.d. for first 2 to 4 days, then 25 mg q.i.d. for balance of first week; 50 mg q.i.d. from second week

on, based on patient tolerance and response. Maximum dose, 300 mg/day.
Children age 1 and older: Initially, 0.75 mg/kg PO in two to four divided doses; gradually increase over 3 to 4 weeks to maximum of 7.5 mg/kg/day in four divided doses or 200 mg/day.

➤ **Hypertensive emergency**
Adults: 10 to 20 mg IM or IV; repeat as needed every 4 to 6 hours. May increase dose to a maximum of 40 mg/dose if necessary. Switch to oral form as soon as possible.
Children: 1.7 to 3.5 mg/kg/day IM or IV divided into four to six doses.

➤ **HF with reduced ejection fraction ♦**
Adults: Initially, 25 to 50 mg PO t.i.d. or q.i.d. in combination with isosorbide dinitrate. Maximum dose is 300 mg daily in divided doses.

ADMINISTRATION
PO
• May give with or without food but giving with food increases absorption. Give consistently with regard to meals.
IV
▼ Give drug as a rapid bolus directly into the vein only when it can't be given orally. Repeat PRN, generally every 4 to 6 hours. It shouldn't be added to infusion solutions.
▼ Drug may discolor upon contact with metal; discolored solutions should be discarded. Use immediately after the vial is opened.
▼ **Incompatibilities:** None.
IM
• Administer undiluted as IM injection.

ACTION
Not fully understood. A direct-acting peripheral vasodilator that relaxes arteriolar smooth muscle.

Route	Onset	Peak	Duration
PO	20–30 min	1–2 hr	2–4 hr
IV	5–20 min	10–80 min	2–6 hr
IM	10–30 min	Within 1 hr	2–6 hr

Half-life: 3 to 7 hours.

ADVERSE REACTIONS
CNS: anxiety, headache, depression, dizziness, peripheral neuritis, *increased ICP*, psychosis, fever. **CV:** angina pectoris, palpitations, tachycardia, orthostatic hypotension, edema, flushing. **EENT:** conjunctivitis, nasal

congestion, lacrimation. **GI:** nausea, vomiting, diarrhea, anorexia, constipation, paralytic ileus. **GU:** difficult urination. **Hematologic:** anemia, *neutropenia, leukopenia, agranulocytosis,* eosinophilia, *thrombocytopenia with or without purpura.* **Musculoskeletal:** muscle cramps, arthralgia. **Respiratory:** dyspnea. **Skin:** diaphoresis, pruritus, urticaria, rash. **Other:** hypersensitivity reactions, chills.

INTERACTIONS
Drug-drug. *Diazoxide, MAO inhibitors:* May cause severe hypotension. Use together cautiously.
Diuretics, other hypotensive drugs: May cause excessive hypotension. Dosage adjustment may be needed.
NSAIDs: May decrease effects of hydralazine. Monitor BP.
Drug-food. *Any food:* Food may increase drug absorption. Encourage patient to take with food.

EFFECTS ON LAB TEST RESULTS
• May decrease Hb level and neutrophil, WBC, granulocyte, platelet, and RBC counts.
• May cause positive ANA titers.

CONTRAINDICATIONS & CAUTIONS
• Contraindicated in patients hypersensitive to drug and in those with CAD or mitral valvular rheumatic heart disease.
• Drug may contain tartrazine and cause allergic reactions, especially in patients hypersensitive to aspirin.
• Drug may produce a clinical picture consistent with SLE.
• Use cautiously in patients with suspected cardiac disease, stroke, or severe renal impairment and in those taking other antihypertensives.
• May cause blood dyscrasias. Discontinue drug if they occur.
Dialyzable drug: Unknown.
⚠ *Overdose S&S:* Hypotension, tachycardia, headache, flushing.

PREGNANCY-LACTATION-REPRODUCTION
• Drug crosses the placental barrier and is associated with fetal toxicity in the third trimester. Use during pregnancy only if expected benefit justifies fetal risk.
• Use cautiously in breastfeeding.

NURSING CONSIDERATIONS
• Frequently monitor patient's BP standing, sitting, and supine; HR; and body weight.
• Drug may be given with diuretics and beta blockers to decrease sodium retention and tachycardia and to prevent angina attacks.
• Older adults may be more sensitive to drug's hypotensive effects.
• Obtain CBC, lupus erythematosus cell preparation, and ANA titer determination before therapy and periodically during long-term therapy.
🔵 *Alert:* Monitor patient closely for signs and symptoms of lupuslike syndrome (sore throat, fever, muscle and joint aches, rash), and notify prescriber immediately if they develop. Long-term steroid therapy may be necessary.
• *Look alike–sound alike:* Don't confuse hydralazine with hydroxyzine.

PATIENT TEACHING
• Instruct patient to take oral form consistently with meals to increase absorption.
• Inform patient that low BP and dizziness upon standing can be minimized by rising slowly and avoiding sudden position changes.
• Tell patient to report all adverse reactions, including unexplained prolonged general tiredness or fever, muscle or joint aching, or chest pain.
• Instruct patient of childbearing potential to notify prescriber of suspected pregnancy.

hydroCHLOROthiazide
hye-droe-klor-oh-THYE-a-zide

Therapeutic class: Diuretics
Pharmacologic class: Thiazide diuretics

AVAILABLE FORMS
Capsules: 12.5 mg
Tablets: 12.5 mg, 25 mg, 50 mg

INDICATIONS & DOSAGES
Adjust-a-dose (for all indications): In patients older than age 65, 12.5 mg daily initially. Adjust in increments of 12.5 mg, if needed.
➤ **Edema**
Adults: 25 to 100 mg PO daily in one to two divided doses.
Children ages 6 months to 12 years: Initially, 1 to 2 mg/kg/day PO in a single dose or two divided doses. May increase to a maximum

of 37.5 mg/day for children ages 6 months to 2 years and 100 mg/day for children ages 2 to 12 years.

Children younger than age 6 months: 1 to 2 mg/kg/day PO in single dose or two divided doses. Doses up to 3 mg/kg/day in two divided doses may be needed. Maximum dose, 37.5 mg/day.

➤ **HTN**

Adults: 12.5 to 50 mg PO daily in one to two divided doses. Increase or decrease daily dose based on BP.

Children ages 6 months to 12 years: Initially, 1 to 2 mg/kg/day PO in a single dose or two divided doses. May increase to a maximum of 37.5 mg/day for children ages 6 months to 2 years and 100 mg/day for children ages 2 to 12 years.

Children younger than age 6 months: 1 to 2 mg/kg/day PO in single dose or two divided doses. Doses up to 3 mg/kg/day in two divided doses may be needed. Maximum dose, 37.5 mg/day.

ADMINISTRATION
PO
• Give with or without food.
• To prevent nocturia, give drug in morning. If second dose is needed, give in early afternoon, preferably not later than 6 p.m.
• Capsules aren't indicated for use in children.

ACTION
Increases sodium and water excretion by inhibiting sodium and chloride reabsorption in distal segment of the nephron.

Route	Onset	Peak	Duration
PO	2–6 hr	1–5 hr	6–12 hr

Half-life: About 6 to 15 hours.

ADVERSE REACTIONS
CNS: dizziness, vertigo, headache, paresthesia, weakness, restlessness, asthenia, fever.
CV: hypotension, vasculitis. **EENT:** blurred vision, yellowing of vision, salivary gland infection. **GI:** *pancreatitis,* anorexia, nausea, epigastric distress, vomiting, abdominal pain, diarrhea, constipation, abdominal cramps. **GU:** *renal failure,* polyuria, frequent urination, glycosuria, interstitial nephritis, erectile dysfunction. **Hematologic:** *aplastic anemia, agranulocytosis, leukopenia, thrombocytopenia,* hemolytic anemia.

Hepatic: jaundice. **Metabolic:** asymptomatic hyperuricemia; hyperglycemia and impaired glucose tolerance; fluid and electrolyte imbalances, including hyponatremia, *hypomagnesemia, hypokalemia,* hypochloremia; metabolic alkalosis; hypercalcemia; volume depletion and dehydration.
Musculoskeletal: muscle spasms. **Respiratory:** *respiratory distress,* pneumonitis.
Skin: dermatitis, photosensitivity reactions, rash, purpura, alopecia, *erythema multiforme,* exfoliative dermatitis, urticaria.
Other: *anaphylactic reactions,* hypersensitivity reactions, gout.

INTERACTIONS
Drug-drug. *Allopurinol:* May increase allopurinol serum concentration and enhance potential for allergic or hypersensitivity reactions to allopurinol. Monitor allopurinol level.
Amphotericin B, corticosteroids, topiramate: May increase risk of hypokalemia. Monitor potassium level closely.
Antidiabetics: May decrease hypoglycemic effects. Adjust dosage if needed. Monitor glucose level.
Antihypertensives: May have additive antihypertensive effect. Use together cautiously.
Barbiturates, opioids: May increase orthostatic hypotensive effect. Monitor patient closely.
Cardiac glycosides: May increase risk of digoxin toxicity from diuretic-induced hypokalemia. Monitor potassium and digoxin levels.
Cholestyramine, colestipol: May decrease intestinal absorption of thiazides. Separate doses by 2 hours.
Diazoxide: May increase antihypertensive, hyperglycemic, and hyperuricemic effects. Use together cautiously.
Dofetilide: May enhance QTc-prolonging effect of dofetilide. Use is contraindicated.
Lithium: May decrease lithium excretion, increasing risk of lithium toxicity. Consider therapy modification.
Multivitamins and minerals (with ADEK, folate, iron): May enhance hypercalcemic effect of these multivitamins and minerals. Monitor patient closely.
NSAIDs: May increase risk of renal failure. May decrease diuretic and antihypertensive effects. Monitor renal function and BP.

H

Drug-herb. *Licorice:* May cause unexpected rapid potassium loss. Discourage use together.

Drug-lifestyle. *Alcohol use:* May increase orthostatic hypotensive effect. Discourage use together.

EFFECTS ON LAB TEST RESULTS
• May increase glucose, cholesterol, triglyceride, calcium, and uric acid levels.
• May decrease potassium, sodium, chloride, magnesium, and serum protein-bound iodine levels.
• May decrease Hb level and granulocyte, WBC, and platelet counts.

CONTRAINDICATIONS & CAUTIONS
• Contraindicated in patients with anuria and patients hypersensitive to other thiazides or other sulfonamide derivatives.
• Drug can cause systemic lupus activation or exacerbation.
• Use cautiously in patients with gout. Drug may reduce clearance of uric acid.
• Use cautiously in children, older adults, and in patients with severe renal disease, gout, diabetes, hypercholesterolemia, impaired hepatic function, or progressive hepatic disease.
Dialyzable drug: Unknown.
⚠ *Overdose S&S:* Electrolyte imbalance, dehydration.

PREGNANCY-LACTATION-REPRODUCTION
• Adequate studies during pregnancy don't exist; use during pregnancy only if clearly needed.
• Drug crosses placental barrier; maternal use may adversely affect fetus.
• Thiazides appear in human milk. Discontinue drug or discontinue breastfeeding, taking into account importance of drug to patient.

NURSING CONSIDERATIONS
• Monitor fluid intake and output, weight, BP, and electrolyte levels; correct electrolyte disturbances before start of therapy.
• Watch for signs and symptoms of hypokalemia, such as muscle weakness and cramps.
• Drug may be used with potassium-sparing diuretic to prevent potassium loss.
• Consult prescriber and dietitian about a high-potassium diet or potassium supplement.

• Monitor creatinine and BUN levels regularly. Cumulative effects of drug may occur with impaired renal function.
• Monitor uric acid level, especially in patients with history of gout.
• Monitor glucose level, especially in patients with diabetes.
• Monitor older adults, who are especially susceptible to excessive diuresis.
• Stop thiazides and thiazide-like diuretics before parathyroid function tests.
• In patients with HTN, therapeutic response may be delayed several weeks.

PATIENT TEACHING
• Instruct patient in safe drug administration.
• Advise patient to report all adverse reactions and to avoid sudden posture changes and to rise slowly to avoid dizziness upon standing quickly.
• Encourage sunblock use to prevent photosensitivity reactions.
• Tell patient to check with prescriber or pharmacist before using OTC drugs.
• Advise patient to report pregnancy, plans to become pregnant, breastfeeding, or plans to breastfeed.

SAFETY ALERT!

HYDROcodone bitartrate
hye-droe-KOE-done

Hysingla ER

Therapeutic class: Opioid analgesics
Pharmacologic class: Opioid analgesics
Controlled substance schedule: II

AVAILABLE FORMS
Capsules (extended-release) ⒸⒾⒸ: 10 mg, 15 mg, 20 mg, 30 mg, 40 mg, 50 mg
Tablets (extended-release) ⒸⒾⒸ: 20 mg, 30 mg, 40 mg, 60 mg, 80 mg, 100 mg, 120 mg

INDICATIONS & DOSAGES
➤ **Management of pain severe enough to require daily, around-the-clock, long-term opioid treatment and for which alternative treatment options are inadequate**
Adults who are opioid naive or who aren't opioid tolerant: Initially, 10 mg extended-release capsule PO every 12 hours. Gradually adjust dosage, preferably in increments of 10 mg every 12 hours every 3 to 7 days, until

---

adequate pain relief and acceptable adverse reactions have been achieved.

Or, 20 mg extended-release tablet PO once daily. Increase dosage in increments of 10 to 20 mg once daily every 3 to 5 days as needed to achieve adequate analgesia.

Adults who are opioid tolerant: Discontinue all other around-the-clock opioids before initiating therapy. Refer to manufacturer's instructions when converting from other oral opioids to hydrocodone; doses aren't equianalgesic.

Adjust-a-dose: In patients with moderate renal impairment to ESRD, start with 50% of the extended-release tablet initial dose or initiate treatment with low-dose extended-release capsule, and monitor patient closely.

For severe hepatic impairment, start with 10 mg extended-release capsule PO every 12 hours or use 50% of initial dose of extended-release tablet. For moderate to severe renal impairment and ESRD, use 50% of initial dose of extended-release tablet.

Monitor patients closely for adverse events such as respiratory depression. Decrease initial dose in older adults, who may be more sensitive to adverse effects.

ADMINISTRATION
PO
Boxed Warning Give capsules and tablets whole. Don't crush, dissolve, or allow patient to chew capsules or tablets because of the risk of rapid release and absorption of a potentially fatal dose of hydrocodone. ∎

• Give capsules or tablets one at a time with enough water to ensure complete swallowing immediately after placing in the mouth.
• Don't presoak, lick, or wet tablets before administration; may increase risk of choking and uncontrolled drug delivery.
• Store at room temperature.

ACTION
Acts as a full agonist primarily at the mu opioid receptor, binding to and activating opioid receptors at various sites in the CNS to produce analgesia.

Route	Onset	Peak	Duration
PO (tablet ER)	Unknown	6–30 hr	Unknown
PO (capsule ER)	Unknown	5 hr	Unknown

Half-life: Tablet ER, 7 to 9 hours; capsule ER, about 8 hours.

ADVERSE REACTIONS
CNS: somnolence, tremor, lethargy, anxiety, depression, insomnia, fatigue, dizziness, drowsiness, headache or migraine, pain, paresthesia, sedation. **CV:** peripheral edema, hot flush, HTN. **EENT:** tinnitus, nasopharyngitis, nasal congestion, oropharyngeal pain, sinusitis, dry mouth. **GI:** constipation, nausea, vomiting, abdominal pain, GERD, decreased appetite, diarrhea, dyspepsia, viral gastroenteritis. **GU:** UTI. **Hepatic:** increased GGT level. **Metabolic:** dehydration, hypercholesterolemia, *hypokalemia.* **Musculoskeletal:** muscle spasms, back pain, foot fracture, joint injury, joint sprain, muscle strain, arthralgia, musculoskeletal pain, myalgia, neck pain, extremity pain, noncardiac chest pain, osteoarthritis. **Respiratory:** URI, bronchitis, cough, dyspnea. **Skin:** pruritus, skin laceration, hyperhidrosis, night sweats, rash. **Other:** fall, flulike syndrome, chills.

INTERACTIONS
Drug-drug. *Anticholinergics:* May increase risk of urine retention, severe constipation, or paralytic ileus. Monitor patient for signs and symptoms of urine retention and constipation in addition to respiratory and CNS depression. Use together cautiously.

Boxed Warning *Benzodiazepines, CNS depressants:* May cause slow or difficult breathing, sedation, and death. Avoid use together. If use together is necessary, limit dosage and duration of each drug to the minimum necessary for desired effect. ∎

Boxed Warning *CYP3A4 inhibitors (amiodarone, erythromycin, ketoconazole, nefazodone, protease inhibitors, ritonavir):* May increase hydrocodone plasma concentration and prolong opioid effects, especially with concomitant CYP3A4 inhibitor use. Monitor patient for respiratory depression and sedation; consider dosage adjustments until drug effects are stable. ∎

Boxed Warning *CYP3A4 inducers (carbamazepine, phenytoin, rifampin):* May induce metabolism and decrease hydrocodone plasma concentration, decreasing efficacy and potentially causing withdrawal symptoms. Monitor patient for effectiveness of drug and for opioid withdrawal symptoms. Consider dosage adjustments until stable. If CYP3A4 inducer is stopped, monitor patient for increased therapeutic and adverse effects, especially respiratory depression. ∎

♣Canada ◇OTC ◆Off-label use ✐Photoguide ⊕Do not crush *Liquid contains alcohol ⌧Genetic

Diuretics (furosemide): May reduce diuretic effect. Monitor patient for clinical effect and increase diuretic dosage as indicated.

Laxatives: May increase GI motility and decrease hydrocodone absorption. Monitor patient for hydrocodone therapeutic effect.

MAO inhibitors: May potentiate effects of opioid analgesics or result in serotonin syndrome. Don't use in patients who have received MAO inhibitors within past 14 days.

Mixed agonist/antagonists (butorphanol, nalbuphine, pentazocine), partial agonists (buprenorphine): May reduce analgesic effect of hydrocodone or precipitate withdrawal symptoms. Avoid concurrent use.

Muscle relaxants: May enhance effects of skeletal muscle relaxants and cause increased respiratory depression. Dosage adjustment may be needed. Monitor patient.

❤ *Alert:* Serotonergic drugs *(amoxapine, antimigraine drugs, buspirone, cyclobenzaprine, dextromethorphan, linezolid, lithium, MAO inhibitors, maprotiline, methylene blue, mirtazapine, nefazodone, SSNRIs, SSRIs, TCAs, trazodone, tryptophan, vilazodone):* May increase risk of serotonin syndrome; may enhance toxic effect of hydrocodone. Use together cautiously. Monitor patient for serotonin syndrome.

Drug-herb. ❤ *Alert: St. John's wort:* May decrease hydrocodone serum concentration. Use together cautiously.

Drug-lifestyle. **Boxed Warning** *Alcohol use:* May increase hydrocodone plasma level and risk of fatal overdose. Patients shouldn't consume alcoholic beverages or use other drugs that contain alcohol. ∎

EFFECTS ON LAB TEST RESULTS
- May increase cholesterol and GGT levels.
- May decrease potassium level.

CONTRAINDICATIONS & CAUTIONS
Boxed Warning Drug exposes patient to risks of addiction, abuse, and misuse even at recommended doses, which can lead to overdose and death. Assess each patient's risk before prescribing, and monitor patients for these behaviors or conditions. ∎

Boxed Warning Accidental ingestion of even one dose of this drug, especially by children, can result in a fatal overdose of hydrocodone. ∎

Boxed Warning Opioids should only be prescribed with benzodiazepines or other CNS depressants to patients for whom alternative treatment options are inadequate. Limit dosages and durations to minimum required. ∎

Boxed Warning The FDA has required a REMS program for this drug. Drug companies with approved opioid analgesic products must make a REMS-compliant education program available to health care providers, who are strongly encouraged to complete the education program; discuss the safe use, serious risks, and proper storage and disposal of opioid analgesics with patients and their caregivers every time these medicines are prescribed; emphasize the importance of reading the Medication Guide every time an opioid analgesic is dispensed to them; and consider using other tools to improve patient, household, and community safety. ∎

❤ *Alert:* Drug should only be prescribed by health care professionals knowledgeable in the use of potent opioids for pain management. Drug should only be used when alternative treatment options are ineffective, not tolerated, or otherwise inadequate to provide sufficient pain management.

- Contraindicated for use as an as-needed analgesic.
- Contraindicated in patients with significant respiratory depression, acute or severe bronchial asthma, known or suspected paralytic ileus, or hypersensitivity to drug or its components.
- Use cautiously in patients with hypersensitivity to morphine, oxycodone, and codeine because cross-reactivity may occur.
- Use cautiously in patients who are cachectic or debilitated; there is potential for crucial respiratory depression even at therapeutic dosages.
- Use cautiously in patients with a history of seizures and adrenal insufficiency.

❤ *Alert:* Drug may lead to rare but serious decrease in adrenal gland cortisol production.

- Use cautiously in older adults and in patients with chronic pulmonary disease, seizure disorder, hypotension or depleted blood volume, or hepatic or renal impairment.

❤ *Alert:* Avoid use in patients with head injuries, increased ICP, brain tumors, impaired consciousness, or coma. Drug reduces respiratory drive, increasing carbon dioxide retention and ICP.

- Drug may reduce sex hormone levels with long-term use.

Reactions in bold italics are *life-threatening*. Interactions may have a *rapid onset* or a ***delayed onset***.

• QTc interval may be prolonged when doses greater than 160 mg daily are used. Use cautiously in patients with HF, bradyarrhythmias, or electrolyte abnormalities, and when patients are using other drugs known to prolong the QTc interval. Don't use in those with congenital long QT syndrome. If QTc-interval prolongation occurs, consider dosage reduction of 33% to 50% or change to another analgesic.

• Esophageal obstruction, dysphagia, and choking have occurred with use of extended-release tablets. Patients with underlying GI disorders or with a small GI lumen are at greater risk. Consider another analgesic in these patients.

• Safety and effectiveness in children younger than age 18 haven't been established. *Dialyzable drug:* Unknown.

⚠ *Overdose S&S:* Respiratory depression, somnolence (can lead to stupor or coma), skeletal muscle flaccidity, cold clammy skin, constricted pupils (although mydriasis rather than miosis may occur due to severe hypoxia in overdose situations), pulmonary edema, bradycardia, hypotension, death.

PREGNANCY-LACTATION-REPRODUCTION

• Use during pregnancy only if benefit outweighs fetal risk.

Boxed Warning Prolonged use during pregnancy can result in neonatal opioid withdrawal syndrome, which may be life-threatening if not recognized and treated according to protocols developed by neonatology experts. ∎

Boxed Warning If opioid use is required for a prolonged period during pregnancy, advise patient of risk of neonatal opioid withdrawal syndrome (poor feeding, diarrhea, irritability, tremor, rigidity, seizures) and assure her that appropriate treatment will be available. ∎

• Don't use during labor and delivery; neonatal respiratory depression may occur.

• Opioids may appear in human milk. Patient should discontinue breastfeeding or discontinue drug.

• Monitor infants exposed to drug through human milk for excess sedation and respiratory depression. Also watch for withdrawal symptoms in infants with discontinuation of maternal opioid analgesic or of breastfeeding.

• Prolonged opioid use may reduce fertility in individuals of reproductive potential. It's unknown whether these effects on fertility are reversible.

NURSING CONSIDERATIONS

• Drug may be targeted for theft, diversion, and misuse.

⏱ *Alert:* When giving first dose, it's preferable to underestimate patient's 24-hour oral hydrocodone requirements and provide rescue medication (immediate-release opioid) than to overestimate the 24-hour oral hydrocodone requirements, which could result in adverse reactions.

Boxed Warning Monitor patients for respiratory depression, especially within first 24 to 72 hours of drug initiation or after dosage increase. Serious, life-threatening, or fatal respiratory depression may occur. ∎

Boxed Warning Monitor patients for abuse or misuse of drug, especially those with a personal or family history of substance abuse (drug or alcohol addiction or abuse, mental illness). Counsel patients about risks and proper use of drug. ∎

⏱ *Alert:* If patient is taking opioids with serotonergic drugs, watch for signs and symptoms of serotonin syndrome (agitation, hallucinations, rapid HR, fever, diaphoresis, shivering or shaking, muscle twitching or stiffness, trouble with coordination, nausea, vomiting, diarrhea), especially when starting treatment or increasing dosages. Signs and symptoms may occur within several hours of coadministration but may also occur later, especially after dosage increase. Discontinue the opioid, serotonergic drug, or both if serotonin syndrome is suspected.

⏱ *Alert:* Monitor patient for signs and symptoms of adrenal insufficiency (nausea, vomiting, loss of appetite, fatigue, weakness, dizziness, low BP). Perform diagnostic testing if adrenal insufficiency is suspected. If adrenal insufficiency is confirmed, treat with corticosteroids and wean patient off opioids if appropriate. Discontinue corticosteroids when clinically appropriate.

• Monitor patient for signs and symptoms of decreased sex hormone levels (low libido, erectile dysfunction, amenorrhea, infertility). If signs and symptoms occur, evaluate patient and obtain lab testing.

⏱ *Alert:* Don't stop drug abruptly; withdraw slowly and individualize the gradual tapering plan to prevent signs and symptoms of withdrawal, worsening pain, and psychological distress in patients who are physically dependent. Refer to manufacturer's label for specific tapering instructions.

⚠ *Alert:* When tapering opioids, monitor patients closely for signs and symptoms of opioid withdrawal (restlessness, lacrimation, rhinorrhea, yawning, perspiration, chills, myalgia, mydriasis, irritability, anxiety, insomnia, backache, joint pain, weakness, abdominal cramps, anorexia, nausea, vomiting, diarrhea, increased BP or HR, increased respiratory rate). Such signs and symptoms may indicate a need to taper more slowly. Also monitor patients for suicidality, use of other substances, and mood changes.

• Patients considered opioid tolerant are those receiving, for 1 week or longer, at least 60 mg morphine per day, 25 mcg/hour transdermal fentanyl, 30 mg oral oxycodone per day, 8 mg oral hydromorphone per day or more, 25 mg oral oxymorphone per day or more, 60 mg oral hydrocodone, or an equianalgesic dose of another opioid.

• Closely monitor patients converting from methadone because methadone has a long half-life and can accumulate in plasma, resulting in significant respiratory depression.

• Closely monitor patients converting from fentanyl patches because of risk of additive effects.

• Older adults receiving drug may become confused and oversedated, especially those with impaired hepatic or renal function. Start with low doses of hydrocodone and observe closely for adverse events such as respiratory depression.

• Watch for decreased bowel motility in patients who have undergone surgery and for biliary spasm in patients with biliary tract disease or acute pancreatitis.

• Monitor patients with history of seizure disorder for worsening seizure control.

• Use lowest initial dose in patients with renal or hepatic impairment, and monitor patients closely for adverse events such as respiratory depression.

• Periodically reevaluate patient's need for therapy.

• *Look alike–sound alike:* Don't confuse hydrocodone ER with hydrocodone standard release. Don't confuse hydrocodone with oxycodone, oxymorphone, or hydromorphone.

PATIENT TEACHING

Boxed Warning Caution patient or caregiver of patient taking an opioid with a benzodiazepine, CNS depressant, or alcohol to seek immediate medical attention for dizziness, light-headedness, extreme sleepiness, slowed or difficult breathing, or unresponsiveness. ■

Boxed Warning Instruct patient to avoid alcoholic beverages, prescription drugs, and OTC products that contain alcohol during treatment. ■

Boxed Warning Instruct patient to swallow drug whole to avoid exposure to a potentially fatal dose of hydrocodone. Crushing, chewing, snorting, or injecting the dissolved product allows uncontrolled delivery of drug and may result in overdose and death. ■

Boxed Warning Inform patient that prolonged use during pregnancy can result in neonatal opioid withdrawal syndrome, which may be life-threatening. ■

⚠ *Alert:* Discuss emergency naloxone treatment for opioid overdose with patient and caregiver. Inform them of ways to obtain naloxone according to their state's prescribing and dispensing guidelines.

⚠ *Alert:* Encourage patient to report all medications being taken, including prescription and OTC medications and supplements.

⚠ *Alert:* Caution patient to immediately report signs and symptoms of serotonin syndrome, adrenal insufficiency, and decreased sex hormone levels.

⚠ *Alert:* Counsel patient not to discontinue opioids without first discussing the need for a gradual tapering regimen with prescriber.

• Caution patient not to share drug and to protect it from theft or misuse.

• Inform patient that potentially serious additive effects may occur if drug is used with other CNS depressants and to avoid such drugs unless supervised by a health care provider.

• Advise patient to report signs and symptoms of respiratory depression (respiratory rate less than 12 breaths/minute, shortness of breath, confusion, excessive drowsiness, nausea, vomiting) and to seek immediate medical attention. Risk of respiratory depression is greatest at drug initiation and dosage increases.

• Warn patient that use of drug, even when taken as recommended, can result in addiction, abuse, and misuse, which can lead to overdose or death.

• Caution patient not to drive or operate dangerous machinery until drug's effects are known.

Reactions in bold italics are *life-threatening*. Interactions may have a *rapid onset* or a ***delayed onset***.

• Warn patient about potential for severe constipation; teach management instructions and when to seek medical attention.

• Inform patient that drug may cause orthostatic hypotension and fainting. Teach how to recognize signs and symptoms of low BP and how to reduce risk of serious consequences of hypotension (e.g., sit or lie down, carefully rise from a sitting or lying position).

• Caution patient to seek medical attention immediately if hypersensitivity reactions, including anaphylaxis, occur.

Boxed Warning Instruct patient to store drug securely and away from children, to dispose of drug properly when no longer needed, and not to throw in regular trash. Accidental ingestion, especially by children, may result in respiratory depression or death. ∎

• Inform patient to dispose of unused capsules through a drug take-back program. If such a program isn't available in patient's area, instruct patient to flush unused capsules down the toilet.

SAFETY ALERT!

HYDROcodone bitartrate–acetaminophen

hye-droe-KOE-done/a-seet-a-MIN-oh-fen

Lortab Elixir

Therapeutic class: Opioid analgesics
Pharmacologic class: Opioid analgesics–para-aminophenol derivatives
Controlled substance schedule: II

AVAILABLE FORMS

Oral solution*: 7.5 mg hydrocodone/325 mg acetaminophen per 15 mL, 10 mg hydrocodone/300 mg acetaminophen per 15 mL
Tablets: 2.5 mg hydrocodone/325 mg acetaminophen, 5 mg hydrocodone/300 mg acetaminophen, 5 mg hydrocodone/325 mg acetaminophen, 7.5 mg hydrocodone/300 mg acetaminophen, 7.5 mg hydrocodone/325 mg acetaminophen, 10 mg hydrocodone/300 mg acetaminophen, 10 mg hydrocodone/325 mg acetaminophen

INDICATIONS & DOSAGES

➤ **Moderate to moderately severe pain**
Adults: 1 to 2 tablets (hydrocodone 2.5 to 5 mg/acetaminophen 300 to 325 mg) PO every 4 to 6 hours as needed or 1 tablet (hydrocodone 7.5 to 10 mg/acetaminophen 300 to 325 mg) PO every 4 to 6 hours as needed. Or, for oral solution, give 15 mL (hydrocodone 7.5 mg/acetaminophen 325 mg) or 11.25 mL (hydrocodone 10 mg/acetaminophen 300 mg) PO every 4 to 6 hours as needed. Refer to manufacturer's instructions for maximum dosages.
Children age 2 and older (solution only): Refer to manufacturer's instructions for specific weight- and age-based dosing.
Adjust-a-dose: Adjust dosage according to severity of pain and patient response. Use a low initial dose in older adults and in patients with hepatic or renal impairment; monitor closely for adverse events, such as respiratory depression and sedation.
Boxed Warning Total acetaminophen intake shouldn't exceed 4,000 mg/day in adults and in children age 14 and older. ∎

ADMINISTRATION
PO

• Give drug with food or milk.

🜂 *Alert:* Ensure accuracy when prescribing, dispensing, and administering oral solution. Dosing errors due to confusion between mg and mL, and among other hydrocodone bitartrate–acetaminophen oral solutions of different concentrations, can result in accidental overdose and death.

• Administer oral solution by a calibrated device such as syringe or dropper.

• Only oral solution is approved for pediatric use.

ACTION

Inhibits synthesis of prostaglandins and binds to opiate receptors in CNS and peripherally blocks pain impulse generation; produces antipyresis by direct action on hypothalamic heat-regulating center; causes cough suppression by direct central action in medulla; may produce generalized CNS depression.

Route	Onset	Peak	Duration
PO (hydrocodone)	10–20 min	1–1.6 hr	4–8 hr
PO (acetaminophen)	Unknown	0.5–1 hr	4–6 hr

Half-life: Hydrocodone, 3.5 to 4.1 hours; acetaminophen, 1.25 to 3 hours.

ADVERSE REACTIONS

CNS: light-headedness, dizziness, sedation, drowsiness, mental clouding, lethargy, impairment of mental and physical performance, anxiety, fear, dysphoria, psychological dependence, mood changes, stupor, *coma.* **CV:** *bradycardia, cardiac arrest, circulatory shock,* hypotension. **EENT:** hearing impairment, permanent hearing loss. **GI:** nausea, vomiting, constipation, abdominal pain, heartburn, peptic ulcer. **GU:** urethral spasms, spasm of vesical sphincters, urine retention, *nephrotoxicity.* **Hematologic:** iron deficiency anemia, prolonged bleeding time, hemolytic anemia, *thrombocytopenia, agranulocytosis.* **Hepatic:** increased LFT values. **Metabolic:** *hypoglycemia.* **Musculoskeletal:** muscle flaccidity. **Respiratory:** *respiratory depression, acute airway obstruction, apnea,* dyspnea. **Skin:** rash, pruritus, diaphoresis, cold and clammy skin, *SJS, TEN.* **Other:** allergic reaction.

INTERACTIONS

Drug-drug. *Anticholinergics:* May increase risk of urine retention, severe constipation, or paralytic ileus. Avoid use together.

Boxed Warning *Antidepressants, antipsychotics, anxiolytics, barbiturates, benzodiazepines or other CNS depressants, other opioids:* May cause slow or difficult breathing, sedation, and death. Avoid use together. If use together is necessary, limit dosage and duration of each drug to minimum necessary for desired effect. ∎

Barbiturates, metyrapone, mipomersen: May increase risk of hepatotoxicity from acetaminophen. Monitor therapy.

Carbamazepine, dasatinib, hydantoins, isoniazid: May increase risk of hepatotoxicity from acetaminophen. Use cautiously together. Consider alternative therapy.

Boxed Warning *CYP3A4 inhibitors (amiodarone, erythromycin, ketoconazole, nefazodone, protease inhibitors, ritonavir):* May increase hydrocodone plasma level and prolong opioid effects, especially if use of CYP3A4 inhibitors is concomitant. These effects may be more pronounced with concomitant use of both CYP3A4 and CYP2D6 inhibitors, particularly when an inhibitor is added after a stable dose is achieved. Monitor patient for respiratory depression and sedation; consider dosage adjustments until drug effects are stable. ∎

Boxed Warning *CYP3A4 inducers (carbamazepine, phenytoin, rifampin):* May decrease hydrocodone plasma level, decreasing efficacy and potentially causing withdrawal symptoms. Monitor patient for effectiveness of drug and for opioid withdrawal symptoms. Consider dosage adjustments until stable. If CYP3A4 inducer is stopped, monitor patient for increased therapeutic and adverse effects, especially respiratory depression. ∎

Diuretics: May reduce effects of diuretics. Monitor clinical response.

MAO inhibitors: May potentiate effects of opioid analgesics. Don't use in patients who have received MAO inhibitors within past 14 days.

Mixed agonist/antagonists (butorphanol, nalbuphine, pentazocine), partial agonists (buprenorphine): May reduce analgesic effect of hydrocodone or precipitate withdrawal symptoms. Avoid concurrent use.

⬩ **Alert:** *Serotonergic drugs (amoxapine, antimigraine drugs, buspirone, cyclobenzaprine, dextromethorphan, linezolid, lithium, MAO inhibitors, maprotiline, methylene blue, mirtazapine, nefazodone, SSNRIs, SSRIs, TCAs, trazodone, tryptophan, vilazodone):* May increase risk of serotonin syndrome. Use together cautiously. Monitor patient for serotonin syndrome.

Sodium oxybate: May increase sleep duration and CNS depression. Consider therapy modification.

Drug-herb. *Kava kava, valerian:* May increase risk of excessive sedation. Avoid use together.

⬩ **Alert:** *St. John's wort:* May decrease hydrocodone serum level. Use together cautiously.

Drug-lifestyle. **Boxed Warning** *Alcohol use:* May increase hydrocodone plasma level and risk of fatal overdose. Patients shouldn't consume alcoholic beverages or use other drugs that contain alcohol. ∎

EFFECTS ON LAB TEST RESULTS

- May increase amylase and lipase levels.
- May decrease thrombocyte and WBC counts.
- Acetaminophen may produce false-positive results on urinary 5-hydroxyindoleacetic acid test.

CONTRAINDICATIONS & CAUTIONS

Boxed Warning Acetaminophen has been associated with acute liver failure, at times

---

Reactions in bold italics are *life-threatening*. Interactions may have a *rapid onset* or a *delayed onset*.

resulting in liver transplant and death. Most liver injury has been associated with the use of acetaminophen at doses exceeding 4,000 mg/day, and often involves more than one acetaminophen-containing product. ▪

Boxed Warning Opioids should only be prescribed with benzodiazepines or other CNS depressants to patients for whom alternative treatment options are inadequate. Limit dosages and durations to minimum required. ▪

Boxed Warning Drug exposes patient to risks of addiction, abuse, and misuse, even at recommended doses, which can lead to overdose and death. Assess each patient's risk before prescribing; monitor patients for these behaviors or conditions. ▪

Boxed Warning The FDA has required a REMS program for this drug. Drug companies with approved opioid analgesic products must make a REMS-compliant education program available to health care providers, who are strongly encouraged to complete the education program; discuss the safe use, serious risks, and proper storage and disposal of opioid analgesics with patients and their caregivers every time these medicines are prescribed; emphasize the importance of reading the Medication Guide every time an opioid analgesic is dispensed to them; and consider using other tools to improve patient, household, and community safety. ▪

Boxed Warning Accidental ingestion of even one dose of this drug, especially by children, can result in a fatal hydrocodone overdose. ▪

• Contraindicated in patients hypersensitive to hydrocodone or acetaminophen and in those with significant respiratory depression, acute or severe bronchial asthma in an unmonitored setting or in the absence of resuscitative equipment, or known or suspected GI obstruction, including paralytic ileus.

Boxed Warning Drug may cause serious, life-threatening, or fatal respiratory depression. ▪

◔ *Alert:* May cause serious, potentially fatal skin reactions, including SJS, TEN, and acute generalized exanthematous pustulosis. Reaction may occur with first or subsequent use when acetaminophen is used as monotherapy or when it's one component of combination drug therapy. Monitor patient for reddening of

the skin, rash, blisters, and detachment of the upper surface of the skin. Stop drug immediately if skin reaction is suspected.

◔ *Alert:* Patients with any of the following conditions are at increased risk for oversedation and respiratory depression and require close monitoring: snoring or sleep apnea, first-time opioid use or previous (nonrecent) opioid use, opioid habituation or need for increased opioid doses, need for prolonged general anesthesia or other sedating drugs, preexisting pulmonary or cardiac disease, or thoracic or other surgical incisions that may impair breathing.

• Use cautiously in patients who are allergic to other opioids because cross-sensitivity may occur.

• Use cautiously in patients with a history of respiratory depression, drug abuse, head injury or increased ICP, seizures, acute abdominal conditions, liver disease, recent anesthesia, pulmonary disease, renal impairment, hypothyroidism, Addison disease, or BPH and urethral stricture.

• Use cautiously in older adults or patients who are debilitated and those sensitive to CNS depressants.

◔ *Alert:* Drug may lead to rare but serious decrease in adrenal gland cortisol production.

• Drug may reduce sex hormone levels with long-term use.

Dialyzable drug: Unknown.

⚠ *Overdose S&S:* Hydrocodone: Loss of consciousness, pinpoint pupils, respiratory depression, stupor, coma, skeletal muscle flaccidity, cold clammy skin, bradycardia, hypotension, apnea, circulatory collapse, cardiac arrest, death. Acetaminophen: Fatal hepatic necrosis, renal tubular necrosis, hypoglycemic coma, thrombocytopenia, nausea, vomiting, diaphoresis, general malaise.

PREGNANCY-LACTATION-REPRODUCTION

• Use during pregnancy only if benefit outweighs fetal risk.

Boxed Warning Prolonged use during pregnancy can result in neonatal opioid withdrawal syndrome, which may be life-threatening if not recognized and treated according to protocols developed by neonatology experts. ▪

Boxed Warning If opioid use is required for a prolonged period during pregnancy, advise patient of risk of neonatal opioid withdrawal syndrome (poor feeding, diarrhea, irritability, tremor, rigidity, seizures) and assure her that appropriate treatment will be available. ∎

• Don't use during labor and delivery; neonatal respiratory depression may occur.

• Opioids may appear in human milk. A decision to breastfeed should take into account benefits to the patient and risks to the infant.

• Monitor infants exposed to drug through human milk for excess sedation and respiratory depression. Also watch for withdrawal symptoms in infants who are breastfed when patient stops an opioid analgesic, or when breastfeeding is stopped.

• Prolonged opioid use may cause reduced fertility in individuals of reproductive potential. It's unknown whether these effects on fertility are reversible.

NURSING CONSIDERATIONS

• Monitor patients closely for an allergic reaction, particularly those who are allergic to other opioids.

• Drug may be targeted for theft, diversion, and misuse.

Boxed Warning Monitor patients for respiratory depression, especially within first 24 to 72 hours of drug initiation or after dosage increase. Serious, life-threatening, or fatal respiratory depression may occur. ∎

Boxed Warning Monitor patients for abuse or misuse of drug, especially those with a personal or family history of substance abuse (drug or alcohol addiction or abuse, mental illness). Counsel patients about risks and proper use of drug. ∎

🕚 *Alert:* Carefully monitor vital signs, pain level, respiratory status, and sedation level in all patients receiving opioids, especially those receiving IV drugs, even those given postoperatively.

🕚 *Alert:* If patient is taking opioids with serotonergic drugs, watch for signs and symptoms of serotonin syndrome (agitation, hallucinations, rapid HR, fever, diaphoresis, shivering or shaking, muscle twitching or stiffness, trouble with coordination, nausea, vomiting, diarrhea), especially when starting treatment or increasing dosages. Signs and symptoms may occur within several hours of coadministration but may also occur later, especially after dosage increase. Discontinue the opioid, serotonergic drug, or both if serotonin syndrome is suspected.

🕚 *Alert:* Monitor patient for signs and symptoms of adrenal insufficiency (nausea,

vomiting, loss of appetite, fatigue, weakness, dizziness, low BP). Perform diagnostic testing if adrenal insufficiency is suspected. If adrenal insufficiency is confirmed, treat with corticosteroids and wean patient off opioids, if appropriate. Discontinue corticosteroids when clinically appropriate.

• Monitor patient for signs and symptoms of decreased sex hormone levels (low libido, erectile dysfunction, amenorrhea, infertility). If signs and symptoms occur, evaluate patient and obtain lab testing.

🕚 *Alert:* Don't stop drug abruptly; withdraw slowly and individualize the gradual tapering plan to prevent signs and symptoms of withdrawal, worsening pain, and psychological distress in patients who are physically dependent. Refer to manufacturer's label for specific tapering instructions.

🕚 *Alert:* When tapering opioids, monitor patients closely for signs and symptoms of opioid withdrawal (restlessness, lacrimation, rhinorrhea, yawning, perspiration, chills, myalgia, mydriasis, irritability, anxiety, insomnia, backache, joint pain, weakness, abdominal cramps, anorexia, nausea, vomiting, diarrhea, increased BP or HR, increased respiratory rate). Such signs and symptoms may indicate a need to taper more slowly. Also monitor patients for suicidality, use of other substances, and mood changes.

• Older adults receiving drug, especially those with impaired hepatic or renal function, may become confused or oversedated. Start with low doses of hydrocodone and observe closely for adverse events such as respiratory depression.

• Monitor patients who have had a head injury.

• Use of opioids in patients with acute abdominal disorders may mask symptoms.

• Monitor patient for constipation; treat aggressively, if present.

• Monitor patients with history of seizure disorder for worsening seizure control.

• Use lowest initial dose in patients with renal or hepatic impairment, and observe closely for adverse events such as respiratory depression.

• Monitor liver and kidney function. Acetaminophen elimination may be increased in patients with hepatic impairment.

• Monitor patient's ability to urinate; report urine retention.

• Monitor BP and pulse regularly.

Reactions in bold italics are *life-threatening*. Interactions may have a *rapid onset* or a ***delayed onset***.

- Periodically reevaluate patient's need for therapy.

PATIENT TEACHING

🔊 *Alert:* Discuss emergency naloxone treatment for opioid overdose with patient and caregiver. Inform them of ways to obtain naloxone according to their state's prescribing and dispensing guidelines.

Boxed Warning Caution patient or caregiver of patient taking an opioid with a benzodiazepine, CNS depressant, or alcohol to seek immediate medical attention for dizziness, light-headedness, extreme sleepiness, slowed or difficult breathing, or unresponsiveness. ∎

Boxed Warning Instruct patient to avoid alcoholic beverages, prescription drugs, and OTC products that contain alcohol during treatment. ∎

Boxed Warning Inform patient that prolonged use of drug during pregnancy can result in neonatal opioid withdrawal syndrome, which may be life-threatening. ∎

Boxed Warning Instruct patient to store drug securely and away from children, to dispose of drug properly when no longer needed, and not to throw in regular trash. Accidental ingestion, especially by children, may result in respiratory depression or death. ∎

🔊 *Alert:* Counsel patient not to discontinue opioids without first discussing the need for a gradual tapering regimen with prescriber.

- Caution patient not to share drug and to protect it from theft or misuse.

- Warn patient that use of drug, even when taken as recommended, can result in addiction, abuse, and misuse, which can lead to overdose or death.

- Inform patient that drug may cause orthostatic hypotension and fainting. Teach patient how to recognize signs and symptoms of low BP and to reduce risk of serious consequences of hypotension by sitting or lying down when symptomatic or by carefully rising from a sitting or lying position.

- Explain the assessment and monitoring process to patient and family. Instruct them to immediately report difficulty breathing or other signs of a potential adverse opioid-related reaction.

- Advise patient that drug may impair judgment and not to operate heavy machinery or drive until drug's effects are known.

- Instruct patient to avoid alcohol while taking drug.

Boxed Warning Warn patient that drug contains acetaminophen (or Tylenol). Caution patient not to take more than 4,000 mg of acetaminophen on a daily basis (including from all medications being taken). Instruct patient to look for "acetaminophen" or "APAP" on package labels, not to use more than one product that contains acetaminophen, and to contact health care provider if patient has taken more than 4,000 mg in a day, even if feeling well. ∎

🔊 *Alert:* Encourage patient to report all medications being taken, including prescription and OTC medications and supplements.

🔊 *Alert:* Caution patient to immediately report signs and symptoms of serotonin syndrome, adrenal insufficiency, and decreased sex hormone levels.

- Teach patient to eat a high-fiber diet, drink plenty of fluids, and use a stool softener or bulk laxative to prevent constipation.

- Tell patient to stop drug and immediately report blurred vision, rash, or yellowing of the skin.

- Inform patient to dispose of unused tablets through a drug take-back program. If such a program isn't available in patient's area, instruct patient to flush unused tablets down the toilet.

🔊 *Alert:* Warn patient to stop drug and seek medical attention immediately if rash or reaction occurs while using acetaminophen.

hydrocortisone (oral, injection, rectal)
hye-droe-KOR-ti-sone

Alkindi Sprinkle, Cortef, Cortenema

hydrocortisone sodium succinate (injection)
Solu-Cortef

Therapeutic class: Corticosteroids
Pharmacologic class: Glucocorticoids

AVAILABLE FORMS
hydrocortisone
Enema: 100 mg/60 mL
Sprinkle capsules ⬤: 0.5 mg, 1 mg, 2 mg, 5 mg
Tablets: 5 mg, 10 mg, 20 mg
hydrocortisone sodium succinate
Injection*: 100-mg vial, 250-mg vial, 500-mg vial, 1,000-mg vial

---

♣Canada ◇OTC ◆Off-label use 🖉Photoguide ⬤Do not crush *Liquid contains alcohol ▨Genetic

INDICATIONS & DOSAGES

➤ **Rheumatic disorders (adjunctive therapy for short-term administration in psoriatic arthritis, RA including juvenile RA, ankylosing spondylitis, acute and subacute bursitis, acute nonspecific tenosynovitis, acute gouty arthritis, posttraumatic osteoarthritis, synovitis of osteoarthritis, epicondylitis); collagen diseases (SLE, acute rheumatic carditis, systemic dermatomyositis); dermatologic diseases (pemphigus, bullous dermatitis herpetiformis, severe erythema multiforme, exfoliative dermatitis, mycosis fungoides, severe psoriasis, severe seborrheic dermatitis)**
Adults: 20 to 240 mg PO daily. Or, initially, 100 to 500 mg succinate IM or IV; repeat every 2, 4, or 6 hours.
➤ **Severe or intractable allergic states (seasonal or perennial allergic rhinitis, bronchial asthma, contact dermatitis, atopic dermatitis, serum sickness, drug hypersensitivity reactions, transfusion reactions)**
Adults: 20 to 240 mg PO daily. Or, initially, 100 to 500 mg succinate IM or IV; repeat every 2, 4, or 6 hours.
Children: 0.56 to 8 mg/kg/day IV or IM in three or four divided doses.
➤ **Severe acute and chronic allergic and inflammatory processes involving the eye and its adnexa (allergic conjunctivitis, keratitis, allergic corneal marginal ulcers, herpes zoster ophthalmicus, iritis and iridocyclitis, chorioretinitis, anterior segment inflammation, diffuse posterior uveitis and choroiditis, optic neuritis, sympathetic ophthalmia)**
Adults: 20 to 240 mg PO daily. Or, initially, 100 to 500 mg succinate IM or IV; repeat every 2, 4, or 6 hours.
➤ **Respiratory diseases (symptomatic sarcoidosis, Loeffler syndrome not manageable by other means, berylliosis, fulminating or disseminated pulmonary TB when used concurrently with appropriate antituberculous chemotherapy, aspiration pneumonitis)**
Adults: 20 to 240 mg PO daily. Or, initially, 100 to 500 mg succinate IM or IV; repeat every 2, 4, or 6 hours.
➤ **Hematologic disorders (ITP in adults [IM form is contraindicated], secondary thrombocytopenia in adults, acquired [autoimmune] hemolytic anemia, erythroblastopenia, congenital [erythroid] hypoplastic anemia)**
Adults: 20 to 240 mg PO daily. Or, initially, 100 to 500 mg succinate IM or IV; repeat every 2, 4, or 6 hours.
➤ **Neoplastic diseases (palliative management of leukemias and lymphomas in adults and acute leukemia of childhood)**
Adults: 20 to 240 mg PO daily. Or, initially, 100 to 500 mg succinate IM or IV; repeat every 2, 4, or 6 hours as needed.
Children older than age 1 month: 0.56 to 8 mg/kg/day IV or IM in three or four divided doses.
➤ **Edematous states (to induce diuresis or remission of proteinuria in nephrotic syndrome, without uremia, of the idiopathic type or that is due to SLE)**
Adults: 20 to 240 mg PO daily. Or, initially, 100 to 500 mg succinate IM or IV; repeat every 2, 4, or 6 hours.
Children older than age 2: 0.56 to 8 mg/kg/day IV or IM in three or four divided doses.
➤ **Nervous system disorders (cerebral edema associated with brain tumors or craniotomy [IV], tuberculous meningitis with subarachnoid block or impending block when used concurrently with appropriate antituberculotics, trichinosis with neurologic or myocardial involvement)**
Adults: 20 to 240 mg PO daily. Or, initially, 100 to 500 mg succinate IM or IV; repeat every 2, 4, or 6 hours.
➤ **Endocrine disorders (adrenal insufficiency, congenital adrenal hyperplasia, nonsuppurative thyroiditis, hypercalcemia associated with cancer)**
Adults: 20 to 240 mg PO daily. Or, initially, 100 to 500 mg succinate IM or IV; repeat every 2, 4, or 6 hours.
➤ **Ulcerative colitis; regional enteritis**
Adults: 20 to 240 mg PO daily. Or, initially, 100 to 500 mg succinate IM or IV; repeat every 2, 4, or 6 hours.
➤ **Adjunctive treatment for ulcerative colitis and proctitis**
Adults: 1 enema (100 mg) PR nightly for 21 days. Or, 1 applicatorful (90-mg foam) PR daily or b.i.d. for 14 to 21 days.
➤ **Replacement therapy in adrenocortical insufficiency**
Children: Initially, 8 to 10 mg/m²/day (sprinkle capsules) t.i.d. in three divided doses. Higher doses may be needed based on child's age and disease symptoms. Individualize to

lowest possible dosage and round dose to nearest 0.5 or 1 mg. In older children, may divide daily dose into two doses b.i.d.

ADMINISTRATION

PO
• Give drug with milk or food when possible. Patient may need another drug to prevent GI irritation.
• Use the same dose when switching from tablets to sprinkle capsules.
• Don't give sprinkle capsule granules through NG or other gastric tube because granules may obstruct tube.
• Don't get sprinkle capsule wet because granules may remain in the capsule.
• To administer: Hold sprinkle capsule with the printed strength at the top; tap capsule to move granules to bottom of capsule. Squeeze bottom of capsule, twist off the top portion, then pour granules onto patient's tongue, or place granules on a spoon or spoonful of soft cold or room temperature food before placing in patient's mouth. Follow with fluid (e.g., water, milk, human milk, or formula). Don't add granules to liquid as this can result in reductions in the dose administered and may result in a bitter taste.

IV
▼ Reconstitute hydrocortisone sodium succinate with no more than 2 mL bacteriostatic water or bacteriostatic saline solution before adding to IV solutions. For doses of 500 mg or more, administer over 10 minutes. For direct injection, inject over 30 seconds to 10 minutes. Give intermittent IV infusion over 20 to 30 minutes.
▼ IV solutions are stable for 4 hours.
▼ **Incompatibilities:** Solutions other than D_5W, NSS, or dextrose 5% in NSS, and other drugs.

IM
• Reconstitute hydrocortisone sodium succinate with no more than 2 mL bacteriostatic water or bacteriostatic saline solution per vial.
• Inject deep into gluteal muscle. Rotate injection sites to prevent muscle atrophy. Avoid IM injection into the deltoid muscle as subcutaneous atrophy and sterile abscesses may occur.
• Injectable forms aren't used for alternate-day therapy.

Rectal
• Have patient lie on the left side during administration and for 30 minutes afterward to allow fluid to distribute throughout the left colon. Have patient try to retain the enema for at least 1 hour but preferably all night.

ACTION
Not clearly defined. Decreases inflammation, mainly by stabilizing leukocyte lysosomal membranes; suppresses immune response; stimulates bone marrow; and influences protein, fat, and carbohydrate metabolism.

Route	Onset	Peak	Duration
PO	Variable	1 hr	Variable
IV, IM, PR	Variable	Variable	Variable

Half-life: Oral, 78 to 128 minutes; IV, 60 to 180 minutes.

ADVERSE REACTIONS
CNS: euphoria, depression, insomnia, psychotic behavior, *pseudotumor cerebri,* vertigo, mood swings, headache, malaise, myasthenia, neuritis, neuropathy, personality changes, paresthesia, fever, syncope, *seizures.* **CV:** *HF,* edema, *arrhythmias,* HTN, thrombophlebitis, *thromboembolism, bradycardia,* tachycardia, vasculitis, cardiomegaly, *circulatory shock.* **EENT:** cataracts, glaucoma, conjunctivitis, otitis media, tonsillitis, pharyngitis, rhinitis. **GI:** abdominal distention, peptic ulceration, GI irritation, increased appetite, hiccups, *pancreatitis,* nausea, vomiting, *GI perforation.* **GU:** menstrual irregularities, increased urine calcium levels. **Hematologic:** easy bruising, leukocytosis. **Metabolic:** *hypokalemia,* hyperglycemia, carbohydrate intolerance, hypercholesterolemia, *hypocalcemia.* **Hepatic:** increased LFT values, hepatomegaly. **Musculoskeletal:** growth suppression in children, muscle weakness, osteoporosis, tendon rupture, vertebral compression fracture. **Respiratory:** URI, *pulmonary edema.* **Skin:** hirsutism, delayed wound healing, acne, atopic dermatitis, atrophic striae, burning sensation, diaphoresis, ecchymosis, erythema, hyperpigmentation or hypopigmentation, rash, thinning hair, urticaria, dry skin, skin eruptions, injection-site atrophy. **Other:** *anaphylaxis, angioedema,* hypersensitivity reactions, cushingoid state, susceptibility to infections, *acute adrenal insufficiency after increased stress or abrupt withdrawal after long-term therapy.*

H

INTERACTIONS

Drug-drug. *Antacids:* May decrease bioavailability of corticosteroids. Separate doses by 2 hours.

Antidiabetics: May increase glucose level and alter antidiabetic needs. Monitor therapy.

Aspirin, indomethacin, other NSAIDs: May increase risk of GI distress and bleeding. Use together cautiously.

Barbiturates: May decrease corticosteroid effect. Increase corticosteroid dosage.

Cyclosporine: May increase toxicity. Monitor patient closely.

CYP3A4 inducers (carbamazepine, efavirenz, nevirapine, oxcarbazepine, phenytoin, phenobarbital, rifabutin, rifampin): May decrease hydrocortisone (systemic) serum level. Increase hydrocortisone dosage.

CYP3A4 inhibitors (erythromycin, itraconazole, ketoconazole, ritonavir): May increase corticosteroid (systemic) serum level. Decrease corticosteroid dosage.

Estrogen-containing products (oral contraceptives, oral estrogen): May reduce effect of hydrocortisone. Increase hydrocortisone dosage as needed.

Live attenuated virus vaccines, other toxoids and vaccines: May decrease antibody response and increase risk of infection and neurologic complications. Avoid using together.

Mifepristone: May cause adrenal insufficiency and require high glucocorticoid doses. Increase glucocorticoid dosage.

NSAIDs: May increase risk of GI adverse effects. Monitor patient closely.

Oral anticoagulants: May alter dosage requirements. Monitor PT and INR closely.

Potassium-depleting drugs (thiazide diuretics): May enhance potassium-wasting effects of hydrocortisone. Monitor potassium level.

Skin-test antigens: May decrease response. Postpone skin testing until after therapy.

Tacrolimus (systemic): May decrease tacrolimus serum level. Conversely, when corticosteroid therapy is discontinued, tacrolimus level may increase. Monitor therapy.

Tacrolimus (topical): May enhance adverse or toxic effect of immunosuppressants. Avoid combination.

Drug-herb. *Echinacea, ginseng:* May diminish therapeutic effect of immunosuppressants. Discourage use together.

EFFECTS ON LAB TEST RESULTS

- May increase glucose and cholesterol levels.
- May decrease potassium and calcium levels.
- May cause decreased ^{131}I uptake and protein-bound iodine levels in thyroid function tests.
- May cause false-negative results in nitro-blue tetrazolium test for systemic bacterial infections.
- May alter reactions to coccidioidin skin tests.

CONTRAINDICATIONS & CAUTIONS

- Contraindicated in patients hypersensitive to drug or its ingredients, in those with systemic fungal infections, and in those receiving immunosuppressive doses together with live-virus vaccines.
- Use with caution in patients with recent MI.
- Use cautiously in patients with GI ulcer, renal disease, HTN, osteoporosis, diabetes, hypothyroidism, cirrhosis, diverticulitis, nonspecific ulcerative colitis, active hepatitis, recent intestinal anastomoses, thromboembolic disorders, seizures, myasthenia gravis, HF, TB, ocular herpes simplex, emotional instability, and psychotic tendencies.
- Drug can cause hypercorticism or suppression of the HPA axis, particularly in younger children or patients receiving high-dose therapy. Withdraw drug slowly.
- Kaposi sarcoma has been reported. Clinical remission may occur after discontinuation of corticosteroids.

Dialyzable drug: Unknown.

PREGNANCY-LACTATION-REPRODUCTION

- Use cautiously during pregnancy and breastfeeding. When essential during pregnancy, use lowest possible dose for the shortest duration. Avoid high doses in first trimester.
- Monitor infants exposed to drug in utero for hypoadrenalism.
- Drug appears in human milk and could cause adverse effects, including growth suppression. Breastfeeding isn't recommended.
- Steroids may alter the motility and number of sperm in some patients.

NURSING CONSIDERATIONS

- Determine whether patient is sensitive to other corticosteroids.
- Most adverse reactions to corticosteroids are dose- or duration-dependent.

Reactions in bold italics are *life-threatening*. Interactions may have a *rapid onset* or a ***delayed onset***.

- For better results and less toxicity, give a once-daily dose in morning.
- ⚠ *Alert:* Salts aren't interchangeable.
- ⚠ *Alert:* Only hydrocortisone sodium succinate can be given IV.
- ⚠ *Alert:* Epidural corticosteroid injections to treat neck and back pain and radiating pain in the arms and legs may result in rare but serious adverse events (vision loss, stroke, paralysis, death). The use of epidural corticosteroid injections isn't approved by the FDA.
- Enema may produce same systemic effects as other forms of hydrocortisone. If enema therapy must exceed 21 days, taper off by giving every other night for 2 to 3 weeks.
- High-dose therapy usually isn't continued beyond 48 hours.
- Always adjust to lowest effective dose.
- Monitor patient's weight, BP, and electrolyte levels.
- Monitor patient for cushingoid effects, including moon face, buffalo hump, central obesity, thinning hair, HTN, and increased susceptibility to infection.
- Unless contraindicated, give a low-sodium diet that's high in potassium and protein. Give potassium supplements.
- Drug may mask or worsen infections, including latent amebiasis.
- Stress (fever, trauma, surgery, and emotional problems) may increase adrenal insufficiency. Increase dosage.
- Watch for depression or psychotic episodes, especially during high-dose therapy.
- Inspect patient's skin for petechiae.
- Patient with diabetes may need increased antidiabetic medication; monitor glucose level.
- Periodic measurement of growth and development may be needed during high-dose or prolonged therapy in children.
- Older adults may be more susceptible to osteoporosis with prolonged use.
- Gradually reduce dosage after long-term therapy.
- Monitor patient for adrenal insufficiency (fatigue, weakness, arthralgia, fever, dizziness, lethargy, depression, fainting, hypotension, dyspnea, anorexia, nausea, vomiting, electrolyte disturbances, hypoglycemia) after abrupt withdrawal or withdrawal after prolonged treatment. Rebound inflammation can also occur. After prolonged use, sudden withdrawal may be fatal.

- ⚠ *Look alike–sound alike:* Don't confuse Solu-Cortef with Solu-Medrol. Don't confuse hydrocortisone with hydrocodone, hydroxychloroquine, or hydrochlorothiazide. Don't confuse Cortef with Coreg or Lortab.

PATIENT TEACHING

- Tell patient not to stop drug abruptly or without prescriber's consent.
- Instruct patient or caregiver in safe drug administration.
- Warn patient on long-term therapy about cushingoid effects (moon face, buffalo hump) and the need to notify prescriber about sudden weight gain or swelling.
- Teach patient signs and symptoms of early adrenal insufficiency: fatigue, muscle weakness, joint pain, fever, anorexia, nausea, shortness of breath, dizziness, and fainting.
- Instruct patient to carry a card with prescriber's name and name and dosage of drug, indicating the need for supplemental systemic glucocorticoids during stress.
- Warn patient about easy bruising.
- Urge patient receiving long-term therapy to consider exercise or physical therapy. Also, tell patient to ask prescriber about vitamin D or calcium supplement.
- Advise patient receiving long-term therapy to have periodic eye exams.
- Caution patient to avoid exposure to infections (such as chickenpox or measles) and to notify prescriber if such exposure occurs.
- ⚠ *Alert:* Counsel patient who receives epidural corticosteroid injections to seek immediate medical attention for vision loss or vision changes; tingling in the arms or legs; sudden weakness or numbness of the face, arm, or leg on one or both sides of the body; dizziness; severe headache; or seizures.
- ⚠ *Alert:* Advise patient to discuss benefits and risks along with other possible treatments with health care provider before patient undergoes epidural corticosteroid injection.

hydrocortisone (topical)
hye-droe-KOR-ti-sone

Ala-Cort, Ala-Scalp, Anusol HC,
Cortizone-10 ◇, Proctocort,
Scalpicin ◇, Texacort

hydrocortisone acetate (topical, rectal)
Anusol HC ◇, Cortaid ◇, Cortifoam,
Micort-HC

hydrocortisone butyrate
Locoid, Locoid Lipocream

hydrocortisone probutate
Pandel

hydrocortisone valerate

Therapeutic class: Corticosteroids
Pharmacologic class: Corticosteroids

AVAILABLE FORMS
hydrocortisone
Cream: 0.5% ◇, 1% ◇, 2.5%
Lotion: 1% ◇, 2%, 2.5%
Ointment: 0.5% ◇, 1% ◇, 2.5%
Rectal cream: 1%, 2.5%
Rectal ointment: 1%
Topical solution: 1% ◇, 2.5%
hydrocortisone acetate
Cream: 1%, 2%, 2.5%, 2.5% ◇
Lotion: 1% ◇, 2%
Rectal foam: 90 mg per application
Rectal suppositories: 25 mg, 30 mg
hydrocortisone butyrate
Cream: 0.1%
Lotion: 0.1%
Ointment: 0.1%
Solution: 0.1%
hydrocortisone probutate
Cream: 0.1%
hydrocortisone valerate
Cream: 0.2%
Ointment: 0.2%

INDICATIONS & DOSAGES
➤ **Inflammation and pruritus from corticosteroid-responsive dermatoses, adjunctive topical management of seborrheic dermatitis of scalp**
Adults and children: Clean area; apply cream, lotion, ointment, or topical solution sparingly daily to q.i.d. as directed until acute phase is controlled; then reduce dosage to one to three times weekly as needed. Give children lowest dose that provides positive results.
➤ **Inflammation from proctitis; adjunctive treatment of chronic ulcerative colitis, cryptitis**
Adults: 1 applicatorful of rectal foam PR daily or b.i.d. for 2 to 3 weeks; then every other day as needed. Or, 1 suppository PR b.i.d. to t.i.d. or 2 suppositories PR b.i.d. for 2 weeks. In factitial proctitis, recommended duration of therapy is 6 to 8 weeks.

ADMINISTRATION
Rectal
• Refer to manufacturer's instructions to properly fill applicator barrel.
• Wash hands before and after application.
• After filling applicator, gently insert tip into anus; push plunger to expel foam; then withdraw applicator.
• Thoroughly clean all applicator parts after each use.
• Avoid excessive handling of suppository, which is designed to melt at body temperature.
• Insert suppository, pointed end first, into rectum using gentle pressure.
Topical
• Gently wash skin before applying. To prevent skin damage, rub in gently, leaving a thin coat. When treating hairy sites, part hair and apply directly to lesions.
• Check individual products or prescription for frequency of administration.
• Avoid applying near eyes or mucous membranes or in ear canal; may be safely used on face, groin, armpits, and under breasts.
• Shake lotion well before use.
• For optimal absorption, apply to moist skin immediately after bathing or after wet soaks.
• Use occlusive dressing only if prescribed.
• Change dressing as prescribed. Stop drug and tell prescriber if skin infection, striae, or atrophy occurs.
• Continue treatment for a few days after lesions clear.

ACTION
Unclear. Diffuses across cell membranes to form complexes with cytoplasmic receptors, showing anti-inflammatory, antipruritic, vasoconstrictive, and antiproliferative activity.

Reactions in bold italics are *life-threatening*. Interactions may have a *rapid onset* or a ***delayed onset***.

Route	Onset	Peak	Duration
Topical, PR	Unknown	Unknown	Unknown

Half-life: Unknown.

ADVERSE REACTIONS
Topical
Skin: burning sensation, pruritus, irritation, dryness, erythema, folliculitis, hypertrichosis, hypopigmentation, acneiform eruptions, allergic contact dermatitis, atrophy, maceration, secondary infection, striae, miliaria with occlusive dressings.
Rectal
GI: local burning, itching, irritation. **Skin:** dryness, folliculitis, hypopigmentation, allergic contact dermatitis, impaired wound healing, fragile skin, petechiae, erythema, diaphoresis. **Other:** secondary infection.

INTERACTIONS
None significant.

EFFECTS ON LAB TEST RESULTS
• May increase glucose level.

CONTRAINDICATIONS & CAUTIONS
• Contraindicated in patients hypersensitive to drug or its components. Rectal formulations are contraindicated in patients with some GI conditions and after surgery. Refer to individual product information.
• Drug can cause hypercorticism or suppression of the HPA axis, which can lead to adrenal crisis.
• Don't use as monotherapy in primary bacterial infections (impetigo, paronychia, erysipelas, cellulitis, angular cheilitis), treatment of rosacea, perioral dermatitis, or acne.
• Drug isn't for ophthalmic use.
Dialyzable drug: Unknown.
⚠ *Overdose S&S:* Systemic effects.

PREGNANCY-LACTATION-REPRODUCTION
• There are no well-controlled studies during pregnancy. Use during pregnancy only if potential benefit justifies fetal risk.
• Use cautiously in breastfeeding.

NURSING CONSIDERATIONS
• If an occlusive dressing is applied and a fever develops, notify prescriber and remove dressing.
• If antifungal or antibiotic combined with corticosteroid fails to provide prompt

improvement, stop corticosteroid until infection is controlled.
• Systemic absorption is likely with use of occlusive dressings, prolonged treatment, or extensive body surface treatment. Watch for symptoms, such as hyperglycemia, glycosuria, and HPA axis suppression.
• Avoid using plastic pants or tight-fitting diapers on treated areas in young children. Children may absorb larger amounts of drug and be more susceptible to systemic toxicity.
• Monitor patient for fluid or electrolyte disturbances (sodium and fluid retention, potassium loss, hypokalemic alkalosis, negative nitrogen balance from catabolism of protein).
• Drug may suppress skin reaction testing.
• *Look alike–sound alike:* Don't confuse hydrocortisone with hydrocodone, hydroxychloroquine, or hydrochlorothiazide.

PATIENT TEACHING
• Teach patient or family member how to apply drug.
• Tell patient to wash hands after application.
• If an occlusive dressing is ordered, advise patient to leave it in place for no longer than 12 hours each day and not to use the dressing on infected or weeping lesions.
• Teach patient how to use rectal foam applicator or suppository if needed.
• Tell patient to stop drug and report signs of systemic absorption, skin irritation or ulceration, hypersensitivity, infection, or lack of improvement.
• For perianal application, instruct patient to place small amount of drug on a tissue and gently rub in.
• Instruct patient to disassemble applicator and clean with warm water after each use.
• Tell patient to stop using this product if condition worsens or if symptoms persist for more than 7 days.

H

HYDROmorphone hydrochloride (dihydromorphinone hydrochloride)

hye-droe-MOR-fone

Dilaudid, Hydromorph Contin ♥

Therapeutic class: Opioid analgesics
Pharmacologic class: Opioids
Controlled substance schedule: II

AVAILABLE FORMS

Capsules (extended-release): 3 mg, 4.5 mg, 6 mg, 9 mg, 10 mg, 12 mg, 18 mg, 20 mg, 24 mg, 30 mg
Injection: 1 mg/mL, 2 mg/mL, 4 mg/mL, 10 mg/mL
Injection (prefilled syringes): 0.2 mg/mL, 0.5 mg/0.5 mL, 1 mg/mL, 2 mg/mL, 4 mg/mL
Oral liquid: 5 mg/5 mL
Suppository: 3 mg
Tablets: 2 mg, 4 mg, 8 mg
Tablets (extended-release) ⓞ: 8 mg, 12 mg, 16 mg, 32 mg

INDICATIONS & DOSAGES

➤ **Management of pain severe enough to require opioid treatment and for which alternative treatment options are inadequate**
Adults: For patients who are opioid naive, 1 to 4 mg immediate-release tablets PO every 4 to 6 hours PRN. Or, 1 to 2 mg IM or subcut every 2 to 3 hours PRN. Or, 0.2 to 1 mg IV (slowly over at least 2 to 3 minutes) every 2 to 3 hours PRN. Or, 2.5 to 10 mg oral liquid every 3 to 6 hours PRN. Or, one suppository every 6 to 8 hours PRN. Or, for adults who are opioid tolerant currently on immediate-release hydromorphone and who require continuous analgesia for an extended period, starting dose of extended-release form is equivalent to total daily dose of immediate-release form. May increase by 4 to 8 mg every 3 to 4 days as needed to achieve adequate analgesia.
Adjust-a-dose: For older adults, use cautiously and reduce initial oral starting dose. Initial IV starting dose for older adults or patients who are debilitated should be 0.2 mg. For those with moderate renal impairment, reduce dose to 50% of usual starting dose. For those with renal or hepatic impairment, reduce dose to 25% to 50% of usual starting dose of immediate-acting forms. For extended-release forms, give patients with moderate hepatic impairment 25% of usual starting dose; give patients with moderate renal impairment 50%, and patients with severe renal impairment 25% of usual starting dose. Use an alternative analgesic for those with severe hepatic impairment.

ADMINISTRATION
PO
• Give drug with food if GI upset occurs.
Boxed Warning Patient should swallow extended-release tablets whole; don't break, chew, dissolve, crush, or inject them. ■
Boxed Warning Ensure accuracy when prescribing, dispensing, and administering oral solution to avoid dosing errors due to confusion between mg and mL, which could result in accidental overdose and death. ■
• For oral solution, use only a calibrated device that can measure and deliver prescribed dose accurately.
IV
Boxed Warning Don't confuse standard hydromorphone for injection with high potency formulation or other opioids; overdose and death could result. ■
▼ Give by direct injection over no less than 2 minutes.
▼ Respiratory depression and hypotension can occur. Give slowly, and monitor patient constantly. Keep resuscitation equipment available.
▼ A slightly yellowish discoloration may develop. Discoloration doesn't indicate loss of potency.
▼ **Incompatibilities:** None listed by manufacturer. Consult a drug incompatibility reference for more information.
IM
• Document administration site.
Subcutaneous
• Rotate injection sites to avoid induration with subcut injection.
PR
• Insert tapered end first.
• Patient must retain suppository.

ACTION
Unknown. Binds with opioid receptors in the CNS, altering perception of and emotional response to pain. Also suppresses the cough reflex by direct action on the cough center in the medulla.

Reactions in bold italics are *life-threatening*. Interactions may have a *rapid onset* or a ***delayed onset***.

Route	Onset	Peak	Duration
PO	15–30 min	30–60 min	3–4 hr
PO (extended-release)	Gradually over 6–8 hr	12–16 hr	13 hr
IV	5 min	10–20 min	3–4 hr
IM	15 min	30–60 min	4–5 hr
PR	Unknown	Unknown	Unknown
Subcut	15 min	30–90 min	4 hr

Half-life: Immediate-release, 2 to 3 hours; PO (extended-release), 11 hours.

ADVERSE REACTIONS

CNS: sedation, somnolence, dizziness, euphoria, light-headedness, insomnia, drug withdrawal syndrome (extended-release form), headache, confusion, syncope, dysgeusia. **CV:** *cardiac arrest,* hypotension, HTN, flushing, *bradycardia,* extrasystoles, palpitations, chest discomfort, edema, tachycardia. **EENT:** blurred vision, diplopia, nystagmus, dry eye syndrome, miosis, tinnitus, dry mouth, rhinorrhea. **GI:** nausea, vomiting, constipation, anorexia, increased appetite, weight loss, diarrhea, ileus, intestinal obstruction, abdominal pain, abdominal distention, eructation, flatulence, gastroenteritis, delayed gastric emptying, biliary colic. **GU:** urine retention, urinary frequency, urinary hesitancy, bladder spasm, ureteral spasm, dysuria, erectile dysfunction, sexual disorder, hypogonadism. **Hepatic:** increased liver enzyme levels. **Musculoskeletal:** arthralgia, muscle contractions. **Respiratory:** oxygen desaturation, hyperventilation, *hypoxia, apnea, respiratory depression, bronchospasm.* **Skin:** diaphoresis, pruritus, hyperhidrosis, rash, urticaria, pain at injection site. **Other:** induration with repeated subcut injections, physical dependence, pain.

INTERACTIONS

Drug-drug. *Anticholinergics:* May increase risk of urine retention or severe constipation. Use together cautiously.

Boxed Warning *Benzodiazepines, CNS depressants:* May cause slow or difficult breathing, sedation, and death. Avoid use together. If use together is necessary, limit dosage and duration of each drug to the minimum necessary for desired effect. ∎

Diuretics: May reduce efficacy of diuretics by inducing release of ADH. Monitor patient.

Droperidol, general anesthetics, minocycline, nabilone, neuromuscular blockers, other opioid analgesics, TCAs, tranquilizers: May cause additive effects. Monitor therapy carefully.

🖖 *Alert: MAO inhibitors:* May manifest as serotonin syndrome or opioid toxicity (e.g., respiratory depression, coma). Use together or within 14 days of MAO inhibitors isn't recommended. If administration with MAO inhibitors is unavoidable, monitor patient carefully for respiratory and CNS depression.

Muscle relaxants: May enhance neuromuscular blocking action of skeletal muscle relaxants and produce an increased degree of respiratory depression. Monitor patient.

Opioids (mixed agonist/antagonist): May diminish analgesic effect of opioid analgesics or cause withdrawal signs and symptoms. Avoid using together.

🖖 *Alert: Serotonergic drugs (amoxapine, antimigraine drugs, buspirone, cyclobenzaprine, dextromethorphan, linezolid, lithium, MAO inhibitors, maprotiline, methylene blue, mirtazapine, nefazodone, SSNRIs, SSRIs, TCAs, trazodone, tryptophan, vilazodone):* May increase risk of serotonin syndrome. Use together cautiously and monitor patient for serotonin syndrome.

Drug-herb. *Kava kava, valerian:* May increase CNS depression. Avoid use together.

🖖 *Alert: St. John's wort:* May increase risk of serotonin syndrome. Use together cautiously and monitor patient for serotonin syndrome.

Drug-lifestyle. Boxed Warning *Alcohol use:* May cause additive effects and risk of fatal overdose. Patients shouldn't consume alcoholic beverages or use other drugs that contain alcohol. ∎

EFFECTS ON LAB TEST RESULTS

• May increase liver enzyme levels.
• May decrease amylase level.
• May interfere with hepatobiliary imaging studies because delayed gastric emptying and contraction of sphincter of Oddi may increase biliary tract pressure.

CONTRAINDICATIONS & CAUTIONS

Boxed Warning Opioids should only be prescribed with benzodiazepines or other CNS depressants to patients for whom alternative treatment options are inadequate. ∎

• Contraindicated in patients hypersensitive to drug; in those with intracranial lesions that cause increased ICP; in those with paralytic ileus or narrowed or obstructed GI tract;

for obstetric analgesia; and in those with depressed ventilation, such as in status asthmaticus, COPD, cor pulmonale, emphysema, and kyphoscoliosis.

Boxed Warning Extended-release form is contraindicated in patients who are opioid naive. It isn't indicated for acute pain or postoperative pain or as a PRN analgesic. Fatal respiratory depression may occur in patients who aren't opioid-tolerant. Accidental intake, especially in children, can cause fatal hydromorphone overdose. ■

Boxed Warning Hydromorphone is an opioid agonist with an abuse liability similar to other opioid agonists, legal or illicit. Risk of abuse is increased in patients with a personal or family history of substance abuse or mental illness. Use with ethanol, other opioids, and other CNS depressants can increase risk of adverse events, including death. ■

Boxed Warning The FDA has required a REMS program for this drug. Drug companies with approved opioid analgesic products must make a REMS-compliant education program available to health care providers, who are strongly encouraged to complete the education program; discuss the safe use, serious risks, and proper storage and disposal of opioid analgesics with patients and their caregivers every time these medicines are prescribed; emphasize the importance of reading the Medication Guide every time an opioid analgesic is dispensed to them; and consider using other tools to improve patient, household, and community safety. ■

Boxed Warning Serious, life-threatening, or fatal respiratory depression may occur. Monitor patients closely, especially at initiation or after a dosage increase. ■

Boxed Warning Accidental ingestion of even one dose of hydromorphone hydrochloride extended-release tablets, especially by children, can result in a fatal overdose of hydromorphone. ■

Boxed Warning Drug may result in neonatal opioid withdrawal syndrome, which may be life-threatening. ■

🜲 *Alert:* Patients with any of the following conditions are at increased risk for oversedation and respiratory depression and require close monitoring: sleep-disordered breathing; first-time opioid use or previous (nonrecent) opioid use; opioid habituation or need for increased opioid doses; need for prolonged general anesthesia or other sedating drugs;

preexisting pulmonary or cardiac disease; or thoracic or other surgical incisions that may impair breathing.

🜲 *Alert:* Drug may lead to rare but serious decrease in adrenal gland cortisol production.
• Drug may reduce sex hormone levels with long-term use.
• Drug may contain a sulfite that can cause allergic-type reactions, including anaphylactic symptoms and life-threatening or less severe asthmatic episodes in certain patients who are susceptible.
• Use cautiously in patients with a history of seizures and adrenal insufficiency.

🜲 *Alert:* Drug may cause severe hypotension, including orthostatic hypotension and syncope, in patients who are ambulatory. Patients with reduced blood volume and those receiving CNS depressants (e.g., phenothiazines or general anesthetics) are at increased risk.

🜲 *Alert:* Drug may reduce respiratory drive and the resultant CO_2 retention may increase ICP. Use cautiously in patients with a head injury.
• Use cautiously in older adults or patients who are debilitated and in those with hepatic or renal disease, hypothyroidism, Addison disease, prostatic hyperplasia, or urethral stricture.
• Safety and effectiveness in children haven't been determined. Drug has been used off label.

Dializable drug: Unknown.

⚠ *Overdose S&S:* Constricted pupils, cold clammy skin, extreme somnolence progressing to stupor or coma, respiratory depression, skeletal muscle flaccidity, bradycardia, hypotension, apnea, cardiac arrest, circulatory collapse, death.

PREGNANCY-LACTATION-REPRODUCTION

🜲 *Alert:* Drug crosses placental barrier. Carefully weigh benefits and risks of using drug during pregnancy.

Boxed Warning Use in pregnancy can cause neonatal withdrawal syndrome, which can be life-threatening, and requires management by neonatology experts. Advise patients of the risk, and assure them that appropriate treatment is available. ■
• Don't use during labor and delivery; neonatal respiratory depression may occur.
• Drug appears in human milk in low concentrations. Monitor infants who are breastfed and exposed to opioids for excess sedation

---

and respiratory depression. Also watch for withdrawal signs and symptoms in infants when maternal administration of an opioid analgesic is stopped, or when breastfeeding is stopped. Breastfeeding isn't recommended during treatment.

• Long-term use can cause hypogonadism and infertility.

NURSING CONSIDERATIONS

⚠ *Alert:* Vial stopper may contain latex.

• Reassess patient's level of pain at least 15 and 30 minutes after administration.

• For better analgesic effect for chronic pain, give drug at regularly scheduled intervals, before patient has intense pain.

Boxed Warning Routinely monitor all patients for signs and symptoms of misuse, abuse, and addiction during treatment. ∎

Boxed Warning Monitor patients for respiratory depression, especially within first 24 to 72 hours of drug initiation and after dosage increase. Serious, life-threatening, or fatal respiratory depression may occur. ∎

⚠ *Alert:* Carefully monitor vital signs, pain level, respiratory status, and sedation level in all patients receiving opioids, especially those receiving IV drugs, even those given postoperatively.

⚠ *Alert:* If patient is taking opioids with serotonergic drugs, watch for signs and symptoms of serotonin syndrome (agitation, hallucinations, rapid HR, fever, diaphoresis, shivering or shaking, muscle twitching or stiffness, trouble with coordination, nausea, vomiting, diarrhea), especially when starting treatment or increasing dosages. Signs and symptoms may occur within several hours of coadministration but may also occur later, especially after dosage increase. Discontinue the opioid, serotonergic drug, or both if serotonin syndrome is suspected.

⚠ *Alert:* Monitor patient for signs and symptoms of adrenal insufficiency (nausea, vomiting, loss of appetite, fatigue, weakness, dizziness, low BP). Perform diagnostic testing if adrenal insufficiency is suspected. If adrenal insufficiency is confirmed, treat with corticosteroids and wean patient off opioids, if appropriate. Discontinue corticosteroids when clinically appropriate.

• Monitor patient for signs and symptoms of decreased sex hormone levels (low libido, erectile dysfunction, amenorrhea, infertility).

If signs and symptoms occur, evaluate patient and obtain lab testing.

⚠ *Alert:* Don't stop drug abruptly; withdraw slowly and individualize the gradual tapering plan to prevent signs and symptoms of withdrawal, worsening pain, and psychological distress in patients who are physically dependent. Refer to manufacturer's label for tapering instructions.

⚠ *Alert:* When tapering opioids, monitor patients closely for signs and symptoms of opioid withdrawal (restlessness, lacrimation, rhinorrhea, yawning, perspiration, chills, myalgia, mydriasis, irritability, anxiety, insomnia, backache, joint pain, weakness, abdominal cramps, anorexia, nausea, vomiting, diarrhea, increased BP or HR, increased respiratory rate). Such signs and symptoms may indicate a need to taper more slowly. Also monitor patient for suicidality, use of other substances, and mood changes.

• Monitor patients with history of seizure disorder for worsening seizure control.

• Patients considered opioid tolerant are those receiving, for 1 week or longer, at least 60 mg morphine per day, 25 mcg/hour transdermal fentanyl, 30 mg oral oxycodone per day, 8 mg oral hydromorphone per day or more, 25 mg oral oxymorphone per day or more, or an equianalgesic dose of another opioid.

• Discontinue all other extended-release opioids before giving extended-release form of hydromorphone.

• Monitor respiratory and circulatory status and bowel function.

• Keep opioid antagonist (naloxone) available.

• Don't use with MAO inhibitor or within 14 days of stopping MAO inhibitor.

• Discontinue use of extended-release form if stopped for more than 3 days.

• Drug may worsen or mask gallbladder pain.

• Drug is a commonly abused opioid.

• Drug may cause constipation. Assess bowel function and need for stool softeners and stimulant laxatives.

• *Look alike–sound alike:* Don't confuse hydromorphone with morphine or oxymorphone. Don't confuse Dilaudid with Dilantin.

PATIENT TEACHING

• Instruct patient to request or take drug before pain becomes intense and to report all adverse reactions.

◐ Alert: Discuss emergency naloxone treatment for opioid overdose with patient and caregiver. Inform them of ways to obtain naloxone according to their state's prescribing and dispensing guidelines.

Boxed Warning Caution patient or caregiver of patient taking an opioid with a benzodiazepine, CNS depressant, or alcohol to seek immediate medical attention for dizziness, light-headedness, extreme sleepiness, slowed or difficult breathing, or unresponsiveness. ∎

Boxed Warning Warn patient that extended-release tablets must be taken whole. Caution patient not to cut, chew, crush, dissolve, or inject them. ∎

◐ Alert: Encourage patient to report all medications being taken, including prescription and OTC medications and supplements.

◐ Alert: Caution patient to immediately report signs and symptoms of serotonin syndrome, adrenal insufficiency, and decreased sex hormone levels.

◐ Alert: Counsel patient not to discontinue opioids without first discussing the need for a gradual tapering regimen with prescriber.

• Warn patient that use of drug, even when taken as recommended, can result in addiction, abuse, and misuse, which can lead to overdose or death. Instruct patient not to discontinue drug without first discussing the need for a tapering regimen with prescriber.

• Inform patient of the risk of severe constipation and measures to prevent it. Advise patient when to seek medical attention if prevention measures are ineffective.

• Instruct patient to use only a calibrated device to measure and deliver prescribed dose of oral solution accurately to prevent accidental overdose.

• Explain the assessment and monitoring process to patient and family. Instruct them to immediately report if patient has any difficulty breathing or any other signs of a potential adverse opioid-related reaction.

• Advise patient to take drug with food if GI upset occurs.

• When drug is used after surgery, encourage patient to turn, cough, and breathe deeply to avoid lung problems.

• Teach patient how to recognize signs and symptoms of low BP and how to reduce risk of serious consequences of hypotension (e.g., by sitting or lying down or by carefully rising from a sitting or lying position).

Boxed Warning Instruct patient to store drug securely and away from children, to dispose of drug properly when no longer needed, and not to throw in regular trash. Accidental ingestion, especially by children, may result in respiratory depression or death. ∎

• Warn outpatient to avoid hazardous activities that require mental alertness until drug's CNS effects are known.

Boxed Warning Inform patient that prolonged use during pregnancy can result in neonatal opioid withdrawal syndrome, which may be life-threatening. ∎

Boxed Warning Instruct patient to avoid alcoholic beverages, prescription drugs, and OTC products that contain alcohol during treatment. ∎

hydroxychloroquine sulfate
hye-droks-ee-KLOR-oh-kwin

Plaquenil

Therapeutic class: Antimalarials
Pharmacologic class: Aminoquinolines

AVAILABLE FORMS
Tablets ⓞⓝⓒ: 100 mg, 200 mg, 300 mg, 400 mg (each 200 mg is equivalent to 155 mg base)

INDICATIONS & DOSAGES
➤ **Suppressive prevention of malaria attacks caused by *Plasmodium vivax*, *Plasmodium malariae*, *Plasmodium ovale*, and susceptible strains of *Plasmodium falciparum***
Adults: 400 mg PO weekly on the same day each week, beginning 2 weeks before entering malaria-endemic area and continuing for 4 weeks after leaving area.
Children weighing 31 kg or more: 6.5 mg/kg PO weekly on the same day each week, beginning 2 weeks before entering malaria-endemic area and continuing for 4 weeks after leaving area. Don't exceed 400 mg weekly.
➤ **Uncomplicated malaria**
Adults: Initially, 800 mg PO, followed by 400 mg at 6 hours, 24 hours, and 48 hours after initial dose.
Children weighing 31 kg or more: Initially, 13 mg/kg (up to 800 mg) PO; then 6.5 mg/kg

---

Reactions in bold italics are ***life-threatening***. Interactions may have a *rapid onset* or a ***delayed onset***.

(up to 400 mg) at 6 hours, 24 hours, and 48 hours after first dose.

➤ **SLE; chronic discoid lupus erythematosus**

Adults: 200 mg PO daily as a single dose or 400 mg PO daily in two divided doses.

➤ **RA**

Adults: Initially, 400 to 600 mg PO daily as a single dose or in two divided doses. When good response occurs, continue at 200 to 400 mg daily in one or two divided doses. Maximum dose is 600 mg or 5 mg/kg per day, whichever is lower.

ADMINISTRATION
PO

🌢 *Alert:* Drug dosage may be discussed in "mg" or "mg base"; be aware of the difference. Hydroxychloroquine sulfate salt 200 mg is equivalent to hydroxychloroquine base 155 mg.

• Give drug with food or milk to minimize GI upset.

• Don't crush or divide film-coated tablets.

• To improve adherence when drug is used for prevention, advise patient to take drug immediately before or after a meal on the same day each week.

ACTION

Concentrates in the acid vesicles of the parasite and inhibits polymerization of heme. Can also inhibit certain enzymes by its interaction with DNA. Mechanisms of the anti-inflammatory and immunomodulatory effects in treatment of RA, chronic discoid lupus erythematosus, and SLE aren't fully known.

Route	Onset	Peak	Duration
PO	Unknown	3–4 hr	Unknown

Half-life: 40 to 50 days.

ADVERSE REACTIONS

CNS: *seizures,* irritability, nightmares, ataxia, psychosis, vertigo, dizziness, hypoactive deep tendon reflexes, headache, fatigue, extrapyramidal disorders, fever, suicidality. **CV:** *cardiomyopathy, HF, QT-interval prolongation, ventricular arrhythmias, torsades de pointes,* bundle-branch block, AV block, *sick sinus syndrome.* **EENT:** blurred vision, retinopathy, difficulty in focusing, reversible corneal changes, typically irreversible nystagmus, tinnitus, deafness. **GI:** decreased appetite, abdominal cramps, diarrhea, nausea, vomiting. **Hematologic:** *agranulocytosis, leukopenia, thrombocytopenia,* anemia, porphyria, *aplastic anemia, hyperleukocytosis.* **Hepatic:** *acute hepatic failure,* abnormal LFT values. **Metabolic:** weight loss, *hypoglycemia.* **Musculoskeletal:** proximal myopathy. **Respiratory:** bronchospasm. **Skin:** pruritus, lichen planus eruptions, skin and mucosal pigmentary changes, pleomorphic skin eruptions, worsened psoriasis, alopecia, photosensitivity, bleaching of hair, urticaria, SCAR. **Other:** *angioedema.*

INTERACTIONS

Drug-drug. *Antacids, kaolin, magnesium:* May decrease GI absorption. Separate dose times by 4 hours.

Antidiabetics, insulin: May enhance effects of a hypoglycemic treatment. An insulin or antidiabetic dosage decrease may be required.

Beta blockers: May increase CV effects of certain beta blockers (metoprolol). Carefully monitor patient. Consider using alternative beta blocker.

Cimetidine: May increase chloroquine exposure. Avoid use together.

Cyclosporine: May increase cyclosporine level. Monitor level closely.

Digoxin: May increase digoxin level. Monitor drug levels; monitor patient for toxicity.

Drugs that prolong QTc interval: May enhance QTc-prolonging effect of highest-risk QTc-prolonging drugs. Avoid combination.

Mefloquine: May increase QTc-interval prolongation and seizure risk when used concurrently. Avoid use together.

Phenothiazines: May increase serum level of phenothiazines. Monitor therapy.

Rifampin: May decrease hydroxychloroquine effect. Avoid use together.

EFFECTS ON LAB TEST RESULTS

• May increase LFT values.

• May decrease Hb level and granulocyte, WBC, and platelet counts.

CONTRAINDICATIONS & CAUTIONS

• Contraindicated in patients hypersensitive to drug.

• Use cautiously in patients with retinal or visual field changes, psoriasis or porphyria, and with long-term treatment in children.

• Daily doses exceeding 5 mg/kg (actual weight) of hydroxychloroquine increase incidence of retinopathy.

• Use cautiously in patients with severe GI, neurologic, or blood disorders.

• Use cautiously in patients with diabetes and in those with low blood glucose levels. Drug may cause hypoglycemia.

• Use cautiously in patients with hepatic disease or alcoholism or when used with hepatotoxic drugs.

▨ Use cautiously in patients with G6PD deficiency. Drug may cause hemolysis.

◑ *Alert:* Use cautiously in patients with cardiac disease or QT-interval prolongation. Drug prolongs QT interval and may cause cardiotoxicity.

◑ *Alert:* Suicidality has been reported in very rare cases.

◑ *Alert:* Drug can't be given to children less than 31 kg because the film-coated tablets can't be crushed or divided.

◑ *Alert:* Safety and effectiveness of drug haven't been established in children for the treatment of RA, chronic discoid lupus erythematosus, or SLE.

Dialyzable drug: Unknown.

⚠ *Overdose S&S:* Headache, drowsiness, visual disturbances, CV collapse, seizures, sudden and early respiratory and cardiac arrest, atrial standstill, nodal rhythm, prolonged intraventricular conduction time, progressive bradycardia leading to ventricular fibrillation or arrest.

PREGNANCY-LACTATION-REPRODUCTION

• Drug doesn't appear to pose a significant risk to the fetus, especially with lower doses.

• Drug appears in human milk. Use cautiously in breastfeeding; infants are extremely sensitive to toxic effects of 4-aminoquinolines such as hydroxychloroquine.

NURSING CONSIDERATIONS

• Before prescribing drug for treatment or prophylaxis of malaria, consult the CDC malaria website (www.cdc.gov/parasites/malaria/).

• Ensure that baseline and periodic ophthalmic exams are performed at baseline and annually. Check periodically for ocular muscle weakness after long-term use. Retinal toxicity is largely dose-related.

• Monitor CBC and LFTs periodically during long-term therapy; if severe blood disorder not caused by disease develops, drug may need to be stopped.

◑ *Alert:* Monitor patient for possible overdose, which can quickly lead to toxic signs or symptoms. Children are extremely susceptible to toxicity.

PATIENT TEACHING

• Teach patient safe drug administration and importance of adherence.

• Advise patient to report adverse reactions, infection, and signs and symptoms of liver failure (dark urine, feeling tired, yellowing of skin or eyes) or bleeding.

• Instruct patient to report changes in medications as many drug interactions exist.

• Tell patient that dizziness may occur and to use caution while driving or performing other tasks that require alertness, coordination, or physical dexterity.

SAFETY ALERT!

hydroxyurea
hye-droks-ee-yoor-EE-a

Droxia, Hydrea, Siklos

Therapeutic class: Antineoplastics
Pharmacologic class: Antimetabolites

AVAILABLE FORMS
Capsules: 200 mg, 300 mg, 400 mg, 500 mg
Tablets: 100 mg, 1,000 mg

INDICATIONS & DOSAGES
Adjust-a-dose (for all indications): Base dosage on patient's actual or ideal weight, whichever is less. Dosage adjustment is recommended in renal impairment. According to manufacturer, if CrCl is less than 60 mL/minute or in patients with ESRD, give 50% of usual dose. If patient is on hemodialysis, give 50% of usual dose after dialysis on dialysis days.

➤ **Carcinoma of the head (excluding lip) and neck, with radiation (Hydrea); resistant chronic myelocytic leukemia (Hydrea)**
Adults: Initially, 1.5 mg/kg PO daily. Individualize treatment regimen based on tumor type, response, and current clinical practice standards.

➤ **To reduce frequency of painful crises and need for blood transfusions in adults with sickle cell anemia with recurrent moderate to severe painful crises (Droxia, Siklos)**

Reactions in bold italics are *life-threatening*. Interactions may have a *rapid onset* or a *delayed onset*.

Adults (Droxia): 15 mg/kg PO once daily. Monitor blood counts every 2 weeks. If blood counts are in acceptable range, may increase dose by 5 mg/kg daily every 12 weeks until maximum tolerated dose or 35 mg/kg daily has been reached. If blood counts are considered toxic, withhold drug until counts recover. Resume treatment after reducing dose by 2.5 mg/kg daily. May titrate up or down every 12 weeks in 2.5-mg/kg/day increments. Patient should be at a stable dose with no hematologic toxicity for 24 weeks. Discontinue drug permanently if hematologic toxicity recurs.

Adults and children age 2 and older (Siklos): 15 mg/kg (adults) or 20 mg/kg (children) PO once daily. Monitor blood counts every 2 weeks. If blood counts are in acceptable range, may increase dosage by 5 mg/kg daily every 8 weeks or if a painful crisis occurs until mild myelosuppression (ANC 2,000 to 4,000/mm³) is achieved, or up to a maximum dose of 35 mg/kg/day. If blood counts are considered toxic, withhold drug until counts recover. Resume treatment after reducing dosage by 5 mg/kg daily. Every 8 weeks thereafter, may adjust dosage up or down in 5-mg/kg daily increments until patient is at a stable, nontoxic dose for 24 weeks. Discontinue permanently if hematologic toxicity develops twice.

➤ **Thrombocythemia ◆**

Adults: 500 to 1,000 mg PO daily. Adjust dosage to maintain platelet count at less than 400,000/mm³.

ADMINISTRATION
PO

- Wear gloves when handling drug or its container, and wash hands before and after contact with bottle or capsule. If powder from capsule is spilled, wipe up immediately with a damp towel. Dispose of towel in a closed container such as a plastic bag. The spill areas should then be cleaned three times using a detergent solution followed by clean water.
- Patient must swallow capsules whole and not open, break, or chew them.
- Patient should take tablets with a glass of water.
- The 1,000-mg tablets have three score lines and can be split into four parts (each 250 mg). The 100-mg tablets can be split into two parts (each 50 mg). Calculate the rounded doses to the nearest 50- or 100-mg strength based on clinical judgment.

- For patients who can't swallow tablets, disperse them immediately before use in a small quantity of water in a teaspoon.

ACTION
May inhibit DNA synthesis.

Route	Onset	Peak	Duration
PO	Unknown	1–4 hr	24 hr

Half-life: 2 to 4 hours.

ADVERSE REACTIONS
CNS: malaise, fever, drowsiness, headache, dizziness, asthenia, fatigue. **CV:** *hemorrhage,* edema. **GI:** anorexia, nausea, vomiting, diarrhea, stomatitis, constipation. **Hematologic:** *leukopenia, thrombocytopenia,* anemia, macrocytosis, megaloblastosis, *bone marrow suppression.* **Metabolic:** hyperuricemia, vitamin D deficiency, weight gain. **Musculoskeletal:** arthralgia, back pain, extremity pain. **Respiratory:** cough, lung disorder, dyspnea. **Skin:** rash, itching, alopecia, dry skin, vasculitic toxicities (including vasculitic ulcerations and gangrene), nail discoloration. **Other:** chills, infection.

INTERACTIONS
Drug-drug. ❸ *Alert: Antiretrovirals (didanosine, stavudine):* May cause hepatotoxicity and hepatic failure, resulting in death. When given with didanosine to patients infected with HIV, severe peripheral neuropathy or fatal pancreatitis may occur. Avoid using with didanosine and stavudine.
Cytotoxic drugs, radiation therapy: May enhance toxicity of hydroxyurea. Use together cautiously.
Interferon: May increase the risk of cutaneous vasculitic toxicities, including vasculitic ulcerations and gangrene. Stop drug.
Live-virus vaccines: May increase risk of vaccine-related adverse reactions, viral replication, and severe infection. Avoid vaccinations during and for 3 months after therapy ends.

EFFECTS ON LAB TEST RESULTS
- May increase BUN, creatinine, hepatic enzyme, and uric acid levels.
- May decrease Hb level and WBC, RBC, and platelet counts.
- May interfere with lactic acid, urea, or uric acid assays, resulting in falsely elevated results.

CONTRAINDICATIONS & CAUTIONS

• Contraindicated in patients hypersensitive to drug or its components.
• Don't initiate treatment if bone marrow function is markedly depressed. Bone marrow suppression may occur, and leukopenia is generally its first and most common manifestation. Thrombocytopenia and anemia occur less often, and are seldom seen without a preceding leukopenia.
• Use cautiously in patients with renal dysfunction and in older adults.
• Safety and effectiveness of Hydrea in children haven't been established.
Dialyzable drug: Yes.
⚠ *Overdose S&S:* Acute mucocutaneous toxicity; soreness, violet erythema on palms and soles followed by scaling of hands and feet; severe generalized hyperpigmentation of the skin; stomatitis.

PREGNANCY-LACTATION-REPRODUCTION

• Drug can cause fetal harm; don't use during pregnancy.
• Verify pregnancy status of patients of childbearing potential before initiating therapy.
• Patients of childbearing potential should use effective contraception during therapy and for at least 6 months after final dose. Males with partners of childbearing potential should use effective contraception during therapy and for at least 6 months (Siklos) or 1 year (Droxia, Hydrea) after final dose.
• Patient should discontinue breastfeeding or discontinue drug.
• Azoospermia or oligospermia, sometimes reversible, has been observed.

NURSING CONSIDERATIONS

Boxed Warning Droxia and Siklos may cause severe myelosuppression. Monitor blood counts at baseline and throughout therapy. Treatment interruption and dosage reductions may be needed. ∎
Boxed Warning Droxia and Siklos are carcinogenic. Monitor patient for malignancies. ∎
• Verify pregnancy status before treatment.
• Routinely measure BUN, uric acid, liver enzyme, and creatinine levels; monitor blood counts every 2 weeks.
• Use fetal Hb (HbF) level to evaluate drug's efficacy in sickle cell anemia. Obtain HbF level every 3 to 4 months. Monitor patient for

an increase in HbF level of at least twofold over baseline.
• Acceptable blood counts during Droxia dosage adjustment for sickle cell anemia are neutrophil count of $2,500/mm^3$ or more, platelet count of $95,000/mm^3$ or more, Hb level more than 5.3 g/dL, and reticulocyte count (if Hb level is below 9 g/dL) at least $95,000/mm^3$. Toxic levels are neutrophil count less than $2,000/mm^3$, platelet count less than $80,000/mm^3$, Hb level less than 4.5 g/dL, and reticulocyte count (if Hb level is below 9 g/dL) less than $80,000/mm^3$.
• Acceptable blood counts during Siklos therapy for sickle cell anemia are neutrophil count of $2,000/mm^3$ or more, platelet count of $80,000/mm^3$ or more, Hb level greater than 5.3 g/dL, and reticulocyte count greater than $80,000/mm^3$ if Hb is less than 9 g/dL. Toxic levels are neutrophil count less than $2,000/mm^3$ (younger patients with lower baseline count may safely tolerate ANC down to $1,250/mm^3$), platelet count less than $80,000/mm^3$, Hb level less than 4.5 g/dL, and reticulocyte count less than $80,000/mm^3$ if Hb level is less than 9 g/dL.
• Hydroxyurea may dramatically lower WBC count in 24 to 48 hours.
⚘ *Alert:* Patients who have received or are currently receiving interferon may be at greater risk for developing cutaneous vasculitic toxicities. Monitor patients closely; discontinue drug if toxicities occur.
⚘ *Alert:* Patients with HIV infection who are also receiving didanosine may be at increased risk for severe peripheral neuropathy and fatal pancreatitis. Avoid this combination.
• Monitor patient for pancreatitis. If it occurs, discontinue drug permanently.
• Drug may increase risk of hyperuricemia. Monitor fluid intake and output; keep patient hydrated.
• To prevent bleeding, avoid all IM injections when platelet count falls below $50,000/mm^3$.
• Blood transfusions may be necessary for cumulative anemia.
• Dosage change may be needed after chemotherapy or radiation therapy.

PATIENT TEACHING

• Tell patient and caregiver to wear gloves when handling drug or its container and to wash their hands before and after contact with the bottle or capsule. If powder from capsule

---

Reactions in bold italics are *life-threatening*. Interactions may have a *rapid onset* or a ***delayed onset***.

is spilled, they should wipe up immediately with a damp towel and dispose of the towel in a closed container such as a plastic bag. The spill areas should then be cleaned three times using a detergent solution followed by clean water.

Boxed Warning Advise patient blood counts must be monitored every 2 weeks throughout therapy to monitor for toxicity. ∎

• Advise patient to watch for signs and symptoms of infection (fever, sore throat, fatigue) and bleeding (easy bruising, nosebleeds, bleeding gums, melena) and to take temperature daily.

• Instruct patient of childbearing potential to use effective contraception during and for at least 6 months after therapy.

• Counsel patient to discontinue breastfeeding.

• Advise male patient with partner of childbearing potential to use effective contraception during and for at least 1 year after therapy ends.

• Inform male patient about the possibility of sperm conservation before start of therapy because azoospermia or oligospermia, sometimes reversible, has occurred.

• Advise patient to inform prescriber if patient has HIV or is taking antiretrovirals.

Boxed Warning Advise patient to use sun protection and that monitoring for development of secondary malignancies will be needed. ∎

hydrOXYzine hydrochloride
hye-DROKS-i-zeen

Atarax ✽

hydrOXYzine pamoate

Therapeutic class: Antihistamines
Pharmacologic class: Piperazine derivatives

AVAILABLE FORMS
hydroxyzine hydrochloride
Injection: 25 mg/mL, 50 mg/mL
Syrup: 10 mg/5 mL
Tablets: 10 mg, 25 mg, 50 mg
hydroxyzine pamoate
Capsules: 25 mg, 50 mg, 100 mg

INDICATIONS & DOSAGES
Adjust-a-dose (for all indications): In older adults, initiate drug at the lower end of dosage range and observe closely.
➤ **Anxiety**
Adults: 50 to 100 mg PO q.i.d. Or, 50 to 100 mg IM t.i.d. or q.i.d.
Children age 6 and older: 50 to 100 mg PO daily in divided doses.
Children younger than age 6: 50 mg PO daily in divided doses.
➤ **Preoperative and postoperative adjunctive therapy for sedation**
Adults: 50 to 100 mg PO.
Children: 0.6 mg/kg/dose PO.
➤ **Preoperative and postoperative and prepartum and postpartum adjunctive therapy to permit reduction in narcotic dosage, allay anxiety, and control emesis**
Adults: 25 to 100 mg IM.
Children: 1.1 mg/kg/dose IM.
➤ **Pruritus**
Adults: 25 mg PO t.i.d. or q.i.d.
Children age 6 and older: 50 to 100 mg PO daily in divided doses.
Children younger than age 6: 50 mg PO daily in divided doses.
➤ **Nausea and vomiting**
Adults: 25 to 100 mg/dose IM.
Children: 1.1 mg/kg/dose IM.

ADMINISTRATION
PO
• Give drug without regard for meals.
• Shake suspension well before giving.
IM
• Parenteral form (hydroxyzine hydrochloride) is for IM use only, preferably by Z-track injection.
🚱 *Alert:* Never give drug IV, subcut, or intra-arterially.
• Aspirate IM injection carefully to prevent inadvertent IV injection. Inject deeply into a large muscle (don't inject into lower and mid-third of upper arm).

ACTION
Suppresses activity in certain essential regions of the subcortical area of the CNS.

Route	Onset	Peak	Duration
PO	15–30 min	2 hr	Varies
IM	Rapid	Unknown	Varies

Half-life: Children ages 1 to 14, 4 to 11 hours; adults, 20 hours; older adults, 29 hours.

ADVERSE REACTIONS
CNS: drowsiness. **GI:** dry mouth. **Respiratory:** *respiratory depression (high doses).*
Skin: pain at IM injection site.

INTERACTIONS
Drug-drug. *Anticholinergics:* May cause additive anticholinergic effects. Use together cautiously.
CNS depressants: May increase CNS depression. Use together cautiously; dosage adjustments may be needed.
QT interval–prolonging drugs: May prolong QT interval and induce torsades de pointes. Monitor ECG.
Drug-lifestyle. *Alcohol use, cannabidiol, cannabis use:* May increase CNS depression. Discourage use together.

EFFECTS ON LAB TEST RESULTS
• May cause false-negative skin allergen tests by reducing or inhibiting the cutaneous response to histamine.
• May cause false-positive serum TCA screen.

CONTRAINDICATIONS & CAUTIONS
• Contraindicated in patients hypersensitive to drug, in those with known hypersensitivity to cetirizine hydrochloride or levocetirizine hydrochloride, and in patients with prolonged QTc interval.
• Drug can prolong QTc interval. Use cautiously in patients with risk factors for QTc-interval prolongation and in patients with conditions that predispose to QTc-interval prolongation and ventricular arrhythmia, as well as in those with recent MI, uncompensated HF, and bradyarrhythmias. Use cautiously during concomitant use of drugs known to prolong QTc interval.
• Use cautiously in older adults and in patients with glaucoma, BPH, urinary stricture, asthma, or COPD.
Dialyzable drug: Unknown.
⚠ *Overdose S&S:* Hypersedation.

PREGNANCY-LACTATION-REPRODUCTION
• Contraindicated during early pregnancy.
• It's unknown if drug appears in human milk. Use during breastfeeding isn't recommended.

NURSING CONSIDERATIONS
• If patient takes other CNS drugs, watch for oversedation.

• Drug may rarely cause acute generalized exanthematous pustulosis (AGEP), a serious skin reaction involving fever, pustules, and large areas of edematous erythema. Discontinue at first sign of rash, worsening of preexisting skin reactions, or other signs or symptoms of hypersensitivity. If signs or symptoms suggest AGEP, don't resume therapy.
• Older adults may be more sensitive to adverse anticholinergic effects; monitor these patients for dizziness, excessive sedation, confusion, hypotension, syncope, and dysuria.
• *Look alike–sound alike:* Don't confuse hydroxyzine with hydroxyurea, Hydrogesic, or hydralazine.

PATIENT TEACHING
• Warn patient to avoid hazardous activities that require alertness and good coordination until effects of drug are known.
• Advise patient against simultaneous use of other CNS depressants, and to avoid use of alcohol during therapy because drug may increase alcohol's effect.
• Tell patient to report all adverse reactions, especially heart palpitations, dizziness, fainting, difficulty breathing, difficulty urinating, or vision changes.

ibandronate sodium
eye-BAN-droh-nate

Boniva

Therapeutic class: Antiosteoporotics
Pharmacologic class: Bisphosphonates

AVAILABLE FORMS
Injection: 3 mg/3 mL prefilled syringes
Tablets ⓞⓣⓒ: 150 mg

INDICATIONS & DOSAGES
Adjust-a-dose (for all indications): In patients with severe renal impairment (CrCl less than 30 mL/minute), drug isn't recommended.
➤ **To treat or prevent postmenopausal osteoporosis**
Women: 150 mg PO once monthly on same day each month. Or, for treatment, 3 mg IV bolus once every 3 months.
➤ **Metastatic bone disease due to breast cancer ♦**
Adults: 6 mg IV over 1 to 2 hours every 3 to 4 weeks for up to 4 years.

Reactions in bold italics are *life-threatening*. Interactions may have a *rapid onset* or a *delayed onset*.

ADMINISTRATION

PO

• Give drug 1 hour before first food or drink of the day and before any other drugs or supplements (including calcium, antacids, or vitamins).

• Make sure patient doesn't lie down for at least 1 hour after receiving drug.

• Give drug with 6 to 8 oz of plain water only; avoid mineral water.

• Patient should swallow tablets whole only. Don't allow patient to chew or suck tablets as this may cause oropharyngeal ulceration.

• Patient shouldn't eat or drink anything except plain water for 1 hour after taking drug; this includes other oral medications.

• If a dose is missed and it's more than 7 days before the next scheduled dose, give dose the next morning; if the next scheduled dose is 7 days or less away, omit the missed dose.

IV

▼ Prefilled syringes are for single use only.

▼ Give undiluted using needle provided with the syringe.

▼ Give by IV bolus over 15 to 30 seconds.

▼ Don't use if drug is discolored or contains particulate matter.

▼ If an IV dose is missed, reschedule missed dose as soon as possible. Schedule subsequent injections once every 3 months from that dose.

▼ Store at room temperature.

▼ **Incompatibilities:** Calcium-containing solutions and other IV drugs.

ACTION

Inhibits bone breakdown and removal to reduce bone loss and increase bone mass.

Route	Onset	Peak	Duration
PO	Unknown	0.5–2 hr	Unknown
IV	Rapid	Unknown	Unknown

Half-life: PO, 37 to 157 hours for the 150-mg dose; IV, about 4.5 to 25.5 hours for the 2- to 4-mg dose.

ADVERSE REACTIONS

CNS: asthenia, dizziness, depression, fatigue, headache, insomnia, vertigo. **CV:** HTN. **EENT:** nasopharyngitis, pharyngitis, tooth disorder. **GI:** dyspepsia, abdominal pain, constipation, diarrhea, gastritis, nausea, vomiting, gastroenteritis. **GU:** cystitis, UTI. **Musculoskeletal:** back pain, arthralgia, arthritis, joint disorder, limb pain, localized osteoarthritis, muscle cramps, myalgia. **Respiratory:** bronchitis, URI, pneumonia. **Skin:** rash. **Other:** allergic reaction, infection, flulike symptoms.

INTERACTIONS

Drug-drug. *Angiogenesis inhibitors (systemic monoclonal antibodies):* May enhance adverse effects of bisphosphonate derivatives, especially risk of osteonecrosis of the jaw. Monitor patient for adverse effects.

Aspirin, NSAIDs: May increase GI irritation and risk of nephrotoxicity. Use together cautiously.

Deferasirox: May enhance adverse effects of deferasirox, especially risk of GI ulceration, irritation, or GI bleeding. Monitor patient for adverse effects.

Drugs that prolong QTc interval: May enhance QTc-prolonging effects. For high-risk QTc-prolonging agents, consider therapy modification. For moderate-risk QTc-prolonging drugs, monitor therapy.

Potassium-competitive acid blockers, PPIs: May decrease ibandronate therapeutic effects. Monitor therapy.

Products containing aluminum, calcium, magnesium, or iron: May decrease ibandronate absorption. Give oral ibandronate 1 hour before vitamins, minerals, or antacids.

Drug-food. *Food, milk, beverages (except water):* May decrease drug absorption. Give oral drug on an empty stomach with plain water.

EFFECTS ON LAB TEST RESULTS

• May decrease calcium level.

• May interfere with bone-imaging agents.

CONTRAINDICATIONS & CAUTIONS

• Contraindicated in patients hypersensitive to drug and in those with uncorrected hypocalcemia.

• Oral form is contraindicated in patients with abnormalities of the esophagus that delay esophageal emptying, such as stricture or achalasia and in those who can't stand or sit upright for 60 minutes.

🕒 *Alert:* There may be an increased risk of atypical fractures of the thigh in patients treated with bisphosphonates.

🕒 *Alert:* Drug may cause osteonecrosis, mainly in the jaw. Avoid invasive dental procedures if possible.

🍁Canada ◇OTC ◆Off-label use ⏀Photoguide ⊜Do not crush *Liquid contains alcohol ▓Genetic

• Drug may cause hypocalcemia, especially if dietary intake of calcium or vitamin D is inadequate.
• Don't give to patients with severe renal impairment (CrCl less than 30 mL/minute).
• Use cautiously in patients with a history of GI disorders.
Dialyzable drug: Yes.
⚠ *Overdose S&S:* Hypocalcemia, hypophosphatemia, hypomagnesemia, upset stomach, dyspepsia, esophagitis, gastritis, ulcer.

PREGNANCY-LACTATION-REPRODUCTION
• There are no adequate studies during pregnancy. Use during pregnancy only if potential benefit justifies fetal risk.
• Not indicated for use in patients of childbearing potential.
• It isn't known if drug appears in human milk. Use cautiously during breastfeeding.

NURSING CONSIDERATIONS
• Correct hypocalcemia or other disturbances of bone and mineral metabolism before therapy.
• Make sure patient has adequate intake of calcium and vitamin D.
• Obtain serum creatinine level and perform an oral exam before each dose in patients receiving IV ibandronate.
• Watch for signs of esophageal irritation (dysphagia, painful swallowing, retrosternal pain, heartburn).
• Monitor patient for bone, joint, and muscle pain, which may be severe and incapacitating and may occur within days, months, or years of start of therapy. When drug is stopped, symptoms may resolve.
• Watch for signs of uveitis and scleritis.
• Use care to avoid intra-arterial or paravenous administration, which can lead to tissue damage; must only be administered IV.

PATIENT TEACHING
• Instruct patient in safe drug administration.
• Advise patient to take calcium and vitamin D supplements as prescribed.
• Tell patient to report any bone, joint, or muscle pain.
• Caution patient to stop drug and immediately report signs and symptoms of esophageal irritation.
• Advise patient to have periodic dental exams to monitor for osteonecrosis of jaw.
• Instruct patient to seek medical attention if severe allergic reaction occurs.

ibrexafungerp
eye-brex-a-FUNJ-erp

Brexafemme

Therapeutic class: Antifungals
Pharmacologic class: Triterpenoid antifungals

AVAILABLE FORMS
Tablets: 150 mg

INDICATIONS & DOSAGES
➤ **Vulvovaginal candidiasis**
Adults and pediatric patients who are postmenarchal: 300 mg (two 150-mg tablets) PO approximately 12 hours apart for 1 day, for a total daily dosage of 600 mg (total of 4 tablets for a course of therapy).
Adjust-a-dose: If concomitantly used with strong CYP3A inhibitor, give one 150-mg tablet approximately 12 hours apart for 1 day (total of 2 tablets for a course of therapy).

ADMINISTRATION
PO
• Give without regard to food.
• Store at 68° to 77° F (20° to 25° C).

ACTION
Inhibits glucan synthase, an enzyme involved in the formation of the fungal cell wall.

Route	Onset	Peak	Duration
PO	Unknown	4–6 hr	Unknown

Half-life: 20 hours.

ADVERSE REACTIONS
CNS: dizziness. **GI:** abdominal pain, diarrhea, flatulence, nausea, vomiting. **GU:** dysmenorrhea, vaginal bleeding. **Hepatic:** elevated transaminase levels. **Musculoskeletal:** back pain. **Skin:** rash. **Other:** hypersensitivity reaction.

INTERACTIONS
Drug-drug. *Strong or moderate CYP3A inducers (bosentan, carbamazepine, efavirenz, etravirine, long-acting barbiturates, phenytoin, rifampin):* May significantly reduce ibrexafungerp level. Avoid use together.
Strong CYP3A inhibitors (itraconazole, ketoconazole): May significantly increase ibrexafungerp level. Reduce ibrexafungerp dosage.

Reactions in bold italics are *life-threatening*. Interactions may have a *rapid onset* or a **delayed onset**.

Drug-herb. *St. John's wort:* May significantly reduce drug level. Discourage use together.

EFFECTS ON LAB TEST RESULTS
• May increase hepatic transaminase levels.

CONTRAINDICATIONS & CAUTIONS
• Contraindicated in patients hypersensitive to drug or its components.
• Safety in patients who are premenarchal hasn't been established.
Dialyzable drug: No.

PREGNANCY-LACTATION-REPRODUCTION
• Drug may cause fetal harm; contraindicated during pregnancy.
• If drug is given during pregnancy or if pregnancy is detected within 4 days after patient takes drug, report drug exposure to Scynexis, Inc. (1-888-982-SCYX [7299]).
• It isn't known if drug appears in human milk or how drug affects milk production or infants who are breastfed. Weigh risk to infant.
• Patients of childbearing potential should use effective contraception during therapy and for 4 days after final dose.

NURSING CONSIDERATIONS
• Verify pregnancy status in patients of childbearing potential before start of therapy.
• If specimens for fungal culture are obtained before therapy, may start antifungal therapy before culture results are known. Adjust therapy once culture result is known.

PATIENT TEACHING
• Tell patient that course of therapy is two doses taken approximately 12 hours apart and that drug can be taken with or without food.
• Instruct patient to report known or suspected pregnancy.
• Tell patient who has inadvertently taken drug during pregnancy that there's a safety study that monitors pregnancy outcomes and to report the pregnancy to Scynexis, Inc. (1-888-982- SCYX [7299]).
• Counsel patient of childbearing potential to use effective contraception during therapy and for 4 days after final dose.
• Advise patient to report if taking other medications, as they may interfere with drug.

---

ibrutinib 🗌
eye-BROO-ti-nib

Imbruvica

Therapeutic class: Antineoplastics
Pharmacologic class: Kinase inhibitors

AVAILABLE FORMS
Capsules 🔘: 70 mg, 140 mg
Tablets 🔘: 140 mg, 280 mg, 420 mg, 560 mg

INDICATIONS & DOSAGES
Adjust-a-dose (for all indications): Recommended dosage for patients with mild hepatic impairment (Child-Pugh class A) is 140 mg daily; for those with moderate hepatic impairment (Child-Pugh class B), recommended dosage is 70 mg daily. Avoid use in patients with severe hepatic impairment (Child-Pugh class C). Refer to manufacturer's instructions for toxicity-related and drug interaction dosage adjustments.

➤ **Mantle cell lymphoma in patients who have received at least one prior therapy**
Adults: 560 mg PO once daily until disease progression or unacceptable toxicity.

➤ **Chronic lymphocytic leukemia (CLL) or small lymphocytic lymphoma (SLL); CLL or SLL with 17p deletion** 🗌
Adults: 420 mg PO once daily as a single agent or in combination with rituximab or obinutuzumab, or in combination with bendamustine and rituximab until disease progression or unacceptable toxicity.

➤ **Waldenström macroglobulinemia**
Adults: 420 mg PO once daily as a single agent or in combination with rituximab until disease progression or unacceptable toxicity occurs.

➤ **Marginal zone lymphoma in patients who have received at least one prior anti-CD20-based therapy**
Adults: 560 mg PO once daily until disease progression or unacceptable toxicity.

➤ **Chronic GVHD**
Adults: 420 mg PO once daily until GVHD progresses, underlying malignancy recurs, unacceptable toxicity occurs, or patient no longer requires treatment.

ADMINISTRATION
PO
- Drug is hazardous; use safe handling precautions.
- Give capsules and tablets whole with a glass of water at approximately same time each day.
- Patient should swallow capsules and tablets whole. Don't break, open, or crush capsules or tablets.
- Consider giving ibrutinib before rituximab or obinutuzumab, if applicable, when given on the same day.
- If a dose is missed, administer as soon as missed dose is remembered on same day; return to normal scheduling the following day. Don't give extra capsules or tablets to make up for missed dose.
- Store at room temperature in original package.

ACTION
Inhibits Bruton tyrosine kinase activity, resulting in decreased malignant B-cell proliferation and survival.

Route	Onset	Peak	Duration
PO	Unknown	1–2 hr	Unknown

Half-life: 4 to 6 hours.

ADVERSE REACTIONS
CNS: dizziness, headache, fatigue, fever, asthenia, insomnia, pain, anxiety. **CV:** atrial fibrillation, atrial flutter, HTN, peripheral edema, *hemorrhage.* **EENT:** blurred vision, decreased visual acuity, dry eye, increased lacrimation, epistaxis, sinusitis, oropharyngeal pain. **GI:** diarrhea, nausea, constipation, abdominal pain, vomiting, stomatitis, dyspepsia, decreased appetite, GERD. **GU:** UTI, hematuria. **Hematologic:** *neutropenia, thrombocytopenia,* anemia. **Metabolic:** dehydration, hyperuricemia, *hypokalemia,* hypoalbuminemia. **Musculoskeletal:** arthropathy, musculoskeletal pain, muscle spasms, arthralgia, weakness. **Respiratory:** URI, pneumonia, dyspnea, cough. **Skin:** skin infections, bruising, rash, petechiae, pruritus. **Other:** chills, *secondary malignancies,* infection, *sepsis.*

INTERACTIONS
Drug-drug. *Anticoagulants, antiplatelet agents, omega-3 fatty acids, vitamin E (systemic):* May increase risk of bleeding. Monitor bleeding risk and patient closely.

Digoxin: May increase digoxin level. Monitor drug concentrations.
Moderate CYP3A inhibitors (amprenavir, aprepitant, atazanavir, ciprofloxacin, crizotinib, darunavir, diltiazem, erythromycin, fluconazole, fosamprenavir, imatinib, verapamil): May increase ibrutinib level. Avoid concurrent use. If ibrutinib must be used, refer to manufacturer's product information for dosage adjustments and monitor patient for toxicities.
Strong CYP3A inducers (carbamazepine, phenytoin, rifampin): May decrease ibrutinib level. Avoid concurrent use and consider agents with less CYP3A induction.
Strong CYP3A inhibitors (clarithromycin, itraconazole, ketoconazole, nefazodone, nelfinavir, posaconazole, ritonavir, saquinavir, voriconazole): May increase ibrutinib level. Avoid concurrent use or withhold ibrutinib for antibiotic or antifungal regimens lasting less than 7 days. Monitor patient closely for toxicities.
Drug-herb. *Flaxseed oil:* May enhance antiplatelet effect. Monitor therapy.
St. John's wort: May decrease ibrutinib level. Avoid use together.
Drug-food. *Grapefruit products, Seville oranges:* May increase ibrutinib level. Avoid use together.

EFFECTS ON LAB TEST RESULTS
- May increase uric acid and creatinine levels.
- May increase lymphocyte count.
- May decrease Hb level and platelet and neutrophil counts.

CONTRAINDICATIONS & CAUTIONS
- Contraindicated in patients hypersensitive to drug or its components.
- Drug may increase risk of renal failure. Fatalities have been reported.
- Avoid use in patients with severe hepatic impairment (Child-Pugh class C).
- Drug may cause cardiac arrythmias and HF, including serious and fatal cases, particularly in patients with cardiac risk factors, HTN, acute infections, or a previous history of arrythmias.
- Use cautiously in older adults because of increased risk of adverse effects.
- Assess baseline risk and monitor patient for TLS; treat as necessary.

Reactions in bold italics are *life-threatening*. Interactions may have a *rapid onset* or a **delayed onset**.

• Drug may increase risk of hemorrhage in patients receiving antiplatelet or anticoagulant therapy. Watch for signs and symptoms of bleeding.

• Safety and effectiveness in children haven't been determined.

Dialyzable drug: Unknown.

PREGNANCY-LACTATION-REPRODUCTION

• Drug may cause fetal harm; avoid use during pregnancy. Patient should avoid pregnancy for 1 month after therapy ends.

• Obtain pregnancy test in patient of childbearing potential before starting drug.

• Male patient should avoid fathering a child during therapy and for 1 month after final dose.

• It isn't known if drug appears in human milk. Patient shouldn't breastfeed during therapy and for 1 week after final dose.

NURSING CONSIDERATIONS

• Verify pregnancy status before treatment.

• Monitor patients for signs and symptoms of hypersensitivity reactions and SJS.

• Fatal bleeding events have occurred. Monitor patients for bleeding and evaluate risk-benefit of use in patients receiving anticoagulants or antiplatelet drugs.

• Consider interrupting therapy for 3 to 7 days before and after surgery, depending on procedure type and risk of bleeding.

• Monitor patients closely for fever and other signs of infection. Serious, sometimes fatal, infections have occurred.

• Monitor blood counts monthly, as indicated.

• Monitor for hyperuricemia and evaluate renal function; maintain hydration.

• Evaluate patients for new malignancy during treatment.

• Monitor patients for HTN and start or adjust antihypertensives as clinically indicated.

• Assess ECG and evaluate patient for arrhythmias and HF at baseline and periodically during therapy. Obtain an ECG for patients who develop arrhythmic signs and symptoms (palpitations, light-headedness, syncope, chest pain) or new-onset dyspnea.

• Assess patient's baseline risk of TLS (high tumor burden) and take appropriate precautions. Monitor patient closely and treat appropriately.

PATIENT TEACHING

• Instruct patient in safe drug administration and handling.

• Caution patient to immediately report signs and symptoms of significant hypersensitivity reaction (wheezing, chest tightness, fever, itching, heavy cough, blue-colored skin, seizures, or swelling of face, lips, tongue, or throat).

• Instruct patient to contact prescriber if palpitations, light-headedness, syncope, chest pain, swelling of extremities, new-onset shortness of breath, diarrhea, nausea, vomiting, abdominal pain, fever, infection, bleeding, or easy bruising occurs.

• Caution patient to avoid becoming pregnant during therapy and for 1 month after therapy ends. Counsel patient to use effective birth control during treatment because drug may cause harm to the fetus.

• Advise male patient to avoid fathering a child during therapy and for 1 month after final dose.

---

ibuprofen ▨
eye-byoo-PROH-fen

Advil ◊, Advil Liqui-Gels ◊, Caldolor, Children's Advil ◊, Children's Motrin Jr Strength ◊, Ibuprofen ◊, Infants' Advil Concentrated Drops ◊, Junior Strength Advil ◊, Novo-Profen✦, pms-Ibuprofen✦

ibuprofen lysine
NeoProfen

Therapeutic class: Anti-inflammatory drugs
Pharmacologic class: NSAIDs

AVAILABLE FORMS
ibuprofen
Capsules: 200 mg ◊
Injection: 800 mg/8 mL (100 mg/mL) in single-dose vials; 800 mg/200 mL in single-dose IV bags
Oral drops: 40 mg/mL ◊
Oral suspension: 40 mg/mL ◊, 100 mg/5 mL ◊
Tablets: 100 mg ◊, 200 mg ◊, 400 mg, 600 mg, 800 mg
Tablets (chewable): 100 mg ◊
ibuprofen lysine
Injection: 10 mg/mL

INDICATIONS & DOSAGES

➤ **RA, osteoarthritis, arthritis**

Adults: 400 to 800 mg PO t.i.d. or q.i.d. Maximum daily dose is 3.2 g.

➤ **Mild to moderate pain; moderate to severe pain as an adjunct to opioid analgesics; fever reduction in children**

Children ages 12 to 17: 400 mg IV every 4 to 6 hours PRN. Infusion time must be at least 10 minutes. Maximum daily dose is 2,400 mg.

Children ages 6 months to younger than 12 years: 10 mg/kg IV up to a maximum single dose of 400 mg every 4 to 6 hours PRN. Infusion time must be at least 10 minutes. Maximum daily dose is 40 mg/kg or 2,400 mg, whichever is less.

➤ **Mild to moderate pain, fever**

Adults: 200 to 400 mg PO every 4 to 6 hours PRN. Or, for pain, 400 to 800 mg IV every 6 hours PRN; for fever, 400 mg IV followed by 400 mg IV every 4 to 6 hours or 100 to 200 mg IV every 4 hours PRN. Infuse over at least 30 minutes. Maximum dose, 3,200 mg/day. Use smallest effective dose.

Children age 12 and older: 200 to 400 mg PO every 4 to 6 hours. Maximum daily dose is 1.2 g. Use smallest effective dose.

Children age 11 weighing 33 to 43 kg: 300 mg chewable tablets or 15 mL (300 mg) oral suspension PO every 6 to 8 hours up to q.i.d.

Children ages 9 to 10 weighing 27 to 32 kg: 250 mg chewable tablets or 12.5 mL (250 mg) oral suspension PO every 6 to 8 hours up to q.i.d.

Children ages 6 to 8 weighing 22 to 27 kg: 200 mg chewable tablets or 10 mL (200 mg) oral suspension PO every 6 to 8 hours up to q.i.d.

Children ages 4 to 5 weighing 16 to 21 kg: 150 mg chewable tablets or 7.5 mL (150 mg) oral suspension PO every 6 to 8 hours up to q.i.d.

Children ages 2 to 3 weighing 11 to 16 kg: 100 mg (5 mL) oral suspension PO every 6 to 8 hours up to q.i.d.

Children ages 12 to 23 months weighing 8 to 10 kg: 75 mg (1.875 mL) oral drops PO every 6 to 8 hours up to q.i.d.

Children ages 6 to 11 months weighing 5 to 8 kg: 50 mg (1.25 mL) oral drops PO every 6 to 8 hours up to q.i.d.

Adjust-a-dose: For children ages 6 months to 11 years, use weight to determine dosage if possible; otherwise, use age. If needed, dose may be repeated every 6 to 8 hours but no more frequently than q.i.d. or a maximum of 30 mg/kg in 24 hours. Consult a health care provider before giving ibuprofen 100 mg chewable tablets to children younger than age 6 or those weighing less than 22 kg, 50 mg chewable tablets to children younger than age 4 or those weighing less than 16 kg, 50 mg oral suspension to children younger than age 2 or those weighing less than 11 kg, or 50 mg oral drops to infants younger than age 6 months or those weighing less than 5 kg. Ibuprofen oral drops should be dosed at 7.5 mg/kg of body weight.

➤ **Relief of signs and symptoms of juvenile arthritis**

Children: Recommended dose is 30 to 40 mg/kg/day of oral suspension PO divided into three or four doses; patients with milder disease may be adequately treated with 20 mg/kg/day. Doses above 50 mg/kg/day aren't recommended because they haven't been studied and may increase risk of serious adverse events. Lower dosage to the smallest dose needed to maintain adequate symptom control when clinical effect is obtained. Maximum single dose, 800 mg; maximum daily dose, 2,400 mg/day.

➤ **Migraine**

Adults: 400 mg (2 capsules) PO at onset of symptoms. Maximum dose, 400 mg in 24 hours unless directed otherwise by health care provider.

➤ **Clinically significant patent ductus arteriosus (PDA) when usual medical management is ineffective (ibuprofen lysine)**

Premature infants weighing between 500 and 1,500 g who are no more than 32 weeks' gestational age: 10 mg/kg IV followed by 5 mg/kg IV 24 hours later followed by a third dose of 5 mg/kg IV 24 hours after second dose. Base doses on birth weight.

Adjust-a-dose: If anuria or marked oliguria (urine output less than 0.6 mL/kg/hour) is evident at the scheduled time of the second or third dose, don't give additional dose until renal function has returned to normal. If the ductus arteriosus closes or is significantly reduced in size after completion of the first course of ibuprofen lysine, no further doses are necessary.

ADMINISTRATION

PO

• Give drug with milk or meals.

- Shake oral suspension and drops well before using.
- Store at room temperature.

IV

▼ Dilute drug with NSS, 5% dextrose, or lactated Ringer solution to 4 mg/mL or less. In adults, give over at least 30 minutes; in children, over at least 10 minutes.

▼ For weight-based dosing at 10 mg/kg, ensure that drug concentration is 4 mg/mL or less.

▼ Diluted solutions are stable for 24 hours at room temperature, except lysine injection.

▼ Give ibuprofen lysine within 30 minutes of preparation and infuse over at least 15 minutes.

▼ Correct dehydration before administering drug.

▼ Store at room temperature. Protect lysine injection vials from light.

▼ **Incompatibilities:** TPN solutions.

ACTION

May inhibit prostaglandin synthesis, to produce anti-inflammatory, analgesic, and antipyretic effects.

Route	Onset	Peak	Duration
PO	Variable	1–2 hr	4–6 hr
IV	Unknown	10–12 min	Unknown

Half-life: 2 to 4 hours; half-life is more than 10 times longer in infants.

ADVERSE REACTIONS

CNS: dizziness, headache, nervousness. **CV:** edema, fluid retention, HTN, hypotension. **EENT:** tinnitus. **GI:** abdominal pain, bloating, constipation, decreased appetite, diarrhea, dyspepsia, epigastric distress, flatulence, heartburn, nausea, vomiting. **GU:** *acute renal failure,* azotemia, cystitis, hematuria, urine retention. **Hematologic:** *agranulocytosis, aplastic anemia, leukopenia, neutropenia, pancytopenia, thrombocytopenia,* anemia, prolonged bleeding time. **Metabolic:** *hypokalemia, hypoglycemia,* hypoproteinemia, hypernatremia, hypoalbuminemia. **Respiratory:** cough, pneumonia. **Skin:** pruritus, rash, injection-site irritation, *wound hemorrhage.* **Other:** *sepsis.*

INTERACTIONS

Drug-drug. *Anticoagulants (warfarin):* May increase risk of serious GI bleeding. Use with extreme caution if concomitant use can't be avoided. Monitor patient closely.

Antihypertensives, furosemide, thiazide diuretics: May decrease the effectiveness of diuretics or antihypertensives. Monitor patient closely.

Aspirin: May negate the antiplatelet effect of low-dose aspirin therapy. Advise patient on the appropriate spacing of doses.

Aspirin, corticosteroids: May cause adverse GI reactions. Avoid using together.

Bisphosphonates: May increase risk of gastric ulceration. Monitor patient for signs of gastric irritation or bleeding.

Cyclosporine: May increase nephrotoxicity of both drugs. Avoid using together.

Digoxin, lithium: May increase levels or effects of these drugs. Monitor patient for toxicity.

Direct thrombin inhibitors (dabigatran, desirudin), factor Xa inhibitors (apixaban, edoxaban, rivaroxaban): May increase risk of bleeding. Coadminister with caution.

Methotrexate: May decrease methotrexate clearance and increase toxicity. Use together cautiously.

Pemetrexed: May increase risk of pemetrexed myelosuppression and kidney and GI toxicity. Consider therapy modification or monitor patient closely if used together.

SSNRIs (desvenlafaxine, duloxetine, venlafaxine), SSRIs (fluoxetine, sertraline): May increase risk of upper GI bleeding. If use together is unavoidable, closely watch for signs and symptoms of GI bleeding. Consider acid suppression therapy.

Triamterene: May increase risk of acute renal failure. Avoid using together; if unavoidable, closely monitor renal function.

Drug-herb. *Dong quai, feverfew, garlic, ginger, ginkgo biloba, horse chestnut, red clover:* May increase risk of bleeding, based on the known effects of components. Discourage use together.

White willow: Herb and drug contain similar components. Discourage use together.

Drug-lifestyle. *Alcohol use:* May cause adverse GI reactions. Discourage use together.

Sun exposure: May cause photosensitivity reactions. Advise patient to avoid excessive sunlight exposure.

EFFECTS ON LAB TEST RESULTS

- May increase BUN, creatinine, ALT, AST, LDH, and potassium levels.

- May decrease glucose, calcium, protein, and albumin levels.
- May decrease Hb level, hematocrit, and neutrophil, WBC, RBC, platelet, and granulocyte counts.

CONTRAINDICATIONS & CAUTIONS

- Contraindicated in patients hypersensitive to drug and in those with history of asthma, urticaria, or other allergic-type reactions to aspirin or other NSAIDs.

Boxed Warning Contraindicated for the treatment of perioperative pain after CABG surgery. ▪

Boxed Warning NSAIDs can increase risk of heart attack or stroke in patients with or without heart disease or risk factors for heart disease. Risk of heart attack or stroke can occur as early as the first weeks of using an NSAID. Risk appears greater at higher doses. Use lowest effective dose for shortest duration possible. ▪

Boxed Warning NSAIDs may increase risk of serious GI adverse events, including bleeding, ulceration, and perforation of the stomach or intestines, which can be fatal. These events can occur at any time during use and without warning symptoms. Older adults are at greater risk for serious GI events. ▪

- Ibuprofen lysine injection is contraindicated in preterm infants with significant renal impairment, proven or suspected untreated infection or necrotizing enterocolitis, thrombocytopenia, coagulation defects, active bleeding, and congenital heart disease in whom patency of the ductus arteriosus is necessary for satisfactory pulmonary or systemic blood flow.

🕛 *Alert:* NSAIDs increase risk of HF.

- Use cautiously in older adults and patients with GI disorders, history of peptic ulcer disease, hepatic or renal disease, cardiac decompensation, HTN, asthma, or intrinsic coagulation defects.
- Long-term NSAID use may result in renal papillary necrosis and other renal injury.
- May increase risk of aseptic meningitis, with fever and coma, particularly in patients with SLE and related connective tissue disease. If signs or symptoms of meningitis occur, consider whether they're related to ibuprofen therapy.

Dialyzable drug: Unknown.

⚠ *Overdose S&S:* Abdominal pain, nausea, vomiting, lethargy, drowsiness, headache, tinnitus, nystagmus, CNS depression, seizures, hypotension, bradycardia, tachycardia, atrial fibrillation, metabolic acidosis, coma, acute renal failure, hyperkalemia, respiratory depression and failure.

PREGNANCY-LACTATION-REPRODUCTION

- There are no adequate studies during pregnancy. Drug can cause fetal harm and is contraindicated in pregnancy starting at 30 weeks' gestation. Before 30 weeks' gestation, use during pregnancy only if potential benefit justifies fetal risk.

🕛 *Alert:* Use of NSAIDs at 20 weeks or later in pregnancy may cause fetal renal dysfunction leading to oligohydramnios and potential neonatal renal impairment; use at 30 weeks or later in pregnancy may increase risk of premature closure of the ductus arteriosus. Avoid use during pregnancy starting at 20 weeks' gestation. If potential benefit justifies fetal risk, use lowest effective dose for the shortest duration. Consider ultrasound monitoring of amniotic fluid if NSAID therapy is longer than 48 hours. Use of 81 mg of low-dose aspirin for certain pregnancy-related conditions under the direction of a prescriber is acceptable.

- Drug appears in human milk. Use cautiously during breastfeeding as directed by prescriber.
- Drug may cause reversible infertility in females.

NURSING CONSIDERATIONS

- Check renal and hepatic function periodically in patients on long-term therapy. Stop drug if abnormalities occur and notify prescriber.
- Monitor BP because drug can lead to new-onset HTN or worsening of preexisting HTN, which may contribute to the increased incidence of CV events.
- Because of their antipyretic and anti-inflammatory actions, NSAIDs may mask signs and symptoms of infection.
- Blurred or diminished vision and changes in color vision may occur.
- Full anti-inflammatory effects may take 1 or 2 weeks to develop.

🕛 *Alert:* Watch for and immediately evaluate signs and symptoms of heart attack (chest pain, shortness of breath or trouble breathing) or stroke (weakness in one part or side of the body, slurred speech).

Reactions in bold italics are *life-threatening*. Interactions may have a *rapid onset* or a *delayed onset*.

Boxed Warning NSAIDs cause an increased risk of serious GI adverse events, including bleeding, ulceration, and perforation of the stomach or intestines, which can be fatal. Older adults are at greater risk. ■

• Monitor patient for signs or symptoms of aseptic meningitis (fever, headache, sensitivity to light, vomiting) and report immediately if they occur.

Boxed Warning NSAIDs may increase the risk of serious thrombotic events, MI, or stroke, which can be fatal. The risk may be greater with longer use or in patients with CV disease or risk factors for CV disease. ■

• Monitor patients for rash, fever, lymphadenopathy, or facial swelling. DRESS syndrome has been reported in patients taking NSAIDs. If signs and symptoms of DRESS syndrome occur, discontinue drug and evaluate patient immediately.

• If patient consumes three or more alcoholic drinks per day, drug may cause stomach bleeding.

PATIENT TEACHING

• Tell patient to take with meals or milk to reduce adverse GI reactions.

◑ Alert: Drug is available OTC. Instruct patient not to exceed 3.2 g daily for adults and children age 12 and older or 30 mg/kg for children ages 6 months to 11 years, not to give to children younger than age 6 months, and not to take for extended periods (longer than 3 days for fever or longer than 10 days for pain) without consulting prescriber.

◑ Alert: Warn patient who is pregnant not to take NSAIDs at 20 weeks' gestation or later unless instructed to do so by prescriber due to fetal risk. Advise patient to discuss taking any OTC medication with a pharmacist or health care provider during pregnancy.

• Tell patient that full therapeutic effect for arthritis may be delayed for 2 to 4 weeks. Although pain relief occurs at low dosage levels, inflammation doesn't improve at dosages less than 400 mg q.i.d.

• Caution patient that use with aspirin, anticoagulants, alcohol, or corticosteroids may increase risk of GI adverse reactions.

• Teach patient to watch for and immediately report to prescriber signs and symptoms of GI bleeding, including blood in vomit, urine, or stool; coffee-ground vomit; and melena.

◑ Alert: Advise patient to seek medical attention immediately if chest pain, shortness of breath or trouble breathing, weakness in one part or side of the body, or slurred speech occurs.

• Tell patient to contact prescriber before using this drug if fluid intake hasn't been adequate or if fluids have been lost as a result of vomiting or diarrhea.

• Warn patient to avoid hazardous activities that require mental alertness until effects on CNS are known.

• Tell patient taking ibuprofen not to take other OTC NSAIDs such as naproxen, as these are in the same class.

• Advise patient to wear sunscreen to avoid hypersensitivity to sunlight.

SAFETY ALERT!

ibutilide fumarate
i-BYOO-ti-lide

Corvert

Therapeutic class: Antiarrhythmics
Pharmacologic class: Methanesulfonanilide derivatives

AVAILABLE FORMS

Injection: 0.1 mg/mL in 10-mL vials

INDICATIONS & DOSAGES

➤ **Rapid conversion of recent-onset atrial fibrillation or atrial flutter to sinus rhythm**

Adults weighing 60 kg or more: 1 mg IV infusion over 10 minutes. May repeat dose if arrhythmia doesn't respond within 10 minutes after completing first dose.

Adults weighing less than 60 kg: 0.01 mg/kg IV infusion over 10 minutes. May repeat dose if arrhythmia doesn't respond within 10 minutes after completing first dose.

ADMINISTRATION

IV

▼ Give drug undiluted or diluted in 50 mL of diluent. May add drug to NSS or D₅W injection before infusion. Add contents of 10-mL vial (0.1 mg/mL) to 50-mL infusion bag to form admixture of about 0.017 mg ibutilide/mL. Use drug with polyvinyl chloride plastic bags or polyolefin bags.

▼ Give drug over 10 minutes.

▼ Stop infusion if arrhythmia is terminated or patient develops ventricular tachycardia or marked prolongation of QT or QTc interval. If arrhythmia doesn't respond within 10 minutes after infusion ends, may repeat dose.

▼ Don't infuse parenteral products that contain particulate matter or are discolored.

▼ **Incompatibilities:** None listed by manufacturer. Consult a drug incompatibility reference for more information.

ACTION

Prolongs action potential in isolated cardiac myocytes and increases atrial and ventricular refractoriness, namely class III electrophysiologic effects.

Route	Onset	Peak	Duration
IV	≤90 min	Unknown	Unknown

Half-life: Averages about 6 hours.

ADVERSE REACTIONS

CNS: headache. **CV:** *sustained polymorphic ventricular tachycardia, AV block, bradycardia, HF,* ventricular extrasystoles, *nonsustained ventricular tachycardia,* hypotension, bundle-branch block, HTN, *prolonged QT interval,* palpitations, tachycardia. **GI:** nausea.

INTERACTIONS

Drug-drug. *Class IA antiarrhythmics (disopyramide, procainamide, quinidine), other class III antiarrhythmics (amiodarone, sotalol):* May increase potential for prolonged refractoriness. Don't give these drugs for at least five half-lives before and 4 hours after ibutilide dose.

Digoxin: Supraventricular arrhythmias may mask cardiotoxicity from excessive digoxin level. Use with caution in patients who may have an increased digoxin therapeutic range.

H_1-receptor antagonists, phenothiazines, TCAs, tetracyclic antidepressants, other drugs that prolong QT interval: May increase risk for proarrhythmia. Monitor patient closely.

EFFECTS ON LAB TEST RESULTS

None reported.

CONTRAINDICATIONS & CAUTIONS

Boxed Warning Administer drug only when the benefits of maintaining sinus rhythm outweigh the immediate risks of ibutilide administration and the risks of maintenance therapy. ■

• Contraindicated in patients hypersensitive to drug or its components.

• Use isn't recommended in patients with history of polymorphic ventricular tachycardia.

• Use cautiously in patients with hepatic or renal dysfunction.

• Safety and effectiveness of drug haven't been established in children.

• Drug's effectiveness hasn't been determined in patients with arrhythmias of more than 90 days' duration.

Dialyzable drug: Unknown.

⚠ *Overdose S&S:* Ventricular ectopy, ventricular tachycardia, third-degree AV block.

PREGNANCY-LACTATION-REPRODUCTION

• Drug causes fetal harm in animals. Use during pregnancy only if clearly needed and potential benefit justifies fetal risk.

• It isn't known if drug appears in human milk. Use isn't recommended during breastfeeding.

NURSING CONSIDERATIONS

Boxed Warning Drug can cause potentially fatal arrhythmias. Only skilled personnel trained in identification and treatment of acute ventricular arrhythmias, particularly polymorphic ventricular tachycardia, should give drug. ■

• Before therapy, correct hypokalemia and hypomagnesemia to reduce risk of proarrhythmia.

Boxed Warning Patients with atrial fibrillation lasting longer than 2 to 3 days must be adequately anticoagulated, generally over at least 2 weeks. ■

• Monitor ECG continuously during administration and for at least 4 hours afterward or until QTc interval returns to baseline; drug can induce or worsen ventricular arrhythmias. Longer monitoring is required if ECG shows arrhythmia or patient has hepatic insufficiency.

• Don't give class IA or other class III antiarrhythmics with infusion or for 4 hours afterward.

PATIENT TEACHING

• Tell patient to report adverse reactions promptly.

• Instruct patient to alert nurse of discomfort at injection site.

Reactions in bold italics are *life-threatening*. Interactions may have a *rapid onset* or a *delayed onset*.

idaruCIZUmab ▧
eye-da-roo-SIZ-uh-mab

Praxbind

Therapeutic class: Antidotes
Pharmacologic class: Humanized mono-clonal antibody fragments

AVAILABLE FORMS
Injection: 2.5 g/50 mL in single-use vials

INDICATIONS & DOSAGES
➤ **To reverse anticoagulant effects of da-bigatran etexilate mesylate (Pradaxa) for emergency surgery or urgent procedures; for life-threatening or uncontrolled bleed-ing**
Adults: 5 g (two 2.5-g vials) as two consec-utive IV infusions by hanging the vials or as two bolus injections, injecting contents of both vials consecutively, one after the other, using syringes.

ADMINISTRATION
IV
▼ Inspect both vials for discoloration and particulate matter before giving. Solution is colorless to slightly yellow and clear to slightly opalescent.
▼ Don't shake vial.
▼ Give drug promptly once removed from vial.
▼ Administer dose undiluted as either an IV bolus via syringe or an infusion by hanging the vials.
▼ Each infusion should take no longer than 5 to 10 minutes.
▼ Administer second vial/infusion within 15 minutes from end of first vial/infusion.
▼ A preexisting IV line may be used for ad-ministration, but line must be flushed with NSS before infusion.
▼ Don't administer other infusions at the same time using the same IV access.
▼ Store vials in refrigerator at 36° to 46° F (2° to 8° C). Don't freeze or shake.
▼ Before use, unopened vial may be kept at room temperature for up to 48 hours if stored in the original package to protect from light, or up to 6 hours when exposed to light.
▼ **Incompatibilities:** Other IV drugs or infusions.

ACTION
A humanized monoclonal antibody frag-ment that binds specifically to dabigatran and its acylglucuronide metabolites with higher affinity than the binding affinity of dabigatran to thrombin, neutralizing dabigatran's antico-agulant effects within minutes.

Route	Onset	Peak	Duration
IV	Rapid	Unknown	24 hr

Half-life: 10.3 hours.

ADVERSE REACTIONS
CNS: headache. **GI:** constipation, nausea.

INTERACTIONS
None reported.

EFFECTS ON LAB TEST RESULTS
• May prolong PTT and ecarin clotting time.

CONTRAINDICATIONS & CAUTIONS
• Hypersensitivity and anaphylactoid reac-tions, such as fever, bronchospasm, hyper-ventilation, rash, and pruritus, may occur. If reactions occur, discontinue drug.
• Reversing dabigatran therapy exposes pa-tients to the thrombotic risk of their under-lying disease. To reduce this risk, consider resumption of anticoagulant therapy as soon as medically appropriate. Dabigatran therapy can be started 24 hours after idarucizumab is given.
▧ Drug contains sorbitol. Use cautiously in patients with hereditary fructose intolerance, as serious and even fatal reactions, including hypoglycemia, hypophosphatemia, metabolic acidosis, increased uric acid level, and acute liver failure, have been reported. The mini-mum amount of sorbitol at which serious ad-verse reactions may occur in these patients isn't known.
• Drug hasn't been studied in patients with hepatic impairment.
• Safety and effectiveness in children haven't been established.
Dialyzable drug: Unknown.

PREGNANCY-LACTATION-REPRODUCTION
• There are no adequate studies during preg-nancy. It isn't known if drug can cause fetal harm or affect reproductive capacity. Use dur-ing pregnancy only if clearly needed.
• It isn't known if drug appears in human milk. Use cautiously during breastfeeding.

I

NURSING CONSIDERATIONS
• For patients with elevated coagulation parameters and reappearance of clinically relevant bleeding, or who require a second emergency surgery or urgent procedure, an additional 5 g of drug may be considered. Safety and effectiveness of repeat treatment haven't been established.
⚱ Assess patient for history of hereditary fructose intolerance before giving drug.
• Monitor patients for hypersensitivity reactions and recurrence of bleeding.
• Monitor patients for signs and symptoms of thrombotic events, including DVT, stroke, and MI. Resume anticoagulant therapy as soon as possible.

PATIENT TEACHING
• Warn patient to immediately report signs and symptoms of hypersensitivity and anaphylactoid reactions (fever, bronchospasm, dyspnea, rash, itching), as drug will need to be discontinued.
• Instruct patient to seek immediate medical attention for signs or symptoms of bleeding.
• Warn patient that reversing dabigatran therapy exposes patient to the thromboembolic risk of the underlying disease. Advise patient that anticoagulant therapy may be resumed as soon as possible to reduce this risk.
⚱ Teach patient with hereditary fructose intolerance to report this condition before receiving drug because drug contains sorbitol and may cause serious and even fatal reactions.

SAFETY ALERT!

idelalisib
eye-del-a-LIS-ib

Zydelig

Therapeutic class: Antineoplastics
Pharmacologic class: Kinase inhibitors

AVAILABLE FORMS
Tablets ⒪ᴛᴄ: 100 mg, 150 mg

INDICATIONS & DOSAGES
➤ **Relapsed chronic lymphocytic leukemia, in combination with rituximab, in patients for whom rituximab alone would be considered appropriate therapy due to other comorbidities**

Adults: 150 mg PO b.i.d. Continue treatment until disease progression or unacceptable toxicity.
Adjust-a-dose: Refer to manufacturer's instructions for toxicity-related dosage adjustments.

ADMINISTRATION
PO
• Drug is considered hazardous; use safe-handling precautions.
• Give without regard for food.
• Patients should swallow tablets whole. Don't crush or split tablets.
• If a dose is missed by less than 6 hours, give missed dose right away and give next dose as usual. If a dose is missed by more than 6 hours, skip missed dose and give next dose at the usual time.

ACTION
Induces apoptosis and inhibits proliferation in cell lines derived from malignant B cells and in primary tumor cell. Also inhibits several cell-signaling pathways to halt movement of B cells to lymph nodes and bone marrow.

Route	Onset	Peak	Duration
PO	Unknown	1.5 hr	Unknown

Half-life: About 8 hours.

ADVERSE REACTIONS
CNS: headache, pain, night sweats, fever, fatigue, asthenia, insomnia. **CV:** peripheral edema. **EENT:** nasal congestion, sinusitis, oral herpes. **GI:** abdominal pain, nausea, vomiting, diarrhea, decreased appetite, GERD, stomatitis, *colitis.* **GU:** UTI. **Hematologic:** anemia, *neutropenia, leukopenia, lymphocytopenia, thrombocytopenia.* **Hepatic:** increased transaminase levels, *hepatotoxicity.* **Metabolic:** dehydration. **Musculoskeletal:** arthralgia. **Respiratory:** pneumonia, *pneumonitis,* cough, dyspnea, bronchitis, URI. **Skin:** rash. **Other:** infection, chills, *sepsis.*

INTERACTIONS
Drug-drug. *CYP3A substrates (alfentanil, cyclosporine, dihydroergotamine, ergotamine, fentanyl, pimozide, quinidine, sirolimus, tacrolimus):* May increase substrate concentration. Avoid use together.
Hepatotoxic drugs: May increase risk of hepatotoxicity. Don't use together.

Reactions in bold italics are *life-threatening*. Interactions may have a *rapid onset* or a ***delayed onset***.

Other drugs that cause diarrhea: May increase risk of diarrhea and toxicity. Avoid use together.
Strong CYP3A inducers (carbamazepine, phenytoin, rifampin): May decrease idelalisib concentration. Avoid use together.
Strong CYP3A inhibitors (ketoconazole, nefazodone, ritonavir): May increase idelalisib level. Monitor patient for toxicity; modify dosage if adverse reactions occur. Use alternative to CYP3A inhibitor if possible.
Vaccines (inactivated): May decrease therapeutic effect of vaccine. Complete all appropriate vaccinations at least 2 weeks before starting idelalisib.
Vaccines (live): May decrease therapeutic effect of vaccine and increase risk of adverse vaccine effects. Avoid use together; give live-attenuated vaccine at least 3 months after idelalisib.
Drug-herb. *Echinacea, St. John's wort:* May decrease idelalisib concentration. Discourage use together.

EFFECTS ON LAB TEST RESULTS

- May increase ALT, AST, and bilirubin levels.
- May decrease sodium level.
- May increase or decrease glucose level.
- May decrease Hb level and neutrophil and platelet counts.
- May increase or decrease lymphocyte count.

CONTRAINDICATIONS & CAUTIONS

- Contraindicated in patients with a history of serious hypersensitivity reactions to drug (including anaphylaxis) and in patients with a history of TEN with any drug.
- Drug isn't indicated and isn't recommended as first-line treatment.
- Severe or life-threatening cutaneous reactions can occur. Discontinue drug for any severe reaction.

Boxed Warning Drug may cause serious or fatal hepatotoxicity, severe diarrhea or colitis, pneumonitis, infections, or intestinal perforation. ■

- Safety and effectiveness in children younger than age 18 haven't been established.

Dialyzable drug: Unknown.

PREGNANCY-LACTATION-REPRODUCTION

- Patients of childbearing potential should avoid becoming pregnant while taking drug. If drug is used during pregnancy, or if patient becomes pregnant while taking drug, apprise patient of potential hazard to a fetus.
- Verify pregnancy status before starting drug.
- Patients of childbearing potential should use effective contraception during treatment and for at least 1 month after final dose.
- Men with partners of childbearing potential should use effective contraception during treatment and for 3 months after final dose.
- It isn't known if drug appears in human milk. Patient shouldn't breastfeed during therapy and for at least 1 month after final dose.

NURSING CONSIDERATIONS

Boxed Warning Monitor AST, ALT, and bilirubin levels because hepatotoxicity may occur; monitor patient carefully and discontinue drug if necessary. Obtain baseline LFTs every 2 weeks for first 3 months of treatment, every 4 weeks for next 3 months, then every 1 to 3 months thereafter. Obtain LFTs weekly to monitor for hepatotoxicity if ALT or AST level rises above 3 × ULN; monitor levels until resolved. Withhold drug if ALT or AST level is greater than 5 × ULN; continue to monitor AST, ALT, and total bilirubin levels weekly until the abnormality is resolved. ■

Boxed Warning Monitor patient carefully for diarrhea, colitis, and intestinal perforation (new or worsening abdominal pain, chills, fever, nausea, or vomiting); discontinue drug if necessary. ■

Boxed Warning Monitor patient for respiratory signs and symptoms (cough, dyspnea, hypoxia, bilateral interstitial infiltrates on X-ray, decrease in oxygen saturation level by more than 5%). If pneumonitis is suspected, interrupt therapy until cause of the pulmonary symptoms has been determined. If pneumonitis is secondary to drug, discontinue drug and treat with corticosteroids. ■

Boxed Warning Serious infections (pneumonia, sepsis, febrile neutropenia), including fatal infections, have occurred. Monitor for signs and symptoms of infection and interrupt drug for grade 3 or higher infection. ■

Alert: Consider *Pneumocystis jiroveci* pneumonia (PJP) prophylaxis. Interrupt treatment in patient with suspected PJP infection of any grade and permanently discontinue drug if PJP infection is confirmed.

Alert: Interrupt treatment for positive CMV infection until infection has resolved. Monitor for CMV reactivation at least monthly if drug is resumed.

• Fatal cases of SJS and TEN have occurred. If SJS or TEN is suspected, interrupt therapy until cause of the reaction has been determined. If SJS or TEN is confirmed, permanently discontinue drug. Other severe or life-threatening (grade 3 or more) cutaneous reactions also have been reported. Monitor patients for development of SCAR and discontinue drug as appropriate.

• DRESS syndrome has occurred; permanently discontinue drug if suspected.

• Monitor CBC, ANC, and platelet count at least every 2 weeks for first 6 months of therapy, and at least weekly in patients whose neutrophil count falls below 1,000 cells/mm^3.

• Drug responds poorly to antimotility agents given for diarrhea.

• Monitor patient for rash.

• Older adults may have increased risk of adverse effects. Monitor these patients carefully.

• Monitor patients for anaphylaxis; discontinue drug if anaphylaxis occurs.

• *Look alike–sound alike:* Don't confuse Zydelig with Zykadia, Zytiga, or Xtandi. Don't confuse idelalisib with copanlisib, duvelisib, ibrutinib, idarubicin, imatinib, or ixazomib.

PATIENT TEACHING

• Instruct patient in safe drug administration and handling.

Boxed Warning Instruct patient to report jaundice, bruising, abdominal pain, or bleeding. ∎

Boxed Warning Caution patient to immediately notify prescriber if the number of bowel movements in a day increases by six or more. ∎

Boxed Warning Warn patient to immediately notify prescriber if severe abdominal pain, chills, fever, nausea, or vomiting occurs, because of risk of colitis and intestinal perforation. ∎

Boxed Warning Advise patient to immediately notify prescriber if fever or signs or symptoms of infection occur. ∎

Boxed Warning Advise patient to report new or worsening respiratory signs and symptoms, including cough or dyspnea. ∎

• Instruct patient that blood tests will be needed periodically, as ordered, to minimize risk of adverse reactions.

• Caution patient that drug may cause SCAR and to notify prescriber immediately if SCAR develops.

• Counsel patient of childbearing potential to avoid pregnancy and to use adequate contraception during therapy and for at least 1 month after therapy ends.

• Counsel male patient with partner of childbearing potential to use effective contraception during treatment and for 3 months after final dose.

• Advise patient to report pregnancy or suspected pregnancy.

• Caution patient not to breastfeed during therapy and for 1 month after final dose.

iloperidone
eye-loe-PER-ih-done

Fanapt

Therapeutic class: Antipsychotics
Pharmacologic class: Dopamine–serotonin antagonists

AVAILABLE FORMS
Tablets: 1 mg, 2 mg, 4 mg, 6 mg, 8 mg, 10 mg, 12 mg

INDICATIONS & DOSAGES
➤ **Schizophrenia**
Adults: Initially, 1 mg PO b.i.d. Increase dosage daily as needed according to the following dosing schedule: 2 mg PO b.i.d. on day 2; 4 mg PO b.i.d. on day 3; 6 mg PO b.i.d. on day 4; 8 mg PO b.i.d. on day 5; 10 mg PO b.i.d. on day 6; 12 mg PO b.i.d. on day 7. Maximum dosage is 12 mg PO b.i.d.
Adjust-a-dose: For patients who are poor metabolizers of CYP2D6 and those taking CYP2D6 inhibitors or CYP3A4 inhibitors, reduce dosage by 50%. Patients with moderate hepatic impairment may need dosage reduction if clinically indicated. Drug shouldn't be used in patients with severe hepatic impairment.

ADMINISTRATION
PO
• Give drug with or without food.
• When restarting drug after dosing interruption of more than 3 days, follow initial titration schedule.

ACTION

Actual mechanism unknown. May antagonize dopamine type 2 (D_2) and serotonin type 2 ($5\text{-}HT_2$) receptors.

Route	Onset	Peak	Duration
PO	Unknown	2–4 hr	Unknown

Half-life: 18 to 37 hours.

ADVERSE REACTIONS

CNS: aggression, delusion, dizziness, extrapyramidal effects, fatigue, lethargy, restlessness, somnolence, tremor. **CV:** hypotension, orthostatic hypotension, palpitations, tachycardia. **EENT:** blurred vision, conjunctivitis, dry mouth, nasal congestion, nasopharyngitis. **GI:** abdominal discomfort, diarrhea, nausea. **GU:** ejaculation failure, erectile dysfunction, urinary incontinence. **Hematologic:** hyperprolactinemia. **Metabolic:** weight gain. **Musculoskeletal:** arthralgia, muscle spasm, musculoskeletal stiffness, myalgia. **Respiratory:** dyspnea, URI. **Skin:** rash.

INTERACTIONS

Drug-drug. *Antihypertensives:* May enhance antihypertensive effects. Use together cautiously.
CNS depressants (barbiturates, droperidol, opioids): May increase depressant effect. Avoid use together. If use together is necessary, limit dosage and duration of each drug to minimum necessary for desired effect.
CYP3A4 or CYP2D6 inhibitors (clarithromycin, fluoxetine, ketoconazole, paroxetine, quinidine): May increase iloperidone level. Reduce dosage by half.
Dextromethorphan: May increase dextromethorphan level. Avoid use together.
Drugs that prolong QT interval (amiodarone, methadone, moxifloxacin, procainamide, quinidine, sotalol, thioridazine): May cause lethal arrhythmias. Avoid use together.
Drug-lifestyle. *Alcohol use:* May increase CNS effects. Discourage use together.

EFFECTS ON LAB TEST RESULTS

• May increase lipid and glucose levels.
• May decrease WBC count and hematocrit.

CONTRAINDICATIONS & CAUTIONS

• Contraindicated in patients hypersensitive to drug or its components; anaphylaxis, angioedema, and other hypersensitivity reactions have been reported.

Boxed Warning *Opioid class warning:* Opioids should only be prescribed with benzodiazepines or other CNS depressants to patients for whom alternative treatment options are inadequate. ■

Boxed Warning Fatal CV events may occur in older adults with dementia. Drug isn't approved for use in patients with dementia-related psychosis. ■

• Avoid use in patients with history of cardiac arrhythmias, QT-interval prolongation, recent acute MI, or uncompensated HF. Discontinue drug for persistent QTc measurement greater than 500 milliseconds.

• Use cautiously in patients with history of stroke, TIA, diabetes, seizures, orthostatic hypotension, NMS, tardive dyskinesia, leukopenia, neutropenia, agranulocytosis, suicidality, or priapism.

• Use cautiously in patients at risk for falls, including those with diseases or conditions or who are taking drugs that may cause somnolence, orthostatic hypotension, or motor or sensory instability.

• Use cautiously in patients with moderate hepatic impairment; these patients may require dosage reduction. Use in patients with severe hepatic impairment isn't recommended.

• Atypical antipsychotics have been associated with metabolic changes, including hyperglycemia, dyslipidemia, and weight gain, that may increase CV and cerebrovascular risk.
Dialyzable drug: Unknown.
⚠ **Overdose S&S:** Prolonged QT interval, drowsiness, extrapyramidal symptoms, sedation, tachycardia, hypotension.

PREGNANCY-LACTATION-REPRODUCTION

• There are no adequate studies during pregnancy. Use during pregnancy only if potential benefit justifies fetal risk.

• Encourage enrollment in the National Pregnancy Registry for Atypical Antipsychotics (1-800-961-2388 or https://womensmentalhealth.org/research/pregnancyregistry/atypicalantipsychotic/).

🔵 *Alert:* Neonates exposed to antipsychotics during the third trimester are at risk for developing extrapyramidal symptoms (repetitive muscle movements of face and body) and withdrawal symptoms (agitation, abnormally increased or decreased muscle tone, tremors,

sleepiness, severe difficulty breathing, difficulty feeding) after delivery.
• It isn't known if drug appears in human milk. Use during breastfeeding isn't recommended.

NURSING CONSIDERATIONS
• Symptom control may be delayed during the first 1 to 2 weeks of treatment compared to other antipsychotics that don't require similar titration.
◑ *Alert:* Obtain baseline BP measurements before starting therapy, and monitor BP regularly. Watch for orthostatic hypotension, especially during first dosage adjustments.
◑ *Alert:* Watch for evidence of NMS (hyperthermia, muscle rigidity, altered mental status, and autonomic instability), which is rare but can be fatal.
◑ *Alert:* Life-threatening hyperglycemia may occur in patients taking atypical antipsychotics. Monitor patients with diabetes regularly. Monitor fasting blood glucose level at drug initiation and periodically during therapy in patients with risk factors for diabetes.
• Monitor patient for tardive dyskinesia, which may occur with prolonged use of drug. If tardive dyskinesia occurs, discontinue drug unless patient's condition warrants continued use.
• Monitor patient for suicidality.
• Complete fall risk assessments when initiating drug and recurrently for patients on long-term therapy, especially for those with diseases or conditions that increase fall risk and in those who are taking other drugs that could increase fall risk.
• Dispense lowest appropriate quantity of drug to reduce the risk of overdose.
• Monitor patient for weight gain.
• Periodically reassess patient to determine continued need for therapy.
• Monitor CBC frequently during the first few months of therapy and discontinue drug if WBC count drops with no other underlying cause.
• Monitor potassium and magnesium levels at baseline and periodically in patients at risk for electrolyte imbalance.
• Drug may lower seizure threshold in patients with a history of seizures; monitor these patients closely.

PATIENT TEACHING
Boxed Warning *Opioid class warning:* Caution patient or caregiver of patient taking an

opioid with a benzodiazepine, CNS depressant, or alcohol to seek immediate medical attention for dizziness, light-headedness, extreme sleepiness, slowed or difficult breathing, or unresponsiveness. ▪
• Instruct patient in safe drug administration and storage.
• Warn patient to avoid driving and other hazardous activities that require mental alertness until the drug's effects are known.
• Warn patient to rise slowly, avoid hot showers, and use other precautions to avoid fainting when starting therapy and to reduce risk of falls.
• Advise patient to avoid becoming overheated or dehydrated.
• Tell patient to notify prescriber about planned, suspected, or known pregnancy.
• Advise patient not to breastfeed during therapy.
• Instruct patient to report symptoms of dizziness, palpitations, or fainting to prescriber.
• Advise patient to avoid alcohol use while taking drug.
• Tell patient to seek emergency medical care if an erection lasts more than 4 hours.
• Warn patient and caregiver about risk of NMS; advise them to seek emergency medical care if symptoms occur.
• Tell patient to notify prescriber about other prescription or OTC drugs that patient is taking or plans to take.

iloprost
EYE-loe-prost

Ventavis

Therapeutic class: Pulmonary vasodilators
Pharmacologic class: Prostacyclin analogues

AVAILABLE FORMS
Inhalation solution: 10 mcg/mL, 20 mcg/mL in single-dose ampules

INDICATIONS & DOSAGES
➤ **PAH in patients with NYHA Class III or IV symptoms**
Adults: Initially, 2.5 mcg inhaled using the I-neb Adaptive Aerosol Delivery (AAD). As tolerated, increase to 5 mcg inhaled

six to nine times daily while patient is awake, as needed, but to no more than every 2 hours. Maximum, 5 mcg nine times daily.

ADMINISTRATION
Inhalational
- Use only I-neb AAD delivery devices, per manufacturer's instructions.
- Don't mix with other medications.
- The 20-mcg/mL concentration is intended for patients receiving the 5-mcg dose who have extended treatment times.
- Discard unused medication.
- Keep drug away from skin and eyes.

ACTION
Lowers pulmonary arterial pressure by dilating systemic and pulmonary arterial vascular beds. Drug also affects platelet aggregation, although effect in PAH treatment isn't known.

Route	Onset	Peak	Duration
Inhalation	Unknown	Within 5 min	30–60 min

Half-life: 20 to 30 minutes.

ADVERSE REACTIONS
CNS: headache, insomnia, syncope. **CV:** hypotension, vasodilation, chest pain, *HF, supraventricular tachycardia,* palpitations, peripheral edema. **EENT:** inability to open jaw (trismus). **GI:** nausea, tongue pain, vomiting. **GU:** *renal failure.* **Hepatic:** increased ALP and GGT levels. **Musculoskeletal:** back pain, muscle cramps. **Respiratory:** cough, dyspnea, hemoptysis, pneumonia. **Other:** flulike syndrome.

INTERACTIONS
Drug-drug. *Anticoagulants, antiplatelet drugs:* May increase risk of bleeding. Monitor patient closely.
Antihypertensives, vasodilators: May increase hypotensive effects of these drugs. Monitor BP.

EFFECTS ON LAB TEST RESULTS
- May increase ALP and GGT levels.

CONTRAINDICATIONS & CAUTIONS
- No known contraindications. Avoid using in patients whose systolic BP is less than 85 mm Hg.

- Use cautiously in older adults, patients with hepatic or renal impairment, and patients with COPD, severe asthma, or acute pulmonary infection.
- Safety and effectiveness in children haven't been established.
- PAH may worsen if drug is withdrawn abruptly or dosages are reduced.
Dialyzable drug: Unknown.
⚠ *Overdose S&S:* Diarrhea, dizziness, flushing, headache, hypotension, nausea, vomiting, jaw or back pain.

PREGNANCY-LACTATION-REPRODUCTION
- There are no adequate studies during pregnancy. Use during pregnancy only if potential benefit justifies fetal risk.
- It isn't known if drug appears in human milk. Patient should discontinue breastfeeding or discontinue drug.

NURSING CONSIDERATIONS
- Monitor patient's vital signs carefully at start of treatment. Monitor patient for syncope.
- If patient develops evidence of pulmonary edema, stop treatment immediately.

PATIENT TEACHING
- Warn patient not to drink drug and that drug is for inhalation only.
- Caution patient to take drug exactly as prescribed.
- Advise patient to keep a backup I-neb AAD in case the original malfunctions.
- Tell patient to keep drug away from skin and eyes and to rinse the area immediately if contact occurs.
- Inform patient that drug may cause dizziness and fainting. Urge patient to stand up slowly from a sitting or lying position and to report to prescriber worsening of symptoms.
- Tell patient to take drug before physical exertion, no more than every 2 hours.
- Tell patient not to expose others, especially those who are pregnant and infants, to drug.
- Teach patient how to clean equipment and safely dispose of used ampules after each treatment. Caution patient not to save or use leftover solution.

imatinib mesylate ⚕
eye-MAT-eh-nib

Gleevec

Therapeutic class: Antineoplastics
Pharmacologic class: Kinase inhibitors

AVAILABLE FORMS
Tablets ⓪: 100 mg, 400 mg

INDICATIONS & DOSAGES
Adjust-a-dose (for all indications): For patients with CrCl of 40 to 59 mL/minute, don't exceed 600 mg daily; if CrCl is 20 to 39 mL/minute, decrease starting dose by 50% and don't exceed 400 mg daily; if CrCl is less than 20 mL/minute, don't exceed 100 mg daily. For patients with severe hepatic impairment, reduce dosage by 25%. If use with a strong CYP3A4 inducer can't be avoided, decrease imatinib dosage by at least 50% and monitor clinical response closely. See manufacturer's package insert for full details on dosage adjustments for children; patients with neutropenia, thrombocytopenia, or hepatotoxicity; and those with adverse reactions.

➤ **Relapsed or refractory Philadelphia chromosome–positive (+) acute lymphoblastic leukemia (ALL)** ⚕
Adults: 600 mg PO daily.

➤ **Newly diagnosed Ph+ ALL in children, in combination with chemotherapy** ⚕
Children age 1 and older: 340 mg/m² PO daily. Maximum dosage is 600 mg daily.

➤ **Aggressive systemic mastocytosis (ASM) without the D816V c-*Kit* mutation or with c-*Kit* mutational status unknown** ⚕
Adults: 400 mg PO daily.
Adjust-a-dose: For patients with ASM associated with eosinophilia, a clonal hematologic disease related to the fusion kinase FIP1L1-PDGFRα, initial dose is 100 mg/day. Increase dose from 100 mg to 400 mg/day if no adverse drug reactions occur and if there is insufficient response to therapy.

➤ **Hypereosinophilic syndrome (HES) or chronic eosinophilic leukemia (CEL), or both** ⚕
Adults: 400 mg PO daily.
Adjust-a-dose: In patients with HES or CEL and demonstrated FIP1L1-PDGFRα fusion kinase, initial dose is 100 mg/day. Increase

dose from 100 mg to 400 mg/day if no adverse drug reactions occur and if there is insufficient response to therapy.

➤ **Myelodysplastic syndrome (MDS) or myeloproliferative disease (MPD) with *PDGFR* gene rearrangements** ⚕
Adults: 400 mg PO daily.

➤ **Unresectable, recurrent, or metastatic dermatofibrosarcoma protuberans**
Adults: 400 mg PO b.i.d. (800 mg/day).

➤ **Chronic myeloid leukemia (CML) in blast crisis, in accelerated phase, or in chronic phase after failure of alfa interferon therapy; newly diagnosed Ph+ chronic-phase CML** ⚕
Adults: For chronic-phase CML, 400 mg PO daily as single dose. For accelerated-phase CML or blast crisis, 600 mg PO daily as single dose. Continue treatment as long as patient continues to benefit. May increase daily dose to 600 mg PO in chronic phase or to 800 mg PO (400 mg PO b.i.d.) in accelerated phase or blast crisis.
Children age 1 and older: For newly diagnosed Ph+ chronic-phase CML only, give 340 mg/m² daily PO. Don't exceed 600 mg/day.

➤ ***Kit* (CD117)-positive or GI stromal tumors (GISTs) after resection** ⚕
Adults: 400 mg PO daily.

➤ ***Kit*-positive unresectable or metastatic malignant GISTs** ⚕
Adults: 400 mg PO daily or b.i.d. May consider a dosage increase up to 800 mg daily (given as 400 mg b.i.d.), as clinically indicated, in patients with clear signs or symptoms of disease progression at a lower dose and in the absence of severe adverse drug reactions.

ADMINISTRATION
PO
• Give with a meal and large glass of water.
• Administer 400-mg or 600-mg dose once daily. Give 800-mg dose as 400 mg b.i.d.
• For daily dosing of 800 mg and above, use the 400-mg tablet to reduce exposure to iron.
• For patients unable to swallow tablets, disperse the tablets in water or apple juice (50 mL for 100-mg tablet and 200 mL for 400-mg tablet). Stir and have patient drink immediately.
• Drug is hazardous. Avoid exposure to crushed tablets.

Reactions in bold italics are *life-threatening*. Interactions may have a *rapid onset* or a ***delayed onset***.

- If dose is missed, give next scheduled dose at its regular time.
- Store at room temperature; protect from moisture.

ACTION

Inhibits the abnormal tyrosine kinase created by the Philadelphia chromosome abnormality in CML; inhibits tumor growth of murine myeloid cells and leukemia lines from patients with CML in blast crisis; also inhibits other kinases for growth and stem cell factors and may inhibit proliferation and induce apoptosis in GIST cells.

Route	Onset	Peak	Duration
PO	Unknown	2–4 hr	Unknown

Half-life: Adults, 18 hours (parent drug), 40 hours (active metabolite); children, 15 hours (parent drug).

ADVERSE REACTIONS

CNS: *cerebral hemorrhage,* fatigue, headache, fever, asthenia, weakness, depression, dizziness, insomnia, anxiety, paresthesia, rigors, peripheral neuropathy, taste alteration. **CV:** *hemorrhage,* edema, fluid retention, HTN, chest pain, palpitations, pericardial effusion, flushing. **EENT:** periorbital edema, increased lacrimation, blurred vision, conjunctivitis, epistaxis, nasopharyngitis, sinusitis, rhinitis, pharyngolaryngeal pain, oropharyngeal pain, dry mouth. **GI:** *GI hemorrhage,* abdominal pain, anorexia, constipation, diarrhea, dyspepsia, nausea, vomiting, gastroenteritis, flatulence, stomatitis, GERD. **Hematologic:** *neutropenia, thrombocytopenia,* anemia, *lymphopenia, pancytopenia,* eosinophilia. **Hepatic:** *hepatotoxicity.* **Metabolic:** *hypokalemia,* weight increase or decrease, hypoproteinemia, increased CK and amylase levels. **Musculoskeletal:** arthralgia, myalgia, muscle cramps, musculoskeletal pain, bone pain, limb pain, back pain, growth suppression in children. **Respiratory:** cough, dyspnea, pneumonia, URI. **Skin:** petechiae, rash, pruritus, alopecia, dry skin, diaphoresis, exfoliative rash, dermatitis, photosensitivity reaction. **Other:** night sweats, flulike symptoms, infection.

INTERACTIONS

Drug-drug. *Alprazolam, certain HMG-CoA reductase inhibitors (simvastatin), cyclosporine, dihydropyridine–calcium channel blockers, pimozide, triazolam:* May increase levels of these drugs. Monitor patient for toxicity, and obtain drug levels, if appropriate.

CYP2D6 substrates with narrow therapeutic window (clonidine, nortriptyline, sotalol): May increase substrate level. Use cautiously together.

CYP3A4 inducers (carbamazepine, dexamethasone, phenobarbital, phenytoin, rifampin): May decrease imatinib level. Avoid concurrent use when possible. If combination must be used, increase imatinib dosage by at least 50%; monitor patient closely.

CYP3A4 inhibitors (clarithromycin, erythromycin, itraconazole, ketoconazole): May decrease metabolism and increase imatinib level. Monitor patient for toxicity.

Levothyroxine: May increase levothyroxine clearance, causing increased TSH levels and symptoms of hypothyroidism. Monitor thyroid function.

Warfarin: May alter metabolism of warfarin. Avoid using together; use standard heparin or a low–molecular-weight heparin.

Drug-herb. *Ginseng:* May increase risk of hepatotoxicity. Avoid use together.

St. John's wort: May decrease drug effects. Discourage use together.

Drug-food. *Grapefruit juice:* May increase imatinib level. Discourage use together.

EFFECTS ON LAB TEST RESULTS

- May increase lipase, glucose, creatinine, bilirubin, ALP, AST, and ALT levels.
- May decrease phosphate, albumin, and sodium levels.
- May increase or decrease potassium level.
- May increase eosinophil count.
- May decrease Hb level and neutrophil and platelet counts.

CONTRAINDICATIONS & CAUTIONS

- Contraindicated in patients hypersensitive to drug or its components.
- Use cautiously in older adults and in patients with hepatic or renal impairment.
- Severe HF and left ventricular dysfunction have occurred in patients taking imatinib. Use cautiously in patients with cardiac disease or risk factors for HF.
- Use cautiously in patients with risk factors for kidney dysfunction, including diabetes, HTN, HF, and preexisting kidney impairment.

• Growth retardation has occurred in children and preadolescents receiving imatinib; long-term effects of prolonged treatment are unknown.

• Safety and effectiveness in children younger than age 1 haven't been established.

Dialyzable drug: Unknown.

⚠ **Overdose S&S:** Muscle cramps; ascites; increased creatinine, AST, ALT, and bilirubin levels; nausea, vomiting, diarrhea, weakness, myalgia.

PREGNANCY-LACTATION-REPRODUCTION

• Drug can harm fetus. Patients of childbearing potential should use highly effective contraception during therapy and for 14 days after final dose.

• Drug appears in human milk. Patient shouldn't breastfeed during treatment and for 1 month after final dose.

NURSING CONSIDERATIONS

▧ In adults with MDS/MPD or ASM, determine *PDGFRB* gene rearrangements status or D816V c-*Kit* mutational status, respectively, before starting therapy.

• Verify pregnancy status before treatment

• Monitor patient closely for possibly severe fluid retention. Older adults may have an increased risk of edema.

• There have been postmarketing reports of severe bullous skin reactions. Monitor patient for skin reactions. Drug may need to be withheld.

• Fatal TLS can occur. Correct dehydration and treat high uric acid levels before starting therapy.

• Monitor weight daily. Report unexpected, rapid weight gain.

• Monitor CBC weekly for first month, every other week for second month, and periodically thereafter.

• Monitor LFTs carefully because hepatotoxicity (occasionally severe) may occur; decrease dosage as needed.

• Monitor kidney function before and periodically during therapy.

• Monitor growth of children being treated with imatinib.

• May increase dosage if no severe adverse reactions or severe non–leukemia-related neutropenia or thrombocytopenia occur in the following circumstances: disease progression, failure to achieve a satisfactory hematologic response after at least 3 months of treatment,

or loss of a previously achieved hematologic response.

▧ In patients with HES and cardiac involvement, cases of cardiogenic shock/left ventricular dysfunction have been associated with the initiation of imatinib therapy. The condition is reversible with administration of systemic steroids and circulatory support measures, and by temporarily withholding imatinib. Monitor echocardiogram and serum troponin in patients with HES/CEL and in patients with MDS/MPD or ASM associated with high eosinophil levels.

▧ Grade 3/4 hemorrhage has been reported in patients with newly diagnosed CML and with GIST. GI tumor sites may be the source of GI bleeds in GIST.

• GI perforations, some fatal, have been reported.

• Monitor TSH level in patients who have had thyroidectomy and receive levothyroxine replacement.

PATIENT TEACHING

• Instruct patient in safe drug administration, handling, and disposal.

• Advise patient to report adverse effects, such as fluid retention and sudden weight gain.

• Advise patient that periodic lab tests will be needed to monitor therapy.

• Inform patient and caregivers that growth retardation has occurred in children and preadolescents receiving imatinib, and that long-term effects of prolonged treatment are unknown. Monitor growth closely.

• Advise patient of the risk of dizziness, blurred vision, or somnolence during treatment and to use caution when driving a car or operating machinery.

• Advise patient of childbearing potential that drug may cause fetal harm. Caution patient to avoid pregnancy during therapy and for 14 days after final dose by using highly effective contraceptives.

• Teach patient to report suspected pregnancy.

• Advise patient not to breastfeed during therapy and for 1 month after final dose.

Reactions in bold italics are *life-threatening*. Interactions may have a *rapid onset* or a ***delayed onset***.

imipenem–cilastatin sodium
i-im-PEN-em/sye-la-STAT-in

Primaxin 500✤, Primaxin IV

Therapeutic class: Antibiotics
Pharmacologic class: Carbapenems–beta-lactams

AVAILABLE FORMS
Powder for injection: 250 mg imipenem/250 mg cilastatin, 500 mg imipenem/500 mg cilastatin

INDICATIONS & DOSAGES
Adjust-a-dose (for all indications): If CrCl is less than 90 mL/minute, adjust dosage and monitor renal function test results. Consult manufacturer's package insert for specific dosage adjustments. For patients on hemodialysis, administer dose after hemodialysis and at intervals timed from the end of that dialysis session. Drug isn't recommended in children with renal impairment who weigh less than 30 kg.

➤ **Serious lower respiratory tract, bone, intra-abdominal, gynecologic, joint, skin, and soft-tissue infections; UTIs; endocarditis; and bacterial septicemia caused by susceptible bacterial species, including** *Acinetobacter, Enterococcus, Staphylococcus aureus, Streptococcus, Escherichia coli, Haemophilus, Klebsiella, Morganella, Proteus, Enterobacter, Pseudomonas aeruginosa,* **or** *Bacteroides,* **including** *B. fragilis*
Adults: For susceptible bacterial species, give 500 mg IV every 6 hours or 1,000 mg IV every 8 hours. For intermediate susceptibility bacterial species, give 1,000 mg IV every 6 hours. Refer to manufacturer's package insert for susceptibility test interpretive criteria. Maximum dosage is 4,000 mg/day.
Children age 3 months and older (except for CNS infections): 15 to 25 mg/kg IV every 6 hours. Maximum daily dose is 4 g.
Infants ages 4 weeks to 3 months weighing 1.5 kg or more (except for CNS infections): 25 mg/kg IV every 6 hours.
Neonates ages 1 to 4 weeks weighing 1.5 kg or more (except for CNS infections): 25 mg/kg IV every 8 hours.
Neonates younger than age 1 week weighing 1.5 kg or more (except for CNS infections): 25 mg/kg IV every 12 hours.

➤ **Neutropenic fever ◆**
Adults: 500 mg IV every 6 hours until patient is afebrile for at least 48 hours and ANC reaches 500 cells/mm^3 and continues to increase.

ADMINISTRATION
IV
▼ Obtain specimens for culture and sensitivity testing before giving first dose. Begin therapy while awaiting results.
🔴 *Alert:* Don't use diluents containing benzyl alcohol to reconstitute drug for administration to neonates; benzyl alcohol has been associated with toxicity in neonates. While toxicity hasn't been demonstrated in children older than age 3 months, small children in this age range may also be at risk for benzyl alcohol toxicity.
▼ Reconstitute powder by adding approximately 10 mL of appropriate diluent to vial; shake until solution is clear. Solution may be colorless to yellow; color variations within this range don't affect drug's potency.
▼ After reconstitution, transfer resulting suspension to 100 mL of an appropriate infusion solution. Repeat transfer of resulting suspension with an additional 10 mL of infusion solution to ensure complete transfer of vial contents to infusion solution. Agitate resulting mixture until clear before administering by IV infusion.
▼ After reconstitution, solution is stable for 4 hours at room temperature and for 24 hours when refrigerated. Don't freeze drug solutions.
▼ Refer to manufacturer's instructions for reconstitution, preparation, and storage instructions for ADD-Vantage vials.
▼ Don't give by direct IV bolus injection.
▼ For adults with normal renal function, give each 500-mg dose by IV infusion over 20 to 30 minutes. Infuse each 1-g dose over 40 to 60 minutes. For adults with renal impairment, refer to manufacturer's instructions for infusion rates.
▼ For children, infuse doses of 500 mg or less over 20 to 30 minutes. Infuse doses greater than 500 mg over 40 to 60 minutes. If nausea occurs, the infusion may be slowed.
▼ **Incompatibilities:** Allopurinol, antibiotics, amiodarone, azithromycin, fluconazole, gemcitabine, lorazepam, meperidine, midazolam, milrinone, sargramostim, sodium bicarbonate.

✤Canada   ◇OTC   ◆Off-label use   🔗Photoguide   ⊜Do not crush   *Liquid contains alcohol   ▧Genetic

ACTION

Inhibits bacterial cell-wall synthesis. Cilastatin prevents renal metabolism of imipenem.

Route	Onset	Peak	Duration
IV	Unknown	Unknown	Unknown

Half-life: 1 hour after IV dose (adults).

ADVERSE REACTIONS

CNS: *seizures.* **CV:** thrombophlebitis, phlebitis, tachycardia. **EENT:** oral candidiasis. **GI:** diarrhea, nausea, vomiting, gastroenteritis. **GU:** urine discoloration, proteinuria, oliguria, increased creatinine level, *anuria.* **Hematologic:** anemia, eosinophilia, *thrombocytopenia.* **Hepatic:** increased ALP level, increased or decreased bilirubin level. **Skin:** injection-site irritation, rash.

INTERACTIONS

Drug-drug. *Cyclosporine:* May increase CNS adverse effects. Use together cautiously.
Ganciclovir: May cause seizures. Avoid using together.
Probenecid: May increase imipenem level. Don't give concurrently.
Valproic acid: May decrease valproic acid level and increase risk of seizures. Use together isn't recommended; consider using an alternative antibiotic. If use together is necessary, consider supplemental anticonvulsant therapy, and monitor patient carefully.

EFFECTS ON LAB TEST RESULTS

- May increase BUN, creatinine, ALT, AST, ALP, bilirubin, chloride, and LDH levels.
- May increase or decrease sodium and bilirubin levels.
- May increase eosinophil count.
- May decrease Hb level, hematocrit, and WBC and platelet counts.
- May interfere with urinary glucose determination by Benedict solution, Fehling solution, or Clinitest.
- May result in a false-positive direct Coombs test.

CONTRAINDICATIONS & CAUTIONS

- Contraindicated in patients hypersensitive to drug or its components and in those with CrCl of 5 mL/minute/1.73 m^2 or less unless hemodialysis is begun within 48 hours.
- Patients with CrCl of 15 to less than 30 mL/minute may have an increased risk of seizures.

- Use cautiously in patients allergic to penicillins or cephalosporins because drug has similar chemical structure. Also use cautiously in patients with a history of sensitivity to multiple allergens. Serious anaphylactic reactions require immediate emergency measures.
- Use cautiously in patients with history of seizure disorders, especially if they also have compromised renal function.
- Drug may cause CDAD, ranging in severity from mild to fatal colitis and occurring even 2 months after drug administration.
- Prolonged use may result in superinfection. Repeated evaluation of patient's condition is essential.
- Use cautiously in children younger than age 3 months. Drug isn't recommended in children with impaired renal function who weigh less than 30 kg.
- Drug isn't indicated in patients with meningitis; safety and effectiveness haven't been established.

Dialyzable drug: Yes.

PREGNANCY-LACTATION-REPRODUCTION

- There are no adequate studies during pregnancy. Use during pregnancy only if potential benefit justifies fetal risk.
- It isn't known if drug appears in human milk. Use cautiously during breastfeeding.

NURSING CONSIDERATIONS

- ⚠ *Alert:* Don't use for CNS infections in children because of seizure risk.
- ⚠ *Alert:* If seizures develop and persist despite anticonvulsant therapy, stop drug.
- For patients receiving hemodialysis, drug is recommended only when benefits outweigh possible risk of seizures.
- Monitor patient for superinfections during and after therapy.
- Monitor organ system functions, including renal, hepatic, and hematopoietic, during prolonged therapy.

PATIENT TEACHING

- Instruct patient to report adverse reactions promptly.
- Tell patient to report discomfort at IV insertion site.
- Urge patient to notify prescriber as soon as possible about loose stools or diarrhea.

Reactions in bold italics are *life-threatening*. Interactions may have a *rapid onset* or a *delayed onset*.

- Advise patient taking valproic acid or divalproex sodium that seizure therapy may need adjustment.

imipramine hydrochloride ⚕
im-IP-ra-meen

Tofranil

imipramine pamoate ⚕

Therapeutic class: Antidepressants
Pharmacologic class: TCAs

AVAILABLE FORMS
imipramine hydrochloride
Tablets: 10 mg, 25 mg, 50 mg
imipramine pamoate
Capsules: 75 mg, 100 mg, 125 mg, 150 mg

INDICATIONS & DOSAGES
➤ **Depression**
Adults: Initially, 75 mg PO daily (outpatients); may increase to 150 mg daily. Don't exceed 200 mg/day. Maintenance outpatient dose is 50 to 150 mg/day. Or, initially 100 mg PO daily (inpatients) in divided doses; gradually increase to 200 mg/day as required. If no response after 2 weeks, increase to 250 to 300 mg/day. Maximum daily dose is 300 mg for patients who are hospitalized.
Adolescents: 30 to 40 mg PO once daily, preferably at bedtime, or in divided doses if necessary. Dosage increases above 100 mg daily are generally unnecessary.
Older adults: Initially, 30 to 40 mg PO daily; maximum shouldn't exceed 100 mg daily.
➤ **Childhood enuresis**
Children age 6 and older: Initially, 25 mg imipramine hydrochloride PO 1 hour before bedtime. If patient doesn't improve within 1 week, increase dose to a maximum of 50 mg if child is younger than age 12; increase dose to a maximum of 75 mg for children age 12 and older. Don't exceed 2.5 mg/kg/day.

ADMINISTRATION
PO
- Give drug without regard for food.
- Give full dose at bedtime if possible. May also give in divided doses.

ACTION
Unknown. Increases norepinephrine, serotonin, or both in the CNS by blocking their reuptake by the presynaptic neurons. Mechanism for enuresis unknown but thought to be separate from drug's antidepressant effects.

Route	Onset	Peak	Duration
PO	Unknown	2–6 hr	Unknown

Half-life: 8 to 21 hours.

ADVERSE REACTIONS
CNS: drowsiness, dizziness, *seizures, stroke,* excitation, tremor, confusion, hallucinations, anxiety, ataxia, fatigue, peripheral neuropathy, restlessness, headache, paresthesia, nervousness, extrapyramidal reactions, agitation, sleep disorders, tiredness, psychosis, taste disturbance, tingling sensation, EEG pattern change. **CV:** orthostatic hypotension, tachycardia, ECG changes, *MI, arrhythmias, heart block,* HTN, *precipitation of HF,* palpitations. **EENT:** blurred vision, mydriasis, angle-closure glaucoma, tinnitus, parotid swelling, black tongue, dry mouth. **GI:** constipation, nausea, vomiting, anorexia, *paralytic ileus,* abdominal cramps, diarrhea. **GU:** urine retention, urinary frequency, urinary tract dilation, impotence, testicular swelling. **Hematologic:** *bone marrow depression, thrombocytopenia.* **Hepatic:** jaundice, altered LFT values. **Metabolic:** *hypoglycemia,* hyperglycemia, weight loss or gain, SIADH. **Skin:** rash, urticaria, photosensitivity reactions, pruritus, diaphoresis, alopecia. **Other:** falls, hypersensitivity reactions, increased or decreased libido, gynecomastia, galactorrhea, breast enlargement.

INTERACTIONS
Drug-drug. *Aclidinium:* May enhance anticholinergic effects. Avoid using together.
Antihypertensives: May potentiate hypotensive effect. Use cautiously together.
Barbiturates, CNS depressants: May enhance CNS depression. Avoid using together.
*Cimetidine, **fluoxetine, fluvoxamine, paroxetine, sertraline:*** May increase imipramine level. Monitor drug levels and patient for signs of toxicity.
Clonidine: May cause life-threatening HTN. Avoid using together.
⚕ *Drugs metabolized by CYP2D6:* May cause higher than usual expected TCA plasma

concentration in poor metabolizers when given usual doses. Monitor therapy. ■

Epinephrine, norepinephrine: May increase hypertensive effect. Use together cautiously.

Linezolid, methylene blue: May cause serotonin syndrome. Use with extreme caution and monitor patient closely.

MAO inhibitors: May cause hyperpyretic crisis, severe seizures, and death. Don't use within 14 days of MAO inhibitor therapy.

QTc-prolonging drugs (quinidine, quinolones): May increase the risk of life-threatening arrhythmias. Avoid using together.

Drug-herb. *SAM-e, St. John's wort, yohimbe:* May cause serotonin syndrome. Discourage use together.

Drug-lifestyle. *Alcohol use:* May enhance CNS depression. Discourage use together.

Smoking: May lower level of drug. Monitor patient for lack of effect.

Sun exposure: May increase risk of photosensitivity reactions. Advise patient to avoid excessive sunlight exposure.

EFFECTS ON LAB TEST RESULTS
• May increase or decrease glucose level.
• May increase LFT values.

CONTRAINDICATIONS & CAUTIONS
Boxed Warning Antidepressants increase risk of suicidality in children, adolescents, and young adults with major depressive disorder and other psychiatric disorders. Imipramine isn't approved for use in children except for those with nocturnal enuresis. ■

• Contraindicated in patients hypersensitive to drug and during acute recovery phase of MI.

🔵 *Alert:* Concomitant use with linezolid or methylene blue can cause serotonin syndrome (fever, mental status changes, muscle twitching, diaphoresis, shivering or shaking, diarrhea, and loss of coordination). Use imipramine with linezolid or methylene blue only for life-threatening or urgent conditions when the potential benefits outweigh the risks of toxicity.

🔵 *Alert:* Use with extreme caution in patients at risk for suicide; in older adults and in patients with history of urine retention, angle-closure glaucoma, or seizure disorders; in patients with increased IOP, CV disease, impaired hepatic function, hyperthyroidism, or

impaired renal function; and in patients receiving thyroid drugs.

🔵 *Alert:* Imipramine pamoate shouldn't be used in children of any age because of increased risk of acute overdose.

Dialyzable drug: No.

⚠ *Overdose S&S:* Cardiac arrhythmias, severe hypotension, seizures, CNS depression, coma, ECG changes, drowsiness, stupor, ataxia, restlessness, agitation, hyperactive reflexes, muscle rigidity, athetoid and choreiform movements, tachycardia, HF, respiratory depression, cyanosis, shock, vomiting, hyperpyrexia, mydriasis, diaphoresis.

PREGNANCY-LACTATION-REPRODUCTION
• There are no adequate studies during pregnancy; however, fetal risk can't be excluded. Use during pregnancy only if potential benefit clearly justifies fetal risk.
• Drug appears in human milk. Use during breastfeeding isn't recommended.

NURSING CONSIDERATIONS
🔵 *Alert:* If linezolid or methylene blue must be given, discontinue imipramine and monitor patient for serotonin toxicity for 2 weeks (5 weeks if fluoxetine was taken) or until 24 hours after the last dose of methylene blue or linezolid, whichever comes first. May resume imipramine 24 hours after last dose of methylene blue or linezolid.
• Don't withdraw drug abruptly due to risk of discontinuation syndrome (GI symptoms, diaphoresis, chills, tremors, sleep disturbances).
• Monitor WBC count during therapy, and monitor patient for fever and sore throat. Discontinue drug if pathologic neutrophil depression occurs.
• Monitor patient for nausea, headache, and malaise after abrupt withdrawal of long-term therapy; these symptoms don't indicate addiction.
• Safety of long-term use as adjunctive therapy for nocturnal enuresis in children age 6 or older hasn't been established. Consider a drug-free period after an adequate therapeutic trial with a favorable response.
• To prevent relapse in children receiving drug for enuresis, withdraw drug gradually.
• Because of hypertensive episodes during surgery in patients receiving TCAs, stop drug gradually several days before surgery.

Reactions in bold italics are *life-threatening*. Interactions may have a *rapid onset* or a ***delayed onset***.

- If signs or symptoms of psychosis occur or increase, expect prescriber to reduce dosage. Monitor mood changes. Monitor patient for suicidality, and allow only a minimum supply of drug.
- Recommend sugarless hard candy or gum to relieve dry mouth. Saliva substitutes may be useful.
- **Alert:** Tofranil may contain tartrazine.
- *Look alike–sound alike:* Don't confuse imipramine with desipramine.

PATIENT TEACHING
Boxed Warning Advise families and caregivers to closely observe patient for increased suicidality. ▪

- **Alert:** Teach patient to recognize and immediately report symptoms of serotonin toxicity (fever, mental status changes, muscle twitching, diaphoresis, shivering or shaking, diarrhea, and loss of coordination).
- Tell patient to take full dose at bedtime whenever possible, but caution patient about possible morning dizziness upon standing up quickly.
- If child is an early-night bed-wetter, tell parents it may be more effective to divide dose and give the first dose earlier in day.
- Tell patient to avoid alcohol while taking this drug.
- Advise patient to consult prescriber before taking other prescription or OTC drugs.
- Warn patient to avoid hazardous activities that require alertness and good coordination until effects of the drug are known. Drowsiness and dizziness usually subside after a few weeks.
- Warn patient not to stop drug suddenly.
- To prevent oversensitivity to the sun, advise patient to use sunblock, wear protective clothing, and avoid prolonged exposure to strong sunlight.

immune globulin intramuscular (gamma globulin, Ig, IGIM)
GamaSTAN

immune globulin intravenous (IGIV) ☒
Asceniv, Bivigam, Flebogamma DIF, Gammagard Liquid, Gammagard S/D, Gammaked, Gammaplex, Gamunex-C, IGIVnex✤, Octagam, Panzyga, Privigen

immune globulin subcutaneous (IGSC, SCIG) ☒
Cutaquig, Cuvitru, Gammagard, Gammaked, Gamunex-C, Hizentra, HyQvia, IGIVnex✤, Xembify

Therapeutic class: Antibodies
Pharmacologic class: Immune serums

AVAILABLE FORMS
immune globulin intramuscular
Injection: 15% to 18% in 2-mL and 10-mL single-dose vials
immune globulin intravenous
Solution for injection (preservative-free): 5% in 20-mL, 50-mL, 100-mL, 200-mL, 500-mL vials; 10% in 10-mL, 20-mL, 25-mL, 50-mL, 100-mL, 200-mL, 300-mL, 400-mL vials
Powder for injection (preservative-free): 5-g, 10-g vials
immune globulin subcutaneous
Solution for injection (kit with hyaluronidase vials): 10% in 25-mL, 50-mL, 100-mL, 200-mL, 300-mL vials
Solution for injection (preservative-free): 10% in 10-mL, 25-mL, 50-mL, 100-mL, 200-mL, 300-mL vials; 16.5% in 6-mL, 10-mL, 12-mL, 20-mL, 24-mL, 48-mL vials; 20% in 5-mL, 10-mL, 20-mL, 40-mL, 50-mL vials and 5-mL, 10-mL, 20-mL prefilled syringes

INDICATIONS & DOSAGES
Boxed Warning Increases risk of thrombosis; don't exceed recommended dosage. ▪
➤ **Primary humoral immunodeficiency (PI)** ☒
Asceniv
Adults and adolescents ages 12 to 17: 300 to 800 mg/kg IV every 3 to 4 weeks. Begin IV infusion at rate of 0.5 mg/kg/minute for first

15 minutes. Increase every 15 minutes, if tolerated, to maximum of 8 mg/kg/minute.

Bivigam
Adults and children age 6 and older: 300 to 800 mg/kg IV every 3 to 4 weeks. Begin IV infusion at a rate of 0.5 mg/kg/minute for first 10 minutes. Increase infusion rate every 20 minutes, if tolerated, by 0.8 mg/kg/minute, to maximum rate of 6 mg/kg/minute.

Cutaquig, Cuvitru
Adults and children age 2 and older: Individualize subcut infusion dose based on patient's pharmacokinetic and clinical response as monitored by IgG trough levels. Infuse at regular intervals from daily to up to every other week. Infusion rate varies by manufacturer based on patient's age, weight volume of solution, and tolerance.

Flebogamma DIF
Adults: 300 to 600 mg/kg 10% solution IV every 3 to 4 weeks. Infuse at 1 mg/kg/minute. After 30 minutes, if tolerated, may gradually increase to maximum rate of 8 mg/kg/minute.
Adults and children age 2 and older: 300 to 600 mg/kg 5% solution IV every 3 to 4 weeks. Infuse at 0.5 mg/kg/minute. After 30 minutes, if tolerated, may gradually increase to maximum rate of 5 mg/kg/minute.

Gammagard Liquid
Adults and children age 2 and older: 300 to 600 mg/kg IV every 3 to 4 weeks. Infuse at 0.8 mg/kg/minute and increase every 30 minutes, if tolerated to 8 mg/kg/minute. May give maintenance therapy weekly by subcut infusion starting 1 week after last IGIV infusion. Initial subcut dose is 1.37 × current IV dose in mg/kg ÷ number of weeks between IV doses. See package insert for dosage adjustments, recommended number of subcut sites, and infusion rates.

Gammagard S/D
Adults and children age 2 and older: 300 to 600 mg/kg IV every 3 to 4 weeks. Initially, infuse in a 5% solution at 0.5 mL/kg/hour; may increase gradually, as tolerated, to maximum rate of 4 mL/kg/hour. Can give patients who tolerate 5% solution 10% solution starting at 0.5 mL/kg/hour and gradually increase to maximum of 8 mL/kg/hour as tolerated.

Gammaked
Adults and children age 2 and older: 300 to 600 mg/kg IV every 3 to 4 weeks. Initially (first 30 minutes): 1 mg/kg/minute. Increase gradually, if tolerated, up to 8 mg/kg/minute. May give maintenance therapy subcut starting

1 week after last IGIV infusion. Initial subcut dose is 1.37 × current IV dose in mg/kg ÷ number of weeks between IV doses. See package insert for dosage adjustments, recommended number of subcut sites, and infusion rates.

Gammaplex
Adults and children age 2 and older: 300 to 800 mg/kg IV every 3 to 4 weeks. Initially, infuse at 0.5 mg/kg/minute for first 15 minutes. Increase every 15 minutes, if tolerated, to 4 mg/kg/minute for 5% solution and 8 mg/kg/minute for 10% solution.

Gamunex-C
Adults and children age 2 and older: 300 to 600 mg/kg IV every 3 to 4 weeks. Initially, infuse at 2 mg/kg/minute for first 30 minutes. Increase gradually, if tolerated, to maximum of 8 mg/kg/minute. May give maintenance therapy subcut starting 1 week after last IGIV infusion. Initial subcut dose is 1.37 × current IV dose in mg/kg ÷ number of weeks between IV doses. See package insert for recommended number of subcut sites and infusion rates.

Hizentra
Adults and children age 2 and older: Calculate initial weekly dose by dividing previous IGIV dose in grams by the number of weeks between doses during patient's IGIV treatment; then multiply this by the dose adjustment factor of 1.37. Or give the same weekly dose in grams as the prior IGSC treatment. Multiply dose in grams by 5 to obtain dose in milliliters. Adjust dose based on clinical response. Give by subcut infusion at regular intervals from daily up to every 2 weeks. See prescribing information for full dosage adjustment guidelines, recommended number of subcut sites, and infusion rates.

HyQvia
Adults: See manufacturer's labeling for initial 7-week subcut infusion ramp-up schedule to increase dose and frequency from a previous 1-week dose to a 3- or 4-week dose. Begin ramp-up 1 week after last infusion of previous treatment.
Patients naive to IgG therapy or switching from another IG subcut therapy: 300 to 600 mg/kg subcut infusion every 3 to 4 weeks, after initial dose ramp-up.
Patients switching from IGIV therapy: Give by subcut infusion at the same dose and frequency as the previous IGIV therapy every 3 to 4 weeks after initial dose ramp-up. For

---

Reactions in bold italics are **life-threatening**. Interactions may have a *rapid onset* or a **delayed onset**.

subsequent dosage adjustments, refer to manufacturer's instructions.

IGIVnex

Adults and children age 1 and older: 100 to 600 mg/kg (1 mL/kg to 6 mL/kg) IV infusion every 3 to 4 weeks individualized to achieve serum IgG level at trough of at least 5 g/L. May give maintenance therapy as weekly subcut infusion. Initial subcut dose is 1.37 × current IV dose in mg/kg ÷ number of weeks between IV doses.

Octagam 5%

Adults and children age 6 and older: 300 to 600 mg/kg IV every 3 to 4 weeks. Start infusion at 0.5 mg/kg/minute for 30 minutes. Increase rate, as tolerated, to 1 mg/kg/minute for 30 minutes, then to 2 mg/kg/minute for 30 minutes. May then increase to maximum rate of 3.33 mg/kg/minute, as tolerated.

Panzyga

Adults and children age 2 and older: 300 to 600 mg/kg IV every 3 to 4 weeks. Start infusion at 1 mg/kg/minute. If tolerated, may increase every 15 to 30 minutes to maximum rate of 14 mg/kg/minute.

Privigen

Adults and children age 3 and older: 200 to 800 mg/kg IV every 3 to 4 weeks. Start infusion at 0.5 mg/kg/minute and increase slowly to 8 mg/kg/minute.

Xembify

Adults and children age 2 and older: Initial weekly dose is the previous IGIV dose in grams divided by the number of weeks between IGIV doses × 1.37. Multiply dose in grams by 5 to obtain dose in milliliters. Or the same weekly dose in grams as the prior IGSC treatment. Adjust dose based on clinical response and IgG trough levels. Give by subcut infusion two to seven times per week. See package insert for full dosage adjustment guidelines, recommended number of subcut sites, and infusion rates.

➤ Measles exposure in patients with PI

IGIV (Flebogamma, Gammagard Liquid, Gamunex-C, Gammagard S/D, Gammaplex, Octagam, Panzyga, Privigen)

Adults and children: If patient has been exposed to measles, consider giving 400 mg/kg IV as soon as possible within 6 days of exposure to provide a measles antibody serum level greater than 240 mIU/mL for at least 2 weeks. If patient is at risk for future measles exposure and receives a dose of less than

530 mg/kg every 3 to 4 weeks, increase dose to at least 530 mg/kg IV to provide a measles antibody serum level of 240 mIU/mL for at least 22 days after infusion.

IVSC (Cutaquig, Cuvitru, Hizentra, HyQvia)

Adults and children: If patient has been exposed to measles, consider giving 400 mg/kg subcut infusion as soon as possible within 6 days of exposure to provide a measles antibody serum level greater than 240 mIU/mL for at least 2 weeks.

Cutaquig: If patient is at risk for future measles exposure and receives a dose of less than 245 mg/kg every week, increase dose to at least 245 mg/kg/week.

Cuvitru: If patient is at risk for future measles exposure and receives a dose of less than 230 mg/kg every week, increase dose to at least 230 mg/kg/week.

HyQvia: If patient is at risk for future measles exposure and receives a dose of less than 530 mg/kg every 3 to 4 weeks, increase dose to at least 530 mg/kg to provide a measles antibody serum level of 240 mIU/mL for at least 22 days after infusion.

➤ Measles exposure (IGIM)

Adults and children: 0.25 mL/kg IM within 6 days after exposure.

Children who are immunocompromised: 0.5 mL/kg IM immediately after exposure. Maximum dosage is 15 mL.

➤ Chronic inflammatory demyelinating polyneuropathy (CIDP)

Gammaked, Gamunex-C, IGIVnex

Adults: 2,000 mg/kg IV in divided doses over 2 to 4 days. May administer as a maintenance infusion of 1,000 mg/kg IV over 1 day every 3 weeks or 500 mg/kg IV on 2 consecutive days every 3 weeks. Recommended initial infusion rate is 2 mg/kg/minute, which may be gradually increased to a maximum of 8 mg/kg/minute for Gammaked or Gamunex-C if infusion is well tolerated. Maximum infusion rate for IGIVnex is 14/mg/kg/minute if infusion is well tolerated.

Hizentra

Adults: For maintenance therapy, begin subcut infusion 1 week after the last IGIV infusion. Give 200 mg/kg/week (1 mL/kg) or 400 mg/kg/week (2 mL/kg) subcut using an infusion pump in one or two sessions over 1 or 2 consecutive days to prevent relapse. Base duration of therapy on clinical response. Refer to package insert for recommended number of subcut sites, infusion rates, and dosage adjustments if symptoms worsen during treatment.

Panzyga

Adults: Give loading dose of 2 g/kg (20 mL/kg) IV divided into two daily doses of 1 g/kg (10 mL/kg) IV on 2 consecutive days. Maintenance dose is 1 to 2 g/kg (10 to 20 mL/kg) IV every 3 weeks divided in two doses over 2 consecutive days. Initial infusion rate is 1 mg/kg/minute for 30 minutes; may gradually increase every 15 to 30 minutes to a maximum of 12 mg/kg/minute if well tolerated.

Privigen

Adults: 2,000 mg/kg IV in divided doses over 2 to 5 days. May give as a maintenance dose of 1,000 mg/kg IV administered in one to two infusions on consecutive days every 3 weeks. Recommended initial infusion rate is 0.5 mg/kg/minute, which may be gradually increased to a maximum of 8 mg/kg/minute if the infusion is well tolerated. Maintenance therapy with Privigen hasn't been studied beyond 6 months.

➤ **Chronic ITP**

Flebogamma DIF 10%, Panzyga

Adults and children age 2 and older: 1 g/kg (10 mL/kg) IV daily for 2 consecutive days. Initial infusion rate is 0.01 mL/kg/minute (1 mg/kg/minute) for first 30 minutes. If tolerated, rate may be gradually increased to 0.04 mL/kg/minute (4 mg/kg/minute) and, if tolerated, gradually increased to a maximum of 0.08 mL/kg/minute (8 mg/kg/minute).

Gammagard S/D

Adults: 1,000 mg/kg IV. May give up to three separate doses on alternate days, if needed, as determined by clinical response and platelet count. Initially, infuse in a 5% solution at 0.5 mL/kg/hour; may increase gradually, as tolerated, to maximum rate of 4 mL/kg/hour. For patients who tolerate 5% solution, can give 10% solution starting at 0.5 mL/kg/hour and gradually increase to maximum of 8 mL/kg/hour, as tolerated.

Gammaked, Gamunex-C, IGIVnex

Adults and children: 2,000 mg/kg IV in two divided doses of 1,000 mg/kg given on 2 consecutive days or 400 mg/kg IV in five doses over 5 consecutive days. Recommended initial infusion rate is 1 mg/kg/minute. If infusion is well tolerated, may gradually increase rate to maximum of 8 mg/kg/minute. If adequate platelet count increase is seen 24 hours after first dose, may withhold second dose.

Gammaplex 5% or 10%

Adults: 1,000 mg/kg IV for 2 consecutive days. Initial infusion rate is 0.5 mg/kg/minute for 15 minutes. If tolerated, may gradually increase rate every 15 minutes to maximum of 4 mg/kg/minute for 5% solution or 8 mg/kg/minute for 10% solution.

Octagam 10%

Adults: 2,000 mg/kg IV in two divided doses of 1,000 mg/kg given on 2 consecutive days. Initial infusion rate is 1 mg/kg/minute for first 30 minutes. If tolerated, may gradually increase rate every 30 minutes to 2 mg/kg/minute, then 4 mg/kg/minute, then 8 mg/kg/minute, then to maximum of 12 mg/kg/minute.

Privigen

Adults and adolescents age 15 and older: 1 g/kg IV daily for 2 consecutive days. Initial infusion rate is 0.5 mg/kg/minute. If tolerated, may gradually increase rate 4 mg/kg/minute.

➤ **Multifocal motor neuropathy (MMN)**

Gammagard Liquid

Adults: 500 to 2,400 mg/kg/month IV based on response. Initial infusion rate is 0.8 mg/kg/minute. If tolerated, may gradually increase rate every 30 minutes to 9 mg/kg/minute.

➤ **Kawasaki syndrome to prevent associated coronary artery aneurysms**

Gammagard S/D

Children: 400 mg/kg IV daily for 4 consecutive days, or a single dose of 1,000 mg/kg. Start 5% infusion at 0.5 mL/kg/hour. May gradually increase rate to maximum of 4 mL/kg/hour, as tolerated. For patients who tolerate 5% solution, can give 10% solution starting at 0.5 mL/kg/hour and gradually increase to maximum of 8 mL/kg/hour, as tolerated. Begin treatment within 7 days of onset of fever. Give with aspirin (80 to 100 mg/kg PO daily in four divided doses).

➤ **Hepatitis A exposure (IGIM)**

Adults and children: 0.1 mL/kg IM as soon as possible after household or institutional exposure. Not indicated in patients with clinical manifestations of hepatitis A or in those exposed more than 2 weeks previously. Before travel to areas where hepatitis A is common, 0.1 mL/kg IM if length of stay will be up to 1 month or 0.2 mL/kg if length of stay will be up to 2 months; repeat every 2 months for longer stays.

Reactions in bold italics are *life-threatening*. Interactions may have a *rapid onset* or a ***delayed onset***.

➤ **Chickenpox (varicella) exposure (IGIM)**
Adults and children: 0.6 to 1.2 mL/kg IM as soon as possible after exposure only if varicella-zoster immune globulin is unavailable.

➤ **Prevention of bacterial infections in patients with acquired hypogammaglobulinemia or recurrent bacterial infections secondary to B-cell chronic lymphocytic leukemia**
Adults and children: 400 mg/kg IV Gammagard S/D every 3 to 4 weeks for patients with hypogammaglobulinemia or recurrent bacterial infections. Initially, infuse in 5% solution at 0.5 mL/kg/hour; may increase gradually, as tolerated, to maximum rate of 4 mL/kg/hour. For patients who tolerate 5% solution, can give 10% solution starting at 0.5 mL/kg/hour and gradually increase to maximum of 8 mL/kg/hour, as tolerated.

✳ *NEW INDICATION:* **Dermatomyositis**
Octagam 10%
Adults: 2 g/kg IV divided in equal doses given over 2 to 5 consecutive days every 4 weeks. Initial infusion rate is 1 mg/kg/minute for first 30 minutes. If tolerated, may gradually increase rate to 2 mg/kg/minute and, if tolerated, may gradually increase to maximum of 4 mg/kg/minute.

⊘ *Alert:* Patients with dermatomyositis are at increased risk for thromboembolic events; don't exceed infusion rate of 4 mg/kg/minute.

➤ **Guillain-Barré syndrome (IGIV)** ◆
Adults: 2,000 mg/kg IV over 2 to 5 days within 2 to 4 weeks of onset.

ADMINISTRATION

• Refer to each product's manufacturer's instructions for reconstitution, dilution, and storage information.

IM

⊘ *Alert:* Verify drug, route, and dose carefully before administration.

• Give in the anterolateral aspects of the upper thigh and the deltoid muscle of the upper arm. Divide doses larger than 10 mL and inject into several muscle sites to reduce pain and discomfort.

• Don't administer IV or subcut because of risk of serious reactions.

• Give drug soon after reconstitution.

• Don't routinely use the gluteal region. If necessary, use only the upper outer quadrant.

IV

▼ Infusion rates vary by manufacturer based on patient's age, weight, volume of solution, and tolerance.

▼ For patients at risk for renal dysfunction or thrombotic events, give at minimum infusion rate practicable.

▼ Inspect each vial for particulate matter and discoloration before administration.

▼ Don't mix products from different manufacturers together.

▼ **Incompatibilities:** Other IV drugs and IV solutions. Don't mix with immune globulin from other manufacturers.

Subcutaneous

• Give IGSC by subcut infusion.

• Refer to each product's manufacturer for instructions on switching between formulations.

• Inspect each vial for particulate matter and discoloration before administration.

• Infusion sites include abdomen, thighs, upper arms, lateral hip, and for Gammagard Liquid, IGIVnex, and Xembify, the lower back.

• May use multiple infusion sites at the same time. Refer to each product's manufacturer's instructions for the number of infusion sites allowed, spacing between sites, amounts to infuse per site, and infusion rate.

• Complete Cuvitru and Xembify infusions within 2 hours to prevent formation of particles in siliconized syringes.

• Don't mix with other products.

• Don't shake vials.

HyQvia only

• Infusion sites include abdomen and thighs.

• If two sites are used simultaneously, the two infusion sites should be on opposite sides of the body.

• Administer components (immune globulin and hyaluronidase) sequentially, beginning with hyaluronidase; don't use either component alone.

• Administer hyaluronidase at an initial rate per site of approximately 1 to 2 mL/minute, or as tolerated.

• Initiate infusion of the full dose of the immune globulin through the same hyaluronidase subcut needle set within approximately 10 minutes of the hyaluronidase infusion.

• Refer to manufacturer's instructions for weight-based initial and subsequent infusion rates.

ACTION

Provides passive immunity by increasing antibody titer. The primary component is IgG. It's unknown how it works for ITP.

Route	Onset	Peak	Duration
IV	Immediate	Immediate	3–4 wk
IM	Unknown	2 days	3–4 wk
Subcut	Unknown	2–5 days	Unknown

Half-life: 26 to 40 days in patients who are immunocompromised.

ADVERSE REACTIONS

CNS: headache, fever, lethargy, malaise, dizziness, fatigue, myasthenia syndrome, asthenia, pain, insomnia, depression, vertigo. **CV:** chest pain, chest tightness, HTN, hypotension, tachycardia, decreased diastolic BP, increased systolic BP, decreased HR, edema, heart murmur, *hemorrhage, thrombosis.* **EENT:** eye irritation, conjunctivitis, eye discharge, ear pain, otitis media, nasal congestion, epistaxis, rhinorrhea, sinusitis, pharyngitis, nasopharyngitis, postnasal drip, sore throat, oropharyngeal pain. **GI:** diarrhea, abdominal pain, nausea, vomiting. **GU:** UTI, vulvovaginal candidiasis, cystitis, dysuria, nephrolithiasis, increased creatinine level. **Hematologic:** anemia, leukopenia. **Hepatic:** increased ALT level, hyperbilirubinemia, increased or decreased ALP level. **Musculoskeletal:** back pain, arthralgia, limb pain, hip pain, muscle cramps, muscle stiffness at injection site. **Respiratory:** dyspnea, wheezing, pneumonia, cough, asthma. **Skin:** erythema, urticaria, purpura, petechiae, pain, local infusion-site reactions, rash, flushing, hematoma, bruise, cellulitis, excoriation, diaphoresis, allergic dermatitis, eczema. **Other:** *anaphylaxis, angioedema, hypersensitivity,* antibody development, infection, chills, rigors, accidental injury, flulike symptoms.

INTERACTIONS

Drug-drug. *Live-virus vaccines:* May decrease therapeutic effect of vaccine. Length of time to wait before giving live-virus vaccinations varies with immune globulin dosage.

EFFECTS ON LAB TEST RESULTS

- May falsely elevate serum glucose level (for IGIV preparations containing maltose such as Octagam).
- May increase ALT, bilirubin, and creatinine levels.
- May increase or decrease ALP level.
- May decrease hematocrit.
- May cause positive Coombs test.
- Gammagard may produce false-positive readings in assays that depend on detection of beta-D-glucans for diagnosis of fungal infections; this may persist during the weeks after infusion of the product.

CONTRAINDICATIONS & CAUTIONS

- Contraindicated in patients hypersensitive to drug or its components and in those with IgA deficiency, especially those who have known antibodies against IgA or history of hypersensitivity.
- Octagam is contraindicated in patients hypersensitive to corn or maltose.
- Hizentra is contraindicated in patients hypersensitive to polysorbate 80 and in patients with hyperprolinemia.
- Privigen is contraindicated in patients with hyperprolinemia.
- HyQvia is contraindicated in patients with known systemic hypersensitivity to hyaluronidase or human albumin.
- GamaSTAN is also contraindicated in patients with severe thrombocytopenia or any coagulation disorder that would contraindicate IM injections.
- Gammaplex 5% is also contraindicated in patients with hereditary intolerance to fructose and in infants and neonates for whom sucrose or fructose tolerance hasn't been established. Gammaplex 10% doesn't contain sucrose or fructose.
- Don't use Flebogamma DIF in patients with hereditary fructose intolerance because it contains sorbitol, which increases risk of adverse reactions.
- Aseptic meningitis syndrome (AMS) may occur with immune globulin treatment administered IV or subcut. AMS may occur more frequently in females. Syndrome usually begins within several hours to 2 days after immune globulin treatment.
- Use IGIV cautiously in patients with a history of CV disease or thrombotic episodes.

Boxed Warning Renal dysfunction and acute renal failure (excluding Cutaquig,

---

Reactions in bold italics are *life-threatening*. Interactions may have a *rapid onset* or a *delayed onset*.

Cuvitru, GamaSTAN, Hizentra, HyQvia, and Xembify). Renal dysfunction, acute renal failure, osmotic nephrosis, and death may occur with IGIV products in patients who are predisposed. Patients at increased risk include those with any degree of preexisting renal insufficiency, diabetes, age greater than 65, volume depletion, sepsis, paraproteinemia, or patients receiving known nephrotoxic drugs. Renal dysfunction and acute renal failure occur more commonly in patients receiving immune globulin IV products containing sucrose. (*Note:* The following IV products don't contain sucrose: Asceniv, Bivigam, Flebogamma 5% DIF, Flebogamma 10% DIF, Gammagard Liquid, Gammagard S/D, Gammaked, Gammaplex, Gamunex-C, Octagam 5%, Octagam 10%, Panzyga, and Privigen.) For patients at risk, administer IGIV products at the minimum concentration dose and infusion rate practicable and ensure adequate hydration. ■

• Subcut and IV formulations can cause hemolysis and hemolytic anemia.
Dialyzable drug: Unknown.

PREGNANCY-LACTATION-REPRODUCTION
• It isn't known if drug can cause fetal harm when used during pregnancy. Use during pregnancy only if clearly needed and potential benefit justifies fetal risk. Refer to individual manufacturer's instructions for use.
• Drug may appear in human milk. Use cautiously during breastfeeding and only if clearly indicated. Refer to individual manufacturer's instructions for use.

NURSING CONSIDERATIONS
Boxed Warning Drug causes increased risk of thrombosis, especially in older adults; those with prolonged immobilization, hypercoagulable conditions, history of venous or arterial thrombosis, hyperviscosity, CV risk factors, or indwelling central venous catheters; and in patients using estrogens. Thrombosis may also occur without these risk factors. Don't exceed recommended dosage. ■
Boxed Warning For patients at increased risk for thrombosis, give minimum concentration available at minimum rate of infusion practicable. ■
Boxed Warning Ensure adequate hydration before administration. ■

Boxed Warning Monitor patients for signs or symptoms of thrombosis (pain or swelling of the extremity with warmth over affected area, discoloration, unexplained dyspnea, chest pain or discomfort that worsens on deep inspiration, tachycardia, chest pain, numbness, or weakness on one side of the body), and assess blood viscosity in patients at risk for hyperviscosity. ■
• Obtain history of allergies and reactions to immunizations. Keep epinephrine available to treat anaphylaxis.
• Monitor patient for signs and symptoms of AMS, including severe headache, nuchal rigidity, drowsiness, fever, photophobia, painful eye movements, nausea, and vomiting. Conduct a thorough neurologic examination on patients exhibiting such signs and symptoms, including CSF studies, to rule out other causes of meningitis.
• IGIV administration may be linked to thrombotic events.
• Transfusion-related lung injury (TRALI) can occur after IGIV treatment and typically appears within 1 to 6 hours after therapy. Monitor patient for severe respiratory distress, hypoxemia, pulmonary edema, and fever with normal LVEF. Provide respiratory support and perform tests for the presence of anti-neutrophil antibodies and anti-human leukocyte antigen antibodies in the product and patient's serum.
• Monitor renal function test results and urine output in patient at risk for developing acute renal failure.
• In patient receiving subcut or IV therapy, monitor CBC and watch for signs and symptoms of hemolysis and hemolytic anemia (weakness, pallor, dark urine, fever, dyspnea, abdominal pain).
• Products made from human plasma may contain infectious agents, such as viruses and, potentially, the Creutzfeldt-Jakob disease agent.
• Hyaluronidase infusion included in the HyQvia kit increases dispersion and absorption of IGSC.

PATIENT TEACHING
🚫 *Alert:* Warn patient of thrombosis risk. Instruct patient to immediately report signs or symptoms.
• Explain to patient and family how drug will be given.

✚Canada   ◇OTC   ◆Off-label use   ✐ Photoguide   ⊜Do not crush   *Liquid contains alcohol   ▓ Genetic

• Teach patient to immediately report all adverse reactions, especially signs and symptoms of hypersensitivity reactions, thrombosis, AMS, TRALI, renal injury, and hemolytic anemia.

• Tell patient that local reactions may occur at injection site. Instruct patient to promptly report adverse reactions that persist or become severe.

• Tell patient that lab blood tests will be needed to monitor therapy.

• Inform patient of possible need for therapy more than once monthly to maintain adequate IgG levels.

• Tell patient to report pregnancy or plans to become pregnant before therapy begins.

• Tell patient who is breastfeeding or planning to breastfeed to discuss breastfeeding before therapy begins.

---

indomethacin
in-doe-METH-a-sin

Indocin, Tivorbex

indomethacin sodium trihydrate

Therapeutic class: Anti-inflammatory drugs
Pharmacologic class: NSAIDs

AVAILABLE FORMS
indomethacin
Capsules: 20 mg, 25 mg, 40 mg, 50 mg
Capsules (extended-release): 75 mg
Injection: 1 mg base/vial
Oral suspension: 25 mg/5 mL
Suppositories: 50 mg, 100 mg ✤
indomethacin sodium trihydrate
Injection: 1 mg base/vial

INDICATIONS & DOSAGES
➤ **Moderate to severe RA or osteoarthritis, ankylosing spondylitis (excluding Tivorbex)**
Adults and children age 15 and older: 25 mg PO b.i.d. or t.i.d. with food or antacids or 25 mg PR b.i.d. or t.i.d.; increase daily dose by 25 or 50 mg every 7 days until satisfactory response is obtained, up to total daily dose of 150 to 200 mg. Or, 75 mg extended-release capsules PO to start, in morning or at bedtime, followed by 75 mg extended-release capsules b.i.d. if needed.

➤ **Acute gouty arthritis (excluding Tivorbex)**
Adults and children age 15 and older: 50 mg PO or PR t.i.d. Reduce dose as soon as possible; then stop therapy. Don't use extended-release form.
➤ **Acute painful shoulders (bursitis or tendinitis) (excluding Tivorbex)**
Adults and children age 15 and older: 75 to 150 mg PO or PR daily in divided doses t.i.d. or q.i.d. for 7 to 14 days. Or, 75 mg (extended-release) PO daily or b.i.d. for 7 to 14 days.
➤ **Mild to moderate acute pain (Tivorbex)**
Adults: 20 mg PO t.i.d. or 40 mg PO b.i.d. or t.i.d.
➤ **To close a hemodynamically significant patent ductus arteriosus in premature neonates**
Neonates older than age 7 days: 0.2 mg/kg IV; then two doses of 0.25 mg/kg at 12- to 24-hour intervals.
Neonates ages 2 to 7 days: 0.2 mg/kg IV; then two doses of 0.2 mg/kg at 12- to 24-hour intervals.
Neonates younger than 48 hours: 0.2 mg/kg IV; then two doses of 0.1 mg/kg IV at 12- to 24-hour intervals.
Adjust-a-dose: If anuria or marked oliguria (urine output less than 0.6 mL/kg/hour) is evident at scheduled time of second or third dose of indomethacin for injection, don't give additional doses until lab studies indicate renal function has returned to normal.

ADMINISTRATION
PO
• Give drug with food, milk, or antacid.
• Patient must swallow extended-release capsules whole; don't crush.
• Shake suspension well before use.
• Measure suspension with oral medication syringe or calibrated cup.
IV
▼ Reconstitute powder for injection with sterile water or NSS. For each 1-mg vial, add 1 or 2 mL of diluent for a solution containing 1 mg/mL or 0.5 mg/mL, respectively. Give over 20 to 30 minutes.
▼ Avoid IV bolus administration or infusion via an umbilical catheter into vessels near the superior mesenteric artery as these may cause vasoconstriction and can compromise blood flow to the intestines.
⊙ *Alert:* Use only preservative-free sterile saline solution or sterile water to prepare.

Reactions in bold italics are *life-threatening*. Interactions may have a *rapid onset* or a **delayed onset**.

Never use diluents containing benzyl alcohol because it has been linked to toxicity in newborns.

▼ Because injection contains no preservatives, reconstitute drug immediately before use and discard unused solution.

▼ Watch carefully for bleeding and for reduced urine output.

▼ **Incompatibilities:** None listed by manufacturer. Consult a drug incompatibility reference for more information.

Rectal

• If suppository is too soft, place in refrigerator for 15 minutes or run under cold water in wrapper.

ACTION

May inhibit prostaglandin synthesis, to produce anti-inflammatory, analgesic, and antipyretic effects.

Route	Onset	Peak	Duration
PO	30 min	2 hr	4–6 hr
IV	Immediate	Immediate	4–6 hr
PR	Unknown	Unknown	4–6 hr

Half-life: Adults (mean), 4.5 hours; neonates, 12 to 20 hours; Tivorbex, 7.5 hours.

ADVERSE REACTIONS

PO and rectal

CNS: headache, dizziness, depression, fatigue, somnolence, syncope, malaise, vertigo.
CV: edema, postprocedural hemorrhage.
EENT: tinnitus. **GI:** abdominal pain, constipation, diarrhea, dyspepsia, nausea, vomiting.
Skin: pruritus, rash, diaphoresis. **Other:** hypersensitivity reactions, hot flush.

INTERACTIONS

Drug-drug. *ACE inhibitors (benazepril, enalaprilat), angiotensin II receptor blockers (candesartan, valsartan):* May reduce antihypertensive effects; may worsen renal function in those with impaired renal function. Monitor patient closely.
Aminoglycosides (amikacin, gentamicin), cyclosporine, methotrexate: May enhance toxicity of these drugs. Avoid using together.
Anticoagulants: May increase bleeding risk. Monitor patient closely.
Antihypertensives: May decrease antihypertensive effect. Monitor patient closely.
Antihypertensives, furosemide, thiazide diuretics: May impair response to both drugs. Avoid using together, if possible.

Aspirin: May increase adverse reactions, including risk of GI toxicity. Avoid using together.
Bisphosphonates: May increase risk of gastric ulceration. Monitor patient for symptoms of gastric irritation or GI bleeding.
Corticosteroids: May increase indomethacin adverse effects. Avoid using together.
Diflunisal, probenecid: May decrease indomethacin excretion. Watch for increased indomethacin adverse effects.
Digoxin: May prolong half-life of digoxin. Use together cautiously.
Dipyridamole: May enhance fluid retention. Avoid using together.
Drospirenone: May increase hyperkalemic effect of drospirenone. Use together cautiously.
Lithium: May increase lithium level. Monitor patient for toxicity.
Methotrexate: May increase methotrexate toxicity. Use together cautiously.
Phenytoin: May increase phenytoin level. Monitor patient closely.
Senna: May inhibit diarrheal effects. Discourage use together.
SSRIs: May increase antiplatelet effect of indomethacin and antidepressant effect of SSRI. Consider alternative to indomethacin or monitor patient for bleeding and decreased antidepressant effect.
Triamterene: May cause nephrotoxicity. Avoid using together.
Drug-herb. *Alfalfa, anise, bilberry, dong quai, garlic:* May cause bleeding. Discourage use together.
White willow: Herb and drug contain similar components. Don't use together.
Drug-lifestyle. *Alcohol use:* May cause GI toxicity. Discourage use together.

EFFECTS ON LAB TEST RESULTS

• May increase potassium level and renal function and LFT values.
• May decrease Hb level and hematocrit.
• May cause false-negative results in dexamethasone suppression test.

CONTRAINDICATIONS & CAUTIONS

• Contraindicated in patients hypersensitive to drug and in those with a history of aspirin- or NSAID-induced asthma, rhinitis, or urticaria.
• Contraindicated in neonates with untreated infection, active bleeding, coagulation defects or thrombocytopenia, congenital heart

disease needing patency of the ductus arteriosus, necrotizing enterocolitis, or significant renal impairment.

Boxed Warning NSAIDs may increase risk of serious thrombotic events, including MI or stroke, which can be fatal. Risk may be greater with longer use or in patients with CV disease or risk factors for CV disease. ∎

Boxed Warning Risk of MI or stroke can occur as early as the first weeks of NSAID use. Risk appears greater at higher doses. Use lowest effective dose for shortest duration possible. ∎

Boxed Warning NSAIDs may increase risk of serious GI adverse events, including bleeding, ulceration, and perforation of the stomach or intestines, which can be fatal. These events can occur at any time during use and without warning symptoms. Older adults and patients with a prior history of peptic ulcer disease or GI bleeding are at greater risk for serious GI events. ∎

🔴 *Alert:* Avoid use in patients with severe HF unless benefits are expected to outweigh risk of worsening HF.

• Suppositories are contraindicated in patients with history of proctitis or recent rectal bleeding.

Boxed Warning Contraindicated for the treatment of perioperative pain after CABG surgery. ∎

• Use cautiously in older adults, patients with a history of GI disease, and those with epilepsy, parkinsonism, hepatic or renal disease, CV disease, infection, and mental illness or depression.

• Safety and effectiveness of oral or suppository formulations in children age 14 and younger (age 17 and younger for Tivorbex) haven't been established.

Dialyzable drug: Unknown.

⚠ *Overdose S&S:* Drowsiness, lethargy, nausea, vomiting, paresthesia, epigastric pain, GI bleeding.

PREGNANCY-LACTATION-REPRODUCTION

🔴 *Alert:* Use of NSAIDs at 20 weeks or later in pregnancy may cause fetal renal dysfunction leading to oligohydramnios and potential neonatal renal impairment; use at 30 weeks or later in pregnancy may increase risk of premature closure of the ductus arteriosus. Avoid use during pregnancy starting at 20 weeks' gestation. If potential benefit justifies fetal risk, use lowest effective dose for the shortest

duration. Consider ultrasound monitoring of amniotic fluid if NSAID therapy is longer than 48 hours. Use of 81 mg of low-dose aspirin for certain pregnancy-related conditions under direction of prescriber is acceptable.

• Drug appears in human milk. Use during breastfeeding isn't recommended by most manufacturers.

• Long-term use of NSAIDs in patients of childbearing potential may be associated with infertility that's reversible upon drug discontinuation.

NURSING CONSIDERATIONS

• Because of the high risk of adverse effects from long-term use, drug shouldn't be used routinely as an analgesic or antipyretic.

🔴 *Alert:* Watch for and immediately evaluate signs and symptoms of heart attack (chest pain, shortness of breath or trouble breathing) or stroke (weakness in one part or side of the body, slurred speech).

• If ductus arteriosus reopens, a second course of one to three doses may be given. If ineffective, surgery may be needed.

• Watch for bleeding in patients receiving anticoagulants, patients with coagulation defects, and neonates.

• Monitor patients for GI adverse effects.

• Because NSAIDs impair synthesis of renal prostaglandins, they can decrease renal blood flow and lead to reversible renal impairment, especially in patients with renal failure, HF, or hepatic dysfunction; in older adults; and in patients taking diuretics. Monitor these patients closely.

• Drug causes sodium retention; watch for weight gain (especially in older adults) and increased BP in patients with HTN.

• Monitor patient for rash and respiratory distress, which may indicate a hypersensitivity reaction.

• Because of their antipyretic and antiinflammatory actions, NSAIDs may mask signs and symptoms of infection.

• Monitor patient on long-term oral therapy for toxicity by conducting regular eye exams, hearing tests, CBCs, and liver and kidney function tests.

PATIENT TEACHING

• Tell patient to take oral dose with food, milk, or antacid to prevent GI upset.

🔴 *Alert:* Advise patient to seek medical attention immediately if chest pain, shortness

---

of breath or trouble breathing, weakness in one part or side of the body, or slurred speech occurs.

⚠ Alert: Warn patient who is pregnant not to take NSAIDs at 20 weeks' gestation or later unless instructed to do so by prescriber due to fetal risk. Advise patient to discuss taking any OTC medication with pharmacist or health care provider during pregnancy.

• Alert patient that using oral form with aspirin, alcohol, other NSAIDs, or corticosteroids may increase risk of adverse GI reactions.

• Teach patient signs and symptoms of GI bleeding (blood in vomit, urine, or stool; coffee-ground vomit; and melena) and to notify prescriber immediately if any of these occurs.

• Tell patient to immediately report signs or symptoms of cardiac events, such as chest pain, shortness of breath, weakness, and slurred speech.

• Warn patient to avoid hazardous activities that require mental alertness until CNS effects are known.

• Tell patient to notify prescriber immediately if visual or hearing changes occur.

• Tell patient to notify prescriber if unexplained weight gain or edema occurs.

BIOSIMILAR DRUG

inFLIXimab
in-FLICKS-ih-mab

Remicade

inFLIXimab-abda
Renflexis

inFLIXimab-axxq
Avsola

inFLIXimab-dyyb
Inflectra

inFLIXimab-qbtx
Ixifi

Therapeutic class: Anti-inflammatory drugs
Pharmacologic class: TNF blockers

AVAILABLE FORMS
Lyophilized powder for injection: 100-mg vials

INDICATIONS & DOSAGES
➤ **Moderately to severely active Crohn disease; reduction in the number of draining enterocutaneous and rectovaginal fistulas and maintenance of fistula closure in adults with fistulizing Crohn disease**
Adults: 5 mg/kg IV infusion over at least 2 hours. Repeat at 2 and 6 weeks, then every 8 weeks thereafter. For patients who respond and then lose their response, consider 10 mg/kg. Patients who don't respond by week 14 are unlikely to respond with continued therapy. In those patients, consider stopping drug.
Children ages 6 to 17: For Crohn disease, 5 mg/kg IV infusion over at least 2 hours. Repeat at 2 and 6 weeks, then every 8 weeks thereafter.
➤ **Moderately to severely active RA (in conjunction with methotrexate)**
Adults: 3 mg/kg IV infusion over at least 2 hours. Repeat at 2 and 6 weeks after first infusion and every 8 weeks thereafter. Dose may be increased up to 10 mg/kg, or doses may be given every 4 weeks if response is inadequate.
➤ **Ulcerative colitis**
Adults: Induction dose, 5 mg/kg IV over at least 2 hours. Repeat at 2 and 6 weeks, then every 8 weeks thereafter.
➤ **Moderate to severe ulcerative colitis in children who have had an inadequate response to conventional therapy**
Children age 6 and older: Initially, 5 mg/kg IV infusion over at least 2 hours at 0, 2, and 6 weeks, followed by a maintenance regimen of 5 mg/kg IV infusion over at least 2 hours every 8 weeks.
➤ **Ankylosing spondylitis**
Adults: 5 mg/kg IV infusion over at least 2 hours. Repeat at 2 and 6 weeks, then every 6 weeks thereafter.
➤ **Psoriatic arthritis, with or without methotrexate**
Adults: 5 mg/kg IV infusion over at least 2 hours. Repeat at 2 and 6 weeks after first infusion, then every 8 weeks thereafter.
➤ **Chronic severe plaque psoriasis**
Adults: 5 mg/kg IV infusion over at least 2 hours. Repeat dose in 2 and 6 weeks, then give 5 mg/kg every 8 weeks thereafter.

ADMINISTRATION

IV

▼ Reconstitute with 10 mL sterile water for injection, using syringe with 21G or smaller needle. Don't shake; gently swirl to dissolve powder. Solution should be colorless to light yellow and opalescent. It may also develop a few translucent particles; don't use if other types of particles develop or discoloration occurs.

▼ Dilute total volume of reconstituted drug to 250 mL with NSS for injection. Infusion concentration ranges from 0.4 to 4 mg/mL.

▼ Use an in-line, sterile, nonpyrogenic, low-protein-binding filter with a pore size smaller than 1.2 microns.

▼ Begin infusion within 3 hours of preparation and give over at least 2 hours.

▼ **Incompatibilities:** Other IV drugs. Don't infuse with other drugs.

ACTION

Binds to human TNF-alpha to neutralize its activity and inhibit its binding with receptors, thereby reducing the infiltration of inflammatory cells and TNF-alpha production in inflamed areas of the intestine.

Route	Onset	Peak	Duration
IV	Unknown	Unknown	Unknown

Half-life: 7 to 12 days.

ADVERSE REACTIONS

CNS: fatigue, fever, headache, pain, systemic and cutaneous vasculitis. **CV:** HTN, chest pain, flushing, tachycardia, *bradycardia.* **EENT:** conjunctivitis, rhinitis, sinusitis, pharyngitis. **GI:** abdominal pain, diarrhea, dyspepsia, nausea. **GU:** UTI. **Hematologic:** *leukopenia, neutropenia,* anemia, hematoma. **Hepatic:** increased ALT level. **Musculoskeletal:** arthralgia, back pain, arthritis, myalgia, bone fracture. **Respiratory:** cough, URI, bronchitis, dyspnea, pneumonia, respiratory tract allergic reaction. **Skin:** rash, pruritus, candidiasis, urticaria, cellulitis, abscess. **Other:** hypersensitivity reactions, infusion reactions, serum sickness, development of antibodies, infection, *sepsis,* candidiasis, *anaphylaxis,* chills, flulike syndrome.

INTERACTIONS

Drug-drug. *CYP450 substrates (cyclosporine, theophylline, warfarin):* May normalize formation of CYP450 enzymes upon initiation or discontinuation of infliximab. Monitor effect or drug concentration; may adjust individual dose of drug product as needed.

Live-virus vaccines: May affect normal immune response. Postpone live-virus vaccine until therapy stops. Withhold live-virus vaccines for at least 6 months in infants born to patients treated with infliximab.

TNF blockers (abatacept, anakinra, golimumab, rilonacept): May increase risk of serious infections and neutropenia. Use together isn't recommended.

Tocilizumab: May increase risk of immunosuppression and infection. Avoid use together.

Drug-herb. *Echinacea:* May diminish therapeutic effect of immunosuppressants. Consider therapy modification.

EFFECTS ON LAB TEST RESULTS

- May increase liver enzyme levels.
- May decrease Hb level, hematocrit, and RBC, WBC, and platelet counts.
- May produce false-negative TB test results.
- May cause false-positive ANA test result.

CONTRAINDICATIONS & CAUTIONS

- Contraindicated in patients hypersensitive to murine proteins or other components of drug. Doses greater than 5 mg/kg are contraindicated in patients with moderate to severe HF.

Boxed Warning Drug increases risk of serious infections that may lead to hospitalization or death, especially in patients taking a concomitant immunosuppressant, such as methotrexate or corticosteroid. Discontinue drug if serious infection or sepsis occurs. ∎

Boxed Warning Carefully consider risks and benefits of treatment before initiating infliximab therapy in patients with long-term or recurrent infection. ∎

Boxed Warning Lymphoma and other malignancies, some fatal, have occurred in children and adolescents treated with TNF blockers, including infliximab. ∎

Boxed Warning Hepatosplenic T-cell lymphoma, a rare type of lymphoma that can be fatal, has occurred in adolescents and young adult males with inflammatory bowel disease treated with TNF blockers, including infliximab. ∎

Boxed Warning Drug increases risk of serious infections, including TB, histoplasmosis, coccidioidomycosis, blastomycosis, bacterial

---

Reactions in bold italics are *life-threatening.* Interactions may have a *rapid onset* or a *delayed onset.*

sepsis, *Listeria, Legionella*, and other opportunistic infections. Patients with histoplasmosis or other invasive fungal infections may present with disseminated rather than localized disease. Antigen and antibody testing for histoplasmosis may be negative in some patients with active infection. Consider antifungal therapy in patients at risk for invasive fungal infections who develop severe systemic illness. ∎

• Depending on the product, each vial contains between 50 and 500 mg of sucrose.

• Use cautiously in older adults; in patients with active infection, history of chronic or recurrent infections, a history of hematologic abnormalities, or preexisting or recent-onset CNS demyelinating or seizure disorders; or in those who have lived in regions where histoplasmosis is endemic.

• Rare cases of severe hepatic reactions (acute liver failure, jaundice, hepatitis, cholestasis) with or without elevations in aminotransferase levels have been reported in postmarketing data. Discontinue drug if signs and symptoms of liver injury occur.

• Use cautiously in patients with hematologic abnormalities. Serious and sometimes fatal cases of leukopenia, neutropenia, thrombocytopenia, and pancytopenia have been reported.
Dialyzable drug: Unknown.

PREGNANCY-LACTATION-REPRODUCTION

• Drug crosses placental barrier but it isn't known if drug can cause fetal harm or can affect reproductive capacity if used during pregnancy. Use during pregnancy only if clearly needed.

• Drug may be present in the serum of infants up to 6 months after birth. Exposed infants may be at increased risk for infection.

• It isn't known if drug appears in human milk. Patient should discontinue breastfeeding or discontinue drug.

NURSING CONSIDERATIONS

• There are no clinically meaningful differences between the biosimilar product and the reference product (Remicade) based on the conditions of their use. However, these drugs aren't considered to be interchangeable and can't be automatically substituted.

• Premedication with antihistamines, acetaminophen, and corticosteroids may be considered at prescriber's discretion to prevent infusion-related reactions.

• Monitor patients for signs and symptoms of hypersensitivity reactions (urticaria, dyspnea, hypotension), which may occur during or within 2 hours of infusion and may be severe. Discontinue drug for severe reactions and treat appropriately.

⚠ *Alert:* Watch for infusion-related reactions, including fever, chills, pruritus, urticaria, dyspnea, hypotension, HTN, and chest pain during administration and for 2 hours afterward. If an infusion-related reaction occurs, stop drug, notify prescriber, and prepare to give acetaminophen, antihistamines, corticosteroids, and epinephrine.

• Don't give live-virus vaccines to infants exposed to drug in utero for at least 6 months after birth because of increased risk of infection, including disseminated infection, which can be fatal.

• Give for Crohn disease and ulcerative colitis only after patient has an inadequate response to conventional therapy.

• Consider stopping treatment in patient who develops significant hematologic abnormalities or CNS adverse reactions.

• Notify prescriber for symptoms of new or worsening HF.

Boxed Warning Discontinue drug if serious infection or sepsis develops. ∎

Boxed Warning Watch for development of lymphoma and infection. Patient with chronic Crohn disease and long-term exposure to immunosuppressants is more likely to develop lymphoma and infection. ∎

• Drug may affect normal immune responses. Patient may develop autoimmune antibodies and lupuslike syndrome; stop drug if this happens. Symptoms should resolve.

Boxed Warning Drug may cause disseminated or extrapulmonary TB and fatal opportunistic infections. ∎

Boxed Warning Evaluate patient for latent TB infection with a tuberculin skin test. Treat latent TB infection before therapy. ∎

Boxed Warning Closely monitor patients for signs and symptoms of infection during and after infliximab treatment, including possible development of TB in patients who tested negative for latent TB infection before start of therapy. ∎

• TNF blockers may increase risk of reactivation of HBV in patients who are chronic carriers. Patients taking concomitant immunosuppressants are at increased risk. Test for HBV infection before therapy begins. Monitor

HBV carriers during and for several months after therapy. If HBV reactivation occurs, discontinue infliximab.

• Monitor patient for hepatotoxicity (jaundice, liver enzyme elevations 5 × ULN or more). Stop drug and closely evaluate patient if these signs or symptoms occur.

• *Look alike–sound alike:* Don't confuse Remicade with Renacidin or Rituxan. Don't confuse infliximab with rituximab or idarucizumab. Don't confuse Inflectra with Injectafer.

PATIENT TEACHING

Boxed Warning Inform patient that testing for TB will be done before therapy and to immediately report signs and symptoms of infection. ■

Boxed Warning Counsel patient about risk of lymphoma and other malignancies. ■

• Tell patient about infusion-reaction symptoms and adverse effects and the need to report them promptly.

• Advise patient to report all adverse reactions and to seek immediate medical attention for signs and symptoms of infection (persistent fever, cough, shortness of breath, fatigue, unusual bleeding or bruising).

• Instruct patient to report pregnancy or plans to become pregnant before start of therapy. Tell patient not to breastfeed during therapy.

• Caution patient who took drug during pregnancy that infant shouldn't receive live-virus vaccines for at least 6 months after birth.

• Tell patient to alert prescriber to therapy before receiving vaccines.

• Advise patient or caregiver to make sure all vaccines are up-to-date before therapy.

SAFETY ALERT!

insulin degludec–liraglutide
IN-su-lin de-GLOO-dek/lir-ah-GLOO-tide

Xultophy 100/3.6

Therapeutic class: Antidiabetics
Pharmacologic class: Insulins–glucagon-like peptide-1 receptor agonists

AVAILABLE FORMS

Injection (prefilled pen): 100 units insulin degludec/3.6 mg liraglutide per mL in 3-mL pens

INDICATIONS & DOSAGES

➤ **Adjunct to diet and exercise to improve glycemic control in patients with type 2 diabetes**

Adults: In patients naive to basal insulin or a glucagon-like peptide-1 (GLP-1) agonist, initially give 10 units (insulin degludec 10 units/liraglutide 0.36 mg) subcut once daily. In patients currently on basal insulin or a GLP-1 agonist, initially give 16 units (insulin degludec 16 units/liraglutide 0.58 mg) subcut once daily. Titrate dosage upwards or downwards by 2 units (insulin degludec 2 units/liraglutide 0.072 mg) every 3 to 4 days until desired fasting plasma glucose level is achieved. Maximum dose, 50 units (insulin degludec 50 units/liraglutide 1.8 mg/day).

Adjust-a-dose: Titrate dosage to minimize risk of hypoglycemia or hyperglycemia; with changes in physical activity, meal patterns, or renal or hepatic function; during acute illness; or when drug is used with other drugs that affect glucose level.

ADMINISTRATION
Subcutaneous

• Discontinue other liraglutide products and basal insulins before start of therapy.

🜂 *Alert:* Pens are for a single patient only; pens should never be shared.

• Dose counter displays numbers for the insulin units.

• Don't mix this product with other insulin products or solutions.

• Give at the same time each day with or without food.

• Visually inspect drug for particulate matter and discoloration before administration.

• Inject subcut into the thigh, upper arm, or abdomen; don't give IV or IM or use in an insulin infusion pump.

• Rotate injection sites within the same region from one injection to the next to reduce risk of lipodystrophy.

• Don't split the dose; give once daily.

• If a dose is missed, omit the missed dose and resume drug at next scheduled dose. Don't give an extra injection or increase dosage to make up for the missed dose.

• If more than 3 days have elapsed since the last dose, reinitiate drug at the starting dose to avoid GI symptoms associated with treatment reinitiation.

Reactions in bold italics are *life-threatening*. Interactions may have a *rapid onset* or a *delayed onset*.

- Before first use, store pens between 36° and 46° F (2° and 8° C) until the expiration date printed on the label. Don't freeze.
- After first use, pens can be stored for 21 days at controlled room temperature (59° to 86° F [15° to 30° C]) or in refrigerator (36° to 46° F [2° to 8° C]); keep all pens away from direct heat and light.

ACTION

Insulin degludec lowers blood glucose level by stimulating peripheral glucose uptake, especially by skeletal muscle and fat, and by inhibiting hepatic glucose production. Insulin also inhibits lipolysis and proteolysis while enhancing protein synthesis. Liraglutide is a GLP-1 receptor agonist that increases glucose-dependent insulin release, decreases glucagon secretion, and slows gastric emptying.

Route	Onset	Peak	Duration
Subcut	Unknown	Unknown	Unknown

Half-life: Insulin degludec, 25 hours; liraglutide, 13 hours.

ADVERSE REACTIONS

CNS: headache. **CV:** peripheral edema. **EENT:** nasopharyngitis. **GI:** nausea, diarrhea, gallbladder disease. **Metabolic:** *hypoglycemia, hypokalemia,* weight gain, increased lipase level. **Respiratory:** URI. **Skin:** injection-site reactions, lipodystrophy. **Other:** antibody formation, hypersensitivity reactions.

INTERACTIONS

Drug-drug. *ACE inhibitors, antidiabetics, ARBs, disopyramide, fibrates, fluoxetine, MAO inhibitors, octreotide, pentoxifylline, pramlintide, salicylates, sulfonamide antibiotics:* May increase hypoglycemia risk. Monitor glucose level closely and adjust Xultophy dosage accordingly.
Atypical antipsychotics (olanzapine, clozapine), corticosteroids, danazol, diuretics, estrogens, glucagon, isoniazid, niacin, oral contraceptives, phenothiazines, progestogens in oral contraceptives, protease inhibitors, somatropin, sympathomimetic agents (albuterol, epinephrine, terbutaline), thyroid hormones: May decrease glucose-lowering effects. Monitor glucose level closely and adjust Xultophy dosage as needed.

Beta blockers, clonidine: May blunt or mask signs and symptoms of hypoglycemia. Monitor glucose level closely.
Beta blockers, clonidine, lithium salts, pentamidine: May increase risk of hypoglycemia or hyperglycemia. Monitor glucose level closely and adjust Xultophy dosage as needed.
Oral medications: May affect gastric absorption of other oral medications taken at the same time. Monitor effectiveness of oral medications.
Peroxisome proliferator-activated receptor (PPAR) gamma agonists (thiazolidinediones [pioglitazone, rosiglitazone]): May cause dose-related fluid retention, which can lead to or exacerbate HF. Discontinue or reduce dosage of PPAR gamma agonist as clinically indicated.
Potassium-lowering drugs (loop and thiazide diuretics, theophylline): May increase risk of hypokalemia. Monitor potassium level.
Drug-lifestyle. *Alcohol use:* May alter glucose level and insulin needs. Discourage use together.

EFFECTS ON LAB TEST RESULTS

- May increase bilirubin, calcitonin, lipase, and amylase levels.
- May decrease potassium level.

CONTRAINDICATIONS & CAUTIONS

Boxed Warning Liraglutide causes dose-dependent and treatment duration–dependent thyroid C-cell tumors at clinically relevant exposures in both genders of rats and mice. It isn't known if drug causes thyroid C-cell tumors, including medullary thyroid carcinoma (MTC), in humans, as the human relevance of liraglutide-induced rodent thyroid C-cell tumors hasn't been determined. ■
Boxed Warning Contraindicated in patients with a personal or family history of MTC and in patients with multiple endocrine neoplasia syndrome type 2 (MEN 2). ■
- Contraindicated during episodes of hypoglycemia and in patients with hypersensitivity to insulin degludec or liraglutide.
- Severe, life-threatening allergic reactions, including anaphylaxis, angioedema and bronchospasm, urticaria, rash, and pruritus, have been reported. If hypersensitivity reactions occur, discontinue drug. Use cautiously in patients with a history of angioedema resulting from use of another GLP-1 receptor agonist.

• Drug isn't recommended as first-line therapy for patients who have inadequate glycemic control with diet and exercise because of the uncertain relevance of the rodent C-cell tumor findings in humans.

• Use cautiously in patients at risk for pancreatitis. Pancreatitis has been observed in patients taking liraglutide. Drug hasn't been studied in patients with a history of pancreatitis; consider other antidiabetic therapies in these patients.

• Use cautiously in patients with visual impairment who may rely on audible clicks to dial their dose.

• Drug isn't indicated for use in patients with type 1 diabetes or diabetic ketoacidosis, or for use in combination with prandial insulin.

• Drug isn't recommended for use in combination with other products containing liraglutide or other GLP-1 receptor agonists.

• Postmarketing reports indicate incidences of acute renal failure and worsening of chronic renal failure, sometimes requiring hemodialysis, in patients treated with liraglutide. In most cases, these events occurred in patients who experienced nausea, vomiting, diarrhea, or dehydration.

• Drug can cause hypokalemia that, if untreated, can cause respiratory paralysis, ventricular arrhythmias, and death.

• Safety and effectiveness in children haven't been established.

• Use cautiously in older adults, as they may be more sensitive to drug's effects.

Dialyzable drug: No.

⚠ *Overdose S&S:* Hypoglycemia, hypokalemia, GI adverse reactions (severe nausea and vomiting).

PREGNANCY-LACTATION-REPRODUCTION

• Animal studies suggest drug may increase fetal adverse events. Use during pregnancy only if potential benefit justifies fetal risk.

• It isn't known if drug appears in human milk. Consider both the potential adverse effects to the infant who is breastfed and the developmental and health benefits of breastfeeding.

NURSING CONSIDERATIONS

• Adjust dosages cautiously and only under medical supervision with frequent glucose monitoring.

• Monitor patients for dehydration. Drug can cause dehydration due to GI adverse reactions; take precautions to avoid fluid depletion.

• Monitor patients for signs and symptoms of pancreatitis (persistent severe abdominal pain that may radiate to the back, with or without vomiting). Discontinue drug if pancreatitis is confirmed.

• Monitor patients for URI and signs and symptoms of gallbladder disease (stomach pain, fever, nausea, vomiting, jaundice).

• Monitor patients for hypersensitivity reactions (urticaria, rash, pruritus, anaphylactic reaction, angioedema).

• Evaluate patients with changes to the thyroid gland or significantly elevated serum calcitonin level.

• Monitor renal function and blood glucose, amylase, and lipase levels.

• Monitor serum potassium level in patients at risk for hypokalemia (patients taking potassium-lowering medication or medications sensitive to potassium levels).

• Monitor patients for lipodystrophy; hyperglycemia may result from alterations at injection site.

• *Look alike–sound alike:* Don't confuse insulin degludec with other insulin products.

PATIENT TEACHING

• Explain that dose counter on pen shows only the number of insulin units to be injected.

• Teach patient how to use dosage pen and how to administer drug, including rotating injection sites.

• Warn patient against sharing pens with other individuals because of the risk of contracting blood-borne pathogens.

• Instruct patient not to take more than 50 units of the pen per day and not to use with other GLP-1 receptor agonists.

• Advise patient not to split doses into two injections and not to mix other insulin or GLP-1 products in the same syringe.

• Emphasize to patient that glucose monitoring will need to be done regularly and that glucose level will need to be checked more carefully with changes in amount of activity, meal patterns, and acute illness.

• Caution patient that dosage changes should only be made under medical supervision.

• Teach patient the signs and symptoms of hypoglycemia (confusion, dizziness, feeling shaky, rapid pulse) and how to manage it.

Reactions in bold italics are *life-threatening*. Interactions may have a *rapid onset* or a *delayed onset*.

• Instruct patient to report all adverse effects and to immediately report edema, chest pain, or palpitations.

Boxed Warning Inform patient of risk of thyroid tumors, including cancer, and to immediately report neck lump or swelling, hoarseness, trouble swallowing, or shortness of breath. ∎

• Warn patient to immediately report severe pain in the abdomen that may or may not radiate to the back (with or without vomiting), as this type of pain may indicate pancreatitis.

• Counsel patient to avoid becoming dehydrated, as acute kidney injury may occur.

SAFETY ALERT!

insulin glargine–lixisenatide
IN-su-lin GLAR-jeen/lix-i-SEN-a-tide

Soliqua 100/33

Therapeutic class: Antidiabetics
Pharmacologic class: Insulins–glucagon-like peptide-1 receptor agonists–long-acting insulins

AVAILABLE FORMS
Injection: insulin glargine 100 units/mL and lixisenatide 33 mcg/mL in 3-mL pens

INDICATIONS & DOSAGES
➤ **Adjunct to diet and exercise to improve glycemic control in patients with type 2 diabetes**
Adults naive to basal insulin or to a glucagon-like peptide-1 (GLP-1) receptor agonist, currently on a GLP-1 receptor agonist, or currently on less than 30 units of basal insulin daily: Initially, 15 units (insulin glargine 15 units/lixisenatide 5 mcg) subcut once daily within the hour before first meal of the day.
Adults inadequately controlled on 30 to 60 units of basal insulin, with or without a GLP-1 receptor agonist: Initially, 30 units (insulin glargine 30 units/lixisenatide 10 mcg) subcut once daily within the hour before first meal of the day.
Adjust-a-dose: Titrate dosage up or down by 2 to 4 units every week based on patient's metabolic needs, blood glucose monitoring results, and glycemic goal until desired fasting glucose level is achieved. Dosage titration may also be needed with changes in activity,

meal patterns, or renal or hepatic function; during acute illness; or when used with other medications that affect glucose level. Use alternative antidiabetic products if patients require a Soliqua 100/33 daily dosage below 15 units or above 60 units. Maximum dose, 60 units (insulin glargine 60 units/lixisenatide 20 mcg) daily.

ADMINISTRATION
Subcutaneous
• Discontinue therapy with a GLP-1 receptor agonist or basal insulin before starting Soliqua 100/33.

• Prefilled pen delivers doses from 15 to 60 units in a single injection.

• Refer to manufacturer's instructions and perform a safety test before each injection to check that pen and needle are working correctly and to ensure that correct dose will be delivered.

• Inspect pen before use. Solution should be clear and colorless to almost colorless.

• Inject into abdominal area, thigh, or upper arm, rotating injection sites within the same region to reduce risk of lipodystrophy.

• Give dose within the hour before first meal of the day.

• Don't administer IV, IM, or via an insulin pump.

• Don't dilute or mix with other insulins or solution.

• Don't administer drug in split doses.

• Remove needle after each injection and store pen without needle attached. Always use a new needle for each injection to prevent contamination.

• If a dose is missed, resume the once-daily regimen as prescribed with the next scheduled dose. Don't administer an extra dose or increase the dose to make up for the missed dose.

🖐 *Alert:* Pen is for single-patient use only because of risk of transmission of blood-borne pathogens even if needle is changed.

• Store drug in refrigerator at 36° to 46° F (2° to 8° C) before first use. Don't freeze. Discard drug if pen has been frozen. Protect from light.

• After first use, store pen at room temperature below 77° F (25° C). Replace pen cap after each use to protect from light. Discard pen 28 days after first use.

ACTION

Insulin glargine lowers blood glucose level by stimulating peripheral glucose uptake and by inhibiting hepatic glucose production. Lixisenatide increases glucose-dependent insulin release, decreases glucagon secretion, and slows gastric emptying.

Route	Onset	Peak	Duration
Subcut	Insulin glargine: 3–4 hr	Insulin glargine: no pronounced peak Lixisenatide: 2.5–3 hr	Insulin glargine: about 24 hr

Half-life: 3 hours (lixisenatide).

ADVERSE REACTIONS

CNS: headache. **CV:** peripheral edema. **EENT:** nasopharyngitis. **GI:** diarrhea, nausea. **Metabolic:** *hypoglycemia, hypokalemia,* weight gain. **Respiratory:** URI. **Skin:** injection-site reactions, lipodystrophy. **Other:** antibody development, hypersensitivity reactions.

INTERACTIONS

Drug-drug. *ACE inhibitors, antidiabetics, ARBs, disopyramide, fibrates, fluoxetine, MAO inhibitors, pentoxifylline, pramlintide, salicylates, somatostatin analogues (octreotide), sulfonamide antibiotics:* May increase risk of hypoglycemia. Monitor glucose level closely and adjust dosage as necessary.

Acetaminophen, antibiotics and other oral medications dependent on threshold concentrations for efficacy: Lixisenatide may reduce rate of absorption of coadministered oral drugs. Give other drugs at least 1 hour before Soliqua 100/33.

Atypical antipsychotics (clozapine, olanzapine), corticosteroids, danazol, diuretics, estrogens, glucagon, isoniazid, niacin, phenothiazines, protease inhibitors, somatropin, sympathomimetic agents (albuterol, epinephrine, terbutaline), thyroid hormones: May decrease blood glucose–lowering effect of Soliqua 100/33. Monitor glucose level closely and adjust Soliqua 100/33 dosage as needed.

Beta blockers, clonidine: May mask signs and symptoms of hypoglycemia. Monitor glucose level closely and adjust Soliqua 100/33 dosage as needed.

Beta blockers, clonidine, lithium salts: May increase or decrease blood glucose–lowering effect of Soliqua 100/33. Monitor glucose level closely and adjust Soliqua 100/33 dosage as necessary.

GLP-1 receptor agonists: May increase risk of overdose and hypoglycemia. Use together isn't recommended.

Oral contraceptives, progesterones: May delay rate of contraceptive absorption. Patient should take contraceptive at least 1 hour before or 11 hours after Soliqua 100/33.

Peroxisome proliferator–activated receptors (PPARs) (fenofibrate, pioglitazone, rosiglitazone): May increase risk of HF. Consider discontinuing drug or reducing dosage of the PPAR-gamma agonist.

Pentamidine: May cause hypoglycemia, which may be followed by hyperglycemia. Monitor glucose level closely and adjust Soliqua 100/33 dosage as needed.

Drug-lifestyle. *Alcohol use:* May increase or decrease blood glucose–lowering effect of Soliqua 100/33. Discourage use together.

Smoking: May decrease insulin absorption and increase insulin resistance. Discourage use together.

EFFECTS ON LAB TEST RESULTS

• May decrease glucose, HbA_{1c}, and potassium levels.

• May cause immunogenicity and antibody positivity.

CONTRAINDICATIONS & CAUTIONS

• Contraindicated during hypoglycemia episodes.

• Contraindicated in patients hypersensitive to either of the active drug substances or their components.

• Rarely, allergic reactions (urticaria, angioedema, anaphylaxis, bronchospasm, hypotension, shock) have been reported. Use cautiously in patients with a history of anaphylaxis or angioedema with use of another GLP-1 receptor agonist.

• Drug isn't indicated for use in patients with type 1 diabetes or for treatment of diabetic ketoacidosis.

• Acute pancreatitis has been reported with GLP-1 receptor agonists. Consider other antidiabetics in patients with a history of pancreatitis.

• Not recommended in patients with ESRD (eGFR less than 15 mL/minute/1.73 m²) or in patients with severe gastroparesis. Consider other antidiabetics.

Reactions in bold italics are *life-threatening*. Interactions may have a *rapid onset* or a ***delayed onset***.

- Use with prandial insulin hasn't been studied.
- Use cautiously in patients with visual impairment who may rely on audible clicks to dial their dose.
- Safety and effectiveness in children haven't been established.
- Use cautiously in older adults. Initial dosing, dose increments, and maintenance dosing should be conservative to avoid hypoglycemia.

Dialyzable drug: Unknown.

⚠ *Overdose S&S:* Insulin glargine: hypoglycemia, hypokalemia. Lixisenatide: increased incidence of GI disorders.

PREGNANCY-LACTATION-REPRODUCTION

- Exposure to lixisenatide during pregnancy may cause fetal harm. Use during pregnancy only if potential benefits justify fetal risk.
- It isn't known if insulin glargine or lixisenatide appears in human milk. Effects on milk production or the infant who is breastfed are unknown. Weigh benefits of breastfeeding and the patient's clinical need for drug against potential adverse effects on the infant.

NURSING CONSIDERATIONS

- Monitor patient for signs and symptoms of hypoglycemia; the long-acting effect of insulin glargine may delay recovery from hypoglycemia.
- Frequently monitor blood glucose level during dosage changes, which may predispose patient to hypoglycemia or hyperglycemia. Adjust concomitant oral antidiabetics as needed.
- Always check insulin label before giving drug, as accidental mix-ups among insulin products have been reported.
- Increase frequency of glucose monitoring with changes to meal pattern or physical activity and in patients with renal or hepatic impairment and hypoglycemia unawareness.
- Monitor patient for signs and symptoms of pancreatitis (persistent severe abdominal pain, sometimes radiating to the back, with or without vomiting). If pancreatitis is suspected, discontinue drug and treat appropriately. If pancreatitis is confirmed, don't restart drug.
- Acute kidney injury and worsening of chronic renal failure have been reported. Monitor renal function and watch for

dehydration due to GI adverse effects when starting drug or increasing dosage in patients with renal impairment and in those reporting severe GI reactions. Assess fluid status closely.
- Monitor patient for worsening glycemic control or failure to achieve targeted glycemic control, significant injection-site reactions, or allergic reactions, as they may indicate antibody formation. Consider alternative antidiabetic therapy.
- Insulin-containing products may cause potassium to shift into the intracellular space, resulting in hypokalemia. Monitor potassium level in patients at risk for hypokalemia (patients using potassium-lowering drugs or drugs sensitive to serum potassium concentrations).
- *Look alike–sound alike:* Don't confuse insulin glargine with other insulin products.

PATIENT TEACHING

- Inform patient that serious hypersensitivity reactions, including anaphylaxis, have been reported. Instruct patient to stop drug and immediately seek medical attention for signs and symptoms of hypersensitivity reactions.
- Advise patient of risk of pancreatitis. Instruct patient to discontinue drug and report persistent abdominal pain, with or without vomiting.
- Teach patient to never share the pen with another person, even if the needle is changed, because of risk of transmission of blood-borne pathogens.
- Inform patient that hypoglycemia is the most common adverse reaction. Teach patient signs and symptoms of hypoglycemia and that regimen changes can predispose patient to hypoglycemia or hyperglycemia.
- Warn patient that hypoglycemia may impair mental alertness and to use caution while driving or operating machinery.
- Advise patient of risk of dehydration due to GI adverse reactions and to take precautions to avoid fluid depletion.
- Inform patient of risk of worsening renal function, which may require dialysis.
- Instruct patient to always check label before each injection to avoid medication errors due to confusion with other insulin products.
- Caution patient that administering more than 60 units of Soliqua 100/33 daily or

concurrent use with other GLP-1 inhibitors can result in lixisenatide overdose.

• Instruct patient on self-management procedures, including glucose monitoring and management of hypoglycemia and hyperglycemia.

• Teach patient how to handle special situations, such as concurrent illness, stress, or emotional disturbances; inadequate or missed insulin dose; inadvertent administration of an increased insulin dose; inadequate food intake; and missed meals.

• Instruct patient on proper administration and handling. Caution patient not to dilute drug or mix drug with other insulin products or solutions.

• Advise patient to report pregnancy, plans to become pregnant, or breastfeeding.

SAFETY ALERT!

Insulins (fixed combinations)

IN-su-lins

insulin lispro protamine–insulin lispro

HumaLOG Mix 50/50, HumaLOG Mix 75/25

isophane insulin suspension–insulin injection combinations

HumuLIN 70/30 ◇, NovoLIN 70/30 ◇

insulin aspart (rDNA origin) protamine suspension–insulin aspart (rDNA origin) injection

NovoLOG Mix 70/30

Therapeutic class: Antidiabetics
Pharmacologic class: Insulins

AVAILABLE FORMS

Injection: Humalog Mix 50/50 (50% insulin lispro protamine suspension and 50% insulin lispro) and 75/25 (75% insulin lispro protamine suspension and 25% insulin lispro) 100 units/mL (U-100) in 10-mL vials, 3-mL prefilled KwikPen syringes
Injection: Humulin 70/30 (70% isophane insulin suspension and 30% regular insulin) 100 units/mL (U-100) in 3-mL and 10-mL vials, 3-mL prefilled pens, 3-mL KwikPen syringes

Injection: Novolog Mix 70/30 (70% insulin aspart protamine suspension and 30% insulin aspart) 100 units/mL (U-100) in 10-mL vials, 3-mL prefilled FlexPen syringes
Injection: Novolin 70/30 (70% isophane insulin suspension and 30% regular insulin) 100 units/mL (U-100) in 10-mL vials, 3-mL prefilled FlexPen syringes

INDICATIONS & DOSAGES

Adjust-a-dose (for all indications): Individualize dosage based on metabolic needs, blood glucose monitoring, and glycemic control goal. Insulin requirements may be altered during acute illness, emotional distress, or stress. Adjust as needed in older adults, in patients with renal or hepatic dysfunction, in patients with obesity, in those with changes in physical activity or meal patterns, during puberty, and in patients concurrently taking drugs that lower blood glucose level. Refer to manufacturer's instructions for dosage adjustments when converting from other insulin regimens and formulations.

➤ **To improve glycemic control in patients with diabetes**

Adults: For Novolog Mix 70/30, individualize dosage and give subcut b.i.d. within 15 minutes before a meal or, in type 2 diabetes, give up to 15 minutes after start of a meal.

Adults: For Humalog Mix 50/50 and 75/25, individualize dosage and give subcut b.i.d. within 15 minutes before a meal.

Adults: For Humulin 70/30, individualize dosage and give subcut b.i.d. about 30 to 45 minutes before a meal.

Adults and children: For Novolin 70/30, individualize dosage and give subcut b.i.d. about 30 to 45 minutes before a meal.

ADMINISTRATION

Subcutaneous

• Inspect vials and syringes. Drug should appear uniformly white and cloudy. Don't use if it looks clear or contains solid particles.

• Administer all insulin mixtures at room temperature.

• Don't freeze vials or pens; discard if frozen.

• Drug is a suspension; administer only subcut, never IV.

• Don't use in insulin infusion pumps.

• Don't mix with other insulins.

• Keep away from direct heat and sunlight.

• Discard insulin exposed to temperatures above 86° F (30° C).

Reactions in bold italics are *life-threatening*. Interactions may have a *rapid onset* or a **delayed onset**.

- Follow product-specific pen device directions for preparation and administration.
- Rotate injection sites to reduce risk of lipodystrophy.
- Give subcut into thighs, arms, buttocks, or abdomen.

⭘ **Alert:** Multidose pens are for single-patient use only. Pens should never be shared even if the needle is changed. Clearly label with patient identifying information where it won't obstruct dosing window, warning, or other product information.

Novolog Mix 70/30
- Keep all unopened Novolog Mix 70/30 refrigerated between 36° and 46° F (2° and 8° C) until expiration date.
- Once vial is opened or has been unopened but stored at room temperature, use within 28 days.
- Once a Novolog Mix 70/30 FlexPen has been punctured, it should be kept at temperatures below 86° F (30° C) for up to 14 days. Don't store a Novolog Mix 70/30 FlexPen that's in use in refrigerator.

Humulin 70/30
- Discard opened or unopened vials stored at room temperature after 31 days.
- Store unopened pen or KwikPen in refrigerator at 36° to 46° F (2° to 8° C). Discard unopened pens stored at room temperature after 10 days.
- Store opened pen or KwikPen at room temperature; discard after 10 days even if syringe contains insulin.

Novolin 70/30
- Store unopened vials in refrigerator at 36° to 46° F (2° to 8° C).
- If refrigeration isn't possible, may keep unopened vials at room temperature for up to 6 weeks (42 days), as long as temperature is at or below 77° F (25° C). Keep unopened vials in carton to protect from light.
- If unopened vials are stored in refrigerator, follow expiration date on label.
- Keep open vials at room temperature.
- Throw away open vial after 6 weeks (42 days) of use, even if insulin remains in vial.

Humalog Mix 75/25 and Humalog Mix 50/50
- Refrigerate vials and pens at 36° to 46° F (2° to 8° C) until ready to use.
- Unrefrigerated (below 86° F [30° C]) vials must be used within 28 days or discarded.

- Unrefrigerated (below 86° F [30° C]) KwikPen and pen must be used within 10 days and then discarded, even if syringe contains insulin.

ACTION

Regulates glucose metabolism by stimulating peripheral glucose uptake and inhibiting hepatic glucose production.

Route	Onset	Peak	Duration
Subcut (Novolog Mix 70/30)	10–20 min	1.8–3.6 hr	Up to 24 hr
Subcut (Humulin 70/30)	30–90 min	2.2 hr	Up to 24 hr
Subcut (Humalog Mix 75/25 and 50/50)	15 min	30 min–4 hr	11–22 hr
Subcut (Novolin 70/30)	30 min	0.8–10 hr	18–24 hr

Half-life: Novolog Mix 70/30, 8 to 9 hours; Humulin 70/30 and Novolin 70/30, unknown; Humalog Mix 50/50 and 75/25, unknown.

ADVERSE REACTIONS

CNS: headache, neuropathy. **CV:** peripheral edema. **EENT:** pharyngitis, rhinitis. **GI:** abdominal pain, diarrhea, nausea, dyspepsia. **Metabolic:** *hypoglycemia, hypokalemia,* weight gain. **Musculoskeletal:** myalgia. **Respiratory:** bronchitis, cough, URI. **Skin:** lipodystrophy, injection-site reactions, rash. **Other:** allergic reactions, insulin antibody production, flulike syndrome, infection.

INTERACTIONS

Drug-drug. *ACE inhibitors, antidiabetics (oral), ARBs, disopyramide, fibrates, fluoxetine,* **MAO inhibitors,** *octreotide, pentoxifylline, pramlintide, salicylates, sulfonamide antibiotics:* May increase risk of hypoglycemia. Monitor glucose level closely and adjust insulin dosage as needed.
Atypical antipsychotics, corticosteroids, danazol, diuretics, estrogens, glucagon, hormonal contraceptives, isoniazid, niacin, phenothiazines, protease inhibitors, sympathomimetics (albuterol, epinephrine, terbutaline), somatropin, thyroid hormones: May decrease blood glucose–lowering effects. Monitor glucose level closely and adjust insulin dosage as needed.

Beta blockers, clonidine: May mask signs and symptoms of hypoglycemia. Avoid concurrent use, if possible, or monitor patient closely.

Beta blockers, clonidine, lithium salts, pentamidine: May cause hypoglycemia or hyperglycemia. Monitor glucose level closely.

Thiazolidinediones (TZDs; pioglitazone, rosiglitazone): May cause fluid retention that can lead to HF. Monitor patient closely and adjust or stop TZDs as clinically indicated.

Drug-herb. *Ginseng:* May increase drug's effects. Discourage use together.

Drug-lifestyle. *Alcohol use:* May cause hyperglycemia or hypoglycemia. Monitor glucose level closely and discourage concurrent use.

EFFECTS ON LAB TEST RESULTS
• May decrease blood glucose and potassium levels.

CONTRAINDICATIONS & CAUTIONS
• Contraindicated during episodes of hypoglycemia or ketoacidosis.
• Contraindicated in patients with a history of hypersensitivity to drug or its components. Severe, life-threatening, generalized allergy, including anaphylaxis, can occur with insulin products.
• Changes in insulin or oral antidiabetic dosages may affect glycemic control and should be made only under medical supervision.
• Use cautiously in patients susceptible to hypokalemia, such as patients who are fasting, are taking potassium-lowering drugs, or are concurrently taking drugs that may affect potassium levels, including IV insulin. Untreated hypokalemia can cause respiratory paralysis, ventricular arrhythmias, and death.
• Hypoglycemia is the most common adverse reaction. Severe hypoglycemia can cause seizures, and may be life-threatening or fatal. Hypoglycemia can occur suddenly, and signs and symptoms may differ. Risk increases with intensity of glycemic control and changes in glycemic treatment, meal patterns, physical activity, or concomitant medications, and in patients with renal or hepatic impairment.
• Use pens cautiously in patients with visual impairment who may rely on audible clicks to dial their dose.
• Use cautiously in older adults, who may be at increased risk for adverse effects. Signs and symptoms of hypoglycemia may be more difficult to recognize in these patients.
• Safety and effectiveness in children haven't been determined except with Novolin 70/30.

Dialyzable drug: Unknown.

⚠ **Overdose S&S:** Hypoglycemia, hypokalemia.

PREGNANCY-LACTATION-REPRODUCTION
• Use cautiously during pregnancy and only if clearly needed.
• Monitor blood glucose levels closely in patients who are pregnant, in patients who have recently given birth, and in patients who are breastfeeding; insulin requirements may change.
• It isn't known if insulin appears in human milk. Use cautiously during breastfeeding.

NURSING CONSIDERATIONS
• The time course of the action of insulin mixtures may vary among patients and in the same patient depending on time of day, injection site, blood supply, temperature, and physical activity.
• Observe injection sites for reactions, such as redness, swelling, itching, or burning. These reactions should resolve within a few days or weeks.
• Assess patient and notify prescriber for signs and symptoms of hypoglycemia (diaphoresis, shaking, trembling, confusion, headache, irritability, hunger, rapid, pulse, nausea) and hyperglycemia (drowsiness, fruity breath odor, frequent urination, thirst).
• Signs and symptoms of hypoglycemia may occur in patients with diabetes regardless of glucose level.
• Symptom awareness may be decreased in patients with long-standing diabetes, diabetic nerve disease, renal disease, or hepatic impairment and in patients who have experienced recurrent hypoglycemia. Treat according to individual facility protocol if necessary.
• May treat mild episodes of hypoglycemia with oral glucose. May treat more severe episodes of hypoglycemia, such as coma, seizure, or neurologic impairment, with IM or subcut glucagon or concentrated IV glucose.
• Monitor blood glucose level and adjust insulin dosages as needed with medical supervision.

• Closely monitor patients also taking other medications because other drugs can mask signs and symptoms of hypoglycemia or cause an increase or decrease in blood glucose level.

• Increase frequency of glucose monitoring in patients who are acutely ill or under emotional stress, or if changes in diet, exercise, or medication regimen occur. These situations may affect rate of insulin absorption.

• Increase frequency of glucose monitoring when initiating therapy or when changes in insulin strength, dosage, manufacturer, or type or method of administration are made. Such changes may affect glycemic control and increase risk of hypoglycemia.

• Monitor potassium levels in patients at risk for hypokalemia (those receiving potassium-depleting drugs or IV insulin).

• Monitor patients for generalized allergic reactions, rash (including pruritus) over entire body, shortness of breath, wheezing, hypotension, rapid pulse, diaphoresis, and anaphylaxis.

• Periodically measure HbA$_{1c}$ levels.

• *Look alike–sound alike:* Don't confuse Novolog with Novolin; don't confuse Humalog with Humulin.

PATIENT TEACHING

• Caution patient not to mix insulin combination products with other insulins.

🛑 *Alert:* Warn patient not to share multidose pen with other people, even if the needle is changed, because of risk of bloodborne pathogen transmission, including HIV and hepatitis.

• Advise patient that hypoglycemic episodes can impair the ability to concentrate and react; advise patient to use caution while driving and operating machinery.

• Instruct patient to keep hard candy or glucose tablets on hand to treat mild cases of hypoglycemia.

• Advise patient to keep a log of glucose levels.

• Instruct patient on long-term sequelae of diabetes if not managed properly.

• Instruct patient to carry identification or wear jewelry indicating that patient has diabetes.

• Advise patient that allergic and hypersensitivity reactions can occur, including injection-site reactions (local pain, redness, or swelling), and to report symptoms to health care provider. Teach patient signs and symptoms of anaphylaxis and to seek emergency medical attention promptly if anaphylaxis occurs.

• Instruct patient on self-management procedures, including glucose monitoring, proper preparation and administration techniques, and management of hypoglycemia and hyperglycemia.

• Warn patient about special situations, such as concurrent conditions (illness, stress, or emotional disturbances), inadequate or skipped insulin dose, inadvertent administration of an increased insulin dose, inadequate food intake, and skipped meals.

• Advise patient to inform prescriber of pregnancy or plans to become pregnant.

• Advise patient that insulin requirements may change during pregnancy and after childbirth.

• Teach patient that alcohol and some other medications may increase or decrease glucose levels. Advise patient to inform prescriber of all medications and supplements being taken.

• Caution patient not to stop insulin abruptly or change amount taken without consulting prescriber.

• Advise patient that any insulin change should be made cautiously and only under medical supervision. Changes in insulin strength, manufacturer, type (regular, NPH, or insulin analogues), species (animal, human), or method of manufacture (rDNA versus animal-source insulin) may result in the need for a dosage change. Dosage of concomitant oral antidiabetic may need adjustment.

• Teach patient to give insulin at appropriate time around a meal, depending on product.

• Instruct patient to rotate injection sites and of the importance of avoiding lipodystrophy.

• Teach patient to store insulin products properly, depending on individual products.

• Explain importance of checking insulin label before each injection as accidental mix-ups among insulin types have been reported.

Insulins (intermediate-acting)

IN-su-lins

isophane insulin suspension (NPH)
HumuLIN N ◇, HumuLIN N KwikPen ◇, NovoLIN N ◇, NovoLIN N FlexPen ◇

Therapeutic class: Antidiabetics
Pharmacologic class: Insulins

AVAILABLE FORMS
Injection: 100 units/mL in 3-mL and 10-mL vials, 3-mL KwikPens (Humulin N); 100 units/mL in 10-mL vials, 3-mL FlexPens (Novolin N)

INDICATIONS & DOSAGES
➤ **Type 1 diabetes; type 2 diabetes that can't be properly controlled by diet, exercise, and weight control**
Adults and children age 12 and older: Individualized dosage given subcut once or twice daily.
Adjust-a-dose: Individualize dosage based on metabolic needs, blood glucose monitoring, and glycemic control goal. Insulin requirements may be altered during acute illness, emotional distress, or stress. Adjust as needed in older adults, patients who have renal or hepatic dysfunction, or have changes in physical activity or meal patterns, and in patients concurrently taking drugs that lower blood glucose level. Refer to manufacturer's instructions for dosage adjustments when converting from other insulin regimens and formulations.

ADMINISTRATION
Subcutaneous
• NPH is an intermediate-acting insulin and must be used concomitantly with rapid- or short-acting insulin.
• Give by subcut injection only; not for IM, IV, or insulin pump administration.
• Give injection in abdominal region, buttocks, thigh, or upper arm. Subcut injection into abdominal wall is generally associated with faster absorption than other injection sites.
• Rotate injection sites within same region to reduce risk of lipodystrophy. A general rule is to not administer within 1 inch (2.5 cm) of same site for 1 month.

• Injection into a lifted skin fold minimizes risk of IM injection.
• Roll vial gently between the hands before each dose to uniformly disperse NPH insulin. Avoid vigorous shaking that may cause air bubbles or foam.
• NPH insulin should be uniformly cloudy or milky after gentle mixing and shouldn't contain particulate matter.
• When mixing NPH insulin with regular insulin, always draw clear regular insulin into syringe first; then administer immediately.
• NPH insulin is typically given within 60 minutes of a meal. However, time of administration depends on patient-specific variables; NPH insulin may be given with mealtime regular or Humalog insulin if indicated.
🔔 *Alert:* Multidose pens are for single patient use only. Pens should never be shared even if the needle is changed. Clearly label with patient identifying information where it won't obstruct dosing window, warning, or other product information.
• Store Humulin N at room temperature, below 86° F (30° C), if not exposed to direct sunlight for 31 days (vial) or 14 days (pen). May store opened vials and unopened vials and pens in refrigerator at 36° to 46° F (2° to 8° C); don't refrigerate opened pens. Discard opened pens after 14 days, even if pen still contains drug. Don't freeze vials or pens.
• Store opened or unopened Novolin N away from direct heat or light at room temperature, below 77° F (25° C) for up to 42 days (vial) or below 86° F (30° C) for up to 28 days (pen). Store unopened Novolin N vials and pens in refrigerator at 36° to 46° F (2° to 8° C) and use until expiration date on label. Don't freeze.

ACTION
Lowers blood glucose level by stimulating peripheral glucose uptake and inhibiting hepatic glucose production; also inhibits lipolysis and proteolysis, and enhances protein synthesis.

Route	Onset	Peak	Duration
Subcut	1–1.5 hr	4–12 hr	Up to 24 hr

Half-life: About 4.4 hours.

ADVERSE REACTIONS
CV: peripheral edema. **EENT:** visual disturbances. **Metabolic:** *hypoglycemia, hypokalemia,* weight gain. **Skin:** injection-site reaction, lipodystrophy, pruritus, rash.

Reactions in bold italics are *life-threatening*. Interactions may have a *rapid onset* or a *delayed onset*.

Other: hypersensitivity reactions, immunogenicity.

INTERACTIONS

Drug-drug. *ACE inhibitors, antidiabetics (oral), ARBs, disopyramide, fibrates, fluoxetine, MAO inhibitors, octreotide, pentoxifylline, pramlintide, salicylates, sulfonamide antibiotics:* May increase risk of hypoglycemia. Monitor glucose level closely and adjust insulin dosage as needed.

Atypical antipsychotics, corticosteroids, danazol, diuretics, estrogens, glucagon, hormonal contraceptives, isoniazid, niacin, phenothiazines, protease inhibitors, sympathomimetics (albuterol, epinephrine, terbutaline), somatropin, thyroid hormones: May decrease blood glucose–lowering effects. Monitor glucose level closely and adjust insulin dosage as needed.

Beta blockers, clonidine: May mask signs and symptoms of hypoglycemia. Avoid concurrent use, if possible, and monitor patient closely.

Beta blockers, clonidine, lithium salts, pentamidine: May cause hypoglycemia or hyperglycemia. Monitor glucose level closely.

Thiazolidinediones (TZDs; pioglitazone, rosiglitazone): May cause fluid retention that can lead to HF. Monitor patient closely and adjust or stop TZDs as clinically indicated.

Drug-lifestyle. *Alcohol use:* May cause hyperglycemia or hypoglycemia. Monitor glucose level closely, and discourage concurrent use.

EFFECTS ON LAB TEST RESULTS

• May decrease blood glucose and potassium levels.

• May develop antibodies that react with human insulin.

CONTRAINDICATIONS & CAUTIONS

• Contraindicated during episodes of hypoglycemia or ketoacidosis.

• Contraindicated in patients with a history of hypersensitivity to drug or its components. Severe, life-threatening, generalized allergy, including anaphylaxis, can occur with insulin products.

• Use cautiously in patients susceptible to hypokalemia, such as patients who are fasting, are taking potassium-lowering drugs, or are concurrently taking drugs that may affect potassium level. Untreated hypokalemia

can cause respiratory paralysis, ventricular arrhythmias, and death.

• Hypoglycemia is the most common adverse reaction. Severe hypoglycemia can cause seizures, and may be life-threatening or fatal. Hypoglycemia can occur suddenly and symptoms may differ. Risk increases with intensity of glycemic control and changes in glycemic treatment, meal patterns, physical activity, and concomitant medications and in patients with renal or hepatic impairment.

• Use cautiously in older adults, who may be at increased risk for adverse effects; signs and symptoms of hypoglycemia may be more difficult to recognize in these patients.

• Safety and effectiveness in children younger than age 12 haven't been established.

Dialyzable drug: Unknown.

⚠ ***Overdose S&S:*** Hypoglycemia, hypokalemia.

PREGNANCY-LACTATION-REPRODUCTION

• Use cautiously in patients who are pregnant and monitor patients closely.

• Monitor blood glucose levels closely in patients who are pregnant, in patients who have recently given birth, and in patients who are breastfeeding; insulin requirements may change.

• It isn't known if insulin appears in human milk. Use cautiously during breastfeeding.

NURSING CONSIDERATIONS

• Monitor blood glucose levels and adjust insulin dosages as needed.

• Monitor patients taking other medications with insulin more closely because other drugs may mask signs and symptoms of hypoglycemia or may cause an increase or decrease in blood glucose level.

• Increase frequency of glucose monitoring in patients who are acutely ill or under emotional stress, or if changes in diet, exercise, or medication regimen occur, as these may affect rate of insulin absorption. Also closely monitor patients after changes to insulin dosage.

• Monitor patients carefully for signs and symptoms of hypoglycemia. Treat according to individual facility policy and procedure if necessary.

• Mild episodes of hypoglycemia may be treated with oral glucose. More severe episodes of hypoglycemia, such as coma, seizure, or neurologic impairment, may be treated with IM or subcut glucagon or concentrated IV glucose.

• Monitor potassium levels in patients at risk for hypokalemia, especially those taking potassium-depleting drugs.
• Assess patient for signs and symptoms of hypoglycemia (seizures, diaphoresis, shaking, trembling, confusion) and hyperglycemia (drowsiness, fruity breath odor, frequent urination, thirst). Notify prescriber if any of these signs or symptoms occur.
• Periodically measure HbA$_{1c}$ levels.
• Monitor patients for generalized allergic reactions, including anaphylaxis.
• *Look alike–sound alike:* Don't confuse Humulin with Humalog; don't confuse Novolin with Novolog.

PATIENT TEACHING

• Instruct patient in self-management, including glucose monitoring; injection preparation, technique, and proper storage of insulin; and recognition and management of hypoglycemia and hyperglycemia.
• Explain to patient that insulin requirements may vary due to illness, stress or emotional disturbance, inadequate food intake, and skipped meals.
• Advise patient that hypoglycemic episodes can impair the ability to concentrate and react; advise patient to use caution while driving and operating machinery.
• Advise patient that allergic and hypersensitivity reactions can occur, including injection-site reactions (local pain, redness, or swelling), and to report signs and symptoms to health care provider. Teach patient signs and symptoms of anaphylaxis and to seek emergency medical attention promptly if anaphylaxis occurs.
• Caution patient to rotate injection sites to avoid developing lipodystrophy.
• *Alert:* Warn patient not to share multidose pen with other people, even if the needle is changed, because of risk of bloodborne pathogen transmission, including HIV and hepatitis.
• Explain importance of checking insulin label before each injection as accidental mix-ups among insulin types have been reported.
• Teach patient that alcohol and some other medications may increase or decrease glucose levels. Advise patient to inform health care provider of all medications and supplements being taken.

• Instruct patient not to stop insulin abruptly or change amount injected without consulting prescriber.
• Advise patient that any insulin changes should be made cautiously and only under medical supervision. Changes in insulin strength, manufacturer, type (regular, NPH, or insulin analogues), species (animal, human), or method of manufacture (rDNA versus animal-source insulin) may result in the need for a dosage change. Dosage of concomitant oral antidiabetic may need adjustment.
• Tell patient to report pregnancy or plans to become pregnant.
• Advise patient who is pregnant or plans to become pregnant of importance of maintaining tight glucose control.
• Inform patient of the change in insulin requirements that may occur during pregnancy and after childbirth.

SAFETY ALERT!

Insulins (long-acting)

IN-su-lins

insulin degludec
Tresiba

insulin detemir (rDNA origin)
Levemir

insulin glargine (rDNA origin)
Basaglar, Lantus, Toujeo

insulin glargine-aglr (rDNA origin)
Rezvoglar

insulin glargine-yfgn (rDNA origin)
Semglee

Therapeutic class: Antidiabetics
Pharmacologic class: Insulins

AVAILABLE FORMS

Injection (degludec): 100 units/mL in 10-mL vials and 3-mL pens, 200 units/mL in 3-mL pens
Injection (detemir): 100 units/mL in 10-mL vials and 3-mL pens
Injection (glargine, glargine-aglr, glargine-yfgn): 100 units/mL in 10-mL vials and

3-mL pens, 200 units/mL in 3-mL pens, 300 units/mL in 1.5-mL and 3-mL pens

INDICATIONS & DOSAGES

Adjust-a-dose (for all indications): Individualize dosage based on metabolic needs, blood glucose monitoring, and glycemic control goal. Insulin requirements may be altered during acute illness, emotional distress, or stress. Adjust dosage as needed in older adults, in patients who have renal or hepatic dysfunction or have changes in physical activity or meal patterns, and in patients who are concurrently taking drugs that lower blood glucose level. Refer to manufacturer's instructions for dosage adjustments when converting from other insulin regimens and formulations.

➤ **To improve glycemic control in patients with type 1 diabetes**

Adults (degludec, detemir, glargine) and children age 2 and older (detemir) or age 6 and older (glargine [except Toujeo]) or age 1 and older requiring 5 units or more daily (degludec): In patients who are insulin naive, initially, approximately one-third (Basaglar, Lantus, Rezvoglar, Semglee) or one-third to one-half (Levemir, Toujeo, Tresiba) of total daily insulin requirements subcut once daily.

Satisfy remainder of the daily insulin requirements with rapid- or short-acting premeal insulin.

➤ **To improve glycemic control in patients with type 2 diabetes**

Adults: Initial insulin degludec dosage is 10 units once daily subcut at any time of day. Initial insulin detemir dosage is 10 units (0.1 to 0.2 unit/kg) subcut once daily in evening or divided into two daily doses in patients inadequately controlled on oral antidiabetics, or once daily in the evening in patients inadequately controlled on a glucagon-like peptide 1 (GLP-1) receptor antagonist. Initial insulin glargine dosage is 0.2 unit/kg (up to 10 units) subcut once daily. Adjust dosage as needed.

Children age 1 and older (degludec only): Initially, in children who are insulin naive, 10 units subcut once daily at same time every day. Or, in children already receiving insulin therapy, start at 80% of the total daily long- or intermediate-acting insulin unit dose to minimize risk of hypoglycemia.

ADMINISTRATION
Subcutaneous
General

• Don't give long-acting insulins by insulin infusion pumps or by IM or IV injection.

• Administer by subcut injection only in the thigh, abdominal wall, or upper arm. Rotate sites within same region (abdomen, thigh, or deltoid) from one injection to the next to reduce risk of lipodystrophy.

• Don't mix or dilute long-acting insulins with other insulins or solutions because the pharmacokinetic and pharmacodynamic profile (onset of action, time to peak effect) of the insulin may be altered unpredictably.

• Inspect visually for particulate matter and discoloration before administration, whenever solution and container permit; use only if solution appears clear and colorless.

• Instructions for priming and using pens vary from one to another, are very detailed, and involve multiple steps. Refer to manufacturer's instructions for use.

ⓘ *Alert:* Multidose pens are for single patient use only. Pens should never be shared even if the needle is changed. Clearly label with patient identifying information where it won't obstruct dosing window, warning, or other product information.

Insulin degludec

• In adults, give insulin degludec once daily at any time of day; in children, give once daily at the same time each day.

• Individualize and titrate dosage every 3 to 4 days based on patient's metabolic needs, blood glucose monitoring results, and glycemic control goal.

• Don't perform dose conversion when using FlexTouch pen. The dose window for both 100-unit and 200-unit pens shows the number of insulin units to be delivered and no conversion is needed.

• In adults with type 1 or type 2 diabetes already on insulin therapy, start insulin degludec at the same unit dose as the total daily long- or intermediate-acting insulin unit dose.

• In children age 1 and older already on insulin therapy, start at 80% of the total daily long- or intermediate-acting insulin unit dose to minimize risk of hypoglycemia.

• For children requiring less than 5 units of drug each day, use the U-100 vials.

• Always use a new needle for each injection to help ensure sterility and prevent blocked needles.
• Store unused pens in refrigerator at 36° to 46° F (2° to 8° C); may be used until expiration date on label. Don't freeze or use if pens have been frozen.
• Store open pen away from heat or light at room temperature, below 86° F (30° C). Discard after 56 days, even if pen still contains insulin and expiration date hasn't passed.

Insulin detemir
• Give insulin detemir once daily or b.i.d. For patients treated with insulin detemir once daily, give dose with evening meal or at bedtime. For patients who require b.i.d. dosing, administer evening dose with evening meal, at bedtime, or 12 hours after morning dose.
• When using insulin detemir with a GLP-1 receptor agonist, give as separate injections; never mix together. Insulin detemir and a GLP-1 receptor agonist may be injected in same body region, but the injections shouldn't be adjacent to each other.
• If converting from insulin glargine or NPH insulin to insulin detemir, maintain the same unit dose. Monitor glucose level closely during transition.
• Store unused (unopened) insulin detemir vials and pens between 36° and 46° F (2° and 8° C). Don't freeze and don't use if vials or pens have been frozen. Keep in carton so that vials or pens stay clean and protected from light.
• If refrigeration isn't possible, unused (unopened) insulin detemir can be kept unrefrigerated at room temperature, below 86° F (30° C), as long as it's kept as cool as possible and away from direct heat and light. Discard unrefrigerated insulin detemir 42 days after it's first kept out of the refrigerator, even if the pen or vial still contains insulin.
• After initial use, store vials in refrigerator; never freeze. If refrigeration isn't possible, the in-use vial can be kept unrefrigerated at room temperature, below 86° F (30° C), as long as it's kept as cool as possible and away from direct heat and light. Discard refrigerated insulin detemir vials 42 days after initial use.
• Pens (in use): After initial use, don't store insulin detemir pen in refrigerator and don't store with the needle in place; keep opened insulin detemir pen away from direct heat

and light at room temperature, below 86° F (30° C). Discard unrefrigerated insulin detemir pens 42 days after they're first kept out of refrigerator.

Insulin glargine
• Give subcut once daily at same time every day, at any time during the day.
• If converting from insulin detemir to insulin glargine, maintain the same unit dose. Monitor glucose level closely during transition.
• Store unopened insulin glargine vials and pens at 36° to 46° F (2° to 8° C). Don't freeze; discard if frozen. If refrigeration isn't possible, the open vial in use can be kept unrefrigerated for up to 28 days away from direct heat and light, as long as the room temperature isn't above 86° F (30° C).
• Opened vials, whether or not refrigerated, must be used within a 28-day period or they must be discarded.
• Opened pens shouldn't be refrigerated but should be kept at room temperature, below 86° F (30° C), away from direct heat and light; discard opened pens kept at room temperature after 28 days.

ACTION

Lowers blood glucose level by stimulating peripheral glucose uptake by binding to insulin receptors on skeletal muscle and in fat cells, and by inhibiting hepatic glucose production; also inhibits lipolysis and proteolysis, and enhances protein synthesis.

Route	Onset	Peak	Duration
Subcut (degludec)	1 hr	9 hr	24+ hr
Subcut (detemir)	3–4 hr	3–9 hr	24 hr
Subcut (glargine)	3–6 hr	Constant	24 hr

Half-life: Degludec, 25 hours; detemir, 5 to 7 hours; glargine, unknown.

ADVERSE REACTIONS

CNS: headache, fever, depression. **CV:** peripheral edema, HTN. **EENT:** cataract, retinopathy, pharyngitis, rhinitis, sinusitis. **GI:** abdominal pain, gastroenteritis, nausea, vomiting, diarrhea. **GU:** UTI. **Metabolic:** *hypoglycemia, hypokalemia,* weight gain. **Musculoskeletal:** back pain, arthralgia, limb pain. **Respiratory:** URI, bronchitis, cough. **Skin:** injection-site reactions, lipodystrophy, pruritus, rash. **Other:** hypersensitivity reactions, flulike symptoms, infection.

Reactions in bold italics are *life-threatening.* Interactions may have a *rapid onset* or a ***delayed onset.***

INTERACTIONS

Drug-drug. *ACE inhibitors, antidiabetics (oral), ARBs, disopyramide, fibrates, fluoxetine, MAO inhibitors, octreotide, pentoxifylline, pramlintide, salicylates, sulfonamide antibiotics:* May increase blood glucose–lowering effect of insulin, increasing risk of hypoglycemia. Monitor glucose level and patient closely. Adjust insulin dosage as necessary.

Antiadrenergics (beta blockers, clonidine): May mask signs and symptoms of hypoglycemia. Avoid concurrent use, if possible, and monitor patient closely.

Atypical antipsychotics, corticosteroids, danazol, diuretics, estrogens, glucagon, hormonal contraceptives, isoniazid, niacin, phenothiazines, protease inhibitors, somatropin, sympathomimetics (albuterol, epinephrine, terbutaline), thyroid hormones: May decrease blood glucose–lowering effect of insulin, increasing risk of hyperglycemia. Monitor glucose level and patient closely. Adjust insulin dosage as necessary.

Beta blockers, clonidine, lithium salts, pentamidine: May increase risk of either hypoglycemia or hyperglycemia. Monitor glucose level closely.

GLP-1 receptor agonists (albiglutide, exenatide, liraglutide): May increase risk of hypoglycemia. Monitor glucose level closely and decrease insulin dosage if necessary.

Thiazolidinediones (TZDs; pioglitazone, rosiglitazone): May cause fluid retention that can lead to HF. Monitor patient closely, and adjust or stop TZD as clinically necessary.

Drug-lifestyle. *Alcohol use:* May cause hyperglycemia or hypoglycemia. Monitor glucose level and discourage concurrent use.

EFFECTS ON LAB TEST RESULTS

• May decrease potassium and blood glucose levels.

CONTRAINDICATIONS & CAUTIONS

• Contraindicated during episodes of hypoglycemia or diabetic ketoacidosis.

• Contraindicated in patients hypersensitive to drug or its components. Severe, life-threatening, generalized allergy, including anaphylaxis, can occur with insulin products.

🔸 **Alert:** Adjust insulin regimen only with appropriate glucose monitoring under medical supervision.

• Use cautiously in patients susceptible to hypokalemia, such as patients who are fasting, are taking potassium-lowering drugs, or are concurrently taking drugs that may affect potassium level. Untreated hypokalemia can cause respiratory paralysis, ventricular arrhythmias, and death.

• Hypoglycemia is the most common adverse reaction. Severe hypoglycemia can cause seizures, and may be life-threatening or fatal. Hypoglycemia can occur suddenly, and symptoms may differ. Risk increases with intensity of glycemic control and changes in glycemic treatment, meal patterns, physical activity, and concomitant medications and in patients with renal or hepatic impairment.

• Use cautiously in older adults, who may be at risk for increased sensitivity to drug's effects. Signs and symptoms of hypoglycemia may be more difficult to recognize in these patients.

• Use prefilled pens cautiously in patients with visual impairment who may rely on audible clicks to dial their dose.

Dialyzable drug: Unknown.

⚠ *Overdose S&S:* Hypoglycemia, hypokalemia, coma, seizure, neurologic impairment.

PREGNANCY-LACTATION-REPRODUCTION

• Use cautiously during pregnancy.

• Closely monitor blood glucose levels during pregnancy, after recent birth, and during breastfeeding; insulin requirements may change.

• It isn't known if insulin appears in human milk. Use cautiously during breastfeeding. Insulin doses may need adjustment.

NURSING CONSIDERATIONS

• Insulin glargine-yfgn (Semglee) and insulin glargine-aglr (Rezvoglar) are biosimilar to the FDA-approved reference product Lantus. There are no clinically meaningful differences between the biosimilar product and the reference product based on the conditions of their use. Semglee is also interchangeable with Lantus and can be substituted without approval of prescriber. Rezvoglar isn't considered interchangeable and can't be automatically substituted.

• Prolonged effect of long-acting insulin may delay recovery from hypoglycemia. Monitor patient carefully.

- Monitor patients taking other medications with insulin more closely because other drugs can mask signs and symptoms of hypoglycemia or cause an increase or a decrease in blood glucose level.
- Adjust dosages regularly, depending on patient-specific glucose measurements.
- Monitor patient carefully for signs and symptoms of hypoglycemia, especially in long-standing disease. Treat according to individual facility policy and procedure if necessary.
- Assess patient for signs and symptoms of hypoglycemia (diaphoresis, shaking, trembling, confusion) and hyperglycemia (drowsiness, fruity breath odor, frequent urination, thirst). Notify prescriber if these signs or symptoms occur.
- Mild episodes of hypoglycemia may be treated with oral glucose. More severe episodes of hypoglycemia, such as coma, seizure, or neurologic impairment, may be treated with IM or subcut glucagon or concentrated IV glucose.
- Periodically measure HbA_{1c} levels.
- Increase frequency of glucose monitoring in patients who are acutely ill or under emotional stress, or if changes in diet, exercise, or medication regimen occur, as these may affect the rate of insulin absorption. Also, closely monitor patient after changes to insulin dosage.
- *Look alike–sound alike:* Don't confuse insulin glargine with insulin glulisine.

PATIENT TEACHING

- Instruct patient in self-management, including glucose monitoring, injection technique, proper storage of insulin, and recognition and management of hypoglycemia and hyperglycemia.
- Explain to patient that insulin requirements may vary due to illness, stress or emotional disturbance, change in activity level, inadequate food intake, and skipped meals.
- Teach patient to watch for signs and symptoms of hypoglycemia (diaphoresis, shaking, trembling, confusion) and hyperglycemia (drowsiness, frequent urination, thirst).
- Advise patient that hypoglycemic episodes may impair the ability to concentrate and react; advise patient to use caution while driving and operating machinery.

- Instruct patient to keep hard candy or glucose tablets on hand to treat mild cases of hypoglycemia.
- Advise patient that allergic and hypersensitivity reactions can occur, including injection-site reactions (local pain, redness, or swelling) and generalized reactions and to report signs or symptoms to health care provider. Teach patient signs and symptoms of anaphylaxis and to seek emergency medical attention promptly if anaphylaxis occurs.
- Instruct patient to rotate injection sites within same region to reduce risk of lipodystrophy.
- **Alert:** Warn patient not to share multidose pen with other people, even if the needle is changed, because of risk of bloodborne pathogen transmission, including HIV and hepatitis.
- Teach patient to store insulin products properly, depending on individual products, and to use only if solution appears clear and colorless.
- Explain importance of checking insulin label before each injection as accidental mix-ups among insulin types have been reported.
- Instruct patient that long-acting insulins shouldn't be diluted or mixed with other insulins or drugs.
- Teach patient that alcohol may affect glucose levels and should be avoided.
- Inform patient that any insulin change should be made cautiously and only under medical supervision. Changes in insulin strength, manufacturer, type (regular, NPH, or insulin analogues), species (animal, human), or method of manufacture (rDNA versus animal-source insulin) may result in the need for a dosage change. Dosage of concomitant oral antidiabetics may need adjustment.
- Instruct patient not to stop insulin abruptly or change amount injected without consulting prescriber.
- Warn patient to report pregnancy or plans to become pregnant.
- Advise patient of the change in insulin requirements that may occur during pregnancy and after childbirth.

SAFETY ALERT!

Insulins (rapid-acting)
IN-su-lins

insulin aspart (rDNA origin)
Fiasp, Kirsty✦, NovoLOG,
NovoRapid✦, Trurapi✦

insulin glulisine (rDNA origin)
Apidra

insulin (human)
Afrezza

insulin (lispro)
Admelog, HumaLOG, Liprelog✦

insulin (lispro-aabc)
Lyumjev

Therapeutic class: Antidiabetics
Pharmacologic class: Insulins

AVAILABLE FORMS
Inhalation powder (Afrezza): 4-unit, 8-unit,
12-unit single-use cartridges
Injection (aspart): 100 units/mL in 10-mL
vials, 3-mL prefilled pens and cartridges
Injection (glulisine): 100 units/mL in 10-mL
vials, 3-mL prefilled pens
Injection (lispro, lispro-aabc): 100 units/mL
in10-mL vials, 3-mL prefilled pens and cartridges; 200 units/mL in 3-mL prefilled pens

INDICATIONS & DOSAGES
Adjust-a-dose (for all indications): Individualize dosage based on metabolic needs, blood
glucose monitoring, and glycemic control
goal. Insulin requirements may be altered during acute illness, emotional distress, or stress.
Adjust as needed in older adults, patients
who have renal or hepatic dysfunction, or
have changes in physical activity or meal patterns, and in those who are concurrently taking drugs that lower blood glucose level. Refer to manufacturer's instructions for dosage
adjustments when converting from other insulin regimens or formulations. Patients with
obesity and children during puberty may need
increased maintenance doses.
➤ **To improve glycemic control in patients
with diabetes (aspart, glulisine, lispro)**
*Adults (lispro-aabc), adults and children age
2 and older (aspart), age 3 and older (lispro),*

age 4 and older (glulisine): For insulin aspart, inject individualized dose subcut at the
start of or within 20 minutes after starting
a meal (Fiasp) or within 5 to 10 minutes before a meal (Novolo). When continuous subcut infusion pump is used, follow health care
provider recommendations when setting basal
and mealtime infusion rates. Usual IV concentration is 0.05 to 1 unit/mL in NSS infused
under close medical supervision.
    For insulin glulisine, inject individual-
ized dose subcut within 15 minutes before or
20 minutes after starting a meal. When continuous subcut infusion pump is used, base
initial dosing on total daily insulin dose of the
previous regimen. Usual IV concentration is
0.05 to 1 unit/mL in NSS infused under close
medical supervision.
    For lispro, inject individualized dose sub-
cut within 15 minutes before a meal or immediately after a meal or, for lispro-aabc, at
the start of a meal or within 20 minutes after starting a meal. When continuous subcut infusion pump is used, follow health care
provider recommendations when setting basal
and mealtime infusion rates. Usual IV concentration is 0.1 to 1 unit/mL in NSS infused
under close medical supervision.
➤ **To improve glycemic control in patients
with diabetes (inhalation)**
Adults: For patients who are insulin naive,
initially 4 units inhaled at beginning of each
meal. To convert to inhaled insulin from subcut mealtime insulin, refer to manufacturer's
instructions. For patients using subcut premixed insulin, estimate mealtime injected
dose by dividing half of total daily injected
premixed insulin dose equally among the
three meals of the day; then convert each estimated injected mealtime dose to an appropriate inhaled dose according to manufacturer's
instructions. Administer half of total daily injected premixed dose as an injected basal insulin dose. Inhaled insulin must be used in
combination with a long-acting insulin in patients with type 1 diabetes.

ADMINISTRATION
General
• Rapid-acting insulins are usually given in a
regimen that includes an intermediate-acting
or a long-acting insulin.
• Don't use if solution is viscous or cloudy;
use only if clear and colorless.

• Multidose pens are for single-patient use only. Pens should never be shared even if the needle is changed. Clearly label with patient identifying information where it won't obstruct dosing window, warning, or other product information.

• Store unopened insulin aspart vials, cartridges, and pens under refrigeration (36° to 46° F [2° to 8° C]) until expiration date or at room temperature of less than 86° F (30° C) for 28 days; don't freeze. Keep away from heat and sunlight. Once opened, may store vials under refrigeration or at room temperature of less than 86° F (30° C); use within 28 days. Store cartridges and pens that have been opened at temperatures less than 86° F (30° C) and use within 28 days; don't freeze or refrigerate.

• Store insulin glulisine under refrigeration at 36° to 46° F (2° to 8° C) and protect from light. Don't store in freezer. Don't allow insulin glulisine to freeze; discard if it has been frozen. Unopened vials and cartridge systems not stored in refrigerator must be used within 28 days. Opened vials, whether or not refrigerated, must be used within 28 days. If refrigeration isn't possible, can keep open vials at room temperature of less than 77° F (25° C) for up to 28 days away from direct heat and light. Don't refrigerate opened cartridge system, but keep below 77° F (25° C) and away from direct heat and light. Discard opened cartridge systems after 28 days. Don't store pen, with or without cartridge system, in refrigerator at any time.

• Store lispro in refrigerator (36° to 46° F [2° to 8° C]), but not in freezer. Protect from direct heat and light. Don't use if frozen. Store unopened vials and pens in refrigerator until expiration date; if stored unopened at room temperature, discard after 28 days. May store opened vials for 28 days under refrigeration or at room temperature; may store opened pens and cartridges for 28 days at room temperature. Discard if exposed to temperatures greater than 98.6° F (37° C).

• **Incompatibilities:** Don't mix with any other insulin except NPH.

IV

▼ Rapid-acting insulin may be administered IV with close monitoring of blood glucose and serum potassium levels under appropriate medical supervision.

▼ Flush IV tubing with priming infusion of 20 mL from insulin infusion whenever new IV tubing set is added to insulin infusion container, to avoid adsorption to IV tubing.

▼ Use NSS and polyvinyl chloride or polypropylene infusion bags for IV infusions.

▼ Always administer IV infusions using an infusion pump.

Subcutaneous

• Administer by subcut injection in abdominal region, buttocks, thigh, or upper arm. Subcut injection into abdominal wall is generally associated with faster absorption than other injection sites.

• Rotate injection sites within same region to reduce risk of lipodystrophy.

• Injection into a lifted skin fold minimizes risk of IM injection.

🛈 *Alert:* Don't transfer 200 unit/mL insulin from a pen to a standard insulin syringe; overdose and severe hypoglycemia can result.

• NovoLog may be diluted with Insulin Diluting Medium for NovoLog for subcut injection. Diluting one part NovoLog to nine parts diluent will yield a concentration one-tenth that of NovoLog (equivalent to U-10). Diluting one part NovoLog to one part diluent will yield a concentration one-half that of NovoLog (equivalent to U-50).

• When used for continuous subcut insulin infusion, replace insulin in the reservoir every 6 days (Fiasp) or 7 days (NovoLog) or according to manufacturer's instructions, whichever is shorter. Change infusion sets and insertion site according to manufacturer's instructions.

• When using for continuous subcut insulin infusion, change insulin glulisine in reservoir and infusion set (reservoirs, tubing, and catheters) every 48 hours or after exposure to temperatures greater than 98.6° F (37° C).

• When using for continuous subcut insulin infusion, change lispro in reservoir at least every 7 days, and change infusion sets and insertion site every 3 days.

• Don't dilute or use mixed insulins in external insulin pumps.

Inhalational

• Administer using a single inhalation per cartridge using Afrezza inhaler only. Inhaler can be used for all cartridge strengths.

• Administer at beginning of a meal.

• Keep inhaler level, with white mouthpiece on top and purple base on bottom, after a cartridge has been inserted into inhaler.

• Loss of drug effect can occur if inhaler is turned upside down, held with mouthpiece

---

Reactions in bold italics are *life-threatening*. Interactions may have a *rapid onset* or a ***delayed onset***.

pointing down, or shaken or dropped after the cartridge has been inserted but before dose has been administered. If any of these occur, replace cartridge before use.

• May mix and match between 4-unit (blue), 8-unit (green), and 12-unit (yellow) cartridges to obtain correct dose.

• Store unused foil packages of inhalation powder until expiration date under refrigeration (36° to 46° F [2° to 8° C]) or if at room temperature, use within 10 days. If in use, unopened blister cards and strips must be used within 10 days and opened strips must be used within 3 days.

• Inhaler can be refrigerated but should be at room temperature before use. Cartridges should be at room temperature for 10 minutes before use.

• Replace inhaler after 15 days of use.

ACTION

Lowers blood glucose level by stimulating peripheral glucose uptake by binding to insulin receptors on skeletal muscle and in fat cells and by inhibiting hepatic glucose production; also inhibits lipolysis and proteolysis, and enhances protein synthesis.

Route	Onset	Peak	Duration
Aspart (IV)	Immediate	Unknown	3–5 hr
Aspart (subcut)	15 min	1–3 hr	3–5 hr
Glulisine (IV)	Immediate	Unknown	5 hr
Glulisine (subcut)	5–15 min	1 hr	5 hr
Lispro (IV)	Immediate	Unknown	Unknown
Lispro (subcut)	15–30 min	30–90 min	≤5 hr
Inhalation	Unknown	12–15 min	180 min

Half-life: Aspart IV, unknown; aspart subcut, 81 minutes; glulisine IV, 13 minutes; glulisine subcut, 42 minutes; lispro IV, 51 to 55 minutes; lispro subcut, 1 hour; inhalation, 28 to 39 minutes.

ADVERSE REACTIONS

CNS: headache, *hypoglycemic seizures,* asthenia, fever, fatigue (inhalation), sensory disturbance. **CV:** HTN, peripheral edema. **EENT:** nasopharyngitis. **GI:** nausea, diarrhea. **GU:** UTI, dysmenorrhea. **Metabolic:** *hypoglycemia, hypokalemia,* weight gain. **Musculoskeletal:** arthralgia, myalgia. **Respiratory:** URI, cough; bronchospasm, throat pain or irritation, bronchitis, decreased pulmonary function (inhaled product). **Skin:** injection- or infusion-site reactions, lipodystrophy,

pruritus, rash. **Other:** *allergic reactions, anaphylaxis,* insulin antibody production, flulike symptoms.

INTERACTIONS

Drug-drug. *ACE inhibitors, antidiabetics (oral), ARBs, disopyramide, fibrates, fluoxetine, MAO inhibitors, octreotide, pentoxifylline, pramlintide, salicylates, sulfonamide antibiotics:* May increase risk of hypoglycemia. Monitor glucose level closely and adjust insulin dosage as needed.

Atypical antipsychotics, corticosteroids, danazol, diuretics, estrogens, glucagon, hormonal contraceptives, isoniazid, niacin, phenothiazines, protease inhibitors, somatropin, sympathomimetics (albuterol, epinephrine, terbutaline), thyroid hormones: May decrease blood glucose–lowering effects. Monitor glucose level closely and adjust insulin dosage as needed.

Beta blockers, clonidine: May mask signs and symptoms of hypoglycemia. Avoid concurrent use, if possible, or monitor patient closely.

Beta blockers, clonidine, lithium salts, pentamidine: May cause hypoglycemia or hyperglycemia. Monitor glucose level closely.

Thiazolidinediones (TZDs; pioglitazone, rosiglitazone): May cause fluid retention that can lead to HF. Monitor patient closely and adjust or stop TZDs as clinically indicated.

Drug-lifestyle. *Alcohol use:* May cause hyperglycemia or hypoglycemia. Monitor glucose level closely and discourage concurrent use.

EFFECTS ON LAB TEST RESULTS

• May decrease glucose and potassium levels.

CONTRAINDICATIONS & CAUTIONS

Boxed Warning Inhaled insulin is contraindicated in patients with chronic lung disease, such as asthma or COPD, as acute bronchospasm has been observed in these patients. ▪

• Contraindicated during episodes of hypoglycemia.

• Contraindicated in patients with a history of hypersensitivity to drug or its components. Severe, life-threatening, generalized allergic reaction, including anaphylaxis, can occur with insulin products.

• Inhaled insulin may increase risk of diabetic ketoacidosis (DKA). Closely monitor

patients at risk for DKA. Change to an alternative route of insulin delivery if needed.
• Inhaled insulin isn't recommended in patients who smoke or who have recently stopped smoking.
• Use cautiously in patients susceptible to hypokalemia, such as patients who are fasting, are taking potassium-lowering drugs, or are concurrently taking drugs that may affect potassium levels. Untreated hypokalemia can cause respiratory paralysis, ventricular arrhythmias, and death.
• Hypoglycemia is the most common adverse reaction. Severe hypoglycemia can cause seizures, and may be life-threatening or fatal. Hypoglycemia can occur suddenly, and symptoms may differ. Risk increases with intensity of glycemic control and changes in glycemic treatment, meal patterns, physical activity, and concomitant medications and in patients with renal or hepatic impairment.
• Use cautiously in older adults, who may be at increased risk for adverse effects. Signs and symptoms of hypoglycemia may be more difficult to recognize in these patients.
• Use prefilled pens cautiously in patients with visual impairment who may rely on audible clicks to dial their dose.
Dialyzable drug: Unknown.
⚠ *Overdose S&S:* Hypoglycemia, hypokalemia.

PREGNANCY-LACTATION-REPRODUCTION
• There are no adequate studies during pregnancy. Poorly controlled diabetes increases maternal and fetal risk of adverse outcomes. Use cautiously during pregnancy.
• Monitor blood glucose levels closely during pregnancy, after recent birth, and during breastfeeding; insulin requirements may change.
• It isn't known if insulin appears in human milk. Refer to manufacturer's instructions for use during breastfeeding.

NURSING CONSIDERATIONS
Boxed Warning Before initiating inhaled insulin, perform a detailed medical history, physical exam, and spirometry (forced expiratory volume in 1 second [FEV_1]) to identify potential lung disease in all patients. ■
• Assess pulmonary function (spirometry) before initiating inhalation product, after 6 months of therapy, and annually, even in the absence of pulmonary symptoms.

• Increase frequency of pulmonary assessment in patients with such symptoms as wheezing, bronchospasm, breathing difficulties, or persistent or recurring cough. Switch to another form of drug for persistent symptoms or decline of 20% or more in FEV_1 from baseline.
• Monitor blood glucose level and adjust insulin dosage as needed.
• Closely monitor patients also taking other medications as other drugs can mask signs and symptoms of hypoglycemia or cause an increase or decrease in blood glucose level.
• Increase frequency of glucose monitoring in patients who are acutely ill or under emotional stress, or if changes in diet, exercise, or medication regimen occur, because these may affect rate of insulin absorption.
• Closely monitor patients at risk for DKA from acute illness or infection; consider changing from inhaled product to alternative route of insulin delivery.
• Increase frequency of glucose monitoring when initiating therapy or when changes in insulin strength, dosage, manufacturer, or type or method of administration are made. Changes may affect glycemic control and increase risk of hypoglycemia.
• Monitor patient carefully for signs and symptoms of hypoglycemia. Symptom awareness may be decreased in patients with long-standing diabetes, diabetic nerve disease, renal disease, or hepatic impairment and in patients who have experienced recurrent hypoglycemia. Treat according to individual facility protocol if necessary.
• Notify prescriber for signs or symptoms of hypoglycemia (diaphoresis, shaking, trembling, confusion) and hyperglycemia (drowsiness, fruity breath odor, frequent urination, thirst).
• Mild episodes of hypoglycemia may be treated with oral glucose. More severe episodes of hypoglycemia, such as coma, seizure, or neurologic impairment, may be treated with IM or subcut glucagon or concentrated IV glucose.
• Monitor potassium levels in patients at risk for hypokalemia (those receiving potassium-depleting drugs or IV insulin).
• Monitor patients for generalized allergic reactions, including anaphylaxis.
• Periodically measure HbA_{1c} levels.

Reactions in bold italics are *life-threatening*. Interactions may have a *rapid onset* or a ***delayed onset***.

• Monitor external pump for malfunction as this may cause a rapid decline in blood glucose level.

• *Look alike–sound alike:* Don't confuse NovoLog with Novolog 70/30. Don't confuse Humalog with Humalog 50/50 or 75/25. Don't confuse insulin glulisine with insulin glargine.

PATIENT TEACHING
General

• Advise patient that hypoglycemic episodes can impair the ability to concentrate and react; advise patient to use caution while driving and operating machinery.

• Instruct patient to keep hard candy or glucose tablets on hand to treat mild cases of hypoglycemia.

• Advise patient to keep a log of glucose levels.

• Instruct patient on the long-term sequelae of diabetes if not managed properly.

• Instruct patient to carry identification or wear jewelry indicating that patient has diabetes.

• Advise patient that allergic and hypersensitivity reactions can occur, including injection-site reactions (local pain, redness, or swelling), and to report symptoms to health care provider. Teach patient signs and symptoms of anaphylaxis and to seek emergency medical attention promptly if anaphylaxis occurs.

• Instruct patient on self-management procedures, including glucose monitoring, proper administration technique, and management of hypoglycemia and hyperglycemia.

• Warn patient that insulin requirements may vary due to illness, stress, emotional disturbances, inadequate or skipped insulin dose, inadvertent administration of an increased insulin dose, inadequate food intake, or skipped meals.

• Instruct patient with diabetes to report pregnancy or plans to become pregnant.

• Advise patient of change in insulin requirements that may occur during pregnancy and after childbirth.

• Teach patient that alcohol and some other medications may increase or decrease glucose levels. Advise patient to inform health care provider of all medications and supplements being taken.

• Caution patient not to stop insulin abruptly or change amount taken without consulting prescriber.

• Advise patient that any change of insulin should be made cautiously and only under medical supervision. Changes in insulin strength, manufacturer, type (regular, NPH, or insulin analogues), species (animal, human), or method of manufacture (rDNA versus animal-source insulin) may result in need for a dosage change. Dosage of concomitant oral antidiabetics may need adjustment.

Injection

• Teach patient to give insulin at appropriate time around a meal, depending on product.

• Instruct patient to rotate injection sites and of the importance of avoiding lipodystrophy.

• Instruct patient that when mixing two types of insulin, to always draw up the shorter-acting insulin first, followed by NPH insulin, and inject immediately.

• Teach patient how to use external insulin pumps properly, to use the appropriate insulin in the pump, not to dilute it or mix it with other insulin formulations, to change the infusion set as directed, to rotate infusion sites, and to follow instructions for patient's specific type of pump.

• Advise patient to have a backup external insulin pump available in case of malfunction.

• Teach patient to store insulin products properly, depending on individual products.

• Explain importance of checking insulin label before each injection; accidental mix-ups among insulin types have been reported.

🕓 *Alert:* Warn patient not to share multidose pen with others, even if the needle is changed, because of risk of blood-borne pathogen transmission, including HIV and hepatitis.

Inhalational

• Instruct patient to read inhaler's medication guide before starting inhalation therapy and to reread it each time the prescription is renewed.

• Caution patient not to open cartridges, place cartridges in mouth, or swallow cartridges.

• Inform patient that inhaled insulin can cause a decline in lung function and that lung function will be evaluated by spirometry before initiation of treatment and periodically during treatment.

• Advise patient to promptly report respiratory difficulty or signs or symptoms of lung cancer (hemoptysis, cough).

• Inform patient that if inhaled product isn't being used, it should be stored in refrigerator. If inhaler is being used, tell patient to leave it at room temperature and use unopened strips within 10 days and opened strips within 3 days.

• Instruct patient never to wash inhaler but to wipe it with a clean, dry cloth.

• Advise patient that inhalers should be discarded and replaced every 15 days.

SAFETY ALERT!

Insulins (short-acting)

IN-su-lins

insulin (regular)

HumuLIN R ◇, HumuLIN R U-500 (concentrated), Myxredlin, NovoLIN R ◇

Therapeutic class: Antidiabetics
Pharmacologic class: Insulins

AVAILABLE FORMS

Infusion: 100 units in 100 mL NSS single-dose container
Injection: 100 units/mL in 3-mL, 10-mL vials; 500 units/mL in 3-mL pens and 20-mL vials

INDICATIONS & DOSAGES

➤ **As adjunct to diet and exercise to improve glycemic control in patients with type 1 and type 2 diabetes**

Adults and children: Inject individualized total daily insulin requirements subcut in three or more divided doses. Initial doses may be lower, and maintenance doses in patients with obesity and children during puberty may be higher. Give 30 minutes before start of a meal. May give IV under medical supervision with close monitoring of blood glucose and potassium levels to avoid hypoglycemia and hypokalemia.

◑ *Alert:* U-500 concentrate is used for the treatment of patients with diabetes who are insulin resistant and require daily doses of more than 200 units because a large dose may be given subcut in a reasonable volume. Don't give U-500 concentrated insulin IV or IM

Adjust-a-dose: Individualize dosage based on metabolic needs, blood glucose monitoring, and glycemic control. Insulin requirements may be altered during acute illness, emotional distress, or stress. Adjust dosage as needed in older adults, in patients with renal or hepatic dysfunction or changes in physical activity or meal patterns, and in patients who are

concurrently taking drugs that lower blood glucose level. Dosage may also need adjustment when switching from another insulin formulation, manufacturer, or strength. IV administration of regular insulin is possible under medical supervision with close monitoring of blood glucose and potassium levels to avoid hypoglycemia and hypokalemia. IV administration of insulin is commonly used in the treatment of diabetic ketoacidosis, perioperative management of diabetes, and maintenance of glycemic control during labor in patients with diabetes.

ADMINISTRATION
General

• Store unopened vials and pens in refrigerator at 36° to 46° F (2° to 8° C). Don't freeze and don't use if vial has been frozen.

◑ *Alert:* Multidose pens are for single patient use only. Pens should never be shared even if the needle is changed. Clearly label with patient identifying information where it won't obstruct dosing window, warning, or other product information.

• Novolin R vials can be kept at room temperature (not greater than 77° F [25° C]), away from heat or light, for up to 42 days; don't refrigerate after first use. Discard after 42 days even if vial is unopened or isn't empty.

• Opened (in use) Humulin R vials can be kept at room temperature (not greater than 86° F [30° C]), away from heat or light, for up to 31 days. Discard after 31 days even if vial is unopened or isn't empty.

• Opened and unopened Humulin R U-500 vials can be kept at room temperature, below 86° F (30° C); discard after 40 days. Also discard opened refrigerated vials after 40 days.

• Opened and unopened Humulin R U-500 pens can be kept at room temperature, below 86° F (30° C); discard after 28 days. Don't store opened pens in refrigerator.

IV

▼ Don't use if solution is viscous or cloudy; use only if clear and colorless.

▼ IV administration requires close monitoring of blood glucose and serum potassium levels. Appropriate medical supervision is required.

▼ Onset of action when administered IV is more rapid in comparison to subcut administration.

▼ For IV use, Humulin R U-100 should be used at a concentration of 0.1 to 1 unit/mL in

---

Reactions in **bold italics** are *life-threatening*. Interactions may have a *rapid onset* or a **delayed onset**.

NSS using polyvinyl chloride infusion bags. Novolin R should be used at concentrations of 0.05 to 1 unit/mL in infusion systems using polypropylene infusion bags and one of the following infusion solutions: NSS, 5% dextrose, or 10% dextrose with potassium chloride 40 mmol/L.

▼ Always administer IV infusions using an infusion pump.

▼ Infusion bags prepared with Humulin R are stable when stored in refrigerator for 48 hours at 36° to 46° F (2° to 8° C) and may be used at room temperature for up to an additional 48 hours.

▼ Infusion bags prepared with Novolin R are stable at room temperature for 24 hours.

▼ Store Myxredlin IV solution at 36° to 46° F (2° to 8° C) in original carton until expiration date. May also store at room temperature up to 77° F (25° C) for up to 30 days; don't return to refrigerator after stored at room temperature. Don't freeze or shake.

▼ **Incompatibilities:** Don't mix regular insulin with any other insulin except NPH; don't mix regular concentrated insulin with any other insulin.

Subcutaneous

• Regular insulin administered by subcut injection should generally be used in regimens that include an intermediate- or long-acting insulin. It may also be used in combination with oral antidiabetics.

• Subcut injection should be followed by a meal within 30 minutes of administration.

• Administer by subcut injection in abdominal region, buttocks, thigh, or upper arm. Subcut injection into abdominal wall is generally associated with faster absorption than other injection sites.

• Injection sites should be rotated within same region to reduce risk of lipodystrophy.

• Injection into a lifted skin fold minimizes risk of IM injection.

• Don't perform dose conversion when using the Humulin R U-500 KwikPen. The dose window of the pen shows the number of units of Humulin R U-500 to be injected, and no dose conversion is required.

• Don't transfer Humulin R U-500 from the pen into a syringe for administration because overdose and severe hypoglycemia can occur.

• Don't use if solution is viscous or cloudy; use only if clear and colorless.

• Don't use regular insulin in external subcut insulin pumps because of precipitation risk.

ACTION

Lowers blood glucose level by stimulating peripheral glucose uptake by binding to insulin receptors on skeletal muscle and in fat cells and by inhibiting hepatic glucose production; also inhibits lipolysis and proteolysis, and enhances protein synthesis.

Route	Onset	Peak	Duration
IV	10–15 min	Unknown	4 hr
U-100 (subcut)	30 min	0.5–2.5 hr	8 hr
U-500 (subcut)	15 min	4–8 hr	13–24 hr

Half-life: IV, 30 to 60 minutes; subcut, 1.5 hours.

ADVERSE REACTIONS

CV: peripheral edema. **Metabolic:** *hypoglycemia, hypokalemia,* weight gain. **Skin:** injection-site reactions, lipodystrophy, pruritus. **Other:** allergic reactions, *anaphylaxis,* insulin antibody production.

INTERACTIONS

Drug-drug. *ACE inhibitors, antidiabetics (oral), ARBs, disopyramide, fibrates, fluoxetine, MAO inhibitors, salicylates, sulfonamide antibiotics, octreotide, pentoxifylline, pramlintide:* May cause hypoglycemia. Monitor glucose level and adjust insulin dosage as needed.

Atypical antipsychotics, corticosteroids, danazol, diuretics, estrogens, glucagon, hormonal contraceptives, isoniazid, niacin, phenothiazines, protease inhibitors, somatropin, sympathomimetics (albuterol, epinephrine, terbutaline), thyroid hormones: May cause hyperglycemia. Monitor glucose level and adjust insulin dosage as needed.

Beta blockers, clonidine: May mask signs and symptoms of hypoglycemia. Avoid concurrent use, if possible, or monitor patient closely.

Beta blockers, clonidine, lithium salts, **pentamidine:** May cause hypoglycemia or hyperglycemia. Monitor glucose level.

Thiazolidinediones (TZDs; pioglitazone, rosiglitazone): May cause fluid retention that can lead to HF. Monitor patient closely, and adjust or stop TZD as clinically necessary.

Drug-lifestyle. *Alcohol use:* May cause hyperglycemia or hypoglycemia. Monitor glucose level closely and discourage concurrent use.

EFFECTS ON LAB TEST RESULTS
• May decrease glucose and potassium levels.
• May develop antibodies that react with human insulin.

CONTRAINDICATIONS & CAUTIONS
• Contraindicated during episodes of hypoglycemia.
• Contraindicated in patients with a history of hypersensitivity to drug or its components. Severe, life-threatening, generalized allergic reactions, including anaphylaxis, can occur with insulin products.
• Use cautiously in patients susceptible to hypokalemia, such as patients who are fasting, are taking potassium-lowering drugs, or are concurrently taking drugs that may affect potassium level. Untreated hypokalemia can cause respiratory paralysis, ventricular arrhythmias, and death.
• Hypoglycemia is the most common adverse reaction. Severe hypoglycemia can cause seizures, and may be life-threatening or fatal. Hypoglycemia can occur suddenly, and symptoms may differ. Risk increases with intensity of glycemic control and changes in glycemic treatment, meal patterns, physical activity, and concomitant medications and in patients with renal or hepatic impairment.
• Human insulin differs from animal-source insulin; change between insulin types cautiously and monitor patient closely.
• Use cautiously in older adults, who may be at increased risk for adverse effects. Signs and symptoms of hypoglycemia may be more difficult to recognize in these patients.
• Use insulin pens cautiously in patients with visual impairment who may rely on audible clicks to dial their dose.
Dialyzable drug: Unknown.
⚠ *Overdose S&S:* Hypoglycemia, hypokalemia.

PREGNANCY-LACTATION-REPRODUCTION
• Use cautiously during pregnancy.
• Monitor blood glucose levels closely during pregnancy, after recent birth, and during breastfeeding; insulin requirements may change.
• It isn't known if insulin appears in human milk. Use cautiously during breastfeeding. Adjust insulin dose as needed.

NURSING CONSIDERATIONS
• Monitor blood glucose level and adjust insulin dosage as needed for patient-specific goals.
• Monitor patient carefully when initiating therapy. Time course of insulins varies with each patient.
• Monitor patient carefully for signs and symptoms of hypoglycemia, especially in long-standing disease. Treat according to individual facility protocol if necessary.
• Mild episodes of hypoglycemia may be treated with oral glucose. More severe episodes of hypoglycemia, such as coma, seizure, or neurologic impairment, may be treated with IM or subcut glucagon or concentrated IV glucose.
• Assess patient and notify prescriber for signs and symptoms of hypoglycemia (diaphoresis, shaking, trembling, confusion) and hyperglycemia (drowsiness, fruity breath odor, frequent urination, thirst).
• Periodically measure HbA_{1c} levels.
• Monitor potassium levels in patients at risk for hypokalemia, including those taking potassium-depleting drugs.
• Increase frequency of glucose monitoring in patients who are acutely ill or under emotional stress, or if changes in diet, exercise, or medication regimen occur because these may affect the rate of insulin absorption. Also monitor patient closely after changes to insulin dosage.
• Monitor patients for generalized allergic reactions, including anaphylaxis.
• Verify product label before giving drug to avoid medication errors.
❶ **Alert:** Medication errors associated with the U-500 vial have resulted in hyperglycemia, hypoglycemia, and death; read labels closely to prevent errors.
❶ **Alert:** Use only a U-500 insulin syringe with U-500 vials to avoid administration errors. Don't use any other type of syringe to administer U-500 insulin.
• *Look alike–sound alike:* Don't confuse Humulin with Humalog. Don't confuse Novolin with NovoLog.

PATIENT TEACHING
• Instruct patient in self-management, including glucose management, injection technique, proper storage of insulin, and recognition and management of hypoglycemia and hyperglycemia.

Reactions in bold italics are *life-threatening*. Interactions may have a *rapid onset* or a ***delayed onset***.

- Teach patient to eat within 30 minutes of injecting short-acting insulin.
- Instruct patient to only use syringes calibrated for their particular concentration of insulin.

🜄 *Alert:* Warn patient not to share multidose pen with other people, even if the needle is changed, because of risk of bloodborne pathogen transmission, including HIV and hepatitis.

- Teach patient to rotate injection sites and the importance of avoiding lipodystrophy.
- Instruct patient that when mixing two types of insulin, to always draw up the shorter-acting insulin first, followed by NPH, and inject immediately.
- Explain importance of checking insulin label before each injection; accidental mix-ups among insulin types have been reported.
- Instruct patient to keep hard candy or glucose tablets on hand to treat mild cases of hypoglycemia.
- Caution patient that hypoglycemic episodes can impair the ability to concentrate and react; advise patient to use caution while driving and operating machinery.
- Advise patient to track glucose levels.
- Instruct patient on long-term risks of diabetes if not managed properly.
- Counsel patient to carry identification or wear jewelry indicating that patient has diabetes.
- Advise patient that allergic reactions, including injection-site reactions (local pain, redness or swelling) and generalized allergic reaction and anaphylaxis (whole-body rash, shortness of breath, wheezing, reduced BP, fast pulse, diaphoresis), can occur. Teach patient to immediately seek emergency medical attention for generalized reactions.
- Warn patient that insulin requirements may vary due to illness, stress, emotional disturbances, inadequate or skipped insulin dose, inadvertent administration of an increased insulin dose, inadequate food intake, skipped meals, or pregnancy.
- Caution patient not to stop insulin abruptly or to change amount injected without consulting prescriber.
- Warn patient that any change in insulin should be made cautiously and only under medical supervision. Changes in insulin strength, manufacturer, type (regular, NPH, or insulin analogues), species (animal, human), or method of manufacture (rDNA, animal-source insulin) may result in the need for a dosage change.
- Caution patient to discuss adjustments to the administration schedule if traveling across more than two time zones.

SAFETY ALERT!

interferon alfa-2b (recombinant) (IFN-alpha 2b)
in-ter-FEER-on

Intron A

Therapeutic class: Antivirals
Pharmacologic class: Biological response modifiers

AVAILABLE FORMS
Powder for injection: 10, 18, and 50 million international units/vial with diluent
Solution for injection: 18 and 25 million international units/vial (6 and 10 million international units/mL)

INDICATIONS & DOSAGES
Adjust-a-dose (for all indications): For all indications except condylomata acuminata, if adverse effects occur, stop drug until they abate; then resume drug at 50% of the previous dose. If intolerance persists, stop drug. See package insert for specific guidance.

➤ **Hairy cell leukemia**
Adults: 2 million international units/m² IM or subcut three times weekly for up to 6 months or more if patient is responding to treatment. Give subcut if platelet count is less than 50,000/mm³.

➤ **AIDS-related Kaposi sarcoma**
Adults: 30 million international units/m² subcut or IM three times weekly. Maintain dose until disease progression or maximal response has been achieved after 16 weeks of treatment. Don't use solution for injection in vials for this indication.

➤ **Chronic HBV infection**
Adults: 30 to 35 million international units IM or subcut weekly, given as 5 million international units daily or 10 million international units three times weekly for 16 weeks.
Children ages 1 to 17: 3 million international units/m² subcut three times weekly for first week; then increase to 6 million international units/m² subcut three times weekly (maximum is 10 million international

units three times weekly) for total of 16 to 24 weeks.

Adjust-a-dose: If WBC count is less than 1.5×10^9/L, granulocyte count is less than 0.75×10^9/L, or platelet count is less than 50×10^9/L, reduce dose by 50%. Permanently discontinue drug if WBC count is less than 1×10^9/L, granulocyte count is less than 0.5×10^9/L, or platelet count is less than 25×10^9/L.

➤ **Chronic HCV infection**

Adults: 3 million international units IM or subcut three times weekly. In patients tolerating therapy with normalization of ALT at 16 weeks of therapy, continue for 18 to 24 months. In patients who haven't normalized the ALT or have persistently high levels of HCV RNA after 16 weeks of therapy, consider stopping therapy.

➤ **Adjunct to surgical treatment in patients with malignant melanoma who are asymptomatic after surgery but at high risk for systemic recurrence for up to 8 weeks after surgery**

Adults: Induction dose, 20 million international units/m^2 by IV infusion over 20 minutes 5 consecutive days weekly for 4 weeks; then maintenance dose of 10 million international units/m^2 subcut three times weekly for 48 weeks. Solution for injection in vials isn't recommended for IV administration and shouldn't be used for the induction phase.

Adjust-a-dose: Withhold dose if severe adverse reactions develop, including granulocyte count more than 250/mm^3 but less than 500/mm^3 or ALT/AST level of more than 5 to $10 \times$ ULN, until adverse reactions abate. Restart at 50% of the previous dose.

➤ **First treatment of clinically aggressive follicular non-Hodgkin lymphoma with chemotherapy containing anthracycline**

Adults: 5 million international units subcut three times weekly for up to 18 months in conjunction with anthracycline-containing chemotherapy regimen.

Adjust-a-dose: For neutrophil count of more than 1,000/mm^3 but less than 1,500/mm^3, decrease dosage by 50%. May resume starting dose if neutrophil count returns to more than 1,500/mm^3. Withhold drug if neutrophil count is less than 1,000/mm^3 or platelet count is less than 50,000/mm^3. Permanently discontinue drug if AST level exceeds $5 \times$ ULN or serum creatinine level is greater than 2 mg/dL.

➤ **Condylomata acuminata (genital or perianal warts)**

Adults: 1 million international units for each lesion (maximum five lesions in a single course) intralesionally three times weekly for 3 weeks. Additional course may be given at 12 to 16 weeks. Don't use the 18-million or 50-million international units powder for injection or the 18-million international units multidose solution for injection for this indication.

ADMINISTRATION

• Reconstitute powder with 1 mL of sterile water; swirl gently. Solution should be clear and colorless to light yellow.

• Reconstituted powder doesn't contain preservative and must be used immediately. Don't reenter vial after withdrawing dose. Discard unused portion.

• Solution in multidose vials should be clear and colorless and may be injected IM, subcut, or intralesionally. Don't give IV.

IV

▼ Prepare infusion solution immediately before use.

▼ Bring solution to room temperature before use.

▼ Based on desired dose, reconstitute appropriate vial strength of drug with diluent provided. Withdraw dose and inject into a 100-mL bag of NSS. Final yield of drug shouldn't be less than 10 million international units/100 mL.

▼ Infuse over 20 minutes.

▼ Give in the evening when possible to enhance tolerability.

▼ Store solution in refrigerator. Store powder before and after reconstitution in refrigerator. Use within 24 hours.

▼ **Incompatibilities:** Dextrose solutions.

IM

• Carefully monitor injection sites in patient with thrombocytopenia. Avoid IM injections if possible.

• Give IM injection in anterior thighs, deltoid, and superolateral buttock.

• In patients whose platelet count falls below 50,000/mm^3, give subcutaneously.

• Give drug at bedtime to minimize daytime drowsiness.

Subcutaneous

• Give subcut injections in thighs, upper outer arms, and abdomen.

Reactions in bold italics are *life-threatening*. Interactions may have a *rapid onset* or a ***delayed onset***.

Intralesional

• For condylomata acuminata intralesional injection, use only 10 million-international unit vial because dilution of other strengths for intralesional use results in a hypertonic solution.

• Don't reconstitute drug in 10 million-international unit vial with more than 1 mL of diluent.

• Use tuberculin or similar syringe and 25G to 30G needle.

• Don't inject too deep beneath lesion or too superficially. As many as five lesions can be treated at one time.

• To ease discomfort, give in evening with acetaminophen.

ACTION

Unknown. May inhibit tumor or viral cell replication and modulate host immune response by enhancing macrophage activity and improving specific lymphocytes' cytotoxicity for target cells.

Route	Onset	Peak	Duration
IV	Unknown	15–60 min	4 hr
IM, subcut	Unknown	3–12 hr	16 hr
Intralesional	Unknown	Unknown	Unknown

Half-life: IV, 2 hours; IM, subcut, 2 to 3 hours.

ADVERSE REACTIONS

CNS: apathy, amnesia, agitation, abnormal dreams, asthenia, depression, difficulty in thinking or concentrating, confusion, dizziness, vertigo, drowsiness, fatigue, insomnia, paresthesia, somnolence, anxiety, aggression, lethargy, nervousness, weakness, abnormal gait, headache, fever, hypothermia, malaise, irritability, taste alteration, smell alteration, voice disorder, dysphagia, emotional lability, pain, *stroke, suicidality.* **CV:** angina, arteritis, arrhythmia, atrial fibrillation, *bradycardia, HF,* cardiomegaly, cardiomyopathy, CAD, chest pain, *cyanosis,* edema, extrasystoles, heart valve disorder, HTN, flushing, hypotension, palpitations, phlebitis, orthostatic hypotension, *PE,* Raynaud disease, tachycardia, *thrombosis, varicose veins.* **EENT:** conjunctivitis, abnormal vision, earache, epistaxis, nasal congestion, rhinorrhea, rhinitis, sinusitis, pharyngitis, gingivitis, dry mouth. **GI:** anorexia, diarrhea, dyspepsia, nausea, vomiting, abdominal pain, constipation, esophagitis, flatulence, stomatitis. **GU:** increased BUN level, decreased libido, impotence, amenorrhea. **Hematologic:** *leukopenia, thrombocytopenia,* anemia, *neutropenia, granulocytopenia.* **Hepatic:** increased LFT values, jaundice, *hepatitis.* **Metabolic:** weight loss, thirst, hypercalcemia, hyperglycemia. **Musculoskeletal:** myalgia, arthralgia, back pain, musculoskeletal pain. **Respiratory:** coughing, dyspnea, bronchitis. **Skin:** alopecia, dryness, injection-site reaction, diaphoresis, pruritus, purpura, rash, dermatitis. **Other:** flulike syndrome, chills, rigors, infection.

INTERACTIONS

Drug-drug. *Aldesleukin, telbivudine:* May enhance adverse or toxic effects of these drugs. Avoid together.

Clozapine: May increase clozapine level and risk of adverse effects, especially neutropenia. Monitor patient closely.

CNS depressants: May increase CNS effects. Avoid using together.

Myelosuppressants (zidovudine): May cause synergistic adverse effects (higher risk of neutropenia). Carefully monitor WBC count.

Ribavirin: May enhance adverse effects, including hemolytic anemia. Monitor therapy.

Theophylline: May reduce theophylline clearance. Monitor theophylline level.

Vitamin K antagonists (warfarin): May increase anticoagulant effect. Monitor PT and INR closely.

EFFECTS ON LAB TEST RESULTS

• May increase calcium, phosphate, AST, ALT, LDH, ALP, triglyceride, creatinine, BUN, and fasting glucose levels.

• May increase or decrease TSH level.

• May increase INR and prolong PT and PTT.

• May decrease Hb level and WBC and platelet counts.

CONTRAINDICATIONS & CAUTIONS

• Contraindicated in patients hypersensitive to drug or its components and in those with autoimmune hepatitis or decompensated liver disease.

• Combination therapy with ribavirin is additionally contraindicated in patients hypersensitive to ribavirin or other components of the product and in those with hemoglobinopathies or CrCl less than 50 mL/minute.

• Use cautiously in older adults and in patients with history of CV disease, cerebrovascular disorders, pulmonary disease, diabetes, coagulation disorders, renal impairment, and severe myelosuppression.

• Depression, psychosis, and suicidality have been linked to drug use; patients with psychotic disorders, especially depression, shouldn't continue drug treatment.

🌙 *Alert:* Neurotoxicity and cardiotoxicity are more common in older adults, especially those with underlying CNS or cardiac impairment.

Dialyzable drug: No.

⚠ *Overdose S&S:* Abnormal liver enzyme levels, renal failure, hemorrhage, MI.

PREGNANCY-LACTATION-REPRODUCTION

• There are no adequate studies during pregnancy. Use during pregnancy only if potential benefit justifies fetal risk.

🌙 *Alert:* Combination therapy with ribavirin is contraindicated during pregnancy and in men whose partners are pregnant.

🌙 *Alert:* Because of fetal risk, warn patients of childbearing potential and male patients with partners of childbearing potential who are receiving combination therapy with ribavirin to use two forms of contraception.

• It isn't known if drug appears in human milk. Patient should discontinue breastfeeding or discontinue drug.

NURSING CONSIDERATIONS

Boxed Warning Alpha interferons cause or aggravate fatal or life-threatening neuropsychiatric, autoimmune, ischemic, and infectious disorders. Monitor patients closely with periodic clinical and lab evaluations. Withdraw patients with persistently severe or worsening signs or symptoms of these conditions from therapy. ■

🌙 *Alert:* Not all dosage forms are appropriate for all indications. Refer to manufacturer's instructions for approved indications before use.

• Verify pregnancy status before treatment.

• Ensure patient is well hydrated, especially at beginning of treatment.

• At start of treatment, monitor patient for flulike signs and symptoms, which tend to diminish with continued therapy. Premedicate patient with acetaminophen to minimize these symptoms.

• Periodically check for adverse CNS reactions, such as decreased mental status and dizziness, during therapy.

• Monitor CBC with differential, platelet count, and blood chemistry and electrolyte studies. Monitor ECG before and during treatment if patient has cardiac disorder or advanced stages of cancer.

• Monitor hepatic function (serum bilirubin, ALT, AST, ALP, and LDH) at 2, 8, and 12 weeks after start of therapy, then every 6 months during therapy. Permanently stop drug for evidence of severe (grade 3) hepatic injury or hepatic decompensation (Child-Pugh classes B and C).

• For patients who develop thrombocytopenia, exercise extreme care in performing invasive procedures; inspect injection site and skin frequently for signs and symptoms of bruising; limit frequency of IM injections; test urine, emesis fluid, stool, and secretions for occult blood.

• Severe adverse reactions may need dosage reduction to half or withholding of drug until reactions subside.

• Use with blood dyscrasia-causing drugs, bone marrow suppressants, or radiation therapy may increase bone marrow suppression. Dosage reduction may be needed.

• For condylomata acuminata, maximum response usually occurs in 4 to 8 weeks.

PATIENT TEACHING

• Advise patient to avoid contact with persons with viral illness; patient is at increased risk for infection during therapy.

• Inform patient that lab tests will be performed before and periodically during therapy.

• Teach patient proper oral hygiene during treatment because bone marrow suppressant effects of interferon may lead to microbial infection, delayed healing, and bleeding gums. Drug also may decrease saliva.

• Advise patient to check with prescriber for instructions after missing a dose.

• Stress need to follow prescriber's instructions about taking and recording temperature and how and when to take acetaminophen.

• Teach patient who will self-administer drug how to prepare injection and how to use and dispose of syringe. Provide information on drug stability.

• Tell patient that drug may cause temporary partial hair loss; hair should return after drug is stopped.

Reactions in bold italics are *life-threatening*. Interactions may have a *rapid onset* or a *delayed onset*.

• Advise patient to report all adverse reactions and to immediately report neuropsychiatric symptoms (depression, mania, psychosis, suicidality).

SAFETY ALERT!

interferon beta-1a
in-ter-FEER-on

Avonex, Rebif

Therapeutic class: Antivirals
Pharmacologic class: Biological response modifiers

AVAILABLE FORMS
Avonex (IM use only)
Injection: 30 mcg (6 million international units)/0.5 mL prefilled syringe or autoinjector
Rebif (subcut use only)
Injection: 8.8 mcg (2.4 million international units)/0.2 mL, 22 mcg (6 million international units)/0.5 mL, 44 mcg (12 million international units)/0.5 mL prefilled syringe or autoinjector

INDICATIONS & DOSAGES
➤ **Relapsing forms of MS, including clinically isolated syndrome, relapsing-remitting disease, and active secondary progressive disease**
Adults age 18 and older: Initially, 7.5 mcg IM (week 1); then increase in increments of 7.5 mcg once weekly (weeks 2 to 4) up to recommended dose (30 mcg once weekly). Or, initially, 4.4 or 8.8 mcg subcut three times weekly for 2 weeks; then increase dose to 11 or 22 mcg three times weekly for another 2 weeks. Then increase to a maintenance dose of 22 or 44 mcg subcut three times weekly.
Adjust-a-dose: For Rebif, in patients with decreased blood counts or elevated LFT values (ALT level greater than 5 × ULN), reduce dosage or withhold drug until toxicity resolves. Stop treatment if jaundice or other signs of hepatic injury occur.

ADMINISTRATION
Subcutaneous
• Visually inspect Rebif for particulate matter and discoloration before administration.
• Rotate sites of injection.

• Administer Rebif at same time on same 3 days at least 48 hours apart each week (late afternoon or evening on Monday, Wednesday, and Friday).
• Use only prefilled syringes for titration to 22 mcg prescribed dose of Rebif.
• Store Rebif in the refrigerator between 36° and 46° F (2° and 8° C). Don't freeze. Rebif may be stored at or below 77° F (25° C) for up to 30 days if away from heat and light but refrigeration is preferred.
IM
🕸 *Alert:* Syringe tip cap contains natural rubber latex, which may cause allergic reactions.
• Rotate injection sites. Don't inject into areas where skin is red, bruised, or irritated.
• Assess injection site after 2 hours for redness, swelling, or tenderness.
• Store Avonex prefilled syringes and autoinjectors in the refrigerator at 36° to 46° F. If refrigeration is unavailable, may store at 77° F for up to 7 days. Once refrigerated, syringes and autoinjectors must not be stored above 77° F. Once removed from refrigerator, warm to room temperature (about 30 minutes). Don't use external heat sources, such as hot water, to warm syringe, or expose to high temperatures. If product has been exposed to conditions other than those recommended after removal from refrigerator, discard product. Don't freeze. Protect from light.
• After giving each dose, discard any remaining product in the syringe or autoinjector.

ACTION
Unknown. Interacts with specific cell receptors found on the surface of cells. Binding of these receptors causes the expression of a number of interferon-induced gene products believed to mediate the biological actions of interferon beta-1a.

Route	Onset	Peak	Duration
Subcut	Unknown	16 hr	Unknown
IM	12 hr	6–36 hr	4 days

Half-life: Subcut, 69 hours; IM, 8 to 54 hours.

ADVERSE REACTIONS
CNS: dizziness, fatigue, asthenia, fever, headache, migraine, pain, depression, *seizures, suicidality,* abnormal coordination, ataxia, hypertonia, malaise, rigors, somnolence. **CV:** chest pain, vasodilation. **EENT:** abnormal vision, dry eyes, sinusitis, toothache, dry mouth. **GI:** abdominal

pain. **GU:** urinary frequency, urinary incontinence, UTI. **Hematologic:** lymphadenopathy, *leukopenia, pancytopenia, thrombocytopenia,* anemia. **Hepatic:** increased transaminase levels, bilirubinemia, hepatic injury. **Metabolic:** hyperthyroidism, hypothyroidism. **Musculoskeletal:** back pain, myalgia, skeletal pain, arthralgia, muscle spasm. **Respiratory:** URI, dyspnea, bronchitis. **Skin:** injection-site reaction, injection-site necrosis, alopecia, ecchymosis at injection site, urticaria, rash, diaphoresis. **Other:** chills, flulike syndrome, infection, hypersensitivity reactions, neutralizing antibodies.

INTERACTIONS
Drug-drug. *Myelosuppressive drugs:* May cause added hematologic toxicities; use cautiously together. Monitor CBC.

EFFECTS ON LAB TEST RESULTS
• May increase liver enzyme levels.
• May increase eosinophil count.
• May decrease Hb level, hematocrit, and WBC and platelet counts.
• May increase or decrease thyroid function test levels.

CONTRAINDICATIONS & CAUTIONS
• Contraindicated in patients hypersensitive to natural or recombinant interferon beta, human albumin, or other components of drug.
• Use cautiously in patients with depression, seizure disorders, severe cardiac conditions, liver disease, or alcohol use disorder.
• Thrombotic microangiopathy (TMA), including thrombotic thrombocytopenic purpura and hemolytic-uremic syndrome, sometimes fatal, has been reported with interferon beta products and may occur several weeks to years after start of therapy.
• Safety and effectiveness of drug in chronic progressive MS or in children younger than age 18 haven't been established.
Dialyzable drug: Unknown.

PREGNANCY-LACTATION-REPRODUCTION
• There are no adequate studies during pregnancy. Use during pregnancy only if potential benefit justifies fetal risk.
• It isn't known if drug appears in human milk. Use cautiously during breastfeeding.

NURSING CONSIDERATIONS
• Monitor patient closely for depression and suicidality. It isn't known if these symptoms are related to the underlying neurologic basis of MS or to the drug.
• Monitor thyroid function tests, WBC count, platelet count, and blood chemistries, including LFTs.
• Monitor patient for TMA and discontinue drug if clinical signs and symptoms and lab findings consistent with TMA occur; manage as clinically indicated.
• Give analgesics or antipyretics to decrease flulike symptoms.
• Monitor patient for hypersensitivity reactions, including anaphylaxis.
• Monitor patient for injection-site reactions, including necrosis. Antibiotics or surgical intervention may be necessary. Don't inject into affected area until completely healed; if multiple lesions occur, may discontinue drug until lesions heal.

PATIENT TEACHING
• Advise patient to read medication guide that comes with drug.
• Teach patient and family member safe drug administration, storage, and needle disposal.
• Instruct patient to keep syringes and needles away from children, not to reuse needles or syringes, and to discard them in a syringe-disposal unit.
• Caution patient not to change dosage or schedule of administration. If a dose is missed, tell patient to take it as soon as remembered and then resume regular schedule. Tell patient not to take two injections within 48 hours of each other.
• Show patient how to store drug.
• Inform patient that flulike signs and symptoms (such as fever, fatigue, muscle aches, headache, chills, and joint pain) aren't uncommon at start of therapy and that analgesics/antipyretics may be prescribed on treatment days to lessen severity of flulike signs and symptoms.
• Advise patient to report depression, suicidality, or other adverse reactions.
• If pregnancy occurs, instruct patient to notify prescriber immediately.

Reactions in bold italics are *life-threatening*. Interactions may have a *rapid onset* or a ***delayed onset***.

interferon beta-1b (recombinant)
in-ter-FEER-on

Betaseron, Extavia

Therapeutic class: Immunomodulators
Pharmacologic class: Biological response modifiers

AVAILABLE FORMS
Powder for injection: 0.3 mg

INDICATIONS & DOSAGES
➤ **Relapsing forms of MS, including clinically isolated syndrome, relapsing-remitting disease, and active secondary progressive disease**
Adults: 0.0625 mg subcut every other day for weeks 1 and 2; then 0.125 mg subcut every other day for weeks 3 and 4; then 0.1875 mg subcut every other day for weeks 5 and 6; then 0.25 mg subcut every other day thereafter.

ADMINISTRATION
Subcutaneous

🚱 *Alert:* The removable rubber cap of the Extavia diluent prefilled syringe contains natural rubber latex, which may cause allergic reactions and shouldn't be handled by latex-sensitive individuals.

• To reconstitute, slowly inject 1.2 mL of supplied diluent (half-NSS for injection) into vial and gently swirl to dissolve drug.

• Don't shake. Discard vial that contains particulates or discolored solution.

• Each mL of reconstituted solution contains 0.25 mg of interferon beta-1b.

• Inject immediately after preparation.

• Rotate injection sites to minimize local reactions and observe site for necrosis. Don't inject into red, sore, or infected skin.

• Give a missed dose as soon as possible; give next injection 48 hours after that dose. Don't give drug on two consecutive days.

• Store at room temperature. After reconstitution, if not used immediately, may refrigerate drug for up to 3 hours. Don't freeze.

ACTION
Exact mechanism unknown. A naturally occurring antiviral and immunoregulatory drug derived from human fibroblasts. Drug attaches to membrane receptors and causes cellular changes, including increased protein synthesis.

Route	Onset	Peak	Duration
Subcut	Unknown	1–8 hr	Unknown

Half-life: 8 minutes to 4.25 hours.

ADVERSE REACTIONS
CNS: depression, asthenia, migraine, headache, pain, malaise, fever, chills, insomnia, incoordination. **CV:** chest pain, peripheral edema, HTN. **GI:** abdominal pain. **GU:** menstrual disorder, urgency, impotence. **Hepatic:** increased transaminase levels. **Hematologic:** *leukopenia, neutropenia, lymphocytopenia,* lymphadenopathy. **Musculoskeletal:** myalgia, hypertonia. **Respiratory:** dyspnea. **Skin:** inflammation, pain, necrosis at injection site, rash, skin disorder. **Other:** flulike syndrome.

INTERACTIONS
None reported.

EFFECTS ON LAB TEST RESULTS
• May increase ALT, AST and bilirubin levels.
• May decrease WBC and neutrophil counts.

CONTRAINDICATIONS & CAUTIONS
• Contraindicated in patients hypersensitive to interferon beta, human albumin, mannitol, or components of drug.
• Use cautiously in patients with HF.
• Drug-induced lupus erythematosus has been reported and has occurred with positive serologic testing (including positive antinuclear or anti-double-stranded DNA antibody testing).
• Thrombotic microangiopathy (TMA), including thrombotic thrombocytopenic purpura and hemolytic-uremic syndrome, sometimes fatal, has been reported with interferon beta products and may occur several weeks to years after start of therapy.
• Seizures have been reported with beta interferon use; however, it's unknown if they're related to a primary seizure disorder, the effects of MS, other causes of seizures (fever), or the use of the drug.
Dialyzable drug: Unknown.

PREGNANCY-LACTATION-REPRODUCTION

- There are no adequate studies during pregnancy; however, spontaneous abortions have been reported in clinical trials. Use during pregnancy only if potential benefit justifies fetal risk.
- It isn't known if drug appears in human milk. Use cautiously during breastfeeding.

NURSING CONSIDERATIONS

⚠️ *Alert:* Serious liver damage, including hepatic failure requiring transplant, can occur. Monitor liver function at 1, 3, and 6 months after therapy starts and periodically thereafter.
- Drug is intended for use under the guidance and supervision of a prescriber. Administer first injection under the supervision of a health care provider. If patients or caregivers are to administer drug, train them in the proper technique for self-administering.
- Monitor patient for signs and symptoms of drug-induced lupus erythematosus (rash, serositis, polyarthritis, nephritis, Raynaud phenomenon); discontinue therapy if they occur.
- Monitor patient for TMA and discontinue drug if clinical signs and symptoms and lab findings consistent with TMA occur; manage as clinically indicated.
- Monitor patient for symptoms of depression and severe psychiatric effects (mania, suicidality, psychosis).
- Monitor CBC and blood chemistries at 1, 3, and 6 months after therapy starts and periodically thereafter.
- Monitor thyroid function tests every 6 months in patients being treated for thyroid disorder.
- Use of analgesics and antipyretics on treatment days may help ameliorate flulike symptoms associated with interferon beta-1b use.
- Monitor patient for injection-site reactions, including necrosis. Antibiotics or surgical intervention may be necessary. Don't inject into affected area until completely healed; if multiple lesions occur, may discontinue drug until lesions heal.

PATIENT TEACHING

- Warn patient about dangers to a fetus and to notify prescriber if pregnancy occurs during therapy.
- Advise patient to read medication guide that comes with drug.

- Teach patient how to perform subcut injections, including solution preparation, aseptic technique, injection-site rotation, and equipment disposal. Periodically reevaluate patient's technique.
- Tell patient to take drug at bedtime to minimize mild flulike symptoms.
- Advise patient to stay well hydrated.
- Tell patient to report sign and symptoms of drug-induced lupus erythematosus.
- Advise patient to report suicidality or depression.
- Urge patient to immediately report signs or symptoms of tissue death at injection site.
- Advise patient of importance of obtaining routine blood tests.

SAFETY ALERT!

ipilimumab ⬥
ip-ih-LIM-yoo-mab

Yervoy

Therapeutic class: Antineoplastics
Pharmacologic class: Monoclonal antibodies

AVAILABLE FORMS

Injection: 50 mg/10 mL (5 mg/mL), 200 mg/40 mL (5 mg/mL) vials

INDICATIONS & DOSAGES

Adjust-a-dose (for all indications): Refer to manufacturer's instructions for toxicity-related dosage adjustments.

➤ **Unresectable or metastatic melanoma**
Adults and children age 12 and older: 3 mg/kg IV infusion over 90 minutes every 3 weeks for a total of four doses. All treatment must be administered within 16 weeks of first dose.

➤ **First-line combination therapy for unresectable or metastatic melanoma**
Adults: 3 mg/kg IV every 3 weeks immediately after nivolumab 1 mg/kg on same day for four combination doses. Continue nivolumab as a single agent until disease progression or unacceptable toxicity.

➤ **Adjuvant treatment of cutaneous melanoma with pathologic involvement of regional lymph nodes of more than 1 mm after complete resection, including total lymphadenectomy**
Adults: 10 mg/kg IV over 90 minutes every 3 weeks for four doses, followed by 10 mg/kg

every 12 weeks for up to 3 years or until documented disease recurrence or unacceptable toxicity.

➤ **Intermediate- or poor-risk, previously untreated advanced renal cell carcinoma in combination with nivolumab**

Adults: 1 mg/kg IV infusion every 3 weeks with nivolumab 3 mg/kg IV infusion every 3 weeks for a maximum of four doses. Then continue nivolumab 240 mg IV over 30 minutes every 2 weeks or 480 mg IV over 30 minutes every 4 weeks as a single agent until disease progression or unacceptable toxicity.

➤ **Microsatellite instability-high or mismatch repair-deficient metastatic colorectal cancer that has progressed following treatment with a fluoropyrimidine, oxaliplatin, and irinotecan, as a single agent or in combination with nivolumab**

Adults and children age 12 and older: 1 mg/kg IV infusion every 3 weeks with nivolumab 3 mg/kg every 3 weeks for up to four doses; then nivolumab 240 mg every 2 weeks or 480 mg every 4 weeks as a single agent until disease progression or unacceptable toxicity.

➤ **Hepatocellular carcinoma in combination with nivolumab following treatment with sorafenib**

Adults: 3 mg/kg IV infusion immediately following nivolumab 1 mg/kg IV infusion given on the same day every 3 weeks for up to four combination doses; then continue nivolumab as a single agent according to manufacturer's prescribing information until disease progression or unacceptable toxicity.

➤ **First-line combination therapy for metastatic NSCLC when tumors express PD-L1 according to FDA-approved testing, with no *EGFR* or *ALK* genomic tumor aberrations** ▨

Adults: 1 mg/kg IV infusion every 6 weeks with nivolumab 360 mg IV infusion every 3 weeks. Continue until disease progression or unacceptable toxicity, or for up to 2 years in patients without disease progression.

➤ **Metastatic or recurrent NSCLC with no *EGFR* or *ALK* genomic tumor aberrations in combination with nivolumab and platinum-doublet chemotherapy** ▨

Adults: 1 mg/kg IV infusion every 6 weeks with nivolumab 360 mg IV infusion every 3 weeks and two cycles of chemotherapy every 3 weeks. Continue until disease progression or unacceptable toxicity, or up to 2 years in patients without disease progression.

➤ **Unresectable malignant pleural mesothelioma in combination with nivolumab**

Adults: 1 mg/kg IV infusion every 6 weeks with nivolumab 360 mg IV infusion every 3 weeks. Continue until disease progression or unacceptable toxicity, or up to 2 years in patients without disease progression.

✷ *NEW INDICATION:* **Unresectable advanced or metastatic esophageal squamous cell carcinoma as first-line treatment, in combination with nivolumab**

Adults: 1 mg/kg IV infusion every 6 weeks with nivolumab 3 mg/kg IV infusion every 2 weeks or 360 mg IV infusion every 3 weeks until disease progression or unacceptable toxicity, or up to 2 years in patients without disease progression.

ADMINISTRATION

IV

▼ Store vials in refrigerator at 36° to 46° F (2° to 8° C). Don't freeze or shake vials. Protect from light.

▼ Visually inspect solution. Solution may be clear to pale yellow. Discard if cloudy or discolored or if particles (other than translucent-to-white, amorphous particles) are present.

▼ Allow vials to come to room temperature for 5 minutes before preparing infusion.

▼ Withdraw required volume of drug and transfer into IV bag of NSS or D_5W. Final concentration should range from 1 to 2 mg/mL. Invert bag gently to mix.

▼ Store diluted solution up to 24 hours under refrigeration or at room temperature (68° to 77° F [20° to 25° C]).

▼ Administer diluted solution over 30 minutes or 90 minutes (for adjuvant melanoma treatment only) through IV line containing a sterile, nonpyrogenic, low-protein-binding in-line filter.

▼ When given in combination with nivolumab, infuse nivolumab first followed by ipilimumab on same day.

▼ After each dose, flush IV line with NSS or D_5W.

▼ Discard unused portion of vial.

▼ **Incompatibilities:** Other IV drugs and solutions other than NSS or D_5W.

ACTION

Binds to the cytotoxic T-lymphocyte–associated antigen 4; this blockade has been shown to augment T-cell–mediated antitumor immune responses.

Route	Onset	Peak	Duration
IV	Rapid	Unknown	Unknown

Half-life: 15.4 days.

ADVERSE REACTIONS

CNS: fatigue, malaise, neuropathy, fever, headache, insomnia. **CV:** HTN, hypotension, edema. **EENT:** dry mouth. **GI:** diarrhea, colitis, enterocolitis, nausea, vomiting, decreased appetite, constipation, stomatitis, abdominal pain. **GU:** nephritis, increased creatinine level. **Hematologic:** anemia, *lymphopenia.* **Hepatic:** ascites, increased transaminase levels, increased ALP level, hyperbilirubinemia, *hepatotoxicity.* **Metabolic:** endocrinopathy (hypothyroidism, hyperthyroidism, *adrenal insufficiency,* hypopituitarism), *hyperkalemia, hypokalemia, hypomagnesemia,* hyperglycemia, hyponatremia, increased lipase and amylase levels, *hypocalcemia,* weight loss. **Musculoskeletal:** pain, arthralgia. **Respiratory:** cough, URI, dyspnea, pneumonitis. **Skin:** pruritus, rash, vitiligo, dermatitis, urticaria. **Other:** flulike symptoms, chills.

INTERACTIONS
None reported.

EFFECTS ON LAB TEST RESULTS
• May increase liver enzymes, ALP, bilirubin, amylase, lipase, and creatinine levels.
• May increase eosinophil count.
• May decrease Hb level.
• May increase or decrease thyroid hormone levels.

CONTRAINDICATIONS & CAUTIONS
• Contraindicated in patients hypersensitive to drug or its components.
• Drug can cause severe and fatal immune-mediated adverse reactions involving any organ system, especially such reactions as enterocolitis, hepatitis, dermatitis (including TEN, SJS, DRESS syndrome), neuropathy, and endocrinopathy. Reactions usually occur during treatment, but may present weeks to months after therapy ends. If severe immune-mediated reactions occur, permanently discontinue ipilimumab and initiate systemic high-dose corticosteroid therapy. Assess patient for these reactions.

• Drug may increase risk of fatal or serious GVHD before or after allogeneic hematopoietic stem cell transplantation. Consider risks and benefits; monitor patient closely.
• Refer to nivolumab prescribing information for additional risk information.
• Safety and effectiveness in children younger than age 12 haven't been determined.
Dialyzable drug: Unknown.

PREGNANCY-LACTATION-REPRODUCTION
• Based on its mechanism of action and data from animal studies, drug can cause fetal harm when given during pregnancy.
• Advise patients of childbearing potential to use effective contraception during treatment and for 3 months after last dose.
• Drug may appear in human milk. Because of the risk of serious adverse reactions in breastfeeding infants, patient shouldn't breastfeed during treatment and for 3 months after final dose.

NURSING CONSIDERATIONS
• Verify pregnancy status before treatment.
• Monitor patient for infusion reactions; interrupt or slow rate of infusion in patients with mild or moderate reactions.
• Assess patients for signs and symptoms of enterocolitis, dermatitis, neuropathy, and endocrinopathy, and evaluate clinical chemistry values, including ACTH level and thyroid function test results, at baseline and before each dose.
• Monitor LFT results and assess patient for signs and symptoms of hepatotoxicity (jaundice, dark urine, nausea, vomiting, right upper quadrant pain, abnormal bleeding or bruising) before each dose.
• Monitor patients for signs and symptoms of enterocolitis and bowel perforation (abdominal pain, fever, ileus, or peritoneal signs and symptoms; increase in stool frequency to seven or more over patient's baseline; fecal incontinence; need for IV hydration for more than 24 hours; GI hemorrhage; GI perforation). Rule out infection and consider endoscopic evaluation for persistent or severe symptoms.
• Monitor patients for signs and symptoms of motor or sensory neuropathy. Withhold ipilimumab in patients with moderate neuropathy. Permanently discontinue drug in patients with severe neuropathy that interferes with daily activities, such as Guillain-Barré–like

---

Reactions in bold italics are *life-threatening*. Interactions may have a *rapid onset* or a ***delayed onset***.

syndromes (unilateral or bilateral weakness, sensory changes, paresthesia).

• Monitor patients for signs and symptoms of dermatitis (rash, pruritus) and consider these symptoms immune-mediated unless an alternative cause is identified. Permanently discontinue ipilimumab in patients with SJS, TEN, or rash complicated by full-thickness dermal ulceration or necrotic, bullous, or hemorrhagic manifestations.

• Monitor patients for signs and symptoms of hypophysitis, adrenal insufficiency (including adrenal crisis), and hyperthyroidism or hypothyroidism (headaches, fatigue, feeling cold, weight gain, changes in mood or behavior, dizziness, or fainting). Endocrinopathies should be considered immune-mediated unless an alternative cause is identified.

• Monitor patients for ocular symptoms (vision changes, eye pain or redness). Administer corticosteroid eyedrops to patients who develop uveitis, iritis, or episcleritis. Permanently discontinue drug in patients with immune-mediated ocular disease unresponsive to local immunosuppressive therapy.

PATIENT TEACHING

• Instruct patient to report history of immune system disorders, such as ulcerative colitis, Crohn disease, lupus, or sarcoidosis; organ transplant; or liver damage.

• Teach patient signs and symptoms of serious immune-mediated adverse reactions, and advise patient to immediately report them to prescriber.

• Advise patient that blood chemistry studies will be needed before start of therapy and before each dose.

• Instruct patient to read the Yervoy Medication Guide before taking each dose.

• Warn patient that ipilimumab can cause fetal harm and to report pregnancy immediately.

• Advise patient of childbearing potential to use effective contraception during treatment and for 3 months after final dose.

• Tell patient not to breastfeed during therapy and for 3 months after final dose.

ipratropium bromide
i-pra-TROE-pee-um

Atrovent HFA, Ipravent ✤

Therapeutic class: Bronchodilators
Pharmacologic class: Anticholinergics

AVAILABLE FORMS

Inhaler: 17 mcg/metered dose
Nasal spray: 0.03% (21 mcg/metered dose), 0.06% (42 mcg/metered dose)
Solution (for inhalation): 0.02% (500 mcg/ vial)

INDICATIONS & DOSAGES

➤ **Bronchospasm in chronic bronchitis and emphysema**
Adults: Usually, 2 inhalations q.i.d.; patient may take additional inhalations as needed but shouldn't exceed 12 inhalations in 24 hours. Or, 500 mcg every 6 to 8 hours via oral nebulizer.
Children age 12 and older: 500 mcg every 6 to 8 hours via oral nebulizer.
➤ **Rhinorrhea caused by allergic and non-allergic perennial rhinitis**
Adults and children age 6 and older: Two 0.03% nasal sprays (42 mcg) per nostril b.i.d. or t.i.d. Total dose, 168 to 252 mcg/day.
➤ **Rhinorrhea caused by the common cold**
Adults and children age 12 and older: Two 0.06% nasal sprays (84 mcg) per nostril t.i.d. or q.i.d. Total dose, 672 mcg/day.
Children ages 5 to 11: Two 0.06% nasal sprays (84 mcg) per nostril t.i.d. Total dose, 504 mcg/day.
➤ **Rhinorrhea caused by seasonal allergic rhinitis**
Adults and children age 5 and older: Two 0.06% nasal sprays (84 mcg) per nostril q.i.d. Total dose is 672 mcg/day.
➤ **Acute asthma exacerbations, in combination with a short-acting beta agonist ♦**
Adults and adolescents age 13 and older: 500 mcg via oral nebulizer every 20 minutes for three doses, then as needed; or 8 inhalations of inhalation aerosol every 20 minutes as needed for up to 3 hours.
Children ages 6 to 12: 250 to 500 mcg via oral nebulizer every 20 minutes for three doses, then as needed; or 4 to 8 inhalations of inhalation aerosol every 20 minutes as needed for up to 3 hours.

Children age 5 and younger: 250 mcg via oral nebulizer every 20 minutes for 1 hour; or 2 inhalations of inhalation aerosol every 20 minutes if needed for 1 hour.

ADMINISTRATION
Inhalational
• Prime inhaler before initial use by releasing 2 test sprays into the air. If inhaler not used for more than 3 days, reprime.
• If more than 1 inhalation is ordered, wait at least 15 seconds between inhalations.
• Use spacer device to improve drug delivery, if appropriate.
• Wash mouthpiece once a week for 30 seconds in warm water only and let air dry.
• Don't puncture inhaler, throw into a fire or incinerator, or use or store near heat or open flame.
• Inhalation solution is for use with oral nebulizer. Refer to manufacturer's instructions for use.
• Protect solution from light. Store unused vials in foil pouch.
• Store inhaler and solution between 59° and 86° F (15° and 30° C).
Intranasal
• Prime nasal spray with 7 sprays of pump before first use; prime with 2 sprays after pump hasn't been used for more than 24 hours.
• Tilt patient's head backward after dose to allow drug to spread to back of nose.
• Store between 59° and 77° F (15° and 25° C); avoid freezing.

ACTION
Inhibits vagally mediated reflexes by antagonizing acetylcholine at muscarinic receptors on bronchial smooth muscle.

Route	Onset	Peak	Duration
Inhalation	15 min	1–2 hr	2–8 hr
Intranasal	15 min	Unknown	Unknown

Half-life: Inhalation, about 2 hours; intranasal, 1.6 hours.

ADVERSE REACTIONS
CNS: dizziness, headache, taste perversion, pain. **CV:** palpitations, chest pain, HTN. **EENT:** blurred vision, epistaxis, rhinitis, pharyngitis, sinusitis, nasal dryness, nasal irritation, nasal congestion, dry mouth. **GI:** nausea, diarrhea, dyspepsia, constipation. **GU:** UTI, urine retention. **Musculoskeletal:** back pain. **Respiratory:** URI, bronchitis, COPD exacerbation, *bronchospasm,* cough, dyspnea, increased sputum. **Skin:** rash. **Other:** flulike symptoms, hypersensitivity reactions.

INTERACTIONS
Drug-drug. *Anticholinergics:* May increase anticholinergic effects. Avoid using together.

EFFECTS ON LAB TEST RESULTS
None reported.

CONTRAINDICATIONS & CAUTIONS
• Contraindicated in patients hypersensitive to drug, atropine, or its derivatives.
• Use cautiously in patients with angle-closure glaucoma, prostatic hyperplasia, or bladder-neck obstruction.
⚠️ **Alert:** Drug isn't indicated for initial treatment of acute episodes of bronchospasm, for which rescue therapy is required for rapid response.
• Safety and effectiveness of intranasal use beyond 4 days in patients with a common cold or 3 weeks in patients with seasonal allergic rhinitis haven't been established.
• Safety and effectiveness of nebulization or inhaler in children younger than age 12 haven't been established.
Dialyzable drug: Unknown.

PREGNANCY-LACTATION-REPRODUCTION
• There are no adequate studies during pregnancy. Use during pregnancy only if clearly needed and if potential benefit justifies fetal risk.
• It isn't known if drug appears in human milk. Use cautiously during breastfeeding.

NURSING CONSIDERATIONS
• If patient uses a face mask for a nebulizer, take care to prevent leakage around the mask because eye pain or temporary blurring of vision may occur.

PATIENT TEACHING
• Warn patient that drug isn't effective for treating acute episodes of bronchospasm when rapid response is needed.
• Teach patient to use metered-dose inhaler (MDI) or oral nebulizer correctly. Refer to manufacturer's instructions for use.

Reactions in bold italics are *life-threatening*. Interactions may have a *rapid onset* or a **delayed onset**.

- Instruct patient to prime inhaler and clean mouthpiece according to manufacturer's instructions.
- Inform patient that use of a spacer device with an MDI may improve drug delivery to lungs.
- Warn patient to avoid accidentally spraying drug into eyes. Temporary blurring of vision may result.
- If more than 1 inhalation is prescribed, tell patient to wait at least 15 seconds before repeating procedure.
- Advise patient who is also using a corticosteroid inhaler to use ipratropium first and then to wait about 5 minutes before using the corticosteroid. This lets the bronchodilator open air passages for maximal effectiveness of the corticosteroid.
- Instruct patient to prime nasal spray as directed by manufacturer and how to safely administer drug.

irbesartan
ir-be-SAR-tan

Avapro♦

Therapeutic class: Antihypertensives
Pharmacologic class: Angiotensin II receptor antagonists

AVAILABLE FORMS
Tablets: 75 mg, 150 mg, 300 mg

INDICATIONS & DOSAGES
Adjust-a-dose (for all indications): For patients who are volume- and sodium-depleted, initially, 75 mg PO daily.
➤ **HTN**
Adults: Initially, 150 mg PO daily, increased to maximum of 300 mg daily, if needed.
➤ **Nephropathy in patients with type 2 diabetes**
Adults: 300 mg PO once daily.

ADMINISTRATION
PO
- Give drug without regard for meals.
- May give with other antihypertensives.

ACTION
Produces antihypertensive effect by competitive antagonist activity at the angiotensin II receptor.

Route	Onset	Peak	Duration
PO	1–2 hr	1.5–2 hr	>24 hr

Half-life: 11 to 15 hours.

ADVERSE REACTIONS
CNS: fatigue, dizziness. **CV:** orthostatic hypotension. **GI:** diarrhea, dyspepsia. **Metabolic:** *hyperkalemia.*

INTERACTIONS
Drug-drug. *ACE inhibitors:* May increase risk of hypotension, renal dysfunction, and hyperkalemia. Use together cautiously; closely monitor BP, renal function, and potassium level.
⊕ *Alert: Aliskiren:* May increase risk of renal impairment, hypotension, and hyperkalemia in patients with diabetes and those with moderate to severe renal impairment (GFR less than 60 mL/minute). Concomitant use is contraindicated in patients with diabetes. Avoid concomitant use in those with moderate to severe renal impairment.
Lithium: May increase lithium concentration, possibly causing toxicity. Monitor lithium serum concentration, and observe patient's clinical response. Adjust lithium dosage as needed.
NSAIDs, selective cyclooxygenase-2 inhibitors (celecoxib): May result in deterioration of renal function. May decrease antihypertensive effect of irbesartan. Periodically monitor renal function during coadministration.
Potassium-sparing diuretics, potassium supplements, trimethoprim: May increase risk of hyperkalemia. Closely monitor serum potassium concentration and adjust treatment as needed.

EFFECTS ON LAB TEST RESULTS
- May lead to false-negative aldosterone-to-renin ratio.

CONTRAINDICATIONS & CAUTIONS
- Contraindicated in patients hypersensitive to drug or its components.
- Use cautiously in older adults and in patients with volume depletion, impaired renal function, HF, and renal artery stenosis.
Dialyzable drug: No.
⚠ *Overdose S&S:* Hypotension, tachycardia, bradycardia.

PREGNANCY-LACTATION-REPRODUCTION

Boxed Warning Use during pregnancy can cause injury and death to the developing fetus. When pregnancy is detected, stop drug as soon as possible. ■
• It isn't known if drug appears in human milk. Use during breastfeeding isn't recommended because of potential for adverse effects on infant.

NURSING CONSIDERATIONS

• Drug may be given with a diuretic or other antihypertensive, if needed, for control of HTN.
• Symptomatic hypotension may occur in patients who are volume- or sodium-depleted (vigorous diuretic use or dialysis). Correct the cause of volume depletion before administration or before a lower dose is used.
• If hypotension occurs, place patient in a supine position and give an IV infusion of NSS, if needed. Once BP has stabilized after a transient hypotensive episode, drug may be continued.
• Dizziness and orthostatic hypotension may occur more frequently in patients with type 2 diabetes and renal disease.

PATIENT TEACHING

• Warn patient of consequences of drug exposure to fetus and to immediately notify prescriber if pregnancy is suspected.
• Teach patient safe drug administration.
• Tell patient to report all adverse reactions and to inform prescriber of other prescription and OTC drugs and supplements being taken.
• Caution patient not to use potassium supplements or salt substitutes containing potassium without consulting prescriber.

SAFETY ALERT!

irinotecan hydrochloride
eye-rye-no-TEE-kan

Camptosar

Therapeutic class: Antineoplastics
Pharmacologic class: DNA topoisomerase inhibitors

AVAILABLE FORMS

Injection: 20 mg/mL in 2-, 5-, 15-, and 25-mL vials

INDICATIONS & DOSAGES

Adjust-a-dose (for all indications): Consider reducing starting dose by at least one level for patients known to be homozygous (*28/*28, *6/*6) or compound heterozygous for the UGT1A1*28 or *6 alleles (*6/*28). Consider reducing starting dose in patients age 65 and older, in those who have received pelvic or abdominal radiation, or in those who have a performance status of 2 or increased bilirubin level. See manufacturer's instructions for details on dosage adjustments due to toxicities.

➤ **Colorectal cancer, metastatic (single-agent regimen)**
Adults: Initially, 125 mg/m^2 by IV infusion over 90 minutes on days 1, 8, 15, and 22; then 2-week rest period. Thereafter, additional courses of treatment may be repeated every 6 weeks with 4 weeks on and 2 weeks off. Subsequent doses may be adjusted to low of 50 mg/m^2 or maximum of 150 mg/m^2 in 25- to 50-mg/m^2 increments based on patient's tolerance. Or, 350 mg/m^2 by IV infusion over 90 minutes once every 3 weeks. May adjust subsequent doses as low as 200 mg/m^2 in 50-mg/m^2 decrements depending on individual patient tolerance. Additional courses may continue indefinitely in patients who respond favorably and in those whose disease remains stable, provided intolerable toxicity doesn't occur.

➤ **Colorectal cancer, metastatic (combination regimen and 5-FU and leucovorin)**
Regimen 1
Adults: 125 mg/m^2 IV infusion on days 1, 8, 15, and 22; then leucovorin 20 mg/m^2 IV bolus on days 1, 8, 15, and 22 and 5-FU 500 mg/m^2 IV bolus on days 1, 8, 15, and 22. Courses are repeated every 6 weeks.
Regimen 2
Adults: 180 mg/m^2 IV infusion on days 1, 15, and 29; then leucovorin 200 mg/m^2 IV over 2 hours on days 1, 2, 15, 16, 29, and 30; then 5-FU 400 mg/m^2 IV bolus on days 1, 2, 15, 16, 29, and 30 and 5-FU 600 mg/m^2 IV infusion over 22 hours on days 1, 2, 15, 16, 29, and 30.

➤ **Esophageal cancer, metastatic or locally advanced ◆**
Adults: 65 mg/m^2 IV infusion on days 1, 8, 15, and 22 of a 6-week cycle (in combination with cisplatin), or 180 mg/m^2 IV infusion every 2 weeks (in combination with leucovorin and 5-FU), or 250 mg/m^2 IV every 3 weeks (in combination with capecitabine).

Reactions in bold italics are *life-threatening*. Interactions may have a *rapid onset* or a **delayed onset**.

➤ **Gastric cancer, metastatic or locally advanced** ◆

Adults: 150 mg/m^2 IV infusion (as a single agent) on days 1 and 15 of a 4-week cycle, or 65 mg/m^2 IV infusion on days 1, 8, 15, and 22 of a 6-week cycle (in combination with cisplatin), or 70 mg/m^2 IV infusion on days 1 and 15 of a 4-week cycle (in combination with cisplatin) for up to six cycles, or 180 mg/m^2 IV infusion over 90 minutes every 2 weeks (in combination with leucovorin and 5-FU), or 250 mg/m^2 IV every 3 weeks (in combination with capecitabine).

➤ **NSCLC, advanced** ◆

Adults: 60 mg/m^2 IV infusion on days 1, 8, and 15 every 4 weeks (in combination with cisplatin).

➤ **Pancreatic cancer, advanced** ◆

Adults: 180 mg/m^2 IV infusion over 90 minutes every 2 weeks (in combination with oxaliplatin, leucovorin, and 5-FU).

➤ **Pancreatic cancer, potentially curable, adjuvant therapy** ◆

Adults: 150 mg/m^2 IV every 2 weeks (in combination with 5-FU, leucovorin, and oxaliplatin; modified FOLFIRINOX [mFOLFIRINOX] regimen) for 24 weeks.

➤ **Small-cell lung cancer, extensive stage** ◆

Adults: 60 mg/m^2 IV infusion on days 1, 8, and 15 every 4 weeks (in combination with cisplatin), or 65 mg/m^2 IV on days 1 and 8 every 3 weeks (in combination with cisplatin), or 175 mg/m^2 IV on day 1 every 3 weeks (in combination with carboplatin), or 50 mg/m^2 IV on days 1, 8, and 15 every 4 weeks (in combination with carboplatin).

➤ **Rhabdomyosarcoma (metastatic or relapsed/progressive) in children** ◆

Children: 50 mg/m^2 (maximum, 100 mg/dose) IV once daily for 5 days during protocol-specific weeks (in combination with ifosfamide, etoposide, vincristine, doxorubicin, cyclophosphamide, dactinomycin, and radiation; high-risk disease) or 50 mg/m^2 IV once daily for 5 days at weeks 1 and 4 (in combination with vincristine).

ADMINISTRATION

IV

▼ Drug packaged in plastic blister to protect against inadvertent breakage and leakage. Inspect vial for damage and signs of leakage before removing blister.

🖒 *Alert:* Drug is hazardous. Follow special handling and disposal procedures. Wear gloves while handling and preparing infusion solutions. If drug contacts skin, wash thoroughly with soap and water. If drug contacts mucous membranes, flush thoroughly with water.

▼ Dilute drug in D$_5$W injection (preferred) or NSS for injection before infusion to yield a final concentration of 0.12 to 2.8 mg/mL.

▼ Administer by IV infusion, usually over 90 minutes.

▼ Prepare infusion solution immediately before use and infuse as soon as possible after preparation. Discard infusion solution if particulates are visible. If infusion solution can't be used immediately, store for up to 24 hours at 35.6° to 46.4°F (2° to 8°C) or discard it.

▼ Premedicate patient with antiemetic drugs on day of treatment starting at least 30 minutes before giving irinotecan.

▼ Watch for irritation and infiltration; extravasation can cause tissue damage. If extravasation occurs, flush site with sterile water and apply ice. Notify prescriber.

▼ Store vial at 59° to 86° F (15° to 30° C). Protect from light. Vials are single use only; discard unused portion.

▼ **Incompatibilities:** Gemcitabine, pemetrexed.

ACTION

Interacts with topoisomerase I, inducing reversible single-strand DNA breaks. Drug binds to the topoisomerase I–DNA complex and prevents religation of these single-strand breaks.

Route	Onset	Peak	Duration
IV	Unknown	1 hr	Unknown

Half-life: About 6 to 12 hours; active metabolite, 10 to 20 hours.

ADVERSE REACTIONS

CNS: asthenia, dizziness, fever, headache, insomnia, pain, akathisia, confusion, somnolence. **CV:** edema, vasodilation, orthostatic hypotension, *thromboembolic event.* **EENT:** rhinitis. **GI:** diarrhea, abdominal cramping, abdominal pain and enlargement, anorexia, constipation, dyspepsia, flatulence, nausea, stomatitis, vomiting. **Hematologic:** anemia, *leukopenia, neutropenia, thrombocytopenia.* **Hepatic:** bilirubinemia, increased ALP and AST levels. **Metabolic:** dehydration, weight loss. **Musculoskeletal:** back pain.

Respiratory: dyspnea, increased cough, pneumonia. **Skin:** alopecia, rash, diaphoresis. **Other:** chills, infection.

INTERACTIONS

Drug-drug. *CYP3A4 inducers (anticonvulsants [carbamazepine, phenobarbital, phenytoin], rifabutin, rifampin):* May significantly decrease irinotecan levels. Avoid use together. For patients requiring anticonvulsant treatment, consider substituting non–enzyme-inducing anticonvulsants at least 2 weeks before start of irinotecan therapy.
CYP3A4 inhibitors (clarithromycin, indinavir, itraconazole, lopinavir, nefazodone, nelfinavir, ritonavir, saquinavir, telaprevir, voriconazole); UGT1A1 inhibitors (atazanavir, gemfibrozil, indinavir): May increase systemic exposure to irinotecan. Discontinue strong CYP3A4 inhibitors at least 1 week before starting irinotecan. Don't give strong CYP3A4 or UGT1A1 inhibitors with irinotecan unless there are no therapeutic alternatives.
Diuretics: May increase risk of dehydration and electrolyte imbalance. Consider stopping diuretic during active periods of nausea and vomiting.
Ketoconazole: May increase irinotecan levels, leading to drug toxicity. Stop ketoconazole at least 1 week before starting irinotecan therapy. Ketoconazole is contraindicated during irinotecan therapy.
Laxatives: May increase risk of diarrhea. Avoid using together.
Live-virus vaccines: May cause serious or fatal infection. Don't give together.
Neuromuscular blockers: May prolong the neuromuscular-blocking effects of succinylcholine, and the neuromuscular blockade of nondepolarizing drugs may be antagonized. Monitor patient for prolonged effects of succinylcholine if given together.
Other antineoplastics: May cause additive adverse effects, such as myelosuppression and diarrhea. Monitor patient closely.
Prochlorperazine: May increase risk of akathisia. Monitor patient closely.
Vaccines (killed or inactivated virus): May diminish response to vaccine. Avoid use together.
Drug-herb. *St. John's wort:* May decrease drug levels. Use together is contraindicated.
Drug-food. *Grapefruit juice:* May increase irinotecan serum concentration. Avoid combination.

EFFECTS ON LAB TEST RESULTS
• May increase ALP, AST, and bilirubin levels.
• May decrease Hb level and platelet, WBC, and neutrophil counts.

CONTRAINDICATIONS & CAUTIONS
• Contraindicated in patients hypersensitive to drug.
⚕ Patients with UGT1A1*28 allele or UGT1A1 *6 alleles (*28/*28, *6/*6) genotype are at increased risk for neutropenia. Consider UGT1A1 genotype testing for the *28 and *6 alleles to determine UGT1A1 metabolizer status. Monitor patients with these alleles for neutropenia during and after treatment.
• Use cautiously in patients with hepatic impairment. See prescribing information for further guidance.
• Early and late diarrhea can occur and late diarrhea can be fatal. Loperamide should be available for management of late diarrhea.
• Fatal interstitial pulmonary disease (IPD) has been reported. Patients with preexisting lung disease, patients taking pulmonary toxic drugs or colony-stimulating factors, and patients receiving radiation therapy are at increased risk. If IPD is diagnosed, all chemotherapy will be discontinued.
• Rare cases of renal impairment and acute renal failure have been identified, usually in patients who became volume-depleted from severe vomiting or diarrhea.
• Safety and effectiveness in children haven't been established.
• Use cautiously in older adults.
Dialyzable drug: Unknown.
⚠ **Overdose S&S:** Severe neutropenia, severe diarrhea.

PREGNANCY-LACTATION-REPRODUCTION
• May cause fetal harm. Patients of childbearing potential should avoid becoming pregnant during therapy.
• Advise patients of childbearing potential to use effective contraception during treatment and for 6 months after final dose.
• Advise male patients with partners of childbearing potential to use condoms during treatment and for 3 months after final dose.
• Drug appears in human milk. Patient shouldn't breastfeed during treatment and for 7 days after final dose.
• Drug may impair fertility.

Reactions in bold italics are *life-threatening*. Interactions may have a *rapid onset* or a **delayed onset**.

NURSING CONSIDERATIONS
• Administer drug under the supervision of a physician experienced with cancer chemotherapy.
• Verify pregnancy before treatment.
Boxed Warning Drug may cause severe myelosuppression. ▪
Boxed Warning Drug can cause severe diarrhea. Treat diarrhea occurring within 24 hours of drug administration with 0.25 to 1 mg atropine IV, unless contraindicated. Treat late diarrhea (occurring more than 24 hours after irinotecan administration) promptly with loperamide. Monitor patient for dehydration, electrolyte imbalance, or sepsis; treat appropriately. Institute antibiotic therapy if ileus, fever, or severe neutropenia develops. Interrupt therapy and reduce subsequent doses if severe diarrhea occurs. Don't begin a new cycle of therapy until treatment-related diarrhea completely resolves. ▪
• Delay subsequent doses until normal bowel function returns for at least 24 hours without an antidiarrheal.
• Pelvic or abdominal irradiation may increase risk of severe myelosuppression. Avoid use of drug in patients undergoing irradiation.
• If neutropenic fever occurs or if ANC falls below 1000/mm^3, temporarily stop therapy. Manage febrile neutropenia promptly with antibiotics.
• A colony-stimulating factor may be helpful in patients with significant neutropenia.
• Monitor WBC count with differential, Hb level, and platelet count before each dose.
• To decrease risk of dehydration, withhold diuretic during treatment and periods of active vomiting or diarrhea.
• Monitor patient for respiratory signs and symptoms (dyspnea, cough, fever) before and during treatment.
• *Look alike–sound alike:* Don't confuse irinotecan with irinotecan liposome or topotecan.

PATIENT TEACHING
• Inform patient about risk of diarrhea and methods to manage it; tell patient to avoid laxatives.
• Instruct patient to report all adverse reactions and to immediately contact prescriber if any of the following occur: diarrhea for the first time during treatment; black or bloody stools; symptoms of dehydration such as light-headedness, dizziness, or faintness;

inability to drink fluids due to nausea or vomiting; inability to control diarrhea within 24 hours; fever or infection; dyspnea or cough.
• Warn patient that hair loss may occur.
• Inform patient that dizziness or visual disturbances may occur within the first 24 hours after treatment.
• Caution patient to avoid pregnancy and breastfeeding during therapy.
• Advise patient of the risk of impaired infertility.

iron sucrose
eye-ern soo-krose

Venofer

Therapeutic class: Iron supplements
Pharmacologic class: Hematinics

AVAILABLE FORMS
Injection: 20 mg/mL of elemental iron in 2.5-mL, 5-mL, and 10-mL single-dose vials

INDICATIONS & DOSAGES
➤ **Iron deficiency anemia in patients who are hemodialysis dependent**
Adults: 100 mg (5 mL) of elemental iron IV directly in the dialysis line by slow injection over 2 to 5 minutes or by infusion of 100 mg diluted in a maximum of 100 mL NSS over 15 minutes per consecutive hemodialysis session. Administer early during each dialysis session. Usual total treatment course is 1,000 mg; may repeat if iron deficiency recurs.
➤ **Iron deficiency anemia in patients with chronic kidney disease not on dialysis**
Adults: 200 mg by undiluted slow IV injection over 2 to 5 minutes, or as an infusion of 200 mg in a maximum of 100 mL NSS over 15 minutes, on five separate occasions in a 14-day period to a total cumulative dose of 1,000 mg; may repeat if needed.
➤ **Iron deficiency anemia in patients with chronic kidney disease dependent on peritoneal dialysis**
Adults: 300 mg IV infusion over 90 minutes on two separate occasions 14 days apart, followed by one 400-mg infusion over 2½ hours 14 days later. Dilute in a maximum of 250 mL NSS; may repeat if needed.

➤ **Maintenance treatment in children with hemodialysis-dependent chronic kidney disease**

Children ages 2 and older: 0.5 mg/kg IV every 2 weeks for 12 weeks. Give undiluted by slow IV injection over 5 minutes or diluted in 25 mL NSS and administered over 5 to 60 minutes. May repeat if necessary. Don't give more than 100 mg/dose.

➤ **Maintenance treatment in children with nondialysis-dependent chronic kidney disease who are receiving erythropoietin or with peritoneal dialysis-dependent chronic kidney disease who are receiving erythropoietin**

Children ages 2 and older: 0.5 mg/kg IV every 4 weeks for 12 weeks. Give undiluted by slow IV injection over 5 minutes or diluted in 25 mL NSS and administered over 5 to 60 minutes. May repeat treatment if necessary. Don't give more than 100 mg per dose.

➤ **Chemotherapy-associated anemia ◆**

Adults: 200 mg IV once every 3 weeks for five doses. Or, 100 mg IV once weekly during weeks 0 to 6, followed by 100 mg IV every other week from weeks 8 to 14. Or, 200 mg IV once a week after each platinum-based chemotherapy cycle for up to six doses. Or, 200 mg IV after each platinum-based chemotherapy cycle for six cycles.

ADMINISTRATION

IV

▼ Inspect drug for particulate matter and discoloration before giving.

▼ For infusion, dilute 100 mg or 200 mg elemental iron in a maximum of 100 mL NSS immediately before infusion, and infuse over at least 15 minutes. Dilute dose 300 mg or greater in a maximum of 250 mL NSS.

▼ Store in original carton at 68° to 77° F (20° to 25° C). Don't freeze.

▼ Syringe remains stable for 7 days at controlled room temperature or under refrigeration. IV admixture remains stable for 7 days at controlled room temperature when added to an infusion bag containing NSS.

▼ **Incompatibilities:** Other IV drugs, parenteral nutrition solutions.

ACTION

Exogenous source of iron that replenishes depleted body iron stores and is essential for Hb synthesis.

Route	Onset	Peak	Duration
IV	Unknown	Unknown	Variable

Half-life: 6 hours.

ADVERSE REACTIONS

CNS: headache, asthenia, dizziness, fever, dysgeusia. **CV:** *HF,* hypotension, chest pain, HTN, fluid retention, edema, graft complications, AV fistula thrombosis. **EENT:** conjunctivitis, ear pain, nasopharyngitis, sinusitis, nasal congestion. **GI:** nausea, vomiting, diarrhea, abdominal pain, peritonitis. **Metabolic:** gout, *hypoglycemia,* hyperglycemia. **Musculoskeletal:** muscle cramps, bone and muscle pain, arthralgia, back pain, limb pain. **Respiratory:** dyspnea, wheezing, cough, URI. **Skin:** rash, pruritus, injection-site reaction. **Other:** accidental injury, pain, *sepsis,* hypersensitivity reactions.

INTERACTIONS

Drug-drug. *Oral iron preparations:* May reduce absorption of oral iron preparations. Avoid using together.

EFFECTS ON LAB TEST RESULTS

None reported.

CONTRAINDICATIONS & CAUTIONS

• Contraindicated in patients with hypersensitivity to drug or its components, evidence of iron overload, or anemia not caused by iron deficiency.

• Use cautiously in older adults.

Dialyzable drug: No.

⚠ *Overdose S&S:* Accumulation of iron in storage sites, potentially leading to hemosiderosis.

PREGNANCY-LACTATION-REPRODUCTION

• Use during pregnancy only if clearly needed.

• Drug appears in human milk. Use cautiously during breastfeeding and monitor infant for constipation and diarrhea.

NURSING CONSIDERATIONS

⚠ *Alert:* Rare but fatal hypersensitivity reactions, characterized by anaphylactic shock, loss of consciousness, collapse, or hypotension, may occur. Monitor patient during infusion and for at least 30 minutes and until clinically stable after completing infusion. Have

---

emergency equipment and therapies readily available.
- Mild to moderate hypersensitivity reactions, with wheezing, dyspnea, hypotension, rash, or pruritus, may occur.
- Infusing drug may reduce hypotension risk.
- Monitor patient for hypotension, dyspnea, headache, vomiting, nausea, dizziness, joint aches, paresthesia, abdominal pain, muscle pain, edema, and CV collapse, which may occur with rapid infusion or total dose administration.
- Transferrin saturation level increases rapidly after IV administration of drug. Obtain iron level at least 48 hours after IV use.
- Monitor ferritin level, transferrin saturation, Hb level, and hematocrit.
- Withhold dose in patient with signs and symptoms of iron overload.
- Keep dose selection in older adults conservative because of decreased hepatic, renal, or cardiac function; other disease; and other drug therapy.

PATIENT TEACHING
- Instruct patient to report all adverse reactions and notify prescriber immediately if symptoms of overdose or allergic reaction occur.

isoniazid (INH, isonicotinic acid hydrazide) ⌀
eye-soe-NYE-a-zid

Therapeutic class: Antituberculotics
Pharmacologic class: Isonicotinic acid hydrazines

AVAILABLE FORMS
Injection: 100 mg/mL
Oral solution: 50 mg/5 mL
Tablets: 100 mg, 300 mg

INDICATIONS & DOSAGES
Adjust-a-dose (for all indications): Give dose after hemodialysis.
➤ **Active TB with other antituberculotics**
Adults and children age 15 and older:
5 mg/kg daily PO or IM in a single daily dose, up to 300 mg/day, with other drugs, continued for 6 months to 2 years. For intermittent multiple-drug regimen, 15 mg/kg (up to 900 mg) PO or IM up to 3 times/week.

Infants and children: 10 to 15 mg/kg PO or IM in a single daily dose, up to 300 mg/day, continued long enough to prevent relapse. Give with at least one other antituberculotic. For intermittent multidrug regimen, 20 to 40 mg/kg (up to 900 mg) PO or IM two or three times weekly.
➤ **Prevention of TB**
Adults weighing more than 30 kg: 300 mg PO daily in a single dose, continued for 6 months to 1 year.
Infants and children: 10 mg/kg PO daily in a single dose, up to 300 mg/day, continued for up to 1 year. In situations in which adherence with daily preventive therapy can't be assured, 20 to 30 mg/kg (not to exceed 900 mg) twice weekly under the direct observation of a health care worker at the time of administration.

ADMINISTRATION
PO
- Don't give with food.
IM
- Solution may crystallize at a low temperature. Warm vial to room temperature before use to redissolve crystals.
- Inject deep IM into a large muscle mass.
- Store at room temperature.

ACTION
May inhibit cell-wall biosynthesis by interfering with lipid and DNA synthesis; bactericidal.

Route	Onset	Peak	Duration
PO, IM	Unknown	1–2 hr	Unknown

Half-life: 0.5 to 5 hours.

ADVERSE REACTIONS
CNS: peripheral neuropathy, *seizures, toxic encephalopathy,* memory impairment, toxic psychosis, fever. **CV:** vasculitis. **EENT:** optic neuritis and atrophy. **GI:** epigastric distress, nausea, vomiting. **Hematologic:** *agranulocytosis, aplastic anemia, thrombocytopenia,* eosinophilia, hemolytic anemia, sideroblastic anemia. **Hepatic:** *hepatitis,* increased transaminase levels, bilirubinemia, jaundice. **Metabolic:** hyperglycemia, *metabolic acidosis.* **Skin:** irritation at injection site, rash, DRESS syndrome. **Other:** gynecomastia, hypersensitivity reactions, pyridoxine deficiency, rheumatic and lupuslike syndromes.

🍁Canada   ◇OTC   ◆Off-label use   ✐Photoguide   ◉Do not crush   *Liquid contains alcohol   ⌀Genetic

INTERACTIONS

Drug-drug. *Acetaminophen:* May inhibit acetaminophen metabolism. Monitor patient closely for hepatotoxicity.

Antacids and laxatives containing aluminum: May decrease isoniazid absorption. Give isoniazid at least 1 hour before antacid or laxative.

Benzodiazepines (diazepam, triazolam): May inhibit metabolic clearance of benzodiazepines that undergo oxidative metabolism, possibly increasing benzodiazepine activity. Monitor for adverse effects.

Carbamazepine: May increase carbamazepine levels. Monitor drug levels closely.

Cycloserine: May increase CNS adverse reactions. Use safety precautions.

Disulfiram: May cause neurologic symptoms, including behavior and coordination changes. Avoid using together.

Enflurane: In rapid acetylators of isoniazid, may cause high-output renal failure because of nephrotoxic inorganic fluoride level. Monitor renal function.

Ketoconazole: May decrease ketoconazole level. Monitor for lack of effectiveness.

Meperidine: May increase CNS adverse reactions and hypotension. Use safety precautions.

Oral anticoagulants: May enhance anticoagulant activity. Monitor PT and INR.

Phenytoin: May inhibit phenytoin metabolism and increase phenytoin level. Monitor patient for phenytoin toxicity.

Rifampin: May increase risk of hepatotoxicity. Monitor LFT values closely.

Theophylline: May increase theophylline level and, in some instances, slightly decrease isoniazid elimination. Monitor theophylline level closely; adjust dosage as appropriate.

Valproate: May increase valproate plasma level. Monitor valproate plasma concentration; adjust dosage as necessary.

Drug-food. *Foods containing histamines (saury, skipjack tuna, other tropical fish):* May cause headache, diaphoresis, palpitations, flushing, diarrhea, itching, wheezing, dyspnea, or hypotension. Patients should avoid these foods during therapy.

Foods containing tyramine (aged cheese, beer, chocolate): May cause hypertensive crisis. Patients should avoid such foods.

Drug-lifestyle. *Alcohol use:* May increase risk of drug-related hepatitis. Discourage use of alcohol.

EFFECTS ON LAB TEST RESULTS

- May increase transaminase, glucose, and bilirubin levels.
- May increase eosinophil count.
- May decrease Hb level and granulocyte and platelet counts.
- May alter result of urine glucose tests that use cupric sulfate method, such as Benedict reagent and Diastix.

CONTRAINDICATIONS & CAUTIONS

Boxed Warning Contraindicated in patients with acute hepatic disease or isoniazid-related liver damage. Severe and sometimes fatal hepatitis associated with drug may occur even after months of treatment but usually occurs during first 3 months of treatment. Risk of developing hepatitis is age-related (increases with age), increases with daily alcohol use, and may be more common in women who are Black or Hispanic, particularly during the postpartum period. If signs or symptoms suggest hepatic damage, discontinue isoniazid because a more severe form of liver damage can occur. ∎

Boxed Warning Defer preventative treatment in patients with acute hepatic disease. ∎

Boxed Warning Treat patients with TB who have isoniazid-related hepatitis with alternative drugs. If isoniazid must be restarted, use only after symptoms and lab abnormalities have resolved. ∎

- Use cautiously in older adults, in patients with chronic non–isoniazid-related liver disease or chronic alcoholism, those with seizure disorders (especially if taking phenytoin), and those with severe renal impairment.

Dialyzable drug: Yes.

⚠ *Overdose S&S:* Nausea, vomiting, dizziness, slurring of speech, blurring of vision, visual hallucinations, respiratory distress, CNS depression progressing from stupor to coma, seizures, severe metabolic acidosis, acetonuria, hyperglycemia.

PREGNANCY-LACTATION-REPRODUCTION

- There are no adequate studies during pregnancy; however, drug should be used as a treatment for active TB during pregnancy because benefit justifies fetal risk.
- Weigh benefit of preventive therapy against fetal risk. Preventive therapy generally should be started after delivery to prevent putting fetus at risk for exposure.

Reactions in bold italics are *life-threatening*. Interactions may have a *rapid onset* or a ***delayed onset***.

• Small amounts of drug in human milk don't produce toxicity in infants who are breastfed. Don't discourage breastfeeding.

NURSING CONSIDERATIONS

⧩ Drug's pharmacokinetics vary among patients because drug is metabolized in the liver by genetically controlled acetylation. Fast acetylators metabolize drug up to 5 times faster than slow acetylators. About 50% of Blacks and Whites are fast acetylators; more than 80% of patients who are Chinese, Japanese, and Inuit are fast acetylators. A report suggests the risk of fatal hepatitis increases in women who are Black or Hispanic and in the postpartum period. The risk of hepatitis increases with daily alcohol use and with age.

⧩ Peripheral neuropathy is more common in patients who are slow acetylators, malnourished, alcoholic, or diabetic. Give pyridoxine to prevent peripheral neuropathy.

Boxed Warning Monitor and interview patients monthly. For those patients older than age 35, also measure hepatic enzyme levels before and periodically throughout treatment. Elevated LFT results occur in about 15% of patients; most abnormalities are mild and transient, but some may persist throughout treatment, and progressive liver dysfunction may occur. If LFT values exceed 3 to 5 × ULN, strongly consider discontinuing treatment. ▪

Boxed Warning Monitor patient for hepatotoxicity. ▪

PATIENT TEACHING

• Instruct patient to take drug exactly as prescribed; warn against stopping drug without prescriber's consent.

• Advise patient that drug shouldn't be taken with food.

Boxed Warning Tell patient to notify prescriber immediately if signs and symptoms of liver impairment occur, such as appetite loss, fatigue, malaise, yellowing of skin or eyes, dark urine, fever of more than 3 days' duration, and abdominal tenderness, particularly of the right upper quadrant. ▪

• Advise patient to avoid alcoholic beverages while taking drug and to avoid certain foods: fish (such as skipjack tuna) and products containing tyramine (such as aged cheese, beer, and chocolate) because drug has some MAO inhibitor activity.

⧩ Caution patient who is a slow acetylator, malnourished, alcoholic, or diabetic to take pyridoxine, as prescribed, to prevent peripheral neuropathy.

• Encourage patient to comply fully with treatment, which may take months or years.

isosorbide dinitrate
eye-soe-SOR-bide

ISDN✤, Isordil

isosorbide mononitrate
Apo-ISMN✤, Imdur✤, Monoket, PMS-ISMN✤, PRO-ISMN✤

Therapeutic class: Antianginals
Pharmacologic class: Nitrates

AVAILABLE FORMS
isosorbide dinitrate
Tablets: 5 mg, 10 mg, 20 mg, 30 mg, 40 mg
Tablets (extended-release) ⓒ: 40 mg
isosorbide mononitrate
Tablets: 10 mg, 20 mg
Tablets (extended-release) ⓒ: 30 mg, 60 mg, 120 mg

INDICATIONS & DOSAGES
➤ **Treatment (immediate-release isosorbide mononitrate only) and prevention of angina pectoris**
Adults (dinitrate): For immediate release, 5 to 20 mg PO b.i.d. to t.i.d., titrated to a maximum of 40 mg PO b.i.d. to t.i.d. For extended-release, usual dose is 40 to 160 mg PO daily.
Adults (mononitrate): For immediate release, 5 to 20 mg PO b.i.d., with the two doses given 7 hours apart. For extended-release, 30 to 60 mg PO daily; titrate every 3 days to 120 mg PO daily. Rarely, 240 mg may be required.
➤ **HF (isosorbide dinitrate)** ◆
Adults: 20 mg immediate-release PO t.i.d. (in combination with hydralazine). Titrate dose every 2 to 4 weeks, as tolerated, to target dose of 40 mg t.i.d. Maximum dose, 120 mg daily in divided doses.

ADMINISTRATION
PO
• Tell patient taking isosorbide dinitrate to swallow oral tablet whole on an empty stomach either 30 minutes before or 1 to 2 hours after meals.

✤Canada ◇OTC ◆Off-label use ✐Photoguide ⓒ Do not crush *Liquid contains alcohol ⧩Genetic

- Store drug in a cool place, in a tightly closed container, and away from light.
- Don't crush or allow patient to chew extended-release tablets.
- Don't give around the clock; allow nitrate-free interval for at least 14 hours for immediate-release products and longer than 18 hours for extended-release products.

ACTION

Thought to reduce cardiac oxygen demand by decreasing preload and afterload. Drug also may increase blood flow through the collateral coronary vessels.

Route	Onset	Peak	Duration
PO	30–45 min	30–60 min	4–8 hr
PO (extended-release)	0.5–4 hr	Unknown	6–12 hr

Half-life: Dinitrate PO, 5 to 6 hours; mononitrate, about 5 hours.

ADVERSE REACTIONS

CNS: headache, fatigue, dizziness, transient light-headedness, weakness, pain, emotional lability, syncope. **CV:** orthostatic hypotension, tachycardia, palpitations, ankle edema, flushing, chest pain, crescendo angina, rebound HTN. **GI:** nausea, abdominal pain. **Respiratory:** URI, cough. **Skin:** cutaneous vasodilation, rash, pruritus. **Other:** hypersensitivity reaction.

INTERACTIONS

Drug-drug. *Antihypertensives:* May increase hypotensive effects. Monitor patient closely during initial therapy.
PDE5 inhibitors (avanafil, sildenafil, tadalafil, vardenafil), riociguat: May cause life-threatening hypotension. Use of nitrates in any form with these drugs is contraindicated.
Drug-lifestyle. *Alcohol use:* May increase hypotension. Discourage use together.

EFFECTS ON LAB TEST RESULTS

- May falsely reduce value in cholesterol tests using the Zlatkis-Zak color reaction.

CONTRAINDICATIONS & CAUTIONS

- Contraindicated in patients with hypersensitivity or idiosyncrasy to nitrates and in those with severe hypotension, increased ICP, shock, or acute MI with low left ventricular filling pressure.

- Nitrates may aggravate angina caused by hypertrophic cardiomyopathy.
- Rarely, methemoglobinemia can occur with drug use.
- Use cautiously in patients with blood volume depletion (such as from diuretic therapy), mild hypotension, or suspected right ventricular infarction.
- Safety and effectiveness in children haven't been established.
Dialyzable drug: Mononitrate, yes; dinitrate, unknown.
⚠ *Overdose S&S:* Venous pooling, decreased cardiac output, hypotension, methemoglobinemia, headache, confusion, vertigo, fever, palpitations, nausea, vomiting (possibly with colic and bloody diarrhea), syncope, air hunger, dyspnea, slow breathing, diaphoresis, flushed skin, heart block, bradycardia, paralysis, coma.

PREGNANCY-LACTATION-REPRODUCTION

- There are no adequate studies during pregnancy. Use during pregnancy only if clearly needed.
- It isn't known if drug appears in human milk. Use cautiously during breastfeeding.

NURSING CONSIDERATIONS

- To prevent tolerance, a nitrate-free interval of 10 to 14 hours per day is recommended. The regimen for isosorbide mononitrate (1 tablet on awakening with the second dose in 7 hours, or 1 extended-release tablet daily) is intended to minimize nitrate tolerance by providing a substantial nitrate-free interval.
- Monitor BP, HR, and intensity and duration of drug response.
- Drug may cause headaches, especially at beginning of therapy. Dosage may be reduced temporarily, but tolerance usually develops. Treat headache with aspirin or acetaminophen.
- Monitor patient for methemoglobinemia, which has occurred with nitrate use. Signs and symptoms are those of impaired oxygen delivery despite adequate cardiac output and adequate arterial partial pressure of oxygen.
- *Look alike–sound alike:* Don't confuse Isordil with Plendil, Isuprel, or Inderal.

PATIENT TEACHING

- Caution patient to take drug as prescribed.

Reactions in bold italics are *life-threatening*. Interactions may have a *rapid onset* or a *delayed onset*.

⟲ Alert: Advise patient that stopping drug abruptly may cause increased angina symptoms and risk of MI.

• Instruct patient in safe drug administration, the need for nitrate-free intervals to minimize tolerance, and storage.

• Tell patient to change to an upright position slowly, to climb stairs carefully, and to lie down at first sign of dizziness.

• Caution patient to avoid alcohol because it may worsen low BP effects.

• Advise patient that use of sildenafil, tadalafil, vardenafil, or avanafil with any nitrate may cause severe low BP. Counsel patient to talk to prescriber before using these drugs together.

ISOtretinoin
eye-so-TRET-i-noyn

Absorica, Absorica LD, Amnesteem, Claravis, Myorisan, Zenatane

Therapeutic class: Antiacne drugs
Pharmacologic class: Retinoic acid derivatives

AVAILABLE FORMS
Capsules: 10 mg, 20 mg, 25 mg, 30 mg, 35 mg, 40 mg
Capsules (Absorica LD): 8 mg, 16 mg, 24 mg, 32 mg

INDICATIONS & DOSAGES
➤ **Severe recalcitrant nodular acne that's unresponsive to conventional therapy**
Adults and adolescents age 12 and older: 0.5 to 1 mg/kg/day PO in two divided doses for 15 to 20 weeks. Or, 0.4 to 0.8 mg/kg/day in two divided doses for 15 to 20 weeks (Absorica LD).
Adjust-a-dose: For adults with very severe disease and scarring or with disease primarily on the trunk, increase to 2 mg/kg/day in two divided doses, or 1.6 mg/kg/day in two divided doses (Absorica LD)
➤ **Moderate acne ◆**
Adults: 20 mg/day (approximately 0.3 to 0.4 mg/kg/day) PO for 6 months, or 0.25 to 0.4 mg/kg daily for 24 weeks.
Children and adolescents ages 12 to 17: 0.25 to 0.4 mg/day PO for 6 to 12 months.
➤ **High-risk neuroblastoma in children, in combination with dinutuximab,**

sargramostim, and aldesleukin, when given after chemotherapy or hematopoietic stem cell transplantation ◆
Children: 80 mg/m^2 every 12 hours on days 15 through 28 of a 28-day cycle for six cycles.

ADMINISTRATION
PO
• Hazardous agent; use safe handling and disposal precautions.

• Before use, have patient read patient information and sign consent form.

• Give drug with or shortly after meals to facilitate absorption, except Absorica or Absorica LD, which may be given without regard to meals.

• Have patient swallow capsule whole with full glass of liquid.

• Absorica isn't substitutable with Absorica LD due to differences in bioavailability.

ACTION
May normalize keratinization, reversibly decrease size of sebaceous glands, and make sebum less viscous and less likely to plug follicles.

Route	Onset	Peak	Duration
PO (Absorica)	Unknown	2.9–6.4 hr	Unknown
PO (Absorica LD)	Unknown	3.5–5 hr	Unknown

Half-life: 18 hours (Absorica); 24 hours (Absorica LD).

ADVERSE REACTIONS
CNS: pseudotumor cerebri, depression, *psychosis, suicidality, aggressive and violent behavior,* hallucinations, emotional instability, headache, fatigue, irritability, pain, dizziness, syncope, drowsiness, insomnia, weakness, lethargy, malaise, nervousness, paresthesia, *seizure, stroke.* **CV:** palpitations, edema, *vascular thrombotic disease,* tachycardia. **EENT:** conjunctivitis, corneal deposits, dry eyes, decreased night vision, visual disturbances, tinnitus, hearing impairment (sometimes irreversible), nasopharyngitis, epistaxis, drying of mucous membranes, dry mouth, dry nose, gum bleeding and inflammation, dry lips, lip inflammation, stye, voice alteration. **GI:** nonspecific GI symptoms, nausea, vomiting, constipation, diarrhea, abdominal pain, anorexia, *acute pancreatitis,* inflammatory bowel disease, esophagitis, esophageal ulceration, colitis. **GU:** abnormal menses, sexual

dysfunction, hematuria, glomerulonephritis. **Hematologic:** increased erythrocyte sedimentation rate, anemia, ***thrombocythemia, thrombocytopenia, neutropenia.*** **Hepatic:** increased liver enzyme levels, ***hepatitis.*** **Metabolic:** hypertriglyceridemia, decreased HDL level, hypercholesterolemia, hyperglycemia, weight loss. **Musculoskeletal:** skeletal hyperostosis, tendon and ligament calcification, premature epiphyseal closure, decreased bone mineral density and other bone abnormalities, back pain, myalgia, arthralgia, stiffness, arthritis, tendinitis. **Respiratory:** ***bronchospasm,*** respiratory tract infections. **Skin:** cheilosis, fragility, rash, dry skin, facial skin desquamation, petechiae, pruritus, nail brittleness, thinning of hair, skin infection, peeling of palms and toes, photosensitivity reaction. **Other:** hypersensitivity reaction, infection, lymphadenopathy.

INTERACTIONS

Drug-drug. *Corticosteroids:* May increase risk of osteoporosis. Use together cautiously. *Fluoride, folate, iron, minerals, multivitamins:* May enhance adverse or toxic effect of retinoic acid derivatives. Avoid combination. *Medicated soaps, cleansers, and cover-ups; preparations containing alcohol; topical resorcinol peeling agents (benzoyl peroxide):* May have cumulative drying effect. Use together cautiously.
Micro-dose progesterone hormonal contraceptives ("minipills") that don't contain estrogen: May decrease effectiveness of contraceptive. Advise patient to use different contraceptive method.
Phenytoin: May increase risk of osteomalacia. Use together cautiously.
Products containing vitamin A: May increase toxic effects of isotretinoin. Avoid using together.
Tetracyclines: May increase risk of pseudotumor cerebri. Avoid using together.
Drug-herb. *St. John's wort:* May decrease effectiveness of hormonal contraceptives. Avoid use together.
Drug-food. *Any high-fat food:* May increase absorption of drug. Advise patient to take drug with milk, a meal, or shortly after a meal.
Drug-lifestyle. *Alcohol use:* May increase risk of hypertriglyceridemia. Discourage use together.

Sun or UV exposure: May increase photosensitivity reaction. Advise patient to avoid excessive sunlight or UV ray exposure.

EFFECTS ON LAB TEST RESULTS
- May increase AST, ALT, ALP, GGT, CK, triglyceride, LDL, LDH, glucose, and uric acid levels.
- May decrease serum HDL level.
- May increase platelet count and erythrocyte sedimentation rate.
- May increase urinary WBC and RBC counts and protein level.

CONTRAINDICATIONS & CAUTIONS
- Contraindicated in patients hypersensitive to parabens (used as preservatives), vitamin A, or other retinoids.
- Use cautiously in patients with a history of mental illness or a family history of psychiatric disorders, asthma, liver disease, diabetes, heart disease, hearing impairment, hypertriglyceridemia, inflammatory bowel disease, osteoporosis, genetic predisposition for age-related osteoporosis, history of childhood osteoporosis, weak bones, anorexia nervosa, osteomalacia, or other disorders of bone metabolism.
- Drug may cause erythema multiforme and SCAR (such as SJS or TEN), which may be serious and result in hospitalization, disability, life-threatening events, or death.
- Rarely, rhabdomyolysis has been reported.
Dialyzable drug: Unknown.
⚠ ***Overdose S&S:*** Vomiting, facial flushing, abdominal pain, headache, dizziness, ataxia.

PREGNANCY-LACTATION-REPRODUCTION
Boxed Warning Contraindicated during pregnancy. There is an extremely high risk of severe birth defects if pregnancy occurs while patient is taking isotretinoin in any amount, even for short periods. Any fetus exposed during pregnancy can be affected; there are no accurate means of determining whether an exposed fetus has been affected. There is an increased risk of spontaneous abortion, and premature births have been reported. ∎
Boxed Warning To minimize risk of fetal exposure, drug is only available through a REMS program (iPLEDGE). ∎
🚱 ***Alert:*** Patient must have negative results from two urine or serum pregnancy tests, one performed in the office when patient is qualified for therapy and the second performed

during the first 5 days of the next normal menstrual period immediately preceding beginning of therapy. A pregnancy test must be repeated every month and must be negative before each course of therapy. For patients with amenorrhea, the second test should be done within 7 days after office visit and immediately preceding beginning of therapy. A pregnancy test must be repeated every month before patient receives the prescription. For patients with irregular cycles, or for those using a contraceptive method that precludes withdrawal bleeding, the second pregnancy test must be done within 7 days after office visit, immediately preceding beginning of therapy, and after patient has used two forms of contraception for 1 month.

Boxed Warning If pregnancy does occur during treatment, discontinue drug immediately and refer patient to an obstetrician-gynecologist experienced in reproductive toxicity. ∎

• It isn't known if drug appears in human milk. Patient should discontinue breastfeeding or discontinue drug.

NURSING CONSIDERATIONS

• If total nodule count has been reduced by more than 70% before patient has completed 15 to 20 weeks of treatment, drug may be discontinued.

• A second course of therapy may begin 8 weeks after completion of first course, if necessary. Improvement may continue after completion of first course.

• Monitor baseline lipid studies, LFTs, and pregnancy tests before therapy and at monthly intervals.

• Regularly monitor glucose levels.

• Monitor patient for tinnitus and hearing loss; discontinue drug and refer patient for further evaluation if they occur.

• Monitor patient for inflammatory bowel disease (abdominal pain, rectal bleeding, severe diarrhea); discontinue drug immediately if signs or symptoms occur.

• Closely watch for and report severe skin reactions. Drug may need to be discontinued.

• Most adverse reactions occur at doses exceeding 1 mg/kg daily. Reactions are generally reversible after dosage reduction or therapy discontinuation.

🔵 *Alert:* If patient experiences headache, nausea and vomiting, or visual disturbances, screen for papilledema. Signs and symptoms

of pseudotumor cerebri require stopping the drug immediately and beginning neurologic interventions promptly.

🔵 *Alert:* Monitor patient for mood disturbance, psychosis, aggressive behavior, or suicidality. Drug may need to be discontinued and patient evaluated.

• Patients may be at increased risk of bone fractures or injury when participating in sports with repetitive impact.

• Spontaneous reports of osteoporosis, osteopenia, bone fractures, and delayed healing of bone fractures have occurred in patients taking drug. To decrease this risk, don't exceed recommended doses and duration.

PATIENT TEACHING

🔵 *Alert:* Warn patient of childbearing potential that if drug is used during pregnancy, severe fetal abnormalities may occur. Patient must commit to either abstain from sex or use two reliable forms of contraception simultaneously for 1 month before, during, and for 1 month after treatment. An isotretinoin medication guide must be given to patient each time isotretinoin is dispensed, as required by law.

• Instruct patient in safe drug administration and handling.

• Tell patient to immediately report visual disturbances, tinnitus, and bone, muscle, or joint pain.

• Warn patient that contact lenses may feel uncomfortable during therapy.

• Advise patient not to drive at night until effect on vision is known. Drug may decrease night vision.

• Warn patient against using abrasives, medicated soaps and cleansers, acne preparations containing peeling drugs, and topical products containing alcohol (including cosmetics, aftershave, cologne) because they may cause cumulative irritation or excessive drying of skin.

• Tell patient to avoid prolonged sun or UV light exposure and to use sunblock and wear protective clothing. Drug may have additive effect if used with other drugs that cause photosensitivity reaction.

• Inform patient that transient exacerbations may occur during therapy.

• Warn patient not to donate blood during therapy and for 1 month after stopping drug because drug could harm fetus of a pregnant recipient.

- Advise patient to consult prescriber before taking OTC medications, vitamins, or herbal supplements.
- Tell patient to report adverse reactions immediately, especially depression, suicidality, persistent headaches, visual disturbances, severe skin reactions, and persistent GI pain.
🕭 *Alert:* Advise patient to read iPLEDGE carefully and to fully understand all information before signing it.

itraconazole
eye-tra-KON-a-zole

Sporanox, Tolsura

Therapeutic class: Antifungals
Pharmacologic class: Synthetic triazoles

AVAILABLE FORMS
Capsules ⬤**C**: 65 mg,100 mg
Oral solution: 10 mg/mL

INDICATIONS & DOSAGES
➤ **Pulmonary and extrapulmonary blastomycosis, nonmeningeal histoplasmosis (capsules)**
Adults: 200 mg PO daily; increase as needed and tolerated by 100 mg to maximum of 400 mg daily. Give dosages exceeding 200 mg PO daily in two divided doses. Continue treatment for at least 3 months. In life-threatening illness, give a loading dose of 200 mg PO t.i.d. for 3 days. Or, 130 mg Tolsura (two 65-mg capsules) PO daily; increase as needed and tolerated by 65 mg to maximum of 260 mg/day. Give dosages exceeding 130 mg PO daily in two divided doses. Continue treatment for at least 3 months. In life-threatening illness, give loading dose of 130 mg t.i.d. for 3 days.
➤ **Aspergillosis (capsules)**
Adults: 200 to 400 mg PO daily for at least 3 months. In life-threatening illness, give loading dose of 200 mg PO t.i.d. for first 3 days of treatment. Or, Tolsura 130 to 260 mg PO daily. Continue treatment for at least 3 months. In life-threatening illness, give loading dose of 130 mg t.i.d. for 3 days.
➤ **Onychomycosis of the toenail (with or without fingernail involvement)**
Adults: 200 mg PO once daily for 12 consecutive weeks.

➤ **Onychomycosis of the fingernail**
Adults: 200 mg PO b.i.d. for 1 week, followed by 3 weeks drug-free. Repeat dosage.
➤ **Oropharyngeal candidiasis**
Adults: 200 mg oral solution swished in mouth vigorously and swallowed daily, for 1 to 2 weeks.
➤ **Oropharyngeal candidiasis in patients unresponsive to fluconazole tablets**
Adults: 100 mg oral solution swished in mouth vigorously and swallowed b.i.d., for 2 to 4 weeks.
➤ **Esophageal candidiasis**
Adults: 100 to 200 mg oral solution swished in mouth vigorously and swallowed daily, for at least 3 weeks. Treatment should continue for 2 weeks after symptoms resolve.

ADMINISTRATION
PO
- Obtain specimen for culture and other relevant lab studies before first dose. Begin therapy while awaiting results.
- Before starting therapy, confirm diagnosis of onychomycosis by sending nail specimens for testing.
- Don't interchange capsules with oral solution.
- Give capsules with a full meal.
- Give oral solution on an empty stomach if possible.
- Patient should swallow capsule whole and not crush, chew, or break it.
- Have patient vigorously swish oral solution in mouth for several seconds and then swallow.
- Store capsules at room temperature; protect from light and moisture.
- Store oral solution at or below 77° F (25° C). Don't freeze. Protect from light and moisture.

ACTION
Interferes with fungal cell-wall synthesis by inhibiting ergosterol formation and increasing cell-wall permeability, leading to osmotic instability.

Route	Onset	Peak	Duration
PO	Unknown	2–5 hr	7–14 days

Half-life: Single dose, 16 to 28 hours; repeated dosing, 34 to 42 hours.

ADVERSE REACTIONS
CNS: headache, fever, dizziness, somnolence, fatigue, malaise, asthenia, pain, tremor,

---

abnormal dreams, anxiety, depression, insomnia, vertigo. **CV: *HF,*** HTN, chest pain, edema, orthostatic hypotension, vasculitis. **EENT:** tinnitus, rhinitis, sinusitis, pharyngitis. **GI:** nausea, vomiting, diarrhea, abdominal pain, anorexia, dyspepsia, flatulence, increased appetite, constipation, gastritis, gastroenteritis, ulcerative stomatitis, gingivitis. **GU:** albuminuria, cystitis, UTI, decreased libido, erectile dysfunction, menstrual disorder. **Hepatic:** impaired hepatic function. **Metabolic:** *hypokalemia,* hypertriglyceridemia, adrenal insufficiency. **Musculoskeletal:** myalgia. **Respiratory:** URI, cough, dyspnea, increased sputum, *Pneumocystis jiroveci* infection. **Skin:** rash, pruritus, diaphoresis. **Other:** gynecomastia, male breast pain, injury, herpes zoster, hypersensitivity reactions.

INTERACTIONS

Consult manufacturer's instructions or drug interactions resource for a full list of interactions.

Drug-drug. *Alprazolam:* May increase and prolong drug levels, CNS depression, and psychomotor impairment. Avoid using together.

*Antacids, carbamazepine, H₂-receptor antagonists, isoniazid, phenobarbital, **phenytoin**, rifabutin, rifampin:* May decrease itraconazole level. Avoid using together.

Boxed Warning *Avanafil , cisapride, disopyramide, dofetilide, dronedarone, eplerenone, ergot alkaloids (such as dihydroergotamine, ergometrine [ergonovine], ergotamine, methylergometrine [methylergonovine]), felodipine, irinotecan, isavuconazole, ivabradine, lomitapide, lovastatin, lurasidone, methadone, naloxegol, nisoldipine, oral midazolam, pimozide, quinidine, ranolazine, simvastatin, ticagrelor, triazolam:* May increase levels of these drugs by CYP450 metabolism, causing serious CV events, including torsades de pointes, QT-interval prolongation, ventricular tachycardia, cardiac arrest, and sudden death. Use together is contraindicated. ∎

Chlordiazepoxide, clonazepam, clorazepate, diazepam, estazolam, flurazepam, quazepam: May increase and prolong drug levels, CNS depression, and psychomotor impairment. Avoid using together.

Ciprofloxacin, clarithromycin, erythromycin: May increase itraconazole levels. Monitor patient for signs of itraconazole toxicity.

Boxed Warning *Colchicine:* May increase colchicine level. Contraindicated in patients with renal or hepatic impairment during and for 2 weeks after itraconazole treatment. Monitor therapy in all other patients and reduce colchicine dosage. ∎

*Cyclosporine, **digoxin**, tacrolimus:* May increase levels of these drugs. Monitor drug levels.

Boxed Warning *Eliglustat:* May increase eliglustat level. Contraindicated in patients who are poor or intermediate metabolizers of CYP2D6 or in those taking strong or moderate CYP2D6 inhibitors. ∎

Boxed Warning *Fesoterodine:* May increase fesoterodine metabolite level. Contraindicated in patients with moderate to severe renal or hepatic impairment during and for 2 weeks after itraconazole treatment. Monitor all other patients for adverse reactions and limit fesoterodine dose. ∎

HMG-CoA reductase inhibitors (atorvastatin, lomitapide, lovastatin, simvastatin): May increase levels and adverse effects of these drugs. Use together is contraindicated during and for 2 weeks after itraconazole treatment except atorvastatin, which may be used at a reduced dosage.

NNRTIs (efavirenz, nevirapine): May decrease itraconazole level. Use together isn't recommended.

Oral anticoagulants: May enhance anticoagulant effect. Monitor PT and INR.

Oral antidiabetics: May cause hypoglycemia, similar to effect of other antifungals. Monitor glucose level. Avoid using together.

PDE5 inhibitors (sildenafil, tadalafil, vardenafil): May increase levels of these drugs, increasing adverse effects. Give PDE5 inhibitors with caution and in reduced doses.

Protease inhibitors (ritonavir, saquinavir): May increase levels of these drugs; ritonavir may increase itraconazole levels. Monitor patient for toxicity and reduce itraconazole dose if necessary.

Boxed Warning *Solifenacin:* May increase solifenacin level. Contraindicated in patients with severe renal or moderate to severe hepatic impairment during and for 2 weeks after itraconazole treatment. Monitor all other patients for adverse effects and limit solifenacin dose. ∎

EFFECTS ON LAB TEST RESULTS
• May increase ALP, ALT, AST, bilirubin, LDH, urea, glucose, triglyceride, and GGT levels.
• May decrease magnesium, calcium, and phosphate levels.
• May increase or decrease potassium level.

CONTRAINDICATIONS & CAUTIONS
Boxed Warning Contraindicated in patients taking certain drugs metabolized by CYP3A4 enzymes. Administration with itraconazole can cause elevated plasma concentrations and may increase or prolong pharmacologic effects and adverse reactions to these drugs. For example, increased plasma concentrations of some of these drugs can lead to QT-interval prolongation and ventricular tachyarrhythmias, including potentially fatal torsades de pointes. ■
• Contraindicated in patients hypersensitive to drug.
• Use cautiously in patients with hypochlorhydria, who may not absorb drug readily. Hypochlorhydria can accompany HIV infection.
Boxed Warning Don't use drug to treat onychomycosis in patients with evidence of ventricular dysfunction, such as HF or history of HF. If signs or symptoms of HF occur while giving oral solution, reassess continued use. If signs or symptoms of HF occur while giving capsules, discontinue use. ■
• Use cautiously in patients receiving other highly bound drugs and in patients with renal or hepatic impairment.
• Drug may cause transient or permanent hearing loss, particularly in older adults.
• Safety and effectiveness in children haven't been determined.
Dialyzable drug: No.

PREGNANCY-LACTATION-REPRODUCTION
• Don't use to treat onychomycosis in patients who are pregnant, contemplating pregnancy, or are of childbearing potential unless they are using effective contraceptive measures and they begin therapy on the second or third day after onset of menses. Effective contraception should be continued throughout therapy and for 2 months after therapy ends.
• Drug may cause maternal or fetal harm. Use to treat systemic fungal infections during pregnancy only if benefit justifies risk.

• Drug appears in human milk. Weigh expected benefits for patient against risk to infant.

NURSING CONSIDERATIONS
• Perform baseline LFTs and monitor results periodically. In patients with baseline hepatic impairment, give drug only if patient's condition is life threatening. If liver dysfunction occurs during therapy, notify prescriber immediately.
• Monitor patient for hearing loss.
• Monitor patient for signs and symptoms of HF during treatment.
• Monitor patient for hypersensitivity reactions.
• Monitor patient for peripheral neuropathy with long-term use.

PATIENT TEACHING
• Teach patient to recognize and report signs and symptoms of liver disease (anorexia, dark urine, pale stools, unusual fatigue, and jaundice) or hearing loss.
• Instruct patient in safe drug administration.
• Urge patient to list other drugs being taken, to avoid drug interactions.
• Advise patient of childbearing potential that an effective form of contraception must be used during therapy and for two menstrual cycles after stopping therapy.

ivabradine
eye-VAB-ra-deen

Corlanor, Lancora ✦

Therapeutic class: CV agents
Pharmacologic class: Cyclic nucleotide-gated channel blockers

AVAILABLE FORMS
Solution: 5 mg/mL
Tablets: 5 mg, 7.5 mg

INDICATIONS & DOSAGES
➤ **To reduce risk of hospitalization for worsening HF in patients with stable, symptomatic chronic HF with LVEF of 35% or less who are in sinus rhythm with resting HR of 70 beats/minute (bpm) or more and either are on maximally tolerated doses of beta blockers or have a contraindication to beta blocker use**

Adults: Initially, 5 mg PO b.i.d. After 2 weeks, adjust dosage to achieve resting HR of 50 to 60 bpm if necessary. Maximum dose is 7.5 mg b.i.d.

Adjust-a-dose: In patients with conduction defects or bradycardia that could lead to hemodynamic compromise, initiate therapy at 2.5 mg b.i.d. before increasing dosage based on HR. If HR is greater than 60 bpm, increase dosage by 2.5 mg b.i.d. up to a maximum of 7.5 mg b.i.d. If HR is less than 50 bpm or patient has signs and symptoms of bradycardia, decrease dosage by 2.5 mg b.i.d.; however, if current dosage is 2.5 mg b.i.d., discontinue therapy.

➤ **Stable symptomatic HF due to dilated cardiomyopathy in patients in sinus rhythm with an elevated HR**

Children age 6 months and older weighing more than 40 kg (tablets): 2.5 mg PO b.i.d. After 2 weeks, adjust dose by 2.5 mg to a target HR reduction of at least 20% based on tolerability. Maximum dose, 7.5 mg b.i.d.

Children age 6 months and older weighing less than 40 kg (oral solution): 0.05 mg/kg/dose b.i.d. Adjust dose at 2-week intervals by 0.05 mg/kg/dose to a target HR reduction of at least 20% based on tolerability. Maximum dose, 0.2 mg/kg/day in children age 6 months to 1 year. Or, 0.3 mg/kg/day to a maximum of 7.5 mg b.i.d. in children age 1 year and older.

Adjust-a-dose: If bradycardia develops, reduce dose to previous titration dose. If bradycardia occurs at initial dose, consider decrease to 0.02 mg/kg b.i.d.

ADMINISTRATION
PO
• Give with meals.
• For oral solution, empty entire contents of ampule(s) into a medication cup; use a calibrated oral syringe to measure prescribed dose from medication cup. Discard unused solution.
• Keep oral solution ampules in original foil pouches until use.
• Store tablets at room temperature.

ACTION
Reduces HR by blocking hyperpolarization-activated cyclic nucleotide-gated channel responsible for the cardiac pacemaker I_f current.

Route	Onset	Peak	Duration
PO	Rapid	1–2 hr	Unknown

Half-life: 6 hours.

ADVERSE REACTIONS
CV: ***bradycardia, conduction disturbances,*** HTN, atrial fibrillation. **EENT:** phosphenes, visual brightness.

INTERACTIONS
Drug-drug. *CYP3A4 inducers (barbiturates, phenytoin, rifampin):* May decrease ivabradine level. Avoid use together.
Drugs that decrease HR (amiodarone, beta blockers, digoxin): May increase risk of bradycardia. Monitor HR.
Moderate CYP3A4 inhibitors (diltiazem, verapamil): May increase ivabradine level, causing bradycardia and conduction disturbances. Avoid use together.
Strong CYP3A4 inhibitors (clarithromycin, HIV protease inhibitors [nelfinavir], itraconazole, nefazodone, telithromycin): May significantly increase ivabradine level, leading to bradycardia and conduction disturbances. Use together is contraindicated.
Drug-herb. *St. John's wort:* May decrease ivabradine level. Discourage use together.
Drug-food. *Grapefruit juice:* May increase ivabradine level, causing bradycardia and conduction disturbances. Discourage use together.

EFFECTS ON LAB TEST RESULTS
None reported.

CONTRAINDICATIONS & CAUTIONS
• Contraindicated in patients hypersensitive to drug or its components and in those with acute decompensated HF, clinically significant hypotension, sick sinus syndrome, SA block, or third-degree AV block unless a functioning demand pacemaker is present; resting HR less than 60 bpm before treatment; severe hepatic impairment; or pacemaker dependence (HR maintained exclusively by the pacemaker).
• Avoid use in patients with second-degree AV block unless a functioning demand pacemaker is present and in those taking diltiazem or verapamil concomitantly.
• Use cautiously in patients with sinus node dysfunction, conduction defects (first- or second-degree AV block, bundle-branch

block), or ventricular dyssynchrony and in those taking other negative chronotropes (digoxin, amiodarone) concomitantly. Drug may increase risk of bradycardia, sinus arrest, and heart block.

• Not recommended in those with demand pacemakers set to rates of 60 bpm or greater. *Dialyzable drug:* Unknown.

⚠ *Overdose S&S:* Severe and prolonged bradycardia.

PREGNANCY-LACTATION-REPRODUCTION

• Based on animal studies drug may cause fetal harm. Avoid use during pregnancy; advise patient of fetal risk. Patients of childbearing potential should use effective contraception during treatment.

• If drug must be used during pregnancy, monitor patients, especially during first trimester, for destabilization of HF that could result from slowing HR. Monitor patients with HF who are in the third trimester for signs and symptoms of preterm birth. Patients who are pregnant with LVEF less than 35% on maximally tolerated doses of beta blockers may be particularly HR-dependent for augmenting cardiac output.

• Drug may appear in human milk. Patient shouldn't breastfeed during therapy.

NURSING CONSIDERATIONS

• Regularly monitor cardiac rhythm. Drug may increase risk of atrial fibrillation. Discontinue drug if atrial fibrillation develops.

• Monitor patient for bradycardia; drug may increase risk of QT-interval prolongation, which may lead to severe ventricular arrhythmias, including torsades de pointes, especially in patients with risk factors such as use of QT-prolonging drugs.

• Monitor patients for phosphenes (transient enhanced brightness in a limited area of the visual field, halos, image decomposition, colored bright lights, or multiple images), which may be triggered by sudden variations in light intensity. Onset is typically within first 2 months of treatment; phosphenes may resolve without discontinuing treatment.

PATIENT TEACHING

• Instruct patient or caregiver in safe drug administration.

• Warn patient of childbearing potential that drug may cause fetal harm. Instruct patient to use effective contraception during treatment

and to report pregnancy or suspected pregnancy.

• Advise patient to avoid breastfeeding during therapy because of risk of fetal harm.

• Caution patient to immediately seek medical attention for significant decreases in HR or such signs and symptoms as dizziness, fatigue, or hypotension.

• Instruct patient to report all adverse reactions and to immediately report signs and symptoms of atrial fibrillation (heart palpitations or racing, chest pressure, worsened shortness of breath).

• Warn patient about possibility of developing luminous phenomena (phosphenes), resulting in transient visual brightness. Advise patient to use caution while driving or operating machinery in situations in which sudden changes in light intensity may occur, especially at night. Inform patient that phosphenes may subside during treatment.

SAFETY ALERT!

ixazomib citrate
ix-AZ-oh-mib

Ninlaro

Therapeutic class: Antineoplastics
Pharmacologic class: Proteasome inhibitors

AVAILABLE FORMS
Capsules ⓄⓃⒸ: 2.3 mg, 3 mg, 4 mg

INDICATIONS & DOSAGES
➤ **Multiple myeloma in combination with lenalidomide and dexamethasone in patients who have received at least one prior therapy**
Adults: 4 mg PO once a week on days 1, 8, and 15 of a 28-day treatment cycle, in combination with lenalidomide 25 mg on days 1 through 21 and dexamethasone 40 mg on days 1, 8, 15, and 22 of a 28-day treatment cycle. Before initiating a new cycle of therapy, ANC should be at least 1,000/mm³, platelet count should be at least 75,000/mm³, and nonhematologic toxicities should generally be recovered to patient's baseline or grade 1 or lower. Continue treatment until disease progression or unacceptable toxicity.
Adjust-a-dose: Reduce starting dose of drug to 3 mg in patients with moderate (total bilirubin level greater than 1.5 and less than

3 × ULN) or severe (total bilirubin level greater than 3 × ULN) hepatic impairment and in patients with severe renal impairment (CrCl of less than 30 mL/minute) or ESRD requiring dialysis. Refer to manufacturer's instructions for toxicity-related dosage adjustments. Refer to lenalidomide prescribing information for dosing recommendations.

ADMINISTRATION
PO
• Hazardous drug: use safe handling and disposal precautions according to facility policy. Use gloves to administer intact capsules.
• Give drug once weekly on the same day, at approximately the same time.
• Give at least 1 hour before or at least 2 hours after food.
• Patient should swallow capsules whole with water and shouldn't chew them. Don't crush or open capsules.
• May give without regard to timing of dialysis.
• If dose is delayed or missed, give only if the next scheduled dose is 72 hours or more away; don't double-dose. Don't repeat dose if patient vomits after taking a dose; resume dosing at the time of the next scheduled dose.
• Store at room temperature. Don't store above 86° F (30° C). Don't freeze.
• Store capsules in original packaging until immediately before use.

ACTION
A reversible proteasome inhibitor that binds and inhibits the chymotrypsin-like activity of the beta 5 subunit of the 20S proteasome, thereby inducing death of multiple myeloma cell lines.

Route	Onset	Peak	Duration
PO	Unknown	1 hr	Unknown

Half-life: 9.5 days.

ADVERSE REACTIONS
CNS: peripheral neuropathy. **CV:** peripheral edema. **EENT:** blurred vision, dry eyes, conjunctivitis. **GI:** diarrhea, constipation, nausea, vomiting. **Hematologic:** *thrombocytopenia, neutropenia.* **Hepatic:** hepatic impairment. **Musculoskeletal:** back pain. **Respiratory:** URI. **Skin:** rash.

INTERACTIONS
Drug-drug. *Strong CYP3A inducers (carbamazepine, phenytoin, rifampin):* May decrease ixazomib concentration. Avoid use together.
Drug-herb. *St. John's wort:* May decrease ixazomib concentration. Avoid use together.
Drug-food. *High-fat meals:* May decrease ixazomib concentration. Patient should take drug at least 1 hour before or at least 2 hours after food.

EFFECTS ON LAB TEST RESULTS
• May increase LFT values.
• May decrease platelet and neutrophil counts.

CONTRAINDICATIONS & CAUTIONS
• Use cautiously in patients with renal or hepatic impairment.
• Bone marrow suppression was commonly reported in clinical trials.
• Thrombocytopenia purpura and TLS can occur rarely. If suspected, stop drug and evaluate. Don't restart unless these conditions have been excluded.
• Drug isn't indicated for use in children.
Dialyzable drug: No.
⚠ **Overdose S&S:** Severe nausea, vomiting, diarrhea, aspiration pneumonia, multiple organ failure, death.

PREGNANCY-LACTATION-REPRODUCTION
• Drug may cause fetal harm; advise patients of risk. Lenalidomide is contraindicated during pregnancy.
• All patients of reproductive potential must use effective contraception during treatment and for 90 days after final dose. Drug is given with dexamethasone, which may decrease effectiveness of hormonal contraceptives.
• It isn't known if drug appears in human milk. Breastfeeding isn't recommended.

NURSING CONSIDERATIONS
• Monitor patients for signs and symptoms of thrombocytopenia (bleeding, bruising). Platelet nadirs typically occur between days 14 and 21 of each 28-day cycle and recover to baseline by the start of the next cycle. Monitor platelet count at least monthly; consider more frequent monitoring during the first three cycles. Adjust dosage and consider platelet transfusions per standard medical guidelines if indicated.

• Monitor patients for GI adverse effects (severe diarrhea, constipation, nausea, vomiting); provide antidiarrheals, antiemetics, and supportive care as needed. Adjust dosage for grade 3 or 4 symptoms.

• Monitor patients for new or worsening peripheral neuropathy. Adjust dosage as clinically indicated.

• Monitor patients for rash; SJS can occur rarely. Provide supportive care or adjust dosage as clinically indicated.

• Monitor patients for peripheral edema. Evaluate for underlying causes and provide supportive care as clinically indicated. Adjust dexamethasone dosage per prescribing information or ixazomib dosage for grade 3 or 4 symptoms.

• Monitor liver enzyme levels regularly and adjust dosage for grade 3 or 4 symptoms.

• *Look alike–sound alike:* Don't confuse ixazomib with carfilzomib, infliximab, or isatuximab.

PATIENT TEACHING

• Instruct patient in safe drug administration and handling. Stress importance of following dosage instructions; overdose has led to death.

• Advise patient to avoid direct contact with the capsule contents: In case of capsule breakage, avoid direct contact of contents with the skin or eyes. If skin contact occurs, wash thoroughly with soap and water. If eye contact occurs, flush thoroughly with water.

• Teach patient to report all adverse reactions and to immediately report bleeding and easy bruising, diarrhea, constipation, nausea and vomiting, rash, abdominal pain, or yellowing of the skin.

• Advise patient to report new or worsening peripheral neuropathy signs and symptoms (tingling, numbness, pain, burning feeling in the feet or hands, weakness in the arms or legs).

• Instruct patient to report unusual extremity swelling or weight gain due to swelling.

• Remind all patients of reproductive potential that it's essential to use effective contraception during treatment and for 90 days after final dose.

• Inform patient of risk to fetus with ixazomib use during pregnancy and to immediately report suspected pregnancy.

• Caution patient not to breastfeed during treatment.

ixekizumab
ix-ee-KIZ-ue-mab

Taltz

Therapeutic class: Immunomodulators
Pharmacologic class: Humanized interleukin-17A antagonists

AVAILABLE FORMS
Injection: 80 mg/mL autoinjector or prefilled syringe

INDICATIONS & DOSAGES

➤ **Moderate to severe plaque psoriasis in patients who are candidates for systemic therapy or phototherapy**
Adults: Initially, 160 mg (two 80-mg injections) subcut at week 0, followed by 80 mg subcut at weeks 2, 4, 6, 8, 10, and 12; then 80 mg every 4 weeks.
Children ages 6 to younger than 18 weighing more than 50 kg: Initially, 160 mg (two 80-mg injections) subcut, followed by 80 mg subcut every 4 weeks.
Children ages 6 to younger than 18 weighing 25 to 50 kg: Initially, 80 mg subcut, followed by 40 mg every 4 weeks.
Children ages 6 to younger than 18 weighing less than 25 kg: Initially, 40 mg subcut, followed by 20 mg every 4 weeks.

➤ **Active psoriatic arthritis**
Adults: Initially, 160 mg (two 80-mg injections) subcut at week 0, followed by 80 mg subcut every 4 weeks. For patients with psoriatic arthritis who have coexistent moderate to severe plaque psoriasis, use the dosing regimen for plaque psoriasis. May be given alone or in combination with a conventional DMARD such as methotrexate.

➤ **Active ankylosing spondylitis**
Adults: Initially, 160 mg (two 80-mg injections) subcut, followed by 80 mg subcut every 4 weeks.

➤ **Active nonradiographic axial spondyloarthritis with objective signs of inflammation**
Adults: 80 mg subcut every 4 weeks.

ADMINISTRATION
Subcutaneous
• Intended for use under guidance of a physician.

• Follow package insert for directions for preparation and administration for children weighing less than 50 kg. Doses of 20 mg or 40 mg must be prepared and given by a health care professional using solution from an 80-mg/mL prefilled syringe.

• Allow medication to reach room temperature for 30 minutes before injection without removing needle cap.

• Inspect solution for particulate matter and discoloration before administration. Solution should be clear and colorless to slightly yellow. Don't use if solution contains particles or is discolored or cloudy. Don't shake.

• Inject the full 1 mL of medication in the autoinjector or prefilled syringe.

• Discard unused portion if any medication remains in the autoinjector or prefilled syringe after injection. Drug doesn't contain preservatives.

• Give each injection in a different location (upper arm, thigh, or abdomen) than previous injection.

• Don't inject into skin that is tender, bruised, erythematous, indurated, or affected by psoriasis.

• If a dose is missed, give as soon as possible; then resume dosing at the regularly scheduled time.

• Store in refrigerator at 36° to 46° F (2° to 8° C). Protect from light. Don't freeze.

ACTION

A humanized monoclonal IgG antibody that binds selectively to IL-17A receptors and inhibits release of proinflammatory cytokines and chemokines.

Route	Onset	Peak	Duration
Subcut	Unknown	4 days	Unknown

Half-life: 13 days.

ADVERSE REACTIONS

EENT: conjunctivitis. **GI:** nausea. **Hematologic:** *neutropenia, thrombocytopenia.* **Respiratory:** URI. **Skin:** injection-site reaction, urticaria. **Other:** tinea infection, infection, flulike symptoms, development of neutralizing antibodies.

INTERACTIONS

Drug-drug. *CYP450 substrates (cyclosporine, warfarin):* May affect substrate levels, especially those with narrow therapeutic

index. Monitor patient for effect and consider dosage modification of substrate.
Live-virus vaccines: May reduce effectiveness of live-virus vaccine. Patients who are immunocompromised may be at increased risk for vaccine-induced infection. Avoid use of live-virus vaccines.

EFFECTS ON LAB TEST RESULTS

• May decrease WBC and platelet counts.

CONTRAINDICATIONS & CAUTIONS

• Contraindicated in patients hypersensitive to drug or its components. Rarely, angioedema and urticaria were reported.

• Contraindicated in patients with active TB. Evaluate patients for TB before initiating treatment and consider providing TB treatment in patients with a history of latent or active TB in whom adequate treatment can't be confirmed.

• Use cautiously in patients at risk for serious infections and in those with Crohn disease or ulcerative colitis.

• Safety in children younger than age 6 hasn't been established.
Dialyzable drug: Unknown.

PREGNANCY-LACTATION-REPRODUCTION

• No data exist on the use of drug during pregnancy. Human IgG is known to cross the placental barrier so it's possible that ixekizumab, a humanized IgG monoclonal antibody, may be transmitted from mother to fetus. Other agents are preferred for treatment of plaque psoriasis during pregnancy.

• Encourage patients who become pregnant during treatment to enroll in Taltz pregnancy registry (1-800-284-1695).

• It isn't known if drug appears in human milk. Weigh benefits to patient against risk to the infant.

NURSING CONSIDERATIONS

• Complete all age-appropriate vaccinations before start of treatment.

• Monitor patients for signs and symptoms of infection, including TB, during and after treatment.

• Monitor patients for hypersensitivity reactions (angioedema, urticaria). If serious reaction occurs, discontinue drug and initiate treatment.

• Monitor patients for onset or exacerbation of Crohn disease and ulcerative colitis.

• *Look alike–sound alike:* Don't confuse ixe-kizumab with infliximab, reslizumab, or rituximab.

PATIENT TEACHING

• Advise patient to report all adverse reactions and to promptly report signs or symptoms of infection (because drug may lower patient's ability to fight infection).
• Warn patient to seek immediate medical attention if signs or symptoms of severe hypersensitivity reaction occur.
• Teach patient and caregivers how to safely use autoinjectors or prefilled syringes.

ketoconazole (oral)

kee-toe-KOE-na-zole

Therapeutic class: Antifungals
Pharmacologic class: Imidazole derivatives

AVAILABLE FORMS

Tablets: 200 mg

INDICATIONS & DOSAGES

Boxed Warning Drug should only be used when other antifungal therapy isn't available or tolerated and potential benefits outweigh risks. ∎

➤ **Fungal infections (coccidioidomycosis, blastomycosis, histoplasmosis, chromomycosis, and paracoccidioidomycosis)**
Adults: Initially, 200 mg PO daily in a single dose. May increase dosage to 400 mg once daily in patients who don't respond. Continue until fungal infection is resolved; usual duration for systemic infection is 6 months. Maximum dosage is 400 mg daily.
Children age 2 and older: 3.3 to 6.6 mg/kg PO daily in a single dose. Continue until fungal infection is resolved; usual duration for systemic infection is 6 months. Maximum dosage is 400 mg daily.
➤ **Prostate cancer, advanced ♦**
Adults: 400 mg PO t.i.d. (in combination with oral hydrocortisone) until disease progression.

ADMINISTRATION

PO

• Give oral tablets 2 hours before antacids, H_2 blockers, or PPIs to prevent decreased absorption due to the high pH of gastric contents. Patients with achlorhydria should take with acidic liquid (e.g., nondiet cola or orange juice).
• A pharmacist can prepare an oral suspension. Shake suspension well before giving.
• Must refrigerate suspension; remains stable for 60 days.

ACTION

Interferes with fungal cell-wall synthesis by inhibiting formation of ergosterol and increasing cell-wall permeability that makes the fungus susceptible to osmotic instability.

Route	Onset	Peak	Duration
PO	Unknown	1–2 hr	Unknown

Half-life: 8 hours.

ADVERSE REACTIONS

CNS: insomnia, nervousness, dizziness, asthenia, headache, fatigue, malaise, paresthesia, somnolence, dysgeusia, weakness, fever, chills. **CV:** orthostatic hypotension, peripheral edema. **EENT:** photophobia, epistaxis, dry mouth. **GI:** nausea, vomiting, upper abdominal pain, diarrhea, constipation, dyspepsia, flatulence, increased appetite, anorexia, tongue discoloration. **GU:** menstrual disorder. **Hematologic:** *thrombocytopenia.* **Hepatic:** *hepatitis,* jaundice. **Metabolic:** hyperlipidemia. **Musculoskeletal:** myalgia. **Skin:** pruritus, rash, *erythema multiforme,* dermatitis, erythema, alopecia, urticaria, xeroderma. **Other:** *anaphylaxis,* hot flush, alcohol intolerance, gynecomastia.

INTERACTIONS

🚫 *Alert:* Ketoconazole can significantly interact with many drugs, especially those metabolized by CYP450 enzyme system. Consult a drug interaction resource or pharmacist for additional information.
Drug-drug. *Alprazolam, eplerenone, ergot alkaloids (dihydroergotamine, ergometrine, ergotamine, methylergometrine), felodipine, irinotecan, lurasidone, oral midazolam, nisoldipine, tolvaptan, triazolam:* May increase levels of these drugs. Use together is contraindicated.
Boxed Warning *Cisapride, disopyramide, dofetilide, dronedarone, methadone, pimozide, quinidine, ranolazine:* May increase levels of these drugs and prolong QT interval. Use together is contraindicated. ∎

Reactions in bold italics are *life-threatening*. Interactions may have a *rapid onset* or a *delayed onset*.

Colchicine: May increase risk of adverse effects in patients with renal or hepatic impairment. Use together is contraindicated.
HMG-CoA reductase inhibitors (atorvastatin, fluvastatin, lovastatin, pravastatin, simvastatin): May increase levels and adverse effects of these drugs. Use together is contraindicated. May coadminister atorvastatin with caution.
Strong CYP3A4 inducers (carbamazepine, efavirenz, isoniazid, nevirapine, rifabutin): May decrease ketoconazole level. Use together isn't recommended. If use is unavoidable, monitor therapy.
Strong CYP3A4 inhibitors (ritonavir): May increase ketoconazole level. Use cautiously together.
Drug-lifestyle. *Alcohol use:* May cause disulfiram-like reaction (flushing, rash, peripheral edema, nausea, headache). Don't use together.

EFFECTS ON LAB TEST RESULTS
• May increase lipid, ALP, ALT, and AST levels.
• May decrease Hb level and platelet count.
• May decrease adrenal function results.

CONTRAINDICATIONS & CAUTIONS
• Contraindicated in patients hypersensitive to drug or its components.
Boxed Warning Drug can cause serious hepatotoxicity that may be fatal or require liver transplantation, even in patients with no obvious risk factors for liver disease. Drug is contraindicated in patients with acute or chronic liver disease. Patient must be informed of risk. ∎
• Drug decreases adrenal corticosteroid secretions at doses of 400 mg. Don't exceed recommended dose of 400 mg.
• Safety and effectiveness in children younger than age 2 haven't been established.
Dialyzable drug: No.

PREGNANCY-LACTATION-REPRODUCTION
• Drug may cause fetal harm based on animal studies. Use in pregnancy only if benefits justify fetal risk.
• Drug may reversibly lower serum testosterone level, causing gynecomastia, impotence, and oligospermia. Testosterone levels are impaired with doses of 800 mg daily and abolished by 1,600 mg daily.
• Drug appears in human milk. Breastfeeding isn't recommended during therapy.

NURSING CONSIDERATIONS
Boxed Warning Because of risk of adverse effects, don't use drug for less serious conditions, such as fungal infections of the skin or nails. ∎
🜂 *Alert:* Monitor patient for signs and symptoms of hepatotoxicity, including elevated liver enzyme levels, nausea that doesn't subside, unusual fatigue, jaundice, dark urine, or pale stool.
• Assess liver function status (AST, ALT, total bilirubin levels), ALP, PT, and INR before starting drug.
• Measure ALT level weekly for duration of treatment. If ALT levels increase above the ULN or 30% above baseline, or if patient develops signs and symptoms of hepatotoxicity, obtain a full set of LFTs. Repeat LFTs to ensure normalization of values. If drug is restarted, monitor patient frequently.
• Monitor adrenal function in patients with adrenal insufficiency or borderline adrenal function and in those experiencing prolonged periods of stress (such as major surgery).
• Review all medications patient is receiving for potential drug interactions with ketoconazole.

PATIENT TEACHING
• Instruct patient in safe drug administration and risk of drug interactions.
• Advise patient to report any new drugs or herbal supplements being taken.
• Make sure patient understands that treatment should continue until all tests indicate that active fungal infection has subsided. If drug is stopped too soon, infection will recur. Treatment for systemic fungal infections may last 6 months.
• Review signs and symptoms of hepatotoxicity with patient. Tell patient to stop drug and notify prescriber if they occur.
• Instruct patient to immediately report irregular heartbeats, palpitations, feeling faint, dizziness, or light-headedness.
• Caution patient to avoid alcohol consumption during treatment.

K

ketoconazole (topical)
kee-toe-KOE-na-zole

Extina, Ketoderm ✤, Ketozole,
Nizoral ◇, Xolegel

Therapeutic class: Antifungals
Pharmacologic class: Imidazoles

AVAILABLE FORMS
Cream: 2%
Foam: 2%
Gel: 2%
Shampoo: 1% ◇, 2%

INDICATIONS & DOSAGES
➤ **Seborrheic dermatitis**
Adults and children age 12 and older: Apply foam to affected area b.i.d. for 4 weeks. Apply gel to affected area once daily for 2 weeks. Apply cream to affected area b.i.d. for 4 weeks or until clearing.
➤ **Tinea corporis, tinea cruris, tinea pedis, tinea versicolor from susceptible organisms; seborrheic dermatitis; cutaneous candidiasis**
Adults: Apply cream to affected and immediate surrounding area once daily for 2 weeks. Patients with tinea pedis need 6 weeks of treatment. For tinea (pityriasis) versicolor, if using 2% shampoo, one application is usually sufficient.
➤ **Scaling caused by dandruff**
Adults and children age 12 and older: Use 1% OTC shampoo every 3 to 4 days for up to 8 weeks; then apply only as needed to control dandruff.
Children younger than age 12: Consult health care provider before use.

ADMINISTRATION
Topical
• For external use only; not for ophthalmic, oral, or intravaginal use. Don't let drug come in contact with eyes or other mucous membranes. Wash hands after application.
• When using foam, dispense into cap of can or other cool surface; don't spray directly onto affected skin or the hands because foam will start to melt. If fingers are warm, rinse them in cold water and dry well; then, using fingertips, gently massage foam into affected areas until it disappears.

• Don't wash areas where gel was applied for at least 3 hours. Have patient wait at least 20 minutes after application before applying makeup or sunscreen to the affected areas.
• When using 1% OTC shampoo, wet hair, lather, and rinse thoroughly; repeat.
• When using 2% shampoo, apply to affected area of damp skin and a side area of surrounding skin, lather, leave on skin for 5 minutes, and rinse.
• Store at room temperature; protect from light.

ACTION
Probably inhibits yeast growth by altering the permeability of the cell membrane.

Route	Onset	Peak	Duration
Topical	Unknown	Unknown	Unknown

Half-life: Unknown.

ADVERSE REACTIONS
Skin: pruritus, application-site reaction, oiliness or dryness of hair and scalp, hair discoloration, change in hair texture with shampoo use; application-site reaction, burning with foam or gel; severe irritation, and stinging or burning with cream. **Other:** hypersensitivity reaction.

INTERACTIONS
None known.

EFFECTS ON LAB TEST RESULTS
None reported.

CONTRAINDICATIONS & CAUTIONS
• Product contains sodium sulfite anhydrous, which may cause severe or life-threatening allergic reactions, including anaphylaxis, in patients with asthma.
Dialyzable drug: No.

PREGNANCY-LACTATION-REPRODUCTION
• There are no adequate studies during pregnancy. Use during pregnancy only if potential benefit justifies fetal risk.
• Drug isn't detectable in plasma with prolonged shampoo use.
• It isn't known if drug appears in human milk. Use cautiously during breastfeeding only if benefits outweigh risk to infant.
• Patients shouldn't apply to breast to avoid direct contact with infants who are breastfeeding.

Reactions in bold italics are *life-threatening*. Interactions may have a *rapid onset* or a **delayed onset**.

NURSING CONSIDERATIONS
• Most patients show improvement soon after treatment begins.
• Treatment of tinea corporis or tinea cruris should continue for at least 2 weeks to reduce possibility of recurrence.

PATIENT TEACHING
• Tell patient to stop drug and notify prescriber if hypersensitivity reaction occurs.
• Advise patient to check with prescriber if condition worsens; drug may have to be stopped and diagnosis reevaluated.
• Tell patient to avoid using shampoo on scalp if skin is broken or inflamed.
• Advise patient that foam and gel are flammable and to avoid fire, flame, and smoking during and immediately after application.
• Instruct patient in safe drug administration and storage.
• Teach patient to wash hands before and after use, unless affected areas are on hands.
• Warn patient that shampoo applied to permanent-waved hair removes curl.
• Tell patient to continue drug for intended duration of therapy, even if signs and symptoms improve soon after starting treatment.

---

ketorolac tromethamine (oral, nasal, injection)
KEE-toe-role-ak

Sprix, Toradol✤

Therapeutic class: Anti-inflammatory drugs
Pharmacologic class: NSAIDs

AVAILABLE FORMS
Injection*: 10 mg/mL ampules ✤, 15 mg/mL single-dose vials and prefilled syringes; 30 mg/mL in single-dose vials, 1- and 2-mL prefilled syringes
Nasal spray: 15.75 mg/spray
Tablets: 10 mg

INDICATIONS & DOSAGES
Boxed Warning Adjust dosage for patients age 65 and older, patients weighing less than 50 kg, and those with moderately elevated serum creatinine level. For these patients, total daily doses shouldn't exceed 60 mg ketorolac injection or 40 mg oral ketorolac. ∎
➤ **Short-term management of moderately severe, acute pain for single-dose treatment**

Adults younger than age 65 and adolescents age 17 and older: 60 mg IM or 30 mg IV.
Adults age 65 and older, patients weighing less than 50 kg, or those with renal impairment: 30 mg IM or 15 mg IV.
➤ **Short-term management of moderately severe, acute pain for multiple-dose treatment**
Adults younger than age 65 and adolescents age 17 and older: 30 mg IM or IV every 6 hours for maximum of 5 days. Maximum daily dose is 120 mg. Or, 31.5 mg (one 15.75-mg spray in each nostril) every 6 to 8 hours; maximum daily dose is 126 mg.
Adults age 65 and older, patients weighing less than 50 kg, or those with renal impairment: 15 mg IM or IV every 6 hours for maximum of 5 days. Maximum daily dose is 60 mg. Or, 15.75 mg (1 spray in only one nostril) every 6 to 8 hours; maximum daily dose is 63 mg.
➤ **Short-term management of moderately severe, acute pain when switching from parenteral to oral administration**
Boxed Warning Oral therapy is indicated only as continuation of IV or IM dosing; never give as initial therapy. ∎
Adults younger than age 65 and adolescents age 17 and older: 20 mg PO as single dose; then 10 mg PO every 4 to 6 hours PRN for maximum of 5 days (combined for both parenteral and oral). Maximum daily dose is 40 mg.
Adults age 65 and older, patients weighing less than 50 kg, or those with renal impairment: 10 mg PO as single dose; then 10 mg PO every 4 to 6 hours PRN for maximum of 5 days (combined for both parenteral and oral). Maximum daily dose is 40 mg.

ADMINISTRATION
Boxed Warning Total treatment duration for combined formulations shouldn't exceed 5 days. ∎
PO
• Give drug with food if GI upset occurs.
IV
▼ Give injection over at least 15 seconds.
▼ Protect from light.
▼ **Incompatibilities:** Solutions that result in a relatively low pH, such as hydroxyzine, meperidine, morphine sulfate, and prochlorperazine.

IM
• When appropriate, give by deep IM injection.
• Patient may feel pain at injection site.
• Put pressure on site for 15 to 30 seconds after injection to minimize local effects.

Intranasal
• Discard nasal spray within 24 hours of first dose, even if bottle still contains medication.
• Each 1.7-g bottle contains eight sprays.
• Activate pump before first use by pumping five times.
• Have patient blow nose gently before use, sit upright or stand, and tilt head slightly forward.
• Insert tip into the nostril, point away from the septum, and spray once while patient holds breath.

ACTION
May inhibit prostaglandin synthesis to produce anti-inflammatory, analgesic, and antipyretic effects.

Route	Onset	Peak	Duration
PO	30–60 min	2–3 hr	4–6 hr
IV, IM	About 30 min	≤2–3 hr	4–6 hr
Intranasal	20 min	45 min	Unknown

Half-life: PO, 2 to 9 hours; IV, 5 to 6 hours; IM, 5 to 6 hours; intranasal, 5 to 6 hours.

ADVERSE REACTIONS
CNS: headache, dizziness, drowsiness. **CV:** edema, HTN. **EENT:** tinnitus. **Nasal spray only:** increased lacrimation, nasal discomfort, rhinalgia, rhinitis, throat irritation. **GI:** abdominal pain, dyspepsia, heartburn, nausea, constipation, diarrhea, flatulence, GI fullness, *GI perforation,* peptic ulceration, stomatitis, vomiting, *GI hemorrhage.* **GU:** renal impairment. **Hematologic:** anemia, decreased platelet adhesion, prolonged bleeding time, purpura. **Hepatic:** increased liver enzyme levels. **Skin:** diaphoresis, pruritus, rash. **Other:** pain at injection site.

INTERACTIONS
Drug-drug. *ACE inhibitors, ARBs:* May cause renal impairment, particularly with volume depletion. May decrease antihypertensive effect. Use together cautiously.
Alprazolam, fluoxetine, thiothixene: May cause hallucinations. Monitor patient closely.

Anticoagulants: May increase anticoagulant levels in the blood. Use together with extreme caution and monitor patient closely.
Antihypertensives, diuretics: May increase risk of nephrotoxicity. May decrease effectiveness of these drugs. Monitor patient closely.
Carbamazepine, phenytoin: May increase risk of seizures. Monitor patient closely.
Lithium: May increase lithium level. Monitor patient closely for lithium toxicity.
Methotrexate: May decrease methotrexate clearance and increase toxicity. Avoid using together.
Boxed Warning *NSAIDs, salicylates:* May increase risk of NSAID-related adverse effects. Use together is contraindicated. ∎
Pentoxifylline: May increase risk of bleeding. Use together is contraindicated.
Probenecid: May increase level and toxicity of ketorolac. Use together is contraindicated.
SSRIs: May increase risk of GI bleeding. Use together cautiously.
Drug-herb. *Dong quai, feverfew, garlic, ginger, horse chestnut, red clover:* May cause bleeding. Discourage use together.
White willow: Herb and drug contain similar components. Discourage use together.
Drug-lifestyle. *Alcohol use:* May increase risk of GI bleeding. Use with caution.
Smoking: May increase risk of GI bleeding. Discourage use together.

EFFECTS ON LAB TEST RESULTS
• May increase ALT and AST levels.
• May decrease Hb level and hematocrit.
• May increase bleeding time.
• May lead to false-positive aldosterone/renin ratio.

CONTRAINDICATIONS & CAUTIONS
Boxed Warning Contraindicated in patients hypersensitive to ketorolac or aspirin or other NSAIDs. Hypersensitivity reactions, ranging from bronchospasm to anaphylactic shock, have occurred and appropriate counteractive measures must be available when first dose of ketorolac injection is given. ∎
Boxed Warning Contraindicated in children younger than age 17, as prophylactic analgesic before major surgery, and intraoperatively when hemostasis is critical; in patients with advanced renal impairment; and in those at risk for renal failure from volume depletion. ∎

Boxed Warning Contraindicated in patients with suspected or confirmed cerebrovascular bleeding, hemorrhagic diathesis, or incomplete hemostasis, and in those at high risk for bleeding because drug inhibits platelet function. ■

Boxed Warning Drug isn't indicated for minor or chronic pain. ■

Boxed Warning NSAIDs can cause peptic ulcers, GI bleeding, or perforation of the stomach or intestines, which can be fatal. These events can occur at any time during therapy and without warning. Contraindicated in patients with active peptic ulcer disease, recent GI bleeding or perforation, and a history of peptic ulcer disease or GI bleeding. Older adults are at greater risk for serious GI events. ■

Boxed Warning Contraindicated for treatment of perioperative pain in patients requiring CABG surgery. ■

Boxed Warning Contraindicated in patients currently receiving aspirin, probenecid, or other NSAIDs because of the cumulative risks of inducing serious NSAID-related adverse reactions. ■

Boxed Warning NSAIDs can increase risk of serious CV thrombotic events, including MI or stroke. Risk of MI or stroke can occur early in treatment and increase with duration of use. Risk appears greater at higher doses. Use lowest effective dose for shortest duration possible. ■

◑ *Alert:* NSAIDs increase risk of HF.

• Use cautiously in older adults and patients with hepatic or renal impairment or cardiac decompensation.

Dialyzable drug: Unlikely.

⚠ *Overdose S&S:* Abdominal pain, nausea, vomiting, peptic ulcers, GI bleeding, renal dysfunction, HTN, lethargy, drowsiness, respiratory depression, coma, anaphylaxis.

PREGNANCY-LACTATION-REPRODUCTION

Boxed Warning Contraindicated during labor and delivery because drug may adversely affect fetal circulation and inhibit uterine contractions. ■

◑ *Alert:* Use of NSAIDs at 20 weeks or later in pregnancy may cause fetal renal dysfunction; use at 30 weeks or later in pregnancy may increase risk of premature closure of the ductus arteriosus. Avoid use during pregnancy starting at 20 weeks' gestation. If potential benefit justifies fetal risk, use lowest

effective dose for the shortest duration. Consider ultrasound monitoring of amniotic fluid if NSAID therapy is longer than 48 hours. Use of 81 mg of low-dose aspirin for certain pregnancy-related conditions under the direction of prescriber is acceptable.

• Prolonged use of NSAIDs in patients of childbearing potential may be associated with infertility that's reversible upon drug discontinuation.

• Low concentrations of drug appear in human milk. Use cautiously during breastfeeding.

NURSING CONSIDERATIONS

• Correct hypovolemia before giving drug.

Boxed Warning Contraindicated for epidural or intrathecal administration because of its alcohol content. ■

◑ *Alert:* Watch for and immediately evaluate signs and symptoms of MI (chest pain, shortness of breath or trouble breathing) or stroke (weakness in one part or side of the body, slurred speech).

• Carefully observe patients with coagulopathies and those taking anticoagulants. Drug inhibits platelet aggregation and can prolong bleeding time.

Boxed Warning NSAIDs may increase the risk of serious thrombotic events, MI, or stroke, which can be fatal. The risk may be greater with longer use or in patients with CV disease or risk factors for CV disease. ■

• NSAIDs may mask signs and symptoms of infection because of their antipyretic and anti-inflammatory actions.

• *Look alike–sound alike:* Don't confuse ketorolac with ketamine or Ketalar.

PATIENT TEACHING

• Instruct patient in safe drug administration.

• Warn patient using nasal spray that transient, mild to moderate nasal irritation may occur that lasts for a few minutes and won't worsen with next dose.

• Advise patient to take a sip of water after using nasal spray to decrease throat sensation.

• Teach patient to read package insert and full directions for use of nasal spray bottle.

• Warn patient not to take ketorolac with other NSAIDs.

◑ *Alert:* Advise patient to seek medical attention immediately for chest pain, shortness of breath or trouble breathing, weakness in one part or side of the body, or slurred speech.

K

• Advise patient to maintain adequate fluid intake.

• Tell patient to promptly report edema and weight gain.

• Teach patient the warning signs and symptoms of hepatotoxicity (nausea, fatigue, lethargy, pruritus, jaundice, right upper quadrant abdominal tenderness, flulike symptoms). Advise patient to stop drug and seek medical help immediately if they occur.

• Instruct patient to immediately report pregnancy.

🜂 **Alert:** Warn patient of risk of NSAID use during pregnancy. Advise patient to discuss OTC medication with a pharmacist or health care provider before use during pregnancy.

• Warn patient receiving drug IM that pain may occur at injection site.

• Teach patient signs and symptoms of GI bleeding (including blood in vomit, urine, or stool; coffee-ground vomit; and melena) and to notify prescriber immediately if any of these occurs.

• Advise patient to take oral medication with food to prevent GI upset.

• Tell patient not to take drug for more than 5 days in a row.

SAFETY ALERT!

labetalol hydrochloride
la-BET-ah-loll

Trandate ✤

Therapeutic class: Antihypertensives
Pharmacologic class: Alpha–beta blockers

AVAILABLE FORMS
Injection: 5 mg/mL in multiple-dose vials and prefilled syringes
Premixed IV solution: 1 mg/mg in 100 mL, 200 mL, 300 mL single-dose bags
Tablets: 100 mg, 200 mg, 300 mg

INDICATIONS & DOSAGES
➤ **HTN**
Adults (inpatients after IV therapy): Once supine diastolic BP has begun to rise, give 200 mg PO, followed by 200 to 400 mg PO in 6 to 12 hours depending on BP response. May increase from 200 mg PO b.i.d. to 400 mg b.i.d., then to 800 mg b.i.d, then to 1,200 mg b.i.d. at 1-day intervals to achieve desired response.

Adults (outpatients): 100 mg PO b.i.d. with or without a diuretic. If needed, dosage is increased to 200 mg b.i.d. after 2 to 3 days. Further increases may be made every 2 to 3 days until optimal response is reached. Usual maintenance dosage is 200 to 400 mg b.i.d. Maximum dose is 2.4 g daily in two divided doses given alone or with a diuretic.

Adjust-a-dose: Usual maintenance dosage for older adults is 100 to 200 mg b.i.d.

➤ **Severe HTN, hypertensive emergencies**
Adults: 2 mg/minute IV infusion until satisfactory response is obtained; then infusion is stopped. Maximum dose is 300 mg.

Or, give by repeated IV injection; initially, 0.25 mg/kg up to maximum of 20 mg IV over 2 minutes. Repeat injections of 40 to 80 mg every 10 minutes until maximum dose of 300 mg is reached, as needed.

ADMINISTRATION
PO
• If dizziness occurs, give dose at bedtime or in smaller doses t.i.d.

• Food increases bioavailability of drug; give in a consistent manner with regard to meals.

IV
▼ Give by slow, direct IV injection over 2 minutes at 10-minute intervals.

▼ For IV infusion, prepare by diluting with D_5W, NSS, or other compatible IV solution (refer to manufacturer's instructions for other compatible solutions) to yield 1 mg/mL (if total volume is 200 mL) or 2 mg/3 mL (if total volume is 250 mL). Infuse at 2 mg/minute.

▼ Further dilution isn't needed for ready-to-use bags.

▼ Give labetalol infusion with an infusion-control device.

▼ Monitor BP during and after completion of infusion or IV injections.

▼ Patient should remain supine during and for 3 hours after infusion. When given IV for hypertensive emergencies, drug produces a rapid, predictable fall in BP within 5 to 10 minutes.

▼ Store at room temperature. Protect from light.

▼ **Incompatibilities:** Alkali solutions, furosemide.

Reactions in bold italics are *life-threatening*. Interactions may have a *rapid onset* or a *delayed onset*.

ACTION

May be related to reduced peripheral vascular resistance, as a result of alpha and beta blockade.

Route	Onset	Peak	Duration
PO	20–120 min	2–4 hr	8–12 hr
IV	2–5 min	5–15 min	16–18 hr

Half-life: IV, about 5.5 hours; oral, 6 to 8 hours.

ADVERSE REACTIONS

CNS: dizziness, fatigue, headache, paresthesia, transient scalp tingling, syncope, vertigo, asthenia, somnolence, taste distortion. **CV:** edema, orthostatic hypotension, flushing, *ventricular arrhythmias.* **EENT:** abnormal vision, nasal congestion. **GI:** nausea, vomiting, dyspepsia. **GU:** sexual dysfunction. **Respiratory:** dyspnea, wheezing. **Skin:** rash, diaphoresis, pruritus.

INTERACTIONS

Drug-drug. *Beta agonists:* May blunt bronchodilator effect of these drugs in patients with bronchospasm. May need to increase dosages of these drugs.
Beta blockers, cardiac glycosides: May increase risk of bradycardia. Monitor therapy.
Calcium channel blockers (verapamil): May increase hypotensive effects. IV coadministration is contraindicated. Use PO forms together cautiously.
Cimetidine: May enhance labetalol's effect. Use together cautiously.
CV drugs, diuretics: May increase hypotensive effects. Monitor BP.
Halothane: May increase hypotensive effect. Monitor BP closely.
Insulin, oral antidiabetics: May alter dosage requirements in previously stabilized patient with diabetes. Monitor patient closely.
Nitroglycerin: May blunt reflex tachycardia produced by nitroglycerin but not the hypotension. Monitor BP if used together.
NSAIDs: May decrease antihypertensive effects. Monitor BP.
TCAs: May increase incidence of tremor. Monitor patient for tremor.
Drug-herb. *Ma huang:* May decrease antihypertensive effects. Discourage use together.

EFFECTS ON LAB TEST RESULTS

• May increase transaminase, creatinine, and urea levels.

• May cause false-positive increase of urine free and total catecholamine levels when measured by a nonspecific trihydroxyindole fluorometric method.
• May cause false-positive test result for amphetamines when screening urine for drugs.

CONTRAINDICATIONS & CAUTIONS

• Contraindicated in patients hypersensitive to drug or its components and in those with bronchial asthma (history of obstructive airway disease), overt HF, greater than first-degree heart block (except in patients with a functioning pacemaker), cardiogenic shock, severe bradycardia, and other conditions that may cause severe and prolonged hypotension.
• Use cautiously in patients with HF, hepatic failure, chronic bronchitis, emphysema, PVD, and pheochromocytoma.
• Inform ophthalmologist of drug use before surgery because drug may cause intraoperative floppy iris syndrome.
• Safety and effectiveness in children haven't been established.
Dialyzable drug: No.
⚠ *Overdose S&S:* Orthostatic hypotension, bradycardia, HF, bronchospasm, seizures.

PREGNANCY-LACTATION-REPRODUCTION

• There are no adequate studies during pregnancy. Use during pregnancy only if potential benefit justifies fetal risk.
• Low amounts of drug appear in human milk and can be detected in the serum of infants who are breastfed. Use cautiously with breastfeeding.

NURSING CONSIDERATIONS

• Monitor BP frequently. Drug masks common signs and symptoms of shock.
• Monitor heart rate and rhythm in patients receiving IV injection.
• Keep patient supine while patient is receiving IV therapy and for up to 3 hours after infusion ends. Monitor BP closely before allowing patient to ambulate.
• In patients with diabetes, monitor glucose level closely because beta blockers may mask certain signs and symptoms of hypoglycemia.
• Monitor patient for HF.
• Abrupt withdrawal may cause or worsen angina.
• Monitor patient for bronchospasm; discontinue drug if it occurs.

• Don't routinely withdraw long-term beta-blocker therapy before surgery.
• Rare occurrences of severe hepatic injury have been reported. Monitor LFTs. Use cautiously in patients with impaired hepatic function, as metabolism of drug may be decreased.
• Monitor patient for hypersensitivity reactions.

PATIENT TEACHING
🛈 *Alert:* Tell patient that stopping drug abruptly can worsen chest pain and trigger a heart attack.
• Caution patient to take drug in a consistent manner with regard to meals.
• Advise patient that dizziness is the most common adverse reaction and tends to occur in the early stages of treatment, in patients taking diuretics, and with higher dosages. Inform patient that dizziness can be minimized by rising slowly and avoiding sudden position changes.
• Warn patient that occasional, harmless scalp tingling may occur, especially when therapy begins.

---

lacosamide
lah-COSS-ah-mide

Vimpat

Therapeutic class: Anticonvulsants
Pharmacologic class: Functionalized amino acids
Controlled substance schedule: V

AVAILABLE FORMS
Injection: 200 mg/20 mL vials
Oral solution: 10 mg/mL
Tablets ⓞⓣⓒ: 50 mg, 100 mg, 150 mg, 200 mg

INDICATIONS & DOSAGES
Adjust-a-dose (for all indications): In patients with mild or moderate hepatic impairment, ESRD, or severe renal impairment (CrCl of 30 mL/minute or less), reduce maximum recommended daily dosage by 25%. Withhold drug in patients with severe hepatic impairment. Dosage supplementation of up to 50% should be considered following a 4-hour hemodialysis treatment. Reduce dosage as needed in patients with hepatic or renal impairment who are taking strong CYP3A4 and

CYP2C9 inhibitors because of increased lacosamide exposure.
➤ **Adjunctive therapy for partial-onset seizures and primary generalized tonic-clonic seizures**
Adults and adolescents age 17 and older: Initially, 50 mg PO b.i.d.; increase by 50 mg b.i.d. at weekly intervals to recommended daily dosage of 100 to 200 mg PO b.i.d. Or, initially 200 mg PO as a single loading dose followed 12 hours later by 100 mg PO b.i.d. for 1 week. Then, increase by 50 mg b.i.d. as needed based on patient response and tolerance up to recommended maintenance dose of 200 mg b.i.d.
Children ages 4 to younger than 17 weighing 50 kg or more: Initially, 50 mg PO b.i.d.; increase as needed by 50 mg b.i.d. at weekly intervals to recommended maintenance dose of 100 to 200 mg PO b.i.d.
Children ages 4 to younger than 17 weighing 30 to less than 50 kg: Initially, 1 mg/kg PO b.i.d.; increase as needed by 1 mg/kg b.i.d. at weekly intervals to recommended maintenance dose of 2 to 4 mg/kg PO b.i.d.
Children ages 4 to younger than 17 weighing 11 to less than 30 kg: Initially, 1 mg/kg PO b.i.d.; increase as needed by 1 mg/kg b.i.d. at weekly intervals to recommended maintenance dose of 3 to 6 mg/kg PO b.i.d.
May give IV at equivalent daily dose and frequency when oral administration isn't feasible.
➤ **Monotherapy for partial-onset seizures**
Adults and adolescents age 17 and older: Initially, 100 mg PO b.i.d.; increase at weekly intervals by 50 mg b.i.d. to recommended daily dosage of 150 to 200 mg PO b.i.d. Or, initially 200 mg PO as a single loading dose followed approximately 12 hours later by 100 mg PO b.i.d. for 1 week. Then, increase by 50 mg b.i.d. as needed based on patient response and tolerance up to recommended maintenance dose of 150 to 200 mg PO b.i.d. When converting from another single antiepileptic, titrate lacosamide to therapeutic dose of 150 to 200 mg PO b.i.d. and maintain for at least 3 days before initiating withdrawal of concomitant drug. Gradually withdraw concomitant drug over at least 6 weeks.
Children ages 4 to younger than 17: In patients weighing 50 kg or more, same dosing as adults; in those weighing 30 to less than 50 kg, initially, 1 mg/kg PO b.i.d.; increase as needed by 1 mg/kg b.i.d. at weekly intervals

---

Reactions in bold italics are *life-threatening*. Interactions may have a *rapid onset* or a ***delayed onset***.

to recommended daily dosage of 2 to 4 mg/kg PO b.i.d.; in those weighing 11 to less than 30 kg, initially, 1 mg/kg PO b.i.d.; increase as needed by 1 mg/kg b.i.d. at weekly intervals to recommended daily dosage of 3 to 6 mg/kg PO b.i.d.

Children ages 1 month to younger than 17 years: In patients weighing 50 kg or more, same dosing as adults; in those weighing 30 to less than 50 kg, initially, 1 mg/kg PO b.i.d.; increase as needed by 1 mg/kg b.i.d. at weekly intervals to recommended daily dosage of 2 to 4 mg/kg PO b.i.d.; in those weighing 11 to less than 30 kg, initially, 1 mg/kg PO b.i.d.; increase as needed by 1 mg/kg b.i.d. at weekly intervals to recommended daily dosage of 3 to 6 mg/kg PO b.i.d.

Children age 1 month and older weighing 6 to less than 11 kg: Initially, 1 mg/kg PO b.i.d.; increase as needed by 1 mg/kg b.i.d. at weekly intervals to recommended daily dosage of 3 to 6 mg/kg PO b.i.d.

Children age 1 month and older weighing less than 6 kg: Initially, 0.66 mg/kg IV t.i.d. Then increase as needed by 0.66 mg/kg IV t.i.d. at weekly intervals to recommended daily dosage of 2.5 to 5 mg/kg IV t.i.d. Or initially, 1 mg/kg PO b.i.d. Then increase by 1 mg/kg PO b.i.d. at weekly intervals to recommended PO dose of 3.75 to 7.5 mg/kg b.i.d.

Adjust-a-dose: May give IV at equivalent daily dose and frequency to patients weighing 6 kg or more when oral administration isn't feasible.

ADMINISTRATION
PO
- Give drug with or without food.
- Use a calibrated measuring device to administer oral solution.
- May also give oral solution by NG or gastrostomy tube.
- Discard unused oral solution remaining after 6 months of first opening bottle.
- Patient should swallow tablets whole; don't divide tablets.

IV
▼ May give solution for injection without further dilution or diluted.
▼ For diluted IV infusion, dilute with NSS, D_5W, or lactated Ringer solution. Discard solution if discolored or if particulate matter is present. Diluted solution is stable for 4 hours at room temperature. May administer without further dilution.

▼ Infuse over 15 to 60 minutes; 30 to 60 minutes is preferred.
▼ Discard unused solution in vial.
▼ IV use hasn't been studied past 5 days of consecutive treatment.
▼ **Incompatibilities:** None listed by manufacturer. Consult a drug incompatibility reference for more information.

ACTION
May selectively enhance slow inactivation of sodium channels, stabilizing hyperexcitable neuronal membranes and inhibiting repetitive neuronal firing.

Route	Onset	Peak	Duration
PO	Unknown	1–4 hr	Unknown
IV	Unknown	30–60 min	Unknown

Half-life: About 13 hours.

ADVERSE REACTIONS
CNS: asthenia, ataxia, balance disorder, abnormal coordination, depression, dizziness, fatigue, gait disturbance, headache, memory impairment, somnolence, paresthesia, oral paresthesia or hypoesthesia, tremor, *seizure.* **CV:** chest pain. **EENT:** blurred vision, diplopia, nystagmus, vertigo. **GI:** diarrhea, nausea, vomiting. **Skin:** pruritus, skin laceration, injection-site pain or discomfort. **Other:** contusion.

INTERACTIONS
Drug-drug. *Drugs that prolong PR interval (beta blockers, calcium channel blockers):* May increase risk of bradycardia or AV block. Monitor patient closely, especially with IV formulation.
Strong CYP2C9 and CYP3A4 inhibitors (clarithromycin, ketoconazole, ritonavir): May increase lacosamide level in patients with renal and hepatic impairment. Consider dosage reductions.
Drug-lifestyle. *Alcohol use:* May cause additive drowsiness. Don't use together.

EFFECTS ON LAB TEST RESULTS
- May increase LFT values.
- May decrease Hb level and neutrophil count.

CONTRAINDICATIONS & CAUTIONS
- Not recommended for patients with severe hepatic impairment.

- Use cautiously in patients with known cardiac conduction problems, depression, myocardial ischemia, or HF and in those with a history of suicidality.
- Drug may predispose patients to atrial fibrillation or flutter, especially patients with diabetic neuropathy or CV disease.
- Use cautiously in patients with phenylketonuria because oral solution contains aspartame, a source of phenylalanine.

Dialyzable drug: 50%.

⚠ *Overdose S&S:* Coma.

PREGNANCY-LACTATION-REPRODUCTION
- There are no adequate studies during pregnancy. Use during pregnancy only if potential benefit justifies fetal risk.
- Patients who are pregnant should enroll in the Antiepileptic Drug Pregnancy Registry (1-888-233-2334 or www.aedpregnancyregistry.org).
- It isn't known if drug appears in human milk. Weigh risk versus benefit of breastfeeding.

NURSING CONSIDERATIONS
🔵 *Alert:* Give loading dose under medical supervision because of increased risk of CNS adverse reactions. Use of a loading dose hasn't been studied in children.

🔵 *Alert:* Monitor patient for syncopal episodes; drug may increase risk of syncope, especially in patients with cardiac disease and in those receiving drugs that slow AV conduction.
- Obtain ECG at baseline and after titrating to maintenance dose in patients with known conduction problems (marked first-degree AV block, second- or third-degree AV block, or sick sinus syndrome without pacemaker), sodium channelopathies (Brugada syndrome), concomitant use of drugs that prolong PR interval, or severe cardiac disease (MI, HF, structural heart disease). Also closely monitor this population when giving IV lacosamide.
- Monitor patient for signs and symptoms of DRESS syndrome, including fever, rash, eosinophilia, hepatitis, nephritis, lymphadenopathy, and myocarditis. If reaction is suspected, discontinue drug and begin alternative treatment.
- Titrate dosage carefully in patients with renal or hepatic impairment.

🔵 *Alert:* Withdraw drug gradually over 1 week to minimize potential for increased seizure activity.

🔵 *Alert:* Drug may increase risk of suicidality. Monitor patient closely for worsening depression, suicidality, and unusual changes in mood or behavior.

PATIENT TEACHING
- Instruct patient in safe drug administration.

🔵 *Alert:* Tell patient, family, and caregivers to report mood changes or suicidality immediately.
- Warn patient to avoid driving and operating heavy machinery until drug's CNS effects are known; drug may cause dizziness and ataxia.
- Advise patient of childbearing potential to report suspected pregnancy or plans to become pregnant or to breastfeed.
- Warn patient not to stop drug abruptly.
- Tell patient to avoid alcohol while taking drug.
- Inform patient with phenylketonuria that a 200-mg dose of oral solution contains 0.32 mg of phenylalanine.
- Advise patient to report blurred vision, dizziness, double vision, nausea, uncoordinated movement, or vertigo.

lamiVUDine (3TC)
lam-ah-VEW-den

Epivir, Epivir-HBV, Heptovir ✷

Therapeutic class: Antiretrovirals
Pharmacologic class: Nucleoside–nucleotide reverse transcriptase inhibitors

AVAILABLE FORMS
lamivudine
Oral solution: 10 mg/mL
Tablets: 150 mg, 300 mg
lamivudine (HBV)
Oral solution: 5 mg/mL
Tablets: 100 mg

INDICATIONS & DOSAGES
Boxed Warning Lamivudine tablets and oral solution used to treat HIV-1 infection contain a higher dose of the active ingredient than do lamivudine tablets and oral solution used to treat chronic HBV infection. Patients infected with HIV-1 should receive only dosing forms appropriate for HIV-1 treatment. ∎

➤ **HIV infection, with other antiretrovirals**

Adults: 300 mg Epivir PO once daily or 150 mg PO b.i.d.

Children ages 3 months and older: 5 mg/kg Epivir solution PO b.i.d. or 10 mg/kg PO once daily. Maximum dose is 300 mg daily.

Children weighing 14 kg or more who can reliably swallow tablets: For 14 to less than 20 kg, give 1 tablet (150 mg) PO once daily or ½ tablet (75 mg) PO b.i.d.; for 20 kg to less than 25 kg, give 1½ tablets (225 mg) PO once daily or ½ tablet (75 mg) PO in morning and 1 tablet (150 mg) PO in evening; for 25 kg or more, give 2 tablets (300 mg) PO once daily or 150 mg PO b.i.d.

Adjust-a-dose: For adults and adolescents weighing 25 kg or more infected with HIV and a CrCl of 30 to 49 mL/minute, give 150 mg Epivir PO daily. If CrCl is 15 to 29 mL/minute, give 150 mg PO on day 1 and then 100 mg daily; if CrCl is 5 to 14 mL/minute, give 150 mg on day 1 and then 50 mg daily; if CrCl is less than 5 mL/minute, give 50 mg on day 1 and then 25 mg daily. Although there are insufficient data to recommend a specific dosage adjustment in children with renal impairment, consider a dosage reduction or an increase in the dosing interval. No additional dosing is needed after routine hemodialysis or peritoneal dialysis.

➤ **Chronic HBV infection with evidence of HBV replication and active liver inflammation**

Adults: 100 mg PO once daily.

Children ages 2 to 17: 3 mg/kg PO once daily, up to a maximum dose of 100 mg daily. Use oral solution for doses less than 100 mg and in patients unable to swallow tablets. Optimum treatment duration isn't known.

Adjust-a-dose: For adults with chronic HBV infection and CrCl of 30 to 49 mL/minute, give first dose of 100 mg lamivudine for HBV; then give 50 mg PO once daily. If CrCl is 15 to 29 mL/minute, give first dose of 100 mg; then give 25 mg PO once daily. If CrCl is 5 to 14 mL/minute, give first dose of 35 mg; then give 15 mg PO once daily. If CrCl is less than 5 mL/minute, give first dose of 35 mg; then give 10 mg PO once daily. There are insufficient data to recommend a specific dosage in children with renal impairment. No additional dosing is needed after routine hemodialysis or peritoneal dialysis.

ADMINISTRATION

PO

• Give without regard for food.

ACTION

A synthetic nucleoside analogue that inhibits HIV and HBV reverse transcription via viral DNA chain termination. Inhibits RNA- and DNA-dependent DNA polymerase activities.

Route	Onset	Peak	Duration
PO	Unknown	1–3 hr	Unknown

Half-life: Adults, 5 to 7 hours; children, 2 hours.

ADVERSE REACTIONS

Adverse reactions may pertain to the combination HIV therapy of lamivudine and zidovudine.

CNS: dizziness, fatigue, fever, headache, insomnia and other sleep disorders, malaise, neuropathy, depressive disorders, paresthesia. **EENT:** nasal symptoms, infections, sore throat. **GI:** anorexia, diarrhea, nausea, vomiting, abdominal cramps, *pancreatitis,* abdominal pain, dyspepsia, stomatitis. **Hematologic:** *neutropenia, thrombocytopenia,* anemia. **Hepatic:** hepatomegaly (children), increased transaminase levels, hyperbilirubinemia. **Metabolic:** *lactic acidosis;* increased lipase, amylase, CK, ALT levels. **Musculoskeletal:** musculoskeletal pain, arthralgia, myalgia. **Respiratory:** cough, abnormal breath sounds (children). **Skin:** rash. **Other:** chills, splenomegaly, lymphadenopathy.

INTERACTIONS

Drug-drug. *Sorbitol:* May decrease lamivudine level. Avoid use together when possible.
Trimethoprim-containing drugs: May increase lamivudine level because of decreased clearance of drug. Monitor patient for toxicity.

EFFECTS ON LAB TEST RESULTS

• May increase ALT, bilirubin, and serum lipase and CK levels.
• May decrease Hb level and neutrophil and platelet counts.

CONTRAINDICATIONS & CAUTIONS

⚠️ *Alert:* Lactic acidosis and severe hepatomegaly with steatosis, including fatal cases, have been reported.
• Contraindicated in patients hypersensitive to drug.

- Use cautiously in patients with renal impairment.
- Don't use with other combination drugs containing lamivudine or emtricitabine.
- Safety and effectiveness of lamivudine haven't been established for treatment of chronic HBV infection in patients dually infected with HIV-1 and HBV. Emergence of HBV variants associated with resistance to lamivudine has also been reported in patients infected with HIV-1 who have received lamivudine-containing antiretroviral regimens in the presence of concurrent HBV infection.
- Use lamivudine for HBV only when an alternative antiviral with a higher genetic barrier to resistance isn't available or appropriate. Drug hasn't been evaluated in patients infected with HBV/HIV-1, HCV, or hepatitis delta virus; in patients with chronic HBV infection with decompensated liver disease; or in recipients of liver transplant.

Boxed Warning Patients with HIV-1 infection should receive only dosage forms appropriate for HIV treatment. ∎

- Drug may increase risk of immune reconstitution syndrome when used in combination antiretroviral therapy.

☽ *Alert:* Use drug cautiously, if at all, in children with history of pancreatitis or other significant risk factors for development of pancreatitis.

Dializable drug: Unknown.

PREGNANCY-LACTATION-REPRODUCTION
- Use during pregnancy only if potential benefit justifies fetal risk.
- Lamivudine is commonly used to treat HIV infection during pregnancy.
- The Antiretroviral Pregnancy Registry monitors maternal-fetal outcomes with exposure to lamivudine. To register, call 1-800-258-4263.
- Because of the potential for HIV transmission, patients with HIV infection shouldn't breastfeed.
- Lamivudine appears in human milk. Use cautiously during breastfeeding.

NURSING CONSIDERATIONS
Boxed Warning Severe acute exacerbations of HBV have been reported in patients who have HBV alone or who are infected with both HBV and HIV-1 and have discontinued drug. Monitor hepatic function closely in patients who discontinue drug. If appropriate, initiate anti-hepatitis B therapy. ∎

☽ *Alert:* Stop treatment immediately and notify prescriber if signs, symptoms, or lab abnormalities suggest pancreatitis. Monitor amylase level.

☽ *Alert:* Lactic acidosis and hepatotoxicity have been reported. Notify prescriber if signs of lactic acidosis or hepatotoxicity occur.

- Scored tablets are the preferred formulation for children infected with HIV-1 who weigh at least 14 kg and for whom a solid dosage form is appropriate because the oral solution has been shown to have lower rates of virologic suppression and lower plasma lamivudine exposure, and patients developed viral resistance more frequently. Monitor HIV-1 viral load more frequently when using oral solution.

Boxed Warning Provide HIV counseling and test patients for HIV before and during therapy because form and dosage of lamivudine for HBV infection aren't appropriate for those infected with both HBV and HIV. If giving lamivudine to patients with HBV and HIV, use the higher dosage indicated for HIV therapy as part of an appropriate combination regimen. If treatment is prescribed for chronic HBV infection in patients with unrecognized or untreated HIV infection, HIV resistance is likely. ∎

- Monitor patient's CBC, platelet count, LFTs, and renal function studies.
- To reduce risk of resistance in patients receiving HBV monotherapy, consider switching to an alternative regimen if serum HBV DNA remains detectable after 24 weeks of treatment. Guide optimal therapy by resistance testing.

PATIENT TEACHING
- Inform patient that long-term effects of drug aren't known.
- Stress importance of taking drug exactly as prescribed.

Boxed Warning Offer HIV counseling and testing to all patients before beginning treatment with lamivudine for HBV and periodically during treatment. ∎

- Inform patient that drug doesn't cure HIV infection, that opportunistic infections and other complications of HIV infection may still occur, and that transmission of HIV to others through sexual contact or blood contamination is still possible.

Reactions in bold italics are *life-threatening*. Interactions may have a *rapid onset* or a **delayed onset**.

• Teach parents or guardians signs and symptoms of pancreatitis. Advise them to report signs and symptoms immediately.

---

lamoTRIgine
la-MO-tri-geen

LaMICtal, Subvenite

Therapeutic class: Anticonvulsants
Pharmacologic class: Phenyltriazines

AVAILABLE FORMS
Tablets: 25 mg, 100 mg, 150 mg, 200 mg
Tablets (chewable dispersible): 2 mg, 5 mg, 25 mg
Tablets (extended-release) ⓓⓝⓒ: 25 mg, 50 mg, 100 mg, 200 mg, 250 mg, 300 mg
Tablets (ODTs): 25 mg, 50 mg, 100 mg, 200 mg

INDICATIONS & DOSAGES
❂ *Alert:* Extended-release formula isn't for use as initial monotherapy or for conversion to monotherapy from two or more concomitant AEDs.

Adjust-a-dose (for all indications): Generally, reduce initial, escalation, and maintenance doses by approximately 25% in patients with moderate and severe hepatic impairment without ascites and 50% in patients with severe hepatic impairment with ascites. May adjust escalation and maintenance doses according to clinical response. In patients with renal impairment, base initial doses on patients' concomitant medications; reduced maintenance doses may be effective for patients with significant renal impairment.

➤ **Conversion to monotherapy using extended-release formula in patients with partial seizures who are receiving treatment with a single enzyme-inducing AED (except valproate)**
Adults and children age 13 and older: Add 50 mg extended-release tablet PO daily to current drug regimen for 2 weeks, followed by 100 mg PO daily for 2 weeks. Then, increase by 100 mg every week until a dosage of 500 mg PO daily is reached. The concomitant enzyme-inducing AED can then be gradually reduced by 20% decrements each week over a 4-week period. Two weeks after completing withdrawal of the enzyme-inducing AED, decrease lamotrigine (extended-release tablet) no faster than 100 mg/day each week to achieve the monotherapy maintenance dosage of 250 to 300 mg/day.

➤ **Conversion to monotherapy using extended-release formula in patients with partial seizures who are receiving adjunctive treatment with valproate**
Adults and children age 13 and older: Add 25 mg extended-release PO every other day for 2 weeks; then increase to 25 mg PO daily for weeks 3 and 4. Increase to 50 mg PO daily for week 5, 100 mg PO daily for week 6, and 150 mg PO daily for week 7. Maintain dosage at 150 mg PO daily while decreasing valproate dosage by no more than 500 mg/day each week until 500 mg/day is achieved; maintain for 1 week. Then, simultaneously increase extended-release tablet to 200 mg/day while decreasing valproate to 250 mg/day; maintain for 1 week. Increase to 250 or 300 mg PO daily as maintenance dosage and discontinue valproate.

➤ **Conversion to monotherapy using extended-release formula in patients with partial seizures who are receiving treatment with a single drug other than an enzyme-inducing AED or valproate**
Adults and children age 13 and older: Add 25 mg extended-release PO daily for 2 weeks; then increase to 50 mg PO daily for weeks 3 and 4. Increase to 100 mg PO daily for week 5. Starting with week 6, continue increasing dosage each week by 50 mg PO daily until a dosage of 250 to 300 mg PO daily is achieved; then withdraw concomitant AED therapy by 20% decrements each week over a 4-week period. No additional lamotrigine (extended-release tablet) adjustment is needed.

➤ **Adjunctive treatment of partial seizures or primary generalized tonic-clonic seizures caused by epilepsy or generalized seizures of Lennox-Gastaut syndrome**
Adults and children older than age 12 taking valproate: 25 mg immediate-release PO every other day for 2 weeks; then 25 mg PO daily for 2 weeks. Continue to increase, as needed, by 25 to 50 mg daily every 1 to 2 weeks until an effective maintenance dosage of 100 to 400 mg daily given in one or two divided doses is reached. When added to valproate alone, the usual daily maintenance dose is 100 to 200 mg.
Adults and children age 13 and older taking valproate: 25 mg extended-release PO every

L

---

other day for 2 weeks; then 25 mg PO daily for 2 weeks; then 50 mg PO daily for 1 week; then 100 mg PO daily for 1 week; then 150 mg PO daily for 1 week. Daily maintenance dose is 200 to 250 mg.

Adults and children age 13 and older not taking carbamazepine, phenytoin, phenobarbital, primidone, or valproate: 25 mg extended-release PO daily for 2 weeks; then 50 mg PO daily for 2 weeks; then 100 mg PO daily for 1 week; then 150 mg PO daily for 1 week; then 200 mg PO daily for 1 week. Daily maintenance dose is 300 to 400 mg.

Adults and children older than age 12 taking anticonvulsant drugs but not carbamazepine, phenytoin, phenobarbital, primidone, or valproate: 25 mg immediate-release PO daily for 1 to 2 weeks; then 50 mg PO daily for another 2 weeks. Continue to increase by 50 mg/day every 1 to 2 weeks until an effective maintenance dose is reached. Daily maintenance dose is 225 to 375 mg PO daily in two divided doses.

Adults and children older than age 12 taking carbamazepine, phenytoin, phenobarbital, or primidone but not valproate: 50 mg immediate-release PO daily for 2 weeks; then 100 mg PO daily in two divided doses for 2 weeks. Increase, as needed, by 100 mg daily every 1 to 2 weeks. Usual maintenance dosage is 300 to 500 mg PO daily in two divided doses.

Adults and children age 13 and older taking carbamazepine, phenytoin, phenobarbital, or primidone but not valproate: 50 mg extended-release PO daily for 2 weeks; then 100 mg PO daily for 2 weeks; then 200 mg PO daily for 1 week; then 300 mg PO daily for 1 week; then 400 mg PO daily for 1 week. Daily maintenance dose is 400 to 600 mg.

Children ages 2 to 12 weighing 6.7 to 40 kg taking valproate: 0.15 mg/kg immediate-release PO daily in one or two divided doses (rounded down to nearest whole tablet) for 2 weeks. Increase to 0.3 mg/kg daily in one or two divided doses for 2 weeks, followed by increasing the daily dose every 1 or 2 weeks with an additional 0.3 mg/kg daily in one or two divided doses. Thereafter, usual maintenance dosage is 1 to 5 mg/kg daily (maximum, 200 mg daily in one to two divided doses). In patients weighing less than 30 kg, maintenance dosage may need to be increased by as much as 50% based on clinical response.

Children ages 2 to 12 weighing 6.7 to 40 kg taking anticonvulsant drugs but not carbamazepine, phenytoin, phenobarbital, primidone, or valproate: 0.3 mg/kg immediate-release PO daily in one or two divided doses (rounded down to the nearest whole tablet) for 2 weeks; then 0.6 mg/kg PO daily in two divided doses for another 2 weeks; then increase the daily dose every 1 to 2 weeks with an additional 0.6 mg/kg PO daily in two divided doses. Thereafter, usual maintenance dose is 4.5 to 7.5 mg/kg PO daily. Maximum dose is 300 mg daily in two divided doses. In patients weighing less than 30 kg, maintenance dosage may need to be increased by as much as 50% based on clinical response.

Children ages 2 to 12 weighing 6.7 to 40 kg taking carbamazepine, phenytoin, phenobarbital, or primidone but not valproate: 0.6 mg/kg immediate-release PO daily in two divided doses (rounded down to nearest whole tablet) for 2 weeks. Increase to 1.2 mg/kg PO daily in two divided doses for 2 weeks; then increase the daily dose every 1 to 2 weeks with an additional 1.2 mg/kg daily in two divided doses. Usual maintenance dosage is 5 to 15 mg/kg PO daily (maximum 400 mg daily in two divided doses). In patients weighing less than 30 kg, maintenance dosage may need to be increased by as much as 50% based on clinical response.

➤ **To convert patients from therapy with an enzyme-inducing AED alone to lamotrigine therapy**

Adults and children age 16 and older: Add 50 mg immediate-release PO once daily to current drug regimen for 2 weeks, followed by 100 mg PO daily in two divided doses for 2 weeks. Then increase daily dosage by 100 mg every 1 to 2 weeks until maintenance dose of 500 mg daily in two divided doses is reached. The concomitant hepatic enzyme-inducing AED can then be gradually reduced by 20% decrements weekly for 4 weeks.

➤ **To convert patients with partial seizures from adjunctive therapy with valproate to therapy with lamotrigine alone**

Adults and children age 16 and older: Add immediate-release form until 200 mg daily is achieved; then gradually decrease valproate to 500 mg daily by decrements of no more than 500 mg daily per week. Maintain these dosages for 1 week, then increase lamotrigine to 300 mg daily while decreasing valproate to 250 mg daily. Maintain these dosages for

1 week, then stop valproate completely while increasing lamotrigine by 100 mg daily every week until a dose of 500 mg daily is reached.

➤ **Bipolar disorder for maintenance treatment to delay time to occurrence of mood episodes (depression, mania, hypomania, mixed episodes) in patients treated for acute mood episodes with standard therapy**

Adults: Initially, 25 mg immediate-release PO once daily for 2 weeks; then 50 mg PO once daily for 2 weeks. Dosage may then be doubled at weekly intervals, to maintenance dosage of 200 mg daily.

Adults taking carbamazepine or other enzyme-inducing drugs without valproate: Initially, 50 mg immediate-release PO once daily for 2 weeks; then 100 mg daily in two divided doses for 2 weeks. Dosage is then increased by 100 mg weekly to maintenance dosage of 400 mg daily, given in two divided doses.

Adults taking valproate: Initially, 25 mg immediate-release PO every other day for 2 weeks; then 25 mg PO once daily for 2 weeks. Dosage may then be doubled at weekly intervals to maintenance dosage of 100 mg daily.

ADMINISTRATION
PO
• Starter and titration kits are available to provide doses consistent with recommended titration schedule for the first 5 weeks of treatment.
• Patient may swallow chewable dispersible tablets whole, chew them, or disperse them in a small amount of water or diluted fruit juice.
• If tablets are chewed, give a small amount of water or diluted fruit juice to aid in swallowing.
• Place ODTs on the tongue and have patient move them around in the mouth.
• Patient may swallow ODTs with or without water and without regard to food.
• Give extended-release tablets once daily with or without food. Patient must swallow tablets whole and must not chew, crush, or divide them.

ACTION
Inhibits release of glutamate (an excitatory neurotransmitter) in the brain via action at voltage-sensitive sodium channels. Is a weak inhibitor of the 5-HT$_3$ receptor.

Route	Onset	Peak	Duration
PO (immediate-release)	Unknown	1–5 hr	Unknown
PO (extended-release)	Unknown	4–11 hr	Unknown

Half-life: 7 to 148 hours, depending on age, dosage schedule, use of other anticonvulsants, and other medical conditions.

ADVERSE REACTIONS
CNS: ataxia, dizziness, drowsiness, headache, migraine, somnolence, fatigue, anxiety, abnormal thinking, amnesia, depression, confusion, dysarthria, emotional lability, fever, incoordination, insomnia, irritability, hypoesthesia, dream abnormality, malaise, pain, asthenia, speech disorder, concentration disturbance, *seizure exacerbation.* **CV:** palpitations, chest pain, edema, *hemorrhage.* **EENT:** blurred vision, diplopia, vision abnormality, nystagmus, rhinitis, epistaxis, dry mouth, pharyngitis, sinusitis. **GI:** nausea, vomiting, abdominal pain, anorexia, constipation, diarrhea, dyspepsia, flatulence, *rectal hemorrhage,* peptic ulcer. **GU:** amenorrhea, dysmenorrhea, urinary frequency, vaginitis, UTI. **Hematologic:** lymphadenopathy. **Metabolic:** weight loss. **Musculoskeletal:** arthralgia, back pain, muscle spasm, neck pain, weakness. **Respiratory:** cough, dyspnea, bronchitis, bronchospasm. **Skin:** rash, pruritus, dermatitis, dry skin, diaphoresis, photosensitivity. **Other:** infection, accidental injury, flulike syndrome.

INTERACTIONS
Drug-drug. *Acetaminophen:* May decrease therapeutic effects of lamotrigine. Monitor patient.

Atazanavir–ritonavir, ethosuximide, lopinavir–ritonavir, oxcarbazepine, phenobarbital, phenytoin, primidone, rifampin: May decrease lamotrigine level. Monitor patient closely; adjust lamotrigine dosage.

Carbamazepine: May decrease effects of lamotrigine while increasing toxicity of carbamazepine. Consider alternative therapy. Adjust doses and monitor patient.

Hormonal contraceptives containing estrogen: May decrease lamotrigine level. Adjust dosage based on individual hormonal product used. By the end of the "pill-free" week, lamotrigine level may double.

Organic cation transporter 2 substrates (dofetilide): May increase lamotrigine or dofetilide plasma level. Don't coadminister.
Strong CYP3A4 inducers (phenytoin, rifampin): May decrease lamotrigine level. Use cautiously together; adjust lamotrigine dosage.
Valproate: May decrease clearance of lamotrigine, which increases lamotrigine level; also decreases valproate level. Monitor patient for toxicity. Reduce lamotrigine dosage if added to a multidrug regimen that includes valproic acid.
Drug-lifestyle. *Sun exposure:* May cause photosensitivity reactions. Advise patient to avoid excessive sun exposure.

EFFECTS ON LAB TEST RESULTS
• May result in false-positive readings in rapid urine drug screens, particularly for phencyclidine.

CONTRAINDICATIONS & CAUTIONS
• Contraindicated in patients hypersensitive to drug or its components.
⚡ *Alert:* Rare, multiorgan hypersensitivity reactions that can be fatal have occurred.
⚡ *Alert:* Drug may cause hemophagocytic lymphohistiocytosis (HLH), a rare and life-threatening immune system reaction.
• Use cautiously in patients with renal, hepatic, or cardiac impairment.
• Drug isn't recommended for treatment of acute manic or mixed episodes of bipolar disorder because effectiveness hasn't been established.
⚡ *Alert:* Use cautiously in patients with structural and functional heart disorders, including HF, valvular heart disease, congenital heart disease, conduction system disease, ventricular arrhythmias, cardiac channelopathies, ischemic heart disease, or multiple risk factors for CAD, especially when used in combination with sodium channel blockers (carbamazepine, phenytoin, topiramate); drug may increase risk of serious or life-threatening arrhythmias. Assess whether potential benefits of lamotrigine outweigh risk of arrhythmia for each patient.
Dialyzable drug: 20%.
⚠ *Overdose S&S:* Ataxia, nystagmus, increased seizures, decreased level of consciousness, coma, intraventricular conduction delay.

PREGNANCY-LACTATION-REPRODUCTION
• Drug may increase risk of congenital malformations in the first trimester. Use during pregnancy only if potential benefit justifies fetal risk.
• Patients should enroll in the North American Antiepileptic Drug Pregnancy Registry (1-888-233-2334 or www.aedpregnancyregistry.org).
• Drug appears in human milk. Use cautiously during breastfeeding. Discontinue breastfeeding if infants develop drug toxicity.

NURSING CONSIDERATIONS
⚡ *Alert:* Closely monitor all patients taking or starting AEDs for changes in behavior indicating worsening of suicidality or depression. Symptoms such as anxiety, agitation, hostility, mania, and hypomania may be precursors to emerging suicidality.
• Don't stop drug abruptly because this may increase seizure frequency. Instead, taper drug over at least 2 weeks.
Boxed Warning Serious rashes, including SJS and TEN, and rash-related death have been reported. Serious rash occurs more frequently in children than in adults, when administered with valproate, or when initial recommended dose or escalation dose is exceeded. Benign rashes may also occur but it's impossible to predict which rash will become serious or life threatening. Stop drug at first sign of rash, unless rash is clearly not drug-related. ∎
Boxed Warning Stopping treatment may not prevent a rash from becoming life-threatening or permanently disabling or disfiguring. ∎
Boxed Warning Extended-release form isn't approved for children younger than age 13. ∎
⚡ *Alert:* Drug may cause aseptic meningitis. Monitor patient for symptoms such as headache, fever, neck stiffness, nausea, vomiting, rash, and photophobia. Discontinue drug if no other cause of meningitis is found.
• Evaluate patients for changes in seizure activity. Check adjunct anticonvulsant level.
⚡ *Alert:* Monitor patient for HLH (persistent fever, hepatosplenomegaly, rash, lymphadenopathy, neurologic symptoms, cytopenias, high serum ferritin level, and liver function and coagulation abnormalities). Evaluate patient with fever or rash promptly, and discontinue drug if HLH or another serious

---

Reactions in bold italics are *life-threatening*. Interactions may have a *rapid onset* or a *delayed onset*.

immune-related reaction is suspected or an alternative cause can't be identified.

• *Look alike–sound alike:* Don't confuse lamotrigine with lamivudine or levothyroxine. Don't confuse Lamictal with Lamisil, labetalol, or Lomotil.

PATIENT TEACHING

❶ Alert: Counsel family member or caregivers to monitor patient for changes in behavior and to immediately report suicidality.

• Instruct patient or caregiver to report worsening of seizures.

• Inform patient that drug may cause rash, especially if administered with valproic acid. Tell patient to report rash or signs or symptoms of hypersensitivity promptly to prescriber; drug may need to be stopped.

• Strongly advise patient to visually inspect tablets with each prescription refill to verify the tablets are correct, to avoid medication errors.

• Caution patient to report all medications being taken or changes to medications, especially oral contraceptives or other hormone products.

• Warn patient not to engage in hazardous activity until drug's CNS effects are known.

• Advise patient to seek immediate medical attention if signs or symptoms of HLH occur, including fever; rash; abdominal pain, tenderness, or swelling; enlarged lymph nodes; yellowing of the skin or eyes; unusual bleeding; seizures; vision changes; or trouble walking.

• Teach patient or caregiver to immediately report headache, fever, mouth ulcers, bruising or petechiae, signs of infection (fever, cough, dyspnea), neck stiffness, nausea, vomiting, rash, drowsiness, confusion, or light sensitivity.

• Warn patient that the drug may trigger sensitivity to the sun and to take precautions until tolerance is determined.

• Warn patient not to stop drug abruptly.

❶ Alert: Advise patient of childbearing potential to discuss drug therapy with prescriber if considering pregnancy.

❶ Alert: Caution patient to seek immediate medical attention for abnormal heart rate or irregular rhythm, or such signs or symptoms as racing heartbeat, skipped or slow heartbeat, shortness of breath, dizziness, or fainting.

lansoprazole
lanz-AH-pray-zol

Prevacid🏷 ◇

Therapeutic class: Antiulcer drugs
Pharmacologic class: PPIs

AVAILABLE FORMS
Capsules (delayed-release) ⓓⓝⓒ: 15 mg ◇, 30 mg
Tablets (ODT delayed-release): 15 mg, 30 mg

INDICATIONS & DOSAGES
Adjust-a-dose (for all indications): Recommended dosage in patients with severe hepatic impairment (Child-Pugh class C) is 15 mg PO daily.

➤ **Short-term treatment of active duodenal ulcer**
Adults: 15 mg PO daily before eating for 4 weeks.

➤ **Maintenance of healed duodenal ulcers**
Adults: 15 mg PO daily.

➤ **Short-term treatment of active benign gastric ulcer**
Adults: 30 mg PO once daily for up to 8 weeks.

➤ **Short-term treatment of erosive esophagitis**
Adults: 30 mg PO daily before eating for up to 8 weeks. If healing doesn't occur, 8 more weeks of therapy may be given. Maintenance dosage for healing is 15 mg PO daily.
Children ages 12 to 17: 30 mg PO once daily for up to 8 weeks.
Children ages 1 to 11 weighing more than 30 kg: 30 mg PO once daily for up to 12 weeks.
Children ages 1 to 11 weighing 30 kg or less: 15 mg PO once daily for up to 12 weeks.

➤ **Long-term treatment of pathologic hypersecretory conditions, including Zollinger-Ellison syndrome**
Adults: Initially, 60 mg PO once daily. Increase dosage, as needed. Give daily amounts above 120 mg in evenly divided doses.

➤ ***Helicobacter pylori* eradication to reduce risk of duodenal ulcer recurrence**
Adults: For patients receiving dual therapy, 30 mg PO lansoprazole with 1 g PO amoxicillin, each given t.i.d. for 14 days. For patients receiving triple therapy, 30 mg PO lansoprazole with 1 g PO amoxicillin and

500 mg PO clarithromycin, all given b.i.d. for 10 to 14 days.

➤ **Short-term treatment of symptomatic GERD**
Adults: 15 mg PO once daily for up to 8 weeks.
Children ages 12 to 17: 15 mg PO once daily for up to 8 weeks.
Children ages 1 to 11 weighing more than 30 kg: 30 mg PO once daily for up to 12 weeks.
Children ages 1 to 11 weighing 30 kg or less: 15 mg PO once daily for up to 12 weeks.
➤ **NSAID-related ulcer in patients who continue NSAID use**
Adults: 30 mg PO daily for 8 weeks.
➤ **To reduce risk of NSAID-related ulcer in patients with history of gastric ulcer who need NSAIDs**
Adults: 15 mg PO daily for up to 12 weeks.
➤ **Dyspepsia** ◆
Adults: 15 or 30 mg once daily for up to 8 weeks.

ADMINISTRATION
PO
• Give before a meal.
• Don't crush or allow patient to chew capsules.
• For patients who have difficulty swallowing capsules, the capsules can be opened and the intact granules sprinkled on 1 tablespoon of applesauce, Ensure pudding, cottage cheese, yogurt, or strained pears and swallowed immediately. Or, capsule contents may be emptied into a small volume (60 mL) of apple, orange, or tomato juice and swallowed.
• Contents of capsule can be mixed with 40 mL of apple juice in a syringe and given within 3 to 5 minutes via an NG or nasojejunal tube. Flush with additional apple juice to give entire dose and maintain patency of the tube.
• Place ODT on patient's tongue and allow it to disintegrate with or without water until the particles can be swallowed.
• To give ODTs using an oral syringe, dissolve a 15-mg tablet in 4 mL water or a 30-mg tablet in 10 mL water and give within 15 minutes. Refill syringe with about 2 mL (15-mg tablet) or 5 mL (30-mg tablet) of water, shake gently, and give any remaining contents.
• To give ODTs through an 8 French or larger NG tube, dissolve a 15-mg tablet in 4 mL water or a 30-mg tablet in 10 mL water and give

within 15 minutes. Refill syringe with about 5 mL of water, shake gently, and flush the NG tube.
• ODTs contain 2.5 mg phenylalanine/ 15-mg tablet and 5.1 mg phenylalanine/ 30-mg tablet.

ACTION
Reduces acid secretion in gastric parietal cells through inhibition of (H^+, K^+)-ATPase enzyme system, inhibiting the final step in gastric acid production.

Route	Onset	Peak	Duration
PO	1–3 hr	1.7 hr	24 hr

Half-life: Less than 2 hours.

ADVERSE REACTIONS
CNS: headache, dizziness. **GI:** abdominal pain, constipation, diarrhea, nausea. **GU:** hematuria.

INTERACTIONS
Drug-drug. *Amoxicillin, clarithromycin:* May increase risk of adverse effects. Monitor patient.
Atazanavir, nelfinavir: May reduce antiviral GI absorption and activity. Don't use together.
Cefuroxime: May reduce cefuroxime absorption. Avoid combination.
Clopidogrel: May decrease clopidogrel serum concentration. Monitor therapy or consider H_2 receptor antagonist (e.g., famotidine).
Digoxin: May increase digoxin level. Monitor digoxin concentration; digoxin dosage adjustment may be needed.
Erlotinib, iron salts, ketoconazole, mycophenolate mofetil: May inhibit absorption of these drugs. Monitor patient closely.
Methotrexate: May increase methotrexate serum level. Monitor methotrexate concentration and adjust dosage as needed.
Rilpivirine: May decrease rilpivirine concentration. Use together is contraindicated.
Strong CYP2C19 or CYP3A inducers (ritonavir): May decrease lansoprazole level. Monitor therapy.
Strong CYP2C19 or CYP3A4 inhibitors (voriconazole): May increase lansoprazole level. Use cautiously together.
Sucralfate: May cause delayed lansoprazole absorption. Give lansoprazole at least 30 minutes before sucralfate.
Tacrolimus: May increase tacrolimus level, especially in patients with a transplant who

---

are intermediate or poor metabolizers of CYP2C19. Monitor tacrolimus level.

Theophylline: May increase theophylline clearance. Adjust theophylline dosage when lansoprazole is started or stopped. Use together cautiously.

Warfarin: May increase bleeding time. Monitor INR and PT.

Drug-herb. *St. John's wort:* May increase risk of sun sensitivity. Advise patient to avoid excessive sunlight exposure.

Drug-food. *Any food:* May decrease rate and extent of GI absorption. Advise patient to take before meals.

EFFECTS ON LAB TEST RESULTS

• May increase LFT values and creatinine, BUN, potassium, lipid, serum urea, gastrin, globulin, and LDH levels.
• May increase or decrease cholesterol or electrolyte levels.
• May decrease Hb level.
• May increase or decrease WBC and platelet counts.
• May cause abnormal RBC count.
• May increase urinary albumin and glucose levels.
• May cause urine crystals.
• May cause positive fecal occult blood result.
• May cause false-positive results in diagnostic investigations for neuroendocrine tumors, urine screening tests for tetrahydrocannabinol, and gastrin secretion in response to secretin stimulation test.

CONTRAINDICATIONS & CAUTIONS

• Contraindicated in patients hypersensitive to drug or its components. Reactions may include anaphylaxis, angioedema, acute interstitial nephritis, and urticaria.

⭘ *Alert:* Prolonged use of PPIs or use with medications such as digoxin or drugs that may cause hypomagnesemia (e.g., diuretics) may require magnesium supplementation and possible discontinuation of drug. Monitor magnesium levels before starting treatment and periodically thereafter.

⭘ *Alert:* Drug may increase risk of hip, wrist, and spine fractures with long-term and multiple daily dose use.

• Acute interstitial nephritis has been observed in patients taking PPIs and may occur at any point during therapy. Discontinue drug if condition develops.

• Prolonged treatment (2 years or more) may cause vitamin B_{12} malabsorption caused by hypochlorhydria or achlorhydria. Observe for clinical signs and symptoms consistent with vitamin B_{12} deficiency.

• Use oral solution cautiously in patients with phenylketonuria.

• Prolonged PPI use beyond 1 year may increase risk of fundic gland polyps. Use the shortest duration of PPI therapy appropriate to the condition being treated.

Dialyzable drug: No.

PREGNANCY-LACTATION-REPRODUCTION

• There are no adequate studies during pregnancy. Use during pregnancy only if clearly needed.

• It isn't known if drug appears in human milk. Evaluate risks and benefits of discontinuing breastfeeding or discontinuing drug.

NURSING CONSIDERATIONS

⭘ *Alert:* Monitor patient for signs and symptoms of low magnesium level, such as abnormal HR or rhythm, palpitations, muscle spasms, tremor, or seizures. In children, abnormal HR may present as fatigue, upset stomach, dizziness, and light-headedness.

• New onset and exacerbation of existing cutaneous lupus erythematosus and SLE have been reported in patients taking PPIs, including lansoprazole. Avoid administering PPIs for longer than medically indicated. Discontinue drug and refer patient to appropriate specialist for evaluation if indicated.

⭘ *Alert:* May increase risk of CDAD. Evaluate for CDAD in patients who develop diarrhea that doesn't improve.

• Patients with severe liver disease may need dosage adjustment, but don't adjust dosage for older adults or patients with renal insufficiency.

• Just because symptoms respond to therapy, gastric malignancy shouldn't be ruled out.

• Monitor patient for hypersensitivity reactions, including SCARs (SJS, TEN, DRESS syndrome, acute generalized exanthematous pustulosis).

• *Look alike–sound alike:* Don't confuse Prevacid with Pepcid, Prilosec, or Prevpac.

PATIENT TEACHING

• Teach patient safe drug administration.
• Inform patient with phenylketonuria that ODTs contain 2.5 mg phenylalanine/15-mg tablet and 5.1 mg phenylalanine/30-mg tablet.

- Advise patient to recognize and report all adverse reactions, especially diarrhea that doesn't improve and signs and symptoms of low magnesium level or SLE.

ledipasvir–sofosbuvir ⌧
LED-i-pas-vir/soe-FOS-bue-vir

Harvoni

Therapeutic class: Antivirals
Pharmacologic class: Antivirals

AVAILABLE FORMS
Pellets: 33.75 mg ledipasvir/150 mg sofosbuvir, 45 mg ledipasvir/200 mg sofosbuvir
Tablets: 45 mg ledipasvir/200 mg sofosbuvir, 90 mg ledipasvir/400 mg sofosbuvir

INDICATIONS & DOSAGES
➤ **Chronic HCV genotype 1 infection in patients who are treatment naive without cirrhosis or with compensated cirrhosis or in patients who are treatment experienced without cirrhosis** ⌧
Adults and children age 3 and older weighing at least 35 kg: One 90 mg/400 mg tablet PO daily for 12 weeks. If pretreatment HCV-RNA is less than 6 million international units/mL in adults without cirrhosis who are treatment naive, may consider treatment course of 8 weeks.
Children age 3 and older weighing 17 to less than 35 kg: 45 mg/200 mg (tablets/pellets) PO once daily for 12 weeks.
Children age 3 and older weighing less than 17 kg: 33.75 mg/150 mg pellets PO once daily for 12 weeks.
➤ **Chronic HCV genotype 1 infection in patients who are treatment experienced with compensated cirrhosis**
Adults and children age 3 and older weighing at least 35 kg: One 90 mg/400 mg tablet PO once daily for 24 weeks.
Children age 3 and older weighing 17 to less than 35 kg: 45 mg/200 mg (tablets/pellets) PO once daily for 24 weeks.
Children age 3 and older weighing less than 17 kg: 33.75 mg/150 mg pellets PO once daily for 24 weeks.
➤ **Chronic HCV genotype 1 infection in patients who are treatment naive or treatment experienced with decompensated cirrhosis, in combination with ribavirin;**

chronic HCV genotype 1 or 4 infection in treatment naive or treatment experienced and received a liver transplant without cirrhosis or with compensated cirrhosis, in combination with ribavirin ⌧
Adults and children age 3 and older weighing at least 35 kg: One 90 mg/400 mg tablet PO once daily with ribavirin for 12 weeks.
Children age 3 and older weighing 17 to less than 35 kg: 45 mg/200 mg (tablets/pellets) PO once daily with ribavirin for 12 weeks.
Children age 3 and older weighing less than 17 kg: 33.75 mg/150 mg pellets PO once daily with ribavirin for 12 weeks.
Adjust-a-dose: Refer to ribavirin manufacturer's information for recommended weight-based dosing schedule and renal impairment dosage.
➤ **Chronic HCV genotype 4, 5, or 6 infection in patients who are treatment naive or treatment experienced without cirrhosis or with compensated cirrhosis** ⌧
Adults and children age 3 and older weighing at least 35 kg: One 90 mg/400 mg tablet PO once daily for 12 weeks.
Children age 3 and older weighing 17 to less than 35 kg: 45 mg/200 mg (tablets/pellets) PO once daily for 12 weeks.
Children age 3 and older weighing less than 17 kg: 33.75 mg/150 mg pellets PO once daily for 12 weeks.

ADMINISTRATION
PO
- May give without regard for food.
- Store at room temperature in original container.
- If giving pellets with food, sprinkle on one or more spoonsful of nonacidic, soft food (pudding, chocolate syrup, mashed potatoes, ice cream) at or below room temperature.
- Give pellets within 30 minutes of mixing with food. Patient shouldn't chew pellets, to avoid bitter taste.
- Give a missed dose within the calendar day as soon as possible. If the calendar day when dose is usually given has passed, omit the missed dose and resume usual dosing schedule.

ACTION
Ledipasvir and sofosbuvir are direct-acting antivirals against HCV. Ledipasvir inhibits the NS5A protein, and sofosbuvir inhibits the

---

NS5B RNA polymerase, both of which are required for viral replication.

Route	Onset	Peak	Duration
PO (ledipasvir)	Unknown	4–4.5 hr	Unknown
PO (sofosbuvir)	Unknown	0.8–1 hr	Unknown

Half-life: Ledipasvir, 47 hours; sofosbuvir, 0.5 hour.

ADVERSE REACTIONS
CNS: fatigue, asthenia, headache, insomnia, irritability, dizziness, depression. **GI:** nausea, diarrhea. **Hepatic:** hyperbilirubinemia. **Metabolic:** increased lipase level. **Musculoskeletal:** myalgia. **Respiratory:** cough, dyspnea.

INTERACTIONS
Drug-drug. ❸ *Alert: Amiodarone:* May increase risk of symptomatic bradycardia. Avoid use together. If use together can't be avoided, advise patient of risk and monitor patient carefully.
Antacids (aluminum hydroxide, magnesium hydroxide): May decrease ledipasvir level. Separate administration of antacids and ledipasvir–sofosbuvir by 4 hours.
Anticonvulsants (carbamazepine, oxcarbazepine, phenobarbital, phenytoin), antimycobacterials (rifabutin, rifampin, rifapentine), P-gp inducers (rifampin): May decrease ledipasvir–sofosbuvir concentrations. Use together isn't recommended.
Atorvastatin: May increase atorvastatin level; may be associated with increased risk of myopathy. Monitor patient closely.
Digoxin: May increase digoxin concentration. Monitor digoxin level.
H₂-receptor antagonists (famotidine): May decrease ledipasvir level. Separate administration by 12 hours or administer simultaneously if H₂-receptor antagonist dose doesn't exceed equivalent of famotidine 40 mg b.i.d.
HIV antiretroviral regimen containing tenofovir disoproxil fumarate (DF), an HIV protease inhibitor (atazanavir, darunavir, lopinavir), and ritonavir: May increase tenofovir-associated adverse reactions. Safety of use together hasn't been established. Consider alternative HCV or antiretroviral therapy or monitor patient closely for tenofovir-associated adverse reactions.
HIV antiretroviral regimen containing tenofovir DF, cobicistat, elvitegravir, and emtricitabine: May increase tenofovir level. Safety of use together hasn't been established; use together isn't recommended.
HIV antiretroviral regimen containing tenofovir DF, efavirenz, and emtricitabine or tenofovir DF without an HIV protease inhibitor, ritonavir, or cobicistat: May increase tenofovir concentration and risk of toxicity. Monitor patient for tenofovir-associated adverse reactions.
HIV antiretroviral regimen containing tipranavir and ritonavir: May decrease ledipasvir–sofosbuvir concentrations and effectiveness. Use together isn't recommended.
HMG-CoA reductase inhibitors (rosuvastatin): May increase concentration of reductase inhibitor and increase risk of myopathy, including rhabdomyolysis. Use together isn't recommended.
Other products containing sofosbuvir: Duplicates therapy. Contraindicated for use together.
PPIs (omeprazole): May decrease ledipasvir level. May give PPI doses equivalent to 20 mg or less of omeprazole simultaneously with ledipasvir–sofosbuvir on an empty stomach.
Simeprevir: May increase ledipasvir–sofosbuvir concentrations. Use together isn't recommended.
Drug-herb. *St. John's wort:* May significantly decrease drug plasma level and reduce effectiveness. Discourage use together.

EFFECTS ON LAB TEST RESULTS
• May increase bilirubin, lipase, and CK levels.

CONTRAINDICATIONS & CAUTIONS
• Contraindicated in patients hypersensitive to either drug or their components.
Boxed Warning Reactivation of HBV may occur in patients infected with HCV and result in fulminant hepatitis, hepatic failure, and death. ∎
❸ *Alert:* Symptomatic bradycardia, including fatal cardiac arrest and cases requiring pacemaker intervention, have been reported when drug is given with amiodarone. Patients taking amiodarone who are also taking beta blockers or have underlying cardiac comorbidities or advanced liver disease may be at increased risk. Symptoms may occur within hours to up to 2 weeks after start of treatment of HCV infection.
Dialyzable drug: Ledipasvir, unlikely; sofosbuvir, 18%.

PREGNANCY-LACTATION-REPRODUCTION
• Use in pregnancy hasn't been well studied. Use cautiously and only if benefits outweigh risk to the fetus.
• If giving drug with ribavirin, the combination regimen is contraindicated in patients who are pregnant and in men whose partners are pregnant.
• It isn't known if drug appears in human milk. Use cautiously during breastfeeding and only if benefits outweigh fetal risk.

NURSING CONSIDERATIONS
Boxed Warning Monitor patient with current or prior HBV infection for hepatitis flare or HBV reactivation with lab testing, and watch for signs and symptoms of liver injury during active and post-treatment follow-up. ∎
⚠ *Alert:* Test all patients for evidence of current or prior HBV infection by measuring HBsAg and hepatitis B core antibody (anti-HBc) before initiating HCV treatment.
⚠ *Alert:* Monitor patients taking amiodarone and those who must start amiodarone or who recently discontinued amiodarone for signs and symptoms of bradycardia (near-fainting or fainting, dizziness, light-headedness, malaise, weakness, excessive fatigue, shortness of breath, chest pain, confusion, or memory problems). Utilize inpatient cardiac monitoring for first 48 hours; continue outpatient or self-monitoring of HR for bradycardia daily through at least first 2 weeks of treatment. Discontinue HCV treatment if signs or symptoms of bradycardia occur.
• Monitor bilirubin, liver enzyme, and serum creatinine levels at baseline and periodically when clinically indicated.
• Monitor serum HCV-RNA level at baseline, during treatment, at end of treatment, during treatment follow-up, and when clinically indicated.

PATIENT TEACHING
Boxed Warning Warn patient to immediately report signs and symptoms of liver injury (fatigue, weakness, loss of appetite, nausea, vomiting, yellow skin or eyes, light-colored stool). ∎
• Instruct patient in safe drug administration.
⚠ *Alert:* Caution patient also taking amiodarone to seek immediate medical attention for signs and symptoms of bradycardia.

• Inform patient that the effect of treatment on HCV transmission isn't known and to follow precautions to prevent transmission.
• Advise patient to report to prescriber all other prescription drugs, OTC medications, vitamins, and herbal supplements being taken because drug interactions are possible.
• Caution patient not to stop drug without first discussing with prescriber.
• Tell patient to report signs and symptoms of adverse reactions (fatigue, nausea, and headache).
• Advise patient to immediately report signs and symptoms of hypersensitivity reactions (wheezing, chest tightness, fever, itching, or swelling of the face, lips, tongue, or throat).

leflunomide
le-FLOO-noh-mide

Arava

Therapeutic class: Antiarthritics
Pharmacologic class: Pyrimidine synthesis inhibitors

AVAILABLE FORMS
Tablets: 10 mg, 20 mg, 100 mg

INDICATIONS & DOSAGES
➤ **Active RA**
Adults: 100 mg PO loading dose every 24 hours for 3 days; then 20 mg (maximum daily dose) PO every 24 hours. Eliminating loading dose may decrease risk of adverse reactions, especially in patients at risk for hematologic or hepatic toxicity. Dose may be decreased to 10 mg daily if higher dose isn't well tolerated.

ADMINISTRATION
PO
⚠ *Alert:* Drug is a hazardous agent; use safe handling precautions according to facility protocol.
• Give drug without regard for food.

ACTION
An immunomodulatory drug that inhibits dihydroorotate dehydrogenase, an enzyme involved in pyrimidine synthesis that has antiproliferative activity and anti-inflammatory effects.

Reactions in bold italics are *life-threatening*. Interactions may have a *rapid onset* or a *delayed onset*.

Route	Onset	Peak	Duration
PO	Unknown	6–12 hr	Unknown

Half-life: Teriflunomide (active metabolite), 18 to 19 days.

ADVERSE REACTIONS

CNS: dizziness, headache, asthenia, somnolence, malaise. **CV:** HTN, chest pain, palpitations, varicose veins, thrombophlebitis. **EENT:** blurred vision, eye disorder, papilledema, retinal disorder, retinal hemorrhage, rhinitis, sore throat, dry mouth, enlarged salivary glands, oral ulcer. **GI:** diarrhea, abdominal pain, anorexia, flatulence, nausea, vomiting. **GU:** vaginal moniliasis. **Hematologic:** leukocytosis, *thrombocytopenia.* **Hepatic:** elevated liver enzyme levels, increased GGT and ALP levels, bilirubinemia, *hepatotoxicity.* **Musculoskeletal:** back pain, tenosynovitis. **Respiratory:** bronchitis, dyspnea. **Skin:** alopecia, rash, pruritus. **Other:** abscess, *anaphylaxis,* allergic reaction, flulike syndrome.

INTERACTIONS

Drug-drug. *Charcoal, cholestyramine:* May decrease leflunomide level. Sometimes used for this effect in leflunomide toxicity.
CYP1A2 substrates (alosetron, duloxetine, theophylline, tizanidine), CYP2C8 substrates (paclitaxel, pioglitazone, repaglinide, rosiglitazone), oral contraceptives (ethinyl estradiol, levonorgestrel): May increase concentration of these drugs. Monitor patient for adverse effects.
HMG-CoA reductase inhibitors (atorvastatin, pravastatin, rosuvastatin, simvastatin): May increase concentration of these drugs. Consider dosage reduction. Rosuvastatin doses shouldn't be greater than 10 mg once daily when given concurrently with leflunomide.
Methotrexate, other hepatotoxic drugs: May increase risk of hepatotoxicity. Monitor liver enzyme levels.
NSAIDs (diclofenac, ibuprofen): May increase NSAID level. Monitor patient.
Rifampin: May increase active leflunomide metabolite level. Use together cautiously.
Tacrolimus: May increase toxic effects of immunosuppressants. Avoid combination.
Tolbutamide: May increase tolbutamide level. Monitor patient.
Vaccines (live-virus): May increase vaccine-related toxic effects. Vaccination with live-virus vaccines isn't recommended. Consider long half-life of drug before giving a live-virus vaccine after stopping drug.
Warfarin: May decrease INR. Monitor therapy.

EFFECTS ON LAB TEST RESULTS

• May increase AST, ALT, GGT, bilirubin glucose, lipid, and CK levels.
• May increase WBC count.
• May decrease platelet count.

CONTRAINDICATIONS & CAUTIONS

• Contraindicated in patients hypersensitive to drug or its components, in patients with severe hepatic impairment, and in those taking teriflunomide.
• Not recommended for patients with evidence of HBV or HBC infection, severe immunodeficiency, bone marrow dysplasia, or severe uncontrolled infections.

Boxed Warning Rare cases of severe and fatal liver injury have occurred during leflunomide therapy. Most cases occur within 6 months of therapy start and in a setting of multiple risk factors for hepatotoxicity. Drug isn't recommended for patients with preexisting liver disease or ALT more than 2 × ULN. ■

Boxed Warning Use cautiously in patients taking other drugs that can cause liver damage. ■

Boxed Warning If confirmed ALT elevations greater than 3 × ULN occur during treatment, stop drug and investigate cause. If ALT elevations are likely leflunomide-induced, start accelerated drug elimination procedure according to manufacturer's instructions; monitor LFTs weekly until normalized. ■

• Use cautiously in patients with renal insufficiency.
• Severe infections including sepsis, which may be fatal, have been reported in patients receiving leflunomide, especially *Pneumocystis jiroveci* pneumonia, TB, and aspergillosis. Most reported cases were confounded by concomitant immunosuppressive therapy or comorbid illness that, in addition to RA, may predispose patients to infection.
• Risk of malignancy, particularly lymphoproliferative disorders, increases with use of some immunosuppressants, including leflunomide.
• Drug isn't recommended in patients younger than age 18.

L

Dialyzable drug: No.

⚠ *Overdose S&S:* Diarrhea, abdominal pain, leukopenia, anemia, elevated LFT results.

PREGNANCY-LACTATION-REPRODUCTION

Boxed Warning Contraindicated during pregnancy and in patients of childbearing potential who aren't using reliable contraception because of the potential for fetal harm. Exclude pregnancy before start of therapy. Stop drug and use accelerated drug elimination procedure if patient becomes pregnant. ■

• Enroll patients in the Leflunomide Pregnancy Registry (1-877-311-8972).

• It isn't known if drug appears in human milk. Patient should discontinue breastfeeding or discontinue drug.

• Patients should avoid pregnancy after drug administration until undetectable serum concentrations (less than 0.02 mg/L) are verified, which may be accomplished by use of the recommended leflunomide removal protocol.

NURSING CONSIDERATIONS

• Before starting leflunomide, evaluate patient for active TB and screen for latent TB infection, check BP, and obtain blood for lab tests, including serum ALT and Hb levels, hematocrit, and WBC and platelet counts; verify pregnancy status.

Boxed Warning Monitor liver enzyme levels at least monthly for 6 months after beginning therapy and every 6 to 8 weeks thereafter. If ALT level rises to more than 3 × ULN, interrupt therapy. If drug is determined to be the cause, start cholestyramine washout (8 g PO t.i.d. for 11 days) or activated charcoal powder (50 g made into a suspension PO every 12 hours for 11 days) and monitor LFT values until normalized. ■

☉ *Alert:* Continue monitoring AST, ALT, and serum albumin levels monthly if treatment includes methotrexate or other potential immunosuppressants.

• Without use of an accelerated drug elimination procedure, it may take up to 2 years to reach undetectable plasma concentrations of teriflunomide (active metabolite of leflunomide) after drug discontinuation.

• Monitor platelet and WBC counts and Hb level or hematocrit at baseline and monthly for 6 months after starting therapy and every 6 to 8 weeks thereafter.

• Monitor patient for peripheral neuropathy as drug may need to be stopped.

• Stop drug and start cholestyramine or charcoal therapy if bone marrow suppression occurs.

• Watch for overlapping hematologic toxicity when switching to another antirheumatic.

• Carefully monitor patient after dose reduction. Because the active metabolite of leflunomide has a prolonged half-life, it may take several weeks for levels to decline.

• Rarely, SJS, TEN, and DRESS syndrome have been reported in patients receiving leflunomide. If patient develops any of these conditions, stop drug and perform an accelerated drug elimination procedure.

• ILD and worsening of preexisting ILD have been reported and can be fatal. Risk increases in patients with a history of ILD. If new-onset or worsening pulmonary symptoms (cough, dyspnea) with or without fever occur, drug may need to be discontinued and the etiology of symptoms investigated as appropriate.

• Monitor BP.

PATIENT TEACHING

• Explain need for and frequency of required blood tests and monitoring.

Boxed Warning Instruct patient to use birth control during course of treatment and until it's been determined that drug is no longer active. ■

• Warn patient to notify prescriber if signs or symptoms of pregnancy (such as late menstrual periods or breast tenderness) occur because of risk of fetal birth defects.

• Advise patient to stop breastfeeding.

• Instruct patient to report all adverse reactions and to immediately report rash or mucous membrane lesions, unusual tiredness, abdominal pain, jaundice, easy bruising, bleeding, fever, recurrent infections, or pallor, which may be warnings of infrequent but serious adverse reactions.

• Inform patient that aspirin, other NSAIDs, and low-dose corticosteroids may continue to be taken during treatment.

• Tell patient that it may take 4 weeks to begin to see improvement from therapy.

• Instruct patient in safe drug handling and administration.

Reactions in bold italics are *life-threatening*. Interactions may have a *rapid onset* or a ***delayed onset***.

lemborexant
lem-boe-REX-ant

Dayvigo

Therapeutic class: Hypnotics
Pharmacologic class: Orexin receptor antagonists
Controlled substance schedule: IV

AVAILABLE FORMS
Tablets: 5 mg, 10 mg

INDICATIONS & DOSAGES
➤ **Insomnia, characterized by difficulties with sleep onset or sleep maintenance**
Adults: 5 mg PO nightly, immediately before bedtime. Increase dose to 10 mg if needed. Maximum dose, 10 mg once daily.
Adjust-a-dose: In patients with moderate hepatic impairment or when used concomitantly with weak CYP3A inhibitors, initial and maximum recommended dose is 5 mg PO once nightly.

ADMINISTRATION
PO
• Give immediately before bedtime; ensure at least 7 hours remain before planned time of awakening.
• May delay sleep onset if drug is given with or soon after a meal.
• Store tablets at 68° to 77° F (20° to 25° C).

ACTION
Blocks orexin receptors, suppressing the system responsible for promoting wakefulness.

Route	Onset	Peak	Duration
PO	Unknown	1–3 hr	Unknown

Half-life: 17 to 19 hours.

ADVERSE REACTIONS
CNS: somnolence, fatigue, headache, nightmares, abnormal dreams, sleep paralysis.

INTERACTIONS
Drug-drug. *CNS depressants (benzodiazepines, opioids, TCAs):* May increase risk of CNS depression. Adjust lemborexant or CNS depressant dosage to limit additive effects.
CYP2B6 substrates (bupropion, methadone): May decrease efficacy of 2B6 substrate.

Monitor for efficacy; consider increased 2B6 substrate dosage if needed.
Other sleep aids: May increase risk of CNS depression. Avoid use together.
Strong or moderate CYP3A inducers (bosentan, carbamazepine, efavirenz, etravirine, modafinil, rifampin): May decrease lemborexant level. Avoid use together.
Strong or moderate CYP3A inhibitors (clarithromycin, fluconazole, itraconazole, verapamil): May increase lemborexant level. Avoid use together.
Weak CYP3A inhibitors (chlorzoxazone, ranitidine): May increase lemborexant level. Don't exceed 5 mg nightly.
Drug-herb. *St. John's wort:* May decrease lemborexant level. Discourage use together.
Drug-food. *High-caloric, high-fat meals:* May delay drug's effect. Patient should avoid ingesting with or soon after a meal.
Drug-lifestyle. *Alcohol use:* May increase CNS depression. Discourage use together.

EFFECTS ON LAB TEST RESULTS
None reported.

CONTRAINDICATIONS & CAUTIONS
• Contraindicated in patients with narcolepsy.
• Use cautiously in patients with moderate hepatic impairment. Not recommended in patients with severe hepatic or renal impairment.
⚠ **Alert:** Use of alcohol or other CNS depressants increases risk of complex sleep behaviors.
• Use in patients with impaired respiratory function, including sleep apnea and COPD, hasn't been studied.
⚠ **Alert:** May worsen depression and increase risk of suicidality. Immediately evaluate patients who report suicidality or exhibit new behavioral changes.
• Use cautiously in patients with history of substance abuse or dependence.
• Safety and effectiveness in children haven't been established.
• Use cautiously in older adults.
Dialyzable drug: No.
⚠ **Overdose S&S:** Increased somnolence.

PREGNANCY-LACTATION-REPRODUCTION
• There are no adequate studies during pregnancy.

• Enroll patients taking drug during pregnancy in the pregnancy exposure registry (1-888-274-2378).

• It isn't known if drug appears in human milk. Weigh benefit to patient against risk to infant. Monitor infants exposed to drug for excessive somnolence.

NURSING CONSIDERATIONS

• Evaluate patient for medical or psychiatric causes of insomnia before drug is prescribed. If insomnia persists for more than 7 to 10 days, reevaluate patient.

• Monitor patient for complex sleep behaviors (preparing and eating food, making phone calls, sleep-walking, sleep-driving while not fully awake); discontinue drug if they occur.

• Monitor patient for daytime somnolence and fall risk, especially older adults.

• Monitor patient for sleep paralysis (inability to move or speak during sleep-wake transitions), hypnagogic/hypnopompic hallucinations (including vivid and disturbing perceptions), and leg weakness.

• Monitor patient for development of dependence on or abuse of drug.

• **Alert:** Be alert for signs and symptoms of depression, suicidality, or behavioral changes.

• **Look alike–sound alike:** Don't confuse Dayvigo with Daypro, Daysee, or Daytrana.

PATIENT TEACHING

• **Alert:** Caution patient, family, or caregiver to immediately report suicidality or new behavioral signs or symptoms.

• Teach patient safe drug administration.

• Warn patient that risk of daytime somnolence increases if drug is taken with less than a full night's sleep. Caution patient against driving and other activities requiring complete mental alertness.

• Explain that CNS depressant effects may persist for several days after discontinuing drug.

• Caution patient that increased drowsiness may increase risk of falls.

• Inform patient and family that drug may cause sleep paralysis, hallucinations, and leg weakness.

• Instruct patient and family to notify prescriber and discontinue drug if complex sleep behaviors occur.

• Advise patient to avoid alcohol or other CNS depressants while taking drug.

• Tell patient not to increase dose without first consulting prescriber.

• Warn patient and family to watch for development of abuse and dependence.

• Tell patient to contact prescriber if insomnia persists for more than 7 to 10 days.

• Advise patient to report pregnancy, plans to become pregnant, or breastfeeding.

SAFETY ALERT!

letrozole
LET-roe-zole

Femara

Therapeutic class: Antineoplastics
Pharmacologic class: Aromatase inhibitors

AVAILABLE FORMS
Tablets: 2.5 mg

INDICATIONS & DOSAGES
Adjust-a-dose (for all indications): In patients with cirrhosis and severe hepatic impairment, give 2.5 mg every other day.

➤ **First-line treatment of hormone receptor–positive or hormone receptor–unknown, locally advanced, or metastatic breast cancer; advanced breast cancer with disease progression after antiestrogen therapy (such as tamoxifen)**
Patients who are postmenopausal: 2.5 mg PO once daily until tumor progression is evident.

➤ **Adjuvant treatment of hormone-positive early breast cancer**
Patients who are postmenopausal: 2.5 mg PO daily. Optimal duration of treatment is unknown.

➤ **Extended adjuvant treatment of early breast cancer following 5 years of adjuvant tamoxifen therapy**
Patients who are postmenopausal: 2.5 mg PO once daily for 5 years.

ADMINISTRATION
PO
• **Alert:** Drug is a hormonal agent and considered a potential teratogen. Follow safe handling procedures.

• Give drug without regard for meals.

ACTION
Inhibits conversion of androgens to estrogens, which decreases tumor mass or delays progression of tumor growth in some patients.

Route	Onset	Peak	Duration
PO	Unknown	2–6 wk (steady-state plasma)	Unknown

Half-life: About 2 days.

ADVERSE REACTIONS
CNS: *stroke,* headache, somnolence, insomnia, dizziness, fatigue, asthenia, mood changes, depression. **CV:** flushing, *MI, thromboembolism,* angina, *HF,* chest pain, edema, HTN. **EENT:** cataract. **GI:** nausea, vomiting, constipation, diarrhea, abdominal pain, anorexia, dyspepsia. **GU:** vaginal bleeding, vaginal irritation, vulvovaginal dryness, UTI. **Hepatic:** hyperbilirubinemia, jaundice. **Metabolic:** hypercholesterolemia, weight gain or loss. **Musculoskeletal:** bone pain, limb pain, back pain, arthralgia, fractures, osteopenia, osteoporosis, myalgia. **Respiratory:** dyspnea, cough, pleural effusion. **Skin:** rash, pruritus, alopecia, diaphoresis, night sweats. **Other:** fall, viral infections, breast pain, hot flashes, *secondary malignancies.*

INTERACTIONS
Drug-drug. *Estrogens:* May produce antagonistic effects with letrozole. Use together isn't recommended.
Methadone: May increase methadone serum concentration. Monitor therapy.
Tamoxifen: May reduce letrozole levels. Monitor therapy.

EFFECTS ON LAB TEST RESULTS
• May increase cholesterol level.
• May decrease lymphocyte count.

CONTRAINDICATIONS & CAUTIONS
• Contraindicated in patients hypersensitive to drug or its components.
• Use drug only in patients who are postmenopausal.
• Use cautiously in patients with severe liver impairment; dosage adjustment isn't needed in those with mild to moderate liver dysfunction.
Dialyzable drug: Unknown.

PREGNANCY-LACTATION-REPRODUCTION
• May cause fetal harm. Contraindicated in patients who are or may become pregnant.
• Patients of childbearing potential should use effective contraception during therapy and for at least 3 weeks after final dose.
• It isn't known if drug appears in human milk. Patient shouldn't breastfeed during therapy and for 3 weeks after final dose.

NURSING CONSIDERATIONS
• Verify pregnancy status before treatment.
• Dosage adjustment isn't needed in patients with CrCl of 10 mL/minute or more.
• Monitor bone density studies.
• *Look alike–sound alike:* Don't confuse Femara with FemHRT.

PATIENT TEACHING
• Teach patient about safe handling of drug.
• Instruct patient to take drug exactly as prescribed.
• Inform patient about potential adverse effects and to report them.
• Advise patient to use caution performing tasks that require alertness, coordination, or dexterity, such as driving, until effects are known.
• Inform patient who is recently menopausal of the need for adequate contraception until postmenopausal status is clinically well established.

SAFETY ALERT!

leuprolide acetate
loo-PROE-lide

Eligard, Fensolvi, Lupron Depot, Lupron Depot-Ped

leuprolide mesylate
Camcevi

Therapeutic class: Antineoplastics
Pharmacologic class: GnRH analogues

AVAILABLE FORMS
leuprolide acetate
Depot injection: 3.75 mg, 7.5 mg, 11.25 mg, 15 mg, 22.5 mg, 30 mg, 45 mg
Injection: 1 mg/0.2 mL
leuprolide mesylate
Depot injection: 42-mg prefilled syringe

INDICATIONS & DOSAGES

➤ **Advanced prostate cancer**
Adults: 1 mg subcut daily. Or, 7.5 mg IM depot injection monthly, 22.5 mg IM depot injection every 3 months, 30 mg IM depot injection every 4 months, or 45 mg IM depot injection every 6 months. Or, 7.5 mg subcut Eligard once monthly, 22.5 mg subcut Eligard every 3 months, 30 mg subcut Eligard every 4 months, or 45 mg subcut Eligard every 6 months. Or, 42 mg subcut Camcevi every 6 months.

➤ **Endometriosis (alone or in combination with norethindrone acetate)**
Adults: 3.75 mg IM depot injection as single injection once monthly for up to 6 months. Or, 11.25 mg IM every 3 months for up to 6 months.

➤ **Central precocious puberty**
Children age 2 and older (Lupron Depot-Ped, Fensolvi): Initially, for child weighing more than 37.5 kg, 15 mg IM once monthly. For child weighing more than 25 to 37.5 kg, 11.25 mg IM once monthly. For child weighing 25 kg or less, 7.5 mg IM once monthly. If clinical suppression isn't achieved with starting dose of Lupron Depot-Ped, increase dosage to next available higher dose in 3.75-mg increments. Or, give 11.25 or 30 mg IM once every 3 months. Or, for 6 month formulation (Fensolvi), give 45 mg subcut every 6 months. Discontinue drug at the appropriate age of puberty onset.

➤ **Anemia related to uterine fibroids (with iron therapy)**
Adults: 3.75 mg IM depot injection once monthly for up to 3 consecutive months. Or 11.25 mg IM depot injection for 1 dose.

➤ **Premenopausal ovarian suppression in patients with breast cancer ◆**
Adults: 3.75 mg IM every 28 days for up to 24 months, or 11.25 mg IM every 3 months for up to 24 months.

ADMINISTRATION

• Products have specific mixing and administration instructions. Read manufacturer's directions closely.
🜂 *Alert:* Hazardous drug; use safe-handling precautions.
🜂 *Alert:* A fractional dose of drug formulated to give every 3, 4, or 6 months isn't equivalent to same dose of once-a-month formulation.
• Store leuprolide acetate powder (depot) and diluent at room temperature; refrigerate unopened vials or syringes of leuprolide acetate or mesylate injection, and protect injection from heat and light.
• Allow refrigerated solution to come to room temperature before use.

IM
• Never give by IV injection.
• Give depot injections under medical supervision.
• Use supplied diluent to reconstitute drug (extra diluent is provided; discard remainder).
• Inject into vial; shake well. Suspension will appear milky. Use immediately.
• Draw appropriate amount into a syringe with a 22G needle.
• For Lupron Depot and Lupron Depot-Ped, use within 2 hours of preparation.
• When using prefilled dual-chamber syringes, prepare for injection according to manufacturer's instructions.
• Gently shake syringe to form a uniform milky suspension. If particles adhere to stopper, tap syringe against your finger.
• Remove needle guard and advance plunger to expel air from syringe. Inject entire contents IM as with a normal injection.

Subcutaneous
• For the two-syringe mixing system, connect the syringes and inject the liquid contents according to manufacturer's instructions.
• Mix product by pushing contents back and forth between syringes for about 45 seconds; shaking the syringes won't mix the contents enough.
• Attach the needle provided in the kit and inject subcut.
• Suspension settles very quickly. Remix if settling occurs. Must be given within 30 minutes.
• Never give by IV injection.

ACTION

Stimulates and then inhibits release of FSH and LH, which suppresses testosterone and estrogen levels.

Route	Onset	Peak	Duration
IM, subcut	Variable	2–6 hr	60–90 days

Half-life: 3 hours.

ADVERSE REACTIONS

CNS: dizziness, depression, headache, migraine, sleep disorder, vertigo, pain, insomnia, paresthesia, asthenia, emotional lability, fatigue, lethargy, anxiety, fever.

Reactions in bold italics are *life-threatening*. Interactions may have a *rapid onset* or a **delayed onset**.

CV: *arrhythmias,* angina, *MI,* peripheral edema, ECG changes, hypotension, HTN, murmur, flushing. **EENT:** nasopharyngitis, sinus congestion. **GI:** nausea, vomiting, anorexia, constipation, diarrhea. **GU:** impotence, vaginitis, urinary frequency, hematuria, UTI, amenorrhea, decreased libido, testicular atrophy. **Hematologic:** anemia. **Metabolic:** weight gain or loss, increased cholesterol level, increased triglyceride levels. **Musculoskeletal:** transient bone pain during first week of treatment, joint disorder, myalgia, neuromuscular disorder, bone loss, back pain, arthralgia. **Respiratory:** dyspnea, URI, cough, *pulmonary fibrosis.* **Skin:** diaphoresis, injection-site reactions, dermatitis, acne, injection-site pain, rash. **Other:** gynecomastia, androgen-like effects, hot flashes, flulike symptoms.

INTERACTIONS
None significant.

EFFECTS ON LAB TEST RESULTS
• May increase bilirubin, cholesterol, triglyceride, BUN, calcium, creatinine, glucose, LDH, phosphorus, AST, ALT, GGT, and uric acid levels.
• May decrease albumin, protein, and potassium levels.
• May increase WBC.
• May decrease Hb level and hematocrit.
• May increase or decrease platelet count.
• May prolong PT and PTT.
• May alter results of pituitary-gonadal system tests during therapy and for 12 weeks after.

CONTRAINDICATIONS & CAUTIONS
• Contraindicated in patients hypersensitive to drug or other GnRH analogues and in patients with undiagnosed vaginal bleeding.
• Androgen deprivation therapy may prolong QT/QTc interval. Consider if benefits of therapy outweigh risks in patients with congenital long QT syndrome, HF, or frequent electrolyte abnormalities, and in patients taking drugs known to prolong QT interval.
• Seizures have been reported in patients taking leuprolide, including those with and without a history of seizures, epilepsy, cerebrovascular disorders, or CNS anomalies or tumors and in patients taking concomitant medications associated with seizures.

• The 30- and 45-mg depot injections are contraindicated in women and children. *Dialyzable drug:* Unknown.

PREGNANCY-LACTATION-REPRODUCTION
• May cause fetal harm; contraindicated in patients who are or may become pregnant during therapy.
• Patients of childbearing potential should use nonhormonal contraception during treatment.
• It isn't known if drug appears in human milk. Use is contraindicated breastfeeding.
• May impair fertility in males of reproductive potential.

NURSING CONSIDERATIONS
• Correct electrolyte abnormalities before starting drug; consider periodic monitoring of ECGs and electrolytes.
• Verify pregnancy status before use.
• With treatment of precocious puberty, increased clinical signs and symptoms of puberty, including vaginal bleeding, may occur during first weeks of therapy or after subsequent doses.
• After starting treatment for central precocious puberty, monitor patient response every 1 to 2 months with a GnRH stimulation test and sex corticosteroid level determinations. Measure bone age for advancement every 6 to 12 months.
• Monitor patient for development or worsening of psychiatric symptoms during treatment (emotional lability, anger, aggression, crying, impatience).
• Monitor children for pseudotumor cerebri (headache, papilledema, vision changes, eye pain, tinnitus, dizziness, nausea).
• *Alert:* During first few weeks of treatment for prostate cancer, signs and symptoms of disease may temporarily worsen or additional signs and symptoms may occur.
• In patients treated with GnRH analogues for prostate cancer, treatment is usually continued upon development of metastatic castration-resistant prostate cancer.
• May increase risk of diabetes and CV events. Monitor patient closely.
• *Look alike–sound alike:* Don't confuse Lupron Depot with Lupron Depot-Ped.

L

PATIENT TEACHING

• Before starting child on treatment for central precocious puberty, make sure parents understand importance of continuous therapy.

• Carefully instruct patient who will self-administer subcut injection about the proper technique. Advise patient to use only the syringes provided by manufacturer.

• Inform patient with history of undesirable effects from other endocrine therapies that leuprolide is easier to tolerate. Advise patient to report all adverse effects.

• Explain that symptoms may worsen at first.

• Advise patient of childbearing potential to use a nonhormonal form of contraception during treatment.

---

levalbuterol hydrochloride
lev-al-BYOO-ter-ol

Xopenex

levalbuterol tartrate
Xopenex HFA

Therapeutic class: Bronchodilators
Pharmacologic class: Beta$_2$ agonists

AVAILABLE FORMS

Inhalation aerosol: 45 mcg per actuation
Solution for inhalation: 0.31 mg, 0.63 mg, or 1.25 mg in 3-mL vials; 1.25 mg/0.5 mL in vials (concentrate)

INDICATIONS & DOSAGES

➤ **To prevent or treat bronchospasm in patients with reversible obstructive airway disease**
Adults and adolescents age 12 and older:
0.63 mg by oral inhalation via nebulizer t.i.d. every 6 to 8 hours. Patients with more severe asthma who don't respond adequately to 0.63 mg t.i.d. may benefit from 1.25 mg t.i.d.
Children ages 6 to 11: 0.31 mg by oral inhalation via nebulizer t.i.d. Routine dosage shouldn't exceed 0.63 mg t.i.d.
Adults and children age 4 and older: 2 inhalations Xopenex HFA (90 mcg) every 4 to 6 hours. In some patients, 1 inhalation (45 mcg) every 4 hours is sufficient.

ADMINISTRATION
Inhalational

• Keep unopened vials of regular solution in foil pouch and use within 2 weeks of opening pouch. Use vials removed from pouch within 1 week and protect from light.

• Use vials of concentrated solution immediately after opening pouch.

• Dilute concentrated solution (1.25 mg/ 0.5 mL) with sterile NSS before administration by nebulizer connected to air compressor. Treatment takes about 5 to 15 minutes. Stop treatment when mist is no longer visible.

• Discard vial if solution isn't colorless.

• Release four test sprays before first use of inhaler or after inhaler has not been used for more than 3 days.

• Shake canister well before use.

• Avoid spraying in the eyes.

• Use a spacer device to improve inhalation, as appropriate.

• Wash actuator with warm water and air-dry thoroughly at least once a week.

• Clean nebulizer according to manufacturer's instructions.

ACTION

Relaxes bronchial smooth muscle by stimulating beta$_2$ receptors; also inhibits release of mediators from mast cells in the airway.

Route	Onset	Peak	Duration
Inhalation	5–15 min	1 hr	3–4 hr

Half-life: 3.25 to 4 hours.

ADVERSE REACTIONS

CNS: dizziness, migraine, nervousness, pain, tremor, anxiety, asthenia, fever, headache, insomnia. **CV:** tachycardia. **EENT:** rhinitis, sinusitis, turbinate edema, pharyngitis. **GI:** dyspepsia, diarrhea, vomiting, abdominal pain. **Musculoskeletal:** leg cramps, myalgia. **Respiratory:** increased cough, asthma, bronchitis. **Skin:** rash, urticaria. **Other:** viral infection, flulike syndrome, accidental injury, lymphadenopathy.

INTERACTIONS

Drug-drug. *Beta blockers:* May block pulmonary effect of the drug and cause severe bronchospasm. Avoid using together, if possible. If use together is unavoidable, consider a cardioselective beta blocker, but use cautiously.

Reactions in bold italics are *life-threatening*. Interactions may have a *rapid onset* or a ***delayed onset***.

Digoxin: May decrease digoxin levels. Monitor digoxin level.

Loop or thiazide diuretics: May cause ECG changes and hypokalemia. Use together cautiously.

MAO inhibitors, TCAs: May potentiate action of levalbuterol on the vascular system. Avoid using within 2 weeks of MAO inhibitor or TCA therapy.

Other short-acting sympathomimetic aerosol bronchodilators, epinephrine: May increase adrenergic adverse effects. Use together cautiously.

EFFECTS ON LAB TEST RESULTS
• May increase glucose level.
• May decrease potassium level.

CONTRAINDICATIONS & CAUTIONS
• Contraindicated in patients hypersensitive to drug or to racemic albuterol.
• Use cautiously in older adults, in patients with CV disorders (especially coronary insufficiency, HTN, and arrhythmias), seizure disorders, hyperthyroidism, or diabetes, and in those who are unusually responsive to sympathomimetic amines.
Dialyzable drug: Unknown.
⚠ *Overdose S&S:* Exaggeration of adverse reactions, hypokalemia, seizures, angina, HTN, hypotension, arrhythmias, muscle cramps, dry mouth, palpitations, nausea, insomnia, cardiac arrest, sudden death.

PREGNANCY-LACTATION-REPRODUCTION
• There are no adequate studies during pregnancy. Use during pregnancy only if potential benefit justifies fetal risk.
• Drug may interfere with uterine contractility. Use to treat bronchospasm during labor only if clearly needed.
• Patients should enroll in MotherToBaby Pregnancy Studies' Asthma & Pregnancy Study (1-877-311-8972 or www.mothertobaby.org/ongoing-study/asthma.)
• It isn't known if drug appears in human milk. Use cautiously during breastfeeding.

NURSING CONSIDERATIONS
🛈 *Alert:* As with other inhaled beta agonists, drug can produce paradoxical bronchospasm or life-threatening CV effects. If this occurs, stop drug immediately and notify prescriber.
• Drug may worsen diabetes and ketoacidosis.

• Monitor potassium level, as drug may temporarily decrease potassium level.
• The compatibility of levalbuterol mixed with other drugs in a nebulizer hasn't been established.

PATIENT TEACHING
• Teach patient safe drug administration and storage.
• Tell patient not to increase dosage or use drug more frequently without consulting prescriber.
• Urge patient to seek medical attention immediately if levalbuterol becomes less effective, if signs and symptoms worsen, or if patient is using drug more frequently than usual.
• Tell patient that the effects of levalbuterol may last up to 8 hours.
• Advise patient to use other inhalational drugs and antiasthmatics only as directed while taking levalbuterol.
• Inform patient that common adverse reactions include palpitations, rapid HR, headache, dizziness, tremor, and nervousness.
• Tell patient to discard inhaler when dose indicator display window shows "0."
• Encourage patient of childbearing potential to report pregnancy or breastfeeding.

levETIRAcetam
lee-vah-tih-RACE-ah-tam

Elepsia XR, Keppra, Keppra XR, Spritam

Therapeutic class: Anticonvulsants
Pharmacologic class: Pyrrolidine derivatives

AVAILABLE FORMS
Injection: 500 mg/5 mL single-use vials
Injection (premixed in NSS): 5 mg/mL in 50-, 100-mL bags; 10 mg/mL in 100-mL bags; 15 mg/mL in 100-mL bags
Oral solution: 100 mg/mL
Tablets 🔵: 250 mg, 500 mg, 750 mg, 1,000 mg
Tablets (extended-release) 🔵: 500 mg, 750 mg, 1,000 mg, 1,500 mg
Tablets for oral suspension: 250 mg, 500 mg, 750 mg, 1,000 mg

INDICATIONS & DOSAGES

Adjust-a-dose (for all indications): For immediate-release and oral solution, in adults with CrCl of 50 to 80 mL/minute, give 500 to 1,000 mg every 12 hours; if CrCl is 30 to 50 mL/minute, give 250 to 750 mg every 12 hours; if CrCl is less than 30 mL/minute, give 250 to 500 mg every 12 hours. For patients on ESRD dialysis, give 500 to 1,000 mg every 24 hours. Give a 250- to 500-mg dose after dialysis.

For extended-release tablets, if CrCl is 50 to 80 mL/minute, give 1,000 mg every 24 hours. If CrCl is 30 to 50 mL/minute, give 500 to 1,500 mg every 24 hours. If CrCl is less than 30 mL/minute, give 500 to 1,000 mg every 24 hours.

➤ **Adjunctive therapy for myoclonic seizures of juvenile myoclonic epilepsy**

Adults and adolescents age 12 and older: Initially, 500 mg PO or IV b.i.d. Increase by 1,000 mg/day every 2 weeks to a dose of 1,500 mg PO or IV b.i.d. (3,000 mg/day).

➤ **Adjunctive therapy for primary generalized tonic-clonic seizures**

Adults and adolescents age 16 and older: Initially, 500 mg PO or IV b.i.d. Increase dose by 500 mg b.i.d. every 2 weeks to dose of 1,500 mg b.i.d.

Children ages 6 to younger than 16: Initially, 10 mg/kg PO or IV b.i.d. Increase dose by 10 mg/kg b.i.d. at 2-week intervals to dose of 30 mg/kg b.i.d. For children weighing more than 20 kg, use either tablets or oral solution. For children weighing 20 kg or less, use oral solution.

➤ **Adjunctive therapy for primary generalized tonic-clonic seizures (Spritam)**

Adults and children age 6 and older weighing more than 40 kg: 500 mg PO b.i.d.; increase as needed and tolerated by 500 mg PO b.i.d. every 2 weeks to a maximum recommended dose of 1,500 mg b.i.d.

Children age 6 and older weighing 20 to 40 kg: 250 mg PO b.i.d.; increase by 250 mg PO b.i.d. every 2 weeks to a maximum of 750 mg b.i.d.

➤ **Adjunctive treatment or monotherapy for partial-onset seizures in patients with epilepsy**

Adults and adolescents age 16 and older: Initially, 500 mg PO or IV b.i.d. Increase dosage by 500 mg b.i.d., as needed, for seizure control at 2-week intervals to maximum of 1,500 mg b.i.d.

Children ages 4 to younger than 16: Initially, 10 mg/kg PO or IV b.i.d. Increase dose by 10 mg/kg b.i.d. at 2-week intervals to recommended dose of 30 mg/kg b.i.d. If patient can't tolerate this dose, reduce it. For children who weigh 20 kg or less, use the oral solution.

Children ages 6 months to younger than 4 years: Initially, 10 mg/kg PO or IV b.i.d. Increase by 10 mg/kg b.i.d. at 2-week intervals to recommended dosage of 25 mg/kg b.i.d. Reduce dosage if patient can't tolerate total daily dose of 50 mg/kg.

Children ages 1 month to 6 months: Initially, 7 mg/kg PO or IV b.i.d. Increase by 7 mg/kg b.i.d. at 2-week intervals to recommended dosage of 21 mg/kg b.i.d.

➤ **Adjunctive treatment for partial-onset seizures in patients with epilepsy (extended-release)**

Adults and children age 12 and older: Initially, 1,000 mg PO once daily. May adjust dosage in increments of 1,000 mg every 2 weeks to maximum of 3,000 mg daily.

➤ **Adjunctive treatment or monotherapy for partial-onset seizures in patients with epilepsy (Spritam)**

Adults and children age 4 and older weighing more than 40 kg: 500 mg PO b.i.d.; increase as needed and tolerated by 500 mg PO b.i.d. every 2 weeks to a maximum recommended dose of 1,500 mg b.i.d.

Children age 4 and older weighing 20 to 40 kg: 250 mg PO b.i.d.; increase by 250 mg PO b.i.d. every 2 weeks to a maximum of 750 mg b.i.d.

➤ **Adjunctive treatment for myoclonic seizures in patients with juvenile myoclonic epilepsy (Spritam)**

Children age 12 and older: 500 mg PO b.i.d.; increase as needed and tolerated by 500 mg PO b.i.d. every 2 weeks to a maximum of 1,500 mg b.i.d.

ADMINISTRATION
PO

- Give drug without regard for food.
- Oral and IV forms are bioequivalent.
- Tablets should be swallowed whole and shouldn't be chewed, broken, or crushed.
- Tablets for oral solution are intended to disintegrate in the mouth. Place tablet on tongue with a dry hand. Follow with a sip of liquid and have patient swallow only after tablet disintegrates; patient shouldn't swallow tablet intact. Or, add whole tablet to a small volume

---

of liquid in a cup (1 tablespoon or enough to cover tablet); allow tablet to disperse, then have patient immediately consume entire contents. Don't give partial tablets.

• Don't push tablets for oral solution through the foil; peel foil from blister by bending up and lifting peel tab around the blister seal.

• For children weighing more than 20 kg, use either tablets or oral solution. For children weighing 20 kg or less, use oral solution.

IV

▼ Dilute drug before giving.

▼ For adults and adolescents receiving adult dosages, dilute 500-mg, 1,000-mg, or 1,500-mg dose in 100 mL NSS, D₅W, or lactated Ringer injection to maximum levetiracetam concentration of 15 mg/mL of diluted solution, and infuse within 4 hours after mixing over 15 minutes.

▼ For children and patients requiring a smaller volume, calculate the amount of diluent to not exceed a maximum levetiracetam concentration of 15 mg/mL of diluted solution; infuse within 4 hours after mixing over 15 minutes.

▼ Drug is compatible with diazepam, lorazepam, and valproate sodium for 4 hours at a controlled room temperature.

▼ Store premixed solution for infusion at 68° to 77° F (20° to 25° C); don't dilute.

▼ Store vials for injection at 77° F (25° C).

▼ **Incompatibilities:** Unknown with other drugs or antiepileptics besides diazepam, lorazepam, and valproate sodium. Consult a drug incompatibility reference for more information.

ACTION

May act by inhibiting simultaneous neuronal firing that leads to seizure activity.

Route	Onset	Peak	Duration
PO (immediate-release), IV	1 hr	1 hr	12 hr
PO (extended-release)	Unknown	4 hr	Unknown

Half-life: About 6 to 8 hours in adults with normal renal function.

ADVERSE REACTIONS

CNS: asthenia, headache, somnolence, amnesia, anxiety, ataxia, depression, dizziness, emotional lability, hostility, aggression, abnormal behavior, irritability, agitation, nervousness, paresthesia, pain, vertigo, hypersomnia, irritability, insomnia, confusion, sedation, abnormal gait, incoordination. **EENT:** diplopia, conjunctivitis, ear pain, rhinitis, sinusitis, nasal congestion, pharyngitis, sore throat. **GI:** anorexia, vomiting, upper abdominal pain, diarrhea, constipation, gastroenteritis. **Hematologic:** *leukopenia, neutropenia.* **Musculoskeletal:** neck pain, joint sprain. **Respiratory:** cough. **Skin:** contusion. **Other:** infection, head injury, flulike symptoms, falls.

INTERACTIONS

Drug-drug. *Antihistamines, benzodiazepines, opioids, other drugs that cause drowsiness, TCAs:* May lead to severe sedation. Avoid using together.

Drug-lifestyle. *Alcohol use:* May lead to severe sedation. Discourage use together.

EFFECTS ON LAB TEST RESULTS

• May alter LFT and renal function results.
• May decrease sodium level.
• May increase eosinophil count.
• May decrease Hb level, hematocrit, and WBC, RBC, platelet, and neutrophil counts.

CONTRAINDICATIONS & CAUTIONS

• Contraindicated in patients hypersensitive to drug.
• Don't use extended-release form in patients with ESRD.
• Anaphylaxis and angioedema may occur after first dose or at any time during treatment.
• Use cautiously in patients with history of psychiatric symptoms, especially psychotic symptoms and behaviors.
• Serious skin reactions, including TEN and SJS, have been reported. Recurrence after a rechallenge is possible.
• Don't abruptly discontinue drug because withdrawal seizures may occur.
• Drug may cause hematologic abnormalities, including decreased RBC, WBC, platelet, and neutrophil counts, decreased Hb level and hematocrit, and increased eosinophil count. Cases of agranulocytosis have been reported in the postmarketing setting.
Dialyzable drug: 50%.
⚠ *Overdose S&S:* Drowsiness, aggression, agitation, coma, depressed level of consciousness, respiratory depression, somnolence.

PREGNANCY-LACTATION-REPRODUCTION

• There are no adequate studies during pregnancy. Use during pregnancy only if potential benefit justifies fetal risk.

• Patients who are pregnant and taking drug should enroll themselves in the North American AED Pregnancy Registry (1-888-233-2334 or https://www.aedpregnancyregistry.org/).

• Drug appears in human milk. Use cautiously during breastfeeding.

NURSING CONSIDERATIONS

• Seizures can occur with abrupt drug stoppage. Tapering is recommended.

• Monitor patients for signs and symptoms of somnolence and fatigue.

• Monitor patients closely for such adverse reactions as dizziness, which may lead to falls.

• Discontinue drug and notify prescriber for signs and symptoms of anaphylaxis (hypotension, hives, rash, respiratory distress), angioedema (swelling of face, lips, mouth, eyes, tongue, throat, feet), and serious dermatologic reaction.

• Monitor renal function as acute kidney injury has been reported.

• Monitor patients ages 1 month to younger than 4 years for increases in diastolic BP.

🝝 *Alert:* Closely monitor all patients taking or starting antiepileptic drugs for changes in behavior indicating psychosis or worsening of suicidality or depression. Symptoms such as anxiety, agitation, hostility, mania, and hypomania may be precursors to emerging suicidality.

• *Look alike–sound alike:* Don't confuse levetiracetam with levofloxacin. Don't confuse Keppra with Kaletra or Keflex.

PATIENT TEACHING

🝝 *Alert:* Tell patient, family, or caregiver to seek medical attention for emerging or worsening depression, suicidality, or unusual changes in mood or behavior.

• Instruct patient in safe drug administration.

• Warn patient to use extra care when sitting or standing to avoid falling.

• Advise patient to seek immediate medical attention for signs and symptoms of anaphylaxis or angioedema.

• Advise patient not to stop drug abruptly because seizure activity may increase.

• Caution patient to call prescriber and not to stop drug suddenly if adverse reactions occur.

• Warn patient that drug may cause dizziness and somnolence and to avoid driving, operating heavy machinery, bike riding, or other hazardous activities until drug's effects are known.

levocetirizine dihydrochloride

LEE-voe-se-TIR-a-zeen

Allergy Relief ◊, Children's Xyzal Allergy 24HR ◊, Xyzal Allergy 24HR ◊

Therapeutic class: Antihistamines
Pharmacologic class: H_1-receptor antagonists

AVAILABLE FORMS

Oral solution: 2.5 mg/5 mL
Tablets: 5 mg

INDICATIONS & DOSAGES

➤ **Seasonal allergic rhinitis (OTC only)**
Adults and children age 12 and older: 5 mg PO once daily in the evening; 2.5 mg PO once daily in the evening may be adequate for some patients.
Children ages 6 to 11: 2.5 mg PO once daily in the evening. Don't exceed 2.5 mg in 4 hours.
Children ages 2 to 5: 1.25 mg (2.5 mL) PO once daily in the evening. Don't exceed 1.25 mg in 24 hours.
Adjust-a-dose: Use in the presence of renal impairment isn't recommended.

➤ **Perennial allergic rhinitis**
Children ages 6 months to 2 years: 1.25 mg (2.5 mL) PO daily in the evening. Don't exceed this dose.
Adjust-a-dose: Use in patients with renal impairment is contraindicated.

➤ **Chronic idiopathic urticaria**
Adults and children age 12 and older: 5 mg once daily in the evening; some patients with less severe symptoms may experience symptom relief with 2.5 mg once daily.
Children ages 6 to 11: 2.5 mg once daily in the evening. Maximum dosage, 2.5 mg/day.
Children ages 6 months to 5 years: 1.25 mg (2.5 mL) once daily in the evening. Maximum dosage, 1.25 mg/day.

Reactions in bold italics are *life-threatening*. Interactions may have a *rapid onset* or a *delayed onset*.

Adjust-a-dose: For patients age 12 and older with CrCl of 50 to 80 mL/minute, give 2.5 mg PO once daily; with CrCl of 30 to 50 mL/minute, give 2.5 mg PO every other day; with CrCl of 10 to 30 mL/minute, give 2.5 mg PO twice weekly (once every 3 to 4 days). Use in patients with ESRD, those undergoing hemodialysis, and children younger than age 12 with any renal impairment is contraindicated.

ADMINISTRATION
PO
• Give drug in the evening without regard for food.
• Use calibrated dosing device for oral solution.

ACTION
H_1-receptor inhibition creates antihistamine effect, relieving allergy symptoms.

Route	Onset	Peak	Duration
PO	1 hr	0.5–1 hr	24 hr

Half-life: Adults, 8 to 9 hours; children, 6 hours.

ADVERSE REACTIONS
CNS: asthenia, fatigue, fever, somnolence. **EENT:** otitis media, epistaxis, dry mouth, nasopharyngitis, pharyngitis. **GI:** diarrhea, vomiting, constipation. **Respiratory:** cough.

INTERACTIONS
Drug-drug. *CNS depressants:* May have additive effects when taken together. Avoid using together.
Ritonavir: May increase serum concentration and half-life of levocetirizine. Use cautiously together.
Theophylline: May decrease the clearance of levocetirizine. Use cautiously together.
Drug-lifestyle. *Alcohol use:* May have additive effect when taken with levocetirizine. Discourage use together.

EFFECTS ON LAB TEST RESULTS
• May prevent, reduce, or mask positive result skin wheal in diagnostic skin test.

CONTRAINDICATIONS & CAUTIONS
• Contraindicated in patients hypersensitive to drug or to cetirizine.
• Contraindicated in patients with CrCl of less than 10 mL/minute, in patients younger than age 12 with impaired renal function, and those undergoing hemodialysis.
• Use cautiously in older adults.
• Use cautiously in patients with predisposing factors for urine retention, such as spinal cord lesion or prostatic hyperplasia. Discontinue drug if urine retention occurs.
• Safety and effectiveness in patients younger than age 6 months haven't been established.
Dialyzable drug: Less than 10%.
⚠ **Overdose S&S:** Drowsiness; initial agitation and restlessness, then drowsiness (in children).

PREGNANCY-LACTATION-REPRODUCTION
• There are no adequate studies during pregnancy. Use only if clearly needed.
• Drug may appear in human milk. Consider benefits of breastfeeding and patient's clinical need for drug. Use only if benefits outweigh risks.

NURSING CONSIDERATIONS
• Monitor renal function in patients with or at risk for renal impairment.

PATIENT TEACHING
• Warn patient not to perform hazardous tasks or those requiring alertness and coordination until CNS effects are known.
• Advise patient to avoid use of alcohol and other CNS depressants while taking this drug.
• Caution patient not to take more than the recommended dose because of increased risk of somnolence at higher doses.

levodopa–carbidopa
lee-voe-DOE-pa/kar-bih-DOE-pa

Dhivy, Duodopa✽, Duopa, Rytary, Sinemet⊘

Therapeutic class: Antiparkinsonian drugs
Pharmacologic class: Decarboxylase inhibitors–dopamine precursors

AVAILABLE FORMS
Capsules (extended-release) ⬤: 95 mg levodopa with 23.75 mg carbidopa, 145 mg levodopa with 36.25 mg carbidopa, 195 mg levodopa with 48.75 mg carbidopa, 245 mg levodopa with 61.25 mg carbidopa
Enteral suspension: levodopa 20 mg/mL with 4.63 mg/mL carbidopa, levodopa

20 mg/mL with 5 mg/mL carbidopa in single-use cassettes♦

Tablets (extended-release) ⓞⓝⓒ: 100 mg levodopa with 25 mg carbidopa, 200 mg levodopa with 50 mg carbidopa
Tablets (immediate-release): 100 mg levodopa with 10 mg carbidopa, 100 mg levodopa with 25 mg carbidopa, 250 mg levodopa with 25 mg carbidopa
Tablets (ODTs): 100 mg levodopa with 10 mg carbidopa, 100 mg levodopa with 25 mg carbidopa, 250 mg levodopa with 25 mg carbidopa

INDICATIONS & DOSAGES

➤ **Idiopathic Parkinson disease, post-encephalitic parkinsonism, and symptomatic parkinsonism resulting from carbon monoxide or manganese intoxication**
Adults: 1 immediate-release tablet of 100 mg levodopa with 25 mg carbidopa PO t.i.d., increased by 1 tablet daily or every other day, as needed, to maximum daily dose of 8 tablets. May use 250 mg levodopa with 25 mg carbidopa or 100 mg levodopa with 10 mg carbidopa tablets, as directed, to obtain maximal response. Optimum daily dose must be determined by careful adjustment for each patient. Or, 1 extended-release capsule of 95 mg levodopa with 23.75 mg carbidopa t.i.d. for 3 days; on day 4, increase to 145 mg levodopa with 36.25 mg carbidopa t.i.d. Adjust dose as needed; may increase dose up to 390 mg levodopa with 97.5 mg t.i.d. May increase frequency of dosing to maximum of five times daily if needed and tolerated. Maximum recommended daily dose is 2,450 mg levodopa with 612.5 mg carbidopa. Or, 1 extended-release tablet of 200 mg levodopa with 50 mg carbidopa b.i.d. at intervals of 6 hours or more. Increase or decrease doses and dosing intervals based on response. Most patients have been adequately treated with a dose that provides 400 to 1,600 mg of levodopa per day (divided doses) at intervals of 4 to 8 hours while awake. Allow at least a 3-day interval between dosage adjustments.

Refer to manufacturer's instructions to convert from immediate-release to extended-release formulations.

➤ **Motor fluctuations in patients with advanced Parkinson disease (Duodopa, Duopa)**
🔵 *Alert:* Before initiating enteral therapy, convert patient from all other forms of levodopa to oral immediate-release levodopa–carbidopa tablets (1:4 ratio).
Adults: Total daily dose (expressed in terms of levodopa) consists of a morning dose, a continuous dose, and extra doses, which can be used to manage acute "off" symptoms not controlled by the morning and continuous dose. Refer to manufacturer's labeling for morning dose and continuous dose calculations and titration instructions. Maximum dose of morning and continuous dose is 2,000 mg of the levodopa component over 16 hours. Maximum of extra doses is one extra dose every 2 hours. Give patient's routine nighttime dosage of oral immediate-release levodopa–carbidopa after discontinuation of daily infusion.
Adjust-a-dose: For dyskinesias or levodopa-related adverse reactions within 1 hour of morning dose on preceding day, decrease morning dose by 1 mL. For dyskinesias or adverse reactions lasting 1 hour or more on preceding day, decrease continuous dose by 0.3 mL/hour. For dyskinesias or adverse reactions lasting for two or more periods of 1 hour or more on preceding day, decrease continuous dose by 0.6 mL/hour.

ADMINISTRATION
PO
• Give drug with food to decrease GI upset, but avoid giving with high-protein meals, which can impair absorption and reduce effectiveness.
• Don't crush or break extended-release form.
• Give ODT immediately after removing from bottle. Place tablet on patient's tongue, where it will dissolve in seconds and be swallowed with saliva. No additional fluid is needed.
• For patients who have difficulty swallowing, capsules may be opened and the entire contents sprinkled on a small amount of applesauce (1 to 2 tablespoons) and then consumed immediately (don't store for future use).
Enteral
• Before use, fully thaw in refrigerator. To ensure controlled thawing, take cartons containing the seven individual cassettes out of the transport box and separate cartons from each other.
• Assign a 12-week, use-by date based on the time the cartons are put into the refrigerator to thaw (may take up to 96 hours to thaw).

Reactions in bold italics are *life-threatening*. Interactions may have a *rapid onset* or a ***delayed onset***.

• Once thawed, individual cartons may be packed in a closer configuration within the refrigerator.

• Remove one cassette from refrigerator 20 minutes before administration (failure to use at room temperature may result in inaccurate dosage).

• Administer through either a nasojejunal tube (temporary administration) or a percutaneous endoscopic gastrostomy-jejunostomy tube (long-term administration) connected to the CADD-Legacy 1400 pump.

• Disconnect tube from the pump at end of infusion and flush tube with room temperature drinking water with a syringe.

• Cassettes are for single use only and should be discarded daily after infusion. Don't reuse opened cassettes.

ACTION

Levodopa, a dopamine precursor, relieves parkinsonian symptoms by being converted to dopamine in the brain. Carbidopa inhibits the decarboxylation of peripheral levodopa, which allows more intact levodopa to travel to the brain.

Route	Onset	Peak	Duration
PO	Unknown	30–120 min	Unknown
Enteral	Unknown	2.5 hr	Unknown

Half-life: 1.5 to 2 hours.

ADVERSE REACTIONS

CNS: syncope, agitation, bradykinetic episodes, dyskinesia, anxiety, confusion, dementia, *suicidality,* dizziness, dream abnormalities, sleep disorder, fever, delusions, hallucinations, depression, headache, insomnia, paresthesia, psychotic episodes, paranoid ideation, somnolence, fatigue, asthenia, taste alterations. **CV:** cardiac irregularities, chest pain, HTN, hypotension, orthostatic hypotension, edema, palpitations, phlebitis, *MI.* **EENT:** oropharyngeal pain, dark saliva, dry mouth. **GI:** anorexia, constipation, duodenal ulcer, diarrhea, dyspepsia, abdominal pain, *GI bleeding,* nausea, vomiting. **GU:** dark urine, urinary frequency, UTI. **Hematologic:** *agranulocytosis,* hemolytic and nonhemolytic anemia, *leukopenia, thrombocytopenia.* **Hepatic:** increased LFT values. **Metabolic:** weight gain or loss. **Musculoskeletal:** back pain, leg pain, muscle cramps, shoulder pain. **Respiratory:** dyspnea, URI, atelectasis. **Skin:** alopecia, rash, diaphoresis, dark sweat, urticaria, pruritus, purpura, bullous lesions. **Other:** increased libido, hypersensitivity, complications of enteral device insertion.

INTERACTIONS

Drug-drug. *Antihypertensives:* May cause additive hypotensive effects. Use together cautiously.

Antipsychotics (butyrophenones, phenothiazines, risperidone): May decrease levodopa activity. Monitor patient closely.

Iron salts (oral): May reduce bioavailability of levodopa–carbidopa. Give iron 2 hours before or after oral levodopa–carbidopa.

Isoniazid: May antagonize antiparkinsonian actions. Use together cautiously. Therapy modification may be necessary.

MAO inhibitors (nonselective [isocarboxazid, phenelzine, tranylcypromine]): May increase risk of severe HTN. Use together is contraindicated. Discontinue MAO inhibitor 2 weeks before start of levodopa–carbidopa.

MAO inhibitors (selective [rasagiline, safinamide, selegiline]): May increase risk of orthostatic hypotension. Monitor patient closely.

Methylphenidate: May increase risk of adverse effects related to levodopa–carbidopa. Monitor patient carefully.

Metoclopramide: May decrease therapeutic effects of levodopa–carbidopa. Monitor therapeutic effects.

Papaverine, phenytoin: May antagonize antiparkinsonian actions. Avoid using together.

Sapropterin: May increase risk of levodopa-related adverse effects. Monitor patient carefully.

TCAs: May cause increase in BP and dyskinesia. Use together cautiously.

Drug-herb. *Kava:* May decrease action of drug. Discourage kava use altogether.

Drug-food. *Foods high in protein:* May decrease levodopa absorption. Don't give levodopa with high-protein foods.

EFFECTS ON LAB TEST RESULTS

• May increase BUN, creatinine, uric acid, ALT, AST, ALP, LDH, glucose, and bilirubin levels.

• May decrease Hb level and hematocrit and WBC, granulocyte, and platelet counts.

• May falsely increase urinary catecholamine level and serum and urinary uric acid levels in colorimetric tests.

• May falsely decrease urinary vanillylmandelic acid level.

• May cause false-positive results in urine ketone tests using sodium nitroprusside reagent and in urine glucose tests using cupric sulfate reagent.

• May cause false-negative urine glucose or false-positive urine acetone results in tests using glucose oxidase.

• May alter results of urine screening tests for phenylketonuria.

• May cause positive Coombs test.

CONTRAINDICATIONS & CAUTIONS

• Contraindicated in patients hypersensitive to drug and in those with angle-closure glaucoma, melanoma, or undiagnosed skin lesions.

• Use cautiously in patients with severe CV, renal, hepatic, endocrine, or pulmonary disorders; orthostatic hypotension; history of peptic ulcer; psychiatric illness; MI with residual arrhythmias; bronchial asthma; emphysema; or well-controlled, chronic open-angle glaucoma.

• Potentially fatal GI complications, including bezoar, ileus, implant-site erosion or ulcer, intestinal hemorrhage, intestinal ischemia, intestinal obstruction, intestinal perforation, pancreatitis, peritonitis, pneumoperitoneum, and postoperative wound infection, may occur in patients receiving enteral therapy.

• May increase risk of impulse-control disorders, dyskinesia, melanoma, orthostatic hypotension, and sudden somnolence.

Dialyzable drug: Unknown.

⚠ *Overdose S&S:* Muscle twitching, blepharospasm.

PREGNANCY-LACTATION-REPRODUCTION

• There are no adequate studies during pregnancy. Use during pregnancy only if potential benefit justifies fetal risk.

• Drug appears in human milk. Use cautiously in breastfeeding.

NURSING CONSIDERATIONS

• Determine optimum daily dose by careful titration in each patient. Therapy should be individualized and adjusted according to the desired therapeutic response.

• Observe patient and monitor vital signs, especially changes in BP, when changing positions and while adjusting dosage. Report significant changes.

• Monitor patient for CV signs and symptoms (chest pain, irregular HR) and neuropathy.

🕒 *Alert:* Because of risk of precipitating a symptom complex resembling NMS (fever, muscular rigidity, altered consciousness, autonomic instability), observe patient closely if levodopa dosage is reduced abruptly or stopped.

• Hallucinations or dyskinesias may require dosage reduction or drug withdrawal.

• Test patients receiving long-term therapy regularly for diabetes and acromegaly, and periodically for hepatic, renal, and hematopoietic function.

🕒 *Alert:* Monitor patient for depression and suicidality.

PATIENT TEACHING

• Instruct patient or caregiver in safe drug administration.

• Warn patient and caregivers not to increase or decrease dosage without prescriber's orders.

🕒 *Alert:* Counsel family member or caregivers to monitor patient for changes in behavior and to immediately report suicidality.

• Advise patient to have skin checks for appearance of melanoma.

• Caution patient about possible dizziness when standing up quickly, especially at start of therapy. Tell patient to change positions slowly and dangle legs before getting out of bed.

• Instruct patient to report adverse reactions (such as somnolence, loss of impulse control) and therapeutic effects.

• Advise patient receiving enteral therapy to immediately report abdominal pain, prolonged constipation, nausea, vomiting, fever, or melena.

• Inform patient that pyridoxine (vitamin B_6) doesn't reverse beneficial effects of levodopa–carbidopa. Multivitamins (without iron) can be taken without reversing levodopa's effects.

levodopa–carbidopa–entacapone
lee-voe-DOE-pa/kar-bih-DOE-pa/
en-ta-KAP-own

Stalevo✔

Therapeutic class: Antiparkinsonian drugs
Pharmacologic class: Dopamine
precursors–decarboxylase inhibitors–
catecholamine-*O*-methyltransferase
inhibitors

AVAILABLE FORMS
Tablets (film-coated) ⓓⓝⓖ: 50 mg levodopa,
12.5 mg carbidopa, and 200 mg entacapone;
75 mg levodopa, 18.75 mg carbidopa, and
200 mg entacapone; 100 mg levodopa,
25 mg carbidopa, and 200 mg entacapone;
125 mg levodopa, 31.25 mg carbidopa, and
200 mg entacapone; 150 mg levodopa,
37.5 mg carbidopa, and 200 mg entacapone;
200 mg levodopa, 50 mg carbidopa, and
200 mg entacapone

INDICATIONS & DOSAGES
➤ **Idiopathic Parkinson disease, to replace individual components at equivalent
strengths; or to replace immediate-release
levodopa–carbidopa for patient who has
end-of-dose "wearing off," who's taking a
total daily levodopa dose of 600 mg or less,
and who has no dyskinesia**
Adults: 1 tablet PO; determine dose and interval by therapeutic response. Maximum,
8 tablets/24 hours for all strengths except
levodopa 200 mg, carbidopa 50 mg, and entacapone 200 mg; for these strengths, give
maximum 6 tablets/24 hours.

ADMINISTRATION
PO
• Don't cut, crush, or allow patient to chew
tablets.
• Give only 1 tablet at each dosing interval.
• Give drug with or without food, but avoid
giving with a high-fat, high-calorie meal by
about 2 hours, which can decrease absorption.

ACTION
Levodopa, a dopamine precursor, relieves
parkinsonian symptoms by converting to
dopamine in the brain. Carbidopa inhibits
the decarboxylation of peripheral levodopa,
which allows more intact levodopa to travel
to the brain. Entacapone is a reversible
catecholamine-*O*-methyltransferase (COMT)
inhibitor that increases levodopa level.

Route	Onset	Peak	Duration
PO	Unknown	1–3.5 hr	Unknown

Half-life: Carbidopa, 1.5 to 2 hours; levodopa, 1 to
3.25 hours; entacapone, 0.75 to 1 hour.

ADVERSE REACTIONS
⚠ *Alert:* Reactions listed are those that occurred more frequently with the addition of
entacapone than with levodopa–carbidopa
alone. Refer to levodopa–carbidopa monograph for less frequent adverse reactions.
CNS: dyskinesia, hyperkinesia, hypokinesia, agitation, anxiety, asthenia, dizziness, fatigue, taste perversion, somnolence. **EENT:**
dry mouth. **GI:** diarrhea, nausea, abdominal pain, constipation, dyspepsia, flatulence,
gastritis, vomiting. **GU:** urine discoloration.
Musculoskeletal: back pain. **Respiratory:**
dyspnea. **Skin:** diaphoresis, purpura. **Other:**
bacterial infection.

INTERACTIONS
Drug-drug. *Ampicillin, chloramphenicol,
cholestyramine, erythromycin, probenecid,
rifampin:* May interfere with entacapone excretion. Use together cautiously.
Antihypertensives: May cause orthostatic hypotension. Adjust antihypertensive dosage as
needed.
CNS depressants: Additive effects. Use together cautiously.
*Dopamine (D2) receptor antagonists (buty-
rophenones, iron salts, isoniazid, metoclopramide, phenothiazines, phenytoin, risperidone):* May decrease levodopa, carbidopa,
and entacapone effects. Monitor patient for
effectiveness.
*Drugs metabolized by COMT (apomor-
phine, dobutamine, dopamine, epinephrine,
isoetharine, isoproterenol, methyldopa, norepinephrine):* May increase HR, arrhythmias,
and excessive BP changes. Use together cautiously.
Iron salts (oral): May reduce bioavailability
of levodopa–carbidopa–entacapone. Separate
drugs by 2 or more hours; monitor therapy.
*MAO inhibitors (nonselective [isocarboxazid,
phenelzine, tranylcypromine]):* May increase
risk of severe HTN. Use together is contraindicated. Discontinue MAO inhibitor

2 weeks before start of levodopa–carbidopa–entacapone.

MAO inhibitors (selective [rasagiline, safinamide, selegiline]): May increase risk of orthostatic hypotension. Monitor patient closely.

Metoclopramide: May increase availability of levodopa and carbidopa by increasing gastric emptying. Monitor patient for adverse effects.

Selegiline: May cause severe hypotension. Use together cautiously, and monitor BP.

TCAs: May increase risk of HTN and dyskinesia. Monitor patient closely.

Drug-food. *Foods high in protein:* May decrease levodopa absorption. Don't give drug with high-protein foods.

Drug-herb. *Kava kava:* May decrease action of drug. Discourage kava kava use altogether.

Drug-lifestyle. *Alcohol use:* May enhance CNS depressant effects. Monitor therapy.

EFFECTS ON LAB TEST RESULTS
● May increase ALP, AST, ALT, LDH, glucose, BUN, and bilirubin levels.
● May decrease Hb level, hematocrit, and platelet and WBC counts.
● May cause false-positive reaction for urinary ketone bodies on a test tape.
● May cause false-negative result for glycosuria with glucose oxidase testing methods.
● May cause abnormal catecholamine and Coombs test.

CONTRAINDICATIONS & CAUTIONS
● Contraindicated in patients hypersensitive to drug or its components.
● Contraindicated in patients with angle-closure glaucoma, suspicious undiagnosed skin lesions, or a history of melanoma.
● Use cautiously in patients with past or current psychosis and in patients with severe pulmonary disease; bronchial asthma; biliary obstruction; peptic ulcer; or renal, hepatic, or endocrine disease.
● Use cautiously in patients with chronic open-angle glaucoma or hepatic impairment.
Dialyzable drug: Unlikely.
⚠ *Overdose S&S:* CNS disturbances, hypotension, tachycardia, rhabdomyolysis, transient renal insufficiency, abdominal pain, loose stools.

PREGNANCY-LACTATION-REPRODUCTION
● There are no adequate studies during pregnancy. Use only if potential benefit justifies fetal risk.
● It isn't known if drug appears in human milk. Use cautiously with breastfeeding.

NURSING CONSIDERATIONS
● Certain CNS effects, such as dyskinesia, may occur at lower dosages and sooner with levodopa–carbidopa–entacapone than with levodopa alone. Dyskinesia may require a reduced dosage.
● Monitor patients for orthostatic hypotension, especially during dosage escalation.
● NMS-like symptoms may develop when levodopa and carbidopa are reduced or stopped, especially in patients taking antipsychotic drugs. Watch patient carefully for fever, hyperthermia, muscle rigidity, involuntary movements, altered consciousness, mental status changes, and autonomic dysfunction.
● During extended therapy, periodically monitor hepatic, hematopoietic, CV, and renal function.
● Diarrhea is common; it usually develops 4 to 12 weeks after treatment starts but may appear as early as the first week or as late as many months after treatment starts.
● *Alert:* Monitor patient for hallucinations, depression, and suicidality.

PATIENT TEACHING
● Instruct patient and caregiver in safe drug administration.
● Teach patient to report a "wearing-off" effect, which may occur at the end of the dosing interval.
● Tell patient that urine, sweat, and saliva may turn dark (red, brown, or black) during treatment.
● Advise patient to notify the prescriber if problems making voluntary movements increase.
● Tell patient that diarrhea is common with this treatment.
● Inform patient that hallucinations may occur.
● Urge patient to immediately report depression, suicidality, or loss of impulse control.
● Explain that patient may become dizzy if rising quickly. Urge patient to use caution when rising.

Reactions in bold italics are *life-threatening*. Interactions may have a *rapid onset* or a ***delayed onset***.

- Tell patient that excessive acidity, iron salts, or a high-fat, high-calorie, or high-protein diet may reduce drug's effectiveness.
- Urge patient to avoid hazardous activities until CNS effects of drug are known.
- Advise patient of childbearing potential to report pregnancy.

levoFLOXacin
lee-voe-FLOX-a-sin

Therapeutic class: Antibiotics
Pharmacologic class: Fluoroquinolones

AVAILABLE FORMS
Infusion (premixed): 250 mg in 50 mL D_5W, 500 mg in 100 mL D_5W, 750 mg in 150 mL D_5W
Ophthalmic solution: 0.5%, 1.5%
Oral solution: 25 mg/mL
Single-use vials: 500 mg, 750 mg
Tablets: 250 mg, 500 mg, 750 mg

INDICATIONS & DOSAGES
Boxed Warning Use in patients with acute bacterial sinusitis, acute bacterial exacerbation of chronic bronchitis, and uncomplicated UTI isn't recommended because of risk of serious adverse effects. Use in these patients only when they have no other treatment options. ■

Adjust-a-dose (for all indications): For patients with CrCl of less than 50 mL/minute, adjust the oral or IV dosage regimen according to the manufacturer's instructions.
➤ **Acute bacterial sinusitis caused by susceptible strains of** *Streptococcus pneumoniae, Moraxella catarrhalis,* **or** *Haemophilus influenzae*
Adults: 500 mg PO or IV infusion over 60 minutes every 24 hours for 10 to 14 days or 750 mg PO or IV over 90 minutes every 24 hours for 5 days.
➤ **Mild to moderate skin and skin-structure infections caused by** *Staphylococcus aureus* **or** *Streptococcus pyogenes*
Adults: 500 mg PO or IV infusion every 24 hours for 7 to 10 days.
➤ **Acute bacterial worsening of chronic bronchitis caused by** *S. aureus, S. pneumoniae, M. catarrhalis, H. influenzae,* **or** *Haemophilus parainfluenzae*
Adults: 500 mg PO or IV infusion every 24 hours for 7 days.

➤ **To prevent inhalation anthrax after confirmed or suspected exposure to** *Bacillus anthracis*
Adults: 500 mg IV infusion or PO every 24 hours for 60 days.
Children age 6 months and older weighing at least 50 kg: 500 mg PO or by slow IV infusion every 24 hours for 60 days.
Children age 6 months and older weighing 30 to less than 50 kg: 250 mg PO or 8 mg/kg (not to exceed 250 mg/dose) oral solution or by slow IV infusion every 12 hours for 60 days.
➤ **Chronic bacterial prostatitis caused by** *Escherichia coli, Enterococcus faecalis,* **or** *Staphylococcus epidermidis*
Adults: 500 mg PO or IV infusion every 24 hours for 28 days.
➤ **Community-acquired pneumonia from** *S. pneumoniae* **(excluding multidrug-resistant strains),** *H. influenzae, H. parainfluenzae, Mycoplasma pneumoniae,* **or** *Chlamydia pneumoniae*
Adults: 750 mg PO or IV infusion every 24 hours for 5 days.
➤ **Community-acquired pneumonia caused by methicillin-susceptible** *S. aureus, S. pneumoniae, H. influenzae, H. parainfluenzae, Klebsiella pneumoniae, M. catarrhalis, C. pneumoniae, Legionella pneumophila,* **or** *M. pneumoniae*
Adults: 500 mg PO or IV infusion every 24 hours for 7 to 14 days.
➤ **Complicated skin and skin-structure infections caused by methicillin-sensitive** *S. aureus, E. faecalis, S. pyogenes,* **or** *Proteus mirabilis*
Adults: 750 mg PO or IV infusion every 24 hours for 7 to 14 days.
➤ **Health care–acquired pneumonia caused by methicillin-susceptible** *S. aureus, Pseudomonas aeruginosa, Serratia marcescens, E. coli, K. pneumoniae, H. influenzae,* **or** *S. pneumoniae*
Adults: 750 mg PO or IV infusion every 24 hours for 7 to 14 days.
➤ **Complicated UTI caused by** *E. faecalis, Enterobacter cloacae, E. coli, K. pneumoniae, P. mirabilis,* **or** *P. aeruginosa;* **acute pyelonephritis caused by** *E. coli*
Adults: 250 mg PO or IV infusion every 24 hours for 10 days.
➤ **Complicated UTI caused by** *E. coli, K. pneumoniae,* **or** *P. mirabilis;* **acute pyelonephritis caused by** *E. coli*

L

Adults: 750 mg PO or IV infusion daily for 5 days.

➤ **Mild to moderate uncomplicated UTI caused by *E. coli, K. pneumoniae,* or *Staphylococcus saprophyticus***
Adults: 250 mg PO daily for 3 days.

➤ **Prophylaxis or treatment of pneumonic and septicemic plague *(Yersinia pestis)***
Adults: 500 mg PO or IV infusion every 24 hours for 10 to 14 days.
Children age 6 months and older weighing 50 kg or more: 500 mg PO or by slow IV infusion every 24 hours for 10 to 14 days.
Children age 6 months and older weighing 30 to less than 50 kg: 250 mg PO or 8 mg/kg (not to exceed 250 mg/dose) oral solution or by slow IV infusion every 12 hours for 10 to 14 days.

➤ **Bacterial conjunctivitis**
Adults and children age 6 and older: On days 1 through 2, instill 1 to 2 drops in affected eye(s) every 2 hours while patient is awake and up to 8 times daily. On days 3 through 7, instill 1 to 2 drops in affected eye(s) every 4 hours while patient is awake up to 4 times daily.

➤ **Corneal ulceration caused by *Corynebacterium* species, *S. aureus, S. epidermidis, S. pneumoniae, Viridans* group streptococci, *P. aeruginosa, S. marcescens***
Adults and children age 6 and older: Instill 1 to 2 drops into affected eye every 30 minutes to 2 hours while awake and 4 to 6 hours after retiring, for 3 days. Then, instill 1 to 2 drops into affected eye every 1 to 4 hours while awake on day 4 until end of treatment based on complete reepithelialization.

➤ **Neutropenia (chemotherapy-induced), antibacterial prophylaxis ◆**
Adults: 500 or 750 mg PO once daily. Some clinicians will provide antibacterial prophylaxis if ANC is anticipated to be less than 500/mm³ for more than 7 days. For hematopoietic cell transplant recipients, begin at the time of stem cell infusion and continue until recovery of neutropenia or until initiation of empirical antibiotic therapy for neutropenic fever.

ADMINISTRATION

PO
• Obtain specimen for culture and sensitivity tests before therapy and as needed to determine if bacterial resistance has occurred.

• Give drug with plenty of fluids to prevent crystalluria.
• Give 2 hours before or 2 hours after antacids, sucralfate, and products containing magnesium, aluminum, iron, or multivitamins with zinc.
• Give oral solution 1 hour before or 2 hours after a meal.

IV
▼ Obtain specimen for culture and sensitivity tests before therapy and as needed to determine if bacterial resistance has occurred.
▼ Give this form only by infusion.
▼ Dilute drug in single-use vials, according to manufacturer's instructions, with D_5W or NSS for injection to a final concentration of 5 mg/mL.
▼ Infuse doses of 500 mg or less over 60 minutes and doses of 750 mg over 90 minutes.
▼ Reconstituted solution should be clear, slightly yellow, and free of particulate matter.
▼ Reconstituted drug is stable for 72 hours at room temperature, for 14 days when refrigerated in plastic containers, and for 6 months when frozen.
▼ Thaw at room temperature or in refrigerator.
▼ **Incompatibilities:** The manufacturer recommends not mixing or infusing other drugs with levofloxacin.

Ophthalmic
• Avoid touching applicator tip to eye or other surfaces.

ACTION

Inhibits bacterial DNA gyrase and prevents DNA replication, transcription, repair, and recombination in susceptible bacteria.

Route	Onset	Peak	Duration
PO, IV	Unknown	1–2 hr	Unknown
Ophthalmic	Unknown	Unknown	Unknown

Half-life: About 6 to 8 hours.

ADVERSE REACTIONS

CNS: dizziness, headache, fever, insomnia, taste disturbance (ophthalmic). **CV:** edema, chest pain. **EENT:** foreign body or burning sensation in eye, eye pain, blurred vision, vision loss, ocular infection, photophobia (ophthalmic). **GI:** abdominal pain, constipation, diarrhea, dyspepsia, nausea, vomiting. **GU:** vaginitis. **Metabolic:** *hypoglycemia.* **Musculoskeletal:** back pain, tendon rupture.

Reactions in bold italics are *life-threatening*. Interactions may have a *rapid onset* or a ***delayed onset***.

Respiratory: allergic pneumonitis, dyspnea. **Skin:** photosensitivity, pruritus, rash, injection-site reaction. **Other:** infection, hypersensitivity reactions.

INTERACTIONS

Drug-drug. *Aluminum hydroxide, aluminum–magnesium hydroxide, calcium carbonate, didanosine, magnesium hydroxide, products containing zinc, sucralfate:* May interfere with GI absorption of levofloxacin. Give levofloxacin 2 hours before or 2 hours after these products.
Antiarrhythmics (Class IA [procainamide, quinidine] or Class III [amiodarone, dofetilide]), chlorpromazine, erythromycin, fluconazole, haloperidol, imipramine, ondansetron, ziprasidone: May increase risk of life-threatening cardiac arrhythmias. Avoid use together.
Antidiabetics: May alter glucose level. Monitor glucose level closely.
Iron salts: May decrease absorption of levofloxacin, reducing anti-infective response. Separate doses by at least 2 hours.
NSAIDs: May increase CNS stimulation. Monitor patient for seizure activity.
Steroids: May increase risk of tendinitis and tendon rupture. Monitor patient for tendon pain or inflammation.
Theophylline: May decrease clearance of theophylline. Monitor theophylline level.
Warfarin and derivatives: May increase effect of oral anticoagulant. Monitor PT and INR.
Drug-lifestyle. *Sun exposure:* May cause photosensitivity reactions. Advise patient to avoid excessive sunlight exposure.

EFFECTS ON LAB TEST RESULTS

• May increase potassium and ALP levels, renal function, and LFT values.
• May increase or decrease glucose level.
• May increase eosinophil count.
• May decrease Hb level and platelet and WBC counts.
• May produce false-positive opioid assay results.

CONTRAINDICATIONS & CAUTIONS

Boxed Warning Drug may cause disabling and potentially irreversible adverse reactions, including tendinitis and tendon rupture, peripheral neuropathy, and CNS effects (hallucinations, anxiety, depression, insomnia, severe headaches, confusion). Discontinue drug with first signs or symptoms of these reactions. ∎

• Risk of tendinitis and tendon rupture increases in patients older than age 60, in patients taking corticosteroids, and in those with heart, kidney, or lung transplants.
Boxed Warning Drug may exacerbate muscle weakness in patients with myasthenia gravis. Avoid use in patients with a history of myasthenia gravis. ∎
☝ *Alert:* Drug is associated with increased incidence of musculoskeletal disorders (arthralgia, arthritis, tendinopathy, and gait abnormality) in children.
☝ *Alert:* Drug may increase risk of aortic dissection or rupture when used systemically. Avoid use in patients with known aortic aneurysm and in patients at risk for an aortic aneurysm, including those with peripheral atherosclerotic vascular diseases, HTN, certain genetic conditions (Marfan syndrome, Ehlers-Danlos syndrome), and older adults. Drug should only be used in these patients if no other treatment options are available.
• Contraindicated in patients hypersensitive to drug, its components, or other fluoroquinolones.
☝ *Alert:* Patients receiving systemic drug have an increased risk of hyperglycemia and hypoglycemia. Hypoglycemia has been reported more frequently in older adults and patients with diabetes.
• Use cautiously in patients with history of seizure disorders or other CNS diseases, such as cerebral arteriosclerosis.
• Use cautiously in patients with personal or family history of QT-interval prolongation, hypokalemia, bradycardia, or recent MI, and in those currently taking antiarrhythmics.
• Use cautiously and with dosage adjustment in patients with renal impairment.
• Drug may increase risk of hypersensitivity reactions, including SCARs, and allergic pneumonitis.
• Drug may rarely cause serious adverse reactions, including vasculitis, arthralgia, myalgia, serum sickness, interstitial nephritis, acute renal insufficiency or renal failure, and blood dyscrasias.
• Drug may cause severe hepatotoxicity. Discontinue immediately if patient develops signs or symptoms of hepatitis.
• Drug is indicated in children (age 6 months and older) only for postexposure inhalational anthrax prevention and for plague.
Dialyzable drug: No.

L

PREGNANCY-LACTATION-REPRODUCTION

• There are no adequate studies during pregnancy. Use during pregnancy only if potential benefit justifies fetal risk.

• Drug likely appears in human milk. Evaluate benefits of continuing therapy and risks of breastfeeding. Manufacturer's information advises patient not to breastfeed during therapy and for 2 days after final dose.

NURSING CONSIDERATIONS

⚠ *Alert:* Monitor patients for signs and symptoms of aortic aneurysm, dissection, and rupture (sudden, severe, and constant pain in the stomach, chest, or back; throbbing in the stomach area, deep pain in the back or side of the stomach; steady, gnawing pain in the stomach that lasts for hours or days; pain in the jaw, neck, back, or chest; coughing or hoarseness; shortness of breath or trouble swallowing). Discontinue drug immediately if any of these aortic disorders are suspected.

• Patients with acute hypersensitivity reactions may need treatment with epinephrine, oxygen, IV fluids, antihistamines, corticosteroids, pressor amines, and airway management.

• Monitor patient for signs and symptoms of peripheral neuropathy (pain, burning, tingling, numbness, weakness, or a change in sensation to light touch, pain, temperature, or sense of body position).

• Most antibacterials can cause pseudomembranous colitis, CDAD. If diarrhea occurs, notify prescriber; drug may be stopped.

• Drug may cause an abnormal ECG.

⚠ *Alert:* Monitor patients receiving systemic drug for symptoms of hypoglycemia (confusion, pounding or rapid heartbeat, dizziness, pale skin, shakiness, diaphoresis, unusual hunger, trembling, headache, weakness, irritability, unusual anxiety). Immediately discontinue drug for blood glucose disturbances, and switch to a nonfluoroquinolone antibiotic if possible.

⚠ *Alert:* Monitor patients receiving systemic drug for psychiatric adverse reactions (disturbances in attention, disorientation, agitation, nervousness, memory impairment, delirium). Discontinue drug for CNS adverse effects, including psychiatric adverse reactions.

⚠ *Alert:* If *P. aeruginosa* is a confirmed or suspected pathogen, use with a beta-lactam.

• Monitor glucose level and results of renal function tests, LFTs, and blood counts.

• *Look alike–sound alike:* Don't confuse levofloxacin with levetiracetam.

PATIENT TEACHING

Boxed Warning Warn patient to immediately notify prescriber for signs and symptoms of serious adverse reactions, including unusual joint or tendon pain, muscle weakness, "pins and needles" tingling or prickling sensation, numbness in the arms or legs, confusion, or hallucinations. ■

⚠ *Alert:* Warn patient to seek immediate medical attention for signs and symptoms of aortic aneurysm, dissection, or rupture.

• Instruct patient to report all adverse reactions.

• Tell patient to take drug as prescribed, even if signs and symptoms disappear.

• Advise patient to take drug with plenty of fluids to prevent crystalluria, and to space antacids, sucralfate, multivitamins with zinc, and products containing magnesium, aluminum, or iron by at least 12 hours before or after oral drug administration.

• Warn patient to avoid hazardous tasks until adverse effects of drug are known.

• Advise patient to avoid excessive sunlight and UV light exposure.

• Tell patient to stop drug and notify prescriber if rash or other signs or symptoms of hypersensitivity develop.

• Instruct patient to notify prescriber of all adverse reactions, including loose stools or diarrhea.

• Tell patient not to take more than one dose in the same day, even if a dose is missed.

• Instruct patient not to use contact lenses during treatment for bacterial conjunctivitis or corneal ulceration.

⚠ *Alert:* Caution patient that significant low blood sugar level can occur. Instruct patient how to manage symptoms and to immediately report any occurrence.

• Advise patient with diabetes that they may need to monitor blood glucose levels more frequently during therapy.

⚠ *Alert:* Inform patients to immediately report psychiatric adverse reactions and that these can occur after just one dose.

• Instruct patient to report diarrhea because of risk of CDAD during and for 2 months or more after treatment.

Reactions in bold italics are *life-threatening*. Interactions may have a *rapid onset* or a *delayed onset*.

levothyroxine sodium
(T₄, L-thyroxine sodium)
lee-voe-thye-ROX-een

Eltroxin✢, Euthyrox, Levo-T,
Levoxyl✐, Synthroid✐, Thyquidity,
Tirosint, Tirosint-Sol, Unithroid

Therapeutic class: Thyroid hormone
replacements
Pharmacologic class: Thyroid hormones

AVAILABLE FORMS
Capsules 🔘: 13 mcg, 25 mcg, 50 mcg,
75 mcg, 88 mcg, 100 mcg, 112 mcg,
125 mcg, 137 mcg, 150 mcg, 175 mcg,
200 mcg
Oral solution: 13 mcg/mL, 20 mcg/mL,
25 mcg/mL, 37.5 mcg/mL, 44 mcg/mL,
50 mcg/mL, 62.5 mcg/mL, 75 mcg/mL,
88 mcg/mL, 100 mcg/mL, 112 mcg/mL,
125 mcg/mL, 137 mcg/mL, 150 mcg/mL,
175 mcg/mL, 200 mcg/mL
Powder for injection: 100 mcg, 200 mcg,
500 mcg
Solution for injection: 20 mcg/mL,
40 mcg/mL, 100 mcg/mL
Tablets: 25 mcg, 50 mcg, 75 mcg, 88 mcg,
100 mcg, 112 mcg, 125 mcg, 137 mcg,
150 mcg, 175 mcg, 200 mcg, 300 mcg

INDICATIONS & DOSAGES
➤ **Thyroid hormone replacement**
Adults age 60 and younger: In otherwise
healthy individuals who have been hypothy-
roid for only a short time (such as a few
months), initiate drug at approximately
1.6 mcg/kg PO once daily. (See individual
manufacturer's instructions.) Monitor TSH
level and adjust dosage every 4 to 6 weeks in
12.5- to 25-mcg increments until patient is
euthyroid and TSH level normalizes.
*Older adults or patients with underlying car-
diac disease:* Initiate dose at 12.5 to 25 mcg
PO daily. Adjust dosage every 6 to 8 weeks,
if needed, until patient is euthyroid and TSH
level normalizes.
*Children in whom growth and puberty are
complete:* 1.6 mcg/kg PO once daily. (See individual manufacturer's instructions.)
*Children older than age 12 in whom growth
and puberty are incomplete:* 2 to 3 mcg/kg
PO daily.

Children ages 6 to 12: 4 to 5 mcg/kg PO
daily.
Children ages 1 to 5: 5 to 6 mcg/kg PO daily.
Children ages 6 months to 1 year: 6 to
8 mcg/kg PO daily.
Children ages 3 to 6 months: 8 to 10 mcg/kg
PO daily.
Infants and neonates birth to age 3 months:
10 to 15 mcg/kg PO daily. In neonates at
risk for cardiac failure, consider a lower initial dose, and increase every 4 to 6 weeks as
needed.
Children at risk for hyperactivity: Initiate at
one-fourth the recommended full replacement dose, and increase weekly by one-fourth
the full recommended replacement dose until the full recommended replacement dose is
reached.
Adjust-a-dose: For children, adjust dosage
based on clinical response and lab parameters.
➤ **Severe, long-standing hypothyroidism**
*Adults and adolescents in whom growth
and puberty are complete:* 12.5 to 25 mcg
PO daily. Increase in increments of 12.5 to
25 mcg every 2 to 4 weeks as needed.
➤ **Myxedema coma**
Adults: Initially, 300 to 500 mcg (0.3 to
0.5 mg) IV as solution followed by 50 to
100 mcg IV once daily until patient is able to
tolerate oral administration. Consider smaller
doses in patients with CV disease and older
adults.
➤ **TSH suppression in well-differentiated
thyroid cancer**
Adults: Dosage is highly individualized. Generally, TSH is suppressed to below 0.1 milli-
international units/L, which usually requires
a dosage greater than 2 mcg/kg/day. However,
in patients with high-risk tumors, target level
for TSH suppression may be lower.

ADMINISTRATION
PO
• Don't crush, break, or allow patient to chew
capsules.
• Give drug at same time each day on an
empty stomach, preferably ½ to 1 hour before
breakfast.
• Give drug at least 4 hours before or after
drugs known to interfere with levothyroxine.
• Give tablets with a full glass of water to prevent difficulty swallowing.
• If necessary, crush tablet and suspend it in
small amount of formula (except soy formula,

which may decrease absorption), human milk, or water, and give by spoon or dropper. Crushed tablet can also be sprinkled over food, except foods containing large amounts of soybean, fiber, or iron.

• Give solution directly into the mouth using a calibrated oral syringe.

IV

▼ Reconstitute powder by adding 5 mL NSS injection only.

▼ Shake vial.

▼ Use immediately after reconstitution.

▼ Give at a rate not to exceed 100 mcg/minute.

▼ Discard any unused portion.

▼ **Incompatibilities:** Don't mix or give with anything other than NSS injection.

ACTION

Synthetic form of thyroxine that affects the growth of tissues, energy expenditure, and the turnover of all substrates.

Route	Onset	Peak	Duration
PO	3–5 days	2–4 hr	Unknown
IV	6–8 hr	Unknown	Unknown

Half-life: 6 to 7 days in euthyroidism; 3 to 4 days in hyperthyroidism; 9 to 10 days in hypothyroidism.

ADVERSE REACTIONS

Adverse reactions are primarily related to hyperthyroidism due to therapeutic overdosage. **CNS:** insomnia, tremor, headache, fever, fatigue, anxiety, emotional lability. **CV:** tachycardia, palpitations, *arrhythmias,* angina pectoris, HTN, *HF.* **GI:** diarrhea, vomiting, abdominal cramps. **GU:** menstrual irregularities. **Metabolic:** weight loss, increased appetite. **Musculoskeletal:** decreased bone density, muscle weakness, tremors. **Respiratory:** dyspnea. **Skin:** allergic skin reactions, diaphoresis, hair loss. **Other:** heat intolerance, impaired fertility, hypersensitivity reaction.

INTERACTIONS

Drug-drug. *Amiodarone, iodide (including iodine-containing radiographic contrast agents), lithium:* May reduce thyroid hormone secretion. Monitor thyroid function studies if used together.

Antacids (aluminum-, magnesium-containing), bile acid sequestrants, calcium carbonate, cholestyramine, colestipol, ferrous sulfate, iron-containing products, orlistat, PPIs, sevelamer, sodium polystyrene

sulfonate, sucralfate: May impair levothyroxine absorption. Separate doses by 4 to 5 hours and monitor therapy.

Beta blockers: May reduce beta-blocker effects. Monitor patient.

Carbamazepine, hydantoins, phenobarbital, rifampin: May increase hepatic metabolism, resulting in hypothyroidism. Monitor patient.

Clofibrate, estrogens, 5-FU, methadone, mitotane, tamoxifen: May decrease thyroid levels. Monitor therapy.

Digoxin: May decrease cardiac glycoside effects. Monitor patient for clinical effect.

Fosphenytoin, phenytoin: May release free thyroid hormone but total and free thyroxine levels may decrease. Monitor thyroxine level.

Insulin, oral antidiabetics: May alter glucose level. Monitor glucose level. Dosage adjustments may be needed.

Ketamine: May produce marked HTN and tachycardia. Use together cautiously.

SSRIs: May increase levothyroxine requirements. Adjust dosage as needed.

Sympathomimetics such as epinephrine: May increase risk of coronary insufficiency. Monitor patient closely.

TCAs, tetracyclic antidepressants: May increase therapeutic effects and toxicity of both drugs. Monitor patient closely.

Theophylline: May decrease theophylline clearance in hypothyroidism; clearance may return to normal when euthyroid state is achieved. Monitor theophylline level.

Warfarin: May increase anticoagulant effects. Monitor patient for bleeding, and check PT and INR closely. Warfarin dosage adjustment may be needed.

Drug-herb. *Horseradish:* May cause abnormal thyroid function. Discourage use in patients undergoing thyroid function tests.

Lemon balm: May have antithyroid effects; may inhibit TSH. Discourage use together.

Drug-food. *Cottonseed meal, dietary fiber, soybean flour, walnuts:* May decrease absorption of drug. Dosage adjustments may be needed.

Grapefruit juice: May delay absorption of drug. Avoid use.

EFFECTS ON LAB TEST RESULTS

• May increase LFT values.

• May decrease thyroid function test results. May alter results of liothyronine, protein-bound iodine, and radioactive ^{131}I uptake studies.

Reactions in bold italics are *life-threatening*. Interactions may have a *rapid onset* or a **delayed onset**.

CONTRAINDICATIONS & CAUTIONS

• Contraindicated in patients hypersensitive to drug and in those with acute MI uncomplicated by hypothyroidism, untreated subclinical or overt thyrotoxicosis, uncorrected adrenal insufficiency, or hypersensitivity to glycerol (Tirosint oral solution).

Boxed Warning Don't use either alone or with other therapeutic agents for treatment of obesity or for weight loss. ∎

Boxed Warning Doses beyond the range of daily hormonal requirements may produce serious or even life-threatening toxicities, especially if given with sympathomimetic amines. ∎

• Use cautiously in older adults and in patients with angina pectoris, HTN, other CV disorders, renal insufficiency, or ischemia.

• Use cautiously in patients with diabetes, diabetes insipidus, or myxedema and during rapid replacement in those with arteriosclerosis.

Dializable drug: No.

⚠ *Overdose S&S:* Signs and symptoms of hyperthyroidism, confusion, disorientation, cerebral embolism, shock, coma, seizures, death.

PREGNANCY-LACTATION-REPRODUCTION

• Drug is safe to use in pregnancy and shouldn't be discontinued during pregnancy.

• Dosage may need to be increased in pregnancy. Measure serum TSH and free T_4 levels as soon as pregnancy is confirmed and, at minimum, during each trimester of pregnancy. Reduce dosage to prepregnancy levels immediately after delivery and measure serum TSH level 4 to 8 weeks postpartum.

• For new-onset hypothyroidism during pregnancy, normalize thyroid function as rapidly as possible. In patients with moderate to severe signs and symptoms, start drug at 1.6 mcg/kg daily. In patients with mild hypothyroidism, start drug at 1 mcg/kg daily. Evaluate serum TSH level every 4 weeks and adjust dosage as indicated.

• Don't use drug for infertility (unless associated with hypothyroidism).

• Drug appears minimally in human milk. Adequate replacement doses of levothyroxine are generally needed to maintain normal lactation in patients with hypothyroidism and should be continued during breastfeeding.

NURSING CONSIDERATIONS

• Patients with diabetes may need increased antidiabetic doses when starting thyroid hormone replacement.

• In patients with CAD who must receive thyroid hormone, observe carefully for possible coronary insufficiency.

• Patients with adult hypothyroidism are unusually sensitive to thyroid hormone. Start at lowest dosage, and adjust to higher dosages according to patient's symptoms and lab data until euthyroid state is reached.

• When changing from levothyroxine to liothyronine, stop levothyroxine and begin liothyronine. Increase dosage in small increments after residual effects of levothyroxine have disappeared. When changing from liothyronine to levothyroxine, start levothyroxine several days before withdrawing liothyronine to avoid relapse. Drugs aren't interchangeable.

• Long-term therapy causes bone loss during premenopause. Consider a basal bone density measurement, and monitor patient closely for osteoporosis.

• Patients taking levothyroxine who need to have ^{131}I uptake studies performed must stop drug 4 weeks before test.

• Patients taking anticoagulants may need their dosage modified and require careful monitoring of coagulation status.

• *Look alike–sound alike:* Don't confuse levothyroxine with lamotrigine or Lanoxin.

PATIENT TEACHING

• Teach patient the importance of consistently taking drug at same time each day (preferably ½ to 1 hour before breakfast) to maintain constant hormone levels.

• Instruct patient or caregiver in safe drug administration.

• Make sure patient understands that replacement therapy is usually for life. The drug should never be stopped unless directed by prescriber.

• Warn patient (especially older patient) to immediately report chest pain, palpitations, diaphoresis, nervousness, shortness of breath, or other signals of overdose or aggravated CV disease.

• Tell patient to report unusual bleeding and bruising or any other adverse reaction.

• Caution patient to tell prescriber about all medications, both OTC and prescription, and herbal products being taken.

- Instruct patient with diabetes to monitor glucose level and report changes.
- Tell patient who plans to have surgery to notify physician or dentist about taking levothyroxine.
- Advise patient to report pregnancy to prescriber because dosage may need adjustment.

SAFETY ALERT!

lidocaine hydrochloride (IV)
LYE-doe-kane

Xylocard ✤

Therapeutic class: Antiarrhythmics
Pharmacologic class: Amide derivatives

AVAILABLE FORMS
Infusion (premixed): 0.2% (2 mg/mL), 0.4% (4 mg/mL), 0.8% (8 mg/mL)
Injection (for direct IV use): 0.5% (5 mg/mL), 1% (10 mg/mL), 2% (20 mg/mL)
Injection (for IV admixtures): 4% (40 mg/mL)

INDICATIONS & DOSAGES
➤ **Ventricular arrhythmias caused by MI, cardiac manipulation, or cardiac glycosides**
Adults: 50 to 100 mg by IV bolus at 25 to 50 mg/minute. Bolus dose is repeated every 5 minutes until arrhythmias subside or adverse reactions develop. Don't exceed 300-mg total bolus during a 1-hour period. Simultaneously, constant infusion of 20 to 50 mcg/kg/minute (1 to 4 mg/minute) is begun. If single bolus has been given, smaller bolus dose may be repeated 15 to 20 minutes after start of infusion to maintain therapeutic level.
Older adults: Reduce dosage and rate of infusion.
➤ **Ventricular arrhythmias; shock-refractory ventricular fibrillation; pulseless ventricular tachycardia ♦**
Children: 1 mg/kg by IV or intraosseous bolus. May repeat infusion, starting more than 15 minutes from first bolus. Start infusion at 20 to 50 mcg/kg/minute.
Adjust-a-dose: For patients with HF, with renal or liver disease, or who weigh less than 50 kg, reduce dosage.

ADMINISTRATION
IV
▼ Give IV bolus at 25 to 50 mg/minute.
▼ Injections (additive syringes and single-use vials) containing 40 to 200 mg/mL are for the preparation of IV infusion solutions only and must be diluted before use.
▼ Prepare IV infusion by adding 1 g (using 25 mL of 4%) to 1 L of D_5W injection to provide a solution containing 1 mg/mL.
▼ Use a more concentrated solution of up to 8 mg/mL in patient with fluid restrictions.
▼ Patients receiving infusions must be on a cardiac monitor and must be attended at all times. Use an infusion control device for giving infusion precisely. Don't exceed 4 mg/minute; faster rate greatly increases risk of toxicity.
▼ Avoid giving injections containing preservatives.
▼ **Incompatibilities:** None listed by manufacturer. Consult a drug incompatibility reference for more information.

ACTION
A class IB antiarrhythmic that decreases the depolarization, automaticity, and excitability in the ventricles during the diastolic phase by direct action on the tissues, especially the Purkinje network.

Route	Onset	Peak	Duration
IV	Rapid	Unknown	15–20 min

Half-life: 1.5 to 2 hours (may be prolonged in patients with HF or hepatic disease).

ADVERSE REACTIONS
CNS: confusion, dizziness, tremor, stupor, restlessness, light-headedness, *seizures,* unconsciousness, lethargy, somnolence, anxiety, euphoria, hallucinations, nervousness, paresthesia, muscle twitching; sensation of cold, heat, or numbness. **CV:** hypotension, *bradycardia, new or worsened arrhythmias, cardiac arrest.* **EENT:** blurred or double vision, tinnitus. **GI:** vomiting. **Respiratory:** *respiratory depression and arrest.* **Skin:** soreness at injection site.

INTERACTIONS
Drug-drug. *Atenolol, metoprolol, nadolol, pindolol, propranolol:* May reduce hepatic metabolism of lidocaine, increasing the risk of toxicity. Give bolus doses of lidocaine at a

---

Reactions in bold italics are *life-threatening*. Interactions may have a *rapid onset* or a **delayed onset**.

slower rate, and monitor lidocaine level and patient closely.

Cimetidine: May decrease clearance of lidocaine, increasing the risk of toxicity. Consider a different H₂-receptor antagonist if possible. Monitor lidocaine level closely.

Ergot-type oxytocic drugs: May cause severe, persistent HTN or stroke. Avoid using together.

Mexiletine: May increase pharmacologic effects. Avoid using together.

Phenytoin, procainamide, propranolol, quinidine: May increase cardiac depressant effects. Monitor patient closely.

Succinylcholine: May prolong neuromuscular blockade. Monitor patient closely.

EFFECTS ON LAB TEST RESULTS
None reported.

CONTRAINDICATIONS & CAUTIONS
• Contraindicated in patients hypersensitive to amide-type local anesthetics.
• Contraindicated in those with Adams-Stokes syndrome, Wolff-Parkinson-White syndrome, and severe degrees of SA, AV, or intraventricular block in the absence of an artificial pacemaker.
• Use cautiously and at reduced dosages in patients with complete or second-degree heart block or sinus bradycardia, in older adults, in those with HF or renal or hepatic disease, and in those weighing less than 50 kg.
Dialyzable drug: No.
⚠ *Overdose S&S:* Circulatory depression, change in level of consciousness, seizures, hypoventilation.

PREGNANCY-LACTATION-REPRODUCTION
• There are no adequate studies with IV lidocaine during pregnancy. Use cautiously if clearly needed, especially during early pregnancy.
• Drug appears in human milk. Use cautiously during breastfeeding.

NURSING CONSIDERATIONS
• Monitor drug level. Therapeutic levels are 1.5 to 5 mcg/mL.
🔔 *Alert:* Monitor patient for toxicity. In many patients who are severely ill, seizures may be the first sign of toxicity, but severe reactions are usually preceded by somnolence, confusion, tremors, and paresthesia. If signs of toxicity occur, stop drug at once and notify

prescriber. Continuing could lead to seizures and coma. Give oxygen through a nasal cannula if not contraindicated. Keep oxygen and CPR equipment available.
• Monitor patient's response, especially BP and electrolytes, BUN, and creatinine levels.
• Correct electrolyte disturbances, especially hypokalemia or hypomagnesemia.
• If arrhythmias worsen or ECG changes occur (for example, QRS complex widens or PR interval substantially prolongs), stop infusion and notify prescriber.

PATIENT TEACHING
• Tell patient to promptly report adverse reactions, such as palpitations, dyspnea, confusion, anxiety, vision changes, dizziness, tinnitus, nausea, and vomiting, because toxicity can occur.

SAFETY ALERT!

linagliptin
lin-a-GLIP-tin

Tradjenta

Therapeutic class: Antidiabetics
Pharmacologic class: DPP-4 inhibitors

AVAILABLE FORMS
Tablets: 5 mg

INDICATIONS & DOSAGES
➤ **Adjunct to diet and exercise to improve glycemic control in adults with type 2 diabetes as monotherapy or as combination therapy with an insulin secretagogue (such as a sulfonylurea) or insulin**
Adults: 5 mg PO daily.
Adjust-a-dose: When used in combination with an insulin secretagogue or insulin, use lower doses of those drugs to decrease the risk of hypoglycemia.

ADMINISTRATION
PO
• Give drug without regard for food.
• Store tablets at 77° F (25° C).

ACTION
Inhibits DPP-4, an enzyme that rapidly inactivates incretin hormones, which play a part in the body's regulation of glucose.

🍁Canada   ◇OTC   ◆Off-label use   ✐Photoguide   ⊕Do not crush   *Liquid contains alcohol   ▨Genetic

Route	Onset	Peak	Duration
PO	Rapid	1.5 hr	Unknown

Half-life: About 12 hours (accumulation).

ADVERSE REACTIONS

CNS: headache. **EENT:** nasopharyngitis. **GI:** diarrhea, constipation. **GU:** UTI. **Metabolic:** hyperlipidemia, weight gain, increased uric acid level, increased lipase level, *hypoglycemia.* **Musculoskeletal:** arthralgia, back pain, myalgia. **Respiratory:** cough, URI.

INTERACTIONS

Drug-drug. *CYP3A4 or P-gp inducers (rifampin):* May decrease linagliptin level. Avoid use together.
Ritonavir: May increase linagliptin effects and risk of adverse effects. Use with caution; monitor response, and adjust dosage as necessary.
Sulfonylureas (glyburide), insulin: May increase risk of hypoglycemia. Monitor glucose level carefully and adjust sulfonylurea or insulin dosage as necessary.
Drug-herb. *St. John's wort:* May decrease concentrations of CYP3A4 substrates. Avoid combination.

EFFECTS ON LAB TEST RESULTS

• May increase lipase, amylase, and uric acid levels.
• May decrease glucose level.

CONTRAINDICATIONS & CAUTIONS

• Contraindicated in patients hypersensitive to drug.
• Drug not for use in patients with type 1 diabetes or for treatment of diabetic ketoacidosis.
• Use cautiously in patients at risk for HF.
• Acute pancreatitis, including fatal cases, has occurred in patients taking linagliptin. It's unknown whether patients with a history of pancreatitis are at increased risk for development of pancreatitis while using linagliptin.
🔔 *Alert:* Drug may cause joint pain that can be severe and disabling. Onset can range from days to years.
• Safety in children hasn't been established.
Dialyzable drug: Unlikely.

PREGNANCY-LACTATION-REPRODUCTION

• There are no adequate studies during pregnancy. Use during pregnancy only if clearly needed.
• It isn't known if drug appears in human milk. Use cautiously in breastfeeding.

NURSING CONSIDERATIONS

• Monitor HbA$_{1c}$ and fasting blood glucose levels periodically.
• Monitor patient for signs and symptoms of hypoglycemia (anxiety, confusion, diaphoresis, tachycardia, paresthesia) and hyperglycemia (excess thirst, urination).
• Insulin and insulin secretagogues are know to cause hypoglycemia; risk increases with linagliptin use.
• Monitor patient for signs and symptoms of pancreatitis (persistent, severe abdominal pain, which may radiate to the back, and vomiting). If pancreatitis is suspected, promptly discontinue linagliptin and initiate appropriate management.
• Monitor patient for signs and symptoms of HF, especially patients with previous history of HF or renal failure.
• Postmarketing cases of bullous pemphigoid requiring hospitalization have been reported in patients taking DPP-4 inhibitors. Monitor patients for signs and symptoms, including blisters or erosions. If bullous pemphigoid is suspected, discontinue linagliptin and refer patient to dermatologist for diagnosis and appropriate treatment.
• Monitor patient for hypersensitivity reactions, including anaphylaxis and SCARs.
• *Look alike–sound alike:* Don't confuse linagliptin with linaclotide.

PATIENT TEACHING

• Inform patient of the risks and benefits of linagliptin and of alternative modes of therapy.
• Instruct patient to take drug only as prescribed. If a dose is missed, advise patient not to double the next dose.
• Explain the importance of proper diet, regular physical activity, and periodic blood glucose monitoring.
• Teach patient to recognize and manage hypoglycemia and hyperglycemia.
• Advise patient to notify the health care provider promptly during periods of stress (such as fever, trauma, infection, or surgery) because medication requirements may change.

Reactions in bold italics are *life-threatening*. Interactions may have a *rapid onset* or a ***delayed onset***.

- Teach patient signs and symptoms of pancreatitis and to immediately contact prescriber if they occur.
- Advise patient to report blisters or erosions, severe joint pain, or signs and symptoms of HF (shortness of breath, edema, weight gain).

linezolid
lih-NEH-zoe-lid

Zyvox

Therapeutic class: Antibiotics
Pharmacologic class: Oxazolidinones

AVAILABLE FORMS
Injection: 2 mg/mL
Powder for oral suspension: 100 mg/5 mL when reconstituted
Tablets: 600 mg

INDICATIONS & DOSAGES
➤ **Vancomycin-resistant** *Enterococcus faecium* **infections, including those with concurrent bacteremia**
Adults and children age 12 and older: 600 mg IV or PO every 12 hours for 14 to 28 days.
Full-term neonates, infants, and children through age 11: 10 mg/kg IV or PO every 8 hours for 14 to 28 days.
Preterm neonates younger than age 7 days (gestational age less than 34 weeks): 10 mg/kg IV or PO every 12 hours for 14 to 28 days. Increase to 10 mg/kg every 8 hours when patient is 7 days old. Consider this dosage increase if neonate has inadequate response.
➤ **Hospital-acquired pneumonia caused by** *Staphylococcus aureus* **(methicillin-susceptible [MSSA] and MRSA strains) or** *Streptococcus pneumoniae* **(including multidrug-resistant strains [MDRSP]); complicated skin and skin-structure infections, including diabetic foot infections without osteomyelitis caused by** *S. aureus* **(MSSA and MRSA),** *Streptococcus pyogenes,* **or** *Streptococcus agalactiae;* **community-acquired pneumonia caused by** *S. pneumoniae* **(including MDRSP), including those with concurrent bacteremia, or** *S. aureus* **(MSSA only)**
Adults and children age 12 and older: 600 mg IV or PO every 12 hours for 10 to 14 days.
Full-term neonates, infants, and children through age 11: 10 mg/kg IV or PO every 8 hours for 10 to 14 days.
Preterm neonates younger than age 7 days (gestational age less than 34 weeks): 10 mg/kg IV or PO every 12 hours for 10 to 14 days. Increase to 10 mg/kg every 8 hours when patient is 7 days old. Consider this dosage increase if neonate has inadequate response.
➤ **Uncomplicated skin and skin-structure infections caused by** *S. aureus* **(MSSA only) or** *S. pyogenes*
Adults: 400 mg PO every 12 hours for 10 to 14 days.
Children ages 12 to 18: 600 mg PO every 12 hours for 10 to 14 days.
Children ages 5 to 11: 10 mg/kg PO every 12 hours for 10 to 14 days.
Full-term neonates, infants, and children younger than age 5: 10 mg/kg PO every 8 hours for 10 to 14 days.
Preterm neonates younger than age 7 days (gestational age less than 34 weeks): 10 mg/kg PO every 12 hours for 10 to 14 days. Increase to 10 mg/kg every 8 hours when patient is 7 days old. Consider this dosage increase if neonate has inadequate response.

ADMINISTRATION
PO
- Give tablets and suspension with or without meals.
- Give one of twice-daily doses after hemodialysis on dialysis days.
- Reconstitute suspension according to manufacturer's instructions.
- Store reconstituted suspension at room temperature and use within 21 days.
IV
▼ Inspect solution for particulate matter and leaks.
▼ Don't inject additives into infusion bag. Give other IV drugs separately or via a separate IV line to avoid incompatibilities. If single IV line is used, flush line before and after infusion with a compatible solution.
▼ Infuse over 30 minutes to 2 hours. Don't infuse drug in a series connection.
▼ Give after hemodialysis on dialysis days.
▼ Store drug at room temperature in its protective overwrap. Solution may turn yellow over time, but this doesn't affect drug's potency.

▼ **Incompatibilities:** Amphotericin B, ceftriaxone, chlorpromazine hydrochloride, diazepam, erythromycin lactobionate, pentamidine isethionate, phenytoin, trimethoprim–sulfamethoxazole.

ACTION

Prevents bacterial protein synthesis by interfering with DNA translation in the ribosomes. Also prevents formation of a functional 70S ribosomal subunit by binding to a site on the bacterial 50S ribosomal subunit; this limits bacterial reproduction.

Route	Onset	Peak	Duration
PO	Unknown	1–2 hr	Unknown
IV	Unknown	30 min	Unknown

Half-life: Adults, 4 to 5 hours; children age 1 week to 11 years, 1.5 to 3 hours.

ADVERSE REACTIONS

CNS: headache, dizziness, fever, altered taste, insomnia; vertigo (children). **GI:** diarrhea, nausea, constipation, oral candidiasis, tongue discoloration, vomiting, abdominal pain. **GU:** vaginal candidiasis. **Hepatic:** increased LFT values. **Hematologic:** *leukopenia, myelosuppression, neutropenia, thrombocytopenia,* eosinophilia, anemia. **Skin:** rash, pruritus. **Other:** fungal infection.

INTERACTIONS

Drug-drug. *Adrenergic drugs (dopamine, epinephrine, pseudoephedrine):* May cause HTN. Monitor BP and HR; start continuous infusions of dopamine and epinephrine at lower doses and titrate to response.
Insulin, oral antidiabetics: May cause symptomatic hypoglycemia. Monitor patient closely.
MAO inhibitors (isocarboxazid, phenelzine): May increase risk of hypertensive crisis or serotonin syndrome. Use within 14 days of MAO inhibitor is contraindicated.
Serotonergic drugs (bupropion, buspirone, opioids, SSNRIs, SSRIs, TCAs, triptans): May cause serotonin syndrome or NMS-like reactions. Avoid use together.
Drug-food. *Foods and beverages high in tyramine (aged cheeses, air-dried meats, red wines, sauerkraut, soy sauce, tap beers):* May increase BP. Provide a list of foods containing tyramine and advise patient that tyramine content of meals shouldn't exceed 100 mg.

EFFECTS ON LAB TEST RESULTS

• May increase ALT, AST, bilirubin, ALP, BUN, creatinine, amylase, lipase, LDH, and BUN levels.
• May decrease glucose level.
• May decrease Hb level and WBC, neutrophil, and platelet counts.

CONTRAINDICATIONS & CAUTIONS

• Contraindicated in patients hypersensitive to drug or its components.
• Use cautiously while monitoring BP in patients with uncontrolled HTN, pheochromocytoma, or thyrotoxicosis and in patients taking sympathomimetics, vasopressors, or dopaminergics.
⚠ *Alert:* Concomitant use with psychiatric drugs or within 2 weeks of taking psychiatric drugs that work through the serotonin system of the brain (SSRIs, SSNRIs, TCAs, MAO inhibitors, and others) can cause serotonin syndrome. Use linezolid with these drugs only for life-threatening or urgent conditions when potential benefits outweigh toxicity risk.
Dialyzable drug: 30%.

PREGNANCY-LACTATION-REPRODUCTION

• There are no adequate studies during pregnancy. Use during pregnancy only if potential benefit justifies fetal risk.
• Drug may appear in human milk. Use cautiously with breastfeeding.

NURSING CONSIDERATIONS

• No dosage adjustment is needed when switching from IV to oral forms.
⚠ *Alert:* Before giving linezolid, stop any serotonergic drug and monitor patient for serotonin toxicity for 2 weeks (5 weeks if fluoxetine was taken) or until 24 hours after the last dose of linezolid, whichever comes first. May resume serotonergic psychiatric drugs 24 hours after last dose of linezolid.
⚠ *Alert:* Nausea and vomiting may be symptoms of lactic acidosis. Monitor patient for unexplained acidosis or low bicarbonate level, and notify prescriber immediately if these occur.
⚠ *Alert:* Monitor platelet count in patients at increased risk for bleeding, those with existing thrombocytopenia, those taking other drugs that may cause thrombocytopenia, and those receiving this drug for longer than 14 days.

Reactions in bold italics are *life-threatening*. Interactions may have a *rapid onset* or a **delayed onset**.

⚠ Alert: Drug may lead to myelosuppression. Monitor CBC weekly.

⚠ Alert: Prolonged use can cause superinfection, including CDAD, which can occur more than 2 months after treatment ends. Consider these diagnoses and take appropriate measures in patients with persistent diarrhea or secondary infections.

⚠ Alert: Drug may cause symptomatic hypoglycemia in patients taking insulin or oral antidiabetics. Monitor patient closely.

• Inappropriate use of antibiotics may lead to development of resistant organisms; carefully consider other drugs before starting therapy, especially in outpatient setting.

• Peripheral and optic neuropathies can occur, especially in patients treated for a longer-than-recommended duration. If these neuropathies occur, drug may need to be discontinued. Patients with vision changes should receive prompt ophthalmic evaluation.

• Use cautiously in patients with seizure disorder.

• **Look alike–sound alike:** Don't confuse Zyvox with Zovirax.

PATIENT TEACHING

• Instruct patient in safe drug administration.

• Stress importance of completing entire course of therapy, even if patient feels better.

• Tell patient to report all adverse reactions promptly.

• Caution patient to report high BP; use of cough or cold preparations, insulin, or oral antidiabetics; or treatment with SSRIs or other antidepressants.

⚠ Alert: Teach patient to recognize and immediately report signs and symptoms of serotonin toxicity (fever, mental status changes, muscle twitching, diaphoresis, shivering or shaking, diarrhea, and loss of coordination).

• Advise patient taking prescribed psychiatric drugs that these drugs may need to be stopped during linezolid therapy but not to stop them without first speaking to prescriber.

• Teach patient to avoid eating large quantities of tyramine-containing foods (aged cheeses, soy sauce, tap beers, red wine) during therapy.

• Inform patient with phenylketonuria that each 5 mL of oral suspension contains 20 mg of phenylalanine. Tablets and injection don't contain phenylalanine.

SAFETY ALERT!

liraglutide
leer-ah-GLOO-tide

Saxenda, Victoza

Therapeutic class: Antidiabetics
Pharmacologic class: Glucagon-like peptide-1 receptor agonists

AVAILABLE FORMS
Injection: 6-mg/mL prefilled multidose pens that deliver doses of 0.6 mg, 1.2 mg, 1.8 mg, 2.4 mg, or 3 mg (Saxenda), or 0.6 mg, 1.2 mg, or 1.8 mg (Victoza)

INDICATIONS & DOSAGES
➤ **As adjunct to diet and exercise to improve glycemic control in patients with type 2 diabetes (Victoza)**
Adults: Initially, 0.6 mg subcut daily; after 1 week, increase dosage to 1.2 mg subcut daily. May increase dosage to 1.8 mg subcut daily if needed to achieve glycemic control.
Children older than age 10: Initially, 0.6 mg subcut daily. After at least 1 week, may increase dosage to 1.2 mg subcut daily to achieve glycemic control. May increase dosage to 1.8 mg subcut daily after at least 1 week if needed.

➤ **To reduce risk of major adverse CV events in patients with type 2 diabetes and established CV disease (Victoza)**
Adults: Initially, 0.6 mg subcut daily; after 1 week, increase dosage to 1.2 mg daily. May increase dosage to 1.8 mg subcut daily if needed to achieve glycemic control.

➤ **As adjunct to diet and exercise for long-term weight management in adults with initial BMI of 30 kg/m² or greater (obese) or 27 kg/m² or greater (overweight) in the presence of at least one weight-related co-morbid condition (HTN, type 2 diabetes, or dyslipidemia) (Saxenda)**
Adults: Initially, 0.6 mg subcut once daily for 1 week. Increase by 0.6 mg/day subcut at weekly intervals to a target dose of 3 mg once daily. If patient can't tolerate an increased dose during titration period, consider delaying dosage escalation for 1 week. Discontinue drug if 3-mg dose isn't tolerated; effectiveness at lower doses hasn't been established.

➤ **As adjunct to diet and exercise for long-term weight management in children**

L

---

weighing more than 60 kg with initial BMI corresponding to 30 kg/m² or greater for adults (obese) by international cut-offs (Saxenda)

Refer to manufacturer's prescribing information for Cole criteria.

Children age 12 and older: Initially, 0.6 mg subcut once daily for 1 week. Increase by 0.6 mg/day subcut at weekly intervals to a target dose of 3 mg once daily. If increased dose isn't tolerated, may lower dose to previous level. Dose escalation for children may take up to 8 weeks.

Adjust-a-dose: For children who don't tolerate Saxenda 3 mg daily, may reduce dose to 2.4 mg daily; discontinue if 2.4 mg daily isn't tolerated.

ADMINISTRATION
Subcutaneous
- Hazardous drug; use safe handling precautions.
- Give drug once daily at any time of day, independently of meals. Inject into abdomen, thigh, or upper arm. Injection site and timing can be changed without dosage adjustment.
- Don't mix drug with insulin for injection or inject liraglutide and insulin in adjacent areas at the same time.
- If a dose is missed, don't double subsequent dose. Resume once-daily regimen. If more than 3 days have elapsed, initiate dose at 0.6 mg daily and, for Victoza, increase as directed by prescriber or, for Saxenda, increase weekly per titration schedule to limit GI adverse reactions.
- Inspect solution before each injection. Use solution only if it is clear, colorless, and contains no particles.
- **Alert:** Multidose pens are for single-patient use only. Pens should never be shared even if the needle is changed. Clearly label with patient identifying information where it won't obstruct dosing window, warning, or other product information.
- Before first use, store drug in refrigerator between 36° and 46° F (2° and 8° C). Discard if pen freezes.
- After initial use of liraglutide pen, pen can be stored for 30 days at room temperature (59° to 86° F [15° to 30° C]) or in refrigerator (36° to 46° F). Keep pen cap on when not in use. Discard pen after 30 days.

ACTION
Stimulates insulin secretion and reduces glucagon secretion; delays gastric emptying.

Route	Onset	Peak	Duration
Subcut	Unknown	8–12 hr	Unknown

Half-life: 13 hours.

ADVERSE REACTIONS
CNS: headache, dizziness, fatigue, insomnia, anxiety, weakness, asthenia, depression. **CV:** increased HR, tachycardia. **EENT:** dry mouth. **GI:** constipation, diarrhea, dyspepsia, nausea, vomiting, abdominal distention or pain, decreased appetite, flatulence, GERD, gastroenteritis. **GU:** UTI. **Hepatic:** cholelithiasis. **Metabolic:** increased lipase level, dyslipidemia, increased CK level, *hypoglycemia.* **Musculoskeletal:** limb pain. **Respiratory:** URI, cough. **Skin:** injection-site reactions, rash. **Other:** anti-liraglutide antibody formation.

INTERACTIONS
Drug-drug. *Insulin, insulin secretagogues (sulfonylureas):* May increase risk of hypoglycemia. Reduce insulin or secretagogue dosage before beginning drug and as needed. *Oral medications:* May impair absorption of oral drugs because of delayed gastric emptying. Use together cautiously.

EFFECTS ON LAB TEST RESULTS
- May increase serum bilirubin, liver enzyme, amylase, and lipase levels and serum calcitonin concentration.
- May decrease blood glucose level.

CONTRAINDICATIONS & CAUTIONS
Boxed Warning Drug causes dose-dependent and treatment duration–dependent thyroid C-cell tumors at clinically relevant exposures in both genders of rats and mice. It isn't known if drug causes thyroid C-cell tumors, including medullary thyroid carcinoma (MTC), in humans, as the human relevance of liraglutide-induced rodent thyroid C-cell tumors hasn't been determined. ∎

Boxed Warning Contraindicated in patients with personal or family history of MTC and in patients with multiple endocrine neoplasia syndrome type 2. ∎
- Contraindicated in patients with a prior serious hypersensitivity reaction to liraglutide or its components.

Reactions in bold italics are *life-threatening*. Interactions may have a *rapid onset* or a ***delayed onset***.

- Avoid Saxenda use in patients with a history of or active suicidality.
- Use cautiously in patients with renal or hepatic impairment and in those with history of pancreatitis.

❸ *Alert:* Acute pancreatitis, including fatal pancreatitis and nonfatal hemorrhagic or necrotizing pancreatitis, has occurred in patients taking liraglutide.

- Victoza isn't a substitute for insulin; don't use for treatment of diabetic ketoacidosis or type 1 diabetes.
- Victoza hasn't been studied in combination with prandial insulin.
- Saxenda isn't indicated for treatment of type 2 diabetes.
- Saxenda and Victoza both contain the same active ingredient and shouldn't be used together.
- Saxenda shouldn't be used in combination with other GLP-1 receptor agonists.
- Saxenda hasn't been studied in patients taking insulin; don't use together.
- Safety and effectiveness of Saxenda in combination with other products intended for weight loss haven't been established.
- Older adults may be more sensitive to drug. Use cautiously.

Dialyzable drug: Unknown.

⚠ *Overdose S&S:* Nausea, vomiting, hypoglycemia.

PREGNANCY-LACTATION-REPRODUCTION

- There are no adequate studies of Victoza during pregnancy. Use during pregnancy only if potential benefit justifies fetal risk.
- Saxenda is contraindicated during pregnancy because weight loss offers no potential benefit to a patient who is pregnant and may result in fetal harm.
- It isn't known if drug appears in human milk. Weigh benefits of therapy against risks.

NURSING CONSIDERATIONS

- Evaluate change in body weight 16 weeks after start of therapy; discontinue Saxenda if body weight loss of at least 4% of baseline hasn't been achieved.
- For children taking Saxenda, evaluate change in body weight 12 weeks after start of therapy; discontinue drug if weight loss of at least 1% of baseline hasn't been achieved.
- Monitor patient closely for signs and symptoms of pancreatitis (persistent, severe abdominal pain, which may radiate to the back,

and vomiting). Discontinue drug promptly if pancreatitis is suspected. Don't restart if pancreatitis is confirmed.

❸ *Alert:* Patients with thyroid nodules found on exam or neck imaging or with elevated serum calcitonin levels should be evaluated by an endocrinologist.

- Drug may increase risk of gallbladder and bile duct disease. If cholelithiasis is suspected, gallbladder studies and appropriate clinical follow-up are indicated.

❸ *Alert:* Monitor patients for emergence or worsening of depression, suicidality, and unusual changes in mood or behavior. Discontinue in patients who experience suicidality.

- Drug isn't recommended for first-line therapy in patients who have inadequate glycemic control with diet and exercise.
- Monitor blood glucose and HbA_{1c} levels. Consider decreasing insulin and insulin secretagogue (such as sulfonylurea) dosage when initiating liraglutide.
- Monitor patient for signs and symptoms of hypoglycemia (tachycardia, palpitations, anxiety, hunger, nausea, diaphoresis, tremors, pallor, restlessness, headache, and speech and motor dysfunction).
- Monitor GI status; drug slows gastric emptying.

PATIENT TEACHING

Boxed Warning Counsel patient regarding risk of MTC and describe signs and symptoms of thyroid tumors (neck mass, dysphagia, dyspnea, persistent hoarseness). ∎

❸ *Alert:* Counsel patient, family member, or caregivers to monitor patent for changes in behavior and to immediately report suicidality.

- Advise patient to report signs and symptoms of acute gallbladder disease or cholelithiasis, including sudden and rapidly intensifying pain in the upper right portion of the abdomen or in the center of the abdomen, just below the breastbone; back pain between the shoulder blades; pain in the right shoulder; nausea; or vomiting.
- Advise patient to stop drug and report persistent, severe abdominal pain that may radiate to the back and may or may not be accompanied by vomiting.

❸ *Alert:* Warn patient not to share multidose pen with other people, even if needle is changed, because of risk of infection, including HIV and hepatitis.

- Emphasize to patient importance of adhering to a diet and exercise program and monitoring glucose and HbA_{1c} levels.
- Advise patient of risk of dehydration; encourage hydration.
- Warn patient of risk of hypersensitivity reactions and advise patient to report reactions should they occur.
- Teach patient how to give subcut injection; instruct patient to rotate sites to prevent injection-site reactions.

lisdexamfetamine dimesylate
lis-DEX-am-FET-a-meen

Vyvanse♦

Therapeutic class: CNS stimulants
Pharmacologic class: Amphetamines
Controlled substance schedule: II

AVAILABLE FORMS
Capsules ⓞⓝⓔ: 10 mg, 20 mg, 30 mg, 40 mg, 50 mg, 60 mg, 70 mg
Tablets (chewable): 10 mg, 20 mg, 30 mg, 40 mg, 50 mg, 60 mg

INDICATIONS & DOSAGES
Adjust-a-dose (for all indications): For patients with severe renal impairment (GFR of 15 mL to less than 30 mL/minute/1.73 m²), maximum dose is 50 mg/day. For those with ESRD (GFR less than 15 mL/minute/1.73 m²), maximum dose is 30 mg/day.
➤ **ADHD**
Adults and children ages 6 to 17: Initially, 30 mg PO once daily in the morning. Increase by 10 or 20 mg at weekly intervals to target dose of 30 to 70 mg/day. Maximum dosage is 70 mg daily.
➤ **Moderate to severe binge eating disorder**
Adults: Initially, 30 mg PO once daily in the morning. Increase by 20 mg at weekly intervals to target dose of 50 to 70 mg/day. Maximum dose is 70 mg/day.

ADMINISTRATION
PO
- Give drug in the morning to prevent insomnia.
- Give drug without regard for meals.
- Have patient swallow capsules whole, or mix capsule contents in yogurt, water, or

orange juice, dissolve completely, and have patient take immediately; don't store.
- For chewable tablets, make sure patient chews tablets thoroughly before swallowing.
- Capsules can be substituted with chewable tablets on a unit/mg basis.
- Don't divide the dose of a single capsule or chewable tablet or give less than one capsule or chewable tablet per day.

ACTION
Increases the release of norepinephrine and dopamine from nerve terminals and blocks their reuptake into the presynaptic neuron.

Route	Onset	Peak	Duration
PO	Rapid	1 hr	8–14 hr

Half-life: Lisdexamfetamine, less than 1 hour; dextroamphetamine, 10 to 13 hours.

ADVERSE REACTIONS
CNS: dizziness, anxiety, fever, irritability, jitteriness, agitation, emotional lability, drowsiness, nightmares, paresthesia, insomnia, tics, tremor. **CV:** tachycardia, palpitations, increased BP. **EENT:** mydriasis, diplopia, dry mouth, oropharyngeal pain. **GI:** constipation, vomiting, decreased appetite, anorexia, diarrhea, nausea, upper abdominal pain, gastroenteritis. **GU:** libido changes, erectile dysfunction, UTI. **Metabolic:** weight loss. **Respiratory:** dyspnea. **Skin:** rash, hyperhidrosis, pruritus.

INTERACTIONS
Drug-drug. *Antihistamines:* May inhibit sedative effects of antihistamines. Monitor patient.
Antihypertensives: May inhibit antihypertensive effects of these drugs. If use together can't be avoided, closely monitor BP when lisdexamfetamine is started or stopped, and adjust antihypertensive dosage as needed.
Buspirone, fentanyl, linezolid, lithium, SSNRIs, SSRIs, tramadol, triptans, tryptophan: May increase risk of serotonin syndrome. Start lisdexamfetamine treatment with lower doses and monitor patients for signs and symptoms of serotonin syndrome, particularly during lisdexamfetamine initiation or dosage increases.
CYP2D6 inhibitors (fluoxetine, paroxetine, quinidine, ritonavir): May increase exposure of dextroamphetamine and increase risk of serotonin syndrome. Start lisdexamfetamine

treatment with lower doses and monitor patient during lisdexamfetamine initiation or dosage increases.

Ethosuximide: May delay absorption of this drug. Monitor patient closely.

Lithium: May inhibit anorectic and CNS stimulant effects of amphetamine. Monitor patient closely.

MAO inhibitors: May cause severe HTN or hypertensive crisis. Use is contraindicated within 14 days of MAO inhibitor therapy.

Norepinephrine: May increase adrenergic effects of norepinephrine. Monitor patient closely.

Phenobarbital, phenytoin: May decrease serum concentration of these drugs. Monitor patient closely.

TCAs: May cause adverse CV effects and increase risk of serotonin syndrome. Avoid use together or monitor patient closely.

Urine acidifiers (ammonium chloride, sodium acid phosphate), methenamine: May decrease serum level due to increased renal excretion of amphetamine. Monitor patient for decreased drug effects.

Urine alkalinizers (sodium bicarbonate): May increase lisdexamfetamine serum level because of decreased renal excretion of amphetamine. Monitor patient for increased drug effects and adjust dosage accordingly.

Drug-herb. *St. John's wort:* May increase risk of serotonin syndrome. Avoid use together.

Drug-food. *Caffeine:* May increase CNS stimulation. Discourage use together.

Drug-lifestyle. *Alcohol use:* May increase CNS depression. Don't use together.

EFFECTS ON LAB TEST RESULTS
• May increase corticosteroid level.
• May interfere with urinary steroid test.

CONTRAINDICATIONS & CAUTIONS
Boxed Warning Drug has a high potential for abuse and dependence. ■

• Contraindicated in patients hypersensitive to sympathomimetic amines or in those with idiosyncratic reactions to them, in patients who are agitated, and in those with a history of drug abuse disorder.

• Anaphylactic reactions, SJS, angioedema, and urticaria have been noted in postmarketing reports.

⚕ *Alert:* Drug isn't indicated or recommended for weight loss.

• Avoid use in patients with advanced arteriosclerosis, hyperthyroidism, symptomatic CV disease, structural cardiac abnormalities, cardiomyopathy, serious heart arrhythmia, moderate to severe HTN, or glaucoma, and those intolerant of changes in HR or BP.

• Use cautiously in patients with a history of arrhythmias, MI, stroke, or seizures.

• Use cautiously in patients with preexisting psychosis, bipolar disorder, aggressive behavior, or Tourette syndrome.

• Drug isn't approved for children younger than age 6.

Dialyzable drug: No.

⚠ *Overdose S&S:* Assaultiveness, confusion, hallucinations, hyperpyrexia, hyperreflexia, panic states, rapid respiration, restlessness, rhabdomyolysis, tremor, fatigue, depression, arrhythmias, circulatory collapse, HTN, hypotension, abdominal cramps, diarrhea, nausea, vomiting, seizures, coma.

PREGNANCY-LACTATION-REPRODUCTION
• There are no adequate studies during pregnancy. Use during pregnancy only if potential benefit justifies fetal risk.

• Drug appears in human milk. Breastfeeding isn't recommended.

NURSING CONSIDERATIONS
• Diagnosis of ADHD must be based on complete history and evaluation of the child with consultation of psychological, educational, and social resources.

• Assess patient for cardiac disease, including a careful history, family history of sudden death or ventricular arrhythmia, and physical exam, before starting therapy.

• Evaluate for bipolar disorder before initiating therapy.

• Give the lowest effective dose in the morning. Afternoon doses may cause insomnia.

Boxed Warning Assess the risk of abuse before initiating therapy, and monitor patient for signs of drug dependence or abuse. Misuse may cause sudden death. ■

⟳ *Alert:* Periodically monitor patients for changes in HR or BP.

• Abruptly stopping the drug can cause severe fatigue and depression.

• Monitor patient closely for adverse CV effects, vision problems, or seizures.

• Monitor BP and pulse routinely.

• Use cautiously in patients taking other drugs that increase risk of serotonin

syndrome. Monitor these patients closely and consider an alternative nonserotonergic drug.
• Carefully observe patient for digital changes because stimulants used to treat ADHD are associated with peripheral vasculopathy, including Raynaud phenomenon.
• Effectiveness of this drug when taken longer than 4 weeks isn't known. Periodically interrupt therapy to determine whether continuation is necessary.
• Growth may be suppressed with long-term stimulant use. Monitor the child for growth and weight gain. Stop treatment if growth is suppressed or if weight gain is lower than expected.
• The drug may trigger Tourette syndrome. Monitor patient, especially at the start of therapy.
• Monitor patient for the appearance or worsening of aggressive behavior or hostility, especially when treatment is initiated.
• May cause psychotic or manic episodes in patients with no prior history or exacerbation of signs and symptoms in patients with preexisting psychosis.

PATIENT TEACHING
• Instruct patient in safe drug administration.
• Warn patient that the misuse of amphetamines can cause serious CV adverse events, including sudden death.
• **Alert:** Instruct patient to immediately report chest pain, shortness of breath, or fainting.
• Tell patient or caregiver that abruptly stopping drug can cause severe fatigue, depression, or general withdrawal reaction.
• Caution patient to avoid activities that require alertness or good psychomotor coordination until CNS effects of drug are known.
• Advise patient taking other drugs that increase risk of serotonin syndrome to immediately report signs and symptoms of serotonin syndrome (confusion, agitation, fever, rapid heartbeat, loss of muscle coordination, vomiting, diaphoresis).
• Warn patient with seizure disorder that drug may decrease seizure threshold. Urge patient to notify prescriber if a seizure occurs.
• Instruct patient or caregiver to report palpitations or visual disturbances.
• Tell patient or caregiver to report worsening aggression, hallucinations, delusions, or mania.
• Advise patient or caregiver that drug may slow growth and cause weight loss

• Instruct patient to immediately report numbness, pain, coolness, skin color change, temperature sensitivity, or unexplained wounds appearing on fingers or toes while taking drug.
• Advise patient to avoid caffeine and alcohol consumption while taking drug.

lisinopril
lye-SIN-oh-pril

Qbrelis, Zestril

Therapeutic class: Antihypertensives
Pharmacologic class: ACE inhibitors

AVAILABLE FORMS
Oral solution: 1 mg/mL
Tablets: 2.5 mg, 5 mg, 10 mg, 20 mg, 30 mg, 40 mg

INDICATIONS & DOSAGES
➤ **HTN**
Adults: Initially, 10 mg PO daily for patients not taking a diuretic. Increase as needed to maximum of 40 mg daily. For patients taking a diuretic, initially, 5 mg PO daily.
Children age 6 and older: Initially, 0.07 mg/kg (up to 5 mg) PO once daily. Increase dosage based on patient response and tolerance. Maximum dose, 0.61 mg/kg (don't exceed 40 mg). Don't use in children with a CrCl of less than 30 mL/minute.
Adjust-a-dose: In adults, if CrCl is 10 to 30 mL/minute, give 5 mg PO daily; if CrCl is less than 10 mL/minute, give 2.5 mg PO daily. May titrate dosage up to 40 mg/day.
➤ **Adjunctive treatment (with diuretics and cardiac glycosides) for HF**
Adults: Initially, 5 mg PO daily; increase as needed to maximum of 40 mg.
Adjust-a-dose: If sodium level is less than 130 mEq/L, serum creatinine level greater than 3 mg/dL, or CrCl less than 30 mL/minute, start treatment at 2.5 mg daily.
➤ **Within 24 hours of acute MI to improve survival in patients who are hemodynamically stable**
Adults: Initially, 5 mg PO; then 5 mg after 24 hours, 10 mg after 48 hours, followed by 10 mg once daily for at least 6 weeks.
Adjust-a-dose: For patients with systolic BP of 120 mm Hg or less during first 3 days after an infarct, decrease dosage to 2.5 mg PO.

Reactions in bold italics are *life-threatening*. Interactions may have a *rapid onset* or a ***delayed onset***.

If systolic BP drops to 100 mm Hg or less, reduce daily maintenance dose of 5 mg to 2.5 mg, if needed. If prolonged systolic BP stays under 90 mm Hg for longer than 1 hour, withdraw drug.

If CrCl is 10 to 30 mL/minute, reduce initial dose to 2.5 mg PO daily and titrate as tolerated to a maximum of 40 mg daily. If patient is on hemodialysis or CrCl is less than 10 mL/minute, start treatment at 2.5 mg PO daily.

ADMINISTRATION
PO
• Give drug without regard for food.
• Oral solution is bioequivalent to lisinopril tablets.
• Store oral solution at room temperature in a tightly closed container. Protect from freezing and excessive heat.
• If tablets are made into a suspension by pharmacist, store at or below 77° F (25° C) for up to 4 weeks; shake before each use.

ACTION
Causes decreased production of angiotensin II and suppression of the RAAS.

Route	Onset	Peak	Duration
PO	1 hr	7 hr	24 hr

Half-life: 12 hours.

ADVERSE REACTIONS
CNS: dizziness, headache, fatigue, asthenia, paresthesia, syncope, vertigo. **CV:** orthostatic hypotension, hypotension, chest pain, flushing, taste disturbance, smell disturbance. **EENT:** vision changes, tinnitus, nasal congestion. **GI:** diarrhea, constipation, flatulence, nausea, dyspepsia. **GU:** impaired renal function, impotence. **Metabolic:** *hyperkalemia,* diabetes, gout, SIADH. **Respiratory:** dyspnea; dry, persistent, tickling, nonproductive cough. **Skin:** rash, diaphoresis, erythema, alopecia, pruritus, photosensitivity, *SJS, TEN,* urticaria.

INTERACTIONS
Drug-drug. *Aliskiren; ACE inhibitors, ARBs (dual therapy):* May increase risk of renal impairment, hypotension, and hyperkalemia. Concomitant use of aliskiren is contraindicated in patients with diabetes. Avoid use together.

Allopurinol: May cause hypersensitivity reaction. Use together cautiously.
Azathioprine: May increase risk of anemia or leukopenia. Monitor hematologic studies if used together.
Cyclooxygenase-2 inhibitors, indomethacin, NSAIDs: May increase risk of renal dysfunction. May reduce hypotensive effects of drug. Adjust dosage as needed.
Diuretics, thiazide diuretics: May cause excessive hypotension with diuretics. Monitor BP closely.
Insulin, oral antidiabetics: May cause hypoglycemia, especially at start of lisinopril therapy. Monitor glucose level.
Lithium: May cause lithium toxicity. Monitor lithium levels.
mTOR inhibitors (everolimus, sirolimus, temsirolimus): May increase risk of angioedema. Monitor patient closely.
Neprilysin inhibitors (sacubitril): May increase risk of angioedema. Use together is contraindicated. Don't give lisinopril within 36 hours of switching to or from sacubitril–valsartan (Entresto).
Phenothiazines: May increase hypotensive effects. Monitor BP closely.
Potassium-sparing diuretics, potassium supplements: May cause hyperkalemia. Monitor lab values.
Sodium aurothiomalate (injectable gold): May increase risk of nitritoid reactions (facial flushing, nausea, vomiting, hypotension). Use cautiously together.
Tizanidine: May cause severe hypotension. Monitor patient.
Drug-herb. *Ma huang:* May decrease antihypertensive effects. Discourage use together.
Drug-food. *Potassium-containing salt substitutes:* May cause hyperkalemia. Monitor lab values.

EFFECTS ON LAB TEST RESULTS
• May increase BUN, creatinine, potassium, and bilirubin levels and LFT values.
• May decrease Hb level and hematocrit.

CONTRAINDICATIONS & CAUTIONS
• Contraindicated in patients hypersensitive to ACE inhibitors and in those with a history of angioedema related to previous treatment with ACE inhibitor.
• Use cautiously in patients with impaired renal function; adjust dosage.

• Use cautiously in patients at risk for hyperkalemia or hypotension and in those with aortic stenosis or hypertrophic cardiomyopathy. The safety and effectiveness of lisinopril on BP control in children younger than age 6 or in children with GFR less than 30 mL/minute hasn't been established.

🜨 Although rare, angioedema, which can be fatal, may occur at any time during treatment, including after first dose; it may involve the head and neck (potentially compromising the airway) or the intestine (presenting with abdominal pain). Patients who are Black and patients with idiopathic or hereditary angioedema may be at increased risk. Patients concurrently receiving mammalian target of rapamycin (mTOR) inhibitor therapy (temsirolimus, sirolimus, everolimus) also may be at increased risk.

Dialyzable drug: Yes.

⚠ *Overdose S&S:* Hypotension.

PREGNANCY-LACTATION-REPRODUCTION

Boxed Warning Drug acts directly on the RAAS and can cause injury and death to a developing fetus. When pregnancy is detected, stop drug as soon as possible. ∎

• It isn't known if drug appears in human milk. Patient should discontinue breastfeeding or discontinue drug.

NURSING CONSIDERATIONS

🜨 Although ACE inhibitors reduce BP in all races, BP reduction is less in patients who are Black taking an ACE inhibitor alone. Patients who are Black should take drug with a thiazide diuretic for a more favorable response.

• Monitor BP frequently. If drug doesn't adequately control BP, diuretics may be added.

• Monitor WBC with differential counts before therapy, every 2 weeks for first 3 months of therapy, and periodically thereafter.

• Monitor serum potassium level periodically.

• Monitor patient for jaundice or significantly increased liver enzyme levels. ACE inhibitors have been associated with hepatic failure.

• *Look alike–sound alike:* Don't confuse lisinopril with fosinopril or Lioresal. Don't confuse Zestril with Zostrix, Zetia, Zebeta, or Zyrtec.

PATIENT TEACHING

🜨 *Alert:* Rarely, facial and throat swelling (including swelling of the larynx) or intestinal swelling may occur, especially after first dose. Advise patient to report abdominal pain, breathing problems, or swelling of face, eyes, lips, or tongue.

• Tell patient that light-headedness can occur, especially during first few days of therapy, to rise slowly to minimize this effect, and to report symptoms to prescriber. If fainting occurs, advise patient to stop drug and call prescriber immediately.

• If unpleasant adverse reactions occur, tell patient not to stop drug suddenly but to notify prescriber.

• Advise patient to report signs and symptoms of infection, such as fever and sore throat.

• Tell patient of childbearing potential to notify prescriber if pregnancy occurs. Drug will need to be stopped.

• Advise patient to report signs and symptoms of hyperkalemia, such as muscle fatigue, weakness, nausea, or abnormal heart rhythm.

• Instruct patient not to use salt substitutes that contain potassium without first consulting prescriber.

• Inform patient that a dry, nonproductive cough may develop during therapy.

---

lisinopril–hydroCHLOROthiazide 🜨
lye-SIN-oh-pril/hye-droe-klor-oh-THYE-a-zide

Zestoretic

Therapeutic class: Antihypertensives
Pharmacologic class: ACE inhibitors–thiazide diuretics

AVAILABLE FORMS
Tablets: 10 mg lisinopril and 12.5 mg hydrochlorothiazide, 20 mg lisinopril and 12.5 mg hydrochlorothiazide, 20 mg lisinopril and 25 mg hydrochlorothiazide

INDICATIONS & DOSAGES
➤ **HTN in patients not adequately controlled on lisinopril or hydrochlorothiazide monotherapy**
Adults: Initially, 10 mg lisinopril and 12.5 mg hydrochlorothiazide or 20 mg lisinopril and 12.5 mg hydrochlorothiazide PO once daily; titrate based on clinical response. Don't increase the hydrochlorothiazide component until 2 to 3 weeks have elapsed. In patients

---

Reactions in bold italics are *life-threatening*. Interactions may have a *rapid onset* or a *delayed onset*.

on adequate pressure control on single-agent hydrochlorothiazide 25 mg PO daily but with significant potassium loss, switch to 10 mg lisinopril and 12.5 mg hydrochlorothiazide tablets. Maximum dosage is 80 mg lisinopril and 50 mg hydrochlorothiazide PO once daily.

Adjust-a-dose: Not for use in patients with CrCl of less than 30 mL/minute/1.73 m². Dosage selection for older adults should be at low end of dosing range.

ADMINISTRATION
PO
- Store at controlled room temperature; protect from excessive light and humidity.
- May give without regard for food.

ACTION
Lisinopril inhibits ACE, leading to decreased angiotensin II production, decreased aldosterone secretion, and increased potassium level. Hydrochlorothiazide inhibits sodium reabsorption in the distal tubules, causing increased excretion of sodium and water as well as potassium and hydrogen ions.

Route	Onset	Peak	Duration
PO (lisinopril)	1 hr	7 hr	24 hr
PO (hydrochloro-thiazide)	2 hr	4 hr	6–12 hr

Half-life: Lisinopril, 12 hours; hydrochlorothiazide, 5.6 to 14.8 hours.

ADVERSE REACTIONS
CNS: dizziness, headache, fatigue, asthenia, paresthesia. **CV:** orthostatic effects, hypotension. **GI:** diarrhea, nausea, vomiting, dyspepsia. **GU:** erectile dysfunction. **Metabolic:** *hypokalemia, hyperkalemia,* hyperglycemia. **Musculoskeletal:** muscle cramps. **Respiratory:** cough, URI. **Skin:** rash.

INTERACTIONS
Drug-drug. *Aliskiren; ACE inhibitors, ARBs (dual therapy):* May increase risk of renal impairment, hypotension, and hyperkalemia. Concomitant use of aliskiren is contraindicated in patients with diabetes. Avoid concomitant use.
Antidiabetics, insulin: May increase blood glucose level. Monitor patient carefully; adjust dosage of antidiabetic as needed.
Barbiturates, opioids: May increase risk of orthostatic hypotension. Avoid use together.

Colestipol resins, cholestyramine: May impair absorption of hydrochlorothiazide. Separate administration times by at least 4 hours.
Corticosteroids, corticotropin: May worsen electrolyte depletion, particularly hypokalemia. Monitor patient carefully.
Cyclooxygenase-2 inhibitors, NSAIDs: May increase risk of renal dysfunction. May diminish antihypertensive effects. Use cautiously together.
Diuretics, other antihypertensives: May increase hypotensive effects. Monitor patient carefully.
Gold injections: May increase risk of nitritoid effects (flushing, nausea, vomiting, hypotension). Avoid use together.
Lithium: May increase lithium level. Monitor patient carefully.
mTOR inhibitors (everolimus, sirolimus, temsirolimus): May increase risk of angioedema. Monitor patient for angioedema.
Neprilysin inhibitors (sacubitril): May increase risk of angioedema. Use together is contraindicated. Don't give lisinopril within 36 hours of switching to or from sacubitril–valsartan (Entresto).
Nondepolarizing skeletal muscle relaxants (tubocurarine): May increase response to muscle relaxant. Avoid use together.
Potassium-sparing diuretics, potassium supplements: May increase risk of hyperkalemia. Avoid use together.
Pressor amines (norepinephrine): May decrease response to pressor amines. Use together cautiously.
Drug-herb. *Capsaicin:* May increase ACE inhibitor–induced cough. Discourage use together.
Ma huang: May decrease antihypertensive effects. Discourage use together.
Drug-food. *Potassium-containing salt substitutes:* May increase risk of hyperkalemia. Discourage use together.
Drug-lifestyle. *Alcohol use:* May increase risk of orthostatic hypotension. Discourage use together.
Sun exposure: May increase risk of photosensitivity. Discourage sun exposure.

EFFECTS ON LAB TEST RESULTS
- May increase glucose, cholesterol, triglyceride, BUN, creatinine, and bilirubin levels and LFT values.
- May decrease calcium, chloride, sodium and magnesium levels.

• May increase or decrease potassium level.
• May decrease Hb level, hematocrit, and WBC count.

CONTRAINDICATIONS & CAUTIONS

▨ Contraindicated in patients hypersensitive to either drug or sulfonamides and in those with history of angioedema related to previous treatment with an ACE inhibitor, hereditary or idiopathic angioedema, or anuria.

• Use cautiously in patients with a history or risk of angioedema, anaphylactoid reactions, salt or volume depletion, collagen vascular disease, obstruction in the outflow tract of the left ventricle, HF, renal artery stenosis, renal disease, jaundice or hepatic disease, asthma, SLE, history of aortic stenosis, hypertrophic cardiomyopathy, existing hyperkalemia or other electrolyte imbalance, or hyperuricemia.

▨ Although rare, angioedema, which can be fatal, may occur at any time during treatment, including after first dose; it may involve the head and neck (potentially compromising the airway) or the intestine (presenting with abdominal pain). Patients who are Black and patients with idiopathic or hereditary angioedema may be at increased risk. Patients concurrently receiving mammalian target of rapamycin (mTOR) inhibitor therapy also may be at increased risk.

Dialyzable drug: Yes (lisinopril); unknown (hydrochlorothiazide).

⚠ *Overdose S&S:* Hypotension, dehydration, electrolyte imbalance.

PREGNANCY-LACTATION-REPRODUCTION

Boxed Warning Drugs that act directly on the RAAS can cause injury and death to a developing fetus. When pregnancy is detected, discontinue drug as soon as possible. ▮

• It isn't known if lisinopril appears in human milk; hydrochlorothiazide does appear in human milk. Patient should discontinue breastfeeding or discontinue drug.

NURSING CONSIDERATIONS

• Drug isn't to be used for initial therapy. Begin combination therapy only after patient has failed to achieve desired effect with monotherapy.
• Consider ACE inhibitor–induced cough if patient develops cough of unknown etiology.

• Correct lisinopril-induced hypotension before major surgery and anesthesia.
• Monitor glucose, electrolyte, and lipid levels during therapy.
• Monitor WBC count in patients with collagen vascular disease or renal disease.
• Monitor patient for jaundice and elevated liver enzyme levels. Discontinue drug and treat appropriately if these occur.
• Drug may cause intestinal angioedema. Monitor patient for abdominal pain.
• Monitor patient for angioedema which may occur at any time during treatment. If symptoms occur, discontinue drug, treat appropriately, and monitor patient until symptoms have resolved.
• Watch for causes of volume depletion (diaphoresis, vomiting, diarrhea, or other causes); volume depletion may cause hypotension.

▨ Patients who are Black may have a more limited response to lisinopril than patients of other races.

PATIENT TEACHING

Boxed Warning Counsel patient of childbearing potential to report possible pregnancy as soon as possible. ▮

• Instruct patient to stop drug and immediately report signs or symptoms suggesting angioedema (abdominal pain; swelling of the face, extremities, eyes, lips, or tongue; difficulty swallowing or breathing).
• Caution patient to report light-headedness, especially during first few days of therapy, and if syncope occurs, to discontinue drug and notify prescriber.
• Tell patient to consult prescriber if fluid losses occur (excessive perspiration, dehydration, vomiting, or diarrhea).
• Advise patient to immediately report signs and symptoms of fluid and electrolyte imbalance (dry mouth, thirst, weakness, lethargy, drowsiness, restlessness, confusion, seizures, muscle pains or cramps, muscle fatigue, decreased urination, rapid heartbeat, nausea, vomiting).
• Instruct patient to promptly report signs and symptoms of infection (sore throat, fever).
• Warn patient to avoid salt substitutes containing potassium.
• Inform patient that a dry, nonproductive cough may develop during therapy.

Reactions in bold italics are *life-threatening*. Interactions may have a *rapid onset* or a *delayed onset*.

lithium carbonate
LITH-ee-um

Carbolith ♣, Lithane ♣, Lithobid

Therapeutic class: Antimanics
Pharmacologic class: Alkali metals

AVAILABLE FORMS
Capsules: 150 mg, 300 mg, 600 mg
Tablets: 300 mg
Tablets (extended-release) ⓓⓝⓒ: 300 mg, 450 mg

INDICATIONS & DOSAGES
Adjust-a-dose (for all indications): In older adults and patients with CrCl of 30 to 89 mL/minute, start at lower doses. Immediate-release lithium isn't recommended in patients with CrCl of less than 30 mL/minute.

➤ **Acute mania in bipolar disorder**
Adults and children age 7 and older weighing more than 30 kg: Initially, 300 mg PO t.i.d. Increase by 300 mg every 3 days to a goal of 600 mg PO b.i.d. or t.i.d.
Children age 7 and older weighing 20 to 30 kg: 300 mg (immediate-release tablets or capsules) PO b.i.d. Increase by 300 mg weekly to a goal of 600 to 1,500 mg PO in divided doses daily.
Adults and children age 12 and older (extended-release tablets): 900 mg PO b.i.d. or 600 mg PO t.i.d.
Adjust-a-dose: Individualize dosage according to serum concentrations and clinical response. Titrate to serum lithium concentrations of 0.8 to 1.2 mEq/L.

➤ **Long-term control in bipolar disorder**
Adults and children age 7 and older weighing more than 30 kg: Usual dose, 300 to 600 mg (immediate-release tablets or capsules) PO b.i.d. or t.i.d.
Children age 7 and older weighing 20 to 30 kg: Usual dose, 600 to 1,200 mg (immediate-release tablets or capsules) PO in divided doses daily.
Adults and children age 12 and older (extended-release tablets): 900 to 1,200 mg/day in divided doses. Usual dose, 600 mg PO b.i.d.
Adjust-a-dose: Individualize dosage according to serum concentrations and clinical response. Titrate immediate-release

formulations to serum lithium concentrations of 0.6 to 1 mEq/L.

ADMINISTRATION
PO
• Give drug after meals with plenty of water to minimize GI upset.
• Don't crush extended-release tablets.

ACTION
Probably alters chemical transmitters in the CNS, possibly by interfering with ionic pump mechanisms in brain cells, and may compete with or replace sodium ions.

Route	Onset	Peak	Duration
PO (immediate-release)	Unknown	30 min–3 hr	Unknown
PO (extended-release)	Unknown	2–6 hr	Unknown

Half-life: 18 to 36 hours.

ADVERSE REACTIONS
CNS: fatigue, lethargy, *coma, seizures,* tremors, drowsiness, headache, confusion, stupor, tongue movements, tics, restlessness, dizziness, vertigo, psychomotor retardation, blackouts, EEG changes, worsened organic mental syndrome, impaired speech, ataxia, incoordination, hypertonicity, fever, choreoathetotic movements, extrapyramidal symptoms, hallucinations, poor memory, dysgeusia. **CV:** *arrhythmias (including Brugada syndrome), bradycardia,* reversible ECG changes, *severe bradycardia,* hypotension, SA node dysfunction. **EENT:** blurred vision, exophthalmos, nystagmus, tinnitus, dry mouth, salivary gland swelling, hypersalivation, dental caries. **GI:** vomiting, anorexia, diarrhea, thirst, nausea, gastritis, abdominal pain, flatulence, indigestion, fecal incontinence. **GU:** polyuria, *renal toxicity with long-term use,* oliguria, glycosuria, decreased CrCl, albuminuria, urinary incontinence, erectile dysfunction. **Hematologic:** leukocytosis. **Metabolic:** transient hyperglycemia, goiter, hypothyroidism, hyponatremia, thirst. **Musculoskeletal:** muscle weakness, muscle hyperirritability, polyarthralgia. **Skin:** pruritus, rash, diminished or absent sensation, drying and thinning of hair, psoriasis, acne, alopecia, folliculitis, DRESS syndrome. **Other:** ankle and wrist edema.

L

INTERACTIONS

Drug-drug. *ACE inhibitors, ARBs:* May increase lithium level. Monitor lithium level; adjust lithium dosage, as needed.

Antiarrhythmics and other drugs that prolong QT interval: May increase risk of life-threatening arrhythmias. Avoid use together.

Antipsychotics (clozapine, haloperidol, risperidone, thioridazine): May increase risk of neurotoxic reactions. Monitor patient closely.

Calcium channel blockers (verapamil): May decrease lithium levels and may increase risk of neurotoxicity. Use together cautiously.

Carbamazepine, fluoxetine, methyldopa, NSAIDs, phenytoin, probenecid: May increase effect of lithium. Monitor patient for lithium toxicity.

Iodide-containing preparations (potassium iodide): May increase risk of hypothyroidism. Monitor thyroid levels.

Metronidazole: May cause lithium toxicity due to reduced lithium renal clearance. Monitor lithium levels.

Neuromuscular blockers (succinylcholine): May cause prolonged paralysis or weakness. Monitor patient closely.

Serotonergic drugs (linezolid, MAO inhibitors, SSNRIs, SSRIs): May increase risk of serotonin syndrome. Use cautiously.

Sodium bicarbonate, theophylline, urine alkalinizers: May increase lithium excretion. Patient should avoid excessive salt. Monitor lithium levels.

Thiazide diuretics: May increase reabsorption of lithium by kidneys, with possible toxic effect. Use with caution, and monitor lithium and electrolyte levels (especially sodium).

Drug-food. *Caffeine:* May decrease lithium level and drug effect. Advise patient who ingests large amounts of caffeine to tell prescriber before stopping caffeine. Adjust lithium dosage, as needed.

Sodium (salt): May change renal elimination of drug if sodium intake changes. Avoid major changes in sodium intake.

EFFECTS ON LAB TEST RESULTS

• May increase glucose, creatinine, and TSH levels.
• May decrease sodium, T_3, T_4, and protein-bound iodine levels.
• May increase WBC and neutrophil counts.
• May increase ^{131}I uptake.

CONTRAINDICATIONS & CAUTIONS

• Contraindicated in patients hypersensitive to drug or if therapy can't be closely monitored.
• Use extreme caution in patients receiving neuromuscular blockers and diuretics; in older adults or patients who are debilitated; and in patients with thyroid disease, seizure disorder, infection, renal or CV disease, dehydration, or sodium depletion.
• Patients with Brugada syndrome (abnormal ECG with increased risk of sudden death) or with risk factors for this condition shouldn't take lithium.

Dialyzable drug: Yes.

⚠ *Overdose S&S:* Diarrhea, vomiting, drowsiness, muscular weakness, lack of coordination, giddiness, ataxia, blurred vision, confusion, tinnitus, large output of dilute urine, slurred speech, loss of consciousness, myoclonic limb movements, agitation, urinary or fecal incontinence, seizures, arrhythmias, hypotension, peripheral vascular collapse, coma.

PREGNANCY-LACTATION-REPRODUCTION

• Drug may cause fetal harm if used during pregnancy. Apprise patient of potential hazard to the fetus.
• If patient decides to continue lithium during pregnancy, monitor serum lithium concentration and adjust dosage if indicated. Two to three days before delivery, decrease lithium dosage or discontinue drug to reduce risk of maternal or neonatal toxicity. Monitor neonate and provide supportive care until lithium is excreted and toxic signs and symptoms disappear, which may take up to 14 days. Consider fetal echocardiography between 16 and 20 weeks' gestation in a patient with first-trimester lithium exposure, due to increased risk of cardiac malformations.
• Drug appears in human milk. Use in breastfeeding isn't recommended. If patient chooses to breastfeed, monitor infant's lithium level.

NURSING CONSIDERATIONS

Boxed Warning Lithium toxicity is closely related to serum lithium levels and can occur at doses close to therapeutic levels. Facilities for prompt and accurate serum lithium determinations should be available before initiation of therapy. ■

• Monitor patient and discontinue drug for signs and symptoms of lithium toxicity (ataxia, drowsiness, weakness, tremor, vomiting).

• When drug level is less than 1.5 mEq/L, adverse reactions are usually mild.

• Obtain baseline ECG, thyroid studies, renal studies, and electrolyte levels.

• Check fluid intake and output, especially when surgery is scheduled.

• Weigh patient daily; monitor patient for edema or sudden weight gain.

• Adjust fluid and salt ingestion to compensate if excessive loss occurs from protracted diaphoresis or diarrhea. Under normal conditions, fluid intake should be 2½ to 3 L daily, and patient should follow a balanced diet with adequate salt intake.

• Monitor urine specific gravity and report level below 1.005, which may indicate diabetes insipidus.

• Drug alters glucose tolerance in patients with diabetes. Monitor glucose level closely.

• Perform outpatient follow-up of thyroid and renal function every 2 to 3 months during 6 months of treatment, then as clinically indicated. Monitor CBC and ECG (patients older than age 40) before therapy and as needed.

• Monitor lithium level twice weekly, 12 hours after the last oral dose, until patient and levels are stable, then every 1 to 2 months or as needed.

• Palpate thyroid to check for enlargement. Monitor weight before and during therapy.

• Monitor cognitive function periodically.

• *Look alike–sound alike:* Don't confuse lithium carbonate with lanthanum carbonate.

PATIENT TEACHING

• Tell patient to take drug with plenty of water and after meals to minimize GI upset.

• Explain the importance of having regular blood tests to determine drug levels and to monitor therapy; even slightly high values can be dangerous.

• Warn patient and caregivers to expect transient nausea, large amounts of urine, thirst, and discomfort during first few days and to watch for evidence of toxicity.

• Instruct patient to withhold one dose and call prescriber immediately if signs and symptoms of toxicity appear, but not to stop drug abruptly.

• Warn patient to avoid hazardous activities that require alertness and good psychomotor coordination until CNS effects are known.

• Tell patient not to switch brands or take other prescription or OTC drugs without prescriber's guidance.

• Advise patient to immediately seek emergency assistance if fainting, light-headedness, abnormal heartbeat, or shortness of breath occurs because these signs and symptoms are associated with a potentially life-threatening heart disorder known as Brugada syndrome.

• Tell patient to wear or carry medical identification at all times.

SAFETY ALERT!

lixisenatide
lix-i-SEN-a-tide

Adlyxin

Therapeutic class: Antidiabetics
Pharmacologic class: Glucagon-like peptide-1 receptor antagonists

AVAILABLE FORMS
Injection: 10 mcg/dose pens; 20 mcg/dose in 3-mL prefilled pens (14 doses)

INDICATIONS & DOSAGES
➤ **Adjunct to diet and exercise to improve glycemic control in patients with type 2 diabetes**
Adults: Initially, 10 mcg subcut once daily for 14 days; then on day 15, increase to maintenance dose of 20 mcg subcut once daily.

ADMINISTRATION
Subcutaneous

• Inspect pen before each use; it should be clear and colorless. Don't use if there is particulate matter or discoloration.

• Administer subcut injection in abdomen, thigh, or upper arm once daily. Rotate injection site with every use.

• Give within 1 hour before first meal of the day, preferably the same meal every day. If a dose is missed, give dose 1 hour before next meal.

• Replace cap after each use. Don't store pen with needle attached.

• Store unused pen in refrigerator at 36° to 46° F (2° to 8° C) in original package; protect from light. After first dose, may store pen at room temperature, below 86° F (30° C). Discard pen after 14 days.

🚯 *Alert:* Use a new needle for each dose. Pens are for single patient use; don't share among patients even if needle is changed, because of risk of blood-borne pathogen transmission.

ACTION

Increases glucose-dependent insulin release, decreases glucagon secretion, and slows gastric emptying.

Route	Onset	Peak	Duration
Subcut	Unknown	1–3.5 hr	Unknown

Half-life: 3 hours.

ADVERSE REACTIONS

CNS: headache, dizziness. **GI:** nausea, vomiting, diarrhea, dyspepsia, constipation, abdominal distention, abdominal pain. **Metabolic:** *hypoglycemia.* **Skin:** injection-site reactions. **Other:** immunogenicity.

INTERACTIONS

Drug-drug. *Basal insulin, sulfonylurea:* May increase risk of hypoglycemia. Reduce basal insulin or sulfonylurea dosage as needed.
Oral contraceptives: May alter concentration of contraceptive. Patient should take contraceptive at least 1 hour before or at least 11 hours after lixisenatide injection.
Oral drugs dependent on threshold concentrations for efficacy (antibiotics) or for which a delay in effect is undesirable (acetaminophen): Lixisenatide causes delayed gastric emptying, which may affect concentrations of other drugs or cause delays in effects. Use together cautiously and give oral drugs 1 hour before lixisenatide injection.

EFFECTS ON LAB TEST RESULTS

• May decrease glucose level.

CONTRAINDICATIONS & CAUTIONS

• Contraindicated in patients hypersensitive to drug or its components.
• Use cautiously in patients with a history of anaphylaxis or angioedema after receiving another GLP-1 receptor agonist.
• May increase risk of pancreatitis, especially in patients with history of cholelithiasis or alcohol abuse.
• Drug hasn't been studied in patients with chronic pancreatitis or a history of unexplained pancreatitis. Consider other antidiabetic therapies.

• May increase risk of acute kidney injury or worsening of renal impairment, especially in patients with nausea, vomiting, diarrhea, or dehydration. Use isn't recommended in patients with ESRD.
• Drug isn't indicated to treat type 1 diabetes or diabetic ketoacidosis.
• Use with short-acting insulin hasn't been studied. Use together isn't recommended.
• Drug hasn't been studied in patients with gastroparesis. Use isn't recommended.
• Antibodies to drug may develop, decreasing glycemic control and increasing risk of injection-site or allergic reactions. Consider alternative therapy if antibodies develop.
• Safety and effectiveness in children haven't been established.
Dialyzable drug: Unknown.
⚠ *Overdose S&S:* Increased GI disorders.

PREGNANCY-LACTATION-REPRODUCTION

• Data are limited concerning use in pregnancy. Use during pregnancy only if benefits outweigh risks.
• It isn't known if drug appears in human milk. Before use, consider clinical needs of the patient and potential adverse effects on the infant.

NURSING CONSIDERATIONS

• Monitor patient for hypersensitivity reactions, including anaphylaxis and angioedema. Discontinue drug and treat appropriately if reaction occurs.
• Monitor glucose level closely to evaluate effectiveness.
• Monitor renal function at beginning of therapy and at dosage escalations in patients with renal impairment or severe GI reactions.
• Monitor patient for signs and symptoms of pancreatitis. Discontinue drug and manage signs and symptoms clinically if pancreatitis is suspected. If pancreatitis is confirmed, don't restart drug.
• *Look alike–sound alike:* Don't confuse lixisenatide with liraglutide.

PATIENT TEACHING

• Tell patient to report all medications being taken before start of therapy.
• Teach patient how to prepare pen, to always use a new needle, and to administer drug according to manufacturer's instructions.

Reactions in bold italics are **life-threatening**. Interactions may have a *rapid onset* or a **delayed onset**.

• Instruct patient to store pen in original container without the needle at room temperature, and to discard pen 14 days after first use.

⊕ Alert: Teach patient not to share pens even if the needle is changed, because of risk of blood-borne pathogen transmission.

• Caution patient to report all adverse reactions, especially signs and symptoms of hypoglycemia (dizziness, confusion, weakness, feeling jittery, diaphoresis), particularly if patient is taking a sulfonylurea or basal insulin, and pancreatitis (persistent, severe abdominal pain that may radiate to the back, with or without vomiting).

• Warn patient to watch for signs and symptoms of hypersensitivity reactions (fever, nausea, difficulty breathing, rash, swelling of the face, lips or tongue) and to stop drug and seek immediate medical attention if they occur.

• Teach patient to report nausea, vomiting, diarrhea, and dehydration promptly, because of risk of kidney injury.

• Advise patient of childbearing potential to report plans to become pregnant or to breast-feed before start of therapy.

---

lofexidine hydrochloride ▒
loe-FEX-i-deen

Lucemyra

Therapeutic class: Opioid cessation drugs
Pharmacologic class: Alpha₂-adrenergic receptor agonists

AVAILABLE FORMS
Tablets: 0.18 mg

INDICATIONS & DOSAGES
➤ **Mitigation of opioid withdrawal symptoms to facilitate abrupt opioid discontinuation**
Adults: Initially, three 0.18-mg tablets PO q.i.d. during the peak withdrawal period (generally 5 to 7 days after last opioid dose). Allow 5 to 6 hours between doses and continue for up to 14 days, with dosing guided by symptoms. Maximum daily dose is 2.88 mg (16 tablets); maximum single dose is 0.72 mg (4 tablets). Discontinue treatment gradually over 2 to 4 days, reducing by 1 tablet per dose every 1 to 2 days.
Adjust-a-dose: For patients with mild hepatic impairment (Child-Pugh score 5 to 6),

give 3 tablets q.i.d. (2.16 mg/day); for those with moderate hepatic impairment (Child-Pugh score 7 to 9), give 2 tablets q.i.d. (1.44 mg/day); for those with severe hepatic impairment (Child-Pugh score greater than 9), give 1 tablet q.i.d. (0.72 mg/day). For patients with mild to moderate renal impairment (eGFR of 30 to 89.9 mL/minute/1.73 m²), give 2 tablets q.i.d. (1.44 mg/day); for those with severe renal impairment, ESRD, or on dialysis (eGFR of less than 30 mL/minute/1.73 m²), give 1 tablet q.i.d. (0.72 mg/day).

ADMINISTRATION
PO
• May give with or without food.
• Store at controlled room temperature 77° F (25° C). Protect from excess moisture and heat. Don't remove desiccant pack from bottle.

ACTION
A central alpha₂-adrenergic agonist that binds to receptors on adrenergic neurons. It inhibits the release of norepinephrine in the central and peripheral nervous systems, reducing the signs and symptoms of opioid withdrawal.

Route	Onset	Peak	Duration
PO	Unknown	3–5 hr	Unknown

Half-life: 11 to 13 hours (first dose); 17 to 22 hours (at steady-state).

ADVERSE REACTIONS
CNS: insomnia, dizziness, somnolence, sedation, syncope. **CV:** orthostatic hypotension, **bradycardia,** hypotension. **EENT:** tinnitus, dry mouth.

INTERACTIONS
Drug-drug. *CNS depressants (barbiturates, benzodiazepines):* May enhance CNS depressant effects. Avoid use together.
CYP2D6 inhibitors (paroxetine): May increase lofexidine concentration. Use cautiously together. Monitor patient for orthostatic hypotension and bradycardia.
Drugs that decrease HR: May increase risk of excessive bradycardia. Avoid use together.
Drugs that increase QT interval (methadone): May further increase QT interval. Use together cautiously and monitor ECGs.
Drugs that lower BP: May increase hypotensive effects. Avoid use together.

Naltrexone: May decrease effectiveness of oral naltrexone if given within 2 hours of lofexidine. Monitor therapy and separate dosing times of drugs by 2 hours.

Drug-lifestyle. *Alcohol use:* May increase CNS depressive effects. Discourage use together.

EFFECTS ON LAB TEST RESULTS
None reported.

CONTRAINDICATIONS & CAUTIONS
• Avoid use in patients with severe coronary insufficiency, recent MI, cerebrovascular disease, chronic renal failure, and marked bradycardia. If drug must be used, monitor ECG, especially in patients with these conditions and electrolyte disturbances.

🕐 *Alert:* Drug causes QT-interval prolongation, especially in patients with renal impairment; prolonged QT interval increases risk of ventricular arrhythmias. Avoid using in patients with congenital long QT syndrome.

• Use cautiously in patients with HF, bradyarrhythmias, and hepatic or renal impairment.

• Use cautiously in outpatient setting. Patients should be capable of self-monitoring for adverse effects.

• Drug may decrease tolerance to opioids and increase the risk of fatal opioid overdose if patient resumes opioid use.

• Use drug for opioid use disorder only with a comprehensive treatment and management program.

🕐 *Alert:* Drug may increase risk of discontinuation symptoms. Don't stop medication abruptly as it can cause a rise in BP, diarrhea, insomnia, chills, hyperhidrosis, and extremity pain.

🕐 Use cautiously in patients who are CYP2D6 poor metabolizers. Monitor patients for orthostatic hypotension and bradycardia.

• Safety and effectiveness in children haven't been established.

• Use cautiously in older adults; consider utilizing dosage adjustments for renal impairment.

Dialyzable drug: Minimal.

⚠️ *Overdose S&S:* Hypotension, bradycardia, sedation.

PREGNANCY-LACTATION-REPRODUCTION
• Safe use in pregnancy hasn't been established. Use only if benefits outweigh fetal risk.

• It isn't known if drug appears in human milk or how drug affects milk production or infants who are breastfed. Use cautiously with breastfeeding.

NURSING CONSIDERATIONS
• Monitor vital signs and watch for bradycardia and hypotension before dosing. Reduce dosage or delay or skip next dose for clinically significant hypotension or bradycardia.

• Monitor ECG in patients with HF, bradycardia, hepatic impairment, or renal impairment and in those taking medications that prolong QT interval, especially if electrolyte disturbances are present.

• Monitor electrolyte levels and correct abnormalities (hypokalemia, hypomagnesemia) before administering drug; monitor ECG when starting drug.

• Monitor patient for drug discontinuation signs and symptoms; manage by resuming previous dose, followed by gradual tapering if signs and symptoms occur.

PATIENT TEACHING
• Teach patient signs and symptoms of hypotension and to rise slowly from a seated or lying position.

• Caution patient to stay hydrated.

• Instruct patient to withhold dose and immediately contact prescriber if signs or symptoms of low BP or slow HR occur (dizziness, light-headedness, feeling faint at rest or when standing up).

• Caution patient to avoid driving or operating heavy machinery until drug's effects are known.

• Advise patient not to abruptly stop drug and to follow instructions for gradual drug discontinuation.

🕐 *Alert:* Inform patient and caregivers of increased risk of overdose if opioids are resumed.

Reactions in bold italics are *life-threatening*. Interactions may have a *rapid onset* or a *delayed onset*.

lopinavir–ritonavir 🕱
low-PIN-ah-ver/ri-TON-ah-veer

Kaletra*🖉

Therapeutic class: Antiretrovirals
Pharmacologic class: Protease inhibitors

AVAILABLE FORMS
Solution: lopinavir 400 mg and ritonavir
100 mg/5 mL (80 mg/mL and 20 mg/mL)*
Tablets 🔵*:* lopinavir 100 mg and ritonavir
25 mg; lopinavir 200 mg and ritonavir
50 mg

INDICATIONS & DOSAGES
➤ **HIV infection, with other antiretrovirals
except efavirenz, nevirapine, or nelfinavir**
Adults: 800 mg lopinavir and 200 mg ritonavir PO once daily (only in patients with less
than three lopinavir resistance–associated
substitutions) or in two evenly divided doses.
Children older than 6 months to 18 years:
230 mg lopinavir and 57.5 mg/m^2 ritonavir
(oral solution) PO b.i.d. with food. Or, if patient weighs more than 35 kg, give four tablets
of lopinavir 100 mg and ritonavir 25 mg PO
b.i.d. If patient weighs between 25 and 35 kg,
give three tablets of lopinavir 100 mg and ritonavir 25 mg PO b.i.d. If patient weighs 15 to
25 kg, give two tablets of lopinavir 100 mg
and ritonavir 25 mg PO b.i.d. Maximum
dosage is lopinavir 400 mg and ritonavir
100 mg PO b.i.d.
Children ages 14 days to 6 months: 16 mg
lopinavir and 4 mg ritonavir/kg oral solution
PO b.i.d. Or, lopinavir 300 mg and ritonavir
75 mg/m^2 PO b.i.d.
Adjust-a-dose: In patients who are pregnant
with no documented lopinavir resistance–
associated substitutions, give 400 mg
lopinavir and 100 mg ritonavir tablets b.i.d.;
avoid oral solution due to ethanol content.
Once-daily dosing isn't recommended. There
are insufficient data to recommend dosing in
patients who are pregnant with documented
lopinavir resistance–associated substitutions.
No dosage adjustment is required during the
postpartum period.
➤ **HIV infection, in combination with
antiretrovirals efavirenz, nevirapine, or
nelfinavir**
Adults: 500 mg lopinavir and 125 mg ritonavir (tablets) PO b.i.d., or 520 mg lopinavir

and 130 mg ritonavir (oral solution) PO b.i.d.
with food.
Children older than 6 months to 18 years:
300 mg lopinavir and 75 mg/m^2 ritonavir
(oral solution) PO b.i.d. with food. Maximum dosage is lopinavir 533 mg and ritonavir
133 mg (oral solution) PO b.i.d. with food.
Or, if patient weighs more than 45 kg, give
five tablets of lopinavir 100 mg and ritonavir
25 mg PO b.i.d. If patient weighs between
30 and 45 kg, give four tablets of lopinavir
100 mg and ritonavir 25 mg PO b.i.d. If patient weighs 20 to 30 kg, give three tablets
of lopinavir 100 mg and ritonavir 25 mg PO
b.i.d. If patient weighs 15 to 20 kg, give two
tablets of lopinavir 100 mg and ritonavir
25 mg PO b.i.d. Maximum dosage is lopinavir
500 mg and ritonavir 125 mg (tablets) PO
b.i.d.

ADMINISTRATION
PO
⚠ *Alert:* Many drug interactions are possible.
Review all drugs patient is taking.
• Give oral solution with food. Give tablets
without regard for food.
• Calculate children's doses based on either
body weight or BSA.
• Tablets must be swallowed whole; don't
crush or divide, and tell patient not to chew.
• Don't use oral solution with polyurethane
feeding tubes because of potential incompatibility with ethanol and propylene glycol. Feeding tubes that are compatible with
ethanol and propylene glycol, such as silicone
and polyvinyl chloride feeding tubes, can be
used.
• Refrigerated solution remains stable until
expiration date on package. If stored at room
temperature, use drug within 2 months.

ACTION
Lopinavir is an HIV protease inhibitor, which
produces immature, noninfectious viral particles. Ritonavir, also an HIV protease inhibitor, slows lopinavir metabolism, thereby
increasing lopinavir level.

Route	Onset	Peak	Duration
PO	Unknown	4 hr	Unknown

Half-life: About 5 to 6 hours.

ADVERSE REACTIONS
CNS: anxiety, fatigue, dizziness, fever,
headache, insomnia, malaise, nervousness,

neuropathy, pain, paresthesia, peripheral neuritis, somnolence, tremors, taste perversion. **CV:** edema, HTN, palpitations. **GI:** *colitis, pancreatitis,* diarrhea, nausea, abdominal pain, anorexia, cholecystitis, constipation, dyspepsia, dysphagia, enterocolitis, esophagitis, flatulence, abdominal distention, gastroenteritis, GERD, hemorrhoids, vomiting. **GU:** erectile dysfunction, menstrual disorder, increased CrCl. **Hematologic:** *leukopenia, neutropenia, thrombocytopenia in children,* anemia. **Hepatic:** *hepatitis,* increased transaminase levels, hyperbilirubinemia. **Metabolic:** decreased glucose tolerance, hypertriglyceridemia, hyperglycemia, hypercholesterolemia, hyperuricemia, hyponatremia in children, hypothyroidism, weight loss; increased amylase, lipase, CK levels. **Musculoskeletal:** arthralgia, back pain, myalgia. **Respiratory:** lower or upper respiratory tract infections, bronchitis, dyspnea, lung edema. **Skin:** dry skin, dermatitis, skin infections, pruritus, rash, night sweats, lipodystrophy. **Other:** hypersensitivity reactions, chills, facial edema, flulike symptoms, gynecomastia, lymphadenopathy, viral infection.

INTERACTIONS

🔶 *Alert:* Drug can significantly interact with many drugs. Consult a drug interaction resource or pharmacist for additional information.

Drug-drug. *Alfuzosin:* Increases hypotension risk. Use together is contraindicated.

Amiodarone, bepridil, lidocaine, quinidine: May increase antiarrhythmic level. Use together cautiously. Monitor levels of these drugs, if possible.

Antiarrhythmics (dronedarone, flecainide, propafenone), pimozide: May increase risk of cardiac arrhythmias. Avoid using together. Dronedarone is contraindicated.

Anticancer agents (ibrutinib, vincristine): May decrease antiviral effects. Refer to prescribing information of individual agent.

Aripiprazole: May enhance adverse effects of ritonavir. Modify therapy.

Atorvastatin: May increase level of this drug and risk of myopathy and rhabdomyolysis. Use lowest possible dose and monitor patient carefully.

Atovaquone, methadone: May decrease levels of these drugs. Consider increasing doses of these drugs.

Avanafil, sildenafil, tadalafil, vardenafil: May increase level of these drugs and adverse effects, such as hypotension and prolonged erection. Monitor patient and adjust dosage according to manufacturer's instructions. Use with sildenafil in PAH treatment is contraindicated.

Bosentan: May increase bosentan level. Consider decreasing bosentan dosage.

Bupropion: May decrease bupropion level and antidepressant effect. Monitor patient for adequate clinical response and adjust bupropion dosage as needed.

Calcium channel blockers (felodipine, nicardipine, nifedipine): May increase levels of these drugs. Use together cautiously.

Carbamazepine, phenobarbital, phenytoin: May decrease lopinavir level. Use together cautiously. Don't use once-daily lopinavir–ritonavir. Consider therapy modification.

Clarithromycin: May increase clarithromycin level in patients with renal impairment. Adjust clarithromycin dosage.

Cobicistat: May enhance therapeutic effects of ritonavir. Avoid use together.

Colchicine: May increase colchicine level. Contraindicated in patients with renal or hepatic impairment. Decrease colchicine dosage if used together in patient with normal renal and hepatic function.

Corticosteroids: May decrease lopinavir level and increase steroid level. Refer to individual product for alternative dosing or alternative product.

Cyclosporine, rapamycin, tacrolimus: May increase levels of these drugs. Monitor therapeutic levels.

Dasatinib, nilotinib: May increase levels of these drugs and risk of adverse events. Adjust dasatinib and nilotinib dosages as needed.

Delavirdine: May increase lopinavir level. Avoid using together.

Didanosine: May decrease absorption of didanosine because lopinavir–ritonavir combination is taken with food. Give didanosine 1 hour before or 2 hours after lopinavir–ritonavir combination.

Disulfiram, metronidazole: May cause disulfiram-like reaction in patients using oral solution (contains alcohol). Avoid use together.

Drugs that prolong PR interval (atazanavir, beta blockers, calcium channel blockers, digoxin): May further prolong PR interval. Use cautiously together.

Drugs that prolong QT interval (amiodarone, flecainide, propafenone): May further

---

Reactions in bold italics are *life-threatening*. Interactions may have a *rapid onset* or a ***delayed onset***.

prolong QT interval and increase risk of ventricular arrhythmias. Avoid use together.

Efavirenz, nelfinavir, nevirapine: May decrease lopinavir level. Consider increasing lopinavir–ritonavir combination dose. Don't use a once-daily regimen of lopinavir–ritonavir combination with these drugs.

Elvitegravir: May increase elvitegravir concentration. Reduce dosages of both drugs and consider modifying therapy.

Ergot derivatives (dihydroergotamine, ergonovine, ergotamine, methylergonovine): May increase risk of ergot toxicity characterized by peripheral vasospasm and ischemia. Use together is contraindicated.

Fentanyl: May increase or prolong sedation or cause respiratory depression. Monitor patient carefully.

Fosamprenavir with ritonavir: May increase rate of adverse reactions. Appropriate doses of the combinations with respect to safety and effectiveness haven't been established.

Hepatitis C antivirals (boceprevir, dasabuvir, elbasvir/grazoprevir, glecaprevir, ombitasvir, paritaprevir, pibrentasvir, simeprevir, sofosbuvir, velpatasvir, voxilaprevir): May increase or decrease drug levels. Use together not recommended.

Hormonal contraceptives (ethinyl estradiol): May decrease effectiveness of contraceptives. Recommend nonhormonal contraceptives.

Itraconazole, ketoconazole: May increase levels of these drugs. Don't give more than 200 mg/day of these drugs.

Lamotrigine, valproic acid: May decrease levels of these drugs. Consider dosage increase of lamotrigine or valproic acid.

Lomitapide: Increases lomitapide exposure, raising hepatotoxicity risk. Use together is contraindicated.

Lovastatin, simvastatin: May increase risk of adverse reactions, such as myopathy and rhabdomyolysis. Use together is contraindicated.

Lurasidone, pimozide, ranolazine: Increases risk of life-threatening reactions. Use together is contraindicated.

Maraviroc: May increase maraviroc blood level. Adjust maraviroc dosage according to its prescribing information.

Methadone: May decrease methadone level. Monitor clinical response and increase methadone dosage as needed.

Midazolam (oral), triazolam: Increases exposure of these drugs and risk of severe sedation or respiratory depression. Use together is contraindicated.

Pitavastatin, pravastatin: May increase statin level and risk of myopathy and rhabdomyolysis. Use together cautiously.

Quetiapine: May increase quetiapine concentration. Consider another antiretroviral or decrease quetiapine dosage to one-sixth of current dose. Monitor patient for adverse effects.

Rifabutin: May increase rifabutin level. Decrease rifabutin dosage by at least 75% or a maximum of 150 mg every other day or three times a week. Monitor patient carefully and adjust dosage as needed.

Rifampin: May decrease effectiveness of Kaletra. Avoid using together.

Rivaroxaban: May increase bleeding risk. Avoid use together.

Rosuvastatin: May increase statin level and risk of myopathy and rhabdomyolysis. Rosuvastatin dosage shouldn't exceed 10 mg daily.

Salmeterol: May increase salmeterol level and risk of CV adverse reactions. Use together isn't recommended.

Saquinavir: May increase levels of these drugs. Avoid using together.

Trazodone: May increase trazodone level and risk of adverse reactions. Consider lower dosage of trazodone.

Warfarin: May affect warfarin level. Monitor INR frequently.

Drug-herb. *Garlic supplements:* May decrease serum concentration of protease inhibitors. Concurrent use isn't recommended. If combination is used, monitor patient closely for signs or symptoms of therapeutic failure.

St. John's wort: May cause loss of virologic response and possible resistance to drug. Discourage use together.

Drug-food. *Any food:* May increase absorption of oral solution. Tell patient to take with food.

EFFECTS ON LAB TEST RESULTS
• May increase glucose, amylase, lipase, cholesterol, bilirubin, sodium, uric acid, and triglyceride levels and LFT values.
• May decrease Hb level and hematocrit and RBC, WBC, neutrophil, and platelet counts.

CONTRAINDICATIONS & CAUTIONS
• Contraindicated in patients hypersensitive to drug or its components.

♣Canada   ◇OTC   ♦Off-label use   ✐Photoguide   ⊜Do not crush   *Liquid contains alcohol   ▧Genetic

• Concomitant use with certain other drugs may result in known or potentially significant drug interactions. Consult full prescribing information before and during treatment for potential drug interactions.

⌧ Genetic or phenotype testing and treatment history should guide use of drug. The number of baseline lopinavir resistance–associated substitutions affects drug's virologic response.

• Avoid use in patients with congenital long QT syndrome or hypokalemia and in those taking drugs that prolong QT interval. Correct potassium abnormalities before starting therapy.

• Use cautiously in patients with a history of pancreatitis, hepatic impairment, HBV or HCV infection, marked elevations in liver enzyme levels, or hemophilia.

• Use cautiously in patients with cardiac conduction abnormalities or underlying cardiac disease.

• Use cautiously in older adults.

• New-onset diabetes, exacerbation of preexisting diabetes, and hyperglycemia have been reported in patients infected with HIV-1 receiving protease inhibitor therapy.

• Oral solution contains 42.4% (volume/volume) alcohol and 15.3% (weight/volume) propylene glycol; use with care, especially in infants and young children. Consider total amounts of alcohol and propylene glycol from all drugs given to children ages 14 days to 6 months to avoid toxicity.

⊙ *Alert:* Safety and effectiveness in neonates younger than age 14 days haven't been established. Use only if benefit outweighs risk. Monitor neonates for toxicity, such as hyperosmolality with or without lactic acidosis, renal toxicity, CNS depression (stupor, coma, apnea), seizures, hypotonia, cardiac arrhythmias, ECG changes, and hemolysis. Toxicity in preterm neonates can be severe or fatal.

Dialyzable drug: Unlikely.

⚠ *Overdose S&S:* Alcohol-related toxicity.

PREGNANCY-LACTATION-REPRODUCTION

• Drug is recommended with dosage adjustments for patients who are pregnant and infected with HIV.

• Avoid use of oral solution during pregnancy because it contains alcohol.

⌧ Once-daily dosing isn't recommended in patients who are pregnant with any

documented lopinavir resistance–associated amino acid substitutions.

• Encourage patient to enroll in the Antiretroviral Pregnancy Registry (1-800-258-4263).

• Patients infected with HIV-1 shouldn't breastfeed, to avoid risk of postnatal transmission of HIV-1.

NURSING CONSIDERATIONS

• Don't administer tablets or oral solution as a once-daily dosing regimen when combined with efavirenz, nevirapine, or nelfinavir.

• Avoid once-daily dosing in children younger than age 18.

• Calculate appropriate dose for each child based on body weight or BSA to avoid underdosing or exceeding the recommended adult dose.

• Assess children for ability to swallow intact tablets before drug is prescribed; use oral solution in a calibrated dosing syringe if a child is unable to reliably swallow a tablet.

• During initial phase of treatment, patients responding to antiretroviral therapy may develop an inflammatory response to indolent or residual opportunistic infections (CMV, MAC, *Pneumocystis jiroveci* pneumonia, TB), which may necessitate further evaluation and treatment. Autoimmune disorders (such as Graves disease, polymyositis, and Guillain-Barré syndrome) have also been reported in the setting of immune reconstitution; however, time to onset is more variable, and onset can occur many months after initiation of antiretroviral treatment.

• Monitor patient for signs of fat redistribution, including central obesity, buffalo hump, peripheral wasting, breast enlargement, and cushingoid appearance.

• Monitor glucose, total cholesterol, and triglyceride levels before starting therapy and periodically thereafter.

• Monitor patient for signs and symptoms of pancreatitis (nausea, vomiting, abdominal pain, or increased lipase and amylase values).

• Monitor patient for signs and symptoms of bleeding (hypotension, rapid HR) and for adverse reactions associated with concomitant drugs.

• Consider potential for drug interactions before and during therapy. Review concomitant medications and monitor patient for adverse reactions associated with the concomitant medications.

Reactions in bold italics are *life-threatening*. Interactions may have a *rapid onset* or a ***delayed onset***.

- *Look alike–sound alike:* Don't confuse Kaletra with Keppra.

PATIENT TEACHING
- Instruct patient or caregiver in safe drug administration.
- Advise patient to report all side effects to prescriber.
- Teach patient signs and symptoms of acute pancreatitis and to seek emergency medical treatment if signs and symptoms occur.
- Tell patient to report all adverse reactions and to immediately report severe nausea, vomiting, or abdominal pain.
- Inform patient that drug doesn't cure HIV infection, that opportunistic infections and other complications of HIV infection may still occur, and that transmission of HIV to others through sexual contact or blood contamination remains possible.
- Advise patient taking an erectile dysfunction drug of the increased risk of adverse effects, including low BP, visual changes, and painful erections, and to promptly report any symptoms to prescriber. Tell patient not to take more often than directed.
- Advise patient to immediately report pregnancy or plans to become pregnant during treatment.
- Warn patient to tell prescriber about other prescription or OTC drugs being taken, including herbal supplements.

SAFETY ALERT!

LORazepam
lor-AZ-e-pam

Ativan✐, Lorazepam Intensol, Loreev XR

Therapeutic class: Anxiolytics
Pharmacologic class: Benzodiazepines
Controlled substance schedule: IV

AVAILABLE FORMS
Capsules (extended-release) ⬭: 1 mg, 1.5 mg, 2 mg, 3 mg
Injection: 2 mg/mL, 4 mg/mL
Oral solution: 2 mg/mL
Tablets: 0.5 mg, 1 mg, 2 mg

INDICATIONS & DOSAGES
➤ **Anxiety**
Adults: 2 to 6 mg PO daily in divided doses, with the largest dose taken before bedtime. Maximum, 10 mg daily. Or extended-release capsule at a dose equal to total daily dose of immediate-release tablets PO daily in the morning.
Adjust-a-dose: If response to extended-release form is inadequate, switch to immediate-release tablets to further titrate dosage; then resume extended-release. If UGT inhibitor is started during use of extended-release capsules, switch to lorazepam tablets to reduce dosage.
Older adults: 1 to 2 mg PO daily in divided doses. Maximum, 10 mg daily.
➤ **Insomnia from anxiety or transient situational stress**
Adults: 2 to 4 mg PO at bedtime.
➤ **Preoperative sedation**
Adults: 2 mg IV total or 0.044 mg/kg IV, whichever is smaller, 15 to 20 minutes before the anticipated operative procedure. Larger doses up to 0.05 mg/kg IV, to total of 4 mg, may be needed. Or, 0.05 mg/kg IM 2 hours before procedure. Total dose shouldn't exceed 4 mg.
➤ **Status epilepticus**
Adults: 4 mg IV at a rate of 2 mg/minute. If seizures continue or recur after 10 to 15 minutes, an additional 4-mg dose may be given. Drug may be given IM if IV access isn't available.

ADMINISTRATION
PO
- Give extended-release capsule in morning without regard for food.
- Don't crush or allow patient to chew extended-release capsule.
- May open capsule and sprinkle entire contents over tablespoon of applesauce; then have patient swallow without chewing and follow with a drink of water. Use within 2 hours of mixing; don't store for later use.
- Use only calibrated dropper provided for oral solution.
- Mix oral solution with liquid or semisolid food, such as water, juices, carbonated beverages, applesauce, or pudding. Gently stir liquid or food for a few seconds and have patient immediately consume entire mixture.

IV

▼ Keep emergency resuscitation equipment and oxygen available.

▼ Give slowly at no more than 2 mg/minute.

▼ Monitor respirations every 5 to 15 minutes and before each IV dose.

▼ Contains benzyl alcohol. Avoid use in neonates.

▼ Refrigerate intact vials and protect from light.

▼ **Incompatibilities:** None listed by manufacturer. Consult a drug incompatibility reference for more information.

IM

• For status epilepticus, may give IM if IV access isn't available.

• For IM use, inject deeply into a muscle. Don't dilute.

• Refrigerate parenteral form to prolong shelf life.

ACTION

Potentiates the effects of GABA, depresses the CNS, and suppresses the spread of seizure activity.

Route	Onset	Peak	Duration
PO	1 hr	2 hr	12–24 hr
IV	5 min	60–90 min	6–8 hr
IM	15–30 min	60–90 min	6–8 hr

Half-life: 10 to 20 hours.

ADVERSE REACTIONS

CNS: drowsiness, sedation, amnesia, hallucinations, confusion, crying, delirium, insomnia, agitation, dizziness, weakness, unsteadiness, depression, asthenia, headache, somnolence, stupor, *coma (injection).* **CV:** hypotension. **EENT:** visual disturbances, nasal congestion. **GI:** abdominal discomfort, nausea, change in appetite. **Respiratory:** *respiratory failure, respiratory depression.* **Other:** pain at injection site.

INTERACTIONS

Drug-drug. *Clozapine:* May cause delirium, sedation, sialorrhea, and ataxia. Don't start simultaneously.

Boxed Warning *Opioids:* May cause slow or difficult breathing, sedation, and death. Avoid use together. If use together is necessary, limit dosage and duration of each drug to the minimum necessary for desired effect. ∎

Oral hormonal contraceptives: May decrease lorazepam level. Monitor closely; lorazepam dosage may need to be increased.

Probenecid: May result in prolonged lorazepam half-life and a decrease in its total clearance. Reduce lorazepam dosage by 50% when coadministered.

Scopolamine: May increase sedation, hallucinations, and irrational behavior with lorazepam injection as preanesthetic. Avoid use together.

Sodium oxybate: May result in additive effects, including increased sleep duration and CNS depression. Use together is contraindicated.

UGT inhibitors (diclofenac, quinidine, ritonavir): May increase lorazepam level. Avoid use with extended-release capsules; switch to immediate-release tablets if needed. Monitor patient.

Valproate: May increase lorazepam plasma concentration. Reduce lorazepam dosage to 50% of normal adult dose when used together.

Drug-herb. *Kava kava:* May enhance adverse or toxic effects of CNS depressants. Monitor therapy.

Yohimbe: May diminish therapeutic effect of antianxiety agents. Monitor therapy.

Drug-lifestyle. *Alcohol use:* May cause additive CNS effects. Discourage use together.

Cannabis: May enhance CNS depressant effect of CNS depressants. Monitor therapy.

EFFECTS ON LAB TEST RESULTS

• May increase LDH level and LFT values.

• May decrease sodium level.

• May decrease WBC count.

CONTRAINDICATIONS & CAUTIONS

• Contraindicated in patients hypersensitive to drug, other benzodiazepines, or the vehicle (including polyethylene glycol, propylene glycol, benzyl alcohol) used in parenteral dosage form, and in patients with acute angle-closure glaucoma. IV administration is contraindicated in patients with sleep apnea and in patients with severe respiratory insufficiency, except those who are mechanically ventilated.

• Contraindicated for intra-arterial administration.

Boxed Warning *Opioid class warning:* Opioids should only be prescribed with benzodiazepines or other CNS depressants to patients

---

Reactions in bold italics are *life-threatening*. Interactions may have a *rapid onset* or a *delayed onset*.

for whom alternative treatment options are inadequate. ■

Boxed Warning Benzodiazepine use exposes patient to risks of abuse, misuse, and addiction, which can lead to overdose or death. Assess each patient's risk of abuse, misuse, and addiction before prescribing and periodically during therapy. ■

🔆 *Alert:* Repeated or lengthy use of general anesthetic and sedation drugs during surgeries or procedures in children younger than age 3 or during the third trimester may affect brain development in children. Weigh benefits of appropriate anesthesia in young children and patients who are pregnant against risks.

• Use cautiously in patients with pulmonary, renal, or hepatic impairment, or history of substance abuse.

• Use cautiously in older adults and in patients who are acutely ill or debilitated.

• Capsules contain FD&C Yellow No. 5 (tartrazine), which may cause allergy reactions.

Dialyzable drug: Unknown.

⚠ *Overdose S&S:* Drowsiness, confusion lethargy, ataxia, hypotonia, hypotension, hypnotic state, stage 1 to 3 coma, death.

PREGNANCY-LACTATION-REPRODUCTION

• May cause fetal harm, including neonatal withdrawal symptoms. Avoid use during pregnancy except in life-threatening situations (status epilepticus) when safer drugs can't be used.

• Drug appears in human milk. Use with breastfeeding isn't recommended.

NURSING CONSIDERATIONS

• Monitor hepatic, renal, and hematopoietic function periodically in patients receiving repeated or prolonged therapy.

Boxed Warning Abrupt discontinuation or rapid dosage reduction of benzodiazepines after continued use may precipitate acute withdrawal reactions, which can be life-threatening. To reduce risk of withdrawal reactions, gradually taper drug to discontinue or reduce dosage. ■

• *Look alike–sound alike:* Don't confuse lorazepam with alprazolam, clonazepam, or Lovaza. Don't confuse Ativan with Atgam.

PATIENT TEACHING

Boxed Warning *Opioid class warning:* Caution patient or caregiver of patient taking an opioid with a benzodiazepine, CNS

depressant, or alcohol to seek immediate medical attention for dizziness, light-headedness, extreme sleepiness, slowed or difficult breathing, or unresponsiveness. ■

Boxed Warning Caution patient that benzodiazepines, even at recommended doses, increase risk of abuse, misuse, and addiction, which can lead to overdose and death, especially when used in combination with other drugs (opioid analgesics), alcohol, or illicit substances. ■

Boxed Warning Inform patient about proper disposal of unused drug and signs and symptoms of benzodiazepine abuse, misuse, and addiction (abdominal pain, amnesia, anorexia, anxiety, aggression, ataxia, blurred vision, confusion, depression, disinhibition, disorientation, dizziness, euphoria, impaired concentration and memory, indigestion, irritability, muscle pain, slurred speech, tremors, vertigo, delirium, paranoia, suicidality, seizures, difficulty breathing, coma). Advise patient to seek emergency medical help if signs and symptoms occur. Advise patient not to take drug at a higher dose, more frequently, or for longer than prescribed. ■

Boxed Warning Tell patient that continued use of drug for several days to weeks may lead to physical dependence and that abrupt discontinuation or rapid dosage reduction may precipitate acute withdrawal reactions (unusual movements, responses, or expressions; seizures; sudden and severe mental or nervous system changes; depression; seeing or hearing things that others don't; homicidal thoughts; extreme increase in activity or talking; losing touch with reality; suicidality), which can be life-threatening. Instruct patient that drug discontinuation or dosage reduction may require a slow taper. ■

Boxed Warning Advise patient about the possibility of developing protracted withdrawal syndrome (anxiety; trouble remembering, learning, or concentrating; depression; problems sleeping; feeling like insects are crawling under the skin; weakness; shaking; muscle twitching; burning or prickling feeling in the hands, arms, legs, or feet; ringing in the ears), with symptoms lasting weeks to more than 12 months. ■

🔆 *Alert:* Discuss with patient who is pregnant the benefits, risks, and appropriate timing of surgery or procedures requiring anesthetic and sedation drugs.

L

• When used before surgery, drug causes substantial preoperative amnesia. Patient teaching requires extra care to ensure adequate recall. Provide written materials or inform a family member, if possible.
• Warn patient to avoid hazardous activities that require alertness or good coordination until effects of drug are known.
• Tell patient to avoid use of alcohol while taking drug.
• Notify patient that smoking may decrease drug's effectiveness.
• Advise patient of childbearing potential to avoid pregnancy during therapy.

---

losartan potassium
low-SAR-tan

Cozaar

Therapeutic class: Antihypertensives
Pharmacologic class: ARBs

AVAILABLE FORMS
Tablets: 25 mg, 50 mg, 100 mg

INDICATIONS & DOSAGES
Adjust-a-dose (for all indications): In adults with mild to moderate hepatic impairment, starting dose is 25 mg once daily.
➤ **HTN**
Adults: Initially, 50 mg PO daily. Maximum daily dose is 100 mg.
Children age 6 and older: 0.7 mg/kg (up to 50 mg) PO daily, adjusted as needed up to 1.4 mg/kg/day (maximum 100 mg).
Adjust-a-dose: For adults with intravascular volume depletion (such as those taking diuretics), initially, 25 mg. Don't use in children with eGFR less than 30 mL/minute/1.73 m^2.
➤ **Nephropathy in patients with type 2 diabetes**
Adults: 50 mg PO once daily. Increase dosage to 100 mg once daily based on BP response.
➤ **To reduce risk of stroke in patients with HTN and left ventricular hypertrophy**
Adults: Initially, 50 mg PO once daily. Adjust dosage based on BP response, adding hydrochlorothiazide 12.5 mg once daily, increasing losartan to 100 mg daily, or both. If further adjustments are required, may increase the daily dosage of hydrochlorothiazide to 25 mg.

ADMINISTRATION
PO
• Give drug without regard for meals.
• If made into suspension by pharmacist, store in refrigerator for up to 4 weeks and shake well before each use.

ACTION
Inhibits vasoconstrictive and aldosterone-secreting action of angiotensin II by blocking angiotensin II receptor on the surface of vascular smooth muscle and other tissue cells.

Route	Onset	Peak	Duration
PO	6 hr	1–2 hr	Unknown

Half-life: Parent drug, about 1.5 to 3 hours; active metabolite, about 4.5 to 10 hours.

ADVERSE REACTIONS
CNS: dizziness, asthenia, fatigue, headache, insomnia. **CV:** edema, chest pain, palpitations, orthostatic hypotension, hypotension. **EENT:** nasal congestion, sinusitis, pharyngitis, sinus disorder. **GI:** abdominal pain, nausea, diarrhea, dyspepsia. **GU:** UTI. **Hematologic:** anemia. **Metabolic:** *hyperkalemia, hypoglycemia.* **Musculoskeletal:** muscle cramps, muscle weakness, myalgia, back or leg pain. **Respiratory:** cough, URI.

INTERACTIONS
Drug-drug. *Aliskiren; ACE inhibitors, ARBs:* May increase risk of renal impairment, hypotension, and hyperkalemia. Concomitant use with aliskiren is contraindicated in patients with diabetes. Avoid use together in patients with renal impairment (GFR less than 60 mL/minute); if must use concomitantly, monitor patient closely.
Amphetamines: May diminish antihypertensive effect. Monitor therapy.
Antifungals (azole derivatives, systemic): May decrease losartan metabolism. Monitor therapy.
Antipsychotics (atypical): May enhance hypotensive effect of these agents. Monitor therapy.
Lithium: May increase lithium level. Monitor lithium level and patient for toxicity.
NSAIDs: May decrease antihypertensive effects. Monitor BP and renal function.
Potassium-sparing diuretics, potassium supplements: May cause hyperkalemia. Monitor patient closely.

Reactions in bold italics are *life-threatening*. Interactions may have a *rapid onset* or a *delayed onset*.

Drug-herb. *Ma huang:* May decrease antihypertensive effects. Discourage use together.
Drug-food. *Salt substitutes containing potassium:* May cause hyperkalemia. Monitor patient closely.

EFFECTS ON LAB TEST RESULTS
• May increase potassium, bilirubin or liver enzyme levels.
• May decrease glucose or sodium level.
• May decrease Hb level.

CONTRAINDICATIONS & CAUTIONS
• Contraindicated in patients hypersensitive to drug.
• Use cautiously in patients with impaired renal or hepatic function.
• Safety and effectiveness in children younger than age 6 haven't been established.
Dialyzable drug: No.
⚠ *Overdose S&S:* Hypotension, tachycardia, bradycardia.

PREGNANCY-LACTATION-REPRODUCTION
Boxed Warning Drugs that act directly on the RAAS can cause fetal injury and death. If pregnancy is suspected, notify prescriber because drug should be stopped as soon as possible. ■
• It isn't known if drug appears in human milk. Patient should discontinue breastfeeding or discontinue drug, taking into account importance of drug to the patient.

NURSING CONSIDERATIONS
• Drug can be used alone or with other antihypertensives.
• Correct fluid volume and sodium depletion before treatment.
🗑 Monitor patient's BP closely to evaluate effectiveness of therapy. When used alone, drug has less of an effect on BP in patients who are Black than in patients of other races.
• Monitor patients who are also taking diuretics for symptomatic hypotension.
• Regularly assess patient's renal function (creatinine and BUN levels).
• Patients with severe HF whose renal function depends on the angiotensin-aldosterone system may develop acute renal failure during therapy. Closely monitor patient's BP, renal function, and potassium levels, especially during first few weeks of therapy and after dosage adjustments.

• *Look alike–sound alike:* Don't confuse Cozaar with Zocor or Colace.

PATIENT TEACHING
• Tell patient to avoid salt substitutes; these products may contain potassium, which can cause high potassium level in patients taking losartan.
• Advise patient to report all adverse reactions and to immediately report swelling of face, eyes, lips, or tongue or breathing difficulty.
• Inform patient of childbearing potential about consequences of taking drug while pregnant and to immediately report suspected pregnancy.
• Advise patient not to breastfeed while taking drug.

lovastatin (mevinolin) 🗑
loe-va-STA-tin

Altoprev

Therapeutic class: Antilipemics
Pharmacologic class: HMG-CoA reductase inhibitors

AVAILABLE FORMS
Tablets: 10 mg, 20 mg, 40 mg
Tablets (extended-release) ⊕: 20 mg, 40 mg, 60 mg

INDICATIONS & DOSAGES
Adjust-a-dose (for all indications): Avoid use of lovastatin with fibrates or niacin at doses greater than 1 g daily. For patients also taking danazol, diltiazem, dronedarone, or verapamil, start lovastatin at 10 mg (immediate-release) and don't exceed 20 mg daily. For patients also taking amiodarone, lovastatin dosage shouldn't exceed 40 mg daily unless clinical benefit is likely to outweigh increased risk of myopathy or rhabdomyolysis. For older adults or patients with CrCl of less than 30 mL/minute, carefully consider dosage increase greater than 20 mg daily and implement cautiously if necessary. For patients requiring smaller reductions in cholesterol levels, use immediate-release lovastatin.
➤ **To prevent and treat CAD; hyperlipidemia**
Adults: Initially, 20 mg (immediate-release) PO once daily with evening meal.

Recommended range is 10 to 80 mg as a single dose or in two divided doses; maximum daily recommended dose is 80 mg. Or, 20 to 60 mg extended-release tablets PO at bedtime.

Make dosage adjustments at intervals of 4 weeks or more.

➤ **Heterozygous familial hypercholesterolemia in adolescents** ⚕

Adolescents ages 10 to 17: Give 10 to 40 mg (immediate-release) PO daily with evening meal. Patients requiring reductions in LDL cholesterol level of 20% or more should start with 20 mg daily. Make dosage adjustments at intervals of 4 weeks or more.

ADMINISTRATION
PO
- Give immediate-release drug with evening meal, which improves absorption and cholesterol biosynthesis. Give extended-release drug at bedtime.
- Don't crush, split, or allow patient to chew extended-release tablets.

ACTION
Inhibits HMG-CoA reductase, an early (and rate-limiting) step in cholesterol biosynthesis.

Route	Onset	Peak	Duration
PO	Unknown	2–4 hr	Unknown
PO (extended-release)	3 days	12–14 hr	Unknown

Half-life: 1.1 to 1.7 hours.

ADVERSE REACTIONS
CNS: headache, dizziness, asthenia, pain. **EENT:** blurred vision, sinusitis. **GI:** abdominal pain or cramps, constipation, diarrhea, dyspepsia, flatulence, heartburn, nausea, vomiting. **GU:** UTI. **Hepatic:** increased transaminase levels. **Metabolic:** increased CK level. **Musculoskeletal:** muscle cramps, back pain, arthralgia, myalgia, myositis, *rhabdomyolysis*. **Skin:** rash. **Other:** flulike syndrome, pain, infection, accidental injury.

INTERACTIONS
Drug-drug. *Amiodarone:* May decrease the metabolism of lovastatin. Avoid combining lovastatin at doses exceeding 40 mg daily with amiodarone unless clinical benefit is likely to outweigh increased risk of myopathy.

Azole antifungals: May cause myopathy and rhabdomyolysis. Avoid using together.
Colchicine: May increase risk of myopathy or rhabdomyolysis. If coadministration can't be avoided, monitor patient for unexplained muscle pain, tenderness, or weakness.
Cyclosporine, gemfibrozil: May cause severe myopathy and rhabdomyolysis. Avoid this combination.
Danazol, diltiazem, dronedarone, verapamil: May cause myopathy and rhabdomyolysis. Don't exceed 20 mg lovastatin daily.
Dronedarone: May increase lovastatin serum concentration. Limit lovastatin to maximum of 20 mg/day (in adults). Increase monitoring for signs and symptoms of lovastatin toxicity (such as myopathy and rhabdomyolysis). Consider therapy modification.
Erythromycin, protease inhibitors (atazanavir, darunavir, fosamprenavir, nefazodone, nelfinavir, ritonavir, saquinavir, tipranavir), strong CYP3A inhibitors (clarithromycin, itraconazole, ketoconazole, posaconazole, voriconazole): Increase risk of myopathy and rhabdomyolysis. Use together is contraindicated.
Macrolides (azithromycin, clarithromycin), nefazodone: May decrease metabolism of HMG-CoA reductase inhibitor, increasing toxicity. Monitor patient for adverse effects and report unexplained muscle pain.
Mifepristone (CYP3A4 inhibitor): May increase lovastatin plasma level, increasing risk of toxicity. Use together is contraindicated.
Niacin, other fibrates: May increase the risk for adverse and toxic effects of lovastatin. Avoid use of lovastatin with fibrates or niacin at doses greater than 1 g daily.
Oral anticoagulants: May increase anticoagulant effect. Monitor patient closely.
Phenytoin: May decrease serum concentration of HMG-CoA reductase inhibitors. Consider therapy modification.
Ranolazine: May increase risk of myopathy and rhabdomyolysis. Consider lovastatin dosage adjustment.
Drug-herb. *Eucalyptus, kava:* May increase risk of hepatotoxicity. Discourage use together.
Red yeast rice: May increase risk of adverse reactions because herb contains compounds similar to those in drug. Discourage use together.
St. John's wort: May increase metabolism of HMG-CoA reductase inhibitors, leading to

---

Reactions in bold italics are *life-threatening*. Interactions may have a *rapid onset* or a ***delayed onset***.

decreased effectiveness of drug's cholesterol-lowering abilities. Consider therapy modification.

Drug-food. *Grapefruit juice:* May increase drug level, increasing risk of adverse effects. Discourage use together.

Drug-lifestyle. *Alcohol use:* May increase risk of hepatotoxicity. Discourage use together.

EFFECTS ON LAB TEST RESULTS
• May increase ALT, AST, bilirubin, and CK levels.
• May cause thyroid function test abnormalities.

CONTRAINDICATIONS & CAUTIONS
• Contraindicated in patients hypersensitive to drug and in those with active liver disease or unexplained persistently increased transaminase level.
• Use cautiously in patients who consume substantial quantities of alcohol or have a history of liver disease.
• Drug may increase risk of rare immune-mediated necrotizing myopathy. Treatment with immunosuppressants may be required.
Dialyzable drug: Unknown.

PREGNANCY-LACTATION-REPRODUCTION
• Drug may cause fetal harm and is contraindicated in most patients who are pregnant or may become pregnant. If patient becomes pregnant during therapy, discontinue drug and apprise patient of potential hazard to the fetus.
• May consider using in patients at high risk for CV events during pregnancy (homozygous familial hypercholesterolemia, established CV disease) on an individual basis.
• It isn't known if drug appears in human milk. Use with breastfeeding is contraindicated.

NURSING CONSIDERATIONS
• Have patient follow a diet restricted in saturated fat and cholesterol during therapy.
• Obtain LFT results at the start of therapy; then monitor results periodically.
▓ Heterozygous familial hypercholesterolemia can be diagnosed in adolescent boys and in girls who are at least 1 year postmenarche and are 10 to 17 years old; if after an adequate trial of diet therapy LDL cholesterol level remains over 189 mg/dL or LDL

cholesterol over 160 mg/dL and patient has a positive family history of premature CV disease or two or more other CV disease risk factors.
• Obtain CK level in patients with unexplained muscle pain.
• Discontinue lovastatin immediately if markedly elevated CK levels occur or myopathy is diagnosed or suspected. Predisposing factors for skeletal muscle effects include advanced age (65 and older), female gender, uncontrolled hypothyroidism, and renal impairment.
• *Look alike–sound alike:* Don't confuse lovastatin with Lotensin.

PATIENT TEACHING
• Instruct patient in safe drug administration and storage.
• Teach patient about proper dietary management of cholesterol and triglycerides. When appropriate, recommend weight control, exercise, and smoking cessation programs.
• Advise patient of risk of myopathy and rhabdomyolysis and to promptly report unexplained muscle pain, tenderness, or weakness, particularly when accompanied by malaise or fever.
• Teach patient about substances that shouldn't be taken with lovastatin and to inform other health care providers about taking lovastatin, especially if a new medication is being prescribed.
• Caution patient to avoid grapefruit juice while taking drug.
🔔 *Alert:* Tell patient of childbearing potential to immediately stop drug and report pregnancy, suspected pregnancy, or breastfeeding.

---

lurasidone hydrochloride
loo-RAS-i-dohne

Latuda🖊

Therapeutic class: Antipsychotics
Pharmacologic class: Dopamine–serotonin receptor antagonists

AVAILABLE FORMS
Tablets: 20 mg, 40 mg, 60 mg, 80 mg, 120 mg

INDICATIONS & DOSAGES
Adjust-a-dose (for all indications): For patients with moderate (CrCl of 30 to less than

50 mL/minute) or severe (CrCl of less than 30 mL/minute) renal impairment or those concomitantly taking a moderate CYP3A4 inhibitor, recommended starting dose is 20 mg and maximum recommended dose is 80 mg. For patients with moderate (Child-Pugh score 7 to 9) or severe (Child-Pugh score 10 to 15) hepatic impairment, recommended starting dose is 20 mg. Maximum recommended dose is 80 mg for patients with moderate hepatic impairment and 40 mg for those with severe hepatic impairment. If moderate CYP3A4 inducer is used concomitantly, it may be necessary to increase lurasidone dosage.

➤ **Schizophrenia**

Adults: Initially, 40 mg PO once daily. May increase to maximum dose of 160 mg daily.

Adolescents ages 13 to 17: 40 mg PO once daily. May increase to maximum dose of 80 mg daily.

➤ **Depressive episodes associated with bipolar I disorder as monotherapy or as adjunctive therapy with lithium or valproate**

Adults: Initially, 20 mg PO once daily. May increase to maximum of 120 mg daily.

➤ **Depressive episodes associated with bipolar I disorder (monotherapy)**

Children ages 10 to 17: 20 mg PO once daily. May increase after 1 week to maximum dose of 80 mg daily.

ADMINISTRATION
PO
• Give with food containing at least 350 calories.

ACTION
Exact mechanism is unknown. Drug's efficacy is mediated through antagonism at the dopamine type 2 and serotonin type 2 receptors.

Route	Onset	Peak	Duration
PO	Unknown	1–3 hr	Unknown

Half-life: 18 to 40 hours.

ADVERSE REACTIONS
CNS: somnolence, akathisia, extrapyramidal symptoms, agitation, dystonia, dizziness, insomnia, abnormal dreams, anxiety, restlessness, fatigue. **CV:** tachycardia. **EENT:** blurred vision, nasopharyngitis, rhinitis, oropharyngeal pain, dry mouth, increased salivation. **GI:** nausea, vomiting, dyspepsia, abdominal pain, diarrhea, dysphagia, increased appetite. **GU:** UTI, increased creatinine level. **Metabolic:** dyslipidemia, hyperglycemia, weight gain. **Musculoskeletal:** back pain. **Respiratory:** URI. **Skin:** rash, pruritus. **Other:** flulike symptoms.

INTERACTIONS
Drug-drug. *Antihypertensives:* May increase risk of hypotension. Monitor orthostatic vital signs and adjust antihypertensive dosage as needed.

Centrally acting drugs: May increase risk of adverse effects (increased cognitive impairment). Avoid use together.

Moderate CYP3A4 inducers (bosentan, efavirenz, etravirine, modafinil, nafcillin): May decrease lurasidone level. Consider increasing lurasidone dosage.

Moderate inhibitors of CYP3A4 (atazanavir, diltiazem, erythromycin, fluconazole, verapamil): May increase lurasidone level. Use together cautiously and reduce lurasidone dosage by 50%. Initial recommended lurasidone dose is 20 mg daily, with maximum dose of 80 mg daily.

Opioids: May cause slow or difficult breathing, sedation, and death. Avoid use together. If use together is necessary, limit dosage and duration of each drug to minimum necessary for desired effect.

Strong inducers of CYP3A4 (carbamazepine, phenytoin, rifampin): May significantly reduce lurasidone level. Don't use together.

Strong inhibitors of CYP3A4 (clarithromycin, ketoconazole, ritonavir, voriconazole): May significantly increase lurasidone level. Use together is contraindicated.

Drug-herb. *Kava kava:* May enhance adverse or toxic effect of CNS depressants. Monitor therapy.

St. John's wort: May significantly reduce lurasidone level. Don't use together.

Drug-food. *Grapefruit, grapefruit juice:* May increase lurasidone level. Patient should avoid grapefruit and grapefruit juice during therapy.

Drug-lifestyle. *Alcohol use, cannabidiol, cannabis:* May increase CNS depressant effect and risk of adverse effects (such as increased cognitive impairment). Discourage use together.

EFFECTS ON LAB TEST RESULTS

• May increase prolactin, total cholesterol, triglyceride, glucose, serum creatinine, AST, ALT, and CK levels.
• May decrease WBC, neutrophil, and granulocyte counts.

CONTRAINDICATIONS & CAUTIONS

• Contraindicated in patients hypersensitive to drug or its components.
⊕ Alert: *Opioid class warning:* Opioids should only be prescribed with benzodiazepines or other CNS depressants to patients for whom alternative treatment options are inadequate.
Boxed Warning Older adults with dementia-related psychosis treated with atypical or conventional antipsychotics are at increased risk for death. Antipsychotics aren't approved for the treatment of dementia-related psychosis. ■
• Use cautiously in patients with hyperlipidemia, diabetes or risk factors for diabetes (family history, obesity), seizures or conditions that lower the seizure threshold (Alzheimer dementia), body temperature dysregulation, major depressive disorder, suicidality, dysphagia, or concomitant illness.
• Use cautiously in patients with known CV disease, cerebrovascular disease, and conditions that cause hypotension (dehydration, hypovolemia, antihypertensive use) and in patients who are antipsychotic-naive because of increased risk of dizziness, tachycardia or bradycardia, and syncope.
• Use cautiously in patients with preexisting low WBC count or a history of drug-induced neutropenia or leukopenia.
• Use cautiously in patients at risk for falls, including those with diseases or conditions or who are taking medications that may cause somnolence, orthostatic hypotension, or motor or sensory instability.
• Safety and effectiveness haven't been established in children with depression.
Dialyzable drug: Unknown.

PREGNANCY-LACTATION-REPRODUCTION

• There are no adequate studies during pregnancy. Use during pregnancy only if clearly needed and potential benefit justifies fetal risk. Drug may cause abnormal muscle movements (extrapyramidal symptoms) or withdrawal symptoms in newborns.
• Enroll patients exposed to lurasidone during pregnancy in the National Pregnancy Registry for Atypical Antipsychotics (1-866-961-2388).
• It isn't known if drug appears in human milk. Patient should discontinue breastfeeding or discontinue drug.

NURSING CONSIDERATIONS

Boxed Warning Antidepressants increase risk of suicidality in children, adolescents, and young adults. Monitor all patients for worsening of depression or emergence of suicidality. ■
• Monitor patients for tardive dyskinesia. Risk increases in older adults and women and with long-term administration. Use the lowest dose for the shortest time possible to minimize risk. Discontinue drug if symptoms occur.
• Monitor patients for extrapyramidal symptoms (bradykinesia, cogwheel rigidity, drooling, extrapyramidal disorder, hypokinesia, muscle rigidity, psychomotor retardation, tremor).
• Monitor patients for orthostatic hypotension, syncope, and excessive sedation.
• Monitor patients for signs and symptoms of NMS, such as fever, diaphoresis, muscle rigidity, altered mental status, irregular pulse or BP, cardiac arrhythmias, increased CK level, rhabdomyolysis, and acute renal failure. Discontinue drug immediately if NMS occurs.
• Monitor CBC, renal function, and prolactin level periodically; discontinue drug if severe neutropenia develops.
• Monitor patients for metabolic changes (such as weight gain and elevated blood glucose, triglyceride, or cholesterol levels), and treat appropriately.
• Complete fall risk assessments at start of therapy and recurrently for patients on long-term therapy, especially for patients with diseases or conditions or who are taking other medications that could exacerbate fall risk.

PATIENT TEACHING

• *Opioid class warning:* Caution patient or caregiver of patient taking an opioid with a benzodiazepine, CNS depressant, or alcohol to seek immediate medical attention for dizziness, light-headedness, extreme sleepiness, slowed or difficult breathing, or unresponsiveness.

Boxed Warning Advise family or caregivers to observe patient closely for worsening of depression or suicidality. Encourage them to report such behaviors to health care provider immediately. ■

• Advise patient to take drug on a regular basis and not to skip doses.

• Inform patient that periodic blood tests will be needed to monitor tolerance to the drug.

• Tell patient to avoid overheating and to maintain adequate hydration.

• Teach patient to monitor weight and maintain a healthy diet because drug may increase weight and blood glucose and cholesterol levels.

• Instruct patient to report all adverse reactions and to immediately report sudden changes in temperature or BP, irregular HR, or severe muscle rigidity.

• Counsel patient of childbearing potential to report pregnancy or breastfeeding before taking drug.

• Tell patient to avoid alcohol and grapefruit products during therapy.

• Warn patient to avoid driving or operating hazardous machinery until drug's effects are known.

SAFETY ALERT!

magnesium sulfate (injection)

Therapeutic class: Electrolyte replacements
Pharmacologic class: Minerals

AVAILABLE FORMS
Injectable: 4%, 8%, 50% in 2-, 10-, 20-, and 50-mL ampules, vials, and prefilled syringes
Injection solution: 1%, 2%, 4%, 8% in pre-mixed single-dose containers

INDICATIONS & DOSAGES
Adjust-a-dose (for all indications): In severe renal impairment, reduce dosage and obtain frequent serum magnesium levels. Dosing recommendations may vary by manufacturer and clinical guidelines. *Note:* 1 g = 8.12 mEq of magnesium.

➤ **Mild hypomagnesemia**
Adults: 1 g IM every 6 hours for four doses, or 1 to 2 g IV over 1 to 2 hours depending on magnesium level.

➤ **Symptomatic severe hypomagnesemia, with magnesium level of 1 mg/dL or less**

Adults: 5 g IV in 1 L of D_5W or NSS over 3 hours; or 4 to 8 g IV over 4 to 24 hours. Base subsequent doses on magnesium level.

➤ **Magnesium supplementation in TPN**
Adults: 8 to 24 mEq IV daily added to TPN solution.
Infants: 2 to 10 mEq/day IV added to TPN solution.

➤ **Seizures in preeclampsia or eclampsia**
Adults: Total initial dose is 10 to 14 g IV. To accomplish this, give 4 to 5 g IV in 250 mL of solution and simultaneously give up to 10 g IM (5 g or 10 mL of the undiluted 50% solution in each buttock). Or, give initial dose of 4 to 6 g IV over 15 minutes. Or, dilute the 50% solution to a 10% to 20% concentration, and give an initial dose of 4 g IV over 3 to 4 minutes. Subsequently, give 4 to 5 g (8 to 10 mL of the 50% solution) IM into alternate buttocks every 4 hours as needed.

After initial IV dose, 1 to 2 g/hour by constant IV infusion. Base subsequent doses on magnesium level; serum magnesium level of 6 mg/100 mL is considered optimal for seizure control. Don't exceed 40 g in a 24-hour period. Maximum dose in patients with severe renal insufficiency is 20 g/48 hours. Administration beyond 7 days isn't recommended.

ADMINISTRATION
IV/IM
• Store between 68° and 77° F (20° and 25° C). Protect from freezing.
• Discard unused portion.
IV
▼ Dilute solution for IV infusion to a concentration of 20% or less.
▼ Visually inspect solution for particulate matter and discoloration; don't give unless solution is clear and colorless to slightly yellow.
▼ Rate of injection by IV push generally shouldn't exceed 150 mg/minute.
▼ Use an infusion pump for continuous infusion to avoid respiratory or cardiac arrest.
▼ For severe hypomagnesemia, watch for respiratory depression and evidence of heart block. Respirations should be better than 16 breaths/minute before giving dose.
▼ **Incompatibilities:** Alcohol (in high concentrations); alkali carbonates, bicarbonates, and hydroxides; barium; calcium chloride; calcium gluconate; cefuroxime; clindamycin; heavy metals; polymyxin B

Reactions in bold italics are *life-threatening*. Interactions may have a *rapid onset* or a **delayed onset**.

sulfate; procaine; salicylates; strontium; tartrates. Magnesium salt precipitate may occur when combined with multiple solutions; consult a drug incompatibility reference for more information.

IM
• Undiluted 50% solutions may be given by deep IM injection to adults. Dilute solutions to 20% or less for use in children.

ACTION

Replaces magnesium and maintains magnesium level; as an anticonvulsant, reduces muscle contractions by interfering with release of acetylcholine at myoneural junction.

Route	Onset	Peak	Duration
IV	Immediate	Unknown	30 min
IM	1 hr	Unknown	3–4 hr

Half-life: Unknown.

ADVERSE REACTIONS

CNS: *CNS depression,* weak or absent deep tendon reflexes, paralysis, drowsiness, stupor. **CV:** *bradycardia, arrhythmias, hypotension, circulatory collapse, flushing.* **EENT:** visual disturbances. **GI:** diarrhea. **Metabolic:** *hypocalcemia,* hypermagnesemia. **Respiratory:** *respiratory distress, pulmonary edema,* decreased respiratory rate. **Skin:** diaphoresis. **Other:** hypothermia.

INTERACTIONS

Drug-drug. *Calcium channel blockers:* May increase magnesium-related adverse effects. Monitor therapy.
Cardiac glycosides: May cause serious cardiac conduction changes. Use together with caution.
CNS depressants: May increase CNS depression. Use together cautiously.
Drugs that induce magnesium loss (amphotericin B, cisplatin, cyclosporine, loop diuretics, thiazide diuretics): May reduce effectiveness of magnesium replacement. Monitor magnesium level closely.
Neuromuscular blockers: May cause increased neuromuscular blockage. Use together cautiously. Closely monitor clinical response.
Drug-lifestyle. *Alcohol use:* May decrease magnesium level. Discourage use together.

EFFECTS ON LAB TEST RESULTS
• May decrease calcium level.

CONTRAINDICATIONS & CAUTIONS
• Contraindicated in patients with myasthenia gravis, myocardial damage, heart block, or diabetic coma.
• Use cautiously in patients with impaired renal function.
⊖ *Alert:* Using magnesium sulfate to stop preterm labor isn't an FDA-approved use of drug; safety and effectiveness of drug for this indication haven't been established.
Dialyzable drug: Yes.
⚠ *Overdose S&S:* Hypotension, facial flushing, feeling of warmth, thirst, nausea, vomiting, lethargy, dysarthria, drowsiness, diminished deep tendon reflexes, shallow respirations, apnea, coma, cardiac arrest, respiratory paralysis, disappearance of patellar reflex.

PREGNANCY-LACTATION-REPRODUCTION
⊖ *Alert:* Drug can cause fetal abnormalities (fetal hypocalcemia, bone abnormalities), especially when given beyond 5 to 7 days to patients who are pregnant. Use during pregnancy only if clearly needed, and inform patient of potential fetal harm.
• When drug is administered by continuous IV infusion (especially for more than 24 hours preceding delivery) to control seizures in patient with eclampsia, the neonate may show signs of magnesium toxicity, including neuromuscular or respiratory depression.
• Drug appears in human milk. Use cautiously during breastfeeding.

NURSING CONSIDERATIONS
• Keep IV calcium available to reverse magnesium intoxication.
• If appropriate, test knee-jerk and patellar reflexes before each additional dose. If absent, notify prescriber and give no more magnesium until reflexes return; otherwise, patient may develop temporary respiratory failure and need cardiopulmonary resuscitation or IV administration of calcium.
• Check magnesium level after repeated doses. Monitor levels hourly in patients with severe hypomagnesemia. Normal plasma magnesium level is 1.5 to 2.5 mEq/L.
• Monitor fluid intake and output. Output should be 100 mL or more during 4-hour period before dose.
• Monitor renal function.
• Drug may contain aluminum. Premature neonates are at higher risk for aluminum

M

toxicity due to immature renal function. Aluminum exposure of more than 4 to 5 mcg/kg/day is associated with CNS and bone toxicity.

• Patients with prolonged exposure to magnesium sulfate who have impaired renal function are at risk for aluminum toxicity.

• *Look alike–sound alike:* Don't confuse magnesium sulfate with manganese sulfate.

PATIENT TEACHING

• Explain use and administration of drug to patient and family.

• Emphasize importance of keeping lab appointments.

• Tell patient about warning signs of high or low magnesium level. Encourage patient to report all adverse effects.

• Instruct patient to report pregnancy or plans to become pregnant during therapy.

mannitol
MAN-i-tole

Osmitrol

Therapeutic class: Diuretics
Pharmacologic class: Osmotic diuretics

AVAILABLE FORMS
Injection: 5%, 10%, 15%, 20%, 25%
Solution for irrigation: 5 g/100 mL

INDICATIONS & DOSAGES

🔆 *Alert:* Dosage, concentration, and rate of administration depend on the age, weight, and condition of patient, including fluid requirement, urine output, and concomitant therapy. The following indications are only general guides to therapy.

➤ **To reduce IOP**
Adults and children: 1.5 to 2 g/kg as a 15% or 20% single-dose solution given IV over at least 30 minutes. For maximum IOP reduction before surgery, give 60 to 90 minutes preoperatively.

➤ **To reduce ICP and treat cerebral edema**
Adults and children: Usually a maximum reduction in ICP in adults can be achieved with a dose of 0.25 g/kg IV over 30 minutes; may repeat every 6 to 8 hours.

Adjust-a-dose: Monitor fluid and electrolyte levels, serum osmolarity, and renal, cardiac, and pulmonary function during and after

infusion. Discontinue if renal, cardiac, or pulmonary status worsens or CNS toxicity develops.

➤ **Irrigating solution during transurethral surgical procedures**
Adults: Irrigate bladder with 5% solution.

ADMINISTRATION
Intravesicular

• Mannitol 5% for irrigation isn't for injection; administer only through transurethral urologic instruments.

• Don't warm above 150° F (66° C).

• Solution contains no preservative; discard unused portion.

• Store at room temperature.

IV

▼ IV infusion through a central venous catheter is preferable.

▼ To redissolve crystallized solution (crystallization occurs at low temperatures or in concentrations higher than 15%), warm containers according to manufacturer's instructions with occasional shaking. Cool to body temperature before giving. Don't use solution with undissolved crystals.

▼ Give as intermittent or continuous infusion at prescribed rate, using an inline filter and an infusion pump. Don't give as direct injection. Don't use polyvinyl chloride bags in series connections.

▼ Give through filtered administration set; use a blood filter set to avoid infusing crystals.

▼ Check patency at infusion site before and during administration.

▼ Monitor patient for signs and symptoms of infiltration; if it occurs, watch for inflammation, edema, and necrosis. Don't give IM or subcut.

▼ Turn off pump before container runs dry.

▼ Discard unused portion.

▼ Store at room temperature; don't freeze.

▼ **Incompatibilities:** Blood products and other drugs.

ACTION

Increases osmotic pressure of glomerular filtrate, thus inhibiting tubular reabsorption of water and electrolytes. Drug elevates plasma osmolality and increases urine output.

Route	Onset	Peak	Duration
IV	0.5–3 hr	20–40 min	3–6 hr

Half-life: 0.5 to 2.5 hours.

Reactions in bold italics are *life-threatening*. Interactions may have a *rapid onset* or a ***delayed onset***.

ADVERSE REACTIONS

CNS: *seizures,* dizziness, confusion, headache, *coma,* lethargy, malaise, asthenia, fever, *rebound increased ICP.* **CV:** edema, thrombophlebitis, hypotension, HTN, *HF,* tachycardia, palpitations, angina pectoris, vascular overload, *cardiac arrest.* **EENT:** blurred vision, dry mouth, rhinitis. **GI:** thirst, nausea, vomiting, diarrhea. **GU:** *acute kidney injury,* urine retention, *anuria,* oliguria, hematuria, osmotic nephrosis, azotemia, polyuria. **Metabolic:** dehydration, fluid and electrolyte imbalance, *metabolic acidosis,* metabolic alkalosis. **Musculoskeletal:** arm pain, myalgia, rigidity. **Respiratory:** *pulmonary edema,* cough. **Skin:** local pain, urticaria, injection-site reaction (erythema, infection), diaphoresis. **Other:** chills, hypersensitivity reactions.

INTERACTIONS

Drug-drug. *Diuretics:* May increase risk of renal toxicity. Avoid use together.
Lithium: May increase urinary excretion of lithium. Monitor lithium level closely.
Nephrotoxic drugs (aminoglycosides, cyclosporine): May increase risk of toxicity and renal failure. Avoid use together.
Neurotoxic drugs (aminoglycosides): May increase risk of CNS toxicity. Avoid use together.
Opioid analgesics: May increase diuretic-related adverse effects and diminish therapeutic effects of diuretics. Monitor therapy.
Sodium phosphates: May enhance nephrotoxic effect of sodium phosphates. Consider therapy modification.
Tobramycin: Mannitol (systemic) may enhance nephrotoxic effect of tobramycin (oral inhalation). Avoid combination.

EFFECTS ON LAB TEST RESULTS

• May increase or decrease sodium, potassium, and other electrolyte levels.
• May interfere with tests for inorganic phosphorus or ethylene glycol level.

CONTRAINDICATIONS & CAUTIONS

• Contraindicated in patients hypersensitive to drug.
• Contraindicated in patients with anuria, severe pulmonary congestion, frank pulmonary edema, active intracranial bleeding (except during craniotomy), or severe hypovolemia.

• Approved for use in children for the reduction of ICP and IOP. Studies haven't defined the optimal dose in children. The safety profile for use in children is similar to that of adults. However, children younger than age 2, particularly preterm and term neonates, may be at higher risk for fluid and electrolyte abnormalities due to decreased GFR and limited ability to concentrate urine.
• Mannitol may increase risk of postoperative bleeding after neurosurgical procedure or traumatic brain injury, due to increased cerebral blood flow.
• Use cautiously in older adults and patients with renal impairment.
Dialyzable drug: Yes.
⚠ *Overdose S&S:* Renal failure, increased electrolyte excretion, orthostatic tachycardia or hypotension, decreased central venous pressure, CNS toxicity (coma, seizures), impaired neuromuscular function, intestinal dilation and ileus, HF, pulmonary edema or water intoxication if urine output is inadequate.

PREGNANCY-LACTATION-REPRODUCTION

• There are no adequate studies during pregnancy. Use during pregnancy only if potential benefit justifies fetal risk.
• It isn't known if drug appears in human milk. Use cautiously during breastfeeding.

NURSING CONSIDERATIONS

• Monitor vital signs, including central venous pressure and fluid intake and output hourly. Report increasing oliguria. Check weight, renal function, fluid balance, and serum and urine sodium and potassium levels daily.
• When treating elevated ICP, also monitor serum osmolarity, electrolyte levels, acid-base balance, osmol gap, and renal, cardiac, and pulmonary function.
• Use urinary catheter in patient with urinary incontinence or coma because therapy requires strict evaluation of fluid intake and output. If patient has urinary catheter, use an hourly urometer collection system to evaluate output accurately.
• To relieve thirst, give frequent oral care or fluids.
• Monitor IV site closely for infiltration and extravasation; drug is a vesicant at concentrations greater than 5%. Extravasation must be treated with hyaluronidase.

- Don't give electrolyte-free solutions with blood. If blood is given simultaneously, add at least 20 mEq of sodium chloride to each liter of drug solution to avoid pseudoagglutination.
- *Look alike–sound alike:* Don't confuse Osmitrol with esmolol.

PATIENT TEACHING

- Tell patient that thirstiness or dry mouth may occur; emphasize importance of drinking only the amount of fluids ordered.
- Instruct patient to promptly report adverse reactions and discomfort at IV site.

maraviroc

mahr-AY-vih-rok

Celsentri✤, Selzentry

Therapeutic class: Antiretrovirals
Pharmacologic class: CCR5 co-receptor antagonists

AVAILABLE FORMS

Oral solution: 20 mg/mL
Tablets ⊙: 25 mg, 75 mg, 150 mg, 300 mg

INDICATIONS & DOSAGES

➤ **Combined with CYP3A4 inhibitors, including protease inhibitors (except tipranavir and ritonavir), delavirdine, elvitegravir–ritonavir, ketoconazole, itraconazole, clarithromycin, other potent CYP3A inhibitors (nefazodone), or boceprevir, to treat only CCR5-tropic HIV-1 infection**
Adults and children age 2 and older weighing more than 40 kg: 150 mg PO b.i.d.
Children age 2 and older weighing 30 to less than 40 kg: 100 mg PO b.i.d.
Children age 2 and older weighing 20 to less than 30 kg: 75 mg (tablets) or 80 mg (oral solution) PO b.i.d.
Children age 2 and older weighing 10 to less than 20 kg: 50 mg PO b.i.d.
Adjust-a-dose: For adults with CrCl of 30 mL/minute or more, no adjustment is needed. Drug is contraindicated in patients with CrCl of less than 30 mL/minute or in those with ESRD on regular hemodialysis.
➤ **Combined with noninteracting concomitant medications (all medications that aren't potent CYP3A inhibitors or inducers), including all NRTIs, dolutegravir,**

tipranavir–ritonavir, nevirapine, raltegravir, or enfuvirtide to treat CCR5-tropic HIV-1 infection
Adults and children age 2 and older weighing 30 kg or more: 300 mg PO b.i.d.
Children weighing 14 to less than 30 kg: 200 mg (10 mL) PO b.i.d.
Children weighing 10 to less than 14 kg: 150 mg (7.5 mL) PO b.i.d.
Children weighing 6 to less than 10 kg: 100 mg (5 mL) PO b.i.d.
Children weighing 4 to less than 6 kg: 40 mg (2 mL) PO b.i.d.
Children weighing 2 to less than 4 kg: 30 mg (1.5 mL) PO b.i.d.
Adjust-a-dose: For adults with renal impairment, no dosage adjustment is needed. If patient with CrCl of less than 30 mL/minute or ESRD on hemodialysis experiences orthostatic hypotension, reduce dosage to 150 mg PO b.i.d.
➤ **Combined with potent CYP3A inducers (without a potent CYP3A inhibitor), including efavirenz, rifampin, etravirine, carbamazepine, phenobarbital, and phenytoin, to treat CCR5-tropic HIV-1 infection**
Adults: 600 mg PO b.i.d.
Adjust-a-dose: Use is contraindicated in patients with CrCl of less than 30 mL/minute and in those with ESRD on regular hemodialysis. Use isn't recommended in children.

ADMINISTRATION

PO

- Give drug without regard for food.
- Patient should swallow tablets whole and not chew them. Use of oral solution is preferred to crushing tablets.
- Use oral solution in patients who can't swallow tablets.
- Use oral dosing syringe for oral solution.
- Give missed dose as soon as possible; don't double next dose or give more than prescribed dose.

ACTION

Blocks viral entry into cells by binding to chemokine receptor type 5 co-receptor and preventing the initiation of HIV replication cycle.

Route	Onset	Peak	Duration
PO	Unknown	30 min–4 hr	Unknown

Half-life: 14 to 18 hours.

Reactions in bold italics are *life-threatening*. Interactions may have a *rapid onset* or a *delayed onset*.

ADVERSE REACTIONS

CNS: anxiety, dizziness, paresthesia, sensory abnormalities, peripheral neuropathy, sleep disturbances, depressive disorders, fever, pain, memory loss, tremor, facial palsy, disturbances in consciousness, *stroke, seizure.* **CV:** unstable angina, *acute cardiac failure,* CAD, endocarditis, *MI,* myocardial ischemia, vascular hypertensive disorders, edema. **EENT:** conjunctivitis, hemianopia, visual field defect, ocular infections, otitis media, ear disorders, nasal congestion, paranasal sinus disorders, sinusitis, rhinitis, esophageal candidiasis. **GI:** abdominal pain, constipation, dyspepsia, stomatitis, appetite disorders, diarrhea, flatulence, bloating abdominal distention, GI atonic and hypomotility disorders, vomiting. **GU:** urinary tract signs and symptoms, anogenital warts, erection and ejaculation disorders. **Hematologic:** anemia, *neutropenia.* **Hepatic:** cirrhosis, *hepatic failure, portal vein thrombosis,* cholestatic jaundice, increased transaminase levels, hyperbilirubinemia. **Metabolic:** lipodystrophies, increased lipase level. **Musculoskeletal:** muscle pains, joint pain, myositis, osteonecrosis, *rhabdomyolysis.* **Respiratory:** URI, lower respiratory infection, bronchitis, cough, pneumonia, breathing abnormalities. **Skin:** rash, folliculitis, pruritus, apocrine and eccrine gland disorders, lithodystrophy, erythema, benign skin neoplasms, nail changes, acne, alopecia. **Other:** herpes infection, bacterial infection, tinea infection, viral infection, immune reconstitution syndrome, influenza.

INTERACTIONS

Drug-drug. *Boceprevir, clarithromycin, CYP3A inhibitors (protease inhibitors except tipranavir–ritonavir), delavirdine, elvitegravir–ritonavir, itraconazole, ketoconazole, nefazodone:* May increase maraviroc level. May need to decrease maraviroc dosage.
CYP3A inducers (carbamazepine, efavirenz, etravirine, phenobarbital, phenytoin, rifampin): May decrease maraviroc level. May need to increase maraviroc dosage.
Drug-herb. *St. John's wort:* May decrease maraviroc level. Discourage use together.

EFFECTS ON LAB TEST RESULTS

• May increase AST, ALT, bilirubin, amylase, lipase, and CK levels.
• May decrease ANC and Hb level.

CONTRAINDICATIONS & CAUTIONS

• Contraindicated in patients hypersensitive to drug or its components.
• Contraindicated in patients with severe renal impairment or ESRD (CrCl of less than 30 mL/minute) who are taking potent CYP3A inhibitors or inducers.
Boxed Warning Hepatotoxicity has been reported with maraviroc use. Severe rash or evidence of a systemic allergic reaction (fever, eosinophilia, or elevated IgE level) before the development of hepatotoxicity may occur. Immediately evaluate patients with signs or symptoms of hepatitis or allergic reaction after drug use. ■
🕓 *Alert:* Before starting drug, test for CCR5 tropism. Outgrowth of preexisting low-level CXCR4- or dual/mixed-tropic HIV-1 not detected by tropism testing at screening has been associated with virologic failure.
• Severe and potentially life-threatening skin and hypersensitivity reactions, including SJS, TEN, and DRESS syndrome, have been reported. Discontinue drug if signs or symptoms of hypersensitivity occur.
• Use cautiously in patients with preexisting liver dysfunction or patients who are infected with HBV or HCV.
• Use cautiously in patients at risk for CV events, with a history of postural hypotension, or taking another medication known to lower BP.
• During initial phase of treatment, patients treated with combination antiretroviral therapy may develop an inflammatory response to indolent or residual opportunistic infections (CMV, MAC, *Pneumocystis jiroveci* pneumonia, TB), which may necessitate further evaluation and treatment. Autoimmune disorders (such as Graves disease, polymyositis, and Guillain-Barré syndrome) have also been reported in the setting of immune reconstitution; however, time to onset is more variable, and onset can occur many months after initiation of antiretroviral treatment.
• Because of immune suppression, risk of malignancy may increase.
• Safety and effectiveness in children younger than age 2 and in children with mild or moderate renal impairment haven't been established.
Dialyzable drug: No.

PREGNANCY-LACTATION-REPRODUCTION
• There are no adequate studies during pregnancy. Use during pregnancy only if potential benefit justifies fetal risk.
• Register patients exposed to drug during pregnancy in the Antiretroviral Pregnancy Registry (1-800-258-4263).
• Patient shouldn't breastfeed while taking drug because of potential for HIV transmission and serious adverse reactions in infants.

NURSING CONSIDERATIONS
• Monitor patient closely for signs and symptoms of infection, hepatic and renal impairment, CV events, and skin and hypersensitivity reactions.
• Monitor patient for malignancy with long-term use.
• Assess viral load, CD4 count, and LFT values before and periodically during treatment.
• Monitor BP for hypotension.

PATIENT TEACHING
• Instruct patient to immediately report signs or symptoms of hepatitis or allergic reaction (rash, yellow eyes or skin, dark urine, vomiting, and abdominal pain).
• Caution patient that drug doesn't cure HIV infection and that patient may still develop HIV-related illness, including opportunistic infections.
• Caution patient that drug doesn't reduce risk of transmission of HIV to others.
• If patient who feels dizzy while taking drug to avoid driving or operating machinery.
• Instruct patient to inform provider of pregnancy or plans to become pregnant while taking drug.
• Counsel patient not to breastfeed during therapy.
• Advise patient to take drug every day as prescribed with other antiretrovirals. Tell patient not to change dose or dosing schedule or stop any antiretroviral without consulting prescriber. Inform patient that missed doses may increase risk of resistance.

medroxyPROGESTERone acetate
me-DROKS-ee-proe-JES-te-rone

Depo-Provera, Depo-subQ Provera 104, Provera◆

Therapeutic class: Estrogens
Pharmacologic class: Progestins

AVAILABLE FORMS
Injection (suspension): 104 mg/0.65 mL, 150 mg/mL, 400 mg/mL
Tablets: 2.5 mg, 5 mg, 10 mg

INDICATIONS & DOSAGES
➤ **Abnormal uterine bleeding caused by hormonal imbalance**
Adults: 5 to 10 mg PO daily for 5 to 10 days beginning on day 16 or 21 of menstrual cycle. If patient also has received estrogen, give 10 mg PO daily for 10 days beginning on day 16 of cycle.
➤ **Secondary amenorrhea**
Adults: 5 to 10 mg PO daily for 5 to 10 days. Start at any time during menstrual cycle (usually during latter half of cycle).
➤ **Endometrial hyperplasia**
Patients who are postmenopausal (intact uterus) receiving conjugated estrogen 0.625 mg: 5 or 10 mg PO daily for 12 to 14 consecutive days per month, beginning day 1 or day 16 of cycle.
➤ **Contraception**
Adults: 150 mg (Depo-Provera) IM once every 3 months. Or, 104 mg Depo-subQ Provera subcut once every 3 months. Give first dose during first 5 days of normal menstrual period; only within first 5 days postpartum if patient isn't breastfeeding; and, if patient is exclusively breastfeeding, only at sixth postpartum week. Refer to manufacturer's instructions when switching from another method of contraception.
➤ **Endometriosis-associated pain**
Adults: 104 mg subcut every 3 months (12 to 14 weeks).

ADMINISTRATION
• Hazardous drug; use safe handling and disposal precautions.
PO
• Giving drug immediately before or after a meal increases its bioavailability.

Reactions in bold italics are *life-threatening*. Interactions may have a *rapid onset* or a ***delayed onset***.

IM

- Only a health care professional should inject drug.
- Shake vigorously before use.
- Give by deep IM injection in the gluteal or deltoid muscle.
- IM injection may be painful. Monitor sites for evidence of sterile abscess. Rotate injection sites to prevent muscle atrophy.

Subcutaneous

- Only health care professional should inject drug.
- Shake vigorously for at least 1 minute before use.
- Give subcut injection over 5 to 7 seconds into the upper anterior thigh or abdomen.
- Rotate injection sites.
- Don't rub injection area.

ACTION

Suppresses ovulation, possibly by inhibiting pituitary gonadotropin secretion, thus preventing follicular maturation and causing endometrial thinning.

Route	Onset	Peak	Duration
PO	Rapid	2–4 hr	3–5 days
IM	Slow	3 wk	3–4 mo
Subcut	Unknown	1 wk	Unknown

Half-life: Oral, 12 to 17 hours; IM, 50 days; subcut, 43 days.

ADVERSE REACTIONS

CNS: anxiety, depression, fatigue, asthenia, insomnia, somnolence, pain, dizziness, headache, nervousness, irritability. **CV:** edema, *thromboembolism.* **EENT:** neuro-ocular lesions. **GI:** bloating, abdominal pain, nausea, diarrhea. **GU:** breakthrough bleeding, dysmenorrhea, amenorrhea, cervical erosion, abnormal secretions, decreased libido, vaginitis, vulvovaginal candidiasis, UTI. **Hepatic:** cholestatic jaundice. **Metabolic:** weight changes, decreased glucose tolerance. **Musculoskeletal:** osteoporosis, arthralgia, back pain, lower limb cramp. **Skin:** rash, induration, sterile abscesses, acne, pruritus, melasma, alopecia, hirsutism, injection-site reaction. **Other:** breast tenderness, enlargement, or secretion; hot flashes.

INTERACTIONS

Drug-drug. *Aminoglutethimide, bosentan, carbamazepine, felbamate, fosphenytoin, oxcarbazepine, phenobarbital, phenytoin,* *rifampin, topiramate:* May decrease progestin effects. Monitor patient for diminished therapeutic response. Tell patient to use a non-hormonal contraceptive during therapy with these drugs.
Anticonvulsants, corticosteroids: These drugs can also reduce bone mass. Monitor patient.
Antidiabetics: May diminish antidiabetic therapeutic effects. Monitor therapy.
NNRTIs, protease inhibitors: May cause significant changes (increase or decrease) in plasma levels of progestins. Monitor patients for diminished progestin response and advise using nonhormonal contraception during therapy.
Strong CYP3A inducers (carbamazepine, phenobarbital, phenytoin, rifabutin, rifampin, rifapentine): May decrease progestin effects. Avoid use together.
Strong CYP3A inhibitors (clarithromycin, itraconazole, ketoconazole, nefazodone, ritonavir, telithromycin, voriconazole): May increase progestin effects. Monitor therapy.
Drug-herb. *St. John's wort:* May decrease progestin effects. Avoid use together.
Drug-food. *Grapefruit:* May increase progestin effects. Monitor therapy.
Drug-lifestyle. *Smoking:* May increase risk of adverse CV effects. If smoking continues, may need alternative therapy.

EFFECTS ON LAB TEST RESULTS

- May increase LFT values, glucose level, thyroid-binding globulin levels, coagulation tests, and prothrombin factors II, VII, VIII, IX, and X.
- May decrease plasma and urinary steroid levels, gonadotropin levels, and sex hormone–binding globulin concentrations.
- May increase or decrease total cholesterol, triglyceride, LDL, and HDL levels.

CONTRAINDICATIONS & CAUTIONS

Boxed Warning Estrogens with progestins increase risk of dementia in patients age 65 and older; risk of DVT, PE, stroke, and MI in patients after menopause; and risk of invasive breast cancer in all. Give estrogens with progestins at lowest effective doses and for shortest duration consistent with treatment goals and risks for the individual patient. ∎

- Contraindicated in patients hypersensitive to drug and in those with active thromboembolic disorders or history of thromboembolic disorders, cerebrovascular

M

disease, stroke, breast cancer, history of breast cancer, known or suspected estrogen- or progesterone-dependent neoplasia, known or suspected pregnancy, undiagnosed abnormal vaginal bleeding, missed abortion, or hepatic dysfunction. Tablets are contraindicated in patients with liver dysfunction.

Boxed Warning Injectable drug shouldn't be used for long-term birth control (more than 2 years) unless other forms of birth control are inadequate. Loss of bone mineral density can occur and may not be reversible. ■

• Use cautiously in patients with diabetes, seizures, migraine, cardiac or renal disease, strong family history of breast cancer, asthma, depression, hypoparathyroidism, porphyria, SLE, hepatic hemangiomas, or breast nodules.

Dialyzable drug: Unknown.

⚠ *Overdose S&S:* Nausea, vomiting, dizziness, breast tenderness, abdominal pain, drowsiness, fatigue, withdrawal bleeding.

PREGNANCY-LACTATION-REPRODUCTION

• Drug is contraindicated in pregnancy or suspected pregnancy, or as a diagnostic test for pregnancy.

• Be alert to the possibility of an ectopic pregnancy in patients using medroxyprogesterone contraceptive injection who become pregnant or complain of severe abdominal pain.

• Drug appears in human milk. Tablets aren't recommended for use during breastfeeding. The manufacturer recommends that the injectable form be used with caution during breastfeeding.

• Ovulation and fertility are likely to be delayed after stopping drug.

NURSING CONSIDERATIONS

Boxed Warning Depo-Provera and Depo-subQ Provera may cause a significant loss of bone mineral density. Loss is greater with increasing duration of use and may not be reversible. In adolescents and young adults, drug may reduce peak bone mass and increase risk of osteoporotic fractures in later life. ■

• Monitor patient for pain, swelling, warmth, or redness in calves; sudden, severe headaches; visual disturbances; numbness in extremities; signs of depression; hypersensitivity reactions; and signs or symptoms of liver dysfunction (abdominal pain, dark urine, jaundice).

• Monitor BP regularly during treatment.

• Monitor patients sensitive to fluid retention, including those with epilepsy, migraines, asthma, and cardiac or renal dysfunction.

• Due to risk of CV disorders, stop drug at least 4 to 6 weeks before any surgery associated with an increased risk of thromboembolism or during periods of prolonged immobilization.

• Drug may decrease glucose tolerance; monitor patient with diabetes carefully.

PATIENT TEACHING

• According to FDA regulations, patient must read package insert explaining possible adverse effects of progestins before receiving first dose. Also, give patient verbal explanation.

• Teach patient that this product doesn't protect against HIV or other sexually transmitted diseases.

• Advise patient to take medication with food if GI upset occurs.

🔔 *Alert:* Tell patient to report unusual symptoms immediately and to stop drug and notify prescriber about visual disturbances or migraine.

• Advise patient of the importance of routine BP monitoring and an annual physical exam, including breasts, abdomen, and pelvic organs.

• Teach patient how to perform routine breast self-exam.

• Instruct patient to immediately report breast abnormalities, vaginal bleeding, swelling, yellowing of skin or eyes, dark urine, clay-colored stools, shortness of breath, chest pain, or pregnancy.

• Advise patient that injection must be given every 3 months to maintain adequate contraceptive effects and that use of injections may be limited to 2 years.

• Tell patient that because this is a long-acting method of birth control, it may take some time for fertility to return after the last injection.

• Inform patient that prolonged use may cause amenorrhea.

• Encourage adequate intake of calcium and vitamin D.

• Inform patient that drug may cause intolerance to contact lenses.

Reactions in bold italics are *life-threatening*. Interactions may have a *rapid onset* or a *delayed onset*.

mefloquine hydrochloride
ME-floe-kwin

Therapeutic class: Antimalarials
Pharmacologic class: Quinine derivatives

AVAILABLE FORMS
Tablets: 250 mg

INDICATIONS & DOSAGES

➤ **Acute malaria infections caused by mefloquine-sensitive strains of *Plasmodium falciparum* or *Plasmodium vivax***

Adults: 1,250 mg (five tablets) PO as a single dose. Or, 750 mg PO followed by 500 mg in 6 to 12 hours.
Children age 6 months and older: 20 to 25 mg/kg PO as a single dose. Maximum dose, 1,250 mg. Dosage may be divided into two doses given 6 to 8 hours apart to reduce the incidence and severity of adverse effects.

➤ **To prevent malaria**

Adults and children age 6 months and older weighing more than 45 kg: 250 mg or approximately 5 mg/kg PO once weekly. Preventive therapy should start 1 week before entering endemic area and continue for 4 weeks after returning. Give subsequent doses on same day of each week, preferably after main meal.
Children age 6 months and older weighing 30 to 45 kg: 187.5 mg (three-quarters of a 250-mg tablet) PO once weekly.
Children age 6 months and older weighing 20 to less than 30 kg: 125 mg (one-half of a 250-mg tablet) PO once weekly.

ADMINISTRATION
PO
• Give with food and at least 240 mL of water.
• May crush tablets and suspend in a small amount of water, milk, or other beverage when giving to small children and other patients unable to swallow tablets whole.
• If patient vomits within 30 minutes of receiving dose, repeat full dose; if within 30 to 60 minutes, give a half dose.

ACTION
May be caused by drug's ability to form complexes with hemin and to raise intravesicular pH in parasite acid vesicles.

Route	Onset	Peak	Duration
PO	Unknown	6–24 hr	Unknown

Half-life: 2 to 4 weeks.

ADVERSE REACTIONS
CNS: fever, dizziness, syncope, headache, fatigue, abnormal dreams, insomnia. **EENT:** tinnitus. **GI:** vomiting, nausea, diarrhea, abdominal discomfort or pain, loss of appetite. **Musculoskeletal:** myalgia. **Skin:** rash. **Other:** chills.

INTERACTIONS
Drug-drug. *Antiarrhythmics or beta blockers, antihistamines or H$_1$-blockers, calcium channel blockers, phenothiazines, TCAs:* May prolong QTc interval and increase risk of life-threatening cardiac arrhythmias. Coadminister with caution.
Carbamazepine, phenobarbital, phenytoin, valproic acid: May decrease drug levels and loss of seizure control at start of mefloquine therapy. Monitor anticonvulsant level.
Chloroquine, quinidine, quinine: May increase risk of seizures and ECG abnormalities. Give mefloquine at least 12 hours after last dose.
CYP3A4 inducers (rifampin): May decrease mefloquine plasma concentration and reduce drug's effect. Use together cautiously.
CYP3A4 inhibitors: May increase mefloquine plasma concentration and risk of adverse reactions. Use together cautiously.
Halofantrine, ketoconazole: May cause fatal prolongation of QTc interval if given with or within 15 weeks of last mefloquine dose. Don't use together.
Live-virus vaccines: May decrease immunization result. Complete vaccination at least 3 days before start of mefloquine.

EFFECTS ON LAB TEST RESULTS
• May increase transaminase levels.
• May decrease hematocrit and WBC and platelet counts.

CONTRAINDICATIONS & CAUTIONS
• Contraindicated in patients hypersensitive to mefloquine or related compounds, in those with a history of seizures, and in patients with active or recent history of depression, generalized anxiety disorder, psychosis, schizophrenia, or other major psychiatric disorders.

M

• Other IV antimalarials should be used to initially treat life-threatening or serious malarial infections. Mefloquine may be used after IV treatment is completed.

Boxed Warning Drug may cause neuropsychiatric adverse reactions that can persist after therapy ends. Drug shouldn't be prescribed for prophylaxis in patients with major psychiatric disorders. ∎

• Use cautiously when treating patients with cardiac disease.

• Cases of agranulocytosis and aplastic anemia have been reported in patients taking mefloquine.

• Use cautiously in patients with hepatic impairment.

Dialyzable drug: No.

PREGNANCY-LACTATION-REPRODUCTION

• Studies during pregnancy have shown no increase in the risk of teratogenic effects after mefloquine use; however, risk to a developing fetus can't be ruled out. Use only if clearly needed.

• Drug appears in human milk in small amounts. Use cautiously during breastfeeding.

NURSING CONSIDERATIONS

• Patients with *P. vivax* infections are at high risk for relapse because drug doesn't eliminate the hepatic-phase exoerythrocytic parasites. Give follow-up therapy with primaquine or other 8-aminoquinolines to avoid relapse after treatment of initial infection.

• Monitor LFT results periodically.

• For suspected overdose, induce vomiting or perform gastric lavage because of risk of cardiotoxicity. Mefloquine has produced cardiac reactions similar to those caused by quinidine and quinine.

⚠ *Alert:* Monitor patient for neurologic signs and symptoms (dizziness, vertigo, tinnitus, seizures, insomnia) or psychiatric signs and symptoms (anxiety, paranoia, hallucinations, depression, restlessness, confusion, behavior changes). Signs and symptoms may be more difficult to detect in children.

Boxed Warning During prophylactic use, if psychiatric or neurologic signs and symptoms occur, drug should be discontinued and an alternative drug prescribed. ∎

• In certain cases, such as when a traveler takes other medications, it may be desirable to start prophylaxis 2 to 3 weeks before departure, to assess drug combination tolerance.

PATIENT TEACHING

• Advise patient taking drug for prevention to take dose immediately before or after a meal on the same day each week (to improve adherence) and to begin treatment 1 week before arrival at endemic area.

• Encourage patient to wear protective clothing and to use insect repellents and bednets in addition to medication for maximum protection.

• Instruct patient in safe drug administration, to read the medication guide, and to always carry the information wallet card during therapy.

• Advise patient to use caution when performing activities that require alertness and coordination because dizziness, disturbed sense of balance, and neuropsychiatric reactions may occur.

⚠ *Alert:* Inform patient that dizziness, vertigo, and tinnitus can occur during treatment, may continue for months or years after treatment, or may be permanent.

⚠ *Alert:* Warn patient to immediately report neurologic or psychiatric signs or symptoms and not to stop drug until discussing with prescriber.

• Counsel patient undergoing long-term therapy to have periodic ophthalmic exams because drug may cause ocular lesions.

• Advise patient of childbearing potential to use reliable contraception during treatment.

SAFETY ALERT!

megestrol acetate
me-JES-trole

Megace ES

Therapeutic class: Antineoplastics
Pharmacologic class: Progestins

AVAILABLE FORMS

Oral suspension: 40 mg/mL
Oral suspension (concentrated): 125 mg/mL
Tablets: 20 mg, 40 mg, 160 mg✲

INDICATIONS & DOSAGES

➤ **Breast cancer (palliative treatment)**
Adults: 40 mg PO q.i.d. for at least 2 months. Use tablets only.
➤ **Endometrial cancer (palliative treatment)**
Adults: 40 to 320 mg PO daily in divided doses for at least 2 months. Use tablets only.

➤ **Anorexia, cachexia, or unexplained significant weight loss in patients with AIDS**
Adults: 400 to 800 mg PO (10 to 20 mL regular oral suspension) or 625 mg PO (5 mL concentrated oral suspension) once daily.

➤ **Cancer-related cachexia ♦**
Adults: 200 to 600 mg PO once daily.

ADMINISTRATION
PO
- Drug is hazardous and considered a teratogen. Follow applicable special handling and disposal procedures.
- Give drug without regard for meals.
- Shake suspension well before pouring.
- The 125-mg/mL and 40-mg/mL strength can't be substituted for each other. Ensure use of correct product for dose.
- Protect tablets and oral suspension from heat; protect tablets from light.

ACTION
Inhibits hormone-dependent tumor growth by inhibiting pituitary and adrenal steroidogenesis. Drug may also have direct cytotoxicity; its appetite-stimulating mechanism is unknown.

Route	Onset	Peak	Duration
PO	Unknown	5 hr (suspension); 1–3 hr (tablets)	Unknown

Half-life: Suspension: 20 to 50 hours. Tablets: mean, 34.2 hours.

ADVERSE REACTIONS
CNS: confusion, *seizures,* depression, headache, neuropathy, insomnia, abnormal thinking, mood changes, fever, asthenia, malaise, pain, paresthesia, hypesthesia.
CV: HTN, *cardiomyopathy,* palpitations, chest pain, edema. **EENT:** amblyopia, pharyngitis, oral moniliasis, increased salivation.
GI: nausea, vomiting, diarrhea, flatulence, constipation, dry mouth, increased appetite, abdominal pain, dyspepsia. **GU:** breakthrough menstrual bleeding, impotence, decreased libido, UTI, urinary incontinence, urinary frequency. **Hematologic:** *leukopenia,* anemia. **Hepatic:** hepatomegaly.
Metabolic: hyperglycemia, weight gain.
Musculoskeletal: carpal tunnel syndrome.
Respiratory: dyspnea, pneumonia, cough, lung disorder. **Skin:** alopecia, rash, diaphoresis, pruritus, herpes lesions. **Other:** gynecomastia, tumor flare, hot flushes.

INTERACTIONS
Drug-drug. *Antidiabetics:* May diminish therapeutic effect of antidiabetics. Monitor therapy.
Dofetilide: May increase dofetilide plasma level, increasing risk of life-threatening cardiac arrhythmias, including torsades de pointes. Avoid use together.
Warfarin: May increase INR. Monitor level closely.
Drug-herb. *Bloodroot, yucca:* May enhance adverse effects of progestins. Monitor therapy.

EFFECTS ON LAB TEST RESULTS
- May increase serum glucose, LDH, and urine albumin levels.
- May decrease WBC count.

CONTRAINDICATIONS & CAUTIONS
- Contraindicated in patients hypersensitive to drug.
- Use cautiously in patients with history of thrombophlebitis or thromboembolism.
- Safety and effectiveness in children haven't been established.
- Use cautiously in older adults.
Dialyzable drug: Unlikely.

PREGNANCY-LACTATION-REPRODUCTION
- Drug may cause fetal harm. Oral solution is contraindicated in pregnancy. If used during pregnancy, or if pregnancy occurs during therapy, apprise patient of potential fetal risk. Patient should avoid pregnancy.
- Drug appears in human milk. Patient shouldn't breastfeed during therapy.

NURSING CONSIDERATIONS
- Evaluate pregnancy status before start of treatment.
- May increase glucose level in patients with diabetes.
- Drug isn't intended for prophylactic use to avoid weight loss. Start treatment with megestrol acetate oral suspension only after treatable causes of weight loss are sought and addressed.
- Two months is an adequate trial period in patients with cancer.
- **Alert:** Drug may cause adrenal insufficiency, which can be fatal. Monitor patient for signs and symptoms, such as hypotension, nausea, vomiting, dizziness, or weakness. Glucocorticoid therapy may be needed.

M

PATIENT TEACHING
• Teach patient safe drug administration and handling.
• Inform patient that therapeutic response isn't immediate. Drug must be taken for at least 2 months to determine effectiveness.
🕓 *Alert:* Tell patient that the ES oral suspension is more concentrated than the regular oral suspension, so a smaller amount is needed if prescription is changed.
• Advise patient to stop breastfeeding during therapy because of risk of toxicity to infant.
• Caution patient of childbearing potential to use an effective form of contraception while receiving drug.
• Tell patient to report all adverse reactions, especially signs and symptoms of adrenal insufficiency.

SAFETY ALERT!

melphalan (L-PAM, phenylalanine mustard)
MEL-fa-lan

Alkeran✳

melphalan hydrochloride
Alkeran✳, Evomela

Therapeutic class: Antineoplastics
Pharmacologic class: Nitrogen mustards

AVAILABLE FORMS
Lyophilized powder for injection: 50 mg
Tablets: 2 mg

INDICATIONS & DOSAGES
➤ **Multiple myeloma (palliative treatment)**
Adults: Initially, 6 mg PO daily for 2 to 3 weeks; then stop drug for up to 4 weeks or until WBC and platelet counts stop dropping and begin to rise again; maintenance dose is 2 mg daily. Or, 10 mg/day for 7 to 10 days, followed by 2 mg/day when WBC is greater than 4,000 cells/mm^3 and platelet count is greater than 100,000 cells/mm^3; dosage is adjusted to between 1 and 3 mg/day depending on hematologic response. Or, 0.15 mg/kg PO daily for 7 days followed by a rest period of 2 to 6 weeks; maintenance dose is 0.05 mg/kg/day or less. Or 0.25 mg/kg/day for 4 consecutive days (or 0.2 mg/kg/day for 5 consecutive days) for a total dose of 1 mg/kg/course; repeat every 4 to 6 weeks.

Or, give IV (Alkeran only) to patients who can't tolerate oral therapy, 16 mg/m^2 given by infusion over 15 to 20 minutes at 2-week intervals for four doses. After patient has recovered from toxicity, give drug at 4-week intervals.
Adjust-a-dose: Withhold drug until recovery for WBC count less than 3,000/mm^3 or platelet count less than 100,000/mm^3. For moderate to severe renal impairment, consider a reduced PO dose initially. For patients with renal insufficiency (BUN level of 30 mg/dL or more), consider reducing IV dose 50%.
➤ **Nonresectable advanced epithelial ovarian cancer (palliative treatment)**
Adults: 0.2 mg/kg PO daily for 5 days. Repeat every 4 to 5 weeks, depending on hematologic tolerance.
Adjust-a-dose: For moderate to severe renal impairment, consider a reduced dose initially.
➤ **Multiple myeloma (conditioning treatment before hematopoietic stem cell transplantation) (Evomela)**
Adults: 100 mg/m^2/day by IV infusion over 30 minutes for 2 consecutive days (day –3 and day –2) before autologous stem cell transplantation (day 0).
Adjust-a-dose: For patients weighing more than 130% of their ideal body weight, calculate BSA based on adjusted ideal body weight.
✳ *NEW INDICATION:* **Neuroblastoma (conditioning treatment before hematopoietic stem cell transplantation)** ♦
Children: 140 mg/m^2 IV infusion in combination with busulfan before transplantation. Or, 180 mg/m^2 IV infusion with prehydration and posthydration 12 to 30 hours before transplantation. Or, 45 mg/m^2/day IV infusion for 4 days starting 8 days before transplantation combined with busulfan or etoposide and carboplatin.
➤ **Amyloidosis, light chain** ♦
Adults: 0.22 mg/kg/day PO for 4 days every 28 days (in combination with oral dexamethasone), or 10 mg/m^2/day PO for 4 days every month (in combination with oral dexamethasone) for 12 to 18 treatment cycles.

ADMINISTRATION
PO
🕓 *Alert:* Hazardous drug; use safe handling and disposal precautions.

Reactions in bold italics are *life-threatening*. Interactions may have a *rapid onset* or a *delayed onset*.

- Give on an empty stomach 1 hour before or 2 hours after meals; food decreases drug absorption.
- Store tablets in refrigerator. Protect from light.

IV

Boxed Warning Preparing and giving this form may be mutagenic, teratogenic, or carcinogenic. Follow facility safe handling protocol to reduce risks. ■

▼ IV drug is available in different formulations, with different indications and preparation and storage instructions.

▼ Monitor infusion carefully; drug is considered a vesicant and extravasation may cause local damage. Administer only through a CVAD. Don't give by direct injection through a peripheral vein. If extravasation occurs, stop infusion immediately, notify prescriber, and follow facility protocol for treatment.

Alkeran

▼ Because drug isn't stable in solution, reconstitute immediately before giving with the 10 mL of sterile diluent supplied by manufacturer, using 20G or larger needle. Shake vigorously until solution appears clear. Resulting solution will contain 5 mg/mL of melphalan. Immediately dilute required dose in NSS for injection to no more than 0.45 mg/mL. Give infusion over at least 15 minutes.

▼ Reconstituted product begins to degrade within 30 minutes. Administration must be finished within 60 minutes of reconstitution.

▼ Don't refrigerate reconstituted product because precipitate will form.

Evomela

▼ Use 8.6 mL NSS as directed to reconstitute and make a 50-mg/10 mL (5-mg/mL) nominal concentration.

▼ Reconstituted drug is stable for 24 hours when refrigerated (41° F [5° C]) without any precipitation because of the high solubility, and is stable for 1 hour at room temperature.

▼ Withdraw required volume needed for dose from vial and add to the appropriate volume of NSS to a final concentration of 0.45 mg/mL.

▼ Admixture solution is stable for 4 hours at room temperature in addition to the 1 hour after reconstitution.

▼ Don't mix Evomela with other melphalan hydrochloride for injection products.

▼ Give into a fast-running IV infusion via CVAD; don't give by direct injection into a peripheral vein.

▼ **Incompatibilities:** Amphotericin B, chlorpromazine, D_5W, lactated Ringer injection. Compatibility with NSS injection depends on the concentration; don't prepare solutions with a concentration exceeding 0.45 mg/mL.

ACTION

Cross-links strands of cellular DNA and interferes with RNA transcription, causing an imbalance of growth that leads to cell death. Not specific to cell cycle.

Route	Onset	Peak	Duration
PO	Unknown	About 1–2 hr	Unknown
IV	Unknown	Unknown	Unknown

Half-life: Oral, about 0.5 to 2.25 hours; IV, about 75 minutes.

ADVERSE REACTIONS

CNS: fatigue, fever, dizziness, abnormal taste. **CV:** vasculitis, edema. **GI:** nausea, vomiting, diarrhea, oral ulceration, stomatitis, decreased appetite, constipation, dyspepsia, abdominal pain, blood in stool. **GU:** amenorrhea, testicular suppression, *renal failure.* **Hematologic:** *thrombocytopenia, leukopenia, bone marrow suppression,* hemolytic anemia. **Hepatic:** *hepatotoxicity.* **Metabolic:** *hypokalemia, hypophosphatemia, febrile neutropenia.* **Respiratory:** *pneumonitis, pulmonary fibrosis.* **Skin:** pruritus, alopecia, urticaria, ulceration at injection site. **Other:** *anaphylaxis,* hypersensitivity reactions.

INTERACTIONS

Drug-drug (IV melphalan only. There are no known drug interactions with oral form). *Anticoagulants, aspirin, NSAIDs:* May increase risk of bleeding. Avoid using together.

Carmustine: May decrease threshold for pulmonary toxicity. Use together cautiously.

Cimetidine: May decrease melphalan level. Monitor patient closely.

Cisplatin: May increase renal impairment, decreasing melphalan clearance. Monitor patient closely.

Clozapine: May increase risk of neutropenia. Monitor WBC count carefully.

M

Cyclosporine: May cause severe renal impairment. Monitor renal function closely.

Immunosuppressants (pimecrolimus): May increase risk of immunosuppression. Avoid concurrent use.

Live-virus vaccines: May increase risk of toxicity from live-virus vaccines. Postpone immunization with live-virus vaccines for at least 3 months after last dose of melphalan.

Nalidixic acid: May cause hemorrhagic ulcerative colitis or intestinal necrosis (children). Monitor therapy.

Drug-herb. *Echinacea:* May alter immune system activity. Consider therapy modification.

Drug-food. *Any food:* May decrease oral drug absorption. Advise patient to take drug on an empty stomach.

EFFECTS ON LAB TEST RESULTS
- May increase BUN level.
- May decrease Hb level and RBC, WBC, and platelet counts.
- May cause a false-positive direct Coombs test.

CONTRAINDICATIONS & CAUTIONS
- Contraindicated in patients hypersensitive to drug and in those with disease resistant to drug.
- Contraindicated in patients with severe leukopenia, thrombocytopenia, or anemia and in those with chronic lymphocytic leukemia.
- Use cautiously in patients receiving radiation and chemotherapy.

Dialyzable drug: No.

⚠ *Overdose S&S:* Vomiting, ulceration of the mouth, diarrhea, GI hemorrhage, bone marrow suppression, decreased consciousness, seizures.

PREGNANCY-LACTATION-REPRODUCTION
- There are no adequate studies during pregnancy, but drug may cause fetal harm. Patient should avoid pregnancy by using an effective contraceptive.
- It isn't known if drug appears in human milk; however, excretion into human milk is likely. Don't give during breastfeeding.
- Drug suppresses ovarian function during premenopause, resulting in amenorrhea in a significant number of patients.
- May damage spermatozoa and testicular tissue, resulting in possible genetic fetal

abnormalities. Reversible and irreversible testicular suppression has also been reported.

NURSING CONSIDERATIONS
Boxed Warning Administer drug only under the supervision of a physician experienced in the use of cancer chemotherapeutic agents. ∎

Boxed Warning Severe bone marrow suppression with resulting bleeding or infection may occur. Controlled trials comparing IV to oral melphalan have shown greater myelosuppression with the IV formulation. ∎

Boxed Warning Drug is leukemogenic. It produces chromosomal aberrations in vitro and in vivo and should be considered potentially mutagenic in humans. ∎

Boxed Warning Hypersensitivity reactions, including anaphylaxis, have occurred in approximately 2% of patients who received the IV formulation. Discontinue drug for serious hypersensitivity reactions. ∎

- Dosage reduction may be needed in patients with renal impairment.
- Monitor uric acid level and CBC. Consider leukocyte growth factor for neutropenia if indicated.
- Monitor patient for bleeding, infection, and secondary malignancies
- To prevent bleeding, avoid all IM injections when platelet count falls below 50,000/mm^3.
- Blood transfusions may be needed for cumulative anemia.
- Drug has moderate emetic potential. Consider prophylactic antiemetic.
- Anaphylaxis may occur. Keep antihistamines and steroids readily available to give if needed.
- *Look alike–sound alike:* Don't confuse melphalan with Mephyton.

PATIENT TEACHING
- Teach patient safe oral drug administration and handling.
- Advise patient to report pain or redness at IV site.
- Instruct patient to report all adverse reactions and to watch for signs and symptoms of infection (fever, sore throat, fatigue) and bleeding (easy bruising, nosebleeds, bleeding gums, melena). Tell patient to take temperature daily.
- Caution patient to stop breastfeeding during therapy because of risk of toxicity to infant.

- Inform patient that drug can interfere with menstrual cycle and stop sperm production in men.
- Advise male patient with sexual partners of childbearing potential to use effective contraception during and after treatment.
- Counsel patient of childbearing potential to avoid pregnancy (which may include use of effective contraceptive methods) during and after treatment.
- Inform patient to report nausea, vomiting, and diarrhea. Antiemetics and antidiarrheals may be prescribed.

---

memantine hydrochloride
me-MAN-teen

Ebixa✦, Namenda✔, Namenda XR✔

Therapeutic class: Anti-Alzheimer drugs
Pharmacologic class: N-methyl-D-aspartate receptor antagonists

AVAILABLE FORMS
Capsules (extended-release) ⓝ: 7 mg, 14 mg, 21 mg, 28 mg
Oral solution: 2 mg/mL
Tablets: 5 mg, 10 mg

INDICATIONS & DOSAGES
➤ **Moderate to severe Alzheimer dementia**
Adults: Initially, 5 mg PO once daily. Increase by 5 mg/day every week until target dose is reached. Maximum, 10 mg PO b.i.d. Doses greater than 5 mg should be given in two divided doses.

Or, for extended-release capsules, initially 7 mg PO once daily. Increase as tolerated by 7-mg increments each week to target dosage of 28 mg PO once daily.
To convert from immediate-release to extended-release form: Patients taking immediate-release 10 mg b.i.d. may switch to extended-release 28 mg once daily the day following the last immediate-release tablet. Patients with severe renal failure taking immediate-release 5 mg b.i.d. may switch to extended-release 14 mg once daily the day following the last immediate-release tablet.
Adjust-a-dose: For patients with severe renal impairment (CrCl of 5 to 29 mL/minute), recommended immediate-release form target dosage is 5 mg b.i.d and extended-release form target dosage is 14 mg/day.

ADMINISTRATION
PO
- Give drug without regard for food.
- Patients may take capsules intact or capsules may be opened, sprinkled on applesauce, then swallowed. Don't allow the patient to divide, chew, or crush capsules.
- Use dosing device provided with the oral solution to withdraw correct dose volume. Slowly squirt dose into the corner of patient's mouth.
- Don't mix oral solution with any other liquid.
- If a single dose is missed, omit it. If several days are missed, may need to resume dosing at a lower dose and retitrate.
- Store at room temperature.

ACTION
Antagonizes N-methyl-D-aspartate receptors, the persistent activation of which seems to increase Alzheimer symptoms.

Route	Onset	Peak	Duration
PO (tablets, solution)	Unknown	3–7 hr	Unknown
PO (capsules)	Unknown	9–12 hr	Unknown

Half-life: 60 to 80 hours.

ADVERSE REACTIONS
CNS: aggressiveness, agitation, anxiety, confusion, depression, dizziness, fatigue, hallucinations, headache, pain, somnolence, drowsiness. **CV:** HTN, hypotension. **GI:** constipation, diarrhea, vomiting, abdominal pain. **GU:** incontinence. **Metabolic:** weight gain. **Musculoskeletal:** back pain. **Respiratory:** coughing, dyspnea. **Other:** flulike symptoms.

INTERACTIONS
Drug-drug. *NMDA antagonists (amantadine, dextromethorphan, ketamine):* Effects of combined use unknown. Use together cautiously.
Urine alkalinizers (carbonic anhydrase inhibitors, sodium bicarbonate): May decrease memantine clearance. Monitor patient for adverse effects.
Drug-food. *Foods that alkalinize urine:* May increase drug level and adverse effects. Use together cautiously.
Drug-lifestyle. *Nicotine:* May alter levels of drug and nicotine. Discourage use together.

M

✦Canada   ◇OTC   ◆Off-label use   ✔Photoguide   ⓝDo not crush   *Liquid contains alcohol   ▦Genetic

EFFECTS ON LAB TEST RESULTS
None reported.

CONTRAINDICATIONS & CAUTIONS
• Contraindicated in patients allergic to drug or its components.
• Use cautiously in patients with seizures, CV disease, or severe hepatic or renal impairment.
• Use cautiously in patients who may have an increased urine pH (from drugs, diet, renal tubular acidosis, or severe UTI).
• Use cautiously in patients with corneal disease because condition may worsen. Periodic ophthalmic exams are recommended.
Dialyzable drug: Unknown.
⚠ *Overdose S&S:* Restlessness, psychosis, visual hallucinations, somnolence, stupor, loss of consciousness, agitation, asthenia, bradycardia, confusion, coma, dizziness, ECG changes, HTN, lethargy, unsteady gait, vertigo, vomiting, weakness.

PREGNANCY-LACTATION-REPRODUCTION
• There are no adequate studies during pregnancy. Use during pregnancy only if potential benefit justifies fetal risk.
• It isn't known if drug appears in human milk. Use cautiously during breastfeeding.

NURSING CONSIDERATIONS
• Monitor patient carefully for adverse reactions as patient may not be able to recognize changes or communicate effectively.
• Monitor cognitive and functional status.

PATIENT TEACHING
• Explain that drug doesn't cure Alzheimer disease but may slow the progression and aid patient to maintain function for a longer period of time.
• Instruct patient in proper drug administration, including missed doses.
• Tell patient or caregiver to report adverse effects.
• To avoid possible interactions, advise patient not to take herbal or OTC products without consulting prescriber and to report all current medicines.

meperidine hydrochloride (pethidine hydrochloride)
me-PER-i-deen

Demerol

Therapeutic class: Opioid analgesics
Pharmacologic class: Opioids
Controlled substance schedule: II

AVAILABLE FORMS
Injection: 25 mg/mL, 50 mg/mL, 75 mg/mL, 100 mg/mL
Solution: 50 mg/5 mL
Tablets: 50 mg

INDICATIONS & DOSAGES
Adjust-a-dose (for all indications): Reduce meperidine dosage by 25% to 50% when administered with phenothiazines or other tranquilizers. Use cautiously and initiate at lower end of dosage range in older adults and patients with hepatic and renal impairment; if needed, titrate dosage slowly.
➤ **Moderate to severe pain that requires an opioid analgesic and for which alternative treatments are inadequate**
Adults: 50 to 150 mg PO, IM, or subcut every 3 to 4 hours PRN.
Children: 1.1 to 1.8 mg/kg PO, or 1.1 to 1.8 mg/kg IM or subcut every 3 to 4 hours. Maximum, 50 to 150 mg every 4 hours PRN.
Adjust-a-dose: For pain uncontrolled with total daily dosage of 600 mg PO, titrate drug off and switch to another analgesic.
➤ **Preoperative analgesia**
Adults: 50 to 100 mg IM or subcut 30 to 90 minutes before beginning of anesthesia.
Children: 1.1 to 2.2 mg/kg IM or subcut up to the adult dose 30 to 90 minutes before anesthesia.
➤ **Adjunct to anesthesia**
Adults: Repeated slow IV injections of fractional doses. Or, continuous IV infusion of a more dilute solution (1 mg/mL) titrated to patient's needs.
➤ **Obstetric analgesia**
Adults: 50 to 100 mg IM or subcut when pain becomes regular; may repeat at 1- to 3-hour intervals.

Reactions in bold italics are *life-threatening*. Interactions may have a *rapid onset* or a *delayed onset*.

ADMINISTRATION
PO
- Solution has local anesthetic effect on mucous membranes if not diluted. Give with a half glass of water.
- Oral dose is less than half as effective as parenteral dose. Give IM if possible. When changing from parenteral to oral route, increase dosage.

Boxed Warning Ensure accuracy when administering solution form. Dosing errors due to confusion between mg and mL can lead to fatal outcomes. ∎

IV
▼ Keep opioid antagonist (naloxone) available.

▼ Give drug by direct injection over 2 to 5 minutes.

▼ Drug may also be given by slow continuous infusion. Drug is compatible with most infusion solutions, including D_5W, NSS, and Ringer or lactated Ringer solutions.

▼ Store at room temperature.

▼ **Incompatibilities:** Aminophyllines, barbiturates, iodide, morphine, phenytoin, sodium bicarbonate.

IM
- Inject deep into large muscle mass.

Subcutaneous
- Subcut injection isn't recommended because it's very painful, but it may be suitable for occasional use. Monitor patient for pain at injection site, local tissue irritation, and induration after subcut injection.

ACTION
Unknown. Binds with opioid receptors in the CNS, altering perception of and emotional response to pain.

Route	Onset	Peak	Duration
PO	10–15 min	60–120 min	2–4 hr
IV	5 min	5–7 min	2–3 hr
IM, subcut	10–15 min	30–50 min	2–4 hr

Half-life: Oral, 3 to 8 hours; injectable, 2 to 5 hours.

ADVERSE REACTIONS
CNS: agitation, incoordination, dizziness, dysphoria, euphoria, delirium, lightheadedness, sedation, somnolence, *seizures,* hallucinations, headache, physical dependence, tremor, confusion, disorientation, syncope. **CV:** *bradycardia, cardiac arrest, shock,* hypotension, tachycardia, palpitations, flushing. **EENT:** visual disturbances, dry mouth.

GI: biliary tract spasms, constipation, ileus, nausea, vomiting. **GU:** urine retention. **Musculoskeletal:** muscle twitching, weakness. **Respiratory:** *respiratory arrest, respiratory depression (central sleep apnea, sleep-related hypoxemia).* **Skin:** diaphoresis, pruritus, urticaria. **Other:** induration, local tissue irritation, pain at injection site, phlebitis after IV delivery, hypersensitivity reactions, *anaphylaxis.*

INTERACTIONS
Drug-drug. *Acyclovir:* Increases meperidine plasma concentration and risk of adverse reactions. Use together cautiously.

Anticholinergics (benztropine, darifenacin, oxybutynin): May increase risk of urine retention, constipation, or paralytic ileus. Monitor patient closely.

Boxed Warning *Benzodiazepines, CNS depressants:* May cause slow or difficult breathing, sedation, and death. Avoid use together. If use together is necessary, limit dosage and duration of each drug to the minimum necessary for desired effect. ∎

Cimetidine: May increase respiratory and CNS depression. Monitor patient closely.

Boxed Warning *CYP3A4 inducers (carbamazepine, phenytoin, rifampin):* May increase meperidine level and increase risk of toxicity if inducers are discontinued. Monitor patient closely when discontinuing an inducer. ∎

Boxed Warning *CYP3A4 inhibitors (erythromycin, ketoconazole, ritonavir):* May increase meperidine plasma concentration, which could increase or prolong adverse reactions; may cause fatal respiratory depression. Monitor patient closely. ∎

Diuretics: May reduce efficacy of diuretics. Monitor therapy.

General anesthetics, phenothiazines, TCAs: May cause respiratory depression, hypotension, profound sedation, or coma. Use together with caution; reduce meperidine dosage.

Boxed Warning *MAO inhibitors (linezolid, phenelzine):* May increase CNS and respiratory depression and hypotension that can be severe or fatal. Use of meperidine within 14 days of an MAO inhibitor is contraindicated. ∎

Oxybate salts (calcium, magnesium, potassium, sodium): May increase CNS depression and sleep duration. Avoid use together. If necessary, use together cautiously and monitor patient closely.

M

♣Canada ◇OTC ◆Off-label use ✐Photoguide ⬤Do not crush *Liquid contains alcohol ▓Genetic

Phenytoin: May decrease meperidine level. Watch for decreased analgesia.

Protease inhibitors: May increase respiratory and CNS depression. Avoid using together.

🜂 *Alert:* *Serotonergic drugs (amoxapine, antiemetics [dolasetron, granisetron, ondansetron, palonosetron], antimigraine drugs, buspirone, cyclobenzaprine, dextromethorphan, linezolid, lithium, maprotiline, methylene blue, mirtazapine, nefazodone, SSNRIs, SSRIs, TCAs, trazodone, tryptophan, vilazodone):* May increase risk of serotonin syndrome. Avoid use together. If necessary, use together cautiously and monitor patient for serotonin syndrome.

Drug-herb. *Kava kava:* May enhance adverse effects of CNS depressants. Monitor therapy.

🜂 *Alert:* *St. John's wort:* May increase risk of serotonin syndrome. Use together cautiously and monitor patient for serotonin syndrome.

Drug-lifestyle. **Boxed Warning** *Alcohol use:* May cause additive CNS and respiratory depressive effects. Don't use together. ∎

EFFECTS ON LAB TEST RESULTS
• May increase amylase level.
• May decrease adrenocorticotropic hormone, cortisol, and LH levels.
• May stimulate prolactin, growth hormone, and pancreatic secretion of insulin and glucagon.

CONTRAINDICATIONS & CAUTIONS
• Contraindicated in patients hypersensitive to drug and in those with significant respiratory depression, acute or severe bronchial asthma in an unmonitored setting or in the absence of resuscitative equipment, and with known or suspected GI obstruction, including paralytic ileus.

Boxed Warning Opioids should only be prescribed with benzodiazepines or other CNS depressants when alternative treatment options are inadequate. ∎

Boxed Warning Oral forms are only available through a REMS program to ensure benefits outweigh risks of addiction, abuse, and misuse. ∎

Boxed Warning Drug may increase risks of opioid addiction, abuse, and misuse, which can lead to overdose and death. Risks increase in patients with a personal or family history of substance abuse or mental illness. Assess risks before drug is prescribed. ∎

🜂 *Alert:* Drug may lead to a rare but serious decrease in adrenal gland cortisol production.
• Drug may cause decreased sex hormone levels with long-term use.

🜂 *Alert:* Patients are at increased risk for oversedation and respiratory depression if they snore or have a history of sleep apnea, haven't used opioids recently or are first-time opioid users, have increased opioid dosage requirements or opioid habituation, have received general anesthesia for longer lengths of time or received other sedating drugs, have preexisting pulmonary or cardiac disease, or have thoracic or other surgical incisions that may impair breathing. Monitor patients carefully.

• Use cautiously in older adults or patients who are debilitated and in those with increased ICP, head injury, asthma and other respiratory conditions, supraventricular tachycardias, seizures, abdominal conditions, decreased bowel motility conditions, hepatic or renal disease, hypothyroidism, Addison disease, urethral stricture, and prostatic hyperplasia.

Dialyzable drug: Unknown.

⚠ *Overdose S&S:* Respiratory depression, somnolence progressing to stupor, coma, bradycardia, hypotension, hypothermia, delirium, skeletal muscle flaccidity, circulatory collapse, death.

PREGNANCY-LACTATION-REPRODUCTION
Boxed Warning Prolonged use of drug during pregnancy can result in neonatal opioid withdrawal syndrome, which may be life-threatening and requires management according to protocols developed by neonatology experts. If prolonged use is needed, advise patient of risks and ensure that appropriate treatment will be available. ∎

• Don't use before labor unless physician determines potential benefits outweigh risks; safe use before labor hasn't been established relative to possible adverse effects on fetal development.

• Drug appears in human milk. Patient should discontinue breastfeeding or discontinue drug.

NURSING CONSIDERATIONS
Boxed Warning Regularly monitor patients for opioid addiction, abuse, and misuse. ∎

Boxed Warning Serious, life-threatening, or fatal respiratory depression can occur.

Reactions in bold italics are *life-threatening*. Interactions may have a *rapid onset* or a *delayed onset*.

Monitor patient closely, especially within first 24 to 72 hours of starting drug and after a dosage increase. ■

Boxed Warning Accidental ingestion of even one dose of drug, especially by children, can be fatal. ■

• In older adults, patients using meperidine for longer than 48 hours, those with preexisting renal or CNS disease, and those taking more than 600 mg/day PO, the active metabolite may accumulate, causing increased adverse CNS reactions, including seizures. Avoid prolonged use.

• Monitor patients with biliary tract disease, including acute pancreatitis, for worsening signs and symptoms.

🔔 *Alert:* Carefully monitor vital signs, pain level, respiratory status, and sedation level in all patients receiving opioids, especially those receiving IV drugs, even those given postoperatively.

🔔 *Alert:* If patient is taking opioids with serotonergic drugs, watch for signs and symptoms of serotonin syndrome (agitation, hallucinations, rapid HR, fever, diaphoresis, shivering or shaking, muscle twitching or stiffness, trouble with coordination, nausea, vomiting, diarrhea), especially when starting treatment or increasing dosages. Signs and symptoms may occur within several hours of coadministration but may also occur later, especially after dosage increase. Discontinue the opioid, serotonergic drug, or both if serotonin syndrome is suspected.

🔔 *Alert:* Monitor patient for signs and symptoms of adrenal insufficiency (nausea, vomiting, loss of appetite, fatigue, weakness, dizziness, low BP). Perform diagnostic testing if adrenal insufficiency is suspected. For confirmed adrenal insufficiency, treat with corticosteroids and wean patient off opioids if appropriate. Discontinue corticosteroids when clinically appropriate.

• Monitor patient for signs and symptoms of decreased sex hormone levels (low libido, erectile dysfunction, amenorrhea, infertility). If signs and symptoms occur, evaluate patient and obtain lab testing.

• When giving drug parenterally, make sure patient is lying down.

• Drug may be used in some patients who are allergic to morphine.

• Reassess patient's level of pain at least 15 and 30 minutes after administration.

• Monitor respiratory and CV status carefully. Don't give if respirations are below 12 breaths/minute, if respiratory rate or depth is decreased, or if change in pupils is noted.

• Monitor bladder function after surgical procedures.

• Monitor bowel function. Patient may need a stimulant laxative and stool softener.

🔔 *Alert:* Don't stop drug abruptly; withdraw slowly and individualize gradual taper plan to prevent signs and symptoms of withdrawal, worsening pain, and psychological distress in patients who are physically dependent. Refer to manufacturer's label for specific tapering instructions.

🔔 *Alert:* When tapering opioids, monitor patient closely for signs and symptoms of opioid withdrawal (restlessness, lacrimation, rhinorrhea, yawning, perspiration, chills, myalgia, mydriasis, irritability, anxiety, insomnia, backache, joint pain, weakness, abdominal cramps, anorexia, nausea, vomiting, diarrhea, increased BP or HR, increased respiratory rate), which may indicate a need to taper more slowly. Also monitor patient for suicidality, use of other substances, or changes in mood.

PATIENT TEACHING

Boxed Warning Caution patient or caregiver of patient taking an opioid with a benzodiazepine, CNS depressant, or alcohol to seek immediate medical attention for dizziness, light-headedness, extreme sleepiness, slowed or difficult breathing, or unresponsiveness. ■

Boxed Warning Advise patient that drug increases risk of opioid addiction, abuse, and misuse, which can lead to overdose and death. Teach patient safe use of drug. ■

Boxed Warning Warn patient to keep drug out of reach of children as accidental ingestion of even one dose can be fatal. ■

🔔 *Alert:* Explain assessment and monitoring process to patient and family. Instruct them to immediately report difficulty breathing or other signs or symptoms of an adverse opioid-related reaction.

🔔 *Alert:* Encourage patient to report all medications being taken, including prescription and OTC medications and supplements.

🔔 *Alert:* Caution patient to immediately report signs and symptoms of serotonin syndrome, adrenal insufficiency, and decreased sex hormone levels.

M

- Encourage patient who has had a surgical procedure to turn, cough, and deep-breathe to prevent lung problems.
- Caution patient who is ambulatory about getting out of bed or walking. Warn outpatient to avoid driving and other potentially hazardous activities that require mental alertness until drug's CNS effects are known.
- Advise patient to avoid alcohol and sleep aids during therapy.
- Caution patient that drug isn't intended for long-term use.
- Teach patient that naloxone is prescribed in conjunction with the opioid when treatment begins or is renewed as a preventive measure to reduce opioid overdose and death.

🕐 **Alert:** Counsel patient not to discontinue opioids without first discussing with prescriber the need for a gradual tapering regimen.

SAFETY ALERT!

mercaptopurine (6-mercaptopurine, 6-MP)
mer-kap-toe-PURE-een

Purinethol❦, Purixan

Therapeutic class: Antineoplastics
Pharmacologic class: Purine antagonists

AVAILABLE FORMS
Oral suspension: 20 mg/mL
Tablets (scored): 50 mg

INDICATIONS & DOSAGES
➤ **Acute lymphoblastic leukemia as part of a combination regimen**
Adults and children: After remission is attained, usual maintenance dose for adults and children is 1.5 to 2.5 mg/kg once daily.

💊 *Adjust-a-dose:* Initial dosage in patients known to have homozygous thiopurine S-methyltransferase (TPMT) or nucleotide diphosphatase (NUDT15) deficiency typically is 10% or less of the recommended dosage. Patients with heterozygous TPMT or NUDT15 deficiency may require dosage reduction based on toxicities. Patients who are heterozygous for both TPMT and NUDT15 may require more substantial dosage reductions. For patients with impaired renal function (CrCl less than 50 mL/minute), begin with the lowest recommended starting dosage

or increase dosing interval to every 36 to 48 hours. For patients with hepatic impairment, begin with the lowest recommended starting dose. If given with allopurinol, reduce mercaptopurine dosage to one-third to one-quarter current dose.

➤ **Acute promyelocytic leukemia, maintenance ◆**
Adults: 60 mg/m²/day for 1 year (in combination with tretinoin and methotrexate).

ADMINISTRATION
PO
🕐 **Alert:** Drug is a hazardous agent; follow safe handling and disposal procedures.
- Give total daily dosage at one time, calculated to the nearest multiple of 25 mg.
- Give consistently with or without food; giving on an empty stomach is preferred.
- Shake oral suspension vigorously for at least 30 seconds to ensure it's well mixed.
- Measure suspension with an oral dosing syringe to ensure proper dosing.
- Once opened, use oral suspension within 8 weeks.
- Omit a missed dose and continue with the next schedule dose.
- Store at room temperature.

ACTION
Inhibits RNA and DNA synthesis.

Route	Onset	Peak	Duration
PO	Unknown	45 min	Unknown

Half-life: Less than 2 hours (tablets); 1.3 hours (suspension).

ADVERSE REACTIONS
CNS: malaise, fever. **EENT:** oral lesions. **GI:** nausea, vomiting, anorexia, diarrhea, *pancreatitis.* **GU:** oligospermia. **Hematologic:** *myelosuppression (leukopenia, neutropenia, thrombocytopenia,* anemia). **Hepatic:** jaundice, *hepatotoxicity,* hyperbilirubinemia. **Metabolic:** hyperuricemia. **Respiratory:** pulmonary fibrosis. **Skin:** rash, hyperpigmentation, alopecia, urticaria. **Other:** infection, secondary malignancies.

INTERACTIONS
Drug-drug. *Allopurinol:* May cause mercaptopurine toxicity. Reduce mercaptopurine dosage if coadministered.
Aminosalicylate derivatives (mesalamine, olsalazine, sulfasalazine): May increase risk

---

Reactions in bold italics are *life-threatening*. Interactions may have a *rapid onset* or a *delayed onset*.

of myelosuppression. Use lowest possible dosages of each drug and monitor patient closely.

Febuxostat: May increase mercaptopurine level. Avoid use together.

Hepatotoxic drugs: May enhance hepatotoxicity of mercaptopurine. Monitor patient for hepatotoxicity.

Inactivated vaccines: May decrease therapeutic effect of vaccine. Complete age-appropriate vaccines before starting therapy, or revaccinate at least 3 months after immunosuppressant discontinuation.

Live-virus vaccines: May increase risk of toxicity from vaccine and infection. Consider therapy modification.

Myelosuppressants (azathioprine): May increase bone marrow suppression when combined with other drugs whose primary or secondary toxicity is myelosuppression. Monitor CBC and adjust dosage if indicated.

Sulfamethoxazole, trimethoprim: May enhance bone marrow suppression. Monitor CBC with differential carefully.

Warfarin: May decrease anticoagulant effect. Monitor PT and INR.

Drug-herb. *Echinacea:* May diminish therapeutic effect of immunosuppressants. Consider therapy modification.

EFFECTS ON LAB TEST RESULTS

• May increase uric acid, transaminase, ALP, and bilirubin levels.
• May decrease Hb level, ANC, and WBC and platelet counts.

CONTRAINDICATIONS & CAUTIONS

• Contraindicated in patients resistant or hypersensitive to drug.
⚕ Patients with TPMT or NUDT15 deficiency are more sensitive to drug's myelosuppressive defects. Consider TPMT phenotype and genotype testing and NUDT15 genotype testing for severe toxicities and excessive myelosuppression.
• Drug can cause myelosuppression and hepatotoxicity and increase risk of secondary neoplasia.
• Use cautiously in older adults.
• Safety and effectiveness in children haven't been determined.

Dialyzable drug: Unlikely.

⚠ **Overdose S&S:** Anorexia, nausea, vomiting, diarrhea, myelosuppression, hepatic dysfunction, gastroenteritis.

PREGNANCY-LACTATION-REPRODUCTION

• Drug may cause fetal harm. Patients of childbearing potential should avoid pregnancy during therapy and for 6 months after final dose.
• Verify pregnancy status before starting drug.
• Males with partners of childbearing potential should use effective contraception during treatment and for 3 months after final dose.
• Drug may appear in human milk. Patient should discontinue breastfeeding during treatment and for 1 week after final dose.
• Drug may impair fertility.

NURSING CONSIDERATIONS

• Monitor CBC and transaminase, ALP, and bilirubin levels weekly during initial therapy and monthly during maintenance to monitor patient for myelosuppression and assess hepatic function.
• Consider modifying dosage after chemotherapy or radiation therapy in patients who have depressed neutrophil or platelet counts.
⊌ *Alert:* Drug may be ordered as "6-mercaptopurine" or as "6-MP." The numeral 6 is part of the drug name and doesn't refer to dosage and should be avoided.
• Leukopenia, thrombocytopenia, or anemia may persist for several days after drug is stopped.
• Watch for signs of bleeding and infection.
⊌ *Alert:* Watch for jaundice, right-sided abdominal tenderness, clay-colored stools, and frothy, dark urine. Hepatic dysfunction is reversible when drug is stopped.
• Anticipate need for blood transfusions because of cumulative anemia.

PATIENT TEACHING

• Teach patient or caregivers on proper handling, storage, administration, and disposal of drug and how to clean up accidental spillage of the solution.
• Instruct patient to watch for signs and symptoms of infection (fever, sore throat, fatigue) and bleeding (easy bruising, nosebleeds, bleeding gums, melena). Tell patient to take temperature daily.
• Advise patient to avoid dental work until blood counts have returned to normal.
• Inform patient of reproductive potential that drug can impair fertility.

M

- Caution patient of childbearing potential not to become pregnant during therapy and for 6 months after final dose.
- Advise male patient with partners of childbearing potential to use effective contraception during therapy and for 3 months after final dose.
- Counsel patient to stop breastfeeding during therapy and for 1 week after final dose because of risk of toxicity to infant.

meropenem
mare-oh-PEN-em

Merrem

Therapeutic class: Antibiotics
Pharmacologic class: Carbapenems

AVAILABLE FORMS
Powder for injection: 500 mg, 1 g

INDICATIONS & DOSAGES
Adjust-a-dose (for all indications): For adults with CrCl of 26 to 50 mL/minute, give usual dose every 12 hours. If CrCl is 10 to 25 mL/minute, give half usual dose every 12 hours; if CrCl is less than 10 mL/minute, give half usual dose every 24 hours.

➤ **Complicated skin and skin-structure infections from** *Staphylococcus aureus* **(methicillin-susceptible isolates only),** *Streptococcus pyogenes, Streptococcus agalactiae,* **viridans group streptococci,** *Enterococcus faecalis* **(excluding vancomycin-resistant isolates),** *Escherichia coli, Proteus mirabilis, Bacteroides fragilis,* **or** *Peptostreptococcus* **species**
Adults and children weighing more than 50 kg: 500 mg IV every 8 hours.
Children age 3 months and older weighing 50 kg or less: 10 mg/kg IV every 8 hours; maximum dose, 500 mg IV every 8 hours.
➤ **Complicated skin and skin-structure infections caused by** *Pseudomonas aeruginosa*
Adults and children weighing more than 50 kg: 1 g IV every 8 hours.
Children age 3 months and older weighing 50 kg or less: 20 mg/kg IV every 8 hours; maximum dose is 1 g IV every 8 hours.
➤ **Complicated intra-abdominal infections (including appendicitis and peritonitis) caused by viridans group streptococci,** *E. coli, Klebsiella pneumoniae, P. aeruginosa,* *B. fragilis, Bacteroides thetaiotaomicron,* **or** *Peptostreptococcus* **species**
Adults and children weighing more than 50 kg: 1 g IV every 8 hours.
Children age 3 months and older weighing 50 kg or less: 20 mg/kg IV every 8 hours; maximum dose is 1 g IV every 8 hours.
Children 32 weeks' or more gestational age (GA) and 14 days or more postnatal age (PNA): 30 mg/kg IV every 8 hours over 30 minutes.
Children 32 weeks' or more GA and less than 14 days PNA: 20 mg/kg IV every 8 hours.
Children less than 32 weeks' GA and 14 days or more PNA: 20 mg/kg IV every 8 hours.
Children less than 32 weeks' GA and less than 14 days PNA: 20 mg/kg IV every 12 hours.
➤ **Bacterial meningitis caused by** *S. pneumoniae, Haemophilus influenzae,* **or** *Neisseria meningitidis*
Children weighing more than 50 kg: 2 g IV every 8 hours.
Children age 3 months and older weighing 50 kg or less: 40 mg/kg IV every 8 hours; maximum dose, 2 g IV every 8 hours.

ADMINISTRATION
IV

▼ Obtain specimen for culture and sensitivity tests before giving first dose. Begin therapy while awaiting results.
🌙 *Alert:* Serious hypersensitivity reactions may occur in patients receiving beta-lactams. Before therapy begins, determine if patient has had previous hypersensitivity reactions to penicillins, cephalosporins, beta-lactams, or other allergens. If an allergic reaction occurs, stop drug and notify prescriber. Serious anaphylactic reactions require emergency treatment.
▼ Use freshly prepared solutions of drug immediately whenever possible. Stability of drug varies with form of drug used (injection vial, infusion vial, or ADD-Vantage container).
▼ For bolus, add 10 mL of sterile water for injection to 500-mg vial or 20 mL to 1-g vial. Shake to dissolve, and let stand until clear. Give over 3 to 5 minutes. May be stored for up to 3 hours at up to 77° F (25° C) or for 13 hours at up to 41° F (5° C).
▼ For infusion, an infusion vial (500 mg/100 mL or 1 g/100 mL) may be directly reconstituted with a compatible infusion fluid. Or, an injection vial may be reconstituted

---

and the resulting solution added to an IV container and further diluted with an appropriate infusion fluid. Don't use ADD-Vantage vials for this purpose. Give over 15 to 30 minutes.

▼ Solutions prepared with NSS at 1 to 20 mg/mL may be stored for 1 hour at up to 77° F (25° C) or 15 hours at up to 41° F (5° C); use solutions prepared with D_5W immediately.

▼ For ADD-Vantage vials, constitute only with half-NSS for injection, NSS for injection, or D_5W in 50-, 100-, or 250-mL Abbott ADD-Vantage flexible diluent containers. Follow manufacturer's guidelines closely when using ADD-Vantage vials.

▼ Don't use flexible container in series connections.

▼ **Incompatibilities:** Compatibility with other drugs hasn't been established. Don't mix with or physically add to solutions containing other drugs.

ACTION

Inhibits cell-wall synthesis in bacteria. Readily penetrates cell wall of most gram-positive and gram-negative bacteria to reach penicillin-binding protein targets.

Route	Onset	Peak	Duration
IV	Unknown	1 hr	Unknown

Half-life: 1 to 1.5 hours.

ADVERSE REACTIONS

CNS: headache, pain, *seizure.* **CV:** peripheral vascular disorder, *shock.* **EENT:** oral candidiasis, glossitis, pharyngitis. **GI:** *CDAD,* GI disorder, constipation, diarrhea, nausea, vomiting. **GU:** hematuria. **Hematologic:** anemia. **Hepatic:** hyperbilirubinemia. **Metabolic:** *hypoglycemia.* **Respiratory:** *apnea,* pneumonia. **Skin:** injection-site inflammation, pruritus, rash. **Other:** *anaphylaxis, sepsis,* hypersensitivity reactions, inflammation, accidental injury.

INTERACTIONS

Drug-drug. *Probenecid:* May decrease renal excretion of meropenem. Avoid using together.
Valproic acid: May decrease valproic acid levels, increasing the risk of seizures. Monitor levels frequently, and observe patient for seizure activity. Consider alternative antibiotic or supplemental anticonvulsant therapy.

EFFECTS ON LAB TEST RESULTS

- May increase ALT, AST, bilirubin, ALP, LDH, creatinine, and BUN levels.
- May increase eosinophil count.
- May decrease Hb level, hematocrit, and WBC count.
- May increase or decrease INR and platelet count.
- May prolong or shorten PT and PTT.
- May produce a positive Coombs test.

CONTRAINDICATIONS & CAUTIONS

- Contraindicated in patients hypersensitive to components of drug or other drugs in same class and in patients who have had anaphylactic reactions to beta-lactams.
- Use cautiously in older adults and in patients with a history of brain lesions, seizure disorders, or impaired renal function.
- SCARs have been reported with meropenem use.

Dialyzable drug: Yes.

⚠ *Overdose S&S:* Exaggerated adverse reactions.

PREGNANCY-LACTATION-REPRODUCTION

- There are no adequate studies during pregnancy. Use during pregnancy only if clearly needed.
- Drug appears in human milk. Use cautiously during breast feeding.

NURSING CONSIDERATIONS

- In patients with CNS disorders, bacterial meningitis, and compromised renal function, drug may cause seizures and other CNS adverse reactions.
- If seizures occur during therapy, stop infusion and notify prescriber. Dosage adjustment may be needed.
- Monitor patient for signs and symptoms of superinfection. Drug may cause overgrowth of nonsusceptible bacteria or fungi.
- Periodically assess organ system functions, including renal, hepatic, and hematopoietic function, during prolonged therapy.
- Monitor patient's fluid balance and weight carefully.
- If patient develops signs and symptoms suggestive of SCAR, stop drug immediately and consider an alternative treatment.
- CDAD may occur up to months after last dose and range from mild diarrhea to fatal colitis. If CDAD occurs, drug will need to be stopped and appropriate treatment begun.

PATIENT TEACHING
• Instruct patient to report adverse reactions or signs and symptoms of superinfection.
• Advise patient to report loose stools to prescriber.
🜛 **Alert:** Advise patient to report rash, peeling skin, trouble swallowing or breathing, or other signs and symptoms of allergic reaction.
• Caution patient that drug can interfere with mental alertness. Caution patient not to operate motorized vehicles or machinery until tolerance is known.

---

mesalamine (mesalazine)
me-SAL-a-meen

Apriso, Asacol HD, Canasa, Delzicol, Lialda, Mezavant❋, Pentasa, Rowasa, Salofalk❋, sfRowasa

Therapeutic class: Anti-inflammatory drugs
Pharmacologic class: Salicylates

AVAILABLE FORMS
Capsules (controlled-release) 🅒🅡🅖: 250 mg, 375 mg, 500 mg
Capsules (delayed-release) 🅒🅡🅖: 400 mg, 800 mg
Rectal suspension: 2 g/60 mL❋, 4 g/60 mL, 1 g/100 mL❋, 4 g/100 mL❋
Suppositories: 500 mg❋, 1,000 mg
Tablets (delayed-release) 🅒🅡🅖: 400 mg❋, 800 mg, 1.2 g

INDICATIONS & DOSAGES
➤ **Active mild to moderate distal ulcerative colitis, proctitis, or proctosigmoiditis**
Adults: 1,000 mg suppository PR once daily at bedtime for 3 to 6 weeks. Or, 4 g retention enema once daily (preferably at bedtime) for 3 to 6 weeks.
➤ **Remission-induction of active, mild to moderate ulcerative colitis in adults**
Lialda
Adults: Two to four 1.2-g tablets (2.4 to 4.8 g) PO once daily for up to 8 weeks.
Children weighing more than 50 kg: Four 1.2-g tablets (4.8 g) PO once daily for 8 weeks.
Children weighing more than 35 to 50 kg: Three 1.2-g tablets (3.6 g) PO once daily for 8 weeks.
Children weighing 24 to 35 kg: Two 1.2-g tablets (2.4 g) PO once daily for 8 weeks.

Pentasa
Adults: Four 250-mg capsules or two 500-mg capsules (1 g) PO q.i.d. for a total dose of 4 g for up to 8 weeks.
Delzicol
Adults: 800 mg t.i.d. (2.4 g) for 6 weeks.
Children age 5 and older weighing 54 to 90 kg: 27 to 44 mg/kg/day PO in two divided doses daily for 6 weeks. Maximum dose, 2.4 g/day.
Children age 5 and older weighing 33 to less than 54 kg: 37 to 61 mg/kg/day PO in two divided doses daily for 6 weeks. Maximum dose, 2 g/day.
Children age 5 and older weighing 17 to less than 33 kg: 36 to 71 mg/kg/day PO in two divided doses daily for 6 weeks. Maximum dose, 1.2 g/day.
➤ **Moderate ulcerative colitis**
Adults: Two 800-mg tablets (1.6 g) Asacol HD t.i.d. for 6 weeks.
➤ **Maintenance of remission of ulcerative colitis in adults**
Adults: 1.5 g Apriso PO once daily in the morning. Or, two 1.2-g Lialda tablets PO once daily. Or, 1 g Pentasa PO q.i.d. Or, 1.6 g Delzicol PO in two to four divided doses.
➤ **Maintenance of remission of ulcerative colitis in children (Lialda)**
Children weighing more than 35 kg: Two 1.2-g tablets (2.4 g) PO once daily.
Children weighing 24 to 35 kg: One 1.2-g tablet (1.2 g) PO once daily.

ADMINISTRATION
PO
• Give Lialda with food.
• Give Apriso with or without food. Don't give with antacids.
• Don't crush or cut delayed-release or controlled-release forms.
• Intact or partially intact tablets may be seen in stool. Notify prescriber if this occurs repeatedly.
• Give Asacol HD on an empty stomach at least 1 hour before or 2 hours after a meal.
• Give Delzicol with or without food. If patient is unable to swallow Delzicol, the capsules can be opened and the contents swallowed whole.
• If patient can't swallow Pentasa capsules whole, they may be opened and the contents sprinkled on applesauce or yogurt and consumed immediately.

Reactions in bold italics are ***life-threatening***. Interactions may have a *rapid onset* or a ***delayed onset***.

Rectal

• Patient should retain rectal enema dosage form overnight (for about 8 hours). Usual course of therapy for rectal form ranges from 3 to 6 weeks.

• Shake suspension well before each use and remove sheath before inserting into rectum.

• Patient should retain suppository for 1 to 3 hours or longer, if possible.

ACTION

An active metabolite of sulfasalazine, drug probably acts topically by inhibiting prostaglandin production in the colon.

Route	Onset	Peak	Duration
PO, PR	Unknown	3–12 hr	Unknown

Half-life: Usually about 25 hours but varies from 1.5 to 296 hours.

ADVERSE REACTIONS

CNS: headache, dizziness, fever, fatigue, paresthesia, pain, vertigo, anxiety. **CV:** HTN. **EENT:** visual disturbance, tinnitus, nasopharyngitis, rhinitis, sinusitis. **GI:** abdominal pain, cramps, discomfort, flatulence, diarrhea, bloody diarrhea, rectal pain, bloating, nausea, vomiting, dyspepsia, constipation, eructation, exacerbation of ulcerative colitis, gastroenteritis, hemorrhoids, *pancreatitis,* tenesmus, *rectal hemorrhage,* sclerosing cholangitis (children), *hemorrhage.* **GU:** interstitial nephritis, hematuria, urinary frequency, nephropathy, *nephrotoxicity.* **Hematologic:** anemia. **Hepatic:** *cholestatic hepatitis,* hepatic insufficiency, increased transaminase levels. **Metabolic:** weight loss (children), increased triglyceride levels. **Musculoskeletal:** arthralgia, arthropathy, myalgia, back pain, lower extremity pain. **Respiratory:** cough, dyspnea. **Skin:** rash, acne, urticaria, hair loss. **Other:** chills, pain, flulike symptoms, infection.

INTERACTIONS

Drug-drug. *Antacids, H₂ antagonists, PPIs:* May cause premature release of delayed- or extended-release products. Avoid concurrent administration. Consider therapy modification.
Azathioprine, mercaptopurine: May cause blood disorders. Monitor blood cell counts and adjust therapy as needed.
Iron supplements: Asacol HD and Delzicol contain iron. Use cautiously in patients at risk for iron overload.

NSAIDs, other nephrotoxic agents: May enhance nephrotoxic effects. Monitor renal function and adverse reactions.
Varicella virus vaccines: May enhance adverse effect of varicella virus–containing vaccines, causing Reye syndrome. Consider therapy modification.
Drug-lifestyle. *Sunlight, UV light exposure:* May cause photosensitivity reactions. Patient should use skin protection and avoid prolonged exposure to sunlight and UV light.

EFFECTS ON LAB TEST RESULTS

• May increase bilirubin, BUN, creatinine, AST, ALT, ALP, LDH, amylase, triglyceride, and lipase levels.
• May decrease CrCl.
• May decrease Hb level and hematocrit and RBC and WBC counts.
• May falsely elevate urine normetanephrine results obtained by liquid chromatography with electrochemical detection.

CONTRAINDICATIONS & CAUTIONS

• Contraindicated in patients allergic to mesalamine, sulfites (including sulfasalazine), any salicylates, or any component of the preparation.

• Avoid use of tablets in patients at risk for upper GI obstruction (pyloric stenosis, upper GI functional disorders) due to delayed release of drug in colon.

• Use cautiously in patients predisposed to pericarditis and myocarditis due to mesalamine-induced cardiac hypersensitivity reactions.

• Use cautiously in older adults, in patients with renal or hepatic impairment, and in those taking nephrotoxic drugs.

Dialyzable drug: Unknown.

⚠ *Overdose S&S:* Confusion, diarrhea, headache, hyperventilation, diaphoresis, tinnitus, vertigo, vomiting.

PREGNANCY-LACTATION-REPRODUCTION

• There are no adequate studies during pregnancy. Drug crosses the placental barrier. Use during pregnancy only if clearly needed.

• Drug appears in human milk. Use cautiously during breastfeeding.

• Drug may cause decreased sperm count, which resolves with drug discontinuation.

M

NURSING CONSIDERATIONS

• Assess renal function before therapy.
• Monitor renal and hepatic function studies and blood cell counts periodically in patients on long-term therapy
• Ensure patients are well hydrated during therapy; mesalamine kidney stones have been reported.
• Monitor patient for hypersensitivity reactions, including those involving organs (hepatitis, myocarditis, pericarditis, nephritis, hematologic abnormalities, pneumonitis).
• Because the mesalamine rectal suspension contains potassium metabisulfite, it may cause hypersensitivity reactions in patients sensitive to sulfites.
• Drug may be associated with an acute intolerance syndrome in which signs and symptoms (abdominal pain, cramping, bloody diarrhea, headache, fever, rash) may be similar to an ulcerative colitis exacerbation. If acute intolerance syndrome is suspected, discontinue drug.
• Apriso contains phenylalanine.
• *Look alike–sound alike:* Don't confuse Asacol with Os-Cal; mesalamine with mecamylamine, megestrol, memantine, metaxalone, or methenamine; Apriso with Apri; or Lialda with Aldara.

PATIENT TEACHING

• Instruct patient to carefully follow instructions supplied with drug for safe drug administration.
• Tell patient not to take drug with antacids.
• Advise patient to drink an adequate amount of fluids.
• Inform patient that intact, partially intact, or tablet shells have been reported in the stool and to contact health care provider if this occurs repeatedly.
• Advise patient to report all adverse reactions and to stop drug if fever or rash occurs. Patient intolerant of sulfasalazine may also be hypersensitive to mesalamine.
• Tell patient to remove foil wrapper from suppositories before inserting into rectum.
• Teach patient about proper use of retention enema.
• Caution patient to wear protective clothing and broad-spectrum sunscreen when exposed to sunlight or UV light and to avoid prolonged exposure.

SAFETY ALERT!

metFORMIN hydrochloride
met-FOR-min

Fortamet, Glumetza, Riomet

Therapeutic class: Antidiabetics
Pharmacologic class: Biguanides

AVAILABLE FORMS

Oral solution: 500 mg/5 mL
Tablets: 500 mg, 625 mg, 750 mg, 850 mg, 1,000 mg
Tablets (extended-release) **OTC**: 500 mg, 750 mg, 1,000 mg

INDICATIONS & DOSAGES

Adjust-a-dose (for all indications): Contraindicated in patients with eGFR below 30 mL/minute/1.73 m^2. Starting drug in patients with eGFR between 30 and 45 mL/minute/1.73 m^2 isn't recommended. If eGFR falls below 45 mL/minute/1.73 m^2 in patients taking drug, assess benefits and risks of continuing treatment. Discontinue if eGFR falls below 30 mL/minute/1.73 m^2. For older adults or patients who are debilitated, use conservative initial and maintenance dosage because of potential decrease in renal function.

➤ **Adjunct to diet to lower glucose level in patients with type 2 diabetes**
Adults: If using immediate-release tablets or oral solution, initially 500 mg PO b.i.d. given with morning and evening meals, or 850 mg PO once daily given with morning meal. Titrate immediate-release forms in increments of 500 mg weekly or 850 mg every other week to maximum dose of 2,550 mg PO daily in divided doses. If using extended-release formulation, start therapy at 500 mg PO once daily with the evening meal. May increase dose as tolerated weekly (every 1 to 2 weeks for Glumetza) in increments of 500 mg daily, up to a maximum dose of 2,000 mg once daily. If higher doses are required, consider a trial of 1,000 mg b.i.d. or use the regular-release formulation up to its maximum dose.
Children ages 10 and older: 500 mg PO b.i.d. using the immediate-release formulation only. Increase dosage in increments of 500 mg weekly up to a maximum of 2,000 mg daily in divided doses.

Reactions in bold italics are *life-threatening*. Interactions may have a *rapid onset* or a **delayed onset**.

➤ **Prevention of type 2 diabetes in patients with prediabetes, especially those with BMI of more than 35 kg/m², those younger than age 60, and patients with prior history of gestational diabetes or polycystic ovary syndrome ♦**

Adults: 850 mg immediate-release tablets PO once daily for 1 month; then increase to 850 mg b.i.d., unless GI adverse effects warrant a longer titration period.

ADMINISTRATION

PO
• Give drug with meals. Maximum doses may be better tolerated if given in three divided doses with meals (immediate-release tablets only).
• Don't cut or crush extended-release tablets.
• Oral solution should be clear.

ACTION

Decreases hepatic glucose production and intestinal absorption of glucose and improves insulin sensitivity (increases peripheral glucose uptake and use).

Route	Onset	Peak	Duration
PO (conventional)	Unknown	2–3 hr	Unknown
PO (extended-release)	Unknown	4–8 hr	Unknown
PO (solution)	Unknown	2.5 hr	Unknown

Half-life: About 4 to 9 hours.

ADVERSE REACTIONS

CNS: asthenia, headache, dizziness, chills, light-headedness, taste disorder. **CV:** chest discomfort, palpitations, flushing. **EENT:** rhinitis. **GI:** diarrhea, nausea, vomiting, indigestion, abdominal bloating, abdominal discomfort, flatulence, anorexia, abnormal stools, constipation, dyspepsia, weight loss. **Metabolic:** vitamin B_{12} deficiency, *hypoglycemia.* **Musculoskeletal:** myalgia, limb pain. **Respiratory:** URI, dyspnea. **Skin:** nail disorder, diaphoresis. **Other:** accidental injury, infection.

INTERACTIONS

Drug-drug. *Beta blockers:* Hypoglycemia may be difficult to recognize in patients using beta blockers. Monitor patient and blood glucose.
Calcium channel blockers, corticosteroids, estrogens, fosphenytoin, hormonal contraceptives, isoniazid, nicotinic acid,

phenothiazines, phenytoin, sympathomimetics, thiazide and other diuretics, thyroid drugs: May produce hyperglycemia. Monitor patient's glycemic control. Metformin dosage may need to be increased.
Carbonic anhydrase inhibitors (acetazolamide, topiramate): May increase risk of lactic acidosis. Monitor patient closely.
Cationic drugs (amiloride, cimetidine, digoxin, morphine, procainamide, quinidine, quinine, triamterene, trimethoprim, vancomycin): May compete for common renal tubular transport systems, which may increase metformin level. Monitor glucose level.
Dolutegravir: Increases metformin exposure. Use alternative drug or limit total daily dose of metformin to 1,000 mg. Closely monitor response to metformin.
Insulin, insulin secretagogues (sulfonylureas): May increase risk of hypoglycemia. Monitor patient closely and adjust insulin or insulin secretagogue dosage as needed.
Nifedipine: May increase metformin level. Monitor patient closely. Metformin dosage may need to be decreased.

Boxed Warning *Radiologic contrast dye:* May cause acute renal failure or lactic acidosis. Withhold metformin at the time of or before procedure and 48 hours after procedure. Restart drug only if kidney function returns to normal. ∎

Drug-herb. *Guar gum:* May decrease hypoglycemic effect. Discourage use together.
Drug-lifestyle. **Boxed Warning** *Alcohol use:* May increase drug effects and potentiate metformin's effect on lactate metabolism. Discourage use together. ∎

EFFECTS ON LAB TEST RESULTS
• May decrease vitamin B_{12} and Hb levels.

CONTRAINDICATIONS & CAUTIONS
• Contraindicated in patients hypersensitive to drug and in those with hepatic disease or metabolic acidosis or lactic acidosis, including diabetic ketoacidosis with or without coma.
• Contraindicated in patients with eGFR below 30 mL/minute/1.73 m². Not recommended in patients with eGFR between 30 and 45 mL/minute/1.73 m².

Boxed Warning Metformin-associated lactic acidosis has resulted in death, hypothermia, hypotension, and resistant

M

bradyarrhythmias. Onset includes nonspecific symptoms, such as malaise, myalgias, respiratory distress, somnolence, and abdominal pain. It's characterized by elevated blood lactate levels (greater than 5 mmol/L), anion gap acidosis (without evidence of ketonuria or ketonemia), an increased lactate/pyruvate ratio, and metformin plasma levels generally above 5 mcg/mL. Metformin decreases liver uptake of lactate, increasing lactate blood levels and risk of lactic acidosis, especially in patients at risk. ∎

Boxed Warning Risk factors for metformin-associated lactic acidosis include renal impairment, concomitant use of certain drugs, age 65 and older, having a radiologic study with contrast, surgery and other procedures, hypoxic states, excessive alcohol intake, and hepatic impairment. ∎

Boxed Warning See manufacturer's instructions for steps to reduce risk and manage lactic acidosis in groups at high risk. ∎

• Discontinue drug in patients with acute HF (particularly when accompanied by hypoperfusion and hypoxemia), CV collapse (shock), acute MI, sepsis, and other conditions associated with hypoxemia that have been linked to lactic acidosis and may cause prerenal azotemia.

• Not indicated for use in patients with type 1 diabetes.

• Use cautiously in older adults and in patients who are debilitated or malnourished.

Dialyzable drug: Yes.

⚠ *Overdose S&S:* Hypoglycemia, lactic acidosis.

PREGNANCY-LACTATION-REPRODUCTION

• Abnormal blood glucose levels during pregnancy may cause fetal harm. Most experts recommend using insulin during pregnancy to maintain blood glucose levels as close to normal as possible. Use metformin during pregnancy only if clearly needed.

• Drug appears in human milk. Patient should discontinue breastfeeding or discontinue drug, taking into account importance of drug to the patient and risk of hypoglycemia in the infant. Consider insulin therapy.

• Metformin tablets increase risk of unintended pregnancy during premenopause because they may cause ovulation in some anovulatory patients.

NURSING CONSIDERATIONS

• Before therapy begins and at least annually thereafter, assess patient's renal function. Assess more frequently in patients at risk for renal impairment.

Boxed Warning For suspected metformin-associated lactic acidosis, immediately discontinue drug and promptly institute supportive measures in a hospital setting. Prompt hemodialysis is recommended. ∎

• Consider more frequent monitoring of patients taking drugs that may increase the risk of metformin-associated lactic acidosis, including drugs that impair renal function, result in significant hemodynamic change, interfere with acid-base balance, or increase metformin accumulation.

• Monitor patient's glucose level regularly to evaluate effectiveness of therapy. Notify prescriber if glucose level increases despite therapy.

• If patient hasn't responded to 4 weeks of therapy with maximum dosage, an oral sulfonylurea can be added while keeping metformin at maximum dosage. If patient still doesn't respond after several months of therapy with both drugs at maximum dosage, prescriber may stop both and start insulin therapy.

• Monitor patient closely during times of increased stress, such as infection, fever, surgery, or trauma. Insulin therapy may be needed in these situations.

• Stop drug at the time of, or before, an iodinated contrast imaging procedure in patients with an eGFR between 30 and 60 mL/minute/1.73 m^2; in patients with a history of hepatic impairment, alcoholism, or HF; or in patients who will be administered intra-arterial iodinated contrast. Reevaluate eGFR 48 hours after the imaging procedure; restart drug if renal function stabilizes.

• Temporarily discontinue drug in patients with restricted food and fluid intake due to surgery or other procedures because of increased risk of volume depletion, hypotension, and renal impairment.

• Monitor patient for evidence of anemia annually. Monitor vitamin B_{12} level every 2 to 3 years. Patients with inadequate vitamin B_{12} or calcium intake or absorption may be predisposed to subnormal vitamin B_{12} level.

- *Look alike–sound alike:* Don't confuse metformin with metronidazole.

PATIENT TEACHING
- Teach patient about diabetes and the importance of adhering to therapeutic regimen, following a specific diet, losing weight, getting exercise, practicing good personal hygiene, and avoiding infection. Explain how and when to monitor glucose level. Teach evidence of low and high glucose levels. Explain emergency measures.

Boxed Warning Instruct patient to stop drug and immediately notify prescriber about unexplained hyperventilation, muscle pain, malaise, dizziness, light-headedness, unusual sleepiness, unexplained stomach pain, feeling of coldness, slow or irregular HR, or other nonspecific symptoms of early lactic acidosis. ■

Boxed Warning Warn patient against excessive alcohol intake while taking drug. ■

- Tell patient not to change drug dosage without prescriber's knowledge. Encourage patient to report abnormal glucose level test results.

🖑 *Alert:* Advise patient not to cut, crush, or chew extended-release tablets; instruct patient to swallow them whole.
- Tell patient that inactive ingredients may be eliminated in the stool as a soft mass resembling the original tablet.
- Advise patient not to take other drugs, including OTC drugs, without first checking with prescriber.
- Instruct patient to carry medical identification at all times.
- Tell patient to report all adverse reactions and that diarrhea, nausea, and upset stomach generally subside over time.
- Discuss risk of unintended pregnancy with patient experiencing premenopause.
- Advise patient to discontinue breastfeeding or discontinue drug.

SAFETY ALERT!

methadone hydrochloride🖉
METH-a-done

Dolophine, Metadol✤, Metadol-D✤, Methadose

Therapeutic class: Opioid analgesics
Pharmacologic class: Opioid agonists
Controlled substance schedule: II

AVAILABLE FORMS
Dispersible tablets and diskets (for methadone maintenance therapy) 🍩: 40 mg
Injection: 10 mg/mL
Oral solution: 1 mg/mL✤, 5 mg/5 mL, 10 mg/5 mL, 10 mg/mL (concentrate)
Tablets: 1 mg✤, 5 mg, 10 mg, 25 mg✤

INDICATIONS & DOSAGES
Adjust-a-dose (for all indications): For older adults and patients with renal or hepatic impairment, reduce initial dose. Refer to manufacturer's instruction for conversion between methadone formulations or between methadone and other opioids.

➤ **Severe chronic pain for which alternative treatment options are inadequate**
Adults: Initiate dosing regimen for each patient individually, taking into account patient's prior analgesic treatment experience and risk factors for addiction, abuse, and misuse. Discontinue all other around-the-clock opioid drugs. Initially, 2.5 mg PO (Dolophine) every 8 to 12 hours, or 2.5 to 10 mg IM, IV, or subcut every 8 to 12 hours. Titrate slowly, no more frequently than every 3 to 5 days, and increase dosage as needed or use rescue drug as needed to maintain analgesia.

➤ **Opioid detoxification; maintenance treatment of opioid addiction**
Adults: Initially, 20 to 30 mg PO daily to suppress withdrawal symptoms (highly individualized; some patients may require a higher dose). Initial dose shouldn't exceed 30 mg. Maintenance dose, 80 to 120 mg PO daily. Adjust dosage as needed.

ADMINISTRATION
- Store all forms at room temperature (59° to 86° F [15° to 30° C]).

PO
- Oral form legally required in maintenance programs.

✤Canada ◇OTC ◆Off-label use 🖉Photoguide 🍩Do not crush *Liquid contains alcohol 🍊Genetic

- Completely dissolve dispersible tablets, disket, or oral solution in 4 oz (120 mL) of water, orange juice, or other acidic fruit beverage. Patient shouldn't chew or swallow tablets before they are dispersed in liquid.
- Dispersible tablets are cross-scored to allow breaking into two 20-mg doses or four 10-mg doses.

IV

▼ Protect from light.

▼ Rate of IV administration not defined by manufacturer.

▼ **Incompatibilities:** None listed by manufacturer. Consult a drug incompatibility reference for more information.

IM

- For parenteral use, IM injection is preferred. Rotate injection sites. Monitor site as local tissue reactions may occur.
- Protect from light.

Subcutaneous

- Monitor patient for pain at injection site, tissue irritation, and induration after injection.
- Protect from light.

ACTION

Unknown. Binds with opioid receptors in the CNS, altering perception of and emotional response to pain.

Route	Onset	Peak	Duration
PO	30–60 min	1–7.5 hr	4–8 hr
IV	Unknown	Unknown	4–8 hr
IM, subcut	10–20 min	1–2 hr	4–8 hr

Half-life: 8 to 59 hours.

ADVERSE REACTIONS

CNS: clouded sensorium, disorientation, dysphoria, hallucinations, dizziness, lightheadedness, sedation, somnolence, *seizures,* agitation, euphoria, asthenia, headache, insomnia, syncope. **CV:** *arrhythmias, bradycardia, prolonged QT interval, cardiac arrest, shock, cardiomyopathy, HF, ECG abnormalities,* flushing, phlebitis, edema, hypotension, palpitations, tachycardia, T-wave inversion. **EENT:** visual disturbances, congenital oculomotor disorders (nystagmus, strabismus), dry mouth, glossitis. **GI:** nausea, vomiting, abdominal pain, anorexia, biliary tract spasm, constipation, ileus. **GU:** decreased libido, urine retention, amenorrhea, sperm abnormalities, reduced seminal vesicle and prostate secretions. **Metabolic:** *hypokalemia, hypomagnesemia, hypoglycemia,*

weight gain. **Respiratory:** *respiratory arrest, respiratory depression, pulmonary edema.* **Skin:** diaphoresis, pruritus, pain at injection site, induration, urticaria, rash. **Other:** physical dependence, tissue irritation, hypersensitivity reaction.

INTERACTIONS

Drug-drug. *Ammonium chloride, other urine acidifiers:* May reduce methadone effect. Watch for decreased pain control.

Anticholinergics (benztropine mesylate, darifenacin, fesoterodine): May increase risk of urine retention or severe constipation. Monitor patient closely.

Boxed Warning *Benzodiazepines, other CNS depressants (antipsychotics, anxiolytics, general anesthetics, hypnotics, MAO inhibitors, muscle relaxants, TCAs, tranquilizers):* May cause respiratory depression, hypotension, profound sedation, coma, or death. If alternative treatment options are inadequate, monitor patient closely and consider delaying or omitting daily methadone dosing for signs and symptoms of respiratory depression and sedation. ■

Boxed Warning *CYP2B6, CYP2C9, CYP2C19, CYP2D6, or CYP3A4 inhibitors (all); CYP2B6, CYP2C9, CYP2C19, or CYP3A4 inducers:* Concomitant use of inhibitors and discontinuation of inducers may cause increased methadone plasma concentrations, resulting in potentially fatal respiratory depression. Monitor patient closely and reduce methadone dosage if necessary. ■

Boxed Warning *CYP2B6, CYP2C9, CYP2C19, or CYP3A4 inducers; CYP2B6, CYP2C9, CYP2C19, CYP2D6, or CYP3A4 inhibitors:* Adding inducers concomitantly with methadone or stopping inhibitors may decrease methadone effect and precipitate a withdrawal syndrome. Monitor patient closely. ■

Diuretics, laxatives, mineralocorticoid hormones: May cause electrolyte disturbances and increase risk of arrhythmias. Monitor patient closely.

MAO inhibitors (linezolid, phenelzine): May increase risk of serotonin syndrome or opioid toxicity. Use within 14 days of MAO inhibitor isn't recommended.

NNRTIs (delavirdine, efavirenz, nevirapine), protease inhibitors (lopinavir–ritonavir, nelfinavir, ritonavir), rifamycins: May increase methadone metabolism, causing opioid

---

Reactions in bold italics are *life-threatening.* Interactions may have a *rapid onset* or a *delayed onset.*

withdrawal symptoms. Monitor patient and adjust dose as needed.

Boxed Warning *Opioids:* May cause slow or difficult breathing, sedation, and death. Avoid use together. If use together is necessary, limit dosage and duration of each drug to the minimum necessary for desired effect. ∎

Protease inhibitors, cimetidine, fluvoxamine: May increase respiratory and CNS depression. Monitor patient closely.

⊌ *Alert:* Serotonergic drugs (amoxapine, antiemetics [dolasetron, granisetron, ondansetron, palonosetron], antimigraine drugs, buspirone, cyclobenzaprine, dextromethorphan, lithium, maprotiline, methylene blue, mirtazapine, nefazodone, SSNRIs, SSRIs, TCAs, trazodone, tryptophan, vilazodone): May increase risk of serotonin syndrome. Use together cautiously and monitor patient for serotonin syndrome.

Boxed Warning *QT interval–prolonging drugs (antiarrhythmics, chlorpromazine, citalopram, dolasetron):* May increase risk of QT-interval prolongation and ventricular arrhythmias. Use with extreme caution. ∎

Drug-herb. ⊌ *Alert: St. John's wort:* May reduce methadone effect and precipitate a withdrawal syndrome. May increase risk of serotonin syndrome. Use together cautiously and monitor patient closely.

Drug-lifestyle. **Boxed Warning** *Alcohol use:* May cause death. Use together is contraindicated. ∎

EFFECTS ON LAB TEST RESULTS
• May increase amylase level.
• May decrease potassium, magnesium, and glucose levels.

CONTRAINDICATIONS & CAUTIONS
• Contraindicated in patients hypersensitive to drug and in those with significant respiratory depression, acute or severe bronchial asthma in an unmonitored setting or in the absence of resuscitative equipment, or known or suspected GI obstruction, including paralytic ileus.

Boxed Warning Respiratory depression, including fatal cases, has been reported during initiation and conversion of patients to methadone, even when drug has been used as recommended and not misused or abused. Proper dosing and titration are essential and drug should only be prescribed by health care professionals knowledgeable in the use of methadone for detoxification and maintenance treatment of opioid addiction. Monitor patient for respiratory depression, especially during initiation or after a dosage increase. ∎

Boxed Warning Accidental ingestion of methadone, especially in children, can result in a fatal overdose of methadone. ∎

Boxed Warning Prolonged QT interval and serious arrhythmia (torsades de pointes) have occurred during methadone treatment. Most cases involve patients being treated for pain with large, multiple daily doses, although cases have been reported in patients receiving doses commonly used for maintenance treatment of opioid addiction. ∎

Boxed Warning Opioids should only be prescribed with benzodiazepines or other CNS depressants to patients for whom alternative treatment options are inadequate. ∎

⊌ *Alert:* Drug may lead to a rare but serious decrease in adrenal gland cortisol production.

⊌ *Alert:* The combined use of medication-assisted treatment (MAT) drugs methadone or buprenorphine with benzodiazepines or other CNS depressants increases the risk of serious adverse effects; however, the harm caused by untreated opioid addiction may outweigh these risks. Patients may require MAT for opioid addiction indefinitely and its use should continue for as long as patients are benefiting and contributes to the intended treatment goals.

• Use cautiously in older adults or patients who are debilitated and in those with severe hepatic or renal impairment, hypothyroidism, Addison disease, prostatic hyperplasia, urethral stricture, head injury, increased ICP, and respiratory conditions.

⊌ *Alert:* Patients are at increased risk for oversedation and respiratory depression if they snore or have a history of sleep apnea, haven't used opioids recently or are first-time opioid users, have increased opioid dosage requirements or opioid habituation, have received general anesthesia for longer lengths of time or received other sedating drugs, have preexisting pulmonary or cardiac disease, or have thoracic or other surgical incisions that may impair breathing. Monitor patients carefully.

⊌ *Alert:* Drug isn't indicated as a PRN analgesic.

Dialyzable drug: No.

M

♣Canada ◇OTC ◆Off-label use ✔Photoguide ⊜Do not crush *Liquid contains alcohol ▓Genetic

⚠ *Overdose S&S:* Miosis, respiratory depression, somnolence, coma, cool clammy skin, skeletal muscle flaccidity, hypotension, apnea, bradycardia, noncardiac pulmonary edema, death.

PREGNANCY-LACTATION-REPRODUCTION

• Use drug during pregnancy only if potential benefit justifies fetal risk. Methadone clearance may increase during pregnancy, particularly during second and third trimesters. Dosage may need to be increased or dosing interval decreased. Use lowest possible dosage.

Boxed Warning Prolonged use during pregnancy can cause neonatal opioid withdrawal syndrome, which can be life-threatening and requires management by neonatology experts. For prolonged use during pregnancy, apprise patient of risk and ensure that appropriate treatment will be available. ■

• Drug appears in human milk. Sedation and respiratory depression in breastfeeding infants have been reported. Monitor infants for respiratory depression and sedation and slowly wean to prevent withdrawal symptoms.

• When methadone is used to treat opioid addiction during breastfeeding, and if additional illicit substances are being abused, patient should express and discard human milk until sobriety is established.

• Long-term opioid use may cause secondary hypogonadism, which may lead to sexual dysfunction or infertility.

• Amenorrhea secondary to substance abuse may resolve after initiation of methadone maintenance treatment. Provide contraception counseling to prevent unplanned pregnancies.

NURSING CONSIDERATIONS

Boxed Warning Methadone is an opioid agonist and Schedule II controlled substance with an abuse liability similar to that of other opioid agonists, legal or illicit. Assess each patient's risk of opioid abuse or addiction before prescribing methadone. Risk of opioid abuse increases in patients with personal or family history of substance abuse (including drug or alcohol abuse or addiction) or mental illness (such as major depressive disorder). Routinely monitor all patients receiving methadone for signs and symptoms of misuse, abuse, and addiction during treatment. ■

Boxed Warning Respiratory depression that can be life-threatening or fatal, QT-interval prolongation, and torsades de pointes have been observed during treatment. Be vigilant during treatment initiation and dosage titration. ■

Boxed Warning Carefully monitor vital signs, pain level, respiratory status, and sedation level in all patients receiving opioids, especially those receiving IV drugs, even when given postoperatively. ■

⟳ *Alert:* If patient is taking opioids with serotonergic drugs, watch for signs and symptoms of serotonin syndrome (agitation, hallucinations, rapid HR, fever, diaphoresis, shivering or shaking, muscle twitching or stiffness, trouble with coordination, nausea, vomiting, diarrhea), especially when starting treatment or increasing dosages. Signs and symptoms may occur within several hours of coadministration but may also occur later, especially after dosage increase. Discontinue the opioid, serotonergic drug, or both if serotonin syndrome is suspected.

⟳ *Alert:* Work with patient to develop strategies to manage the use of prescribed or illicit benzodiazepines or other CNS depressants when starting MAT. Taper benzodiazepine or CNS depressant to discontinuation if possible.

⟳ *Alert:* If patient is receiving prescribed benzodiazepines or other CNS depressants for anxiety or insomnia, verify the diagnosis and consider other treatment options for these conditions if possible.

⟳ *Alert:* Coordinate care to ensure other prescribers are aware of patient's MAT.

⟳ *Alert:* Monitor patient for illicit drug use, including urine or blood screening.

⟳ *Alert:* Monitor patient for signs and symptoms of adrenal insufficiency (nausea, vomiting, loss of appetite, fatigue, weakness, dizziness, low BP). Perform diagnostic testing if adrenal insufficiency is suspected. For confirmed adrenal insufficiency, treat with corticosteroids and wean patient off opioids if appropriate. Discontinue corticosteroids when clinically appropriate.

• Monitor patient for signs and symptoms of decreased sex hormone levels (low libido, erectile dysfunction, amenorrhea, infertility). If signs and symptoms occur, evaluate patient and obtain lab testing.

• Reassess patient's level of pain at least 15 and 30 minutes after parenteral administration and 30 minutes after oral administration.

Reactions in bold italics are *life-threatening*. Interactions may have a *rapid onset* or a ***delayed onset***.

Boxed Warning When used for detoxification and maintenance of opioid dependence, treatment products in oral form shall be dispensed only by opioid treatment programs. Administer in accordance with treatment standards cited in 42 CFR (Code of Federal Regulations) Section 8, including limitations on unsupervised administration. Dispensing hospitals and pharmacies are approved by the FDA and designated state authorities. ■

• Use an around-the-clock regimen to manage severe, chronic pain.

• Give an additional analgesic to patient being treated in a methadone maintenance program if needed to control pain.

• Monitor patient closely because drug has cumulative effect; marked sedation can occur after repeated doses.

• Monitor circulatory status and bladder and bowel function. Patient may need a stool softener and stimulant laxative.

⚠ *Alert:* Respiratory depressant effects may last longer than analgesic effects. Monitor patient's respiratory status closely.

• When used as an adjunct in the treatment of opioid addiction (maintenance), withdrawal is usually delayed and mild.

⚠ *Alert:* Use caution when dosing. Confusion has occurred between milliliter and milligram doses.

⚠ *Alert:* Don't stop drug abruptly; withdraw slowly and individualize gradual taper plan to prevent signs and symptoms of withdrawal, worsening pain, and psychological distress in patients who are physically dependent. Refer to manufacturer's label for specific tapering instructions.

⚠ *Alert:* When tapering opioids, monitor patient closely for signs and symptoms of opioid withdrawal (restlessness, lacrimation, rhinorrhea, yawning, perspiration, chills, myalgia, mydriasis, irritability, anxiety, insomnia, backache, joint pain, weakness, abdominal cramps, anorexia, nausea, vomiting, diarrhea, increased BP or HR, increased respiratory rate), which may indicate a need to taper more slowly. Also monitor patient for suicidality, use of other substances, or changes in mood.

• *Look alike–sound alike:* Don't confuse methadone with methylphenidate, dexmethylphenidate, or Mephyton.

PATIENT TEACHING

⚠ *Alert:* Explain assessment and monitoring process to patient and family. Instruct them to immediately report difficulty breathing or other signs or symptoms of a potential adverse opioid-related reaction.

Boxed Warning Instruct patient on proper administration of oral forms to decrease risk of respiratory depression. ■

Boxed Warning Caution patient or caregiver of patient taking an opioid with a benzodiazepine, CNS depressant, or alcohol to seek immediate medical attention for dizziness, light-headedness, extreme sleepiness, slowed or difficult breathing, or unresponsiveness. ■

⚠ *Alert:* Encourage patient to report all medications being taken, including prescription and OTC medications and supplements.

⚠ *Alert:* Caution patient to immediately report signs and symptoms of serotonin syndrome, adrenal insufficiency, and decreased sex hormone levels.

⚠ *Alert:* Teach patient not to take nonprescribed benzodiazepines, sedatives, or alcohol when taking MAT due to the increased risk of overdose and death.

⚠ *Alert:* Advise patient to notify all prescribers of MAT and not to stop MAT or other prescribed drugs without first consulting prescriber.

• Caution patient who is ambulatory about getting out of bed or walking. Warn outpatient to avoid hazardous activities that require mental alertness until drug's CNS effects are known.

Boxed Warning Advise patient to keep drug out of reach of children. Accidental ingestion can result in fatal methadone overdose. ■

• Instruct patient to increase fluid and fiber in diet, if not contraindicated, to combat constipation.

• Teach patient who is breastfeeding to monitor infant for respiratory depression and sedation; advise patient when to contact health care provider for emergency care.

• Inform patient that prolonged opioid use may reduce fertility; it isn't known if effects are reversible. Advise patient about contraceptive use if needed.

• Teach patient that naloxone is prescribed in conjunction with the opioid when beginning and renewing treatment as a preventive measure to reduce opioid overdose and death.

⚠ *Alert:* Counsel patient not to discontinue opioids without first discussing with prescriber the need for a gradual tapering regimen.

M

♣Canada   ◇OTC   ◆Off-label use   ✐Photoguide   ⊜Do not crush   *Liquid contains alcohol   ▓Genetic

methIMAzole ⚕

meth-IM-a-zole

Tapazole ✦

Therapeutic class: Antihyperthyroid drugs
Pharmacologic class: Thyroid hormone antagonists

AVAILABLE FORMS
Tablets: 5 mg, 10 mg, 20 mg ✦

INDICATIONS & DOSAGES
➤ **Hyperthyroidism**
Adults: If mild, 15 mg PO daily in three divided doses given at 8-hour intervals. If moderately severe, 30 to 40 mg daily in three divided doses given at 8-hour intervals. If severe, 60 mg daily in three divided doses given at 8-hour intervals. Maintenance dosage ranges, 5 to 15 mg daily.
Children: 0.4 mg/kg/day PO in three divided doses given at 8-hour intervals. Maintenance dosage is 0.2 mg/kg/day in three divided doses daily.

ADMINISTRATION
PO
• Hazardous drug; use gloves to administer intact tablets.
• Omit a missed dose and give next scheduled dose as usual.
• Store at room temperature.

ACTION
Inhibits synthesis of thyroid hormones.

Route	Onset	Peak	Duration
PO	Rapid	1–2 hr	36–72 hr

Half-life: 4 to 6 hours.

ADVERSE REACTIONS
CNS: headache, drowsiness, vertigo, paresthesia, neuritis, CNS stimulation, loss of taste, fever. **CV:** edema. **GI:** nausea, vomiting, salivary gland enlargement, epigastric distress. **Hematologic:** *agranulocytosis, leukopenia, thrombocytopenia, aplastic anemia.* **Hepatic:** jaundice, hepatic dysfunction, *hepatitis.* **Metabolic:** hypothyroidism, *hypoglycemic coma.* **Musculoskeletal:** arthralgia, myalgia. **Skin:** rash, urticaria, discoloration, pruritus, lupuslike syndrome, abnormal hair loss. **Other:** lymphadenopathy.

INTERACTIONS
Drug-drug. *Beta blockers:* Beta-blocker clearance may be enhanced by hyperthyroidism. Dosage of beta blocker may need to be reduced when patient becomes euthyroid.
Cardiac glycosides (digitalis): May increase cardiac glycoside level. Cardiac glycoside dosage may need to be reduced.
Theophylline: May decrease theophylline clearance. Dosage adjustment may be needed.
Warfarin: May alter dosage requirements. Monitor PT and INR, and adjust warfarin dosage as needed.

EFFECTS ON LAB TEST RESULTS
• May increase LFT values and PT.
• May decrease Hb level and granulocyte, WBC, and platelet counts.
• May alter thyroid uptake of ^{123}I or ^{131}I.

CONTRAINDICATIONS & CAUTIONS
• Contraindicated in patients hypersensitive to drug and in those with history of acute pancreatitis after methimazole use.
• Drug may cause hypoprothrombinemia and bleeding. Monitor patient for bleeding.
• Drug may rarely cause vasculitis, including cutaneous vasculitis, glomerulonephritis, pulmonary hemorrhage, CNS vasculitis, and neuropathy. If vasculitis is suspected, discontinue drug and initiate appropriate therapy.
⚕ Patients with hereditary galactose intolerance, Lapp lactase deficiency, or glucose-galactose malabsorption shouldn't receive methimazole formulations that contain lactose.
Dialyzable drug: No.
⚠ **Overdose S&S:** Nausea, vomiting, epigastric distress, headache, fever, joint pain, pruritus, edema, aplastic anemia, agranulocytosis, hepatitis, nephrotic syndrome, exfoliative dermatitis, neuropathies, CNS stimulation or depression.

PREGNANCY-LACTATION-REPRODUCTION
• Drug may cause fetal harm, particularly in first trimester; consider other agents during this time. Drug crosses the placental barrier and can cause goiter and hypothyroidism in the fetus. Use cautiously during pregnancy.

Reactions in bold italics are *life-threatening*. Interactions may have a *rapid onset* or a *delayed onset*.

• If drug is used during pregnancy or if patient becomes pregnant during therapy, apprise patient of fetal risk.

• Patients who are pregnant may need lower doses as pregnancy progresses, and drug may be stopped during last few weeks of pregnancy. Monitor thyroid function studies closely.

• Drug appears in human milk. Use cautiously and administer after breastfeeding and in divided doses.

NURSING CONSIDERATIONS

• Monitor CBC periodically to detect impending leukopenia, thrombocytopenia, aplastic anemia, and agranulocytosis; also monitor hepatic function. Stop drug if liver abnormality occurs.

⚠ *Alert:* Drug may increase risk of agranulocytosis, which can be life-threatening. Monitor patient for sore throat, fever, and general malaise and report symptoms promptly.

• Monitor PT, especially before invasive procedures.

• Monitor thyroid function tests and watch for evidence of hypothyroidism (mental depression, cold intolerance, and hard, nonpitting edema); notify prescriber because patient may need dosage adjustment.

⚠ *Alert:* Stop drug and notify prescriber if severe rash or enlarged lymph nodes develop.

• *Look alike–sound alike:* Don't confuse methimazole with methazolamide, metolazone, or metronidazole.

PATIENT TEACHING

• Instruct patient in safe drug administration, handling, and storage.

• Warn patient to report fever, sore throat, mouth sores, skin eruptions, anorexia, itching, right upper quadrant pain, yellow skin or eyes, blood in the urine, decreased urine output, shortness of breath, or coughing up blood.

• Tell patient to ask prescriber about eating iodine-rich foods, including iodized salt, bread, dairy products, and shellfish, because the iodine in these foods may make drug less effective.

• Warn patient that drug may cause drowsiness; advise patient to use caution when operating machinery or a vehicle.

• Teach patient to watch for evidence of hypothyroidism (unexplained weight gain,

fatigue, cold intolerance) and to notify prescriber if it arises.

• Caution patient to report pregnancy or plans to become pregnant during therapy.

SAFETY ALERT!

methotrexate (amethopterin)
meth-oh-TREKS-ate

Otrexup, Rasuvo, RediTrex, Xatmep

methotrexate sodium
Trexall, Metoject ✽

Therapeutic class: Antineoplastics
Pharmacologic class: Folate antagonists

AVAILABLE FORMS

Injection (autoinjector, prefilled syringe):
7.5 mg, 10 mg, 12.5 mg, 15 mg, 17.5 mg, 20 mg, 22.5 mg, 25 mg, 30 mg
Injection: 10 mg/1 mL ✽, 25 mg/mL preservative-free vials; 25 mg/mL vials*
Lyophilized powder: 1,000-mg preservative-free vials
Oral solution: 2.5 mg/mL
Tablets: 2.5 mg, 5 mg, 7.5 mg, 10 mg, 15 mg

INDICATIONS & DOSAGES

Adjust-a-dose (for all indications): Reduce dosage in patients with impaired renal function.

➤ **Trophoblastic tumors (choriocarcinoma, hydatidiform mole)**
Adults: 15 to 30 mg PO or IM daily for 5 days. Repeat after 1 or more weeks, based on response or toxicity. Number of courses is three to maximum of five.

➤ **Low risk gestational trophoblastic neoplasia (GTN)**
Adults: 30 to 200 mg/m^2 or 0.4 to 1 mg/kg IV or IM.

➤ **High risk GTN**
Adults: 300 mg/m^2 IV infusion over 12 hours as part of multidrug regimen.

➤ **Acute lymphocytic leukemia (except Otrexup, Rasuvo)**
Adults and children: For induction, 3.3 mg/m^2 daily PO (tablets), IV, or IM with 60 mg/m^2 prednisone daily for 4 to 6 weeks or until remission occurs; then 30 mg/m^2 PO or IM weekly in two divided doses or 2.5 mg/kg IV every 14 days. Or, 10 to 5,000 mg/m^2

IV as part of multidrug regimen. Or, 20 to 30 mg/m^2/week IM as part of multidose regimen. Or, 20 mg/m^2 Trexall PO once weekly. Or, for oral solution use in children, 20 mg/m^2 once weekly.

Adjust-a-dose: Individualize dose and schedule of IV or IM injection based on disease state, patient risk category, concurrent drugs used, phase of treatment, and treatment response.

➤ **Meningeal leukemia**

Adults and children age 3 and older: 12 to 15 mg intrathecally every 2 days or more, up to twice weekly.

Children ages 3 to younger than 9: 12 mg intrathecally every 2 days or more, up to twice weekly.

Children ages 2 to younger than 3: 10 mg intrathecally every 2 days or more, up to twice weekly.

Children ages 1 to younger than 2: 8 mg intrathecally every 2 days or more, up to twice weekly.

Children younger than age 1: 6 mg intrathecally every 2 days or more, up to twice weekly.

Adjust-a-dose: Administration interval of less than 1 week may increase toxicity. Continue treatment until CSF cell count falls within normal range.

➤ **Lymphoma (Burkitt tumor stage I, II)**

Adults: 10 to 25 mg PO daily for 4 to 8 days, with 7- to 10-day rest intervals; commonly given with other agents.

➤ **Lymphosarcoma (stage III)**

Adults: 0.625 to 2.5 mg/kg daily PO, IM, or IV; commonly given with other agents.

➤ **Non-Hodgkin lymphoma**

Adults: Dosage varies from 10 to 8,000 mg/m^2 IV based on treatment regimen. Single-agent use may be 8,000 mg/m^2 IV for CNS direct therapy infused over 4 hours, or 5 to 75 mg IV for cutaneous forms of lymphoma.

Combination therapy dosage is 1,000 to 3,000 mg/m^2 IV followed by leucovorin rescue. Or, 25 mg Trexall PO two to four times a week as part of metronomic combination chemotherapy.

➤ **Osteosarcoma**

Adults: Typically, 12 g/m^2 IV (maximum dose, 20 g) as 4-hour infusion as part of combination chemotherapy regimen. Give with leucovorin rescue regimen.

➤ **Mycosis fungoides**

Adults: 5 to 50 mg PO or IM once weekly; if poor response, may increase to 15 to 37.5 mg IM twice weekly. Or, 25 to 75 mg Trexall PO once weekly as monotherapy or 10 mg/m^2 PO twice weekly as part of combination chemotherapy.

Adjust-a-dose: Dosage reductions or cessation is guided by patient response and hematologic monitoring.

➤ **Psoriasis**

Adults: 10 to 25 mg PO, IM, IV, or subcut as single weekly dose; or 2.5 to 5 mg PO every 12 hours for three doses weekly. Dosage shouldn't exceed 30 mg/week.

➤ **RA**

Adults: Initially, 7.5 mg PO, IM, or subcut weekly, either in single dose or divided as 2.5 mg PO every 12 hours for three doses once weekly. Dosage may be gradually increased to maximum of 20 mg weekly.

➤ **Polyarticular course, juvenile RA**

Children and adolescents age 2 to 16: 10 mg/m^2 PO, IM, or subcut once weekly. Or, 20 to 30 mg/m^2/week IM or subcut.

➤ **Breast cancer**

Adults: 40 mg/m^2 IV as component of cyclophosphamide and 5-FU–based regimen.

➤ **Squamous cell carcinoma of head and neck**

Adults: 40 to 60 mg/m^2 IV once weekly.

➤ **Moderate to severe Crohn disease ◆**

Adults: Initially, 12.5 to 15 mg IM or subcut once weekly. May gradually increase to maximum of 25 mg IM or subcut once weekly; may reduce to 15 mg once weekly if steroid-free remission is maintained for 4 months.

➤ **SLE (moderate to severe) ◆**

Adults: 5 to 15 mg once weekly; may increase by 2.5-mg increments every 4 weeks to maximum of 25 mg once weekly, in combination with prednisone.

ADMINISTRATION
PO

🔴 *Alert:* Drug is cytotoxic; follow special handling and disposal procedures.

• Give on an empty stomach.

• Use an accurate measuring device to measure oral solution.

• May store oral solution at room temperature for up to 60 days or refrigerate. Don't freeze.

IV

🔴 *Alert:* Preparing and giving parenteral drug may be mutagenic, teratogenic, or carcinogenic. Follow facility protocol to reduce risks.

▼ Dilution of drug depends on product, and infusion guidelines vary, depending on dose.

Reactions in bold italics are *life-threatening*. Interactions may have a *rapid onset* or a *delayed onset*.

▼ For methotrexate therapy with leucovorin rescue, patients should be well hydrated. Administer 1 L/m² of IV fluids over 6 hours before initiation of methotrexate infusion. Continue hydration at 125 mL/m²/hour during the methotrexate infusion and for 2 days after infusion has been completed.

▼ May use IV formulations containing benzyl alcohol IV, IM, or subcut. Use preservative-free formulation for intrathecal use and for treatment of neonates or low-birth-weight infants.

▼ **Incompatibilities:** None listed by manufacturer. Consult a drug incompatibility reference for more information.

IM

🔃 *Alert:* Preparing and giving parenteral drug may be mutagenic, teratogenic, or carcinogenic. Follow facility protocol to reduce risks.

Subcutaneous

• Administer subcutaneously in the abdomen or thigh only.

• Otrexup, RediTrex, and Rasuvo are single-dose syringes for once-weekly subcut use only and are available in specific dosage strengths. Use another formulation for dosing by other routes, doses less than 7.5 mg/week, doses more than 25 or 30 mg/week, high-dose regimens, or dosage adjustments between the available doses.

Intrathecal

• Preparing and giving parenteral drug may be mutagenic, teratogenic, or carcinogenic. Follow facility protocol to reduce risks.

Boxed Warning Use preservative-free form for intrathecal or high-dose administration. ∎

• Reconstitute to 1 mg/mL concentration with preservative-free NSS.

ACTION

Reversibly binds to dihydrofolate reductase, blocking reduction of folic acid to tetrahydrofolate, a cofactor necessary for purine, protein, and DNA synthesis.

Route	Onset	Peak	Duration
PO	Unknown	45 min–6 hr	Unknown
IV	Immediate	Immediate	Unknown
IM	Unknown	30 min–1 hr	Unknown
Subcut	Unknown	1–2 hr	Unknown
Intrathecal	Unknown	Unknown	Unknown

Half-life: For doses below 30 mg/m², about 3 to 10 hours (adults), 0.7 to 5.8 hours (children); for doses of 30 mg/m² and above, 8 to 15 hours.

ADVERSE REACTIONS

CNS: demyelination, malaise, fatigue, dizziness, headache, aphasia, hemiparesis, fever. **CV:** *thromboembolic events,* chest pain, hypotension, pericardial effusion, pericarditis. **EENT:** blurred vision, pharyngitis. **GI:** gingivitis, stomatitis, diarrhea, GI ulceration, *GI bleeding,* enteritis, nausea, vomiting. **GU:** nephropathy, tubular necrosis, *renal failure,* menstrual dysfunction, abortion, cystitis. **Hematologic:** *leukopenia, pancytopenia, anemia, neutropenia, thrombocytopenia.* **Hepatic:** *acute toxicity, chronic toxicity,* including cirrhosis, *hepatic fibrosis,* increased liver enzyme levels. **Metabolic:** weight loss, hyperuricemia. **Musculoskeletal:** arthralgia, myalgia, osteoporosis in children on long-term therapy. **Respiratory:** *interstitial pneumonitis,* cough, *PE.* **Skin:** urticaria, pruritus, hyperpigmentation, erythematous rashes, ecchymoses, rash, photosensitivity reactions, alopecia, acne, psoriatic lesions aggravated by exposure to sun. **Other:** chills, reduced resistance to infection, lymphadenopathy, *sepsis.*

INTERACTIONS

Drug-drug. *Acitretin (vitamin A derivative):* May increase risk of hepatitis. Avoid using together.

Folic acid derivatives: Antagonizes methotrexate effect. Avoid using together, except for leucovorin rescue with high-dose methotrexate therapy.

Fosphenytoin, phenytoin: May decrease phenytoin and fosphenytoin levels. Monitor drug levels closely.

Hepatotoxic drugs: May increase risk of hepatotoxicity. Monitor patient closely.

Nitrous oxide: Potentiates effect of methotrexate, increasing risk of methotrexate adverse reactions. Avoid use together.

Boxed Warning *NSAIDs, salicylates:* May increase methotrexate toxicity. Avoid using together. ∎

Oral antibiotics: May decrease absorption of methotrexate. Monitor patient closely.

Penicillins, sulfonamides, trimethoprim: May increase methotrexate level. Monitor patient for methotrexate toxicity.

Probenecid: May impair excretion of methotrexate, causing increased level, effect, and toxicity of methotrexate. Monitor methotrexate level closely and adjust dosage accordingly.

◑ Alert: *PPIs:* May cause methotrexate toxicity, especially when high doses of methotrexate are given. Use cautiously.

◑ Alert: *Theophylline:* May increase theophylline level. Monitor theophylline level closely.

Thiopurines: May increase thiopurine level. Monitor patient closely.

Vaccines: May make immunizations ineffective; may cause risk of disseminated infection with live-virus vaccines. Postpone immunization, if possible.

Drug-food. *Any food:* May delay absorption and reduce peak level of methotrexate. Instruct patient to take drug on an empty stomach.

Drug-lifestyle. *Alcohol use:* May increase hepatotoxicity. Discourage use together.

Sun exposure: May cause photosensitivity reactions. Advise patient to avoid excessive sunlight exposure.

EFFECTS ON LAB TEST RESULTS
- May increase uric acid level and LFT values.
- May decrease Hb level and WBC, RBC, and platelet counts.
- May alter results of lab assay for folate, which interferes with detection of folic acid deficiency.

CONTRAINDICATIONS & CAUTIONS
Boxed Warning Contraindicated in patients hypersensitive to drug. ∎
- Contraindicated in patients with psoriasis or RA who also have alcoholism, alcoholic liver, chronic liver disease, immunodeficiency syndromes, or blood dyscrasias.

Boxed Warning Use drug only in patients with life-threatening neoplastic diseases and in those with severe psoriasis or RA not adequately responsive to other therapy; deaths have occurred. Closely monitor patients for bone marrow, liver, lung, and kidney toxicities. ∎

Boxed Warning Methotrexate given with radiotherapy may increase the risk of soft-tissue necrosis and osteonecrosis. ∎

Boxed Warning Unexpectedly severe (sometimes fatal) bone marrow suppression, aplastic anemia, and GI toxicity have been reported with concomitant administration of methotrexate (usually in high dosage) with some NSAIDs. ∎

Boxed Warning Use cautiously and at modified dosage in patients with impaired hepatic or renal function, bone marrow suppression, aplasia, leukopenia, thrombocytopenia, or anemia. ∎
- Use cautiously in very young patients, older adults, or patients who are debilitated and in those with infection, peptic ulceration, or ulcerative colitis.

Dialyzable drug: Yes (using a high-flux dialyzer).

⚠ Overdose S&S: Leukopenia, thrombocytopenia, anemia, pancytopenia, bone marrow suppression, mucositis, stomatitis, oral ulceration, nausea, vomiting, GI ulceration, GI bleeding, sepsis or septic shock, renal failure, aplastic anemia, headache, seizures, acute toxic encephalopathy, cerebellar herniation associated with increased ICP, death.

PREGNANCY-LACTATION-REPRODUCTION
Boxed Warning Contraindicated during pregnancy for nonneoplastic disease. Don't use in patients of childbearing potential with neoplasms unless benefits outweigh risks. ∎
- Contraindicated during breastfeeding.

Boxed Warning If either partner is receiving methotrexate, they should avoid conception during and for a minimum of 3 months after therapy for males, and during and for 6 months after therapy for females. ∎
- Drug has been reported to cause impaired fertility, oligospermia, and menstrual dysfunction during therapy and for a short period after therapy ends.

NURSING CONSIDERATIONS
Boxed Warning Methotrexate should be used only by health care providers whose knowledge and experience include the use of antimetabolite therapy. ∎

Boxed Warning Drug can cause severe and fatal toxicities. Modify dosage or discontinue drug for bone marrow suppression, infection, and renal, GI, pulmonary, and dermatologic toxicities or hypersensitivity. ∎

Boxed Warning Methotrexate-induced lung disease, including acute or chronic interstitial pneumonitis, is a potentially dangerous lesion that may occur at any time during therapy. It isn't always fully reversible. Pulmonary symptoms (especially a dry, nonproductive cough) may require interruption of treatment and careful investigation. ∎

Boxed Warning Diarrhea and ulcerative stomatitis require interruption of therapy; hemorrhagic enteritis and death from intestinal perforation may occur. ∎

Reactions in bold italics are *life-threatening*. Interactions may have a *rapid onset* or a *delayed onset*.

Nursing2024
DRUG HANDBOOK®

Photoguide to tablets and capsules

This photoguide includes 415 tablets and capsules that are among the most commonly prescribed or important to identify generic and trade name drugs. Organized alphabetically by generic name, each pill is shown in actual size and color along with its imprint code and dosage strength. Page numbers indicate where to find additional information within the book.

INDEX OF TRADE NAMES IN PHOTOGUIDE TO TABLETS AND CAPSULES

ALENDRONATE SODIUM

Fosamax
(Page 95)

70 mg

ALFUZOSIN HYDROCHLORIDE

Uroxatral
(Page 1702)

10 mg

ALLOPURINOL

Zyloprim
(Page 99)

100 mg   300 mg

ALPRAZOLAM

Xanax
(Page 106)

0.25 mg   0.5 mg   1 mg

2 mg

AMLODIPINE BESYLATE

Norvasc
(Page 123)

2.5 mg   5 mg

ANASTROZOLE

Arimidex
(Page 136)

1 mg

APIXABAN

Eliquis
(Page 139)

 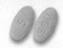

2.5 mg   5 mg

ARIPIPRAZOLE

Abilify
(Page 147)

10 mg

15 mg

30 mg

ATAZANAVIR SULFATE

Reyataz
(Page 157)

200 mg

ATENOLOL

Tenormin
(Page 162)

25 mg

50 mg

100 mg

ATOMOXETINE HYDROCHLORIDE

Strattera
(Page 164)

10 mg

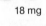

18 mg

25 mg

40 mg

60 mg

ATORVASTATIN CALCIUM

Lipitor
(Page 166)

10 mg

20 mg

40 mg

80 mg

AZITHROMYCIN

Zithromax
(Page 181)

250 mg

500 mg

BENAZEPRIL HYDROCHLORIDE

Lotensin
(Page 195)

20 mg

40 mg

BREXPIPRAZOLE

Rexulti
(Page 217)

0.5 mg

1 mg

2 mg

3 mg

BUMETANIDE

Bumex
(Page 227)

0.5 mg

1 mg

2 mg

BUPROPION HYDROCHLORIDE

Wellbutrin SR
(Page 235)

100 mg

150 mg

200 mg

CANDESARTAN CILEXETIL

Atacand
(Page 255)

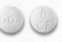 4 mg

 8 mg

 16 mg

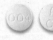

 32 mg

CARVEDILOL

Coreg
(Page 273)

 3.125 mg

6.25 mg

12.5 mg

 25 mg

Coreg CR
(Page 273)

 10 mg

 20 mg

 40 mg

 80 mg

CELECOXIB

CeleBREX
(Page 301)

 100 mg

 200 mg

CIPROFLOXACIN

Cipro
(Page 320)

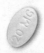

250 mg   500 mg

CITALOPRAM HYDROBROMIDE

CeleXA
(Page 328)

20 mg   40 mg

CLONAZEPAM

KlonoPIN
(Page 341)

0.5 mg   1 mg   2 mg

CLOPIDOGREL BISULFATE

Plavix
(Page 347)

75 mg

CLOZAPINE

Clozaril
(Page 350)

25 mg   100 mg

COLCHICINE

Colcrys
(Page 360)

0.6 mg

DABIGATRAN ETEXILATE MESYLATE

Pradaxa
(Page 373)

75 mg   150 mg

DESLORATADINE

Clarinex
(Page 1725)

5 mg

DESVENLAFAXINE SUCCINATE

Pristiq
(Page 405)

50 mg

100 mg

DEXLANSOPRAZOLE

Dexilant
(Page 1726)

30 mg

60 mg

DEXMETHYLPHENIDATE HYDROCHLORIDE

Focalin XR
(Page 410)

5mg

10 mg

15 mg

20 mg

30 mg

40 mg

DIAZEPAM

Valium
(Page 418)

2 mg

5 mg

10 mg

DIGOXIN

Lanoxin
(Page 429)

0.125 mg

0.25 mg

DILTIAZEM HYDROCHLORIDE

Cardizem
(Page 433)

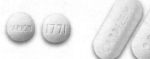

30 mg   90 mg

Cardizem CD
(Page 433)

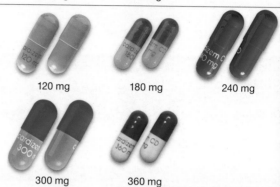

120 mg   180 mg   240 mg

300 mg   360 mg

Cardizem LA
(Page 433)

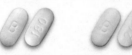

180 mg   240 mg   360 mg

DIVALPROEX SODIUM

Depakote
(Page 1517)

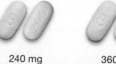

125 mg   250 mg   500 mg

Depakote Sprinkle
(Page 1517)

125 mg

DONEPEZIL HYDROCHLORIDE

Aricept
(Page 447)

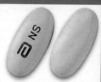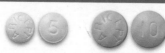

5 mg   10 mg

DOXAZOSIN MESYLATE

Cardura
(Page 451)

1 mg

2 mg

4 mg

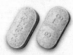
8 mg

DULOXETINE HYDROCHLORIDE

Cymbalta
(Page 477)

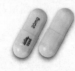
20 mg

30 mg

60 mg

DUTASTERIDE

Avodart
(Page 480)

0.5 mg

ELETRIPTAN HYDROBROMIDE

Relpax
(Page 490)

20 mg

40 mg

ENALAPRIL MALEATE

Vasotec
(Page 509)

2.5 mg

5 mg

10 mg

20 mg

ERYTHROMYCIN BASE

Eryc
(Page 546)

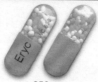

250 mg

Ery-Tab
(Page 546)

333 mg

ESCITALOPRAM OXALATE

Lexapro
(Page 548)

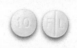

10 mg   20 mg

ESOMEPRAZOLE MAGNESIUM

Nexium
(Page 555)

20 mg   40 mg

ESTROGENS (CONJUGATED)

Premarin
(Page 573)

0.3 mg   0.45 mg   0.625 mg

0.9 mg   1.25 mg

ESZOPICLONE

Lunesta
(Page 575)

1 mg   2 mg   3 mg

EZETIMIBE

Zetia
(Page 601)

10 mg

EZETIMIBE—SIMVASTATIN

Vytorin
(Page 1665)

10 mg/10 mg   10 mg/20 mg   10 mg/40 mg

10 mg/80 mg

FAMOTIDINE

Pepcid
(Page 604)

20 mg   40 mg

FENOFIBRATE

TriCor
(Page 609)

48 mg   145 mg

FINASTERIDE

Propecia
(Page 623)

1 mg

Proscar
(Page 623)

5 mg

FLUCONAZOLE

Diflucan
(Page 630)

50 mg

100 mg

150 mg

200 mg

FLUOXETINE HYDROCHLORIDE

Prozac
(Page 640)

10 mg

20 mg

40 mg

FROVATRIPTAN SUCCINATE

Frova
(Page 666)

2.5 mg

FUROSEMIDE

Lasix
(Page 669)

20 mg

40 mg

80 mg

GABAPENTIN

Neurontin
(Page 672)

100 mg

300 mg

400 mg

GEMFIBROZIL

Lopid
(Page 679)

600 mg

GLIMEPIRIDE

Amaryl
(Page 688)

1 mg   2 mg   4 mg

GLIPIZIDE

Glucotrol XL
(Page 689)

2.5 mg   5 mg   10 mg

IRBESARTAN

Avapro
(Page 807)

75 mg   150 mg   300 mg

LAMIVUDINE—ZIDOVUDINE

Combivir
(Page 1667)

150 mg/300 mg

LANSOPRAZOLE

Prevacid
(Page 845)

15 mg   30 mg

LEVODOPA—CARBIDOPA

Sinemet
(Page 863)

100 mg/10 mg   250 mg/25 mg

LEVODOPA—CARBIDOPA—ENTACAPONE

Stalevo
(Page 867)

| 50 mg/12.5 mg/ | 100 mg/25 mg/ | 150 mg/37.5 mg/ |
| 200 mg | 200 mg | 200 mg |

LEVOTHYROXINE SODIUM

Levoxyl
(Page 873)

| 25 mcg | 50 mcg | 75 mcg |

| 88 mcg | 100 mcg | 112 mcg |

| 125 mcg | 137 mcg | 150 mcg |

| 175 mcg | 200 mcg |

Synthroid
(Page 873)

   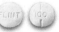

| 25 mcg | 50 mcg | 75 mcg |

| 88 mcg | 100 mcg | 112 mcg |

| 125 mcg | 150 mcg | 175 mcg |

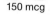

| 200 mcg | 300 mcg |

LISDEXAMFETAMINE DIMESYLATE

Vyvanse
(Page 884)

20 mg

30 mg

40 mg

50 mg

60 mg

70 mg

LISINOPRIL

Zestril
(Page 886)

2.5 mg

5 mg

10 mg

20 mg

40 mg

LOPINAVIR–RITONAVIR

Kaletra
(Page 897)

200 mg/50 mg

LORAZEPAM

Ativan
(Page 901)

0.5 mg

1 mg

2 mg

LOSARTAN POTASSIUM

Cozaar
(Page 904)

25 mg

50 mg

LUBIPROSTONE

Amitiza
(Page 1642)

24 mcg

LURASIDONE HYDROCHLORIDE

Latuda
(Page 907)

20 mg

40 mg

80 mg

MEDROXYPROGESTERONE ACETATE

Provera
(Page 916)

2.5 mg

5 mg

10 mg

MELOXICAM

Mobic
(Page 1752)

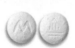

7.5 mg

15 mg

MEMANTINE HYDROCHLORIDE

Namenda
(Page 925)

5 mg

10 mg

Namenda XR
(Page 925)

7 mg

14 mg

21 mg

28 mg

METHADONE HYDROCHLORIDE

(Page 939)

5 mg

10 mg

METHYLPHENIDATE HYDROCHLORIDE

Concerta
(Page 953)

18 mg

36 mg

54 mg

Ritalin
(Page 953)

5 mg

10 mg

20 mg

METHYLPREDNISOLONE

Medrol
(Page 957)

4 mg   16 mg

METOPROLOL SUCCINATE

Toprol-XL
(Page 966)

50 mg   100 mg   200 mg

METOPROLOL TARTRATE

Lopressor
(Page 966)

 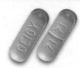

50 mg   100 mg

MILNACIPRAN HYDROCHLORIDE

Savella
(Page 981)

12.5 mg   25 mg   50 mg

MODAFINIL

Provigil
(Page 994)

 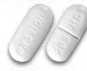

100 mg   200 mg

MONTELUKAST SODIUM

Singulair
(Page 999)

4 mg   5 mg   10 mg

NAPROXEN

Naprosyn
(Page 1026)

500 mg

NIFEDIPINE

Procardia XL
(Page 1050)

30 mg   60 mg   90 mg

NITROFURANTOIN MACROCRYSTALS

Macrodantin
(Page 1054)

25 mg   50 mg   100 mg

NITROGLYCERIN

Nitrostat
(Page 1056)

0.4 mg

NORTRIPTYLINE HYDROCHLORIDE

Pamelor
(Page 1071)

10 mg   25 mg   50 mg

75 mg

OLANZAPINE

Zyprexa
(Page 1086)

2.5 mg   5 mg   7.5 mg

10 mg   15 mg   20 mg

OLMESARTAN MEDOXOMIL

Benicar
(Page 1093)

20 mg   40 mg

OLMESARTAN MEDOXOMIL—HYDROCHLOROTHIAZIDE

Benicar HCT
(Page 1664)

20 mg/12.5 mg   40 mg/12.5 mg   40 mg/25 mg

OMEGA-3–FATTY ACIDS

Lovaza
(Page 1101)

1 g

OSELTAMIVIR PHOSPHATE

Tamiflu
(Page 1116)

30 mg   45 mg   75 mg

OXYCODONE HYDROCHLORIDE

OxyCONTIN
(Page 1134)

10 mg

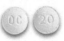

20 mg

40 mg

80 mg

PANTOPRAZOLE SODIUM

Protonix
(Page 1164)

20 mg

40 mg

PHENYTOIN SODIUM (EXTENDED RELEASE)

Dilantin
(Page 1202)

30 mg

100 mg

PIOGLITAZONE HYDROCHLORIDE

Actos
(Page 1209)

15 mg

30 mg

45 mg

POTASSIUM CHLORIDE

Klor-Con
(Page 1226)

8 mEq

10 mEq

PRASUGREL HYDROCHLORIDE

Effient
(Page 1232)

5 mg

10 mg

PREGABALIN

Lyrica
(Page 1244)

25 mg

50 mg

75 mg

100 mg

150 mg

200 mg

225 mg

300 mg

PROPRANOLOL HYDROCHLORIDE

Inderal LA
(Page 1260)

60 mg

80 mg

120 mg

160 mg

QUETIAPINE FUMARATE

Seroquel
(Page 1264)

25 mg　　　　　50 mg　　　　　100 mg

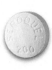

200 mg　　　　　300 mg　　　　　400 mg

QUINAPRIL HYDROCHLORIDE

Accupril
(Page 1268)

5 mg　　　　　10 mg　　　　　20 mg

40 mg

RABEPRAZOLE SODIUM

Aciphex
(Page 1270)

20 mg

RALOXIFENE HYDROCHLORIDE

Evista
(Page 1272)

60 mg

RANOLAZINE

Ranexa
(Page 1283)

500 mg

RASAGILINE MESYLATE

Azilect
(Page 1285)

0.5 mg   1 mg

RISEDRONATE SODIUM

Actonel
(Page 1312)

35 mg

RISPERIDONE

RisperDAL
(Page 1314)

0.25 mg   0.5 mg   1 mg

2 mg   3 mg   4 mg

RIVAROXABAN

Xarelto
(Page 1324)

15 mg   20 mg

RIVASTIGMINE TARTRATE

(Page 1328)

1.5 mg   3 mg   4.5 mg

6 mg

ROFLUMILAST

Daliresp
(Page 1330)

250 mg   500 mg

ROSUVASTATIN CALCIUM

Crestor
(Page 1335)

5 mg   10 mg   20 mg

40 mg

SAXAGLIPTIN

Onglyza
(Page 1350)

2.5 mg   5 mg

SERTRALINE HYDROCHLORIDE

Zoloft
(Page 1365)

50 mg   100 mg

SILDENAFIL CITRATE

Viagra
(Page 1369)

25 mg   50 mg   100 mg

SIMVASTATIN

Zocor
(Page 1373)

5 mg

10 mg

20 mg

40 mg

SITAGLIPTIN PHOSPHATE

Januvia
(Page 1378)

100 mg

SOLIFENACIN SUCCINATE

VESIcare
(Page 1389)

5 mg   10 mg

SPIRONOLACTONE

Aldactone
(Page 1397)

25 mg   50 mg   100 mg

SUCRALFATE

Carafate
(Page 1401)

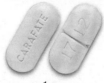

1 g

SULFAMETHOXAZOLE—TRIMETHOPRIM

Bactrim DS
(Page 1406)

800 mg/160 mg

SUMATRIPTAN SUCCINATE

Imitrex
(Page 1410)

25 mg   50 mg

SUNITINIB MALATE

Sutent
(Page 1412)

12.5 mg   25 mg   50 mg

TADALAFIL

Cialis
(Page 1419)

2.5 mg   5 mg   10 mg

20 mg

TAMSULOSIN HYDROCHLORIDE

Flomax
(Page 1423)

0.4 mg

TAPENTADOL HYDROCHLORIDE

Nucynta
(Page 1777)

50 mg   100 mg

Nucynta ER
(Page 1777)

100 mg

TELMISARTAN

Micardis
(Page 1428)

20 mg 40 mg 80 mg

TEMAZEPAM

Restoril
(Page 1429)

7.5 mg 15 mg 30 mg

TENOFOVIR DISOPROXIL FUMARATE

Viread
(Page 1432)

300 mg

TICAGRELOR

Brilinta
(Page 1453)

90 mg

TOLTERODINE TARTRATE

Detrol
(Page 1472)

1 mg 2 mg

TOPIRAMATE

Topamax
(Page 1476)

15 mg

25 mg

25 mg

50 mg

100 mg

200 mg

TRAMADOL HYDROCHLORIDE—ACETAMINOPHEN

Ultracet
(Page 1658)

37.5 mg/325 mg

VALACYCLOVIR HYDROCHLORIDE

Valtrex
(Page 1516)

500 mg

1,000 mg

VALSARTAN

Diovan
(Page 1521)

40 mg

80 mg

160 mg

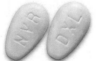

320 mg

VALSARTAN—HYDROCHLOROTHIAZIDE

Diovan HCT
(Page 1665)

80 mg/12.5 mg   160 mg/12.5 mg   160 mg/25 mg

320 mg/12.5 mg   320 mg/25 mg

VENLAFAXINE HYDROCHLORIDE

Effexor XR
(Page 1532)

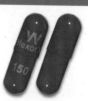

75 mg   150 mg

VERAPAMIL HYDROCHLORIDE

Verelan
(Page 1535)

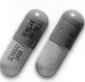

120 mg   180 mg   240 mg

VILAZODONE HYDROCHLORIDE

Viibryd
(Page 1542)

10 mg   20 mg   40 mg

ZAFIRLUKAST

Accolate
(Page 1564)

10 mg   20 mg

ZIDOVUDINE

Retrovir
(Page 1567)

100 mg

ZIPRASIDONE HYDROCHLORIDE

Geodon
(Page 1569)

20 mg

40 mg

60 mg

80 mg

ZOLPIDEM TARTRATE

Ambien
(Page 1577)

5 mg

10 mg

Boxed Warning Malignant lymphomas may occur in patients receiving low-dose methotrexate and may regress upon discontinuing drug. ■

Boxed Warning Methotrexate may induce TLS in patients with rapidly growing tumors. ■

Boxed Warning Severe, occasionally fatal skin reactions have been reported following single or multiple doses of methotrexate. Reactions have occurred within days of methotrexate administration. Recovery has been reported with discontinuation of therapy. ■

Boxed Warning Potentially fatal opportunistic infections, especially *Pneumocystis jiroveci* pneumonia, may occur with methotrexate therapy. ■

Boxed Warning The high-dose regimens for osteosarcoma require meticulous care. ■

🕄 *Alert:* Drug may be given daily or once weekly, depending on the disease. To avoid administration errors, know patient's dosing schedule.

• Monitor pulmonary function tests periodically.

• Monitor fluid intake and output daily. Encourage fluid intake of 2 to 3 L daily.

• Delayed drug elimination may occur with impaired renal function, third space effusion (ascites), or other disorders, increasing systemic level and risk of toxicity.

🕄 *Alert:* Alkalinize urine by giving sodium bicarbonate tablets or fluids to prevent precipitation of drug, especially at high doses. Maintain urine pH above 7.

Boxed Warning It's essential to monitor CBC with differential, platelet count, and liver and renal function periodically. Watch for increases in AST, ALT, and ALP levels, which may signal hepatic dysfunction. Periodic liver biopsies are recommended for patients with psoriasis who are receiving long-term treatment. Monitor patients at risk for impaired drug elimination (renal dysfunction, pleural effusions, ascites) more frequently. ■

• WBC and platelet count nadirs usually occur on day 7.

• Watch for signs and symptoms of bleeding (especially GI) and infection.

• To prevent bleeding, avoid all IM injections when platelet count is below 50,000/mm³.

• Give blood transfusions for cumulative anemia. Patient may receive injections of RBC colony-stimulating factors to promote RBC production and decrease need for blood transfusions.

• Leucovorin rescue is needed with doses of more than 100 mg and starts 24 hours after therapy starts. Leucovorin is continued until methotrexate level falls below 5×10^{-8} M. Consult specialized references for specific recommendations for leucovorin dosage. Monitor methotrexate level and adjust leucovorin dose.

• Monitor patient for neurotoxicity with intrathecal administration. Acute chemical arachnoiditis causes headache, back pain, nuchal rigidity, and fever. Paraparesis or paraplegia is present with subacute myelopathy.

• Transient acute stroke-like syndrome can occur with high-dose infusions (confusion, hemiparesis, transient blindness, seizure, coma).

PATIENT TEACHING

• Advise patient to watch for signs and symptoms of infection (fever, sore throat, fatigue) and bleeding (easy bruising, nosebleeds, bleeding gums, melena). Tell patient to take temperature daily.

Boxed Warning Fully inform patient of the risks involved with methotrexate therapy. ■

• Instruct patient of childbearing potential of the fetal risk and to inform prescriber of known or suspected pregnancy.

• Counsel patient of childbearing potential to use effective contraception during treatment and for 6 months after final dose.

• Advise male patient of reproductive potential to use effective contraception during treatment and for 3 months after final dose.

• Caution patient to stop breastfeeding during therapy.

• Teach and encourage diligent mouth care to reduce risk of superinfection in the mouth.

• Inform caregivers to always use an accurate measuring device when administering the oral solution.

• Instruct patient how to take leucovorin. Stress importance of taking as directed.

• Tell patient to use highly protective sunblock and wear protective clothing when exposed to sunlight.

SAFETY ALERT!

methyldopa
meth-il-DOE-pa

Therapeutic class: Antihypertensives
Pharmacologic class: Centrally acting antiadrenergics

AVAILABLE FORMS
Tablets: 125 mg, 250 mg, 500 mg

INDICATIONS & DOSAGES
➤ **HTN**
Adults: Initially, 250 mg PO b.i.d. to t.i.d. in first 48 hours. Limit initial daily dose to 500 mg/day when given with antihypertensives other than thiazide diuretics. Adjust dosage at no less than 48-hour intervals. Maintenance dosage is 500 mg to 2 g daily in two to four divided doses. Maximum recommended PO daily dose is 3 g.
Children: Initially, 10 mg/kg/day PO daily in two to four divided doses. Maximum daily dose is 65 mg/kg or 3 g, whichever is less.
Adjust-a-dose: Adjust dosage if other antihypertensives are added to or deleted from therapy.

ADMINISTRATION
PO
• Increase dosage in the evening to minimize sedation.
• Store pharmacy-made suspension in refrigerator or in the dark at room temperature for up to 14 days; shake well before each use.
• Store at room temperature; protect from light.

ACTION
May inhibit the central vasomotor centers, decreasing sympathetic outflow to the heart, kidneys, and peripheral vasculature.

Route	Onset	Peak	Duration
PO	4–6 hr	Unknown	12–48 hr

Half-life: About 105 minutes.

ADVERSE REACTIONS
CNS: decreased mental acuity, sedation, headache, weakness, asthenia, dizziness, paresthesia, parkinsonism, Bell's palsy, involuntary choreoathetoid movements, psychic disturbances, depression, nightmares. **CV:** orthostatic hypotension, edema, *bradycardia, HF, myocarditis,* aggravated angina, carotid sinus hypersensitivity. **EENT:** nasal congestion, salivary gland inflammation, sore or "black" tongue, dry mouth. **GI:** *pancreatitis,* nausea, vomiting, diarrhea, constipation, flatus, abdominal distention, colitis. **GU:** amenorrhea, impotence. **Hematologic:** *thrombocytopenia, leukopenia, bone marrow depression,* hemolytic anemia. **Hepatic:** *hepatitis,* jaundice. **Metabolic:** hyperprolactinemia, weight gain. **Musculoskeletal:** arthralgia, myalgia. **Skin:** TEN, rash. **Other:** drug-induced fever, breast enlargement, gynecomastia, lactation.

INTERACTIONS
Drug-drug. *Amphetamines, pseudoephedrine, SNRIs, TCAs:* May decrease antihypertensive effects. Monitor patient closely.
Anesthetics: May need lower doses of anesthetics. Use together cautiously.
Antihypertensives: May increase risk of hypotension. Use cautiously.
Barbiturates: May decrease actions of methyldopa. Monitor patient closely.
Ferrous sulfate or gluconate: May decrease bioavailability of methyldopa. Separate doses.
Levodopa: May increase hypotensive effects, which may increase adverse CNS reactions. Monitor patient closely.
Lithium: May increase lithium level. Watch for increased lithium level and signs and symptoms of toxicity.
MAO inhibitors: May increase adverse effects of methyldopa. Use together is contraindicated.

EFFECTS ON LAB TEST RESULTS
• May increase BUN and creatinine levels and LFT values.
• May decrease Hb level, hematocrit, and platelet and WBC counts.
• May interfere with results of urinary uric acid testing, serum creatinine test, and AST test.
• May cause positive Coombs test result.
• May falsely increase urine catecholamine level, interfering with the diagnosis of pheochromocytoma.

CONTRAINDICATIONS & CAUTIONS
• Contraindicated in patients hypersensitive to drug and in those with active hepatic disease (such as acute hepatitis) or active cirrhosis.

Reactions in bold italics are *life-threatening*. Interactions may have a *rapid onset* or a *delayed onset*.

• Contraindicated in those whose previous methyldopa therapy caused liver problems and in those taking MAO inhibitors.
• Use cautiously in older adults and patients with history of impaired hepatic function or sulfite sensitivity.
Dialyzable drug: Yes.
⚠ *Overdose S&S:* Sedation, acute hypotension, weakness, bradycardia, dizziness, constipation, abdominal distention, flatus, diarrhea, nausea, vomiting, light-headedness.

PREGNANCY-LACTATION-REPRODUCTION

• There are no well-controlled studies in the first trimester. Use during pregnancy only if clearly needed. Available data show use during pregnancy doesn't cause fetal harm and may improve fetal outcomes compared to untreated HTN.
• Drug appears in human milk. Use cautiously during breastfeeding.

NURSING CONSIDERATIONS

• Monitor BP regularly. Older adults are more likely to experience hypotension, syncope, and sedation.
• Occasionally, tolerance may occur, usually between the second and third months of therapy. Adding a diuretic or adjusting dosage may be needed. If patient's response changes significantly, notify prescriber.
• After dialysis, monitor patient for HTN and notify prescriber, if needed. Patient may need an extra dose of drug.
• Monitor CBC with differential counts before therapy and periodically thereafter.
• Monitor LFT values periodically during first 12 weeks or if jaundice with or without fever occurs.
• Patients who need blood transfusions should have direct and indirect Coombs tests to prevent cross-matching problems.
• Monitor Coombs test results before therapy and at 6 and 12 months after start of therapy. In patients who have received drug for several months, positive reaction to direct Coombs test may indicate hemolytic anemia.
• Monitor patient for involuntary twitching or writhing (choreoathetoid) movements; discontinue drug if they occur.

PATIENT TEACHING

• If unpleasant adverse reactions occur, advise patient not to suddenly stop taking drug but to notify prescriber.

• Instruct patient to report signs and symptoms of infection, yellowing of the skin, flu-like symptoms, and muscle aches.
• Sodium and water retention may occur but can be relieved with diuretics.
• Warn patient that, particularly at the start of therapy, drug may impair ability to perform tasks that require mental alertness.
• Inform patient that low BP and dizziness upon rising can be minimized by rising slowly and avoiding sudden position changes and that dry mouth can be relieved by chewing gum or sucking on hard candy or ice chips.
• Tell patient that urine may turn dark if left sitting in toilet bowl or if toilet bowl has been treated with bleach.

methylnaltrexone bromide
meth-il-nal-TREKS-one

Relistor

Therapeutic class: GI drugs
Pharmacologic class: Opioid antagonists

M

AVAILABLE FORMS

Injection: 8 mg/0.4 mL, 12 mg/0.6 mL prefilled syringe; 12 mg/0.6 mL in single-use vial
Tablets: 150 mg

INDICATIONS & DOSAGES

➤ **Opioid-induced constipation (OIC) in those receiving palliative care for advanced illness when response to laxatives is insufficient**
Adults weighing more than 114 kg: 0.15 mg/kg subcut every other day, as needed.
Adults weighing 62 to 114 kg: 12 mg subcut every other day, as needed.
Adults weighing 38 to less than 62 kg: 8 mg subcut every other day, as needed.
Adults weighing less than 38 kg: 0.15 mg/kg subcut every other day, as needed.
Adjust-a-dose: In patients with CrCl of less than 60 mL/minute who weigh more than 114 kg, give 0.075 mg/kg; if weight is 62 to 114 kg, give 6 mg; if weight is 38 to less than 62 kg, give 4 mg; if weight is less than 38 kg, give 0.075 mg/kg subcut every other day.
➤ **OIC in patients with chronic noncancer pain**
Adults: 450 mg PO or 12 mg subcut once daily. Discontinue maintenance laxative

therapy before starting methylnaltrexone. May resume laxative after patient has taken methylnaltrexone for 3 days if OIC symptoms persist. Reevaluate need for drug when opioid regimen is changed.

Adjust-a-dose: For CrCl of less than 60 mL/ minute, 150 mg PO once daily or 6 mg subcut once daily. For moderate or severe hepatic impairment, 150 mg PO once daily. Or, for moderate or severe hepatic impairment in patient weighing more than 114 kg, 0.075 mg/kg subcut; 62 to 114 kg, 6 mg subcut; 38 to less than 62 kg, 4 mg subcut; less than 38 kg, 0.075 mg/kg subcut.

ADMINISTRATION
PO
• Give tablets with water on an empty stomach at least 30 minutes before first meal of the day.
Subcutaneous
• Inspect solution; don't give if particulate matter or discoloration is present.
• Give no more than one dose within 24 hours.
• To determine injection volume for the 0.15 mg/kg dose, multiply patient's weight in pounds by 0.0034 and round up to the nearest 0.1 mL, or multiply patient's weight in kilograms by 0.0075 and round up to the nearest 0.1 mL.
• Store drug at room temperature, away from light.
• After drawn into a syringe as directed, drug is stable at room temperature for 24 hours. Vials are for single use only.
• Give injections subcutaneously into the abdomen, thighs, or upper arms; rotate injection sites. Don't inject into bruised, tender, red, or hard areas.

ACTION
Antagonizes GI mu-opioid receptors, preventing opioid-induced slowing of GI motility and transit time.

Route	Onset	Peak	Duration
PO	Unknown	1.5 hr	Unknown
Subcut	Unknown	30 min	Unknown

Half-life: PO, 15 hours.

ADVERSE REACTIONS
CNS: dizziness, tremor, headache, anxiety. **EENT:** rhinorrhea. **GI:** abdominal pain, abdominal distention, flatulence, nausea, diarrhea, vomiting. **Musculoskeletal:** muscle spasms. **Skin:** hyperhidrosis. **Other:** chills, hot flushes.

INTERACTIONS
Drug-drug. *Opioid antagonists:* May increase risk of opioid withdrawal. Avoid combination.

EFFECTS ON LAB TEST RESULTS
None reported.

CONTRAINDICATIONS & CAUTIONS
🔴 *Alert:* Contraindicated in patients hypersensitive to drug, in patients with known or suspected GI obstruction, and in those at increased risk for recurrent obstruction because of increased risk of GI perforation.
🔴 *Alert:* Use cautiously in patients with peptic ulcer disease, Ogilvie syndrome, diverticular disease, infiltrative GI tract malignancies, or peritoneal metastases because of increased risk of GI perforation.
• Use cautiously in patients with peritoneal catheters.
• Patients with disruptions to the blood-brain barrier may be at increased risk for opioid withdrawal or reduced analgesia. Consider overall risk-benefit profile.
• Drug hasn't been studied in patients with ESRD requiring dialysis.
• Safety and effectiveness in children haven't been established.
Dialyzable drug: Unknown.
⚠ *Overdose S&S:* Orthostatic hypotension, signs and symptoms of opioid withdrawal.

PREGNANCY-LACTATION-REPRODUCTION
• Don't use during pregnancy unless benefits outweigh fetal risk. Use in pregnancy may cause opioid withdrawal in a fetus.
• It isn't known if drug appears in human milk. Patient should discontinue breastfeeding or discontinue drug.

NURSING CONSIDERATIONS
🔴 *Alert:* Watch for symptoms of perforation (severe, persistent, or worsening abdominal pain). If symptoms occur, stop drug and evaluate patient.
• Monitor patient for opioid withdrawal and analgesia effectiveness during coadministration.
• Discontinue drug if treatment with the opioid pain medication is also discontinued.

PATIENT TEACHING

• Advise patient that drug may be effective within a few minutes to a few hours after administration and to remain near toilet facilities after receiving drug.
• Instruct patient to discontinue drug and notify prescriber if severe, persistent, or worsening abdominal pain or diarrhea or rash occurs.
• Teach patient or caregiver safe PO or subcut drug administration and syringe disposal.
• Inform patient that vial is for single-use.
• Advise patient to report loss of analgesia or signs and symptoms of opioid withdrawal (hyperhidrosis, chills, diarrhea, abdominal pain, anxiety, yawning).
• Warn patient to report all adverse reactions, to immediately report severe, worsening, or persistent abdominal pain, and to discontinue drug for severe or persistent diarrhea.

---

methylphenidate hydrochloride
meth-il-FEN-i-date

Adhansia XR, Aptensio XR, Biphentin ✣, Concerta✔, Cotempla XR-ODT, Jornay PM, Methylin, QuilliChew ER, Quillivant XR, Relexxii, Ritalin✔, Ritalin LA

methylphenidate transdermal system
Daytrana

Therapeutic class: CNS stimulants
Pharmacologic class: Piperidine derivatives
Controlled substance schedule: II

AVAILABLE FORMS

Oral solution: 5 mg/5 mL, 10 mg/5 mL
Tablets (chewable): 2.5 mg, 5 mg, 10 mg
Tablets (Ritalin): 5 mg, 10 mg, 20 mg
Extended-release
Capsules ⓓⓝⓒ: 10 mg, 15 mg, 20 mg, 25 mg, 30 mg, 35 mg, 40 mg, 45 mg, 50 mg, 55 mg, 60 mg, 70 mg, 80 mg, 85 mg, 100 mg
Oral suspension: 25 mg/5 mL
Tablets ⓓⓝⓒ: 18 mg, 27 mg, 36 mg, 54 mg, 72 mg
Tablets (chewable) ⓓⓝⓒ: 20 mg, 30 mg, 40 mg
Tablets (ODTs) ⓓⓝⓒ: 8.6 mg, 17.3 mg, 25.9 mg
Sustained-release
Tablets (Ritalin-SR) ⓓⓝⓒ: 20 mg

Transdermal system
Patch: 10 mg/9 hours, 15 mg/9 hours, 20 mg/9 hours, 30 mg/9 hours

INDICATIONS & DOSAGES
➤ **ADHD**
Methylin
Adults: 20 to 30 mg (immediate-release) PO b.i.d. or t.i.d. Dosage varies; maximum dosage is 60 mg daily.
Children age 6 and older: Initially, 5 mg PO b.i.d. immediate-release form before breakfast and lunch, increasing by 5 to 10 mg at weekly intervals, as needed, until an optimum daily dose of 2 mg/kg is reached, not to exceed 60 mg/day.

To use Ritalin-SR tablets in place of immediate-release methylphenidate tablets, calculate methylphenidate dosage in 8-hour intervals.
Concerta, Relexxii
Adults ages 18 to 65 not taking methylphenidate, or for patients taking other stimulants: Initially, 18 or 36 mg PO daily. May increase dosage in 18-mg increments at weekly intervals to maximum of 72 mg daily.
Adolescents ages 13 to 17 not currently taking methylphenidate, or for patients taking other stimulants: 18 mg PO extended-release once daily in the morning. Adjust dosage by 18 mg at weekly intervals to a maximum of 72 mg PO once daily in the morning.
Children ages 6 to 12 not currently taking methylphenidate, or for patients taking other stimulants: 18 mg extended-release PO once daily every morning. Adjust dosage by 18 mg at weekly intervals to a maximum of 54 mg daily every morning.
Adults and adolescents age 13 to 17 currently taking methylphenidate: If previous methylphenidate dosage was 5 mg b.i.d. or t.i.d., give 18 mg PO every morning. If previous dosage was 10 mg b.i.d. or t.i.d., give 36 mg PO every morning. If previous dosage was 15 mg b.i.d. or t.i.d., give 54 mg PO every morning. If previous dosage was 20 mg b.i.d. or t.i.d., give 72 mg every morning.
Children age 6 to 12 currently taking methylphenidate: If previous methylphenidate dosage was 5 mg b.i.d. or t.i.d., give 18 mg PO every morning. If previous dosage was 10 mg b.i.d. or t.i.d., give 36 mg PO every morning. If previous dosage was 15 mg b.i.d. or t.i.d., give 54 mg PO every morning. Maximum conversion daily dose is 54 mg.

M

✣Canada   ◇OTC   ◆Off-label use   ✔Photoguide   ⓓⓝⓒDo not crush   *Liquid contains alcohol   ▩Genetic

Aptensio XR, Biphentin
Adults and children age 6 and older: Initially, 10 mg PO daily in the morning. Increase dosage weekly in increments of 10 mg to maximum of 60 mg daily.

Ritalin LA
Adults and children age 6 and older: Initially, 10 to 20 mg PO once daily. Increase by 10 mg at weekly intervals to a maximum of 60 mg daily. To replace current b.i.d. methylphenidate dosage, give total daily dosage PO once daily. For example, if previous methylphenidate dosage was 10 mg b.i.d., give 20 mg PO once daily.

Daytrana
Adults and children ages 6 to 17: Initially, apply one 10-mg patch daily. Apply 2 hours before desired effect and remove 9 hours later. Increase dosage weekly by 5 mg as needed to maximum of 30 mg daily. Base final dose and wear time on patient response.

Quillivant XR
Adults and children age 6 and older: Initially, 10 to 20 mg PO once daily in a.m. May titrate weekly in dosages of 10 to 20 mg. Maximum dose, 60 mg daily.

QuilliChew ER
Adults and children age 6 and older: Initially, 20 mg PO once daily in the morning. Titrate dose up or down weekly in increments of 10 mg, 15 mg, or 20 mg. Maximum dose, 60 mg daily.

Cotempla XR-ODT
Children age 6 and older: Initially, 17.3 mg PO daily in the morning. May increase dosage weekly in increments of 8.6 to 17.3 mg per day. Don't exceed a daily dosage of 51.8 mg.

Jornay PM
Adults and children age 6 and older: Initially, 20 mg PO once daily in the evening. May adjust timing of administration between 6:30 p.m. and 9:30 p.m. May titrate weekly in dosages of 20 mg. Maximum dose, 100 mg daily.

Adhansia XR
Adults and children age 6 and older: Initially, 25 mg PO once daily in the morning. May titrate dosages of 10 to 15 mg in intervals of at least 5 days. Maximum dose, 85 mg daily in adults and 70 mg in children.

➤ **Narcolepsy (Methylin, Ritalin-SR only)**
Adults: 10 mg immediate-release PO b.i.d. or t.i.d. 30 to 45 minutes before meals. Dosage varies; maximum dose is 60 mg/day.

Children age 6 and older: Initially, 5 mg immediate-release PO b.i.d. (before breakfast and lunch). Increase dosage, if needed, by 5 to 10 mg weekly. Maximum dose is 60 mg.

To use Ritalin-SR tablets in place of immediate-release methylphenidate tablets, calculate the dose of methylphenidate in 8-hour intervals.

ADMINISTRATION
PO
- Give chewable tablet with at least 240 mL of water or other liquid.
- Give immediate-release tablets, chewable tablets, and oral solution in divided doses b.i.d. or t.i.d., preferably 30 to 45 minutes before meals. Give last daily dose before 6 p.m. to prevent insomnia (except for Jornay PM).
- Give Jornay PM between 6:30 p.m. and 9:30 p.m. Give consistently with or without food.
- Adhansia XR, Aptensio XR, Biphentin, Jornay PM, or Ritalin LA may be swallowed whole, or the contents of the capsule may be sprinkled onto a small amount of cool applesauce and taken immediately. Give with or without food.
- Extended-release and sustained-release tablets (Ritalin-SR) must be swallowed whole and never crushed, chewed, or divided.
- Concerta and Relexxii may be taken with or without food and must be swallowed whole. Don't crush, divide, or allow patient to chew Concerta tablets.
- Vigorously shake oral suspension bottle for 10 seconds before administering dose. Use oral dosing dispenser to measure dose. May give with or without food. Suspension remains stable for up to 4 months after reconstitution.
- For ODT, remove tablet with dry hands from blister pack and immediately place on patient's tongue. Allow it to disintegrate and be swallowed without chewing or crushing; no liquid is needed. Give consistently with or without food.

Transdermal
- Apply to clean, dry, nonirritated skin on the hip. Avoid placing the patch on the waistline or where tight clothing may rub it off. If possible, alternate sides of the body daily.
- Don't cut patches.
- Press patch firmly in place with palm of hand for about 30 seconds to ensure good contact. Don't apply with dressing or tape.

Reactions in bold italics are **life-threatening**. Interactions may have a *rapid onset* or a ***delayed onset***.

• If patch doesn't fully adhere or partially or fully detaches, replace with a new patch at a different site; ensure total wear time doesn't exceed 9 hours.

• Upon removal, fold patch in half, sticking adhesive sides together; then flush patch down toilet or place in appropriate lidded container.

ACTION

Releases nerve terminal stores of norepinephrine, promoting nerve impulse transmission. At high doses, effects are mediated by dopamine.

Route	Onset	Peak	Duration
PO (Methylin, Ritalin)	Unknown	2 hr	Unknown
PO (Ritalin-SR)	Unknown	5 hr	8 hr
PO (Aptensio XR)	Unknown	2 hr; 8 hr	Unknown
PO (Ritalin LA)	Unknown	1–3 hr; 4–7 hr	Unknown
PO (Adhansia XR)	Unknown	1–4 hr; 8–14 hr	Unknown
PO (Jornay PM)	Unknown	14 hr	Unknown
PO (Concerta, Relexxii)	Unknown	6–10 hr	Unknown
PO (QuilliChew XR, Quillivant XR)	Unknown	5 hr	Unknown
PO (Cotempla XR-ODT)	Unknown	4.5–5 hr	Unknown
Transdermal	2 hr	8–10 hr	Unknown

Half-life: Conventional, 3 to 6 hours; extended-release (Ritalin-SR), 3 to 8 hours; (Concerta, Ritalin LA), 3.5 hours; (Aptensio XR), 5 hours; (Adhansia XR), 4 to 7 hours; (Jornay PM), 5.9 hours; (Quillivant XR), 6 hours; (QuilliChew XR), 5 hours; (Relexxii), 3.6 hours; (Cotempla XR-ODT), 3.5 to 5.5 hours; transdermal, 4 to 5 hours.

ADVERSE REACTIONS

CNS: nervousness, headache, insomnia, *seizures*, tics, dizziness, akathisia, dyskinesia, drowsiness, mood swings, anxiety, irritability, depression, tremor, vertigo, confusion, sedation, fever. **CV:** palpitations, tachycardia, increased BP. **EENT:** blurred vision, eye pain, pharyngitis, sinusitis, bruxism, dry mouth, oropharyngeal pain. **GI:** nausea, abdominal pain, anorexia, decreased appetite, vomiting, constipation, dyspepsia, diarrhea. **GU:** decreased libido, dysmenorrhea. **Metabolic:** weight loss. **Musculoskeletal:** back pain. **Respiratory:** cough, URI. **Skin:** rash, excoriation, application-site irritation (redness,

swelling, papules), hyperhidrosis, bruising. **Other:** motion sickness.

INTERACTIONS

Drug-drug. *Antacids, H₂ antagonists, PPIs:* May interfere with normal release of extended-release forms. Monitor therapy.
Anticonvulsants (such as phenobarbital, phenytoin, primidone), SSRIs, TCAs (clomipramine, desipramine, imipramine), warfarin: May increase levels of these drugs. Monitor patient for adverse reactions, and decrease dose of these drugs as needed. Monitor drug levels (or coagulation times if patient is also taking warfarin).
Antihypertensives: May decrease antihypertensive effect. Monitor BP.
Centrally acting alpha₂ agonists, clonidine: May cause serious adverse events. Avoid using together.
Halogenated anesthetics (desflurane, enflurane, halothane, isoflurane): May suddenly increase BP and HR during surgery. Avoid use of methamphetamine on day of surgery.
MAO inhibitors (linezolid, selegiline): May cause severe HTN or hypertensive crisis. Use together is contraindicated. Avoid using within 14 days of MAO inhibitor therapy.
Risperidone: May increase risk of extrapyramidal symptoms. Monitor patient closely.
Drug-food. *Caffeine:* May increase amphetamine and related amine effects. Discourage use together.
Drug-lifestyle. *Alcohol use:* May increase methylphenidate concentration, causing toxicity. Discourage use together.

EFFECTS ON LAB TEST RESULTS

• May increase transaminase levels.
• May decrease Hb level and hematocrit and platelet and WBC counts.

CONTRAINDICATIONS & CAUTIONS

• Contraindicated in patients hypersensitive to drug. Some formulations are contraindicated in patients with glaucoma, motor tics, family history or diagnosis of Tourette syndrome, or history of marked anxiety, tension, or agitation. Refer to individual manufacturer's instructions.
• Avoid use in patients with structural cardiac abnormalities, cardiomyopathy, CAD, and serious arrhythmias.

M

🜄 *Alert:* Drug may increase risk of prolonged, painful erection (priapism) in males of any age, with or without sexual stimulation. Incidence is rare, but if not treated immediately, priapism may lead to permanent damage to the penis.

• Because they don't dissolve, Concerta and Relexxii aren't recommended in patients with a history of peritonitis or with severe GI narrowing (such as small-bowel inflammatory disease, short-gut syndrome caused by adhesions or decreased transit time, cystic fibrosis, chronic intestinal pseudo-obstruction, or Meckel diverticulum).

• Use cautiously in patients with a history of emotional disorder, preexisting psychosis or bipolar disorder, seizures, EEG abnormalities, or HTN, and in patients whose underlying medical conditions might be compromised by increases in BP or HR, such as those with preexisting HTN, HF, recent MI, or hyperthyroidism.

Boxed Warning Drug has a high potential for abuse and dependence. Use cautiously in patients with a history of drug dependence or alcoholism. Long-term abusive use can lead to tolerance and psychological dependence. Psychotic episodes can occur. Monitor patient for severe depression and the effects of chronic overactivity during drug withdrawal. ■

• Chewable tablets contain phenylalanine.

• The transdermal patch may cause irreversible chemical leukoderma (loss of skin color) at patch application site and other areas of the body. Although not harmful, if hypopigmentation occurs, consider alternative treatments.

Dialyzable drug: Unknown.

⚠ *Overdose S&S:* Agitation, cardiac arrhythmias, confusion, seizures, coma, delirium, dryness of mucous membranes, euphoria, flushing, hallucinations, headache, hyperpyrexia, hyperreflexia, HTN, muscle twitching, mydriasis, palpitations, diaphoresis, tachycardia, tremors, vomiting.

PREGNANCY-LACTATION-REPRODUCTION

• There are no adequate studies during pregnancy. Use during pregnancy only if potential benefit justifies fetal risk.

• Stimulants cause vasoconstriction and decrease placental perfusion. Premature delivery and low-birth-weight infants have been reported.

• Prescribers are encouraged to register patients in the National Pregnancy Registry for ADHD Medication (1-866-961-2388 or www.womensmentalhealth.org/pregnancyregistry).

• Drug appears in human milk. Use cautiously during breastfeeding and monitor infant closely.

NURSING CONSIDERATIONS

• Don't use drug to prevent fatigue or treat severe depression.

• Before starting drug, assess for the presence of cardiac disease by performing a careful history, family history of sudden death or ventricular arrhythmia, and physical exam.

Boxed Warning Assess risk of abuse before prescribing; monitor patients for signs and symptoms of abuse and dependence during therapy. ■

• Maintain careful prescription records. Monitor patient for signs and symptoms of abuse and overdose and periodically reevaluate need for use.

• Drug may trigger Tourette syndrome in children. Monitor patient, especially at start of therapy.

• Observe patient for signs of excessive stimulation. Monitor BP.

• Check CBC, differential, and platelet counts with long-term use, particularly if patient shows signs or symptoms of hematologic toxicity (fever, sore throat, easy bruising).

• Monitor height and weight in children on long-term therapy. Drug may delay growth spurt, but children will attain normal height when drug is stopped.

• Carefully observe patient for digital changes because stimulants used to treat ADHD are associated with peripheral vasculopathy, including Raynaud phenomenon.

• If ADHD hasn't improved after a 1-month period at the appropriate dose, prescriber may discontinue drug.

• Monitor patients using patch for chemical leukoderma. Report skin changes to prescriber.

• *Look alike–sound alike:* Don't confuse methylphenidate with methadone. Don't confuse Ritalin with ritodrine or Rifadin. Don't confuse Ritalin-SR with Ritalin LA.

Reactions in bold italics are *life-threatening*. Interactions may have a *rapid onset* or a ***delayed onset***.

PATIENT TEACHING
• Instruct patient or caregiver in proper administration, storage, and handling of prescribed formulation.
• Advise patient to avoid alcohol and caffeine during therapy.
• Caution patient with phenylketonuria that the chewable tablets contain phenylalanine.
⚠️ *Alert:* Inform male patient of any age and caregivers of the rare but possible risk of priapism. Caution patient to seek medical attention if priapism or an erection lasting longer than 4 hours occurs.
• Instruct patient and caregiver to watch for signs of chemical leukoderma, especially under skin patch site, and to report any skin changes to prescriber. Caution patient not to stop treatment without first consulting prescriber.
• Caution patient to avoid activities that require alertness or good psychomotor coordination until CNS effects of drug are known.
• Warn patient with seizure disorder that drug may decrease seizure threshold and to notify prescriber if seizure occurs.
• If the applied patch is missing, have caregiver ask the child when or how the patch came off. Teach child that patch shouldn't be shared or removed except by caregiver or health care provider.
• Encourage caregiver to use the application chart provided with patch carton to keep track of application and removal.
• Tell caregiver to remove patch sooner than 9 hours if the child has decreased evening appetite or has difficulty sleeping.
• Inform patient or caregiver the effects of patch last for several hours after its removal.
• Warn patient and caregiver to avoid exposing patch to direct external heat sources, such as heating pads, electric blankets, and heated water beds.
• Tell caregiver to notify prescriber if the child develops bumps, swelling, or blistering at the patch application site or is experiencing blurred vision or other serious side effects.

methylPREDNISolone
meth-il-pred-NIS-oh-lone

Medrol🔊

methylPREDNISolone acetate
Depo-Medrol

methylPREDNISolone sodium succinate
Solu-Medrol

Therapeutic class: Corticosteroids
Pharmacologic class: Glucocorticoids

AVAILABLE FORMS
methylprednisolone
Tablets: 2 mg, 4 mg, 8 mg, 16 mg, 32 mg
methylprednisolone acetate
Injection (suspension): 20 mg/mL,
40 mg/mL, 80 mg/mL
methylprednisolone sodium succinate
Injection*: 40 mg, 125 mg, 500 mg,
1,000 mg, 2,000 mg vials

INDICATIONS & DOSAGES
➤ **Severe inflammation or immunosuppression**
Adults and children: 4 to 48 mg PO daily depending on the disease treated. After favorable response is noted, determine maintenance dosage by decreasing until lowest dosage that will maintain adequate clinical response is achieved. Or, 4 to 120 mg acetate IM daily, or 10 to 40 mg succinate IM or IV, with subsequent doses dictated by patient's clinical response and condition. Or, 4 to 10 mg acetate into small joints, 10 to 40 mg acetate into medium joints, or 20 to 80 mg acetate into larger joints. Intralesional use is usually 20 to 60 mg acetate. Repeat intralesional and intra-articular injections every 1 to 5 weeks.
Children: 0.11 to 1.6 mg/kg/day PO, IM, or IV in three to four divided doses (sodium succinate).

ADMINISTRATION
PO
• Give drug with milk or food when possible. Patients who are critically ill may need to take drug with an antacid or H_2-receptor antagonist.

IV

▼ Use only methylprednisolone sodium succinate, never the acetate form.

▼ Reconstitute according to manufacturer's directions using supplied diluent, or use bacteriostatic water for injection with benzyl alcohol.

◑ *Alert:* Don't use formulations containing benzyl alcohol in neonates, which can cause potentially fatal toxicity.

▼ Compatible solutions include D_5W, NSS, and dextrose 5% in NSS.

▼ For direct injection, inject diluted drug into vein or free-flowing compatible IV solution over at least 1 minute.

▼ For IV infusion, dilute solution according to manufacturer's instructions and give over prescribed duration.

▼ For doses greater than 0.5 g, give IV over at least 30 to 60 minutes to prevent arrhythmias and circulatory collapse. Recommended infusion rate is giving over at least 30 minutes.

▼ Discard reconstituted solution after 48 hours.

▼ **Incompatibilities:** Don't dilute or mix with other solutions. Consult a drug incompatibility reference for more information.

IM

• Give injection deeply into gluteal muscle. Avoid injection into the deltoid muscle. Avoid subcut injection because atrophy and sterile abscesses may occur.

• Dermal atrophy may occur with large doses of acetate form. Use several small injections rather than a single large dose, and rotate injection sites.

Intra-articular

• Don't dilute or mix methylprednisolone acetate with other solutions.

• Exclude septic joint process before injection.

• Avoid injection or leakage into the dermis.

ACTION

Not clearly defined. Decreases inflammation, mainly by stabilizing leukocyte lysosomal membranes; suppresses immune response; stimulates bone marrow; and influences protein, fat, and carbohydrate metabolism.

Route	Onset	Peak	Duration
PO	Rapid	2–3 hr	30–36 hr
IV	1 hr	Immediate	12 hr
IM	6–48 hr	4–8 days	4–8 days
Intra-articular	1 wk	Unknown	1–5 wk

Half-life: 2 to 36 hours.

ADVERSE REACTIONS

CNS: euphoria, insomnia, psychotic behavior, *pseudotumor cerebri*, vertigo, headache, depression, personality changes, paresthesia, *seizures*, malaise, emotional lability, insomnia, syncope. **CV:** *arrhythmias, HF, cardiomyopathy*, HTN, *bradycardia*, tachycardia, *myocardial rupture after MI*, edema, thrombophlebitis, *thromboembolism, cardiac arrest, CV collapse*. **EENT:** cataracts, glaucoma, IOP, exophthalmoses, rhinitis. **GI:** peptic ulceration, GI irritation, increased appetite, *pancreatitis*, nausea, vomiting, abdominal distention. **GU:** menstrual irregularities. **Hematologic:** leukocytosis. **Metabolic:** *hypokalemia*, hyperglycemia, diabetes, sodium and water retention, carbohydrate intolerance, hypercholesterolemia, negative nitrogen balance, *hypocalcemia*. **Musculoskeletal:** growth suppression in children, muscle weakness, osteoporosis, myopathy, vertebral compression fractures, pathologic fracture of long bones, tendon rupture, aseptic necrosis; calcium deposit in soft tissue, postinjection flare (intra-articular. **Respiratory:** *pulmonary edema*. **Skin:** hirsutism, delayed wound healing, petechiae, ecchymoses, facial erythema, diaphoresis, fragile skin, acne, skin eruptions, cutaneous and subcutaneous atrophy. **Other:** cushingoid state, susceptibility to infections, *acute adrenal insufficiency after increased stress or abrupt withdrawal after long-term therapy, hypersensitivity reactions.*

INTERACTIONS

Drug-drug. *Aminoglutethimide:* May decrease methylprednisolone's therapeutic effects. Monitor therapy.

Anticholinesterases: May produce severe weakness in patients with myasthenia gravis. If possible, withdraw anticholinesterase agents at least 24 hours before methylprednisolone therapy.

Antidiabetics: May increase glucose concentrations. Antidiabetic dosage adjustment may be needed.

Reactions in bold italics are *life-threatening*. Interactions may have a *rapid onset* or a *delayed onset*.

Aspirin, indomethacin, other NSAIDs: May increase risk of GI distress and bleeding. Use together cautiously.

Barbiturates, carbamazepine, phenytoin, rifampin: May decrease corticosteroid effect. Increase corticosteroid dosage.

Cyclosporine: May increase toxicity. Monitor patient closely.

Estrogens (oral contraceptives): May decrease methylprednisolone clearance. Monitor therapy.

Ketoconazole and macrolide antibiotics: May decrease methylprednisolone clearance. Decreased dose may be required.

Mifepristone: May diminish methylprednisolone's therapeutic effects. Avoid combination.

Oral anticoagulants: May alter dosage requirements. Monitor PT and INR closely.

Potassium-depleting drugs (amphotericin B, thiazide diuretics): May enhance potassium-wasting effects of methylprednisolone. Monitor potassium level.

Salicylates: May decrease salicylate levels. Monitor patient for lack of salicylate effectiveness.

Skin-test antigens: May decrease response. Postpone skin testing until after therapy.

Toxoids, vaccines: May decrease antibody response and may increase risk of complications. Avoid using together.

Drug-herb. *Echinacea:* May decrease therapeutic effects of immunosuppressants. Discourage use together.

EFFECTS ON LAB TEST RESULTS
• May increase glucose, cholesterol, ALT, AST, ALP, sodium, and urine calcium levels.
• May decrease potassium and calcium levels.
• May alter reactions to skin tests.

CONTRAINDICATIONS & CAUTIONS
• Contraindicated in patients hypersensitive to drug or its components, in those with systemic fungal infections (except intra-articular), in premature infants (acetate and succinate containing benzyl alcohol), and in patients receiving immunosuppressive doses together with live-virus vaccines.
• IM injections are contraindicated in patients with idiopathic thrombocytopenia purpura.
• Intrathecal use is contraindicated.
• Use cautiously in older adults and patients with GI ulceration or renal disease, HTN, osteoporosis, diabetes, hypothyroidism,

cirrhosis, diverticulitis, nonspecific ulcerative colitis, recent intestinal anastomoses, thromboembolic disorders, seizures, active hepatitis, myasthenia gravis, HF, TB, ocular herpes simplex, cataracts, glaucoma, emotional instability, and psychotic tendencies.
• Prolonged use may increase risk of infection, mask signs of infection, and activate latent infections.
Dialyzable drug: Unknown.

PREGNANCY-LACTATION-REPRODUCTION
• There are no adequate studies during pregnancy. Drug crosses the placental barrier. Use during pregnancy only if potential benefit justifies fetal risk. Use lowest effective dose for shortest duration.
• Monitor infants born to mothers who received corticosteroids during pregnancy for hypoadrenalism.
• Drug appears in human milk. Patient should discontinue breastfeeding or discontinue drug.

NURSING CONSIDERATIONS
⚕ *Alert:* Epidural corticosteroid injections to treat neck and back pain and radiating pain in the arms and legs may result in rare but serious adverse events (loss of vision, stroke, paralysis, death). The use of epidural corticosteroid injections isn't approved by the FDA.
⚕ *Alert:* Drug may cause suppression of the HPA axis, which can lead to adrenal crisis. Younger children and patients receiving high doses are at increased risk. Withdrawal from corticosteroids should be done slowly and with careful patient monitoring.
• Medrol may contain tartrazine. Watch for allergic reaction to tartrazine in patients with sensitivity to aspirin.
• Drug may be used for alternate-day therapy.
• Most adverse reactions to corticosteroids are dose- or duration-dependent. For better results and less toxicity, give a once-daily dose in the morning.
⚕ *Alert:* Different salts aren't interchangeable.
• If immediate onset of action is needed, don't use acetate form.
• Always adjust to lowest effective dose.
• Monitor weight, BP, electrolyte level, and sleep patterns. Euphoria may initially interfere with sleep, but patients typically adjust to therapy in 1 to 3 weeks.

M

- Monitor patient for cushingoid effects, including moon facies, supraclavicular fat pad, central obesity, thinning hair, HTN, and increased susceptibility to infection.
- Measure growth and development periodically in children during high-dose or prolonged treatment.
- Watch for depression or psychotic episodes, especially in high-dose therapy.
- Patients with diabetes may need increased insulin; monitor glucose level.
- Watch for an enhanced response to drug in patients with hypothyroidism or cirrhosis.
- Unless contraindicated, give low-sodium diet that's high in potassium and protein. Give potassium supplements as needed.
- Older adults may be more susceptible to osteoporosis with prolonged use.
- Taper off dosage after long-term therapy.
- **Look alike–sound alike:** Don't confuse Solu-Medrol with Solu-Cortef. Don't confuse methylprednisolone with medroxyprogesterone or methyltestosterone.

PATIENT TEACHING

⚠️ **Alert:** Counsel patient to discuss benefits and risks and other possible treatments with health care provider before undergoing epidural corticosteroid injection.
- Tell patient not to stop drug abruptly or without prescriber's consent.
- Instruct patient to take oral form of drug with milk or food.
- Teach patient signs and symptoms of early adrenal insufficiency: fatigue, muscle weakness, joint pain, fever, anorexia, nausea, shortness of breath, dizziness, and fainting.
- Instruct patient to carry or wear medical identification indicating the need for supplemental systemic glucocorticoids during stress. This card should contain prescriber's name, name of drug, and dosage taken.
- Warn patient on long-term therapy about cushingoid effects and the need to report sudden weight gain or swelling.
- Advise patient receiving long-term therapy to consider exercise or physical therapy. Also, tell patient to ask prescriber about vitamin D or calcium supplement.
- Instruct patient to avoid exposure to infections (such as chickenpox or measles) and to contact prescriber if such exposure occurs.

methylTESTOSTERone
meth-il-tes-TOS-te-rone

Methitest

Therapeutic class: Androgens
Pharmacologic class: Androgens
Controlled substance schedule: III

AVAILABLE FORMS
Capsules: 10 mg
Tablets: 10 mg

INDICATIONS & DOSAGES
➤ **Metastatic breast cancer**
Patients 1 to 5 years after menopause: 50 to 200 mg PO daily.
➤ **Hypogonadism; delayed puberty in carefully selected males**
Men and adolescents: 10 to 50 mg PO daily for 4 to 6 months.

ADMINISTRATION
PO
⚠️ **Alert:** Drug is hazardous; use safe handling and disposal precautions.
- Give without regard for food.
- Store at room temperature; protect from light, heat, and moisture.

ACTION
Stimulates target tissues to develop normally in androgen-deficient men. May have some antiestrogen properties, making it useful in treating certain estrogen-dependent breast cancers.

Route	Onset	Peak	Duration
PO	Unknown	Unknown	Unknown

Half-life: Varies from 10 to 100 minutes.

ADVERSE REACTIONS
CNS: headache, anxiety, depression, paresthesia, *stroke.* **CV:** edema, *HF, venous thromboembolism, MI.* **GI:** irritation of oral mucosa with buccal administration, nausea. **GU:** oligospermia, decreased ejaculatory volume, priapism, amenorrhea, altered libido. **Hematologic:** *suppression of clotting factors,* polycythemia. **Hepatic:** abnormal LFT values, reversible jaundice, *cholestatic hepatitis.* **Metabolic:** hypernatremia, *hyperkalemia,* hyperphosphatemia, hypercholesterolemia, hypercalcemia. **Skin:** hirsutism,

---

Reactions in bold italics are *life-threatening*. Interactions may have a *rapid onset* or a *delayed onset*.

acne, male-pattern baldness. **Other:** hypersensitivity reactions, androgenic effects in women, gynecomastia, hypoestrogenic effects in women, excessive hormonal effects in men.

INTERACTIONS

Drug-drug. *Cyclosporine (systemic):* May increase cyclosporine-associated hepatotoxicity. Consider therapy modification.
Hepatotoxic drugs: May increase risk of hepatotoxicity. Monitor liver function closely.
Insulin, oral antidiabetics: May decrease glucose level; may alter dosage requirements. Monitor glucose level in patients with diabetes.
Oxyphenbutazone: May increase oxyphenbutazone serum level. Monitor patient.
Vitamin K antagonist (warfarin): May increase sensitivity to oral anticoagulants; may alter dosage requirements. Monitor PT and INR.
Drug-herb. *Saw palmetto:* May cause hormone-like effects. Don't use together.

EFFECTS ON LAB TEST RESULTS

• May increase sodium, potassium, phosphate, liver enzyme, lipid, and calcium levels.
• May decrease thyroxine-binding globulin and total T_4 levels.
• May increase RBC count and resin uptake of T_3 and T_4.

CONTRAINDICATIONS & CAUTIONS

• Contraindicated in men with breast or prostate cancer.
• Drug isn't indicated to enhance athletic performance.
• Use cautiously in older adults; patients with cardiac, renal, or hepatic disease or diabetes; and healthy males with delayed puberty.
Dialyzable drug: Unknown.
⚠ *Overdose S&S:* Nausea, edema.

PREGNANCY-LACTATION-REPRODUCTION

• Contraindicated in patients who are or may become pregnant. Use during pregnancy may cause virilization of the female fetus. If pregnancy occurs during therapy, apprise patient of potential fetal hazard.
• It isn't known if drug appears in human milk. Patient should discontinue breastfeeding or discontinue drug.

NURSING CONSIDERATIONS

• In children, obtain X-rays of wrist bones before therapy begins to establish bone maturation level. During treatment, bones may mature more rapidly than they grow in length. Review X-rays every 6 months to monitor bone maturation.
• Drug is typically used only for intermittent therapy. Because of potential hepatotoxicity, watch closely for jaundice.
• Promptly report evidence of virilization in women, such as deepening of the voice, increased hair growth, acne, or baldness.
• Watch for hypoestrogenic effects in women (flushing, diaphoresis, vaginal bleeding, nervousness, emotional lability, menstrual irregularities, and vaginitis, including itching, dryness, and burning).
• Watch for excessive hormonal effects in men. If patient is prepubertal, watch for premature epiphyseal closure, acne, priapism, growth of body and facial hair, and phallic enlargement. If patient is postpubertal, watch for testicular atrophy, oligospermia, decreased ejaculatory volume, impotence, gynecomastia, and epididymitis.
• Unless contraindicated, use with high-calorie, high-protein diet. Give small, frequent meals.
• Periodically check cholesterol, calcium, and Hb levels, hematocrit, and cardiac and LFT results.
• Check weight regularly. Control edema with sodium restriction or diuretics.
• In patients with breast cancer, therapeutic response usually occurs within 3 months. If disease appears to progress, stop drug.
• Report signs of hypercalcemia. In metastatic breast cancer, hypercalcemia may indicate progression of bone metastases.
⚠ *Alert:* Drug has potential for abuse. Monitor patient for nontherapeutic uses.
• *Look alike–sound alike:* Testosterone and methyltestosterone aren't interchangeable. Don't confuse methyltestosterone with medroxyprogesterone.

PATIENT TEACHING

• Ensure patient understands importance of using effective contraception during therapy.
• Teach patient about potential adverse reactions and to report them.
• Tell patient of childbearing potential to report menstrual irregularities and to stop drug while awaiting exam.

- Warn patient of fetal risk and to stop drug immediately and notify prescriber if pregnancy is suspected.
- Tell female patient to immediately report evidence of virilization, such as acne, swelling, weight gain, increased hair growth, hoarseness, clitoral enlargement, decreased breast size, deepening of voice, changes in libido, male pattern baldness, and oily skin or hair.
- Teach patient signs and symptoms of low glucose level (hypoglycemia) and method for checking glucose level; drug enhances hypoglycemia. Instruct patient to report signs or symptoms of hypoglycemia immediately.
- Advise adolescent and parents about the potential adverse effect on bone maturation before start of therapy.

---

metoclopramide hydrochloride ℞
met-oh-KLOE-pra-mide

Gimoti, Reglan

Therapeutic class: GI stimulants
Pharmacologic class: Dopamine antagonists

AVAILABLE FORMS
Injection: 5 mg/mL
Nasal spray: 15 mg/actuation
Oral solution: 5 mg/5 mL
Tablets: 5 mg, 10 mg
Tablets (ODTs): 5 mg, 10 mg

INDICATIONS & DOSAGES
℞ *Adjust-a-dose (for all indications):* Refer to manufacturer's product information for dosage adjustments, if indicated, for older adults, for patients with hepatic or renal impairment or ESRD, in CYP2D6 poor metabolizers, and with concomitant use with strong CYP2D6 inhibitors.

➤ **To prevent or reduce nausea and vomiting from emetogenic cancer chemotherapy**
Adults: 1 to 2 mg/kg IV 30 minutes before chemotherapy; repeat every 2 hours for two doses, then every 3 hours for three doses.

➤ **To prevent or reduce postoperative nausea and vomiting**
Adults: 10 to 20 mg IM near end of surgical procedure.

➤ **To facilitate small-bowel intubation**
Adults and children older than age 14: 10 mg IV as a single dose over 1 to 2 minutes.
Children ages 6 to 14: 2.5 to 5 mg IV as a single dose slowly over 1 to 2 minutes.
Children younger than age 6: 0.1 mg/kg IV as a single dose slowly over 1 to 2 minutes.

➤ **To aid in radiologic exam**
Adults: 10 mg IV as a single dose over 1 to 2 minutes.

➤ **Delayed gastric emptying secondary to diabetic gastroparesis**
Adults: 10 mg PO q.i.d. for mild symptoms for 2 to 8 weeks depending on response. Maximum daily dosage, 40 mg. Or, 1 nasal spray (15 mg) in one nostril q.i.d. for 2 to 8 weeks depending on response. Or, 10 mg IM or by slow IV push over 1 to 2 minutes 30 minutes before each meal and at bedtime for up to 10 days for severe symptoms; then may start PO dose and continue for 2 to 8 weeks.
Older adults: 5 mg PO q.i.d. for 2 to 8 weeks depending on response. Or, may switch patients on a stable 10-mg dose on another form to nasal spray (15 mg) in one nostril q.i.d. for 2 to 8 weeks depending on response.

➤ **GERD**
Adults: 10 to 15 mg PO q.i.d. continuously for up to 12 weeks. Or, up to 20 mg PO PRN before provoking situation.

ADMINISTRATION
PO
- Give drug 30 minutes before each meal and at bedtime.

PO (ODT)
- Give drug at least 30 minutes before eating and at bedtime.
- Give immediately after opening sealed blister. If the tablet breaks or crumbles, throw it away and obtain a new one.
- Place tablet on patient's tongue. Tell patient to let it melt for approximately 1 minute and then swallow.
- Don't repeat dose if inadvertently given with food.

IV
▼ Drug is compatible with D_5W, NSS for injection, dextrose 5% in half-NSS, Ringer injection, and lactated Ringer injection. NSS is the preferred diluent; drug is most stable in this solution.
▼ Give doses of 10 mg or less by direct injection over 1 to 2 minutes. Dilute doses

---

larger than 10 mg in 50 mL of compatible diluent, and infuse over at least 15 minutes. Monitor BP closely.

▼ There is no need to protect drug from light if infusion mixture is given within 24 hours. If protected from light and refrigerated, it's stable for 48 hours.

▼ **Incompatibilities:** Cephalothin, chloramphenicol, sodium bicarbonate.

IM
• Inspect for particulate matter and discoloration. If either is present, don't use.
• Inject into a large muscle.

Intranasal
• Prime pump with 10 sprays into the air before first use.
• Give 30 minutes before each meal and at bedtime.
• Have patient lean head slightly forward and aim nozzle toward back of the nose; use index finger to close other nostril. Spray while patient inhales slowly. If uncertain that spray entered the nose, don't repeat dose; give next dose as scheduled.
• Omit missed dose and give next dose as scheduled.
• Nasal spray isn't recommended for initial therapy.
• Discard bottle after 4 weeks after opening, even if bottle contains unused drug.

ACTION
Stimulates motility of upper GI tract, increases lower esophageal sphincter tone, and blocks dopamine receptors at the chemoreceptor trigger zone.

Route	Onset	Peak	Duration
PO	30–60 min	1–2 hr	1–2 hr
IV	1–3 min	Unknown	1–2 hr
IM	10–15 min	Unknown	1–2 hr
Intranasal	Unknown	0.5–3.5 hr	1–2 hr

Half-life: 4 to 6 hours; ODT, 7 hours; nasal spray, 8.1 hours.

ADVERSE REACTIONS
CNS: anxiety, depression, drowsiness, dystonic reactions, fatigue, lassitude, restlessness, *seizures, suicidality,* akathisia, confusion, depression, dizziness, extrapyramidal symptoms, fever, hallucinations, headache, insomnia, tardive dyskinesia, NMS, dysgeusia (nasal spray). **CV:** *bradycardia, supraventricular tachycardia, AV block,* hypotension, fluid retention, transient HTN,

flushing, *HF.* **EENT:** visual disturbance. **GI:** bowel disorders, diarrhea, nausea. **GU:** amenorrhea, incontinence, urinary frequency, erectile dysfunction. **Skin:** rash, urticaria. **Other:** loss of libido, prolactin secretion, gynecomastia, hypersensitivity reaction, including *bronchospasm*.

INTERACTIONS
Drug-drug. *Anticholinergics, antidiarrheals, opioid analgesics:* May antagonize GI motility effects of metoclopramide. Use together cautiously.
Antiparkinsonian drugs (dopamine agonists): May decrease therapeutic effects of antiparkinsonian drugs. Monitor therapy.
Antipsychotics: May increase toxic effects of antipsychotics. Don't use together.
CNS depressants: May cause additive CNS effects. Avoid using together.
Cyclosporine: May increase cyclosporine absorption. Monitor therapy.
CYP2D6 inhibitors (bupropion, fluoxetine, paroxetine, quinidine): May increase metoclopramide level. Adjust metoclopramide dosage as indicated. Recommended dosage adjustment: 5 mg q.i.d. before each meal and at bedtime or 10 mg t.i.d.
Digoxin: May diminish digoxin absorption. Monitor therapy.
Insulin: May increase GI motility and food delivery to intestines, increasing blood glucose level. Monitor blood glucose level.
MAO inhibitors: May increase release of catecholamines in patients with HTN. Use together cautiously.
Mivacurium, succinylcholine: Inhibits plasma cholinesterase level, leading to enhanced neuromuscular blockade. Monitor patient closely.
Phenothiazines: May increase risk of extrapyramidal effects. Monitor patient closely.
Drug-lifestyle. *Alcohol use:* May cause additive CNS effects. Discourage use together.

EFFECTS ON LAB TEST RESULTS
• May increase LFT values and aldosterone and prolactin levels.
• May decrease neutrophil and granulocyte counts.

CONTRAINDICATIONS & CAUTIONS
• Contraindicated in patients hypersensitive to drug and in those with pheochromocytoma

M

or other catecholamine-releasing paragangliomas, tardive dyskinesia, or seizure disorders.
• Contraindicated in patients for whom stimulation of GI motility might be dangerous (those with hemorrhage, obstruction, or perforation).

Boxed Warning Drug can cause irreversible tardive dyskinesia, even after drug is stopped. Risk increases with duration of therapy and total cumulative dose; there is no treatment. Discontinue drug if signs and symptoms occur. Except in rare cases, avoid treatment for longer than 12 weeks. ∎

• In addition to tardive dyskinesia, drug may cause other extrapyramidal signs and symptoms, parkinsonian symptoms, and motor restlessness.
• Metoclopramide isn't recommended for use in children due to the risk of tardive dyskinesia and other extrapyramidal signs and symptoms as well as the risk of methemoglobinemia in neonates.
• Nasal spray isn't recommended in patients with moderate or severe hepatic or renal impairment and patients concurrently using strong CYP2D6 inhibitors.
• Galactorrhea, amenorrhea, gynecomastia, and impotence have been reported with prolactin-elevating drugs, including metoclopramide.
🕛 *Alert:* NMS has occurred rarely and may be fatal. If signs and symptoms develop (fever, CNS symptoms, irregular pulse, cardiac arrhythmias, or abnormal BP), discontinue drug.
• Use cautiously in patients with history of depression, Parkinson disease, or HTN.
Dialyzable drug: No.
⚠ *Overdose S&S:* Drowsiness, disorientation, extrapyramidal reactions; seizures, lethargy (in infants and children).

PREGNANCY-LACTATION-REPRODUCTION
• There are no adequate studies during pregnancy. Use during pregnancy only if clearly needed.
• Drug appears in human milk. Use cautiously during breastfeeding. Monitor neonate for extrapyramidal signs and symptoms and methemoglobinemia.

NURSING CONSIDERATIONS
• Monitor bowel sounds.
• Drug may cause tardive dyskinesia, parkinsonian symptoms, and motor restlessness.

Monitor patient for involuntary movements of face, tongue, and extremities, which may indicate tardive dyskinesia or other extrapyramidal adverse effects.
• Monitor patient for fever, CNS symptoms, irregular pulse, cardiac arrhythmias, or abnormal BP, which may indicate NMS.
• Monitor patient for dizziness, headache, or nervousness after metoclopramide is stopped; these may indicate withdrawal.
• Diphenhydramine or benztropine may be used to counteract extrapyramidal adverse effects from high doses.

PATIENT TEACHING
• Teach patient proper drug administration for prescribed formulation.
• Tell patient to avoid activities that require alertness for 2 hours after doses.
• Urge patient to report persistent or serious adverse reactions promptly.
• Teach patient signs and symptoms of tardive dyskinesia, other extrapyramidal signs and symptoms, and NMS. Advise patient to discontinue drug and to seek immediate medical attention if such signs and symptoms occur.
• Advise patient not to drink alcohol during therapy.
• Instruct patient to report pregnancy or breastfeeding.

met0Lazone
me-TOLE-a-zone

Therapeutic class: Diuretics
Pharmacologic class: Thiazide-like diuretics

AVAILABLE FORMS
Tablets: 2.5 mg, 5 mg, 10 mg

INDICATIONS & DOSAGES
➤ **Edema in HF or renal disease**
Adults: 5 to 20 mg PO once daily. Use lowest effective dose for maintenance therapy.
➤ **HTN**
Adults: 2.5 to 5 mg PO once daily. Base maintenance dosage on BP.

ADMINISTRATION
PO
• Give drug in the morning without regard for meals.

Reactions in bold italics are *life-threatening*. Interactions may have a *rapid onset* or a ***delayed onset***.

ACTION
Increases sodium and water excretion by inhibiting sodium reabsorption in ascending loop of Henle.

Route	Onset	Peak	Duration
PO	1 hr	8 hr	≥24 hr

Half-life: 6 to 20 hours.

ADVERSE REACTIONS
CNS: dizziness, headache, fatigue, vertigo, syncope, paresthesia, weakness, restlessness, drowsiness, anxiety, depression, nervousness. **CV:** orthostatic hypotension, palpitations, chest pain, *venous thrombosis.* **EENT:** blurred vision. **GI:** *pancreatitis,* anorexia, nausea, epigastric pain, vomiting, abdominal pain, diarrhea, constipation, dry mouth. **GU:** nocturia, polyuria, impotence. **Hematologic:** *aplastic anemia, agranulocytosis, leukopenia.* **Hepatic:** jaundice, *hepatitis.* **Metabolic:** hyperglycemia, *hypokalemia, hypomagnesemia,* hyponatremia, hypochloremia, metabolic alkalosis, hypercalcemia, volume depletion and dehydration, gout. **Musculoskeletal:** muscle cramps. **Skin:** dermatitis, photosensitivity reactions, rash, pruritus, urticaria, skin necrosis, purpura, *SJS, TEN,* cutaneous vasculitis.

INTERACTIONS
Drug-drug. *Amphotericin B, corticosteroids:* May increase risk of hypokalemia. Monitor potassium level closely.
Anticoagulants: May decrease anticoagulant response. Monitor PT and INR.
Antidiabetics: May alter glucose level and require dosage adjustment of antidiabetics. Monitor glucose level.
Antihypertensives: May increase hypotensive effect. Monitor therapy.
Barbiturates, opioids: May increase orthostatic hypotensive effect. Monitor patient closely.
Calcium salts: May decrease calcium excretion. Monitor therapy.
Carbamazepine: May increase risk of hyponatremia. Monitor therapy.
Cholestyramine, colestipol: May decrease intestinal absorption of thiazides. Separate doses.
Diazoxide: May increase antihypertensive, hyperglycemic, and hyperuricemic effects. Use together cautiously.

Diuretics (bumetanide, ethacrynic acid, furosemide, torsemide): May cause excessive diuretic response, resulting in serious electrolyte imbalances or dehydration. Adjust dosages carefully, and monitor patient closely for signs and symptoms of excessive diuretic response.
Levodopa–carbidopa: May increase risk of hypotension. Monitor therapy.
Lithium: May decrease lithium clearance, increasing risk of lithium toxicity. Monitor lithium level.
Methenamine: May decrease effectiveness of methenamine. Monitor therapy.
NSAIDs: May increase risk of renal failure. May decrease diuretic and antihypertensive effects. Monitor renal function and BP.
QT-interval-prolonging drugs: May increase risk of QT-interval prolongation and ventricular arrhythmias. Avoid use together.
Drug-herb. *Licorice:* May cause hypokalemia. Discourage use together.
Drug-lifestyle. *Alcohol use:* May increase orthostatic hypotensive effect. Discourage use together.
Sun exposure: May cause photosensitivity reaction. Advise patient to avoid excessive sunlight exposure.

EFFECTS ON LAB TEST RESULTS
• May increase glucose, calcium, cholesterol, BUN, uric acid, and triglyceride levels.
• May decrease potassium, sodium, magnesium, phosphate, and chloride levels.
• May decrease Hb level and granulocyte and WBC counts.

CONTRAINDICATIONS & CAUTIONS
• Contraindicated in patients hypersensitive to thiazides, other sulfonamide-derived drugs, or metolazone and in those with anuria, hepatic coma, or precoma.
• Use cautiously in patients with impaired renal or hepatic function, electrolyte imbalances, hyperuricemia, SLE, diabetes, or gout.
Dialyzable drug: Unlikely.
⚠ **Overdose S&S:** Orthostatic hypotension, dizziness, drowsiness, lethargy, syncope, CNS depression, electrolyte abnormalities, hemoconcentration, depressed respirations, GI irritation and hypermotility.

PREGNANCY-LACTATION-REPRODUCTION
• There are no adequate studies during pregnancy. Use during pregnancy only if clearly needed.
• Drug appears in human milk. Patient should discontinue breastfeeding or discontinue drug.

NURSING CONSIDERATIONS
• Monitor fluid intake and output, weight, BP, and electrolyte levels.
• Watch for signs and symptoms of hypokalemia, such as muscle weakness and cramps. Drug may be used with potassium-sparing diuretic to prevent potassium loss.
• Consult dietitian about a high-potassium diet.
• Monitor glucose level, especially in patients with diabetes.
• Monitor uric acid level, especially in patients with history of gout.
• Monitor older adults, who are especially susceptible to excessive diuresis.
• In patients with HTN, therapeutic response may be delayed several weeks.
• Monitor BP. Add another antihypertensive for inadequate response.
• Metolazone and furosemide may be used together to enhance diuretic effect.
• Unlike thiazide diuretics, metolazone is effective in patients with decreased renal function.
• Stop thiazides and thiazide-like diuretics before parathyroid function tests.
• *Look alike–sound alike:* Don't confuse metolazone with methadone, metoclopramide, metoprolol, methimazole, or methazolamide.

PATIENT TEACHING
• Tell patient to take drug in morning to prevent need to urinate at night.
• Advise patient to avoid sudden posture changes and to rise slowly to avoid dizziness upon standing quickly.
• Instruct patient to use sunblock and protective clothing to prevent photosensitivity reactions.
• Educate patient to increase dietary intake of potassium-containing foods.
• Teach patient about adverse reactions and to report them promptly.

metoprolol succinate
me-toe-PROE-lole

Kapspargo Sprinkle, Toprol-XL◆

metoprolol tartrate
Lopressor◆

Therapeutic class: Antihypertensives
Pharmacologic class: Selective beta-adrenergic blockers

AVAILABLE FORMS
metoprolol succinate
Capsules (extended-release): 25 mg, 50 mg, 100 mg, 200 mg
Tablets (extended-release) ⓒ*:* 25 mg, 50 mg, 100 mg, 200 mg
metoprolol tartrate
Injection: 1 mg/mL
Tablets: 25 mg, 37.5 mg, 50 mg, 75 mg, 100 mg
Tablets (extended-release) ⓒ*:* 100 mg✽, 200 mg✽

INDICATIONS & DOSAGES
➤ **HTN**
Adults: Initially, 50 mg PO b.i.d. or 100 mg PO once daily; then up to 100 to 400 mg daily in two or three divided doses. Or, 25 to 100 mg extended-release tablets (tartrate equivalent) PO once daily. Adjust dosage as needed and tolerated at intervals of not less than 1 week to maximum of 400 mg (extended-release) daily or 450 mg (immediate-release) daily.
Children older than age 6 (metoprolol succinate): Initially, 1 mg/kg PO once daily, not to exceed 50 mg PO daily. Adjust dosage based on BP response. Doses greater than 2 mg/kg or in excess of 200 mg/day haven't been studied.
➤ **Early intervention in acute MI**
Adults: 5 mg metoprolol tartrate IV bolus every 2 minutes for three doses. Then, starting 15 minutes after the last IV dose, 25 to 50 mg PO every 6 hours for 48 hours. Maintenance dosage is 100 mg PO b.i.d.
➤ **Late intervention in acute MI**
Adults: 100 mg PO b.i.d. as soon as clinical condition allows in patients with contraindications for or intolerance to early intervention. Continue for at least 3 months.

➤ **Angina pectoris**

Adults: Initially, 100 mg PO daily as a single dose or in two equally divided doses; increased at weekly intervals until an adequate response or a pronounced decrease in HR is seen. Effects of daily dose beyond 400 mg aren't known. Or, 100 mg extended-release tablets (tartrate equivalent) once daily. Adjust dosage as needed and tolerated at intervals of not less than 1 week to maximum of 400 mg daily.

➤ **Stable symptomatic HF (NYHA Class II) resulting from ischemia, HTN, or cardiomyopathy**

Adults: 25 mg metoprolol succinate PO once daily for 2 weeks. Double the dose every 2 weeks, as tolerated, to a maximum of 200 mg daily.

Adjust-a-dose: In patients with more severe HF, start with 12.5 mg Toprol-XL PO once daily for 2 weeks. Kapspargo isn't suitable for doses of less than 25 mg daily.

ADMINISTRATION
PO
- Give drug with or immediately after meal.
- Extended-release tablets may be cut in half on scored line, but never crushed or chewed.
- Patient may swallow extended-release capsules whole or may open capsules and sprinkle contents over soft foods (applesauce, pudding, yogurt). Patient should swallow drug and food mixture within 60 minutes.
- If a dose is missed, omit the missed dose and give the next scheduled dose without doubling it.

IV
▼ Give drug undiluted by direct injection in an intensive care setting at a rate of 5 mg over 1 to 2 minutes.

▼ Store drug at room temperature and protect from light. Discard solution if it's discolored or contains particles.

▼ **Incompatibilities:** None listed by manufacturer. Consult a drug incompatibility reference for more information.

ACTION
A selective beta blocker that selectively blocks beta$_1$ receptors; decreases cardiac output, peripheral resistance, and cardiac oxygen consumption; and depresses renin secretion.

Route	Onset	Peak	Duration
PO	15 min	1 hr	6–12 hr
PO (extended-release)	15 min	6–12 hr	24 hr
IV	5 min	20 min	5–8 hr

Half-life: 3 to 10 hours.

ADVERSE REACTIONS
CNS: fatigue, dizziness, depression, headache, insomnia, mental confusion, nightmares, short-term memory loss, hallucinations, vertigo, *stroke*. **CV:** hypotension, *bradycardia, HF,* edema, palpitations, Raynaud syndrome, cold extremity, first-degree AV block. **EENT:** blurred vision, tinnitus, rhinitis, dry mouth. **GI:** nausea, diarrhea, constipation, heartburn, flatulence, gastric pain, vomiting. **GU:** decreased libido, erectile dysfunction. **Respiratory:** dyspnea, wheezing, *bronchospasm.* **Skin:** rash, pruritus, gangrene (IV). **Other:** accidental injury.

INTERACTIONS
Drug-drug. *Amiodarone:* May increase bradycardic effects. Monitor therapy.
Barbiturates: May reduce metoprolol effect. Monitor therapy.
Calcium channel blockers: May increase hypotensive effects. Monitor therapy.
Cardiac glycosides: May cause excessive bradycardia and increased depressant effect on myocardium. Use together cautiously.
Catecholamine-depleting drugs (MAO inhibitors): May have additive effect. Monitor patient for hypotension and bradycardia.
Clonidine: May increase risk of bradycardia. If clonidine and a beta blocker are coadministered, withdraw the beta blocker several days before the gradual withdrawal of clonidine.
CYP2D6 inhibitors (fluoxetine, paroxetine, propafenone, quinidine): May increase metoprolol level. Monitor vital signs carefully. Metoprolol dosage reduction may be needed.
Epinephrine: May blunt epinephrine effect during treatment of allergic reaction. Monitor therapy.
Hydralazine: May increase levels and effects of both drugs. Monitor patient closely. May need to adjust dosage.
Indomethacin, NSAIDs: May decrease antihypertensive effect. Monitor BP and adjust dosage.

M

Insulin, oral antidiabetics: May alter dosage requirements in previously stabilized patients with diabetes. Monitor patient closely.

IV lidocaine: May reduce hepatic metabolism of lidocaine, increasing risk of toxicity. Give bolus doses of lidocaine at a slower rate, and monitor lidocaine level closely.

Theophylline: May decrease bronchodilatory effects of theophylline. Monitor patient.

Verapamil: May increase effects of both drugs. Monitor cardiac function closely, and decrease dosages as needed.

Drug-herb. *Ma huang:* May decrease antihypertensive effects. Discourage use together.

Drug-food. *Any food:* May increase absorption. Encourage patient to take drug with food.

EFFECTS ON LAB TEST RESULTS
• May increase transaminase, ALP, and LDH levels.

CONTRAINDICATIONS & CAUTIONS
• Contraindicated in patients hypersensitive to drug or other beta blockers.
• Contraindicated in patients with sinus bradycardia, greater than first-degree heart block, cardiogenic shock, sick sinus syndrome (unless a permanent pacemaker is in place), or overt HF when used to treat HTN or angina. When used to treat MI, drug is contraindicated in patients with HR less than 45 beats/minute, greater than first-degree heart block, PR interval of 0.24 second or longer with first-degree heart block, systolic BP less than 100 mm Hg, or moderate to severe cardiac failure.
• Use cautiously in patients with HF, diabetes, or bronchospastic or hepatic disease.
• Use cautiously in patients with pheochromocytoma and only after alpha blocker has been initiated to avoid paradoxical increase in BP.
• Avoid initiating high-dose, extended-release drug in patients undergoing noncardiac surgery because drug has been associated with bradycardia, hypotension, stroke, and death.
• Don't routinely withdraw long-term beta-blocker therapy before surgery.

Dialyzable drug: Yes.

⚠ **Overdose S&S:** Bradycardia, nausea, hypotension, bronchospasm, HF, cardiac arrest, coma, AV block, vomiting.

PREGNANCY-LACTATION-REPRODUCTION
• There are no adequate studies during pregnancy. Drug crosses the placental barrier. Use during pregnancy only if clearly needed. Monitor fetal growth.
• Drug appears in human milk in very small quantities. Consider possible infant exposure with use during breastfeeding.

NURSING CONSIDERATIONS
• Always check patient's apical pulse rate before giving drug. If it's slower than 60 beats/minute, withhold drug and contact prescriber immediately to verify dose.
• In patients with diabetes, monitor glucose level closely because drug masks common signs and symptoms of hypoglycemia.
• Monitor BP frequently; drug masks common signs and symptoms of shock.
• Beta blockers may mask tachycardia caused by hyperthyroidism. In patients with suspected thyrotoxicosis, taper off beta blocker to avoid thyroid storm.

Boxed Warning When stopping long-term therapy, taper dosage over 1 to 2 weeks. Abrupt discontinuation may cause exacerbations of angina or MI. Don't discontinue therapy abruptly even in patients treated only for HTN. Restart metoprolol, at least temporarily, if angina markedly worsens or acute coronary insufficiency occurs. ■
• Beta selectivity is lost at higher doses. Watch for peripheral side effects.
• *Look alike–sound alike:* Don't confuse metoprolol succinate with metoprolol tartrate. Don't confuse metoprolol with metaproterenol, misoprostol, or metolazone. Don't confuse Toprol-XL with Topamax, Tegretol, or Tegretol-XR.

PATIENT TEACHING
• Instruct patient to take drug exactly as prescribed and with meals.
• Caution patient to avoid driving and other tasks requiring mental alertness until response to therapy has been established.
• Advise patient to inform dentist or prescriber about use of this drug before procedures or surgery.
• Tell patient to report all adverse reactions, especially weight gain and shortness of breath.

Boxed Warning Instruct patient not to stop drug suddenly but to notify prescriber about unpleasant adverse reactions. ■

Reactions in bold italics are *life-threatening*. Interactions may have a *rapid onset* or a *delayed onset*.

metroNIDAZOLE (oral, injection) ⚥

met-roe-NYE-da-zole

Flagyl R

metroNIDAZOLE hydrochloride ⚥

Therapeutic class: Antiprotozoals
Pharmacologic class: Nitroimidazoles

AVAILABLE FORMS

Capsules: 375 mg, 500 mg✤
Injection: 500 mg/100 mL in ready-to-use (RTU) minibags
Tablets: 250 mg, 500 mg

INDICATIONS & DOSAGES

Boxed Warning Use metronidazole only for the conditions for which it's indicated because it may be carcinogenic. Avoid unnecessary use. ∎

Adjust-a-dose (for all indications): For severe hepatic impairment (Child-Pugh class C), reduce dosage of tablets and IV infusion by 50%.

➤ **Amebic liver abscess**
Adults: 500 to 750 mg PO t.i.d. for 5 to 10 days.
Children: 35 to 50 mg/kg PO daily in three divided doses for 7 to 10 days.
Adjust-a-dose: For severe hepatic impairment (Child-Pugh class C), reduce dosage to 375 mg (capsules) PO every 8 hours for 5 to 10 days.

➤ **Intestinal amebiasis**
Adults: 750 mg PO t.i.d. for 7 to 10 days.
Children: 35 to 50 mg/kg PO daily in three divided doses for 7 to 10 days. IV form may be necessary for severe infection or extraintestinal disease.
Adjust-a-dose: For severe hepatic impairment (Child-Pugh class C), reduce dose to 375 mg (capsules) PO every 8 hours for 5 to 10 days.

➤ **Trichomoniasis**
Adults: One 250-mg tablet PO t.i.d. for 7 days, or 2 g PO in single dose (may give the 2-g dose in two 1-g doses, both on the same day); wait 4 to 6 weeks before repeating course. Or, one 375-mg capsule PO b.i.d. for 7 days.
Adjust-a-dose: For severe hepatic impairment (Child-Pugh class C), reduce dosage to 375 mg (capsules) PO once daily.

➤ **Bacterial infections caused by anaerobic microorganisms**
Adults: Loading dose, 15 mg/kg IV infused over 1 hour. Maintenance dose, 7.5 mg/kg IV or 500 mg PO every 6 hours for 7 to 10 days; infections involving bone, joint, lower respiratory tract, and endocardium may require longer treatment. Give first maintenance dose 6 hours after loading dose. Maximum dose shouldn't exceed 4 g daily.

➤ **To prevent postoperative infection in contaminated or potentially contaminated colorectal surgery**
Adults: Infuse 15 mg/kg IV over 30 to 60 minutes and complete about 1 hour before surgery. Then, infuse 7.5 mg/kg IV over 30 to 60 minutes at 6 and 12 hours after first dose.

ADMINISTRATION

● Obtain specimen for culture and sensitivity before giving first dose, if possible. Begin therapy while awaiting results.
PO
● Give tablets and capsules with food if GI upset occurs.
● Give missed dose as soon as possible unless it's close to time for next dose.
IV
▼ IV RTU minibags need no preparation.
▼ Don't give by IV push. Infuse over 30 to 60 minutes.
▼ Store at room temperature. Don't remove overwrap until ready to use.
▼ **Incompatibilities:** Other IV drugs. Avoid contact of drug solution with equipment containing aluminum.

ACTION

Direct-acting trichomonacide and amebicide that works inside and outside the intestines. It's thought to enter the cells of microorganisms that contain nitroreductase, forming unstable compounds that bind to DNA and inhibit synthesis, causing cell death.

Route	Onset	Peak	Duration
PO	Unknown	1–2 hr	Unknown
IV	Immediate	1 hr	Unknown

Half-life: 6 to 8 hours.

ADVERSE REACTIONS

CNS: headache, *seizures,* fever, vertigo, ataxia, dizziness, syncope, incoordination, confusion, irritability, depression, weakness, somnolence, insomnia, *encephalopathy,*

M

aseptic meningitis, peripheral neuropathy. **CV:** *prolonged QT interval,* flattened T wave, chest pain, edema, flushing, thrombophlebitis after IV infusion. **EENT:** nystagmus, optic neuropathy, rhinitis, sinusitis, dry mouth, pharyngitis. **GI:** nausea, abdominal pain, stomatitis, epigastric distress, vomiting, anorexia, diarrhea, constipation, proctitis, metallic taste, *pancreatitis.* **GU:** vaginitis, darkened urine, polyuria, dysuria, cystitis, dyspareunia, dryness of vagina and vulva, vaginal candidiasis, genital pruritus, *UTI,* dysmenorrhea, decreased libido. **Hematologic:** *leukopenia, agranulocytosis, neutropenia, thrombocytopenia, eosinophilia.* **Hepatic:** jaundice, increased liver enzyme levels. **Musculoskeletal:** transient joint pains, myalgia, muscle spasms. **Respiratory:** dyspnea, URI. **Skin:** rash, SCARs, pruritus, urticaria, diaphoresis, erythema. **Other:** overgrowth of nonsusceptible organisms, *candidiasis,* flulike symptoms, hypersensitivity reactions, including *anaphylaxis.*

INTERACTIONS

Drug-drug. *Busulfan:* May increase busulfan toxicity. Avoid using together.

Cimetidine: May increase risk of metronidazole toxicity because of inhibited hepatic metabolism. Monitor for toxicity.

CYP3A4 substrates (amiodarone, aripiprazole, dofetilide, lomitapide, pimozide): May increase substrate level. Monitor therapy.

🜋 *Alert: Disulfiram:* May cause acute psychosis and confusion. Avoid giving metronidazole within 2 weeks of disulfiram.

5-FU: May increase 5-FU level and toxicity. Use cautiously together.

Lithium: May increase lithium level, which may cause toxicity. Monitor lithium level.

Mebendazole: May increase risk of SJS or TEN. Consider therapy modification.

Phenobarbital, phenytoin: May decrease metronidazole effectiveness; may reduce total phenytoin clearance. Monitor patient.

QT-interval-prolonging drugs: May increase risk of QT-interval prolongation and ventricular arrhythmias. Avoid use together.

Vecuronium: May potentiate neuromuscular blocking effects of vecuronium. Use cautiously together.

Warfarin: May increase anticoagulant effects and risk of bleeding. Reduce warfarin as needed.

Drug-lifestyle. *Alcohol use:* May cause disulfiram-like reaction, including nausea, vomiting, headache, cramps, and flushing. Warn patient to avoid alcohol during and for 3 days after completing drug therapy.

EFFECTS ON LAB TEST RESULTS

• May increase LFT values.
• May falsely decrease triglyceride and aminotransferase levels.
• May decrease WBC, platelet, and neutrophil counts.
• May interfere with ALT, AST, glucose, and LDH testing.

CONTRAINDICATIONS & CAUTIONS

• Contraindicated in patients hypersensitive to drug or other nitroimidazole derivatives.
🜋 Contraindicated in patients with Cockayne syndrome. Irreversible hepatotoxicity may occur.
• The use of disulfiram within 2 weeks of metronidazole therapy and the use of alcohol or propylene glycol products during treatment and for 3 days after treatment ends are contraindicated.
• Use cautiously in patients with history of blood dyscrasia, seizure disorder, or retinal or visual field changes.
• Use cautiously in patients who take hepatotoxic drugs or have hepatic disease, alcoholism, or renal impairment.
• Each RTU bag contains 14 mEq of sodium.
• Prolonged use may cause superinfections, including CDAD and pseudomembranous colitis, which may occur more than 2 months after therapy ends.

Dialyzable drug: Yes.

⚠ *Overdose S&S:* Nausea, vomiting, ataxia, neurotoxicity.

PREGNANCY-LACTATION-REPRODUCTION

• Drug crosses the placental barrier. Consult current guidelines for appropriate use during pregnancy.
• Drug appears in human milk. Patient should discontinue breastfeeding or discontinue drug. Or, patient may express and discard human milk during metronidazole therapy and for 24 hours after final dose.

NURSING CONSIDERATIONS

• Monitor LFT results carefully in older adults and patients with hepatic impairment.

Reactions in bold italics are *life-threatening.* Interactions may have a *rapid onset* or a *delayed onset.*

- Observe patient for edema, especially if patient is receiving corticosteroids; IV form may cause sodium retention.
- Record number and character of stools when drug is used to treat amebiasis. Give drug only after confirming *Trichomonas vaginalis* infection by wet smear or culture or identifying *Entamoeba histolytica*.
- Sexual partners of patients being treated for *T. vaginalis* infection, even if asymptomatic, must also be treated to avoid reinfection.
- *Look alike–sound alike:* Don't confuse metronidazole with metformin.

PATIENT TEACHING
- Inform patient with trichomoniasis of need for sexual partners to be treated simultaneously to avoid reinfection.
- Tell patient to avoid alcohol and alcohol-containing drugs during and for at least 3 days after treatment course.
- Alert patient that a metallic taste and dark or red-brown urine may occur.
- Tell patient to report signs and symptoms of candidal overgrowth.
- Caution patient to report all adverse reactions immediately, especially neurologic symptoms (seizures, peripheral neuropathy).
- Advise patient to report pregnancy or plans to become pregnant.

metroNIDAZOLE (topical, vaginal)
me-troe-NI-da-zole

MetroCream, MetroGel, MetroLotion, Noritate, Nuvessa, Rosadan, Vandazole

Therapeutic class: Antibacterials (topical)
Pharmacologic class: Nitroimidazoles

AVAILABLE FORMS
Topical cream: 0.75%, 1%
Topical gel: 0.75%, 1%
Topical lotion: 0.75%
Vaginal gel: 0.75%, 1.3%

INDICATIONS & DOSAGES
➤ **Inflammatory papules and pustules of acne rosacea**
Adults: If using a 0.75% preparation, apply thin film to affected area b.i.d., morning and evening. If using a 1% preparation, apply thin film to affected area once daily. After response is seen (usually within 3 weeks), adjust frequency and duration of therapy.
➤ **Bacterial vaginosis**
Adults and children who are postmenarchal: One applicatorful of 0.75% (approximately 37.5 mg) vaginally daily or b.i.d. for 5 days. For once-daily use, give at bedtime.
Adults and children age 12 and older: One applicatorful (approximately 65 mg) of 1.3% vaginal gel intravaginally once as a single dose at bedtime.

ADMINISTRATION
Topical
- Clean area thoroughly before use; then wait 15 to 20 minutes before applying drug to minimize risk of local irritation. Avoid contact with eyes.
- Patient should wait at least 5 minutes after using lotion before applying cosmetics.
Vaginal
- Screw the end of the applicator onto the tube and squeeze slowly. The plunger will stop when the applicator is full.
- Insert gently into the vagina as far as possible without causing discomfort.
- Wash plunger and barrel in warm, soapy water and rinse thoroughly. Dry before reassembling.

ACTION
Unknown. May cause bactericidal effect by interacting with bacterial DNA. Drug is active against many anaerobic gram-negative bacilli, anaerobic gram-positive cocci, *Gardnerella vaginalis*, and *Campylobacter fetus*.

Route	Onset	Peak	Duration
Topical	Unknown	8–12 hr	Unknown
Vaginal	Unknown	6–12 hr	Unknown

Half-life: Unknown.

ADVERSE REACTIONS
Topical form
CNS: headache. **CV:** HTN. **GU:** UTI. **Respiratory:** URI. **Skin:** transient redness, dryness, mild burning, stinging, contact dermatitis, pruritus, rash, exacerbation of rosacea.
Vaginal form
CNS: headache, dizziness, dysgeusia, depression. **EENT:** pharyngitis. **GI:** cramps, GI distress, nausea, loose stools, pain, vomiting, diarrhea, decreased appetite. **GU:** metrorrhagia, dysmenorrhea, cervicitis, vaginitis, perineal

M

and vulvovaginal itching, vaginal burning, vaginal discharge, pelvic discomfort. **Musculoskeletal:** muscle cramps. **Skin:** transient redness, dryness, mild burning, stinging, rash, pruritus. **Other:** overgrowth of nonsusceptible organisms, breast pain.

INTERACTIONS
Drug-drug. *Disulfiram:* May cause disulfiram-like reaction when used with vaginal form of metronidazole. Don't use together, and wait 2 weeks after stopping disulfiram before starting metronidazole vaginal therapy.
Lithium: May increase lithium level in patients taking high doses of lithium. Use cautiously together. Consider monitoring lithium level.
Lopinavir: May enhance adverse and toxic effects of lopinavir and result in a disulfiram-like reaction. Monitor therapy.
Oral anticoagulants: May increase anticoagulant effect. Monitor patient for adverse reactions.
Tipranavir: May enhance adverse effect of tipranavir. Monitor therapy.
Warfarin: May increase PT. Monitor therapy.
Drug-lifestyle. *Alcohol use:* May cause disulfiram-like reaction when used with vaginal form. Don't use together or for at least 24 hours after vaginal treatment.

EFFECTS ON LAB TEST RESULTS
• May interfere with AST, ALT, LDH, triglyceride, and glucose levels.
• May increase or decrease WBC count.

CONTRAINDICATIONS & CAUTIONS
• Contraindicated in patients hypersensitive to drug or its ingredients, such as parabens, and other nitroimidazole derivatives.
• Use cautiously in patients with history or evidence of blood dyscrasia and in those with hepatic impairment.
• Use vaginal gel cautiously in patients with history of CNS diseases. Oral form may cause seizures and peripheral neuropathy.
• Prolonged use of vaginal form can lead to fungal or bacterial superinfection.
Dialyzable drug: Unknown.

PREGNANCY-LACTATION-REPRODUCTION
• There are no adequate studies during pregnancy. Use during pregnancy only if clearly needed and benefit justifies fetal risk.

• Drug may appear in human milk after vaginal or topical use because some of drug is absorbed systemically. Patient should discontinue breastfeeding or discontinue drug.

NURSING CONSIDERATIONS
• Topical therapy hasn't been linked to the adverse effects observed with parenteral or oral therapy, but some drug may be absorbed after topical use.
• Don't use vaginal form in patients who have taken disulfiram within past 2 weeks.
• Monitor patient for worsening symptoms.

PATIENT TEACHING
• Teach patient safe drug administration.
• Instruct patient to avoid use of topical gel around eyes.
• If local reactions occur, advise patient to apply drug less frequently or stop using it and notify prescriber.
• Advise patient to avoid sexual intercourse and use of other vaginal products (tampons, douches) while using vaginal preparation.
• Caution patient to avoid alcohol while being treated with vaginal preparation.

micafungin sodium
mi-ka-FUN-gin

Mycamine

Therapeutic class: Antifungals
Pharmacologic class: Echinocandins

AVAILABLE FORMS
Lyophilized powder for injection: 50 mg, 100 mg in single-use vials

INDICATIONS & DOSAGES
➤ **Candidemia, acute disseminated candidiasis, and *Candida* peritonitis and abscesses**
Adults: 100 mg IV daily for 10 to 47 days (mean duration, 15 days).
Children age 4 months and older: 2 mg/kg IV once daily. Maximum dosage is 100 mg daily.
➤ **To treat candidemia, acute disseminated candidiasis, *Candida* peritonitis, and abscesses without meningoencephalitis, ocular dissemination, or both**
Children younger than age 4 months: 4 mg/kg IV once daily.

Reactions in bold italics are *life-threatening*. Interactions may have a *rapid onset* or a ***delayed onset***.

➤ **Esophageal candidiasis**
Adults: 150 mg IV daily for 10 to 30 days (mean duration, 15 days).
Children age 4 months and older weighing more than 30 kg: 2.5 mg/kg IV once daily. Maximum dosage is 150 mg daily.
Children age 4 months and older weighing 30 kg or less: 3 mg/kg IV once daily.
➤ **To prevent candidal infection in hematopoietic stem cell transplant recipients**
Adults: 50 mg IV daily for 6 to 51 days (mean duration, 19 days).
Children age 4 months and older: 1 mg/kg IV once daily. Maximum dosage is 50 mg daily.

ADMINISTRATION
IV

▼ Reconstitute each 50-mg or 100-mg vial with 5 mL of NSS without a bacteriostatic agent or D_5W for injection. To minimize foaming, dissolve powder by swirling the vial; don't shake it. Don't use solution if precipitation or foreign matter is present.
▼ For adult, dilute dose in 100 mL of NSS or D_5W for injection.
▼ For children's doses: Add reconstituted drug to NSS or D_5W IV infusion bag or syringe. Ensure that final concentration of solution is between 0.5 and 4 mg/mL. To minimize risk of infusion reactions, administer concentrations of greater than 1.5 mg/mL via central catheter.
▼ Flush line with NSS for injection before infusing drug.
▼ Infuse drug over 1 hour.
▼ Reconstituted product and diluted infusion may be stored for up to 24 hours at room temperature.
▼ Protect diluted solution from light.
▼ Drug is preservative-free; discard partially used vials.
▼ **Incompatibilities:** Don't mix or confuse with other medications. Drug may precipitate when mixed with commonly used drugs.

ACTION

Inhibits synthesis of an essential component of fungal cell walls. Drug is active against *Candida albicans, C. glabrata, C. guilliermondii, C. krusei, C. parapsilosis*, and *C. tropicalis.*

Route	Onset	Peak	Duration
IV	Unknown	Unknown	Unknown

Half-life: 11 to 21 hours.

ADVERSE REACTIONS
CNS: headache, insomnia, anxiety, dizziness, fever, rigors, delirium, *seizures, intracranial hemorrhage.* **CV:** atrial fibrillation, bradycardia, cardiac disorders, HTN, hypotension, tachycardia, vascular disorders, phlebitis, *injection-site thrombosis,* edema, *cardiac arrest, MI, pericardial effusion.* **EENT:** epistaxis. **GI:** abdominal pain, abdominal distention, diarrhea, nausea, vomiting, anorexia, dyspepsia, mucositis, constipation. **GU:** decreased urine output, hematuria, *renal failure.* **Hematologic:** *leukopenia, neutropenia, thrombocytopenia,* anemia, *coagulopathy, pancytopenia.* **Hepatic:** elevated LFT values, hepatic injury, hepatomegaly, hyperbilirubinemia, jaundice, *hepatic failure.* **Metabolic:** *hypocalcemia, hypokalemia, hypomagnesemia,* hypophosphatemia, hyperglycemia, *hypoglycemia, hyperkalemia,* hypernatremia. **Respiratory:** cough, dyspnea. **Skin:** infusion-site inflammation, pruritus, rash, urticaria. **Other:** hypersensitivity reactions.

INTERACTIONS
Drug-drug. *Sirolimus:* May increase sirolimus level. Monitor patient for evidence of toxicity, and decrease sirolimus dose if needed.

EFFECTS ON LAB TEST RESULTS
• May increase ALP, ALT, AST, bilirubin, BUN, creatinine, sodium, and LDH levels.
• May decrease calcium, magnesium, phosphorus, and potassium levels.
• May decrease Hb level and hematocrit and neutrophil and platelet counts.

CONTRAINDICATIONS & CAUTIONS
• Contraindicated in patients hypersensitive to drug or other echinocandins.
• Drug may increase risk of hepatic disorder.
Dialyzable drug: No.

PREGNANCY-LACTATION-REPRODUCTION
• There are no adequate studies during pregnancy. Use during pregnancy only if potential benefit justifies fetal risk.
• It isn't known if drug appears in human milk. Use cautiously during breastfeeding.

NURSING CONSIDERATIONS
• Injection-site reactions occur more often in patients receiving drug by peripheral IV.

M

• To reduce the risk of histamine-mediated reactions, infuse drug over at least 1 hour.

Alert: If patient develops signs of serious hypersensitivity reaction, including shock, stop infusion and notify prescriber immediately.

• Monitor hepatic and renal function during therapy.

• Monitor patient for hemolysis and hemolytic anemia.

PATIENT TEACHING

• Advise patient to report pain or redness at infusion site.

• Teach patient about adverse reactions and to report them immediately.

• Tell patient lab tests will most likely be needed to monitor hematologic, renal, and hepatic function.

miconazole

my-KON-a-zole

Oravig

miconazole nitrate

Desenex ◇, Fungoid Tincture ◇, Lotrimin AF ◇, Micaderm, Micatin ◇, Micozole🍁 ◇, Monistat ◇, M-Zole 3 ◇, Vagistat-3 ◇, Zeasorb-AF ◇

Therapeutic class: Antifungals
Pharmacologic class: Imidazoles

AVAILABLE FORMS

Aerosol powder: 2% ◇
Aerosol spray: 2% ◇
Buccal tablets DNC: 50 mg
Powder: 2% ◇
Topical ointment: 2% ◇
Topical solution: 2% ◇
Vaginal cream: 2% ◇, 4% ◇
Vaginal suppositories: 100 mg ◇, 200 mg ◇, 400 mg🍁 ◇, 1,200 mg ◇

INDICATIONS & DOSAGES

➤ **Tinea corporis, tinea cruris, tinea pedis, cutaneous candidiasis, common dermatophyte infections**

Adults and children older than age 2: Apply sparingly b.i.d. for 2 weeks (tinea cruris) to 4 weeks (tinea pedis and corporis). Powder or spray can be used liberally over affected area. In children younger than age 2, use only under the direction and supervision of a physician.

➤ **Vulvovaginal candidiasis**

Adults and children age 12 and older: One applicatorful 2% or 100-mg suppository vaginally at bedtime for 7 days; repeat course, if needed. Or, one applicatorful 4% or 200-mg suppository vaginally at bedtime for 3 days. Or, one 1,200-mg suppository vaginally at bedtime for 1 day. May apply topical cream sparingly to affected area b.i.d. for 7 days or as needed for external symptoms.

➤ **Oropharyngeal candidiasis**

Adults and children age 16 and older: One 50-mg buccal tablet to the upper gum region once daily for 14 consecutive days.

ADMINISTRATION

PO

• Apply buccal tablet to the gum in the morning with dry hands after patient has brushed teeth.

• Place the rounded surface of the tablet against the gum just above the incisor. Apply slight pressure over the upper lip for 30 seconds to ensure adhesion.

• Alternate sides of the mouth for each dose.

• Patient shouldn't crush, chew, or swallow buccal tablets.

• If a buccal tablet that has been in place for at least 6 hours and dislodges or patient swallows it, don't apply a new tablet until the next regularly scheduled dose.

Topical

• Cleanse and thoroughly dry area before application

• Don't use occlusive dressings.

• For tinea pedis, pay special attention to spaces between toes.

Vaginal

• Suppository is inserted high into vagina with applicator provided.

• Store between 59° and 86° F (15° and 30° C).

ACTION

Fungicidal; disrupts fungal cell membrane permeability.

Route	Onset	Peak	Duration
PO	Unknown	7 hr	15 hr
Topical, vaginal	Unknown	Unknown	Unknown

Half-life: 24 hours (terminal).

ADVERSE REACTIONS

CNS: headache, fatigue, pain, dysgeusia, ageusia. **EENT:** dry mouth, oral discomfort, toothache. **GI:** diarrhea, nausea, upper abdominal pain, vomiting (buccal tablets), gastroenteritis. **GU:** pelvic cramps, pruritus and irritation with vaginal cream; vulvovaginal burning. **Hematologic:** anemia, *lymphopenia, neutropenia.* **Hepatic:** increased GGT level (buccal tablets). **Respiratory:** cough, URI. **Skin:** allergic contact dermatitis, burning, irritation, maceration, pain, edema.

INTERACTIONS

Drug-drug. *Fosphenytoin, phenytoin, sulfonylureas:* Buccal form may increase levels of these drugs. Monitor therapy.
Progesterone: Vaginal form of drug may diminish progesterone effects. Avoid use together.
Warfarin: Buccal form of drug may enhance anticoagulant effect. Monitor PT and INR, and observe patient for bleeding. Oral form of drug may increase warfarin concentration. Monitor therapy.
Drug-herb. *Saccharomyces boulardii:* Antifungals may decrease therapeutic effect. Consider alternative therapy.

EFFECTS ON LAB TEST RESULTS

• May increase GGT level.

CONTRAINDICATIONS & CAUTIONS

• Contraindicated in patients hypersensitive to drug or its components. Cross-sensitivity to imidazole antifungals may occur.
• Buccal tablets are contraindicated in patients hypersensitive to milk protein concentrate.
• Use buccal tablets cautiously in patients with hepatic impairment.
• Safety and effectiveness of Oravig haven't been established for children younger than age 16; don't use in younger children because of risk of choking.
Dialyzable drug: Unknown.

PREGNANCY-LACTATION-REPRODUCTION

• There are no adequate studies during pregnancy. Use oral form during pregnancy only if potential benefit justifies fetal risk.
⚠ *Alert:* Vaginal preparation shouldn't be used during first trimester and should be used during pregnancy only if recommended by prescriber.
• It isn't known if drug appears in human milk. Topical and vaginal administration

should result in low systemic absorption. Use cautiously during breastfeeding.
• Vaginal form can weaken latex condoms and diaphragms.

NURSING CONSIDERATIONS

• Carefully monitor patients with hepatic impairment who are taking oral form.
• Monitor patients for hypersensitivity and adverse reactions.

PATIENT TEACHING

• Advise patient that vaginal form is for perineal or vaginal use only and to keep drug out of eyes.
• Caution patient that frequent or persistent yeast infections may suggest a more serious medical problem.
• Tell patient that drug may stain clothing.
• Warn patient to stop drug if sensitivity or chemical irritation occurs.
• Tell patient to use drug for full treatment period prescribed and to notify prescriber if symptoms persist or worsen despite therapy.
• Advise patient to avoid tampons and sexual intercourse during vaginal treatment.
• Show patient how to properly administer prescribed formulation.
• Emphasize that patient can eat and drink with the buccal tablet in place but to avoid chewing gum.

SAFETY ALERT!

midazolam hydrochloride
MID-aye-zoe-lam

Nayzilam, Seizalam

Therapeutic class: Anxiolytics
Pharmacologic class: Benzodiazepines
Controlled substance schedule: IV

AVAILABLE FORMS

Injection: 1 mg/mL, 5 mg/mL
Injection (preservative-free): 1 mg/mL, 5 mg/mL
Nasal spray: 5 mg/0.1 mL
Syrup: 2 mg/mL

INDICATIONS & DOSAGES

➤ **Preoperative sedation (to induce sleepiness or drowsiness and relieve apprehension)**
Adults age 60 and older: 0.02 to 0.05 mg/kg IM 30 to 60 minutes before surgery.

Adults younger than age 60: 0.07 to 0.08 mg/kg IM 30 to 60 minutes before surgery. Usual dose is 5 mg.

➤ **Moderate sedation before short diagnostic or endoscopic procedures**

Adults age 60 or older and patients who are debilitated or chronically ill: 0.5 to 1.5 mg IV over at least 2 minutes. Incremental doses shouldn't exceed 1 mg. A total dose of up to 3.5 mg is usually sufficient.

Adults younger than age 60: Initially, small dose not to exceed 2.5 mg IV given slowly over at least 2 minutes; wait at least 2 minutes to evaluate sedative effect. Then repeat in 2 minutes PRN, in small increments of first dose over at least 2 minutes each to achieve desired effect. Total dose of up to 5 mg may be used. Additional doses to maintain desired level of sedation may be given by slow titration in increments of 25% of dose used to first reach the sedative end point.

➤ **To induce sleepiness and amnesia and to relieve apprehension before anesthesia or before and during procedures**

PO

Children ages 6 to 16 who are cooperative: 0.25 to 0.5 mg/kg PO as a single dose, up to 20 mg.

Infants and children ages 6 months to 5 years or less cooperative, older children: 0.25 to 1 mg/kg PO as a single dose, up to 20 mg.

IV

Children ages 12 to 16: Initially, no more than 2.5 mg IV given slowly; repeat in 2 minutes, if needed, in small increments of first dose over at least 2 minutes to achieve desired effect. Total dose of up to 10 mg may be used. Additional doses to maintain desired level of sedation may be given by slow titration in increments of 25% of dose used to first reach the sedative end point.

Children ages 6 to 12: 0.025 to 0.05 mg/kg IV over 2 to 3 minutes. Additional doses may be given in small increments after 2 to 3 minutes. Total dose of up to 0.4 mg/kg, not to exceed 10 mg, may be used.

Children ages 6 months to 5 years: 0.05 to 0.1 mg/kg IV over 2 to 3 minutes. Additional doses may be given in small increments after 2 to 3 minutes. Total dose of up to 0.6 mg/kg, not to exceed 6 mg, may be used.

IM

Children: 0.1 to 0.15 mg/kg IM. Use up to 0.5 mg/kg in patients who are more anxious. May use total dose of up to 10 mg.

Adjust-a-dose: For children who are obese, base dose on ideal body weight. Children who are at high risk or debilitated and children receiving other sedatives need lower doses.

➤ **To induce general anesthesia**

Adults older than age 55: 0.3 mg/kg IV infusion over 20 to 30 seconds if patient hasn't received premedication, or 0.2 mg/kg IV infusion over 20 to 30 seconds if patient has received a sedative or opioid premedication. Allow 2 minutes for effect. Additional increments of 25% of first dose may be needed to complete induction.

Adults younger than age 55: 0.3 to 0.35 mg/kg IV infusion over 20 to 30 seconds if patient hasn't received premedication, or 0.25 mg/kg IV infusion over 20 to 30 seconds if patient has received a sedative or opioid premedication. Allow 2 minutes for effect. Additional increments of 25% of first dose may be needed to complete induction.

Adjust-a-dose: For patients who are debilitated, initially, 0.2 to 0.25 mg/kg. As little as 0.15 mg/kg may be needed.

➤ **As continuous infusion to sedate patients in critical care unit who are intubated**

Adults: Initially, 0.01 to 0.05 mg/kg may be given IV over several minutes, repeated at 10- to 15-minute intervals until adequate sedation is achieved. To maintain sedation, usual initial infusion rate is 0.02 to 0.1 mg/kg/hour. Higher loading dose or infusion rates may be needed in some patients. Use the lowest effective rate.

Children: Initially, 0.05 to 0.2 mg/kg may be given IV over 2 to 3 minutes or longer; then continuous infusion at rate of 0.06 to 0.12 mg/kg/hour. Increase or decrease infusion to maintain desired effect.

Neonates more than 32 weeks' gestational age: Initially, 0.06 mg/kg/hour IV. Adjust rate, as needed, using lowest possible rate.

Neonates less than 32 weeks' gestational age: Initially, 0.03 mg/kg/hour IV. Adjust rate, as needed, using lowest possible rate.

➤ **Status epilepticus (Seizalam)**

Adults: 10 mg IM once.

➤ **Acute treatment of intermittent, stereotypic episodes of frequent seizure activity (distinct from patient's usual seizure pattern) (Nayzilam)**

Adults and children older than age 12: 1 spray (5-mg dose) into one nostril; may repeat in opposite nostril after 10 minutes if no response. Don't use more than two doses per

---

Reactions in bold italics are *life-threatening*. Interactions may have a *rapid onset* or a *delayed onset*.

seizure cluster, no more than one episode in 3 days, and no more than five episodes in a month.

➤ **Status epilepticus** ♦

Infants, children, and adolescents: For patients weighing more than 40 kg, 10 mg IM once; for those weighing 13 to 40 kg, 5 mg IM once. Or, 0.2 mg/kg intranasally; maximum dose, 10 mg. Or, 0.1 mg/kg IV; maximum dose, 10 mg.

ADMINISTRATION
PO

Boxed Warning Midazolam syrup has been associated with respiratory depression and respiratory arrest, especially when used in noncritical-care settings. Restrict use to hospital or ambulatory care settings that can provide continuous respiratory and cardiac function monitoring. ∎

• Give drug without regard for food. Dispense syrup directly into the mouth and don't mix with any liquid before dispensing.

• Refer to manufacturer's instructions for use of oral dispenser and press-in bottle dispenser.

IV

Boxed Warning IV midazolam has been associated with respiratory depression and respiratory arrest, especially when used in noncritical-care settings. Restrict use to hospital or ambulatory care settings that can provide continuous monitoring of cardiac and respiratory function. Ensure availability of resuscitative drugs and equipment and personnel trained in their use and skilled in airway management. ∎

▼ Drug may be mixed in the same syringe with morphine sulfate, meperidine, atropine, or scopolamine.

▼ When mixing infusion, use 5-mg/mL vial and dilute to 0.5 mg/mL with D₅W or NSS.

Boxed Warning Give slowly over at least 2 minutes, and wait at least 2 minutes when initiating or titrating doses to fully evaluate therapeutic effect. Initial adult dose shouldn't exceed 2.5 mg. Lower initial doses are necessary for adults age 60 and older, for patients who are debilitated, and for those receiving concomitant opioids or other CNS depressants. ∎

Boxed Warning Calculate pediatric dosages using mg/kg and titrate all dosages slowly. Initial pediatric dose depends on child's age, procedure, and route of administration. ∎

Boxed Warning Avoid rapid injection (less than 2 minutes) in neonate because rapid injection has been associated with severe hypotension and seizures, particularly when neonate has also received fentanyl. ∎

▼ **Incompatibilities:** None listed by manufacturer. Consult a drug incompatibility reference for more information.

IM

• Inject deeply into a large muscle.
• Inject Seizalam in mid-outer thigh.

Intranasal

• Don't test or prime nasal spray unit before use.

• Remove nasal spray unit from blister pack carefully. Hold nasal spray unit with thumb on the plunger and middle and index fingers on each side of the nozzle.

• Place the tip of the nozzle into one nostril until the fingers on either side of the nozzle touch the bottom of the nose; press plunger firmly to deliver dose.

ACTION

May potentiate the effects of GABA, depress the CNS, and suppress the spread of seizure activity.

Route	Onset	Peak	Duration
PO	10–20 min	45–60 min	2–6 hr
IV	90 sec–5 min	Rapid	2–6 hr
IM	15 min	15–60 min	2–6 hr
Intranasal	10 min	8–28 min	2–4 hr

Half-life: 2 to 6 hours.

ADVERSE REACTIONS

CNS: oversedation, drowsiness, amnesia, headache, *seizures,* postictal state, involuntary movements, paresthesia, hallucinations, confusion, dreaming during emergence, insomnia, nightmares, dizziness, paradoxical behavior or excitement, fever, difficulty speaking. **CV:** variations in BP and pulse rate, *arrhythmias.* **EENT:** nystagmus, increased tearing, nasal discomfort, rhinorrhea, congestion, throat irritation, excessive salivation. **GI:** nausea, retching, vomiting, hiccups. **GU:** *acute renal failure.* **Respiratory:** *respiratory depression, apnea,* hyperventilation, shallow respirations, dyspnea, *hypoxia,* rhonchi, coughing, wheezing, *upper airway obstruction.* **Skin:** rash, injection-site reaction. **Other:** hypersensitivity reactions.

INTERACTIONS

Drug-drug. *CNS depressants:* May cause apnea. Use together cautiously. Adjust dosage of midazolam if used with opiates or other CNS depressants.

CYP3A4 inducers (carbamazepine, phenytoin, rifampin): May decrease midazolam level. Use cautiously and adjust dosage as needed.

CYP3A4 inhibitors (calcium channel blockers, cimetidine, fluconazole, itraconazole, ketoconazole, macrolide antibiotics [erythromycin]): May increase and prolong midazolam level, CNS depression, and psychomotor impairment. Avoid using together. If must be given together, monitor patient closely.

Hormonal contraceptives: May prolong half-life of midazolam. Use together cautiously.

Boxed Warning *Opioids:* May cause slow or difficult breathing, sedation, and death. Avoid use together. If use together is necessary, limit dosage and duration of each drug to minimum necessary for desired effect. ■

Protease inhibitors (ritonavir, saquinavir): May increase midazolam level and prolong sedation. Use together cautiously. Consider lower midazolam doses with combined use.

Theophylline: May antagonize sedative effect of midazolam. Use together cautiously.

Drug-herb. *Ginkgo biloba, St. John's wort:* May decrease drug level. Discourage use together.

Drug-food. *Grapefruit juice:* May increase bioavailability of oral drug. Don't use together.

Drug-lifestyle. *Alcohol use:* May cause additive CNS effects. Don't use together.

EFFECTS ON LAB TEST RESULTS

None reported.

CONTRAINDICATIONS & CAUTIONS

• Contraindicated in patients hypersensitive to drug or its components and in those with acute narrow-angle glaucoma, shock, coma, or acute alcohol intoxication.

• Intrathecal or epidural injection of parenteral forms containing benzyl alcohol is contraindicated.

◑ **Alert:** Drug should only be used with individualization of the dosage.

• Use cautiously in older adults or patients who are debilitated; in patients with uncompensated acute illness, HF, impaired gag reflex, or respiratory, renal, or hepatic disease; and in patients at risk for falls.

• Benzodiazepines are associated with paradoxical reactions (agitation, aggressive behavior, involuntary movements) and anterograde amnesia.

Boxed Warning Midazolam should only be administered by persons specifically trained in the use of anesthetics and management of effects of anesthetics, including resuscitation of patients in the age-group being treated. The appropriate emergency equipment must be immediately available. ■

Boxed Warning Opioids should only be prescribed with benzodiazepines or other CNS depressants to patients for whom alternative treatment options are inadequate. ■

Boxed Warning Benzodiazepine use exposes patient to risks of abuse, misuse, and addiction, which can lead to overdose or death. Assess each patient's risk of abuse, misuse, and addiction before prescribing and periodically during therapy. ■

Boxed Warning Abrupt discontinuation or rapid dosage reduction of benzodiazepines after continued use may precipitate acute withdrawal reactions, which can be life-threatening. To reduce risk of withdrawal reactions, gradually taper drug to discontinue or reduce dosage. ■

• When overdose is suspected, flumazenil may be used as a reversal agent.

• Risk of suicidality is increased with intranasal form.

◑ **Alert:** Repeated or lengthy use of general anesthetics and sedation drugs during surgeries or procedures in children younger than age 3 and in patients during the third trimester may affect the development of children's brains; weigh benefits against risks.

Dialyzable drug: Unknown.

⚠ *Overdose S&S:* Excessive sedation, somnolence, confusion, impaired coordination, diminished reflexes, coma, altered vital signs.

PREGNANCY-LACTATION-REPRODUCTION

• Drug crosses the placental barrier. Several studies suggest an increased risk of congenital malformations associated with benzodiazepine use. Use during pregnancy isn't recommended.

• Drug appears in human milk. Use cautiously during breastfeeding.

Reactions in bold italics are *life-threatening*. Interactions may have a *rapid onset* or a **delayed onset**.

NURSING CONSIDERATIONS

Boxed Warning A qualified individual, other than the practitioner performing the procedure, should monitor patient throughout procedure. Have oxygen and resuscitation equipment available in case of severe respiratory depression. Excessive amounts and rapid infusion have been linked to respiratory arrest. Continuously monitor patient, including children taking syrup form, for life-threatening respiratory depression. ■

• Monitor BP, HR and rhythm, respirations, airway integrity, and pulse oximetry during procedure.

• For status epilepticus, continuously monitor respiratory and cardiac function until condition stabilizes. Have airway management and resuscitation equipment available.

PATIENT TEACHING

• Teach patient about drug's use and potential adverse reactions; advise patient to immediately report difficulty breathing.

Boxed Warning Caution patient or caregivers of patient taking an opioid with a benzodiazepine, CNS depressant, or alcohol to seek immediate medical attention for dizziness, light-headedness, extreme sleepiness, slowed or difficult breathing, or unresponsiveness. ■

Boxed Warning Caution patient that benzodiazepines, even at recommended doses, increase the risk of abuse, misuse, and addiction, which can lead to overdose and death, especially when used in combination with other drugs (opioid analgesics), alcohol, or illicit substances. ■

Boxed Warning Inform patient about signs and symptoms of benzodiazepine abuse, misuse, and addiction (abdominal pain, amnesia, anorexia, anxiety, aggression, ataxia, blurred vision, confusion, depression, disinhibition, disorientation, dizziness, euphoria, impaired concentration and memory, indigestion, irritability, muscle pain, slurred speech, tremors, vertigo, delirium, paranoia, suicidality, seizures, difficulty breathing, coma) and to seek emergency medical care if they occur. Explain proper disposal of unused drug. Advise patient not to take drug at a higher dose, more frequently, or for longer than prescribed. ■

Boxed Warning Tell patient that continued use of drug for several days to weeks may lead to physical dependence and that abrupt discontinuation or rapid dosage reduction may precipitate acute withdrawal reactions (unusual movements, responses, or expressions; seizures; sudden and severe mental or nervous system changes; depression; seeing or hearing things that others don't; homicidal thoughts; extreme increase in activity or talking; losing touch with reality; suicidality), which can be life-threatening. Instruct patient that discontinuation or dosage reduction may require a slow taper. ■

Boxed Warning Advise patient about the possibility of developing protracted withdrawal syndrome (anxiety; trouble remembering, learning, or concentrating; depression; problems sleeping; feeling like insects are crawling under the skin; weakness; shaking; muscle twitching; burning or prickling feeling in the hands, arms, legs, or feet; ringing in the ears), with symptoms lasting weeks to more than 12 months. ■

• Because drug diminishes patient's recall of events around the time of surgery, provide written information, family member instructions, and follow-up contact.

⚠ **Alert:** Discuss with parents or caregivers of child younger than age 3 and with patient who is pregnant the benefits, risks, and appropriate timing of surgery or procedures requiring anesthetics and sedation drugs.

• Warn patient to avoid hazardous activities that require alertness or good coordination until effects of drug are known.

---

miglitol
MIG-li-tol

Glyset

Therapeutic class: Antidiabetics
Pharmacologic class: Alpha-glucosidase inhibitors

AVAILABLE FORMS
Tablets: 25 mg, 50 mg, 100 mg

INDICATIONS & DOSAGES
➤ **Adjunct to diet in patients with type 2 diabetes, alone or with a sulfonylurea**
Adults: 25 mg PO t.i.d. May start with 25 mg PO daily and increase gradually to t.i.d. to minimize GI upset; dosage may be increased after 4 to 8 weeks to 50 mg PO t.i.d. Dosage may then be further increased after 3 months,

based on HbA$_{1c}$ level, to maximum of 100 mg PO t.i.d.

ADMINISTRATION
PO
• Give drug with first bite of each main meal.

ACTION
Lowers glucose level by inhibiting enzymes in the small intestine, which delays the digestion of carbohydrates after a meal, resulting in a smaller increase in postprandial glucose level.

Route	Onset	Peak	Duration
PO	Unknown	2–3 hr	Unknown

Half-life: About 2 hours.

ADVERSE REACTIONS
GI: abdominal pain, diarrhea, flatulence.
Skin: rash.

INTERACTIONS
Drug-drug. *Digoxin, propranolol:* May decrease bioavailability of these drugs. Monitor clinical response and adjust dosage.
Insulin, sulfonylureas: May increase risk of hypoglycemia. Consider decreasing dosages of miglitol, insulin, and sulfonylureas.
Intestinal adsorbents (charcoal), digestive enzyme preparations (amylase, pancreatin): May reduce effect of miglitol. Avoid using together.
MAO inhibitors, salicylates, SSRIs: May enhance hypoglycemic effect. Monitor therapy.
Thiazide and thiazide-like diuretics (hydrochlorothiazide, indapamide): May decrease therapeutic effect of antidiabetics. Monitor therapy.

EFFECTS ON LAB TEST RESULTS
• May decrease iron level.

CONTRAINDICATIONS & CAUTIONS
• Contraindicated in patients hypersensitive to drug or its components and in those with diabetic ketoacidosis, inflammatory bowel disease, colonic ulceration, partial intestinal obstruction, chronic intestinal diseases with marked disorders of digestion or absorption, or conditions that may deteriorate because of increased gas formation in the intestine, and in patients predisposed to intestinal obstruction.

• Drug isn't recommended in patients with CrCl of less than 25 mL/minute or if serum creatinine level is more than 2 mg/dL.
• Fever, trauma, infection, or surgery can cause a temporary loss of blood glucose control; temporary insulin therapy may be needed.
• Safety and effectiveness in children haven't been established.
Dialyzable drug: Unknown.
⚠ *Overdose S&S:* Transient increases in flatulence, diarrhea, and abdominal discomfort.

PREGNANCY-LACTATION-REPRODUCTION
• Safe use in pregnancy hasn't been established. Abnormal blood glucose levels during pregnancy may cause harm to the fetus. Most experts recommend insulin be used during pregnancy to maintain blood glucose levels. Don't use miglitol during pregnancy unless clearly needed.
• Drug appears in human milk. Use during breastfeeding isn't recommended.

NURSING CONSIDERATIONS
• In patients also taking insulin or a sulfonylurea, dosage adjustment of these drugs may be needed. Monitor patient for hypoglycemia.
• Diabetes management should include diet control, an exercise program, and regular testing of urine and glucose level.
• Monitor glucose level regularly, especially during situations of increased stress, such as infection, fever, surgery, or trauma.
• Monitor HbA$_{1c}$ level every 3 months to evaluate long-term glycemic control.
• Treat mild to moderate hypoglycemia with a ready form of sugar, such as glucose tablets or gel. Severe hypoglycemia may necessitate IV glucose or glucagon.
• Monitor patient for adverse GI effects.

PATIENT TEACHING
• Instruct patient in safe drug administration.
• Stress importance of adhering to diet, weight reduction, and exercise instructions. Urge patient to have glucose and HbA$_{1c}$ levels tested regularly.
• Inform patient that drug treatment relieves symptoms but doesn't cure diabetes.
• Teach patient how to recognize high and low glucose levels.
• Instruct patient to have a source of glucose readily available to treat hypoglycemia.

Reactions in bold italics are *life-threatening*. Interactions may have a *rapid onset* or a **delayed onset**.

• Advise patient that sucrose (table sugar, cane sugar) or fruit juices shouldn't be used to treat low-glucose reactions with this drug. Oral glucose (dextrose) or glucagon is necessary to increase glucose.

• Caution patient to seek medical advice promptly during periods of stress, such as fever, trauma, infection, or surgery, because dosage may have to be adjusted.

• Show patient how and when to monitor glucose level.

• Advise patient that adverse GI effects are most common during first few weeks of therapy and should improve over time.

• Urge patient to carry medical identification at all times.

milnacipran hydrochloride
mil-NAY-ci-pran

Savella⚕

Therapeutic class: Antifibromyalgia drugs
Pharmacologic class: SSNRIs

AVAILABLE FORMS
Tablets: 12.5 mg, 25 mg, 50 mg, 100 mg

INDICATIONS & DOSAGES
➤ **Fibromyalgia**
Adults: Initially, 12.5 mg PO once daily; increase dosage to 12.5 mg b.i.d. on days 2 and 3, followed by 25 mg b.i.d. on days 4 to 7. Increase to 50 mg b.i.d. after day 7. May increase to 100 mg PO b.i.d. based on individual response; recommended dosage is 50 mg b.i.d.
Adjust-a-dose: For patients with CrCl of 5 to 29 mL/minute, give 25 mg b.i.d. May increase to 50 mg b.i.d. based on individual tolerance.

ADMINISTRATION
PO
• Give drug with or without food, but giving with food may improve tolerability.

ACTION
Unclear. Milnacipran is a potent inhibitor of neuronal norepinephrine and serotonin reuptake; however, it doesn't affect the uptake of dopamine or other transmitters.

Route	Onset	Peak	Duration
PO	Unknown	2–4 hr	36–48 hr

Half-life: 6 to 8 hours; active metabolite, 8 to 10 hours.

ADVERSE REACTIONS
CNS: anxiety, depression, dizziness, falls, fatigue, fever, hypoesthesia, irritability, insomnia, migraine, paresthesia, stress, somnolence, headache, tremors, dysgeusia. **CV:** chest discomfort, chest pain, flushing, HTN, palpitations, peripheral edema, tachycardia. **EENT:** blurred vision, dry mouth. **GI:** abdominal distention, abdominal pain, constipation, decreased appetite, diarrhea, flatulence, GERD, dyspepsia, nausea, vomiting. **GU:** cystitis, UTI; in men—dysuria, ejaculation disorder, ejaculation failure, erectile dysfunction, libido decrease, prostatitis, scrotal pain, testicular pain, testicular swelling, urethral pain, urinary hesitation, urine retention, urine flow decrease. **Metabolic:** hypercholesterolemia, weight loss or gain. **Respiratory:** dyspnea, URI. **Skin:** hyperhidrosis, pruritus, rash. **Other:** chills, contusion, hot flush, night sweats.

INTERACTIONS
Drug-drug. *Amphetamines, antipsychotics (risperidone), buspirone, cyclobenzaprine, dopamine antagonists (metoclopramide):* May cause serotonin syndrome (diarrhea, dysreflexia, fever, hallucinations, loss of coordination, nausea, tachycardia). If use together can't be avoided, closely monitor patient for signs and symptoms of serotonin syndrome.
🕙 *Alert: Aspirin, NSAIDs, platelet inhibitors, warfarin:* May increase risk of bleeding. Use together cautiously.
Clomipramine: May cause euphoria and orthostatic hypotension when switching from clomipramine to milnacipran. Use together may also increase risk of serotonin syndrome. Monitor patient closely.
Clonidine: May decrease antihypertensive effect of clonidine. Monitor therapy.
Digoxin: May cause orthostatic hypotension and tachycardia and digoxin-related adverse effects. Avoid use of digoxin IV; when using oral digoxin and drug together, monitor patient closely.
Epinephrine, norepinephrine: May cause paroxysmal HTN and arrhythmia. Use cautiously together.

M

Linezolid, methylene blue: May cause CNS toxicity and serotonin syndrome. Avoid use together.

Lithium, other serotonergic drugs (SSNRIs, SSRIs, TCAs, tramadol, triptans): May cause serotonin syndrome. Avoid use together.

MAO inhibitors: May cause serotonin syndrome. Avoid using drug within 2 weeks after MAO inhibitor therapy; wait at least 5 days after stopping milnacipran or before starting MAO inhibitor.

Drug-herb. *Herbs with anticoagulant properties (alfalfa, anise, bilberry):* May increase risk of bleeding. Use together cautiously.

St. John's wort: May increase risk of serotonin syndrome. Avoid using together.

Drug-lifestyle. *Alcohol use:* May enhance psychomotor impairment and aggravate pre-existing liver disease. Don't administer to patients using alcohol or with chronic liver disease.

EFFECTS ON LAB TEST RESULTS
• May increase LFT values.
• May decrease sodium level.

CONTRAINDICATIONS & CAUTIONS
• Contraindicated in patients hypersensitive to drug or its components.

� *Alert:* Pupillary dilation that occurs after drug use may trigger an angle-closure attack in patients with anatomically narrow angles who don't have a patent iridectomy.

� *Alert:* Serotonin syndrome, a potentially life-threatening condition, may occur, particularly with concomitant use of serotonergic drugs (including triptans and tramadol) and drugs that impair serotonin metabolism (including MAO inhibitors). Signs and symptoms of serotonin syndrome include mental status changes (agitation, coma, hallucinations), autonomic instability (hyperthermia, labile BP, tachycardia), neuromuscular aberrations (hyperreflexia, incoordination), and diarrhea, nausea, and vomiting.

• Use cautiously in patients with a history of mania, seizures, severe hepatic impairment, or dysuria; in patients who consume substantial amounts of alcohol; and in those with HTN or controlled angle-closure glaucoma.

Boxed Warning Drug may increase risk of suicidality in children, adolescents, and young adults with major depressive disorder or other psychiatric disorder. Drug isn't approved for use in children. ∎

Dialyzable drug: Unlikely.

⚠ *Overdose S&S:* HTN, cardiac arrest, decreased level of consciousness, confusion, dizziness, elevated LFT results.

PREGNANCY-LACTATION-REPRODUCTION
• There are no adequate studies during pregnancy. Use during pregnancy only if potential benefit justifies fetal risk. Neonates exposed to SSRIs or SSNRIs late in the third trimester have developed complications requiring prolonged hospitalization, respiratory support, and tube feeding.

• Manufacturer advises patients who are pregnant to enroll in the Savella Pregnancy Registry (1-877-643-3010).

• Drug appears in human milk. Use cautiously during breastfeeding.

NURSING CONSIDERATIONS
• Monitor patient closely for worsening depression or suicidality, especially during the first few months of therapy and with dosage adjustments.

• To prevent withdrawal signs and symptoms, decrease dosage gradually, and watch for signs and symptoms that may arise when drug is stopped, such as dysphoria, irritability, agitation, dizziness, sensory disturbances, anxiety, confusion, headache, lethargy, emotional lability, insomnia, hypomania, tinnitus, and seizures.

• Carefully monitor HR and BP.

• Monitor patient for signs and symptoms of hyponatremia (headache, difficulty concentrating, memory impairment, confusion, weakness, unsteadiness, hallucination, syncope, seizures, coma, respiratory arrest).

• Monitor LFT values and sodium level before and during therapy.

PATIENT TEACHING
Boxed Warning Warn families and caregivers to immediately report signs and symptoms of worsening depression (such as agitation, irritability, insomnia, hostility, and impulsivity) and suicidality. ∎

• Advise patient to avoid taking NSAIDs and aspirin while taking drug to reduce risk of bleeding.

• Tell patient to avoid alcohol while taking drug.

• Instruct patient to have frequent HR and BP monitoring.

Reactions in bold italics are *life-threatening*. Interactions may have a *rapid onset* or a ***delayed onset***.

• Tell patient to report urinary hesitation or urine retention or signs and symptoms of sexual dysfunction.

• Instruct patient to report pregnancy, plans to become pregnant, or breastfeeding.

• Warn patient not to stop drug suddenly.

• Tell patient to consult prescriber before taking other prescription or OTC drugs or herbal supplements.

• Warn patient to avoid hazardous activities that require alertness and good coordination until drug's effects are known.

• Teach patient safe drug administration.

SAFETY ALERT!

milrinone lactate
MIL-ri-none

Therapeutic class: Inotropes
Pharmacologic class: Bipyridine phosphodiesterase inhibitors

AVAILABLE FORMS
Injection: 1 mg/mL vial
Injection (premixed): 200 mcg/mL in D_5W

INDICATIONS & DOSAGES
➤ **Short-term treatment of acutely decompensated HF**
Adults: Give first loading dose of 50 mcg/kg IV slowly over 10 minutes; then give continuous IV infusion of 0.375 to 0.75 mcg/kg/minute (0.59 to 1.13 mg/kg/day). Titrate infusion dose based on clinical and hemodynamic responses. Don't exceed 1.13 mg/kg/day.
Adjust-a-dose: If CrCl is 50 mL/minute, infusion rate is 0.43 mcg/kg/minute; if 40 mL/minute, infusion rate is 0.38 mcg/kg/minute; if 30 mL/minute, infusion rate is 0.33 mcg/kg/minute; if 20 mL/minute, infusion rate is 0.28 mcg/kg/minute; if 10 mL/minute, infusion rate is 0.23 mcg/kg/minute; and if 5 mL/minute, infusion rate is 0.2 mcg/kg/minute.

ADMINISTRATION
IV

▼ Give loading dose undiluted as a direct injection over 10 minutes.

▼ For continuous IV infusion, dilute vials labeled as containing 10, 20, or 50 mg of milrinone with 40, 80, or 200 mL, respectively, of ½ NSS, NSS, or D_5W to provide solutions containing approximately 200 mcg/mL

of milrinone. Don't dilute 200-mcg/mL commercially available bags.

▼ Visually inspect solution. Discard if discoloration or particulate matter is present.

▼ Don't use premixed containers in series connections or administer with blood because of risk of air embolism.

▼ **Incompatibilities:** None listed by manufacturer. Consult a drug incompatibility reference for more information.

ACTION
Produces inotropic action by increasing cellular levels of cAMP and vasodilation by relaxing vascular smooth muscle.

Route	Onset	Peak	Duration
IV	5–15 min	Unknown	Unknown

Half-life: 2.4 hours.

ADVERSE REACTIONS
CNS: headache. **CV:** *ventricular arrhythmias,* ventricular ectopic activity, *ventricular tachycardia,* hypotension, nonsustained ventricular tachycardia, chest pain.

INTERACTIONS
None significant.

EFFECTS ON LAB TEST RESULTS
• May cause abnormal LFT results.
• May cause electrolyte changes.

CONTRAINDICATIONS & CAUTIONS
• Contraindicated in patients hypersensitive to drug.
🔇 *Alert:* Use of milrinone for more than 48 hours in patients with HF hasn't been shown to be safe or effective.
🔇 *Alert:* Drug has been associated with increased frequency of ventricular arrhythmias, including nonsustained ventricular tachycardia and supraventricular tachycardia and ventricular fibrillation in the high-risk population. Closely monitor patient.
• Drug isn't recommended for use in patients with severe aortic or pulmonic valvular disease in place of surgery and during acute phase after an MI.
• Use cautiously in patients with atrial flutter or fibrillation because drug may increase ventricular response rate.
• Safety and effectiveness in children haven't been established.

M

Dialyzable drug: Unknown.
⚠ *Overdose S&S:* Hypotension.

PREGNANCY-LACTATION-REPRODUCTION

• There are no adequate studies during pregnancy. Use during pregnancy only if potential benefit justifies fetal risk.
• It isn't known if drug appears in human milk. Use cautiously during breastfeeding.

NURSING CONSIDERATIONS

• Monitor cardiac rhythm during infusion.
• In patients with atrial flutter or fibrillation, drug is typically given with digoxin and diuretics.
• Improved cardiac output may increase urine output. Reduce diuretic dosage when HF improves. Potassium loss may cause digitalis toxicity.
• Monitor fluid and electrolyte status, BP, HR, and renal function during therapy. Excessive decrease in BP requires stopping or slowing rate of infusion.
• Correct hypoxemia and electrolyte imbalances, especially hypokalemia and hypomagnesemia, before use and throughout therapy.

PATIENT TEACHING

• Instruct patient to report adverse reactions promptly, especially angina or palpitations.
• Tell patient that drug may cause headache, which can be treated with analgesics.
• Teach patient to report discomfort at IV insertion site.

---

minocycline hydrochloride
mi-noe-SYE-kleen

Minocin, Minolira, Solodyn, Ximino

Therapeutic class: Antibiotics
Pharmacologic class: Tetracyclines

AVAILABLE FORMS

Capsules 🔵*:* 50 mg, 75 mg, 100 mg
Capsules (extended-release): 45 mg, 90 mg, 135 mg
Injection: 100-mg vial
Tablets: 50 mg, 75 mg, 100 mg
Tablets (extended-release) 🔵*:* 45 mg, 55 mg, 65 mg, 80 mg, 90 mg, 105 mg, 115 mg, 135 mg

INDICATIONS & DOSAGES

Adjust-a-dose (for all indications): Decrease dosage or increase dosing interval in patients with renal impairment. Don't exceed 200 mg (immediate-release) in 24 hours.

➤ **Infections caused by susceptible gram-negative and gram-positive organisms (including *Haemophilus ducreyi*, *Yersinia pestis*, and *Campylobacter fetus*), other organisms (including *Rickettsiae* species, *Mycoplasma pneumoniae*, *Chlamydia trachomatis*, and *Clostridioides* species)**
Adults: 200 mg PO or IV initially; then 100 mg PO or IV every 12 hours. May use 100 or 200 mg PO initially; then 50 mg q.i.d. Maximum dosage is 400 mg/day.
Children older than age 8: Initially, 4 mg/kg PO or IV; then, 2 mg/kg PO or IV every 12 hours. Maximum dose is 100 mg/dose or 200 mg/dose for the loading dose.

➤ **Gonorrhea in patients allergic to penicillin**
Adults: Initially, 200 mg PO or IV; then 100 mg PO or IV every 12 hours for at least 4 days. Obtain samples for follow-up cultures within 2 to 3 days after treatment.

➤ **Syphilis in patients allergic to penicillin**
Adults: Initially, 200 mg PO or IV; then 100 mg PO or IV every 12 hours for 10 to 15 days.

➤ **Meningococcal carrier state**
Adults: 100 mg PO every 12 hours for 5 days.

➤ **Uncomplicated urethral, endocervical, or rectal infection caused by *C. trachomatis* or *Ureaplasma urealyticum***
Adults: 100 mg PO every 12 hours for at least 7 days. Or, 200 mg IV initially; then 100 mg IV every 12 hours, not to exceed 400 mg in 24 hours.

➤ **Uncomplicated gonococcal urethritis**
Men: 100 mg PO every 12 hours for 5 days.

➤ **Treatment of inflammatory lesions of nonnodular moderate to severe acne vulgaris**
Adults and children age 12 and older: 1 mg/kg extended-release tablets PO once daily for 12 weeks.

➤ **Acne vulgaris**
Adults: Initially, 200 mg (immediate-release) PO; then 100 mg PO every 12 hours. Or, initially 100 to 200 mg (immediate-release) PO followed by 50 mg PO every 6 hours.
Children age 8 and older: Initially, 4 mg/kg (immediate-release) PO followed by 2 mg/kg PO every 12 hours. Maximum is 200 mg for

---

the loading dose and 100 mg/dose for additional doses.

ADMINISTRATION
PO
• Obtain specimen for culture and sensitivity tests before first dose. Begin therapy while awaiting results.
• Give drug with a full glass of water. Patient may take with food to help decrease esophageal irritation.
• Drug shouldn't be given within 1 hour of bedtime, to avoid esophageal irritation or ulceration.
• Give capsules and extended-release tablets at the same time each day, with or without food.
• Patient must swallow capsules and extended-release tablets whole and not crush, chew, or split them; however, Minolira extended-release tablets may be split on the score line.
• Don't expose drug to light, heat, or moisture.

IV
▼ Reconstitute powder with 5 mL sterile water for injection; further dilute to 100 to 1,000 mL with sodium chloride injection, dextrose injection, or dextrose and sodium chloride injection, or to 250 to 1,000 mL with Ringer injection or lactated Ringer injection. (Don't use solutions containing calcium except for lactated Ringer, because a precipitate may form.)
▼ Infuse over 60 minutes, avoid rapid administration, and don't administer with other drugs.
▼ Use parenteral therapy only when oral therapy is inadequate or isn't tolerated. Institute oral therapy as soon as possible.
▼ **Incompatibilities:** Other drugs.

ACTION
May be bacteriostatic by binding to microorganism's ribosomal subunits, inhibiting protein synthesis; may also alter the cytoplasmic membrane of susceptible microorganisms.

Route	Onset	Peak	Duration
PO	Unknown	1–4 hr	Unknown
PO (extended-release)	Unknown	3.5–4 hr	Unknown
IV	Unknown	Unknown	Unknown

Half-life: PO, 11.1 to 22.1 hours; IV, 15 to 23 hours.

ADVERSE REACTIONS
CNS: headache, light-headedness, dizziness, vertigo, fatigue, mood alterations, somnolence, *seizure,* malaise, drowsiness, fever, paresthesia, hypesthesia, sedation. **CV:** vasculitis, thrombophlebitis. **EENT:** tooth disorder, tinnitus, dry mouth, oral candidiasis, glossitis. **GI:** anorexia, diarrhea, nausea, dysphagia, vomiting, dyspepsia, *pancreatitis,* stomatitis, enterocolitis, *pseudomembranous colitis.* **GU:** interstitial nephritis, vulvovaginitis. **Hematologic:** *neutropenia, thrombocytopenia,* eosinophilia, hemolytic anemia. **Hepatic:** jaundice, *hepatotoxicity.* **Musculoskeletal:** arthralgia, myalgia, joint swelling, arthritis. **Respiratory:** *bronchospasm,* cough, dyspnea, asthma exacerbation, pneumonitis. **Skin:** maculopapular and erythematous rashes; pruritus; urticaria; alopecia; hyperpigmentation of nails, skin, and mucous membranes; injection-site reaction. **Other:** superinfection, discolored secretions, hypersensitivity reactions.

INTERACTIONS
Drug-drug. *Antacids (including sodium bicarbonate) and laxatives containing aluminum, magnesium, or calcium; antidiarrheals:* May decrease antibiotic absorption. Give antibiotic 1 hour before or 2 hours after these drugs.
Ergot alkaloids and their derivative: May increase risk of liver toxicity. Avoid use together.
Ferrous sulfate and other iron products, zinc: May decrease iron absorption and minocycline level. Give drug 2 hours before or 3 hours after iron.
Hormonal contraceptives: May decrease contraceptive effectiveness and increase risk of breakthrough bleeding. Advise patient to use nonhormonal contraceptive.
Isotretinoin: May increase ICP. Don't use together.
Live-virus vaccines: May decrease vaccine effectiveness. Avoid administering together.
Methoxyflurane: May cause renal toxicity. Avoid use together.
Oral anticoagulants: May increase anticoagulant effect. Monitor PT and INR, and adjust dosage.
Penicillins: May disrupt bactericidal action of penicillins. Avoid using together.
Retinoids: May increase risk of pseudotumor cerebri. Avoid administering together.

M

Drug-lifestyle. *Sun or UV light exposure:* May cause photosensitivity reactions. Advise patient to avoid excessive sunlight or UV exposure.

EFFECTS ON LAB TEST RESULTS
• May increase BUN and liver enzyme levels.
• May increase eosinophil count.
• May decrease Hb level and platelet and neutrophil counts.
• May falsely elevate fluorometric test results for urine catecholamines.

CONTRAINDICATIONS & CAUTIONS
• Contraindicated in patients hypersensitive to drug or other tetracyclines.
⚠ *Alert:* Severe and fatal cases of hypersensitivity reactions (including anaphylaxis, serious skin reactions [SJS, erythema multiforme, DRESS syndrome]) have been reported.
⚠ *Alert:* Some products may contain tartrazine, which can cause allergy-type reactions (including bronchial asthma). Although incidence of this sensitivity is low, these reactions are frequently seen in patients who are also sensitive to aspirin.
• Use cautiously in patients with impaired renal or hepatic function.
• Use of these drugs during last half of pregnancy and in children younger than age 8 may cause permanent discoloration of teeth, enamel defects, and bone growth retardation.
• Drug may cause superinfection. If overgrowth of nonsusceptible organisms occurs, discontinue drug and begin appropriate therapy.
• Increases in ICP and pseudotumor cerebri have been reported. If visual disturbances occur, a prompt ophthalmologic exam is needed.
Dialyzable drug: No.
⚠ *Overdose S&S:* Dizziness, nausea, vomiting.

PREGNANCY-LACTATION-REPRODUCTION
• There are no adequate studies during pregnancy. Drug may cause fetal harm. Avoid use in pregnancy.
• If pregnancy occurs during therapy, stop drug immediately and apprise patient of potential fetal hazard.
• Drug appears in human milk. Patient should discontinue breastfeeding or discontinue drug.
• Drug shouldn't be used to treat acne in patients attempting to conceive a child.

NURSING CONSIDERATIONS
• Monitor renal function and LFT results.
⚠ *Alert:* Check expiration date. Outdated or deteriorated drug may cause reversible nephrotoxicity (Fanconi syndrome).
• If large doses are given, therapy is prolonged, or patient is at high risk, monitor patient for signs and symptoms of superinfection.
• Drug may cause mild to severe CDAD, which can occur up to 2 months after therapy ends. If diarrhea occurs, evaluate patient for CDAD. Drug may need to be discontinued and appropriate therapy begun.
• Check patient's tongue for signs of candidal infection. Stress good oral hygiene.
• Drug may discolor teeth in older children and young adults, more commonly when used as long-term treatment. Watch for brown pigmentation, and notify prescriber if it occurs.
• Photosensitivity reactions may occur within a few minutes to several hours after exposure. Photosensitivity lasts after therapy ends.
• Monitor patient for hypersensitivity reactions. Discontinue drug immediately if reaction occurs.
• *Look alike–sound alike:* Don't confuse Minocin with niacin or minoxidil.

PATIENT TEACHING
• Tell patient to take entire amount of drug exactly as prescribed, even if feeling better.
• Instruct patient how to properly administer prescribed formulation.
• Teach patient about potential adverse reactions and to report them promptly.
• Warn patient to avoid driving or other hazardous tasks because of possible adverse CNS effects.
• Caution patient to avoid direct sunlight and UV light, wear protective clothing, and use sunscreen.
• Warn patient that diarrhea may occur up to 2 months after last dose. Tell patient to report diarrhea to prescriber.
• Tell patient not to take drug if pregnant or trying to become pregnant because of potential fetal hazard.
• Warn patient that drug can decrease hormonal contraceptive effectiveness. Advise the use of a nonhormonal method.

mirabegron
mir-a-BEG-ron

Myrbetriq

Therapeutic class: Bladder antispasmodics
Pharmacologic class: Beta-3 adrenergic agonists

AVAILABLE FORMS
Granules (extended-release oral suspension):
8 mg/mL (after reconstitution)
Tablets (extended-release) ⓄⓃⒸ: 25 mg, 50 mg

INDICATIONS & DOSAGES
Adjust-a-dose (for all indications): For patients with severe renal impairment (CrCl of 15 to 29 mL/minute) or moderate hepatic impairment (Child-Pugh class B), give no more than 25 mg daily. Drug isn't recommended for patients with ESRD (CrCl of less than 15 mL/minute) or for patients with severe hepatic impairment (Child-Pugh class C). Refer to manufacturer's instructions for recommended dosing in children age 3 and older weighing less than 35 kg with renal or hepatic impairment.

➤ **Overactive bladder with symptoms of urge incontinence, urgency, and frequency**
Adults: Initially, 25 mg PO once daily. Drug is effective within 8 weeks. Based on individual patient effectiveness and tolerability, may increase dosage to 50 mg once daily after 4 to 8 weeks.

➤ **Overactive bladder with symptoms of urge incontinence, urgency, and frequency in combination with solifenacin succinate**
Adults: Initially, mirabegron 25 mg PO once daily with solifenacin 5 mg PO once daily. May increase mirabegron to 50 mg PO once daily with solifenacin 5 mg PO once daily after 4 to 8 weeks if necessary.

➤ **Neurogenic detrusor overactivity**
Children age 3 and older weighing 35 kg or more (extended-release tablets): 25 mg PO once daily. After 4 to 8 weeks, may increase to maximum dose of 50 mg once daily.
Children age 3 and older weighing 35 kg or more (extended-release granules): Initially, 6 mL (48 mg) PO once daily. After 4 to 8 weeks, may increase to maximum dose of 10 mL (80 mg) once daily.
Children age 3 and older weighing 22 to less than 35 kg (extended-release granules):
Initially, 4 mL (32 mg) PO once daily. After 4 to 8 weeks, may increase to maximum dose of 8 mL (64 mg) once daily.
Children age 3 and older weighing 11 to less than 22 kg (extended-release granules): Initially, 3 mL (24 mg) PO once daily. After 4 to 8 weeks, may increase to maximum dose of 6 mL (48 mg) once daily.

ADMINISTRATION
PO
- May give tablets without regard to food.
- Patient should swallow tablets whole with water; don't crush or divide tablets.
- Give granule suspension with food.
- Granule dosing for adults hasn't been determined.
- For suspension: Measure 100 mL of water and add the total volume to the bottle; immediately shake vigorously for 1 minute. Let stand for 10 to 30 minutes. Shake vigorously again for 1 to 2 minutes until granules have dispersed.
- Give suspension with an appropriate dosing device.
- Store reconstituted suspension at room temperature for up to 28 days. Discard unused portion after 28 days.
- Give missed dose as soon as possible unless more than 12 hours have elapsed; then omit missed dose and give next scheduled dose.

ACTION
Relaxes the detrusor smooth muscle during storage phase of the urinary bladder fill-void cycle, increasing bladder capacity.

Route	Onset	Peak	Duration
PO	Unknown	3.5 hr	Unknown

Half-life: Adults, 50 hours; children, 26 to 31 hours.

ADVERSE REACTIONS
CNS: headache, fatigue, dizziness. **CV:** HTN, tachycardia. **EENT:** nasopharyngitis, dry mouth, sinusitis. **GI:** constipation, nausea, diarrhea, abdominal pain, gastroenteritis. **GU:** UTI, cystitis, urine retention. **Musculoskeletal:** arthralgia, back pain. **Respiratory:** URI, cough. **Other:** flulike symptoms.

INTERACTIONS
Drug-drug. *Digoxin:* May increase digoxin level. Monitor digoxin level and titrate mirabegron to lowest effective dosage.

M

Drugs metabolized by CYP2D6 (desipramine, flecainide, metoprolol, propafenone, thioridazine): May increase levels of these drugs. Monitor patient for adverse events; adjust dosage as needed.

Ketoconazole: May increase mirabegron concentration. Monitor patient response.

Metoprolol: May alter metoprolol concentration. Monitor BP closely.

Muscarinic antagonists (solifenacin): May increase risk of urine retention. Use cautiously together.

Rifampin: May decrease mirabegron concentration. Monitor patient response.

Warfarin: May increase warfarin level. Monitor INR; adjust warfarin dosage as necessary.

EFFECTS ON LAB TEST RESULTS
- May increase ALT, AST, GGT, and LDH levels.

CONTRAINDICATIONS & CAUTIONS
- Contraindicated in patients hypersensitive to drug or its components.
- Drug isn't recommended for use in patients with severe, uncontrolled HTN (systolic BP 180 mm Hg or higher or diastolic BP 110 mm Hg or higher) or severe renal impairment.
- Use cautiously in patients with HTN or bladder outlet obstruction.
- Safety and effectiveness in children younger than age 3 haven't been established.

Dialyzable drug: Unknown.

⚠ **Overdose S&S:** Palpitations, increased HR, increased BP.

PREGNANCY-LACTATION-REPRODUCTION
- There are no adequate studies during pregnancy. Use during pregnancy only if potential benefit justifies fetal risk.
- It isn't known if drug appears in human milk. Patient should discontinue breastfeeding or discontinue drug.

NURSING CONSIDERATIONS
- Monitor BP and pulse regularly, especially in patients with HTN or atrial fibrillation.
- Monitor patient for angioedema of the face, lips, tongue, or larynx, which may be life-threatening and can occur after first dose. Promptly discontinue drug if airway involvement occurs, and ensure a patent airway.
- Monitor patient closely for urine retention and bladder obstruction, especially in those already taking bladder antispasmodics.

- Monitor LFT values periodically.
- Monitor patients for rash or pruritus.

PATIENT TEACHING
- Teach patient or caregiver safe drug administration for formulation prescribed.
- Warn patient that drug may cause an increase in BP or pulse. Teach patient to monitor BP and pulse at home and to report increases to the health care provider.
- Advise patient that difficulty in emptying the bladder and infrequent bladder infections may occur and to report concerns to health care provider.
- Tell patient to report rash or itching, which may indicate an allergy or a serious adverse reaction.
- Advise patient to immediately report signs and symptoms of a significant reaction (fast heartbeat, palpitations, back pain, bloody urine, chills, severe dizziness, passing out, severe headache, wheezing, chest tightness, fever, bad cough, blue skin, seizures, or swelling of face, lips, tongue, or throat).
- Teach patient to report pregnancy to health care provider as soon as possible.

mirtazapine
mir-TAZ-a-peen

Remeron, Remeron SolTab

Therapeutic class: Antidepressants
Pharmacologic class: Tetracyclic antidepressants

AVAILABLE FORMS
Tablets: 7.5 mg, 15 mg, 30 mg, 45 mg
Tablets (ODTs) ⬛: 15 mg, 30 mg, 45 mg

INDICATIONS & DOSAGES
➤ **Major depressive disorder**
Adults: Initially, 15 mg PO at bedtime. Maintenance dose is 15 to 45 mg daily. Adjust dosage at intervals of at least 1 week.

ADMINISTRATION
PO
- Give drug without regard for food.
- Remove ODT from blister pack and immediately place on patient's tongue.
- ODT may be given with or without water. Tablet disintegrates in saliva.
- Don't split or crush ODT.

ACTION
Thought to enhance central noradrenergic and serotonergic activity.

Route	Onset	Peak	Duration
PO	Unknown	2 hr	Unknown

Half-life: About 20 to 40 hours.

ADVERSE REACTIONS
CNS: somnolence, dizziness, asthenia, abnormal dreams, abnormal thinking, tremors, confusion, drowsiness, agitation, amnesia, anxiety, apathy, depression, hypoesthesia, malaise, myasthenia, paresthesia, twitching, vertigo, thirst. **CV:** edema, peripheral edema, HTN, vasodilation. **EENT:** angle-closure glaucoma, dry mouth, sinusitis. **GI:** increased appetite, constipation, abdominal pain, anorexia, vomiting, nausea. **GU:** urinary frequency, UTI. **Metabolic:** weight gain. **Musculoskeletal:** myalgia, weakness, back pain, myasthenia, arthralgia. **Respiratory:** dyspnea, cough. **Skin:** pruritus, rash. **Other:** flulike syndrome.

INTERACTIONS
Drug-drug. *Cimetidine:* May increase mirtazapine level. Consider therapy modification. *CYP2D6, CYP3A4 inhibitors (clarithromycin, ketoconazole):* May increase mirtazapine level. Consider therapy modification. *CYP3A4 inducers (carbamazepine, phenytoin, rifampin):* May decrease mirtazapine level. Consider therapy modification. *Diazepam, other CNS depressants:* May cause additive CNS effects. Avoid using together.
◑ **Alert:** *Linezolid, methylene blue:* May cause serotonin syndrome. Use together is contraindicated.
◑ **Alert:** *MAO inhibitors:* May increase risk of serotonin syndrome. Use within 14 days of MAO inhibitor therapy is contraindicated.
QT interval–prolonging agents (antiarrhythmics, fluoroquinolones, macrolides): May cause additive QT interval–prolonging effects. Use cautiously together.
Serotonergic drugs (antidepressants, antiemetics [5-HT$_3$ antagonists], buspirone, fentanyl, lithium, TCAs, tramadol, triptans, tryptophan): May increase risk of serotonin syndrome. Monitor therapy.
Warfarin: May increase anticoagulant effect. Closely monitor INR when mirtazapine is started or stopped, and adjust warfarin dosage as needed.
Drug-herb. *St. John's wort:* May increase risk of serotonin syndrome. Use together cautiously and monitor patient closely for adverse reactions.
Drug-lifestyle. *Alcohol use:* May cause additive CNS effects. Discourage use together.

EFFECTS ON LAB TEST RESULTS
• May increase cholesterol and triglyceride levels and LFT values.
• May decrease sodium level.
• May decrease ANC.

CONTRAINDICATIONS & CAUTIONS
• Contraindicated in patients hypersensitive to drug.
◑ **Alert:** Concomitant use with MAO inhibitors, linezolid, or methylene blue can cause serotonin syndrome (fever, mental status changes, muscle twitching, diaphoresis, shivering or shaking, diarrhea, or loss of coordination). Use together is contraindicated.
Boxed Warning Drug may increase risk of suicidality in children, adolescents, and young adults with major depressive or other psychiatric disorders. Drug isn't approved for use in children. ∎
• Use cautiously in patients with CV or cerebrovascular disease, seizure disorders, suicidality, hepatic or renal impairment, or history of mania or hypomania.
• Use cautiously in patients with conditions that predispose them to hypotension, such as dehydration, hypovolemia, or antihypertensive therapy.
• Use may trigger angle-closure glaucoma attack due to pupil dilation in patients with anatomically narrow angles.
• Give drug cautiously to older adults; decreased clearance has occurred in this age-group.
Dialyzable drug: Unknown.
▲ **Overdose S&S:** Disorientation, drowsiness, impaired memory, tachycardia.

PREGNANCY-LACTATION-REPRODUCTION
• There are no adequate studies during pregnancy. Use during pregnancy only if clearly needed.
• Drug may appear in human milk. Use cautiously during breastfeeding.
• Register patients who are pregnant in the National Pregnancy Registry for

M

Antidepressants at 1-844-405-6185 or https://womensmentalhealth.org/clinical-and-research-programs/pregnancyregistry/antidepressants/

NURSING CONSIDERATIONS

⚕ *Alert:* If linezolid or methylene blue must be given, mirtazapine must be stopped and patient should be monitored for serotonin toxicity for 2 weeks, or until 24 hours after the last dose of methylene blue or linezolid, whichever comes first. Treatment with mirtazapine may be resumed 24 hours after last dose of methylene blue or linezolid.

Boxed Warning Appropriately monitor and closely observe patients of all ages who are started on antidepressants for clinical worsening, mood changes, suicidality, or unusual changes in behavior. ■

• Monitor patient for distressing restlessness and need to move, which occurs most frequently during first few weeks of treatment.
• Although agranulocytosis occurs rarely, stop drug and monitor patient closely if a sore throat, fever, stomatitis, or other signs and symptoms of infection with a low WBC count develop.
• Lower dosages tend to be more sedating than higher dosages.

PATIENT TEACHING

Boxed Warning Advise families and caregivers to closely observe patient for increasing suicidality. ■

⚕ *Alert:* Teach patient to recognize and immediately report signs and symptoms of serotonin toxicity.
• Caution patient to avoid hazardous activities if feeling too sleepy.
• Tell patient to report signs and symptoms of infection, such as fever, chills, sore throat, mucous membrane irritation, or flulike syndrome.
• Instruct patient not to use alcohol or other CNS depressants while taking drug.
• Instruct patient not to take other drugs or stop drug abruptly without prescriber's approval.
• Tell patient of childbearing potential to report suspected pregnancy immediately and to notify prescriber if breastfeeding.
• Instruct patient how to properly administer prescribed formulation.

---

mitoMYcin (mitomycin-C)
mye-toe-MYE-sin

Mutamycin

Therapeutic class: Antineoplastics
Pharmacologic class: Antineoplastic antibiotics

AVAILABLE FORMS
Powder for injection: 5-mg, 20-mg, 40-mg vials

INDICATIONS & DOSAGES
Dosage and indications vary. Check treatment protocol with prescriber.

➤ **Disseminated adenocarcinoma of stomach or pancreas in combination with other chemotherapeutic agents**
Adults: 20 mg/m^2 IV as a single dose at 6- to 8-week intervals if patient has full hematologic recovery. Fully evaluate patient after each cycle and reduce dosage if toxicities occur. Discontinue drug if disease progresses after two courses of therapy.
Adjust-a-dose: Refer to manufacturer's instructions for toxicity-related dosage instructions.

➤ **Anal cancer** ◆
Adults: 10 mg/m^2 IV on days 1 and 29 (maximum dose, 20 mg/dose) in combination with 5-FU and radiation therapy. Or, 10 mg/m^2 IV on day 1 (maximum dose, 15 mg/dose) in combination with capecitabine and radiation therapy. Or, 12 mg/m^2 IV on day 1 (maximum dose, 20 mg/dose) in combination with capecitabine and radiation therapy. Or, 12 mg/m^2 or 15 mg/m^2 on day 1 in combination with 5-FU and radiation therapy.

➤ **Bladder cancer (muscle invasive)** ◆
Adults: 12 mg/m^2 IV on day 1 in combination with 5-FU and radiation therapy.

ADMINISTRATION
IV
⚕ *Alert:* Don't give to patients with serum creatinine level greater than 1.7 mg/dL.
⚕ *Alert:* Preparing and giving drug may be mutagenic, teratogenic, or carcinogenic. Use safe handling and disposal precautions.
▼ Drug is a vesicant. Never give drug IM or subcut. Consider using a CVAD.

▼ Using sterile water for injection, reconstitute drug in 5-mg vials with 10 mL, 20-mg vials with 40 mL, and 40-mg vials with 80 mL. Solution will appear clear to pale blue. Protect from light.

▼ Give drug by slow IV push (1.5 mg/mL/minute) or slow IV infusion (over 15 to 30 minutes) into side arm of a free-flowing IV line.

▼ When reconstituted with sterile water, solution is stable for 14 days under refrigeration and for 7 days at room temperature, if protected from light.

▼ Stop infusion immediately and notify prescriber if extravasation occurs because of potential for severe ulceration and necrosis. Initiate dimethyl sulfate antidote.

▼ **Incompatibilities:** None listed by manufacturer. Consult a drug incompatibility reference for more information.

ACTION

Similar to an alkylating drug, cross-linking strands of DNA and causing an imbalance of cell growth, leading to cell death.

Route	Onset	Peak	Duration
IV	Unknown	Unknown	Unknown

Half-life: About 17 minutes.

ADVERSE REACTIONS

CNS: neurologic abnormalities, fatigue, fever. **GI:** mucositis, nausea, vomiting, anorexia, stomatitis. **GU:** *renal toxicity, hemolytic-uremic syndrome.* **Hematologic:** *thrombocytopenia, leukopenia, microangiopathic hemolytic anemia.* **Respiratory:** dyspnea, nonproductive cough. **Skin:** injection-site reaction, reversible alopecia.

INTERACTIONS

None reported.

EFFECTS ON LAB TEST RESULTS

• May increase BUN and creatinine levels.
• May decrease Hb level and WBC and platelet counts.

CONTRAINDICATIONS & CAUTIONS

• Contraindicated in patients hypersensitive to drug and in those with thrombocytopenia, coagulation disorders, or an increased bleeding tendency from other causes.
• Don't give to patients with serum creatinine level greater than 1.7 mg/dL.

• Safety and effectiveness in children haven't been determined.
• Use cautiously in older adults.
Dialyzable drug: Unknown.

PREGNANCY-LACTATION-REPRODUCTION

• Drug can cause fetal harm. If used during pregnancy, or pregnancy occurs during therapy, apprise patient of fetal risk and the potential for pregnancy loss.
• It isn't known if drug appears in human milk. Patient should discontinue breastfeeding or discontinue drug.

NURSING CONSIDERATIONS

Boxed Warning Administer drug under the supervision of a prescriber experienced with cancer chemotherapeutic agents. ∎

Boxed Warning Bone marrow suppression (thrombocytopenia and leukopenia), which may contribute to overwhelming infections in patient who is already compromised, is the most common and severe toxic effect. ∎

• Reevaluate patient fully after each course of mitomycin, and reduce dosage if patient has experienced toxicities.

🕒 *Alert:* Pulmonary toxicity, which may be severe and life-threatening, has been reported infrequently. Signs and symptoms may include dyspnea with a nonproductive cough and pulmonary infiltrates on X-ray. Drug may need to be discontinued.

🕒 *Alert:* Extravasation may occur, causing cellulitis, ulceration, and tissue slough. If signs or symptoms of these conditions occur, stop infusion immediately and notify prescriber. Withdraw 3 to 5 mL of blood; then remove infusion needle. If skin necrosis develops, skin grafting may be necessary.

• Leukopenia may occur up to 8 weeks after therapy; continue CBC and blood studies at least 8 weeks after therapy stops. Leukopenia and thrombocytopenia are cumulative. If WBC count falls below 2,000/mm^3 or granulocyte count falls below 1,000/mm^3, follow facility protocol for controlling infection in patients who are immunocompromised.

• Anticipate need for blood transfusions to combat anemia.

• Monitor renal function tests.

Boxed Warning Drug can cause hemolytic-uremic syndrome (hemolytic anemia, thrombocytopenia, and irreversible renal failure). The syndrome may occur at any time during systemic therapy with mitomycin; however, most cases occur at doses of 60 mg or more. Blood product transfusion may exacerbate symptoms associated with this syndrome. ∎

PATIENT TEACHING
• Advise patient to report all adverse reactions and to immediately report pain or burning at injection site during or after administration.
• Warn patient to watch for signs and symptoms of infection (fever, sore throat, fatigue), bleeding (easy bruising, nosebleeds, bleeding gums, melena), and pulmonary toxicity (dyspnea with nonproductive cough). Tell patient to take temperature daily.
• Inform patient that hair loss may occur but that it's usually reversible.
• Advise patient of the potential for fetal harm if drug is used during pregnancy.

SAFETY ALERT!

mitoXANTRONE hydrochloride
mye-toe-ZAN-trone

Therapeutic class: Antineoplastics
Pharmacologic class: DNA-reactive drugs–anthracenediones

AVAILABLE FORMS
Injection: 2 mg/mL

INDICATIONS & DOSAGES
➤ **Combination initial therapy for acute nonlymphocytic leukemia (ANLL)**
Adults: Induction begins with 12 mg/m^2 IV daily on days 1 to 3, with 100 mg/m^2 daily of cytarabine on days 1 to 7 as a continuous 24-hour infusion. A second induction with mitoxantrone for 2 days and cytarabine for 5 days may be given if response isn't adequate. Consolidation therapy: 12 mg/m^2 IV infusion daily on days 1 and 2 and cytarabine 100 mg/m^2 for 5 days given as a continuous 24-hour infusion on days 1 through 5. The first course is given approximately 6 weeks after the final induction course; the second is generally given 4 weeks after the first. Severe myelosuppression has occurred with this regimen.
➤ **To reduce neurologic disability and frequency of relapse in chronic progressive, progressive relapsing, or worsening relapsing-remitting MS**

Adults: 12 mg/m^2 IV over 5 to 15 minutes every 3 months. Maximum cumulative lifetime dose is 140 mg/m^2.
➤ **Advanced hormone-refractory prostate cancer**
Men: 12 to 14 mg/m^2 as a short IV infusion every 21 days. Drug is given as an adjunct to corticosteroid therapy.

ADMINISTRATION
IV
▼ Preparing and giving drug may be mutagenic, teratogenic, or carcinogenic. Follow facility protocol to reduce risks.
▼ Dilute dose in at least 50 mL of NSS for injection or D$_5$W injection. Don't mix with other drugs. Can further dilute in D$_5$W, NSS, or D$_5$NSS; use immediately if further diluted.
Boxed Warning Give slowly into a free-flowing IV infusion of NSS or D$_5$W injection over at least 3 minutes. ∎
Boxed Warning Never give subcutaneously, intra-arterially, intramuscularly, or intrathecally. ∎
Boxed Warning Severe local tissue damage may result if extravasation occurs. ∎
▼ If extravasation occurs, stop infusion immediately and notify prescriber. Place ice packs over the area intermittently.
▼ Once vial is penetrated, undiluted solution may be stored for 7 days at room temperature or 14 days in refrigerator. Don't freeze.
▼ **Incompatibilities:** Other drugs.

ACTION
Reacts with DNA, producing cytotoxic effect. Probably not specific to cell cycle.

Route	Onset	Peak	Duration
IV	Unknown	Unknown	Unknown

Half-life: Terminal half-life, 23 to 215 hours.

ADVERSE REACTIONS
CNS: fever, headache, *seizures,* asthenia, pain, fatigue, anxiety, depression. **CV:** *arrhythmias,* ECG abnormalities, *HF, ischemia,* decreased LVEF, HTN, tachycardia, edema, *hemorrhage.* **EENT:** conjunctivitis, blurred vision, sinusitis, pharyngitis, rhinitis. **GI:** abdominal pain, *GI hemorrhage,* constipation, diarrhea, mucositis, nausea, stomatitis, vomiting, dyspepsia, anorexia. **GU:** amenorrhea, menstrual disorder, UTI, *renal failure,* hematuria, decreased libido,

---

Reactions in bold italics are *life-threatening*. Interactions may have a *rapid onset* or a ***delayed onset***.

proteinuria, impotence, sterility. **Hematologic:** *myelosuppression,* anemia. **Hepatic:** jaundice, abnormal transaminase levels. **Metabolic:** hyperuricemia, *hypocalcemia, hypokalemia,* hyponatremia, weight gain or loss. **Musculoskeletal:** back pain. **Respiratory:** cough, dyspnea, URI, pneumonia. **Skin:** alopecia, ecchymoses, local irritation or phlebitis, petechiae, diaphoresis, nail bed changes. **Other:** chills, fungal infections, infection, *sepsis.*

INTERACTIONS
Drug-drug. *Clozapine:* May increase risk of neutropenia. Monitor patient closely.
Cyclosporine: May increase effects of mitoxantrone. Monitor patient closely.
Live-virus vaccines: May increase risk of vaccine-induced adverse reactions. Defer vaccination until mitoxantrone therapy has been completed.
Natalizumab, tofacitinib: May increase risk of immunosuppression. Avoid use together.
Palifermin: May increase severity of oral mucositis. Don't give palifermin within 24 hours before or after mitoxantrone dose.
Pimecrolimus, tacrolimus (topical): May enhance adverse or toxic effect of mitoxantrone. Avoid use together.
Trastuzumab: May increase risk of trastuzumab-induced cardiac dysfunction. Monitor patient closely for signs and symptoms of cardiac dysfunction.

EFFECTS ON LAB TEST RESULTS
• May increase creatinine, BUN, ALT, AST, bilirubin, GGT, uric acid, and urine protein levels.
• May decrease calcium, potassium, and sodium levels.
• May decrease Hb level and hematocrit and platelet, WBC, and granulocyte counts.

CONTRAINDICATIONS & CAUTIONS
• Contraindicated in patients hypersensitive to drug.
• Drug contains sodium metabisulfite, which may cause an allergic reaction, especially in patients with asthma.
Boxed Warning Present or history of CV disease, radiotherapy to mediastinal or pericardial area, previous therapy with other anthracyclines or anthracenediones, or use of other cardiotoxic drugs may increase risk of cardiotoxicity. ∎

• Patients who are significantly myelosuppressed shouldn't receive drug unless benefits outweigh risks.
• Use cautiously in patients with hepatic impairment.
Dialyzable drug: No.
⚠ *Overdose S&S:* Severe leukopenia.

PREGNANCY-LACTATION-REPRODUCTION
• Drug may cause fetal harm. Patient should avoid pregnancy during therapy. If used during pregnancy or if pregnancy occurs during therapy, apprise patient of fetal risk.
• Patients with MS who are biologically capable of becoming pregnant even if they are using contraception should have a pregnancy test before each dose, and results should be known before drug administration.
• Drug appears in human milk. Patient should discontinue breastfeeding before starting drug.
• Drug may affect fertility.

NURSING CONSIDERATIONS
Boxed Warning Administer under the supervision of a prescriber experienced with cytotoxic chemotherapy. ∎
Boxed Warning Except when used to treat ANLL, mitoxantrone should generally not be given to patients with baseline neutrophil counts less than 1,500 cells/mm³. Frequently monitor peripheral blood cell counts for all patients using drug. ∎
Boxed Warning Assess all patients for cardiac signs and symptoms by history, physical exam, LVEF, and ECG before therapy. Assess patients with MS for cardiac signs and symptoms by history, physical exam, and ECG before each dose. ∎
Boxed Warning Patients with MS shouldn't receive a cumulative mitoxantrone dose greater than 140 mg/m². ∎
Boxed Warning Drug can cause potentially fatal HF during therapy or months to years after therapy. All patients should have baseline quantitative evaluation of LVEF. In patients with MS, evaluate LVEF before initiating treatment and before administering each dose of mitoxantrone. Patients with MS with a baseline LVEF below the lower limit of normal shouldn't be treated with mitoxantrone. All patients with MS who have finished treatment should receive yearly, quantitative LVEF evaluation to detect late-occurring cardiotoxicity. Additional doses of mitoxantrone

shouldn't be given to patients with MS who have experienced either a drop in LVEF to below the lower limit of normal or a clinically significant reduction in LVEF during mitoxantrone therapy. ■

Boxed Warning Use of drug has been associated with cardiotoxicity; risk of cardiotoxicity increases with cumulative dose of 140 mg/m^2, although toxicities may occur at any dose. Continue ongoing cardiac monitoring to detect late occurring cardiotoxicity. ■

• Closely monitor hematologic and chemistry results, including LFT values. Obtain CBC and platelet counts before each course of treatment. Patient may require blood transfusion or RBC or WBC colony-stimulating factors.

• Avoid all IM injections in patients with thrombocytopenia.

• If severe nonhematologic toxicity occurs during first course, delay second course until patient recovers.

Boxed Warning Secondary acute myelocytic leukemia has been reported with mitoxantrone therapy. ■

• Verify pregnancy status before treatment in all patients of childbearing potential, with results known before administration.

PATIENT TEACHING

• Advise patient to immediately report injection-site discomfort.

• Tell patient that urine may appear blue-green within 24 hours after receiving drug and that the whites of the eyes may turn blue. These effects are not harmful but may persist during therapy.

• Teach patient about potential adverse reactions and tell patient to report them. Advise patient to watch for signs and symptoms of bleeding and infection.

• Advise patient of childbearing potential to use appropriate contraceptive method to avoid pregnancy during therapy.

• Inform patient of potential effects on fertility.

modafinil
moe-DAF-i-nil

Alertec✦, Provigil✑

Therapeutic class: CNS stimulants
Pharmacologic class: Analeptics
Controlled substance schedule: IV

AVAILABLE FORMS
Tablets: 100 mg, 200 mg

INDICATIONS & DOSAGES
➤ **To improve wakefulness in patients with excessive daytime sleepiness caused by narcolepsy, obstructive sleep apnea-hypopnea syndrome, and shift-work sleep disorder**
Adults: 200 mg PO daily, as a single dose in the morning. Patients with shift-work sleep disorder should take dose about 1 hour before the start of their shift.
Adjust-a-dose: In patients with severe hepatic impairment, give 100 mg PO daily as a single dose in the morning. Consider lower doses and close monitoring in older adults.

ADMINISTRATION
PO
• Give drug without regard for food; however, food may delay effect of drug.
• Store at room temperature.

ACTION
Unknown. Similar to action of sympathomimetics, including amphetamines, but drug is structurally distinct from amphetamines and doesn't alter release of dopamine or norepinephrine.

Route	Onset	Peak	Duration
PO	Unknown	2–4 hr	Unknown

Half-life: 15 hours.

ADVERSE REACTIONS
CNS: headache, nervousness, dizziness, drowsiness, insomnia, depression, anxiety, paresthesia, hypertonia, hyperkinesia, confusion, emotional lability, vertigo, tremor, dyskinesia, agitation, thirst, taste perversion. **CV:** HTN, vasodilation, chest pain, palpitations, tachycardia, edema. **EENT:** abnormal vision, epistaxis, rhinitis, dry mouth, mouth ulcer, pharyngitis. **GI:** nausea, diarrhea, anorexia, gingivitis, dyspepsia, constipation,

flatulence, decreased appetite, abdominal pain. **GU:** abnormal urine. **Hematologic:** eosinophilia. **Hepatic:** abnormal LFT values. **Metabolic:** weight loss. **Musculoskeletal:** back or neck pain. **Respiratory:** *asthma.* **Skin:** diaphoresis. **Other:** chills.

INTERACTIONS
Drug-drug. *Cyclosporine, theophylline:* May reduce levels of these drugs. Use together cautiously.

CYP2C19 substrates (diazepam, phenytoin, propranolol): May inhibit CYP2C19, causing higher levels of drugs metabolized by this enzyme. Use together cautiously; adjust dosage as needed.

CYP3A4 inducers (carbamazepine, phenobarbital, rifampin): May alter modafinil level. Monitor patient closely.

CYP3A4/5 substrates (cyclosporine, midazolam, triazolam): May decrease level of the substrate. Adjust substrate dosage as needed.

Dextroamphetamine, methylphenidate: May cause 1-hour delay in modafinil absorption. Separate dosing times.

Hormonal contraceptives: May reduce contraceptive effectiveness. Advise patient to use alternative or additional method of contraception during modafinil therapy and for 1 month after final dose.

MAO inhibitors: May increase risk of hypertensive crisis. Use cautiously together.

Warfarin: May increase warfarin level. Monitor patient closely for toxicity.

TCAs: May increase TCA level. Reduce dosage of these drugs.

Drug-lifestyle. *Alcohol use:* Coadministration hasn't been studied. Avoid using together.

EFFECTS ON LAB TEST RESULTS
• May increase glucose, GGT, and ALP levels.
• May increase eosinophil count.

CONTRAINDICATIONS & CAUTIONS
• Contraindicated in patients hypersensitive to modafinil or armodafinil or its inactive ingredients.
• Drug isn't recommended in patients with a history of left ventricular hypertrophy or ischemic ECG changes, chest pain, arrhythmias, or other evidence of mitral valve prolapse linked to CNS stimulant use.

• Use cautiously in patients with recent MI or unstable angina and in those with history of psychosis or mania.
• Use cautiously and give reduced dosage to patients with severe hepatic impairment, with or without cirrhosis.
• Safety and effectiveness in patients with severe renal impairment haven't been determined.
• Modafinil isn't approved for use in children. *Dialyzable drug:* Unknown.
⚠ *Overdose S&S:* Agitation or excitation, insomnia, slight or moderate elevations in hemodynamic parameters, aggressiveness, anxiety, confusion, shortened PT, diarrhea, irritability, nausea, nervousness, palpitations, sleep disturbances, tremor, bradycardia, chest pain, HTN, tachycardia, hallucination, restlessness.

PREGNANCY-LACTATION-REPRODUCTION
• There are no adequate studies during pregnancy. Use during pregnancy only if potential benefit justifies fetal risk.
• Prescribers are encouraged to register patients who are pregnant, or patients may self-enroll, in the Provigil Pregnancy Registry (1-866-404-4106).
• Caution patient that use of hormonal contraceptives (including depot or implantable contraceptives) with modafinil may reduce contraceptive effectiveness. Recommend an alternative method of contraception during therapy and for 1 month after therapy ends.
• It isn't known if drug appears in human milk. Use cautiously during breastfeeding.

NURSING CONSIDERATIONS
• Life-threatening angioedema, SJS, TEN, and DRESS syndrome can occur. Monitor patient for rash, dysphagia, bronchospasm, fever, and organ dysfunction. Stop drug and begin appropriate treatment.
• Monitor patient for emergence or exacerbation of psychiatric signs and symptoms, and HTN.
• *Look alike–sound alike:* Don't confuse Provigil with Nuvigil; don't confuse Alertec with Arthrotec.

PATIENT TEACHING
ⓘ *Alert:* Advise patient to stop drug and notify prescriber if rash, peeling skin, trouble swallowing or breathing, or other symptoms of allergic reaction occur.

• Caution patient to report planned, suspected, or known pregnancy, or breastfeeding.
• Tell patient to avoid alcohol while taking drug.
• Warn patient to avoid activities that require alertness or good coordination until CNS effects of drug are known.

mometasone furoate
moe-MET-a-sone

Asmanex HFA, Asmanex Twisthaler, Elocon✦

mometasone furoate monohydrate
Nasonex

Therapeutic class: Anti-inflammatory drugs
Pharmacologic class: Glucocorticoids

AVAILABLE FORMS
Cream: 0.1%
Inhalation aerosol: 50 mcg/actuation, 100 mcg/actuation, 200 mcg/actuation, 400 mcg/actuation✦
Inhalation powder: 110 mcg/inhalation, 220 mcg/inhalation
Lotion: 0.1%
Nasal spray: 50 mcg/spray ◊
Ointment: 0.1%

INDICATIONS & DOSAGES
➤ **Maintenance therapy for asthma; asthma in patients who take an oral corticosteroid**
Asmanex Twisthaler
Adults and children age 12 and older who previously used a bronchodilator or inhaled corticosteroid: Initially, 220 mcg by oral inhalation every day in the evening. Maximum, 440 mcg/day.
Adults and children age 12 and older who previously received an oral corticosteroid: 440 mcg by oral inhalation b.i.d. Maximum, 880 mcg/day.
Children ages 4 to 11 regardless of prior therapy: 110 mcg by oral inhalation once daily in the evening.
Adjust-a-dose: For patients on long-term oral corticosteroid therapy, reduce oral prednisone dosage by no more than 2.5 mg/day at weekly intervals, beginning at least 1 week after starting mometasone. After stopping oral

corticosteroid, reduce mometasone dosage to lowest effective amount. Carefully monitor patient for signs and symptoms of asthma instability and adrenal insufficiency.
Asmanex HFA
Adults and children age 12 and older who previously used a medium-dose inhaled corticosteroid: Using a 100-mcg inhaler, 2 inhalations b.i.d. (morning and evening). Maximum, 800 mcg/day.
Adults and children age 12 and older who previously used a high-dose inhaled corticosteroid: Using a 200-mcg inhaler, 2 inhalations b.i.d. (morning and evening). Maximum, 800 mcg/day.
Adults and children age 12 and older who previously received an oral corticosteroid: 200 mcg by oral inhalation b.i.d. (morning and evening). Maximum, 800 mcg/day.
Children age 5 to younger than age 12: Using a 50-mcg inhaler, 2 inhalations b.i.d. (morning and evening). Maximum, 200 mcg/day.
Adjust-a-dose: For patients currently receiving long-term oral corticosteroid therapy, wean prednisone slowly, beginning after at least 1 week of Asmanex HFA therapy. Carefully monitor patient for signs and symptoms of asthma instability and adrenal insufficiency. If a dosage regimen fails to provide adequate asthma control, reevaluate the therapeutic regimen and consider additional therapeutic options, such as replacing the current strength of inhaler with a higher strength, initiating an inhaled corticosteroid and LABA combination product, or initiating oral corticosteroids.
➤ **Allergic rhinitis; nasal congestion associated with seasonal allergic rhinitis**
Adults and children age 12 and older: 2 sprays (50 mcg/spray) in each nostril once daily.
Children ages 2 to 11: 1 spray (50 mcg/spray) in each nostril once daily.
➤ **Prophylaxis of seasonal allergic rhinitis**
Adults and children age 12 and older: 2 sprays (50 mcg/spray) in each nostril once daily 2 to 4 weeks before anticipated start of pollen season.
➤ **Nasal polyps**
Adults: 2 sprays (50 mcg/spray) in each nostril once daily to b.i.d.
➤ **Dermatoses**
Adults: Apply thin film of cream or ointment to affected areas once daily. Or, apply a few drops of lotion to affected areas and massage

---

Reactions in bold italics are *life-threatening*. Interactions may have a *rapid onset* or a ***delayed onset***.

lightly. Discontinue when control is achieved. If no improvement is seen within 2 weeks, reassess diagnosis.

Children age 12 and older: Apply a few drops of lotion to affected areas once daily and massage lightly. Discontinue when control is achieved. If no improvement is seen within 2 weeks, reassess diagnosis.

Children age 2 and older: Apply thin film of cream or ointment to affected areas once daily. Discontinue when control is achieved. If no improvement is seen within 2 weeks, reassess diagnosis.

ADMINISTRATION

Inhalational aerosol

• Shake well before each inhalation.
• Prime before first use by releasing four test sprays into the air, away from the face, shaking well before each spray.
• If the inhaler hasn't been used for more than 5 days, prime inhaler again with four test sprays.
• Have patient rinse mouth with water without swallowing after administration.

Inhalational powder

• Give once-daily dosing in the evening.
• Have patient exhale fully before bringing Twisthaler up to the mouth, placing between lips, and inhaling quickly and deeply.
• Patient shouldn't breathe out through inhaler but should remove inhaler and hold breath for 10 seconds if possible.
• Have patient rinse mouth after administration.
• Discard 45 days after opening foil pouch or when dose counter reads "00."

Intranasal

• Before initial use, prime nasal spray pump 10 times or until fine spray appears.
• Pump may be stored for 1 week without repriming. If unused for more than 1 week, reprime two times or until a fine spray appears.
• Shake well before each use.

Topical

• Drug is for topical use only; not for oral, ophthalmic, or intravaginal use. Avoid use on axillae, groin, or face.
• Don't use with occlusive dressings or in diaper area if child still requires diapers or plastic pants unless directed by prescriber.

ACTION

Unknown, although corticosteroids inhibit many cells and mediators involved in inflammation and the asthmatic response.

Route	Onset	Peak	Duration
Inhalation	Unknown	1–2.5 hr	Unknown
Intranasal	Unknown	Unknown	Unknown
Topical	8 hr	Unknown	Unknown

Half-life: Oral, 5 hours; nasal and topical, unknown.

ADVERSE REACTIONS

CNS: headache, depression, fatigue, insomnia, pain, paresthesia. **CV:** chest pain. **EENT:** increased IOP, earache, otitis media, epistaxis, nasal irritation, allergic rhinitis, pharyngitis, sinus congestion, sinusitis, dry throat, oral candidiasis, dysphonia. **GI:** abdominal pain, anorexia, dyspepsia, flatulence, gastroenteritis, nausea, vomiting, thrush. **GU:** dysmenorrhea, menstrual disorder, UTI. **Metabolic:** decreased glucocorticoid levels. **Musculoskeletal:** arthralgia, back pain, myalgia. **Respiratory:** URI, cough, bronchitis, wheezing, respiratory disorder. **Skin:** burning, pruritus, skin atrophy, furunculosis, folliculitis, skin depigmentation, taut and shiny skin, telangiectasia, candidiasis, bacterial infection, bruise. **Other:** flulike symptoms, infection, fever.

INTERACTIONS

Drug-drug. *Esketamine:* May decrease therapeutic effect of esketamine nasal spray. Give mometasone intranasal at least 1 hour before esketamine.

Strong CYP3A4 inhibitors (atazanavir, clarithromycin, cobicistat-containing products, itraconazole, ketoconazole, nefazodone, nelfinavir, ritonavir, saquinavir): May increase systemic exposure to mometasone and increase risk of systemic adverse effects, especially with long-term use. Use together cautiously.

Drug-lifestyle. *Smoking:* Smoking tobacco may decrease effect of inhaled mometasone. Discourage smoking and monitor therapy.

EFFECTS ON LAB TEST RESULTS

None reported.

CONTRAINDICATIONS & CAUTIONS

• Contraindicated in patients hypersensitive to drug or its components, in those hypersensitive to milk proteins (Asmanex Twisthaler

M

only), and in those with status asthmaticus or other acute forms of asthma or bronchospasm (as primary treatment).

• Use cautiously in patients at high risk for decreased bone mineral content (those with a family history of osteoporosis, prolonged immobilization, long-term use of drugs that reduce bone mass), patients switching from a systemic to an inhaled corticosteroid, and patients with active or dormant TB, untreated systemic infections, cataracts, glaucoma, ocular herpes simplex, diabetes, myasthenia, MI, thyroid disease, psychiatric disturbances, or immunosuppression.

• Drug may cause HPA axis suppression with potential for glucocorticosteroid insufficiency during treatment or after treatment withdrawal. Evaluate patient periodically for HPA suppression.

◔ *Alert:* Children treated with topical corticosteroids are at greater risk than adults for HPA axis suppression and Cushing syndrome. Don't use in treatment of diaper dermatitis.

• If patient develops allergic contact dermatitis, usually diagnosed by a failure to heal, drug should be discontinued.

• If skin infections are present or develop, topical drug may need to be discontinued until infection is controlled.

Dialyzable drug: Unknown.

⚠ *Overdose S&S:* Hypercorticism with long-term overdose.

PREGNANCY-LACTATION-REPRODUCTION

• There are no adequate studies during pregnancy. Use during pregnancy only if clearly needed and use justifies fetal risk.

• Systemically administered corticosteroids appear in human milk and could suppress growth, interfere with endogenous corticosteroid production, or cause other untoward effects. Use cautiously during breastfeeding.

NURSING CONSIDERATIONS

◔ *Alert:* Don't use inhalation form for acute bronchospasm. Life-threatening paradoxical bronchospasm can occur after inhalation. Stop drug and use a fast-acting bronchodilator.

• Wean patients slowly from a systemic corticosteroid after they switch to mometasone. Monitor pulmonary function tests, beta-agonist use, and asthma symptoms.

◔ *Alert:* If patient is switching from an oral corticosteroid to an inhaled form, watch closely for evidence of adrenal insufficiency, such as fatigue, lethargy, weakness, nausea, vomiting, and hypotension.

• After an oral corticosteroid is withdrawn, HPA function may not recover for months. Patient experiencing trauma, stress, infection, or surgery during this HPA recovery period is particularly vulnerable to adrenal insufficiency or adrenal crisis.

• Because inhaled and topical corticosteroids can be systemically absorbed, watch for cushingoid effects.

• Assess patient for bone loss during long-term use.

• Monitor children's growth periodically with long-term inhaler use.

• Watch for evidence of localized mouth infections, vision changes, loss of glucose control, and immunosuppression.

• If patient has taken a corticosteroid during pregnancy, monitor neonate for hypoadrenalism.

• Monitor older adults for increased sensitivity to drug effects.

PATIENT TEACHING

• Instruct patient on proper use and routine care of the inhaler or nasal spray pump.

• Tell patient to use drug regularly as prescribed.

• Caution patient not to use inhalers for immediate relief of an asthma attack or bronchospasm. Verify patient has a rescue inhaler prescribed.

• Instruct patient to rinse mouth after using inhaler to prevent thrush.

• Inform patient that maximal benefits of inhaler might not occur for 1 to 2 weeks or longer after therapy starts. Instruct patient to notify prescriber if condition fails to improve or worsens.

• Tell patient that if bronchospasm occurs after using inhaler, to immediately use a fast-acting bronchodilator. Urge patient to contact prescriber immediately if bronchospasm doesn't respond to the fast-acting bronchodilator.

◔ *Alert:* Urge patient who has been weaned from an oral corticosteroid to contact prescriber immediately if an asthma attack occurs or if patient experiences a period of stress. The oral corticosteroid may need to be resumed.

Reactions in bold italics are *life-threatening*. Interactions may have a *rapid onset* or a ***delayed onset***.

- Warn patient to avoid exposure to chickenpox or measles and to notify prescriber if such contact occurs.
- Long-term use of an inhaled corticosteroid may increase risk of cataracts or glaucoma; tell patient to report vision changes.
- Advise patient to write the date on a new inhaler on the day inhaler is opened and to discard the inhaler after 45 days or when the dose counter reads "00."
- Instruct patient not to use topical form with occlusive dressings or diapers unless instructed by prescriber.

montelukast sodium
mon-te-LOO-kast

Singulair

Therapeutic class: Antiasthmatics
Pharmacologic class: Leukotriene-receptor antagonists

AVAILABLE FORMS
Oral granules: 4-mg packet
Tablets (chewable): 4 mg, 5 mg
Tablets (film-coated): 10 mg

INDICATIONS & DOSAGES
➤ **Asthma**
Adults and children age 15 and older: 10 mg PO once daily in evening.
Children ages 6 to 14: 5-mg chewable tablet PO once daily in evening.
Children ages 2 to 5: 4-mg chewable tablet or 1 packet of 4-mg oral granules PO once daily in evening.
Children ages 12 to 23 months: 1 packet of 4-mg oral granules PO once daily in the evening.
➤ **Seasonal allergic rhinitis, perennial allergic rhinitis**
Adults and children age 15 and older: 10 mg PO once daily in evening.
Children ages 6 to 14: 5-mg chewable tablet PO once daily in evening.
Children ages 2 to 5: 4-mg chewable tablet or 1 packet of 4-mg oral granules PO once daily in evening.
Children ages 6 to 23 months (perennial allergic rhinitis only): 1 packet of 4-mg oral granules PO once daily in evening.

➤ **Prevention of exercise-induced bronchoconstriction**
Adults and children age 15 and older: 10 mg PO at least 2 hours before exercise. Patients already taking a daily dose shouldn't take an additional dose. Also, an additional dose shouldn't be taken within 24 hours of a previous dose.
Children ages 6 to 14: 5 mg PO at least 2 hours before exercise (1 chewable tablet). Patients already taking a daily dose shouldn't take an additional dose; an additional dose shouldn't be taken within 24 hours of a previous dose.

ADMINISTRATION
PO
- Give oral granules directly in the mouth, dissolved in 5 mL of cold or room-temperature baby formula or human milk, or mixed with a spoonful of cold or room-temperature soft foods (use only applesauce, carrots, rice, or ice cream). Use within 15 minutes of opening the packet.
- May be given without regard to food.
- For patients with both asthma and allergic rhinitis, give only one dose daily in the evening.
- If a dose is missed, omit the dose; give next dose at regularly scheduled time.

ACTION
Reduces early and late-phase bronchoconstriction from antigen challenge.

Route	Onset	Peak	Duration
PO (chewable, granules)	Unknown	2–2.5 hr	24 hr
PO (film-coated)	Unknown	3–4 hr	24 hr

Half-life: 2.75 to 5.5 hours.

ADVERSE REACTIONS
CNS: headache, asthenia, dizziness, fatigue, fever, somnolence, weakness. **EENT:** conjunctivitis, otitis media, ear pain, rhinorrhea, nasal congestion, epistaxis, laryngitis, sinusitis, pharyngitis, rhinitis, tonsillitis, dental pain. **GI:** abdominal pain, dyspepsia, gastroenteritis, nausea, diarrhea. **GU:** pyuria. **Hematologic:** systemic eosinophilia. **Hepatic:** increased transaminase levels. **Respiratory:** URI, cough, wheezing, pneumonia, bronchitis. **Skin:** rash, dermatitis, urticaria, eczema. **Other:** flulike symptoms, trauma, varicella, viral infection.

M

INTERACTIONS
Drug-drug. *Gemfibrozil:* May increase montelukast level. Monitor therapy.
Lumacaftor–ivacaftor: May decrease montelukast level. Monitor therapy.

EFFECTS ON LAB TEST RESULTS
• May increase ALT and AST levels.
• May increase urinary WBC count.

CONTRAINDICATIONS & CAUTIONS
• Contraindicated in patients hypersensitive to drug or its components.
• Avoid use with aspirin and other NSAIDs in patients with known aspirin sensitivity because drug hasn't been shown to affect the bronchoconstrictor response to aspirin and other NSAIDs in patients with asthma who are aspirin-sensitive.
• Patients with asthma may present with systemic eosinophilia that may manifest as clinical features of vasculitis consistent with Churg-Strauss syndrome. Churg-Strauss syndrome is often treated with systemic corticosteroid therapy. These reactions have sometimes been associated with reduction of oral corticosteroid dosage. Be alert to development of eosinophilia, vasculitic rash, worsening pulmonary symptoms, cardiac complications, or neuropathy.
• Use cautiously and with appropriate monitoring in patients whose dosages of systemic corticosteroids are reduced.
Boxed Warning Serious neuropsychiatric events have been reported in patients taking montelukast. The benefits may not outweigh the risk of neuropsychiatric symptoms in patients with allergic rhinitis; reserve use for patients who have an inadequate response or intolerance to alternative therapies. Discuss risks with patients and caregivers. ∎
Boxed Warning The neuropsychiatric events reported in patients taking montelukast include, but aren't limited to, agitation, aggressive behavior or hostility, anxiousness, depression, disorientation, disturbance in attention, dream abnormalities, hallucinations, insomnia, irritability, memory impairment, restlessness, somnambulism, suicidality (including suicide), and tremor. ∎
• Use cautiously in patients with hepatic disease, jaundice, or hepatitis.
Dialyzable drug: Unknown.

⚠ *Overdose S&S:* Headache, vomiting, psychomotor hyperactivity, thirst, somnolence, hyperkinesia, abdominal pain.

PREGNANCY-LACTATION-REPRODUCTION
• There are no adequate studies during pregnancy. Use during pregnancy only if clearly needed.
• Drug reportedly appears in human milk. Use cautiously during breastfeeding.

NURSING CONSIDERATIONS
• Assess patient's underlying condition; monitor patient for effectiveness.
🔷 *Alert:* Don't abruptly substitute drug for inhaled or oral corticosteroids. Dose of inhaled corticosteroids may be reduced gradually.
🔷 *Alert:* Drug isn't indicated for use in patients with acute asthmatic attacks, status asthmaticus, or as monotherapy for management of exercise-induced bronchospasm. Continue appropriate rescue drug for acute worsening.
Boxed Warning Monitor patients for neuropsychiatric symptoms. Discontinue drug immediately if neuropsychiatric symptoms occur. ∎

PATIENT TEACHING
• Explain how to properly administer drug in prescribed formulation.
• Advise patient to take drug daily, even if asymptomatic, and to contact prescriber if asthma isn't well controlled.
• Warn patient not to reduce or stop taking other prescribed antiasthmatics without prescriber's approval.
• Advise patient to seek medical attention if short-acting inhaled bronchodilators are needed more often than usual during drug therapy.
• Warn patient that drug isn't beneficial in acute asthma attacks or in acute exercise-induced bronchospasm. Advise patient to keep appropriate rescue drugs available.
Boxed Warning Advise patient and caregivers of the risk of neuropsychiatric symptoms and to immediately report symptoms if they occur. ∎
• Advise patient with known aspirin sensitivity to continue to avoid using aspirin and NSAIDs during drug therapy.
🔷 *Alert:* Advise patient with phenylketonuria that chewable tablet contains phenylalanine.

Reactions in bold italics are *life-threatening*. Interactions may have a *rapid onset* or a *delayed onset*.

morphine hydrochloride
MOR-feen

Doloral ♣

morphine sulfate
Duramorph PF, Infumorph, M-Eslon ♣, Mitigo, MS Contin, Statex ♣

Therapeutic class: Opioid analgesics
Pharmacologic class: Opioids
Controlled substance schedule: II

AVAILABLE FORMS
morphine hydrochloride
Syrup: 1 mg/mL* ♣, 5 mg/mL* ♣
morphine sulfate
Capsules (extended-release microgranules [M-Eslon]) ⓄⓃⒸ: 10 mg ♣, 15 mg ♣, 30 mg ♣, 60 mg ♣, 100 mg ♣, 200 mg ♣
Capsules (extended-release pellets) ⓄⓃⒸ: 10 mg, 20 mg, 30 mg, 40 mg, 45 mg, 50 mg, 60 mg, 75 mg, 80 mg, 90 mg, 100 mg, 120 mg, 200 mg
Injection with preservative: 0.5 mg/mL, 1 mg/mL, 2 mg/mL, 5 mg/mL, 10 mg/mL, 15 mg/mL, 50 mg/mL
Injection without preservative (Duramorph, Infumorph): 0.5 mg/mL, 1 mg/mL, 10 mg/mL, 25 mg/mL
Injection without preservative (Carpuject and prefilled syringes and vials): 2 mg/mL, 4 mg/mL, 8 mg/mL, 10 mg/mL, 15 mg/mL
Oral solution: 10 mg/5 mL, 20 mg/5 mL, 20 mg/mL (concentrate), 100 mg/5 mL (concentrate)
Suppositories: 5 mg, 10 mg, 20 mg, 30 mg
Tablets: 5 mg ♣, 10 mg ♣, 15 mg, 20 mg ♣, 25 mg ♣, 30 mg ♣, 50 mg ♣
Tablets (extended-release) ⓄⓃⒸ: 15 mg, 30 mg, 60 mg, 100 mg, 200 mg
Tablets (extended-release, abuse deterrent) ⓄⓃⒸ: 15 mg, 30 mg, 60 mg, 100 mg

INDICATIONS & DOSAGES
🜊 *Alert:* Initiate dosing for each patient individually and use the lowest effective dosage for the shortest duration consistent with individual treatment goals.
➤ **Moderate to severe pain**
Adults: Initially, 10 mg (based on 70 kg individual) IM or 0.1 to 0.2 mg/kg IV every 4 hours PRN. Or, 15 to 30 mg (immediate-release tablets) PO, or 10 to 20 mg (oral solution) PO, or 10 to 20 mg PR every 4 hours PRN.

For extended-release tablet, give 15 or 30 mg PO every 8 to 12 hours.

For epidural injection, give 5 mg by epidural catheter; then, if pain isn't relieved adequately in 1 hour, give supplementary doses of 1 to 2 mg at intervals sufficient to assess effectiveness. Maximum total epidural dose shouldn't exceed 10 mg/24 hours.

For intrathecal injection, a single dose of 0.2 to 1 mg may provide pain relief for 24 hours (only in the lumbar area). Don't repeat injections.
➤ **Moderate to severe pain requiring continuous, around-the-clock oral opioid**
Adults: For patients receiving other oral morphine formulations, may convert to extended-release capsules by administering patient's total daily oral morphine dose as extended-release capsules once daily or by administering one-half of patient's total daily oral morphine dose b.i.d. Patient's 24-hour morphine requirement may also be divided every 8 hours and given as extended-release tablets. Initial dosage in patients who are opioid-naive or opioid-nontolerant is 15 mg extended-release tablets PO every 8 or 12 hours. Don't give extended-release capsules more frequently than every 12 hours.

ADMINISTRATION
PO
Boxed Warning Take care when administering morphine oral solution to avoid dosing errors because of confusion among different concentrations and between milligrams and milliliters, which could result in accidental overdose and death. The 20-mg/mL concentration is indicated for use only in patients who are opioid-tolerant because of the risk of fatal respiratory depression in patients who are opioid-naive. It's packaged with a calibrated oral syringe for accurate dosing. ∎
Boxed Warning Instruct patient to swallow extended-release or long-acting morphine sulfate oral formulations whole, without crushing, chewing, or dissolving, which may cause rapid, uncontrolled release and absorption of a potentially fatal dose of morphine. If necessary, extended-release capsules may be carefully opened and entire contents poured into cool, soft foods such as applesauce and swallowed immediately without chewing. ∎

M

- Give morphine sulfate without regard to food.
- May give extended-release capsules through a gastrostomy tube; flush tube with water, sprinkle contents of capsules in 10 mL of water, and flush through tube. Don't give through an NG tube.

IV

▼ For direct IV injection, give slowly over 4 to 5 minutes.

▼ For continuous infusion, mix drug with D_5W to yield 0.1 to 1 mg/mL, and give by a continuous infusion device.

▼ In adults with severe, chronic pain, maintenance IV infusion is 0.8 to 80 mg/hour; sometimes higher doses are needed.

▼ Make sure an opioid antagonist is immediately available before administering IV.

▼ Infumorph and Duramorph are supplied in sealed ampules. Treat accidental dermal exposure to these drugs by removing contaminated clothing and rinsing affected area with water.

▼ Inspect parenteral drug products for particulate matter before opening the amber ampule and again for color after removing contents from ampule. Don't use if solution in the unopened ampule contains a precipitate that doesn't disappear upon shaking. After removal, don't use unless solution is colorless or pale yellow.

▼ **Incompatibilities:** None listed by manufacturer. Consult a drug incompatibility reference for more information.

IM

- Document injection site.
- Store injection solution at room temperature and protect from light.
- Solution may darken with age. Don't use if injection appears darker than pale yellow, is discolored, or contains precipitate.

Epidural/intrathecal

- Document injection site; limit to lumbar area.
- ⚠ *Alert:* Intrathecal dosage is usually one-tenth that of epidural dosage.
- Verify proper placement of needle or catheter in the intrathecal or epidural space before injecting drug.
- Inspect for particulate matter and discoloration before administration. Don't use if it's darker than pale yellow, discolored in any other way, or contains a precipitate.
- Store injection solution at room temperature until ready to use; discard unused portion.
- Protect from light; don't freeze or heat sterilize.

Rectal

- Refrigeration of rectal suppository isn't needed.

ACTION

Unknown. Binds with opioid receptors in the CNS, altering perception of and emotional response to pain.

Route	Onset	Peak	Duration
PO	30 min	1–2 hr	3–5 hr
PO (extended-release)	1–2 hr	3–4 hr	8–24 hr
IV	5–10 min	20 min	4–5 hr
IM	10–30 min	30–60 min	4–5 hr
PR	20–60 min	20–60 min	3–7 hr
Epidural	10–60 min	15–60 min	24 hr
Intrathecal	15–60 min	30–60 min	24 hr

Half-life: Immediate release, 2 to 4 hours; extended release, 11 to 24 hours; epidural, 39 to 249 minutes; intrathecal (CSF), 42 to 136 minutes; IV/IM, 1.5 to 4.5 hours.

ADVERSE REACTIONS

CNS: dizziness, drowsiness, headache, euphoria, light-headedness, myoclonus, nightmares, abnormal dreams, amnesia, apathy, ataxia, confusion, decreased cough reflex, sedation, hypoesthesia, paresthesia, insomnia, lethargy, somnolence, *seizures,* depression, hallucinations, nervousness, agitation, slurred speech, physical dependence, fever, vertigo, syncope, anxiety, tremor, asthenia, voice disorder, withdrawal syndrome. **CV:** *bradycardia, cardiac arrest, shock,* HTN, hypotension, tachycardia, palpitations, peripheral circulatory collapse, peripheral edema, chest pain, syncope, flushing, atrial fibrillation, vasodilation. **EENT:** miosis, blurred vision, conjunctivitis, diplopia, nystagmus, rhinitis, dry mouth. **GI:** constipation, nausea, vomiting, anorexia, biliary tract spasms, dry mouth, ileus, flatulence, abdominal pain, delayed gastric emptying, diarrhea, dysphagia, gastric atony, GERD, hiccups. **GU:** urine retention, urinary hesitancy, decreased libido, amenorrhea, impotence, prolonged labor. **Hematologic:** *thrombocytopenia, anemia, leukopenia.* **Metabolic:** hyponatremia, SIADH. **Musculoskeletal:** back pain, footdrop, ostealgia. **Respiratory:** *apnea, respiratory arrest, respiratory depression,* atelectasis, dyspnea, *hypoxia.* **Skin:** diaphoresis, pallor, rash, edema, pruritus, skin flushing,

---

Reactions in bold italics are *life-threatening*. Interactions may have a *rapid onset* or a **delayed onset**.

pain at injection site. **Other:** gynecomastia, flulike symptoms.

INTERACTIONS

Drug-drug. *Alvimopan:* May enhance adverse or toxic effects of alvimopan. Alvimopan is contraindicated in patients receiving therapeutic doses of opioids for more than 7 consecutive days immediately before alvimopan initiation. Consider therapy modification.
Anticholinergics (benztropine, darifenacin, oxybutynin): Increased risk of urine retention, constipation, and paralytic ileus. Use cautiously together.
Boxed Warning *Benzodiazepines, CNS depressants:* May cause slow or difficult breathing, sedation, and death. Avoid use together. If use together is necessary, limit dosage and duration of each drug to the minimum necessary for desired effect. ■
Diuretics: May reduce efficacy of diuretics. Monitor therapy.
General anesthetics, hypnotics, muscle relaxants, other opioid analgesics, TCAs: May cause respiratory depression, hypotension, profound sedation, or coma. Use together with caution, reduce morphine dose, and monitor patient response.
MAO inhibitors: May increase risk of serotonin syndrome or opioid toxicity. Don't use morphine within 14 days of MAO inhibitor. Consider use of alternative opioid with careful monitoring and small doses.
Mixed agonist/antagonist, partial agonist opioid analgesics: May reduce effect of morphine or precipitate withdrawal symptoms. Avoid use together; if use together is necessary, monitor patient closely.
P2Y12 inhibitors (clopidogrel, prasugrel, ticagrelor): May decrease absorption and peak concentration of oral P2Y12 inhibitors when used with IV morphine sulfate and delay onset of antiplatelet effect. Consider use of a parenteral antiplatelet agent in the setting of ACS requiring coadministration of IV morphine.
Alert: *Serotonergic drugs (amoxapine, antiemetics [dolasetron, granisetron, ondansetron, palonosetron], antimigraine drugs, buspirone, cyclobenzaprine, dextromethorphan, linezolid, lithium, maprotiline, methylene blue, mirtazapine, nefazodone, SSNRIs, SSRIs, TCAs, trazodone, tryptophan, vilazodone):* May increase risk of serotonin syndrome. Use together cautiously and monitor patient for serotonin syndrome.
Drug-herb. **Alert:** *St. John's wort:* May increase risk of serotonin syndrome. Use together cautiously and monitor patient for serotonin syndrome.
Drug-lifestyle. **Boxed Warning** *Alcohol use:* May cause additive CNS effects and fatal overdose. Warn patient to avoid alcohol and products containing alcohol. ■

EFFECTS ON LAB TEST RESULTS

- May increase amylase level.
- May decrease sodium level.
- May decrease Hb level (morphine sulfate) and platelet count.
- May cause abnormal LFT values (morphine sulfate).

CONTRAINDICATIONS & CAUTIONS

- Contraindicated in patients hypersensitive to drug and in those with conditions that would preclude IV administration of opioids (acute bronchial asthma or upper airway obstruction).

Boxed Warning To ensure the benefits of opioid analgesics outweigh the risks of addiction, abuse, and misuse, the FDA requires REMS programs for these products. ■
Boxed Warning Opioids should only be prescribed with benzodiazepines or other CNS depressants to patients for whom alternative treatment options are inadequate. ■
Boxed Warning Use of extended-release or long-acting morphine sulfate forms may increase the risk of addiction, abuse, and misuse, even at recommended doses, and has a greater risk of overdose and death. Reserve their use for patients for whom alternative treatment options are ineffective, not tolerated, or are otherwise insufficient to provide adequate pain management. ■
Boxed Warning Accidental ingestion of even one dose of extended-release or long-acting forms of morphine sulfate, especially by children, can result in a fatal overdose. Keep out of reach of children. ■
Alert: Drug may lead to a rare but serious decrease in adrenal gland cortisol production.
- Drug may cause decreased sex hormone levels with long-term use.

Alert: Patients are at increased risk for oversedation and respiratory depression if they snore or have a history of sleep apnea, haven't used opioids recently or are first-time

M

opioid users, have increased opioid dosage requirements or opioid habituation, have received general anesthesia for longer lengths of time or received other sedating drugs, have preexisting pulmonary or cardiac disease, or have thoracic or other surgical incisions that may impair breathing. Monitor patients carefully.

• Contraindicated in patients with GI obstruction.

• Use with caution in older adults or patients who are debilitated and in those with head injury, increased ICP, seizures, chronic pulmonary disease, prostatic hyperplasia, severe hepatic or renal disease, acute abdominal conditions, hypothyroidism, Addison disease, and urethral stricture.

• Use with caution in patients with circulatory shock, biliary tract disease, CNS depression, toxic psychosis, acute alcoholism, delirium tremens, and seizure disorders.

• Morphine hydrochloride syrup isn't indicated for use in children.

Dialyzable drug: Yes.

⚠ *Overdose S&S:* Miosis, CNS depression, respiratory depression, apnea, flaccid skeletal muscles, bradycardia, hypotension, circulatory collapse, cardiac arrest, respiratory arrest, death.

PREGNANCY-LACTATION-REPRODUCTION

🜀 *Alert:* Carefully weigh risks and benefits of using drug during pregnancy. Use in pregnancy only if need for opioid analgesia clearly outweighs fetal risk.

Boxed Warning Prolonged use of opioids during pregnancy can result in neonatal opioid withdrawal syndrome, which may be life-threatening if not recognized and treated, and requires management according to protocols developed by neonatology experts. If opioid use is required for a prolonged period, apprise patient who is pregnant of risk to the neonate and ensure appropriate treatment will be available. ∎

• Because of the potential for serious adverse reactions in breastfeeding infants, including respiratory depression, sedation, and possibly withdrawal symptoms upon cessation of morphine to the mother, patient should discontinue breastfeeding or discontinue drug, taking into account importance of drug to the mother.

• If morphine use is necessary in patient who is breastfeeding, use cautiously. Limit use and supplement with nonopioid agents. Monitor infant for increased sleepiness, difficulty feeding or breathing, and limpness.

• Prolonged opioid use may cause reduced fertility.

NURSING CONSIDERATIONS

Boxed Warning Assess each patient's risk of addiction, abuse, or misuse before prescribing extended-release or long-acting forms of morphine sulfate, and monitor all patients regularly for development of these behaviors. ∎

Boxed Warning Monitor patients for respiratory depression, especially during initiation of extended-release or long-acting morphine sulfate or after a dosage increase. Serious, life-threatening, or fatal respiratory depression may occur. ∎

🜀 *Alert:* If patient is taking opioids with serotonergic drugs, watch for signs and symptoms of serotonin syndrome (agitation, hallucinations, rapid HR, fever, diaphoresis, shivering or shaking, muscle twitching or stiffness, trouble with coordination, nausea, vomiting, diarrhea), especially at start of treatment and at dosage increases. Signs and symptoms may occur within several hours of coadministration but may also occur later, especially after dosage increase. Discontinue the opioid, serotonergic drug, or both if serotonin syndrome is suspected.

🜀 *Alert:* Monitor patient for signs and symptoms of adrenal insufficiency (nausea, vomiting, loss of appetite, fatigue, weakness, dizziness, low BP). Perform diagnostic testing if adrenal insufficiency is suspected. If adrenal insufficiency is confirmed, treat with corticosteroids and wean patient off opioids if appropriate. Discontinue corticosteroids when clinically appropriate.

• Monitor patient for signs and symptoms of decreased sex hormone levels (low libido, erectile dysfunction, amenorrhea, infertility). If signs and symptoms occur, evaluate patient and obtain lab testing.

🜀 *Alert:* Carefully monitor vital signs, pain level, respiratory status, and sedation level in all patients receiving opioids, especially those receiving IV drugs, even those given postoperatively.

• Reassess patient's level of pain at least 15 and 30 minutes after giving parenterally and 30 minutes after giving orally.

🜀 *Alert:* Keep opioid antagonist (naloxone) and resuscitation equipment available.

Reactions in bold italics are *life-threatening*. Interactions may have a *rapid onset* or a *delayed onset*.

• Monitor circulatory, respiratory, bladder, and bowel functions carefully. Drug may cause hypotension, urine retention, nausea, vomiting, ileus, or altered level of consciousness regardless of the route.

🔔 *Alert:* Intrathecal dosage is usually one-tenth of epidural dosage.

Boxed Warning Life-threatening respiratory depression may occur with morphine use, even when drug has been used as recommended and not misused or abused. Morphine should only be prescribed by health care providers knowledgeable in the use of potent opioids for management of long-term pain. Monitor patients for respiratory depression, especially during initiation of morphine or after a dosage increase. ∎

• If respirations drop below 12 breaths/minute, withhold dose and notify prescriber.

Boxed Warning Morphine has an abuse liability similar to other opioid analgesics and may be misused, abused, or diverted. ∎

🔔 *Alert:* Extended-release tablets and capsules aren't for use on an as-needed basis for mild or acute pain or for postoperative pain, unless patient has already been receiving long-term opioid therapy before surgery or if postoperative pain is expected to be moderate to severe and persist for an extended period.

• Preservative-free preparations are available for epidural and intrathecal use.

• Epidural administration has been associated with less potential for immediate or late adverse effects than intrathecal administration; use epidural route whenever possible.

• A constant IV infusion of naloxone, 0.6 mg/hour, for 24 hours after intrathecal injection may reduce potential adverse effects.

Boxed Warning When the epidural or intrathecal route is used, observe patients in a fully equipped and staffed environment for at least 24 hours after the initial dose. ∎

• Infumorph isn't recommended for single-dose IV, IM, or subcut administration.

• Improper or erroneous substitution of Infumorph 200 or 500 (10 or 25 mg/mL, respectively) for regular Duramorph (0.5 or 1 mg/mL) is likely to result in serious overdose, leading to seizures, respiratory depression, and possibly fatal outcome.

• When drug is given epidurally, monitor patient closely for respiratory depression up to 24 hours after the injection. Check respiratory rate and depth every 30 to 60 minutes for 24 hours. Watch for pruritus and skin flushing.

• Morphine is drug of choice in relieving MI pain; may cause transient decrease in BP.

• An around-the-clock regimen best manages severe, chronic pain. Verify patient has a breakthrough pain medication prescribed in addition to the around-the-clock medication.

• Morphine may worsen or mask gallbladder pain.

• Constipation is commonly severe with maintenance dose. Ensure that stool softener or stimulant laxative is ordered.

• Taper morphine sulfate therapy gradually when stopping therapy.

Boxed Warning Each ampule of Infumorph and Duramorph contains a large amount of a potent opioid that has been associated with abuse and dependence among health care providers. Due to the limited indications for this product, risk of overdose, and risk of its diversion and abuse, special measures should be taken to control this product within the hospital or clinic. Infumorph and Duramorph should be subject to rigid accounting, rigorous control of wastage, and restricted access. ∎

Boxed Warning Accidental consumption of morphine, especially by children, can result in a fatal overdose of morphine. ∎

🔔 *Alert:* Don't stop drug abruptly; withdraw slowly and individualize gradual taper plan to prevent signs and symptoms of withdrawal, worsening pain, and psychological distress in patients who are physically dependent. Refer to manufacturer's label for specific tapering instructions.

🔔 *Alert:* When tapering opioids, monitor patient closely for signs and symptoms of opioid withdrawal (restlessness, lacrimation, rhinorrhea, yawning, perspiration, chills, myalgia, mydriasis, irritability, anxiety, insomnia, backache, joint pain, weakness, abdominal cramps, anorexia, nausea, vomiting, diarrhea, increased BP or HR, increased respiratory rate), which may indicate a need to taper more slowly. Also monitor patient for suicidality, use of other substances, or changes in mood.

• *Look alike–sound alike:* Don't confuse morphine with hydromorphone. Don't confuse MS Contin with Oxycontin.

PATIENT TEACHING

Boxed Warning Caution patient or caregiver of patient taking an opioid with a benzodiazepine, CNS depressant, or alcohol to seek immediate medical attention for dizziness,

M

light-headedness, extreme sleepiness, slowed or difficult breathing, or unresponsiveness. ■

• Emphasize to patient and caregivers importance of reading the medication guide provided by the pharmacist.

Boxed Warning Instruct patient and caregivers on safe use, serious risks, and storage and disposal of morphine products. ■

Boxed Warning Tell patient to keep morphine oral preparations out of the reach of children. In case of accidental ingestion, advise patient to immediately seek emergency medical help. ■

⟳ *Alert:* Explain assessment and monitoring process to patient and family. Instruct them to immediately report difficulty breathing or other signs or symptoms of a potential adverse opioid-related reaction.

• Encourage patient to report all medications being taken, including prescription and OTC medications and supplements.

• Warn patient that morphine can cause constipation.

⟳ *Alert:* Caution patient to immediately report signs and symptoms of serotonin syndrome, adrenal insufficiency, and decreased sex hormone levels.

• When drug is used after surgery, encourage patient to turn, cough, and deep-breathe to prevent lung problems.

• Caution patient who is ambulatory about getting out of bed or walking. Warn outpatient to avoid driving and other potentially hazardous activities that require mental alertness until drug's adverse CNS effects are known.

Boxed Warning Drinking alcohol or taking drugs containing alcohol while taking extended-release capsules may cause additive CNS effects and potentially fatal overdose. Warn patient to read labels on OTC drugs carefully for alcohol content and not to use alcohol in any form. ■

• Teach patient that naloxone is prescribed in conjunction with the opioid when treatment is started or renewed as a preventive measure to reduce opioid overdose and death.

⟳ *Alert:* Counsel patient not to discontinue opioids without first discussing with prescriber the need for a gradual tapering regimen.

⟳ *Alert:* Warn patient not to crush, break, or chew extended-release forms.

moxifloxacin hydrochloride
mox-i-FLOKS-a-sin

Moxeza, Vigamox

Therapeutic class: Antibiotics
Pharmacologic class: Fluoroquinolones

AVAILABLE FORMS
Injection: 400 mg/250 mL
Ophthalmic solution: 0.5%
Tablets (film-coated): 400 mg

INDICATIONS & DOSAGES
Boxed Warning Use in patients with acute bacterial sinusitis or acute bacterial exacerbation of bronchitis isn't recommended due to risk of serious adverse effects. Use drug in these patients only when they have no other treatment options. ■

➤ **Acute bacterial sinusitis caused by** *Streptococcus pneumoniae, Haemophilus influenzae,* **or** *Moraxella catarrhalis*
Adults: 400 mg PO or IV every 24 hours for 10 days.

➤ **Complicated skin and skin-structure infections caused by methicillin-susceptible** *Staphylococcus aureus, Escherichia coli, Klebsiella pneumoniae,* **or** *Enterobacter cloacae*
Adults: 400 mg PO or IV every 24 hours for 7 to 21 days.

➤ **Complicated intra-abdominal infection caused by** *E. coli, Bacteroides fragilis, Streptococcus anginosus, Streptococcus constellatus, Enterococcus faecalis, Proteus mirabilis, Clostridium perfringens, Bacteroides thetaiotaomicron,* **or** *Peptostreptococcus* **species**
Adults: 400 mg PO or IV every 24 hours for 5 to 14 days. Start with the IV form; switch to PO when appropriate.

➤ **Community-acquired pneumonia from multidrug-resistant** *S. pneumoniae* **(resistance to two or more of the following antibiotics: penicillin, second-generation cephalosporins, macrolides, sulfamethoxazole–trimethoprim, tetracyclines),** *S. aureus, M. catarrhalis, H. influenzae, K. pneumoniae, Chlamydia pneumoniae,* **or** *Mycoplasma pneumoniae*
Adults: 400 mg PO or IV every 24 hours for 7 to 14 days.

Reactions in bold italics are *life-threatening.* Interactions may have a *rapid onset* or a ***delayed onset.***

➤ **Acute bacterial exacerbation of chronic bronchitis caused by *S. pneumoniae, H. influenzae, H. parainfluenzae, K. pneumoniae, S. aureus,* or *M. catarrhalis***
Adults: 400 mg PO or IV every 24 hours for 5 days.

➤ **Uncomplicated skin-structure or skin infection caused by *S. aureus* or *Streptococcus pyogenes***
Adults: 400 mg PO or IV every 24 hours for 7 days.

➤ **Plague (pneumonic and septicemic) caused by susceptible isolates of *Yersinia pestis***
Adults: For prophylaxis and treatment, 400 mg PO or IV every 24 hours for 10 to 14 days.

➤ **Bacterial conjunctivitis caused by susceptible strains of aerobic gram-positive and gram-negative organisms and *Chlamydia trachomatis***
Adults and children: 1 drop into affected eye(s) t.i.d. for 7 days.
Adults and children age 4 months and older (Moxeza): 1 drop into affected eye(s) b.i.d. for 7 days.

ADMINISTRATION
PO
• Give drug without regard for food. Give at same time each day.
• Give dose 4 hours before or 8 hours after antacids, sucralfate, multivitamins, didanosine buffered tablets for oral suspension or pediatric powder for oral solution, and other products containing aluminum, magnesium, iron, and zinc, to avoid decreasing drug's therapeutic effects.
• Store drug at controlled room temperature.
• If a dose is missed more than 8 hours before the next scheduled dose, give the dose. If less than 8 hours remain before the next dose, omit the missed dose; then continue with the next scheduled dose. Don't double the dose to compensate for a missed dose.
IV
▼ Don't refrigerate. Product precipitates if refrigerated.
▼ Don't use if particulate matter is visible.
▼ Flush IV line with a compatible solution such as D₅W, NSS, or lactated Ringer solution before and after use.
▼ Give only by infusion over 1 hour. Avoid rapid or bolus infusion.
▼ **Incompatibilities:** Other IV drugs.

Ophthalmic
• Place gentle pressure on lacrimal duct for 1 to 2 minutes after instilling drop.
• Solution isn't for injection subconjunctivally or into anterior chamber of the eye.

ACTION
Interferes with action of enzymes needed for bacterial replication. Inhibits topoisomerases I (DNA gyrase) and IV, impairing bacterial DNA replication, transcription, repair, and recombination.

Route	Onset	Peak	Duration
PO, IV	Unknown	1–3 hr	Unknown
Ophthalmic	Unknown	Unknown	Unknown

Half-life: PO, 11.5 to 15.6 hours; IV, 8.2 to 15.4 hours; ophthalmic, 13 hours.

ADVERSE REACTIONS
CNS: dizziness, headache, insomnia, fever. **EENT:** with ophthalmic use: conjunctivitis; dry eyes; increased lacrimation; keratitis; ocular discomfort, pain, or pruritus; reduced visual acuity; subconjunctival hemorrhage; otitis media; pharyngitis; rhinitis. **GI:** abdominal pain, anorexia, constipation, diarrhea, dyspepsia, nausea, vomiting. **Hematologic:** anemia, neutrophilia, prolonged PT. **Hepatic:** abnormal LFT values. **Metabolic:** *hypokalemia, hypoglycemia,* hyperchloremia, hyperalbuminemia, decreased amylase level. **Respiratory:** *hypoxia.*

INTERACTIONS
Drug-drug. *Aluminum hydroxide, aluminum–magnesium hydroxide, calcium carbonate, didanosine, magnesium hydroxide, multivitamins, products containing zinc:* May interfere with GI absorption of moxifloxacin. Give moxifloxacin 4 hours before or 8 hours after these products.
Antidiabetics: May cause hyperglycemia and hypoglycemia. Monitor blood glucose control.
Class IA antiarrhythmics (procainamide, quinidine), class III antiarrhythmics (amiodarone, sotalol); drugs that prolong QT interval (antipsychotics, erythromycin, TCAs): May have additive QT-interval prolongation effect. Avoid using together.
Live-virus vaccines: May decrease effectiveness of live-virus vaccines. Don't give live-virus vaccines during therapy.

M

NSAIDs: May increase risk of CNS stimulation and seizures. Monitor patient and adjust treatment as needed.

Boxed Warning *Steroids:* May increase risk of tendinitis and tendon rupture. Monitor patient for tendon pain or inflammation. ∎

Sucralfate: May decrease absorption of moxifloxacin, reducing anti-infective response. If use together can't be avoided, take oral form 4 hours before or 8 hours after sucralfate.

Warfarin: May increase anticoagulant effects. Monitor PT and INR closely.

Drug-lifestyle. *Sun or UV light exposure:* May cause moderate to severe photosensitivity reactions. Advise patient to avoid excessive sunlight or UV light exposure.

EFFECTS ON LAB TEST RESULTS
• May increase ALT, ionized calcium, chloride, globulin, and albumin levels.
• May decrease potassium and amylase levels and oxygen partial pressure.
• May increase or decrease bilirubin and glucose levels.
• May increase WBC count and PT and INR.
• May decrease Hb level and hematocrit and RBC, eosinophil, and basophil counts.
• May increase or decrease neutrophil count.

CONTRAINDICATIONS & CAUTIONS
Boxed Warning Drug is associated with increased risk of tendinitis and tendon rupture, especially in patients older than age 60, patients taking corticosteroids, and those with heart, kidney, or lung transplants. ∎

☾ *Alert:* Drug may increase risk of aortic dissection or rupture when used systemically. Avoid use in patients with known aortic aneurysm and patients at risk for an aortic aneurysm, including those with peripheral atherosclerotic vascular diseases, HTN, or certain genetic conditions (Marfan syndrome, Ehlers-Danlos syndrome), and older adults. Drug should only be used in these patients if no other treatment options are available.

☾ *Alert:* Patients receiving systemic drug have an increased risk of hypoglycemia, which can result in coma. Hypoglycemia has been reported more frequently in older adults and in patients with diabetes.

• Contraindicated in patients hypersensitive to drug or other fluoroquinolones.

☾ *Alert:* Drug can prolong QT interval in some patients. Use cautiously in patients with ongoing proarrhythmic conditions, such as clinically significant bradycardia or acute myocardial ischemia.

• Discontinue drug at first sign of rash, jaundice, or other signs or symptoms of hypersensitivity.

• Seizures, increased ICP, and pseudotumor cerebri have been reported in patients taking fluoroquinolones. Drug may cause CNS events (including agitation, anxiety, confusion, depression, insomnia and, rarely, suicidality), which may occur after first dose. Use cautiously in patients who may have CNS disorders or risk factors for seizures. Drug may need to be discontinued.

Boxed Warning Drug may exacerbate muscle weakness in patients with myasthenia gravis. Avoid use of fluoroquinolones in patients with known history of myasthenia gravis. ∎

• Drug may cause CDAD, ranging in severity from mild diarrhea to fatal colitis, which can occur more than 2 months after therapy. If CDAD is suspected or confirmed, drug may need to be discontinued and appropriate therapy initiated.

• Safety and effectiveness of PO and IV formulations in children haven't been established.

Dialyzable drug: Minimal.

PREGNANCY-LACTATION-REPRODUCTION
• There are no adequate studies during pregnancy. Use during pregnancy only if potential benefit justifies fetal risk.
• Drug may appear in human milk. Patient should discontinue breastfeeding or discontinue drug.

NURSING CONSIDERATIONS
Boxed Warning Monitor patient for tendinitis and tendon rupture, peripheral neuropathy, and CNS effects (seizures, toxic psychoses, increased ICP, pseudotumor cerebri, tremors, restlessness, anxiety, light-headedness, confusion, hallucinations, paranoia, depression, nightmares, insomnia and, rarely, suicidality). If any of these serious adverse reactions occur, discontinue drug immediately. ∎

Boxed Warning Monitor patient for signs and symptoms of peripheral neuropathy (pain, burning, tingling, numbness, weakness, or change in sensation to light touch, pain or temperature, or sense of body position) and immediately report them. ∎

Reactions in bold italics are *life-threatening*. Interactions may have a *rapid onset* or a *delayed onset*.

• Monitor patient for hypersensitivity reactions, including anaphylaxis.

• If diarrhea develops during therapy, send stool specimen for *Clostridioides difficile* test.

• Patient with signs or symptoms of conjunctivitis shouldn't wear contact lenses.

• Rupture of the Achilles and other tendons is linked to fluoroquinolone use. If pain, inflammation, or tendon rupture occurs, stop drug and notify prescriber.

🔴 *Alert:* Monitor patient for signs and symptoms of aortic aneurysm, dissection, and rupture (sudden, severe, constant pain in the stomach, chest, or back; throbbing in the stomach area; deep pain in the back or side of the stomach; steady, gnawing pain in the stomach that lasts for hours or days; pain in the jaw, neck, back, or chest; coughing or hoarseness; shortness of breath; trouble swallowing). Discontinue drug immediately if any of these aortic disorders are suspected.

🔴 *Alert:* Monitor patients receiving systemic drug for symptoms of hypoglycemia (confusion, pounding or rapid heartbeat, dizziness, pale skin, shakiness, diaphoresis, unusual hunger, trembling, headache, weakness, irritability, unusual anxiety). Immediately discontinue drug for blood glucose disturbances and switch to a nonfluoroquinolone antibiotic if possible.

🔴 *Alert:* Monitor patients receiving systemic drug for psychiatric adverse reactions (disturbances in attention, disorientation, agitation, nervousness, memory impairment, delirium). Discontinue drug for CNS adverse effects, including psychiatric adverse reactions.

• *Look alike–sound alike:* Don't confuse Vigamox with Amoxil.

PATIENT TEACHING

Boxed Warning Warn patient to immediately report signs and symptoms of serious adverse reactions, including unusual joint or tendon pain, muscle weakness, "pins and needles" tingling or prickling sensation, numbness in the arms or legs, confusion, or hallucinations. ∎

🔴 *Alert:* Warn patient to seek immediate medical attention for signs and symptoms of aortic aneurysm.

• Instruct patient in proper drug administration for the formulation prescribed.

• Tell patient to finish entire course of therapy, even if symptoms are relieved.

🔴 *Alert:* Caution patient that significantly low blood glucose levels can occur. Instruct patient how to manage signs and symptoms of low glucose level and to immediately report signs and symptoms to prescriber.

🔴 *Alert:* Advise patient with diabetes that more frequent blood glucose monitoring may be needed during therapy.

🔴 *Alert:* Inform patient to immediately report psychiatric adverse reactions, which can occur after just one dose.

• Instruct patient to contact prescriber and stop drug if allergic reaction, rash, heart palpitations, fainting, or persistent diarrhea occurs.

• Direct patient to contact prescriber, stop drug, rest, and refrain from exercise if pain, inflammation, or tendon rupture occurs.

• Warn patient that drug may cause dizziness and light-headedness. Tell patient to avoid hazardous activities, such as driving or operating machinery, until effects of drug are known.

• Instruct patient to avoid excessive sunlight exposure and UV light and to report photosensitivity reactions to prescriber.

• Tell patient not to wear contact lenses during ophthalmic treatment.

• Instruct patient not to touch ophthalmic dropper tip to anything, including eyes and fingers.

mupirocin
myoo-PEER-oh-sin

Centany

Therapeutic class: Antibacterials (topical)
Pharmacologic class: Antibiotics

AVAILABLE FORMS
Topical cream: 2%
Topical ointment: 2%

INDICATIONS & DOSAGES
➤ **Impetigo (topical ointment)**
Adults and children age 2 months and older: Apply to affected areas t.i.d. Reevaluate patient in 3 to 5 days; may cover affected area with gauze dressing, if needed.

➤ Traumatic skin lesions infected with *Staphylococcus aureus* or *Streptococcus pyogenes* (cream)

Adults and children age 3 months and older: Apply thin film with cotton swab or gauze pad t.i.d. for 10 days; may cover with gauze dressing, if needed. Reevaluate patient if improvement doesn't occur in 3 to 5 days.

➤ To eradicate nasal colonization by MRSA in adults and health care workers (intranasal ointment)

Adults and children age 12 and older: Divide ointment in single-use tube between nostrils (half tube per nostril) b.i.d. for 5 days. After application, close nostrils by pressing together and releasing sides of nose repeatedly for 1 minute to spread ointment throughout nares.

ADMINISTRATION
Topical
• Apply topical ointment and cream with gauze pad or cotton swab to avoid contamination.
• Don't apply topical ointment or cream to the eye or in the nose.
• Patient should not use cosmetics and other skin products on treated area.
Intranasal
• Don't use other nasal products with intranasal ointment.
• Don't apply to the eyes.

ACTION
Inhibits bacterial protein synthesis by reversibly and specifically binding to bacterial isoleucyl transfer-RNA synthetase.

Route	Onset	Peak	Duration
Topical, intranasal	Unknown	Unknown	Unknown

Half-life: 17 to 36 minutes.

ADVERSE REACTIONS
CNS: taste perversion, headache. **EENT:** rhinitis, pharyngitis, burning or stinging with intranasal use. **GI:** nausea. **Respiratory:** respiratory tract congestion, cough with intranasal use. **Skin:** localized burning, erythema with topical use, pain, pruritus, rash, stinging.

INTERACTIONS
None.

EFFECTS ON LAB TEST RESULTS
None reported.

CONTRAINDICATIONS & CAUTIONS
• Contraindicated in patients hypersensitive to drug or its components.
• Use cautiously in patients with burns or large open wounds.
• Use in patients with impaired renal function hasn't been studied.
Dialyzable drug: Unknown.

PREGNANCY-LACTATION-REPRODUCTION
• There are no adequate studies during pregnancy. Use during pregnancy only if clearly needed.
• It isn't known if drug appears in human milk. Use cautiously during breastfeeding.

NURSING CONSIDERATIONS
• Drug isn't for ophthalmic or internal use.
• Prolonged use may cause overgrowth of nonsusceptible bacteria and fungi.
• Prolonged use may cause CDAD, ranging in severity from mild diarrhea to fatal colitis, which can occur more than 2 months after therapy ends. For suspected or confirmed CDAD, drug may need to be discontinued and appropriate therapy initiated.
• Discontinue drug if sensitization or severe local irritation occurs.

PATIENT TEACHING
• Tell patient to notify prescriber immediately if condition doesn't improve or gets worse in 3 to 5 days.
• Advise patient to avoid contact with eyes and if accidental contact occurs, to rinse well with water.
• Urge patient to immediately report diarrhea.
• Tell patient not to use other nasal products with intranasal ointment.
• Warn patient about local adverse reactions related to drug use.
• Caution patient not to use cosmetics or other skin products on treated area.

Reactions in bold italics are *life-threatening*. Interactions may have a *rapid onset* or a ***delayed onset***.

mycophenolate mofetil
my-koe-FIN-oh-late

CellCept

mycophenolate mofetil hydrochloride
CellCept, CellCept Intravenous

mycophenolic acid (mycophenolate sodium)
Myfortic

Therapeutic class: Immunosuppressants
Pharmacologic class: Mycophenolic acid derivatives

AVAILABLE FORMS
mycophenolate mofetil
Capsules 📵: 250 mg
Powder for oral suspension: 200 mg/mL
Tablets: 500 mg
mycophenolate mofetil hydrochloride
Injection: 500 mg/vial
mycophenolic acid
Tablets (extended-release) 📵: 180 mg, 360 mg

INDICATIONS & DOSAGES
Adjust-a-dose (for all indications): If neutropenia develops (ANC less than $1.3 \times 10^3/\mu L$), stop drug or reduce dosage.

➤ **To prevent organ rejection in patients receiving allogeneic renal transplants**
Adults: 1 g IV or PO (regular-release) b.i.d. with corticosteroids and cyclosporine. Or, 720 mg extended-release tablets PO b.i.d.
Children ages 5 to 16 (extended-release): 400 mg/m² BSA PO b.i.d. Maximum dose, 720 mg PO b.i.d. Or, for patients with BSA of 1.19 to 1.58 m², give 540 mg PO b.i.d. If BSA is greater than 1.58 m², give 720 mg PO b.i.d. Extended-release formulation isn't recommended for BSA of less than 1.19 m².
Children ages 3 months to 18 years: For oral suspension, give 600 mg/m² PO b.i.d.; maximum dose is 1 g b.i.d. Or, for patients with BSA of 1.25 to 1.5 m², give 750 mg (capsules) PO b.i.d. If BSA is greater than 1.5 m², give 1 g (tablets or capsules) PO b.i.d.
Adjust-a-dose: For patients with severe chronic renal impairment (GFR less than 25 mL/minute/1.73 m²) outside of immediate

posttransplant period, avoid doses above 1 g b.i.d.

➤ **To prevent organ rejection in patients receiving allogeneic cardiac transplant, in combination with cyclosporine and corticosteroids**
Adults: 1.5 g PO or IV b.i.d.
Children age 3 months to 18 years: For oral suspension, 600 mg/m² PO b.i.d. If well tolerated, may increase maintenance dose to 900 mg/m² b.i.d. Or, for patients with BSA of 1.25 to 1.5 m², 750 mg (capsules) PO b.i.d. If BSA is greater than 1.5 m², give 1 g (tablets or capsules) PO b.i.d.

➤ **To prevent organ rejection in patients receiving allogeneic hepatic transplant, in combination with cyclosporine and corticosteroids**
Adults: 1 g IV b.i.d. or 1.5 g PO b.i.d.
Children age 3 months to 18 years: For oral suspension, 600 mg/m² PO b.i.d. If well tolerated, may increase maintenance dose to 900 mg/m² b.i.d. Or, for patients with BSA of 1.25 to 1.5 m², 750 mg (capsules) PO b.i.d. If BSA is greater than 1.5 m², give 1 g (tablets or capsules) PO b.i.d.

ADMINISTRATION
PO
🚫 *Alert:* Drug is considered a potential mutagen and teratogen. Follow safe-handling procedures when preparing, administering, or dispensing.
• Don't crush tablets; don't open or crush capsules.
• Give on an empty stomach (1 hour before or 2 hours after a meal). In patients who are stable after renal transplant, may give with food if necessary.
• Avoid inhaling powder in capsule or having it contact skin or mucous membranes. If contact occurs, wash skin thoroughly with soap and water, and rinse eyes with water.
• The extended-release tablets are not interchangeable with other forms.
• Suspension may be administered via NG tube with a minimum size 8 French catheter (at least 1.7-mm interior diameter).
IV
▼ Reconstitute using 14 mL of D_5W. Further dilute to 6 mg/1 mL: 1-g doses in 140 mL of D_5W and 1.5-g doses in 210 mL of D_5W.
▼ Never give by rapid or bolus IV injection. Infuse drug over at least 2 hours.

M

▼ Use within 4 hours of reconstitution and dilution.

▼ **Incompatibilities:** Other IV drugs or solutions.

ACTION
Inhibits proliferative response of T and B lymphocytes, suppresses antibody formation by B lymphocytes, and may inhibit recruitment of leukocytes into sites of inflammation and graft rejection.

Route	Onset	Peak	Duration
PO	Unknown	1–1.5 hr	7–18 hr
PO (extended-release)	Unknown	1.5–2.75 hr	8–17 hr
IV	Unknown	Unknown	10–17 hr

Half-life: Oral, 8 to 18 hours; IV, 17 hours.

ADVERSE REACTIONS
CNS: asthenia, fever, headache, pain, tremor, dizziness, insomnia, depression, psychosis, anxiety. **CV:** chest pain, edema, HTN, hypotension, tachycardia, phlebitis, *thrombosis.* **EENT:** conjunctivitis, visual disturbance, ear pain, deafness, pharyngitis. **GI:** abdominal pain, constipation, diarrhea, dyspepsia, nausea, anorexia, oral candidiasis, vomiting, flatulence. **GU:** hematuria, increased creatinine level, increased BUN level, UTI. **Hematologic:** anemia, *leukopenia, thrombocytopenia,* hypochromic anemia, leukocytosis. **Hepatic:** increased liver enzyme levels. **Metabolic:** hyperlipidemia, hyperglycemia, *hyperkalemia, hypokalemia, hypomagnesemia, hypocalcemia,* hyperuricemia, hypophosphatemia, increased LDH level. **Musculoskeletal:** arthralgia, back pain. **Respiratory:** cough, dyspnea, pleural effusion, bronchitis, pneumonia. **Skin:** acne, rash, alopecia, skin carcinoma, ecchymosis. **Other:** infection, *sepsis.*

INTERACTIONS
Drug-drug. *Acyclovir, ganciclovir, valacyclovir, valganciclovir, other drugs that undergo renal tubular secretion:* May increase risk of toxicity for both drugs. Monitor patient closely.
Antacids with magnesium and aluminum hydroxides: May decrease mycophenolate absorption. Give at least 2 hours after mycophenolate.

Azathioprine: May increase risk of bone marrow suppression. Don't use together.
Bile acid sequestrants, cholestyramine, oral activated charcoal, trimethoprim–sulfamethoxazole, other drugs that interfere with enterohepatic recirculation: May interfere with enterohepatic recirculation, reducing mycophenolate bioavailability. Avoid using together.
Cyclosporine, drugs that alter normal GI flora (amoxicillin plus clavulanic acid, ciprofloxacin), rifamycins (rifampin): May decrease mycophenolate level. Monitor response to therapy and increase dosage if necessary.
Drug that modulate glucuronidation (isavuconazole, telmisartan): May increase or decrease mycophenolate level. Monitor patient for efficacy and adverse reactions.
Hormonal contraceptives: May decrease effectiveness of contraceptive. Recommend addition of barrier form of contraception during treatment and for 6 weeks after treatment ends.
Immunosuppressants (sirolimus, tacrolimus): May increase immunosuppression. Monitor patient closely.
Live-virus vaccines: May decrease vaccine effectiveness. Avoid using together.
Norfloxacin and metronidazole: Combined use may decrease mycophenolate level. No effect is seen when given separately. Don't combine with mycophenolate.
PPIs (lansoprazole, pantoprazole): May decrease mycophenolate level. Monitor patient for mycophenolate efficacy.
Probenecid, salicylates: May increase mycophenolate level. Monitor patient closely.
Sevelamer, other calcium-free phosphate binders: May decrease mycophenolate level. Avoid using together. If concomitant use is unavoidable, give 2 hours after mycophenolate to minimize impact on absorption.
Drug-herb. *Cat's claw, echinacea:* May increase immunostimulation. Discourage use together.
Drug-food. *Any food:* May delay absorption of extended-release form. Advise patient to take on an empty stomach 1 hour before or 2 hours after a meal.
Drug-lifestyle. *Sunlight, UV light exposure:* May increase risk of skin cancer. Patient should limit sunlight or UV light exposure.

Reactions in bold italics are *life-threatening*. Interactions may have a *rapid onset* or a *delayed onset*.

EFFECTS ON LAB TEST RESULTS
• May increase cholesterol, BUN, creatinine, LDH, liver enzyme, and glucose levels.
• May decrease phosphorus, calcium, and magnesium levels.
• May increase or decrease potassium level.
• May decrease Hb level and platelet count.
• May increase or decrease WBC count.

CONTRAINDICATIONS & CAUTIONS
• Contraindicated in patients hypersensitive to drug, its ingredients, or mycophenolic acid and in patients sensitive to polysorbate 80.
• Use cautiously in patients with GI disorders. Bleeding and perforation may occur.
• Oral suspension contains aspartame; use cautiously in patients with phenylketonuria.
• Use cautiously in patients with severe renal impairment, diabetes, or liver disease.
• Immunosuppression can lead to increased risk of other infection.
• Determine drug concentrations before and after changes to immunosuppressive therapy are made or when adding or discontinuing concomitant medications.
Dialyzable drug: No.
⚠ *Overdose S&S:* Nausea, vomiting, diarrhea, neutropenia.

PREGNANCY-LACTATION-REPRODUCTION
Boxed Warning Use during pregnancy is associated with increased risk of first-trimester pregnancy loss and congenital malformations. Patients of childbearing potential must be counseled regarding pregnancy prevention and planning and to use acceptable contraception during therapy and for 6 weeks after final dose. ■
• For patients using drug at any time during pregnancy and those becoming pregnant within 6 weeks of discontinuing therapy, prescriber should report pregnancy to the Mycophenolate Pregnancy Registry (1-800-617-8191).
• It isn't known if drug appears in human milk. Breastfeeding isn't recommended during therapy.
• Sexually active male patients or their partners of childbearing potential should use effective contraception during treatment of the male patient and for at least 90 days after final dose.
• Based on animal data, patients shouldn't donate semen during therapy and for 90 days after final dose.

NURSING CONSIDERATIONS
Boxed Warning Increased risk of infection and lymphoma may result from immunosuppression. ■
• Monitor CBC weekly during first month, twice monthly for second and third months, then monthly through first year.
Boxed Warning Drug should only be used by health care providers experienced in immunosuppressive therapy and management of patients with renal, cardiac, or hepatic transplantation and in facilities equipped and staffed with adequate lab and supportive medical resources. ■
• Start drug therapy within 24 hours after transplantation. Use IV form in patients unable to take oral forms.
• IV form can be given for up to 14 days; switch patient to capsules or tablets as soon as oral drugs can be tolerated.
• Monitor liver and renal function.
🕒 *Alert:* Polyomavirus-associated nephropathy, PML, CMV infections, and reactivation of HBV or HCV infection have been reported in patients treated with immunosuppressants. Consider reducing immunosuppressant dosage in patients who develop evidence of new or reactivated viral infections.
🕒 *Alert:* Drugs causing immunosuppression increase the risk of opportunistic infections, including activation of latent viral infections such as BK virus-associated neuropathy, which may lead to serious outcomes, including kidney graft loss.
🕒 *Alert:* Pure red cell aplasia (PRCA) has occurred in patients treated with this drug in combination with other immunosuppressants. Patients may experience fatigue, lethargy, or pallor. PRCA may be reversible with dose reduction or stopping drug. However, this may put graft at risk.

PATIENT TEACHING
• Teach patient safe drug administration and handling for prescribed formulation.
• Stress importance of following treatment as prescribed.
• Inform patient of the importance of follow-up visits and ongoing lab tests during therapy.
• Tell patient of childbearing potential pregnancy testing will be done 1 week before therapy begins and then again 8 to 10 days later. Inform patient that repeat tests should be performed during routine follow-up visits.

M

- Instruct patient to use two forms of contraception during therapy and for 6 weeks after final dose, even if there's a history of infertility. Tell patient to immediately report suspected pregnancy.
- Caution patient not to breastfeed during therapy.
- Tell male patient with partner of childbearing potential to use effective contraception during treatment and for at least 90 days after final dose.
- Advise patient not to donate semen during therapy and for 90 days after final dose.
- Instruct patient not to donate blood during therapy and for at least 6 weeks after final dose because the blood or blood products might be administered to a patient of childbearing potential or during pregnancy.

Boxed Warning Warn patient of the increased risk of infection and lymphoma and other malignancies. ■

- Caution patient to promptly report signs and symptoms of infection (fever, cough, malaise, erythema, wound drainage, pain).
- Advise patient not to drive or operate heavy machinery if somnolence, confusion, dizziness, tremor, or hypotension occurs.
- Instruct patient with increased risk of skin cancer to limit exposure to sunlight and UV light by wearing protective clothing and using a broad-spectrum sunscreen with a high protection factor.

nadolol
nay-DOE-lol

Corgard

Therapeutic class: Antihypertensives, antianginals
Pharmacologic class: Nonselective beta blockers

AVAILABLE FORMS
Tablets: 20 mg, 40 mg, 80 mg, 160 mg❦

INDICATIONS & DOSAGES
Adjust-a-dose (for all indications): If CrCl is 31 to 50 mL/minute, change dosing interval to every 24 to 36 hours; if CrCl is 10 to 30 mL/minute, every 24 to 48 hours; and if CrCl is less than 10 mL/minute, every 40 to 60 hours.

Boxed Warning Abruptly stopping drug may worsen angina and cause MI. Reduce dosage gradually over 1 to 2 weeks. ■

➤ **Angina pectoris**
Adults: 40 mg PO once daily. Increase in 40- to 80-mg increments at 3- to 7-day intervals until optimal response occurs. Usual maintenance dose is 40 to 80 mg once daily; up to 240 mg once daily may be needed.

➤ **HTN**
Adults: 40 mg PO once daily. Increase in 40- to 80-mg increments until optimal response occurs. Usual maintenance dose is 40 to 80 mg once daily. Doses up to 320 mg daily may be needed.

ADMINISTRATION
PO
- Give drug without regard for food.
- Store at room temperature and avoid heat. Protect from light.
- Check apical pulse before giving drug. If slower than 60 beats/minute, withhold drug and call prescriber.

ACTION
Reduces cardiac oxygen demand by blocking catecholamine-induced increases in HR, BP, and force of myocardial contraction. Depresses renin secretion.

Route	Onset	Peak	Duration
PO	Unknown	3–4 hr	17–24 hr

Half-life: About 20 to 24 hours.

ADVERSE REACTIONS
CNS: fatigue, dizziness, drowsiness.
CV: *bradycardia, HF,* hypotension, rhythm and conduction disturbances, peripheral vascular insufficiency (Raynaud phenomenon).

INTERACTIONS
Drug-drug. *Acetylcholinesterase inhibitors, amiodarone, dipyridamole, ivabradine, midodrine:* May enhance bradycardic effect. Monitor HR.
Amphetamine, methylphenidate: May decrease antihypertensive effect. Monitor BP.
Anilidopiperidine opioids: May increase bradycardic and hypotensive effects. Monitor HR and BP.
Antihypertensives: May increase antihypertensive effect. Monitor BP closely.

Reactions in bold italics are *life-threatening*. Interactions may have a *rapid onset* or a *delayed onset*.

Antipsychotics (second-generation atypicals), MAO inhibitors, phenothiazines: May enhance hypotensive effect. Monitor BP.

Barbiturates, calcium channel blockers, diazoxide, duloxetine, levodopa, methoxyflurane, pentoxifylline, PDE5 inhibitors, prostacyclin analogues, quinagolide: May enhance hypotensive effect. Monitor BP.

Beta$_2$ agonists: May diminish bronchodilatory effect. Avoid combination.

Bretylium: May increase bradycardic and AV blockade effects. Monitor HR and BP.

Cardiac glycosides: May cause excessive bradycardia and additive effects on AV conduction. Use together cautiously.

Ceritinib: May increase bradycardic effect. Avoid use together. If use together is necessary, monitor BP and HR.

Cholinergic agonists: May increase potential for cardiac conduction abnormalities and bronchoconstriction. Administer with caution; monitor patient for conduction disturbances.

Disopyramide: May increase bradycardic and negative inotropic effects. Monitor HR and BP.

Dronedarone: May enhance bradycardic effect and increase nadolol serum concentration. Use lower initial nadolol dosage and monitor therapy.

Epinephrine: May decrease patient response to epinephrine for treatment of an allergic reaction. Monitor patient closely for decreased clinical effect.

Ergot derivatives: May increase vasoconstricting effect. Consider other therapies.

Fingolimod: May enhance bradycardic effect. Avoid concomitant use. If not possible, patient should have overnight continuous ECG monitoring after first fingolimod dose. Monitor HR.

Floctafenine, methacholine: May enhance adverse or toxic effect. Avoid combination.

General anesthetics: May increase hypotensive effects. Consider stopping nadolol before surgery.

Insulin, oral antidiabetics: May mask symptoms of hypoglycemia (such as tachycardia), as a result of beta blockade. May also alter dosage requirements in patients with diabetes who are stabilized. Monitor glucose level closely and use with caution in patients with diabetes.

IV lidocaine: May reduce hepatic metabolism of lidocaine, increasing the risk of toxicity. Give bolus doses of lidocaine at a slower rate and monitor lidocaine level closely.

Lacosamide: May enhance AV blockade effect. Monitor patient.

NSAIDs: May decrease antihypertensive effect. Monitor BP and adjust dosage.

Obinutuzumab: May enhance hypotensive effect. Consider withholding nadolol for 12 hours before to 1 hour after infusion of obinutuzumab.

Prazosin: May increase risk of orthostatic hypotension in the early phases of use together. Assist patient to stand slowly until effects are known.

Reserpine: May increase hypotension or bradycardia. Monitor patient for adverse effects, such as dizziness, syncope, and postural hypotension.

Verapamil: May increase effects of both drugs. Monitor cardiac function closely and decrease dosages as necessary.

Drug-herb. *Dong quai, ephedra, garlic, ginseng, licorice, yohimbe:* May worsen HTN or affect fluid and electrolytes. Avoid use.

Drug-food. *Green tea:* May decrease nadolol serum concentration. Discourage use together.

EFFECTS ON LAB TEST RESULTS
• May lead to false-positive aldosterone/renin ratio.

CONTRAINDICATIONS & CAUTIONS
• Contraindicated in patients with bronchial asthma, sinus bradycardia and greater than first-degree heart block (except in patients with functional pacemaker), cardiogenic shock, and overt (uncompensated) HF.
• Use cautiously in patients with HF, chronic bronchitis, emphysema, renal or hepatic impairment, myasthenia gravis, PVD, psoriasis, or psychiatric disease and in patients undergoing major surgery involving general anesthesia. Drug shouldn't be routinely withdrawn before major surgery.
• Generally, patients with bronchospastic disease shouldn't receive beta blockers because they may block bronchodilation.
• Use cautiously in patients with diabetes because beta blockers may mask certain signs and symptoms of hypoglycemia.
• Drug may mask certain signs and symptoms (tachycardia) of hyperthyroidism and precipitate thyroid storm with abrupt

N

withdrawal in patients with suspected thyrotoxicosis.
Dialyzable drug: Yes.
⚠ *Overdose S&S:* Bradycardia, cardiac failure, hypotension, bronchospasm.

PREGNANCY-LACTATION-REPRODUCTION
• Use cautiously during pregnancy and only if benefit justifies fetal risk.
• Monitor fetal growth during pregnancy.
• Monitor neonate exposed to nadolol in utero for bradycardia, respiratory depression, and hypoglycemia.
• Drug appears in human milk. Patient should discontinue breastfeeding or discontinue drug.

NURSING CONSIDERATIONS
• Monitor BP and HR frequently. If patient develops severe hypotension, give vasopressors, as prescribed.
• Drug masks signs and symptoms of shock, hypoglycemia, and hyperthyroidism.
Boxed Warning Abrupt withdrawal of drug may exacerbate ischemic heart disease and in some cases cause MI. If discontinuing nadolol after long-term administration, gradually reduce dosage over 1 to 2 weeks and monitor patient closely. If angina worsens or acute coronary insufficiency develops, temporarily restart nadolol and take other measures to manage unstable angina. Because CAD is common and may be unrecognized, don't discontinue nadolol abruptly in patients treated only for HTN. ∎
• *Look alike–sound alike:* Don't confuse Corgard with Coreg or Cognex.

PATIENT TEACHING
• Explain importance of taking drug as prescribed even when patient feels well.
Boxed Warning Warn patient not to stop drug suddenly. ∎
• Teach patient how to check pulse rate and to check it before each dose. If pulse rate is below 60 beats/minute, tell patient to notify prescriber. Signs or symptoms of slow HR may include dizziness or light-headedness.
• Advise patient with diabetes that drug can mask normal signs or symptoms of low blood glucose level.
• Counsel patient to report pregnancy or plans to become pregnant or to breastfeed.

nafcillin sodium
naf-SIL-in

Therapeutic class: Antibiotics
Pharmacologic class: Penicillinase-resistant penicillins

AVAILABLE FORMS
Infusion: 1-g, 2-g single-dose containers
Infusion or injection: 1-g, 2-g single-dose vials; 10-g multidose vials

INDICATIONS & DOSAGES
Adjust-a-dose (for all indications): In patients with concomitant renal failure and hepatic insufficiency, measure nafcillin serum levels and adjust dosage accordingly. Duration of therapy depends on type and severity of the infection and overall condition of patient. In severe infection, continue for at least 14 days. Continue for at least 48 hours after patient is afebrile and asymptomatic and cultures are negative. Treatment of endocarditis and osteomyelitis may require a longer duration of therapy.
➤ **Systemic infection caused by susceptible organisms (methicillin-sensitive *Staphylococcus aureus*)**
Adults: 500 mg IV every 4 hours, or 500 mg IM every 4 to 6 hours. For severe infections, 1 g IV or IM every 4 hours.
Infants and children weighing less than 40 kg: 25 mg/kg IM b.i.d.
Neonates: 10 mg/kg IM b.i.d.

ADMINISTRATION
• Before giving drug, ensure patient isn't allergic to penicillins or cephalosporins.
• Obtain specimen for culture and sensitivity tests before giving first dose. Begin therapy while awaiting results.
IV
▼ Check container for leaks, cloudiness, or precipitate before use. Discard if present.
▼ Reconstitute and dilute drug according to manufacturer's instructions. Final concentration shouldn't exceed 40 mg/mL.
▼ Give drug by intermittent IV infusion over 30 to 60 minutes, or by direct IV injection over 5 to 10 minutes.
▼ Drug is a vesicant; ensure proper needle or catheter placement before and during infusion.

Reactions in bold italics are ***life-threatening***. Interactions may have a *rapid onset* or a ***delayed onset***.

▼ Reconstituted vials of 10 to 40 mg/mL are stable for 24 hours at room temperature.
▼ **Incompatibilities:** Other drugs.

IM
• Reconstitute with sterile water for injection, NSS for injection, or bacteriostatic water for injection according to manufacturer's instructions. Add 3.4 mL to 1-g vial or 6.6 mL to 2-g vial. Reconstituted vials contain 250 mg/mL.
• For neonates, use sterile water for injection or NSS for injection to avoid the administration of benzyl alcohol.
• Administer clear solution by deep intragluteal IM injection immediately after reconstitution; rotate sites.
• Solutions are stable for 3 days at room temperature, for 7 days if refrigerated, and 90 days if frozen.

ACTION
Inhibits cell-wall synthesis during bacterial multiplication.

Route	Onset	Peak	Duration
IV	Immediate	Immediate	Unknown
IM	Unknown	30–60 min	Unknown

Half-life: About 33 to 61 minutes.

ADVERSE REACTIONS
CNS: *neurotoxicity.* **CV:** thrombophlebitis, vein irritation. **GI:** nausea, *pseudomembranous colitis,* diarrhea, vomiting, CDAD. **GU:** renal tubular damage, interstitial nephritis. **Hematologic:** *agranulocytosis, leukopenia, neutropenia, thrombocytopenia,* anemia, eosinophilia. **Hepatic:** elevated transaminase levels, cholestasis. **Skin:** severe tissue necrosis (with subcutaneous extravasation), injection-site pain and reactions. **Other:** *anaphylaxis,* hypersensitivity reactions.

INTERACTIONS
Drug-drug. *Aminoglycosides:* May have synergistic effect; drugs are chemically and physically incompatible. Don't combine in same IV solution.
Antivirals: May decrease serum concentration of antivirals. Avoid combination.
Bedaquiline: May decrease bedaquiline serum concentration. Avoid combination.
Clozapine: May decrease clozapine serum concentration. Monitor therapy.
Cyclosporine: May cause subtherapeutic cyclosporine levels. Monitor cyclosporine levels.

CYP3A4 substrates: May decrease serum concentration of the substrates. Use with caution.
Deflazacort: May decrease serum concentration of active metabolite(s) of deflazacort. Avoid combination.
Fentanyl: May decrease fentanyl serum concentration. Monitor pain level and watch for withdrawal signs and symptoms.
Guanfacine: May decrease guanfacine serum concentration. Increase guanfacine dosage by up to double when initiating concomitant therapy. Increase guanfacine dosage gradually over 1 to 2 weeks if nafcillin therapy is just starting.
Hormonal contraceptives: May decrease contraceptive effectiveness. Advise use of additional form of contraception during therapy.
Hydrocodone: May decrease hydrocodone serum concentration. Monitor pain level.
Live-virus vaccines: May reduce effectiveness of live-virus vaccine. Don't use concurrently.
Lurasidone: May decrease lurasidone serum concentration. Monitor patient for decreased lurasidone effects.
Methotrexate: May cause methotrexate toxicity. Monitor patient closely.
Probenecid: May increase nafcillin level. Probenecid may be used for this purpose.
Ranolazine: May decrease ranolazine serum concentration. Avoid combination.
Tetracycline: May decrease nafcillin's effectiveness. Avoid concurrent use.
Warfarin: May decrease effects of warfarin. Monitor PT and INR closely.
Zolpidem: May decrease zolpidem serum concentration. Monitor patient.

EFFECTS ON LAB TEST RESULTS
• May increase liver transaminase levels.
• May decrease Hb level and hematocrit and neutrophil, WBC, eosinophil, granulocyte, and platelet counts.
• May cause false-positive Coombs test and false-positive urinary and serum protein levels with sulfosalicylic acid testing, but not with dipstick testing.

CONTRAINDICATIONS & CAUTIONS
• Contraindicated in patients hypersensitive to drug or other penicillins.
• Use cautiously in patients with asthma, GI distress, hepatic impairment, or renal dysfunction and in those with other drug allergies

N

(especially to cephalosporins) because of possible cross-sensitivity.
• Use cautiously in patients with diseases that can be affected by sodium level such as HF; drug may contain a significant amount of sodium.
• Superinfection and CDAD can occur during therapy and up to 2 months after therapy ends. Drug may need to be discontinued and appropriate treatment initiated.
• Drug may infrequently cause renal tubular damage and interstitial nephritis, especially with large IV doses.
• Safety and effectiveness of IV nafcillin in children haven't been determined.
Dialyzable drug: No.
⚠ *Overdose S&S:* Neurotoxic reactions.

PREGNANCY-LACTATION-REPRODUCTION
• Use during pregnancy only if clearly needed.
• Penicillins appear in human milk. Use cautiously during breastfeeding.

NURSING CONSIDERATIONS
• Bacterial or fungal superinfection may occur with large doses or prolonged therapy, especially in older adults and patients who are debilitated or immunosuppressed.
• Serious and fatal hypersensitivity reactions can occur, including anaphylactic reactions requiring treatment with epinephrine. Obtain complete drug allergy history and monitor patient during and after drug administration.
• Obtain samples for urinalysis and BUN and creatinine values before and periodically during therapy.
• Obtain LFTs before and periodically during therapy, especially when using high nafcillin doses.
• Monitor WBC counts twice weekly in patients receiving drug for longer than 2 weeks. Neutropenia commonly occurs in the third week.
• Monitor patient for signs and symptoms of interstitial nephritis (abnormal urinalysis results, rash, fever, eosinophilia, hematuria, proteinuria, renal insufficiency).
• Monitor IV site; skin sloughing from subcutaneous extravasation may occur.

PATIENT TEACHING
• Tell patient to report burning or irritation at the IV site.

• Caution patient to take drug exactly as directed. Skipping doses or not completing full course may decrease effectiveness and increase likelihood that bacteria will develop resistance.
• Advise patient to notify prescriber of all adverse reactions, especially rash or signs and symptoms of superinfection (recurring fever, chills, malaise) or CDAD (unexplained diarrhea).

SAFETY ALERT!

nalbuphine hydrochloride
NAL-byoo-feen

Nubain✦

Therapeutic class: Opioid analgesics
Pharmacologic class: Opioid agonist-antagonists–opioid partial agonists

AVAILABLE FORMS
Injection: 10 mg/mL, 20 mg/mL

INDICATIONS & DOSAGES
Adjust-a-dose (for all indications): In patients with renal or hepatic impairment, decrease dosage.
➤ **Moderate to severe pain (non-opioid-tolerant patients)**
Adults: For patient weighing about 70 kg, 10 to 20 mg subcut, IM, or IV every 3 to 6 hours PRN. Maximum, 160 mg daily. Adjust dosage according to the severity of pain, physical status, and other drugs patient is receiving.
➤ **Adjunct to balanced anesthesia; preoperative and postoperative analgesia; obstetric analgesia during labor and delivery**
Adults: 0.3 to 3 mg/kg IV over 10 to 15 minutes; then maintenance dose of 0.25 to 0.5 mg/kg in single IV dose PRN.

ADMINISTRATION
IV
▼ Inject slowly over at least 2 to 3 minutes into a vein or into an IV line containing a compatible, free-flowing IV solution, such as D_5W, NSS, or lactated Ringer solution. Administer larger doses (0.3 to 3 mg/kg) over 10 to 15 minutes.
▼ Respiratory depression can be reversed with naloxone. Keep oxygen and resuscitation and intubation equipment available, particularly when giving IV.

Reactions in bold italics are *life-threatening*. Interactions may have a *rapid onset* or a *delayed onset*.

▼ Store at room temperature; protect from excessive light.

▼ **Incompatibilities:** None listed by manufacturer. Consult a drug incompatibility reference for more information.

IM
• Document injection site.
• Store vial in carton to protect from light.

Subcutaneous
• Document injection site.
• Store vial in carton to protect from light.

ACTION

Unknown. Binds with opioid receptors in the CNS, altering perception of and emotional response to pain. Drug is an agonist at kappa opioid receptors and an antagonist at mu opioid receptors.

Route	Onset	Peak	Duration
IV	2–3 min	2–3 min	3–6 hr
IM, subcut	<15 min	<15 min	3–6 hr

Half-life: 5 hours.

ADVERSE REACTIONS

CNS: dizziness, headache, sedation, vertigo. **CV:** *bradycardia,* hypotension. **EENT:** dry mouth. **GI:** nausea, vomiting. **Respiratory:** *respiratory depression.* **Skin:** clamminess, diaphoresis.

INTERACTIONS

Drug-drug. *Anticholinergics:* May increase risk of adverse effects. Monitor patient for urine retention and constipation.

Boxed Warning *Benzodiazepines, CNS depressants, opioids:* May cause respiratory depression, profound sedation, coma, and death. Avoid use together unless alternative treatment options are inadequate. If use together is necessary, limit dosage and duration of each drug to minimum necessary for desired effect. Monitor patient response closely. ∎

Diuretics: May reduce efficacy of diuretics. Monitor therapy.

MAO inhibitors (linezolid, phenelzine, tranylcypromine): May increase risk of serotonin syndrome or opioid toxicity. Avoid using MAO inhibitors during treatment and don't use drug within 14 days of MAO inhibitor therapy.

Naltrexone: May result in opioid withdrawal signs and symptoms and decreased opioid effectiveness. Avoid combination.

🍵 *Alert: Serotonergic drugs (amoxapine, antiemetics [dolasetron, granisetron, ondansetron, palonosetron], antimigraine drugs, buspirone, cyclobenzaprine, dextromethorphan, lithium, maprotiline, methylene blue, mirtazapine, nefazodone, SSNRIs, SSRIs, TCAs, trazodone, tryptophan, vilazodone):* May increase risk of serotonin syndrome. Use together cautiously. Monitor patient for serotonin syndrome.

Drug-lifestyle. **Boxed Warning** *Alcohol use:* May cause additive effects. Avoid use together. ∎

🍵 *Alert: St. John's wort:* May increase risk of serotonin syndrome. Use together cautiously. Monitor patient for serotonin syndrome.

EFFECTS ON LAB TEST RESULTS

• May interfere with enzymatic methods for detection of opioids.

CONTRAINDICATIONS & CAUTIONS

• Contraindicated in patients hypersensitive to drug or its components and in those with significant respiratory depression, known or suspected GI obstruction (including paralytic ileus), and acute or severe asthma in an unmonitored setting or in the absence of resuscitative equipment.

• Use cautiously and at low doses in patients with preexisting respiratory compromise.

🍵 *Alert:* Drug should only be administered as a supplement to general anesthesia by those specifically trained in the use of IV anesthetics and management of respiratory effects of potent opioids. Naloxone hydrochloride and emergency resuscitative equipment should be readily available.

🍵 *Alert:* Patients are at increased risk for oversedation and respiratory depression if they snore or have a history of sleep apnea, haven't used opioids recently or are first-time opioid users, have increased opioid dosage requirements or opioid habituation, have received general anesthesia for longer lengths of time or received other sedating drugs, have preexisting pulmonary or cardiac disease, or have thoracic or other surgical incisions that may impair breathing. Monitor patients carefully.

🍵 *Alert:* Drug may lead to a rare but serious decrease in adrenal gland cortisol production.

• Drug may cause decreased sex hormone levels with long-term use.

N

• Use cautiously in patients with history of drug abuse, in patients with cachexia or debilitation, in older adults, and in those with emotional instability, head injury, increased ICP, impaired ventilation, MI accompanied by nausea and vomiting, upcoming biliary surgery, seizure disorders, or hepatic, renal, or adrenal insufficiency.

• Drug may cause mood disorders and osteoporosis.

🔸 *Alert:* Certain commercial preparations contain sodium metabisulfite.

Dialyzable drug: Unknown.

⚠ *Overdose S&S:* Sleepiness, mild dysphoria.

PREGNANCY-LACTATION-REPRODUCTION

• There are no adequate studies during pregnancy. Use only if clearly needed.

🔸 *Alert:* When used for pain relief during labor, fetal bradycardia can occur. Monitor fetuses and newborns for bradycardia.

• Prolonged use of drug during pregnancy can result in neonatal withdrawal syndrome, which may be life-threatening and which requires management according to neonatology expert protocols.

• Use cautiously during breastfeeding.

• Monitor infant for excess sedation and respiratory depression. Withdrawal signs and symptoms can occur with stoppage of maternal opioid use or stoppage of breastfeeding.

• Long-term opioid use can cause secondary hypogonadism, infertility, and sexual dysfunction.

NURSING CONSIDERATIONS

• Reassess pain level at least 15 and 30 minutes after parenteral administration.

🔸 *Alert:* Carefully monitor vital signs, pain level, respiratory status, and sedation level in all patients receiving opioids, especially those receiving IV drugs, even those given postoperatively.

Boxed Warning Concomitant use of opioids with benzodiazepines or other CNS depressants, including alcohol, may result in profound sedation, respiratory depression, coma, and death. ▪

Boxed Warning Drug can cause life-threatening or fatal respiratory depression. Monitor patient for respiratory depression, especially within first 24 to 72 hours of the start of therapy and after dosage increase. ▪

• Before starting drug, assess patient's risk of opioid abuse, misuse, and addiction.

Regularly monitor patients for development of these behaviors or conditions.

🔸 *Alert:* If patient is taking opioids with serotonergic drugs, watch for signs and symptoms of serotonin syndrome (agitation, hallucinations, rapid HR, fever, diaphoresis, shivering or shaking, muscle twitching or stiffness, trouble with coordination, nausea, vomiting, diarrhea), especially at start of therapy and after dosage increase. Signs and symptoms may occur within several hours of coadministration but may also occur later, especially after dosage increase. Discontinue opioid, serotonergic drug, or both if serotonin syndrome is suspected.

🔸 *Alert:* Monitor patient for signs and symptoms of adrenal insufficiency (nausea, vomiting, loss of appetite, fatigue, weakness, dizziness, low BP). Perform diagnostic testing if adrenal insufficiency is suspected. For confirmed adrenal insufficiency, treat with corticosteroids and wean patient off opioids if appropriate. Discontinue corticosteroids when clinically appropriate.

• Monitor patient for signs and symptoms of decreased sex hormone levels (low libido, erectile dysfunction, amenorrhea, infertility). If signs and symptoms occur, evaluate patient and obtain lab testing.

🔸 *Alert:* Don't stop drug abruptly; withdraw slowly and individualize the gradual tapering plan to prevent signs and symptoms of withdrawal, worsening pain, and psychological distress in patients who are physically dependent. Refer to manufacturer's label for specific tapering instructions.

🔸 *Alert:* When tapering opioids, monitor patient closely for signs and symptoms of opioid withdrawal (restlessness, lacrimation, rhinorrhea, yawning, perspiration, chills, myalgia, mydriasis, irritability, anxiety, insomnia, backache, joint pain, weakness, abdominal cramps, anorexia, nausea, vomiting, diarrhea, increased BP or HR, increased respiratory rate); such symptoms may indicate a need to taper more slowly. Also monitor patient for suicidality, use of other substances, and mood changes.

• For patients who have received long-term therapy, taper dose by 25% to 50% every 2 to 4 days. If signs or symptoms of withdrawal occur, increase dosage to the previous level; then taper more slowly.

• Monitor circulatory and respiratory status and bladder and bowel function. If

---

Reactions in bold italics are *life-threatening*. Interactions may have a *rapid onset* or a *delayed onset*.

respirations are shallow or rate is below 12 breaths/minute, withhold dose and notify prescriber.

• Severe constipation commonly occurs with maintenance therapy. Make sure stool softener or other stimulant laxative is ordered.

• Monitor patient with a history of seizures for worsening of seizure control.

• Psychological and physical dependence may occur with prolonged use.

• *Look alike–sound alike:* Don't confuse Nubain with Navane or Nebcin. Don't confuse nalbuphine with naloxone.

PATIENT TEACHING

🔵 *Alert:* Encourage patient to report all medications being taken, including prescription and OTC medications and supplements.

🔵 *Alert:* Counsel patient not to discontinue opioids without first discussing with prescriber the need for a gradual tapering regimen.

Boxed Warning Caution patient or caregiver of patient taking an opioid with a benzodiazepine, CNS depressant, or alcohol to seek immediate medical attention for dizziness, light-headedness, extreme sleepiness, slowed or difficult breathing, or unresponsiveness. ■

🔵 *Alert:* Caution patient to immediately report signs and symptoms of serotonin syndrome.

• Caution patient who is ambulatory about getting out of bed or walking. Warn outpatient to avoid driving and other hazardous activities that require mental alertness until drug's CNS effects are known.

• Teach patient that naloxone is prescribed in conjunction with the opioid when treatment is started or renewed as a preventive measure to reduce opioid overdose and death.

• Ensure someone close to patient knows how to administer naloxone.

• Teach patient to report adverse effects and how to manage troublesome adverse effects such as constipation.

• Tell patient to report pregnancy or plans to become pregnant or to breastfeed.

naloxone hydrochloride
nal-OX-one

Kloxxado, Narcan, S.O.S. Naloxone ✦, Zimhi

Therapeutic class: Antidotes
Pharmacologic class: Opioid antagonists

AVAILABLE FORMS

Injection: 0.4 mg/mL, 1 mg/mL
Injection (autoinjector): 10 mg/0.4 mL
Injection (prefilled syringe): 5 mg/0.5 mL, 2 mg/2 mL
Nasal spray: 2 mg/0.1 mL, 4 mg/0.1 mL, 8 mg/0.1 mL

INDICATIONS & DOSAGES

➤ **Known or suspected opioid-induced respiratory depression, including that caused by pentazocine, methadone, nalbuphine, and butorphanol**

Adults: 0.4 to 2 mg IV, IM, or subcut. Repeat dose every 2 to 3 minutes PRN. If patient doesn't respond after 10 mg have been given, question diagnosis of opioid-induced toxicity. After reversal, additional dose(s) may be needed at a later interval (e.g., 20 to 60 minutes) depending on type and duration of opioid.

Children age 1 month and older: 0.01 mg/kg IV; then, second dose of 0.1 mg/kg IV, if needed. If IV route isn't available, drug may be given IM or subcut in divided doses.

Neonates: 0.01 mg/kg IV, IM, or subcut. Repeat dose every 2 to 3 minutes PRN.

➤ **Postoperative opioid depression**

Adults: 0.1 to 0.2 mg IV every 2 to 3 minutes PRN. Repeat doses may be required within 1- or 2-hour intervals depending on amount, type (short- or long-acting), and time interval since last administration. Supplemental IM doses have produced a longer-lasting effect.

Children: 0.005 to 0.01 mg IV repeated every 2 to 3 minutes PRN.

➤ **Emergency treatment of known or suspected opioid overdose**

Adults and children: 0.4 to 2 mg, or 5 mg/ 0.5 mL (Zimhi) IM or subcut. If desired response doesn't occur after 2 or 3 minutes, may give another dose. If still no response and additional doses are available, give every 2 or 3 minutes until emergency medical assistance arrives.

N

Or, contents of 1 nasal spray (4 mg or 8 mg) intranasally as a single dose; may repeat dose every 2 to 3 minutes in alternating nostrils until emergency medical assistance arrives. In neonates with known or suspected exposure to maternal opioid use, consider using another form to allow dosing according to weight and titration to effect.

Adjust-a-dose: Restrict prescription of naloxone 2-mg nasal spray to patients who are opioid-dependent and expected to be at risk for severe opioid withdrawal in situations in which there is low risk of accidental or intentional opioid exposure by household contacts.

➤ **Temporary prophylaxis of respiratory or CNS depression in military personnel and chemical incident responders entering area contaminated with high-potency opioids**

Adults: 10 mg (contents of one autoinjector) IM or subcut as a single dose immediately before entering area with suspected contamination; may repeat for prolonged exposure.

➤ **Emergency treatment of respiratory or CNS depression caused by suspected chemical weapon use of high-potency opioids**

Adults and children age 12 and older: 10 mg (contents of one autoinjector) IM or subcut as a single dose; may repeat as needed until emergency medical assistance arrives.

➤ **Opioid-induced pruritus ◆**

Adults: 0.25 mcg/kg/hour IV. Monitor pain control; verify that drug isn't reversing analgesia.

ADMINISTRATION

IV

▼ Give IV push undiluted over 30 seconds.

▼ Give continuous infusion to control adverse effects of epidural morphine.

▼ For continuous infusion, dilute 2 mg of drug in 500 mL D_5W or NSS to yield a concentration of 0.004 mg/mL; use within 24 hours.

▼ Titrate rate to patient's response.

▼ **Incompatibilities:** Alkaline solutions, amphotericin B cholesteryl sulfate, preparations containing bisulfite, sulfite, long-chain or high-molecular-weight anions.

IM

• May give IM into large muscle, such as upper arm, buttocks, or thigh.

• Use mixtures within 24 hours. After 24 hours, discard.

• Use prefilled syringe or autoinjector, if available, to administer drug into anterolateral thigh, through clothing if necessary. In children younger than age 1, pinch thigh muscle while administering.

• Refer to manufacturer's instructions for directions for specific device.

Intranasal

• Don't prime or test the device before administration.

• Each container contains a single intranasal spray; don't reuse.

• To administer nasal spray, place patient in the supine position and support the back of the neck to allow the head to tilt back. After administration, turn patient on side.

• If repeat administration is necessary, use a new container and alternate nostrils.

Subcutaneous

• May give undiluted or, if necessary, diluted in sterile water for injection to obtain weight-based dose.

• Use prefilled syringe or autoinjector, if available, to administer drug into anterolateral thigh, through clothing if necessary. In children younger than age 1, pinch thigh muscle while administering.

ACTION

May displace opioid analgesics from their receptors (competitive antagonism); drug has no pharmacologic activity of its own.

Route	Onset	Peak	Duration
IV	1–2 min	5–15 min	Variable
IM, subcut	2–5 min	5–15 min	Variable
Intranasal	8–13 min	20–30 min	Variable

Half-life: IV, IM, or subcut, 30 to 81 minutes in adults, 3 hours in neonates; intranasal, about 2 hours.

ADVERSE REACTIONS

CNS: *seizures,* tremors, headache, dizziness, light-headedness, asthenia, presyncope, agitation, irritability, tremor, nervousness, paresthesia, restlessness, shivering, pain, coma, confusion, fever, yawning, *encephalopathy,* hallucination; excessive crying, hyperreflexia in neonates. **CV:** *ventricular fibrillation, ventricular tachycardia,* increased BP, hypotension, tachycardia. **EENT:** nasal dryness, edema, congestion, inflammation, rhinalgia, rhinitis, rhinorrhea, sneezing, toothache. **GI:** nausea, vomiting, constipation, abdominal pain, abdominal cramps. **GU:** elevated

---

Reactions in bold italics are *life-threatening*. Interactions may have a *rapid onset* or a *delayed onset*.

bilirubin level. **Musculoskeletal:** pain, muscle spasm. **Respiratory:** *pulmonary edema.* **Skin:** diaphoresis, piloerection, injection-site pain and erythema, dry skin. **Other:** hot flash, withdrawal symptoms in patients who are opioid-dependent.

INTERACTIONS

Drug-drug. *Methylnaltrexone, naldemedine, naloxegol:* May enhance risk of opioid withdrawal. Avoid combination.

Partial opioid agonists, mixed opioid agonists-antagonists (buprenorphine, pentazocine): May cause incomplete reversal or require repeated dosing of naloxone due to long duration of action and slow binding rate of these drugs. Monitor patient for continued respiratory depression.

EFFECTS ON LAB TEST RESULTS

None reported.

CONTRAINDICATIONS & CAUTIONS

• Contraindicated in patients hypersensitive to drug.

🜂 *Alert:* Use cautiously in patients with cardiac irritability or opioid addiction. Abrupt reversal of opioid-induced CNS depression may result in sudden opioid withdrawal signs and symptoms (such as nausea, vomiting, diaphoresis, tachycardia, CNS excitement, and increased BP).

🜂 *Alert:* In infants younger than age 4 weeks, sudden opioid withdrawal can be life-threatening. Signs and symptoms include excessive crying, increased reflexes, and seizures.

• Use cautiously in patients with a history of seizures; avoid use in meperidine-induced seizures.

Dialyzable drug: Unknown.

PREGNANCY-LACTATION-REPRODUCTION

• Use during pregnancy only if there's a clear indication for its use. Don't withhold drug because of fears of teratogenicity.

• Drug crosses the placental barrier and may precipitate withdrawal in the fetus and the opioid-dependent mother. Monitor fetus for distress.

• It isn't known if drug appears in human milk. Use cautiously; however, because drug is used for opioid reversal, consider the opioid concentration in the milk during breastfeeding and potential transfer of the opioid to the infant.

NURSING CONSIDERATIONS

• Duration of action of the opioid may exceed that of naloxone, and patients may relapse into respiratory depression. Monitor patients closely and repeat dose if needed.

• Respiratory rate increases within 1 to 2 minutes.

• Abrupt postoperative reversal of opioid depression may result in adverse CV effects; monitor patients closely.

🜂 *Alert:* Drug only reverses respiratory depression caused by opioids; it doesn't reverse other drug-induced respiratory depression, including that caused by benzodiazepines.

• Monitor patients, especially infants younger than age 4 weeks, for opioid withdrawal signs and symptoms.

• Patients who receive drug to reverse opioid-induced respiratory depression may exhibit tachypnea.

• Monitor respiratory depth and rate. Provide oxygen, ventilation, and other resuscitation measures.

• Carefully observe administration site for signs or symptoms of infection after the opioid emergency.

• *Look alike–sound alike:* Don't confuse naloxone with naltrexone.

PATIENT TEACHING

• Reassure family that patient will be monitored closely until effects of opioid resolve.

• Teach patient and family about signs and symptoms of opioid toxicity emergency (unusual sleepiness or inability to awaken the person, breathing problems, pinpoint pupils).

• Counsel family to give naloxone immediately for suspected overdose.

• Advise person who will be administering intranasal drug to read instructions carefully before use. Remind the person that the spray is single-use only; if signs and symptoms of an opioid emergency return, a second container must be used.

• Instruct person who will be administering drug to seek emergency help immediately after giving first dose and to give additional doses every 2 to 3 minutes if patient doesn't respond or relapses into respiratory depression before emergency assistance arrives.

• Warn patient and caregivers that naloxone administration can precipitate acute opioid withdrawal symptoms, which can be fatal in neonates.

N

naltrexone
nal-TREX-one

Vivitrol

naltrexone hydrochloride
Revia✦

Therapeutic class: Antidotes
Pharmacologic class: Opioid antagonists, antidotes

AVAILABLE FORMS
naltrexone
Injection: 380-mg vial dose kit
naltrexone hydrochloride
Tablets: 25 mg, 50 mg, 100 mg

INDICATIONS & DOSAGES
➤ **Adjunct for maintaining opioid-free state in patients who are detoxified**
Adults: Initially, 25 mg PO. If no withdrawal signs or symptoms occur after initiation, may start patient on 50 mg every 24 hours the following day. Or, 50 mg PO every weekday with a 100-mg dose on Saturday, 100 mg every other day, or 150 mg every third day. Or, 380 mg IM in gluteal muscle every 4 weeks or once a month.
➤ **Alcohol dependence**
Adults: 50 mg PO once daily for up to 12 weeks, or 380 mg IM in gluteal muscle every 4 weeks or once monthly.

ADMINISTRATION
• Don't give to patients who haven't been opioid free for at least 7 to 10 days. May consider a naloxone challenge test.
PO
• Keep container tightly closed and protect from light.
• Give without regard to meals; give with food if GI upset occurs.
IM
• Vivitrol must be prepared and administered by a health care provider.
• Use only the diluent, needles, and other components supplied with the dose kit. Don't substitute.
• Allow drug to reach room temperature before administering (about 45 minutes).
• Administer IM into gluteal muscle, alternating buttocks for each subsequent administration. Avoid giving IV, subcut, or inadvertently into fatty tissue. Monitor injection site.
• Store in refrigerator or up to 7 days at controlled room temperature. Don't freeze.
• Give missed dose as soon as possible.

ACTION
Probably reversibly blocks the effects of exogenous opioids by competitively occupying opiate receptors in the brain. Mechanism of action in alcohol dependence is unknown; however, may be related to the endogenous system.

Route	Onset	Peak	Duration
PO	15–30 min	1 hr	24–72 hr
IM	Unknown	2 hr	>30 days

Half-life: PO, about 4 hours; IM, 5 to 10 days.

ADVERSE REACTIONS
CNS: insomnia, anxiety, nervousness, headache, depression, dizziness, fatigue, somnolence, syncope, low energy, increased energy, irritability, nervousness, suicidality, depression. **CV:** HTN. **EENT:** dry mouth, nasopharyngitis, toothache. **GI:** nausea, diarrhea, vomiting, abdominal pain, anorexia, constipation, increased thirst, decreased appetite. **GU:** delayed ejaculation, decreased potency. **Hepatic:** hepatic enzyme abnormalities. **Musculoskeletal:** muscle and joint pain, muscle cramps, back pain. **Skin:** injection-site reaction, rash. **Other:** chills, flulike symptoms.

INTERACTIONS
Drug-drug. *Bremelanotide:* May decrease naltrexone's effects. Avoid use together.
Methylnaltrexone, naldemedine, naloxegol: May enhance adverse effects; increases risk of opioid withdrawal. Avoid use together.
Products that contain opioids (including certain cough medications, antidiarrheals): May decrease effect of opioid. Avoid using together.
Thioridazine: May cause lethargy and somnolence. Monitor patient closely.

EFFECTS ON LAB TEST RESULTS
• May increase AST and ALT levels.
• May increase WBC count.
• May interfere with enzymatic methods for detecting opioids in urine.

Reactions in bold italics are *life-threatening*. Interactions may have a *rapid onset* or a ***delayed onset***.

CONTRAINDICATIONS & CAUTIONS

• Contraindicated in patients hypersensitive to drug or components of the diluent, those currently dependent on opioids, those receiving opioid analgesics, those who fail the naloxone challenge test or who have a positive urine screen for opioids, or those in acute opioid withdrawal.

• Drug may precipitate opioid withdrawal.

• Fatal overdose may occur if patient uses opioids at the end of a dosing interval, after missing a dose, or after discontinuing treatment. Attempts by patient to overcome blockade may also lead to fatal overdose.

• Dose-related hepatic injury may occur. Use cautiously in patients with mild hepatic disease or history of recent hepatic disease.

• Administer IM injection cautiously to patients with thrombocytopenia or coagulation disorders (hemophilia and severe liver failure).

• Suicidality and depression have been noted in postmarketing reports.

• Drug should be part of a comprehensive treatment plan that includes psychosocial support.

• Safety and effectiveness in children haven't been evaluated.

Dialyzable drug: Unknown.

⚠ *Overdose S&S:* Injection-site reaction, nausea, abdominal pain, somnolence, dizziness.

PREGNANCY-LACTATION-REPRODUCTION

• Use during pregnancy only if potential benefit justifies fetal risk.

• Drug may appear in human milk. Use cautiously during breastfeeding.

NURSING CONSIDERATIONS

🜨 *Alert:* Patient must be completely free from opioids before taking naltrexone or severe withdrawal symptoms may occur. Patients who have been addicted to short-acting opioids, such as heroin and meperidine, must wait at least 7 days after last opioid dose before starting drug. Patients who have been addicted to longer-acting opioids such as methadone should wait at least 10 days.

• Don't begin treatment for opioid dependence until patient receives naloxone challenge, a test of opioid dependence. If signs and symptoms of opioid withdrawal persist after naloxone challenge, don't give drug.

• In an emergency, patient may be given an opioid analgesic, but dose must be higher than usual to overcome naltrexone's effect. Watch for respiratory depression from the opioid; it may be longer and deeper.

🜨 *Alert:* Discontinue drug if patient develops signs or symptoms of acute hepatitis.

• Monitor patient for depression and suicidality.

• Patients expected to be nonadherent because of history of opioid dependence may benefit from flexible maintenance-dose regimen of 100 mg on Monday and Wednesday and 150 mg on Friday.

• Monitor patient for an injection-site reaction, including pain, tenderness, swelling, erythema, bruising, or pruritus. In some cases, an injection-site reaction may be very severe, with induration, cellulitis, hematoma, abscess, sterile abscess, and necrosis.

• Use drug only as part of a comprehensive rehabilitation program.

• *Look alike–sound alike:* Don't confuse naltrexone with naloxone or methylnaltrexone.

PATIENT TEACHING

• Advise patient to carry medical identification and to inform medical personnel about taking naltrexone.

• Tell patient that drug can block the effects of opioids and opioid-like drugs, including heroin, pain medicine, antidiarrheals, or cough medicine.

🜨 *Alert:* Warn patient that using large doses of heroin or any other opioid can cause serious injury, coma, or death.

• Advise patient who previously used opioids that patient may be more sensitive to lower doses of opioids after naltrexone therapy.

• Warn patient of risk of hepatic injury and to seek medical attention if signs or symptoms of acute hepatitis occur.

🜨 *Alert:* Tell caregiver of patient dependent on alcohol to monitor patient closely for signs of depression or suicidality and to report this immediately to prescriber.

• Provides names of nonopioid drugs that patient can continue to take for pain, diarrhea, or cough.

• Tell patient to report pain, swelling, tenderness, induration, bruising, pruritus, or redness at the injection site.

• Advise patient to immediately report signs and symptoms of allergic reaction, including

N

hives, dyspnea, coughing, trouble swallowing or talking, wheezing, or facial swelling.
• Counsel patient to report pregnancy or plans to become pregnant.

naproxen
na-PROX-en

EC-Naprosyn, Naprosyn

naproxen sodium
Aleve ◇, Anaprox DS, Flanax Pain Relief ◇, Maxidol ◇, Mediproxen ◇, Motrimax ◇, Naprelan

Therapeutic class: NSAIDs
Pharmacologic class: NSAIDs

AVAILABLE FORMS
naproxen
Oral suspension: 125 mg/5 mL
Tablets: 250 mg, 375 mg, 500 mg
Tablets (delayed-release) DNC: 375 mg, 500 mg, 750 mg
naproxen sodium
Capsules: 220 mg ◇
Tablets (extended-release) DNC: 375 mg, 500 mg, 750 mg
Tablets (film-coated) DNC: 220 mg ◇, 275 mg, 550 mg
Note: 220 mg of naproxen sodium contains 200 mg of naproxen

INDICATIONS & DOSAGES
Adjust-a-dose (for all indications): Consider lower dosage in older adults and patients with renal or hepatic impairment. Not recommended for patients with moderate or severe renal impairment (CrCl less than 30 mL/minute).
➤ **Temporary relief of minor aches and pains; fever reduction (naproxen sodium)**
Adults and children age 12 and older: 220 mg immediate-release PO every 8 to 12 hours while symptoms last. May give 440 mg within first hour. Maximum dosage, 440 mg in any 8- to 12-hour period and 660 mg in a 24-hour period.
➤ **Acute gout**
Adults: 750 mg naproxen PO; then 250 mg every 8 hours until attack subsides. Or, 825 mg naproxen sodium PO; then 275 mg every 8 hours until attack subsides. Or, 1,000 to 1,500 mg extended-release tablets PO on day 1, followed by 1,000 mg daily until attack subsides.
➤ **Acute tendinitis, bursitis, pain, primary dysmenorrhea**
Adults: 550 mg naproxen sodium PO, then 550 mg PO every 12 hours or 275 mg every 6 to 8 hours. Initial total daily dose shouldn't exceed 1,375 mg; thereafter, total daily dose shouldn't exceed 1,100 mg. Or, 500 mg naproxen PO followed by 500 mg PO every 12 hours or 250 mg PO every 6 to 8 hours. Total daily dose shouldn't exceed 1,250 mg on day 1, or 1,000 mg thereafter. Or, 1,000 mg extended-release tablets PO once daily for a limited time.
➤ **Ankylosing spondylitis, osteoarthritis, RA**
Adults: 275 to 550 mg naproxen sodium PO b.i.d. Or, 250 to 500 mg naproxen tablet or suspension PO b.i.d. Or, 375 or 500 mg naproxen delayed-release tablet PO b.i.d. Or, 750 to 1,000 mg extended-release tablets PO once daily. During long-term administration, may adjust naproxen dose up or down depending on clinical response. In patients who tolerate lower doses well, may increase dose to 1,500 mg/day when a higher level of anti-inflammatory or analgesic activity is required.
➤ **Juvenile idiopathic arthritis**
Children age 2 and older: 10 mg/kg naproxen suspension PO daily in two divided doses. Don't exceed 15 mg/kg/day.

ADMINISTRATION
PO
Alert: Different dosage strengths and formulations (e.g., tablets, suspension) aren't interchangeable. Consider this difference when changing strengths or formulations.
• Give drug with food, milk, or antacids to minimize GI upset. Have patient drink a full glass of water or other liquid with each dose.
• Shake suspension well.
• Make sure patient swallows delayed-release, extended-release, and film-coated tablets whole and doesn't break, crush, or chew them.

ACTION
May inhibit prostaglandin synthesis to produce anti-inflammatory, analgesic, and antipyretic effects.

Route	Onset	Peak	Duration
PO (immediate-release)	30–60 min	2–4 hr (naproxen) 1–2 hr (naproxen sodium)	<12 hr
PO (delayed-release)	30–60 min	4–6 hr	<12 hr
PO (suspension)	60 min	1–4 hr	<12 hr

Half-life: 12 to 17 hours.

ADVERSE REACTIONS

CNS: dizziness, drowsiness, headache, vertigo, paresthesia, insomnia, asthenia, pain, fever. **CV:** edema, palpitations, chest pain, HTN. **EENT:** visual disturbances, tinnitus, auditory disturbances, pharyngitis, rhinitis, sinusitis. **GI:** abdominal pain, constipation, diarrhea, dyspepsia, dysphasia, flatulence, epigastric pain, heartburn, nausea, occult blood loss, peptic ulceration, stomatitis, thirst, vomiting. **GU:** UTI, cystitis. **Hematologic:** ecchymoses, increased bleeding time, anemia. **Musculoskeletal:** arthralgia, arthropathy, cramps, myalgia, tendinopathy, back pain. **Respiratory:** dyspnea, cough, bronchitis. **Skin:** diaphoresis, pruritus, purpura, rash. **Other:** flulike syndrome.

INTERACTIONS

Drug-drug. *Antacids, cholestyramine:* May delay naproxen absorption. Avoid concomitant use.
Anticoagulants (warfarin), antiplatelets (aspirin), corticosteroids, other NSAIDs, salicylates, TCAs: May cause adverse GI reactions and bleeding. Avoid use together.
Antihypertensives (ACE inhibitors, ARBs, beta blockers), diuretics: May decrease effect of these drugs. Monitor patient.
ARBs, ACE inhibitors, tacrolimus: May cause renal impairment. Use together cautiously.
Cyclosporine: May increase risk of nephrotoxicity. Monitor renal function; consider therapy modification.
Digoxin: May increase serum digoxin level. Monitor levels.
Lithium: May increase lithium level. Observe patient for toxicity and monitor level. Adjustment of lithium dosage may be required.
Methotrexate: May cause toxicity. Monitor patient closely.
Oral anticoagulants, NSAIDs, SSNRIs, SSRIs, other sulfonylureas, highly protein-bound drugs: May cause toxicity. Monitor patient closely.
Pemetrexed: May result in pemetrexed toxicity (myelosuppression, renal toxicity, and GI toxicity). Consider therapy modification.
Potassium-sparing diuretics: May reduce antihypertensive effects and enhance hyperkalemic effects. Monitor patient closely.
Probenecid: May decrease elimination of naproxen. Monitor patient for toxicity.
Drug-herb. *Alfalfa, anise, bilberry, dong quai, feverfew, garlic, ginger, ginkgo, horse chestnut, licorice, red clover:* May cause bleeding, based on the known effects of components. Discourage use together.
White willow: Herb and drug contain similar components. Discourage use together.
Drug-lifestyle. *Alcohol use, smoking:* May cause GI irritation and bleeding. Avoid use together.

EFFECTS ON LAB TEST RESULTS

• May increase BUN, creatinine, ALT, AST, and potassium levels.
• May increase bleeding time.
• May interfere with urinary 5-hydroxyindoleacetic acid and 17-hydroxycorticosteroid determinations.

CONTRAINDICATIONS & CAUTIONS

• Contraindicated in patients hypersensitive to drug and in those with the syndrome of aspirin-sensitive asthma, rhinitis, and nasal polyps.
• Drug can cause serious skin reactions (SJS, TEN). Stop drug at first sign of rash or hypersensitivity.
Boxed Warning Naproxen is contraindicated for the treatment of perioperative pain after CABG. ■
• Use cautiously in older adults and in patients with HTN, hyperkalemia, renal disease, CV disease, GI disorders, hepatic disease, or history of peptic ulcer disease.
• Drug may increase risk of aseptic meningitis, especially in patients with lupus and mixed connective tissue disorders.
• Drug isn't a substitute for low-dose aspirin for CV protection.
Dialyzable drug: No.
⚠ *Overdose S&S:* Drowsiness, heartburn, indigestion, nausea, vomiting, seizures.

N

PREGNANCY-LACTATION-REPRODUCTION

⚠ *Alert:* Use of NSAIDs at 20 weeks or later in pregnancy may cause fetal renal dysfunction leading to oligohydramnios and potential neonatal renal impairment. Use at 30 weeks or later in pregnancy may increase risk of premature closure of the ductus arteriosus. Avoid use during pregnancy starting at 20 weeks' gestation. If potential benefit justifies fetal risk, use lowest effective dose for the shortest duration. Consider ultrasound monitoring of amniotic fluid when NSAID therapy exceeds 48 hours. Use of 81 mg of low-dose aspirin for certain pregnancy-related conditions under the direction of a prescriber is acceptable.

• Use cautiously during breastfeeding.

• NSAIDs may cause reversible infertility in women. Consider discontinuing drug in patients having difficulty conceiving.

NURSING CONSIDERATIONS

• Because NSAIDs impair synthesis of renal prostaglandins, they can decrease renal blood flow and lead to reversible renal impairment, especially in patients with renal failure, HF, or liver dysfunction; in older adults; and in those taking diuretics. Monitor these patients closely.

• Before starting therapy, correct volume status in patients with dehydration or hypovolemia.

• Monitor CBC and renal and hepatic function every 4 to 6 months during long-term therapy.

• Monitor patient for neurologic effects (drowsiness, dizziness, blurred vision), which may impair physical or mental abilities.

⚠ *Alert:* Watch for and immediately evaluate signs and symptoms of heart attack (chest pain, shortness of breath or trouble breathing), or stroke (weakness in one part or side of the body, slurred speech).

Boxed Warning NSAIDs cause an increased risk of serious GI adverse events, including bleeding, ulceration, and perforation of the stomach or intestines, which can be fatal. Older adults are at greater risk. These events may occur at any time during therapy without warning. ■

Boxed Warning NSAIDs may increase the risk of serious thrombotic events, MI, or stroke, which can be fatal. The risk may be greater with longer use or in patients with CV disease or risk factors for CV disease. ■

• Because of their antipyretic and anti-inflammatory actions, NSAIDs may mask signs and symptoms of infection.

• Drug may prolong bleeding time and anemias can occur.

• *Look alike–sound alike:* Don't confuse Anaprox with Anaspaz or Avapro. Don't confuse Naprelan with Naprosyn.

PATIENT TEACHING

⚠ *Alert:* Drug is available without prescription (naproxen sodium, 220 mg). Instruct adult not to take more than 440 mg of naproxen sodium in any 8- to 12-hour period or 660 mg of naproxen sodium in a 24-hour period.

• Advise patient to take drug with food or milk to minimize GI upset and to drink a full glass of water or other liquid with each dose.

• Tell patient taking prescription doses for arthritis that full therapeutic effect may be delayed 2 to 4 weeks.

• Warn patient against taking naproxen and naproxen sodium at the same time.

⚠ *Alert:* Advise patient to seek medical attention immediately if chest pain, shortness of breath or trouble breathing, weakness in one part or side of the body, or slurred speech occurs.

• Teach patient signs and symptoms of GI bleeding (including blood in vomit, urine, or stool; coffee-ground vomit; and melena) and to notify prescriber immediately if any of these occurs.

• Advise patient to stop drug immediately and contact prescriber if rash or fever develops.

• Caution patient that use with aspirin, alcohol, other NSAIDs, or corticosteroids may increase risk of adverse GI reactions.

• Warn patient against hazardous activities that require mental alertness until CNS effects are known.

⚠ *Alert:* Warn patient against taking NSAIDs at 20 weeks' gestation or later unless instructed to do so by prescriber due to fetal risk. Advise patient to discuss taking OTC medications with a pharmacist or health care provider during pregnancy.

naratriptan hydrochloride
nar-ah-TRIP-tan

Amerge

Therapeutic class: Antimigraine drugs
Pharmacologic class: Serotonin 5-HT$_1$ receptor agonists

AVAILABLE FORMS
Tablets: 1 mg, 2.5 mg

INDICATIONS & DOSAGES
➤ **Acute migraine attacks with or without aura**
Adults: 1 or 2.5 mg PO as a single dose as soon as symptoms appear. If headache returns or responds only partially, may repeat dose after 4 hours. Maximum, 5 mg in 24 hours.
Adjust-a-dose: For patients with mild to moderate renal or hepatic impairment, 1 mg starting dose, not to exceed 2.5 mg in 24 hours.

ADMINISTRATION
PO
• Give drug without regard for food.
• Store suspension in refrigerator for up to 90 days; shake well before each use.

ACTION
May act as an agonist at serotonin receptors on extracerebral intracranial blood vessels, which constricts the affected vessels, inhibits neuropeptide release, and reduces pain transmission in the trigeminal pathways.

Route	Onset	Peak	Duration
PO	1–2 hr	2–3 hr	Unknown

Half-life: 6 hours.

ADVERSE REACTIONS
CNS: paresthesia, dizziness, drowsiness, fatigue, vertigo, pain, sensation of pressure (chest, neck, throat, jaw). **EENT:** ear, nose, and throat infection; photophobia, pharynx constriction, dry mouth. **GI:** nausea, hyposalivation, vomiting. **Musculoskeletal:** neck pain. **Other:** sensations of warmth, cold, pressure, tightness, or heaviness.

INTERACTIONS
Drug-drug. *Antiemetics (5-HT$_3$ antagonists), antipsychotics, bromocriptine, linezolid, MAO inhibitors, methylene blue, methylphenidate, opioids, SSNRIs, SSRIs, TCAs, tedizolid, tramadol:* May increase risk of serotonin syndrome. Monitor therapy.
Drugs that prolong QT interval (antiarrhythmics, arsenic trioxide, chlorpromazine, dolasetron, droperidol, mefloquine, mesoridazine, moxifloxacin, pentamidine, pimozide, tacrolimus, thioridazine, ziprasidone): May cause an additive effect and prolong QT interval. Monitor patient closely.
Ergot-containing or ergot-type drugs (dihydroergotamine, methysergide), other 5-HT$_1$ agonists: May prolong vasospastic reactions. Use within 24 hours of naratriptan is contraindicated.
Hormonal contraceptives: May slightly increase naratriptan level. Monitor patient.
Drug-herb. *St. John's wort:* May increase serotonergic effect. Discourage use together.
Drug-lifestyle. *Smoking:* May increase naratriptan clearance. Discourage smoking.

EFFECTS ON LAB TEST RESULTS
None reported.

CONTRAINDICATIONS & CAUTIONS
• Contraindicated in patients hypersensitive to drug or its components and in those with prior or current cardiac ischemia, Wolff-Parkinson-White syndrome, vasospastic CAD, arrhythmias associated with accessory conduction pathways, cerebrovascular (stroke, TIA) or peripheral vascular syndromes, hemiplegic or basilar migraines, ischemic bowel disease, or uncontrolled HTN.
• Contraindicated in older adults, patients with severe renal impairment (CrCl less than 15 mL/minute), patients with severe hepatic impairment (Child-Pugh class C), and patients who have used ergot-containing, ergot-type, or other 5-HT$_1$ agonists within 24 hours.
🜂 *Alert:* Coronary artery spasm, transient ischemia, MI, ventricular tachycardia, and ventricular fibrillation and death have been reported within a few hours of administration. Discontinue drug if these occur. If signs or symptoms of angina occur after dose, evaluate patient for CAD or Prinzmetal angina before additional doses are given and monitor ECG.
• Use cautiously in patients with risk factors for CAD, such as HTN, hypercholesterolemia, obesity, diabetes, smoking, strong family history of CAD, women after menopause, and men older than age 40,

N

unless patient is free from cardiac disease. Monitor patient closely after first dose.
• Use cautiously in patients with renal or hepatic impairment.
• Drug isn't indicated for prevention of migraine attacks.
• Safety and effectiveness in patients younger than age 18 or when treating cluster headaches or more than four migraines in a 30-day period haven't been established.
Dialyzable drug: Unknown.
⚠ *Overdose S&S:* Chest pain, ischemic ECG changes, increased BP resulting in lightheadedness, neck tension, tiredness, loss of coordination.

PREGNANCY-LACTATION-REPRODUCTION
• There are no adequate studies during pregnancy. Use only if potential benefit justifies fetal risk.
• It isn't known if drug appears in breast milk. Use cautiously during breastfeeding.

NURSING CONSIDERATIONS
• Patients with risk factors for CAD should have cardiac evaluation to rule out CAD before starting drug and periodically during therapy.
• Drug can cause significant BP elevations, including in patients with no history of HTN. Monitor BP.
• Use drug only when patient has a clear diagnosis of migraine.
• Overuse of acute migraine drugs may lead to medication overuse headache, which may present as migrainelike daily headaches or as a marked increase in frequency of migraine attacks.
🕒 *Alert:* Combining drug with other serotonin-modulating drugs may cause serotonin syndrome. Symptoms include restlessness, hallucinations, loss of coordination, fast heartbeat, rapid changes in BP, increased body temperature, hyperreflexia, nausea, vomiting, and diarrhea. Serotonin syndrome is more likely to occur when starting or increasing the dose of naratriptan, the SSRI, or the SSNRI.
• *Look alike–sound alike:* Don't confuse Amerge with Altace or Amaryl.

PATIENT TEACHING
• Instruct patient to take drug only as prescribed and to read the accompanying patient instruction leaflet before using drug.

• Tell patient to seek immediate medical care for chest pain, difficulty breathing, irregular heartbeat, weakness, swelling of the face, rash or hives, or slurring of speech.
• Caution patient not to take other prescription or OTC drugs or herbal preparations without first consulting prescriber.
• Inform patient that somnolence and dizziness can occur with naratriptan use. Instruct patient to evaluate ability to perform complex tasks while taking drug.
• Tell patient that drug is intended to relieve, not prevent, migraines.
• Instruct patient to take dose soon after headache starts. If no response occurs with first tablet, tell patient to seek medical approval before taking second tablet.
• Advise patient to increase fluid intake.
• Counsel patient not to use drug during known or suspected pregnancy without discussing with prescriber.
• Advise patient to notify prescriber of breastfeeding or plans to breastfeed.
• Tell patient to alert prescriber about adverse effects.
• Encourage patient to keep a headache diary record of headache frequency and medication use.

---

natalizumab
nah-tah-LIZ-yoo-mab

Tysabri

Therapeutic class: Immunomodulators
Pharmacologic class: Monoclonal antibodies

AVAILABLE FORMS
Injection: 300 mg/15 mL single-use vials

INDICATIONS & DOSAGES
➤ **As monotherapy for the treatment of patients with relapsing forms of MS; to induce and maintain clinical response and remission in patients with moderately to severely active Crohn disease with evidence of inflammation who have had an inadequate response to, or are unable to tolerate, conventional therapies and inhibitors of TNF-α**
Adults: 300 mg IV over 1 hour every 4 weeks.

Reactions in bold italics are *life-threatening*. Interactions may have a *rapid onset* or a **delayed onset**.

ADMINISTRATION

IV

▼ Dilute 300 mg in 100 mL NSS to final concentration of 2.6 mg/mL.

▼ Invert IV bag gently to mix solution; don't shake.

▼ Infuse over 1 hour; don't give by IV push or bolus.

▼ Flush IV line with NSS after infusion is complete.

▼ Refrigerate solution and use within 8 hours if not used immediately.

▼ Refrigerate single-dose vials between 36° and 46° F (2° and 8° C). Don't shake or freeze; protect from light.

▼ **Incompatibilities:** Don't mix or infuse with other drugs. Don't use any diluent other than NSS.

ACTION

May block interaction between adhesion molecules on inflammatory cells and receptors on endothelial cells of vessel walls.

Route	Onset	Peak	Duration
IV	Unknown	Unknown	Unknown

Half-life: 3 to 17 days.

ADVERSE REACTIONS

CNS: depression, dysesthesia, fatigue, headache, vertigo, somnolence, tremor, syncope. **CV:** chest discomfort, peripheral edema. **EENT:** tooth infections, toothache, sinusitis, pharyngolaryngeal pain, tonsillitis. **GI:** abdominal discomfort, diarrhea, gastroenteritis, nausea, dyspepsia, constipation, flatulence, stomatitis. **GU:** UTI, vaginitis, amenorrhea, dysmenorrhea, irregular menstruation, urinary frequency, urinary urgency, ovarian cyst. **Hepatic:** abnormal LFT values, cholelithiasis. **Metabolic:** weight increase or decrease. **Musculoskeletal:** arthralgia, extremity pain, muscle cramps, swollen joints, back pain. **Respiratory:** upper and lower respiratory tract infection, cough. **Skin:** rash, dermatitis, pruritus, dry skin, urticaria, night sweats, thermal injury, skin laceration. **Other:** hypersensitivity reaction, infusion-related reaction, herpes infection, viral infection, rigors, seasonal allergy, flulike symptoms.

INTERACTIONS

Drug-drug. *Corticosteroids, immunosuppressants, TNF inhibitors:* May increase risk of infection. Avoid using together.

Live-virus vaccines: May cause reduced effectiveness of the vaccine. Defer vaccine administration until immune function has returned.

Drug-herb. *Echinacea:* May decrease effectiveness of natalizumab. Consider therapy modification.

EFFECTS ON LAB TEST RESULTS

● May increase LFT values.

● May increase lymphocyte, monocyte, eosinophil, basophil, and nucleated RBC counts.

● May decrease platelet count.

● May cause transient decrease in Hb level.

CONTRAINDICATIONS & CAUTIONS

● Contraindicated in patients hypersensitive to drug or its components or in those with current or history of progressive multifocal leukoencephalopathy (PML). Use with other immunosuppressants or TNF-α inhibitors isn't recommended.

Boxed Warning Natalizumab increases risk of PML; risk increases with duration of therapy, number of infusions, prior use of immunosuppressants, and presence of anti–JC virus antibodies. Consider these factors with expected benefit when initiating and continuing treatment. ∎

● Safety and effectiveness in children and patients with chronic progressive MS haven't been established.

Dialyzable drug: Unknown.

PREGNANCY-LACTATION-REPRODUCTION

● Drug crosses the placental barrier. Use in pregnancy only if benefit justifies fetal risk.

● Obtain CBC in neonates exposed to drug in utero to assess for thrombocytopenia and anemia.

● Drug appears in human milk. Effects on infants are unknown.

NURSING CONSIDERATIONS

Boxed Warning Only prescribers registered in the TOUCH Prescribing Program may prescribe drug. ∎

● Report PML and serious opportunistic and atypical infections to Biogen Idec (1-800-456-2255).

● Safety and effectiveness of natalizumab treatment beyond 2 years are unknown. When used for Crohn disease, discontinue drug after

N

12 weeks if patient hasn't experienced therapeutic benefit.

Boxed Warning Monitor patient for PML. Withhold drug immediately at the first signs or symptoms suggestive of PML. Symptoms include clumsiness; progressive weakness; and visual, speech, and sometimes personality changes. Gadolinium-enhanced MRI and CSF analysis for JC viral DNA are recommended for diagnosis. ■

• Obtain a baseline brain MRI scan before starting therapy.

⚠ *Alert:* Watch for evidence of hypersensitivity reaction during and for 1 hour after infusion, which may include dizziness, urticaria, fever, rash, rigors, pruritus, nausea, flushing, hypotension, dyspnea, and chest pain.

• If hypersensitivity reaction occurs, stop drug and notify prescriber.

⚠ *Alert:* Drug increases risk of developing encephalitis, acute retinal necrosis, and meningitis caused by herpes simplex and varicella zoster viruses. Monitor patient for signs and symptoms of these conditions. Discontinue drug if any of these signs and symptoms occur and initiate appropriate treatment.

• Other serious infections, including opportunistic infections, have occurred. Concurrent use of antineoplastics, immunosuppressants, or immunomodulating agents may increase the risk. Discontinue therapy until successful resolution of the infection.

• For patients who start therapy while on long-term corticosteroids, begin steroid taper as soon as a therapeutic benefit has occurred. If corticosteroids can't be tapered within 6 months, discontinue drug.

• Patients who develop antibodies to drug have an increased risk of infusion-related reaction.

• Discontinue drug in patients with jaundice or other evidence of significant liver injury. Elevated serum hepatic enzymes and elevated total bilirubin levels may occur as early as 6 days after the first dose.

• Monitor patient for thrombocytopenia (easy bruising, abnormal bleeding, petechiae, abnormally heavy menstrual periods). Discontinue drug and evaluate patient immediately if thrombocytopenia occurs.

PATIENT TEACHING

• Inform patient that drug use requires enrollment in and adherence with the TOUCH program.

• Tell patient to read the "Medication Guide for Tysabri" before each infusion.

• Urge patient to immediately report progressively worsening symptoms persisting over several days, including changes in eyesight, balance, strength, and thinking, memory, and orientation leading to confusion and personality changes.

• Advise patient to inform all health care providers about receiving this drug.

• Urge patient to immediately report rash, hives, dizziness, fever, shaking chills, or itching while drug is infusing or up to 1 hour afterward.

• Tell patient about the potential for liver injury and low platelet count.

• Inform patient that drug may affect ability to fight infections. Instruct patient to report signs and symptoms of infection and to use caution when around people who are ill.

• Instruct patient to report pregnancy or plans to become pregnant.

SAFETY ALERT!

nateglinide ⚕
na-te-GLYE-nide

Therapeutic class: Antidiabetics
Pharmacologic class: Meglitinide derivatives

AVAILABLE FORMS
Tablets: 60 mg, 120 mg

INDICATIONS & DOSAGES
➤ **Type 2 diabetes as an adjunct to diet and exercise to improve glycemic control**
Adults: 120 mg PO t.i.d before meals. Patients near goal HbA$_{1c}$ level at start of treatment may receive 60 mg PO t.i.d.

ADMINISTRATION
PO
• Give drug 1 to 30 minutes before a meal.
• If patient plans to skip a meal, skip the dose to reduce risk of hypoglycemia.

ACTION
Lowers glucose level by stimulating insulin secretion from pancreatic beta cells.

Route	Onset	Peak	Duration
PO	20 min	1 hr	4 hr

Half-life: About 1.5 hours.

ADVERSE REACTIONS
CNS: dizziness. **GI:** diarrhea. **Metabolic:** *hypoglycemia,* hyperuricemia, weight gain. **Musculoskeletal:** back pain, arthropathy. **Respiratory:** URI, bronchitis, cough. **Other:** flulike symptoms, accidental trauma.

INTERACTIONS
Drug-drug. *Androgens, antidiabetics, glucomannan, guanethidine, MAO inhibitors, nonselective beta blockers, NSAIDs, pegvisomant, quinolones, salicylates, SSRIs, thioacetic acid:* May increase hypoglycemic action of nateglinide. Monitor glucose level closely. Consider dosage reduction.

Beta blockers, clonidine, guanethidine, reserpine: May mask signs and symptoms of hypoglycemia. Increase frequency of glucose monitoring.

Ceritinib, eltrombopag: May increase nateglinide serum concentration. Monitor glucose level closely.

Corticosteroids, rifamycins, somatostatin analogues, somatropin, sympathomimetics, thiazides, thyroid products: May decrease hypoglycemic action of nateglinide. Monitor glucose level closely. Consider dosage increase.

CYP2C9 inducers (phenytoin, rifampin): May decrease hypoglycemic action of nateglinide. Monitor glucose level closely. Consider dosage increase.

CYP2C9 inhibitors (amiodarone, fluconazole, sulfinpyrazone, voriconazole): May increase hypoglycemic action of nateglinide. Monitor glucose level closely. Consider dosage reduction.

Mifepristone: May increase nateglinide serum concentration. Use lowest recommended dosage of nateglinide. Monitor patient closely for adverse effects during and for 2 weeks after mifepristone treatment.

Drug-herb. *Gymnema sylvestre:* May increase hypoglycemic action of nateglinide. Monitor glucose level closely.

St. John's wort: May decrease hypoglycemic action of nateglinide. Monitor glucose level closely.

Drug-lifestyle. *Alcohol use:* May increase hypoglycemic action of nateglinide. Monitor glucose level closely.

EFFECTS ON LAB TEST RESULTS
• May increase uric acid level.

CONTRAINDICATIONS & CAUTIONS
• Contraindicated in patients hypersensitive to drug and in those with type 1 diabetes or diabetic ketoacidosis.
• Use cautiously in patients with moderate to severe liver dysfunction or adrenal or pituitary insufficiency, in older adults, and patients who are malnourished.
▨ Patients known to be poor metabolizers of CYP2C9 substrates may need dosage reductions and increased glucose monitoring.
• Safety and effectiveness in children haven't been established.
Dialyzable drug: No.
⚠ **Overdose S&S:** Hypoglycemic symptoms.

PREGNANCY-LACTATION-REPRODUCTION
• It isn't known if drug can cause fetal harm when administered during pregnancy. Use during pregnancy only if the potential benefit justifies fetal risk.
• It isn't known if drug appears in human milk. Patient should discontinue breastfeeding or discontinue drug.

NURSING CONSIDERATIONS
• Refer to manufacturer's or FDA guidelines regarding which antidiabetics may be used together and which may not.
• Monitor glucose level regularly to evaluate drug's effectiveness.
• Observe patient for signs and symptoms of hypoglycemia. To minimize risk of hypoglycemia, make sure patient has a meal immediately after dose. If hypoglycemia occurs and patient remains conscious, give patient an oral form of glucose. If unconscious, treat patient with IV glucose.
• Risk of hypoglycemia increases with strenuous exercise, alcohol ingestion, insufficient caloric intake, changes in meal pattern, and changes to coadministered medications.
• Symptoms of hypoglycemia may be masked in patients with autonomic neuropathy and in those who use beta blockers, clonidine, or guanethidine.
• Insulin therapy may be needed for glycemic control in patients with fever, infection, or trauma and in those undergoing surgery.
• Monitor glucose level closely when other drugs are started or stopped, to detect possible drug interactions.
• Periodically monitor HbA_{1c} level.
• Drug's effectiveness may decrease over time.

N

• Usually, no special dosage adjustments are necessary in older adults, but some in this age-group may have greater sensitivity to glucose-lowering effect.

PATIENT TEACHING
• Teach patient safe drug administration.
• Instruct patient on risk of hypoglycemia, its signs and symptoms (diaphoresis, rapid pulse, trembling, confusion, headache, irritability, and nausea), and ways to treat these symptoms by eating or drinking something containing sugar.
• Teach patient how to monitor and log glucose levels to evaluate diabetes control.
• Advise patient to notify prescriber for persistent low or high glucose level.
• Instruct patient to adhere to prescribed diet and exercise regimen.
• Explain possible long-term complications of diabetes and importance of regular preventive therapy.
• Encourage patient to wear a medical identification bracelet.
• Inform patient of potential drug-drug interactions with nateglinide.
• Advise patient to report pregnancy or planned pregnancy.
• Caution patient that breastfeeding isn't recommended while taking drug.

SAFETY ALERT!

necitumumab
ne-si-TOOM-oo-mab

Portrazza

Therapeutic class: Antineoplastics
Pharmacologic class: Epidermal growth factor receptor antagonists

AVAILABLE FORMS
Injection: 800 mg/50 mL in single-dose vials

INDICATIONS & DOSAGES
➤ **First-line treatment of metastatic squamous cell NSCLC in combination with gemcitabine and cisplatin**
Adults: 800 mg IV infusion on days 1 and 8 of each 3-week cycle given before gemcitabine and cisplatin infusions. Continue until disease progression or unacceptable toxicity occurs.
Adjust-a-dose: **Boxed Warning** For grade 3 or 4 electrolyte abnormalities (such as

hypomagnesemia, hypocalcemia, or hypokalemia), withhold drug and replace electrolytes as medically indicated. Resume subsequent cycles after electrolyte abnormalities improve to grade 2 or less. ∎

Refer to manufacturer's instructions for other toxicity-related dosage adjustments and premedication instructions.

ADMINISTRATION
IV
▼ Inspect solution for particulate matter and discoloration. If present, discard solution.
▼ Dilute to a final volume of 250 mL in NSS. Don't use solutions containing dextrose.
▼ Gently invert to ensure mixing; don't shake.
▼ Store diluted infusions up to 24 hours at 36° to 46° F (2° to 8° C) or up to 4 hours at room temperature (up to 77° F [25° C]).
▼ Discard vial with any unused portion.
▼ Administer via infusion pump over 60 minutes through a separate infusion line. Flush line with NSS at end of infusion.
▼ Give drug before gemcitabine and cisplatin.
▼ Refrigerate vials at 36° to 46° F (2° to 8° C); don't freeze. Protect from light.
▼ **Incompatibilities:** Dextrose, electrolytes, other drugs.

ACTION
A recombinant human IgG1 monoclonal antibody that binds to human epidermal growth factor receptor (EGFR) and blocks binding of EGFR to ligands, inhibiting angiogenesis and malignant progression, and allowing apoptosis.

Route	Onset	Peak	Duration
IV	Unknown	Unknown	Unknown

Half-life: 14 days.

ADVERSE REACTIONS
CNS: headache. **CV:** *cardiopulmonary arrest or sudden death, arterial thromboembolism, PE, venous thromboembolism,* phlebitis. **EENT:** conjunctivitis, oropharyngeal pain. **GI:** vomiting, diarrhea, stomatitis, dysphagia. **Metabolic:** weight loss, *hypomagnesemia, hypokalemia, hypocalcemia,* hypophosphatemia. **Musculoskeletal:** muscle spasms. **Respiratory:** hemoptysis. **Skin:** rash, dermatitis, acneiform rash, acne, pruritus, dry

---

Reactions in bold italics are *life-threatening*. Interactions may have a *rapid onset* or a *delayed onset*.

skin, skin fissures, erythema, paronychia, skin toxicity. **Other:** infusion reaction.

INTERACTIONS
Drug-lifestyle. *Sun exposure:* May increase photosensitivity. Patient should avoid sun exposure.

EFFECTS ON LAB TEST RESULTS
• May decrease magnesium, potassium, calcium, and phosphorus levels.

CONTRAINDICATIONS & CAUTIONS
Boxed Warning Drug may increase risk of cardiopulmonary arrest and sudden death when used in combination with gemcitabine and cisplatin. Closely monitor electrolyte levels, including magnesium, potassium, and calcium. ∎
• Drug isn't indicated for nonsquamous NSCLC.
• Drug increases risk of VTE and arterial thromboembolism (ATE), which can be fatal. Discontinue drug for serious or life-threatening VTE or ATE.
• Safety and effectiveness in children haven't been established.
• Use cautiously in older adults, because they may have increased risk of adverse reactions. *Dialyzable drug:* Unknown.

PREGNANCY-LACTATION-REPRODUCTION
• Contraindicated during pregnancy; drug may cause fetal harm. Advise patients to use effective contraception during therapy and for 3 months after therapy ends.
• There are no data about breastfeeding. Patient shouldn't breastfeed during treatment and for 3 months after final dose.

NURSING CONSIDERATIONS
Boxed Warning Closely monitor electrolyte levels, including magnesium, potassium, and calcium, before each dose and for at least 8 weeks after final dose. Aggressively replace electrolytes as indicated. ∎
• Monitor patients for infusion reaction.
• Monitor patients for skin reactions, which may be severe and usually develop within first 2 weeks of treatment; drug may need to be withheld or discontinued, or dosage reduced.
• Monitor patients for signs and symptoms of ATE (pain, pallor, pulselessness, loss of function, coldness) and VTE (pain, swelling, erythema, dyspnea, hypotension, tachycardia).

• *Look alike–sound alike:* Don't confuse necitumumab with bevacizumab, nivolumab, pembrolizumab, or ramucirumab. Don't confuse Portrazza with Arzerra.

PATIENT TEACHING
• Teach patient about adverse reactions and to immediately report them.
• Explain that drug may reduce blood levels of magnesium, calcium, and potassium and that these levels must be carefully monitored. Advise patient to take any supplements prescribed.
• Advise patient that lab monitoring will be needed to monitor for adverse reactions to treatment.
• Teach patient signs and symptoms of infusion reactions (fever, chills, difficulty breathing) and to report them immediately.
• Warn patient of childbearing potential to use contraception during therapy and for 3 months after final dose.
• Instruct patient not to breastfeed during therapy and for 3 months after final dose.
• Caution patient to minimize sun exposure, wear protective clothing, and use sunscreen.

---

nelfinavir mesylate
nell-FIN-ah-veer

Viracept

Therapeutic class: Antiretrovirals
Pharmacologic class: Protease inhibitors

N

AVAILABLE FORMS
Tablets: 250 mg, 625 mg

INDICATIONS & DOSAGES
➤ **HIV infection, in combination with other antiretrovirals**
Adults and children age 13 and older: 1,250 mg PO b.i.d. or 750 mg PO t.i.d. Maximum dosage is 2,500 mg/day.
Children ages 2 to 12: 45 to 55 mg/kg PO b.i.d. or 25 to 35 mg/kg PO t.i.d.; don't exceed 2,500 mg/day (b.i.d. dosing) or 2,250 mg/day (t.i.d. dosing).

ADMINISTRATION
PO
• Give with a meal.
• May dissolve tablets in a small amount of water; mix well. Give the cloudy liquid

immediately, rinse the glass, and give the rinse to patient to ensure entire dose is consumed.

• Give a missed dose as soon as possible; then resume regular schedule. Don't double dose.

ACTION

An HIV-1 protease inhibitor, which prevents cleavage of the viral polyprotein, resulting in the production of immature, noninfectious virus.

Route	Onset	Peak	Duration
PO	Unknown	2–4 hr	Unknown

Half-life: 3.5 to 5 hours.

ADVERSE REACTIONS

CNS: *seizures, suicidality,* anxiety, asthenia, depression, dizziness, emotional lability, headache, hyperkinesia, insomnia, malaise, migraine, paresthesia, sleep disorder, somnolence, fever. **EENT:** acute iritis, eye disease, pharyngitis, rhinitis, sinusitis. **GI:** diarrhea, *pancreatitis,* flatulence, nausea, abdominal pain, anorexia, dyspepsia, epigastric pain, GI bleeding, mouth ulceration, vomiting. **GU:** sexual dysfunction, urine abnormality. **Hematologic:** *leukopenia, thrombocytopenia,* anemia. **Hepatic:** *hepatitis,* abnormal LFT values. **Metabolic:** *hypoglycemia,* hyperglycemia, dehydration, diabetes, hyperlipidemia, hyperuricemia. **Musculoskeletal:** arthralgia, arthritis, back pain, cramps, myasthenia, myopathy. **Respiratory:** dyspnea. **Skin:** rash, dermatitis, folliculitis, fungal dermatitis, pruritus, diaphoresis, urticaria. **Other:** redistribution or accumulation of body fat, allergic reaction, accidental injury.

INTERACTIONS

♻ *Alert:* Consult full prescribing information for potential drug interactions before and during treatment.

Drug-drug. *Alfuzosin, amiodarone, cisapride, ergot derivatives, lurasidone, oral midazolam, pimozide, quinidine, triazolam:* May increase levels of these drugs, causing increased risk of life-threatening adverse events. Use together is contraindicated.

Anticoagulants (warfarin): May affect warfarin concentration. Monitor INR.

♻ *Alert: Atorvastatin, rosuvastatin:* May increase statin level and risk of myopathy and rhabdomyolysis. Atorvastatin dosage shouldn't exceed 40 mg/day. Rosuvastatin dosage shouldn't exceed 10 mg/day.

Azithromycin: May increase azithromycin level. Monitor patient for liver and hearing impairment.

Bosentan: May increase bosentan level. Decrease bosentan dosage.

Carbamazepine, phenobarbital: May reduce the effectiveness of nelfinavir. Use together cautiously.

Colchicine: May cause increased colchicine plasma concentration and increased risk of toxicity. Avoid combination.

Cyclosporine, sirolimus, tacrolimus: May increase levels of these immunosuppressants. Use together cautiously.

Delavirdine: May decrease delavirdine serum concentration and increase nelfinavir serum concentration. Consider therapy modification.

Didanosine: May decrease didanosine absorption. Take nelfinavir with food at least 2 hours before or 1 hour after didanosine.

Drugs that prolong QT interval: May increase risk of life-threatening cardiac arrhythmias such as torsades de pointes. Monitor patient and ECG closely.

Ethinyl estradiol, norethindrone: May decrease contraceptive level and effectiveness. Advise patient to use alternative contraceptive measures during therapy.

Fluticasone: May increase fluticasone plasma concentration. Use cautiously; consider alternatives for long-term use.

HIV protease inhibitors (saquinavir): May increase levels of protease inhibitors. Use together cautiously.

♻ *Alert: Lovastatin, simvastatin:* May increase statin level and risk of myopathy and rhabdomyolysis. Use together is contraindicated.

Methadone, phenytoin: May decrease levels of these drugs. Adjust dosage of these drugs accordingly.

Omeprazole: May decrease nelfinavir level. Concomitant use may lead to loss of virologic response and development of resistance.

Quetiapine: May increase quetiapine level. Consider alternative antiretroviral therapy. If coadministration is necessary, reduce quetiapine dose to one-sixth of current dose and monitor patient closely. Refer to quetiapine prescribing information.

Rifabutin: May increase rifabutin level and decrease nelfinavir level. Reduce dosage of

---

Reactions in bold italics are *life-threatening*. Interactions may have a *rapid onset* or a *delayed onset*.

rifabutin to half the usual dose and increase nelfinavir to 1,250 mg b.i.d.

Rifampin: May decrease nelfinavir level. Use together is contraindicated.

Sildenafil, tadalafil, vardenafil: May increase adverse effects of these drugs. Caution patient not to exceed 25 mg of sildenafil in a 48-hour period, 2.5 mg of vardenafil in 24 hours, or 10 mg of tadalafil in 72 hours. Contraindicated when used for treatment of PAH.

Trazodone: May increase trazodone plasma concentration. Use with caution and consider a lower trazodone dose.

Drug-herb. *St. John's wort:* May decrease drug level. Use together is contraindicated.

EFFECTS ON LAB TEST RESULTS

• May increase ALT, AST, ALP, bilirubin, GGT, amylase, LDH, CK, uric acid, and lipid levels.
• May increase or decrease glucose level.
• May decrease Hb level and WBC and platelet counts.

CONTRAINDICATIONS & CAUTIONS

• Contraindicated in patients hypersensitive to drug or its components and in those with moderate or severe hepatic impairment.
• Contraindicated with drugs that are highly dependent on CYP3A for clearance (alfuzosin, amiodarone, ergot derivatives, rifampin, lovastatin, simvastatin, pimozide, quinidine, sildenafil used for pulmonary HTN, oral midazolam, triazolam).
• Use cautiously in patients with mild hepatic dysfunction or hemophilia types A or B.
• Hyperglycemia requiring treatment with insulin or oral antidiabetics has been reported in postmarketing reports. A causal relationship hasn't been established.
• Immune reconstitution syndrome has been reported in patients treated with combination antiretroviral therapy. During initial treatment, patients whose immune system responds may develop inflammatory response to indolent or residual opportunistic infections, which may require further evaluation and treatment. Autoimmune disorders have also been reported in the setting of immune reconstitution and can occur many months after initiation of treatment.

Dialyzable drug: Unlikely.

PREGNANCY-LACTATION-REPRODUCTION

• Consider alternative antiretrovirals during pregnancy. Drug may cause hepatic adverse events. Use only if potential benefit justifies fetal risk.
• Enroll patients who are pregnant taking nelfinavir in the Antiretroviral Pregnancy Registry (1-800-258-4263).
• Patients shouldn't breastfeed because of risk of transmitting HIV to infant.
• Patients using estrogen-based oral contraception should use alternative or additional contraception.

NURSING CONSIDERATIONS

• Drug may increase bleeding risk in patients with hemophilia. Monitor patients closely.
• Monitor glucose levels carefully.
• Monitor LFT, viral load CD4$^+$ count, and triglyceride and cholesterol levels.
• Monitor patient for opportunistic infections.
• *Look alike–sound alike:* Don't confuse nelfinavir with nevirapine. Don't confuse Viracept with Viramune or Viramune XR.

PATIENT TEACHING

• Instruct patient in safe drug administration, to take drug every day at the same time as prescribed, and not to alter dose or stop drug without medical approval.
• Inform patient that drug doesn't cure HIV infection.
• Tell patient that long-term effects of drug are unknown and that there are no data stating that nelfinavir reduces risk of HIV transmission.
• Tell patient that diarrhea is the most common adverse effect and that it can be controlled with loperamide, if needed.
• Instruct patient taking hormonal contraceptives to use alternative or additional contraceptive measures while taking nelfinavir.
• Advise patient to report pregnancy or breastfeeding.
• *Alert:* Caution patient taking sildenafil, vardenafil, or tadalafil for erectile dysfunction about an increased risk of adverse events related to these drugs, including low BP, visual changes, and painful erections. Tell patient to promptly report signs and symptoms and not to exceed recommended dosage and frequency.

N

• Advise patient to report use of other prescribed or OTC drugs or herbal products because of possible drug interactions.

neomycin sulfate
nee-o-MYE-sin

Therapeutic class: Antibiotics
Pharmacologic class: Aminoglycosides

AVAILABLE FORMS
Tablets: 500 mg

INDICATIONS & DOSAGES
➤ **To suppress intestinal bacteria before surgery**
Adults: As part of bowel preparation regimen, 1 g neomycin PO at 1 p.m., 2 p.m., and 11 p.m. on day before 8 a.m. surgery. May give in combination with other oral and IV antibiotics.

ADMINISTRATION
PO
• For preoperative bowel preparation, provide a low-residue or clear liquid diet starting on preoperative day 3.

ACTION
Inhibits protein synthesis by binding directly to the 30S ribosomal subunit; bactericidal.

Route	Onset	Peak	Duration
PO	Unknown	1–4 hr	48–72 hr

Half-life: 2 to 3 hours.

ADVERSE REACTIONS
CNS: *neuromuscular blockade.* **EENT:** ototoxicity. **GI:** nausea, vomiting, diarrhea, malabsorption syndrome, CDAD. **GU:** *nephrotoxicity.* **Respiratory:** *respiratory paralysis.*

INTERACTIONS
Drug-drug. **Boxed Warning** *Acyclovir, amphotericin B, cephalosporins, cidofovir, cisplatin, methoxyflurane, vancomycin, other aminoglycosides:* May increase nephrotoxicity. Monitor renal function test results. ■
Boxed Warning *Anesthetics, neuromuscular blockers (decamethonium, succinylcholine, tubocurarine):* May increase effects of nondepolarizing muscle relaxants, including prolonged respiratory depression and respiratory

paralysis. Use together only when necessary, and expect to reduce dosage of nondepolarizing muscle relaxants. Mechanical ventilation may be needed. ■
Digoxin: May decrease digoxin absorption. Monitor digoxin level.
5-FU, methotrexate, penicillin V, vitamin B_{12} (oral): May inhibit GI absorption of these drugs. Monitor therapy.
Boxed Warning *IV loop diuretics (ethacrynic acid, furosemide):* May increase ototoxicity. Monitor patient's hearing. ■
Oral anticoagulants: May inhibit vitamin K–producing bacteria; may increase anticoagulant effect. Monitor PT and INR.

EFFECTS ON LAB TEST RESULTS
• May increase BUN, creatinine, and nonprotein nitrogen levels.
• May increase urine protein, casts, and cell counts.
• May decrease urine specific gravity.

CONTRAINDICATIONS & CAUTIONS
• Contraindicated in patients hypersensitive to neomycin or other aminoglycosides and in those with intestinal obstruction or inflammatory or ulcerative GI disease.
• Use cautiously in older adults and in patients with impaired renal function or neuromuscular disorders.
• Prolonged use can cause superinfection including CDAD, which can occur 2 months after therapy ends.
• Drug's ototoxic and nephrotoxic effects limit its usefulness. Use for hepatic coma (encephalopathy) is no longer recommended.
• Safety and effectiveness of oral neomycin sulfate in patients younger than age 18 haven't been established.
Dialyzable drug: Yes.
⚠ *Overdose S&S:* Neurotoxicity, ototoxicity, nephrotoxicity.

PREGNANCY-LACTATION-REPRODUCTION
• Drug may cause fetal harm. Use during pregnancy only if clearly needed.
• Patient should discontinue breastfeeding or discontinue drug.

NURSING CONSIDERATIONS
Boxed Warning Due to increased risk of nephrotoxicity, monitor renal function: urine output, specific gravity, urinalysis, BUN and creatinine levels, and creatinine clearance.

Reactions in bold italics are *life-threatening*. Interactions may have a *rapid onset* or a *delayed onset*.

Report evidence of declining renal function to prescriber. ■

Boxed Warning Due to increased risk of neurotoxicity and ototoxicity, evaluate patient's hearing before and during prolonged therapy. Notify prescriber if patient has tinnitus, vertigo, or hearing loss. Deafness may start several weeks after drug is stopped. ■

Boxed Warning Don't use with other aminoglycosides or neurotoxic or nephrotoxic drugs; risk of toxicities increase. ■

• If renal insufficiency develops during therapy, consider reducing dosage or discontinuing therapy.

• Watch for signs and symptoms of superinfection (chills, fever, diarrhea), including CDAD, which can occur more than 2 months after therapy ends.

Boxed Warning Neuromuscular blockade and respiratory paralysis have been reported after administration of aminoglycosides. Monitor patient closely. ■

PATIENT TEACHING

• Instruct patient to report all adverse reactions promptly, especially fever, chills, diarrhea, changes in hearing, changes in urine amount, or dark urine.

• Encourage patient to maintain adequate fluid intake.

• Caution patient to take drug exactly as directed. Skipping doses or not completing full course may decrease effectiveness and increase likelihood that bacteria will develop resistance.

• Advise patient to report pregnancy or plans to become pregnant.

SAFETY ALERT!

neratinib 🗑
ner-A-ti-nib

Nerlynx

Therapeutic class: Antineoplastics
Pharmacologic class: Tyrosine kinase inhibitors

AVAILABLE FORMS
Tablets 🔵*:* 40 mg

INDICATIONS & DOSAGES
Adjust-a-dose (for all indications): For severe hepatic impairment (Child-Pugh class C),

reduce dosage to 80 mg once daily. Refer to manufacturer's instructions for toxicity-related adjustments.

➤ **Extended adjuvant treatment of early-stage HER2-overexpressed or amplified breast cancer, after adjuvant trastuzumab-based therapy** 🗑
Adults: 240 mg (6 tablets) PO once daily. May initiate therapy with dosage escalation: 120 mg (3 tablets) daily week 1 (days 1 to 7), 160 mg daily (4 tablets) week 2 (days 8 to 14), then 240 mg daily day 15 and onwards. Give continuously until disease recurrence or for up to 1 year.

➤ **Advanced or metastatic HER2-positive breast cancer in combination with capecitabine in patients who have received two or more prior anti-HER2-based regimens in the metastatic setting**
Adults: 240 mg (6 tablets) PO once daily on days 1 to 21 of a 21-day cycle plus capecitabine (750 mg/m^2 PO b.i.d.) on days 1 to 14 of a 21-day cycle. Or, may initiate therapy with dosage escalation: 120 mg (3 tablets) daily week 1 (days 1 to 7), 160 mg daily (4 tablets) week 2 (days 8 to 14), then 240 mg daily day 15 and onwards. Continue until disease progression or unacceptable toxicity.

ADMINISTRATION
PO

• Give antidiarrheal prophylaxis during first two cycles of treatment; initiate with first dose of drug. Patient should receive loperamide as follows when not using dose escalation: For weeks 1 and 2 (days 1 to 14), give loperamide 4 mg t.i.d.; for weeks 3 to 8 (days 15 to 56), give loperamide 4 mg b.i.d.; for weeks 9 to 52 (days 57 to 365), give loperamide 4 mg as needed, not to exceed 16 mg/day; titrate dosing to achieve one to two bowel movements per day.

• If diarrhea occurs despite prophylaxis, treat with additional antidiarrheals, fluids, and electrolytes as clinically indicated. Therapy interruptions and dosage reductions may also be required to manage diarrhea.

• Give with food at the same time each day.

• Patient must swallow tablets whole and not crush, chew, or split them.

• If a dose is missed, skip the missed dose and resume normal schedule.

• Store at room temperature (68° to 77° F [20° to 25° C]).

N

♣Canada   ◇OTC   ◆Off-label use   ✐ Photoguide   Do not crush   *Liquid contains alcohol   🗑 Genetic

ACTION

A kinase inhibitor that irreversibly binds to epidermal growth factor receptor, HER2, and HER4, inhibiting their activity and causing antitumor activity.

Route	Onset	Peak	Duration
PO	Unknown	2–8 hr	Unknown

Half-life: 7 to 17 hours.

ADVERSE REACTIONS

CNS: fatigue, malaise, dizziness. **EENT:** epistaxis, dry mouth. **GI:** diarrhea, nausea, abdominal pain, vomiting, stomatitis, decreased appetite, tongue burning, mucosal inflammation, dyspepsia, abdominal distention. **GU:** UTI, dysuria, *renal impairment.* **Hepatic:** increased ALT and AST levels, *hepatotoxicity.* **Metabolic:** weight loss, dehydration. **Musculoskeletal:** muscle spasms, back pain, arthralgia. **Respiratory:** URI. **Skin:** rash, dermatitis, dry skin, nail disorders, skin fissures. **Other:** flulike symptoms.

INTERACTIONS

Drug-drug. *Antacids:* May decrease neratinib level. Give neratinib 3 hours after antacids.
H₂-receptor antagonists: May decrease neratinib level. Give neratinib at least 2 hours before or 10 hours after H₂-receptor antagonists.
Moderate and strong CYP3A4 inducers (bosentan, carbamazepine, efavirenz, phenytoin, rifampin): May decrease neratinib level. Avoid use together.
Moderate and strong CYP3A4 inhibitors (aprepitant, clarithromycin, ciprofloxacin, diltiazem, ketoconazole, ritonavir): May increase neratinib level. Avoid use together.
P-gp substrates (dabigatran, digoxin, fexofenadine): May increase P-gp substrate level and increase risk of substrate-related adverse reactions. Adjust P-gp substrate dosage, if clinically indicated.
PPIs: May decrease neratinib level. Avoid use together.
Drug-herb. *St. John's wort:* May decrease neratinib level. Discourage use together.
Drug-food. *Grapefruit juice:* May increase neratinib level. Discourage use together.

EFFECTS ON LAB TEST RESULTS

• May increase AST and ALT levels.

CONTRAINDICATIONS & CAUTIONS

• Use cautiously in patients with severe hepatic impairment (Child-Pugh class C).
• Safety and effectiveness in children haven't been established.
• Use cautiously in older adults because of increased severity of adverse reactions.
Dialyzable drug: Unknown.
⚠ **Overdose S&S:** Diarrhea, nausea, vomiting, dehydration.

PREGNANCY-LACTATION-REPRODUCTION

• Drug may cause fetal harm. Verify pregnancy status before treatment.
• Patients of childbearing potential should use effective contraception during treatment and for at least 1 month after final dose.
• Male patients with partners of childbearing potential should use effective contraception during treatment and for 3 months after last dose.
• Serious adverse reactions may occur in infants who are breastfed. Advise patient not to breastfeed during treatment and for at least 1 month after final dose.

NURSING CONSIDERATIONS

• Verify pregnancy status before treatment.
• Measure total bilirubin, AST, ALT, and ALP levels at baseline, monthly for the first 3 months, then every 3 months during treatment and as clinically indicated.
• Monitor patients for sign and symptoms of hepatotoxicity (worsening fatigue, nausea, vomiting, right upper quadrant tenderness, fever, rash, eosinophilia). Therapy may need to be interrupted, dosage reduced, or drug permanently discontinued.
• Monitor patients for diarrhea, vomiting, and dehydration, especially older adults. For severe diarrhea, administer fluid and electrolytes as needed, interrupt treatment, and reduce subsequent doses. Perform stool cultures as clinically indicated to exclude infectious causes of grade 3 or 4 diarrhea or diarrhea of any grade with complicating features (dehydration, fever, neutropenia).

PATIENT TEACHING

• Caution patient of childbearing potential that drug can cause fetal harm and that a pregnancy test will be performed before therapy begins.
• Advise patient of childbearing potential to use effective contraception during treatment

and for at least 1 month after last dose. Male patient with partner of childbearing potential should use effective contraception during treatment and for at least 3 months after final dose.

• Counsel patient not to breastfeed during therapy and for at least 1 month after final dose.

• Tell patient that lab tests will be needed during therapy.

• Stress importance of antidiarrheal prophylaxis with loperamide. Remind patient to immediately report severe episodes of diarrhea.

• Caution patient to report all adverse reactions, especially signs and symptoms of liver toxicity, such as worsening fatigue, nausea, vomiting, right upper quadrant tenderness, fever, or rash.

nevirapine
neh-VEER-ah-pine

Viramune, Viramune XR

Therapeutic class: Antiretrovirals
Pharmacologic class: NRTIs

AVAILABLE FORMS
Oral suspension: 50 mg/5 mL
Tablets: 200 mg
Tablets (extended-release) ⊙: 100 mg, 400 mg

INDICATIONS & DOSAGES
➤ **HIV-1, in combination with other antiretrovirals**
⊙ *Alert:* Adhere strictly to 14-day lead-in period with nevirapine 200-mg daily dosing to decrease risk of rash.
Adults: 200 mg (immediate-release) PO daily for the first 14 days; then 200 mg PO b.i.d. Or, 400 mg (extended-release) PO once daily after 14-day lead-in period with 200-mg (immediate-release) daily dosing.

If patient has already completed the lead-in period and is on a b.i.d. regimen of immediate-release formulation, another lead-in period isn't required to switch to extended-release.
Children and adolescents, infants 15 days and older (immediate-release): 150 mg/m²/dose (maximum dose, 200 mg/dose) PO once daily for first 14 days; then increase to

150 mg/m²/dose (maximum, 200 mg/dose) PO b.i.d.
Children age 6 and older with BSA of 1.17 m² or greater (extended-release): Initially, 150 mg/m² (immediate-release) PO once daily for 14 days. Then increase to 400 mg (extended-release) PO once daily. Maximum dose, 400 mg/day.

If child has already completed the lead-in period and is on a b.i.d. regimen of immediate-release formulation, another lead-in period isn't required.
Adjust-a-dose: Don't increase immediate-release lead-in dose if patient experiences mild to moderate rash without constitutional symptoms during 14-day lead-in period of 200 mg/day (150 mg/m²/day in children) until rash has resolved. If rash is present beyond 14-day lead-in period with immediate-release formulation, don't begin extended-release drug.

For patients on dialysis, give an additional 200-mg (immediate-release) dose after each dialysis treatment. Extended-release formula hasn't been studied in patients with renal impairment.

ADMINISTRATION
PO
⊙ *Alert:* Drug is a hazardous agent; use safe handling and disposal precautions per facility protocol.

• Use drug with at least one other antiretroviral.

• Administer with or without food, antacid, or didanosine.

• Extended-release tablets must be swallowed whole and shouldn't be crushed, chewed, or divided.

• Shake suspension gently before administering. An oral dosing syringe is recommended. If using a dosing cup, rinse the cup and administer the rinse also.

• Don't continue immediate-release lead-in dosing beyond 28 days.

• If dosing interruption exceeds 7 days, restart 14-day lead-in dosing.

ACTION
Binds directly to reverse transcriptase and blocks RNA-dependent and DNA-dependent DNA polymerase activities by disrupting the enzyme's catalytic site.

N

Route	Onset	Peak	Duration
PO (immediate-release)	Unknown	4 hr	Unknown
PO (extended-release)	Unknown	24 hr	Unknown

Half-life: 25 to 30 hours.

ADVERSE REACTIONS

CNS: fever, headache, fatigue. **GI:** nausea, abdominal pain, diarrhea. **Hematologic:** *neutropenia, thrombocytopenia,* anemia. **Hepatic:** *hepatitis,* elevated liver enzyme levels. **Metabolic:** increased cholesterol level, increased LDL level. **Musculoskeletal:** myalgia, arthralgia. **Skin:** blistering, rash, *SJS.*

INTERACTIONS

Drug-drug. *Amiodarone, artemether, calcium channel blockers, carbamazepine, cyclophosphamide, ergotamine, fentanyl, immunosuppressants:* May decrease exposure of these drugs. Monitor therapy effectiveness.
Atazanavir: May increase risk of virologic failure due to decreased atazanavir exposure; may increase risk of nevirapine toxicity. Avoid combination.
Boceprevir, telaprevir: May decrease boceprevir or telaprevir level. Don't use together.
Clarithromycin: May decrease clarithromycin level. Consider alternative to clarithromycin such as azithromycin.
Delavirdine, etravirine, rilpivirine: May alter nevirapine concentration. Don't use together, as combination hasn't proved beneficial.
Drugs extensively metabolized by CYP450: May lower levels of these drugs. Dosage adjustment of these drugs may be needed.
Efavirenz: May decrease efavirenz concentration and increase adverse reactions. Concurrent use isn't recommended.
Fluconazole, voriconazole: May increase nevirapine exposure. Monitor patient for increased adverse effects; consider therapy modification.
Fosamprenavir: May decrease fosamprenavir plasma concentration. Don't give concurrently unless ritonavir is part of the treatment regimen.
Itraconazole, ketoconazole: May decrease itraconazole or ketoconazole level. Avoid using together.

Lopinavir–ritonavir: May decrease lopinavir level. Adjust dosage based on lopinavir manufacturer's instructions.
Methadone: May decrease methadone level. Increased methadone dosage may be required to prevent signs and symptoms of opiate withdrawal.
Protease inhibitors, hormonal contraceptives: May decrease levels of these drugs. Use together cautiously.
Rifabutin: May increase rifabutin level. Dosage adjustment may be needed. Monitor patient closely.
Rifampin: May decrease nevirapine level and effectiveness. Avoid concomitant use.
Saquinavir: May decrease saquinavir level. Avoid use together.
Warfarin: May increase anticoagulant effect of warfarin. Monitor INR and adjust warfarin dose as needed.
Drug-herb. *St. John's wort:* May decrease drug level. Don't use together.

EFFECTS ON LAB TEST RESULTS

• May increase ALT, AST, GGT, bilirubin, LDL, amylase, and serum cholesterol levels.
• May decrease serum phosphate level.
• May decrease Hb level and neutrophil count.

CONTRAINDICATIONS & CAUTIONS

• Contraindicated in patients hypersensitive to drug.
• Contraindicated in patients with moderate or severe hepatic impairment or as part of occupational or nonoccupational postexposure prophylaxis regimens.

Boxed Warning Severe and fatal hepatotoxicity, particularly in the first 18 weeks, has been reported in patients treated with nevirapine. In some cases, patients presented with nonspecific prodromal signs or symptoms of hepatitis and progressed to hepatic failure. These events are often associated with rash and fever. ■

Boxed Warning Women and patients with higher CD4+ cell counts at start of therapy are at increased risk for life-threatening hepatotoxicity. Women with CD4+ cell counts higher than 250/mm^3, including patients who are pregnant receiving drug in combination with other antiretrovirals for treatment of HIV-1 infection, are at greatest risk. However, hepatotoxicity associated with nevirapine use

---

Reactions in bold italics are *life-threatening*. Interactions may have a *rapid onset* or a *delayed onset*.

can occur in both genders, at all CD4$^+$ cell counts, and at any time during treatment. ∎

Boxed Warning Severe, life-threatening, sometimes fatal skin reactions have occurred, including SJS, TEN, and hypersensitivity reactions characterized by rash, constitutional findings, and organ dysfunction. ∎

• Use cautiously in patients with mild hepatic impairment; pharmacokinetics haven't been evaluated in these patients.

• Unless benefit outweighs risk, drug isn't indicated in adult females with CD4$^+$ cell counts greater than 250 cells/mm^3 or adult males with CD4$^+$ cell counts greater than 400 cells/mm^3.

• Immune reconstitution syndrome has been reported in patients treated with combination antiretroviral therapy. During the initial treatment, patients whose immune system responds may develop inflammatory response to indolent or residual opportunistic infections. Autoimmune disorders have also been reported in the setting of immune reconstitution and can occur many months after initiation of treatment.

Dialyzable drug: Yes.

⚠ *Overdose S&S:* Edema, erythema nodosum, fatigue, fever, headache, insomnia, nausea, pulmonary infiltrates, rash, vertigo, vomiting, weight decrease.

PREGNANCY-LACTATION-REPRODUCTION

• Use cautiously during pregnancy due to increased risk of severe hepatic events. Encourage patient to participate in the Antiretroviral Pregnancy Registry (1-800-258-4263).

• Patients with HIV infection shouldn't breastfeed.

• Drug may reduce fertility in patients of childbearing potential, based on animal studies.

NURSING CONSIDERATIONS

• Monitor CBC, viral load, and renal function tests before therapy and regularly throughout.

Boxed Warning Monitor patient intensively during first 18 weeks of therapy to detect potentially life-threatening hepatotoxicity or skin reactions. Use extra vigilance during first 6 weeks of therapy when risk of these reactions peaks. ∎

• Assess LFT values at baseline, before dosage escalation, 2 weeks after dosage escalation, and periodically during therapy.

❸ *Alert:* Monitor patient for blistering, oral lesions, conjunctivitis, muscle or joint aches, or general malaise. Especially look for severe rash or rash accompanied by fever. Immediately report these signs and symptoms to prescriber.

❸ *Alert:* Be vigilant for signs or symptoms of hepatitis, such as fatigue, malaise, anorexia, nausea, jaundice, bilirubinuria, acholic stools, liver tenderness, or hepatomegaly. Consider diagnosis of hepatotoxicity in this setting, even if transaminase levels are initially normal or alternative diagnoses are possible.

Boxed Warning Check AST and ALT levels immediately if patient has signs or symptoms suggestive of hepatitis or hypersensitivity reaction. Check these levels for all patients who develop a rash in first 18 weeks of treatment. ∎

Boxed Warning Patients with signs or symptoms of hepatitis or with increased ALT or AST levels combined with rash or other systemic symptoms, including hypersensitivity reactions, must stop drug and immediately seek medical evaluation. ∎

Boxed Warning Don't restart drug after clinical hepatitis, elevated transaminase levels combined with rash or other systemic symptoms, or after severe rash or hypersensitivity reactions. In some cases, hepatic injury has progressed despite discontinuation of treatment. ∎

• Antiretroviral therapy may be changed if disease progresses during nevirapine therapy. Drug shouldn't be used as monotherapy for HIV infection because of the rapid emergence of resistance.

• Drug may cause body-fat redistribution.

• *Look alike–sound alike:* Don't confuse nevirapine with nelfinavir. Don't confuse Viramune with Viracept.

PATIENT TEACHING

• Inform patient that drug doesn't cure HIV and that illnesses from advanced HIV infection still may occur. Explain that drug doesn't reduce risk of HIV transmission.

• Instruct patient to report rash immediately and to stop drug until told to resume.

• Tell patient with signs or symptoms of hepatitis (such as fatigue, malaise, anorexia, nausea, jaundice, liver tenderness or hepatomegaly, with or without initially abnormal transaminase levels) to stop drug and seek medical evaluation immediately.

N

• Instruct patient that clinical and lab monitoring is essential, especially during the first 18 weeks of therapy, to detect potentially life-threatening hepatotoxicity and skin reactions.
• Stress importance of taking drug exactly as prescribed.
• Advise patient that if therapy interruption exceeds 7 days, the 14-day lead-in dosages must be repeated.
• Tell patient not to use other drugs or herbal products unless approved by prescriber.
• Advise patient of childbearing potential who is on an antiretroviral regimen to discuss hormonal contraceptives with prescriber.
• Teach patient to immediately report signs or symptoms of infection.
• Inform patient that redistribution or accumulation of fat may occur.

niCARdipine hydrochloride
nye-KAR-de-peen

Cardene IV

Therapeutic class: Antihypertensives, antianginals
Pharmacologic class: Calcium channel blockers

AVAILABLE FORMS
Capsules: 20 mg, 30 mg
Injection: 2.5 mg/mL vials; 20 mg/200 mL, 40 mg/200 mL in premixed bags

INDICATIONS & DOSAGES
➤ **Chronic stable angina (used alone or with other antianginals)**
Adults: Initially, 20 mg capsule PO t.i.d. Adjust dosage no sooner than every 3 days based on patient response. Usual range, 20 to 40 mg t.i.d.
➤ **HTN**
Adults: Initially, 20 mg capsule PO t.i.d.; range, 20 to 40 mg t.i.d. Adjust dosage every 3 days based on patient response. Or, to initiate therapy in patient who can't take oral nicardipine, give 5 mg/hour IV infusion; then increase by 2.5 mg/hour every 5 minutes for rapid control or every 15 minutes for gradual control to maximum of 15 mg/hour. After achieving BP goal, decrease infusion rate to 3 mg/hour. Or, as a substitute for oral nicardipine therapy, if patient takes 20 mg PO every 8 hours, give 0.5 mg/hour IV infusion; if

patient takes 30 mg PO every 8 hours, give 1.2 mg/hour IV infusion; if patient takes 40 mg PO every 8 hours, give 2.2 mg/hour IV infusion.
Adjust-a-dose: For patients with renal impairment, use starting dose of 20 mg PO t.i.d. with slow titration. For patients with hepatic impairment, use starting dose of 20 mg b.i.d. with slow titration. For patients with hypotension or tachycardia, discontinue infusion; may restart at lower dose when BP and HR stabilize.

ADMINISTRATION
PO
• Give drug with or without food, but avoid giving with high-fat meal.
IV
▼ Dilute 25-mg vial with 240 mL D$_5$W, dextrose 5% in NSS or half-NSS, or NSS or half-NSS to a concentration of 0.1 mg/mL. Injection remains stable in polyvinyl chloride container for 24 hours at controlled room temperature.
▼ Check premixed bags for leaks, solution clarity, and intact seal. Don't add other drugs to bag.
▼ Closely monitor BP during and after completion of infusion.
▼ Administer via central line or through a large peripheral vein. To minimize risk of peripheral venous irritation, change infusion site every 12 hours.
▼ Don't combine premixed or injection with any product in the same IV line or premixed container.
▼ Don't use plastic containers in series connections. Doing so may result in air embolism.
▼ When switching to oral form, give first dose of t.i.d. regimen 1 hour before stopping infusion. If using a different oral drug, start it when infusion ends.
▼ If solution is kept at room temperature, protect from light and use within 24 hours.
▼ **Incompatibilities:** Sodium bicarbonate (5%) injection, lactated Ringer injection. Consult a drug incompatibility reference for other possible incompatibilities.

ACTION
Inhibits calcium ion influx across cardiac and smooth muscle cells but is more selective to vascular smooth muscle than cardiac muscle. Drug also dilates coronary arteries and arterioles.

Reactions in bold italics are *life-threatening*. Interactions may have a *rapid onset* or a ***delayed onset***.

Route	Onset	Peak	Duration
PO	0.5–2 hr	1–2 hr	<8 hr
IV	Immediate	45 min	<8 hr

Half-life: 8.6 (PO); 14 hours (IV).

ADVERSE REACTIONS

CNS: headache, dizziness, light-headedness, asthenia, drowsiness, paresthesia, somnolence. **CV:** angina, peripheral edema, palpitations, flushing, hypotension, tachycardia. **EENT:** dry mouth. **GI:** nausea, vomiting, abdominal discomfort, dyspepsia. **Musculoskeletal:** myalgia. **Skin:** rash, diaphoresis, injection-site reaction, pain at injection site.

INTERACTIONS

Drug-drug. *Antihypertensives, protease inhibitors:* May increase antihypertensive effect. Monitor BP closely.
Cimetidine: May decrease metabolism of calcium channel blockers. Monitor patient for increased pharmacologic effect.
Cyclosporine, tacrolimus: May increase plasma levels of these drugs. Monitor patient for toxicity.
Fentanyl: May cause severe hypotension. Closely monitor BP.
Drug-food. *Grapefruit and grapefruit juice:* May increase bioavailability of nicardipine. Discourage use together.
High-fat foods: May decrease absorption of nicardipine. Discourage use together.

EFFECTS ON LAB TEST RESULTS

None reported.

CONTRAINDICATIONS & CAUTIONS

• Contraindicated in patients hypersensitive to drug and in those with advanced aortic stenosis.
• Use cautiously in patients with hypotension or impaired hepatic or renal function and in older adults.
• Avoid systemic hypotension when administering drug to patients who have sustained an acute cerebral infarction or hemorrhage.
• Consider lower dosages and closely monitor responses in patients with hepatic impairment or reduced hepatic blood flow.
• Titrate gradually in patients with renal impairment.
• MI and increased angina have been noted when calcium channel blockers have been started or doses titrated. Abrupt withdrawal

can cause rebound angina in patients with CAD.
• Use cautiously in patients with HF due to increased risk of worse outcomes.
• Safety and effectiveness in patients younger than age 18 haven't been established.
Dialyzable drug: No.
⚠ *Overdose S&S:* Hypotension, bradycardia, palpitations, flushing, drowsiness, confusion, slurred speech.

PREGNANCY-LACTATION-REPRODUCTION

• There are no adequate studies during pregnancy. Use during pregnancy only if potential benefits outweigh fetal risk.
• Use cautiously during breastfeeding, and monitor infant for adverse effects. Some manufacturers recommend that patient avoid breastfeeding during therapy.

NURSING CONSIDERATIONS

• Closely monitor BP and HR. Drug can cause symptomatic hypotension or tachycardia. Measure BP frequently during initial therapy.
🖑 *Alert:* Only immediate-release form is approved for treatment of angina.
• To reduce risk of venous thrombosis, phlebitis, and vascular impairment, don't use small veins, such as those on the dorsum of the hand or wrist. Use extreme care to avoid intra-arterial administration or extravasation.
• *Look alike–sound alike:* Don't confuse nicardipine with niacinamide, nifedipine, or nimodipine. Don't confuse Cardene with Cardura, Cardizem, or codeine.

PATIENT TEACHING

• Instruct patient in safe drug administration and to take oral form exactly as prescribed.
• Teach patient to report injection-site pain.
• Advise patient to immediately report chest pain. An increase in frequency, severity, or duration of chest pain may occur at start of therapy or during dosage adjustments.
• Caution patient to get up from a sitting or lying position slowly to avoid dizziness caused by a decrease in BP.
• Advise patient to discuss pregnancy or plans to become pregnant with prescriber.

N

nicotine
NIK-oh-teen

Habitrol ◇, Nicoderm CQ ◇, Nicotine Transdermal System Patch Kit ◇, Nicotrol, Nicotrol NS

nicotine polacrilex
Commit ◇, Habitrol ◇, Nicorelief ◇, Nicorette ◇, Nicorette Mini ◇

Therapeutic class: Smoking cessation aids
Pharmacologic class: Nicotinic agonists

AVAILABLE FORMS
Gum: 2 mg ◇, 4 mg per piece ◇
Lozenges: 2 mg ◇, 4 mg ◇
Nasal spray: 10 mg/mL (0.5 mg/actuation)
Oral inhaler: 10-mg cartridge (4 mg delivered)
Transdermal patch: 7 mg ◇, 14 mg ◇, 21 mg ◇

INDICATIONS & DOSAGES
➤ **As an aid to smoking cessation for the relief of nicotine withdrawal signs and symptoms as part of a comprehensive behavioral smoking cessation program**
Adults: For gum, initially patient should slowly chew 1 piece every 1 to 2 hours weeks 1 to 6, then 1 piece every 2 to 4 hours weeks 7 to 9, then 1 piece every 4 to 8 hours weeks 10 to 12. Maximum dosage is 24 pieces/day. Patient who smokes first cigarette more than 30 minutes after waking up should use 2-mg pieces; patient who smokes first cigarette within 30 minutes of waking up should use 4-mg pieces. For best results, at least 9 pieces should be chewed per day for first 6 weeks.

For oral inhaler, patient should use 6 to 16 cartridges/day weeks 1 to 12; initially, at least 6 cartridges/day for the first 3 to 6 weeks and adjust dosage based on signs or symptoms of nicotine withdrawal or excess. After 12 weeks, taper dosage over 6 to 12 additional weeks. Use beyond 6 months isn't recommended.

For lozenge, patient who smokes within 30 minutes of waking up should use 4-mg lozenge; patient who smokes first cigarette more than 30 minutes after waking up should use 2-mg lozenge. Weeks 1 to 6, 1 lozenge every 1 to 2 hours; weeks 7 to 9, 1 lozenge every 2 to 4 hours; weeks 10 to 12, 1 lozenge every 4 to 8 hours. Patient should use at least 9 lozenges/day during the first 6 weeks. Maximum, 5 lozenges in 6 hours or 20 lozenges/day.

For nasal spray, initially one or two doses per hour (one dose is 1 spray in each nostril); may increase to a maximum recommended dose of 40 mg (80 sprays)/day. For best results, at least eight doses per day are recommended. Don't exceed five doses per hour or 40 doses per day. Treat for 3 months. Use selected dosage for up to 8 weeks; then discontinue over the next 4 to 6 weeks by using such strategies as using only one-half a dose (1 spray) at a time, using spray less frequently, tallying daily usage, skipping a dose, or setting a planned "quit date." Use beyond 6 months isn't recommended.

For transdermal patch (Habitrol) in patients who smoke more than 10 cigarettes a day, apply one 21-mg patch daily during weeks 1 to 4; during weeks 5 to 6, decrease patch strength to 14 mg; during weeks 7 to 8, decrease patch strength to 7 mg, then discontinue. If patient smokes 10 or fewer cigarettes per day, start with 14-mg patch daily for 6 weeks, then 7-mg patch for 2 weeks, then discontinue. Patch may be worn for 24 hours.

For transdermal patch (Nicoderm CQ) in patients who smoke more than 10 cigarettes a day, apply one 21-mg patch daily during weeks 1 to 6; during weeks 7 to 8, decrease patch strength to 14 mg; during weeks 9 to 10, decrease patch strength to 7 mg, then discontinue. If patient smokes 10 or fewer cigarettes per day, start with 14-mg patch daily for 6 weeks, then 7-mg patch for 2 weeks, then discontinue. Patch may be worn for 16 or 24 hours. If vivid dreams occur, patient should remove patch before bedtime. May move to higher dose if patient is experiencing withdrawal symptoms or lower dose if adverse effects occur.

ADMINISTRATION
● Hazardous drug; use safe handling and disposal precautions.
Buccal (gum)
● Patient shouldn't eat or drink for 15 minutes before chewing or while chewing a piece of nicotine gum.
● Patient should chew the gum slowly until it tingles, then place it between cheek and gum.

When the tingle is gone, patient should begin chewing again until the tingle returns. This process should be repeated until most of the tingle is gone (about 30 minutes).
- Store at room temperature.
- Wrap used pieces of gum in paper and discard.

Buccal (lozenge)
- Patient shouldn't eat or drink 15 minutes before using lozenge or while lozenge is in mouth.
- Patient should place lozenge in mouth and allow lozenge to slowly dissolve (about 20 to 30 minutes); there may be a warm or tingling sensation. Patient should minimize swallowing and not chew or swallow lozenge.
- Occasionally patient should move lozenge from one side of mouth to the other until it's completely dissolved (about 20 to 30 minutes).
- Patient shouldn't use more than one lozenge at a time or continuously use one lozenge after another because GI adverse effects may occur.
- Patient who slips and has a cigarette should continue use.
- Store at room temperature; protect from light.

Inhalational
- Follow manufacturer's directions for assembling inhaler.
- Patient shouldn't inhale into the lungs like a cigarette but instead, inhale deeply into back of throat or puff in short breaths.
- Each cartridge may be used multiple times to provide a total of about 20 minutes of active puffing time. When not in use, keep mouthpiece in locked position out of reach of children and pets.
- Store mouthpiece in plastic storage case. Clean regularly with soap and water.
- Store and use at room temperature; protect from light.

Intranasal (spray)
- See manufacturer's instructions for use of device.
- Give with patient's head tilted back slightly; patient shouldn't sniff, swallow, or inhale through the nose during actuation.
- Patient shouldn't blow nose for 2 to 3 minutes after administration.
- Avoid contact with solution. If skin, lips, mouth, eyes, or ears come in contact with nicotine solution, immediately rinse with water.

Transdermal (patch)
- Apply one new patch every 24 hours on dry, clean, and hairless skin on upper body or outer arm. Save pouch for patch disposal after use.
- Remove backing from patch and immediately press onto skin for 10 seconds. After handling patch, wash hands.
- Don't cut patch or use a patch that's damaged on opening protective pouch.
- Don't apply patch to skin that is oily, burned, broken out, cut, or irritated. Avoid using soaps, lotions, oils, or creams that contain aloe, lanolin, or glycerin moisturizers on skin where the patch will be applied.
- Apply patch at the same time each day and rotate application sites. Allow at least 1 week before applying to previously used skin.
- Patient shouldn't wear more than one patch at a time and patches shouldn't be left on for more than 24 hours; patches lose potency after 24 hours and increased skin irritation may occur.
- Throw away the patch by folding sticky ends together. Replace in pouch and discard.

ACTION

Binds to nicotinic-cholinergic receptors in the adrenal medulla, neuromuscular junctions, and in the brain, causing stimulation and reward effects. Replaces endogenous nicotine effects obtained from smoking or other forms of tobacco. When appropriate doses are used, reduces withdrawal symptoms, including nicotine craving associated with quitting smoking.

Route	Onset	Peak	Duration
Buccal (gum, lozenge)	Unknown	About 30 min	Unknown
Inhalation	Unknown	Within 15 min	Unknown
Intranasal	Rapid	10–20 min	Unknown
Transdermal	Unknown	2–8 hr	Unknown

Half-life: Inhaler and nasal spray, 1 to 2 hours; transdermal patch, 4 hours.

ADVERSE REACTIONS

CNS: impaired concentration, confusion, fever, headache, nervousness, pain, tremor, incoordination, increased dreaming, apathy, withdrawal signs and symptoms (dizziness, anxiety, restlessness, cravings, sleep disorder, depression, drug dependence, fatigue), paresthesia. **CV:** tachycardia, HTN, palpitations,

N

chest discomfort or tightness, facial flushing (nasal spray). **EENT:** Gum: gum problems, tooth disorder, stomatitis, glossitis. Inhaler: mouth and throat irritation, taste disturbance, rhinitis, sinusitis, tooth disorder. Nasal spray: transient epistaxis, transient changes in sense of smell and taste, earache, numbness of nose or mouth, burning of nose or eyes, hoarseness, watery eyes, sneezing or runny nose, nasal mucosa irritation, ulcer, or blister. **GI:** dyspepsia, flatulence, hiccups, nausea, constipation, diarrhea, increased appetite. **GU:** menstrual disorder. **Metabolic:** weight gain. **Musculoskeletal:** back pain, arthralgia, jaw or neck pain (inhaler, gum), myalgia. **Respiratory:** cough (inhaler), bronchitis, dyspnea. **Skin:** rash, acne, application-site reaction, diaphoresis, pruritus. **Other:** allergic reaction, flulike symptoms.

INTERACTIONS

Drug-drug. *Acetaminophen, adrenergic antagonists (labetalol, prazosin), beta blockers (propranolol and others), imipramine, oxazepam, pentazocine, theophylline:* May cause a deinduction of hepatic enzymes on smoking cessation with or without nicotine replacement. A decrease in dosage of these drugs after smoking cessation may be needed. Monitor patient closely.

Adenosine: May enhance AV-blocking and tachycardic effects of adenosine. Monitor therapy.

Adrenergic agonists (isoproterenol, phenylephrine): May decrease circulating catecholamines with smoking cessation with or without nicotine replacement. An increase in dosage of these drugs after cessation of smoking may be needed. Monitor patient.

Cimetidine: May increase nicotine concentration. Monitor therapy.

Insulin: May increase subcutaneous absorption of insulin. A decrease in insulin dosage after cessation of smoking may be needed. Monitor patient closely.

Nasal vasoconstrictors (xylometazoline): May delay time to onset and peak nicotine concentration of nasal formulation. Advise patient of delay in nicotine effect.

Niacin: May increase flushing and dizziness. Use cautiously together.

TCAs: May affect pharmacokinetics of TCAs with smoking cessation with or without nicotine replacement. Monitor patient and adjust TCA dosage as necessary.

Drug-herb. *Lobelia:* May result in additive nicotine effects. Discourage use together.

Drug-food. *Acidic foods and beverages:* May decrease absorption of lozenge. Discourage use together.

Caffeine: May increase caffeine's effects after smoking cessation. Monitor patient.

Drug-lifestyle. *Smoking:* May have additive nicotine effect and increase risk of toxicity. Discourage smoking.

EFFECTS ON LAB TEST RESULTS

None reported.

CONTRAINDICATIONS & CAUTIONS

• Contraindicated in patients with known hypersensitivity or allergy to nicotine or components of the products, including menthol (inhaler) or soy (lozenges).

• Nicotine from any source can be toxic and addictive; dependence on nicotine replacements has occurred.

• Use cautiously in patients with recent MI, serious arrhythmias, CAD, severe or worsening angina, HTN, vasospastic diseases, or PVD.

• Use oral inhaler cautiously in patients with bronchospastic disease because of potential for airway irritation. Other forms of nicotine replacement may be preferred.

• Nasal spray isn't recommended in patients with chronic allergy, rhinitis, nasal polyps, sinusitis, or severe reactive airway disease.

• Use patch cautiously in patients with skin problems and in those allergic to adhesive tape.

• Use cautiously in patients with type 1 diabetes, hyperthyroidism, pheochromocytoma, severe renal or hepatic impairment, or history of seizures.

• Use cautiously in patients with oropharyngeal inflammation, history of esophagitis, or peptic ulcer disease because healing of GI disorders may be delayed.

• Nicotine gum may cause severe occlusal stress due to its heavier viscosity compared to ordinary chewing gum. The gum may loosen inlays or fillings, damage oral mucosa and natural teeth, and stick to dentures.

• Use gum cautiously in patients receiving a sodium-restricted diet.

🕚 *Alert:* Nicotine exposure by children and pets may cause poisoning and is potentially fatal.

• Use in children hasn't been studied.

Reactions in bold italics are **life-threatening**. Interactions may have a *rapid onset* or a **delayed onset**.

• Use cautiously in older adults; consider initiating treatment at the low end of the dosage range.

Dialyzable drug: Unknown.

⚠ *Overdose S&S:* Lethargy, pallor, cold sweat, nausea, salivation, vomiting, abdominal pain, diarrhea, headache, dizziness, disturbed hearing and vision, tremor, mental confusion, and weakness, ataxia, hypotension, seizures, arrhythmias, vascular collapse, central respiratory paralysis, coma.

PREGNANCY-LACTATION-REPRODUCTION

• Nicotine may cause fetal harm, including spontaneous abortion. Encourage patients who are pregnant to attempt smoking cessation through nonpharmacologic means. Use during pregnancy only under medical supervision and if the likelihood of smoking cessation justifies risk of nicotine use by patient who might continue to smoke during pregnancy.

• Nicotine appears in human milk; however, the amount of nicotine from nicotine replacement products in human milk isn't known. Encourage patients who are breastfeeding not to smoke. Weigh risk of exposure of the infant to nicotine from nicotine replacement therapy against risks associated with the patient's use of replacement therapy and continued smoking.

NURSING CONSIDERATIONS

• Connect patients who smoke with programs to assist with smoking cessation, such as government-based quit lines.

• Successful smoking cessation programs are individualized and include frequent supportive care.

• Monitor patients for withdrawal signs and symptoms (craving, nervousness, restlessness, irritability, mood lability, anxiety, drowsiness, sleep disturbances, impaired concentration, increased appetite, headache, myalgia, constipation, fatigue, weight gain).

• Monitor patients for tachycardia and other arrhythmias. Discontinue drug if CV signs and symptoms occur.

• Monitor patients for signs and symptoms of toxicity and overuse (nausea, abdominal pain, vomiting, diarrhea, diaphoresis, flushing, dizziness, disturbed hearing and vision, confusion, weakness, palpitations, altered respiration, hypotension); ensure that drug is used only as directed.

• Monitor patients for temporomandibular joint dysfunction and pain due to excessive chewing of gum.

• Discontinue patch if skin redness caused by the patch doesn't resolve after 4 days or if inflammation or rash occurs.

• OTC products aren't for sale to individuals younger than age 18.

• *Look alike–sound alike:* Don't confuse nicotine brand names.

PATIENT TEACHING

• Emphasize that patient should stop smoking completely while on nicotine replacement therapy to avoid additive nicotine levels higher than smoking alone.

• Teach patient how to properly apply or use products.

• Warn patient to adhere to maximum dosage ranges for these products.

• Advise patient to read all patient education material that comes with each product being used.

• Inform patient using nasal spray that nasal irritation is likely to occur but may lessen with continued use.

• Tell patient that onset of nasal spray's effect may be delayed if patient has a cold or rhinitis.

• Advise patient using gum to report jaw or tooth pain.

• Alert patient using gum that gum can stick to and damage dentures and dental work.

• Instruct patient to use hard, sugarless candy between doses of gum to help provide oral stimulation.

• Advise patient that participating in a comprehensive smoking cessation program improves success.

• Discuss benefits and risks of nicotine replacement versus smoking with patient who is or plans to become pregnant or breastfeed.

• Caution patient that smoking cessation may affect drug pharmacokinetics so dosage adjustments may be needed for other prescribed drugs.

🛈 *Alert:* Advise patient to keep all nicotine products, including used inhaler cartridges, nasal spray bottles, and patches, out of reach of children and pets.

N

NIFEdipine
nye-FED-i-peen

Adalat OROS✤, Procardia XL🖉

Therapeutic class: Antihypertensives,
antianginals
Pharmacologic class: Calcium channel
blockers

AVAILABLE FORMS
Capsules ⓞ: 10 mg, 20 mg
Tablets (extended-release) ⓞ: 20 mg✤,
30 mg, 60 mg, 90 mg

INDICATIONS & DOSAGES
Adjust-a-dose (for all indications): For older
adults and patients with renal and hepatic impairment, initiate drug at the low end of the
dosing range.
➤ **Vasospastic angina (Prinzmetal or variant angina), classic chronic stable angina
pectoris**
Adults: Initially, 10 mg short-acting capsule
PO t.i.d. Usual effective dosage range is 10
to 20 mg t.i.d. Some patients may require
up to 30 mg q.i.d. Maximum daily dose is
180 mg/day. Adjust dosage over 7 to 14 days
to evaluate response. Or, 30 to 60 mg
(extended-release tablets) PO once daily.
Maximum daily dose is 120 mg. Adjust
dosage over 7 to 14 days to evaluate response.
Use doses of more than 90 mg cautiously and
only when clinically warranted.
➤ **HTN**
Adults: Initially, 30 or 60 mg extended-
release tablet PO once daily, adjusted over 7
to 14 days. Maximum dose is 120 mg/day.
➤ **Raynaud phenomenon ♦**
Adults: Initially, 30 mg extended-release
tablet once daily. If needed, may increase
gradually, usually once every 4 weeks, but
not more frequently than once every 7 to
10 days; monitor BP closely with each
dosage increase. Usual effective dose, 30 to
120 mg/day.

ADMINISTRATION
PO
• May give immediate-release form with or
without food. If flushing occurs, may give
with a low-fat meal.

⊘ **Alert:** Don't use capsules SL to rapidly reduce severe high BP because result may be
fatal. Give capsules whole.
• Give extended-release tablets whole; don't
split, crush, or allow patient to chew tablets.
• Protect capsules from direct light and moisture and store at room temperature.

ACTION
Thought to inhibit calcium ion influx across
cardiac and smooth muscle cells, decreasing
contractility and oxygen demand. Drug may
also dilate coronary arteries and arterioles.

Route	Onset	Peak	Duration
PO	20 min	30–60 min	4–8 hr
PO (extended-release)	20 min	2.5–5 hr	24 hr

Half-life: 2 to 5 hours.

ADVERSE REACTIONS
CNS: dizziness, fatigue, light-headedness,
giddiness, headache, weakness, drowsiness,
insomnia, pain, paresthesia, nervousness,
mood changes, shakiness, sleep disturbances,
fever, balance difficulties, tremor. **CV:** flushing, heat sensation, peripheral edema, palpitations, transient hypotension, pulmonary
edema. **EENT:** blurred vision, nasal congestion, sore throat, dry mouth. **GI:** nausea,
heartburn, diarrhea, constipation, cramps,
flatulence, abdominal pain, dyspepsia. **GU:**
impotence, polyuria. **Musculoskeletal:** muscle cramps, arthralgia, inflammation, joint
stiffness. **Respiratory:** dyspnea, cough,
wheezing, chest congestion, shortness of
breath, pleuritic chest pain. **Skin:** dermatitis,
pruritus, urticaria, diaphoresis, rash. **Other:**
chills, sexual difficulties, inflammation.

INTERACTIONS
Drug-drug. *ACE inhibitors (benazepril):*
May increase hypotensive effects. Monitor
BP and adjust nifedipine dosage as needed.
Alpha$_1$ blockers (doxazosin): May increase
nifedipine plasma concentration. Monitor BP
and adjust nifedipine dosage as needed.
Beta blockers (propranolol): May cause hy-
potension and HF and exacerbate angina. Use
together cautiously.
Cimetidine: May increase nifedipine level.
Use together cautiously.
Cyclosporine, tacrolimus: May increase
serum levels of these drugs and increase risk

Reactions in bold italics are *life-threatening*. Interactions may have a *rapid onset* or a **delayed onset**.

of toxicity. Monitor serum levels and adjust dosage as needed.

CYP3A4 inhibitors (azole antifungals, erythromycin, nefazodone, ritonavir, verapamil), diltiazem: May increase effects of nifedipine. Monitor BP closely; decrease nifedipine dosage as needed.

Digoxin: May cause elevated digoxin level. Monitor digoxin level.

Diuretics, fentanyl: May increase hypotensive effects. Monitor BP.

PDE5 inhibitors (sildenafil): Increases risk of hypotension. Monitor BP and adjust nifedipine dosage if needed.

Quinidine: May decrease levels and effects of quinidine while increasing effects of nifedipine. Monitor HR and adjust nifedipine dose as needed.

Strong CYP3A4 inducers (carbamazepine, dexamethasone, phenytoin, rifabutin, rifampin): May decrease nifedipine level. Use together is contraindicated.

Vincristine: May increase risk of vincristine toxicity. Monitor therapy.

Warfarin: May increase PT. Monitor coagulation parameters and adjust warfarin dosage as needed.

Drug-herb. *Melatonin, St. John's wort:* May interfere with antihypertensive effect. Discourage use together.

Drug-food. *Grapefruit juice:* May increase bioavailability of drug. Avoid use together.

EFFECTS ON LAB TEST RESULTS
• May increase ALT, AST, ALP, CK, and LDH levels.

CONTRAINDICATIONS & CAUTIONS
• Contraindicated in patients hypersensitive to drug, in those taking strong CYP450 inducers (rifampin), and in patients with cardiogenic shock, ACS, ST-segment elevation MI, or essential hypertension.
• Angina exacerbation and MI have occurred at start of therapy or with dosage titration of dihydropyridine calcium channel blockers. Reflex tachycardia may occur, resulting in angina or MI in patients with obstructive coronary disease, especially in the absence of concurrent beta blockade.
• BP must be lowered at a rate appropriate for patient's clinical condition to avoid symptomatic hypotension with or without syncope. Use of immediate-release nifedipine in hypertensive emergencies and urgencies isn't safe or effective. Serious adverse events (death, cerebrovascular ischemia, syncope, stroke, acute MI, fetal distress) have been reported. Don't use immediate-release nifedipine for acute BP reduction or to manage primary HTN.
• Avoid use in patients with HF; drug may worsen symptoms.
• Use with extreme caution in patients with severe aortic stenosis. Drug may reduce coronary perfusion, resulting in ischemia.
• Use cautiously in patients with hypertrophic cardiomyopathy and outflow tract obstruction because reduction in afterload may worsen symptoms.
• Use cautiously before major surgery. Cardiopulmonary bypass, intraoperative blood loss, or vasodilating anesthesia may result in severe hypotension or increased fluid requirements. Consider withdrawing nifedipine more than 36 hours before surgery if possible.
• Rare reversible elevations in BUN and serum creatinine levels have been reported in patients with preexisting chronic renal insufficiency.
• Use cautiously in patients with hepatic impairment. Clearance of nifedipine is reduced in patients with cirrhosis; monitor patient and consider dosage adjustments.
• **Alert:** Immediate-release drug is considered a high-risk drug for older adults because of the potential for hypotension and increased risk of precipitating myocardial ischemia in this population. Avoid use.
• **Alert:** Use extended-release form cautiously because of an increased risk of serious GI obstruction in patients both with and without risk factors. (Risk factors for GI obstruction include altered GI anatomy, GI hypomotility related to GERD, colon cancer, ileus, obesity, hypothyroidism, diabetes, and concomitant use of H_2 blockers, NSAIDs, laxatives, anticholinergic agents, and levothyroxine.)
• Safety and effectiveness in children haven't been established.
Dialyzable drug: Unlikely.
⚠ **Overdose S&S:** Hypotension, dizziness, palpitations, flushing, nervousness.

PREGNANCY-LACTATION-REPRODUCTION
• Drug crosses the placental barrier. Oral nifedipine is a preferred agent for treating chronic HTN during pregnancy. Immediate-release nifedipine is recommended for

N

managing acute-onset, severe HTN during pregnancy and postpartum.

• Drug appears in human milk. Base decision to continue or discontinue breastfeeding during therapy on benefit to patient and risk and benefit to infant.

NURSING CONSIDERATIONS

• Monitor BP and HR regularly, especially in patients who take beta blockers or other antihypertensives.

• Watch for signs and symptoms of HF.

• Monitor patient for peripheral edema; carefully differentiate between adverse effect and HF symptom.

• Don't give immediate-release capsules within 1 week of acute MI, or in ACS.

• *Look alike–sound alike:* Don't confuse nifedipine with nimodipine, nisoldipine, or nicardipine. Don't confuse Procardia XL with Cartia XT.

PATIENT TEACHING

• If patient is kept on nitrate therapy during nifedipine dosage adjustment, urge continued adherence. Patient may take SL nitroglycerin, as needed, for acute chest pain.

• Tell patient that chest pain may worsen briefly as therapy starts or dosage increases.

• Instruct patient in safe drug administration.

• Tell patient not to abruptly stop drug unless directed by prescriber. Abrupt withdrawal may cause rebound angina in patients with CAD.

• Reassure patient taking the extended-release tablet that the wax mold may be passed in the stools. Assure patient that drug has already been completely absorbed.

SAFETY ALERT!

niraparib ⌧
nye-RAP-a-rib

Zejula

Therapeutic class: Antineoplastics
Pharmacologic class: Poly (ADP-ribose) polymerase inhibitors

AVAILABLE FORMS
Capsules ⒪ⓃⒸ: 100 mg

INDICATIONS & DOSAGES

Adjust-a-dose (for all indications): Refer to manufacturer's instructions for toxicity-related dosage adjustments. For patients with moderate hepatic impairment, give 200 mg/day; reduce dosage further for hepatic toxicity, if needed.

➤ **Maintenance treatment of recurrent epithelial ovarian, fallopian tube, or primary peritoneal cancer in patients who are in complete or partial response to platinum-based chemotherapy**

Adults: 300 mg (3 capsules) PO once daily beginning no later than 8 weeks after most recent platinum-containing regimen. Continue treatment until disease progression or unacceptable toxicity occurs.

➤ **Advanced ovarian, fallopian tube, or primary peritoneal cancer in patients who have been treated with three or more prior chemotherapy regimens and whose cancer is associated with homologous recombination deficiency positive status defined by either a deleterious or suspected deleterious *BRCA* mutation or genomic instability and who have progressed more than 6 months after response to the last platinum-based chemotherapy** ⌧

Adults: 300 mg (3 capsules) PO once daily until disease progression or unacceptable toxicity occurs.

➤ **Maintenance treatment of patients with advanced epithelial ovarian, fallopian tube, or primary peritoneal cancer who are in a complete or partial response to first-line platinum-based chemotherapy**

Adults weighing less than 77 kg or with a platelet count less than 150×10^9/L: 200 mg (2 capsules) PO once daily beginning no later than 12 weeks after most recent platinum-containing regimen and continuing until disease progression or unacceptable toxicity occurs.

Adults weighing 77 kg or more and with a platelet count of 150×10^9/L or more: 300 mg (3 capsules) PO once daily beginning no later than 12 weeks after most recent platinum-containing regimen and continuing until disease progression or unacceptable toxicity occurs.

ADMINISTRATION
PO
• Hazardous drug; use safe handling and disposal precautions.

- May give with or without food.
- Give at approximately same time each day; administer antiemetic to prevent nausea and vomiting. Bedtime administration may also help diminish nausea.
- Patients should swallow capsules whole.
- If dose is missed or vomited, don't make up dose; resume at next scheduled time.

ACTION

An inhibitor of poly (ADP-ribose) polymerase (PARP) enzymes PARP-1 and PARP-2, which have a role in DNA repair. Inhibition of PARP enzymatic activity and increased formation of PARP–DNA complexes result in DNA damage, apoptosis, and cell death.

Route	Onset	Peak	Duration
PO	Unknown	3 hr	Unknown

Half-life: 36 hours.

ADVERSE REACTIONS

CNS: fatigue, headache, dizziness, insomnia, anxiety, depression, dysgeusia, asthenia. **CV:** palpitations, HTN, tachycardia, peripheral edema. **EENT:** conjunctivitis, epistaxis, nasopharyngitis, dry mouth. **GI:** nausea, constipation, intestinal obstruction, vomiting, abdominal pain, abdominal distention, mucositis, stomatitis, diarrhea, dyspepsia, decreased appetite. **GU:** UTI, acute kidney injury. **Hematologic:** anemia, *neutropenia, leukopenia, thrombocytopenia.* **Hepatic:** increased liver enzyme levels. **Metabolic:** weight loss, hyperglycemia, *hypokalemia, hypomagnesemia.* **Musculoskeletal:** myalgia, arthralgia, back pain. **Respiratory:** dyspnea, cough, bronchitis. **Skin:** rash.

INTERACTIONS

None reported. Formal drug interaction studies haven't been performed.

EFFECTS ON LAB TEST RESULTS

- May increase ALP, GGT, AST, ALT, glucose, and creatinine levels.
- May decrease potassium, sodium, albumin, and magnesium levels.
- May decrease Hb level, ANC, and platelet and WBC counts.

CONTRAINDICATIONS & CAUTIONS

- Contraindicated in patients hypersensitive to drug or its components.

- Capsules contain FD&C Yellow No. 5 (tartrazine), which may cause allergic-type reactions. Use cautiously in patients with aspirin hypersensitivity, who may have increased sensitivity.
- Drug may increase risk of bone marrow suppression, myelodysplastic syndrome (MDS), or acute myeloid leukemia (AML). Discontinue drug if MDS or AML is confirmed.
- HTN and hypertensive crisis have occurred in patients treated with drug. Closely monitor patients with CV disorders.
- Use in severe renal disease, ESRD, and in moderate to severe hepatic impairment hasn't been studied.
- Safety and effectiveness in children haven't been established.

Dialyzable drug: Unknown.

PREGNANCY-LACTATION-REPRODUCTION

- Drug may cause fetal harm. Advise patients of childbearing potential to use appropriate contraception during and for at least 6 months after final dose.
- It isn't known if drug appears in human milk. Advise against breastfeeding during treatment and for 1 month after final dose.
- Drug may impair male fertility.

NURSING CONSIDERATIONS

- Assess CBC before treatment; don't give drug until hematologic toxicity from previous chemotherapy has resolved.
- Monitor CBC weekly for first month, then monthly for 11 months, then periodically.
- Monitor BP and HR weekly for first 2 months, then monthly for 1 year and periodically thereafter. Manage HTN with medication and dosage adjustments as clinically indicated. Closely monitor patients with cardiac disorders.
- Monitor all patients for PRES (seizure, headache, visual disturbances, altered mental status, HTN). If confirmed by MRI, discontinue drug.
- Obtain pregnancy test before start of treatment.
- *Look alike–sound alike:* Don't confuse niraparib with enasidenib, neratinib, nilotinib, nintedanib, olaparib, rucaparib, or talazoparib. Don't confuse Zejula with Zydelig or Zytiga.

N

PATIENT TEACHING

• Teach patient safe drug administration and handling.
• Explain that lab testing will be needed to monitor treatment.
• Advise patient to report all adverse reactions.
• Teach patient how to manage nausea.
• Warn patient of risk of blood disorders and to report weakness, fatigue, fever, weight loss, frequent infections, bruising, bleeding easily, blood in urine or stool, and breathlessness.
• Inform patient that BP and HR will be monitored during therapy.
• Advise patient of childbearing potential that a pregnancy test will be needed before therapy begins and that drug can cause fetal harm. Advise patient to use contraception during treatment and for 6 months after final dose.
• Inform male patient that drug may impair fertility.
• Caution patient not to breastfeed during therapy and for 1 month after final dose.

---

nitrofurantoin macrocrystals ⚛
nye-troh-fyoo-RAN-toyn

Furadantin, Macrodantin✒

nitrofurantoin monohydrate/ macrocrystals ⚛
Macrobid

Therapeutic class: Antibiotics
Pharmacologic class: Nitrofurans

AVAILABLE FORMS
Capsules: 25 mg, 50 mg, 100 mg
Oral suspension: 25 mg/5 mL

INDICATIONS & DOSAGES
➤ **UTIs caused by susceptible *Escherichia coli*, *Staphylococcus aureus*, enterococci, or certain strains of *Klebsiella* and *Enterobacter* species**
Adults and children older than age 12: 50 to 100 mg PO q.i.d. with meals and at bedtime. Continue for 1 week or for at least 3 days after sterility of urine is obtained. Or, 100 mg Macrobid PO every 12 hours for 7 days.
Children ages 1 month to 12 years: 5 to 7 mg/kg PO daily in four divided doses. Continue for 1 week or for at least 3 days after sterility of urine is obtained.

➤ **UTI prophylaxis**
Adults: 50 to 100 mg PO daily at bedtime.
Children: 1 to 2 mg/kg PO daily in a single dose at bedtime or divided into two doses given every 12 hours.

ADMINISTRATION
PO
• Obtain urine specimen for culture and sensitivity tests before giving. Repeat as needed. Begin therapy while awaiting results.
• Shake suspension well before use. May mix suspension with water, milk, fruit juice, or infant formula.
• Give with food or milk to minimize GI distress and improve absorption.
• Don't open monohydrate/macrocrystals capsule; may open macrocrystals capsule and mix contents with food or juice for immediate use.
• Protect from light. Oral suspension should be dispensed in amber glass bottles.

ACTION
May interfere with bacterial enzyme systems and bacterial cell-wall formation.

Route	Onset	Peak	Duration
PO	Unknown	Unknown	Unknown

Half-life: 20 minutes to 1 hour.

ADVERSE REACTIONS
CNS: headache. **GI:** nausea, flatulence. **Hematologic:** decreased Hb level, eosinophilia. **Hepatic:** increased transaminase levels. **Metabolic:** hyperphosphatemia. **Other:** hypersensitivity reactions.

INTERACTIONS
Drug-drug. *Antacids containing magnesium trisilicate:* May decrease nitrofurantoin absorption. Avoid combination.
Dapsone (topical), nitric oxide, prilocaine, sodium nitrite, tetracaine (topical): May enhance nitrofurantoin adverse effects. Monitor therapy.
Eplerenone: May enhance hyperkalemic effect. Monitor potassium level.
Live vaccines (BCG, cholera, typhoid): May diminish therapeutic effect of live vaccines. Avoid combination.
Probenecid, sulfinpyrazone: May inhibit excretion of nitrofurantoin, increasing drug levels and risk of toxicity. The resulting

---

Reactions in bold italics are *life-threatening*. Interactions may have a *rapid onset* or a ***delayed onset***.

decreased urinary levels could lessen antibacterial effects. Avoid using together.

Drug-food. *Any food:* May increase absorption. Advise patient to take drug with food or milk.

EFFECTS ON LAB TEST RESULTS
• May increase AST, ALT, bilirubin, phosphorus, and ALP levels.
• May increase eosinophil count.
• May decrease Hb level and WBC, granulocyte, and platelet counts.
• May cause false-positive results in urine glucose tests using cupric sulfate (Benedict reagent, Fehling solution).

CONTRAINDICATIONS & CAUTIONS
• Contraindicated in infants age 1 month and younger; in patients with anuria, oliguria, or CrCl less than 60 mL/minute; in patients with a history of cholestatic jaundice or hepatic dysfunction associated with nitrofurantoin use; and in patients with a known hypersensitivity to drug.
• Use cautiously in patients with renal impairment, asthma, anemia, diabetes, electrolyte abnormalities, vitamin B deficiency, or debilitating disease. These diseases may increase the risk of peripheral neuropathy.
• Chronic, subacute, or acute pulmonary hypersensitivity reactions may occur. Patients on continuous treatment for 6 months or longer are at highest risk. If not recognized early, pulmonary function may be permanently impaired.
• Peripheral neuropathy, which may become severe or irreversible, has occurred.
• Optic neuritis has been reported rarely in postmarketing experience with nitrofurantoin formulations.
▨ Patients with G6PD deficiency have an increased risk of developing hemolytic anemia. This deficiency is found in 10% of Blacks and a small percentage of ethnic groups of Mediterranean and Near-Eastern origin. If hemolytic anemia occurs, discontinue drug. Hemolysis ceases when drug is stopped.
Dialyzable drug: Yes.
⚠ *Overdose S&S:* Vomiting.

PREGNANCY-LACTATION-REPRODUCTION
• Contraindicated during pregnancy at 38 to 42 weeks' gestation, during labor and delivery, and when onset of labor is imminent due to possible hemolytic anemia in the neonate.

• There are no well-controlled studies during pregnancy. Use during pregnancy before 38 weeks for shortest effective course only if clearly needed.
• Because of possible serious adverse reactions in infants younger than age 1 month, patient should discontinue breastfeeding or discontinue drug.
• High doses may halt sperm production, which is reversible when drug is discontinued.

NURSING CONSIDERATIONS
• Monitor fluid intake and output carefully. Treatment may turn urine brown or dark yellow.
• Monitor LFT values, because of risk of fatal hepatic reactions. Stop drug immediately if hepatitis occurs, and treat appropriately.
• Monitor CBC, renal function, and pulmonary status regularly.
⚠ *Alert:* Monitor patient for signs and symptoms of superinfection, which can occur up to 2 months after therapy ends. Use of nitrofurantoin may result in growth of nonsusceptible organisms, especially *Pseudomonas* species, or cause fungal or bacterial superinfection, such as CDAD and pseudomembranous colitis.
• Monitor patient for pulmonary sensitivity reactions, including cough, chest pain, fever, chills, dyspnea, ECG changes, and pulmonary infiltration with consolidation or effusions.
⚠ *Alert:* Hypersensitivity may develop when drug is used for long-term therapy.
• Some patients may experience fewer adverse GI effects with nitrofurantoin macrocrystals.
• Dual-release capsules (25 mg nitrofurantoin macrocrystals combined with 75 mg nitrofurantoin monohydrate) enable patients to take drug only twice daily.
• *Look alike–sound alike:* Don't confuse nitrofurantoin with Neurontin. Don't confuse Macrobid with Micro-K.

PATIENT TEACHING
• Instruct patient to take drug for as long as prescribed, exactly as directed, even after feeling better.
• Tell patient to take drug with food or milk to minimize stomach upset.
• Instruct patient to report adverse reactions, especially peripheral neuropathy

N

(burning sensation, numbness, tingling) and pulmonary signs and symptoms (malaise, dyspnea, cough, fever), which can become severe or irreversible.

• Advise patient to immediately report diarrhea, bloody stools with or without stomach cramps, and fever during or as late as 2 or more months after treatment ends.

• Alert patient that drug may turn urine dark yellow or brown.

• Counsel patient to report pregnancy, plans to become pregnant, or breastfeeding.

• Advise patient not to use antacid preparations containing magnesium trisilicate.

SAFETY ALERT!

nitroglycerin (glyceryl trinitrate)
nye-troe-GLIH-ser-in

Nitro-Bid, Nitro-Dur, Nitroject✤, Nitrolingual, NitroMist, Nitrostat⬦, Rectiv, Rho-Nitro Pumpspray✤, Trinipatch✤

Therapeutic class: Vasodilators, antianginals
Pharmacologic class: Nitrates

AVAILABLE FORMS
Aerosol (translingual): 0.4 mg/metered spray
Injection: 5-mg/mL vial; 100 mcg/mL, 200 mcg/mL, 400 mcg/mL premixed in glass containers
Ointment: 2%
Rectal ointment: 0.4%
Tablets (SL) ⓞⓉⒸ*:* 0.3 mg (1/200 grain), 0.4 mg (1/150 grain), 0.6 mg (1/100 grain)
Transdermal patch: 0.1 mg/hour, 0.2 mg/hour, 0.3 mg/hour, 0.4 mg/hour, 0.6 mg/hour, 0.8 mg/hour release rate

INDICATIONS & DOSAGES
➤ **To prevent chronic anginal attacks**
Adults: For 2% ointment: Start dosage with ½ inch ointment, increasing by ½-inch increments until desired results are achieved. Range of dosage with ointment is ½ inch to 5 inches (1.25 to 12.7 cm). Usual dose is 1 to 2 inches (2.5 to 5.08 cm) every 6 to 8 hours. Transdermal patch: Starting dose is 0.2 to 0.4 mg/hour once daily applied for 12 to 14 hours a day (with a patch-off period of 10 to 12 hours).

➤ **Acute angina pectoris; to prevent or minimize anginal attacks before stressful events**
Adults: 1 SL tablet dissolved under the tongue or in the buccal pouch as soon as angina begins. Repeat every 5 minutes, if needed, to a maximum of three doses within a 15-minute period. May be used prophylactically 5 to 10 minutes before activities that might precipitate an acute angina attack. Or, 1 or 2 metered-dose sprays Nitrolingual into mouth, preferably onto or under the tongue. Repeat every 3 to 5 minutes, if needed, to a maximum of 3 sprays within a 15-minute period. May use prophylactically 5 to 10 minutes before activities that might precipitate an acute angina attack.

➤ **Perioperative HTN, HF after MI, angina pectoris in acute situations; to produce controlled hypotension during surgery**
Adults: Initially, 5 mcg/minute IV infusion, increasing as needed by 5 mcg/minute every 3 to 5 minutes until response occurs. If a 20-mcg/minute rate doesn't produce a response, increase dosage by as much as 20 mcg/minute every 3 to 5 minutes. Maximum dosage, 200 mcg/minute.

➤ **Moderate to severe pain from chronic anal fissure**
Adults: 1 inch (2.5 cm) of ointment PR every 12 hours for up to 3 weeks.

ADMINISTRATION
IV
▼ Dilute with D_5W or NSS for injection. Concentration shouldn't exceed 400 mcg/mL.
▼ Always give with an infusion control device and titrate to desired response.
▼ Regular polyvinyl chloride tubing can absorb drug, making it necessary to infuse higher dosages. A special nonabsorbent polyvinyl chloride tubing is available. Always mix in glass bottles and avoid using a filter.
▼ Use the same type of infusion set when changing lines.
▼ When changing the concentration of infusion, flush the administration set with 15 to 20 mL of the new concentration before use. This will clear the line of the old drug solution.
▼ **Incompatibilities:** Other drugs.

Reactions in bold italics are *life-threatening*. Interactions may have a *rapid onset* or a ***delayed onset***.

Topical

• To apply ointment, measure prescribed amount on the application paper; then place the paper on any nonhairy area and tape in place. Don't rub in.

• Cover with plastic film to aid absorption and to protect clothing. Remove all excess ointment from previous site before applying the next dose. Avoid getting ointment on fingers.

Rectal

• Cover a finger with plastic wrap, disposable surgical glove, or a finger cot.

• Apply 1 inch of ointment onto the covered finger.

• Gently insert the ointment into the anal canal using the covered finger no further than the first finger joint. Wash hands after use.

Transdermal

• Apply patch to any nonhairy part of the skin except distal parts of the arms or legs. (Absorption won't be maximal at distal sites.)

• Remove patch after 12 to 14 hours; wash skin with soap and water. Rotate patch sites.

• A cardioverter-defibrillator shouldn't be discharged through a paddle electrode that overlies a nitroglycerin patch.

• Remove patch before defibrillation. Because of the aluminum backing on the patch, the electric current may cause arcing that can damage the paddles and burn patient.

• When stopping transdermal treatment of angina, gradually reduce the dosage and frequency of application over 4 to 6 weeks.

Sublingual

• Give tablet at first sign of attack. Patient should wet the tablet with saliva and place it under tongue until absorbed. Dose may be repeated every 5 minutes for a maximum of three doses. If drug doesn't provide relief, obtain prompt medical attention.

• Don't crush or allow patient to chew or swallow tablet.

Buccal

• The tablet should be placed between the lip and gum above the incisors or between the cheek and gum. Tablets shouldn't be swallowed or chewed.

Translingual

• Don't shake container. Prime pump before use. If pump isn't used frequently, reprime before use. Follow manufacturer's instructions.

• Patient using translingual aerosol form shouldn't inhale the spray but should release it onto or under the tongue, then wait about 10 seconds or so before swallowing. Patient shouldn't rinse or spit for 5 to 10 minutes after a dose.

ACTION

Reduces cardiac oxygen demand by decreasing left ventricular end-diastolic pressure (preload) and, to a lesser extent, systemic vascular resistance (afterload). Also increases blood flow through the collateral coronary vessels.

Route	Onset	Peak	Duration
IV	Immediate	Immediate	3–5 min
Topical	15–30 min	1 hr	7 hr
Transdermal	30 min	2 hr	10–12 hr
SL	1–3 min	5–7 min	25 min
Buccal	3 min	Unknown	3–5 hr
Translingual	1–3 min	4–15 min	25 min
PR	Immediate	Unknown	Unknown

Half-life: About 1 to 4 minutes.

ADVERSE REACTIONS

CNS: headache, paresthesia, dizziness, syncope, weakness. **CV:** hypotension, bradycardia, flushing, palpitations, peripheral edema. **EENT:** pharyngitis, rhinitis, SL burning. **GI:** nausea, vomiting, abdominal pain. **Respiratory:** dyspnea, diaphoresis. **Skin:** contact dermatitis, rash. **Other:** hypersensitivity reactions.

INTERACTIONS

Drug-drug. *Alteplase:* May decrease tissue plasminogen activator antigen level. Avoid using together; if unavoidable, use lowest effective dose of nitroglycerin.

Antihypertensives, barbiturates: May increase hypotensive effect. Monitor BP closely.

Avanafil, sildenafil, tadalafil, vardenafil: May cause severe hypotension. Use of nitrates in any form with these drugs is contraindicated.

Ergotamine, ergot derivatives: May diminish vasodilatory effect of nitroglycerin. Avoid combination.

Heparin: IV nitroglycerin may interfere with anticoagulant effect of heparin. Monitor PTT.

Nitric oxide: May increase risk of methemoglobinemia. Monitor therapy.

Rilmenidine, riociguat: May cause hypotension. Use together is contraindicated.

Drug-lifestyle. *Alcohol use:* May increase hypotension. Discourage use together.

EFFECTS ON LAB TEST RESULTS
• IV nitroglycerin may falsely elevate triglyceride assay results with some tests.

CONTRAINDICATIONS & CAUTIONS
• Contraindicated in patients hypersensitive to nitrates.
• Contraindicated in patients who are taking PDE5 inhibitors for erectile dysfunction or PAH.
• Contraindicated in patients with early MI (sublingual), severe anemia, acute circulatory failure or shock, increased ICP, angle-closure glaucoma, orthostatic hypotension, or allergy to adhesives (transdermal).
• IV nitroglycerin is contraindicated in patients hypersensitive to IV form and in those with cardiac tamponade, restrictive cardiomyopathy, or constrictive pericarditis.
• Use cautiously in patients with hypotension or volume depletion.
Dialyzable drug: Unknown.
⚠ *Overdose S&S:* Vasodilation, decreased cardiac output, venous pooling, severe hypotension, methemoglobinemia.

PREGNANCY-LACTATION-REPRODUCTION
• Nitroglycerin crosses the placental barrier. There are no adequate studies during pregnancy. Use only if clearly needed.
• It isn't known if drug appears in human milk. Use cautiously during breastfeeding.

NURSING CONSIDERATIONS
• Closely monitor vital signs, particularly BP, during infusion, especially in patient with an MI. Excessive hypotension can worsen ischemia.
• Monitor BP and intensity and duration of drug response.
• Drug may cause headaches, especially at beginning of therapy. Dosage may be reduced temporarily, but tolerance usually develops. Treat headache with NSAIDs or acetaminophen.
• Tolerance to drug can be minimized with a 10- to 12-hour nitrate-free interval. To achieve this, remove the transdermal system in the early evening and apply a new system the next morning or omit the last daily dose of a buccal, sustained-release, or ointment form. Check with the prescriber for alterations in dosage regimen if tolerance is suspected.

• Wipe off nitroglycerin paste or remove patch before defibrillation to avoid patient burns.
• *Look alike–sound alike:* Don't confuse nitroglycerin with nitroprusside or nitrofurantoin.

PATIENT TEACHING
• Caution patient to take nitroglycerin regularly, as prescribed, and to have it accessible at all times.
• *Alert:* Advise patient that stopping drug abruptly may cause coronary artery spasm.
• Teach patient how to give the prescribed form of nitroglycerin.
• Tell patient to take nitroglycerin at first sign of attack. If drug doesn't provide relief, patient should obtain medical help promptly.
• Advise patient who complains of a tingling sensation with SL drug to try holding tablet in cheek.
• Instruct patient to take an additional oral dose before anticipated stress or at bedtime if chest pain occurs at night.
• Urge patient using skin patches to dispose of them carefully because enough medication remains after normal use to be hazardous to children and pets.
• If patients using skin patches are scheduled for an MRI scan, advise them to notify the facility that they are wearing a patch.
• Advise patient to avoid alcohol.
• To minimize dizziness when standing up, advise patient to rise slowly, to go up and down stairs carefully, and to lie down at the first sign of dizziness.
• *Alert:* Advise patient that use of avanafil, sildenafil, tadalafil, or vardenafil with any nitrate may cause life-threatening low BP. Use together is contraindicated.
• Tell patient to store SL tablets in cool, dark place in a tightly closed container.
• Tell patient to store SL tablets in original container or other container specifically approved for this use and to carry the container in a jacket pocket or purse, not in a pocket close to the body.

---

nitroprusside sodium
nye-troe-PRUSS-ide

Nipride ✤, Nipride RTU

Therapeutic class: Antihypertensives
Pharmacologic class: Vasodilators

AVAILABLE FORMS
Injection: 25 mg/mL, 20 mg/100 mL,
50 mg/100 mL

INDICATIONS & DOSAGES
➤ **To lower BP quickly in hypertensive emergencies; to produce controlled hypotension to reduce bleeding during surgery; treatment of acute HF**
Adults and children: Begin infusion at
0.3 mcg/kg/minute IV and gradually titrate every few minutes (no less than 5 minutes) until achieving desired effect, or until reaching maximum dose of 10 mcg/kg/minute (whichever occurs first). BP can't be further reduced without compromising vital organ perfusion.
Adjust-a-dose: Patients also taking other antihypertensives are extremely sensitive to nitroprusside. Titrate dosage accordingly. If GFR is less than 30 mL/minute/1.73 m², titrate dose to less than 3 mcg/kg/minute. In patients with anuria, limit mean dose to 1 mcg/kg/minute.

ADMINISTRATION
IV
▼ Prepare solution by dissolving 50 mg in 2 to 3 mL of D_5W injection or according to manufacturer's instructions.
Boxed Warning Drug isn't for direct injection and must be further diluted before infusion. Further dilute concentration in 250, 500, or 1,000 mL of D_5W to provide solutions with 200, 100, or 50 mcg/mL, respectively. ∎
Boxed Warning Immediately discontinue infusion if adequate BP reduction isn't obtained within 10 minutes at maximum dose. ∎
▼ Reconstitute ADD-Vantage vials labeled as containing 50 mg of drug according to manufacturer's directions.
▼ Because drug is sensitive to light, wrap solution in foil or other opaque material; it's not necessary to wrap the tubing. Fresh solution has a faint brownish tint. Discard if solution is discolored, particulate matter is visible, or if it's been 24 hours since dilution.
⊕ *Alert:* Use an infusion pump. Drug is best given via piggyback through a peripheral line with no other drug. Don't titrate rate of main IV line while drug is being infused. Even a small bolus can cause severe hypotension.
Boxed Warning Use drug only when available equipment and personnel allow BP to be continuously monitored using either a continually reinflated sphygmomanometer or (preferably) an intra-arterial pressure sensor. ∎
▼ When used to treat HF, guide drug titration using results of invasive hemodynamic monitoring and simultaneous urine output monitoring.
▼ Confirm drug's effect at any infusion rate after an additional 5 minutes before titrating to a higher dose to achieve desired BP.
▼ If severe hypotension occurs, stop infusion; effects of drug quickly reverse. Notify prescriber.
▼ **Incompatibilities:** Other drugs.

ACTION
Relaxes arteriolar and venous smooth muscle.

Route	Onset	Peak	Duration
IV	Immediate	1–2 min	10 min

Half-life: 2 minutes.

ADVERSE REACTIONS
CNS: headache, dizziness, *increased ICP,* loss of consciousness, apprehension, restlessness. **CV:** *bradycardia,* hypotension, tachycardia, palpitations, ECG changes, flushing, venous streaking, retrosternal discomfort. **GI:** nausea, abdominal pain, ileus. **Hematologic:** *methemoglobinemia,* decreased platelet aggregation. **Metabolic:** acidosis, hypothyroidism. **Musculoskeletal:** muscle twitching. **Skin:** diaphoresis, pink color, rash. **Other:** *thiocyanate toxicity, cyanide toxicity,* irritation at IV site.

INTERACTIONS
Drug-drug. *Amphetamines, methylphenidate:* May decrease antihypertensive effect. Monitor BP.
Antipsychotics (second-generation, atypical), barbiturates, brimonidine (topical),

N

diazoxide, duloxetine, ganglionic blockers, general anesthetics, levodopa, lormetazepam, negative inotropic drugs, pentoxifylline, prostacyclin analogues, other antihypertensives: May cause additive effects. Monitor BP closely.

Dapsone (topical), nitric oxide, prilocaine, sodium nitrite, tetracaine (topical): May enhance adverse or toxic effects. Monitor patient closely for hypoxia and cyanosis.

PDE5 inhibitors (sildenafil, vardenafil), riociguat: May increase hypotensive effects. Use together is contraindicated.

EFFECTS ON LAB TEST RESULTS

• May increase serum cyanide and creatinine levels.
• May decrease RBC and WBC counts.

CONTRAINDICATIONS & CAUTIONS

• Contraindicated in patients hypersensitive to drug.
• Contraindicated in patients with compensatory HTN (such as in arteriovenous shunt or coarctation of the aorta), inadequate cerebral circulation, acute HF with reduced peripheral vascular resistance (high-output HF in endotoxic sepsis), congenital optic atrophy, or tobacco-induced amblyopia, and in patients who are moribund coming to emergency surgery.
• Use with extreme caution in patients with increased ICP.
• Use cautiously in patients with hypothyroidism, hepatic or renal disease, hyponatremia, or low vitamin B level and in those who are poor surgical risks.
• Drug may increase methemoglobinemia risk. Evaluate and treat patients with impaired oxygenation despite adequate cardiac output and oxygen saturation level.
Dialyzable drug: Yes.
⚠ *Overdose S&S:* Hypotension, acidosis, cyanide or thiocyanate toxicity.

PREGNANCY-LACTATION-REPRODUCTION

• There are no adequate studies during pregnancy. Use only if clearly needed. Animal studies have demonstrated fetal harm. Advise patient of fetal risk.
• It isn't known if drug appears in human milk. Patient should discontinue breastfeeding or discontinue drug.

NURSING CONSIDERATIONS

Boxed Warning Drug can cause severe hypotension, which can lead to ischemic injuries or death. Use drug only when available equipment and personnel allow BP to be continuously monitored. Hypotension should resolve within 10 minutes after discontinuing drug. ∎
• Obtain baseline vital signs before giving drug; ascertain parameters prescriber wants to achieve. Monitor BP continuously. Patients receiving other antihypertensives may be more sensitive to drug.
• Keep patient in supine position when starting therapy or titrating drug.
Boxed Warning Dose-related cyanide toxicity can occur and may be lethal. Patient's ability to buffer cyanide will be exceeded in less than 1 hour at the maximum dose rate of 10 mcg/kg/minute. Limit maximum infusion rate to as short a duration as possible. Hepatic dysfunction increases risk of cyanide toxicity. ∎
• An early sign of cyanide toxicity is increasing dosage requirement to maintain BP control.
Boxed Warning Although acid-base balance and venous oxygen concentration should be monitored and may indicate cyanide toxicity, these lab tests provide imperfect guidance. ∎
⊘ *Alert:* Monitor patient for cyanide toxicity (venous hyperoxemia with bright red venous blood, profound hypotension, metabolic acidosis, dyspnea, bradycardia, headache, tinnitus, confusion, seizure, loss of consciousness, ataxia, or vomiting). Stop drug immediately and notify prescriber if toxicity occurs.
• *Look alike–sound alike:* Don't confuse nitroprusside with nitroglycerin.

PATIENT TEACHING

• Instruct patient to report all adverse reactions promptly, especially signs and symptoms of hypotension and cyanide toxicity.
• Tell patient to alert nurse if discomfort occurs at IV insertion site.
• Inform patient who is pregnant of fetal risk.

SAFETY ALERT!

nivolumab ⚕
neh-VOL-you-mab

Opdivo

Therapeutic class: Antineoplastics
Pharmacologic class: Monoclonal antibodies

AVAILABLE FORMS
Injection: 40 mg/4 mL, 100 mg/10 mL, 120 mg/12 mL, 240 mg/24 mL single-dose vials

INDICATIONS & DOSAGES
Adjust-a-dose (for all indications): Refer to manufacturer's instructions for dosage adjustments for adverse reactions and treatment-related toxicities.

➤ **Unresectable or metastatic melanoma; adjuvant treatment of melanoma with lymph node involvement or metastatic disease in patients who have undergone complete resection**
Adults: 240 mg IV infusion every 2 weeks or 480 mg every 4 weeks until disease progression or unacceptable toxicity occurs.

➤ **Unresectable or metastatic melanoma, in combination with ipilimumab**
Adults: 1 mg/kg IV infusion followed by ipilimumab 3 mg/kg IV infusion on the same day, every 3 weeks for a maximum of four doses or until unacceptable toxicity; then nivolumab 240 mg IV infusion every 2 weeks or 480 mg every 4 weeks until disease progression or unacceptable toxicity occurs.

➤ **Metastatic NSCLC with progression on or after platinum-based chemotherapy; patients with epidermal growth factor receptor (*EGFR*) or *ALK* genomic tumor aberrations should have disease progression on therapy for these aberrations before nivolumab ⚕**
Adults: 240 mg IV infusion every 2 weeks or 480 mg every 4 weeks until disease progression or unacceptable toxicity occurs.

➤ **First-line combination therapy for metastatic NSCLC when tumors express PD-L1 with no *EGFR* or *ALK* genomic tumor aberrations**
Adults: 360 mg IV infusion every 3 weeks followed by ipilimumab 1 mg/kg IV on the same day every 6 weeks. Continue until disease progression or unacceptable toxicity occurs, or up to 2 years in patients without disease progression.

➤ **First-line combination treatment of metastatic or recurrent NSCLC with no *EGFR* or *ALK* genomic aberrations ⚕**
Adults: 360 mg IV infusion every 3 weeks followed by ipilimumab 1 mg/kg IV on the same day every 6 weeks and two cycles of platinum-doublet chemotherapy every 3 weeks. Continue nivolumab and ipilimumab until disease progression or unacceptable toxicity occurs or up to 2 years in patients without disease progression.

✳ *NEW INDICATION:* **Neoadjuvant treatment of resectable NSCLC (tumors of at least 4 cm or node-positive), in combination with platinum-doublet chemotherapy**
Adults: 360 mg IV infusion followed by platinum-doublet chemotherapy on the same day every 3 weeks for three cycles.

➤ **Advanced renal carcinoma in patients who have received prior antiangiogenic therapy**
Adults: 240 mg IV infusion once every 2 weeks or 480 mg every 4 weeks until disease progression or unacceptable toxicity occurs.

➤ **Intermediate or poor risk, previously untreated advanced renal cell carcinoma, in combination with ipilimumab**
Adults: 3 mg/kg IV infusion followed by ipilimumab 1 mg/kg IV infusion on the same day every 3 weeks for four doses; then nivolumab 240 mg as a single-agent IV infusion every 2 weeks or 480 mg every 4 weeks over 30 minutes until disease progression or unacceptable toxicity occurs.

➤ **Advanced renal cell carcinoma as first-line treatment, in combination with cabozantinib**
Adults: 240 mg IV infusion once every 2 weeks or 480 mg every 4 weeks until disease progression or unacceptable toxicity occurs, or up to 2 years with cabozantinib 40 mg PO daily without food until disease progression or unacceptable toxicity.

➤ **Classical Hodgkin lymphoma that has relapsed or progressed after autologous hematopoietic stem cell transplantation (HSCT) and posttransplantation brentuximab vedotin; after three or more lines of systemic therapy that includes autologous HSCT; recurrent or metastatic squamous cell carcinoma of the head and neck with**

N

disease progression on or after platinum-based therapy
Adults: 240 mg IV infusion every 2 weeks or 480 mg every 4 weeks until disease progression or unacceptable toxicity occurs.

➤ **Locally advanced or metastatic urothelial carcinoma in patients with disease progression during or after platinum-containing chemotherapy, or who have disease progression within 12 months of neoadjuvant or adjuvant treatment with a platinum-containing chemotherapy**
Adults: 240 mg IV infusion every 2 weeks or 480 mg every 4 weeks until disease progression or unacceptable toxicity occurs.

✳ *NEW INDICATION:* **Adjuvant treatment of urothelial carcinoma in patients at high risk for recurrence after undergoing radical resection**
Adults: 240 mg IV infusion every 2 weeks or 480 mg IV infusion every 4 weeks until disease recurrence or unacceptable toxicity occurs, or up to 1-year treatment.

➤ **Microsatellite instability-high (MSI-H) or mismatch repair deficient (dMMR) metastatic colorectal cancer that has progressed following treatment with a fluoropyrimidine, oxaliplatin, and irinotecan**
Adults and children age 12 and older weighing 40 kg or more: 240 mg IV infusion every 2 weeks or 480 mg every 4 weeks until disease progression or unacceptable toxicity occurs.
Adults and children age 12 and older weighing less than 40 kg: 3 mg/kg IV infusion every 2 weeks.

➤ **MSI-H or dMMR metastatic colorectal cancer that has progressed after treatment with a fluoropyrimidine, oxaliplatin, and irinotecan in combination with ipilimumab**
Adults and children age 12 and older weighing 40 kg or more: 3 mg/kg IV infusion over 30 minutes followed by ipilimumab 1 mg/kg IV infusion on the same day, every 3 weeks for four doses; then nivolumab 240 mg as a single-agent IV infusion over 30 minutes every 2 weeks or 480 mg every 4 weeks until disease progression or unacceptable toxicity occurs.
Adults and children age 12 and older weighing less than 40 kg: 3 mg/kg IV infusion followed by ipilimumab 1 mg/kg IV infusion on the same day, every 3 weeks for four doses; then nivolumab 3 mg/kg as a single-agent IV infusion over 30 minutes every 2 weeks until

disease progression or unacceptable toxicity occurs.

➤ **Hepatocellular carcinoma in patients previously treated with sorafenib**
Adults: 1 mg/kg IV infusion every 3 weeks followed by ipilimumab 3 mg/kg IV infusion on the same day for four doses; then nivolumab 240 mg as a single-agent IV infusion every 2 weeks or 480 mg every 4 weeks until disease progression or unacceptable toxicity occurs.

➤ **Unresectable advanced, recurrent, or metastatic esophageal squamous cell carcinoma after prior fluoropyrimidine- and platinum-based chemotherapy**
Adults: 240 mg IV infusion every 2 weeks or 480 mg every 4 weeks until disease progression or unacceptable toxicity occurs.

➤ **Advanced or metastatic gastric cancer, gastroesophageal junction cancer, and esophageal adenocarcinoma, in combination with fluoropyrimidine- and platinum-containing chemotherapy**
Adults: 360 mg IV infusion every 3 weeks with fluoropyrimidine- and platinum-containing chemotherapy every 3 weeks; or 240 mg IV infusion every 2 weeks with fluoropyrimidine- and platinum-containing chemotherapy every 2 weeks until disease progression or unacceptable toxicity occurs, or up to 2 years in patients without disease progression.

➤ **Adjuvant treatment of completely resected esophageal or gastroesophageal junction cancer with residual pathologic disease in patients who have received neoadjuvant chemoradiotherapy**
Adults: 240 mg IV infusion every 2 weeks, or 480 mg IV infusion every 4 weeks until disease progression or unacceptable toxicity occurs or up to 1 year of treatment.

✳ *NEW INDICATION:* **Unresectable advanced or metastatic esophageal squamous cell carcinoma as first-line treatment, in combination with fluoropyrimidine- and platinum-containing chemotherapy**
Adults: 240 mg IV infusion every 2 weeks or 480 mg IV infusion every 4 weeks in combination with chemotherapy. Continue nivolumab until disease progression or unacceptable toxicity occurs, or up to 2 years.

✳ *NEW INDICATION:* **Unresectable advanced or metastatic esophageal squamous cell carcinoma as first-line treatment, in combination with ipilimumab**

Adults: 3 mg/kg IV infusion every 2 weeks or 360 mg IV infusion every 3 weeks with ipilimumab 1 mg/kg IV infusion every 6 weeks until disease progression or unacceptable toxicity occurs, or up to 2 years.

➤ **Unresectable malignant pleural mesothelioma, in combination with ipilimumab**

Adults: 360 mg IV every 3 weeks followed by ipilimumab 1 mg/kg IV on the same day every 6 weeks. Continue until disease progression or unacceptable toxicity occurs, or up to 2 years in patients without disease progression.

ADMINISTRATION

IV

▼ When administering with ipilimumab, infuse nivolumab first followed by ipilimumab on the same day. Use separate infusion bags and filters for each infusion. Refer to ipilimumab manufacturer's instructions for administration information.

▼ Visually inspect for particulate matter and discoloration (solution should be clear to opalescent, colorless to pale yellow).

▼ Store vial refrigerated at 36° to 46° F (2° to 8° C). Don't freeze.

▼ Protect from light by storing in original package until time of use.

▼ To prepare: Withdraw required volume of nivolumab, transfer to IV container, and dilute with NSS or 5% dextrose injection to yield a final concentration of 1 to 10 mg/mL. Don't exceed total volume of 160 mL. For patients weighing less than 40 kg, the total volume mustn't exceed 4 mL/kg of body weight. Mix by gentle inversion; don't shake.

▼ Discard all partially used or empty vials.

▼ Diluted solution remains stable at room temperature for no more than 8 hours, including room temperature storage of infusion in the IV container and time for administration of infusion.

▼ Diluted solution remains stable under refrigeration (36° to 46° F [2° to 8° C]) for no more than 24 hours from time of infusion preparation. Don't freeze.

▼ Give through IV line containing a sterile, nonpyrogenic, low-protein-binding in-line filter (pore size, 0.2 to 1.2 microns) over 30 minutes.

▼ Flush IV line at end of infusion.

▼ **Incompatibilities:** Don't administer with other drugs through same IV line.

ACTION

A humanized monoclonal antibody that binds to the PD1 receptor found on the surface of T cells, reversing T-cell suppression and resulting in decreased tumor growth.

Route	Onset	Peak	Duration
IV	Unknown	Unknown	Unknown

Half-life: About 25 days.

ADVERSE REACTIONS

CNS: dizziness, peripheral and sensory neuropathy, fatigue, headache, neuritis, asthenia, fever. **CV:** peripheral edema, *ventricular arrhythmia,* HTN, chest pain. **EENT:** iridocyclitis. **GI:** abdominal pain, colitis, nausea, vomiting, constipation, diarrhea, stomatitis, decreased appetite. **GU:** renal dysfunction, nephritis, renal insufficiency. **Hematologic:** anemia, *lymphopenia, thrombocytopenia, neutropenia.* **Hepatic:** increased AST, ALT, bilirubin, and ALP levels; *hepatitis.* **Metabolic:** hyponatremia, *hyperkalemia, hypokalemia,* hyperglycemia, hypercalcemia, *hypocalcemia, hypomagnesemia,* hypothyroidism, hyperthyroidism, increased triglyceride and cholesterol levels, weight loss. **Musculoskeletal:** pain, arthralgia. **Respiratory:** cough, URI, dyspnea, pneumonitis, *ILD,* pleural effusion. **Skin:** rash, pruritus, erythema, exfoliative dermatitis, *erythema multiforme,* psoriasis, skin depigmentation. **Other:** infusion-related reactions, thyroiditis.

INTERACTIONS

Drug-drug. *Immunosuppressants:* May diminish therapeutic effect of nivolumab. Consider therapy modification.

EFFECTS ON LAB TEST RESULTS

• May increase creatinine, total bilirubin, amylase, lipase, ALT, AST, ALP, glucose, triglyceride, and cholesterol levels.

• May decrease sodium and magnesium levels.

• May increase or decrease thyroid function and potassium and calcium levels.

• May decrease RBC, lymphocyte, neutrophil, and platelet counts.

CONTRAINDICATIONS & CAUTIONS

• Contraindicated in patients hypersensitive to drug or its components.

N

◔ *Alert:* If nivolumab is withheld for an adverse reaction, also withhold ipilimumab.

◔ *Alert:* Drug can cause severe immune-mediated pneumonitis or ILD, which can be fatal.

• Drug can cause the following immune-mediated conditions: colitis, hepatitis, nephritis, renal dysfunction, hypothyroidism and hyperthyroidism, life-threatening rash, encephalitis, and other serious adverse reactions.

• Drug can cause hypophysitis and adrenal insufficiency.

• Nivolumab shouldn't be used for the treatment of multiple myeloma. Use in combination with a thalidomide analogue plus dexamethasone increased risk of mortality in clinical trials. This combination isn't recommended outside the setting of a clinical trial.

• Drug hasn't been studied in patients with severe hepatic impairment.

• Safety and effectiveness haven't been established in children younger than age 12 with MSI-H or dMMR metastatic colorectal cancer or in patients younger than age 18 for the other approved indications.

Dialyzable drug: Unknown.

PREGNANCY-LACTATION-REPRODUCTION

◔ *Alert:* Use cautiously during pregnancy. Drug may cause fetal harm and increase risk of abortion and premature infant death.

• Patients of childbearing potential should use effective contraception during treatment and for at least 5 months after final dose.

• Verify pregnancy status before starting therapy.

• It isn't known if drug appears in human milk. Patient should discontinue breastfeeding during treatment and for 5 months after final dose because of possible serious adverse effects in infants who are breastfed.

NURSING CONSIDERATIONS

• Infusion-related reactions, which can be severe or life-threatening, can occur. Discontinue drug for severe or life-threatening reactions. For mild to moderate reactions, either interrupt infusion or decrease infusion rate.

• Drug can cause type 1 diabetes. Monitor glucose levels and withhold drug for severe hyperglycemia until metabolic control is achieved; permanently discontinue for life-threatening hyperglycemia.

• Monitor patients for acute GVHD and hepatic veno-occlusive disease. Transplant-related mortality has occurred.

• Monitor patient for signs and symptoms of immune-mediated severe pneumonitis or ILD (fever, cough, dyspnea, chest pain) or colitis (fever, abdominal pain, diarrhea, bloody stools). Adjust dosage or discontinue drug as needed. Refer to manufacturer's instructions for corticosteroid treatment if indicated.

• Obtain LFT values at baseline and monitor periodically during treatment because of risk of immune-mediated hepatitis. Adjust dosages or discontinue drug as needed. Refer to manufacturer's instructions for corticosteroid treatment if indicated.

• Obtain serum creatinine level at baseline and monitor periodically during treatment because of risk of immune-mediated nephritis and renal dysfunction. Adjust dosages or discontinue drug as needed. Refer to manufacturer's instructions for corticosteroid treatment if indicated.

• Monitor thyroid function at baseline and periodically during treatment because of risk of immune-mediated hypothyroidism and hyperthyroidism. Administer hormone replacement therapy for hypothyroidism, or initiate medical management for control of hyperthyroidism. There are no recommended nivolumab dosage adjustments for hypothyroidism or hyperthyroidism.

• Monitor patient for other immune-mediated adverse reactions, which may occur during or after nivolumab has been discontinued. Rule out other causes of reactions first. Based on severity of reaction, withhold drug, administer corticosteroids, or initiate hormone-replacement therapy, if appropriate.

• *Look alike–sound alike:* Don't confuse nivolumab with other monoclonal antibodies.

PATIENT TEACHING

• Instruct patient to inform prescriber if patient has known disease that affects the immune system, lungs, liver, or kidney or has had an organ transplant.

• Educate patient and family to recognize and immediately report signs and symptoms of pneumonitis (new or worsening cough, chest pain, shortness of breath), colitis (diarrhea, bloody stools, melena, severe abdominal pain or tenderness), hepatic dysfunction (dark urine, yellowing of eyes, nausea, vomiting, right-sided abdominal pain, lethargy,

---

Reactions in bold italics are *life-threatening*. Interactions may have a *rapid onset* or a *delayed onset*.

easy bruising or bleeding), renal dysfunction (decreased urine output, blood in urine, edema, loss of appetite), hormone gland problems (weight gain or loss, feeling hot or cold, constipation, persistent or unusual headaches, extreme fatigue, changes in mood or behavior, dizziness, hair loss, deepening voice), rash, vision changes, severe or persistent muscle or joint pains, or severe muscle weakness.

◐ Alert: Warn patient who is pregnant of fetal risk. Advise patient of childbearing potential to use effective contraception during and for at least 5 months after last dose.

• Advise patient to report known or suspected pregnancy to prescriber.

• Caution patient not to breastfeed while taking drug and for 5 months after last dose.

• Reinforce importance of lab tests and instruct patient to keep follow-up appointments to monitor drug's safety and effectiveness.

norelgestromin–ethinyl estradiol transdermal system
nor-el-JES-troe-min/ETH-i-nill ess-tra-DYE-ole

Evra♣, Xulane, Zafemy

Therapeutic class: Contraceptives
Pharmacologic class: Estrogen–progestin combinations

AVAILABLE FORMS
Transdermal patch: norelgestromin 4.86 mg and ethinyl estradiol 0.53 mg per patch, delivering 150 mcg norelgestromin and 35 mcg ethinyl estradiol daily; norelgestromin 6 mg and ethinyl estradiol 0.60 mg per patch delivering 200 mcg norelgestromin and 35 mcg ethinyl estradiol daily♣

INDICATIONS & DOSAGES
➤ **Contraception**
Patients of childbearing potential with a BMI less than 30 kg/m² : Apply 1 patch weekly for 3 weeks (21 total days). Apply each new patch on the same day of the week. Week 4 is patch-free, and withdrawal bleeding is expected. On the day after week 4 ends, apply a new patch to start a new 4-week cycle. The patch-free interval between cycles should never be longer than 7 days.

ADMINISTRATION
Transdermal
• Hazardous agent; follow special handling and disposal procedures.

• Apply patch to a clean, dry area of the skin on the buttocks, abdomen, upper outer arm, or upper torso. Don't apply to the breasts or to skin that is red, irritated, or cut, or on the same location as the previous patch.

• Patient shouldn't apply makeup, creams, lotions, powders, or other topical products at application site.

• Press patch down firmly onto the skin using palm of the hand; apply pressure for 10 seconds. Run fingers over entire surface area to smooth out any wrinkles in the patch.

• Check patch daily to ensure all edges are sticking. Don't use tape or wraps to hold patch in place.

• Don't cut, damage, or alter the size of the patch, as contraception may be impaired.

• If skin becomes irritated, remove patch and apply a new patch at a different site.

ACTION
Combination hormonal contraceptives act by suppressing gonadotropins. The primary mechanism of this action is ovulation inhibition. However, changes in cervical mucus increase the difficulty of sperm entry into the uterus, and changes in the endometrium decrease the likelihood of implantation.

Route	Onset	Peak	Duration
Transdermal	Rapid	2 days	Unknown

Half-life: Norelgestromin, 28 hours; ethinyl estradiol, about 17 hours.

ADVERSE REACTIONS
CNS: headache, emotional lability, dizziness, fatigue, migraine, insomnia, anxiety. **CV:** increased BP, *PE.* **EENT:** contact lens intolerance, changes in corneal curvature. **GI:** nausea, diarrhea, abdominal pain, vomiting, abdominal distention, cholestatic jaundice. **GU:** dysmenorrhea, vaginal bleeding and menstrual disorders, vulvovaginal candidiasis, genital discharge, uterine spasm, vaginal dryness, vulvar dryness, premenstrual syndrome, libido changes. **Metabolic:** weight changes, fluid retention, lipid disorders. **Musculoskeletal:** muscle spasms. **Skin:** application-site reaction, melasma, pruritus, acne, dermatitis, erythema. **Other:** breast tenderness, enlargement, or secretion.

N

INTERACTIONS

Drug-drug. *Acetaminophen, clofibric acid, morphine, salicylic acid, temazepam:* May decrease levels or increase clearance of these drugs. Monitor patient for lack of effect.

Anticoagulants: May increase or decrease effect of anticoagulant. Monitor patient and lab values.

Ascorbic acid, atorvastatin, etravirine, rosuvastatin: May increase hormone levels. Use together cautiously.

Barbiturates, felbamate, griseofulvin, oxcarbazepine, tetracyclines, topiramate: May reduce contraceptive effectiveness, resulting in unintended pregnancy or breakthrough bleeding. Encourage backup contraception if used together.

Cyclosporine, prednisolone, theophylline, tizanidine, voriconazole: May increase levels of these drugs. Monitor patient for adverse reactions.

CYP3A4 inducers (bosentan, carbamazepine, phenytoin, rifampin): May reduce contraceptive effectiveness, resulting in unintended pregnancy or breakthrough bleeding. Encourage backup contraception if used together.

CYP3A4 inhibitors (fluconazole, itraconazole): May increase hormone levels. Use together cautiously.

HIV protease inhibitors: May increase or decrease contraceptive level. Use together cautiously.

Ombitasvir, paritaprevir, ritonavir: May cause elevated ALT level. Use is contraindicated.

Sugammadex: May decrease contraceptive effectiveness. Patient should use backup contraception while using sugammadex and for 7 days after.

Drug-herb. *St. John's wort:* May reduce effectiveness of drug. Don't use together.

Drug-food. *Grapefruit juice:* May increase plasma hormone concentrations. Avoid use.

Drug-lifestyle. **Boxed Warning** *Smoking:* May increase risk of CV adverse effects, related to age and number of cigarettes smoked daily. Urge patient not to smoke. ∎

EFFECTS ON LAB TEST RESULTS

• May increase circulating total thyroid hormone, triglyceride, other binding proteins, sex hormone–binding globulin, total circulating endogenous sex steroid, corticoid, and factor VII, VIII, IX, and X levels.

• May decrease antithrombin III and folate levels.

• May decrease free T_3 resin uptake and glucose tolerance.

CONTRAINDICATIONS & CAUTIONS

Boxed Warning Cigarette smoking increases the risk of serious adverse cardiac effects from hormonal contraceptive use. Risk increases with age, especially in women older than age 35, and with the number of cigarettes smoked. Hormonal contraceptives are contraindicated in women older than age 35 who smoke. ∎

☻ *Alert:* There is an increased risk of VTE in patients ages 15 to 44 using the norelgestromin–ethinyl estradiol transdermal system compared to patients using oral contraceptives.

☻ *Alert:* The contraceptive patch has higher steady-state concentrations and lower peak concentrations than oral contraceptives. It's unknown whether the risk of serious adverse events is higher with oral contraceptives containing ethinyl estradiol 30 to 35 mcg. Increased estrogen exposure may increase the risk of adverse events, including VTE.

Boxed Warning Contraindicated in patients with a BMI of 30 kg/m^2 or more. Risk of venous thromboembolic events in these patients may be greater compared to risk in patients with a BMI less than 30 kg/m^2. ∎

• Contraindicated in patients hypersensitive to components of drug; in those with history of DVT or related disorder; in patients at high risk for arterial or venous thrombotic diseases or with current or past history of cerebrovascular disease or CAD; in those with uncontrolled HTN and inherited or acquired hypercoagulopathies; and in patients with headaches with focal neurologic conditions, migraine headaches with aura, or migraine headaches if older than age 35.

• Contraindicated in patients with past or current known or suspected breast cancer or other known or suspected estrogen- or progestin-sensitive neoplasia and in those with hepatic adenoma or cancer.

• Contraindicated in patients with thrombophlebitis, thromboembolic disorders, valvular heart disease with complications, diabetes with vascular involvement, major surgery with prolonged immobilization, undiagnosed abnormal genital bleeding,

---

Reactions in bold italics are *life-threatening*. Interactions may have a *rapid onset* or a *delayed onset*.

cholestatic jaundice of pregnancy or jaundice with previous hormonal contraceptive use, benign or malignant liver tumors or liver disease, or acute or chronic hepatocellular disease with abnormal hepatic function.

• Contraindicated with hepatitis C drug combinations containing ombitasvir–paritaprevir–ritonavir, with or without dasabuvir, due to potential for ALT elevations.

• Use cautiously in patients with CV disease risk factors, conditions that might be aggravated by fluid retention, or history of depression.

• Use cautiously in patients with prediabetes or diabetes; drug may decrease glucose tolerance.

• Use cautiously in patients with personal or family history of hypertriglyceridemia; drug may increase risk of pancreatitis.

• Drug may increase lipid levels. Consider alternative drug for patient with uncontrolled dyslipidemia.

Dialyzable drug: Unknown.

⚠ *Overdose S&S:* Nausea, vomiting, withdrawal uterine bleeding.

PREGNANCY-LACTATION-REPRODUCTION

• Contraindicated with known or suspected pregnancy. Discontinue if pregnancy occurs.

• Patient should use alternative contraceptive method during breastfeeding until the infant weans completely.

• In patients who choose not to breastfeed, don't begin drug until 4 weeks after childbirth.

NURSING CONSIDERATIONS

🚫 *Alert:* Patients taking combination hormonal contraceptives may be at increased risk for thrombophlebitis, venous thrombosis with or without embolism, PE, MI, cerebral hemorrhage, cerebral thrombosis, HTN, gallbladder disease, hepatic adenomas, benign liver tumors, mesenteric thrombosis, and retinal thrombosis.

• Increased risk of MI occurs primarily in smokers and women with HTN, hypercholesterolemia, morbid obesity, and diabetes.

• Encourage women with a history of HTN or renal disease to use a different contraceptive. If this drug is used, monitor BP closely and stop use if HTN occurs.

• Drug may be less effective in patients who weigh 90 kg or more.

• The risk of thromboembolic disease increases if therapy is used postpartum or postabortion.

• Rule out pregnancy if withdrawal bleeding fails to occur for two consecutive cycles.

• Stop drug and notify prescriber at least 4 weeks before and for 2 weeks after an elective surgery that increases the risk of thromboembolism, and during and after prolonged immobilization. Teach patient about alternative methods of contraception during this time.

• Stop drug and notify prescriber if patient has headaches, vision loss, proptosis, diplopia, papilledema, retinal vascular lesions, jaundice, or depression.

PATIENT TEACHING

• Emphasize the importance of having regular annual physical exams to check for adverse effects or developing contraindications.

• Tell patient that drug doesn't protect against HIV and other sexually transmitted diseases.

• Advise patient to notify prescriber immediately for unrelieved leg pain, sudden shortness of breath, pain or pressure in the chest, severe headache, weakness or numbness in an arm or leg, trouble speaking, or yellowing of the skin or eyes.

• Advise patient to use a backup method of contraception for the first 7 days of use.

• Tell patient switching from estrogen–progestin oral contraceptives to apply first patch on the first day of withdrawal bleeding. If no bleeding occurs within 5 days of last hormonally active pill, advise patient to obtain a pregnancy test.

• Instruct patient in safe drug administration and handling. Tell patient to carefully fold used patch in half so that it sticks to itself before discarding and to discard out of reach of children and pets.

• Warn patient to immediately stop use for confirmed pregnancy.

• Tell patient who wears contact lenses to report visual changes or changes in lens tolerance.

• Advise patient not to smoke while using the patch.

• Counsel patient who is unsure what to do about mistakes with patch use to use a backup method of birth control and contact health care provider.

• Tell patient undergoing an MRI scan to alert facility that she's using a transdermal patch.

N

• Instruct patient to report all drugs and supplements being taken, as some can decrease contraceptive effectiveness; a backup contraceptive method may be needed.

• Advise patient receiving thyroid hormone replacement therapy that increased doses of thyroid hormone may be needed.

SAFETY ALERT!

norepinephrine bitartrate (levarterenol bitartrate, noradrenaline acid tartrate)
nor-ep-i-NEF-rin

Levophed

Therapeutic class: Vasopressors
Pharmacologic class: Alpha/beta agonists

AVAILABLE FORMS
Injection: 1 mg/mL ampule or vial; 4 mg/250 mL, 8 mg/250 mL premixed container

INDICATIONS & DOSAGES
➤ **To restore BP in acute hypotension**
Adults: Initially, 8 to 12 mcg/minute by IV infusion; then titrate to maintain systolic BP at 80 to 100 mm Hg in patients who were previously normotensive and 40 mm Hg below preexisting systolic BP in patients who were previously hypertensive. Average maintenance dose is 2 to 4 mcg/minute.
Adjust-a-dose: Gradually reduce infusion rate while expanding blood volume with IV fluids when discontinuing norepinephrine.

ADMINISTRATION
IV
▼ Premixed containers require no additional dilution. Be aware there are two different concentrations.

▼ Infuse into a large vein to minimize risk of extravasation. Avoid infusion into leg veins of older adults or patients with occlusive vascular disease of the legs.

▼ Add 4 mg to 1,000 mL D_5W alone or D_5W in NSS for injection. Use continuous infusion pump to regulate infusion flow rate. Avoid using a catheter tie-in technique.

▼ Never leave patient unattended during infusion. Check BP every 2 minutes until stabilized; then check every 5 minutes.

▼ During infusion, frequently monitor ECG, cardiac output, central venous pressure, pulmonary artery occlusion pressure, pulse rate, urine output, and color and temperature of limbs. Titrate infusion rate based on findings and prescriber guidelines.

🕑 *Alert:* Check site frequently for signs and symptoms of extravasation. If they appear, stop infusion immediately and call prescriber. To prevent sloughing and necrosis, use a fine hypodermic needle to infiltrate area with 5 to 10 mg phentolamine in 10 to 15 mL of NSS as soon as possible. Immediate local hyperemic changes will occur if area is infiltrated within 12 hours. Also, check for blanching along course of infused vein, which may progress to superficial sloughing.

▼ Protect drug from light. Discard discolored solution or solution that contains precipitate. Solution will deteriorate after 24 hours.

▼ If prolonged therapy is needed, change injection site frequently.

▼ Avoid mixing with alkaline solutions, oxidizing drugs, or iron salts. The use of NSS alone isn't recommended because of the lack of oxidation protection.

▼ **Incompatibilities:** Alkalis, drotrecogin alfa, iron salts, oxidizers, regular insulin, thiopental.

ACTION
Stimulates alpha and beta$_1$ receptors in the sympathetic nervous system, causing vasoconstriction and cardiac stimulation.

Route	Onset	Peak	Duration
IV	Immediate	Immediate	1–2 min after infusion

Half-life: About 1 minute.

ADVERSE REACTIONS
CNS: headache, anxiety. **CV:** *bradycardia, severe HTN, arrhythmias, ischemic injury.* **Respiratory:** respiratory difficulties, *pulmonary edema.* **Skin:** irritation with extravasation, necrosis and gangrene secondary to extravasation. **Other:** *anaphylaxis.*

INTERACTIONS
Drug-drug. *Alpha blockers:* May antagonize drug effects. Monitor perfusion and BP.
Antidiabetics: May decrease insulin sensitivity and increase glucose level. Monitor glucose level and adjust dosages if needed.

Reactions in bold italics are *life-threatening*. Interactions may have a *rapid onset* or a **delayed onset**.

Antihistamines, atropine, ergot alkaloids, guanethidine, imipramine, linezolid, MAO inhibitors, methyldopa, oxytocics, TCAs: May cause severe, prolonged HTN. Use together with extreme caution.

Atomoxetine: May enhance hypertensive and tachycardic effects. Monitor BP and HR.

Inhaled anesthetics (cyclopropane, halothane): May increase risk of arrhythmias. Don't use together.

EFFECTS ON LAB TEST RESULTS
None reported.

CONTRAINDICATIONS & CAUTIONS
• Avoid use in patients with mesenteric or peripheral vascular thrombosis (unless drug is deemed necessary as a life-saving procedure), profound hypoxia, hypercarbia, or hypotension resulting from blood volume deficit (except as an emergency measure).
• Use cautiously in patients with sulfite sensitivity and older adults.
• Safety and effectiveness in children haven't been established.
Dialyzable drug: Unknown.
⚠ *Overdose S&S:* Headache, severe HTN, reflex bradycardia, increased peripheral resistance, decreased cardiac output.

PREGNANCY-LACTATION-REPRODUCTION
• Safe use in pregnancy hasn't been established. Use during pregnancy only if clearly needed.
• It isn't known if drug appears in human milk. Use cautiously during breastfeeding.

NURSING CONSIDERATIONS
• Drug isn't a substitute for blood or fluid replacement therapy. If patient has volume deficit, replace fluids before giving vasopressors.
• Keep emergency drugs on hand to reverse effects of drug: atropine for reflex bradycardia, phentolamine to decrease vasopressor effects, and propranolol for arrhythmias.
• Notify prescriber immediately of decreased urine output.
• When stopping drug, gradually slow infusion rate. Continue monitoring vital signs, watching for possible severe drop in BP.
🔔 *Alert:* Monitor infusion site carefully as extravasation can cause tissue necrosis.
• *Look alike–sound alike:* Don't confuse norepinephrine with epinephrine.

PATIENT TEACHING
• Tell patient to report adverse reactions promptly.
• Advise patient that vital signs will be monitored frequently and to immediately report discomfort at IV insertion site.

---

norethindrone
nor-ETH-in-drone

Camila, Errin, Heather, Incassia, Jencycla, Lyleq, Movisse ✤, Nor-QD

norethindrone acetate
Norlutate ✤

Therapeutic class: Contraceptives
Pharmacologic class: Progestins

AVAILABLE FORMS
norethindrone
Tablets: 0.35 mg
norethindrone acetate
Tablets: 5 mg

INDICATIONS & DOSAGES
➤ **Amenorrhea, abnormal uterine bleeding**
Adults: 2.5 to 10 mg norethindrone acetate PO daily for 5 to 10 days, beginning in the assumed latter half of the menstrual cycle.
➤ **Endometriosis**
Adults: 5 mg norethindrone acetate PO daily for 14 days; then increased by 2.5 mg/day every 2 weeks, up to 15 mg daily. Therapy may continue for 6 to 9 months or until breakthrough bleeding warrants temporary termination.
➤ **Contraception**
Patients of childbearing potential and patients who are menarchal: Initially, 0.35 mg norethindrone PO on first day of menstruation; then 0.35 mg daily.

ADMINISTRATION
PO
• Drug is hazardous agent; follow applicable special handling and disposal procedures.
• Give without regard to meals. May give with food if GI upset occurs.
• When used for contraception, give drug at same time every day, continuously, with no interruption between pill packs.

N

• When drug is used to prevent pregnancy, patient should use a backup method of contraception for 48 hours after a missed dose or a dose taken 3 or more hours after scheduled dose. If vomiting occurs soon after giving a dose, patient should use backup contraception for 48 hours.

ACTION

Suppresses ovulation, possibly by inhibiting pituitary gonadotropin secretion, and forms thick cervical mucus.

Route	Onset	Peak	Duration
PO	Unknown	2 hr	Unknown

Half-life: 8 to 9 hours.

ADVERSE REACTIONS

CNS: depression, headache, mood swings, dizziness, fatigue, insomnia, migraine, nervousness. **CV:** edema, *thromboembolism.* **EENT:** optic neuritis. **GI:** bloating, abdominal pain or cramping, nausea, vomiting. **GU:** breakthrough bleeding, menstrual irregularities, cervical erosion, abnormal secretions. **Hepatic:** cholestatic jaundice, *hepatitis.* **Metabolic:** weight changes. **Musculoskeletal:** limb pain. **Skin:** melasma, rash, acne, pruritus, alopecia, hirsutism, hemorrhagic skin eruptions. **Other:** breast tenderness, enlargement, or secretion; suppressed lactation, premenstrual-like syndrome, *anaphylactic reactions.*

INTERACTIONS

Drug-drug. *Barbiturates:* May decrease progestin effects. Monitor patient for diminished therapeutic response.
Cyclosporine: May increase cyclosporine level. Use together cautiously.
CYP3A4 inducers (bosentan, carbamazepine, phenobarbital, phenytoin, rifampin): May decrease effectiveness of contraceptive hormones. Consider alternative nonhormonal contraception.
CYP3A5 inhibitors (itraconazole, ketoconazole), NNRTIs (etravirine, ritonavir), protease inhibitors: May increase progestin level. Monitor therapy.
Ulipristal: May decrease effectiveness of both drugs. Avoid norethindrone within 5 days of using ulipristal.
Drug-herb. *St. John's wort:* May decrease effectiveness of contraceptive hormones.

Discourage use together. Patient should use alternative nonhormonal contraception.
Drug-lifestyle. *Smoking:* May increase risk of adverse CV effects. If smoking continues, may need alternative therapy.

EFFECTS ON LAB TEST RESULTS

• May increase LFT values and lipase level.
• May decrease HDL level.
• May decrease sex hormone-binding globulin concentrations.
• May alter thyroid function test results and decrease metyrapone test results.

CONTRAINDICATIONS & CAUTIONS

• Contraindicated in patients hypersensitive to drug and in those with breast cancer, undiagnosed abnormal vaginal bleeding, impaired liver function or hepatic disease, benign or malignant liver tumors, current or recent thromboembolic disorders (stroke, MI), or active DVT, PE, or history of these conditions.
• Use cautiously in patients with seizures, migraines, cardiac or renal disease, asthma, and depression.
• Use cautiously in patients with risk factors for arterial vascular disease (HTN, diabetes, tobacco use, hypercholesterolemia, obesity) or venous thromboembolism (VTE) (personal or family history of VTE, SLE).
• Use cautiously in patients with diabetes; drug may decrease glucose tolerance but insulin requirements generally don't change.
⊕ *Alert:* Norethindrone acetate may cause visual abnormalities due to papilledema or retinal vascular lesions. If these occur, discontinue drug.
Dialyzable drug: Unknown.

PREGNANCY-LACTATION-REPRODUCTION

• Contraindicated during pregnancy or as a diagnostic test for pregnancy; may cause fetal harm.
• Drug appears in human milk. Use cautiously during breastfeeding. Patient who breastfeeds exclusively may start progestin-only pills (POPs) 6 weeks after delivery. Patient who partially breastfeeds may start pills 3 weeks after delivery.

NURSING CONSIDERATIONS

• If switching from combined oral contraceptives to POPs, patient should take the first POP the day after the last active combined pill.

Reactions in bold italics are *life-threatening*. Interactions may have a *rapid onset* or a *delayed onset*.

• If switching from POPs to combined pills, patient should take the first active combined pill on the first day of menstruation, even if the POP pack isn't finished.

🚱 *Alert:* Norethindrone acetate is twice as potent as norethindrone. Norethindrone acetate shouldn't be used for contraception.

• Patients with menstrual disorders usually need preliminary estrogen treatment.

• Watch patient closely for signs of edema.

• Monitor BP.

PATIENT TEACHING

• According to FDA regulations, patient must read package insert explaining possible adverse effects before receiving first dose. Also, give patient verbal explanation.

• Teach patient safe drug administration and handling.

🚱 *Alert:* Advise patient to report unusual signs and symptoms immediately and to stop drug and report visual disturbances or migraine, or pain or numbness in the arms or legs.

• Teach patient how to perform routine breast self-exam.

• Tell patient to report suspected pregnancy to prescriber.

• Encourage patient to stop or reduce smoking because of the risk of CV complications.

• Tell patient with diabetes that drug may effect glucose levels and to closely monitor levels.

• Warn patient that drug doesn't protect against HIV or other sexually transmitted diseases.

---

nortriptyline hydrochloride ⌘
nor-TRIP-ti-leen

Aventyl ♣, Pamelor ✐

Therapeutic class: Antidepressants
Pharmacologic class: TCAs

AVAILABLE FORMS

Capsules: 10 mg, 25 mg, 50 mg, 75 mg
Oral solution: 10 mg/5 mL*

INDICATIONS & DOSAGES

➤ **Depression**

Adults: 25 mg PO t.i.d. or q.i.d., gradually increased to maximum of 150 mg daily. Or, give total daily dose at bedtime.

Older adults and adolescents: 30 to 50 mg PO daily given once or in divided doses.

ADMINISTRATION
PO

• Give drug without regard for food.

• Use medication measuring device for solution.

ACTION

Unknown. Increases the amount of norepinephrine, serotonin, or both in the CNS by blocking reuptake by the presynaptic neurons.

Route	Onset	Peak	Duration
PO	Unknown	4–9 hr	Unknown

Half-life: 14 to 51 hours.

ADVERSE REACTIONS

CNS: *stroke,* numbness, tingling, paresthesia of extremities, incoordination, ataxia, tremors, peripheral neuropathy, extrapyramidal symptoms, *seizures,* alteration in EEG, confusional states with hallucinations, delusions, disorientation, panic, anxiety, restlessness, agitation, insomnia, nightmares, hypomania, exacerbation of psychosis, drowsiness, dizziness, weakness, fatigue, headache. **CV:** edema, hypotension, HTN, tachycardia, palpitations, *MI,* arrhythmias, *heart block,* flushing. **EENT:** blurred vision, disturbance of accommodation, mydriasis, angle-closure glaucoma, tinnitus, dry mouth. **GI:** constipation, paralytic ileus, nausea and vomiting, anorexia, epigastric distress, diarrhea, peculiar taste, stomatitis, abdominal cramps, black tongue. **GU:** urine retention, delayed micturition, dilation of the urinary tract, erectile dysfunction, testicular swelling, urinary frequency, nocturia, increased or decreased libido. **Hematologic:** bone marrow depression, eosinophilia, purpura, *thrombocytopenia.* **Hepatic:** jaundice, altered liver function. **Metabolic:** weight gain or loss, SIADH. **Skin:** rash, petechiae, urticaria, itching, photosensitivity, alopecia, diaphoresis. **Other:** drug fever, gynecomastia, breast enlargement and galactorrhea in women.

INTERACTIONS

Drug-drug. *Anticholinergics:* May increase anticholinergic adverse effects (urine retention, constipation). Monitor patient.
Barbiturates, CNS depressants: May enhance CNS depression. Avoid using together.
Buspirone, fentanyl, lithium, SSNRIs, SSRIs, TCAs, tramadol, triptans: May increase

N

---

risk of serotonin syndrome. Monitor patient closely.

Cimetidine, TCAs (fluoxetine, fluvoxamine, paroxetine, sertraline): May increase nortriptyline level. Monitor drug levels and patient for signs of toxicity.

Drugs that prolong QT interval: May increase risk of life-threatening cardiac arrhythmias, including torsades de pointes. Monitor patient and ECG.

Epinephrine, norepinephrine: May increase hypertensive effect. Use together cautiously.

Linezolid, methylene blue: May cause serotonin syndrome. Use extreme caution and monitor patient closely.

MAO inhibitors: May increase risk of serotonin syndrome. Concurrent use is contraindicated. Avoid using within 14 days of MAO inhibitor therapy.

Quinolones: May increase the risk of life-threatening arrhythmias. Avoid using together.

Reserpine: May produce a stimulating effect in some patients. Monitor patient.

Drug-herb. *Evening primrose oil:* May cause additive or synergistic effect, lowering seizure threshold and increasing the risk of seizure. Discourage use together.

St. John's wort, SAM-e, yohimbe: May cause serotonin syndrome and reduced drug level. Discourage use together.

Drug-lifestyle. *Alcohol use:* May enhance CNS depression. Discourage use together.

Sun exposure: May increase risk of photosensitivity reactions. Advise patient to avoid excessive sunlight exposure.

EFFECTS ON LAB TEST RESULTS
• May increase LFT values.
• May increase or decrease glucose level.
• May increase eosinophil count.
• May decrease WBC, RBC, granulocyte, and platelet counts.

CONTRAINDICATIONS & CAUTIONS
• Contraindicated in patients hypersensitive to drug and during acute recovery phase of MI.

Boxed Warning Drug may increase risk of suicidality in children, adolescents, and young adults with major depressive disorder or other psychiatric disorder. Nortriptyline isn't approved for use in children. ∎

🕚 *Alert:* Concomitant use with linezolid or methylene blue can cause serotonin syndrome

(fever, mental status changes, muscle twitching, diaphoresis, shivering or shaking, diarrhea, loss of coordination). Use drug with linezolid or methylene blue only for life-threatening or urgent conditions when the potential benefits outweigh the risks of toxicity.

▨ Patients who are poor metabolizers of CYP2D6 have higher plasma concentration when given usual doses. Approximately 7% to 10% of whites are poor metabolizers.

• Drug isn't approved for use in patients with bipolar depression. Screen for bipolar depression before starting drug.

• Use with extreme caution in patients with glaucoma, suicidality, history of urine retention or seizures, CV disease, or hyperthyroidism and in those receiving thyroid drugs.

Dialyzable drug: No.

⚠ **Overdose S&S:** Cardiac arrhythmias, severe hypotension, shock, HF, pulmonary edema, seizures, CNS depression, coma, ECG changes, confusion, restlessness, disturbed concentration, transient visual hallucinations, dilated pupils, agitation, hyperactive reflexes, stupor, drowsiness, muscle rigidity, vomiting, hypothermia, hyperpyrexia.

PREGNANCY-LACTATION-REPRODUCTION
• Nortriptyline crosses the placental barrier. Neonates may experience irritability, jitteriness, and seizures.

• Safe use during pregnancy and breastfeeding hasn't been established. Weigh potential benefits against possible hazards.

• Encourage enrollment in the National Pregnancy Registry for Antidepressants (1-866-691-2388).

• Monitor patient during pregnancy and infants who are breastfeeding for adverse reactions.

NURSING CONSIDERATIONS
Boxed Warning Monitor all patients for clinical worsening, suicidality, or unusual changes in behavior. ∎

🕚 *Alert:* If linezolid or methylene blue must be given, stop nortriptyline and monitor patient for serotonin toxicity for 2 weeks or until 24 hours after the last dose of methylene blue or linezolid, whichever comes first. Treatment with nortriptyline may resume 24 hours after the last dose of methylene blue or linezolid.

• To withdraw drug, gradually taper dosage and monitor patient for reemerging symptoms.

• Because patients using TCAs may suffer hypertensive episodes during surgery, stop drug gradually several days before surgery.
• If signs or symptoms of psychosis occur or increase, expect to reduce dosage. Record mood changes. Monitor patient for suicidality; allow patient only a minimum supply of drug.
• *Look alike–sound alike:* Don't confuse nortriptyline with amitriptyline. Don't confuse Pamelor with Tambocor.

PATIENT TEACHING
Boxed Warning Advise families and caregivers to closely observe patient for increased suicidality. ■
• Instruct patient in safe drug administration.
• Teach patient to recognize and immediately report signs and symptoms of serotonin syndrome (fever, mental status changes, muscle twitching, diaphoresis, shivering or shaking, diarrhea, loss of coordination).
• Warn patient to avoid activities that require alertness and good coordination until effects of drug are known. Drowsiness and dizziness usually subside after a few weeks.
• Recommend use of sugarless hard candy or gum to relieve dry mouth. Saliva substitutes may be needed.
• Tell patient to consult prescriber before taking other prescription or OTC drugs.
• Warn patient not to stop drug suddenly.
• To prevent oversensitivity to the sun, advise patient to use sun block, wear protective clothing, and avoid prolonged exposure to strong sunlight.
• Advise patient to immediately report pregnancy or plans to become pregnant or breastfeed during treatment.

nystatin
nye-STAT-in

Nyaderm❦, Nyamyc, Nystop

Therapeutic class: Antifungals
Pharmacologic class: Polyene macrolides

AVAILABLE FORMS
Cream: 25,000 units/g❦, 100,000 units/g
Ointment: 100,000 units/g
Oral suspension: 100,000 units/mL
Powder: 100,000 units/g
Tablets: 500,000 units

INDICATIONS & DOSAGES
➤ **Intestinal candidiasis**
Adults: 500,000 to 1 million units PO as tablets t.i.d.
➤ **Fungal infections (cutaneous and mucocutaneous)**
Adults and children: Apply cream or ointment and gently massage into affected areas b.i.d. Or, apply powder to lesions b.i.d. to t.i.d. until lesions have healed.
➤ **Oral candidiasis (thrush)**
Adults and children: 400,000 to 600,000 units PO as oral suspension q.i.d. for up to 14 days.
Infants: 200,000 units PO as oral suspension q.i.d.

ADMINISTRATION
PO
• To treat oral candidiasis, after patient's mouth is clean of food debris, have patient hold suspension in mouth for several minutes before swallowing. When treating infants, use dropper to place one-half of dose in each side of the mouth and avoid feedings for 5 to 10 minutes after administration.
• Shake suspension well before use.
• Suspension made with bulk powder contains no preservatives. Use immediately. Don't store.
Topical
• Store at room temperature.
• For fungal infection of the feet, apply the powder to feet and all footwear.

ACTION
Probably binds to sterols in fungal cell membrane, altering cell permeability and allowing leakage of intracellular components.

Route	Onset	Peak	Duration
PO, topical	24–72 hr	Unknown	Unknown

Half-life: Unknown.

ADVERSE REACTIONS
GI: transient nausea, vomiting, diarrhea, GI upset. **GU:** irritation, sensitization. **Skin:** rash.

INTERACTIONS
Drug-drug. *Saccharomyces boulardii:* Systemic antifungal agents may diminish therapeutic effect of *Saccharomyces boulardii.* Avoid combination.

N

EFFECTS ON LAB TEST RESULTS
None reported.

CONTRAINDICATIONS & CAUTIONS
• Contraindicated in patients hypersensitive to drug.
• Rarely, SJS has been reported.
• Don't use topical powder for the treatment of systemic, oral, intravaginal, or ophthalmic infections.
• Although approved by the FDA for treatment of intestinal candidiasis, the drug isn't recommended by the Infectious Diseases Society of America.
Dialyzable drug: Unknown.
⚠ *Overdose S&S:* Nausea, GI upset.
• *Look alike–sound alike:* Don't confuse nystatin with atorvastatin, fluvastatin, or any other statins.

PREGNANCY-LACTATION-REPRODUCTION
• Use cautiously during pregnancy and only when clearly needed.
• It's unknown if drug appears in human milk; absorption is poor after oral ingestion. Use cautiously in breastfeeding.

NURSING CONSIDERATIONS
• Drug isn't effective against systemic infections.
• Monitor patient for rash.
• Avoid skin contact when applying.

PATIENT TEACHING
• Advise patient to continue taking drug for at least 2 days after signs and symptoms resolve.
• Instruct patient to report redness, swelling, or irritation.
• Tell patient that overusing mouthwash or wearing poorly fitting dentures may promote infection.
• Teach patient wearing dentures to remove dentures and clean them to avoid reinfection.
• For fungal foot infections, teach patient to dust powder freely on the feet and footwear.

obinutuzumab
oh-bi-nue-TOOZ-ue-mab

Gazyva

Therapeutic class: Antineoplastics
Pharmacologic class: Monoclonal antibodies

AVAILABLE FORMS
Injection: 1,000 mg/40 mL (25 mg/mL) single-dose vial

INDICATIONS & DOSAGES
Adjust-a-dose (for all indications): Refer to manufacturer's instructions for toxicity-related dosage adjustments, including infusion rate changes for infusion reactions.
➤ **Chronic lymphocytic leukemia previously untreated, in combination with chlorambucil**
Adults: Each cycle lasts 28 days. Cycle 1, day 1: 100 mg IV at 25 mg/hour over 4 hours; don't increase infusion rate. Cycle 1, day 2: 900 mg IV at 50 mg/hour; may increase infusion rate in increments of 50 mg/hour every 30 minutes to maximum rate of 400 mg/hour. Cycle 1, days 8 and 15: If no infusion reaction occurred during previous infusion and final infusion rate was 100 mg/hour or faster, give 1,000 mg IV at 100 mg/hour; may increase infusion rate by 100 mg/hour every 30 minutes to maximum rate of 400 mg/hour. For cycles 2 to 6 on day 1 only, give 1,000 mg every 28 days for five doses: If no infusion reaction occurred during previous infusion and final infusion rate was 100 mg/hour or faster, give 1,000 mg IV at 100 mg/hour; may increase infusion rate in increments of 100 mg/hour every 30 minutes to maximum of 400 mg/hour.

If appropriate, patients who don't complete the day-1, cycle-1 dose may proceed to the day-2, cycle-1 dose.
➤ **Follicular lymphoma, in combination with bendamustine followed by obinutuzumab monotherapy in patients who relapsed after, or are refractory to, a rituximab-containing regimen**
Adults: Each cycle lasts 28 days. Cycle 1, day 1: 1,000 mg IV at 50 mg/hour; may increase infusion rate in increments of 50 mg/hour every 30 minutes to maximum rate of 400 mg/hour. Cycle 1, days 8 and

---

15: If no infusion reaction occurred during previous infusion and final infusion rate was 100 mg/hour or faster, give 1,000 mg IV at 100 mg/hour; may increase infusion rate by 100 mg/hour every 30 minutes to maximum rate of 400 mg/hour.

For cycles 2 to 6 or 2 to 8 on day 1 only: If no infusion reaction occurred during previous infusion and final infusion rate was 100 mg/hour or faster, give 1,000 mg IV at 100 mg/hour; may increase infusion rate in increments of 100 mg/hour every 30 minutes to maximum rate of 400 mg/hour. Or, for patients who don't experience a grade 3 or higher infusion reaction during cycle 1, may give over 90 minutes on day 1 of cycles 2 to 6 and during monotherapy as 100 mg/hour for 30 minutes, then 900 mg/hour for approximately 60 minutes.

Patients who achieve stable disease, complete response, or partial response to the initial 6 cycles of obinutuzumab in combination with bendamustine should continue on obinutuzumab 1,000 mg as monotherapy once every 2 months for 2 years, beginning approximately 2 months after last dose during the induction phase. During monotherapy, maintain original dosing schedule for subsequent doses.

➤ **Previously untreated stage II bulky, III, or IV follicular lymphoma in combination with chemotherapy, followed by obinutuzumab monotherapy in patients achieving at least a partial remission**

Adults: Cycle 1, day 1: 1,000 mg IV at 50 mg/hour; may increase infusion rate in increments of 50 mg/hour every 30 minutes to maximum rate of 400 mg/hour. Cycle 1, days 8 and 15: If no infusion reaction occurred during previous infusion and final infusion rate was 100 mg/hour or faster, give 1,000 mg IV at 100 mg/hour; may increase infusion rate by 100 mg/hour every 30 minutes to maximum rate of 400 mg/hour.

For cycles 2 to 6 or 2 to 8, on day 1 only: If no infusion reaction occurred during previous infusion and final infusion rate was 100 mg/hour or faster, give 1,000 mg IV at 100 mg/hour; may increase infusion rate in increments of 100 mg/hour every 30 minutes to maximum rate of 400 mg/hour. Or, for patients who don't experience a grade 3 or higher infusion reaction during cycle 1, may give over 90 minutes on day 1 of cycles 2 to 6 or 2 to 8 and during monotherapy as 100 mg/hour for 30 minutes, then 900 mg/hour for approximately 60 minutes.

Treat concurrently with one of the following chemotherapy regimens: six 28-day cycles in combination with bendamustine; or six 21-day cycles in combination with cyclophosphamide, doxorubicin, vincristine, and prednisone, followed by two additional 21-day cycles of obinutuzumab alone; or eight 21-day cycles in combination with cyclophosphamide, vincristine, and prednisone.

Patients who achieve a complete response or partial response to the initial six or eight cycles of obinutuzumab should continue on obinutuzumab 1,000 mg as monotherapy once every 2 months, maintaining the original dosing schedule for up to 2 years.

ADMINISTRATION

IV

🖐 *Alert:* Premedicate all patients with acetaminophen and an antihistamine (such as diphenhydramine) at least 30 minutes before infusion and a glucocorticoid (dexamethasone or methylprednisolone) at least 1 hour before each infusion to reduce infusion-related reactions. Refer to manufacturer's instructions for premedication dosage instructions.

▼ Store vials in refrigerator at 36° to 46° F (2° to 8° C).

▼ Protect vials from light; don't freeze or shake vials.

▼ Administer through a dedicated IV line; don't administer as an IV push or bolus.

▼ If a dose is missed, give missed dose as soon as possible and adjust future doses accordingly to maintain the time interval between chemotherapy cycles.

▼ Solution should be used immediately but is stable in refrigerator for up to 24 hours followed by 48 hours (including infusion time) at room temperature.

▼ **Incompatibilities:** Don't mix with other drugs or solutions, other than NSS.

ACTION

Binds to the CD20 antigen on pre-B and mature B lymphocytes, mediating lysis of both normal and malignant B cells.

Route	Onset	Peak	Duration
IV	Unknown	Unknown	Unknown

Half-life: 25.5 to 35.3 days.

ADVERSE REACTIONS

CNS: fever, fatigue, headache, insomnia.
CV: *worsening of cardiac conditions, hemorrhagic event.* **EENT:** sinusitis, nasopharyngitis, nasal congestion. **GI:** nausea, vomiting, dyspepsia, diarrhea, constipation, decreased appetite. **GU:** UTI. **Hematologic:** *neutropenia, lymphopenia, leukopenia, thrombocytopenia,* anemia. **Hepatic:** elevated ALT, AST, and ALP levels. **Metabolic:** *hypocalcemia, hypokalemia, hyperkalemia,* hyponatremia, hypophosphatemia, hyperbilirubinemia, hypoalbuminemia. **Musculoskeletal:** bone and muscle pain, arthralgia, extremity pain, weakness. **Respiratory:** cough, URI, pneumonia. **Skin:** pruritus. **Other:** infusion-related reaction, *TLS, sepsis,* herpesvirus infection.

INTERACTIONS

Drug-drug. *Vaccines:* Immunization with live or attenuated viral vaccines during or after therapy hasn't been studied. Avoid immunization with live-virus vaccines during treatment and until B-cell recovery.

EFFECTS ON LAB TEST RESULTS

- May increase creatinine, uric acid, ALP, bilirubin, AST, and ALT levels.
- May decrease calcium, sodium, phosphate, and albumin levels.
- May increase or decrease potassium level.
- May decrease CrCl.
- May decrease Hb level and WBC, lymphocyte, and platelet counts.
- May diminish diagnostic effect of coccidioidin skin test.

CONTRAINDICATIONS & CAUTIONS

- Contraindicated in patients hypersensitive to drug or its components and in those who experienced serum sickness with prior obinutuzumab use.

Boxed Warning HBV reactivation, including fulminant hepatitis, hepatic failure, and death, may occur. Screen all patients for HBV infection before starting therapy and monitor carriers for active HBV infection during and for several months after therapy is complete. Discontinue therapy and any concomitant chemotherapy if HBV reactivates and treat appropriately. The decision to restart therapy should be discussed with physician experienced in treating HBV infection. ∎

Boxed Warning JC virus infection, resulting in PML, has been reported. Monitor patients for new-onset neurologic symptoms or change in existing neurologic symptoms. Discontinue therapy and reduce or stop concomitant chemotherapy or immunosuppressive therapy in patients who develop PML. ∎

- Use cautiously in patients with history of recurring or chronic infections.
- Patients with severe and long-lasting neutropenia (lasting more than 1 week) should receive antimicrobial prophylaxis throughout treatment. Also consider antiviral and antifungal prophylaxis and G-CSFs.
- Consider withholding other drugs that may increase bleeding risk.
- May cause severe infusion reactions, including bronchospasm, shortness of breath, tachycardia, hypotension, HTN, nausea, vomiting, diarrhea, headache, and chills. Delayed reactions (up to 24 hours) may occur. Premedicate appropriately and consider infusion rate reduction, interruption of therapy, or discontinuation if reactions persist.
- Give in a facility with access to resuscitative emergency equipment.
- Use cautiously in patients with cardiac or pulmonary conditions; these patients may be at increased risk for serious infusion reactions.
- Consider temporarily withholding antihypertensives for 12 hours before, during, and for 1 hour after administration due to risk of hypotension.
Dialyzable drug: Unknown.

PREGNANCY-LACTATION-REPRODUCTION

- There are no adequate studies during pregnancy. Based on drug's mechanism of action and findings in animals, B-cell depletion may occur in infants exposed to drug in utero. Advise patients of fetal risk.
- Advise patients of childbearing potential to use effective contraception during treatment and for 6 months after final dose.
- It isn't known if drug appears in human milk. Because of the potential of serious adverse reactions in the infant, advise against breastfeed during treatment and for 6 months after final dose.

NURSING CONSIDERATIONS

⚠ *Alert:* Monitor patient for infusion reactions (hypotension, tachycardia, dyspnea, respiratory symptoms, nausea, vomiting,

---

Reactions in bold italics are *life-threatening*. Interactions may have a *rapid onset* or a ***delayed onset***.

diarrhea, HTN, flushing headache, fever, chills), which can be fatal. Symptoms may occur up to 24 hours after infusion.

• Cases of TLS with fatalities have been reported. Acute renal failure, hyperkalemia, hypocalcemia, hyperuricemia, or hyperphosphatemia may occur. Administer prophylaxis (antihyperuricemic therapy [allopurinol] and hydration) in patients at high risk or with high tumor burden or renal impairment before therapy. Correct electrolyte abnormalities and monitor renal function and hydration.

• Patient may develop detectable antibodies to obinutuzumab.

• Regularly monitor blood counts. If neutropenia occurs, consider prophylaxis with antiviral and antifungal agents. Neutropenia may occur 28 days or more after end of treatment and last for more than 28 days.

• Monitor patient for bleeding and thrombocytopenia. Transfuse blood products if appropriate.

• Regularly monitor renal function and electrolyte and uric acid levels.

• Monitor patient for clinical and lab signs and symptoms of hepatitis or HBV reactivation during and for several months after treatment.

• Monitor BP before, during, and after infusion. Consider withholding antihypertensives for 12 hours before, during, and for 1 hour after infusion if appropriate.

• *Look alike–sound alike:* Don't confuse obinutuzumab with blinatumomab, dinutuximab, obiltoxaximab, ocrelizumab, ofatumumab, olaratumab, omalizumab, or rituximab.

PATIENT TEACHING

• Teach patient to seek immediate medical attention for infusion-related reactions, such as dizziness, nausea, chills, fever, vomiting, diarrhea, breathing problems, or chest pain.

• Instruct patient to seek immediate medical attention for signs and symptoms of TLS, such as nausea, vomiting, diarrhea, and lethargy.

• Tell patient to report signs and symptoms of infection, including fever and cough.

• Inform patient of the need for periodic monitoring of blood work.

• Advise patient to avoid vaccinations with live-virus vaccines.

• Caution patient of childbearing potential of fetal risk from exposure and to use effective contraception during treatment and for 6 months after final dose.

• Advise patient not to breastfeed during treatment and for 6 months after final dose.

Boxed Warning Instruct patient to report signs and symptoms of hepatitis, such as worsening fatigue or yellowing of skin or eyes and that patient will be monitored for hepatitis reactivation and treated appropriately. ■

Boxed Warning Advise patient to immediately report new or changed neurologic signs and symptoms, such as confusion, dizziness or loss of balance, difficulty talking or walking, or vision problems. ■

ocrelizumab
oh-kre-LIZ-ue-mab

Ocrevus

Therapeutic class: MS drugs
Pharmacologic class: Monoclonal antibodies

AVAILABLE FORMS
Injection: 300 mg/10 mL preservative-free vials

INDICATIONS & DOSAGES
➤ **Relapsing or primary progressive MS**
Adults: Initially, 300 mg IV infusion on day 1 followed by 300 mg IV infusion 2 weeks later. Then, 600 mg IV infusion every 6 months beginning 6 months after first 300-mg dose.

Before each infusion, premedicate with 100 mg IV methylprednisolone (or equivalent corticosteroid) 30 minutes before infusion and an antihistamine such as diphenhydramine 30 to 60 minutes before infusion. May also add an antipyretic such as acetaminophen.

Adjust-a-dose: For life-threatening or disabling infusion reactions, immediately stop infusion, provide supportive treatment, and permanently discontinue drug. For mild, moderate, and severe infusion reactions, refer to manufacturer's instructions for interrupting therapy and IV infusion rates.

ADMINISTRATION
🚫 *Alert:* Screen for HBV and review quantitative serum Ig test results before first dose.

IV

▼ For 300-mg dose, withdraw 10 mL of drug and dilute into an infusion bag containing 250 mL NSS. For 600-mg dose, withdraw 20 mL of drug and dilute into 500 mL NSS.

▼ Use infusion solution immediately or store up to 24 hours in refrigerator at 36° to 46° F (2° to 8° C) or up to 8 hours at room temperature (up to 77° F [25° C]), including infusion time. Discard any excess solution that's not used the same day.

▼ Inspect for particulate matter or discoloration before use.

▼ Administer diluted solution through a dedicated line using an infusion set with a 0.2- or 0.22-micron in-line filter. No incompatibilities with polyvinyl chloride or polyolefin bags and IV administration sets have been observed.

▼ Administer infusion when solution is at room temperature.

▼ Begin 300-mg dose infusion at 30 mL/hour and increase by 30 mL/hour every 30 minutes to a maximum rate of 180 mL/hour. Duration of infusion is 2.5 hours or longer.

▼ Begin 600-mg dose infusion at 40 mL/hour and increase by 40 mL/hour every 30 minutes to a maximum rate of 200 mL/hour. Duration of infusion is 3.5 hours or longer.

▼ If a dose is missed, administer as soon as possible and reset the dose schedule to give the next dose 6 months later. Doses must be separated by at least 5 months.

▼ Keep vials in the carton to protect from light and store in refrigerator at 36° to 46° F (2° to 8° C). Don't freeze or shake vials.

▼ **Incompatibilities:** Don't give with solutions other than NSS.

ACTION

A recombinant humanized monoclonal antibody directed against CD20-expressing B cells, which causes antibody-dependent cellular cytolysis and complement-mediated lysis.

Route	Onset	Peak	Duration
IV	14 days	Unknown	27–175 wk

Half-life: 26 days.

ADVERSE REACTIONS

CNS: depression. **CV:** peripheral edema. **GI:** diarrhea. **Musculoskeletal:** back pain, limb pain. **Respiratory:** URI, lower respiratory tract infections, cough. **Skin:** skin infections. **Other:** infusion reactions, herpes infections.

INTERACTIONS

Drug-drug. *Immunosuppressants and immune-modulating therapies (corticosteroids, daclizumab, fingolimod, mitoxantrone, natalizumab, teriflunomide):* May increase risk of immunosuppression when used in combination or when switching from listed drugs to ocrelizumab. Use cautiously together.

Other MS drugs: Use of ocrelizumab with other MS drugs hasn't been studied. Consider the potential for increased immunosuppressive effects.

Tacrolimus (topical): May enhance adverse effects of immunosuppressants. Avoid combination.

Vaccines (live-attenuated or live-virus): May decrease vaccine's effects or increase infection risk. Vaccines aren't recommended during treatment or until B-cell recovery occurs. Give all necessary live vaccine immunizations according to immunization guidelines at least 4 weeks before and all necessary nonlive vaccines at least 2 weeks before drug initiation.

Drug-herb. *Echinacea:* May decrease therapeutic effect of immunosuppressants. Avoid combination.

EFFECTS ON LAB TEST RESULTS

● May decrease total Ig level.
● May decrease neutrophil count.
● May decrease effect of *Coccidioides immitis* skin test.

CONTRAINDICATIONS & CAUTIONS

● Contraindicated in patients with a history of life-threatening infusion reaction to ocrelizumab or active HBV infection.

🔆 *Alert:* Screen patient for HBV infection before therapy begins. For patients who are negative for HBsAg and positive for HB core antibody (HBcAb+) or are carriers of HBV (HBsAg+), consult a liver disease specialist before therapy begins and during treatment.

● Drug may increase frequency of herpes and other infections.

● Drug may cause an increase in malignancy, including breast cancer. Follow standard cancer screening guidelines.

● Safety and effectiveness in children haven't been established.

Dialyzable drug: Unknown.

Reactions in bold italics are *life-threatening*. Interactions may have a *rapid onset* or a **delayed onset**.

PREGNANCY-LACTATION-REPRODUCTION

• Drug hasn't been studied during pregnancy. Immunoglobulins cross the placental barrier. Infants born to mothers exposed to other anti-CD20 antibodies experienced transient peripheral B-cell depletion and lymphocytopenia.

• Encourage participation in pregnancy exposure registry (1-833-872-4370 or www.ocrevuspregnancyregistry.com).

• Patients of childbearing potential should use contraception during therapy and for 6 months after final infusion.

• Drug may appear in human milk. Risk of infant harm during breastfeeding is unknown. Consider patient's clinical need for drug along with potential adverse reactions in the infant.

NURSING CONSIDERATIONS

• Administer drug under supervision of an experienced health care provider with access to supportive measures to manage severe reactions.

• Before every infusion, monitor patient for signs and symptoms of infection (fever, chills, persistent cough, herpes [cold sores, shingles, genital sores]). Delay infusion until an active infection resolves.

• Drug may decrease Ig levels and increase risk of infections. Monitor serum Ig levels during and after treatment until B-cell repletion, especially in the setting of recurrent serious infections.

• Monitor patient for infusion reactions during and for at least 1 hour after completion of the infusion. Reactions include pruritus, rash, urticaria, erythema, bronchospasm, throat irritation, oropharyngeal pain, dyspnea, pharyngeal or laryngeal edema, flushing, hypotension, fever, fatigue, headache, dizziness, nausea, and tachycardia. Infusion reactions can occur up to 24 hours after the infusion. If infusion reaction occurs, interrupt or discontinue infusion or decrease rate depending on severity of reaction.

• PML has occurred in patients treated with other MS drugs and can lead to severe disability or death. Monitor patient for new or worsening signs or symptoms of neurologic function changes (problems with thinking, clumsiness, vision changes, personality changes, weakness on one side of the body). At first sign or symptom, withhold drug and obtain an appropriate diagnostic evaluation, including an MRI.

• *Look alike–sound alike:* Don't confuse ocrelizumab with eculizumab, obiltoxaximab, obinutuzumab, ofatumumab, omalizumab, or rituximab.

PATIENT TEACHING

• Advise patient to undergo standard cancer screenings because drug may increase the risk of malignancy, including breast cancer.

• Educate patient to immediately report signs and symptoms of an infusion reaction; teach patient that signs and symptoms can occur 24 hours after the infusion ends.

• Instruct patient to immediately report signs and symptoms of infection (fever, chills, cough, herpes [including cold sores, shingles, or genital sores]).

• Teach patient to immediately report signs and symptoms associated with PML.

• Remind patient of childbearing potential to use contraception during therapy and for 6 months after final infusion.

• Caution patient to report pregnancy or breastfeeding before therapy begins.

• Inform patient that drug can cause reactivation of HBV infection, that testing for HBV will be performed before therapy begins, and that monitoring is required if patient is at risk.

• Inform patient that all necessary vaccinations should be completed at least 4 weeks before therapy begins. Advise patient that live-virus or live-attenuated vaccines aren't recommended during therapy.

octreotide acetate
ok-TREE-oh-tide

Bynfezia, Mycapssa, Octreotide Acetate Omega ✦, Sandostatin, Sandostatin LAR Depot

Therapeutic class: Endocrine-metabolic agents
Pharmacologic class: Somatostatin analogues

AVAILABLE FORMS

Capsules (delayed-release) ⓘ: 20 mg
Injection: 50 mcg/mL, 100 mcg/mL, 500 mcg/mL single-dose ampule, vial, or prefilled syringe
Injection (multidose): 200 mcg/mL, 1,000 mcg/mL vials; 2,500 mcg/mL in 2.8 mL single-patient-use pen

Injection for LAR (powder for suspension):
10 mg/6 mL, 20 mg/6 mL, 30 mg/6 mL

INDICATIONS & DOSAGES

➤ **Flushing and diarrhea from carcinoid tumors**

Adults: 100 to 600 mcg subcut or IV daily in two to four divided doses for first 2 weeks of therapy. Usual daily dosage is 450 mcg but can range from 50 to 1,500 mcg/day. Base subsequent dosage on individual response. Or, LAR Depot 20 mg IM (intragluteally) at 4-week intervals for 2 months. If switching from octreotide solution, continue subcut for 2 weeks at same dosage they were taking before the switch. After 2 months, adjust dosage based on symptoms.

➤ **Watery diarrhea from vasoactive intestinal polypeptide–secreting tumors (VIPomas)**

Adults: 200 to 300 mcg subcut or IV daily in two to four divided doses for first 2 weeks of therapy. Base subsequent dosage on individual response. Range is 150 to 750 mcg/day, but usually shouldn't exceed 450 mcg daily. Or, LAR Depot 20 mg IM (intragluteally) at 4-week intervals for 2 months. If switching from octreotide solution, continue subcut for 2 weeks at same dosage they were taking before the switch. After 2 months, adjust dosage based on symptoms.

➤ **Acromegaly**

Adults: Initially, 50 mcg subcut or IV t.i.d.; then adjust based on insulin-like growth factor 1 (IGF-1) (somatomedin C) level every 2 weeks. Or, may obtain multiple growth hormone levels at 0 to 8 hours after octreotide administration to permit more rapid dose titration.

Usual dosage is 100 mcg subcut or IV t.i.d.; some patients require up to 500 mcg t.i.d. Or, LAR Depot 20 mg IM (intragluteally) at 4-week intervals for 3 months; then adjust dosage based on growth hormone and somatomedin C levels and symptoms. See manufacturer's instructions for a detailed dosing schedule. For depot injection, drug should be withdrawn yearly for 4-week interval in patients who have received irradiation.

For long-term maintenance in patients who responded to and tolerated octreotide or lanreotide injections, may switch to 20-mg capsules PO b.i.d.; increase in increments of 20 mg every 2 weeks based on IGF-1 level

and signs and symptoms. Maximum dosage, 80 mg daily.

Adjust-a-dose: In patients with cirrhosis of the liver or renal failure requiring dialysis, starting dose of LAR Depot is 10 mg IM every 4 weeks. In patients with kidney failure, initate capsules at 20 mg daily and titrate as tolerated.

➤ **Gastroesophageal variceal hemorrhage** ◆

Adults: 500 mcg as an IV bolus, followed by a continuous IV infusion of 50 mcg/hour for 2 to 5 days. May repeat a bolus within the first hour of treatment if hemorrhage isn't controlled.

➤ **Gastroenteropancreatic neuroendocrine tumors (metastatic)** ◆

Adults: 30 mg IM every 4 weeks until tumor progression or death. Or, initially, 20 to 30 mg IM every 28 days; titrate by 10 mg every 4 weeks or maintain same dose and reduce dosing interval to every 3 weeks if frequent supplemental subcut doses are needed. IM range is 20 to 60 mg every 28 days.

➤ **High-output gastroenteropancreatic fistula** ◆

Adults: 100 mcg subcut three times daily; discontinue and consider alternative agents if fistula output doesn't decrease after 3 to 5 days.

ADMINISTRATION
PO
• Give with a glass of water on an empty stomach at least 1 hour before or 2 hours after a meal.
• Patient must swallow capsules whole and not crush or chew them.
• Refrigerate unopened wallets of capsules at 36° to 46° F (2° to 8° C). After first use, may store opened wallets at room temperature for 1 month.

IV
▼ Dilute in 50 to 200 mL D_5W or NSS and infuse over 15 to 30 minutes.
▼ May be given by IV push over 3 minutes.
▼ Store solution in refrigerator between 36° and 46° F (2° and 8° C). May store at room temperature of 70° to 86° F (20° to 30° C) for up to 14 days. Discard multidose vials within 14 days after initial entry.
▼ Solution is stable for 24 hours as a parenteral admixture.
▼ Protect from light.
▼ **Incompatibilities:** TPN.

Reactions in bold italics are *life-threatening*. Interactions may have a *rapid onset* or a ***delayed onset***.

IM

- For IM route, use LAR Depot suspension only.
- **Alert:** Never give injectable suspension by IV or subcut routes.
- May give as initial therapy or as alternative to prior subcut therapy.
- Don't use if particulates or discoloration are observed.
- Follow the mixing instructions included in the packaging and give immediately after mixing.
- For LAR Depot suspension: Before dilution, store refrigerated between 36° and 46° F (2° and 8° C). May store at room temperature of 68° to 77° F (20° to 25° C) for up to 10 days.
- Depot kit should remain at room temperature for 30 to 60 minutes before preparation of the drug suspension.
- Rotate injection sites.
- Administer into gluteal area only; avoid deltoid muscle injections due to significant pain and discomfort at injection site.

Subcutaneous

- Don't use if particulates or discoloration is observed.
- Rotate injection sites. Avoid multiple injections at the same site within a short period of time.

ACTION

Mimics action of naturally occurring somatostatin.

Route	Onset	Peak	Duration
IV	Rapid	Unknown	Up to 12 hr
IM (LAR)	Unknown	1 hr	Unknown
Subcut	30 min	24 min	Up to 12 hr

Half-life: 1.7 to 1.9 hours, increased in older adults and patients with cirrhosis and renal impairment; long-acting, unknown.

ADVERSE REACTIONS

CNS: confusion, dizziness, fatigue, headache, light-headedness, depression, weakness, pain. **CV:** *arrhythmias, bradycardia,* conduction abnormalities, peripheral edema, HTN. **EENT:** blurred vision, hearing loss, sinusitis, nasopharyngitis. **GI:** abdominal pain or discomfort, diarrhea, loose stools, nausea, *pancreatitis,* constipation, fat malabsorption, flatulence, abdominal distention, vomiting, dyspepsia, intestinal polyp. **GU:** urinary frequency, UTI. **Hepatic:** gallbladder abnormalities, cholelithiasis. **Metabolic:** *hypoglycemia,* hyperglycemia, hypothyroidism, suppressed secretion of growth hormone and gastroenterohepatic peptides (gastrin, VIP, insulin, glucagon, secretin, motilin, and pancreatic polypeptide). **Musculoskeletal:** backache, joint pain, osteoarthritis. **Respiratory:** URI. **Skin:** alopecia, erythema or pain at injection site, flushing, wheal, bruising, hair loss, pruritus, diaphoresis. **Other:** cold symptoms, flulike symptoms, pain or burning at subcut injection site.

INTERACTIONS

Drug-drug. *Androgens, MAO inhibitors, quinolone antibiotics, salicylates, SSRIs:* May increase risk of hypoglycemia. Monitor patient closely.
Antacids, H$_2$-receptor antagonists, PPIs: May decrease absorption of capsules. Increase octreatide dosage if necessary.
Beta blockers (propranolol) and other drugs that may cause bradycardia, ivabradine: May have additive effect and further lower HR. Decrease beta blocker dosage as needed.
Bromocriptine: May increase bromocriptine availability. Monitor therapy.
Codeine: May decrease codeine metabolism and decrease morphine formation. Monitor therapy.
Cyclosporine: May decrease cyclosporine level. Consider therapy modification; monitor patient closely.
Drugs that prolong QT interval (antiarrhythmics, SSRIs, TCAs): May increase risk of life-threatening cardiac arrhythmias, including torsades de pointes. Monitor patient and ECG.
Insulin, oral antidiabetics: May inhibit secretion of insulin and glucagon. Monitor patient and adjust dosage of antidiabetics as needed.
Lacosamide: May increase risk of AV-blocking effect of lacosamide. Monitor patient closely.
Levonorgestrel: May decrease effect of oral contraceptive or increase breakthrough bleeding. If used together, patient should use alternative nonhormonal contraceptive or backup method.
Quinidine, terfenadine, rifampin: May decrease excretion of these drugs. Use with caution and reduce dosage as needed.

Drug-food. *Any food:* May alter absorption of dietary fats. Administer injections between meals to decrease GI effects.

EFFECTS ON LAB TEST RESULTS
• May increase or decrease glucose level.
• May decrease vitamin B_{12} level.
• May alter LFT and TSH values.
• May affect Schilling test results.

CONTRAINDICATIONS & CAUTIONS
• Contraindicated in patients hypersensitive to drug or its components.
• Use cautiously in older adults, who may be more sensitive to drug.
• Use cautiously in patients with pancreatitis, gallbladder or bile disorders, cardiac abnormalities, diabetes, hypothyroidism, or nutritional disorders; octreotide may cause or exacerbate these conditions.
• Use cautiously in patients with renal impairment requiring dialysis or hepatic cirrhosis. Dosage adjustment may be needed.
Dialyzable drug: Unknown.
⚠ **Overdose S&S:** Hypoglycemia, flushing, dizziness, nausea, hypotension, arrhythmia, hepatic steatosis, pancreatitis, lethargy, weakness, lactic acidosis.

PREGNANCY-LACTATION-REPRODUCTION
• Drug crosses placental barrier. Use cautiously during pregnancy only if clearly needed and benefit justifies fetal risk.
• Drug may restore fertility in women with acromegaly. Patients of childbearing potential should use contraception during treatment.
• Obtain pregnancy test before LAR treatment to minimize fetal risk.
• Patients planning pregnancy should discontinue long-acting formulation approximately 2 months before planned pregnancy; patients may use short-acting formulation until conception.
• Drug appears in human milk. Use cautiously during breastfeeding.

NURSING CONSIDERATIONS
• Monitor baseline thyroid function tests.
• Monitor somatomedin C levels every 2 weeks. Dosage adjustments are based on this level.
• Periodically monitor lab tests, such as thyroid function, glucose, urine 5-hydroxyindoleacetic acid, plasma serotonin, vitamin B_{12} level, and plasma substance P (for carcinoid tumors).
• Monitor patient regularly for gallbladder disease. Therapy may be related to the development of cholelithiasis because of its effect on gallbladder motility or fat absorption.
• Monitor patient closely for signs and symptoms of glucose imbalance. Patients with type 1 diabetes and those receiving oral antidiabetics or oral diazoxide may need dosage adjustments during therapy. Monitor glucose level.
• Monitor patient closely for bradycardia, arrhythmias, conduction abnormalities, and other ECG changes (e.g., prolonged QT interval).
• Drug may alter fluid and electrolyte balance; other therapies may need adjusting.
• Half-life may be altered in patients with ESRD who are receiving dialysis.
• Monitor patient for breakthrough signs and symptoms with LAR Depot; patient may require supplemental subcut octreotide.
• *Look alike–sound alike:* To avoid giving drug by the wrong route, don't confuse octreotide acetate injection with injectable depot suspension product.
• *Look alike–sound alike:* Don't confuse Sandostatin with Sandimmune, Sandoglobulin, Sandostatin LAR, sargramostim, or simvastatin.

PATIENT TEACHING
• Urge patient to report signs and symptoms of abdominal discomfort immediately.
• Stress importance of the need for periodic lab testing during octreotide therapy.
• Counsel patient to immediately report pregnancy, plans to become pregnant, breastfeeding, or plans to breastfeed during treatment.
• Advise patient with diabetes to monitor blood glucose level closely and to discuss results with prescriber before making dosage changes.

ofloxacin (oral)
oh-FLOKS-a-sin

Therapeutic class: Antibiotics
Pharmacologic class: Fluoroquinolones

AVAILABLE FORMS
Tablets: 200 mg, 300 mg, 400 mg

INDICATIONS & DOSAGES

Boxed Warning Use in patients with acute bacterial exacerbation of bronchitis and uncomplicated UTIs isn't recommended because of risk of serious adverse effects. Use drug in these patients only when they have no other treatment options. ∎

Adjust-a-dose (for all indications): For patients with CrCl of 20 to 50 mL/minute, give first dose as recommended; then give usual maintenance dose every 24 hours. For patients with CrCl less than 20 mL/minute, give 50% of recommended dose every 24 hours. For patients with severe hepatic impairment, don't exceed 400 mg/day.

➤ **Acute bacterial worsening of chronic bronchitis, uncomplicated skin and skin-structure infections, and community-acquired pneumonia**
Adults: 400 mg PO every 12 hours for 10 days.

➤ **Acute, uncomplicated urethral and cervical gonorrhea**
Adults: 400 mg PO as a single dose.

➤ **Mixed infection of the urethra and cervix due to *Chlamydia trachomatis* and *Neisseria gonorrhoeae*; nongonococcal cervicitis or urethritis due to *C. trachomatis***
Adults: 300 mg PO every 12 hours for 7 days.

➤ **Uncomplicated cystitis caused by *Escherichia coli*, *Klebsiella pneumoniae*, or other organisms**
Adults: 200 mg PO every 12 hours for 3 days (*E. coli* or *K. pneumoniae*) or 200 mg PO every 12 hours for 7 days (other organisms).

➤ **Complicated UTI**
Adults: 200 mg PO every 12 hours for 10 days.

➤ **Prostatitis from *E. coli***
Adults: 300 mg PO every 12 hours for 6 weeks.

➤ **Acute pelvic inflammatory disease due to *C. trachomatis* and *N. gonorrhoeae***
Adults: 400 mg PO every 12 hours with metronidazole for 10 to 14 days.

ADMINISTRATION
PO
• Give drug with or without food but don't give within 2 hours of antacids and vitamins.
• Give drug with plenty of fluids.

ACTION
Interferes with DNA gyrase, which is needed for synthesis of bacterial DNA. Spectrum of action includes many gram-positive and gram-negative aerobic bacteria, including *Enterobacteriaceae* and *Pseudomonas aeruginosa*.

Route	Onset	Peak	Duration
PO	Unknown	60–120 min	Unknown

Half-life: 4 to 5 hours.

ADVERSE REACTIONS
CNS: dizziness, fatigue, fever, headache, insomnia, lethargy, nervousness, sleep disorders, somnolence. **CV:** chest pain, phlebitis. **EENT:** visual disturbances, pharyngitis. **GI:** nausea, *pseudomembranous colitis,* abdominal pain or cramps, anorexia, constipation, diarrhea, dry mouth, dysgeusia, flatulence, vomiting, decreased appetite. **GU:** external genital pruritus in women, glycosuria, hematuria, proteinuria, vaginal discharge, vaginitis. **Hematologic:** *leukopenia, neutropenia,* neutrophilia, anemia, eosinophilia, leukocytosis, *thrombocytopenia,* thrombocytosis, lymphocytosis, lymphocytopenia. **Musculoskeletal:** body pain, myalgia. **Skin:** pruritus, rash. **Other:** hypersensitivity reactions.

INTERACTIONS
Drug-drug. *Aluminum hydroxide, aluminum-magnesium hydroxide, calcium carbonate, magnesium hydroxide:* May decrease effects of ofloxacin. Give antacid at least 2 hours before or 2 hours after ofloxacin.
Antidiabetics: May affect glucose level, causing hypoglycemia or hyperglycemia. Monitor patient closely.
Didanosine (chewable or buffered tablets or pediatric powder for oral solution): May interfere with GI absorption of ofloxacin. Separate doses by 2 hours.
Drugs that prolong QT interval (antiarrhythmics, pimozide, ziprasidone): May increase risk of life-threatening ventricular arrhythmias. Avoid use together.
Iron salts: May decrease absorption of ofloxacin, reducing anti-infective response. Separate doses by at least 2 hours.
NSAIDs: May enhance seizure-potentiating effect of ofloxacin. Monitor therapy closely.
Sevelamer: May decrease absorption of quinolones. Give oral quinolones at least 2 hours before or 6 hours after sevelamer. Consider therapy modification.

Boxed Warning *Steroids:* May increase risk of tendinitis and tendon rupture. Monitor patient for tendon pain or inflammation. ■

Sucralfate: May decrease absorption of ofloxacin, reducing anti-infective response. If use together can't be avoided, give ofloxacin 2 hours before or 6 hours after sucralfate.

Theophylline: May increase theophylline level. Monitor patient closely and adjust theophylline dosage as needed.

Warfarin: May prolong PT and INR. Monitor PT and INR.

Drug-lifestyle. *Sunlight or UV light exposure:* May cause photosensitivity reactions. Advise patient to avoid excessive sunlight or UV light exposure.

EFFECTS ON LAB TEST RESULTS

• May increase BUN, creatinine, and liver enzyme levels.
• May increase or decrease serum glucose level.
• May increase urinary glucose and protein levels and pH.
• May increase presence of pus and blood cells in urine.
• May decrease urine specific gravity.
• May increase erythrocyte sedimentation rate, band forms, and eosinophil count.
• May decrease Hb level, hematocrit, and neutrophil count.
• May increase or decrease WBC and platelet counts.
• May produce false-positive urine screen results for opiates.

CONTRAINDICATIONS & CAUTIONS

Boxed Warning Drug is associated with increased risk of tendinitis and tendon rupture, especially in patients older than age 60, patients taking corticosteroids, and those with heart, kidney, or lung transplants. ■

Boxed Warning Drug may exacerbate muscle weakness in patients with myasthenia gravis. Avoid use in patients with a known history of myasthenia gravis. ■

• Contraindicated in patients hypersensitive to drug or other fluoroquinolones.
• Avoid use in patients with known QT interval prolongation or uncorrected hypokalemia and those taking drugs that prolong QT interval due to risk of further QT interval prolongation and torsades de pointes.

🌙 *Alert:* Serious, even fatal, hypersensitivity reactions can occur, even after first dose.

Discontinue drug at first sign of rash or hypersensitivity. Emergency treatment with epinephrine and resuscitative measures may be needed.

• Use cautiously in patients with seizure disorders, CNS diseases such as cerebral arteriosclerosis, or hepatic or renal impairment.

🌙 *Alert:* Patients receiving systemic drug have an increased risk of hypoglycemia, which can result in coma. Hypoglycemia has been reported more frequently in older adults and patients with diabetes.

• Mild to life-threatening CDAD can occur during therapy and up to 2 months after therapy ends. Monitor patient for diarrhea as drug may need to be discontinued and other therapy begun.

🌙 *Alert:* Drug may increase risk of aortic dissection or rupture when used systemically. Avoid use in patients with known aortic aneurysm and patients at risk for an aortic aneurysm, including those with peripheral atherosclerotic vascular diseases, HTN, certain genetic conditions (Marfan syndrome, Ehlers-Danlos syndrome), and older adults. Use drug in these patients only if no other treatment options are available.

• Safety and effectiveness in children younger than age 18 haven't been established.

Dialyzable drug: No.

⚠ *Overdose S&S:* Nausea, vomiting, seizures, vertigo, dysgeusia, psychosis, dizziness, drowsiness, hot and cold flushes, facial swelling and numbness, slurred speech, mild to moderate disorientation.

PREGNANCY-LACTATION-REPRODUCTION

• There are no adequate studies during pregnancy. Drug does cross the placental barrier. Use only if potential benefit justifies fetal risk.

• Drug appears in human milk in levels similar to those found in plasma. Patient should discontinue breastfeeding or discontinue drug.

NURSING CONSIDERATIONS

Boxed Warning Fluoroquinolones have been associated with disabling and potentially irreversible serious adverse reactions that have occurred together, including tendinitis and tendon rupture, peripheral neuropathy, and CNS effects (seizures, toxic psychoses, increased ICP, pseudotumor cerebri, tremors, restlessness, anxiety, light-headedness,

---

Reactions in bold italics are *life-threatening*. Interactions may have a *rapid onset* or a *delayed onset*.

confusion, hallucinations, paranoia, depression, nightmares, insomnia and, rarely, suicidality). If any of these serious adverse reactions occur, discontinue drug immediately. ■

Boxed Warning Monitor patient for signs and symptoms of peripheral neuropathy (pain, burning, tingling, numbness, weakness, or a change in sensation to light touch, pain, temperature, or the sense of body position) and report them immediately. Signs and symptoms can occur at any time during treatment and can last for months or years or be permanent. ■

⊙ *Alert:* Patients treated for gonorrhea should be tested for syphilis. Drug isn't effective against syphilis, and treating gonorrhea may mask or delay syphilis symptoms.

• Periodically assess organ system functions during prolonged therapy.

• Monitor patient for overgrowth of nonsusceptible organisms.

• Monitor renal and hepatic studies and CBC in prolonged therapy.

• Test for *Clostridioides difficile* if patient develops diarrhea.

⊙ *Alert:* Monitor patients receiving systemic drug for signs and symptoms of hypoglycemia (confusion, pounding or rapid heartbeat, dizziness, pale skin, shakiness, diaphoresis, unusual hunger, trembling, headache, weakness, irritability, unusual anxiety). Immediately discontinue drug for blood glucose disturbances and switch to a nonfluoroquinolone antibiotic, if possible.

⊙ *Alert:* Monitor patients receiving systemic drug for psychiatric adverse reactions (disturbances in attention, disorientation, agitation, nervousness, memory impairment, delirium). Discontinue drug for CNS adverse effects, including psychiatric adverse reactions.

• Monitor patient for adverse CNS effects, including dizziness, headache, seizures, or depression. Stop drug and notify prescriber if these effects occur.

• Monitor patient for hypersensitivity reactions. Stop drug and initiate supportive therapy, as indicated.

⊙ *Alert:* Monitor patient for signs and symptoms of aortic aneurysm, dissection, and rupture (sudden, severe, and constant pain in the stomach, chest, or back; throbbing in the stomach area; deep pain in the back or side of the stomach; steady, gnawing pain in the stomach that lasts for hours or days;

pain in the jaw, neck, back, or chest; coughing or hoarseness; shortness of breath or trouble swallowing). Discontinue drug immediately if any of these aortic disorders are suspected.

PATIENT TEACHING

• Instruct patient in safe drug administration and to take drug exactly as prescribed even if feeling better.

Boxed Warning Warn patient to immediately report signs and symptoms of serious adverse reactions, including unusual joint or tendon pain, muscle weakness, "pins and needles" tingling or prickling sensation, numbness in the arms or legs, confusion, or hallucinations. ■

• Tell patient to drink plenty of fluids during drug therapy and to finish the entire prescription, even after starting to feel better.

⊙ *Alert:* Caution patient that significantly low blood glucose level can occur. Show patient how to manage signs and symptoms of low blood glucose level and to immediately report such occurrences to prescriber.

⊙ *Alert:* Advise patient with diabetes that more frequent monitoring of blood glucose levels may be needed during therapy.

⊙ *Alert:* Inform patient to immediately report psychiatric adverse reactions and warn that these can occur after just one dose.

• Warn patient that dizziness and lightheadedness may occur. Advise caution when driving or operating hazardous machinery until effects of drug are known.

• Warn patient that hypersensitivity reactions may follow first dose. Advise patient to stop drug at first sign of rash or other allergic reaction and call prescriber immediately.

• Advise patient to avoid prolonged exposure to direct sunlight or UV light and to use a sunscreen and protective clothing when outdoors.

• Advise patient to report severe bloody diarrhea.

⊙ *Alert:* Warn patient to seek immediate medical attention for signs and symptoms of aortic aneurysm.

OLANZapine
oh-LAN-za-peen

Zyprexa✦, Zyprexa Zydis

OLANZapine pamoate
Zyprexa Relprevv

Therapeutic class: Antipsychotics
Pharmacologic class:
Thienobenzodiazepines

AVAILABLE FORMS
Injection: 10 mg
Injection (extended-release suspension):
210 mg/vial, 300 mg/vial, 405 mg/vial
Tablets: 2.5 mg, 5 mg, 7.5 mg, 10 mg, 15 mg,
20 mg
Tablets (ODTs): 5 mg, 10 mg, 15 mg, 20 mg

INDICATIONS & DOSAGES
➤ **Schizophrenia**
Adults: Initially, 5 to 10 mg PO once daily
with the goal to be at 10 mg daily within several days of starting therapy. Adjust dose in
5-mg increments at intervals of 1 week or
more. Most patients respond to 10 to 15 mg
daily. Safety of dosages greater than 20 mg
daily hasn't been established. Or, for maintenance dosing, 150 mg (extended-release)
IM every 2 weeks, or 300 mg (extended-
release) IM every 2 or 4 weeks, or 210 mg
(extended-release) IM every 2 weeks, or
405 mg (extended-release) IM every 4 weeks.
Children age 13 and older: 2.5 or 5 mg PO
once daily. Adjust dose as needed in increments of 2.5 or 5 mg. Maintenance dose,
10 mg/day. Safety hasn't been established for
doses exceeding 20 mg daily.
Adjust-a-dose: In older adults, patients who
are debilitated, patients predisposed to hypotensive reactions, and patients who may
metabolize olanzapine more slowly than
usual (nonsmoking women older than age 65)
or may be more pharmacodynamically sensitive to olanzapine, initially, 5 mg PO or
150 mg IM every 4 weeks. Increase dosage
cautiously.
➤ **Short-term treatment of acute manic
episodes linked to bipolar I disorder**
Adults: Initially, 10 to 15 mg PO daily. Adjust
dosage as needed in 5-mg daily increments
at intervals of 24 hours or more. Maximum,
20 mg PO daily. Duration of treatment is usually 2 weeks.
Children age 13 and older: 2.5 or 5 mg PO
once daily. Adjust dose as needed in increments of 2.5 or 5 mg. Maintenance dose is
10 mg/day. Maximum dose is 20 mg/day.
➤ **Short-term treatment, with lithium
or valproate, of acute mixed or manic
episodes linked to bipolar I disorder**
Adults: 10 mg PO once daily. Dosage range
is 5 to 20 mg daily. Duration of treatment is
6 weeks.
➤ **Maintenance treatment of bipolar I
disorder**
Adults: 5 to 20 mg PO daily.
Children age 13 and older: 2.5 or 5 mg PO
once daily. Adjust dosage as needed in increments of 2.5 or 5 mg. Maintenance dose is
10 mg/day. Maximum dose is 20 mg/day.
Adjust-a-dose: In older adults, patients who
are debilitated, patients predisposed to hypotensive reactions, and patients who may
metabolize olanzapine more slowly than
usual (nonsmoking women older than age 65)
or may be more pharmacodynamically sensitive to olanzapine, initially, 5 mg PO. Increase
dosage cautiously.
➤ **Agitation caused by schizophrenia and
bipolar I mania**
Adults: 10 mg IM (short-acting) (range, 2.5 to
10 mg). May give subsequent doses of up to
10 mg 2 hours after first dose or 4 hours after
second dose, up to 30 mg IM daily. Maximum
of three doses of 10 mg 2 to 4 hours apart. If
maintenance therapy is required, convert patient to 5 to 20 mg PO daily.
Adjust-a-dose: In older adults, give 5 mg IM.
In patients who are debilitated, in those predisposed to hypotension, and in patients sensitive to effects of drug, give 2.5 mg IM.
➤ **Depressive episodes associated with
bipolar I disorder**
Adults: 5 mg PO with fluoxetine 20 mg PO
once daily in the evening. Dosage adjustments can be made based on effectiveness and
tolerability within ranges of olanzapine 5 to
12.5 mg and fluoxetine 20 to 50 mg.
Children age 10 and older: 2.5 mg PO
with 20 mg fluoxetine PO once daily in the
evening. Adjust dosage based on effectiveness and tolerability. Doses above 12 mg
(olanzapine) with fluoxetine doses above
50 mg haven't been evaluated.

Reactions in bold italics are *life-threatening*. Interactions may have a *rapid onset* or a *delayed onset*.

> **Treatment-resistant depression**
Adults: 5 mg PO with 20 mg fluoxetine PO once daily in the evening. Dosage adjustments can be made based on effectiveness and tolerability within ranges of olanzapine 5 to 20 mg and fluoxetine 20 to 50 mg.

> **Preventing chemotherapy-associated acute and delayed nausea or vomiting ◆**
Adults: 5 or 10 mg PO on day of chemotherapy (day 1) followed by 5 or 10 mg once daily on days 2 to 4 (in combination with dexamethasone and palonosetron on day 1 only).

> **Chemotherapy-associated breakthrough nausea or vomiting ◆**
Adults: 5 or 10 mg PO once daily for 3 days.
Children age 3 and older: 0.1 to 0.14 mg/kg/dose ODT PO once or twice daily. Round dose to nearest 1.25 mg.

ADMINISTRATION
PO
• Give drug without regard for food.
• Don't push tablet through foil backing; remove foil from package, then remove tablet.
• Place ODT on patient's tongue immediately after opening package.
• ODT may be given without water.

IM
• Be aware that there are two different IM formulations, a short-acting and a long-acting formulation, with different dosing schedules.
• Inspect IM solution for particulate matter and discoloration before administration.
• To reconstitute IM injection, dissolve contents of one vial with 2.1 mL of sterile water for injection to yield a clear yellow 5 mg/mL solution. Store at room temperature and give within 1 hour of reconstitution. Discard any unused solution.
• For Zyprexa Relprevv extended-release injection, follow specific manufacturer's instructions for the appropriate diluent to add for each dosage. After drug is suspended in the solution, may hold at room temperature for 24 hours.
• Olanzapine extended-release formula is intended for deep gluteal IM injection only.
🚫 *Alert:* Injection is for IM use only. Don't administer IV or subcut.

ACTION
May block dopamine and 5-HT$_2$ receptors.

Route	Onset	Peak	Duration
PO	1–6 wk	6 hr	Unknown
IM	10–15 min	15–45 min	Unknown
IM (extended-release)	Unknown	1 wk	Months

Half-life: 21 to 54 hours; extended release, 30 days.

ADVERSE REACTIONS
CNS: somnolence, insomnia, parkinsonism, dizziness, *NMS, suicide attempt,* abnormal gait, asthenia, personality disorder, auditory hallucinations, restlessness, fatigue, akathisia, headache, tremor, articulation impairment, tardive dyskinesia, fever, extrapyramidal events (IM), hypertonia. **CV:** *prolonged QT interval,* orthostatic hypotension, tachycardia, chest pain, HTN, ecchymosis, peripheral edema, hypotension (IM). **EENT:** amblyopia, conjunctivitis, rhinitis, nasal congestion, pharyngitis, sore throat. **GI:** constipation, dry mouth, dyspepsia, increased appetite, increased salivation, vomiting, thirst, flatulence. **GU:** hematuria, metrorrhagia, urinary incontinence, UTI, amenorrhea, vaginitis, vaginal discharge. **Hematologic:** *leukopenia.* **Hepatic:** increased liver enzyme levels. **Metabolic:** hyperglycemia, dyslipidemia, weight gain. **Musculoskeletal:** joint pain, extremity pain, back pain, neck rigidity, twitching, muscle spasm, stiffness. **Respiratory:** increased cough, dyspnea, URI. **Skin:** diaphoresis, ecchymosis, acne, injection-site reaction, injection-site pain (IM). **Other:** flu-like syndrome, viral infection, injury.

INTERACTIONS
Drug-drug. *Amphetamines:* May decrease stimulatory effect of amphetamines. Monitor therapy.
Anticholinergics: May increase adverse effects of anticholinergics, including severe GI hypermotility. Monitor therapy.
Antihypertensives: May potentiate hypotensive effects. Monitor BP closely.
Carbamazepine, omeprazole, rifampin: May increase clearance of olanzapine. Monitor patient.
Centrally acting drugs: May potentiate CNS effects. Avoid combination.
Ciprofloxacin: May increase olanzapine level. Monitor patient for increased adverse effects.
Diazepam: May increase CNS effects (orthostatic hypotension). Monitor patient.
Dopamine agonists, levodopa: May antagonize activity of these drugs. Monitor patient.

Fluoxetine: May increase olanzapine level. Use together cautiously.

Fluvoxamine: May increase olanzapine level. May need to reduce olanzapine dose.

Lamotrigine: May increase sedative effect of olanzapine. Monitor patient.

Opioid agonists: May cause slow or difficult breathing, sedation, and death. Avoid use together. If use together is necessary, limit dosage and duration of each drug to minimum necessary for desired effect.

QT-prolonging agents: May enhance QTc-prolonging effect of QT-prolonging agents. Consider therapy modification.

Drug-herb. *Kava kava:* May increase adverse or toxic effect of olanzapine. Monitor patient.

St. John's wort: May decrease drug level. Discourage use together.

Drug-lifestyle. *Alcohol use:* May increase CNS effects. Don't use together.

Smoking: May increase drug clearance. Urge patient to quit smoking.

EFFECTS ON LAB TEST RESULTS

- May increase AST, ALT, GGT, CK, glucose, triglyceride, uric acid, and prolactin levels.
- May decrease bilirubin level.
- May increase eosinophil count.
- May decrease WBC count.

CONTRAINDICATIONS & CAUTIONS

- Contraindicated in patients hypersensitive to drug.

Boxed Warning Sedation (including coma) or delirium have been reported following injections of olanzapine extended-release formula. This drug must be administered in a registered health care facility with ready access to emergency response services. After each injection, a health care provider must observe patient for at least 3 hours. Olanzapine extended-release is available only through the restricted Zyprexa Relprevv Patient Care Program (1-877-772-9390). ■

Boxed Warning Drug may increase risk of CV or infection-related death in older adults with dementia. Olanzapine isn't approved to treat patients with dementia-related psychosis. ■

- Opioids should only be prescribed with benzodiazepines or other CNS depressants to patients for whom alternative treatment options are inadequate.

- In postmarketing experience, risk of severe adverse reactions (including fatalities) increased with concomitant use of anticholinergics.
- Use cautiously in patients with a current diagnosis or history of urine retention, clinically significant prostatic hypertrophy, constipation, or history of paralytic ileus or related conditions.
- Use cautiously in patients with heart disease, cerebrovascular disease, conditions that predispose patient to hypotension, history of seizures or conditions that might lower the seizure threshold, and hepatic impairment.
- Use cautiously in older adults, patients with a history of paralytic ileus, and those at risk for aspiration pneumonia, prostatic hyperplasia, or angle-closure glaucoma.
- Use cautiously during initiation of therapy in patients at high risk for suicide.
- Impaired core body temperature regulation may occur. Patient should use caution with strenuous exercise, heat exposure, and dehydration.
- Safety and effectiveness of olanzapine pamoate long-acting formulation in children haven't been established.

Dialyzable drug: No.

⚠ Overdose S&S: Agitation, aggressiveness, dysarthria, tachycardia, extrapyramidal symptoms, reduced level of consciousness, aspiration, cardiopulmonary arrest, cardiac arrhythmias, delirium, NMS, respiratory depression or arrest, seizures, HTN, hypotension.

PREGNANCY-LACTATION-REPRODUCTION

- There are no adequate studies during pregnancy. Use only if potential benefit justifies fetal risk. Use during pregnancy should be individualized.
- **Alert:** Neonates exposed to antipsychotics during the third trimester are at risk for developing extrapyramidal signs and symptoms (repetitive muscle movements of the face and body) and withdrawal signs and symptoms (agitation, abnormally increased or decreased muscle tone, tremors, sleepiness, severe difficulty breathing, difficulty feeding) after delivery and may require intensive care support.
- Enroll patients exposed to drug during pregnancy in the National Pregnancy Registry for Atypical Antipsychotics (1-866-961-2388).
- Drug appears in human milk. Breastfeeding isn't recommended.

• Drug may reversibly decrease female fertility.

NURSING CONSIDERATIONS

🔵 *Alert:* Watch for evidence of NMS (hyper-congestion, muscle rigidity, altered mental status, autonomic instability), which is rare but commonly fatal. Stop drug immediately; monitor and treat patient as needed.

🔵 *Alert:* Drug may cause hyperglycemia. Monitor patients with diabetes regularly. In patients with risk factors for diabetes, obtain fasting blood glucose test results at baseline and periodically.

• Monitor patient for symptoms of metabolic syndrome (significant weight gain and in-creased BMI, HTN, hyperglycemia, hyper-cholesterolemia, and hypertriglyceridemia).

🔵 *Alert:* Monitor patient for DRESS syn-drome, which can be fatal. DRESS syndrome consists of three or more of the following signs and symptoms: cutaneous reaction, eosinophilia, fever, and lymphadenopathy, plus one or more of the following systemic complications: hepatitis, myocarditis, peri-carditis, nephritis, and pneumonia. Discon-tinue drug immediately if DRESS syndrome is suspected and provide supportive care.

Boxed Warning When using olanzapine and fluoxetine in combination, also refer to the suicidality Boxed Warning section of the package insert for Symbyax. ∎

🔵 *Alert:* Drug may increase risk of suicidal-ity in young adults ages 18 to 24 during first 2 months of treatment.

• ODTs contain phenylalanine.

• Monitor patient for abnormal body tem-perature regulation, especially if patient exer-cises, is exposed to extreme heat, takes anti-cholinergics, or is dehydrated.

• Obtain baseline and periodic LFT results.

• Monitor patient for mental status changes, sedation, coma, or delirium.

• Monitor patient for tardive dyskinesia, which may occur after prolonged use. It may not appear until months or years later and may disappear spontaneously or persist for life, despite stopping drug.

• Periodically reevaluate the long-term use-fulness of olanzapine.

• Patient who feels dizzy or drowsy after an IM injection should remain recumbent until assessment for orthostatic hypotension and bradycardia can be done. Patient should rest until the feeling passes.

• Taper dosage slowly when discontinuing.

🔵 *Alert:* Monitor patient receiving extended-release injection for postinjection delirium sedation syndrome (PDSS). Signs and symp-toms that may be consistent with overdose and PDSS include sedation, coma, delirium, confusion, disorientation, agitation, anxi-ety, and other cognitive impairment. Other possible signs and symptoms of PDSS in-clude dysarthria, ataxia, aggression, dizzi-ness, weakness, HTN, and seizures.

🔵 *Alert:* After receiving extended-release in-jection and after postinjection observation period, patients must be alert, oriented, and absent of signs or symptoms of PDSS before release. Patients must be accompanied to their destination upon leaving the facility. If PDSS is suspected, patients must remain under med-ical supervision.

• *Look alike–sound alike:* Don't confuse olan-zapine with olsalazine or quetiapine. Don't confuse Zyprexa with Zyrtec, Zestril, or Celexa. Don't confuse Zyprexa Zydis with Zelapar or zolpidem.

PATIENT TEACHING

• Teach patient safe drug administration for prescribed formulation.

🔵 *Alert:* Caution patient or caregiver of pa-tient taking an opioid with a benzodiazepine, CNS depressant, or alcohol to seek imme-diate medical attention for dizziness, light-headedness, extreme sleepiness, slowed or difficult breathing, or unresponsiveness.

🔵 *Alert:* Inform patient of risk of DRESS syn-drome and importance of reporting symptoms immediately.

• Caution patient against exposure to extreme heat; drug may impair body's ability to reduce temperature.

• Inform patient of potential for weight gain.

• Advise patient to avoid alcohol.

• Tell patient to rise slowly to avoid dizziness upon standing up quickly.

• Inform patient that ODTs contain pheny-lalanine.

• Instruct patient with diabetes to closely monitor blood glucose level. Drug may cause hyperglycemia.

• Urge patient to report pregnancy, suspected pregnancy, or plans to become pregnant.

• Advise patient not to breastfeed during therapy.

🔵 *Alert:* Warn patient not to drive or oper-ate heavy machinery for rest of day after

O

receiving extended-release injection and to seek medical attention if signs and symptoms of PDSS occur.

SAFETY ALERT!

oliceridine 🔒
oh-li-SER-i-deen

Olinvyk

Therapeutic class: Opioid analgesics
Pharmacologic class: Opioid agonists
Controlled substance schedule: II

AVAILABLE FORMS
Injection: 1 mg/mL single-dose vials; 1 mg/1 mL single-patient-use vials for PCA

INDICATIONS & DOSAGES
Boxed Warning Because of the risk of addiction, abuse, and misuse of opioids, reserve use for patients for whom alternative treatments (nonopioid analgesics or opioid combination products) haven't been tolerated, aren't expected to be tolerated, didn't provide adequate analgesia, or aren't expected to provide adequate analgesia. ∎

🖢 *Alert:* Initiate dosing for each patient individually and use the lowest effective dose for the shortest duration consistent with individual treatment goals.

➤ **Acute pain severe enough to require an IV opioid analgesic when alternative treatments are inadequate**
Adults: Initially, 1.5 mg IV with supplemental doses of 0.75 mg beginning 1 hour after initial dose and hourly thereafter as needed. For PCA, initial dose can be followed by demand doses of 0.35 mg with a 6-minute lockout; may increase to 0.5 mg. Individual single doses greater than 3 mg haven't been evaluated. Maximum daily dose is 27 mg. If maximum daily dose is met and analgesia is still required, use alternative analgesics until oliceridine can be resumed the next day.
Adjust-a-dose: For patients with mild or moderate hepatic impairment, less frequent dosing may be required. For those with severe hepatic impairment, consider reducing initial dose; administer subsequent doses after reviewing pain severity and clinical status. For patients with central sleep apnea (CSA) and sleep-related hypoxemia, consider decreasing dose.

If CYP3A4 inducers are used concomitantly, consider increased oliceridine dose. If discontinuing CYP3A4 inducer, monitor patient for respiratory depression and sedation and consider decreasing oliceridine dose.
🖢 Patients who are normal CYP2D6 metabolizers taking a CYP2D6 inhibitor and a strong CYP3A4 inhibitor or who are discontinuing a CYP3A4 inducer may require less frequent dosing. Patients who are known CYP2D6 poor metabolizers taking a CYP3A4 inhibitor or discontinuing a CYP3A4 inducer may require less frequent dosing.

ADMINISTRATION
IV
▼ For PCA use, transfer drug directly from vial into PCA syringe or IV bag without diluting.
▼ Inspect for particulate matter and discoloration. Don't use if particles or discoloration is present.
▼ Store at room temperature (68° to 77° F [20° to 25° C]). Don't freeze. Protect from light.
▼ **Incompatibilities:** None listed by manufacturer. Consult a drug incompatibility reference for more information.

ACTION
Unknown. Binds with opioid receptors in the CNS, altering perception of and emotional response to pain.

Route	Onset	Peak	Duration
IV	2–5 min	Unknown	Unknown

Half-life: 1.3 to 3 hours; metabolites, 44 hours.

ADVERSE REACTIONS
CNS: anxiety, dizziness, fever, headache, insomnia, restlessness, sedation, somnolence. **CV:** flushing, HTN, hypotension, tachycardia. **EENT:** dry mouth. **GI:** constipation, diarrhea, dyspepsia, flatulence, nausea, vomiting. **Hematologic:** anemia. **Hepatic:** elevated ALT level. **Metabolic:** *hypocalcemia, hypokalemia, hypomagnesemia,* hypophosphatemia. **Musculoskeletal:** back pain, muscle spasms. **Respiratory:** cough, decreased oxygen saturation, dyspnea, *hypoxia.* **Skin:** hyperhidrosis, infusion-site extravasation, pruritus, rash.

Reactions in bold italics are *life-threatening*. Interactions may have a *rapid onset* or a *delayed onset*.

INTERACTIONS

Drug-drug. *Anticholinergics (atropine, benztropine, hyoscyamine, solifenacin, tolterodine):* May increase risk of urine retention or severe constipation, which may lead to paralytic ileus. Monitor patient closely.

Boxed Warning *Benzodiazepines, CNS depressants (antipsychotics, anxiolytics, general anesthetics, hypnotics, muscle relaxants, other opioids, sedatives, tranquilizers):* May cause profound sedation, respiratory depression, coma, and death. Avoid use together. If used together, limit dose and duration of each drug to the minimum necessary for desired effect. Monitor patient for respiratory depression and sedation. ∎

CNS depressants (general anesthetics, phenothiazines): May cause severe hypotension, orthostatic hypotension, and syncope. Monitor patient closely.

CYP3A4 inducers (carbamazepine, phenytoin, rifampin): May decrease oliceridine level and efficacy. Monitor patient closely for increased pain or opioid withdrawal. Consider supplemental oliceridine doses. If discontinuing CYP3A4 inducer, consider reducing oliceridine dose and monitor patient for respiratory depression.

Diuretics: May reduce diuretic efficacy. Monitor patient for diminished diuresis or effect on BP; increase diuretic dose as needed.

Mixed opioid agonist-antagonists (butorphanol, nalbuphine, pentazocine) or partial agonist (buprenorphine) analgesics: May reduce analgesic effect and precipitate withdrawal symptoms. Avoid use together.

Moderate to strong CYP2D6 inhibitors (bupropion, fluoxetine, paroxetine, quinidine) or CYP3A4 inhibitors (azole antifungals [itraconazole, ketoconazole], macrolide antibiotics [erythromycin], protease inhibitors [ritonavir, telaprevir], SSRIs): May increase oliceridine level, resulting in increased or prolonged opioid effects or adverse reactions. Patients taking a CYP2D6 inhibitor and a CYP3A4 inhibitor are at increased risk. Consider less frequent oliceridine dosing. Monitor patient for respiratory depression and sedation. If discontinuing CYP2D6 or CYP3A4 inhibitor, may need to increase oliceridine dose. Monitor patient for opioid withdrawal.

Muscle relaxants: May enhance relaxant effect and respiratory depression. Monitor patient and decrease dose of oliceridine or muscle relaxant as necessary.

Serotonergic drugs (drugs that affect the serotonin neurotransmitter system [mirtazapine, tramadol, trazodone], 5-HT$_3$ receptor antagonists, MAO inhibitors [isocarboxazid, linezolid, methylene blue, phenelzine], muscle relaxants [cyclobenzaprine, metaxalone], SSNRIs, SSRIs, TCAs, triptans): May increase risk of serotonin syndrome. Use together cautiously. Discontinue oliceridine if serotonin syndrome is suspected.

Drug-lifestyle. **Boxed Warning** *Alcohol use, illicit drugs:* May cause profound sedation, respiratory depression, coma, and death. Discourage use together. If used together, monitor patient for signs and symptoms of respiratory depression and sedation. ∎

EFFECTS ON LAB TEST RESULTS

- May increase ALT and amylase levels.
- May decrease calcium, magnesium, phosphate, and potassium levels.
- May decrease RBC count.

CONTRAINDICATIONS & CAUTIONS

- Contraindicated in patients hypersensitive to oliceridine and in those with significant respiratory depression, acute or severe bronchial asthma in an unmonitored setting or in the absence of resuscitative equipment, or known or suspected GI obstruction, including paralytic ileus.

Boxed Warning Individualize dose based on severity of pain, patient response, prior analgesic experience, and risk factors for addiction, abuse, and misuse. ∎

Boxed Warning Oliceridine increases risk of opioid addiction, abuse, and misuse, which can lead to overdose and death. Assess individual's risk (personal or family history of substance abuse, mental illness [major depression]) and monitor patient for development of these conditions. Addiction can occur in patients appropriately prescribed and if drug is misused or abused. ∎

Boxed Warning Serious, life-threatening, or fatal respiratory depression may occur. Monitor patients for respiratory depression, especially during initiation or after dosage increase. ∎

Boxed Warning Concomitant use with benzodiazepines or other CNS depressants may result in profound sedation, respiratory depression, coma, and death. Reserve concomitant use for patients for whom alternative treatments are inadequate; limit doses and durations to the minimum required; and monitor patients for signs and symptoms of respiratory depression and sedation. ■

• Opioids can cause sleep-related breathing disorders, including CSA and sleep-related hypoxemia; the risk increases with increased dosages. For patients with CSA, consider decreasing opioid dosage using best practices for opioid taper.

• Use cautiously in older adults, in patients who are cachectic or debilitated, and in patients with substantially decreased respiratory reserve, COPD, cor pulmonale, hypoxia, hypercapnia, or preexisting respiratory depression, due to risk of life-threatening respiratory depression. Monitor patient closely and consider use of nonopioid analgesics.

• Use cautiously in patients at risk for intracranial effects of CO_2 retention (increased ICP, brain tumors, head injury) due to reduction of respiratory drive and increase in ICP.

• Avoid use in patients with head injury, impaired consciousness, or coma; drug may mask clinical changes.

• Use cautiously in patients with biliary tract disease or acute pancreatitis. Drug may cause increased serum amylase level and worsening of symptoms.

• Use cautiously in patients with severe hepatic impairment, QT-interval prolongation, and adrenal insufficiency.

• Avoid total daily dose above 27 mg due to increased risk of QT-interval prolongation.

• Use cautiously in patients with seizure disorders. Drug may worsen seizure control.

• Use cautiously in patients with compromised ability to maintain BP due to reduced blood volume or use of certain CNS depressants (general anesthetics, phenothiazines). Monitor BP closely. Avoid use in patients with circulatory shock due to risk of further vasodilation.

▨ Use cautiously in patients with decreased CYP2D6 function due to an increased risk of prolonged opioid adverse reactions and exacerbated respiratory depression. Closely monitor patient for respiratory depression and sedation; consider less frequent dosing.

• Safety of use beyond 48 hours hasn't been established.

• Safety and effectiveness in children haven't been established.

Dialyzable drug: Unlikely.

⚠ *Overdose S&S:* Respiratory depression, somnolence progressing to stupor or coma, skeletal muscle flaccidity, cold and clammy skin, constricted pupils. In some cases, marked pupil dilation (may be seen with severe hypoxia), pulmonary edema, bradycardia, hypotension, partial or complete airway obstruction, atypical snoring, death.

PREGNANCY-LACTATION-REPRODUCTION

Boxed Warning Prolonged use during pregnancy can result in neonatal opioid withdrawal syndrome, which may be life-threatening and requires management by neonatology experts. If prolonged opioid use is required, advise patient who is pregnant of the risk and ensure that appropriate treatment will be available. ■

• Oliceridine isn't recommended for use immediately before or during labor. If used, monitor infant for excess sedation and respiratory depression.

• It isn't known if drug causes major birth defects and miscarriage.

• It isn't known if drug appears in human milk. When deciding if patient should breastfeed, consider risks versus benefits to patient and infant. Monitor infant who is breastfed for excess sedation and respiratory depression. Withdrawal symptoms can occur in infants when breastfeeding is stopped or drug is discontinued.

• Prolonged opioid use may reduce fertility in patients of reproductive potential. It's unknown if effects on fertility are reversible.

NURSING CONSIDERATIONS

Boxed Warning Assess each patient's risk of addiction, abuse, and misuse, and monitor patient regularly for the development of these behaviors or conditions. ■

Boxed Warning Monitor patient closely for respiratory depression, especially 24 to 48 hours after initiating therapy and after dosage increases; adjust dosage accordingly. Management of respiratory depression may include close observation, supportive measures, or use of opioid antagonists. ■

• If pain level increases after dosage stabilization, attempt to identify source of increased pain before increasing oliceridine dosage.

⟳ *Alert:* Monitor patient for adrenal insufficiency (nausea, vomiting, anorexia, fatigue, weakness, dizziness, hypotension). If confirmed, wean patient off oliceridine and treat

---

Reactions in bold italics are *life-threatening*. Interactions may have a *rapid onset* or a *delayed onset*.

with corticosteroids until adrenal function recovers. If necessary, try other opioids.
• Monitor patient for severe hypotension, orthostatic hypotension, and syncope, especially after dosage initiation or titration.
🔊 **Alert:** Don't abruptly discontinue drug in patient physically dependent on opioids. If discontinuing drug, gradually taper dose while monitoring patient for signs and symptoms of withdrawal (restlessness, lacrimation, rhinorrhea, yawning, perspiration, chills, myalgia, mydriasis, irritability, anxiety, backache, joint pain, weakness, abdominal cramps, insomnia, nausea, anorexia, vomiting, diarrhea; increased BP, respiratory rate, or HR). If withdrawal occurs, increase dosage to previous level and taper more slowly.

PATIENT TEACHING
Boxed Warning Warn patient not to drive or operate dangerous machinery until drug's effects are known. Caution patient to avoid use with other CNS depressants, including alcohol. ▪
Boxed Warning Teach patient about risk of physical dependence on opioids and risk of withdrawal symptoms if drug is stopped abruptly. ▪
Boxed Warning Warn patient and family members of risk of serious, life-threatening, or fatal respiratory depression, especially during drug initiation or after dosage increases and with concomitant use of benzodiazepines or other CNS depressants. Tell patient to seek immediate medical attention if respiratory depression occurs. ▪
Boxed Warning Inform patient that prolonged use of drug during pregnancy can result in neonatal opioid withdrawal syndrome, which may be life-threatening. ▪
🔊 **Alert:** Advise patient taking other drugs that increase risk of serotonin syndrome to immediately report signs and symptoms of serotonin syndrome (confusion, agitation, fever, rapid heartbeat, loss of muscle coordination, vomiting, diaphoresis) and to seek medical attention right away.
• Advise patient about risk of severe constipation, how to manage it, and when to inform prescriber.

---

olmesartan medoxomil ▧
ol-ma-SAR-tan

Benicar🔊, Olmetec🍁

Therapeutic class: Antihypertensives
Pharmacologic class: Angiotensin II receptor antagonists

AVAILABLE FORMS
Tablets: 5 mg, 10 mg🍁, 20 mg, 40 mg

INDICATIONS & DOSAGES
➤ **HTN**
Adults: 20 mg PO once daily if patient has no volume depletion. May increase dosage to 40 mg PO once daily if BP isn't reduced after 2 weeks of therapy.
Children ages 6 to 16 weighing 35 kg or more: Initially, 20 mg PO daily, with maintenance dosage of 20 to 40 mg daily.
Children ages 6 to 16 weighing 20 to less than 35 kg: Initially, 10 mg PO daily, with maintenance dosage of 10 to 20 mg daily.
Adjust-a-dose: In patients with possible depletion of intravascular volume (those with impaired renal function who are taking diuretics), consider a lower starting dose. Use cautiously in patients with CrCl less than 20 mL/minute.

ADMINISTRATION
PO
• Give drug without regard for food.
• Drug may be made into suspension by pharmacist if patient is unable to swallow pills.
• Refrigerate suspension, which may be stored for up to 28 days.
• Shake suspension well before use.

ACTION
Blocks vasoconstrictor and aldosterone-secreting effects of angiotensin II by selectively blocking the binding of angiotensin II to the angiotensin I, or AT_1, receptor in the vascular smooth muscle.

Route	Onset	Peak	Duration
PO	Rapid	1–2 hr	24 hr

Half-life: 13 hours.

ADVERSE REACTIONS
CNS: headache, dizziness. **EENT:** pharyngitis, rhinitis, sinusitis. **GI:** diarrhea.

GU: hematuria. **Metabolic:** hyperglycemia, hypertriglyceridemia. **Musculoskeletal:** back pain. **Respiratory:** bronchitis, URI. **Other:** flulike symptoms.

INTERACTIONS

Drug-drug. *ACE inhibitors:* May increase risk of hyperkalemia and decrease renal function. Consider monotherapy; if coadministration can't be avoided, monitor renal function and serum potassium level.

🔔 *Alert: Aliskiren:* May increase risk of renal impairment, hypotension, and hyperkalemia in patients with diabetes and those with moderate to severe renal impairment (GFR less than 60 mL/minute). Concomitant use is contraindicated in patients with diabetes. Avoid concomitant use in patients with moderate to severe renal impairment.

Colesevelam: Reduces olmesartan level. Give olmesartan at least 4 hours before colesevelam.

Cyclo-oxygenase-2 inhibitors, NSAIDs: May decrease antihypertensive effects of olmesartan. Coadministration in older adults, patients who are volume-depleted, or those with compromised renal function may result in deterioration of renal function, including possible acute renal failure. Monitor BP and renal function periodically.

Heparin: May increase serum potassium level. Monitor serum potassium level.

Lithium: May increase serum lithium level and risk of toxicity. Closely monitor serum lithium level and adjust dosage as needed.

Potassium: May increase risk of hyperkalemia, possibly with cardiac arrhythmias or arrest. Closely monitor serum potassium level and renal function; adjust therapy as needed.

Potassium-sparing diuretics: May increase risk of hyperkalemia. Closely monitor serum potassium level.

Trimethoprim: May increase risk of hyperkalemia, especially in older adults. If use together can't be avoided, closely monitor potassium level.

Drug-herb. *Yohimbe:* May decrease antihypertensive effect of olmesartan. Closely monitor patient.

EFFECTS ON LAB TEST RESULTS
• May increase potassium, glucose, triglyceride, uric acid, liver enzyme, bilirubin, and CK levels.
• May decrease Hb level and hematocrit.

• May lead to false-negative aldosterone/renin ratio.

CONTRAINDICATIONS & CAUTIONS
• Contraindicated in patients hypersensitive to drug or its components and in patients with diabetes who are also taking aliskiren.
• Avoid use in patients who experienced angioedema with other ARBs and in those with renal impairment who are also taking aliskiren.
• Use cautiously in patients who are volume- or sodium-depleted, those whose renal function depends on the RAAS (such as patients with severe HF), and those with unilateral or bilateral renal artery stenosis.

🔔 *Alert:* Drug can cause spruelike enteropathy (severe chronic diarrhea with substantial weight loss).
• Effectiveness in children younger than age 6 hasn't been proven.

Dialyzable drug: Unknown.

⚠ *Overdose S&S:* Hypotension, tachycardia, bradycardia.

PREGNANCY-LACTATION-REPRODUCTION
Boxed Warning Drug may cause fetal and neonatal complications and death. If patient becomes pregnant, stop drug immediately. ∎
• It isn't known if drug appears in human milk. Patient should discontinue breastfeeding or discontinue drug.

NURSING CONSIDERATIONS
• Symptomatic hypotension may occur in patients who are volume- or sodium-depleted, especially those being treated with high doses of a diuretic. If hypotension occurs, place patient supine and treat supportively. Treatment may continue once BP is stabilized.
• If BP isn't adequately controlled, a diuretic or other antihypertensive drugs also may be prescribed.
• Closely monitor patients with HF for oliguria, azotemia, and acute renal failure.
• Watch for signs and symptoms of angioedema.
• Monitor serum potassium level; drug can cause hyperkalemia.
• Monitor BUN and creatinine level in patients with unilateral or bilateral renal artery stenosis.
▨ The antihypertensive effects of ACE inhibitors and ARBs are reduced in patients who are Black; use of these drugs as initial

---

Reactions in bold italics are *life-threatening*. Interactions may have a *rapid onset* or a *delayed onset*.

antihypertensive therapy in these patients isn't recommended.

PATIENT TEACHING

• Tell patient to take drug exactly as prescribed and not to stop taking it, even if feeling better.

• Teach patient or caregiver safe drug administration for formulation prescribed.

• Advise patient to promptly report all adverse reactions, especially light-headedness and fainting.

• Teach patient to avoid potassium supplements and potassium-containing salt substitutes.

• Educate patient to report signs and symptoms of angioedema (wheezing, swelling of face, lips, tongue, or throat).

🕔 *Alert:* Tell patient to contact prescriber if severe chronic diarrhea with substantial weight loss develops, even if months to years have elapsed before symptoms occur.

• Advise patient of childbearing potential that drug can cause fetal harm and to immediately report pregnancy to health care provider.

• Inform patient with diabetes that glucose readings may rise and that dosage of diabetes drugs may need adjustment.

• Warn patient that inadequate fluid intake, excessive perspiration, diarrhea, or vomiting may lead to an excessive drop in BP, light-headedness, and possibly fainting.

• Instruct patient that other antihypertensives can have additive effects. Patient should inform prescriber of all medications being taken, including OTC drugs and herbal products.

olodaterol
OH-loe-DA-ter-ol

Inspiolto Respimat✤ , Striverdi Respimat

Therapeutic class: Bronchodilators
Pharmacologic class: Long-acting selective beta$_2$-adrenergic agonists

AVAILABLE FORMS
Inhalation aerosol: 2.5 mcg/actuation

INDICATIONS & DOSAGES
➤ **Long-term maintenance treatment of airway obstruction in patients with COPD,** **including chronic bronchitis and emphysema**

Adults: 2 inhalations once daily. Maximum dose is 2 inhalations in 24 hours.

ADMINISTRATION
Inhalational

• Prime inhaler by spraying toward ground until aerosol cloud is seen; then repeat spray three more times before first use or if inhaler hasn't been used for more than 21 days. If not used for more than 3 days, spray once toward ground to prime.

• To administer dose, have patient breathe in slowly through the mouth and press the dose release button. Patient should then continue to breathe in slowly as long as possible and then hold breath for 10 seconds if possible. Repeat for the second inhalation.

• While patient is inhaling dose, have patient hold inhaler flat; make sure patient doesn't cover air vents on the mouthpiece.

• Give at same time each day.

• Store at 68° to 77° F (20° to 25° C); avoid freezing. Discard 3 months after cartridge has been inserted into inhaler.

ACTION

Binds and activates beta$_2$ adrenoceptors in the lungs, resulting in relaxation of smooth muscle cells and bronchodilation.

Route	Onset	Peak	Duration
Inhalation	5 min	10–20 min	24 hr

Half-life: 7.5 hours.

ADVERSE REACTIONS
CNS: fever, dizziness. **EENT:** nasopharyngitis. **GI:** constipation. **GU:** UTI. **Musculoskeletal:** back pain, arthralgia. **Respiratory:** URI, bronchitis, pneumonia, cough. **Skin:** rash.

INTERACTIONS
Drug-drug. *Atomoxetine, linezolid:* May have additive tachycardic effect. Monitor patient carefully.
Beta blockers: May diminish effect of both drugs and increase risk of bronchospasm. Avoid combination if possible.
Cannabinoid-containing products: May increase tachycardic effect of olodaterol. Monitor therapy closely.
Corticosteroids, non-potassium-sparing diuretics, xanthine derivatives (theophylline):

May increase risk of hypokalemia. Monitor potassium level.

Drugs that prolong QT interval (antiarrhythmics, droperidol, haloperidol, mifepristone, TCAs, thioridazine): May increase risk of life-threatening cardiac arrhythmias. Use together cautiously.

Loop diuretics, thiazide and thiazide-like diuretics: May increase hypokalemic effect of diuretics. Monitor potassium level.

MAO inhibitors, TCAs: May increase CV effects. Use together cautiously.

Other beta₂ agonists (long-acting): May have additive risk of toxic adverse effects. Use together is contraindicated.

Tedizolid: May increase hypertensive and tachycardic effects of olodaterol. Monitor therapy closely.

Drug-food. *Caffeine:* May increase risk of hypokalemia. Discourage use together.

EFFECTS ON LAB TEST RESULTS
• May increase glucose level.
• May decrease potassium level.

CONTRAINDICATIONS & CAUTIONS
• Use of a LABA, including olodaterol, without an inhaled corticosteroid is contraindicated in patients with asthma. Drug isn't indicated for use in asthma.
• **Alert:** Rare, paradoxical, life-threatening bronchospasm has been reported. Discontinue drug immediately and treat emergently.
• Discontinue drug if hypersensitivity reactions such as angioedema occur.
• Don't initiate drug in patients with acute deterioration of COPD.
• Contraindicated as rescue therapy for acute symptoms.
• Use cautiously in patients with extreme sensitivity to other sympathomimetics, CV conditions (coronary insufficiency, cardiac arrhythmias, hypertrophic obstructive cardiomyopathy, HTN), seizure disorders, diabetes, or thyrotoxicosis.
• Use cautiously in patients with known or suspected prolongation of QT interval.
• Safety and effectiveness in children haven't been established.

Dialyzable drug: Unknown.

⚠ Overdose S&S: CV toxicity, HTN or hypotension, tachycardia, arrhythmias, palpitations, dizziness, nervousness, insomnia, anxiety, headache, tremor, dry mouth, muscle spasms, nausea, fatigue, malaise, hypokalemia, hyperglycemia, metabolic acidosis.

PREGNANCY-LACTATION-REPRODUCTION
• There are no adequate studies during pregnancy. Use during pregnancy only if potential benefit justifies fetal risk.
• It isn't known if drug appears in human milk but it's likely. Use cautiously during breastfeeding.

NURSING CONSIDERATIONS
• Patient must also be prescribed a short-acting inhaled beta₂ agonist to provide symptomatic relief.
• Monitor patient for increased use of inhaled beta₂ agonist and decreased control of symptoms of bronchospasm. Evaluate for deterioration of disease.
• Monitor FEV₁, FVC, and other pulmonary function tests; serum potassium and serum glucose levels; and BP and HR.
• **Alert:** Excessive use of drug by using more frequently, increasing the number of inhalations, or using in combination with other medications containing LABAs may cause CV effects and death.
• Monitor patient for hypokalemia (which may increase risk of cardiac arrhythmias) and hyperglycemia.
• **Look alike–sound alike:** Don't confuse olodaterol with olopatadine. Don't confuse Striverdi Respimat with Combivent Respimat.

PATIENT TEACHING
• Warn patient that drug isn't approved for treatment of asthma. Advise patient that using a LABA, including olodaterol, without an inhaled corticosteroid is contraindicated in patients with asthma.
• Teach patient how to use the inhaler device; then ask patient to demonstrate its use.
• Advise patient to take medication at same time each day.
• Explain that drug has a long-acting effect and should never be used as a "rescue medication" to relieve acute symptoms. Advise patient to always carry a rescue inhaler.
• Advise patient to report worsening signs or symptoms of COPD, increased frequency of rescue medication use, and decrease in effectiveness of rescue medication.
• Warn patient not to use drug with other LABAs and not to regularly use short-acting

---

beta₂ agonists. Short-acting beta₂ agonists should only be used for acute symptoms.
- Instruct patient to report palpitations, chest pain, rapid heartbeat, muscle spasms, weakness, tremor or nervousness, URI, confusion, flushed dry skin, excessive thirst, urination, or hunger.
- Teach patient to seek emergency medical care for serious allergic reactions (breathing problems, rash, hives, or swelling of the face, mouth, or tongue).
- Caution patient not to stop drug without first discussing with prescriber.
- Instruct patient to consult prescriber before starting new prescription or OTC medications or herbal or nutritional supplements.
- Advise patient to report pregnancy, plans to become pregnant, or breastfeeding.

omadacycline
oh-MAD-a-sye-kleen

Nuzyra

Therapeutic class: Antibiotics
Pharmacologic class: Tetracyclines

AVAILABLE FORMS
Injection: 100 mg single-dose vial
Tablets: 150-mg base

INDICATIONS & DOSAGES
➤ **Treatment of community-acquired bacterial pneumonia (CABP) caused by** *Streptococcus pneumoniae, Staphylococcus aureus* **(methicillin-susceptible isolates),** *Haemophilus influenzae, Haemophilus parainfluenzae, Klebsiella pneumoniae, Legionella pneumophila, Mycoplasma pneumoniae,* **and** *Chlamydophila pneumoniae*
Adults: Initially, 200 mg IV infusion over 60 minutes once or 100 mg IV infusion over 30 minutes b.i.d. on day 1; then 100 mg IV infusion over 30 minutes once daily or 300 mg PO once daily. Or, initially, 300 mg PO b.i.d. on day 1; then 300 mg PO once daily. Treat for 7 to 14 days.
➤ **Treatment of acute bacterial skin and skin-structure infections caused by** *S. aureus* **(methicillin-susceptible and methicillin-resistant isolates),** *Staphylococcus lugdunensis, Streptococcus pyogenes, Streptococcus anginosus* **group (includes** *S. anginosus, S. intermedius, S. constellatus*), *Enterococcus faecalis, Enterobacter cloacae,* **and** *K. pneumoniae*
Adults: Initially, 200 mg IV infusion over 60 minutes once or 100 mg IV infusion over 30 minutes b.i.d. on day 1; then 100 mg IV infusion over 30 minutes once daily. Or, initially, 450 mg PO once daily on days 1 and 2; then 300 mg PO once daily beginning on day 3. Treat for 7 to 14 days.

ADMINISTRATION
PO
- Patient should fast for at least 4 hours before dose; then take with water.
- Patient shouldn't eat or drink (except water) for 2 hours after dose or ingest dairy products, antacids, or multivitamins for 4 hours after dose.

IV
▼ Reconstitute each 100-mg vial with 5 mL sterile water, NSS, or D₅W for injection.
▼ Gently swirl contents and let stand until drug cake dissolves completely and foam disperses. Don't shake.
▼ Reconstituted solution should be yellow to dark orange; if not, discard it. Visually inspect vial for particulate matter and discoloration before further dilution and administration. If necessary, invert vial to dissolve remaining powder and swirl gently to prevent foaming.
▼ Within 1 hour of reconstitution, withdraw 5 mL or 10 mL of solution and further dilute in a 100-mL bag of NSS or D₅W, for a final concentration of either 1 mg/mL or 2 mg/mL. Discard any unused portion of solution.
▼ Infuse diluted solution within 24 hours if kept at room temperature or within 7 days when refrigerated. Don't freeze.
▼ Remove from refrigerator and allow solution to warm to room temperature 60 minutes before use.
▼ Administer through a dedicated line or Y-site. If the same IV line is used for infusion of other drugs, flush the line with NSS or D₅W before and after infusion of omadacycline.
▼ Administer infusion over 60 minutes for 200-mg dose or 30 minutes for 100-mg dose.
▼ Store vials at room temperature.
▼ **Incompatibilities:** Don't administer solutions containing multivalent cations

(calcium, magnesium) through the same IV line. Infusion with other medications and infusion solutions other than NSS or D₅W hasn't been studied.

ACTION

A tetracycline antibiotic that exerts its bacteriostatic effect by inhibiting bacterial protein synthesis.

Route	Onset	Peak	Duration
PO	Unknown	2.5 hr	Unknown
IV	Unknown	30 min	Unknown

Half-life: 15 to 17 hours.

ADVERSE REACTIONS

CNS: insomnia, headache, fatigue, lethargy, vertigo. **CV:** HTN, tachycardia, atrial fibrillation. **EENT:** oral candidiasis, oral pharyngeal pain. **GI:** vomiting, constipation, nausea, diarrhea, abdominal pain, dyspepsia, dysgeusia. **GU:** vulvovaginal mycotic infection. **Hematologic:** anemia, thrombocytosis. **Hepatic:** elevated LFT values. **Skin:** pruritus, erythema, sweating, urticaria. **Other:** infusion-site reaction, hypersensitivity.

INTERACTIONS

Drug-drug. *Antacids containing aluminum, calcium, magnesium, bismuth subsalicylate; iron-containing preparations; iron supplements:* May decrease omadacycline absorption. Separate doses by at least 4 hours before and 4 hours after omadacycline.
Anticoagulants (warfarin): May increase anticoagulant effects. Monitor patient closely and decrease anticoagulant dosage if needed.
Drug-food. *Dairy products:* May decrease omadacycline absorption. Separate dairy product use by at least 4 hours before and 4 hours after omadacycline.
Food, nondairy drinks (except water): May decrease omadacycline absorption. Avoid for at least 4 hours before and 2 hours after omadacycline.
Drug-lifestyle. *Sun exposure:* May cause photosensitivity. Advise patient to avoid sun exposure and to wear sun-protective clothing and sunscreen.

EFFECTS ON LAB TEST RESULTS

• May increase ALT, AST, GGT, CK, bilirubin, ALP, and lipase levels.

CONTRAINDICATIONS & CAUTIONS

• Contraindicated in patients hypersensitive to drug or its components or tetracycline class drugs.
• Use only to treat or prevent infections proven or strongly suspected to be caused by susceptible bacteria to reduce development of drug-resistance.
⚠ *Alert:* In clinical trials, when drug was used to treat CABP, there was a higher mortality rate than for patients treated with moxifloxacin. All deaths occurred in patients older than age 65 and most had multiple comorbid conditions. The cause of the mortality imbalance isn't known.
⚠ *Alert:* CDAD has been reported and may range from mild diarrhea to fatal colitis.
• Use of tetracycline class drugs during the last half (second or third trimester) of pregnancy, during infancy, and in children younger than age 8 may cause permanent yellow-gray-brown discoloration of the teeth or tooth enamel hypoplasia, and may cause reversible inhibition of bone growth.
• Use cautiously in older adults.
• Safety and effectiveness in patients younger than age 18 haven't been established. Use in children younger than age 8 isn't recommended.
Dialyzable drug: 8.9%.

PREGNANCY-LACTATION-REPRODUCTION

• Drug may cause fetal harm. Advise patients of childbearing potential to use contraception during therapy.
• Tetracyclines appear in human milk. Breastfeeding isn't recommended during treatment and for 4 days after final dose.
• Based on animal studies, drug may affect fertility.

NURSING CONSIDERATIONS

• Confirm that patients don't have an allergy to any tetracycline class drug before starting therapy.
• Monitor patients for hypersensitivity reactions, including anaphylaxis.
• Monitor patients for signs and symptoms of CDAD (watery or bloody stools [with or without stomach cramps or fever]) during and for several months after treatment with antibacterial drugs. If CDAD is suspected or confirmed, antibiotic use other than for treatment of *Clostridioides difficile* may need to

---

Reactions in bold italics are *life-threatening*. Interactions may have a *rapid onset* or a *delayed onset*.

be discontinued. Initiate appropriate treatment.

• Monitor patients for tetracycline class adverse reactions, including photosensitivity, pseudotumor cerebri, and antianabolic activity (increased BUN level, azotemia, acidosis, hyperphosphatemia, pancreatitis, abnormal LFT values). Discontinue drug if any of these are suspected.

• *Look alike–sound alike:* Don't confuse omadacycline with omacetaxine.

PATIENT TEACHING

• Warn patient that antibacterial drugs should only be used to treat bacterial infections and shouldn't be used to treat viral infections such as the common cold.

• Advise patient to report all adverse reactions.

• Caution patient to seek immediate medical attention for serious allergic reactions.

• Teach patient safe drug administration.

• Caution patient to take drug exactly as directed even if feeling better. Stress importance of not skipping doses and completing therapy as prescribed.

• Warn patient that nonadherence may decrease effectiveness of treatment and risk that the bacteria will develop resistance and not be treatable by antibacterial drugs in the future.

⟲ *Alert:* Instruct patient to immediately report watery or bloody stools (with or without stomach cramps or fever) as these may indicate CDAD.

• Advise patient that drug can cause photosensitivity and to avoid sun exposure and wear sun-protective clothing and sunscreen during treatment.

• Advise patient of childbearing potential of fetal risk if drug is used during pregnancy. Caution patient to use contraceptives during treatment and to immediately report suspected pregnancy.

• Teach patient that breastfeeding isn't recommended during treatment and for 4 days after final dose.

---

omalizumab
oh-mah-lye-ZOO-mab

Xolair

Therapeutic class: Antiasthmatics
Pharmacologic class: Monoclonal antibodies

AVAILABLE FORMS
Powder for injection: 150 mg in single-dose vials
Prefilled syringe: 75 mg/0.5 mL (0.5 mL), 150 mg/mL (1 mL)

INDICATIONS & DOSAGES
➤ **Moderate to severe persistent asthma in patients with positive skin test or in vitro reactivity to a perennial aeroallergen and whose symptoms aren't adequately controlled by inhaled corticosteroids**
Adults and children age 6 and older: 75 to 375 mg subcut every 2 or 4 weeks. Dose and frequency vary with pretreatment IgE level (international units/mL) and patient weight. (Refer to manufacturer's instructions.)
➤ **Nasal polyps as add-on maintenance treatment in patients with inadequate response to nasal corticosteroids**
Adults: 75 to 600 mg subcut every 2 or 4 weeks. Dosage and frequency vary with pretreatment IgE level (international units/mL) and patient weight. (Refer to manufacturer's instructions.)
➤ **Chronic idiopathic urticaria in patients who are symptomatic despite H_1 antihistamine treatment**
Adults and adolescents age 12 and older: 150 to 300 mg subcut every 4 weeks. Dosing isn't dependent on serum IgE level or body weight. Periodically reassess need for continued therapy; treatment duration hasn't been evaluated.

ADMINISTRATION
Subcutaneous
• Reconstitute with 1.4 mL of sterile water for injection only. Swirl gently, don't shake. Continue to swirl for 5 to 10 seconds approximately every 5 minutes until there are no visible gel-like particles in the solution.
• The lyophilized product takes 15 to 20 minutes to dissolve completely. Don't use if vial's contents don't dissolve completely by 40 minutes.

- The fully reconstituted product will appear clear or slightly opalescent and may have a few small bubbles or foam around edge of vial.
- Use 18G needle to draw medication into syringe, then replace with a 25G needle for administration.
- Because solution is slightly viscous, it may take 5 to 10 seconds to administer.
- Give at least first three doses in a health care setting under the guidance of a health care provider.
- Divide doses of more than 150 mg between two or more injection sites.
- Don't give more than one injection per site. Choose a different injection site for each new injection that's at least 1 inch from other injection sites.
- Use reconstituted solution within 4 hours if at room temperature or within 8 hours if refrigerated. Protect from sunlight.
- Recommended injection sites are upper arm, stomach, or front and middle of the thighs for lyophilized powder, or upper arm and front and middle of the thighs for prefilled syringe.
- Don't inject into moles, scars, bruises, tender areas, or broken skin.
- Store vials before reconstitution and prefilled syringes under refrigeration at 36° to 46° F (2° to 8° C).

ACTION

Inhibits binding of IgE to high-affinity receptor on surface of mast cells and basophils, which limits release of allergic response mediators.

Route	Onset	Peak	Duration
Subcut	Slow	7–8 days	Unknown

Half-life: About 24 to 26 days.

ADVERSE REACTIONS

CNS: anxiety, headache, dizziness, fatigue, pain, migraine, fever. **CV:** *MI, PE, thrombosis,* angina pectoris, peripheral edema. **EENT:** otitis media, earache, pharyngitis, sinusitis. **GI:** abdominal pain, gastroenteritis, toothache. **GU:** UTI. **Musculoskeletal:** arm pain, arthralgia, fracture, leg pain. **Respiratory:** URI, cough, asthma. **Skin:** injection-site reaction, dermatitis, pruritus, bleeding, bruising, burning, redness, pain, inflammation, stinging, swelling, warmth. **Other:** viral and fungal infections, alopecia.

INTERACTIONS

Drug-drug. *Loxapine (inhalation only):* May enhance adverse or toxic effect of loxapine. Avoid combination.

EFFECTS ON LAB TEST RESULTS

- May increase IgE level, which may remain elevated for up to 1 year after treatment ends.
- May increase eosinophil count.

CONTRAINDICATIONS & CAUTIONS

- Contraindicated in patients severely hypersensitive to drug or its ingredients.

Boxed Warning Anaphylaxis presenting as bronchospasm, hypotension, syncope, urticaria, or angioedema of the throat or tongue has been reported after administration as early as the first dose and even after a year of treatment. ▪

Boxed Warning Initiate therapy in a health care setting because of anaphylaxis risk. After deeming therapy safe, prescriber may determine that patient or caregiver can safely administer drug using a prefilled syringe. ▪

⚉ *Alert:* Drug isn't indicated for other allergic conditions or other forms of urticaria.

- Safety and effectiveness in children younger than age 6 haven't been established. *Dialyzable drug:* Unknown.

PREGNANCY-LACTATION-REPRODUCTION

- Drug may increase risk of low birth weight in infants, and there are pregnancy risks associated with poorly or moderately controlled asthma during pregnancy. Use only if clearly needed.
- Encourage enrollment in the MotherToBaby Pregnancy Studies for asthma (1-866-626-6847 or http://mothertobaby.org).
- It isn't known if drug appears in human milk. Use cautiously during breastfeeding.

NURSING CONSIDERATIONS

⚉ *Alert:* Don't use this drug to treat acute bronchospasm or status asthmaticus.

- Don't abruptly stop systemic or inhaled corticosteroid when omalizumab therapy starts; taper the dose gradually and under supervision.
- Injection-site reactions, such as bruising, redness, warmth, burning, stinging, itching, hives, pain, induration, and inflammation, may occur, usually within 1 hour after the injection. These reactions last fewer than 8 days

---

Reactions in bold italics are *life-threatening*. Interactions may have a *rapid onset* or a ***delayed onset***.

and decrease in frequency with subsequent injections.

Boxed Warning Observe patient for an appropriate time period after the injection, and keep drugs available to respond to anaphylactic reactions (such as bronchospasm, hypotension, syncope, urticaria, or angioedema of the throat or tongue). These reactions usually occur within 2 hours of subcut injection; however, delayed reactions may occur up to 24 hours after administration. Anaphylaxis has also occurred beyond 1 year after beginning regularly administered treatment. If patient has a severe hypersensitivity reaction, stop treatment. ∎

🖐 *Alert:* Drug may slightly increase risk of CV and cerebrovascular events (TIA, MI, chest pain, pulmonary HTN, DVT, PE). Periodically reassess the need for continued therapy based on disease severity and asthma control.

• Drug increases IgE level, so it can't be used to determine appropriate dosage during therapy or for 1 year after therapy ends.

• Monitor pulmonary function test results for signs and symptoms of infection.

• The needle cover on the prefilled syringe contains dry natural rubber (a derivative of latex), which may cause allergic reactions in individuals sensitive to latex.

• *Look alike–sound alike:* Don't confuse omalizumab with obinutuzumab or ofatumumab.

PATIENT TEACHING
• Advise patient to review Medication Guide given with each dose.
• Tell patient not to stop or reduce the dosage of other asthma drugs unless directed by prescriber.
• Explain that patient may not notice an immediate improvement in asthma after therapy starts.
• Show adult, adolescent age 12 and older with adult supervision, or caregiver how to administer the subcut prefilled syringe and assess ability to inject subcut to ensure proper administration.
Boxed Warning Teach patient signs and symptoms of anaphylaxis and to seek immediate medical care if symptoms occur. ∎

omega-3–fatty acids
oh-MEG-a-three/FAT-tee-AS-ids

Lovaza🖌, Vascepa

Therapeutic class: Antilipemics
Pharmacologic class: Fatty acids

AVAILABLE FORMS
Capsules 🔘: 0.5 g, 1 g

INDICATIONS & DOSAGES
➤ **Adjunct to diet to reduce triglyceride levels 500 mg/dL or higher**
Adults: 4 g PO once daily (Lovaza only) or divided as 2 g PO b.i.d.
➤ **Adjunct to maximally tolerated statin therapy to reduce risk of MI, stroke, coronary revascularization, and unstable angina requiring hospitalization in adults with elevated triglyceride levels (150 mg/dL or higher) and established CV disease or diabetes and two or more additional risk factors for CV disease (Vascepa)**
Adults: 2 g PO b.i.d.

ADMINISTRATION
PO
• Give with meals.
• Make sure patient swallows capsules whole and doesn't chew, crush, dissolve, or extract contents of capsule.
• If a dose is missed, give missed dose as soon as possible; don't double dose.

ACTION
May reduce hepatic formation of triglycerides because two components of drug are poor substrates for the necessary enzymes. These components also block formation of other fatty acids.

Route	Onset	Peak	Duration
PO	Unknown	5–9 hr	Unknown

Half-life: Eicosapentaenoic acid, about 37 to 89 hours; docosahexaenoic acid, about 46 hours.

ADVERSE REACTIONS
CNS: altered taste. **CV:** peripheral edema, atrial fibrillation, atrial flutter. **EENT:** oropharyngeal pain. **GI:** abdominal pain, belching, dyspepsia, diarrhea, nausea. **Metabolic:** gout. **Musculoskeletal:** arthralgia, back pain. **Skin:** rash.

🍁Canada ◇OTC ◆Off-label use 🖌Photoguide 🔘Do not crush *Liquid contains alcohol ▨ Genetic

INTERACTIONS
Drug-drug. *Anticoagulants, antiplatelet drugs:* May prolong bleeding time. Monitor patient.
Ibrutinib: May enhance antiplatelet effect of ibrutinib. Monitor therapy.

EFFECTS ON LAB TEST RESULTS
• May increase bleeding time and ALT, AST, triglyceride, and LDL cholesterol levels.

CONTRAINDICATIONS & CAUTIONS
• Contraindicated in patients hypersensitive to drug or its components.
• Use cautiously in patients with known hypersensitivity to fish or shellfish.
• Use cautiously in patients with coagulopathy and in those receiving therapeutic anticoagulation or antiplatelet therapy because of risk of prolonged bleeding time.
• Effect of drug on risk of pancreatitis hasn't been determined.
• May increase risk of atrial fibrillation or atrial flutter.
• Safety and effectiveness in children haven't been established.
Dialyzable drug: Unknown.

PREGNANCY-LACTATION-REPRODUCTION
• There are no adequate studies during pregnancy. Use cautiously and only if benefit justifies possible risks to the fetus.
• Drug may appear in human milk. Use cautiously during breastfeeding.

NURSING CONSIDERATIONS
• Assess patient for conditions that contribute to increased triglycerides, such as diabetes and hypothyroidism, before treatment.
• Monitor patient for changes in INR after drug initiation and after omega-3–fatty acid dosage changes in patients receiving warfarin.
• Evaluate patient's current drug regimen for any drugs known to sharply increase triglyceride levels, including estrogen therapy, thiazide diuretics, and beta blockers. Stopping these drugs, if appropriate, may negate the need for drug.
• Continue diet and lifestyle modifications during treatment.
• Obtain baseline triglyceride levels to confirm that they're consistently abnormal before therapy; then recheck periodically during treatment. If patient has an inadequate response after 2 months, stop drug.

• Monitor LDL level to make sure it doesn't increase excessively during treatment.
• Periodically monitor hepatic transaminase levels in patients with hepatic impairment.
• **Look alike–sound alike:** Don't confuse Lovaza with lorazepam or lovastatin.

PATIENT TEACHING
• Explain that taking drug doesn't reduce the importance of following the recommended diet and exercise plan.
• Remind patient of the need for follow-up blood work to evaluate progress.
• Instruct patient in safe drug administration for prescribed formulation.
• Advise patient to notify prescriber about bothersome side effects.
• Tell patient to report planned or suspected pregnancy.

---

omeprazole ▨
oh-MEP-ra-zole

Losec ✢

omeprazole magnesium
Losec ✢, Prilosec OTC ◇, Prilosec Packets

Therapeutic class: Antiulcer drugs
Pharmacologic class: PPIs

AVAILABLE FORMS
Capsules (delayed-release) ⓞⓣⓒ: 10 mg, 20 mg, 40 mg
Powder (for delayed-release oral suspension): 2.5 mg/packet, 10 mg/packet
Suspension: 2 mg/mL
Tablets (delayed-release) ⓞⓣⓒ: 20 mg ◇

INDICATIONS & DOSAGES
➤ **Symptomatic GERD without esophageal lesions**
Adults: 20 mg PO, as delayed-release form or oral suspension, daily for 4 weeks for patients who respond poorly to customary medical treatment, usually including an adequate course of H$_2$-receptor antagonists.
Children ages 1 to 16 weighing 20 kg or more: 20 mg PO daily for up to 4 weeks.
Children ages 1 to 16 weighing 10 to less than 20 kg: 10 mg PO daily for up to 4 weeks.
Children ages 1 to 16 weighing 5 to less than 10 kg: 5 mg PO daily for up to 4 weeks.

Reactions in bold italics are *life-threatening*. Interactions may have a *rapid onset* or a *delayed onset*.

➤ **Erosive esophagitis (EE)** ▨
Adults: 20 mg PO daily. For recurrent EE or GERD signs and symptoms, treat for up to 12 months.
Adjust-a-dose: When drug is used for maintenance of healing of EE, dosage reduction to 10 mg once daily is recommended for patients with hepatic impairment (Child-Pugh class A, B, or C) and patients of Asian descent.
Children ages 1 to 16 weighing 20 kg or more: 20 mg PO daily for 4 to 8 weeks; continue up to 12 months for maintenance of healing.
Children ages 1 to 16 weighing 10 to less than 20 kg: 10 mg PO daily for 4 to 8 weeks; continue up to 12 months for maintenance of healing.
Children ages 1 to 16 weighing 5 to less than 10 kg: 5 mg PO daily for 4 to 8 weeks; continue up to 12 months for maintenance of healing.
Infants weighing 3 to less than 5 kg: 2.5 mg once daily for up to 6 weeks.
➤ **Pathologic hypersecretory conditions (such as Zollinger-Ellison syndrome)**
Adults: Initially, 60 mg PO daily; adjust dosage based on patient response. If daily dose exceeds 80 mg, give in divided doses. Doses up to 120 mg t.i.d. have been given. Continue therapy as long as clinically indicated.
➤ **Duodenal ulcer (short-term treatment)**
Adults: 20 mg PO, as delayed-release form or oral suspension, daily for 4 weeks.
➤ *Helicobacter pylori* **infection and duodenal ulcer disease, to eradicate** *H. pylori* **with clarithromycin (dual therapy)**
Adults: 40 mg PO every morning with clarithromycin 500 mg PO t.i.d. for 14 days. For patients with an ulcer at start of therapy, give another 14 days of omeprazole 20 mg PO once daily.
➤ *H. pylori* **infection and duodenal ulcer disease, to eradicate** *H. pylori* **with clarithromycin and amoxicillin (triple therapy)**
Adults: 20 mg PO with clarithromycin 500 mg PO and amoxicillin 1,000 mg PO, each given b.i.d. for 10 days. For patients with an ulcer at start of therapy, give another 18 days of omeprazole 20 mg PO once daily.
➤ **Short-term treatment of active benign gastric ulcer**
Adults: 40 mg PO once daily for 4 to 8 weeks.
➤ **Frequent heartburn (2 or more days a week)**

Adults: 20 mg Prilosec OTC PO once daily before breakfast for 14 days. May repeat the 14-day course every 4 months.
➤ **Dyspepsia** ♦
Adults: 20 mg once daily for 4- to 8-week trial; may continue longer if signs and symptoms improve.

ADMINISTRATION
PO
• Don't crush tablets or capsules. For patients who have difficulty swallowing, capsules may be opened and contents mixed with 15 mL of applesauce. Follow with water to ensure complete swallowing of pellets.
• Give drug at least 30 to 60 minutes before meals; best if taken before breakfast. If administering twice daily, give first dose before breakfast and second dose before evening meal.
• For oral suspension, empty contents of 2.5-mg packet into container containing 5 mL water; empty contents of 10-mg packet into container containing 15 mL water. Stir and leave for 2 to 3 minutes to thicken. Stir and administer within 30 minutes. If material remains after drinking, add more water, stir, and give immediately.
• For patients with an NG or gastric tube in place, add 5 mL water to catheter-tipped syringe; then add contents of 2.5-mg packet (or 15 mL water for 10-mg packet). Immediately shake syringe and leave for 2 to 3 minutes to thicken. Shake syringe and inject through NG or gastric tube, #6 French or larger, into stomach within 30 minutes. Refill syringe with an equal amount of water. Shake and flush any remaining contents from NG or gastric tube into stomach.
• May give concomitantly with antacids.
• If a dose is missed, give missed dose as soon as possible unless close to next scheduled dose. Don't give two doses to make up for missed dose.

ACTION
Inhibits proton pump activity by binding to hydrogen–potassium adenosine triphosphatase, located at secretory surface of gastric parietal cells, to suppress gastric acid secretion.

Route	Onset	Peak	Duration
PO	1 hr	30 min–2 hr	<3 days

Half-life: 30 to 60 minutes.

ADVERSE REACTIONS

CNS: asthenia, dizziness, headache. **GI:** abdominal pain, constipation, diarrhea, flatulence, nausea, vomiting, acid regurgitation. **Musculoskeletal:** back pain, weakness. **Respiratory:** cough, URI. **Skin:** rash.

INTERACTIONS

Drug-drug. *Ampicillin esters, azole antifungals (such as ketoconazole), erlotinib, iron derivatives, nilotinib:* May cause poor bioavailability of these drugs because they need a low gastric pH for optimal absorption. Avoid using together.

Atazanavir, nelfinavir: May decrease plasma concentrations of these drugs and therapeutic effect. Avoid use together.

Benzodiazepines (metabolized by hepatic oxidation), fosphenytoin, phenytoin, warfarin: May decrease hepatic clearance and increase levels of these drugs. Monitor drug levels.

Bisphosphonates: May decrease therapeutic effect of bisphosphonates. Monitor therapy.

Calcium salts: May decrease GI absorption of calcium salts. Closely monitor clinical response and increase calcium dosage if needed.

Cilostazol: May increase cilostazol level. Reduce cilostazol dosage.

Clopidogrel: May decrease antiplatelet activity. Avoid use together.

Cyclosporine: May increase cyclosporine serum concentration. Monitor cyclosporine level closely.

Digoxin: May increase digoxin level, causing toxicity. Monitor digoxin level.

Drugs that induce CYP2C19 or CYP3A4 (rifampin): May substantially decrease omeprazole concentration. Avoid concomitant use.

Fluvoxamine: May increase omeprazole level. Monitor patient for increased adverse reactions.

Fosphenytoin, phenytoin: May increase levels of these drugs. Monitor therapy closely.

Iron salts: May interfere with iron absorption. Omeprazole may need to be temporarily stopped, or parenteral iron may be given as an alternative.

Mycophenolate: May decrease mycophenolate serum concentration; may reduce formation of active metabolite for mycophenolate. Monitor therapy.

Methotrexate: May increase methotrexate level, causing toxicity. Monitor patient closely.

Saquinavir: May increase saquinavir serum concentration, resulting in increased toxicity. Monitor therapy.

Tacrolimus: May increase tacrolimus level and risk of toxicity. Monitor tacrolimus trough concentration when omeprazole is started and stopped.

Voriconazole: May increase serum concentrations of both drugs. Consider reducing omeprazole dosage by 50%; monitor therapy.

Warfarin: May increase INR and PT, leading to abnormal bleeding and death. Monitor INR and PT and adjust warfarin dosage, if needed.

Drug-herb. *St. John's wort:* May substantially decrease omeprazole concentration. Avoid concomitant use.

Drug-food. *Vitamin B_{12}:* Prolonged treatment with omeprazole (2 years or longer) may lead to malabsorption of dietary vitamin B_{12}. Avoid concomitant use.

EFFECTS ON LAB TEST RESULTS

• May increase LFT values.
• May falsely elevate serum chromogranin A (CgA) level.
• May decrease magnesium, sodium, glucose, and vitamin B_{12} levels.

CONTRAINDICATIONS & CAUTIONS

• Contraindicated in patients hypersensitive to drug or its components and in patients receiving rilpivirine-containing products.
• SCARs, including SJS, TEN, DRESS syndrome, and acute generalized exanthematous pustulosis, have been reported. If reaction occurs, discontinue drug and refer patient to specialist for evaluation.
◐ *Alert:* High-dose, long-term PPI therapy may be associated with an increased risk of hip, wrist, and spine fractures.
▧ Bioavailability is increased in patients of Asian descent, and reduced dosages are recommended when used for healing EE.
• Use cautiously in patients with hypokalemia and respiratory alkalosis and in patients on a low-sodium diet.
• Risk of fundic gland polyps increases with long-term use, especially beyond 1 year.
• Use of PPIs may increase risk of CDAD. Consider CDAD diagnosis in patients with persistent diarrhea that doesn't improve.
• New onset or exacerbation of existing cutaneous and systemic lupus erythematosus may occur; discontinue therapy and refer patient to specialist for evaluation.

Reactions in bold italics are *life-threatening*. Interactions may have a *rapid onset* or a ***delayed onset***.

Dialyzable drug: Unlikely.
⚠ *Overdose S&S:* Confusion, drowsiness, blurred vision, tachycardia, nausea, vomiting, diaphoresis, flushing, headache, dry mouth.

PREGNANCY-LACTATION-REPRODUCTION

• Use during pregnancy only if potential benefit justifies fetal risk. When treating GERD during pregnancy, PPIs may be used when necessary; however, lifestyle modification is the initial treatment.
• Drug appears in human milk. Use cautiously during breastfeeding.

NURSING CONSIDERATIONS

Alert: May increase risk of CDAD. Evaluate for CDAD in patients who develop diarrhea that doesn't improve.
Alert: Watch for new or worsening rash or worsening signs and symptoms of cutaneous or systemic lupus erythematosus. If suspected, discontinue drug and notify prescriber.
• False-positive results in diagnostic investigations for neuroendocrine tumors may occur due to increased CgA level. Temporarily stop omeprazole treatment at least 14 days before assessing CgA level and consider repeating the test if initial CgA level is high. If serial tests are performed (e.g., for monitoring), the same commercial lab should be used for testing, as reference ranges between tests may vary.
• Long-term therapy may cause vitamin B_{12} absorption problems. Assess patient for signs and symptoms of cyanocobalamin deficiency (weakness, heart palpitations, dyspnea, paresthesia, pale skin, smooth tongue, CNS changes, loss of appetite).
• Because risk of fundic gland polyps increases with long-term use, especially beyond 1 year, use drug for shortest duration appropriate to the condition being treated.
• Periodically assess patient for osteoporosis.
• Monitor patient for signs and symptoms of acute interstitial nephritis. If suspected, discontinue drug and evaluate patient.
• Drug increases its own bioavailability with repeated doses. Drug is unstable in gastric acid; less drug is lost to hydrolysis because drug increases gastric pH.
• Gastrin level rises in most patients during the first 2 weeks of therapy.
Alert: Prolonged use of PPIs may cause low magnesium levels. Monitor magnesium levels before starting treatment and periodically thereafter.
Alert: Monitor patients for signs and symptoms of low magnesium level, such as abnormal HR or rhythm, palpitations, muscle spasms, tremors, or seizures. In children, an abnormal HR may present as fatigue, upset stomach, dizziness, and light-headedness. Magnesium supplementation or drug discontinuation may be required.
• *Look alike–sound alike:* Don't confuse Prilosec OTC with Prevacid, prednisone, Pristiq, Prozac, or prilocaine. Don't confuse omeprazole with aripiprazole, esomeprazole, or fomepizole.

PATIENT TEACHING

• Teach patient safe drug administration.
• Advise patient to immediately report severe skin reactions with blistering, peeling, or bleeding on any part of the skin.
• Caution patient to avoid hazardous activities if dizziness occurs.
• Advise patient that Prilosec OTC isn't intended to treat infrequent heartburn (one episode of heartburn a week or less), or for those who want immediate relief of heartburn.
• Inform patient that Prilosec OTC may take 1 to 4 days for full effect, although some patients may get complete relief of symptoms within 24 hours.
• Teach patient to recognize and report signs and symptoms of low magnesium levels.
• Advise patient or caregiver to report diarrhea that doesn't improve.
• Instruct patient or caregiver to report fractures, especially of the hip, wrist, or spine.

onabotulinumtoxinA

oh-nuh-BOT-yoo-lin-num-TOKS-in aye

Botox

onabotulinumtoxinA (cosmetic)

Botox Cosmetic

Therapeutic class: Neuromuscular transmission blockers
Pharmacologic class: Acetylcholine release inhibitors

AVAILABLE FORMS

onabotulinumtoxinA
Injection: 100 units/vial, 200 units/vial

onabotulinumtoxinA (cosmetic)
Injection: 50 units/vial, 100 units/vial

INDICATIONS & DOSAGES
Adjust-a-dose (for all indications): When adults are being treated for one or more indications, maximum cumulative dose generally shouldn't exceed 400 units in a 3-month interval (Botox) or 360 units in a 3-month interval (Botox Cosmetic).

➤ **Overactive bladder signs and symptoms (urge urinary incontinence, urgency, and frequency) in patients with inadequate response to or intolerant of anticholinergic medication (Botox)**
Adults: Recommended total dose is 100 units, given as 0.5 mL (5 units) IM across 20 sites into the detrusor muscle. Give prophylactic antibiotics (except aminoglycosides) 1 to 3 days before treatment, on treatment day, and 1 to 3 days after treatment to reduce likelihood of procedure-related UTI. Discontinue antiplatelet therapy at least 3 days before administration. Consider retreatment no sooner than 12 weeks from prior injection.

➤ **Urinary incontinence due to detrusor overactivity associated with a neurologic condition, such as spinal cord injury or MS, after inadequate response to or intolerance of anticholinergic medication (Botox)**
Adults: Recommended total dose is 200 units, given as 30 injections of 1 mL (6.7 units) each (total volume of 30 mL) IM across 30 sites into the detrusor muscle. For the final injection, inject approximately 1 mL of sterile NSS to ensure that the remaining medication in the needle is delivered to the bladder. Give prophylactic antibiotics (except aminoglycosides) 1 to 3 days before treatment, on treatment day, and 1 to 3 days after treatment to reduce likelihood of procedure-related UTI. Consider retreatment no sooner than 12 weeks from prior injection. Discontinue antiplatelet therapy at least 3 days before administration.

➤ **Neurogenic detrusor overactivity in children with inadequate response to or intolerance of anticholinergics (Botox)**
Children age 5 and older weighing 34 kg or more: 200 units given as 20 injections (each injection, 0.5 mL for a total volume of 10 mL) into the detrusor muscle, spaced approximately 1 cm apart. For the final injection, inject approximately 1 mL of sterile NSS to ensure remaining medication in needle is delivered to the bladder. Refer to manufacturer's instructions for dilution.
Children age 5 and older weighing less than 34 kg: 6 units/kg given as 20 injections (each injection, 0.5 mL for a total volume of 10 mL) into the detrusor muscle, spaced approximately 1 cm apart. For the final injection, inject approximately 1 mL of sterile NSS to ensure remaining medication in needle is delivered to the bladder. Refer to manufacturer's instructions for dilution and dosages.

➤ **Prophylaxis of headaches in patients with chronic migraine (15 days per month or more, with headache lasting 4 hours a day or longer) (Botox)**
Adults: Recommended total dose is 155 units, given as 0.1 mL (5 units), IM divided across seven head/neck muscles every 12 weeks. Injections should be equally divided and administered bilaterally into 31 total sites. Refer to manufacturer's instructions for injection-site diagrams.

➤ **Upper limb spasticity (Botox)**
Adults: 5 to 50 units per site IM. Up to 200 units divided into four sites for biceps brachii. The lowest recommended starting dose should be used. Tailor dosing in initial and sequential treatment sessions to the individual based on the size, number, and location of muscles involved; severity of spasticity; presence of local muscle weakness; and patient's response to previous treatment or adverse event history with onabotulinumtoxinA. Administer no more than 50 units per site. Refer to manufacturer's instructions for specific sites and dosages. Consider retreatment no sooner than 12 weeks from prior injection.
Children age 2 and older: 3 to 6 units/kg IM divided among affected muscles to a maximum of 6 units/kg or 200 units, whichever is lower. Use lowest recommended starting dose. Tailor initial dose and sequential treatments to the individual based on size, number, and location of muscles involved; severity of spasticity; presence of local muscle weakness; and patient's response to previous treatment or adverse event history with onabotulinumtoxinA. Refer to manufacturer's instructions for specific sites and dosages.

➤ **Lower limb spasticity (Botox)**
Adults: 300 to 400 units IM divided among five muscles (gastrocnemius, soleus, tibialis posterior, flexor hallucis longus, and flexor digitorum longus). Use lowest recommended

starting dose and administer no more than 50 units per site. Individualize dosing in initial and sequential treatment sessions based on size, number, and location of muscles involved; severity of spasticity; presence of local muscle weakness; and patient's response to previous treatment or adverse event history with onabotulinumtoxinA. Refer to manufacturer's instructions for specific sites and dosages. May repeat therapy no sooner than 12 weeks, with appropriate dosage based on clinical condition of patient at time of retreatment.

Children age 2 and older: 4 to 8 units/kg IM divided among the affected muscles to a maximum of 8 units/kg or 300 units, whichever is lower. Tailor initial dose and sequential treatments to the individual based on size, number, and location of muscles involved; severity of spasticity; presence of local muscle weakness; and patient's response to previous treatment or adverse event history with onabotulinumtoxinA. Refer to manufacturer's instructions for specific sites and dosages.

➤ **Lower limb spasticity, excluding spasticity caused by cerebral palsy (Botox)**
Children ages 2 to 17: 4 to 8 units/kg body weight IM divided among four muscles (gastrocnemius medial head, gastrocnemius lateral head, soleus, and tibialis posterior). Use lowest recommended starting dose and give no more than 8 units/kg body weight or 300 units per treatment session, whichever is lower. Maximum dose in a 3-month period is 10 units/kg body weight or 340 units when treating both lower limbs or the upper and lower limbs in combination.

Individualize dosing in initial and sequential treatment sessions based on size, number, and location of muscles involved; severity of spasticity; presence of local muscle weakness; and patient's response to previous treatment or adverse event history with onabotulinumtoxinA. Refer to manufacturer's instructions for specific sites and dosages. May repeat therapy no sooner than 12 weeks, with appropriate dosage based on patient's clinical condition at time of retreatment.

🛈 *Alert:* When treating both lower limbs, or the upper and lower limbs in combination, total pediatric dosage shouldn't exceed 10 units/kg or 340 units (whichever is lower) in a 3-month interval.

➤ **Cervical dystonia to reduce severity of abnormal head position and neck pain (Botox)**
Adults and children age 16 and older: Adjust initial and subsequent dosing based on patient's head and neck position, localization of pain, muscle hypertrophy, patient response, and adverse event history. Use lower initial dose in patients who are botulinum toxin–naive. Administer no more than 50 units per site. See prescribing information for mean doses and ranges used in studies.

➤ **Severe axillary hyperhidrosis inadequately managed by topical agents (Botox)**
Adults: 50 units (2 mL) injected intradermally in 0.1- to 0.2-mL aliquots to each axilla, evenly distributed in 10 to 15 sites approximately 1 to 2 cm apart. May administer repeat injections when clinical effect of a previous injection diminishes.

➤ **Blepharospasm associated with dystonia (Botox)**
Adults and children age 12 and older: 1.25 to 2.5 units (0.05 to 0.1 mL volume at each site) IM into medial and lateral pretarsal orbicularis oculi of upper lid and into lateral pretarsal orbicularis oculi of lower lid. Cumulative dose in a 30-day period shouldn't exceed 200 units.

➤ **Strabismus (Botox)**
Adults and children age 12 and older: It's recommended that several drops of local anesthetic and an ocular decongestant be given several minutes before injection.

For vertical muscles, and for horizontal strabismus of less than 20 prism diopters: 1.25 to 2.5 units in any one muscle. For horizontal strabismus of 20 to 50 prism diopters: 2.5 to 5 units in any one muscle. Maximum dose is 25 units for any one muscle. For reexamination and subsequent dosing, see prescribing information. For persistent cranial nerve VI palsy lasting 1 month or longer: 1.25 to 2.5 units IM in medial rectus muscle.

➤ **Temporary improvement in appearance of moderate to severe glabellar lines associated with corrugator or procerus muscle activity (Botox Cosmetic)**
Adults: Inject 4 units (0.1 mL) IM into each of five sites, two in each corrugator muscle and one in the procerus muscle for a total dose of 20 units; administer no more frequently than every 3 to 4 months. An effective dose for facial lines is determined by gross

observation of patient's ability to activate the superficial muscles injected.

➤ **Temporary improvement in appearance of moderate to severe lateral canthal lines associated with orbicularis oculi activity (Botox Cosmetic)**

Adults: Inject 4 units (0.1 mL) IM into each of three sites per side (six total injection points) in the lateral orbicularis oculi muscle for a total of 24 units (0.6 mL) (12 units per side); administer no more frequently than every 3 months. For simultaneous treatment with glabellar lines, dose is 24 units for lateral canthal lines and 20 units for glabellar lines, with total dose of 44 units.

➤ **Temporary improvement in appearance of moderate to severe forehead lines associated with frontalis muscle activity (Botox Cosmetic)**

Adults: 4 units (0.1 mL) IM into each of five forehead line sites (20 units) with 4 units (0.1 mL) IM into each of five glabellar line sites (20 units). Recommended total dose for forehead lines and glabellar lines together is 40 units. Administer no more frequently than every 3 months.

ADMINISTRATION
IM, intradermal

🔆 *Alert:* Don't use Botox and contact Allergan (1-800-890-4345) if carton labeling doesn't contain an intact tamper-evident seal.

• Store unopened vials refrigerated at 36° to 46° F (2° to 8° C) for up to 36 months or until expiration date.

• Reconstitute each vial with sterile, nonpreserved NSS for injection by drawing up proper amount of diluent (see manufacturer's instructions) in appropriate-sized syringe (see manufacturer's instructions) and slowly injecting diluent into vial.

• Discard vial if a vacuum doesn't pull the diluent into the vial.

• Gently mix drug with the NSS by rotating vial.

• Administer within 24 hours after reconstitution; store in refrigerator until administration.

ACTION

Blocks neuromuscular transmission by inhibiting release of acetylcholine. IM doses chemically denervate muscle, reducing muscular activity either temporarily or permanently. Intradermal administration causes temporary chemical denervation of sweat glands, resulting in local reduction in sweating. Intradetrusor injection affects detrusor muscle activity via inhibition of acetylcholine release.

Route	Onset	Peak	Duration
IM, intradermal	Varies by site	Varies by site	Varies by site

Half-life: Unknown.

ADVERSE REACTIONS
Overactive bladder symptoms

GU: UTI, dysuria, urine retention, bacteriuria, residual urine volume, hematuria. **Other:** injection-site soreness or ***hemorrhage***.

Intradetrusor injection

GI: constipation. **GU:** UTI, dysuria, urine retention, hematuria, bacteriuria, leukocyturia. **Musculoskeletal:** weakness, muscle spasm, gait disturbance, falls. **Other:** injection-site soreness or ***hemorrhage***.

Chronic migraine headache prophylaxis

CNS: headache, worsening migraine. **CV:** HTN. **EENT:** ptosis, facial paresis. **Musculoskeletal:** neck pain, weakness, stiffness, myalgia, muscle spasm. **Respiratory:** bronchitis. **Other:** injection-site pain.

Upper and lower limb spasticity

CNS: fatigue. **GI:** nausea. **Musculoskeletal:** extremity pain, weakness. **Respiratory:** bronchitis, URI. **Other:** injection-site soreness or ***hemorrhage***.

Cervical dystonia

CNS: headache, dizziness, fever, speech disorder, numbness, asthenia, drowsiness. **EENT:** ptosis, diplopia, blepharoptosis, rhinitis, oral dryness. **GI:** nausea, dysphagia. **Musculoskeletal:** neck pain, back pain, stiffness, hypertonia. **Respiratory:** URI, increased cough, dyspnea. **Other:** flulike syndrome, injection-site soreness, antibody formation.

Severe axillary hyperhidrosis

CNS: headache, fever, anxiety, dizziness. **EENT:** pharyngitis. **GI:** nausea. **Metabolic:** nonaxillary sweating. **Musculoskeletal:** neck or back pain. **Skin:** pruritus. **Other:** flulike syndrome, injection-site pain, injection-site bleeding, infection.

Blepharospasm associated with dystonia

EENT: ptosis, superficial punctate keratitis, eye dryness, irritation, tearing, lagophthalmos, photophobia, ectropion, keratitis, diplopia, entropion, local swelling of eyelid

---

Reactions in bold italics are *life-threatening*. Interactions may have a *rapid onset* or a ***delayed onset***.

skin. **Skin:** diffuse rash. **Other:** injection-site soreness or *hemorrhage*.

Strabismus

EENT: vertical deviation due to effect on adjacent extraocular muscles, ptosis. **Other:** injection-site soreness or *hemorrhage*.

Persistent cranial nerve VI palsy

Other: injection-site soreness or *hemorrhage*.

Glabellar lines

CNS: facial paresis. **EENT:** eyelid ptosis. **Musculoskeletal:** muscular weakness. **Other:** facial pain.

Lateral canthal lines

EENT: eyelid edema.

Forehead lines

CNS: headache. **EENT:** eyelid ptosis. **Skin:** brow ptosis, skin tightness.

INTERACTIONS

Drug-drug. *Aminoglycosides, neuromuscular blockers (curare or curare-like compounds):* May increase effect of toxin and risk of respiratory depression. Use cautiously together.

Anticholinergics: May increase systemic anticholinergic effects. Avoid use together.

Anticoagulants, antiplatelet drugs: May increase risk of bleeding. Discontinue antiplatelet therapy at least 3 days before injection procedure; monitor patients on anticoagulant therapy carefully.

Muscle relaxants, other botulinum neurotoxin products: May cause excessive neuromuscular weakness. Avoid use together.

EFFECTS ON LAB TEST RESULTS
• May increase urinary RBC, leukocyte, and bacteria counts.

CONTRAINDICATIONS & CAUTIONS
Boxed Warning The effects of onabotulinumtoxinA and all botulinum toxin products may spread from the injection area to produce signs and symptoms consistent with botulinum toxin effects. These may include asthenia, generalized muscle weakness, diplopia, ptosis, dysphagia, dysphonia, dysarthria, urinary incontinence, and breathing difficulties, which have reportedly occurred hours to weeks after injection. Swallowing and breathing difficulties can be life-threatening; deaths have been reported. Risk of symptoms developing is probably greatest in children treated for spasticity, but symptoms can also occur in adults treated for

spasticity and other conditions, particularly in those with an underlying condition predisposing them to these symptoms. In unapproved uses and in approved indications, cases of spread of effect have been reported at doses comparable to those used to treat cervical dystonia and at lower doses. ■

🕒 *Alert:* If overdose occurs, antitoxin against botulinum toxin is available from the CDC but won't reverse botulinum toxin-induced effects already apparent by the time of antitoxin administration. In the event of suspected or actual cases of botulinum toxin poisoning, contact your local or state health department to process a request for antitoxin through the CDC. If you don't receive a response within 30 minutes, contact the CDC directly at 1-800-232-4636.

• Contraindicated in known hypersensitivity to botulinum toxin and in patient with infection at injection sites.

• Contraindicated in patients being treated for overactive bladder with UTIs and in patients with overactive bladder or detrusor overactivity associated with a neurologic condition who have postvoid residual urine volume greater than 200 mL but don't self-catheterize routinely.

• Use cautiously in patients with bleeding disorders and in those receiving anticoagulation therapy.

• Use cautiously in patients with inflammation at the proposed injection site or when excessive weakness or atrophy presents in the target muscle.

• Use cautiously in patients with preexisting neuromuscular disorders, compromised respiratory function, or corneal exposure and ulceration due to reduced blinking.

Dialyzable drug: Unknown.

⚠ *Overdose S&S:* Neuromuscular weakness, aspiration pneumonia, respiratory muscle paralysis, respiratory failure, death.

PREGNANCY-LACTATION-REPRODUCTION
• There are no adequate studies during pregnancy. Use only if benefit justifies risks to the fetus.

• It isn't known if drug appears in human milk. Use cautiously during breastfeeding.

NURSING CONSIDERATIONS
🕒 *Alert:* Signs and symptoms of overdose usually don't occur immediately after injection. Should accidental injection or oral

ingestion occur or overdose be suspected, patient should be medically supervised for several weeks for signs and symptoms of systemic muscular weakness, which could be local or distant from the injection.

Boxed Warning Monitor patient for swallowing and breathing difficulties, which can lead to death. ■

• Prescribers administering the drug must understand the relevant neuromuscular or orbital anatomy and any alterations to that anatomy due to prior surgical procedures.

• Treatment of strabismus and upper limb spasticity requires an understanding of standard electromyographic techniques and may be useful when treating cervical dystonia.

• Botox and Botox Cosmetic contain the same active ingredient in the same formulation but aren't interchangeable.

• Drug isn't interchangeable with other preparations of botulinum toxin products and can't be converted into units of other botulinum toxin products.

• When giving bladder injections, give prophylactic antibiotics (except aminoglycosides) 1 to 3 days before treatment, on the day of treatment, and 1 to 3 days after treatment to reduce likelihood of procedure-related UTI. Or, patients receiving general anesthesia or conscious sedation may receive one dose of IV prophylactic antibiotics (except aminoglycosides) before injections on the day of treatment.

• Start treatment at lowest recommended dosage.

• Watch for bronchitis and URI in patients being treated for upper limb spasticity.

• Discontinue antiplatelet therapy at least 3 days before the injection procedure; patients on anticoagulant therapy need to be managed appropriately to decrease bleeding risk.

• Repeat treatment may be administered when effect of previous injection has diminished, but generally no sooner than 12 weeks after previous injection.

• Degree or pattern of muscle spasticity at the time of reinjection may necessitate alterations in dosage and of muscles to be injected.

• To prepare eye for injection, several drops of a local anesthetic and an ocular decongestant are instilled several minutes before injection.

• Monitor patient for retrobulbar hemorrhages and compromised retinal circulation after eye injections.

PATIENT TEACHING

Boxed Warning Caution patient to seek immediate medical attention if serious side effects occur, such as difficulty swallowing, speaking, or breathing. These side effects can occur hours, days, or even weeks after injection and can be fatal. ■

• Teach patient to report signs and symptoms of botulism toxicity, such as loss of strength or muscle weakness, double vision, blurred vision, drooping eyelids, hoarseness, change in or loss of voice, trouble speaking clearly, or loss of bladder control. Inform patient that, if these side effects occur, patient shouldn't drive a car, operate machinery, or perform other dangerous activities.

• Advise patient that onabotulinumtoxinA injections may cause reduced blinking or reduced effectiveness of blinking, and to seek immediate medical attention if eye pain or irritation occurs after treatment.

• Instruct patient to report voiding difficulties after bladder injections for urinary incontinence.

ondansetron
on-DAN-sah-tron

ondansetron hydrochloride

Therapeutic class: Antiemetics
Pharmacologic class: Selective serotonin
(5-HT$_3$) receptor antagonists

AVAILABLE FORMS

Injection: 2 mg/mL
Oral solution: 4 mg/5 mL
Tablets: 4 mg, 8 mg, 24 mg
Tablets (ODTs): 4 mg, 8 mg

INDICATIONS & DOSAGES

Adjust-a-dose (for all indications): For patients with severe hepatic impairment (Child-Pugh class C), total daily dose shouldn't exceed 8 mg.

➤ **To prevent nausea and vomiting from highly emetogenic chemotherapy**
Adults: 24 mg PO as a single dose or 8 mg PO b.i.d. for two doses 30 minutes before chemotherapy. Or, three successive 8-mg PO doses (ODT) 30 minutes before start of single-day highly emetogenic chemotherapy.

If patient can't take oral form, give 0.15 mg/kg IV over 15 minutes beginning 30 minutes before chemotherapy. Give a second 0.15-mg/kg IV dose 4 hours later, then a third 0.15-mg/kg IV dose 8 hours after first dose. Don't exceed 16 mg/dose.

Children ages 6 months to 18 years: 0.15 mg/kg IV over 15 minutes beginning 30 minutes before chemotherapy. Give second dose of 0.15 mg/kg IV over 15 minutes 4 hours after first dose. Give third 0.15-mg/kg IV dose 8 hours after first dose. No single IV dose should exceed 16 mg.

➤ **To prevent nausea and vomiting from moderately emetogenic chemotherapy**

Adults: Administer in combination with neurokinin 1 receptor antagonist and dexamethasone for carboplatin-based regimens or in combination with dexamethasone for non-carboplatin-based regimens. Give 8 mg PO 30 minutes before chemotherapy. Then, 8 mg PO 8 hours after first dose. Then, 8 mg PO every 12 hours for 1 to 2 days after completion of chemotherapy. Or, one dose of 0.15 mg/kg IV. No single IV dose should exceed 16 mg.

Children ages 12 and older: 8 mg PO (ODT, tablet, solution) 30 minutes before chemotherapy, then 8 mg PO 4 hours and 8 hours after first dose. Then, 8 mg every 8 hours for 1 to 2 days after completion of chemotherapy.

Children ages 4 to 11: Give 4 mg PO 30 minutes before chemotherapy. Then, 4 mg PO 4 and 8 hours after first dose. Then, 4 mg PO every 8 hours for 1 to 2 days after completion of chemotherapy.

Infants and children ages 6 months to 18 years: Three doses of 0.15 mg/kg IV. Give first dose 30 minutes before chemotherapy; give subsequent doses 4 and 8 hours after first dose. Infuse drug over 15 minutes. No single IV dose should exceed 16 mg.

➤ **To prevent postoperative nausea and vomiting**

Adults: 4 mg undiluted solution for injection IM or IV over 2 to 5 minutes at end of surgery. Or, 8 mg ODT PO as a single dose 30 to 60 minutes before surgery.

Children ages 1 month to 12 years weighing more than 40 kg: 4 mg IV as a single dose over 2 to 5 minutes.

Children ages 1 month to 12 years weighing 40 kg or less: 0.1 mg/kg IV as a single dose over 2 to 5 minutes. Maximum dose is 4 mg/dose.

➤ **To prevent nausea and vomiting from radiation therapy in patients receiving total body irradiation, single high-dose fraction radiation therapy to abdomen, or daily fractionated radiation therapy to abdomen**

Adults: For patients receiving total body irradiation, give 8 mg PO ODT 1 to 2 hours before each fraction of radiation therapy each day. May administer b.i.d. Give in combination with dexamethasone. For patients receiving single high-dose fraction radiation therapy to the abdomen, give 8 mg PO ODT 1 to 2 hours before therapy, then every 8 hours for 1 to 2 days after completion of therapy. For patients receiving daily fractionated radiation therapy, give 8 mg PO ODT 1 to 2 hours before therapy, then every 8 hours for each day therapy is given.

ADMINISTRATION
PO
• Open blister of ODT just before use by peeling backing off. Don't push ODT through foil blister.
• Protect 4-mg tablets and oral solution from light.

IV

◑ *Alert:* No single IV dose should exceed 16 mg due to the risk of QT-interval prolongation.

▼ If precipitate is noted in vial, shake vigorously until dissolved.
▼ Dilute drug in 50 mL of D_5W injection or NSS for injection.
▼ Don't use diluted solution beyond 24 hours; diluents typically don't contain preservatives.
▼ Infuse over 15 minutes.
▼ Store vials between 36° and 86° F (2° and 30° C). Protect from light.
▼ **Incompatibilities:** Alkaline solutions.

IM
• Document injection site.
• If precipitate is noted in vial, shake vigorously until dissolved.
• Give IM injection undiluted.

ACTION
May block 5-HT$_3$ in the CNS in the chemoreceptor trigger zone and in the peripheral nervous system on nerve terminals of the vagus nerve.

Route	Onset	Peak	Duration
PO	30 min	1–2 hr	Unknown
IV	Immediate	Unknown	Unknown
IM	Unknown	Unknown	Unknown

Half-life: About 3 to 6 hours.

ADVERSE REACTIONS
CNS: dizziness, fatigue, headache, malaise, sedation, extrapyramidal syndrome, fever, agitation, anxiety, pain. **CV:** chest pain. **GI:** constipation, diarrhea. **GU:** gynecologic disorders, urine retention. **Hepatic:** increased transaminase levels. **Respiratory:** *hypoxia*. **Skin:** pruritus, rash. **Other:** chills, injection-site reaction.

INTERACTIONS
Drug-drug. 🌑 *Alert: Apomorphine:* May cause profound hypotension and loss of consciousness. Use together is contraindicated.
Drugs (such as cimetidine) that alter hepatic drug-metabolizing enzymes, phenobarbital, rifampin: May change pharmacokinetics of ondansetron, but there is no need to adjust dosage based on clinical data.
Drugs that prolong QTc interval (antiarrhythmics, antipsychotics, antidepressants): May result in ventricular arrhythmias. Use cautiously and avoid combination with drugs at highest risk for QTc-interval prolongation.
SSNRIs, SSRIs: May result in serotonin syndrome. Use cautiously and monitor patient.
Tramadol: May decrease tramadol effects. Monitor patient to ensure effective pain control.
Drug-herb. *Horehound:* May enhance serotonergic effects. Discourage use together.
St. John's wort: May decrease ondansetron serum concentration. Consider therapy modification.

EFFECTS ON LAB TEST RESULTS
• May increase ALT and AST levels.

CONTRAINDICATIONS & CAUTIONS
• Use is contraindicated in patients hypersensitive to drug.
• ECG changes, including prolonged QT interval and torsades de pointes, have been reported. Avoid use in patients with congenital long QT syndrome.
• Use cautiously in patients with hepatic impairment.
Dialyzable drug: Unlikely.
⚠ *Overdose S&S:* Sudden transient blindness, severe constipation, hypotension, faintness, heart block, somnolence, agitation, tachycardia, tachypnea, HTN, flushing, mydriasis, diaphoresis, myoclonic movements, horizontal nystagmus, hyperreflexia, seizure.

PREGNANCY-LACTATION-REPRODUCTION
• There are no adequate studies during pregnancy. Drug crosses placental barrier during first trimester. Use only if clearly needed.
• It isn't known if drug appears in human milk. Use cautiously during breastfeeding.

NURSING CONSIDERATIONS
🌑 *Alert:* Drug may increase the risk of prolonged QT interval and torsades de pointes. Monitor ECG in patients with congenital long QT syndrome, in those with HF or bradyarrhythmias, and in those taking other medications that can prolong the QT interval.
🌑 *Alert:* Correct electrolyte abnormalities (hypokalemia or hypomagnesemia) before infusing drug.
• Monitor patients for decreased bowel activity, especially those at risk for GI obstruction; drug may mask progressive ileus or gastric distention.
🌑 *Alert:* Monitor patients for signs and symptoms of myocardial ischemia during and immediately after IV administration.
• Monitor LFT results.
• Monitor patients for signs and symptoms of serotonin syndrome (mental status changes, tachycardia, diaphoresis, flushing, nausea, vomiting, tremors, muscle rigidity).
• May give drug in combination with neurokinin-1 receptor antagonist, dexamethasone, and olanzapine according to chemotherapy antiemetic treatment guidelines.
• *Look alike–sound alike:* Don't confuse ondansetron with dolasetron, granisetron, or palonosetron.

PATIENT TEACHING
• Instruct patient in safe drug administration.
🌑 *Alert:* Caution patient to immediately report a syncopal episode (fainting, loss of consciousness) or signs and symptoms of abnormal HR or rhythm, such as palpitations, dyspnea, dizziness, or light-headedness.
• Tell patient that an ECG may be necessary to monitor HR and rhythm.
• Instruct patient to immediately report difficulty breathing after drug administration.
• Tell patient receiving drug IV to report discomfort at insertion site.

---

opicapone
oh-PIK-a-pone

Ongentys

Therapeutic class: Antiparkinsonians
Pharmacologic class: Catechol-O-
methyltransferase inhibitors

AVAILABLE FORMS
Capsules: 25 mg, 50 mg

INDICATIONS & DOSAGES
➤ **Adjunctive treatment to levodopa–carbidopa in patients with Parkinson disease experiencing "off" episodes**
Adults: 50 mg PO daily at bedtime.
Adjust-a-dose: For patients with moderate hepatic impairment (Child-Pugh class B), reduce dose to 25 mg PO at bedtime. Avoid use in patients with severe (Child-Pugh class C) hepatic impairment.

ADMINISTRATION
PO
• Give 1 hour before and at least 1 hour after food.
• If a dose is missed, resume scheduled dosing next day; don't double dose.
• Store capsules below 86° F (30° C).

ACTION
Inhibits catechol-O-methyltransferase (COMT), a metabolizing enzyme of levodopa, resulting in higher levels of levodopa.

Route	Onset	Peak	Duration
PO	Unknown	1–4 hr	5+ days

Half-life: 1 to 2 hours.

ADVERSE REACTIONS
CNS: dyskinesia, dizziness, hallucinations, insomnia, impulse control disorder, syncope. **CV:** hypotension, HTN. **EENT:** dry mouth. **GI:** constipation. **Metabolic:** increased CK level, weight loss.

INTERACTIONS
Drug-drug. *Drugs metabolized by COMT (dobutamine, dopamine, epinephrine, isoproterenol, norepinephrine):* May increase risk of arrhythmias, increase HR, and cause excessive changes in BP. Use together cautiously.

Levodopa: Potentiates effects of levodopa, causing dyskinesia or exacerbating preexisting dyskinesia. Reduce dosage of levodopa or other dopaminergic drugs as indicated.
⚠ *Alert: Nonselective MAO inhibitors (isocarboxazid, phenelzine, tranylcypromine):* May increase risk of arrhythmias, increase HR, or cause excessive changes in BP due to increased levels of catecholamines. Concomitant use is contraindicated.

EFFECTS ON LAB TEST RESULTS
• May increase CK level.

CONTRAINDICATIONS & CAUTIONS
• Contraindicated in patients with history of pheochromocytoma, paraganglioma, or other catecholamine-secreting neoplasms.
• Avoid use in patients with severe hepatic impairment (Child-Pugh class C).
• Avoid use in patients with major psychotic disorders because of risk of psychosis exacerbation.
• Use cautiously in patients with suspected or diagnosed dopamine dysregulation syndrome. Consider stopping drug, as indicated.
• Safety and effectiveness in children haven't been established.
Dialyzable drug: Unlikely.

PREGNANCY-LACTATION-REPRODUCTION
• There are no studies during pregnancy. Use only if benefit outweighs fetal risk.
• It isn't known if drug appears in human milk or how drug affects infants who are breastfed or milk production. Consider benefit to patient against possible risk to infant.

NURSING CONSIDERATIONS
⚠ *Alert:* Monitor patient treated with opicapone and drugs metabolized by COMT for arrhythmias, increased HR, and excessive changes in BP regardless of route of administration, including inhalation, of the concomitant drug.
⚠ *Alert:* Before starting drug, assess patient for factors that may increase risk of somnolence with dopaminergic therapy (concomitant sedating medications, sleep disorders).
• Monitor patient for daytime somnolence during activities that require full attention (driving, conversation, eating). If daytime somnolence occurs, consider discontinuing drug or adjusting dosage of other dopaminergic or sedating drugs.

O

• Monitor patient for development of impulse control or compulsive disorders (intense urge to gamble or spend money, increased sexual urge, binge eating, inability to control these urges). Reevaluate current therapy for Parkinson disease and consider stopping drug if these signs or symptoms develop.

• Monitor patient for hypotension (orthostatic and nonorthostatic); if it occurs, discontinue drug or adjust dosage of other drugs that lower BP.

• Observe patient for development of dyskinesia or exacerbation of preexisting dyskinesia. Consider reducing daily levodopa dose or other dopaminergic drug if dyskinesia occurs.

• Monitor patient for hallucinations (auditory, visual, mixed), delusions, agitation, or aggressive behavior. Consider stopping drug if hallucinations or psychotic-like behaviors develop.

• When discontinuing drug, monitor patient for a symptom complex resembling NMS (elevated temperature, muscular rigidity, altered consciousness, autonomic instability). Adjust other dopaminergic agents as needed.

• *Look alike–sound alike:* Don't confuse opicapone with entacapone or tolcapone. Don't confuse Ongentys with Onglyza.

PATIENT TEACHING

🕒 *Alert:* Warn patient and caregiver about daytime somnolence. Caution patient not to operate hazardous machinery, including motor vehicles, if daytime somnolence occurs while taking drug.

• Counsel patient to report dizziness, lightheadedness, or fainting.

• Warn patient that drug may cause dyskinesia (sudden, uncontrolled movements) or exacerbate preexisting dyskinesia. Contact prescriber if dyskinesia occurs.

• Advise patient to report hallucinations, delusions, or aggressive behavior.

• Counsel patient to report intense uncontrollable urges to gamble, spend money, or binge eat, or if increased sexual or other intense urges occur.

• Advise patient to consult prescriber before stopping drug and to inform prescriber if fever, confusion, or severe muscle stiffness develops after stopping drug.

oritavancin diphosphate
or-it-a-VAN-sin

Kimyrsa, Orbactiv

Therapeutic class: Antibiotics
Pharmacologic class: Lipoglycopeptides

AVAILABLE FORMS
Powder for injection: 400-mg, 1,200-mg vial

INDICATIONS & DOSAGES
➤ **Acute bacterial skin and skin-structure infections caused or suspected to be caused by susceptible gram-positive bacteria, including** *Staphylococcus aureus* **(methicillin-sensitive and methicillin-resistant);** *Streptococcus* **species, including** *S. pyogenes, S. agalactiae, S. dysgalactiae, S. anginosus, S. intermedius,* **and** *S. constellatus;* **and vancomycin-susceptible** *Enterococcus faecalis*
Adults: A single dose of 1,200 mg IV.

ADMINISTRATION
IV
▼ Obtain specimen for culture and sensitivity testing before giving.

▼ Prepare three 400-mg vials for a single 1,200-mg IV dose.

▼ Reconstitute each 400 mg vial with 40 mL of sterile water for injection to provide a solution containing 10 mg/mL/vial. Reconstitute each 1,200-mg vial with 40 mL sterile water for injection to provide a solution containing 30 mg/mL/vial.

▼ Gently swirl vial to avoid foaming and ensure that all powder is completely reconstituted in solution. Inspect for particulate matter. Solution should be clear and colorless to pale yellow (Orbactiv) or pink (Kimyrsa).

▼ For infusion, further dilute Orbactiv in 1,000 mL D_5W; withdraw 120 mL from 1,000-mL D_5W bag and add 120 mL Orbactiv reconstituted solution. Or, further dilute Kimyrsa in 250 mL NSS or D_5W; withdraw 40 mL from a 250-mL IV bag and add 40 mL Kimyrsa reconstituted solution.

▼ Infuse Orbactiv over 3 hours. If IV line is also used to infuse other drugs, flush it with D_5W before and after each infusion.

▼ Infuse Kimyrsa over 1 hour. If IV line is also used to infuse other drugs, flush it with NSS or D_5W before and after each infusion.

Reactions in bold italics are *life-threatening*. Interactions may have a *rapid onset* or a ***delayed onset***.

▼ Refrigerate Orbactiv solution after reconstitution and use within 12 hours or within 6 hours when stored at room temperature, including 3-hour infusion time.

▼ Refrigerate Kimyrsa solution after reconstitution and use within 12 hours or within 4 hours when stored at room temperature, including 1-hour infusion time.

▼ **Incompatibilities:** NSS (Orbactiv). Basic or neutral pH drugs.

ACTION

Disrupts bacterial cell-wall synthesis and bacterial membrane integrity.

Route	Onset	Peak	Duration
IV	Unknown	Unknown	Unknown

Half-life: 245 hours.

ADVERSE REACTIONS

CNS: headache, dizziness. **CV:** tachycardia, peripheral edema, injection-site phlebitis, *leukocytoclastic vasculitis.* **GI:** nausea, vomiting, diarrhea. **Hematologic:** anemia, eosinophilia. **Hepatic:** elevated ALT, AST, and bilirubin levels. **Metabolic:** *hypoglycemia,* hyperuricemia. **Musculoskeletal:** tenosynovitis, myalgia, osteomyelitis. **Respiratory:** *bronchospasm,* wheezing. **Skin:** infusion-site erythema, extravasation, induration, pruritus, limb and subcutaneous abscesses, rash, urticaria, *erythema multiforme,* cellulitis. **Other:** infusion reaction, hypersensitivity, *angioedema.*

INTERACTIONS

Drug-drug. *Dextromethorphan, midazolam:* May decrease concentrations of these drugs. Monitor patient for effectiveness.
Omeprazole: May increase omeprazole level. Monitor patient for omeprazole toxicity.
Unfractionated heparin sodium (IV): May falsely elevate PTT test results for up to 120 hours (5 days). Heparin use is contraindicated for 120 hours after oritavancin administration.
Warfarin: May increase warfarin level and risk of bleeding. Monitor INR and patient for bleeding.

EFFECTS ON LAB TEST RESULTS

• May increase AST, ALT, uric acid, and total bilirubin levels.
• May decrease glucose level.

• May artificially prolong PTT for up to 120 hours, prolong PT and increase INR for up to 12 hours, and prolong activated clotting time for up to 24 hours after dose is given.
• May elevate D-dimer for up to 72 hours after dose is given.
• May cause positive indirect and direct antiglobulin tests. Positive indirect test may interfere with cross-matching for blood transfusions.

CONTRAINDICATIONS & CAUTIONS

• Contraindicated in patients hypersensitive to drug or its components.
• Use of unfractionated heparin IV is contraindicated for 120 hours after oritavancin administration.
• Use cautiously in patients with history of hypersensitivity to glycopeptides (vancomycin, telavancin, dalbavancin); serious hypersensitivity reactions have been reported. If acute reaction occurs, discontinue drug and treat immediately.
• Drug can cause superinfection, including CDAD and pseudomembranous colitis, which can occur more than 2 months after therapy ends.
• Drug may increase risk of osteomyelitis; an alternative antibacterial therapy may be needed.
• Drug hasn't been studied in patients with severe renal or hepatic impairment.
• Safety and effectiveness in children haven't been established.
Dialyzable drug: No.

PREGNANCY-LACTATION-REPRODUCTION

• There are no adequate studies during pregnancy. Use only if potential benefit justifies fetal risk.
• It isn't known if drug appears in human milk. Use cautiously during breastfeeding.

NURSING CONSIDERATIONS

• Monitor patient for signs and symptoms of CDAD (frequent, watery stools) and osteomyelitis (fever, erythema, edema, pain).
• Monitor patient for infusion-related reactions (pruritus, rash, urticaria, flushing, chest pain, back pain, chills, tremor). Slow rate or interrupt infusion if reaction develops.
• If patient needs anticoagulation, consider using anticoagulants that don't require PTT or INR monitoring.

O

- *Look alike–sound alike:* Don't confuse Orbactiv with Activase or Vibativ. Don't confuse oritavancin with telavancin or dalbavancin.

PATIENT TEACHING
- Explain that antibiotics can change normal intestinal flora and that patient should report severe watery or bloody diarrhea as this may indicate a more serious intestinal infection.
- Instruct patient to report discomfort at IV insertion site.
- Warn patient that allergic reactions, including serious allergic reactions, can occur and require immediate treatment.

---

oseltamivir phosphate ☒
oh-sel-TAM-i-ver

Tamiflu♥

Therapeutic class: Antivirals
Pharmacologic class: Selective neuraminidase inhibitors

AVAILABLE FORMS
Capsules: 30 mg, 45 mg, 75 mg
Oral suspension: 6 mg/mL after reconstitution

INDICATIONS & DOSAGES
➤ **To prevent influenza A and B**
Adults and adolescents age 13 and older:
75 mg PO (capsule or 12.5 mL suspension) once daily for 1 week after last exposure if vaccinated or 2 weeks if unvaccinated. In patients who are immunocompromised, may continue drug for up to 12 weeks.
Children ages 1 to 12 weighing 40.1 kg or more: 75 mg (12.5 mL suspension) PO once daily for 10 days.
Children ages 1 to 12 weighing 23.1 to 40 kg: 60 mg (10 mL suspension) PO once daily for 10 days.
Children ages 1 to 12 weighing 15.1 to 23 kg: 45 mg (7.5 mL suspension) PO once daily for 10 days.
Children ages 1 to 12 weighing 15 kg or less: 30 mg (5 mL suspension) PO once daily for 10 days.
Adjust-a-dose: For adults and adolescents with CrCl of 30 to 60 mL/minute, reduce dosage to 30 mg PO once daily. For CrCl of 10 to 30 mL/minute, reduce dosage to 30 mg every other day. For patients on hemodialysis (CrCl less than 10 mL/minute), give 30 mg PO immediately, then 30 mg after every hemodialysis session for 5 days. For patients on continuous ambulatory peritoneal dialysis (CrCl less than 10 mL/minute), give 30 mg PO immediately and 30 mg once weekly.
➤ **To treat influenza**
Adults and adolescents age 13 and older:
75 mg PO b.i.d. (capsule or 12.5 mL suspension) for 5 days. Begin treatment within 2 days of onset of influenza symptoms.
Children ages 1 to 12 weighing 40.1 kg or more: 75 mg (12.5 mL suspension) PO b.i.d. for 5 days.
Children ages 1 to 12 weighing 23.1 to 40 kg: 60 mg (10 mL) PO b.i.d. for 5 days.
Children ages 1 to 12 weighing 15.1 to 23 kg: 45 mg (7.5 mL) PO b.i.d. for 5 days.
Children ages 1 to 12 weighing 15 kg or less: 30 mg (5 mL) PO b.i.d. for 5 days.
Children ages 2 weeks to younger than 1 year: 3 mg/kg PO b.i.d. for 5 days. Begin treatment within 2 days of influenza onset.
Adjust-a-dose: For adults and adolescents with CrCl of 30 to 60 mL/minute, reduce dosage to 30 mg PO b.i.d. for 5 days. For CrCl of 10 to 30 mL/minute, reduce dosage to 30 mg PO once daily for 5 days. For patients on hemodialysis (CrCl less than 10 mL/minute), give 30 mg PO immediately after hemodialysis, then 30 mg after each hemodialysis cycle. Don't exceed treatment duration of longer than 5 days. For patients on continuous ambulatory peritoneal dialysis (CrCl less than 10 mL/minute), give a single dose of 30 mg PO immediately after dialysis exchange.

ADMINISTRATION
PO
- Give drug with meals to decrease GI adverse effects.
- Store at room temperature (59° to 86° F [15° to 30° C]).
- May open capsules and mix contents with sweetened liquids, such as regular or sugar-free chocolate syrup, corn syrup, caramel topping, or light brown sugar (dissolved in water).
- Oral suspension is preferred for patients who can't swallow capsules.
- Shake oral suspension well before use.
- In an emergency, pharmacists can compound an oral suspension (6 mg/mL) from capsules.

Reactions in bold italics are *life-threatening*. Interactions may have a *rapid onset* or a ***delayed onset***.

• May give via NG or orogastric tube. Dissolve powder from capsule in 20 mL sterile water and inject in tube; follow with 10-mL sterile water flush.

• Once reconstituted, store oral suspension in refrigerator at 36° to 46° F (2° to 8° C) or at room temperature. Use within 10 days of preparation if stored at room temperature or within 17 days of preparation if stored under refrigeration.

• If a dose is missed, give missed dose as soon as possible. If next dose is due within 2 hours, skip missed dose and give next dose on schedule.

ACTION

Inhibits influenza A and B virus enzyme neuraminidase, which is thought to play a role in viral particle aggregation and release from the host cell and appears to interfere with viral replication.

Route	Onset	Peak	Duration
PO	Unknown	Unknown	Unknown

Half-life: 1 to 10 hours.

ADVERSE REACTIONS

CNS: headache, pain. **GI:** nausea, vomiting, diarrhea (infants). **Skin:** diaper rash (infants).

INTERACTIONS

Drug-drug. *Live attenuated influenza virus vaccine:* May decrease effect of live attenuated influenza virus vaccine. Avoid oseltamivir 48 hours before vaccination and 2 weeks after.

EFFECTS ON LAB TEST RESULTS

None reported.

CONTRAINDICATIONS & CAUTIONS

• Contraindicated in patients hypersensitive to drug or its components.

⊠ Oral suspension contains 2 g of sorbitol, which is above the maximum limit for patients with hereditary fructose intolerance and may cause dyspepsia and diarrhea.

• Use cautiously in patients with renal failure, chronic cardiac or respiratory diseases, or any medical condition that may require imminent hospitalization.

• Safety and effectiveness of repeated treatment courses haven't been established.
Dialyzable drug: Yes.
⚠ **Overdose S&S:** Nausea, vomiting.

PREGNANCY-LACTATION-REPRODUCTION

• Drug is recommended to treat or prevent influenza during pregnancy and up to 2 weeks postpartum. It shouldn't be used as a substitute for vaccination during pregnancy.

• Drug appears in human milk in small amounts. According to the CDC, patient may continue oseltamivir while breastfeeding.

NURSING CONSIDERATIONS

• Drug must be given within 2 days of onset of symptoms.

• Initiate postexposure prophylaxis within 48 hours after close contact with an infected individual. Initiate seasonal prophylaxis during a community outbreak.

⚠ *Alert:* Closely monitor patients with influenza for neuropsychiatric symptoms, such as hallucinations, delirium, and abnormal behavior. Risks and benefits of continuing drug should be evaluated.

• Monitor patient for secondary bacterial infections. Drug is only effective against influenza viruses.

• *Look alike–sound alike:* Don't confuse Tamiflu with Thera-Flu.

PATIENT TEACHING

• Instruct patient to begin treatment as soon as possible after appearance of flu symptoms.

• Inform patient that drug may be taken with or without meals. If nausea or vomiting occurs, patient can take drug with food or milk.

• Advise patient to complete the full course of treatment, even if symptoms resolve.

• Alert patient that drug isn't a replacement for the annual influenza vaccination. Patients for whom vaccine is indicated should continue to receive the vaccine each fall.

• Advise patient or caregivers of the risk of neuropsychiatric events and to report abnormal behavior.

• Caution patient or caregivers of the risk of severe allergic reactions (including anaphylaxis) or serious skin reactions. Instruct patient or caregivers to stop drug and seek immediate medical attention if a reaction occurs or is suspected.

⊠ Inform patient with hereditary fructose intolerance that oral suspension contains sorbitol in an amount above the daily maximum limit of sorbitol and may cause dyspepsia and diarrhea.

O

osilodrostat
oh-sil-oh-DROE-stat

Isturisa

Therapeutic class: Endocrine-metabolic agents
Pharmacologic class: Cortisol synthesis inhibitors

AVAILABLE FORMS
Tablets: 1 mg, 5 mg, 10 mg

INDICATIONS & DOSAGES
➤ **Cushing disease in patients for whom pituitary surgery isn't an option or hasn't been curative**
Adults: Initially, 2 mg PO b.i.d. Increase by 1 to 2 mg PO b.i.d. every 2 weeks based on cortisol change, tolerability, and clinical response. Refer to manufacturer's instructions for dosage titration and modification. Usual maintenance dose is 2 to 7 mg PO b.i.d. Maximum dose is 30 mg PO b.i.d.
Adjust-a-dose: For patients with moderate hepatic impairment (Child-Pugh class B), start at 1 mg PO b.i.d. For patients with severe hepatic impairment (Child-Pugh class C), start at 1 mg PO once daily in the evening.

ADMINISTRATION
PO
• Give without regard to meals.
• If a dose is missed, give at next scheduled time.
• Store tablets at 68° to 77° F (20° to 25° C).

ACTION
Inhibits the enzyme responsible for cortisol biosynthesis in the adrenal gland.

Route	Onset	Peak	Duration
PO	Unknown	1 hr	Unknown

Half-life: 4 hours.

ADVERSE REACTIONS
CNS: fatigue, headache, dizziness, fever, insomnia, anxiety, depression, malaise, syncope. **CV:** *prolonged QT interval,* edema, hypotension, HTN, tachycardia. **EENT:** nasopharyngitis. **GI:** nausea, vomiting, diarrhea, abdominal pain, decreased appetite, dyspepsia, gastroenteritis. **GU:** UTI. **Hematologic:** anemia, decreased ANC. **Hepatic:** elevated

transaminase levels. **Metabolic:** hypocortisolism, *adrenal insufficiency, hypokalemia,* altered pituitary corticotroph tumor volume, increased testosterone level. **Musculoskeletal:** arthralgia, back pain, myalgia. **Respiratory:** cough. **Skin:** rash, hirsutism, acne, alopecia. **Other:** flulike symptoms.

INTERACTIONS
Drug-drug. *CYP1A2, CYP2C19 substrates with a narrow therapeutic index (theophylline, tizanidine):* May increase levels of substrate. Use together cautiously.
Drugs that prolong QT interval: May further prolong QT interval, increasing risk of cardiac arrhythmia. Avoid use together.
Strong CYP2B6, CYP3A4 inducers (carbamazepine, phenobarbital, rifampin): May decrease osilodrostat level and reduce its efficacy. Osilodrostat dosage increase may be necessary. When inducers are discontinued, reduce osilodrostat dosage as needed.
Strong CYP3A4 inhibitors (clarithromycin, itraconazole): May increase osilodrostat level and adverse reactions. Reduce osilodrostat dosage by 50%.

EFFECTS ON LAB TEST RESULTS
• May increase AST, ALT, androgen, cortisol and aldosterone precursors (11-deoxycortisol, 11-deoxycorticosterone), corticotropin, and testosterone levels.
• May decrease potassium and cortisol levels.
• May decrease ANC and RBC count.

CONTRAINDICATIONS & CAUTIONS
• Drug may increase risk of hypocortisolism, leading to life-threatening adrenal insufficiency.
• Drug may cause dose-dependent prolonged QT interval and cardiac arrhythmias. Use cautiously in patients at risk (congenital long QT syndrome, HF, bradyarrhythmia, uncorrected electrolyte abnormalities, concomitant drugs that prolong QT interval).
• Use caution when interpreting urine free cortisol levels in patients with moderate to severe renal impairment due to reduced urine free cortisol excretion.
• Safety and effectiveness in children haven't been established.
Dialyzable drug: Unknown.
⚠ **Overdose S&S:** Hypocortisolism (nausea, vomiting, fatigue, hypotension, abdominal pain, loss of appetite, dizziness, syncope).

Reactions in bold italics are *life-threatening*. Interactions may have a *rapid onset* or a *delayed onset*.

PREGNANCY-LACTATION-REPRODUCTION
- Information is insufficient to recommend use during pregnancy.
- It isn't known if drug appears in human milk. Patient shouldn't breastfeed during therapy and for 1 week after final dose.

NURSING CONSIDERATIONS
- Obtain baseline QTc interval before initiating therapy and repeat within 1 week. Thereafter, monitor ECG periodically; consider more frequent monitoring in patients at risk for prolonged QTc interval. Consider temporary discontinuation of drug if QTc interval is greater than 480 msec.
- Obtain baseline potassium and magnesium levels, and correct abnormalities before initiating drug, if necessary. Monitor levels periodically thereafter.
- Give oral or IV potassium supplement to patient with hypokalemia. If hypokalemia persists, osilodrostat reduction or discontinuation or administration of mineralocorticoid antagonists may be necessary.
- Monitor patient for worsening HTN, edema, and signs and symptoms of hypocortisolism (nausea, vomiting, fatigue, abdominal pain, loss of appetite). Also evaluate for precipitating causes of hypocortisolism (infection, physical stress).
- Monitor cortisol levels every 1 to 2 months once maintenance dose is achieved. Patients with hepatic impairment may require more frequent monitoring during dosage titration.
- Decrease dosage or temporarily discontinue drug if urine free cortisol level decreases below target range, cortisol level rapidly decreases, or patient reports signs and symptoms of hypocortisolism.
- Stop drug and administer glucocorticoid replacement therapy if serum or plasma cortisol levels are below target range and patient has signs and symptoms of adrenal insufficiency (hypotension, hypoglycemia, abnormal electrolyte levels).
- When urine cortisol and serum or plasma cortisol levels are within target range and signs and symptoms resolve, reinitiate drug at lower dose.
- Monitor female patient for development of signs and symptoms of hyperandrogenism (hirsutism, hypertrichosis, acne).
- *Look alike–sound alike:* Don't confuse osilodrostat with orlistat.

PATIENT TEACHING
- Teach patient signs and symptoms of hypocortisolism and advise patient to contact prescriber if they occur.
- Advise female patient to report signs and symptoms associated with hyperandrogenism.
- Instruct patient of the importance of lab monitoring and adhering to visits with prescriber.
- Tell patient an ECG is needed before starting drug and periodically thereafter. Advise patient to immediately report signs and symptoms of QT-interval prolongation (irregular heartbeat).
- Educate patient on importance of contacting prescriber if worsening edema or HTN occurs.
- Advise patient to report pregnancy or plans to become pregnant during therapy.
- Caution patient not to breastfeed during therapy and for 1 week after final dose.
- Tell patient to report all drug changes to prescriber.

SAFETY ALERT!

osimertinib mesylate ▒
oh-sim-ER-ti-nib

Tagrisso

Therapeutic class: Antineoplastics
Pharmacologic class: Tyrosine kinase inhibitors

AVAILABLE FORMS
Tablets ⊕*:* 40 mg, 80 mg

INDICATIONS & DOSAGES
Adjust-a-dose (for all indications): Refer to manufacturer's instructions for toxicity-related dosage adjustments. If drug must be given with a strong CYP3A4 inducer, increase osimertinib dosage to 160 mg daily. Resume osimertinib at 80 mg daily 3 weeks after discontinuing the strong CYP3A4 inducer.
➤ **Metastatic epidermal growth factor receptor (EGFR) T790M mutation-positive NSCLC in patients who have progressed on or after EGFR tyrosine kinase inhibitor therapy** ▒
Adults: 80 mg PO once daily until disease progression or unacceptable toxicity.

➤ **First-line treatment of metastatic NSCLC in patients whose tumors have *EGFR* exon 19 deletions or exon 21 L858R mutations**

Adults: 80 mg PO once daily until disease progression or unacceptable toxicity occurs.

➤ **Adjuvant therapy after tumor resection in patients with NSCLC whose tumors have *EGFR* exon 19 deletions or exon 21 L858R mutations**

Adults: 80 mg PO once daily until disease recurs or unacceptable toxicity develops, or for up to 3 years.

ADMINISTRATION

PO

⚠ *Alert:* Hazardous drug; use safe handling and disposal precautions. Use single gloves to administer intact tablets. Avoid exposure to crushed tablets.

- May give with or without food.
- Don't make up for a missed dose. Resume dosing at next scheduled dose.
- If patient is unable to swallow solids, disperse tablet in approximately 60 mL of non-carbonated water. Stir until tablet is completely dispersed into small pieces and have patient swallow immediately. Rinse container with 120 to 240 mL of water and give to patient immediately.
- To give through an NG tube, disperse tablet in 15 mL noncarbonated water and use an additional 15 mL of water to transfer any residual to the syringe. Give through the NG tube followed by a 30 mL water flush.
- Prepare oral liquid in a controlled device using double gloves and protective gown. Don't crush or heat during preparation.
- If a dose is missed, omit the missed dose. Don't make up the missed dose, but give the next dose at the scheduled time.
- Store at room temperature (68° to 77° F [20° to 25° C]).

ACTION

A kinase inhibitor of EGFR that binds irreversibly to select mutant forms of *EGFR*, including T790M, L858R, and exon 19 deletion. In vitro, drug also inhibited the activity of HER2, HER3, HER4, ACK1, and BLK at clinically relevant concentrations.

Route	Onset	Peak	Duration
PO	Unknown	6 hr	Unknown

Half-life: 48 hours.

ADVERSE REACTIONS

CNS: headache, fever, fatigue, dizziness. **CV:** *prolonged QTc-interval,* reduced LVEF, *cardiomyopathy.* **EENT:** nasopharyngitis, epistaxis, keratitis. **GI:** diarrhea, nausea, decreased appetite, constipation, stomatitis, vomiting, abdominal pain. **GU:** UTI, increased BUN level. **Hematologic:** *lymphopenia, thrombocytopenia,* anemia, *neutropenia.* **Hepatic:** increased AST, ALT, and bilirubin levels. **Metabolic:** hypermagnesemia, hyponatremia, *hypokalemia,* hyperglycemia. **Musculoskeletal:** musculoskeletal pain. **Respiratory:** cough, pneumonia, URI, interstitial pneumonitis, *PE.* **Skin:** rash, dry skin, pruritus, urticaria, hand-foot syndrome, alopecia, nail toxicity.

INTERACTIONS

Drug-drug. *BCRP (rosuvastatin, sulfasalazine, topotecan), P-gp substrates:* Use together may increase exposure to the BCRP or substrate and risk of exposure-related toxicity. Monitor patient for adverse reactions.
Cyclosporine: May increase cyclosporine level. Monitor therapy.
Drugs that prolong QT interval (amiodarone, chlorpromazine, disopyramide, moxifloxacin, procainamide, quinidine, sotalol, thioridazine, ziprasidone): May cause additive QT-interval prolongation and increased risk of cardiac arrhythmia. Avoid use together.
Strong CYP3A inducers (carbamazepine, phenytoin, rifampin): May decrease osimertinib plasma concentration. Avoid use together.
Drug-herb. *St. John's wort:* May decrease osimertinib plasma concentration. Discourage use together.

EFFECTS ON LAB TEST RESULTS

- May increase AST, ALT, bilirubin, magnesium, and blood glucose levels.
- May decrease sodium and potassium levels.
- May decrease Hb level and lymphocyte, platelet, and neutrophil counts.

CONTRAINDICATIONS & CAUTIONS

- Use cautiously in patients with congenital long QTc syndrome, HF, or electrolyte abnormalities and in those taking medications known to prolong QTc interval.
- ILD and cardiomyopathy (cardiac failure, pulmonary edema, decreased ejection

---

*Reactions in bold italics are **life-threatening**. Interactions may have a rapid onset or a **delayed onset**.*

fraction, stress cardiomyopathy) may occur with treatment.
• Safety and effectiveness in children haven't been established.
Dializable drug: Unknown.

PREGNANCY-LACTATION-REPRODUCTION
• Based on animal study data, drug may cause fetal harm. Advise patients of childbearing potential of fetal risk and to use effective contraception during therapy and for up to 6 weeks after last dose.
• Men should use contraception during therapy and for up to 4 months after last dose.
• It isn't known if drug appears in human milk. Because of potential for adverse effects in the infant, patients shouldn't breastfeed during therapy and for 2 weeks after final dose.
• Drug may impair fertility in patients of reproductive potential. It isn't known if the effects are reversible.

NURSING CONSIDERATIONS
⌧ Confirm T790M, exon 19 deletions, or exon 21 L858R *EGFR* mutations in tumor or plasma specimens, as appropriate, before initiation of treatment.
• Verify pregnancy status before starting drug.
• Assess LVEF by echocardiogram or MUGA before therapy begins and every 3 months during therapy.
• Monitor ECG and electrolyte levels in patients with congenital long QTc syndrome, HF, or electrolyte abnormalities and in those taking medications known to prolong QTc interval.
• Monitor patient for signs and symptoms of ILD (dyspnea, cough, fever, worsening respiratory symptoms). Interrupt treatment and promptly evaluate for ILD. Discontinue drug if ILD is confirmed.
• Monitor patient for signs and symptoms of keratitis (eye inflammation, light sensitivity, lacrimation, vision changes, pain); if they occur, refer patient to an ophthalmologist for evaluation.
• Monitor patient for skin toxicity (rash, nail changes, dry skin, itching); drug may increase risk of erythema multiforme, cutaneous vasculitis, and SJS.
• *Look alike–sound alike:* Don't confuse osimertinib with olaparib or ospemifene. Don't confuse Tagrisso with Targretin or Tasigna.

PATIENT TEACHING
• Instruct patient in safe drug handling and administration.
• Teach patient to promptly report all adverse reactions, especially new or worsening cough, trouble breathing, shortness of breath, fever or symptoms of keratitis.
• Advise patient to seek medical attention for rapid heartbeat or heart pounding, swollen feet or ankles, dizziness, light-headedness, or faintness.
• Inform patient of the risks of severe or fatal ILD, including pneumonitis, and to immediately report new or worsening respiratory signs or symptoms.
• Teach patient the signs and symptoms of QTc-interval prolongation (dizziness, light-headedness, and syncope).
• Inform patient of the risk of cardiomyopathy and to immediately report signs or symptoms of HF.
• Advise patient to immediately report signs or symptoms of keratitis, such as eye inflammation, lacrimation, light sensitivity, eye pain, red eye, or vision changes.
• Inform patient of the risk of SJS, cutaneous vasculitis, or erythema multiforme and to immediately report development of target lesions or severe blistering or peeling of the skin.
• Advise patient not to breastfeed during therapy and for up to 2 weeks after therapy ends.
• Warn patient of childbearing potential of fetal risk, and to use contraception during therapy and for 6 weeks after therapy ends. Teach men to use contraception during therapy and for 4 months after therapy ends.
• Caution patient to report pregnancy or suspected pregnancy during treatment.

ospemifene
os-PEM-i-feen

Osphena

Therapeutic class: Selective estrogen receptor modulators
Pharmacologic class: Selective estrogen agonists–antagonists

AVAILABLE FORMS
Tablets: 60 mg

INDICATIONS & DOSAGES

➤ **Moderate to severe dyspareunia due to vulvar and vaginal atrophy of menopause**
Adults: 60 mg PO once daily.

➤ **Moderate to severe vaginal dryness, a symptom of vulvar and vaginal atrophy, due to menopause**
Adults: 60 mg PO once daily.

ADMINISTRATION

PO

🕛 *Alert:* Hazardous drug; use safe handling and disposal precautions, including single gloving for administration.

• Give with food.

• Store medication at room temperature.

ACTION

Binds to estrogen receptors, activating estrogenic pathways in some tissues (agonism) and blocking estrogenic pathways in others (antagonism).

Route	Onset	Peak	Duration
PO	12 wk	2 hr	Unknown

Half-life: 26 hours.

ADVERSE REACTIONS

CNS: headache. **CV:** hot flushes. **GU:** vaginal hemorrhage, vaginal discharge, endometrial hyperplasia. **Musculoskeletal:** muscle spasms. **Skin:** hyperhidrosis, night sweats.

INTERACTIONS

Drug-drug. *CYP2C9, CYP2C19, CYP3A4 inducers (rifampin):* May decrease ospemifene level, decreasing therapeutic effect. Avoid use together.
CYP2C9, CYP2C19, CYP3A4 inhibitors (fluconazole, ketoconazole, omeprazole): May increase ospemifene level, increasing risk of ospemifene-related adverse effects. Avoid use together.
Estrogen agonists–antagonists, estrogens: Safety of concomitant use hasn't been established. Don't use together.
Highly protein-bound drugs (phenytoin, tolbutamide): May increase exposure of ospemifene or highly protein-bound drug, increasing adverse reactions. Monitor clinical response when either drug is started or stopped.
Drug-herb. *St. John's wort:* May decrease drug level and therapeutic effect. Avoid use together.

EFFECTS ON LAB TEST RESULTS

None reported.

CONTRAINDICATIONS & CAUTIONS

• Contraindicated in women hypersensitive to drug or its components; in women with undiagnosed abnormal genital bleeding or known or suspected estrogen-dependent neoplasm; and in those with active or previous DVT or PE or active or previous arterial thromboembolic disease (stroke, MI).

Boxed Warning Estrogen-alone therapy increases the risk of stroke and DVT. Ospemifene should be prescribed for the shortest duration according to treatment goals and patient's individual risk factors. ∎

• Don't use in patients with known or suspected breast cancer or in those with a history of breast cancer. Drug hasn't been studied in this population.

• Don't use in patients with severe hepatic impairment.

• Use cautiously in patients with an increased risk of CV disorders, arterial vascular disease, or venous thromboembolism (obesity, SLE, family history, personal history).
Dialyzable drug: Unknown.

PREGNANCY-LACTATION-REPRODUCTION

• Drug may cause fetal harm and is contraindicated in patients who are or may become pregnant.

• It isn't known if drug appears in human milk.

NURSING CONSIDERATIONS

Boxed Warning Drug causes increased risk of endometrial cancer in patients with a uterus who use unopposed estrogens; consider adding a progestin in these patients. Patients without a uterus don't need a progestin. Evaluate patient for uterine cancer if patient experiences persistent or recurrent abnormal genital bleeding. ∎

• Discontinue drug immediately if a venous thromboembolism or thromboembolic or hemorrhagic stroke is suspected or occurs.

• Discontinue drug at least 4 to 6 weeks before surgery that's associated with an increased risk of thromboembolism or during periods of extended immobilization.

• Monitor patient for signs and symptoms of PE or cardiac event (sudden onset of shortness of breath and chest pain).

Reactions in bold italics are *life-threatening*. Interactions may have a *rapid onset* or a *delayed onset*.

- *Look alike–sound alike:* Don't confuse ospemifene with osimertinib, raloxifene, or toremifene.

PATIENT TEACHING

- Instruct patient to take drug with food for better absorption.
- Inform patient that drug may initiate or worsen hot flashes.
- Advise patient to immediately report all adverse reactions, especially unusual vaginal discharge or bleeding.
- Caution patient that drug may increase risk of blood clots, stroke, or heart attack. To decrease risk, drug may need to be discontinued at least 4 to 6 weeks before elective surgery or during prolonged immobilization.
- Instruct patient to seek immediate care if weakness on one side of the body, trouble speaking or thinking, change in balance, droop on one side of the face, or blurred eyesight develops.

SAFETY ALERT!

oxaliplatin
ox-AL-i-pla-tin

Therapeutic class: Antineoplastics
Pharmacologic class: Platinum-containing compounds

AVAILABLE FORMS
Solution for injection: 5 mg/mL

INDICATIONS & DOSAGES
Adjust-a-dose (for all indications): For patients with severe renal impairment (CrCl less than 30 mL/minute), initial recommended dose is 65 mg/m². Refer to manufacturer's instructions for toxicity-related dosage adjustments.

➤ **First-line treatment of advanced colorectal cancer with 5-FU and leucovorin (5-FU/LV)**
Adults: On day 1, give 85 mg/m² oxaliplatin IV in 250 to 500 mL D₅W and leucovorin 200 mg/m² IV in D₅W simultaneously over 120 minutes, in separate bags using a Y-line, followed by 5-FU 400 mg/m² IV bolus over 2 to 4 minutes, followed by 600 mg/m² 5-FU IV infusion in 500 mL D₅W over 22 hours.

On day 2, give 200 mg/m² leucovorin IV infusion over 120 minutes, followed by 400 mg/m² 5-FU IV bolus over 2 to

4 minutes, followed by 600 mg/m² 5-FU IV infusion in 500 mL D₅W over 22 hours.

Repeat cycle every 2 weeks until disease progression or unacceptable toxicity occurs.

➤ **With 5-FU/LV for the adjuvant treatment of stage III colon cancer in patients who have had complete resection of the primary tumor**
Adults: On day 1, give oxaliplatin, 85 mg/m² IV in 250 to 500 mL D₅W and 200 mg/m² leucovorin IV infusion in D₅W, both over 120 minutes at the same time, in separate bags, using a Y-line. Follow with 400 mg/m² 5-FU IV bolus over 2 to 4 minutes, then 600 mg/m² 5-FU in 500 mL D₅W as a 22-hour continuous infusion.

On day 2, give leucovorin, 200 mg/m² IV infused over 120 minutes, followed by 400 mg/m² 5-FU as an IV bolus over 2 to 4 minutes, then 600 mg/m² 5-FU in 500 mL D₅W as a 22-hour infusion.

Repeat cycle every 2 weeks for up to 12 cycles.

➤ **Esophageal cancer ◆**
CAPOX regimen
Adults: 130 mg/m² IV on day 1 every 3 weeks (in combination with capecitabine and nivolumab) until disease progression or unacceptable toxicity.

FLOT regimen
Adults: 85 mg/m² IV on day 1 every 2 weeks (in combination with 5-FU, leucovorin, and docetaxel) for four preoperative and four postoperative cycles; or eight cycles in advanced or metastatic disease.

FOLFOX4 regimen
Adults: 85 mg/m² IV on day 1 every 2 weeks (in combination with 5-FU and leucovorin and radiation) for three cycles, then without radiation for three more cycles.

mFOLFOX regimen
Adults: 85 mg/m² IV on day 1 every 2 weeks (in combination with 5-FU, leucovorin, and nivolumab) until disease progression or unacceptable toxicity.

➤ **Gastric cancer ◆**
CAPOX regimen
Adults: 130 mg/m² IV on day 1 every 3 weeks (in combination with capecitabine) for eight cycles or (in combination with capecitabine and nivolumab) until disease progression or unacceptable toxicity.

FLOT regimen
Adults: 85 mg/m² IV on day 1 every 2 weeks (in combination with 5-FU, leucovorin, and

O

docetaxel) for four preoperative and four postoperative cycles; or for eight cycles in advanced or metastatic disease.

mFOLFOX regimen
Adults: 85 mg/m² IV on day 1 every 2 weeks (in combination with 5-FU, leucovorin, and nivolumab) until disease progression or unacceptable toxicity.

➤ **Pancreatic cancer, adjuvant therapy ♦**
Adults: 85 mg/m² IV every 2 weeks (in combination with 5-FU, leucovorin, and irinotecan; modified FOLFIRINOX regimen) for 24 weeks.

➤ **Pancreatic cancer, advanced or metastatic ♦**
Adults: 85 mg/m² IV every 2 weeks (in combination with 5-FU, leucovorin, and irinotecan; FOLFIRINOX regimen) for up to 6 months, or 110 to 130 mg/m² IV on day 1 every 3 weeks (in combination with capecitabine) until disease progression or unacceptable toxicity.

ADMINISTRATION

IV
🌢 *Alert:* Preparing and giving drug may be mutagenic, teratogenic, or carcinogenic. Follow facility recommendations to reduce risks. Facilities typically recommend wearing a single glove during receiving, unpacking, and placing in storage. Double gloving and gown are required during administration.

▼ Reconstitute powder using sterile water for injection or D_5W. Add 10 mL to a 50-mg vial or 20 mL to a 100-mg vial, for a yield of 5 mg/mL. Never reconstitute with sodium chloride solution or other solution containing chloride.

▼ Reconstituted solutions must be further diluted in an infusion solution of 250 to 500 mL of D_5W.

▼ Inspect bag for particulate matter and discoloration before giving, and discard if present.

▼ Don't use needles or IV administration sets that contain aluminum because it displaces the platinum, causing it to lose potency and form a black precipitate.

▼ Premedicate with antiemetics, with or without dexamethasone.

▼ Give oxaliplatin and leucovorin over 2 hours at the same time in separate bags, using a Y-line. Extend the infusion time to 6 hours to decrease acute toxicities.

▼ When used in combination with 5-FU, infuse oxaliplatin first.

▼ Store unopened vials at room temperature. Reconstituted solutions are stable if refrigerated (36° to 46° F [2° to 8° C]) for up to 24 hours. After final dilution, solutions are stable for 6 hours at room temperature and up to 24 hours under refrigeration.

▼ **Incompatibilities:** Alkaline solutions or drugs such as 5-FU. Flush infusion line with D_5W before giving any other drugs simultaneously.

ACTION

Inhibits cell replication and transcription by forming platinum complexes that cross-link with DNA molecules. Not specific to cell cycle.

Route	Onset	Peak	Duration
IV	Unknown	Unknown	Unknown

Half-life: 391 hours (long, terminal phase).

ADVERSE REACTIONS

CNS: pain, peripheral neuropathy, fatigue, headache, dizziness, insomnia, fever, taste perversion, sensory disturbance, anxiety, depression. **CV:** chest pain, *thromboembolism,* edema, flushing, peripheral edema, hypotension. **EENT:** abnormal lacrimation, conjunctivitis, abnormal vision, epistaxis, rhinitis, pharyngolaryngeal dysesthesias, pharyngitis, dry mouth. **GI:** nausea, vomiting, diarrhea, stomatitis, abdominal pain, anorexia, constipation, dyspepsia, gastroesophageal reflux, flatulence, mucositis, dysphagia. **GU:** dysuria, hematuria, urinary frequency, increased serum creatinine level. **Hematologic:** *febrile neutropenia,* anemia, *leukopenia, thrombocytopenia.* **Hepatic:** increased AST, ALT, ALP, and bilirubin levels. **Metabolic:** *hypokalemia, hypocalcemia,* hyperglycemia, hypoalbuminemia, hyponatremia, dehydration, weight gain. **Musculoskeletal:** back pain, arthralgia, myalgia. **Respiratory:** dyspnea, cough, URI, hiccups, *pulmonary toxicity.* **Skin:** injection-site reaction, rash, alopecia, dry skin, pruritus, diaphoresis. **Other:** *hypersensitivity reactions,* hand-foot syndrome, infection, rigors.

INTERACTIONS

Drug-drug. *Anticoagulants:* May increase risk of hemorrhage. Monitor patient closely.

Bacille Calmette-Guérin vaccine (BCG): May diminish therapeutic effect of BCG (intravesical). Avoid combination.

Clozapine: May increase risk of agranulocytosis. Avoid use together.

Deferiprone: May increase risk of neutropenia. Avoid combination.

Denosumab: May increase risk of serious infections. Monitor therapy.

Drugs that prolong QT interval (Class IA and III antiarrhythmics): May further prolong QT interval, increasing risk of cardiac arrhythmia. Avoid use together.

Fosphenytoin, phenytoin: May decrease serum concentration of fosphenytoin and phenytoin. Monitor therapy.

Leflunomide: May increase risk of pancytopenia, agranulocytosis, or thrombocytopenia. Consider not using a leflunomide loading dose in patients receiving other immunosuppressants. Monitor patient for bone marrow suppression at least monthly. Consider therapy modification.

Live-virus vaccines, pimecrolimus, tacrolimus (topical): May enhance adverse or toxic effects of these drugs. Avoid combination.

Natalizumab: May enhance adverse or toxic effect of natalizumab; specifically, may increase risk of concurrent infection. Avoid combination.

Nephrotoxic drugs (such as gentamicin): May decrease elimination of these drugs and increase gentamicin level. Monitor patient for toxicity.

Roflumilast: May enhance immunosuppressive effect of roflumilast. Consider therapy modification.

Sipuleucel-T: May diminish sipuleucel-T therapeutic effect. Monitor therapy.

Taxane derivatives: May enhance myelosuppressive effect of taxane derivatives. Administer taxane derivative before platinum derivative when given as sequential infusions to limit toxicity. Consider therapy modification.

Tofacitinib: May enhance immunosuppressive effect of tofacitinib. Avoid combination.

Topotecan: May enhance adverse or toxic effect of topotecan. Consider therapy modification.

Trastuzumab: May increase neutropenia. Monitor therapy.

Vaccines (inactivated): May diminish therapeutic effect of inactivated vaccines. Monitor therapy.

EFFECTS ON LAB TEST RESULTS
• May increase glucose, creatinine, bilirubin, ALP, AST, and ALT levels.
• May decrease potassium, albumin, calcium, and sodium levels.
• May decrease Hb level and neutrophil, WBC, and platelet counts.

CONTRAINDICATIONS & CAUTIONS
Boxed Warning Serious and fatal hypersensitivity adverse reactions, including anaphylaxis, can occur. Oxaliplatin is contraindicated in patients with hypersensitivity reactions to oxaliplatin and other platinum-based drugs. Immediately and permanently discontinue oxaliplatin for hypersensitivity reactions and administer appropriate treatment. ▌

• Oxaliplatin may cause early-onset (occurs within hours or 1 to 2 days) or persistent (greater than 14 days) peripheral sensory neuropathy.
• Oxaliplatin has been associated with rare, sometimes fatal, pulmonary fibrosis and rhabdomyolysis.
• Extravasation of oxaliplatin can cause tissue necrosis. If extravasation occurs, stop infusion and notify health care provider immediately.
• Severe myelosuppression with sepsis, neutropenic sepsis, and septic shock have occurred in patients receiving oxaliplatin with 5-FU and leucovorin.
• Use cautiously in patients with renal impairment or peripheral sensory neuropathy.
• Use cautiously in patients with CV disease and avoid use in patients with congenital long QT syndrome. May cause QT-interval prolongation and ventricular arrhythmias.

Dialyzable drug: Unknown.

⚠ *Overdose S&S:* Thrombocytopenia, dyspnea, wheezing, paresthesia, vomiting, chest pain, respiratory failure, bradycardia, dysesthesia, laryngospasm, myelosuppression, nausea, diarrhea, neurotoxicity.

PREGNANCY-LACTATION-REPRODUCTION
• Drug may cause fetal harm. If used during pregnancy or if patient becomes pregnant while using oxaliplatin, drug may cause harm to the fetus.
• Patients of childbearing potential should use effective contraception during therapy and for at least 9 months after final dose.

- Men with partners of childbearing potential should use effect contraception during therapy and for 6 months after final dose.
- It isn't known if drug appears in human milk. Patient should discontinue breastfeeding or discontinue drug.
- Drug may impair fertility.

NURSING CONSIDERATIONS

- Administer drug under the supervision of a physician experienced in the use of cancer chemotherapeutic agents.

Boxed Warning Monitor patient for anaphylactic reactions, which may occur within minutes of administration. Immediately and permanently discontinue drug if reactions develop; manage reactions as clinically indicated. ∎

- Premedication with antiemetics, including 5-HT$_3$ receptor antagonists with or without dexamethasone, is recommended.
- Drug doesn't require patient prehydration.
- Drug clearance is reduced in patients with renal impairment.
- Monitor CBC, platelet count, LFTs, and kidney function tests before each chemotherapy cycle.
- Monitor ECG in patients with known prolonged QT interval.
- Monitor electrolyte levels and correct abnormalities at baseline and periodically during treatment.
- Monitor patient for injection-site reaction; extravasation with necrosis may occur. If extravasation occurs, stop infusion immediately and disconnect; gently aspirate extravasated solution; remove needle; and elevate extremity.
- Monitor patient for neuropathy. Acute neuropathy is reversible; it occurs within 2 days of dosing and resolves within 14 days. Persistent peripheral neuropathy occurs more than 14 days after dosing and causes paresthesia, dysesthesia, hypoesthesia, and other neurologic impairments that can interfere with daily activities (such as walking or swallowing).
- Monitor patient for pulmonary toxicity. Evaluate unexplained respiratory signs and symptoms while withholding treatment. Discontinue drug for confirmed ILD or pulmonary fibrosis.
- Monitor patient for PRES (headache, altered mental function, seizures, vision changes, HTN). Confirm with MRI;

permanently discontinue drug if diagnosis confirmed.
- Monitor patient for bleeding, especially when drug is used in combination with 5-FU or leucovorin.
- Monitor patient for rhabdomyolysis (muscle pain, weakness, fever, red-brown urine, decrease urine output).
- Avoid ice and cold exposure during infusion of drug because cold temperatures can worsen acute neurologic symptoms. Cover patient with a blanket during infusion.
- Diarrhea, dehydration, hypokalemia, and fatigue may occur more frequently in older adults.
- *Look alike–sound alike:* Don't confuse oxaliplatin with carboplatin or cisplatin.

PATIENT TEACHING

- Inform patient of potential serious adverse reactions and of need to report them promptly.
- Tell patient to avoid exposure to cold or cold objects (such as cold drinks or ice cubes), which can bring on or worsen acute symptoms of peripheral neuropathy. Advise patient to drink warm drinks, wear warm clothing, and cover any exposed skin (hands, face, and head).
- Advise patient to immediately report trouble breathing or signs and symptoms of an allergic reaction, such as rash, hives, swelling of lips or tongue, or sudden cough.
- Instruct patient to report fever, signs and symptoms of infection, persistent vomiting, diarrhea, or signs and symptoms of dehydration (thirst, dry mouth, light-headedness, and decreased urination).
- Warn patient of childbearing potential of the risk of harm to the fetus if oxaliplatin is used during pregnancy. Advise use of effective contraception.
- Advise patient of reproductive potential desiring children to consider fertility preservation before therapy.
- Caution patient not to breastfeed during treatment and for 3 months after final dose.
- Advise patient that dizziness and vision abnormalities may affect patient's ability to drive and use machinery.

oxazepam
oks-A-ze–pam

Therapeutic class: Anxiolytics
Pharmacologic class: Benzodiazepines
Controlled substance schedule: IV

AVAILABLE FORMS
Capsules: 10 mg, 15 mg, 30 mg

INDICATIONS & DOSAGES
➤ **Alcohol withdrawal, severe anxiety**
Adults: 15 to 30 mg PO t.i.d. or q.i.d.
➤ **Mild to moderate anxiety**
Adults and children older than age 12: 10 to 15 mg PO t.i.d. or q.i.d.
➤ **Severe anxiety syndromes; agitation; anxiety associated with depression**
Adults and children older than age 12: 15 to 30 mg PO t.i.d. or q.i.d.
➤ **Anxiety, tension, irritability, agitation**
Older adults: 10 mg PO t.i.d. May increase cautiously to 15 mg t.i.d. or q.i.d.

ADMINISTRATION
PO
• Give drug without regard for meals.

ACTION
May stimulate GABA receptors in the ascending reticular activating system.

Route	Onset	Peak	Duration
PO	Unknown	3 hr	Unknown

Half-life: About 8 hours.

ADVERSE REACTIONS
CNS: drowsiness, lethargy, dizziness, vertigo, headache, syncope, tremor, slurred speech, changes in EEG patterns. **CV:** edema. **GI:** nausea. **GU:** altered libido. **Skin:** rash.

INTERACTIONS
Drug-drug. *Clozapine:* May enhance toxic effect of clozapine. Consider decreasing oxazepam dosage.
CNS depressants: May increase CNS depression. Use together cautiously.
Melatonin: May enhance sedative effect of benzodiazepines. Use with caution.
Boxed Warning *Opioids:* May cause slow or difficult breathing, sedation, and death. Avoid use together. If use together is

necessary, limit dosage and duration of each drug to minimum necessary for desired effect. ■
Drug-herb. *Cannabinoid-containing products, kava kava, kratom:* May increase sedation. Discourage use together.
Yohimbe: May decrease effect of oxazepam. Discourage use together.
Drug-lifestyle. *Alcohol use:* May cause additive CNS effects. Don't use together.

EFFECTS ON LAB TEST RESULTS
• May increase LFT values.
• May decrease WBC count.

CONTRAINDICATIONS & CAUTIONS
• Contraindicated in patients hypersensitive to drug and in those with psychoses.
Boxed Warning Opioids should only be prescribed with benzodiazepines or other CNS depressants to patients for whom alternative treatment options are inadequate. ■
Boxed Warning Benzodiazepine use exposes patient to risks of abuse, misuse, and addiction, which can lead to overdose or death. Assess each patient's risk of abuse, misuse, and addiction before prescribing and periodically during therapy. ■
Boxed Warning Abrupt discontinuation or rapid dosage reduction of benzodiazepines after continued use may precipitate acute withdrawal reactions, which can be lifethreatening. To reduce risk of withdrawal reactions, gradually taper drug to discontinue or reduce dosage. ■
• Use cautiously in older adults and in patients at risk for falls.
• Use cautiously in patients with respiratory disease or history of substance abuse and in patients in whom a decrease in BP might lead to cardiac problems.
• Safety and effectiveness in children younger than age 6 haven't been established. Absolute dosage for children ages 6 to 12 isn't established.
Dialyzable drug: No.
⚠ **Overdose S&S:** Drowsiness, confusion, lethargy, ataxia, hypotonia, hypotension, hypnotic state, coma, death.

PREGNANCY-LACTATION-REPRODUCTION
• Drug crosses placental barrier and may adversely affect the fetus (premature birth, low birth weight, hypoglycemia, respiratory problems), especially in first and third trimesters.

Use during pregnancy should almost always be avoided.

• Drug appears in human milk. Drowsiness, lethargy, or weight loss may occur in breastfed infants. Breastfeeding isn't recommended.

NURSING CONSIDERATIONS
• Monitor hepatic, renal, and hematopoietic function periodically in patients receiving repeated or prolonged therapy.

Boxed Warning Concomitant use of benzodiazepines and opioids may result in profound sedation, respiratory depression, coma, and death. Limit dosages and durations to the minimum required. Monitor patients for signs and symptoms of respiratory depression and sedation. ■

• Monitor patients closely for fall risk.
• *Look alike–sound alike:* Don't confuse oxazepam with oxaprozin, oxcarbazepine, or quazepam.

PATIENT TEACHING
Boxed Warning Caution patient or caregiver of patient taking an opioid with a benzodiazepine, CNS depressant, or alcohol to seek immediate medical attention if patient experiences dizziness, light-headedness, extreme sleepiness, slowed or difficult breathing, or unresponsiveness. ■

Boxed Warning Caution patient that benzodiazepines, even at recommended doses, increase risk of abuse, misuse, and addiction, which can lead to overdose and death, especially when used in combination with other drugs (opioid analgesics), alcohol, or illicit substances. ■

Boxed Warning Inform patient on proper disposal of unused drug and about signs and symptoms of benzodiazepine abuse, misuse, and addiction (abdominal pain, amnesia, anorexia, anxiety, aggression, ataxia, blurred vision, confusion, depression, disinhibition, disorientation, dizziness, euphoria, impaired concentration and memory, indigestion, irritability, muscle pain, slurred speech, tremors, vertigo, delirium, paranoia, suicidality, seizures, difficulty breathing, coma) and to seek emergency medical help if they occur. Advise patient not to take drug at a higher dose, more frequently, or for longer than prescribed. ■

Boxed Warning Tell patient that continued use of drug for several days to weeks may lead to physical dependence and that abrupt discontinuation or rapid dosage reduction may precipitate acute withdrawal reactions (unusual movements, responses, or expressions; seizures; sudden and severe mental or nervous system changes; depression; seeing or hearing things that others don't; homicidal thoughts; extreme increase in activity or talking; losing touch with reality; suicidality), which can be life-threatening. Instruct patient that discontinuation or dosage reduction may require a slow taper. ■

Boxed Warning Advise patient about the risk of protracted withdrawal syndrome (anxiety; trouble remembering, learning, or concentrating; depression; problems sleeping; feeling like insects are crawling under the skin; weakness; shaking; muscle twitching; burning or prickling feeling in the hands, arms, legs, or feet; ringing in the ears), with symptoms lasting weeks to more than 12 months. ■

• Warn patient to avoid hazardous activities that require alertness or good coordination until effects of drug are known.
• Tell patient to avoid use of alcohol.
• Notify patient that smoking may decrease drug's effectiveness.
• Warn patient of childbearing potential to avoid use during pregnancy.

OXcarbazepine ⚥
ox-car-BAZ-e-peen

Oxtellar XR, Trileptal

Therapeutic class: Anticonvulsants
Pharmacologic class: Carboxamide derivatives

AVAILABLE FORMS
Oral suspension: 300 mg/5 mL (60 mg/mL)
Tablets (extended-release) ⓄTC: 150 mg, 300 mg, 600 mg
Tablets (film-coated): 150 mg, 300 mg, 600 mg

INDICATIONS & DOSAGES
Adjust-a-dose (for all indications): If CrCl is less than 30 mL/minute, start therapy at 150 mg PO b.i.d immediate-release or 300 mg PO daily extended-release (one-half usual starting dose) and increase slowly to achieve desired response. In patients with ESRD on

---

dialysis, use immediate-release formulation instead of extended-release formulation.

➤ **Adjunctive treatment of partial seizures in patients with epilepsy**

Immediate-release

Adults: Initially, 300 mg immediate-release tablets or suspension PO b.i.d. Increase by a maximum of 600 mg daily (300 mg PO b.i.d.) at weekly intervals. Maximum recommended daily dose is 1,200 mg PO in two divided doses.

Children ages 4 to 16 (immediate-release): Initially, 8 to 10 mg/kg PO daily in two divided doses, not to exceed 600 mg daily. The target maintenance dose depends on patient's weight and should be divided into two doses. If patient weighs between 20 and 29 kg, target maintenance dose is 900 mg daily in two divided doses. If patient weighs between 29.1 and 39 kg, target maintenance dose is 1,200 mg daily in two divided doses. If patient weighs more than 39 kg, target maintenance dose is 1,800 mg daily in two divided doses. Target doses should be achieved over 2 weeks.

Children ages 2 to younger than 4 (immediate-release): Initially, 8 to 10 mg/kg PO daily in two divided doses, not to exceed 600 mg daily. If patient weighs less than 20 kg, a starting dose of 16 to 20 mg/kg may be considered. Maximum maintenance dosage should be achieved over 2 to 4 weeks and shouldn't exceed 60 mg/kg/day in a two-dose divided regimen.

Extended-release

Adults: 600 mg extended-release tablets PO daily. May increase at weekly intervals in 600-mg/day increments. Usual dosage, 1,200 to 2,400 mg daily.

Children ages 6 to 17 (extended-release): 8 to 10 mg/kg PO once daily, not to exceed 600 mg daily in first week. May increase at weekly intervals in 8- to 10-mg/kg increments once daily, not to exceed 600 mg. Target daily dose in patients weighing more than 39 kg is 1,800 mg/day; from 29.1 to 39 kg, 1,200 mg/day; and from 20 to 29 kg, 900 mg/day.

Older adults: When using extended-release tablets, consider a lower starting dose (300 or 450 mg/day). Dosage increases can be made at weekly intervals in increments of 300 to 450 mg/day.

Adjust-a-dose: If drug is used concomitantly with strong CYP3A4 enzyme inducers or UGT inducers, which include certain antiepileptic drugs, consider initiating dosage of extended-release formulation at 900 mg once daily in adults and 12 to 15 mg/kg once daily in children. Refer to Interactions section and product insert for more information.

➤ **To change from multidrug to single-drug treatment of partial seizures in patients with epilepsy**

Adults: Initially, 300 mg immediate-release tablets or suspension PO b.i.d., while reducing dose of concomitant anticonvulsant. Increase oxcarbazepine by a maximum of 600 mg daily at weekly intervals over 2 to 4 weeks. Recommended daily dose is 2,400 mg PO in two divided doses. Withdraw other anticonvulsant completely over 3 to 6 weeks.

Children ages 4 to 16: Initially, 8 to 10 mg/kg immediate-release tablets or suspension PO daily in two divided doses, while reducing dose of concomitant anticonvulsant. Increase oxcarbazepine by a maximum of 10 mg/kg daily at weekly intervals to achieve the recommended daily dose by weight listed in the manufacturer's instructions. Withdraw other anticonvulsant completely over 3 to 6 weeks. See manufacturer's instructions for weight-based maintenance dosing with oxcarbazepine monotherapy.

➤ **Monotherapy for partial-onset seizures**

Immediate-release

Adults: Initially, 300 mg immediate-release tablets or suspension PO b.i.d. Increase dosage by 300 mg daily every third day to a daily dose of 1,200 mg in two divided doses. Or, 600 mg extended-release tablets PO daily. May increase at weekly intervals in 600-mg/day increments. Usual dosage is 1,200 to 2,400 mg once daily.

Children ages 4 to 16: Initially, 8 to 10 mg/kg immediate-release tablets or suspension PO daily in two divided doses, increasing dosage by 5 mg/kg daily every third day to the recommended daily dose range by weight in the manufacturer's instructions.

Extended-release

Adults: Initially, 600 mg extended-release tablets PO daily. May increase at weekly intervals in 600-mg/day increments. Usual dosage is 1,200 to 2,400 mg daily.

Children ages 6 to 17: Initially, 8 to 10 mg/kg extended-release tablets PO daily, not to exceed 600 mg daily in first week. May increase at weekly intervals in increments of 8 to 10 mg/kg once daily, not to exceed 600 mg.

O

Target daily dose in patients weighing more than 39 kg is 1,800 mg/day; from 29.1 to 39 kg, 1,200 mg/day; and from 20 to 29 kg, 900 mg/day.

Adjust-a-dose: If drug is used concomitantly with strong CYP3A4 enzyme inducers or UGT inducers, which include certain antiepileptic drugs, consider initiating dosage of extended-release formulation at 900 mg once daily in adults and 12 to 15 mg/kg once daily in children. Refer to Interactions section and product insert for more information.

ADMINISTRATION
PO
- For suspension, firmly insert plastic adapter provided with the bottle. Cover adapter with child-resistant cap when not in use.
- Shake bottle for at least 10 seconds, remove child-resistant cap, and insert oral dosing syringe provided to withdraw appropriate dose.
- May give dose directly from oral syringe or may mix in a small glass of water immediately before patient swallows it.
- Rinse syringe with warm water after use and allow to dry thoroughly.
- Use suspension within 7 weeks of first opening container.
- Give immediate-release tablets and oral suspension without regard for food.
- Give extended-release tablets on an empty stomach (at least 1 hour before or 2 hours after a meal). Don't cut, crush, or allow patient to chew tablets. For ease of swallowing, use multiple lower-strength tablets for appropriate dose.
- When converting from immediate-release to extended-release form, higher doses may be needed.
- Oral tablets and suspension may be interchanged at equal doses.

ACTION
Thought to prevent seizure spread in the brain by blocking voltage-sensitive sodium channels and to produce anticonvulsant effects by increasing potassium conduction and modulating high-voltage activated calcium channels.

Route	Onset	Peak	Duration
PO	Unknown	Immediate-release: 3–13 hr (adults), 1 hr (children); extended-release: 7 hr (adults)	Unknown

Half-life: Immediate-release: About 2 hours for drug; about 9 hours for the active metabolite (adults). Children ages 2 to 5, 4.8 to 6.7 hours for active metabolite; children ages 6 to 8, 7.2 to 9.3 hours for active metabolite. Extended-release: 7 to 11 hours for drug.

ADVERSE REACTIONS
CNS: abnormal gait, ataxia, dizziness, drowsiness, fatigue, headache, tremor, vertigo, *seizures,* abnormal coordination, agitation, amnesia, anxiety, asthenia, confusion, emotional lability, feeling abnormal, fever, hypoesthesia, impaired concentration, insomnia, somnolence, nervousness, speech disorder, falls, thirst, taste perversion, abnormal EEG. **CV:** chest pain, edema, hypotension. **EENT:** abnormal vision, diplopia, nystagmus, abnormal accommodation, ear pain, ear infection, epistaxis, rhinitis, sinusitis, toothache, dry mouth, pharyngitis. **GI:** abdominal pain, nausea, vomiting, rectal hemorrhage, anorexia, constipation, diarrhea, dyspepsia, gastritis. **GU:** urinary frequency, UTI, vaginitis. **Hematologic:** lymphadenopathy. **Metabolic:** hyponatremia, weight gain. **Musculoskeletal:** back pain, muscular weakness. **Respiratory:** URI, bronchitis, pulmonary infection, coughing, pneumonia. **Skin:** acne, bruising, hot flashes, diaphoresis, purpura, rash. **Other:** allergic reaction, infection, hot flash.

INTERACTIONS
Drug-drug. *Carbamazepine, rifampin, valproic acid, verapamil:* May decrease oxcarbazepine level. Monitor patient and level closely.
CYP3A4 substrates (cyclosporine, itraconazole, rivaroxaban): May decrease serum concentrations of substrates. Substrate dosage modifications may be needed.
Dolutegravir, elvitegravir, ledipasvir, rilpivirine, simeprevir, sofosbuvir, tenofovir, ulipristal: May decrease serum concentration of these drugs. Avoid combination.
Hormonal contraceptives: May decrease levels of ethinyl estradiol and levonorgestrel, reducing hormonal contraceptive effectiveness.

Reactions in bold italics are *life-threatening.* Interactions may have a *rapid onset* or a **delayed onset.**

Caution patients of childbearing potential to use alternative forms of contraception.
Phenobarbital, phenytoin: May decrease oxcarbazepine level. May decrease ox-carbazepine level. Monitor patient closely.
Selegiline: May enhance serotonergic effect of selegiline. Avoid combination.
Thiazide and thiazide-like diuretics: May increase risk of hyponatremia. Monitor therapy.
Drug-lifestyle. *Alcohol use:* May increase CNS depression. Discourage use together.

EFFECTS ON LAB TEST RESULTS
• May decrease sodium level.
• May decrease serum T_4 without affecting T_3 or TSH levels.

CONTRAINDICATIONS & CAUTIONS
• Contraindicated in patients hypersensitive to drug or its components or to eslicarbazepine acetate.
⊙ *Alert:* SCARs have been reported in both children and adults in association with oxcarbazepine use. Reactions may be life-threatening and require hospitalization. Recurrence of serious skin reactions after rechallenge with oxcarbazepine has also been reported.
▨ Screen patients of Asian ancestry for the human leukocyte antigen allele (HLA-B*1502) before therapy; these patients may be at increased risk for SJS or TEN with oxcarbazepine therapy.
• May increase risk of suicidality.
Dialyzable drug: Unknown.

PREGNANCY-LACTATION-REPRODUCTION
• There are no adequate studies during pregnancy; drug may cause fetal harm. Use cautiously during pregnancy and only if benefit justifies fetal risk.
• Patients exposed to drug during pregnancy are encouraged to enroll themselves in the North American AED Pregnancy Registry (1-888-233-2334).
• Plasma levels of the active metabolite of oxcarbazepine may gradually decrease throughout pregnancy and increase after delivery. Monitor patient carefully during pregnancy and postpartum period.
• Drug and its active metabolite appear in human milk in small amounts. Patient should discontinue breastfeeding or discontinue drug.

NURSING CONSIDERATIONS
⊙ *Alert:* Patients with history of hypersensitivity reaction to carbamazepine may develop hypersensitivities to oxcarbazepine. Ask patient about carbamazepine hypersensitivity and stop drug immediately if signs or symptoms of hypersensitivity occur.
⊙ *Alert:* Closely monitor all patients taking or starting antiepileptic drugs for changes in behavior indicating worsening of suicidality or depression. Symptoms such as anxiety, agitation, hostility, mania, and hypomania may be precursors to emerging suicidality.
⊙ *Alert:* Withdraw drug gradually to minimize risk of increased seizure activity.
• Watch for signs and symptoms of hyponatremia, including nausea, malaise, headache, lethargy, confusion, and decreased sensation.
• Monitor sodium level in patients receiving oxcarbazepine for maintenance treatment, especially patients receiving other therapies that may decrease sodium levels.
• Oxcarbazepine use has been linked to several nervous system-related adverse reactions, including psychomotor slowing, difficulty with concentration, speech or language problems, somnolence, fatigue, and coordination abnormalities, such as ataxia and gait disturbances.
⊙ *Alert:* Rare serious and sometimes fatal dermatologic reactions can occur. If skin reactions occur, discontinue drug.
• Monitor patient for DRESS syndrome (fever, rash, lymphadenopathy, facial edema, organ system disorders, such as hepatitis, nephritis, myocarditis, myositis, hematologic abnormalities). Evaluate patient immediately and discontinue drug if alternative cause isn't determined.
• *Look alike–sound alike:* Don't confuse oxcarbazepine with carbamazepine, oxazepam, or oxaprozin. Don't confuse Trileptal with TriLipix.

PATIENT TEACHING
• Teach patient safe drug administration.
• Tell patient to contact prescriber before interrupting or stopping drug.
• Advise patient not to discontinue drug abruptly because of the risk of increasing seizure frequency.
• Instruct patient to report signs and symptoms of low sodium in the blood, such as nausea, malaise, headache, lethargy, and confusion.

◑ *Alert:* DRESS syndrome hypersensitivity reactions may occur. Tell patient to report fever and swollen lymph nodes to prescriber.

◑ *Alert:* Serious skin reactions, including SJS and TEN, can occur. Advise patient to immediately report rashes to prescriber.

• Caution patient to avoid driving and other potentially hazardous activities that require mental alertness until effects of drug are known.

• Instruct patient using hormonal contraceptives to use alternative form of contraception during therapy.

• Tell patient to avoid alcohol during therapy.

oxybutynin
oks-i-BYOO-ti-nin

Oxytrol, Oxytrol for Women ◇

oxybutynin chloride
Ditropan XL, Gelnique

Therapeutic class: Urinary antispasmodics
Pharmacologic class: Antimuscarinics

AVAILABLE FORMS
oxybutynin
Transdermal patch: 36-mg patch delivering 3.9 mg/day ◇
oxybutynin chloride
Syrup: 5 mg/5 mL
Tablets: 5 mg
Tablets (extended-release) ⓄⓉⒸ*:* 5 mg, 10 mg, 15 mg
Topical gel: 10% in 1 g single-dose sachets

INDICATIONS & DOSAGES
➤ **Overactive bladder**
Adults: 5 mg (immediate-release tablet) PO b.i.d. to t.i.d.; maximum, 5 mg q.i.d. Or, 5 to 10 mg (extended-release tablet) PO once daily. Dosage adjustments may be made weekly in 5-mg increments, as needed, to maximum of 30 mg PO daily. Or, apply one patch twice weekly (every 3 to 4 days) to dry, intact skin on the abdomen, hip, or buttock. Or, 1 g topical gel (10%) once daily.
Older adults: A lower initial starting dose of 2.5 mg (immediate-release) PO b.i.d. or t.i.d. is recommended.
➤ **Symptoms of detrusor overactivity associated with a neurologic condition (e.g., spina bifida)**

Children age 5 and older (immediate-release): 5 mg PO b.i.d. or t.i.d.
Children age 6 and older (extended-release): 5 mg once daily; adjust in 5-mg increments at weekly intervals. Maximum daily dose, 20 mg/day.

ADMINISTRATION
PO
• Don't crush extended-release tablets.
• Give without regard for food.
• Measure syrup dose with a liquid medication dispenser or syringe.
Topical (gel)
• Use immediately after sachets are opened.
• Apply to dry, intact skin on the abdomen, upper arms or shoulders, or thighs.
• Don't apply to recently shaved skin.
• Rotate application sites.
• Patient shouldn't bathe, shower, or swim for 1 hour after gel application.
• Cover treated area with clothing after gel has dried to prevent transfer of medication to others.
Transdermal
• Apply immediately after removing from protective pouch.
• Apply to dry, intact skin on the abdomen, hip, or buttock.
• Don't apply to areas with cuts, scrapes, or irritation.
• Avoid reapplication to the same site within 7 days.
• Don't expose patch to sunlight.
• Don't cut the patch.
• Contact with water while bathing, swimming, showering, or exercising won't change the effect; however, rubbing of the patch area should be avoided during these activities.

ACTION
Relaxes smooth muscle of bladder by antagonizing muscarinic receptors, relieving symptoms of overactive bladder.

Route	Onset	Peak	Duration
PO	30–60 min	60 min	6–10 hr
PO (extended-release)	Unknown	4–6 hr	24 hr
Topical (gel)	Unknown	Unknown	Unknown
Transdermal	Unknown	24–48 hr	96 hr

Half-life: Tablets or oral solution, 2 to 3 hours; extended-release tablets, 12 to 13 hours; patch, 64 hours.

Reactions in bold italics are *life-threatening*. Interactions may have a *rapid onset* or a ***delayed onset***.

ADVERSE REACTIONS
PO
CNS: dizziness, insomnia, nervousness, drowsiness, restlessness, asthenia, fever, headache, somnolence, confusion, dygeusia, thirst. **CV:** palpitations, flushing, peripheral edema, increased or decreased BP. **EENT:** blurred vision, dry eyes, eye irritation, sinus or nasal congestion, nasopharyngitis, hoarseness, dry mouth, sore throat, coated tongue. **GI:** constipation, diarrhea, nausea, vomiting, dyspepsia, decreased GI motility, flatulence, dysphagia, belching, abdominal pain. **GU:** dysuria, urinary hesitancy, urine retention, urinary frequency, impotence, UTI, cystitis. **Metabolic:** fluid retention, *hypoglycemia.* **Musculoskeletal:** back pain, arthralgia, limb pain. **Respiratory:** URI, bronchitis, cough, *asthma.* **Skin:** rash, dry skin, pruritus. **Other:** fungal infection, fall.

Topical (gel)
CNS: dizziness, fatigue, headache. **EENT:** dry mouth, nasopharyngitis. **GI:** viral gastroenteritis, constipation. **GU:** UTI. **Metabolic:** increased serum glucose level. **Respiratory:** URI. **Skin:** application-site reaction, pruritus.

Transdermal patch
EENT: abnormal vision, dry mouth. **GI:** diarrhea, constipation. **GU:** dysuria. **Skin:** pruritus, erythema, vesicles, macules, rash, burning at application site.

INTERACTIONS
Drug-drug. *Amantadine, anticholinergics:* May increase anticholinergic effects (dry mouth, constipation, blurred vision, somnolence). Use together cautiously.
Cannabinoid-containing products: May enhance tachycardic effect of cannabinoid-containing products. Monitor therapy closely.
CNS depressants: May increase CNS effects. Use together cautiously.
CYP3A4 inhibitors (clarithromycin, erythromycin, itraconazole, ketoconazole, miconazole): May increase oxybutynin concentration. Use together cautiously.
Ipratropium (oral inhalation): May increase anticholinergic effects (dry mouth, constipation, blurred vision, somnolence). Avoid combination.
Opioid agonists (buprenorphine): May increase risk of constipation and urine retention. Monitor therapy closely.
Drug-lifestyle. *Alcohol use:* May increase CNS effects. Discourage use together.

Exercise, hot weather: May cause heatstroke. Advise patient to use with caution in hot weather.

EFFECTS ON LAB TEST RESULTS
• May decrease glucose level.
• May suppress the wheal and flare reactions to skin test antigens.

CONTRAINDICATIONS & CAUTIONS
• Contraindicated in patients hypersensitive to drug or its components and in those with conditions that decrease GI motility, uncontrolled narrow-angle glaucoma, urine or gastric retention, or obstructive uropathy.
• Angioedema may occur after a single dose.
• Use cautiously in older adults and in patients with autonomic neuropathy, reflux esophagitis, myasthenia gravis, Parkinson disease, or hepatic or renal disease.
• Use cautiously in patients with preexisting dementia treated with a cholinesterase inhibitor.
• Extended-release form isn't recommended for children who can't swallow the tablet whole without chewing, dividing, or crushing or for children younger than age 6.
• Use extended-release form cautiously in patients with bladder outflow obstruction, gastric obstruction, ulcerative colitis, intestinal atony, myasthenia gravis, or gastroesophageal reflux and in those taking drugs that worsen esophagitis (bisphosphonates).
Dialyzable drug: Unknown.
⚠ **Overdose S&S:** Restlessness, tremors, irritability, seizures, delirium, hallucinations, flushing, fever, dehydration, cardiac arrhythmias, vomiting, urine retention, hypotension or HTN, respiratory failure, paralysis, coma.

PREGNANCY-LACTATION-REPRODUCTION
• Use cautiously during pregnancy and only if benefit justifies fetal risk.
• It isn't known if drug appears in human milk. Use cautiously during breastfeeding.
• Lactation suppression has been reported.

NURSING CONSIDERATIONS
• Drug may aggravate symptoms of hyperthyroidism, CAD, HF, arrhythmias, tachycardia, HTN, or prostatic hyperplasia.
• Monitor patient for anticholinergic effects (confusion, dry mouth, dizziness, blurred vision, tachycardia). If anticholinergic effects occur, consider dosage reduction or discontinuation.

• Monitor patient for episodes of incontinence and postvoid residual.
• *Look alike–sound alike:* Don't confuse Ditropan with Detrol, diazepam, Diprivan, or dithranol. Don't confuse oxybutynin with OxyCONTIN.

PATIENT TEACHING
• Teach patient safe drug administration for formulation prescribed.
• Warn patient to avoid hazardous activities, such as operating machinery or driving, until CNS effects of drug are known.
• Caution patient that using drug during very hot weather may cause fever or heatstroke because it suppresses sweating.
• Warn patient to only wear one patch at a time.
• Tell patient to dispose of old patches carefully in the trash in a manner that prevents accidental application or ingestion by children and pets.
• Tell patient to remove patch before undergoing an MRI scan.
• Gel contains alcohol. Caution patient to avoid open flames or smoking until gel has dried.
• Advise patient to avoid alcohol while taking drug.
• Tell patient that drug may cause dry mouth.
• Advise patient of risk of angioedema (swelling of the tongue or throat, difficulty breathing) and to seek immediate medical attention if symptoms occur.

SAFETY ALERT!

oxyCODONE
oks-i-KOE-done

Xtampza ER

oxyCODONE hydrochloride
Oxaydo, OxyCONTIN✲, Oxy.IR✲, OxyNEO✦, Roxicodone, Roxybond, Supeudol✦

Therapeutic class: Opioid analgesics
Pharmacologic class: Opioids
Controlled substance schedule: II

AVAILABLE FORMS
oxycodone
Capsules (extended-release, 12-hour abuse deterrent): 9-mg base, 13.5-mg base, 18-mg base, 27-mg base, 36-mg base

oxycodone hydrochloride
Capsules: 5 mg
Oral solution: 5 mg/5 mL
Oral solution (concentrate): 20 mg/mL
Tablets (extended-release, 12-hour abuse-deterrent) **ONC**: 10 mg, 15 mg, 20 mg, 30 mg, 40 mg, 60 mg, 80 mg
Tablets (immediate-release): 5 mg, 7.5 mg, 10 mg, 15 mg, 20 mg, 30 mg

INDICATIONS & DOSAGES
Boxed Warning Use in patients for whom alternative treatments are ineffective, not tolerated, or inadequate. ■
➤ **Moderate to severe pain**
Adults: 5 to 15 mg immediate-release PO every 4 to 6 hours. Titrate dosage based on response. For acute pain, use for up to 7 days. For control of severe, chronic pain, give on a regularly scheduled basis every 4 to 6 hours.
➤ **Moderate to severe pain in patients who need a continuous, around-the-clock analgesic for an extended period of time**
Adults who aren't opioid-tolerant: 10 mg extended-release tablets or 9 mg extended-release capsules PO every 12 hours. May increase dose every 1 to 2 days until desired pain control is achieved.
Adults who are opioid-tolerant: Refer to manufacturer's instructions for extended-release tablets or capsules or concentrated oral solution (20 mg/mL) for conversion from other formulations and drugs.
Children age 11 and older who are opioid-tolerant (extended-release tablets): Refer to manufacturer's recommendations.
Adjust-a-dose: For older adults, patients who are debilitated, and those with hepatic or renal impairment, or if patient is receiving CNS depressants, decrease initial starting dose by one-third to one-half.

ADMINISTRATION
PO
• To minimize GI upset, give drug after meals or with milk.
Boxed Warning Patient must swallow extended-release tablets whole. ■
❂ *Alert:* The 60- and 80-mg extended-release tablets, or a single 40-mg dose, or a total daily dose of more than 80 mg is limited to patients who are opioid-tolerant.
Boxed Warning Oxycodone concentrated oral solution, available as a 20-mg/mL

Reactions in bold italics are *life-threatening*. Interactions may have a *rapid onset* or a ***delayed onset***.

concentration, is indicated for use in patients who are opioid-tolerant only. ■

Boxed Warning Use care when administering oxycodone concentrated oral solution, to avoid dosing errors due to confusion between milligram and milliliter and among other oxycodone solutions with different concentrations. Such confusion could result in accidental overdose and death. Ensure that the proper dose is communicated and dispensed. ■

◐ **Alert:** Oxycodone extended-release capsules aren't bioequivalent to oxycodone hydrochloride extended-release tablets.

ACTION

Unknown. Binds with opioid receptors in the CNS, altering perception of and emotional response to pain.

Route	Onset	Peak	Duration
PO (immediate-release)	10–15 min	0.5–1 hr	3–6 hr
PO (extended-release)	Unknown	4–5 hr	12 hr

Half-life: 3 to 4 hours. Extended-release tablets, 4.5 hours; extended-release capsules, 5.6 hours.

ADVERSE REACTIONS

CNS: clouded sensorium, dizziness, euphoria, light-headedness, physical dependence, withdrawal syndrome, sedation, somnolence, headache, asthenia, fever, abnormal dreams, insomnia, confusion, irritability, migraine, tremor. **CV:** *bradycardia,* hypotension, edema, flushing, HTN, tachycardia. **EENT:** blurred vision, pharyngitis, rhinitis, sinusitis, oropharyngeal pain. **GI:** constipation, nausea, vomiting, ileus, diarrhea, anorexia, gastritis, GERD, abdominal pain. **GU:** urine retention. **Hematologic:** anemia; decreased Hb level, platelet count, RBC count. **Hepatic:** increased ALT level. **Metabolic:** hypochloremia, hyponatremia, hyperglycemia. **Musculoskeletal:** weakness, arthralgia, myalgia, back pain, tremor. **Respiratory:** *respiratory depression,* cough, dyspnea. **Skin:** diaphoresis, pruritus. **Other:** chills.

INTERACTIONS

Drug-drug. *Alvimopan:* May enhance alvimopan-related toxicity. Alvimopan is contraindicated in patients receiving opioids for more than 7 consecutive days before starting alvimopan.

Anticholinergic agents: May increase risk of constipation and urine retention. Monitor therapy closely.

Boxed Warning *Benzodiazepines, CNS depressants:* May cause slow or difficult breathing, sedation, and death. Avoid use together. If use together is necessary, limit dosage and duration of each drug to minimum necessary for desired effect. ■

Boxed Warning *CYP3A4 inducers (such as carbamazepine, phenytoin, rifampin):* May increase oxycodone level and cause oxycodone-related adverse reactions if inducer is discontinued. Taper inducers cautiously and adjust oxycodone dosage as needed. ■

Boxed Warning *CYP3A4 inhibitors such as azole antifungals (ketoconazole), macrolide antibiotics (erythromycin), protease inhibitors (ritonavir):* May increase oxycodone level, increase or prolong adverse effects, and cause fatal respiratory depression. Carefully monitor patient over extended period of time and adjust oxycodone dosage as needed. ■

General anesthetics, hypnotics, MAO inhibitors, TCAs: May cause additive adverse effects (e.g., CNS or respiratory depression). Use together with caution. Reduce oxycodone dose and monitor patient response.

◐ **Alert:** *Serotonergic drugs (amoxapine, antiemetics [dolasetron, granisetron, ondansetron, palonosetron], antimigraine drugs, buspirone, cyclobenzaprine, dextromethorphan, linezolid, lithium, MAO inhibitors, maprotiline, methylene blue, mirtazapine, nefazodone, SSNRIs, SSRIs, TCAs, trazodone, tryptophan, vilazodone):* May increase risk of serotonin syndrome. Use together cautiously and monitor patient for serotonin syndrome.

Drug-herb. *Cannabinoid-containing products, kava kava:* May enhance adverse effects of CNS depressants. Monitor therapy carefully.

◐ **Alert:** *St. John's wort:* May increase risk of serotonin syndrome. May decrease oxycodone serum concentration. Use together cautiously.

Drug-lifestyle. **Boxed Warning** *Alcohol use:* May increase risk of profound sedation, respiratory depression, coma, and death. Don't use together. ■

O

EFFECTS ON LAB TEST RESULTS
• May increase blood glucose and ALT levels.
• May decrease serum chloride and sodium levels.
• May decrease Hb level and RBC and platelet counts.
• Quinolones (levofloxacin, ofloxacin) may cause a false-positive urine screen result for opioids.

CONTRAINDICATIONS & CAUTIONS
Boxed Warning Drug is only available through a REMS program. Health care providers should complete a REMS-compliant education program and counsel patients or caregivers, with every prescription, on safe use, serious risks, storage, and disposal of these products; emphasize to patients and caregivers the importance of reading the Medication Guide every time it's provided by the pharmacist, and consider other tools to improve patient, household, and community safety. ▪

Boxed Warning Opioids should only be prescribed with benzodiazepines or other CNS depressants to patients for whom alternative treatment options are inadequate. ▪

⚠ *Alert:* Patients are at increased risk for oversedation and respiratory depression if they snore or have a history of sleep apnea, haven't used opioids recently or are first-time opioid users, have increased opioid dosage requirements or opioid habituation, have received general anesthesia for longer lengths of time or received other sedating drugs, have preexisting pulmonary or cardiac disease, or have thoracic or other surgical incisions that may impair breathing. Monitor patients carefully.

⚠ *Alert:* Drug may lead to rare but serious decrease in adrenal gland cortisol production.
• Drug may cause decreased sex hormone levels with long-term use.
• Contraindicated in patients hypersensitive to drug.
• Contraindicated in known or suspected paralytic ileus, significant respiratory depression, and acute or severe bronchial asthma.
• Use cautiously in older adults, in patients who are debilitated, and in those with head injury, increased ICP, seizures, asthma, COPD, prostatic hyperplasia, severe hepatic or renal disease, acute abdominal conditions, urethral stricture, hypothyroidism, Addison disease, and arrhythmias.

Boxed Warning Serious, life-threatening, or fatal respiratory depression may occur with use of extended-release oxycodone. Monitor patient for respiratory depression, especially during initiation of therapy and after a dosage increase. Crushing, dissolving, or chewing extended-release tablets can cause rapid release and absorption of a potentially fatal dose of oxycodone. ▪

Boxed Warning Accidental ingestion of even one dose of drug, especially by children, can result in a fatal oxycodone overdose. ▪

Boxed Warning Patients must be screened for increased risk of opioid abuse (personal or family history of substance abuse or mental illness) before being prescribed opioids. ▪

• Oxycodone extended-release tablets are indicated for moderate to severe pain, when an around-the-clock opioid analgesic is needed for an extended period. They aren't intended for use as as-needed analgesics.

Dialyzable drug: Unknown.

⚠ *Overdose S&S:* CNS depression, respiratory depression, apnea, flaccid skeletal muscles, bradycardia, hypotension, circulatory collapse, cardiac arrest, respiratory arrest, death.

PREGNANCY-LACTATION-REPRODUCTION
⚠ *Alert:* Carefully weigh risks and benefits of using drug during pregnancy.

Boxed Warning Prolonged use of extended-release oxycodone during pregnancy can result in neonatal opioid withdrawal syndrome, which may be life-threatening if not recognized and treated and requires management according to protocols developed by neonatology experts. If prolonged use is required, advise patient of risks and ensure appropriate treatment is available. ▪

• There are no adequate studies during pregnancy. Use only if potential benefit justifies fetal risk.
• Drug isn't recommended for use during or immediately before labor as uterine contractions may be adversely affected.
• Naloxone should be available to reverse opioid-induced respiratory depression in the neonate.
• Drug appears in human milk. Breastfeeding isn't recommended.

• Long-term opioid use may cause secondary hypogonadism, which may lead to sexual dysfunction or infertility.

NURSING CONSIDERATIONS

Boxed Warning Serious, life-threatening or fatal respiratory depression can occur. Monitor patient closely, especially within first 24 to 72 hours of starting drug and after a dosage increase. ■

Boxed Warning Routinely monitor all patients on opioids for signs and symptoms of misuse, abuse, and addiction. ■

⚕ *Alert:* Carefully monitor vital signs, pain level, respiratory status, and sedation level in all patients receiving opioids, especially those receiving IV drugs, even when given postoperatively.

• Reassess patient's level of pain at least 15 and 30 minutes after administration.

• For full analgesic effect, give drug before patient has intense pain.

• Keep opioid antagonist (naloxone) and resuscitation equipment available.

⚕ *Alert:* If patient is taking opioids with serotonergic drugs, watch for signs and symptoms of serotonin syndrome (agitation, hallucinations, rapid HR, fever, diaphoresis, shivering or shaking, muscle twitching or stiffness, trouble with coordination, nausea, vomiting, diarrhea), especially at start of treatment or with dosage increases. Signs and symptoms may occur within several hours of coadministration but may also occur later, especially after dosage increase. Discontinue opioid, serotonergic drug, or both if serotonin syndrome is suspected.

⚕ *Alert:* Monitor patient for signs and symptoms of adrenal insufficiency (nausea, vomiting, loss of appetite, fatigue, weakness, dizziness, low BP). Perform diagnostic testing if adrenal insufficiency is suspected. If adrenal insufficiency is confirmed, treat with corticosteroids and wean patient off opioids if appropriate. Discontinue corticosteroids when clinically appropriate.

• Monitor patient for signs and symptoms of decreased sex hormone levels (low libido, erectile dysfunction, amenorrhea, infertility). If signs and symptoms occur, evaluate patient and obtain lab testing.

• Patients taking extended-release form around-the-clock may need to take immediate-release form for worsening of pain

or prevention of incident or breakthrough pain.

• Single-drug oxycodone solution or tablets are especially useful for patients who shouldn't take aspirin or acetaminophen.

• Monitor circulatory and respiratory status closely, especially within the first 24 to 72 hours of initiation of therapy. Withhold dose and notify prescriber if respirations are shallow or if respiratory rate falls below 12 breaths/minute.

• Monitor patient's bladder and bowel patterns. Patient may need a stimulant laxative because drug has a constipating effect.

Boxed Warning Drug is potentially addictive, even at recommended doses, and if drug is misused. Chewing, crushing, snorting, or injecting it can lead to overdose and death. ■

• OxyCONTIN has been formulated to prevent immediate access to full-dose oxycodone by cutting, chewing, or breaking the tablet. Attempts to dissolve tablets will result in a gummy substance that can't be drawn up into a syringe or injected.

⚕ *Alert:* Don't stop drug abruptly; withdraw slowly and individualize gradual taper plan to prevent signs and symptoms of withdrawal, worsening of pain, and psychological distress in patients who are physically dependent. Refer to manufacturer's label for specific tapering instructions.

⚕ *Alert:* When tapering opioids, monitor patients closely for signs and symptoms of opioid withdrawal (restlessness, lacrimation, rhinorrhea, yawning, perspiration, chills, myalgia, mydriasis, irritability, anxiety, insomnia, backache, joint pain, weakness, abdominal cramps, anorexia, nausea, vomiting, diarrhea; increased BP or HR and increased respiratory rate), which may indicate a need to taper more slowly. Also monitor patients for suicidality, use of other substances, or changes in mood.

• *Look alike–sound alike:* Don't confuse oxycodone with hydrocodone, OxyCONTIN, or oxymorphone. Don't confuse OxyCONTIN with MS Contin or oxybutynin, or Roxicodone with Roxybond.

PATIENT TEACHING

Boxed Warning Caution patient or caregiver of patient taking an opioid with a benzodiazepine, CNS depressant, or alcohol to seek immediate medical attention if patient experiences dizziness, light-headedness, extreme

sleepiness, slowed or difficult breathing, or unresponsiveness. ■
• Advise patient to avoid alcohol during therapy.
Boxed Warning Advise patient that drug increases risk of opioid addiction, abuse, and misuse, which can lead to overdose and death. Teach patient proper use of drug. ■
• Teach patient or caregiver safe drug administration, storage, and disposal.
• Instruct patient to take drug before pain is intense.
• Explain assessment and monitoring process to patient and family. Instruct them to immediately report difficulty breathing or other signs or symptoms of a potential adverse opioid-related reaction.
• Tell patient to take drug with milk or after eating.
Boxed Warning Instruct patient or caregiver to keep drug out of the reach of children because accidental ingestion of even one dose can result in a fatal oxycodone overdose. Advise patient or caregiver that if accidental ingestion occurs, to seek emergency medical help immediately. ■
◑ *Alert:* Encourage patient to report all medications being taken, including prescription and OTC medications and supplements.
◑ *Alert:* Caution patient to immediately report symptoms of serotonin syndrome, adrenal insufficiency, and decreased sex hormone levels.
• Caution patient who is ambulatory about getting out of bed or walking. Warn outpatient to avoid driving and other hazardous activities that require mental alertness until drug's CNS effects are known.
• Inform patient that urine drug testing and review of state prescription drug monitoring program will be done periodically.
• Teach patient that naloxone is prescribed in conjunction with the opioid when treatment begins or is renewed as a preventive measure to reduce opioid overdose and death.
◑ *Alert:* Counsel patient not to discontinue opioids without first discussing with prescriber the need for a gradual tapering regimen.

SAFETY ALERT!

oxyCODONE hydrochloride-acetaminophen
oks-i-KOE-done/a-seet-a-MIN-oh-fen

Endocet, Nalocet, Percocet, Prolate

Therapeutic class: Opioid analgesics
Pharmacologic class: Opioid agonists–para-aminophenol derivatives
Controlled substance schedule: II

AVAILABLE FORMS
Oral solution: 5 mg oxycodone hydrochloride/325 mg acetaminophen, 10 mg oxycodone hydrochloride/300 mg acetaminophen per 5 mL
Tablets: 2.5 mg oxycodone hydrochloride/300 mg acetaminophen, 5 mg oxycodone hydrochloride/300 mg acetaminophen, 7.5 mg oxycodone hydrochloride/300 mg acetaminophen, 10 mg oxycodone hydrochloride/300 mg acetaminophen, 2.5 mg oxycodone hydrochloride/325 mg acetaminophen, 5 mg oxycodone hydrochloride/325 mg acetaminophen, 7.5 mg oxycodone hydrochloride/325 mg acetaminophen, 10 mg oxycodone hydrochloride/325 mg acetaminophen

INDICATIONS & DOSAGES
◑ *Alert:* Use in patients for whom alternative treatments are ineffective, not tolerated, or are inadequate.
➤ **Moderate to moderately severe pain; initial dose based on oxycodone content; maximum daily dose based on acetaminophen**
Adults: Oxycodone 2.5 to 10 mg and acetaminophen 325 mg PO every 6 hours as needed for pain. Adjust dosage based on pain severity and patient response. Maximum daily doses shouldn't exceed 60 mg oxycodone or 4 g acetaminophen.
Adjust-a-dose: Consider decreased dosage in patients with renal or hepatic impairment, chronic alcoholics, older adults, and patients overly sensitive to effects of opioids. Gradually taper dosage if therapy lasts for more than a few weeks.

ADMINISTRATION
PO
• Give without regard to food.

Reactions in bold italics are *life-threatening*. Interactions may have a *rapid onset* or a **delayed onset**.

- Give oral solution with an accurate measuring device (calibrated oral syringe or measuring cup).
- Store at room temperature.

ACTION

Oxycodone binds with opioid receptors in the CNS, altering perception of and emotional response to pain. Acetaminophen is thought to produce analgesia by inhibiting prostaglandin and other substances that sensitize pain receptors. The combination reduces pain more effectively than acetaminophen alone.

Route	Onset	Peak	Duration
PO (acetaminophen)	<1 hr	10–60 min	4–6 hr
PO (oxycodone)	10–15 min	30 min–1 hr	3–6 hr

Half-life: Acetaminophen, 1.25 to 3 hours; oxycodone, 3.5 to 4 hours.

ADVERSE REACTIONS

CNS: paresthesia, hypoesthesia, dizziness, drowsiness, fatigue, headache, dysphoria, insomnia. **CV:** peripheral edema, flushing, circulatory depression, hypotension, *shock.* **EENT:** dry mouth. **GI:** constipation, dyspepsia, nausea, vomiting, diarrhea. **GU:** dysuria. **Hematologic:** *hemolytic anemia, neutropenia, pancytopenia, thrombocytopenia.* **Hepatic:** increased liver enzyme levels. **Respiratory:** cough, *apnea, respiratory arrest,* respiratory depression. **Skin:** pruritus, erythema, erythematous dermatitis, excoriation, rash.

INTERACTIONS

Drug-drug. *Anticholinergics (atropine, dicyclomine, scopolamine):* May increase risk of paralytic ileus. Monitor patient closely.

Boxed Warning *Benzodiazepines, CNS depressants:* May cause slow or difficult breathing, sedation, and death. Avoid use together. If use together is necessary, limit dosage and duration of each drug to minimum necessary for desired effect. ∎

Beta blockers (propranolol): May inhibit acetaminophen metabolism. Use together carefully.

Boxed Warning *CYP3A4 inducers (carbamazepine, phenytoin, rifampin):* May increase oxycodone level and cause oxycodone-related adverse reactions if inducer is discontinued. Taper inducers cautiously and adjust oxycodone dosage as needed. ∎

Boxed Warning *CYP3A4 inhibitors (such as azole antifungals [ketoconazole]):* May increase oxycodone level, increase or prolong adverse effects, and cause fatal respiratory depression. Carefully monitor patient over extended period and adjust oxycodone dosage as needed. ∎

Desmopressin: May increase desmopressin-related toxicity. Monitor therapy.
General anesthetics, neuromuscular blockers: May increase CNS depression. Use together cautiously, decreasing dosage of one or both agents.
Lamotrigine, loop diuretics, zidovudine: May decrease effects of these drugs when used with acetaminophen. Use together cautiously.
Mixed opioid agonist–antagonist combinations: May decrease effects of oxycodone and precipitate withdrawal. Use together carefully.
Oral contraceptives: May decrease acetaminophen half-life. Use together cautiously.
Probenecid: May increase effectiveness of acetaminophen. Use together cautiously.

🔵 *Alert:* Serotonergic drugs (amoxapine, antiemetics [dolasetron, granisetron, ondansetron, palonosetron], antimigraine drugs, buspirone, cyclobenzaprine, dextromethorphan, linezolid, lithium, MAO inhibitors, maprotiline, methylene blue, mirtazapine, nefazodone, SSNRIs, SSRIs, TCAs, trazodone, tryptophan, vilazodone): May increase risk of serotonin syndrome. Use together cautiously and monitor patient for serotonin syndrome.

Drug-herb. *Cannabinoid-containing products, kava kava:* May enhance adverse effects of CNS depressants. Monitor therapy carefully.

🔵 *Alert: St. John's wort:* May increase risk of serotonin syndrome. May decrease oxycodone serum concentration. Use together cautiously.

Drug-lifestyle. Boxed Warning *Alcohol use:* May increase risk of profound sedation, respiratory depression, coma, and death. Don't use together. ∎

EFFECTS ON LAB TEST RESULTS

- May increase potassium, amylase, bilirubin, or liver enzyme levels.
- May increase or decrease blood glucose level.
- May decrease platelet count.
- May cause cross-reactivity with urinary assays used to detect cocaine and marijuana.

- Quinolones (levofloxacin, ofloxacin) may cause a false-positive urine screen result for opioids.
- Acetaminophen may cause false-positive result for urinary 5-hydroxyindoleacetic acid.

CONTRAINDICATIONS & CAUTIONS

Boxed Warning Drug is only available through a REMS program. Health care providers should complete a REMS-compliant education program and counsel patients or caregivers, with every prescription, on safe use, serious risks, storage, and disposal of these products; emphasize to patients and caregivers the importance of reading the Medication Guide every time it's provided by the pharmacist, and consider other tools to improve patient, household, and community safety. ∎

- Contraindicated in patients hypersensitive to components of drug and in those with significant respiratory depression, acute or severe bronchial asthma, hypercarbia, or known or suspected GI obstruction, including paralytic ileus.

Boxed Warning Acetaminophen may increase risk of acute liver failure, liver transplant, and death. Liver injury is generally associated with use of acetaminophen at doses exceeding 4,000 mg/day and the use of more than one acetaminophen-containing product. ∎

Boxed Warning Serious, life-threatening, or fatal respiratory depression may occur with use of oxycodone–acetaminophen. Monitor patient for respiratory depression, especially during initiation of therapy and after a dosage increase. ∎

Boxed Warning Accidental ingestion of even one dose of oxycodone–acetaminophen, especially by children, can result in a fatal overdose of oxycodone. ∎

Boxed Warning Patients must be screened for increased risk of opioid abuse (personal or family history of substance abuse or mental illness) before being prescribed opioids. ∎

Boxed Warning Opioids should only be prescribed with benzodiazepines or other CNS depressants to patients for whom alternative treatment options are inadequate. ∎

⚠ *Alert:* Patients are at increased risk for oversedation and respiratory depression if they snore or have a history of sleep apnea, haven't used opioids recently or are first-time opioid users, have increased opioid dosage requirements or opioid habituation, have received general anesthesia for longer lengths of time or received other sedating drugs, have preexisting pulmonary or cardiac disease, or have thoracic or other surgical incisions that may impair breathing. Monitor patients carefully.

⚠ *Alert:* May cause serious, potentially fatal skin reactions, including SJS, TEN, and acute generalized exanthematous pustulosis. Reaction may occur with first or subsequent use when acetaminophen is used as monotherapy or when it's one component of combination drug therapy. Monitor for reddening of the skin, rash, blisters, and detachment of the upper surface of the skin. Stop drug immediately if skin reaction is suspected.

⚠ *Alert:* Drug may lead to rare but serious decrease in adrenal gland cortisol production.

- Drug may cause decreased sex hormone levels with long-term use.
- Use cautiously in patients with increased sensitivity to codeine, head injury, increased ICP, intracranial lesions, seizures, alcoholism, delirium tremens, biliary disease including pancreatitis, liver disease, COPD, preexisting respiratory impairment, or cor pulmonale.
- Use cautiously in acute abdominal conditions because this drug may obscure diagnostic signs or markedly increase respiratory depression or CSF pressure.
- Use cautiously in patients who are hypotensive, in older adults, in patients who are debilitated, and in those with severe renal or hepatic impairment, hypothyroidism, urethral stricture, or Addison disease.
- Safety and effectivess in children haven't been established.

Dialyzable drug: Oxycodone, unknown; acetaminophen, unknown.

⚠ *Overdose S&S:* Oxycodone: Pinpoint pupils, respiratory depression, loss of consciousness, somnolence, stupor, coma, skeletal muscle flaccidity, cold and clammy skin, bradycardia, hypotension, apnea, circulatory collapse, cardiac arrest, death. Acetaminophen: Nausea, vomiting, diaphoresis, general malaise, hepatic necrosis, renal tubular necrosis, hypoglycemic coma, coagulation defects.

Reactions in bold italics are *life-threatening*. Interactions may have a *rapid onset* or a ***delayed onset***.

PREGNANCY-LACTATION-REPRODUCTION

⚉ *Alert:* Carefully weigh risks and benefits of using drug during pregnancy.

Boxed Warning Prolonged use of oxycodone–acetaminophen during pregnancy can result in neonatal opioid withdrawal syndrome, which may be life-threatening if not recognized and treated and requires management according to protocols developed by neonatology experts. If prolonged use is required, advise patient of risks and ensure appropriate treatment is available. ■

• Don't use immediately before labor.

• Use during breastfeeding isn't recommended.

NURSING CONSIDERATIONS

• Initiate dosing regimen for each patient individually, taking into account patient's severity of pain, patient response, prior analgesic treatment experience, and risk factors for addiction, abuse, and misuse.

⚉ *Alert:* Carefully monitor vital signs, pain level, respiratory status, and sedation level in all patients receiving opioids, especially those receiving IV drugs, even those given postoperatively.

• Keep opioid antagonist (naloxone) and resuscitation equipment available.

• The lowest effective dosage should be prescribed for the shortest period of time. Inform patients of risks and signs and symptoms of morphine toxicity.

Boxed Warning Assess patients identified as being at increased risk for abuse; drug should be prescribed with extreme care. Drug may cause physical dependence and tolerance with long-term therapy. Routinely monitor all patients using opioids for signs and symptoms of misuse, abuse, and addiction. ■

Boxed Warning Drug is potentially addictive. Chewing, crushing, dissolving, or injecting it can lead to overdose and death. ■

Boxed Warning Serious, life-threatening or fatal respiratory depression can occur. Monitor patient closely, especially within first 24 to 72 hours of starting drug and after a dosage increase. ■

Boxed Warning Accidental ingestion of even one dose of drug, especially by children, can be fatal. ■

⚉ *Alert:* If patient is taking opioids with serotonergic drugs, watch for signs and symptoms of serotonin syndrome (agitation, hallucinations, rapid HR, fever, diaphoresis, shivering or shaking, muscle twitching or stiffness, trouble with coordination, nausea, vomiting, diarrhea), especially at start of treatment and at dosage increases. Signs and symptoms may occur within several hours of coadministration but may also occur later, especially after dosage increase. Discontinue opioid, serotonergic drug, or both if serotonin syndrome is suspected.

⚉ *Alert:* Monitor patient for signs and symptoms of adrenal insufficiency (nausea, vomiting, loss of appetite, fatigue, weakness, dizziness, low BP). Perform diagnostic testing if adrenal insufficiency is suspected. If adrenal insufficiency is confirmed, treat with corticosteroids and wean patient off opioids if appropriate. Discontinue corticosteroids when clinically appropriate.

• Monitor patient for signs and symptoms of decreased sex hormone levels (low libido, erectile dysfunction, amenorrhea, infertility). If signs and symptoms occur, evaluate patient and obtain lab testing.

• Monitor patients for orthostatic hypotension.

• Monitor patients with head injury carefully. Oxycodone's effects on pupillary response and consciousness may mask worsening of neurologic status.

• Monitor patients with acute abdominal conditions closely. Drug may mask signs and symptoms in these patients.

• Observe for seizures in patients with convulsive disorders.

• Monitor bowel motility postoperatively, especially after intra-abdominal surgery.

⚉ *Alert:* Don't stop drug abruptly; withdraw slowly and individualize gradual taper plan to prevent signs and symptoms of withdrawal, worsening of pain, and psychological distress in patients who are physically dependent. Refer to manufacturer's label for specific tapering instructions.

⚉ *Alert:* When tapering opioids, monitor patients closely for signs and symptoms of opioid withdrawal (such as restlessness, lacrimation, rhinorrhea, yawning, perspiration, chills, myalgia, mydriasis, irritability, anxiety, insomnia, backache, joint pain, weakness, abdominal cramps, anorexia, nausea, vomiting, diarrhea; increased BP or HR and increased respiratory rate), which may indicate a need to taper more slowly. Also monitor patients

for suicidality, use of other substances, or changes in mood.
• **Look alike–sound alike:** Don't confuse oxycodone and acetaminophen with hydrocodone and acetaminophen. Don't confuse Percocet with Fioricet or Percodan.

PATIENT TEACHING

Boxed Warning Caution patient or caregiver of patient taking an opioid with a benzodiazepine, CNS depressant, or alcohol to seek immediate medical attention if patient experiences dizziness, light-headedness, extreme sleepiness, slowed or difficult breathing, or unresponsiveness. ∎
• Warn patient to avoid alcohol and other CNS depressants.

Boxed Warning Teach patient to look for acetaminophen on labels of all prescriptions and OTC medications being taken and to not use more than one product containing acetaminophen. Warn patient to seek medical attention if acetaminophen intake exceeds 4,000 mg/day even if feeling well. ∎

Boxed Warning Advise patient that drug increases risk of opioid addiction, abuse, and misuse which can lead to overdose and death. Teach patient proper use of drug. ∎
• Explain assessment and monitoring process to patient and family. Instruct them to immediately report difficulty breathing or other signs or symptoms of a potential adverse opioid-related reaction.

Boxed Warning Instruct patient or caregiver to keep drug out of the reach of children because accidental ingestion of even one dose can result in a fatal overdose of oxycodone. Advise patient or caregiver that if accidental ingestion occurs, to seek emergency medical help immediately. ∎
● **Alert:** Encourage patient to report all medications being taken, including prescription and OTC medications and supplements.
● **Alert:** Caution patient to immediately report signs and symptoms of serotonin syndrome, adrenal insufficiency, and decreased sex hormone levels.
● **Alert:** Warn patient to stop drug and seek medical attention immediately if rash or reaction occurs while using acetaminophen.
• Inform patient with severe hepatic or renal disease that serial blood tests will be needed.
• Advise patient not to drive a car or operate heavy machinery while taking this drug.

Boxed Warning Caution patient that oxycodone may be habit-forming and to take drug only as long as prescribed in the amounts prescribed. Advise patient that if drug is taken for more than a few weeks, it should be tapered off gradually. ∎
• Caution patient who is breastfeeding not to use drug because it can cause morphine toxicity (sleepiness, difficulty breastfeeding, breathing difficulties, limpness) in infants.
• Inform patient that urine drug testing and review of state prescription drug monitoring program will be done periodically.
• Teach patient that naloxone is prescribed in conjunction with the opioid when treatment begins or is renewed as a preventive measure to reduce opioid overdose and death.
● **Alert:** Counsel patient not to discontinue opioids without first discussing with prescriber the need for a gradual tapering regimen.

SAFETY ALERT!

oxyMORphone hydrochloride
oks-i-MOR-fone

Therapeutic class: Opioid analgesics
Pharmacologic class: Opioids
Controlled substance schedule: II

AVAILABLE FORMS
Tablets (extended-release): 5 mg, 7.5 mg, 10 mg, 15 mg, 20 mg, 30 mg, 40 mg
Tablets (immediate-release): 5 mg, 10 mg

INDICATIONS & DOSAGES
Adjust-a-dose (for all indications): For older adults or patients with mild hepatic impairment or CrCl less than 50 mL/minute, start with the lowest possible dose and slowly increase as tolerated. For patients receiving CNS depressants, begin at one-third to one-half of usual dose.

Refer to manufacturer's product information for instructions about converting to immediate-release tablets from other opioids and extended-release formulation.
● **Alert:** Use in patients for whom alternative treatments are ineffective, not tolerated, or inadequate.
➤ **Acute pain severe enough to require an opioid analgesic and for which alternative treatments are inadequate**

Reactions in bold italics are *life-threatening*. Interactions may have a *rapid onset* or a ***delayed onset***.

Adults: In patients who are opioid-naive, 5 to 10 mg immediate-release PO every 4 to 6 hours. Adjust dosage based on patient response.

➤ **Chronic pain**
Adults: 5 mg extended-release PO every 12 hours. Adjust dosage based on patient response.

ADMINISTRATION
PO
• Give 1 hour before or 2 hours after a meal.
Boxed Warning Patient should swallow extended-release tablets whole. Don't break, crush, dissolve, or allow patient to chew tablets, which can cause rapid release and can be fatal. ∎

ACTION
May bind with opioid receptors in the CNS, altering perception of and emotional response to pain.

Route	Onset	Peak	Duration
PO	Varies	Varies	Varies

Half-life: Immediate-release, 7 to 9 hours; extended-release, 9 to 11 hours.

ADVERSE REACTIONS
CNS: clouded sensorium, dizziness, euphoria, headache, sedation, drowsiness, somnolence, fatigue, lethargy, *seizures,* dysphoria, light-headedness, hallucinations, physical dependence, fever, confusion, anxiety, insomnia, depression. **CV:** hypotension, HTN, *bradycardia,* palpitations, tachycardia, flushing, edema. **EENT:** blurred vision, diplopia, miosis, dry mouth. **GI:** constipation, nausea, vomiting, diarrhea, ileus, abdominal pain, decreased appetite, dyspepsia, flatulence. **GU:** urine retention. **Metabolic:** dehydration, weight loss. **Respiratory:** dyspnea, *respiratory depression, laryngeal edema, bronchospasm.* **Skin:** diaphoresis, pruritus.

INTERACTIONS
Drug-drug. *Agonist or antagonist analgesics (mixed or partial):* May reduce analgesic effect or precipitate withdrawal symptoms. Don't use together.
Anticholinergics: May increase risk of urine retention or severe constipation, leading to paralytic ileus. Monitor patient for abdominal pain or distention.

Boxed Warning *Benzodiazepines, CNS depressants:* May cause slow or difficult breathing, sedation, and death. Avoid use together. If use together is necessary, limit dosage and duration of each drug to minimum necessary for desired effect. ∎
Cimetidine: May increase CNS reactions. Monitor patient closely.
Eluxadoline: May increase constipation. Avoid combination.
MAO inhibitors: May cause severe opioid potentiation. Don't use opioids if patient has received MAO inhibitors within 14 days. Avoid combination.
Propofol: May increase bradycardia risk. Monitor ECG closely.
Alert: *Serotonergic drugs (amoxapine, antiemetics [dolasetron, granisetron, ondansetron, palonosetron], antimigraine drugs, buspirone, cyclobenzaprine, dextromethorphan, linezolid, lithium, MAO inhibitors, maprotiline, methylene blue, mirtazapine, nefazodone, SSNRIs, SSRIs, TCAs, trazodone, tryptophan, vilazodone):* May increase risk of serotonin syndrome. Use together cautiously and monitor patient for serotonin syndrome.
Drug-herb. *Cannabinoid-containing products, kava kava:* May enhance adverse effects of CNS depressants. Monitor therapy closely.
Alert: *St. John's wort:* May increase risk of serotonin syndrome. Use together cautiously and monitor patient for serotonin syndrome.
Drug-lifestyle. Boxed Warning *Alcohol use:* Alcoholic beverages or medications containing alcohol may cause additive effects and result in a potentially fatal oxymorphone overdose. Don't use together. ∎

EFFECTS ON LAB TEST RESULTS
• May increase amylase and lipase levels.
• Some quinolones (most consistently levofloxacin and ofloxacin) may produce false-positive urine screening results for opioids using commercially available immunoassay kits.

CONTRAINDICATIONS & CAUTIONS
Boxed Warning Drug is only available through a REMS program. Health care providers should complete a REMS-compliant education program and counsel patients or caregivers, with every prescription, on safe use, serious risks, storage, and disposal of these products; emphasize to patients

and caregivers the importance of reading the Medication Guide every time it's provided by the pharmacist, and consider other tools to improve patient, household, and community safety. ■

• Contraindicated in patients hypersensitive to drug; in those with acute or severe bronchial asthma in an unmonitored setting or in the absence of resuscitative equipment, severe respiratory depression, upper airway obstruction, or GI obstruction, including paralytic ileus; and in those with moderate to severe hepatic impairment. ■

Boxed Warning Opioids should only be prescribed with benzodiazepines or other CNS depressants to patients for whom alternative treatment options are inadequate. ■

Boxed Warning Accidental ingestion of even one dose of oxymorphone, especially by children, can result in a fatal oxymorphone overdose. ■

Boxed Warning Patients must be screened for increased risk of opioid abuse (personal or family history of substance abuse or mental illness) before being prescribed opioids. ■

○ *Alert:* Drug may lead to rare but serious decrease in adrenal gland cortisol production.

• Drug may cause decreased sex hormone levels with long-term use.

○ *Alert:* Patients are at increased risk for oversedation and respiratory depression if they snore or have a history of sleep apnea, haven't used opioids recently or are first-time opioid users, have increased opioid dosage requirements or opioid habituation, have received general anesthesia for longer lengths of time or received other sedating drugs, have preexisting pulmonary or cardiac disease, or have thoracic or other surgical incisions that may impair breathing. Monitor patients carefully.

• Use cautiously in older adults, in patients who are debilitated, and in those with head injury, increased ICP, seizures, asthma, COPD, acute abdominal conditions, biliary tract disease (including pancreatitis), acute alcoholism, delirium tremens, prostatic hyperplasia, renal or mild hepatic impairment, urethral stricture, respiratory depression, hypothyroidism, Addison disease, and arrhythmias.

Dialyzable drug: Unknown.

⚠ *Overdose S&S:* Miosis, CNS depression, respiratory depression, apnea, flaccid skeletal muscles, bradycardia, hypotension, circulatory collapse, cardiac arrest, respiratory arrest, death.

PREGNANCY-LACTATION-REPRODUCTION

• Opioids cross the placental barrier. During pregnancy, use minimum effective dose and only if benefit justifies fetal risk.

• Use cautiously during labor as uterine contractions and fetal HR may be affected.

Boxed Warning Prolonged use of oxymorphone during pregnancy can result in neonatal opioid withdrawal syndrome, which may be life-threatening if not recognized and treated and requires management according to protocols developed by neonatology experts. If drug is used for a prolonged period during pregnancy, advise patient of risk of withdrawal and ensure appropriate treatment will be available. ■

○ *Alert:* Use cautiously during breastfeeding. Use the lowest dose for the shortest duration of time, and only if drug is needed. Monitor infants for apnea and sedation.

NURSING CONSIDERATIONS

• Keep opioid antagonist (naloxone) and resuscitation equipment available.

Boxed Warning Monitor circulatory and respiratory status closely, especially within the first 24 to 72 hours of initiation of therapy or after a dosage increase. Withhold dose and notify prescriber for signs or symptoms of respiratory depression. ■

Boxed Warning Assess patients identified as being at increased risk for abuse; drug should be prescribed with extreme care. Drug may cause physical dependence and tolerance with long-term use. Routinely monitor all patients using opioids for signs and symptoms of misuse, abuse, and addiction. ■

Boxed Warning Drug is potentially addictive. Chewing, crushing, snorting, or injecting it can lead to overdose and death. ■

○ *Alert:* Carefully monitor vital signs, pain level, respiratory status, and sedation level in all patients receiving opioids.

○ *Alert:* If patient is taking opioids with serotonergic drugs, watch for signs and symptoms of serotonin syndrome (agitation, hallucinations, rapid HR, fever, diaphoresis, shivering or shaking, muscle twitching or stiffness, trouble with coordination, nausea, vomiting, diarrhea), especially at start of treatment or after dosage increases. Signs and symptoms may occur within several hours of

---

Reactions in bold italics are *life-threatening*. Interactions may have a *rapid onset* or a *delayed onset*.

coadministration but may also occur later, especially after dosage increase. Discontinue opioid, serotonergic drug, or both if serotonin syndrome is suspected.

◑ *Alert:* Monitor patient for signs and symptoms of adrenal insufficiency (nausea, vomiting, loss of appetite, fatigue, weakness, dizziness, low BP). Perform diagnostic testing if adrenal insufficiency is suspected. If adrenal insufficiency is confirmed, treat with corticosteroids and wean patient off opioids if appropriate. Discontinue corticosteroids when clinically appropriate.

• Monitor patient for signs and symptoms of decreased sex hormone levels (low libido, erectile dysfunction, amenorrhea, infertility). If signs and symptoms occur, evaluate patient and obtain lab testing.

• Use of this drug may worsen gallbladder pain.

• Drug isn't for mild pain. For better effect, give drug before patient has intense pain.

• Monitor bladder and bowel function. Patient may need a stimulant laxative.

◑ *Alert:* Closely monitor neonate whose mother received opioid analgesics during labor for signs and symptoms of respiratory depression. A specific opioid antagonist, such as naloxone or nalmefene, should be available for reversal of opioid-induced respiratory depression in a neonate.

◑ *Alert:* Don't stop drug abruptly; withdraw slowly and individualize gradual taper plan to prevent signs and symptoms of withdrawal, worsening of pain, and psychological distress in patients who are physically dependent. Refer to manufacturer's label for specific tapering instructions.

◑ *Alert:* When tapering opioids, monitor patients closely for signs and symptoms of opioid withdrawal (such as restlessness, lacrimation, rhinorrhea, yawning, perspiration, chills, myalgia, mydriasis, irritability, anxiety, insomnia, backache, joint pain, weakness, abdominal cramps, anorexia, nausea, vomiting, diarrhea; increased BP or HR and increased respiratory rate), which may indicate a need to taper more slowly. Also monitor patients for suicidality, use of other substances, or changes in mood.

• *Look alike–sound alike:* Don't confuse oxymorphone with hydromorphone, oxymetholone, or oxycodone.

PATIENT TEACHING

◑ *Alert:* Encourage patient to report all medications being taken, including prescription and OTC medications and supplements.

◑ *Alert:* Caution patient to immediately report signs and symptoms of serotonin syndrome, adrenal insufficiency, and decreased sex hormone levels.

• Instruct patient to ask for drug before pain is intense.

• Explain the assessment and monitoring process to patient and family. Instruct them to immediately report difficulty breathing or other signs of a potential adverse opioid-related reaction.

Boxed Warning Caution patient or caregiver of patient taking an opioid with a benzodiazepine, CNS depressant, or alcohol to seek immediate medical attention if patient experiences dizziness, light-headedness, extreme sleepiness, slowed or difficult breathing, or unresponsiveness. ∎

Boxed Warning Inform patient that the use of oxymorphone, even when taken as recommended, can result in addiction, abuse, and misuse, which can lead to overdose or death. ∎

• Instruct patient not to share oxymorphone with others and to take steps to protect oxymorphone from theft or misuse.

• Caution patient who is ambulatory about getting out of bed or walking. Warn outpatient to avoid driving and other hazardous activities that require mental alertness until drug's CNS effects are known.

Boxed Warning Caution patient not to consume alcohol or take any prescription or OTC drug containing alcohol with oral form as this can lead to an overdose. ∎

• Tell patient to take tablets 1 hour before or 2 hours after a meal.

Boxed Warning Advise patient to swallow ER tablets whole and not to break, crush, dissolve, or chew them. ∎

Boxed Warning Instruct patient to keep tablets in a child-resistant container and in a safe place out of the reach of children. Accidental ingestion of even one dose by a child can result in death. In case of accidental ingestion, seek emergency medical help immediately. ∎

• Teach patient that naloxone is prescribed in conjunction with the opioid when treatment begins or is renewed as a preventive measure to reduce opioid overdose and death.

⚫ *Alert:* Counsel patient not to discontinue opioids without first discussing with prescriber the need for a gradual tapering regimen.

SAFETY ALERT!

oxytocin (synthetic injection)
oks-i-TOE-sin

Pitocin

Therapeutic class: Oxytocics
Pharmacologic class: Exogenous hormones

AVAILABLE FORMS
Injection: 10 units/mL

INDICATIONS & DOSAGES
➤ **To induce or stimulate labor**
Adults: Initially, 0.5 to 1 milliunit/minute IV infusion. Increase rate by 1 to 2 milliunits/minute at 30- to 60-minute intervals until normal contraction pattern is established. Decrease rate when labor is firmly established. Rates exceeding 9 to 10 milliunits/minute are rarely required.
➤ **To reduce postpartum bleeding after expulsion of placenta**
Adults: 10 to 40 units IV infused at rate needed to sustain uterine contraction and control uterine atony. Also, may give 10 units IM after delivery of placenta.
➤ **Incomplete, inevitable, or elective abortion**
Adults: 10 units IV infusion at 10 to 20 milliunits (20 to 40 drops)/minute. Don't exceed 30 units in 12 hours.

ADMINISTRATION
IV
▼ Never give drug simultaneously by more than one route.
▼ To induce or stimulate labor, dilute drug by adding 10 units to 1 L of NSS or lactated Ringer solution.
▼ To produce intense uterine contractions and reduce postpartum bleeding, dilute drug by adding 10 to 40 units to 1,000 mL of NSS or lactated Ringer solution.
▼ To treat abortion, add 10 units to 500 mL NSS or D₅W.

▼ Don't give bolus injection; use an infusion pump. Give drug only by piggyback infusion so that it may be stopped without interrupting IV line.
▼ **Incompatibilities:** None listed by manufacturer. Consult a drug incompatibility reference for more information.
IM
● Drug isn't recommended for routine IM use, but 10 units may be given IM after delivery of placenta to control postpartum uterine bleeding.
● Never give drug simultaneously by more than one route.

ACTION
Causes potent and selective stimulation of uterine and mammary gland smooth muscle.

Route	Onset	Peak	Duration
IV	1 min	Unknown	1 hr
IM	3–5 min	Unknown	2–3 hr

Half-life: 1 to 6 minutes.

ADVERSE REACTIONS
Maternal
CNS: *subarachnoid hemorrhage, seizures, coma.* **CV:** *arrhythmias,* HTN, PVCs, hypotension, tachycardia. **GI:** nausea, vomiting. **GU:** *abruptio placentae,* tetanic uterine contractions, *postpartum hemorrhage, uterine rupture,* impaired uterine blood flow, pelvic hematoma, increased uterine motility. **Hematologic:** *afibrinogenemia, possibly related to postpartum bleeding, pelvic hematoma.* **Other:** *anaphylaxis, death from oxytocin-induced water intoxication,* hypersensitivity reactions.
Fetal or neonate
CNS: *brain damage, seizures.* **CV:** *bradycardia, arrhythmias,* PVCs. **EENT:** neonatal retinal hemorrhage. **Hepatic:** neonatal jaundice. **Other:** *low Apgar scores at 5 minutes, death.*

INTERACTIONS
Drug-drug. *Carboprost tromethamine:* May enhance adverse effect of oxytocin. Avoid combination.
Cyclopropane anesthetics: May cause less pronounced bradycardia and hypotension. Use together cautiously.

Reactions in bold italics are *life-threatening*. Interactions may have a *rapid onset* or a ***delayed onset***.

Dinoprostone: May enhance oxytocic effects of oxytocin. Concomitant use isn't recommended. If used sequentially, monitor uterine activity closely. Administer oxytocin 30 minutes after removing dinoprostone vaginal insert and 6 to 12 hours after application of dinoprostone gel.

Drugs that prolong QT interval (azithromycin, clofazimine, ondansetron): May increase risk of life-threatening cardiac arrhythmias, including torsades de pointes. Use together cautiously.

Misoprostol: May increase oxytocin adverse effects. Don't use together.

Vasoconstrictors: May cause severe HTN if oxytocin is given within 3 to 4 hours of vasoconstrictor in patient receiving caudal block anesthetic. Avoid using together.

EFFECTS ON LAB TEST RESULTS
None reported.

CONTRAINDICATIONS & CAUTIONS
• Contraindicated in patients hypersensitive to drug.
• Contraindicated when vaginal delivery isn't advised (placenta previa, vasa previa, invasive cervical carcinoma, genital herpes), when cephalopelvic disproportion is present, or when delivery requires conversion, as in transverse lie.
• Contraindicated in fetal distress when delivery isn't imminent, in prematurity, in other obstetric emergencies, and in patients with severe toxemia or hypertonic uterine patterns.
• Use cautiously, if at all, in patients with invasive cervical cancer and in those with previous cervical or uterine surgery (including cesarean section), grand multiparity, uterine sepsis, traumatic delivery, or overdistended uterus.
❸ *Alert:* May cause antidiuretic effect and risk of severe water intoxication, seizures, or death, particularly with large doses or when given by slow infusion over 24 hours and if patient is receiving fluids by mouth.
Dialyzable drug: Unknown.
⚠ *Overdose S&S:* Uterine hypersensitivity, tumultuous labor, uterine rupture, cervical and vaginal lacerations, postpartum hemorrhage, uteroplacental hypoperfusion, variable deceleration of fetal HR, fetal hypoxia, hypercapnia, perinatal hepatic necrosis, water intoxication, seizures, death.

PREGNANCY-LACTATION-REPRODUCTION
Boxed Warning Drug is only indicated for the medical, rather than the elective, induction of labor. ∎
• Use cautiously during first and second stages of labor because uterine hypertonicity, tetanic contraction, cervical laceration, uterine rupture, and maternal and fetal death have been reported.
• Drug wouldn't be expected to cause fetal abnormalities when used as indicated. Use cautiously during pregnancy or breastfeeding. Administration of exogenous oxytocin may disrupt initiation of breastfeeding.

NURSING CONSIDERATIONS
❸ *Alert:* All patients receiving oxytocin IV must be under continuous observation by trained personnel who have a thorough knowledge of the drug and are qualified to identify complications.
❸ *Alert:* Discontinue oxytocin infusion immediately if uterine hyperactivity or fetal distress occurs. Administer oxygen to the mother. Mother and fetus must be evaluated by the responsible physician.
• Drug is used to induce or reinforce labor only when pelvis is known to be adequate, when vaginal delivery is indicated, when fetal maturity is assured, and when fetal position is favorable. Use drug only in hospital where critical care facilities and prescriber are immediately available.
• Monitor fluid intake and output. Antidiuretic effect may lead to fluid overload, seizures, and coma from water intoxication.
• Monitor and record uterine contractions, HR, BP, intrauterine pressure, fetal HR, and character of blood loss at least every 15 minutes.

PATIENT TEACHING
• Explain use and administration of drug to patient and family.
• Instruct patient to promptly report adverse reactions (site irritation, nausea, bleeding, blurred vision, difficulty speaking, wheezing, itching, swelling, heartbeat that doesn't feel normal, trouble passing urine, bad belly pain, or weakness on one side of the body).

PACLitaxel (conventional)
pac-li-TAKS-el

Therapeutic class: Antineoplastics
Pharmacologic class: Taxoids

AVAILABLE FORMS
Injection: 6 mg/mL in 5-mL, 16.7-mL, 25-mL, 50-mL vials

INDICATIONS & DOSAGES
Adjust-a-dose (for all indications): Refer to manufacturer's instructions for toxicity-related and hepatic impairment dosage adjustments and management. Treatment isn't recommended if transaminase levels are $10 \times$ ULN or greater or bilirubin levels are greater than $5 \times$ ULN for 3-hour infusion, or if transaminase levels are $10 \times$ ULN or greater or bilirubin levels are greater than 7.5 mg/dL for 24-hour infusion.

➤ **AIDS-related Kaposi sarcoma**
Adults: 135 mg/m² IV over 3 hours every 3 weeks, or 100 mg/m² IV over 3 hours every 2 weeks.
Adjust-a-dose: Reduce dexamethasone dose for premedication to 10 mg PO.

➤ **First-line and subsequent therapy for advanced ovarian cancer**
Adults (previously untreated): 175 mg/m² IV over 3 hours every 3 weeks, followed by cisplatin 75 mg/m²; or 135 mg/m² IV over 24 hours every 3 weeks, followed by cisplatin 75 mg/m² every 3 weeks.
Adults (previously treated): 135 or 175 mg/m² IV over 3 hours every 3 weeks.

➤ **Metastatic or relapsed breast cancer**
Adults: 175 mg/m² IV over 3 hours every 3 weeks.

➤ **Adjuvant treatment of node-positive breast cancer**
Adults: 175 mg/m² IV over 3 hours every 3 weeks for four cycles given after completion of a doxorubicin-containing combination chemotherapy.

➤ **First treatment of advanced NSCLC in patients who aren't candidates for curative surgery or radiation**
Adults: 135 mg/m² IV infusion over 24 hours, followed by cisplatin 75 mg/m². Repeat cycle every 3 weeks.

ADMINISTRATION
IV
⚠ *Alert:* Preparing and giving drug may be mutagenic, teratogenic, or carcinogenic. Follow institutional safe handling and disposal policies to reduce risks.

Boxed Warning To reduce risk or severity of hypersensitivity, patients must receive pretreatment with antihistamines and corticosteroids. Both H_1-receptor antagonists such as diphenhydramine and H_2-receptor antagonists, such as famotidine or cimetidine, may be used. Fatal reactions have occurred despite premedication. ∎

▼ Prepare and store infusion solutions in glass containers or polypropylene bottles, or use polypropylene or polyolefin bags. Undiluted concentrate shouldn't contact polyvinyl chloride IV bags or tubing.

▼ Dilute concentrate before infusion. Compatible solutions include NSS for injection, D_5W, 5% dextrose in NSS for injection, and 5% dextrose in lactated Ringer injection. Dilute to yield 0.3 to 1.2 mg/mL. Diluted solutions are stable for 27 hours at room temperature. Prepared solution may appear hazy.

▼ Give through polyethylene-lined administration sets, and use an in-line 0.22-micron filter.

⚠ *Alert:* Watch for irritation and infiltration; extravasation can cause tissue damage and necrosis. Administration of hyaluronidase may be needed.

▼ Closely monitor patient and vital signs during infusion, especially during the first hour.

⚠ *Alert:* When indicated, cisplatin dose should follow paclitaxel dose.

▼ **Incompatibilities:** Y-site incompatibilities: amiodarone, amphotericin B cholesteryl sulfate, amphotericin conventional, amphotericin B liposomal, chlorpromazine, diazepam, digoxin, gemtuzumab ozogamicin, hydroxyzine, idarubicin, indomethacin, labetalol, methylprednisolone sodium succinate, phenytoin, propranolol. Consult a drug incompatibility reference for additional information.

ACTION
Prevents depolymerization of cellular microtubules, inhibiting normal reorganization of microtubule network needed for mitosis and other vital cellular functions.

Reactions in bold italics are *life-threatening*. Interactions may have a *rapid onset* or a ***delayed onset***.

Route	Onset	Peak	Duration
IV	Unknown	Unknown	Unknown

Half-life: 13.1 to 52.7 hours.

ADVERSE REACTIONS

CNS: peripheral neuropathy, asthenia, fever. **CV:** *bradycardia,* tachycardia, HTN, hypotension, edema, flushing, abnormal ECG, *arrhythmias,* syncope, *venous thrombosis.* **GI:** nausea, vomiting, diarrhea, mucositis. **Hematologic:** *neutropenia, leukopenia, thrombocytopenia,* anemia, *bleeding.* **Hepatic:** elevated LFT values. **Musculoskeletal:** myalgia, arthralgia. **Respiratory:** dyspnea. **Skin:** alopecia, rash, injection-site reaction, nail changes. **Other:** hypersensitivity reactions, *anaphylaxis,* infections.

INTERACTIONS

Drug-drug. *Cisplatin:* May cause additive myelosuppressive effects. Give paclitaxel before cisplatin to increase paclitaxel clearance. *CYP2C8 and CYP3A4 inducers (carbamazepine, phenobarbital):* May decrease paclitaxel serum concentration. Monitor therapy. *CYP2C8 and CYP3A4 inhibitors (clarithromycin, cyclosporine, dexamethasone, diazepam, etoposide, felodipine,* **ketoconazole,** *quinidine, retinoic acid, teniposide, testosterone, verapamil, vincristine):* May increase paclitaxel level. Monitor patient for toxicity. *Doxorubicin:* May increase plasma levels of doxorubicin and its active metabolite, doxorubicinol. Use together cautiously. *Live-virus vaccines:* May increase risk of vaccine-induced adverse reactions. Use together isn't recommended. Patients with malignancies who are in remission can receive live-virus vaccines 3 months after completion of chemotherapy.

EFFECTS ON LAB TEST RESULTS

• May increase ALP, ALT, AST, and bilirubin levels.
• May decrease Hb level and neutrophil, WBC, and platelet counts.

CONTRAINDICATIONS & CAUTIONS

• Contraindicated in patients hypersensitive to drug or other drugs formulated with polyoxyethylated castor oil.

Boxed Warning Patients who experience hypersensitivity reactions shouldn't be rechallenged with drug. ■

Boxed Warning Contraindicated in those with baseline neutrophil counts below 1,500/mm³ and platelet counts below 100,000/mm³, or in those with AIDS-related Kaposi sarcoma with baseline neutrophil counts below 1,000/mm³. ■

• Use cautiously in patients with hepatic impairment.
• Use cautiously in older adults, who may be at higher risk for severe adverse effects.
• Safety and effectiveness in children haven't been determined.

Dialyzable drug: No.

⚠ *Overdose S&S:* Bone marrow suppression, sensory neurotoxicity, mucositis, acute ethanol toxicity (in children), CNS toxicity (in children).

PREGNANCY-LACTATION-REPRODUCTION

• Drug may cause fetal harm. Patients should avoid pregnancy during therapy. Men shouldn't father a child during therapy.
• Drug may appear in human milk. Patient should discontinue breastfeeding or discontinue drug.

NURSING CONSIDERATIONS

Boxed Warning Administer drug under the supervision of a prescriber experienced with cancer chemotherapeutic agents and only when adequate diagnostic and treatment facilities are readily available to manage complications. ■

• Patient may experience peripheral neuropathies, which may be cumulative and dose related. Patients with severe symptoms may need dosage reduction.

Boxed Warning Monitor blood counts before and during therapy. Bone marrow toxicity is the most common and dose-limiting toxicity. Institute bleeding precautions, as indicated. ■

• Monitor vital signs closely during infusion, especially during the first hour.
• Monitor infusion site for extravasation.
• If patient develops significant cardiac conduction abnormalities, use indicated therapy and continuous cardiac monitoring during therapy and subsequent infusions.
• *Look alike–sound alike:* Don't confuse paclitaxel with paroxetine or with paclitaxel protein-bound particles.

P

♣Canada ◇OTC ◆ Off-label use ✐ Photoguide ⓒ Do not crush *Liquid contains alcohol ▧ Genetic

PATIENT TEACHING

- Advise patient to report any pain or burning at site of injection.
- Urge patient to report fever, sore throat, fatigue, easy bruising, nosebleeds, bleeding gums, or melena. Tell patient to take temperature daily.
- Instruct patient to immediately report trouble breathing; swelling of the face, lips, tongue, or throat; trouble swallowing; hives; or rash.
- Teach patient to report tingling or burning sensation or numbness in limbs immediately.
- Warn patient that reversible hair loss will probably occur.
- Caution patient of childbearing potential to avoid pregnancy or breastfeeding during therapy. Recommend consulting prescriber before becoming pregnant.
- Counsel male patient not to father a child during therapy.

SAFETY ALERT!

PACLitaxel protein-bound particles

pac-li-TAKS-el

Abraxane

Therapeutic class: Antineoplastics
Pharmacologic class: Taxoids

AVAILABLE FORMS

Lyophilized powder for injection: 100 mg in single-use vials

INDICATIONS & DOSAGES

➤ **Metastatic breast cancer after failure of combination chemotherapy or relapse within 6 months of adjuvant chemotherapy (previous therapy should have included an anthracycline unless clinically contraindicated at the time)**
Adults: 260 mg/m^2 IV over 30 minutes every 3 weeks.
Adjust-a-dose: For patients with moderate hepatic impairment (serum bilirubin level greater than 1.5 to 3 × ULN and AST level less than 10 × ULN) and patients with severe hepatic impairment (serum bilirubin level greater than 3 to 5 × ULN and AST level less than 10 × ULN), recommended dosage is 200 mg/m^2/dose initially; may increase dosage to 260 mg/m^2/dose in subsequent

courses if patient tolerates reduced dosage for two cycles. Don't give to patients with very severe hepatic impairment (serum bilirubin level more than 5 × ULN or AST level more than 10 × ULN).
Refer to manufacturer's instructions for toxicity-related dosage adjustments.
➤ **NSCLC as first-line treatment in combination with carboplatin in patients who aren't candidates for curative surgery or radiation therapy**
Adults: 100 mg/m^2 IV over 30 minutes on days 1, 8, and 15 of each 21-day cycle. Give carboplatin immediately after paclitaxel protein-bound particles dose on day 1 of each 21-day cycle. Refer to manufacturer's instructions for carboplatin dosage.
Adjust-a-dose: For patients with moderate hepatic impairment (serum bilirubin level greater than 1.5 to 3 × ULN and AST level less than 10 × ULN) and severe hepatic impairment (serum bilirubin level greater than 3 to 5 × ULN and AST level less than 10 × ULN), recommended dosage is 80 mg/m^2/dose; may increase dosage to 100 mg/m^2/dose in subsequent courses if patient tolerates reduced dosage for two cycles. Don't give to patients with very severe hepatic impairment (serum bilirubin level more than 5 × ULN or AST level more than 10 × ULN).
Refer to manufacturer's instructions for toxicity-related dosage adjustments.
➤ **Metastatic pancreatic adenocarcinoma as first-line treatment in combination with gemcitabine**
Adults: 125 mg/m^2 IV over 30 to 40 minutes on days 1, 8, and 15 of each 28-day cycle. Give gemcitabine IV immediately after each paclitaxel dose. Refer to manufacturer's instructions for gemcitabine dosage.
Adjust-a-dose: Drug isn't recommended for patients with serum bilirubin level greater than 1.5 and AST level less than 10 × ULN; or very severe hepatic impairment with serum bilirubin level more than 5 × ULN or AST level more than 10 × ULN.
Refer to manufacturer's instructions for toxicity-related dosage adjustments.

ADMINISTRATION

IV
⚠️ *Alert:* Hazardous drug; use safe handling and disposal precautions.

Reactions in bold italics are *life-threatening*. Interactions may have a *rapid onset* or a ***delayed onset***.

▼ Reconstitute the vial with 20 mL of NSS to yield 5 mg/mL of drug. Direct the stream slowly, over at least 1 minute, onto the inside wall of the vial to avoid foaming. Let the vial sit for 5 minutes to ensure proper wetting of the powder. Gently swirl or turn the vial for at least 2 minutes until completely dissolved. If foaming occurs, let the solution stand for 15 minutes for the foam to subside. If particles are visible, gently invert the vial again to ensure complete resuspension. The solution should appear milky and uniform. Inject the correct dose into an empty polyvinyl chloride-type IV bag and use immediately.

▼ Visually inspect reconstituted suspension in IV bag for proteinaceous strands, particulate matter, or discoloration before administration; discard suspension if present.

▼ Give drug over 30 minutes (breast cancer and NSCLC) or over 30 to 40 minutes (pancreatic adenocarcinoma).

▼ The suspension for infusion, when prepared in an infusion bag, can be stored at 36° to 46° F (2° to 8° C), protected from bright light, for up to 24 hours.

▼ Store unopened vials at room temperature in the original package. Store reconstituted vials at 36° to 46° F (2° to 8° C) for up to 24 hours, protected from light.

▼ The total combined refrigerated storage time of reconstituted solution in vial and infusion bag is 24 hours. This may be followed by storage in infusion bag at ambient temperature and lighting conditions for a maximum of 4 hours.

▼ **Incompatibilities:** None listed by manufacturer. Consult a drug compatibility reference for more information.

ACTION

Prevents depolymerization of cellular microtubules, inhibiting reorganization of the microtubule network and disrupting mitosis and other vital cell functions.

Route	Onset	Peak	Duration
IV	Unknown	Unknown	Unknown

Half-life: 13 to 27 hours.

ADVERSE REACTIONS

CNS: asthenia, depression, peripheral neuropathy, headache, fatigue, sensory neuropathy, fever, dysgeusia. **CV:** abnormal ECG, edema, HTN, hypotension, *severe CV*

event, bleeding. **EENT:** visual disturbances, epistaxis. **GI:** anorexia, diarrhea, nausea, constipation, oral candidiasis, vomiting, mucositis. **GU:** increased serum creatinine level, UTI. **Hematologic:** anemia, *neutropenia, thrombocytopenia, bleeding, myelosuppression.* **Hepatic:** elevated liver enzyme levels. **Metabolic:** dehydration. **Musculoskeletal:** arthralgia, myalgia. **Respiratory:** cough, dyspnea, pneumonia, respiratory tract infection. **Skin:** alopecia, rash, injection-site reactions. **Other:** infections, hypersensitivity reactions, dehydration, *sepsis.*

INTERACTIONS

Drug-drug. *Clozapine:* May increase risk of agranulocytosis. Avoid use together.
CYP2C8 and CYP3A4 inducers: May decrease serum paclitaxel concentration. Use cautiously together.
CYP2C8 and CYP3A4 inhibitors: May increase serum paclitaxel concentration. Use cautiously together.
Live-virus vaccines: May increase vaccine-related adverse effects. Avoid use together. Don't give vaccines for at least 3 months after immunosuppressants.
Vaccines (inactivated): May diminish vaccine therapeutic effects. Monitor therapy.

EFFECTS ON LAB TEST RESULTS

• May increase ALP, AST, bilirubin, creatinine, and GGT levels.
• May decrease Hb level and neutrophil and platelet counts.

CONTRAINDICATIONS & CAUTIONS

Boxed Warning Contraindicated in patients with baseline neutrophil count of less than 1,500/mm^3. ▪

• Contraindicated in patients hypersensitive to drug or its components; severe and sometimes fatal hypersensitivity reactions can occur. Don't rechallenge patients who experience a hypersensitivity reaction.
• Use cautiously in patients hypersensitive to other taxanes; cross-hypersensitivity can occur.
• Use cautiously in patients with hepatic impairment; increased exposure and toxicity can occur.
• Use isn't recommended in patients with metastatic pancreatic adenocarcinoma who have moderate to severe hepatic impairment.
• Use hasn't been studied in patients with creatinine level less than 30 mL/minute.

• Drug contains human albumin; although rare, viruses and Creutzfeldt-Jakob disease may be transmitted.
• Safety and effectiveness in children haven't been established.
Dialyzable drug: Unknown.
⚠ *Overdose S&S:* Bone marrow suppression, sensory neurotoxicity, acute ethanol toxicity (in children), CNS toxicity (in children).

PREGNANCY-LACTATION-REPRODUCTION
• Patients of childbearing potential should avoid pregnancy during therapy and for at least 6 months after final dose. Males shouldn't father a child during therapy and for at least 3 months after final dose.
• Drug may impair fertility.
• Drug appears in human milk. Patient shouldn't breastfeed during therapy and for 2 weeks after final dose.

NURSING CONSIDERATIONS
◔ *Alert:* Give only under supervision of practitioner experienced in using chemotherapy in a facility that can manage associated complications.
◔ *Alert:* Don't substitute Abraxane for other forms of paclitaxel.
Boxed Warning Monitor CBC frequently to evaluate for neutropenia, which may be severe and may result in infection. ∎
• Don't repeat dose until neutrophil count recovers to more than 1,500/mm³ and platelet count recovers to more than 100,000/mm³.
• Obtain CBC before dosing on day 1 for metastatic breast cancer and before days 1, 8, and 15 for NSCLC or pancreatic cancer.
• If patient becomes febrile regardless of ANC, initiate treatment with broad-spectrum antibiotics.
• Watch for pneumonitis in patients receiving drug in combination with gemcitabine. Interrupt treatment for suspected pneumonitis (sudden onset of dry, persistent cough; dyspnea). For confirmed pneumonitis, permanently discontinue treatment with paclitaxel and gemcitabine.
• Assess for severe hematologic, neurologic, cutaneous, or GI toxicities, which may require dosage reductions or drug discontinuation.
• Monitor patient for hypersensitivity reactions; don't rechallenge patients with severe reactions.
• Assess patient for symptoms of sensory neuropathy and severe neutropenia.

• Monitor LFT and renal function test results.
• Monitor infusion site closely for extravasation and infiltration.
• Verify pregnancy status before treatment.

PATIENT TEACHING
• Warn patient that alopecia commonly occurs but is reversible after therapy.
• Teach patient to recognize signs of neuropathy, such as tingling, burning, and numbness in arms and legs.
• Tell patient to report signs and symptoms of infection, pneumonitis, hypersensitivity reactions, severe abdominal pain, or severe diarrhea.
• Advise patient to contact prescriber if nausea and vomiting persist or interfere with adequate nutrition. Reassure patient that an antiemetic can be prescribed.
• Explain that many patients experience weakness and fatigue, so it's important to rest.
• To reduce or prevent mouth sores, remind patient to perform proper oral hygiene.
• Tell patient to avoid pregnancy during therapy and for at least 6 months after final dose and not to breastfeed during therapy and for 2 weeks after final dose.
• Advise male patient to avoid fathering a child during therapy and for at least 3 months after final dose.
• Advise patient of reproductive potential that drug may impair fertility.

SAFETY ALERT!

palbociclib ▨
pal-boe-SYE-klib

Ibrance

Therapeutic class: Antineoplastics
Pharmacologic class: Kinase inhibitors

AVAILABLE FORMS
Capsules ⓝⓖ: 75 mg, 100 mg, 125 mg
Tablets ⓝⓖ: 75 mg, 100 mg, 125 mg

INDICATIONS & DOSAGES
➤ **Hormone receptor (HR)–positive, HER2-negative advanced or metastatic breast cancer, as initial endocrine-based therapy in men or patients who are postmenopausal, in combination with an aromatase inhibitor, or in combination with**

fulvestrant in patients with disease progression after endocrine therapy 🔬

Adults: 125 mg PO daily for 21 consecutive days followed by 7 days off to complete a cycle of 28 days. When given with an aromatase inhibitor, refer to prescribing information for the inhibitor being used. When given with fulvestrant, recommended dosage of fulvestrant is 500 mg PO on days 1, 15, and 29, and once monthly thereafter; refer to full prescribing information for fulvestrant.

Patients who are premenopausal and perimenopausal treated with the combination of palbociclib and fulvestrant should be treated with luteinizing hormone-releasing hormone (LHRH) agonists according to current standards.

For men treated with combination palbociclib plus aromatase inhibitor therapy, consider treatment with an LHRH agonist according to current clinical practice standards.

Adjust-a-dose: If concomitant use of strong CYP3A inhibitors is unavoidable, decrease palbociclib dosage to 75 mg daily. If strong inhibitor is discontinued, increase palbociclib dosage after three to five half-lives have passed from CYP3A inhibitor dose. Refer to manufacturer's instructions for toxicity-related dosage adjustments.

ADMINISTRATION
PO

🜂 *Alert:* Hazardous drug; use safe handling and disposal precautions.
- Give tablets without regard to food.
- Give capsules whole with food.
- Capsules and tablets shouldn't be crushed, chewed, or opened before they are swallowed; or ingested if they are broken, cracked, or otherwise not intact.
- If patient vomits after taking a dose or misses a dose, give the next prescribed dose at the usual time.

ACTION

Inhibits cyclin-dependent kinase 4 and 6. Reduces cellular proliferation of ER-positive breast cancer cell line by blocking progression of cell from G_1 to S phase of the cell cycle, resulting in decreased phosphorylation and decreased tumor growth.

Route	Onset	Peak	Duration
PO	N/A	4–12 hr	N/A

Half-life: 24 to 34 hours.

ADVERSE REACTIONS

CNS: asthenia, fatigue, fever, dysgeusia.
EENT: blurred vision, dry eyes, epistaxis.
GI: decreased appetite, stomatitis, nausea, diarrhea, vomiting. **Hematologic:** *neutropenia, febrile neutropenia, leukopenia,* anemia, *thrombocytopenia.* **Hepatic:** increased transaminase levels. **Skin:** alopecia, rash, dry skin. **Other:** infections.

INTERACTIONS

Drug-drug. *Alfentanil, cyclosporine, dihydroergotamine, ergotamine, everolimus, fentanyl, midazolam, pimozide, quinidine, sirolimus, tacrolimus:* May increase concentrations of these drugs. Dosages of these drugs may need to be decreased.
Strong or moderate CYP3A inducers (rifampin, phenytoin): May decrease palbociclib concentration. Avoid concurrent use.
Strong CYP3A inhibitors (clarithromycin, itraconazole): May increase palbociclib concentration. Avoid use together; if unavoidable, decrease palbociclib dosage.
Drug-herb. *St. John's wort:* May decrease palbociclib concentration. Discourage use together.
Drug-food. *Grapefruit, grapefruit juice:* May increase palbociclib concentration. Discourage use together.

EFFECTS ON LAB TEST RESULTS
- May increase ALT and AST levels.
- May decrease Hb level and WBC, neutrophil, lymphocyte, and platelet counts.

CONTRAINDICATIONS & CAUTIONS
- Contraindicated in patients hypersensitive to drug or its components.
- 🜂 *Alert:* May cause severe or fatal ILD and pneumonitis.
- May cause neutropenia and increase risk of infection.
- Drug hasn't been studied in children.
- Use cautiously in older adults, who may experience a greater sensitivity to drug's effects.
Dialyzable drug: Unknown.

PREGNANCY-LACTATION-REPRODUCTION
- Contraindicated during pregnancy due to risk of fetal harm. Patients of childbearing potential should use effective contraception during treatment and for at least 3 weeks after final dose.

P

- Patients shouldn't breastfeed during treatment and for 3 weeks after final dose.
- Male patients with partners of childbearing potential should use effective contraception during treatment and for 3 months after final dose.
- Drug may cause infertility in males. Men should consider sperm preservation before treatment.

NURSING CONSIDERATIONS
- Monitor CBC before start of therapy, at beginning of each cycle, on day 15 of first two cycles, and as clinically indicated. Interrupt therapy and adjust dosage as necessary.
- Monitor patient for myelosuppression or infection; treat appropriately.
- Verify pregnancy status before treatment.
- **Alert:** Monitor patients for new or worsening pulmonary symptoms; if they occur, interrupt therapy immediately and evaluate patient. If infection, neoplasm, and other causes are excluded, permanently discontinue treatment in patients with severe ILD or pneumonitis.

PATIENT TEACHING
- **Alert:** Warn patient to immediately report difficulty or discomfort with breathing or shortness of breath while at rest or with low activity; these may be symptoms of ILD or pneumonitis.
- Instruct patient in safe drug administration and handling.
- Teach patient to report signs and symptoms of decreased bone marrow function and infection (fever, chills, shortness of breath, weakness, abnormal bleeding or bruising).
- Instruct patient to tell prescriber of all medications being taken, including prescription and OTC drugs and herbal products.
- Caution patient to avoid grapefruit and grapefruit juice.
- Advise patient of fetal risk and to use effect contraception.
- Inform male patient of reproductive potential of infertility risk. Advise him to consider sperm preservation before treatment.

paliperidone
pal-ee-PER-i-done

Invega

paliperidone palmitate
Invega Hafyera, Invega Sustenna, Invega Trinza

Therapeutic class: Antipsychotics
Pharmacologic class: Benzisoxazole derivatives

AVAILABLE FORMS
Injection: 39 mg/0.25 mL, 78 mg/0.5 mL, 117 mg/0.75 mL, 156 mg/mL, 234 mg/1.5 mL, 273 mg/0.88 mL, 410 mg/1.32 mL, 546 mg/1.75 mL, 819 mg/2.63 mL, 1,092 mg/3.5 mL; 1,560 mg/5 mL single-dose prefilled syringe
Tablets (extended-release) ⊙: 1.5 mg, 3 mg, 6 mg, 9 mg

INDICATIONS & DOSAGES
Adjust-a-dose (for all indications): In patients with CrCl of 50 to less than 80 mL/minute, initial dosage is 3 mg PO once daily and maximum dosage is 6 mg once daily; in patients with CrCl of 10 to 49 mL/minute, initial dosage is 1.5 mg PO once daily and maximum dosage is 3 mg once daily; in patients with CrCl less than 10 mL/minute, use isn't recommended. If using injectable form (Invega Sustenna) and CrCl is 50 to less than 80 mL/minute, give 156 mg IM on day 1 and 117 mg IM 1 week later, followed by monthly injections of 78 mg IM. If using injectable 3-month form (Invega Trinza) and CrCl is 50 to less than 80 mL/minute, adjust dosage and stabilize patient using the monthly IM injection, then transition to the 3-month IM injection. Invega Trinza isn't recommended in patients with CrCl of less than 50 mL/minute.

➤ **Schizophrenia and schizoaffective disorder**
Adults: 6 mg PO once daily in the morning; may increase or decrease dose in 3-mg increments not sooner than every 4 days in schizoaffective disorder or every 5 days in schizophrenia to a range of 3 to 12 mg daily; maximum dose is 12 mg/day. Or, 234 mg IM on treatment day 1 and 156 mg IM 1 week later, both administered in deltoid muscle.

Reactions in bold italics are *life-threatening*. Interactions may have a *rapid onset* or a ***delayed onset***.

Recommended maintenance dosage is 117 mg IM monthly (range, 39 to 234 mg based on tolerability and efficacy) given in the deltoid or gluteal muscle. Adjustments may be made monthly. Maximum recommended monthly dose is 234 mg. See manufacturer's instructions for missed dosage schedules.

➤ **Schizophrenia**

Adults: Use 3-month IM paliperidone (Invega Trinza) only after monthly IM paliperidone (Invega Sustenna) has been established as adequate treatment for at least 4 months. The last two doses of monthly IM paliperidone should be the same dosage strength before starting 3-month IM paliperidone. Initiate 3-month IM paliperidone with next scheduled monthly IM paliperidone. Base 3-month dose on the previous monthly dose, using the equivalent 3.5 times higher dose. May adjust dosage of 3-month paliperidone every 3 months in increments ranging from 273 to 819 mg based on response and tolerability.

Use 6-month IM paliperidone (Invega Hafyera) only after monthly IM paliperidone (Invega Sustenna) has been established as adequate treatment for at least 4 months and at same dosage for at least 2 months, or after IM 3-month paliperidone (Invega Trinza) has been established as adequate treatment for at least one 3-month cycle. Initiate with the next scheduled once-a-month injection, or up to 1 week before or after, or with the next scheduled every-3-month injection, or up to 2 weeks before or after. Base dosage on dosage of previous product. If last dose of once-a-month product was 156 mg, give 1,092 mg of 6-month product; if last dose of once-a-month product was 234 mg, give 1,560 mg of 6-month product. If last dose of 3-month product was 546 mg, give 1,092 mg of 6-month product; if last dose of 3-month product was 819 mg, give 1,560 mg of 6-month product.

Because of long-acting nature of Invega Trinza and Invega Hafyera, patient's response to adjusted dose may not be apparent for several months. See manufacturer's instructions for missed dosage schedules.

Adolescents ages 12 to 17: Initially, 3 mg PO daily. May increase dosage by 3 mg/day every 5 days based on clinical response. Maximum dose is 12 mg/day for patients weighing 51 kg or more and 6 mg/day for patients weighing less than 51 kg.

ADMINISTRATION

PO

• Give tablet whole with or without food; don't crush or break.

IM

• Inspect for particulate matter and discoloration.

• Don't give IV or subcut.

• For Invega Sustenna, shake syringe vigorously for at least 10 seconds to ensure a homogenous suspension before administration. Only use needle provided in kit.

• For Invega Trinza, shake syringe vigorously for at least 15 seconds within 5 minutes of administration.

• For Invega Hafyera, shake syringe vigorously for at least 15 seconds, rest briefly, then shake again for 15 seconds within 5 minutes of administration.

• For Invega Trinza or Invega Hafyera, use the thin-wall needles provided. Don't use needles from the 1-month pack or other commercially available needles, to reduce the risk of blockage.

• Inject slowly and deeply into deltoid or gluteal muscle.

• Injection is for single use only. Don't administer dose in divided injections.

• Administer first two doses of Invega Sustenna into deltoid muscle. After second dose, can give monthly maintenance doses in deltoid or gluteal muscle.

• If incomplete administration occurs, don't reinject the dose remaining in the syringe. Don't administer another dose.

• Alternate injection sites at each administration.

• May give monthly or 3-month IM paliperidone maintenance doses within 7 days before or after next monthly dose date.

• Refer to manufacturer's instructions for missed dose management and switching from other antipsychotics.

• Store at room temperature.

ACTION

Exact mechanism remains unclear. May antagonize both central dopamine (D_2) and serotonin type 2 receptors, as well as alpha$_1$, alpha$_2$, and H$_1$ receptors. Drug is a major active metabolite of risperidone.

P

Route	Onset	Peak	Duration
PO	Unknown	24 hr	Unknown
IM (Sustenna)	1 day	13 days	126 days
IM (Trinza)	1 day	30–33 days	Up to 18 months
IM (Hafyera)	1 day	29–32 days	Up to 18 months

Half-life: 23 hours (oral); 25 to 49 days (IM, monthly, Sustenna); 84 to 139 days (IM, 3-month, Trinza); 148 to 159 days (IM, Hafyera).

ADVERSE REACTIONS

CNS: akathisia, headache, parkinsonism, somnolence, agitation, anxiety, asthenia, dizziness, dystonia, extrapyramidal disorder, fatigue, hypertonia, lethargy, nightmares, psychosis, fever, sedation, sleep disorder, tremor, dyskinesia, hyperkinesia, insomnia. **CV:** HTN, orthostatic hypotension, edema, palpitations, sinus arrhythmia, bradycardia, tachycardia, *AV block,* bundle-branch block. **EENT:** blurred vision, eye movement disorder, epistaxis, nasopharyngitis, rhinitis, dry mouth, salivary hypersecretion, sore throat, tongue paralysis, swollen tongue. **GI:** abdominal pain, dyspepsia, nausea, vomiting, diarrhea, constipation, increased or decreased appetite. **GU:** amenorrhea, irregular menses, galactorrhea, decreased male libido, erectile dysfunction, UTI. **Metabolic:** blood insulin increases, hyperprolactinemia, weight gain. **Musculoskeletal:** back pain, extremity pain, musculoskeletal stiffness, myalgia. **Respiratory:** cough, URI. **Skin:** pruritus, rash, injection-site reaction. **Other:** breast tenderness, gynecomastia.

INTERACTIONS

⚠️ *Alert:* Paliperidone can significantly interact with many drugs. Consult a drug interaction resource or pharmacist for additional information.

Drug-drug. *Anticholinergics:* May worsen adverse effects. Use cautiously together.

Antihypertensives, drugs that induce hypotension: May worsen orthostatic hypotension. Monitor patient closely.

Centrally acting drugs: May worsen CNS adverse effects. Use cautiously together.

Divalproex sodium, valproate: Increases paliperidone concentration. Consider paliperidone dosage reduction.

Drugs that prolong QTc interval, such as antiarrhythmics (amiodarone, procainamide, *quinidine, sotalol), antipsychotics (chlorpromazine, thioridazine), quinolone antibiotics (moxifloxacin):* May further prolong QTc interval. Avoid using together.

Levodopa, other dopamine agonists: May antagonize effects of these drugs. Use cautiously together.

Opioid agonists: Opioids may cause slow or difficult breathing, sedation, and death. Avoid use together. If use together is necessary, limit dosage and duration of each drug to minimum necessary for desired effect.

Risperidone: May increase toxic effects of paliperidone. Use alternative combination if possible.

Serotonin modulators: May increase risk of NMS and serotonin syndrome. Monitor therapy.

Strong CYP3A and P-gp inducers: May decrease paliperidone concentration. Dosage may need to be increased or decreased depending on use. Avoid using inducers with extended-release IM formulation, if possible. If inducer is necessary, consider using paliperidone extended-release tablets.

Drug-herb. *St. John's wort:* May increase serum concentration of paliperidone. Consider therapy modification.

Drug-lifestyle. *Alcohol use:* May worsen CNS side effects. Discourage use together.

EFFECTS ON LAB TEST RESULTS

• May increase blood glucose, lipid, and prolactin levels.
• May decrease HDL level.
• May decrease WBC count.

CONTRAINDICATIONS & CAUTIONS

• Contraindicated in patients hypersensitive to paliperidone or risperidone.

Boxed Warning Older adults with dementia-related psychosis treated with atypical or conventional antipsychotics are at increased risk for death. Antipsychotics aren't approved for the treatment of dementia-related psychosis. ■

• Avoid use in patients with congenital long QT syndrome or history of cardiac arrhythmias.

• Oral drug isn't recommended in patients with preexisting severe GI narrowing.

• Use cautiously in patients with a history of seizures, conditions that lower the seizure threshold, or Parkinson disease; in those at risk for aspiration pneumonia or impaired

---

Reactions in bold italics are *life-threatening*. Interactions may have a *rapid onset* or a ***delayed onset***.

temperature regulation; and in those with bradycardia, hypokalemia, hypomagnesemia, CV disease, cerebrovascular disease, dehydration, or hypovolemia, and older adults.
• Use cautiously in patients with diabetes or risk factors for diabetes (obesity, family history of diabetes).
• Use cautiously in patients with history of suicidality.
• Somnolence, orthostatic hypotension, and motor and sensory instability may lead to falls and fall-related injuries.
• Rare cases of priapism (requiring surgery) have been reported.
Dialyzable drug: Unknown.
⚠ *Overdose S&S:* Extrapyramidal symptoms, unsteady gait, drowsiness, sedation, tachycardia, hypotension, prolonged QT interval.

PREGNANCY-LACTATION-REPRODUCTION
• Use in pregnancy only if potential benefit justifies fetal risk.
• Patients exposed to drug during pregnancy should enroll in the National Pregnancy Registry for Atypical Antipsychotics (1-866-961-2388 or online at http://womensmentalhealth.org/clinical-and-research-programs/pregnancyregistry/).
◑ *Alert:* Neonates exposed to antipsychotics during the third trimester are at increased risk for developing extrapyramidal signs and symptoms and withdrawal signs and symptoms after delivery.
• Drug appears in human milk. The known benefits of breastfeeding should outweigh the unknown risks of infant's exposure to paliperidone. Monitor infants exposed to drug for sedation, failure to thrive, jitteriness, tremors, and abnormal muscle movements.
• Drug may inhibit reproductive function.

NURSING CONSIDERATIONS
• Establish tolerability with oral paliperidone or oral risperidone before initiating treatment with paliperidone injection.
◑ *Alert:* Monitor patient for atypical ventricular tachycardia, such as torsades de pointes, and ECG changes, particularly lengthening of the QT interval.
• Obtain baseline BP before starting therapy, and monitor BP regularly. Watch for orthostatic hypotension.
◑ *Alert:* Watch for evidence of NMS, a rare but deadly complication.

• Monitor patient for tardive dyskinesia; it may disappear spontaneously or persist for life despite discontinuing drug. Seek smallest dosage and shortest duration of treatment that produce a satisfactory clinical response.
◑ *Alert:* Drug may cause hyperglycemia, dyslipidemia, weight gain, and other metabolic changes. Monitor patient with diabetes regularly. In patient with risk factors for diabetes, obtain fasting blood glucose test results at baseline and periodically.
• Monitor patient for seizure activity.
• Assess patient for dysphagia.
• Monitor patient for abnormal body temperature regulation, especially if patient exercises, is exposed to extreme heat, takes anticholinergics, or becomes dehydrated.
• Monitor patient for somnolence and sedation. Antipsychotics, including paliperidone, have the potential to impair judgment, thinking, or motor skills.
• Assess fall risk at start of treatment and recurrently during long-term therapy.
• Dispense lowest appropriate quantity of drug, to reduce risk of overdose.

PATIENT TEACHING
• Advise patient to seek immediate medical care for signs and symptoms of NMS (fever, muscle rigidity, altered mental status, irregular pulse or BP, tachycardia, diaphoresis, or cardiac arrhythmia).
• Teach patient safe drug administration.
• Caution patient or caregiver of patient taking an opioid with a benzodiazepine, CNS depressant, or alcohol to seek immediate medical attention if patient experiences dizziness, light-headedness, extreme sleepiness, slowed or difficult breathing, or unresponsiveness.
• Advise patient to avoid alcohol during therapy.
• Tell patient that remains of the tablet coating may appear in feces.
• Instruct patient not to perform activities that require mental alertness until effects of drug are known.
• Advise patient that drug may cause somnolence, orthostatic hypotension, and motor and sensory instability, which may lead to falls and fall-related injuries.
• Warn patient to use caution in performing excessively strenuous activities because body temperature may be disrupted.
• Advise patient that drug may lower BP and to change positions slowly.

P

- Inform patient with a preexisting low WBC count or a history of drug-induced leukopenia or neutropenia that CBC monitoring will be needed during therapy.
- Instruct patient to seek medical attention for amenorrhea, galactorrhea, erectile dysfunction, or gynecomastia.
- Advise patient to seek medical attention for an erection lasting more than 4 hours.
- Caution patient to contact prescriber before taking other drugs, to avoid potential interactions.
- Advise patient to report pregnancy or plans to breastfeed.

palonosetron hydrochloride
pal-oh-NOE-se-tron

Therapeutic class: Antiemetics
Pharmacologic class: Selective serotonin (5-HT$_3$) receptor antagonists

AVAILABLE FORMS
Injection: 0.25 mg in 2-mL, 0.25 mg in 5-mL single-use vials; 0.25 mg in 5-mL prefilled syringe

INDICATIONS & DOSAGES
➤ **Prevention of chemotherapy-induced nausea and vomiting (moderate to highly emetogenic regimen)**
Adults: 0.25 mg given IV over 30 seconds, 30 minutes before chemotherapy starts.
➤ **Prevention of chemotherapy-induced nausea and vomiting (including highly emetogenic chemotherapy)**
Children age 1 month to younger than 17 years: Infuse 20 mcg/kg IV over 15 minutes beginning approximately 30 minutes before chemotherapy starts. Maximum dosage, 1.5 mg.
➤ **Prevention of postoperative nausea and vomiting (PONV) for up to 24 hours after surgery**
Adults: 0.075 mg IV over 10 seconds immediately before anesthesia induction.

ADMINISTRATION
IV
▼ Flush with NSS before and after injection.
▼ Inspect for particulate matter and discoloration; solution should be clear and colorless.

▼ Give by rapid IV injection through a peripheral or central IV line.
▼ Don't use prefilled syringe to give dose of less than 0.25 mg.
▼ Store at room temperature. Protect from light.
▼ **Incompatibilities:** Don't mix with other drugs.

ACTION
Antagonizes 5-HT$_3$ receptors in the GI tract and brain, which inhibits emesis caused by chemotherapy.

Route	Onset	Peak	Duration
IV	30 min	Unknown	5 days

Half-life: 40 hours (adults); 20 to 30 hours (children).

ADVERSE REACTIONS
CNS: dizziness, headache, weakness. **CV:** *bradycardia, QT-interval prolongation (PONV).* **GI:** constipation, diarrhea. **GU:** urine retention.

INTERACTIONS
Drug-drug. *Antiarrhythmics or other drugs that prolong the QTc interval, diuretics that induce electrolyte abnormalities, high-dose anthracycline:* May increase risk of prolonged QTc interval. Use together cautiously.
Apomorphine: May cause profound hypotension and loss of consciousness. Use together is contraindicated.
Fentanyl, 5-HT$_3$ receptor antagonists, IV methylene blue, lithium, MAO inhibitors, mirtazapine, SSNRIs, SSRIs, tramadol: May increase risk of serotonin syndrome. Avoid use together.

EFFECTS ON LAB TEST RESULTS
- May increase glucose, ALT, AST, and bilirubin levels.
- May increase or decrease potassium level.

CONTRAINDICATIONS & CAUTIONS
- Contraindicated in patients hypersensitive to palonosetron or its ingredients.
- Use cautiously in patients hypersensitive to other 5-HT$_3$ antagonists, in those taking drugs that affect cardiac conduction, and in those with cardiac conduction abnormalities, hypokalemia, or hypomagnesemia.
Dializable drug: Unlikely.

Reactions in bold italics are *life-threatening*. Interactions may have a *rapid onset* or a ***delayed onset***.

PREGNANCY-LACTATION-REPRODUCTION
- Use in pregnancy only if clearly needed.
- It isn't known if drug appears in human milk. Consider risk of infant exposure when deciding to discontinue breastfeeding during therapy.

NURSING CONSIDERATIONS
- Before giving this drug, check patient's potassium level.
- Consider adding corticosteroids to the antiemetic regimen, particularly for patients receiving highly emetogenic chemotherapy.
- Monitor patient for hypersensitivity reactions.
- Make sure patient has additional antiemetics for breakthrough nausea or vomiting.
- If patient has cardiac conduction abnormalities, assess ECG before giving drug.
- Monitor patient for serotonin syndrome (mental status changes with or without GI symptoms).

PATIENT TEACHING
- Instruct patient to seek immediate medical attention for signs or symptoms of hypersensitivity reaction.
- Advise patient to take a different antiemetic for breakthrough nausea or vomiting at the first sign of nausea rather than waiting until symptoms become severe.
- Inform patient of risk of serotonin syndrome and to seek immediate medical attention if signs or symptoms occur.
- Urge patient with a history of cardiac conduction abnormalities to report any changes in drug regimen, such as adding or stopping an antiarrhythmic.

---

pamidronate disodium
pa-mi-DROE-nate

Therapeutic class: Antiosteoporotics
Pharmacologic class: Bisphosphonates

AVAILABLE FORMS
Powder for injection: 30 mg/vial, 60 mg/vial, 90 mg/vial
Solution for injection: 3 mg/mL, 6 mg/mL, 9 mg/mL in 10-mL vials

INDICATIONS & DOSAGES
➤ **Moderate to severe hypercalcemia from cancer (with or without bone metastases)**

Adults: Dosage depends on severity of hypercalcemia. Correct calcium level for albumin. Corrected calcium (CCa) level is calculated using this formula:

$$\underset{\text{(mg/dL)}}{\text{CCa}} = \underset{\text{(mg/dL)}}{\text{serum calcium}} + \underset{\text{(g/dL)}}{0.8\,(4 - \text{serum albumin})}$$

Give patients with CCa levels of 12 to 13.5 mg/dL 60 to 90 mg by IV infusion as a single dose over 2 to 24 hours. Give patients with CCa levels greater than 13.5 mg/dL 90 mg by IV infusion over 2 to 24 hours. Allow at least 7 days before retreatment to permit full response to first dose.
➤ **Moderate to severe Paget disease**
Adults: 30 mg IV as a 4-hour infusion on 3 consecutive days for total dose of 90 mg. Repeat cycle as needed.
➤ **Osteolytic bone metastases of breast cancer with standard antineoplastic therapy**
Adults: 90 mg IV infusion over 2 hours every 3 to 4 weeks.
➤ **Osteolytic bone lesions of multiple myeloma**
Adults: 90 mg IV over 4 hours once monthly.

ADMINISTRATION
IV
🜂 *Alert:* Hazardous drug; use safe handling and disposal precautions.
▼ Reconstitute powder with 10 mL of sterile water for injection. After drug is completely dissolved, add to 250 mL (2-hour infusion), 500 mL (4-hour infusion), or 1,000 mL (up to 24-hour infusion) of half-NSS or NSS for injection or D_5W.
▼ Inspect solution for precipitate before use.
▼ Give drug only by IV infusion. Injecting a bolus may cause nephropathy.
▼ Infusions longer than 2 hours may reduce the risk of renal toxicity, particularly in patients with preexisting renal insufficiency.
▼ Solution remains stable for 24 hours at room temperature.
▼ Store reconstituted drug at 36° to 46° F (2° to 8° C) for up to 24 hours.
▼ **Incompatibilities:** Calcium-containing infusion solutions, such as Ringer injection. Give in a line separate from all other drugs.

ACTION
An antihypercalcemic that inhibits resorption of bone but apparently not bone formation.

Adsorbs to hydroxyapatite crystals in bone and may directly block calcium phosphate dissolution and mature osteoclast formation.

Route	Onset	Peak	Duration
IV	Unknown	Unknown	Unknown

Half-life: 21 to 35 hours.

ADVERSE REACTIONS

CNS: asthenia, fatigue, somnolence, fever, headache, psychosis, anxiety, insomnia, drowsiness, syncope, pain. **CV:** atrial fibrillation/flutter, tachycardia, HTN, edema, fluid overload, HF. **EENT:** sinusitis, rhinitis. **GI:** abdominal pain, anorexia, dyspepsia, constipation, diarrhea, nausea, stomatitis, vomiting, *GI hemorrhage.* **GU:** renal dysfunction, UTI, uremia. **Hematologic:** *leukopenia, thrombocytopenia,* anemia. **Hepatic:** elevated live enzyme levels. **Metabolic:** hypophosphatemia, *hypokalemia, hypomagnesemia, hypocalcemia.* **Musculoskeletal:** arthralgia, back pain, myalgia, skeletal pain, weakness. **Respiratory:** cough, dyspnea, pleural effusions, URI. **Skin:** infusion-site reaction, pain at infusion site. **Other:** metastases, hypothyroidism, candidiasis.

INTERACTIONS

Nephrotoxic drugs, thalidomide: May increase risk of renal dysfunction. Use with caution.

EFFECTS ON LAB TEST RESULTS

• May increase creatinine level.
• May decrease phosphate, potassium, magnesium, and calcium levels.
• May decrease Hb level and WBC and platelet counts.
• May interfere with technetium-99m diphosphonate imaging agents.

CONTRAINDICATIONS & CAUTIONS

• Contraindicated in patients hypersensitive to drug or other bisphosphonates.
🔴 *Alert:* There may be an increased risk of atypical fractures of the thigh and osteonecrosis of the jaw in patients treated with bisphosphonates.
• Use cautiously in patients with renal impairment.
Dialyzable drug: Yes.
⚠ *Overdose S&S:* High fever, hypotension, taste perversion, hypocalcemia.

PREGNANCY-LACTATION-REPRODUCTION

• Drug may cause fetal harm. Use during pregnancy isn't recommended.
• It isn't known if drug appears in human milk. Patient should discontinue breastfeeding or discontinue drug.

NURSING CONSIDERATIONS

• Assess hydration before treatment. Use drug only after patient has been vigorously hydrated with NSS. In patients with mild to moderate hypercalcemia, hydration alone may be sufficient.
• Because drug can cause electrolyte imbalances, carefully monitor electrolyte levels, especially calcium, phosphate, and magnesium. Short-term use of calcium may be needed in patients with severe hypocalcemia.
• Monitor CBC and differential count, creatinine and Hb levels, and hematocrit.
• Carefully monitor patients with preexisting anemia, leukopenia, or thrombocytopenia during first 2 weeks of therapy.
• Monitor patient's temperature. Patient may experience a slight elevation for 24 to 48 hours after therapy.
🔴 *Alert:* Because renal dysfunction may lead to renal failure, single doses shouldn't exceed 90 mg.
• Monitor creatinine level before each treatment.
• In patients treated for bone metastases who have kidney dysfunction, withhold dose until kidney function returns to baseline. Treating bone metastases in patients with severe kidney disease isn't recommended. For other indications, determine whether the potential benefit outweighs the risk.
• Severe musculoskeletal pain may occur within several days to several months of start of therapy. Symptoms may resolve partially or completely with drug stoppage.
• Bisphosphonates can interfere with bone-imaging agents.
🔴 *Alert:* Patients should have a dental exam with appropriate preventive dentistry before taking drug, especially those with risk factors, including cancer, chemotherapy, corticosteroid therapy, and poor oral hygiene. These patients should avoid dental procedures, if possible, during therapy.

PATIENT TEACHING

• Explain use and administration of drug to patient and family.

Reactions in bold italics are *life-threatening*. Interactions may have a *rapid onset* or a *delayed onset*.

• Instruct patient to report adverse reactions promptly.

• Tell patient to immediately report groin or thigh pain.

• Instruct patient to take vitamin D and calcium supplements, as prescribed.

• Caution patient to maintain good oral hygiene and have regular dental checkups.

• Advise patient to report pregnancy or breastfeeding.

pancrelipase
pan-kre-LYE-pase

Creon, Pancreaze, Pertzye, Viokace, Zenpep

Therapeutic class: Digestive enzymes
Pharmacologic class: Pancreatic enzymes

AVAILABLE FORMS
Creon
Capsules (delayed-release) ⓓⓝⓒ: 3,000 units lipase, 9,500 units protease, 15,000 units amylase; 6,000 units lipase, 19,000 units protease, 30,000 units amylase; 12,000 units lipase, 38,000 units protease, 60,000 units amylase; 24,000 units lipase, 76,000 units protease, 120,000 units amylase; 36,000 units lipase, 114,000 units protease, 180,000 units amylase

Pancreaze
Capsules (delayed-release) ⓓⓝⓒ: 2,600 units lipase, 8,800 units protease, 15,200 units amylase; 4,200 units lipase, 14,200 units protease, 24,600 units amylase; 10,500 units lipase, 35,500 units protease, 61,550 units amylase; 16,800 units lipase, 56,800 units protease, 98,400 units amylase; 21,000 units lipase, 54,700 units protease, 83,900 units amylase; 37,000 units lipase, 97,300 units amylase; 149,900 units amylase

Pertzye
Capsules (delayed-release) ⓓⓝⓒ: 4,000 units lipase, 14,375 units protease, 15,125 units amylase; 8,000 units lipase, 28,750 units protease, 30,250 units amylase; 16,000 units lipase, 57,500 units protease, 60,500 units amylase; 24,000 units lipase, 86,250 units protease, 90,750 units amylase

Viokace
Tablets ⓓⓝⓒ: 10,440 units lipase, 39,150 units protease, 39,150 units amylase; 20,880 units

lipase, 78,300 units protease, 78,300 units amylase

Zenpep
Capsules (enteric-coated beads) ⓓⓝⓒ:
3,000 units lipase, 10,000 units protease, 14,000 units amylase; 5,000 units lipase, 17,000 units protease, 24,000 units amylase; 10,000 units lipase, 32,000 units protease, 42,000 units amylase; 15,000 units lipase, 47,000 units protease, 63,000 units amylase; 20,000 units lipase, 63,000 units protease, 84,000 units amylase; 25,000 units lipase, 79,000 units protease, 105,000 units amylase; 40,000 units lipase, 126,000 units protease, 168,000 units amylase

INDICATIONS & DOSAGES
➤ **Pancreatic insufficiency due to cystic fibrosis and other conditions**
Adults and children older than age 4: 500 lipase units/kg PO per meal to a maximum of 2,500 lipase units/kg per meal (or 10,000 lipase units/kg per day) or less than 4,000 lipase units/g fat ingested per day.
Children older than age 12 months to 4 years: 1,000 lipase units/kg PO per meal up to maximum dose of 2,500 lipase units/kg per meal, 10,000 lipase units/kg daily, or 4,000 lipase units/g of fat ingested daily.
Infants up to age 12 months: 2,000 to 4,000 lipase units PO per 120 mL of formula or per breastfeeding.
➤ **Exocrine pancreatic insufficiency due to chronic pancreatitis or pancreatectomy (Creon)**
Adults: 72,000 lipase units PO per meal while consuming at least 100 g of fat per day. Or, 500 lipase units/kg per meal. Adjust dosage to patient's response.
➤ **Exocrine pancreatic insufficiency due to chronic pancreatitis or pancreatectomy, with a PPI (Viokace)**
Adults: 500 lipase units/kg PO per meal to a maximum of 2,500 lipase units/kg per meal (or 10,000 lipase units/kg/day) or less than 4,000 lipase units/g fat ingested per day. Adjust dosage to patient's response.

ADMINISTRATION
PO
• Give drug before or with meals and snacks.
• Don't crush or allow patient to chew capsules. May open capsules containing enteric-coated microspheres and sprinkle capsule contents on a small quantity of soft food at

room temperature. Have patient swallow immediately, without chewing, and follow dose with glass of water or juice to avoid mucosal irritation.

• For infants, mix capsule contents with applesauce and give within 15 minutes of each feeding. Follow with 120 mL of formula or human milk. Don't mix directly with formula or human milk. Capsule contents may be administered directly into infant's mouth before feeding. Avoid contact with or inhalation of powder because it may be highly irritating. Older children may swallow capsules with food.

• Viokace tablets aren't enteric-coated; therefore, patient should take with a PPI. Ensure patient swallows entire tablet with sufficient fluid; mucosal irritation could result from retained drug.

• Consult manufacturer's guidance on gastrostomy tube administration.

• Give half the prescribed dose at start of a meal and the second half in the middle of the meal; for snacks, give half the prescribed mealtime dose with each snack.

• Total daily dose should reflect about three meals plus two or three snacks per day.

• If a dose is missed, omit the missed dose and give next dose with the next meal or snack. Don't double dose.

ACTION
Replaces endogenous exocrine pancreatic enzymes and aids digestion of starches, fats, and proteins.

Route	Onset	Peak	Duration
PO	Variable	Variable	Variable

Half-life: Unknown.

ADVERSE REACTIONS
CNS: headache, dizziness. **CV:** edema. **EENT:** nasopharyngitis. **GI:** abdominal pain, abnormal feces, nausea, diarrhea with high doses, dyspepsia, vomiting, weight loss, flatulence, anal pruritus, early satiety. **Hematologic:** anemia, lymphadenopathy. **Hepatic:** biliary tract stones, hydrocholecystis. **Metabolic:** hyperglycemia, *hypoglycemia.* **Respiratory:** cough. **Skin:** contusion. **Other:** infection, ascites.

INTERACTIONS
Drug-drug. *Oral iron supplement:* May decrease iron response. Monitor patient for decreased effectiveness.

EFFECTS ON LAB TEST RESULTS
• May increase uric acid level.

CONTRAINDICATIONS & CAUTIONS
• Use cautiously in patients with a known allergy to proteins of porcine origin.
• Use cautiously in patients with gout, renal impairment, or hyperuricemia.
⚠ *Alert:* High-dose use of pancreatic enzymes has been associated with fibrosing colonopathy. Use cautiously when doses exceed 2,500 lipase units/kg/meal (or are greater than 10,000 lipase units/kg/day).
Dialyzable drug: Unknown.
⚠ *Overdose S&S:* Transient intestinal upset, diarrhea.

PREGNANCY-LACTATION-REPRODUCTION
• Use cautiously during pregnancy and only if clearly needed. Nutrition should be optimized during pregnancy.
• It isn't known if drug appears in human milk; however, it's unlikely since drug isn't absorbed systemically. Use cautiously during breastfeeding.

NURSING CONSIDERATIONS
⚠ *Alert:* Use drug only for confirmed exocrine pancreatic insufficiency. It isn't effective in GI disorders unrelated to enzyme deficiency.
• Monitor patient's stools. Adequate replacement decreases number of bowel movements and improves stool consistency.
• Individual products aren't bioequivalent and shouldn't be interchanged without prescriber supervision.
• Dosage varies with degree of maldigestion and malabsorption, amount of fat in diet, and enzyme activity of individual preparations.

PATIENT TEACHING
• Instruct patient or caregiver in safe drug administration.
• Advise patient to take drug with food and generous amounts of liquid.
• Instruct patient to consult prescriber before changing brands.
• Advise patient to report unusual or severe stomach area pain, bloating, trouble passing

---

Reactions in bold italics are *life-threatening*. Interactions may have a *rapid onset* or a *delayed onset*.

stool, nausea, vomiting, or diarrhea, which may indicate fibrosing colonopathy.
• Instruct patient to report pregnancy or plans to become pregnant.

SAFETY ALERT!

pancuronium bromide
pan-kyoo-ROE-nee-um

Therapeutic class: Skeletal muscle relaxants
Pharmacologic class: Nondepolarizing neuromuscular blockers

AVAILABLE FORMS
Injection: 1 mg/mL

INDICATIONS & DOSAGES
➤ **Adjunct to anesthesia to relax skeletal muscle, facilitate intubation, and assist with mechanical ventilation**
Adults and children age 1 month and older:
Initially, 0.04 to 0.1 mg/kg IV; then 0.01 mg/kg IV every 25 to 60 minutes. For ET intubation, a bolus dose of 0.06 to 0.1 mg/kg IV is recommended. Conditions satisfactory for intubation are usually present within 2 to 3 minutes.
Neonates: Individualize dosage. It's recommended that a test dose of 0.02 mg/kg IV be given first to measure responsiveness.

ADMINISTRATION
IV
Boxed Warning This drug should be administered by adequately trained individuals familiar with its actions, characteristics, and hazards. ■
▼ Only staff skilled in airway management should use drug.
▼ Drug has no known effect on consciousness, pain threshold, or cerebration. To avoid patient distress, don't induce neuromuscular blockade before unconsciousness.
▼ Keep ET equipment, ventilator, oxygen, atropine, edrophonium, epinephrine, and neostigmine immediately available.
▼ Store in refrigerator. The 10-mL vial will maintain full clinical potency for up to 6 months at room temperature.
▼ Compatible in solution with NSS, dextrose 5%, dextrose 5% and sodium chloride, and lactated Ringer solution.
▼ When mixed with approved solutions in glass or plastic containers, drug will remain stable in solution for 48 hours with no alteration in potency or pH.
▼ May administer undiluted by rapid IV injection.
▼ **Incompatibilities:** Alkaline solutions, barbiturates, diazepam, thiopental sodium. Consult a drug compatibility reference for additional information.

ACTION
Prevents acetylcholine from binding to receptors on the motor end plate, blocking neuromuscular transmission.

Route	Onset	Peak	Duration
IV	30–45 sec	3–4.5 min	35–65 min

Half-life: 89 to 161 minutes.

ADVERSE REACTIONS
CV: tachycardia, increased BP, flushing.
EENT: excessive salivation. **Musculoskeletal:** residual muscle weakness. **Respiratory:** *prolonged respiratory insufficiency or apnea.* **Skin:** transient rashes. **Other:** allergic or idiosyncratic hypersensitivity reactions.

INTERACTIONS
Drug-drug. *Aminoglycosides (amikacin, gentamicin, neomycin, streptomycin, tobramycin):*
May increase the effects of pancuronium, including prolonged respiratory depression. Use together only when necessary. Dose of pancuronium may need to be reduced.
Azathioprine: May reverse neuromuscular blockade induced by pancuronium. Monitor patient.
Calcium channel blockers, clindamycin, general anesthetics (enflurane, halothane, isoflurane), ketamine, lincomycin, magnesium salts, polymyxin antibiotics (colistin, polymyxin B sulfate), procainamide, quinidine, quinine: May enhance neuromuscular blockade, increasing skeletal muscle relaxation and prolonging effect of pancuronium. Use together cautiously during and after surgery.
Carbamazepine, phenytoin: May decrease effects of pancuronium. May need to increase pancuronium dose.
Diuretics: May cause electrolyte imbalance or alter neuromuscular blockade. Monitor electrolytes before giving drug.
Lithium, opioid analgesics: May enhance neuromuscular blockade, increasing skeletal muscle relaxation and possibly causing

P

respiratory paralysis. Use cautiously, and reduce dose of pancuronium.
Succinylcholine: May increase intensity and duration of neuromuscular blockade. Allow effects of succinylcholine to subside before giving pancuronium.
Theophylline: May produce a dose-dependent reversal of neuromuscular blocking effects. Monitor patient for clinical effect.

EFFECTS ON LAB TEST RESULTS
None reported.

CONTRAINDICATIONS & CAUTIONS
• Contraindicated in patients hypersensitive to pancuronium, bromides, or components of the formulation.
• Use cautiously in older adults or patients who are debilitated; in patients with renal, hepatic, or pulmonary impairment; and in those with respiratory depression, myasthenia gravis, myasthenic syndrome related to lung cancer, dehydration, thyroid disorders, CV disease, collagen diseases, porphyria, electrolyte disturbances, hyperthermia, severe obesity, and toxemic states. Also, use large doses cautiously in patients undergoing cesarean section.
🡒 *Alert:* Some formulations contain benzyl alcohol, which has been associated with fatal gasping syndrome in premature neonates.
Dialyzable drug: Unknown.
⚠ *Overdose S&S:* Residual neuromuscular blockade (skeletal muscle weakness, decreased respiratory reserve, low tidal volume, apnea).

PREGNANCY-LACTATION-REPRODUCTION
• It isn't known if drug can cause fetal harm. Use during pregnancy only if benefit justifies fetal risk.
• There is no information on the use of drug during breastfeeding.

NURSING CONSIDERATIONS
• Dosage depends on anesthetic used, individual needs, and response. Dosages are representative and must be adjusted.
• Allow succinylcholine effects to subside before giving this drug.
• Monitor baseline electrolyte determinations (electrolyte imbalance can potentiate neuromuscular effects) and vital signs, especially respirations and HR.

• Measure fluid intake and output; renal dysfunction may prolong duration of action because 25% of drug is excreted unchanged in the urine.
• A nerve stimulator and train-of-four monitoring are recommended to confirm antagonism of neuromuscular blockade and recovery of muscle strength. Make sure there's some evidence of spontaneous recovery before attempting pharmacologic reversal with neostigmine.
• Monitor respirations closely until patient recovers fully from neuromuscular blockade, as indicated by tests of muscle strength (hand grip, head lift, and ability to cough).
• After spontaneous recovery starts, neuromuscular blockade may be reversed with an anticholinesterase (such as neostigmine or edrophonium), which is usually given with an anticholinergic (such as atropine).
• Drug doesn't cause histamine release or hypotension, but it may raise HR and BP.
• Give analgesics for pain.
🡒 *Alert:* Careful dosage calculation is essential. Always verify dosage with another health care professional.

PATIENT TEACHING
• Explain all events and procedures to patient because patient can still hear.

pantoprazole sodium
pan-TOE-pray-zol

Pantoloc🍁, Protonix🗲, Protonix IV

Therapeutic class: Antiulcer drugs
Pharmacologic class: PPIs

AVAILABLE FORMS
Granules for delayed-release suspension ⓞⓝⓒ:
40 mg/packet
Injection: 40 mg/vial
Tablets (delayed-release) ⓞⓝⓒ: 20 mg, 40 mg
Tablets (enteric-coated) ⓞⓝⓒ: 20 mg🍁,
40 mg🍁

INDICATIONS & DOSAGES
🡒 **Maintenance of healing of erosive esophagitis**
Adults: 40 mg PO once daily.
🡒 **Short-term treatment of erosive esophagitis associated with GERD**

Adults: 40 mg PO once daily for up to
8 weeks. For patients who haven't healed after
8 weeks of treatment, another 8-week course
may be considered. Or, 40 mg IV once daily
for 7 to 10 days. Switch to PO form when patient can take orally.

*Children age 5 and older weighing 40 kg or
more:* 40 mg PO once daily for up to 8 weeks.
*Children age 5 and older weighing 15 to less
than 40 kg:* 20 mg PO once daily for up to
8 weeks.

Adjust-a-dose: Consider dosage reduction in
children who are poor CYP2C19 metabolizers.

➤ **Long-term maintenance of healing erosive esophagitis and reduction in relapse
rates of daytime and nighttime heartburn
symptoms in patients with GERD**
Adults: 40 mg PO once daily.

➤ **Treatment of pathologic hypersecretion
conditions, including Zollinger-Ellison syndrome**
Adults: Individualize dosage. Usual dosage
is 40 mg PO b.i.d. Usual IV dose is 80 mg
IV every 12 hours for no more than 6 days.
For those needing a higher dose, 80 mg every
8 hours is expected to maintain acid output
below 10 mEq/hour. Maximum daily dose is
240 mg/day. When converting from IV to PO
form, ensure continuity of suppression of acid
secretion.

➤ **Dyspepsia ◆**
Adults: 20 to 40 mg PO once daily for 4 to
8 weeks.

➤ **Uncomplicated peptic ulcer ◆**
Adults: 40 mg PO once daily for 4 to 8 weeks.

➤ **Active peptic ulcer bleeding ◆**
Adults: 40 mg IV b.i.d. for at least 72 hours
before transitioning to oral dosing. After
14 days, decrease to 20 mg PO once daily.

ADMINISTRATION
PO
• Give tablets without regard for food and
make sure patient swallows them whole.
• May give with antacids.
• Don't crush or split tablets. Don't allow patient to chew granules (delayed-release oral
suspension).
• Give 30 to 60 minutes before a meal. For
twice-daily dosing, give first dose before
breakfast and second dose before dinner.
• Give delayed-release granules for oral suspension in 1 tsp applesauce or 1 tsp (5 mL)
apple juice 30 minutes before a meal by
mouth. To give via NG tube, mix with 10 mL

apple juice; then flush tube twice with 10 mL
apple juice. Don't give in water or other liq-
uids or foods.
• Delayed-release granule packets can't be
divided to make a smaller dose.
IV
▼ Safety and effectiveness of the IV form
for GERD and in patients with a history of
erosive esophagitis for more than 10 days
are unknown.
▼ Reconstitute each vial with 10 mL of
NSS.
▼ Compatible diluents for infusion include
NSS, D₅W, and lactated Ringer solution for
injection.
▼ For patients with GERD, further dilute
with 100 mL of diluent to yield 0.4 mg/mL.
▼ For patients with hypersecretion, combine
two reconstituted vials and further dilute
with 80 mL of diluent to a total volume of
100 mL, to yield 0.8 mg/mL.
▼ Infuse diluted solutions over 15 minutes at
a rate of about 7 mL/minute.
▼ For a 2-minute infusion, give the reconstituted vials (final yield of about 4 mg/mL)
over at least 2 minutes.
▼ Reconstituted 15-minute infusion
(0.4 mg/mL) may be stored for up to 6 hours
and the diluted solutions for up to 24 hours
at room temperature.
▼ Reconstituted 2-minute solution
(4 mg/mL) may be stored for up to 24 hours
at room temperature before infusion.
▼ **Incompatibilities:** Midazolam, zinc-
containing products or solutions. Don't give
another infusion simultaneously through the
same line.

ACTION
Inhibits proton pump activity by binding
to hydrogen-potassium adenosine triphosphatase, located at secretory surface of gastric parietal cells, to suppress gastric acid
secretion.

Route	Onset	Peak	Duration
PO	Unknown	2.5 hr	>24 hr
IV	15–30 min	Unknown	24 hr

Half-life: 1 hour.

ADVERSE REACTIONS
CNS: asthenia, dizziness, headache, depression, vertigo, fever. **CV:** edema, thrombophlebitis (IV). **EENT:** blurred vision, otitis media, pharyngitis, rhinitis, sinusitis, dry

mouth. **GI:** abdominal pain, constipation, diarrhea, flatulence, nausea, vomiting. **Hematologic:** *leukopenia, thrombocytopenia.* **Hepatic:** elevated liver enzyme levels. **Metabolic:** hyperglycemia, hypertriglyceridemia. **Musculoskeletal:** arthralgia, myalgia, back pain, hypertonia, neck pain. **Respiratory:** URI. **Skin:** rash, pruritus, urticaria. **Other:** flulike syndrome, infection, injection-site reaction, photosensitivity reactions, hypersensitivity reaction.

INTERACTIONS

Drug-drug. *Ampicillin esters, dasatinib, erlotinib, iron salts, ketoconazole, mycophenolate, nilotinib:* May decrease absorption of these drugs. Monitor patient closely and separate doses.

Azole antifungals (itraconazole, ketoconazole): May decrease plasma levels of these drugs. Avoid this combination if possible.

Methotrexate: May increase methotrexate concentration and risk of toxicity. Closely monitor methotrexate concentration, and watch for signs and symptoms of methotrexate toxicity.

Protease inhibitors (atazanavir, nelfinavir): May reduce antiviral activity of these drugs. Adjust dosage as needed; administration of atazanavir or nelfinavir with pantoprazole isn't recommended.

Rilpivirine: May decrease antiviral effect and increase risk of drug resistance. Concomitant use is contraindicated.

Salicylates: Enteric-coated salicylates may dissolve more rapidly, increasing gastric adverse reactions. Monitor patient.

Warfarin: May increase INR and prolong PT. Monitor patient and lab values.

Drug-lifestyle. *Sun exposure:* May increase risk of sunburn. Advise patient to avoid excessive sunlight exposure.

EFFECTS ON LAB TEST RESULTS

• May increase glucose, CK, and triglyceride levels.
• May decrease B_{12} and magnesium levels.
• May increase LFT values.
• May cause false-positive urine screen test for tetrahydrocannabinol.
• May increase serum chromogranin A level, causing a false-positive result in diagnostic investigation for neuroendocrine tumors.

CONTRAINDICATIONS & CAUTIONS

• Contraindicated in patients hypersensitive to components of the formulation.
• PPI therapy may be associated with an increased risk of osteoporosis-related fractures. Patients should use lowest dose and shortest duration of therapy appropriate to condition being treated.
• May increase risk of acute tubulointerstitial nephritis (TIN), which may occur at any point during PPI therapy.
• PPI use is associated with increased risk of fundic gland polyps that increases with long-term use, especially beyond 1 year.
• Cutaneous lupus erythematosus (CLE) and SLE have been reported, occurring as both new onset and an exacerbation of existing autoimmune disease in patients of all ages within weeks to years after continuous drug therapy.
• IV formulation contains edetate disodium, a chelator of zinc. Consider zinc supplements in patients at risk for zinc deficiency.
• Prolonged oral use (over 3 years) may lead to vitamin B_{12} deficiency.
Dialyzable drug: No.

PREGNANCY-LACTATION-REPRODUCTION

• There are no adequate studies during pregnancy. Use cautiously and only if clearly needed.
• Drug appears in human milk in limited amount. Use cautiously during breastfeeding.

NURSING CONSIDERATIONS

• Symptomatic response to therapy doesn't preclude the presence of gastric malignancy.
⚕ *Alert:* Prolonged use of PPIs may cause low magnesium levels. Monitor magnesium levels before start of treatment and periodically thereafter.
⚕ *Alert:* Monitor patient for signs and symptoms of low magnesium level, such as abnormal HR or rhythm, palpitations, muscle spasms, tremor, or seizures. In children, abnormal HR may present as fatigue, upset stomach, dizziness, and light-headedness. Magnesium supplementation or drug discontinuation may be required.
⚕ *Alert:* May increase risk of CDAD. Evaluate for CDAD in patients who develop diarrhea that doesn't improve.
• If signs or symptoms consistent with CLE or SLE are noted, discontinue drug and refer patient to the appropriate specialist for

evaluation. Most patients improve with discontinuation of the PPI alone in 4 to 12 weeks.
- Monitor patient for TIN (symptomatic hypersensitivity reactions, nonspecific symptoms of decreased renal function [malaise, nausea, anorexia]). Discontinue drug and evaluate patient with suspected acute TIN.
- Monitor patient for hypersensitivity reactions, including SCARs; discontinue drug if present.
- *Look alike–sound alike:* Don't confuse Protonix with Prilosec, Prozac, or Prevacid. Don't confuse pantoprazole with aripiprazole.

PATIENT TEACHING
- Teach patient or caregiver safe drug administration.
- Instruct patient to take exactly as prescribed and at about the same time every day.
- Tell patient that antacids don't affect drug absorption.
- Advise patient to immediately report diarrhea that doesn't improve.
- Instruct patient to report fractures, especially of the hip, wrist, or spine.
- Teach patient to report all adverse reactions and to recognize and report signs and symptoms of low magnesium level.
- Advise patient of childbearing potential to report known or suspected pregnancy.

PARoxetine hydrochloride
pa-ROKS-e-teen

Paxil, Paxil CR

PARoxetine mesylate
Pexeva

Therapeutic class: Antidepressants
Pharmacologic class: SSRIs

AVAILABLE FORMS
paroxetine hydrochloride
Suspension: 10 mg/5 mL
Tablets ⓓ: 10 mg, 20 mg, 30 mg, 40 mg
Tablets (controlled-release) ⓓ: 12.5 mg, 25 mg, 37.5 mg
paroxetine mesylate
Capsules: 7.5 mg
Tablets ⓓ: 10 mg, 20 mg, 30 mg

INDICATIONS & DOSAGES
Adjust-a-dose (for all indications): For older adults and patients who are debilitated and those with renal or hepatic impairment taking immediate-release form, initially, 10 mg PO daily, preferably in morning. If patient doesn't respond after full antidepressant effect has occurred, increase dose in 10-mg/day increments at intervals of at least 1 week to a maximum of 40 mg daily. If using controlled-release form, start therapy at 12.5 mg daily. Don't exceed 50 mg daily.

➤ **Major depressive disorder (excluding capsules)**
Adults: Initially, 20 mg PO daily, preferably in morning, as indicated. If patient doesn't improve, increase dose by 10 mg daily at intervals of at least 1 week to a maximum of 50 mg daily. If using controlled-release form, initially, 25 mg PO daily. Increase dose in 12.5-mg/day increments at intervals of at least 1 week to a maximum of 62.5 mg daily.

➤ **OCD (Paxil and Pexeva only)**
Adults: Initially, 20 mg PO daily, preferably in morning. Increase dose in 10-mg day increments at intervals of at least 1 week. Maximum daily dose is 60 mg.

➤ **Panic disorder (excluding capsules)**
Adults: Initially, 10 mg PO daily. Increase dose in 10-mg/day increments at intervals of at least 1 week, up to a maximum of 60 mg daily. Or, 12.5 mg Paxil CR PO as a single daily dose. Increase dose in 12.5-mg/day increments at intervals of at least 1 week, up to a maximum of 75 mg daily.

➤ **Social anxiety disorder (Paxil and Paxil CR only)**
Adults: Initially, 20 mg PO daily. Dosage range is 20 to 60 mg daily. Adjust dosage to maintain patient on lowest effective dose. Or, 12.5 mg Paxil CR PO as a single daily dose. Increase dose in 12.5-mg/day increments at intervals of at least 1 week, up to a maximum of 37.5 mg daily.

➤ **Generalized anxiety disorder (Paxil and Pexeva only)**
Adults: 20 mg PO daily initially. Increase dose in 10-mg/day increments at intervals of at least 1 week, up to a maximum of 50 mg daily. Doses greater than 20 mg/day don't appear to have an added benefit.

➤ **PTSD (Paxil only)**
Adults: Initially, 20 mg PO daily. Increase dose in 10-mg/day increments at intervals of

P

at least 1 week. Maximum daily dose is 50 mg
PO.
➤ **Premenstrual dysphoric disorder
(PMDD) (Paxil CR only)**
Adults: Initially, 12.5 mg Paxil CR PO as
a single daily dose. May be given daily
throughout menstrual cycle or daily during
the luteal phase of menstrual cycle. Dose
changes should occur at intervals of at least
1 week. Maximum dose is 25 mg PO daily.
➤ **Moderate to severe vasomotor symptoms associated with menopause (capsules
only)**
Adults: 7.5 mg capsule PO daily at bedtime.

ADMINISTRATION
PO
• Give drug in the morning without regard for
food (excluding capsules). Give capsules at
bedtime.
• Don't split or crush controlled-release
tablets.
• Shake oral suspension well before each use.
Measure with oral syringe or calibrated mea-
suring device.

ACTION
Thought to be linked to drug's inhibition of
CNS neuronal uptake of serotonin.

Route	Onset	Peak	Duration
PO	Unknown	3–8 hr	Unknown
PO (controlled-release)	Unknown	6–10 hr	Unknown

Half-life: Paroxetine, 21 hours; controlled-release,
15 to 20 hours; paroxetine mesylate, 33.2 hours.

ADVERSE REACTIONS
CNS: asthenia, dizziness, fatigue, headache,
insomnia, somnolence, tremor, nervousness,
anxiety, paresthesia, confusion, agitation,
dysgeusia. **CV:** palpitations, vasodilation,
HTN, tachycardia, chest pain. **EENT:** blurred
vision, tinnitus, lump or tightness in throat,
dry mouth, pharyngitis, rhinitis, sinusitis.
GI: nausea, constipation, diarrhea, flatulence,
vomiting, dyspepsia, decreased appetite, abdominal pain. **GU:** ejaculatory disturbances,
sexual dysfunction, decreased libido, urinary
frequency, other urinary disorders, dysmenorrhea, female genital tract disease. **Metabolic:**
weight gain. **Musculoskeletal:** myopathy,
myalgia, myasthenia, back pain. **Respiratory:** dyspnea. **Skin:** diaphoresis, rash, pruritus. **Other:** yawning.

INTERACTIONS
Drug-drug. *Anticoagulants, platelet in-
hibitors:* May impair platelet aggregation and
increase risk of bleeding. Monitor patient for
signs and symptoms of bleeding.
Atomoxetine: May alter atomoxetine level.
Initiate atomoxetine at a reduced dosage.
Barbiturates (phenobarbital), phenytoin:
May alter pharmacokinetics of both drugs.
Dosage adjustments may be needed.
Cimetidine: May decrease hepatic
metabolism of paroxetine, leading to risk of
adverse reactions. Dosage adjustments may
be needed.
Digoxin: May decrease digoxin level. Use together cautiously.
*Drugs metabolized by CYP2D6 (desipramine,
dextromethorphan, flecainide, metoprolol,
propafenone):* May increase CYP2D6 substrate level. Adjust substrate dosage.
*Drugs that prolong QT interval (antiarrhyth-
mics [amiodarone, bretylium, disopyramide,
dofetilide, procainamide, quinidine, sotalol],
arsenic trioxide, chlorpromazine, cisapride,
dolasetron, droperidol, mefloquine, mesoridazine, moxifloxacin, pentamidine, pimozide,
tacrolimus, ziprasidone):* May increase risk
of life-threatening cardiac arrhythmias, including torsades de pointes. Monitor patient
closely.
Fosamprenavir, ritonavir: May decrease
paroxetine plasma level. Adjust dosage as
needed.
Galantamine: May alter oral bioavailability
of galantamine. Use together cautiously.
Linezolid, methylene blue: May cause serotonin syndrome. Allow at least 2 weeks after
stopping linezolid before giving paroxetine.
*MAO inhibitors (phenelzine, selegiline,
tranylcypromine):* May cause serotonin syndrome and signs and symptoms resembling
NMS. Avoid using within 14 days of MAO
inhibitor therapy.
NSAIDs: May increase risk of GI bleeding. If
possible, avoid concurrent use. If coadministration can't be avoided, consider shorten-
ing NSAID treatment duration, decreasing
dosage, or switching to acetaminophen or a
TCA.
Pimozide, thioridazine: May increase levels
of these drugs. Use together is contraindicated.
Risperidone: May increase risperidone level,
increasing risk of adverse reactions; serotonin
syndrome may occur. Use together cautiously.

Reactions in bold italics are *life-threatening*. Interactions may have a *rapid onset* or a ***delayed onset***.

Serotonergic agents (amphetamines, buspirone, lithium, SNRIs, SSRIs, tramadol, triptans): May increase risk of serotonin syndrome. Monitor patient closely.

Sympathomimetics: May increase sensitivity to the effect of sympathomimetics and increase risk of serotonin syndrome. Monitor patient.

Tamoxifen: May reduce plasma concentration of active tamoxifen metabolite. Avoid combination.

TCAs: May increase plasma concentration and elimination half-life of TCAs. TCA dosage reduction may be needed.

Warfarin: May increase anticoagulant effect. Monitor therapy.

Drug-herb. *SAM-e:* May increase risk of serotonin syndrome. Avoid use together.

St. John's wort: May increase sedative-hypnotic effects and risk of serotonin syndrome. Discourage use together.

Drug-lifestyle. *Alcohol use:* May alter psychomotor function. Discourage use together.

EFFECTS ON LAB TEST RESULTS
• May increase LFT values.
• May decrease sodium level.
• May decrease Hb level.

CONTRAINDICATIONS & CAUTIONS
• Contraindicated in patients hypersensitive to drug or its components; some formulations contain polysorbate 80.

Boxed Warning Antidepressants increase the risk of suicidality in children, adolescents, and young adults with depression and other psychiatric disorders. Health professionals considering the use of paroxetine in a child, adolescent, or young adult must balance this risk with the clinical need. Paroxetine isn't approved for use in children. ■

⚠ Alert: Use with linezolid or methylene blue can cause serotonin syndrome (fever, mental status changes, muscle twitching, diaphoresis, shivering or shaking, diarrhea, loss of coordination). Use drug with linezolid or methylene blue only for life-threatening or urgent conditions when the potential benefits outweigh the risks of toxicity.

• Angle-closure glaucoma has occurred in patients with untreated anatomically narrow angles.

• Hepatic and renal impairment increases plasma levels; use cautiously and reduce dosage if needed.

• Use cautiously in patients with history of seizure disorders or mania and in those with other severe, systemic illness.

• Use cautiously in patients at risk for volume depletion and monitor them appropriately.

Dialyzable drug: Unlikely.

⚠ Overdose S&S: Coma, confusion, dizziness, nausea, somnolence, tachycardia, tremor, vomiting, acute renal failure, aggressive reactions, bradycardia, dystonia, hepatic necrosis, HTN, hypotension, jaundice, manic reactions, mydriasis, myoclonus, rhabdomyolysis, seizures, serotonin syndrome, stupor, hepatic impairment, syncope, urine retention, ventricular arrhythmias.

PREGNANCY-LACTATION-REPRODUCTION
• Drug can cause fetal harm, especially if taken in the first trimester. Manufacturer suggests discontinuing drug or switching to another antidepressant unless benefits justify continuing treatment. Consider other treatment options for patients planning pregnancy.
• Contraindicated for treatment of vasomotor symptoms during pregnancy.
• Drug appears in human milk. Use during breastfeeding only if benefit of treating postpartum depression with this drug outweighs risk. Monitor infants for growth.

NURSING CONSIDERATIONS
• Patients taking Paxil CR for PMDD should be periodically reassessed to determine the need for continued treatment.
• If signs or symptoms of psychosis occur or increase, expect prescriber to reduce dosage. Record mood changes. Monitor patient for suicidality, and allow only a minimum supply of drug.

Boxed Warning Drug may increase the risk of suicidality in children, adolescents, and young adults ages 18 to 24 during the first 2 months of treatment, especially in those with major depressive disorder or other psychiatric disorder. ■

Boxed Warning Monitor patients starting antidepressant therapy for clinical worsening, suicidality, or unusual changes in behavior. ■

⚠ Alert: If linezolid or methylene blue must be given, stop paroxetine and monitor patient for serotonin toxicity for 2 weeks or until 24 hours after the last dose of methylene blue or linezolid, whichever comes first. Treatment with paroxetine may be resumed 24 hours after the last dose of methylene blue or linezolid.

• Monitor patient for complaints of sexual dysfunction. In men, they include anorgasmia, erectile difficulties, and delayed ejaculation or orgasm; in women, they include anorgasmia or difficulty with orgasm.

⚠ *Alert:* Don't stop drug abruptly. Withdrawal or discontinuation syndrome may occur if drug is stopped abruptly. Symptoms include headache, myalgia, lethargy, and general flu-like symptoms. Taper drug slowly over 1 to 2 weeks.

⚠ *Alert:* Combining triptans with an SSRI or an SSNRI may cause serotonin syndrome or NMS-like reactions. Signs and symptoms of serotonin syndrome may include restlessness, hallucinations, loss of coordination, fast heartbeat, rapid changes in BP, increased body temperature, overactive reflexes, nausea, vomiting, and diarrhea. Serotonin syndrome may be more likely to occur when starting or increasing the dose of triptan, SSRI, or SSNRI.

• *Look alike–sound alike:* Don't confuse paroxetine with fluoxetine or paclitaxel. Don't confuse Paxil with Doxil, paclitaxel, or Plavix.

PATIENT TEACHING

Boxed Warning Advise families and caregivers to closely observe patient for increased suicidality. ∎

⚠ *Alert:* Teach patient to recognize and immediately report signs and symptoms of serotonin toxicity.

• Teach patient safe drug administration.

• Warn patient to avoid activities that require alertness and good coordination until effects of drug are known.

• Advise patient to report sexual dysfunction and to consult prescriber for management strategies.

• Advise patient of childbearing potential to report pregnancy, plans to become pregnant, or breastfeeding during therapy.

• Tell patient to avoid alcohol and to consult prescriber before taking other prescription or OTC drugs or herbal medicines.

• Instruct patient not to stop taking drug abruptly.

SAFETY ALERT!

pegaspargase (PEG-L-asparaginase)
peg-AHS-per-jays

Oncaspar

Therapeutic class: Antineoplastics
Pharmacologic class: Modified L-asparaginases

AVAILABLE FORMS
Injection: 3,750 international units/5-mL solution in single-use vial (750 international units/mL)

INDICATIONS & DOSAGES
➤ **As part of a multidrug chemotherapy regimen in first-line treatment of acute lymphoblastic leukemia, and acute lymphoblastic leukemia with hypersensitivity to native forms of l-asparaginase**
Adults older than age 21: 2,000 international units/m^2 IV or IM every 14 days.
Adults and children age 21 and younger: 2,500 international units/m^2 IV or IM every 14 days.
Adjust-a-dose: Refer to manufacturer's product information for dosage adjustments due to adverse reactions.

ADMINISTRATION
• Premedicate with acetaminophen, an H$_1$ receptor blocker (such as diphenhydramine), and an H$_2$ receptor blocker (such as famotidine) 30 to 60 minutes before treatment to decrease risk and severity of infusion and hypersensitivity reactions.

• Don't freeze or use drug that has been frozen; freezing destroys drug's effectiveness.

• Don't use if stored at room temperature for longer than 48 hours. Keep refrigerated at 36° to 46° F (2° to 8° C).

• Don't use if drug has been shaken or vigorously agitated.

IV

▼ Give IV only if IM route is contraindicated.

▼ Give IV over 1 to 2 hours in 100 mL of NSS or D$_5$W through an infusion that's already running.

▼ Drug may be a contact irritant, and solution must be handled and given with care.

Reactions in bold italics are *life-threatening*. Interactions may have a *rapid onset* or a **delayed onset**.

Wear gloves. Avoid inhalation of vapors and contact with skin or mucous membranes, especially in the eyes. If contact occurs, wash with generous amounts of water for at least 15 minutes.

▼ Don't use if cloudy or contains precipitate. Avoid excessive agitation of drug; don't shake.

▼ Discard unused portions. Use only one dose per vial; don't reenter vial.

▼ **Incompatibilities:** None listed by manufacturer. Don't infuse other drugs through same IV line as pegaspargase. Consult a drug incompatibility reference for more information.

IM
• IM is the preferred route and is associated with lower incidence of adverse effects.
• When giving IM, limit volume given at a single injection site to 2 mL. If volume to be given exceeds 2 mL, use multiple injection sites.
• Administer as deep IM injection into a large muscle.

ACTION
A modified version of the enzyme L-asparaginase that exerts cytotoxic effects by inactivating the amino acid asparagine, which tumor cells need to synthesize proteins.

Route	Onset	Peak	Duration
IV	Unknown	Unknown	2–4 wk
IM	Unknown	5 days	21 days

Half-life: IV, about 5.3 days; IM, about 5.8 days.

ADVERSE REACTIONS
CNS: *stroke.* **GI:** *pancreatitis.* **Hematologic:** *coagulopathy, febrile neutropenia.* **Hepatic:** abnormal LFT values. **Metabolic:** hyperglycemia, hypertriglyceridemia, hypoalbuminemia. **Other:** hypersensitivity reactions, antibody development.

INTERACTIONS
Drug-drug. *Dexamethasone:* May increase glucocorticoid toxicities, including osteonecrosis. Use cautiously together.
Oral contraceptives: May enhance thrombogenic effect of asparaginase products. Patient should use nonhormonal contraception.

EFFECTS ON LAB TEST RESULTS
• May increase BUN, creatinine, amylase, lipase, bilirubin, ALT, AST, uric acid, and ammonia levels.
• May increase or decrease glucose level.
• May increase INR.
• May decrease fibrinogen level and antithrombin III, WBC, RBC, platelet, neutrophil, and granulocyte counts.
• May prolong PT and PTT.

CONTRAINDICATIONS & CAUTIONS
• Contraindicated in patients with pancreatitis or history of pancreatitis with prior L-asparaginase therapy, in those who have had significant thrombosis or hemorrhagic events related to previous treatment with L-asparaginase, and in those with severe hepatic impairment.
• Contraindicated in patients with history of serious allergic reactions to drug, such as generalized urticaria, bronchospasm, laryngeal edema, hypotension, or other unacceptable adverse reactions.
• Discontinue drug in patients with serious thrombotic events.
• Use cautiously in patients with mild or moderate hepatic impairment.
• Use cautiously in patients with a history of diabetes.
Dializable drug: Unknown.
⚠ *Overdose S&S:* Elevated liver enzyme levels, rash.

PREGNANCY-LACTATION-REPRODUCTION
• Drug may cause fetal harm. Use only if clearly needed.
• Patients of childbearing potential should use effective nonhormonal contraceptive methods during treatment and for at least 3 months after final dose.
• It isn't known if drug appears in human milk. Patient should discontinue breastfeeding during treatment and for 1 month after final dose.

NURSING CONSIDERATIONS
• Take preventive measures (including adequate hydration) before starting treatment. Hyperuricemia may result from rapid lysis of leukemic cells.
• Verify pregnancy status before treatment.
❂ *Alert:* Monitor patients closely for hypersensitivity (including life-threatening anaphylaxis). Observe patient for 1 hour after

P

giving drug and have emergency equipment and other drugs needed to treat anaphylaxis readily available. Moderate to life-threatening hypersensitivity requires stopping L-asparaginase.

• To assess effects of therapy, monitor patient's peripheral blood count and bone marrow. A drop in circulating lymphoblasts is often noted after therapy starts, sometimes accompanied by a marked rise in uric acid level.

• Obtain frequent amylase and lipase determinations and evaluate patient with abdominal pain to detect pancreatitis.

• Monitor patient's glucose level during therapy to detect hyperglycemia.

• Monitor patient for liver dysfunction when using drug with hepatotoxic chemotherapeutic drugs.

• Drug may affect several plasma proteins; monitor fibrinogen, PT, INR, and PTT at baseline and periodically during and after treatment.

• *Look alike–sound alike:* Don't confuse pegaspargase with asparaginase.

PATIENT TEACHING

• Inform patient of risk of hypersensitivity reactions and importance of reporting them immediately.

• Tell patient not to take other drugs, including OTC preparations, until approved by prescriber because pegaspargase use with drugs such as aspirin increases the risk of bleeding. Drug may also increase toxicity of other drugs.

• Advise patient to use an electric razor and soft toothbrush to minimize bleeding.

• Urge patient to report all adverse reactions and signs and symptoms of infection (fever, chills, and malaise); drug may suppress the immune system. Advise patient to avoid crowds, if possible, and people who are sick.

• Advise patient to report signs and symptoms of thrombosis (severe headache, arm or leg swelling, acute shortness of breath, and chest pain).

• Tell patient to report severe abdominal pain, which may indicate pancreatitis.

• Teach patient to report excessive thirst or an increase in the volume or frequency of urination.

• Encourage patient to drink plenty of fluids every 24 hours (unless instructed not to).

• Caution patient of childbearing potential to avoid pregnancy and breastfeeding during therapy.

SAFETY ALERT!
BIOSIMILAR DRUG

pegfilgrastim
peg-fil-GRA-stim

Neulasta, Neulasta Onpro Kit

pegfilgrastim-apgf
Nyvepria

pegfilgrastim-bmez
Ziextenzo

pegfilgrastim-cbqv
Udenyca

pegfilgrastim-jmdb
Fulphila

pegfilgrastim-pbbk
Fylnetra

Therapeutic class: Colony-stimulating factors
Pharmacologic class: Hematopoietics

AVAILABLE FORMS
Injection: 6 mg/0.6 mL prefilled syringe

INDICATIONS & DOSAGES

➤ **To reduce incidence of infection in patients with nonmyeloid malignancies receiving myelosuppressive chemotherapy that may cause febrile neutropenia**
Adults and children weighing more than 45 kg: 6 mg subcut once per chemotherapy cycle. Don't give in period between 14 days before and 24 hours after administration of cytotoxic chemotherapy.
Children: Give once per chemotherapy cycle, beginning 24 hours after completion of chemotherapy. Children weighing 31 to 44 kg, give 4 mg subcut. Children weighing 21 to 30 kg, give 2.5 mg subcut. Children weighing 10 to 20 kg, give 1.5 mg subcut. Children weighing less than 10 kg, give 0.1 mg/kg subcut.

➤ **To increase survival in patients acutely exposed to myelosuppressive doses of radiation (Neulasta)**

Reactions in bold italics are *life-threatening*. Interactions may have a *rapid onset* or a **delayed onset**.

Adults and children weighing 45 kg or more:
6 mg subcut as soon as possible after suspected or confirmed exposure. Repeat 1 week after first dose.

Children: Give as soon as possible after suspected or confirmed exposure. Repeat 1 week after first dose. *Children weighing 31 to 44 kg,* give 4 mg subcut. *Children weighing 21 to 30 kg,* give 2.5 mg subcut. *Children weighing 10 to 20 kg,* give 1.5 mg subcut. *Children weighing less than 10 kg,* give 0.1 mg/kg subcut.

ADMINISTRATION
Subcutaneous

☝ *Alert:* Don't use prefilled syringe for patients requiring less than 6 mg (0.6 mL), as syringe doesn't have graduated markings for smaller doses. Transfer drug to appropriately marked syringe to measure dose of less than 0.6 mL.

☝ *Alert:* Needle cap contains dry natural rubber derived from latex; persons with latex allergies shouldn't administer the drug.

• Allow drug to come to room temperature as directed by manufacturer before giving; protect from light.

• Don't shake.

• Don't use if visible discoloration or particulate matter is present.

• Refer to manufacturer's instructions for storage and stability information; requirements vary by product.

• Refer to manufacturer's instructions for administering drug using the Neulasta Onpro Kit with sterile on-body injector (OBI) and for its removal and disposal.

• After a missed dose due to failure or leakage of OBI for Neulasta, give a new dose manually by single-dose prefilled syringe as soon as possible.

ACTION
Binds cell receptors to stimulate proliferation, differentiation, commitment, and end-cell function of neutrophils.

Route	Onset	Peak	Duration
Subcut	Unknown	Unknown	Unknown

Half-life: 15 to 80 hours, adults; 20 to 38 hours, children.

ADVERSE REACTIONS
Musculoskeletal: bone pain, extremity pain.

INTERACTIONS
Drug-drug. *Belotecan:* May increase neutropenic effect of belotecan. Don't give G-CSF for at least 24 hours after belotecan; monitor patient closely.

Bleomycin, topotecan: May increase pulmonary toxicity of these drugs. Monitor therapy.

Tisagenlecleucel: May increase risk of adverse effects of tisagenlecleucel. Avoid combination.

EFFECTS ON LAB TEST RESULTS
• May increase granulocyte count.
• May decrease platelet count.
• May cause transient positive bone imaging changes.

CONTRAINDICATIONS & CAUTIONS
• Contraindicated in patients hypersensitive to filgrastim or components of the drug.

• Drug isn't indicated for peripheral blood progenitor cell mobilization in hematopoietic stem cell transplantation.

• Myelodysplastic syndrome (MDS) and acute myeloid leukemia (AML) have been associated with the use of pegfilgrastim products in conjunction with chemotherapy or radiotherapy in patients with breast and lung cancer. Monitor patients for signs and symptoms of MDS and AML in these settings.

• G-CSF drugs may act as growth factor for any tumor type.

• Use cautiously in patients with sickle cell disease, those receiving chemotherapy causing delayed myelosuppression, and those receiving radiation therapy.

• Neulasta OBI isn't recommended for acute radiation exposure or for use in children.

• Neulasta OBI uses acrylic adhesive; use cautiously in patients with reactions to acrylic adhesive.

Dialyzable drug: Unknown.

⚠ *Overdose S&S:* Leukocytosis, bone pain, edema, dyspnea, pleural effusions.

PREGNANCY-LACTATION-REPRODUCTION
• There are no adequate studies during pregnancy. Use only if potential benefit justifies fetal risk.

• It isn't known if drug appears in human milk. Use cautiously during breastfeeding.

NURSING CONSIDERATIONS

🛈 *Alert:* Splenic rupture may occur rarely. Assess patient who experiences signs or symptoms of left upper abdominal or shoulder pain for an enlarged spleen or splenic rupture.

• Obtain CBC and platelet count before therapy and monitor during therapy.

• Monitor patient for allergic-type reactions, including anaphylaxis, rash, and urticaria, which can occur with first or subsequent treatment.

• Evaluate patient with fever, lung infiltrates, or respiratory distress for ARDS. Notify prescriber if respiratory status worsens.

• Keep patient with sickle cell disease well hydrated, and monitor for symptoms of sickle cell crisis. Discontinue use if sickle cell crisis occurs.

• Monitor patient for capillary leak syndrome (hypotension, hypoalbuminemia, edema, hemoconcentration) and manage with symptomatic treatment, if necessary.

🛈 *Alert:* After acute radiation exposure, obtain a baseline CBC but don't delay drug administration if a CBC isn't readily available. Estimate patient's absorbed radiation dose (level of radiation exposure) based on information from public health authorities, biodosimetry if available, or clinical findings, such as time to onset of vomiting or lymphocyte depletion kinetics.

• Monitor patient for aortitis (fever, abdominal pain, malaise, back pain, increased C-reactive protein and WBC count), which may occur as early as the first week of treatment. Discontinue drug if aortitis is suspected.

• Monitor patient for signs and symptoms of glomerulonephritis (azotemia, hematuria, proteinuria).

• *Look alike–sound alike:* Don't confuse Neulasta with Neumega, Neupogen, or Lunesta.

PATIENT TEACHING

• Advise patient to report all adverse reactions.

• Tell patient to report signs and symptoms of allergic reactions, fever, or breathing problems.

🛈 *Alert:* Rarely, splenic rupture may occur. Advise patient to immediately report upper left abdominal or shoulder tip pain.

• Tell patient with sickle cell disease to keep drinking fluids and report signs or symptoms of sickle cell crisis.

• Instruct patient or caregiver how to give drug if it's to be given at home, including danger of reusing syringes and proper syringe disposal.

• Instruct patient using OBI not to expose injector to oxygen-rich environments (hyperbaric chamber), MRI, X-ray (including airport X-ray), CT scan, or ultrasound (may damage injector system).

• Instruct patient to keep OBI at least 4 inches (10 cm) away from electrical equipment, including cell phones, cordless phones, microwaves, and other common appliances (injector may not work properly).

• Advise patient to avoid activities, such as traveling, driving, or operating machinery, for 26 to 29 hours after using OBI.

• Caution patient to report OBI device failure immediately to determine need for replacement dose.

---

peginterferon alfa-2a ⌧
peg-in-ter-FEER-on

Pegasys

Therapeutic class: Antivirals
Pharmacologic class: Interferons

AVAILABLE FORMS

Injection:* 180 mcg/1 mL single-dose vial; 180 mcg/0.5 mL prefilled syringe

INDICATIONS & DOSAGES

Adjust-a-dose (for all indications): Refer to manufacturer's instructions for toxicity-related dosage adjustments. In adults with CrCl less than 30 mL/minute, including patients on hemodialysis, decrease dosage to 135 mcg once weekly. There are no recommendations for children with renal impairment.

➤ **Chronic HCV infection with compensated hepatic disease in patients not previously treated with interferon alfa, in combination with other HCV antiviral drugs** ⌧
Adults with HCV genotype 1 or 4: 180 mcg subcut in abdomen or thigh once weekly as monotherapy or combination therapy with ribavirin for 48 weeks. Refer to prescribing information of the other HCV antiviral for duration of entire treatment regimen. If used with ribavirin with or without other HCV antivirals, treatment duration is 48 weeks.

Reactions in bold italics are *life-threatening*. Interactions may have a *rapid onset* or a ***delayed onset***.

Adults with HCV genotype 2 or 3: 180 mcg subcut in abdomen or thigh once weekly. Refer to prescribing information of the other HCV antiviral for duration of entire treatment regimen. If used with ribavirin with or without other HCV antivirals, treatment duration is 24 weeks.

Children age 5 and older: 180 mcg/1.73 m² × BSA subcut once weekly in combination with ribavirin. Treat patients with genotype 2 or 3 for 24 weeks, other genotypes for 48 weeks. Maximum dose is 180 mcg once weekly.

➤ **Chronic HCV infection (regardless of genotype) in patients with HIV-1 infection who haven't previously been treated with interferon alfa**
Adults: 180 mcg subcut in abdomen or thigh once weekly. When used with ribavirin, treatment duration is 48 weeks. When used with other HCV antivirals, refer to prescribing information of the other HCV antiviral for treatment duration.

➤ **Chronic HBV infection in patients with compensated liver disease and evidence of viral replication and liver inflammation**
Adults: 180 mcg subcut in abdomen or thigh once weekly for 48 weeks.

➤ **Hepatitis B e-antigen (HBeAg)-positive chronic HBV infection in noncirrhotic children who have evidence of viral replication and elevation in serum ALT level**
Children age 3 and older: 180 mcg/1.73 m² × BSA subcut once weekly in combination with ribavirin. Maximum recommended dosage is 180 mcg weekly; recommended duration of therapy is 48 weeks. Patients who turn age 18 during therapy should maintain the recommended pediatric dosage through completion of therapy.

ADMINISTRATION
Subcutaneous
• Vials and prefilled syringes are for single use only. Discard unused portion.
• Don't shake. Allow to reach room temperature before use, but don't leave out of refrigerator for more than 24 hours. Don't freeze.
• Protect from light.
• For children, use 180-mcg/mL vial to withdraw appropriate dose and give using a 1-mL tuberculin syringe. Use of a prefilled syringe isn't recommended.
• Visually inspect drug for particulate matter and discoloration before administration; don't

use if particulate matter is visible or product is discolored.
• Give in abdomen or thigh; rotate injection site.
• Give on same day and at approximately same time each week.

ACTION
Causes reversible decreases in leukocyte and platelet counts, partially through stimulation of production of effector proteins in vitro. Inhibits HCV RNA replication.

Route	Onset	Peak	Duration
Subcut	Unknown	3–4 days	<1 wk

Half-life: 160 hours (range, 84 to 353 hours).

ADVERSE REACTIONS
CNS: depression, dizziness, headache, insomnia, irritability, fever, anxiety, asthenia, concentration impairment, memory impairment, mood alteration, nervousness, rigors, pain. **EENT:** blurred vision, epistaxis, nasopharyngitis, dry mouth. **GI:** abdominal pain, anorexia, diarrhea, nausea, vomiting. **Hematologic:** *neutropenia, thrombocytopenia,* anemia, *lymphopenia.* **Hepatic:** increased transaminase levels. **Metabolic:** weight loss. **Musculoskeletal:** arthralgia, myalgia, back pain. **Respiratory:** cough, dyspnea, URI. **Skin:** alopecia, pruritus, dermatitis, diaphoresis, rash, dry skin, eczema. **Other:** injection-site reaction, hypothyroidism, flulike syndrome, growth inhibition.

INTERACTIONS
Drug-drug. *Methadone:* May increase methadone level. Monitor patient closely and decrease methadone dosage as needed.
NRTIs: May cause severe and potentially fatal hepatic decompensation. If used together in patients coinfected with HIV who are taking NRTIs, monitor for toxicities.
Ribavirin: May cause additive hematologic toxicity. Monitor hematologic function.
Telbivudine: May increase risk of peripheral neuropathy. Avoid use together.
Theophylline, other drugs metabolized by CYP1A2: May increase theophylline level and may interact with other drugs metabolized by this enzyme system. Monitor theophylline level and adjust dosage as needed.
Zidovudine: May enhance adverse or toxic effect of zidovudine; may decrease zidovudine metabolism. Monitor therapy.

EFFECTS ON LAB TEST RESULTS

• May increase triglyceride, AST, and ALT levels.
• May decrease Hb level, hematocrit, ANC, and WBC and platelet counts.
• May increase or decrease thyroid function test values.

CONTRAINDICATIONS & CAUTIONS

• Contraindicated in patients hypersensitive to interferon alfa-2a or any components of formulation.
• Contraindicated in patients with autoimmune hepatitis or decompensated liver disease (with monoinfection or coinfection with HIV) before or during treatment with drug.
• Contraindicated in neonates and infants due to benzyl alcohol content.
• Use cautiously in patients with a history of depression.
• Use cautiously in patients with baseline neutrophil counts less than 1,500/mm³, baseline platelet counts less than 90,000/mm³, or baseline Hb level less than 10 g/dL.
• Use cautiously in patients with CrCl less than 50 mL/minute.
• Use cautiously in patients with cardiac disease or HTN, thyroid disease, autoimmune disorders, pulmonary disorders, colitis, pancreatitis, and ophthalmologic disorders.
• Use cautiously in older adults because they may be at increased risk for adverse reactions.
🔷 **Alert:** Use cautiously in patients also taking ribavirin. Ribavirin is also known to cause hemolytic anemia, which may worsen cardiac disease.
• Drug may inhibit growth in children.
• Safety and effectiveness haven't been established in patients who have failed to respond to other interferon alfa treatments, in solid organ transplant recipients, in patients with HBV infection also infected with HCV or HIV, or in patients with hepatitis C also infected with HBV or HIV with a CD4+ cell count less than 100 cells/mm³.
Dialyzable drug: No.
⚠ **Overdose S&S:** Fatigue, elevated liver enzyme levels, neutropenia, thrombocytopenia.

PREGNANCY-LACTATION-REPRODUCTION

• There are no adequate studies of drug used as monotherapy during pregnancy. Use drug as monotherapy only if potential benefit justifies fetal risk and only in patients of childbearing potential when they are using effective contraception. Some professional guidelines discourage use during pregnancy.
• Combination therapy with ribavirin may cause fetal birth defects or death and is contraindicated during pregnancy. Regular pregnancy testing is required before, monthly during, and for 6 months after treatment in patients and partners of male patients on combination therapy with ribavirin. Patients of childbearing potential and men with partners of childbearing potential must use two forms of effective contraception during therapy and for at least 6 months after therapy ends.
• Prescribers are encouraged to enroll patients or partners of male patients who become pregnant during combination therapy with ribavirin in the Ribavirin Pregnancy Registry (1-800-593-2214).
• It isn't known if drug appears in human milk. Patient should discontinue breastfeeding or discontinue drug.
• Drug may disrupt the menstrual cycle. It isn't known if drug impairs fertility.

NURSING CONSIDERATIONS

Boxed Warning Alpha interferons may cause or aggravate fatal or life-threatening neuropsychiatric (aggressive behavior, psychoses, hallucinations, bipolar disorders, mania), autoimmune (hepatitis, ITP, RA, interstitial nephritis, SLE), ischemic, and infectious disorders. Monitor patients closely with periodic clinical and lab evaluations. Withdraw patients with persistently severe or worsening signs or symptoms of these conditions from therapy. ■
• Obtain CBC before treatment and monitor counts routinely during therapy. Stop drug in patients who develop severe decrease in neutrophil or platelet counts.
• Monitor patient for hypersensitivity reactions (including angioedema and anaphylaxis) and severe skin reactions (including SJS and exfoliative dermatitis).
• Stop drug if uncontrollable thyroid disease, hyperglycemia, hypoglycemia, or diabetes occurs during treatment.
• If persistent or unexplained pulmonary infiltrates or pulmonary dysfunction occur, stop drug.
• Stop drug if signs and symptoms of colitis occur, such as abdominal pain, bloody diarrhea, and fever. Symptoms should resolve within 1 to 3 weeks.

• Stop drug if signs and symptoms of pancreatitis occur, including fever, malaise, and abdominal pain.

• Obtain baseline eye exam and periodically monitor eye exams during treatment. Stop drug if new or worsening disorders occur.

• Monitor kidney function, liver function, and uric acid and TSH levels.

• Verify negative pregnancy status before, monthly during, and for 6 months after combined therapy with ribavirin. Verify negative pregnancy status in partners of male patients on combined therapy with ribavirin monthly during treatment and for at least 6 months after treatment.

• *Look alike–sound alike:* Don't confuse peginterferon alfa-2a with interferon alfa-2a, interferon alfa-2b, or interferon alfa-n3.

PATIENT TEACHING

• Advise patient to read medication guide that comes with drug.

• Teach patient proper way to give drug and dispose of needles and syringes, if appropriate.

• Instruct patient to immediately report depression or suicidality.

• Tell patient to report signs and symptoms of pancreatitis, colitis, eye disorders, or respiratory disorders.

• Advise patient who feels dizzy, tired, confused, or sleepy to avoid driving or operating machinery.

• Caution patient not to switch to another brand of interferon without consulting health care provider.

• Tell patient that flulike symptoms commonly occur, including tiredness, weakness, fever, chills, muscle aches, joint pain, and headaches. Inform patient that injecting in the evening may lessen symptoms.

• Advise patient of childbearing potential that drug may alter menstrual cycles and impair fertility.

🛈 *Alert:* When drug is used with ribavirin, tell patient and partners to take extreme care to avoid pregnancy during treatment with ribavirin and for 6 months after treatment ends.

SAFETY ALERT!

pembrolizumab ⚭
pem-broe-LIZ-ue-mab

Keytruda

Therapeutic class: Antineoplastics
Pharmacologic class: Monoclonal antibodies

AVAILABLE FORMS

Injection: 25 mg/mL (4 mL) solution in single-use vial

INDICATIONS & DOSAGES

🛈 *Alert:* Refer to manufacturer's instructions for additional treatment criteria by diagnosis, dosing information of drugs used in combination therapy regimens, and treatment duration.

Adjust-a-dose (for all indications): Refer to manufacturer's instructions for toxicity-related dosage adjustments.

➤ **Unresectable or metastatic melanoma**
Adults: 200-mg IV infusion over 30 minutes every 3 weeks, or 400-mg IV infusion every 6 weeks, until disease progression or unacceptable toxicity.

➤ **Adjuvant treatment of melanoma with lymph node involvement after complete resection**
Adults: 200-mg IV infusion over 30 minutes every 3 weeks, or 400-mg IV infusion every 6 weeks.
Children age 12 and older: 2 mg/kg IV over 30 minutes every 3 weeks up to maximum dose of 200 mg.

➤ **Head and neck squamous cell carcinoma**
Adults: 200-mg IV infusion every 3 weeks, or 400-mg IV infusion every 6 weeks.

➤ **NSCLC** ⚭
Adults: 200-mg IV infusion every 3 weeks, or 400-mg IV infusion every 6 weeks.

➤ **Classical Hodgkin lymphoma**
Adults: 200-mg IV infusion every 3 weeks, or 400-mg IV infusion every 6 weeks.
Children age 12 and older: 2 mg/kg IV over 30 minutes every 3 weeks up to maximum dose of 200 mg.

➤ **Primary mediastinal large B-cell lymphoma (PMBCL)**
Adults: 200-mg IV infusion every 3 weeks, or 400-mg IV infusion every 6 weeks.

P

🍁 Canada ◇ OTC ◆ Off-label use 🖉 Photoguide ⊛ Do not crush *Liquid contains alcohol ⚭ Genetic

Children age 12 and older: 2 mg/kg IV over 30 minutes every 3 weeks up to maximum dose of 200 mg.

➤ **Urothelial carcinoma**
Adults: 200-mg IV infusion every 3 weeks, or 400-mg IV infusion every 6 weeks.

➤ **Microsatellite instability-high (MSI-H) or mismatch repair deficient solid tumors** ⌧
Adults: 200-mg IV infusion every 3 weeks, or 400-mg IV infusion every 6 weeks.
Children age 2 and older: 2 mg/kg (up to maximum of 200 mg/dose) IV infusion every 3 weeks.

➤ **MSI-H or mismatch repair deficient colorectal cancer** ⌧
Adults: 200-mg IV infusion every 3 weeks, or 400-mg IV infusion every 6 weeks.

➤ **MSI-H or mismatch repair deficient endometrial carcinoma** ⌧
Adults: 200-mg IV infusion every 3 weeks, or 400-mg IV infusion every 6 weeks.

➤ **Gastric cancer**
Adults: 200-mg IV infusion every 3 weeks, or 400-mg IV infusion every 6 weeks.

➤ **Esophageal carcinoma**
Adults: 200-mg IV infusion every 3 weeks, or 400-mg IV infusion every 6 weeks, until disease progression or unacceptable toxicity occurs, or up to 24 months in patients without disease progression.

➤ **Cervical cancer**
Adults: 200-mg IV infusion every 3 weeks, or 400-mg IV infusion every 6 weeks.

➤ **Hepatocellular carcinoma**
Adults: 200-mg IV infusion every 3 weeks, or 400-mg IV infusion every 6 weeks.

➤ **Recurrent locally advanced or metastatic Merkel cell carcinoma**
Adults: 200-mg IV infusion every 3 weeks, or 400-mg IV infusion every 6 weeks.
Children: 2 mg/kg/dose to maximum of 200 mg/dose IV infusion every 3 weeks.

➤ **Advanced renal cell carcinoma, in combination with axitinib or lenvatinib**
Adults: 200-mg IV infusion every 3 weeks, or 400-mg IV infusion every 6 weeks, in combination with 5 mg axitinib PO b.i.d. or lenvatinib 20 mg PO daily.

➤ **Endometrial carcinoma that isn't MSI-H or mismatch repair deficient, in combination with lenvatinib** ⌧
Adults: 200-mg IV infusion every 3 weeks, or 400-mg IV infusion every 6 weeks, in combination with lenvatinib 20 mg PO once daily.

➤ **Tumor mutational burden-high (TMB-H) solid tumors** ⌧
Adults: 200-mg IV infusion every 3 weeks, or 400-mg IV infusion every 6 weeks.
Children age 2 and older: 2 mg/kg IV infusion to maximum dose of 200 mg every 3 weeks.

➤ **Cutaneous squamous cell carcinoma**
Adults: 200-mg IV infusion every 3 weeks, or 400-mg IV infusion every 6 weeks.

➤ **Triple-negative breast cancer (TNBC), in combination with chemotherapy (neoadjuvant and adjuvant)**
Adults: Neoadjuvant treatment in combination with chemotherapy for 24 weeks (eight doses of 200-mg IV infusion every 3 weeks, or four doses of 400-mg IV infusion every 6 weeks), followed by adjuvant treatment as a single agent for up to 27 weeks (nine doses of 200-mg IV infusion every 3 weeks, or five doses of 400-mg IV infusion every 6 weeks). Give before chemotherapy when given on same day.

➤ **TNBC, in combination with chemotherapy**
Adults: 200-mg IV infusion every 3 weeks, or 400-mg IV infusion every 6 weeks. Give before chemotherapy when given on same day.

ADMINISTRATION

IV
▼ Don't give as IV push or bolus.
▼ Visually inspect solution for particulate matter and discoloration. Solution appears clear to slightly opalescent, colorless to slightly yellow. Discard if particles are visible.
▼ Dilute to yield 1 to 10 mg/mL in bag of NSS or D_5W. Gently invert bag to mix solution.
▼ Discard unused portion left in vial.
▼ Administer infusion over 30 minutes using an IV line with a nonpyrogenic, low-protein-binding 0.2- to 5-micron filter.
▼ Diluted solution remains stable for 96 hours if refrigerated and for 6 hours at room temperature. Don't freeze.
▼ **Incompatibilities:** Don't infuse other drugs through same infusion line.

ACTION

A humanized monoclonal antibody that binds to the PD1 receptor found on the surface of T cells, reversing T-cell suppression and resulting in decreased tumor growth.

Reactions in bold italics are *life-threatening*. Interactions may have a *rapid onset* or a ***delayed onset***.

Route	Onset	Peak	Duration
IV	Unknown	Unknown	Unknown

Half-life: 22 days.

ADVERSE REACTIONS
CNS: asthenia, fatigue, fever, confusion, peripheral neuropathy, weakness, headache, dizziness, insomnia. **CV:** peripheral edema, HTN, pericarditis, *MI, arrhythmia, cardiac tamponade,* pericardial effusion. **EENT:** uveitis, nasopharyngitis. **GI:** nausea, constipation, diarrhea, vomiting, abdominal pain, colitis, stomatitis. **GU:** *renal failure,* nephritis, UTI. **Hematologic:** anemia, *lymphocytopenia, thrombocytopenia, neutropenia.* **Hepatic:** *hepatitis.* **Metabolic:** decreased appetite, hypophysitis, hyperthyroidism, hypothyroidism, hyperglycemia, *hyponatremia, hyperkalemia, hypokalemia, hypomagnesemia,* hypoalbuminemia, hypertriglyceridemia, hypercholesterolemia, decreased bicarbonate level, hypercalcemia, *hypocalcemia, increased INR,* increased AST, ALT, and ALP levels. **Musculoskeletal:** arthralgia, back pain, musculoskeletal pain, myalgia, myositis, immune-mediated arthritis. **Respiratory:** cough, dyspnea, URI, pneumonitis, pneumonia, pleural effusion, *respiratory failure.* **Skin:** pruritus, rash, immune-mediated rash, vitiligo. **Other:** antibody development, flulike symptoms, infection, chills, *sepsis.*

INTERACTIONS
Drug-drug. *Thalidomide:* May increase mortality in patients with multiple myeloma when used with pembrolizumab and dexamethasone. This combination isn't recommended.

EFFECTS ON LAB TEST RESULTS
• May increase glucose, triglyceride, cholesterol, creatinine, ALP, ALT, and AST levels.
• May decrease bicarbonate, sodium, magnesium, and albumin levels.
• May increase or decrease potassium, calcium, and thyroid hormone levels.
• May decrease Hb level and lymphocyte, platelet, and WBC counts.

CONTRAINDICATIONS & CAUTIONS
• Contraindicated in patients hypersensitive to drug or its components.
⚠ *Alert:* Patients with *EGFR* or *ALK* genomic tumor aberrations should have disease progression on FDA-approved therapy for these aberrations before receiving pembrolizumab.
⚠ *Alert:* Drug can cause immune-mediated reactions (such as pneumonitis, pericarditis, myelitis, hepatitis, endocrinopathies, colitis, nephritis, and renal dysfunction); drug may need to be withheld or permanently discontinued.
• Severe, life-threatening infusion-related reactions have occurred in patients receiving drug. Stop infusion immediately and administer supportive care.
• Use cautiously in patients who receive allogeneic hematopoietic stem cell transplantation before or after treatment with a PD-1/PD-L1 blocking antibody. Serious or fatal complications have occurred, including GVHD, hepatic veno-occlusive disease, and steroid-requiring febrile syndrome. Monitor patient closely if benefits outweigh risks.
• Use hasn't been studied in patients with moderate or severe hepatic impairment.
• Safety and effectiveness have been established in children younger than age 18 with cHL, PMBCL, MSI-H cancer, and TMB-H cancer. Safety and effectiveness in children haven't been established in the other approved indications.
Dialyzable drug: Unknown.

PREGNANCY-LACTATION-REPRODUCTION
• Drug may cause fetal harm. Don't use during pregnancy. Patients of childbearing potential should use highly effective contraception during therapy and for 4 months after final dose.
• It isn't known if drug appears in human milk. Patient shouldn't breastfeed during therapy and for 4 months after final dose.

NURSING CONSIDERATIONS
• Verify pregnancy status in patients of childbearing potential before initiation.
• Monitor patient closely for signs and symptoms of hypersensitivity or infusion reactions. Stop infusion and have drugs, such as epinephrine, antihistamines, and corticosteroids, available for immediate treatment of such a reaction.
• Assess for signs and symptoms of immune-mediated reactions. Thyroid disorders, liver toxicity, and hypophysitis typically occur early in treatment. Pulmonary, renal, and GI toxicity may develop after 6 months of treatment.

P

• Monitor patient for immune-mediated pneumonitis (shortness of breath, chest pain, new or worsening cough). Evaluate radiographically, give corticosteroids if clinically indicated, and withhold or discontinue drug based on grade.

• Monitor patient for signs and symptoms of immune-mediated colitis (increased frequency of bowel movements or diarrhea; abdominal pain or tenderness; melena). Give corticosteroids as clinically indicated and withhold or discontinue drug based on toxicity grade.

• Monitor patient for signs and symptoms of immune-mediated hepatitis (elevated liver enzyme levels, jaundice, tea-colored urine, nausea, vomiting, anorexia, right upper quadrant abdominal pain, abnormal bleeding or bruising). Give corticosteroids as clinically indicated and withhold or discontinue drug based on toxicity grade.

• Monitor patient for signs and symptoms of hypophysitis, the immune-mediated inflammation of the pituitary gland (persistent or unusual headaches, extreme weakness, dizziness, fainting, vision changes). Give corticosteroids and hormone replacement as clinically indicated and withhold or discontinue drug based on toxicity grade.

• Monitor patient for signs and symptoms of immune-mediated endocrine disorders (hypothyroidism, hyperthyroidism, adrenal insufficiency), which may include tachycardia, weight loss or gain, edema, and hair loss. Assess hormone levels at baseline, periodically during treatment, and as clinically indicated. Give corticosteroids and hormone replacement as clinically indicated and withhold or discontinue drug based on toxicity grade.

• Be aware of potential for less common immune-mediated adverse reactions, such as exfoliative dermatitis, uveitis, arthritis, myositis, pancreatitis, hemolytic anemia, and partial seizures in patients with inflammatory foci in the brain. Based on severity of adverse reaction, withhold drug and administer corticosteroids.

PATIENT TEACHING

• Caution patient about the risk of immune-mediated adverse effects that may require corticosteroid treatment and interruption of therapy or discontinuation of drug.

• Teach patient signs and symptoms of lung problems (dyspnea, chest pain, cough), colitis (diarrhea; melena; abdominal pain), liver problems (yellowing of the skin or eyes, dark urine, nausea or vomiting, decreased appetite, abdominal pain, bleeding or bruising), hormone gland problems (rapid heartbeat, weight loss, diaphoresis, weight gain, hair loss, feeling cold), renal problems (changes in the amount or color of urine), and other problems (rash, vision changes, muscle or joint pain, muscle weakness) and to report them to prescriber.

• Advise patient to report pregnancy, plans to become pregnant, or breastfeeding.

• Teach patient of childbearing potential of potential hazard to the fetus and to use contraception during therapy and for 4 months after final dose.

• Advise patient to stop breastfeeding during therapy and for 4 months after final dose.

• Instruct patient to keep lab test appointments as requested by prescriber to monitor drug's safety and effectiveness.

SAFETY ALERT!

PEMEtrexed disodium ⌧

pem-e-TREKS-ed

Alimta, Pemfexy

Therapeutic class: Antineoplastics
Pharmacologic class: Folate antagonists

AVAILABLE FORMS

Injection (lyophilized powder for solution): 100 mg, 500 mg in single-use vials
Solution for injection: 500 mg (25 mg/mL) multidose vial

INDICATIONS & DOSAGES

Adjust-a-dose (for all indications): Refer to manufacturer's instructions for toxicity-related dosage adjustments.

➤ **Malignant pleural mesothelioma in patients whose disease is unresectable or who aren't candidates for curative surgery, in combination with cisplatin**

Adults: 500 mg/m² IV infusion on day 1 of each 21-day cycle before cisplatin. Refer to full prescribing information for cisplatin.

➤ **Locally advanced or metastatic NSCLC after prior chemotherapy; as single-agent maintenance therapy for patients whose disease hasn't progressed after four cycles of platinum-based first-line chemotherapy**

Adults: 500 mg/m² IV infusion on day 1 of each 21-day cycle.

➤ **In combination with cisplatin for initial treatment of patients with locally advanced or metastatic, nonsquamous NSCLC**

Adults: 500 mg/m² IV infusion administered before cisplatin on day 1 of each 21-day cycle for up to six cycles in the absence of disease progression or unacceptable toxicity. Refer to full prescribing information for cisplatin.

➤ **Initial treatment of metastatic nonsquamous NSCLC with no *EGFR* or *ALK* genomic tumor aberrations, in combination with pembrolizumab and platinum chemotherapy** ▨

Adults: 500 mg/m² IV infusion administered after pembrolizumab and before carboplatin or cisplatin on day 1 of each 21-day cycle for four cycles. After completion of platinum-based therapy, may give pemetrexed as maintenance therapy, alone or with pembrolizumab, until disease progression or unacceptable toxicity occurs. Refer to the full prescribing information for pembrolizumab and carboplatin or cisplatin.

ADMINISTRATION

IV

⊙ *Alert:* Hazardous drug; use safe handling and disposal precautions.

▼ Premedicate with folic acid 400 to 1,000 mcg PO once daily beginning 7 days before first dose of drug and continue during therapy and for 21 days after last dose.

▼ Premedicate with vitamin B₁₂ 1 mg IM 1 week before first dose of pemetrexed and every three cycles thereafter. Don't substitute PO vitamin B₁₂ for IM. After the first cycle, may give vitamin B₁₂ injections on the first day of the cycle.

▼ Premedicate with dexamethasone 4 mg PO b.i.d. the day before, the day of, and the day after pemetrexed administration.

▼ Reconstitute 100-mg vial with 4.2 mL or 500-mg vial with 20 mL of preservative-free NSS to yield 25 mg/mL.

▼ Swirl vial gently until powder is completely dissolved. Solution should be clear and colorless to yellow or yellow-green. If particulate matter is observed, discard vial.

▼ Calculate appropriate dose, and further dilute with NSS so total volume of solution is 100 mL.

▼ Give over 10 minutes.

▼ Reconstituted solution and dilution are stable for 24 hours refrigerated.

▼ Dilute Pemfexy solution with D₅W to a total volume of 100 mL. Don't use diluents other than D₅W.

▼ **Incompatibilities:** Calcium-containing diluents, including Ringer or lactated Ringer for injection; other drugs or diluents. Consult a compatibility reference for full details.

ACTION

Disturbs cell replication by inhibiting several folate-dependent enzymes involved in nucleotide synthesis.

Route	Onset	Peak	Duration
IV	Unknown	Unknown	Unknown

Half-life: 3.5 hours.

ADVERSE REACTIONS

CNS: depression, fatigue, fever, neuropathy, taste disturbance. **CV:** *cardiac ischemia,* edema, thrombosis. **EENT:** conjunctivitis, increased lacrimation, pharyngitis. **GI:** anorexia, constipation, diarrhea, dyspepsia, nausea, stomatitis, vomiting. **GU:** elevated creatinine level, *renal failure.* **Hematologic:** anemia, *leukopenia, neutropenia, febrile neutropenia, thrombocytopenia.* **Hepatic:** increased transaminase levels, increased ALP level. **Metabolic:** dehydration, hyperglycemia, hypoalbuminemia, *hyponatremia,* hypophosphatemia, *hypocalcemia, hyperkalemia, hypokalemia.* **Musculoskeletal:** arthralgia, myalgia. **Respiratory:** cough, dyspnea. **Skin:** alopecia, rash, pruritus, erythema multiforme. **Other:** allergic reaction, infection.

INTERACTIONS

Drug-drug. *Ibuprofen:* May decrease pemetrexed clearance in patients with mild to moderate renal insufficiency (CrCl between 45 and 79 mL/minute). Avoid ibuprofen for 2 days before, during, and 2 days after pemetrexed therapy. Monitor patient for myelosuppression and assess renal and GI toxicity status more frequently if ibuprofen use can't be avoided.

Nephrotoxic drugs, probenecid: May delay pemetrexed clearance. Monitor patient.

Vaccines, inactivated: May decrease therapeutic effect of vaccines. Complete age-appropriate vaccinations at least 2 weeks before start of drug therapy, or if vaccine is

given within 2 weeks, revaccinate at least 3 months after drug is discontinued.
Vaccines, live: May increase adverse effects and decrease therapeutic effect of vaccine. Avoid use during and for 3 months after drug therapy.

EFFECTS ON LAB TEST RESULTS
• May increase glucose, ALT, AST, ALP, and creatinine levels.
• May decrease albumin, sodium, phosphate, and calcium levels.
• May increase or decrease potassium level.
• May decrease Hb level, hematocrit, ANC, and platelet and WBC counts.

CONTRAINDICATIONS & CAUTIONS
• Contraindicated in patients with a history of severe hypersensitivity reaction to drug.
• Don't use in patients with CrCl of less than 45 mL/minute.
• Drug can cause severe myelosuppression requiring transfusions, which may lead to neutropenic infection, serious interstitial pneumonitis (including fatal cases), and radiation recall in patients who received radiation weeks to years previously.
Dialyzable drug: Unknown.
⚠ *Overdose S&S:* Neutropenia, anemia, thrombocytopenia, mucositis, rash, infection with or without fever, diarrhea.

PREGNANCY-LACTATION-REPRODUCTION
• Drug can cause fetal harm. Avoid use during pregnancy. Patients of childbearing potential should use effective contraception during therapy and for 6 months after final dose. Males with partners of childbearing potential should use contraception during treatment and for 3 months after final dose.
• If used during pregnancy or if patient becomes pregnant during therapy, inform patient that drug may harm fetus.
• It isn't known if drug appears in human milk. Patient shouldn't breastfeed during and for 1 week after treatment.
• Drug may impair male fertility. It's unknown if effects are reversible.

NURSING CONSIDERATIONS
• Patient shouldn't start a new cycle of treatment unless ANC is 1,500/mm³ or more, platelet count is 100,000/mm³ or more, and CrCl is 45 mL/minute or more.
• Verify pregnancy status before treatment.

• Monitor patient for hypersensitivity reactions.
• Monitor patient for new-onset or worsening of pulmonary symptoms (dyspnea, cough, fever). Evaluate patient for pneumonitis if they occur.
• Monitor renal function, CBC, platelet count, Hb level, hematocrit, and LFT values.
• Assess patient for neurotoxicity, mucositis, and diarrhea. Severe symptoms may warrant dosage adjustment.
• Monitor patient for infections and skin toxicity (SJS, TEN).
• To reduce the occurrence and severity of pemetrexed toxicity, give a corticosteroid, such as dexamethasone 4 mg PO b.i.d., the day before, the day of, and the day after giving this drug.
🕭 *Alert:* To reduce toxicity, patient should take folic acid daily and receive IM vitamin B₁₂.
• *Look alike–sound alike:* Don't confuse pemetrexed with methotrexate or pralatrexate.

PATIENT TEACHING
• Stress importance of taking prescribed premedications to reduce risk of treatment-related toxicity.
• Inform patient that blood cell counts may drop during therapy. Instruct patient to report infection, fever, bleeding, or signs and symptoms of anemia (fatigue, shortness of breath, cold hands and feet, pallor).
• Tell patient who has received prior radiation about the risk of radiation recall. Advise patient to immediately report inflammation or blisters in a previously irradiated area.
• Urge patient to report adverse effects, especially fever, sore throat, infection, diarrhea, fatigue, bleeding, cough, shortness of breath, and limb pain.
• Advise patient of childbearing potential and male patient with partners of childbearing potential of fetal risk and the need for effective contraception.
• Caution patient not to breastfeed during treatment and for 1 week after final dose.

Reactions in bold italics are *life-threatening*. Interactions may have a *rapid onset* or a *delayed onset*.

penicillin G benzathine (benzathine benzylpenicillin)
pen-i-SILL-in

Bicillin L-A

Therapeutic class: Antibiotics
Pharmacologic class: Natural penicillins

AVAILABLE FORMS
Injection: 600,000 units/syringe (1 mL);
1,200,000 units/syringe (2 mL);
2,400,000 units/syringe (4 mL)

INDICATIONS & DOSAGES
➤ **Congenital syphilis**
Children ages 2 to 12: Follow CDC guidelines.
Children younger than age 2: 50,000 units/kg to maximum of 2.4 million units IM as a single dose.
➤ **Group A streptococcal URIs**
Adults: 1.2 million units IM as a single injection.
Children weighing 27 kg or more: 900,000 units IM as a single injection.
Infants and children weighing less than 27 kg: 300,000 to 600,000 units IM as a single injection.
➤ **To prevent poststreptococcal rheumatic fever and glomerulonephritis**
Adults and children weighing 27 kg or more: 1.2 million units IM once monthly or 300,000 units IM every 2 weeks.
➤ **Syphilis (primary, secondary, and latent)**
Adults: 2.4 million units IM as a single dose.
➤ **Syphilis (tertiary and neurosyphilis)**
Adults: 2.4 million units IM once every 7 days for 3 weeks.
➤ **Yaws, bejel, and pinta**
Adults: 1.2 million units IM as a single injection.

ADMINISTRATION
IM
Boxed Warning Inadvertent IV use may cause cardiac arrest and death. ■
• Before giving drug, ask patient about allergic reactions to penicillin.
• Obtain specimen for culture and sensitivity tests before giving first dose. Begin therapy while awaiting results.
• Warm to room temperature before giving to lessen injection-site pain.
• Shake well before injecting.
• Inspect visually for particulate matter and discoloration before administration.
• Inject deep into upper outer quadrant of buttocks or ventrogluteal site in adults and in midlateral thigh in infants and small children. Rotate injection sites. Avoid injection into or near major nerves or blood vessels to prevent permanent neurovascular damage.
• Inject at a slow, steady rate to prevent needle occlusion.
• Injection may be painful, but ice applied to the site may ease discomfort.
• Store in refrigerator at 36° to 46° F (2° to 8° C); don't freeze.

ACTION
Inhibits cell-wall synthesis during bacterial multiplication.

Route	Onset	Peak	Duration
IM	Unknown	12–24 hr	1–4 wk

Half-life: Unknown.

ADVERSE REACTIONS
CNS: neuropathy, headache. **GI:** *pseudomembranous colitis,* enterocolitis, nausea, vomiting, blood in stool, CDAD. **GU:** nephropathy. **Hematologic:** *agranulocytosis, leukopenia, thrombocytopenia,* eosinophilia, hemolytic anemia. **Skin:** hypersensitive skin reactions. **Other:** *anaphylaxis,* hypersensitivity reactions, sterile abscess at injection site.

INTERACTIONS
Drug-drug. *Aminoglycosides (amikacin, gentamicin, tobramycin):* May decrease aminoglycoside level. Monitor therapy.
Live-virus vaccines: May decrease effectiveness of live-virus vaccines. Avoid concurrent use.
Methotrexate: May increase risk of methotrexate toxicity. Monitor patient closely.
Probenecid: May increase penicillin level. Probenecid may be used for this purpose.
Tetracycline: May antagonize penicillin G benzathine effects. Avoid using together.
Warfarin: May increase anticoagulant effects. Monitor therapy.

P

EFFECTS ON LAB TEST RESULTS
• May increase BUN, creatinine, and AST levels.
• May decrease Hb level and platelet, WBC, and granulocyte counts.
• May cause positive Coombs test results.
• May cause false-positive CSF protein test results.
• May alter urine glucose testing using cupric sulfate (Benedict reagent).

CONTRAINDICATIONS & CAUTIONS
• Contraindicated in patients hypersensitive to drug or other penicillins.
Boxed Warning Not for IV use or to be mixed with other IV solutions. Risk of cardiorespiratory arrest and death. ∎
• Inadvertent intravascular administration, including inadvertent direct intra-arterial injection or injection immediately adjacent to arteries, has resulted in severe neurovascular damage, including transverse myelitis with permanent paralysis, gangrene requiring amputation of digits and more proximal portions of extremities, and necrosis and sloughing at and surrounding the injection site.
• Use cautiously in patients allergic to other drugs, especially to cephalosporins, because of possible cross-sensitivity.
• Use cautiously in older adults and patients with a history of significant allergies or asthma.
• Drug may cause CDAD ranging in severity from mild diarrhea to fatal colitis. For suspected or confirmed CDAD, discontinue drug and start CDAD treatment.
• Drug may cause SCARs, including SJS, DRESS syndrome, and TEN. Monitor patient closely.
Dialyzable drug: Yes.
⚠ *Overdose S&S:* Neuromuscular hyperexcitability, seizures.

PREGNANCY-LACTATION-REPRODUCTION
• There are no adequate studies during pregnancy; however, fetal adverse effects haven't been reported. Use only if clearly needed.
• Drug appears in human milk. Use cautiously during breastfeeding.

NURSING CONSIDERATIONS
⚕ *Alert:* Bicillin L-A is the only penicillin G benzathine product indicated for sexually transmitted infections. Don't substitute Bicillin C-R because it may not be effective.

• Monitor patient for diarrhea and severe skin reactions. Drug may need to be stopped.
• Drug's extremely slow absorption time makes allergic reactions difficult to treat.
• Large doses or prolonged therapy may cause bacterial or fungal superinfection, especially in older adults or patients who are debilitated or immunosuppressed.
• Monitor patients with syphilis for Jarisch-Herxheimer reactions (fever, chills, myalgia, headache, exacerbation of skin lesions, tachycardia, hyperventilation, flushing, mild hypotension). Reactions occur 1 to 2 hours after initial treatment and resolve within 12 to 24 hours.
• *Look alike–sound alike:* Don't confuse penicillin G benzathine with penicillamine or the various other types of penicillin.

PATIENT TEACHING
• Tell patient to report adverse reactions promptly.
• Advise patient that watery and bloody stools with or without stomach cramps and fever may occur during and up to 2 months or more after antibiotic use. Instruct the patient to report these symptoms as soon as possible.
• Warn patient that IM injection may be painful but that ice applied to the site may ease discomfort.
• Tell patient to take entire quantity of drug exactly as prescribed, even if feeling better.

penicillin G potassium (benzylpenicillin potassium)
pen-i-SILL-in

Pfizerpen

Therapeutic class: Antibiotics
Pharmacologic class: Natural penicillins

AVAILABLE FORMS
Injection: 1 million units, 5 million units, 20 million units
Premixed injection: 1 million units/50 mL, 2 million units/50 mL, 3 million units/50 mL

INDICATIONS & DOSAGES
Adjust-a-dose (for all indications): For patients who are uremic with a CrCl greater than 10 mL/minute/1.73 m², give full loading dose followed by one-half of loading dose

---

every 4 to 5 hours. If CrCl is less than 10 mL/minute/1.73 m^2, give full loading dose followed by one-half of loading dose every 8 to 10 hours. Make additional dosage modification in patients with hepatic disease and renal impairment.

➤ **Actinomycosis**
Adults: For cervicofacial infections, 1 to 6 million units/day in divided doses IM or IV every 4 to 6 hours. For thoracic or abdominal infections, 10 to 20 million units/day in divided doses IM or IV every 4 to 6 hours or by continuous IV infusion.

➤ **Anthrax**
Adults: 8 million units/day in divided doses IM or IV every 6 hours; higher doses may be required depending on susceptibility of the organism.

➤ **Clostridial infections (botulism, gas gangrene, tetanus)**
Adults: 20 million units/day in divided doses IM or IV every 4 to 6 hours.

➤ **Diphtheria**
Adults: 2 to 3 million units/day in divided doses IM or IV every 4 to 6 hours for 10 to 12 days.
Children: 150,000 to 250,000 units/kg/day in equal doses IM or IV every 6 hours for 7 to 10 days.

➤ **Disseminated gonococcal infections**
Adults: 10 million units/day in divided doses IM or IV every 4 to 6 hours. Duration depends on type of infection.
Children weighing 45 kg or more with arthritis, endocarditis, or meningitis: 10 million units/day in four equally divided doses IM or IV, with duration of therapy depending on type of infection.
Children weighing less than 45 kg with arthritis: 100,000 units/kg/day in four equally divided doses IM or IV for 7 to 10 days.
Children weighing less than 45 kg with endocarditis: 250,000 units/kg/day in equal doses IM or IV every 4 hours for 4 weeks.
Children weighing less than 45 kg with meningitis: 250,000 units/kg/day in equal doses IM or IV every 4 hours for 10 to 14 days.

➤ ***Erysipelothrix* endocarditis**
Adults: 12 to 20 million units/day in divided doses IM or IV every 4 to 6 hours for 4 to 6 weeks.

➤ **Fusospirochetosis**
Adults: 5 to 10 million units/day in divided doses IM or IV every 4 to 6 hours.

➤ **Haverhill fever; rat bite fever**
Adults: 12 to 20 million units/day in divided doses IM or IV every 4 to 6 hours for 3 to 4 weeks.

➤ **Haverhill fever (with endocarditis caused by *Streptobacillus moniliformis*); rat bite fever**
Children: 150,000 to 250,000 units/kg/day in equal doses every 4 hours for 4 weeks.

➤ ***Listeria monocytogenes* endocarditis or meningitis**
Adults: 15 to 20 million units/day in divided doses IM or IV every 4 to 6 hours. Treat for 2 weeks for meningitis and 4 weeks for endocarditis.

➤ **Meningococcal meningitis or septicemia**
Adults: 24 million units/day as 2 million units IM or IV every 2 hours.

➤ **Meningitis caused by susceptible strains of pneumococcus and meningococcus**
Children: 250,000 units/kg/day in equal doses IM or IV every 4 hours for 7 to 14 days, depending on infecting organism. Maximum dosage, 12 to 20 million units/day.

➤ **Neurosyphilis**
Adults: 12 to 24 million units/day (2 to 4 million units every 4 hours) IM or IV for 10 to 14 days. Many experts recommend penicillin G benzathine 2.4 million units IM weekly for 3 weeks following completion of this regimen.

➤ **Syphilis (congenital and neurosyphilis) after newborn period**
Children: 200,000 to 300,000 units/kg/day (given as 50,000 units/kg IV every 4 to 6 hours) for 10 to 14 days.

➤ ***Pasteurella multocida* bacteremia or meningitis**
Adults: 4 to 6 million units/day in divided doses IM or IV every 4 to 6 hours for 2 weeks.

➤ **Serious staphylococcal infections**
Adults: 5 to 24 million units/day in equally divided doses IM or IV every 4 to 6 hours.

➤ **Serious streptococcal infections**
Adults: 12 to 24 million units/day in equally divided doses IM or IV every 4 to 6 hours.

➤ **Serious streptococcal infections, such as pneumonia and endocarditis (*Streptococcus pneumoniae*), and meningococcal infections**
Children: 150,000 to 300,000 units/kg/day in equal doses IM or IV every 4 to 6 hours. Duration of therapy depends on infecting organism and type of infection.

P

➤ **Leptospirosis** ◆
Adults: 1.5 million units IV every 6 hours for 7 days.

ADMINISTRATION

- Obtain specimen for culture and sensitivity tests before giving first dose. Begin therapy while awaiting results.
- Before giving, ask patient about allergic reactions to penicillin.
- May give IM or by continuous IV infusion for dosages of 500,000, 1 million, or 5 million units. Drug is also suitable for intrapleural, intra-articular, intrathecal, and other local instillations.
- Administer 20 million unit dosage form by IV infusion only.
- ⚠️ *Alert:* Don't use in children requiring less than 1 million units/dose.

IV
▼ Reconstitute drug with sterile water for injection or NSS for injection. Volume of diluent varies with manufacturer.
▼ Reconstituted solution may be stored in refrigerator for up to 7 days.
▼ For continuous infusion, add reconstituted drug to 1 to 2 L of compatible solution. Determine how much fluid is needed and what the rate should be for a 24-hour period; then, add the drug to this fluid.
▼ Don't administer premixed solutions to patients requiring less than 1 million units per dose.
▼ Intermittent IV infusions have been administered over 15 to 30 minutes for infants and children and over 1 to 2 hours for adults.
▼ Thaw frozen bags at room temperature. May keep at room temperature for 24 hours or under refrigeration for 14 days. Don't refreeze thawed antibiotics.
▼ **Incompatibilities:** None listed by manufacturer. Consult a drug incompatibility reference for more information.

IM
- Vials containing 20 million units aren't intended for IM use.
- IM is the preferred route. Keep total volume of injection small.
- Give deep into large muscle; injection may be extremely painful.
- IM injection may be painful, but ice applied to the site may help alleviate discomfort.

ACTION

Inhibits cell-wall synthesis during bacterial multiplication.

Route	Onset	Peak	Duration
IV	Immediate	Immediate	Unknown
IM	Unknown	15–30 min	Unknown

Half-life: 31 to 50 minutes.

ADVERSE REACTIONS

CNS: *seizures, coma,* agitation, anxiety, confusion, depression, dizziness, fatigue, hallucinations, lethargy, hyperreflexia, myoclonic twitches, neuropathy. **CV:** local thrombophlebitis or phlebitis, *cardiac arrest, arrhythmias.* **GI:** *pseudomembranous colitis,* enterocolitis, nausea, vomiting, *CDAD.* **GU:** interstitial nephritis, nephropathy. **Hematologic:** *agranulocytosis, leukopenia, thrombocytopenia,* anemia, eosinophilia, hemolytic anemia. **Metabolic:** *hyperkalemia.* **Musculoskeletal:** arthralgia, myalgia. **Skin:** exfoliative dermatitis, maculopapular eruptions, pain at injection site. **Other:** *anaphylaxis,* hypersensitivity reactions, overgrowth of nonsusceptible organisms.

INTERACTIONS

Drug-drug. *Aminoglycosides (amikacin, gentamicin, tobramycin):* May decrease aminoglycoside level. Monitor therapy.
Aspirin, furosemide, indomethacin, sulfonamides, thiazide diuretics: May compete with penicillin for renal tubular secretion, prolonging penicillin half-life. Monitor patient.
Bacteriostatic antibacterial agents (chloramphenicol, macrolide antibiotics, sulfonamides, tetracyclines): May decrease bactericidal effect of penicillin. Avoid use together.
Heparin: May increase risk of bleeding. Closely monitor patient and adjust heparin dosage as needed.
Hormonal contraceptives: May decrease hormonal contraceptive effectiveness. Advise use of additional form of contraception during therapy.
Live-virus vaccines: May decrease effectiveness of live-virus vaccines. Don't use together.
Methotrexate: May increase risk of methotrexate toxicity. Monitor patient closely.
Oral anticoagulants: May increase or decrease anticoagulant effects. Monitor PT and INR.

Reactions in bold italics are *life-threatening*. Interactions may have a *rapid onset* or a ***delayed onset***.

Potassium-sparing diuretics: May increase risk of hyperkalemia. Avoid using together.
Probenecid: May increase penicillin level. Probenecid may be used for this purpose.

EFFECTS ON LAB TEST RESULTS
• May increase potassium level.
• May decrease Hb level and platelet, WBC, and granulocyte counts.
• May cause positive Coombs test result.
• May cause false-positive CSF protein test result.
• May alter urine glucose testing using cupric sulfate (Benedict reagent, Fehling solution, or Clinitest tablet).

CONTRAINDICATIONS & CAUTIONS
• Contraindicated in patients hypersensitive to drug or other penicillins.
• Use cautiously in patients with other drug allergies, especially to cephalosporins, because of possible cross-sensitivity.
• Use cautiously in older adults and patients with renal impairment, significant allergies, or asthma.
• Drug may cause CDAD ranging in severity from mild diarrhea to fatal colitis. If CDAD is suspected or confirmed, drug may need to be discontinued and treatment initiated.
• SCARs (SJS, TEN, DRESS syndrome, acute generalized exanthematous pustulosis) have been reported.
Dialyzable drug: Yes.
⚠ *Overdose S&S:* Agitation, confusion, asterixis, hallucinations, stupor, coma, multifocal myoclonus, seizures, encephalopathy, hyperkalemia.

PREGNANCY-LACTATION-REPRODUCTION
• There are no adequate studies during pregnancy. Use only if clearly needed.
• Penicillins appear in human milk. Use cautiously during breastfeeding.

NURSING CONSIDERATIONS
• Monitor IV site for phlebitis.
• Monitor renal function closely. Patients with poor renal function may have increased levels of penicillin and are at increased risk for adverse effects.
• Due to increased risk of electrolyte imbalances, monitor potassium and sodium levels closely in patients receiving more than 10 million units IV daily.

• Monitor liver function and CBC periodically during therapy.
• Observe patient closely. With large doses and prolonged therapy, bacterial or fungal superinfection may occur, especially in older adults or patients who are debilitated or immunosuppressed.
• For most acute infections, continue treatment for at least 48 to 72 hours after patient becomes asymptomatic. For group A beta-hemolytic streptococcal infections, maintain treatment for at least 10 days to reduce risk of rheumatic fever.
• Monitor patients with syphilis or other spirochetal infections (Lyme disease, relapsing fever) for Jarisch-Herxheimer reactions (fever, chills, myalgia, headache, exacerbation of skin lesions, tachycardia, hyperventilation, flushing, mild hypotension). Reactions occur 1 to 2 hours after initial treatment and resolve within 12 to 24 hours.
• *Look alike–sound alike:* Don't confuse penicillin G potassium with Polycillin, penicillamine, or the various other types of penicillin.

PATIENT TEACHING
• Tell patient to notify prescriber if rash, fever, or chills develop. A rash is the most common allergic reaction.
• Warn patient that IM injection may be painful but that ice applied to the site may help alleviate discomfort.
• Advise patient that watery and bloody stools with or without stomach cramps and fever may occur during and for up to 2 months or more after antibiotic use. Instruct patient to report these symptoms as soon as possible.

penicillin G procaine (benzylpenicillin procaine)
pen-i-SILL-in

Therapeutic class: Antibiotics
Pharmacologic class: Natural penicillins

AVAILABLE FORMS
Injection: 600,000 units/mL in 1-mL and 2-mL syringes

INDICATIONS & DOSAGES
➤ **Cutaneous anthrax**
Adults: 600,000 to 1 million units/day IM.

➤ **Inhalational anthrax (postexposure)**
Adults: 1.2 million units IM every 12 hours. Available safety data for penicillin G procaine at this dose would best support a duration of therapy of 2 weeks or less.
Children: 25,000 units/kg (maximum, 1.2 million units) IM every 12 hours.
Note: Treatment of inhalational anthrax (postexposure) must be continued for a total of 60 days. Consider risks and benefits of continuing administration of penicillin G procaine for more than 2 weeks or switching to an effective alternative treatment.

➤ **Bacterial endocarditis (group A streptococci), only in extremely sensitive infections**
Adults: 600,000 to 1 million units/day IM.

➤ **Adjunctive therapy for diphtheria with antitoxin**
Adults: 300,000 to 600,000 units/day IM for 14 days.

➤ **Diphtheria carrier state**
Adults: 300,000 units/day IM for 10 days.

➤ **Erysipeloid**
Adults: 600,000 to 1 million units/day IM.

➤ **Fusospirochetosis (Vincent infection)**
Adults: 600,000 to 1 million units/day IM.

➤ **Pneumonia (pneumococcal), moderately severe (uncomplicated)**
Adults: 600,000 to 1 million units/day IM for a minimum of 10 days.

➤ **Rat bite fever (*Streptobacillus moniliformis* and *Spirillum minus*)**
Adults: 600,000 to 1 million units/day IM.

➤ **Staphylococcal infections, moderately severe to severe**
Adults: 600,000 to 1 million units/day IM for a minimum of 10 days.

➤ **Streptococcal infections (group A), including moderately severe to severe tonsillitis, erysipelas, scarlet fever, URI, and skin and soft-tissue infections**
Adults: 600,000 to 1 million units/day IM for minimum of 10 days.

➤ **Syphilis (primary, secondary, and latent syphilis with negative spinal fluid)**
Adults and children older than age 12: 600,000 units/day IM for 8 days; total, 4.8 million units.

➤ **Late syphilis (tertiary syphilis, neurosyphilis, and latent syphilis with positive spinal fluid exam or no spinal fluid exam)**
Adults: 600,000 units/day IM for 10 to 15 days; total, 6 to 9 million units.

➤ **Congenital syphilis**
Children weighing less than 31.7 kg: 50,000 units/kg/day IM for 10 days. Maximum dosage, 2.4 million units/day.

➤ **Yaws, bejel, pinta**
Adults: Treatment as for syphilis in the corresponding stage of disease.

ADMINISTRATION
IM
● Before giving drug, ask patient about allergic reactions to penicillin.
● Obtain specimen for culture and sensitivity tests before giving first dose. Begin therapy while awaiting results.
● Give deep in upper outer quadrant of buttocks or ventrogluteal site in adults and in midlateral thigh in neonates, infants, and small children. Rotate injection sites. Don't give subcut. Don't massage injection site. Avoid injection near major nerves or blood vessels.
● Inject at a slow, steady rate to avoid needle blockage caused by high concentration of suspended material in product.
❶ *Alert:* Inadvertent IV, intravascular, or intraarterial administration may cause severe or permanent neurovascular damage.
● IM injection may be painful, but ice applied to the site may help alleviate discomfort.
● Inspect for particulate matter and discoloration before administration.
● Store at 36° to 46° F (2° to 8° C); don't freeze.

ACTION
Inhibits cell-wall synthesis during bacterial multiplication.

Route	Onset	Peak	Duration
IM	Unknown	1–4 hr	15–24 hr

Half-life: Unknown.

ADVERSE REACTIONS
CNS: depression, dizziness, fatigue, lethargy, fever. **GI:** *pseudomembranous colitis,* enterocolitis, nausea, vomiting. **Musculoskeletal:** arthralgia. **Skin:** rash, SCARs. **Other:** *anaphylaxis,* hypersensitivity reactions, chills, overgrowth of nonsusceptible organisms.

INTERACTIONS
Drug-drug. *Aminoglycosides (amikacin, gentamicin, tobramycin):* May decrease aminoglycoside level. Monitor therapy.

Reactions in bold italics are *life-threatening*. Interactions may have a *rapid onset* or a **delayed onset**.

Hormonal contraceptives: May decrease hormonal contraceptive effectiveness. Advise use of additional form of contraception during therapy.

Live-virus vaccines: May decrease vaccine effectiveness. Avoid concurrent use.

Methotrexate: May increase risk of methotrexate toxicity. Monitor patient closely.

Oral anticoagulants (warfarin): May increase or decrease effects of warfarin. Monitor coagulation status and adjust warfarin dosage as needed.

Probenecid: May increase penicillin level. Probenecid may be used for this purpose.

Tetracycline: May decrease bactericidal effect of penicillin. Avoid concurrent use of these drugs.

EFFECTS ON LAB TEST RESULTS

• May decrease Hb level and platelet, WBC, and granulocyte counts.

CONTRAINDICATIONS & CAUTIONS

• Contraindicated in patients hypersensitive to drug or other penicillins.

• Use cautiously in patients with other drug allergies, especially to cephalosporins, because of possible cross-sensitivity. Some formulations contain sulfites, which may cause allergic reactions in sensitive people.

• In patients with a history of hypersensitivity to procaine, administer intradermal test with 0.1 mL of 1% or 2% procaine solution and observe for wheal, flare, or eruption. If these occur, don't use drug and treat sensitivity supportively.

⚕ Use cautiously in patients with G6PD deficiency, congenital or idiopathic methemoglobinemia, cardiac or pulmonary compromise, or exposure to oxidizing agents and in infants younger than age 6 months due to increased risk of methemoglobinemia related to procaine.

• Drug may cause CDAD ranging in severity from mild diarrhea to fatal colitis. If CDAD is suspected or confirmed, drug may need to be discontinued and treatment initiated.

Dialyzable drug: Yes.

⚠ *Overdose S&S:* Neuromuscular hyperexcitability, seizures.

PREGNANCY-LACTATION-REPRODUCTION

• Penicillin G crosses the placental barrier; however, there are no adequate studies during pregnancy and there is no human evidence of adverse effects on the fetus if drug is used during pregnancy. Use only when clearly needed.

• Drug appears in human milk. Use cautiously during breastfeeding.

NURSING CONSIDERATIONS

⚠ *Alert:* Continue postexposure treatment for inhalation anthrax for 60 days. Prescriber should consider the risk-benefit ratio of continuing penicillin longer than 2 weeks, compared with switching to another drug.

• Monitor patient for diarrhea and initiate therapeutic measures as needed. Drug may need to be stopped.

• Allergic reactions are hard to treat because of drug's slow absorption rate.

• Monitor patient for SCARs. Stop drug immediately if SCARs are suspected.

• Monitor patients for procaine neuropsychiatric reaction (anxiety, confusion, agitation, depression, weakness, seizure, hallucination, combativeness, expressed "fear of impending death"), especially after a large single dose. Reactions are transient and last 15 to 30 minutes.

• Monitor patients who are at risk for methemoglobinemia (cyanosis, headache, tachycardia, shortness of breath, light-headedness, fatigue). Signs and symptoms may occur immediately after exposure or hours later.

• Monitor renal and hematopoietic function periodically with prolonged use.

• Monitor patients for fibrosis and atrophy from repeated IM injections.

• Monitor patients with syphilis for Jarisch-Herxheimer reactions (fever, chills, myalgia, headache, exacerbation of skin lesions, tachycardia, hyperventilation, flushing, mild hypotension). Reactions occur 1 to 2 hours after initial treatment and resolve within 12 to 24 hours.

• If large doses are given or if therapy is prolonged, bacterial or fungal superinfection may occur, especially in older adults and patients who are debilitated or immunosuppressed.

• Treatment duration depends on site and cause of infection.

• *Look alike–sound alike:* Don't confuse penicillin G procaine with Polycillin, penicillamine, or the various other types of penicillin.

P

PATIENT TEACHING

• Tell patient to report adverse reactions promptly. A rash is the most common allergic reaction.
• Warn patient that IM injection may be painful but that ice applied to the site may help alleviate discomfort.
• Advise patient that watery and bloody stools with or without stomach cramps and fever may occur during and for up to 2 months or more after antibiotic use. Instruct patient to report these symptoms as soon as possible.

penicillin G sodium (benzylpenicillin sodium)
pen-i-SILL-in

Therapeutic class: Antibiotics
Pharmacologic class: Natural penicillins

AVAILABLE FORMS
Injection: 5 million-unit vial

INDICATIONS & DOSAGES
Adjust-a-dose (for all indications): If CrCl is less than 10 mL/minute, give the full loading dose followed by 50% of the loading dose every 8 to 10 hours. If patient is uremic and CrCl is more than 10 mL/minute, give full loading dose; then give half the loading dose every 4 to 5 hours for additional doses. Make additional dosage adjustments in patients with hepatic disease and renal impairment.

➤ **Actinomycosis**
Adults: For cervicofacial infections, 1 to 6 million units/day in divided doses IM or IV every 4 to 6 hours. For thoracic or abdominal infections, 10 to 20 million units/day in divided doses every 4 to 6 hours.

➤ **Anthrax**
Adults: 8 million units/day in divided doses IM or IV every 6 hours; higher dosages may be required depending on susceptibility of the organism.

➤ **Clostridial infections (botulism, gas gangrene, tetanus)**
Adults: 20 million units/day in divided doses IM or IV every 4 to 6 hours.

➤ **Diphtheria**
Adults: 2 to 3 million units/day in divided doses IM or IV every 4 to 6 hours for 10 to 12 days.

➤ *Erysipelothrix* **endocarditis**
Adults: 12 to 20 million units/day in divided doses IM or IV every 4 to 6 hours for 4 to 6 weeks.

➤ **Fusospirochetosis**
Adults: 5 to 10 million units/day in divided doses IM or IV every 4 to 6 hours.

➤ **Haverhill fever; rat bite fever**
Adults: 12 to 20 million units/day in divided doses IM or IV every 4 to 6 hours for 3 to 4 weeks.

➤ *Listeria monocytogenes* **infections, including endocarditis or meningitis**
Adults: 15 to 20 million units/day in divided doses IM or IV every 4 to 6 hours. Treat for 2 weeks for meningitis and 4 weeks for endocarditis.

➤ **Meningococcal meningitis or septicemia**
Adults: 24 million units/day as 2 million units IM or IV every 2 hours.

➤ **Neurosyphilis**
Adults: 12 to 24 million units/day (2 to 4 million units IM or IV every 4 hours) for 10 to 14 days. Many experts recommend benzathine penicillin G 2.4 million units IM weekly for 3 weeks following completion of this regimen.

➤ *Pasteurella multocida* **infections, including bacteremia or meningitis**
Adults: 4 to 6 million units/day in divided doses IM or IV every 4 to 6 hours for 2 weeks.

➤ **Serious staphylococcal and streptococcal infections**
Adults: 5 to 24 million units/day in equally divided doses IM or IV every 4 to 6 hours.

ADMINISTRATION
🔔 *Alert:* Don't use in patients requiring less than 1 million units/dose.
• Obtain specimen for culture and sensitivity tests before giving first dose. Begin therapy while awaiting results.
• Before giving, ask patient about allergic reactions to penicillin.
• Reconstitute drug with sterile water for injection, NSS for injection, or D_5W. Check manufacturer's instructions for volume of diluent necessary to produce desired drug level.
• May refrigerate reconstituted solution for 3 days.

IV

▼ Give by intermittent infusion: Dilute drug in 50 to 100 mL, and give over 30 minutes to 2 hours every 4 to 6 hours.

▼ Sterile reconstituted solution may be kept in refrigerator for up to 3 days.

▼ **Incompatibilities:** None listed by manufacturer. Consult a drug incompatibility reference for more information.

IM

• IM is the preferred route.

• Injection may be painful, but ice applied to site may help alleviate discomfort.

• Give deep in upper outer quadrant of buttocks in adults and in midlateral thigh in small children. Rotate injection sites. Don't give subcut.

ACTION

Inhibits cell-wall synthesis during bacterial multiplication.

Route	Onset	Peak	Duration
IV	Immediate	Immediate	Unknown
IM	Unknown	15–30 min	Unknown

Half-life: 31 to 50 minutes.

ADVERSE REACTIONS

CNS: neuropathy. **CV:** phlebitis or thrombophlebitis from IV, *HF.* **GI:** enterocolitis, ischemic colitis, nausea, vomiting, *pseudomembranous colitis, CDAD.* **GU:** renal tubular damage, *interstitial nephritis.* **Hematologic:** hemolytic anemia, *agranulocytosis, leukopenia, thrombocytopenia,* anemia, eosinophilia. **Metabolic:** electrolyte disturbances. **Musculoskeletal:** arthralgia. **Other:** hypersensitivity reactions, *anaphylaxis,* overgrowth of nonsusceptible organisms, injection-site pain.

INTERACTIONS

Drug-drug. *Aminoglycosides (amikacin, gentamicin, tobramycin):* May decrease aminoglycoside level. Monitor therapy.

Aspirin, furosemide, indomethacin, sulfonamides, thiazide diuretics: May compete with penicillin for renal tubular secretion, prolonging the half-life of penicillin. Monitor patient.

Bacteriostatic antibacterial agents (chloramphenicol, macrolide antibiotics, sulfonamides, tetracyclines): May decrease bactericidal effect of penicillin. Avoid concomitant use.

Hormonal contraceptives: May decrease hormonal contraceptive effectiveness. Advise use of additional form of contraception during penicillin therapy.

Live-virus vaccines: May decrease effectiveness of live-virus vaccines. Avoid concurrent use.

Methotrexate: May increase risk of methotrexate toxicity. Monitor patient closely.

Oral anticoagulants: May increase or decrease anticoagulant effects. Monitor PT and INR.

Probenecid: May increase penicillin level. Probenecid may be used for this purpose.

Tetracyclines: May interfere with bactericidal action of penicillins. Avoid coadministration.

EFFECTS ON LAB TEST RESULTS

• May decrease Hb level and platelet, WBC, granulocyte, and RBC counts.

• May cause positive Coombs test result.

• May cause false-positive CSF protein test result.

• May alter urine glucose testing using cupric sulfate (Benedict reagent, Fehling solution, or Clinitest tablet).

CONTRAINDICATIONS & CAUTIONS

• Contraindicated in patients hypersensitive to drug or other penicillins and in those on sodium-restricted diets.

• Use cautiously in patients with renal impairment.

• Drug may cause CDAD ranging in severity from mild diarrhea to fatal colitis. If CDAD is suspected or confirmed, drug may need to be discontinued and treatment initiated.

• Use cautiously in patients with other drug allergies, especially to cephalosporins, because of possible cross-sensitivity.

• Drug may cause renal tubular damage, interstitial nephritis, HF, and electrolyte imbalance when given in high doses.

Dialyzable drug: Yes.

⚠ *Overdose S&S:* Neuromuscular hyperexcitability, agitation, confusion, hallucinations, stupor, coma, encephalopathy, hypernatremia, seizures.

PREGNANCY-LACTATION-REPRODUCTION

• There are no adequate studies during pregnancy. Use only if clearly needed.

• Drug appears in human milk. Use cautiously during breastfeeding.

NURSING CONSIDERATIONS

• Drug may alter normal colon flora. Monitor patient for diarrhea, and initiate therapeutic measures as needed. Drug may need to be stopped.

• Observe patient closely. With large doses and prolonged therapy, bacterial or fungal superinfection may occur, especially in older adults or patients who are debilitated or immunosuppressed.

• Antibiotic use can cause overgrowth of nonsusceptible organisms (superinfection). Monitor patient for infection.

• For most acute infections, continue treatment for at least 48 to 72 hours after patient becomes asymptomatic. Maintain antibiotic therapy for group A beta-hemolytic streptococcal infections for at least 10 days to reduce risk of rheumatic fever.

• Give high doses (above 10 million units) by IV slowly because of the potential adverse effects of electrolyte imbalance from the sodium content, which is 1.68 mEq of sodium per million units.

• Monitor patients for renal tubular damage and interstitial nephritis (fever, rash, eosinophilia, proteinuria, eosinophiluria, hematuria, increased serum urea nitrogen level).

• Monitor patients with syphilis or other spirochetal infections (Lyme disease, relapsing fever) for Jarisch-Herxheimer reactions (fever, chills, myalgia, headache, exacerbation of skin lesions, tachycardia, hyperventilation, flushing, mild hypotension). Reactions occur 1 to 2 hours after initial treatment and resolve within 12 to 24 hours.

• *Look alike–sound alike:* Don't confuse penicillin G sodium with penicillamine or the various other types of penicillin.

PATIENT TEACHING

• Tell patient to report adverse reactions promptly, especially hypersensitivity reactions and diarrhea.

• Instruct patient to report discomfort at IV site.

• Warn patient receiving IM injection that the injection may be painful but that ice applied to site may help alleviate discomfort.

• Advise patient that watery and bloody stools with or without stomach cramps and fever may occur during and for up to 2 months or more after antibiotic use. Instruct patient to report these symptoms as soon as possible.

penicillin V potassium (phenoxymethyl penicillin potassium)
pen-i-SIL-in

Penicillin-VK

Therapeutic class: Antibiotics
Pharmacologic class: Natural penicillins

AVAILABLE FORMS
Oral suspension: 125 mg/5 mL, 250 mg/5 mL (after reconstitution)
Tablets: 250 mg, 500 mg

INDICATIONS & DOSAGES
➤ **Fusospirochetosis (Vincent infection) and staphylococcal infections**
Adults and children age 12 and older: 250 to 500 mg PO every 6 to 8 hours.
➤ **Pneumococcal infections**
Adults and children age 12 and older: 250 to 500 mg PO every 6 hours until patient has been afebrile for at least 2 days.
➤ **Streptococcal infections**
Adults and children age 12 and older: 125 to 250 mg PO every 6 to 8 hours for 10 days.
➤ **Group A beta-hemolytic streptococcal pharyngitis**
Adults and children age 12 and older: 500 mg PO b.i.d. to t.i.d., or 250 mg PO q.i.d. for 10 days.
➤ **To prevent recurrent rheumatic fever or chorea**
Adults and children age 12 and older: 125 to 250 mg PO b.i.d.
➤ **Bacterial endocarditis prophylaxis in patients with congenital heart disease or rheumatic or other acquired valvular heart disease**
Adults and children age 12 and older weighing more than 27.2 kg: 2 g PO 1 hour before dental or upper respiratory tract surgical procedure, followed by 1 g 6 hours later.
Children age 12 and older weighing less than 27.2 kg: 1 g PO 1 hour before dental or upper respiratory tract surgical procedure, followed by 500 mg 6 hours later.

ADMINISTRATION
PO
• Before giving drug, ask patient about allergic reactions to penicillins.

- Obtain specimen for culture and sensitivity tests before giving first dose. Begin therapy while awaiting results.
- Give on an empty stomach 1 hour before or 2 hours after meals, to enhance absorption.
- Give drug with food if patient has stomach upset.
- Store oral solution in refrigerator. Discard any portion after 14 days.

ACTION

Inhibits cell-wall synthesis during bacterial multiplication.

Route	Onset	Peak	Duration
PO	Unknown	30–60 min	Unknown

Half-life: 30 minutes.

ADVERSE REACTIONS

CNS: fever. **EENT:** oral candidiasis. **GI:** epigastric distress, nausea, diarrhea, black hairy tongue, vomiting. **Hematologic:** *leukopenia, thrombocytopenia,* eosinophilia, hemolytic anemia. **Skin:** skin eruptions, urticaria. **Other:** *anaphylaxis,* hypersensitivity reactions, overgrowth of nonsusceptible organisms.

INTERACTIONS

Drug-drug. *Aminoglycosides (amikacin, gentamicin, tobramycin):* May decrease aminoglycoside level. Monitor therapy.
Methotrexate: May increase risk of methotrexate toxicity. Monitor patient closely.
Probenecid: May increase penicillin level. Probenecid may be used for this purpose.
Tetracyclines: May impair bactericidal effects of penicillin V. Avoid use together.
Warfarin: May increase anticoagulant effects. Monitor therapy.

EFFECTS ON LAB TEST RESULTS

- May increase eosinophil count.
- May decrease Hb level and platelet, WBC, and granulocyte counts.
- May alter results of turbidimetric test methods using sulfosalicylic acid, acetic acid, trichloroacetic acid, and nitric acid.

CONTRAINDICATIONS & CAUTIONS

- Contraindicated in patients hypersensitive to drug or other penicillins.
- Drug may cause CDAD ranging in severity from mild diarrhea to fatal colitis. If CDAD is

suspected or confirmed, drug may need to be discontinued and treatment initiated.
- Use cautiously in patients with GI disturbances, seizure disorder, or renal impairment and in those with other drug allergies, especially to cephalosporins, because of possible cross-sensitivity.
Dialyzable drug: Unknown.
⚠ **Overdose S&S:** Neuromuscular hyperexcitability, seizures.

PREGNANCY-LACTATION-REPRODUCTION

- May use cautiously during pregnancy.
- Drug appears in human milk. Use cautiously during breastfeeding.

NURSING CONSIDERATIONS

- Drug may alter normal colon flora. Monitor patient for diarrhea, and initiate therapeutic measures as needed. Drug may need to be stopped.
- Periodically assess renal and hematopoietic function in patients receiving long-term therapy.
- If large doses are given or if therapy is prolonged, bacterial or fungal superinfection may occur, especially in older adults and patients who are debilitated or immunosuppressed.
- After treatment for streptococcal infections, reculture patient to determine whether streptococci have been eradicated.
- Amoxicillin is preferred over other antibiotics for endocarditis prophylaxis; however, penicillin V can be used as an alternative, if necessary.
- *Look alike–sound alike:* Don't confuse penicillin V potassium with penicillamine or the various other types of penicillin.

PATIENT TEACHING

- Instruct patient to take entire quantity of drug exactly as prescribed, even after feeling better.
- Tell patient to take drug with food if stomach upset occurs.
- Advise patient that antibiotics can cause diarrhea, which commonly resolves after therapy.
- Instruct patient to discard any unused reconstituted suspension after 14 days.
- Advise patient to notify prescriber if rash, fever, or chills develop. A rash is the most common allergic reaction.

P

pentamidine isethionate
pen-TAM-i-deen

NebuPent, Pentam

Therapeutic class: Antiprotozoals
Pharmacologic class: Diamidine derivatives

AVAILABLE FORMS
Aerosol, powder for solution: 300-mg vial
Injection: 300-mg vial

INDICATIONS & DOSAGES
➤ *Pneumocystis jiroveci* pneumonia
(Pentam)
Adults and children age 4 months and older:
4 mg/kg IV over 1 to 2 hours or IM once daily
for 14 to 21 days.
➤ **To prevent *P. jiroveci* pneumonia in pa-
tients at high risk (NebuPent)**
Adults: 300 mg by inhalation using a Respir-
gard II nebulizer once every 4 weeks.

ADMINISTRATION
IV
▼ Reconstitute drug with 3 to 5 mL sterile
water for injection or D₅W.
▼ Dilute reconstituted drug in 50 to 250 mL
D₅W. Reconstituted solution is stable for
48 hours.
▼ Infuse over 60 to 120 minutes.
▼ IV infusion solutions prepared in D₅W
are stable at room temperature for up to
24 hours.
▼ To minimize risk of hypotension, infuse
drug slowly with patient lying down. Closely
monitor BP.
🕒 *Alert:* Closely monitor infusion. Extravasation may cause ulceration, tissue necrosis,
or sloughing and may require surgical debridement and skin grafting. If extravasation
occurs, discontinue infusion immediately
and manage symptoms.
▼ **Incompatibilities:** None listed by manufacturer. Consult a drug incompatibility
reference for more information.
IM
● Reconstitute drug with 3 mL sterile water
for a solution containing 100 mg/mL.
● Give deep into muscle.
● Rotate injection sites.
● Solution is stable for 48 hours after reconstitution. Store at room temperature to avoid
crystallization.

Inhalational
🕒 *Alert:* Hazardous drug; use safe handling
and disposal precautions.
● Give aerosol form only by Respirgard II
nebulizer. Dosage recommendations are
based on particle size and delivery rate of this
device. Deliver dose until nebulizer chamber
is empty (about 30 to 45 minutes).
● To give aerosol, mix contents of one vial
in 6 mL sterile water for injection. Don't use
NSS. Don't mix with other drugs.
● Don't use the Respirgard II to administer a
bronchodilator because there may be an incompatibility between pentamidine and the
bronchodilator.
● Don't use low-pressure (less than 20 pounds
per square inch [PSI]) compressors. The flow
rate should be 5 to 7 L/minute from 40- to
50-PSI air or oxygen source.
● Solution remains stable for 48 hours after
reconstitution when kept in original vial at
room temperature, protected from light.

ACTION
May interfere with biosynthesis of DNA,
RNA, phospholipids, and proteins in suscepti-
ble organisms.

Route	Onset	Peak	Duration
IV, IM, inhalation	Unknown	Unknown	Unknown

Half-life: IV, about 5 to 8 hours; IM, 7 to 11 hours;
inhalation, unknown.

ADVERSE REACTIONS
CNS: confusion, hallucinations, headache,
fatigue, dizziness, fever. **CV:** chest pain, hypotension. **EENT:** pharyngitis, sinusitis. **GI:**
nausea, metallic taste, diarrhea, anorexia.
GU: azotemia, impaired renal function.
Hematologic: *leukopenia, thrombocytopenia,* anemia. **Hepatic:** elevated liver function
test results. **Metabolic:** *hypoglycemia.* **Respiratory:** cough, wheezing, dyspnea, bronchitis, URI, *bronchospasm.* **Skin:** rash; sterile abscess or necrosis, pain, or induration at
site of IM injection. **Other:** night sweats, infection.

INTERACTIONS
Drug-drug. *Amphotericin B, capreomycin,
cisplatin, methoxyflurane, polymyxin B, vancomycin:* May increase risk of nephrotoxicity.
Monitor renal function test results closely.

Reactions in bold italics are *life-threatening*. Interactions may have a *rapid onset* or a ***delayed onset***.

Antidiabetics: May initially cause hypoglycemia, then hyperglycemia, because pentamidine may harm pancreatic cells. Monitor blood glucose levels and adjust dosages when needed.

Antineoplastics: May cause additive bone marrow suppression. Use together cautiously; monitor hematologic study results.

Drugs that prolong the QT interval (antipsychotics; antiarrhythmics, such as amiodarone, disopyramide, procainamide, quinidine, sotalol; fluoroquinolones; macrolides; TCAs): May cause additive effect. Use together cautiously; monitor patient for adverse cardiac effects.

EFFECTS ON LAB TEST RESULTS

• May increase BUN, creatinine, and potassium levels and LFT values.
• May increase or decrease glucose level.
• May decrease Hb level, hematocrit, and WBC and platelet counts.

CONTRAINDICATIONS & CAUTIONS

• Contraindicated in patients with history of anaphylactic reaction or hypersensitivity to drug.
• Fatalities due to severe hypotension, hypoglycemia, acute pancreatitis, and cardiac arrhythmias have been reported.
• Use cautiously in patients with HTN, hypotension, ventricular tachycardia, hypoglycemia, hyperglycemia, hypocalcemia, leukopenia, thrombocytopenia, anemia, diabetes, pancreatitis, SJS, or hepatic or renal dysfunction.
🔊 *Alert:* Severe hypotension may occur after a single IV or IM dose, and is more likely with rapid IV administration. Monitor patients closely.

Dialyzable drug: No.

⚠ *Overdose S&S:* Renal and hepatic impairment, hypotension, cardiopulmonary arrest.

PREGNANCY-LACTATION-REPRODUCTION

• It isn't known if drug causes fetal harm. Use during pregnancy only if potential benefits justify unknown risks and only if clearly needed.
• It isn't known if drug appears in human milk. Use cautiously during breastfeeding and only if potential benefits justify unknown risks.

NURSING CONSIDERATIONS

🔊 *Alert:* Monitor glucose, creatinine, and BUN levels daily. After parenteral administration, glucose level may decrease initially; hypoglycemia may be severe in 5% to 10% of patients. After several months of therapy, this may be followed by hyperglycemia and type 1 diabetes, which may be permanent.
• Monitor CBC with platelet count, renal function, LFT results, calcium level, and ECG before, during, and after therapy.
🔊 *Alert:* Monitor BP during and after infusion because of increased risk of severe hypotension with IV or IM administration.
• Extravasation can lead to ulceration, tissue necrosis, or sloughing at injection site. Monitor IV site closely.
• Inhalation drug may cause bronchospasm or cough, especially in patients with a history of asthma or smoking. Use of an inhaled bronchodilator before each inhaled pentamidine dose may minimize symptom recurrence.
• Use of aerosolized drug has been associated with acute pancreatitis. Discontinue drug if signs or symptoms of acute pancreatitis occur.
• In patients with AIDS, drug may produce less severe adverse reactions than sulfamethoxazole–trimethoprim.

PATIENT TEACHING

• Instruct patient to use the aerosol device until the chamber is empty, which may take up to 45 minutes.
• Warn patient that IM injection is painful.
• Instruct patient to complete the full course, even if feeling better.
• Tell patient to report signs and symptoms of pulmonary infection, such as shortness of breath, fever, or cough.

SAFETY ALERT!

pertuzumab 🧬
per-TU-zoo-mab

Perjeta

Therapeutic class: Antineoplastics
Pharmacologic class: Monoclonal antibodies

AVAILABLE FORMS

Injection: 420 mg/14 mL (30 mg/mL) in single-use vials

INDICATIONS & DOSAGES

Adjust-a-dose (for all indications): Refer to manufacturer's information for adjustments related to missed or delayed doses and for complete information on drugs used in combination with pertuzumab.

➤ **HER2-positive metastatic breast cancer with trastuzumab and docetaxel in patients who haven't received prior anti-HER2 therapy or chemotherapy for metastatic disease** ⚲

Adults: Initial loading dose of 840 mg IV as a 60-minute infusion in combination with trastuzumab 8 mg/kg and docetaxel 75 mg/m². Administer a maintenance regimen every 3 weeks with pertuzumab 420 mg IV as a 30- to 60-minute infusion in combination with trastuzumab 6 mg/kg or trastuzumab hyaluronidase-oysk (600 mg trastuzumab/10,000 units hyaluronidase) subcut over 2 to 5 minutes and docetaxel (may increase docetaxel dose to 100 mg/m² if initial dose is tolerated).

➤ **Neoadjuvant treatment of HER2-positive, locally advanced, inflammatory, or early-stage breast cancer in combination with other drugs** ⚲

Adults: Initial loading dose of 840 mg IV as a 60-minute infusion, then a maintenance regimen every 3 weeks with pertuzumab 420 mg IV as a 30- to 60-minute infusion in combination with either four preoperative cycles with trastuzumab or trastuzumab hyaluronidase-oysk and docetaxel followed by three postoperative cycles of 5-FU, epirubicin, and cyclophosphamide (FEC); or three or four preoperative cycles of FEC alone followed by three or four preoperative cycles of pertuzumab in combination with docetaxel and trastuzumab or trastuzumab hyaluronidase-oysk; or six preoperative cycles of pertuzumab in combination with docetaxel, carboplatin, and trastuzumab (TCH) or trastuzumab hyaluronidase-oysk; or four preoperative cycles of dose-dense doxorubicin and cyclophosphamide (ddAC) alone followed by four preoperative cycles of pertuzumab in combination with paclitaxel and trastuzumab or trastuzumab hyaluronidase-oysk. After surgery, continue trastuzumab or trastuzumab hyaluronidase-oysk to complete 1 year of treatment, up to 18 cycles.

➤ **Adjuvant treatment of patients with HER2-positive early breast cancer at high risk for recurrence as part of a complete regimen for breast cancer, including anthracycline or taxane-based chemotherapy**

Adults: Initial loading dose, 840 mg IV as a 60-minute infusion in combination with trastuzumab 8 mg/kg or trastuzumab hyaluronidase-oysk (600 mg trastuzumab/10,000 units hyaluronidase) subcut over 2 to 5 minutes starting day 1 of first taxane-containing cycle. Administer a maintenance regimen every 3 weeks with pertuzumab 420 mg IV as a 30- to 60-minute infusion in combination with trastuzumab 6 mg/kg. Continue maintenance regimen for a total of 1 year (up to 18 cycles) or until disease recurrence or unmanageable toxicity, whichever occurs first. Withhold or discontinue pertuzumab if trastuzumab or trastuzumab hyaluronidase-oysk is withheld or discontinued.

ADMINISTRATION

IV

⚠️ *Alert:* Hazardous drug; use safe handling and disposal precautions.

▼ Don't administer as IV push or bolus.

▼ Refrigerate vials. Store in outer carton to protect from light.

▼ Inspect solution for particulates and discoloration. Solution should be clear to slightly opalescent and colorless to pale brown.

▼ Withdraw appropriate amount of pertuzumab and dilute in 250 mL NSS in a PVC or non-PVC polyolefin infusion bag.

▼ Invert bag gently to mix solution; don't shake. Administer immediately.

▼ May store diluted solution, refrigerated, for up to 24 hours.

▼ Administer pertuzumab sequentially. Pertuzumab and trastuzumab or trastuzumab hyaluronidase-oysk can be given in any order. Give docetaxel after pertuzumab and trastuzumab or trastuzumab hyaluronidase-oysk. Observe patient for 30 to 60 minutes after infusing pertuzumab before administering the other drugs.

▼ **Incompatibilities:** Other drugs. Only mix with NSS.

ACTION

Binds to HER2 protein receptor, causing inhibition of signaling pathways, which results in cell growth arrest and apoptosis.

Route	Onset	Peak	Duration
IV	Unknown	Unknown	Unknown

Half-life: 18 days.

ADVERSE REACTIONS

CNS: fatigue, asthenia, fever, peripheral neuropathy, headache, dizziness, insomnia, dysgeusia. **CV:** peripheral edema, *left ventricular dysfunction.* **EENT:** increased tearing, nasopharyngitis, oropharyngeal pain. **GI:** diarrhea, nausea, vomiting, constipation, stomatitis, decreased appetite, abdominal pain. **Hematologic:** *neutropenia,* anemia, *leukopenia, febrile neutropenia, thrombocytopenia.* **Hepatic:** elevated liver enzyme levels. **Metabolic:** *hypokalemia,* hyperuricemia, hyperphosphatemia. **Musculoskeletal:** myalgia, arthralgia. **Respiratory:** URI, dyspnea, cough, pleural effusion. **Skin:** alopecia, hand-foot syndrome, rash, pruritus, dry skin, paronychia, nail disorder, infusion-site reaction. **Other:** mucosal inflammation, infusion-related hypersensitivity, immunogenicity.

INTERACTIONS

None reported.

EFFECTS ON LAB TEST RESULTS

• May increase liver enzyme, phosphate, and uric acid levels.
• May decrease potassium level.
• May decrease platelet, WBC, and RBC counts.

CONTRAINDICATIONS & CAUTIONS

Boxed Warning Pertuzumab can cause subclinical and clinical cardiac failure. Evaluate LVEF in all patients before and during treatment. Discontinue drug treatment for a confirmed clinically significant decrease in left ventricular function. ∎
• Contraindicated in patients hypersensitive to drug or its components.
• Use cautiously in patients with a history of HF or reduced LVEF and in those with severe renal impairment. Prior exposure to radiotherapy may increase risk of left ventricular dysfunction.
Dialyzable drug: Unknown.

PREGNANCY-LACTATION-REPRODUCTION

Boxed Warning Exposure to drug during pregnancy can result in embryo or fetal death,

delayed renal development, and other birth defects. Verify pregnancy status before starting drug. Advise patients of risks and the need for effective contraception during therapy and for 7 months after therapy ends. ∎
• If patient becomes pregnant during therapy, monitor closely. If oligohydramnios occurs, perform fetal testing.
• It isn't known if drug appears in human milk. Patient should discontinue breastfeeding or discontinue drug. Consider drug's extended half-life when making breastfeeding decisions after therapy ends.

NURSING CONSIDERATIONS

☒ Verify HER2 status with reputable lab. Drug is only useful in patients with HER2 protein overexpression.
Boxed Warning Assess LVEF before starting treatment and every 3 months during treatment for metastatic disease or every 6 weeks during neoadjuvant treatment. ∎
• Withhold or discontinue pertuzumab if trastuzumab is withheld or discontinued. If docetaxel is discontinued, treatment with pertuzumab and trastuzumab may continue.
• Monitor patient for hypersensitivity or infusion reactions for 60 minutes after first infusion and for 30 minutes after subsequent infusions. For significant infusion-related reactions, slow or interrupt infusion and treat symptoms. If severe reactions occur, consider permanently discontinuing drug.
• Monitor CBC regularly.
• Monitor patients for fever or infection.
☒ An increased incidence of febrile neutropenia has occurred in patients of Asian descent.
• Verify pregnancy status of patient of childbearing potential before starting drug.

PATIENT TEACHING

Boxed Warning Inform patient of childbearing potential that drug may cause fetal harm. Counsel patient to use reliable birth control methods while taking this drug and for 7 months after therapy ends. ∎
• Teach patient that hair loss (alopecia) and skin and nail adverse reactions are common during treatment.
• Instruct patient to immediately report fever or other signs and symptoms of infection.
• Caution patient to immediately report shortness of breath, unusual edema, weight gain, or excessive fatigue.

P

♣Canada   ◇OTC   ♦Off-label use   ✒Photoguide   ⊕Do not crush   *Liquid contains alcohol   ☒Genetic

• Advise patient to immediately report signs or symptoms of LVEF dysfunction, including worsening shortness of breath, cough, palpitations, weight gain of more than 5 lb in 24 hours, dizziness or loss of consciousness, swelling of the ankles, legs, or face.
• Tell patient that regular monitoring of cardiac function will be needed.

phentermine hydrochloride
FEN-ter-meen

Adipex-P, Lomaira

Therapeutic class: Anorexiants
Pharmacologic class: Sympathomimetic amines
Controlled substance schedule: IV

AVAILABLE FORMS
Capsules: 15 mg, 30 mg, 37.5 mg
Tablets: 8 mg, 37.5 mg
Tablets (ODTs): 15 mg, 30 mg, 37.5 mg

INDICATIONS & DOSAGES
➤ **Short-term adjunct in exogenous obesity for patients with an initial BMI of 30 kg/m^2 or more, or of 27 kg/m^2 or more in the presence of other risk factors (e.g., controlled HTN, diabetes, hyperlipidemia)**
Adults and children age 16 and older: 15 to 37.5 mg PO daily as a single dose or two divided doses. Or, 15 to 37.5 mg ODT PO daily.
Adults (Lomaira): 8 mg PO t.i.d. 30 minutes before meals.
Adjust-a-dose: Individualize dosage to obtain adequate response with lowest effective dose. Maximum dose of Adipex-P is 15 mg daily for patients with severe renal impairment (eGFR of 15 to 29 mL/minute/1.73 m^2).

ADMINISTRATION
PO
• Tablets are scored and may be split to achieve lower dose.
• Give Adipex-P before breakfast or 1 to 2 hours after breakfast. Give Lomaira 30 minutes before meals. Give ODT in the morning with or without food.
• Avoid giving in the late evening, to prevent insomnia.
• Using dry hands, immediately place ODT on top of the tongue to dissolve; then have patient swallow with or without water.

ACTION
Unknown. Phentermine is a sympathomimetic amine with pharmacologic properties similar to amphetamines. The mechanism of action in reducing appetite may be secondary to CNS effects, including stimulation of the hypothalamus to release norepinephrine.

Route	Onset	Peak	Duration
PO	Unknown	3–4.4 hr	Unknown

Half-life: About 20 hours.

ADVERSE REACTIONS
CNS: insomnia, overstimulation, headache, restlessness, euphoria, dysphoria, dizziness, tremor, psychosis, dysgeusia. **CV:** palpitations, tachycardia, ischemic events, increased BP. **GI:** dry mouth, constipation, diarrhea, other GI disturbances. **GU:** erectile dysfunction, altered libido. **Skin:** urticaria.

INTERACTIONS
Drug-drug. *Acetazolamide, antacids, sodium bicarbonate:* May increase renal reabsorption. Monitor patient for enhanced effects.
Adrenergic neuron blockers: May reduce hypotensive effect. Monitor patient for cardiac changes.
Ammonium chloride, ascorbic acid: May decrease level and increase renal excretion of phentermine. Monitor patient for decreased phentermine effects.
Dexfenfluramine, fenfluramine: May increase risk of primary pulmonary HTN and valvular heart disease. Monitor patient closely.
Insulin, oral antidiabetics: May alter antidiabetic requirements. Monitor glucose level.
MAO inhibitors: May cause severe HTN or hypertensive crisis. Contraindicated within 14 days of MAO inhibitor therapy.
Other products for weight loss: Effects of coadministration are unknown. Use together isn't recommended.
Serotonin uptake inhibitors (fluoxetine, fluvoxamine, paroxetine, sertraline): May increase risk of serotonin syndrome. Use together isn't recommended.
Drug-food. *Alcohol use:* May increase risk of adverse drug reactions. Monitor patient.
Caffeine: May increase CNS stimulation. Discourage use together.

EFFECTS ON LAB TEST RESULTS
None reported.

Reactions in bold italics are *life-threatening*. Interactions may have a *rapid onset* or a **delayed onset**.

CONTRAINDICATIONS & CAUTIONS
• Contraindicated in patients hypersensitive to sympathomimetic amines, in those with idiosyncratic reactions to them, in patients who are agitated, and within 14 days after taking an MAO inhibitor.
• Contraindicated in patients with history of drug abuse, hyperthyroidism, CV disease (heart disease, stroke, CAD, HF, arrhythmias, moderate to severe or uncontrolled HTN, advanced arteriosclerosis), or glaucoma.
• Rare cases of valvular heart disease have been reported in patients who have taken phentermine alone.
• Avoid Adipex-P in patients with eGFR less than 15 mL/minute/1.73 m^2 or ESRD requiring dialysis.
• Use cautiously in older adults and patients with HTN (even mild HTN), renal impairment, or seizure disorders.
• Safety and effectiveness in children younger than age 16 haven't been determined.
Dialyzable drug: Unknown.
⚠ *Overdose S&S:* Restlessness, tremor, hyperreflexia, rapid respiration, confusion, assaultiveness, hallucinations, panic states, fatigue, depression, arrhythmias, HTN, hypotension, circulatory collapse, nausea, vomiting, diarrhea, abdominal cramps, seizures, coma.

PREGNANCY-LACTATION-REPRODUCTION
• Contraindicated during pregnancy and breastfeeding.

NURSING CONSIDERATIONS
• Use drug with a weight-reduction program.
• Monitor patient for tolerance, dependence, or potential abuse. Drug is chemically related to amphetamines, which carry a high abuse potential.
• Monitor BP.
• Don't stop drug abruptly; taper dosage.
• *Look alike–sound alike:* Don't confuse phentermine with phentolamine or phenytoin.

PATIENT TEACHING
• Counsel patient in use of effective contraception and to immediately report pregnancy.
• Instruct patient to immediately report shortness of breath or dyspnea, which could be an early sign of a serious adverse effect such as primary pulmonary HTN.

• Advise patient to avoid products that contain caffeine and to report evidence of excessive stimulation.
• Warn patient that fatigue may result as drug effects wear off and that patient will need more rest.
• Caution patient to avoid operating hazardous machinery, including automobiles, until drug's effects are known.
• Warn patient that drug may lose its effectiveness over time.
• Advise patient not to stop drug abruptly. Remind patient that drug is for short-term use (usually a few weeks).
⚠ *Alert:* Caution patient to keep drug in a safe place and protect it from theft.
⚠ *Alert:* Advise patient never to give drug to anyone else because it can cause harm or death.
• Stress importance of eating healthy and other healthy lifestyle choices.

phentermine hydrochloride–topiramate
FEN-ter-meen/toe-PIE-rah-mate

Qsymia

Therapeutic class: Anorexiants–anticonvulsants
Pharmacologic class: Sympathomimetic amines–sulfamate-substituted monosaccharides
Controlled substance schedule: IV

AVAILABLE FORMS
Capsules (extended-release) ⓓⓝⓒ: 3.75 mg phentermine/23 mg topiramate, 7.5 mg phentermine/46 mg topiramate, 11.25 mg phentermine/69 mg topiramate, 15 mg phentermine/92 mg topiramate

INDICATIONS & DOSAGES
➤ **Chronic weight management, as an adjunct to diet and increased physical activity in patients with initial BMI of 30 kg/m^2 or greater (obese) or 27 kg/m^2 or greater (overweight) and at least one weight-related comorbidity, such as HTN, type 2 diabetes, or dyslipidemia**
Adults: Initially, 3.75 mg phentermine/23 mg topiramate extended-release PO every morning for 14 days; then increase to 7.5 mg

phentermine/46 mg topiramate extended-release every morning. Evaluate weight loss after 12 weeks of treatment. If patient hasn't lost at least 3% of baseline body weight, discontinue drug or escalate dosage to 11.25 mg phentermine/69 mg topiramate extended-release every morning for 14 days, followed by 15 mg phentermine/92 mg topiramate extended-release every morning. Evaluate weight loss 12 weeks after dosage escalation. If patient hasn't lost at least 5% of baseline body weight, discontinue drug by decreasing dosage to every other day for at least 1 week before stopping treatment altogether.

Adjust-a-dose: For patients with moderate renal impairment (CrCl of 30 to less than 50 mL/minute), severe renal impairment (CrCl less than 30 mL/minute), or moderate hepatic impairment (Child-Pugh class B), don't exceed 7.5 mg phentermine/46 mg topiramate once daily.

✷ *NEW INDICATION:* **Chronic weight management, as an adjunct to diet and increased physical activity in children with BMI in the 95th percentile or more standardized for age and sex**
Children age 12 and older: Initially, 3.75 mg phentermine/23 mg topiramate PO every morning for 14 days; then increase to 7.5 mg phentermine/46 mg topiramate every morning. Evaluate weight loss after 12 weeks of therapy. If child hasn't lost at least 3% of baseline BMI, escalate dosage to 11.25 mg phentermine/69 mg topiramate every morning for 14 days, followed by 15 mg phentermine/92 mg topiramate every morning. Evaluate BMI 12 weeks after dosage escalation. If patient hasn't lost at least 5% of baseline BMI, discontinue drug by decreasing dose to every other day for at least 1 week before stopping therapy.

Adjust-a-dose: If child's weight loss exceeds 0.9 kg/week, consider dosage reduction. For patients with moderate renal impairment (CrCl of 30 to less than 50 mL/minute), severe renal impairment (CrCl less than 30 mL/minute), or moderate hepatic impairment (Child-Pugh class B), don't exceed 7.5 mg phentermine/46 mg topiramate once daily.

ADMINISTRATION
PO
• Give drug in morning with or without food. Don't give in evening due to risk of insomnia.
• Don't open, cut, or crush capsules.

ACTION
Phentermine: Unknown. Drug is a sympathomimetic amine with pharmacologic properties similar to amphetamines. Mechanism of action in reducing appetite may be secondary to CNS effects, including stimulation of the hypothalamus to release norepinephrine. Topiramate: Unknown in weight management. May involve appetite suppression and satiety enhancement via a variety of neurotransmitter or enzymatic effects.

Route	Onset	Peak	Duration
PO	Unknown	6 hr (phentermine); 9 hr (topiramate)	Unknown

Half-life: Phentermine, 20 hours; topiramate, 65 hours.

ADVERSE REACTIONS
CNS: paresthesia, headache, dizziness, dysgeusia, hypoesthesia, disturbance in attention or memory, cognitive disorder, insomnia, depression, anxiety, fatigue, fever, irritability, thirst. **CV:** palpitations, chest discomfort, increased HR. **EENT:** blurred vision, eye pain, dry eye, ear infection, nasal congestion, nasopharyngitis, sinusitis, sinus congestion, oral paresthesia, pharyngolaryngeal pain, dry mouth. **GI:** constipation, nausea, diarrhea, dyspepsia, GERD, gastroenteritis, decreased appetite, abdominal pain. **GU:** UTI, dysmenorrhea, increased creatinine level. **Metabolic:** hyperammonemia, *hypokalemia, metabolic acidosis, hypoglycemia.* **Musculoskeletal:** arthralgia, back pain, extremity pain, muscle spasms, musculoskeletal pain, neck pain, ligament sprain, decreased bone mineral density (children), slowed height growth (children). **Respiratory:** cough, bronchitis, URI. **Skin:** alopecia, rash. **Other:** procedural pain, flulike symptoms.

INTERACTIONS
Drug-drug. *Amitriptyline:* May increase amitriptyline level. Monitor therapy.
Anticholinergics (atropine, benztropine): May increase risk of heat-related disorders, such as decreased sweating and increased body temperature. Use together cautiously.
Carbamazepine, phenytoin: May decrease topiramate plasma concentration. Use together cautiously.
Carbonic anhydrase inhibitors (acetazolamide, methazolamide, zonisamide): May increase risk of metabolic acidosis and kidney

---

Reactions in bold italics are *life-threatening*. Interactions may have a *rapid onset* or a *delayed onset*.

stones. May also increase risk of heat-related disorders, such as decreased sweating and increased body temperature. Avoid concurrent use.

CNS depressants (barbiturates, benzodiazepines, sleep medications): May increase CNS depressant effects. Avoid use together.

Diltiazem: May decrease diltiazem level and increase topiramate level. Use together cautiously.

Lithium: High topiramate dosage may increase lithium level. Monitor lithium level.

MAO inhibitors: May increase risk of hypertensive crisis. Use is contraindicated during or within 14 days of MAO inhibitor administration.

Non-potassium-sparing diuretics (loop and thiazide diuretics): May increase risk of hypokalemia. Monitor potassium level.

Oral antidiabetics, insulin: May increase risk of hypoglycemia. Monitor glucose level closely.

Oral contraceptives (progestins): May decrease contraceptive effectiveness. Consider therapy modification and adding an additional, nonhormonal contraceptive method.

Other weight-loss drugs: Use with other weight-loss drugs hasn't been studied. Avoid use together.

Pioglitazone: May decrease pioglitazone level. Monitor glucose level closely.

Serotonin uptake inhibitors (fluoxetine, fluvoxamine, paroxetine, sertraline): May increase risk of serotonin syndrome. Use together isn't recommended.

Valproic acid: May increase risk of hyperammonemia and encephalopathy. Monitor patient and measure blood ammonia level if symptoms develop.

Drug-herb. *Weight-loss supplements:* Use with other weight-loss products hasn't been studied. Avoid use together.

Drug-food. *Ketogenic diet (high-protein, low-carbohydrate):* May increase risk of kidney stones. Use together cautiously.

Drug-lifestyle. *Alcohol use:* May increase CNS depressant effects. Discourage use together.

EFFECTS ON LAB TEST RESULTS
• May increase creatinine and ammonium levels.
• May decrease sodium bicarbonate, potassium, and glucose levels.

CONTRAINDICATIONS & CAUTIONS
• Contraindicated in patients hypersensitive to drug or its components or with idiosyncrasy to the sympathomimetic amines; in those with glaucoma or hyperthyroidism; and during or within 14 days after administration of MAO inhibitors.
• Avoid use in patients with severe hepatic impairment or ESRD and in those with a history of or active suicidality or suicide attempts.
• Use cautiously in patients with increased resting HR, especially those with cardiac or cerebrovascular disease (history of MI or stroke in the past 6 months, life-threatening arrhythmias, HF), in patients with depression or suicidality; in older adults; and in those at risk for development of metabolic acidosis or kidney stones.
• Use cautiously in patients with a history of depression.
⚠ *Alert:* Drug is a controlled substance because it can be abused, leading to drug dependence.
• Drug is only available through certified pharmacies that are enrolled in the Qsymia certified pharmacy network; see www.qsymiarems.com or call 1-888-998-4887.
Dialyzable drug: Phentermine, no; topiramate, yes.
⚠ *Overdose S&S:* Phentermine: Restlessness, tremor, rapid respiration, confusion, hallucinations, arrhythmias, changes in BP, nausea, vomiting, diarrhea. Topiramate: Metabolic acidosis, seizures, drowsiness, speech disturbance, blurred vision, hypotension, abdominal pain, agitation, dizziness, depression.

PREGNANCY-LACTATION-REPRODUCTION
• Contraindicated during pregnancy and breastfeeding.
• Assess for pregnancy before and monthly during treatment. Patients of childbearing potential should use effective contraception during therapy.
• Prescribers and patients should report pregnancies that occur during therapy to the Qsymia Pregnancy Surveillance Program (1-888-998-4887).
• For patients taking combined oral contraceptives (COCs), use of drug may cause irregular bleeding. Patients should continue taking the COC and contact health care provider.

NURSING CONSIDERATIONS
• Verify pregnancy status of patients of child-bearing potential before and monthly during therapy.
• Gradually decrease dosage when discontinuing drug to lower risk of seizures. If it's necessary to stop drug immediately, monitor patient closely.
• Monitor patient for mood disorders and insomnia; if present, decrease dosage or discontinue drug.
• Monitor patient for emergence or worsening of depression, suicidality, or unusual changes in mood or behavior. Discontinue drug in patients who experience suicidality.
• Monitor resting HR. If sustained tachycardia occurs, decrease dosage or stop drug.
• Assess electrolyte, glucose, and bicarbonate levels before and periodically during treatment.
• Drug causes decreased sweating, which can predispose patients to heat-related disorders. Monitor fluid loss, especially in hot weather.
• Monitor BP regularly, especially in patients with history of HTN.
• Monitor patient for ocular changes (acute myopia, severe and persistent eye pain, vision changes, anterior chamber shallowing, redness, increased IOP, mydriasis). Discontinue drug immediately if any of these symptoms occur.
• Monitor patient for potential abuse of drug. Phentermine has a known potential for abuse.
• Phentermine is related chemically and pharmacologically to amphetamines.

PATIENT TEACHING
• Advise patient to take drug once daily in the morning and to avoid nighttime dosing because of insomnia.
• Inform patient that drug is only available through certified pharmacies that are enrolled in the Qsymia certified pharmacy network.
🔔 *Alert:* Tell patient to keep drug in a safe place and protect it from theft. Advise patient never to give drug to anyone else because it can cause harm or death and is against the law.
• Warn patient not to increase dosage without first discussing with prescriber.
• Advise patient of childbearing potential of fetal risk and that pregnancy testing will be done before start of therapy and monthly during therapy.

• Counsel patient to use effective contraception and to immediately report pregnancy.
• Instruct patient to tell all health care providers about all medications, nutritional supplements, and vitamins (including weight-loss products) that are being taken or may be taken during therapy.
• Caution patient to report sustained periods of heart pounding or racing while at rest; mood changes, depression, or suicidality; prolonged diarrhea; scheduled surgery; occurrence or history of seizures; or use of a high-protein, low-carbohydrate diet.
• Teach patient to immediately report severe and persistent eye pain or significant vision changes.
• Instruct patient to report changes in attention, concentration, memory, or difficulty finding words.
• Tell patient to avoid operating hazardous machinery, including automobiles, until effects of drug are known.
• Advise patient with diabetes to monitor glucose level closely and to report episodes of hypoglycemia. Medication regimen may need adjustment.
• Caution patient to watch for decreased sweating or increased body temperature during physical activity, especially during hot weather.
• Warn patient not to stop drug abruptly as seizures may result.
• Advise patient to increase fluid intake to prevent kidney stones and to report severe side or back pain or blood in urine.

phenytoin (diphenylhydantoin) ☒
FEN-i-toe-in

Dilantin-125, Dilantin Infatabs

phenytoin sodium
Dilantin✐, Phenytek

Therapeutic class: Anticonvulsants
Pharmacologic class: Hydantoin derivatives

AVAILABLE FORMS
phenytoin
Oral suspension: 125 mg/5 mL*
Tablets (chewable): 50 mg
phenytoin sodium
Injection: 50 mg/mL

Reactions in bold italics are *life-threatening*. Interactions may have a *rapid onset* or a **delayed onset**.

phenytoin sodium (extended)
Capsules (extended-release): 30 mg, 100 mg, 200 mg, 300 mg

INDICATIONS & DOSAGES

➤ **To control tonic-clonic (grand mal) and psychomotor (temporal lobe) seizures**
Adults: Highly individualized. Initially, 100 mg (immediate-release, extended-release) PO t.i.d. Adjust dosage at no less than 7- to 10-day intervals until desired response is obtained. Usual range is 300 to 600 mg daily. If patient is stabilized on 100-mg extended-release capsules t.i.d., once-daily dosing with 300-mg extended-release capsules is possible as an alternative. Or, 125 mg oral solution t.i.d. in patients without previous treatment. May increase to 625 mg daily.
Children: 5 mg/kg/day in two to three equally divided doses. Adjust dosage at no less than 7- to 10-day intervals. Usual maintenance dose range is 4 to 8 mg/kg daily. Maximum dose is 300 mg/day.

➤ **To control tonic-clonic (grand mal) and psychomotor (temporal lobe) seizures in patients requiring a loading dose**
Adults: Initially, 1 g (extended-release) PO divided into three doses, which are given at 2-hour intervals with careful monitoring. Begin maintenance dosage of 100 mg (extended-release) PO t.i.d. to q.i.d. 24 hours after loading dose.

➤ **Generalized tonic-clonic status epilepticus; prevention and treatment of seizures during neurosurgery**
Adults: Loading dose of 10 to 15 mg/kg IV (1 to 1.5 g may be needed) at a rate not exceeding 50 mg/minute; then maintenance dosage of 100 mg PO or IV every 6 to 8 hours.
Children: Loading dose of 15 to 20 mg/kg IV, at a rate not exceeding 1 to 3 mg/kg/minute or 50 mg/minute, whichever is slower; then highly individualized maintenance dosages.

ADMINISTRATION

⚠ *Alert:* Hazardous drug; use safe handling and disposal precautions.
PO
• Give divided doses with or after meals to decrease adverse GI reactions.
• If daily dose can't be divided equally, give larger dose before bedtime.

• For chewable tablets, patient may chew thoroughly before swallowing or may swallow whole.
• Shake suspension well before use. Administer dose using a calibrated oral dosing syringe.
• Different oral forms aren't interchangeable.
• Don't crush or allow patient to chew extended-release capsules.
• For oral suspension, withhold enteral feedings for 1 to 2 hours before and 1 to 2 hours after giving drug, if possible, to improve absorption.
IV
▼ Clear tubing with NSS. Use only clear solution for injection. A slight yellow color is acceptable.
▼ To give as an infusion, dilute in NSS to a final concentration of phenytoin sodium in the solution of no less than 5 mg/mL. Begin infusion immediately after mixture has been prepared; infusion should run through an 0.22- to 0.55-micron in-line filter. Infusion must be completed within 4 hours.
▼ Check patency of catheter before giving. Monitor site for extravasation because it can cause severe tissue damage.
Boxed Warning Drug must be administered slowly. In adults, don't exceed 50 mg/minute IV. In children, administer drug at a rate not exceeding 1 to 3 mg/kg/minute or 50 mg/minute, whichever is slower because of the risk of severe hypotension and cardiac arrhythmias. Continuous monitoring of BP and ECG during IV administration is essential. ∎
▼ Follow each injection with injection of sterile NSS through the same needle or catheter.
▼ If possible, don't give by IV push into veins on back of hand to avoid purple glove syndrome. Inject into larger veins or central venous catheter, if available.
▼ Discard 4 hours after preparation. Don't refrigerate.
▼ **Incompatibilities:** Amikacin, aminophylline, amphotericin B, bretylium, cephapirin, ciprofloxacin, D_5W, diltiazem, dobutamine, enalaprilat, fat emulsions, hydromorphone, insulin (regular), levorphanol, lidocaine, lincomycin, meperidine, morphine sulfate, nitroglycerin, norepinephrine, other IV drugs or infusion solutions, pentobarbital sodium, potassium chloride, procaine, propofol, streptomycin, sufentanil

P.

citrate, theophylline, vitamin B complex with C. If giving as an infusion, don't mix drug with D_5W because it will precipitate. Consult a compatibility drug reference for additional details.

IM

• Give IM only if dosage adjustments are made; IM dose is 50% greater than oral dose.

• Be aware that drug isn't ordinarily given IM because drug may precipitate at injection site; cause pain, necrosis, or abscess formation; and be absorbed erratically.

• Don't give by IM route for treatment of status epilepticus as peak plasma levels may not be attained for up to 24 hours.

ACTION

May stabilize neuronal membranes and limit seizure activity either by increasing efflux or decreasing influx of sodium ions across cell membranes in the motor cortex during generation of nerve impulses.

Route	Onset	Peak	Duration
PO	Unknown	1.5–3 hr	Unknown
PO (extended-release)	Unknown	4–12 hr	Unknown
IV	Immediate	1–2 hr	Unknown
IM	Unknown	Unknown	Unknown

Half-life: Varies with dose, formulation, and concentration changes.

ADVERSE REACTIONS

CNS: ataxia, decreased coordination, mental confusion, slurred speech, dizziness, headache, insomnia, nervousness, twitching, peripheral neuropathy, vertigo. **CV:** *brady-cardia,* periarteritis nodosa, hypotension, *CV arrest.* **EENT:** diplopia, nystagmus, blurred vision, gingival hyperplasia. **GI:** nausea, vomiting, constipation. **Hematologic:** *agranulocytosis, leukopenia, pancytopenia, thrombocytopenia,* macrocythemia, megaloblastic anemia. **Hepatic:** *toxic hepatitis, acute hepatic failure.* **Metabolic:** hyperglycemia. **Musculoskeletal:** osteomalacia. **Skin:** *SCARs,* bullous or purpuric dermatitis, discoloration of skin if given by IV push in back of hand, exfoliative dermatitis, hypertrichosis, inflammation at injection site, necrosis, pain, photosensitivity reactions, scarlatiniform or morbilliform rash. **Other:** hypersensitivity reactions, lymphadenopathy, SLE, thickening of facial features.

INTERACTIONS

⊘ *Alert:* Phenytoin can significantly interact with many drugs. Consult a drug interaction resource or pharmacist for additional information.

Drug-drug. *Acetaminophen:* May decrease the therapeutic effects of acetaminophen and increase the incidence of hepatotoxicity. Monitor for toxicity.

Amiodarone, antihistamines, chloramphenicol, **cimetidine,** *cycloserine,* **fluconazole, isoniazid,** *metronidazole, omeprazole, phenylbutazone, salicylates,* **sulfonamides, ticlopidine:** May increase phenytoin activity and toxicity. Monitor patient for toxicity and adjust dosage as needed.

Antacids: May decrease phenytoin absorption. Separate dosing times.

Atracurium, cisatracurium, pancuronium, rocuronium, vecuronium: May decrease the effects of nondepolarizing muscle relaxant. May need to increase the nondepolarizing muscle relaxant dose.

Barbiturates, carbamazepine, dexamethasone, diazepam, diazoxide, folic acid, rifampin, theophylline, vigabatrin: May decrease phenytoin activity. Monitor phenytoin level.

Carbamazepine, cardiac glycosides, doxycycline, quinidine, theophylline: May decrease effects of these drugs. Monitor patient.

Colesevelam: May impair phenytoin absorption. Administer phenytoin 4 hours prior to colesevelam.

Corticosteroids: May decrease phenytoin level and corticosteroid effects. Measure phenytoin level and adjust phenytoin and corticosteroid dosages as needed.

Cyclosporine: May decrease cyclosporine levels, risking organ rejection. Monitor cyclosporine levels closely and adjust dosage as needed.

CYP2C9 substrates: May increase serum drug level. Use cautiously in patients who are intermediate or poor metabolizers of CYP2C9 substrates. Monitor patient for toxicity and decrease dosage as appropriate.

Disulfiram: May increase toxic effects of phenytoin. Monitor phenytoin level closely and adjust dosage as needed.

Efavirenz: May increase phenytoin level and decrease efavirenz level. Monitor patient and adjust dosages of either or both drugs if needed.

Reactions in bold italics are *life-threatening*. Interactions may have a *rapid onset* or a *delayed onset*.

Erlotinib: May increase phenytoin level and decrease erlotinib level. Monitor patient response.

Hormonal contraceptives: May increase phenytoin level and decrease contraceptive effectiveness. Monitor phenytoin level and adjust dosage if needed. Alternative form of contraception is recommended during therapy.

Isoniazid: May increase phenytoin level. Monitor phenytoin level and patient for toxicity.

Lithium: May increase toxicity of lithium, despite normal lithium levels. Monitor patient for adverse effects.

Methylphenidate: May increase phenytoin level. Monitor phenytoin level and adjust phenytoin dosage as needed.

NNRTIs (delavirdine, efavirenz, rilpivirine): May cause loss of virologic response. Use with delavirdine is contraindicated. Monitor patient closely.

Phenobarbital, valproate: May increase or decrease phenytoin level and worsen valproate-associated hyperammonemia. Monitor therapy.

Protease inhibitors (fosamprenavir, lopinavir–ritonavir): May decrease levels of both drugs. Measure phenytoin level and adjust dosage of phenytoin or protease inhibitor as needed.

Warfarin: May increase effects of warfarin and increase phenytoin level. Monitor patient for bleeding.

Drug-herb. *St. John's wort:* May decrease phenytoin level. Monitor phenytoin level.

Drug-food. *Enteral tube feedings:* May interfere with absorption of oral drug. Monitor serum drug level more frequently.

Drug-lifestyle. *Alcohol use (acute):* May increase phenytoin level. Discourage use together.

Alcohol use (long-term): May decrease drug's activity. Strongly discourage use together.

EFFECTS ON LAB TEST RESULTS
• May increase ALP, GGT, and glucose levels.
• May decrease T_3 and T_4 levels.
• May decrease Hb level, hematocrit, and platelet, WBC, RBC, and granulocyte counts.
• May falsely reduce protein-bound iodine or free T_4 level test results.
• May cause lower than normal dexamethasone and metyrapone test results.

CONTRAINDICATIONS & CAUTIONS
• Contraindicated in patients hypersensitive to hydantoins and in those with a history of prior acute hepatotoxicity attributable to phenytoin. Parenteral phenytoin is also contraindicated in patients with sinus bradycardia, SA block, second- or third-degree AV block, or Adams-Stokes syndrome.
• Use cautiously in patients with hepatic or renal dysfunction, hypotension, hypoalbuminemia, myocardial insufficiency, diabetes, porphyria, or respiratory depression; in older adults or patients who are debilitated; and in those receiving other hydantoin derivatives.
• Older adults tend to metabolize drug slowly and may need reduced dosages.
Dialyzable drug: Yes.
⚠ **Overdose S&S:** Ataxia, dysarthria, nystagmus, hyperreflexia, lethargy, nausea, slurred speech, tremor, vomiting, coma, hypotension, circulatory and respiratory depression.

PREGNANCY-LACTATION-REPRODUCTION
• Drug may cause fetal harm. Prenatal exposure may increase risk of congenital malformations and other adverse outcomes. Avoid use during pregnancy when possible; if necessary, use as monotherapy. Dosage adjustments may be needed to maintain clinical response because therapeutic dose needs usually increase during pregnancy.
• A potentially life-threatening bleeding disorder related to decreased levels of vitamin K–dependent clotting factors that may occur in neonates exposed to phenytoin in utero can be prevented with vitamin K administration to the mother before delivery and to the neonate after birth.
• Drug may interact with hormone-containing contraceptives; use of nonhormonal contraceptives is recommended.
• Patients exposed to drug during pregnancy should enroll in the North American AED Pregnancy Registry (1-888-233-2334).
• Drug appears in human milk. Breastfeeding isn't recommended.

NURSING CONSIDERATIONS
Boxed Warning Carefully monitor cardiac status during and after IV administration. CV toxicity may increase with infusion rates above those recommended. Toxicity has also been reported at or below the recommended infusion rate. Reduction in administration rate or discontinuation of dosing may be needed. ∎

P

⚕ Patients of Asian descent who have tested positive for the allele HLA-B*1502 have an increased risk of SCARs, including SJS and TEN. Monitor these patients carefully.

• If rash appears, stop drug. If rash is scarlatiniform or morbilliform, resume drug after rash clears. If rash reappears, stop therapy. If rash is exfoliative, purpuric, or bullous, don't resume drug.

• Monitor patient for hypersensitivity reactions, including angioedema.

• Don't stop drug suddenly because this may worsen seizures. Call prescriber immediately if adverse reactions develop.

• Monitor drug level. Total phenytoin therapeutic level ranges from 10 to 20 mcg/mL in adults and children and 8 to 15 mcg/mL in neonates. Free phenytoin therapeutic level ranges from 1 to 2 mcg/mL.

• Monitor the unbound fraction of phenytoin in patients with renal or hepatic impairment or hypoalbuminemia. The fraction of unbound phenytoin increases in these patients.

• Long-term use may decrease bone mineral density. Vitamin D and calcium supplements may be needed.

• Because of the risks of cardiac and local toxicity with parenteral phenytoin, use oral form when possible.

• Monitor CBC and calcium level every 6 months, and periodically monitor hepatic function. Prescriber may prescribe folic acid and vitamin B_{12} for evident megaloblastic anemia.

• Maintain seizure precautions, as needed.

🔔 *Alert:* Closely monitor all patients for changes in behavior that may indicate worsening suicidality or depression.

• Watch for gingival hyperplasia, especially in children.

• After seizures become controlled with divided doses, once-daily dosing may be considered.

• *Look alike–sound alike:* Don't confuse phenytoin with mephenytoin, fosphenytoin, phenelzine, phentermine, or phenobarbital. Don't confuse Dilantin with Dilaudid, diltiazem, or Dipentum.

PATIENT TEACHING

• Tell patient to report all adverse reactions and to notify prescriber if rash develops.

• Advise patient and caregivers to immediately report changes in behavior that may indicate worsening suicidality or depression.

• Caution patient to avoid driving and other potentially hazardous activities that require mental alertness until drug's CNS effects are known.

• Advise patient not to change brands or dosage forms once stabilized on therapy.

• Dilantin capsules are the only oral form that can be given once daily. Toxic levels may result if any other brand or form is given once daily. Dilantin tablets and oral suspension should never be taken once daily.

• Tell patient not to use capsules that are discolored.

• Advise patient to avoid alcohol.

• Warn patient and parents not to stop drug abruptly.

• Stress importance of good oral hygiene and regular dental exams. Surgical removal of excess gum tissue may be needed periodically if dental hygiene is poor.

• Advise patient of childbearing potential who isn't planning a pregnancy to use effective contraception; warn patient about potential for decreased hormonal contraceptive efficacy.

• Instruct patient to report pregnancy, plans to become pregnant, breastfeeding, or plans to breastfeed during therapy.

• Advise patient that drug may cause an increase in blood glucose levels.

pilocarpine hydrochloride (oral)
pye-loe-KAR-peen

Salagen

Therapeutic class: Cholinergic agonists
Pharmacologic class: Cholinergic agonists

AVAILABLE FORMS
Tablets: 5 mg, 7.5 mg

INDICATIONS & DOSAGES
Adjust-a-dose (for all indications): For patients with moderate hepatic impairment, initial dose is 5 mg PO b.i.d. Adjust dosage based on tolerance.

➤ **Xerostomia from salivary gland hypofunction caused by radiotherapy for cancer of head and neck**
Adults: 5 mg PO t.i.d.; may increase to 10 mg PO t.i.d. as needed.

➤ **Dry mouth in patients with Sjögren syndrome**
Adults: 5 mg PO q.i.d.

ADMINISTRATION

PO
• Don't give drug with a high-fat meal.
• Store at room temperature.

ACTION

Cholinergic parasympathomimetic that increases secretion of salivary glands, eliminating dryness.

Route	Onset	Peak	Duration
PO	20 min	1 hr	3–5 hr

Half-life: 45 minutes to 1.35 hours.

ADVERSE REACTIONS

CNS: asthenia, dizziness, fever, headache, tremor, pain, somnolence, taste perversion. **CV:** flushing, HTN, tachycardia, edema, palpitations. **EENT:** abnormal vision, lacrimation, amblyopia, conjunctivitis, tinnitus, epistaxis, rhinitis, sinusitis, pharyngitis, voice alteration, increased salivation, glossitis. **GI:** nausea, dyspepsia, diarrhea, constipation, abdominal pain, flatulence, stomatitis, vomiting, dysphagia. **GU:** urinary frequency, urinary incontinence, UTI, vaginitis. **Musculoskeletal:** myalgia, weakness, back pain. **Skin:** diaphoresis, rash, pruritus. **Other:** chills, flu-like syndrome, infection, hypersensitivity reaction.

INTERACTIONS

Drug-drug. *Beta blockers:* May increase risk of conduction disturbances. Use together cautiously.
Drugs with anticholinergic effects (atropine, inhaled ipratropium): May antagonize anticholinergic effects. Use together cautiously.
Drugs with parasympathomimetic effects: May result in additive pharmacologic effects. Monitor patient closely.
Drug-food. *High-fat meals:* May reduce drug absorption. Discourage patient from eating high-fat meals.

EFFECTS ON LAB TEST RESULTS
None reported.

CONTRAINDICATIONS & CAUTIONS
• Contraindicated in patients hypersensitive to pilocarpine, in those with uncontrolled asthma, and in those for whom miosis is undesirable, as in acute iritis or angle-closure glaucoma.
• Use in severe hepatic impairment isn't recommended.
• Use cautiously in patients with CV disease, controlled asthma, chronic bronchitis, COPD, cholelithiasis, biliary tract disease, nephrolithiasis, moderate hepatic impairment, or cognitive or psychiatric disturbances.
• Safety and effectiveness in children haven't been established.
Dialyzable drug: Unknown.
⚠ *Overdose S&S:* Exaggerated parasympathetic effects, CV depression, bronchoconstriction, death.

PREGNANCY-LACTATION-REPRODUCTION
• There are no adequate studies during pregnancy. Use only if potential benefit justifies fetal risk.
• It isn't known if drug appears in human milk. Patient should discontinue breastfeeding or discontinue drug.

NURSING CONSIDERATIONS
• Monitor patient for signs and symptoms of toxicity: headache, visual disturbance, lacrimation, diaphoresis, respiratory distress, GI spasm, nausea, vomiting, diarrhea, AV block, tachycardia, bradycardia, hypotension, HTN, shock, mental confusion, arrhythmia, and tremors. Immediately report suspected toxicity.
• Monitor patient for dehydration from diaphoresis and poor fluid intake.
• *Look alike–sound alike:* Don't confuse Salagen with selegiline.

PATIENT TEACHING
• Warn patient that driving ability may be impaired, especially at night, by drug-induced visual disturbances.
• Advise patient to drink plenty of fluids to prevent dehydration.
• Tell older adults with Sjögren syndrome that this age-group may be especially prone to urinary frequency, diarrhea, and dizziness.
• Advise patient not to take drug with a high-fat meal.
• Instruct patient to report changes in eyesight and eye pain or irritation.

P

pimecrolimus
py-meck-roh-LY-mus

Elidel

Therapeutic class: Immunosuppressants (topical)
Pharmacologic class: Topical immunomodulators

AVAILABLE FORMS
Cream: 1%*

INDICATIONS & DOSAGES
➤ **Atopic dermatitis (mild to moderate) as second-line therapy for short and non-continuous prolonged treatment in patients who are nonimmunocompromised and in whom use of other conventional therapies is deemed inadvisable, or in patients with inadequate response to or intolerance of conventional therapies**
Adults and children age 2 and older: Apply a thin layer to the affected skin b.i.d. and rub in gently and completely. Discontinue therapy when signs and symptoms (itch, rash, redness) resolve. If signs and symptoms persist beyond 6 weeks, reevaluate patient.

ADMINISTRATION
Topical
• Drug may be used on all skin surfaces, including the head, neck, and intertriginous areas.
Boxed Warning Limit application to areas of involvement. ▪
• Clear infections at treatment sites before using.
• Don't use with occlusive dressing.

ACTION
Unknown. Inhibits T-cell activation and prevents the release of inflammatory cytokines and mediators from mast cells.

Route	Onset	Peak	Duration
Topical	Unknown	Unknown	Unknown

Half-life: Unknown.

ADVERSE REACTIONS
CNS: headache, fever. **EENT:** eye infection, conjunctivitis, earache, otitis media, epistaxis, nasopharyngitis, sinusitis, nasal congestion, pharyngitis, rhinorrhea, sinus congestion, rhinitis, tonsillitis, toothache. **GI:** gastroenteritis, abdominal pain, vomiting, diarrhea, nausea, constipation, loose stools. **GU:** dysmenorrhea. **Musculoskeletal:** back pain, arthralgias. **Respiratory:** URI, bronchitis, cough, *asthma,* pneumonia, wheezing, dyspnea. **Skin:** application-site reaction (burning, irritation, erythema, pruritus), skin infections, impetigo, folliculitis, molluscum contagiosum, herpes simplex, varicella, papilloma, urticaria, acne. **Other:** flulike illness, hypersensitivity, bacterial infection, viral infection.

INTERACTIONS
Drug-drug. *CYP3A4 inhibitors (calcium channel blockers, erythromycin, fluconazole, itraconazole, ketoconazole):* May decrease metabolism of pimecrolimus. Use together cautiously.
Immunosuppressants: May enhance adverse or toxic effect of immunosuppressants. Avoid use together.
Drug-lifestyle. *Natural or artificial sun exposure:* May worsen atopic dermatitis. Advise patient to avoid or minimize sunlight exposure.

EFFECTS ON LAB TEST RESULTS
None reported.

CONTRAINDICATIONS & CAUTIONS
• Contraindicated in patients hypersensitive to drug or its components, in patients with Netherton syndrome, and in patients who are immunocompromised, including those on systemic immunosuppressants.
Boxed Warning Long-term safety of topical calcineurin inhibitors hasn't been established. ▪
Boxed Warning Although a causal relationship hasn't been established, rare cases of malignancy (e.g., skin malignancy, lymphoma) have been reported in patients treated with topical calcineurin inhibitors, including pimecrolimus. ▪
• Contraindicated in patients with active cutaneous viral infections or infected atopic dermatitis.
• Avoid use on malignant or premalignant skin conditions.
• Use cautiously in patients with varicella zoster virus infection, HSV infection, or eczema herpeticum.
Boxed Warning Not indicated for use in children younger than age 2. ▪
Dialyzable drug: Unknown.

Reactions in bold italics are *life-threatening*. Interactions may have a *rapid onset* or a *delayed onset*.

PREGNANCY-LACTATION-REPRODUCTION
• There are no adequate studies during pregnancy. Use only if potential benefit justifies fetal risk.
• It's unknown if drug appears in human milk. Serious adverse reactions may occur in infants who are breastfed and exposed to drug. Patient should discontinue breastfeeding or discontinue drug.

NURSING CONSIDERATIONS
🛈 *Alert:* Use drug only after other therapies have failed because of the risk of cancer.
Boxed Warning Avoid continuous long-term use of drug and limit application to areas of involvement of atopic dermatitis. ∎
• May cause local symptoms such as skin burning. Most local reactions start within 1 to 5 days after treatment, are mild to moderately severe, and last no longer than 5 days.
• Monitor patient for lymphadenopathy. If lymphadenopathy occurs and its cause is unknown, or if patient develops acute infectious mononucleosis, consider stopping drug.
• Drug use may cause papillomas or warts. Consider stopping drug if papillomas worsen or don't respond to conventional treatment.
• *Look alike–sound alike:* Don't confuse pimecrolimus with tacrolimus.

PATIENT TEACHING
• Inform patient that drug is for external use only and to use it as directed.
• Tell patient to report adverse reactions.
• Caution patient not to use with an occlusive dressing.
• Instruct patient and caregivers to wash hands before and after application and that skin should be dry before applying cream.
• Tell patient to stop therapy after signs and symptoms have resolved. If signs and symptoms persist longer than 6 weeks, advise patient to contact prescriber.
• Teach patient to resume treatment at first signs of recurrence.
• Stress that patient should minimize or avoid exposure to natural or artificial sunlight (including tanning beds and UVA-UVB treatment) while using this drug.
• Tell patient to expect application-site reactions but to notify prescriber if reaction is severe or persists for longer than 1 week.

pioglitazone hydrochloride
pye-oh-GLI-ta-zone

Actos⟡

Therapeutic class: Antidiabetics
Pharmacologic class: Thiazolidinediones

AVAILABLE FORMS
Tablets: 15 mg, 30 mg, 45 mg

INDICATIONS & DOSAGES
➤ **Type 2 diabetes, alone or with a sulfonylurea, metformin, or insulin as an adjunct to diet and exercise to improve glycemic control**
Adults: Initially, 15 or 30 mg PO once daily. Titrate in 15-mg increments to maximum of 45 mg daily based on HbA_{1c}.
Adjust-a-dose: For patients taking pioglitazone with insulin, reduce insulin by 10% to 25% if patient reports hypoglycemia. Maximum recommended dose of pioglitazone is 15 mg when used with gemfibrozil or other strong CYP2C8 inhibitors. Start with 15 mg in patients with NYHA Class I or II HF.

ADMINISTRATION
PO
• Give drug without regard for meals.
• For missed dose, omit missed dose and resume regular schedule the following day; don't double dose.

ACTION
Lowers glucose level by decreasing insulin resistance and hepatic glucose production. Improves sensitivity of insulin in muscle and adipose tissue.

Route	Onset	Peak	Duration
PO	30 min	≤2 hr	Unknown

Half-life: 3 to 7 hours.

ADVERSE REACTIONS
CNS: headache, dizziness. **CV:** edema, *HF, HTN,* chest pain. **EENT:** macular edema, sinusitis, pharyngitis, tooth disorder. **GI:** diarrhea, flatulence. **GU:** UTI. **Hematologic:** anemia. **Metabolic:** *hypoglycemia,* weight gain. **Musculoskeletal:** myalgia, fractures, back pain. **Respiratory:** URI.

P

INTERACTIONS

Drug-drug. *Atorvastatin:* May decrease atorvastatin and pioglitazone levels. Monitor patient and glucose level.

CYP2C8 inducers (rifampin): May decrease pioglitazone concentration. Don't exceed maximum recommended pioglitazone dose of 45 mg.

Hormonal contraceptives: May decrease level of hormonal contraceptives, reducing contraceptive effectiveness. Advise patient taking drug and hormonal contraceptives to consider additional birth control measures.

Insulin: May increase incidence of edema and HF and may cause additive or synergistic pharmacologic effects. If hypoglycemia occurs, decrease insulin dosage. If edema or HF occurs, decrease pioglitazone dosage.

Ketoconazole: May increase pioglitazone level. Monitor glucose level more frequently.

Strong CYP2C8 inhibitors (gemfibrozil): May increase pioglitazone level. Monitor patient and glucose level. Maximum pioglitazone dose is 15 mg.

Sulfonylureas: May increase risk of hypoglycemia. If hypoglycemia occurs, reduce sulfonylurea dosage.

Topiramate: May decrease pioglitazone level. Monitor glycemic control.

Drug-herb. *Eucalyptus:* May increase hypoglycemic effects. Discourage use together.

Drug-lifestyle. *Alcohol use:* May alter glycemic control and increase risk of hypoglycemia. Discourage use together.

EFFECTS ON LAB TEST RESULTS

• May increase LFT values and CK, HDL, and total cholesterol levels.
• May decrease glucose and triglyceride levels.
• May decrease Hb level and hematocrit.

CONTRAINDICATIONS & CAUTIONS

Boxed Warning Contraindicated in patients with NYHA Class III or IV HF; not recommended in those with symptomatic HF. ■

• Contraindicated in patients hypersensitive to drug or its components and in those with active bladder cancer.
• Don't use in patients with type 1 diabetes and diabetic ketoacidosis; use cautiously in those with active liver disease.
• Safety and effectiveness in children haven't been established.

Dialyzable drug: Unknown.

PREGNANCY-LACTATION-REPRODUCTION

• Use during pregnancy only if benefit justifies fetal risk. Insulin is preferred antidiabetic during pregnancy.
• It isn't known if drug appears in human milk. Patient should discontinue breastfeeding or discontinue drug.

NURSING CONSIDERATIONS

⚠ *Alert:* Measure liver enzyme levels before start of therapy. In patients with liver disorder, monitor LFT values periodically during treatment. Obtain LFT results in patients who develop signs and symptoms of liver dysfunction, such as nausea, vomiting, abdominal pain, fatigue, anorexia, or dark urine. Stop drug if patient develops jaundice or if LFT results show ALT level greater than 3 × ULN with bilirubin level greater than 2 × ULN.

Boxed Warning Drug can cause fluid retention, leading to or worsening HF. Observe patients carefully for signs and symptoms of HF (including excessive, rapid weight gain; dyspnea; and edema). If these signs and symptoms develop, the HF should be managed according to the current standards of care. Also, stopping or reducing dose of pioglitazone must be considered. ■

• Hb level and hematocrit may drop, usually during first 4 to 12 weeks of therapy.
• Management of type 2 diabetes should include diet control. Because caloric restrictions, weight loss, and exercise help improve insulin sensitivity and help make drug therapy effective, these measures are essential for proper diabetes management.

⚠ *Alert:* Watch for hypoglycemia, especially in patients receiving combination therapy. Dosage adjustments of these drugs may be needed.

• Monitor glucose level regularly, especially during situations of increased stress, such as infection, fever, surgery, and trauma.

⚠ *Alert:* Drug may be associated with an increased risk of bladder cancer when used for more than 1 year. Monitor patients for signs and symptoms of bladder cancer (such as blood in urine or abdominal pain). If considering use in patients with a history of bladder cancer, weigh benefits of blood glucose control with drug against unknown risks of cancer recurrence.

• Monitor patient for blurred vision or decreased visual acuity. Refer patient with symptoms to an ophthalmologist for macular edema evaluation.

• Long-term treatment increases risk of fractures (forearm, hand, wrist, foot, ankle, fibula, and tibia) in females. Give only if risk outweighs benefits.

• *Look alike–sound alike:* Don't confuse pioglitazone with rosiglitazone. Don't confuse Actos with Actidose or Actonel.

PATIENT TEACHING

• Instruct patient in safe drug administration.
• Instruct patient to adhere to dietary instructions and to have glucose and HbA$_{1c}$ levels tested regularly.
• Teach patient taking pioglitazone with insulin or oral antidiabetics the signs and symptoms of hypoglycemia.
• Advise patient to notify prescriber during periods of stress, such as fever, trauma, infection, or surgery, because dosage may need adjustment.
• Instruct patient how and when to monitor glucose level.
• Notify patient that blood tests of liver function will be performed before therapy starts and, if appropriate, periodically thereafter.
• Tell patient to immediately report all adverse reactions, especially unexplained nausea, vomiting, abdominal pain, fatigue, anorexia, and dark urine, because these symptoms may indicate liver problems.
• Warn patient to report signs or symptoms of HF (unusually rapid weight gain, swelling, or shortness of breath).
• Advise patient with insulin resistance who is anovulatory and premenopausal that therapy may cause resumption of ovulation; recommend using contraception.
• Tell patient to have regular eye exams and to report any visual changes immediately.
• Advise patient to report blood in the urine, red-colored urine, new or worsening urge to urinate, or pain when urinating; these symptoms may indicate bladder cancer.

piperacillin sodium–tazobactam sodium
pi-PER-a-sil-in/ta-zoe-BAK-tam

Zosyn

Therapeutic class: Antibiotics
Pharmacologic class: Extended-spectrum penicillins–beta-lactamase inhibitors

AVAILABLE FORMS

Powder for injection: 2 g piperacillin and 0.25 g tazobactam per vial, 3 g piperacillin and 0.375 g tazobactam per vial, 4 g piperacillin and 0.5 g tazobactam per vial
Premixed, frozen solution for injection: 2 g piperacillin and 0.25 g tazobactam per 50-mL container, 3 g piperacillin and 0.375 g tazobactam per 50-mL container, 4 g piperacillin and 0.5 g tazobactam per 100-mL container

INDICATIONS & DOSAGES

➤ **Moderate to severe infections from piperacillin-resistant, piperacillin-tazobactam–susceptible, beta-lactamase–producing strains of microorganisms in appendicitis (complicated by rupture or abscess) and peritonitis caused by** *Escherichia coli, Bacteroides fragilis, B. ovatus, B. thetaiotaomicron,* **or** *B. vulgatus;* **skin and skin-structure infections caused by** *Staphylococcus aureus;* **postpartum endometritis or pelvic inflammatory disease caused by** *E. coli;* **moderately severe community-acquired pneumonia caused by** *Haemophilus influenzae*
Adults: 3.375 g (3 g piperacillin/0.375 g tazobactam) every 6 hours by IV infusion for 7 to 10 days.
Adjust-a-dose: If CrCl is 20 to 40 mL/minute, give 2.25 g (2 g piperacillin/0.25 g tazobactam) every 6 hours; if CrCl is less than 20 mL/minute, give 2.25 g (2 g piperacillin/0.25 g tazobactam) every 8 hours. In patients on continuous ambulatory peritoneal dialysis (CAPD), give 2.25 g (2 g piperacillin/0.25 g tazobactam) every 12 hours. In patients on hemodialysis, give 2.25 g (2 g piperacillin/0.25 g tazobactam) every 12 hours with a supplemental dose of 0.75 g (0.67 g piperacillin/0.08 g tazobactam) after each dialysis period.

➤ **Appendicitis, peritonitis**

Children weighing more than 40 kg with normal renal function: 3.375 g (3 g piperacillin/0.375 g tazobactam) every 6 hours by IV infusion for 7 to 10 days.

Children age 9 months and older weighing 40 kg or less with normal renal function: 100 mg piperacillin/12.5 mg tazobactam per kg of body weight every 8 hours by IV infusion for 7 to 10 days.

Children age 2 to 9 months: 80 mg piperacillin/10 mg tazobactam per kg of body weight every 8 hours by IV infusion for 7 to 10 days.

➤ **Moderate to severe health care–associated pneumonia caused by piperacillin-resistant, beta-lactamase–producing strains of *S. aureus* or by piperacillin-tazobactam–susceptible *Acinetobacter baumannii*, *H. influenzae*, *Klebsiella pneumoniae*, and *Pseudomonas aeruginosa***

Adults and children weighing more than 40 kg with normal renal function: 4.5 g (4 g piperacillin/0.5 g tazobactam) IV every 6 hours with aminoglycoside. Patients with *P. aeruginosa* should continue aminoglycoside or antipseudomonal fluoroquinolone treatment; if *P. aeruginosa* isn't isolated, aminoglycoside or fluoroquinolone treatment may be stopped. Duration of treatment is usually 7 to 14 days.

Children age 9 months and older weighing 40 kg or less with normal renal function: 100 mg piperacillin/12.5 mg tazobactam per kg of body weight every 6 hours by IV infusion for 7 to 10 days.

Children age 2 to 9 months: 80 mg piperacillin/10 mg tazobactam per kg of body weight every 6 hours by IV infusion for 7 to 10 days.

Adjust-a-dose: In adults, if CrCl is 20 to 40 mL/minute, give 3.375 g (3 g piperacillin/0.375 g tazobactam) every 6 hours; if CrCl is less than 20 mL/minute, give 2.25 g (2 g piperacillin/0.25 g tazobactam) every 6 hours. In patients with CAPD, give 2.25 g (2 g piperacillin/0.25 g tazobactam) every 8 hours. In patients on hemodialysis, give 2.25 g (2 g piperacillin/0.25 g tazobactam) every 8 hours with a supplemental dose of 0.75 g (0.67 g piperacillin/0.08 g tazobactam) after each dialysis period.

ADMINISTRATION

IV

▼ Before giving drug, ask patient about allergic reactions to penicillins, cephalosporins, or beta-lactamase inhibitors.

▼ Obtain specimen for culture and sensitivity tests before giving first dose. Therapy may begin while awaiting results.

▼ Reconstitute each gram (based on piperacillin content) with 5 mL of diluent, such as sterile or bacteriostatic water for injection, NSS for injection, bacteriostatic NSS for injection, D_5W, dextrose 5% in NSS for injection, or dextran 6% in NSS for injection.

▼ Shake until dissolved.

▼ Further dilute to 50 to 150 mL before infusion.

▼ Use drug immediately after reconstitution.

▼ Stop any primary infusion during administration, if possible.

▼ Infuse over at least 30 minutes.

▼ Discard unused drug in single-dose vials after 24 hours if stored at room temperature or 48 hours if refrigerated.

▼ Diluted drug remains stable in IV bags for 24 hours at room temperature or for 1 week refrigerated.

▼ Store premixed, frozen solution containers at or below –4° F (–20° C).

▼ Thaw frozen container at room temperature (68° to 77° F [20° to 25° C]) or under refrigeration (36° to 46° F [2° to 8° C]). Don't force-thaw by immersion in water baths or by microwave irradiation.

▼ Check for minute leaks by squeezing container firmly. If leaks are detected, discard solution as sterility may be impaired.

▼ Visually inspect solution, which may precipitate while frozen but will dissolve upon reaching room temperature with little or no agitation. If, after visual inspection, solution remains cloudy, an insoluble precipitate is noted, or if any seals or outlet ports aren't intact, discard container.

▼ Don't use plastic containers in series connections.

▼ **Incompatibilities:** Other drugs.

ACTION

Inhibits cell-wall synthesis during bacterial multiplication.

Route	Onset	Peak	Duration
IV	Immediate	Immediate	Unknown

Half-life: About 0.7 to 1.2 hours.

ADVERSE REACTIONS

CNS: headache, insomnia, fever, *seizures,* agitation, anxiety, dizziness, pain. **CV:** chest pain, edema, HTN, hypotension, tachycardia, phlebitis at IV site, thrombophlebitis. **EENT:** rhinitis, oral candidiasis. **GI:** diarrhea, constipation, nausea, abdominal pain, dyspepsia, stool changes, vomiting. **GU:** candidiasis, interstitial nephritis, increased BUN and creatinine levels. **Hematologic:** *leukopenia, neutropenia, thrombocythemia,* anemia, eosinophilia. **Hepatic:** abnormal LFT values. **Skin:** pruritus, rash. **Other:** hypersensitivity reactions, inflammation.

INTERACTIONS

Drug-drug. *Aminoglycosides (amikacin, gentamicin, streptomycin, tobramycin):* Penicillins may decrease serum concentration of aminoglycosides. Consider therapy modification.
Anticoagulants, heparin: May prolong effectiveness and increase risk of bleeding. Monitor PT and INR closely.
Hormonal contraceptives: May decrease contraceptive effectiveness. Advise using another form of contraception.
Live-virus vaccines: May decrease vaccine effectiveness. Don't use together.
Methotrexate: May increase risk of methotrexate toxicity. Monitor closely.
Probenecid: May increase piperacillin level. Probenecid may be used for this purpose.
Vancomycin: May increase nephrotoxicity. Monitor therapy.
Vecuronium: May prolong neuromuscular blockade. Monitor patient closely.

EFFECTS ON LAB TEST RESULTS

• May increase serum sodium level because of sodium content in drug.
• May increase BUN, creatinine, ALP, ALT, and AST levels.
• May increase eosinophil count.
• May decrease Hb level and neutrophil and WBC counts.
• May increase or decrease platelet count.
• May prolong PTT and PT.

• May cause false-positive result for urine glucose tests using copper reduction method such as Clinitest.
• May cause false-positive test for *Aspergillus*.

CONTRAINDICATIONS & CAUTIONS

• Contraindicated in patients hypersensitive to drug, other penicillins, cephalosporins, or beta-lactamase inhibitors.
• Drug can cause CDAD. Consider possibility of CDAD in all patients who present with diarrhea after antibiotic use.
• Use cautiously in patients with renal impairment or seizure disorders. Penicillins can cause neuromuscular excitability or seizures.
• Use cautiously in patients who are critically ill and in patients with bleeding tendencies, uremia, hypokalemia, and allergies to other drugs.
Dialyzable drug: Yes.
⚠ **Overdose S&S:** Neuromuscular hyperexcitability, seizures.

PREGNANCY-LACTATION-REPRODUCTION

• There are no adequate studies during pregnancy. Piperacillin and tazobactam cross the placental barrier in humans. Use only if clearly needed.
• Drug appears in low concentrations in human milk. Use cautiously if breastfeeding.

NURSING CONSIDERATIONS

• Drug may cause CDAD ranging in severity from mild diarrhea to fatal colitis. Monitor patient for diarrhea and initiate therapeutic measures as needed. Drug may need to be stopped.
• Studies have shown that drug is an independent risk factor for renal failure and delayed renal function recovery in patients who are critically ill. Alternative treatments should be considered; if alternative treatment options are inadequate or unavailable, monitor renal function during therapy.
• SCARs can occur. If rash develops, monitor patient closely and discontinue drug if lesion progresses.
• Hemodialysis removes 30% to 40% of a dose in 4 hours. Additional doses may be needed after each dialysis period.
• If large doses are given or if therapy is prolonged, bacterial or fungal superinfection may occur, especially in older adults or patients who are debilitated or immunosuppressed.

P

- Drug contains 2.84 mEq (65 mg) sodium per gram of piperacillin. Monitor sodium intake and electrolyte levels.
- Monitor hematologic and coagulation parameters.
- **Alert:** Monitor patient for hemophagocytic lymphohistiocytosis (fever, rash, lymphadenopathy, hepatosplenomegaly, cytopenia), a life-threatening excessive immune activation syndrome that occurs most often in infants younger than age 18 months. Discontinue drug immediately for such signs or symptoms.
- Monitor patient with cystic fibrosis for fever and rash.
- **Look alike–sound alike:** Don't confuse Zosyn with Zyvox.

PATIENT TEACHING
- Tell patient to report allergic and other adverse reactions promptly.
- Instruct patient to report discomfort at IV site.
- Advise patient that watery and bloody stools with or without stomach cramps and fever may occur during and for up to 2 months or more after antibiotic use. Instruct patient to report these symptoms as soon as possible.

---

pitavastatin ▧
pih-tav-a-STAT-in

Livalo, Zypitamag

Therapeutic class: Antilipemics
Pharmacologic class: HMG-CoA reductase inhibitors

AVAILABLE FORMS
Tablets: 1 mg, 2 mg, 4 mg

INDICATIONS & DOSAGES
Adjust-a-dose (for all indications): For adults with moderate and severe renal impairment (GFR of 15 to 59 mL/minute/1.73 m^2) and those with ESRD who are on hemodialysis, start with 1 mg PO daily; maximum dosage is 2 mg daily.

➤ **Primary hyperlipidemia or mixed dyslipidemia as adjunctive therapy with diet to decrease total cholesterol (TC), LDL cholesterol (LDL-C), and apolipoprotein B (apo B) triglyceride levels, and to increase HDL cholesterol level**

Adults: Initially, 2 mg PO daily. May increase dosage as needed, to maximum of 4 mg PO daily.
➤ **Heterozygous familial hypercholesterolemia (HeFH) in children to reduce elevated TC, LDL-C, and apo B levels (Livalo)** ▧
Children age 8 and older: Initially, 2 mg PO daily. May increase as needed, to maximum of 4 mg daily.

ADMINISTRATION
PO
- May give without regard to food at same time each day.

ACTION
Inhibits HMG-CoA reductase, a hepatic enzyme that's needed for cholesterol biosynthesis.

Route	Onset	Peak	Duration
PO	Unknown	1 hr	Unknown

Half-life: 12 hours.

ADVERSE REACTIONS
CNS: headache. **EENT:** nasopharyngitis. **GI:** constipation, diarrhea. **Musculoskeletal:** back pain, myalgia, extremity pain. **Other:** flulike symptoms, hypersensitivity reactions.

INTERACTIONS
Drug-drug. *Colchicine:* May cause myopathy, including rhabdomyolysis. Use cautiously together.
Cyclosporine: May increase pitavastatin level. Use together is contraindicated.
Erythromycin: May increase pitavastatin levels. Don't exceed 1 mg pitavastatin daily.
Fibrates (gemfibrozil), niacin: May increase risk of myopathy. Use together cautiously; consider reducing pitavastatin dosage when combined with niacin.
Rifampin: May increase pitavastatin levels. Don't exceed 2 mg pitavastatin daily.
Vitamin K antagonists (warfarin): May enhance anticoagulant effect. Monitor therapy.
Drug-herb. *Herbal cholesterol-lowering products:* May increase pitavastatin levels. Discourage using together.
Drug-food. *Grapefruit juice:* May increase pitavastatin levels and increase risk of adverse effects, including rhabdomyolysis and myopathy. Avoid using together.

Reactions in bold italics are *life-threatening*. Interactions may have a *rapid onset* or a ***delayed onset***.

EFFECTS ON LAB TEST RESULTS
• May increase AST, ALT, CK, bilirubin, HbA_{1c}, and glucose levels.

CONTRAINDICATIONS & CAUTIONS
• Contraindicated in patients hypersensitive to drug or its components and in those with active liver disease, which may include unexplained persistent elevations of hepatic transaminase levels.
• Use cautiously in older adults and in patients with renal impairment, inadequately treated hypothyroidism, or a history of myopathy or rhabdomyolysis.
• Statin therapy should be interrupted if patient shows signs of serious liver injury, hyperbilirubinemia, or jaundice. The drug shouldn't be restarted if another cause can't be found.
• Drug hasn't been studied in Fredrickson Type I, III, and V dyslipidemias.
• Safety and effectiveness of Livalo in children younger than age 8 with HeFH or in children with other types of hyperlipidemia haven't been established. Safety and effectiveness of Zypitamag in children haven't been established.
Dialyzable drug: Unlikely.

PREGNANCY-LACTATION-REPRODUCTION
• May cause fetal harm. Use during pregnancy is contraindicated unless benefits to patient outweigh fetal risk.
• Drug should be discontinued before conception. If pregnancy occurs during therapy, apprise patient of fetal risks with continued use.
• Drug is contraindicated during breastfeeding.

NURSING CONSIDERATIONS
• Start pitavastatin only after diet and other nondrug therapies have proved ineffective.
• Monitor LFT results and CK levels before therapy, 12 weeks after therapy initiation, after a dosage change, and periodically thereafter.
• Monitor lipid levels at baseline, 4 weeks after start of therapy, and at titration; adjust dosage accordingly.
• Discontinue drug if myopathy develops or if CK level markedly increases. Doses greater than 4 mg once daily were associated with an increased risk of severe myopathy in pre-

marketing clinical studies. Don't exceed 4 mg once daily.
• Temporarily withhold drug if patient develops sepsis; hypotension; dehydration; severe metabolic, endocrine, or electrolyte disorders; uncontrolled seizures; or trauma or if patient requires major surgery. These conditions may predispose patient to myopathy or rhabdomyolysis.
• *Look alike–sound alike:* Don't confuse pitavastatin with atorvastatin, fluvastatin, lovastatin, nystatin, pravastatin, rosuvastatin, or simvastatin.

PATIENT TEACHING
• Instruct patient in safe drug administration.
• Explain the importance of controlling serum lipid levels. Teach appropriate dietary management (restricting saturated fat and cholesterol intake), weight control, and exercise.
• Advise patient of childbearing potential to use contraception during therapy and to discuss future pregnancy and breastfeeding plans with health care provider.
• Warn patient to report unexplained muscle pain, tenderness, or weakness, especially if accompanied by fever or malaise.
• Teach patient that blood tests to check liver enzyme levels will be needed after start of therapy, after a dosage increase, and periodically thereafter.
• Tell patient that drug may increase blood glucose level; however, the CV benefits are thought to outweigh blood glucose level increase.

plecanatide
ple-KAN-a-tide

Trulance

Therapeutic class: Laxatives
Pharmacologic class: Guanylate cyclase-C agonists

AVAILABLE FORMS
Tablets: 3 mg

INDICATIONS & DOSAGES
➤ **Chronic idiopathic constipation or IBS with constipation**
Adults: 3 mg PO daily.

ADMINISTRATION
PO
- May give with or without food.
- Patient should swallow tablets whole, if possible.
- For patients with swallowing difficulties, may crush tablet and mix with 1 tsp of room temperature applesauce; give immediately.
- May dissolve tablet by placing whole tablet in a cup and adding 30 mL of room temperature water; swirl for at least 10 seconds. Give mixture immediately. To give any portion left in cup, add an additional 30 mL of water and swirl for at least 10 seconds. Give immediately; don't store mixture.
- If giving dissolved tablet by NG or gastric feeding tube, place tablet in 30 mL of water and swirl for at least 15 seconds. Draw up mixture using an appropriate syringe and administer. Flush tube with 30 mL of water before and at least 10 mL of water after administration.
- Skip a missed dose and give next dose at regularly scheduled time. Don't double dose.
- Store in dry place at room temperature. Keep drug in its original bottle with supplied desiccant.

ACTION
Plecanatide and its active metabolite bind to guanylate cyclase-C and act locally on the luminal surface of the intestinal epithelium, resulting in increased secretion of chloride and bicarbonate into the intestinal lumen, resulting in increased intestinal fluid and accelerated transit.

Route	Onset	Peak	Duration
PO	Unknown	Unknown	Unknown

Half-life: Unknown due to negligible systemic absorption.

ADVERSE REACTIONS
CNS: dizziness. **EENT:** sinusitis, nasopharyngitis. **GI:** diarrhea, abdominal distention, flatulence, abdominal tenderness, nausea. **GU:** UTI. **Hepatic:** elevated liver enzyme levels. **Respiratory:** URI.

INTERACTIONS
None reported.

EFFECTS ON LAB TEST RESULTS
- May increase AST and ALT levels.

CONTRAINDICATIONS & CAUTIONS
Boxed Warning Contraindicated in patients younger than age 6 because of risk of serious dehydration. ■
Boxed Warning Safety and effectiveness in patients younger than age 18 haven't been established. Avoid use in patients age 6 to younger than age 18. ■
- Contraindicated in patients with known or suspected mechanical GI obstruction.
- Don't administered to patients with severe diarrhea. Diarrhea is the most common adverse effect of plecanatide.
- Use cautiously in older adults.
Dialyzable drug: Unlikely.

PREGNANCY-LACTATION-REPRODUCTION
- Drug isn't absorbed systemically; use during pregnancy isn't expected to result in fetal exposure.
- Drug isn't expected to appear in human milk because it isn't absorbed systemically. Use cautiously during breastfeeding.

NURSING CONSIDERATIONS
- Monitor patient for diarrhea. If severe diarrhea occurs, withhold drug and rehydrate patient.
- *Look alike–sound alike:* Don't confuse Trulance with Trulicity.

PATIENT TEACHING
- Teach patient safe drug administration.
- Instruct patient to stop taking drug if severe diarrhea occurs and to contact prescriber.
- *Alert:* Warn patient to securely store drug away from children. Accidental ingestion may cause severe diarrhea and dehydration.

SAFETY ALERT!

polatuzumab vedotin-piiq
poe-la-TOOZ-ue-mab ve-DOE-tin

Polivy

Therapeutic class: Antineoplastics
Pharmacologic class: Antibodies–drug conjugates

AVAILABLE FORMS
Injection: 30 mg, 140 mg single-dose vial

INDICATIONS & DOSAGES

➤ **Relapsed or refractory diffuse large B-cell lymphoma, not otherwise specified, in combination with bendamustine and a rituximab product, after at least two prior therapies**

Adults: 1.8 mg/kg IV infusion every 21 days for six cycles in combination with bendamustine and a rituximab product in any order on day 1 of each cycle. Recommended bendamustine dose is 90 mg/m²/day on days 1 and 2 when administered with polatuzumab vedotin and a rituximab product. Recommended dose of the rituximab product is 375 mg/m² IV on day 1 of each cycle.

Adjust-a-dose: Refer to manufacturer's instructions for toxicity-related dosage adjustments.

ADMINISTRATION

IV

▼ If patient isn't already premedicated, administer an antihistamine and antipyretic 30 to 60 minutes before infusion.

◑ *Alert:* Drug is cytotoxic; use safe handling and disposal precautions.

▼ Reconstitute each vial immediately before use with 7.2 mL of sterile water for injection if using 140-mg vial and 1.8 mL if using 30-mg vial. Direct stream toward the inside wall of the vial to obtain a concentration of 20 mg/mL.

▼ Gently swirl vial until completely dissolved. Don't shake.

▼ Inspect reconstituted solution for discoloration and particulate matter. Solution should be colorless to slightly brown, clear to slightly opalescent. Don't use if solution is discolored, cloudy, or contains visible particulates. Don't freeze or expose to direct sunlight.

▼ Store unused reconstituted solution refrigerated at 36° to 46° F (2° to 8° C) for up to 48 hours or at room temperature for up to 8 hours before dilution. Discard vial when cumulative storage time before dilution exceeds 48 hours.

▼ Dilute drug to a final concentration of 0.72 to 2.7 mg/mL in an IV infusion bag with a minimum volume of 50 mL NSS, ½ NSS, or D₅W.

▼ Gently mix IV bag by slowly inverting the bag. Don't shake. Inspect for particulates and discard if present.

▼ Limit agitation of diluted product during preparation and transportation to administration site. Don't transport diluted product through an automated system, such as a pneumatic tube or automated cart.

▼ Administer via a dedicated line with a nonpyrogenic, low-protein-binding in-line or add-on filter (0.2- or 0.22-micron pore size) and catheter.

▼ If patient tolerates initial infusion over 90 minutes, may give subsequent infusions over 30 minutes.

▼ If not used immediately, store the diluted solution as specified in the manufacturer's information. Discard if storage time exceeds these limits. Don't freeze or expose to direct sunlight.

▼ Give missed dose as soon as possible. Adjust the administration schedule to maintain a 21-day interval between doses.

▼ Store vials refrigerated at 36° to 46° F (2° to 8° C) in original carton to protect from light. Don't freeze or shake.

▼ **Incompatibilities:** Don't mix with or administer as an infusion with other drugs.

ACTION

An antibody-drug conjugate that binds to CD79b (a B-cell surface protein), resulting in death of dividing cells through inhibition of cell division and apoptosis.

Route	Onset	Peak	Duration
IV	Unknown	Unknown	Unknown

Half-life: About 12 days.

ADVERSE REACTIONS

CNS: peripheral neuropathy, dizziness, fever, fatigue. **EENT:** blurred vision. **GI:** diarrhea, vomiting, decreased appetite. **Hematologic:** *neutropenia, thrombocytopenia,* anemia, *lymphopenia, pancytopenia.* **Hepatic:** transaminase elevation. **Metabolic:** *hypokalemia,* weight loss, hypoalbuminemia, *hypocalcemia,* hypophosphatemia, increased lipase level, increased amylase level. **Musculoskeletal:** arthralgia. **Respiratory:** pneumonia, URI, pneumonitis, lower respiratory tract infection, dyspnea. **Other:** infusion-related reaction, *sepsis,* herpesvirus infection, CMV infection.

INTERACTIONS

Drug-drug. *Strong CYP3A inducers (rifampin):* May decrease effectiveness of

P

polatuzumab vedotin. Monitor patient for therapeutic effectiveness.

Strong CYP3A inhibitors (ketoconazole): May increase toxicity of polatuzumab vedotin. Monitor patient for toxicity.

EFFECTS ON LAB TEST RESULTS
• May increase ALT, AST, lipase, amylase, and creatinine levels.
• May decrease potassium, albumin, calcium, and phosphorus levels.
• May decrease Hb level and neutrophil, platelet, and lymphocyte counts.

CONTRAINDICATIONS & CAUTIONS
• Peripheral neuropathy, including severe cases, may occur as early as the first cycle of treatment and is a cumulative effect. Exacerbation of preexisting peripheral neuropathy may also occur.
• Infusion-related reactions, including severe cases, may occur. Delayed infusion-related reactions have occurred as late as 24 hours after drug administration.
• Treatment can cause serious or severe myelosuppression, including neutropenia, thrombocytopenia, and anemia.
• Fatal or serious infections, including opportunistic infections such as sepsis, pneumonia (including *Pneumocystis jiroveci* and other fungal pneumonia), herpesvirus infection, and CMV infection, have occurred.
• PML has been reported after treatment.
• Drug may cause TLS. Use cautiously in patients with high tumor burden and rapidly proliferative tumor; these patients are at increased risk.
• Serious cases of hepatotoxicity consistent with hepatocellular injury have occurred. Use cautiously in patients with preexisting liver disease or elevated baseline liver enzyme levels and in those taking concomitant medications.
• Safety and effectiveness in children haven't been established.
Dialyzable drug: Unknown.

PREGNANCY-LACTATION-REPRODUCTION
• Drug may cause fetal harm. Advise patient of fetal risk.
• Test patients of childbearing potential for pregnancy before starting treatment.
• Patients of childbearing potential should use effective contraception during treatment and for at least 3 months after final dose.

• Male patients with partners of childbearing potential should use effective contraception during treatment and for at least 5 months after final dose.
• It isn't known if drug appears in human milk. Patient shouldn't breastfeed during treatment and for at least 2 months after final dose.
• Drug may impair male fertility; reversal of this effect is unknown.

NURSING CONSIDERATIONS
• Verify pregnancy status in patients of childbearing potential before starting drug.
• Monitor patients for infusion-related reactions during each infusion and for a minimum of 90 minutes after completion of a 90-minute infusion and 30 minutes after a 30-minute infusion.
• If an infusion-related reaction occurs, interrupt the infusion and institute appropriate medical management.
• Monitor CBC throughout treatment. Cytopenias may require a therapy interruption, dosage reduction, or drug discontinuation. Consider prophylactic granulocyte colony stimulating factor administration for neutropenia.
• Closely monitor patients during treatment for signs and symptoms of infection. Administer prophylaxis for *P. jiroveci* pneumonia and herpesvirus infection.
• Monitor patients for new or worsening neurologic, cognitive, or behavioral changes. Withhold drug and any concomitant chemotherapy if PML is suspected; permanently discontinue drug if the diagnosis is confirmed.
• Monitor patients for TLS and administer TLS prophylaxis for patients at increased risk for TLS.
• Monitor patients for new or worsening peripheral neuropathy (hypoesthesia, hyperesthesia, paresthesia, dysesthesia, neuropathic pain, burning sensation, weakness, gait disturbance). Interrupt therapy, reduce dosage, or discontinue drug as clinically indicated.
• Monitor liver enzyme and bilirubin levels throughout treatment.
• *Look alike–sound alike:* Don't confuse polatuzumab vedotin-piiq with other monoclonal antibodies.

PATIENT TEACHING

• Advise patient that drug can cause peripheral neuropathy and to report numbness or tingling of the hands or feet or muscle weakness to prescriber.

• Tell patient to report signs and symptoms of infusion reactions (fever, chills, rash, or breathing problems) within 24 hours of infusion.

• Counsel patient to immediately report signs or symptoms of bleeding.

• Instruct patient to contact prescriber for a fever (temperature of 100.4° F [38° C] or greater) or other evidence of infection (chills, cough, pain on urination).

• Inform patient that lab blood work will be needed periodically to monitor for adverse effects.

• Advise patient to seek immediate medical attention for signs and symptoms of PML (new-onset or changes in neurologic signs and symptoms, including confusion, dizziness, loss of balance, difficulty talking or walking, changes in vision).

• Direct patient to seek immediate medical attention for signs and symptoms of TLS (nausea, vomiting, diarrhea, lethargy).

• Tell patient to report signs and symptoms of liver injury (fatigue, anorexia, right upper abdominal discomfort, dark urine, jaundice).

• Warn patient of childbearing potential of the fetal risk and that pregnancy testing will be performed before therapy. Advise patient to report known or suspected pregnancy during therapy.

• Instruct patient of childbearing potential to use effective contraception during treatment and for at least 3 months after final dose.

• Teach male patient with partner of childbearing potential to use effective contraception during treatment and for 5 months after final dose.

• Counsel patient not to breastfeed during therapy and for at 2 months after final dose.

ponesimod
poe-NES-i-mod

Ponvory

Therapeutic class: MS drugs
Pharmacologic class: Sphingosine
1-phosphate receptor modulators

AVAILABLE FORMS
Tablets ⬤: 2 mg, 3 mg, 4 mg, 5 mg, 6 mg, 7 mg, 8 mg, 9 mg, 10 mg, 20 mg

INDICATIONS & DOSAGES
➤ **Relapsing forms of MS, including clinically isolated syndrome, relapsing-remitting disease, and active secondary progressive disease**
Adults: Initially, 1 tablet PO daily from starter pack for days 1 to 14: days 1 and 2, 2 mg; days 3 and 4, 3 mg; days 5 and 6, 4 mg; day 7, 5 mg; day 8, 6 mg; day 9, 7 mg; day 10, 8 mg; day 11, 9 mg; days 12 to 14, 10 mg; then begin maintenance dose, 20 mg PO daily starting on day 15.

ADMINISTRATION
PO
• Give without regard to food.

• Patient should swallow tablets whole.

• Give first dose in appropriate setting with resources to manage symptomatic bradycardia.

• If patient has missed fewer than four consecutive titration doses, resume treatment with first missed titration dose and continue titration schedule.

• If patient has missed fewer than four consecutive maintenance doses, resume treatment with maintenance dose.

• If patient has missed four or more consecutive daily doses during titration or maintenance, reinitiate with day 1 of titration regimen with a new starter pack and complete first-dose monitoring in patients for whom it's recommended.

• Store tablets at 68° to 77° F (20° to 25° C) in original package; protect from moisture.

ACTION
Decreases ability of lymphocytes to leave the lymph nodes, reducing number of lymphocytes in peripheral blood that migrate into the CNS.

Route	Onset	Peak	Duration
PO	Unknown	2–4 hr	Unknown

Half-life: 33 hours.

ADVERSE REACTIONS

CNS: depression, dizziness, fatigue, fever, insomnia, migraine, somnolence, vertigo, *seizures.* **CV:** AV conduction delay, *brady-cardia,* chest discomfort, HTN, peripheral edema. **EENT:** macular edema, rhinitis, sinusitis, dry mouth. **GI:** dyspepsia. **GU:** UTI. **Hematologic:** elevated C-reactive protein level, *lymphopenia.* **Hepatic:** increased LFT values. **Metabolic:** hyperlipidemia, *hyper-kalemia.* **Musculoskeletal:** back pain, extremity pain, joint swelling. **Respiratory:** cough, dyspnea, pneumonia, URI. **Other:** infection, herpes zoster.

INTERACTIONS

Drug-drug. *Alemtuzumab:* May prolong effects of alemtuzumab and have additive immunosuppressive effects. Don't initiate ponesimod therapy after alemtuzumab.

Immune-modulating, immunosuppressive, or antineoplastic therapies: May have additive immunosuppressive effects. Use together cautiously. When switching from drugs with prolonged immune effects, consider their half-life and mode of action.

Beta blockers (atenolol, carvedilol, labetalol, metoprolol): May have additive HR-lowering effects. Use cautiously together; beta blocker dose interruption may be necessary. May initiate beta blockers in patients receiving stable doses of ponesimod.

Beta interferon, glatiramer acetate: May have additive immunosuppressive effects. May start ponesimod immediately after discontinuation of these drugs.

🌓 *Alert:* Drugs that prolong QT interval (Class IA [procainamide, quinidine] and Class III [amiodarone, sotalol]) antiarrhythmics, diltiazem, verapamil, other drugs that may decrease HR (digoxin): May have additive effects on HR. Consult cardiologist before use together.

Drugs that slow HR or AV conduction: May have additive effects. Monitor patient closely and consult cardiologist as appropriate.

Strong CYP3A4 and UGT1A1 inducers (carbamazepine, phenytoin, rifampin): May decrease ponesimod level. Avoid use together.

Vaccines: May decrease effectiveness of vaccine during therapy and for 2 weeks after final dose of ponesimod. Live attenuated vaccines may increase risk of infection; administer at least 1 month before starting ponesimod. Avoid live vaccines during ponesimod therapy and for 2 weeks after final dose.

Drug-lifestyle. *Sun exposure:* May increase risk of skin cancer. Limit exposure to sunlight and UV light.

EFFECTS ON LAB TEST RESULTS

• May increase transaminase, bilirubin, C-reactive protein, cholesterol, and potassium levels.
• May decrease lymphocyte count.

CONTRAINDICATIONS & CAUTIONS

• Contraindicated in patients with history of MI, unstable angina, stroke, TIA, decompensated HF requiring hospitalization, or Class III or IV HF during last 6 months.
• Contraindicated in patients with Mobitz type II second- or third-degree AV block or sick sinus syndrome, or SA block, unless patient has a functioning pacemaker.
• Avoid use in patients with moderate or severe hepatic impairment (Child-Pugh class B or C).
• Use cautiously in patients with preexisting heart and cerebrovascular conditions, HTN, arrhythmias, prolonged QTc interval, risk of prolonged QTc interval, or concomitant drug therapy that slows HR or AV conduction or prolongs QTc interval after consulting cardiologist on monitoring strategy.
• Use cautiously in patients with sinus bradycardia (HR less than 55 beats/minute), in those with first- or second-degree (Mobitz type I) AV block, or in patients in stable condition with history of MI or HF with onset greater than 6 months before drug initiation. Consult cardiologist and perform first-dose monitoring in these patients.
• Use cautiously in patients with pulmonary fibrosis, asthma, and COPD. Dose-dependent reductions in respiratory function were seen in patients treated with drug.
• Use cautiously in patients with macular edema and in those at increased risk for macular edema (diabetes, uveitis).
• Avoid use in patients receiving concomitant phototherapy (UV-B radiation or PUVA-photochemotherapy).

Reactions in bold italics are *life-threatening*. Interactions may have a *rapid onset* or a **delayed onset**.

• Drug increases risk of life-threatening and fatal infections.

• Drug may cause severe exacerbation of MS, including disease rebound, after discontinuation.

• Safety and effectiveness in children haven't been established.

• Use cautiously in older adults.

Dialyzable drug: No.

⚠ *Overdose S&S:* Bradycardia, AV conduction block.

PREGNANCY-LACTATION-REPRODUCTION

• Based on animal studies, drug may cause fetal harm. Advise patients who are pregnant of the fetal risk.

• It isn't known if drug appears in human milk or how drug affects milk production or infants who are breastfed. Consider benefits and risk before use during breastfeeding.

• Patients of childbearing potential should use effective contraception during therapy and for 1 week after final dose.

NURSING CONSIDERATIONS

• Obtain baseline ECG for preexisting conduction abnormalities. If present, consult cardiologist.

• Administer first dose in a setting where resources to appropriately manage symptomatic bradycardia are available for patients at risk. After first dose, monitor patient for 4 hours for bradycardia with hourly HR and BP measurement. Obtain ECG before dose and after 4-hour observation period. If abnormalities occur, follow manufacturer's prescribing instructions to determine additional required monitoring.

• Review recent (within 6 months) CBC before starting drug. Delay therapy in patients with active infection until it resolves.

• Obtain transaminase and bilirubin levels (within 6 months) before starting therapy. If liver dysfunction is suspected during therapy, recheck transaminase and bilirubin levels. Discontinue drug if significant liver injury is confirmed.

• Obtain ophthalmic evaluation of the fundus, including macula at baseline, with a reported vision change, and periodically in patients at increased risk.

• Obtain antibody test for varicella zoster virus (VZV) in patient without confirmed history of varicella or without documentation of a full course of vaccination against VZV

before therapy. Give varicella vaccine in patient who is antibody-negative and delay start of ponesimod for 4 weeks.

• Monitor patient for active infection. Consider interrupting therapy for serious infection.

• Monitor patient for signs and symptoms of cryptococcal meningitis (headache, fever, neck pain, nausea, vomiting, sensitivity to light, confusion) and disseminated cryptococcal infections (fever, cough, hemoptysis, chest pain, night sweats, weight loss). If infection is diagnosed, suspend therapy and begin appropriate treatment.

🔵 *Alert:* Monitor patient for signs and symptoms or MRI findings suggestive of progressive multifocal leukoencephalopathy (progressive weakness on one side of the body or clumsiness of limbs, vision disturbances, changes in thinking, memory, and orientation leading to confusion and personality changes). If suspected, suspend therapy; if confirmed, discontinue drug.

🔵 *Alert:* Monitor patient for signs and symptoms of PRES (cognitive deficits, behavioral changes, cortical visual disturbances, other neurologic cortical signs and symptoms; increased ICP; accelerated neurologic deterioration). Promptly perform a physical and neurologic exam and consider MRI. Delay in diagnosis and treatment may lead to permanent neurologic deficit. If PRES is suspected, discontinue drug.

• Obtain spirometric evaluation of respiratory function in patient with pulmonary fibrosis, asthma, and COPD during therapy as clinically indicated.

• Monitor BP periodically during therapy. Treat elevations appropriately.

• Obtain periodic skin exams for malignancies.

• Monitor patient for infection during therapy and for 2 weeks after stopping drug. Give other immunosuppressants cautiously during this time.

• Monitor patient for exacerbation of MS, including disease rebound after drug is stopped. Initiate appropriate treatment as indicated.

PATIENT TEACHING

• Teach patient about safe drug administration, reporting a missed dose, and not to discontinue drug without first discussing with prescriber.

• Tell patient about increased risk of infection during therapy and for 2 weeks after stopping drug. Advise patient to report signs and symptoms of infection (fever, fatigue, body aches, chills, nausea, vomiting, headache with neck stiffness, light sensitivity, confusion).

• Advise patient to avoid vaccines 1 month before starting drug, during therapy, and for 2 weeks after stopping drug.

• Inform patient that use of other drugs to suppress the immune system may increase risk of infection.

• Counsel patient that drug initiation may cause transient bradycardia. Inform patient with certain cardiac conditions that a cardiology consult is necessary with monitoring after first dose of drug and after dose interruption or drug discontinuation.

• Instruct patient to report signs and symptoms of bradycardia (dizziness, lightheadedness, palpitations, shortness of breath, confusion, chest pain, tiredness).

• Tell patient to report new-onset or worsening breathing difficulties.

• Instruct patient to report unexplained nausea, vomiting, abdominal pain, fatigue, anorexia, jaundice, or dark urine.

• Inform patient that drug may increase risk of skin cancer. Tell patient to limit exposure to sunlight and UV light by wearing protective clothing and using sunscreen with high protection factor, and to report suspicious skin lesions.

• Advise patient of childbearing potential to use effective contraception during therapy and for 1 week after final dose.

• Tell patient to report blurriness, shadows or blind spot in the center of vision, light sensitivity, or unusually colored vision.

• Instruct patient to immediately report signs and symptoms of PRES (sudden onset of severe headache, altered mental status, visual disturbances, seizure). Emphasize that delayed treatment could lead to permanent neurologic sequelae.

• Advise patient to report worsening MS symptoms after stopping drug.

posaconazole ☒
poe-sa-KON-a-zole

Noxafil, Posanol ✦

Therapeutic class: Antifungals
Pharmacologic class: Triazole antifungals

AVAILABLE FORMS
Injection: 300 mg (18 mg/mL) single-dose vial
Oral suspension: 40 mg/mL
Powder for oral suspension (delayed-release): 300 mg
Tablets (delayed-release) ⓄⓉⒸ*:* 100 mg

INDICATIONS & DOSAGES
➤ **Prevention of invasive *Aspergillus* and *Candida* infections in patients who are immunocompromised and at high risk until recovered from neutropenia or immunosuppression**
Adults: 200 mg (5 mL) oral suspension PO t.i.d. Or, 300 mg delayed-release tablet PO with food b.i.d. on first day, then 300 mg once daily. Or, 300 mg IV b.i.d. on first day, then 300 mg once daily.
Children ages 2 to younger than 18 weighing more than 40 kg: 6 mg/kg up to maximum of 300 mg IV infusion b.i.d. on first day, then 6 mg/kg to maximum of 300 mg once daily. Or, 300 mg delayed-release tablet PO b.i.d. on first day, then 300 mg PO once daily.
Children ages 2 to younger than 18 weighing 40 kg or less: 6 mg/kg up to maximum of 300 mg IV infusion b.i.d. on first day, then 6 mg/kg to maximum of 300 mg once daily.
➤ **Oropharyngeal candidiasis**
Adults and children age 13 and older: 100 mg (2.5 mL) PO oral suspension b.i.d. on first day, then 100 mg (2.5 mL) once daily for 13 days.
➤ **Oropharyngeal candidiasis resistant to itraconazole or fluconazole treatment**
Adults and children age 13 and older: 400 mg (10 mL) PO oral suspension b.i.d.; duration of treatment is based on severity of underlying disease and patient response.
➤ **Treatment of invasive aspergillosis**
Adults and children ages 13 to 17: 300 mg delayed-release tablet PO or IV b.i.d. on first day, then 300 mg PO or IV once daily for 6 to 12 weeks. May switch between IV and

---

Reactions in bold italics are *life-threatening*. Interactions may have a *rapid onset* or a **delayed onset**.

delayed-release tablets; no loading dose is required when switching between formulations.

ADMINISTRATION
PO
• Delayed-release tablets and oral suspension aren't to be used interchangeably because of differences in the dosing of each formulation.
PO (suspension)
• Give with a full meal, liquid nutritional supplement, or an acidic carbonated beverage (e.g., ginger ale).
• Shake well before giving it.
• Measure doses using calibrated spoon provided with the drug, which has two markings, one for 2.5 mL and one for 5 mL. After patient takes dose, fill spoon with water and have patient drink it to ensure a full dose.
• Store at room temperature.
PO (delayed-release tablets)
• Administer with or without food.
• Patient should swallow tablets whole; don't divide, crush, or allow patient to chew tablets.
• Delayed-release oral formulation is preferred for prophylaxis due to higher plasma drug exposures.
IV
▼ Bring refrigerated vial to room temperature.
▼ To prepare, transfer one vial of drug to IV bag or bottle of half-NSS, NSS, D_5W, D_5W half-NSS, D_5W NSS, or D_5W with 20 mEq potassium chloride to achieve a final concentration that's between 1 and 2 mg/mL. Solution may be colorless to yellow.
▼ Use mixture immediately after preparation, or it can be stored up to 24 hours refrigerated (36° to 46° F [2° to 8° C]).
⏿ *Alert:* When multiple dosing is required, administer via central venous catheter (CVC). Infuse over 90 minutes. Don't give by IV push or bolus.
▼ If a CVC isn't available, administer only once through peripheral venous catheter over 30 minutes in advance of CVC insertion or to bridge during CVC replacement or use for another IV treatment; multiple peripheral infusions given through the same vein may result in infusion-site reactions.
▼ An in-line filter (0.22-micron polyethersulfone or polyvinylidene difluoride) must be used during infusion.
▼ **Incompatibilities:** Diluents, including lactated Ringer solution, 5% dextrose with lactated Ringer solution, 4.2% sodium bicarbonate. Consult a drug incompatibility reference for more information.

ACTION
Blocks the synthesis of ergosterol, a vital component of the fungal cell membrane.

Route	Onset	Peak	Duration
PO (suspension)	Unknown	3–5 hr	Unknown
PO (tablets)	Unknown	4–5 hr	Unknown
IV	Unknown	Unknown	Unknown

Half-life: Suspension, 20 to 66 hours; tablets, 26 to 31 hours; injection, 27 hours.

ADVERSE REACTIONS
CNS: dizziness, fatigue, fever, headache, insomnia, weakness, paresthesia. **CV:** edema, HTN, hypotension, tachycardia, thrombophlebitis at IV site, *PE.* **EENT:** blurred vision, epistaxis, pharyngitis, oral stomatitis, oral candidiasis. **GI:** abdominal pain, constipation, diarrhea, dyspepsia, mucositis, nausea, vomiting, *pancreatitis.* **GU:** *vaginal hemorrhage, acute renal failure.* **Hematologic:** anemia, petechiae, *febrile neutropenia, neutropenia, thrombocytopenia, hemolytic-uremic syndrome.* **Hepatic:** bilirubinemia, *hepatic insufficiency,* increased liver enzyme levels, jaundice, *hepatitis.* **Metabolic:** anorexia, hyperglycemia, *hypokalemia, hypomagnesemia, hypocalcemia, adrenocortical insufficiency,* weight loss, dehydration. **Musculoskeletal:** arthralgia, back pain, musculoskeletal pain. **Respiratory:** cough, dyspnea, URI, pneumonia. **Skin:** petechiae, pruritus, rash, diaphoresis. **Other:** bacteremia, CMV infection, herpes simplex, rigors, chills, hypersensitivity reaction.

INTERACTIONS
Drug-drug. *Atazanavir, ritonavir:* May increase plasma concentrations of these drugs. Frequently monitor for adverse effects and toxicity during coadministration.
Calcium channel blockers, phenytoin: May increase levels of these drugs. Reduce dosages, increase monitoring of levels, and observe patient for adverse effects.
Cimetidine, phenytoin: May decrease level and effectiveness of posaconazole. Avoid using together.
Cyclosporine: May increase cyclosporine level. Reduce cyclosporine dosage to about three-fourths original dose at start of posaconazole therapy and monitor

P

cyclosporine level. Adjust cyclosporine dosage accordingly at end of posaconazole therapy.

CYP3A4 substrates (astemizole, cisapride, halofantrine, pimozide, quinidine, terfenadine): May lead to QT-interval prolongation and torsades de pointes. Use together is contraindicated.

Digoxin: May increase digoxin level. Monitor digoxin level.

Efavirenz: May significantly decrease posaconazole plasma concentration. Avoid use together unless benefit outweighs risks.

Ergot alkaloids (dihydroergotamine, ergotamine): May increase ergot level. Use together is contraindicated.

Fosamprenavir: May decrease posaconazole level. Monitor patient closely for breakthrough fungal infection.

HMG-CoA reductase inhibitors metabolized through CYP3A4: May increase levels of these drugs. Use with posaconazole is contraindicated.

Metoclopramide: May decrease posaconazole level when used with posaconazole suspension. (No such effect when used with posaconazole tablets.) Monitor patient for breakthrough fungal infections.

Midazolam: May significantly increase midazolam concentration and potentiate or prolong sedative or hypnotic effects. Reversal agents should be readily available.

PPIs: May decrease posaconazole level. Consider therapy modification.

QTc interval–prolonging drugs: May enhance prolongation of QTc interval. When used with moderate QTc interval–prolonging drugs, monitor therapy. Avoid use with high-risk QTc interval–prolonging drugs; if use together is unavoidable, monitor QTc interval and cardiac rhythm closely.

Rifabutin: May decrease level and effectiveness of posaconazole while increasing rifabutin level and risk of toxicity. Avoid using together. If unavoidable, monitor patient for uveitis, leukopenia, and other adverse effects.

Sirolimus: May increase sirolimus level, resulting in sirolimus toxicity. Use together is contraindicated.

Tacrolimus: May increase tacrolimus level. Reduce tacrolimus dosage to about one-third original dose when starting posaconazole and monitor tacrolimus trough level. Adjust tacrolimus dosage accordingly at end of posaconazole therapy.

Venetoclax: May increase venetoclax level and risk of toxicity. Coadministration during initiation and ramp-up phase is contraindicated in patients with chronic lymphocytic leukemia or small lymphocytic lymphoma due to risk of TLS.

Vinca alkaloids (vincristine, vinblastine): May increase plasma concentrations of vinca alkaloids, leading to neurotoxicity and other serious adverse reactions. Don't use together unless there are no alternative antifungal treatment options.

Drug-food. *Any food, liquid nutritional supplements:* May greatly enhance absorption of drug. Always give drug with liquid supplement or food.

EFFECTS ON LAB TEST RESULTS
• May increase AST, ALT, bilirubin, creatinine, ALP, and glucose levels.
• May decrease potassium, magnesium, and calcium levels.
• May decrease WBC, RBC, and platelet counts.

CONTRAINDICATIONS & CAUTIONS
• Contraindicated in patients hypersensitive to drug or its components.
▓ Powder for delayed-release oral suspension is contraindicated in patients with known or suspected hereditary fructose intolerance (HFI).
• Use cautiously in patients hypersensitive to other azole antifungals, patients with potentially proarrhythmic conditions, and patients with hepatic or renal insufficiency.
• May cause electrolyte disturbances.
⊙ *Alert:* Drug may prolong QT interval and increase risk of torsades de pointes.
Dialyzable drug: No.

PREGNANCY-LACTATION-REPRODUCTION
• There are no adequate studies during pregnancy. Drug may cause fetal harm. Use only if potential benefit outweighs fetal risk.
• It isn't known if drug appears in human milk. Patient should discontinue breastfeeding or discontinue drug.

NURSING CONSIDERATIONS
• Use IV route only when oral administration isn't possible.
• Avoid IV route in patients with moderate or severe renal impairment (eGFR less than 50 mL/minute), unless benefit vs. risk to

patient justifies its use. Closely monitor serum creatinine level; if increases occur, consider changing to oral therapy.

⌧ Assess for history of HFI (nausea, vomiting, abdominal pain with ingestion of sorbitol, fructose, or sucrose). Monitor children receiving oral suspension closely; HFI may have not yet been diagnosed.

• Correct electrolyte imbalances, especially potassium, magnesium, and calcium imbalances, before therapy.

• Monitor patient for signs and symptoms of electrolyte imbalance, including a slow, weak, or irregular pulse; ECG change; nausea; neuromuscular irritability; and tetany.

• Obtain baseline LFTs, including bilirubin level, before therapy and periodically during treatment. Notify prescriber if patient develops signs or symptoms of hepatic dysfunction.

• Monitor patient weighing more than 120 kg closely for breakthrough fungal infections because of lower plasma drug exposure.

• Monitor patient who has severe vomiting or diarrhea for breakthrough fungal infection.

• *Look alike–sound alike:* Don't confuse posaconazole with fluconazole, ketoconazole, itraconazole, or voriconazole. Don't confuse Noxafil with minoxidil.

PATIENT TEACHING

• Instruct patient in safe drug administration. Tell patient or caregiver to measure doses using spoon provided with drug. Household spoons vary in size and may yield an incorrect dose.

• Instruct patient who can't take a liquid supplement or eat a full meal to notify prescriber. A different anti-infective may be needed, or monitoring may need to be increased.

• Tell patient to report irregular heartbeat, fainting, or severe diarrhea or vomiting.

• Explain the signs and symptoms of liver dysfunction, including abdominal pain, yellowing skin or eyes, pale stools, and dark urine.

• Urge patient to contact the prescriber or pharmacist before taking other prescription or OTC drugs, herbal supplements, or dietary supplements.

• Tell patient of childbearing potential that drug may cause fetal harm.

⌧ Inform patient and caregivers that Noxafil PowderMix for delayed-release oral suspension contains sorbitol and can be life-threatening in patients with HFI.

potassium acetate

Therapeutic class: Potassium supplements
Pharmacologic class: Potassium salts

AVAILABLE FORMS

Injection: 2 mEq/mL in 20-mL, 50-mL, and 100-mL vials

INDICATIONS & DOSAGES

➤ **To correct or prevent hypokalemia**
Adults: Individualize dosage and give by IV infusion; normal daily requirements are 40 to 80 mEq/24 hours.
Children: Individualize dosage and give by IV infusion; normal daily requirements are 2 to 3 mEq/kg/24 hours. For newborns, normal daily requirement is 2 to 6 mEq/kg/24 hours.

ADMINISTRATION

IV

▼ Use only when oral replacement isn't feasible.

▼ Don't give undiluted potassium. Maximum infusion rate is 1 mEq/kg/hour.

▼ Don't add potassium to a hanging bag. Mix well to avoid layering.

▼ To prevent pain, use largest peripheral vein and a well-placed small-bore needle.

▼ Give only by infusion, never IV push or IM. Watch for pain and redness at infusion site.

▼ Give slowly as diluted solution; rapid infusion may cause fatal hyperkalemia.

▼ May give by intraosseous infusion if necessary.

▼ **Incompatibilities:** None listed by manufacturer. Consult a drug incompatibility reference for more information.

ACTION

Replaces potassium and maintains potassium level.

Route	Onset	Peak	Duration
IV	Immediate	Immediate	Unknown

Half-life: Unknown.

ADVERSE REACTIONS

CNS: paresthesia of limbs, listlessness, mental confusion, weakness or heaviness of legs, flaccid paralysis. **CV:** *arrhythmias, cardiac arrest, heart block,* ECG changes,

P

hypotension. **Metabolic:** *hyperkalemia.* **Skin:** redness at infusion site.

INTERACTIONS

Drug-drug. *ACE inhibitors, aldosterone blockers, ARBs, potassium-sparing diuretics:* May increase risk of hyperkalemia. Use together with caution.

Eplerenone: May increase hyperkalemia risk. Use together is contraindicated when eplerenone is used to treat HTN.

Heparin: May enhance hyperkalemic effects of potassium salts. Monitor therapy.

Drug-food. *Potassium-containing salt substitutes:* May increase risk of hyperkalemia. Use together cautiously.

EFFECTS ON LAB TEST RESULTS

• May increase potassium and bicarbonate levels.

CONTRAINDICATIONS & CAUTIONS

• Contraindicated in patients with severe renal impairment with oliguria, anuria, or azotemia.

• Contraindicated in patients with adrenal insufficiency and in those with diseases that cause high potassium levels.

• Use cautiously in patients with cardiac disease, severe hepatic insufficiency, or renal impairment.

🜂 *Alert:* Product contains aluminum and may reach toxic levels with prolonged parenteral administration in patients with renal impairment. Premature neonates are particularly at risk.

Dialyzable drug: Yes

⚠ *Overdose S&S:* Paresthesia, flaccid paralysis, listlessness, confusion, weakness and heaviness of legs, hypotension, cardiac arrhythmias, heart block, ECG changes, cardiac arrest.

PREGNANCY-LACTATION-REPRODUCTION

• Safe use during pregnancy hasn't been established. Use only if benefit justifies fetal risk.

• It isn't known if drug appears in human milk. Use cautiously during breastfeeding.

NURSING CONSIDERATIONS

• During therapy, monitor ECG, renal function, fluid intake and output, and potassium, creatinine, and BUN levels. Never give potassium postoperatively until urine flow is established.

• Monitor patient for adverse reactions due to hyperkalemia, including muscle weakness or paralysis, and cardiac conduction abnormalities (heart block, ventricular arrhythmias, asystole).

• Monitor IV site carefully for extravasation.

🜂 *Alert:* Consider a separate storage area for concentrated IV potassium. Fatal outcomes are possible if concentrated potassium is administered by IV push.

• Carefully give solutions containing acetate ions to patients with metabolic or respiratory alkalosis and to those with conditions such as hepatic impairment in which the acetate levels may be increased or the utilization of the ion may be impaired.

• *Look alike–sound alike:* Potassium preparations aren't interchangeable; verify preparation before use.

PATIENT TEACHING

• Explain use and administration to patient and family.

• Tell patient to report adverse effects, especially pain at insertion site.

• Advise patient to immediately report signs and symptoms of hyperkalemia (arrhythmia, bradycardia, weakness).

SAFETY ALERT!

potassium chloride
Klor-Con🜂, Klor-Con 10, Klor-Con M10, Klor-Con M15, Klor-Con M20, Klor-Con Sprinkle, K-Tab

Therapeutic class: Potassium supplements
Pharmacologic class: Potassium salts

AVAILABLE FORMS

Capsules (extended-release) ⓞⓡⓖ: 8 mEq, 10 mEq
Injection concentrate: 2 mEq/mL
Injection for IV infusion: 0.1 mEq/mL, 0.2 mEq/mL, 0.4 mEq/mL; 20 mEq/L, 30 mEq/L, 40 mEq/L in various solutions
Oral liquid: 20 mEq/15 mL, 40 mEq/15 mL
Powder for oral administration: 20 mEq/packet
Tablets (extended-release) ⓞⓡⓖ: 8 mEq, 10 mEq, 15 mEq, 20 mEq

---

Reactions in bold italics are *life-threatening*. Interactions may have a *rapid onset* or a ***delayed onset***.

INDICATIONS & DOSAGES
➤ To prevent hypokalemia
Adults: Initially, 20 mEq of potassium supplement PO daily. Adjust dosage, as needed, based on potassium levels. Patient should take no more than 20 mEq at a single dose; divide dose if patient requires more than 20 mEq/day.
➤ Hypokalemia
Adults: 40 to 100 mEq PO in two to five divided doses daily. Patient should take no more than 20 mEq at a single dose. Maximum dose of diluted IV potassium chloride is 40 mEq/L at 10 mEq/hour. Don't exceed 200 mEq daily. Further doses are based on potassium levels and blood pH. Give IV potassium replacement only with monitoring of ECG and potassium level.
➤ Severe hypokalemia
Adults: Dilute potassium chloride in a suitable IV solution to achieve 20 to 40 mEq/L, and give at no more than 40 mEq/hour.

Further doses are based on potassium level. Don't exceed 400 mEq IV daily. Give IV potassium replacement only with monitoring of ECG and potassium level.

ADMINISTRATION
PO
• Make sure powders are completely dissolved before giving.
• Give with meals and a full glass of water or other liquid to minimize GI irritation.
• Enteric-coated tablets are not recommended because of increased risk of GI bleeding and small-bowel ulcerations.
• Tablets in wax matrix may lodge in the esophagus and cause ulceration in patients with esophageal compression from an enlarged left atrium. Use sugar-free liquid form in these patients and in those with esophageal stasis or obstruction. Have patient sip slowly to minimize GI irritation.
• Don't crush extended-release forms.
• For patients with difficulty swallowing whole tablets, may break some extended-release tablets (Klor-Con M) in half. Or, may place a whole tablet in 120 mL water and allow to disintegrate over about 2 minutes; stir for about 30 seconds to create a suspension. Have patient swallow suspension immediately. Add 30 mL water to glass, swirl, and have patient drink immediately; then repeat to ensure entire dose is consumed.

• For extended-release capsules, may open capsules and sprinkle contents on a spoonful of applesauce or pudding. Have patient swallow immediately without chewing; follow with a full glass of water or juice. Don't add to hot foods or save mixture for later.
• Dissolve powder for oral solution in at least 120 mL cold water or other beverage. Increase dilution if GI irritation occurs.
IV
▼ Use only when oral replacement isn't feasible or when hypokalemia is life-threatening.
▼ Give by infusion only, never IV push or IM. Give slowly as dilute solution; rapid infusion may cause fatal hyperkalemia.
▼ Administer high concentrations (200 to 400 mEq/L) exclusively via a central route and infusion pump at maximum rate of 40 mEq/hour.
▼ If burning occurs during infusion, decrease rate.
▼ Drug is a vesicant/irritant (at concentrations greater than 0.1 mEq/mL); ensure proper needle or catheter placement before and during infusion. Avoid extravasation.
▼ **Incompatibilities:** None listed by manufacturer. Consult a drug incompatibility reference for more information.

ACTION
Replaces potassium and maintains potassium level.

Route	Onset	Peak	Duration
PO	Unknown	Unknown	Unknown
IV	Immediate	Immediate	Unknown

Half-life: Unknown.

ADVERSE REACTIONS
CNS: paresthesia of limbs, listlessness, confusion, weakness or heaviness of limbs, flaccid paralysis. **CV:** *arrhythmias, heart block, cardiac arrest,* ECG changes, hypotension, phlebitis or venous thrombosis at injection site. **GI:** nausea, vomiting, abdominal pain, diarrhea, flatulence. **Metabolic:** hypovolemia, *hyperkalemia.* **Respiratory:** *respiratory paralysis.* **Skin:** injection-site reactions, extravasation, febrile response.

INTERACTIONS
Drug-drug. *ACE inhibitors, ARBs, digoxin, heparins, potassium-sparing diuretics:* May

P

cause hyperkalemia. Use together with extreme caution. Monitor potassium level.
Eplerenone: May increase hyperkalemia risk. Use together is contraindicated when eplerenone is used to treat HTN.
NSAIDs: May cause potassium retention. Closely monitor potassium level in patients taking NSAIDs.

EFFECTS ON LAB TEST RESULTS
• May increase potassium and chloride levels.

CONTRAINDICATIONS & CAUTIONS
• Contraindicated in patients hypersensitive to potassium chloride or components of the formulation, in patients with renal failure, and in those with conditions in which potassium retention is present.
• Use cautiously in patients with cardiac disease, renal impairment, and acid-base disorders.
Dialyzable drug: Yes.
⚠ *Overdose S&S:* ECG changes, weakness, flaccidity, respiratory paralysis, cardiac arrhythmias, death.

PREGNANCY-LACTATION-REPRODUCTION
• It isn't known if drug causes fetal harm. Use only if clearly needed.
• It isn't known if drug appears in human milk. Use cautiously during breastfeeding.

NURSING CONSIDERATIONS
• Patients at increased risk for GI lesions when taking oral potassium include those with scleroderma, diabetes, mitral valve replacement, cardiomegaly, or esophageal strictures, and older adults or patients who are immobile.
• Drug is commonly used orally with potassium-wasting diuretics to maintain potassium levels.
• Monitor continuous ECG and electrolyte levels during therapy.
• Monitor renal function. After surgery, don't give drug until urine flow is established.
• Monitor patient for hyperkalemia (palpitations, shortness of breath, chest pain, nausea, vomiting).
• Patient may be sensitive to tartrazine in some of these products.
🛑 *Alert:* Consider a separate storage area for concentrated IV potassium. Fatal outcomes are possible if concentrated potassium is administered by IV push.

• *Look alike–sound alike:* Potassium preparations aren't interchangeable; verify preparation before use and don't switch products. Don't confuse KCl with HCl or KlorCon with Klaron.

PATIENT TEACHING
• Teach patient safe drug administration.
• Inform patient of signs and symptoms of hyperkalemia, and tell patient to notify prescriber if they occur.
• Tell patient to report discomfort at IV insertion site.
• Warn patient not to use salt substitutes concurrently, except with prescriber's permission.
• Tell patient not to be concerned if wax matrix appears in stool because the drug has already been absorbed.

---

pramipexole dihydrochloride
pram-ah-PEX-ole

Mirapex ER

Therapeutic class: Antiparkinsonian drugs
Pharmacologic class: Nonergot dopamine agonists

AVAILABLE FORMS
Tablets: 0.125 mg, 0.25 mg, 0.5 mg, 0.75 mg, 1 mg, 1.5 mg
Tablets (extended-release) ⚫: 0.375 mg, 0.75 mg, 1.5 mg, 2.25 mg, 3 mg, 3.75 mg, 4.5 mg

INDICATIONS & DOSAGES
➤ **Parkinson disease**
Adults: Initially, 0.375 mg PO daily in three divided doses. Adjust doses slowly (not more often than every 5 to 7 days) over several weeks until desired therapeutic effect is achieved. Maintenance dosage is 1.5 to 4.5 mg daily in three divided doses. Or, 0.375 mg (extended-release form) PO once daily. May titrate dosage gradually (not more often than every 5 days), first to 0.75 mg PO daily, then by 0.75-mg increments to maximum recommended dosage of 4.5 mg/day.
Adjust-a-dose: For patients with CrCl over 50 mL/minute, first dosage of immediate-release tablets is 0.125 mg PO t.i.d., up to 1.5 mg t.i.d. For those with CrCl of 30 to 50 mL/minute, first dosage is 0.125 mg PO b.i.d., up to 0.75 mg t.i.d. For those with CrCl

---

of 15 mL/minute to less than 30 mL/minute, first dosage is 0.125 mg PO daily, up to 1.5 mg daily. If using extended-release tablets, in patients with CrCl of 30 to 50 mL/minute, initially give dose every other day. Use caution and assess response and tolerability before increasing to daily dosing after 1 week and before titration. Titrate dosage in 0.375-mg increments up to 2.25 mg/day, no more frequently than at weekly intervals. Don't use extended-release tablets in patients with CrCl of less than 30 mL/minute or in patients on hemodialysis.

➤ **Moderate to severe primary restless legs syndrome (immediate-release only)**
Adults: 0.125 mg PO daily. May increase after 4 to 7 days to 0.25 mg PO daily, as needed. May increase again after 4 to 7 days to 0.5 mg PO daily, if needed.
Adjust-a-dose: For patients with CrCl of 20 to 60 mL/minute, increase the duration between titration steps to 14 days.

ADMINISTRATION
PO
• Give drug with or without food; giving with food may reduce nausea.
• Don't allow patient to chew, crush, or divide extended-release tablets; patient should swallow whole.
• If a significant interruption in therapy occurs, retitration of therapy may be warranted.
• For restless legs syndrome, give 2 to 3 hours before bedtime.
• Give a missed dose as soon as possible, but no later than 12 hours after regularly scheduled time. After 12 hours, skip missed dose and give next dose on the following day at regularly scheduled time.

ACTION
Exact action is unknown; thought to stimulate dopamine receptors.

Route	Onset	Peak	Duration
PO	Rapid	2 hr	Unknown
PO (extended-release)	Unknown	6 hr	Unknown

Half-life: About 8 to 12 hours.

ADVERSE REACTIONS
CNS: asthenia, confusion, dizziness, dream abnormalities, new or worsening dyskinesia, extrapyramidal syndrome, hallucinations, insomnia, somnolence, amnesia, akathisia, drowsiness, delusions, dystonia, gait abnormalities, hypoesthesia, hypertonia, tremor, myoclonus, paranoid reaction, malaise, sleep disorders, thought abnormalities, depression, vertigo, fever, equilibrium disturbance, impulse control disorders. **CV:** orthostatic hypotension, chest pain, edema. **EENT:** accommodation abnormalities, diplopia, vision abnormalities, rhinitis, nasal congestion, excessive salivation, dry mouth. **GI:** constipation, diarrhea, nausea, anorexia, increased appetite, dysphagia, vomiting, abdominal distress. **GU:** erectile dysfunction, decreased libido, urinary frequency, UTI, urinary incontinence. **Metabolic:** weight loss. **Musculoskeletal:** arthritis, bursitis, myasthenia, twitching, limb pain, muscle spasm. **Respiratory:** dyspnea, cough, pneumonia. **Skin:** skin disorders. **Other:** accidental injury, flulike symptoms.

INTERACTIONS
Drug-drug. *Antipsychotics (typical [fluphenazine, haloperidol, thioridazine]):* May diminish therapeutic effects of pramipexole. Avoid use together if possible; if use together is unavoidable, monitor therapy carefully.
Cimetidine, diltiazem, quinidine, quinine, triamterene, verapamil: May decrease pramipexole clearance. Adjust dosage as needed.
Dopamine antagonists (metoclopramide, prochlorperazine, promethazine): May reduce pramipexole effectiveness. Monitor patient closely.
Drug-lifestyle. *Alcohol use:* May increase sedative effects. Avoid use together.

EFFECTS ON LAB TEST RESULTS
• May increase CK level.

CONTRAINDICATIONS & CAUTIONS
• Contraindicated in patients hypersensitive to drug or its components.
• Use cautiously in patients with renal impairment or hypotension and in older adults.
• Use cautiously in patients with a known major psychotic disorder due to risk of exacerbating psychosis.
• Drug may cause or exacerbate dyskinesia.
• Drug may cause postural deformities, including antecollis (forward head and neck flexion), bent spine syndrome (forward trunk flexion), and Pisa syndrome (lateral trunk

P

flexion). Dosage reduction or drug discontinuation may be necessary.
Dialyzable drug: Unknown.

PREGNANCY-LACTATION-REPRODUCTION
• There are no studies during pregnancy. Use only if benefit clearly justifies fetal risk.
• It isn't known if drug appears in human milk. Drug inhibits prolactin secretion and may inhibit lactation. Patient should discontinue breastfeeding or discontinue drug.

NURSING CONSIDERATIONS
• Drug should be tapered off at a rate of 0.75 mg/day until daily dose has been reduced to 0.75 mg. Thereafter, dose may be reduced by 0.375 mg/day.
• Drug may cause orthostatic hypotension, especially during dosage increases. Monitor patient closely.
• Drug may cause intense impulse control and compulsive behaviors. Monitor patient for problems with impulse control (such as gambling urges, intense sexual urges, binge eating).
• Adjust dosage gradually to achieve maximal therapeutic effect, balanced against the main adverse effects of dyskinesia, hallucinations, somnolence, and dry mouth.
• Assess patients for preexisting sleep disorder and monitor for daytime sleepiness and for episodes of falling asleep without warning. Drug may need to be discontinued.
• Monitor patients for hallucinations (visual, auditory, or mixed) and new or worsening psychotic-like behaviors (paranoia, delusions, agitation, disorientation, aggressive behavior, agitation, delirium). Drug may need to be discontinued.
• Monitor patients for rhabdomyolysis and postural deformity.
• *Look alike–sound alike:* Don't confuse Mirapex with Hiprex, Mifeprex, or MiraLax.

PATIENT TEACHING
• Teach patient safe drug administration.
• Instruct patient not to rise rapidly after sitting or lying down because of risk of dizziness.
• Tell patient about potential for daytime sleepiness and falling asleep without warning and to report episodes to prescriber. Caution patient to avoid hazardous activities until CNS response to drug is known.

• Advise patient to use caution before taking drug with other CNS depressants.
• Tell patient (especially older adults) to immediately report hallucinations and changes in impulse control behaviors.
• Instruct patient to take drug with food if nausea develops.
• Caution patient to report pregnancy or plans to become pregnant or to breastfeed.
• Inform patient that it may take 4 weeks for effects of drug to be noticed because of slow adjustment schedule.
• Instruct patient that drug should be tapered gradually and not stopped abruptly.
• Advise patient to report problems with muscle control (dyskinesias).
• Inform patient that residue resembling a swollen tablet or pieces of original tablet may appear in stool.
• Alert patient and caregivers that patient may experience intense urges to spend money or to gamble, increased sexual urges, binge eating, or other intense urges and that patient may not be able to control these urges.

pramlintide acetate
PRAM-lin-tide

SymlinPen 60, SymlinPen 120

Therapeutic class: Antidiabetics
Pharmacologic class: Human amylin analogues

AVAILABLE FORMS
Injection: 1000 mcg/mL in 1.5-mL and 2.7-mL multidose pen injectors

INDICATIONS & DOSAGES
➤ **Adjunct to insulin in patients with type 1 diabetes**
Adults: Initially, 15 mcg subcut before major meals. Reduce mealtime insulin doses, including premixed insulins, by 50%. Increase pramlintide dose by 15-mcg increments every 3 days if no nausea occurs, to a maintenance dose of 30 to 60 mcg. Adjust insulin dose as needed.
Adjust-a-dose: If significant nausea at 45 or 60 mcg persists, decrease to 30 mcg. If nausea persists at 30 mcg, consider stopping.
➤ **Adjunct to insulin in patients with type 2 diabetes**

Adults: Initially, 60 mcg subcut immediately before major meals. Reduce mealtime insulin doses, including premixed insulins, by 50%. Increase pramlintide dose to 120 mcg if no significant nausea occurs for at least 3 days. Adjust insulin dose as needed.

Adjust-a-dose: If significant nausea persists at 120 mcg, decrease to 60 mcg.

ADMINISTRATION
Subcutaneous
• Allow medication to reach room temperature before injecting.
• Give each dose subcut into abdomen or thigh. Rotate injection sites.
• Administer immediately before each major meal consisting of 250 kcal or more or containing 30 g or more of carbohydrates.
• Always administer pramlintide and insulin as separate injections. The injection site for pramlintide should be distinct from the site for concomitant insulin injection.
• Don't transfer drug to syringe for administration. Don't mix with any type of insulin.
⊙ *Alert:* Multidose pens are for single-patient use only. Pens should never be shared, even if the needle is changed. Clearly label with patient identifying information where it won't obstruct the dosing window, warning, or other product information.
• For a missed dose, wait until the next scheduled dose time and give usual amount.
• Use 1.5-mL injector for 15-, 30-, 45-, or 60-mcg doses. Use 2.7-mL injector for 60- or 120-mcg doses.
• After initial use, may keep refrigerated or at room temperature (86° F [30° C]).
• Discard after 30 days; protect from light.

ACTION
Slows rate at which food leaves the stomach, reducing the initial postprandial increase in glucose level. Decreases hyperglycemia by reducing postprandial glucagon level and reduces total caloric intake by reducing appetite.

Route	Onset	Peak	Duration
Subcut	Unknown	19–21 min	3 hr

Half-life: Parent drug and metabolite, about 48 minutes each.

ADVERSE REACTIONS
CNS: dizziness, fatigue, headache. **EENT:** pharyngitis. **GI:** abdominal pain, anorexia, nausea, vomiting. **Metabolic:** *hypoglycemia.* **Musculoskeletal:** arthralgia. **Respiratory:** cough. **Skin:** injection-site reaction. **Other:** allergic reaction, accidental injury.

INTERACTIONS
Drug-drug. *ACE inhibitors, disopyramide, fibrates, fluoxetine, MAO inhibitors, oral antidiabetics, pentoxifylline, propoxyphene, salicylates, sulfonamide antibiotics:* May increase risk of hypoglycemia. Monitor glucose level closely.
Alpha-glucosidase inhibitors (acarbose), anticholinergics (atropine, benztropine, TCAs): May alter GI motility and slow intestinal absorption. Avoid using together.
Beta blockers, clonidine, guanethidine, reserpine: May mask signs of hypoglycemia. Monitor glucose level closely.
Oral drugs dependent on rapid onset of action (such as analgesics, antibiotics, oral contraceptives): May delay absorption because of slowed gastric emptying. If rapid effect is needed, give oral drug 1 hour before or 2 hours after pramlintide.

EFFECTS ON LAB TEST RESULTS
None reported.

CONTRAINDICATIONS & CAUTIONS
• Contraindicated in patients hypersensitive to drug or its components, including metacresol, and in patients with gastroparesis or hypoglycemia unawareness.
• Don't use in patients nonadherent with current insulin and glucose monitoring regimen, patients with an HbA_{1c} level greater than 9%, patients with recurrent severe hypoglycemia during the previous 6 months, and patients who take drugs that stimulate GI motility.
• Use cautiously in patients with visual or dexterity impairment.
• Pramlintide alone doesn't cause hypoglycemia but is indicated for use with insulin and may be used with other antidiabetics, such as sulfonylurea or metformin, which may increase risk of hypoglycemia. Close monitoring and insulin dosage adjustments are necessary to manage risk.
• Safe use in children hasn't been established.
• Use cautiously in older adults.
Dialyzable drug: Unknown.
⚠ *Overdose S&S:* Severe nausea, vomiting, diarrhea, vasodilation, dizziness.

P

PREGNANCY-LACTATION-REPRODUCTION
• There are no adequate studies during pregnancy. Use only if potential benefit justifies fetal risk. Other agents are currently recommended to treat diabetes in patients who are pregnant.
• It isn't known if drug appears in human milk. Use during breastfeeding only if benefit clearly outweighs risk to infant.

NURSING CONSIDERATIONS
• Before starting drug, review patient's HbA$_{1c}$ level, recent blood glucose monitoring data, hypoglycemic episodes, current insulin regimen, and body weight.
Boxed Warning When used with insulin, drug may increase risk of insulin-induced severe hypoglycemia, particularly in patients with type 1 diabetes. Risk of severe hypoglycemia is highest within first 3 hours after an injection. Serious injuries may occur if severe hypoglycemia develops while patient is operating a motor vehicle or heavy machinery or engaging in other high-risk activities. ∎
Boxed Warning Appropriate patient selection, careful patient instruction, and insulin dosage adjustments are critical elements for reducing risk of hypoglycemia. ∎
• Symptoms of hypoglycemia may be masked in patients with a long history of diabetes, diabetic nerve disease, or intensified diabetes control.
• Notify prescriber of severe nausea and vomiting. A reduced dose may be needed.
• If patient has persistent nausea or recurrent, unexplained hypoglycemia that requires medical assistance, stop drug.
• Monitor patient for local reaction at injection site (erythema, edema, pruritus). Minor reactions usually resolve in a few days to weeks.
• If patient doesn't adhere to glucose monitoring or drug dosage adjustments, drug will need to be stopped.

PATIENT TEACHING
• Instruct patient in safe drug administration and storage.
• Teach patient how to take drug exactly as prescribed, at mealtimes. Explain that it doesn't replace daily insulin but may lower the amount of insulin needed.
• Explain that a meal is considered more than 250 calories or 30 g of carbohydrates.

• Caution patient not to change doses of pramlintide or insulin without consulting prescriber.
⊙ **Alert:** Warn patient not to share the multidose pen with other people, even if the needle is changed, because of the risk of bloodborne pathogen transmission, including HIV and hepatitis virus.
Boxed Warning Tell patient to refrain from driving, operating heavy machinery, or performing other risky activities that may cause harm to patient or others until drug's effects on glucose level are known. ∎
Boxed Warning Caution patient about possibility of severe hypoglycemia, particularly within 3 hours after injection. ∎
• Teach patient and family members the signs and symptoms of hypoglycemia, including hunger, headache, diaphoresis, tremor, irritability, and difficulty concentrating.
• Instruct patient and family members what to do if patient develops hypoglycemia.
• Tell patient to report severe nausea and vomiting to prescriber.
• Advise patient of childbearing potential to report known or suspected pregnancy or plans to become pregnant.
• Teach patient how to handle unplanned situations, such as illness or stress, low or forgotten insulin dose, accidental use of too much insulin or drug, not enough food, or missed meals.

SAFETY ALERT!

prasugrel hydrochloride
PRA-soo-grel

Effient⬦

Therapeutic class: Antiplatelet drugs
Pharmacologic class: Adenosine diphosphate–induced platelet aggregation inhibitors

AVAILABLE FORMS
Tablets: 5 mg, 10 mg

INDICATIONS & DOSAGES
➤ **To reduce thrombotic events in patients with ACS (unstable angina and non-ST-elevation MI) managed with PCI; to reduce thrombotic events in patients with ACS (ST-elevation MI) managed with primary or delayed PCI**

Adults: Initially, single 60-mg loading dose; then 10 mg PO once daily. Patient should also take aspirin 75 to 325 mg PO daily.
Adjust-a-dose: For adults weighing less than 60 kg, consider reducing dosage to 5 mg PO once daily.

ADMINISTRATION
PO
• May give drug with or without food.
• Don't break tablets. In an emergent primary PCI setting, crushing tablets (using a commercially available syringe crusher) and mixing with 25 mL water led to faster absorption and a quicker, more potent antiplatelet effect (seen as early as 30 minutes). Also, tablets may be chewed and swallowed (bitter to taste) or crushed and mixed in food or liquid (applesauce, juice, water) and immediately given by mouth or gastric tube.
• Administration via an enteral tube that bypasses the acidic environment of the stomach may result in reduced bioavailability of prasugrel.

ACTION
Inhibits platelet activation and aggregation through irreversible binding of its active metabolite to the $P2Y_{12}$ class of ADP receptors on platelets.

Route	Onset	Peak	Duration
PO	Rapid	30 min	5–9 days

Half-life: 7 hours (range, 2 to 15 hours).

ADVERSE REACTIONS
CNS: dizziness, fatigue, headache, fever. **CV:** atrial fibrillation, *bradycardia,* HTN or hypotension, peripheral edema, *hemorrhage.* **EENT:** epistaxis. **GI:** *GI bleeding,* nausea, diarrhea. **Hematologic:** anemia, *leukopenia.* **Metabolic:** hypercholesterolemia, hyperlipidemia. **Musculoskeletal:** back pain, extremity pain, noncardiac chest pain. **Respiratory:** cough, dyspnea. **Skin:** rash.

INTERACTIONS
Drug-drug. *Direct factor Xa inhibitors (rivaroxaban), direct thrombin inhibitors (dabigatran, desirudin), fibrinolytics (tenecteplase), heparin, low-molecular-weight heparin, NSAIDs (long-term use), platelet inhibitors, warfarin:* May increase the risk of bleeding. Use together cautiously.

Opioids: Delay absorption of prasugrel due to slowed gastric emptying. Consider therapy modification.
Vitamin E (systemic): May enhance antiplatelet effect of agents with antiplatelet properties. Monitor therapy.
Drug-herb. *Fish oil, garlic, ginger, ginkgo, omega-3 fatty acids:* Inhibit platelet aggregation. Use cautiously together; monitor patient for signs and symptoms of bleeding.

EFFECTS ON LAB TEST RESULTS
• May increase cholesterol and lipid levels.
• May increase Hb level.
• May decrease WBC and platelet counts.

CONTRAINDICATIONS & CAUTIONS
Boxed Warning Contraindicated in patients with pathologic bleeding (such as peptic ulcer or intracranial hemorrhage) and in those with a history of TIA or stroke. ■
Boxed Warning Drug isn't recommended in patients age 75 and older because of the increased risk of intracranial and fatal bleeding and uncertain benefit, except in high-risk situations (patients with diabetes or a history of prior MI). In these situations, drug's effect appears to be greater and its use may be considered. ■
Boxed Warning Don't start drug in patients likely to undergo urgent CABG. ■
Boxed Warning Use cautiously in patients who weigh less than 60 kg and in those with a propensity to bleed or who are using drugs that increase bleeding risk (warfarin, heparin, fibrinolytic therapy, long-term NSAID use) because of increased risk of bleeding. ■
• Contraindicated in patients with hypersensitivity to prasugrel, its components, or to other thienopyridines. Angioedema can occur.
• Use cautiously in patients at risk for increased bleeding from trauma, surgery, or other pathologic conditions and in those with severe hepatic impairment.
Dialyzable drug: Unlikely.
⚠ **Overdose S&S:** Bleeding due to impaired clotting ability.

PREGNANCY-LACTATION-REPRODUCTION
• There are no adequate studies during pregnancy. Use during pregnancy and breastfeeding only if maternal benefit justifies fetal risk.

NURSING CONSIDERATIONS

Boxed Warning Drug may cause significant, sometimes fatal, bleeding. Suspect bleeding in patient who is hypotensive and has recently undergone PCI, CABG, or other surgical procedure. Manage bleeding without stopping drug, if possible. Stopping drug within first few weeks after ACS occurrence increases the risk of further CV events. ■

• Monitor patient for unusual bleeding or bruising and hypersensitivity reactions.

Boxed Warning If possible, discontinue drug 7 days before CABG or any surgery. ■

• Bleeding associated with CABG may be treated with transfusion of blood products, such as RBCs and platelets; however, platelets may be ineffective if given within 6 hours of loading dose or within 4 hours of maintenance dose.

🕔 *Alert:* Drug may cause fatal thrombotic thrombocytopenic purpura (thrombocytopenia, hemolytic anemia, neurologic signs and symptoms, renal dysfunction, and fever) that requires urgent treatment, including plasmapheresis.

• *Look alike–sound alike:* Don't confuse prasugrel with pravastatin or propranolol.

PATIENT TEACHING

• Instruct patient in safe drug administration.
• Inform patient that bruising will occur more easily and that it may take longer than usual to stop bleeding.
• Teach patient to report prolonged or excessive bleeding, bruising, blood in the stool or urine, or fever, fatigue, low urine output, or neurologic signs and symptoms.
• Advise patient to inform health care providers, including dentists, of prasugrel use before scheduling surgery or taking new drugs.
• Inform patient that duration of therapy may be determined by the type of stent used and not to discontinue drug without first consulting prescriber.

pravastatin sodium (eptastatin)▨
prah-va-STA-tin

Therapeutic class: Antilipemics
Pharmacologic class: HMG-CoA reductase inhibitors

AVAILABLE FORMS
Tablets: 10 mg, 20 mg, 40 mg, 80 mg

INDICATIONS & DOSAGES
Adjust-a-dose (for all indications): In patients with renal dysfunction, start with 10 mg PO daily. In patients taking immunosuppressants, begin with 10 mg PO at bedtime and adjust to higher dosages with caution. Most patients treated with the combination of immunosuppressants and pravastatin receive up to 20 mg pravastatin daily. In patients taking clarithromycin, limit dose to 40 mg once daily.

➤ **Primary and secondary prevention of coronary events; hyperlipidemia**
Adults: Initially, 40 mg PO once daily at the same time each day, with or without food. Adjust dosage every 4 weeks, based on patient tolerance and response; maximum daily dose is 80 mg. Dosage range is 10 to 80 mg daily.

➤ **Heterozygous familial hypercholesterolemia** ▨
Adolescents ages 14 to 18: 40 mg PO once daily. Maximum dose is 40 mg daily.
Children ages 8 to 13: 20 mg PO once daily. Maximum dose is 20 mg daily.

ADMINISTRATION
PO
• Give drug without regard for meals.
• If patient is also taking a bile acid resin (cholestyramine, colestipol), administer pravastatin 1 hour before or 4 hours after the resin.

ACTION
Inhibits HMG-CoA reductase, an early (and rate-limiting) step in cholesterol biosynthesis.

Route	Onset	Peak	Duration
PO	Unknown	60–90 min	Unknown

Half-life: 1.8 hours.

ADVERSE REACTIONS
CNS: dizziness, fatigue, headache, fever, sleep disturbance, anxiety, paresthesia.

Reactions in bold italics are *life-threatening*. Interactions may have a *rapid onset* or a *delayed onset*.

CV: chest pain, edema. **EENT:** rhinitis, pharyngitis, sinus abnormality, vision disturbance. **GI:** nausea, abdominal pain, abdominal distention, constipation, diarrhea, flatulence, heartburn, vomiting. **GU:** UTI. **Hepatic:** elevated liver enzyme levels. **Metabolic:** weight gain or loss, increased CK level. **Musculoskeletal:** pain, muscle cramp, myalgia. **Respiratory:** URI, cough, tracheobronchitis, pulmonary infection. **Skin:** rash. **Other:** viral infection, flulike symptoms.

INTERACTIONS

Drug-drug. *Cholestyramine, colestipol:* May decrease pravastatin level. Give pravastatin 1 hour before or 4 hours after these drugs.
Clarithromycin: May increase pravastatin level. Limit pravastatin to 40 mg once daily.
Colchicine: May increase risk of myopathy or rhabdomyolysis. Consider therapy modification.
Cyclosporine: May increase pravastatin level and pravastatin-related adverse reactions. If concomitant use can't be avoided, limit pravastatin to 20 mg daily.
◆ *Alert: Darunavir and ritonavir, lopinavir– ritonavir:* May increase pravastatin level and risk of myopathy and rhabdomyolysis. Use together cautiously.
Erythromycin: May increase pravastatin level. Monitor therapy.
Fibrates (fenofibrate): May increase risk of muscle pain and weakness. Avoid combination unless there are no other options.
Gemfibrozil: May increase risk of myopathy or rhabdomyolysis. Avoid use together.
Hepatotoxic drugs: May increase risk of hepatotoxicity. Avoid using together.
Niacin: May increase skeletal muscle effects. Consider pravastatin dosage reduction.
Protease inhibitors (ritonavir, saquinavir): May reduce pravastatin level. Monitor clinical response.
Rifampin: May decrease pravastatin levels. Carefully monitor clinical response.
Warfarin: May increase anticoagulative effect of warfarin. Monitor therapy.
Drug-herb. *Kava kava:* May increase risk of hepatotoxicity. Discourage use together.
Red yeast rice: May increase risk of adverse reactions because herb contains compounds similar to those in drug. Discourage use together.

Drug-food. *Oat bran:* May decrease effectiveness of pravastatin. Separate administration times as much as possible.
Drug-lifestyle. *Alcohol use:* May increase risk of hepatotoxicity. Discourage use together.

EFFECTS ON LAB TEST RESULTS
• May increase ALT, AST, CK, ALP, HbA$_{1c}$, fasting glucose, and bilirubin levels.
• May alter thyroid function test values.

CONTRAINDICATIONS & CAUTIONS
• Contraindicated in patients hypersensitive to drug and in those with active liver disease or conditions that cause unexplained, persistent elevations of transaminase levels.
• Use cautiously in patients who consume large quantities of alcohol or have a history of liver disease or renal failure.
• Interrupt statin therapy if patient shows signs of serious liver injury, hyperbilirubinemia, or jaundice. Don't restart drug if another cause can't be found.
• Statins may rarely cause rhabdomyolysis with acute renal failure and immune-mediated necrotizing myopathy.
• Withhold drug temporarily for acute or serious conditions predisposing patient to renal failure secondary to rhabdomyolysis, including sepsis, hypotension, major surgery, trauma, uncontrolled epilepsy, or severe metabolic, endocrine. or electrolyte disorder.
• Statins may alter blunt adrenal or gonadal steroid hormone levels.
• Safety and effectiveness in children younger than age 8 haven't been established.
Dialyzable drug: Unknown.

PREGNANCY-LACTATION-REPRODUCTION
• May cause fetal harm. Use during pregnancy is contraindicated unless benefits to patient outweigh fetal risk. Discontinue drug before conception. If pregnancy occurs during therapy, apprise patient of fetal risks with continued use during pregnancy.
• Drug appears in human milk. Contraindicated during breastfeeding.

NURSING CONSIDERATIONS
• Patient should follow a diet restricted in saturated fat and cholesterol during therapy.
▨ Use in children with heterozygous familial hypercholesterolemia if LDL cholesterol level is at least 190 mg/dL, or if LDL cholesterol is at least 160 mg/dL and patient has either

a positive family history of premature CV disease or two or more other CV disease risk factors.
• Obtain LFT results at start of therapy and then periodically. A liver biopsy may be performed if elevated liver enzyme levels persist.
• Monitor patient for fatigue and severe signs or symptoms affecting muscles. Evaluate patient for conditions that increase risk of muscle problems and obtain CK and creatinine levels and urinalysis for myoglobinuria. Drug may need to be withheld or discontinued.
• *Look alike–sound alike:* Don't confuse pravastatin with nystatin, pitavastatin, or prasugrel.

PATIENT TEACHING
• Instruct patient in safe drug administration.
• Tell patient to report adverse reactions.
• Inform patient that LFTs will be performed before and periodically throughout treatment.
• Tell patient to promptly report signs and symptoms of liver injury, including fatigue, anorexia, right upper quadrant discomfort, dark urine, or jaundice.
• Teach patient to promptly report any unexplained muscle pain, tenderness, or weakness, especially if accompanied by malaise or fever or if symptoms persist after discontinuing drug.
• Inform patient that the drug may increase blood sugar levels; however, the CV benefits are thought to outweigh the slight increase in risk.
• Teach patient about proper dietary management of cholesterol and triglycerides. When appropriate, recommend weight control, exercise, and smoking cessation programs.
• Inform patient that it may take up to 4 weeks to achieve full therapeutic effect.
• *Alert:* Tell patient of childbearing potential to stop drug and immediately report known or suspected pregnancy or breastfeeding.

---

prazosin hydrochloride
PRA-zoh-sin

Minipress

Therapeutic class: Antihypertensives
Pharmacologic class: Alpha blockers

AVAILABLE FORMS
Capsules: 1 mg, 2 mg, 5 mg

INDICATIONS & DOSAGES
➤ HTN
Adults: Initially, 1 mg PO b.i.d. or t.i.d. Dosage may be increased slowly. Maximum daily dose is 20 mg. Maintenance dosage is 6 to 15 mg daily in divided doses. Some patients need larger dosages (up to 40 mg daily in divided doses).
Adjust-a-dose: If other antihypertensives or diuretics are added to therapy, decrease prazosin dosage to 1 or 2 mg t.i.d. and retitrate to maintenance dosage.

ADMINISTRATION
PO
• Give drug without regard for meals.

ACTION
Unknown. Thought to act by blocking alpha-adrenergic receptors.

Route	Onset	Peak	Duration
PO	30–90 min	2–4 hr	10–24 hr

Half-life: 2 to 3 hours.

ADVERSE REACTIONS
CNS: dizziness, syncope, headache, drowsiness, nervousness, weakness, depression, vertigo, lack of energy. **CV:** orthostatic hypotension, palpitations, edema. **EENT:** blurred vision, reddened sclera, epistaxis, nasal congestion, dry mouth. **GI:** vomiting, diarrhea, nausea, constipation. **GU:** urinary frequency. **Respiratory:** dyspnea. **Skin:** rash.

INTERACTIONS
Drug-drug. *Antihypertensives, diuretics:* May increase hypotension. Reduce prazosin dosage to 1 or 2 mg t.i.d. and retitrate as needed.
PDE5 inhibitors (avanafil, sildenafil, tadalafil, vardenafil): May increase frequency of hypotensive effect or syncope with loss of consciousness. Initiate PDE5 inhibitor at the lowest dose.
Verapamil: May increase prazosin level. Monitor patient closely.
Drug-herb. *Ma huang:* May decrease antihypertensive effects. Discourage use together.
Yohimbe: May reduce prazosin effect. Discourage use together.

EFFECTS ON LAB TEST RESULTS
• May increase LFT values.
• May cause positive ANA titer.

Reactions in bold italics are *life-threatening*. Interactions may have a *rapid onset* or a **delayed onset**.

• May alter results of screening tests for pheochromocytoma by increasing urinary metabolite of norepinephrine and vanillyl-mandelic acid.

CONTRAINDICATIONS & CAUTIONS
• Contraindicated in patients hypersensitive to drug or its components, quinazolines, or other alpha blockers.
• Use cautiously in patients receiving other antihypertensives.
• Not approved for use in children.
• Intraoperative floppy iris syndrome has been observed during cataract surgery in some patients treated with alpha$_1$ blockers.
• May cause syncope with sudden loss of consciousness.
• Prolonged erections and priapism have been reported with alpha-1 blockers.
Dialyzable drug: No.
⚠ *Overdose S&S:* Profound drowsiness, depressed reflexes, hypotension.

PREGNANCY-LACTATION-REPRODUCTION
• There are no adequate studies during pregnancy. Use only if maternal benefits justify maternal and fetal risk.
• Drug appears in human milk. Use cautiously during breastfeeding.

NURSING CONSIDERATIONS
• Monitor BP and pulse rate frequently.
• Older adults may be more sensitive to drug's hypotensive effects.
• Adherence might be improved with twice-daily dosing. Discuss dosing change with prescriber if adherence problems are suspected.
🕚 *Alert:* If first dose is more than 1 mg, first-dose syncope may occur.
• *Look alike–sound alike:* Don't confuse prazosin with prednisone.

PATIENT TEACHING
• Warn patient that dizziness may occur with first dose. If dizziness occurs, tell patient to sit or lie down. Reassure patient that this effect disappears with continued dosing. Dizziness may also occur with alcohol use, prolonged standing, exercise, or during hot weather.
• Caution patient to avoid driving or performing hazardous tasks for the first 24 hours after starting this drug or increasing the dose.

• Tell patient not to suddenly stop taking drug, but to notify prescriber if unpleasant adverse reactions occur.
• Advise patient to minimize low BP and dizziness upon standing by rising slowly and avoiding sudden position changes.
• Priapism may occur. Advise patient to seek emergency treatment for erections lasting longer than 4 hours.
• Advise patient of childbearing potential to report pregnancy, plans to become pregnant, or breastfeeding.

prednisoLONE
pred-NISS-oh-lone

prednisoLONE sodium phosphate
Orapred ODT, Pediapred

Therapeutic class: Corticosteroids
Pharmacologic class: Glucocorticoids–mineralocorticoids

AVAILABLE FORMS
prednisolone
Syrup: 15 mg/5 mL
Tablets: 5 mg
prednisolone sodium phosphate
Oral solution: 5 mg/5 mL, 10 mg/5 mL, 15 mg/5 mL, 20 mg/5 mL, 25 mg/5 mL
Tablets (ODTs) 🅖: 10 mg, 15 mg, 30 mg

INDICATIONS & DOSAGES
➤ **Severe inflammation, disorders requiring immunosuppression**
Adults: 5 to 60 mg PO daily.
Children: 0.14 to 2 mg/kg/day PO in three or four divided doses (4 to 60 mg/m^2/day).
Adjust-a-dose: Dosage requirements vary and must be individualized based on disease being treated and patient response.
➤ **Uncontrolled asthma in those taking inhaled corticosteroids and long-acting bronchodilators**
Children: 0.14 to 2 mg/kg/day prednisolone sodium phosphate in single or divided doses. Continue short course (or "burst" therapy) until child achieves a peak expiratory flow rate of 80% of personal best, or until symptoms resolve. This usually requires 3 to 10 days of treatment but can take longer. Tapering the dose after improvement doesn't necessarily prevent relapse.

➤ **Acute exacerbations of MS**
Adults and children: 200 mg/day prednisolone sodium phosphate PO as single or divided dose for 7 days; then 80 mg every other day for 1 month.

➤ **Nephrotic syndrome**
Children: 60 mg/m² prednisolone sodium phosphate PO in three divided doses daily for 4 weeks, followed by 4 weeks of single-dose alternate-day therapy at 40 mg/m²/day.

ADMINISTRATION
PO
• Give drug with food or milk to reduce GI irritation. Patient may need another drug to prevent GI irritation.
• Don't cut or crush ODTs.
• Don't remove ODTs from blister pack until right before dosing.
• Patient may swallow ODT whole or allow to dissolve in mouth with or without water.

ACTION
Not clearly defined. Decreases inflammation, mainly by stabilizing leukocyte lysosomal membranes; suppresses immune response; stimulates bone marrow; and influences protein, fat, and carbohydrate metabolism.

Route	Onset	Peak	Duration
PO	Rapid	1–2 hr	18–36 hr

Half-life: 2 to 4 hours.

ADVERSE REACTIONS
CNS: euphoria, insomnia, *pseudotumor cerebri, seizures,* psychotic behavior, vertigo, headache, paresthesia, mood swings, neuropathy, neuritis, paraparesis, paresthesia, personality change, sensory disturbance. **CV:** *arrhythmias, bradycardia, cardiac enlargement, circulatory collapse, fat embolism, HF, thromboembolism,* HTN, edema, *pulmonary edema,* syncope, tachycardia, thrombophlebitis, vasculitis. **EENT:** cataracts, glaucoma, exophthalmos, increased IOP. **GI:** peptic ulceration, *pancreatitis,* abdominal distention, GI irritation, increased appetite, nausea, vomiting. **GU:** menstrual irregularities, altered motility and number of sperm, increased urine calcium level. **Hepatic:** elevated liver enzyme levels, hepatomegaly. **Metabolic:** *hypokalemia,* hyperglycemia, hypernatremia, carbohydrate intolerance, hypercholesterolemia, *hypocalcemia,* latent diabetes, weight gain, protein catabolism (negative nitrogen balance). **Musculoskeletal:** growth suppression in children, muscle weakness, osteoporosis, aseptic necrosis of femoral and humeral heads, loss of muscle mass, pathologic long bone fractures, myopathy, tendon rupture, vertebral compression fractures. **Skin:** diaphoresis, dry scalp, ecchymoses, petechiae, pigmentation changes, striae, thin fragile skin, facial erythema, hirsutism, delayed wound healing, acne, various skin eruptions. **Other:** hypersensitivity reactions; after increased stress—*acute adrenal insufficiency,* susceptibility to infections, cushingoid state; withdrawal symptoms (rebound inflammation, fatigue, weakness, arthralgia, fever, dizziness, depression, fainting, orthostatic hypotension, dyspnea, nausea, anorexia *hypoglycemia*).

INTERACTIONS
Drug-drug. *Anticholinesterase agents (donepezil, rivastigmine):* May cause severe weakness in patients with myasthenia gravis. If possible, withdraw anticholinesterase agent at least 24 hours before corticosteroid therapy.
Antidiabetics: May increase glucose level. Adjust antidiabetic dosage as necessary.
Aspirin, indomethacin, other NSAIDs: May increase risk of GI distress and bleeding. Use together cautiously.
Cyclosporine: May increase toxicity and risk of seizures. Monitor patient closely.
CYP3A4 inducers (barbiturates, carbamazepine, fosphenytoin, phenytoin, rifampin): May decrease corticosteroid effect. Increase corticosteroid dosage.
CYP3A4 inhibitors (azole antifungals, macrolide antibiotics): May decrease corticosteroid metabolism and increase risk of toxicity. Reduce steroid dosage as needed.
Drugs that deplete potassium (thiazide diuretics, amphotericin B): May enhance potassium-wasting effects of prednisolone. Monitor potassium level.
Estrogens: May increase pharmacologic and toxic effects of prednisolone. Monitor patient closely.
Oral anticoagulants (warfarin): May alter anticoagulant dosage requirements. Monitor PT and INR closely.
Salicylates: May decrease salicylate level. Monitor patient for lack of salicylate effectiveness.

Reactions in bold italics are *life-threatening*. Interactions may have a *rapid onset* or a *delayed onset*.

Skin-test antigens: May decrease response. Postpone skin testing until therapy is completed.
Toxoids, vaccines: May decrease antibody response and may increase risk of organism replication in some live attenuated vaccines. Avoid using together.

EFFECTS ON LAB TEST RESULTS

- May increase glucose and cholesterol levels and LFT values.
- May decrease T_3, T_4, potassium, and calcium levels.
- May decrease ^{131}I uptake and protein-bound iodine levels in thyroid function tests.
- May alter skin test results.
- May cause false-negative results in nitroblue tetrazolium test for systemic bacterial infections.

CONTRAINDICATIONS & CAUTIONS

- Contraindicated in patients hypersensitive to drug or its ingredients, in those with systemic fungal infections or cerebral malaria, and in those receiving immunosuppressive doses together with live-virus vaccines.
- Use cautiously in patients with recent MI, GI ulcer, renal disease, HTN, osteoporosis, diabetes, hypothyroidism, cirrhosis, active hepatitis, diverticulitis, nonspecific ulcerative colitis, recent intestinal anastomoses, thromboembolic disorders, seizures, myasthenia gravis, HF, TB, ocular herpes simplex, emotional instability, and psychotic tendencies.

Alert: Prolonged use can increase incidence of secondary infection, activate latent infections, prolong viral infections, and mask infections.

- Drug can suppress HPA axis, which can lead to adrenal crisis. Always withdraw drug slowly and carefully.
- Drug may increase risk of Kaposi sarcoma. Discontinuing drug may result in clinical improvement.

Dialyzable drug: Unknown.
Overdose S&S: Abnormal fat deposits, accentuated menopausal symptoms, acne, adrenal insufficiency, decreased glucose tolerance, decreased resistance to infection, dry scaly skin, ecchymosis, excessive appetite, fluid retention, fractures, headache, hypertrichosis, hypokalemia, increased BP, diaphoresis, menstrual disorder, mental symptoms, moon face, negative nitrogen balance with delayed bone and wound healing, neuropathy, osteoporosis, peptic ulcer, pigmentation, striae, tachycardia, thinning scalp hair, thrombophlebitis, weakness, weight gain; hepatomegaly, abdominal distention (in children).

PREGNANCY-LACTATION-REPRODUCTION

- Drug can cause fetal harm. If drug is used during pregnancy, or if patient becomes pregnant during therapy, advise patient about fetal risk.
- Observe infants born to mothers who have received corticosteroids during pregnancy for signs and symptoms of hypoadrenalism.
- Drug appears in human milk and could suppress growth, interfere with endogenous corticosteroid production, or cause other untoward effects in the infant. Use cautiously during breastfeeding. Refer to manufacturer's instructions for each product.

NURSING CONSIDERATIONS

- Determine whether patient is hypersensitive to other corticosteroids.
- Always adjust to lowest effective dose.
- Most adverse reactions to corticosteroids are dose- or duration-dependent.
- Monitor patient's weight, BP, and electrolyte level.
- Monitor patient for cushingoid effects, including moon face, buffalo hump, central obesity, thinning hair, HTN, and increased susceptibility to infection.
- Watch for depression or psychotic episodes, especially during high-dose therapy.
- Patients with diabetes may need increased antidiabetic dosage; monitor glucose level.
- Give patient low-sodium diet that's high in potassium and protein. Give potassium supplements as needed.
- Older adults may be more susceptible to osteoporosis with long-term use.
- Monitor patient for acute myopathy with high-dose therapy; monitor CK level.
- Gradually reduce dosage after long-term therapy to prevent withdrawal symptoms.
- **Look alike–sound alike:** Don't confuse prednisolone with prednisone.

PATIENT TEACHING

- Instruct patient in safe drug administration and to take drug exactly as prescribed.
- Tell patient not to stop drug abruptly or without prescriber's consent.

P

- Teach patient signs and symptoms of early adrenal insufficiency: fatigue, muscle weakness, joint pain, fever, anorexia, nausea, shortness of breath, dizziness, and fainting.
- Instruct patient to carry medical identification that includes prescriber's name and name, dosage of drug, and the need for supplemental systemic glucocorticoids during stress.
- Warn patient on long-term therapy about cushingoid effects and the need to notify prescriber about sudden weight gain or swelling.
- Tell patient to report slow healing.
- Advise patient receiving long-term therapy to consider exercise or physical therapy and to ask prescriber about vitamin D or calcium supplement.
- Instruct patient to avoid exposure to infections and to notify prescriber if exposure occurs.
- Tell patient to avoid immunizations while taking drug.
- Advise patient of childbearing potential to report pregnancy, plans to become pregnant, or breastfeeding.

---

prednisoLONE acetate (ophthalmic suspension)
pred-NISS-oh-lone

Pred Forte, Pred Mild

prednisoLONE sodium phosphate (solution)

Therapeutic class: Anti-inflammatory drugs (ophthalmic)
Pharmacologic class: Corticosteroids

AVAILABLE FORMS
prednisolone acetate
Ophthalmic suspension: 0.12%, 1%
prednisolone sodium phosphate
Ophthalmic solution: 1%

INDICATIONS & DOSAGES
➤ **Inflammation of palpebral and bulbar conjunctiva, cornea, and anterior segment of globe**
prednisolone acetate
Adults: 1 or 2 drops into affected eye b.i.d. to q.i.d. In severe conditions, may increase dosing frequency during initial 24 to 48 hours, if needed. If signs and symptoms fail to improve

after 2 days, reevaluate. In chronic conditions, taper doses gradually.
prednisolone sodium phosphate
Adults: 1 or 2 drops into conjunctival sac hourly during the day and every 2 hours at night until response is observed. May reduce to 1 drop every 4 hours, then 1 drop t.i.d. to q.i.d. as needed for adequate response. In chronic conditions, taper doses gradually.

ADMINISTRATION
Ophthalmic
- Shake suspension and check dosage before giving to ensure correct strength. Store in tightly covered container.
- Apply light finger pressure on lacrimal sac for 1 to 2 minutes after instillation.
- Don't touch dropper tip to eyelids or other surfaces when placing drops in eyes.
- May contain benzalkonium chloride, which may be absorbed by soft contact lenses. Have patient remove contacts before using drops and wait 15 minutes before reinserting.

ACTION
Suppresses edema, fibrin deposition, capillary dilation, leukocyte migration, capillary proliferation, and collagen deposition.

Route	Onset	Peak	Duration
Ophthalmic	Unknown	Unknown	Unknown

Half-life: Unknown.

ADVERSE REACTIONS
EENT: cataracts, corneal ulceration, discharge, discomfort, foreign body sensation, glaucoma worsening, increased IOP, secondary corneal infection, interference with corneal wound healing, optic nerve damage with excessive or long-term use, visual acuity and visual field defects. **Other:** adrenal suppression with excessive or long-term use, systemic effects.

INTERACTIONS
None significant.

EFFECTS ON LAB TEST RESULTS
None reported.

CONTRAINDICATIONS & CAUTIONS
- Contraindicated in patients hypersensitive to prednisolone or components of the formulation, after uncomplicated removal of a superficial corneal foreign body, and in patients

---

with acute, untreated, purulent ocular infections; acute superficial herpes simplex (dendritic keratitis); vaccinia, varicella, or other viral or fungal eye diseases; or ocular TB.

• Use cautiously in patients with corneal thinning or corneal abrasions that may be contaminated (especially with herpes).

• Use after cataract surgery may delay healing and increase the incidence of bleb formation.

• Use in the presence of thin corneal or thin scleral tissue may lead to perforation.

• Withdraw drug by gradually tapering dosage in patients with chronic conditions.

• Prolonged use may result in glaucoma and cataracts.

Dialyzable drug: Unknown.

PREGNANCY-LACTATION-REPRODUCTION

• There are no adequate studies during pregnancy. The amount of drug that crosses the placental barrier through ophthalmic drops isn't known. Use only if potential benefit justifies fetal risk.

• It isn't known if drug appears in human milk. Use cautiously during breastfeeding.

NURSING CONSIDERATIONS

• IOP can increase with prolonged use. Use cautiously in patients with glaucoma. Monitor IOP and visual acuity in patients receiving treatment for 10 days or longer.

• Monitor patient for irritation and secondary infections; drug may need to be discontinued.

• *Look alike–sound alike:* Don't confuse prednisolone with prednisone.

PATIENT TEACHING

• Teach patient how to safely instill drops and to wash hands before and after instillation. Warn patient not to touch tip of dropper to eye or surrounding area.

• Advise patient to remove contact lenses before administration and wait 15 minutes before reinserting.

• Tell patient on long-term therapy to have IOP tested frequently.

• Tell patient not to share drug, washcloths, or towels with family members and to notify prescriber if anyone develops the same signs or symptoms.

• Stress importance of adherence with recommended therapy.

• Tell patient to notify prescriber if improvement doesn't occur within several days or if pain, itching, or swelling of eye occurs.

• Warn patient not to use leftover drug for new eye inflammation because serious problems may occur.

---

predniSONE
PRED-ni-sone

Prednisone Intensol*, Rayos, Winpred✦

Therapeutic class: Corticosteroids
Pharmacologic class: Adrenocorticoids

AVAILABLE FORMS

Oral solution: 5 mg/5 mL*, 5 mg/mL (concentrate)*
Tablets: 1 mg, 2.5 mg, 5 mg, 10 mg, 20 mg, 50 mg
Tablets (delayed-release) ⓓⓒ: 1 mg, 2 mg, 5 mg

INDICATIONS & DOSAGES

➤ **Severe inflammation, disorders requiring immunosuppression, endocrine deficiency disorders (immediate-release, delayed-release)**

Adults and children: Initially, 5 to 60 mg PO daily in single dose or as two to four divided doses. Maintenance dosage is given daily or every other day (immediate-release only). Use lowest dose that will maintain adequate clinical response. Dosage must be individualized, and constant monitoring is needed.

➤ **Acute exacerbations of MS (immediate-release)**

Adults: 200 mg PO daily for 7 days; then 80 mg PO every other day for 1 month.

ADMINISTRATION
PO

• Unless contraindicated, give drug with food to reduce GI irritation. Patient may need another drug to prevent GI irritation.

• May dilute solution in juice or other flavored diluent or semisolid food such as applesauce before using.

• Make sure patient swallows delayed-release tablets whole and doesn't break, chew, or divide them.

• Discard opened bottle of solution after 90 days. Administer only using the provided calibrated dropper.

✦Canada   ◇OTC   ◆Off-label use   ✔Photoguide   ⓓDo not crush   *Liquid contains alcohol   ▨Genetic

ACTION
Not clearly defined. Decreases inflammation, mainly by stabilizing leukocyte lysosomal membranes; suppresses immune response; stimulates bone marrow; and influences protein, fat, and carbohydrate metabolism.

Route	Onset	Peak	Duration
PO (immediate-release)	Variable	2 hr	Variable
PO (delayed-release)	4 hr	6–6.5 hr	Unknown

Half-life: 2 to 3 hours.

ADVERSE REACTIONS
CNS: euphoria, malaise, fever, insomnia, psychotic behavior, behavior and mood changes, *pseudotumor cerebri,* vertigo, syncope, headache, paresthesia, abnormal sensory symptoms, arachnoiditis, neuropathy, paraplegia. **CV:** *HF, pulmonary edema,* HTN, edema, *arrhythmias, bradycardia,* tachycardia, thrombophlebitis, *fat embolism, thromboembolism,* cardiac enlargement, vasculitis. **EENT:** cataracts, glaucoma, blurred vision, oral candidiasis. **GI:** peptic ulceration, ulcerative esophagitis, perforation of the intestine, *pancreatitis,* GI irritation, increased appetite, nausea, vomiting, constipation, diarrhea, abdominal distention. **GU:** menstrual irregularities, increased urine calcium level. **Hematologic:** anemia, *neutropenia.* **Hepatic:** hepatomegaly. **Metabolic:** *hypokalemia,* hypernatremia, hyperglycemia, carbohydrate and glucose intolerance, diabetes, hypercholesterolemia, *hypocalcemia,* weight gain, protein catabolism (negative nitrogen balance). **Musculoskeletal:** growth suppression in children, muscle weakness, osteopenia, osteoporosis, arthralgia, aseptic necrosis of femoral and humeral head, pathologic long bone fracture, tendon rupture, vertebral compression fractures. **Skin:** hirsutism, delayed wound healing, acne, various skin eruptions, diaphoresis, thin fragile skin, thinning hair, striae, facial erythema, pigmentation changes, urticaria. **Other:** cushingoid state, abnormal fat deposits, susceptibility to infections, hypersensitivity reaction; *acute adrenal insufficiency* after increased stress or abrupt withdrawal after long-term therapy, withdrawal symptoms (rebound inflammation, fatigue, weakness, arthralgia, fever, dizziness, lethargy, depression, fainting, orthostatic hypotension, dyspnea, anorexia, *hypoglycemia*).

INTERACTIONS
Drug-drug. *Aminoglutethimide:* May lead to loss of corticosteroid-induced adrenal suppression. Use cautiously together.
Antidiabetics: May increase blood glucose concentration. Adjust antidiabetic dosage as necessary.
Aspirin, indomethacin, other NSAIDs: May increase risk of GI distress and bleeding. Use together cautiously.
Cardiac glycosides: May increase risk of arrhythmias due to hypokalemia. Monitor patient closely.
Cholestyramine: May increase clearance of corticosteroids. Monitor therapy.
Cyclosporine: May increase toxicity and cause seizures. Monitor patient closely.
CYP3A4 inducers (barbiturates, carbamazepine, fosphenytoin, phenobarbital, phenytoin, rifampin): May decrease corticosteroid effect. Increase corticosteroid dosage.
CYP3A4 inhibitors (ketoconazole, macrolides, troleandomycin): May inhibit metabolism of corticosteroids and decrease their clearance. Titrate corticosteroid dosage to avoid toxicity.
Isoniazid: May decrease isoniazid serum concentration. Monitor therapy.
Oral anticoagulants: May alter dosage requirements. Monitor PT and INR closely.
Potassium-depleting drugs (thiazide diuretics, amphotericin B): May enhance potassium-wasting effects of prednisone. Monitor potassium level.
Salicylates: May decrease salicylate level. Monitor patient for lack of salicylate effectiveness.
Skin-test antigens: May decrease response. Postpone skin testing until therapy is completed.
Toxoids, live or attenuated vaccines: May decrease antibody response and may increase risk of neurologic complications. Avoid using together.

EFFECTS ON LAB TEST RESULTS
• May increase glucose and cholesterol levels.
• May decrease T_3, T_4, potassium, and calcium levels.
• May decrease ^{131}I uptake and protein-bound iodine values in thyroid function tests.
• May cause false-negative results in nitro-blue tetrazolium test for systemic bacterial infections.
• May alter reactions to skin tests.

Reactions in bold italics are *life-threatening*. Interactions may have a *rapid onset* or a *delayed onset*.

CONTRAINDICATIONS & CAUTIONS

• Contraindicated in patients hypersensitive to drug or its components; in those with systemic fungal infections (immediate-release only), cerebral malaria, or active ocular herpes simplex; and in those receiving immunosuppressive doses together with live-virus vaccines.

• Use cautiously in patients with recent MI, GI ulcer, renal disease, HTN, osteoporosis, diabetes, seizures, hypothyroidism, cirrhosis, active hepatitis, diverticulitis, nonspecific ulcerative colitis, recent intestinal anastomoses, thromboembolic disorders, myasthenia gravis, HF, TB, ocular herpes simplex, and psychiatric disturbances.

❸ Alert: Patients are more susceptible to infections (from mild to fatal) during therapy. Drug can also mask signs and symptoms of infection.

• Drug can cause cataracts or glaucoma.

❸ Alert: High-dose therapy is associated with acute myopathy that most often occurs in patients receiving neuromuscular drugs or in those with diseases such as myasthenia gravis.

Dialyzable drug: Unknown.

PREGNANCY-LACTATION-REPRODUCTION

• May cause fetal harm. Use only if potential benefits justify fetal risk.

• Monitor infants born to mothers who received substantial amounts of drug during pregnancy for signs and symptoms of hypoadrenalism.

• Drug appears in human milk. Patient should discontinue breastfeeding or discontinue drug.

• Drug may increase or decrease motility and number of sperm.

NURSING CONSIDERATIONS

• Determine if patient is hypersensitive to other corticosteroids.

• Immediate-release drug may be used for alternate-day therapy.

• Always adjust to lowest effective dose.

• Most adverse reactions to corticosteroids are dose- or duration-dependent.

• For better results and less toxicity, give a once-daily dose in the morning.

• Monitor BP, sleep patterns, and potassium level.

• If therapy lasts 6 weeks, monitor IOP.

• Weigh patient daily; report sudden weight gain to prescriber.

• Drug can cause HPA axis suppression and result in corticosteroid insufficiency if withdrawn. Reduce dosage gradually and reinstitute corticosteroid therapy if needed.

• Monitor patient for HPA axis suppression and cushingoid effects, including moon face, buffalo hump, central obesity, thinning hair, HTN, and increased susceptibility to infection.

• Watch for depression or psychotic episodes, especially during high-dose therapy.

• Patient with diabetes may need increased insulin; monitor glucose level.

• Older adults may be more susceptible to osteoporosis with long-term use.

• Patients with thyroid status changes may need dosage adjustment.

• Drug can cause osteoporosis at any age. Monitor bone density in patients on long-term therapy and bone growth in children. Institute bone-loss prevention measures if therapy is expected to last 3 months or more.

• Monitor growth in children on long-term therapy.

• Monitor patient for signs and symptoms of infection. Drug may mask or worsen infections, including latent amebiasis.

• Unless contraindicated, give low-sodium diet that's high in potassium and protein. Give potassium supplements as needed.

• Gradually reduce dosage after long-term therapy.

• *Look alike–sound alike:* Don't confuse prednisone with prednisolone or primidone.

PATIENT TEACHING

• Instruct patient in safe drug administration.

• Tell patient not to stop drug abruptly or without prescriber's consent.

• Advise patient to report all adverse reactions.

• Teach patient signs and symptoms of early adrenal insufficiency: fatigue, muscle weakness, joint pain, fever, anorexia, nausea, shortness of breath, dizziness, and fainting.

• Instruct patient to carry or wear medical identification indicating the need for supplemental systemic glucocorticoids during stress. It should include prescriber's name and name and dosage of drug.

• Warn patient on long-term therapy about cushingoid effects (moon face, buffalo hump) and the need to notify prescriber about sudden weight gain or swelling.

• Advise patient receiving long-term therapy to consider exercise or physical therapy. Also, tell patient to ask prescriber about vitamin D or calcium supplement.

• Tell patient to report slow healing.

• Advise patient receiving long-term therapy to have periodic eye exams.

• Instruct patient to report infection, to avoid exposure to infections, and to contact prescriber if exposure occurs.

pregabalin
pre-GAB-a-lin

Lyrica✦, Lyrica CR

Therapeutic class: Anticonvulsants
Pharmacologic class: CNS drugs
Controlled substance schedule: V

AVAILABLE FORMS
Capsules: 25 mg, 50 mg, 75 mg, 100 mg, 150 mg, 200 mg, 225 mg, 300 mg
Oral solution: 20 mg/mL
Tablets (extended-release) ⓘ: 82.5 mg, 165 mg, 330 mg

INDICATIONS & DOSAGES
Adjust-a-dose (for all indications): Refer to specific product information for guidelines regarding dosing in patients with renal impairment.

➤ **Fibromyalgia**
Adults (immediate-release and oral solution): 75 mg PO b.i.d. (150 mg/day). May increase to 150 mg b.i.d. (300 mg/day) within 1 week, based on patient response. If pain relief insufficient with 300 mg/day, increase to 225 mg b.i.d. (450 mg/day).

➤ **Diabetic peripheral neuropathy**
Adults: Initially, 50 mg PO t.i.d. May increase to 100 mg PO t.i.d. within 1 week based on patient response. Maximum dose is 300 mg/day. Or, initially 165 mg (extended-release) PO once daily after an evening meal. Increase to 330 mg within 1 week, based on patient response. Maximum dose is 330 mg once daily.

➤ **Neuropathic pain associated with spinal cord injury**
Adults: Initially, 75 mg POb.i.d. (150 mg/day). May increase to 150 mg b.i.d. (300 mg/day) within 1 week based on patient response. If

pain relief is insufficient after 2 to 3 weeks, increase to 300 mg b.i.d. Maximum dose is 600 mg/day.

➤ **Postherpetic neuralgia**
Adults: Initially, 75 mg PO b.i.d. or 50 mg PO t.i.d. May increase to 300 mg/day in two or three equally divided doses within 1 week based on patient response. If pain relief insufficient after 2 to 4 weeks, may increase to 300 mg b.i.d. or 200 mg t.i.d. Or, initially 165 mg (extended-release) PO once daily after an evening meal. Increase to 330 mg within 1 week, based on patient response. If pain relief is insufficient after 2 to 4 weeks and patient tolerates drug, may increase up to 660 mg. Maximum dose is 660 mg once daily.

➤ **Partial-onset seizures (adjunctive therapy)**
Adults: Initially, 75 mg PO b.i.d. or 50 mg PO t.i.d. Range, 150 to 600 mg/day. Dosage may be increased to maximum 600 mg/day.
Children ages 4 to 16 weighing 30 kg or more: 2.5 mg/kg/day PO in two or three divided doses. May increase weekly up to 10 mg/kg/day (maximum, 600 mg/day).
Children ages 4 to 16 weighing less than 30 kg: 3.5 mg/kg/day PO in two or three divided doses. May increase to 14 mg/kg/day.
Children ages 1 month to younger than 4 years: 3.5 mg/kg/day PO in three divided doses. May increase to 14 mg/kg/day.

ADMINISTRATION
PO
• Give immediate-release form without regard for food.

• Give extended-release form after an evening meal. Don't crush, split, or allow patient to chew extended-release tablets.

• Give a missed immediate-release dose as soon as possible unless it's almost time for the next dose; then skip missed dose and give next dose as regularly scheduled.

• If an extended-release dose is missed after the evening meal, give before bedtime after a snack. If dose is missed before bedtime, give in the morning with a meal. If dose is missed in the morning, wait until the evening meal to give the next scheduled dose.

• Don't stop drug abruptly. Instead, taper gradually over at least 1 week.

• Follow manufacturer's instructions when switching from immediate-release to extended-release.

• Store Lyrica CR in original container.

Reactions in bold italics are *life-threatening*. Interactions may have a *rapid onset* or a *delayed onset*.

ACTION

May contribute to analgesic and anticonvulsant effects by binding to sites in CNS.

Route	Onset	Peak	Duration
PO (immediate-release)	Unknown	0.7–1.5 hr	Unknown
PO (extended-release)	Unknown	5–12 hr	Unknown

Half-life: Adults, 6.3 hours. Children up to age 6, 3 to 4 hours; children age 7 up to 17, 4 to 6 hours.

ADVERSE REACTIONS

CNS: ataxia, dizziness, somnolence, tremor, abnormal gait, abnormal thinking, amnesia, anxiety, asthenia, balance disorder, confusion, fatigue, depersonalization, euphoria, headache, hyperesthesia, hypertonia, incoordination, myoclonus, nervousness, nystagmus, pain, paresthesia, stupor, twitching, vertigo. **CV:** edema, chest pain, HTN, hypotension. **EENT:** blurred or abnormal vision, conjunctivitis, diplopia, eye disorder, otitis media, tinnitus, dry mouth, nasopharyngitis, sinusitis. **GI:** abdominal pain, constipation, flatulence, gastroenteritis, increased appetite, vomiting, nausea. **GU:** anorgasmia, impotence, decreased libido, urinary incontinence, urinary frequency, UTI. **Hematologic:** *thrombocytopenia.* **Hepatic:** increased transaminase levels. **Metabolic:** *hypoglycemia,* weight gain, increased or decreased appetite. **Musculoskeletal:** arthralgia, back and chest pain, leg cramps, myalgia, myasthenia, neuropathy. **Respiratory:** bronchitis, dyspnea, cough. **Skin:** ecchymosis, pruritus, contact dermatitis. **Other:** accidental injury, infection, flulike syndrome, hypersensitivity reaction.

INTERACTIONS

Drug-drug. *ACE inhibitors:* May increase risk of angioedema with concomitant use. Monitor patient.
🛈 *Alert: CNS depressants:* May increase risk of respiratory depression. Use lowest effective dose of pregabalin and monitor patient response.
Pioglitazone, rosiglitazone: May cause additive fluid retention and weight gain. Monitor patient closely.
Drug-lifestyle. 🛈 *Alert: Alcohol use:* May increase risk of CNS depression and respiratory difficulties. Discourage use together.

EFFECTS ON LAB TEST RESULTS

• May increase CK, ALK, and AST levels.
• May decrease platelet count.

CONTRAINDICATIONS & CAUTIONS

• Contraindicated in patients hypersensitive to drug or its components.
• Use cautiously in patients with NYHA Class III or IV HF.
🛈 *Alert:* May cause life-threatening and fatal respiratory depression in older adults and in patients with respiratory risk factors (CNS depressant or opioid use, COPD). Begin treatment at lowest dose and monitor patient closely.
🛈 *Alert:* Use cautiously in patients with depression. Drug may increase risk of suicidality.
🛈 *Alert:* Use cautiously in patients with history of substance abuse. Drug may cause physical and psychological dependence.
• Drug may prolong QT interval; however, clinical trial data didn't show an increase in related adverse effects.
Dialyzable drug: Yes.
⚠ *Overdose S&S:* Exaggerated adverse effects.

PREGNANCY-LACTATION-REPRODUCTION

• There are no adequate studies during pregnancy. Drug may cause fetal harm. Use in pregnancy only if potential benefit clearly justifies fetal risk.
• Patients exposed to drug during pregnancy should enroll in the North American AED Pregnancy Registry (1-888-233-2334).
• Drug appears in human milk. Patient should discontinue breastfeeding or discontinue drug.

NURSING CONSIDERATIONS

🛈 *Alert:* Monitor patient for signs and symptoms of hypersensitivity reactions (hives, rash, dyspnea, wheezing, angioedema). Signs and symptoms of angioedema include swelling of the face, mouth, and neck, which may compromise breathing. Discontinue drug immediately if angioedema occurs.
🛈 *Alert:* Monitor patient for worsening depression, suicidality, or unusual mood or behavior changes.
• Monitor patient's weight and fluid status, especially if patient has HF.
• Check for changes in vision.

P

• Withdraw drug gradually over 1 week, especially in patients with seizure disorder.
🕭 *Alert:* Watch for signs of rhabdomyolysis, such as dark, red, or cola-colored urine; muscle tenderness; generalized weakness; or muscle stiffness or aching.
• *Look alike–sound alike:* Don't confuse Lyrica with Lopressor or Hydrea.

PATIENT TEACHING
• Instruct patient in safe drug administration.
• Warn patient not to stop drug abruptly and that it should be tapered over at least 1 week.
🕭 *Alert:* Caution patient or caregiver to seek immediate medical attention for confusion or disorientation; unusual dizziness or lightheadedness; lethargy; extreme sleepiness; slow, shallow, or difficult breathing; unresponsiveness; or cyanosis of the lips, fingers, or toes.
• Advise patient that drug may cause angioedema, with swelling of the face, mouth (lip, gum, and tongue), and neck (larynx and pharynx) that can lead to life-threatening respiratory compromise. Instruct patient to discontinue drug and immediately seek medical care if these symptoms occur.
• Tell patient to seek immediate medical care for a hypersensitivity reaction, such as blisters, dyspnea, hives, rash, or wheezing.
🕭 *Alert:* Counsel patient, caregiver, and family about risk of suicidality. Advise them of the need to be alert for the emergence or worsening of symptoms of depression, unusual changes in mood or behavior, or the emergence of suicidality or thoughts about self-harm and to immediately report behaviors of concern to health care provider.
• Caution patient to avoid hazardous activities until drug's effects are known.
• Instruct patient to watch for weight changes and water retention.
• Advise patient to report vision changes and malaise or fever accompanied by muscle pain, tenderness, or weakness.
• Tell male patient taking pregabalin who plans to father a child to consult prescriber about fetal risk because of male-mediated teratogenicity.
• Advise patient of childbearing potential to report pregnancy, plans to become pregnant, or breastfeeding.
• Urge patient with diabetes to inspect skin closely for ulcer formation.
• Advise patient to avoid alcohol.

SAFETY ALERT!

procainamide hydrochloride
proe-KANE-a-myed

Therapeutic class: Antiarrhythmics
Pharmacologic class: Procaine derivatives

AVAILABLE FORMS
Injection: 100 mg/mL, 500 mg/mL

INDICATIONS & DOSAGES
➤ **Life-threatening ventricular arrhythmias**
Adults: Loading dose: 100 mg every 5 minutes by slow IV push, no faster than 50 mg/minute, until arrhythmias disappear, adverse effects develop, or 500 mg has been given. Or, give a loading dose of 500 to 600 mg IV infusion over 25 to 30 minutes. Maximum total dose given by repeated bolus injections or loading infusion is 1 g. Maintenance infusion: To maintain therapeutic levels, give continuous infusion of 2 to 6 mg/minute based on clinical response and patient condition; monitor closely.

For patients with less-threatening arrhythmias but who are nauseated, vomiting, or are ordered to receive nothing by mouth, give 50 mg/kg IM divided into fractional doses of one-eighth to one-fourth every 3 to 6 hours. If more than three injections are given, prescriber may wish to assess patient factors, such as age and renal function, clinical response and, if available, blood levels of procainamide and *N*-acetylprocainamide (NAPA) in adjusting further dosages for that patient. For arrhythmias occurring during surgery, give 100 to 500 mg IM.
Adjust-a-dose: For patients with renal or hepatic dysfunction, decrease dosage or increase dosing interval, as needed.

ADMINISTRATION
IV
▼ Vials for IV injection contain 1 g of drug: 100 mg/mL (10 mL) or 500 mg/mL (2 mL).
▼ Direct injection into a vein or into tubing of an established IV line should be done slowly at a rate not to exceed 50 mg/minute.
▼ For loading dose infusion, dilute with compatible IV solution, such as D₅W injection (1 g diluted to 50 mL), and give with patient supine at a rate not exceeding 25 to

---

Reactions in bold italics are *life-threatening*. Interactions may have a *rapid onset* or a *delayed onset*.

50 mg/minute. Keep patient supine during IV administration.

▼ For IV infusion to maintain therapeutic levels, dilute 1 g procainamide in 500 or 250 mL D$_5$W and administer at 2 to 6 mg/minute based on patient response and clinical condition.

▼ Attend patient receiving infusion at all times. Use an infusion-control device to give infusion precisely.

◑ *Alert:* Monitor BP and ECG continuously during IV administration. Watch for prolonged QTc intervals and widening of the QRS complexes, heart block, or increased arrhythmias. If such reactions occur, withhold drug, obtain rhythm strip, and notify prescriber immediately. If drug is given too rapidly, hypotension can occur. Watch closely for adverse reactions during infusion, and notify prescriber if they occur.

▼ Solution may turn slightly yellow upon standing. Discard solutions that are slightly darker than yellow or discolored in any other way.

▼ **Incompatibilities:** 5% dextrose in normal saline, esmolol, milrinone, phenytoin sodium.

IM

• Use IM route only if IV route isn't feasible. IM injection may be painful and can increase CK level.

ACTION

Decreases excitability, conduction velocity, automaticity, and membrane responsiveness with prolonged refractory period. Larger than usual doses may induce AV block.

Route	Onset	Peak	Duration
IV	Immediate	Immediate	Unknown
IM	10–30 min	15–60 min	Unknown

Half-life: About 3 to 4 hours.

ADVERSE REACTIONS

CNS: psychosis with hallucination, giddiness, confusion, depression, dizziness, weakness, bitter taste. **CV:** flushing, hypotension, *bradycardia, AV block, ventricular fibrillation, ventricular asystole.* **GI:** abdominal pain, nausea, vomiting, anorexia, diarrhea. **Skin:** maculopapular rash, urticaria, pruritus. **Other:** lupuslike syndrome, *angioneurotic edema.*

INTERACTIONS

Drug-drug. *Amiodarone:* May increase procainamide level and toxicity and have additive effects on QTc interval and QRS complex. Avoid using together.

Antiarrhythmics: May enhance antiarrhythmic and hypotensive effects. Avoid using together.

Anticholinergics: May increase antivagal effects. Monitor patient closely.

Cimetidine: May increase procainamide level. Avoid using together if possible. Monitor procainamide level closely and adjust the dosage as necessary.

Macrolides and related antibiotics (azithromycin, clarithromycin, erythromycin, telithromycin): May prolong the QT interval. Use with caution. Avoid use with telithromycin.

Neuromuscular blockers: May increase skeletal muscle relaxant effect. May need to decrease dosage of neuromuscular blocker.

Quinolones: Life-threatening arrhythmias, including torsades de pointes, can occur. Avoid using together; sparfloxacin is contraindicated.

Thioridazine, ziprasidone: May prolong QTc interval. Avoid using together.

Trimethoprim: May increase procainamide level. Watch for toxicity.

Drug-herb. *Licorice:* May prolong QTc interval. Urge caution.

Drug-lifestyle. *Alcohol use:* May reduce drug level. Discourage use together.

EFFECTS ON LAB TEST RESULTS

• May increase ALT, AST, ALP, LDH, and bilirubin levels.

• May decrease Hb level, hematocrit, and WBC and platelet counts.

• May cause positive ANA titers and positive direct antiglobulin (Coombs) tests.

CONTRAINDICATIONS & CAUTIONS

• Contraindicated in patients hypersensitive to this drug and related drugs.

• Drug contains sulfite, which can cause allergic-type reactions, including anaphylaxis. Sensitivity to sulfites may be more frequent in patients with asthma.

• Contraindicated in patients with complete heart block in the absence of an artificial pacemaker. Also contraindicated in those with SLE or atypical ventricular tachycardia (torsades de pointes).

P

• Use with extreme caution in patients with ventricular tachycardia during coronary occlusion.

• Use cautiously in patients with HF or other conduction disturbances, such as bundle-branch heart block, first-degree heart block, sinus bradycardia, or digoxin intoxication, and in those with hepatic or renal insufficiency.

• Avoid use in patients with second-degree heart block or some types of hemiblock unless ventricular rate is controlled by a pacemaker.

• Use cautiously in patients with myasthenia gravis; drug may worsen symptoms.

Boxed Warning Use cautiously in patients with blood dyscrasias or bone marrow suppression. ∎

Dialyzable drug: Procainamide, 20 to 50%; metabolite NAPA, less than 5%.

⚠ *Overdose S&S:* Progressive widening of QRS complex, prolonged QT and PR intervals, lowered R and T waves, increasing AV block, ventricular ectopy, ventricular tachycardia, hypotension, CNS depression, tremor, respiratory depression.

PREGNANCY-LACTATION-REPRODUCTION

• Use during pregnancy only if clearly needed. It isn't known if drug can harm the fetus.

• Procainamide and metabolite NAPA appear in human milk. Patient should discontinue breastfeeding or discontinue drug.

NURSING CONSIDERATIONS

Boxed Warning Because of its proarrhythmic effects, procainamide should be reserved for patients with life-threatening ventricular arrhythmias. ∎

• Digitalize or cardiovert patients with atrial flutter or fibrillation before therapy with procainamide to prevent ventricular rate acceleration in patient.

• Monitor level of drug and its active metabolite NAPA.

• Monitor ECG closely. If QRS widens more than 25% or marked prolongation of the QTc interval occurs, check for overdosage.

• Hypokalemia predisposes patient to arrhythmias. Monitor electrolytes, especially potassium level.

• Older adults may be more likely to develop hypotension. Monitor BP carefully.

Boxed Warning Agranulocytosis, bone marrow depression, neutropenia, hypoplastic anemia, and thrombocytopenia have been noted in patients during the first 12 weeks of therapy. It is recommended that CBCs be performed at weekly intervals for the first 3 months of therapy and periodically thereafter. ∎

Boxed Warning Perform CBCs promptly if patient develops signs of infection, bruising, or bleeding. If hematologic disorder is identified, discontinue drug. Blood counts usually return to normal within 1 month of discontinuation. ∎

Boxed Warning Positive ANA titer is common in about 60% of patients who don't have symptoms of lupuslike syndrome. This response seems to be related to prolonged use, not dosage. If positive ANA titer develops, assess the benefits and risks of continued therapy. ∎

• Discontinue IV therapy if persistent conduction disturbances or hypotension develops. As soon as cardiac rhythm is stabilized, start oral antiarrhythmic maintenance therapy 3 to 4 hours after last IV dose.

PATIENT TEACHING

• Instruct patient to report all adverse reactions and to immediately report fever, rash, muscle pain, diarrhea, bleeding, bruises, pleuritic chest pain, or signs and symptoms of infection.

• Advise patient to report sulfite sensitivity before receiving drug.

SAFETY ALERT!

procarbazine hydrochloride
pro-KAR-ba-zeen

Matulane

Therapeutic class: Antineoplastics
Pharmacologic class: Methylhydrazine derivatives

AVAILABLE FORMS
Capsules: 50 mg

INDICATIONS & DOSAGES
Adjust-a-dose (for all indications): Base dosage on actual weight. In patient with obesity or weight gain due to fluid retention, use estimated lean body mass.

Reactions in bold italics are *life-threatening*. Interactions may have a *rapid onset* or a **delayed onset**.

➤ **Single-agent therapy or adjunctive treatment of Hodgkin lymphoma (stages III and IV) and other cancers using nitrogen mustard, vincristine, procarbazine, prednisone (MOPP) regimen**

Adults: For single-agent therapy, give 2 to 4 mg/kg/day PO in single dose or divided doses for first week. Then, 4 to 6 mg/kg/day until WBC count falls below 4,000/mm^3, platelet count falls below 100,000/mm^3, or maximum response is obtained. Maintenance dose is 1 to 2 mg/kg/day after bone marrow recovery.

Children: The prescribing information provides this dosage schedule as a guideline only: For single-agent therapy, give 50 mg/m^2/day PO for first week; then 100 mg/m^2/day until response or toxicity occurs. Maintenance dose is 50 mg/m^2/day PO after bone marrow recovery.

➤ **CNS tumors, anaplastic oligodendroglioma/oligoastrocytoma ◆**
PCV regimen

Adults: 60 mg/m^2 PO on days 8 to 21 every 6 weeks (in combination with lomustine and vincristine beginning within 4 weeks after radiotherapy) for six cycles, or 75 mg/m^2 PO on days 8 to 21 every 6 weeks (in combination with lomustine and vincristine, followed by radiotherapy) for up to four cycles.

➤ **CNS tumors (low-grade gliomas) ◆**
PCV regimen

Adults: 60 mg/m^2 PO on days 8 to 21 every 8 weeks (after radiotherapy; in combination with lomustine and vincristine) for six cycles.

TPCV regimen

Children younger than age 10: 50 mg/m^2 PO every 6 hours for four doses (at hours 60, 66, 72, and 78) during a 42-day cycle (in combination with thioguanine, vincristine, and lomustine) for a total of eight cycles.

ADMINISTRATION
PO

🚯 *Alert:* Hazardous drug; use safe handling and disposal precautions.

• Give drug with or after meals. May give once daily or in two to three divided doses.

• Some protocols advise administering in the evening; refer to specific protocol for details.

ACTION

Unknown. Thought to inhibit DNA, RNA, and protein synthesis.

Route	Onset	Peak	Duration
PO	Rapid	60 min	Unknown

Half-life: About 1 hour.

ADVERSE REACTIONS

CNS: ataxia, hallucinations, *coma,* confusion, depression, dizziness, headache, insomnia, nervousness, neuropathy, nightmares, paresthesia, syncope, tremors, fever, lethargy, drowsiness, weakness, slurred speech, *seizures.* **CV:** flushing, hypotension, tachycardia, edema. **EENT:** nystagmus, photophobia, retinal hemorrhage, diplopia, inability to focus, papilledema, hearing loss, dry mouth. **GI:** nausea, vomiting, abdominal pain, anorexia, constipation, diarrhea, dysphagia, *hematemesis, melena,* stomatitis. **GU:** hematuria, nocturia, urinary frequency. **Hematologic:** anemia, *pancytopenia, leukopenia, thrombocytopenia,* eosinophilia, hemolytic anemia, bleeding tendency (petechiae, purpura, epistaxis, hemoptysis). **Hepatic:** *hepatotoxicity,* jaundice. **Musculoskeletal:** myalgia, arthralgia, foot drop. **Respiratory:** pleural effusion, cough, pneumonitis. **Skin:** herpes lesions, dermatitis, hyperpigmentation, pruritus, rash, reversible alopecia, diaphoresis. **Other:** *secondary malignancies,* allergic reaction, falls, gynecomastia, infections, hoarseness.

INTERACTIONS

Drug-drug. *Antihistamines, hypotensive agents, phenothiazines:* May cause additive CNS depression effect. Use together cautiously.

CNS depressants: May cause additive depressant effects. Avoid using together.

Drugs high in tyramine, local anesthetics, MAO inhibitors, sympathomimetics, TCAs: May cause hypertensive crisis or serotonin syndrome. Avoid use together.

Drug-food. *Caffeine:* May result in arrhythmias and severe HTN. Discourage caffeine intake.

Foods high in tyramine (cheese, cured meats, fava or broad bean pods, soy products, bananas): May cause hypertensive crisis or serotonin syndrome. Monitor patient closely; advise patient to avoid or limit intake.

Drug-lifestyle. 🚯 *Alert: Alcohol use:* Mild disulfiram-like reaction may cause flushing, headache, nausea, and hypotension. Warn patient to avoid alcoholic beverages.

P

EFFECTS ON LAB TEST RESULTS
• May increase LFT values.
• May increase eosinophil count.
• May decrease Hb level and platelet, RBC, and WBC counts.

CONTRAINDICATIONS & CAUTIONS
• Contraindicated in patients hypersensitive to drug and in those with inadequate bone marrow reserve as shown by bone marrow aspiration.
• Consider hospitalization for the initial course of treatment when appropriate for patients with renal or hepatic impairment, as toxicity can occur.
• Drug may increase risk of secondary malignancy.
Dialyzable drug: Unknown.
⚠ *Overdose S&S:* Nausea, vomiting, diarrhea, enteritis, hypotension, tremors, seizures, coma.

PREGNANCY-LACTATION-REPRODUCTION
• Drug can cause fetal harm. Patients of childbearing potential should avoid pregnancy during therapy.
• Patients shouldn't breastfeed during therapy.
• Drug may decrease fertility.

NURSING CONSIDERATIONS
Boxed Warning Give drug only under the supervision of a physician experienced with potent antineoplastic drugs. Adequate clinical and lab facilities should be available for treatment monitoring. ∎
• Obtain baseline lab data before starting therapy. Monitor hematologic status at least every 3 or 4 days, including Hb level, hematocrit, and WBC, differential, reticulocyte, and platelet counts.
🕔 *Alert:* Prompt discontinuation of therapy is recommended if patient develops CNS signs or symptoms, such as paresthesia, neuropathies, or confusion; leukopenia (WBC count less than 4,000 cell/mm³); thrombocytopenia (platelet count less than 100,000/mm³); hypersensitivity reaction; stomatitis; diarrhea; or hemorrhage or bleeding tendencies.
• Bone marrow depression begins 2 to 8 weeks after the start of treatment.
• Avoid all IM injections when platelet count is below 50,000/mm³.

• Evaluate hepatic and renal function before starting therapy. Monitor urinalysis, ALT, AST, ALP, and BUN levels at least weekly.
• Drug has high emetic potential; give antiemetics to prevent nausea and vomiting.
• The manufacturer recommends that if radiation or chemotherapeutic agents with bone marrow depressant activity have been used, give patient a 1-month interval without such therapy before beginning procarbazine therapy.
• Monitor patient for hypertensive crisis (HTN, headache, seizure, blurred vision, confusion, chest pain, shortness of breath) and serotonin syndrome (fever, headache, neurologic changes, HTN, diaphoresis, nausea, vomiting); drug exhibits some MAO inhibitory activity.
• *Look alike–sound alike:* Don't confuse procarbazine with dacarbazine.

PATIENT TEACHING
• To decrease nausea and vomiting, advise patient to take drug at bedtime and in divided doses and to take antiemetics as prescribed.
• Tell patient to watch for fever, sore throat, fatigue, easy bruising, nosebleeds, bleeding gums, or melena. Tell patient to take temperature daily.
• Advise patient not to consume alcohol or alcohol-containing products during therapy, and to discontinue tobacco use.
• Instruct patient to avoid OTC medications that contain antihistamines and sympathomimetics and to avoid foods and drinks high in tyramine, such as wine, tea, coffee, cola, cheese, and bananas.
• Warn patient to avoid hazardous activities that require alertness and good motor coordination until CNS effects of drug are known.
• Caution patient of childbearing potential to avoid becoming pregnant during therapy and to consult prescriber before becoming pregnant.

Reactions in bold italics are *life-threatening*. Interactions may have a *rapid onset* or a ***delayed onset***.

prochlorperazine
proe-klor-PER-a-zeen

Compro

prochlorperazine edisylate

prochlorperazine maleate
Prochlorazine✤, Procomp

Therapeutic class: Antiemetics
Pharmacologic class: Dopamine antagonists

AVAILABLE FORMS
prochlorperazine
Suppositories: 25 mg
prochlorperazine edisylate
Injection: 5 mg/mL
prochlorperazine maleate
Tablets: 5 mg, 10 mg

INDICATIONS & DOSAGES
➤ **To control preoperative nausea**
Adults: 5 to 10 mg IM 1 to 2 hours before induction of anesthesia; repeat once in 30 minutes, if needed. Or, 5 to 10 mg IV at no more than 5 mg/minute 15 to 30 minutes before induction of anesthesia; repeat once, if needed. Maximum IM and IV dose is 40 mg/day.
➤ **Severe nausea and vomiting**
Adults: 5 to 10 mg PO t.i.d. or q.i.d.; 25 mg PR b.i.d.; or 5 to 10 mg IM, repeated every 3 to 4 hours, as needed. Maximum IM dose is 40 mg daily. Or, 2.5 to 10 mg IV at no more than 5 mg/minute. Maximum IV dose is 40 mg daily.
Children weighing 18 to 39 kg: 2.5 mg PO t.i.d.; or 5 mg PO b.i.d. Maximum, 15 mg daily. Or, 0.132 mg/kg by deep IM injection t.i.d. to q.i.d. Control is usually achieved with one dose.
Children weighing 14 to 17 kg: 2.5 mg PO b.i.d. or t.i.d. Maximum, 10 mg daily. Or, 0.132 mg/kg by deep IM injection t.i.d. to q.i.d. Control is usually achieved with one dose.
Children weighing 9 to 13 kg: 2.5 mg PO once daily or b.i.d. Maximum, 7.5 mg daily. Or, 0.132 mg/kg by deep IM injection t.i.d. to q.i.d. Control is usually achieved with one dose.

➤ **Schizophrenia**
Adults: Treatment guidelines may not include drug as recommended therapy for this indication. According to prescribing information, for mild conditions, 5 or 10 mg PO t.i.d. or q.i.d. For moderate to severe conditions, start with 10 mg PO t.i.d. or q.i.d.; increase by small increments every 2 or 3 days until symptoms are controlled or adverse reactions become bothersome. Patients may respond on 50 to 75 mg/day in divided doses. For severe conditions, 100 to 150 mg PO daily. Or, for severe symptoms, 10 to 20 mg by deep IM injection. Repeat the initial IM dose every 2 to 4 hours (or, in resistant cases, every hour) to gain control of patient, as necessary. More than three or four IM doses are seldom necessary. If, in rare cases, parenteral therapy is needed for a prolonged period, give 10 to 20 mg IM every 4 to 6 hours. After control is achieved, switch patient to an oral form of drug at same dosage level or higher.
Children ages 2 to 12: Initially, 2.5 mg PO b.i.d. or t.i.d., not to exceed 10 mg on the first day. Increase dosage according to patient response. Maximum dose is 20 mg/day (ages 2 to 5) or 25 mg/day (ages 6 to 12). Or, 0.132 mg/kg IM as a single dose. Don't exceed 10 mg/day on first day of therapy.
➤ **Nonpsychotic anxiety**
Adults: Treatment guidelines may not include drug as recommended therapy for this indication. According to prescribing information, give 5 mg PO t.i.d. or q.i.d. Maximum dose is 20 mg/day for no longer than 12 weeks.

ADMINISTRATION
PO
• Administer without regard to meals.
IV
▼ Give undiluted or diluted in isotonic solution by slow IV injection or infusion at a rate not to exceed 5 mg/minute. Don't exceed 10 mg in a single dose or total IV dose of 40 mg/day.
▼ Don't give by bolus injection.
▼ To prevent contact dermatitis, avoid getting injection solution on hands or clothing.
▼ Protect from light.
▼ **Incompatibilities:** Other IV drugs.
IM
• For IM use, inject deeply into upper outer quadrant of gluteal region.
• Don't give by subcut route or mix in syringe with another drug.

P

- To prevent contact dermatitis, avoid getting injection solution on hands or clothing.
- Store in light-resistant container. Slight yellowing doesn't affect potency; discard extremely discolored solutions.

Rectal

- Don't remove from wrapper until ready to use.
- Moisten suppository with water before insertion.
- If suppository is too soft because of warm storage, chill in refrigerator for 30 minutes or run cold water over it before removing wrapper.

ACTION

Acts on the chemoreceptor trigger zone to inhibit nausea and vomiting; in larger doses, it partially depresses vomiting center.

Route	Onset	Peak	Duration
PO	30–60 min	Unknown	3–4 hr
IV	Unknown	Unknown	Unknown
IM	10–20 min	Unknown	3–4 hr
PR	1 hr	Unknown	3–12 hr

Half-life: PO, 6 to 10 hours (single dose); 14 to 22 hours (repeated dosing). IV, 6 to 10 hours.

ADVERSE REACTIONS

CNS: extrapyramidal reactions, dizziness, EEG changes, pseudoparkinsonism, sedation, drowsiness, motor restlessness, dystonia, tardive dyskinesia. **CV:** orthostatic hypotension, ECG changes, tachycardia, edema. **EENT:** blurred vision, ocular changes, dry mouth. **GI:** constipation, obstipation, increased appetite, intestinal obstruction, nausea, vomiting. **GU:** urine retention, dark urine, inhibited ejaculation, priapism, menstrual irregularities. **Hematologic:** *agranulocytosis, transient leukopenia,* hemolytic anemia, eosinophilia. **Hepatic:** cholestatic jaundice. **Metabolic:** weight gain. **Skin:** mild photosensitivity reactions, allergic reactions, exfoliative dermatitis, contact dermatitis, urticaria, eczema. **Other:** hypersensitivity reactions, gynecomastia, hyperprolactinemia.

INTERACTIONS

Drug-drug. *Antacids:* May inhibit absorption of oral phenothiazines. Separate antacid and phenothiazine doses by at least 2 hours.
Anticholinergics, including antidepressants and antiparkinsonian drugs: May increase anticholinergic activity and may aggravate parkinsonian symptoms. Use together cautiously.
Anticoagulants: May decrease anticoagulant effects. Monitor PT and INR, and adjust dosage as needed.
Anticonvulsants: May lower seizure threshold; dosage adjustments of anticonvulsants may be needed.
Barbiturates: May decrease phenothiazine effect. Monitor patient for decreased antiemetic effect.
CNS depressants (anesthetics, opioids): May intensify or prolong action of these drugs. Monitor patient. Contraindicated with high doses of CNS depressants.
Loop diuretics, thiazides: May add to orthostatic hypotension caused by prochlorperazine. Monitor BP.
Nitroglycerin: May impair absorption of SL nitroglycerin tablets. Monitor therapy.
Propranolol: May increase plasma levels of both drugs. Observe for increased adverse effects.
Drug-herb. *Kava kava:* May increase risk of dystonic reactions. Discourage use together.
Drug-lifestyle. *Alcohol use:* May increase CNS depression, particularly psychomotor skills. Strongly discourage use together.

EFFECTS ON LAB TEST RESULTS

- May increase LFT values.
- May decrease platelet, RBC, WBC, and granulocyte counts.
- May cause false-positive results for phenylketonuria and pregnancy tests.

CONTRAINDICATIONS & CAUTIONS

- Contraindicated in patients hypersensitive to phenothiazines and in patients with CNS depression, including those in a coma.
- Contraindicated during pediatric surgery and in children younger than age 2 or weighing less than 9 kg.

Boxed Warning Drug isn't approved for the treatment of older adults with dementia-related psychosis due to an increased risk of death. ▮

- Use cautiously in patients with impaired CV function, glaucoma, seizure disorders, and Parkinson disease; in those who have been exposed to extreme heat or who are debilitated or appear emaciated; and in children with acute illness.

Reactions in bold italics are *life-threatening*. Interactions may have a *rapid onset* or a ***delayed onset***.

❸ Alert: Potentially irreversible tardive dyskinesia and potentially fatal NMS have been reported with antipsychotic use.

Dialyzable drug: No.

⚠ Overdose S&S: Dystonic reactions, CNS depression, agitation, restlessness, seizures, ECG changes, cardiac arrhythmias, fever, hypotension, dry mouth, ileus.

PREGNANCY-LACTATION-REPRODUCTION

• Safe use during pregnancy hasn't been established. Use only if potential benefit justifies fetal risk.

❸ Alert: Neonates exposed to antipsychotics in the third trimester are at risk for extrapyramidal or withdrawal symptoms after delivery that may range in severity from mild to severe and may require intensive care support.

• Drug may appear in human milk. Use cautiously during breastfeeding.

NURSING CONSIDERATIONS

• Watch for orthostatic hypotension, especially when giving drug IV.

• To reduce hypotension risk, patients receiving IV drug must remain supine and be observed for at least 30 minutes after administration.

• Monitor CBC, electrolyte levels, fasting glucose level, lipid panel, and LFT values during long-term therapy.

❸ Alert: Use drug only when vomiting can't be controlled by other measures or when only a few doses are needed. If more than four doses are needed in 24 hours, notify prescriber.

• Immediately report signs and symptoms of tardive dyskinesia (involuntary rhythmic movements of the face, tongue, or jaw) as drug may need to be discontinued.

• Immediately report signs and symptoms of NMS (high fever, confusion, muscle rigidity, unstable vital signs) as drug should be discontinued and supportive therapy begun.

• *Look alike–sound alike:* Don't confuse prochlorperazine with chlorpromazine.

PATIENT TEACHING

• Advise patient to report all adverse reactions and to immediately report signs and symptoms of tardive dyskinesia and NMS.

• Tell patient to avoid extreme heat because drug may interfere with the body's thermoregulatory mechanisms.

• Advise patient to avoid alcohol while taking drug because of increased CNS depression.

• Tell patient to call prescriber if more than prescribed doses are needed within 24 hours.

SAFETY ALERT!

promethazine hydrochloride
proe-METH-a-zeen

Histantil✿, Phenergan, Promethegan

Therapeutic class: Antiemetics
Pharmacologic class: Phenothiazines

AVAILABLE FORMS

Injection: 25 mg/mL, 50 mg/mL
Suppositories: 12.5 mg, 25 mg, 50 mg
Syrup: 6.25 mg/5 mL*
Tablets: 12.5 mg, 25 mg, 50 mg

INDICATIONS & DOSAGES

➤ **Motion sickness**

Adults: 25 mg PO or PR taken 30 minutes to 1 hour before departure. May repeat dose 8 to 12 hours later PRN. Then, 25 mg PO b.i.d. on successive travel days on rising and again before the evening meal.

Children age 2 and older: 12.5 to 25 mg PO or PR 30 minutes to 1 hour before departure. May repeat dose 8 to 12 hours later PRN.

➤ **Nausea and vomiting**

Adults: 12.5 to 25 mg PO, IM, IV, or PR every 4 to 6 hours PRN.

Children age 2 and older: 0.25 to 1 mg/kg PO or PR every 4 to 6 hours PRN. Or, 0.132 mg/kg IM.

➤ **Rhinitis, allergy symptoms**

Adults: 25 mg PO or PR at bedtime; or, 12.5 mg PO or PR t.i.d. and at bedtime. Or, 25 mg deep IM or IV. May repeat dose within 2 hours if needed. Use oral dosing as soon as possible.

Children age 2 and older: Maximum dose is 25 mg PO or PR at bedtime; or, 6.25 to 12.5 mg PO or PR t.i.d. Use lowest effective dose and avoid other respiratory depressants.

➤ **Nighttime sedation**

Adults: 25 to 50 mg PO, IM, or PR at bedtime. Or, 25 mg IV at bedtime.

Children age 2 and older: 0.5 to 1.1 mg/kg/dose (maximum, 25 mg) PO or PR at bedtime. Manufacturer doesn't provide exact dosage of parenteral promethazine. Use lowest possible effective dose.

P

➤ **Adjunct to analgesics for routine preoperative or postoperative sedation**

Adults: 25 to 50 mg IM, PO, or PR. Or, 25 mg IV in combination with an appropriately reduced dose of opioid or barbiturate and the required amount of a belladonna alkaloid.

Children age 2 and older: 0.5 to 1.1 mg/kg PO, IM, or PR in combination with an appropriately reduced dose of opioid or barbiturate and the appropriate dose of an atropine-like drug.

➤ **Obstetric sedation**

Adults: 25 to 50 mg deep IM or IV in the early stages of labor. When labor is definitely established, may give 25 to 75 mg IM or IV with an appropriately reduced dose of desired opioid. If necessary, may repeat once or twice at 4-hour intervals. Maximum dose is 100 mg/24 hours.

ADMINISTRATION

PO

• Reduce GI distress by giving drug with food or milk.

IV

▼ If solution is discolored or contains a precipitate, discard.

▼ Give injection through a free-flowing IV line; consider giving over 10 to 15 minutes to minimize risk of phlebitis.

Boxed Warning Be alert for extravasation. Severe chemical irritation and damage can result. ∎

⚫ *Alert:* Don't give at a concentration above 25 mg/mL or a rate above 25 mg/minute.

Boxed Warning Don't give IV solution subcutaneously or intra-arterially. ∎

▼ **Incompatibilities:** None listed by manufacturer. Consult a drug incompatibility reference for more information.

IM

Boxed Warning IM injection is the preferred parenteral route. Inject deep IM into large muscle mass. ∎

• Rotate injection sites.

Rectal

• If suppository is too soft, place wrapped in refrigerator for 15 minutes or run under cold water.

• Store in refrigerator between 36° and 46° F (2° and 8° C).

ACTION

Phenothiazine derivative that competes with histamine for H_1-receptor sites on effector cells. Prevents, but doesn't reverse, histamine-mediated responses. At high doses, drug also has local anesthetic effects.

Route	Onset	Peak	Duration
PO	15–60 min	Unknown	<12 hr
IV	3–5 min	Unknown	<12 hr
IM, PR	20 min	Unknown	<12 hr

Half-life: Approximately 9 to 19 hours depending on route and formulation.

ADVERSE REACTIONS

CNS: drowsiness, sedation, confusion, sleepiness, dizziness, disorientation, extrapyramidal symptoms, insomnia, nightmares, agitation, lassitude, incoordination, fatigue, tremors, *seizures,* catatonic-like state, hysteria. **CV:** hypotension, HTN, *bradycardia,* tachycardia. **EENT:** blurred vision, diplopia, tinnitus, nasal stuffiness, dry mouth, tongue protrusion. **GI:** nausea, vomiting. **GU:** urine retention. **Hematologic:** *leukopenia, thrombocytopenia, agranulocytosis.* **Hepatic:** jaundice. **Metabolic:** hyperglycemia. **Respiratory:** asthma, *respiratory depression, apnea.* **Skin:** photosensitivity, rash, urticaria, injection-site reaction, dermatitis. **Other:** *angioneurotic edema.*

INTERACTIONS

Drug-drug. *Anticholinergics, TCAs:* May increase anticholinergic effects. Avoid using together.

Antipsychotics: May increase risk of NMS. Monitor patient; discontinue promethazine if interaction is suspected.

CNS depressants: May increase sedation. Use together cautiously. If used together, reduce CNS depressant dosage.

Epinephrine: May block or reverse effects of epinephrine. Use other pressor drugs instead.

MAO inhibitors: May increase extrapyramidal effects. Avoid using together.

Drug-lifestyle. *Alcohol use:* May increase sedation. Discourage use together.

Sun exposure: May cause photosensitivity reactions. Advise patient to avoid extensive sunlight exposure and to use sun block.

EFFECTS ON LAB TEST RESULTS

• May increase blood glucose level.

• May decrease WBC, platelet, and granulocyte counts.

• May prevent, reduce, or mask positive result in diagnostic skin test.

Reactions in bold italics are *life-threatening.* Interactions may have a *rapid onset* or a ***delayed onset.***

- May cause false-positive or false-negative pregnancy test result.
- May cause false-positive or false-negative with urine detection of amphetamine and methamphetamine.

CONTRAINDICATIONS & CAUTIONS

- Contraindicated in patients hypersensitive to drug, in those who have experienced adverse reactions to phenothiazines, and in patients who are comatose and for treatment of lower respiratory tract symptoms, including asthma.

Boxed Warning Contraindicated in children younger than age 2 because of the potential for fatal respiratory depression. Use the lowest effective dose in children older than age 2 and avoid administering with drugs that can cause respiratory depression. ■

- Use cautiously in patients with a history of seizures and in those taking drugs that affect the seizure threshold as drug can lower the seizure threshold.
- Use cautiously in patients with pulmonary, hepatic, or CV disease; acutely ill or dehydrated children; and in those with intestinal obstruction, prostatic hyperplasia, bladderneck obstruction, angle-closure glaucoma, seizure disorders, CNS depression, bone marrow depression, or stenosing or peptic ulcerations.

Dialyzable drug: No.

⚠ *Overdose S&S:* Hypotension, respiratory depression, ataxia, athetosis, positive Babinski reflex, unconsciousness, hyperreflexia, hypertonia, dry mouth, fixed dilated pupils, flushing, GI symptoms, seizures, sudden death; hyperexcitability, nightmares (in children).

PREGNANCY-LACTATION-REPRODUCTION

- There are no adequate studies during pregnancy. Use only if potential benefit justifies fetal risk.
- Use of drug within 2 weeks of delivery may inhibit platelet aggregation in the newborn.
- It isn't known if drug appears in human milk. Patient should discontinue breastfeeding or discontinue drug.

NURSING CONSIDERATIONS

Boxed Warning Perivascular extravasation, unintentional intra-arterial injection, or intraneuronal or perineuronal infiltration of the drug may result in irritation and tissue

damage. Adverse reactions include burning, pain, thrombophlebitis, tissue necrosis, and gangrene. ■

- Monitor patient for NMS: altered mental status, autonomic instability, muscle rigidity, and hyperpyrexia.
- Stop drug 4 days before diagnostic skin testing because antihistamines can prevent, reduce, or mask positive skin test response.
- Drug is used as an adjunct to analgesics, usually to increase sedation; it has no analgesic activity.
- *Look alike–sound alike:* Don't confuse promethazine with chlorpromazine or prednisone.

PATIENT TEACHING

- Teach patient safe drug administration.
- When treating motion sickness, tell patient to take first dose 30 to 60 minutes before travel; dose may be repeated in 8 to 12 hours, if necessary. On succeeding days of travel, patient should take dose upon arising and with evening meal.
- Warn patient to avoid alcohol and hazardous activities that require alertness until CNS effects of drug are known.
- Tell patient to report all adverse reactions promptly.
- Warn patient about possible photosensitivity reactions. Advise patient to avoid sun, sunlamps, and tanning beds; use sun block; and wear protective clothing and eyewear.
- Advise patient to report discomfort at IV site immediately.
- Instruct patient to report involuntary muscle movements.

P

propafenone hydrochloride
proe-PAF-a-non

Rythmol SR

Therapeutic class: Antiarrhythmics
Pharmacologic class: Sodium channel antagonists

AVAILABLE FORMS

Capsules (extended-release) ⓓⓝⓒ: 225 mg, 325 mg, 425 mg
Tablets (immediate-release): 150 mg, 225 mg, 300 mg

INDICATIONS & DOSAGES

Adjust-a-dose (for all indications): Consider reducing dosage in patients with hepatic impairment, significant widening of the QRS complex, or second- or third-degree AV block. Reduce dosage in older adults.

➤ **To treat life-threatening ventricular arrhythmias such as sustained ventricular tachycardia; to prolong time to recurrence of paroxysmal supraventricular tachycardia (PSVT) and paroxysmal atrial fibrillation or flutter in patients without structural heart disease**

Adults: Initially, 150 mg immediate-release tablet PO every 8 hours. May increase dosage every 3 or 4 days to 225 mg every 8 hours. If needed, may increase dosage to 300 mg every 8 hours. Maximum daily dose, 900 mg.

➤ **To prolong time until recurrence of symptomatic atrial fibrillation (AF) in patients with episodic AF who don't have structural heart disease**

Adults: Initially, 150-mg immediate-release tablet PO every 8 hours. May increase dosage after 3 to 4 days to 225- to 300-mg immediate-release tablet PO every 8 hours. Maximum dosage is 900 mg/day. Or, 225 mg extended-release capsule PO every 12 hours. May increase dose after 5 days to 325 mg PO every 12 hours. May increase dose to 425 mg every 12 hours.

ADMINISTRATION
PO

- Give without regard to food.
- Don't crush or open the extended-release capsules.
- Skip a missed dose. Don't double the dose but give next dose at the usual time.

ACTION

Reduces inward sodium current in cardiac cells, prolongs refractory period in AV node, and decreases excitability, conduction velocity, and automaticity in cardiac tissue.

Route	Onset	Peak	Duration
PO (immediate-release)	Unknown	3.5 hr	Unknown
PO (extended-release)	Unknown	3–8 hr	Unknown

Half-life: 2 to 10 hours.

ADVERSE REACTIONS

CNS: dizziness, anxiety, asthenia, ataxia, drowsiness, fatigue, headache, insomnia, syncope, tremor, weakness, unusual taste. **CV: *HF, bradycardia, arrhythmias, ventricular tachycardia, PVCs, ventricular fibrillation,*** AF, bundle-branch block, angina, chest pain, edema, first-degree AV block, hypotension, prolonged QRS complex, intraventricular conduction delay, palpitations, murmur. **EENT:** blurred vision, dry mouth. **GI:** nausea, vomiting, constipation, diarrhea, dyspepsia, anorexia, flatulence. **Respiratory:** dyspnea, rales, URI, wheezing. **Skin:** rash, diaphoresis.

INTERACTIONS

Drug-drug. *Antiarrhythmics, fluoxetine, paroxetine, sertraline:* May increase risk of prolonged QTc interval and arrhythmias. Avoid use together.

Beta blockers (metoprolol, propranolol): May decrease metabolism of these drugs. Adjust dosage of beta blocker as needed and monitor therapy.

Cardiac glycosides (digoxin, digitoxin): May increase glycoside level. Reduce glycoside dosage and monitor patient closely.

Cimetidine: May increase propafenone levels. Monitor patient for adverse effects and toxicity.

Cyclosporine: May increase cyclosporine level, causing toxicity. Monitor patient closely; dosage adjustment may be necessary.

CYP2D6 inhibitors (paroxetine, ritonavir, sertraline), CYP3A4 inhibitors (erythromycin, ketoconazole, saquinavir): May increase propafenone level. Avoid use together.

Desipramine, imipramine, venlafaxine: May decrease metabolism of these drugs. Monitor patient closely.

Lidocaine: May decrease lidocaine metabolism. Monitor patient for increased CNS adverse effects and lidocaine toxicity.

Local anesthetics: May increase risk of CNS toxicity. Monitor patient closely.

Mexiletine: May decrease mexiletine metabolism, increasing level and adverse reactions. Monitor mexiletine level and patient closely.

Orlistat: May reduce fraction of propafenone available for absorption. Abrupt discontinuation of orlistat can result in severe adverse events. Use together with caution.

Phenobarbital, rifampin: May increase propafenone clearance. Watch for decreased antiarrhythmic effect.

Reactions in bold italics are *life-threatening*. Interactions may have a *rapid onset* or a **delayed onset**.

QTc interval–prolonging drugs (haloperidol, quinidine): Use together may enhance QTc-interval prolongation and risk of ventricular arrhythmias. Monitor patient closely and consider therapy modification.

Ritonavir: May increase propafenone level, causing life-threatening arrhythmias. Avoid using together.

SSRIs, TCAs: May increase risk of cardiac arrhythmias. Avoid use together.

Theophylline: May decrease theophylline metabolism. Monitor theophylline level and ECG closely.

Warfarin: May increase warfarin level. Monitor PT and INR closely, and adjust warfarin dose as needed.

Drug-food. *Grapefruit, grapefruit juice:* May increase drug level. Discourage use together.

Drug-lifestyle. *Smoking:* May increase propafenone level and risk of cardiac arrhythmias.

EFFECTS ON LAB TEST RESULTS
• May increase urine ketone, glucose, LDH, uric acid, ALP, ALT, and AST levels.
• May decrease potassium level.
• May cause positive ANA titers.

CONTRAINDICATIONS & CAUTIONS
• Contraindicated in patients hypersensitive to drug and in those with severe or uncontrolled HF; cardiogenic shock; SA, AV, or intraventricular disorders of impulse conduction without a pacemaker; bradycardia; Brugada syndrome; marked hypotension; bronchospastic disorders and severe obstructive pulmonary disease; or electrolyte imbalances.

Boxed Warning Class 1C antiarrhythmics, including propafenone, may significantly increase risk of adverse effects in patients with structural heart disease. ∎

Boxed Warning Because of propafenone's proarrhythmic effects, reserve its use for patients with life-threatening ventricular arrhythmias. ∎

• Drug has caused new or worsened arrhythmias. Monitor ECG before and during therapy.

• Use cautiously in patients with a history of HF because drug may weaken the contraction of the heart.

• Use cautiously in patients taking other cardiac depressants and in those with hepatic or renal impairment.

• Use cautiously in patients with myasthenia gravis; may cause exacerbation.

Dialyzable drug: Unlikely.

⚠ *Overdose S&S:* Hypotension, somnolence, bradycardia, intra-atrial and intraventricular conduction disturbance.

PREGNANCY-LACTATION-REPRODUCTION
• There are no adequate studies during pregnancy. Use only if potential benefit justifies fetal risk.
• Drug appears in human milk. Use drug cautiously during breastfeeding if clearly needed.

NURSING CONSIDERATIONS
↻ *Alert:* Perform continuous cardiac monitoring at start of therapy and during dosage adjustments. If PR interval or QRS complex increases by more than 25%, reduce dosage.
• Monitor HR and BP.
• Monitor electrolyte levels and correct abnormalities before and during therapy.
• If using with digoxin, frequently monitor ECG and digoxin level.
• Pacing and sensing thresholds of artificial pacemakers may change; monitor pacemaker function.
• Agranulocytosis may develop during first 2 to 3 months of therapy. If patient has an unexplained fever, monitor leukocyte count. WBC count usually normalizes 14 days after drug is discontinued.

PATIENT TEACHING
• Instruct patient in safe drug administration. Stress importance of taking drug exactly as prescribed.
• Advise patient to report all adverse reactions promptly, including fever, sore throat, chills, and other signs and symptoms of infection.
• Tell patient to report palpitations, dizziness, passing out, swelling in arms or legs, trouble breathing, or sudden weight gain.
• Instruct patient to report prolonged diarrhea, diaphoresis, vomiting, or loss of appetite or thirst, any of which may cause an electrolyte imbalance.
• Instruct patient to report changes in OTC, prescription, and supplement use.

SAFETY ALERT!

propofol
PROE-po-fole

Diprivan

Therapeutic class: Sedative-hypnotics
Pharmacologic class: Phenol derivatives

AVAILABLE FORMS
Injection: 10 mg/mL*

INDICATIONS & DOSAGES
➤ **To induce general anesthesia**
Adults younger than age 55 classified as American Society of Anesthesiologists (ASA) Physical Status (PS) category I or II: 2 to 2.5 mg/kg IV. Give in 40-mg boluses every 10 seconds until desired response is achieved.
Children ages 3 to 16 classified as ASA PS I or II: 2.5 to 3.5 mg/kg IV over 20 to 30 seconds.
Adjust-a-dose: In older adults and patients who are debilitated, hypovolemic, or classified as ASA PS III or IV, give 1 to 1.5 mg/kg, in 20-mg boluses, every 10 seconds. For cardiac anesthesia, give 20 mg (0.5 to 1.5 mg/kg) every 10 seconds until desired response is achieved. For patients undergoing neurosurgery, give 20 mg (1 to 2 mg/kg) every 10 seconds until desired response is achieved.
➤ **To maintain anesthesia**
Healthy adults younger than age 55: 0.1 to 0.2 mg/kg/minute (6 to 12 mg/kg/hour) IV. Or, 25- to 50-mg intermittent boluses PRN.
Healthy children ages 2 months to 16 years: Initially, 200 to 300 mcg/kg/minute for 30 minutes, then 125 to 150 mcg/kg/minute (7.5 to 9 mg/kg/hour) IV titrated to achieve desired clinical effect. Younger children may require higher maintenance infusion rates than older children.
Adjust-a-dose: In older adults and patients who are debilitated, hypovolemic, or classified as ASA PS III or IV, give half the usual maintenance dose (0.05 to 0.1 mg/kg/minute or 3 to 6 mg/kg/hour). For cardiac anesthesia with secondary opioid, 100 to 150 mcg/kg/minute; low dose with primary opioid, 50 to 100 mcg/kg/minute. For patients undergoing neurosurgery, give 100 to 200 mcg/kg/minute (6 to 12 mg/kg/hour).
➤ **Monitored anesthesia care**
Healthy adults younger than age 55: Initially, 100 to 150 mcg/kg/minute (6 to

9 mg/kg/hour) IV for 3 to 5 minutes or a slow injection of 0.5 mg/kg over 3 to 5 minutes. For maintenance dose, give infusion of 25 to 75 mcg/kg/minute (1.5 to 4.5 mg/kg/hour) for first 10 to 15 minutes, then reduce dosage to 25 to 50 mcg/kg/minute or incremental 10- or 20-mg boluses.
Adjust-a-dose: In older adults and patients who are debilitated or classified as ASA PS III or IV, give 80% of usual adult maintenance dose. Don't use rapid bolus.
➤ **To sedate patients in the ICU who are intubated**
Adults: Initially, 5 mcg/kg/minute (0.3 mg/kg/hour) IV for 5 minutes. Increments of 5 to 10 mcg/kg/minute (0.3 to 0.6 mg/kg/hour) over 5 to 10 minutes may be used until desired sedation is achieved. Maintenance rate, 5 to 50 mcg/kg/minute (0.3 to 3 mg/kg/hour). Maximum dosage, 4 mg/kg/hour unless benefits outweigh risks.

ADMINISTRATION
IV
⚠ *Alert:* Maintain strict aseptic technique when handling solution. Drug can support growth of microorganisms; don't use if solution might be contaminated. Don't access vial more than once or use on multiple patients.
▼ Shake well.
▼ Don't use if emulsion shows evidence of separation.
▼ Don't infuse through a filter with a pore size smaller than 5 microns. Give via larger veins in arms to decrease injection-site pain.
▼ Titrate drug daily to maintain minimum effective level. Allow 3 to 5 minutes between dosage adjustments to assess effects.
▼ Discard tubing and unused portions of drug after 12 hours.
▼ Store between 40° and 77° F (4° and 25° C); don't freeze.
▼ **Incompatibilities:** Other IV drugs, blood and plasma.

ACTION
Unknown. Rapid-acting IV sedative-hypnotic.

Route	Onset	Peak	Duration
IV	<40 sec	Unknown	10–15 min

Half-life: Initial, 40 minutes; terminal, 4 to 7 hours and up to 3 days after 10-day infusion.

Reactions in bold italics are *life-threatening*. Interactions may have a *rapid onset* or a **delayed onset**.

ADVERSE REACTIONS

CNS: dystonic or choreiform movement.
CV: *bradycardia, arrhythmia,* hypotension, HTN, decreased cardiac output, tachycardia. **Metabolic:** hypertriglyceridemia. **Respiratory:** *apnea, respiratory acidosis.* **Skin:** rash, pruritus. **Other:** burning or stinging at injection site.

INTERACTIONS

Drug-drug. *Inhaled anesthetics (enflurane, halothane, isoflurane), opioids (alfentanil, fentanyl, meperidine, morphine), sedatives (barbiturates, benzodiazepines, chloral hydrate, droperidol):* May increase anesthetic and sedative effects and further decrease BP and cardiac output. Monitor patient closely.
Valproate: May increase propofol level. Reduce propofol dosage and monitor patient closely.

EFFECTS ON LAB TEST RESULTS

• May increase serum triglyceride levels.

CONTRAINDICATIONS & CAUTIONS

• Contraindicated in patients hypersensitive to drug or its components (soybean oil, glycerol, egg lecithin, disodium edetate, sodium hydroxide); in patients with allergies to eggs, egg products, soybeans, or soy products; and in those unable to undergo general anesthesia or sedation.
◑ Alert: Repeated or lengthy use of general anesthetic and sedation drugs during surgeries or procedures in children younger than age 3 or in patients during the third trimester may affect the development of children's brains. Weigh benefits of appropriate anesthesia in young children and patients who are pregnant against risks.
• Use cautiously in older adults, patients who are hemodynamically unstable or who have seizures, and in those with respiratory disease, disorders of lipid metabolism, or increased ICP.
Dialyzable drug: Unknown.
⚠ Overdose S&S: Cardiorespiratory depression.

PREGNANCY-LACTATION-REPRODUCTION

• There are no adequate studies during pregnancy. Use only if clearly needed.
• Drug isn't recommended for obstetric uses, including cesarean deliveries, as it may cause neonatal CNS and respiratory depression.
• Drug appears in human milk. Avoid use during breastfeeding.

NURSING CONSIDERATIONS

• If drug is used for prolonged sedation in ICU, urine may turn green.
• For general anesthesia or monitored anesthesia care sedation, trained staff not involved in the surgical or diagnostic procedure should give drug. For ICU sedation, persons skilled in managing patients who are critically ill and trained in cardiopulmonary resuscitation and airway management should give drug.
• Continuously monitor vital signs.
◑ Alert: The FDA issued an alert after receiving reports of chills, fever, and body aches in several clusters of patients shortly after patients received propofol for sedation or general anesthesia. Various lots of the drug were tested, but no toxins, bacteria, or other signs of contamination were found. The FDA advises all health care providers to carefully follow the handling and use sections of the prescribing information for this drug. They recommend that all patients be evaluated for possible reactions following use of the drug, and that anyone experiencing signs of acute febrile reactions be evaluated for possible bacterial sepsis. They ask that any adverse events after the use of propofol be reported to the FDA MedWatch.
• Monitor patient at risk for hyperlipidemia for elevated triglyceride levels.
• Drug contains 0.1 g of fat (1.1 kcal)/mL. Reduce other lipid products if given together.
• Some formulations contain ethylenediaminetetraacetic acid, a strong metal chelator. Consider supplemental zinc during prolonged therapy and in patients predisposed to zinc deficiency (those with burns, sepsis, or diarrhea).
• Some formulations contain sodium metabisulfite, a sulfite, which may cause allergic-type reactions, including anaphylactic signs and symptoms and life-threatening or less severe asthmatic episodes, in certain susceptible people.
• When giving drug in the ICU, assess patient's CNS function daily to determine minimum dose needed.
• Stop drug gradually to prevent abrupt awakening and increased agitation.
• Drug may be misused. Manage drug to prevent risk of diversion.

PATIENT TEACHING

• Advise patient that performance of activities requiring mental alertness may be impaired for some time after drug use.
• Tell patient that abnormal dreams or anesthesia awareness may occur.
�£ Alert: Discuss with parents or caregivers of child younger than age 3 and with patients who are pregnant the benefits, risks, and appropriate timing of surgery or procedures requiring anesthetic and sedation drugs.

SAFETY ALERT!

propranolol hydrochloride ☒
proe-PRAN-oh-lol

Hemangeol, Inderal LA✦, Inderal XL, InnoPran XL

Therapeutic class: Antihypertensives
Pharmacologic class: Nonselective beta blockers

AVAILABLE FORMS

Capsules (extended-release) ☐: 60 mg, 80 mg, 120 mg, 160 mg
Injection: 1 mg/mL
Oral solution: 4 mg/mL, 4.28 mg/mL, 8 mg/mL
Tablets: 10 mg, 20 mg, 40 mg, 60 mg, 80 mg

INDICATIONS & DOSAGES

➤ **Angina pectoris**
Adults: Total doses of 80 to 320 mg/day (immediate-release) PO in two to four divided doses. Or, one 80-mg extended-release capsule daily. Increase dosage at 3- to 7-day intervals until optimal response is obtained or a maximum of 320 mg PO daily has been given.

➤ **To decrease risk of death after MI**
Adults: Initially, 40 mg PO t.i.d. After 1 month, titrate to 60 to 80 mg t.i.d. as tolerated. Maintenance dose is 180 to 240 mg/day in divided doses b.i.d., t.i.d., or q.i.d.

➤ **Supraventricular, ventricular, and atrial arrhythmias; tachyarrhythmias caused by excessive catecholamine action during anesthesia, hyperthyroidism, or pheochromocytoma**
Adults: 1 to 3 mg by slow IV push, not to exceed 1 mg/minute. After 3 mg have been given, another dose may be given in 2 minutes; subsequent doses, no sooner than every

4 hours. Transfer to oral therapy as soon as possible. Usual maintenance dose is 10 to 30 mg PO t.i.d. or q.i.d.

➤ **HTN**
Adults: Initially, 80 mg PO daily in two divided doses or extended-release form once daily. Increase at 3- to 7-day intervals to maximum daily dose of 640 mg (immediate-release or LA extended-release). Usual maintenance dose is 120 to 240 mg daily or 120 to 160 mg daily as extended-release. For Inderal XL or InnoPran XL, dose is 80 mg PO once daily at bedtime. Give consistently with or without food. Adjust to maximum of 120 mg daily if needed. Full effects are seen in about 2 to 3 weeks.

➤ **Essential tremor**
Adults: 40 mg (tablets or oral solution) PO b.i.d. Usual maintenance dose is 120 to 320 mg daily in three divided doses.

➤ **Hypertrophic subaortic stenosis**
Adults: 20 to 40 mg PO t.i.d. or q.i.d. before meals and at bedtime, or 80 to 160 mg LA extended-release capsules once daily.

➤ **Adjunctive therapy in pheochromocytoma**
Adults: 60 mg PO daily in divided doses with an alpha blocker 3 days before surgery.

➤ **Prevention of migraine**
Adults: Initially, 80 mg PO in divided doses (immediate-release) or daily (LA extended-release). May increase to 160 to 240 mg/day.

➤ **Proliferating infantile hemangioma requiring systemic therapy (Hemangeol)**
Infants ages 5 weeks to 5 months: Initially, 0.6 mg/kg PO b.i.d. for 1 week. Increase to 1.1 mg/kg PO b.i.d. after 1 week. Increase to maintenance dose of 1.7 mg/kg PO b.i.d. after 2 weeks of treatment and maintain for 6 months. Administer doses at least 9 hours apart during or after feeding.
Adjust-a-dose: Readjust dosage periodically for changes in child's weight.

ADMINISTRATION
PO

• Give immediate-release tablets on an empty stomach. Give extended-release capsules consistently with or without food. Food may increase absorption of propranolol.
• Adherence may be improved by giving drug twice daily or as extended-release capsules. Check with prescriber.

Reactions in bold italics are *life-threatening*. Interactions may have a *rapid onset* or a **delayed onset**.

• Check BP and apical pulse before giving drug. If hypotension or extremes in pulse rate occur, withhold drug and notify prescriber.
• Monitor HR and BP for 2 hours after first dose and when increasing Hemangeol dosage.
• Give Hemangeol during or right after a feeding. Skip dose if child isn't eating or is vomiting. Don't shake before use.
• Give Hemangeol directly into child's mouth using the oral dosing syringe. If needed, may dilute with a small quantity of milk or fruit juice and give in baby's bottle.
• Don't substitute extended-release form for immediate-release on a milligram-for-milligram basis. Retitration may be necessary.

IV

▼ For direct injection, give into a large vessel or into the tubing of a free-flowing, compatible IV solution; don't give by continuous IV infusion.
▼ Drug is compatible with D_5W, half-NSS, NSS, and lactated Ringer solution.
▼ Infusion rate shouldn't exceed 1 mg/minute.
▼ Double-check dose and route. IV doses are much smaller than oral doses.
▼ Monitor BP, ECG, central venous pressure, and HR and rhythm frequently, especially during IV administration. If patient develops severe hypotension, notify prescriber; a vasopressor may be prescribed.
▼ For overdose, give IV isoproterenol, IV atropine, or glucagon; refractory cases may require a pacemaker.
▼ **Incompatibilities:** None.

ACTION
Reduces cardiac oxygen demand by blocking catecholamine-induced increases in HR, BP, and force of myocardial contraction. Drug depresses renin secretion and prevents vasodilation of cerebral arteries.

Route	Onset	Peak	Duration
PO	30 min	1–4 hr	12 hr
PO (Hemangeol)	Rapid	1–4 hr	Unknown
PO (extended-release)	Unknown	6–14 hr	24 hr
IV	Immediate	1 min	5 min

Half-life: About 3 to 6 hours; 8 hours for InnoPran XL; 3 to 6 hours for Hemangeol.

ADVERSE REACTIONS
CNS: fatigue, lethargy, vivid dreams, agitation, hallucinations, disorientation, short-term memory loss, emotional lability, mental depression, light-headedness, dizziness, insomnia, sleep disorder. **CV:** hypotension, Raynaud syndrome (arterial insufficiency), *bradycardia, HF, intensification of AV block, mesenteric arterial thrombosis.* **EENT:** dry eyes, visual disturbances. **GI:** abdominal cramping, constipation, diarrhea, decreased appetite, nausea, vomiting, *ischemic colitis.* **GU:** impotence, Peyronie disease. **Hematologic:** *agranulocytosis,* purpura. **Respiratory:** bronchitis, bronchiolitis (infants), *bronchospasm.* **Skin:** rash, alopecia. **Other:** SLE, hypersensitivity reactions.

INTERACTIONS
Drug-drug. *ACE inhibitors, alpha blockers, antiarrhythmics (amiodarone), calcium channel blockers (diltiazem, verapamil):* May increase risk of hypotension and other cardiac adverse effects. Use together cautiously.
Aminophylline: May antagonize beta-blocking effects of propranolol. Use together cautiously.
Cardiac glycosides (digoxin): May reduce the positive inotrope effect of the glycoside. Monitor patient for clinical effect.
Cimetidine, ciprofloxacin, fluconazole, fluoxetine, paroxetine: May inhibit metabolism of propranolol. Watch for increased beta-blocking effect.
Dobutamine, isoproterenol: May decrease effects of these drugs. Monitor therapy.
Epinephrine: May cause severe vasoconstriction. Monitor BP and observe patient carefully.
Glucagon: May antagonize propranolol effect. May be used therapeutically and in emergencies.
Haloperidol: May cause cardiac arrest. Avoid using together.
Insulin, oral antidiabetics: May alter requirements for these drugs in previously stabilized diabetics. Monitor patient for hypoglycemia.
Lidocaine: May reduce clearance of lidocaine. Monitor lidocaine level closely.
MAO inhibitors, TCAs: May increase hypotensive effect. Monitor therapy.
NSAIDs: May blunt antihypertensive effect. Monitor therapy.
Phenothiazines (chlorpromazine, thioridazine): May increase risk of serious adverse reactions

P

to either drug. Use with thioridazine is contraindicated. If chlorpromazine must be used, monitor pulse rate and BP and decrease propranolol dosage as needed.

Propafenone, quinidine: May increase propranolol level. Monitor cardiac function, and adjust propranolol dose as needed.

Reserpine: May increase risk of hypotension, bradycardia, vertigo, or syncope. Monitor therapy.

Theophylline: May decrease theophylline clearance by 30% to 52% and diminish bronchodilatory effect. Consider therapy modification.

Warfarin: May increase warfarin level. Monitor PT and INR.

Drug-herb. *Ma huang:* May decrease antihypertensive effects. Discourage use together.

Drug-lifestyle. *Alcohol use:* May increase or decrease propranolol level. Discourage alcohol use.

Smoking: May decrease propranolol level. Monitor clinical response and adjust dosage as needed. Discourage smoking.

EFFECTS ON LAB TEST RESULTS
- May increase T_4, BUN, transaminase, ALP, potassium, and LDH levels.
- May decrease T_3 level.
- May decrease granulocyte count.

CONTRAINDICATIONS & CAUTIONS
⚠️ *Alert:* Abrupt withdrawal of drug may cause exacerbation of angina or MI. To discontinue drug, gradually reduce dosage over 1 to 2 weeks. If angina worsens or acute coronary insufficiency develops, resume therapy at least temporarily. Because CAD may be unrecognized, don't discontinue drug abruptly, even when taken for other indications.

- Contraindicated in patients with known hypersensitivity to drug, bronchial asthma, sinus bradycardia and heart block greater than first-degree, cardiogenic shock, and overt and decompensated HF (unless failure is secondary to a tachyarrhythmia that can be treated with propranolol).

- Hemangeol is contraindicated in infants weighing less than 2 kg, premature infants with corrected age younger than 5 weeks, infants with an HR less than 80 beats/minute or BP lower than 50/30 mm Hg, and in infants with greater than first-degree heart block, decompensated HF, asthma, pheochromocytoma, or history of bronchospasm.

- Use cautiously in patients with hepatic or renal impairment, Wolff-Parkinson-White syndrome, nonallergic bronchospastic diseases, or hepatic disease and in those taking other antihypertensives.

- Use cautiously in patients who have diabetes because drug masks some symptoms of hypoglycemia.

- Use cautiously in patients with renal insufficiency due to increased risk of hypoglycemia.

- In patients with thyrotoxicosis, use drug cautiously because it may mask the signs and symptoms. Abrupt withdrawal may exacerbate symptoms of hyperthyroidism, including thyroid storm.

- Older adults may experience enhanced adverse reactions and may need dosage adjustment.

Dialyzable drug: No.

⚠️ *Overdose S&S:* Bradycardia, hypotension.

PREGNANCY-LACTATION-REPRODUCTION
- There are no adequate studies during pregnancy. Use only if potential benefit justifies fetal risk.

- Drug is associated with fetal intrauterine growth retardation and neonatal bradycardia, hypoglycemia, and respiratory depression. If drug is used during pregnancy, ensure adequate monitoring of infants is available at birth.

- Drug appears in human milk. Use cautiously during breastfeeding. Monitor infants for signs and symptoms of beta blockade and hypoglycemia.

NURSING CONSIDERATIONS
- Drug masks common signs and symptoms of shock and hypoglycemia.

- Monitor HR and BP.

▧ Some antihypertensives are less effective in lowering BP when used as monotherapy in patients who are Black. Monitor these patients for expected therapeutic effects; dosage and therapy adjustments may be necessary.

⚠️ *Alert:* Don't stop drug before surgery for pheochromocytoma. Before any surgical procedure, tell anesthesiologist that patient is receiving propranolol.

- *Look alike–sound alike:* Don't confuse propranolol with prasugrel. Don't confuse Inderal with Isordil, Adderall, or Imuran.

Reactions in bold italics are *life-threatening*. Interactions may have a *rapid onset* or a *delayed onset*.

PATIENT TEACHING
- Instruct patient in safe drug administration.
- Caution patient to continue taking drug as prescribed, even if feeling well, and to promptly report adverse reactions.
- Advise patient that propranolol may interfere with glaucoma screening because it can reduce IOP.
- Teach caregiver to skip Hemangeol dose if child isn't eating or is vomiting.
- ◑ *Alert:* Caution patient not to stop drug without advice from prescriber because abruptly stopping drug can worsen chest pain or cause an MI.
- Advise patient to avoid smoking and alcohol.
- Inform patient or caregivers of risk of hypoglycemia, especially in children with prolonged physical exertion.

pyridostigmine bromide
peer-id-oh-STIG-meen

Mestinon*, Regonol*

Therapeutic class: Muscle stimulants
Pharmacologic class: Cholinesterase inhibitors

AVAILABLE FORMS
Injection: 5 mg/mL
Syrup: 60 mg/5 mL*
Tablets: 30 mg, 60 mg
Tablets (extended-release) ⓓ: 180 mg

INDICATIONS & DOSAGES
Adjust-a-dose (for all indications): Smaller doses may be required in patients with renal disease. Adjust dosage to achieve desired effect.
➤ **Antidote for nondepolarizing neuromuscular blockers**
Adults: 0.1 to 0.25 mg/kg IV. Immediately before or with dose, also give atropine sulfate 0.6 to 1.2 mg IV or an equipotent dose of glycopyrrolate.
➤ **Myasthenia gravis**
Adults: 60 to 120 mg immediate-release PO every 3 or 4 hours. Average dosage is 600 mg daily, but dosages up to 1,500 mg daily may be needed. Dosage must be adjusted for each patient, based on response and tolerance. Or, 180 to 540 mg extended-release tablets PO daily or b.i.d., with at least 6 hours between doses.

ADMINISTRATION
PO
- Don't crush extended-release tablets.
- If patient has trouble swallowing, give syrup form. If patient can't tolerate sweet flavor, give over ice chips.
IV
◑ *Alert:* Drug should only be administered by individuals familiar with its actions, characteristics, and hazards.
▼ Don't use solution if it contains particulate matter or appears discolored.
▼ Position patient to ease breathing. Keep atropine injection available, and be prepared to give it immediately.
▼ Monitor vital signs frequently, especially respirations. Provide respiratory support as needed.
▼ Give injection no faster than 1 mg/minute. Rapid infusion may cause bradycardia and seizures.
▼ **Incompatibilities:** Alkaline solutions.

ACTION
Inhibits acetylcholinesterase, blocking destruction of acetylcholine from the parasympathetic and somatic efferent nerves. Acetylcholine accumulates, promoting increased stimulation of the receptors.

Route	Onset	Peak	Duration
PO	20–30 min	2 hr	3–4 hr
PO (extended-release)	30–60 min	1–2 hr	6–12 hr
IV	2–5 min	Unknown	2–3 hr

Half-life: 1 to 3 hours depending on route.

ADVERSE REACTIONS
CNS: headache with high doses, weakness, syncope, hyperesthesia. **CV:** *bradycardia, cardiac arrest,* hypotension, thrombophlebitis. **EENT:** miosis, amblyopia, epistaxis, rhinorrhea, increased salivation. **GI:** nausea, vomiting, abdominal cramps, diarrhea, increased peristalsis. **GU:** urinary frequency, urinary urgency, dysmenorrhea. **Musculoskeletal:** muscle cramps, muscle fasciculations, muscle weakness, tingling in extremities, myalgia, neck pain. **Respiratory:** *bronchospasm, bronchoconstriction,* increased bronchial secretions. **Skin:** rash, diaphoresis, dry skin.

P

INTERACTIONS

Drug-drug. *Aminoglycosides, anticholinergics, atropine, corticosteroids, general or local anesthetics, magnesium, procainamide, quinidine, tetracyclines:* May antagonize cholinergic effects. Observe patient for lack of drug effect.

Beta blockers: May increase bradycardia risk. Monitor therapy.

Ganglionic blockers: May increase risk of hypotension. Monitor patient closely.

Succinylcholine: May prolong the phase I block of the depolarizing muscle relaxant. Avoid using together.

EFFECTS ON LAB TEST RESULTS

None reported.

CONTRAINDICATIONS & CAUTIONS

• Contraindicated in patients hypersensitive to anticholinesterases or bromides and in those with mechanical obstruction of the intestinal or urinary tract.

• Use cautiously in patients with bronchial asthma, bradycardia, arrhythmias, epilepsy, recent coronary occlusion, vagotonia, renal impairment, hyperthyroidism, glaucoma, or peptic ulcer.

• Safety and effectiveness in children haven't been established.

Dialyzable drug: Unknown.

PREGNANCY-LACTATION-REPRODUCTION

• Drug may cross placental barrier. Use during pregnancy only if potential benefits justify maternal and fetal hazards.

• Drug appears in human milk. Use cautiously during breastfeeding.

NURSING CONSIDERATIONS

• Stop all other cholinergics before giving this drug.

• Monitor and document patient's response after each dose. Optimum dosage is difficult to judge.

• Monitor ECG, BP, and HR, especially when giving drug IV.

• Monitor patient for cholinergic reactions (nausea, vomiting, diarrhea, increased salivation). Use atropine immediately to treat cholinergic crisis.

🛈 **Alert:** Regonol contains benzyl alcohol preservative, which may cause toxicity in neonates.

• Mestinon syrup contains 5% alcohol.

• *Look alike–sound alike:* Don't confuse pyridostigmine with physostigmine. Don't confuse Regonol with Reglan or Renagel.

PATIENT TEACHING

• Advise patient to report all adverse reactions.

• When giving drug for myasthenia gravis, stress importance of taking exactly as prescribed, on time, in evenly spaced doses.

• Explain that patient may have to take drug for life.

• Advise patient to wear or carry medical identification that indicates patient has myasthenia gravis.

QUEtiapine fumarate

kwe-TYE-a-peen

Seroquel❤, Seroquel XR

Therapeutic class: Antipsychotics
Pharmacologic class: Dibenzothiazepine derivatives

AVAILABLE FORMS

Tablets: 25 mg, 50 mg, 100 mg, 200 mg, 300 mg, 400 mg
Tablets (extended-release) 🔲*:* 50 mg, 150 mg, 200 mg, 300 mg, 400 mg

INDICATIONS & DOSAGES

Adjust-a-dose (for all indications): Use slower titration rates and lower target doses in older adults and patients who are debilitated or who are predisposed to hypotension. Begin older adults on 50 mg/day (immediate-release or extended-release) and increase by 50 mg/day as needed depending on clinical response and tolerability.

Patients with hepatic impairment should begin immediate-release with 25 mg/day and increase by 25 to 50 mg/day to an effective dose, or begin extended-release with 50 mg/day and increase by 50 mg/day to an effective dose, depending on clinical response and tolerability.

Adjust dosage when drug is used in combination with CYP3A4 inducers and inhibitors.

➤ **Schizophrenia**

Adults: Initially, 25 mg (immediate-release) PO b.i.d., with increases in increments of 25 to 50 mg b.i.d. or t.i.d. on days 2 and 3, as tolerated. Target range is 300 to 400 mg

---

daily divided into two or three doses by day 4. Further dosage adjustments, if indicated, should occur at intervals of not less than 2 days. Dosage can be increased or decreased by 25 to 50 mg b.i.d. Effect generally occurs at 150 to 750 mg daily. Maximum dosage is 750 mg/day for acute therapy, or 800 mg/day for maintenance treatment.

Or, initially, 300 mg/day (extended-release) PO once daily, preferably in the evening. Titrate within a dose range of 400 to 800 mg/day, depending on the response and tolerance of the individual. Increase at intervals as short as 1 day and in increments of up to 300 mg/day. Maximum dose is 800 mg/day (extended-release).

Adolescents ages 13 to 17: Initially, 25 mg (immediate-release) PO b.i.d. on day 1; 50 mg b.i.d. on day 2; 100 mg b.i.d. on day 3; 150 mg b.i.d. on day 4; and 200 mg b.i.d. on day 5. Adjust dosage by no more than 100 mg/day. Usual dosage for immediate-release tablets is 400 to 800 mg/day, divided into two or three doses depending on response and tolerability; maximum dosage, 800 mg/day. Or initially, 50 mg/day (extended-release) PO on day 1; 100 mg/day on day 2; 200 mg/day on day 3; 300 mg/day on day 4; and 400 mg/day on day 5. Make adjustments in increments of no greater than 100 mg/day. Usual extended-release dosage is 400 to 800 mg/day; maximum dosage, 800 mg/day.

➤ **Monotherapy and adjunctive therapy with lithium or divalproex for the short-term treatment of acute manic episodes associated with bipolar I disorder; adjunctive maintenance therapy with lithium or divalproex**

Adults: Initially, 50 mg (immediate-release) PO b.i.d. on day 1; 100 mg b.i.d. on day 2; 150 mg b.i.d. on day 3; and 200 mg b.i.d. on day 4. Further dosage adjustments after day 4 should be no greater than 200 mg daily to a maximum daily dose of 800 mg. Usual dose is 400 to 800 mg daily. For maintenance therapy with lithium or divalproex, continue treatment at the dosage required to maintain symptom remission.

Or, start with 300 mg (extended-release) PO on day 1 and 600 mg PO on day 2 once daily in the evening. Dosage may be adjusted based on response and tolerability to maximum dosage of 800 mg/day.

➤ **Bipolar I disorder, acute manic episodes**
Children and adolescents ages 10 to 17: Total daily dosage for initial 5 days of therapy is 50 mg PO on day 1, then 100 mg on day 2, then 200 mg on day 3, then 300 mg on day 4, and 400 mg on day 5, given in divided doses b.i.d. or t.i.d. (immediate-release) or daily (extended-release). After day 5, adjust dosage in increments of no more than 100 mg/day within the recommended range of 400 to 600 mg/day. Maximum dosage, 600 mg/day.

➤ **Bipolar depression**
Adults: Initially, 50 mg PO once daily at bedtime; increase on day 2 to 100 mg; increase on day 3 to 200 mg; increase on day 4 to maintenance dose of 300 mg/day. Maximum dosage, 300 mg/day (immediate- or extended-release).

➤ **Major depressive disorder, adjunctive therapy with antidepressants**
Adults: 50 mg PO (extended-release) once daily in the evening on days 1 and 2. On day 3, may increase dosage to 150 mg PO once daily in the evening. Dosages ranging from 150 to 300 mg/day have proved effective.

ADMINISTRATION
PO
• Don't crush or allow patient to chew extended-release tablets.
• Give immediate-release tablets without regard for food; give extended-release tablets without food or with a light meal (about 300 calories), preferably in the evening.
• Patients who are currently being treated with divided doses of the immediate-release form may be switched to extended-release tablets at the equivalent total daily dose taken once daily. Individual dosage adjustments may be necessary.

ACTION
Blocks dopamine type 2 (D_2) and serotonin type 2A ($5-HT_{2A}$) receptors. Its action may be mediated through this antagonism.

Route	Onset	Peak	Duration
PO	Unknown	1.5 hr	Unknown
PO (extended-release)	Unknown	6 hr	Unknown

Half-life: 6 hours; extended-release, 7 to 12 hours.

ADVERSE REACTIONS
CNS: dizziness, headache, drowsiness, somnolence, hypertonia, dysarthria, asthenia,

agitation, extrapyramidal reaction, fatigue, lethargy, hypersomnia, pain, change in dreams, anxiety, schizophrenia, paresthesia, irritability, restlessness, migraine, ataxia, confusion, disorientation, fever, depression, attention disturbance, thirst. **CV:** orthostatic hypotension, tachycardia, palpitations, peripheral edema, hypotension, HTN, syncope. **EENT:** blurred vision, amblyopia, ear pain, epistaxis, nasal congestion, pharyngitis, rhinitis, sinusitis, dry mouth, toothache. **GI:** dyspepsia, abdominal pain, constipation, nausea, vomiting, increased or decreased appetite, diarrhea, gastroenteritis, dysphagia, gastroesophageal reflux. **GU:** UTI, decreased libido, urinary frequency. **Hematologic:** *leukopenia, neutropenia, agranulocytosis.* **Metabolic:** weight gain, hyperglycemia, hyperlipidemia, increased ALT level. **Musculoskeletal:** back pain, neck pain, arthralgia, myalgia, weakness, tremor, dyskinesia, akathisia, restless leg syndrome, muscle spasms. **Respiratory:** increased cough, dyspnea. **Skin:** rash, diaphoresis, pallor, acne. **Other:** flulike syndrome, *accidental overdose.*

INTERACTIONS

Drug-drug. *Anticholinergics:* May increase anticholinergic effects. Use together cautiously; monitor patient for urine retention.
Antihypertensives: May increase effects of antihypertensives. Monitor BP.
CNS depressants: May increase CNS effects. Use together cautiously.
Dopamine agonists, levodopa: May antagonize the effects of these drugs. Monitor patient.
Lorazepam: May decrease lorazepam clearance and increase CNS depression. Monitor patient for increased CNS effects.
Opioids: May cause slow or difficult breathing, sedation, and death. Avoid use together if possible. If use together is necessary, limit dosage and duration of each drug to minimum necessary for desired effect. Consider therapy modification.
QTc interval–prolonging drugs: May enhance QTc-interval prolongation and risk of ventricular arrhythmias. Avoid use in patients at highest risk; monitor therapy for those at lower risk.
Strong CYP3A4 inducers (carbamazepine, phenobarbital, phenytoin, rifampin, thioridazine): May decrease quetiapine serum concentration. Increase quetiapine dosage up to fivefold of the original dose when used in combination with prolonged treatment (greater than 7 to 14 days); titrate based on clinical response and tolerability. When the CYP3A4 inducer is discontinued, reduce quetiapine dosage to the original level within 7 to 14 days.
Strong CYP3A4 inhibitors (erythromycin, fluconazole, itraconazole, ketoconazole, nefazodone, ritonavir): May increase quetiapine serum concentration. Reduce quetiapine dosage to one-sixth of original dose when used together. When the CYP3A4 inhibitor is discontinued, increase quetiapine dosage by sixfold.
Voriconazole: May decrease quetiapine metabolism. Consider therapy modification.
Drug-herb. *St. John's wort:* May increase risk of serotonin syndrome and decrease quetiapine serum concentration. Consider therapy modification.
Drug-lifestyle. *Alcohol use, cannabis/cannabidiol:* May increase CNS effects. Discourage use together.

EFFECTS ON LAB TEST RESULTS

- May increase liver enzyme, prolactin, TSH, cholesterol, triglyceride, and glucose levels.
- May decrease T_4 level.
- May decrease WBC count.
- May cause false-positive results in urine enzyme immunoassays for methadone and TCAs.

CONTRAINDICATIONS & CAUTIONS

- Contraindicated in patients hypersensitive to drug or its ingredients.

Boxed Warning The risk of cerebrovascular adverse events (stroke, transient ischemic attack) and death is increased in older adults with dementia-related psychosis. Quetiapine isn't approved for the treatment of patients with dementia-related psychosis. ∎

Boxed Warning Suicidality may occur in children, adolescents, and young adults (younger than age 24) who are taking quetiapine. Watch for clinical worsening and suicidality in patients of all ages who are started on antidepressant therapy. Quetiapine isn't approved for use in children younger than age 10. ∎

- Avoid use when risk of torsades de pointes or sudden death may be increased, including in patients with a history of cardiac

---

Reactions in bold italics are *life-threatening.* Interactions may have a *rapid onset* or a *delayed onset.*

arrhythmias such as bradycardia, hypokalemia, or hypomagnesemia. Also avoid use with other drugs that prolong the QTc interval and in patients with congenital prolongation of the QT interval.

- Use cautiously in patients with increased risk of QT-interval prolongation, such as those with CV disease, family history of QT-interval prolongation, HF, or heart hypertrophy, and in older adults.
- Use cautiously in patients at risk for falls, including those with diseases, conditions, or who are taking medications that may cause somnolence, orthostatic hypotension, or motor or sensory instability.
- Use cautiously in patients with CV disease, cerebrovascular disease, conditions that predispose to hypotension, a history of seizures or conditions that lower the seizure threshold, urine retention, clinically significant prostatic hypertrophy, or constipation, and conditions in which core body temperature may be elevated.
- Rare cases of NMS have been reported. Monitor patients for mental status changes, fever, muscle rigidity, or autonomic instability.
- Drug may cause extrapyramidal signs and symptoms. Consider stopping drug for signs or symptoms of tardive dyskinesia.
- Use cautiously in patients with renal disease; experience is limited.
- Use cautiously in patients at risk for aspiration pneumonia.
- Use cautiously in patients with preexisting low WBC count or history of drug-induced leukopenia or neutropenia. Drug may cause leukopenia, neutropenia, and agranulocytosis, including fatal cases. Monitor CBC frequently during first few months; discontinue therapy at first sign of decline in WBC count.
Dialyzable drug: Unknown.
⚠ Overdose S&S: Drowsiness, hypotension, sedation, tachycardia, hypokalemia, delirium, QTc-interval prolongation, first-degree heart block.

PREGNANCY-LACTATION-REPRODUCTION

⊙ Alert: Neonates exposed to antipsychotics during the third trimester are at risk for developing extrapyramidal signs and symptoms (repetitive muscle movements of the face and body) and withdrawal signs and symptoms (agitation, abnormally increased or decreased muscle tone, tremors, sleepiness, severe difficulty breathing, difficulty feeding) after

delivery. Use in pregnancy only if potential benefit justifies fetal risk.

- Enroll patients exposed to drug during pregnancy in the National Pregnancy Registry for Atypical Antipsychotics (1-866-961-2388 or www.womensmentalhealth.org/research/pregnancy registry).
- Drug appears in human milk. Breastfeeding isn't recommended.
- Drug may reversibly decrease fertility in patients of childbearing potential.

NURSING CONSIDERATIONS

⊙ Alert: Watch for evidence of NMS (extrapyramidal effects, hyperthermia, autonomic disturbance), which is rare but deadly.

- Complete fall risk assessments when initiating antipsychotic treatment and recurrently for patients on long-term therapy, especially for patients with diseases, conditions, or who are taking other drugs that could exacerbate fall risk.
- Monitor patient for tardive dyskinesia, which may occur after prolonged use. It may not appear until months or years later and may disappear spontaneously or persist for life, despite ending drug. Antipsychotic treatment may suppress signs and symptoms of tardive dyskinesia and may mask the underlying process. Consider discontinuing therapy if signs or symptoms of tardive dyskinesia occur.
- Hyperglycemia may occur in patients taking drug. Monitor patients with diabetes regularly. All patients should be monitored for signs and symptoms of hyperglycemia and undergo a fasting blood glucose test if signs or symptoms develop during treatment.
- Monitor BP before and periodically during therapy. Hypotension in all patients and HTN in children and adolescents can occur.
- Monitor patient with signs and symptoms of infection for neutropenia. Treat promptly if signs and symptoms of neutropenia occur; discontinue drug for ANC less than 1,000/mm^3.
- Monitor patient for weight gain by checking waist circumference and BMI.
⊙ Alert: Monitor patient for symptoms of metabolic syndrome (significant weight gain and increased BMI, HTN, hyperglycemia, hypercholesterolemia, and hypertriglyceridemia).
- Monitor patient for hyperprolactinemia (galactorrhea, amenorrhea, gynecomastia, impotence, decreased bone density).

• Drug use may cause cataract formation with long-term use. Obtain baseline ophthalmologic exam and reassess every 6 months.

• Gradually reduce dosage when discontinuing drug and monitor patient for withdrawal signs and symptoms (insomnia, nausea, vomiting, headache, dizziness, irritability).

PATIENT TEACHING

Boxed Warning Suicidality may occur in children, adolescents, and young adults (younger than age 24) taking quetiapine. Advise families and caregivers of the need for close observation and communication with prescriber if suicidality occurs. ∎

• Advise patient and caregiver to use caution when quetiapine is being taken with other centrally acting drugs because of the risk of increased CNS effects.

• Caution patient to avoid alcohol, cannabis, and cannabidiol while taking drug.

• Tell patient to report other prescription or OTC drugs being taken.

• Warn patient about risk of dizziness when standing up quickly. The risk is greatest during the 3- to 5-day period of first dosage adjustment, when resuming treatment, and when increasing dosages.

• Tell patient to avoid becoming overheated or dehydrated.

• Advise patient to report signs and symptoms of hyperglycemia (excessive thirst, excessive urination, excessive hunger or weakness).

• Warn patient to avoid activities that require mental alertness until effects of drug are known, especially during first dosage adjustment or dosage increases.

• Remind patient to have an eye exam at start of therapy and every 6 months during therapy to check for cataracts.

• Tell patient of childbearing potential to report planned, suspected, or known pregnancy.

• Advise patient not to breastfeed during therapy.

• Instruct patient in proper drug administration.

• Tell patient and caregivers to report all adverse reactions and to be alert for fever, muscle rigidity, repetitive muscle movements of the face, anxiety, agitation, panic attacks, insomnia, irritability, hostility, aggressiveness, impulsivity, motor restlessness, hypomania, mania, other unusual changes in behavior, worsening of depression, and suicidality.

• Advise patient that drug may cause somnolence, orthostatic hypotension, and motor and sensory instability, which may lead to falls, fractures, or other injuries.

• Tell patient not to stop medication abruptly.

quinapril hydrochloride ☒
KWIN-a-pril

Accupril✱

Therapeutic class: Antihypertensives
Pharmacologic class: ACE inhibitors

AVAILABLE FORMS
Tablets: 5 mg, 10 mg, 20 mg, 40 mg

INDICATIONS & DOSAGES
➤ **HTN**
Adults: Initially, 10 to 20 mg PO daily. May adjust dosage based on patient response at intervals of at least 2 weeks. Most patients are controlled at 20 to 80 mg daily as a single dose or in two equally divided doses. If patient is taking a diuretic, start therapy with 5 mg daily.

Older adults: For patients age 65 and older, start therapy at 10 mg PO daily and titrate to optimal response.

Adjust-a-dose: For adults with CrCl over 60 mL/minute, give 10 mg once daily initially; for CrCl of 30 to 60 mL/minute, 5 mg PO daily initially; for CrCl of 10 to 30 mL/minute, 2.5 mg PO daily initially.

➤ **HF**
Adults: 5 mg PO b.i.d. initially. Dosage may be increased at weekly intervals. Usual effective dose is 20 to 40 mg daily in two equally divided doses.

Adjust-a-dose: For patients with CrCl over 30 mL/minute, first dose is 5 mg PO daily. If tolerated, increase to b.i.d. dosing the next day. Adjust dosage at weekly intervals thereafter. If CrCl is 10 to 30 mL/minute, first dose is 2.5 mg PO daily. If tolerated, increase to b.i.d. dosing the next day. Adjust dosage at weekly intervals thereafter.

ADMINISTRATION
PO
• Don't give drug with a high-fat meal because this may decrease absorption of drug.

ACTION

Prevents conversion of angiotensin I to angiotensin II, a potent vasoconstrictor. Less angiotensin II decreases peripheral arterial resistance, decreasing aldosterone secretion, which reduces sodium and water retention and lowers BP.

Route	Onset	Peak	Duration
PO	1 hr	1–4 hr	24 hr

Half-life: Quinapril, 0.8 hour; quinaprilat, 3 hours.

ADVERSE REACTIONS

CNS: headache, dizziness, fatigue. **CV:** hypotension, chest pain. **GI:** abdominal pain, vomiting, nausea, diarrhea. **Metabolic:** elevated creatinine and BUN levels, *hyperkalemia.* **Musculoskeletal:** back pain, myalgia. **Respiratory:** cough, dyspnea. **Skin:** rash.

INTERACTIONS

Drug-drug. ● *Alert: Aliskiren:* May increase risk of renal impairment, hypotension, and hyperkalemia in patients with diabetes and those with moderate to severe renal impairment (GFR less than 60 mL/minute). Concomitant use is contraindicated in patients with diabetes. Avoid concomitant use in patients with moderate to severe renal impairment.

Diuretics, other antihypertensives: May cause excessive hypotension. Stop diuretic or reduce dose of quinapril, as needed.

Lithium: May increase lithium level and lithium toxicity. Monitor lithium level.

Neprilysin inhibitors (sacubitril, sacubitril–valsartan): May increase risk of angioedema. Use together is contraindicated.

NSAIDs: May decrease antihypertensive effects. Monitor BP. Combination may result in a significant decrease in renal function. Monitor renal function.

Potassium-sparing diuretics, potassium supplements: May cause hyperkalemia. Monitor patient closely.

Tetracycline: May decrease absorption if taken with quinapril. Separate dosing times by at least 2 hours if used together. Consider therapy modification.

Drug-herb. *Yohimbe:* May decrease antihypertensive effects. Discourage use together.

Drug-food. *Salt substitutes containing potassium:* May cause hyperkalemia. Discourage use together.

EFFECTS ON LAB TEST RESULTS

• May increase potassium, BUN, and creatinine levels, and LFT values.
• May decrease sodium level.
• May decrease granulocyte and platelet counts.
• May lead to false-negative aldosterone/renin ratio.

CONTRAINDICATIONS & CAUTIONS

• Contraindicated in patients hypersensitive to ACE inhibitors and in those with a history of angioedema related to treatment with an ACE inhibitor.
• Contraindicated when used within 36 hours of switching to or from a neprilysin inhibitor, such as sacubitril or the combination drug sacubitril–valsartan.
• Use cautiously in patients with impaired renal function.
• Acute renal failure and hypertensive crisis have been reported.
• Safety and effectiveness in children haven't been established.

Dialyzable drug: No.

⚠ *Overdose S&S:* Severe hypotension.

PREGNANCY-LACTATION-REPRODUCTION

Boxed Warning Use of drugs that act directly on the RAAS can cause injury and death to a developing fetus. Stop drug as soon as possible for confirmed pregnancy. ▮
• Drug appears in human milk. Use cautiously during breastfeeding.

NURSING CONSIDERATIONS

• Monitor patient for angioedema, including of the head, neck, and extremities (stridor, edema of the face, tongue, glottis) and of the intestines (abdominal pain with or without nausea or vomiting). If there is airway involvement, treat emergently, including epinephrine 1:1,000 (0.3 to 0.5 mL) if necessary.
• Assess renal and hepatic function before and periodically throughout therapy.
• Monitor BP for effectiveness of therapy. When adjusting dosage, measure BP before giving dose (trough) and 2 to 6 hours after dosing (peak).
• Monitor potassium level. Risk factors for hyperkalemia include renal insufficiency, diabetes, and concomitant use of drugs that raise potassium level.

Q

⌧ Although ACE inhibitors reduce BP in all races, they reduce it less in Blacks taking an ACE inhibitor alone. Patients who are Black should take drug with a thiazide diuretic for a better response.

⌧ ACE inhibitors appear to increase risk of angioedema in patients who are Black.

• Other ACE inhibitors have caused agranulocytosis and neutropenia. Monitor CBC with differential counts before therapy and periodically thereafter.

PATIENT TEACHING

• Advise patient to report signs of infection, such as fever and sore throat.

🜚 *Alert:* Facial and throat swelling (including swelling of the tongue and larynx) may occur, especially after first dose. Advise patient to report signs or symptoms of breathing difficulty or swelling of face, eyes, lips, or tongue.

• Light-headedness can occur, especially during first few days of therapy. Tell patient to rise slowly to minimize effect and to report signs and symptoms to prescriber. If fainting occurs, patient should stop taking drug and call prescriber immediately.

• Inform patient that inadequate fluid intake, vomiting, diarrhea, and excessive perspiration can lead to light-headedness and fainting. Tell patient to use caution in hot weather and during exercise.

• Tell patient to avoid salt substitutes. These products may contain potassium, which can cause high potassium level in patients taking quinapril.

• Advise patient of childbearing potential about potential fetal hazards and to immediately report pregnancy. Drug will need to be stopped.

• Tell patient to avoid taking with a high-fat meal because this may decrease absorption of drug.

RABEprazole sodium
ra-BEP-ra-zole

Aciphex ✦

Therapeutic class: Antiulcer drugs
Pharmacologic class: PPIs

AVAILABLE FORMS

Tablets (delayed-release) ⓞⓣⓒ: 20 mg

INDICATIONS & DOSAGES

➤ **Healing of erosive or ulcerative GERD**
Adults: 20 mg PO daily for 4 to 8 weeks. Additional 8-week course may be considered, if needed.

➤ **Maintenance of healing of erosive or ulcerative GERD**
Adults: 20 mg PO daily for up to 12 months.

➤ **Healing of duodenal ulcers**
Adults: 20 mg PO daily after morning meal for up to 4 weeks.

➤ **Pathologic hypersecretory conditions, including Zollinger-Ellison syndrome**
Adults: Initially, 60 mg PO daily; may increase, as needed, to 100 mg PO daily or 60 mg PO b.i.d.

➤ **Symptomatic GERD, including daytime and nighttime heartburn**
Adults: 20 mg PO daily for 4 weeks. May consider additional 4-week course, if needed.
Children age 12 and older: 20 mg PO daily for up to 8 weeks.

➤ *Helicobacter pylori* **eradication, to reduce risk of duodenal ulcer recurrence**
Adults: 20 mg PO b.i.d., combined with amoxicillin 1,000 mg PO b.i.d. and clarithromycin 500 mg PO b.i.d., for 7 days with morning and evening meals.

ADMINISTRATION
PO

• Don't crush, split, or allow patient to chew tablets.

• Give tablets without regard for food but if used for treatment of duodenal ulcers, give after a meal; when used for *H. pylori* eradication, give with food.

ACTION

Blocks proton pump activity and gastric acid secretion by inhibiting gastric hydrogen–potassium adenosine triphosphatase (an enzyme) at secretory surface of gastric parietal cells.

Route	Onset	Peak	Duration
PO	<1 hr	1–6.5 hr	24 hr

Half-life: 1 to 2 hours.

ADVERSE REACTIONS

CNS: headache, pain, dizziness. **CV:** peripheral edema. **EENT:** dry mouth, pharyngitis. **GI:** abdominal pain, constipation, diarrhea, flatulence, nausea, vomiting, taste perversion. **Hepatic:** elevated liver enzyme levels, *hepatitis, hepatic encephalopathy.* **Musculoskeletal:** arthralgia, myalgia. **Other:** infection.

INTERACTIONS

Drug-drug. *Antiretrovirals (atazanavir, nelfinavir, saquinavir):* May increase or decrease exposure of antiretrovirals. Refer to antiretroviral prescribing information.

Clarithromycin: May increase rabeprazole level. Monitor patient closely.

Cyclosporine: May inhibit cyclosporine metabolism. Use together cautiously.

Dabigatran: May decrease dabigatran serum concentration. Monitor therapy.

Digoxin: May increase digoxin level. Monitor digoxin levels.

Ketoconazole, other gastric pH-dependent drugs: May reduce absorption of these drugs because of rabeprazole's effect on reducing intragastric acidity. Monitor patient closely.

Methotrexate: May increase methotrexate level and risk of toxicity. Closely monitor methotrexate level, and watch for signs and symptoms of methotrexate toxicity. Rabeprazole may need to be suspended or stopped in patients taking high-dose methotrexate.

Rilpivirine-containing products: May reduce antiviral effect and promote drug resistance. Use together is contraindicated.

Tacrolimus: May increase tacrolimus level. Monitor tacrolimus level; adjust dosage as indicated.

Warfarin: May inhibit warfarin metabolism. Monitor PT and INR.

EFFECTS ON LAB TEST RESULTS

• May decrease magnesium and B_{12} levels.
• Can cause false-positive in the diagnosis of neuroendocrine tumors and gastrinoma.
• Can cause false-positive for tetrahydrocannabinol urine screening tests.

CONTRAINDICATIONS & CAUTIONS

• Contraindicated in patients hypersensitive to drug, other benzimidazoles (lansoprazole, omeprazole), or components of these formulations.
• In *H. pylori* eradication, clarithromycin is contraindicated in patients hypersensitive to macrolides and in those taking pimozide; amoxicillin is contraindicated in patients hypersensitive to penicillin or cephalosporins.

• Avoid use in patients with severe hepatic impairment. If necessary, monitor for adverse reactions.
• Long-term (1 year or more) and multiple daily-dose rabeprazole therapy may be associated with an increased risk of osteoporosis-related fractures of the hip, wrist, or spine. Use lowest dosage and shortest duration of therapy appropriate to condition being treated. May consider vitamin D and calcium supplementation and following appropriate guidelines to reduce risk of fractures in patients at risk.
• Acute interstitial nephritis has been observed in patients taking rabeprazole and may occur at any point during therapy. Discontinue drug if this condition develops.
• Vitamin B_{12} malabsorption and deficiency have been reported in patients receiving prolonged daily treatment (longer than 3 years) with acid suppressants.
• Cutaneous lupus erythematosus (CLE) and SLE have been reported, occurring as both new onset and an exacerbation of existing autoimmune disease in patients of all ages within weeks to years after continuous drug therapy.
• Long-term use (1 year or more) may increase risk of fundic gland polyps. Use lowest dosage and shortest duration of therapy appropriate to condition being treated.

Dialyzable drug: No.

PREGNANCY-LACTATION-REPRODUCTION

• There are no adequate studies during pregnancy. Use only if potential benefit justifies fetal risk.
• In *H. pylori* eradication, clarithromycin is contraindicated during pregnancy.
• It isn't known if drug appears in human milk. Use cautiously during breastfeeding.

NURSING CONSIDERATIONS

• Consider additional courses of therapy if duodenal ulcer or GERD isn't healed after first course of therapy.
• If *H. pylori* eradication is unsuccessful, do susceptibility testing. If patient is resistant to clarithromycin or susceptibility testing isn't possible, expect to start therapy using a different antimicrobial.
• **Alert:** Prolonged use of PPIs (longer than 3 months) may cause low magnesium levels, especially if patient is on concurrent magnesium-lowering drugs, such as digoxin

R

and diuretics. Monitor magnesium levels before starting treatment and periodically thereafter.

🔶 Alert: Monitor patients for signs and symptoms of low magnesium level, such as abnormal HR or rhythm, palpitations, muscle spasms, tremor, or seizures. In children, abnormal HR may present as fatigue, upset stomach, dizziness, and light-headedness. Magnesium supplementation or drug discontinuation may be needed.

• Symptomatic response to therapy doesn't preclude presence of gastric malignancy.

🔶 Alert: Patients treated for *H. pylori* eradication have developed pseudomembranous colitis with nearly all antibiotics, including clarithromycin and amoxicillin. Monitor patient closely.

🔶 Alert: May increase CDAD. Evaluate for CDAD in patients who develop diarrhea that doesn't improve. Use lowest dosage and shortest duration appropriate to condition being treated.

• If signs or symptoms of CLE or SLE appear, discontinue drug and refer patient to the appropriate specialist for evaluation. Most patients improve with discontinuation of the PPI alone in 4 to 12 weeks.

• Drug may cause false-positive in the diagnosis of neuroendocrine tumors and gastrinoma. Temporarily stop treatment at least 14 days before testing.

• *Look alike–sound alike:* Don't confuse Aciphex with Accupril or Aricept. Don't confuse rabeprazole with aripiprazole.

PATIENT TEACHING

• Instruct patient in safe drug administration. Explain importance of taking drug exactly as prescribed.

• Inform patient that drug may increase the risk of osteoporosis-related fractures of the hip, wrist, or spine with multiple daily doses that are continued for longer than 1 year.

• Teach patient to recognize and report signs and symptoms of low magnesium levels.

raloxifene hydrochloride
ral-OKS-i-feen

Evista⬦

Therapeutic class: Antiosteoporotics
Pharmacologic class: Selective estrogen receptor modulators

AVAILABLE FORMS
Tablets: 60 mg

INDICATIONS & DOSAGES

➤ **To prevent or treat osteoporosis; to reduce risk of invasive breast cancer in patients who are postmenopausal who have osteoporosis or are at high risk for invasive breast cancer**
Adults: 60 mg PO once daily.

ADMINISTRATION
PO
• Give drug without regard for food.
• Stop drug at least 72 hours before prolonged immobilization and resume only after patient is fully mobilized.

ACTION
Reduces resorption of bone and decreases overall bone turnover. Also has estrogen antagonist activity to block some estrogen effects in breast and uterine tissues.

Route	Onset	Peak	Duration
PO	Unknown	Unknown	Unknown

Half-life: 27.5 to 32.5 hours.

ADVERSE REACTIONS
CNS: depression, insomnia, fever, migraine, headache, vertigo, neuralgia, hyperesthesia. **CV:** chest pain, peripheral edema, varicose veins, syncope, ***thromboembolism.*** **EENT:** conjunctivitis, sinusitis, rhinitis, pharyngitis, laryngitis. **GI:** nausea, diarrhea, dyspepsia, vomiting, flatulence, gastroenteritis, GI disorder, abdominal pain. **GU:** vaginitis, UTI, cystitis, leukorrhea, uterine disorder, endometrial disorder, vaginal bleeding, urinary tract disorder. **Metabolic:** weight gain. **Musculoskeletal:** arthralgia, myalgia, arthritis, tendon disorder, leg cramps, muscle spasms. **Respiratory:** increased cough, pneumonia, bronchitis. **Skin:** rash, diaphoresis. **Other:** infection, flulike syndrome, hot flashes, breast pain.

Reactions in bold italics are *life-threatening*. Interactions may have a *rapid onset* or a **delayed onset**.

INTERACTIONS

Drug-drug. *Bile acid sequestrants (cholestyramine):* May cause significant reduction in absorption of raloxifene. Avoid using together.

Highly protein-bound drugs (clofibrate, diazepam, diazoxide, ibuprofen, lidocaine, naproxen): May interfere with binding sites. Use together cautiously.

Levothyroxine: May decrease levothyroxine absorption. Consider therapy modification.

Ospemifene: May increase adverse toxic effects of both drugs. Avoid combination.

Systemic estrogens: Safety of concomitant use hasn't been established. Use together isn't recommended.

Warfarin: May decrease PT. Monitor PT and INR closely.

EFFECTS ON LAB TEST RESULTS

• May increase triglyceride level.

CONTRAINDICATIONS & CAUTIONS

Boxed Warning Increased risk of venous thromboembolism and death from stroke. Contraindicated in patients with a history of, or active, venous thromboembolism, including DVT, PE, and retinal vein thrombosis. Consider risk-benefit balance in patients at risk for stroke, including those with documented CAD or who are at increased risk for major coronary events. ■

• Raloxifene shouldn't be used for primary or secondary prevention of CV disease.

• Use cautiously in patients with moderate or severe hepatic or renal impairment.

• Safety and effectiveness of drug in men haven't been evaluated.

• Safety of use with systemic estrogens and use in patients who are premenopausal haven't been established. Use isn't recommended.

Dialyzable drug: Unknown.

⚠ **Overdose S&S:** Leg cramps, dizziness, ataxia, flushing, rash, tremors, vomiting, elevated ALP level.

PREGNANCY-LACTATION-REPRODUCTION

• Contraindicated during pregnancy. Drug isn't indicated for use in patients who may become pregnant; drug may cause fetal harm. If drug is used during pregnancy or if pregnancy occurs during therapy, apprise patient of fetal risk.

• Contraindicated during breastfeeding.

NURSING CONSIDERATIONS

• Watch for signs of blood clots. Greatest risk of thromboembolic events occurs during first 4 months of treatment.

• Watch for breast abnormalities; drug doesn't eliminate risk of breast cancer.

• Conduct breast exams and obtain mammograms before starting, and regularly during therapy.

• Monitor bone mineral density at baseline and every 1 to 3 years thereafter.

• Effect on bone mineral density beyond 2 years of drug treatment isn't known.

• Measure height and weight annually.

• Monitor serum calcium and vitamin D levels at baseline and at 3 and 6 months to assess treatment response and adherence to therapy.

• For osteoporosis treatment, add supplemental calcium (average of 1,500 mg daily) and vitamin D (400 to 800 units daily) to the diet if daily intake is inadequate.

• Monitor triglyceride level if previous treatment with estrogen caused elevation.

PATIENT TEACHING

• Teach patient safe drug administration.

• Advise patient to avoid long periods of restricted movement (such as during traveling) because of increased risk of venous thromboembolic events.

• Inform patient that hot flashes or flushing may occur and that drug doesn't aid in reducing them.

• Instruct patient to practice other bone loss-prevention measures, including taking supplemental calcium and vitamin D if dietary intake is inadequate, performing weight-bearing exercises, and stopping alcohol consumption and smoking.

• Advise patient to report unexplained uterine bleeding or breast abnormalities during therapy.

• Explain adverse reactions and instruct patient to read patient information insert before starting therapy and each time prescription is renewed.

R

raltegravir potassium
ral-TEG-ra-vir

Isentress, Isentress HD

Therapeutic class: Antiretrovirals
Pharmacologic class: HIV integrase strand transfer inhibitors

AVAILABLE FORMS
Powder for oral suspension: 100-mg packets
Tablets (chewable): 25 mg, 100 mg
Tablets (film-coated) ☐: 400 mg, 600 mg

INDICATIONS & DOSAGES
➤ **HIV-1 infection, with other antiretrovirals**

Adults and children weighing 40 kg or more who are treatment-naive or virologically suppressed on an initial regimen of raltegravir 400-mg tablet b.i.d.: 1,200 mg (two 600-mg tablets) PO once daily or 400-mg tablet PO b.i.d. or 300 mg chewable tablets b.i.d. if child can't swallow a tablet.

Adults who are treatment-experienced: 400-mg tablet PO b.i.d.

Adults: When administered concomitantly with rifampin, give 800 mg (two 400-mg tablets) PO b.i.d.

Children weighing 28 to less than 40 kg: 400-mg tablet b.i.d. or 200 mg chewable tablets PO b.i.d. if child can't swallow a tablet.

Children weighing 25 to less than 28 kg: 400-mg tablet b.i.d. or 150 mg chewable tablets PO b.i.d. if child can't swallow a tablet.

Children at least age 4 weeks weighing 20 to less than 25 kg: 150 mg chewable tablets PO b.i.d.

Children at least age 4 weeks weighing 14 to less than 20 kg: 100 mg chewable tablets or 100 mg oral suspension (10 mL) PO b.i.d.

Children at least age 4 weeks weighing 10 to less than 14 kg: 75 mg chewable tablets or 80 mg oral suspension (8 mL) PO b.i.d.

Children at least age 4 weeks weighing 8 to less than 10 kg: 50 mg chewable tablets or 60 mg oral suspension (6 mL) PO b.i.d.

Children at least age 4 weeks weighing 6 to less than 8 kg: 50 mg chewable tablets or 40 mg oral suspension (4 mL) PO b.i.d.

Children at least age 4 weeks weighing 4 to less than 6 kg: 25 mg chewable tablet or 30 mg oral suspension (3 mL) PO b.i.d.

Children at least age 4 weeks weighing 3 to less than 4 kg: 20 mg chewable tablet or 25 mg oral suspension (2.5 mL) PO b.i.d.

Full-term neonate (birth to 28 days): Refer to manufacturer's instructions for dosage based on weight and age.

ADMINISTRATION
PO
• Don't substitute chewable tablets or oral suspension for film-coated tablets.
• Give drug without regard for meals.

Tablets and chewable tablets
• Maximum dosage of chewable tablets is 300 mg b.i.d.
• Patient must swallow film-coated tablets whole.
• The 100-mg chewable tablet can be broken into two equal halves.
• Chewable tablets can be chewed or swallowed whole.

Oral suspension
• Maximum dosage of oral suspension is 100 mg b.i.d.
• Patients can continue oral suspension as long as weight remains below 20 kg.
• To administer, open foil packet of drug (100 mg). Measure 10 mL of water in provided mixing cup. Pour packet contents into the water, close lid, and swirl for 45 seconds. Don't shake or turn mixing cup upside down. Final concentration, 10 mg/mL.
• When mixed, measure recommended suspension dose into the oral syringe provided.
• Give within 30 minutes of mixing with water. Discard any remaining suspension in the trash.
• If patient received drug 2 to 24 hours before delivery, give neonate's first dose between 24 and 48 hours after birth.
• See detailed "Instructions for Use" that come with the oral suspension.
• If a dose is missed, give missed dose as soon as possible; don't double the next dose.

ACTION
Inhibits HIV-1 integrase, an enzyme required for HIV-1 replication.

Route	Onset	Peak	Duration
PO	Rapid	3 hr	Unknown

Half-life: About 9 hours.

Reactions in bold italics are *life-threatening*. Interactions may have a *rapid onset* or a ***delayed onset***.

ADVERSE REACTIONS

CNS: headache, fatigue, dizziness, insomnia, asthenia, abnormal dreams, depression, nightmares. **GI:** nausea, abdominal pain, vomiting, diarrhea, flatulence, decreased appetite. **Hematologic:** anemia, *neutropenia, thrombocytopenia.* **Hepatic:** increased LFT values. **Metabolic:** hyperglycemia, increased lipase level, increased CK level, increased lipid levels. **Musculoskeletal:** myopathy, *rhabdomyolysis.* **Skin:** rash.

INTERACTIONS

Drug-drug. *Antacids containing aluminum, magnesium, or calcium carbonate:* Ingestion with raltegravir at any time may significantly decrease raltegravir plasma level. Coadministration or staggered administration isn't recommended.

Etravirine, tipranavir with ritonavir: May decrease serum concentration of raltegravir HD. Coadministration isn't recommended.

Fibric acid derivatives, HMG-CoA reductase inhibitors: May increase risk of rhabdomyolysis. Monitor therapy.

Strong inducers of drug-metabolizing enzymes (carbamazepine, phenobarbital, phenytoin): May affect raltegravir metabolism. Coadministration isn't recommended.

UGT1A1 inducers (rifampin): May decrease raltegravir level. Adjust raltegravir dosage to 800 mg b.i.d. when giving with rifampin. Use with 600-mg tablets isn't recommended. Use together in children hasn't been studied.

EFFECTS ON LAB TEST RESULTS

• May increase serum creatinine, bilirubin, AST, ALT, ALP, amylase, lipase, glucose, cholesterol, triglyceride, and CK levels.
• May decrease Hb level and neutrophil and platelet counts.

CONTRAINDICATIONS & CAUTIONS

🚯 *Alert:* Severe, potentially life-threatening and fatal skin reactions have been reported, including SJS and TEN. Hypersensitivity reactions, including rash; organ dysfunction, including hepatic failure; and general malaise, muscle or joint aches, edema, conjunctivitis, facial edema, angioedema, oral blisters, and eosinophilia have also been reported. Discontinue drug immediately if signs or symptoms of SCARs or hypersensitivity reactions occur.

🚯 *Alert:* Use cautiously in older adults, especially those with hepatic, renal, and cardiac insufficiency.
Dialyzable drug: Unknown.

PREGNANCY-LACTATION-REPRODUCTION

• There are no adequate during pregnancy. Use only if potential benefit outweighs fetal risk.
• Enroll patients who are pregnant and exposed to drug in the Antiretroviral Pregnancy Registry (1-800-258-4263).
• Patients infected with HIV-1 shouldn't breastfeed to avoid risking postnatal HIV-1 transmission.

NURSING CONSIDERATIONS

• Obtain lab tests, including viral load, CD4 count, CBC, platelet count, and LFTs, before therapy and regularly throughout therapy.
• Use drug with at least one other antiretroviral.
• Watch for signs and symptoms of myopathy or rash.
• Monitor patient for signs and symptoms of depression and suicidality.
• Monitor patient for immune reconstitution syndrome (inflammatory response to indolent or residual opportunistic infections [CMV, MAC, *Pneumocystis jiroveci* pneumonia, TB]), which may necessitate further evaluation and treatment.
• Autoimmune disorders (such as Graves disease, polymyositis, and Guillain-Barré syndrome) have been reported in the setting of immune reconstitution; time to onset varies, and can occur many months after initiation treatment.
• Avoid dosing before a dialysis session because the extent to which drug may be dialyzable is unknown.

PATIENT TEACHING

• Inform patient that drug doesn't cure HIV infection, that patient may continue to develop opportunistic infections and other complications of HIV infection, and transmit HIV to others through sexual contact or blood contamination.
• Advise patient to use barrier protection during sexual intercourse.
• Tell patient that breastfeeding isn't recommended.
• Instruct patient in safe drug preparation and administration.

R

• Advise patient to immediately report worsening symptoms or unexplained muscle pain, tenderness, or weakness while taking the drug.

• Instruct patient to avoid missing any doses to decrease the risk of developing HIV resistance.

• Instruct patient to immediately stop taking raltegravir and seek medical attention if a rash associated with any of the following signs or symptoms develops: fever; generally ill feeling; extreme tiredness; muscle or joint aches; blisters; oral lesions; eye inflammation; facial swelling; swelling of the eyes, lips, or mouth; breathing difficulty; or signs and symptoms of liver problems (such as yellowing of the skin or whites of the eyes, dark or tea-colored urine, pale-colored stools or bowel movements, nausea, vomiting, loss of appetite, pain, aching or sensitivity on the right side below the ribs).

• Advise patient with phenylketonuria that the 25-mg and 100-mg chewable tablets contain phenylalanine.

• Advise patient to report use of other drugs, including OTC drugs; this drug interacts with other drugs.

• Remind patient or caregiver to use calibrated syringe to administer dose.

ramelteon
ra-MEL-tee-on

Rozerem

Therapeutic class: Hypnotics
Pharmacologic class: Melatonin receptor agonists

AVAILABLE FORMS
Tablets ⓞⓣⓒ: 8 mg

INDICATIONS & DOSAGES
➤ **Insomnia characterized by trouble falling asleep**
Adults: 8 mg PO within 30 minutes of bedtime. Maximum dose is 8 mg daily.

ADMINISTRATION
PO
• Don't give drug with or immediately after a high-fat meal.
• Give drug within 30 minutes of bedtime.

• Don't break, crush, or allow patient to chew tablets. Patient should swallow tablets whole.

ACTION
Acts on receptors believed to maintain the circadian rhythm underlying the normal sleep-wake cycle.

Route	Onset	Peak	Duration
PO	Rapid	0.5–1.5 hr	Unknown

Half-life: Parent compound, 1 to 2.6 hours; metabolite M-II, 2 to 5 hours.

ADVERSE REACTIONS
CNS: depression, dizziness, fatigue, headache, somnolence, worsened insomnia.
GI: nausea.

INTERACTIONS
Drug-drug. *CNS depressants:* May cause excessive CNS depression. Use together cautiously.
Donepezil, doxepin: May increase ramelteon level. Monitor patient closely.
Opioids: May cause slow or difficult breathing, sedation, and death. Avoid use together. If use together is necessary, limit dosage and duration of each drug to minimum necessary for desired effect.
Strong CYP enzyme inducer (rifampin): May decrease ramelteon level. Monitor patient for lack of effect.
Strong CYP1A2 inhibitor (fluvoxamine): May increase ramelteon level. Use together is contraindicated.
Strong CYP2C9 inhibitor (fluconazole), strong CYP3A4 inhibitor (ketoconazole), weak CYP1A2 inhibitors: May increase ramelteon level. Use together cautiously.
Drug-food. *Food (especially high-fat meals):* May delay time to peak drug effect. Tell patient to take drug on an empty stomach.
Drug-lifestyle. *Alcohol use:* May cause excessive CNS depression. Discourage alcohol use.

EFFECTS ON LAB TEST RESULTS
• May increase prolactin level.
• May decrease testosterone level.

CONTRAINDICATIONS & CAUTIONS
• Contraindicated in patients hypersensitive to drug or its components. Don't use in patients with severe hepatic impairment, severe sleep apnea, or severe COPD.

Reactions in bold italics are *life-threatening*. Interactions may have a *rapid onset* or a **delayed onset**.

- Opioids should only be prescribed with benzodiazepines or other CNS depressants to patients for whom alternative treatment options are inadequate.
- Use cautiously in patients with depression or moderate hepatic impairment.
- Drug is associated with abnormal thinking and behavior changes, including worsening depression, hallucinations, aggression, bizarre behavior, agitation, mania, amnesia, anxiety, and other neuropsychiatric symptoms, which may occur unpredictably.

Dialyzable drug: No.

PREGNANCY-LACTATION-REPRODUCTION

- There are no adequate studies during pregnancy. Drug may cause fetal harm. Use only if clearly needed and potential benefit justifies fetal risk.
- Drug appears in human milk. Use cautiously during breastfeeding.
- Drug has been associated with decreased testosterone levels and increased prolactin levels. Effects on reproduction are unknown.

NURSING CONSIDERATIONS

⚠️ *Alert:* Anaphylaxis and angioedema may occur as early as the first dose. Monitor patient closely. Emergency treatment may be needed.
- Thoroughly evaluate the cause of insomnia before starting drug.
- Assess patient for behavioral or cognitive disorders.
- Failure of insomnia to resolve after 7 to 10 days of treatment may indicate the presence of a primary psychiatric or medical illness that should be evaluated.

⚠️ *Alert:* Monitor patient for signs and symptoms of depression, worsening of depression, and suicidality.
- Drug doesn't cause physical dependence.
- *Look alike–sound alike:* Don't confuse Rozerem with Razadyne or Remeron. Don't confuse ramelteon with Remeron.

PATIENT TEACHING

- Instruct patient in safe drug administration.
- Caution patient or caregiver of patient taking an opioid with a benzodiazepine, CNS depressant, or alcohol to seek immediate medical attention for dizziness, light-headedness, extreme sleepiness, slowed or difficult breathing, or unresponsiveness.

⚠️ *Alert:* Warn patient that drug may cause allergic reactions, facial swelling, and complex sleep-related behaviors, such as driving, eating, and making phone calls while asleep. Advise patient to report these and all adverse effects.
- Advise patient and caregiver to report signs and symptoms of depression, worsening of depression, suicidality, nightmares, or hallucinations.
- Caution against performing activities that require mental alertness or physical coordination after taking drug.
- Caution patient to avoid alcohol while taking drug.
- Tell patient to consult prescriber if insomnia worsens or behavior changes.
- Urge patient to consult prescriber if menses stops or, for both genders, if libido decreases or galactorrhea or fertility problems develop.

---

ramipril 🗶
RA-mi-pril

Altace

Therapeutic class: Antihypertensives
Pharmacologic class: ACE inhibitors

AVAILABLE FORMS

Capsules ⬤: 1.25 mg, 2.5 mg, 5 mg, 10 mg

INDICATIONS & DOSAGES

➤ **HTN**
Adults: Initially, 2.5 mg PO once daily for patients not taking a diuretic, and 1.25 mg PO once daily for patients taking a diuretic. Increase dosage, if needed, based on patient response. Maintenance dose is 2.5 to 20 mg daily as a single dose or in divided doses.
Adjust-a-dose: For patients with CrCl less than 40 mL/minute, give 1.25 mg PO daily. Adjust dosage gradually based on response. Maximum daily dose is 5 mg.

➤ **HF after MI**
Adults: Initially, 2.5 mg PO b.i.d. If hypotension occurs, decrease dosage to 1.25 mg PO b.i.d. Adjust as tolerated, with dosage increase (as tolerated) at 1 week and subsequent increases about 3 weeks apart, to target dosage of 5 mg PO b.i.d.
Adjust-a-dose: For patients with CrCl less than 40 mL/minute, give 1.25 mg PO daily.

R

Adjust dosage gradually based on response. Maximum dosage is 2.5 mg b.i.d.

➤ **To reduce risk of MI, stroke, and death from CV causes**
Adults age 55 and older: 2.5 mg PO once daily for 1 week, then 5 mg PO once daily for 3 weeks. Increase as tolerated to a maintenance dose of 10 mg PO once daily.
Adjust-a-dose: In patients who are hypertensive or who have recently had an MI, daily dose may be divided.

ADMINISTRATION
PO
• Give drug without regard for meals.
• Patient should swallow capsules whole.
• If patient can't swallow capsules, open capsule and sprinkle contents on a small amount of applesauce (4 oz) or mix with 120 mL of water or apple juice. May store for up to 24 hours at room temperature or up to 48 hours under refrigeration if not given immediately.

ACTION
Prevents conversion of angiotensin I to angiotensin II, a potent vasoconstrictor. Less angiotensin II decreases peripheral arterial resistance, decreasing aldosterone secretion, which reduces sodium and water retention and lowers BP.

Route	Onset	Peak	Duration
PO	1–2 hr	2–4 hr	24 hr

Half-life: 13 to 17 hours.

ADVERSE REACTIONS
CNS: headache, dizziness, fatigue, vertigo, syncope. **CV:** *HF,* MI, hypotension, angina pectoris. **GI:** nausea, vomiting, diarrhea. **GU:** renal dysfunction. **Metabolic:** *hyperkalemia.* **Respiratory:** dyspnea; dry, persistent, tickling, nonproductive cough.

INTERACTIONS
Drug-drug. ⚙ *Alert: Aliskiren:* May increase risk of renal impairment, hypotension, and hyperkalemia in patients with diabetes and those with moderate to severe renal impairment (GFR less than 60 mL/minute). Concomitant use is contraindicated in patients with diabetes. Avoid concomitant use in those with moderate to severe renal impairment.
Diuretics: May cause excessive hypotension, especially at start of therapy. Stop diuretic at

least 3 days before therapy begins, increase sodium intake, or reduce starting dose of ramipril.
Insulin, oral antidiabetics: May cause hypoglycemia, especially at start of ramipril therapy. Monitor glucose level closely.
Iron dextran: May increase risk of anaphylactic-type reaction. If drugs must be given concurrently, have resuscitation equipment and trained personnel on hand before iron dextran administration and the use of a test dose before first therapeutic dose.
Lanthanum: May decrease ramipril serum concentration. Give ramipril at least 2 hours before or after lanthanum.
Lithium: May increase lithium level. Use together cautiously and monitor lithium level.
mTOR inhibitors (temsirolimus), neprilysin inhibitors (sacubitril, sacubitril–valsartan): May increase risk of angioedema. Use together is contraindicated.
NSAIDs: May decrease antihypertensive effects and increase risk of renal dysfunction. Monitor BP and renal function.
Potassium-sparing diuretics, potassium supplements: May cause hyperkalemia; ramipril attenuates potassium loss. Monitor potassium level closely.
Salicylates (aspirin): May decrease antihypertensive effects of ramipril and increase nephrotoxic effect. Ramipril dosage increase or aspirin dosage decrease may be needed.
Telmisartan: May increase risk of renal dysfunction. Avoid use together.
Tizanidine: May cause severe hypotension. Use cautiously and monitor BP closely.
Drug-herb. *Capsaicin:* May cause cough. Discourage use together.
Grass pollen allergen extract (5 grass extract): May increase risk of severe allergic reaction to 5 grass extract. Don't use together.
Ma huang: May decrease antihypertensive effects. Discourage use together.
Drug-food. *Salt substitutes containing potassium:* May cause hyperkalemia; ramipril attenuates potassium loss. Discourage use of salt substitutes during therapy.

EFFECTS ON LAB TEST RESULTS
• May increase BUN, creatinine, bilirubin, liver enzyme, glucose, and potassium levels.
• May decrease Hb level and hematocrit.
• May decrease RBC and platelet counts.

Reactions in bold italics are *life-threatening*. Interactions may have a *rapid onset* or a *delayed onset*.

CONTRAINDICATIONS & CAUTIONS

• Contraindicated in patients hypersensitive to ACE inhibitors and in those with a history of angioedema related to ACE inhibitor use.
• Use cautiously in patients with renal or hepatic impairment.
• Anaphylactoid reactions have been reported in patients dialyzed with high-flux membranes and also treated with ACE inhibitors and in those undergoing LDL apheresis with dextran sulfate absorption.

Dialyzable drug: Unknown.

⚠ *Overdose S&S:* Hypotension.

PREGNANCY-LACTATION-REPRODUCTION

Boxed Warning Use during pregnancy can cause injury and death to the developing fetus. Stop drug as soon as pregnancy is detected. ■

• Drug may appear in human milk. Use during breastfeeding isn't recommended.

NURSING CONSIDERATIONS

• Monitor BP regularly for drug effectiveness.
• Correct fluid and electrolyte imbalances before starting therapy.
• Closely assess renal function in patients during first few weeks of therapy, then regularly thereafter. Dosage reduction or drug stoppage may be necessary.
▧ Although ACE inhibitors reduce BP in all races, they reduce it less in patients who are Black taking the ACE inhibitor alone. These patients should use drug in combination therapy for a more favorable response.
▧ ACE inhibitors appear to increase risk of angioedema in patients who are Black.
• Discontinue drug if patient develops jaundice or significant hepatic enzyme elevation (rare).
• Monitor CBC with differential counts before therapy and periodically thereafter.
• Drug may reduce Hb and WBC, RBC, and platelet counts, especially in patients with impaired renal function or collagen vascular diseases (SLE or scleroderma).
• Monitor potassium level. Risk factors for hyperkalemia include renal insufficiency, diabetes, and concomitant use of drugs that raise potassium level.
• *Look alike–sound alike:* Don't confuse ramipril with Amaryl or enalapril. Don't confuse Altace with alteplase.

PATIENT TEACHING

• Teach patient safe drug administration.
• Tell patient to report adverse reactions. Dosage adjustment or stoppage of drug may be needed.
ⓘ *Alert:* Rarely, swelling of the face and throat (including swelling of the larynx) may occur, especially after first dose. Advise patient to report breathing difficulty or swelling of face, eyes, lips, or tongue.
• Inform patient that light-headedness can occur, especially during first few days of therapy. Tell patient to rise slowly to minimize this effect and to report light-headedness to prescriber. If fainting occurs, advise patient to stop drug and call prescriber immediately.
• Advise patient to report signs and symptoms of infection, such as fever and sore throat.
• Tell patient to avoid salt substitutes. These products may contain potassium, which can cause high potassium level in patients taking ramipril.
Boxed Warning Tell patient of childbearing potential to report pregnancy. Drug will need to be stopped. ■

SAFETY ALERT!

ramucirumab ▧
ra-mue-SIR-ue-mab

Cyramza

Therapeutic class: Antineoplastics
Pharmacologic class: Monoclonal antibodies

R

AVAILABLE FORMS

Injection: 10-mg/mL single-dose vial

INDICATIONS & DOSAGES

Adjust-a-dose (for all indications): Refer to manufacturer's instructions for toxicity-related dosage.
➤ **Advanced gastric cancer or gastro-esophageal junction adenocarcinoma, as a single agent or in combination with paclitaxel, after prior fluoropyrimidine- or platinum-containing chemotherapy**
Adults: 8 mg/kg IV over 60 minutes every 2 weeks. Continue until disease progression or unacceptable toxicity. When given in combination, administer ramucirumab before paclitaxel.

➡Canada   ◇OTC   ◆Off-label use   ℘Photoguide   ⓜDo not crush   *Liquid contains alcohol   ▧Genetic

➤ **Metastatic NSCLC in combination with docetaxel in patients with disease progression on or after platinum-based chemotherapy. (Patients with *EGFR* or *ALK* genomic tumor aberrations should have shown disease progression on FDA-approved therapy for these before treatment with ramucirumab.)** ▧

Adults: 10 mg/kg IV on day 1 of a 21-day cycle before docetaxel infusion. Continue until disease progression or unacceptable toxicity.

➤ **First-line treatment, in combination with erlotinib, for metastatic NSCLC with *EGFR* exon 19 deletions or exon 21 (L858R) mutations** ▧

Adults: 10 mg/kg IV infusion every 2 weeks. Continue until disease progression or unacceptable toxicity occurs. Refer to manufacturer's instructions for erlotinib prescribing information.

➤ **Colorectal cancer in combination with FOLFIRI (irinotecan, folinic acid, and 5-FU) in patients with disease progression on or after therapy with bevacizumab, oxaliplatin, and a fluoropyrimidine**

Adults: 8 mg/kg IV every 2 weeks before FOLFIRI administration. Continue until disease progression or unacceptable toxicity.

➤ **Hepatocellular carcinoma in patients who have an alpha-fetoprotein of at least 400 ng/mL and have been treated with sorafenib**

Adults: 8 mg/kg IV infusion every 2 weeks. Continue until disease progression or unacceptable toxicity.

ADMINISTRATION

IV

⚠️ *Alert:* Drug is a hazardous agent; use safe handling and disposal precautions.

▼ If patient tolerates first infusion over 60 minutes, may administer subsequent infusions over 30 minutes.

▼ For each infusion, premedicate with IV histamine (H_1) antagonist (diphenhydramine). For patients with prior grade 1 or 2 infusion-related reaction (IRR), also premedicate with dexamethasone or equivalent and acetaminophen before each infusion.

▼ Dilute drug with NSS to final volume of 250 mL. Diluted solution remains stable for 24 hours if refrigerated or 4 hours at room temperature. Gently invert container; don't shake.

▼ Inspect solution for particles and discoloration before administration.

▼ Give infusion through separate infusion line using a protein-sparing 0.22-micron filter. Flush line with NSS at end of infusion.

▼ Store vials in refrigerator at 36° to 46° F (2° to 8° C) until ready to use. Keep vial in outer carton to protect from light. Don't freeze or shake vial.

▼ **Incompatibilities:** Dextrose solutions, electrolytes, other medications.

ACTION

A vascular endothelial growth factor receptor 2 antagonist that inhibits proliferation and migration of human endothelial cells, angiogenesis, and tumor growth.

Route	Onset	Peak	Duration
IV	Unknown	Unknown	Unknown

Half-life: 14 days.

ADVERSE REACTIONS

CNS: headache, fatigue, insomnia, fever. **CV:** HTN, peripheral edema, *arterial thromboembolic events, hemorrhage.* **EENT:** increased tearing, epistaxis, gingival bleeding. **GI:** diarrhea, intestinal obstruction, stomatitis, *GI hemorrhage, GI perforation,* decreased appetite, abdominal pain, ascites, vomiting. **GU:** proteinuria. **Hematologic:** anemia, *neutropenia, thrombocytopenia.* **Hepatic:** increased LFT values. **Metabolic:** hyponatremia, hypoalbuminemia, *hypokalemia, hypocalcemia.* **Musculoskeletal:** back pain. **Skin:** rash, alopecia. **Other:** *sepsis,* infections, antibody development, hypothyroidism, infusion-related reaction.

INTERACTIONS

None reported.

EFFECTS ON LAB TEST RESULTS

• May increase TSH and urine protein levels.
• May decrease sodium, calcium, potassium, and albumin levels.
• May decrease Hb level and RBC, neutrophil, and platelet counts.

CONTRAINDICATIONS & CAUTIONS

• Drug increases risk of hemorrhage, including severe and sometimes fatal hemorrhagic events. Permanently discontinue drug in patients who experience severe bleeding.

Reactions in bold italics are *life-threatening*. Interactions may have a *rapid onset* or a *delayed onset*.

- Withhold drug 28 days before surgery. Resume at least 2 weeks after the surgical intervention based on clinical judgment of adequate wound healing. If patient develops wound-healing complications during therapy, discontinue drug until wound is fully healed.
- Permanently discontinue drug in patients who experience GI perforation, a potentially fatal event.
- Use cautiously in patients with cirrhosis (Child-Pugh class B or C). Use in patients with hepatic impairment (Child-Pugh class B or C) only if potential benefits outweigh risks.
⚠ *Alert:* Rare and sometimes fatal RPLS has been reported.
- Safety and effectiveness in children haven't been established.
Dialyzable drug: Unknown.

PREGNANCY-LACTATION-REPRODUCTION
- Drug may cause fetal harm. Patients of childbearing potential should use effective contraception during and for at least 3 months after last ramucirumab dose.
- It isn't known if drug appears in human milk. Because of the risk of serious adverse reactions in infants who are breastfed, breastfeeding isn't recommended during treatment.
- Based on animal data, drug may impair fertility in women.

NURSING CONSIDERATIONS
⚠ *Alert:* Serious, sometimes fatal, arterial thromboembolic events, including MI, cardiac arrest, stroke, and cerebral ischemia, have occurred. Monitor patient closely, and permanently discontinue drug in patients who experience a severe embolic event.
- Assess BP every 2 weeks or more frequently as clinically indicated. Control HTN before start of therapy. If severe HTN occurs, withhold drug until controlled. Discontinue drug permanently if HTN can't be controlled, in hypertensive crisis, or in hypertensive encephalopathy.
- Premedicate before each infusion, and monitor patient for IRR.
⚠ *Alert:* Assess patient for signs and symptoms of GI perforation (severe abdominal pain, nausea, vomiting, fever).
⚠ *Alert:* Monitor recent wounds for complications during therapy. For wound healing complications, withhold drug until wound is fully healed.

- Monitor patients with cirrhosis (Child-Pugh class B or C) for new-onset or worsening encephalopathy, ascites, or hepatorenal syndrome.
- Monitor patient for signs and symptoms of RPLS (HTN, headache, visual disturbances, altered consciousness, seizures). Confirm diagnosis with MRI; discontinue drug and provide supportive care.
- Monitor thyroid function.
- *Look alike–sound alike:* Don't confuse Cyramza with Cimzia.

PATIENT TEACHING
⚠ *Alert:* Inform patient that drug can cause severe bleeding. Advise patient to contact prescriber for bleeding or symptoms of bleeding, including light-headedness.
- Warn patient of increased risk of embolic events.
- Advise patient to undergo routine BP monitoring and to contact health care provider if BP is elevated or if signs and symptoms of HTN (severe headache, light-headedness, or neurologic symptoms) occur.
⚠ *Alert:* Caution patient to notify health care provider for severe diarrhea, vomiting, or severe abdominal pain.
⚠ *Alert:* Warn patient that drug may impair wound healing. Instruct patient not to undergo surgery without first discussing risk with health care provider.
- Teach patient about risk of maintaining pregnancy, risk to fetus, and risk to postnatal infant development during and after treatment with ramucirumab. Discuss the need to avoid pregnancy, including use of adequate contraception, for at least 3 months after last dose.
- Advise patient of childbearing potential that drug may impair fertility.
- Counsel patient on the need to discontinue breastfeeding during treatment.

R

BIOSIMILAR DRUG

ranibizumab
RA-ni-BIZ-oo-mab

Lucentis, Susvimo

ranibizumab-nuna
Byooviz

Therapeutic class: Vascular endothelial growth factor A inhibitors
Pharmacologic class: Monoclonal antibodies

AVAILABLE FORMS
Intravitreal infusion via ocular implant: 100 mg/mL single-dose vial
Intravitreal injection: 6 mg/mL, 10 mg/mL in single-use glass vials or prefilled syringes

INDICATIONS & DOSAGES
➤ **Neovascular (wet) age-related macular degeneration or macular edema after retinal vein occlusion**
Adults: 0.5 mg (0.05 mL of 10-mg/mL solution) by intravitreal injection once a month (approximately 28 days between doses).
Adjust-a-dose: May start less frequent dosing after 3 or 4 monthly doses, although less frequent dosing is less effective. Assess patients regularly.
➤ **Neovascular (wet) age-related macular degeneration (Susvimo)**
Adults: 2 mg (0.02 mL of 100 mg/mL solution) continuous delivery by ocular implant with refills every 24 weeks.
Adjust-a-dose: May give supplemental intravitreal injection to the affected eye with ocular implant in place if needed.
➤ **Diabetic macular edema; diabetic retinopathy (except Byooviz)**
Adults: 0.3 mg (0.05 mL of 6-mg/mL solution) by intravitreal injection once a month (approximately 28 days between doses).
➤ **Myopic choroidal neovascularization**
Adults: 0.5 mg (0.05 mL of 10-mg/mL solution) by intravitreal injection once a month (approximately 28 days between doses) for up to 3 months. May retreat if needed.

ADMINISTRATION
Ophthalmic intravitreal injection
• Store vials in original carton under refrigeration until use. Don't freeze.

• Protect from light.
• Withdraw vial contents through a 5-micron, 19G filter needle attached to a 1-mL tuberculin syringe; discard filter needle after withdrawal of vial contents.
• Replace filter needle with a sterile 30G × ½-inch needle for the intravitreal injection. Expel contents until 0.05 mL remains in syringe.
• Follow manufacturer's instructions for use of the prefilled syringe.
• Carry out intravitreal injection procedure under aseptic conditions with adequate anesthesia and a broad-spectrum microbicide given before injection.
Ophthalmic ocular implant
• Initial fill and refill-exchange must be performed under sterile conditions by a practitioner experienced in ophthalmic surgery following manufacturer's instructions.
• A 34G needle with integrated filter is included with drug; a 5-micron, sterile 19G × 1.5-inch needle and a 1-mL syringe are needed but not included.
• Refrigerate drug; don't freeze or shake vial.

ACTION
Binds to the receptor-binding site of active forms of vascular endothelial growth factor A, reducing endothelial cell proliferation, vascular leakage, and new blood vessel formation.

Route	Onset	Peak	Duration
Intravitreal injection	Unknown	1 day	Unknown
Ocular implant	Unknown	26 days	Unknown

Half-life: Injection, 9 days; implant, unknown.

ADVERSE REACTIONS
CNS: headache, peripheral neuropathy. **CV:** atrial fibrillation, peripheral edema, *arterial thromboembolic events.* **EENT:** conjunctival hemorrhage, eye pain, vitreous floaters, increased IOP, eye hypotony, vitreous detachment, intraocular inflammation, cataract, foreign body sensation in eyes, eye irritation, increased lacrimation, blepharitis, dry eye, visual disturbance or blurred vision, eye pruritus, ocular hyperemia, retinal disorder, maculopathy, retinal degeneration, ocular discomfort, conjunctival hyperemia, posterior capsule opacification, injection-site hemorrhage, iritis, conjunctival bleb, vitreous hemorrhage, conjunctival edema, corneal abrasion, corneal edema, nasopharyngitis, sinusitis.

Reactions in bold italics are *life-threatening*. Interactions may have a *rapid onset* or a *delayed onset*.

GI: nausea, constipation, GERD. **GU:** *renal failure,* chronic renal failure. **Hematologic:** anemia. **Metabolic:** hypercholesterolemia. **Musculoskeletal:** arthralgia. **Respiratory:** URI, bronchitis, COPD, cough. **Skin:** wound healing complications. **Other:** seasonal allergy, flulike symptoms, antibody formation.

INTERACTIONS
None reported.

EFFECTS ON LAB TEST RESULTS
• May increase cholesterol level.
• May decrease Hb level.

CONTRAINDICATIONS & CAUTIONS
• Contraindicated in patients with known hypersensitivity to drug or its components and in patients with ocular or periocular infections.
• May increase risk of arterial thromboembolic events (nonfatal stroke, nonfatal MI, vascular death, or death of unknown cause), especially in patients with diabetes.
• May cause serious intraocular inflammation if drug is given within 9 days after verteporfin photodynamic therapy.
• May increase risk of endophthalmitis, retinal detachment, and increased IOP both before and after injection.
Dialyzable drug: Unknown.

PREGNANCY-LACTATION-REPRODUCTION
• Use during pregnancy hasn't been studied. Based on its mechanism of action, drug may pose a risk to embryo-fetal development. Use only if clearly needed.
• It isn't known if drug appears in human milk. Use cautiously in during breastfeeding.
• Based on its mechanism of action, drug may affect fertility.

NURSING CONSIDERATIONS
• Before and 30 minutes after intravitreal injection, monitor patient for elevated IOP using tonometry.
• Check for perfusion of the optic nerve head immediately after injection.
• Use one vial per treatment of a single eye. If second eye treatment is necessary, use new vial and reestablish sterile field.
• Monitor patient for hypersensitivity reactions, which may present as severe intraocular inflammation.

• Monitor patient for signs and symptoms suggestive of endophthalmitis (eye redness, sensitivity to light, eye pain, vision changes).
• Monitor patient for arterial thromboembolic events.

PATIENT TEACHING
• Instruct patient to seek immediate care from the ophthalmologist for eye redness, sensitivity to light, eye pain, or vision changes.

ranolazine
ra-NOE-la-zeen

Aspruzyo Sprinkle, Ranexa◆

Therapeutic class: Antianginals
Pharmacologic class: CV drugs

AVAILABLE FORMS
Granules (extended-release) ⊚*:* 500 mg, 1,000 mg
Tablets (extended-release) ⊚*:* 500 mg, 1,000 mg

INDICATIONS & DOSAGES
➤ **Chronic angina**
Adults: Initially, 500 mg PO b.i.d. Increase, if needed, to maximum of 1,000 mg b.i.d.
Adjust-a-dose: Limit maximum dose to 500 mg b.i.d. in patients on moderate CYP3A inhibitors. Avoid concomitant use of Aspruzyo Sprinkle with strong CYP3A inhibitors and CYP3A inducers.

ADMINISTRATION
PO
• Give without regard for meals.
• Give whole; don't crush or cut tablets.
• Don't crush or allow patient to chew granules.
• Sprinkle granules on 1 tablespoon of soft food and have patient consume immediately.
• If a dose is missed, give at next scheduled time; don't double a dose.

ACTION
May result from increased efficiency of myocardial oxygen use when myocardial metabolism is shifted away from fatty acid oxidation toward glucose oxidation. Antianginal and anti-ischemic properties

R

don't decrease HR or BP and don't increase myocardial work.

Route	Onset	Peak	Duration
PO	Rapid	2–5 hr	Unknown

Half-life: 7 hours.

ADVERSE REACTIONS

CNS: dizziness, headache, weakness, syncope, vertigo. **CV:** palpitations, ***bradycardia,*** peripheral edema, hypotension. **EENT:** blurred vision, tinnitus, dry mouth. **GI:** abdominal pain, constipation, nausea, vomiting, dyspepsia, anorexia. **GU:** hematuria. **Respiratory:** dyspnea. **Skin:** hyperhidrosis.

INTERACTIONS

Drug-drug. *CYP2D6 substrates (antipsychotics, TCAs):* May increase levels of these drugs. Substrate dosage reduction may be needed.

CYP3A inducers (carbamazepine, phenobarbital, phenytoin, rifabutin, rifampin, rifapentine): May reduce ranolazine plasma concentration to subtherapeutic levels. Avoid use together.

Digoxin: May increase digoxin level. Monitor digoxin level periodically; digoxin dosage may need to be reduced.

Drugs that prolong QT interval (antiarrhythmics [dofetilide, quinidine, sotalol], antipsychotics [chlorpromazine, ziprasidone]): May increase risk of prolonged QT interval and ventricular arrhythmia. Use cautiously together.

Metformin: May increase metformin level when given with ranolazine 1,000 mg b.i.d. Limit metformin dosage to 1,700 mg/day and monitor blood glucose level.

Moderate CYP3A inhibitors (diltiazem, erythromycin, verapamil): May increase ranolazine level. Limit maximum ranolazine dosage to 500 mg b.i.d.

P-gp inhibitors (amiloride, atorvastatin, cyclosporine, felodipine): May increase ranolazine level. Use cautiously together and titrate ranolazine dosage based on clinical response.

Simvastatin: May increase simvastatin level. Limit simvastatin dosage to 20 mg once daily, and monitor patient for adverse effects.

Strong CYP3A inhibitors (clarithromycin, itraconazole, ketoconazole, nefazodone, nelfinavir, ritonavir, saquinavir): May increase ranolazine level. Avoid use together.

Drug-herb. *St. John's wort:* May reduce ranolazine plasma concentration to subtherapeutic levels. Discourage use together.

Drug-food. *Grapefruit products:* May increase drug level and prolong QT interval. Discourage use together.

EFFECTS ON LAB TEST RESULTS

• May increase potassium, creatinine, and BUN levels.
• May decrease HbA_{1c} level.

CONTRAINDICATIONS & CAUTIONS

• Contraindicated in patients with liver cirrhosis.
• Use cautiously in patients with renal impairment. Discontinue drug if acute renal failure develops.

🔱 *Alert:* Drug prolongs QT interval according to dose. Use cautiously in patients taking QT interval–prolonging drugs and in those with a family history of long QT syndrome, congenital long QT syndrome, or acquired QT-interval prolongation. Clinical studies didn't show an increased risk of proarrhythmia or sudden death.
• Drug isn't indicated for ACS.
Dialyzable drug: Unlikely.

PREGNANCY-LACTATION-REPRODUCTION

• There are no adequate studies during pregnancy. Use only if potential benefit justifies fetal risk.
• It isn't known if drug appears human milk. Patient should discontinue breastfeeding or discontinue drug.

NURSING CONSIDERATIONS

• Obtain baseline ECG and monitor subsequent ECG for prolonged QT interval. Measure QTc interval regularly.
• If patient has renal insufficiency, monitor BP closely.
• Monitor electrolyte levels, especially potassium, and correct abnormalities.

PATIENT TEACHING

• Teach patient about drug's potential to affect heart rhythm. Advise patient to immediately report palpitations or fainting.
• Urge patient to report all other prescription or OTC drugs or herbal supplements being taken.
• Tell patient to keep taking other drugs prescribed for angina.

- Instruct patient that drug may be taken with or without food.
- Caution patient to avoid grapefruit products while taking drug.
- Advise patient that if a dose is missed, to take it at the next scheduled time and not to double the dose.

🜚 *Alert:* Warn patient that tablets must be swallowed whole and not crushed, broken, or chewed.

- Explain that drug won't stop a sudden anginal attack. Advise patient to keep other treatments, such as SL nitroglycerin, readily available.
- Tell patient to avoid activities that require mental alertness until drug's effects are known.

rasagiline mesylate
ra-SA-ji-leen

Azilect⬧

Therapeutic class: Antiparkinsonian drugs
Pharmacologic class: Irreversible, selective MAO inhibitors type B

AVAILABLE FORMS
Tablets: 0.5 mg, 1 mg

INDICATIONS & DOSAGES
➤ **Idiopathic Parkinson disease, as monotherapy or with levodopa**
Adults: As monotherapy, 1 mg PO once daily. As adjunctive therapy, initial dose is 0.5 mg PO once daily. May increase to 1 mg PO once daily based on tolerance and clinical response.
Adjust-a-dose: If patient has mild hepatic impairment or takes a CYP1A2 inhibitor such as ciprofloxacin, give 0.5 mg once daily.

ADMINISTRATION
PO
- Give drug without regard to meals.
- If a dose is missed, omit the missed dose and give next dose as scheduled; don't double dose.

ACTION
Unknown. May increase extracellular dopamine level in the CNS, improving neurotransmission and relieving signs and symptoms of Parkinson disease.

Route	Onset	Peak	Duration
PO	Variable	1 hr	1 wk

Half-life: 3 hours.

ADVERSE REACTIONS
Monotherapy
CNS: headache, depression, fever, hallucinations, malaise, paresthesia, vertigo. **EENT:** conjunctivitis, rhinitis. **GI:** dyspepsia, gastroenteritis. **GU:** albuminuria. **Musculoskeletal:** arthralgia, arthritis, neck pain. **Skin:** ecchymosis. **Other:** falls, flulike syndrome.
Adjunctive therapy
CNS: insomnia, dizziness, headache, abnormal dreams, amnesia, ataxia, dyskinesia, dystonia, hallucinations, paresthesia, somnolence. **CV:** bundle-branch block, edema, orthostatic hypotension, *hemorrhage.* **EENT:** epistaxis, dry mouth, gingivitis. **GI:** nausea, abdominal pain, anorexia, constipation, diarrhea, dyspepsia, dysphagia, vomiting, *GI hemorrhage.* **GU:** albuminuria, hematuria, urinary incontinence. **Hematologic:** anemia. **Metabolic:** weight loss. **Musculoskeletal:** arthralgia, arthritis, back pain, bursitis, hernia, leg cramps, myasthenia, neck pain, tenosynovitis. **Respiratory:** dyspnea, cough, URI. **Skin:** ecchymosis, rash, diaphoresis. **Other:** infection, accidental injury, falls.

INTERACTIONS
Drug-drug. *Ciprofloxacin and other CYP1A2 inhibitors:* May double rasagiline level. Decrease rasagiline dosage to 0.5 mg daily.
Cyclobenzaprine: May enhance serotonergic effects. Concomitant use is contraindicated.
Dextromethorphan: May cause episodes of psychosis or bizarre behavior. Concomitant use is contraindicated.
Dopamine antagonists (antipsychotics, metoclopramide): May decrease effectiveness of rasagiline. Avoid use together.
Levodopa: May increase rasagiline level. Watch for dyskinesia, dystonia, hallucinations, and hypotension, and reduce levodopa dosage if needed.
MAO inhibitors: May cause serotonin syndrome. Contraindicated with or within 14 days of other MAO inhibitors.
Opiate agonists (fentanyl, meperidine, methadone, tramadol): May cause severe, sometimes fatal, serotonin syndrome. Concomitant use is contraindicated.

R

SSNRIs, SSRIs, TCAs, tetracyclic antidepressants, triazolopyridine antidepressants: May cause serotonin syndrome. Stop rasagiline for at least 14 days before starting an antidepressant. Stop fluoxetine for 5 weeks before starting rasagiline.

Sympathomimetics (decongestants): May cause severe hypertensive reaction. Use together cautiously.

Drug-herb. *St. John's wort:* May cause severe reaction. Use together is contraindicated.

Drug-food. *Foods with very high levels of tyramine (more than 150 mg), such as aged cheeses, cured meats, fava beans:* May cause hypertensive reaction. Urge patient to avoid foods high in tyramine.

EFFECTS ON LAB TEST RESULTS
None reported.

CONTRAINDICATIONS & CAUTIONS
• Exacerbation of HTN may occur during treatment, which may require medication adjustment if sustained.
• Somnolence and falling asleep without prior warning while engaged in ADLs (including operating motor vehicles) have been reported in some patients. Evaluate patient for factors that may increase these risks.
• Use cautiously in patients with mild hepatic impairment. Use in patients with moderate or severe hepatic impairment isn't recommended.

Dialyzable drug: Unknown.

⚠ **Overdose S&S:** Drowsiness, dizziness, faintness, irritability, hyperactivity, agitation, severe headache, hallucinations, trismus, opisthotonos, seizures, coma, rapid and irregular pulse, HTN, hypotension and vascular collapse, precordial pain, respiratory depression and failure, hyperpyrexia, diaphoresis, cool and clammy skin.

PREGNANCY-LACTATION-REPRODUCTION
• There are no adequate studies during pregnancy. Use only if potential benefit justifies fetal risk.
• It isn't known if drug appears in human milk. Use cautiously during breastfeeding.

NURSING CONSIDERATIONS
• Orthostatic hypotension occurs most frequently during first 2 months of therapy; help patient to rise from a reclining position.
• Monitor patient for new-onset HTN or HTN that isn't adequately controlled after starting drug.
• Monitor patient for serotonin syndrome (confusion, hypomania, hallucinations, agitation, delirium, headache, coma).
• Monitor patient for drowsiness, significant daytime sleepiness, or episodes of falling asleep during activities that require active participation. Discontinue drug if these symptoms occur.
• Ask patient or caregiver about new or worsening impulsive or compulsive behaviors, such as new or increased gambling urges, sexual urges, uncontrolled spending, or other urges; patient may not recognize these behaviors as abnormal.
• Monitor patient for dyskinesia and dopaminergic adverse effects when drug is used as an adjunct to levodopa. Drug may also exacerbate preexisting dyskinesia.
• Examine patient's skin periodically for possible melanoma because patients with Parkinson disease have a higher risk of skin cancer.
• Monitor patient for withdrawal-related signs and symptoms (elevated temperature, muscle rigidity, altered level of consciousness, autonomic instability), especially after rapid dosage reduction or withdrawal or change in drugs.
• Notify prescriber if patient is having elective surgery; drug should be stopped at least 2 weeks before.
• *Look alike–sound alike:* Don't confuse Azilect with Aricept.

PATIENT TEACHING
• Explain the risk of hypertensive crisis if patient ingests foods containing very high levels of tyramine while taking rasagiline. Give patient a list of these foods and products.
• Advise patient to rise slowly after prolonged sitting or lying down.
• Caution patient to immediately report confusion, hallucinations, agitation, delirium, syncope, shivering, diaphoresis, high fever, tachycardia, nausea, diarrhea, muscle rigidity or twitching, or tremors.
• Advise patient that drug may cause patient to fall asleep during activities that require active participation and to report if drowsiness,

---

Reactions in bold italics are *life-threatening*. Interactions may have a *rapid onset* or a ***delayed onset***.

significant daytime sleepiness, or episodes of falling asleep during such activities occur.
• Tell patient to report difficulty controlling impulsive or compulsive behaviors, such as new or increased gambling urges, sexual urges, uncontrolled spending, or other urges.
• Urge patient to watch for skin changes that could suggest melanoma and to have periodic skin exams.
• Instruct patient to maintain usual dosage schedule if a dose is missed and not to double the next dose.
• Tell patient to report plans to become pregnant or to breastfeed.
• Advise patient to contact prescriber before discontinuing rasagiline.

SAFETY ALERT!

relugolix
re-loo-GOE-lix

Orgovyx

Therapeutic class: Endocrine drugs
Pharmacologic class: GnRH receptor antagonists

AVAILABLE FORMS
Tablets ⓓⓝⓒ: 120 mg

INDICATIONS & DOSAGES
➤ **Advanced prostate cancer**
Adults: 360 mg PO on day 1, then 120 mg PO once daily.
Adjust-a-dose: For patients taking combined P-gp and strong CYP3A inducers, increase relugolix dosage to 240 mg once daily. After discontinuing the combined P-gp and strong CYP3A inducer, resume 120 mg daily relugolix dosage.

ADMINISTRATION
PO
• Give without regard to food and at same time each day.
• Patient must swallow capsules whole; don't crush or allow patient to chew capsules.
• Give missed dose as soon as possible. If more than 12 hours has elapsed since the missed dose, skip the dose and resume regular schedule the next day.
• If therapy is interrupted beyond 7 days, restart drug at 360 mg on day 1, then continue with 120 mg once daily.

• Store at room temperature. Don't store above 86° F (30° C).

ACTION
Reduces release of LH, FSH, and testosterone by binding to pituitary GnRH receptors.

Route	Onset	Peak	Duration
PO	Unknown	2.25 hr	Unknown

Half-life: 60.8 hours.

ADVERSE REACTIONS
CNS: fatigue. **GI:** constipation, diarrhea. **Hematologic:** decreased Hb level. **Hepatic:** elevated AST and ALT levels. **Metabolic:** hyperglycemia, hypertriglyceridemia. **Musculoskeletal:** musculoskeletal pain. **Other:** hot flushes.

INTERACTIONS
Drug-drug. *Combined P-gp and strong CYP3A inducers (carbamazepine, dexamethasone, rifampin):* May decrease relugolix level and effectiveness. Avoid use together. If unable to avoid use together, increase relugolix dosage.
Drugs that prolong QTc interval (ciprofloxacin, haloperidol, lithium, methadone, procainamide, SSRIs, TCAs): May increase risk of prolonged QTc interval. Monitor patient closely.
Oral P-gp inhibitors (amiodarone, erythromycin, ketoconazole, saquinavir): May increase relugolix level. Avoid use together. If unable to avoid use together, give inhibitor at least 6 hours after relugolix and monitor patient frequently for adverse reactions. May interrupt relugolix therapy for up to 2 weeks if a short course of P-gp inhibitor therapy is required.
Drug-herb. *St John's wort:* May decrease relugolix level and effectiveness. Discourage use together.

EFFECTS ON LAB TEST RESULTS
• May increase PSA, testosterone, glucose, triglyceride, ALT, and AST levels.
• May decrease Hb level.

CONTRAINDICATIONS & CAUTIONS
• Androgen deprivation therapy may prolong QT interval. Weigh benefits of therapy against risk in patients with congenital long QT syndrome, HF, or frequent electrolyte

R

abnormalities, and in patients taking drugs known to prolong QT interval.
• Safety and effectiveness in females and children haven't been established.
Dialyzable drug: Unknown.

PREGNANCY-LACTATION-REPRODUCTION
• Drug may cause fetal harm and loss of pregnancy.
• It isn't known if drug appears in human milk or how drug affects milk production or infants who are breastfed.
• Male patients with partners of childbearing potential should use effective contraception during therapy and for 2 weeks after final dose.
• Drug may impair fertility in male patients of reproductive potential.

NURSING CONSIDERATIONS
• Monitor patient for signs and symptoms of prolonged QT interval.
• Obtain ECG and electrolyte levels at baseline and periodically during therapy. Correct electrolyte abnormalities, as necessary.
• Monitor PSA level periodically. If PSA level increases, obtain serum testosterone concentration.
• Monitor patient for signs and symptoms of hyperglycemia.
• Obtain LFT values at baseline and periodically during therapy.
• Monitor patient for signs and symptoms of anemia.

PATIENT TEACHING
• Teach patient how to properly take and store drug.
• Instruct patient about signs and symptoms of prolonged QT interval (palpitations, chest pain, dizziness, fainting) and to immediately report if they occur.
• Inform patient about adverse reactions related to androgen deprivation therapy, including hot flushes, increased weight, decreased sex drive, and difficulties with erectile function.
• Warn patient that drug may cause fetal harm and loss of pregnancy.
• Advise male patient with partner of childbearing potential to use effective contraception during therapy and for 2 weeks after final dose.
• Inform male patient that drug may cause infertility.

relugolix–estradiol–norethindrone acetate
re-loo-GOE-lix/ess-tra-DYE-ole/nor-ETH-in-drone

Myfembree

Therapeutic class: Hormones
Pharmacologic class: GnRH receptor antagonists–estrogens–progestins

AVAILABLE FORMS
Tablets: relugolix 40 mg, estradiol 1 mg, norethindrone acetate 0.5 mg

INDICATIONS & DOSAGES
Adjust-a-dose (for all indications): If use with oral P-gp inhibitors can't be avoided, give Myfembree first and separate dosing by at least 6 hours.
➤ **Management of heavy menstrual bleeding associated with uterine leiomyomas (fibroids) in patients who are premenopausal**
Adults: 1 tablet PO daily for up to 24 months.
✳ *NEW INDICATION:* **Management of moderate to severe pain associated with endometriosis**
Adults: 1 tablet PO daily for up to 24 months.

ADMINISTRATION
PO
• Give at approximately same time each day, without regard to meals.
• Start drug after onset of menses but no later than 7 days after onset.
• If a dose is missed, give missed dose as soon as possible the same day and resume regular schedule the next day at usual time.
• Store tablets at room temperature.

ACTION
Nonpeptide GnRH receptor antagonist that binds to pituitary GnRH receptors, reduces release of LH and FSH, decreases serum levels of estradiol and progesterone, and reduces bleeding associated with uterine fibroids. Estradiol may reduce bone loss that can occur with relugolix, and norethindrone may protect uterus from the adverse effects of unopposed estrogen.

Route	Onset	Peak	Duration
PO	Unknown	1–7 hr	Unknown

Half-life: 10.9 to 61.5 hours.

Reactions in bold italics are *life-threatening*. Interactions may have a *rapid onset* or a ***delayed onset***.

ADVERSE REACTIONS

CNS: anxiety, depression, irritability, mood disorders. **CV:** HTN. **GI:** dyspepsia. **GU:** abnormal uterine bleeding, decreased libido. **Musculoskeletal:** bone loss. **Skin:** alopecia, hyperhidrosis, night sweats. **Other:** hot flush, breast cyst, hypersensitivity.

INTERACTIONS

Drug-drug. *Combined P-gp and strong CYP3A inducers (rifampin):* May decrease relugolix, estradiol, or norethindrone level. Avoid use together.
Estrogen-containing contraceptives: May increase estrogen level and risk of estrogen-associated adverse events. May decrease efficacy of relugolix, estradiol, and norethindrone. Avoid use together.
P-gp inhibitors (erythromycin): May increase relugolix level. Avoid use together. If concomitant use is necessary, separate doses by 6 hours and monitor patient for adverse reactions.
Drug-herb. *St. John's wort:* May decrease relugolix, estradiol, or norethindrone level. Discourage use together.
Drug-lifestyle. **Boxed Warning** *Smoking:* May increase risk of CV events, especially in patients older than age 35. Use together is contraindicated. ∎

EFFECTS ON LAB TEST RESULTS

• May increase hepatic transaminase, binding protein (thyroid-binding globulin, corticosteroid-binding globulin), angiotensinogen-renin substrate, alpha-1 antitrypsin, ceruloplasmin, glucose, total cholesterol, LDL, and triglyceride levels.
• May decrease free thyroid, corticosteroid hormone, and free testosterone levels.
• May increase platelet count, fibrinogen plasminogen antigen, and clotting factor.
• May increase bleeding times.
• May decrease antithrombin III and anti-factor Xa levels.

CONTRAINDICATIONS & CAUTIONS

Boxed Warning Drug increases risk of thrombotic or thromboembolic disorders, including PE, DVT, stroke, and MI, especially in patients at increased risk for these events. ∎
Boxed Warning Contraindicated in patients with current or history of thrombotic or thromboembolic disorders, in patients older than age 35 who smoke, and in patients with uncontrolled HTN, dyslipidemia, vascular disease, or obesity. ∎
• Contraindicated in patients at high risk for arterial, venous thrombotic, or thromboembolic disorder (cerebrovascular disease, CAD, PVD, thrombogenic valvular or thrombogenic rhythm diseases of the heart, inherited or acquired hypercoagulopathies, or headaches with focal neurologic symptoms or migraine headaches with aura if older than age 35).
• Contraindicated in patients hypersensitive to drug or its components.
• Contraindicated in patients with known osteoporosis; current or history of breast cancer or other hormone-sensitive malignancies; increased risk of hormone-sensitive malignancies; known hepatic impairment or disease; or undiagnosed abnormal uterine bleeding.
• Stop drug immediately if arterial or venous thrombotic, CV, or cerebrovascular event occurs, or if hormone-sensitive malignancy is diagnosed.
• Stop drug if sudden unexplained partial or complete vision loss, proptosis, diplopia, papilledema, or retinal vascular lesions occur. Evaluate patient immediately for retinal vein thrombosis.
• Therapy duration is limited to 24 months. Drug may cause decreases in bone mineral density (BMD) that may not be completely reversible. Baseline and periodic BMD assessments are recommended. Assess risks and benefits for patients with additional risk factors for bone loss.
• Drug may contribute to depression, mood disorders, or suicidal ideation.
• Use cautiously in patients with well-controlled HTN; monitor BP and stop drug if BP rises significantly.
• Use cautiously in patients with history of cholestatic jaundice related to past estrogen use or pregnancy.
• Use cautiously in patients with prediabetes, diabetes, or hypertriglyceridemia. Drug may decrease glucose tolerance and increase cholesterol and triglyceride levels.
• Drug may cause uterine fibroid prolapse or expulsion.
• Drug may cause alopecia. Stop drug if hair loss becomes a concern.
• Safety and effectiveness in children haven't been established.
Dialyzable drug: Unknown.

R

⚠ *Overdose S&S:* Nausea, vomiting, breast tenderness, abdominal pain, drowsiness, fatigue, withdrawal bleeding.

PREGNANCY-LACTATION-REPRODUCTION
• Drug is contraindicated during pregnancy and may cause early pregnancy loss. Exclude pregnancy before starting therapy.
• Drug may delay ability to recognize pregnancy because it alters menstrual bleeding. If pregnancy is suspected, perform testing; stop drug if pregnancy is confirmed.
• Enroll patients exposed to drug during pregnancy in Myfembree Pregnancy Exposure Registry (1-855-428-0707).
• Patients of childbearing potential should use effective nonhormonal contraception during therapy and for 1 week after final dose. Avoid use with hormonal contraceptives.
• Drug may appear in human milk. Weigh benefits against risk to infant.

NURSING CONSIDERATIONS
• Verify pregnancy status before start of therapy. Monitor patient for pregnancy.
• Monitor patient for hypersensitivity reaction; immediately stop drug if reaction occurs.
• Monitor patient for signs and symptoms of hepatic impairment or gallbladder disease. Periodically obtain LFTs.
• Monitor patient for development of impaired glucose tolerance or hyperlipidemia.
• Monitor patient for development of thromboembolic disorders, including DVT.
• Assess patient for mood changes and signs and symptoms of depression during therapy. Reevaluate benefits and risk of continued therapy if changes occur. Refer patient with new or worsening signs or symptoms to a mental health professional, as appropriate.
• Monitor patient for HTN.
• Obtain dual-energy X-ray absorptiometry at baseline and periodically during therapy.
• Monitor standard of care surveillance breast exams and mammography.
• Monitor patient for severe uterine bleeding and cramping.
• Stop drug 4 to 6 weeks before surgery that's associated with an increased risk of thromboembolism, or during periods of prolonged immobilization.

PATIENT TEACHING
• Instruct patient to start drug as soon as possible after onset of menses but no later than 7 days after start of menses.
• Advise patient that using estrogen and progestin combinations may increase risk of venous and arterial thrombotic or thromboembolic events, especially in patients at high risk.
• Instruct patient to seek medical attention for severe uterine bleeding because drug may cause uterine fibroid prolapse or expulsion.
• Inform patient about risk of bone loss and that calcium and vitamin D supplements may be beneficial if dietary intake isn't adequate. Advise patient not to take oral iron supplements at the same time as calcium and vitamin D.
• Tell patient that depression, mood disorders, and suicidality may occur while taking drug and to promptly seek medical attention if new-onset or worsening depression, anxiety, or other mood changes occur.
• Advise patient to promptly seek medical attention for signs or symptoms of liver injury occur (jaundice, right upper abdominal pain).
• Advise patient that drug may delay recognition of pregnancy because it may reduce duration and amount of menstrual bleeding. Tell patient to use effective nonhormonal contraception during therapy and to stop drug if pregnancy is confirmed.
• Tell patient who is pregnant about registry that monitors outcomes in patients exposed to drug during pregnancy.
• Inform patient that alopecia, hair loss, and hair thinning may occur during therapy, and may not reverse after stopping drug. Advise patient to contact health care provider about concerns or changes regarding hair.
• Advise patient to report use of other prescription or OTC drugs or dietary supplements; concomitant use may decrease drug's therapeutic effects.

Reactions in bold italics are *life-threatening*. Interactions may have a *rapid onset* or a ***delayed onset***.

remdesivir

rem-DE-si-vir

Veklury

Therapeutic class: Antivirals
Pharmacologic class: SARS-CoV-2
nucleotide analogue RNA polymerase
inhibitors

AVAILABLE FORMS
Injection: 100 mg/20 mL single-dose vial
Powder for injection: 100 mg single-dose vial

INDICATIONS & DOSAGES
➤ **Coronavirus disease 2019 (COVID-19)
requiring hospitalization**
Adults and children age 12 and older weighing 40 kg or more: 200 mg IV infusion on day 1 followed by maintenance dose of 100 mg IV infusion once daily starting on day 2 for 5 days in patients not requiring invasive mechanical ventilation or extracorporeal membrane oxygenation (ECMO); if no clinical improvement, may extend therapy 5 additional days. Therapy duration for patients requiring invasive mechanical ventilation or ECMO is 10 days.
Children age 28 days and older weighing 3 to less than 40 kg: Initiate therapy as soon as possible after diagnosis with 5 mg/kg IV infusion on day 1, followed by maintenance dose of 2.5 mg/kg IV infusion once daily on day 2 for 5 days in patients not requiring invasive mechanical ventilation or ECMO; if no clinical improvement, may extend therapy 5 additional days. Give for 10 days to patients requiring invasive mechanical ventilation or ECMO.
Adjust-a-dose: Consider discontinuing drug if ALT level increases to greater than 10 × ULN. Discontinue if ALT elevation is accompanied by signs or symptoms of liver inflammation.
✳ **NEW INDICATION: Nonhospitalized patients with mild to moderate COVID-19 at high risk for progression to severe COVID-19, including hospitalization or death**
Adults and children age 12 and older weighing 40 kg or more: Initiate therapy as soon as possible after diagnosis and within 7 days of symptom onset with 200 mg IV infusion on day 1, followed by 100 mg IV infusion once daily on days 2 and 3.
Children age 28 days and older weighing 3 to less than 40 kg: Initiate therapy as soon as possible and within 7 days of symptom onset with 5 mg/kg IV infusion on day 1, followed by 2.5 mg/kg IV infusion once daily on days 2 and 3.
Adjust-a-dose: Consider discontinuing drug if ALT level increases to greater than 10 × ULN. Discontinue if ALT elevation accompanies signs or symptoms of liver inflammation.

ADMINISTRATION
IV
▼ Remdesivir lyophilized powder is the only form approved for use in children weighing less than 40 kg.
▼ Prepare diluted solution on same day as administration.
▼ Let single-dose solution vial reach room temperature (68° to 77° F [20° to 25° C]). Sealed vials can remain at room temperature for up to 12 hours before dilution.
▼ Reconstitute powder with 19 mL sterile water for injection. Immediately shake for 30 seconds; allow contents to settle for 2 to 3 minutes. If contents aren't dissolved, repeat as necessary. Shake until dissolution. Discard vial if contents don't dissolve completely.
▼ Inspect solution for particulates and discoloration. Discard vial if the reconstituted powder or solution contains particulate matter or discoloration. Before dilution, solution should be clear or slightly yellow.
▼ For patient weighing at least 40 kg: Immediately further dilute reconstituted powder in 100 or 250 mL NSS or dilute the solution in 250 mL NSS. From NSS infusion bag, withdraw (and discard) 40 mL for 200-mg dose or 20 mL for 100-mg dose. Inject desired dose of drug into infusion bag and gently invert bag 20 times to mix solution. Don't shake.
▼ For children weighing 3 to less than 40 kg: Immediately further dilute 100 mg/20 mL reconstituted solution to a concentration of 1.25 mg/mL in NSS with the volume required based on weight-based dose.
▼ Give infusion over 30 to 120 minutes.
▼ Prepared solution is stable for 24 hours at room temperature or for 48 hours refrigerated at 36° to 46° F (2° to 8° C).

R

♣Canada ◇OTC ♦Off-label use ✐Photoguide ⊕Do not crush *Liquid contains alcohol ⊠Genetic

▼ Store vials of powder below 86° F (30° C). Refrigerate vials of solution at 36° to 46° F (2° to 8° C).

▼ **Incompatibilities:** Other medications or solutions; use only NSS for the final dilution.

ACTION
Inhibits viral replication.

Route	Onset	Peak	Duration
IV	Unknown	40 min	Unknown

Half-life: 1 hour.

ADVERSE REACTIONS
GI: nausea. **GU:** *acute kidney injury,* decreased GFR. **Hematologic:** decreased Hb, increased PT, *lymphocytopenia.* **Hepatic:** elevated transaminase levels, hyperbilirubinemia. **Metabolic:** hyperglycemia. **Skin:** administration-site extravasation, injection-site erythema, rash. **Other:** hypersensitivity reactions, infusion reaction.

INTERACTIONS
Drug-drug. *Chloroquine phosphate, hydroxychloroquine:* May decrease antiviral activity. Don't use together.
Other drugs: Interaction studies of drug with other concomitant medications haven't been conducted in humans. Monitor patient closely.

EFFECTS ON LAB TEST RESULTS
• May increase ALT, AST, bilirubin, and glucose levels.
• May decrease potassium level, CrCl, and eGFR.
• May increase or decrease creatinine level.
• May prolong PT and PTT.
• May increase urinary glucose and protein levels.
• May decrease Hb level and lymphocyte count.

CONTRAINDICATIONS & CAUTIONS
• Contraindicated in patients with clinically significant hypersensitivity reactions to drug or its components.
• Drug isn't recommended for patients with eGFR less than 30 mL/minute.
• Hypersensitivity, including infusion-related and anaphylactic reactions, has been observed during and after administration.
Dialyzable drug: Unknown.

PREGNANCY-LACTATION-REPRODUCTION
• It isn't known if drug increases risk of major birth defects, miscarriage, or adverse maternal or fetal outcomes. Use only if potential benefit justifies the risk.
• A pregnancy exposure registry is available at https://covid-pr.pregistry.com or 1-800-616-3791.
• It isn't known if drug appears in human milk or how drug affects milk production or infants who are breastfed. Use cautiously during breastfeeding.
• Patients with COVID-19 should follow clinical guidelines to avoid exposing infant to virus.

NURSING CONSIDERATIONS
• Drug should only be administered in a setting capable of providing acute care for severe infusion or hypersensitivity reactions and to activate the emergency medical system, as necessary.
• Obtain baseline eGFR before starting drug and monitor renal function as appropriate during therapy.
• Obtain baseline LFT values and PT before starting drug and monitor as appropriate during therapy.
• Monitor patient for hypersensitivity reactions (hypotension, HTN, tachycardia, bradycardia, hypoxia, fever, dyspnea, wheezing, angioedema, rash, nausea, diaphoresis, shivering). Consider slower infusion time up to 120 minutes to prevent hypersensitivity reaction. If significant hypersensitivity reaction occurs, immediately discontinue drug and initiate appropriate treatment.

PATIENT TEACHING
• Advise patient that hypersensitivity reaction may occur and to report changes in HR, fever, shortness of breath, wheezing, rash, nausea, diaphoresis, shivering, or swelling of lips, face, or throat.
• Caution patient that drug may increase risk of renal and hepatic dysfunction. Advise patient to immediately report signs or symptoms of liver inflammation (dark urine, fatigue, upset stomach or stomach pain, light-colored stools, vomiting, or jaundice).
• Instruct patient to immediately report pregnancy.
• Advise patient who is breastfeeding to discuss alternative feeding options with prescriber.

Reactions in bold italics are *life-threatening*. Interactions may have a *rapid onset* or a **delayed onset**.

repaglinide
re-PAG-li-nide

Therapeutic class: Antidiabetics
Pharmacologic class: Meglitinides

AVAILABLE FORMS
Tablets: 0.5 mg, 1 mg, 2 mg

INDICATIONS & DOSAGES
➤ **Type 2 diabetes, as adjunct to diet and exercise**
Adults: For patients not previously treated or whose HbA_{1c} level is below 8%, starting dose is 0.5 mg PO before each meal. For patients previously treated with glucose-lowering drugs and whose HbA_{1c} is 8% or more, first dose is 1 to 2 mg PO before each meal. Recommended dosage range is 0.5 to 4 mg before meals b.i.d., t.i.d., or q.i.d. Maximum daily dose is 16 mg.

Determine dosage by glucose response. May double dosage up to 4 mg before each meal until satisfactory glucose response is achieved. At least 1 week should elapse between dosage adjustments to assess response to each dose.

Adjust-a-dose: In patients with severe renal impairment (CrCl of 20 to 40 mL/minute), starting dosage is 0.5 mg. Gradually titrate dosage, if needed, to achieve glycemic control. Use cautiously in patients with impaired liver function and allow longer intervals between dosage adjustments to allow full assessment of response. Dosage adjustment is recommended with concomitant use of strong CYP3A4 or CYP2C8 inhibitors or inducers.

ADMINISTRATION
PO
• Give drug within 30 minutes before meals.
• If patient skips a meal, skip the scheduled dose to reduce the risk of hypoglycemia.

ACTION
Stimulates insulin release from beta cells in the pancreas by closing adenosine triphosphate (ATP)-dependent potassium channels in beta cell membranes, which causes calcium channels to open. Increased calcium influx induces insulin secretion; the overall effect is to lower glucose level.

Route	Onset	Peak	Duration
PO	15–60 min	1 hr	6 hr

Half-life: 1 hour.

ADVERSE REACTIONS
CNS: headache, paresthesia. **CV:** angina. **EENT:** rhinitis, sinusitis, tooth disorder. **GI:** constipation, diarrhea, dyspepsia, nausea, vomiting. **GU:** UTI. **Metabolic:** *hypoglycemia,* hyperglycemia. **Musculoskeletal:** arthralgia, back pain. **Respiratory:** bronchitis, URI. **Other:** hypersensitivity reaction.

INTERACTIONS
Drug-drug. *Barbiturates, carbamazepine, rifampin, similar inducers of CYP2C8 and CYP3A4:* May decrease repaglinide level. Monitor glucose level and increase repaglinide dosage as necessary.
Beta blockers, chloramphenicol, coumarin derivatives, MAO inhibitors, NSAIDs, other drugs that are highly protein bound, probenecid, salicylates, sulfonamides: May increase hypoglycemic action of repaglinide. Monitor glucose level.
Calcium channel blockers, corticosteroids, estrogens, fosphenytoin, hormonal contraceptives, isoniazid, nicotinic acid, phenothiazines, phenytoin, sympathomimetics, thiazides and other diuretics, thyroid products: May produce hyperglycemia, resulting in a loss of glycemic control. Monitor glucose level.
Clarithromycin: May increase repaglinide levels. Adjust repaglinide dosage.
Clopidogrel: May increase repaglinide level. Start repaglinide at 0.5 mg before each meal. Maximum dosage is 4 mg/day. Avoid use together if possible.
Cyclosporine: May increase repaglinide serum concentration. Don't exceed repaglinide dosage of 6 mg/day; monitor glucose level closely.
Erythromycin, itraconazole, ketoconazole, miconazole, similar inhibitors of CYP2C8 and CYP3A4: May increase repaglinide level. Monitor glucose level and reduce repaglinide dosage as necessary.
Gemfibrozil: Significantly increases repaglinide level. Use together is contraindicated.
Statins (atorvastatin, simvastatin): May increase repaglinide level. Monitor glucose level.

R

Thiazolidinediones (pioglitazone, rosiglitazone): May increase risk of hypoglycemia, edema, and weight gain. Monitor patient.

Drug-herb. *Burdock:* May increase hypoglycemic effects. Discourage use together. *St. John's wort:* May decrease repaglinide level and its therapeutic effect. Don't use together.

Drug-food. *Grapefruit juice:* May inhibit metabolism of drug. Discourage use together.

Drug-lifestyle. *Alcohol use:* May alter glycemic control, most commonly causing hypoglycemia. Discourage use together.

EFFECTS ON LAB TEST RESULTS
• May increase or decrease glucose level.

CONTRAINDICATIONS & CAUTIONS
• Contraindicated in patients hypersensitive to drug or its inactive ingredients and in those with type 1 diabetes or diabetic ketoacidosis with or without coma.
• Drug isn't indicated for use in combination with NPH insulin due to risk of serious CV adverse events.
• Use cautiously in older adults and in patients with debilitation, malnourishment, or hepatic, adrenal, or pituitary insufficiency.
Dialyzable drug: Unknown.
⚠ *Overdose S&S:* Hypoglycemia, severe hypoglycemic reactions (coma, seizures, neurologic impairment).

PREGNANCY-LACTATION-REPRODUCTION
• Safety during pregnancy hasn't been established. Use only if clearly needed.
• Abnormal blood glucose levels during pregnancy may cause fetal harm. Most experts recommend insulin during pregnancy to maintain blood glucose levels as close to normal as possible.
• It isn't known if drug appears in human milk. Patient should discontinue breastfeeding or discontinue drug.

NURSING CONSIDERATIONS
• Increase dosage carefully in patients with renal dysfunction.
• Monitor glucose and HbA_{1c} levels for loss of glycemic control, especially during stress, such as fever, trauma, infection, or surgery.
• Hypoglycemia may be difficult to recognize in patients with longstanding diabetes or diabetic nerve disease, in older adults, and in patients taking beta blockers.

• When switching to a different oral antidiabetic, begin new drug on day after last dose of repaglinide.

PATIENT TEACHING
• Stress importance of diet and exercise with drug therapy.
• Discuss symptoms of hypoglycemia with patient and family.
• Encourage patient to keep regular appointments and have HbA_{1c} level checked every 3 months to determine long-term glucose control.
• Teach patient safe drug administration.
• Instruct patient to monitor glucose level carefully. Teach patient what to do when ill, undergoing surgery, or under added stress.
• Advise patient planning pregnancy to first consult prescriber. Insulin may be needed during pregnancy and breastfeeding.
• Teach patient to carry candy or other simple sugars to treat mild hypoglycemia episodes. Patient experiencing severe episode may need emergency treatment.
• Advise patient to avoid alcohol, which lowers glucose level.

reslizumab
res-LIZ-ue-mab

Cinqair

Therapeutic class: Immunomodulators
Pharmacologic class: Interleukin-5 antagonist monoclonal antibodies

AVAILABLE FORMS
Injection: 100 mg/10 mL single-use vial

INDICATIONS & DOSAGES
➤ **Add-on maintenance treatment of patients with severe asthma with an eosinophilic phenotype**
Adults: 3 mg/kg IV infusion once every 4 weeks.

ADMINISTRATION
IV
▼ Don't give as IV push or bolus.
▼ Visually inspect for particulate matter and discoloration. Solution should be clear to slightly hazy, opalescent, colorless to slightly yellow. Particles that appear as translucent-to-white amorphous particulates

may be present. Discard if solution appears discolored or if other foreign particulates are present.

▼ To minimize foaming, don't shake.

▼ Discard any unused portion. Drug doesn't contain preservative.

▼ Slowly inject required volume into a 50-mL NSS infusion bag of polyvinyl chloride or polyolefin. Gently invert bag. Don't shake. Don't mix or dilute with other drugs.

▼ Time between preparation and administration shouldn't exceed 16 hours. If not used immediately, store diluted reslizumab solution in refrigerator at 36° to 46° F (2° to 8° C) or at room temperature (up to 77° F [25° C]), protected from light, for up to 16 hours.

▼ If refrigerated before administration, allow diluted solution to warm to room temperature.

▼ Use an infusion set with an in-line, low-protein-binding, 0.2-micron polyethersulfone, polyvinylidene fluoride nylon, or cellulose acetate in-line infusion filter.

▼ Infuse over 20 to 50 minutes (depending on the volume to be infused based on patient weight); then flush IV administration set with NSS to ensure that all reslizumab has been administered.

▼ **Incompatibilities:** Physical and biochemical compatibility studies haven't been conducted. Don't infuse with other drugs or solutions other than NSS.

ACTION
Binds to interleukin-5, reducing production and survival of eosinophils, which limits inflammation, a component of the pathogenesis of asthma; however, its exact mechanism in asthma hasn't been established.

Route	Onset	Peak	Duration
IV	Unknown	Unknown	Unknown

Half-life: 24 days.

ADVERSE REACTIONS
EENT: oropharyngeal pain. **Musculoskeletal:** myalgia, musculoskeletal chest pain, neck pain, muscle spasm, extremity pain, muscle fatigue, musculoskeletal pain. **Other:** antibody development.

INTERACTIONS
None reported.

EFFECTS ON LAB TEST RESULTS
- May increase CK level.
- May decrease blood eosinophil count.

CONTRAINDICATIONS & CAUTIONS
Boxed Warning Anaphylaxis has occurred in patients receiving reslizumab and was reported as early as the second dose. Give only in a health care setting prepared to manage anaphylactic reactions. Discontinue if patient experiences anaphylaxis. ■

- Contraindicated in patients hypersensitive to drug or its components.
- Drug isn't indicated for status asthmaticus, acute bronchospasm, or acute asthma exacerbations.
- Drug isn't indicated for eosinophilic conditions other than severe asthma with an eosinophilic phenotype.
- Safety and effectiveness in children haven't been established.

Dialyzable drug: Unlikely.

PREGNANCY-LACTATION-REPRODUCTION
- Use in pregnancy hasn't been studied. Weigh risks to the developing fetus against risks of the mother's poorly controlled asthma.
- Monoclonal antibodies such as reslizumab are known to cross the placental barrier, so drug may affect a fetus. Risk appears to be greater during the second and third trimesters. Closely monitor asthma control in patients who are pregnant; adjust reslizumab dosage as necessary to maintain optimal control.
- It isn't known if reslizumab appears in human milk; however, human IgG is known to appear in human milk. Weigh risks to the infant who is breastfed against patient's need for drug.

NURSING CONSIDERATIONS
Boxed Warning Monitor patient for signs and symptoms of anaphylaxis (dyspnea, decreased oxygen saturation, wheezing, vomiting, urticaria) during infusion and for an appropriate amount of time after infusion has been completed. Discontinue drug immediately if severe systemic reaction occurs. ■

- If patient has preexisting parasitic infection, treat infection before initiating reslizumab. If patient becomes infected with parasites while receiving drug and doesn't respond to antiparasitic treatment, discontinue reslizumab until infection resolves.

R

- Don't abruptly discontinue systemic or inhaled corticosteroids upon initiation of reslizumab. If appropriate, decrease corticosteroid dosage gradually.
- *Look alike–sound alike:* Don't confuse reslizumab with infliximab, ixekizumab, or rituximab.

PATIENT TEACHING

Boxed Warning Teach patient signs and symptoms of anaphylaxis (mucosal swelling, airway compromise, reduced BP, rash, hives, itching). Instruct patient to immediately report signs and symptoms of an allergic reaction that occur during or after receiving a reslizumab infusion. ∎

- Explain to patient that reslizumab doesn't treat acute asthma symptoms or exacerbations. Advise patient to seek medical attention if asthma remains uncontrolled or worsens after initiation of reslizumab.
- Inform patient that there is a small risk of malignancy associated with reslizumab therapy.
- Warn patient not to discontinue systemic or inhaled corticosteroids except under medical supervision. Inform patient that reducing corticosteroid dosage may be associated with signs and symptoms of systemic withdrawal or may unmask conditions previously suppressed by corticosteroid therapy.
- Tell patient to notify health care provider for an existing or developing parasitic infection.
- Teach patient to report all adverse reactions to prescriber.

---

ribavirin
rye-ba-VYE-rin

Ibavyr✢, Virazole

Therapeutic class: Antivirals
Pharmacologic class: Nucleosides–nucleotides

AVAILABLE FORMS
Capsules ⓞⓝⓒ: 200 mg
Powder for inhalation solution: 6 g in 100-mL glass vial
Tablets: 200 mg, 400 mg✢

INDICATIONS & DOSAGES
Adjust-a-dose (for all indications): Refer to manufacturer's instructions for each formulation for dosage adjustments in patients with impaired renal function or hematologic toxicities. Some formulations are contraindicated in patients with CrCl of less than 50 mL/minute or in patients with hepatic decompensation (Child-Pugh classes B and C).

➤ **Hospitalized infants and young children infected by RSV**
Infants and young children: Solution in concentration of 20 mg/mL delivered via the Viratek Small Particle Aerosol Generator (SPAG-2) and mechanical ventilator, oxygen hood, oxygen tent, or face mask. Treatment is given for 12 to 18 hours/day for at least 3 days, and no longer than 7 days.

➤ **Chronic HCV monoinfection in combination with interferon alfa-2b (capsules)**
Adults weighing more than 105 kg: 1,400 mg PO daily in two divided doses, 600 mg in the morning and 800 mg in the evening.
Adults weighing more than 81 to 105 kg: 1,200 mg PO daily in two divided doses, 600 mg in the morning and 600 mg in the evening.
Adults weighing 66 to 80 kg: 1,000 mg PO daily in two divided doses, 400 mg in the morning and 600 mg in the evening.
Adults weighing less than 66 kg: 800 mg PO daily in two divided doses, 400 mg in the morning and 400 mg in the evening.
Adjust-a-dose: Individualize therapy duration for 24 or 48 weeks based on genotype or prior treatment failure.

➤ **Chronic HCV monoinfection in children, in combination with interferon alfa-2b (capsules)**
Children age 3 and older weighing more than 73 kg: 1,200 mg PO daily in two divided doses, 600 mg in the morning and 600 mg in the evening.
Children age 3 and older weighing 60 to 73 kg: 1,000 mg PO daily in two divided doses, 400 mg in the morning and 600 mg in the evening.
Children age 3 and older weighing 47 to 59 kg: 800 mg PO daily in two divided doses, 400 mg in the morning and 400 mg in the evening.
Adjust-a-dose: For children with HCV genotypes 2 or 3, recommended therapy duration is 24 weeks; for genotype 1, therapy duration is 48 weeks.

➤ **Chronic HCV monoinfection in combination with peginterferon alfa-2a (tablets)**
Adults with genotype 1 or 4 weighing 75 kg or more: 1,200 mg PO daily in two divided doses for 48 weeks.

Reactions in bold italics are *life-threatening*. Interactions may have a *rapid onset* or a ***delayed onset***.

Adults with genotype 1 or 4 weighing less than 75 kg: 1,000 mg daily in two divided doses for 48 weeks.

Adults with genotype 2 or 3: 800 mg PO daily in two divided doses for 24 weeks.

Adolescents and children age 5 and older weighing 75 kg or more: 1,200 mg PO daily in two divided doses, 600 mg in the morning and 600 mg in the evening.

Adolescents and children age 5 and older weighing 60 to 74 kg: 1,000 mg PO daily in two divided doses, 400 mg in the morning and 600 mg in the evening.

Adolescents and children age 5 and older weighing 47 to 59 kg: 800 mg PO daily in two divided doses, 400 mg in the morning and 400 mg in the evening.

Adolescents and children age 5 and older weighing 34 to 46 kg: 600 mg PO daily in two divided doses, 200 mg in the morning and 400 mg in the evening.

Adolescents and children age 5 and older who weigh 23 to 33 kg: 400 mg PO daily in two divided doses, 200 mg in the morning and 200 mg in the evening.

Treatment duration for children and adolescents with genotype 2 or 3 is 24 weeks and for all other genotypes is 48 weeks.

➤ **Chronic HCV infection (regardless of genotype) in patients with HIV infection, in combination with peginterferon alfa-2a**
Adults: 800 mg (tablets) PO daily in two divided doses for 48 weeks.

ADMINISTRATION
⚠ *Alert:* Drug is a hazardous agent. Use appropriate precautions for handling and disposal.

Inhalational
• Give by the Viratek SPAG-2 only. Don't use any other aerosol-generating device.
• Administer in a well-ventilated room (at least six air changes/hour).
• Use sterile USP water for injection, not bacteriostatic water. Water used to reconstitute this drug must not contain any antimicrobial product. Follow manufacturer's instructions for preparation.
• Discard solutions placed in the SPAG-2 unit at least every 24 hours before adding newly reconstituted solution.
• Don't give with other aerosolized medications.
• Store reconstituted solutions at room temperature for 24 hours.

PO
• Give drug with food and at the same time every day.
⚠ *Alert:* Capsules should never be opened, crushed, or broken.

ACTION
Inhibits viral activity by an unknown mechanism, possibly by inhibiting RNA and DNA synthesis by depleting intracellular nucleotide pools.

Route	Onset	Peak	Duration
Inhalation	Unknown	Unknown	Unknown
PO	Unknown	2 hr	Unknown

Half-life: First phase, 9.25 hours; second phase, 40 hours.

ADVERSE REACTIONS
CNS: fatigue, anxiety, depression, dizziness, headache, insomnia, agitation, rigors, chills, emotional lability, lack of concentration, memory impairment, pain, asthenia, taste perversion, irritability, nervousness, fever, malaise, aggressive or hostile behaviors, *suicidality.* **CV:** chest pain, flushing; hypotension, digoxin toxicity, tachycardia, *bradycardia, cardiac arrest (inhalation).* **EENT:** blurred vision, conjunctivitis, rhinitis, sinusitis, pharyngitis, dry mouth. **GI:** anorexia, diarrhea, nausea, vomiting, weight loss, abdominal pain, dyspepsia, constipation. **GU:** menstrual disorder. **Hematologic:** anemia, hemolytic anemia, *leukopenia, neutropenia, thrombocytopenia,* reticulocytosis. **Hepatic:** hyperbilirubinemia, hepatomegaly, *hepatic decompensation.* **Metabolic:** hyperuricemia, weight loss, hypothyroidism. **Musculoskeletal:** myalgia, arthralgia, back pain, limb pain, pediatric growth retardation. **Respiratory:** dyspnea, URI, cough; worsening of pulmonary status, *bronchospasm, pulmonary edema,* hypoventilation, pneumonia, *pneumothorax, apnea,* atelectasis, ventilator dependence (inhalation). **Skin:** alopecia, dermatitis, eczema, dermatologic disorder, pruritus, rash, dry skin, diaphoresis. **Other:** viral infection, flulike illness, bacterial infection.

INTERACTIONS
Drug-drug. *Azathioprine:* May induce severe pancytopenia and increase risk of myelotoxicity (neutropenia, thrombocytopenia, anemia). Monitor closely for signs of myelosuppression. Consider an alternative agent if possible.

R

Didanosine: May increase toxicity. Coadministration is contraindicated.

Influenza vaccine (live): May decrease therapeutic effect of vaccine. Avoid giving antiviral 48 hours before and up to 2 weeks after vaccination.

Lamivudine, stavudine, zidovudine: May decrease antiretroviral activity and enhance hepatotoxic effects. Use together cautiously; consider therapy modification.

NRTIs (abacavir, emtricitabine, lamivudine, tenofovir): May increase risk of hepatic impairment and anemia. Consider discontinuing NRTI. Reduce dosage or discontinue interferon, ribavirin, or both for worsening clinical toxicity.

Warfarin: May decrease anticoagulation effect. Monitor PT and INR.

EFFECTS ON LAB TEST RESULTS
• May increase TSH, uric acid, ALT, AST, and bilirubin levels.
• May increase reticulocyte count.
• May decrease Hb level and WBC and platelet counts.

CONTRAINDICATIONS & CAUTIONS
Boxed Warning Monotherapy is ineffective for treatment of chronic HCV infection; drug shouldn't be used alone for this indication. ■
Boxed Warning Aerosol form isn't indicated for use in adults. ■
Boxed Warning Ribavirin may cause hemolytic anemia and worsen cardiac disease, leading to potentially fatal MI. Patients with a history of significant or unstable cardiac disease shouldn't be treated with ribavirin. ■
• Aerosol form is contraindicated in patients hypersensitive to drug.
• Oral form is contraindicated in patients with known hypersensitivity to ribavirin or its components, autoimmune hepatitis, or hemoglobinopathies.
• Capsules are contraindicated in patients with CrCl of less than 50 mL/minute.
• Ribavirin tablets and peginterferon alfa-2a combination therapy is contraindicated in hepatic decompensation (Child-Pugh score greater than 6; class B and C) in patients with cirrhosis and chronic HCV monoinfection before treatment and in hepatic decompensation (Child-Pugh score of 6 or greater) in patients with cirrhosis and chronic HCV infection coinfected with HIV before treatment.

Boxed Warning In infants, aerosolized ribavirin has been associated with sudden deterioration of respiratory function. Monitor respiratory function carefully and stop treatment if sudden respiratory deterioration occurs. Reinstitute only with extreme caution, continuous monitoring, and consideration of concomitant administration of bronchodilators. ■
• Use cautiously in older adults and patients with hepatic or renal insufficiency.
• Patients who initiate oral treatment before their 18th birthday should maintain pediatric dosing through completion of therapy.
Dialyzable drug: 50%.
⚠ *Overdose S&S:* Increased severity of adverse reactions.

PREGNANCY-LACTATION-REPRODUCTION
Boxed Warning Contraindicated in patients who are pregnant and in men whose partners are pregnant; significant teratogenic and embryocidal effects have occurred in all animal species exposed to ribavirin. ■
Boxed Warning Women receiving ribavirin and men receiving ribavirin who have partners of childbearing potential should use extreme care to avoid pregnancy during therapy and should use at least two reliable forms of effective contraception during therapy and during 6-month (tablets) and 9-month (capsules) posttreatment follow-up. ■
• If pregnancy occurs during therapy or during 6 months (tablets) or 9 months (capsules) after therapy ends, advise patient of teratogenic fetal risk.
• Patients of childbearing potential must have a negative pregnancy test immediately before start of therapy. Pregnancy tests must be performed monthly during therapy and for 6 months (tablets) or 9 months (capsules) after therapy ends.
• Advise health care workers who are pregnant to avoid unnecessary exposure to aerosol form.
• It isn't known if drug appears in human milk. Patient should discontinue breastfeeding or discontinue drug, taking into account importance of drug to the mother.

NURSING CONSIDERATIONS
Aerosol form
⊕ *Alert:* The long-term and cumulative effects in health care personnel exposed to this form aren't known. Eye irritation and headache may occur.

Reactions in bold italics are *life-threatening*. Interactions may have a *rapid onset* or a *delayed onset*.

Boxed Warning Use in patients on ventilators should only be undertaken by health care providers and staff familiar with this mode of administration and the specific ventilator used. Experienced providers and staff should use procedures that minimize accumulation of drug precipitate, which can result in ventilator dysfunction and increases in pulmonary pressures. ■

• This form is indicated only for severe lower respiratory tract infection caused by RSV. Although you should begin treatment while awaiting test results, an RSV infection must be documented eventually.

• Most infants and children with RSV infection don't require treatment with antivirals because the disease is commonly mild and self-limiting. Premature infants or those with cardiopulmonary disease experience RSV in its most severe form and benefit most from treatment with ribavirin aerosol.

Oral form

• Don't start therapy until a negative pregnancy test is confirmed in patient or partner of patient; pregnancy test is required every month during therapy and for 6 months (tablets) to 9 months (capsules) afterward.

• Monitor hematologic status, liver and renal function, and TSH level at baseline and throughout therapy.

• Combination therapy has been observed to inhibit growth in children ages 5 to 17. Monitor child's height and weight during therapy.

🚯 *Alert:* Monitor patient for suicidality, severe depression, hemolytic anemia, bone marrow suppression, autoimmune and infective disorders, ophthalmic disorders, CV disorders, pulmonary dysfunction, pancreatitis, and diabetes.

• Stop drug if pulmonary infiltrates or severe pulmonary impairment or pancreatitis occurs.

• In patients receiving azathioprine with ribavirin, monitor CBC, including platelet counts, weekly for first month, twice monthly for second and third months of treatment, then monthly or more frequently if dosage or other therapy changes are necessary.

• Monitor HCV-RNA level. If patients who have been previously treated have a detectable HCV-RNA level at week 12 or 24 of treatment, sustained virologic response is unlikely; consider therapy discontinuation.

PATIENT TEACHING

• Inform parents of need for drug, and answer any questions.

• Teach patient safe drug administration and handling.

• Advise patient and caregivers to seek immediate medical attention if suicidality and worsening of depression occur.

• Encourage parents to immediately report any subtle change in child.

• Warn patient of childbearing potential that drug is a teratogen, and provide contraception counseling. Advise patient that extreme care must be taken to avoid pregnancy during therapy and for 6 or 9 months after completion of treatment.

• Advise patient to immediately report a pregnancy.

• Caution patient to be well hydrated, especially during initial stages of treatment.

SAFETY ALERT!

ribociclib ▨
RYE-boe-sye-klib

Kisqali

Therapeutic class: Antineoplastics
Pharmacologic class: Cyclin-dependent kinase inhibitors

AVAILABLE FORMS

Tablets ⓄⓃⒸ: 200 mg

INDICATIONS & DOSAGES

Adjust-a-dose (for all indications): Refer to manufacturer's instructions for toxicity-related dosage adjustment. For patients with moderate (Child-Pugh class B) or severe (Child-Pugh class C) hepatic impairment, reduce starting dose to 400 mg once daily. For patients with severe renal impairment, reduce starting dose to 200 mg PO once daily. If giving with strong CYP3A inhibitor, reduce ribociclib dose to 400 mg once daily; allow 5 half-lives of the inhibitor after discontinuation of the inhibitor before returning to the initial ribociclib dose.

➤ **Initial endocrine-based therapy in patients who are premenopausal, perimenopausal, or postmenopausal for treatment of hormone receptor–positive, HER2–negative advanced or metastatic breast cancer, in combination with**

R

aromatase inhibitor or with fulvestrant in patients who are postmenopausal as initial endocrine-based therapy or after disease progression on endocrine therapy ≋

Women: 600 mg (three 200-mg tablets) PO once daily for 21 consecutive days followed by 7 days off therapy. Letrozole 2.5 mg once daily is given throughout the 28-day cycle. For dosing and administration with other aromatase inhibitors, refer to the respective prescribing information.

Or, when given with fulvestrant, the recommended fulvestrant dose is 500 mg PO on days 1, 15, and 29 and once monthly thereafter. Refer to the full prescribing information of fulvestrant.

Treat patients who are premenopausal or perimenopausal with a luteinizing hormone-releasing hormone agonist, according to current clinical practice standards.

✳ *NEW INDICATION:* Hormone receptor-positive, HER-2 negative advanced or metastatic breast cancer in combination with an aromatase inhibitor or with fulvestrant as initial endocrine-based therapy or following disease progression on endocrine therapy for men ≋

Men: 600 mg (three 200-mg tablets) PO once daily for 21 consecutive days followed by 7 days off therapy. Give letrozole 2.5 mg once daily throughout the 28-day cycle. For dosing and administration with other aromatase inhibitors, refer to the respective prescribing information. When combined with fulvestrant, give 500 mg fulvestrant PO on days 1, 15, and once monthly thereafter. Refer to full fulvestrant prescribing information.

Men should also be treated with a luteinizing hormone-releasing hormone agonist, according to current clinical practice standards.

ADMINISTRATION
PO

⚠ *Alert:* Hazardous drug; use safe handling and disposal precautions.

• May give with or without food.

• Patients should swallow tablets whole and not chew, crush, or split them before swallowing. Don't use cracked, broken, or damaged tablets.

• Give medication at the same time each day, preferably in the morning.

• Skip a missed dose or a dose lost due to vomiting after intake. Give the next dose at its usual time.

ACTION

A cyclin-dependent kinase inhibitor that prevents progression through the cell cycle, resulting in arrest in the G1 phase. The combination of ribociclib and an aromatase inhibitor causes increased inhibition of tumor growth compared to each agent alone. The combination of ribociclib and fulvestrant results in tumor growth inhibition in estrogen receptor-positive breast cancer models.

Route	Onset	Peak	Duration
PO	Unknown	1–4 hr	Unknown

Half-life: 30 to 55 hours.

ADVERSE REACTIONS

CNS: headache, insomnia, fatigue, dizziness, vertigo, fever. **CV:** peripheral edema, *prolonged QT interval,* syncope. **GI:** nausea, diarrhea, vomiting, constipation, stomatitis, abdominal pain, decreased appetite. **GU:** UTI. **Hematologic:** *neutropenia, leukopenia, lymphopenia,* anemia. **Hepatic:** abnormal LFT values. **Musculoskeletal:** back pain, arthralgia. **Respiratory:** dyspnea, ILD, pneumonitis. **Skin:** alopecia, rash, pruritus.

INTERACTIONS

Drug-drug. *CYP3A substrates with narrow therapeutic index (alfentanil, cyclosporine, dihydroergotamine, ergotamine, everolimus, fentanyl, midazolam, pimozide, quinidine, sirolimus, tacrolimus):* May increase exposure to these drugs. Decrease substrate dosage when concomitant use with ribociclib is necessary.

Drugs that prolong QT interval (amiodarone, bepridil, chloroquine, clarithromycin, disopyramide, haloperidol, methadone, moxifloxacin, ondansetron, pimozide, procainamide, quinidine, sotalol): May increase risk of prolonged QT interval and ventricular arrhythmias. Avoid use together.

Strong CYP3A4 inducers (carbamazepine, phenytoin, rifampin): May decrease ribociclib level. Avoid use together.

Strong CYP3A4 inhibitors (clarithromycin, conivaptan, itraconazole, ketoconazole, lopinavir–ritonavir, nefazodone, nelfinavir, posaconazole, ritonavir, saquinavir, voriconazole): May increase ribociclib level. Avoid use together. If coadministration is unavoidable, decrease ribociclib dosage. If strong inhibitor is discontinued, resume prior

---

Reactions in bold italics are *life-threatening*. Interactions may have a *rapid onset* or a **delayed onset**.

ribociclib dosage after at least five half-lives of the CYP3A inhibitor.

Drug-herb. *St. John's wort:* May decrease ribociclib level. Discourage use together.

Drug-food. *Grapefruit or grapefruit juice, pomegranates or pomegranate juice:* May increase ribociclib plasma concentration. Don't use together.

EFFECTS ON LAB TEST RESULTS

• May increase ALT, AST, GGT, and serum creatinine levels.
• May decrease phosphorus, glucose, albumin, and potassium levels.
• May decrease Hb level and leukocyte, neutrophil, lymphocyte, and platelet counts.

CONTRAINDICATIONS & CAUTIONS

⚠ *Alert:* Cyclin-dependent kinase 4/6 (CDK4/6) inhibitors may cause rare but severe or fatal interstitial lung disease (ILD) and pneumonitis.

• Drug may prolong QT interval. Avoid use in patients with long QT syndrome, uncontrolled or significant cardiac disease (recent MI, HF, unstable angina, bradyarrhythmias), or electrolyte abnormalities and in those taking drugs known to prolong the QTc interval.

• Drug may increase risk of hepatobiliary toxicity, SCARs, and neutropenia.

Dialyzable drug: Unknown.

PREGNANCY-LACTATION-REPRODUCTION

• Drug may cause fetal harm; avoid use during pregnancy. Obtain a pregnancy test before start of therapy. Patients of childbearing potential should use effective contraception during therapy and for at least 3 weeks after final dose.

• It isn't known if drug appears in human milk. Patients shouldn't breastfeed during therapy and for at least 3 weeks after final dose.

• Drug may impair fertility in males.

NURSING CONSIDERATIONS

⚠ *Alert:* Monitor patients for new or worsening pulmonary symptoms (hypoxia, cough, dyspnea, interstitial infiltrates on radiologic images); if they occur, interrupt therapy immediately and evaluate the patient. If infection, neoplasm, and other causes are excluded, permanently discontinue treatment in patients with severe ILD or pneumonitis.

• Monitor LFTs before start of therapy, every 2 weeks for the first two cycles, then at the beginning of each subsequent four cycles, and as clinically indicated because of the risk of hepatobiliary toxicity. Interrupt therapy, reduce dosage, or discontinue drug based on LFT values as directed in manufacturer's instructions.

• Monitor electrolyte levels (potassium, calcium, phosphorus, magnesium) before start of therapy, at the beginning of the first six cycles, and as clinically indicated. Correct electrolyte abnormalities before therapy begins.

• Assess ECG before treatment. Initiate treatment only in patients with a baseline QTcF (QT interval corrected for HR via Fridericia's method) of less than 450 msec. Repeat ECG on day 14 of the first cycle, at the beginning of the second cycle, and as clinically indicated. Interrupt therapy, reduce dosage, or discontinue drug based on QT-interval prolongation as directed in manufacturer's instructions.

• Assess CBC before start of therapy, every 2 weeks for the first two cycles, at the beginning of each subsequent four cycles, then as clinically indicated. Interrupt therapy, reduce dosage, or discontinue drug based on CBC results as directed in manufacturer's instructions.

• Monitor patient closely for hepatobiliary toxicity and neutropenia.

• Monitor patient for SCARs, including SJS, TEN, drug-induced hypersensitivity syndrome, and DRESS syndrome. Withhold treatment and consult a dermatologist if signs and symptoms occur.

• Verify pregnancy status before treatment.

PATIENT TEACHING

⚠ *Alert:* Warn patients to immediately report difficulty or discomfort with breathing or shortness of breath while at rest or with low activity; these may be symptoms of ILD or pneumonitis.

• Teach patient to immediately report signs and symptoms related to QT-interval prolongation (fast or irregular heartbeat, dizziness, syncope).

• Advise patient to immediately report signs and symptoms of liver dysfunction (jaundice, dark or brown urine, fatigue, loss of appetite, upper abdominal pain, bleeding or bruising more easily than usual), skin reactions, and infection (fever, chills, pain, malaise).

• Inform patient of childbearing potential of the fetal risk and to use effective contraception

R

during therapy and for at least 3 weeks after final dose.

• Advise patient not to breastfeed during therapy and for at least 3 weeks after final dose.

rifAMPin (rifampicin)
rif-AM-pin

Rifadin, Rofact✽

Therapeutic class: Antituberculotics
Pharmacologic class: Semisynthetic rifamycins

AVAILABLE FORMS
Capsules: 150 mg, 300 mg
Powder for injection: 600 mg/vial

INDICATIONS & DOSAGES
➤ **Pulmonary TB, with other antituberculotics**
Adults: 10 mg/kg PO or IV daily in single dose. Maximum daily dose is 600 mg.
Children: 10 to 20 mg/kg PO or IV daily in single dose. Maximum daily dose is 600 mg.
➤ **Meningococcal carriers**
Adults: 600 mg PO or IV every 12 hours for 2 days.
Children ages 1 month to 12 years: 10 mg/kg PO or IV every 12 hours for 2 days, not to exceed 600 mg/day.
Neonates: 5 mg/kg PO or IV every 12 hours for 2 days.
➤ **Cholestatic pruritus ♦**
Adults: 150 to 300 mg PO b.i.d.

ADMINISTRATION
PO
• For pulmonary TB, give drug with other antituberculotics.
• For best absorption, give capsules 1 hour before or 2 hours after a meal with a full glass of water.
• For patients who can't tolerate capsules on an empty stomach or those who have difficulty swallowing capsules or when lower doses are needed, consult pharmacist for preparation of an oral suspension.
IV
▼ Reconstitute drug with 10 mL of sterile water for injection to yield 60 mg/mL.
▼ Add to 100 mL of D_5W and infuse over 30 minutes, or add to 500 mL of D_5W and infuse over 3 hours.

▼ When dextrose is contraindicated, dilute with NSS for injection. Once prepared, dilutions in D_5W remain stable for up to 4 hours and dilutions in NSS remain stable for up to 24 hours at room temperature.
▼ **Incompatibilities:** Diltiazem, other IV solutions.

ACTION
Inhibits DNA-dependent RNA polymerase, which impairs RNA synthesis; bactericidal.

Route	Onset	Peak	Duration
PO	Unknown	2–4 hr	<24 hr
IV	Unknown	Unknown	<24 hr

Half-life: 3 to 4 hours (adults). Varies with repeated administration and age.

ADVERSE REACTIONS
CNS: headache, fatigue, drowsiness, behavioral changes, dizziness, mental confusion, inability to concentrate, generalized numbness, ataxia, fever. **CV:** flushing, *shock.* **EENT:** visual disturbances, conjunctivitis, sore mouth or tongue, tooth discoloration. **GI:** *pseudomembranous colitis,* epigastric distress, heartburn, anorexia, nausea, vomiting, abdominal pain, diarrhea, flatulence. **GU:** menstrual disturbances. **Hematologic:** *thrombocytopenia, transient leukopenia,* eosinophilia, hemolytic anemia, vitamin-K coagulation disorder. **Hepatic:** jaundice, *hepatotoxicity.* **Metabolic:** hyperuricemia. **Musculoskeletal:** muscular weakness, pain in extremities. **Respiratory:** shortness of breath, wheezing. **Skin:** pruritus, urticaria, rash. **Other:** flulike syndrome, discoloration of body fluids, porphyria exacerbation, hypersensitivity reactions.

INTERACTIONS
⚠ *Alert:* Rifampin can significantly interact with many drugs. Consult a drug interaction resource or pharmacist for additional information.
Drug-drug. *Amiodarone, analgesics, anticonvulsants, barbiturates, bazedoxifene, beta blockers, bosentan, cardiac glycosides, chloramphenicol, citalopram, clofibrate,* **corticosteroids, cyclosporine,** *dapsone, delavirdine, diazepam, digoxin, disopyramide, doxycycline, enalapril, fluoroquinolones, hydantoins, losartan, methadone, mexiletine, midazolam, nifedipine, ondansetron, opioids, propafenone, quinidine,* **ritonavir,**

Reactions in bold italics are *life-threatening*. Interactions may have a *rapid onset* or a **delayed onset**.

*rosiglitazone, sulfonylureas, **tacrolimus**, TCAs, theophylline, tocainide, triazolam, verapamil, zolpidem:* May decrease effectiveness of these drugs. Monitor effectiveness.

Anticoagulants (warfarin): May increase requirements for anticoagulant. Monitor PT and INR closely, and adjust dosage of anticoagulants.

Atazanavir, boceprevir, darunavir, fosamprenavir, saquinavir, tipranavir: May decrease plasma concentrations of antivirals, resulting in loss of antiviral efficacy or development of viral resistance. Use together is contraindicated.

Daclatasvir, simeprevir, sofosbuvir, telaprevir: May decrease levels of these hepatitis C antivirals. Avoid use together.

Efavirenz, zidovudine: May decrease levels of these antiretrovirals. Avoid use together.

Halothane: May increase risk of hepatotoxicity. Monitor LFT results.

Hormonal contraceptives (estrogens, progestins): May decrease hormone exposure. Patient should use nonhormonal contraceptives during rifampin therapy.

Isoniazid: May increase risk of hepatotoxicity. Monitor LFT results.

Ketoconazole, para-aminosalicylate sodium: May interfere with absorption of rifampin. Separate doses by 8 to 12 hours.

Macrolide antibiotics, protease inhibitors: May inhibit rifampin metabolism but increase metabolism of other drug. Monitor patient for clinical and adverse effects.

Probenecid: May increase rifampin levels. Use together cautiously.

Saquinavir: May increase risk of severe hepatocellular toxicity. Use together is contraindicated.

Voriconazole: May decrease voriconazole's therapeutic effects while increasing the risk of rifampin adverse effects. Use together is contraindicated.

Drug-lifestyle. *Alcohol use:* May increase risk of hepatotoxicity. Discourage use together.

EFFECTS ON LAB TEST RESULTS
• May increase ALT, AST, ALP, bilirubin, BUN, and uric acid levels.
• May increase eosinophil count.
• May decrease Hb level and platelet and WBC counts.
• May alter standard folate and vitamin B_{12} assay results.

CONTRAINDICATIONS & CAUTIONS
• Contraindicated in patients hypersensitive to rifampin or related drugs.
• Drug isn't indicated for treatment of meningococcal disease, only for short-term treatment of asymptomatic carrier states.
• Use cautiously in patients with liver disease or diabetes.
• Hypersensitivity reactions, including erythema multiforme, SJS, TEN, and DRESS syndrome, have occurred. Discontinue drug for SCAR signs or symptoms.
Dialyzable drug: Poorly.
⚠ **Overdose S&S:** Nausea; vomiting; abdominal pain; pruritus; headache; increasing lethargy; unconsciousness; transient increases in liver enzyme or bilirubin levels; brownish red or orange discoloration of skin, urine, sweat, saliva, tears, and feces; facial or periorbital edema; hypotension; tachycardia; ventricular arrhythmias; seizures; cardiac arrest; liver enlargement; jaundice.

PREGNANCY-LACTATION-REPRODUCTION
• There are no adequate studies during pregnancy. Drug may cross placental barrier and cause fetal harm. Use only if clearly needed and potential benefit justifies fetal risk.
• Drug can cause postnatal hemorrhages in the mother and infant when given during last few weeks of pregnancy; treatment with vitamin K may be indicated.
• Drug appears in human milk. Patient should discontinue breastfeeding or discontinue drug.

NURSING CONSIDERATIONS
• Monitor hepatic function, hematopoietic studies, and uric acid level. Drug's systemic effects may asymptomatically raise LFT values and uric acid level. In patients with existing impaired hepatic function, monitor LFT values, especially AST and ALT, before therapy, then every 2 to 4 weeks during therapy.
• Watch for and report signs and symptoms of hepatic impairment.
• For TB, a three-drug regimen of rifampin, isoniazid (INH), and pyrazinamide is recommended in the initial phase of short-course therapy, which is usually continued for 2 months. Guidelines also recommend that either streptomycin or ethambutol be added as a fourth drug if community rates of INH resistance are 4% or greater. After the initial phase, continue treatment for at least

4 months or longer if sputum culture remains positive, if resistant organisms are present, or if patient tests positive for HIV.
• Monitor patients on intermittent therapy for adherence.
• *Look alike–sound alike:* Don't confuse rifampin with rifabutin, rifaximin, or rifapentine.

PATIENT TEACHING
• Instruct patient on safe drug administration.
• Warn patient that drowsiness may occur and that drug can turn body fluids red-orange and permanently stain contact lenses.
• Advise patient to use nonhormonal contraception.
• Caution patient to report fever, loss of appetite, malaise, nausea, vomiting, dark urine, or yellowing of eyes or skin.
• Advise patient to avoid alcohol during drug therapy.
• Instruct patient on importance of not missing any doses and completing full course of therapy.

rifapentine
rif-a-PEN-teen

Priftin

Therapeutic class: Antituberculotics
Pharmacologic class: Synthetic rifamycins

AVAILABLE FORMS
Tablets (film-coated): 150 mg

INDICATIONS & DOSAGES
❸ *Alert:* Give drug as directly observed therapy for all indications.
➤ **Pulmonary TB, with at least one other antituberculotic to which the isolate is susceptible**
Adults and children age 12 and older: During initial phase of short-course therapy, 600 mg PO twice weekly for 2 months, with an interval between doses of at least 3 days (72 hours). During continuation phase of short-course therapy, 600 mg PO once weekly for 4 months, combined with isoniazid or another drug to which the isolate is susceptible.
Older adults: Begin therapy at low end of dosing range.
➤ **Latent TB infection caused by *Mycobacterium tuberculosis*, in combination with**

isoniazid, in patients at high risk for progression to TB disease
Adults and children age 12 and older: Base rifapentine dosage on patient's weight and administer PO once weekly. If patient weighs more than 50 kg, give 900 mg; if patient weighs 32.1 to 50 kg, give 750 mg; if patient weighs 25.1 to 32 kg, give 600 mg; if patient weighs 14.1 to 25 kg, give 450 mg; if patient weighs 10 to 14 kg, give 300 mg. Maximum dose, 900 mg once weekly. Recommended isoniazid dose is 15 mg/kg (rounded to nearest 50 or 100 mg) up to maximum of 900 mg once weekly for 12 weeks.
Children ages 2 to 11: Base rifapentine dosage on patient's weight and administer PO once weekly. If patient weighs more than 50 kg, give 900 mg; if patient weighs 32.1 to 50 kg, give 750 mg; if patient weighs 25.1 to 32 kg, give 600 mg; if patient weighs 14.1 to 25 kg, give 450 mg; if patient weighs 10 to 14 kg, give 300 mg. Maximum dose, 900 mg once weekly. Recommended isoniazid dose is 25 mg/kg (rounded to nearest 50 or 100 mg) up to maximum of 900 mg once weekly for 12 weeks.

ADMINISTRATION
PO
• Give drug with meals to increase oral bioavailability and possibly reduce the incidence of GI upset, nausea, and vomiting.
• For patients who can't swallow tablets, tablets may be crushed and added to small amount of semisolid food and consumed immediately.
❸ *Alert:* Give drug with appropriate daily companion drugs. Compliance with all drug regimens, especially with daily companion drugs on the days when rifapentine isn't given, is crucial for early sputum conversion and protection from relapse of TB.

ACTION
Inhibits DNA-dependent RNA polymerase in susceptible strains of *M. tuberculosis.* Demonstrates bactericidal activity against the organism both intracellularly and extracellularly.

Route	Onset	Peak	Duration
PO	Unknown	3–10 hr	Unknown

Half-life: 17 hours.

Reactions in bold italics are *life-threatening*. Interactions may have a *rapid onset* or a ***delayed onset***.

ADVERSE REACTIONS

CNS: headache, dizziness, fever. **CV:** chest pain. **EENT:** conjunctivitis, epistaxis. **GI:** anorexia, nausea, vomiting, dyspepsia, diarrhea, abdominal pain. **GU:** uremia, pyuria, proteinuria, hematuria, urinary casts, increased BUN level. **Hematologic:** *leukopenia, leukocytosis, neutropenia,* anemia, *thrombocythemia, thrombocytopenia,* lymphadenopathy. **Hepatic:** increased transaminase levels. **Musculoskeletal:** arthralgia, back pain. **Respiratory:** hemoptysis, cough. **Skin:** diaphoresis, rash, pruritus, acne, maculopapular rash.

INTERACTIONS

Drug-drug. *Antiarrhythmics (disopyramide, mexiletine, quinidine, tocainide), antibiotics (chloramphenicol, clarithromycin, dapsone, doxycycline, fluoroquinolones), anticonvulsants (phenytoin), antifungals (fluconazole, itraconazole, ketoconazole), barbiturates, benzodiazepines (diazepam), beta blockers, calcium channel blockers (diltiazem, nifedipine, verapamil), cardiac glycosides, clofibrate,* **corticosteroids,** *haloperidol, HIV protease inhibitors (nelfinavir, ritonavir, saquinavir),* **immunosuppressants (cyclosporine, tacrolimus),** *levothyroxine, opioid analgesics (methadone), oral anticoagulants (warfarin), oral antidiabetics (sulfonylureas), progestins, quinine, reverse transcriptase inhibitors (delavirdine, zidovudine), sildenafil, TCAs (amitriptyline, nortriptyline), theophylline:* May decrease activity of these drugs because of cytochrome P-450 enzyme metabolism. May need to adjust dosage.
Hormonal contraceptives: May reduce effectiveness of contraceptive. Patient should use nonhormonal contraceptives during therapy.
Ritonavir: May decrease ritonavir levels. Carefully monitor patient's response.

EFFECTS ON LAB TEST RESULTS

- May increase uric acid, ALT, and AST levels.
- May decrease blood glucose level.
- May increase platelet count.
- May decrease Hb level and neutrophil and WBC counts.
- May alter folate and vitamin B_{12} assay results.

CONTRAINDICATIONS & CAUTIONS

- Contraindicated in patients hypersensitive to rifamycins (rifapentine, rifampin, or rifabutin).

- May cause hypersensitivity reactions, including anaphylaxis (flulike illness, hypotension, urticaria, angioedema, bronchospasm, conjunctivitis, thrombocytopenia, neutropenia). If signs or symptoms occur, stop drug and notify prescriber.
- SCARs, including SJS and DRESS syndrome, have been reported with rifapentine use. Discontinue drug at first appearance of rash, mucosal lesions, or other signs and symptoms of hypersensitivity.
- Patients with abnormal LFT values or liver disease and those initiating treatment for active pulmonary TB should receive rifapentine only in cases of necessity and under strict medical supervision.
- For patients with active pulmonary TB who are infected with HIV, don't use drug once weekly in the continuation phase regimen in combination with isoniazid because of a higher rate of failure or relapse with rifampin-resistant organisms. Rifapentine hasn't been studied as part of the initial phase treatment regimen in patients with active pulmonary TB who are infected with HIV.
- Rule out active TB disease before starting treatment for latent TB infection.
- Patients considered at high risk for progression to TB disease include those in close contact with patients with active TB or recent conversion to a positive result on tuberculin skin test, patients with pulmonary fibrosis on X-ray, and patients with HIV infection.
- Rifapentine in combination with isoniazid isn't recommended for patients presumed to be exposed to rifamycin- or isoniazid-resistant *M. tuberculosis.*
- Use cautiously in patients with cavitary pulmonary lesions or positive sputum cultures after initial treatment phase and in patients with bilateral pulmonary disease; higher relapse rates may occur in these patients.
- CDAD has been reported, ranging from mild diarrhea to fatal colitis, and can occur more than 2 months after therapy ends. Drug may need to be discontinued and appropriate measures initiated.
- Avoid using drug in patients with porphyria.
Dialyzable drug: Unlikely.
⚠ **Overdose S&S:** Hematuria, neutropenia, hyperglycemia, hyperuricemia, arthritis, increased ALT level, pruritus.

R

🍁Canada   ◇OTC   ◆Off-label use   𝒫Photoguide   ⓓⓝⓒDo not crush   *Liquid contains alcohol   ▓Genetic

PREGNANCY-LACTATION-REPRODUCTION
• There are no adequate studies during pregnancy. Drug may cause fetal harm. Use only if potential benefit justifies fetal risk.
• Drug may cause postnatal hemorrhages in the mother and infant when another rifamycin (rifampin) is given during last few weeks of pregnancy. Monitor PT in patients who are pregnant and neonates exposed to rifapentine during last few weeks of pregnancy. Treatment with vitamin K may be indicated.
• It isn't known if drug appears in human milk. Use cautiously during breastfeeding. If used, monitor infant for hepatotoxicity.

NURSING CONSIDERATIONS
• Monitor patient for signs and symptoms of hypersensitivity reaction; if they occur, use supportive measures and discontinue drug.
• Rifamycin antibiotics may cause hepatotoxicity. In patients with abnormal LFT values or liver disease and patients starting treatment for active pulmonary TB, obtain serum transaminase levels before start of therapy and every 2 to 4 weeks during therapy. Discontinue drug if evidence of liver injury occurs.
• Monitor patient for CDAD.
• *Look alike–sound alike:* Don't confuse rifapentine with rifabutin or rifampin.

PATIENT TEACHING
• Teach patient safe drug administration and storage.
• Stress importance of strict adherence to this drug regimen and that of daily companion drugs, as well as needed follow-up visits and lab tests.
• Advise patient of childbearing potential to use nonhormonal contraceptives.
• Caution mother of infant exposed to rifapentine through human milk to watch for signs and symptoms of hepatotoxicity (irritability, prolonged unexplained crying, jaundice, loss of appetite, vomiting, darkened urine, lightened stool).
• Instruct patient to report all adverse reactions, especially fever, appetite loss, malaise, nausea, vomiting, darkened urine, yellowish skin and eyes, joint pain or swelling, skin or mucosal lesions, or excessive loose stools or diarrhea.
• Tell patient that drug may turn body fluids red-orange and permanently stain dentures or contact lenses. Instruct patient to remove soft contact lenses during therapy.

rifAXIMin
rif-AX-i-min

Xifaxan

Therapeutic class: Antibiotics
Pharmacologic class: Rifamycin antibacterials

AVAILABLE FORMS
Tablets: 200 mg, 550 mg

INDICATIONS & DOSAGES
➤ **Traveler's diarrhea from noninvasive strains of** *Escherichia coli*
Adults and children age 12 and older: 200 mg PO t.i.d. for 3 days.
➤ **To reduce risk of overt hepatic encephalopathy recurrence**
Adults: 550 mg PO b.i.d.
➤ **IBS with diarrhea**
Adults: 550 mg PO t.i.d. for 14 days. May repeat regimen twice if symptoms recur.

ADMINISTRATION
PO
• Give drug without regard for food.

ACTION
Binds to the beta-subunit of bacterial DNA-dependent RNA polymerase, which inhibits bacterial RNA synthesis and kills *E. coli*.

Route	Onset	Peak	Duration
PO	Unknown	1 hr	Unknown

Half-life: 1.8 to 6 hours.

ADVERSE REACTIONS
CNS: depression, dizziness, fatigue, fever, headache, insomnia. **CV:** peripheral edema. **EENT:** nasopharyngitis. **GI:** ascites, abdominal pain, nausea, *CDAD.* **Hematologic:** anemia. **Hepatic:** increased ALT level. **Musculoskeletal:** arthralgia, muscle spasms, myalgia. **Respiratory:** dyspnea. **Skin:** rash, pruritus.

INTERACTIONS
Drug-drug. *P-gp inhibitors (cyclosporine, diltiazem, ketoconazole, PPIs, saquinavir):*

Reactions in bold italics are *life-threatening.* Interactions may have a *rapid onset* or a *delayed onset.*

May increase systemic exposure of rifaximin. Use together cautiously.

Warfarin: May interfere with effect on INR. Monitor INR and PT closely.

EFFECTS ON LAB TEST RESULTS
- May increase CK and ALT levels.
- May decrease Hb level.

CONTRAINDICATIONS & CAUTIONS
- Contraindicated in patients hypersensitive to rifaximin or its components, rifamycin, or other antimicrobial agents.
- Hypersensitivity reactions, including exfoliative dermatitis, angioneurotic edema, and anaphylaxis have occurred.
- Use of drug for traveler's diarrhea without proven or strongly suspected bacterial infection or as prophylaxis isn't likely to be beneficial and increases risk of development of drug-resistant bacteria.
- Use with caution in patients with severe hepatic impairment.

Dialyzable drug: Unknown.

PREGNANCY-LACTATION-REPRODUCTION
- Safety during pregnancy hasn't been established; some animal studies have demonstrated adverse events. Because of limited absorption of rifaximin in patients with normal hepatic function, fetal exposure to drug is expected to be low.
- It isn't known if drug appears in human milk. Use cautiously during breastfeeding.

NURSING CONSIDERATIONS
- Don't use drug in patients whose illness may be caused by *Campylobacter jejuni*, *Shigella*, or *Salmonella*.
- **Alert:** Don't use drug in patients with blood in the stool, diarrhea with fever, or diarrhea from pathogens other than *E. coli*.
- Stop drug if diarrhea worsens or lasts longer than 24 to 48 hours. Patient may need a different antibiotic.
- Patients who have diarrhea after antibiotic therapy may have CDAD, which may range from mild to life-threatening.
- Monitor patient for overgrowth of nonsusceptible organisms.
- *Look alike–sound alike:* Don't confuse rifaximin with rifampin.

PATIENT TEACHING
- Teach patient safe drug administration.

- Tell patient to take all the prescribed drug, even if feeling better before drug is finished.
- Advise patient to notify prescriber if diarrhea worsens or lasts longer than 1 or 2 days after starting treatment. A different treatment may be needed.
- Caution patient that CDAD (watery and bloody stools with or without stomach cramps and fever) may occur as late as 2 or more months after the last dose of antibiotic. Advise patient to report signs or symptoms of CDAD as soon as possible.
- Explain that this drug is only for treating diarrhea caused by contaminated foods or beverages while traveling and not for any other type of infection.
- Caution patient not to share drug with others.

rilpivirine hydrochloride
ril-pi-VIR-een

Edurant

Therapeutic class: Antiretrovirals
Pharmacologic class: NNRTIs

AVAILABLE FORMS
Tablets: 25 mg

INDICATIONS & DOSAGES
➤ **HIV-1 infection in patients who are antiretroviral-naive with HIV-1 RNA 100,000 copies/mL or less at start of therapy, in combination with other antiretrovirals**

Adults and adolescents age 12 and older weighing at least 35 kg: 25 mg PO once daily.

Adjust-a-dose: For patients concomitantly receiving rifabutin, increase rilpivirine dosage to 50 mg once daily. When rifabutin is stopped, decrease rilpivirine to 25 mg once daily.

For patients who are pregnant and were already on a stable regimen before pregnancy and who are virologically suppressed (HIV-1 RNA less than 50 copies/mL), recommended dosage is 25 mg once daily.

➤ **In combination with cabotegravir for short-term treatment of HIV-1 infection in patients who are virologically suppressed (HIV-1 RNA less than 50 copies/mL) on a stable regimen as an oral lead-in to assess tolerability of rilpivirine before use**

R

of cabotegravir–rilpivirine (Cabenuva) extended-release injectable suspensions

Adults and adolescents age 12 and older weighing at least 35 kg: 25 mg PO once daily in combination with cabotegravir 30 mg PO once daily. Use oral lead-in dose for at least 28 days.

➤ **In combination with cabotegravir for short-term treatment of HIV-1 infection in patients with HIV-1 RNA less than 50 copies/mL who are on a stable oral therapy regimen but who will miss scheduled injections with cabotegravir–rilpivirine (Cabenuva) extended-release injectable suspensions by more than 7 days to up to 2 consecutive months**

Adults and adolescents age 12 and older weighing at least 35 kg: One 25-mg tablet PO once daily in combination with cabotegravir 30 mg PO once daily at approximately the same time each day with a meal starting about 1 month after the last injection and continuing until the day injection dosing is restarted. Refer to Cabenuva prescribing information for dosing instructions.

Adjust-a-dose: For oral therapy with rilpivirine and cabotegravir lasting more than 2 months, an alternative oral regimen, which may include rilpivirine, is recommended.

ADMINISTRATION
PO
- Give drug with a normal to high-calorie meal.
- Patient should swallow tablets whole with water.
- Don't give a missed dose if next scheduled dose is within 12 hours.
- Store tablets at room temperature and in the original bottle to protect from light.

ACTION
Inhibits HIV-1 replication by noncompetitive inhibition of HIV-1 reverse transcriptase but doesn't inhibit the human cellular DNA polymerases alpha, beta, and gamma.

Route	Onset	Peak	Duration
PO	Rapid	4–5 hr	Unknown

Half-life: 50 hours.

ADVERSE REACTIONS
CNS: abnormal dreams, dizziness, fatigue, headache, insomnia, *depressive disorders.*
GI: nausea, vomiting, abdominal pain. **Skin:** rash.

INTERACTIONS
Drug-drug. *Antacids (aluminum or magnesium hydroxide, calcium carbonate):* May significantly decrease rilpivirine level. Give antacids either 2 hours before or at least 4 hours after rilpivirine.
Anticonvulsants (carbamazepine, oxcarbazepine, phenobarbital, phenytoin): May decrease rilpivirine level, decrease response, and increase risk of resistance to NNRTIs. Use together is contraindicated.
Azole antifungals (fluconazole, itraconazole, ketoconazole, posaconazole, voriconazole): May increase rilpivirine level and decrease antifungal level. Monitor effectiveness of antifungal.
Delavirdine: May increase rilpivirine level. Don't use together.
Didanosine (buffered): May decrease rilpivirine level. Administer didanosine at least 2 hours before or 4 hours after rilpivirine.
Drugs that prolong QT interval: May increase risk of torsades de pointes. Use together cautiously.
H₂-receptor antagonists (cimetidine, famotidine, nizatidine, ranitidine): May significantly decrease rilpivirine level. Give H_2-receptor antagonists at least 12 hours before or 4 hours after rilpivirine.
Macrolide antibiotics (clarithromycin, erythromycin): May increase rilpivirine level and risk of torsades de pointes. When possible, consider an alternative such as azithromycin.
Methadone: May decrease levels of both drugs. Monitor effectiveness of methadone and adjust methadone dosage as needed.
Other NNRTIs (efavirenz, etravirine, nevirapine): May decrease rilpivirine level. Don't use together.
PPIs (esomeprazole, lansoprazole, pantoprazole, rabeprazole): May decrease rilpivirine level, decrease virologic response, and increase risk of resistance to NNRTIs. Use together is contraindicated.
Rifamycins (rifampin, rifapentine): May decrease rilpivirine level, decrease virologic response, and increase risk of resistance to NNRTIs. Use together is contraindicated.
Rifabutin: May decrease rilpivirine level. Increase rilpivirine dose to 50 mg once daily during coadministration. Use with cabotegravir–rilpivirine injections is contraindicated.

Reactions in bold italics are *life-threatening.* Interactions may have a *rapid onset* or a **delayed onset.**

Systemic glucocorticoids (dexamethasone): May decrease rilpivirine level and virologic response, and increase risk of resistance to NNRTIs. Use together is contraindicated.

Drug-herb. *St. John's wort:* May decrease rilpivirine level and virologic response, and increase risk of resistance to NNRTIs. Use together is contraindicated.

Drug-food. *Grapefruit products:* May inhibit metabolism of rilpivirine. Avoid use during therapy.

EFFECTS ON LAB TEST RESULTS
• May increase AST, ALT, bilirubin, creatinine, total cholesterol, HDL, LDL, and triglyceride levels.
• May decrease cortisol level.

CONTRAINDICATIONS & CAUTIONS
• Contraindicated in patients hypersensitive to drug or its components.
• Use cautiously when administering with drugs known to prolong QT interval, in older adults, and in patients with severe renal impairment, ESRD, or severe hepatic impairment.
• Redistribution or accumulation of body fat, including central obesity, dorsocervical fat enlargement (buffalo hump), peripheral wasting, facial wasting, breast enlargement, and "cushingoid appearance," has occurred in patients receiving antiretroviral therapy. The mechanism and long-term consequences of these events are currently unknown. A causal relationship hasn't been established.
• Hepatic adverse events have been reported. Patients with underlying HBV or HCV infection or marked elevations in transaminase levels before treatment may be at increased risk for worsening or development of transaminase elevations.
• Severe skin and hypersensitivity reactions have been reported, including severe rash or rash accompanied by fever, blisters, mucosal involvement, conjunctivitis, facial edema, angioedema, hepatitis, eosinophilia, or DRESS syndrome. Most rashes occurred within first 4 to 6 weeks of therapy. Discontinue drug if hypersensitivity reaction or rash develops.
• Use in combination with cabotegravir only in patients with no history of treatment failure and no known or suspected resistance to either cabotegravir or rilpivirine.

• Safety and effectiveness in children younger than age 12 or weighing less than 35 kg haven't been established.
Dialyzable drug: Unlikely.

PREGNANCY-LACTATION-REPRODUCTION
• Enroll patients exposed to drug during pregnancy in the Antiretroviral Pregnancy Registry (1-800-258-4263).
• Use cautiously during pregnancy. Monitor viral load closely.
• It isn't known if drug appears in human milk. Patients shouldn't breastfeed during therapy.
• The CDC recommends that a patient with HIV not breastfeed to avoid postnatal transmission of HIV.

NURSING CONSIDERATIONS
• Patients should take drug with a regular meal and not with a protein drink; taking drug with a protein-rich nutritional drink alone may lower the exposure of rilpivirine by 50%.
• Always use rilpivirine in combination with other antiretrovirals.
• Drug isn't a cure for HIV infection. Patients must stay on continuous antiretroviral therapy to control HIV infection and decrease HIV-related illnesses.
• Monitor patient for severe rash or rash accompanied by fever, blisters, mucosal involvement, conjunctivitis, facial edema, angioedema, hepatitis, eosinophilia, or DRESS syndrome. Discontinue drug if hypersensitivity reaction or rash develops; initiate appropriate therapy.
• Assess patient for redistribution or accumulation of body fat.
• Monitor patients for reemergence of infections, such as *Mycobacterium avium*, cytomegalovirus, *Pneumocystis jiroveci* pneumonia, and TB, during initial phase of combination treatment. Treat infections appropriately.
• Monitor patients for autoimmune disorders (such as Graves disease, polymyositis, and Guillain-Barré syndrome, and autoimmune hepatitis) that have also been reported to occur with immune reconstitution; however, the time to onset varies, and can occur many months after initiation of treatment.
• Monitor patients for depressive disorders (depressed mood, dysphoria, negative thoughts, suicidality). Weigh risks of continued therapy against benefits of treatment.

R

• Monitor liver enzyme levels before and during treatment for patients with underlying hepatic disease, including HBV or HCV infection, and for patients with marked transaminase elevations. Consider monitoring liver enzyme levels for patients without preexisting hepatic dysfunction or other risk factors. Monitor patients with severe renal impairment or ESRD for adverse reactions during treatment.

PATIENT TEACHING
• Advise patient that rilpivirine isn't a cure for HIV infection or AIDS and that patient must stay on continuous antiretroviral therapy to control HIV infection.
• Tell patient to report all medications and supplements being taken because many of them may interact with rilpivirine.
• Instruct patient in safe drug administration.
• Warn patient that rilpivirine may cause depressed or altered mood and to report mood changes or symptoms of depression immediately.
• Advise patient to immediately report hypersensitivity reaction or rash.
• Tell patient to report pregnancy immediately. Also advise patient not to breastfeed.

---

risankizumab-rzaa
RIS-an-KIZ-ue-mab

Skyrizi

Therapeutic class: Immunomodulators
Pharmacologic class: Interleukin-23 receptor antagonists

AVAILABLE FORMS
Injection (IV): 600 mg/10 mL vial
Injection (subcut): 75 mg/0.83 mL, 150 mg/mL prefilled syringes; 150 mg/mL prefilled pen; 360/234 mL prefilled cartridge with on-body injector

INDICATIONS & DOSAGES
➤ **Moderate to severe plaque psoriasis in patients who are candidates for systemic therapy or phototherapy**
Adults: 150 mg subcut at week 0, week 4, and every 12 weeks thereafter.
✷ *NEW INDICATION:* **Active psoriatic arthritis**

Adults: 150 mg subcut at week 0, week 4, and every 12 weeks thereafter, alone or in combination with nonbiologic DMARDs.
✷ *NEW INDICATION:* **Moderate to severe Crohn disease**
Adults: 600-mg IV infusion over at least 1 hour at weeks 0, 4, and 8, then 360 mg subcut at week 12 and every 8 weeks thereafter.

ADMINISTRATION
IV
▼ Withdraw 10 mL of solution from vial and inject into 100, 250, or 500 mL IV bag or glass bottle of D_5W for final concentration of 1.2 to 6 mg/mL.
▼ Don't shake vial or diluted solution.
▼ Allow diluted solution to warm to room temperature if stored in refrigerator before start of infusion.
▼ Infuse over at least 1 hour. Complete infusion within 8 hours of dilution if stored at room temperature.
▼ Refrigerate diluted solution for up to 20 hours at 36° to 46° F (2° to 8° C).
▼ Store vials at 36° to 46° F (2° to 8° C), protected from light.
▼ **Incompatibilities:** Don't infuse in same IV line with other drugs.
Subcutaneous
• For each dose, administer injections at different locations, such as thighs, abdomen or, if given by health care professional or caregiver, the upper outer arm.
• Don't inject into areas where skin is tender, bruised, erythematous, indurated, or affected by psoriasis.
• If giving two 75 mg/0.83 mL injections for a 150-mg dose, give in two different anatomic locations.
• Keep in original carton to protect from light until use.
• Allow solution to warm to room temperature out of direct sunlight in the carton for 15 to 30 minutes for prefilled syringes, 30 to 90 minutes for prefilled pens, and 45 to 90 minutes for prefilled cartridge before use.
• Inspect solution for particulate matter and discoloration before use. Don't administer if solution contains large particles or is cloudy or discolored.
• Don't use if the syringe has been shaken, dropped, or damaged or if the tray seal is broken or missing.

Reactions in bold italics are *life-threatening*. Interactions may have a *rapid onset* or a **delayed onset**.

• Give a missed dose as soon as possible; then resume dosing at the regular scheduled time.

• Store refrigerated at 36° to 46° F (2° to 8° C). Don't use if the liquid has been frozen.

ACTION

An IgG1 monoclonal antibody that selectively binds to the p19 subunit of IL-23, thereby inhibiting its interaction with the IL-23 receptor, which inhibits the release of proinflammatory cytokines and chemokines.

Route	Onset	Peak	Duration
Subcut	Unknown	3–14 days	Unknown

Half-life: About 28 days.

ADVERSE REACTIONS

CNS: headache, fatigue, fever. **GI:** abdominal pain. **GU:** UTI. **Musculoskeletal:** arthralgia, back pain, arthropathy. **Respiratory:** URI. **Skin:** injection-site reactions, tinea infections, infection, antibody development.

INTERACTIONS

Drug-drug. *Live vaccines:* It isn't known if drug affects response to live or inactive vaccines. Avoid use together.

EFFECTS ON LAB TEST RESULTS

None reported.

CONTRAINDICATIONS & CAUTIONS

• Drug may increase risk of infection. Don't start drug in patients with clinically active infection until the infection resolves or is adequately treated.

• Use cautiously in patients with chronic infection or a history of recurrent infections.

• Evaluate patients for TB before initiating treatment. Don't give to patients with active TB. Consider anti-TB therapy in patients with a history of latent or active TB in whom adequate treatment can't be confirmed.

• Drug may increase risk of liver injury in patients with Crohn disease. Consider other treatment options in patients with liver cirrhosis.

• Safety and effectiveness in children haven't been established.
Dialyzable drug: Unknown.

PREGNANCY-LACTATION-REPRODUCTION

• Data are insufficient to evaluate pregnancy risk. Human IgG crosses the placental barrier and drug may be transferred from the mother to the developing fetus.

• Encourage patients who are pregnant to enroll in the Pregnancy Exposure Registry by calling 1-877-302-2161.

• It isn't known if drug appears in human milk. Maternal IgG is present in human milk. Before use in a patient who is breastfeeding, consider the benefits of breastfeeding along with potential adverse effects to the infant.

NURSING CONSIDERATIONS

• Evaluate patients for TB before, during, and after therapy. Anti-TB therapy may be required.

• Complete all age-appropriate immunizations according to current guidelines and schedules before initiating therapy.

• Obtain baseline LFT values in patients with Crohn disease and monitor values during induction, for at least up to 12 weeks of treatment, and periodically thereafter.

• Monitor patients for signs and symptoms of infection (fever, diaphoresis, chills, cough, dyspnea, bloody phlegm, muscle aches, weight loss, diarrhea or stomach pain, frequent urination, burning pain with urination, warm, red, or painful skin sores that aren't psoriasis). If infection occurs or isn't responding to therapy, withhold drug until infection resolves.

PATIENT TEACHING

• Tell patient to report all adverse reactions.

• Instruct patient and caregivers on proper injection technique and needle and syringe disposal; supervise initial self-injection.

• Warn patient that drug may lower the ability of the immune system to fight infections. Stress the importance of reporting history of infections to prescriber and to immediately report signs and symptoms of infection.

• Teach patient with a history of TB or active TB that treatment for TB may be needed before therapy begins.

• Instruct patient to seek immediate medical attention for signs and symptoms of hepatic dysfunction (rash, nausea, vomiting, abdominal pain, fatigue, anorexia, jaundice, dark urine).

• Counsel patient to become up-to-date with appropriate vaccines before therapy begins.

• Advise patient to report pregnancy, plans to become pregnant, breastfeeding, or plans to breastfeed before therapy begins.

R

risedronate sodium

ris-ED-roe-nate

Actonel✐, Atelvia

Therapeutic class: Antiosteoporotics
Pharmacologic class: Bisphosphonates

AVAILABLE FORMS

Tablets ⒹⓃⒸ: 5 mg, 30 mg, 35 mg, 75 mg,
150 mg
Tablets (delayed-release) ⒹⓃⒸ: 35 mg

INDICATIONS & DOSAGES

➤ **To prevent and treat postmenopausal
osteoporosis**
Women: 5-mg immediate-release tablet PO
once daily. Or, 35-mg immediate-release
tablet PO once weekly. Or, 75 mg immediate-
release tablet PO on 2 consecutive days for a
total of 150 mg each month. Or, one 150-mg
immediate-release tablet PO once monthly.
➤ **To treat postmenopausal osteoporosis**
Women: 35-mg delayed-release tablet PO
once weekly.
➤ **To increase bone mass in men with osteoporosis**
Men: One 35-mg immediate-release tablet PO
once weekly.
➤ **To prevent or treat glucocorticoid-
induced osteoporosis in patients taking
7.5 mg or more of prednisone or equivalent
glucocorticoid daily**
Adults: 5 mg immediate-release tablet PO
daily.
➤ **Paget disease (immediate-release)**
Adults: 30 mg PO daily for 2 months. If relapse occurs or ALP level doesn't normalize, may repeat treatment course 2 months or
more after completing first treatment course.

ADMINISTRATION
PO
• Give immediate-release tablets at least
30 minutes before the first food, drink, or
medication of the day, other than water. Give
with 8 oz of plain water while patient sits or
stands.
• Patient shouldn't eat or drink anything except plain water or take other medications for
at least 30 minutes after taking immediate-
release risedronate.
• Give delayed-release tablet in the morning
immediately after breakfast and not under

fasting conditions because of a higher risk
of abdominal pain if taken when fasting. Give
with 8 oz of plain water while patient sits or
stands.
• Warn patient against lying down for
30 minutes after taking drug.
• Make sure patient doesn't chew, crush, cut,
or suck tablets.
• Refer to manufacturer's instructions for
missed doses.

ACTION

Reverses the loss of bone mineral density by
reducing bone turnover and bone resorption.
In patients with Paget disease, drug causes
bone turnover to return to normal.

Route	Onset	Peak	Duration
PO	1 hr	1 hr	Unknown
PO (delayed-release)	Unknown	3 hr	Unknown

Half-life: Immediate-release, 23 hours; delayed-
release, 561 hours.

ADVERSE REACTIONS

CNS: asthenia, headache, depression, dizziness, insomnia. **CV:** HTN, arrhythmia, chest
pain, peripheral edema. **EENT:** cataract,
pharyngitis, rhinitis. **GI:** nausea, diarrhea, abdominal pain, vomiting, dyspepsia, flatulence,
gastritis, GERD, GI disease, constipation.
GU: UTI, BPH, nephrolithiasis. **Hematologic:** ecchymosis, anemia. **Musculoskeletal:** arthralgia, neck pain, back pain, extremity pain, myalgia, bone pain, muscle cramps.
Respiratory: URI, bronchitis. **Skin:** rash,
pruritus. **Other:** infection, flulike symptoms.

INTERACTIONS

Drug-drug. *Aspirin, NSAIDs:* May increase
risk of upper GI adverse events. Use cautiously together.
*Calcium supplements; antacids that contain
calcium, magnesium, or aluminum:* May interfere with risedronate absorption. Advise
patient to separate dosing times.
H₂ antagonists, PPIs: May affect enteric
coating on delayed-release tablets, increasing bioavailability. Use together isn't recommended.
Drug-food. *Any food:* May interfere with
absorption of drug. Advise patient to take
immediate-release tablets at least 30 minutes
before first food or drink of the day (other
than water).

Reactions in bold italics are *life-threatening*. Interactions may have a *rapid onset* or a ***delayed onset***.

EFFECTS ON LAB TEST RESULTS
• May increase parathyroid hormone level.
• May decrease calcium and phosphorus levels.

CONTRAINDICATIONS & CAUTIONS
• Contraindicated in patients hypersensitive to components of the product, in patients with hypocalcemia or conditions that delay esophageal emptying, and in those who can't stand or sit upright for 30 minutes after administration.
• Use cautiously in patients with renal impairment. Drug isn't recommended for use in patients with CrCl less than 30 mL/minute.
• Hypersensitivity and skin reactions have been reported, including angioedema, generalized rash, bullous skin reactions, SJS, and TEN.
◑ *Alert:* Drug may increase risk of thigh fractures.
• Drug increases risk of osteonecrosis of the jaw, which can occur spontaneously. For patients requiring invasive dental procedures, discontinuing bisphosphonate treatment may reduce risk.
• Use cautiously in patients with upper GI disorders, such as dysphagia, esophagitis, and esophageal or gastric ulcers.
• Treat hypocalcemia and other disturbances of bone and mineral metabolism before starting treatment.
• Immediate-release and delayed-release formulations contain the same active ingredient and must not be given together.
Dialyzable drug: Unknown.
⚠ *Overdose S&S:* Hypocalcemia, hypophosphatemia.

PREGNANCY-LACTATION-REPRODUCTION
• There are no adequate studies during pregnancy but fetal exposure to drug is likely. Discontinue drug for confirmed pregnancy.
• It isn't known if drug appears in human milk. Patient should discontinue breastfeeding or discontinue drug.

NURSING CONSIDERATIONS
• Assess sex steroid hormonal status of both men and women with glucocorticoid-induced osteoporosis; hormone replacement may be appropriate.
• Monitor patient for osteonecrosis of the jaw. Associated risk factors include invasive dental procedures, cancer diagnosis, concomitant treatment such as chemotherapy and steroids,

poor oral hygiene, and preexisting dental disease. If signs or symptoms occur, stop drug and refer patient to oral surgeon.
◑ *Alert:* Drug may cause dysphagia, esophagitis, and esophageal or gastric ulcers. Monitor patient for symptoms of esophageal disease.
• Severe musculoskeletal pain has been associated with bisphosphonate use and may occur within days, months, or years of start of therapy. When drug is stopped, symptoms may resolve partially or completely.
• Give supplemental calcium and vitamin D if dietary intake is inadequate. Because calcium supplements and drugs containing calcium, aluminum, or magnesium may interfere with risedronate absorption, separate dosing times.
• Periodically evaluate need for continued therapy in all patients. Consider discontinuation of therapy in patients at low risk for fracture after 3 to 5 years of use.
• Periodically evaluate risk of fracture in patients who discontinue therapy.
• Monitor patient for eye inflammation. Refer patient for ophthalmologic evaluation if inflammation occurs.
• Bisphosphonates can interfere with bone-imaging agents.
• *Look alike–sound alike:* Don't confuse Actonel with Actos.

PATIENT TEACHING
• Explain that drug may reverse bone loss by stopping more bone loss and increasing bone strength.
• Stress importance of adhering to special dosing instructions, including staying in an upright position for 30 minutes after taking drug with plain water and to avoid taking other medications for at least 30 minutes after a risedronate dose.
• Tell patient not to chew, cut, crush, or suck the tablet because doing so may irritate the mouth.
• Advise patient to immediately report GI discomfort (such as difficulty or pain when swallowing, retrosternal pain, or severe heartburn).
• Tell patient that Actonel and Atelvia contain the same active ingredient and must not be taken together.
• Advise patient to take calcium and vitamin D if dietary intake is inadequate, but to take them at a different time than risedronate.

R

• Advise patient to stop smoking and drinking alcohol, as appropriate. Also, advise patient to perform weight-bearing exercise.

risperiDONE
ris-PEER-i-dohn

Perseris, RisperDAL✲, RisperDAL Consta

Therapeutic class: Antipsychotics
Pharmacologic class: Benzisoxazole derivatives

AVAILABLE FORMS
Injection (IM): 12.5 mg, 25 mg, 37.5 mg, 50 mg
Injection (subcut): 90 mg, 120 mg
Oral solution: 1 mg/mL
Tablets: 0.25 mg, 0.5 mg, 1 mg, 2 mg, 3 mg, 4 mg
Tablets (ODTs): 0.25 mg, 0.5 mg, 1 mg, 2 mg, 3 mg, 4 mg

INDICATIONS & DOSAGES
Adjust-a-dose (for all indications): When oral formulations are administered with a CYP3A4 inducer, such as carbamazepine, phenytoin, rifampin, or phenobarbital, increase risperidone dosage up to double patient's usual dosage; decrease dosage when the enzyme inducer is discontinued. When administered with a CYP3A4 inhibitor, such as fluoxetine or paroxetine, reduce risperidone dosage; titrate slowly and don't exceed 8 mg/day in adults. It may be necessary to increase risperidone dosage when the enzyme inhibitor is discontinued.
➤ **Schizophrenia**
Adults: May give drug PO once daily or b.i.d. Initial dosing is generally 2 mg PO daily. Increase dosage at intervals not less than 24 hours, in increments of 1 to 2 mg/day, as tolerated, to a recommended dose of 4 to 8 mg/day. Periodically reassess to determine the need for maintenance treatment with an appropriate dose. Maximum dose is 16 mg/day.
Adjust-a-dose: In older adults, patients with hypotension, and those with CrCl of less than 30 mL/minute or severe hepatic impairment, use lower starting dosage of 0.5 mg PO b.i.d. May increase in increments of 0.5 mg or less

b.i.d. Increase to dosages above 1.5 mg b.i.d. at intervals of at least 1 week.
Adolescents ages 13 to 17: Start treatment with 0.5 mg PO once daily, given as a single daily dose in either the morning or evening. Adjust dose, if indicated, at intervals of not less than 24 hours, in increments of 0.5 or 1 mg/day, as tolerated, to a recommended dose of 3 mg/day. Reassess periodically to determine need for maintenance treatment with an appropriate dose. Maximum dose is 6 mg/day.
➤ **Parenteral maintenance therapy for schizophrenia or bipolar I disorder (as monotherapy or as combination therapy with lithium or valproate)**
Adults: Establish tolerance to oral risperidone before giving IM. Give 25 mg deep IM every 2 weeks.

Adjust dose no sooner than every 4 weeks. Maximum, 50 mg IM every 2 weeks. Continue oral antipsychotic for 3 weeks after first IM injection, then stop oral therapy. Continue therapy at lowest dose needed. Periodically reevaluate long-term risks and benefits of drug for the individual patient.

For subcut dosing, inject 90 or 120 mg once monthly where Perseris 90 mg corresponds to 3 mg/day oral risperidone and Perseris 120 mg corresponds to 4 mg/day oral risperidone.
Adjust-a-dose: In patients with hepatic or renal impairment, titrate slowly to 2 mg PO daily for 1 week. If tolerated, give 25 mg IM every 2 weeks, or may consider initial dose of 12.5 mg IM. Continue oral form of risperidone (or another antipsychotic) with the first injection and for 3 subsequent weeks to maintain therapeutic drug levels.

At initiation of therapy with carbamazepine or other known CYP3A4 hepatic enzyme inducers, closely monitor patient during first 4 to 8 weeks. A dosage increase or additional oral risperidone may need to be considered. On discontinuation of carbamazepine or other CYP3A4 inducers, reevaluate risperidone injection dosage and, if necessary, decrease dosage. Patients may be placed on a lower risperidone injection dosage between 2 and 4 weeks before the planned discontinuation of carbamazepine or other CYP3A4 inducers to adjust for the expected increase in risperidone plasma concentration.
➤ **Monotherapy or combination therapy with lithium or valproate for 3-week**

---

treatment of acute manic or mixed episodes from bipolar I disorder

Adults: Initially, 2 to 3 mg PO once daily. Adjust dose by 1 mg daily. Dosage range is 1 to 6 mg daily. Or, 25 mg IM every 2 weeks. Some patients may benefit from a higher dose of 37.5 or 50 mg.

Adjust-a-dose: In older adults, patients with hypotension, and those with severe renal or hepatic impairment, start with 0.5 mg PO b.i.d. Increase dosage by 0.5 mg b.i.d. Increase in dosages above 1.5 mg b.i.d. should occur at least 1 week apart. Subsequent switches to once-daily dosing may be made after patient is on a twice-daily regimen for 2 to 3 days at the target dose.

Children and adolescents ages 10 to 17: 0.5 mg PO as a single daily dose in either the morning or evening. Adjust dose, if indicated, at intervals not less than 24 hours, in increments of 0.5 or 1 mg/day, as tolerated, to a recommended dose of 2.5 mg/day.

➤ **Irritability, including aggression, self-injury, and temper tantrums, associated with an autistic disorder**

Adolescents and children ages 5 to 17 weighing 20 kg or more: Initially, 0.5 mg PO once daily or in two divided doses. After 4 days, increase dose to 1 mg. Increase dosage further in 0.5-mg increments at intervals of at least 2 weeks.

Children ages 5 to 17 weighing more than 15 and less than 20 kg: Initially, 0.25 mg PO once daily or in two divided doses. After 4 days, increase dose to 0.5 mg. Increase dosage further in 0.25-mg increments at intervals of at least 2 weeks.

ADMINISTRATION
PO
- Give drug without regard for meals.
- Oral solution isn't compatible with cola or tea.
- Open package for ODTs immediately before giving by peeling off foil backing with dry hands. Don't push tablets through the foil. ODTs can be swallowed with or without liquid.

IM
- Drug should be administered by a health care professional.
- Continue oral therapy for the first 3 weeks of IM injection therapy until injections take effect, then stop oral therapy.

- Bring injection to room temperature for at least 30 minutes before reconstitution (don't warm any other way).
- To reconstitute IM injection, inject premeasured diluent into vial and shake vigorously for at least 10 seconds. Suspension appears uniform, thick, and milky; particles are visible, but no dry particles remain. Use drug immediately after reconstitution. If more than 2 minutes pass before injection, shake vigorously again. See manufacturer's package insert for more detailed instructions.
- Use injection kit with 1-inch needle for deltoid muscle injection and kit with 2-inch needle for gluteal muscle injection.
- Inject deep IM into gluteal or deltoid muscle every 2 weeks, alternating injections between the two buttocks or two arms.
- Refrigerate IM injection kit and protect it from light. Drug can be stored at temperature less than 77° F (25° C) for no more than 7 days before administration.

Subcutaneous
- For abdominal subcut injection only. Don't give by any other route.
- Only a health care professional should administer drug.
- Allow package to come to room temperature for at least 15 minutes before preparation.
- Prepare medication immediately before administration.
- Give a missed dose as soon as possible.

ACTION
Blocks dopamine, 5-HT$_2$, alpha$_1$ and alpha$_2$ adrenergic, and H$_1$ histaminergic receptors in the brain.

Route	Onset	Peak	Duration
PO	Unknown	1 hr	Unknown
IM	3 wk	4–6 wk	7 wk
Subcut	Unknown	4–6 hr	4 wk

Half-life: PO, 3 to 20 hours; IM, 3 to 6 days; subcut, 9 to 11 days.

ADVERSE REACTIONS
CNS: akathisia, sedation, somnolence, dystonia, headache, insomnia, agitation, anxiety, pain, parkinsonism, abnormal gait, ataxia, dizziness, fever, hallucination, mania, impaired concentration, abnormal thinking and dreaming, tremor, hypoesthesia, fatigue, depression, nervousness, vertigo, syncope.
CV: tachycardia, bradycardia, bundle-branch

R

---

block, ECG changes, chest pain, hypotension, edema, palpitations, HTN. **EENT:** abnormal vision, conjunctivitis, decreased visual acuity, ear disorder (IM), rhinorrhea, nasal congestion, epistaxis, rhinitis, sinusitis, pharyngitis, dry mouth, increased saliva, toothache. **GI:** constipation, nausea, vomiting, dyspepsia, abdominal pain, anorexia, increased appetite, diarrhea. **GU:** urinary incontinence, increased urination, abnormal orgasm, decreased libido, vaginal dryness, amenorrhea, menstrual disorder, cystitis, erectile dysfunction, UTI. **Metabolic:** weight gain or loss, hyperglycemia. **Musculoskeletal:** arthralgia, back pain, leg pain, myalgia, muscle rigidity, muscle spasm. **Respiratory:** cough, dyspnea, bronchitis, pneumonia, URI. **Skin:** rash, eczema, pruritus, dry skin, photosensitivity reactions, acne; injection-site pain, reaction, or infection (IM, subcut). **Other:** increased thirst, galactorrhea, gynecomastia, hypersensitivity reaction, viral infection, falls, injury.

INTERACTIONS

Drug-drug. *Antihypertensives, drugs with hypotensive effects:* May enhance hypotensive effects. Monitor BP.

Clozapine: May decrease risperidone clearance, increasing toxicity. Monitor patient closely.

CNS depressants: May cause additive CNS depression. Use together cautiously.

CYP3A4 inducers (carbamazepine, phenobarbital, phenytoin, rifampin): May increase risperidone clearance and decrease effectiveness. Monitor patient closely.

Dopamine agonists, levodopa: May antagonize effects of these drugs. Use together cautiously and monitor patient.

Fluoxetine, paroxetine: May increase the risk of risperidone's adverse effects, including serotonin syndrome. Monitor patient closely and decrease risperidone dose as needed.

Methylphenidate: May increase risk of extrapyramidal symptoms with change in dosage of either medication. Monitor patient closely.

Boxed Warning *Opioids:* May cause slow or difficult breathing, sedation, and death. Avoid use together. If use together is necessary, limit dosage and duration of each drug to minimum necessary for desired effect. ■

QTc interval–prolonging drugs (dofetilide, procainamide, sotalol): May increase risk of QTc-interval prolongation and risk of

life-threatening ventricular arrhythmias. Use together cautiously unless contraindicated.

Drug-lifestyle. *Alcohol use:* May cause additive CNS depression. Discourage use together.

EFFECTS ON LAB TEST RESULTS

• May increase AST, ALT, blood glucose, cholesterol, triglyceride, GGT, and prolactin levels.

• May decrease Hb level, hematocrit, and WBC count.

CONTRAINDICATIONS & CAUTIONS

• Contraindicated in patients hypersensitive to drug.

• Opioids should only be prescribed with benzodiazepines or other CNS depressants to patients for whom alternative treatment options are inadequate.

Boxed Warning Older adults with dementia-related psychosis treated with antipsychotics are at increased risk for death. Drug isn't approved to treat older adults with dementia-related psychosis. ■

• Use cautiously in patients with CV disease, cerebrovascular disease, dehydration, hypovolemia, history of seizures, or conditions that could affect metabolism or hemodynamic responses.

• Use cautiously in patients exposed to extreme heat.

• Use caution in patients at risk for aspiration pneumonia.

• Use IM or subcut injection cautiously in patients with hepatic or renal impairment.

• Somnolence, orthostatic hypotension, and motor and sensory instability have been reported, which may lead to falls and fall-related injuries.

Dialyzable drug: Unknown.

⚠ *Overdose S&S:* Drowsiness, sedation, tachycardia, hypotension, extrapyramidal symptoms, QT-interval prolongation, seizures, torsades de pointes.

PREGNANCY-LACTATION-REPRODUCTION

⚠ *Alert:* Neonates exposed to antipsychotics during the third trimester are at risk for developing extrapyramidal signs and symptoms (repetitive muscle movements of the face and body) and withdrawal signs and symptoms (agitation, abnormally increased or decreased muscle tone, tremors, sleepiness, severe difficulty breathing, difficulty feeding) after

---

Reactions in bold italics are *life-threatening*. Interactions may have a *rapid onset* or a ***delayed onset***.

delivery. Use in patients who are pregnant only if potential benefit justifies fetal risk.

• Enroll patients exposed to drug during pregnancy in the National Pregnancy Registry for Atypical Antipsychotics (1-866-961-2388).

• Drug appears in human milk. Patient should discontinue breastfeeding or discontinue drug.

• Drug may cause hyperprolactinemia, which may decrease reproductive function in both men and women.

NURSING CONSIDERATIONS

⟳ *Alert:* Obtain baseline BP measurements before starting therapy, and monitor BP regularly. Watch for orthostatic hypotension, especially during first dosage adjustment.

• Monitor patient for tardive dyskinesia, which may occur after prolonged use. It may not appear until months or years later and may disappear spontaneously or persist for life, despite stopping drug.

⟳ *Alert:* Watch for evidence of NMS (extrapyramidal effects, hyperthermia, autonomic disturbance), which is rare but can be fatal.

⟳ *Alert:* Life-threatening hyperglycemia may occur in patients taking atypical antipsychotics. Monitor patients with diabetes regularly.

• Monitor patient for symptoms of metabolic syndrome (significant weight gain and increased BMI, HTN, hyperglycemia, hypercholesterolemia, and hypertriglyceridemia).

• Periodically reevaluate drug's risks and benefits, especially during prolonged use.

• Patients experiencing persistent somnolence may benefit from administering half the daily PO dose b.i.d.

• Monitor CBC in patients with preexisting low WBC count or history of drug-induced leukopenia or neutropenia.

• Assess fall risk when initiating treatment and recurrently for patients on long-term therapy, especially for older adults and patients with diseases, conditions, or other drug regimens that could increase fall risk.

• *Look alike–sound alike:* Don't confuse risperidone with reserpine or ropinirole. Don't confuse Risperdal with Restoril.

PATIENT TEACHING

• Instruct patient in safe drug administration.

• Warn patient to avoid activities that require alertness until effects of drug are known.

• Caution patient or caregiver of patient taking an opioid with a benzodiazepine, CNS depressant, or alcohol to seek immediate medical attention for dizziness, light-headedness, extreme sleepiness, slowed or difficult breathing, or unresponsiveness.

• Warn patient to rise slowly, and use other precautions to avoid fainting when starting therapy.

• Advise patient that drug may increase fall risk due to somnolence, orthostatic hypotension, and motor and sensory instability.

• Advise patient to use caution in hot weather to prevent heatstroke.

• Inform male patient of the possibility of prolonged or painful penile erections, and to seek immediate medical attention if they occur.

• Inform patient with phenylketonuria that ODT contains phenylalanine.

• Advise patient to avoid alcohol during therapy.

ritonavir
ri-TOE-na-veer

Norvir

Therapeutic class: Antiretrovirals
Pharmacologic class: Protease inhibitors

AVAILABLE FORMS
Oral powder: 100-mg packet
Oral solution: 80 mg/mL*
Tablets ⓭*:* 100 mg

INDICATIONS & DOSAGES
➤ **HIV infection, with other antiretrovirals**
Adults: 600 mg PO b.i.d. with meals. To reduce adverse GI effects, begin with 300 mg PO b.i.d. and increase by 100 mg b.i.d. at 2- to 3-day intervals.
Children older than age 1 month: 350 to 400 mg/m² PO b.i.d.; don't exceed 600 mg PO b.i.d. Initially, start with 250 mg/m² b.i.d. and increase by 50 mg/m² PO b.i.d. at 2- to 3-day intervals. If children can't reach b.i.d. doses of 400 mg/m² because of adverse effects, consider alternative therapy.
Adjust-a-dose: Dosage reduction is necessary when drug is used with other protease inhibitors: atazanavir, darunavir, fosamprenavir, saquinavir, and tipranavir. Consult full

R

prescribing information for dosage modification.

ADMINISTRATION
PO
• Give drug with meals.
• Don't administer ritonavir oral solution to neonates until postmenstrual age (first day of the mother's last menstrual period to birth plus the time elapsed after birth) reaches 44 weeks.
• Oral solution may be mixed with chocolate milk or enteral nutrition therapy liquids, such as Ensure or Advera, within 1 hour of dosing. Shake well.
• When giving oral solution to children, use a calibrated dosing syringe, if possible.
• Don't use polyurethane feeding tubes with oral solution due to potential incompatibility. Feeding tubes compatible with ethanol and propylene glycol, such as silicone and polyvinyl chloride feeding tubes, can be used for oral solution.
• Don't use oral powder for doses less than 100 mg or for incremental doses between 100-mg intervals; use oral solution instead.
• Mix oral powder with soft food, such as applesauce or vanilla pudding, or with liquid, such as water, chocolate milk, or infant formula, to lessen bitter aftertaste of oral powder. Give within 2 hours of preparation; discard and prepare new dose if more than 2 hours have elapsed since preparation.
• Make sure patient swallows tablets whole and doesn't break, crush, or chew them.
• Give a missed dose as soon as possible; then return to the normal schedule. Don't double the next dose.

ACTION
An HIV-1 protease inhibitor. Drug binds to the protease-active site and inhibits activity of the enzyme, preventing cleavage of the viral polyproteins and causing formation of immature, noninfectious viral particles.

Route	Onset	Peak	Duration
PO	Unknown	2–4 hr	Unknown

Half-life: 3 to 5 hours.

ADVERSE REACTIONS
CNS: anxiety, paresthesia, confusion, depression, dizziness, fatigue, headache, pain, peripheral neuropathy, somnolence, syncope, taste perversion, thinking abnormality.
CV: HTN, hypotension, edema, flushing.
EENT: blurred vision, oropharyngeal pain.
GI: diarrhea, nausea, vomiting, *pancreatitis*, abdominal pain, GERD, *GI bleeding*, dyspepsia, flatulence. **GU:** urinary frequency.
Hematologic: anemia, *neutropenia, thrombocytopenia.* **Hepatic:** increased LFT values, *hepatitis.* **Metabolic:** electrolyte imbalance due to severe diarrhea, gout, hyperglycemia, lipid disorders. **Musculoskeletal:** arthralgia, myalgia, myopathy. **Respiratory:** cough. **Skin:** pruritus, rash, acne, lipodystrophy. **Other:** hypersensitivity reactions.

INTERACTIONS
⚠ *Alert:* Ritonavir can significantly interact with many drugs. Consult a drug interaction resource or pharmacist for additional information.
Drug-drug. *Amiodarone, dronedarone, flecainide, propafenone, quinidine:* May cause cardiac arrhythmias. Use together is contraindicated.
Apixaban: May increase apixaban concentration. Refer to manufacturer's instructions for possible dosage reductions.
Atazanavir, darunavir, fosamprenavir, saquinavir, tipranavir: Protease inhibitors may increase the serum concentration of other protease inhibitors. Ritonavir dosage reduction is necessary when ritonavir is used with other protease inhibitors. Consult full prescribing information and clinical study information of these protease inhibitors if they are administered with a reduced ritonavir dosage.
⚠ *Alert: Atorvastatin, pitavastatin, pravastatin, rosuvastatin:* May increase statin level and risk of myopathy and rhabdomyolysis. Use together cautiously at the recommended dosage for the statin given in combination with ritonavir. Refer to prescribing information for statin drug dosage limitations.
Atovaquone, divalproex, lamotrigine, phenytoin: May decrease levels of these drugs. Use together cautiously and monitor drug levels closely.
Beta blockers, disopyramide, fluoxetine, mexiletine, nefazodone: May increase levels of these drugs, causing cardiac and neurologic events. Use together cautiously.
Bupropion, buspirone, calcium channel blockers, carbamazepine, clonazepam, clorazepate, cyclosporine, desipramine, dexamethasone, diazepam, **digoxin**, *dronabinol, estazolam, ethosuximide, flurazepam, lidocaine,*

Reactions in bold italics are *life-threatening*. Interactions may have a *rapid onset* or a **delayed onset**.

methamphetamine, metoprolol, perphenazine, prednisone, quinine, risperidone, sirolimus, SSRIs, tacrolimus, TCAs, thioridazine, timolol, tramadol, zolpidem: May increase levels of these drugs. Use cautiously together and consider decreasing the dosage of these drugs by almost 50%. Monitor therapeutic levels.

Clarithromycin: May increase clarithromycin level. If CrCl ranges from 30 to 60 mL/minute, reduce clarithromycin dosage by 50%. If CrCl is less than 30 mL/minute, reduce clarithromycin dosage by 75%.

Clozapine, piroxicam: May increase levels and toxicity of these drugs. Avoid using together.

Colchicine: May increase risk of serious or life-threatening reactions in patients with renal or hepatic impairment. Use together is contraindicated.

Delavirdine: May increase ritonavir level. Adjusted dose recommendations aren't established. Use together cautiously.

Disulfiram, metronidazole: May increase risk of disulfiram-like reactions because ritonavir formulations contain alcohol. Monitor patient.

Drugs that prolong QT interval (antiarrhythmics, encorafenib, ivosidenib, levofloxacin): May have additive QT-interval prolonging effect. Use cautiously together.

Edoxaban: May increase edoxaban serum concentration. Consider dosage adjustment if using for venous thromboembolism. (Dosage adjustment isn't needed for atrial fibrillation).

Ethinyl estradiol: May decrease ethinyl estradiol level. Use an alternative or additional method of birth control.

Fluticasone: May significantly increase fluticasone exposure, significantly decreasing cortisol concentrations and causing systemic corticosteroid effects (including Cushing syndrome). Don't use together, if possible.

HMG-CoA reductase inhibitors: May cause large increase in statin levels, resulting in myopathy. Use cautiously with atorvastatin and rosuvastatin, using lowest doses possible; monitor patient carefully. Consider using fluvastatin or pravastatin.

Itraconazole, ketoconazole: May increase levels of these drugs. Don't exceed 200 mg/day of these drugs.

◊ *Alert: Lovastatin, simvastatin:* May increase statin level and risk of myopathy and rhabdomyolysis. Use together is contraindicated.

Meperidine: May increase meperidine level. Dosage increases and long-term use together

aren't recommended because of CNS effects. Use cautiously together.

Methadone: May decrease methadone levels. Consider increasing methadone dosage.

PDE5 inhibitors (sildenafil, tadalafil, vardenafil): May increase levels of PDE5 inhibitor, causing hypotension, syncope, visual changes, or prolonged erection. Use together cautiously and increase monitoring for adverse reactions. Tell patient not to exceed 25 mg of sildenafil in a 48-hour period, 10 mg of tadalafil in a 72-hour period, or 2.5 mg of vardenafil in a 72-hour period.

Quinine: May increase quinine level. Consider decreased quinine dosage when used together.

Rifabutin: May increase rifabutin levels. Monitor patient and reduce rifabutin daily dosage by at least 75% of usual dose.

Rifampin, rifapentine: May decrease ritonavir levels. Consider using rifabutin.

Rivaroxaban: May lead to risk of increased bleeding. Avoid use together.

Boxed Warning *Several classes of drugs, including sedative-hypnotics, antiarrhythmics, ergot alkaloids (alfuzosin, apalutamide, bepridil, ergot derivatives, flecainide, lomitapide, lurasidone, methylergonovine, oral midazolam, pimozide, propafenone, quinidine, ranolazine, sildenafil [Revatio when used to treat PAH], simvastatin, triazolam):* May cause life-threatening adverse reactions due to possible effects of ritonavir on hepatic metabolism of these drugs. Use together is contraindicated. ■

Theophylline: May decrease theophylline levels. Increase dose based on blood levels.

Trazodone: May increase trazodone level, causing nausea, dizziness, hypotension, and syncope. Avoid using together. If unavoidable, use cautiously and lower trazodone dose.

Voriconazole: Decreases voriconazole level and reduces antifungal response. Voriconazole is contraindicated with ritonavir doses of 400 mg every 12 hours or greater.

Warfarin: May affect INR. Monitor patient frequently after initiating coadministration and adjust warfarin dosage as needed.

Drug-herb. *St. John's wort:* May substantially reduce drug levels. Use together is contraindicated.

Drug-lifestyle. *Smoking:* May decrease drug levels. Discourage smoking.

R

EFFECTS ON LAB TEST RESULTS
- May increase ALT, AST, GGT, amylase, bilirubin, glucose, triglyceride, lipid, CK, and uric acid levels.
- May decrease Hb level, hematocrit, and WBC, RBC, platelet, and neutrophil counts.

CONTRAINDICATIONS & CAUTIONS
Boxed Warning Administration with sedative-hypnotics, antiarrhythmics, or ergot alkaloid preparations may result in potentially serious or life-threatening adverse events because of possible effects on the hepatic metabolism of certain drugs. Review medications taken by patients before administering ritonavir or when administering other medications to patients already taking ritonavir. ■
- Contraindicated in patients hypersensitive to drug or its components.
- **Alert:** Consult full prescribing information before and during treatment for potential drug interactions.
- Use cautiously in patients with hepatic disease, liver enzyme abnormalities, or hepatitis and in those with signs or symptoms of pancreatitis.
- **Alert:** Patients with advanced HIV infection may have increased risk of elevated triglyceride levels and in some cases fatal pancreatitis.
- Hyperglycemia requiring treatment has been reported in patients receiving protease inhibitors. Use cautiously in patients with diabetes.
- Use cautiously in patients with hemophilia A or B. Drug may increase risk of bleeding events. Additional factor VIII may be needed.
- Safety and effectiveness in children younger than age 1 month haven't been established.
- May cause toxicity in preterm neonates. Don't use oral solution in preterm neonates in the immediate postnatal period. A safe and effective dose in this patient population hasn't been established.
Dialyzable drug: Unlikely.
⚠ *Overdose S&S:* Paresthesia, renal failure with eosinophilia, alcohol-related toxicity with oral solution.

PREGNANCY-LACTATION-REPRODUCTION
- There are no adequate studies during pregnancy. Use only if potential benefit justifies fetal risk.
- Enroll patients who are pregnant and exposed to drug in the Antiretroviral Pregnancy Registry (1-800-258-4263).
- Avoid using oral solution during pregnancy because it contains alcohol.
- Breastfeeding is contraindicated because of the potential for postnatal HIV-1 transmission.

NURSING CONSIDERATIONS
- Consult full prescribing information and clinical trial information when using ritonavir with other protease inhibitors.
- Monitor patient for immune reconstitution syndrome. During initial phase of treatment, patients responding to antiretroviral therapy may develop an inflammatory response to indolent or residual opportunistic infections (CMV, MAC, *Pneumocystis jiroveci* pneumonia, TB), which may necessitate further evaluation and treatment. Autoimmune disorders (such as Graves disease, polymyositis, and Guillain-Barré syndrome) have also been reported in the setting of immune reconstitution; however, time to onset is more variable, and can occur many months after initiation of antiretroviral treatment.
- Patients beginning regimens with ritonavir and nucleosides may improve GI tolerance by starting ritonavir alone and then adding nucleosides before completing 2 weeks of ritonavir.
- In patients with liver disease, monitor liver enzyme and triglyceride levels frequently, especially during the first 3 months of treatment.
- Monitor lipid levels before and periodically during therapy.
- Monitor patient for redistribution or accumulation of body fat, which has been observed with antiretroviral therapy.
- Monitor total amounts of alcohol and propylene glycol from all drugs given to children ages 1 to 6 months, to avoid alcohol-related toxicity.
- *Look alike–sound alike:* Don't confuse ritonavir with Retrovir. Don't confuse Norvir with Norvasc.

PATIENT TEACHING
- Explain that drug doesn't cure HIV infection and that opportunistic infections and other complications of HIV infection may continue to develop. Drug hasn't been shown to reduce the risk of transmitting HIV to others through sexual contact or blood contamination.
- Teach patient safe drug administration.
- Caution patient to take drug as prescribed and not to adjust dosage or stop therapy without first consulting prescriber.

• Advise patient taking a PDE5 inhibitor for erectile dysfunction to promptly report hypotension, dizziness, visual changes, and prolonged erection to prescriber. Caution against exceeding the recommended reduced dosage.

• Advise patient using hormonal contraceptives to use an alternative contraceptive or an additional barrier method during therapy.

• Caution patient to report signs and symptoms of pancreatitis (nausea, vomiting, and abdominal pain) immediately.

• Counsel patient that ritonavir must always be taken in combination with other antiretrovirals.

• Advise patient to report use of other drugs, including OTC drugs; this drug interacts with many drugs.

SAFETY ALERT!
BIOSIMILAR DRUG

riTUXimab
ri-TUK-si-mab

Rituxan

riTUXimab-abbs
Truxima

riTUXimab-arrx
Riabni

riTUXimab-pvvr
Ruxience

Therapeutic class: Antineoplastics
Pharmacologic class: Monoclonal antibodies

AVAILABLE FORMS
Injection: 10 mg/mL in 10-mL and 50-mL single-use, sterile vials

INDICATIONS & DOSAGES
➤ **Maintenance therapy for patients with previously untreated follicular, CD20-positive, B-cell non-Hodgkin lymphoma (NHL) who achieved complete or partial response to rituximab in combination with chemotherapy**
Adults: 375 mg/m^2 IV as single agent every 8 weeks for 12 doses beginning 8 weeks after completion of combination therapy.

➤ **Wegener granulomatosis (WG); microscopic polyangiitis (MPA) in combination with glucocorticoids**
Adults: 375 mg/m^2 IV once weekly for 4 weeks. Give methylprednisolone 1,000 mg/day IV for 1 to 3 days followed by oral prednisone 1 mg/kg/day (not to exceed 80 mg/day and tapered per clinical need) to treat severe vasculitis symptoms. This regimen should begin within 14 days before or with the initiation of rituximab and may continue during and after the 4-week course of rituximab treatment.
Children ages 2 to 17: 375 mg/m^2 IV once weekly for 4 weeks. Give IV methylprednisolone 30 mg/kg (not to exceed 1 g/day) once daily for 3 days. Refer to manufacturer's instructions for follow-up treatment dosing for adults and children.

➤ **Previously untreated, follicular CD20-positive, B-cell NHL with cyclophosphamide-vincristine-prednisolone (CVP) chemotherapy regimen**
Adults: 375 mg/m^2 IV given on day 1 of each CVP cycle, for up to eight doses.

➤ **Previously untreated low-grade, CD20-positive, B-cell NHL following first-line treatment with CVP chemotherapy**
Adults: For patients who fail to progress after six to eight cycles of CVP chemotherapy, give 375 mg/m^2 IV once weekly for 4 doses every 6 months for up to 16 doses.

➤ **CD20-positive chronic lymphocytic leukemia (CLL) in combination with fludarabine and cyclophosphamide**
Adults: 375 mg/m^2 IV given day before combination treatment. Then give 500 mg/m^2 IV on day 1 of cycles two through six in combination with fludarabine and cyclophosphamide (every 28 days).

➤ **Relapsed or refractory low-grade or follicular, CD20-positive, B-cell NHL**
Adults: Initially, 375 mg/m^2 IV once weekly for four or eight doses. Retreatment for patients with progressive disease, 375 mg/m^2 IV infusion once weekly for four doses.

➤ **With ibritumomab tiuxetan (Zevalin) for relapsed or refractory low-grade, follicular or transformed B-cell NHL**
Adults: 250 mg/m^2 IV 4 hours before indium-111 Zevalin infusion. Repeat in 7 to 9 days, 4 hours before yttrium-90 Zevalin infusion. Refer to ibritumomab prescribing information.

➤ **With methotrexate to reduce the signs and symptoms of moderate to severely**

R

active RA in patients who have had an in-adequate response to one or more TNF an-tagonists

Adults: Two 1,000-mg IV infusions 2 weeks apart. To reduce the incidence and sever-ity of infusion reactions, give methylpred-nisolone 100 mg IV, or its equivalent, 30 min-utes before each infusion. May give addi-tional courses every 24 weeks or based on clinical evaluation but no sooner than every 16 weeks.

➤ **Diffuse large B-cell, CD20-positive NHL, given with cyclophosphamide-Adriamycin (doxorubicin)-Oncovin (vincristine)-prednisone (CHOP) chemotherapy regimen or other anthracycline-based chemotherapy regimens**

Adults: 375 mg/m^2 IV on day 1 of each chemotherapy cycle for up to eight infusions.

➤ **Moderate to severe pemphigus vulgaris (Rituxan only)**

Adults: Initially, give two 1,000-mg IV infu-sions separated by 2 weeks in combination with a tapering course of glucocorticoids; then use a maintenance schedule of rituximab 500-mg IV infusion at month 12 and every 6 months thereafter or based on clinical eval-uation. If patient relapses, give rituximab 1,000-mg IV infusion with consideration to resuming or increasing the dosage of the glu-cocorticoid based on clinical evaluation. Al-low at least 16 weeks between rituximab in-fusions. Methylprednisolone 100 mg IV or equivalent glucocorticoid is recommended 30 minutes before each rituximab infusion.

✳ *NEW INDICATION:* **Previously untreated, advanced stage, CD20-positive, diffuse large B-cell lymphoma, Burkitt lymphoma, Burkitt-like lymphoma, or mature B-cell leukemia, in combination with chemother-apy**

Children ages 6 months and older: 375 mg/m^2 IV infusion in combination with systemic Lymphome Malin B chemotherapy. Give drug on day 1 and day 2 (48 hours apart) of each induction course, and on day 1 of each of the two consolidation courses. Give prednisone component of regimen before rituximab. Re-fer to manufacturer's instructions for addi-tional dosing information.

➤ **Burkitt lymphoma ◆**

Adults: 375 mg/m^2 IV on days 1 and 11 of cycles one and three and days 2 and 8 of cy-cles two and four. Or, 375 mg/m^2 IV at start of each chemotherapy cycle, followed by two

additional doses 3 and 6 weeks after comple-tion of chemotherapy. Or, 50 mg/m^2 IV on day 8 and 375 mg/m^2 IV on days 10 and 12 of cycle two, followed by 375 mg/m^2 IV on day 8 of cycles three to seven.

ADMINISTRATION

IV

▼ Premedicate with acetaminophen and an antihistamine before each infusion.

▼ Protect vials from direct sunlight.

▼ Dilute to yield 1 to 4 mg/mL in bag of D$_5$W or NSS. Gently invert bag to mix so-lution.

▼ Give as an infusion; don't give as IV push or bolus.

▼ Begin infusion at rate of 50 mg/hour. If no hypersensitivity or infusion-related events occur, increase rate by 50 mg/hour every 30 minutes, to maximum of 400 mg/hour. Start subsequent infusions at 100 mg/hour and increase by 100 mg/hour every 30 min-utes, to maximum of 400 mg/hour as toler-ated.

▼ For previously untreated follicular NHL and diffuse large B-cell NHL, patients may receive a 90-minute infusion in cycle 2 with a glucocorticoid-containing chemotherapy regimen if they didn't experience a grade 3 or 4 infusion-related adverse event during cycle 1. Refer to manufacturer's instructions.

▼ Discard unused portion left in vial.

▼ Store diluted solutions in refrigerator at 36° to 46° F (2° to 8° C) because they don't contain a preservative.

▼ **Incompatibilities:** Other IV drugs.

ACTION

A murine and human monoclonal antibody directed against CD20 antigen found on the surface of normal and malignant B lympho-cytes. Binding to this antigen mediates the lysis of the B cells.

Route	Onset	Peak	Duration
IV	Variable	Variable	6–12 mo

Half-life: Varies widely, possibly because of dif-ferences in tumor burden among patients and changes in CD20-positive B-cell populations on repeated therapy.

ADVERSE REACTIONS

CNS: asthenia, fever, headache, agitation, dizziness, fatigue, hypesthesia, hypertonia, insomnia, malaise, anxiety, pain, paresthesia,

peripheral neuropathy, taste perversion.
CV: hypotension, chest pain, edema, flushing, HTN, peripheral edema, *serious CV event.* **EENT:** conjunctivitis, epistaxis, rhinitis, sinusitis, throat irritation, oral candidiasis. **GI:** nausea, abdominal pain or enlargement, anorexia, diarrhea, dyspepsia, vomiting. **GU:** UTI. **Hematologic:** *leukopenia, neutropenia, thrombocytopenia, lymphopenia,* anemia. **Hepatic:** hepatobiliary disease, increased transaminase levels. **Metabolic:** hyperglycemia, hyperuricemia, increased LDH level, hypophosphatemia, *hypocalcemia,* weight gain. **Musculoskeletal:** back pain, myalgia, arthralgia, muscle spasms. **Respiratory:** *bronchospasm,* bronchitis, URI, cough increase, dyspnea, *pulmonary toxicity.* **Skin:** pruritus, rash, pain at injection site, urticaria, night sweats. **Other:** chills, rigors, *angioedema, infusion reaction,* infection, antibody development.

INTERACTIONS
Drug-drug. *Certolizumab, denosumab, tocilizumab:* May increase risk of serious infection. Avoid use together.
Cisplatin: May cause renal toxicity. Monitor renal function tests.
Leflunomide: May increase risk of hematologic toxicity. Monitor patient for bone marrow suppression at least monthly if both medications are needed.
❂ *Alert: Live-virus vaccines:* Virus replication may occur. Avoid vaccination with live-virus vaccines within 4 weeks before or during treatment.

EFFECTS ON LAB TEST RESULTS
• May increase glucose, potassium, uric acid, ALT, and LDH levels.
• May decrease calcium level.
• May increase or decrease phosphate level.
• May decrease Hb level and WBC, platelet, and neutrophil counts.

CONTRAINDICATIONS & CAUTIONS
Boxed Warning HBV reactivation, including fulminant hepatitis, hepatic failure, and death, may occur in patients treated with rituximab. ∎
❂ *Alert:* Consult hepatitis expert when screening identifies patients at risk for HBV reactivation due to prior HBV infection.
• Use cautiously in patients with a history of arrhythmia or angina.

• Drug isn't recommended for use in patients with severe, active infections.
Dializable drug: Unknown.

PREGNANCY-LACTATION-REPRODUCTION
• Verify pregnancy status before treatment.
• Based on human data, drug can cause adverse developmental outcomes, including B-cell lymphocytopenia, in infants exposed to drug in utero. Advise patients who are pregnant of the fetal risk. Monitor exposed newborns and infants for infection.
• Patients of childbearing potential should use effective contraception during therapy and for 12 months after therapy ends.
• It isn't known if drug appears in human milk. Patient should discontinue breastfeeding during and for 6 months after treatment.

NURSING CONSIDERATIONS
Boxed Warning Deaths from infusion reactions have occurred; most fatal reactions are associated with the first infusion. Monitor patient for infusion reaction complex, including hypoxia, pulmonary infiltrates, ARDS, MI, or cardiogenic shock. Interrupt infusion or slow infusion rate until symptoms improve; then continue infusion at no more than one-half the previous rate. Closely monitor patient. Discontinue rituximab infusion for severe reactions and administer medical treatment for grade 3 or 4 infusion reactions. ∎
• Monitor BP closely during infusion. If hypotension, bronchospasm, or angioedema occurs, stop infusion and restart at half the rate when symptoms resolve.
• If serious or life-threatening arrhythmias occur, stop infusion. If patient develops significant arrhythmias, monitor cardiac function during and after subsequent infusions.
• *Pneumocystis jiroveci* pneumonia and antiherpetic viral prophylaxis is recommended for patients with CLL during and for up to 12 months after treatment ends; with WG and MPA during and for up to 6 months after treatment; and should be considered for pemphigus vulgaris during and after treatment.
Boxed Warning Screen all patients for HBV infection before treatment by measuring HBsAg and hepatitis B core antibody. Monitor patients with evidence of current or prior HBV infection during and for several months after therapy. If HBV reactivation occurs, discontinue rituximab and

R

concomitant chemotherapy and begin appropriate treatment. ∎
• Monitor patients for bacterial, fungal, and new or reactivated viral infections.
• Monitor patients with WG and MPA carefully for signs and symptoms of infection (fever, pain, cold or flu symptoms, erythema) if biological agents or DMARDs are used concomitantly.
• Ensure patient is up-to-date with all immunizations in agreement with current immunization guidelines before starting drug, if possible. Give non-live vaccines at least 4 weeks before a course of rituximab.

Boxed Warning Severe mucocutaneous reactions (including TEN, SJS, paraneoplastic pemphigus, and lichenoid or vesiculobullous dermatitis) may occur, with variable onset. Avoid further infusions and promptly start treatment of the skin reaction. ∎
• Infusion-related reactions are most severe with the first infusion. Subsequent infusions are generally well tolerated.
◐ *Alert:* Acute renal failure requiring dialysis has been reported in the setting of TLS after treatment of patients with NHL.
• Patients at high risk for TLS may receive prophylactic allopurinol and hydration to correct hyperuricemia. Monitor renal function and fluid balance, and correct electrolyte abnormalities.

Boxed Warning JC virus infection resulting in PML has been reported in patients within 12 months of their last rituximab infusion. Monitor patient for new-onset neurologic manifestations. ∎
• Obtain CBC at regular intervals and more frequently in patients in whom cytopenias develop.
• Monitor patient for abdominal pain. Bowel obstruction and perforation have occurred with chemotherapy.
• *Look alike–sound alike:* Don't confuse rituximab with infliximab.

PATIENT TEACHING
• Provide patient with medication guide to read before each treatment session.
• Tell patient to report signs and symptoms of hypersensitivity, such as itching, rash, chills, or rigor, during and after infusion.
• Urge patient to report all adverse reactions, especially fever, sore throat, fatigue, easy bruising, nosebleeds, bleeding gums,

abdominal pain, or melena and to take temperature daily.
• Advise patient of childbearing potential to use effective contraception during therapy and for 12 months after final dose.
• Advise patient to avoid breastfeeding during and for 6 months after therapy ends.

SAFETY ALERT!

rivaroxaban ▨
riv-a-ROX-a-ban

Xarelto⌀

Therapeutic class: Anticoagulants
Pharmacologic class: Factor Xa inhibitors

AVAILABLE FORMS
Granules for oral suspension: 1 mg/mL after reconstitution
Tablets: 2.5 mg, 10 mg, 15 mg, 20 mg

INDICATIONS & DOSAGES
➤ **Prophylaxis of DVT that may lead to PE in patients undergoing knee or hip replacement surgery**
Adults: 10 mg PO once daily, 6 to 10 hours after surgery once hemostasis has been established. Treat for 35 days after hip replacement surgery and 12 days after knee replacement surgery.
Adjust-a-dose: If CrCl is less than 15 mL/minute, avoid use. Use cautiously in patients with moderate renal impairment (CrCl ranging from 30 to less than 50 mL/minute).
➤ **Treatment of DVT or PE**
Adults: 15 mg PO b.i.d. with food for 21 days; then 20 mg PO once daily for remainder of treatment.
Adjust-a-dose: If CrCl is less than 15 mL/minute, avoid use.
➤ **To decrease risk of recurrent DVT or PE after initial 6 months of treatment**
Adults: 10 mg PO once daily with or without food.
Adjust-a-dose: If CrCl is less than 15 mL/minute, avoid use.
➤ **Stroke and systemic embolism risk reduction in patients with nonvalvular atrial fibrillation**
Adults: 20 mg once daily with evening meal.
Adjust-a-dose: In patients with CrCl of 15 to 50 mL/minute, reduce dosage to 15 mg once daily.

➤ **To reduce risk of major CV events in patients with chronic CAD or peripheral artery disease (PAD), in combination with aspirin**

Adults: 2.5 mg PO b.i.d., with or without food, in combination with aspirin (75 to 100 mg) once daily.

➤ **Venous thromboembolism (VTE) prophylaxis in patients who are acutely ill and at risk for thromboembolic complications but aren't at high risk for bleeding**

Adults: 10 mg PO once daily for total duration of 31 to 39 days.

Adjust-a-dose: If CrCl is less than 15 mL/minute, avoid use.

➤ **To reduce risk of major thrombotic vascular events in patients with PAD, including patients after recent lower extremity revascularization due to symptomatic PAD once hemostasis is established**

Adults: 2.5 mg PO b.i.d. in combination with aspirin (75 to 100 mg) once daily.

✻ *NEW INDICATION:* **VTE and to reduce risk of recurrent VTE after at least 5 days of initial parenteral anticoagulant therapy**

Children from birth to younger than age 18, weighing 50 kg or more: 20 mg oral suspension or tablets PO daily.

Children from birth to younger than age 18 weighing 30 to 49.9 kg: 15 mg oral suspension or tablets PO daily.

Children from birth to younger than age 18 weighing 12 to 29.9 kg: 5 mg oral suspension PO b.i.d.

Children from birth to younger than age 18 weighing 10 to 11.9 kg: 3 mg oral suspension PO t.i.d.

Children from birth to younger than age 18 weighing 9 to 9.9 kg: 2.8 mg oral suspension PO t.i.d.

Children from birth to younger than age 18 weighing 8 to 8.9 kg: 2.4 mg oral suspension PO t.i.d.

Children from birth to younger than age 18 weighing 7 to 7.9 kg: 1.8 mg oral suspension PO t.i.d.

Children from birth to younger than age 18 weighing 5 to 6.9 kg: 1.6 mg oral suspension PO t.i.d.

Children from birth to less than age 18 weighing 4 to 4.9 kg: 1.4 mg oral suspension PO t.i.d.

Children from birth to younger than age 18 weighing 3 to 3.9 kg: 0.9 mg oral suspension PO t.i.d.

Children from birth to younger age 18 weighing 2 to 2.9 kg: 0.8 mg oral suspension PO t.i.d.

Adjust-a-dose: Children younger than age 6 months should have been at least 37 weeks of gestation at birth, have had at least 10 days of oral feeding, and weigh 2.6 kg or more at time of dosing. Continue therapy for at least 3 months and up to 12 months, when necessary. In children younger than age 2 with catheter-related thrombosis, continue therapy for at least 1 month and up to 3 months, when necessary. Avoid use in children age 1 and older with moderate or severe renal impairment (eGFR less than 50 mL/minute/1.72 m²). Refer to manufacturer's instructions for renal impairment in children younger than age 1 and for recommendations for switching to and from other anticoagulants.

✻ *NEW INDICATION:* **Thromboprophylaxis in patients with congenital heart disease after Fontan procedure**

Children age 2 and older weighing 50 kg or more: 10 mg oral suspension or tablets PO daily.

Children age 2 and older weighing 30 to 49.9 kg: 7.5 mg oral suspension PO daily.

Children age 2 and older weighing 20 to 29.9 kg: 2.5 mg oral suspension PO b.i.d.

Children age 2 and older weighing 12 to 19.9 kg: 2 mg oral suspension PO b.i.d.

Children age 2 and older weighing 10 to 11.9 kg: 1.7 mg oral suspension PO b.i.d.

Children age 2 and olde, weighing 8 to 9.9 kg: 1.6 mg oral suspension PO b.i.d.

Children age 2 and older weighing 7 to 7.9 kg: 1.1 mg oral suspension PO b.i.d.

Adjust-a-dose: Avoid use in children age 1 and older with moderate or severe renal impairment (eGFR less than 50 mL/minute/1.73m²). Refer to manufacturer's instructions for renal impairment in children younger than age 1 and for recommendations for switching to and from other anticoagulants.

ADMINISTRATION
PO

• Give 2.5- or 10-mg tablets without regard for food. Give 15- and 20-mg tablets with food. For nonvalvular atrial fibrillation, give with evening meal.

• For patients unable to swallow tablets whole, crush tablet and mix with applesauce immediately before use; administer

R

orally. Immediately follow administration of a crushed 15- or 20-mg tablet with food.

• For administration via NG or gastric feeding tube, crush tablet and suspend in 50 mL of water; confirm gastric placement and administer within 4 hours. Delivery of drug into the small intestine will result in reduced absorption. Immediately follow administration of a crushed 15- or 20-mg tablet with an enteral feeding.

• May give suspension via NG or gastric feeding tube. Flush tube with water after administration. For children with recurrent VTE, immediately follow with enteral feeding to increase absorption.

• Oral suspensions should be prepared by a pharmacist, stored at room temperature, and used within 60 days of preparation.

• For adults, if 2.5-mg b.i.d. dose is missed, give single dose at next scheduled time. If 15-mg b.i.d. dose is missed, give dose immediately to ensure intake of 30 mg/day; may give two 15-mg tablets at once. If daily 10-mg, 15-mg, or 20-mg dose is missed, give the missed dose immediately; don't double dose within the same day to make up for a missed dose.

• For children, give a missed daily dose as soon as possible but only on the same day. If not possible, skip the missed dose and continue the next day as prescribed. Give a missed morning dose of b.i.d. dosing as soon as possible; may give together with evening dose. Give a missed evening dose only in the same evening. Skip a missed t.i.d. dose and resume regular dosing at the next scheduled time without compensating for the missed dose.

ACTION

Selectively blocks the active site of factor Xa, which is necessary for coagulation.

Route	Onset	Peak	Duration
PO	Unknown	2–4 hr	Unknown

Half-life: 5 to 9 hours.

ADVERSE REACTIONS

CNS: syncope, fatigue, dizziness, anxiety, depression, insomnia. **EENT:** epistaxis, oropharyngeal pain, sinusitis. **GI:** abdominal pain, dyspepsia, gastroenteritis, *GI hemorrhage,* vomiting. **GU:** UTI. **Hematologic:** *bleeding events (including hemorrhage, intracranial hemorrhage).* **Musculoskeletal:** extremity

pain, muscle spasm, back pain. **Respiratory:** cough. **Skin:** wound secretion, pruritus, blister.

INTERACTIONS

Drug-drug. *Anticoagulants (warfarin), antithrombotic agents, aspirin, fibrinolytics, NSAIDs, P2Y12 platelet aggregation inhibitors, thienopyridines, SSNRIs, SSRIs:* May increase bleeding risk. Avoid use together. Monitor patient carefully for bleeding if drugs must be given together.

Combined P-gp and strong CYP3A4 inducers (carbamazepine, phenytoin, rifampin): May significantly decrease rivaroxaban level. Avoid use together.

Combined P-gp and strong CYP3A4 inhibitors (conivaptan, itraconazole, ketoconazole, lopinavir–ritonavir, ritonavir): May significantly increase rivaroxaban level. Avoid use together.

Combined P-gp and weak or moderate CYP3A4 inhibitors (amiodarone, azithromycin, diltiazem, dronedarone, erythromycin, felodipine, quinidine, ranolazine, verapamil): May increase rivaroxaban level. Use together only if benefit outweighs risk.

Mifepristone: May increase risk of bleeding. Avoid use together.

Drug-herb. *Herbs with anticoagulant or antiplatelet properties (alfalfa, anise, bilberry):* May enhance adverse effects of anticoagulants; bleeding may occur. Avoid use together.

St. John's wort: May significantly decrease rivaroxaban level. Avoid use together.

EFFECTS ON LAB TEST RESULTS

• May decrease granulocyte and platelet counts.

CONTRAINDICATIONS & CAUTIONS

Boxed Warning There is an increased risk of epidural or spinal hematomas, possibly resulting in long-term or permanent paralysis, in patients who have received anticoagulants and are receiving neuraxial anesthesia or undergoing spinal puncture. Patients at increased risk include those with indwelling epidural catheters; concomitant use of other drugs that affect hemostasis, such as NSAIDs, platelet inhibitors, and other anticoagulants; history of traumatic or repeated epidural or spinal punctures; and history of spinal deformity or spinal surgery. Monitor patients frequently for neurologic

---

Reactions in bold italics are *life-threatening*. Interactions may have a *rapid onset* or a *delayed onset*.

impairment. Urgent treatment is needed for neurologic compromise. Consider risks and benefits before neuraxial procedures in patients who have received anticoagulants for thromboprophylaxis. ∎

Boxed Warning Discontinuing rivaroxaban places patients at increased risk for thrombotic events. If anticoagulation with rivaroxaban must be discontinued for a reason other than pathological bleeding or completion of a course of therapy, consider coverage with another anticoagulant. ∎

• Contraindicated in patients hypersensitive to drug and in those with active major bleeding.

① Alert: Patients who are acutely ill and with the following conditions are at increased risk for bleeding with the use of rivaroxaban for primary VTE prophylaxis: history of bronchiectasis, pulmonary cavitation, or pulmonary hemorrhage; active cancer (i.e., undergoing acute, in-hospital cancer treatment); active gastroduodenal ulcer in the 3 months before treatment; history of bleeding in the 3 months before treatment; or dual antiplatelet therapy. Rivaroxaban isn't for use for primary VTE prophylaxis in these hospitalized patients who are acutely ill and at high risk for bleeding.

• Use isn't recommended in patients with prosthetic heart valves.

• Don't use in patients with triple positive antiphospholipid syndrome due to increased risk of recurrent thrombotic events compared to vitamin K antagonist therapy.

• Use cautiously in conditions associated with increased risk of hemorrhage, and in older adults.

• Avoid use in patients with CrCl of less than 15 mL/minute who are taking drug for PE or DVT treatment or recurrence prophylaxis or prophylaxis of DVT after hip or knee replacement surgery.

• In patients with nonvalvular atrial fibrillation, assess renal function more frequently in situations in which renal function may decline and adjust therapy accordingly. Consider dosage adjustment or drug discontinuation in patients who develop acute renal failure.

• Avoid use in patients with moderate or severe hepatic impairment (Child-Pugh class B or C) and in those with hepatic disease associated with coagulopathy.

▨ Use cautiously in patients of Japanese descent because drug exposure in these patients may be increased up to 40% when compared to other ethnicities, but differences are reduced when values are corrected for body weight.

• Safety and effectiveness in children haven't been established.

Dialyzable drug: No.

⚠ Overdose S&S: Hemorrhage.

PREGNANCY-LACTATION-REPRODUCTION

• There are no adequate studies during pregnancy. Use cautiously and only if potential benefit justifies fetal risk because of the potential for pregnancy-related hemorrhage or emergent delivery with use of an anticoagulant that isn't readily reversible.

• Drug appears in human milk; however, the effects on infants who are breastfed are unknown.

NURSING CONSIDERATIONS

Boxed Warning Monitor patient frequently for signs and symptoms of neurologic impairment. Urgent treatment is necessary for neurologic compromise. ∎

Boxed Warning Consider the benefits and risks before neuraxial intervention in patients anticoagulated or to be anticoagulated for thromboprophylaxis. Optimal timing between rivaroxaban administration and neuraxial procedures isn't known. ∎

• Don't remove an epidural catheter earlier than 18 hours after last administration of drug, and don't give next dose until 6 hours after catheter removal unless traumatic puncture occurred; if puncture has occurred, wait 24 hours before giving next dose.

• Monitor patient carefully for bleeding, which can occur at any site during therapy.

• If an anticoagulant must be discontinued to reduce risk of bleeding with surgical or other procedures, stop drug at least 24 hours before procedure. When deciding whether to delay a procedure until 24 hours after last dose, weigh the increased risk of bleeding against the urgency of intervention. Restart drug after procedure when adequate hemostasis has been established, as the time to onset of therapeutic effect is short.

① Alert: Watch for signs and symptoms of blood loss. Search for a bleeding site if an unexplained fall in hematocrit or BP occurs. Patients with moderate renal failure (CrCl ranging from 30 to less than 50 mL/minute) are at increased risk.

R

PATIENT TEACHING
• Instruct patient to take drug only as directed and not to discontinue drug without consulting prescriber.
• Tell patient how to manage a missed dose.
🕔 *Alert:* If patient has had neuraxial anesthesia or spinal puncture, especially if taking concomitant NSAIDs or platelet inhibitors, advise patient to watch for signs and symptoms of spinal or epidural hematoma (midline back pain, tingling, numbness of the limbs, muscular weakness, bowel or bladder dysfunction). If any of these signs and symptoms occur, advise patient to contact prescriber immediately.
• Advise patient to watch for bleeding risks, especially if patient had a spinal catheter or is currently taking drugs or supplements that increase bleeding risk.
• Instruct patient to report pregnancy and plans to become pregnant or to breastfeed.
• Caution patient to report changes in medications or herbal supplements or unusual bleeding or bruising.
• Instruct patient to inform all health care providers that patient is taking rivaroxaban before scheduling invasive procedures (including dental procedures).

---

rivastigmine
ri-va-STIG-meen

Exelon Patch

rivastigmine tartrate✎

Therapeutic class: Anti-Alzheimer drugs
Pharmacologic class: Cholinesterase inhibitors

AVAILABLE FORMS
Capsules 🆗*:* 1.5 mg, 3 mg, 4.5 mg, 6 mg
Transdermal patch: 4.6 mg/24 hours, 9.5 mg/24 hours, 13.3 mg/24 hours

INDICATIONS & DOSAGES
Adjust-a-dose (for all indications): Patients with moderate to severe renal impairment (GFR less than 50 mL/minute) or mild to moderate hepatic impairment (Child-Pugh score of 5 to 9) may be able to only tolerate lower doses of oral drug. For patients with mild to moderate hepatic impairment, consider using 4.6 mg/24 hours transdermal patch for both initial and maintenance dose. For patients weighing less than 50 kg, watch for toxicities (nausea, vomiting) and if they occur, consider reducing maintenance dose; reduce dose of transdermal patch to 4.6 mg/24 hours.

➤ **Mild to moderate Alzheimer dementia**
Adults: Initially, 1.5 mg PO b.i.d. If tolerated, may increase to 3 mg b.i.d. after 2 weeks. After 2 weeks at this dose, may increase to 4.5 mg b.i.d. and to 6 mg b.i.d., as tolerated. Effective dosage range is 6 to 12 mg daily; maximum, 12 mg daily. Or, 4.6 mg/24 hours transdermal patch once daily. After 4 weeks, if tolerated, increase to 9.5 mg/24 hours transdermal patch for as long as therapeutic benefit persists; if needed after at least 4 weeks, increase to 13.3 mg/24 hours transdermal patch. Maximum dose is 13.3 mg/24 hours.

➤ **Severe Alzheimer dementia (transdermal patch only)**
Adults: Initially, 4.6 mg/24 hours transdermal patch once daily. After 4 weeks, if tolerated, increase to 9.5 mg/24 hours transdermal patch; then, if tolerated after an additional 4 weeks, increase to 13.3 mg/24 hours transdermal patch.

➤ **Mild to moderate dementia associated with Parkinson disease**
Adults: Initially, 1.5 mg PO b.i.d. May increase, as tolerated, to 3 mg b.i.d., then to 4.5 mg b.i.d., and finally to 6 mg b.i.d. after a minimum of 4 weeks at each dose; maximum dose is 12 mg daily.

Or, 4.6 mg/24 hours transdermal patch once daily. After 4 weeks, if tolerated, increase to 9.5 mg/24 hours transdermal patch for as long as therapeutic benefit persists; if needed after at least 4 weeks, increase to 13.3 mg/24 hours transdermal patch. Maximum dose is 13.3 mg/24 hours.

➤ **Neuropsychiatric symptoms associated with Lewy body dementia ♦**
Adults: Initially, 1.5 mg PO b.i.d.; increase as tolerated by 1.5 mg b.i.d. every 2 weeks to a maximum of 6 mg b.i.d.

ADMINISTRATION
PO
• Give drug with food in the morning and evening.
• Patient should swallow capsule whole.
• If therapy is interrupted for more than 3 days, restart with 1.5 mg b.i.d. and retitrate.

Transdermal

• Apply patch once daily to clean, dry, hairless skin on the upper or lower back, upper arm, or chest, in a place not rubbed by tight clothing. Press down firmly for 30 seconds until edges stick well.

• Change the site daily, and don't use the same site within 14 days. Avoid exposing patch to external heat sources (sauna, excess sunlight).

• Avoid eye contact; wash hands with soap and water after removing patch. In case of contact with eyes or if eyes become red after handling patch, rinse immediately with plenty of water. Seek medical advice if symptoms don't resolve.

ACTION

Thought to increase acetylcholine level by inhibiting cholinesterase enzyme, which causes acetylcholine hydrolysis.

Route	Onset	Peak	Duration
PO	Rapid	1 hr	8–10 hr
Transdermal	30–60 min	8–16 hr	24 hr

Half-life: Oral, 1.5 hours; transdermal, 3 hours.

ADVERSE REACTIONS

CNS: headache, dizziness, syncope, fatigue, asthenia, malaise, somnolence, tremor, insomnia, confusion, depression, anxiety, hallucinations, aggressive reaction, psychomotor hyperactivity, vertigo, agitation, nervousness, gait disturbance. **CV:** HTN. **EENT:** excess salivation. **GI:** nausea, vomiting, diarrhea, anorexia, abdominal pain, dyspepsia. **GU:** UTI, incontinence. **Metabolic:** weight loss. **Musculoskeletal:** bradykinesia, dyskinesia, hypokinesia, weakness, cogwheel rigidity. **Respiratory:** URI, cough, bronchitis. **Skin:** diaphoresis, rash, application-site pruritus or erythema. **Other:** falls.

INTERACTIONS

Drug-drug. *Anticholinergics:* May decrease effectiveness of rivastigmine. Monitor patient for expected therapeutic effects.
Beta blockers, bradycardia-inducing drugs: May worsen bradycardia. Use together isn't recommended.
Bethanechol, succinylcholine or cholinergic antagonists: May increase effects of these drugs. Monitor patient closely.

Metoclopramide: May enhance risk of extrapyramidal reactions. Concomitant use isn't recommended.
Neuromuscular-blockers: May decrease neuromuscular blocking effect. Monitor patient closely.
NSAIDs: May increase gastric acid secretions. Monitor patient for symptoms of active or occult GI bleeding.
Drug-lifestyle. *Smoking:* May increase drug clearance. Discourage smoking.

EFFECTS ON LAB TEST RESULTS

None reported.

CONTRAINDICATIONS & CAUTIONS

• Contraindicated in patients hypersensitive to drug, other carbamate derivatives, or other components of drug.
• Isolated cases of disseminated allergic dermatitis, irrespective of administration route (oral or transdermal), have been reported. Discontinue drug if allergic dermatitis occurs.
• Contraindicated in patients with history of transdermal patch application-site reaction suggestive of allergic contact dermatitis.
• Use cautiously in patients with history of CV disease, GI bleeding, seizure disorder, GU conditions, asthma, or obstructive pulmonary disease.
Dialyzable drug: No.
⚠ **Overdose S&S:** Nausea, vomiting, excessive salivation, diaphoresis, bradycardia, hypotension, respiratory depression, syncope, seizures, muscle weakness.

PREGNANCY-LACTATION-REPRODUCTION

• There are no adequate studies during pregnancy. Use only if clearly needed.
• It isn't known if drug appears in human milk. Patient should discontinue breastfeeding or discontinue drug.

NURSING CONSIDERATIONS

• Expect significant GI adverse effects (such as nausea, vomiting, anorexia, and weight loss), which may lead to dehydration. These effects are less common during maintenance doses.
• Monitor patient for evidence of active or occult GI bleeding.
• Dramatic memory improvement is unlikely. As disease progresses, the benefits of drug may decline.

• Carefully monitor patient with a history of GI bleeding, NSAID use, arrhythmias, seizures, or pulmonary conditions for adverse effects.

• If adverse reactions, such as diarrhea, loss of appetite, nausea, or vomiting, occur with transdermal patch, stop use for several days, then restart at the same or lower dose. If treatment is interrupted for more than several days, restart patch at the lowest dose and retitrate.

• Patients weighing less than 50 kg may experience more adverse reactions when using the transdermal patch.

• Application-site reactions may occur with the transdermal patch. Discontinue treatment if application-site reaction spreads beyond the patch size, if there's evidence of a more intense local reaction (increasing erythema, edema, papules, vesicles), and if symptoms don't significantly improve within 48 hours after patch removal.

• When switching from oral form to the transdermal patch, patients on a total daily dose of less than 6 mg can be switched to 4.6 mg/24 hours. Patients taking 6 to 12 mg PO can switch to the 9.5 mg/24 hour patch. The patch should be applied on the day after the last oral dose.

PATIENT TEACHING

• Teach patient and caregiver safe drug administration.

• Advise patient that memory improvement may be subtle and that drug more likely slows future memory loss.

• Tell patient to report nausea, vomiting, or diarrhea.

• Advise patient to consult prescriber before using OTC drugs.

• Advise patient to remove used patch, place in previously saved pouch and discard in trash (away from pets or children), and then wash hands with soap and water. In case of contact with eyes or if eyes become red after handling patch, tell patient to rinse immediately with plenty of water and seek medical advice if symptoms don't resolve.

roflumilast
roe-FLUE-mi-last

Daliresp✇

Therapeutic class: Miscellaneous respiratory drugs
Pharmacologic class: Selective phosphodiesterase inhibitors

AVAILABLE FORMS
Tablets: 250 mcg, 500 mcg

INDICATIONS & DOSAGES
➤ **To reduce risk of COPD exacerbations in patients with severe COPD associated with chronic bronchitis and a history of exacerbations**
Adults: 250 mcg once daily for 4 weeks; then increase to 500 mcg PO daily (maintenance dose).

ADMINISTRATION
PO
• Give drug without regard to food.

ACTION
Selectively inhibits phosphodiesterase-4 (PDE_4), which is a cAMP-metabolizing enzyme in the lung tissue. Inhibition of PDE_4 leads to accumulation of intracellular cAMP. Effects of drug are thought to be related to the increased intracellular cAMP in lung cells.

Route	Onset	Peak	Duration
PO	Unknown	1–2 hr	Unknown

Half-life: 17 hours; N-oxide metabolite, 30 hours.

ADVERSE REACTIONS
CNS: anxiety, depression, headache, insomnia, dizziness, tremor. **EENT:** rhinitis, sinusitis. **GI:** abdominal pain, diarrhea, dyspepsia, gastritis, nausea, vomiting, decreased appetite. **GU:** UTI. **Metabolic:** weight loss. **Musculoskeletal:** back pain, muscle spasms. **Other:** flulike symptoms.

INTERACTIONS
Drug-drug. *Ciprofloxacin (systemic):* May increase roflumilast serum concentration. Monitor therapy.
CYP450 inducers (carbamazepine, phenobarbital, phenytoin, rifampin): May decrease

---

Reactions in bold italics are *life-threatening*. Interactions may have a *rapid onset* or a ***delayed onset***.

the effectiveness of roflumilast. Avoid use together.

CYP450 inhibitors (cimetidine, erythromycin, fluvoxamine, ketoconazole): May increase roflumilast concentration and risk of adverse reactions. Use together cautiously.

Immunosuppressants (except short-term corticosteroids, beclomethasone [oral inhalation], cytarabine [liposomal], fluticasone [oral inhalation]): May enhance immunosuppressive effect. Consider therapy modification.

Oral contraceptives containing gestodene and ethinyl estradiol: May increase roflumilast exposure and result in increased adverse effects. Weigh risk of concurrent use against benefit.

EFFECTS ON LAB TEST RESULTS
None reported.

CONTRAINDICATIONS & CAUTIONS
• Contraindicated in patients hypersensitive to drug or its components and in those with moderate to severe hepatic impairment (Child-Pugh class B or C).
• Use cautiously in patients with history of depression or suicidality.
Dialyzable drug: Unlikely.

PREGNANCY-LACTATION-REPRODUCTION
• There are no adequate studies during pregnancy. Use only if potential benefit justifies fetal risk.
• Don't use during labor and delivery.
• Drug may appear in human milk. Patient should discontinue breastfeeding or discontinue drug.

NURSING CONSIDERATIONS
• Drug isn't a bronchodilator and isn't indicated for the relief of acute bronchospasm.
• Monitor patients for signs and symptoms of psychiatric adverse events, including insomnia, anxiety, depression, suicidality, and suicide attempts. If events occur, evaluate the risks versus benefits of continuing drug.
• Monitor weight regularly; if unexplained or significant weight loss occurs, evaluate cause and consider stopping drug.

PATIENT TEACHING
• Teach patient that drug isn't a bronchodilator and isn't to be used for the relief of acute bronchospasm.

• Advise patient, family, and caregivers to watch for signs and symptoms of psychiatric adverse events, including insomnia, anxiety, depression, suicidality, and suicide attempts, and to report any occurrences to the health care provider.
• Tell patient to report unexplained or significant weight loss.

rolapitant hydrochloride
roe-LA-pi-tant

Varubi

Therapeutic class: Antiemetics
Pharmacologic class: Substance P and neurokinin-1 receptor antagonists

AVAILABLE FORMS
Tablets: 90 mg

INDICATIONS & DOSAGES
➤ **Prevention of delayed nausea and vomiting associated with emetogenic chemotherapy (in combination with other antiemetics)**
Adults: 180 mg PO. Administer within 2 hours of chemotherapy on day 1. Give dexamethasone 20 mg on day 1, 30 minutes before chemotherapy and then 8 mg PO b.i.d. on days 2, 3, and 4. Also give a 5-HT_3 receptor antagonist on day 1. Refer to manufacturer's instructions for appropriate dosing information.
➤ **Prevention of delayed nausea and vomiting associated with anthracycline and cyclophosphamide–based or moderately emetogenic chemotherapy, in combination with other antiemetics**
Adults: 180 mg PO. Administer within 2 hours of chemotherapy on day 1. Give dexamethasone 20 mg PO 30 minutes before chemotherapy on day 1. Also give a 5-HT_3 receptor antagonist on day 1. Refer to manufacturer's instructions for appropriate dosing information.

ADMINISTRATION
PO
• Give drug before each scheduled chemotherapy cycle.
• Give no more frequently than every 2 weeks.
• Give without regard to meals.
• Store at room temperature.

R

ACTION

A selective and competitive antagonist of human substance P/neurokinin-1 receptors in the brain. Appears to be synergistic with 5-HT$_3$ antagonists and corticosteroids.

Route	Onset	Peak	Duration
PO	30 min	4 hr	Unknown

Half-life: About 7 days.

ADVERSE REACTIONS

CNS: dizziness. **GI:** abdominal pain, decreased appetite, dyspepsia, stomatitis. **GU:** UTI. **Hematologic:** *neutropenia,* anemia. **Respiratory:** hiccups.

INTERACTIONS

Drug-drug. *BCRP substrates with a narrow therapeutic index (irinotecan, methotrexate, rosuvastatin, topotecan):* May increase plasma concentrations of BCRP substrates and risk of BCRP-related adverse reactions. Monitor patient. Use lowest effective rosuvastatin dose.
CYP2D6 substrates (dextromethorphan, TCAs): May increase plasma concentrations of CYP2D6 substrates for at least 28 days after rolapitant dose. Monitor patient closely for increased adverse effects.
CYP2D6 substrates with a narrow therapeutic index (pimozide, thioridazine): May increase pimozide and thioridazine level and risk of QT-interval prolongation. Use is contraindicated.
Dabigatran, edoxaban: May increase serum concentration of anticoagulant. Consider therapy modification.
P-gp substrates with a narrow therapeutic index (digoxin): May increase plasma concentrations of substrates and risk of adverse reactions. Monitor drug levels and watch for increased adverse reactions if concomitant use can't be avoided.
Strong CYP3A4 inducers (rifampin): May decrease plasma concentration and therapeutic effect of rolapitant. Avoid concomitant use, if possible.
Warfarin: May increase warfarin level. Monitor INR and PTT; adjust doses as needed to maintain target INR.

EFFECTS ON LAB TEST RESULTS

• May decrease Hb level and neutrophil count.

CONTRAINDICATIONS & CAUTIONS

• Contraindicated in patients hypersensitive to drug or its components, including soybean oil.
• Drug hasn't been studied in patients with severe hepatic impairment (Child-Pugh class C); avoid use. Monitor closely for adverse reactions if use can't be avoided.
• Safety and effectiveness in children haven't been established. Drug is contraindicated in children younger than age 2 because of irreversible sexual development impairment and infertility observed in rats.
Dialyzable drug: Unlikely.

PREGNANCY-LACTATION-REPRODUCTION

• There are no data regarding use during pregnancy. Use only if benefits outweigh fetal risk.
• It isn't known if drug appears in human milk. Give only if benefits outweigh risks to infant who is breastfed.

NURSING CONSIDERATIONS

⚠ *Alert:* Before giving drug, assess patient's current drug list for potential drug-drug interactions.
• Drug is used to prevent, not treat, nausea and vomiting.
• Always use drug in combination with a corticosteroid and a 5-HT$_3$ inhibitor.
• *Look alike–sound alike:* Don't confuse rolapitant with aprepitant or fosaprepitant. Don't confuse Varubi with valrubicin.

PATIENT TEACHING

• Remind patient that rolapitant is taken in combination with a corticosteroid and a 5-HT$_3$ inhibitor.
• Inform patient that rolapitant prevents nausea and vomiting; it doesn't treat them. Advise patient to take other antiemetics for breakthrough nausea and vomiting.
• Remind patient to take drug 1 to 2 hours before scheduled chemotherapy.
• Inform patient that rolapitant is associated with drug-drug interactions and that it's important to report all medications being taken, including OTC drugs and supplements, before starting therapy.
• Advise patient to inform prescriber and pharmacist of dosage changes or new prescription drug therapy because drug interactions can be delayed after rolapitant is discontinued.

Reactions in bold italics are *life-threatening*. Interactions may have a *rapid onset* or a *delayed onset*.

• Advise patient to report pregnancy, plans to become pregnant, or breastfeeding.

rOPINIRole hydrochloride
roe-PIN-i-role

Therapeutic class: Antiparkinsonian drugs
Pharmacologic class: Nonergot dopamine agonists

AVAILABLE FORMS
Tablets: 0.25 mg, 0.5 mg, 1 mg, 2 mg, 3 mg, 4 mg, 5 mg
Tablets (extended-release) ⓒ: 2 mg, 4 mg, 6 mg, 8 mg, 12 mg

INDICATIONS & DOSAGES
Adjust-a-dose (for all indications): For patients with ESRD on hemodialysis using immediate-release formula, give 0.25 mg PO t.i.d. for Parkinson disease and 0.25 mg PO daily for restless legs syndrome. Base further dosage escalations on tolerability and need for efficacy. Recommended maximum total daily dose in patients receiving regular dialysis is 18 mg/day for Parkinson disease and 3 mg daily for restless legs syndrome. Supplemental doses after dialysis aren't required. No dosage adjustment is necessary in patients with moderate renal impairment (CrCl of 30 to 50 mL/minute).

For patients with ESRD on hemodialysis using extended-release formula, give 2 mg once daily initially. May titrate dosage upward for a maximum dose of 18 mg/day if needed. Supplemental doses after dialysis aren't required.

➤ **Parkinson disease**
Adults: Initially, 0.25 mg PO t.i.d. Increase dose by 0.25 mg t.i.d. at weekly intervals for 4 weeks. After week 4, daily dosage may be increased by 1.5 mg/day on a weekly basis up to a dose of 9 mg/day, and then by up to 3 mg/day weekly to a total dose of 24 mg/day (8 mg t.i.d.). For extended-release form, starting dosage is 2 mg PO once daily for 1 to 2 weeks. May increase by 2 mg/day at 1-week or longer intervals. Although the maximum dosage is 24 mg/day, patients with advanced Parkinson disease should generally be maintained at 8 mg or lower daily and patients with early Parkinson disease should generally be maintained at 12 mg or lower daily. To switch

from immediate-release to extended-release tablets, refer to manufacturer's instructions.
Older adults: Adjust dosages individually, according to patient response; clearance may be reduced in these patients.
➤ **Moderate to severe restless legs syndrome (immediate-release)**
Adults: Initially, 0.25 mg PO 1 to 3 hours before bedtime. May increase dose as needed and tolerated after 2 days to 0.5 mg, then to 1 mg by the end of the first week. May further increase dose as needed and tolerated as follows: Week 2, give 1 mg once daily. Week 3, give 1.5 mg once daily. Week 4, give 2 mg once daily. Week 5, give 2.5 mg once daily. Week 6, give 3 mg once daily. Week 7, give 4 mg once daily. Maximum dosage is 4 mg/day. Patient should take all doses 1 to 3 hours before bedtime.

ADMINISTRATION
PO
• Give drug with food if nausea occurs.
• Patient must swallow extended-release tablets whole; they mustn't be chewed, crushed, or divided.
• Don't double dose after a missed dose.

ACTION
Thought to stimulate dopamine (D_2) receptors.

Route	Onset	Peak	Duration
PO (immediate-release)	Unknown	1–2 hr	6 hr
PO (extended-release)	Unknown	6–10 hr	Unknown

Half-life: 6 hours.

ADVERSE REACTIONS
Early Parkinson disease (without levodopa)
CNS: dizziness, fatigue, somnolence, syncope, hallucinations, aggravated Parkinson disease, headache, confusion, hyperkinesia, hypesthesia, vertigo, amnesia, impaired concentration, malaise, asthenia, pain. **CV:** orthostatic hypotension, orthostatic symptoms, HTN, edema, chest pain, extrasystoles, atrial fibrillation, palpitations, tachycardia, flushing. **EENT:** abnormal vision, eye abnormality, xerophthalmia, dry mouth, pharyngitis, rhinitis, sinusitis. **GI:** nausea, vomiting, dyspepsia, flatulence, abdominal pain, anorexia, constipation. **GU:** UTI, erectile dysfunction. **Musculoskeletal:** back pain. **Respiratory:** bronchitis, dyspnea, yawning. **Skin:** diaphoresis.

R

Other: viral infection, peripheral ischemia.
Advanced Parkinson disease (with levodopa)
CNS: dizziness, somnolence, headache, hallucinations, aggravated parkinsonism, insomnia, abnormal dreaming, confusion, tremor, anxiety, nervousness, amnesia, paresis, paresthesia, syncope, pain. **CV:** hypotension, HTN.
EENT: diplopia. **GI:** nausea, abdominal pain, dry mouth, vomiting, constipation, diarrhea, dysphagia, flatulence, increased saliva. **GU:** UTI, pyuria, urinary incontinence. **Hematologic:** anemia. **Metabolic:** weight decrease, suppressed prolactin. **Musculoskeletal:** dyskinesia, arthralgia, arthritis, hypokinesia, back pain. **Respiratory:** URI, dyspnea.
Skin: diaphoresis. **Other:** falls, injury, viral infection.
Restless legs syndrome
CNS: fatigue, somnolence, dizziness, vertigo, paresthesia. **CV:** peripheral edema.
EENT: nasopharyngitis, nasal congestion. **GI:** nausea, vomiting, diarrhea, dyspepsia, dry mouth. **Musculoskeletal:** arthralgia, muscle cramps, extremity pain, back pain. **Respiratory:** cough. **Skin:** diaphoresis. **Other:** flulike symptoms.

INTERACTIONS
Drug-drug. *BP-lowering agents:* May enhance hypotensive effect. Monitor BP carefully.
Cimetidine, ciprofloxacin, fluvoxamine, inhibitors or substrates of CYP1A2, ritonavir: May alter ropinirole clearance. Adjust ropinirole dosage if other drugs are started or stopped during treatment.
CNS depressants: May increase CNS effects. Use together cautiously.
Dopamine antagonists (neuroleptics), metoclopramide: May decrease ropinirole effects. Avoid using together.
Estrogens: May decrease ropinirole clearance. Adjust ropinirole dosage if estrogen therapy is started or stopped during treatment.
Drug-lifestyle. *Alcohol use:* May increase sedative effect. Discourage use together.
Smoking: May increase drug clearance. Discourage use together.

EFFECTS ON LAB TEST RESULTS
• May increase ALP level.
• May decrease Hb level.

CONTRAINDICATIONS & CAUTIONS
• Contraindicated in patients hypersensitive to drug.

• Use cautiously in patients with severe hepatic or renal impairment.
Dialyzable drug: 30%.
⚠ *Overdose S&S:* Nausea, dizziness, visual hallucinations, hyperhidrosis, claustrophobia, chorea, palpitations, asthenia, nightmares, vomiting, increased coughing, fatigue, syncope, vasovagal syncope, dyskinesia, agitation, chest pain, orthostatic hypotension, somnolence, confusion.

PREGNANCY-LACTATION-REPRODUCTION
• There are no adequate studies during pregnancy. Use only if potential benefit justifies fetal risk.
• Drug inhibits prolactin secretion and could potentially inhibit lactation. It isn't known if drug appears in human milk. Use cautiously during breastfeeding.

NURSING CONSIDERATIONS
⊕ **Alert:** Monitor patient carefully for orthostatic hypotension, especially during dosage increases.
• Drug may potentiate the adverse effects of levodopa and may cause or worsen dyskinesia. Dosage may be decreased.
• Although not reported with ropinirole, other adverse reactions reported with dopaminergic therapy include hyperpyrexia, fibrotic complications, and confusion, which may occur with rapid dosage reduction or withdrawal of drug.
• Patient may have syncope, with or without bradycardia. Monitor patient carefully, especially for 4 weeks after start of therapy and with dosage increases.
• Rapid dosage reduction or withdrawal of drug can cause signs and symptoms resembling NMS (elevated temperature, muscular rigidity, altered consciousness, autonomic instability). When used for Parkinson disease, withdraw drug gradually over 7 days. For immediate-release form, reduce frequency from t.i.d. to b.i.d. for 4 days; then, for next 3 days, reduce frequency to once daily before complete withdrawal.
• Withdraw extended-release form gradually over 7 days.
• When used for restless legs syndrome, gradual reduction of the daily dose is recommended.
• Drug can cause somnolence and sudden episodes of falling asleep. Continually reassess patient for drowsiness or sleepiness

and for factors that could contribute to sleepiness.

• Avoid use in patients with major psychotic disorders. Drug may cause changes in or worsening of mental status, abnormal thinking, and behavioral changes, which may be severe and include paranoid ideation, delusions, hallucinations, confusion, psychotic-like behavior, disorientation, aggressive behavior, agitation, and delirium.

• Augmentation (an increase in symptoms or earlier onset of symptoms in the evening or even the afternoon, or spread of symptoms to other extremities) and early-morning rebound symptoms (onset of symptoms in the early morning) have been observed in a postmarketing trial in restless legs syndrome. Review use of drug, adjust dosage, or discontinue treatment if augmentation or early-morning rebound symptoms occur.

• Ask patient about development or worsening of impulsive or compulsive behaviors, such as new or increased gambling urges, sexual urges, uncontrolled spending, or other urges, because patient may not recognize these behaviors as abnormal.

• Patients with Parkinson disease have an increased risk of melanoma. Monitor patient for melanoma development during periodic dermatologic screenings.

• *Look alike–sound alike:* Don't confuse ropinirole with risperidone.

PATIENT TEACHING
• Teach patient about safe drug administration.

• Advise patient to inform prescriber if starting or stopping medications, OTC drugs or herbs, or smoking.

• Tell patient (especially older adult) to contact prescriber if paranoid ideation, delusions, hallucinations, confusion, psychotic-like behavior, disorientation, aggressive behavior, agitation, or delirium occurs.

• Instruct patient not to rise rapidly after sitting or lying down because of risk of dizziness, which may occur more frequently early in therapy or when dosage increases.

• Sleepiness and sudden episodes of falling asleep can occur, sometimes without warning. Warn patient to minimize hazardous activities until CNS effects of drug are known.

• Tell patient to contact prescriber if experiencing difficulty controlling impulsive or compulsive behaviors, such as new or

increased gambling urges, sexual urges, uncontrolled spending, or other urges.

• Advise patient to avoid alcohol.

• Tell patient to notify prescriber about planned, suspected, or known pregnancy or breastfeeding.

rosuvastatin calcium ✂
roe-SOO-va-STAT-tin

Crestor✿, Ezallor Sprinkle

Therapeutic class: Antilipemics
Pharmacologic class: HMG-CoA reductase inhibitors

AVAILABLE FORMS
Capsules ⓓⓝⓒ: 5 mg, 10 mg, 20 mg, 40 mg
Tablets: 5 mg, 10 mg, 20 mg, 40 mg

INDICATIONS & DOSAGES
Adjust-a-dose (for all indications): If CrCl is less than 30 mL/minute/1.73 m^2 initially, give 5 mg once daily; don't exceed 10 mg once daily.
✂ For patients of Asian descent, initial dose is 5 mg.
➤ **Risk reduction in patients without clinical evidence of CAD but with multiple risk factors**
Adults: Initially, 10 mg tablets PO once daily; 5 mg PO once daily in patients needing less aggressive LDL cholesterol reduction. For aggressive lipid reduction (LDL greater than 190 mg/dL) initially, 20 mg PO once daily. Increase as needed to maximum of 40 mg PO daily. May titrate dosage every 2 to 4 weeks based on lipid levels.
➤ **Children with heterozygous familial hypercholesterolemia to reduce total cholesterol, LDL cholesterol, and apolipoprotein B levels after failing an adequate trial of diet therapy when LDL cholesterol is more than 190 mg/dL, or more than 160 mg/dL and there is a positive family history of premature CV disease or two or more other CV disease risk factors ✂**
Children ages 10 to 17: 5 to 20 mg tablets PO daily.
Children ages 8 to younger than 10: 5 to 10 mg tablets PO daily.
Adjust-a-dose: May titrate dosage every 4 weeks or more based on lipid levels.

R

➤ **Children with homozygous familial hypercholesterolemia to reduce LDL cholesterol, total cholesterol, non-HDL cholesterol, and apolipoprotein B levels after failing an adequate trial of diet therapy** ⚕

Children ages 7 to 17: 20 mg tablets PO once daily either alone or with other lipid-lowering treatments.

➤ **Adjunct to diet to reduce LDL cholesterol, total cholesterol, apolipoprotein B, non-HDL cholesterol, and triglyceride (TG) levels and to increase HDL cholesterol level in patients with primary hypercholesterolemia (heterozygous familial and nonfamilial) and mixed dyslipidemia (Fredrickson types IIa and IIb); adjunct to diet to treat elevated TG level (Fredrickson type IV)** ⚕

Adults: Initially, 10 mg tablets PO once daily; 5 mg PO once daily in patients needing less aggressive LDL cholesterol reduction or those predisposed to myopathy. For aggressive lipid lowering when LDL is greater than 190 mg/dL, initially, 20 mg PO once daily. Increase as needed to maximum of 40 mg PO daily. May titrate dosage every 2 to 4 weeks based on lipid levels.

➤ **Adjunct to diet to treat primary dysbetalipoproteinemia (type III hyperlipoproteinemia)** ⚕

Adults: Initially, 10 mg tablets or capsules PO once daily; 5 mg PO once daily in patients needing less aggressive LDL cholesterol reduction or those predisposed to myopathy. For aggressive lipid lowering when LDL level is greater than 190 mg/dL, initially, 20 mg PO once daily. Increase as needed to maximum of 40 mg PO daily. May titrate dosage every 2 to 4 weeks based on lipid levels.

➤ **Adjunct to diet to treat hypertriglyceridemia**

Adults: Initially, 10 to 20 mg capsules PO once daily. May titrate dosage every 2 to 4 weeks based on lipid levels. Maximum, 40 mg daily.

➤ **Adjunct to diet to slow atherosclerosis progression in patients with elevated cholesterol**

Adults: Initially, 10 mg tablets PO daily. Increase as needed every 2 to 4 weeks based on lipid levels to maximum of 40 mg daily.

➤ **Adjunct to lipid-lowering therapies; to reduce LDL cholesterol, apolipoprotein B,** and total cholesterol levels in homozygous familial hypercholesterolemia ⚕

Adults: Initially, 20 mg tablets or capsules PO once daily. Maximum, 40 mg once daily.

ADMINISTRATION
PO
• Give drug without regard for meals.
• Patient should swallow tablets and capsules whole; don't crush capsule.
• May open capsules and sprinkle contents on a tsp of soft food, such as applesauce or pudding. Give within 60 minutes of preparation. Patient shouldn't chew mixtures.
• For NG administration, empty contents of capsule into a 60-mL catheter-tipped syringe, add 40 mL water, replace plunger, and shake syringe vigorously for 15 seconds. Immediately attach syringe to NG tube and administer contents. Flush NG tube with additional 20 mL water.

ACTION
Inhibits HMG-CoA reductase, increases LDL receptors on liver cells, and inhibits hepatic synthesis of very–low-density lipoprotein.

Route	Onset	Peak	Duration
PO	1 wk	3–5 hr	Unknown

Half-life: About 19 hours.

ADVERSE REACTIONS
CNS: asthenia, dizziness, headache. **GI:** abdominal pain, constipation, diarrhea, dyspepsia, nausea, vomiting. **GU:** cystitis. **Hematologic:** anemia, ecchymosis. **Hepatic:** elevated ALT level. **Metabolic:** diabetes. **Musculoskeletal:** arthralgia, myalgia, neck pain.

INTERACTIONS
Drug-drug. *Antacids:* May decrease rosuvastatin level. Give antacids at least 2 hours after rosuvastatin.

Atazanavir, atazanavir–ritonavir, lopinavir–ritonavir, simeprevir: May increase rosuvastatin level and risk of myopathy and rhabdomyolysis. Rosuvastatin dosage shouldn't exceed 10 mg daily.

Colchicine: May increase risk of myopathy and rhabdomyolysis. Avoid use together. If use together is necessary, monitor patient for signs and symptoms of myopathy and elevated CK level during use and after dosage increases.

Reactions in bold italics are *life-threatening*. Interactions may have a *rapid onset* or a *delayed onset*.

Coumarin anticoagulants (warfarin): May prolong INR. Achieve stable INR before starting drug; monitor INR frequently.

Cyclosporine, darolutamide: May increase rosuvastatin level and risk of myopathy or rhabdomyolysis. Don't exceed 5 mg of rosuvastatin daily. Watch for evidence of toxicity.

Daptomycin: May increase risk of rhabdomyolysis. Withhold rosuvastatin temporarily or monitor patient and CK level closely during coadministration.

Eltrombopag: May increase rosuvastatin level and risk of toxicity. Consider reducing rosuvastatin dosage.

Fenofibrate: May increase rosuvastatin level and risk of myopathy or rhabdomyolysis. Use together cautiously.

Gemfibrozil: May significantly increase rosuvastatin level and risk of myopathy or rhabdomyolysis. Avoid use together. If used together, don't exceed 10 mg/day of rosuvastatin.

Hormonal contraceptives: May increase ethinyl estradiol and norgestrel levels. Watch for adverse effects.

Niacin: May increase risk of myopathy or rhabdomyolysis. Monitor patient closely.

Regorafenib: May increase rosuvastatin exposure and risk of myopathy. Don't exceed 10 mg rosuvastatin once daily.

Drug-herb. *Red yeast rice:* May enhance adverse or toxic effects of HMG-CoA reductase inhibitors (statins). Discourage use together.

Drug-lifestyle. *Alcohol use:* May increase risk of hepatotoxicity. Discourage use together.

EFFECTS ON LAB TEST RESULTS

• May increase HbA_{1c}, fasting blood sugar, CK, ALT, AST, glucose, glutamyl transpeptidase, ALP, and bilirubin levels.
• May cause thyroid function abnormalities, dipstick-positive proteinuria, and microscopic hematuria.

CONTRAINDICATIONS & CAUTIONS

• Contraindicated in patients hypersensitive to rosuvastatin or its components, patients with active liver disease, and those with unexplained persistently increased transaminase levels.
• Use cautiously in patients who drink substantial amounts of alcohol or have a history of liver disease and in those at increased risk

for myopathies, such as those with renal impairment, advanced age, or hypothyroidism.
⚡ Use cautiously in patients of Asian descent because they have a greater risk of elevated drug levels.
• Rare postmarketing reports of cognitive impairment (memory loss, forgetfulness, amnesia, memory impairment, confusion) have been associated with statin use. These reported symptoms are generally not serious and are reversible upon statin discontinuation, with variable times to symptom onset (1 day to years) and symptom resolution (median of 3 weeks).
• Ezallor capsules aren't approved for use in children.

Dialyzable drug: No.

⚠ **Overdose S&S:** Unexplained muscle pain, tenderness, or weakness, especially with malaise or fever.

PREGNANCY-LACTATION-REPRODUCTION

• May cause fetal harm. Use during pregnancy is contraindicated unless benefits outweigh fetal risk. Discontinue drug before conception. If pregnancy occurs during therapy, apprise patient of potential fetal risks with continued use during pregnancy.
• Advise patients of childbearing potential to use effective contraception during therapy.
• Drug may appear in human milk. Use while breastfeeding is contraindicated.

NURSING CONSIDERATIONS

• Before therapy starts, assess patient for underlying causes of hypercholesterolemia, including poorly controlled diabetes, hypothyroidism, nephrotic syndrome, dyslipoproteinemias, obstructive liver disease, drug interaction, and alcoholism.
• Before therapy starts, advise patient to control hypercholesterolemia with diet, exercise, and weight reduction.
• Interrupt statin therapy if patient shows signs or symptoms of serious liver injury, hyperbilirubinemia, or jaundice. Don't restart drug if another cause can't be found.
• Monitor LFTs at baseline and with any indication of hepatotoxicity.
⚠ **Alert:** Rarely, rhabdomyolysis with acute renal failure has developed in patients taking drugs in this class, including rosuvastatin.
• Monitor lipid panel at baseline and a fasting lipid profile within 4 to 12 weeks after

R

initiation or dosage adjustment and every 3 to 12 months thereafter.
• Patients who are age 65 or older, have hypothyroidism, or have renal insufficiency may be at a greater risk for developing myopathy while receiving a statin.
• Notify prescriber if CK level becomes markedly elevated or myopathy is suspected, or if routine urinalysis shows persistent proteinuria and patient is taking 40 mg daily.
• Withhold drug temporarily if patient becomes predisposed to myopathy or rhabdomyolysis because of sepsis, hypotension, major surgery, trauma, uncontrolled seizures, or severe metabolic, endocrine, or electrolyte disorders.
• Rare cases of immune-mediated necrotizing myopathy have been reported.

PATIENT TEACHING
• Instruct patient to take drug exactly as prescribed.
• Teach patient about diet, exercise, and weight control.
• Inform patient that rare instances of memory loss and confusion have occurred with statin use. These reported events were generally not serious and resolved when drug was discontinued.
• Advise patient that drug may increase blood glucose level but that the CV benefits are thought to outweigh the slight increase in risk.
• Tell patient to immediately report unexplained muscle pain, tenderness, or weakness (especially if accompanied by malaise or fever) and loss of appetite, upper abdominal pain, dark-colored urine, or yellowing of skin or eyes.
• Instruct patient to take drug at least 2 hours before taking aluminum- or magnesium-containing antacids.
◐ *Alert:* Tell patient to immediately report known or suspected pregnancy or if breastfeeding.

rucaparib camsylate ⊗
roo-KAP-a-rib

Rubraca

Therapeutic class: Antineoplastics
Pharmacologic class: Poly (ADP-ribose) polymerase (PARP) inhibitors

AVAILABLE FORMS
Tablets: 200 mg, 250 mg, 300 mg

INDICATIONS & DOSAGES
Adjust-a-dose (for all indications): To manage any adverse reaction, interrupt therapy or consider dosage reduction. First dosage reduction, 500 mg b.i.d.; second dosage reduction, 400 mg b.i.d.; third dosage reduction, 300 mg b.i.d. For prolonged hematologic toxicities, interrupt therapy and monitor blood counts weekly until recovery. If levels haven't recovered to grade 1 or less after 4 weeks, refer patient to hematologist for further investigation.
➤ **Maintenance treatment of patients with recurrent epithelial ovarian, fallopian tube, or primary peritoneal cancer who are in a complete or partial response to platinum-based chemotherapy**
Adults: 600 mg PO b.i.d. Continue treatment until disease progression or unacceptable toxicity occurs.
➤ **Deleterious *BRCA* mutation (germline or somatic)–associated metastatic castration-resistant prostate cancer in patients who have been treated with androgen receptor–directed therapy and a taxane-based chemotherapy** ⊗
Adults: 600 mg (two 300-mg tablets) PO b.i.d., for a total daily dose of 1,200 mg. Patient should also receive a GnRH analogue concurrently or should have had bilateral orchiectomy. Continue treatment until disease progression or unacceptable toxicity occurs.

ADMINISTRATION
PO
• May give without regard for food.
• Omit a missed dose and give next dose at its scheduled time. Don't replace vomited doses.
• Store at 68° to 77° F (20° to 25° C).

Reactions in bold italics are *life-threatening*. Interactions may have a *rapid onset* or a ***delayed onset***.

ACTION

Induces cytotoxicity by inhibiting PARP enzyme activity and increased formation of PARP–DNA complexes, resulting in DNA damage, apoptosis, and cell death.

Route	Onset	Peak	Duration
PO	Unknown	1.9 hr	Unknown

Half-life: 26 hours.

ADVERSE REACTIONS

CNS: fatigue, dizziness, fever, depression, dysgeusia. **CV:** peripheral edema. **EENT:** nasopharyngitis. **GI:** nausea, vomiting, constipation, decreased appetite, diarrhea, abdominal pain or distention, dyspepsia, stomatitis. **GU:** increased creatinine level. **Hematologic:** anemia, *thrombocytopenia, neutropenia, febrile neutropenia.* **Hepatic:** increased LFT values. **Metabolic:** increased cholesterol level, increased triglyceride levels, hyponatremia. **Respiratory:** URI, dyspnea. **Skin:** rash, photosensitivity reaction, pruritus, hand-foot syndrome.

INTERACTIONS

Drug-drug. *CYP450 substrates:* May increase systemic substrate exposure and toxicity risk. Dosage adjustments may be needed. *Warfarin:* May increase warfarin level. Monitor PT and INR.

Drug-lifestyle. *Sun exposure:* May cause photosensitivity. Patient should use appropriate sun protection to avoid sunburn.

EFFECTS ON LAB TEST RESULTS

• May increase creatinine, ALT, AST, ALP, triglyceride, and cholesterol levels.
• May decrease sodium level.
• May decrease Hb level, ANC, and lymphocyte and platelet counts.

CONTRAINDICATIONS & CAUTIONS

• Use cautiously in patients with renal or liver impairment; starting dosage adjustments haven't been established for patients with CrCl of less than 30 mL/minute, for those on dialysis, or for patients with moderate to severe hepatic impairment (bilirubin level greater than 1.5 × ULN).
• Drug may increase risk of myelodysplastic syndrome (MDS) or acute myeloid leukemia (AML). For confirmed MDS or AML, discontinue drug.

• Safety and effectiveness in children haven't been established.
• Use cautiously in older adults.
Dialyzable drug: Unknown.

PREGNANCY-LACTATION-REPRODUCTION

• Drug can cause fetal harm. Patients of childbearing potential should use effective contraception during therapy and for 6 months after final dose.
• Male patients with partners of childbearing potential or who are pregnant should use effective contraception during treatment and for 3 months after final dose.
• Advise patients not to breastfeed during therapy and for 2 weeks after final dose.

NURSING CONSIDERATIONS

⚗ Patients should be tested for *BRCA* mutation (germline or somatic) before treatment. Information on tests may be found at https://www.fda.gov/medical-devices/vitro-diagnostics/list-cleared-or-approved-companion-diagnostic-devices-vitro-and-imaging-tools.
• Monitor CBC at baseline and monthly thereafter. Don't start therapy until patient has recovered from hematologic toxicity caused by prior chemotherapy (grade 1 or less).
• Verify pregnancy status before therapy.

PATIENT TEACHING

• Instruct patient in safe drug administration and handling.
• Advise patient of childbearing potential to use effective contraception during treatment and for 6 months after final dose. Tell patient that pregnancy testing will be performed before treatment begins.
• Caution patient not to breastfeed during treatment and for 2 weeks after final dose.
• Advise male patient with partner of childbearing potential or who is pregnant to use effective contraception during treatment and for 3 months after final dose.
• Warn patient that drug may cause photosensitivity and to use appropriate sun protection.
• Advise patient to report all adverse reactions, especially weakness, fatigue, fever, weight loss, frequent infections, bruising, easy bleeding, dyspnea, blood in urine or stool, nausea, and vomiting.

R

sacubitril–valsartan ⬚
sak-UE-bi-tril/val-SAR-tan

Entresto

Therapeutic class: Antihypertensives
Pharmacologic class: Neprilysin inhibitors–
ARBs

AVAILABLE FORMS
Tablets: 24 mg sacubitril/26 mg valsartan,
49 mg sacubitril/51 mg valsartan, 97 mg
sacubitril/103 mg valsartan

INDICATIONS & DOSAGES
Adjust-a-dose (for all indications): For patients not currently taking an ACE inhibitor
or ARB, or previously taking a low dose of
these agents, and patients with severe renal impairment (estimated GFR less than
30 mL/minute/1.73 m^2) or moderate hepatic
impairment (Child-Pugh class B), reduce initial dose to half the usual starting dose, then
follow the recommended dosage escalation.
Initiate patients weighing 40 to 50 kg who
meet these criteria at 0.8 mg/kg PO b.i.d.
➤ **To reduce risk of CV death and hospitalization for HF in patients with chronic
HF (NYHA Class II to IV) and reduced
ejection fraction**
Adults: Initially, 49 mg sacubitril/51 mg valsartan PO b.i.d. Increase after 2 to 4 weeks
to target maintenance dose of 97 mg sacubi-
tril/103 mg valsartan, as tolerated.
➤ **Symptomatic HF in children with systemic left ventricular systolic dysfunction**
*Children age 1 year and older weighing at
least 50 kg:* Initially, 49 mg sacubitril/51 mg
valsartan PO b.i.d. If tolerated, may increase
to 72 mg sacubitril/78 mg valsartan after
2 weeks, then increase to 97 mg sacubitril/
103 mg valsartan after 2 additional weeks.
*Children age 1 year and older weighing at
least 40 kg to less than 50 kg:* Initially, 24 mg
sacubitril/26 mg valsartan PO b.i.d. If tolerated, may increase to 49 mg sacubitril/51 mg
valsartan after 2 weeks, then increase to
72 mg sacubitril/78 mg valsartan after 2 additional weeks.
*Children age 1 year and older weighing less
than 40 kg:* Use oral suspension and the recommended mg/kg doses of the combined
amount of both sacubitril and valsartan. Initially, 1.6 mg/kg PO b.i.d. If tolerated, may

increase to 2.3 mg/kg after 2 weeks, then increase to 3.1 mg/kg after 2 additional weeks.

ADMINISTRATION
PO
• If patient is switching to or from an ACE
inhibitor, allow a washout period of 36 hours
between giving the two drugs.
• May give with or without food.
• Give a missed dose as soon as possible on
the same day; then resume twice-daily dosing.
Omit missed dose if close to the scheduled
next dose.
• An oral suspension may be prepared by a
pharmacist for patients unable to swallow
tablets. Suspension can be stored for up to
15 days, but not above 77° F (25° C); don't
refrigerate. Shake before use.

ACTION
Inhibits neprilysin and angiotensin II, enhancing the protective neurohormonal systems of
the heart (natriuretic peptide system) while
suppressing the harmful RAAS.

Route	Onset	Peak	Duration
PO	Unknown	0.5–2 hr	Unknown

Half-life: Sacubitril, 1.4 hours; valsartan, 9.9 hours.

ADVERSE REACTIONS
CNS: dizziness. **CV:** *hypotension.* **GU:** *renal
failure.* **Hematologic:** anemia. **Metabolic:**
hyperkalemia. **Respiratory:** cough. **Other:**
falls.

INTERACTIONS
Drug-drug. *ACE inhibitors:* May increase
risk of angioedema. Use together is contraindicated. Don't give sacubitril–valsartan
within 36 hours of switching from or to an
ACE inhibitor.
Aliskiren: May increase risk of renal failure. Contraindicated for use together in
patients with diabetes. Avoid use in patients with renal impairment (GFR less than
60 mL/minute/1.73 m^2).
ARBs: Will cause dual blockade of the
RAAS. Avoid concurrent use as product contains valsartan.
Canagliflozin: May enhance hyperkalemic
and hypotensive effects. Monitor potassium
level and BP carefully.
Cyclooxygenase-2 inhibitors, NSAIDs: May
increase risk of renal failure. Monitor renal
function closely.

Reactions in bold italics are *life-threatening*. Interactions may have a *rapid onset* or a **delayed onset**.

Lithium: May increase lithium level and risk of lithium toxicity. Monitor serum lithium level.

Potassium-sparing diuretics (amiloride, spironolactone, triamterene), potassium supplements: May increase serum potassium level. Use cautiously and monitor patient closely.

Sodium phosphates: May enhance risk of acute phosphate nephropathy. Seek alternatives to oral sodium phosphate bowel preparations.

EFFECTS ON LAB TEST RESULTS

• May increase serum creatinine and potassium levels.
• May decrease Hb level and hematocrit.

CONTRAINDICATIONS & CAUTIONS

• Contraindicated in patients with a history of angioedema related to previous ACE or ARB therapy and in patients hypersensitive to components of drug.
• Use in patients with severe hepatic impairment (Child-Pugh class C) isn't recommended.
▨ Drug may cause angioedema requiring emergency treatment and which can be fatal. Risk is greater in patients who are Black than in patients of other ethnicities.
• Drug lowers BP and may cause symptomatic hypotension.
• ACE inhibitors and ARBs have been associated with oliguria, progressive azotemia, acute renal failure, hyperkalemia, and death. Monitor patient closely.
Dialyzable drug: Unlikely.
⚠ *Overdose S&S:* Hypotension.

PREGNANCY-LACTATION-REPRODUCTION

Boxed Warning Use during pregnancy can cause injury and death to the developing fetus from effects on the RAAS. Stop drug as soon as pregnancy is detected. ∎
• Use during pregnancy only if there is no appropriate alternative therapy and if drug is considered lifesaving for patient. Advise patients who are pregnant of fetal risk.
• It isn't known if drug appears in human milk. Because of the potential for serious reactions in the infant, patient shouldn't breastfeed during therapy.

NURSING CONSIDERATIONS

• Drug is usually given with other HF therapies, in place of an ACE inhibitor or other ARB.
• To help prevent hypotension, correct volume or salt depletion before start of therapy.
• Monitor patients for hypotension. Patients who are volume- or salt-depleted, such as those on high-dose diuretics, may be at increased risk. Consider dosage adjustment of diuretics and concomitant antihypertensives and treat other cause of hypotension such as hypovolemia. Reduce dosage or temporarily discontinue sacubitril–valsartan for persistent hypotension.
▨ Monitor all patients, especially patients who are Black, for angioedema (swelling of the face, tongue, throat, and lips; airway compromise; dyspnea). Discontinue drug and treat emergently.
• Monitor renal function and reduce dosage or temporarily interrupt therapy in patients who develop clinically significant decreased renal function.
• Monitor serum potassium level periodically and treat appropriately. Patients with severe renal impairment, diabetes, hypoaldosteronism, or a high-potassium diet may be at increased risk for hyperkalemia. Reduce dosage or interrupt therapy as clinically indicated.

PATIENT TEACHING

• Explain to patient that drug is usually used with other HF therapies, in place of an ACE inhibitor or other ARB therapy.
• Advise patient to report all adverse reactions, especially signs and symptoms of angioedema and allergic reaction (swelling of the face, lips, tongue, or throat; trouble breathing). Advise patient to seek immediate emergency medical help if they occur.
• Instruct patient to take drug exactly as prescribed and not to take within 36 hours of an ACE inhibitor.
• Tell patient to report pregnancy as drug can cause fetal harm. Caution patient not to breastfeed during therapy.
• Caution patient to report dizziness, lightheadedness, or extreme fatigue.

S

safinamide mesylate
sa-FIN-a-mide

Xadago

Therapeutic class: Antiparkinsonian drugs
Pharmacologic class: MAO-B inhibitors

AVAILABLE FORMS
Tablets: 50 mg, 100 mg

INDICATIONS & DOSAGES
➤ **Parkinson disease in patients experiencing "off" episodes as adjunctive treatment to levodopa–carbidopa**
Adults: 50 mg PO once daily. After 2 weeks, may increase to 100 mg daily based on individual need and tolerability.
Adjust-a-dose: For patients with moderate hepatic impairment (Child-Pugh class B), maximum recommended dosage is 50 mg once daily. If patient progresses to severe hepatic impairment, discontinue drug. When discontinuing drug, taper 100-mg dose before stopping drug by decreasing dosage to 50 mg for 1 week.

ADMINISTRATION
PO
• May give with or without food.
• Give at the same time each day.
• If a dose is missed, patient should take the next dose at same time the next day.
• Store at room temperature.

ACTION
An inhibitor of MAO-B. Blockade of MAO-B is thought to result in an increase in dopamine levels by blocking the catabolism of dopamine, which then increases dopaminergic activity in the brain.

Route	Onset	Peak	Duration
PO	Unknown	2–3 hr	Unknown

Half-life: 20 to 26 hours.

ADVERSE REACTIONS
CNS: dyskinesia, insomnia, anxiety. **CV:** orthostatic hypotension, HTN. **GI:** nausea, dyspepsia. **Respiratory:** cough. **Other:** fall.

INTERACTIONS
Drug-drug. *Cold remedies; nasal, oral, and ophthalmic decongestants; sympathomimetic medications (amphetamine, methylphenidate):* May increase risk of hypertensive crisis. Use together is contraindicated.
Cyclobenzaprine, MAO inhibitor class drugs or other drugs that are potent inhibitors of MAO (linezolid, MAO-B inhibitors), opioids (meperidine and derivatives, methadone, propoxyphene, tramadol), SSNRIs, TCAs, tetracyclic antidepressants, triazolopyridine: May increase risk of serotonin syndrome. Use together is contraindicated. Allow at least 14 days to lapse after discontinuing safinamide and starting these drugs.
Dextromethorphan: May cause episodes of psychosis or bizarre behavior. Use together is contraindicated.
Dopamine antagonists (antipsychotics, metoclopramide): May decrease effectiveness of safinamide and exacerbate Parkinson symptoms. Monitor therapy.
Isoniazid: Isoniazid has some MAO-inhibiting activity. Watch for HTN and reaction to dietary tyramine in patients taking both drugs.
SSRIs: May cause serotonin syndrome. Monitor patient for signs and symptoms of serotonin syndrome; use lowest effective dosage of SSRI with safinamide.
Drug-herb. *St John's wort:* May increase risk of serotonin syndrome. Discourage use together. Allow 14 days to lapse between discontinuing safinamide and starting St. John's wort.
Drug-food. *Tyramine-containing foods (aged, fermented, cured, pickled, or smoked food):* May increase risk of HTN. Avoid these types of food. Monitor patient closely.
Drug-lifestyle. *Alcohol use:* May increase sedative effects. Don't use together.

EFFECTS ON LAB TEST RESULTS
• May increase ALT and AST levels.

CONTRAINDICATIONS & CAUTIONS
• Contraindicated in patients hypersensitive to drug or its components and in patients with severe hepatic impairment (Child-Pugh class C).
• Use cautiously in patients with moderate hepatic impairment (Child-Pugh class B).
• Use cautiously in patients with major psychotic disorder; drug may exacerbate psychosis. Consider dosage reduction or drug discontinuation if patient develops hallucinations or psychotic-like behaviors.

Reactions in bold italics are *life-threatening*. Interactions may have a *rapid onset* or a *delayed onset*.

- Safinamide isn't effective alone for the treatment of Parkinson disease. Patients should take levodopa–carbidopa with this drug.
- Safety and effectiveness in children haven't been studied.

Dialyzable drug: Unknown.

PREGNANCY-LACTATION-REPRODUCTION

- There are no adequate or well-controlled studies during pregnancy. Developmental toxicity and teratogenic effects were observed in animal studies. Other Parkinson disease agents may be preferred. Use only if benefits outweigh fetal risk.
- It isn't known if drug appears in human milk. Use cautiously during breastfeeding if benefits outweigh risk of infant exposure.

NURSING CONSIDERATIONS

- Monitor patients for hypersensitivity reactions, including dyspnea and swelling of the tongue and oral mucosa.
- Monitor patients for new-onset HTN or uncontrolled HTN.
- Monitor patients for serotonin syndrome (mental status changes [including agitation, hallucinations, delirium, coma], tachycardia, labile BP, dizziness, diaphoresis, flushing, hyperthermia, rigidity, monoclonus, hyperreflexia, incoordination, seizures, nausea, vomiting, diarrhea).
- Monitor LFT values and discontinue drug if patient develops severe hepatic impairment.
- Patients may experience excessive drowsiness and fall asleep suddenly without warning. Monitor patients for daytime sleepiness or falling asleep during activities (driving, talking, eating). Drug may need to be discontinued.
- Monitor patients for new-onset or exacerbated dyskinesia. Reducing levodopa or other dopaminergic drug dosage may be needed.
- A withdrawal syndrome (elevated temperature, muscular rigidity, confusion, altered consciousness, autonomic instability) resembling NMS may occur with rapid dosage reduction, drug withdrawal, or changes in drug regimen that increase central dopaminergic tone. Adjust dosage carefully and taper dosage before discontinuation.
- Drug may exacerbate psychotic behaviors and cause hallucinations or psychotic-like behaviors. If signs and symptoms occur, dosage

reduction or drug discontinuation may be needed.

- Drug may cause impulse control or compulsive behaviors. Monitor patients for new or increased gambling urges, sexual urges, uncontrolled spending, binge eating, or other intense urges and the inability to control these urges. If signs or symptoms occur, dosage reduction or drug discontinuation may be needed.
- Periodically monitor for visual changes in patients with a history of retinal or macular degeneration, uveitis, personal or family history of retinal disease, albinism, retinitis pigmentosa, diabetic retinopathy, or other retinopathy.

PATIENT TEACHING

- Tell patient to report all adverse reactions to prescriber.
- Inform patient that drug may elevate BP. Advise patient to monitor BP and report elevations.
- Teach patient signs and symptoms of serotonin syndrome and to report them should they occur.
- Explain that drug can cause sleepiness and patient can fall asleep suddenly during daily activities. Caution patient not to drive, operate heavy machinery, work in high places, or engage in other dangerous activities until drug's effects are known.
- Advise patient to avoid foods that contain large amounts of tyramine (aged, fermented, cured, smoked, or pickled foods) because of the potential for substantial increases in BP.
- Warn patient not to discontinue drug rapidly; drug should be tapered to avoid withdrawal.
- Explain that drug may cause retinal changes. Tell patient to notify prescriber if visual changes occur.
- Advise patient to immediately report hallucinations, psychotic behavior, compulsive behaviors, or problems with impulse control (gambling, spending money, sexual urges, binge eating).
- Caution patient to immediately report pregnancy, plans to become pregnant, breastfeeding, or plans to breastfeed during treatment.

S

salmeterol xinafoate
sal-ME-te-role

Serevent Diskus

Therapeutic class: Bronchodilators
Pharmacologic class: Long-acting selective beta₂ agonists

AVAILABLE FORMS
Inhalation powder: 50 mcg/dose

INDICATIONS & DOSAGES
➤ **Long-term maintenance of asthma; to prevent bronchospasm only as concomitant therapy with an inhaled corticosteroid (ICS) in patients with reversible obstructive airway disease, including nocturnal asthma**
Adults and children age 4 and older: 1 inhalation (50 mcg) b.i.d. in the morning and evening, about 12 hours apart.
➤ **To prevent exercise-induced bronchospasm**
Adults and children age 4 and older: 1 inhalation (50 mcg) at least 30 minutes before exercise. Additional doses shouldn't be taken for at least 12 hours.
➤ **COPD, emphysema, or chronic bronchitis**
Adults: 1 inhalation (50 mcg) b.i.d. in the morning and evening, about 12 hours apart.

ADMINISTRATION
Inhalational
• Inhaler must be used in a level, flat position.
• Patient should hold breath for about 10 seconds after inhaling, then breathe out fully.
• Give drug 30 minutes before exercise to prevent exercise-induced bronchospasm.
• Don't use a spacer device with this drug.
• Don't wash the inhaler and always keep it in a dry place.
• Discard inhaler 6 weeks after opening foil pouch or when counter reads "0."

ACTION
Unclear. Selectively activates beta₂ receptors, which results in bronchodilation; also, blocks the release of allergic mediators from mast cells lining the respiratory tract.

Route	Onset	Peak	Duration
Inhalation	30–120 min	20 min	12 hr

Half-life: 5.5 hours.

ADVERSE REACTIONS
CNS: anxiety, headache, dizziness, tremor, nervousness, paresthesia, sleep disturbance, fever. **CV:** tachycardia, palpitations, HTN, edema. **EENT:** conjunctivitis, keratitis, nasal congestion, sinusitis, rhinitis, pharyngitis, candidiasis of mouth or throat, hyposalivation, throat irritation, dental discomfort, tracheitis. **GI:** nausea, vomiting, dyspepsia. **Metabolic:** hyperglycemia. **Musculoskeletal:** joint and back pain, myalgia, muscle cramps, arthralgia, articular rheumatism. **Respiratory:** bronchitis, URI, cough, viral respiratory infection, *asthma.* **Skin:** rash, urticaria, photodermatitis. **Other:** hypersensitivity reactions, flulike symptoms.

INTERACTIONS
Drug-drug. *Antiarrhythmics (amiodarone, disopyramide, sotalol), chlorpromazine, dolasetron, droperidol, moxifloxacin, pentamidine, pimozide, tacrolimus, thioridazine, ziprasidone:* May prolong QT interval and increase risk of life-threatening cardiac arrhythmias. Monitor QT interval closely.
Beta agonists, other methylxanthines, theophylline: May cause adverse cardiac effects with excessive use. Monitor patient.
Beta blockers (nonselective): May diminish bronchodilatory effects. Use cardioselective beta blockers if therapy is indicated.
CYP3A4 inhibitors (atazanavir, clarithromycin, itraconazole, ketoconazole, ritonavir): May increase cardiac effects. Avoid use together.
Diuretics (non-potassium-sparing): May worsen hypokalemia and ECG changes. Use cautiously together.
MAO inhibitors: May cause risk of severe adverse CV effects. Avoid use within 14 days of MAO inhibitor therapy.
TCAs: May cause risk of moderate to severe adverse CV effects. Avoid use together within 14 days.

EFFECTS ON LAB TEST RESULTS
• May decrease potassium and glucose levels.

CONTRAINDICATIONS & CAUTIONS
• Contraindicated in patients hypersensitive to drug, its ingredients, or milk proteins.
⚠ *Alert:* Contraindicated as the primary treatment for acute episodes of asthma or COPD.
Boxed Warning Contraindicated for treatment of asthma without an ICS. Using

---

without an ICS may increase the risk of asthma-related death. ∎

Boxed Warning Only use salmeterol as additional therapy for patients whose condition isn't adequately controlled on other medications or patients whose disease severity warrants initiation of treatment with two maintenance therapies. Don't use salmeterol for patients whose asthma is adequately controlled on low- or medium-dose ICS. ∎

• Clinical trial data don't suggest an increased risk of death with the use of salmeterol in patients with COPD.

• Paradoxical bronchospasm that may be life-threatening may occur; distinguish from inadequate response. Discontinue salmeterol and start alternative treatment if paradoxical bronchospasm occurs.

◑ *Alert:* Don't use drug with other medications containing LABAs.

• Use cautiously in patients unusually responsive to sympathomimetics and those with coronary insufficiency, arrhythmias, HTN, other CV disorders, thyrotoxicosis, hepatic impairment, diabetes, or seizure disorders. *Dializable drug:* Unknown.

⚠ *Overdose S&S:* Exaggeration of adverse reactions, hypokalemia, seizures, angina, HTN, hypotension, dry mouth, muscle cramps, dizziness, fatigue, insomnia, tachycardia, ventricular arrhythmias, cardiac arrest, sudden death.

PREGNANCY-LACTATION-REPRODUCTION

• There are no adequate studies during pregnancy, but drug may be teratogenic. Use only if potential benefit justifies fetal risk.

• It isn't known if drug appears in human milk. Use cautiously during breastfeeding.

NURSING CONSIDERATIONS

Boxed Warning LABAs may increase risk of asthma-related hospitalization in children and adolescents. For children and adolescents with asthma who require addition of a LABA to an ICS, a fixed-dose combination product containing both should be used to ensure adherence with both drugs. ∎

• Drug isn't indicated for acute bronchospasm.

◑ *Alert:* Monitor patient for rash and urticaria, which may signal a hypersensitivity reaction.

• Monitor patient for hypokalemia and hyperglycemia.

PATIENT TEACHING

Boxed Warning Teach parents of child or adolescent who requires the use of a separate ICS and a LABA that appropriate steps must be taken to ensure adherence with both treatment components, because of the increased risk of asthma-related death. If adherence can't be ensured, a fixed-dose combination product containing both drugs is recommended. ∎

• Instruct patient in safe drug administration.

• Remind patient to take drug at about 12-hour intervals for optimal effect and to take drug even when feeling better.

• Advise patient that immediate hypersensitivity reactions (such as urticaria, angioedema, rash, bronchospasm, and hypotension, including anaphylaxis) may occur after administration of this drug and to seek immediate medical attention if such reactions occur.

◑ *Alert:* Tell patient drug shouldn't be used to treat acute bronchospasm. Patient must use a short-acting beta$_2$ agonist, such as albuterol, to treat worsening symptoms.

• Tell patient to contact prescriber if the short-acting agonist no longer provides sufficient relief or if patient needs more than 4 inhalations daily. This may be a sign that the asthma symptoms are worsening. Tell patient not to increase the dosage of salmeterol.

• If patient takes an ICS, patient should continue to use it regularly. Warn patient not to take other drugs without prescriber's consent.

• Advise patient to report pregnancy during therapy.

SAFETY ALERT!

sargramostim (GM-CSF; granulocyte-macrophage colony-stimulating factor)
sar-GRAM-oh-stim

Leukine

Therapeutic class: Hematopoietics
Pharmacologic class: Colony-stimulating factors

AVAILABLE FORMS
Powder for injection: 250 mcg

S

INDICATIONS & DOSAGES

➤ **To accelerate hematopoietic reconstitution after autologous or allogeneic bone marrow transplantation in patients with non-Hodgkin lymphoma or acute lymphoblastic leukemia or in patients with Hodgkin lymphoma**

Adults and children age 2 and older:
250 mcg/m^2 daily given as 2-hour IV infusion beginning 2 to 4 hours after bone marrow transplantation and not less than 24 hours after last dose of chemotherapy or radiotherapy. Don't give until post–marrow infusion ANC falls below 500 cells/mm^3. Continue until ANC exceeds 1,500 cells/mm^3 for 3 consecutive days.

Adjust-a-dose: Discontinue immediately if blast cells appear or disease progression occurs. Temporarily discontinue or reduce dosage by 50% if a severe adverse reaction occurs. Interrupt therapy or reduce dosage by 50% if ANC exceeds 20,000 cells/mm^3 or WBC count exceeds 50,000 cells/mm^3.

➤ **Neutrophil recovery after induction chemotherapy in acute myelogenous leukemia (AML)**

Adults age 55 and older: Initially, 250 mcg/m^2 IV once daily over 4 hours beginning day 11 or 4 days after completion of induction therapy; initiate only if bone marrow is hypoplastic with less than 5% blasts on day 10. If a second induction cycle is needed, begin sargramostim 4 days after completing chemotherapy and only if bone marrow is hypoplastic with less than 5% blasts. Continue until the ANC exceeds 1,500 cells/mm^3 for 3 consecutive days or for a maximum of 42 days.

Adjust-a-dose: Discontinue immediately if leukemic regrowth occurs. Reduce dosage by 50% or temporarily discontinue if a severe adverse reaction occurs. Interrupt therapy or reduce dosage by 50% if ANC exceeds 20,000 cells/mm^3.

➤ **Mobilization of peripheral blood progenitor cells (PBPCs)**

Adults: 250 mcg/m^2 by continuous IV infusion over 24 hours or by subcut injection once daily. Continue through PBPC collection.

Adjust-a-dose: If WBC count exceeds 50,000 cells/mm^3, reduce dosage by 50%. If adequate numbers of cells aren't collected, consider other mobilization therapy.

➤ **Post-PBPC transplantation**

Adults: 250 mcg/m^2 by continuous IV infusion over 24 hours or by subcut injection once daily beginning immediately after PBPC infusion; continue until ANC exceeds 1,500 cells/mm^3 for 3 consecutive days.

➤ **Bone marrow transplantation failure or engraftment delay**

Adults and children age 2 and older:
250 mcg/m^2 as a 2-hour IV infusion daily for 14 days. This course of therapy may be repeated after 7 days of no therapy. If engraftment still hasn't occurred, a third course of 500 mcg/m^2 daily IV for 14 days may be attempted after another therapy-free 7 days.

Adjust-a-dose: Stimulation of marrow precursors may result in rapid rise of WBC count. If blast cells appear or increase to 10% or more of WBC count or if the underlying disease progresses, stop therapy. If WBC count exceeds 50,000 cells/mm^3 or ANC exceeds 20,000 cells/mm^3, temporarily stop drug or reduce dose by 50%.

➤ **To increase survival in patients acutely exposed to myelosuppressive doses of radiation (hematopoietic syndrome of acute radiation syndrome) given as soon as possible after suspected or confirmed exposure to radiation doses greater than 2 gray**

Adults and children weighing more than 40 kg: 7 mcg/kg subcut once daily. Continue until ANC remains more than 1,000 cells/mm^3 for three consecutive CBCs obtained every third day, or exceeds 10,000 cells/mm^3 after a radiation-induced nadir.

Children weighing 15 to 40 kg: 10 mcg/kg subcut once daily. Continue until ANC remains more than 1,000 cells/mm^3 for three consecutive CBCs obtained every third day, or exceeds 10,000 cells/mm^3 after a radiation-induced nadir.

Children weighing less than 15 kg: 12 mcg/kg subcut once daily. Continue until ANC remains more than 1,000 cells/mm^3 for three consecutive CBCs obtained every third day, or exceeds 10,000 cells/mm^3 after a radiation-induced nadir.

➤ **Neuroblastoma in children at high risk ◆**

Children and adolescents: 250 mcg/m^2 subcut or IV once daily for 14 days, beginning 3 days before administration of dinutuximab (each cycle is 28 days); sargramostim is administered during cycles 1, 3, and 5 (regimen also includes dinutuximab, isotretinoin, and aldesleukin).

Reactions in bold italics are *life-threatening*. Interactions may have a *rapid onset* or a **delayed onset**.

ADMINISTRATION

IV

▼ Reconstitute powder for injection with 1 mL of sterile or bacteriostatic water for injection. Direct stream of sterile water against side of vial and gently swirl contents to minimize foaming. Avoid excessive or vigorous agitation or shaking.

▼ Further dilute in NSS. If drug yield falls below 10 mcg/mL, add human albumin at final concentration of 0.1% to NSS before adding sargramostim to prevent adsorption to components of the delivery system. To yield 0.1% human albumin, add 1 mg human albumin to each milliliter of NSS (dilute 1 mL of 5% human albumin in 50 mL of NSS).

▼ Don't use in-line filter.

▼ Give as soon as possible after mixing and no later than 6 hours after reconstituting.

▼ **Incompatibilities:** Other IV drugs, unless specific compatibility data are available.

Subcutaneous

● Reconstitute powder for injection with 1 mL sterile or bacteriostatic water for injection. Direct stream of sterile or bacteriostatic water against side of vial and gently swirl contents to minimize foaming. Avoid excessive or vigorous agitation or shaking.

ACTION

Induces cellular responses by binding to specific receptors on surfaces of target cells.

Route	Onset	Peak	Duration
IV	15 min	Immediate	Unknown
Subcut	15 min	2.5–4 hr	Unknown

Half-life: IV, about 1 hour; subcut, about 4 hours.

ADVERSE REACTIONS

CNS: asthenia, CNS disorders, fever, headache, malaise, anxiety, insomnia, paresthesia. **CV:** *hemorrhage,* edema, peripheral edema, HTN, supraventricular arrhythmias, chest pain, pericardial effusion, tachycardia. **EENT:** retinal hemorrhage, epistaxis, pharyngitis, rhinitis. **GI:** anorexia, diarrhea, dysphagia, abdominal pain, GI disorders, nausea, stomatitis, vomiting, *GI hemorrhage.* **GU:** urinary tract disorder, abnormal kidney function, increased creatinine level, increased BUN level. **Hematologic:** blood dyscrasias, *thrombocytopenia, leukopenia.* **Hepatic:** liver damage, bilirubinemia, increased ALT level. **Metabolic:** hyperglycemia, decreased albumin level, *hypomagnesemia.* **Musculoskeletal:** arthralgias, bone pain. **Respiratory:** dyspnea, lung disorders, pleural effusion. **Skin:** alopecia, pruritus, rash. **Other:** mucous membrane disorder, chills, *sepsis,* antisargramostim antibodies.

INTERACTIONS

Drug-drug. *Bleomycin, cyclophosphamide:* May enhance risk of pulmonary toxicity. Monitor patient closely.

Corticosteroids, lithium: May increase myeloproliferative effects of sargramostim. Use cautiously together.

EFFECTS ON LAB TEST RESULTS

● May increase BUN, creatinine, AST, ALT, ALP, bilirubin, and glucose levels.

● May decrease calcium, magnesium, and albumin levels.

● May decrease leukocyte and platelet counts.

CONTRAINDICATIONS & CAUTIONS

● Contraindicated in patients hypersensitive to drug or its components or to yeast-derived products and in those with excessive leukemic myeloid blasts in bone marrow or peripheral blood.

● Infusion-related reactions (respiratory distress, hypoxia, flushing, hypotension, syncope, and tachycardia) may occur after administration of the first dose.

● Concomitant use within 24 hours of chemotherapy or radiation is contraindicated.

● Lyophilized powder reconstituted with bacteriostatic water contains benzyl alcohol, which has been associated with fatal gasping syndrome in neonates. Don't administer to neonates.

● Use cautiously in patients with cardiac disease, hypoxia, fluid retention, pulmonary infiltrates, HF, or impaired renal or hepatic function because these conditions may be worsened.

● Drug may interfere with bone imaging studies; increased hematopoietic activity of the bone marrow may appear as transient positive bone imaging changes.

● Safety and effectiveness haven't been established in children younger than age 2 or for autologous peripheral blood progenitor cells and bone marrow transplantation, allogeneic bone marrow transplantation, and treatment of delayed neutrophil recovery or graft failure.

S

Dialyzable drug: Unknown.

⚠ *Overdose S&S:* Dyspnea, malaise, nausea, fever, rash, sinus tachycardia, headache, chills.

PREGNANCY-LACTATION-REPRODUCTION

• There are no adequate studies during pregnancy. Use only if clearly needed. If needed during pregnancy, use only lyophilized powder reconstituted with preservative-free sterile water due to the risk posed by benzyl alcohol.

• It isn't known if drug appears in human milk. Patients shouldn't breastfeed during treatment and for at least 2 weeks after final dose.

NURSING CONSIDERATIONS

• If severe adverse reactions occur, reduce dose by 50% or temporarily stop drug and notify prescriber. Resume therapy when reactions decrease. Transient rash and local reactions at injection site may occur.

• Monitor patient for infusion-related reactions (respiratory distress, hypoxia, flushing, hypotension, syncope, and tachycardia), which may occur after administration of the first dose. If patient exhibits signs of dyspnea, reduce rate of infusion by 50%; if symptoms persist or worsen, discontinue infusion.

• Rapidly dividing progenitor cells may be sensitive to cytotoxic therapies, making the drug ineffective; don't give within 24 hours of last dose of chemotherapy or radiotherapy.

• Monitor CBC with differential, including exam for presence of blast cells, biweekly.

• Monitor body weight and hydration status; drug may increase risk of effusions and capillary leak syndrome.

• Monitor patients for supraventricular arrhythmias, especially those with preexisting cardiac disease.

• Drug accelerates myeloid recovery in patients receiving bone marrow that is either unpurged or purged by anti-B cell monoclonal antibodies more than in those who receive bone marrow that is chemically purged.

• Drug may produce a limited response in patients with transplants who have received extensive radiotherapy or who have received other myelotoxic drugs.

• Drug can act as a growth factor for any tumor type, particularly myeloid malignant disease.

PATIENT TEACHING

• Review administration schedule with patient and caregivers, and address their concerns.

• Urge patient to report all adverse reactions promptly.

---

sarilumab
sar-IL-ue-mab

Kevzara

Therapeutic class: Antirheumatics
Pharmacologic class: Monoclonal antibodies

AVAILABLE FORMS

Injection: 150 mg/1.14 mL, 200 mg/1.14 mL single-dose prefilled syringes and pens

INDICATIONS & DOSAGES

➤ **Moderately to severely active RA in patients who have had an inadequate response or intolerance to one or more DMARDs, as monotherapy or in combination with methotrexate or other conventional DMARDs**

Adults: 200 mg subcut once every 2 weeks.

Adjust-a-dose: Reduce dosage to 150 mg every 2 weeks for management of neutropenia, thrombocytopenia, and elevated liver enzyme levels. Refer to manufacturer's instructions for specific toxicity-related dosage adjustments.

ADMINISTRATION
Subcutaneous

• Allow prefilled syringe to sit at room temperature for 30 minutes or prefilled pen to sit at room temperature for 60 minutes before subcut injection; don't warm in any other way.

• Inspect solution before use. Don't use if solution is cloudy, discolored, or contains particles, or if any part of prefilled syringe appears to be damaged.

• Inject the full amount in the syringe or pen (1.14 mL).

• Rotate injection sites with each injection. Don't inject into bruises, scars, or tender or damaged skin.

• Keep unused syringes or pens in original carton to protect from light and store in refrigerator between 36° and 46° F (2° and 8° C); don't freeze, heat, or shake.

• May store drug at room temperature up to 77° F (25° C) for up to 14 days in carton. Use within 14 days after removing from refrigerator.

ACTION

An interleukin 6 (IL-6) receptor antagonist that binds to both soluble and membrane-bound IL-6 receptors causing an anti-inflammatory effect that leads to a reduction in C-reactive protein levels.

Route	Onset	Peak	Duration
Subcut	Unknown	2–4 days	28 days (150-mg dose), 43 days (200-mg dose)

Half-life: 150-mg dose, 8 days; 200-mg dose, 10 days.

ADVERSE REACTIONS

EENT: nasopharyngitis, oral herpes simplex. **GU:** UTI. **Hematologic:** *neutropenia, leukopenia, thrombocytopenia.* **Hepatic:** increased ALT and AST levels. **Metabolic:** hypertriglyceridemia. **Respiratory:** URI. **Skin:** injection-site erythema, pruritus, or reaction. **Other:** infection, immunosuppression, hypersensitivity reactions, antibody development.

INTERACTIONS

Drug-drug. *Biological DMARDs (anti-CD20 monoclonal antibodies, IL-1R antagonists, selective costimulation modulators, TNF antagonists):* May increase risk of immunosuppression and infection. Avoid use together.
Corticosteroids: May increase risk of immunosuppression and infection. Monitor patient closely.
Corticosteroids, NSAIDs: May increase risk of GI perforation. Avoid concurrent use.
CYP450 substrates (atorvastatin, lovastatin, oral contraceptives, theophylline, warfarin): May alter substrate concentrations. Use cautiously together. Monitor substrate levels if possible and adjust substrate dosage as needed.
Live-virus vaccines: May increase risk of infection. Avoid use together.

EFFECTS ON LAB TEST RESULTS

• May increase AST, ALT, LDL, HDL, cholesterol, and triglyceride levels.
• May decrease ANC and neutrophil and platelet counts.

CONTRAINDICATIONS & CAUTIONS

• Contraindicated in patients with hypersensitivity to drug or its components.
Boxed Warning Serious infections leading to hospitalization or death, including bacterial, viral, invasive fungal, TB, and other opportunistic infections, can occur. Avoid use in patients with an active infection. ∎
• Consider risks and benefits of use in patients with chronic or recurrent infection, a history of serious or opportunistic infections, underlying conditions in addition to RA that may predispose them to infections, exposure to TB, or a history of living or traveling to areas of endemic TB or mycoses.
• Risk of GI perforation may increase in patients with concurrent diverticulitis or use of NSAIDs or corticosteroids.
• Drug isn't recommended in patients with active hepatic disease, hepatic impairment (ALT or AST level more than $1.5 \times$ ULN), ANC less than 2,000 cells/mm^3, or platelet count less than 150,000 cells/mm^3.
• Drug may increase risk of viral reactivation, including herpes zoster.
• Drug may increase risk of malignancies.
• Drug use hasn't been studied in patients with hepatic impairment or severe renal impairment.
• Safety and effectiveness in children haven't been established.
• Use cautiously in patients age 65 and older because of increased risk of infections.
Dialyzable drug: Unknown.

PREGNANCY-LACTATION-REPRODUCTION

• Effect of drug on a fetus is unknown; however, monoclonal antibodies cross the placental barrier in the third trimester and drug may affect immune response in infants exposed in utero. Use in pregnancy only if potential benefit justifies fetal risk.
• It isn't known if drug appears in human milk. Consider benefits and risks of drug before patient starts breastfeeding.
• Enroll patients exposed to drug during pregnancy in a pregnancy registry to monitor outcomes by calling 1-877-311-8972.

NURSING CONSIDERATIONS

Boxed Warning Monitor patients for infection during treatment. Interrupt treatment if serious or opportunistic infection occurs; don't restart drug until infection is controlled. ∎

• Perform prompt and complete testing to evaluate a new infection during treatment and initiate appropriate antimicrobial therapy while closely monitoring patient.

Boxed Warning Assess patient for TB risk factors and test for latent TB before drug initiation. If positive, start treatment for TB before beginning therapy. Consider anti-TB therapy for patients with a history of TB in whom an adequate course of treatment can't be confirmed and in patients who test negatively for latent TB but have risk factors for TB. ∎

• Monitor neutrophil and platelet counts before therapy, 4 to 8 weeks after start of therapy, and every 3 months thereafter.

• Monitor ALT and AST levels before therapy, 4 to 8 weeks after start of therapy, and every 3 months thereafter. Assess bilirubin level or other LFT values as clinically indicated.

• Monitor lipid parameters (LDL, HDL, triglycerides) 4 to 8 weeks after start of therapy and every 6 months thereafter.

• Monitor patients for hypersensitivity reactions (injection-site rash, generalized rash, urticaria). If anaphylaxis or other severe hypersensitivity reaction occurs, stop drug immediately.

• Monitor patients with concurrent diverticulitis and those who are taking corticosteroids or NSAIDs for GI perforation. Promptly evaluate acute abdominal signs and symptoms.

• *Look alike–sound alike:* Don't confuse sarilumab with sirolimus. Don't confuse Kevzara with Keppra.

PATIENT TEACHING
Boxed Warning Warn patient that drug may lower resistance to infection and to contact prescriber immediately if signs and symptoms of infection appear, to ensure rapid evaluation and appropriate treatment. ∎

• Assess patient for the ability to self-administer drug. Instruct patient or caregivers in injection technique and syringe disposal.

• Advise patient to seek immediate medical attention for signs or symptoms of serious allergic reactions (shortness of breath, chest pain, dizziness, moderate or severe stomach pain or vomiting, or swelling of the lips, tongue, or face).

• Caution patient (especially if taking NSAIDs or steroids or with a history of tears of the stomach or intestines) of increased risk of GI perforation. Instruct patient to seek

medical attention immediately for severe, persistent abdominal pain.

• Tell patient to discuss plans for surgery or a medical procedure with prescriber.

• Instruct patient to keep carton in an insulated bag with an ice pack when traveling.

• Caution patient to immediately report pregnancy that occurs during treatment.

---

sAXagliptin
sax-a-GLIP-tin

Onglyza⬧

Therapeutic class: Antidiabetics
Pharmacologic class: DPP-4 enzyme inhibitors

AVAILABLE FORMS
Tablets ᴼᵀᶜ: 2.5 mg, 5 mg

INDICATIONS & DOSAGES
➤ **Adjunct to diet and exercise to improve glycemic control in type 2 diabetes**
Adults: 2.5 or 5 mg PO once daily.
Adjust-a-dose: For patient with eGFR of 45 mL/minute/1.73 m^2 or less, ESRD requiring hemodialysis, or if patient is taking strong CYP3A4/5 inhibitors, give 2.5 mg PO once daily. If patient requires hemodialysis, give 2.5 mg once daily after treatment.

ADMINISTRATION
PO
• Give drug with or without food.
• Don't split or cut tablets.

ACTION
Inhibits DPP-4, an enzyme that rapidly inactivates incretin hormones, which play a part in the body's regulation of glucose. By increasing active incretin levels, drug helps to increase insulin release and decrease circulating glucose.

Route	Onset	Peak	Duration
PO	Unknown	2 hr	24 hr

Half-life: 2.5 hours.

ADVERSE REACTIONS
CNS: headache. **CV:** peripheral edema. **GU:** UTI. **Metabolic:** *hypoglycemia.* **Respiratory:** URI. **Other:** hypersensitivity reaction.

Reactions in bold italics are *life-threatening*. Interactions may have a *rapid onset* or a ***delayed onset***.

INTERACTIONS
Drug-drug. *Insulin, sulfonylurea hypoglycemics (chlorpropamide, glimepiride, glipizide, glyburide, tolbutamide):* May increase risk of hypoglycemia. Decrease dosage of insulin or sulfonylurea drugs if used together.
Strong CYP3A4/5 inhibitors (atazanavir, clarithromycin, itraconazole, ketoconazole, nefazodone, nelfinavir, ritonavir, saquinavir): May increase saxagliptin level. Reduce dosage to 2.5 mg PO daily.

EFFECTS ON LAB TEST RESULTS
• May decrease glucose level.
• May decrease lymphocyte count.

CONTRAINDICATIONS & CAUTIONS
• Contraindicated in patients hypersensitive to drug or its components.
• Hypersensitivity reactions, including anaphylaxis, angioedema, and exfoliative skin conditions such as bullous pemphigoid, have occurred within the first 3 months of therapy initiation. Discontinue drug for suspected hypersensitivity.
• Use cautiously in patients with a history of angioedema to another DPP-4 inhibitor because it's unknown if such patients will be predisposed to angioedema with saxagliptin.
❸ *Alert:* Use cautiously in patients with a history of HF or renal disease. Drug may increase risk of HF in these patients.
• Rare cases of acute pancreatitis have been reported. Discontinue drug for suspected pancreatitis.
• Drug isn't indicated to treat type 1 diabetes or diabetic ketoacidosis.
• Safety and effectiveness in children haven't been established.
• Use cautiously in older adults.
Dialyzable drug: 23%.

PREGNANCY-LACTATION-REPRODUCTION
• There are no adequate studies during pregnancy. Use only if clearly needed.
• It isn't known if drug appears in human milk. Use cautiously during breastfeeding.

NURSING CONSIDERATIONS
❸ *Alert:* Drug may cause joint pain that can be severe and disabling. Report severe and persistent joint pain to prescriber as drug may need to be discontinued.
❸ *Alert:* Monitor patient for signs and symptoms of HF (dyspnea, orthopnea, tiredness, weakness, fatigue, weight gain, peripheral or abdominal edema). Drug may need to be discontinued and other antidiabetics may be required.
• Monitor blood glucose level and watch for signs and symptoms of hypoglycemia.
• Monitor HbA$_{1c}$ level periodically to assess long-term glycemic control.
• Assess renal function before starting drug and periodically thereafter.
• Monitor patient for skin blistering or erosions. Discontinue drug if bullous pemphigoid is suspected and consider referral to a dermatologist.
• Management of type 2 diabetes should also include diet control and exercise. Because calorie restriction, weight loss, and exercise help improve insulin sensitivity and help make drug therapy effective, these measures are essential for proper diabetes management.
• *Look alike–sound alike:* Don't confuse saxagliptin with sitagliptin.

PATIENT TEACHING
• Instruct patient in safe drug administration.
• Tell patient to stop drug and seek immediate medical attention for signs and symptoms of hypersensitivity, including rash, flaking or peeling skin, itching, or swelling of the skin, face, lips, tongue, or throat.
❸ *Alert:* Instruct patient to immediately report signs and symptoms of HF to prescriber. Patient should not stop drug without first discussing with prescriber.
❸ *Alert:* Instruct patient to report severe and persistent joint pain to prescriber as drug may need to be discontinued.
• Advise patient that drug isn't a substitute for diet and exercise and that it's important to follow a prescribed dietary and physical activity routine and to monitor glucose levels.
• Inform patient and family members of the signs and symptoms of hypoglycemia and hyperglycemia and the steps to take should these occur, including notifying the prescriber.
• Tell patient to notify prescriber during periods of stress, such as fever, infection, or surgery, because dosage may need adjustment.
• Teach patient to stop drug if signs and symptoms of pancreatitis (persistent severe abdominal pain, sometimes radiating to the back; vomiting) occur.
• Advise patient to immediately report skin blisters or erosions.

S

scopolamine
skoe-POL-a-meen

Transderm Scop

Therapeutic class: Antiemetics
Pharmacologic class: Belladonna alkaloids–antimuscarinics

AVAILABLE FORMS
Transdermal patch: 1 mg/3 days

INDICATIONS & DOSAGES
➤ **To prevent postoperative nausea and vomiting**
Adults: Apply 1 transdermal patch to the skin behind the ear the evening before scheduled surgery. To minimize exposure of a newborn to drug, apply patch 1 hour before cesarean birth. Keep patch in place for 24 hours after surgery; then remove and discard.
➤ **To prevent nausea and vomiting from motion sickness**
Adults: Apply 1 transdermal patch to the skin behind the ear at least 4 hours before antiemetic is needed. Remove and place a new patch behind other ear if needed for longer than 3 days.

ADMINISTRATION
Transdermal
- Keep in foil wrapper until ready to use.
- Wear gloves to apply or remove patch.
- Place patch behind ear, on clean, dry, hairless area.
- If patch is dislodged, replace with a new one.
- Don't cut patch in any way.
- Don't apply more than one patch at a time.
- After patch removal, wash application site thoroughly.
- Fold patch in half after removal to avoid accidental contact with drug; then discard.

ACTION
Inhibits muscarinic actions of acetylcholine on autonomic effectors innervated by postganglionic cholinergic neurons. May affect neural pathways originating in the inner ear to inhibit nausea and vomiting.

Route	Onset	Peak	Duration
Transdermal	4 hr	24 hr	72 hr

Half-life: 9.5 hours.

ADVERSE REACTIONS
CNS: dizziness, somnolence, agitation, confusion. **EENT:** dilated pupils, visual impairment, dry mouth, pharyngitis. **Skin:** rash, contact dermatitis with transdermal patch.

INTERACTIONS
Drug-drug. *Amantadine, antihistamines, antiparkinsonian drugs, disopyramide, meperidine, muscle relaxants, phenothiazines, procainamide, quinidine, TCAs:* May increase risk of adverse CNS reactions. Avoid using together.
Anticholinergics (benztropine, cyclopentolate, darifenacin): May increase risk of intestinal obstruction, urine retention, or other CNS adverse reactions. Monitor patient closely.
CNS depressants: May increase risk of CNS depression. Monitor patient closely.
Glucagon: May enhance adverse effects of glucagon, especially GI effects. Use together cautiously.
Glycopyrrolate (oral inhalation): May enhance adverse and anticholinergic effects. Avoid concurrent use.
Drug-lifestyle. *Alcohol use:* May increase risk of CNS depression. Discourage use together.

EFFECTS ON LAB TEST RESULTS
- May interfere with the gastric secretion test.

CONTRAINDICATIONS & CAUTIONS
- Contraindicated in patients hypersensitive to scopolamine, other belladonna alkaloids, or components in the formulation or delivery system and in patients with angle-closure glaucoma.
- Use cautiously in patients with open-angle glaucoma, history of seizures, risk factors for seizures or psychosis, pyloric obstruction, urinary bladder neck obstruction, impaired renal or hepatic function, and patients suspected of having intestinal obstruction.
- Use cautiously in patients taking oral medications; absorption of oral medications may be decreased due to decreased gastric motility and delayed gastric emptying.
- Drug isn't recommended for use in children because a safe and effective dose hasn't been established and children are particularly susceptible to the adverse effects of belladonna.

Reactions in bold italics are ***life-threatening***. Interactions may have a *rapid onset* or a ***delayed onset***.

• Use cautiously in older adults because of the increased likelihood of CNS effects, such as hallucinations, confusion, and dizziness.

• Use cautiously in patients in hot or humid environments; drug can cause heatstroke.

Dialyzable drug: Unknown.

⚠ *Overdose S&S:* Lethargy, somnolence, coma, confusion, agitation, hallucinations, leukocytosis, seizures, visual disturbances, dry flushed skin, dry mouth, decreased bowel sounds, urine retention, tachycardia, HTN, supraventricular arrhythmias, circulatory or respiratory collapse, death.

PREGNANCY-LACTATION-REPRODUCTION

• Use during pregnancy only if potential benefit justifies risk to mother and fetus.

• Eclamptic seizures have been reported during pregnancy, with severe preeclampsia soon after injection of IV and IM scopolamine. Avoid use of transdermal scopolamine in patients with severe preeclampsia.

• Drug appears in human milk. Use cautiously during breastfeeding.

NURSING CONSIDERATIONS

• Monitor patient because some patients become temporarily excited or disoriented and some develop amnesia or become drowsy. Reorient patient as needed.

• Monitor patient for new or worsening psychiatric signs or symptoms (acute psychosis, agitation, speech disorder, hallucinations, paranoia, delusion).

• Monitor patient for decreased GI motility and urine retention.

• Stop drug if patient experiences signs and symptoms of angle-closure glaucoma or has difficulty urinating.

• Monitor patient for withdrawal signs and symptoms (dizziness, nausea, vomiting, abdominal cramps, diaphoresis, headache, confusion, weakness, bradycardia, hypotension) when drug is discontinued after several days of use. Withdrawal signs and symptoms usually present 24 hours or more after patch removal.

• Tolerance may develop when therapy is prolonged.

• Atropine-like toxicity may cause dose-related adverse reactions. Individual tolerance varies greatly.

🔹 *Alert:* Overdose may cause curare-like effects such as respiratory paralysis. Keep emergency equipment available.

• Remove patch before MRI to prevent skin burns.

PATIENT TEACHING

• Instruct patient in safe drug administration, including to wash and dry hands thoroughly before and after applying transdermal patch and before touching the eye to avoid temporary pupil dilation and blurred vision.

• Advise patient that the transdermal method releases a controlled therapeutic amount of drug. Transderm Scop is effective if applied at least 4 hours before experiencing motion.

• Remind patient to remove one patch before applying another and to not apply more than one patch at a time.

• Alert patient to possible withdrawal signs and symptoms when transdermal system is used for longer than 72 hours.

• Advise patient that eyes may be more sensitive to light while wearing patch. Advise patient to wear sunglasses for comfort.

• Warn patient to avoid activities that require alertness until CNS effects of drug are known.

• Instruct patient to read the brochure that comes with the transdermal product.

• Instruct patient requiring an MRI to inform facility about wearing a transdermal patch.

• Urge patient to report urinary hesitancy or urine retention.

selegiline
se-LE-ji-leen

Emsam

selegiline hydrochloride
(L-deprenyl hydrochloride)
Zelapar

Therapeutic class: Antiparkinsonian drugs
Pharmacologic class: MAO inhibitors

S

AVAILABLE FORMS
selegiline
Transdermal system: 6 mg/24 hours, 9 mg/24 hours, 12 mg/24 hours
selegiline hydrochloride
Capsules: 5 mg
Tablets: 5 mg
Tablets (ODTs): 1.25 mg

♣Canada ◇OTC ◆ Off-label use 🖉 Photoguide ⓓⓓ Do not crush *Liquid contains alcohol ▒ Genetic

INDICATIONS & DOSAGES
➤ **Adjunctive treatment with levodopa–carbidopa in managing signs and symptoms of Parkinson disease**
Adults: For capsules and tablets, 10 mg PO daily divided as 5 mg at breakfast and 5 mg at lunch. After 2 or 3 days, gradual decrease of levodopa–carbidopa dosage may be needed. Or, if using ODTs, start with 1.25 mg PO once daily. Increase to 2.5 mg daily after at least 6 weeks, if tolerated and needed. Maximum dose is 10 mg/day for tablets and capsules and 2.5 mg once daily for ODTs.
Adjust-a-dose: For adults with mild to moderate hepatic impairment (Child Pugh class A or B), reduce the ODT dose to 1.25 mg once daily depending on clinical response and tolerability.
➤ **Major depressive disorder (Emsam)**
Adults: Apply one patch daily. Initially, use 6 mg/day. Increase, if needed, in increments of 3 mg/day at intervals of 2 or more weeks. Maximum daily dose, 12 mg.
Adults age 65 and older: 6 mg transdermal patch daily.

ADMINISTRATION
PO
• Don't give food or liquids for 5 minutes before and after giving ODTs.
• Don't push ODTs through the foil backing; peel the backing off and gently remove the tablet.
• Place tablet on top of tongue.
Transdermal
• Apply patch to dry, intact skin on the upper torso, upper thigh, or outer surface of the upper arm once every 24 hours.
• Apply at the same time each day and rotate application sites.
• Don't cut the transdermal patch into smaller pieces.

ACTION
May inhibit MAO type B (mainly found in the brain) and dopamine metabolism. At higher-than-recommended doses, drug nonselectively inhibits MAO, including MAO type A (mainly found in the intestine). May also directly increase dopaminergic activity by decreasing the reuptake of dopamine into nerve cells.

Route	Onset	Peak	Duration
PO (tablet, capsule)	Unknown	40–90 min	Unknown
PO (ODT)	5 min	10–15 min	Unknown
Transdermal	Unknown	Unknown	24 hr

Half-life: Selegiline, 2 to 10 hours; N-desmethyl deprenyl, 2 hours; L-amphetamine, 17.75 hours; L-methamphetamine, 20.5 hours.

ADVERSE REACTIONS
Oral form
CNS: anxiety, dizziness, loss of balance, depression, increased bradykinesia, dyskinesia, headache, confusion, hallucinations, vivid dreams, insomnia, lethargy, somnolence, tremor, ataxia, pain. **CV:** HTN, palpitations, chest pain. **EENT:** pharyngitis, rhinitis, dry mouth, tooth disorder. **GI:** constipation, nausea, abdominal pain, diarrhea, stomatitis, dyspepsia, vomiting, flatulence. **GU:** urine retention. **Metabolic:** weight loss, *hypokalemia.* **Musculoskeletal:** aches, leg cramps, myalgia, back pain. **Respiratory:** dyspnea. **Skin:** rash, ecchymosis.
Transdermal form
CNS: headache, insomnia. **CV:** orthostatic hypotension. **EENT:** sinusitis, dry mouth, pharyngitis. **GI:** diarrhea, dyspepsia. **GU:** abnormal ejaculation. **Metabolic:** weight gain, weight loss. **Skin:** application-site reaction, rash.

INTERACTIONS
Drug-drug. *Bupropion, cyclobenzaprine, mirtazapine, MAO inhibitors, sympathomimetic amines (including amphetamines, cold products, and weight-loss preparations containing vasoconstrictors), TCAs:* May cause hypertensive crisis. Separate use by at least 14 days.
Carbamazepine, oxcarbazepine: May increase selegiline levels. Use together is contraindicated.
Citalopram, duloxetine, fluoxetine, fluvoxamine, nefazodone, paroxetine, sertraline, venlafaxine: May cause serotonin syndrome (CNS irritability, shivering, and altered consciousness). Separate use by at least 2 weeks (5 weeks if switching to or from fluoxetine).
Dextromethorphan: May increase risk of psychosis or bizarre behavior. Use together is contraindicated.
Hormonal contraceptives: May increase plasma selegiline level and increase adverse reactions. Monitor patient closely.

Reactions in bold italics are *life-threatening*. Interactions may have a *rapid onset* or a ***delayed onset***.

Linezolid, methylene blue: May cause serotonin syndrome. Don't administer within 14 days of each other.

Opioids (meperidine, methadone, tramadol): May increase risk of serotonin syndrome. Separate use by at least 14 days.

Drug-herb. *St. John's wort:* May cause increased serotonergic effects. Warn against using together.

Drug-food. ❸ *Alert: Foods high in tyramine (aged cheese or meats, fava beans, herring, sauerkraut, unpasteurized beer):* May cause hypertensive crisis, especially at increased doses. Provide patient with a list of foods to avoid beginning on first day of transdermal daily dose of 9 mg or 12 mg and for 2 weeks after dosage reduction to 6 mg daily, or after discontinuation of 9- or 12-mg daily dose.

Drug-lifestyle. *Alcohol use:* May increase risk of adverse effects. Discourage use together.

EFFECTS ON LAB TEST RESULTS

• May cause positive result for amphetamine on urine drug screen.

CONTRAINDICATIONS & CAUTIONS

• Contraindicated in patients hypersensitive to drug, and in patients with pheochromocytoma (transdermal patch).

Boxed Warning Transdermal patch is contraindicated in patients younger than age 12 because of risk of hypertensive crisis. ∎

❸ *Alert:* Concomitant use with linezolid or methylene blue can cause serotonin syndrome (fever, mental status changes, muscle twitching, diaphoresis, shivering or shaking, diarrhea, loss of coordination). Use drug with linezolid or methylene blue only for life-threatening or urgent conditions when the potential benefits outweigh the risks of toxicity.

• Don't use oral drug with the transdermal system.

• ODTs aren't recommended in patients with severe hepatic or renal impairment or ESRD.

• Orthostatic hypotension may occur during first 2 months of therapy or after dosage increases, especially in older adults.

• Somnolence and falling asleep without warning while engaged in ADLs (including operating motor vehicles) have been reported in some patients. Evaluate patients for factors that may increase these risks, such as older adults with sleep disorders and patients taking sedatives.

• Avoid use in patients with major psychotic disorders. Drug may cause changes in or worsening of mental status, abnormal thinking, and behavioral changes, which may be severe and include paranoid ideation, delusions, hallucinations, confusion, psychotic-like behavior, disorientation, aggressive behavior, agitation, and delirium. Drug isn't approved for bipolar depression.

• Reevaluate patients receiving transdermal patch for extended periods for continued effectiveness.

• Hypertensive reactions have been reported in patients who ingested tyramine-containing foods while receiving oral selegiline.

Dialyzable drug: Unknown.

⚠ *Overdose S&S:* Drowsiness, dizziness, faintness, irritability, hyperactivity, agitation, severe headache, hallucinations, trismus, opisthotonos, seizures, coma, rapid and irregular pulse, HTN, hypotension and vascular collapse, precordial pain, respiratory depression and failure, hyperpyrexia, diaphoresis, cool and clammy skin.

PREGNANCY-LACTATION-REPRODUCTION

• There are no adequate studies during pregnancy. Use only if potential benefit justifies fetal risk.

• It isn't known if drug appears in human milk. Because of risk of serious adverse reactions, including hypertensive reactions, patient shouldn't breastfeed during and for 7 days after final dose.

NURSING CONSIDERATIONS

❸ *Alert:* Some patients experience new or increased adverse reactions to levodopa, such as dyskinesia, when it's used with selegiline. These patients need a 10% to 30% reduction of levodopa–carbidopa dosage.

Boxed Warning Transdermal system used to treat depression may increase risk of suicidality in children, adolescents, and young adults ages 18 to 24, especially during the first few months of treatment, especially in those with major depressive or other psychiatric disorder. ∎

❸ *Alert:* If linezolid or methylene blue must be given, stop selegiline and monitor patient for serotonin toxicity for 2 weeks, or until 24 hours after the last dose of methylene blue or linezolid, whichever comes first. May resume selegiline 24 hours after last dose of methylene blue or linezolid.

- Monitor patients with major depressive disorder for worsening of symptoms and of suicidality, especially during the first few weeks of treatment and during dosage changes.
- ⚠️ *Alert:* Monitor patient carefully for orthostatic hypotension, especially during first 2 months of treatment and after dosage increases. Help patient rise from a reclining position.
- Monitor patient for new-onset HTN or HTN that isn't adequately controlled after starting drug.
- Monitor patient taking antidepressants and selegiline concomitantly for serotonin syndrome and hyperpyrexia.
- Monitor patient for drowsiness, significant daytime sleepiness, or episodes of falling asleep during activities that require active participation. Discontinue drug if present.
- Monitor patient for psychotic-like behavior, changes in or worsening of mental status, abnormal thinking, and behavioral changes.
- Ask patient about the development or worsening of impulsive or compulsive behaviors, such as new or increased gambling urges, sexual urges, binge eating, uncontrolled spending, or other urges, because patient may not recognize these behaviors as abnormal.
- Examine patient's skin periodically for possible melanoma, because of risk of skin cancer associated with drug and with Parkinson disease.
- Examine patient's mouth for irritation or ulceration; be aware of patient complaints of swallowing or mouth pain when taking ODTs.

PATIENT TEACHING
- Instruct patient in safe drug administration.
- ⚠️ *Alert:* Teach patient to recognize and immediately report signs and symptoms of serotonin toxicity (fever, mental status changes, muscle twitching, diaphoresis, shivering or shaking, diarrhea, loss of coordination).
- Advise patient not to take drug in the evening because doing so may cause insomnia.
- Explain risk of hypertensive crisis if patient ingests foods or beverages containing tyramine during therapy; if using a 9-mg/day or higher transdermal system, patient should avoid these products altogether. Give patient a list of tyramine-containing foods and products.
- ⚠️ *Alert:* Warn patient about the many drugs, including OTC drugs, that may interact with

this drug and about the need to consult a pharmacist or prescriber before using them.
- Teach patient and family the signs and symptoms of hypertensive crisis, including severe headache, sore or stiff neck, nausea, vomiting, diaphoresis, rapid heartbeat, dilated pupils, and photophobia.
- Instruct patient not to rise rapidly after sitting or lying down because of risk of dizziness, which may occur more frequently early in therapy or after dosage increases.
- Advise patient taking antidepressants concomitantly with selegiline to immediately report such signs and symptoms as confusion, hallucinations, agitation, delirium, syncope, shivering, diaphoresis, high fever, tachycardia, nausea, diarrhea, muscle rigidity or twitching, or tremors.
- Explain that drug may cause patient to fall asleep during activities that require active participation. Advise patient to contact prescriber if drowsiness, significant daytime sleepiness, or episodes of falling asleep during such activities occur.
- Tell patient to report paranoid ideation, delusions, hallucinations, confusion, psychotic-like behavior, disorientation, aggressive behavior, agitation, or delirium.
- Tell patient to contact prescriber if experiencing difficulty controlling impulsive or compulsive behaviors, such as new or increased gambling urges, sexual urges, binge eating, uncontrolled spending, or other urges.
- Urge patient to watch for skin changes that could suggest melanoma and to have periodic skin exams by a health professional.
- Advise patient taking ODTs to report mouth pain, pain when swallowing, or ulcerations.
- Caution patient to contact prescriber before discontinuing selegiline.
- Tell patient that each ODT contains 1.25 mg phenylalanine.

Boxed Warning Advise family members of patient using transdermal system to watch for and immediately report new or worsening suicidality. ■
- Tell patient to avoid exposing transdermal system to direct external heat sources, such as heating pads, electric blankets, hot tubs, heated water beds, and prolonged sunlight.
- Inform patient that MAO inhibitors may need to be stopped 10 days before surgery requiring general anesthesia and to discuss MAO inhibitor use with surgeon.

Reactions in bold italics are *life-threatening*. Interactions may have a *rapid onset* or a *delayed onset*.

• Advise patient planning pregnancy or breastfeeding to first contact prescriber.

SAFETY ALERT!

selpercatinib ⌘
sel-per-KA-ti-nib

Retevmo

Therapeutic class: Antineoplastics
Pharmacologic class: Kinase inhibitors

AVAILABLE FORMS
Capsules ⃝: 40 mg, 80 mg

INDICATIONS & DOSAGES
Adjust-a-dose (for all indications): Refer to manufacturer's instructions for toxicity-related dosage adjustments. For patients with severe hepatic impairment taking either 120 mg or 160 mg b.i.d., reduce dosage to 80 mg b.i.d. For patients unable to avoid taking a strong CYP3A inhibitor, reduce selpercatinib 120 mg b.i.d. to 40 mg b.i.d., and reduce selpercatinib 160 mg b.i.d. to 80 mg b.i.d. For patients unable to avoid taking a moderate CYP3A inhibitor, reduce selpercatinib 120 mg b.i.d. to 80 mg b.i.d. and reduce selpercatinib 160 mg b.i.d. to 120 mg b.i.d. After the CYP3A inhibitor has been discontinued, wait three to five elimination half-lives; then resume selpercatinib at the dose taken before initiating the CYP3A inhibitor.
➤ **Metastatic,** *RET* **fusion-positive NSCLC** ⌘
Adults weighing 50 kg or more: 160 mg PO b.i.d. until disease progression or unacceptable toxicity.
Adults weighing less than 50 kg: 120 mg PO b.i.d. until disease progression or unacceptable toxicity.
➤ **Advanced or metastatic** *RET***-mutant medullary thyroid cancer** ⌘
Adults and children age 12 and older weighing 50 kg or more: 160 mg PO b.i.d. until disease progression or unacceptable toxicity.
Adults and children age 12 and older weighing less than 50 kg: 120 mg PO b.i.d. until disease progression or unacceptable toxicity.
➤ **Advanced or metastatic** *RET* **fusion-positive thyroid cancer** ⌘
Adults and children age 12 and older weighing 50 kg or more: 160 mg PO b.i.d. until disease progression or unacceptable toxicity.

Adults and children age 12 and older weighing less than 50 kg: 120 mg PO b.i.d. until disease progression or unacceptable toxicity.

ADMINISTRATION
PO
• Give approximately every 12 hours.
• May give without regard to food. If given concomitantly with a PPI, give with food.
• Give 2 hours before or 10 hours after an H_2 receptor antagonist.
• Give 2 hours before or 2 hours after a locally acting antacid or buffered medication.
• Patient must swallow capsules whole; don't crush or allow patient to chew capsules.
• Don't give a missed dose unless it's more than 6 hours until the next scheduled dose.
• If patient vomits after administration, don't give an additional dose but resume dose at the next scheduled time.
• Store capsules at 68° to 77° F (20° to 25° C).

ACTION
Decreases cell proliferation of tumor cell lines.

Route	Onset	Peak	Duration
PO	Unknown	2 hr	Unknown

Half-life: 32 hours.

ADVERSE REACTIONS
CNS: fatigue, headache, fever. **CV:** edema, HTN, *hemorrhage, prolonged QT interval.* **EENT:** dry mouth. **GI:** abdominal pain, constipation, diarrhea, nausea, vomiting. **GU:** increased creatinine level. **Hematologic:** *leukopenia, thrombocytopenia.* **Hepatic:** *hepatotoxicity.* **Metabolic:** hypothyroidism, hyperglycemia, hypoglycemia, *hypocalcemia,* hypercholesterolemia, hyponatremia, *hypomagnesemia, hyperkalemia.* **Respiratory:** cough, dyspnea, pneumonia. **Skin:** rash. **Other:** hypersensitivity reaction.

INTERACTIONS
Drug-drug. *Buffered medication, locally acting antacids (antacids containing aluminum, magnesium, or calcium; simethicone):* May decrease selpercatinib level and antitumor activity. Avoid use together. If unable to avoid use together, give selpercatinib 2 hours before or 2 hours after buffered medication or locally acting antacid.
CYP2C8 and CYP3A substrates (midazolam, repaglinide): May increase level of these

S

substrates and increase risk of their adverse reactions. Avoid use together. If unable to avoid use together, modify substrate dosage as recommended in substrate's approved product labeling.

Drugs that prolong QT interval (amiodarone, ciprofloxacin, haloperidol, lithium, methadone, procainamide, SSRIs, TCAs), thioridazine: May increase risk of prolonged QTc interval. Monitor QT interval by ECG frequently.

H₂ receptor antagonists (famotidine, ranitidine): May decrease selpercatinib level and antitumor activity. Avoid use together. If unable to avoid use together, give selpercatinib 2 hours before or 10 hours after H₂ receptor antagonist.

Moderate CYP3A inducers (bosentan, efavirenz), strong CYP3A inducers (rifampin): May decrease selpercatinib level and antitumor activity. Avoid use together.

Moderate CYP3A inhibitors (diltiazem, fluconazole, verapamil), strong CYP3A inhibitors (itraconazole): May increase selpercatinib level and risk of adverse reactions, including prolonged QTc interval. Avoid use together. If unable to avoid use together, monitor QT interval by ECG more frequently and reduce selpercatinib dosage.

PPIs (dexlansoprazole, esomeprazole, lansoprazole, omeprazole): May decrease selpercatinib level and antitumor activity. Avoid use together. If unable to avoid use together, give selpercatinib with food.

Drug-herb. *St. John's wort:* May decrease selpercatinib level and antitumor activity. Discourage use together.

EFFECTS ON LAB TEST RESULTS

• May increase AST, ALT, creatinine, ALP, total cholesterol, potassium, and bilirubin levels.
• May decrease albumin, calcium, sodium, and magnesium levels.
• May increase or decrease glucose level.
• May decrease leukocyte and platelet counts.

CONTRAINDICATIONS & CAUTIONS

• Use cautiously in patients with hepatic impairment, HTN, or hypersensitivity to drug and in those at risk for developing prolonged QTc interval (known long QT syndromes, significant bradyarrhythmias, severe or uncontrolled HF).

• Drug may impair wound healing. Safety of resuming drug after resolution of wound-healing complications hasn't been established.
• TLS has been reported in patients with medullary thyroid carcinoma receiving drug. Patients at increased risk have rapidly growing tumors, high tumor burden, renal dysfunction, or dehydration.
• Don't initiate drug in patients with uncontrolled HTN.
• Recommended dosage hasn't been established for patients with severe renal impairment or ESRD.
• Drug may cause elevated serum creatinine levels. If elevated levels persist, consider alternative markers for evaluating renal function.
• Safety and effectiveness in children younger than age 12 haven't been established.
⚠ *Alert:* Infrequent but fatal adverse reactions have occurred, including sepsis, cardiac arrest, and respiratory failure.
Dialyzable drug: Unknown.

PREGNANCY-LACTATION-REPRODUCTION

• Drug may cause fetal harm. Advise patients of childbearing potential to avoid pregnancy during therapy.
• Determine pregnancy status before starting drug.
• Patients of childbearing potential or male patients with partners of childbearing potential should use effective contraception during therapy and for 1 week after final dose.
• It isn't known if drug appears in human milk. Because of possible adverse effects on the infant, patient shouldn't breastfeed during therapy and for 1 week after final dose.
• Drug may impair fertility in women and men.

NURSING CONSIDERATIONS

• Obtain ALT and AST levels before therapy, every 2 weeks during the first 3 months, then monthly and as clinically indicated. Withhold drug, reduce dosage, or permanently discontinue drug based on severity of hepatotoxicity.
▨ Verify that genetic testing has been obtained before starting drug.
• Verify pregnancy status before starting drug.
• Assess QT interval and electrolyte and TSH levels at baseline, periodically during therapy;

adjust frequency of assessment based on risk factors.
• Correct hypokalemia, hypomagnesemia, and hypocalcemia before starting drug and during therapy as needed.
• Optimize BP before initiating drug. Monitor BP 1 week after initiation, monthly thereafter, and as clinically indicated. Initiate or adjust antihypertensives as appropriate.
• Monitor patient for signs and symptoms of liver toxicity (jaundice, tea-colored urine, drowsiness, abnormal bleeding or bruising, anorexia, nausea, vomiting, upper right quadrant abdominal pain).
• Closely monitor patient at risk for developing prolonged QTc interval. Monitor QT interval more frequently when giving drug with strong and moderate CYP3A inhibitors or drugs known to prolong QT interval. Withhold drug, reduce dosage, or permanently discontinue drug based on severity.
🌓 *Alert:* Monitor patient for hemorrhagic events (cerebral hemorrhage, tracheostomy site hemorrhage, hemoptysis). Permanently discontinue drug in patient with severe or life-threatening hemorrhage.
• Monitor patient for hypersensitivity reactions, including fever, rash, arthralgias, or myalgias with concurrent decreased platelet counts or transaminitis. Withhold drug, reduce dosage, or permanently discontinue drug based on severity and manage with corticosteroids. Continue steroids until patient reaches target dose; then taper. Permanently discontinue selpercatinib for recurrent hypersensitivity.
• Monitor patient for impaired wound healing. Withhold drug for 7 days before elective surgery. Don't administer for at least 2 weeks after major surgery and until adequate wound healing has occurred.
• Monitor patient for TLS. Consider prophylaxis with hydration in patient at risk and treat as clinically indicated.
• *Look alike–sound alike:* Don't confuse Retevmo with Retrovir. Don't confuse selpercatinib with selumetinib or tucatinib.

PATIENT TEACHING
• Tell patient that genetic testing is necessary before starting drug.
• Instruct patient in safe drug administration.
• Inform patient that lab testing and physical exams will be performed before and during therapy.

• Advise patient to report all adverse reactions, including increased BP (confusion, headaches, shortness of breath, dizziness, chest pain), irregular heartbeat, liver toxicity (jaundice, fatigue, abnormal bleeding or bruising, pain in upper right abdomen), bleeding, and allergic reactions (especially in first month of treatment).
• Tell patient about risk of impaired wound healing and to inform prescriber of planned surgical procedures.
• Caution patient of childbearing potential that drug can cause fetal harm and pregnancy testing is required before therapy starts.
• Advise patient of childbearing potential and male patient with a partner of childbearing potential to use effective contraception during therapy and for at least 1 week after final dose.
• Caution patient not to breastfeed during therapy and for at least 1 week after final dose.
• Inform patient that drug may impair fertility.

semaglutide
sem-a-GLOO-tide

Ozempic, Rybelsus, Wegovy

Therapeutic class: Antidiabetics
Pharmacologic class: Human glucagon-like peptide-1 receptor agonists

AVAILABLE FORMS
Injection: prefilled pen injectors delivering 0.25 mg, 0.5 mg, 1 mg, 1.7 mg, 2 mg, 2.4 mg per injection
Tablets ⬤: 3 mg, 7 mg, 14 mg

INDICATIONS & DOSAGES
➤ **Adjunct to diet and exercise to improve glycemic control in patients with type 2 diabetes; to reduce risk of major adverse CV events (CV death, nonfatal MI or nonfatal stroke) in patients with type 2 diabetes and established CV disease (Ozempic only)**
Adults: Initially, 0.25 mg subcut once weekly for 4 weeks; then increase to 0.5 mg once weekly. After 4 weeks, if needed, may increase to 1 mg once weekly. After 4 weeks, if needed, increase to 2 mg once weekly. Maximum dose, 2 mg once weekly.

Or, initially, 3 mg PO once daily for 30 days. After 30 days, increase to 7 mg PO once daily. After 30 days, if needed, may increase to 14 mg PO once daily.

➤ **Adjunct to diet and exercise for long-term weight management in patients with initial BMI of at least 30 kg/m², or at least 27 kg/m² and at least one weight-related comorbid condition (HTN, type 2 diabetes, or dyslipidemia) (Wegovy only)**
Adults: Initially, 0.25 mg subcut once weekly for 4 weeks, then increase to 0.5 mg for 4 weeks, then 1 mg for 4 weeks, then 1.7 mg for 4 weeks, then to 2.4 mg weekly maintenance dose.
Adjust-a-dose: If any dose isn't initially tolerated, delay dose escalation for 4 weeks. If 2.4-mg dose isn't tolerated, temporarily decrease to 1.7 mg for 4 weeks, then reescalate. If 2.4 mg isn't tolerated after reescalation, discontinue drug.

ADMINISTRATION
PO
- Patient should take on an empty stomach at least 30 minutes before first food, beverage, or other oral medications of the day with no more than 4 oz (120 mL) of water only.
- Patient should swallow tablets whole and not split, crush, or chew them.
- Use 3-mg dose for initiating treatment. It isn't effective for glycemic control.
- Giving two 7-mg tablets to achieve a 14-mg dose isn't recommended.
- If a dose is missed, skip the missed dose and give the next dose the following day.
- Patients on 0.5 mg weekly of subcut semaglutide can be transitioned to oral semaglutide 7 mg or 14 mg. Patients can start oral semaglutide up to 7 days after the last subcut injection. There is no equivalent oral dose for 1 mg subcut semaglutide.
- Patients taking 14 mg PO daily can be transitioned to subcut semaglutide at a dose of 0.5 mg once weekly. Patients can start the subcut injection the day after the last oral dose.

Subcutaneous
- Semaglutide solution appears clear and colorless. Don't use if particulate matter or coloration is seen.
- Use 0.25-mg dose for initiating treatment only. It isn't effective for glycemic control.

- Give drug once weekly on the same day each week at any time of day, without regard to meals.
- Administer subcut in the abdomen, thigh, or upper arm. Rotate injection sites.
- Administer insulin as a separate injection; never mix the products. May inject semaglutide and insulin in the same body region but don't inject in sites adjacent to one another.
- May change the day of weekly administration if the time between two doses is at least 48 hours.
- Give a missed Ozempic dose as soon as possible within 5 days after the missed dose. If more than 5 days have passed, skip the missed dose and give the next dose on the regularly scheduled day.
- Give a missed Wegovy dose as soon as possible if more than 48 hours before the next scheduled dose. Omit the missed dose if less than 48 hours until the next scheduled dose.
- ⚠️ *Alert:* Device is for single patient use. Never share this device with others, even if the needle has been changed, since it could transmit blood-borne pathogens.
- Store pen capped without a needle attached. Always use a new needle for each use. After each use, always remove and safely discard needle.
- Before first use, refrigerate Ozempic and Wegovy pens between 36° and 46° F (2° and 8° C). Don't store in freezer or directly adjacent to the refrigerator cooling element.
- After first use, store Ozempic pen for up to 56 days at controlled room temperature (59° to 86° F [15° to 30° C]) or refrigerated (36° to 46° F [2° to 8° C]); don't freeze. Protect from excessive heat and sunlight.
- May keep Wegovy pen at 46° to 86° F (8° to 30° C) for up to 28 days before cap removal, if needed.

ACTION
Stimulates the release of insulin and lowers glucagon secretion in the presence of elevated glucose levels. It also causes a minor delay in gastric emptying in the early postprandial phase.

Route	Onset	Peak	Duration
PO	Unknown	1 hr	Unknown
Subcut	Unknown	1–3 days	Unknown

Half-life: About 1 week.

Reactions in bold italics are *life-threatening*. Interactions may have a *rapid onset* or a ***delayed onset***.

ADVERSE REACTIONS

CNS: headache, fatigue, dizziness. **CV:** increased HR, hypotension. **EENT:** diabetic retinopathy complications. **GI:** nausea, vomiting, diarrhea, abdominal pain, constipation, dyspepsia, eructation, flatulence, GERD, gastritis, gastroenteritis, cholelithiasis, decreased appetite (PO), abdominal distension. **Hematologic:** *hypoglycemia.* **Metabolic:** increased amylase level, increased lipase level. **Skin:** hair loss, injection-site reaction. **Other:** immunogenicity.

INTERACTIONS

Drug-drug. *Insulin, insulin secretagogues (glipizide, repaglinide):* May increase risk of hypoglycemia. A reduced insulin or insulin secretagogue dosage may be required.
Oral medications: May change therapeutic effect of oral drugs because semaglutide delays gastric emptying. Monitor patient closely.
Other weight loss drugs: Safety and effectiveness of coadministration are unknown. Use together isn't recommended.
Drug-herb. *Herbal products for weight loss:* Safety and effectiveness of coadministration are unknown. Discourage use together.

EFFECTS ON LAB TEST RESULTS

• May increase amylase and lipase levels.

CONTRAINDICATIONS & CAUTIONS

• Contraindicated in patients hypersensitive to drug or its components.
• Drug isn't indicated for type 1 diabetes or the treatment of diabetic ketoacidosis, or as a substitute for insulin.
Boxed Warning Semaglutide caused thyroid adenomas and carcinomas after lifetime exposure in rodents. It isn't known whether drug causes thyroid C-cell tumors, including medullary thyroid carcinoma (MTC). ◼
Boxed Warning Contraindicated in patients with a personal or family history of MTC and in patients with multiple endocrine neoplasia syndrome type 2 (MEN 2). ◼
• Use cautiously in patients with a history of diabetic retinopathy. Rapid improvement in glucose control has been associated with temporary worsening of diabetic retinopathy. The effect of long-term improved glucose control using this drug and diabetic retinopathy hasn't been studied.
• Use cautiously in patients with a history of chronic renal failure; worsening of renal

function has been reported, particularly in patients who experienced nausea, vomiting, and diarrhea.
• Cases of pancreatitis have occurred. For suspected pancreatitis, discontinue drug and treat appropriately. For confirmed pancreatitis, don't restart drug.
• Use in patients with a history of pancreatitis hasn't been studied. Consider use of other antidiabetics.
• Avoid Wegovy in patients with a history of suicide attempts or active suicidality. Suicidality has been reported with other weight management products.
• Safety and effectiveness in children haven't been determined.
Dialyzable drug: Unknown.

PREGNANCY-LACTATION-REPRODUCTION

• Based on animal studies, drug may adversely affect a fetus. Poorly controlled diabetes, especially in patients who are pregnant, carries many risks. Use of glucagon-like peptide-1 receptor agonists isn't recommended for patients with type 2 diabetes planning pregnancy.
• Appropriate weight gain during pregnancy, even in patients who are overweight or obese, is recommended.
• Patients planning pregnancy should discontinue drug at least 2 months before conception.
• Register patients exposed to Wegovy during pregnancy at 1-800-727-6500.
• It isn't known if drug appears in human milk or how it affects an infant or milk production. Breastfeeding isn't recommended during treatment with oral semaglutide. Consider mother's clinical need and risks to the infant during treatment with injectable semaglutide.

NURSING CONSIDERATIONS

Boxed Warning Monitor patients for MTC or MEN 2. It isn't known if routine monitoring of serum calcitonin level or thyroid ultrasound can detect these cancers early. Further evaluate patients with elevated serum calcitonin level or thyroid nodules on physical exam or neck imaging. ◼
◔ *Alert:* Monitor patients for hypersensitivity reactions, including anaphylaxis and angioedema. Discontinue drug and treat appropriately if reaction occurs. Use cautiously in

patients with a history of hypersensitivity to another glucagon-like peptide-1 agonist.
• Monitor patients for pancreatitis (persistent severe abdominal pain that may radiate to the back or be accompanied by vomiting). For suspected pancreatitis, discontinue drug.
• Monitor patients for acute gallbladder disease. Rapid or substantial weight loss can increase the risk.
• Monitor patients with a history of diabetic retinopathy for disease progression.
• Monitor patients for acute kidney injury. Assess renal function at baseline and during dosage adjustments. Assess for nausea, vomiting, diarrhea, or dehydration, which are associated with worsening of renal function.
• Monitor glucose level and HbA$_{1c}$.
• Monitor glucose level before and periodically during treatment for weight loss in patients with type 2 diabetes.
• Monitor patients for signs and symptoms of hypoglycemia (confusion, irritability, shakiness, diaphoresis, hunger, palpitations, pallor, speech and motor dysfunction).
• Monitor HR periodically; drug may need to be discontinued for sustained increase in resting HR.
• Monitor patients taking drug for weight management for new or worsening depression, suicidality, or unusual changes in mood or behavior.
• *Look alike–sound alike:* Don't confuse semaglutide with sitagliptin.

PATIENT TEACHING
• Instruct patient to report all adverse reactions.
• Teach patient proper drug administration and storage.
• Tell patient how to manage missed doses.
• *Alert:* Caution patient never to share injection pen with another person, even if the needle is changed, due to risk of blood-borne pathogen transmission.
Boxed Warning Counsel patient on the risk of MTC and MEN 2 and to report signs and symptoms of thyroid tumors (neck mass, dysphagia, dyspnea, persistent hoarseness). ■
• Caution patient to discontinue drug and seek immediate medical attention for hypersensitivity reactions (difficulty breathing, throat or tongue swelling).
• Advise patient taking Wegovy to report new or worsening depression, suicidality, and other unusual changes in mood or behavior and to discontinue drug.

• Caution patient to immediately report signs and symptoms of pancreatitis and to discontinue drug.
• Instruct patient to report vision changes.
• Inform patient of the risk of kidney injury. Risk increases with risk of dehydration due to GI adverse effects. Instruct patient to take precautions to avoid fluid depletion and to report nausea, vomiting, diarrhea, or dehydration to prescriber. Advise patient that worsening renal impairment may require dialysis.
• Caution patient about the use of drug during pregnancy and while breastfeeding. Advise patient not to breastfeed while taking oral semaglutide. Encourage patient to discuss drug with prescriber before a planned pregnancy.
• Stress importance of adhering to proper diet and regular physical activity and that glucose and HbA$_{1c}$ levels and other lab tests will be monitored during therapy.
• Teach patient to recognize and manage hypoglycemia. Caution patient who is also taking insulin or insulin secretagogues about the increased risk of hypoglycemia.
• Tell patient to immediately report stresses to the body (fever, surgery, trauma, infection) because drug requirements may change.
• Tell patient that nausea, vomiting, and diarrhea are common at start of therapy but decrease over time for most patients.

serdexmethylphenidate–dexmethylphenidate
ser-dex-meth-il-FEN-i-date/
dex-meth-il-FEN-i-date

Azstarys

Therapeutic class: CNS stimulants
Pharmacologic class: Norepinephrine and dopamine reuptake inhibitors
Controlled substance schedule: II

AVAILABLE FORMS
Capsules: serdexmethylphenidate/dexmethylphenidate: 26.1 mg/5.2 mg, 39.2 mg/7.8 mg, 52.3 mg/10.4 mg

INDICATIONS & DOSAGES
➤ **ADHD**
Adults and children age 13 and older: Initially, serdexmethylphenidate 39.2 mg/dexmethylphenidate 7.8 mg PO once daily

in the morning. May increase after 1 week to maximum dosage of serdexmethylphenidate 52.3 mg/dexmethylphenidate 10.4 mg PO daily.

Children ages 6 to 12: Initially, serdexmethylphenidate 39.2 mg/dexmethylphenidate 7.8 mg PO once daily in the morning. May increase dose after 1 week, serdexmethylphenidate 52.3 mg/dexmethylphenidate 10.4 mg PO once daily, or decrease dose, serdexmethylphenidate 26.1 mg/dexmethylphenidate 5.2 mg PO daily, depending on response and tolerability. Maximum dosage, serdexmethylphenidate 52.3 mg/dexmethylphenidate 10.4 mg PO daily.

Adjust-a-dose: Reduce dosage or discontinue drug if paradoxical aggravation of ADHD symptoms or other adverse reactions occur. Periodically discontinue drug to assess child's condition. If no improvement after dosage adjustment over 1 month, discontinue drug.

ADMINISTRATION
PO
- Give without regard to meals.
- Have patient swallow capsule whole or mix capsule contents in 50 mL water or 2 tablespoons applesauce. Give entire mixture within 10 minutes. Don't store.
- If switching from another methylphenidate drug, discontinue that drug and initiate this drug using the dosage schedule above.
- Store at room temperature.

ACTION
Exact mechanism unknown.

Route	Onset	Peak	Duration
PO	Unknown	2–4.5 hr	Unknown

Half-life: Serdexmethylphenidate, 5.7 hours; dexmethylphenidate, 11.7 hours.

ADVERSE REACTIONS
CNS: anxiety, dizziness, dyskinesia, emotional lability, fever, insomnia, irritability. **CV:** chest pain, chest tightness, increased BP, palpitations, tachycardia. **GI:** abdominal pain, decreased appetite, dyspepsia, nausea, vomiting. **GU:** priapism. **Hematologic:** *pancytopenia, thrombocytopenia, thrombotic thrombocytopenic purpura.* **Hepatic:** increased liver enzyme levels. **Metabolic:** weight loss. **Musculoskeletal:** growth suppression. **Other:** hypersensitivity reactions.

INTERACTIONS
Drug-drug. *Antihypertensives (ACE inhibitors, ARBs, beta blockers, calcium channel blockers, centrally acting alpha-2 receptor agonists, potassium-sparing and thiazide diuretics):* May decrease effectiveness of antihypertensives. Monitor BP and adjust antihypertensive dosage as needed.

MAO inhibitors (isocarboxazid, linezolid, methylene blue, phenelzine, selegiline, tranylcypromine): May cause hypertensive crisis. Avoid use together or within 14 days of discontinuing MAO inhibitor.

Halogenated anesthetics (desflurane, enflurane, halothane, isoflurane, sevoflurane): May increase risk of sudden HTN and tachycardia during surgery. Avoid use on day of surgery.

Risperidone: May increase risk of extrapyramidal reaction when dosage of either drug is changed. Monitor patient for extrapyramidal reaction.

Serotonergic drugs (opioids, SSNRIs, SSRIs, TCAs): May increase risk of serotonin syndrome. Use together cautiously.

EFFECTS ON LAB TEST RESULTS
- May increase ALP, bilirubin, and liver enzyme levels.
- May decrease platelet count.
- May increase or decrease WBC count.

CONTRAINDICATIONS & CAUTIONS
Boxed Warning Drug and other CNS stimulants (methylphenidate-containing products, amphetamines) have high potential for abuse and dependence. Use cautiously in patients with history of drug dependence. ■
- Contraindicated in patients hypersensitive to drug or its components.
- Avoid use in patients with structural cardiac abnormalities, cardiomyopathy, heart rhythm abnormalities, CAD, or other serious heart problems. Sudden death, stroke, and MI have been reported with CNS stimulants.
- Drug may cause peripheral vasculopathy, including Raynaud phenomenon. Dosage may need to be reduced or drug discontinued.
- Drug may exacerbate signs and symptoms of behavior disturbance and thought disorder in patients with a preexisting psychotic disorder. Use cautiously.
- Drug may induce manic or mixed mood episode in patients with bipolar disorder. Use cautiously.

S

• Drug may cause psychotic or manic signs or symptoms in patients with no history of psychotic disorder. If signs or symptoms occur, consider discontinuing drug.

• Drug may increase risk of prolonged and painful erection (priapism), sometimes requiring surgical intervention.

• Drug may cause weight loss and slowed growth rates in children. Interrupt or discontinue therapy if these occur.

• Don't substitute drug for other methylphenidate products.

• Long-term efficacy of methylphenidate use in children hasn't been established.

• Safety and effectiveness in children younger than age 6 haven't been established.

• Drug hasn't been studied in patients age 65 and older.

Dialyzable drug: Unknown.

⚠ *Overdose S&S:* Nausea, vomiting, diarrhea, restlessness, anxiety, agitation, tremors, hyperreflexia, muscle twitching, seizures (may be followed by coma), euphoria, confusion, hallucinations, delirium, sweating, flushing, headache, hyperpyrexia, tachycardia, palpitations, cardiac arrhythmias, HTN, hypotension, tachypnea, mydriasis, dryness of mucous membranes, rhabdomyolysis.

PREGNANCY-LACTATION-REPRODUCTION

• There are no studies of use during pregnancy. It isn't known if drug increases risk of major birth defects, miscarriage, or adverse maternal or fetal outcomes.

• Use of CNS stimulants during pregnancy can cause vasoconstriction and decreased placental perfusion. Premature delivery and low birth weight have been reported in amphetamine-dependent patients.

• Enroll patients exposed to drug during pregnancy in the National Pregnancy Registry for Psychostimulants (1-866-961-2388).

• It isn't known if drug appears in human milk, or how drug affects milk production or infants who are breastfed. Before using during breastfeeding, consider benefits of therapy and risks to the infant.

NURSING CONSIDERATIONS

Boxed Warning Abuse and misuse may lead to addiction. Addiction may develop even when patient takes drug as prescribed. Monitor patient for signs and symptoms of abuse and dependence during therapy (increased HR, respiratory rate, BP; sweating; dilated pupils; hyperactivity; restlessness; insomnia; decreased appetite; loss of coordination; tremors; flushed skin; vomiting; abdominal pain). Anxiety, psychosis, hostility, aggression, and suicidality or homicidal ideation have also been observed. Maintain careful prescription records and periodically reevaluate need for use. ∎

Boxed Warning Drug may produce withdrawal syndrome during abrupt cessation, rapid dosage reduction, or administration of an antagonist. Withdrawal signs and symptoms include dysphoric mood; depression; fatigue; vivid, unpleasant dreams; insomnia or hypersomnia; increased appetite; and psychomotor retardation or agitation. ∎

• Assess patient for cardiac abnormalities (family history of sudden death, ventricular arrhythmia, cardiomyopathy).

• Screen patient for history of depressive symptoms, depression, bipolar disorder, and family history of suicide.

• Monitor patient for tolerance to drug.

• Monitor patient for HTN and tachycardia.

• Monitor patient for exertional chest pain, unexplained syncope, or arrhythmias.

• Carefully observe patient for digital changes and signs and symptoms of peripheral vasculopathy, including Raynaud phenomenon. Refer patient to rheumatologist if indicated.

• Monitor height and weight in children.

PATIENT TEACHING

Boxed Warning Warn patient and caregiver that drug is a federally controlled substance. Stress drug's potential for abuse or dependence. ∎

• Instruct patient on proper drug administration and storage.

• Instruct patient and caregiver to dispose of remaining, unused, or expired drug in accordance with local requirements or drug take-back programs.

• Tell patient not to give drug to anyone else.

• Advise patient and caregiver about serious CV risks (sudden death, MI, stroke) and to immediately report exertional chest pain or unexplained syncope.

• Inform patient about risk of increased HR and BP and need for frequent monitoring during therapy.

• Tell patient about risk of peripheral vasculopathy, including Raynaud phenomenon, and to report new numbness, pain, skin color

---

change, sensitivity to temperature in fingers or toes, or unexplained wounds on fingers or toes.

• Inform patient and caregiver that at recommended doses, drug can cause psychotic or manic symptoms, even in patients with no history of psychotic disorders or mania. Tell patient to report new or worsening symptoms, such as mania, hearing voices, or seeing or believing things that aren't real.

• Inform male patient and caregiver of possible risk of priapism and to seek immediate medical attention if this occurs.

• Advise child and caregiver of risk of weight loss and slow growth rate.

• Instruct patient of childbearing potential to report pregnancy or plans to become pregnant during therapy.

• Tell patient who is breastfeeding to monitor infant for agitation, poor feeding, and reduced weight gain.

• Inform patient and caregiver that therapy may be stopped periodically to assess ADHD symptoms.

sertraline hydrochloride
SIR-trah-leen

Zoloft🔎

Therapeutic class: Antidepressants
Pharmacologic class: SSRIs

AVAILABLE FORMS
Capsules 🅾🅽🅲: 150 mg, 200 mg
Oral concentrate*: 20 mg/mL
Tablets: 25 mg, 50 mg, 100 mg

INDICATIONS & DOSAGES
Adjust-a-dose (for all indications): If dosage changes are needed, increase by 25 to 50 mg (except when used for premenstrual dysmorphic disorder) at intervals of no less than 1 week. For patients with mild hepatic impairment (Child-Pugh score 5 or 6), both the recommended starting dosage and therapeutic range are half the recommended daily dosage.

➤ **Depression**
Adults: 50 mg tablet or oral concentrate PO daily. Adjust dosage weekly as needed and tolerated; dosage ranges from 50 to 200 mg daily. May switch to capsule form when dosage is 150 or 200 mg daily.

➤ **OCD**
Adults: 50 mg tablet or oral concentrate PO once daily. If patient doesn't improve, increase dosage weekly, up to 200 mg daily. May switch to capsule form when dosage is 150 or 200 mg daily.
Children ages 6 to 17: Initially, 25 mg tablet or oral concentrate PO daily in children ages 6 to 12, or 50 mg PO daily in adolescents ages 13 to 17. Increase dosage weekly, as needed, up to 200 mg daily. May switch to capsule form when dosage is 150 or 200 mg daily.

➤ **Panic disorder**
Adults: Initially, 25 mg tablet or oral concentrate PO daily for 3 to 7 days; then increase to 50 mg PO daily. If patient doesn't improve, increase dose to maximum of 200 mg daily.

➤ **PTSD**
Adults: Initially, 25 mg PO once daily. Increase to 50 mg PO once daily after 1 week. Increase as needed at weekly intervals to a maximum of 200 mg daily. Maintain patient on lowest effective dose.

➤ **Premenstrual dysphoric disorder**
Adults: Initially, 50 mg PO daily either continuously or only during the luteal phase of the menstrual cycle. If patient doesn't respond, may increase dose 50 mg per menstrual cycle, up to 150 mg daily for continuous use or up to 100 mg daily for luteal-phase doses. If a 100-mg daily dose has been established with luteal-phase dosing, give 50 mg daily for 2 to 3 days at the beginning of each luteal phase before increasing to 100 mg.

➤ **Social anxiety disorder**
Adults: Initially, 25 mg PO once daily. Increase dosage to 50 mg PO once daily after 1 week of therapy. Dose range is 50 to 200 mg daily. Adjust to the lowest effective dosage and periodically reassess patient to determine the need for long-term treatment.

➤ **Generalized anxiety disorder ♦**
Adults: Initially, 25 mg once daily. May increase based on response and tolerability in increments of 25 to 50 mg at intervals of 1 to 2 weeks or more. Usual dose, 50 to 150 mg/day. Maximum dose, 200 mg/day.

ADMINISTRATION
PO
• Give drug without regard for food.
• Don't use oral concentrate dropper, which is made of rubber, for patient with latex allergy.

S

• Dilute oral concentrate before administration. Mix oral concentrate with 4 oz (120 mL) of water, ginger ale, lemon-lime soda, lemonade, or orange juice only, and give immediately.

• Patient must swallow capsules whole. Don't crush, open, or allow patient to chew capsules.

ACTION

Thought to be linked to drug's inhibition of CNS neuronal reuptake of serotonin.

Route	Onset	Peak	Duration
PO	1 wk	4–8 hr	Unknown

Half-life: 62 to 104 hours.

ADVERSE REACTIONS

CNS: fatigue, headache, tremor, dizziness, insomnia, somnolence, anxiety, agitation, hyperkinesia, aggression. **CV:** palpitations. **EENT:** visual disturbances, blurred vision, mydriasis, dry mouth, epistaxis. **GI:** nausea, diarrhea, dyspepsia, vomiting, constipation, thirst, flatulence, anorexia, abdominal pain, decreased appetite. **GU:** male sexual dysfunction, decreased libido (both genders), urinary incontinence. **Metabolic:** weight loss. **Musculoskeletal:** myalgia, arthralgia. **Skin:** rash, pruritus, diaphoresis, alopecia, purpura.

INTERACTIONS

Drug-drug. *Agents with antiplatelet properties (NSAIDs, P2Y12 inhibitors, SSRIs), aspirin, clopidogrel, heparin:* May enhance antiplatelet effect and bleeding risk. Monitor therapy.

Amphetamines, buspirone, dextromethorphan, dihydroergotamine, lithium salts, meperidine, other SSRIs or SSNRIs (duloxetine, venlafaxine), sumatriptan, TCAs, tramadol, trazodone, tryptophan: May increase the risk of serotonin syndrome. Avoid combinations of drugs that increase the availability of serotonin in the CNS; monitor patient closely if used together.

Apixaban, dabigatran, edoxaban, rivaroxaban: May increase bleeding risk. Monitor patient carefully.

Cimetidine: May decrease clearance of sertraline. Monitor patient closely.

CYP2D6 substrates (atomoxetine, desipramine, dextromethorphan, flecainide, metoprolol, nebivolol, perphenazine, propafenone, thioridazine, tolterodine, venlafaxine): May increase exposure of the substrate. If concurrent use is needed, decrease the substrate dosage. If sertraline is discontinued, an increased substrate dosage may be needed.

Disulfiram: Oral concentrate contains alcohol, which may react with drug. Use together is contraindicated.

Diuretics: May increase risk of hyponatremia. Monitor patient closely.

Drugs that prolong QTc interval (amiodarone, droperidol, erythromycin, methadone, moxifloxacin, procainamide, sotalol, tacrolimus, ziprasidone): May increase risk of QTc-interval prolongation or ventricular arrhythmias, including torsades de pointes. Avoid use together.

Fosphenytoin, phenytoin: May increase phenytoin concentration. Monitor phenytoin level and reduce phenytoin dosage if needed.

Linezolid, methylene blue: May cause serotonin syndrome. Use extreme caution and monitor patient closely. If treatment is necessary, discontinue sertraline before treatment with linezolid or methylene blue.

MAO inhibitors (phenelzine, selegiline, tranylcypromine): May cause serotonin syndrome or signs and symptoms resembling NMS. Use of sertraline with or within 2 weeks of an MAO inhibitor is contraindicated.

Pimozide: May increase risk of QT-interval prolongation and ventricular arrhythmias. Use together is contraindicated.

Triptans: May cause serotonin syndrome (restlessness, hallucinations, loss of coordination, fast heartbeat, rapid changes in BP, increased body temperature, hyperreflexia, nausea, vomiting, and diarrhea) or NMS-like reactions. Use cautiously, with close monitoring, especially at the start of treatment and during dosage adjustments.

Warfarin, other highly protein-bound drugs: May increase level of sertraline or other highly protein-bound drug. May prolong PT or increase INR. Monitor patient closely; monitor PT and INR.

Drug-herb. *Alfalfa, anise, bilberry:* May increase risk of bleeding. Consider alternative agents.

St. John's wort: May cause additive effects and serotonin syndrome. Discourage use together.

Drug-lifestyle. *Alcohol use:* May increase psychomotor impairment. Discourage use together.

Reactions in bold italics are *life-threatening*. Interactions may have a *rapid onset* or a ***delayed onset***.

EFFECTS ON LAB TEST RESULTS
• May increase cholesterol, TSH, ALT, and AST levels.
• May decrease sodium level.
• May increase or decrease glucose level.
• May show false-positive urine immunoassay screening tests for benzodiazepines.

CONTRAINDICATIONS & CAUTIONS
• Contraindicated in patients hypersensitive to drug or its components.
• Use cautiously in patients at risk for suicide and in those with seizure disorders, major affective disorder, or diseases or conditions that affect metabolism or hemodynamic responses.
• Screen patients for bipolar disorder, as drug may activate manic or hypomanic states.
• Use cautiously in older adults and patients who are volume-depleted. Drug may increase risk of hyponatremia.
• Avoid use in patients with angle-closure glaucoma.
• Use cautiously in patients at risk for QT-interval prolongation.
❸ *Alert:* Sertraline isn't approved for use in children except those with OCD.
❸ *Alert:* Drug may increase risk of bleeding, especially with concomitant use of aspirin, NSAIDs, other antiplatelet drugs, warfarin, and other anticoagulants.
Dialyzable drug: Unknown.
⚠ *Overdose S&S:* Somnolence, vomiting, tachycardia, nausea, dizziness, agitation, tremor, bradycardia, bundle-branch block, coma, seizures, delirium, hallucinations, HTN, hypotension, manic reactions, pancreatitis, prolonged QT interval, serotonin syndrome, stupor, syncope.

PREGNANCY-LACTATION-REPRODUCTION
• There are no adequate studies during pregnancy. Use only if potential benefit justifies fetal risk.
• Neonates exposed to sertraline and other SSRIs or SSNRIs late in the third trimester have developed complications requiring prolonged hospitalization, respiratory support, and tube feeding.
• Neonates exposed to SSRIs during pregnancy may be at increased risk for persistent pulmonary HTN of the newborn.
• Enroll patients exposed to drug during pregnancy in the National Pregnancy Registry for Antidepressants (1-866-961-2388 or https://womensmentalhealth.org/research/pregnancyregistry/antidepressants/).
• It isn't known if drug appears in human milk. Use cautiously during breastfeeding.

NURSING CONSIDERATIONS
• Record mood changes. Monitor patient for suicidality, and allow only a minimum supply of drug.
Boxed Warning Drug may increase the risk of suicidality in children, adolescents, and young adults with major depressive disorder or other psychiatric disorder. ■
Boxed Warning Closely monitor all patients being treated with antidepressants for clinical worsening, suicidality, and unusual changes in behavior, especially during initial few months of treatment or at times of dosage increases or decreases. ■
• Assess patients for sexual dysfunction at baseline and periodically during treatment. SSRIs may cause signs and symptoms of sexual dysfunction and patients may not spontaneously report changes in sexual function.
• Monitor patients for hyponatremia (headache, difficulty concentrating, memory impairment, confusion, weakness, unsteadiness, falls, hallucinations, seizure, respiratory arrest).
❸ *Alert:* If linezolid or methylene blue must be given, stop sertraline and monitor patient for serotonin toxicity for 2 weeks, or until 24 hours after the last dose of methylene blue or linezolid, whichever comes first. May resume sertraline 24 hours after last dose of methylene blue or linezolid.
❸ *Alert:* Combining triptans with an SSRI or an SSNRI may cause serotonin syndrome or NMS-like reactions. Signs and symptoms of serotonin syndrome may include restlessness, hallucinations, loss of coordination, fast heartbeat, rapid changes in BP, increased body temperature, overactive reflexes, nausea, vomiting, and diarrhea. Serotonin syndrome may be more likely to occur when starting or increasing the dose of triptan, SSRI, or SSNRI.
• Gradual dosage reduction is recommended when stopping treatment. Monitor patient for discontinuation syndrome (nausea, diaphoresis, dysphoric mood, agitation, dizziness, paresthesia, tremor, insomnia, tinnitus, seizures, lethargy, confusion), especially after abrupt end of treatment.
• *Look alike–sound alike:* Don't confuse sertraline with cetirizine.

S

♣Canada   ◇OTC   ♦Off-label use   ✐Photoguide   ⊜Do not crush   *Liquid contains alcohol   ▩ Genetic

PATIENT TEACHING

Boxed Warning Advise families and caregivers to closely observe patient for increased suicidality. ∎

• Instruct patient in safe drug administration.

❂ *Alert:* Teach patient to recognize and immediately report signs and symptoms of serotonin syndrome.

• Advise patient to use caution when performing hazardous tasks that require alertness.

• Tell patient to avoid alcohol and to consult prescriber before taking OTC drugs.

• Advise patient to avoid stopping drug abruptly and to discuss a gradual taper plan with prescriber.

---

sevelamer carbonate
se-VEL-a-mer

Renvela

sevelamer hydrochloride
Renagel

Therapeutic class: Hypophosphatemics
Pharmacologic class: Polymeric phosphate binders

AVAILABLE FORMS
sevelamer carbonate
Oral suspension: 0.8-g, 2.4-g packets
Tablets (film-coated) ⬛: 800 mg
sevelamer hydrochloride
Tablets (film-coated) ⬛: 400 mg, 800 mg

INDICATIONS & DOSAGES
➤ **To control phosphorus level in patients with chronic kidney disease on dialysis**
Adults not taking a phosphate binder: Initially, 800 to 1,600 mg (one to two 800-mg tablets, or two to four 400-mg tablets, or one to two 0.8-g packets) PO with each meal, based on phosphorus level. If phosphorus level is greater than 5.5 mg/dL and less than 7.5 mg/dL, start with 800 mg t.i.d. with meals. If phosphorus level is greater than or equal to 7.5 mg/dL and less than 9 mg/dL, start with two 800-mg tablets t.i.d., or three 400-mg tablets t.i.d. with meals. If phosphorus level is 9 mg/dL or more, start with 1,600 mg t.i.d. (two 800-mg tablets, or four 400-mg tablets, or two 0.8-g packets) with meals.

Adults switching from calcium acetate: Initially, if taking one 667-mg calcium acetate tablet per meal, start with 800 mg PO per meal. If taking two 667-mg calcium acetate tablets per meal, start with two 800-mg tablets, or three 400-mg tablets, or two 0.8-g packets per meal. If taking three 667-mg calcium acetate tablets per meal, start with three 800-mg tablets, or five 400-mg tablets, or one 2.4-g packet per meal.

Adjust-a-dose: If phosphorus level is greater than 5.5 mg/dL, increase by one tablet per meal at 2-week intervals. If phosphorus level is 3.5 to 5.5 mg/dL, maintain current dose. If phosphorus level is less than 3.5 mg/dL, decrease dose by one tablet per meal.

Children age 6 and older not taking a phosphate binder (Renvela only): Initially, 800 to 1,600 mg PO t.i.d. with meals, based on BSA. For BSA of 0.75 m^2 to less than 1.2 m^2, give 800 mg per meal or snack. Increase or decrease by 400 mg/dose at 2-week intervals as needed to achieve target levels. For BSA of 1.2 m^2 or greater, give 1,600 mg per meal or snack. Increase or decrease by 800 mg/dose at 2-week intervals as needed to achieve target levels.

ADMINISTRATION
PO
• Don't cut, crush, or allow patient to chew tablets.

• Mix powder packets with appropriate amount of water as directed. Stir mixture vigorously (it doesn't dissolve) and have patient drink entire preparation within 30 minutes.

• May also premix entire contents of powder packet with a small amount of food or beverage and have patient consume within 30 minutes as part of a meal. Don't heat or add to heated foods or liquids.

• Give drug with meals.

• Drug may bind to other drugs and decrease their bioavailability. Give other drugs 1 hour before or 3 hours after this drug.

ACTION
Inhibits intestinal phosphate absorption and decreases phosphorus levels.

Route	Onset	Peak	Duration
PO	Unknown	Unknown	Unknown

Half-life: Unknown.

Reactions in bold italics are *life-threatening*. Interactions may have a *rapid onset* or a ***delayed onset***.

ADVERSE REACTIONS

GI: diarrhea, dyspepsia, vomiting, nausea, constipation, flatulence, abdominal pain; peritonitis (patients on peritoneal dialysis).

INTERACTIONS

Drug-drug. *Ciprofloxacin, other quinolones:* May decrease effectiveness of ciprofloxacin or other quinolones. Give quinolones either 2 hours before or 6 hours after sevelamer.
Mycophenolate: May decrease mycophenolic acid plasma concentration, decreasing effectiveness. Administer sevelamer 2 hours after mycophenolate.
Thyroid hormones (levothyroxine): May decrease effectiveness of hormones. Separate administration times by at least several hours. Consider therapy modification.

EFFECTS ON LAB TEST RESULTS

• May decrease phosphorus level.

CONTRAINDICATIONS & CAUTIONS

• Contraindicated in patients hypersensitive to drug or its components and in those with hypophosphatemia or bowel obstruction.
• Use cautiously in patient with dysphagia, swallowing disorders, severe GI motility disorders, or major GI tract surgery.
• May reduce absorption of vitamins D, E, and K and folic acid.
Dializable drug: Unknown.

PREGNANCY-LACTATION-REPRODUCTION

• There are no adequate studies during pregnancy. Use only if potential benefit justifies fetal risk. Drug isn't absorbed systemically.
• Drug may decrease serum levels of fat-soluble vitamins and folic acid in patients who are pregnant. Consider supplementation if clinically indicated.
• No information is available regarding use in breastfeeding.

NURSING CONSIDERATIONS

• Monitor serum chemistries, including phosphorus, calcium, and bicarbonate levels.
• Monitor parathyroid hormone level.
• *Look alike–sound alike:* Don't confuse Renvela with Renagel.

PATIENT TEACHING

• Instruct patient to take with meals and to adhere to prescribed diet.

🛈 *Alert:* Inform patient that tablets must be taken whole because contents expand in water. Warn patient not to cut, crush, or chew tablets.
• Advise patient to take reconstituted oral suspension immediately or within 30 minutes.
• Tell patient to check with pharmacist before taking other drugs at the same time as sevelamer.
• Inform patient about common adverse reactions, including constipation that, if left untreated, may lead to severe complications.

---

sildenafil citrate
sil-DEN-a-fill

Revatio, Viagra🔗

Therapeutic class: Erectile dysfunction drugs
Pharmacologic class: PDE5 inhibitors

AVAILABLE FORMS

Injection: 10 mg/12.5 mL single-use vials
Oral suspension (Revatio): 10 mg/mL
Tablets (Revatio): 20 mg
Tablets (Viagra): 25 mg, 50 mg, 100 mg

INDICATIONS & DOSAGES

➤ **Erectile dysfunction (Viagra only)**
Adult men younger than age 65: 50 mg PO, as needed, 30 minutes to 4 hours (usually about 1 hour) before sexual activity. Dosage range is 25 to 100 mg based on effectiveness and tolerance. Maximum is one dose daily.
Adult men age 65 and older: 25 mg PO, as needed, about 1 hour before sexual activity. Dosage may be adjusted based on patient response.
Adjust-a-dose: For adults with hepatic or severe renal impairment (CrCl less than 30 mL/minute), 25 mg PO about 1 hour before sexual activity. May adjust dosage based on patient response.
➤ **To improve exercise ability and delay clinical worsening in patients with WHO Group 1 PAH (Revatio only)**
Adults: 5 or 20 mg PO t.i.d., 4 to 6 hours apart. Or, 2.5 or 10 mg IV bolus t.i.d.

ADMINISTRATION

🛈 *Alert:* Don't substitute Viagra for Revatio because there isn't an equivalent dose.

S

PO

- Give without regard for food.
- Don't give to patients taking nitrates.
- Follow manufacturer's directions for reconstitution of powder for oral suspension.
- Shake suspension for at least 10 seconds before use; don't mix with other medications.
- Label Revatio suspension with expiration date, which is 60 days from date of reconstitution.

IV

▼ Inspect solution visually for particulate matter and discoloration before administering.

▼ Don't give to patients taking nitrates.

▼ Ten-mg IV dose is equivalent to 20-mg oral dose (Revatio).

▼ **Incompatibilities:** None listed by manufacturer. Consult a drug incompatibility reference for more information.

ACTION

When used for erectile dysfunction, drug increases effect of nitric oxide by inhibiting PDE5. When sexual stimulation causes local release of nitric oxide, inhibition of PDE5 by sildenafil causes increased levels of cyclic guanosine monophosphate (cGMP) in the corpus cavernosum, resulting in smooth muscle relaxation and inflow of blood to the corpus cavernosum. In PAH, drug increases cGMP level by preventing its breakdown by phosphodiesterase, prolonging smooth muscle relaxation of the pulmonary vasculature, which leads to vasodilation.

Route	Onset	Peak	Duration
PO	15–30 min	30–120 min	4 hr
IV	Unknown	Unknown	Unknown

Half-life: 4 hours.

ADVERSE REACTIONS

CNS: headache, *seizures,* anxiety, dizziness, insomnia, somnolence, paresthesia, fever.
CV: flushing. **EENT:** visual disturbance (temporary vision loss, diplopia, photophobia, altered color perception, blurred vision), nasal congestion, epistaxis, rhinitis, sinusitis.
GI: dyspepsia, diarrhea, gastritis, nausea.
GU: UTI. **Musculoskeletal:** back pain, myalgia. **Respiratory:** dyspnea. **Skin:** erythema, rash.

INTERACTIONS

Drug-drug. *Alpha blockers:* May cause symptomatic hypotension. Consider dosage reduction.

Amyl nitrate: May increase vasodilatory effects. Don't use together.
Antihypertensives: May increase hypotension. Use cautiously.
Bosentan: May decrease sildenafil level and increase bosentan level. Monitor patient closely for bosentan adverse reactions.
CYP3A inhibitors (erythromycin, itraconazole, ketoconazole, protease inhibitors, ritonavir, saquinavir): May increase sildenafil level, increasing risk of adverse events, including hypotension, visual changes, and priapism. Reduce Viagra starting dose to 25 mg when used with itraconazole, ketoconazole, erythromycin, or protease inhibitors. When used with ritonavir, atazanavir, or darunavir, maximum Viagra dose is 25 mg in a 48-hour period. Use with Revatio isn't recommended.
CYP450 inducers, rifampin: May reduce sildenafil level. Monitor effect.
Guanylate cyclase (GC) stimulators (riociguat): May potentiate hypotensive effects of GC stimulators. Use together is contraindicated.
Hepatic isoenzyme inhibitors (cimetidine, erythromycin, itraconazole, ketoconazole): May reduce sildenafil clearance. Avoid using together.
Isosorbide, nitroglycerin: May cause severe hypotension. Use of nitrates in any form with sildenafil is contraindicated.
Other PDE5 inhibitors: May increase risk of hypotension. Don't use together.
Vitamin K antagonists: May increase risk of bleeding (primarily epistaxis). Monitor patient.
Drug-herb. *St. John's wort:* May decrease sildenafil level. Don't use together.
Drug-food. *Grapefruit:* May increase drug level, while delaying absorption. Advise patient to avoid using together.
Drug-lifestyle. *Alcohol use:* Excessive alcohol intake may increase risk of hypotension. Advise patient to avoid or limit alcohol consumption.

EFFECTS ON LAB TEST RESULTS

- May increase sodium, uric acid, and liver enzyme levels.
- May increase or decrease glucose level.

CONTRAINDICATIONS & CAUTIONS

- Contraindicated in patients hypersensitive to drug or its components.

Reactions in bold italics are *life-threatening.* Interactions may have a *rapid onset* or a *delayed onset.*

• Use cautiously in patients age 65 and older; in patients with hepatic or severe renal impairment, retinitis pigmentosa, bleeding disorders, or active peptic ulcer disease; in those who have suffered an MI, stroke, or life-threatening arrhythmia within past 6 months; in those with history of cardiac failure, CAD, uncontrolled high or low BP, or anatomic deformation of the penis (such as angulation, cavernosal fibrosis, or Peyronie disease); and in those with conditions that may predispose them to priapism (such as sickle cell anemia, multiple myeloma, or leukemia).

• Vision loss, including permanent loss of vision, has been reported in patients taking drug for erectile dysfunction and may be a sign of nonarteritic anterior ischemic optic neuropathy (NAION). Risk may increase with history of vision loss. Other risk factors for NAION include low cup-to-disk ratio ("crowded disk"), CAD, diabetes, HTN, hyperlipidemia, smoking, and age older than 50.

• Pulmonary vasodilators used to treat PAH can worsen the CV status of patients with pulmonary veno-occlusive disease (PVOD). Use in patients with PVOD isn't recommended. If pulmonary edema occurs after drug is administered for PAH, consider the possibility of PVOD.

• Safe and effective use of drug to treat PAH in patients with sickle cell anemia hasn't been established. Drug may increase risk of vaso-occlusive crises requiring hospitalization in patients with sickle cell disease.

• Safe use of drug to treat PAH in children hasn't been established. Use isn't recommended, particularly prolonged use, due to increased mortality.

• Decreased hearing and hearing loss with or without tinnitus and dizziness have been reported. Obtain prompt medical attention for hearing loss.

Dialyzable drug: Unlikely.

PREGNANCY-LACTATION-REPRODUCTION

• Viagra isn't indicated for use in women. There are no adequate studies during pregnancy or breastfeeding.

• Information regarding use of drug to treat PAH during pregnancy is limited. Current guidelines recommend that women with PAH use effective contraception and avoid pregnancy.

• It isn't known if Revatio appears in human milk. Use cautiously during breastfeeding.

NURSING CONSIDERATIONS

⚠️ *Alert:* Systemic vasodilatory properties cause transient decreases in supine BP and cardiac output (about 2 hours after ingestion).

• The serious CV events linked to this drug's use in erectile dysfunction mainly involve patients with underlying CV disease who are at increased risk for cardiac effects related to sexual activity.

• Patients with PAH caused by connective tissue disease are more prone to epistaxis during therapy than those with primary pulmonary HTN.

• IV use is for patients with PAH temporarily unable to take oral medications.

• *Look alike–sound alike:* Don't confuse Viagra with Allegra.

PATIENT TEACHING

• Instruct patient in safe drug administration.

• Caution patient to take drug only as prescribed.

• Advise patient that drug shouldn't be used with nitrates or GC stimulators under any circumstances. Revatio and Viagra or other PDE5 inhibitors used for erectile dysfunction shouldn't be used together.

• Advise patient of potential cardiac risk of sexual activity, especially in presence of CV risk factors. Instruct patient to notify prescriber and refrain from further activity if such symptoms as chest pain, dizziness, or nausea occur when starting sexual activity.

• Warn patient that erections lasting longer than 4 hours and priapism (painful erections lasting longer than 6 hours) may occur; tell patient to seek immediate medical attention if either of these occurs. Penile tissue damage and permanent loss of potency may result if priapism isn't treated immediately.

• Inform patient that drug used for erectile dysfunction doesn't protect against sexually transmitted diseases; advise patient to use protective measures such as condoms.

• Advise patient receiving HIV medications of the increased risk of sildenafil adverse events, including low BP, visual changes, and priapism, and to promptly report such symptoms to prescriber. Tell patient not to exceed 25 mg of sildenafil.

• Inform patient that maximum benefit can be expected less than 2 hours after ingestion.

• Inform patient that impairment of color discrimination (blue, green) may occur and to avoid hazardous activities that rely on color discrimination.

S

• Instruct patient to immediately report vision or hearing changes.

---

silodosin
SI-lo-doe-sin

Rapaflo

Therapeutic class: BPH drugs
Pharmacologic class: Alpha₁ blockers

AVAILABLE FORMS
Capsules ⓞⓝⓒ: 4 mg, 8 mg

INDICATIONS & DOSAGES
➤ **To improve symptoms of BPH**
Men: 8 mg PO once daily.
Adjust-a-dose: For patients with CrCl of 30 to 50 mL/minute, give 4 mg PO once daily.

ADMINISTRATION
PO
• Give drug once daily with a meal.
• For patients who can't swallow capsules, contents of capsule may be sprinkled on a tablespoonful of applesauce (not hot), swallowed within 5 minutes without chewing, and followed with 8 oz (240 mL) of cool water to ensure complete swallowing of the powder. Don't store for future use.

ACTION
Causes relaxation of smooth muscles in the prostate and bladder tissues by antagonizing postsynaptic alpha₁ adrenoreceptors, thereby improving urine flow and reducing signs and symptoms of BPH.

Route	Onset	Peak	Duration
PO	Unknown	3 hr	Unknown

Half-life: About 13 hours.

ADVERSE REACTIONS
CNS: asthenia, dizziness, headache, insomnia. **CV:** orthostatic hypotension. **EENT:** nasal congestion, nasopharyngitis, rhinorrhea, sinusitis. **GI:** abdominal pain, diarrhea. **GU:** retrograde ejaculation.

INTERACTIONS
Drug-drug. *Alpha blockers:* May increase risk of symptomatic hypotension. Avoid use together.

Antihypertensives: May cause dizziness and orthostatic hypotension. Use together cautiously and monitor patient for adverse reactions.
Moderate CYP3A4 inhibitors (diltiazem, erythromycin, verapamil): May increase silodosin level. Use together cautiously.
PDE5 inhibitors (sildenafil, tadalafil): May cause symptomatic hypotension. Monitor patient closely.
Strong CYP3A4 inhibitors (clarithromycin, itraconazole, ketoconazole, ritonavir): May increase silodosin level. Use together is contraindicated.
Strong P-gp/ABCB1 inhibitors (cyclosporine, ketoconazole, ritonavir, verapamil): May increase silodosin level. Use together isn't recommended.
Drug-herb. *St. John's wort:* May decrease silodosin level and its effects. Consider modifying therapy.

EFFECTS ON LAB TEST RESULTS
• May increase PSA level.

CONTRAINDICATIONS & CAUTIONS
• Contraindicated in patients hypersensitive to drug or its components and in those with severe renal or hepatic impairment.
• Drug isn't indicated to treat HTN.
• Safety and effectiveness in children haven't been established.
Dialyzable drug: Unlikely.
⚠ *Overdose S&S:* Orthostatic hypotension.

PREGNANCY-LACTATION-REPRODUCTION
• Drug isn't approved for use in women.
• Drug may cause reversible decrease in male fertility based on animal studies.

NURSING CONSIDERATIONS
• Because BPH and prostate cancer cause similar signs and symptoms, prostate cancer should be ruled out before the start of silodosin therapy.
• Monitor patient for orthostatic hypotension. Carefully monitor older adults for hypotension; risk of orthostatic hypotension increases with age.
• Current or previous use of an alpha blocker may predispose patient to floppy-iris syndrome during cataract surgery.

Reactions in bold italics are *life-threatening*. Interactions may have a *rapid onset* or a ***delayed onset***.

PATIENT TEACHING
• Instruct patient in safe drug administration.
• Warn patient about possible hypotension, and explain that it may cause dizziness.
• Caution patient against driving or operating hazardous machinery until drug's effects are known.
• Advise patient who needs cataract surgery to inform ophthalmologist about taking silodosin.
• Inform patient about the possibility of retrograde ejaculation, which is reversible upon drug discontinuation and doesn't pose a safety concern.

---

simvastatin ☒
sim-va-STAT-in

FloLipid, Zocor🖉

Therapeutic class: Antilipemics
Pharmacologic class: HMG-CoA reductase inhibitors

AVAILABLE FORMS
Oral suspension: 20 mg/5 mL, 40 mg/5 mL
Tablets: 5 mg, 10 mg, 20 mg, 40 mg, 80 mg

INDICATIONS & DOSAGES
Adjust-a-dose (for all indications): In patients with severe renal insufficiency, start with 5 mg PO daily.
➤ **To reduce risk of death from CV disease and CV events in patients at high risk for coronary events; to reduce total and LDL cholesterol, apolipoprotein B, and triglyceride levels and increase HDL cholesterol level in patients with primary hyperlipidemia and mixed dyslipidemia; to reduce triglyceride levels; to reduce triglyceride levels and VLDL cholesterol level in patients with dysbetalipoproteinemia**
Adults: Initially, 10 to 20 mg PO daily in evening. In patients at high risk for a CAD event due to existing CAD, diabetes, PVD, or history of stroke, the recommended initial dose is 40 mg PO daily. Adjust dosage every 4 weeks based on patient tolerance and response. Patients unable to achieve their LDL-cholesterol goals utilizing simvastatin 40 mg shouldn't be titrated to 80-mg dose but should be placed on alternative LDL-cholesterol lowering treatment.

➤ **To reduce total and LDL cholesterol levels in patients with homozygous familial hypercholesterolemia** ☒
Adults: 40 mg PO daily in evening.
➤ **Heterozygous familial hypercholesterolemia in boys and postmenarchal girls** ☒
Children ages 10 to 17: Give 10 mg PO once daily in the evening. Maximum, 40 mg daily.

ADMINISTRATION
PO
• Give drug in the evening.
• Give oral suspension in the evening on an empty stomach. Shake bottle well for 20 seconds before using.

ACTION
Inhibits HMG-CoA reductase, an early (and rate-limiting) step in cholesterol biosynthesis.

Route	Onset	Peak	Duration
PO	Unknown	1–2 hr	Unknown

Half-life: Unknown.

ADVERSE REACTIONS
CNS: asthenia, headache, insomnia, vertigo. **CV:** edema, atrial fibrillation. **EENT:** sinusitis. **GI:** abdominal pain, constipation, gastritis, nausea. **GU:** UTI. **Metabolic:** diabetes. **Hepatic:** increased transaminase levels. **Musculoskeletal:** myalgia. **Respiratory:** URI, bronchitis. **Skin:** eczema.

INTERACTIONS
Drug-drug. *Amiodarone, amlodipine, ranolazine:* May increase risk of myopathy and rhabdomyolysis. Don't exceed 20 mg simvastatin daily.
Azole antifungals (fluconazole, itraconazole, ketoconazole), **macrolides (azithromycin, clarithromycin, erythromycin):** May increase simvastatin level and adverse effects. Avoid using together or, if it can't be avoided, suspend simvastatin therapy for course of treatment.
Bile acid sequestrants (cholestyramine, colestipol): May decrease GI absorption of simvastatin. Separate administration times by at least 4 hours.
Colchicine: May increase risk of myopathy and rhabdomyolysis. Monitor patient closely.
Cyclosporine, danazol, gemfibrozil: May increase risk of myopathy and rhabdomyolysis. Use together is contraindicated.

S

Daptomycin: May increase risk of myopathy and rhabdomyolysis. Temporarily suspend simvastatin for course of daptomycin treatment.

Digoxin: May slightly increase digoxin level. Closely monitor digoxin levels at the start of simvastatin therapy.

Dronedarone, diltiazem, verapamil: May increase risk of myopathy and rhabdomyolysis. Don't exceed 10 mg simvastatin daily.

Efavirenz, rifampin: May decrease simvastatin level. Monitor effectiveness.

Fibrates (other than gemfibrozil): Increase risk of myopathy. Use cautiously together.

Hepatotoxic drugs: May increase risk for hepatotoxicity. Avoid using together.

Lomitapide: May increase risk of myopathy or rhabdomyolysis. Reduce simvastatin dosage by 50% when starting lomitapide; don't exceed simvastatin 20 mg/day (or 40 mg/day for patients who previously tolerated simvastatin 80 mg/day for 1 year or more without muscle toxicity).

☒ *Niacin:* May increase risk of myopathy and rhabdomyolysis with niacin dose of 1 g/day or more. Patients of Chinese descent and possibly others of Asian descent shouldn't receive simvastatin with lipid-modifying dose of niacin-containing products.

Strong CYP3A4 inhibitors (nefazodone, protease inhibitors [amprenavir, atazanavir, darunavir, fosamprenavir, lopinavir-ritonavir, nelfinavir, ritonavir, saquinavir]): May inhibit metabolism of simvastatin and increase risk of adverse effects, including rhabdomyolysis. Use together is contraindicated.

Warfarin: May slightly enhance anticoagulant effect. Monitor PT and INR when therapy starts or dose is adjusted.

Drug-herb. *Eucalyptus, kava kava:* May increase risk of hepatotoxicity. Discourage use together.

Red yeast rice: May increase risk of rhabdomyolysis. Discourage use together.

St. John's wort: May decrease simvastatin level. Discourage use together.

Drug-food. *Grapefruit juice:* Large amounts (greater than 1 quart/day [1 L/day]) may increase drug levels, increasing risk of adverse effects, including myopathy and rhabdomyolysis. Discourage use together.

Drug-lifestyle. *Alcohol use:* May increase risk of hepatotoxicity. Discourage use together.

EFFECTS ON LAB TEST RESULTS
• May increase HbA$_{1c}$, fasting blood glucose, ALT, AST, ALP, GGT, and CK levels.

CONTRAINDICATIONS & CAUTIONS
• Simvastatin occasionally causes myopathy manifested as muscle pain, tenderness, or weakness, with CK level more than 10 × ULN. Myopathy sometimes takes the form of rhabdomyolysis with or without acute renal failure secondary to myoglobinuria, and rare fatalities have occurred. The risk of myopathy, including rhabdomyolysis, is dose related. Predisposing factors for myopathy include advanced age (age 65 and older), female gender, uncontrolled hypothyroidism, and renal impairment.

• Contraindicated in patients hypersensitive to drug and in those with active liver disease or conditions that cause unexplained persistent elevations of transaminase levels.

• Contraindicated for use at its highest dosage (80 mg/day) in patients not previously prescribed simvastatin or in patients who have had prior muscle toxicity. Patients who can't reach their goal LDL cholesterol level on 40-mg dose should be switched to an alternative agent. Only patients who have tolerated the 80-mg dose without muscle toxicity for more than 12 months should continue taking 80 mg daily.

• Immune-mediated necrotizing myopathy (IMNM) (proximal muscle weakness, persistent CK elevation even after statin is stopped, positive anti–HMG CoA reductase antibody, biopsy positive for necrotizing myopathy) has been reported rarely with statin use. Treat IMNM with immunosuppressants.

• Use cautiously in older adults and patients who consume large amounts of alcohol or have a history of liver disease.

• Rare reports of cognitive impairment (memory loss, forgetfulness, amnesia, memory impairment, confusion) have been associated with statin use. These reported symptoms are generally not serious and are reversible upon statin discontinuation, with variable times to symptom onset (1 day to years) and symptom resolution (median of 3 weeks).

Dialyzable drug: Unknown.

PREGNANCY-LACTATION-REPRODUCTION
• May cause fetal harm. Use during pregnancy is contraindicated unless benefits

---

outweigh fetal risk. Discontinue drug before conception.
• If pregnancy occurs during therapy, apprise patient of fetal risks with continued use during pregnancy.
• Contraindicated during breastfeeding.

NURSING CONSIDERATIONS
• Obtain LFT results before initiation of treatment and thereafter when clinically indicated. Obtain lipid determinations after 4 weeks of therapy and periodically thereafter.
• Monitor all patients for myopathy (unexplained muscle pain, weakness, or tenderness). Periodic CK determinations may be considered in patients starting therapy or in patients whose dosage is being increased, but there's no assurance that such monitoring will prevent myopathy.
• Statin may increase HbA_{1c} and fasting glucose levels.
• Interrupt statin therapy if patient shows signs or symptoms of serious liver injury, hyperbilirubinemia, or jaundice. Don't restart drug if another cause can't be found.
• A daily dose of 40 mg significantly reduces risk of death from CAD, nonfatal MI, stroke, and revascularization procedures.
• *Look alike–sound alike:* Don't confuse Zocor with Cozaar.

PATIENT TEACHING
• Instruct patient in safe drug administration.
• Teach patient about proper dietary management of cholesterol and triglycerides. When appropriate, recommend weight control, exercise, and smoking cessation programs.
• Inform patient that rare instances of memory loss and confusion have occurred with statin use. These reported events were generally not serious and resolved when drug was discontinued.
• Tell patient that drug may increase blood glucose level, but the CV benefits are thought to outweigh the slight increase in risk.
• Caution patient to immediately report unexplained muscle pain, tenderness, or weakness (especially if accompanied by malaise or fever) and loss of appetite, upper abdominal pain, dark-colored urine, or yellowing of skin or eyes.
• *Alert:* Tell patient to stop drug and immediately report pregnancy or breastfeeding.

sirolimus ⚕
sir-OH-li-mus

Rapamune

Therapeutic class: Immunosuppressants
Pharmacologic class: MTOR inhibitors

AVAILABLE FORMS
Oral solution: 1 mg/mL
Tablets ⓄⓉⒸ: 0.5 mg, 1 mg, 2 mg

INDICATIONS & DOSAGES
➤ **With cyclosporine and corticosteroids, to prevent organ rejection in patients receiving renal transplants**
Adults and children age 13 and older with low-to-moderate immunogenic risk: Initially, 6 mg PO for patients with low-to-moderate immunologic risk weighing 40 kg or more or 3 mg/m² for patients weighing less than 40 kg as one-time dose as soon as possible after transplantation but 4 hours after administration of cyclosporine; then maintenance dose of 2 mg PO once daily for patients weighing 40 kg or more or 1 mg/m² PO once daily for patients weighing less than 40 kg.
Adults with high immunogenic risk: May give up to 15 mg PO on day 1 after transplantation, then 5 mg/day PO beginning on day 2 after transplantation. Obtain trough concentration between days 5 and 7 and adjust dosage as needed.

Maximum daily dose shouldn't exceed 40 mg. If a daily dose exceeds 40 mg due to a loading dose, give the loading dose over 2 days. Monitor trough concentrations at least 3 to 4 days after a loading dose.
Adjust-a-dose: When adjusting maintenance dosage, continue patient on the new maintenance dosage for at least 7 to 14 days before further dosage adjustments with concentration monitoring because drug has a long half-life.

For patients with mild to moderate hepatic impairment, reduce maintenance dose by about one-third, and by about one-half in patients with severe hepatic impairment. It isn't necessary to reduce loading dose. Two to 4 months after transplant in patients with low-to-moderate risk of graft rejection, taper off cyclosporine over 4 to 8 weeks. While tapering cyclosporine, adjust sirolimus dose

S

every 1 to 2 weeks to obtain levels between 16 and 24 nanograms/mL. Base dosage adjustments on clinical status, tissue biopsies, and lab findings.

➤ **Lymphangioleiomyomatosis**

Adults: Initially, 2 mg PO daily consistently with or without food at same time each day. Measure trough concentration in 10 to 20 days and adjust dosage to achieve sirolimus trough level of between 5 and 15 nanograms/mL, allowing at least 7 to 14 days on new dose before further dosage adjustment. Once a stable dosage is achieved, perform therapeutic drug monitoring at least every 3 months.

ADMINISTRATION
PO
🔔 *Alert:* Drug is a hazardous agent; use safe handling and disposal precautions.
• Give drug consistently either with or without food.
• Patients should swallow tablets whole. Don't crush or split tablets.
• Dilute oral solution before use. After dilution, use immediately and discard oral solution syringe.
• When diluting oral solution, empty correct amount into glass or plastic (not Styrofoam) container holding at least 2 oz (60 mL) of either water or orange juice. Don't use grapefruit juice or any other liquid. Stir vigorously and have patient drink immediately. Refill container with at least 4 oz (120 mL) of water or orange juice, stir again, and have patient drink all contents.
• Oral solution may develop a slight haze during refrigeration, which doesn't affect potency of drug. If haze develops, bring to room temperature and shake until haze disappears.
• Store oral solution away from light, and refrigerate at 36° to 46° F (2° to 8° C). After opening bottle, use contents within 1 month. If needed, store bottles and pouches at room temperature (up to 77° F [25° C]) for several days. Oral solution may be kept in oral amber syringe for 24 hours at room temperature.
• Store tablets between 68° and 77° F (20° and 25° C). Protect from light.

ACTION
Inhibits T-cell activation and proliferation that occurs in response to antigenic and cytokine stimulation. Also inhibits antibody formation.

Route	Onset	Peak	Duration
PO	Unknown	1–3 hr (solution); 1–6 hr (tablet)	Unknown

Half-life: Adults, about 46 to 78 hours; children, 13.7 ± 6.2 hours.

ADVERSE REACTIONS
CNS: fever, headache, pain, dizziness. **CV:** chest pain, edema, HTN, peripheral edema, tachycardia, *venous thromboembolism.* **GI:** abdominal pain, constipation, diarrhea, nausea, ascites, stomatitis. **GU:** UTI, pyelonephritis, nephrotic syndrome, menstrual disorder. **Hematologic:** anemia, *thrombocytopenia, leukopenia,* ecchymosis, *thrombotic thrombocytopenic purpura, hemolytic-uremic syndrome.* **Hepatic:** *hepatotoxicity.* **Metabolic:** hypercholesteremia, *hyperkalemia,* hyperlipidemia, *hypokalemia,* hypophosphatemia, hypertriglyceridemia, *hypoglycemia, acidosis,* diabetes, dehydration, hyperglycemia. **Musculoskeletal:** arthralgia, bone necrosis, myalgia. **Respiratory:** URI, pneumonia. **Skin:** acne, rash, fungal dermatitis, pruritus, *melanoma, squamous cell carcinoma, basal cell carcinoma.* **Other:** *sepsis,* abnormal healing, infection, lymphadenopathy, herpes simplex, herpes zoster, *malignancy.*

INTERACTIONS
Drug-drug. *ACE inhibitors (captopril, enalapril, lisinopril):* May increase risk of angioedema. Use together cautiously.
Aminoglycosides, amphotericin B, other nephrotoxic drugs: May increase risk of nephrotoxicity. Use with caution.
Calcineurin inhibitors (CNI) (cyclosporine, pimecrolimus, tacrolimus): May increase risk of CNI-induced hemolytic-uremic syndrome, thrombotic thrombocytopenic purpura, or thrombotic microangiopathy. Monitor patient closely.
Cyclosporine: May increase sirolimus level and toxicity. Give sirolimus 4 hours after cyclosporine. If cyclosporine is stopped, higher doses of sirolimus are needed; monitor level and adjust dosage as needed.
CYP3A4 inducers (carbamazepine, phenobarbital, phenytoin, rifabutin, rifapentine): May decrease sirolimus blood level. Monitor patient closely.
CYP3A4 inhibitors (amiodarone, bromocriptine, cimetidine, clarithromycin, clotrimazole, danazol, erythromycin, fluconazole,

---

Reactions in bold italics are *life-threatening*. Interactions may have a *rapid onset* or a *delayed onset*.

itraconazole, metoclopramide, nicardipine, posaconazole, ritonavir, verapamil, voriconazole): May increase sirolimus blood level. Monitor sirolimus level closely.

Diltiazem: May increase sirolimus levels. Monitor sirolimus level, as needed.

HMG-CoA reductase inhibitors or fibrates: May increase risk of rhabdomyolysis with the combination of sirolimus and cyclosporine. Monitor patient closely.

Ketoconazole: May increase rate and extent of sirolimus absorption. Avoid using together.

Live-virus vaccines: May reduce vaccine effectiveness. Avoid using together.

Rifampin: May decrease sirolimus level. Alternative therapy to rifampin should be prescribed.

Verapamil: May increase verapamil level. Use together cautiously.

Drug-herb. *St. John's wort:* May decrease sirolimus levels. Discourage use together.

Drug-food. *Grapefruit juice:* May decrease drug metabolism. Discourage use together.

Drug-lifestyle. *Sun exposure:* May increase risk of skin cancer. Advise patient to avoid sunlight exposure.

EFFECTS ON LAB TEST RESULTS

• May increase urine protein, creatinine, glucose, LDH, liver enzyme, cholesterol, and lipid levels.
• May decrease phosphate and potassium, levels.
• May increase RBC count.
• May decrease platelet count.
• May increase or decrease WBC count.

CONTRAINDICATIONS & CAUTIONS

• Contraindicated in patients hypersensitive to active drug, its derivatives, or components of product.
• Use cautiously in patients with hyperlipidemia and impaired liver or renal function.
• Cases of ILD, including pneumonitis, bronchiolitis obliterans organizing pneumonia, and pulmonary fibrosis (some fatal), have occurred. ILD may be associated with pulmonary HTN and risk may increase with higher trough levels. ILD may resolve with reduced doses or with drug discontinuation.

Boxed Warning Fatal bronchial anastomotic dehiscence has been reported in patients with lung transplants when sirolimus has been used as part of an immunosuppressive regimen. Safety and effectiveness of

sirolimus as immunosuppressive therapy haven't been established in patients with liver or lung transplants. Use in these patients isn't recommended. ∎

Boxed Warning Patients taking drug are more susceptible to infection, lymphoma, and other malignancies. ∎

Dialyzable drug: No.

⚠ *Overdose S&S:* Exaggerated adverse effects.

PREGNANCY-LACTATION-REPRODUCTION

• There are no adequate studies during pregnancy; drug may cause fetal harm. Patient must use effective contraception before and during therapy and for 12 weeks after therapy ends. Use during pregnancy only if potential benefit outweighs fetal risk.
• It isn't known if drug appears in human milk. Patient should discontinue breastfeeding or discontinue drug.
• Drug affects male and female fertility. In most cases, azoospermia has been reversible when drug is discontinued.

NURSING CONSIDERATIONS

Boxed Warning Using this drug with tacrolimus or cyclosporine may cause hepatic artery thrombosis, leading to graft loss and death in patients with liver transplants. ∎

Boxed Warning Only those experienced in immunosuppressive therapy and management of patients with kidney transplants should prescribe drug. Manage patients receiving drug in facilities equipped and staffed with adequate lab and supportive medical resources. ∎

⚡ *Alert:* Drugs causing immunosuppression increase the risk of opportunistic infections, including activation of latent viral infections such as BK virus–associated neuropathy, which may lead to serious outcomes, including kidney graft loss.

⚡ *Alert:* Drug has been associated with hypersensitivity reactions, including anaphylactic reactions, angioedema, exfoliative dermatitis, and hypersensitivity vasculitis. Monitor patient closely.

• Use drug in regimen with cyclosporine and corticosteroids. After 2 to 4 months of combined therapy in patients who are at low-to-moderate risk, wean off cyclosporine as cyclosporine inhibits the metabolism and transport of sirolimus. Sirolimus concentration

may decrease when cyclosporine is discontinued unless the sirolimus dosage is increased.
⚠ Cyclosporine withdrawal in patients with high risk of graft rejection isn't recommended. This includes patients with Banff grade III acute rejection or vascular rejection before cyclosporine withdrawal, those who are dialysis dependent, those with serum creatinine level greater than 4.5 mg/dL, patients who are Black, patients with retransplants or multiorgan transplants, and patients with high panel of reactive antibodies.
• After transplantation, give antimicrobial prophylaxis for *Pneumocystis jiroveci* for 1 year and for CMV for 3 months.
• Monitor renal function tests, including urine protein levels. Adjustment of immunosuppressive regimen may be needed.
• Monitor cholesterol and triglyceride levels. Treatment with lipid-lowering drugs during therapy isn't uncommon. If hyperlipidemia is detected, additional interventions, such as diet and exercise, should begin.
• Assess for rhabdomyolysis.
• Monitor drug levels closely in patients age 13 and older who weigh less than 40 kg, patients with hepatic impairment, those also receiving drugs that induce or inhibit CYP3A4, and patients in whom cyclosporine dosing is markedly reduced or stopped.
• Monitor patient for impaired or delayed wound healing (including wound dehiscence), fluid accumulation (including edema, lymphedema, pleural effusion, ascites, pericardial effusion), and malignancies (including skin carcinoma).

PATIENT TEACHING
• Teach patient how to properly store, dilute, and give drug.
• Advise patient to report adverse effects and that drug may increase risk of infections and certain cancers.
• Alert patient about risks during pregnancy and to use effective contraception before and during therapy and for 12 weeks after final dose.
• Inform patient that drug may impair fertility.
• Caution patient to wash area with soap and water if drug solution touches skin or mucous membranes.
• Advise patient to limit UV light and sun exposure because of the increased risk of skin cancer.

SITagliptin phosphate
sit-a-GLIP-tin

Januvia◆

Therapeutic class: Antidiabetics
Pharmacologic class: DPP-4 enzyme inhibitors

AVAILABLE FORMS
Tablets: 25 mg, 50 mg, 100 mg

INDICATIONS & DOSAGES
➤ **To improve glycemic control in addition to diet and exercise in patients with type 2 diabetes, alone or in combination therapy**
Adults: 100 mg PO once daily.
Adjust-a-dose: For patients with eGFR of 30 to less than 45 mL/minute/1.73 m^2, give 50 mg once daily; for patients with eGFR less than 30 mL/minute/1.73 m^2 or ESRD with hemodialysis or peritoneal dialysis, give 25 mg once daily. Give without regard to timing of dialysis session.

ADMINISTRATION
PO
• Give drug without regard for food.

ACTION
Inhibits DPP-4, an enzyme that rapidly inactivates incretin hormones, which play a part in the body's regulation of glucose. By increasing and prolonging active incretin levels, the drug helps to increase insulin release and decrease circulating glucose.

Route	Onset	Peak	Duration
PO	Rapid	1–4 hr	Unknown

Half-life: About 12.5 hours.

ADVERSE REACTIONS
CNS: headache. **CV:** edema. **EENT:** nasopharyngitis. **GI:** abdominal pain, nausea, diarrhea. **Metabolic:** *hypoglycemia.* **Respiratory:** URI.

INTERACTIONS
Drug-drug. *Digoxin:* Causes a slight increase in digoxin peak. Monitor patient when used together.
Insulin, insulin secretagogues: May increase risk of hypoglycemia. Dosage adjustment of these drugs may be required.

Reactions in bold italics are *life-threatening*. Interactions may have a *rapid onset* or a ***delayed onset***.

EFFECTS ON LAB TEST RESULTS
• May increase creatinine level.
• May increase WBC count.

CONTRAINDICATIONS & CAUTIONS
• Contraindicated in patients with type 1 diabetes or diabetic ketoacidosis.
• Consider risk and benefits before initiating drug in patients at risk for HF.
• Contraindicated in patients with a history of hypersensitivity to sitagliptin. Angioedema, anaphylaxis, and exfoliative skin conditions such as SJS have been reported, some after first dose or up to 3 months after drug initiation.
• Bullous pemphigoid has been reported in patients taking DPP-4 inhibitors.
• Use cautiously in older adults, in patients with moderate to severe renal insufficiency, and in those taking other antidiabetics.
• Drug may increase risk of pancreatitis. Safe use in patients with a history of pancreatitis hasn't been evaluated.
• Safety and effectiveness in children haven't been evaluated.
Dialyzable drug: 13.5%.

PREGNANCY-LACTATION-REPRODUCTION
• There are no adequate studies during pregnancy. Use only if clearly needed.
• Report prenatal exposure to the Januvia Pregnancy Registry (1-800-986-8999).
• It isn't known if drug appears in human milk. Use cautiously during breastfeeding.

NURSING CONSIDERATIONS
• Assess renal function before start of therapy and periodically thereafter.
• Monitor HbA$_{1c}$ level periodically to assess long-term glycemic control.
• Management of type 2 diabetes should include diet control. Because caloric restrictions, weight loss, and exercise help improve insulin sensitivity and help make drug therapy effective, these measures are essential for proper diabetes management.
• Watch for hypoglycemia, especially in patients receiving combination therapy.
• Monitor patient for pancreatitis (persistent abdominal pain with or without vomiting). Discontinue drug for suspected pancreatitis.
• Monitor patient for skin blistering or erosions. Discontinue drug for suspected bullous pemphigoid and consider referral to a dermatologist.

• Drug may cause joint pain that can be severe and disabling. Report severe and persistent joint pain to prescriber; drug may need to be discontinued.
• *Look alike–sound alike:* Don't confuse sitagliptin with saxagliptin.

PATIENT TEACHING
• Tell patient that drug isn't a substitute for diet and exercise and that it's important to follow a prescribed dietary and physical activity routine and to monitor glucose level.
• Instruct patient to immediately report persistent, severe abdominal pain that may radiate to the back, with or without vomiting.
• Inform patient and family members of the signs and symptoms of hyperglycemia and hypoglycemia and the steps to take if these symptoms occur.
• Advise patient to report all adverse reactions, and to immediately report signs and symptoms of hypersensitivity (rash, swelling of the face).
• Teach patient signs and symptoms of HF and to notify prescriber if signs or symptoms develop, including shortness of breath, rapid weight increase, or swelling of the feet.
• Instruct patient that during periods of stress (such as fever, trauma, infection, or surgery), medication requirements may change and dosage adjustments may be needed. Advise patient to seek medical advice promptly.
• Advise patient to immediately report new or worsening joint pain that's severe and persistent because drug may need to be discontinued.
• Provide patient with information on complications associated with diabetes and ways to assess for them.
• Tell patient drug may be taken without regard for food.

sodium ferric gluconate complex
Ferrlecit

Therapeutic class: Iron supplements
Pharmacologic class: Macromolecular iron complexes–hematinics

AVAILABLE FORMS
Injection: 62.5 mg elemental iron (12.5 mg/mL) in 5-mL ampules*

INDICATIONS & DOSAGES

➤ **Iron deficiency anemia in patients with chronic kidney disease receiving long-term hemodialysis and supplemental erythropoietin**

Adults and children older than age 15: 10 mL (125 mg elemental iron) IV over 1 hour per dialysis session. Most patients need minimum cumulative dose of 1 g elemental iron given over more than eight sequential dialysis treatments to achieve a favorable Hb or hematocrit response.

Children ages 6 to 15: 1.5 mg/kg (maximum 125 mg/dose) IV over 1 hour per dialysis session. Maximum dosage is 125 mg per dose.

ADMINISTRATION

IV

▼ Drug contains benzyl alcohol. Don't use in neonates.

▼ For adults, dilute in 100 mL NSS; for children, dilute in 25 mL NSS. Give immediately over 1 hour.

▼ Alternatively, give to adults undiluted at a rate not to exceed 1 mL/minute (12.5 mg/minute) per dialysis session.

▼ **Incompatibilities:** Other IV drugs. Don't add drug to parenteral nutrition solutions for infusion.

ACTION

Restores total body iron content, which is critical for normal Hb synthesis and oxygen transport.

Route	Onset	Peak	Duration
IV	Unknown	Varies	Unknown

Half-life: 1 hour in healthy, iron-deficient adults.

ADVERSE REACTIONS

CNS: asthenia, headache, fatigue, malaise, dizziness, paresthesia, agitation, somnolence, syncope, pain, fever, light-headedness, weakness. **CV:** hypotension, HTN, tachycardia, *bradycardia*, angina, chest pain, *MI*, edema, flushing, *thrombosis*. **EENT:** conjunctivitis, abnormal vision, rhinitis, pharyngitis. **GI:** anorexia, nausea, vomiting, diarrhea, rectal disorder, dyspepsia, eructation, flatulence, melena, abdominal pain. **GU:** UTI. **Hematologic:** anemia, abnormal erythrocytes. **Metabolic:** *hyperkalemia, hypoglycemia, hypokalemia,* hypervolemia. **Musculoskeletal:** myalgia, arthralgia, back pain, arm pain, cramps. **Respiratory:** dyspnea, coughing,

URI, pneumonia, pulmonary edema. **Skin:** pruritus, diaphoresis, rash, injection-site reaction. **Other:** infection, chills, rigors, flulike syndrome, *sepsis, carcinoma,* lymphadenopathy.

INTERACTIONS

Drug-drug. *ACE inhibitors:* May increase risk of adverse effects, including sensitivity reactions. Monitor patient closely.

Oral iron preparations: May reduce absorption of oral iron preparations. Avoid using together.

EFFECTS ON LAB TEST RESULTS

• May increase serum ferritin level and transferrin saturation.
• May decrease glucose level.
• May increase or decrease potassium level.
• May increase Hb level and hematocrit.
• May decrease leukocyte count.

CONTRAINDICATIONS & CAUTIONS

• Contraindicated in patients hypersensitive to drug or its components (such as benzyl alcohol) and in those with iron overload or anemias not related to iron deficiency.
• Don't use in patients with elevated ferritin levels.
• Use cautiously in older adults.
• Safety and effectiveness in children younger than age 6 haven't been established.
Dialyzable drug: No.

PREGNANCY-LACTATION-REPRODUCTION

• There are no adequate studies during pregnancy. Drug may increase fetal risk due to hypersensitivity reactions and benzyl alcohol exposure. Use only if clearly needed.
• It isn't known if drug appears in human milk and drug contains benzyl alcohol. Use alternative iron replacement therapy during breastfeeding.

NURSING CONSIDERATIONS

⚠ **Alert:** Dosage is expressed in milligrams of elemental iron.
⚠ **Alert:** Before administering, assess patients for history of reactions to iron products.
⚠ **Alert:** Life-threatening hypersensitivity reactions, such as CV collapse, cardiac arrest, bronchospasm, oral or pharyngeal edema, dyspnea, angioedema, urticaria, and pruritus (sometimes linked to pain and muscle spasm of the chest or back) may occur during

---

Reactions in bold italics are *life-threatening*. Interactions may have a *rapid onset* or a **delayed onset**.

infusion. Monitor patients closely during infusion and for at least 30 minutes after infusion until clinically stable. Ensure that emergency measures to treat anaphylaxis are immediately available.

⚊ *Alert:* Closely monitor patients during and after drug administration for profound hypotension with flushing, light-headedness, malaise, fatigue, weakness, or severe chest, back, flank, or groin pain; these symptoms may or may not be associated with hypersensitivity reactions and usually resolve within 1 to 2 hours.

⚊ *Alert:* Drug contains benzyl alcohol, which is associated with adverse events and death in neonates and infants, including fatal gasping syndrome. The minimum amount of benzyl alcohol that may cause toxicity isn't known.

• Drug shouldn't be used in patients with iron overload, which often occurs in hemoglobinopathies and other refractory anemias.

• Monitor ferritin level, iron saturation, Hb level, and hematocrit.

• In patients on hemodialysis, adverse reactions may be related to dialysis itself or to chronic renal failure.

• Check with patient about other potential sources of iron, such as OTC iron preparations and iron-containing multiple vitamins with minerals.

PATIENT TEACHING
• Teach patient to immediately report all adverse reactions, especially those occurring during and after the infusion.

• Abdominal pain, diarrhea, vomiting, drowsiness, and rapid breathing may indicate iron poisoning. Urge patient to notify prescriber immediately.

---

sodium zirconium cyclosilicate
SOE-dee-um zir-KOE-nee-um SYE-kloe-sil-i-kate

Lokelma

Therapeutic class: Antidotes
Pharmacologic class: Potassium binders

AVAILABLE FORMS
Powder for oral suspension: 5-g, 10-g packets

INDICATIONS & DOSAGES
➤ **Hyperkalemia**
Adults: Initially, 10 g PO t.i.d. for up to 48 hours. For continued treatment after 48 hours, give 10 g PO once daily. Maintenance dosage range is 5 g PO every other day to 15 g PO once daily.

Adjust-a-dose: Monitor serum potassium level and adjust dosage based on target potassium level range. During maintenance treatment, up-titrate dosage based on potassium level at intervals of 1 week or longer and in increments of 5 g. Decrease dosage or stop drug if potassium level falls below desired target range.

For patients on long-term hemodialysis, recommended starting dose is 5 g once daily on non-dialysis days. Consider a starting dose of 10 g once daily on non-dialysis days in patients with serum potassium level greater than 6.5 mEq/L. Monitor serum potassium level and adjust dosage based on the predialysis serum potassium value after the long interdialytic interval and desired target range. During initiation and after a dosage adjustment, assess serum potassium level after 1 week. Recommended maintenance dosage range is 5 to 15 g once daily, on non-dialysis days. Discontinue drug or decrease dosage if serum potassium level falls below desired target range based on the predialysis value after the long interdialytic interval, or patient develops clinically significant hypokalemia.

ADMINISTRATION
PO
• Empty entire contents of packet(s) into a glass containing at least 3 tablespoons of water or more if desired, stir well, and have patient drink immediately. If powder remains in the glass, add water, stir, and have patient drink immediately. Repeat until no powder remains.

• Give other oral medications at least 2 hours before or 2 hours after giving sodium zirconium cyclosilicate.

• Store at 59° to 86° F (15° to 30° C).

ACTION
A potassium binder that preferentially exchanges potassium for hydrogen and sodium. Increases fecal potassium excretion through the binding of potassium in the lumen of the GI tract; reduces concentration of free

S

potassium in the GI lumen and lowers serum potassium levels.

Route	Onset	Peak	Duration
PO	1 hr	Unknown	Unknown

Half-life: Unknown.

ADVERSE REACTIONS
CV: edema. **Metabolic:** *hypokalemia.*

INTERACTIONS
Drug-drug. *Drugs with pH-dependent solubility (atorvastatin, clopidogrel, dabigatran, furosemide):* May increase or decrease efficacy of coadministered drugs that have pH-dependent solubility. Separate drug administration from other oral medications by at least 2 hours.

EFFECTS ON LAB TEST RESULTS
• May increase bicarbonate level.
• May decrease potassium level.

CONTRAINDICATIONS & CAUTIONS
⚠ *Alert:* Drug shouldn't be used as an emergency treatment for life-threatening hyperkalemia because of its delayed onset of action.
• Drug hasn't been studied in patients with motility disorders (severe constipation, bowel obstruction or impaction, postoperative bowel motility disorders). Avoid use in these patients as drug may be ineffective and may worsen GI conditions.
• Safety and effectiveness in children haven't been established.
Dialyzable drug: No.
⚠ *Overdose S&S:* Hypokalemia.

PREGNANCY-LACTATION-REPRODUCTION
• Drug isn't absorbed systemically and isn't expected to result in fetal exposure.
• Breastfeeding isn't expected to result in exposure of infant to drug.

NURSING CONSIDERATIONS
• Monitor potassium level and adjust dosage based on serum potassium level and desired target range.
• Monitor patient for signs and symptoms of edema, especially in patients who should restrict sodium intake or are prone to fluid overload (HF, renal disease). Each 5-g dose contains 400 mg of sodium. Adjust dietary sodium, if appropriate, and increase diuretic dosage as needed.

• Drug has radio-opaque properties and may appear like an imaging agent during abdominal X-ray procedures.

PATIENT TEACHING
• Teach patient to report all adverse reactions.
• Stress importance of drinking the entire dose.
• Advise patient taking other oral medications to separate dosing of drug by at least 2 hours (before or after).
• Instruct patient to adjust dietary sodium, if appropriate.

sofosbuvir ⚗
soe-FOS-bue-vir

Sovaldi

Therapeutic class: Antivirals
Pharmacologic class: Nucleotide analogue NS5B polymerase inhibitors

AVAILABLE FORMS
Oral pellets: 150 mg, 200 mg
Tablets: 200 mg, 400 mg

INDICATIONS & DOSAGES
Adjust-a-dose (for all indications): Sofosbuvir dosage reduction isn't recommended. Discontinue sofosbuvir if concomitant antivirals are stopped. Adjust concomitant ribavirin or peginterferon alfa dosage if GFR is less than 50 mL/minute or hepatic decompensation or adverse reactions occur. Refer to manufacturer's instructions for ribavirin or peginterferon alfa dosage adjustments.
➤ **Chronic HCV infection (genotype 1 or 4) with or without HIV coinfection, as component of combination antiviral regimen in patients who are treatment-naive without cirrhosis or with compensated cirrhosis (Child-Pugh class A)** ⚗
Adults: 400 mg PO daily with peginterferon alfa and ribavirin for 12 weeks. For patients with HCV genotype 1 who can't receive interferon, give 400 mg PO daily with ribavirin for 24 weeks.
➤ **Chronic HCV infection (genotype 2) with or without HIV coinfection, as part of combination antiviral regimen in patients who are treatment-naive or treatment-experienced without cirrhosis or with compensated cirrhosis (Child-Pugh class A)** ⚗

Adults and children age 3 and older weighing at least 35 kg: 400 mg PO daily with ribavirin for 12 weeks.

Children age 3 and older weighing 17 to less than 35 kg: 200 mg PO daily with ribavirin for 12 weeks.

Children age 3 and older weighing less than 17 kg: 150 mg PO daily with ribavirin for 12 weeks.

➤ **Chronic HCV infection (genotype 3) with or without HIV coinfection, as part of combination antiviral regimen in patients who are treatment-naive or treatment-experienced without cirrhosis or with compensated cirrhosis (Child-Pugh class A)** ▧

Adults and children age 3 and older weighing at least 35 kg: 400 mg PO daily with ribavirin for 24 weeks.

Children age 3 and older weighing 17 to less than 35 kg: 200 mg PO daily with ribavirin for 24 weeks.

Children age 3 and older weighing less than 17 kg: 150 mg PO daily with ribavirin for 24 weeks.

➤ **Chronic HCV infection with hepatocellular carcinoma in patients awaiting liver transplant**

Adults and children age 3 and older: 400 mg PO daily with ribavirin for 48 weeks or until liver transplant.

ADMINISTRATION
PO
• Give without regard for food.
• Children unable to swallow tablets can use the pellet formulation.
• Patients shouldn't chew oral pellets. If giving without food, pour entire contents of packet directly in the mouth. Patients may drink water after swallowing pellets if needed. If giving with food, sprinkle pellets on one or more spoonfuls of nonacidic food (pudding, chocolate syrup, mashed potatoes, ice cream) at or below room temperature. Gently mix and give within 30 minutes. Patients should swallow entire contents without chewing to avoid a bitter aftertaste.

ACTION
Inhibits HCV NS5B RNA polymerase, inhibiting viral replication.

Route	Onset	Peak	Duration
PO	Unknown	0.5–2 hr	Unknown

Half-life: 0.4 hour.

ADVERSE REACTIONS
CNS: headache, insomnia, asthenia, fever, fatigue, irritability. **GI:** nausea, diarrhea, decreased appetite. **Hematologic:** anemia, ***neutropenia, thrombocytopenia.*** **Hepatic:** hyperbilirubinemia. **Metabolic:** increased CK level. **Musculoskeletal:** myalgia. **Skin:** pruritus, rash. **Other:** flulike illness, chills.

INTERACTIONS
Drug-drug. ⟲ *Alert: Amiodarone:* May increase risk of symptomatic bradycardia, including cardiac arrest and cases requiring pacemaker intervention. Avoid use together. If use together can't be avoided, advise patient of risk and monitor carefully.

Anticonvulsants (carbamazepine, oxcarbazepine, phenobarbital, phenytoin, primidone), antimycobacterials (rifabutin, rifampin, rifapentine), HIV protease inhibitors (tipranavir, ritonavir): May decrease sofosbuvir level. Avoid use together.

Drug-herb. *St. John's wort:* May decrease sofosbuvir plasma concentration. Don't use together.

EFFECTS ON LAB TEST RESULTS
• May increase CK, bilirubin, and lipase levels.
• May decrease Hb level and neutrophil and platelet counts.

CONTRAINDICATIONS & CAUTIONS
• Contraindicated in patients hypersensitive to drug or its components.
• Refer to prescribing information for peginterferon alfa and ribavirin for contraindications when drug is given in these combination regimens.

Boxed Warning Reactivation of HBV may occur in patients coinfected with HCV and result in fulminant hepatitis, hepatic failure, and death. Screen all patients for current or prior HBV infection before treatment by measuring HBsAg and anti-HBc; if patient is positive for HBV infection, assess baseline HBV DNA. ▮

⟲ *Alert:* Symptomatic bradycardia, including fatal cardiac arrest and cases requiring pacemaker intervention, has been reported when sofosbuvir is administered with amiodarone. Patients taking amiodarone who are also taking beta blockers or who have underlying cardiac comorbidities or advanced liver disease may be at increased risk. Signs and symptoms

S

may occur within hours to up to 2 weeks after start of HCV therapy.

• Safety and effectiveness of drug haven't been studied in patients with eGFR of less than 30 mL/minute, ESRD, or decompensated cirrhosis.

• Using in combination with other products containing sofosbuvir isn't recommended.

• Safety and effectiveness in children younger than age 3 with HCV genotype 2 or 3 and children with genotype 1 or 4 haven't been established.

Dialyzable drug: 18%.

PREGNANCY-LACTATION-REPRODUCTION

• Combination therapy with ribavirin is contraindicated in patients who are pregnant and in men whose partners are pregnant. Obtain baseline negative pregnancy test before start of therapy.

• Patients of childbearing potential and male patients with partners of childbearing potential must use two forms of effective nonhormonal contraception while receiving treatment regimens that include ribavirin and for 9 months for female patients or 6 months for male patients after therapy ends.

• Patients who are pregnant, are coinfected with HCV/HIV-1, and are taking concomitant antiretrovirals should enroll in the Antiretroviral Pregnancy Registry (1-800-258-4263).

• Combination therapy with ribavirin is contraindicated with breastfeeding. Patients must discontinue breastfeeding or discontinue drug.

NURSING CONSIDERATIONS

• Sofosbuvir isn't recommended as monotherapy. Always use as part of combination regimen.

Boxed Warning Monitor patient with current or prior HBV infection for hepatitis flare or HBV reactivation with lab testing; watch for signs and symptoms of liver injury during active and posttreatment follow-up. ∎

⏱ *Alert:* Monitor patients who must take amiodarone and those who must start amiodarone or who recently discontinued amiodarone for signs and symptoms of bradycardia (near-fainting or fainting, dizziness, light-headedness, malaise, weakness, excessive fatigue, shortness of breath, chest pain, confusion or memory problems). Inpatient cardiac monitoring should be utilized for first 48 hours, then outpatient monitoring or self-monitoring of HR for bradycardia should

continue daily through at least first 2 weeks of treatment. Discontinue HCV treatment if signs or symptoms occur.

• Refer to ribavirin or peginterferon alfa prescribing information for complete guidance on their concomitant use.

• Monitor blood counts and bilirubin, liver enzyme, and serum creatinine levels at baseline and periodically when clinically indicated.

• Monitor serum HCV-RNA level at baseline, during treatment, at end of treatment, during treatment follow-up, and when clinically indicated.

• Verify pregnancy status according to ribavirin prescribing information during and after treatment.

• Treatment response varies based on patient and viral factors. Monitor patient carefully.

PATIENT TEACHING

• Advise patient that using drug as single agent isn't recommended. Sofosbuvir must always be used as part of combination regimen with ribavirin or peginterferon and ribavirin.

Boxed Warning Warn patient to immediately report signs and symptoms of liver injury (fatigue, weakness, loss of appetite, nausea, vomiting, yellowing of skin or eyes, light-colored stool). ∎

• Teach patient to immediately report signs and symptoms of hypersensitivity reaction (wheezing, chest tightness, fever, itching, heavy cough, blue-colored skin, seizures, or swelling of face, lips, tongue, or throat) and to seek medical attention.

⏱ *Alert:* Caution patient to seek immediate medical attention for signs and symptoms of bradycardia.

• Explain to patient and partner the risk of birth defects, contraception requirements, and pregnancy testing related to therapy.

• Teach patient to report all signs and symptoms of adverse reactions, such as headache, dyspepsia, and insomnia.

• Caution patient not to use other medications while taking this drug without first notifying prescriber.

• Teach patient to keep drug in original container.

• Advise patient to report liver problems (other than HCV infection), history of liver transplant, severe kidney problems or dialysis, positive HIV status, or other medical conditions.

Reactions in bold italics are *life-threatening*. Interactions may have a *rapid onset* or a *delayed onset*.

- Warn patient not to breastfeed while taking drug.
- Instruct patient not to discontinue drug without first discussing with prescriber.

sofosbuvir–velpatasvir ☒
soe-FOS-bue-vir/vel-PAT-as-vir

Epclusa

Therapeutic class: Antivirals
Pharmacologic class: Nucleotide analogue NS5B polymerase inhibitors/HCV NS5A inhibitors

AVAILABLE FORMS
Oral pellets: 150 mg sofosbuvir and 37.5 mg velpatasvir, 200 mg sofosbuvir and 50 mg velpatasvir
Tablets: 200 mg sofosbuvir and 50 mg velpatasvir, 400 mg sofosbuvir and 100 mg velpatasvir

INDICATIONS & DOSAGES
➤ **Chronic HCV genotype 1, 2, 3, 4, 5, or 6 infection without cirrhosis or with compensated cirrhosis (Child-Pugh class A) or with decompensated cirrhosis (Child-Pugh class B or C) in combination with ribavirin** ☒
Adults and children age 3 and older weighing at least 30 kg: 400 mg sofosbuvir and 100 mg velpatasvir PO once daily for 12 weeks. Refer to manufacturer's instructions for ribavirin weight-based dosing.
Children age 3 and older weighing 17 to less than 30 kg: 200 mg sofosbuvir and 50 mg velpatasvir PO once daily for 12 weeks. Refer to manufacturer's instructions for ribavirin weight-based dosing.
Children age 3 and older weighing less than 17 kg: 150 mg sofosbuvir and 37.5 mg velpatasvir PO once daily for 12 weeks. Refer to manufacturer's instructions for ribavirin weight-based dosing.

ADMINISTRATION
PO
- Keep tablets in original container.
- May give with or without food.
- Oral pellets can be taken directly in the mouth or given with food to increase palatability.
- Sprinkle oral pellets on one or more spoonfuls of nonacidic soft food (pudding,

chocolate syrup, ice cream) at or below room temperature and give within 15 minutes of gently mixing.
- To avoid bitter aftertaste, patient shouldn't chew pellets.
- Store below 86° F (30° C).

ACTION
Sofosbuvir and velpatasvir are direct-acting antivirals that inhibit viral replication of HCV.

Route	Onset	Peak	Duration
PO (sofosbuvir)	Unknown	0.5–1 hr	Unknown
PO (velpatasvir)	Unknown	3 hr	Unknown

Half-life: Sofosbuvir, 0.5 hour; velpatasvir, 15 hours.

ADVERSE REACTIONS
CNS: headache, fatigue, asthenia, insomnia, irritability, depression. **GI:** nausea, diarrhea. **Hematologic:** anemia. **Metabolic:** CK elevations, increased lipase level. **Skin:** rash.

INTERACTIONS
Drug-drug. *Antacids (aluminum hydroxide, magnesium hydroxide):* May decrease velpatasvir level. Separate antacid and drug administration by 4 hours.
🖒 *Alert: Amiodarone:* May result in serious symptomatic bradycardia. Use together isn't recommended but if coadministration is necessary, cardiac monitoring is recommended.
Anticonvulsants (carbamazepine, oxcarbazepine, phenobarbital, phenytoin), antimycobacterial drugs (rifabutin, rifampin, rifapentine): May decrease levels of both antivirals. Avoid use together.
Atorvastatin, rosuvastatin: May significantly increase statin level and increase risk of rhabdomyolysis. Use together cautiously and monitor patient closely. Don't exceed a 10-mg dose of rosuvastatin if given with sofosbuvir and velpatasvir.
Digoxin: May increase digoxin level. Monitor digoxin level and adjust digoxin dosage as needed.
Efavirenz: May decrease velpatasvir level. Use together isn't recommended.
H$_2$ antagonists (famotidine): May decrease velpatasvir level. Give H$_2$ antagonist simultaneously or 12 hours apart from drug at a dose that doesn't exceed an equivalent of famotidine 40 mg b.i.d.
Moderate to potent CYP2B6, CYP2C8, or CYP3A4 inducers (carbamazepine, rifampin),

S

P-gp inducers: May significantly decrease sofosbuvir or velpatasvir level, reducing therapeutic effect. Use together isn't recommended.

PPIs (omeprazole): May decrease velpatasvir level. Avoid use together, but if coadministration is necessary, give drug 4 hours before omeprazole 20 mg.

Tenofovir: May increase tenofovir level. Monitor patient for tenofovir-associated adverse reactions.

Tipranavir/ritonavir: May decrease levels of both antivirals. Avoid use together.

Topotecan: May increase topotecan level. Avoid use together.

Drug-herb. *St. John's wort:* May decrease antiviral levels and therapeutic effects. Use together isn't recommended.

EFFECTS ON LAB TEST RESULTS

• May increase lipase, CK, and indirect bilirubin levels.
• May decrease Hb level.

CONTRAINDICATIONS & CAUTIONS

• Combination regimen with ribavirin is contraindicated in patients for whom ribavirin is contraindicated. Refer to ribavirin manufacturer's instructions for contraindications.
• Warnings and precautions for ribavirin apply when used in combination with Epclusa. Refer to ribavirin prescribing information.
Boxed Warning Reactivation of HBV infection may occur in patients coinfected with HCV and result in fulminant hepatitis, hepatic failure, and death. Screen all patients for current or prior HBV infection by measuring HBsAg and anti-hepatitis B core antibody (anti-HBc) before treatment and if positive for HBV infection, assess baseline HBV DNA level. ∎

🜂 *Alert:* Serious symptomatic bradycardia may occur in patients taking amiodarone, particularly in patients also taking beta blockers, in those with underlying cardiac comorbidities, and in patients with advanced liver disease.
• Safety and effectiveness in children younger than age 3 haven't been established.
Dialyzable drug: Sofosbuvir active metabolite, 53%; velpatasvir, unlikely.

PREGNANCY-LACTATION-REPRODUCTION

• Use of sofosbuvir and velpatasvir in pregnancy hasn't been studied.

• Combination regimen with ribavirin is contraindicated in patients who are pregnant and in men whose partners are pregnant.
• Advise patients using combination treatment with ribavirin to use two effective forms of contraception during treatment and for 6 months (males) or 9 months (females) after therapy ends. Refer to ribavirin manufacturer's instructions for pregnancy testing before, during, and after therapy and for information about breastfeeding.
• It isn't known if sofosbuvir and velpatasvir and their metabolites appear in human milk or how they affect human milk production or the infant who is breastfed. Use cautiously, weighing benefits for the patient and risk of breastfeeding for the infant.

NURSING CONSIDERATIONS

Boxed Warning Monitor patient with current or prior HBV infection for hepatitis flare or HBV reactivation with lab testing. Watch for signs and symptoms of liver injury during active therapy and posttreatment follow-up. ∎
🜂 *Alert:* For patients taking amiodarone (with or without beta blockers) who have no other treatment options and must begin Epclusa, cardiac monitoring in an inpatient setting for first 48 hours of coadministration is recommended, followed by outpatient or self-monitoring of HR daily for at least 2 weeks. Patients who discontinue amiodarone just before starting Epclusa and those who must begin amiodarone while taking Epclusa should also undergo similar cardiac monitoring.
• Monitor patient for bradycardia (near-fainting, syncope, dizziness, light-headedness, malaise, weakness, excessive fatigue, shortness of breath, chest pain, confusion, memory problems) and report it immediately.
• Clinical and hepatic lab monitoring, including direct bilirubin, is recommended for patients with decompensated cirrhosis taking Epclusa plus ribavirin.
• Monitor patient for anemia.

PATIENT TEACHING

Boxed Warning Warn patient to immediately report signs and symptoms of liver injury (fatigue, weakness, loss of appetite, nausea, vomiting, yellowing of skin or eyes, and light-colored stool). ∎

- Advise patient to report other prescription or OTC medications or herbal products being taken, including St. John's wort.
- Inform patient that it's important not to miss or skip doses and to take this medication for as long as recommended by prescriber.
- Advise patient to avoid pregnancy during combination treatment with ribavirin and to contact prescriber immediately if pregnancy occurs.

🌙 *Alert:* Counsel patient who is also taking amiodarone about the risk of symptomatic bradycardia. Teach patient to self-monitor HR. Caution patient to seek medical attention for signs and symptoms of bradycardia.

sofosbuvir–velpatasvir–voxilaprevir ☒

soe-FOS-bue-vir/vel-PAT-as-vir/vox-i-LA-pre-vir

Vosevi

Therapeutic class: Antivirals
Pharmacologic class: Nucleotide analogue HCV NS5B polymerase inhibitors—NS5A inhibitors—NS3/4A protease inhibitors

AVAILABLE FORMS
Tablets: 400 mg sofosbuvir/100 mg velpatasvir/100 mg voxilaprevir

INDICATIONS & DOSAGES
➤ **Chronic HCV infection without cirrhosis or with compensated cirrhosis (Child-Pugh class A) in patients who have genotype 1, 2, 3, 4, 5, or 6 infection and have previously been treated with an HCV regimen containing an NS5A inhibitor, or in patients who have genotype 1a or 3 infection who have previously been treated with an HCV regimen containing sofosbuvir without an NS5A inhibitor** ☒
Adults: 1 tablet PO daily for 12 weeks.

ADMINISTRATION
PO
- Give with food to increase drug absorption.
- Store below 86° F (30° C) in original container.

ACTION
Sofosbuvir inhibits HCV NS5B RNA-dependent RNA polymerase, velpatasvir inhibits HCV NS5A protein, and voxilaprevir is a protease inhibitor. All three work together to halt HCV viral replication.

Route	Onset	Peak	Duration
PO	Unknown	2 hr (sofosbuvir); 4 hr (velpatasvir, voxilaprevir)	Unknown

Half-life: Sofosbuvir, 0.5 hour; velpatasvir, 17 hours; voxilaprevir, 33 hours.

ADVERSE REACTIONS
CNS: headache, insomnia, asthenia, depression, fatigue. **GI:** diarrhea, nausea. **Hepatic:** hyperbilirubinemia. **Metabolic:** lipase elevation, CK elevation. **Skin:** rash.

INTERACTIONS
Drug-drug. 🌙 *Alert: Amiodarone:* May increase risk of symptomatic bradycardia, including cardiac arrest and cases requiring pacemaker intervention. Avoid use together. If administration can't be avoided, advise patient of risk and monitor carefully.
Antacids: May decrease velpatasvir concentration. Separate antacids and drug by 4 hours.
Atazanavir, cyclosporine, lopinavir: May increase voxilaprevir level. Use together isn't recommended.
Atorvastatin, fluvastatin, lovastatin, simvastatin: May increase statin concentration. Avoid use together. If necessary, give lowest necessary statin dose based on risks and benefits.
Dabigatran: May increase dabigatran concentration, especially in patient with moderate renal impairment. Use cautiously together, monitor patient closely, and refer to dabigatran prescribing information for dosage adjustments.
Digoxin: May increase digoxin concentration. Use cautiously together and monitor digoxin level.
Efavirenz: May decrease velpatasvir and voxilaprevir plasma concentrations. Use together isn't recommended.
H_2-receptor antagonists (famotidine): May decrease velpatasvir concentration. Limit concurrent H_2 antagonist to equivalent of famotidine 40 mg b.i.d.
Moderate to potent inducers of CYP2B6, CYP2C8, or CYP3A4 (carbamazepine, oxcarbazepine, phenobarbital, phenytoin, rifabutin, rifapentine), P-gp inducers: May significantly

S

decrease sofosbuvir–velpatasvir–voxilaprevir plasma concentration. Use together isn't recommended.
Pitavastatin, rosuvastatin: May increase rosuvastatin and pitavastatin levels and risk of myopathy and rhabdomyolysis. Use together isn't recommended.
PPIs (omeprazole and others): May decrease velpatasvir concentration. Limit omeprazole to a dose of 20 mg. Other PPIs haven't been studied.
Pravastatin: May increase pravastatin level and risk of myopathy and rhabdomyolysis. Limit pravastatin dose to 40 mg.
Rifampin: May significantly alter sofosbuvir–velpatasvir–voxilaprevir plasma concentration. Use together is contraindicated.
Substrates of BCRP, OATP1B1, OATP1B3, OATP2B1, P-gp (imatinib, irinotecan, lapatinib, methotrexate, mitoxantrone, sulfasalazine, topotecan): May decrease concentrations of these substrates. Use together isn't recommended.
Tenofovir disoproxil fumarate: May increase tenofovir concentration, especially in patients with renal impairment. Monitor patient for tenofovir-associated adverse reactions; refer to tenofovir prescribing information for dosage adjustments.
Tipranavir/ritonavir: May decrease sofosbuvir and velpatasvir plasma concentrations. Use together isn't recommended.
Drug-herb. *St. John's wort:* May significantly decrease sofosbuvir, velpatasvir, or voxilaprevir plasma concentration. Discourage use together.
Drug-food. *Any food:* Increases drug concentrations. Give concurrently with food.

EFFECTS ON LAB TEST RESULTS

- May increase lipase, CK, and total bilirubin levels.

CONTRAINDICATIONS & CAUTIONS

Boxed Warning HBV reactivation has been reported, in some cases resulting in fulminant hepatitis, hepatic failure, and death. Test all patients for evidence of current or prior HBV infection before initiation of HCV treatment. ■

Alert: Use cautiously in patients with risk factors for liver failure (hepatocellular carcinoma, alcohol abuse).

Alert: Symptomatic bradycardia, including fatal cardiac arrest and cases requiring pacemaker intervention, has been reported when amiodarone has been administered with a sofosbuvir-containing regimen. Patients taking amiodarone who are also taking beta blockers, or who have underlying cardiac comorbidities or advanced liver disease, may be at increased risk. Signs and symptoms may occur within hours to up to 2 weeks after start of HCV therapy.

- Drug isn't recommended in patients with moderate or severe hepatic impairment (Child-Pugh class B or C).
- Dosage adjustment isn't recommended in patients with renal impairment, including patients on dialysis.
- Safety and effectiveness in children haven't been established.

Dialyzable drug: Sofosbuvir metabolite, yes; velpatasvir and voxilaprevir, unlikely.

PREGNANCY-LACTATION-REPRODUCTION

- Drug hasn't been studied during pregnancy. Use during pregnancy isn't recommended.
- It isn't known if drug or its metabolites appear in human milk, affect milk production, or affect an infant who is breastfed. Consider benefits and risks before use during breastfeeding.

NURSING CONSIDERATIONS

Boxed Warning Before initiating HCV treatment, test all patients for current or prior HBV infection by measuring HBsAg and hepatitis B core antibody (anti-HBc). ■

Boxed Warning Monitor patients coinfected with HCV or HBV for HBV reactivation and hepatitis flare during HCV treatment and posttreatment follow-up. Manage HBV infection as clinically indicated. ■

Alert: Monitor closely for liver failure and discontinue drug in patients who develop signs and symptoms of decompensation or as clinically indicated.

Alert: Administration with amiodarone isn't recommended. If these drugs must be used together or if amiodarone has been discontinued just before beginning HCV therapy, monitor patient for signs and symptoms of bradycardia (near-fainting, fainting, dizziness, light-headedness, malaise, weakness, excessive fatigue, shortness of breath, chest pain, confusion, or memory problems). Utilize inpatient cardiac monitoring for first 48 hours; then outpatient monitoring or self-monitoring of HR for bradycardia should continue daily for at least first 2 weeks of treatment. Discontinue drug if signs or symptoms of bradycardia occur.

• Verify pregnancy status before treatment.
• *Look alike–sound alike:* Don't confuse sofosbuvir–velpatasvir combination with sofosbuvir–velpatasvir–voxilaprevir combination.

PATIENT TEACHING

• Advise patient to report a history of HBV infection before therapy begins.

Boxed Warning Warn patient that therapy can increase risk of HBV reactivation and that lab testing for HBV exposure will be needed before therapy begins. ■

• Explain that for therapy to be effective, patient needs to take drug exactly as prescribed for the entire duration.
• Caution patient not to stop treatment without first discussing with prescriber.
● *Alert:* Caution patient to seek immediate medical attention for signs and symptoms of bradycardia.
● *Alert:* Warn patient to immediately report signs and symptoms of liver injury (fatigue, weakness, loss of appetite, nausea, vomiting, yellowing of skin or eyes, light-colored stool).
• Caution patient to immediately report pregnancy or breastfeeding to prescriber.

---

solifenacin succinate
sole-ah-FEN-ah-sin

VESIcare✔, VESIcare LS

Therapeutic class: Urinary antispasmodics
Pharmacologic class: Antimuscarinics

AVAILABLE FORMS
Oral suspension: 1 mg/mL
Tablets (film-coated) ⓖ: 5 mg, 10 mg

INDICATIONS & DOSAGES
➤ **Overactive bladder with urinary urgency, frequency, and urge incontinence**
Adults: 5 mg PO once daily. May increase to 10 mg once daily if 5-mg dose is well tolerated.
Adjust-a-dose: For patients with CrCl less than 30 mL/minute or moderate hepatic impairment (Child-Pugh class B), or if drug is taken concurrently with CYP3A4 inhibitors, maximum dose is 5 mg.

➤ **Neurogenic detrusor overactivity**
Children age 2 and older weighing 60 kg or more: Initially, 5 mL PO once daily. May titrate to lowest effective dose; maximum daily dose, 10 mL.
Children age 2 and older weighing more than 45 to 60 kg: Initially, 4 mL PO once daily. May titrate to lowest effective dose; maximum daily dose, 8 mL.
Children age 2 and older weighing more than 30 to 45 kg: Initially, 3 mL PO once daily. May titrate to lowest effective dose; maximum daily dose, 6 mL.
Children age 2 and older weighing more than 15 to 30 kg: Initially, 3 mL PO once daily. May titrate to lowest effective dose; maximum daily dose, 5 mL.
Children age 2 and older weighing 9 to 15 kg: Initially, 2 mL PO once daily. May titrate to lowest effective dose; maximum daily dose, 4 mL.
Adjust-a-dose: Don't exceed the recommended initial dose in children with severe renal impairment (CrCl less than 30 mL/minute/1.73 m^2) or moderate hepatic impairment (Child-Pugh class B), or in those taking concomitant CYP3A4 inhibitors.

ADMINISTRATION
PO
• Give drug without regard for food.
• Patient should swallow tablet whole with water.
• Follow oral suspension dose with liquid, such as water or milk.

ACTION
Relaxes smooth muscle of bladder by antagonizing muscarinic receptors, relieving symptoms of overactive bladder.

Route	Onset	Peak	Duration
PO	Unknown	3–8 hr (tablets); 2–6 hr (oral suspension)	Unknown

Half-life: Tablets, 45 to 68 hours; oral suspension, 26 hours.

ADVERSE REACTIONS
CNS: depression, dizziness, fatigue. **CV:** HTN, leg swelling. **EENT:** blurred vision, dry eyes, dry mouth, pharyngitis. **GI:** constipation, dyspepsia, nausea, upper abdominal pain, vomiting. **GU:** urine retention, UTI. **Respiratory:** cough. **Other:** influenza.

S

INTERACTIONS

Drug-drug. *Drugs that prolong QT interval:* May increase risk of serious cardiac arrhythmias. Monitor patient and ECG closely.

Potassium chloride (solid oral dosage forms only): May increase ulcer risk. Avoid using solid oral dosage forms of potassium chloride.

Strong CYP3A4 inducers (carbamazepine, phenobarbital, phenytoin): May decrease solifenacin concentration. Monitor therapy.

Strong CYP3A4 inhibitors (ketoconazole): May increase solifenacin level. Don't exceed solifenacin starting dose when used together.

EFFECTS ON LAB TEST RESULTS

None reported.

CONTRAINDICATIONS & CAUTIONS

- Contraindicated in patients hypersensitive to drug or its components and in patients with urine or gastric retention or uncontrolled narrow-angle glaucoma.
- Drug isn't recommended for use in patients with severe hepatic impairment (Child-Pugh class C).
- Angioedema has been reported, including after first dose.
- Use cautiously in older adults and in patients with a history of prolonged QT interval, those being treated for angle-closure glaucoma, and those with bladder outflow obstruction, decreased GI motility, renal insufficiency, or moderate hepatic impairment.
- CNS anticholinergic effects can occur, including headache, confusion, hallucinations, and somnolence.

Dialyzable drug: Unknown.

⚠ **Overdose S&S:** Anticholinergic effects (fixed and dilated pupils, blurred vision, failure of heel-to-toe exam, tremors, dry skin).

PREGNANCY-LACTATION-REPRODUCTION

- There are no adequate studies during pregnancy. Use only if potential benefit justifies fetal risk.
- It isn't known if drug appears in human milk. Use cautiously during breastfeeding after considering risks to the infant.

NURSING CONSIDERATIONS

- Assess bladder function, and monitor drug effects.
- Watch for urine retention in patient with bladder outlet obstruction.
- Monitor patient for decreased gastric motility and constipation.
- Monitor patient for signs and symptoms of anticholinergic CNS effects (including headache, confusion, hallucinations, and somnolence), particularly after beginning treatment or increasing dosage. If patient experiences anticholinergic CNS effects, consider dosage reduction or drug discontinuation.

PATIENT TEACHING

- Explain that drug may cause blurred vision and drowsiness. Tell patient not to drive, operate heavy machinery, or perform hazardous activities or tasks until effects of the drug are known.
- Discourage use of other drugs that may cause dry mouth, constipation, urine retention, or blurred vision.
- Teach patient safe drug administration.
- Urge patient to report all adverse reactions, especially swelling in the face, lips, or tongue or abdominal pain or constipation that lasts 3 days or longer.
- Tell patient that drug decreases the ability to sweat normally, and advise cautious use in hot environments or during strenuous activity.

somatropin 🔲
soe-ma-TROE-pin

Genotropin, Genotropin MiniQuick, Humatrope, Norditropin FlexPro, Nutropin AQ NuSpin, Omnitrope, Saizen, Serostim, Zomacton, Zorbtive

Therapeutic class: Growth hormones
Pharmacologic class: Anterior pituitary hormones

AVAILABLE FORMS

Genotropin injection: 5 mg and 12 mg in two-chamber cartridges
Genotropin MiniQuick injection: 0.2 mg, 0.4 mg, 0.6 mg, 0.8 mg, 1 mg, 1.2 mg, 1.4 mg, 1.6 mg, 1.8 mg, 2 mg prefilled syringes
Humatrope injection: 5 mg vial; 6 mg, 12 mg, 24 mg cartridges
Norditropin injection: 5 mg/1.5 mL, 10 mg/1.5 mL, 15 mg/1.5 mL, 30 mg/3 mL prefilled pens

Nutropin AQ injection: 5 mg/2-mL device,
10 mg/2-mL device or pen, 20 mg/2-mL
device or pen
Omnitrope injection: 5.8 mg/vial; 5 mg/
1.5 mL, 10 mg/1.5 mL injection cartridge
Saizen injection: 5 mg, 8.8 mg vials
Serostim injection: 5 mg, 6 mg single-dose
vials; 4 mg multidose vial
Zomacton* injection: 5 mg, 10 mg vials
Zorbtive injection: 8.8 mg vials

INDICATIONS & DOSAGES
➤ **Long-term treatment of growth failure
in children with inadequate secretion of
endogenous growth hormone (GH)**
Children: 0.18 to 0.3 mg/kg/week Humatrope subcut, divided into equal doses given
six to seven times weekly. Or, up to 0.3 mg/kg
Nutropin AQ subcut weekly in daily divided
doses; in patients who are pubertal, a weekly
dosage of up to 0.7 mg/kg (Nutropin AQ) in
daily divided doses may be used. Or, Saizen
0.18 mg/kg/week subcut divided into equal
doses given on 3 alternate days six times
per week or daily. Or, Norditropin 0.024 to
0.034 mg/kg/day subcut given on 6 or
7 days each week. Or, 0.16 to 0.24 mg/kg
Genotropin or Omnitrope subcut weekly
divided into six or seven doses. Or, 0.18 to
0.3 mg/kg/week Zomacton divided into equal
doses given 3, 6, or 7 days per week.
➤ **Growth failure from chronic renal insufficiency up to time of renal transplantation**
Children: Up to 0.35 mg/kg/week Nutropin
AQ subcut divided into daily doses.
➤ **Long-term treatment of short stature
from Turner syndrome**
Children: Up to 0.375 mg/kg/week Humatrope or Nutropin AQ subcut, divided
into equal doses given three to seven times
weekly. Or, up to 0.375 mg/kg/week Zomacton subcut divided into equal doses given
three, six, or seven times weekly. Or, up to
0.067 mg/kg/day Norditropin subcut given on
6 or 7 days each week. Or, 0.33 mg/kg/week
Genotropin or Omnitrope divided into six or
seven once-daily subcut injections per week.
➤ **Short stature in children with Noonan
syndrome (Norditropin only)**
Children: Up to 0.46 mg/kg subcut weekly,
divided into six or seven equal daily doses.
➤ **Long-term treatment of growth failure
in children with Prader-Willi syndrome diagnosed by genetic testing**

Children: 0.24 mg/kg Genotropin,
Norditropin, or Omnitrope subcut weekly
divided into six or seven equal daily doses.
Individualize dosage based on growth
response.
➤ **Replacement of endogenous GH in
adults with GH deficiency**
Adults: Initially, not more than 0.006 mg/kg
Humatrope or Zomacton subcut daily. May
increase to maximum of 0.0125 mg/kg Humatrope or Zomacton daily. Or, initially
0.004 mg/kg Norditropin subcut daily.
May increase Norditropin to maximum of
0.016 mg/kg daily after about 6 weeks. Or,
initially, 0.2 mg Norditropin or Zomacton
subcut daily (range 0.15 to 0.3 mg/day);
may increase by 0.1 to 0.2 mg/day every
1 to 2 months based on clinical response and
insulin-like growth factor-1 concentration.

Or, initially, not more than 0.006 mg/kg
Nutropin AQ subcut daily. May increase
dosage to maximum of 0.025 mg/kg
daily in patients younger than age 35 or
0.0125 mg/kg daily in patients older than
age 35. Or, starting dosages not exceeding
0.04 mg/kg Genotropin or Omnitrope subcut
weekly divided into six or seven equal doses;
may increase at 4- to 8-week intervals to a
maximum dose of 0.08 mg/kg subcut weekly
divided into six or seven equal doses. Or,
initially, not more than 0.005 mg/kg Saizen
subcut daily. May increase after 4 weeks to a
maximum dose of 0.01 mg/kg daily based on
patient tolerance and clinical response.
➤ **HIV wasting or cachexia (Serostim only)**
*Adults and children weighing more than
55 kg:* 6 mg subcut daily at bedtime.
Adults and children weighing 45 to 55 kg:
5 mg subcut daily at bedtime.
Adults and children weighing 35 to 45 kg:
4 mg subcut daily at bedtime.
Adults and children weighing less than 35 kg:
0.1 mg/kg/day subcut daily at bedtime.
➤ **Long-term treatment of growth failure
in children born small for gestational age
(SGA) who don't catch up by age 2**
Children: 0.48 mg/kg Genotropin or Omnitrope subcut weekly divided into six or seven
doses.
➤ **Short stature in children born SGA who
don't catch up by age 2 to 4**
Children: Up to 0.067 mg/kg/day Norditropin
or Humatrope subcut given on 6 or 7 days
each week.

➤ Idiopathic short stature
Children: Up to 0.37 mg/kg Humatrope subcut weekly divided into six or seven equal doses or Zomacton divided into three, six, or seven equal doses. Or, up to 0.47 mg/kg/week Genotropin, Omnitrope, or Norditropin subcut divided into six or seven equal doses. Or, up to 0.3 mg/kg/week Nutropin AQ subcut divided into equal daily doses.

➤ Short bowel syndrome (Zorbtive only)
Adults: 0.1 mg/kg/day subcut daily for 4 weeks. Maximum dosage, 8 mg/day.
Adjust-a-dose: For moderate toxicity, treat symptomatically with analgesics or reduce dosage to 0.05 mg/kg/day; maximum dosage, 4 mg/day).

➤ Treatment of short stature or growth failure in children with short stature homeobox-containing (*SHOX*) gene deficiency (Humatrope or Zomacton) ▨
Children: 0.35 mg/kg subcut weekly divided into equal doses 3 (Zomacton only), 6, or 7 days/week.

ADMINISTRATION
• Refer to product insert for brand-specific reconstitution instructions.

Subcutaneous
• To prepare solution, inject supplied diluent into vial containing drug by aiming stream of liquid against wall of glass vial. Then swirl vial gently until contents are completely dissolved. Don't shake vial.
⚠ *Alert:* Don't use vials containing benzyl alcohol in neonates or if patient has a known benzyl alcohol sensitivity.
⚠ *Alert:* When administering to newborn, reconstitute with sterile water for injection.
• After reconstitution, make sure solution is clear. Don't inject solution if it's cloudy or contains particles.
• For patients on hemodialysis, give drug before bedtime or at least 3 to 4 hours after dialysis. For long-term cycling peritoneal dialysis, give drug in the morning after completion of dialysis. For long-term ambulatory peritoneal dialysis, give drug in the evening at the time of the overnight exchange.
• Rotate injection sites to avoid tissue atrophy.
• Store reconstituted drug in refrigerator; use within manufacturer's recommended time frame for each drug.
• If patient develops sensitivity to diluent, reconstitute drug with sterile water for injection. When drug is reconstituted in this way, use only one reconstituted dose per vial, refrigerate solution if it isn't used immediately after reconstitution, use reconstituted dose within 24 hours, and discard unused portion.

ACTION
Purified GH of recombinant DNA origin that stimulates skeletal, linear, muscle, and organ growth.

Route	Onset	Peak	Duration
Subcut	Unknown	Varies by brand	18–20 hr

Half-life: Varies by brand. Refer to manufacturer's drug label.

ADVERSE REACTIONS
CNS: headache, pain, hypoesthesia, paresthesia, fatigue, fever, depression, insomnia. **CV:** edema, chest pain, HTN. **EENT:** periorbital edema, otitis media, pharyngitis, sinusitis, tonsillitis. **GI:** nausea, vomiting, flatulence, abdominal pain. **GU:** UTI. **Hematologic:** eosinophilia, anemia. **Metabolic:** mild hyperglycemia, hypothyroidism, impaired glucose tolerance, hyperlipidemia, new or worsening diabetes. **Musculoskeletal:** arthralgia, carpal tunnel syndrome, myalgia, new or exacerbated scoliosis, limb pain, bone pain, stiffness of extremities, abnormal bone growth. **Respiratory:** URI, bronchitis, dyspnea. **Skin:** injection-site pain or reaction, diaphoresis, hematoma, melanocytic nevus, rash, acne. **Other:** antibodies to GH, infection, flulike syndrome, gynecomastia.

INTERACTIONS
Drug-drug. *Corticotropin, corticosteroids:* Long-term use may inhibit growth response to GH. Monitor patient for lack of effect.
Estrogen replacement: May decrease somatropin level in adult women. Increase somatropin dosage as necessary.
Insulin, oral antidiabetics: Somatropin may decrease insulin sensitivity. Antidiabetic dosage may need adjustment.

EFFECTS ON LAB TEST RESULTS
• May increase cholesterol, triglyceride, phosphorus, AST, ALT, ALP, HbA_{1c}, IGF-1, TSH, and parathyroid hormone levels.
• May increase or decrease glucose level.
• May decrease eosinophil count.

Reactions in bold italics are *life-threatening*. Interactions may have a *rapid onset* or a **delayed onset**.

CONTRAINDICATIONS & CAUTIONS

• Contraindicated in patients with hypersensitivity to somatropin or its excipients.

• Contraindicated in children with closed epiphyses and in patients with active proliferative or severe nonproliferative diabetic retinopathy or an active underlying intracranial lesion.

• Contraindicated in patients with active malignancy. An increased risk of second neoplasm has been reported in childhood cancer survivors treated with somatropin. Patients with HIV and children with short stature (genetic cause) have increased baseline risk of developing malignancies. Consider risk and benefits before initiating therapy; monitor these patients carefully.

• Contraindicated in patients with Prader-Willi syndrome who are severely obese, have a history of upper airway obstruction or sleep apnea, or have severe respiratory impairment.

• For patients hypersensitive to either metacresol or glycerin, don't use supplied diluent to reconstitute Humatrope.

• Contraindicated in patients with acute critical illness due to complications following open heart or abdominal surgery, trauma, or acute respiratory failure. Safety of continuing somatropin treatment in patients receiving replacement doses for approved indications who concurrently develop acute critical illnesses hasn't been established. Weigh potential benefit of treatment continuation against risks.

• Serious systemic hypersensitivity reactions, including anaphylactic reactions and angioedema, have been reported.

• Use cautiously in children with hypothyroidism and in those with GH deficiency caused by intracranial lesion.

• Use cautiously in patients with diabetes.

• May increase risk of pancreatitis. Monitor patient for persistent abdominal pain with or without vomiting.

• Patients receiving somatropin who have or are at risk for pituitary hormone deficiency may be at risk for reduced serum cortisol levels or unmasking of central (secondary) hypoadrenalism. Also, patients treated with glucocorticoid replacement for previously diagnosed hypoadrenalism may require an increase in maintenance or stress doses once somatropin therapy begins.

Dialyzable drug: Unknown.

⚠ *Overdose S&S:* Fluid retention, hypoglycemia followed by hyperglycemia, glucose intolerance, gigantism, acromegaly.

PREGNANCY-LACTATION-REPRODUCTION

• There are no adequate studies during pregnancy. Use only if clearly needed.

• It isn't known if drug appears in human milk. Use cautiously during breastfeeding.

NURSING CONSIDERATIONS

• Frequently examine children with hypothyroidism and those whose GH deficiency is caused by an intracranial lesion for progression or recurrence of underlying disease.

• Obtain hip X-rays to check for slipped capital femoral epiphysis or femoral avascular necrosis before starting somatropin in patients with growth failure secondary to chronic kidney disease.

• Watch for slipped capital femoral epiphysis (limb, hip, or knee pain) or progression of scoliosis in patients with rapid growth.

🚫 *Alert:* In patients with Prader-Willi syndrome who are morbidly obese and in those with a history of respiratory impairment, sleep apnea, or unidentified respiratory infection, therapy may be life-threatening. Assess patients with Prader-Willi syndrome for sleep apnea and upper airway obstruction before treatment. Interrupt treatment if signs of upper airway obstruction occur.

• Monitor patient with Prader-Willi syndrome for signs of respiratory infection.

• Monitor child's height regularly. Regular checkups, including monitoring of blood and radiologic studies, are also needed.

• Monitor patient's glucose level regularly because GH may induce a state of insulin resistance or new-onset diabetes.

• Transient fluid retention may occur in adults, including arthralgia, myalgia, or nerve compression syndromes such as carpal tunnel syndrome, in addition to edema.

• Excessive glucocorticoid therapy inhibits somatropin's growth-promoting effect. Patients with coexisting corticotropin deficiency should have their glucocorticoid replacement dosage carefully adjusted to avoid growth inhibition.

• Monitor results of periodic thyroid function tests for hypothyroidism; condition may need thyroid hormone treatment.

• Patient should have ophthalmic exams to assess for intracranial HTN (IH) before and

S

periodically during therapy. Monitor patient for signs and symptoms of IH (papilledema, visual changes, headache, nausea, vomiting). Patients with Turner syndrome may be at increased risk.

• Monitor patients with preexisting tumors or growth failure secondary to an intracranial lesion for recurrence or progression of underlying disease; discontinue therapy with evidence of recurrence.

• Monitor all patients for increased growth, or potential malignant changes, of skin lesions.

• Monitor patients for signs and symptoms of serious systemic hypersensitivity reactions.

• Only adults with GH deficiency alone or together with multiple hormone deficiencies from pituitary or hypothalamic disease, surgery, radiation, or trauma or those who were GH deficient as children and have been confirmed GH deficient as adults can take Saizen.

• *Look alike–sound alike:* Don't confuse somatropin with somatrem or sumatriptan or Humatrope with homatropine.

PATIENT TEACHING

• Inform parents that child with endocrine disorders (including GH deficiency) may have an increased risk of slipped capital epiphyses. Tell parents to notify prescriber if they notice their child limping.

• Advise parents to be alert for limping or complaints of hip or knee pain in children.

• Instruct patient with diabetes to monitor glucose level closely and report changes to prescriber.

• Instruct patient or parents in appropriate injection technique and needle disposal. Tell them to rotate injection sites.

• Advise patient or parents that serious systemic hypersensitivity reactions, including anaphylaxis and angioedema, can occur and to seek immediate medical attention if an allergic reaction occurs.

• Stress importance of close follow-up care and of reporting all adverse reactions.

sotalol hydrochloride
SOE-ta-lole

Betapace, Betapace AF, Sorine, Sotylize

Therapeutic class: Antiarrhythmics
Pharmacologic class: Nonselective beta blockers

AVAILABLE FORMS
Oral solution: 5 mg/mL
Solution for injection: 15 mg/mL
Tablets: 80 mg, 120 mg, 160 mg, 240 mg
Tablets (AF): 80 mg, 120 mg, 160 mg

INDICATIONS & DOSAGES
Boxed Warning Calculate CrCl before dosing; adjust dosing interval based on CrCl. Don't initiate therapy with IV sotalol or oral solution if baseline QTc exceeds 450 msec. ∎
Boxed Warning *Adjust-a-dose (for all indications):* If QT interval prolongs to 500 msec or greater, reduce dosage, lengthen dosing interval, or discontinue drug. ∎
➤ **Documented, life-threatening ventricular arrhythmias**
Adults: Initially, 80 mg PO b.i.d. Increase dosage gradually (increments of 80 mg/day for Sotylize) every 3 days as needed and tolerated. Most patients respond to 160 to 320 mg/day, although some patients with refractory arrhythmias need up to 640 mg/day. Or, 75 mg IV once daily or b.i.d. based on CrCl. After 3 days, dosage may be increased to 75 to 150 mg IV once daily or every 12 hours based on CrCl. For refractory life-threatening arrhythmias, dosage may be increased to 225 to 300 mg IV once daily or every 12 hours.
Children age 2 and older with normal renal function: Initially, 1.2 mg/kg PO t.i.d. Titrate dosage to a maximum of 2.4 mg/kg (equivalent to 320 mg total daily dose for adults). Guide titration by clinical response, HR, and QTc interval. Allow at least 36 hours between dose increments.
Children younger than age 2 with normal renal function: Calculate dosage according to age factor plotted on a logarithmic scale found in manufacturer's instructions.
Adjust-a-dose: Adults: For oral route, if CrCl is 30 to 60 mL/minute, increase dosage interval to every 24 hours; if CrCl is 10 to

---

Reactions in bold italics are *life-threatening*. Interactions may have a *rapid onset* or a **delayed onset**.

29 mL/minute, increase interval to every 36 to 48 hours; and if CrCl is less than 10 mL/minute, individualize dosage. For IV route, if CrCl is 40 to 59 mL/minute, give IV drug once daily; don't give if CrCl is less than 40 mL/minute.

Children: Use in any age-group with decreased renal function should be at lower dosages or at increased intervals between doses. Use of sotalol in children with renal impairment hasn't been investigated.

➤ **To maintain normal sinus rhythm or to delay recurrence of atrial fibrillation or atrial flutter in patients with symptomatic atrial fibrillation or flutter who are currently in sinus rhythm**

Adults: 80 mg PO b.i.d. (Don't use if baseline QT interval exceeds 450 msec.) Increase dosage as needed to 120 mg PO b.i.d. after 3 days if the QTc interval is less than 500 msec. Maximum dosage is 160 mg PO b.i.d. Or, 75 mg IV once daily or every 12 hours based on CrCl. After 3 days, dosage may be increased to 112.5 to 150 mg IV once daily or every 12 hours based on clearance.

Children age 2 and older with normal renal function: Initially, 1.2 mg/kg PO t.i.d. Titrate dosage to a maximum of 2.4 mg/kg (equivalent to 320 mg total daily dose for adults). Guide titration by clinical response, HR, and QTc interval. Allow at least 36 hours between dose increments.

Children younger than age 2 with normal renal function: Initially, 1.2 mg/kg PO t.i.d. multiplied by age factor plotted on a logarithmic scale found in manufacturer's instructions.

Adjust-a-dose: Adults: For oral route, if CrCl is 40 to 60 mL/minute, increase dosage interval to every 24 hours; if CrCl is less than 40 mL/minute, use is contraindicated. For IV route, if CrCl is 40 to 59 mL/minute, give IV drug once daily; don't give if CrCl is less than 40 mL/minute.

Children: Use in any age-group with decreased renal function should be at lower dosages or at increased intervals between doses. Use of sotalol in children with renal impairment hasn't been investigated.

ADMINISTRATION
PO
• May give without regard for food, but patient should take the same way each time.

• Give 2 hours before or 2 hours after antacids.
• Skip a missed dose and give next dose at the usual time. Don't double the dose or shorten dosing interval.

IV
▼ Dilute drug with NSS, D_5W, or lactated Ringer solution in a volume of 120 to 250 mL to compensate for dead space in the infusion set.
▼ Give loading dose over 1 hour.
▼ Use an infusion pump to administer drug at a constant rate over 5 hours.
▼ **Incompatibilities:** None listed by manufacturer. Consult a drug incompatibility reference for more information.

ACTION
Depresses sinus HR, slows AV conduction, decreases cardiac output, and lowers systolic and diastolic BP. Drug also has class III antiarrhythmic properties and can prolong duration of the cardiac action potential.

Route	Onset	Peak	Duration
PO	1–2 hr	2–4 hr	Unknown
IV	5–10 min	Unknown	Unknown

Half-life: Adults, 12 hours; children, 9.5 hours.

ADVERSE REACTIONS
CNS: asthenia, headache, dizziness, weakness, fatigue. **CV:** chest pain, palpitations, *bradycardia, AV block, prolonged QT interval, proarrhythmic events (including polymorphic ventricular tachycardia, PVCs, ventricular fibrillation),* edema, ECG abnormalities, hypotension. **EENT:** visual disturbance. **GI:** nausea, vomiting, diarrhea, abdominal pain. **Musculoskeletal:** pain. **Respiratory:** dyspnea. **Skin:** diaphoresis.

INTERACTIONS
Drug-drug. *Antacids containing aluminum oxide and magnesium hydroxide:* May reduce bradycardic effect. Avoid sotalol administration within 2 hours of antacid.
Antihypertensives, catecholamine-depleting drugs (guanethidine, reserpine): May increase hypotensive effects or cause marked bradycardia. Monitor BP and pulse closely.
Beta$_2$-agonists (albuterol, isoproterenol, terbutaline): May diminish the bronchodilatory effect. Dosage increase may be needed.

S

Clonidine: May enhance rebound effect after withdrawal of clonidine. Stop sotalol several days before withdrawing clonidine.

Drugs that prolong QT interval (Class I and III antiarrhythmics, bepridil, macrolide antibiotics, phenothiazines, quinolones, TCAs): May cause excessive QT prolongation. Monitor QT interval.

General anesthetics: May increase myocardial depression. Monitor patient closely.

Insulin, oral antidiabetics: May cause hyperglycemia and may mask signs and symptoms of hypoglycemia. Adjust dosage accordingly.

Negative chronotropes (beta blockers [metoprolol], calcium channel blockers [diltiazem, verapamil], cardiac glycosides): May increase risk of bradycardia and hypotension. Monitor patient closely.

Prazosin: May increase the risk of orthostatic hypotension. Assist patient to stand slowly until effects are known.

Theophylline: May decrease bronchodilating effects. Avoid using together.

EFFECTS ON LAB TEST RESULTS
• May increase glucose level.
• May cause false-positive catecholamine level.

CONTRAINDICATIONS & CAUTIONS
• Contraindicated in patients hypersensitive to drug.
• Contraindicated in those with severe sinus node dysfunction, sinus bradycardia, second- and third-degree AV block unless patient has a pacemaker, congenital or acquired long QT-interval syndrome, cardiogenic shock, uncontrolled HF, CrCl of less than 40 mL/minute, and bronchial asthma.
• Contraindicated in patients with hypokalemia or hypomagnesemia before correction of imbalance.
• Use of beta blockers in patients with bronchospastic diseases (chronic bronchitis, emphysema) isn't recommended. If used, give smallest effective dose.

Boxed Warning Sotalol can cause life-threatening ventricular tachycardia associated with QT-interval prolongation. ∎

• Use cautiously in patients with renal impairment, hypothyroidism, or diabetes (beta blockers may mask signs and symptoms of hypoglycemia).
• Use cautiously in patients with a history of allergic reactions, including anaphylaxis.

Patients taking beta blockers may have more severe reactions and be less responsive to epinephrine.

• Use of beta blockers may increase risk of general anesthesia and surgical procedures; however, beta blockers shouldn't routinely be withheld before major surgery.

Dialyzable drug: Yes.

⚠ *Overdose S&S:* Bradycardia, bronchospasm, HF, hypoglycemia, hypotension, asystole, QT-interval prolongation, torsades de pointes, ventricular tachycardia, death.

PREGNANCY-LACTATION-REPRODUCTION
• There are no adequate studies during pregnancy. Use only if potential benefit justifies fetal risk. Drug crosses placental barrier and appears in amniotic fluid.
• Drug appears in human milk. Patient should discontinue breastfeeding or discontinue drug.

NURSING CONSIDERATIONS
Boxed Warning Because proarrhythmic events may occur at the start of therapy and during dosage adjustments, patients should be hospitalized for a minimum of 3 days in a facility that can provide calculations of CrCl, continuous ECG monitoring, and cardiac resuscitation. Calculate CrCl before dosing; adjust the dosing interval based on CrCl. ∎

Boxed Warning The baseline QTc interval must be less than or equal to 450 msec before starting sotalol IV or oral suspension. If QT interval is 500 msec or more, dosage or frequency must be decreased or drug discontinued. ∎

• Assess patient for new or worsened symptoms of HF.
• Monitor BP closely.
• Although patients receiving IV lidocaine may start sotalol therapy without ill effects, withdraw other antiarrhythmics before therapy begins. Sotalol therapy typically is delayed until two or three half-lives of the withdrawn drug have elapsed. After withdrawing amiodarone, give sotalol only after QT interval normalizes.
• Adjust dosage slowly, allowing 3 days between dosage increments for adequate monitoring of QT intervals and for drug levels to reach a steady-state level.
• Monitor electrolytes regularly, especially if patient is receiving diuretics. Electrolyte imbalances, such as hypokalemia or

hypomagnesemia, may enhance QT-interval prolongation and increase the risk of serious arrhythmias such as torsades de pointes.

• Abrupt withdrawal of beta blockers may exacerbate angina and increase risk of MI. Gradually reduce dosage over 1 to 2 weeks after long-term use. Monitor patient closely.

• Beta blockers may mask signs and symptoms of hyperthyroidism (tachycardia). Abrupt withdrawal of beta blockers in patients with thyroid disease may exacerbate signs and symptoms of hyperthyroidism, including thyroid storm.

• *Look alike–sound alike:* Don't confuse sotalol with Sudafed.

PATIENT TEACHING

• Explain that patient will need to be hospitalized for initiation of drug therapy.

• Instruct patient in safe drug administration.

• Warn patient to report all adverse reactions and to immediately report fast, irregular heartbeat; light-headedness; or fainting.

• Encourage patient to report severe diarrhea, unusual sweating, vomiting, anorexia, or excessive thirst as these conditions could lead to electrolyte changes.

• Stress need to take drug as prescribed, even when feeling well. Caution patient against stopping drug suddenly.

• Caution patient against using OTC drugs and decongestants while taking drug.

• Advise patient to report pregnancy or plans to become pregnant or to breastfeed.

---

spironolactone
speer-on-oh-LAK-tone

Aldactone⚕, CaroSpir

Therapeutic class: Diuretics
Pharmacologic class: Potassium-sparing diuretics–aldosterone receptor antagonists

AVAILABLE FORMS
Oral suspension: 25 mg/5 mL
Tablets: 25 mg, 50 mg, 100 mg

INDICATIONS & DOSAGES
➤ **Edema due to HF, hepatic cirrhosis, or nephrotic syndrome (except CaroSpir)**
Adults: Initially, 100 mg PO (tablets) daily as a single dose or in divided doses. When used as the only agent for diuresis, give drug

for at least 5 days before increasing dosage to obtain desired dose. Usual dosage ranges from 25 to 200 mg PO daily. When given for cirrhosis, initiate drug in a hospital setting and titrate slowly.
➤ **Edema from hepatic cirrhosis (CaroSpir)**
Adults: Initially, 75 mg suspension PO daily in either single or divided doses. Initiate therapy in a hospital setting and slowly titrate. When used as the only agent for diuresis, give for at least 5 days before increasing dosage. If patient requires more than 100 mg, use another formulation.
➤ **HTN**
Adults: Initially, 25 to 50 mg (tablets) PO daily or in divided doses. Or, 20 to 75 mg suspension PO daily in single or divided doses. May titrate dosage at 2-week intervals. Dosages higher than 75 (suspension) or 100 (tablets) mg/day generally don't provide additional BP reductions.
➤ **To manage primary hyperaldosteronism (except CaroSpir)**
Adults: 100 to 400 mg (tablets) PO daily. Use lowest effective dose.
➤ **Severe HF (class III or IV), usually as adjunct to other HF therapies (except CaroSpir)**
Adults: 25 mg (tablets) PO daily in patients with serum potassium level of 5.0 mEq/L or less and eGFR greater than 50 mL/minute/1.73 m². May increase to 50 mg (tablets) PO daily as clinically indicated.
Adjust-a-dose: Patients who don't tolerate 25 mg daily may have dosage decreased to every other day. In patients with eGFR between 30 and 50 mL/minute/1.73m², consider initiating at 25 mg every other day.
➤ **NYHA HF (class III or IV) with other HF therapies (CaroSpir)**
Adults: Initially, 20 mg suspension PO once daily in patients with serum potassium level of 5.0 mEq/L or less and eGFR greater than 50 mL/minute/1.73 m². May increase dosage to 37.5 mg if 20-mg dose is tolerated.
Adjust-a-dose: In patients with eGFR between 30 and 50 mL/minute/1.73 m², consider initial dose of 10 mg, because of risk of hyperkalemia. If patient develops hyperkalemia on 20-mg once-daily therapy, reduce dosage to 20 mg every other day.

ADMINISTRATION
PO
• Drug is a hazardous agent; use safe handling and disposal precautions.
• CaroSpir suspension isn't therapeutically equivalent to Aldactone tablets.
• May give tablets or suspension with or without food but give consistently with respect to food.

ACTION
Antagonizes aldosterone in the distal tubules, increasing sodium and water excretion.

Route	Onset	Peak	Duration
PO (tablets)	Unknown	3–4 hr	2–3 days
PO (suspension)	Unknown	2.5–5 hr	Unknown

Half-life: Tablets, 1.25 hours; suspension, 1 to 2 hours.

ADVERSE REACTIONS
CNS: headache, drowsiness, lethargy, confusion, ataxia, fever. **CV:** vasculitis. **GI:** diarrhea, *gastric bleeding*, ulceration, cramping, gastritis, nausea, vomiting. **GU:** *renal failure*, erectile dysfunction, menstrual disturbances, postmenopausal bleeding, decreased libido. **Hematologic:** *agranulocytosis, thrombocytopenia.* **Hepatic:** *hepatotoxicity.* **Metabolic:** *hyperkalemia,* hypovolemia, hyponatremia, mild acidosis, hyperuricemia. **Musculoskeletal:** leg cramps. **Skin:** alopecia, urticaria, hirsutism, maculopapular eruptions, *DRESS syndrome, SJS, TEN.* **Other:** *anaphylaxis,* gynecomastia, breast soreness.

INTERACTIONS
Drug-drug. *ACE inhibitors, ARBs:* May increase risk of severe hyperkalemia. Use together with caution and monitor potassium levels.
Aspirin and other salicylates: May block diuretic effect of spironolactone. Watch for diminished spironolactone response.
Cholestyramine: May increase risk of metabolic acidosis and hyperkalemia. Monitor therapy.
Digoxin: May alter digoxin clearance, increasing risk of toxicity. Monitor digoxin level.
◑ *Alert: Eplerenone:* May increase risk of severe hyperkalemia. Use together is contraindicated.

Heparin, low-molecular-weight heparins: May increase risk of hyperkalemia. Use cautiously and monitor potassium level.
Lithium: May reduce lithium renal clearance and increase risk of lithium toxicity. Monitor patient closely.
NSAIDs: May decrease diuretic effect and increase potassium level. Monitor patient closely.
Potassium-sparing diuretics, potassium supplements: May result in hyperkalemia. Don't use together.
Trimethoprim: May increase risk of hyperkalemia. Use together cautiously.
Warfarin: May decrease anticoagulant effect. Monitor PT and INR, especially with dosage change.
Drug-herb. *Licorice:* May block ulcer-healing and aldosterone-like effects of herb; may increase risk of hypokalemia. Discourage use together.
Drug-food. *Potassium-rich foods, such as citrus fruits and tomatoes, salt substitutes containing potassium:* May increase risk of hyperkalemia. Urge caution.

EFFECTS ON LAB TEST RESULTS
• May increase glucose, uric acid, BUN, and potassium levels.
• May decrease sodium, magnesium, and calcium levels.
• May decrease granulocyte count.
• May cause hypochloremic alkalosis.
• May alter fluorometric determinations of plasma and urinary 17-hydroxycorticosteroid levels.

CONTRAINDICATIONS & CAUTIONS
• Use spironolactone only for those conditions for which it's indicated. Drug has been shown to be tumorigenic in long-term toxicity studies in rats. Avoid unnecessary use.
• Contraindicated in patients hypersensitive to drug and in those with anuria, acute or progressive renal insufficiency, Addison disease, or hyperkalemia.
• Use cautiously in patients with fluid or electrolyte imbalances and in those with impaired renal or hepatic function.
• Drug isn't recommended for primary treatment of HTN.
• Drug should be initiated in a hospital setting for patients with hepatic disease with cirrhosis and ascites. Drug can cause fluid and electrolyte disturbances, impair neurologic

---

Reactions in bold italics are *life-threatening*. Interactions may have a *rapid onset* or a **delayed onset**.

function, and worsen hepatic encephalopathy and coma.
• Safety and effectiveness in children haven't been established.

⚠ *Overdose S&S:* Drowsiness, confusion, rash, nausea, vomiting, dizziness, diarrhea, hyperkalemia.

PREGNANCY-LACTATION-REPRODUCTION
• Use of diuretics to treat edema during normal pregnancies isn't appropriate. Drug may cause fetal harm because of its antiandrogenic activity; avoid use in first trimester. Use during pregnancy only if clearly needed and potential benefit justifies fetal risk.
• A major metabolite of drug appears in human milk. Use cautiously during breastfeeding, taking into account importance of drug to patient, benefits of breastfeeding, and risk of exposure to infant.

NURSING CONSIDERATIONS
• Drug increases serum potassium level and may be useful for treating edema when use of other diuretics has caused hypokalemia.
• Monitor electrolyte levels (especially potassium), renal function, fluid intake and output, weight, and BP closely.
• Monitor older adults closely as this age-group is more susceptible to excessive diuresis.
• Inform lab that patient is taking spironolactone because drug may interfere with tests that measure digoxin level.
• Drug is less potent than thiazide and loop diuretics and is useful as an adjunct to other diuretic therapy. Diuretic effect is delayed 2 to 3 days when used alone.
• Maximum antihypertensive response may be delayed for up to 2 weeks.
• Watch for hyperchloremic metabolic acidosis, especially in patients with hepatic cirrhosis.
• *Look alike–sound alike:* Don't confuse Aldactone with Aldactazide.

PATIENT TEACHING
• Instruct patient in safe drug administration and handling.
• Tell patient to report all adverse reactions.
🔔 *Alert:* To prevent serious hyperkalemia, warn patient to avoid excessive ingestion of potassium-rich foods (such as citrus fruits, tomatoes, bananas, dates, and apricots), salt substitutes containing potassium, and potassium supplements.
• Caution patient not to perform hazardous activities if adverse CNS reactions occur.
• Advise patient about possible breast tenderness or enlargement.
• Instruct patient to immediately report pregnancy, plans to become pregnant, breastfeeding, or plans to breastfeed during treatment.

SAFETY ALERT!

succinylcholine chloride (suxamethonium chloride) ▨
suks-in-il-KOE-leen

Anectine, Quelicin

Therapeutic class: Skeletal muscle relaxants
Pharmacologic class: Depolarizing neuromuscular blockers

AVAILABLE FORMS
Injection: 20 mg/mL

INDICATIONS & DOSAGES
➤ **Adjunct to anesthesia to facilitate tracheal intubation; to provide skeletal muscle relaxation during surgery or mechanical ventilation**
Adults: 0.6 mg/kg IV given over 10 to 30 seconds. Dosage range is 0.3 to 1.1 mg/kg. For longer response, give 1 mg/mL solution as a continuous infusion at 0.5 to 10 mg/minute, or give an initial IV injection of 0.3 to 1.1 mg/kg followed by further injections of 0.04 to 0.07 mg/kg, as needed, to maintain relaxation. Or, 3 to 4 mg/kg IM. Maximum IM dose is 150 mg.
Children: 1 to 2 mg/kg IV or 3 to 4 mg/kg IM. Maximum IM dose is 150 mg.

ADMINISTRATION
IV
▼ Only staff skilled in airway management should use drug.
▼ Give test dose of 5 to 10 mg after patient has been anesthetized. If no respiratory depression occurs or transient depression lasts for up to 5 minutes, then patient can metabolize drug, and it is safe to continue. Don't give if patient develops respiratory paralysis sufficient to need ET intubation. (Recovery should occur within 30 to 60 minutes.)

S

▼ Use within 24 hours after reconstitution.
▼ Store injectable form in refrigerator.
▼ **Incompatibilities:** Alkaline solutions, barbiturates, nafcillin, sodium bicarbonate, solutions with pH above 8.5, thiopental sodium.

IM
• Inject deeply, preferably high into deltoid muscle. Use IM route only when IV access isn't available.
• Store injectable form in refrigerator.

ACTION
Binds with a high affinity to cholinergic receptors, prolonging depolarization of the motor end plate and ultimately producing muscle paralysis.

Route	Onset	Peak	Duration
IV	30–60 sec	1–2 min	4–6 min
IM	2–3 min	Unknown	10–30 min

Half-life: Unknown.

ADVERSE REACTIONS
CV: *arrhythmias, bradycardia, cardiac arrest,* tachycardia, HTN, hypotension, flushing. **EENT:** increased IOP, excessive salivation. **Metabolic:** *hyperkalemia.* **Musculoskeletal:** postoperative muscle pain, muscle fasciculation, jaw rigidity, *rhabdomyolysis with acute renal failure.* **Respiratory:** *apnea, bronchoconstriction, prolonged respiratory depression.* **Skin:** rash. **Other:** allergic or idiosyncratic hypersensitivity reactions, *anaphylaxis, malignant hyperthermia.*

INTERACTIONS
Drug-drug. *Aminoglycosides, anticholinesterases (echothiophate, edrophonium, neostigmine, physostigmine, pyridostigmine), aprotinin, general anesthetics (enflurane, halothane, isoflurane), glucocorticoids, hormonal contraceptives, lidocaine, lithium, magnesium, metoclopramide, oxytocin, polymyxin antibiotics (colistin, polymyxin B sulfate), procainamide, quinine:* May enhance neuromuscular blockade, increasing skeletal muscle relaxation and potentiating effect. Use together cautiously during and after surgery.
Cardiac glycosides: May increase risk of arrhythmias. Use together cautiously.
Cyclophosphamide, lithium, MAO inhibitors: May enhance neuromuscular blockade and prolong apnea. Use together cautiously.

Opioid analgesics: May enhance neuromuscular blockade, increasing skeletal muscle relaxation and possibly causing respiratory paralysis. Use together cautiously.
Parenteral magnesium sulfate: May enhance neuromuscular blockade, may increase skeletal muscle relaxation, and may cause respiratory paralysis. Use together cautiously, preferably at reduced doses.

EFFECTS ON LAB TEST RESULTS
• May increase myoglobin and potassium levels.

CONTRAINDICATIONS & CAUTIONS
⚠ Contraindicated in patients hypersensitive to drug and in those with personal or family history of malignant hyperthermia.
• Contraindicated in patients with skeletal muscle myopathies and after the acute phase of injury following acute major burns, multiple trauma, skeletal muscle denervation, or upper motor neuron injury.
• Drug increases IOP. Use only when potential benefit outweighs risk when an increase in IOP is undesirable, such as in narrow-angle glaucoma or penetrating eye injury.
⚠ Use carefully in patients with reduced plasma cholinesterase activity due to risk of prolonged neuromuscular block. Plasma cholinesterase activity may be diminished in the presence of genetic abnormalities of plasma cholinesterase, pregnancy, severe liver or kidney disease, malignant tumors, infections, burns, anemia, decompensated heart disease, peptic ulcer, myxedema, and certain drugs and chemicals.
• Use cautiously in older adults or patients who are debilitated; in patients receiving quinidine or cardiac glycoside therapy; in patients with hepatic, renal, or pulmonary impairment; and in those with respiratory depression, severe burns or trauma, electrolyte imbalances, hyperkalemia, paraplegia, spinal CNS injury, stroke, degenerative or dystrophic neuromuscular disease, myasthenia gravis, myasthenic syndrome related to lung cancer, dehydration, thyroid disorders, collagen diseases, porphyria, fractures, muscle spasms, dislocations, eye surgery, and pheochromocytoma.
Dialyzable drug: Unknown.
⚠ **Overdose S&S:** Prolonged neuromuscular blockade (skeletal muscle weakness,

decreased respiratory reserve, low tidal volume, apnea).

PREGNANCY-LACTATION-REPRODUCTION
• There are no adequate studies during pregnancy. Use only if clearly needed.
• Use large doses cautiously in patients undergoing cesarean section and monitor neonate for apnea and flaccidity.
• It isn't known if drug appears in human milk. Use cautiously during breastfeeding.

NURSING CONSIDERATIONS
• Drug has no known effect on consciousness, pain threshold, or cerebration. To avoid patient distress, don't induce neuromuscular blockade before unconsciousness.
• Dosage depends on anesthetic used, individual needs, and response. Recommended dosages must be individually adjusted. Drug should only be administered by experienced personnel trained in its use.

Boxed Warning Drug may cause acute rhabdomyolysis with hyperkalemia followed by ventricular arrhythmias, cardiac arrest, and death after administration to apparently healthy children who have undiagnosed skeletal muscle myopathy, most frequently Duchenne muscular dystrophy. Institute treatment for hyperkalemia when a healthy-appearing infant or child develops cardiac arrest soon after administration of succinylcholine. In children, drug should be reserved for use in emergency intubation, for instances when securing the airway is necessary, or for IM use when a suitable vein is inaccessible. ■

▧ Assess patients for personal or family history of malignant hyperthermia as drug is contraindicated in these patients.
• Children may be less sensitive to drug than adults.
• May cause a transient increase in ICP, and may increase intragastric pressure, which could result in regurgitation and possible aspiration of stomach contents.
• Monitor baseline electrolyte determinations and vital signs. Check respirations every 5 to 10 minutes during infusion.
• Monitor respirations closely until tests of muscle strength (hand grip, head lift, and ability to cough) indicate full recovery from neuromuscular blockade.

◑ *Alert:* Don't use reversing drugs. Unlike nondepolarizing drugs, neostigmine or edrophonium may worsen neuromuscular blockade if given before succinylcholine is metabolized by cholinesterase.
• Repeated or continuous infusions aren't advisable; they may cause reduced response or prolonged muscle relaxation and apnea.
• Give analgesics for pain.
• Keep airway clear. Have emergency respiratory support equipment (ET equipment, ventilator, oxygen, atropine, and epinephrine) immediately available.

◑ *Alert:* Carefully calculate dosage and always verify dosage with another health care professional.

PATIENT TEACHING
• Explain all events and procedures to patient because patient can still hear.
• Reassure patient that postoperative stiffness is normal and will soon subside.

---

sucralfate
soo-KRAL-fayt

Carafate◑

Therapeutic class: Antiulcer drugs
Pharmacologic class: GI protectants

AVAILABLE FORMS
Suspension: 1 g/10 mL
Tablets: 1 g

INDICATIONS & DOSAGES
Adjust-a-dose (for all indications): Dosage selection for older adults should be cautious, usually starting at the low end of the dosing range; monitor renal function.

➤ **Short-term treatment of duodenal ulcer**
Adults: 1 g PO q.i.d. 1 hour before meals and at bedtime. Continue for 4 to 8 weeks unless healing has been demonstrated by X-ray or endoscopic exam.

➤ **Maintenance therapy for duodenal ulcer (tablets only)**
Adults: 1 g PO b.i.d.

ADMINISTRATION
PO
• Shake suspension well before pouring.
• Give suspension with an accurate measuring device (calibrated oral syringe or measuring cup).

S

- After administration, flush NG tube with water to ensure passage into stomach.
- Give drug on an empty stomach 1 hour before meals.

ACTION

Selectively forms a coating that acts locally to protect the gastric lining against peptic acid, pepsin, and bile salts.

Route	Onset	Peak	Duration
PO	Unknown	Unknown	6 hr

Half-life: Unknown.

ADVERSE REACTIONS

GI: constipation.

INTERACTIONS

Drug-drug. *Antacids:* May decrease binding of drug to gastroduodenal mucosa, impairing effectiveness. Separate doses by 30 minutes.
Cimetidine, digoxin, fosphenytoin, furosemide (oral), ketoconazole, phenytoin, quinidine, ranitidine, tetracycline, theophylline: May decrease absorption of these drugs. Separate doses by at least 2 hours.
Ciprofloxacin, levofloxacin, moxifloxacin, ofloxacin: May decrease absorption of these drugs, reducing anti-infective response. If use together can't be avoided, give 2 hours before sucralfate.
Warfarin: May decrease anticoagulant effect. Monitor effectiveness and adjust dosage as necessary.

EFFECTS ON LAB TEST RESULTS

- May increase glucose level.

CONTRAINDICATIONS & CAUTIONS

- Contraindicated in patients with known hypersensitivity reactions to the active substance or to the components.
- Use cautiously in patients with chronic renal failure; toxic reactions may be greater in patients with impaired renal function.
- Safety and effectiveness in children haven't been established.
Dialyzable drug: Unknown.
⚠ *Overdose S&S:* Dyspepsia, abdominal pain, nausea, vomiting.

PREGNANCY-LACTATION-REPRODUCTION

- There are no adequate studies during pregnancy. Use only if clearly needed.

- It isn't known if drug appears in human milk. Use cautiously during breastfeeding.

NURSING CONSIDERATIONS

- Drug causes few adverse reactions because it's minimally absorbed.
- Monitor patient for severe, persistent constipation.
- Drug is as effective as cimetidine in healing duodenal ulcer.
- Drug contains aluminum but isn't classified as an antacid. Monitor patient with renal insufficiency for aluminum toxicity.
- Hyperglycemia has been reported in patients with diabetes who are taking suspension. Closely monitor blood glucose level and adjust dosage of antidiabetics if indicated.

PATIENT TEACHING

- Teach patient safe medication administration.
- Instruct patient to continue prescribed regimen to ensure complete healing. Pain and other ulcer signs and symptoms may subside within first few weeks of therapy.
- Urge patient to avoid cigarette smoking, which may increase gastric acid secretion and worsen disease.
- Antacids may be used while taking drug, but separate doses by 30 minutes.

SAFETY ALERT!

SUFentanil

soo-FEN-ta-nil

Dsuvia

Therapeutic class: Opioid analgesics
Pharmacologic class: Opioid agonists
Controlled substance schedule: II

AVAILABLE FORMS

Tablets (SL): 30 mcg

INDICATIONS & DOSAGES

➤ **Management of acute pain severe enough to require an opioid analgesic and for which alternative treatments are inadequate**
Adults: 30 mcg SL as needed with a minimum of 1 hour between doses. Maximum cumulative dose is 360 mcg/day (12 tablets). Don't use for more than 72 hours.

Reactions in bold italics are *life-threatening*. Interactions may have a *rapid onset* or a *delayed onset*.

ADMINISTRATION
Sublingual
Boxed Warning Drug is only to be administered by a health care professional in a medically certified health care setting. ■

• Drug is packaged as a single-use product. Don't reuse. Don't use if pouch is broken or single-dose applicator (SDA) is damaged.

🖐 *Alert:* Wear gloves when administering drug and dispose of SDA in biohazard waste.

• Follow manufacturer's instructions for use of delivery applicator.

• If patient has excessively dry mouth, provide ice chips before giving drug.

• Patient should allow drug to dissolve under the tongue and not chew or swallow the tablet.

• Patient should minimize talking and not eat or drink for 10 minutes after each dose.

• Visually confirm SL tablet placement.

• Store at 68° to 77° F (20° to 25° C) in a secure, limited-access location in accordance with institutional procedures for Schedule II products.

ACTION
An opioid agonist that is relatively selective for the mu-opioid receptor, although it can bind to other opioid receptors at higher doses. The analgesia and sedation effects are thought to be mediated through opioid-specific receptors throughout the CNS, with no ceiling effect to analgesia.

Route	Onset	Peak	Duration
SL	Unknown	1 hr	Unknown

Half-life: 13.4 hours.

ADVERSE REACTIONS
CNS: dizziness, headache. **CV:** hypotension. **GI:** nausea, vomiting. **Respiratory:** *respiratory depression,* decreased oxygen saturation.

INTERACTIONS
Drug-drug. *Anticholinergics:* May increase risk of urine retention or severe constipation, which may lead to paralytic ileus. Monitor patient for signs and symptoms of urine retention or reduced gastric motility.

Boxed Warning *Benzodiazepines, CNS depressants:* May increase risk of hypotension, respiratory depression, sedation, coma, and death. Use together only in patients with no alternative treatment options, and limit dosages and durations to the minimum

required. Monitor patients closely for signs or symptoms of respiratory depression and sedation. ■

Boxed Warning *CYP3A4 inducers (carbamazepine, phenytoin, rifampin):* May decrease sufentanil level and lead to decreased efficacy or withdrawal symptoms in patients who have developed physical dependence. If use together is necessary, consider an alternative medication that permits dosage titration. Monitor patient for opioid withdrawal. If the CYP3A4 inducer is discontinued, consider decreasing sufentanil dosage and monitor patient for signs and symptoms of respiratory depression. ■

Boxed Warning *CYP3A4 inhibitors (erythromycin, ketoconazole, ritonavir):* May increase sufentanil level, leading to increased or prolonged opioid effects. Monitor patient for respiratory depression and sedation. If use together is necessary, consider an alternative medication that permits dosage titration. If the CYP3A4 inhibitor is discontinued, consider increasing sufentanil dosage until stable drug effects are achieved and monitor patient for opioid withdrawal symptoms. ■

Diuretics: May decrease the effects of diuretics by inducing the release of ADH. Monitor patients for signs and symptoms of diminished diuresis or effects on BP and increase the diuretic dosage as needed.

MAO inhibitors (linezolid, phenelzine, tranylcypromine): May increase risk of serotonin syndrome or opioid toxicity. Use of sufentanil isn't recommended for patients taking MAO inhibitors or within 14 days of stopping MAO inhibitor treatment.

Mixed agonist/antagonist and partial opioid analgesics (buprenorphine, butorphanol, nalbuphine, pentazocine): May reduce analgesic effect of sufentanil or precipitate withdrawal symptoms. Avoid use together.

Muscle relaxants: May enhance neuromuscular blocking action of skeletal muscle relaxants and produce increased respiratory depression. Monitor patient for signs and symptoms of respiratory depression, decrease dosage of the skeletal muscle relaxant, or consider discontinuing sufentanil.

Serotonergic drugs (mirtazapine, SSNRIs, SSRIs, TCAs, tramadol, trazodone, triptans): May increase risk of serotonin syndrome. If use together is necessary, monitor patient closely, especially during treatment initiation

S

and dosage adjustment. Discontinue sufentanil if serotonin syndrome is suspected.

Drug-lifestyle. **Boxed Warning** *Alcohol use:* May increase risk of hypotension, respiratory depression, sedation, coma, and death. Don't use together. ▪

EFFECTS ON LAB TEST RESULTS
• May increase amylase level.

CONTRAINDICATIONS & CAUTIONS
• Contraindicated in patients with significant respiratory depression, acute or severe bronchial asthma in an unmonitored setting or in the absence of resuscitative equipment, known or suspected GI obstruction (including paralytic ileus), or known hypersensitivity to sufentanil or its components.

Boxed Warning Accidental exposure to or ingestion of sufentanil, even a single dose, can result in respiratory depression and death, especially in children. ▪

Boxed Warning Because of the potential for life-threatening respiratory depression due to accidental exposure, sufentanil is only available through a REMS program. Drug may only be dispensed in a certified medically supervised health care setting and drug must be discontinued before discharge or transfer from that setting. ▪

Boxed Warning Serious, life-threatening, or fatal respiratory depression has been reported with the use of opioids, even when used as recommended. Unrecognized respiratory depression may lead to respiratory arrest and death. Risk is greatest during the initiation of therapy but can occur at any time. ▪

Boxed Warning Sufentanil is a Schedule II controlled substance and exposes users to the risks of addiction, abuse, and misuse, including overdose and death. ▪

• Opioids can cause sleep-related breathing disorders, including central sleep apnea (CSA) and sleep-related hypoxemia. Opioid use increases risk of CSA in a dose-dependent fashion. In patients with CSA, consider minimizing sufentanil use and monitor patients for signs or symptoms of respiratory depression.

• Use cautiously in patients with chronic pulmonary disease, in older adults, and in patients who are cachectic or debilitated, as they are at increased risk for respiratory depression, even at recommended doses. Consider nonopioid analgesics whenever possible.

• Drug may cause severe hypotension, including orthostatic hypotension and syncope in patients who are ambulatory. Use cautiously in patients with hypovolemia or CV disease and in those taking drugs that may exaggerate hypotensive effects. Avoid use in patients with circulatory shock.

• Avoid use in patients with impaired consciousness or coma. Sufentanil isn't suitable for use in patients who aren't alert and able to follow directions.

• Drug may mask clinical changes in patients with head injury.

• Drug may increase the frequency of seizures in patients with seizure disorders and may increase the risk of seizures occurring in other clinical settings associated with seizures.

• Use cautiously in patients with bradyarrhythmias; drug may lower HR.

• Drug isn't approved for use in children, for use long-term, or for home use.

Dialyzable drug: Unknown.

⚠ *Overdose S&S:* Respiratory depression, somnolence, stupor, coma, skeletal muscle flaccidity, cold and clammy skin, constricted pupils, pulmonary edema, bradycardia, hypotension, partial or complete airway obstruction, atypical snoring, marked hypoxia-related mydriasis, death.

PREGNANCY-LACTATION-REPRODUCTION
🔆 *Alert:* Prolonged use of opioids during pregnancy can cause neonatal opioid withdrawal syndrome, which may be life-threatening. If prolonged opioid therapy is required during pregnancy, ensure protocols for management by neonatology experts are available and warn patient of risk to the neonate.

• Opioids cross the placental barrier and may produce respiratory depression and psychophysiologic effects in neonates. Sufentanil shouldn't be used during or immediately before labor when other analgesics are more appropriate.

• Infants exposed to sufentanil through human milk should be monitored for excess sedation and respiratory depression. Withdrawal symptoms can occur in breastfed infants when maternal administration of an opioid analgesic is stopped or when breastfeeding is stopped.

• Long-term use of opioids may reduce fertility in females and males of reproductive

---

potential. It isn't known if these effects on fertility are reversible.

NURSING CONSIDERATIONS

Boxed Warning Monitor patients closely for respiratory depression, sedation, and hypotension, especially during initiation of therapy. Ensure opioid antagonist (naloxone) and emergency equipment are readily available. ∎
Boxed Warning Assess patients' risk of addiction, abuse, and misuse before prescribing sufentanil, and monitor patients regularly for these behaviors and conditions. Risk increases in patients with a personal or family history of substance abuse or mental illness. ∎

• Watch for serotonin syndrome in patient who is taking concomitant serotonergic drugs. Assess for mental status changes (agitation, hallucinations, coma), autonomic instability (tachycardia, labile BP, hyperthermia), neuromuscular abnormalities (hyperreflexia, loss of coordination, rigidity), and GI signs and symptoms (nausea, vomiting, diarrhea). Discontinue sufentanil for suspected serotonin syndrome.
• Use cautiously in patients with hepatic and severe renal impairment and monitor patients closely for respiratory depression, sedation, and hypotension.
• Monitor patients with a history of seizure disorders for worsened seizure control.
• Monitor patients for adrenal insufficiency (nausea, vomiting, anorexia, fatigue, weakness, dizziness, hypotension). If adrenal insufficiency is diagnosed, treat with physiologic replacement of corticosteroids, and wean patient from the opioid.
• Monitor patients for hypotension, especially for changes in HR, particularly when initiating therapy.
• Monitor patients with biliary tract disease (acute pancreatitis) for worsening symptoms.
• Use cautiously in patients susceptible to the intracranial effects of carbon dioxide retention, such as those with brain tumors or increased ICP. Drug may decrease respiratory drive. Monitor patients for sedation and respiratory depression.
• Monitor neonates exposed to opioids during labor for excess sedation and respiratory depression. Monitor neonates with prolonged exposure in utero for opioid withdrawal syndrome (irritability, hyperactivity, abnormal

sleep pattern, high-pitched cry, tremor, vomiting, diarrhea, failure to gain weight).
Boxed Warning Drug must be discontinued before patient leaves the certified medically supervised setting. Don't use for more than 72 hours. ∎
• *Look alike–sound alike:* Don't confuse Dsuvia with Duavee.

PATIENT TEACHING

Boxed Warning Inform patient that accidental exposure may result in respiratory depression or death, especially in children, and that the risk is greatest at start of therapy but can occur at any time. ∎
Boxed Warning Inform patient that the use of sufentanil can result in addiction, abuse, and misuse, even when taken as recommended. ∎

• Teach patient safe drug administration and handling.
• Teach patient to report all adverse reactions.
• Warn patient that hypersensitivity reactions, including anaphylaxis, have been reported. Advise patient to immediately report signs and symptoms of hypersensitivity reactions.
• Caution patient that sufentanil may cause orthostatic hypotension and syncope. Teach patient how to recognize signs and symptoms of low BP and how to reduce the risk of serious consequences should hypotension occur.
• Inform patient that opioids can cause adrenal insufficiency, and to report signs and symptoms of adrenal insufficiency if they occur.
• Teach patient that naloxone is prescribed in conjunction with the opioid when treatment is started or renewed as a preventive measure to reduce opioid overdose and death.
• Warn patient with a history of seizure disorder that drug can increase risk of seizures.
• Inform patient of childbearing potential that sufentanil can cause fetal harm and to report known or suspected pregnancy.
• Advise patient who is breastfeeding to monitor infant for increased sleepiness (more than usual), breathing difficulties, or limpness. Instruct patient to seek immediate medical care if these signs or symptoms occur.

S

sulfamethoxazole–trimethoprim ⚘

sul-fa-meth-OX-a-zole/tri-meth-O-prim

Bactrim, Bactrim DS✐, Septra,
Septra DS, Sulfatrim*

Therapeutic class: Antibiotics
Pharmacologic class: Sulfonamides–folate
antagonists

AVAILABLE FORMS
Injection: sulfamethoxazole 80 mg/mL and
trimethoprim 16 mg/mL in 5-mL vials*
Oral suspension: sulfamethoxazole 200 mg
and trimethoprim 40 mg/5 mL*
Tablets (double-strength): sulfamethoxazole
800 mg and trimethoprim 160 mg
Tablets (single-strength): sulfamethoxazole
100 mg and trimethoprim 20 mg ✲, sulfamethoxazole 400 mg and trimethoprim 80 mg

INDICATIONS & DOSAGES
Adjust-a-dose (for all indications): For patients with CrCl of 15 to 30 mL/minute, reduce daily dose by 50%. Don't give to those
with CrCl less than 15 mL/minute.
➤ **Shigellosis, or UTIs caused by susceptible strains of** *Escherichia coli,* *Proteus* **(in-
dole positive or negative),** *Klebsiella,* *Morganella morganii,* **or** *Enterobacter* **species**
Adults: 800 mg sulfamethoxazole/160 mg
trimethoprim PO every 12 hours for 10 to
14 days in UTIs and for 5 days in shigellosis. If indicated, give 8 to 10 mg/kg/day IV,
based on trimethoprim component, in two to
four divided doses every 6, 8, or 12 hours for
5 days for shigellosis or up to 14 days for severe UTIs. Maximum daily dose is 60 mL
trimethoprim.
Children age 2 months and older: 8 mg/kg/
day PO, based on trimethoprim component, in two divided doses every 12 hours for
10 days for UTIs and 5 days for shigellosis.
If indicated, give 8 to 10 mg/kg/day IV, based
on trimethoprim component, in two to four divided doses every 6, 8, or 12 hours for up to
14 days for severe UTIs and 5 days for shigellosis. Don't exceed adult dose.
➤ **Otitis media in patients with penicillin
allergy or penicillin-resistant infection**
Children age 2 months and older: 8 mg/kg/
day PO, based on trimethoprim component, in
two divided doses every 12 hours for 10 days.

➤ **Chronic bronchitis, URIs**
Adults: 800 mg sulfamethoxazole/160 mg
trimethoprim PO every 12 hours for 14 days.
➤ **Traveler's diarrhea**
Adults: 800 mg sulfamethoxazole/160 mg
trimethoprim PO b.i.d. for 5 days.
➤ *Pneumocystis jiroveci* **pneumonia**
Adults and children older than age 2 months:
15 to 20 mg/kg/day IV or PO, based on
trimethoprim component, in equally divided
doses every 6 hours (PO) or in divided doses
every 6 to 8 hours (IV) for 14 days. Some
guidelines recommend treatment duration of
21 days.
➤ *P. jiroveci* **pneumonia prophylaxis in patients who are immunosuppressed**
Adults: 800 mg sulfamethoxazole/160 mg
trimethoprim every 24 hours.
Children older than age 2 months:
750 mg/m^2 sulfamethoxazole with trimethoprim 150 mg/m^2 daily in equally divided
doses b.i.d., on 3 consecutive days per week.

ADMINISTRATION
PO
● Before giving drug, ask if patient is allergic
to sulfa drugs.
● Obtain specimen for culture and sensitiv-
ity tests before giving. Begin therapy while
awaiting results.
● Give without regard to meals.
● Give drug with 8 oz (240 mL) of water.
● Shake suspension well before using.
IV
▼ Before giving drug, ask patient if patient
is allergic to sulfa drugs.
▼ Obtain specimen for culture and sensitiv-
ity tests before giving. Begin therapy while
awaiting results.
▼ Don't give by rapid infusion or bolus injection.
▼ Dilute each 5 mL of concentrate in 75 to
125 mL of D$_5$W. Don't mix with other drugs
or solutions.
▼ Infuse slowly over 60 to 90 minutes.
▼ Don't refrigerate; use within 6 hours if diluted in 125 mL, within 4 hours if diluted
in 100 mL, and within 2 hours if diluted in
75 mL.
▼ Discard solution if it's cloudy or crystallized.
▼ Never give drug IM.
▼ **Incompatibilities:** None listed by manufacturer. Consult a drug incompatibility
reference for more information.

Reactions in bold italics are *life-threatening*. Interactions may have a *rapid onset* or a **delayed onset**.

ACTION

Sulfamethoxazole inhibits formation of di-hydrofolic acid from PABA; trimethoprim inhibits dihydrofolate reductase formation. Both decrease bacterial folic acid synthesis and are bactericidal.

Route	Onset	Peak	Duration
PO	Unknown	1–4 hr	Unknown
IV	Immediate	Unknown	Unknown

Half-life: Sulfamethoxazole, 9 to 12 hours; trimethoprim, 6 to 11 hours.

ADVERSE REACTIONS

CNS: *seizures,* apathy, aseptic meningitis, ataxia, depression, fatigue, hallucinations, headache, insomnia, nervousness, peripheral neuritis, vertigo. **CV:** thrombophlebitis, polyarteritis nodosa. **EENT:** tinnitus. **GI:** *pancreatitis, pseudomembranous colitis,* diarrhea, nausea, vomiting, abdominal pain, anorexia, stomatitis. **GU:** *toxic nephrosis with oliguria and anuria,* crystalluria, hematuria, interstitial nephritis, *renal failure.* **Hematologic:** *agranulocytosis, aplastic anemia,* eosinophilia, *leukopenia, neutropenia, thrombocytopenia,* hemolytic anemia, megaloblastic anemia, ITP, methemoglobinemia. **Hepatic:** *hepatotoxicity,* jaundice. **Metabolic:** *hyperkalemia, hypoglycemia,* hyponatremia. **Musculoskeletal:** arthralgia, muscle weakness, myalgia. **Respiratory:** pulmonary infiltrates, cough, shortness of breath. **Skin:** generalized skin eruption, *erythema multiforme, SJS, TEN,* exfoliative dermatitis, photosensitivity reactions, pruritus, urticaria, rash. **Other:** *anaphylaxis, DRESS syndrome,* hypersensitivity reactions.

INTERACTIONS

Drug-drug. *Antiarrhythmics (amiodarone, bretylium, disopyramide, quinidine, sotalol), arsenic trioxide, chlorpromazine, dolasetron, droperidol, mefloquine, mesoridazine, moxifloxacin, pentamidine, pimozide, tacrolimus, thioridazine, ziprasidone, other drugs that prolong QT interval:* May prolong QT interval and increase risk of life-threatening cardiac arrhythmias, including torsades de pointes. Use together with caution unless contraindicated. Consult pharmacist as necessary. *Cyclosporine:* May decrease cyclosporine level and increase nephrotoxicity risk. Avoid using together.

Digoxin: May increase digoxin level. Monitor digoxin level.
Diuretics: May increase incidence of thrombocytopenia with purpura in older adults receiving certain diuretics, mainly thiazides. Avoid concomitant use.
Dofetilide: May increase dofetilide level and effects. May increase risk of prolonged QT-interval syndrome and fatal ventricular arrhythmias. Contraindicated for use together.
Indomethacin: May increase sulfamethoxazole blood level. Avoid concomitant use.
Methotrexate: May increase methotrexate level. Monitor methotrexate level.
Oral antidiabetics: May increase hypoglycemic effect. Monitor glucose level.
Phenytoin: May inhibit hepatic metabolism of phenytoin. Monitor phenytoin level.
Procainamide: May prolong QT interval. Closely monitor patient for clinical and ECG signs of toxicity.
Pyrimethamine: May increase risk of megaloblastic anemia. Avoid use together.
TCAs: May decrease efficacy of TCAs. Monitor therapeutic response to TCAs and adjust dosage accordingly.
Warfarin: May increase anticoagulant effect. Monitor patient for bleeding; monitor PT and INR.
Zidovudine: May increase myelotoxicity. Monitor patient closely.

Drug-herb. *St. John's wort:* May decrease drug level. Consider therapy modification.

Drug-lifestyle. *Sun exposure:* May increase risk of photosensitivity reactions. Advise patient to avoid excessive sunlight exposure.

EFFECTS ON LAB TEST RESULTS

- May increase aminotransferase, bilirubin, potassium, BUN, and creatinine levels.
- May decrease sodium and glucose levels.
- May decrease Hb level and granulocyte, platelet, and WBC counts.

CONTRAINDICATIONS & CAUTIONS

- Contraindicated in patients hypersensitive to trimethoprim or sulfonamides and in patients with a history of trimethoprim or sulfonamide drug-induced immune thrombocytopenia.
- Severe, life-threatening, and fatal cases of thrombocytopenia have been reported and may be immune-mediated. Once drug is discontinued, thrombocytopenia usually resolves within 1 week.

S

- Contraindicated in those with CrCl less than 15 mL/minute, porphyria, megaloblastic anemia from folate deficiency, or marked hepatic damage.
- Contraindicated in infants younger than age 2 months.
- Some forms may contain benzyl alcohol, which, in newborn infants, has been associated with an increased incidence of neurologic and other complications that are sometimes fatal. Avoid use in neonates.
- Use cautiously and in reduced dosages in patients with CrCl of 15 to 30 mL/minute, severe allergy or bronchial asthma, or blood dyscrasia.
- ⚕ Use cautiously in patients with G6PD deficiency as hemolytic anemia can result.
- May cause CDAD ranging from mild diarrhea to fatal colitis.

Dialyzable drug: Moderately.

⚠ *Overdose S&S:* Headache, drowsiness, unconsciousness, fever, depression, confusion, anorexia, colic, nausea, vomiting, diarrhea, hematuria, crystalluria; blood dyscrasias and jaundice (late signs).

PREGNANCY-LACTATION-REPRODUCTION
- There are no well-controlled studies during pregnancy; drug may cause fetal harm. Use only if potential benefit justifies fetal risk.
- Contraindicated during breastfeeding because of risk of bilirubin displacement and kernicterus.

NURSING CONSIDERATIONS
- ⚕ *Alert:* Double-check dosage, which may be written as trimethoprim component.
- ⚕ *Alert:* "DS" product means "double strength."
- Monitor renal function, CBC, potassium level, and LFT results.
- Promptly report rash, sore throat, fever, cough, mouth sores, or iris lesions—early signs and symptoms of erythema multiforme, which may progress to life-threatening SJS, or blood dyscrasias.
- Watch for signs and symptoms of superinfection, such as fever, chills, and increased pulse.
- ⚕ *Alert:* Adverse reactions, especially hypersensitivity reactions, rash, and fever, occur much more frequently in patients with AIDS.
- Monitor patient for CDAD. Discontinue drug and provide supportive treatment for suspected or confirmed CDAD.

PATIENT TEACHING
- Instruct patient in safe drug administration.
- Tell patient to take drug as prescribed, even if feeling better.
- Encourage patient to drink plenty of fluids to prevent crystalluria and kidney stone formation.
- Tell patient to report adverse reactions promptly, especially diarrhea, fever, rash, bruising, bleeding, and throat or other pain.
- Instruct patient receiving drug IV to report discomfort at IV insertion site.
- Advise patient to avoid prolonged sun exposure, wear protective clothing, and use sunscreen.

sulfaSALAzine (salazosulfapyridine, sulphasalazine) ⚕
sul-fuh-SAL-uh-zeen

Azulfidine, Azulfidine EN-tabs, Salazopyrin ♣, Salazopyrin EN-Tabs ♣

Therapeutic class: Anti-inflammatory drugs
Pharmacologic class: Sulfonamide salicylates

AVAILABLE FORMS
Tablets: 500 mg
Tablets (delayed-release) ⓞⓣⓒ*:* 500 mg

INDICATIONS & DOSAGES
➤ **Mild to moderate ulcerative colitis, adjunctive therapy in severe ulcerative colitis, prolongation of remission period between acute ulcerative colitis attacks**
Adults: Initially, 3 to 4 g PO daily in evenly divided doses not exceeding 8 hours apart; may start with 1 to 2 g, with gradual increase to minimize adverse effects. Usual maintenance dose is 2 g PO daily.
Children age 6 and older: Initially, 40 to 60 mg/kg PO daily, divided into three to six doses; may start at lower dose if GI intolerance occurs. Maintenance dose is 30 mg/kg in each 24-hour period, divided into four doses.
➤ **RA in patients who have responded inadequately to salicylates or NSAIDs**
Adults (delayed-release tablets): 2 g PO daily in two evenly divided doses. To reduce possible GI intolerance, start at 0.5 to 1 g daily.

May increase to 3 g PO daily if clinical response after 12 weeks is inadequate.

➤ **Polyarticular-course juvenile RA in patients who have responded inadequately to salicylates or other NSAIDs**

Children age 6 and older (delayed-release tablets): 30 to 50 mg/kg PO daily in two evenly divided doses. Maximum dose is 2 g daily. To reduce possible GI intolerance, start with one-quarter to one-third of planned maintenance dose and increase weekly until reaching maintenance dose at 1 month.

ADMINISTRATION
PO
- Give drug with food to decrease GI irritation.
- Patient must swallow delayed-release tablets whole and mustn't crush, chew, or split them.
- An oral suspension may be made by a pharmacist. Shake well before use.

ACTION
May be related to observed anti-inflammatory or immunomodulatory properties.

Route	Onset	Peak	Duration
PO	Unknown	3–12 hr	Unknown

Half-life: 4 to 11 hours.

ADVERSE REACTIONS
CNS: *seizures,* dizziness, headache, depression, hallucinations, fever. **GI:** nausea, vomiting, abdominal pain, gastric distress, anorexia, stomatitis, dyspepsia. **GU:** oligospermia, infertility. **Hematologic:** *agranulocytosis, leukopenia, thrombocytopenia, hemolytic anemia.* **Hepatic:** abnormal LFT values. **Skin:** rash, urticaria, pruritus, cyanosis.

INTERACTIONS
Drug-drug. *Digoxin:* May reduce absorption of digoxin. Monitor patient closely.
Folic acid: May decrease absorption of folic acid. Monitor patient.
Methotrexate: May enhance hepatotoxic effect of methotrexate. Monitor patient for hematologic toxicity and adverse GI events, especially nausea.
Prilocaine: May increase risk of significant methemoglobinemia. Monitor patient. Avoid lidocaine and prilocaine in infants receiving such agents.

Thiopurines (azathioprine, mercaptopurine): May increase leukopenia. Monitor WBC count closely.
Warfarin: May alter anticoagulant effect. Monitor therapy.
Drug-herb. *Dong quai, St. John's wort:* May also cause photosensitization. Avoid use together.

EFFECTS ON LAB TEST RESULTS
- May increase ALT and AST levels.
- May decrease Hb level and granulocyte, platelet, and WBC counts.
- May interfere with measurements, by liquid chromatography, of urinary normetanephrine and cause false-positive test results in patients exposed to sulfasalazine or its metabolite.

CONTRAINDICATIONS & CAUTIONS
- Contraindicated in patients hypersensitive to drug, its metabolites, sulfonamides, or salicylates and in those with porphyria or intestinal and urinary obstruction.
- Use cautiously and in reduced doses in patients with impaired hepatic or renal function, severe allergy, or bronchial asthma.
- ▨ Use cautiously in patients with G6PD deficiency as hemolytic anemia can result.
- SCARs, some fatal, including DRESS syndrome, exfoliative dermatitis, SJS, and TEN, have been reported. Patients are at highest risk for SCARs early in therapy, with most events occurring within first month of treatment. Discontinue drug at first appearance of rash or mucosal lesions.
- Serious CNS reactions can occur, including seizures, meningitis, spinal cord disorders, peripheral neuropathy, hearing loss, ataxia, and hallucinations.

Dialyzable drug: Yes.

⚠ **Overdose S&S:** Nausea, gastric distress, abdominal pain, drowsiness, seizures.

PREGNANCY-LACTATION-REPRODUCTION
- There are no adequate studies during pregnancy. Use only if clearly needed.
- Drug and its active metabolite appear in human milk. Use cautiously during breastfeeding; monitor infant for kernicterus and diarrhea or bloody stools.
- Oligospermia and infertility have been observed in men treated with drug; stopping drug may reverse these effects.

S

♣Canada ◇OTC ◆Off-label use ✐Photoguide ⊕Do not crush *Liquid contains alcohol ▨Genetic

NURSING CONSIDERATIONS

• Therapeutic response in patients with RA may occur as soon as 4 weeks after starting therapy, but it may take up to 12 weeks in others.

• Drug may cause urine discoloration.

⚠ *Alert:* Stop drug immediately and notify prescriber if patient shows signs and symptoms of hypersensitivity.

• Maintain adequate fluid intake to prevent crystalluria and stone formation.

• Obtain CBCs, including differential WBC count and LFT values, before start of treatment and every second week during first 3 months of therapy, monthly during the second 3 months, once every 3 months thereafter, and as clinically indicated. Obtain a urinalysis with careful microscopic exam and an assessment of renal function periodically during treatment.

• Serum sulfapyridine levels greater than 50 mcg/mL appear to be associated with an increased incidence of adverse reactions.

✂ Observe patients with G6PD deficiency closely for signs and symptoms of hemolytic anemia.

• *Look alike–sound alike:* Don't confuse sulfasalazine with sulfisoxazole, salsalate, or sulfadiazine.

PATIENT TEACHING

• Instruct patient in safe drug administration and to drink plenty of water.

• Advise patient that drug may produce an orange-yellow discoloration of skin and urine and may cause contact lenses to turn yellow.

• Teach patient about adverse reactions and to report them. Advise patient of the need for careful medical supervision. A sore throat, fever, pallor, purpura, or jaundice may indicate a serious blood disorder.

• Advise patient that blood and urine tests will be needed to monitor treatment and that it's important to keep lab and physician appointments.

SUMAtriptan succinate
sue-mah-TRIP-tan

Imitrex✦, Imitrex STATdose, Onzetra Xsail, Tosymra, Zembrace SymTouch

Therapeutic class: Antimigraine drugs
Pharmacologic class: Serotonin 5-HT$_1$ receptor agonists

AVAILABLE FORMS

Injection: 4 mg/0.5 mL, 6 mg/0.5 mL pre-filled syringes; 6 mg/0.5 mL vials; 3 mg/0.5 mL, 4 mg/0.5 mL, 6 mg/0.5 mL single-dose autoinjector
Nasal powder: 11 mg (base)/disposable nosepiece
Nasal solution: 5 mg, 10 mg, 20 mg per actuation
Tablets ⓞⓝⓒ: 25 mg, 50 mg, 100 mg (base)

INDICATIONS & DOSAGES

➤ **Acute migraine attacks (with or without aura)**
Adults: 1 to 6 mg subcut depending on product; maximum dose is 12 mg in 24 hours, separated by at least 1 hour. Or 25 to 100 mg PO, initially. If desired response isn't achieved in 2 hours, may give second dose of 25 to 100 mg. Additional doses may be used in at least 2-hour intervals. Maximum daily oral dose, 200 mg.

For nasal spray, give 5 mg, 10 mg, or 20 mg once in one nostril; may repeat once after 2 hours, for maximum daily dose of 40 mg. Or, Tosymra 10 mg given as a single spray in one nostril. Maximum recommended dose within 24 hours is 30 mg, with doses separated by at least 1 hour. May also give at least 1 hour after another sumatriptan product.

For nasal powder, one 11 mg nosepiece in each nostril (22 mg total), using the Xsail breath-powered delivery device. If desired response isn't achieved in 2 hours, or migraine returns after a transient improvement, may give second dose of 22 mg. Maximum recommended dose within 24 hours is two doses (44 mg/4 nosepieces) or one dose of 22 mg and one dose of another sumatriptan product, separated by at least 2 hours.

Reactions in bold italics are *life-threatening*. Interactions may have a *rapid onset* or a *delayed onset*.

Adjust-a-dose: In patients with mild to moderate hepatic impairment, the maximum single oral dose shouldn't exceed 50 mg.

➤ **Cluster headache (except Zembrace)**
Adults: 6 mg subcut. Maximum recommended dose is two 6-mg injections in 24 hours, separated by at least 1 hour.

ADMINISTRATION
PO
• Give drug without regard for food.
• Give drug whole; don't crush or break tablet.
Subcutaneous
• Redness or pain at injection site should subside within 1 hour after injection.
• Use injection site with adequate skin and subcutaneous tissue thickness to accommodate length of needle.
Intranasal spray
• Have patient blow nose before use.
• Give medication for inhalation in one nostril, while blocking the other nostril.
• Patient should keep head upright and breathe gently for 10 to 20 seconds after administration.
Intranasal powder
• Use with the Xsail device only; insert disposable nosepiece into the device body.
• Pierce capsule inside nosepiece by pressing and releasing the white piercing button one time on the device body.
• Insert nosepiece into one nostril, ensuring a tight seal; rotate device, place mouthpiece into mouth, and blow forcefully through mouthpiece for 2 to 3 seconds to deliver powder into the nasal cavity.
• Remove and discard nosepiece; repeat in other nostril, using a second nosepiece.

ACTION
May act as an agonist at serotonin receptors on extracerebral intracranial blood vessels, which constricts the affected vessels, inhibits neuropeptide release, and reduces pain transmission in the trigeminal pathways.

Route	Onset	Peak	Duration
PO	30 min	2–2.5 hr	Unknown
Subcut	10 min	12 min	Unknown
Intranasal spray	15–30 min	5–23 min	Unknown
Intranasal powder	Unknown	45 min	Unknown

Half-life: About 2 hours; intranasal, about 3 hours.

ADVERSE REACTIONS
CNS: dizziness, vertigo, drowsiness, headache, malaise, fatigue, pain, paresthesia, tingling sensation, warm or hot sensation, burning sensation; heaviness, pressure, or tightness; tight feeling in head, cold sensation, numbness, dysgeusia. **CV:** flushing, pressure or tightness in chest. **EENT:** altered vision; discomfort of throat, nasal cavity or sinus, mouth, jaw, or tongue; rhinorrhea, rhinitis, pharyngeal edema. **GI:** abdominal discomfort, dysphagia, diarrhea, nausea, vomiting, unusual or bad taste (nasal spray). **Musculoskeletal:** myalgia, muscle cramps, neck pain. **Respiratory:** *bronchospasm,* upper respiratory tract inflammation and dyspnea (PO). **Skin:** injection-site or application-site reaction, diaphoresis.

INTERACTIONS
Drug-drug. *Ergot and ergot derivatives, other 5-HT$_1$ agonists (triptans):* May prolong vasospastic effects. Don't use within 24 hours of sumatriptan therapy.
MAO inhibitors: May reduce sumatriptan clearance. Use with or within 2 weeks of MAO inhibitor is contraindicated.
Serotonergic drugs (methylene blue, SNRIs, SSRIs, TCAs): May cause serotonin syndrome. Monitor patient closely if use together can't be avoided.
Drug-herb. *St. John's wort:* May increase serotonin levels. Use together cautiously.

EFFECTS ON LAB TEST RESULTS
• May increase liver enzyme levels.

CONTRAINDICATIONS & CAUTIONS
• Contraindicated in patients with hypersensitivity to drug or its components and in those with history, symptoms, or signs of ischemic cardiac, cerebrovascular (such as stroke or TIA), or peripheral vascular syndromes (such as ischemic bowel disease); hemiplegic or basilar migraine; significant underlying CV diseases, including angina pectoris, MI, and silent myocardial ischemia; Wolff-Parkinson-White syndrome or arrhythmias associated with other cardiac accessory conduction pathway disorders; uncontrolled HTN; or severe hepatic impairment.
• Use cautiously in patients with risk factors for CAD, such as patients who are postmenopausal, men older than age 40, or patients with HTN, hypercholesterolemia,

S

obesity, diabetes, smoking, or family history of CAD.

• Noncoronary vasospastic reactions may occur with use of 5-HT$_1$ agonists, including peripheral vascular ischemia, GI ischemia and infarction (abdominal pain, bloody diarrhea), splenic infarction, Raynaud syndrome, or transient or permanent blindness.

• Before use, exclude other neurologic conditions in patients not previously diagnosed with migraine or cluster headaches and in those with atypical symptoms.

Dialyzable drug: Unknown.

PREGNANCY-LACTATION-REPRODUCTION

• There are no adequate studies during pregnancy. Use only if potential benefit justifies fetal risk.

• Drug appears in human milk after subcut administration. Refer to individual manufacturer's instructions regarding breastfeeding.

NURSING CONSIDERATIONS

◆ *Alert:* When giving drug to patient at risk for CAD, give first dose in presence of other medical personnel. Rarely, serious adverse cardiac effects can follow administration.

◆ *Alert:* Combining drug with serotonergic drugs may cause serotonin syndrome. Symptoms include restlessness, hallucinations, loss of coordination, fast heartbeat, rapid changes in BP, increased body temperature, hyperreflexia, nausea, vomiting, and diarrhea. Serotonin syndrome may occur when starting or increasing the dose of drug, TCAs, MAO inhibitors, SSRIs, or SSNRIs.

• Monitor BP; significant BP elevations have occurred even in patients without a history of HTN.

• Monitor patient for seizures. Seizures have been reported in patients with and without a history of seizures.

• After subcut injection, most patients experience relief in 1 to 2 hours.

• *Look alike–sound alike:* Don't confuse sumatriptan with somatropin.

PATIENT TEACHING

• Inform patient that drug is intended only to treat migraine attacks, not to prevent them or reduce their occurrence.

• Teach safe drug administration.

• Advise patient to take drug only as prescribed. Medication overuse headaches or increased frequency of migraine attacks may occur.

• Caution patient who is pregnant or may become pregnant not to use drug but to discuss with prescriber risks and benefits of using drug during pregnancy.

• Tell patient that drug may be taken at any time during a migraine attack, as soon as signs or symptoms appear.

◆ *Alert:* Tell patient to report all adverse reactions and to immediately report persistent or severe chest pain. Warn patient to stop using drug and to call prescriber if pain or tightness in the throat, wheezing, heart throbbing, rash, lumps, hives, or swollen eyelids, face, or lips develop.

SAFETY ALERT!

SUNItinib malate
su-NIT-e-nib

Sutent✏

Therapeutic class: Antineoplastics
Pharmacologic class: Protein-tyrosine kinase inhibitors

AVAILABLE FORMS

Capsules: 12.5 mg, 25 mg, 37.5 mg, 50 mg

INDICATIONS & DOSAGES

Adjust-a-dose (for all indications): Refer to manufacturer's instructions for toxicity-related dosage adjustments.

➤ **GI stromal tumor after disease progression on or intolerance to imatinib; advanced renal cell carcinoma**

Adults: 50 mg PO once daily for 4 weeks, followed by 2 weeks off the drug. Repeat cycle until disease progression or unacceptable toxicity.

Adjust-a-dose: Increase or decrease dosage in 12.5-mg increments based on individual safety and tolerability. If drug must be administered with a strong CYP3A4 inhibitor, reduce dosage to a minimum of 37.5 mg/day. If drug must be administered with a CYP3A4 inducer, consider increasing dosage to 87.5 mg daily; carefully monitor patient for toxicity.

➤ **Progressive, well-differentiated pancreatic neuroendocrine tumors in patients with unresectable locally advanced, or metastatic disease**

Reactions in bold italics are *life-threatening*. Interactions may have a *rapid onset* or a *delayed onset*.

Adults: 37.5 mg PO once daily given continuously without a scheduled off-treatment period. Maximum recommended dosage is 50 mg daily. Continue until disease progression or unacceptable toxicity.

Adjust-a-dose: Increase or decrease in 12.5-mg increments based on patient tolerance and safety. If drug must be administered with a strong CYP3A4 inhibitor, consider decreasing dosage to 25 mg daily. If drug must be administered with a CYP3A4 inducer, consider increasing dosage to 62.5 mg daily and carefully monitor patient for toxicity.

➤ **Adjuvant treatment of patients at high risk for recurrent renal cell carcinoma after nephrectomy**
Adults: 50 mg PO once daily, on a schedule of 4 weeks on treatment followed by 2 weeks off treatment for a maximum of nine 6-week cycles.

Adjust-a-dose: Increase or decrease dosage in 12.5-mg increments based on individual safety and tolerability. If drug must be administered with a strong CYP3A4 inhibitor, reduce dosage to a minimum of 37.5 mg/day. If drug must be administered with a CYP3A4 inducer, consider increasing dosage to 87.5 mg daily; carefully monitor patient for toxicity.

ADMINISTRATION
PO

◑ *Alert:* Hazardous agent; use safe handling and disposal. Avoid contact with broken capsules.

• Give drug without regard for meals.
• If a dose is missed by less than 12 hours, give missed dose right away. If a dose is missed by more than 12 hours, skip missed dose and give next scheduled dose at its regular time.

ACTION
A multi-kinase inhibitor targeting several receptor tyrosine kinases, which are involved in tumor growth, pathologic angiogenesis, and metastatic progression of cancer.

Route	Onset	Peak	Duration
PO	Unknown	6–12 hr	Unknown

Half-life: 40 to 60 hours; primary metabolite, 80 to 110 hours.

ADVERSE REACTIONS
CNS: altered taste, asthenia, dizziness, fatigue, fever, headache, insomnia, depression. **CV:** *decreased LVEF,* HTN, peripheral edema, chest pain. **EENT:** dry mouth, nasopharyngitis, oral pain. **GI:** abdominal pain, anorexia, GERD, constipation, diarrhea, dyspepsia, flatulence, mucositis, nausea, stomatitis, vomiting, hemorrhoids. **Hematologic:** *bleeding, lymphopenia, neutropenia, thrombocytopenia,* anemia. **Hepatic:** elevated LFT values. **Metabolic:** hypernatremia, hyperuricemia, *hypokalemia, hyperkalemia,* hyponatremia, hypercalcemia, *hypocalcemia, hypomagnesemia,* hypophosphatemia, hypothyroidism, increased lipase level, weight loss. **Musculoskeletal:** arthralgia, back pain, limb pain, myalgia. **Respiratory:** cough, dyspnea, URI. **Skin:** alopecia, dry skin, hair color changes, hand-foot syndrome, rash, erythema, pruritus, skin discoloration. **Other:** flulike symptoms, chills.

INTERACTIONS
Drug-drug. *Bevacizumab:* May enhance hypertensive effect of sunitinib and increase risk of microangiopathic hemolytic anemia. Avoid use together.

QTc interval–prolonging drugs (antiarrhythmics [amiodarone, disopyramide, dofetilide, procainamide, quinidine, sotalol], arsenic trioxide, chlorpromazine, cisapride, dolasetron, droperidol, mefloquine, mesoridazine, moxifloxacin, pentamidine, pimozide, tacrolimus, thioridazine, ziprasidone): May increase risk of QTc-interval prolongation and ventricular arrhythmias. Carefully monitor ECG and QT interval. Consider therapy modification.

Strong CYP3A4 inducers (carbamazepine, dexamethasone, phenobarbital, phenytoin, rifabutin, rifampin, rifapentine): May decrease sunitinib level and effects. If use together can't be avoided, increase sunitinib dosage.

Strong CYP3A4 inhibitors (atazanavir, clarithromycin, itraconazole, ketoconazole, nefazodone, nelfinavir, ritonavir, saquinavir, voriconazole): May increase sunitinib level and toxicity. If use together can't be avoided, decrease sunitinib dosage.

Drug-herb. *Echinacea, St. John's wort:* May cause an unpredictable decrease in drug level. Discourage use together.

Drug-food. *Grapefruit:* May increase drug level. Discourage use together.

EFFECTS ON LAB TEST RESULTS
• May increase AST, ALT, ALP, total and indirect bilirubin, amylase, lipase, creatinine, uric acid, and TSH levels.

S

- May decrease phosphorus, magnesium, and albumin levels.
- May increase or decrease potassium, calcium, glucose, and sodium levels.
- May decrease Hb level, hematocrit, and RBC, neutrophil, lymphocyte, WBC, and platelet counts.

CONTRAINDICATIONS & CAUTIONS

- Contraindicated in patients hypersensitive to drug or its components.
- Use cautiously in patients with electrolyte imbalance or a history of HTN, QT-interval prolongation, concurrent antiarrhythmic use, bradycardia, MI, angina, CABG, symptomatic HF, stroke, TIA, or PE.
- Thrombotic microangiopathy (TMA), including thrombotic thrombocytopenic purpura and hemolytic-uremic syndrome, sometimes leading to renal failure or a fatal outcome, has been reported. Discontinue if TMA develops.
- Proteinuria and nephrotic syndrome have been reported, and some cases have resulted in renal failure and fatal outcomes. Monitor patient for development or worsening of proteinuria.
- SCARs have been reported, including erythema multiforme, SJS, and TEN, some of which were fatal. If patient develops signs or symptoms of a progressive rash, often with blisters or mucosal lesions, discontinue drug. If a diagnosis of SJS or TEN is suspected, don't restart drug.
- Necrotizing fasciitis, including of the perineum and secondary to fistula formation, sometimes fatal, has been reported. Discontinue drug if necrotizing fasciitis develops.
- Drug has been associated with symptomatic hypoglycemia, which may result in loss of consciousness or require hospitalization. Blood glucose level reductions may be worse in patients with diabetes. Check blood glucose levels regularly during and after discontinuation of treatment. Assess if antidiabetic dosage needs adjustment to minimize risk of hypoglycemia.

Dialyzable drug: No.

PREGNANCY-LACTATION-REPRODUCTION

- Drug can cause fetal harm when used during pregnancy. Patients of childbearing potential should avoid pregnancy during therapy. If drug is used during pregnancy, or if patient becomes pregnant while taking drug, apprise patient of fetal risk.
- Patients of childbearing potential should use effective contraception during treatment and for at least 4 weeks after final dose.
- Male patients with partners of childbearing potential should use effective contraception during treatment and for 7 weeks after final dose.
- It isn't known if drug appears in human milk. Patient should discontinue breastfeeding or discontinue drug.
- Sunitinib treatment may compromise male and female fertility.

NURSING CONSIDERATIONS

Boxed Warning Drug may cause severe, sometimes fatal, hepatotoxicity. Monitor liver function before and during each cycle of therapy. ∎

- Obtain LFT values at baseline, before each treatment cycle, and when clinically indicated.
- Verify pregnancy status before treatment.
- **Alert:** Drug may cause CV events, including HF, myocardial disorders, and cardiomyopathy, which may be fatal. Monitor CV status closely.
- Obtain baseline evaluation of LVEF in all patients before treatment. If patient had a cardiac event in the year before treatment, check LVEF periodically.
- Interrupt therapy or decrease dosage in patients with LVEF less than 50% and more than 20% below baseline.
- Monitor patient's BP closely. If severe HTN occurs, notify prescriber. Drug may need to be withheld until BP is controlled.
- Monitor patient for signs and symptoms of HF, especially if there is a history of heart disease.
- Obtain CBC with platelet count and serum chemistries, including phosphate, magnesium, and calcium levels, before each treatment cycle.
- Obtain urinalysis at baseline and periodically during treatment, with follow-up measurement of 24-hour urine protein as clinically indicated to evaluate patient for nephrotic syndrome.
- Check blood glucose level regularly during and after discontinuation of treatment. Assess if antidiabetic dosage needs adjustment to minimize risk of hypoglycemia.
- Thyroid dysfunction (hypothyroidism, hyperthyroidism, thyroiditis) may occur. Monitor thyroid function at baseline and closely

---

Reactions in bold italics are *life-threatening*. Interactions may have a *rapid onset* or a **delayed onset**.

monitor patients for signs and symptoms suggestive of thyroid dysfunction.

• For patients with ESRD on hemodialysis, no starting dosage adjustment is recommended. However, given the decreased exposure compared to patients with normal renal function, may increase subsequent doses gradually up to twofold based on safety and tolerability.

• Patient who has seizures may have reversible posterior leukoencephalopathy syndrome. Signs and symptoms include HTN, headache, decreased alertness, altered mental functioning, and vision loss. Stop treatment temporarily.

• Impaired wound healing has been reported during therapy. Temporarily interrupt therapy in patients undergoing major surgical procedures. May resume drug when health care provider determines patient has recovered.

• Provide antiemetics or antidiarrheals as needed for adverse GI effects.

• Monitor patient with renal cell carcinoma or GI stromal tumor with high tumor burden closely and treat as clinically indicated because of the risk of TLS. Correct dehydration and high uric acid levels before treatment.

• Osteonecrosis of the jaw has been reported. Consider preventive dentistry before treatment with sunitinib. If possible, avoid invasive dental procedures, particularly in patients receiving IV bisphosphonate therapy.

🔵 Alert: Drug may cause bleeding in GI tract, urinary tract, respiratory tract, and brain, which may be fatal. Monitor patient and CBC closely.

• Drug may cause GI perforation in patients with intra-abdominal malignancies. Monitor patient closely.

PATIENT TEACHING

• Advise patient to keep appointments for blood tests and periodic heart function evaluations.

• Teach patient safe drug administration and handling.

• Tell patient about common adverse effects, such as diarrhea, nausea, vomiting, fatigue, mouth pain, and taste disturbance, and to report all adverse reactions.

• Advise patient that severe hypoglycemia can occur. Inform patient of the signs, symptoms, and risks associated with hypoglycemia.

• Inform patient about changes that may occur in skin and hair, including color changes and dry, red, blistering skin of the hands and feet.

• Urge patient to tell prescriber about all prescribed and OTC drugs or herbal supplements.

• Warn patient not to consume grapefruit products during therapy.

• Tell patient to notify prescriber about unusual bleeding, trouble breathing, fainting, light-headedness, and heart palpitations, wheezing, severe or prolonged diarrhea or vomiting, or swelling of the hands or lower legs.

• Advise patient of childbearing potential to use effective contraception during treatment and for at least 4 weeks after final dose.

• Caution male patient with partner of childbearing potential to use effective contraception during treatment and for 7 weeks after final dose.

suvorexant
soo-voe-REX-ant

Belsomra

Therapeutic class: Hypnotics
Pharmacologic class: Orexin receptor antagonists
Controlled substance schedule: IV

AVAILABLE FORMS
Tablets: 5 mg, 10 mg, 15 mg, 20 mg

INDICATIONS & DOSAGES
➤ **Insomnia characterized by difficulties with sleep onset or sleep maintenance**
Adults: 10 mg PO daily within 30 minutes of going to bed. If 10-mg dose is tolerated but not effective, increase to a maximum of 20 mg PO daily. Don't exceed more than one dose per night.
Adjust-a-dose: For patients taking concomitant moderate CYP3A4 inhibitors, give 5 mg PO daily at night. Maximum dose is 10 mg daily.

ADMINISTRATION
PO
• Give drug within 30 minutes of bedtime and ensure at least 7 hours remain before planned time of awakening.

S

• May give with or without food; however, the time to drug's effect is delayed if drug is taken with or soon after a meal.

ACTION

Blocks orexin receptors, suppressing the system responsible for promoting wakefulness.

Route	Onset	Peak	Duration
PO	30 min	2 hr	Unknown

Half-life: 12 hours.

ADVERSE REACTIONS

CNS: somnolence, headache, dizziness, abnormal dreams. **EENT:** dry mouth. **GI:** diarrhea. **Respiratory:** cough, URI.

INTERACTIONS

Drug-drug. *CNS depressants, including other drugs that treat insomnia:* May cause excessive CNS depression. Use together isn't recommended.

Digoxin: May decrease digoxin metabolism. Monitor digoxin level.

Moderate CYP3A4 inhibitors (amprenavir, aprepitant, atazanavir, ciprofloxacin, diltiazem, erythromycin, fluconazole, fosamprenavir, imatinib, verapamil): May decrease suvorexant metabolism. Decrease initial suvorexant daily dose to 5 mg; don't exceed a dose of 10 mg.

Opioids: May cause slow or difficult breathing, sedation, and death. Avoid use together. If use together is necessary, limit dosage and duration of each drug to minimum necessary for desired effect.

Strong CYP3A4 inducers (carbamazepine, phenytoin, rifampin): May decrease clinical effect of suvorexant. Monitor patient for reduced therapeutic effect.

Strong CYP3A4 inhibitors (clarithromycin, conivaptan, itraconazole, ketoconazole, nefazodone, nelfinavir, posaconazole, ritonavir, saquinavir, telaprevir): May increase risk of additive toxicity. Avoid use together.

Drug-food. *Grapefruit juice:* May decrease drug metabolism and increase drug level. Decrease suvorexant dosage.

Drug-lifestyle. *Alcohol use:* May cause excessive CNS depression. Discourage use together.

EFFECTS ON LAB TEST RESULTS

• May increase cholesterol level.

CONTRAINDICATIONS & CAUTIONS

• Contraindicated in patients hypersensitive to drug or its components and in those with narcolepsy.

• Opioids should only be prescribed with benzodiazepines or other CNS depressants to patients for whom alternative treatment options are inadequate.

• Not recommended for use in patients with severe hepatic impairment.

⚠ **Alert:** Drug may increase risk of suicidality. Immediately evaluate patients who report suicidality or exhibit new behavioral signs or symptoms.

• Use cautiously in patients with compromised respiratory status (obstructive sleep apnea, COPD) or a history of drug abuse or dependence.

• Drug can cause drowsiness. Patients, especially older adults, are at higher risk for falls.

• Safety and effectiveness in children haven't been studied.

Dialyzable drug: Unknown.

⚠ **Overdose S&S:** Increased frequency and duration of somnolence.

PREGNANCY-LACTATION-REPRODUCTION

• Drug hasn't been studied in pregnancy. Use cautiously during pregnancy and only if benefits outweigh fetal risk.

• It isn't known if drug appears in human milk. Use cautiously during breastfeeding.

NURSING CONSIDERATIONS

• Use the smallest effective dosage in all patients. Lower dosages may be necessary in obese or female patients because a higher incidence of adverse effects have been observed.

• Complex behaviors, such as sleepwalking, "sleep driving" (driving while not fully awake), preparing and eating food, making phone calls, or having sex with subsequent amnesia of the event, have been reported. These behaviors may occur after the first or any subsequent use of the drug, with or without the concomitant use of alcohol or CNS depressants, which increase the risk. Discontinue drug for complex sleep behavior.

• Monitor patient for daytime somnolence. Decrease dosage or discontinue drug if daytime somnolence develops in patients who drive.

Reactions in bold italics are *life-threatening*. Interactions may have a *rapid onset* or a **delayed onset**.

• Carefully evaluate patient for physical or psychiatric causes of sleep disturbances before drug is prescribed. If insomnia persists for more than 7 to 10 days, reevaluate patient.

• Monitor patients for sleep paralysis (inability to move or speak during sleep-wake transitions), hallucinations, and mild cataplexy signs and symptoms (periods of leg weakness).

⚠ *Alert:* Worsening of depression or suicidality may occur. Be alert for signs and symptoms of depression or behavioral changes.

PATIENT TEACHING

• Teach patient safe drug administration.

• Instruct patient not to increase dosage without first consulting prescriber.

• Caution patient or caregiver of patient taking an opioid with a benzodiazepine, CNS depressant, or alcohol to seek immediate medical attention for dizziness, light-headedness, extreme sleepiness, slowed or difficult breathing, or unresponsiveness.

• Advise patient to avoid alcohol and other drugs that cause sleepiness while taking suvorexant.

• Advise patient that increased drowsiness may increase the risk of falls in some patients, especially older adults.

• Tell patient to notify prescriber if abnormal thoughts and behavior, symptoms of depression (changes in mood, excessive tiredness), or insomnia that persists for more than 7 to 10 days occurs.

⚠ *Alert:* Caution patient to immediately report suicidality or new behavioral signs or symptoms.

• Inform patient that sleep paralysis (inability to move or speak during sleep-wake transitions), vivid and disturbing perceptions, and temporary leg weakness can occur.

• Advise patient that daytime somnolence can occur and to avoid performing activities that require mental alertness or physical coordination (such as driving) until fully awake.

• Warn patient of the risk of performing complex behaviors, such as driving, eating, and making phone calls, while asleep and to report if these symptoms occur.

• Advise patient to report pregnancy, plans to become pregnant, or to breastfeed.

tacrolimus (topical)
tack-ROW-lim-us

Protopic

Therapeutic class: Immunomodulators
Pharmacologic class: Calcineurin inhibitors

AVAILABLE FORMS
Ointment: 0.03%, 0.1%

INDICATIONS & DOSAGES
➤ **Moderate to severe atopic dermatitis in patients unresponsive to other therapies or unable to use other therapies because of risks**
Adults and children age 16 and older: Thin layer of 0.03% or 0.1% strength applied to affected areas b.i.d. and rubbed in completely.
Children ages 2 to 15: Thin layer of 0.03% strength applied to affected areas b.i.d. and rubbed in completely.

ADMINISTRATION
Topical
⚠ *Alert:* Hazardous drug; use safe handling and disposal precautions.

• In patients with infected atopic dermatitis, clear infections at treatment site before using drug.

• Don't use with occlusive dressings.

• Stop drug when signs and symptoms resolve.

• If signs and symptoms of atopic dermatitis don't improve within 6 weeks, refer patient for reevaluation by a health care provider to confirm the diagnosis.

ACTION
Unknown. Probably acts as an immune system modulator in the skin by inhibiting T-lymphocyte activation, which causes immunosuppression. Drug also inhibits the release of mediators from mast cells and basophils in skin.

Route	Onset	Peak	Duration
Topical	Unknown	Unknown	Unknown

Half-life: Unknown.

ADVERSE REACTIONS
CNS: headache, hyperesthesia, asthenia, insomnia, fever, depression, pain, paresthesia.
CV: peripheral edema, HTN, facial edema.

EENT: conjunctivitis, otitis media, ear pain, pharyngitis, rhinitis, sinusitis, periodontal abscess, tooth disorder. **GI:** diarrhea, vomiting, nausea, abdominal pain, gastroenteritis, dyspepsia. **GU:** dysmenorrhea, UTI. **Musculoskeletal:** back pain, arthralgia, myalgia. **Respiratory:** increased cough, *asthma,* pneumonia, bronchitis. **Skin:** alopecia, burning, cellulitis, pruritus, erythema, infection, herpes simplex, eczema herpeticum, pustular rash, folliculitis, urticaria, maculopapular rash, fungal dermatitis, acne, sunburn, tingling, benign skin neoplasm, vesiculobullous rash, dry skin, varicella zoster, herpes zoster, eczema, exfoliative dermatitis, contact dermatitis. **Other:** flulike symptoms, accidental injury, infection, alcohol intolerance, cyst, allergic reaction.

INTERACTIONS
Drug-drug. *CYP3A4 inhibitors (calcium channel blockers, cimetidine, erythromycin, fluconazole, itraconazole, ketoconazole, protease inhibitors):* May increase tacrolimus level if systemic absorption occurs. Use together cautiously.
Immunosuppressants: May enhance adverse effects of other immunosuppressants. Avoid use together.
Tacrolimus (systemic): May increase toxicity. Use together cautiously and decrease dosage as needed.
Drug-food. *Grapefruit juice:* May increase tacrolimus level if absorbed systemically. Monitor therapy.
Drug-lifestyle. *Alcohol use:* May cause flushing. Discourage use together.
Sun exposure: May cause phototoxicity. Advise patient to avoid excessive sunlight or artificial ultraviolet light exposure.

EFFECTS ON LAB TEST RESULTS
None reported.

CONTRAINDICATIONS & CAUTIONS
• Contraindicated in patients hypersensitive to drug.
Boxed Warning Don't use in children younger than age 2. Only 0.03% ointment is indicated for children ages 2 to 15. ■
• Don't use in patients who are immunocompromised or in patients with skin conditions with a skin barrier defect in which there is a potential for increased systemic absorption,

such as Netherton syndrome or generalized erythroderma.
• Safety hasn't been established beyond 1 year of noncontinuous use.
• Renal insufficiency has been reported in patients who were prescribed ointment for application to large BSAs. Use cautiously in patients with predisposed renal impairment.
🕙 *Alert:* Use only after other therapies have failed or aren't advisable.
Dialyzable drug: Unknown.

PREGNANCY-LACTATION-REPRODUCTION
• There are no adequate topical tacrolimus studies in pregnancy, and experience is too limited to assess its safe use during pregnancy. Drug crosses the placental barrier with systemic use. Use only if potential benefit justifies fetal risk.
• Drug appears in human milk. Patient should discontinue breastfeeding or discontinue drug.

NURSING CONSIDERATIONS
Boxed Warning Long-term safety of topical calcineurin inhibitors such as tacrolimus hasn't been established. Use drug only for short-term or intermittent long-term therapy. Limit application to areas of involvement with atopic dermatitis. Rare cases of malignancy have been reported without confirmation of causal relationship. ■
• Ensure that bacterial or viral skin infections of the treatment area have resolved before starting tacrolimus.
• Use of this drug may increase the risk of varicella zoster, HSV, and eczema herpeticum.
• Consider stopping drug in patients with lymphadenopathy if cause is unknown or acute mononucleosis is diagnosed.
• Monitor all cases of lymphadenopathy until resolution.
• Local adverse effects are most common during the first few days of treatment.
• Avoid use on areas of skin affected by premalignant and malignant skin conditions.

PATIENT TEACHING
• Teach patient safe drug administration and handling.
• Tell patient to wash hands before and after applying drug and to avoid applying drug to wet skin.

- Urge patient not to use bandages or other occlusive dressings.
- Tell patient not to bathe, shower, or swim immediately after application because doing so could wash the ointment off.
- Inform patient that a moisturizer can be applied after topical tacrolimus.
- Tell patient to stop treatment when the signs and symptoms resolve.
- Instruct patient to report if symptoms worsen or don't improve.
- Advise patient to avoid or minimize exposure to natural or artificial sunlight.
- Caution patient not to use drug for any disorder other than that for which it was prescribed.
- Encourage patient to report adverse reactions.
- Tell patient to store the ointment at room temperature.

tadalafil ⚕
tah-DAL-ah-fill

Adcirca, Alyq, Cialis✐

Therapeutic class: Erectile dysfunction drugs
Pharmacologic class: PDE5 inhibitors

AVAILABLE FORMS
Tablets (film-coated): 2.5 mg, 5 mg, 10 mg, 20 mg

INDICATIONS & DOSAGES
➤ **Erectile dysfunction (Cialis)**
Adults: 10 mg PO as a single dose, as needed, at least 30 minutes before sexual activity. Base range of 5 to 20 mg on effectiveness and tolerance. Maximum is one dose daily. Or 2.5 mg PO once daily without regard to timing of sexual activity. May increase to 5 mg PO daily.
Adjust-a-dose: If CrCl ranges from 30 to 50 mL/minute, begin 5 mg once daily; maximum dose, 10 mg once every 48 hours. If CrCl falls below 30 mL/minute or patient requires hemodialysis, maximum is 5 mg once every 72 hours as needed; daily use isn't recommended. Use cautiously in patients with mild or moderate hepatic impairment (Child-Pugh class A or B); don't exceed 10 mg daily. Patients taking potent CYP3A4 inhibitors shouldn't exceed one 10-mg dose every

72 hours if taken as needed; the once-daily dose shouldn't exceed 2.5 mg.
➤ **BPH (Cialis)**
Adults: 5 mg PO once daily taken at approximately the same time every day. When used with finasteride, recommended dose of Cialis is 5 mg once daily taken at approximately the same time every day for up to 26 weeks.
Adjust-a-dose: In patients with CrCl of 30 to 50 mL/minute, starting dose is 2.5 mg PO daily. May increase to 5 mg PO daily based on individual response. Not recommended for patients with CrCl less than 30 mL/minute or in patients on hemodialysis.
➤ **BPH and erectile dysfunction (Cialis)**
Adults: 5 mg PO once daily taken at approximately the same time every day, without regard to the timing of sexual activity.
Adjust-a-dose: In patients with CrCl of 30 to 50 mL/minute, starting dose is 2.5 mg PO daily. May increase to 5 mg PO daily based on individual response. Not recommended for patients with CrCl less than 30 mL/minute or in patients on hemodialysis.
➤ **PAH (Adcirca, Alyq)**
Adults: 40 mg (two 20-mg tablets) PO once daily.
Adjust-a-dose: For patients with CrCl of 31 to 80 mL/minute, start with 20 mg PO once daily. Increase to 40 mg once daily if tolerated. Avoid use in patients with CrCl of 30 mL/minute or less and in those on hemodialysis. Consider starting dose of 20 mg PO once daily in patients with mild or moderate hepatic impairment (Child-Pugh class A or B).

In patients receiving ritonavir for at least 1 week, start at 20 mg PO once daily and increase to 40 mg as tolerated. Don't use Adcirca or Alyq when starting ritonavir; stop Adcirca or Alyq at least 24 hours before starting ritonavir. After at least 1 week, may give 20 mg PO once daily and increase to 40 mg as tolerated.

ADMINISTRATION
PO
- Give drug without regard for food.
- Don't split Cialis tablets. Give entire dose as prescribed.
- Dividing 40-mg PAH dose over the course of the day isn't recommended.

ACTION
Inhibits PDE5 enzyme, which leads to increased cyclic guanosine monophosphate

T

levels, prolonged smooth muscle relaxation, and increased blood flow into the corpus cavernosum and pulmonary arteries. Effect is also seen in the smooth muscle of the prostate and bladder and their vascular supply.

Route	Onset	Peak	Duration
PO	Within 1 hr	0.5–6 hr	Up to 36 hr

Half-life: 15 to 17.5 hours; PAH (in patients not receiving bosentan), 35 hours.

ADVERSE REACTIONS
CNS: dizziness, headache. **CV:** flushing, HTN. **EENT:** nasal congestion, nasopharyngitis. **GI:** dyspepsia, abdominal pain, diarrhea, GERD, gastroenteritis, nausea. **GU:** UTI. **Musculoskeletal:** back pain, limb pain, myalgia. **Respiratory:** cough, respiratory tract infection.

INTERACTIONS
Drug-drug. *Alpha blockers:* May increase risk of hypotension. For erectile dysfunction, patient should be on stable dose before starting tadalafil at lowest recommended dosage. Use with tadalafil for BPH treatment isn't recommended; stop alpha blocker at least 1 day before starting tadalafil.
Antihypertensives (amlodipine, ARBs, enalapril, metoprolol): May increase hypotensive effect. Monitor patient closely.
Guanylate cyclase stimulators (riociguat): May increase hypotension. Use together is contraindicated.
Nitrates: May enhance hypotensive effects. Use together is contraindicated. If patient requires nitrates, wait at least 48 hours after last tadalafil dose.
Other PDE5 inhibitors (sildenafil, vardenafil): Use together hasn't been studied. Discourage use together.
Potent CYP3A4 inhibitors (ketoconazole, protease inhibitors, ritonavir): May increase tadalafil level. For erectile dysfunction, don't exceed a 10-mg dose of Cialis every 72 hours if taken as needed or 2.5 mg as the once-daily dose. For PAH, avoid use together.
Rifampin, other CYP450 inducers: May decrease tadalafil level. Avoid use together for PAH. For erectile dysfunction or BPH, monitor patient closely.
Drug-food. *Grapefruit:* May increase drug level. Discourage use together.
Drug-lifestyle. *Alcohol use:* May increase risk of headache, dizziness, orthostatic hypotension, and increased HR. Discourage use together.
Inhaled street drugs ("poppers," amyl nitrate, butyl nitrate, nitrite): May enhance hypotensive effects, causing dizziness, syncope, MI, or stroke. Use together is contraindicated.

EFFECTS ON LAB TEST RESULTS
None reported.

CONTRAINDICATIONS & CAUTIONS
• Contraindicated in patients hypersensitive to drug or its components and in those taking nitrates or GC stimulators.
• Use cautiously in patients with mild or moderate hepatic impairment (Child-Pugh class A or B).
• Drug isn't recommended for patients with severe hepatic impairment (Child-Pugh class C), severe renal impairment, unstable angina, angina that occurs during sexual intercourse, NYHA Class II or greater HF within past 6 months, uncontrolled arrhythmias, hypotension (lower than 90/50 mm Hg), uncontrolled HTN (higher than 170/100 mm Hg), stroke within past 6 months, or an MI within past 90 days.
• Use cautiously in patients with left ventricular outflow obstruction, autonomic dysfunction, or preexisting hypotension. Use in patients with pulmonary veno-occlusive disease isn't recommended.
▧ Drug isn't recommended for patients whose cardiac status makes sexual activity inadvisable or for those with known hereditary degenerative retinal disorders.
• Nonarteritic anterior ischemic optic neuropathy (NAION), a rare cause of decreased vision, including permanent vision loss, has been reported with all PDE5 inhibitors; a causal relationship hasn't been established. Most, but not all, of these patients had underlying risk factors for NAION.
• Use cautiously in patients with bleeding disorders, significant peptic ulceration, or renal impairment.
• Use cautiously in patients with conditions predisposing them to priapism (sickle cell anemia, multiple myeloma, and leukemia) and in those with anatomic penis abnormalities.
• Safety and effectiveness in children with PAH haven't been established.
• Use cautiously in older adults.
Dialyzable drug: No.

Reactions in bold italics are *life-threatening*. Interactions may have a *rapid onset* or a ***delayed onset***.

PREGNANCY-LACTATION-REPRODUCTION

- There are no adequate studies during pregnancy. Tadalafil crosses the placental barrier. Untreated PAH during pregnancy increases risk of HF, stroke, preterm delivery, and maternal and fetal death.
- It isn't known if drug appears in human milk. If tadalafil is required for PAH, consider risks and benefits to the infant.
- Tadalafil is only indicated for PAH in women.

NURSING CONSIDERATIONS

⚠️ *Alert:* Sexual activity may increase cardiac risk. Evaluate patient's cardiac risk before starting drug.
- Before drug initiation, assess patient for underlying causes of erectile dysfunction.
- Transient decreases in supine BP may occur. Monitor patient for orthostatic hypotension.
- Prolonged erections and priapism may occur.
- Monitor patients for (rare) vision or hearing loss and report immediately.
- *Look alike–sound alike:* Don't confuse tadalafil with sildenafil or vardenafil. Don't confuse Alyq with Alli.

PATIENT TEACHING

- Warn patient that taking drug with nitrates or guanylate cyclase stimulators could cause a serious drop in BP, which increases the risk of heart attack or stroke.
- Tell patient to seek immediate medical attention if chest pain develops after taking the drug.
- Inform patient that drug doesn't protect against sexually transmitted diseases and to use protective measures.
- Urge patient to seek emergency medical care for an erection lasting more than 4 hours.
- Tell patient to take drug about 30 to 60 minutes before anticipated sexual activity if using as needed. Explain that drug has no effect without sexual stimulation.
- Warn patient not to change dosage unless directed by prescriber.
- Caution patient against drinking large amounts of alcohol while taking drug.
- Instruct patient to report vision or hearing changes, especially sudden loss of vision in one or both eyes.

tamoxifen citrate
ta-MOX-i-fen

Nolvadex-D ♣, Soltamox

Therapeutic class: Antineoplastics
Pharmacologic class: Nonsteroidal antiestrogens

AVAILABLE FORMS
Oral solution: 10 mg/5 mL*
Tablets: 10 mg, 20 mg

INDICATIONS & DOSAGES
➤ **Estrogen receptor–positive metastatic breast cancer**
Adults: 20 to 40 mg PO daily; divide doses of more than 20 mg/day into two doses.
➤ **Adjuvant treatment of early-stage estrogen–receptor-positive breast cancer; to reduce occurrence of contralateral breast cancer**
Adults: 20 mg PO daily for 5 to 10 years.
➤ **To reduce breast cancer occurrence**
High-risk adults: 20 mg PO daily for 5 years.
➤ **Ductal carcinoma in situ (DCIS) after breast surgery and radiation to reduce risk of invasive breast cancer**
Adults: 20 mg PO daily for 5 years.
➤ **Prevention or treatment of antiandrogen-associated gynecomastia in patients with prostate cancer ♦**
Adults: 20 mg PO daily for up to 12 months.

ADMINISTRATION
PO
⚠️ *Alert:* Hazardous drug with potential teratogenic effects; follow safe-handling and disposal precautions.
- Give drug without regard to food.
- Use supplied dosing cup for oral solution.
- Store at room temperature. Protect from light and excessive heat.
- Don't freeze or refrigerate oral solution; use within 3 months of opening.

ACTION
Competes with estrogen for estrogen receptor–positive breast cancer cells, thereby preventing their growth.

♣Canada ◇OTC ♦ Off-label use ✐ Photoguide 🌐Do not crush *Liquid contains alcohol ▩ Genetic

Route	Onset	Peak	Duration
PO	Unknown	5 hr	Several wk

Half-life: Terminal phase, 5 to 7 days for tamoxifen and 14 days for the metabolite.

ADVERSE REACTIONS

CNS: sleepiness, headache, fatigue, depression, insomnia, dizziness, anxiety, mood changes, paresthesia, pain. **CV:** fluid retention, chest pain, HTN, edema, flushing, ischemic heart disease, lymphedema, vasodilation, *thromboembolism.* **EENT:** corneal changes, cataracts, retinopathy, pharyngitis. **GI:** nausea, vomiting, diarrhea, constipation, dyspepsia, GI disorder, abdominal cramps, abdominal pain, anorexia. **GU:** amenorrhea, irregular menses, vaginal discharge, vaginal dryness, vaginitis, vulvovaginitis, ovarian cysts, vaginal bleeding. **Hematologic:** anemia, *leukopenia, thrombocytopenia.* **Hepatic:** elevated liver enzyme levels. **Metabolic:** weight gain or loss, hypercholesterolemia. **Musculoskeletal:** bone pain, arthralgia, arthritis, osteoporosis, fracture, arthrosis, myalgia. **Respiratory:** *PE,* cough, dyspnea, bronchitis. **Skin:** skin changes, rash, diaphoresis, alopecia. **Other:** tumor pain, hot flashes, infection, flulike syndrome, neoplasm, breast pain.

INTERACTIONS

Drug-drug. *Aromatase inhibitors (anastrozole, letrozole):* May decrease aromatase inhibitor serum concentration. Avoid use together.
Coumarin-type anticoagulants (warfarin): May significantly increase anticoagulant effect. Monitor patient, PT, and INR closely. Tamoxifen is contraindicated when used to reduce risk of breast cancer in high-risk patients and patients with DCIS.
Cytotoxic drugs: May increase risk of thromboembolic events. Monitor patient.
Drugs that prolong QTc interval: May increase risk of life-threatening cardiac arrhythmias. Use together cautiously.
Strong CYP2D6 inhibitors (fluoxetine, paroxetine, sertraline): May decrease serum level of active metabolite(s) of tamoxifen and decrease tamoxifen's therapeutic effects. Avoid use together.
Strong CYP3A4 inducers (rifampin): May decrease tamoxifen level. Monitor patient for clinical effects.

Drug-herb. *St. John's wort:* May decrease tamoxifen serum concentration. Avoid use together.
Drug-food. *Grapefruit, grapefruit juice:* May decrease tamoxifen metabolism. Avoid use together.

EFFECTS ON LAB TEST RESULTS

• May increase serum creatinine, calcium, T_4, cholesterol, bilirubin, lipid, and liver enzyme levels.
• May decrease WBC and platelet counts.

CONTRAINDICATIONS & CAUTIONS

• Contraindicated in patients hypersensitive to drug.
• Contraindicated as therapy to reduce risk of breast cancer in high-risk patients and patients with DCIS who concurrently are taking coumarin-type anticoagulants or in patients with history of VTE.

Boxed Warning Serious and life-threatening events associated with tamoxifen include uterine malignancies, stroke, and PE. Discuss potential benefits versus risks with patients at high risk for breast cancer and patients with DCIS who are considering tamoxifen to reduce their risks of developing breast cancer. Benefits of drug outweigh its risks in patients already diagnosed with breast cancer. ∎
• Use cautiously in patients with leukopenia, thrombocytopenia, or bone marrow suppression.
• Drug increases risk of endometrial changes, including hyperplasia, polyps, endometrial cancer, and uterine cancer.
• Drug may increase risk of fatty liver, cholestasis, hepatitis, hepatic necrosis, and liver cancer.
Dialyzable drug: No.
⚠ *Overdose S&S:* Tremors, hyperreflexia, unsteady gait, dizziness, seizures, prolonged QT interval.

PREGNANCY-LACTATION-REPRODUCTION

• May cause fetal harm when used during pregnancy. Fetal risks include the potential long-term risk of a diethylstilbestrol (DES)-like syndrome. Sexually active patients should use barrier or nonhormonal contraceptives during treatment and for 2 months after final dose.
• Rule out pregnancy before therapy.
• Drug may cause infertility in women.

Reactions in bold italics are *life-threatening*. Interactions may have a *rapid onset* or a *delayed onset*.

• Breastfeeding is contraindicated during therapy and for 3 months after final dose.

NURSING CONSIDERATIONS
• Verify pregnancy status before treatment.
• Monitor lipid levels during long-term therapy in patients with hyperlipidemia.
• Monitor calcium level. At start of therapy, drug may compound hypercalcemia related to bone metastases.
• Monitor patient for signs and symptoms of venous thromboembolism.
• Monitor bone mineral density in patients who are premenopausal.
• Patients should have baseline and periodic gynecologic exams because of a slight increased risk of endometrial cancer.
• Women should have periodic eye exams because of increased risk of cataracts, retinal vein thrombosis, and retinopathy.
• Monitor CBC closely in patients with leukopenia or thrombocytopenia.
• Monitor liver function periodically.
• Patient may initially experience worsening symptoms.
• Karyopyknotic index of vaginal smears and estrogen effect of Papanicolaou smears may vary in patients after menopause.
• **Look alike–sound alike:** Don't confuse tamoxifen with tamsulosin.

PATIENT TEACHING
• Teach patient safe drug administration and handling.
• Reassure patient that acute worsening of bone pain during therapy usually indicates drug will produce good response. Give analgesics to relieve pain.
• Strongly encourage patients who are taking or have taken drug to have regular gynecologic exams because drug may increase risk of uterine cancer.
• Encourage patients to have mammograms and breast exams as recommended.
• Advise patient to use a barrier form of contraception because short-term therapy induces ovulation in patients who are premenopausal.
• Instruct patient to report vaginal bleeding or changes in menstrual cycle.
• Caution patient to use effective nonhormonal contraception during treatment and for 2 months after final dose. Advise patient to consult prescriber before becoming pregnant.
• Tell patient to report all adverse reactions, especially signs and symptoms of stroke

(headache, vision changes, confusion, difficulty speaking, weakness of face, arm, or leg, especially on one side of the body), PE (chest pain, difficulty breathing, rapid breathing, diaphoresis, fainting), and DVT (leg swelling, tenderness).
• Advise patient to report vision changes.

tamsulosin hydrochloride
tam-soo-LOE-sin

Flomax✎, Flomax CR♣

Therapeutic class: BPH drugs
Pharmacologic class: Alpha blockers

AVAILABLE FORMS
Capsules ⊙: 0.4 mg

INDICATIONS & DOSAGES
➤ **BPH**
Adults: 0.4 mg PO once daily, given 30 minutes after same meal each day. If no response after 2 to 4 weeks, increase dosage to 0.8 mg PO once daily.
➤ **Ureteral stone expulsion** ◆
Adults: 0.4 mg PO daily until expulsion of stones or for up to 4 weeks for medical expulsive therapy of stones at least 5 to 10 mm. Or, 0.4 mg daily starting immediately after lithotripsy for 2 weeks to 3 months.

ADMINISTRATION
PO
• Don't crush, open, or allow patient to chew capsules.
• Give drug about 30 minutes after same meal each day.
• If a dose is missed, give missed dose as soon as possible. If 1 day elapses without a dose, continue with the next regularly scheduled dose. If dose is missed for several days, consult prescriber.
• If treatment is interrupted for several days, restart with 0.4 mg daily.

ACTION
Selectively blocks alpha receptors in the prostate, leading to relaxation of smooth muscles in the bladder neck and prostate, improving urine flow and reducing symptoms of BPH.

T

Route	Onset	Peak	Duration
PO	Unknown	4–7 hr	9–15 hr

Half-life: 9 to 13 hours.

ADVERSE REACTIONS

CNS: dizziness, headache, asthenia, insomnia, somnolence, syncope, vertigo. **CV:** chest pain, orthostatic hypotension. **EENT:** rhinitis, pharyngitis, sinusitis, tooth disorder. **GI:** diarrhea, nausea. **GU:** decreased libido, abnormal ejaculation. **Musculoskeletal:** back pain. **Respiratory:** increased cough. **Other:** infection.

INTERACTIONS

Drug-drug. *Alpha blockers:* May interact with tamsulosin. Avoid using together.
Cimetidine: May decrease tamsulosin clearance. Use together cautiously.
Moderate CYP3A4 inhibitors (erythromycin): May decrease tamsulosin metabolism. Use cautiously and monitor therapy.
Moderate and strong CYP2D6 inhibitors (paroxetine, terbinafine): May increase tamsulosin level. Monitor therapy.
PDE5 inhibitors: May cause symptomatic hypotension. Use together cautiously.
Strong CYP3A4 inhibitors (ketoconazole): May increase tamsulosin serum concentration. Avoid use together.
Warfarin: Limited studies are inconclusive. Use together cautiously.
Drug-herb. *St. John's wort:* May decrease tamsulosin serum concentration. Consider therapy modification.

EFFECTS ON LAB TEST RESULTS
None reported.

CONTRAINDICATIONS & CAUTIONS
• Contraindicated in patients hypersensitive to drug or its components.
• Use cautiously in patients with serious or life-threatening sulfa allergy.
• Intraoperative floppy iris syndrome has been observed during cataract and glaucoma surgery in some patients who are taking or had previously taken alpha₁ blockers, including tamsulosin, which may increase risk of eye complications during and after surgery. Avoid initiating therapy in patients scheduled for cataract or glaucoma surgery.
• Not indicated in children.
Dialyzable drug: Unlikely.

⚠ *Overdose S&S:* Severe headache, hypotension.

PREGNANCY-LACTATION-REPRODUCTION
• Drug isn't indicated for use in women.
• Don't use drug for off-label indication during pregnancy or breastfeeding.

NURSING CONSIDERATIONS
• Monitor patient for decreases in BP. Drug may cause orthostatic hypotension and syncope, especially with first dose.
• Symptoms of BPH and prostate cancer are similar; screen for prostate cancer before starting therapy and at regular intervals during therapy.
• Rare but serious priapism can occur and must be treated urgently.
• *Look alike–sound alike:* Don't confuse Flomax with Fosamax, Flonase, or Flovent.

PATIENT TEACHING
• Instruct patient in safe drug administration.
• Advise patient that drug may cause sudden drop in BP, especially after first dose or when changing doses. Tell patient to rise slowly from a chair or bed when starting therapy and to avoid situations in which injury could result from fainting.
• Instruct patient not to drive or perform hazardous tasks for 12 hours after first dose or changes in dose until response can be monitored.
• Warn patient that rarely priapism can occur and to report it immediately.
• Advise patient considering cataract or glaucoma surgery to inform the ophthalmologist about taking drug.

tasimelteon
TAS-i-MEL-tee-on

Hetlioz, Hetlioz LQ

Therapeutic class: Hypnotics
Pharmacologic class: Melatonin receptor agonists

AVAILABLE FORMS
Capsules 🅞🅝🅒: 20 mg
Oral suspension: 4 mg/mL

Reactions in bold italics are *life-threatening*. Interactions may have a *rapid onset* or a **delayed onset**.

INDICATIONS & DOSAGES

➤ **Non-24-hour sleep-wake disorder**
Adults: 20 mg PO at same time each night before bedtime.

➤ **Nighttime sleep disturbances in Smith-Magenis syndrome**
Adults and children age 16 and older: 20 mg PO 1 hour before bedtime.
Children ages 3 to 15 weighing more than 28 kg: 20 mg oral suspension PO 1 hour before bedtime.
Children ages 3 to 15 weighing 28 kg or less: 0.7 mg/kg oral suspension PO 1 hour before bedtime.

ADMINISTRATION
PO
• Give drug without food.
• Give capsule whole; don't open or crush.
• Shake oral suspension for at least 30 seconds before administration. Remove seal and insert press-in bottle adapter (included in package) into neck of bottle until a tight seal is made. Turn bottle upside down and withdraw prescribed amount from bottle. Leave press-in bottle adapter in place on bottle neck and replace cap.
• Give at same time each night. If patient can't take dose at approximately the same time on a given night, skip that dose.
• After administration, patient should limit activities to preparing for sleep.
• Capsules and oral suspension can't be substituted for each other.
• Store capsules at room temperature.
• Refrigerate oral suspension. After opening, discard 48-mL bottle after 5 weeks and 158-mL bottle after 8 weeks.

ACTION
Binds to melatonin receptors in the brain, resulting in regulation of sleep-wake cycle.

Route	Onset	Peak	Duration
PO (capsules)	Unknown	0.5–3 hr	Unknown
PO (suspension)	Unknown	15–30 min	Unknown

Half-life: 1 to 2 hours.

ADVERSE REACTIONS
CNS: headache, nightmares, abnormal dreams. **GU:** UTI. **Hepatic:** elevated transaminase levels. **Respiratory:** URI.

INTERACTIONS
Drug-drug. *Beta-adrenergic receptor antagonists (acebutolol, metoprolol):* May reduce tasimelteon efficacy when antagonist is given at night. Monitor therapy.
Strong CYP3A4 inducers (carbamazepine, primidone, rifampin): May decrease exposure to tasimelteon, resulting in decreased efficacy. Avoid use together.
Strong CYP1A2 inhibitors (fluvoxamine): May increase exposure to tasimelteon, increasing risk of adverse events. Avoid use together.
Drug-herb. *St. John's wort:* May decrease drug level and decrease effectiveness. Consider therapy modification.
Drug-food. *Alcohol use:* May cause additive effect of tasimelteon. Discourage use together.
Drug-lifestyle. *Smoking:* May decrease tasimelteon exposure by 40% compared to nonsmokers. Discourage use together.

EFFECTS ON LAB TEST RESULTS
• May increase ALT level.

CONTRAINDICATIONS & CAUTIONS
• Contraindicated in patients hypersensitive to drug or its components.
• Use in patients with severe hepatic impairment (Child-Pugh class C) hasn't been studied and isn't recommended.
• Use cautiously in older adults. Drug may have up to twofold increase in exposure, increasing risk of adverse events in these patients.
Dialyzable drug: Yes.

PREGNANCY-LACTATION-REPRODUCTION
• There are no adequate studies during pregnancy. Use only if benefits outweigh fetal risk.
• It isn't known if drug appears in human milk. Use cautiously during breastfeeding.

NURSING CONSIDERATIONS
• Females have a 20% to 30% greater overall exposure to tasimelteon than males.
• Drug's effects may not occur for weeks or months because of individual differences in circadian rhythms.

PATIENT TEACHING
• Tell patient to swallow capsule whole at bedtime.

- Counsel patient to shake oral suspension for at least 30 seconds before taking.
- Instruct patient to take drug at the same time every night. If patient can't take dose at approximately the same time on a given night, patient should skip dose.
- Warn patient to limit activities after taking drug, since drug decreases mental alertness.
- Caution patient against performing tasks that require mental alertness, such as operating machinery or driving.
- Advise patient that drug may take several weeks or months to become effective.
- Caution patient to avoid alcohol because of additive effects.
- Inform patient that smoking decreases effects of drug and should be avoided.

telavancin
tell-uh-VAN-sin

Vibativ

Therapeutic class: Antibiotics
Pharmacologic class: Lipoglycopeptides

AVAILABLE FORMS
Lyophilized powder for injection: 750-mg single-use vials

INDICATIONS & DOSAGES
Adjust-a-dose (for all indications): For patients with CrCl of 30 to 50 mL/minute, give 7.5 mg/kg every 24 hours; if CrCl ranges from 10 to 29 mL/minute, give 10 mg/kg every 48 hours.
➤ **Complicated skin and skin-structure infections caused by susceptible gram-positive organisms, such as *Staphylococcus aureus*, MRSA, *Streptococcus pyogenes*, *Streptococcus agalactiae*, *Streptococcus anginosus* group, or *Enterococcus faecalis* (vancomycin-susceptible isolates only)**
Adults: 10 mg/kg IV infusion once every 24 hours for 7 to 14 days.
➤ **Hospital-acquired and ventilator-associated bacterial pneumonia caused by susceptible isolates of *S. aureus* (including methicillin-susceptible and methicillin-resistant isolates)**
Adults: 10 mg/kg IV once every 24 hours for 7 to 21 days.

ADMINISTRATION
IV
▼ Reconstitute 750-mg vial with 45 mL sterile water, D_5W, or NSS for injection. Mix thoroughly but don't shake; reconstitution may take up to 20 minutes. Resultant solution has a concentration of 15 mg/mL.
▼ Further dilute doses of 150 to 800 mg in 100 to 250 mL of D_5W, NSS, or lactated Ringer solution before infusion. Further dilute doses less than 150 mg or greater than 800 mg to a final concentration of 0.6 to 8 mg/mL.
▼ Inspect for particulate matter before infusion.
▼ Infuse drug over 60 minutes.
▼ Reconstituted solution is stable for 12 hours at room temperature or 7 days if refrigerated.
▼ Diluted IV solution remains stable for 12 hours at room temperature or 7 days if refrigerated, including reconstituted time. Diluted solution in the infusion bag may be frozen for up to 32 days.
▼ **Incompatibilities:** Other IV drugs. If line is used for other IV drugs, flush with D_5W, NSS, or lactated Ringer solution before and after infusion.

ACTION
Inhibits bacterial cell-wall synthesis by binding to the bacterial cell membrane and disrupting its function.

Route	Onset	Peak	Duration
IV	Unknown	Unknown	Unknown

Half-life: About 6.6 to 9.6 hours.

ADVERSE REACTIONS
CNS: taste disturbance, dizziness. **GI:** abdominal pain, decreased appetite, diarrhea, nausea, vomiting. **GU:** foamy urine, new-onset or worsening renal impairment, *acute renal failure.* **Skin:** generalized pruritus, infusion-site pain, infusion-site reaction, localized erythema, rash. **Other:** rigors.

INTERACTIONS
Drug-drug. *Drugs that prolong QTc interval (erythromycin, sotalol, thioridazine):* May enhance QTc-prolonging effect. Avoid such combinations when possible. Use should be accompanied by close monitoring for evidence of QT prolongation or other cardiac rhythm alterations.

Reactions in bold italics are *life-threatening*. Interactions may have a *rapid onset* or a ***delayed onset***.

Heparin: May artificially prolong PTT, which could lead to incorrect decrease of heparin dosage. Concomitant use with IV unfractionated heparin is contraindicated.

Vaccines (cholera, live attenuated Ty21a strain of typhoid): May diminish vaccine's effect. Avoid cholera vaccine within 14 days of oral or parenteral antibiotics; don't give typhoid vaccine until at least 3 days after stopping antibiotic.

EFFECTS ON LAB TEST RESULTS
• May increase factor Xa and INR.
• May falsely prolong PT, PTT, and activated clotting time.
• May falsely affect urine qualitative dipstick protein assays and quantitative dye methods, such as pyrogallol red-molybdate.

CONTRAINDICATIONS & CAUTIONS
⚠️ *Alert:* Reserve drug for treatment of pneumonia when alternative treatments aren't suitable.

⚠️ *Alert:* Contraindicated in patients hypersensitive to drug or its components. Serious and potentially fatal hypersensitivity reactions, including anaphylactic reactions, may occur after first or subsequent doses. Use cautiously in patients with known hypersensitivity to vancomycin.

⚠️ *Alert:* Concomitant use of IV unfractionated heparin sodium is contraindicated because PTT test results may be artificially prolonged for 0 to 18 hours after administration.
• Avoid use in patients with prolonged QTc interval, uncompensated HF, or severe left ventricular hypertrophy.

Boxed Warning Patients with preexisting moderate to severe renal impairment (CrCl of 50 mL/minute or less) treated with telavancin for hospital-acquired bacterial pneumonia or ventilator-associated bacterial pneumonia have demonstrated higher mortality than those treated with vancomycin. Use drug in such patients only when anticipated benefit outweighs risk. ∎

Boxed Warning New-onset and worsening renal impairment has been reported. Monitor renal function. ∎

• Drug has been less effective in patients with moderate to severe preexisting renal impairment when used to treat skin and skin-structure infections. Consider alternative therapy.

• Older adults are more likely to have reduced renal function; use cautiously and base dosage on renal function.
• Safety and effectiveness in children haven't been established.
Dialyzable drug: 5.9%.

PREGNANCY-LACTATION-REPRODUCTION
Boxed Warning May cause fetal harm. Adverse outcomes have been observed in animal studies. ∎

Boxed Warning Verify pregnancy status before starting drug in patients of childbearing potential. Advise patients who are pregnant of fetal risk. Patients of childbearing potential should use effective contraception during treatment and for 2 days after final dose. ∎

• It isn't known if drug appears in human milk. Use cautiously during breastfeeding.
• Drug may impair male fertility.

NURSING CONSIDERATIONS
Boxed Warning Monitor renal function before and during therapy. ∎

⚠️ *Alert:* Rapid IV infusion may cause "red-man syndrome" (flushing of the upper body, urticaria, pruritus, or rash on the face, neck, trunk, or upper extremities). Infuse over at least 60 minutes.
• If diarrhea develops, evaluate patient for CDAD, which can be fatal and can occur more than 2 months after final dose.
• Watch for signs and symptoms of superinfection, such as continued fever, chills, and increased pulse rate.
• Obtain blood samples for PT, INR, PTT, activated clotting time, and coagulation-based factor X activity as close as possible to the next telavancin dose.
• Monitor patient for hypersensitivity reactions, including anaphylaxis, which may occur at any time during therapy. Stop drug at first sign of hypersensitivity reaction.
• *Look alike–sound alike:* Don't confuse telavancin with telithromycin.

PATIENT TEACHING
Boxed Warning Advise patients of childbearing potential to use an effective method of contraception during therapy and for 2 days after final dose. ∎

• Tell patient to report a history of kidney problems, heart problems (including QTc-interval prolongation), or diabetes before starting drug.

• Instruct patient to report all adverse reactions, especially diarrhea that develops during treatment or within 2 months of completing treatment.

---

telmisartan
tell-mah-SAR-tan

Micardis✣

Therapeutic class: Antihypertensives
Pharmacologic class: ARBs

AVAILABLE FORMS
Tablets: 20 mg, 40 mg, 80 mg

INDICATIONS & DOSAGES
Adjust-a-dose (for all indications): In patients with biliary obstructive disorders or hepatic insufficiency, initiate at low doses and up titrate slowly.
➤ **HTN**
Adults: 40 mg PO once daily. BP response is dose-related over a range of 20 to 80 mg once daily.
➤ **CV risk reduction in patients at high risk and unable to take ACE inhibitors**
Adults age 55 and older: 80 mg PO once daily.

ADMINISTRATION
PO
• Give drug without regard for food.
• Remove tablet from blister pack immediately before administration.
• Give missed dose as soon as possible. If it's close to the time for the next dose, omit the missed dose. Give the next dose at the regular time.

ACTION
Blocks vasoconstricting and aldosterone-secreting effects of angiotensin II by preventing angiotensin II from binding to the angiotensin I receptor.

Route	Onset	Peak	Duration
PO	3 hr	30–60 min	24 hr

Half-life: 24 hours.

ADVERSE REACTIONS
CNS: dizziness, pain, fatigue, headache. **CV:** chest pain, HTN, peripheral edema, intermittent claudication. **EENT:** pharyngitis, sinusitis.

GI: nausea, abdominal pain, diarrhea, dyspepsia. **GU:** UTI. **Musculoskeletal:** back pain, myalgia. **Respiratory:** cough, URI. **Skin:** ulceration. **Other:** flulike symptoms.

INTERACTIONS
Drug-drug. *ACE inhibitors:* May affect renal function and cause acute renal failure. Consider therapy modification.
Aliskiren: Increases risk of renal impairment, hypotension, and hyperkalemia. Use together is contraindicated in patients with diabetes. Avoid coadministration in patients with moderate to severe renal impairment (GFR less than 60 mL/minute).
COX-2 inhibitors, NSAIDs: May result in worsening renal function. May decrease antihypertensive effect. Monitor BP and renal function periodically.
Digoxin: May increase digoxin level. Monitor digoxin level closely.
Lithium: May cause reversible increase in lithium level and toxicity. Monitor lithium level, and adjust lithium dose as needed.
Ramipril, ramiprilat: May increase levels of these drugs and decrease telmisartan level. Avoid use together.
Drug-food. *Salt substitutes containing potassium:* May cause hyperkalemia. Discourage use together.

EFFECTS ON LAB TEST RESULTS
• May increase BUN, potassium, serum creatinine, and liver enzyme levels.
• May decrease Hb level.

CONTRAINDICATIONS & CAUTIONS
• Contraindicated in patients hypersensitive to drug or its components.
• Use cautiously in patients with hypotension, biliary obstruction disorders, or renal and hepatic insufficiency and in those with an activated RAAS, such as patients who are volume- or sodium-depleted (for example, those being treated with high doses of diuretics).
• Safety and effectiveness in children haven't been determined.
Dialyzable drug: No.
⚠ *Overdose S&S:* Hypotension, dizziness, tachycardia, bradycardia.

PREGNANCY-LACTATION-REPRODUCTION
Boxed Warning Use during pregnancy can cause injury and death to a developing

---

Reactions in bold italics are **life-threatening**. Interactions may have a *rapid onset* or a **delayed onset**.

fetus because drug acts directly on the RAAS. Stop drug as soon possible after detecting pregnancy. ∎

• It isn't known if drug appears in human milk. Patient shouldn't breastfeed during therapy.

NURSING CONSIDERATIONS

• Monitor patient for hypotension after starting drug. Place patient supine if hypotension occurs, and give IV NSS, if needed.

• If possible, correct volume and sodium depletion before first dose.

• Monitor potassium level periodically during therapy.

• Most of the antihypertensive effect occurs within 2 weeks. Maximal BP reduction is usually reached after 4 weeks. Diuretic may be added if BP isn't controlled by drug alone.

⏺ *Alert:* In patients whose renal function may depend on the activity of the RAAS (such as those with severe HF), drug may cause oliguria or progressive azotemia and (rarely) acute renal failure or death.

• Drug isn't removed by hemodialysis. Patients undergoing dialysis may develop orthostatic hypotension. Closely monitor BP.

• Monitor patients with impaired hepatic function or biliary obstruction carefully.

• Monitor patient for hypersensitivity reactions. Angioedema has been reported rarely. If signs or symptoms of angioedema (swelling of head and neck) occur, discontinue drug immediately.

• Rhabdomyolysis has been reported rarely. Monitor patient for myalgia, stiffness, and muscle weakness.

PATIENT TEACHING

• Instruct patient in safe drug administration.

• Inform patient of childbearing potential of the consequences of second- and third-trimester exposure to drug and to immediately report pregnancy.

• Advise patient not to breastfeed during therapy.

• Tell patient that if dizziness or low BP occurs on standing, to lie down, rise slowly from a lying to standing position, and climb stairs slowly.

• Tell patient to report all OTC drugs being taken before starting drug and to report all adverse reactions.

• Caution patient not to use salt substitutes containing potassium.

SAFETY ALERT!

temazepam
te-MAZ-e-pam

Restoril ✐

Therapeutic class: Hypnotics
Pharmacologic class: Benzodiazepines
Controlled substance schedule: IV

AVAILABLE FORMS
Capsules: 7.5 mg, 15 mg, 22.5 mg, 30 mg

INDICATIONS & DOSAGES
➤ **Short-term treatment (7 to 10 days) of insomnia**
Adults: 7.5 to 30 mg PO at bedtime.
Older adults or patients who are debilitated: Initially, 7.5 mg PO at bedtime until individualized response is determined.

ADMINISTRATION
PO
• Give drug without regard for food.

ACTION
Potentiates GABA neuronal inhibition in the CNS.

Route	Onset	Peak	Duration
PO	10–20 min	1.5 hr	Unknown

Half-life: Terminal, 3.5 to 18.4 hours.

ADVERSE REACTIONS
CNS: drowsiness, dizziness, hangover effect, lethargy, disturbed coordination, daytime sedation, confusion, nightmares, vertigo, euphoria, weakness, headache, fatigue, nervousness, anxiety, depression. **EENT:** blurred vision, dry mouth. **GI:** abdominal discomfort, diarrhea, nausea.

INTERACTIONS
Drug-drug. *Clozapine:* May cause delirium, sedation, sialorrhea, and ataxia. Don't start drugs simultaneously, and monitor patient carefully.
CNS depressants: May increase CNS depression. Use together cautiously.
Boxed Warning *Opioids:* May cause slow or difficult breathing, sedation, and death. Avoid use together. If use together is necessary, limit dosage and duration of each drug to minimum necessary for desired effect. ∎

Drug-herb. *Calendula, kava kava, lemon balm, passion flower, skullcap, valerian:* May enhance sedation. Don't use together.
Drug-lifestyle. *Alcohol use:* May cause additive CNS depressant effects. Discourage use together.

EFFECTS ON LAB TEST RESULTS
• May increase LFT values.

CONTRAINDICATIONS & CAUTIONS
• Contraindicated in patients hypersensitive to drug or other benzodiazepines.
Boxed Warning Opioids should only be prescribed with benzodiazepines or other CNS depressants to patients for whom alternative treatment options are inadequate. ■
Boxed Warning Benzodiazepine use exposes patient to risks of abuse, misuse, and addiction, which can lead to overdose or death. Assess patient's risk of abuse, misuse, and addiction before and periodically during therapy. ■
Boxed Warning Abrupt discontinuation or rapid dosage reduction of benzodiazepines after continued use may precipitate acute withdrawal reactions, which can be life-threatening. To reduce risk of withdrawal reactions, gradually taper drug to discontinue or reduce dosage. ■
• Use cautiously in patients with chronic pulmonary insufficiency, impaired hepatic or renal function, severe or latent depression, suicidality, and history of drug abuse.
• Use cautiously in patients who are debilitated, those age 65 and older, and others at increased risk for oversedation, dizziness, confusion, ataxia, and falls.
🛈 *Alert:* Drug may cause rare but serious injury, including death, due to complex sleep behaviors, such as sleepwalking, sleep driving, and engaging in other activities while not fully awake. These behaviors can occur even at the lowest recommended doses and after just one dose.
Dialyzable drug: Unknown.
⚠ *Overdose S&S:* Somnolence, impaired coordination, slurred speech, confusion, coma, decreased reflexes, hypotension, seizures, respiratory depression, apnea.

PREGNANCY-LACTATION-REPRODUCTION
• Contraindicated in patients who are or may become pregnant; may cause fetal harm. If used during pregnancy, or if patient becomes pregnant during therapy, apprise patient of fetal risk.
• It isn't known if drug appears in human milk. Use cautiously during breastfeeding; monitor infants for possible drowsiness, lethargy, or weight loss.

NURSING CONSIDERATIONS
🛈 *Alert:* Monitor patient closely. Anaphylaxis and angioedema may occur as early as the first dose (rare).
• Assess mental status before starting therapy and reduce dosages in older adults, who may be more sensitive to drug's adverse CNS effects.
• Take precautions to prevent drug hoarding by patients who are depressed, suicidal, or drug-dependent or who have a history of drug abuse.
• To discontinue drug, follow a gradual dosage-tapering schedule and monitor patient for withdrawal signs and symptoms (cramps, seizures, tremor, diaphoresis).
• *Look alike–sound alike:* Don't confuse Restoril with Risperdal or Vistaril. Don't confuse temazepam with flurazepam.

PATIENT TEACHING
🛈 *Alert:* Warn patient that drug may cause allergic reactions (rare), facial swelling (rare), and complex sleep-related behaviors, such as driving, eating, and making phone calls while asleep. Advise patient to report these adverse effects.
Boxed Warning Caution patient or caregiver of patient taking an opioid with a benzodiazepine, CNS depressant, or alcohol to seek immediate medical attention if patient experiences dizziness, light-headedness, extreme sleepiness, slowed or difficult breathing, or unresponsiveness. ■
Boxed Warning Caution patient that benzodiazepines, even at recommended doses, increase risk of abuse, misuse, and addiction, which can lead to overdose and death, especially when used in combination with other drugs (opioid analgesics), alcohol, or illicit substances. ■
• Tell patient to avoid alcohol.
• Teach patient proper handling and disposal of unused drug.
• Advise patient not to take drug at a higher dose, more frequently, or for longer than prescribed.

Boxed Warning Tell patient that continued use of drug for several days to weeks may lead to physical dependence and that abrupt discontinuation or rapid dosage reduction may precipitate acute withdrawal reactions, which can be life-threatening. Instruct patient that discontinuation or dosage reduction may require a slow taper. ■

• Advise patient about the possibility of developing protracted withdrawal syndrome (anxiety; trouble remembering, learning, or concentrating; depression; problems sleeping; feeling like insects are crawling under the skin; weakness; shaking; muscle twitching; burning or prickling feeling in the hands, arms, legs, or feet; ringing in the ears), with symptoms lasting weeks to more than 12 months.

• Caution patient that drug increases risk of falls and to avoid performing activities that require mental alertness or physical coordination.

🕭 *Alert:* Warn patient of risk of injury or death related to complex sleep behaviors. Direct patient to stop drug and immediately report an episode of complex sleep behavior or not remembering activities performed while taking drug.

• Instruct patient to stop drug before becoming pregnant.

• Tell patient to not take drug unless patient can stay in bed a full night (7 to 8 hours) before becoming active again.

SAFETY ALERT!

tenecteplase
teh-NEK-ti-plaze

TNKase

Therapeutic class: Thrombolytics
Pharmacologic class: Recombinant tissue plasminogen activators

AVAILABLE FORMS
Injection: 50 mg/vial

INDICATIONS & DOSAGES
➤ **To reduce risk of death from an acute MI**
Adults weighing 90 kg or more: 50 mg (10 mL) by IV bolus over 5 seconds.
Adults weighing 80 to less than 90 kg: 45 mg (9 mL) by IV bolus over 5 seconds.

Adults weighing 70 to less than 80 kg: 40 mg (8 mL) by IV bolus over 5 seconds.
Adults weighing 60 to less than 70 kg: 35 mg (7 mL) by IV bolus over 5 seconds.
Adults weighing less than 60 kg: 30 mg (6 mL) by IV bolus over 5 seconds. Maximum dose is 50 mg.

ADMINISTRATION
IV

▼ Give IV only. Don't give IM or subcut.

▼ Use syringe prefilled with 10 mL sterile water for injection (don't use bacteriostatic water for injection), and inject the entire contents into drug vial. Gently swirl solution once mixed. Don't shake. Visually inspect product for particulate matter before administration.

▼ Draw up the appropriate dose needed from the reconstituted vial with the syringe and discard any unused portion. Give drug immediately, or refrigerate at 36° to 46° F (2° to 8° C) and use within 8 hours.

▼ Give drug in a designated line. Flush dextrose-containing lines with NSS before administration.

▼ Give the drug rapidly over 5 seconds.

▼ Store vial in refrigerator at 36° to 46° F (2° to 8° C).

▼ **Incompatibilities:** Solutions containing dextrose, other IV drugs.

ACTION
Promotes fibrinolysis by binding to fibrin and converting plasminogen to plasmin.

Route	Onset	Peak	Duration
IV	Immediate	Immediate	Unknown

Half-life: 90 to 130 minutes.

ADVERSE REACTIONS
CNS: *stroke.* **CV:** *bleeding.* **EENT:** pharyngeal bleeding, epistaxis. **GI:** *GI bleeding.* **GU:** hematuria. **Skin:** hematoma. **Other:** bleeding at puncture site.

INTERACTIONS
Drug-drug. *Anticoagulants (direct thrombin inhibitors, heparin, vitamin K antagonists), drugs that alter platelet function (aspirin, dipyridamole, glycoprotein IIb/IIIa inhibitors [abciximab, eptifibatide, tirofiban], NSAIDs, P2Y12 inhibitors, SSRIs):* May increase risk of bleeding when used before, during, or after tenecteplase use. Use together cautiously.

Drug-herb. *Alfalfa, anise, bilberry:* May increase bleeding risk. Consider therapy modification.

EFFECTS ON LAB TEST RESULTS
- May increase INR.
- May prolong PT and PTT.

CONTRAINDICATIONS & CAUTIONS
- Contraindicated in patients with hypersensitivity to drug; active internal bleeding; history of stroke; ischemic stroke within 3 months; prior intracranial hemorrhage; suspected aortic dissection; intracranial or intraspinal surgery or trauma during previous 2 months; intracranial neoplasm, aneurysm, or arteriovenous malformation; severe uncontrolled HTN; bleeding diathesis; or significant closed head or facial trauma within 3 months.
- Use cautiously in patients who have had recent major surgery (such as CABG), organ biopsy, obstetric delivery, or previous puncture of noncompressible vessels.
- Use cautiously in patients age 75 and older and patients with recent trauma, recent GI or GU bleeding, high risk of left ventricular thrombus, acute pericarditis, systolic BP 180 mm Hg or higher or diastolic BP 110 mm Hg or higher, severe hepatic dysfunction, hemostatic defects, subacute bacterial endocarditis, septic thrombophlebitis, occluded AV cannula at seriously infected site, diabetic hemorrhagic retinopathy, or cerebrovascular disease.
- Safety and effectiveness in children haven't been established.

Dialyzable drug: Unknown.

PREGNANCY-LACTATION-REPRODUCTION
- There are no adequate studies during pregnancy. Use only if potential benefit justifies fetal risk.
- It isn't known if drug appears in human milk. Use cautiously during breastfeeding.

NURSING CONSIDERATIONS
- Begin therapy as soon as possible after onset of MI symptoms.
- Avoid noncompressible arterial punctures and internal jugular and subclavian venous punctures. Minimize all arterial and venous punctures during treatment.
- Avoid IM injections and nonessential patient handling for first few hours after treatment.
- Give heparin as prescribed but not in the same IV line.
- Monitor patient for bleeding. If serious bleeding occurs, stop heparin and antiplatelet drugs immediately.

Alert: Use exact patient weight for dosage. An overestimation in patient weight can lead to significant increase in bleeding or intracerebral hemorrhage.
- Monitor ECG for reperfusion arrhythmias.
- Life-threatening cholesterol embolism has been rarely reported in patients treated with thrombolytics. Signs and symptoms may include livedo reticularis (purple toe syndrome), acute renal failure, gangrenous digits, HTN, pancreatitis, MI, cerebral infarction, spinal cord infarction, retinal artery occlusion, bowel infarction, and rhabdomyolysis.
- ***Look alike–sound alike:*** Don't confuse tenecteplase with alteplase or reteplase. Don't confuse TNKase with Activase.

PATIENT TEACHING
- Tell patient to immediately report all adverse reactions, including bleeding.
- Explain use of drug to patient and family.

tenofovir alafenamide
te-NOE-fo-veer

Vemlidy

tenofovir disoproxil fumarate
Viread✐

Therapeutic class: Antiretrovirals
Pharmacologic class: NRTIs

AVAILABLE FORMS
tenofovir alafenamide
Tablets: 25 mg
tenofovir disoproxil fumarate
Oral powder: 40 mg. One level scoop delivers 1 g of powder containing tenofovir 40 mg
Tablets: 150 mg, 200 mg, 250 mg, 300 mg

INDICATIONS & DOSAGES
➤ **Chronic HBV infection (tenofovir alafenamide)**
Adults: 25 mg PO daily.
➤ **HIV-1 infection, with other antiretrovirals; chronic HBV infection (tenofovir disoproxil fumarate)**

Tablets

Adults and children age 2 and older weighing 35 kg or more: 300 mg PO once daily.

Adults and children age 2 and older weighing 17 to less than 35 kg and able to swallow intact tablet: 8 mg/kg PO once daily up to maximum of 300 mg. Refer to product insert for specific weight-based dosing.

Powder

Adults and children age 2 and older weighing at least 10 kg and unable to swallow tablet: 8 mg/kg PO once daily. Maximum dosage is 300 mg/day. See product insert for weight-based dosing.

Adjust-a-dose: For adults with CrCl of 30 to 49 mL/minute, 300 mg PO every 48 hours. For CrCl of 10 to 29 mL/minute, 300 mg PO every 72 to 96 hours. For patients receiving hemodialysis, 300 mg PO every 7 days or after a total of about 12 hours of hemodialysis. There are no recommendations for patients with CrCl of less than 10 mL/minute not receiving hemodialysis or for children with renal impairment.

ADMINISTRATION
PO

• Give tenofovir alafenamide with food. Give tenofovir disoproxil fumarate without regard to food.

• For patients receiving dialysis, give dose after session.

• Monitor weight periodically and adjust dosage accordingly.

• For patients receiving tenofovir powder, measure only with supplied dosing scoop. Mix with 2 to 4 oz of soft food not requiring chewing (such as applesauce, baby food, or yogurt). Patient should ingest entire mixture immediately to avoid bitter taste. Don't mix in a liquid because the powder may float on top of the liquid, even after stirring.

ACTION

Hydrolyzed to produce tenofovir, a nucleoside analogue of adenosine monophosphate that yields tenofovir diphosphate. Tenofovir diphosphate inhibits HIV replication by inhibiting viral RNA-dependent DNA polymerase. Tenofovir inhibits replication of HBV by inhibiting HBV polymerase.

Route	Onset	Peak	Duration
PO (alafen-amide)	Unknown	0.5 hr	Unknown
PO (disoproxil fumarate)	Unknown	36–144 min	Unknown

Half-life: Alafenamide, 0.5 hour; disoproxil fumarate, 17 hours.

ADVERSE REACTIONS
tenofovir alafenamide

CNS: headache, fatigue. **GI:** abdominal pain, nausea, diarrhea, dyspepsia, vomiting, flatulence. **GU:** glycosuria. **Hepatic:** increased transaminase levels. **Metabolic:** increased amylase, CK, LDL, and triglyceride levels. **Musculoskeletal:** back pain, arthralgia, decreased bone mineral density. **Respiratory:** cough. **Skin:** rash.

tenofovir disoproxil fumarate

CNS: asthenia, headache, pain, fever, peripheral neuropathy, insomnia, dizziness, depression, anxiety, fatigue. **CV:** chest pain. **EENT:** sinusitis, nasopharyngitis. **GI:** nausea, abdominal pain, dyspepsia, diarrhea, vomiting, anorexia, flatulence. **GU:** hematuria. **Hematologic:** *neutropenia.* **Hepatic:** increased ALP and transaminase levels. **Metabolic:** hyperglycemia; increased cholesterol, triglyceride, and CK levels; weight loss. **Musculoskeletal:** arthralgia, back pain, myalgia, decreased bone mineral density. **Respiratory:** URI, pneumonia. **Skin:** rash, pruritus, diaphoresis. **Other:** lipodystrophy.

INTERACTIONS

Drug-drug. *Adefovir:* May diminish therapeutic effect of tenofovir; may increase serum concentration of both drugs, resulting in additive nephrotoxicity. Avoid combination.

Atazanavir: May decrease atazanavir level, causing resistance. Give both drugs with ritonavir.

Atazanavir with ritonavir, darunavir with ritonavir, lopinavir–ritonavir: May increase tenofovir-associated adverse reactions. Monitor patient carefully.

Carbamazepine: May decrease tenofovir alafenamide level. Increase tenofovir alafenamide dosage to 50 mg once daily.

Drugs that reduce renal function or compete for renal tubular secretion (acyclovir, aminoglycosides, cidofovir, ganciclovir, NSAIDs, valacyclovir, valganciclovir): May increase levels of tenofovir or other renally eliminated drugs. Monitor patient for adverse effects.

Ledipasvir–sofosbuvir: May increase tenofovir exposure. When given with tenofovir without an HIV-1 protease inhibitor/ritonavir or an HIV-1 protease inhibitor/cobicistat combination, monitor patient for adverse reactions associated with tenofovir. When given with tenofovir and an HIV-1 protease inhibitor/ritonavir or an HIV-1 protease inhibitor/cobicistat combination, consider modifying therapy. If use together is necessary, monitor patient for tenofovir-associated adverse effects.

Oxcarbazepine, phenobarbital, phenytoin: May decrease tenofovir alafenamide level. Use together isn't recommended.

Rifabutin, rifampin, rifapentine: May decrease tenofovir alafenamide level. Use together isn't recommended.

Sofosbuvir–velpatasvir: May increase tenofovir exposure. Monitor patient for tenofovir-associated adverse effects.

Drug-herb. *St. John's wort:* May decrease tenofovir alafenamide level. Discourage use together.

Drug-food. *Fatty meals:* May increase tenofovir bioavailability. Monitor patient for adverse effects.

EFFECTS ON LAB TEST RESULTS
• May increase amylase, lipase, AST, ALT, ALP, CK, serum and urine glucose, creatinine, phosphate, cholesterol, and triglyceride levels.
• May decrease neutrophil count.

CONTRAINDICATIONS & CAUTIONS
• Contraindicated in patients hypersensitive to components of drug.
• Use very cautiously in patients with risk factors for liver disease or with hepatic impairment.
• Use cautiously in patients with renal impairment; avoid use with concurrent or recent nephrotoxic therapy.
• Immune reconstitution syndrome has been reported in patients with HIV-1 treated with combination antiretroviral therapy.
• Use cautiously in patients at higher risk for decreased renal function, including older adults and patients with recent or concurrent use of nephrotoxic drugs.
• Lactic acidosis and severe hepatomegaly with steatosis, including fatal cases, have been reported with the use of nucleoside analogues.

• Don't use tenofovir as monotherapy for the treatment of HIV-1 infection.
• Don't use tenofovir for the treatment of HIV-1 infection in combination with the fixed-dose combination products that also contain tenofovir, such as Complera, Descovy, Genvoya, or Truvada. Don't administer tenofovir with adefovir.

Dialyzable drug: Yes.

PREGNANCY-LACTATION-REPRODUCTION
• There are no adequate studies during pregnancy. Use only if clearly needed.
• Register patients exposed to drug during pregnancy in the Antiretroviral Pregnancy Registry (1-800-258-4263).
• The CDC recommends that patients with HIV-1 infection not breastfeed to avoid risking postnatal transmission of HIV-1.
• Tenofovir is present in human milk. Use cautiously during breastfeeding in patients with HBV infection.

NURSING CONSIDERATIONS
• Before starting drug, test patient for HBV infection and HIV-1 infection. Don't use tenofovir alone in patients with HIV-1 infection.
• **Alert:** Drug may cause lactic acidosis and hepatomegaly with steatosis, even fatal cases. These effects may occur without elevated transaminase levels. Risk factors include long-term antiretroviral use, obesity, and being female. Monitor all patients closely.
• Assess estimated CrCl and serum creatinine, urine glucose, and urine protein levels at baseline and during therapy as clinically appropriate in all patients. In patients with chronic kidney disease, also assess serum phosphorus level.

Boxed Warning Severe acute exacerbations of hepatitis have been reported in patients infected with HBV after anti-HBV therapy has stopped. Monitor hepatic function closely for at least several months. Resumption of therapy may be warranted. ∎
• Drug may be linked to osteomalacia and decreased bone mineral density, increased creatinine and BUN levels, and phosphaturia. Monitor patient carefully.
• Drug may lead to decreased HIV-RNA level and CD4+ cell counts.
• Monitor patient for immune reconstitution syndrome, an inflammatory response to indolent or residual opportunistic infections, which may require further evaluation and

---

Reactions in bold italics are *life-threatening*. Interactions may have a *rapid onset* or a *delayed onset*.

treatment. Autoimmune disorders have also been reported.

PATIENT TEACHING
- Instruct patient in safe drug administration.
- Inform patient that drug doesn't cure HIV infection, that opportunistic infections and other complications of HIV infection may still occur, and that transmission of HIV to others through sexual contact or blood contamination is still possible.
- Advise patient to obtain all ordered lab tests to assess safety of treatment regimen.
- Tell patient to report adverse effects, including nausea, vomiting, diarrhea, flatulence, and headache.
- Instruct patient to consult prescriber before taking OTC or other prescription medications or supplements, vitamins, or herbal supplements.
- Advise patient to discuss pregnancy and breastfeeding risks with prescriber.

terazosin hydrochloride
ter-AY-zoe-sin

Therapeutic class: Antihypertensives
Pharmacologic class: Alpha blockers

AVAILABLE FORMS
Capsules: 1 mg, 2 mg, 5 mg, 10 mg

INDICATIONS & DOSAGES
➤ HTN
Adults: Initially, 1 mg PO at bedtime. May increase dosage gradually based on response. Usual dosage range is 1 to 5 mg daily. Maximum recommended dosage is 20 mg daily. If response is substantially diminished at 24 hours, consider a dosage increase or use of a twice-daily regimen.
➤ Symptomatic BPH
Adults: Initially, 1 mg PO at bedtime. Dosage may be titrated stepwise to 2, 5, or 10 mg once daily to achieve optimal response. Most patients need 10 mg daily for optimal response. Maximum recommended dosage is 20 mg/day.

ADMINISTRATION
PO
- Give drug without regard for meals.
- Give twice-daily regimen doses 12 hours apart.

- If drug is discontinued for several days or longer, restart drug with the initial dosing regimen.

ACTION
Improves urine flow in patients with BPH by blocking alpha-adrenergic receptors in the bladder neck and prostate, relieving urethral pressure. Drug also reduces peripheral vascular resistance and BP via arterial and venous dilation.

Route	Onset	Peak	Duration
PO	15 min	1 hr	24 hr

Half-life: About 12 hours.

ADVERSE REACTIONS
CNS: anxiety, headache, dizziness, fever, insomnia, asthenia, syncope, nervousness, paresthesia, drowsiness, somnolence, vertigo. **CV:** chest pain, edema, palpitations, orthostatic hypotension, tachycardia, arrhythmia, vasodilation. **EENT:** conjunctivitis, blurred vision, tinnitus, nasal congestion, epistaxis, sinusitis, pharyngitis, rhinitis, dry mouth. **GI:** nausea, abdominal pain, constipation, dyspepsia, flatulence, vomiting. **GU:** erectile dysfunction, urinary frequency, urinary incontinence, UTI. **Metabolic:** gout. **Musculoskeletal:** arthralgia, arthritis, back pain, joint disorder, limb pain, myalgia. **Respiratory:** dyspnea, cough, bronchitis. **Skin:** pruritus, rash, diaphoresis. **Other:** flulike syndrome, cold symptoms.

INTERACTIONS
Drug-drug. *Antihypertensives, antipsychotics, calcium channel blockers, PDE5 inhibitors (tadalafil, vardenafil):* May increase hypotensive effect. Use together cautiously.
Drug-herb. *Yohimbe:* May diminish antihypertensive effect of drug. Monitor therapy.

EFFECTS ON LAB TEST RESULTS
- May decrease total protein, albumin, total cholesterol, and combined LDL and VLDL levels.
- May decrease Hb level, hematocrit, and WBC and platelet counts.

CONTRAINDICATIONS & CAUTIONS
- Contraindicated in patients hypersensitive to drug.
- May cause marked lowering of BP, especially orthostatic hypotension, and syncope

T

in association with first dose or first few days of therapy. A similar effect can be expected if therapy is interrupted for several days then restarted, dosage is rapidly increased, or when another antihypertensive is introduced. Always initiate treatment with a 1-mg dose at bedtime.

• Intraoperative floppy iris syndrome has been observed during cataract and glaucoma surgery in some patients who are taking or had previously taken alpha$_1$ blockers, which may increase risk of eye complications during and after surgery. Don't initiate drug in patients scheduled for cataract or glaucoma surgery.

• May cause CNS depression and impair mental alertness.

• Rare cases of priapism have been reported.

Dialyzable drug: 10%.

⚠ *Overdose S&S:* Hypotension.

PREGNANCY-LACTATION-REPRODUCTION

• Safety use during pregnancy hasn't been established. Use only if potential benefit justifies fetal risk.

• It isn't known if drug appears in human milk. Use cautiously during breastfeeding.

NURSING CONSIDERATIONS

• Monitor BP frequently. Evaluate patient for signs and symptoms of hypotension, such as dizziness or palpitations.

• Symptoms of BPH and prostate cancer are similar. Rule out prostate cancer before starting therapy.

PATIENT TEACHING

• Tell patient not to stop drug suddenly but to notify prescriber if adverse reactions occur.

• Inform patient about the rare but serious possibility of priapism and to report it immediately.

• Warn patient to avoid hazardous activities that require mental alertness, such as driving or operating heavy machinery, for 12 hours after first dose.

• Tell patient that light-headedness from hypotension can occur. Advise patient to rise slowly and to report signs and symptoms to prescriber.

• Advise patient considering cataract or glaucoma surgery to inform ophthalmologist about taking terazosin.

terbinafine hydrochloride (oral)
ter-BIN-ah-feen

Therapeutic class: Antifungals
Pharmacologic class: Synthetic allylamine derivatives

AVAILABLE FORMS
Tablets: 250 mg

INDICATIONS & DOSAGES
➤ **Fingernail and toenail onychomycosis caused by dermatophytes (tinea unguium)**
Adults: 250 mg PO once daily for 6 weeks for fingernail infection and 12 weeks for toenail infection.

ADMINISTRATION
PO
• Confirm diagnosis with nail specimen testing (potassium hydroxide preparation, fungal culture, or nail biopsy).

• Give tablets without regard for food.

• Give missed dose as soon as possible unless it's less than 4 hours before the next scheduled dose.

• Store tablets at room temperature; protect from light.

ACTION
Prevents biosynthesis of ergosterol, causing a deficiency of this essential component of fungal cell membranes.

Route	Onset	Peak	Duration
PO	Unknown	≤2 hr	Unknown

Half-life: Adults, 36 hours; children, 27 to 31 hours.

ADVERSE REACTIONS
CNS: headache, taste disturbances. **EENT:** vision disturbances. **GI:** diarrhea, dyspepsia, nausea, abdominal pain, flatulence. **Hematologic:** *neutropenia.* **Hepatic:** liver enzyme elevations. **Skin:** rash, pruritus, urticaria.

INTERACTIONS
Drug-drug. *Caffeine:* May decrease caffeine clearance. Use cautiously together.
Cimetidine: May decrease clearance of terbinafine. Avoid using together.
Codeine: May decrease serum concentration of codeine's active metabolite. Monitor therapy.

Reactions in bold italics are *life-threatening*. Interactions may have a *rapid onset* or a **delayed onset**.

Cyclosporine: May decrease cyclosporine level. Monitor cyclosporine level.

CYP2C9, CYP3A4 enzyme inhibitors (amiodarone, fluconazole): May substantially increase systemic exposure of terbinafine. Use together cautiously.

CYP2D6 substrates (class 1C antiarrhythmics [flecainide], beta blockers, MAO inhibitors Type B, SSRIs [paroxetine, venlafaxine], TCAs): May inhibit substrate metabolism. Dosage adjustment may be needed. Monitor therapy.

Rifampin: Significantly increases terbinafine clearance. Avoid use together.

Tamoxifen: May decrease serum concentration of tamoxifen's active metabolite. Consider alternative to terbinafine.

Tramadol: May decrease serum concentration of tramadol's active metabolite. Monitor patient closely.

Warfarin: May alter anticoagulation effect. Monitor PT.

Drug-lifestyle. *Sunlight, UV light:* May increase risk of photosensitivity reactions. Patient should minimize exposure.

EFFECTS ON LAB TEST RESULTS
• May increase AST and ALT levels.
• May decrease platelet, neutrophil, and lymphocyte counts.

CONTRAINDICATIONS & CAUTIONS
• Contraindicated in patients hypersensitive to drug or its components.
• *Alert:* Contraindicated in patients with chronic or active liver disease.
• Cases of liver failure, some leading to liver transplant or death, have occurred in patients with and without preexisting liver disease.
• Disturbances of taste and smell have been reported and may last up to 1 year or become permanent.
• Depressive signs and symptoms have occurred during postmarketing use.
• Serious skin reactions (SJS, TEN, and others) and hypersensitivity reactions have occurred. If these occur, discontinue drug.
• Thrombotic microangiopathy (TMA), including thrombotic thrombocytopenic purpura and hemolytic-uremic syndrome, can occur and fatalities have been reported.
• There have been postmarketing reports of new and worsened cases of cutaneous lupus erythematosus and SLE. Discontinue drug in patients with signs and symptoms suggestive of SLE.
• Safety and effectiveness in children haven't been established.
• Use cautiously in older adults.
Dialyzable drug: Unknown.
⚠ Overdose S&S: Abdominal pain, dizziness, frequent urination, headache, nausea, rash, vomiting.

PREGNANCY-LACTATION-REPRODUCTION
• There are no adequate studies during pregnancy. Because treatment can be postponed until after pregnancy, it's recommended that terbinafine not be initiated during pregnancy.
• Drug appears in human milk. Use during breastfeeding isn't recommended.

NURSING CONSIDERATIONS
• Obtain liver function test results before treatment to screen for chronic or active liver disease.
• Monitor LFT values periodically during treatment. Stop drug if evidence of liver injury develops.
• Monitor CBC in patients taking drug for longer than 6 weeks, especially those with known or suspected immunodeficiency or signs or symptoms of secondary infection. Stop drug for neutrophil count of 1,000 cells/mm³ or less.
• Monitor and evaluate patients who develop unexplained thrombocytopenia and anemia for TMA. Discontinue drug if clinical signs and symptoms and lab findings consistent with TMA occur.
• Monitor patient for depression or changes in taste or smell. Discontinue drug if taste or smell disturbance occurs.
• *Look alike–sound alike:* Don't confuse terbinafine with terbutaline.

PATIENT TEACHING
• Inform patient that successful treatment may take 12 weeks for toenail infections and 6 weeks for fingernail infections.
• Instruct patient in proper drug administration.
• Tell patient to immediately report depression; smell, taste, or vision disturbances (changes in the ocular lens and retina may occur); and signs or symptoms of liver injury (persistent nausea, anorexia, fatigue, vomiting, right upper quadrant pain, jaundice, dark urine, or pale stools).

T

- Advise patient to minimize exposure to sunlight with sunscreen and protective clothing and to avoid UV light (tanning beds, UVA/B treatment).

---

terconazole
ter-CONE-uh-zole

Therapeutic class: Antifungals
Pharmacologic class: Triazole derivatives

AVAILABLE FORMS
Vaginal cream: 0.4%*, 0.8%*
Vaginal suppositories: 80 mg

INDICATIONS & DOSAGES
➤ **Vulvovaginal candidiasis**
Adults: One applicatorful of cream or 1 suppository inserted into vagina at bedtime; 0.4% cream used for 7 consecutive days; 0.8% cream or 80-mg suppository for 3 consecutive days. Repeat course, if needed, after reconfirmation of diagnosis by smear or culture.

ADMINISTRATION
Vaginal
- Insert drug high in vagina (except during pregnancy) at bedtime.
- Use applicator supplied by the manufacturer.
- Wash applicator after each use and allow it to dry thoroughly.
- Store drug at room temperature.

ACTION
May increase *Candida* cell membrane permeability.

Route	Onset	Peak	Duration
Vaginal	Unknown	5–10 hr	Unknown

Half-life: 6.4 to 8.5 hours.

ADVERSE REACTIONS
CNS: headache, fever, pain. **GI:** abdominal pain. **GU:** dysmenorrhea, vulvovaginal discomfort (burning, irritation, itching). **Other:** chills.

INTERACTIONS
None significant.

EFFECTS ON LAB TEST RESULTS
None reported.

CONTRAINDICATIONS & CAUTIONS
- Contraindicated in patients hypersensitive to drug or its inactive ingredients.
- Safety and effectiveness in children haven't been determined.
Dialyzable drug: Unknown.

PREGNANCY-LACTATION-REPRODUCTION
- Because drug is absorbed from the vagina, it shouldn't be used in the first trimester unless prescriber considers it essential to patient's welfare.
- May use during second and third trimesters if potential benefit outweighs fetal risk.
- It isn't known if drug appears in human milk. Patient should discontinue breastfeeding or discontinue drug.

NURSING CONSIDERATIONS
- Menstruation or hormonal contraceptives don't impact drug's therapeutic effect.
- Assess patient's ability to self-administer. Self-administration may be difficult in patients with arthritis or limited range of motion.
- *Look alike–sound alike:* Don't confuse terconazole with tioconazole.

PATIENT TEACHING
- Instruct patient in safe drug administration.
- Advise patient to continue treatment during menstrual period. However, advise not to use tampons.
- Instruct patient on self-administration of drug; remind patient to insert drug high in vagina (except during pregnancy).
- Tell patient to use drug for full treatment period prescribed. Explain how to prevent reinfection.
- Instruct patient to notify prescriber and stop drug if fever, chills, other flulike signs and symptoms, irritation, or sensitivity develops.
- Caution patient to refrain from sexual intercourse during treatment.
- Tell patient that the suppository formulation may react with latex or rubber, weakening condoms and diaphragms. Use of condoms or diaphragms during treatment isn't recommended.
- Advise patient that male partner also may need treatment if symptomatic.
- Inform patient of pregnancy and breastfeeding risks.

Reactions in bold italics are *life-threatening*. Interactions may have a *rapid onset* or a *delayed onset*.

teriparatide (rDNA origin)
tehr-ih-PAHR-uh-tide

Forteo

Therapeutic class: Antiosteoporotics
Pharmacologic class: Recombinant human parathyroid hormones

AVAILABLE FORMS
Injection: 20 mcg/dose in multidose prefilled pen

INDICATIONS & DOSAGES
➤ **Osteoporosis in patients who are post-menopausal and at high risk for fracture; primary or hypogonadal osteoporosis in men at high risk for fracture; glucocorticoid-induced osteoporosis in men and women**
Adults: 20 mcg subcut once daily for up to 2 years. May consider treatment beyond 2 years for patients who remain at or have returned to having a high risk for fracture.

ADMINISTRATION
Subcutaneous
• Give drug without regard to meals or time of day.
• Keep refrigerated; minimize time out of refrigerator during use. Don't freeze.
• After each use, safely remove the needle, recap the delivery device, and put it back in the refrigerator right away.
• Inspect solution before giving.
• Drug is a colorless, clear liquid. Don't use if solid particles are present or if solution appears cloudy or colored.
• Give while patient is sitting or lying down to avoid orthostatic hypotension.
• Give in the thigh or abdomen. Rotate administration sites.
• Discard pen after 28-day use, even if some unused solution remains.

ACTION
Promotes new bone formation, skeletal bone mass, and bone strength by regulating calcium and phosphorus metabolism in bones and kidneys.

Route	Onset	Peak	Duration
Subcut	Rapid	30 min	3 hr

Half-life: 1 hour.

ADVERSE REACTIONS
CNS: asthenia, depression, dizziness, headache, insomnia, pain, syncope, vertigo, anxiety. **CV:** angina pectoris, HTN, orthostatic hypotension. **EENT:** pharyngitis, rhinitis, tooth disorder. **GI:** constipation, diarrhea, dyspepsia, gastritis, GI disorder, nausea, vomiting. **Metabolic:** hypercalcemia, hyperuricemia. **Musculoskeletal:** arthralgia, leg cramps, neck pain. **Respiratory:** dyspnea, increased cough, pneumonia. **Skin:** rash, diaphoresis. **Other:** herpes zoster.

INTERACTIONS
Drug-drug. *Digoxin:* May predispose patient who is hypercalcemic to digitalis toxicity. Use together cautiously.

EFFECTS ON LAB TEST RESULTS
• May increase calcium (transient) and uric acid levels.
• May increase urinary calcium and phosphorus excretion.
• May decrease phosphorus level.

CONTRAINDICATIONS & CAUTIONS
• Contraindicated in patients hypersensitive to drug or its components.
• Drug increases risk of osteosarcoma. Avoid use in patients at increased risk for osteosarcoma, such as those with Paget disease or unexplained ALP elevations, children and young adults with open epiphyses, hereditary disorders predisposing to osteosarcoma, bone metastases or a history of skeletal malignancies, and patients who have had skeletal radiation.
• Drug hasn't been studied in patients with preexisting hypercalcemia; drug may cause hypercalcemia or exacerbate hypercalcemia. Avoid use in patients with underlying hypercalcemic disorder (primary hyperparathyroidism).
• Calciphylaxis and worsening of previously stable cutaneous calcification have been reported with use of drug. Risk factors for calciphylaxis include underlying autoimmune disease, kidney failure, and concomitant warfarin or systemic corticosteroid use. Discontinue drug in patients who develop new or worsening cutaneous calcification.
• Use cautiously in patients with active or recent urolithiasis; hepatic, renal, or cardiac disease; or hypotension.
Dialyzable drug: Unknown.

T.

⚠ *Overdose S&S:* Hypercalcemia, orthostatic hypotension, nausea, vomiting, dizziness, headache.

PREGNANCY-LACTATION-REPRODUCTION
• There are no adequate studies during pregnancy. Consider discontinuing drug in confirmed pregnancy. Use only if potential benefit justifies fetal risk.
• It isn't known if drug appears in human milk. Patient should discontinue breastfeeding or discontinue drug.

NURSING CONSIDERATIONS
• If patient may have urolithiasis or hypercalciuria, measure urinary calcium excretion before treatment.
• Monitor patient for orthostatic hypotension.
• Monitor calcium level. If persistent hypercalcemia develops, stop drug and evaluate possible cause.
• Monitor dietary intake. Patient may need supplemental calcium and vitamin D for inadequate dietary intake.
• *Look alike–sound alike:* Don't confuse Forteo with Forfivo XL.

PATIENT TEACHING
• Instruct patient on proper use and disposal of prefilled pen.
• Tell patient not to share pen with others.
• Teach patient to discard pen after 28-day use period, even if unused solution remains.
• Advise patient to remain in a sitting position while taking drug to prevent orthostatic hypotension.
• Caution patient to sit or lie down if drug causes a fast heartbeat, light-headedness, or dizziness. Tell patient to report persistent or worsening symptoms.
• Urge patient to report persistent symptoms of hypercalcemia, which include nausea, vomiting, constipation, lethargy, and muscle weakness.
• Encourage adequate calcium and vitamin D intake in the diet or by supplementation.

testosterone
tes-TOS-te-rone

Natesto, Testopel

testosterone cypionate
Depo-Testosterone

testosterone enanthate
Xyosted

testosterone undecanoate
Aveed, Jatenzo, Kyzatrex, Tlando

Therapeutic class: Androgens
Pharmacologic class: Androgens
Controlled substance schedule: III

AVAILABLE FORMS
testosterone
Nasal gel (metered): 5.5 mg/actuation
Pellets (subcut implant): 12.5 mg, 25 mg, 37.5 mg, 50 mg, 75 mg, 100 mg, 200 mg
testosterone cypionate
Injection (in oil): 100 mg/mL*, 200 mg/mL*
testosterone enanthate
Autoinjector: 50 mg/0.5 mL, 75 mg/0.5 mL, 100 mg/0.5 mL
Injection (in oil): 200 mg/mL
testosterone undecanoate
Capsules: 100 mg, 112.5 mg, 150 mg, 158 mg, 198 mg, 200 mg, 237 mg
Injection (in oil): 250 mg/mL

INDICATIONS & DOSAGES
➤ **Hypogonadism**
Men: 50 to 400 mg cypionate or enanthate in oil IM every 2 to 4 weeks. Or, 75 mg enanthate autoinjector subcut in abdominal region once a week. Or, initially, 750 mg undecanoate in oil IM and 4 weeks later; then 750 mg IM every 10 weeks thereafter. Or, initially, 200 or 237 mg undecanoate capsules PO b.i.d. Or, 150 to 450 mg (2 to 6 pellets) implanted subcut every 3 to 6 months. Or, 11 mg (2 pump actuations; 1 actuation per nostril) intranasally t.i.d., once in the morning, once in the afternoon, and once in the evening (6 to 8 hours apart), preferably at same time each day for a total daily dose of 33 mg.
Adjust-a-dose: When total testosterone concentration consistently exceeds 1,050 ng/dL, discontinue nasal spray therapy. If total

---

Reactions in bold italics are *life-threatening*. Interactions may have a *rapid onset* or a *delayed onset*.

testosterone concentration is consistently below 300 ng/dL, consider alternative treatment. Adjust dosage as indicated in product inserts and periodic measurement of serum testosterone concentration.

➤ **Delayed puberty**
Men and boys: 50 to 200 mg enanthate IM every 2 to 4 weeks for 4 to 6 months. Or, 150 to 450 mg pellets implanted subcut every 3 to 6 months for a limited duration, such as 4 to 6 months.

➤ **Metastatic breast cancer**
Patients 1 to 5 years after menopause: 200 to 400 mg enanthate IM every 2 to 4 weeks.

ADMINISTRATION
⟁ *Alert:* Hazardous drug; use safe handling and disposal precautions.
PO
• Give with food.
IM
• Store IM preparations at room temperature. If crystals appear, warm and shake bottle to disperse them.
• Inject deep into upper outer quadrant of gluteal muscle. Rotate injection sites; report soreness at site.
Subcutaneous
• In most men, the pellets are implanted in an area on the anterior abdominal wall.
• Number of pellets implanted depends on the required dose.
• Enanthate autoinjector isn't for IM or IV administration.
• Don't use autoinjector if liquid is cloudy, if visible particles are present, or if the seal is broken.
• Don't use autoinjector within 2 inches of the navel; where skin is tender, bruised, red, scaly, or hard; and in areas with scars, tattoos, or stretch marks.
Intranasal
• Prime pump before first use by inverting then depressing pump 10 times (discard this portion of product into sink).
• Have patient blow nose before application.
• To administer, insert actuator into nostril until pump reaches base of nose; tilt so tip is in contact with lateral wall of nostril. Depress slowly until pump stops, then remove from nose while wiping tip to transfer gel to lateral side of nostril.
• After administration, press on nostrils just below bridge of nose and lightly massage.

• Make sure patient refrains from blowing nose or sniffing for 1 hour after administration.
• If gel gets on hands, wash with warm soap and water.

ACTION
Stimulates target tissues to develop normally in androgen-deficient men. May have some antiestrogen properties, making it useful in treating certain estrogen-dependent breast cancers.

Route	Onset	Peak	Duration
PO	Unknown	2–4 hr	Unknown
IM	Unknown	4–42 days	2–10 wk
Subcut (implant)	Unknown	Unknown	3–6 mo
Subcut (enanthate)	Unknown	6–168 hr	Unknown
Intranasal	Unknown	40 min	Unknown

Half-life: 10 to 100 minutes; cypionate, about 8 days.

ADVERSE REACTIONS
Refer to manufacturer's prescribing information for each product for additional adverse reactions not listed here.
CNS: headache, anxiety, depression, paresthesia, sleep apnea, mood swings, aggressive behavior, irritability, bitter taste. **CV:** edema, HTN. **EENT:** nasal discomfort, nasopharyngitis, rhinorrhea, epistaxis, rhinomia, nasal dryness or congestion, nasal scabbing, gum or mouth irritation; gum pain, tenderness, or edema. **GI:** nausea, diarrhea. **GU:** amenorrhea, oligospermia, decreased ejaculatory disorder, increased or decreased libido, priapism, prostatitis, increased PSA level. **Hematologic:** polycythemia, *suppression of clotting factors.* **Hepatic:** altered LFT values, reversible jaundice, *cholestatic hepatitis.* **Metabolic:** hypernatremia, *hyperkalemia,* hypercalcemia, hyperphosphatemia, hypercholesterolemia, weight gain. **Musculoskeletal:** back pain, arthralgia. **Respiratory:** cough, URI. **Skin:** pain, implantation- or injection-site reaction, induration at injection site, local edema, acne, hyperhidrosis, hirsutism, male pattern baldness. **Other:** androgenic effects in women, gynecomastia, hypersensitivity reactions, hypoestrogenic effects in women, excessive hormonal effects in men.

T

INTERACTIONS

Drug-drug. *Corticosteroids:* May increase risk of edema. Use together cautiously, especially in patients with cardiac, hepatic, or renal disease.

Cyclosporine: Androgens may enhance hepatotoxic effects. Consider therapy modification.

Drugs that increase BP (NSAIDs, pseudoephedrine): May increase risk of HTN. Monitor therapy.

Hepatotoxic drugs: May increase risk of hepatotoxicity. Monitor liver function closely.

Insulin, oral antidiabetics: May decrease glucose level; may alter dosage requirements. Monitor glucose level in patients with diabetes.

Oral anticoagulants (warfarin): May increase sensitivity; may alter dosage requirements. Monitor PT and INR; decrease anticoagulant dose if necessary.

Drug-food. *Licorice:* May decrease testosterone level. Avoid use.

EFFECTS ON LAB TEST RESULTS

• May increase LFT values and sodium, potassium, phosphate, cholesterol, calcium, creatinine, CK, and serum PSA levels.
• May increase resin uptake of T_3 and T_4.
• May increase Hb level, hematocrit, and RBC count.
• May decrease thyroxine-binding globulin, total T_4, and 17-ketosteroid levels.
• May decrease leukocyte count.
• May cause abnormal glucose tolerance test results.

CONTRAINDICATIONS & CAUTIONS

• Contraindicated in patients hypersensitive to drug or its components and in those with hypercalcemia or cardiac, hepatic, or renal decompensation.
• Contraindicated in men with breast cancer or known or suspected prostate cancer.
• Venous thromboembolic events (VTEs), including DVT and PE, have been reported in patients using testosterone products.

Boxed Warning Serious pulmonary oil microembolism reactions, involving urge to cough, dyspnea, throat tightening, chest pain, dizziness, and episodes of anaphylaxis, including life-threatening reactions, have been reported to occur during or immediately after administration of testosterone undecanoate injection. These reactions can occur after any injection during therapy, including after first dose. Observe patients for 30 minutes after each dose. Drug is available only through the Aveed REMS program. ■

Boxed Warning Oral and subcutaneous testosterone products can increase BP, increasing the risk of major adverse CV events, including nonfatal MI, nonfatal stroke, and CV death. Before initiating drug, consider evaluating patient's baseline CV risk and ensure adequate BP control. ■

🕒 *Alert:* Drug has potential for abuse, usually at doses higher than those prescribed and usually in conjunction with other anabolic androgenic steroids (AASs). Abuse is associated with serious safety risks, such as MI, HF, stroke, depression, hostility, aggression, liver toxicity, and male infertility. Withdrawal signs and symptoms (depression, fatigue, irritability, loss of appetite, decreased libido, and insomnia) can occur in patients abusing high testosterone doses.

🕒 *Alert:* Contraindicated in men with age-related low testosterone signs and symptoms only. Testosterone replacement therapy is only approved for men with primary or secondary hypogonadism resulting from certain medical conditions and with low testosterone levels confirmed by lab testing.

• Prolonged use of high doses of androgens has been associated with peliosis hepatis and hepatic neoplasms, including hepatocellular carcinoma.
• Use cautiously in older adults.
• Intranasal form isn't recommended for use with nasally administered drugs other than sympathomimetic decongestants or for use in patients with mucosal inflammatory disorders, sinus disease or history of nasal disorders, nasal or sinus surgery, nasal fracture within previous 6 months, or nasal fracture that caused a deviated anterior nasal septum.
• Use cautiously in patients with sleep apnea or those with risk factors for sleep apnea (obesity, chronic lung disease).

Dialyzable drug: Unknown.

⚠ *Overdose S&S:* Stroke (with enanthate injection).

PREGNANCY-LACTATION-REPRODUCTION

• Drug is teratogenic and may cause fetal harm. Use is contraindicated during pregnancy. If pregnancy occurs during therapy, apprise patient of potential hazard to the fetus.

Reactions in bold italics are *life-threatening*. Interactions may have a *rapid onset* or a *delayed onset*.

- Contraindicated during breastfeeding because of potential for virilization in infants who are breastfed.
- Large doses may suppress spermatogenesis and cause irreversible infertility in males.

NURSING CONSIDERATIONS

- Verify pregnancy status before treatment.
- Cypionate, enanthate, and undecanoate are long-acting solutions.

⚠ Alert: If testosterone abuse is suspected, check serum testosterone concentrations to ensure they are within therapeutic range. Consider possibility of testosterone and AAS abuse in patients who present with serious CV or psychiatric adverse events.

Boxed Warning Starting about 6 weeks after initiating subcut therapy or 3 weeks after initiating PO therapy, periodically monitor patient for and treat new-onset or worsening HTN and reevaluate whether benefits of drug outweigh its risks in patients who develop CV risk factors or CV disease during treatment. Use subcut and PO testosterone only for the treatment of men with hypogonadal conditions associated with structural or genetic conditions. ∎

- If patient experiences severe rhinitis, temporarily discontinue intranasal therapy until signs and symptoms resolve. If signs and symptoms persist, an alternative testosterone replacement therapy is recommended.
- Monitor patient's liver function, and check PSA, cholesterol, and HDL levels periodically.
- Check Hb and hematocrit levels periodically.

⚠ Alert: Confirm low testosterone levels on at least two mornings before initiating therapy. Avoid measuring testosterone level later in the day when levels can be low, even in patients who don't have hypogonadism.

- Monitor testosterone levels after initial dosage titration, and periodically as described in prescribing information for each product. Adjust dosage if needed.
- Evaluate patients who report pain, edema, or warmth and erythema in lower extremity for DVT; evaluate those who present with acute shortness of breath for PE. For suspected VTE, discontinue drug and initiate appropriate workup and management.
- In patients with metastatic breast cancer, hypercalcemia usually indicates progression

of bone metastases. Report signs and symptoms of hypercalcemia.

- Report evidence of virilization in women. Androgenic effects include acne, edema, weight gain, increased hair growth, hoarseness, clitoral enlargement, decreased breast size, changes in libido, male pattern baldness, and oily skin or hair.
- Watch for hypoestrogenic effects in women (flushing; diaphoresis; vaginitis, including itching, drying, and burning; vaginal bleeding; menstrual irregularities).
- Watch for excessive hormonal effects in men and boys. In a boy during prepuberty, watch for premature epiphyseal closure, acne, priapism, growth of body and facial hair, and phallic enlargement. In men after puberty, watch for testicular atrophy, oligospermia, decreased ejaculatory volume, impotence, gynecomastia, and epididymitis.
- Drug may increase risk of depression and suicidality. Evaluate patients with new-onset or worsening depression, anxiety, mood changes, or suicidality.
- Monitor patient's weight and BP routinely.
- Monitor prepubertal boys by X-ray for rate of bone maturation.
- Using testosterone esters to treat males with hypogonadism may potentiate sleep apnea. Monitor patients with risk factors such as obesity or chronic lung diseases.

⚠ Alert: Therapeutic response in breast cancer is usually apparent within 3 months. If disease progresses, stop drug.

- Androgens may alter results of lab studies during therapy and for 2 to 3 weeks after therapy ends.

⚠ Alert: Testosterone salts aren't interchangeable.

- **Look alike–sound alike:** Don't confuse testosterone with testolactone.

PATIENT TEACHING

- Make sure patient understands importance of using an effective contraceptive during therapy.
- Show patient how to safely administer drug.
- Instruct patient to report suspected pregnancy and to stop drug immediately.

⚠ Alert: Warn patient to seek immediate medical attention for signs and symptoms of heart attack (chest pain, shortness of breath, trouble breathing) or stroke (weakness in one part or side of the body, slurred speech).

• Advise patient and caregiver to seek medical attention for manifestations of new-onset or worsening depression, suicidality, anxiety, or other mood changes.

• Review signs and symptoms of virilization. Instruct patient to notify prescriber if they occur.

• Advise patient to wear cotton underwear and to wash after intercourse to decrease risk of vaginitis.

• Instruct male patient to report priapism, reduced ejaculatory volume, or gynecomastia.

• Warn patient with diabetes to be alert for hypoglycemia and to notify prescriber if it occurs.

• Instruct boys using testosterone for delayed puberty to have X-rays of hand and wrist obtained every 6 months during treatment.

• Tell patient to report sudden weight gain.

• Warn patient that drug shouldn't be used to enhance athletic performance.

---

testosterone transdermal
tes-TOS-te-rone

Androderm, AndroGel, Fortesta, Testim, Vogelxo

Therapeutic class: Androgens
Pharmacologic class: Androgens

AVAILABLE FORMS
1% gel*: 25 mg, 50 mg per unit dose; 12.5 mg per pump actuation
1.62% gel*: 20.25 mg, 40.5 mg per unit dose; 20.25 mg per pump actuation
2% gel: 10 mg per pump actuation
Transdermal solution*: 30 mg per metered-dose pump
Transdermal system: 2 mg/day, 4 mg/day

INDICATIONS & DOSAGES
➤ **Primary or hypogonadotropic hypogonadism**
Men: One Androderm 4 mg/day system (don't use two 2-mg/day patches) applied to back, abdomen, upper arm, or thigh nightly. After 2 weeks, may increase dosage to 6 mg once daily or may decrease to 2 mg once daily, depending on morning serum testosterone levels.

Or, initially, 50 mg of AndroGel 1% (two 25-mg packets or one 50-mg packet) applied every morning to shoulders, upper arms, or

abdomen. Check testosterone level after about 2 weeks. If response is inadequate, may increase AndroGel to 75 mg daily. Then, adjust to 100 mg if needed.

Or, 50 mg of Testim (1 tube) applied once daily in the morning to shoulders and upper arms. Don't apply to genitals or abdomen. May increase dosage to a maximum 100 mg/day, if needed, based on testosterone levels.

Or, initially, 40.5 mg (2 pumps or one 40.5-mg packet)) of AndroGel 1.62% applied once daily in the morning to upper arms or shoulders. May adjust dosage between a minimum of 20.25 mg (1 pump or one 20.25-mg packet) and a maximum of 81 mg (4 pumps or two 40.5-mg packets) titrated based on the predose morning serum testosterone concentration at about 14 days and 28 days after starting treatment or the last dosage adjustment.

Or, initially 40 mg (4 pumps) of Fortesta once daily to the thighs in the morning. May adjust dosage between 10 mg and maximum of 70 mg based on testosterone concentration drawn 2 hours after application approximately 14 days and 35 days after start of treatment and the last dosage adjustment.

Or, initially 60 mg (2 pumps) of solution, one actuation to each axilla, once daily. May adjust dosage between 30 mg (1 actuation) and a maximum of 120 mg (4 actuations) based on serum testosterone concentration drawn 2 to 8 hours after application and at least 14 days after starting treatment or the last dosage adjustment. For doses of more than 60 mg daily, alternate axillae, allowing them to dry completely before applying next actuation.

Or, 50 mg of Vogelxo once daily to shoulders or upper arms. If serum testosterone concentration falls below normal range, increase dose to a maximum of 100 mg of testosterone.

ADMINISTRATION
⚠ *Alert:* Hazardous drug; use safe handling and disposal precautions according to facility policy.
Transdermal
• Wear gloves when handling patches. Fold used patches with adhesive sides together to discard.
• Apply patch immediately after opening the pouch and removing the protective liner.
• Apply patch nightly to clean, dry, intact skin of the back, abdomen, upper arms, or

---

thighs only. Press firmly in place to ensure good contact. Rotate sites; don't reuse a site for 7 days.

• Don't apply to bony areas or parts of the body subject to prolonged pressure while sleeping or sitting; don't apply to oily, damaged, or irritated skin.

• Reapply patch if it falls off. If patch can't be reapplied and has been worn at least 12 hours, apply a new patch at the next scheduled application time.

• Patient should avoid swimming, showering, or washing the administration site for at least 3 hours after application.

Topical

• AndroGel 1.62% and AndroGel 1% and topical solution aren't interchangeable.

• Fully prime the pumps according to manufacturer's instructions. Discard this portion of the product.

• Wear gloves to apply gel to clean, dry, intact skin as directed for each product. Don't apply to the genitals or bony prominences.

• Application in the morning is preferable. Allow application sites to dry before dressing. Cover the application sites with clothing.

• Patient should avoid swimming or washing the administration site for 2 to 5 hours after application, depending on product.

• Gel contains alcohol and is flammable. Patient should avoid fire, flames, or smoking until gel has dried.

• Apply topical solution, using the applicator provided, to clean, dry, intact skin of the axilla as directed. Don't use the fingers or hand to rub the solution into the skin.

• Patient should apply deodorant or antiperspirant (stick or roll-on) at least 2 minutes before applying the solution.

ACTION

Releases testosterone, which stimulates target tissues to develop normally in androgen-deficient men.

Route	Onset	Peak	Duration
Transdermal, topical	Unknown	4–24 hr	24 hr–10 days

Half-life: 10 to 100 minutes.

ADVERSE REACTIONS

CNS: abnormal dreams, asthenia, depression, headache, sleep apnea, smell disorder, aggressive behavior, mood swings, fatigue, insomnia, irritability, nervousness, taste disorder. **CV:** HTN, edema. **GI:** *GI bleeding,* diarrhea, increased appetite, vomiting. **GU:** prostatitis, prostate abnormalities, UTI, ejaculation disorder, erectile dysfunction, polyuria, decreased libido, pelvic pain, urinary incontinence, increased PSA level. **Hematologic:** polycythemia. **Hepatic:** reversible jaundice. **Metabolic:** hypernatremia, *hypokalemia,* hypercalcemia, hyperphosphatemia, hypercholesterolemia, weight gain. **Skin:** alopecia; application-site pruritus, blister, erythema, vesicles, burning, induration; acne irritation; allergic contact dermatitis; hyperhidrosis. **Other:** gynecomastia, breast tenderness, flulike syndrome, hot flash.

INTERACTIONS

Drug-drug. *Corticosteroids:* May increase risk of edema. Use together cautiously, especially in patients with renal, cardiac, or hepatic disease.

Cyclosporine: Androgens may enhance hepatotoxic effect. Consider therapy modification.

Hepatotoxic drugs: May increase risk of hepatotoxicity. Monitor liver function closely.

Insulin, oral antidiabetics: May enhance hypoglycemic effect and alter dosage requirements of listed drugs. Monitor glucose level in patients with diabetes.

Oral anticoagulants (warfarin): May alter anticoagulant dosage requirements. Monitor PT and INR.

EFFECTS ON LAB TEST RESULTS

• May increase PSA, sodium, phosphate, cholesterol, liver enzyme, calcium, creatinine, and TSH levels.

• May decrease glucose, potassium, HDL, and total T_4 levels.

• May increase Hb level, hematocrit, and RBC count.

• May increase resin uptake of T_3 and T_4.

CONTRAINDICATIONS & CAUTIONS

• Contraindicated in patients hypersensitive to drug, in women, and in men with known or suspected breast or prostate cancer.

🜚 *Alert:* Contraindicated in men with age-related low testosterone symptoms only. Testosterone replacement therapy is only approved for men with primary or secondary hypogonadism resulting from certain medical conditions and with low testosterone levels confirmed by lab testing.

• Use cautiously in patients with cancer at risk for hypercalcemia (and associated hypercalciuria).

🜄 *Alert:* Drug has potential for abuse, usually at doses higher than those prescribed and usually in conjunction with other anabolic androgenic steroids (AASs). Abuse is associated with serious safety risks, such as MI, HF, stroke, depression, hostility, aggression, liver toxicity, and male infertility. Withdrawal signs and symptoms (depression, fatigue, irritability, loss of appetite, decreased libido, and insomnia) can occur in patients abusing high testosterone doses.

🜄 *Alert:* Drug may increase risk of heart attack and stroke.

• Venous thromboembolic events (VTEs), including DVT and PE, have been reported in patients using testosterone products.

• Prolonged use of high doses of androgens has been associated with development of peliosis hepatis and hepatic neoplasms, including hepatocellular carcinoma.

• Use cautiously in older adults.

Dialyzable drug: Unknown.

PREGNANCY-LACTATION-REPRODUCTION

• Drug isn't indicated for use in women. Apprise patients who are pregnant of risk of virilization of a female fetus with transfer of testosterone from men undergoing treatment.

• Drug is teratogenic; may cause fetal harm.

• Contraindicated in patients who are breastfeeding because of potential for virilization in the infant.

NURSING CONSIDERATIONS

Boxed Warning Virilization in children can occur after secondary exposure to transdermal application sites on men. Children should avoid contact with unwashed or unclothed application sites. ■

• Monitor serum calcium concentrations in patients with cancer at risk for hypercalcemia (and associated hypercalciuria).

🜄 *Alert:* For suspected testosterone abuse, check serum testosterone concentrations to ensure they fall within therapeutic range. Consider testosterone and anabolic androgenic steroid abuse in patients who present with serious CV or psychiatric adverse events.

• Treatment of men who are hypogonadal with testosterone esters may increase risk of

sleep apnea. Monitor patients with risk factors, such as obesity or chronic lung diseases.

• Periodically assess LFT results, lipid profiles, Hb level, hematocrit (with long-term use), and levels of prostatic acid phosphatase and PSA.

🜄 *Alert:* Confirm low testosterone levels on at least two mornings before initiating therapy. Avoid measuring testosterone level later in the day when levels can be low, even in men who don't have hypogonadism. Refer to manufacturer's instructions for product-specific recommendations.

• Watch for excessive hormonal effects.

• Evaluate patients who report pain, edema, or warmth and erythema in lower extremity for DVT; evaluate those who present with acute shortness of breath for PE. If VTE is suspected, discontinue treatment and initiate appropriate workup and management.

• Remove topical patch before an MRI because patch contains aluminum.

PATIENT TEACHING

• Teach patient how to prime pumps and to self-administer drug according to individual manufacturer's instructions.

Boxed Warning Instruct patient to strictly adhere to recommended instructions for use to avoid secondary exposure in children. ■

Boxed Warning Tell patient to wash hands thoroughly after using product and to cover treated area with clothing. ■

• Instruct patient to thoroughly wash application site with soap and water if anticipating direct skin-to-skin contact.

• Warn patient with diabetes that drug may decrease glucose level and to be alert for hypoglycemia.

🜄 *Alert:* Warn patient to seek immediate medical attention for signs and symptoms of heart attack (chest pain, shortness of breath, trouble breathing) or stroke (weakness in one part or side of the body, slurred speech).

• Advise patient to report persistent erections, nausea, vomiting, changes in skin color, ankle swelling, or sudden weight gain to prescriber.

• Tell patient that Androderm doesn't have to be removed during sexual intercourse or while showering.

• Caution patient undergoing an MRI to alert the facility about using a transdermal patch.

Reactions in bold italics are *life-threatening*. Interactions may have a *rapid onset* or a ***delayed onset***.

tetracycline hydrochloride
tet-ra-SYE-kleen

Therapeutic class: Antibiotics
Pharmacologic class: Tetracyclines

AVAILABLE FORMS
Capsules: 250 mg, 500 mg

INDICATIONS & DOSAGES
Adjust-a-dose (for all indications): Decrease recommended dosages or extend dosing intervals in patients with renal impairment.
➤ **Infections caused by susceptible organisms, such as *Haemophilus ducreyi, Yersinia pestis, Campylobacter fetus, Rickettsiae* species, *Mycoplasma pneumoniae, Chlamydia psittaci, Chlamydia trachomatis, Entamoeba* species, *Actinomyces* species, *Bacillus anthracis, Vibrio cholerae, Listeria monocytogenes, Fusobacterium fusiforme, Haemophilus influenzae, Treponema* species, *Francisella tularensis, Clostridioides* species, *Escherichia coli, Enterobacter aerogenes, Shigella* species, *Klebsiella* species, *Borrelia* species, *Streptococcus pneumoniae, Streptococcus pyogenes, and Staphylococcus aureus***
Adults: 1 to 2 g/day PO in two or four divided doses depending on the severity of infection.
Children older than age 8: 25 to 50 mg/kg PO daily, in divided doses every 6 hours.
➤ **Uncomplicated urethral, endocervical, or rectal infections caused by *C. trachomatis***
Adults: 500 mg PO q.i.d. for at least 7 days.
➤ **Brucellosis**
Adults: 500 mg PO q.i.d. for 3 weeks in combination with streptomycin.
➤ **Uncomplicated gonorrhea in patients allergic to penicillin**
Adults: 500 mg PO q.i.d. for 7 days.
➤ **Syphilis in patients allergic to penicillin**
Adults and adolescents: 500 mg PO q.i.d. for 15 days. If infection has lasted 1 year or longer, treat for 30 days.
➤ **Acne (moderate to severe; long-term therapy) as adjunct to topical therapy**
Adults and adolescents: Initially, 1 g PO daily in divided doses. For maintenance, 125 to 500 mg daily. (Alternate-day or intermittent therapy may be adequate in some patients.)

ADMINISTRATION
PO
• Obtain specimen for culture and sensitivity tests before giving first dose. Begin therapy while awaiting results.
• For streptococcal infections, continue therapy for 10 days.
• Milk or other dairy products, antacids, or iron products interfere with drug absorption, reducing its effectiveness. For best drug absorption, give drug with a full glass of water on an empty stomach, at least 1 hour before or 2 hours after meals.
• Give drug with adequate amount of fluid at least 1 hour before bedtime to prevent esophageal irritation or ulceration.
• Store at room temperature. Protect from light.
🕔 *Alert:* Be careful not to administer outdated drug because of the highly increased risk of nephrotoxicity and Fanconi syndrome.

ACTION
May exert bacteriostatic effect by binding to the 30S and possibly 50S ribosomal subunits of microorganisms, thus inhibiting protein synthesis. May also alter the cytoplasmic membrane of susceptible microorganisms.

Route	Onset	Peak	Duration
PO	Unknown	2–4 hr	Unknown

Half-life: 6 to 11 hours.

ADVERSE REACTIONS
CNS: headache. **EENT:** black, hairy tongue; glossitis; oral candidiasis; sore throat. **GI:** diarrhea, epigastric distress, nausea, anorexia, dysphagia, enterocolitis, esophagitis, esophageal ulceration, vomiting. **GU:** inflammatory lesions in anogenital region (candida overgrowth). **Hematologic:** hemolytic anemia, *neutropenia, thrombocytopenia,* eosinophilia. **Hepatic:** hepatotoxicity. **Musculoskeletal:** bone growth retardation in children younger than age 8. **Skin:** increased pigmentation, maculopapular and erythematous rash, photosensitivity reactions, urticaria. **Other:** enamel defects, hypersensitivity reactions, permanent discoloration of teeth.

INTERACTIONS
Drug-drug. *Antacids, laxatives, and multivitamins containing aluminum, magnesium, or calcium; antidiarrheals containing bismuth subsalicylate:* May decrease antibiotic

absorption. Give antibiotic 1 hour before or 2 hours after these drugs.

Ferrous sulfate and other iron products, sodium bicarbonate, zinc: May decrease antibiotic absorption. Give tetracycline 2 hours before or 3 hours after these products.

Hormonal contraceptives: May decrease contraceptive effectiveness and increase risk of breakthrough bleeding. Advise patient to use nonhormonal contraceptive.

Isotretinoin: May increase risk of pseudotumor cerebri. Avoid use together.

⊕ Alert: *Methoxyflurane:* May cause fatal nephrotoxicity. Avoid using together.

Oral anticoagulants: May increase anticoagulant effects. Monitor PT and INR, and adjust anticoagulant dosage.

Penicillins: May interfere with bactericidal action of penicillins. Avoid use together.

Drug-food. *Dairy products:* May decrease antibiotic absorption. Give antibiotic 1 hour before or 2 hours after eating or drinking dairy products.

Drug-lifestyle. *Sun exposure:* May cause photosensitivity reactions. Advise patient to avoid excessive sunlight exposure.

EFFECTS ON LAB TEST RESULTS
• May increase BUN and liver enzyme levels.
• May increase eosinophil count.
• May decrease RBC, platelet, and neutrophil counts.

CONTRAINDICATIONS & CAUTIONS
• Contraindicated in patients hypersensitive to drug or other tetracyclines.
• Some tetracyclines may contain sulfites and are contraindicated in patients with sulfite hypersensitivity.
• CDAD, ranging in severity from mild diarrhea to fatal colitis, has been reported with use of nearly all antibacterial drugs, including tetracyclines.
• Use cautiously in patients with renal or hepatic impairment. Avoid using or use cautiously in children younger than age 8 because drug may cause permanent discoloration of teeth, enamel defects, and bone growth retardation.

Dialyzable drug: No.

⚠ Overdose S&S: Dizziness, nausea, vomiting.

PREGNANCY-LACTATION-REPRODUCTION
• Don't use during pregnancy unless absolutely necessary. May have toxic effects on the developing fetus (often related to retardation of skeletal development and discoloration of teeth). If used during pregnancy or if patient becomes pregnant during therapy, apprise patient of fetal risk.
• Patients who are pregnant and have renal disease may be more prone to developing tetracycline-associated liver failure.
• Drug appears in human milk. Patient should discontinue breastfeeding or discontinue drug.

NURSING CONSIDERATIONS
• For suspected or confirmed CDAD, discontinue ongoing use of antibacterial drugs not directed at *Clostridioides difficile.* Institute appropriate fluid and electrolyte management, protein supplementation, and antibacterial treatment of *C. difficile.*
• If large doses are given, therapy is prolonged, or patient is at high risk, monitor patient for signs and symptoms of superinfection.
• Pseudotumor cerebri (benign intracranial HTN) in adults has been associated with tetracycline use. Monitor patient for clinical manifestations, including headache, blurred vision, diplopia, and vision loss; papilledema can be found on funduscopy.
• In patients with renal or hepatic impairment, monitor renal function tests and LFT values.
• Assess tongue for signs of candidal infection. Emphasize good oral hygiene.
• For suspected coexistent syphilis, perform dark field exam before therapy and monitor blood serology monthly for at least 4 months.
• Drug isn't indicated for treatment of neurosyphilis.
• Photosensitivity reactions may occur within a few minutes to several hours after sun or UV light exposure. Photosensitivity lasts after therapy ends. Discontinue drug at first sign of skin erythema.

PATIENT TEACHING
• Instruct patient in safe drug administration.
• Tell patient to take drug exactly as prescribed, even after feeling better, and to take entire amount prescribed.
• Instruct patient to check drug's expiration date and not to use if outdated.
• Advise patient to promptly report all adverse reactions and to immediately report headache, blurred vision, diplopia, vision loss, watery diarrhea, abdominal cramping and pain, fever, or blood or pus in the stool.

Reactions in bold italics are *life-threatening*. Interactions may have a *rapid onset* or a **delayed onset**.

- Warn patient that use of tetracyclines with oral contraceptives may make contraceptives less effective.
- Warn patient to avoid direct sunlight and ultraviolet light and to use sun protection.

SAFETY ALERT!

thiotepa (TESPA, triethyl-enethiophosphoramide, TSPA) ▨
thye-oh-TEP-a

Tepadina

Therapeutic class: Antineoplastics
Pharmacologic class: Alkylating drugs

AVAILABLE FORMS
Injection: 15 mg, 100 mg per vial

INDICATIONS & DOSAGES
➤ **Breast or ovarian adenocarcinoma**
Adults: 0.3 to 0.4 mg/kg IV every 1 to 4 weeks. Adjust maintenance dose weekly based on blood counts; don't give more often than weekly.
➤ **Superficial papillary bladder carcinoma**
Adults: 60 mg in 30 to 60 mL of NSS instilled in bladder and retained for 2 hours once weekly for 4 weeks. May repeat course as necessary with caution; bone-marrow depression may be increased with second and third courses.
➤ **Neoplastic effusions**
Adults: 0.6 to 0.8 mg/kg intracavitarily every 1 to 4 weeks. Adjust maintenance dose weekly based on blood counts; don't give more often than weekly.
➤ **To reduce risk of graft rejection when used in conjunction with high-dose busulfan and cyclophosphamide as a preparative regimen for allogeneic hematopoietic progenitor (stem) cell transplantation (HSCT) for children with class 3 beta-thalassemia** ▨
Children older than age 1 month: Two doses of 5 mg/kg IV approximately 12 hours apart on the 6th day before allogeneic HSCT (in combination with high-dose busulfan and cyclophosphamide).

ADMINISTRATION
⏺ *Alert:* Hazardous drug; use safe-handling and disposal precautions.

- Reconstitute with 1.5 mL of sterile water for injection in 15-mg vial to yield 10 mg/mL or with 10 mL of sterile water for injection in 100-mg vial to yield 10 mg/mL. Don't reconstitute with other solutions. Mix manually by repeated inversions.
- Reconstituted solution remains stable for 8 hours when refrigerated.
IV
▼ Further dilute reconstituted solution in 500 mL NSS if dose is 250 to 500 mg, or in 1,000 mL if dose is greater than 500 mg. If dose is less than 250 mg, dilute with NSS to a final concentration of 0.5 to 1 mg/mL.
▼ After dilution, solution remains stable for 24 hours when refrigerated or for 4 hours at room temperature. Microbiologically, the product should be used immediately.
▼ If solution appears grossly opaque or has a precipitate, discard it. Make sure solution appears clear to slightly opaque.
▼ Infuse via a central venous catheter over 3 hours using an infusion set equipped with a 0.2-micron in-line filter. Before and after infusion, flush catheter with approximately 5 mL NSS.
▼ If pain occurs at insertion site, dilute drug further or use a local anesthetic to reduce pain. Make sure drug doesn't infiltrate.
▼ Refrigerate and protect dry powder from direct sunlight to avoid possible drug breakdown. Don't freeze.
▼ **Incompatibilities:** None listed by manufacturer. Consult a drug incompatibility reference for more information.
Intravesical
- Recommended dose is 60 mg in 30 to 60 mL of NSS instilled into bladder by catheter; ask patient to retain solution for 2 hours. If discomfort is too great with 60 mL, reduce volume to 30 mL. Reposition patient every 15 minutes for maximum area contact.
Intracavitary
- For intracavitary instillation, drug may be given through the same tubing used to remove the fluid from the cavity involved.

ACTION
Cross-links strands of cellular DNA and interferes with RNA transcription, causing an imbalance of growth that leads to cell death. Not specific to cell cycle.

Route	Onset	Peak	Duration
IV	Unknown	Unknown	Unknown

Half-life: Adults, 1.4 to 3.7 hours; active metabolite, 4.9 to 17.6 hours. Children, 1.7 hours; active metabolite, 4 hours.

ADVERSE REACTIONS

CNS: headache, dizziness, fatigue, weakness, fever. **EENT:** blurred vision, conjunctivitis. **GI:** diarrhea, nausea, vomiting, abdominal pain, anorexia, mucositis, stomatitis, *hemorrhage*. **GU:** amenorrhea, hematuria, decreased spermatogenesis, dysuria, urine retention, cystitis, hemorrhagic cystitis (with intravesical administration). **Hematologic:** *leukopenia, thrombocytopenia, neutropenia,* anemia. **Hepatic:** elevated liver enzyme levels, hyperbilirubinemia. **Respiratory:** *laryngeal edema, asthma,* wheezing, pneumonia. **Skin:** dermatitis, alopecia, skin depigmentation, injection-site pain, urticaria, rash. **Other:** GVHD, infection, CMV infection, hypersensitivity reactions, including *anaphylaxis*.

INTERACTIONS

Drug-drug. *Anticoagulants, aspirin, NSAIDs:* May increase risk of bleeding. Avoid using together.
Live-virus or attenuated virus vaccines: May increase risk of infection or decrease effect of vaccine. Use together is contraindicated until resolution of immunosuppressive effects.
Myelosuppressive agents: May increase myelosuppression. Monitor patient.
Neuromuscular blockers: May prolong muscular paralysis. Monitor patient.
Other alkylating drugs, irradiation therapy: May intensify toxicity rather than enhance therapeutic response. Avoid using together.
Strong CYP3A4 inducers (phenytoin, rifampin): May increase serum concentrations of active metabolite(s) of thiotepa. Avoid using together; if use together is unavoidable, monitor patient for adverse effects.
Strong CYP3A4 inhibitors (clarithromycin, itraconazole, ritonavir): May decrease serum concentrations of active metabolite(s) of thiotepa. Avoid using together; if use together is unavoidable, monitor patient for adverse effects and decreased efficacy.
Drug-herb. *Echinacea:* May decrease therapeutic effect of drug. Avoid using together.

EFFECTS ON LAB TEST RESULTS

• May increase AST, ALT, and bilirubin levels.
• May decrease Hb level and lymphocyte, platelet, WBC, RBC, and neutrophil counts.

CONTRAINDICATIONS & CAUTIONS

• Contraindicated in patients hypersensitive to drug.
• Generally contraindicated in patients with existing hepatic or renal dysfunction or bone marrow suppression or damage. However, if need outweighs risk in such patients, may use drug cautiously in low dosage, and accompanied by hepatic, renal, and hematopoietic function tests.

Boxed Warning May cause severe bone marrow suppression, and high doses may cause marrow ablation with resulting infection or bleeding. Monitor hematologic lab parameters. HSCT is required to prevent potentially fatal complications of the prolonged myelosuppression after high doses of drug. ∎

Boxed Warning Drug may be carcinogenic in humans. ∎

• Myelodysplastic syndromes and acute non-lymphocytic leukemia have been reported in patients treated with thiotepa.
• Death has occurred after intravesical administration, caused by bone marrow depression from systemically absorbed drug, and from septicemia and hemorrhage as a direct result of hematopoietic depression.
• Fatal encephalopathy has occurred with high doses of drug. Don't exceed recommended dosage.
Dialyzable drug: Yes.
⚠ *Overdose S&S:* Hematopoietic toxicity, bleeding.

PREGNANCY-LACTATION-REPRODUCTION

• Drug can cause fetal harm when used during pregnancy. If used during pregnancy, or if pregnancy occurs during therapy, apprise patient and patient's partner of fetal risk.
• Verify pregnancy status before starting drug.
• Patients of childbearing potential should use highly effective contraception during treatment and for at least 6 months after therapy ends. Males with partners of childbearing potential should use effective contraception during treatment and for at least 1 year after therapy ends.

Reactions in bold italics are *life-threatening*. Interactions may have a *rapid onset* or a *delayed onset*.

- It isn't known if drug appears in human milk. Patient should discontinue breastfeeding or discontinue drug.
- May interfere with spermatogenesis.

NURSING CONSIDERATIONS

- Monitor CBC weekly for at least 3 weeks after last dose.
- Drug is excreted through the skin of patients receiving high-dose therapy and may cause skin discoloration and reactions. Skin discoloration, pruritus, blistering, desquamation, and peeling may be more severe in the groin, axillae, skinfolds, and neck area, and under dressings.
- Patients should shower or bathe with water at least twice daily for 48 hours after administration. Change occlusive dressing and clean the covered skin at least twice daily for 48 hours after administration. Change bed linens daily during treatment.
- Hepatic veno-occlusive disease may occur in patients who have received high-dose therapy in conjunction with busulfan and cyclophosphamide. Monitor patient by physical exam and by observing serum transaminase and bilirubin levels daily through bone marrow transplant day +28.
- If WBC count drops below 3,000/mm³ or if platelet count falls below 150,000/mm³, stop drug and notify prescriber.
- Therapeutic effects are commonly accompanied by toxicity.
- Give blood transfusions for cumulative anemia.
- Doses of 300 mg/m² or greater are associated with high emetic potential in children. Antiemetics are recommended to prevent nausea and vomiting.
- Monitor patient for CNS toxicity (headache, apathy, psychomotor retardation, disorientation, confusion, amnesia, hallucinations, drowsiness, somnolence, seizures, coma, inappropriate behaviors, forgetfulness). Discontinue drug for severe or life-threatening CNS toxicity.
- Monitor patient for secondary malignancies.
- *Look alike–sound alike:* Don't confuse thiotepa with thioguanine.

PATIENT TEACHING

- Instruct patient to shower or bathe with water, change the occlusive dressing, and clean the covered skin at least twice daily through 48 hours after the drug has been administered to prevent skin toxicities.

- Instruct patient to change bed sheets daily during therapy.
- Advise patient to watch for signs and symptoms of infection (fever, sore throat, fatigue) and bleeding (easy bruising, nosebleeds, bleeding gums, melena). Tell patient to take temperature daily and to report even mild infections.
- Tell patient to immediately report signs and symptoms of CNS toxicity.
- Instruct patient to avoid OTC products containing aspirin or NSAIDs.
- Advise patient to stop breastfeeding during therapy because of risk of toxicity to infant.
- Advise patient of childbearing potential to use highly effective contraception during treatment and for at least 6 months after therapy ends. Advise male patient with partner of childbearing potential to use effective contraception during treatment and for at least 1 year after therapy ends.

tiaGABine hydrochloride
tye-AG-ah-been

Gabitril

Therapeutic class: Anticonvulsants
Pharmacologic class: GABA enhancers

AVAILABLE FORMS
Tablets: 2 mg, 4 mg, 12 mg, 16 mg

INDICATIONS & DOSAGES
➤ **Adjunctive treatment of partial seizures**
Adults taking enzyme-inducing anticonvulsants: Initially, 4 mg PO once daily. Total daily dose may be increased by 4 to 8 mg at weekly intervals until clinical response or up to 56 mg daily. Give total daily dose in two to four divided doses.
Children ages 12 to 18 taking enzyme-inducing anticonvulsants: Initially, 4 mg PO once daily. Total daily dose may be increased by 4 mg at beginning of week 2 and thereafter by 4 to 8 mg per week until clinical response or up to 32 mg daily. Give total daily dose in two to four divided doses.
Adjust-a-dose: Consider dosage adjustment when there is an addition, discontinuation, or dosage change in the enzyme-inducing drug (carbamazepine, phenytoin, primidone, phenobarbital).
  For patients with hepatic impairment, reduce first and maintenance doses or increase

T

dosing intervals. For patients who are non-induced (taking only non-enzyme-inducing anticonvulsants), reduce dosage and, if necessary, titrate slowly.

ADMINISTRATION
PO
• Give drug with food.
• If a dose is missed, don't attempt to make up for the missed dose by increasing the next dose. If more than one dose has been missed, drug may need to be retitrated.

ACTION
Unknown. May act by facilitating the effects of the inhibitory neurotransmitter GABA. By binding to recognition sites linked to GABA uptake carrier, drug may make more GABA available.

Route	Onset	Peak	Duration
PO	Rapid	45 min (fasting)	Unknown

Half-life: 2 to 5 hours when given with enzyme inducers; 7 to 9 hours when given without enzyme inducers.

ADVERSE REACTIONS
CNS: asthenia, dizziness, nervousness, somnolence, abnormal gait, agitation, ataxia, confusion, depression, difficulty with concentration and attention, difficulty with memory, emotional lability, hostility, insomnia, language problems, paresthesia, speech disorder, tremor, pain, malaise, syncope, paranoia, migraine, hallucination. **CV:** vasodilation, chest pain, HTN, palpitations, tachycardia, edema, lymphadenopathy. **EENT:** amblyopia, nystagmus, abnormal vision, ear pain, otitis media, tinnitus, epistaxis, mouth ulceration, pharyngitis. **GI:** nausea, abdominal pain, diarrhea, increased appetite, vomiting, gingivitis, stomatitis. **GU:** UTI, dysmenorrhea, dysuria, metrorrhagia, urinary incontinence, vaginitis. **Metabolic:** weight gain or loss. **Musculoskeletal:** generalized weakness, myasthenia, neck pain, arthralgia, myalgia, hyperkinesia, hypokinesia. **Respiratory:** increased cough, bronchitis, dyspnea, pneumonia. **Skin:** pruritus, rash, ecchymosis, alopecia, dry skin, diaphoresis. **Other:** accidental injury, flulike syndrome, infection, allergic reaction, chills.

INTERACTIONS
Drug-drug. *Carbamazepine, phenobarbital, phenytoin, other CYP3A4 inducers:* May increase tiagabine clearance. Monitor patient closely.
CNS depressants (benzodiazepines, muscle relaxants, opioids, SSRIs): May enhance CNS effects. Avoid use together if possible.
CYP3A4 inhibitors (including conivaptan): May decrease tiagabine metabolism. Monitor therapy.
Drug-herb. *Kava kava:* May enhance adverse CNS effects of tiagabine. Monitor patient closely.
St. John's wort: May enhance tiagabine metabolism. Monitor patient closely.
Drug-lifestyle. *Alcohol use:* May enhance CNS effects. Use together cautiously and monitor therapy.

EFFECTS ON LAB TEST RESULTS
None reported.

CONTRAINDICATIONS & CAUTIONS
• Contraindicated in patients hypersensitive to drug or its components.
⚠ Alert: Drug may cause new-onset seizures and status epilepticus in patients without a history of epilepsy. In these patients, stop drug and evaluate for underlying seizure disorder. Drug shouldn't be used for off-label uses.
• Use cautiously in patients with psychiatric symptoms and hepatic impairment.
• Safety and effectiveness haven't been established for any indication other than as adjunctive therapy for partial seizures in adults and children age 12 and older.
Dialyzable drug: Unlikely.
⚠ Overdose S&S: Somnolence, impaired consciousness, agitation, confusion, speech difficulty, hostility, depression, weakness, seizures.

PREGNANCY-LACTATION-REPRODUCTION
• Drug may cause fetal harm, but there are no adequate studies during pregnancy. Use only if clearly needed.
• Patients taking drug during pregnancy should enroll in the North American AED (Antiepileptic Drug) Pregnancy Registry (1-888-233-2334 or www.aedpregnancyregistry.org).
• It isn't known if drug or its metabolites appear in human milk. Use during breastfeeding only if benefit clearly outweighs risks.

NURSING CONSIDERATIONS
⚠ Alert: Closely monitor all patients taking or starting antiepileptic drugs for changes in

---

behavior indicating worsening of suicidality or depression. Symptoms such as anxiety, agitation, hostility, mania, and hypomania may be precursors to emerging suicidality.

• Withdraw drug gradually unless safety concerns require a more rapid withdrawal because sudden withdrawal may cause more frequent seizures.

🟡 *Alert:* Use of anticonvulsants, including tiagabine, may cause status epilepticus and sudden unexpected death in patients with and without epilepsy.

• Monitor patient for cognitive and neuropsychiatric symptoms, including impaired concentration, speech or language problems, confusion, somnolence, and fatigue.

• Drug may cause moderately severe to incapacitating generalized weakness, which resolves after dosage is reduced or drug stopped.

• Monitor LFT values periodically, especially in patients with moderate hepatic impairment.

• Monitor tiagabine level.

• Monitor patient for serious rash, including SJS.

• *Look alike–sound alike:* Don't confuse tiagabine with tizanidine; both have 4-mg starting doses.

PATIENT TEACHING

🟡 *Alert:* Advise patient, caregivers, and family to immediately report new-onset or worsening depression, emergence of suicidality, thoughts of self-harm, or other unusual changes in mood or behavior.

• Teach patient safe drug administration and to take drug only as prescribed.

• Warn patient that drug may cause dizziness, somnolence, and other signs and symptoms of CNS depression. Advise patient to avoid driving and other potentially hazardous activities that require mental alertness until drug's CNS effects are known.

• Tell patient of childbearing potential to report pregnancy or plans to become pregnant during therapy.

• Instruct patient of childbearing potential to report plans to breastfeed because it isn't known if drug appears in human milk.

• Caution patient not to discontinue drug abruptly because of risk of seizures.

• Advise patient not to drink alcohol while taking drug.

SAFETY ALERT!

ticagrelor
TYE-ka-GREL-or

Brilinta🥄

Therapeutic class: Antiplatelet drugs
Pharmacologic class: P2Y$_{12}$ platelet inhibitors

AVAILABLE FORMS
Tablets: 60 mg, 90 mg

INDICATIONS & DOSAGES

➤ **ACS or a history of MI to reduce rate of CV death, MI, and stroke; after stent placement for treatment of ACS to reduce rate of thrombosis**

Adults: Initially, 180 mg PO as a loading dose; then, a maintenance dose of 90 mg PO b.i.d. during first year after an ACS event. After 1 year, give 60 mg b.i.d. Give daily maintenance dose with 75 to 100 mg of aspirin daily.

➤ **To reduce risk of a first MI or stroke in patients with CAD at high risk**

Adults: 60 mg b.i.d. in combination with aspirin (75 to 100 mg daily). Continue ticagrelor and aspirin indefinitely.

➤ **To reduce risk of stroke in patients with acute ischemic stroke (NIH Stroke Scale score of 5 or less) or high-risk TIA**

Adults: Initially, 180 mg PO as a loading dose; then, a maintenance dose of 90 mg PO b.i.d. for up to 30 days. Use in combination with a loading dose of aspirin (300 to 325 mg) and a daily maintenance dose of aspirin (75 to 100 mg).

ADMINISTRATION
PO

• Give drug without regard to food.

• For patients unable to swallow tablets whole, tablets can be crushed, mixed with water, and drunk. The mixture can also be given via an NG tube.

• Omit a missed dose and give next dose at its scheduled time; don't give an extra dose to make up for the missed dose.

• Store at room temperature in the original container. Keep away from moisture and humidity.

T

ACTION

Inhibits platelet aggregation by reversibly interacting with the $P2Y_{12}$ ADP receptor.

Route	Onset	Peak	Duration
PO	Rapid	1–5 hr	8 hr

Half-life: 7 hours (ticagrelor), 9 hours (active metabolite).

ADVERSE REACTIONS

CNS: headache, dizziness. **CV:** *bleeding,* bradyarrhythmias, abnormal ECG. **GI:** nausea, diarrhea. **GU:** increased creatinine level. **Respiratory:** dyspnea.

INTERACTIONS

Drug-drug. *Anticoagulants, antiplatelet agents, fibrinolytics, long-term NSAIDs, omega-3 fatty acids, vitamin E:* May increase risk of bleeding. Use cautiously together.

Boxed Warning *Aspirin:* Maintenance doses of aspirin greater than 100 mg/day may decrease ticagrelor effectiveness and increase risk of bleeding. Maintenance doses of aspirin shouldn't exceed 100 mg/day. ∎

Digoxin: May increase digoxin level. Monitor digoxin level at start of treatment and with any changes to treatment.

Opioids (morphine): May decrease ticagrelor exposure. Consider using parenteral antiplatelet agent in patients with ACS who require coadministration of morphine or other opioid.

Other $P2Y_{12}$ platelet inhibitors: Increases risk of bleeding. Use together is contraindicated.

Statins: May increase levels of these drugs. Don't exceed 40 mg of simvastatin or lovastatin with concurrent ticagrelor use.

Strong CYP3A4 inducers (carbamazepine, dexamethasone, phenobarbital, phenytoin, rifampin): May significantly decrease ticagrelor and active metabolite levels, and therapeutic effect. Avoid use together.

Strong CYP3A4 inhibitors (atazanavir, clarithromycin, itraconazole, ketoconazole, nefazodone, nelfinavir, ritonavir, saquinavir, telithromycin): May significantly increase ticagrelor level and risk of adverse reactions. Avoid use together.

Drug-herb. *Alfalfa, anise, bilberry:* May increase risk of bleeding. Avoid using together.

St. John's wort: May increase metabolism of ticagrelor and decrease drug's effectiveness. Avoid using together.

Drug-food. *Grapefruit juice:* May increase ticagrelor level. Monitor therapy closely.

EFFECTS ON LAB TEST RESULTS

• May increase uric acid and creatinine levels.
• May cause false-negative functional tests for heparin-induced thrombocytopenia.

CONTRAINDICATIONS & CAUTIONS

Boxed Warning Drug can cause serious, sometimes fatal bleeding. Contraindicated in patients with history of intracranial hemorrhage or active pathologic bleeding (including peptic ulcer). ∎

Boxed Warning Don't start ticagrelor in patients who will undergo planned urgent CABG. If possible, discontinue ticagrelor at least 5 days before any surgery. ∎

• Contraindicated in patients hypersensitive to drug. Avoid use in those with severe hepatic impairment.
• Use isn't recommended in patients with an NIH Stroke Scale score greater than 5 receiving thrombolysis.
• Use cautiously in patients with moderate hepatic failure, older adults, patients with history of a bleeding disorder, and patients who have had percutaneous invasive procedures.

⚕ *Alert:* Drug can cause ventricular pauses. Bradyarrhythmias, including AV block, have been reported. Patients with a history of sick sinus syndrome, second- or third-degree AV block, or bradycardia-related syncope (without pacemakers) weren't studied.

Dialyzable drug: No.

⚠ *Overdose S&S:* Bleeding, nausea, vomiting, diarrhea, ventricular pauses.

PREGNANCY-LACTATION-REPRODUCTION

• There are no adequate studies during pregnancy. Use only if potential benefit justifies fetal risk.
• It isn't known if drug or its active metabolites appear in human milk. Patient should discontinue breastfeeding or discontinue drug.

NURSING CONSIDERATIONS

Boxed Warning If possible, manage bleeding without discontinuing ticagrelor; premature discontinuation of treatment increases risk of MI, stent thrombosis, or death. If drug must be temporarily stopped, restart as soon as possible. ∎

• Monitor patient for bleeding.
• Monitor patient for respiratory effects, including dyspnea, sleep apnea, and Cheyne-Stokes respiration. Rule out underlying

---

Reactions in bold italics are *life-threatening*. Interactions may have a *rapid onset* or a ***delayed onset***.

conditions that require treatment in patients with new, prolonged, or worsened difficulty breathing.

• Dyspnea secondary to ticagrelor therapy is usually mild to moderate, and often self-limiting with continued treatment. If ticagrelor is discontinued for intolerable dyspnea, consider another antiplatelet agent.

• Ticagrelor can be given to patients with ACS who have already been given a loading dose of clopidogrel.

PATIENT TEACHING

Boxed Warning Tell patient not to take more than 100 mg of aspirin per day. Warn that other OTC products may also contain aspirin. ■

• Instruct patient in safe drug administration.

• Inform patient that bleeding or bruising may occur more easily and it will take longer for the bleeding to stop. Tell patient to immediately report unexpected, prolonged, or excessive bleeding, or blood in the urine or stool.

• Warn patient not to stop drug without consulting prescriber.

• Caution patient to notify all health care providers about taking ticagrelor before any scheduled surgery or dental appointment. Advise patient to discuss with original prescriber recommendations by other providers to stop taking ticagrelor.

• Tell patient that ticagrelor may cause mild to moderate shortness of breath and to report unexpected shortness of breath, especially if it's severe.

• Advise patient to report pregnancy or plans to become pregnant before using drug.

• Warn patient taking drug not to breastfeed.

---

tiotropium bromide
tye-oh-TROH-pee-um

Spiriva HandiHaler, Spiriva Respimat

Therapeutic class: Bronchodilators
Pharmacologic class: Anticholinergics

AVAILABLE FORMS

Capsules (powder for inhalation): 18 mcg
Spray inhaler (Respimat): 1.25 mcg/actuation, 2.5 mcg/actuation

INDICATIONS & DOSAGES

➤ **To reduce COPD exacerbations; maintenance treatment of bronchospasm in COPD, including chronic bronchitis and emphysema**

Adults: 2 oral inhalations of 1 capsule (18 mcg) once daily using HandiHaler inhalation device. Or, 2 inhalations (2.5 mcg each) of spray once daily.

➤ **Long-term maintenance treatment of asthma (Spiriva Respimat)**

Adults and children age 6 and older: 2 inhalations of 1.25 mcg/actuation spray once daily; total dose equals 2.5 mcg of tiotropium. Maximum benefits in lung function may take up to 4 to 8 weeks of dosing.

ADMINISTRATION
Inhalational
Capsules

• Give capsules only by oral inhalation with the HandiHaler device; don't store in device.

• Open capsule blister immediately before use. One capsule contains two inhalations.

• Capsules aren't for oral ingestion.

Respimat spray inhaler

• Before first use, insert cartridge into the inhaler.

• Prime the unit before using it for the first time by actuating the inhaler toward the ground until an aerosol cloud is visible; then repeat the process three more times.

• If not used for more than 3 days, the inhaler should be actuated once to prepare it for use. If not used for more than 21 days, the inhaler should be actuated until an aerosol cloud is visible; then repeat the process three more times.

• When the labeled number of actuations (28 or 60) has been dispensed from the Respimat inhaler, a locking mechanism engages to prevent further actuations.

ACTION

Competitive, reversible inhibition of muscarinic receptors in smooth muscle leads to bronchodilation.

Route	Onset	Peak	Duration
Inhalation	Unknown	5–7 min	>24 hr

Half-life: COPD, 25 hours; asthma, 44 hours.

ADVERSE REACTIONS

CNS: depression, paresthesia, headache, dizziness, fever, insomnia. **CV:** *angina* *pectoris,* chest pain, edema, palpitations, HTN. **EENT:** cataract, epistaxis, dry mouth, sinusitis, laryngitis, dysphonia, pharyngitis, rhinitis, oropharyngeal candidiasis. **GI:** abdominal pain, constipation, dyspepsia, GERD, stomatitis, vomiting, diarrhea. **GU:** UTI. **Metabolic:** hypercholesterolemia, hyperglycemia. **Musculoskeletal:** arthritis, leg pain, myalgia, skeletal pain. **Respiratory:** URI, cough, bronchitis. **Skin:** rash, pruritus. **Other:** allergic reaction, candidiasis, flulike syndrome, herpes zoster, infections.

INTERACTIONS

Drug-drug. *Anticholinergics:* May increase the risk of adverse reactions. Avoid using together.

Glucagon: May increase risk of GI adverse effects. Avoid combination.

Opioids: May increase risk of constipation and urine retention. Monitor patient closely.

Potassium chloride: May increase ulcer risk. Avoid combination.

EFFECTS ON LAB TEST RESULTS

• May increase cholesterol and glucose levels.

CONTRAINDICATIONS & CAUTIONS

• Contraindicated in patients hypersensitive to atropine, its derivatives, ipratropium, or components of the product.

• Immediate hypersensitivity reactions can occur, including urticaria, angioedema, rash, itching, and anaphylaxis.

• Use cautiously in patients with CrCl of less than 60 mL/minute, and in patients with angle-closure glaucoma, prostatic hyperplasia, or bladder neck obstruction due to increased risk of anticholinergic effects.

• Use capsule cautiously in patients with severe hypersensitivity to milk protein.

Dialyzable drug: Unknown.

⚠ *Overdose S&S:* Change in mental status, tremors, abdominal pain, severe constipation.

PREGNANCY-LACTATION-REPRODUCTION

• There are no adequate studies during pregnancy. Use only if potential benefit justifies fetal risk.

• It isn't known if drug appears in human milk. Use cautiously during breastfeeding.

NURSING CONSIDERATIONS

🔔 *Alert:* Use drug for maintenance treatment of COPD or asthma, not for acute bronchospasm.

• Watch for evidence of hypersensitivity (especially angioedema) and paradoxical bronchospasm. Discontinue drug immediately.

• Monitor patient for anticholinergic effects (dry mouth, constipation, tachycardia, blurred vision, new or worsening glaucoma, dysuria, urine retention).

• *Look alike–sound alike:* Don't confuse Spiriva with Inspra.

PATIENT TEACHING

• Inform patient that drug is for maintenance treatment of COPD or asthma and not for immediate relief of breathing problems.

• Explain that capsules are for inhalation and shouldn't be swallowed.

• Instruct patient in proper drug administration and storage.

• Provide full instructions for the HandiHaler device or the Respimat spray inhaler. Demonstrate use and observe return demonstration from patient.

• Tell patient not to get powder or spray in eyes.

• Review signs and symptoms of hypersensitivity (especially angioedema) and paradoxical bronchospasm. Tell patient to stop the drug and contact prescriber if they occur.

• Advise patient to report eye pain, blurred vision, visual halos, colored images, or red eyes immediately.

tipranavir
tih-PRAN-uh-veer

Aptivus

Therapeutic class: Antiretrovirals
Pharmacologic class: Protease inhibitors

AVAILABLE FORMS

Capsules ⓞⓝⓒ: 250 mg*
Oral solution: 100 mg/mL

INDICATIONS & DOSAGES

➤ **HIV-1 in patients with viral replication who are highly treatment-experienced and have HIV-1 strains resistant to multiple protease inhibitors, in combination with ritonavir and other antiretrovirals**

Adults: 500 mg PO b.i.d. with 200 mg of ritonavir b.i.d.

Children ages 2 to 18: 14 mg/kg with ritonavir 6 mg/kg (or tipranavir 375 mg/m^2 with ritonavir 150 mg/m^2) b.i.d., not to exceed dosage of tipranavir 500 mg with ritonavir 200 mg b.i.d.

Adjust-a-dose: For children who develop intolerance or toxicity, consider decreasing dosage to tipranavir 12 mg/kg with ritonavir 5 mg/kg (or tipranavir 290 mg/m^2 with ritonavir 115 mg/m^2) b.i.d. provided the virus isn't resistant to multiple protease inhibitors.

Discontinue if asymptomatic AST or ALT elevations greater than 10 × ULN occur. Also discontinue if AST or ALT elevations greater than 5 to 10 × ULN occur concurrently with total bilirubin level greater than 2.5 × ULN.

ADMINISTRATION

PO

- Give with ritonavir and other antiretrovirals.
- Make sure patient swallows capsules whole and doesn't break, crush, or chew them.
- When given with ritonavir tablets, drug must only be taken with meals; when given with ritonavir capsules or solution, drug can be taken with or without meals.
- Don't freeze or refrigerate oral solution.
- Store unopened capsule bottle in refrigerator; store opened capsule bottle at room temperature.
- Use within 60 days of opening capsule bottle or oral solution bottle.

ACTION

Inhibits virus-specific processing of polyproteins in HIV-1 infected cells, preventing formation of mature virions.

Route	Onset	Peak	Duration
PO	Unknown	3 hr	Unknown

Half-life: Adults, 6 hours; children age 2 to younger than age 6, 8.1 hours; children age 6 to younger than age 12, 7.1 hours; children ages 12 to 18, 5.2 hours.

ADVERSE REACTIONS

CNS: dizziness, fatigue, headache, insomnia, malaise, peripheral neuropathy, fever, sleep disorder, somnolence. **EENT:** epistaxis. **GI:** anorexia, diarrhea, *pancreatitis,* abdominal distention, abdominal pain, dyspepsia, flatulence, GERD, nausea, vomiting. **GU:** renal insufficiency. **Hematologic:** *neutropenia,* *thrombocytopenia,* anemia. **Hepatic:** *hepatic failure, hepatitis.* **Metabolic:** decreased appetite, dehydration, diabetes, facial wasting, hyperglycemia, hyperlipidemia, hypertriglyceridemia, weight loss. **Musculoskeletal:** muscle cramps, myalgia. **Respiratory:** cough, dyspnea. **Skin:** rash, acquired lipodystrophy, exanthem, lipoatrophy, lipohypertrophy, pruritus. **Other:** flulike illness, hypersensitivity.

INTERACTIONS

Refer to manufacturer's prescribing information for complete list of drug interactions.

Drug-drug. *Alfuzosin:* May increase alfuzosin serum concentration. Use together is contraindicated.

Amiodarone, bepridil, flecainide, propafenone, quinidine: May increase levels of these drugs and risk of life-threatening arrhythmias. Use together is contraindicated.

Anticoagulants: May increase anticoagulant effect. Monitor patient closely.

🕔 *Alert: Atorvastatin:* May increase levels of both drugs and risk of myopathy and rhabdomyolysis. Avoid use together.

Bosentan: May decrease tipranavir serum concentration; may increase bosentan serum concentration. Use bosentan 62.5 mg/day or every other day in adults taking tipranavir/ritonavir for at least 10 days. Temporarily stop bosentan (for at least 36 hours) before starting tipranavir/ritonavir; wait at least 10 days before restarting bosentan. Consider therapy modification.

Calcium channel blockers (diltiazem, felodipine, nicardipine, nisoldipine, verapamil): May cause unpredictable interaction. Use together cautiously and monitor patient closely.

Cisapride: May increase risk of cardiac arrhythmias. Use together is contraindicated.

Clarithromycin: May increase levels of both drugs. If CrCl ranges from 30 to 60 mL/minute, decrease clarithromycin dose by 50%. If CrCl falls below 30 mL/minute, decrease clarithromycin dose by 75%.

Clozapine: May increase clozapine serum concentration. Monitor patient closely.

Codeine: May decrease effectiveness of codeine. Consider therapy modification.

Colchicine: May increase risk of life-threatening and fatal colchicine toxicity. Use together is contraindicated in patients with renal or hepatic impairment. In patients with healthy renal and hepatic function, reduce

T

colchicine dosage according to manufacturer's instructions.

Contraceptives (progestins and estrogens): May decrease contraceptive effectiveness. Patient should use alternative or additional contraceptive method.

Cyclosporine, sirolimus, tacrolimus: May cause unpredictable interaction. Monitor drug levels closely until they've stabilized.

CYP3A4 inducers: May increase metabolism of protease inhibitors. Consider therapy modification. Administration with strong inducers is contraindicated.

Desipramine: May increase desipramine level. Decrease dose and monitor desipramine level.

Didanosine: May decrease didanosine level. Separate dosing by at least 2 hours.

Disulfiram, metronidazole: May cause disulfiram-like reaction when used with capsules. Use together cautiously.

Ergot derivatives (dihydroergotamine, ergonovine, ergotamine, methylergonovine): May cause acute ergot toxicity, including peripheral vasospasm and ischemia of extremities. Use together is contraindicated.

Estrogen-based hormone therapy: May decrease estrogen level, and rash may occur. Monitor patient carefully. Advise using nonhormonal contraception.

Fluoxetine, paroxetine, sertraline: May increase levels of these drugs. Adjust dosages as needed.

Glimepiride, glipizide, glyburide, pioglitazone, repaglinide, tolbutamide: May affect glucose levels. Monitor glucose level carefully.

⚠ *Alert:* *Lovastatin, simvastatin:* May increase risk of myopathy and rhabdomyolysis. Use together is contraindicated.

Lurasidone: May increase risk of serious or life-threatening reactions. Use together is contraindicated.

Meperidine: May increase normeperidine metabolite. Avoid using together.

Methadone: May decrease methadone level by 50%. Consider increasing methadone dosage.

Midazolam, triazolam: May cause prolonged or increased sedation or respiratory depression. Use together is contraindicated.

Pimozide: May cause life-threatening arrhythmias. Use together is contraindicated.

Rifabutin: May increase rifabutin level. Decrease rifabutin dose by 75%.

Rifampin: May lead to loss of virologic response and resistance to tipranavir and other protease inhibitors. Use together is contraindicated.

Sildenafil, tadalafil, vardenafil: May increase levels of these drugs. Use together cautiously. Tell patient not to exceed 25 mg sildenafil in 48 hours, 10 mg tadalafil every 72 hours, or 2.5 mg vardenafil every 72 hours when used for erectile dysfunction. Use of sildenafil (Revatio) for treatment of PAH is contraindicated. See prescribing information for administration with tadalafil for PAH.

Tamoxifen: May decrease serum concentration of active metabolite of tamoxifen. Avoid combination.

Trazodone: May increase trazodone serum concentration. Use together cautiously and consider a lower trazodone dose.

Valproic acid: May reduce valproic acid plasma level. Use with caution.

Vitamin E: May cause vitamin E toxicity if supplemental vitamin E dose is greater than a standard multivitamin when used with oral solution. Oral solution contains 116 international units/mL of vitamin E. Use cautiously together.

Warfarin: May cause unpredictable reaction. Check INR often.

Drug-herb. *Garlic:* May decrease serum concentration of protease inhibitors. Use together isn't recommended.

St. John's wort: May lead to loss of virologic response and resistance to tipranavir and other antiretrovirals. Use together is contraindicated.

EFFECTS ON LAB TEST RESULTS

• May increase total cholesterol, triglyceride, blood glucose, amylase, lipase, bilirubin, GGT, CK, ALT, and AST levels.

• May decrease Hb level, hematocrit, and WBC, neutrophil, and platelet counts.

CONTRAINDICATIONS & CAUTIONS

Boxed Warning Tipranavir use has been associated with fatal and nonfatal intracranial hemorrhage, clinical hepatitis, and hepatic decompensation. ■

• Contraindicated in patients hypersensitive to ingredients of the product; patients with moderate or severe (Child-Pugh class B or C) hepatic insufficiency; and patients taking drugs that are potent CYP3A inducers, that depend on CYP3A for clearance, or are contraindicated for use with ritonavir.

Reactions in bold italics are *life-threatening*. Interactions may have a *rapid onset* or a *delayed onset*.

🖐 *Alert:* Don't give drug to patients who are treatment-naive.

• Use cautiously in patients with bleeding risk, sulfonamide allergy, diabetes, liver disease, HBV or HCV infection, or hemophilia A or B.

• Use cautiously in older adults, who are more likely to have decreased organ function, multidrug therapy, and other illnesses.

Dialyzable drug: No.

PREGNANCY-LACTATION-REPRODUCTION

• There are no adequate studies in pregnancy. Tipranavir crosses the placental barrier. Use only if potential benefit justifies fetal risk.

• To monitor maternal-fetal outcomes, register patients exposed to drug in the Antiretroviral Pregnancy Registry (1-800-258-4263).

• The CDC recommends that patients with HIV-1 infection not breastfeed to avoid risking postnatal transmission of HIV-1.

NURSING CONSIDERATIONS

Boxed Warning Patients with chronic HBV or HCV infection are at increased risk for hepatotoxicity; fatalities have been reported. ▮

• Assess for evidence of hepatitis, such as fatigue, malaise, anorexia, nausea, jaundice, bilirubinemia, acholic stools, liver tenderness, and hepatomegaly. If patient develops signs or symptoms of hepatitis, notify prescriber.

• To be effective, drug must be given with ritonavir and with other antiretrovirals.

🖐 *Alert:* Monitor patient for signs and symptoms of intracranial hemorrhage, including headache, nausea, vomiting, change in mental status, speech or balance difficulties, and seizures.

🖐 *Alert:* Obtain thorough patient drug history. Many drugs may interact with tipranavir. Consider potential for drug interactions before and during therapy; review concomitant medications during therapy; and monitor patient for adverse reactions associated with concomitant medications.

• Monitor LFTs at start of treatment and often during treatment.

• Monitor glucose level closely. New-onset diabetes, worsening of preexisting diabetes, and hyperglycemia may occur.

• Obtain baseline cholesterol and triglyceride levels at start of and periodically during therapy.

• Monitor patient for cushingoid symptoms, such as central obesity, buffalo hump, peripheral wasting, facial wasting, and breast enlargement.

• Monitor patient for severe rash.

• Monitor patient for immune reconstitution syndrome (inflammatory response to indolent or residual opportunistic infections, such as CMV, TB, *Pneumocystis jiroveci* pneumonia, herpes simplex, or herpes zoster).

PATIENT TEACHING

• Explain that drug doesn't cure HIV infection and doesn't reduce the risk of transmitting the virus to others.

🖐 *Alert:* Many drugs may interfere with this drug. Urge patient to report all prescription and OTC drugs and herbal products being taken.

• Teach patient safe drug administration and storage.

• Instruct patient taking oral solution not to take supplemental vitamin E in a dose greater than a standard multivitamin.

• Tell patient that drug is effective only when taken with ritonavir and other antiretrovirals.

• Instruct patient taking ritonavir tablets to take them with meals; patient taking ritonavir capsules or solution can take them with or without meals.

• Urge patient to report all adverse reactions and to stop drug and contact prescriber if signs and symptoms of hepatitis or intracranial hemorrhage occur.

• If patient of childbearing potential uses hormonal contraceptives, advise use of barrier contraception.

• Tell patient that redistribution or accumulation of body fat may occur.

• Advise patient that breastfeeding isn't recommended to avoid transmission of HIV-1 infection.

tirbanibulin
tir-ban-i-BUE-lin

Klisyri

Therapeutic class: Antineoplastics
Pharmacologic class: Microtubule inhibitors

AVAILABLE FORMS
Ointment: 1% single-dose packet

INDICATIONS & DOSAGES
➤ **Actinic keratosis on the face or scalp**
Adults: Apply ointment evenly to affected area once daily for 5 consecutive days.

ADMINISTRATION
Topical
• For topical use only; not for oral or ophthalmic use.
• Use one single-dose packet per application; discard packet and unused ointment after use.
• Don't apply to a treatment area of more than 25 cm².
• Don't apply occlusive dressings to affected area.
• Wash hands immediately with soap and water after applying drug.
• Avoid washing and touching treated area for approximately 8 hours after application; after 8 hours, may wash the area with a mild soap.
• Avoid getting drug near and around the mouth, lips, and periocular area. If ocular exposure occurs, flush with water.
• Store at 68° to 77° F (20° to 25° C). Don't refrigerate or freeze.

ACTION
Unknown.

Route	Onset	Peak	Duration
Topical	Unknown	7 hr	Unknown

Half-life: Unknown.

ADVERSE REACTIONS
Skin: application-site pruritus, application-site pain, crusting, erosion, erythema, flaking, pustulation, scaling, swelling, vesiculation, ulceration.

INTERACTIONS
None reported.

EFFECTS ON LAB TEST RESULTS
None reported.

CONTRAINDICATIONS & CAUTIONS
• Safety and effectiveness in children haven't been established.
• Older adults may have greater sensitivity to drug.
Dialyzable drug: Unknown.

PREGNANCY-LACTATION-REPRODUCTION
• There are no studies during pregnancy. It's unknown if drug increases risk of major birth defects, miscarriage, or adverse patient or fetal outcomes.
• It isn't known if drug appears in human milk or how drug affects milk production or

infants who are breastfed. Consider benefits and risk to the infant.

NURSING CONSIDERATIONS
• Monitor patient for local skin reactions of the treated area.
• Monitor patient for eye irritation.
• Flush patient's eye if accidental exposure occurs and notify prescriber.
• Don't use ointment if skin hasn't healed from previous drug, procedure, or surgical treatment.
• Avoid using occlusive dressings.
• *Look alike–sound alike:* Don't confuse tirbanibulin with eribulin, terbinafine, or terbutaline.

PATIENT TEACHING
• Instruct patient on proper drug application and potential adverse effects.
• Tell patient to flush eye with water and notify prescriber if accidental contact with eye occurs.
• Instruct patient to wash hands well after applying drug.
• Caution patient to avoid inadvertent transfer of drug to other areas of the body, or to another person.

---

tiZANidine hydrochloride
tis-AN-i-deen

Zanaflex

Therapeutic class: Skeletal muscle relaxants
Pharmacologic class: Centrally acting alpha₂-adrenergic agonists

AVAILABLE FORMS
Capsules: 2 mg, 4 mg, 6 mg
Tablets: 2 mg, 4 mg

INDICATIONS & DOSAGES
➤ **Management of spasticity**
Adults: Initially, 2 mg PO every 6 to 8 hours, as needed, to maximum of three doses in 24 hours. Dosage can be increased gradually in 2- to 4-mg increments, with 1 to 4 days between increases. Maximum, 36 mg daily.
Adjust-a-dose: Use cautiously and reduce dosage during titration in patients with hepatic impairment or renal insufficiency (CrCl of less than 25 mL/minute). If higher dosages are needed, increase individual doses rather than frequency.

Reactions in bold italics are *life-threatening*. Interactions may have a *rapid onset* or a *delayed onset*.

ADMINISTRATION
PO
- Give drug consistently as either tablets or capsules and with or without food for same absorption rate and effect.

🝚 *Alert:* Capsules and tablets are bioequivalent only when taken on an empty stomach.

ACTION
Central alpha₂ agonist that may reduce spasticity by increasing presynaptic inhibition of motor neurons at the level of the spinal cord.

Route	Onset	Peak	Duration
PO	Unknown	1–2 hr	3–6 hr

Half-life: 2.5 hours; metabolites, 20 to 40 hours.

ADVERSE REACTIONS
CNS: somnolence, sedation, asthenia, weakness, tiredness, dizziness, speech disorder, dyskinesia, nervousness, hallucinations, delusions. **CV:** hypotension, *bradycardia.* **EENT:** amblyopia, dry mouth, visual field defect, pharyngitis, rhinitis, sinusitis. **GI:** constipation, vomiting, dyspepsia. **GU:** UTI, urinary frequency. **Hepatic:** hepatic injury. **Other:** infection, flulike syndrome.

INTERACTIONS
Drug-drug. *Antihypertensives, other alpha agonists (clonidine):* May cause hypotension. Monitor patient closely. Avoid use with other alpha agonists.

Baclofen, benzodiazepines, cannabis, dronabinol, magnesium sulfate, other CNS depressants: May have additive CNS depressant effects. Avoid using together.

CYP1A2 inhibitors (amiodarone, acyclovir, cimetidine, famotidine, fluoroquinolones, mexiletine, propafenone, ticlopidine, verapamil, zileuton): May significantly increase tizanidine level. Avoid use together. If use together is unavoidable, reduce tizanidine dosage.

Drugs that prolong QTc interval: May increase QTc interval and risk of ventricular arrhythmias. Monitor therapy.

Opioids: May cause slow or difficult breathing, sedation, and death. Avoid use together. If use together is necessary, limit dosage and duration of each drug to minimum necessary for desired effect.

Oral contraceptives: May decrease tizanidine clearance. Reduce tizanidine dosage.

Strong CYP1A2 inhibitors (ciprofloxacin, fluvoxamine): May increase tizanidine level and risk of adverse effects. Use together is contraindicated.

Drug-herb. *Kava kava:* May enhance adverse CNS effects. Monitor patient closely.

Drug-lifestyle. *Alcohol use:* May increase CNS depression. Discourage use together.

EFFECTS ON LAB TEST RESULTS
- May increase AST and ALT levels.

CONTRAINDICATIONS & CAUTIONS
- Contraindicated in patients hypersensitive to drug.
- *Opioid class warning:* Opioids should only be prescribed with benzodiazepines or other CNS depressants to patients for whom alternative treatment options are inadequate.
- Use cautiously in patients with renal or hepatic impairment or psychiatric disorders and in older adults.
- May cause sedation, which may interfere with everyday activities.
- Safety and effectiveness in children haven't been established.

Dialyzable drug: Unlikely.

⚠ *Overdose S&S:* Lethargy, somnolence, confusion, coma, bradycardia, hypotension, respiratory depression, depressed cardiac function.

PREGNANCY-LACTATION-REPRODUCTION
- Drug hasn't been studied during pregnancy. Animal data suggest fetal risk. Use only if potential benefit justifies fetal risk.
- It isn't known if drug appears in human milk. Use cautiously during breastfeeding.

NURSING CONSIDERATIONS
- Due to its short duration of therapeutic effect, reserve drug for daily activities and times when relief of spasticity is most important.
- Obtain LFT results before treatment, 1 month after maximum dose is achieved, and if liver injury is suspected.
- Monitor renal function, especially in older adults and patients with renal insufficiency.
- May prolong QT interval, and cause bradycardia and hypotension. Closely monitor vital signs, especially in patients receiving maximum recommended dosage and those taking other drugs that prolong QT interval.

T

• Monitor patient for signs and symptoms of excess sedation if patient is taking drug along with another CNS depressant.

• Consider discontinuing drug in patients who develop hallucinations.

🔵 *Alert:* Stop drug gradually, especially in patients taking high doses (20 to 28 mg daily) for a prolonged period (9 weeks or more) and in those taking concomitant opioids. Decrease dosage slowly by 2 to 4 mg/day to minimize the potential for rebound HTN, tachycardia, and hypertension.

• *Look alike–sound alike:* Don't confuse tizanidine with tiagabine. Don't confuse Zanaflex with Xiaflex.

PATIENT TEACHING

• *Opioid class warning:* Caution patient or caregiver of patient taking an opioid with a benzodiazepine, CNS depressant, or alcohol to seek immediate medical attention for dizziness, light-headedness, extreme sleepiness, slowed or difficult breathing, or unresponsiveness.

• Caution patient to avoid alcohol and activities that require alertness, such as driving or operating machinery, until drug's effects are known. Drug may cause drowsiness.

• Inform patient that dizziness upon standing quickly can be minimized by rising slowly.

🔵 *Alert:* Advise patient that tizanidine absorption varies depending on whether drug is taken with or without food and that it should always be taken the same way to reduce risk of changes in efficacy and adverse reactions.

• Instruct patient to inform the health care provider and pharmacist when medications are added or removed from patient's regimen.

• Advise patient not to suddenly stop taking medication.

tobramycin
toe-bra-MYE-sin

Tobrex

tobramycin sulfate
Bethkis, Kitabis Pak, TOBI, TOBI Podhaler

Therapeutic class: Antibiotics
Pharmacologic class: Aminoglycosides

AVAILABLE FORMS

Capsules (for inhalation): 28 mg

Multidose vials: 10 mg/mL (pediatric), 40 mg/mL
Nebulizer solution (for inhalation): 300 mg/ 4 mL, 300 mg/5 mL
Ophthalmic ointment: 0.3%
Ophthalmic solution: 0.3%
Powder for injection: 1.2-g vial

INDICATIONS & DOSAGES

➤ **Serious infection caused by sensitive strains of *Escherichia coli, Proteus, Klebsiella, Enterobacter, Serratia, Morganella morganii, Staphylococcus aureus, Citrobacter, Pseudomonas,* or *Providencia***
Adults: 3 mg/kg/day IM or IV in three equal doses every 8 hours. For life-threatening infections, give up to 5 mg/kg/day in divided doses every 6 to 8 hours; reduce to 3 mg/kg daily as soon as clinically indicated.
Children older than age 1 week: 6 to 7.5 mg/kg/ day IM or IV, in three or four divided doses.
Neonates younger than age 1 week or preterm infants: Up to 4 mg/kg/day IV or IM in two equal doses every 12 hours.
Adjust-a-dose: For patients with renal impairment, give loading dose of 1 mg/kg; then give decreased doses at 8-hour intervals or same dose at prolonged intervals. For patients on hemodialysis, adjust dosage based on dialysis method, filter type, and flow rate; give after dialysis and adjust according to serum concentrations. For patients with severe cystic fibrosis, initially give 10 mg/kg/day IV or IM in four divided doses. For patients who are obese, calculate dose using estimated lean body weight plus 40% of excess weight.
➤ **To manage patients with cystic fibrosis and *Pseudomonas aeruginosa* infection**
Adults and children age 6 and older: 300 mg via nebulizer every 12 hours for 28 days. Or, using TOBI Podhaler device, have patient inhale contents of four 28-mg (112 mg) capsules every 12 hours for 28 days. Stop therapy for 28 days; then repeat and continue cycles of 28 days on drug and 28 days off.
➤ **External ocular infections by susceptible bacteria**
Adults and children age 2 months and older: In mild to moderate infections, instill 1 or 2 drops into affected eye(s) every 4 hours, or apply ½-inch (1.27-cm) ribbon of ointment every 8 to 12 hours. In severe infections, instill 2 drops into infected eye(s) every 60 minutes until condition improves; then reduce frequency. Or, apply -inch ribbon of ointment

---

Reactions in bold italics are *life-threatening*. Interactions may have a *rapid onset* or a *delayed onset*.

every 3 to 4 hours until condition improves; then reduce frequency to b.i.d. to t.i.d.

ADMINISTRATION

• For IV, IM, and inhalational use, obtain specimen for culture and sensitivity tests before giving. Begin therapy while awaiting results.

IV

▼ For adults, dilute in 50 to 100 mL of NSS or D₅W; use a smaller volume for children.

▼ Keep reconstituted solution in refrigerator and use within 96 hours or keep at room temperature for 24 hours.

▼ Infuse over 20 to 60 minutes.

▼ After infusion, flush line with NSS or D₅W.

▼ Obtain blood for peak level 30 minutes after infusion stops; draw blood for trough level just before next dose. Don't collect blood in a heparinized tube because of incompatibility.

▼ **Incompatibilities:** Don't mix with other drugs; administer separately.

IM

• Obtain blood for peak level 1 hour after IM injection; draw blood for trough level just before next dose. Don't collect blood in a heparinized tube because of incompatibility.

• Withdraw appropriate dose directly from vial.

Inhalational

• Capsules aren't for oral ingestion.

• Give nebulizer solution over 15 minutes using handheld Pari LC Plus reusable nebulizer. Refer to manufacturer's instructions for recommended compressor.

• Give capsules only by oral inhalation using Podhaler device. A new Podhaler device is supplied with each weekly pack of capsules. Use only for 7 days; then discard.

• Store capsules in blister packs at room temperature and remove immediately before use.

• Give doses as close to 12 hours apart as possible. Doses shouldn't be taken less than 6 hours apart.

• If several inhaled medications and chest physiotherapy have been prescribed, follow prescriber's recommendations for when to administer them in relation to each other; guidelines recommend giving the Podhaler last.

• Don't dilute or mix with other drugs, including dornase alfa, in a nebulizer.

• Unrefrigerated inhalation solution normally appears slightly yellow but may darken with age, which doesn't affect quality.

• Store solution in refrigerator until expiration date or at room temperature for up to 28 days. Protect from light.

Ophthalmic

⚠ *Alert:* Tobramycin ophthalmic solution isn't for injection.

• When two different ophthalmic solutions are used, allow at least 10 minutes between instillations.

• Apply light finger pressure on lacrimal sac for 1 minute after drops are instilled.

• Apply ointment to conjunctiva. Don't let tube touch eye.

ACTION

Generally bactericidal. Inhibits protein synthesis by binding directly to the 30S ribosomal subunit.

Route	Onset	Peak	Duration
IV	Immediate	30 min	8 hr
IM	Unknown	30–60 min	8 hr
Inhalation	Unknown	60 min	Unknown
Ophthalmic	Unknown	Unknown	Unknown

Half-life: IV, 2 hours. Adults: inhalation, 3 to 4.4 hours. Adults with impaired renal function, 5 to 70 hours. Neonates weighing 1,200 g or less, 11 hours; neonates weighing more than 1,200 g, 2 to 9 hours. Infants, 3 to 5 hours. Children and adolescents, 0.5 to 3 hours.

ADVERSE REACTIONS

CNS: headache, lethargy, confusion, disorientation, fever, dizziness, vertigo; taste perversion (inhalation). **EENT:** blurred vision (ophthalmic); hearing loss, tinnitus, ototoxicity; dysphonia, epistaxis, laryngitis, pharyngitis, tonsillitis (inhalation). **GI:** vomiting, nausea, diarrhea. **GU:** *nephrotoxicity,* possible increase in urinary excretion of casts. **Hematologic:** anemia, eosinophilia, *leukopenia, thrombocytopenia, agranulocytosis.* **Metabolic:** electrolyte imbalances. **Musculoskeletal:** muscle twitching, chest pain. myalgia. **Respiratory:** cough, dyspnea, bronchitis, decreased forced expiratory volume, hemoptysis, rales, wheezing, increased sputum (inhalation). **Skin:** rash, urticaria, pruritus, dermatitis, pain at injection site.

INTERACTIONS

Drug-drug. **Boxed Warning** *Acyclovir, amphotericin B, cephalosporins, cidofovir, cisplatin, colistin, methoxyflurane, polymyxin B, vancomycin, other aminoglycosides:* May increase nephrotoxicity or neurotoxicity when used with injectable tobramycin formulation. Monitor renal function. ∎

Atracurium, pancuronium, rocuronium, vecuronium: May increase effects of nondepolarizing muscle relaxants, including prolonged respiratory depression. Use together only when necessary, and expect to reduce dosage of nondepolarizing muscle relaxant.

Boxed Warning *Cyclosporine , foscarnet, NSAIDs:* May increase risk of nephrotoxicity. Avoid combination. ∎

General anesthetics: May increase neuromuscular blockade. Monitor patient for increased clinical effects.

Boxed Warning *IV loop diuretics (ethacrynic acid, furosemide):* May increase ototoxicity when used with injectable tobramycin. Monitor patient's hearing. ∎

Parenteral penicillins: May inactivate tobramycin in vitro. Don't mix together.

EFFECTS ON LAB TEST RESULTS

• May increase AST, ALT, LDH, bilirubin, BUN, creatinine, nonprotein nitrogen, and urine urea levels.
• May decrease calcium, magnesium, sodium, and potassium levels.
• May increase eosinophil count, Ig levels, and RBC sedimentation rate (inhalation).
• May decrease Hb level, hematocrit, and platelet count.
• May increase or decrease WBC count.

CONTRAINDICATIONS & CAUTIONS

• Contraindicated in patients hypersensitive to drug or other aminoglycosides.

Boxed Warning Use tobramycin injection cautiously in premature infants and neonates because of their renal immaturity and resulting prolongation of drug's serum half-life. ∎

Boxed Warning For injectable tobramycin, neurotoxicity manifested as both auditory and vestibular ototoxicity can occur. Auditory changes are irreversible, are usually bilateral, and may be partial or total. Other manifestations of neurotoxicity may include numbness, skin tingling, muscle twitching, and seizures. Risk of hearing loss increases with degree of exposure to either high peak or high trough serum concentrations; other factors that may increase patient risk are advanced age and dehydration. Patients who develop cochlear damage may not have symptoms during therapy to warn them of eighth-nerve toxicity, and partial or total irreversible bilateral

deafness may continue to develop after drug discontinuation. ∎

🔄 *Alert:* Avoid concurrent or sequential use with other drugs with neurotoxic, nephrotoxic, or ototoxic potential.
• Use cautiously in patients with impaired renal function or neuromuscular disorders and in older adults.

Boxed Warning For injectable tobramycin, neuromuscular blockade can occur. Closely monitor patients at high risk, including patients with underlying neuromuscular disorders (e.g., myasthenia gravis) and those concomitantly receiving neuromuscular blockers. Neuromuscular blockade is reversible but may require treatment. ∎

Dialyzable drug: Yes.

⚠️ *Overdose S&S:* Nephrotoxicity, dizziness, tinnitus, vertigo, loss of high-tone hearing acuity, neuromuscular blockade, respiratory failure, respiratory paralysis (systemic); punctate keratitis, erythema, tearing, edema, eyelid itching (ophthalmic).

PREGNANCY-LACTATION-REPRODUCTION

Boxed Warning Aminoglycosides can cause fetal harm when given during pregnancy.
• There are no adequate studies during pregnancy. If used during pregnancy, or if patient becomes pregnant during therapy, apprise patient of fetal risk.
• Amount of drug that appears in human milk isn't known. Because of the potential for adverse effects in the infant, patient should discontinue breastfeeding or discontinue drug.

NURSING CONSIDERATIONS

• It's recommended that dosage be determined by appropriate pharmacokinetic methods and patient-specific parameters.
• Monitor peak and trough levels to determine dosage in patients with burns or cystic fibrosis; these patients may have reduced drug serum concentrations. Reserve higher peak levels for patients with cystic fibrosis, who need greater lung penetration.
• Don't obtain blood samples by fingerstick to monitor tobramycin concentration; skin contaminated with the drug may falsely elevate drug level.
• Follow facility protocol for obtaining peak and trough levels; guidelines recommend obtaining blood samples for peak level 30 minutes after IV infusion or 1 hour after

---

Reactions in bold italics are *life-threatening*. Interactions may have a *rapid onset* or a ***delayed onset***.

IM injection, trough level at 8 hours or just before the next scheduled dose.

Boxed Warning Peak levels over 12 mcg/mL and trough levels over 2 mcg/mL may increase risk of toxicity. Periodically monitor peak and trough serum concentrations. ■

• If ophthalmic tobramycin is given with systemic tobramycin, carefully monitor levels.

• Weigh patient and review renal function studies before therapy.

◑ *Alert:* If patient complains of tinnitus, vertigo, or hearing loss, notify prescriber.

Boxed Warning Monitor patient for signs and symptoms of neurotoxicity, including numbness, skin tingling, muscle twitching, and seizures. ■

Boxed Warning Closely monitor patient for ototoxicity and nephrotoxicity. ■

Boxed Warning If possible, obtain serial audiograms in patients old enough to be tested, particularly patients at high risk. Evidence of impaired renal, vestibular, or auditory function requires drug discontinuation or dosage adjustment. ■

Boxed Warning Due to increased risk of nephrotoxicity, monitor renal function: urine output, specific gravity, urinalysis, serum creatinine, CrCl, and BUN. Notify prescriber about signs and symptoms of decreasing renal function. Advanced age and dehydration may increase risk of nephrotoxicity. ■

• Watch for signs and symptoms of superinfection, such as continued fever, chills, and increased pulse rate.

• Monitor electrolyte levels.

• If no response occurs in 3 to 5 days, therapy may be stopped and new specimens obtained for culture and sensitivity testing.

• *Look alike–sound alike:* Don't confuse Tobrex with TobraDex.

PATIENT TEACHING

◑ *Alert:* Explain that capsules are for inhalation only and shouldn't be swallowed.

• Provide full instructions on inhalation or ophthalmic drug administration and storage.

• Advise patient not to wear contact lenses during treatment of ophthalmic infections.

• Teach patient how to use and maintain nebulizer and compressor.

• Instruct patient to report all adverse reactions promptly.

• Caution patient not to perform hazardous activities if adverse CNS reactions occur.

• Encourage patient to maintain adequate fluid intake.

---

tocilizumab ⬚
toe-sih-LIZ-oo-mab

Actemra

Therapeutic class: Antiarthritics
Pharmacologic class: Interleukin-6 receptor inhibitors

AVAILABLE FORMS

Injection (for IV use): 80 mg/4 mL, 200 mg/10 mL, 400 mg/20 mL in single-use vials
Injection (for subcut use): 162 mg/0.9 mL in prefilled syringe or autoinjector

INDICATIONS & DOSAGES

Adjust-a-dose (for all indications): Refer to manufacturer's instructions for toxicity-related dosage adjustments.

➤ **Systemic juvenile idiopathic arthritis (SJIA) alone or in combination with methotrexate** ⬚

Children age 2 and older weighing 30 kg or more: 8 mg/kg IV infusion once every 2 weeks. Or, 162 mg subcut once each week.

Children age 2 and older weighing less than 30 kg: 12 mg/kg IV infusion once every 2 weeks. Or, 162 mg subcut once every 2 weeks.

Adjust-a-dose: If appropriate, concomitant methotrexate or other medications should be dose-modified or stopped and tocilizumab dosage adjusted until the clinical situation has been evaluated. In SJIA, the decision to discontinue tocilizumab for a lab abnormality should be based on medical assessment of the individual patient.

➤ **As monotherapy or with methotrexate or other nonbiologic DMARDs for moderately to severely active RA when response to one or more DMARDs is inadequate**

Adults: Initially, 4 mg/kg IV infusion every 4 weeks. May increase dosage to 8 mg/kg every 4 weeks based on clinical response. Maximum dose is 800 mg per infusion. Or, for patients weighing 100 kg or more, 162 mg subcut once each week. Or, for patients weighing less than 100 kg, 162 mg subcut every other week, followed by an increase to every week based on clinical response.

T

➤ **Polyarticular juvenile idiopathic arthritis (PJIA) alone or in combination with methotrexate** ☒

Children age 2 and older weighing 30 kg or more: 8 mg/kg IV infusion once every 4 weeks. Or, 162 mg subcut once every 2 weeks.
Children age 2 and older weighing less than 30 kg: 10 mg/kg IV infusion once every 4 weeks. Or, 162 mg subcut once every 3 weeks.

Adjust-a-dose: Don't change dose based on a single-visit weight as weight may fluctuate. If appropriate, concomitant methotrexate or other medications should be dose-modified or stopped and tocilizumab dosage adjusted until the clinical situation has been evaluated. In PJIA, the decision to discontinue tocilizumab for a lab abnormality should be based on medical assessment of the individual patient.

➤ **Giant cell arteritis (GCA)** ☒

Adults: 6 mg/kg IV infusion every 4 weeks in combination with a tapering course of glucocorticoids. Maximum dose is 600 mg per infusion. Or, 162 mg subcut once each week in combination with a tapering course of glucocorticoids. Or, 162 mg subcut once every other week in combination with a tapering course of glucocorticoids as clinically indicated. May continue tocilizumab after glucocorticoids are stopped.

➤ **Chimeric antigen receptor (CAR) T cell–induced severe or life-threatening cytokine release syndrome (CRS), alone or in combination with corticosteroids**

Adults and children age 2 and older weighing 30 kg or more: 8 mg/kg IV infusion. May repeat infusion up to three more doses at least 8 hours apart if no clinical improvement in signs and symptoms of CRS. Maximum dose is 800 mg per infusion.
Adults and children age 2 and older weighing less than 30 kg: 12 mg/kg IV. May repeat infusion up to three more doses at least 8 hours apart if no clinical improvement in signs and symptoms of CRS. Maximum dose is 800 mg per infusion.

➤ **To slow decline in pulmonary function in patients with systemic sclerosis-associated interstitial lung disease (SSc-ILD)**

Adults: 162 mg subcut once each week. Subcut administration with the prefilled autoinjector hasn't been studied in this indication.

ADMINISTRATION

IV

▼ Check body weight before calculating each dose. For patients weighing 30 kg or more, dilute to 100 mL in NSS or half-NSS for IV infusion following manufacturer's instructions. For patients weighing less than 30 kg, dilute to 50 mL in NSS or half-NSS for IV infusion following manufacturer's instructions. Allow diluted solutions to reach room temperature before infusing.

▼ Don't use solution if it's discolored or contains particulate matter.

▼ Store NSS infusion solutions at 36° to 46° F (2° to 8° C) or at room temperature for up to 24 hours, or half-NSS infusion solutions at 36° to 46° F for up to 24 hours or at room temperature for up to 4 hours. Protect all solutions from light.

▼ Administer infusion over 60 minutes; infusion must be administered with infusion set. Don't administer as IV push or bolus.

▼ **Incompatibilities:** Don't infuse in same line with other IV drugs.

Subcutaneous

• When transitioning from IV therapy to subcut administration, administer the first subcut dose instead of the next scheduled IV dose.

• Dosing interruption or reduction in administration frequency of subcut dose from every week to every other week is recommended for management of certain dose-related lab changes, including elevated liver enzyme levels, neutropenia, and thrombocytopenia.

• Remove prefilled syringe from refrigerator 30 minutes before use or autoinjector 45 minutes before use. Don't warm in any other way.

• Don't use if product contains particulate matter or is cloudy or discolored, or if any part of syringe or autoinjector is damaged.

• Inject full amount in the syringe or autoinjector (0.9 mL).

• Rotate injection sites with each injection; never give into moles, scars, or areas where skin is tender, bruised, red, hard, or not intact. Don't rub injection site.

ACTION

Inhibits interleukin-6–mediated inflammatory processes by decreasing inflammatory markers such as C-reactive protein, rheumatoid factor, and erythrocyte sedimentation rate.

Reactions in bold italics are *life-threatening*. Interactions may have a *rapid onset* or a *delayed onset*.

Route	Onset	Peak	Duration
IV	Unknown	Unknown	Unknown
Subcut	Unknown	3–4.5 days	Unknown

Half-life: IV, 11 to 13 days; subcut, 5 to 13 days.

ADVERSE REACTIONS

CNS: dizziness, headache. **CV:** HTN, peripheral edema. **EENT:** nasopharyngitis, oral mucosa ulcer. **GI:** gastritis, stomatitis, upper abdominal pain, gastric ulcer, diarrhea. **Hematologic:** *thrombocytopenia, neutropenia.* **Hepatic:** elevated LFT values. **Metabolic:** elevated lipid levels, weight gain. **Respiratory:** bronchitis, URI. **Skin:** pruritus, rash, urticaria, injection-site reactions. **Other:** anti-tocilizumab antibody development, infection, infusion-related reactions.

INTERACTIONS

Drug-drug. *Biological DMARDs (anti-CD20 monoclonal antibodies, interleukin-1 receptor antagonists, selective costimulation modulators, TNF antagonists):* May increase risk of serious infection. Don't use together.
Cyclosporine, theophylline, warfarin: May decrease drug levels. Monitor levels closely and adjust dosage as needed.
CYP3A4 substrates (atorvastatin, lovastatin, omeprazole, simvastatin): May decrease levels of these drugs. Avoid use together.
Hormonal contraceptives: May decrease effects of contraceptives. Consider nonhormonal alternatives for contraception.
Live-virus vaccines: No data are available on secondary transmission of infection from live-virus vaccine. Avoid using together.
Drug-herb. *Echinacea:* May decrease effect of immunosuppressants. Avoid combination.

EFFECTS ON LAB TEST RESULTS

• May increase bilirubin, ALT, AST, and lipid levels.
• May decrease leukocyte, platelet, and neutrophil counts.

CONTRAINDICATIONS & CAUTIONS

Boxed Warning Risks and benefits of treatment with tocilizumab should be carefully considered before start of therapy in patients with chronic or recurrent infection. ■
Boxed Warning Patients treated with tocilizumab are at increased risk for developing serious infections (active pulmonary or extrapulmonary TB; invasive fungal infections [candidiasis, aspergillosis, pneumocystis]; or bacterial, viral, and other infections caused by opportunistic pathogens) that may lead to hospitalization or death. Most patients who developed these infections were taking concomitant immunosuppressants, such as methotrexate or corticosteroids. ■
• Contraindicated in patients hypersensitive to drug or its components.
• Months to years after treatment, serious cases of hepatic injury have been observed in patients taking drug IV or subcut, some cases resulting in liver transplant or death. Avoid use in patients with active hepatic disease or hepatic impairment.
• Don't initiate drug in patients with ANC less than 2,000/mm^3 or platelet count less than 100,000/mm^3, or in those with ALT or AST level more than $1.5 \times$ ULN.
🜚 *Alert:* Use cautiously in patients who have been exposed to TB, in those with history of chronic or recurrent infection, serious or opportunistic infection, or underlying conditions that increase risk of infection. Use cautiously in those who have resided or traveled in areas with endemic TB or mycosis.
🜚 *Alert:* Patients with severe or life-threatening CRS frequently have cytopenias or elevated ALT or AST level due to chemotherapy or CRS. Before start of therapy, consider the potential benefit of treating the CRS versus the risks of short-term treatment with tocilizumab.
• Use cautiously in patients at risk for GI perforation.
• Use cautiously in patients with preexisting CNS demyelinating disorders such as MS.
• Drug may increase risk of malignancy.
• For patients older than age 65 being treated with tocilizumab, give drug cautiously because serious infections are more common in this population.
Dialyzable drug: Unknown.

PREGNANCY-LACTATION-REPRODUCTION

• Based on animal data, there may be a risk to the fetus. Use during pregnancy only if benefit outweighs risk to the fetus.
• Encourage patients taking drug during pregnancy to register with the OTIS Autoimmune Diseases in Pregnancy Study (1-877-311-8972).

T

• It isn't known if drug appears in human milk. Patient should discontinue breastfeeding or discontinue drug.

NURSING CONSIDERATIONS

Boxed Warning Serious infections, including TB and bacterial, invasive fungal, viral, and other opportunistic infections, may occur. Monitor patient closely for signs and symptoms of infection during and after treatment. Drug may need to be discontinued if infection occurs during treatment. ■

Boxed Warning Patient should be evaluated and treated, if necessary, for latent TB before start of therapy. Monitor patient for possible TB development during therapy, even if patient tested negative before therapy. ■

• Before starting drug, screen patient for prior HBV infection due to risk of viral reactivation.

• Monitor patient for hypersensitivity reactions, including anaphylaxis.

• Suspect GI perforation in patient with new-onset abdominal symptoms.

• Monitor lipid levels and neutrophil and platelet counts at baseline and every 4 to 8 weeks during therapy.

• For patients with RA, GCA, and SSc-ILD, obtain LFTs before starting drug, every 4 to 8 weeks after start of therapy for first 6 months of treatment, and every 3 months thereafter. Monitor neutrophil and platelet counts before starting drug, every 4 to 8 weeks after start of therapy, and every 3 months thereafter. Monitor lipid levels at baseline and 4 to 8 weeks after starting therapy. Check subsequent levels according to clinical guidelines.

• For patients with PJIA and SJIA, monitor LFTs at the time of second administration and thereafter every 4 to 8 weeks for patients with PJIA and every 2 to 4 weeks for patients with SJIA.

• Measure LFT values promptly in patients with signs and symptoms of liver injury, such as fatigue, anorexia, right upper abdominal discomfort, dark urine, or jaundice.

• Ensure supportive measures are available to treat hypersensitivity reaction.

• Monitor patient closely for signs and symptoms of demyelinating disorders.

• Recommended immunizations (except live-virus vaccines) should be brought up-to-date before beginning therapy.

• Subcut injection is intended for use under the guidance of a health care practitioner.

After proper training, patient may self-inject drug or patient's caregiver may administer drug if a health care practitioner determines that it's appropriate. Assess suitability of patient for subcut home use.

PATIENT TEACHING

🔵 *Alert:* Warn patient to seek immediate medical attention for abdominal pain, fatigue, anorexia, dark urine, jaundice, or signs and symptoms of infection (fever, chills, muscle aches) or hypersensitivity reaction (rash; shortness of breath; swelling of the lips, tongue, or face; chest pain; feeling faint; abdominal pain; vomiting).

• Inform patient that prescriber will order blood tests before and during therapy.

• Teach patient or caregiver proper subcut injection technique and to follow directions in manufacturer's instructions. Caution patient to inform prescriber before administering next dose if signs or symptoms of allergic reaction occur.

• Instruct patient that TB and hepatitis B screening will be needed before therapy begins.

• Advise patient to report pregnancy or plans to breastfeed.

• Tell patient to avoid exposure to infections.

• Remind patient to contact prescriber before scheduling surgery.

• Caution patient to avoid live-virus vaccines during therapy.

• Recommend that patient use nonhormonal contraception during therapy.

tofacitinib citrate 🔳
toe-fa-SYE-ti-nib

Xeljanz, Xeljanz XR

Therapeutic class: Antirheumatics
Pharmacologic class: Janus kinase inhibitors

AVAILABLE FORMS
Oral solution: 1 mg/mL
Tablets: 5 mg, 10 mg
Tablets (extended-release) 🔵: 11 mg, 22 mg

INDICATIONS & DOSAGES
Adjust-a-dose (for all indications): Refer to manufacturer's instructions for toxicity-related dosage adjustments.

➤ **Moderately to severely active RA after inadequate response or intolerance to one or more TNF blockers**
Adults: 5 mg (immediate-release) PO b.i.d. Or, 11 mg (extended-release) once daily.
Adjust-a-dose: Reduce dosage to 5 mg (immediate-release) once daily in patients with moderate or severe renal insufficiency or moderate hepatic impairment, in those receiving concurrent potent CYP3A4 inhibitors, and in those receiving a moderate CYP3A4 inhibitor with a potent CYP2C19 inhibitor.

➤ **Active psoriatic arthritis after inadequate response or intolerance to one or more TNF blockers, in combination with nonbiologic DMARDs**
Adults: 5 mg (immediate-release) PO b.i.d. Or, 11 mg (extended-release) once daily.
Adjust-a-dose: Reduce dosage to 5 mg (immediate-release) once daily in patients with moderate or severe renal insufficiency or moderate hepatic impairment, in those receiving concurrent potent CYP3A4 inhibitors, and in those receiving a moderate CYP3A4 inhibitor with a potent CYP2C19 inhibitor.

➤ **Moderately to severely active ulcerative colitis after inadequate response or intolerance to one or more TNF blockers**
Adults: 10 mg (immediate-release) PO b.i.d. or 22 mg (extended-release) for at least 8 weeks followed by 5 or 10 mg (immediate-release) b.i.d. or 11 or 22 mg (extended-release) once daily depending on therapeutic response. Use lowest effective dose to maintain response. Discontinue after 16 weeks of treatment with 10 mg b.i.d. (immediate-release) or 22 mg once daily (extended-release) if adequate therapeutic benefit isn't achieved.
Adjust-a-dose: In patients with moderate or severe renal insufficiency or moderate hepatic impairment, in those receiving concurrent potent CYP3A4 inhibitors, and in those receiving a moderate CYP3A4 inhibitor with a potent CYP2C19 inhibitor: If patient is taking 10 mg b.i.d. (immediate-release), reduce dosage to 5 mg b.i.d. or, if patient is taking 5 mg b.i.d., reduce dosage to 5 mg once daily. If patient is taking 22 mg (extended-release) once daily, reduce to 11 mg once daily; if patient is taking 11 mg (extended-release) once daily, reduce to 5 mg (immediate-release) once daily.

➤ **Polyarticular course juvenile idiopathic arthritis (pcJIA) after inadequate response or intolerance to one or more TNF blockers**

Children age 2 and older weighing 40 kg or more: 5 mg (tablet or 5 mL oral solution) PO b.i.d.
Children age 2 and older weighing 20 to less than 40 kg: 4 mg (4 mL) oral solution PO b.i.d.
Children age 2 and older weighing 10 to less than 20 kg: 3.2 mg (3.2 mL) oral solution PO b.i.d.
Adjust-a-dose: In patients receiving strong CYP3A4 inhibitors or a moderate CYP3A4 inhibitor with a strong CYP2C19 inhibitor and in those with moderate or severe renal impairment or moderate hepatic impairment, reduce to once-daily dosing.

✴ *NEW INDICATION:* **Ankylosing spondylitis after inadequate response or intolerance to one or more TNF blockers**
Adults: 5 mg (immediate-release) PO b.i.d. Or, 11 mg (extended-release) PO once daily.
Adjust-a-dose: Reduce dosage to 5 mg (immediate-release) PO daily in patients with moderate to severe renal impairment or moderate hepatic impairment, in those receiving concurrent potent CYP3A4 inhibitors, and in those receiving a moderate CYP3A4 inhibitor with a strong CYP2C19 inhibitor.

ADMINISTRATION
PO
• May give with or without food.
• Make sure patient swallows extended-release tablets whole and intact. Don't crush, split, or allow patient to chew tablets.
• May switch patients treated with 5-mg immediate-release tablets b.i.d. to 11-mg extended-release tablets once daily the day after last 5-mg dose. May switch patients treated with 10-mg immediate-release tablets b.i.d. to 22-mg extended-release tablets once daily the day after the last 10-mg dose.
• May switch patients treated with 5 mL oral solution to a 5-mg immediate-release tablet.
• Give oral solution using the included press-in bottle adapter and oral dosing syringe.
• For patients on hemodialysis, give dose after dialysis session. If patient took a dose before dialysis, don't give a supplemental dose after dialysis.
• Store at room temperature. Store oral solution in original bottle and carton to protect from light. Use within 60 days of opening bottle or discard.

T

ACTION
Inhibits activity of Janus kinases, preventing activation of certain intracellular activities that influence immune cell function.

Route	Onset	Peak	Duration
PO (immediate-release)	Unknown	0.5–1 hr	Unknown
PO (extended-release)	Unknown	4 hr	Unknown

Half-life: Immediate-release, 3 hours; extended-release, 6 to 8 hours.

ADVERSE REACTIONS
CNS: headache, paresthesia, insomnia, fever, fatigue. **CV:** HTN, peripheral edema. **EENT:** nasopharyngitis, sinus congestion. **GI:** diarrhea, abdominal pain, dyspepsia, vomiting, gastritis, gastroenteritis, nausea, diverticulitis. **GU:** UTI, increased creatinine level. **Hematologic:** anemia. **Hepatic:** hepatic steatosis, elevated ALT level. **Metabolic:** dehydration, elevated lipid levels, increased CK level. **Musculoskeletal:** muscle and bone pain, arthralgia, tendon disorder, joint swelling. **Respiratory:** URI, dyspnea, cough. **Skin:** rash, erythema, pruritus, cancer, acne, cellulitis. **Other:** infection, herpes zoster.

INTERACTIONS
Drug-drug. *Conivaptan:* May increase tofacitinib serum concentration. Avoid combination.
Immunosuppressants (azathioprine, cyclosporine, corticosteroids, methotrexate, tacrolimus): May increase risk of immunosuppression and serious infection. Use together isn't recommended.
Live-virus vaccines: May increase adverse effects of vaccines. Avoid using together; don't give live-attenuated vaccines for at least 3 months with immunosuppressants.
Moderate CYP3A4 inhibitors plus strong CYP2C19 inhibitors (fluconazole), strong CYP3A4 inhibitors (ketoconazole): May increase tofacitinib plasma level. Decrease tofacitinib dosage per manufacturer's instructions.
Strong CYP3A4 inducers (rifampin): May decrease tofacitinib plasma level. Use together isn't recommended.
Drug-herb. *Echinacea:* May diminish therapeutic effect of immunosuppressants. Avoid combination.

St. John's wort: May decrease serum concentration of CYP3A4 substrates. Consider therapy modification.

EFFECTS ON LAB TEST RESULTS
• May increase creatinine, CK, liver enzyme, and lipid levels.
• May decrease Hb level and lymphocyte and neutrophil counts.

CONTRAINDICATIONS & CAUTIONS
• Contraindicated in patients hypersensitive to drug or its components.
• Use in patients with severe hepatic impairment isn't recommended.
🌢 *Alert:* Use cautiously in patients at risk for serious infection (including those who have resided or traveled in areas of endemic TB or mycoses), those at risk for GI perforation (history of diverticulitis), and those with known malignancy.

Boxed Warning Serious infections leading to hospitalization or death, including TB and bacterial, invasive fungal, viral, and other opportunistic infections, have occurred in patients receiving tofacitinib, especially patients on concomitant immunosuppressants, such as methotrexate or corticosteroids. Evaluate risk before starting therapy in patients with chronic or recurrent infection. If a serious infection develops, interrupt therapy until infection is controlled. ∎

Boxed Warning Lymphoma and other malignancies have been observed in patients treated with tofacitinib. In patients with RA, a higher rate of malignancies was observed compared to those treated with TNF blockers. Patients who are current or past smokers are at increased risk for lymphomas and lung cancers. ∎

Boxed Warning Epstein-Barr virus–associated post-transplant lymphoproliferative disorder has been increasingly observed in patients with renal transplant treated with tofacitinib and concomitant immunosuppressants. ∎

Boxed Warning Patients age 50 and older with RA and at least one CV risk factor treated with tofacitinib have an increased risk of major adverse CV events (CV death, MI, stroke) and thrombosis (PE, venous, and arterial) when compared to use of other TNF blockers in patients with RA. ∎

• When treating patients with ulcerative colitis, use lowest effective dose for shortest

---

duration needed to achieve and maintain therapeutic response.

• Patients shouldn't receive live-virus vaccines during therapy. Update immunizations according to current guidelines before starting drug.

• Use cautiously when giving extended-release formulation to patients with preexisting severe GI narrowing (pathologic or iatrogenic). There have been rare reports of obstructive signs and symptoms in patients with known strictures in association with ingestion of other drugs utilizing a nondeformable extended-release formulation.

• Consider risks and benefits of treatment before initiating therapy in patients with a known malignancy other than a successfully treated nonmelanoma skin cancer or when considering continuing tofacitinib in patients who develop a malignancy.

• Safety and efficacy of oral solution in children for indications other than pcJIA or of extended-release tablets in children haven't been established.

• Effectiveness of tofacitinib as monotherapy hasn't been studied in patients with psoriatic arthritis.

• Use cautiously in patients with a history of chronic lung disease or in those who develop ILD, patients with diabetes, and patients older than age 65 because of increased risk of serious infection.

Dialyzable drug: Unknown.

PREGNANCY-LACTATION-REPRODUCTION

• There are no adequate studies during pregnancy, but drug may cause fetal harm. Use only if clearly needed and potential benefit justifies fetal risk.

• Encourage enrollment in pregnancy exposure registry (1-877-311-8972).

• It isn't known if drug appears in human milk. Patient shouldn't breastfeed while taking drug and for at least 18 hours after final dose of immediate-release form or 36 hours after final dose of extended-release form.

• Based on animal studies, drug may reduce fertility in patients of childbearing potential. It isn't known if this effect is reversible.

NURSING CONSIDERATIONS

Boxed Warning Before therapy, patients should be tested for latent TB. If test is positive, treatment for TB should begin before start of tofacitinib therapy. Monitor all patients for active TB during treatment, even if initial latent TB test is negative. ▪

Boxed Warning Monitor patients for thrombosis, including PE, DVT, and arterial thrombosis. Promptly evaluate patients if signs or symptoms occur and discontinue drug. ▪

▓ Drug may reactivate viral infections such as herpes zoster. Risk of reactivation of herpes zoster appears to be higher in patients treated in Japan and Korea.

• The impact of drug on chronic viral hepatitis reactivation is unknown. Screen for viral hepatitis in accordance with clinical guidelines before starting therapy.

• Monitor patient during and after treatment for signs and symptoms of infection. Interrupt treatment if serious infection occurs; don't restart until infection is resolved.

• Monitor lymphocyte count at baseline and every 3 months thereafter.

• Monitor neutrophil count, platelet, and Hb level at baseline, after 4 to 8 weeks of treatment, and every 3 months thereafter.

• Don't initiate therapy if lymphocyte count falls below $500/mm^3$, ANC falls below $1,000/mm^3$, or Hb level falls below 9 g/dL.

• Monitor LFT results regularly, especially in patients with history of taking DMARDs such as methotrexate. For suspected drug-induced liver injury, stop drug until drug cause is ruled out.

• Assess lipid levels 4 to 8 weeks after drug initiation and then periodically; manage appropriately as needed.

• Monitor patients for GI perforation. Promptly evaluate patients with sudden new-onset abdominal pain or other GI signs and symptoms, especially those also taking NSAIDs.

• Perform periodic skin exam of patients who are at increased risk for skin cancer.

• May cause HTN; monitor BP.

PATIENT TEACHING

Boxed Warning Inform patient that drug may increase risk of major CV events, including MI, stroke, and CV death. ▪

Boxed Warning Warn patient to stop drug and immediately report signs and symptoms of thrombosis (sudden shortness of breath, chest pain that worsens with breathing, swelling of the leg or arm, leg pain or tenderness, red or discolored skin in an affected extremity). ▪

- Advise patient to inform prescriber of all adverse reactions, especially signs and symptoms of infection, abdominal pain, or illness.
- Caution patient to obtain lab tests (CBC, liver enzymes, lipids) regularly as directed.
- Instruct patient to report pregnancy or plans to become pregnant.
- Warn patient to avoid live-virus vaccines.

tolterodine tartrate ℞
toll-TEAR-oh-deen

Detrol✏, Detrol LA

Therapeutic class: Urinary antispasmodics
Pharmacologic class: Antimuscarinics

AVAILABLE FORMS
Capsules (extended-release) ⒹⓃⒸ: 2 mg, 4 mg
Tablets: 1 mg, 2 mg

INDICATIONS & DOSAGES
➤ **Overactive bladder in patients with symptoms of urinary frequency, urgency, or urge incontinence**
Adults: 2-mg tablet PO b.i.d. or 4-mg extended-release capsule PO once daily. Dose may be reduced to 1-mg tablet PO b.i.d. or 2-mg extended-release capsule PO once daily, based on patient response and tolerance.
Adjust-a-dose: For patients with significantly reduced renal function (CrCl of 10 to 30 mL/minute) or those taking a potent CYP3A4 inhibitor, give 1-mg tablet PO b.i.d. or 2-mg extended-release capsule PO daily. For patients with mild to moderate hepatic impairment (Child-Pugh class A or B), give 2-mg extended-release capsule PO daily. For patients with significant hepatic impairment (Child-Pugh class C), give 1-mg tablet PO b.i.d.

ADMINISTRATION
PO
- Give extended-release capsules with liquid because they must be swallowed whole. Don't crush or allow patient to chew capsules.
- Give without regard to meals.

ACTION
Relaxes smooth muscle of bladder by antagonizing muscarinic receptors, relieving symptoms of overactive bladder.

Route	Onset	Peak	Duration
PO	Unknown	1–2 hr	Unknown
PO (extended-release)	Unknown	2–6 hr	Unknown

Half-life: Immediate-release tablet, 2 to 11 hours; extended-release capsule, about 18 hours.

ADVERSE REACTIONS
CNS: headache, fatigue, vertigo, dizziness, somnolence, drowsiness, anxiety. **CV:** chest pain. **EENT:** abnormal vision, dry eyes, sinusitis, dry mouth. **GI:** abdominal pain, constipation, diarrhea, dyspepsia. **GU:** dysuria, urine retention. **Metabolic:** weight gain. **Musculoskeletal:** arthralgia. **Respiratory:** bronchitis. **Skin:** dry skin. **Other:** flulike syndrome, infection.

INTERACTIONS
Drug-drug. *Anticholinergics (ipratropium, tiotropium):* Coadministration may increase frequency or severity of anticholinergic adverse reactions (such as blurred vision, constipation, dry mouth, or somnolence). Monitor patient closely.
Antifungals (itraconazole, ketoconazole, miconazole), CYP3A4 inhibitors (clarithromycin, erythromycin): May increase tolterodine level. Don't give more than 1-mg tablet b.i.d. or 2-mg extended-release capsule once daily of tolterodine if used together.
Class IA (procainamide, quinidine), Class III (amiodarone, sotalol) antiarrhythmics; CYP2D6 or CYP3A4 inhibitors (fluoxetine, ketoconazole): May increase risk of QT-interval prolongation. Use cautiously together.
Drug-food. *Grapefruit juice:* May increase drug level. Monitor patient.

EFFECTS ON LAB TEST RESULTS
None reported.

CONTRAINDICATIONS & CAUTIONS
- Contraindicated in patients hypersensitive to drug or its components or to fesoterodine fumarate extended-release tablets and in those with uncontrolled angle-closure glaucoma or urine or gastric retention.
- Use cautiously in patients with significant bladder outflow obstruction, GI obstructive disorders (such as pyloric stenosis), controlled angle-closure glaucoma, myasthenia gravis, and hepatic or renal impairment.

Reactions in bold italics are *life-threatening*. Interactions may have a *rapid onset* or a ***delayed onset***.

Alert: Anaphylaxis and angioedema requiring hospitalization and emergency medical treatment have occurred with the first or subsequent doses of tolterodine. Discontinue drug and promptly initiate appropriate therapy if difficulty breathing, upper airway obstruction, or fall in BP occurs.

• An additive effect of tolterodine with other drugs that prolong the QT interval cannot be excluded, which increases risk of life-threatening cardiac arrhythmias. Consider this when tolterodine is prescribed to patients with known history of QT-interval prolongation or those who are taking other drugs that prolong the QT interval, such as Class IA (procainamide, quinidine) or Class III (amiodarone, sotalol) antiarrhythmics.

May increase risk of QT-interval prolongation in poor CYP2D6 metabolizers.

• Extended-release capsules aren't recommended for use in patients with severe hepatic impairment (Child-Pugh class C) or those with CrCl of less than 10 mL/minute.

• Effectiveness in children hasn't been established.

Dialyzable drug: Unknown.

Overdose S&S: Dry mouth, severe central anticholinergic effects, QT-interval prolongation.

PREGNANCY-LACTATION-REPRODUCTION

• There are no adequate studies during pregnancy. Use only if potential benefit justifies fetal risk.

• It isn't known if drug appears in human milk. Use cautiously during breastfeeding, taking into consideration benefits of treatment and risk of infant exposure.

NURSING CONSIDERATIONS

• Assess baseline bladder function and monitor therapeutic effects.

• Monitor patient for residual urine after voiding.

• Monitor relevant lab values in patients with hepatic or renal impairment.

• *Look alike–sound alike:* Don't confuse tolterodine with fesoterodine or Detrol with Ditropan.

PATIENT TEACHING

• Advise patient to avoid driving or other potentially hazardous activities until effects of drug are known.

• Instruct patient to immediately report all adverse reactions and signs and symptoms

of infection, urine retention, GI problems, or difficulty breathing.

• Tell patient taking extended-release form to swallow capsule whole and to take with liquids.

• Caution patient to immediately report pregnancy, plans to become pregnant, breastfeeding, or plans to breastfeed during treatment.

---

tolvaptan
tol-VAP-tan

Jinarc ✤, Jynarque, Samsca

Therapeutic class: Vasopressin antagonists
Pharmacologic class: Selective vasopressin receptor antagonists

AVAILABLE FORMS
Tablets: 15 mg, 30 mg, 45 mg, 60 mg, 90 mg

INDICATIONS & DOSAGES
➤ **Hypervolemic and euvolemic hyponatremia (serum sodium level less than 125 mEq/L or symptomatic hyponatremia that has resisted correction with fluid restriction), including patients with HF and SIADH (Samsca only)**
Adults: Initially, 15 mg PO once daily. After at least 24 hours, may increase to 30 mg PO once daily, to maximum dosage of 60 mg PO once daily for no more than 30 days. Titrate dosage at 24-hour intervals to desired serum sodium concentration.

➤ **To slow kidney function decline in patients at risk for rapidly progressing autosomal dominant polycystic kidney disease (ADPKD) (Jynarque only)**
Adults: Initially, 60 mg PO daily as 45 mg taken on waking and 15 mg taken 8 hours later. Titrate to 60 mg plus 30 mg, then to 90 mg plus 30 mg per day if tolerated, with at least weekly intervals between titrations. May be down-titrated based on tolerability.

Adjust-a-dose: When administered with a moderate CYP3A inhibitor, reduce Jynarque dosage per manufacturer's instructions. Use with strong CYP3A inhibitors is contraindicated.

ADMINISTRATION
PO
• Give drug with or without food.

- For patients with hyponatremia, avoid restricting fluids during the first 24 hours of therapy.
- Make sure patient drinks water when thirsty and throughout the day and night if awake.
- Give a missed Samsca dose as soon as possible unless it's near the next scheduled dose; then skip the missed dose and give the next scheduled dose.
- Skip a missed Jynarque dose and give the next dose at its scheduled time.

ACTION

Antagonizes the effect of vasopressin, causing an increase in urine excretion, which results in an increase in free water clearance, a decrease in urine osmolality, and ultimately an increase in serum sodium level.

Route	Onset	Peak	Duration
PO	2–4 hr	2–4 hr	Unknown

Half-life: Dose-dependent, 3 to 12 hours.

ADVERSE REACTIONS

CNS: asthenia, fatigue, dizziness, fever, *stroke,* thirst. **CV:** *intracardiac thrombus, PE, ventricular fibrillation, DVT,* palpitations. **EENT:** dry mouth. **GI:** anorexia, constipation, nausea, *GI bleeding,* abdominal distention, *ischemic colitis,* diarrhea, dyspepsia. **GU:** polyuria, urinary frequency or urgency, urethral hemorrhage, *vaginal hemorrhage,* nocturia. **Hematologic:** *DIC.* **Metabolic:** fluid imbalance, hyperglycemia, hyperuricemia, *diabetic ketoacidosis.* **Musculoskeletal:** *rhabdomyolysis.* **Respiratory:** *respiratory failure.* **Skin:** dry skin, rash.

INTERACTIONS

Drug-drug. *ACE inhibitors, ARBs, potassium-sparing diuretics:* May increase hyperkalemic effect of these drugs. Monitor potassium level closely.
CYP3A inducers (barbiturates, carbamazepine, phenytoin, rifabutin, rifampin, rifapentine): May decrease tolvaptan level. Avoid concomitant use with strong inducers if possible; monitor patient response and adjust dosage as needed.
Digoxin: May increase digoxin level. Monitor patient; adjust digoxin dosage as needed.
Hypertonic sodium chloride solution: May increase risk of a too-rapid increase in serum sodium concentrations. Avoid using together.

Moderate CYP3A inhibitors (aprepitant, conivaptan, diltiazem, erythromycin, fluconazole, verapamil): May increase tolvaptan level. Avoid using together or adjust tolvaptan dosage as needed.
Strong CYP3A inhibitors (ketoconazole): May significantly increase tolvaptan level. Use together is contraindicated.
V_2-agonists (desmopressin): May decrease therapeutic effect of desmopressin. Avoid using with a V_2-agonist.
Drug-herb. *St John's wort:* May decrease drug level. Don't use together.
Drug-food. *Grapefruit juice:* May increase drug level. Don't use together.

EFFECTS ON LAB TEST RESULTS

- May increase glucose, potassium, uric acid, ALT, AST, and bilirubin levels.
- May prolong PT.

CONTRAINDICATIONS & CAUTIONS

Boxed Warning Tolvaptan can cause serious and potentially fatal liver injury. Acute liver failure requiring liver transplantation has been reported.
Boxed Warning Samsca is contraindicated for use in ADPKD outside of the FDA-approved REMS program. Tolvaptan can cause serious and potentially fatal liver injury and shouldn't be prescribed or used outside of the FDA-approved REMS program. Jynarque is available only through the Jynarque REMS program. In Canada, Jinarc is available only through a controlled hepatic safety monitoring and distribution program.
Boxed Warning Samsca should be initiated and reinitiated only in a hospital setting where serum sodium level can be monitored closely.
- Contraindicated in patients hypersensitive to drug or its components.
- Contraindicated in patients with hypovolemia or hyponatremia, and in those who require urgent rise in serum sodium level, are anuric, or are unable to sense or appropriately respond to thirst.
- Jynarque and Jinarc are contraindicated in patients with a history or signs or symptoms of significant liver impairment or injury (doesn't apply to uncomplicated polycystic liver disease).
- Jynarque is contraindicated in patients with uncorrected abnormal blood sodium

concentrations, or uncorrected urinary out-flow obstruction.

• Use cautiously in patients with dehydration; avoid use in those receiving hypertonic saline solution.

• Avoid use in patients with underlying liver disease, including cirrhosis, because the ability to recover from liver injury may be impaired; use not recommended in patients with CrCl of less than 10 mL/minute.

Dialyzable drug: Unlikely.

⚠ *Overdose S&S:* Polyuria, thirst, dehydration, hypovolemia, hypernatremia.

PREGNANCY-LACTATION-REPRODUCTION

• There are no adequate studies during pregnancy. Use only if potential benefit justifies fetal risk.

• It isn't known if drug appears in human milk. Patient shouldn't breastfeed during therapy due to potential for serious adverse reactions in the infant.

NURSING CONSIDERATIONS

Boxed Warning Don't correct hyponatremia (for example, more than 12 mEq/L/24 hours) too rapidly; doing so may cause osmotic demyelination resulting in dysarthria, mutism, dysphagia, lethargy, affective changes, spastic quadriparesis, seizures, coma, and death. Slower correction may be necessary in patients who are susceptible, including those with severe malnutrition, alcoholism, or advanced liver disease. ■

Boxed Warning To reduce risk of significant or irreversible liver injury, perform ALT, AST, and bilirubin blood testing before start of ADPKD treatment, at 2 and 4 weeks after initiation, monthly for 18 months, and every 3 months thereafter. Monitor patient for concurrent signs and symptoms that may indicate liver injury. Prompt action in response to lab abnormalities or signs and symptoms indicative of hepatic injury can mitigate, but not eliminate, risk of serious hepatotoxicity. ■

🕙 *Alert:* Monitor LFT values and assess liver function promptly in patients reporting fatigue, anorexia, right upper abdominal discomfort, dark urine, or jaundice. For suspected liver injury, stop drug immediately, initiate treatment, and investigate cause. Don't reinitiate drug unless the cause for liver injury is definitively unrelated to tolvaptan therapy.

• Immediately discontinue Jynarque for signs or symptoms consistent with hepatic injury or if ALT, AST, or bilirubin level increases to greater than 2 × ULN. Obtain repeat tests within 48 to 72 hours, and continue testing as appropriate. If lab abnormalities stabilize or resolve, restart drug with more frequent monitoring as long as ALT and AST levels remain below 3 × ULN. Don't restart drug in patients who experience signs or symptoms consistent with hepatic injury or whose ALT or AST level exceeds 3 × ULN at any time during treatment, unless there's another explanation for liver injury and the injury has resolved.

• In patients taking Jynarque who have a stable, low baseline AST or ALT level, an increase above 2 × baseline, even if less than 2 × ULN, may indicate early liver injury. Such elevations may warrant treatment suspension and prompt (48 to 72 hours) reevaluation of LFT trends before reinitiation of therapy with more frequent monitoring.

• During Jynarque therapy, if serum sodium level increases above normal range or patient becomes hypovolemic or dehydrated and fluid intake can't be increased, suspend drug until serum sodium level, hydration status, and volume status are within normal range.

• Monitor serum electrolyte levels, volume status, and neurologic status when therapy is begun, during dosage titration, and regularly during therapy.

• Monitor potassium level in patients with potassium level greater than 5 mEq/L and in those who are taking drugs known to increase potassium level.

• After treatment for hyponatremia has ended, patients should resume fluid restriction. Monitor patients for changes in serum sodium level and volume status.

• Monitor patients for weight loss, tachycardia, and hypotension, which may signal dehydration.

PATIENT TEACHING

• Instruct patient in proper drug administration.

• Advise patient to promptly report all adverse reactions, especially difficulty speaking or swallowing, drowsiness, mood changes, trouble controlling body movement, seizures, fatigue, anorexia, right upper abdominal discomfort, dark urine, or jaundice.

T

- Teach patient to inform prescriber of all drugs, herbs, and supplements being taken because of the potential for interactions.
- Advise patient to continue ingestion of fluid in response to thirst during therapy and to resume previous fluid restriction after tolvaptan is discontinued.
- Caution patient to prevent dehydration.
- Tell patient not to stop or restart drug without first consulting prescriber; Samsca should only be restarted in the hospital where sodium level can be monitored closely.
- Inform patient that Samsca should be stopped after 30 days to decrease risk of liver injury.
- Caution patient to report pregnancy or plans to become pregnant.
- Advise patient not to breastfeed.

---

topiramate ⚠
toe-PIE-rah-mate

Eprontia, Qudexy XR, Topamax♦, Trokendi XR

Therapeutic class: Anticonvulsants
Pharmacologic class: Sulfamate-substituted monosaccharides

AVAILABLE FORMS
Capsules, sprinkles: 15 mg, 25 mg
Capsules (extended-release) ⓒ: 25 mg, 50 mg, 100 mg, 150 mg, 200 mg
Oral solution: 25 mg/mL
Tablets ⓒ: 25 mg, 50 mg, 100 mg, 200 mg

INDICATIONS & DOSAGES
Adjust-a-dose (for all indications): For adults, if CrCl is less than 70 mL/minute/1.73 m², reduce dosage by 50%. For patients at high risk for renal insufficiency, obtain an estimated CrCl before dosing. For patients on hemodialysis, supplemental doses may be needed during rapid drops in drug level during prolonged dialysis treatment.

➤ **Initial monotherapy for partial-onset or primary generalized tonic-clonic seizures**
Adults and children age 10 or older: Recommended daily dose is 400 mg (immediate-release) PO in two divided doses (morning and evening). To achieve this dosage, adjust as follows: first week, 25 mg PO b.i.d.; second week, 50 mg PO b.i.d.; third week, 75 mg PO b.i.d.; fourth week, 100 mg PO b.i.d.;

fifth week, 150 mg PO b.i.d.; and sixth week, 200 mg PO b.i.d. Or, using extended-release capsules, initially 50 mg PO once daily. Increase dosage weekly by increments of 50 mg for first 4 weeks, then 100 mg for weeks 5 and 6 to recommended 400 mg once daily.
Children ages 2 to younger than 10 (immediate-release, Qudexy XR extended-release) or children ages 6 to younger than 10 (Trokendi XR extended-release): During titration period, initially 25 mg/day (immediate-release or extended-release) PO nightly for first week. Based on tolerability, can increase to 50 mg/day (once daily for extended-release or 25 mg PO b.i.d. for immediate-release) in the second week. Can increase by 25 to 50 mg/day each subsequent week as tolerated. Attempt titration to the minimum maintenance dosage over 5 to 7 weeks of the total titration period. Based on tolerability and seizure control, can attempt additional titration to a higher dosage (up to the maximum maintenance dosage) at 25 to 50 mg/day in weekly increments. Total daily dosage shouldn't exceed the maximum maintenance dosage for each range of body weight.

Give maintenance doses of extended-release form once daily; give maintenance doses of immediate-release form in two equally divided PO doses daily. If patient weighs up to 11 kg, maintenance dosage range is 150 mg/day to a maximum of 250 mg/day. If patient weighs 12 to 22 kg, maintenance dosage range is 200 mg/day to a maximum of 300 mg/day. If patient weighs 23 to 31 kg, maintenance dosage range is 200 mg/day to a maximum of 350 mg/day. If patient weighs 32 to 38 kg, maintenance dosage range is 250 mg/day to a maximum of 350 mg/day. If patient weighs more than 38 kg, maintenance dosage range is 250 mg/day to a maximum of 400 mg/day.
➤ **Adjunctive treatment for partial-onset or primary generalized tonic-clonic seizures or Lennox-Gastaut syndrome**
Adults and children age 17 and older: Initially, 25 to 50 mg PO daily; increase gradually by 25 to 50 mg/week until an effective daily dose is reached. Adjust to recommended daily dose of 200 to 400 mg PO in two divided doses of immediate-release or once daily of extended-release for adults with partial-onset seizures or Lennox-Gastaut syndrome, or 400 mg PO in two divided doses of immediate-release or once daily of

---

extended-release for adults with primary generalized tonic-clonic seizures.

Children ages 6 to 16 (Trokendi XR) or ages 2 to 16 (Qudexy XR): Initially, 25 mg PO daily at bedtime (based on range of 1 to 3 mg/kg once daily) for first week. Increase dosage at 1- or 2-week intervals by increments of 1 to 3 mg/kg daily. Guide dosage titration by clinical outcome. Recommended daily dose is 5 to 9 mg/kg once daily.

Children ages 2 to 16 (immediate-release): Initially, 25 mg/day (or less, based on a range of 1 to 3 mg/kg/day) PO given at bedtime for 1 week. Increase at 1- or 2-week intervals by 1 to 3 mg/kg daily (given in two divided doses) to achieve optimal response. Guide titration by clinical outcome. Recommended daily dose is 5 to 9 mg/kg, in two divided doses. Maximum, 400 mg/day.

➤ **To prevent migraine headache**
Adults and adolescents age 12 and older: For immediate-release, initially, 25 mg PO daily in evening for first week. Then, 25 mg PO b.i.d. in morning and evening for second week. For third week, 25 mg PO in morning and 50 mg PO in evening. For fourth week, 50 mg PO b.i.d. in morning and evening. Recommended total daily dose is 100 mg.

For extended-release, initially, 25 mg PO once daily. After 1 week, increase to 50 mg daily, then weekly by 25 mg daily until recommended daily dose of 100 mg is reached. Guide dosage and titration rate according to clinical outcome. Allow longer intervals between dosage adjustments if needed.

ADMINISTRATION
PO
• Give drug without regard for food.
• Immediate-release and Qudexy XR capsules may be opened and contents sprinkled on a teaspoon of soft food. Patient should swallow immediately without chewing.
• Patient should swallow Trokendi XR capsules whole and intact. Don't sprinkle capsule contents on food or allow patient to chew or crush capsules; doing so may disrupt the triphasic release properties.
• Don't break tablets, due to bitter taste.
• Use a calibrated measuring device for the oral solution.
• Discard unused portion of oral solution after 60 days.

ACTION
Unknown. May block a sodium channel and potentiate the activity of GABA while inhibiting glutamate and carbonic anhydrase.

Route	Onset	Peak	Duration
PO (immediate-release)	Unknown	0.5–2 hr	Unknown
PO (extended-release)	Unknown	About 20 hr (Qudexy XR); 24 hr (Trokendi XR)	Unknown

Half-life: Immediate-release, 21 hours; extended-release, 31 to 56 hours.

ADVERSE REACTIONS
CNS: anxiety, asthenia, ataxia, confusion, dizziness, fatigue, insomnia, nervousness, paresthesia, psychomotor slowing, somnolence, speech tremor, abnormal coordination, gait abnormality, aggressive reaction, agitation, depression, emotional lability, fever, hyperkinesia, hypertonia, hypoesthesia, personality disorder, vertigo, taste perversion; difficulty with concentration, memory, attention, mood, or language. **CV:** chest pain, flushing. **EENT:** abnormal vision, diplopia, nystagmus, conjunctivitis, secondary angle-closure glaucoma, epistaxis, pharyngitis, sinusitis, rhinitis, dry mouth, increased salivation. **GI:** anorexia, nausea, abdominal pain, constipation, diarrhea, dyspepsia, gastroenteritis, gingivitis, vomiting, gastritis. **GU:** decreased libido, hematuria, impotence, intermenstrual bleeding, menstrual disorder, menorrhagia, urinary frequency, renal calculi, urinary incontinence, UTI, vaginitis, *vaginal hemorrhage,* cystitis. **Hematologic:** anemia. **Hepatic:** increased GGT level. **Metabolic:** weight gain or loss, metabolic acidosis. **Musculoskeletal:** arthralgia, back or leg pain, cramps, muscle weakness, myalgia. **Respiratory:** URI, bronchitis, coughing, dyspnea, pneumonia. **Skin:** acne, alopecia, decreased sweating, pruritus, rash. **Other:** body odor, breast pain, flulike syndrome, hot flashes, infection.

INTERACTIONS
Drug-drug. *Amitriptyline:* May increase amitriptyline level. Monitor response and adjust amitriptyline dosage as needed.
Cannabidiol, cannabis: May enhance CNS depressant effect of topiramate. Monitor therapy.

Carbamazepine: May decrease topiramate level. Monitor patient.

Carbonic anhydrase inhibitors (acetazolamide, dichlorphenamide): May increase risk of metabolic acidosis and cause renal calculus formation. Avoid using together.

CNS depressants (including opioids), magnesium sulfate: May cause CNS depression and other adverse cognitive and neuropsychiatric events. Use together cautiously.

Fosphenytoin, phenytoin: May decrease topiramate level and increase phenytoin level. Monitor levels.

Hormonal contraceptives: May decrease effectiveness. Report changes in menstrual patterns. Advise patient to use another contraceptive method.

Hydrochlorothiazide: May increase topiramate level. Monitor patient and decrease topiramate dosage as needed.

Lithium: May increase serum lithium level. Monitor patient and lithium level closely.

Pioglitazone: May increase pioglitazone level. Monitor patient closely.

Salicylates: May enhance toxicity of both agents. Avoid using together.

Valproic acid: May decrease valproic acid and topiramate level. May increase risk of hypothermia and hyperammonemia. Monitor patient.

Warfarin: May decrease anticoagulation effect. Monitor PT and INR.

Drug-herb. *Kava kava:* May increase CNS depressant effects. Avoid using together.

Drug-food. *Ketogenic diet:* May increase possibility of acidosis or kidney stones. Monitor patient for adverse effects.

Drug-lifestyle. *Alcohol use:* May cause CNS depression and other adverse cognitive and neuropsychiatric events. Discourage use together. Patient shouldn't take Trokendi 6 hours before or after alcohol use.

EFFECTS ON LAB TEST RESULTS
• May increase liver enzyme and ammonia levels.
• May decrease bicarbonate level.
• May decrease Hb level and hematocrit.

CONTRAINDICATIONS & CAUTIONS
• Contraindicated in patients hypersensitive to drug or its components.
• Use cautiously in patients with hepatic and renal impairment.
• Bioequivalence hasn't been demonstrated between Trokendi XR and Qudexy XR.

• Acute myopia associated with secondary angle-closure glaucoma has been reported in adults and children receiving topiramate. Such symptoms as acute-onset decreased visual acuity or ocular pain typically occur within 1 month of therapy initiation. Discontinue drug as rapidly as possible, according to judgment of health care provider.
• Serious skin reactions (SJS and TEN) have been reported. Discontinue drug at first sign of rash, unless not drug related.
• Use cautiously with other drugs that predispose patients to heat-related disorders, including other carbonic anhydrase inhibitors and anticholinergics.
▓ Use cautiously in patients with inborn errors of metabolism or reduced hepatic mitochondrial activity, which may increase risk of hyperammonemia with or without encephalopathy. Risk increases with coadministration of valproic acid.

Dialyzable drug: Yes.

⚠ **Overdose S&S:** Abdominal pain, abnormal coordination, agitation, blurred vision, seizures, depression, diplopia, dizziness, drowsiness, hypotension, lethargy, impaired mentation, speech disturbance, stupor, severe metabolic acidosis.

PREGNANCY-LACTATION-REPRODUCTION
⊕ Alert: Drug may cause fetal harm, including birth defects. Use during pregnancy only if potential benefit outweighs fetal risk. Consider alternative medications with a lower risk of adverse outcomes for these patients. Patients of childbearing potential who aren't planning a pregnancy should use effective contraception while taking this drug.
• Patients who become pregnant during therapy should register with the North American Antiepileptic Drug (AED) Pregnancy Registry (1-888-233-2334).
• Although drug's effect on labor and delivery hasn't been established, development of topiramate-induced metabolic acidosis in the mother or fetus may result in adverse effects and fetal death.
• Tell patients of childbearing potential that drug may decrease effectiveness of hormonal contraceptives. Advise patients using hormonal contraceptives to report change in menstrual patterns.
• Drug appears in human milk, but effect of exposure in infants isn't known. Use cautiously during breastfeeding.

Reactions in bold italics are *life-threatening*. Interactions may have a *rapid onset* or a ***delayed onset***.

NURSING CONSIDERATIONS

🛈 *Alert:* Closely monitor all patients taking or starting antiepileptic drugs for changes in behavior indicating worsening of suicidality or depression. Symptoms such as anxiety, agitation, hostility, mania, and hypomania may be precursors to emerging suicidality.

• Monitor patient for cognitive and neuropsychiatric adverse reactions, including behavior disturbances, somnolence, fatigue, confusion, psychomotor slowing, or difficulty with concentration, memory, speech, or language.

• If needed, withdraw anticonvulsant (including topiramate) gradually to minimize risk of increased seizure activity.

• Monitoring topiramate level isn't necessary.

• Monitor patient for hyperammonemia (unexplained lethargy, vomiting, mental status changes), especially patient taking valproic acid.

• Drug may infrequently cause oligohidrosis and hyperthermia, mainly in children. Monitor patient closely, especially in hot weather.

• Drug may cause metabolic acidosis from renal bicarbonate loss. Factors that may predispose patients to acidosis, such as renal disease, severe respiratory disorders, status epilepticus, diarrhea, surgery, ketogenic diet, or drugs, may add to topiramate's bicarbonate-lowering effects.

• Measure baseline and periodic bicarbonate levels. Monitor patient for signs and symptoms of metabolic acidosis, including hyperventilation, fatigue, anorexia, cardiac arrhythmias, and stupor. If metabolic acidosis develops and persists, consider reducing the dosage, gradually stopping the drug, or offering alkali treatment.

• Drug increases risk of kidney stones; increased fluid intake lowers risk.

• Monitor renal function, electrolyte and ammonia levels, and weight.

• Monitor patient for SCARs, including SJS and TEN. Discontinue drug at first sign of rash, unless clearly not drug related.

• Drug is rapidly cleared by dialysis. A prolonged period of dialysis may cause low drug level and seizures. A supplemental dose may be needed.

• Stop drug if patient experiences acute myopia and secondary angle-closure glaucoma.

• *Look alike–sound alike:* Don't confuse Topamax with Toprol-XL, Tegretol, or Tegretol-XR.

PATIENT TEACHING

• Instruct patient in proper drug administration.

• Tell patient not to consume alcohol within 6 hours before to 6 hours after taking Trokendi XR form.

• Instruct patient to report all adverse reactions and to immediately seek medical attention if blurred vision, visual disturbances, or eye pain occurs, to reduce risk of permanent vision loss.

• Advise patient to immediately report high or persistent fever or decreased sweating.

• Tell patient to use appropriate caution when engaging in activities in which loss of consciousness could result in serious danger to patient or others nearby. Some patients with epilepsy will continue to have unpredictable seizures and may need to avoid such activities entirely.

• Caution patient to drink plenty of fluids during therapy to minimize risk of forming kidney stones.

• Teach patient that a ketogenic diet may increase kidney stone or acidosis risk.

• Advise patient not to drive or operate hazardous machinery until CNS effects of drug are known. Drug can cause sleepiness, dizziness, confusion, and concentration problems.

🛈 *Alert:* Teach patient of childbearing potential to use effective contraception during treatment, and explain about the drug's effect on fetal development. Tell patient to report pregnancy or plans to become pregnant during therapy.

• Caution patient not to stop drug abruptly, to prevent onset of seizures.

SAFETY ALERT!

topotecan hydrochloride
toh-poh-TEE-ken

Hycamtin

Therapeutic class: Antineoplastics
Pharmacologic class: DNA topoisomerase inhibitors

AVAILABLE FORMS

Capsules 🚫*:* 0.25 mg, 1 mg
Injection (lyophilized powder): 4 mg single-dose vial
Injection (solution): 1 mg/mL, 4 mg/4 mL vial

INDICATIONS & DOSAGES
Adjust-a-dose (for all indications): Refer to manufacturer's instructions for toxicity-related dosage adjustments.

➤ **Relapsed small-cell lung cancer (SCLC) in patients with a prior complete or partial response who are at least 45 days from the end of first-line chemotherapy**
Adults: 2.3 mg/m^2/day PO once daily for 5 consecutive days, starting on day 1 of a 21-day cycle. Repeat cycle every 21 days. Round the calculated dose to the nearest 0.25 mg.
Adjust-a-dose: For patients with moderate renal impairment (CrCl 30 to 49 mL/minute), give 1.5 mg/m^2/day. For patients with severe renal impairment (CrCl less than 30 mL/minute), give 0.6 mg/m^2/day.

➤ **With cisplatin, stage IV-B, recurrent, or persistent cervical cancer unresponsive to surgery or radiation**
Adults: 0.75 mg/m^2 by IV infusion on days 1, 2, and 3, followed by 50 mg/m^2 cisplatin by IV infusion on day 1. Maximum recommended topotecan dosage is 4 mg. Repeat cycle every 21 days. Adjust subsequent doses of drug based on hematologic toxicities.

➤ **Metastatic ovarian cancer after failure of first or subsequent chemotherapy; SCLC in patients with platinum-sensitive disease who progressed at least 60 days after initiation of first-line chemotherapy**
Adults: 1.5 mg/m^2 IV infusion daily for 5 consecutive days, starting on day 1 of a 21-day cycle. Maximum recommended dosage is 4 mg. For ovarian cancer, continue until disease progression or unacceptable toxicity.
Adjust-a-dose: For patients with CrCl of 20 to 39 mL/minute, decrease dosage to 0.75 mg/m^2.

ADMINISTRATION
☙ *Alert:* Verify dosage using BSA before administration. Calculate CrCl with Cockcroft-Gault method using ideal body weight.

PO
☙ *Alert:* Hazardous drug; avoid direct contact with capsule contents.
• Give drug without regard to food.
• Don't crush, divide, or allow patient to chew capsules.
• If patient misses a dose or vomits after taking a dose, don't give a replacement dose.

IV
☙ *Alert:* Hazardous drug; use safe handling and disposal precautions.

▼ Reconstitute each 4-mg vial of lyophilized powder with 4 mL sterile water for injection.
▼ Further dilute appropriate volume of solution or reconstituted solution in either NSS or D$_5$W before giving.
▼ Lyophilized form contains no antibacterial preservative; use reconstituted product immediately. Discard any unused portion.
▼ Infuse over 30 minutes and monitor insertion site during infusion. If extravasation occurs, immediately discontinue infusion and notify prescriber.
▼ When giving topotecan with cisplatin, always give topotecan first.
▼ If stored at 68° to 77° F (20° to 25° C) and exposed to normal lighting, reconstituted drug is stable for 24 hours. Protect unopened vials from light.
▼ **Incompatibilities:** Many drugs are incompatible with topotecan. Consult a drug incompatibility reference for information.

ACTION
Interacts with topoisomerase I, inducing reversible single-strand DNA breaks. Drug binds to the topoisomerase I–DNA complex and prevents repair of these single-strand breaks.

Route	Onset	Peak	Duration
PO	Unknown	1–2 hr	Unknown
IV	Unknown	Unknown	Unknown

Half-life: Oral, 3 to 6 hours; IV, 2 to 3 hours.

ADVERSE REACTIONS
CNS: asthenia, fatigue, fever, pain. **EENT:** pharyngitis. **GI:** abdominal pain, anorexia, constipation, diarrhea, nausea, intestinal obstruction, stomatitis, vomiting. **Hematologic:** anemia, *leukopenia, neutropenia, thrombocytopenia.* **Hepatic:** elevated liver enzyme levels, hyperbilirubinemia, *hepatotoxicity.* **Metabolic:** weight gain or loss. **Musculoskeletal:** weakness. **Respiratory:** coughing, dyspnea, pneumonia. **Skin:** alopecia, diaphoresis, rash. **Other:** chills, infection, *sepsis.*

INTERACTIONS
Drug-drug. *BCRP inhibitors (cyclosporine, eltrombopag), P-gp inhibitors (cyclosporine, ketoconazole, ritonavir):* May increase systemic exposure to oral topotecan. Avoid concomitant use.

Reactions in bold italics are *life-threatening*. Interactions may have a *rapid onset* or a ***delayed onset***.

Cisplatin, cytotoxic agents: May increase severity of myelosuppression. Use together with extreme caution. Dosage reductions may be needed.

Fosphenytoin, phenytoin: May decrease topotecan serum concentration. Consider using alternative agent to phenytoin.

G-CSF: May increase myelosuppression and risk of ILD. If G-CSF is to be used, don't start it until 24 hours after last dose of IV topotecan treatment each cycle.

Drug-herb. *Echinacea:* May diminish therapeutic effect of topotecan. Avoid use together.

EFFECTS ON LAB TEST RESULTS
• May increase ALT, AST, and bilirubin levels.
• May decrease Hb level and WBC, platelet, and neutrophil counts.

CONTRAINDICATIONS & CAUTIONS
⊕ *Alert:* Administer drug under the supervision of a health care provider experienced in the use of chemotherapeutic agents. Ensure that appropriate diagnostic and treatment facilities are readily available.
• Contraindicated in patients hypersensitive to drug or its components.
• Use cautiously in patients with renal impairment and in patients with a history of ILD, pulmonary fibrosis, lung cancer, thoracic radiation, and use of pneumotoxic drugs.
• Safety and effectiveness of drug in children haven't been established.
Dialyzable drug: Unknown.
⚠ *Overdose S&S:* Bone marrow suppression.

PREGNANCY-LACTATION-REPRODUCTION
• Drug can cause fetal harm. If used during pregnancy, or if patient becomes pregnant during therapy, apprise patient of potential hazard to a fetus.
• Patient of childbearing potential should use highly effective contraception during treatment and for at least 6 months after final dose.
• Drug may damage spermatozoa, possibly resulting in genetic and fetal abnormalities. Advise males with partners of childbearing potential to use effective contraception during and for 3 months after final dose.
• It isn't known if drug appears in human milk. Advise patient not to breastfeed during treatment and for 1 week after final dose.
• Drug may have both acute and long-term adverse effects on male and female fertility. Patient should seek counseling on fertility

and family planning options before starting treatment.

NURSING CONSIDERATIONS
Boxed Warning Before starting the first course of therapy, patient must have baseline neutrophil count of 1,500/mm^3 or more and platelet count of 100,000/mm^3 or more. Perform peripheral blood counts frequently to monitor patient for bone marrow suppression, primarily neutropenia, which may be severe and result in infection and death. ■
• Don't give subsequent courses until neutrophil count recovers to more than 1,000/mm^3, platelet count recovers to more than 100,000/mm^3, and Hb level recovers to 9 g/dL (with transfusion, if needed).
• WBC colony-stimulating factors may promote cell growth and decrease risk for infection.
⊕ *Alert:* Fatalities due to neutropenic colitis have been reported. Consider possibility of neutropenic colitis in patients presenting with fever, neutropenia, and a compatible pattern of abdominal pain.
⊕ *Alert:* Drug may cause ILD, which may be fatal. Monitor patient for cough, fever, dyspnea, and hypoxia; stop drug if they occur.
• Monitor CBC with differential and platelet count, renal function tests, and bilirubin level before each infusion and regularly during therapy.
• Verify pregnancy status of patients of childbearing potential before therapy.
• If extravasation occurs, discontinue infusion immediately and manage appropriately. Ensure proper needle and catheter placement before and during infusion.
• Monitor patient taking oral topotecan for diarrhea; manage with antidiarrheals at first sign of diarrhea. Withhold drug and reduce dosage based on severity.
• *Look alike–sound alike:* Don't confuse topotecan with irinotecan. Don't confuse Hycamtin with Mycamine.

PATIENT TEACHING
• Instruct patient in proper administration and handling of capsules.
• Urge patient to promptly report all adverse reactions, especially sore throat, fever, chills, or unusual bleeding or bruising.
• Advise patient that although diarrhea is common, it may become severe and should be reported to health care provider.

T

• Caution patient to avoid contact with people with infections.
• Inform patient of potential hazard to the fetus if drug is used during pregnancy, or if patient becomes pregnant while taking drug.
• Advise patient of childbearing potential to use highly effective contraception during treatment and for at least 6 months after final dose and to report known or suspected pregnancy.
• Counsel male patient with a partner of childbearing potential to use effective contraception during and for 3 months after therapy ends.
• Caution patient to avoid breastfeeding during therapy and for 1 week after final dose.
• Teach patient and family about drug's adverse reactions and need for frequent monitoring of blood counts.

---

torsemide ℞
TOR-seh-mide

Soaanz

Therapeutic class: Diuretics
Pharmacologic class: Loop diuretics

AVAILABLE FORMS
Tablets: 5 mg, 10 mg, 20 mg, 40 mg, 60 mg, 100 mg

INDICATIONS & DOSAGES
➤ **Diuresis in patients with HF**
Adults: Initially, 10 to 20 mg PO once daily. If response is inadequate, double dose until desired effect is achieved. Maximum, 200 mg daily.
➤ **Diuresis in patients with chronic renal failure**
Adults: Initially, 20 mg PO once daily. If response is inadequate, double dose until response is obtained. Maximum, 200 mg daily.
➤ **Diuresis in patients with hepatic cirrhosis (except Soaanz)**
Adults: Initially, 5 to 10 mg PO once daily with an aldosterone antagonist or a potassium-sparing diuretic. If response is inadequate, double dose until desired effect is achieved. Maximum, 40 mg daily.
➤ **HTN (except Soaanz)**
Adults: Initially, 5 mg PO daily. Increase to 10 mg if needed and tolerated after 4 to 6 weeks. Add another antihypertensive if response is still inadequate.

ADMINISTRATION
PO
• May give with or without food.
• To prevent nocturia, give drug in the morning.

ACTION
Enhances excretion of sodium, chloride, and water by acting on the ascending loop of Henle.

Route	Onset	Peak	Duration
PO	1 hr	1–2 hr	6–8 hr

Half-life: 3.5 hours.

ADVERSE REACTIONS
CNS: asthenia, dizziness, headache, nervousness, insomnia, weakness. **CV:** ECG abnormalities, chest pain, edema, orthostatic hypotension. **EENT:** rhinitis, sore throat. **GI:** excessive thirst, diarrhea, constipation, nausea, dyspepsia. **GU:** excessive urination, impotence, increased BUN and creatinine levels. **Metabolic:** electrolyte imbalances, including *hypokalemia* and *hypomagnesemia; dehydration*; hypochloremic alkalosis; hyperuricemia; increased glucose level. **Musculoskeletal:** arthralgia, myalgia. **Respiratory:** cough.

INTERACTIONS
Drug-drug. *ACE inhibitors, ARBs:* May increase risk of hypotension and renal impairment. Use together cautiously.
Aminoglycoside antibiotics (gentamycin), cisplatin: May increase ototoxicity. Avoid use together if possible.
Amphotericin B, corticosteroids, metolazone: May increase risk of hypokalemia. Monitor potassium level.
Antidiabetics: May decrease hypoglycemic effect, resulting in higher glucose level. Monitor glucose level.
Chlorothiazide, chlorthalidone, hydrochlorothiazide, indapamide, metolazone: May cause excessive diuretic response, resulting in serious electrolyte abnormalities or dehydration. Adjust doses carefully, and monitor patient closely for signs and symptoms of excessive diuretic response.
Cholestyramine: May decrease absorption of torsemide. Give torsemide at least 1 hour before or 4 to 6 hours after cholestyramine.
CYP2C9 inducers (rifampin): May increase torsemide clearance and decrease plasma

---

Reactions in bold italics are *life-threatening*. Interactions may have a *rapid onset* or a **delayed onset**.

concentrations. Monitor patient closely and adjust torsemide dosage if indicated.

CYP2C9 inhibitors (amiodarone, fluconazole, miconazole, oxandrolone): May decrease torsemide clearance and increase plasma concentrations. Monitor patient closely and adjust torsemide dosage if indicated.

CYP2C9 substrates (sensitive ones such as celecoxib and those with a narrow therapeutic range, such as warfarin or phenytoin): May affect efficacy and safety of substrate. Monitor patient and adjust dosages if necessary.

Digoxin: Electrolyte imbalance caused by diuretic may lead to digoxin-induced arrhythmia. Use together cautiously.

Lithium: May increase lithium level and cause toxicity. Use together cautiously and monitor lithium level.

Methotrexate: May increase methotrexate serum concentration; may diminish therapeutic effects of torsemide. Consider therapy modification.

NSAIDs: May decrease effects of loop diuretics and increase risk of renal failure. Use together cautiously.

Probenecid: May decrease diuretic effect. Avoid using together.

Radiocontrast agents: May increase risk of renal toxicity. Use together cautiously.

Salicylates: May decrease excretion, possibly leading to salicylate toxicity. Avoid using together.

Drug-herb. *Licorice:* May cause unexpected rapid potassium loss. Discourage use together.

Yohimbe: May decrease antihypertensive effect of torsemide. Monitor therapy closely.

EFFECTS ON LAB TEST RESULTS

- May increase BUN, creatinine, cholesterol, glucose, AST, ALT, GGT, and uric acid levels.
- May decrease vitamin B_1, calcium, sodium, potassium, and magnesium levels.
- May decrease RBC, WBC, and platelet counts.
- Can cause false-negative aldosterone/renin ratios.

CONTRAINDICATIONS & CAUTIONS

- Contraindicated in patients hypersensitive to drug, other sulfonamide derivatives, or povidone and in those with anuria or hepatic coma.
- Use cautiously in patients with hepatic disease and related cirrhosis and ascites; sudden changes in fluid and electrolyte balance may precipitate hepatic coma in these patients.
- SCARs (including SJS and TEN), leukopenia, thrombocytopenia, pancreatitis, tinnitus, and ototoxicity have been reported with torsemide use.
- ☙ The antihypertensive effects of torsemide are, on average, greater in patients who are Black than in other patients.
- Safety and effectiveness in children haven't been determined.

Dialyzable drug: No.

⚠ **Overdose S&S:** Dehydration, hypovolemia, hypotension, hypokalemia, hypochloremic alkalosis, hemoconcentration.

PREGNANCY-LACTATION-REPRODUCTION

- There are no adequate studies during pregnancy. Use only if clearly needed.
- It isn't known if drug appears in human milk. Diuretics can suppress lactation. Use cautiously during breastfeeding.

NURSING CONSIDERATIONS

- Monitor fluid intake and output, renal function, electrolyte levels, BP, weight, and pulse rate during rapid diuresis and routinely with long-term use. Drug can cause profound diuresis and water and electrolyte depletion.
- Watch for signs of hypokalemia, such as muscle weakness and cramps.
- Monitor glucose level periodically.
- Consult prescriber and dietitian about providing a high-potassium diet or potassium supplement. Foods rich in potassium include citrus fruits, bananas, and dates.
- Monitor older adults, who are especially susceptible to excessive diuresis with potential for circulatory collapse and thromboembolic complications.
- Monitor patient for tinnitus and hearing loss, which are usually reversible. Higher than recommended doses, severe renal impairment, and hypoproteinemia may increase risk.
- **Look alike–sound alike:** Don't confuse torsemide with furosemide.

PATIENT TEACHING

- Tell patient to take drug in morning to prevent the need to urinate at night.
- Advise patient to change positions slowly to prevent dizziness and to limit alcohol intake and strenuous exercise in hot weather to prevent dizziness.

• Instruct patient to immediately report ringing in ears because it may indicate toxicity.
• Tell patient to report weakness, cramping, nausea, and dizziness.
• Advise patient to check with prescriber or pharmacist before taking OTC drugs.

traMADol hydrochloride
TRAM-uh-dohl

ConZip, Durela✤, Qdolo, Ralivia✤, Tridural✤, Ultram, Zytram XL✤

Therapeutic class: Analgesics
Pharmacologic class: Synthetic centrally active analgesics
Controlled substance schedule: IV

AVAILABLE FORMS
Capsules (extended-release) ⓄⓃⒸ: 100 mg, 200 mg, 300 mg
Solution: 5 mg/mL
Tablets: 50 mg, 100 mg
Tablets (extended-release) ⓄⓃⒸ: 75 mg✤, 100 mg, 150 mg✤, 200 mg, 300 mg, 400 mg✤

INDICATIONS & DOSAGES
⏺ *Alert:* Initiate dosing regimen for each patient individually, taking into account patient's severity of pain, response, prior analgesic treatment experience, and risk factors for addiction, abuse, and misuse. Use lowest effective dosage for shortest duration consistent with individual patient treatment goals.

➤ **Moderate to moderately severe chronic pain**
Adults age 17 and older: Initially, 25 mg (immediate-release) PO in the morning. Adjust by 25 mg every 3 days to 100 mg/day (25 mg q.i.d.). Thereafter, adjust by 50 mg every 3 days to reach 200 mg/day (50 mg q.i.d.). Thereafter, give 50 to 100 mg PO every 4 to 6 hours PRN. Maximum, 400 mg daily.
Adults age 18 and older not taking immediate-release tablets: 100 mg extended-release form PO once daily. Titrate by 100 mg every 5 days to relieve pain. Do not exceed 300 mg/day.
Adults age 18 and older currently taking immediate-release tablets: Calculate the 24-hour tramadol immediate-release dose and initiate a total daily dose of extended-release product rounded down to the next lowest 100-mg increment. Subsequently, individualize

according to patient need. Maximum dose is 300 mg daily.
Adjust-a-dose: For immediate-release form, if CrCl is less than 30 mL/minute, increase dose interval to every 12 hours; maximum is 200 mg daily. For patients with severe hepatic impairment, give 50 mg (immediate-release) every 12 hours. For patients older than age 75, maximum is 300 mg (immediate-release) daily in divided doses. Don't use extended-release form in patients with severe hepatic or renal impairment.

ADMINISTRATION
PO
• Give drug without regard for meals in a consistent manner.
• Extended-release capsules and tablets must be swallowed whole; don't break or crush tablets.

Boxed Warning Avoid dosing errors when giving oral solution; don't confuse "mg" and "mL," which could result in accidental overdose and death. ▮

• Use an oral dosing device or calibrated syringe for solution to correctly measure prescribed amount.
• Patient undergoing dialysis can receive the regular dose on the day of dialysis.

ACTION
Unknown. Thought to bind to opioid receptors and inhibit reuptake of norepinephrine and serotonin.

Route	Onset	Peak	Duration
PO	1 hr	2–3 hr	Unknown
PO (extended-release)	Unknown	10–12 hr	Unknown

Half-life: 7.6 hours; extended-release, 8 to 10 hours.

ADVERSE REACTIONS
CNS: dizziness, headache, somnolence, drowsiness, vertigo, anxiety, asthenia, hypoesthesia, lethargy, CNS stimulation, confusion, coordination disturbance, ataxia, depersonalization, euphoria, malaise, nervousness, sleep disorder, insomnia, fever, paresthesia, tremor, hypertonia, depression, agitation, apathy, pain, restlessness. **CV:** vasodilation, flushing, chest pain, orthostatic hypotension, HTN, peripheral edema. **EENT:** visual disturbances, dry mouth, sore throat, nasal or sinus congestion, rhinorrhea, nasopharyngitis,

---

Reactions in bold italics are *life-threatening*. Interactions may have a *rapid onset* or a ***delayed onset***.

pharyngitis, rhinitis, sinusitis. **GI:** constipation, nausea, vomiting, abdominal pain, anorexia, diarrhea, dyspepsia, flatulence, viral gastroenteritis. **GU:** menopausal symptoms, proteinuria, urinary frequency, urine retention, pelvic pain, UTI, prostate disorder. **Metabolic:** weight loss, hyperglycemia. **Musculoskeletal:** arthralgia, neck pain, back pain, limb pain, myalgia. **Respiratory:** bronchitis, URI. **Skin:** diaphoresis, dermatitis, pruritus, rash. **Other:** chills, hot flash, withdrawal syndrome, accidental injury, fall, flulike symptoms.

INTERACTIONS

Drug-drug. *Anticholinergics (atropine, benztropine, cyclopentolate, darifenacin, fesoterodine):* May increase risk of urine retention or severe constipation and paralytic ileus. Monitor patient closely.

Boxed Warning *Benzodiazepines, CNS depressants:* May cause slow or difficult breathing, sedation, and death. Avoid use together. If use together is necessary, limit dosage and duration of each drug to minimum necessary for desired effect. ∎

Carbamazepine: May decrease tramadol level, decrease effect of carbamazepine, and increase CNS depression. Avoid use together.

CNS depressants, opioids: May cause additive effects. Use together cautiously; tramadol dosage may need to be reduced.

Cyclobenzaprine, neuroleptics, other opioids, SSNRIs, SSRIs, TCAs: May increase risk of seizures. Monitor patient closely.

Boxed Warning *CYP2D6 inhibitors (bupropion, fluoxetine, quinidine):* May decrease therapeutic effect of tramadol. Monitor patient closely for withdrawal signs and symptoms, seizures, and serotonin syndrome. If inhibitor is discontinued, monitor patient for opioid toxicity, including respiratory depression. ∎

Boxed Warning *CYP3A4 inducers:* May decrease tramadol serum concentration. Monitor therapy closely. If inducer is discontinued, consider decreasing tramadol dosage and monitor patient for seizures, serotonin syndrome, sedation, and respiratory depression. ∎

Boxed Warning *CYP3A4 inhibitors :* May increase tramadol serum concentration. Monitor therapy closely. If inhibitor is discontinued, consider increasing tramadol dosage, and monitor patient for opioid withdrawal. ∎

Digoxin: May increase risk of digoxin toxicity. Monitor therapy.

Diuretics: May decrease effectiveness of diuretic. Monitor therapy.

MAO inhibitors: May increase risk of serotonin syndrome. Concomitant use or use with 14 days of MAO inhibitor therapy is contraindicated.

Mixed agonist/antagonist and partial agonist opioid analgesics (buprenorphine, butorphanol, nalbuphine, pentazocine): May reduce analgesic effect of tramadol and precipitate withdrawal symptoms. Avoid use together.

⚠ *Alert:* Serotonergic drugs (amoxapine, antiemetics [dolasetron, granisetron, ondansetron, palonosetron], antimigraine drugs, buspirone, cyclobenzaprine, dextromethorphan, linezolid, lithium, maprotiline, methylene blue, mirtazapine, nefazodone, SSNRIs, SSRIs, TCAs, trazodone, tryptophan, vilazodone):* May increase risk of serotonin syndrome. Use together cautiously and monitor patient for serotonin syndrome.

Vitamin K antagonists (warfarin): May increase anticoagulant effects. Monitor therapy closely.

Drug-herb. *Kava kava:* May increase CNS depression. Monitor therapy closely.

⚠ *Alert: St. John's wort:* May increase risk of serotonin syndrome. Use together cautiously and monitor patient for serotonin syndrome.

Drug-lifestyle. **Boxed Warning** *Alcohol use:* May have additive effects. Don't use together. ∎

EFFECTS ON LAB TEST RESULTS

• May increase BUN, creatinine, GGT, and liver enzyme levels.

• May decrease Hb, sodium, and glucose levels.

CONTRAINDICATIONS & CAUTIONS

Boxed Warning To ensure that the benefits of opioid analgesics outweigh the risks of addiction, abuse, and misuse, the FDA has required a REMS for these products. Under the requirements of the REMS, drug companies with approved opioid analgesic products must make REMS-compliant education programs available to health care providers. Further information on the Opioid Analgesic REMS program is available by calling 1-800-503-0784 or at www.opioidanalgesicrems.com. ∎

• Contraindicated in patients hypersensitive to drug or opioids, in patients with severe renal or hepatic impairment, in patients who are suicidal, and in those with acute intoxication from alcohol, hypnotics, centrally acting analgesics, opioids, or psychotropic drugs.

• Contraindicated in patients with GI obstruction, including paralytic ileus.

• Contraindicated in patients with significant respiratory depression or acute or severe bronchial asthma or hypercapnia in unmonitored settings or where resuscitative equipment isn't available.

Boxed Warning Contraindicated in children younger than age 12 and for postoperative management in children younger than age 18 after tonsillectomy or adenoidectomy. ■

Boxed Warning May cause fatal respiratory depression, especially during initiation or dosage increase. ■

Boxed Warning The effects of concomitant use or discontinuation of CYP3A4 inducers or inhibitors, or CYP2D6 inhibitors with tramadol are complex and require careful consideration of the effects on parent drug, tramadol, and the active metabolite, M1. ■

Boxed Warning Opioids should only be prescribed with benzodiazepines or other CNS depressants to patients for whom alternative treatment options are inadequate. ■

◆ *Alert:* Serious hypersensitivity reactions can occur, usually after the first dose. Patients with history of anaphylactic reaction to codeine and opioids may be at increased risk.

◆ *Alert:* Patients are at increased risk for oversedation and respiratory depression if they snore or have a history of sleep apnea, haven't used opioids recently or are first-time opioid users, have increased opioid dosage requirements or opioid habituation, have received general anesthesia for longer lengths of time or received other sedating drugs, have preexisting pulmonary or cardiac disease, or have thoracic or other surgical incisions that may impair breathing. Monitor patients carefully.

• Use cautiously in patients at risk for seizures or respiratory depression; in patients with increased ICP or head injury, acute abdominal conditions; or renal or hepatic impairment; and in patients with physical dependence on opioids. Withdrawal symptoms may occur if drug is abruptly discontinued.

◆ *Alert:* Drug can cause life-threatening serotonin syndrome.

◆ *Alert:* Use cautiously in patients who are experiencing depression or an emotional disturbance because of the increased risk of suicide.

◆ *Alert:* Drug may lead to rare but serious decrease in adrenal gland cortisol production.

• Drug may cause decreased sex hormone levels with long-term use.

Boxed Warning Avoid use in adolescents ages 12 to 18 with obesity or such conditions as obstructive sleep apnea or severe lung disease or other risk factors that may increase their sensitivity to tramadol's respiratory depressant effects. ■

Boxed Warning Patients who are CYP2D6 ultrarapid metabolizers shouldn't use tramadol because of the risk of life-threatening or fatal respiratory depression. ■

• Use with extreme caution in older adults and in patients with cachexia or debilitation.

Dialyzable drug: 7%.

⚠ *Overdose S&S:* Lethargy, somnolence, stupor, coma, seizures, skeletal muscle flaccidity, respiratory depression, cool clammy skin, miosis, bradycardia, hypotension, cardiac arrest, death.

PREGNANCY-LACTATION-REPRODUCTION

• Safe use during pregnancy hasn't been established. Use only if potential benefit justifies fetal risk.

Boxed Warning Prolonged use during pregnancy can result in neonatal opioid withdrawal syndrome, which may be life-threatening if not recognized and treated according to neonatology expert protocols. If opioid use is required for a prolonged period during pregnancy, advise patient of the risk of neonatal opioid withdrawal syndrome; ensure that appropriate treatment will be available. ■

• Use during breastfeeding isn't recommended due to the risk of serious adverse reactions in breastfed infants, such as excess sleepiness, difficulty breastfeeding, or serious breathing problems that could result in death.

NURSING CONSIDERATIONS

Boxed Warning Monitor patient taking an opioid with a benzodiazepine, CNS depressant, or alcohol for signs and symptoms of respiratory depression, including dizziness, light-headedness, extreme sleepiness, slowed or difficult breathing, or unresponsiveness. ■

Boxed Warning Tramadol exposes patients to the risk of addiction, abuse, and misuse, which can lead to overdose and death. Assess each patient's risk before prescribing; monitor patient regularly for development of abnormal behaviors. ∎

• Reassess patient's level of pain after administration.

• Monitor CV and respiratory status, especially within first 24 to 72 hours of therapy initiation and after dosage increases; adjust dosage accordingly. Withhold dose and notify prescriber if respirations are shallow or rate is below 12 breaths/minute.

☻ *Alert:* Carefully monitor vital signs, pain level, respiratory status, and sedation level in all patients receiving opioids, especially those receiving IV drugs, even those given postoperatively.

• Monitor bowel and bladder function. Anticipate need for stimulant laxative.

• For better analgesic effect, give drug before onset of intense pain.

• Monitor patients at risk for seizures. Drug may reduce seizure threshold.

• In the case of an overdose, naloxone may also increase risk of seizures. Assess the potential need for access to naloxone.

• Monitor patient for drug dependence. Drug can produce dependence similar to that of codeine and thus has potential for abuse.

• Monitor patient for hyponatremia (confusion, disorientation), especially when initiating therapy. Females older than age 65 may be at higher risk.

• Monitor patient, especially patient with predisposing risk factors (diabetes), for hypoglycemia. Monitor blood glucose level and discontinue drug if appropriate.

☻ *Alert:* Don't stop drug abruptly; withdraw slowly and individualize the gradual tapering plan to prevent signs and symptoms of withdrawal, worsening pain, and psychological distress in patients who are physically dependent. Refer to manufacturer's label for specific tapering instructions.

☻ *Alert:* When tapering opioids, monitor patient closely for signs and symptoms of opioid withdrawal (restlessness, lacrimation, rhinorrhea, yawning, perspiration, chills, myalgia, mydriasis, irritability, anxiety, insomnia, backache, joint pain, weakness, abdominal cramps, anorexia, nausea, vomiting, diarrhea, increased BP or HR, increased respiratory rate). Such signs and symptoms may indicate a need to taper more slowly. Also monitor

patient for suicidality, use of other substances, and mood changes.

☻ *Alert:* If patient is taking opioids with serotonergic drugs, watch for signs and symptoms of serotonin syndrome (agitation, hallucinations, rapid HR, fever, diaphoresis, shivering or shaking, muscle twitching or stiffness, trouble with coordination, nausea, vomiting, diarrhea), especially when starting treatment or increasing dosages. Signs and symptoms may occur within several hours of coadministration but may also occur later, especially after dosage increase. Discontinue the opioid, serotonergic drug, or both if serotonin syndrome is suspected.

☻ *Alert:* Monitor patient for signs and symptoms of adrenal insufficiency (nausea, vomiting, loss of appetite, fatigue, weakness, dizziness, low BP). Perform diagnostic testing if adrenal insufficiency is suspected. If adrenal insufficiency is confirmed, treat with corticosteroids and wean patient off opioids if appropriate. Discontinue corticosteroids when clinically appropriate.

• Monitor patient for signs and symptoms of decreased sex hormone levels (low libido, erectile dysfunction, amenorrhea, infertility). If signs and symptoms occur, further evaluate patient.

• *Look alike–sound alike:* Don't confuse tramadol with trazodone or trandolapril.

PATIENT TEACHING

Boxed Warning Caution patient or caregiver of patient taking an opioid with a benzodiazepine, CNS depressant, or alcohol to seek immediate medical attention if patient experiences dizziness, light-headedness, extreme sleepiness, slowed or difficult breathing, or unresponsiveness. ∎

Boxed Warning Advise patient that crushing, chewing, or dissolving extended-release form can cause rapid release of the drug and a potentially fatal dose. ∎

Boxed Warning Tell patient to keep drug away from children. Accidental ingestion of even one dose of tramadol, especially in children, can result in fatal overdose. ∎

☻ *Alert:* Warn patient and caregivers of patient taking tramadol to watch for slow or shallow breathing, difficulty or noisy breathing, confusion, excessive sleepiness, trouble breastfeeding, or limpness. If any of these signs or symptoms occur, tell them to stop drug and seek immediate emergency medical attention.

♻ *Alert:* Discuss with patient and caregiver the availability of naloxone for the emergency treatment of opioid overdose.

• Explain assessment and monitoring process to patient and family. Instruct them to immediately report difficulty breathing or other signs or symptoms of a potential adverse opioid-related reaction.

• Tell patient to take drug as prescribed and not to increase dose or dosage interval unless ordered by prescriber.

• Caution patient who is ambulatory to be careful when rising and walking. Warn outpatient to avoid driving and other potentially hazardous activities that require mental alertness until drug's CNS effects are known.

• Advise patient to check with prescriber before taking OTC drugs because drug interactions can occur.

♻ *Alert:* Counsel patient not to discontinue opioids without first discussing the need for a gradual tapering regimen with prescriber.

♻ *Alert:* Encourage patient to report all medications being taken, including prescription and OTC medications and supplements because drug interactions can occur.

• Advise patient that drug may cause constipation.

♻ *Alert:* Caution patient to immediately report signs and symptoms of serotonin syndrome, adrenal insufficiency, and decreased sex hormone levels.

SAFETY ALERT!

trastuzumab ▨
trass-too-ZOO-mab

Herceptin

trastuzumab-anns
Kanjinti

trastuzumab-dkst
Ogivri

trastuzumab-dttb
Ontruzant

trastuzumab-pkrb
Herzuma

trastuzumab-qyyp
Trazimera

Therapeutic class: Antineoplastics
Pharmacologic class: Monoclonal antibodies

AVAILABLE FORMS
Lyophilized powder for injection: 150-mg single-dose vial, 420-mg multiple-dose vial

INDICATIONS & DOSAGES
Adjust-a-dose (for all indications): If LVEF decreased 16% or more from baseline or if LVEF is below normal limits with a 10% or more decrease from baseline, withhold treatment for at least 4 weeks and repeat LVEF every 4 weeks. May resume treatment if LVEF returns to normal within 4 to 8 weeks and remains at 15% or less decrease from baseline. Discontinue drug permanently for persistent (more than 8 weeks) LVEF decline or for more than three incidents of treatment interruptions for cardiomyopathy.

➤ **HER2-overexpressing metastatic gastric or gastroesophageal junction adenocarcinoma in patients not previously treated for metastatic disease in combination with cisplatin and capecitabine or 5-FU** ▨
Adults: Initially, 8 mg/kg IV infusion. Then, 6 mg/kg IV every 3 weeks until disease progression or intolerable toxicity develops.

➤ **Metastatic breast cancer in patients whose tumors overexpress HER2 protein** ▨
Adults: Loading dose of 4 mg/kg IV infusion. If tolerated, continue with 2 mg/kg IV infusion weekly. If patient hasn't previously received one or more chemotherapy regimens for their metastatic disease, drug is given with paclitaxel.

➤ **After surgical resection of HER2-overexpressing node-positive, node-negative (ER/PR negative or with one high-risk feature) breast cancer** ▨
Adults: During treatment with paclitaxel, docetaxel, or docetaxel–carboplatin, give loading dose of 4 mg/kg IV infusion. Then, 2 mg/kg IV weekly during chemotherapy for the first 12 weeks (paclitaxel or docetaxel) or 18 weeks (docetaxel–carboplatin). One week after the last weekly dose, continue trastuzumab 6 mg/kg IV every 3 weeks for a total of 52 weeks.

Reactions in bold italics are *life-threatening*. Interactions may have a *rapid onset* or a **delayed onset**.

➤ As single agent after surgical resection of HER2-overexpressing breast cancer within 3 weeks of completion of multimodality, anthracycline-based chemotherapy ▨

Adults: Initial dose, 8 mg/kg IV infusion. Then, 6 mg/kg IV every 3 weeks for a total of 52 weeks.

➤ Neoadjuvant treatment of HER2-positive locally advanced, inflammatory, or early breast cancer ▨ ◆

Adults: Initially, 8 mg/kg IV (cycle 1) followed by 6 mg/kg IV every 3 weeks for a total of four neoadjuvant cycles; postoperatively, administer three cycles of adjuvant FEC (5-FU, epirubicin, and cyclophosphamide) chemotherapy and continue trastuzumab to complete 1 year of treatment.

➤ HER2-positive metastatic breast cancer (in combination with pertuzumab and docetaxel) in patients without prior anti-HER2 therapy or chemotherapy to treat metastatic disease ▨ ◆

Adults: Initially, 8 mg/kg IV followed by a maintenance dose of 6 mg/kg IV every 3 weeks until disease progression or unacceptable toxicity.

➤ HER2-positive metastatic breast cancer (in combination with either docetaxel or vinorelbine) ▨ ◆

Adults: Initially, 8 mg/kg IV followed by a maintenance dose of 6 mg/kg IV every 3 weeks until disease progression or unacceptable toxicity (in combination with docetaxel or vinorelbine), or 4 mg/kg IV loading dose followed by a maintenance dose of 2 mg/kg IV weekly until disease progression (in combination with docetaxel).

➤ HER2-positive, hormone receptor–positive metastatic breast cancer (in combination with an aromatase inhibitor) when chemotherapy isn't immediately indicated ▨ ◆

Adults: Initially, 4 mg/kg IV followed by a maintenance dose of 2 mg/kg IV weekly until disease progression (in combination with anastrozole).

➤ HER2-overexpressing metastatic breast cancer (in combination with lapatinib) that had progressed on prior trastuzumab-containing therapy ▨ ◆

Adults: Initially, 4 mg/kg IV followed by a maintenance dose of 2 mg/kg IV every week.

ADMINISTRATION
IV

🜟 *Alert:* Hazardous drug; use safe handling and disposal precautions.

▼ Reconstitute drug with bacteriostatic water for injection, according to manufacturer's instructions for vial size, to yield a multidose solution containing 21 mg/mL. Don't shake vial during reconstitution. Make sure reconstituted preparation appears colorless to pale yellow and free of particulates.

▼ After reconstitution, use single-dose solution without preservative immediately or label multidose vial containing benzyl alcohol with expiration 28 days from date of reconstitution and refrigerate at 36° to 46° F (2° to 8° C).

▼ Discard unused portion in single-dose vial. Avoid use of other reconstitution diluents.

▼ Determine dose and calculate volume of 21-mg/mL solution needed. Withdraw this amount from vial and add it to an infusion bag containing 250 mL of NSS. Don't use D_5W or dextrose-containing solutions. Gently invert bag to mix solution. Store diluted solution in infusion bag containing NSS at 36° to 46° F (2° to 8° C) for no more than 24 hours before use. Don't freeze.

▼ If using 150-mg vial, reconstitute with 7.4 mL of sterile water for injection to yield a concentration of 21 mg/mL; add to 250-mL NSS infusion bag. Use immediately or refrigerate at 36° to 46° F (2° to 8° C) for no more than 24 hours.

▼ Don't give as IV push or bolus.

▼ Infuse loading dose over 90 minutes. If well tolerated, infuse maintenance doses over 30 to 90 minutes.

▼ If patient misses a dose by 1 week or less, give usual maintenance dose as soon as possible; don't wait until next planned cycle. Give subsequent maintenance doses 7 or 21 days later according to the weekly or 3-weekly schedules, respectively. If patient misses a dose by more than 1 week, give a reloading dose as soon as possible followed by maintenance doses 7 or 21 days later according to the weekly or 3-weekly schedules.

▼ Before reconstitution, store vials in refrigerator at 36° to 46° F (2° to 8° C).

▼ **Incompatibilities:** Other IV drugs or dextrose solutions.

T

♣Canada   ◇OTC   ◆ Off-label use   🖉 Photoguide   ⊜Do not crush   *Liquid contains alcohol   ▨ Genetic

ACTION
A recombinant DNA-derived monoclonal antibody that selectively binds to HER2, inhibiting proliferation of tumor cells that overexpress HER2.

Route	Onset	Peak	Duration
IV	Unknown	Unknown	Unknown

Half-life: Unknown.

ADVERSE REACTIONS
CNS: asthenia, dizziness, fever, headache, insomnia, pain, depression, neuropathy, paresthesia, peripheral neuritis, fatigue, dysgeusia. **CV:** peripheral edema, edema, *HF,* HTN, arrhythmias, tachycardia, decreased LVEF, palpitations. **EENT:** epistaxis, dysphagia, pharyngitis, rhinitis, sinusitis, nasopharyngitis, sore throat. **GI:** abdominal pain, anorexia, diarrhea, nausea, vomiting, constipation, dyspepsia, stomatitis, mucosal inflammation. **GU:** UTI, *renal failure.* **Hematologic:** *leukopenia,* anemia, *neutropenia, thrombocytopenia.* **Metabolic:** weight loss, *hypokalemia.* **Musculoskeletal:** back pain, weakness, arthralgia, bone pain, muscle spasm, myalgia. **Respiratory:** dyspnea, cough, URI. **Skin:** rash, acne, nail disorder, pruritus. **Other:** *anaphylaxis,* chills, flulike syndrome, herpes simplex, infection, allergic reaction, infusion-related reaction, accidental injury.

INTERACTIONS
Drug-drug. **Boxed Warning** *Anthracyclines (daunorubicin, doxorubicin):* May increase risk of cardiac dysfunction. Avoid anthracycline-based therapy for up to 7 months after stopping trastuzumab–hyaluronidase. If used together, carefully monitor patient's cardiac function. ■
Myelosuppressive chemotherapy: May increase neutropenic effect of myelosuppressants. Monitor therapy closely.

EFFECTS ON LAB TEST RESULTS
• May decrease potassium level.
• May decrease Hb level and platelet and WBC counts.

CONTRAINDICATIONS & CAUTIONS
• Contraindicated in patients hypersensitive to drug.
• Use cautiously in older adults and in patients with cardiac dysfunction.

Boxed Warning Drug can cause serious and fatal infusion reactions and pulmonary toxicity. ■
• Use with extreme caution in patients with pulmonary compromise, symptomatic intrinsic pulmonary disease (such as asthma, COPD), or extensive tumor involvement of the lungs.
Boxed Warning Drug can cause subclinical and clinical HF, with greatest risk when administered concurrently with anthracyclines. ■
• Safety and effectiveness in children haven't been established.
Dialyzable drug: Unknown.

PREGNANCY-LACTATION-REPRODUCTION
Boxed Warning Exposure to drug during pregnancy can result in oligohydramnios, in some cases complicated by pulmonary hypoplasia, skeletal abnormalities, and neonatal death. Advise patient of these risks and the need for effective contraception. ■
• Verify pregnancy status before start of therapy.
• Advise patient of childbearing potential to use effective contraception during treatment and for 7 months after final dose.
• If drug is used during pregnancy, or if patient becomes pregnant during therapy or within 7 months after final dose, fetal harm can occur. Immediately report Herceptin exposure to the Genentech Adverse Event Line (1-888-835-2555).
• It isn't known if drug appears in human milk. Patient should discontinue breastfeeding or discontinue drug.

NURSING CONSIDERATIONS
Boxed Warning Evaluate LVEF before and during treatment. Discontinue drug in patients receiving adjuvant therapy and withhold drug in those with metastatic disease for clinically significant decreases in LVEF. ■
• Assess LVEF by echocardiogram or MUGA scan before therapy, every 3 months during therapy, and when therapy ends.
• Repeat LVEF measurement at 4-week intervals if drug is withheld for significant left ventricular cardiac dysfunction.
• Assess LVEF every 6 months for 2 years after therapy ends when drug is used in adjuvant therapy.
• Monitor patient receiving both drug and chemotherapy closely for cardiac dysfunction

---

Reactions in bold italics are *life-threatening*. Interactions may have a *rapid onset* or a *delayed onset*.

or failure, anemia, renal toxicity, leukopenia, diarrhea, and infection.

⌧ Drug is only indicated in tumors with HER2 protein overexpression or HER2 gene amplification. Assessment of tumor specimens should be performed using FDA-approved tests specific for breast or gastric cancers by labs with demonstrated proficiency to obtain reliable results.

Boxed Warning Signs and symptoms of serious infusion reactions and pulmonary toxicity usually occur during or within 24 hours of infusion. Interrupt infusion if patient experiences dyspnea or clinically significant hypotension and monitor patient until signs and symptoms completely resolve. Discontinue drug for anaphylaxis, angioedema, interstitial pneumonitis, or ARDS. ∎

• Assess for first-infusion symptom complex, commonly consisting of chills or fever. Other signs or symptoms include nausea, vomiting, pain, rigors, headache, dizziness, dyspnea, hypotension, rash, and asthenia and occur infrequently with subsequent infusions.

• For mild to moderate infusion reaction, decrease infusion rate. For dyspnea and hypotension, interrupt infusion. For severe infusion reaction, discontinue drug.

• *Look alike–sound alike:* Don't confuse trastuzumab with ado-trastuzumab emtansine.

PATIENT TEACHING

• Tell patient about risk of first-dose infusion-related adverse reactions and to report all adverse reactions to prescriber.

• Urge patient to notify prescriber immediately if signs or symptoms of heart problems occur, such as shortness of breath, increased cough, or swelling in arms or legs. Tell patient that these effects can occur after therapy ends.

• Advise patient to stop breastfeeding during therapy and for 7 months after last dose.

Boxed Warning Advise patient of the fetal risks of drug exposure and the need for effective contraception. ∎

• Tell patient to avoid pregnancy during therapy and for 7 months after last dose and to notify prescriber immediately if pregnancy occurs during this time.

SAFETY ALERT!

trastuzumab–hyaluronidase-oysk ⌧
tras-TOOZ-ue-mab/hye-al-ur-ON-i-dase

Herceptin Hylecta

Therapeutic class: Antineoplastics
Pharmacologic class: Monoclonal antibodies–endoglycosidases

AVAILABLE FORMS
Injection: 600 mg trastuzumab and 10,000 units hyaluronidase/5 mL in single-dose vial

INDICATIONS & DOSAGES
Adjust-a-dose (for all indications): Withhold drug for at least 4 weeks if there is a 16% or more absolute decrease in LVEF from pretreatment values or if LVEF is below institutional limits of normal and there is a 10% or more absolute decrease in LVEF from pretreatment values. May resume therapy within 4 to 8 weeks if LVEF returns to normal limits and the absolute decrease in LVEF from baseline is 15% or less. Permanently discontinue therapy for a persistent (more than 8 weeks) LVEF decline or for suspension of therapy on more than three occasions for cardiomyopathy.

➤ **Adjuvant treatment of HER2 overexpressing node-positive or node-negative (ER/PR-negative or with one high-risk feature) breast cancer as part of a treatment regimen consisting of doxorubicin, cyclophosphamide, and either paclitaxel or docetaxel; as part of a treatment regimen with docetaxel and carboplatin; or as a single agent after multimodality anthracycline-based therapy** ⌧
Adults: 600 mg trastuzumab/10,000 units hyaluronidase subcut once every 3 weeks for 52 weeks or until disease recurrence. Extending treatment in adjuvant breast cancer beyond 1 year isn't recommended.

➤ **First-line treatment of HER2-overexpressing metastatic breast cancer in combination with paclitaxel or as a single agent for treatment of HER2-overexpressing breast cancer in patients who have received one or more chemotherapy regimens for metastatic disease** ⌧

T

Adults: 600 mg trastuzumab/10,000 units hyaluronidase subcut once every 3 weeks until disease progression.

ADMINISTRATION
Subcutaneous
🛈 *Alert:* Hazardous drug; use safe handling and disposal precautions.

- Don't administer intravenously.
- Drug isn't interchangeable with conventional trastuzumab products or ado-trastuzumab emtansine.
- Drug should be administered by a health care professional.
- Inspect visually for particulate matter and discoloration before administration; don't use vial if abnormalities are present.
- Discard any unused portion remaining in vial; vial is for single use only.
- To avoid needle clogging, attach the hypodermic injection needle to the syringe immediately before administration. Drug is compatible with syringes made with polypropylene and polycarbonate and with stainless steel transfer and injection needles.
- Withdraw solution from the vial and into the syringe; replace the transfer needle with a syringe closing cap. Label the syringe with the peel-off sticker.
- Alternate injection site between left and right thigh.
- Give new injections at least 1 inch (2.5 cm) from the old previous site on healthy skin and never into areas where the skin is red, bruised, tender, or hard, or where there are moles or scars.
- Administer dose subcut over approximately 2 to 5 minutes.
- Can store the prepared syringe in the refrigerator at 36° to 46° F (2° to 8° C) for up to 24 hours and subsequently at 68° to 77° F (20° to 25° C) for up to 4 hours. Protect from light. Don't shake or freeze.
- If one dose is missed, give the next dose as soon as possible. The interval between doses shouldn't be less than 3 weeks.

ACTION
Trastuzumab is a HER2/neu receptor antagonist that inhibits the proliferation of human tumor cells that overexpress HER2. Hyaluronidase is an enzyme shown to increase the absorption rate of a trastuzumab product into the systemic circulation.

Route	Onset	Peak	Duration
Subcut (trastuzumab)	Unknown	3 days	Unknown
Subcut (hyaluronidase)	Unknown	Unknown	24–48 hr

Half-life: trastuzumab, unknown; hyaluronan, 0.5 day.

ADVERSE REACTIONS
CNS: asthenia, fatigue, headache, fever, chills, dizziness, dysgeusia, insomnia, neuropathy, peripheral neuritis, paresthesia, pain, depression. **CV:** HTN, left ventricular dysfunction, *HF,* flushing, arrhythmia, tachycardia, edema. **EENT:** epistaxis, nasal inflammation/discomfort, sinusitis, pharyngitis, rhinitis. **GI:** nausea, diarrhea, vomiting, stomatitis, constipation, mucosal inflammation, abdominal pain, dyspepsia, decreased appetite. **GU:** UTI, irregular menstruation, amenorrhea. **Hematologic:** *neutropenia,* anemia, *leukopenia, granulocytopenia, febrile neutropenia.* **Hepatic:** abnormal LFT values. **Musculoskeletal:** myalgia, arthralgia, back pain, extremity pain, bone pain. **Respiratory:** cough, dyspnea, URI, bronchitis. **Skin:** alopecia, rash, radiation skin injury, incision-site pain and complications, cellulitis, nail disorder, pruritus, skin discoloration, acne, injection-site reactions, erythema. **Other:** accidental injury, *hypersensitivity reactions,* herpes simplex, viral infection, infection, flulike syndrome.

INTERACTIONS
Drug-drug. `Boxed Warning` *Anthracyclines (daunorubicin, doxorubicin):* May increase risk of cardiac dysfunction. Avoid anthracycline-based therapy for up to 7 months after stopping trastuzumab–hyaluronidase. If used together, carefully monitor patient's cardiac function. ∎
Myelosuppressive chemotherapy: May increase neutropenic effect of myelosuppressants. Monitor therapy closely.

EFFECTS ON LAB TEST RESULTS
- May increase ALT level.
- May decrease WBC and RBC counts.

CONTRAINDICATIONS & CAUTIONS
`Boxed Warning` Drug can cause subclinical and clinical HF, with greatest risk when administered concurrently with anthracyclines. ∎

Reactions in bold italics are *life-threatening*. Interactions may have a *rapid onset* or a **delayed onset**.

Boxed Warning Drug can cause serious and fatal pulmonary toxicity, including dyspnea, interstitial pneumonitis, pulmonary infiltrates, pleural effusions, noncardiogenic pulmonary edema, pulmonary insufficiency and hypoxia, ARDS, and pulmonary fibrosis. Patients with symptomatic intrinsic lung disease or with extensive tumor involvement of the lungs, resulting in dyspnea at rest, appear to have more severe toxicity.

• May exacerbate chemotherapy-induced neutropenia.

• Severe administration-related reactions, including hypersensitivity and anaphylaxis, have been reported. Patients experiencing dyspnea at rest due to complications of advanced malignancy and comorbidities may be at increased risk for a severe or fatal administration-related reaction.

• Safety and effectiveness in children haven't been studied.

• Patients age 65 and older are at increased risk for cardiac dysfunction.

Dialyzable drug: Unknown.

PREGNANCY-LACTATION-REPRODUCTION

Boxed Warning Drug can cause fetal harm (oligohydramnios and pulmonary hypoplasia, skeletal abnormalities) and neonatal death. Verify pregnancy status before start of treatment. Apprise patients who are pregnant and patients of childbearing potential that exposure to these drugs during pregnancy or within 7 months before conception can result in fetal harm.

Boxed Warning Patients of childbearing potential should use effective contraception during treatment and for 7 months after final dose.

• If drug is administered during pregnancy, or if patient becomes pregnant while receiving drug or within 7 months after the final dose, health care providers and patient should immediately report exposure to Genentech pregnancy pharmacovigilance program (1-888-835-2555).

• There is no information regarding the presence of trastuzumab or hyaluronidase in human milk, the effects on the infant who is breastfed, or the effects on milk production during therapy or within 7 months of therapy.

NURSING CONSIDERATIONS

• Verify pregnancy status before start of treatment.

⊕ Alert: Monitor patients for systemic hypersensitivity reactions, especially during the first dose. Permanently discontinue drug in patients who experience anaphylaxis or severe hypersensitivity reactions. Medications and emergency equipment should be immediately available.

Boxed Warning Monitor patients for pulmonary toxicity, which usually occurs during or within 24 hours of administration. Discontinue drug for anaphylaxis, angioedema, interstitial pneumonitis, or ARDS and monitor patient until symptoms completely resolve.

Boxed Warning Evaluate LVEF before and during treatment. Discontinue drug in patients receiving adjuvant therapy; withhold drug in patients with metastatic disease for clinically significant decreases in LVEF.

• Obtain thorough baseline cardiac assessment, including history, physical exam, and determination of LVEF by echocardiogram or MUGA scan. Obtain baseline LVEF measurement immediately before initiation of therapy, then every 3 months during and upon completion of therapy. Repeat LVEF measurement at 4-week intervals if therapy is withheld for significant left ventricular cardiac dysfunction. Obtain LVEF measurements every 6 months for at least 2 years after completion of therapy as a component of adjuvant therapy.

• *Look alike–sound alike:* Don't confuse trastuzumab–hyaluronidase-oysk with ado-trastuzumab emtansine or intravenous trastuzumab.

PATIENT TEACHING

Boxed Warning Advise patient to immediately report signs and symptoms of cardiotoxicity, including new-onset or worsening shortness of breath, cough, swelling of the ankles or legs, swelling of the face, palpitations, weight gain of more than 5 pounds in 24 hours, dizziness, or loss of consciousness.

Boxed Warning Warn patient who is pregnant and patient of childbearing potential of the fetal risk from exposure to drug during pregnancy or within 7 months before conception.

Boxed Warning Caution patient of childbearing potential to use effective contraception during treatment and for 7 months after the final dose.

• Teach patient that pregnancy testing will be needed before therapy begins and to immediately report known or suspected pregnancy.

T

• Advise patient to immediately report signs and symptoms of hypersensitivity and administration-related reactions, including dizziness, nausea, chills, fever, vomiting, diarrhea, urticaria, angioedema, breathing problems, or chest pain.

traZODone hydrochloride
TRAYZ-oh-dohn

Therapeutic class: Antidepressants
Pharmacologic class: Serotonin reuptake inhibitor

AVAILABLE FORMS
Tablets ⓄⓃⒸ: 50 mg, 100 mg, 150 mg, 300 mg

INDICATIONS & DOSAGES
➤ **Major depressive disorder**
Adults: Initially, 150 mg PO daily in divided doses; then increased by 50 mg daily every 3 to 4 days, as needed. Dose ranges from 150 to 400 mg daily. Maximum, 600 mg daily for inpatients and 400 mg daily for outpatients.
Adjust-a-dose: After achieving adequate response, may gradually reduce dosage depending on therapeutic response.

ADMINISTRATION
PO
• Give drug shortly after meals or a light snack for optimal absorption and to decrease risk of dizziness.
• If drowsiness occurs, may give a large portion of the dose at bedtime.
• Make sure patient swallows tablets whole or breaks them along the score lines. Tablets shouldn't be chewed or crushed.

ACTION
Unknown. Inhibits CNS neuronal uptake of serotonin; not a tricyclic derivative.

Route	Onset	Peak	Duration
PO	Unknown	1–2 hr	Unknown

Half-life: 5 to 9 hours.

ADVERSE REACTIONS
CNS: drowsiness, dizziness, nervousness, fatigue, confusion, decreased concentration, malaise, tremor, headache, insomnia, syncope, disorientation, incoordination. **CV:** orthostatic hypotension, HTN, edema. **EENT:** blurred vision, red or itchy eyes, tinnitus, dry mouth, nasal congestion. **GI:** constipation, nausea, vomiting, anorexia, diarrhea. **Hematologic:** anemia. **Metabolic:** weight gain or loss. **Musculoskeletal:** aches, pains. **Skin:** rash, urticaria, diaphoresis.

INTERACTIONS
Drug-drug. *Amphetamines, antipsychotics, buspirone, dextromethorphan, dihydroergotamine, lithium salts, meperidine, opioid analgesics, SSRIs or SSNRIs (duloxetine, venlafaxine), sumatriptan (and other 5-HT₃ antagonists), TCAs, tramadol, tryptophan:* May increase the risk of serotonin syndrome. Avoid combining drugs that increase the availability of serotonin in the CNS; monitor patient closely if used together.
Anticoagulants (aspirin, clopidogrel, dabigatran, NSAIDs, rivaroxaban), antiplatelet agents: May increase risk of bleeding. Monitor patient closely.
Antihypertensives: May increase hypotensive effect of trazodone. Antihypertensive dosage may need to be decreased.
Clonidine, CNS depressants: May enhance CNS depression. Avoid using together.
CYP3A4 inducers (carbamazepine, phenytoin, rifampin): May reduce trazodone level. Monitor patient closely; may need to increase trazodone dose.
CYP3A4 inhibitors (clarithromycin, conivaptan, ketoconazole): May slow the clearance of trazodone and increase trazodone level. May cause nausea, hypotension, and fainting. Consider decreasing trazodone dose. Avoid combination with conivaptan.
Digoxin, fosphenytoin, phenytoin: May increase levels of these drugs. Watch for toxicity.
Drugs that prolong QTc interval (antiarrhythmics [amiodarone, disopyramide, procainamide, quinidine, sotalol], chlorpromazine, gatifloxacin, thioridazine, ziprasidone): May increase QTc-interval prolonging effect and risk of ventricular arrhythmias. Consider therapy modification.
Linezolid, methylene blue: May cause serotonin syndrome. Don't use together.
⚠ *Alert:* MAO inhibitors (isocarboxazid, methylene blue, selegiline): Serious and sometimes fatal reactions have occurred. Allow at least 14 days between discontinuing an MAO inhibitor and starting trazodone and at least 14 days after stopping trazodone before starting an MAO inhibitor.

Reactions in bold italics are *life-threatening*. Interactions may have a *rapid onset* or a *delayed onset*.

Protease inhibitors (amprenavir, atazanavir, fosamprenavir, lopinavir–ritonavir, nelfinavir, ritonavir, saquinavir): May increase trazodone levels and adverse effects. Monitor patient and adjust trazodone dose, as needed.
Warfarin: May increase risk of bleeding. Monitor INR closely.
Drug-herb. *Ginkgo biloba:* May cause sedation. Discourage use together.
St. John's wort: May cause serotonin syndrome. Discourage use together.
Drug-lifestyle. *Alcohol use:* May enhance CNS depression. Discourage use together.

EFFECTS ON LAB TEST RESULTS
• May increase amylase, bilirubin, ALT, and AST levels.
• May decrease sodium level.
• May decrease Hb level.
• May increase WBC count.
• May cause false-positive urine test for amphetamine/methamphetamine.

CONTRAINDICATIONS & CAUTIONS
• Contraindicated in patients hypersensitive to drug.
• Avoid use in patients with a history of arrhythmias, symptomatic bradycardia, hypokalemia, hypomagnesemia, or known QT-interval prolongation; in combination with drugs that prolong QT interval; or during initial recovery phase of MI. Drug may increase risk of arrhythmias and prolong QTc interval.
◑ Alert: Concomitant use with linezolid or methylene blue can cause serotonin syndrome. Use drug with linezolid or methylene blue only for life-threatening or urgent conditions when the potential benefits outweigh the risks of toxicity.
• Use cautiously in patients at risk for suicide, in patients with renal or hepatic impairment, in those with a history of seizures, and with medications that may lower seizure threshold.
• Drug may increase risk of mixed-manic episodes. Screen patients for personal or family history of bipolar disorder, mania, or hypomania before starting therapy.
• May cause mild pupillary dilation, which may trigger an angle-closure attack in patient with anatomically narrow angles who doesn't have a patent iridectomy.
Dialyzable drug: Unlikely.
⚠ Overdose S&S: Priapism, respiratory arrest, seizures, ECG changes, drowsiness, vomiting.

PREGNANCY-LACTATION-REPRODUCTION
• There are no adequate studies during pregnancy. Use only if clearly needed and potential benefit justifies fetal risk.
• Encourage patients exposed to antidepressants during pregnancy to enroll in the National Pregnancy Registry for Antidepressants (844-405-6185 or https://womensmentalhealth.org/clinical-and-research-programs/pregnancyregistry/antidepressants/).
• Drug may appear in human milk. Use cautiously during breastfeeding.

NURSING CONSIDERATIONS
• Monitor patient for signs and symptoms of serotonin syndrome (mental status changes, tachycardia, labile BP, hyperreflexia, incoordination, nausea, vomiting, diarrhea) or NMS (hyperthermia, muscle rigidity, rapidly fluctuating vital signs, mental status change). If these signs and symptoms occur, immediately discontinue trazodone and any other serotonergic, antidopaminergic, or antipsychotic drugs.
• Using trazodone for depression in a patient who is bipolar can trigger a mixed-manic episode. If patient develops manic symptoms, withhold trazodone and initiate appropriate therapy.
◑ Alert: If linezolid or methylene blue must be given, stop trazodone and monitor patient for serotonin toxicity for 2 weeks, or until 24 hours after the last dose of methylene blue or linezolid, whichever comes first. May resume trazodone 24 hours after last dose of methylene blue or linezolid.
• Record mood changes. Monitor patient for suicidality and allow only minimum supply of drug.
Boxed Warning Drug may increase risk of suicidality in children, adolescents, and young adults ages 18 to 24, especially during the first few months of treatment, especially those with major depressive disorder or other psychiatric disorder. Drug isn't approved for use in children. ▪
• Consider evaluating patients who haven't had an iridectomy for narrow-angle glaucoma risk factors.
• *Look alike–sound alike:* Don't confuse trazodone hydrochloride with tramadol hydrochloride. Don't confuse trazodone with ziprasidone.

PATIENT TEACHING
• Instruct patient in safe drug administration.
● *Alert:* Tell patient to report a persistent, painful erection (priapism); immediate intervention may be needed.
● *Alert:* Advise patient to immediately report signs and symptoms of serotonin toxicity and NMS.
• Warn patient to avoid activities that require alertness and good coordination until effects of drug are known.
Boxed Warning Teach caregivers to recognize and report suicidality. ■
• Tell patient that it might take up to 6 weeks to see therapeutic effect if used for depression.
• Advise patient not to stop drug abruptly in order to avoid withdrawal symptoms.
• Caution patient to avoid alcohol because it will increase sedation.
• Instruct patient to report pregnancy, plans to become pregnant, breastfeeding, or plans to breastfeed during therapy.

tretinoin (retinoic acid, vitamin A acid)
TRET-i-noyn

Altreno, Atralin, Avita, Renova, Retin-A, Retin-A Micro, StieVA-A✤

Therapeutic class: Antiacne drugs
Pharmacologic class: Retinoids

AVAILABLE FORMS
Cream: 0.01%✤, 0.02%, 0.025%, 0.05%, 0.1%
Gel: 0.01%, 0.025%, 0.04%, 0.05%
Lotion: 0.05%
Microsphere gel: 0.04%, 0.06%, 0.08%, 0.1%

INDICATIONS & DOSAGES
➤ **Acne vulgaris (except Renova)**
Adults: Clean affected area and lightly apply once daily at bedtime.
Children age 12 and older (Retin-A Micro, StieVA-A): Clean affected area and lightly apply once daily at bedtime.
Children age 10 and older (Atralin): Clean affected area and lightly apply once daily at bedtime.
Children age 9 and older (Altreno): Apply a thin layer to the affected areas once daily.

➤ **Adjunctive use in the mitigation of fine facial wrinkles in patients who use comprehensive skin care and sunlight avoidance programs (Renova)**
Adults: Apply a small, pea-size amount (¼ inch or 5 mm in diameter) to cover the entire face lightly, once daily in the evening.

ADMINISTRATION
Topical
● *Alert:* Hazardous drug; use safe handling and disposal precautions.
• Clean area thoroughly before application, and avoid getting drug in eyes, mouth, paranasal creases, or mucous membranes.
• Patients using Renova should gently wash their faces with a mild soap, pat the skin dry, and wait 20 to 30 minutes before applying medication.

ACTION
Inhibits comedones by increasing epidermal cell mitosis and turnover.

Route	Onset	Peak	Duration
Topical	Unknown	Unknown	Unknown

Half-life: Unknown.

ADVERSE REACTIONS
Skin: dry skin, feeling of warmth, slight stinging, local erythema, pruritus, local skin exfoliation or desquamation, application-site pain, chapping, swelling, blistering, crusting, temporary hyperpigmentation or hypopigmentation, burning sensation, skin irritation, dermatitis, photosensitivity.

INTERACTIONS
Drug-drug. *Multivitamins:* May increase adverse effects of retinoic acid. Avoid combination.
Topical drugs containing benzoyl peroxide, resorcinol, salicylic acid, or sulfur: May increase risk of skin irritation. Avoid using together.
Topical minoxidil or photosensitizing drugs (fluoroquinolones, phenothiazines, sulfonamides, tetracyclines, thiazides): May increase risk of skin irritation. Avoid using together.
Drug-food. *Vitamin A:* Vitamin A supplementation can cause toxicity. Avoid excessive intake of vitamin A (cod liver oil, halibut fish oil).

Reactions in bold italics are *life-threatening*. Interactions may have a *rapid onset* or a ***delayed onset***.

Drug-lifestyle. *Abrasive cleansers, cream depilatories, medicated cosmetics, skin preparations containing alcohol, waxes:* May increase risk of skin irritation. Discourage use together.

Sun exposure, tanning lamps: May increase photosensitivity reaction. Advise patient to avoid excessive exposure.

EFFECTS ON LAB TEST RESULTS
None reported.

CONTRAINDICATIONS & CAUTIONS
• Contraindicated in patients hypersensitive to drug or its components and in those with sunburn.
• Use cautiously in patients with eczema.
• Use Atralin gel and Altreno lotion with caution in patients with known sensitivities or allergies to fish because gel contains soluble fish proteins.
• Use cautiously in patients with significant sun exposure (such as occupation-related) and in patients inherently sensitive to sunlight.
Dialyzable drug: Unknown.
⚠ *Overdose S&S:* Marked redness, skin peeling, skin discomfort.

PREGNANCY-LACTATION-REPRODUCTION
⚠ *Alert:* Don't use if patient is pregnant, attempting to become pregnant, or at high risk for pregnancy.
• There are no adequate studies during pregnancy. Use only if potential benefit justifies fetal risk.
• It isn't known if drug appears in human milk. Use cautiously during breastfeeding.

NURSING CONSIDERATIONS
• Initially, drug may be applied every 2 to 3 days using a lower concentration to reduce irritation.
• After satisfactory response, consider less frequent applications or use of other formulations.
• *Look alike–sound alike:* Don't confuse tretinoin with trientine, triamcinolone, or isotretinoin.

PATIENT TEACHING
• Instruct patient in safe drug application and handling.
• Teach patient to wash hands after application.

• Warn patient against using strong or medicated cosmetics, soaps, or other skin cleansers. Also advise patient to avoid topical products containing alcohol, astringents, spices, and lime because they may interfere with drug's actions.
• Caution patient not to apply to sunburned skin.
• Tell patient using drug for treatment of fine wrinkles to avoid washing face or applying another skin product or cosmetic for 1 hour after application. Advise patient to apply skin moisturizer at least every morning to protect treated areas from dryness.
• Inform patient that normal use of cosmetics is allowed.
• Advise patient not to stop drug if temporary worsening of inflammatory lesions occurs. If severe local irritation develops, advise patient to stop drug temporarily and notify prescriber. Dosage will be readjusted when application is resumed. Some redness and scaling are normal reactions.
• Warn patient that increased sensitivity to wind or cold temperatures may occur.
• Instruct patient to minimize exposure to sunlight or ultraviolet rays during treatment. If a sunburn develops, advise patient to delay therapy until sunburn subsides. Tell patient who can't avoid exposure to sunlight to use SPF-15 sunblock and to wear protective clothing.
• Warn patient that a temporary increase in lesions may occur, which will improve in 2 to 3 weeks.
• Tell patient not to use drug if pregnant or trying to become pregnant. Advise patient to stop drug and report suspected pregnancy.

triamcinolone acetonide (injection)
trye-am-SIN-oh-lone

Kenalog-10*, Kenalog-40*, Kenalog-80*, Triesence, Xipere, Zilretta

Therapeutic class: Corticosteroids
Pharmacologic class: Glucocorticoids

AVAILABLE FORMS
Injection (extended-release powder): 32 mg per vial

T

Injection (suspension): 10 mg/mL, 40 mg/mL, 80 mg/mL

Injection (intravitreal): 40 mg/mL

Injection (suprachoroidal): 40 mg/mL

INDICATIONS & DOSAGES

➤ **Severe inflammation, immunosuppression**

Adults: 60 mg IM, then 20 to 100 mg IM as needed every 6 weeks, if possible. Or, individualize initial intralesional dose depending on the specific disease and lesion. For maintenance, use the lowest dosage and time intervals to maintain an adequate clinical response. Or, initially, 2.5 to 15 mg into joints (depending on joint size) or soft tissue; then may increase to 10 mg for smaller areas and 40 mg for larger areas. Maximum dose (several joints at one time) is 80 mg. A local anesthetic is commonly injected with triamcinolone into the joint.

Children: Dosage may vary depending on the specific disease. Range of initial dose is 0.11 to 1.6 mg/kg/day IM in three or four divided doses (3.2 to 48 mg/m² BSA/day). Or, 2.5 to 5 mg for smaller joints and from 5 to 15 mg for larger joints, depending on the specific disease.

➤ **Management of osteoarthritis pain of the knee (Zilretta extended-release)**

Adults: 32 mg (5 mL) as a single intra-articular injection. Drug isn't intended for repeat administration.

➤ **Ophthalmic diseases (sympathetic ophthalmia, temporal arteritis, uveitis, ocular inflammatory conditions unresponsive to topical corticosteroids)**

Adults and children: 4 mg (100 mcL of 40 mg/mL suspension) injected intravitreally, with subsequent doses as needed during treatment.

➤ **Visualization during vitrectomy**

Adults and children: 1 to 4 mg (25 to 100 mcL of 40 mg/mL suspension) injected intravitreally.

✳ *NEW INDICATION:* **Macular edema associated with uveitis (Xipere)**

Adults: 4 mg as a single suprachoroidal injection.

ADMINISTRATION

IM (Kenalog-40 or Kenalog-80)

• Give deep into gluteal muscle. Rotate injection sites to prevent muscle atrophy.

• Don't use 10 mg/mL strength for this route.

• Shake well before use and ensure there's no clumping.

• Administer immediately after withdrawal to prevent settling in the syringe.

• Don't administer IV or via epidural or intrathecal route.

Intra-articular

• Prepare extended-release product only using the diluent supplied in the kit. Refer to manufacturer labeling for preparation instructions and administration techniques.

• Promptly inject after preparation.

• If needed, may store in vial for up to 4 hours at ambient conditions. Gently swirl vial to resuspend any settled microspheres before preparing syringe for injection.

• Extended-release form isn't interchangeable with other formulations of injectable triamcinolone acetonide.

• Strict aseptic technique is mandatory.

• Prior use of a local anesthetic may be desirable.

• Refrigerate extended-release product before use. If unable to refrigerate, store sealed, unopened kits at or below 77° F (25° C) for up to 6 weeks; then discard.

Intralesional (Kenalog-10)

• Strict aseptic technique is mandatory.

• Inject directly into the lesion intradermally or subcutaneously.

• It is preferable to use a tuberculin syringe and small-bore needle (23G to 25G).

Intravitreal

• Before injecting, give adequate anesthesia and a broad-spectrum microbicide.

• Shake vial vigorously for 10 seconds to ensure a uniform suspension. Inspect suspension for clumping or granules. If present, don't use.

• Inject drug without delay under controlled aseptic conditions.

• Each vial is for the treatment of a single eye only.

• Protect from light. Don't freeze. Store between 39° and 77° F (4° and 25° C).

Suprachoroidal

• Before injecting, give adequate anesthesia and a broad-spectrum microbicide.

• Shake vial vigorously for 10 seconds to ensure a uniform suspension. Inspect suspension for clumping or granules. If present, don't use.

• Inject only using SCS Microinjector under aseptic conditions. Administer injection without delay to prevent settling.

Reactions in bold italics are *life-threatening*. Interactions may have a *rapid onset* or a *delayed onset*.

- Each vial is for treatment of a single eye only.
- Protect from light. Don't freeze. Store between 59° and 77° F (15° and 25° C).

ACTION
Not clearly defined. Decreases inflammation, mainly by stabilizing leukocyte lysosomal membranes; suppresses immune response; stimulates bone marrow; influences protein, fat, and carbohydrate metabolism; and suppresses adrenal function at high doses.

Route	Onset	Peak	Duration
IM, intra-articular, intralesional	12–48 hr	Unknown	30–42 days
Intra-articular (extended-release)	Unknown	7 hr	Unknown
Intravitreal, supra-choroidal	Unknown	Unknown	Unknown

Half-life: 300 minutes; intravitreal, 13 to 24 days.

ADVERSE REACTIONS
Systemic reactions associated with corticosteroid therapy are possible. Refer to manufacturer's prescribing information for additional adverse reactions not listed here.
CNS: euphoria, insomnia, *pseudotumor cerebri, seizures,* headache, paresthesia, psychotic behavior, vertigo, *stroke.* **CV:** *arrhythmias, HF, thromboembolism,* HTN, edema, thrombophlebitis. **EENT:** cataracts, dry eye, photophobia, vitreous floaters, uveitis, punctate keratitis, conjunctival edema, eyelid ptosis, glaucoma, increased IOP, eye pain and inflammation, conjunctival hemorrhage, reduced visual acuity, sinusitis; injection-site reactions with ophthalmic injections. **GI:** *pancreatitis,* peptic ulceration, GI irritation, increased appetite, nausea, vomiting. **GU:** menstrual irregularities, increased urine calcium level. **Metabolic:** *hypokalemia,* hyperglycemia and carbohydrate intolerance, hypercholesterolemia, hypocalcemia. **Musculoskeletal:** growth suppression in children, muscle weakness, osteoporosis, acute myopathy, joint swelling. **Respiratory:** cough. **Skin:** hirsutism, delayed wound healing, acne, various skin eruptions, contusions. **Other:** *acute adrenal insufficiency,* cushingoid state, susceptibility to infections after increased stress or abrupt withdrawal after long-term therapy.

INTERACTIONS
Drug-drug. *Anticholinesterase drugs (ambenonium, neostigmine):* May cause severe weakness in patients with myasthenia gravis. Withdraw anticholinesterase drug at least 24 hours before corticosteroid therapy, if possible.
Antidiabetics: May increase blood glucose level. Adjust dosage of antidiabetics as needed.
Aspirin, indomethacin, other NSAIDs: May increase risk of GI distress and bleeding. Use together cautiously.
Barbiturates, carbamazepine, fosphenytoin, phenytoin, rifampin: May decrease corticosteroid effect. Increase corticosteroid dosage.
Cyclosporine: May increase toxicity and seizures. Monitor patient closely.
CYP3A4 inhibitors (clarithromycin, ketoconazole, nefazodone, ritonavir), macrolide antibiotics: May increase corticosteroid adverse effects. Use cautiously together and monitor patient for adverse effects.
Estrogens, hormonal contraceptives: May decrease hepatic metabolism of some corticosteroids. Monitor therapy.
Isoniazid: May decrease isoniazid level and antituberculin effect. Monitor therapy.
Oral anticoagulants: May alter dosage requirements. Monitor PT and INR closely.
Potassium-depleting drugs, such as thiazide and loop diuretics and amphotericin B: May enhance potassium-wasting effects of triamcinolone. Monitor potassium level.
Salicylates: May decrease salicylate level. Monitor patient for lack of salicylate effectiveness.
Skin-test antigens: May decrease response. Postpone skin testing until after therapy.
Toxoids, vaccines: May decrease antibody response and increase risk of neurologic complications. Defer routine administration of vaccines or toxoids until corticosteroid therapy is discontinued, if possible.
Drug-herb. *Echinacea:* May decrease therapeutic effect of immunosuppressants. Avoid combination.

EFFECTS ON LAB TEST RESULTS
- May increase sodium and glucose levels.
- May decrease potassium and calcium levels.
- May alter reactions to skin tests.

CONTRAINDICATIONS & CAUTIONS

• Contraindicated in patients hypersensitive to drug or its ingredients, in patients with cerebral malaria, in those with systemic fungal infections, and in those receiving immunosuppressive doses together with live-virus vaccines.

• IM injections are contraindicated in patients with ITP.

• Intravitreal injections are contraindicated in patients with active ocular herpes simplex virus.

• Suprachoroidal injections are contraindicated in patients with active or suspected ocular or periocular infections, including most viral diseases of the cornea and conjunctiva, active epithelial herpes simplex keratitis, vaccinia, varicella, mycobacterial infections, and fungal diseases.

• Extended-release form is for intra-articular use only for osteoarthritis pain of the knee as a one-time injection; repeat dosing hasn't been studied.

• Safety and effectiveness of extended-release and suprachoroidal forms in children haven't been established.

• Use cautiously in patients with recent MI, GI ulcer, renal disease, HTN, osteoporosis, diabetes, hypothyroidism, cirrhosis, diverticulitis, nonspecific ulcerative colitis, recent intestinal anastomoses, thromboembolic disorders, seizures, myasthenia gravis, active hepatitis, lactation, HF, TB, ocular herpes simplex, emotional instability, or psychotic tendencies.

⚠ *Alert:* Use of corticosteroids increases risk of cataracts.

Dialyzable drug: Unknown.

PREGNANCY-LACTATION-REPRODUCTION

• Some manufacturers report that human studies show that triamcinolone acetonide can cause fetal harm. Use only if potential benefit justifies fetal risk.

• Carefully observe infants born to patients who have received corticosteroids during pregnancy for signs and symptoms of hypoadrenalism.

• Drug appears in human milk and could suppress infant growth, interfere with endogenous corticosteroid production, or cause other untoward effects. Use cautiously during breastfeeding.

NURSING CONSIDERATIONS

• Determine whether patient is sensitive to other corticosteroids.

• Drug isn't used for alternate-day therapy.

• Always adjust to lowest effective dose.

• Most adverse reactions to corticosteroids are dose- or duration-dependent.

• Monitor patient's weight, BP, and glucose and electrolyte levels. If used for more than 6 weeks, monitor IOP.

• Monitor patient for cushingoid effects, such as moon face, buffalo hump, central obesity, thinning hair, HTN, and increased susceptibility to infection.

• Watch for depression or psychotic episodes, especially during high-dose therapy.

• Patient with diabetes may need increased insulin dosage; monitor glucose level.

• Drug may mask or worsen infections, including latent amebiasis.

• Older adults may be more susceptible to osteoporosis with long-term use.

• Unless contraindicated, give low-sodium diet that's high in potassium and protein. Give potassium supplements as needed.

• Gradually reduce dosage after long-term (more than 10 to 14 days) therapy. Drug may affect patient's sleep.

⚠ *Alert:* Ophthalmic injections must be performed under mandatory aseptic technique, which includes the use of sterile gloves, sterile drape, and sterile eyelid speculum.

⚠ *Alert:* Monitor patients receiving ophthalmic injections for increased IOP, which can lead to glaucoma and damage to the optic nerve.

• Intra-articular injection may be complicated by joint infection; increased pain accompanied by local swelling, further restriction of joint motion, fever, and malaise suggest septic arthritis. For confirmed septic arthritis, institute appropriate antimicrobial therapy.

• *Look alike–sound alike:* Don't confuse triamcinolone with Triaminic. Don't confuse Kenalog with Ketalar.

PATIENT TEACHING

• Tell patient not to stop drug abruptly or without prescriber's consent.

• Teach patient signs and symptoms of early adrenal insufficiency: fatigue, muscle weakness, joint pain, fever, anorexia, nausea, shortness of breath, dizziness, and fainting.

• Instruct patient to carry medical identification that includes prescriber's name and

---

Reactions in bold italics are *life-threatening*. Interactions may have a *rapid onset* or a *delayed onset*.

drug's name and dosage and indicates patient's need for supplemental systemic glucocorticoids during stress.

• Warn patient on long-term therapy about cushingoid effects (moon face, buffalo hump) and the need to notify prescriber about sudden weight gain and swelling.

• Tell patient to report slow wound healing.

• Advise patient receiving long-term therapy to consider exercise or physical therapy. Also, tell patient to ask prescriber about vitamin D or calcium supplement.

• Instruct patient to avoid exposure to infections and to notify prescriber if exposure occurs.

• Tell patient to report ophthalmic signs and symptoms (eye pain, redness, sensitivity to light, vision loss or disturbance) to prescriber and to seek immediate care from an ophthalmologist if these occur.

triamcinolone acetonide (intranasal)
trye-am-SIN-oh-lone

GoodSense Nasal Allergy ◇, Nasacort Allergy 24 Hour ◇, Nasacort AQ✚ ◇

Therapeutic class: Corticosteroids
Pharmacologic class: Corticosteroids

AVAILABLE FORMS
Nasal spray: 55 mcg/spray

INDICATIONS & DOSAGES
➤ **Nasal symptoms of seasonal and perennial allergic rhinitis**
Adults and children age 12 and older: 2 sprays in each nostril once daily while sniffing gently; may decrease to 1 spray in each nostril once daily after symptom control. Adjust to minimum effective dosage.
Children ages 6 to 11: 1 spray in each nostril once daily while sniffing gently. Maximum dosage is 2 sprays in each nostril once daily. Adjust to minimum effective dosage.
Children ages 2 to 5: 1 spray in each nostril once daily while sniffing gently.
Adjust-a-dose: Start older adults at lower end of dosing range.

ADMINISTRATION
Intranasal
• Shake well before each use.

• Release 5 sprays into the air to prime before first use. Reprime with 1 spray if not used for 2 weeks or more.

• Patient should gently blow nose to clear nostrils.

• Insert nozzle into nostril, pointing away from septum. Hold other nostril closed and have patient sniff gently while spraying.

• Patient should avoid blowing nose for 15 minutes after use.

ACTION
Controls the rate of protein synthesis, depresses the migration of polymorphonuclear leukocytes and fibroblasts, reverses capillary permeability, and stabilizes lysosomal membranes at the cellular level.

Route	Onset	Peak	Duration
Intranasal	Unknown	1.5–4 hr	Unknown

Half-life: About 3 hours.

ADVERSE REACTIONS
CNS: headache, bitter taste. **EENT:** nasal irritation, burning, epistaxis, nasal and sinus congestion, rhinitis, nasopharyngitis, oral candidiasis, sinusitis, sneezing, stinging, throat pain, rhinorrhea, excoriation, tooth disorder. **GI:** dyspepsia, nausea, vomiting, upper abdominal pain, diarrhea. **Respiratory:** *asthma symptoms,* cough, bronchitis. **Skin:** rash. **Other:** flulike syndrome.

INTERACTIONS
None significant.

EFFECTS ON LAB TEST RESULTS
None reported.

CONTRAINDICATIONS & CAUTIONS
• Contraindicated in patients hypersensitive to drug or its components and in those with untreated mucosal infection.

• Use with caution, if at all, in patients with active or quiescent tuberculous infection of respiratory tract, glaucoma, cataracts, increased IOP, ocular herpes simplex, eye infection, or untreated fungal, bacterial, or systemic viral infection.

• Use cautiously in patients already receiving systemic corticosteroids because of increased likelihood of HPA axis suppression.

• Use cautiously in patients with recent nasal septal ulcers, nasal surgery, or trauma because drug may inhibit wound healing.

T

• Use cautiously in patients with severe or recurrent nosebleeds.
• Drug isn't indicated for use in children younger than age 2 when used for self-medication.
Dialyzable drug: Unknown.
⚠ *Overdose S&S:* GI upset, nasal irritation, headache.

PREGNANCY-LACTATION-REPRODUCTION
• There are no adequate studies during pregnancy. Use only if potential benefit justifies fetal risk.
• It isn't known if drug appears in human milk. Use cautiously during breastfeeding.

NURSING CONSIDERATIONS
⚠ *Alert:* Excessive doses may cause signs and symptoms of hyperadrenocorticism and adrenal axis suppression; stop drug slowly.
• To decrease risk of adverse effects, individualize drug dosage and titrate to minimum effective dosage.
• Monitor growth rate in children, which may be slower while using this product, especially if child needs to use spray for longer than 2 months a year.
• Discontinue drug if symptom relief hasn't occurred after 1 week of treatment.
• *Look alike–sound alike:* Don't confuse triamcinolone with Triaminic.

PATIENT TEACHING
• Teach patient how to use nasal spray, including how to prime pump.
• Instruct patient to avoid getting aerosol in eyes or mouth. If this occurs, tell patient to rinse with copious amounts of cool tap water.
• Tell patient not to blow nose for 15 minutes after use.
• Stress importance of using drug on a regular schedule because its effectiveness depends on regular use. Warn patient not to exceed prescribed dosage.
• Tell patient to notify prescriber if signs and symptoms don't diminish or if condition worsens in 1 week.
• Warn patient to avoid exposure to chickenpox or measles and, if exposed, to notify prescriber.
• Instruct patient to watch for and report signs and symptoms of nasal infection. Drug may need to be stopped.

triamcinolone acetonide (topical)
trye-am-SIN-oh-lone

Aristocort✤, Kenalog, Oracort✤, Oralone, Trianex, Triderm, Tritocin

Therapeutic class: Corticosteroids
Pharmacologic class: Corticosteroids

AVAILABLE FORMS
Aerosol*: 0.2 mg/2-second spray (0.147 mg/g)
Cream: 0.025%, 0.1%, 0.5%
Dental paste: 0.1%
Lotion: 0.025%, 0.1%
Ointment: 0.025%, 0.05%, 0.1%, 0.5%

INDICATIONS & DOSAGES
➤ **Inflammation and pruritus from corticosteroid-responsive dermatoses**
Adults and children: Clean area; apply aerosol, cream, lotion, or ointment sparingly b.i.d. to q.i.d. Rub in lightly. Or, 3 or 4 applications of spray daily.
➤ **Symptom relief from oral inflammatory and ulcerative oral lesions**
Adults and children: Apply paste at bedtime and, if needed, b.i.d. to q.i.d., preferably after meals.

ADMINISTRATION
Topical
• Gently wash skin before applying. To avoid skin damage, rub in gently, leaving a thin coat. When treating hairy sites, part hair and apply directly to lesions.
• Don't apply near eyes or in ear canal.
• When using aerosol near the face, cover patient's eyes and warn against inhaling spray. Aerosol contains alcohol and may cause irritation or burning when used on open lesions. Spray at a distance of 3 to 6 inches (7.6 to 15.25 cm) from affected area.
• Occlusive dressings may be used in severe or resistant dermatoses.
• Apply small amount of paste to oral lesion without rubbing; press to lesion until thin film develops.
• Patient shouldn't rinse after using dental paste and should avoid eating or drinking for 30 minutes after application of dental paste.

Reactions in bold italics are *life-threatening*. Interactions may have a *rapid onset* or a *delayed onset*.

ACTION
Unclear. Diffuses across cell membranes to form complexes with cytoplasmic receptors, showing anti-inflammatory, antipruritic, vasoconstrictive, and antiproliferative activity.

Route	Onset	Peak	Duration
Topical	Several hr	Unknown	1 wk

Half-life: Biologic, 18 to 36 hours.

ADVERSE REACTIONS
EENT: oral mucosa changes; oral burning, itching, irritation, dryness, blistering or peeling. **GU:** glycosuria. **Metabolic:** hyperglycemia. **Skin:** burning, pruritus, irritation, dryness, erythema, folliculitis, hypertrichosis, hypopigmentation, acneiform eruptions, perioral dermatitis, allergic contact dermatitis, maceration, desquamation, secondary infection, atrophy, striae, miliaria with occlusive dressings. **Other:** *HPA axis suppression,* Cushing syndrome.

INTERACTIONS
Drug-drug. *Aldesleukin:* Corticosteroids may decrease antineoplastic effect. Avoid combination.

EFFECTS ON LAB TEST RESULTS
• May increase glucose level.

CONTRAINDICATIONS & CAUTIONS
• Contraindicated in patients hypersensitive to drug or its components.
• Contraindicated in the presence of fungal, viral, or bacterial infections of the mouth or throat (paste).
• Don't use as monotherapy in primary bacterial infections (impetigo, paronychia, erysipelas, cellulitis, angular cheilitis), treatment of rosacea, perioral dermatitis, or acne.
• Considered a medium-potency (0.025% and 0.1% cream, ointment, lotion) and high-potency (0.5% cream, ointment) drug, according to vasoconstrictive properties.
• Don't use very-high-potency or high-potency agents on the face, groin, or axilla areas.
• Drug isn't for ophthalmic use.
• Prolonged corticosteroid therapy may interfere with growth and development in children.
• Use cautiously in older adults because of age-related changes in skin integrity and risks associated with systemic absorption.

Dialyzable drug: Unknown.
⚠ *Overdose S&S:* Systemic effects (including reversible HPA axis suppression, Cushing syndrome, hyperglycemia, glycosuria).

PREGNANCY-LACTATION-REPRODUCTION
• There are no adequate studies during pregnancy. Use only if potential benefit justifies fetal risk. Don't use in large amounts or for prolonged periods in patients who are pregnant.
• It isn't known if drug appears in human milk. Use cautiously during breastfeeding.

NURSING CONSIDERATIONS
• Stop drug and tell prescriber if skin infection, striae, or atrophy occur.
• If antifungal or antibiotic combined with corticosteroid fails to provide prompt improvement, stop corticosteroid until infection is controlled.
• Systemic absorption is more likely with the use of occlusive dressings, prolonged treatment, or extensive body surface treatment.
• Avoid using plastic pants or tight-fitting diapers on treated areas in young children. Children may absorb larger amounts of drug and be more susceptible to systemic toxicity.
• Monitor skin integrity.
• If used for prolonged time and on large skin areas, monitor patient for HPA axis suppression and fungal or bacterial superinfection.
• When used in oral cavity, reevaluate if no improvement in 7 days.
• When using aerosol solution, reevaluate if no improvement in 2 weeks.

PATIENT TEACHING
• Teach patient or family member how to apply drug.
• Advise patient not to use an occlusive dressing unless instructed to. If an occlusive dressing is ordered, advise patient to leave it in place for no longer than 12 hours each day and not to use the dressing on infected or weeping lesions.
• Caution patient that aerosol is flammable. Patient should avoid heat, flames, and smoking when applying aerosol.
• Tell patient to stop drug and report signs of systemic absorption, skin irritation or ulceration, hypersensitivity, infection, or lack of improvement.

T

triamterene–hydroCHLOROthiazide

try-AM-tur-een/hye-droe-klor-oh-THYE-a-zide

Maxzide, Maxzide-25

Therapeutic class: Antihypertensives–diuretics
Pharmacologic class: Thiazide diuretics–potassium-sparing diuretics

AVAILABLE FORMS

Capsules: triamterene 37.5 mg/hydrochlorothiazide 25 mg
Tablets: triamterene 37.5 mg/hydrochlorothiazide 25 mg, triamterene 75 mg/hydrochlorothiazide 50 mg

INDICATIONS & DOSAGES

➤ **HTN or edema in patients who develop hypokalemia on hydrochlorothiazide alone, or who require a thiazide diuretic and in whom development of hypokalemia can't be risked**
Adults: Triamterene 37.5 mg/hydrochlorothiazide 25 mg PO one or two tablets or capsules daily as a single dose. Or, triamterene 75 mg/hydrochlorothiazide 50 mg PO daily.

ADMINISTRATION

PO
• May give without regard to meals. Give drug with food to minimize GI upset.
• To prevent nocturia, give drug in the morning.
• Giving two tablets or capsules in divided doses may increase risk of electrolyte imbalance and renal dysfunction; give as a single dose once daily.

ACTION

Triamterene works on distal tubule and collecting duct to inhibit reabsorption of sodium in exchange for potassium and hydrogen; hydrochlorothiazide increases excretion of sodium, chloride, potassium, hydrogen, and water by inhibiting reabsorption in distal segment of the nephron.

Route	Onset	Peak	Duration
PO (triamterene)	2–4 hr	1 hr	7–9 hr
PO (hydrochloro-thiazide)	2 hr	4 hr	6–12 hr

Half-life: Triamterene, 1.5 to 2.5 hours; hydrochlorothiazide, 6 to 15 hours.

ADVERSE REACTIONS

CNS: weakness, fatigue, dizziness, fever, headache, drowsiness, insomnia, depression, anxiety, vertigo, restlessness, paresthesia, taste alteration. **CV:** arrhythmia, orthostatic hypotension, chest pain, tachycardia. **EENT:** xanthopsia, transient blurred vision, dry mouth, sialadenitis. **GI:** diarrhea, nausea, vomiting, constipation, abdominal pain, *pancreatitis,* change in appetite, anorexia, gastric irritation, cramping. **GU:** erectile dysfunction, *acute renal failure,* glycosuria, interstitial nephritis, renal calculi, urine discoloration. **Hematologic:** *leukopenia, thrombocytopenia,* purpura, anemia, *agranulocytosis.* **Hepatic:** jaundice, altered LFT results. **Metabolic:** diabetes, *hyperkalemia,* hyperglycemia, hyperuricemia, *hypokalemia,* hyponatremia, *metabolic acidosis,* hypochloremic alkalosis, hypercalcemia, *hypomagnesemia.* **Musculoskeletal:** muscle cramps. **Respiratory:** shortness of breath, *pulmonary edema.* **Skin:** rash, urticaria, photosensitivity. **Other:** hypersensitivity reaction, *anaphylaxis.*

INTERACTIONS

Drug-drug. *ACE inhibitors and ARBs, potassium-containing medications (such as penicillin G potassium), potassium supplements:* May increase risk of hyperkalemia. Avoid concurrent use.
Adrenocorticotropic hormone, amphotericin B, beta$_2$-agonists, corticosteroids: May increase electrolyte depletion, particularly potassium. Use together carefully.
Amiloride, spironolactone, triamterene-containing agents: May increase risk of hyperkalemia. Use together is contraindicated.
Antidiabetics (oral agents and insulin): May increase or decrease blood glucose level. Dosage adjustment of antidiabetic may be required.
Antigout drugs: May increase uric acid level. Increase dosage of antigout medication if indicated.
Barbiturates, opioids: May increase risk of orthostatic hypotension. Use together cautiously.
Bile acid sequestrants: May decrease absorption of thiazide diuretics. Consider therapy modification.
Calcium salts, multivitamins: May decrease calcium excretion. Monitor therapy closely.

Reactions in bold italics are *life-threatening*. Interactions may have a *rapid onset* or a **delayed onset**.

Dofetilide: May increase QTc interval–prolonging effect of dofetilide. Avoid combination.

Laxatives: May increase potassium loss. Avoid use together.

Lithium: May increase lithium level, especially in patients with renal insufficiency. Avoid use together.

NSAIDs: May diminish antihypertensive effects and increase risk of acute renal failure. Use together cautiously.

Oral anticoagulants: May decrease anticoagulant effect. Adjust anticoagulant dosage as necessary.

Other antihypertensives: May increase risk of hypotension. Use together carefully and adjust dosage as appropriate.

Polystyrene, other exchange resins: May reduce potassium level, increase sodium retention, and increase edema. Avoid use together unless in setting of hyperkalemia.

Skeletal muscle relaxants, nondepolarizing (tubocurarine): May increase responsiveness to muscle relaxant. Avoid concurrent use.

Vitamin D analogues (calcipotriene, calcitriol, ergocalciferol, paricalcitol): May increase hypercalcemic effect of vitamin D. Monitor therapy closely.

Drug-herb. *Yohimbe:* May decrease antihypertensive effect of hydrochlorothiazide. Monitor therapy closely.

Drug-food. *Salt substitutes with potassium:* May increase risk of hyperkalemia. Discourage use together.

Drug-lifestyle. *Alcohol use:* May increase risk of orthostatic hypotension. Discourage use together.

Sun exposure: May increase risk of photosensitivity. Discourage sun exposure.

EFFECTS ON LAB TEST RESULTS

- May increase BUN, creatinine, liver enzyme, calcium, uric acid, cholesterol, and triglyceride levels.
- May increase urine glucose level.
- May decrease sodium, chloride, magnesium, and phosphate levels.
- May increase or decrease potassium or blood glucose level.
- May decrease protein-bound iodine level without signs of thyroid imbalance.
- May decrease leukocyte and platelet counts.
- May interfere with quinidine assays and parathyroid function tests.

CONTRAINDICATIONS & CAUTIONS

Boxed Warning Abnormal elevation of serum potassium levels (5.5 mEq/L or more) can occur and is more likely in patients with renal impairment or diabetes (even without concurrent renal impairment), in older adults, and in patients with severe illness. ■

- Contraindicated in patients hypersensitive to either drug or to sulfonamides and in those with preexisting hyperkalemia, anuria, acute and chronic renal insufficiency, or significant renal impairment.
- Use cautiously in patients with impaired hepatic function, electrolyte imbalance, or lupus and in those with a history of kidney stones or gout.
- Use cautiously in patients at risk for metabolic or respiratory acidosis. Monitor acid-base balance and electrolyte levels closely.
- Safety and effectiveness in children haven't been established.

Dialyzable drug: Unlikely.

⚠ *Overdose S&S:* Hyperkalemia or hypokalemia, dehydration, nausea, vomiting, weakness, hypotension, lethargy, GI irritation, coma.

PREGNANCY-LACTATION-REPRODUCTION

- There are no adequate studies during pregnancy. Use only if potential benefit justifies fetal risk.
- Both drugs may appear in human milk. Patient should discontinue breastfeeding or discontinue drug.

NURSING CONSIDERATIONS

Boxed Warning Monitor potassium level at initiation of therapy, with dosage changes, and with any illness that may influence renal function. ■

- Warning signs and symptoms of hyperkalemia include paresthesia, muscular weakness, fatigue, flaccid paralysis, bradycardia, and shock.
- Fixed-dose combinations aren't to be used for initial therapy except in patients in whom development of hyperkalemia can't be risked (patients taking cardiac glycosides and those with history of cardiac arrhythmias).
- Monitor potassium level carefully in patients using this combination; if hyperkalemia is suspected, obtain ECG and monitor levels.
- If hyperkalemia is present, stop combination and use thiazide alone.

• For potassium level greater than 6.5 mEq/L, consider IV calcium chloride, sodium bicarbonate, glucose, or sodium polystyrene sulfonate; consider dialysis if no improvement.
• Monitor patient for infection (sore throat, fever), which could be a sign of leukopenia, or for bruising, which could be a sign of thrombocytopenia.
• Monitor patient for acute myopia and secondary angle-closure glaucoma (acute vision changes, ocular pain usually within hours to weeks of drug ingestion), especially in patient with a history of possible sulfonamide or penicillin allergy. Discontinue drug as soon as possible if symptoms occur.
• Monitor patient for hyperuricemia or acute gout. Antigout drug dosages may need adjustment.
• Thiazides may alter calcium and phosphate levels. Discontinue drug before testing parathyroid function.
• Monitor patients with diabetes for changes in antidiabetic or insulin requirements. Patients with latent diabetes may become fully diabetic during therapy.
• Monitor BP, fluid balance, LFT values, and electrolyte levels.

PATIENT TEACHING

• Teach patient to report light-headedness, especially during first few days of therapy. Warn patient to discontinue drug and notify prescriber if syncope occurs.
• Caution patient to notify prescriber if fluid loss occurs from excessive perspiration, dehydration, vomiting, or diarrhea.
• Advise patient not to use salt substitutes containing potassium.
• Instruct patient to promptly report signs and symptoms of infection (sore throat, fever) or bruising.
• Inform patient that to be effective, drug must be taken daily as prescribed, and to continue to take drug even if feeling well.
• Advise patient to avoid taking drug at bedtime, to prevent nighttime diuresis.
• Teach patient the warning signs and symptoms of fluid and electrolyte imbalance (decreased urine production, drowsiness, dry mouth, fast HR, fatigue, low BP, muscular fatigue, muscle pain or cramps, restlessness, stomach disturbances, thirst, and weakness).
• Advise patient to keep follow-up appointments to monitor electrolyte levels.
• Warn patient to avoid sun exposure.

• Caution patient to avoid alcohol, to decrease risk of a sudden drop in BP.
• Instruct patient to consult prescriber before taking other prescription or OTC medications, herbal products, or vitamin and mineral supplements.

SAFETY ALERT!

triazolam
trye-AY-zoe-lam

Halcion

Therapeutic class: Hypnotics
Pharmacologic class: Benzodiazepines
Controlled substance schedule: IV

AVAILABLE FORMS
Tablets: 0.125 mg, 0.25 mg

INDICATIONS & DOSAGES
➤ **Short-term treatment (7 to 10 days) of insomnia**
Adults: 0.25 PO at bedtime. May increase to maximum of 0.5 mg if inadequate response to a lower dose.
Older adults, patients with low body weight, and patients who are debilitated: 0.125 mg PO at bedtime. Maximum dose is 0.25 mg.

ADMINISTRATION
PO
• Don't give drug with or right after a meal.

ACTION
Unknown. Probably acts on the limbic system, thalamus, and hypothalamus of the CNS to produce hypnotic effects by increasing levels of inhibitory neurotransmitter GABA.

Route	Onset	Peak	Duration
PO	15–30 min	<2 hr	6–7 hr

Half-life: 1.5 to 5.5 hours.

ADVERSE REACTIONS
CNS: drowsiness, ataxia, dizziness, headache, nervousness, light-headedness. **GI:** nausea, vomiting.

INTERACTIONS
Drug-drug. *Anticonvulsants, antihistamines, CNS depressants, dronabinol, magnesium sulfate, psychotropics:* May cause excessive CNS depression. Use together cautiously.

Reactions in bold italics are *life-threatening*. Interactions may have a *rapid onset* or a *delayed onset*.

Cimetidine, fluvoxamine, isoniazid, macrolide antibiotics (clarithromycin, erythromycin), oral contraceptives, ranitidine: May increase triazolam level. Monitor patient closely and consider triazolam dosage reduction.

CYP3A4 inducers: May decrease triazolam serum concentration. Consider alternative drug (strong inducers) or monitor therapy closely (moderate inducers).

Diltiazem (moderate CYP3A inhibitors): May increase CNS depression and prolong effects of triazolam. Reduce triazolam dose.

Boxed Warning *Opioids:* May cause slow or difficult breathing, sedation, coma, and death. Avoid use together. If use together is necessary, limit dosage and duration of each drug to minimum necessary for desired effect. ■

Strong CYP3A inhibitors (azole antifungals [fluconazole, itraconazole, ketoconazole, miconazole], lopinavir, nefazodone, nelfinavir, ritonavir, saquinavir): May increase and prolong triazolam level. Use together is contraindicated.

Drug-herb. *Calendula, hops, kava kava, lemon balm, passion flower, skullcap, valerian:* May enhance sedative effect of drug. Discourage use together.

St. John's wort: May decrease triazolam serum concentration. Consider therapy modification.

Yohimbe: May decrease effect of antianxiety agents. Monitor therapy closely.

Drug-food. *Grapefruit:* May delay onset and increase drug effects. Discourage use together.

Drug-lifestyle. ☯ *Alert: Alcohol use:* May cause additive CNS effects. Discourage use together. ■

EFFECTS ON LAB TEST RESULTS
• May increase LFT values.

CONTRAINDICATIONS & CAUTIONS
• Contraindicated in patients hypersensitive to drug or other benzodiazepines.

Boxed Warning Benzodiazepine use exposes patient to risks of abuse, misuse, and addiction, which can lead to overdose or death. Assess each patient's risk for abuse, misuse, and addiction before prescribing and periodically during therapy. ■

• Prescription should be written for short-term use of 7 to 10 days, with quantities limited to a 1-month supply.

Boxed Warning Abrupt discontinuation or rapid dosage reduction of benzodiazepines after continued use may precipitate acute withdrawal reactions, which can be life-threatening. To reduce risk of withdrawal reactions, gradually taper drug to discontinue or reduce dosage. ■

Boxed Warning Opioids should only be prescribed with benzodiazepines or other CNS depressants to patients for whom alternative treatment options are inadequate. Assess patient's risk of abuse, misuse, and addiction. ■

• Use cautiously in patients with impaired hepatic or renal function, chronic pulmonary insufficiency, sleep apnea, mental depression, suicidality, or history of drug abuse.

Dialyzable drug: Unlikely.

⚠ *Overdose S&S:* Somnolence, impaired coordination, slurred speech, confusion, coma, decreased reflexes, hypotension, seizures, respiratory depression, apnea, death.

PREGNANCY-LACTATION-REPRODUCTION
• Drug may cause fetal harm. Patient should stop drug before becoming pregnant. If patient becomes pregnant, apprise patient of fetal risk.

• Data collection on pregnancy exposure is ongoing at the National Pregnancy Registry for Psychiatric Medications (1-866-961-2388).

• Monitor infants exposed to drug during pregnancy for respiratory depression, sedation, withdrawal, and feeding problems.

• Drug may appear in human milk. Use during breastfeeding isn't recommended.

NURSING CONSIDERATIONS
☯ *Alert:* Anaphylaxis and angioedema may occur as early as the first dose; monitor patient closely.

• Assess mental status before starting therapy, and reduce doses in older adults.

• Use the lowest effective dose, as there are significant dose-related adverse reactions.

• Use of drug for more than 3 weeks requires patient evaluation for primary psychiatric or medical conditions, which may be causing insomnia.

• Monitor patient for abnormal thinking and behavior changes, including aggressiveness, extroversion, bizarre behavior, agitation, hallucinations, depersonalization, and worsening of depression.

T

- Take precautions to prevent hoarding or overdosing by patients who are depressed, suicidal, or drug-dependent or who have history of drug abuse.
- Minor changes in EEG patterns (usually low-voltage fast activity) may occur during and after therapy.
- Monitor patient for increased daytime anxiety.
- *Look alike–sound alike:* Don't confuse triazolam with alprazolam. Don't confuse Halcion with Haldol or halcinonide.

PATIENT TEACHING

Boxed Warning Caution patient or caregiver of patient taking an opioid with a benzodiazepine, CNS depressant, or alcohol to seek immediate medical attention if patient experiences dizziness, light-headedness, extreme sleepiness, slowed or difficult breathing, or unresponsiveness. ■

Boxed Warning Caution patient that benzodiazepines, even at recommended doses, increase the risk of abuse, misuse, and addiction, which can lead to overdose and death, especially when used in combination with other drugs (opioid analgesics), alcohol, or illicit substances. ■

Boxed Warning Inform patient about signs and symptoms of benzodiazepine abuse, misuse, and addiction (abdominal pain, amnesia, anorexia, anxiety, aggression, ataxia, blurred vision, confusion, depression, disinhibition, disorientation, dizziness, euphoria, impaired concentration and memory, indigestion, irritability, muscle pain, slurred speech, tremors, vertigo, delirium, paranoia, suicidality, seizures, difficulty breathing, coma) and to seek emergency medical help if they occur. Instruct patient on proper disposal of unused drug. ■

- Advise patient not to take drug at a higher dose, more frequently, or for longer than prescribed.

Boxed Warning Tell patient that continued use of drug for several days to weeks may lead to physical dependence and that abrupt discontinuation or rapid dosage reduction may precipitate acute withdrawal reactions (unusual movements, responses, or expressions; seizures; sudden and severe mental or nervous system changes; depression; seeing or hearing things that others don't; homicidal thoughts; extreme increase in activity or talking; losing touch with reality; suicidality),

which can be life-threatening. Instruct patient that discontinuation or dosage reduction may require a slow taper. ■

Boxed Warning Advise patient about the possibility of developing protracted withdrawal syndrome (anxiety; trouble remembering, learning, or concentrating; depression; problems sleeping; feeling like insects are crawling under the skin; weakness; shaking; muscle twitching; burning or prickling feeling in the hands, arms, legs, or feet; ringing in the ears), with symptoms lasting weeks to more than 12 months. ■

♦ *Alert:* Warn patient that drug may cause allergic reactions, facial swelling, and complex sleep-related behaviors (driving, eating, and making phone calls while asleep). Advise patient to report these effects.

- Warn patient not to take more than prescribed amount; overdose can occur at total daily dose of 2 mg (or four times highest recommended amount).
- Tell patient to avoid alcohol use while taking drug.
- Caution patient to avoid performing activities that require mental alertness or physical coordination.
- Inform patient that drug doesn't tend to cause morning drowsiness.
- Tell patient that rebound insomnia may occur for 1 or 2 nights after stopping therapy.
- Tell patient to avoid pregnancy and breastfeeding while taking drug.
- Advise patient to take drug immediately before bedtime and not with, or immediately after, a meal.
- Instruct patient to consult prescriber before taking other prescription or OTC medications or herbal products.

---

trospium chloride
TROZ-pee-um

Trosec ♦

Therapeutic class: Urinary antispasmodics
Pharmacologic class: Antimuscarinics

AVAILABLE FORMS
Capsules (extended-release): 60 mg
Tablets: 20 mg

Reactions in bold italics are *life-threatening*. Interactions may have a *rapid onset* or a ***delayed onset***.

INDICATIONS & DOSAGES
➤ **Overactive bladder (urinary urge incontinence, urgency, frequency)**
Adults: 20 mg (immediate-release) tablet PO b.i.d. Or, 60 mg extended-release capsule PO once daily in morning.
Adjust-a-dose: For adults age 75 and older, reduce dosage to 20 mg (immediate-release) PO once daily based on patient tolerance. For CrCl of less than 30 mL/minute, give 20 mg (immediate-release) PO once daily at bedtime. Extended-release form isn't recommended if CrCl falls below 30 mL/minute.

ADMINISTRATION
PO
• Give tablets at least 1 hour before meals or on an empty stomach.
• Give extended-release form in the morning with water on an empty stomach at least 1 hour before meal.

ACTION
Relaxes smooth muscle of bladder by antagonizing muscarinic receptors, relieving symptoms of overactive bladder.

Route	Onset	Peak	Duration
PO	Unknown	5–6 hr	Unknown

Half-life: About 20 hours (immediate-release); 35 hours (extended-release).

ADVERSE REACTIONS
CNS: fatigue, headache. **EENT:** dry eyes, mouth, and nose; nasopharyngitis. **GI:** constipation, abdominal pain and distention, dyspepsia, flatulence, nausea. **GU:** urine retention, UTI. **Other:** flulike symptoms.

INTERACTIONS
Drug-drug. *Anticholinergics:* May increase dry mouth, constipation, or other adverse effects. Monitor patient.
Metformin, morphine, procainamide, pancuronium, tenofovir, vancomycin: May alter elimination of these drugs or trospium, increasing levels. Monitor patient closely.
Opioid analgesics: May increase risk of constipation and urine retention. Monitor therapy closely.
Prokinetic GI agents: May decrease therapeutic effect of GI prokinetic agents. Monitor therapy closely.

Drug-food. *High-fat foods:* May significantly decrease absorption. Give drug at least 1 hour before meals or on an empty stomach.
Drug-lifestyle. *Alcohol use:* May increase drowsiness. Use of alcoholic beverages within 2 hours of taking extended-release capsules isn't recommended. Discourage use together.

EFFECTS ON LAB TEST RESULTS
None reported.

CONTRAINDICATIONS & CAUTIONS
• Contraindicated in patients hypersensitive to the drug or any of its ingredients and in those with or at risk for urine retention, gastric retention, or uncontrolled narrow-angle glaucoma.
• Use cautiously in patients with significant bladder outflow obstruction, obstructive GI disorders, ulcerative colitis, intestinal atony, myasthenia gravis, renal insufficiency, moderate or severe hepatic impairment, or controlled narrow-angle glaucoma.
• Safety and effectiveness in children haven't been determined.
Dialyzable drug: Unknown.
⚠ *Overdose S&S:* Severe anticholinergic effects, tachycardia, mydriasis.

PREGNANCY-LACTATION-REPRODUCTION
• There are no adequate studies during pregnancy. Use only if potential benefit justifies fetal risk.
• It isn't known if drug appears in human milk. Use during breastfeeding only if potential benefit justifies risk to the infant.

NURSING CONSIDERATIONS
• Assess patient to determine baseline bladder function, and monitor patient for therapeutic effects.
• Angioedema of the face, lips, tongue, or larynx, which may be life-threatening, can occur after first dose. Discontinue drug and promptly provide treatment to ensure a patent airway.
• Various CNS anticholinergic effects have been reported, including dizziness, confusion, hallucinations, and somnolence. Monitor patients for signs and symptoms of anticholinergic CNS effects, particularly after beginning treatment or increasing dosage. Dosage may need to be reduced or drug discontinued.

- If patient has bladder outflow obstruction, watch for evidence of urine retention.
- Monitor patient for decreased gastric motility and constipation.
- Monitor renal and hepatic function periodically during therapy.

PATIENT TEACHING

- Teach patient safe drug administration.
- Caution patient of risk of angioedema and to seek immediate medical care for swelling of the tongue or throat or difficulty breathing.
- Discourage use of other drugs that may cause dry mouth, constipation, blurred vision, or urine retention.
- Tell patient that alcohol use may increase drowsiness and fatigue. Discourage alcohol consumption. Advise patient not to use alcohol within 2 hours of taking extended-release capsules.
- Explain that drug may decrease sweating and increase the risk of heatstroke when used in hot environments or during strenuous activities.
- Urge patient to avoid activities that are hazardous or require mental alertness until drug's effects are known.

---

ulipristal acetate ⚠
UE-li-PRIS-tal

ella

Therapeutic class: Contraceptives
Pharmacologic class: Progesterone agonists–antagonists

AVAILABLE FORMS
Tablets: 30 mg

INDICATIONS & DOSAGES
➤ **Prevention of pregnancy following unprotected intercourse or a known or suspected contraceptive failure**
Women and postmenarchal adolescents:
30 mg (1 tablet) PO as soon as possible within 120 hours (5 days) after unprotected intercourse or a known or suspected contraceptive failure.

ADMINISTRATION
PO
⚠ *Alert:* Hazardous drug; use safe-handling and disposal precautions.

- May give without regard for food.
- If vomiting occurs within 3 hours of tablet ingestion, may repeat dose.
- May give at any time during the menstrual cycle.

ACTION
Inhibits or delays ovulation and alters endometrium to avoid egg implantation; prevents progestin from binding to progesterone receptor.

Route	Onset	Peak	Duration
PO	Unknown	1 hr	Unknown

Half-life: 32 to 38 hours.

ADVERSE REACTIONS
CNS: headache, fatigue, dizziness. **GI:** nausea, abdominal pain. **GU:** dysmenorrhea, intermenstrual bleeding, irregular menses.

INTERACTIONS
Drug-drug. *CYP3A4 inducers (barbiturates, bosentan, carbamazepine, efavirenz, felbamate, griseofulvin, oxcarbazepine, phenytoin, rifampin, topiramate):* May decrease effectiveness of contraceptive. Avoid concurrent use.
CYP3A4 inhibitors (itraconazole, ketoconazole): May increase serum ulipristal levels and risk of adverse reactions. Monitor patient.
Hormonal contraceptives: May impair ability of ulipristal to delay ovulation or decrease effectiveness of regular hormonal contraceptives. Hormonal contraceptives shouldn't be resumed until 5 days after patient takes ulipristal.
Progestins: May decrease effect of progestins. Patient should use reliable barrier method of contraception until next menstrual period.
Drug-herb. *St. John's wort:* May decrease effectiveness of contraceptive. Avoid concurrent use.

EFFECTS ON LAB TEST RESULTS
None reported.

CONTRAINDICATIONS & CAUTIONS
- Contraindicated for use with known or suspected pregnancy.
- Contraindicated in females who are prepubescent or postmenopausal.
- Drug isn't indicated for termination of an existing pregnancy or as routine contraception.

Reactions in bold italics are *life-threatening*. Interactions may have a *rapid onset* or a ***delayed onset***.

- Safety and effectiveness of repeated use within the same menstrual cycle aren't known; repeat use isn't recommended.
⧄ Drug exposure in patients of South Asian descent may exceed that in patients who are White or Black; however, no difference in effectiveness and safety was observed.
Dialyzable drug: Unknown.

PREGNANCY-LACTATION-REPRODUCTION

- There are no adequate studies during pregnancy. Drug is contraindicated during pregnancy.
- Drug appears in human milk. Effect of drug exposure on newborns or infants hasn't been studied; risk to infants who are breastfed can't be excluded. The CDC recommends discarding human milk for 24 hours after drug is taken.

NURSING CONSIDERATIONS

- Exclude pregnancy before use.
- Perform follow-up physical and pelvic exam if there is concern about patient's health or pregnancy status after drug administration.
- Ulipristal won't terminate existing pregnancy.
- Exclude ectopic pregnancy in patients who become pregnant or complain of lower abdominal pain 3 to 5 weeks after ulipristal use.
- Fertility returns rapidly after drug administration; routine contraceptives should be initiated or continued as soon as possible but not sooner than 5 days after emergency contraception.
- Drug may reduce effectiveness of regular hormonal contraceptives; additional use of a barrier method is recommended for subsequent intercourse during the same menstrual cycle.
- After drug administration, menses can occur a few days earlier or later than usual. For menses delayed beyond 1 week, rule out pregnancy.
- Drug doesn't protect against HIV infection (AIDS) or other sexually transmitted infections.
- *Look alike–sound alike:* Don't confuse ulipristal with ursodiol.

PATIENT TEACHING

- Teach patient that drug isn't intended for routine use as a contraceptive, won't terminate an existing pregnancy, and should only be used once per menstrual cycle.
- Advise patient not to take additional levonorgestrel emergency contraceptive pills within 5 days of ulipristal acetate.

- Instruct patient to take as soon as possible and not more than 120 hours after unprotected intercourse or known suspected contraceptive failure.
- Warn patient not to use ulipristal during pregnancy or to breastfeed for 24 hours after taking drug.
- Tell patient to contact prescriber if vomiting occurred within 3 hours of taking drug.
- Advise patient to report lower abdominal pain immediately.
- Instruct patient to resume routine contraceptives no sooner than 5 days after ulipristal and to use a barrier method during the same menstrual cycle.
- Advise patient that after drug administration, menses can occur a few days earlier or later than usual. Tell patient to report late menses beyond 1 week because testing will be necessary to rule out pregnancy.
- Warn patient that drug doesn't protect against HIV infection (AIDS) or other sexually transmitted infections.

ursodiol
ur-soe-DYE-ol

Reltone, Urso Forte, Urso 250

Therapeutic class: Miscellaneous GI drugs
Pharmacologic class: Bile acids

AVAILABLE FORMS
Capsules: 200 mg, 400 mg
Tablets: 250 mg, 500 mg

INDICATIONS & DOSAGES
➤ **Gallstone dissolution (capsules only)**
Adults: 8 to 10 mg/kg daily PO in two or three divided doses.
➤ **Gallstone prevention in patients undergoing rapid weight loss (capsules only)**
Adults: 600 mg PO daily or 300 mg PO b.i.d.
➤ **Primary biliary cholangitis (PBC) (tablets only)**
Adults: 13 to 15 mg/kg PO daily in two to four divided doses.

ADMINISTRATION
PO
- Give capsules without regard for food.
- Give tablets with food.

U

• May break scored tablets in half to achieve recommended dose. Don't use tablet segments that break incorrectly.
• Due to bitter taste, store halved tablets separately from whole tablets.
• Store at room temperature.

ACTION

Decreases secretion of cholesterol from the liver, reabsorbs cholesterol by the intestine, and subsequently decreases cholesterol content of bile stones. Increases bile acid level and displaces toxic levels of endogenous hydrophobic bile acids that accumulate in cholestatic liver disease.

Route	Onset	Peak	Duration
PO	Unknown	3 wk	Unknown

Half-life: Unknown.

ADVERSE REACTIONS

CNS: dizziness, fatigue, headache, insomnia. **CV:** chest pain. **EENT:** allergy, pharyngitis, rhinitis, sinusitis. **GI:** abdominal pain, constipation, diarrhea, dyspepsia, flatulence, GI disorder, nausea, peptic ulcer, vomiting. **GU:** increased creatinine level, UTI, dysmenorrhea. **Hematologic:** *leukopenia, thrombocytopenia.* **Hepatic:** cholecystitis. **Metabolic:** increased glucose level. **Musculoskeletal:** arthralgia, arthritis, back pain, musculoskeletal pain, myalgia. **Respiratory:** bronchitis, cough, URI. **Skin:** alopecia, rash. **Other:** flu-like symptoms, viral infection.

INTERACTIONS

Drug-drug. *Aluminum-based antacids:* May reduce ursodiol absorption. Avoid use together.
Bile acid sequestrants (cholestyramine, colestipol): May reduce ursodiol absorption. Avoid use together.
Clofibrate, estrogens, oral contraceptives: May counteract effect of ursodiol. Avoid use together.

EFFECTS ON LAB TEST RESULTS

• May decrease AST and ALT levels in the presence of liver disease.
• May increase LFT values and glucose and creatinine levels.
• May decrease WBC and platelet counts.

CONTRAINDICATIONS & CAUTIONS

• Capsules are contraindicated in patients with calcified cholesterol stones, radiopaque stones, and radiolucent bile pigment stones, which ursodiol can't dissolve.
• Capsules are contraindicated in patients with compelling reasons for cholecystectomy, including unremitting acute cholecystitis, cholangitis, biliary obstruction, gallstone pancreatitis, or biliary GI fistula.
• Tablets are contraindicated in patients with biliary obstruction.
• Contraindicated in patients with hypersensitivity or intolerance to ursodiol or bile acids.
• Use cautiously for gallstone indications in patients with chronic liver disease and in patients with a nonvisualizing gallbladder.
• Patients with variceal bleeding, hepatic encephalopathy, or ascites and those in need of an urgent liver transplant should receive appropriate specific treatment.
• Safety and effectiveness in children haven't been established.
• Use cautiously in older adults.
Dialyzable drug: Unlikely.

PREGNANCY-LACTATION-REPRODUCTION

• Available data show drug may be used cautiously during pregnancy, especially second and third trimesters.
• Drug may appear in human milk. Use cautiously during breastfeeding.

NURSING CONSIDERATIONS

• Monitor LFTs at baseline, every month for 3 months, then every 6 months in patients with PBC.
• Monitor AST and ALT levels at baseline and as clinically indicated in patients receiving drug for gallstones.
• Obtain gallbladder ultrasounds every 6 months for first year of therapy to monitor gallstone response. If gallstones have dissolved, continue therapy and obtain repeat ultrasound within 1 to 3 months to confirm dissolution. If partial stone dissolution isn't seen by 12 months of therapy, likelihood of success is greatly reduced.

PATIENT TEACHING

• Instruct patient in safe drug administration.
• Caution patient to avoid aluminum-based antacids.
• Advise patient that gallstone dissolution requires months of therapy, that complete

---

Reactions in bold italics are *life-threatening*. Interactions may have a *rapid onset* or a *delayed onset*.

dissolution doesn't occur in all patients, and recurrence of stones within 5 years has been observed in 50% of patients.

• Inform patient that gallbladder ultrasounds will be obtained to monitor therapy.

• Explain that most patients who achieve complete stone dissolution showed complete or partial dissolution on the first treatment evaluation.

ustekinumab
us-te-KIN-ue-mab

Stelara

Therapeutic class: Immunomodulators
Pharmacologic class: Monoclonal antibodies

AVAILABLE FORMS
Injection: 45 mg/0.5 mL, 90 mg/mL prefilled syringes; 45 mg/0.5 mL in single-dose vials
IV infusion: 130 mg/26 mL in single-dose vials

INDICATIONS & DOSAGES
➤ **Moderate to severe plaque psoriasis in patients who are candidates for phototherapy or systemic therapy**
Adults and children age 6 and older weighing more than 100 kg: Initially, 90 mg subcut; repeat dose in 4 weeks, followed by maintenance dose of 90 mg subcut every 12 weeks.
Adults weighing 100 kg or less and children age 6 and older weighing 60 to 100 kg: Initially, 45 mg subcut; repeat dose in 4 weeks, followed by maintenance dose of 45 mg subcut every 12 weeks.
Children age 6 and older weighing less than 60 kg: Initially, 0.75 mg/kg subcut; repeat dose in 4 weeks, followed by maintenance dose of 0.75 mg/kg subcut every 12 weeks.
➤ **Psoriatic arthritis as monotherapy or in combination with methotrexate**
Adults: Initially, 45 mg subcut; repeat in 4 weeks. Then maintenance dose of 45 mg subcut every 12 weeks.
Children age 6 and older weighing 60 kg or more: Initially, 45 mg subcut; repeat dose in 4 weeks, followed by maintenance dose of 45 mg subcut every 12 weeks.
Children age 6 and older weighing less than 60 kg: Initially, 0.75 mg/kg subcut; repeat

dose in 4 weeks, followed by maintenance dose of 0.75 mg/kg subcut every 12 weeks.
➤ **Psoriatic arthritis with coexistent moderate to severe plaque psoriasis as monotherapy or in combination with methotrexate**
Adults and children age 6 and older weighing more than 100 kg: Initially, 90 mg subcut; repeat dose in 4 weeks. Then maintenance dose of 90 mg subcut every 12 weeks.
➤ **Moderately to severely active ulcerative colitis or Crohn disease**
Adults weighing more than 85 kg: Initially, 520 mg IV infusion; then after 8 weeks begin maintenance dose of 90 mg subcut every 8 weeks.
Adults weighing from 55 to 85 kg: Initially, 390 mg IV infusion; then after 8 weeks begin maintenance dose of 90 mg subcut every 8 weeks.
Adults weighing 55 kg or less: Initial dosage is 260 mg IV infusion, then after 8 weeks, begin maintenance dose 90 mg subcut every 8 weeks.

ADMINISTRATION
IV
▼ Refrigerate vials upright at 36° to 46° F (2° to 8° C) and protected from light; don't freeze or shake.
▼ After calculating dosage and volume, withdraw an equal amount of fluid from 250-mL bag of NSS or 0.45% NSS and discard. Add drug to the NSS bag or 0.45% NSS and gently mix.
▼ Each vial is for single use only. Discard any remaining solution.
▼ May store diluted solution up to 7 hours at room temperature.
▼ Inspect diluted solution before infusion; don't use if particulate matter or discoloration is present.
▼ Infuse over at least 1 hour using an in-line 0.2-micron, low-protein-binding filter.
▼ **Incompatibilities:** Don't infuse in same IV line with other drugs.
Subcutaneous
• Refrigerate vials (upright) and syringes at 36° to 46° F (2° to 8° C) and protected from light; don't freeze or shake.
• May store prefilled syringes at room temperature for 30 days or less in original container protected from light. Once syringes are at room temperature, don't put back into refrigerator. Discard within 30 days if not used.

U

• Discard any unused portion.
• Before administration, inspect for particulate matter and discoloration. Drug appears colorless to light yellow and may contain a few small translucent or white particles. Don't use if discolored or cloudy or if other particulate matter is present.

🔔 *Alert:* Needle cover on the prefilled syringe contains a latex derivative. Persons sensitive to latex shouldn't handle needle cover.

• Give each subcut injection at a different anatomic location (such as upper arms, gluteal regions, top of thighs, or any quadrant of abdomen) than the previous injection; don't administer into areas with psoriasis or where skin is tender, bruised, erythematous, or indurated.

• Drug should only be administered under the guidance and supervision of a health care provider and to patients who will be closely monitored and have regular follow-up visits with a health care provider.

ACTION

Antagonizes interleukin 12 and 23 cytokines by binding to an interleukin-specific P40 protein subunit that disrupts interleukin-based inflammatory and immune responses.

Route	Onset	Peak	Duration
Subcut	Unknown	7–13.5 days	Unknown
IV	Unknown	Unknown	Unknown

Half-life: 10 to 126 days (psoriasis); 19 days (ulcerative colitis or Crohn disease).

ADVERSE REACTIONS

CNS: depression, dizziness, fatigue, headache, asthenia, fever. **EENT:** nasopharyngitis, pharyngolaryngeal pain, sinusitis, dental infection. **GI:** diarrhea, nausea, vomiting, abdominal pain. **GU:** vulvovaginal candidiasis or mycotic infection, UTI. **Musculoskeletal:** back pain, myalgia, arthralgia. **Respiratory:** URI, bronchitis. **Skin:** injection-site erythema, pruritus, acne. **Other:** *malignancies,* antibody development, flulike symptoms, infection.

INTERACTIONS

Drug-drug. *Allergen immunotherapy:* May increase risk of allergic reaction. Use cautiously together.
CYP450 substrates (cyclosporine, warfarin): May alter drug concentrations. Monitor

patient for clinical effects and adjust dosage as needed.
Inactivated vaccines: May not elicit an immune response sufficient to prevent disease. Revaccination may be required.
Live-virus vaccines: May transmit infection. Use together is contraindicated.
Pimecrolimus, tacrolimus (topical): May enhance adverse effect of ustekinumab. Avoid combination.
Drug-herb. *Echinacea:* May decrease therapeutic effect of ustekinumab. Consider therapy modification.

EFFECTS ON LAB TEST RESULTS
None reported.

CONTRAINDICATIONS & CAUTIONS
• Contraindicated in patients with clinically significant hypersensitivity to drug or its components. Hypersensitivity reactions, including anaphylaxis and angioedema, have been reported.
• Drug may increase risk of infections and reactivation of latent infections, including serious bacterial, fungal, and viral infections.
• Drug is contraindicated in patients with a clinically important active infection. Don't administer ustekinumab until the infection resolves or is adequately treated. Exercise caution when considering the use of ustekinumab in patients with a chronic infection or a history of recurrent infection.
• Don't administer to patients with active TB. Initiate treatment of latent TB before administering ustekinumab. Consider anti-TB therapy before initiation of ustekinumab in patients with a history of latent or active TB in which an adequate course of treatment can't be confirmed.
• Drug may increase the risk of malignancy. Safety of ustekinumab hasn't been evaluated in patients with a history of malignancy or a known malignancy.
• Safety of use in combination with other immunosuppressants or phototherapy hasn't been evaluated in psoriasis studies.
• Drug may decrease the protective effect of allergen immunotherapy, which may increase the risk of an allergic reaction to a dose of allergen immunotherapy. Use cautiously in patients receiving or who have received allergen immunotherapy, particularly for anaphylaxis.

Reactions in bold italics are *life-threatening*. Interactions may have a *rapid onset* or a *delayed onset*.

- The rapid appearance of multiple cutaneous squamous cell carcinomas in patients with preexisting risk factors for developing nonmelanoma skin cancer has been reported.
- Drug may cause PRES. Signs and symptoms include headache, seizures, confusion, and visual disturbances. For suspected PRES, discontinue drug and administer appropriate treatment.
- Cases of interstitial pneumonia, eosinophilic pneumonia, and cryptogenic organizing pneumonia have been reported with serious outcomes, including respiratory failure and prolonged hospitalization.
Dialyzable drug: Unknown.

PREGNANCY-LACTATION-REPRODUCTION
- Drug hasn't been studied during pregnancy. Use only if potential benefit outweighs fetal risk.
- Drug may appear in human milk. Use cautiously during breastfeeding.

NURSING CONSIDERATIONS
- Evaluate patients for TB before initiating drug. Closely monitor patients receiving drug for signs and symptoms of active TB (fever, cough, night sweats, fatigue, and unexplained weight loss) during and after treatment.
- Patients should receive all immunizations appropriate for age as recommended by current immunization guidelines before starting treatment. Patients being treated with ustekinumab shouldn't receive live-virus vaccines. Don't give bacillus Calmette-Guérin vaccines for 1 year before initiating treatment, during treatment, or for 1 year after discontinuation of treatment.
- In adolescents, it's recommended that drug be administered by a health care provider.
- Use caution when administering live-virus vaccines to household contacts of patient receiving drug because of the risk of shedding from the household contact and transmission to patient.
- Monitor patients for signs and symptoms of infection (fever, fatigue, sore throat, erythema, pain, cough). If infection develops, withhold drug and treat infection.
- Monitor patient for signs and symptoms of PRES (headache, seizures, confusion, visual disturbances).
- Monitor all patients for nonmelanoma skin cancer. Closely follow patients older than

age 60, those with a medical history of prolonged immunosuppressive therapy, and those with a history of psoralen–UVA treatment.
- Monitor patient for cough, dyspnea, and interstitial infiltrates after one to three doses. For confirmed noninfectious pneumonia, discontinue drug and institute appropriate treatment.
- After proper training in subcut injection technique, patient may self-inject.
- *Look alike–sound alike:* Don't confuse ustekinumab with infliximab or rituximab.

PATIENT TEACHING
- Instruct patient or caregiver to follow directions provided in the Medication Guide.
- Caution patient to immediately report signs or symptoms of PRES or pneumonia.
- Inform patient that drug may lower the ability of the immune system to fight infections. Stress importance of communicating any history of infections to health care provider and reporting signs or symptoms of infection.
- Advise patient to seek immediate medical attention if signs or symptoms of serious allergic reactions occur (wheezing, chest tightness, fever, itching, cough, blue skin color, seizures, facial swelling).
- Instruct patient or caregiver in injection techniques. Assess their ability to inject subcutaneously to ensure proper administration. The first self-injection should be performed under the supervision of a qualified health care professional.
- Advise patient that the needle cover on the prefilled syringe contains a latex derivative, which may cause allergic reactions in latex-sensitive individuals.
- Instruct patient or caregiver in proper technique for syringe and needle disposal. Advise patient not to reuse or share needles or syringes.
- Caution patient to avoid live-virus vaccines during and after therapy.
- Warn patient that drug may increase the risk of malignancy.
- Advise patient of childbearing potential to report pregnancy, plans to become pregnant, breastfeeding, or plans to breastfeed.

U

valACYclovir hydrochloride
val-ah-SYE-kloe-vir

Valtrex🍁

Therapeutic class: Antivirals
Pharmacologic class: Nucleosides–
nucleotides

AVAILABLE FORMS
Tablets: 500 mg, 1 g

INDICATIONS & DOSAGES
➤ **Herpes zoster infection (shingles)**
Adults: 1 g PO t.i.d. for 7 days.
Adjust-a-dose: For patients with CrCl of
30 to 49 mL/minute, give 1 g PO every
12 hours; if CrCl is 10 to 29 mL/minute,
give 1 g PO every 24 hours; if CrCl is less
than 10 mL/minute, give 500 mg PO every
24 hours.
➤ **First episode of genital herpes**
Adults: 1 g PO b.i.d. for 10 days.
Adjust-a-dose: For patients with CrCl of 10 to
29 mL/minute, give 1 g PO every 24 hours; if
CrCl is less than 10 mL/minute, give 500 mg
PO every 24 hours.
➤ **Recurrent genital herpes in immunocompetent patients**
Adults: 500 mg PO b.i.d. for 3 days, given at
the first sign or symptom of an episode.
Adjust-a-dose: For patients with CrCl of
29 mL/minute or less, give 500 mg PO every
24 hours.
➤ **Long-term suppression of recurrent
genital herpes**
Adults: 1 g PO once daily. In patients with a
history of nine or fewer recurrences per year,
use alternative dose of 500 mg once daily.
Adjust-a-dose: For patients with CrCl of
29 mL/minute or less, give 500 mg PO every
24 hours (every 48 hours if patient has nine or
fewer occurrences per year).
➤ **Long-term suppression of recurrent
genital herpes in patients with HIV and
CD4+ cell count of 100/mm³ or greater**
Adults: 500 mg PO b.i.d.
Adjust-a-dose: For patients with CrCl of
29 mL/minute or less, give 500 mg PO every
24 hours (every 48 hours if patient has nine or
fewer occurrences per year).
➤ **Cold sores (herpes labialis)**
Adults and children age 12 and older: 2 g PO
b.i.d. for 1 day taken 12 hours apart.

Adjust-a-dose: For patients with CrCl of 30
to 49 mL/minute, give 1 g every 12 hours
for two doses; if CrCl is 10 to 29 mL/minute,
give 500 mg every 12 hours for two doses; if
CrCl is less than 10 mL/minute, give 500 mg
as a single dose.
➤ **To reduce transmission of genital herpes
in patients with history of nine or fewer
occurrences per year**
Adults: 500 mg PO daily for source partner.
➤ **Chickenpox**
Children ages 2 to younger than 18: 20 mg/kg
PO t.i.d. for 5 days. Maximum dose is 1 g t.i.d.

ADMINISTRATION
PO
• Give drug without regard for meals.
• An oral suspension may be compounded by
a pharmacist if needed.
• Suspension must be refrigerated then shaken
before each dose. Discard unused portion
after 28 days.
• Give after hemodialysis on dialysis days.

ACTION
Rapidly converts to acyclovir, which in
turn becomes incorporated into viral DNA,
thereby terminating growth of the DNA
chain; inhibits viral DNA polymerase, causing inhibition of viral replication.

Route	Onset	Peak	Duration
PO	30 min	1.4–2.6 hr	Unknown

Half-life: 2.5 to 3.25 hours.

ADVERSE REACTIONS
CNS: headache, depression, dizziness, fatigue, fever. **EENT:** nasopharyngitis, rhinorrhea. **GI:** nausea, abdominal pain, diarrhea,
vomiting. **GU:** dysmenorrhea. **Hematologic:**
thrombocytopenia, neutropenia. **Hepatic:**
increased ALT and AST levels. **Metabolic:**
dehydration. **Musculoskeletal:** arthralgia.
Respiratory: URI. **Skin:** rash. **Other:** herpes simplex.

INTERACTIONS
Drug-drug. *Nephrotoxic drugs (aminoglycosides, contrast dye, cyclosporine, lithium):*
May increase risk of acute renal failure. Use
cautiously together.

EFFECTS ON LAB TEST RESULTS
• May increase ALP, ALT, AST, and creatinine levels.

Reactions in bold italics are *life-threatening*. Interactions may have a *rapid onset* or a **delayed onset**.

• May decrease Hb level and platelet and WBC counts.

CONTRAINDICATIONS & CAUTIONS
• Contraindicated in patients hypersensitive to valacyclovir, acyclovir, or components of the formulation.
🛈 *Alert:* Thrombotic thrombocytopenic purpura (TTP) and hemolytic-uremic syndrome (HUS) may occur in allogeneic bone marrow or renal transplant recipients and patients with advanced HIV at doses of 8 g/day. Discontinue drug if signs or symptoms or lab findings of TTP or HUS occur.
• Use cautiously in older adults or patients with dehydration, in those with renal impairment, and in those receiving other nephrotoxic drugs. CNS effects, such as agitation, hallucinations, confusion, delirium, seizures, and encephalopathy, can occur in patients with normal or abnormal renal function.
• Safety and effectiveness of therapy beyond 12 months (beyond 6 months in patients infected with HIV-1) or beyond 8 months in reduction of transmission of genital herpes haven't been established.
• Safety and effectiveness in prepubertal children haven't been established except for in chickenpox.
Dializable drug: 33%.

PREGNANCY-LACTATION-REPRODUCTION
• There are no adequate studies during pregnancy. Use only if potential benefits outweigh fetal risk.
• Drug appears in human milk. Use cautiously during breastfeeding.

NURSING CONSIDERATIONS
• Start treatment for herpes zoster infection at earliest signs or symptoms. It's most effective when started within 48 hours of onset of rash.
• Monitor renal function; give appropriate dose adjusted for renal status.
• If renal failure and anuria occur, hemodialysis may be beneficial until renal function returns.
• Monitor patient for CNS changes (agitation, hallucinations, confusion, delirium, seizures, and encephalopathy). Discontinue drug if changes occur.
• *Look alike–sound alike:* Don't confuse valacyclovir (Valtrex) with valganciclovir (Valcyte) or acyclovir. Don't confuse Valtrex with Keflex or Zovirax.

PATIENT TEACHING
• Instruct patient in safe drug administration.
• Teach patient signs and symptoms of herpes infection (rash, tingling, itching, and pain), and to notify prescriber immediately if they occur. Treatment should begin as soon as possible after symptoms appear, preferably within 48 hours of the onset of zoster rash.
• Caution patient to immediately report CNS changes, kidney problems, and any adverse reactions.
• Tell patient that drug isn't a cure for herpes but may decrease length and severity of symptoms.
• Advise patient with genital herpes to use safe sex practices in combination with suppressive therapy, even if no symptoms appear.
• Caution patient to maintain adequate hydration.

valproate sodium 🈺
val-PROH-ayt

valproic acid

divalproex sodium
Depakote✐, Depakote ER, Depakote Sprinkle✐, Epival✤

Therapeutic class: Anticonvulsants
Pharmacologic class: Carboxylic acid derivatives

AVAILABLE FORMS
The strengths of valproate sodium and divalproex sodium are expressed in terms of valproic acid.
valproate sodium
Injection: 100 mg/mL
valproic acid
Capsules 🚫: 250 mg
Syrup: 250 mg/5 mL
divalproex sodium
Capsules (delayed-release sprinkle) 🚫: 125 mg
Tablets (delayed-release) 🚫: 125 mg, 250 mg, 500 mg
Tablets (extended-release) 🚫: 250 mg, 500 mg

INDICATIONS & DOSAGES
Adjust-a-dose (for all indications): For older adults, start at lower dosage. Increase dosage more slowly and with regular monitoring of

V

fluid and nutritional intake, and watch for dehydration, somnolence, and other adverse reactions.

➤ **Simple and complex absence seizures, mixed seizure types (including absence seizures)**
Adults and children age 2 and older: Initially, 10 to 15 mg/kg PO (valproic acid) or IV daily, or 15 mg/kg sprinkles, extended-release, or delayed-release PO daily; then increase by 5 to 10 mg/kg daily at weekly intervals up to maximum of 60 mg/kg daily. Don't use Depakote ER in children younger than age 10.

➤ **Complex partial seizures**
Adults and children age 10 and older: 10 to 15 mg/kg PO or valproate sodium IV daily; then increase by 5 to 10 mg/kg daily at weekly intervals, up to 60 mg/kg daily.

➤ **Mania**
Adults: Initially, 750 mg delayed-release PO daily in divided doses, or 25 mg/kg extended-release PO once daily. Adjust dosage based on patient's response; maximum dose for either form is 60 mg/kg daily.

➤ **To prevent migraine headache**
Adults: Initially, 250 mg delayed-release divalproex sodium PO b.i.d. Some patients may need up to 1,000 mg daily. Or, 500 mg extended-release PO daily for 1 week; then 1,000 mg PO daily. Maximum recommended dosage is 60 mg/kg/day.

ADMINISTRATION

⚠ *Alert:* Hazardous agent; use safe-handling and disposal precautions.

PO
• Don't crush delayed- or extended-release tablets.
• Give drug with food or milk to reduce adverse GI effects.
• Don't give syrup to patients who need sodium restriction. Check with prescriber.
• Sprinkle capsules may be swallowed whole or opened and contents sprinkled on a teaspoonful of soft food. Patient should swallow immediately without chewing.
• Give a missed dose as soon as possible unless it's almost time for the next scheduled dose.

IV
▼ IV use is indicated only in patients who can't take drug orally. Switch patient to oral form as soon as feasible; effects of IV use for longer than 14 days are unknown.

▼ Dilute valproate sodium injection with at least 50 mL of a compatible diluent. It's physically compatible and chemically stable in D_5W, NSS, and lactated Ringer solution for 24 hours at room temperature. Discard unused portion left in vial.
▼ Infuse drug over 60 minutes at no more than 20 mg/minute and at the same frequency as oral dosage.
▼ Monitor drug level, and adjust dosage as needed.
▼ **Incompatibilities:** None listed by manufacturer. Consult a drug incompatibility reference for more information.

ACTION

Hasn't been established. Activity in epilepsy is thought to be related to increased brain concentrations of GABA.

Route	Onset	Peak	Duration
PO	Unknown	Variable	Unknown
IV	Unknown	1 hr	Unknown

Half-life: Adults, 9 to 16 hours; children, 3.5 to 67 hours based on age.

ADVERSE REACTIONS

CNS: asthenia, dizziness, headache, insomnia, pain, paresthesia, tardive dyskinesia, nervousness, somnolence, vertigo, tremor, agitation, abnormal gait, dysarthria, hallucinations, hypertonia, abnormal thinking, amnesia, ataxia, depression, emotional lability, catatonic reactions, malaise, confusion, fever, abnormal dreams, personality disorder, psychosis, speech disorder, taste perversion. **CV:** *arrhythmia,* chest pain, edema, HTN, hypotension, vasodilation, tachycardia, palpitations. **EENT:** blurred vision, diplopia, dry eyes, photophobia, conjunctivitis, eye pain, nystagmus, deafness, ear pain, tinnitus, epistaxis, rhinitis, dry mouth, gum hemorrhage, oral ulcerations, pharyngitis, periodontal abscess. **GI:** abdominal pain, anorexia, diarrhea, fecal incontinence, flatulence, gastroenteritis, glossitis, stomatitis, dyspepsia, nausea, vomiting, hematemesis, eructation, *pancreatitis,* constipation, increased appetite. **GU:** vaginitis, dysmenorrhea, dysuria, cystitis, urinary frequency, urinary incontinence. **Hematologic:** *hemorrhage, leukopenia, thrombocytopenia,* anemia. **Hepatic:** increased transaminase levels. **Metabolic:** weight gain or loss, hypoproteinemia. **Musculoskeletal:** back and neck pain, arthralgia, leg cramps, twitching, myasthenia. **Respiratory:** bronchitis, cough, dyspnea, hiccups, pneumonia. **Skin:** alopecia, diaphoresis, ecchymosis, petechiae, discoid lupus erythematosus, dry skin, furunculosis, seborrhea, rash, pruritus; injection-site pain, inflammation, or reaction. **Other:** flulike syndrome, infection, chills, accidental injury.

INTERACTIONS

❸ Alert: Drug can significantly interact with many drugs. Consult a drug interaction resource or pharmacist for additional information.

Drug-drug. *Aspirin, erythromycin, felbamate:* May cause valproic acid toxicity. Use together cautiously and monitor drug level.

Benzodiazepines, other CNS depressants: May cause excessive CNS depression. Avoid using together.

Carbamazepine: May cause carbamazepine CNS toxicity; may decrease valproic acid level and cause loss of seizure control. Use together cautiously, if at all. Monitor patient for seizure activity and toxicity during therapy and for at least 1 month after stopping either drug.

Carbapenem antibiotics (ertapenem, imipenem, meropenem): May decrease valproic acid level and cause loss of seizure control. Consider alternative antimicrobial agent. Monitor levels closely.

Clonazepam: May increase risk of absence seizures in patients with a history of absence seizures. Monitor patient closely.

Estrogen-containing hormonal contraceptives: May decrease valproate concentration and increase seizure frequency. Monitor valproate level and clinical response.

Ethosuximide: May increase ethosuximide level. Monitor patient closely.

Fosphenytoin, phenytoin: May increase or decrease phenytoin level; may decrease valproate level. Monitor patient closely.

Lamotrigine: May increase lamotrigine level and decrease valproate level; serious skin reactions may occur. Monitor levels closely.

Phenobarbital: May increase phenobarbital level; may increase clearance of valproate. Monitor patient closely.

Propofol: May increase propofol level. Reduce propofol dosage.

Rifampin: May decrease valproate level. Monitor level of valproate.

Rufinamide: May increase rufinamide serum concentration. Begin valproate therapy at a low dosage, and titrate to a clinically effective dosage.

TCAs (amitriptyline, nortriptyline): May increase TCA level. Monitor drug level.

Topiramate: May cause hyperammonemia with and without encephalopathy. Concomitant use has been associated with hypothermia. Check blood ammonia levels in patients reporting hypothermia.

Warfarin: May displace warfarin from binding sites. Monitor PT and INR.

Zidovudine: May decrease zidovudine clearance. Avoid using together.

Drug-lifestyle. *Alcohol use:* May cause excessive CNS depression. Discourage use together.

EFFECTS ON LAB TEST RESULTS

• May increase ammonia, ALT, and AST levels.

• May increase eosinophil count and bleeding time.

• May decrease platelet, RBC, and WBC counts.

• May cause false-positive results for urine ketone levels.

• May alter thyroid function test results.

CONTRAINDICATIONS & CAUTIONS

• Contraindicated in patients hypersensitive to drug and in those with hepatic disease or significant hepatic dysfunction, and in patients with a urea cycle disorder (UCD).

▓ **Boxed Warning** Patients with hereditary neurometabolic syndromes caused by DNA mutations of the mitochondrial DNA polymerase gamma (*POLG*) gene such as Alpers-Huttenlocher syndrome are at high risk for acute liver failure and fatalities. Drug is contraindicated in patients known to have mitochondrial disorders caused by *POLG* mutations and in children younger than age 2 who are suspected of having a mitochondrial disorder. In patients older than age 2 who are clinically suspected of having a hereditary mitochondrial disease, use only after other anticonvulsants have failed. ■

Boxed Warning Cases of life-threatening pancreatitis have been reported in children and adults receiving valproate shortly after initial use as well as after several years of use. ■

• Safety and effectiveness of Depakote ER in children younger than age 10 haven't been established.

Dialyzable drug: 20%.
⚠ *Overdose S&S:* Somnolence, heart block, deep coma, hypernatremia.

PREGNANCY-LACTATION-REPRODUCTION

Boxed Warning Avoid use in patients who may become pregnant. Valproate can cause teratogenic effects, such as neural tube defects and other organ system malformations. Drug is contraindicated for prevention of migraines during pregnancy. ■

Boxed Warning Children born to patients who took drug during pregnancy have an increased risk of lower cognitive test scores. Consider alternative medication during pregnancy unless use of drug is essential. Patients of childbearing potential should use effective contraception during therapy. ■

Boxed Warning Use during pregnancy in patients with epilepsy or bipolar disorder only if other drugs have failed to control symptoms. Drug is contraindicated for use in pregnancy for reversible conditions not associated with permanent injury or death. ■

• To prevent major seizures, patients with epilepsy who are pregnant shouldn't discontinue drug abruptly.

• Patients taking valproate during pregnancy may develop hepatic failure or clotting abnormalities, including thrombocytopenia, hypofibrinogenemia, or decrease in other coagulation factors, which may result in hemorrhagic complications in the neonate, including death.

• Offer prenatal diagnostic testing to patient who is pregnant and using drug, to detect neural tube and other defects.

• Male infertility has been reported.

• Hypoglycemia in neonates and fatal cases of hepatic failure in infants after maternal use during pregnancy have been reported.

• Patients who are pregnant should enroll in the North American AED (Antiepileptic Drug) Pregnancy Registry (1-888-233-2334 or http://www.aedpregnancyregistry.org/).

• Drug appears in human milk. Use cautiously during breastfeeding.

• Monitor infants who are breastfed for liver damage (jaundice, unusual bruising, bleeding).

NURSING CONSIDERATIONS

▓ **Boxed Warning** During treatment, closely monitor patients older than age 2 who are suspected of having a mitochondrial disorder for development of acute liver injury; perform regular clinical assessments and serum liver testing. Perform *POLG* mutation screening in accordance with current clinical practice. ■

Boxed Warning Fatal hepatotoxicity may follow nonspecific signs and symptoms, such as malaise, fever, anorexia, facial edema, vomiting, weakness, and lethargy. If these signs and symptoms occur during therapy, notify prescriber immediately because patient might be developing hepatic dysfunction and must stop drug. Monitor LFT values before therapy and at frequent intervals, especially during first 6 months. ■

Boxed Warning Patients at high risk for fatal hepatotoxicity include those with congenital metabolic disorders, mental retardation, or organic brain disease; those taking multiple anticonvulsants; and children younger than age 2. In children younger than age 2, use with extreme caution and as a sole agent, weighing benefits of therapy against risks. ■

🕒 *Alert:* Closely monitor all patients taking or starting antiepileptic drugs for changes in behavior indicating worsening of suicidality or depression. Symptoms such as anxiety, agitation, hostility, mania, and hypomania may be precursors to emerging suicidality.

🕒 *Alert:* Dose-related thrombocytopenia can occur. Monitor CBC, platelet count, PT, and INR before starting therapy and at frequent intervals. Decrease dose or discontinue drug if hemorrhage, bruising, or coagulation disorder occurs.

🕒 *Alert:* Monitor patients and immediately report symptoms of DRESS syndrome (rash, fever, swollen glands). Discontinue drug for suspected DRESS syndrome.

• Monitor valproate and concomitant drug levels closely when introducing or withdrawing enzyme-inducing drugs.

• Adverse reactions may not be caused by valproic acid alone because it's usually used with other anticonvulsants.

• When converting adults and children age 10 and older with seizures from Depakote to Depakote ER, make sure the extended-release dose is 8% to 20% higher than the regular dose taken previously. See manufacturer's package insert for more details.

• Never withdraw drug suddenly because sudden withdrawal may worsen seizures.

Reactions in bold italics are *life-threatening*. Interactions may have a *rapid onset* or a *delayed onset*.

Call prescriber at once if adverse reactions
develop.
• Notify prescriber if tremors occur; a dosage
reduction may be needed.
• Monitor drug level. Therapeutic level
ranges from 50 to 100 mcg/mL for seizure
control and 50 to 125 mcg/mL for mania.
• When converting patients from a brand-
name drug to a generic drug, use caution because breakthrough seizures may
occur.
🚺 *Alert:* Sometimes fatal, hyperammonemic
encephalopathy may occur when starting valproate therapy in patients with UCD. Evaluate
patients with UCD risk factors before starting valproate therapy. Patients who develop
symptoms of unexplained hyperammonemic encephalopathy during valproate therapy
should stop drug, undergo prompt appropriate treatment, and be evaluated for underlying
UCD.
• *Look alike–sound alike:* Don't confuse
Depakote with Depakote ER.

PATIENT TEACHING
🚺 *Alert:* Tell patient and caregivers that drug
may increase risk of suicidality and to immediately report the emergence or worsening of
depression, unusual changes in mood or behavior, emergence of suicidality, or thoughts
about self-harm.
• Teach patient safe drug administration and
handling.
• Advise patient and parents to keep drug out
of children's reach.
• Warn patient and parents not to stop drug
therapy abruptly.
🚺 *Alert:* Tell patient to immediately report rash (with or without blisters), fever,
swollen lymph nodes, mouth ulcers, or skin
shedding.
Boxed Warning Warn patients and caregivers that abdominal pain, nausea, vomiting,
and anorexia can be symptoms of pancreatitis
that require prompt medical evaluation. ▮
• Advise patient to avoid driving and other
potentially hazardous activities that require
mental alertness until drug's CNS effects are
known.
• Instruct patient or parents to call prescriber
if malaise, weakness, lethargy, facial swelling,
loss of appetite, or vomiting occurs.
• Tell patient to report pregnancy or plans
to become pregnant or to breastfeed during
therapy.

valsartan
val-SAR-tan

Diovan🖉

Therapeutic class: Antihypertensives
Pharmacologic class: ARBs

AVAILABLE FORMS
Solution: 4 mg/mL
Tablets: 40 mg, 80 mg, 160 mg, 320 mg

INDICATIONS & DOSAGES
➤ **HTN (used alone or with other antihypertensives)**
Adults: Initially, 80 or 160 mg tablets PO once
daily, or 40 to 80 mg oral solution b.i.d. Expect to see a reduction in BP in 2 to 4 weeks.
If additional antihypertensive effect is needed,
may increase dosage to 160 or 320 mg daily.
Usual dosage range is 80 to 320 mg daily.
Children ages 6 to 16: Initially, 0.65 mg/kg
oral solution b.i.d. (up to 40 mg total). Adjust
dosage according to patient response and tolerability, up to 1.35 mg/kg b.i.d. or 160 mg
daily.
Children ages 1 to 16: Initially, 1 mg/kg tablet
PO once daily (up to 40 mg total), or consider
a starting dose of 2 mg/kg in select patients
when greater BP reduction is needed. Adjust
dosage according to patient response and tolerability, up to 4 mg/kg or 160 mg daily.
➤ **NYHA Class II to IV HF**
Adults: Initially, 40 mg PO b.i.d.; increase as
tolerated to 80 mg b.i.d., and then to target
dose of 160 mg b.i.d.
➤ **To reduce CV death in patients with left
ventricular failure or dysfunction who are
stable after MI**
Adults: 20 mg PO b.i.d. Initial dose may be
given as soon as 12 hours after MI. Increase
dose to 40 mg b.i.d. within 7 days. Increase
subsequent doses, as tolerated, to target dose
of 160 mg b.i.d.
Adjust-a-dose: Consider dosage reduction for
symptomatic hypotension or renal dysfunction.

ADMINISTRATION
PO
• Give drug without regard for food.
• Pharmacists may prepare a suspension
from tablets for children ages 1 to 5, patients
older than age 5 unable to swallow pills, and

V

♣Canada   ◇OTC   ◆Off-label use   🖉Photoguide   ⬬Do not crush   *Liquid contains alcohol   ▨Genetic

children for whom the calculated dose doesn't correspond to an available tablet strength.
• Shake suspension at least 10 seconds before pouring. Store suspension at room temperature for 30 days or in refrigerator for 75 days.
• Oral solution and suspension aren't therapeutically equivalent to the tablet formulation; peak concentration is higher. When switching between formulations, expect to adjust valsartan dosage.
• If a dose is missed, give as soon as remembered. If it's close to the next dose, don't give the missed dose. Give the next scheduled dose.

ACTION

Blocks the binding of angiotensin II to receptor sites in vascular smooth muscle and the adrenal gland, which inhibits the pressor effects of the RAAS.

Route	Onset	Peak	Duration
PO (solution)	Unknown	0.7–3.7 hr	24 hr
PO (tablets)	2 hr	2–4 hr	24 hr

Half-life: 6 hours.

ADVERSE REACTIONS

CNS: dizziness, headache, fatigue, vertigo, syncope. **CV:** edema, hypotension, orthostatic hypotension. **EENT:** blurred vision, rhinitis, sinusitis, pharyngitis. **GI:** abdominal pain, diarrhea, nausea. **GU:** renal impairment. **Hematologic:** *neutropenia.* **Metabolic:** *hyperkalemia.* **Musculoskeletal:** arthralgia, back pain. **Respiratory:** URI, cough. **Other:** viral infection.

INTERACTIONS

Drug-drug. *ACE inhibitors:* May increase risk of renal dysfunction, hypotension, and hyperkalemia. Avoid use together but, if necessary, closely monitor BP, serum potassium level, and renal function.
Aliskiren: May increase risk of renal impairment, hypotension, and hyperkalemia in patients with diabetes and in those with moderate to severe renal impairment (GFR less than 60 mL/minute). Concomitant use is contraindicated in patients with diabetes. Avoid concomitant use in those with moderate to severe renal impairment.
Antihepaciviral combination products: May increase valsartan serum concentration. Consider therapy modification or decrease valsartan dosage and monitor patient for hypotension and worsening renal function.

Lithium: May increase lithium level. Monitor lithium level and patient for toxicity.
NSAIDs: May result in deterioration of renal function in older adults, patients who are volume-depleted, and in those with compromised renal function. Monitor renal function. May also decrease antihypertensive effect. Monitor BP.
Potassium supplements, potassium-sparing diuretics, other angiotensin II blockers: May increase potassium level. May also increase creatinine level in patients with HF. Avoid using together.
Trimethoprim: May increase risk of hyperkalemia, especially in older adults. Closely monitor serum potassium level.
Drug-food. *Salt substitutes containing potassium:* May increase potassium level. May also increase creatinine level in patients with HF. Discourage use together.

EFFECTS ON LAB TEST RESULTS

• May increase potassium, BUN, and creatinine levels.
• May decrease neutrophil count.

CONTRAINDICATIONS & CAUTIONS

• Contraindicated in patients hypersensitive to drug or its components.
• Angioedema, a rare life-threatening reaction, has been reported. Discontinue drug immediately and treat emergently if angioedema occurs. Don't give drug to patients with history of angioedema.
• Use cautiously in patients with renal or severe hepatic disease.
• Safety and effectiveness haven't been established in children younger than age 6 and in children of any age with GFR less than 30 mL/minute/1.73 m^2.
Dialyzable drug: No.
⚠ **Overdose S&S:** Hypotension, tachycardia, bradycardia, decreased level of consciousness, circulatory collapse, shock.

PREGNANCY-LACTATION-REPRODUCTION

Boxed Warning Drugs that act directly on the RAAS can cause injury and death to the developing fetus. When pregnancy is detected, stop drug as soon as possible. ▉
• It isn't known if drug appears in human milk. Patient should discontinue breastfeeding or discontinue drug.

NURSING CONSIDERATIONS
• Monitor BP and watch for hypotension. Excessive hypotension can occur when drug is given with high doses of diuretics.
• Correct volume and sodium depletions before starting drug.
• Monitor serum BUN, creatinine, and potassium levels.

PATIENT TEACHING
• Instruct patient in safe drug administration.
• Advise patient to report all adverse effects, especially dizziness upon standing or other signs and symptoms of hypotension.
• Tell patient of childbearing potential to report pregnancy. Drug will need to be stopped.

---

vancomycin hydrochloride
van-koh-MYE-sin

Firvanq, Vancocin

Therapeutic class: Antibiotics
Pharmacologic class: Glycopeptides

AVAILABLE FORMS
Capsules: 125 mg, 250 mg
Powder for injection: 500-mg, 750-mg, 1-g, 1.25-g, 1.5-g. 5-g, 10-g vials
Powder for oral solution: 25 mg/mL, 50 mg/mL concentration after dilution
Premixed for injection: 500 mg, 750 mg, 750 mg, 1 g, 1.25 g, 1.5 g, 1.75 g, 2 g, 2.5 g

INDICATIONS & DOSAGES
Adjust-a-dose (for all indications): In renal insufficiency, adjust dosage based on degree of renal impairment, drug level, severity of infection, and susceptibility of causative organism. Initially, give 15 mg/kg, and adjust subsequent doses as needed. In patients who are anephric, an initial dose of 15 mg/kg should be followed with a dose of 1.9 mg/kg/24 hours.
➤ **Serious or severe infections when other antibiotics are ineffective or contraindicated, including those caused by MRSA, *Staphylococcus epidermidis*, or diphtheroid organisms**
Adults: 500 mg IV every 6 hours or 1 g IV every 12 hours.
Children: 10 mg/kg IV every 6 hours.
Neonates and young infants: 15 mg/kg IV loading dose; then 10 mg/kg IV every

12 hours if child is younger than age 1 week or 10 mg/kg IV every 8 hours if older than 1 week but younger than 1 month.
Older adults: 15 mg/kg IV loading dose. Subsequent doses are based on renal function and drug levels.
➤ **CDAD**
Adults: 125 mg PO every 6 hours for 10 days.
Children: 40 mg/kg/day PO in three or four divided doses for 7 to 10 days. Maximum daily dose is 2 g.
➤ **Staphylococcal enterocolitis**
Adults: 500 mg to 2 g PO in three or four divided doses daily for 7 to 10 days.
Children: 40 mg/kg/day PO in three or four divided doses for 7 to 10 days. Maximum daily dose is 2 g.

ADMINISTRATION
⚠ *Alert:* Obtain specimen for culture and sensitivity tests before giving. Because of the emergence of vancomycin-resistant enterococci, reserve use for treatment of serious infections caused by gram-positive bacteria resistant to beta-lactam anti-infectives.
PO
• Powder for oral solution must be reconstituted by the pharmacist before use.
⚠ *Alert:* Oral form is ineffective for systemic infections.
IV
▼ This route is ineffective for CDAD and staphylococcal enterocolitis.
▼ Reconstitute with sterile water for injection to provide a solution containing 50 mg/mL.
▼ Refrigerate solution after reconstitution and use within 96 hours.
▼ For infusion, further dilute with NSS for injection or D_5W to a final concentration of no more than 5 mg/mL and infuse as soon as possible at no faster than 30 minutes for every 500 mg or over at least 60 minutes, whichever is longer.
▼ Drug is an irritant; give by secure IV route and ensure proper needle or catheter placement before and during infusion. Pain, tenderness, and necrosis may occur with extravasation. Can minimize frequency and severity of thrombophlebitis by slow infusion of drug and rotation of venous access sites.
▼ Drug is available premixed in NSS or D_5W solution in a variety of volumes.

V

▼ Thawed, premixed solution remains stable for 72 hours at room temperature or for 30 days in refrigerator. Don't refreeze.

🕒 *Alert:* Rapid infusion (over several minutes) has been associated with hypotension, shock and, rarely, cardiac arrest.

▼ Check site daily for phlebitis and irritation. Severe irritation and necrosis can result from extravasation.

▼ **Incompatibilities:** Beta-lactam antibiotics, many other drugs (vancomycin has a low pH). Consult a drug incompatibility reference for more information.

ACTION

Hinders bacterial cell-wall synthesis, damaging the bacterial plasma membrane and making the cell more vulnerable to osmotic pressure. Also interferes with RNA synthesis.

Route	Onset	Peak	Duration
PO	Unknown	Unknown	Unknown
IV	Immediate	Immediate	Unknown

Half-life: 4 to 6 hours (longer in patients with renal impairment).

ADVERSE REACTIONS

CNS: fever, pain, headache, fatigue, dizziness, malaise, vertigo, depression, insomnia. **CV:** hypotension, chest pain, edema, flushing, phlebitis at injection site. **EENT:** ototoxicity, tinnitus. **GI:** *pseudomembranous colitis,* nausea, abdominal pain, vomiting, diarrhea, constipation, flatulence. **GU:** *nephrotoxicity,* interstitial nephritis, renal tubular necrosis, UTI. **Hematologic:** *leukopenia, neutropenia,* eosinophilia, *thrombocytopenia,* anemia. **Metabolic:** *hypokalemia (PO).* **Musculoskeletal:** myalgia, back pain. **Respiratory:** dyspnea, wheezing. **Skin:** dermatitis, erythema, injection-site reaction or pain. **Other:** hypersensitivity reaction, chills, superinfection.

INTERACTIONS

Drug-drug. *Anesthetics:* May cause erythema, histamine-like flushing, and anaphylactoid reaction. Monitor patient closely.
Nephrotoxic drugs (aminoglycosides, amphotericin B, bacitracin, cisplatin, colistin, piperacillin, polymyxin B, viomycin), neurotoxic drugs: May increase risk of nephrotoxicity or ototoxicity. Monitor renal function and hearing function test results.

Nondepolarizing muscle relaxants: May enhance neuromuscular blockade. Monitor patient closely.
NSAIDs: May increase vancomycin serum concentration. Monitor therapy.

EFFECTS ON LAB TEST RESULTS

• May increase BUN and creatinine levels.
• May decrease potassium level.
• May increase eosinophil count.
• May decrease neutrophil and WBC counts.

CONTRAINDICATIONS & CAUTIONS

• Contraindicated in patients hypersensitive to drug or its components.
• Use cautiously in patients receiving other neurotoxic, nephrotoxic, or ototoxic drugs; in patients older than age 60; and in those with impaired hepatic or renal function, hearing loss, or allergies to other antibiotics.
Dialyzable drug: Poorly dialyzable.

PREGNANCY-LACTATION-REPRODUCTION

• It isn't known if drug causes fetal harm. Use during pregnancy only if clearly needed.
Boxed Warning Verify pregnancy status before using IV formulations containing polyethylene glycol and N-acetyl-D-alanine. Fetal malformations have occurred in animal studies using these formulations. If vancomycin is needed during the first or second trimester, use other available formulations. ∎
• Drug appears in human milk. Patient should discontinue breastfeeding or discontinue drug.

NURSING CONSIDERATIONS

• Obtain hearing evaluation before and during prolonged therapy.
• Monitor patient's fluid balance and watch for oliguria and cloudy urine.
• Monitor patient carefully for vancomycin flushing syndrome (red-man syndrome), which can occur with rapid drug infusion. Signs and symptoms include maculopapular rash on face, neck, trunk, and limbs and pruritus and hypotension caused by histamine release. If wheezing, urticaria, or pain and muscle spasm of the chest and back occur, stop infusion and notify prescriber.
• Assess renal function (BUN, creatinine level and CrCl, urinalysis, and urine output) before and during therapy.
• Carefully monitor vancomycin serum concentrations to adjust IV dosage requirements.

Reactions in bold italics are *life-threatening*. Interactions may have a *rapid onset* or a *delayed onset*.

• Monitor patient for hypersensitivity reactions, including skin reactions.
• Monitor IV site for irritation, phlebitis, and extravasation.
• Periodically monitor leukocyte count during IV therapy.
• Monitor patient for signs and symptoms of superinfection. CDAD can occur up to 2 months after therapy ends.
• *Look alike–sound alike:* Don't confuse vancomycin with clindamycin, gentamicin, or Vibramycin.

PATIENT TEACHING
• Advise patient to take entire amount of drug exactly as directed, even after feeling better.
• Instruct patient receiving drug IV to report discomfort at IV insertion site.
• Tell patient to report ringing in ears.
• Advise patient to report adverse reactions to prescriber immediately.
• Caution patient to immediately report pregnancy.

vardenafil hydrochloride
var-DEN-ah-fill

Therapeutic class: Erectile dysfunction drugs
Pharmacologic class: PDE5 inhibitors

AVAILABLE FORMS
Tablets (film-coated): 2.5 mg, 5 mg, 10 mg, 20 mg
Tablets (ODTs) : 10 mg

INDICATIONS & DOSAGES
➤ **Erectile dysfunction**
Adults: 10 mg PO as a single dose, as needed, 1 hour before sexual activity. Dosage range is 5 to 20 mg, based on formulation, effectiveness, and tolerance. Maximum, 10 mg/day for ODT or 20 mg once daily for tablets.
Adjust-a-dose: For patients with moderate hepatic impairment (Child-Pugh class B) and patients age 65 and older, first dose is 5 mg daily, as needed. Don't exceed 10 mg daily in patients with hepatic impairment. Dosage adjustment may be needed in patients taking potent CYP3A4 inhibitors. Consult manufacturer's instructions for drug-interaction dosage adjustments.

ADMINISTRATION
PO
• Tablets and ODTs aren't interchangeable.
• Give drug without regard for food.
• Don't split or crush ODTs.
• Place ODT on the tongue to disintegrate. Have patient take without water or other liquid.
• Don't remove ODT from blister pack until ready to use.

ACTION
Increases cyclic guanosine monophosphate levels, prolongs smooth muscle relaxation, and promotes blood flow into the corpus cavernosum by inhibiting PDE5.

Route	Onset	Peak	Duration
PO	60 min	30–120 min	Unknown

Half-life: 4 to 6 hours.

ADVERSE REACTIONS
CNS: headache, dizziness. **CV:** flushing, hypotension, tachycardia. **EENT:** rhinitis, sinusitis, nasal congestion. **GI:** dyspepsia, nausea. **Metabolic:** increased CK level. **Musculoskeletal:** back pain. **Other:** flulike syndrome.

INTERACTIONS
Drug-drug. *Alpha blockers:* May enhance hypotensive effects. Start concomitant treatment at reduced dosage only if patient is stable on alpha-blocker therapy.
Antiarrhythmics of Class IA (quinidine, procainamide) and Class III (amiodarone, sotalol): May prolong QTc interval. Avoid using together.
Guanylate cyclase (GC) stimulators (riociguat), nitrates: May enhance hypotensive effects. Use together is contraindicated.
Strong and moderate CYP3A4 inhibitors (erythromycin, itraconazole, ketoconazole, ritonavir): May increase vardenafil level. Reduce vardenafil dosage and extend dosing interval according to manufacturer's instructions. Use with ODTs is contraindicated.
Drug-food. *Grapefruit, grapefruit juice:* May increase vardenafil level. Avoid use together.
High-fat meals: May reduce peak level of drug. Discourage use with a high-fat meal.
Drug-lifestyle. *Alcohol use:* May increase risk of hypotension and orthostasis. Discourage use together.

V

EFFECTS ON LAB TEST RESULTS
• May increase CK and liver transaminase levels.

CONTRAINDICATIONS & CAUTIONS
• Contraindicated in patients hypersensitive to drug or its components and in those taking nitrates, nitric oxide donors, or GC stimulators.
• Not recommended in patients with unstable angina, hypotension (systolic less than 90 mm Hg), uncontrolled HTN (over 170/110 mm Hg), stroke, life-threatening arrhythmia, an MI within past 6 months, severe cardiac failure, severe hepatic impairment (Child-Pugh class C), ESRD requiring dialysis, congenital QTc-interval prolongation, or hereditary degenerative retinal disorders.
• Don't use ODTs in patients with moderate or severe hepatic impairment (Child-Pugh class B or C) or in those requiring dialysis.
• Use cautiously in patients with bleeding disorders or significant peptic ulceration.
• Use cautiously in those with anatomic penis abnormalities or conditions that predispose patient to priapism (such as sickle cell anemia, multiple myeloma, or leukemia).
• May cause vision loss and visual disturbances. Use cautiously in patients with or at increased risk for nonarteritic ischemic optic neuropathy, "crowded optic disc."
• May cause sudden decreased or loss of hearing, tinnitus, and dizziness.
Dialyzable drug: Unlikely.
⚠ *Overdose S&S:* Back pain or myalgia, abnormal vision.

PREGNANCY-LACTATION-REPRODUCTION
• Drug isn't indicated for use in women.

NURSING CONSIDERATIONS
🕲 *Alert:* Sexual activity may increase cardiac risk. Evaluate patient's cardiac risk before start of therapy.
• Before patient starts drug, assess for underlying causes of erectile dysfunction.
• Transient decreases in supine BP may occur.
• Prolonged erections and priapism may occur.

PATIENT TEACHING
• Instruct patient in safe drug administration.
• Tell patient that drug doesn't protect against sexually transmitted diseases and to use protective measures.
• Urge patient to seek immediate medical care if erection lasts more than 4 hours.

• Explain that drug has no effect without sexual stimulation.
• Warn patient not to change dosage unless directed by prescriber.
• Tell patient to stop drug and seek medical attention for sudden vision loss in one or both eyes or sudden decrease in or loss of hearing.

varenicline tartrate
vah-RENN-ih-kleen

Chantix

Therapeutic class: Smoking cessation aids
Pharmacologic class: Nicotinic acetylcholine receptor partial agonists

AVAILABLE FORMS
Tablets: 0.5 mg, 1 mg

INDICATIONS & DOSAGES
➤ **Smoking cessation**
Adults: Start dosing 1 week before patient stops smoking. Or, patient can begin dosing, then stop smoking between days 8 and 35 of treatment. Give 0.5 mg PO once daily on days 1 through 3. Days 4 through 7, give 0.5 mg PO b.i.d. Day 8 through the end of week 12, give 1 mg PO b.i.d. If patient successfully stops smoking, give an additional 12-week course to help with long-term success.
Adjust-a-dose: Consider dosage reduction in patients who can't tolerate adverse effects. In patients with severe renal impairment, 0.5 mg PO once daily. Adjust as needed to maximum of 0.5 mg b.i.d. In patients with ESRD undergoing dialysis, 0.5 mg once daily.

ADMINISTRATION
PO
• Give drug with full glass of water after a meal.

ACTION
Blocks the effects of nicotine by binding at alpha₄ beta₂ neuronal nicotinic acetylcholine receptors. Drug also increases dopamine activity, decreasing craving and withdrawal symptoms.

Route	Onset	Peak	Duration
PO	4 days	3–4 hr	24 hr

Half-life: 24 hours.

Reactions in bold italics are *life-threatening*. Interactions may have a *rapid onset* or a *delayed onset*.

ADVERSE REACTIONS
CNS: abnormal dreams, headache, insomnia, altered attention or emotions, asthenia, depression, drowsiness, fatigue, irritability, lethargy, anxiety, agitation, tension, hostility, malaise, nightmares, sleep disorder, somnolence, altered taste, *suicidality*. **CV:** angina, chest pain, edema, hot flush, HTN. **EENT:** epistaxis, rhinorrhea, dry mouth. **GI:** nausea, abdominal pain, constipation, diarrhea, dyspepsia, flatulence, GERD, vomiting, increased or decreased appetite. **GU:** polyuria. **Respiratory:** dyspnea, URI. **Skin:** rash, hyperhidrosis. **Other:** flulike symptoms.

INTERACTIONS
Drug-drug. *Nicotine-replacement therapy:* May increase nausea, vomiting, dizziness, dyspepsia, and fatigue. Monitor patient closely.
Drug-lifestyle. ☉ *Alert: Alcohol use:* May decrease alcohol tolerance, with symptoms of increased drunkenness, unusual or aggressive behavior, or amnesia. Caution patient to reduce amount of alcohol consumed until ability to tolerate alcohol is known.

EFFECTS ON LAB TEST RESULTS
• May increase LFT values.

CONTRAINDICATIONS & CAUTIONS
• Contraindicated in patients hypersensitive to drug or its components.
• Consider risks versus benefits before use. Drug increases the likelihood of abstinence from smoking for as long as 1 year. Health benefits of quitting smoking are immediate and substantial.
☉ *Alert:* Serious neuropsychiatric events, including suicidality, have been reported with use of this drug. Carefully weigh risks versus benefits of smoking cessation. Somnambulism has been reported.
☉ *Alert:* Drug may be associated with increased risk of CV events (stroke, angina, MI, need for coronary revascularization, new diagnosis of PVD, or admission for a procedure to treat PVD) in patients who have CV disease. Consider risks and benefits before prescribing.
☉ *Alert:* Drug may increase risk of seizures. Use cautiously in patients with a history of seizures or who are at increased risk for seizures.
• Hypersensitivity reactions, including angioedema, SJS, and erythema multiforme, have been reported. Stop drug at first sign or symptom of hypersensitivity reaction.

• Use cautiously in older adults and in patients with severe renal impairment or preexisting psychiatric illness.
• Not recommended for use in children age 16 or younger.
Dialyzable drug: Yes.

PREGNANCY-LACTATION-REPRODUCTION
• There are no adequate studies during pregnancy. Use only if potential benefit justifies fetal risk.
• It isn't known if drug appears in human milk. Patient should discontinue breastfeeding or discontinue drug.

NURSING CONSIDERATIONS
• Assess patient's readiness and motivation to stop smoking.
• For patients who are sure they aren't able or willing to quit abruptly, consider a gradual approach by initiating drug and reducing smoking simultaneously until complete abstinence by 12 weeks. Then continue drug for additional 12 weeks.
• Encourage patient who is motivated to quit but didn't succeed during prior therapy or who relapsed after treatment, to make another attempt after contributing factors to the failed attempt have been identified and addressed.
☉ *Alert:* Monitor patient for changes in behavior, agitation, depressed mood, hostility, suicidality, and worsening of preexisting psychiatric illness and report immediately.
• Notify prescriber if patient develops intolerable adverse reactions such as nausea; dosage reduction may be needed.
• Monitor patient for hypersensitivity reactions. Discontinue drug for such signs and symptoms as swelling of the face, mouth, neck, or extremities or rash with mucosal lesions.
• Temporarily monitor levels of drugs (theophylline, warfarin, and insulin) after patient stops smoking to be sure levels are still within therapeutic range.

PATIENT TEACHING
• Teach patient safe drug administration and to take as directed.
• Provide patient with educational materials and needed counseling.
• Cases of sleepwalking have been reported in patients taking varenicline. Some patients have described harmful behavior to self, others, or property. Instruct patient to

V

discontinue drug and notify prescriber if such behaviors occur.

• Instruct patient to choose a date to stop smoking and to begin treatment 1 week before this date. Or, patient can begin drug, then quit smoking between days 8 and 35.

⦿ *Alert:* Caution patient that drug can affect reaction to alcohol. Advise patient to reduce amount of alcohol consumed until patient's alcohol tolerance is known.

⦿ *Alert:* Warn patient to stop drug and seek medical attention if seizures occur.

• Advise patient to discontinue drug and seek immediate medical care if swelling of the face, mouth, extremities, and neck or a rash with mucosal lesions develops.

• Explain that nausea and insomnia are common and usually temporary. Urge patient to contact prescriber if adverse effects are persistently troubling; a dosage reduction may help.

• Urge patient to continue trying to abstain from smoking if early lapses occur after successfully quitting.

• Tell patient that dosages of other drugs being taken may need adjustment when patient stops smoking.

• Advise patient to use caution when driving or operating machinery until effects of drug are known.

⦿ *Alert:* Instruct patient and family to monitor patient for changes in behavior and mood, including agitation, depression, hostility, suicidality, and worsening of preexisting psychiatric illness; stop drug and report changes to health care provider immediately.

• If patient plans to become pregnant or to breastfeed, explain the risks of smoking and the risks and benefits of taking drug to aid smoking cessation.

SAFETY ALERT!

vasopressin
vay-soe-PRESS-in

Vasostrict

Therapeutic class: Antidiuretic hormones
Pharmacologic class: Posterior pituitary hormones

AVAILABLE FORMS
Injection (ready to use): 20 units/100 mL, 40 units/100 mL, 60 units/100 mL single-dose vials

Injection (solution for dilution): 20 units/mL single-dose vials; 200 units/10 mL multiple-dose vials

INDICATIONS & DOSAGES
➤ **Vasodilatory shock in patients who remain hypotensive despite fluids and catecholamines**
Adults: For postcardiotomy shock, begin IV infusion at 0.03 unit/minute; for septic shock begin IV infusion at 0.01 unit/minute. If target BP isn't achieved, titrate dosage up by 0.005 unit/minute at 10- to 15-minute intervals. After target BP has been maintained for 8 hours (without use of catecholamines), taper drug by 0.005 unit/minute every hour as tolerated to maintain BP. Maximum dosage for postcardiotomy shock is 0.1 unit/minute and for septic shock, 0.07 unit/minute.

ADMINISTRATION
IV

▼ For IV infusion with solution for dilution, dilute in NSS or D_5W to a concentration of 0.1 to 1 unit/mL. For patients with fluid restrictions, mix 5 mL (100 units) in 100 mL; for patients with no fluid restrictions, mix 2.5 mL (50 units) in 500 mL.

▼ Inspect for particulate matter and discoloration before use.

▼ Titrate to lowest dosage compatible with a clinically acceptable response. Monitor BP every 10 to 15 minutes.

▼ Administer by CVAD if possible, using an infusion pump.

▼ Intact vials can be stored at 68° to 77° F (20° to 25° C) for up to 12 months or refrigerated until manufacturer's original expiration date.

▼ Discard unused diluted solution after 18 hours at room temperature or 24 hours under refrigeration. Discard vials 48 hours after first entry.

▼ **Incompatibilities:** None listed by manufacturer. Consult a drug incompatibility reference for more information.

ACTION
Causes contraction of smooth muscle in the vascular bed and increases systemic vascular resistance and mean arterial BP and decreases HR and cardiac output.

Route	Onset	Peak	Duration
IV	Rapid	15 min	20 min

Half-life: Less than 10 minutes.

ADVERSE REACTIONS

CV: *hemorrhagic shock, HF,* atrial fibrillation, *bradycardia, myocardial ischemia, decreased cardiac output, distal limb ischemia, intractable bleeding.* **GI:** *mesenteric ischemia.* **GU:** *acute renal insufficiency.* **Hematologic:** *thrombocytopenia.* **Hepatic:** hyperbilirubinemia. **Metabolic:** *hyponatremia,* diabetes insipidus. **Skin:** ischemic lesions.

INTERACTIONS

Drug-drug. *Catecholamines:* Causes additive effect on mean arterial pressure and other hemodynamic parameters. Adjust vasopressin dosage as needed.

Drugs suspected of causing diabetes insipidus (clozapine, demeclocycline, foscarnet, lithium): May decrease pressor and antidiuretic effects. Adjust vasopressin dosage as needed.

Drugs suspected of causing SIADH (chlorpropamide, cyclophosphamide, enalapril, felbamate, haloperidol, ifosfamide, methyldopa, pentamidine, SSRIs, TCAs, vincristine): May increase pressor and antidiuretic effects. Adjust vasopressin dosage as needed.

Ganglionic blockers: May increase sensitivity to pressor effects. Monitor patient and BP. Adjust vasopressin dosage as needed.

Indomethacin: May prolong effect on cardiac index and systemic vascular resistance. Adjust vasopressin dosage as needed.

EFFECTS ON LAB TEST RESULTS

• May increase bilirubin level.
• May decrease sodium level.
• May decrease platelet count.

CONTRAINDICATIONS & CAUTIONS

• Contraindicated in patients allergic or hypersensitive to 8-arginine vasopressin. Multidose vial is also contraindicated in patients allergic to chlorobutanol.
• Use in patients with impaired cardiac response may worsen cardiac output.
• Reversible diabetes insipidus, manifested by the development of polyuria, diluted urine, and hypernatremia, may occur after cessation of treatment. Some patients may require readministration of vasopressin or administration of desmopressin to correct fluid and electrolyte shifts.
• Use cautiously in older adults.
• Safety and effectiveness in children haven't been established.

Dialyzable drug: Unknown.

⚠ *Overdose S&S:* Hyponatremia, ventricular arrhythmias, rhabdomyolysis, nonspecific GI symptoms; peripheral, mesenteric, or coronary ischemia.

PREGNANCY-LACTATION-REPRODUCTION

• There are no adequate studies during pregnancy, and it isn't known whether drug can cause fetal harm. Drug may produce tonic uterine contractions that could threaten continuation of pregnancy.
• Because of increased clearance during the second and third trimesters, dosage may need to be increased.
• It isn't known if drug appears in human milk.

NURSING CONSIDERATIONS

🕛 *Alert:* Extravasation may result in severe tissue damage. Ensure proper IV catheter placement before and during infusion and monitor patient closely.
• Monitor patient for hypersensitivity reactions.
• Monitor BP and hemodynamic parameters every 10 to 15 minutes during therapy.
• Monitor urine specific gravity and fluid intake and output to aid evaluation of drug effectiveness.
• Monitor serum electrolyte levels, fluid status, and urine output during and after therapy.
• Monitor ECG.
• Monitor patients for bleeding, palpitations, or signs and symptoms of ischemia (chest pain, limb peripheral pain, paresthesia, coldness, decreased or absent pulses, abdominal pain, nausea, vomiting).
• *Look alike–sound alike:* Don't confuse vasopressin with desmopressin.

PATIENT TEACHING

• Tell patient to immediately report all adverse reactions, especially bleeding, chest pain, palpitations, limb pain, limb coldness and pallor, paresthesia, nausea, vomiting, or abdominal pain.
• Advise patient to immediately report signs or symptoms of hypersensitivity reactions

V

(breathing difficulty, wheezing, hives, nausea, vomiting, or swelling of the face, lips, or tongue).
• Teach patient to immediately report infusion-site symptoms.

SAFETY ALERT!

venetoclax
ven-ET-oh-klax

Venclexta

Therapeutic class: Antineoplastics
Pharmacologic class: BCL-2 inhibitors

AVAILABLE FORMS
Tablets ⓄⓉⒸ: 10 mg, 50 mg, 100 mg

INDICATIONS & DOSAGES
Adjust-a-dose (for all indications): Refer to manufacturer's instructions for TLS, drug interaction, and toxicity-related dosage adjustments and management. Reduce daily dose by 50% for patients with severe hepatic impairment (Child-Pugh class C); monitor patients closely for signs and symptoms of toxicity.
➤ **Chronic lymphocytic leukemia (CLL) or small lymphocytic lymphoma (SLL)**
Adults: Initially, 20 mg PO once daily week 1; increase to 50 mg PO once daily week 2; increase to 100 mg PO once daily week 3; increase to 200 mg PO once daily week 4; then increase to 400 mg PO once daily week 5 and thereafter. Continue until disease progression or unacceptable toxicity occurs.

If drug is used in combination with rituximab or obinutuzumab, refer to manufacturer's instructions.
➤ **Newly diagnosed acute myeloid leukemia (AML) in combination with azacitidine or decitabine or low-dose cytarabine in patients age 75 or older, or in patients who have comorbidities that preclude use of intensive induction chemotherapy**
Adults taking venetoclax in combination with azacitidine or decitabine: Initially, on day 1 give 100 mg PO once daily; on day 2 increase to 200 mg PO once daily; on day 3 increase to 400 mg PO once daily and then give 400 mg PO once daily thereafter. Continue until disease progression or unacceptable toxicity occurs.
Adults taking venetoclax in combination with low-dose cytarabine: Initially, on day 1 give 100 mg PO once daily; on day 2 increase to 200 mg PO once daily; on day 3 increase to 400 mg PO once daily; on day 4 increase to 600 mg PO once daily and then give 600 mg PO once daily thereafter. Continue until disease progression or unacceptable toxicity occurs.

ADMINISTRATION
PO
⚠ *Alert:* Hazardous drug; use safe handling and disposal precautions. Wear gloves to handle tablet.
• Give with a meal and water at approximately the same time each day.
• If patient misses a dose and it's within 8 hours of the usual dosing time, give missed dose as soon as possible and resume normal daily dosing schedule. If it has been more than 8 hours, don't give missed dose and resume usual dosing schedule the next day.
• If patient vomits after administration of a dose, don't give additional doses that day; give next dose at the usual time.
• Tablets must be swallowed whole; don't crush, break, or allow patient to chew tablets.
• Store at or below 86° F (30° C).

ACTION
An inhibitor of B-cell lymphoma 2 (BCL-2), an antiapoptotic protein. Overexpression of BCL-2 has been demonstrated in CLL cells and has been associated with resistance to chemotherapeutic agents. Venetoclax helps restore apoptosis by binding directly to the BCL-2 protein, displacing proapoptotic proteins and restoring the apoptotic process.

Route	Onset	Peak	Duration
PO	Unknown	5–8 hr	Unknown

Half-life: 26 hours.

ADVERSE REACTIONS
CNS: fatigue, headache, fever. **CV:** edema. **GI:** diarrhea, nausea, vomiting, constipation, mucositis. **GU:** UTI. **Hematologic:** *neutropenia*, anemia, *thrombocytopenia*, *febrile neutropenia*, *autoimmune hemolytic anemia*. **Hepatic:** increased AST level. **Metabolic:** *hyperkalemia*, hypoalbuminemia, hyperglycemia, hyperphosphatemia, hypophosphatemia, *hypokalemia, hypocalcemia*, hyperuricemia, *TLS*. **Musculoskeletal:** back pain. **Respiratory:** URI, lower

---

respiratory tract infection, cough, pneumonia. **Skin:** rash. **Other:** *sepsis.*

INTERACTIONS
Drug-drug. *Live attenuated vaccines:* Safety and effectiveness haven't been studied and vaccines may be less effective. Don't give vaccines before, during, or after treatment until B-cell recovery occurs.
Moderate CYP3A inducers (bosentan, efavirenz, etravirine, modafinil, nafcillin), strong CYP3A inducers (carbamazepine, phenytoin, rifampin): May decrease venetoclax level. Avoid use together.
Moderate CYP3A inhibitors (ciprofloxacin, diltiazem, dronedarone, erythromycin, fluconazole, verapamil), P-gp inhibitors (amiodarone, azithromycin, captopril, carvedilol, cyclosporine, felodipine, quinidine, ranolazine, ticagrelor): May increase venetoclax level and risk of TLS. Consider alternative treatments. If a moderate inhibitor must be used, reduce venetoclax dosage by at least 50%; monitor patient closely. Resume venetoclax dose that was used before initiating the inhibitor 2 to 3 days after discontinuing inhibitor.
P-gp substrates (digoxin, everolimus, sirolimus): May inhibit absorption of P-gp substrates. Avoid administration of narrow therapeutic index P-gp substrates with venetoclax. If substrate must be used, patient should take it at least 6 hours before venetoclax.
Strong CYP3A inhibitors (clarithromycin, conivaptan, itraconazole, ketoconazole, lopinavir, posaconazole, ritonavir, telaprevir, voriconazole): May increase venetoclax level and risk of TLS. Use during initiation and ramp-up phase is contraindicated. For patients who have completed ramp-up phase and are on a steady daily dose of venetoclax, reduce venetoclax dosage by at least 75% when used concomitantly with strong CYP3A inhibitors. If using posaconazole, dosage shouldn't exceed 70 mg daily. Resume venetoclax dose that was used before initiating the CYP3A inhibitor 2 to 3 days after discontinuing inhibitor.
Warfarin: May increase INR. Monitor INR closely.
Drug-herb. *St. John's wort:* May decrease venetoclax level. Don't use together.
Drug-food. *Grapefruit products, Seville oranges, starfruit:* May increase venetoclax level. Discourage use together.

EFFECTS ON LAB TEST RESULTS
- May increase ALP, bilirubin, uric acid, and glucose levels.
- May decrease calcium, sodium, and albumin levels.
- May increase or decrease potassium and phosphate levels.
- May decrease Hb level, hematocrit, and neutrophil, lymphocyte, and platelet counts.

CONTRAINDICATIONS & CAUTIONS
- Contraindicated in patients hypersensitive to drug or its components.
- Contraindicated with strong CYP3A inhibitors at initiation and during ramp-up phase due to the potential for increased risk of TLS.
- **Alert:** Drug may cause a rapid reduction in tumor volume and increases the risk of TLS and renal failure (requiring dialysis); fatalities have been reported. Risk of TLS increases with high tumor burden, concomitant use of CYP3A or P-gp inhibitors, and comorbidities (reduced renal function, type of malignancy, splenomegaly in patients with CLL or SLL). The 5-week ramp-up dosing schedule is designed to gradually reduce tumor burden and decrease risk of TLS.
- Use cautiously in patients with hepatic impairment. Reduce dosage in patients with severe impairment. Adverse events may increase; monitor patients closely for toxicity, especially during initiation and ramp-up period.
- Use cautiously in patients with renal impairment. Patients with decreased renal function (CrCl of less than 80 mL/minute) are at increased risk for TLS and may require more intensive TLS prophylaxis and monitoring during treatment initiation and dosage escalation.
- Some studies have shown increased mortality in patients with multiple myeloma when venetoclax is used in combination with bortezomib and dexamethasone.
- **Alert:** Drug may cause bone marrow suppression (neutropenia, thrombocytopenia, anemia). Grade 3 and 4 neutropenia occurs in 50% of patients taking drug.
- Fatal and serious infections, such as pneumonia and sepsis, have occurred in patients treated with venetoclax.
- Safety and effectiveness in children haven't been established.
Dialyzable drug: Unlikely.

V

♣Canada ◇OTC ◆Off-label use ✏Photoguide ⊛Do not crush *Liquid contains alcohol ⚹ Genetic

PREGNANCY-LACTATION-REPRODUCTION
• Drug may cause fetal harm. Patients of childbearing potential should have pregnancy testing before therapy and use effective contraception during and for at least 30 days after treatment ends. Apprise patients who become pregnant while taking venetoclax of fetal risk.
• Based on animal data, venetoclax may compromise fertility in males.
• It isn't known if drug appears in human milk. Because of the potential for serious adverse reactions in the infant, patient should discontinue breastfeeding during and for 1 week after final dose.

NURSING CONSIDERATIONS
• Patients at high risk for TLS may require hospitalization at treatment initiation.
• Assess patient for risk of TLS before treatment (radiographic evaluation; assessment of potassium, uric acid, phosphorus, calcium, and creatinine levels and renal function). Give prophylactic hydration and antihyperuricemics before first dose of venetoclax as clinically indicated. See prescribing information for recommended TLS prophylaxis and monitoring.
• Monitor serum chemistry values. Changes due to TLS can occur as soon as 6 to 8 hours after first dose and at each dosage increase.
• Monitor CBC with differential throughout treatment; treatment interruption and dosage reduction may be required. Consider WBC growth factor support as clinically indicated.
• Monitor patient for infection, including neutropenic fever. Treat with antimicrobials as appropriate. Withhold drug for grade 3 and higher infection.
• *Look alike–sound alike:* Don't confuse venetoclax with vandetanib, vemurafenib, venlafaxine, or vismodegib. Don't confuse Venclexta with venlafaxine.

PATIENT TEACHING
• Teach patient safe drug administration and handling.
• Explain that treatment may be interrupted, dosage decreased, or treatment stopped due to adverse effects. Tell patient to report all adverse reactions promptly.
• Advise patient of risk of TLS, particularly at treatment initiation and during ramp-up phase, and to immediately report TLS signs and symptoms (fever, chills, nausea, vomiting, confusion, shortness of breath, seizures,

irregular heartbeat, dark or cloudy urine, unusual tiredness, muscle pain, joint discomfort).
• Inform patient that it may be necessary to take drug under direct medical supervision to allow for monitoring for TLS.
• Advise patient to maintain adequate hydration to reduce risk of TLS. Recommended intake is 6 to 8 glasses (56 oz) beginning 2 days before treatment, on first day of treatment, and each time dosage is increased.
• Warn patient to immediately report fever or signs and symptoms of infection.
• Remind patient of importance of keeping scheduled appointments for blood work or other lab tests to monitor for adverse effects.
• Caution patient that venetoclax may interact with other drugs. Advise patient to report the use of prescription and OTC medications and supplements and not to start new medications or supplements without first discussing with prescriber.
• Instruct patient to avoid consuming grapefruit products, Seville oranges, or starfruit during treatment.
• Advise patient to avoid vaccination with live-virus vaccines during treatment.
• Caution patient of childbearing potential to use effective contraception during and for at least 30 days after therapy ends.
• Instruct patient to immediately report known or suspected pregnancy or plans to become pregnant.
• Warn patient not to breastfeed during treatment and for 1 week after final dose.
• Advise male patient of risk of infertility due to treatment and of the option of sperm banking.

venlafaxine hydrochloride
ven-la-FAX-een

Effexor XR♦

Therapeutic class: Antidepressants
Pharmacologic class: SSNRIs

AVAILABLE FORMS
Capsules (extended-release) ⬤*:* 37.5 mg, 75 mg, 150 mg
Tablets: 25 mg, 37.5 mg, 50 mg, 75 mg, 100 mg
Tablets (extended-release) ⬤*:* 37.5 mg, 75 mg, 150 mg, 225 mg

INDICATIONS & DOSAGES

Adjust-a-dose (for all indications): For patients with mild to moderate renal impairment (CrCl 30 to 89 mL/minute), reduce daily amount by 25% in patients taking immediate-release tablets. Reduce by 25% to 50% in those taking extended-release form. For those with severe renal impairment (CrCl less than 30 mL/minute) or on hemodialysis, reduce total daily dose by 50% or more and withhold dose until dialysis is completed. For patients with mild to moderate hepatic impairment (Child-Pugh score 5 to 9), reduce daily amount by 50%. For patients with severe hepatic impairment (Child-Pugh score 10 to 15) or cirrhosis, reduce total daily dose by 50% or more.

➤ **Major depressive disorder**

Adults: Initially, 75 mg (immediate-release) PO daily in two or three divided doses with food. Increase as tolerated and needed by 75 mg daily every 4 days. For outpatients who are moderately depressed, usual maximum is 225 mg daily; in certain patients who are severely depressed, dose may be as high as 375 mg daily. For extended-release capsules or tablets, 75 mg PO daily in a single dose. For some patients, it may be desirable to start at 37.5 mg PO daily for 4 to 7 days before increasing to 75 mg daily. Dosage may be increased by 75 mg daily every 4 days to maximum of 225 mg daily.

May switch immediate-release formulation to extended-release formulation by using the nearest equivalent dose in mg/day. For example, may switch 37.5 mg immediate-release b.i.d. to 75 mg extended-release daily.

➤ **Generalized anxiety disorder**

Adults: Initially, 75 mg extended-release capsule PO daily in a single dose. For some patients, it may be desirable to start at 37.5 mg PO daily for 4 to 7 days before increasing to 75 mg daily. Dosage may be increased by 75 mg daily every 4 days to maximum of 225 mg daily.

➤ **Panic disorder**

Adults: Initially, 37.5 mg extended-release capsule PO daily for 1 week, then increase dose to 75 mg daily. If patient isn't responding, may increase dose by up to 75 mg/day in no less than weekly intervals, as needed, to a maximum dose of 225 mg daily.

➤ **Social anxiety disorder**

Adults: Initially, 75 mg extended-release capsule or tablet PO daily as a single dose. Maximum dose, 75 mg/day.

➤ **Vasomotor signs and symptoms of menopause** ◆

Adults: Initially, 37.5 mg once daily; may increase after 1 week based on response and tolerability to 75 mg once daily for extended-release forms or 75 mg/day in two to three divided doses for immediate-release form.

ADMINISTRATION
PO

• Give drug with food and a full glass of water at approximately the same time each day.
• For extended-release capsules and tablets, don't divide, crush, place in water, or allow patient to chew.
• May give pellet-filled capsules by carefully opening capsule and sprinkling the pellets on a spoonful of applesauce. Patient should swallow applesauce immediately without chewing, then follow with a glass of water to ensure that all pellets are swallowed.
• Give a missed dose as soon as possible unless it's almost time for the next scheduled dose. Don't give two doses at the same time.

ACTION

Potent and selective inhibitor of neuronal serotonin and norepinephrine reuptake and weak inhibitor of dopamine reuptake.

Route	Onset	Peak	Duration
PO (immediate-release)	Unknown	2 hr	Unknown
PO (extended-release)	Unknown	5.5 hr	Unknown

Half-life: Immediate-release, 3 to 7 hours; extended-release, 7.5 to 14 hours.

ADVERSE REACTIONS

CNS: asthenia, headache, somnolence, dizziness, nervousness, insomnia, anxiety, tremor, abnormal dreams, paresthesia, agitation, weakness, syncope, taste alteration, apathy, confusion. **CV:** HTN, hypotension, tachycardia, vasodilation, palpitations, chest pain. **EENT:** blurred vision, mydriasis, visual disturbance, tinnitus, dry mouth. **GI:** nausea, constipation, anorexia, vomiting, diarrhea, dyspepsia, flatulence, bruxism. **GU:** abnormal ejaculation, erectile dysfunction, anorgasmia, urinary frequency, impaired urination, heavy menstrual bleeding, decreased libido. **Metabolic:** weight gain, weight loss, increased appetite, hypercholesterolemia. **Respiratory:** yawning. **Skin:** diaphoresis,

V

alopecia, pruritus, photosensitivity, urticaria, ecchymosis, rash. **Other:** chills.

INTERACTIONS
Drug-drug. *Anticoagulants, aspirin, NSAIDs:* May increase antiplatelet effect of aspirin and NSAIDs and anticoagulant effect of anticoagulants. Monitor patient for increased risk of bleeding.
Cimetidine: May increase venlafaxine level. Use together cautiously.
Linezolid, methylene blue (IV): May cause serotonin syndrome. Use together is contraindicated.
MAO inhibitors (phenelzine, selegiline, tranylcypromine): May cause serotonin syndrome and signs and symptoms resembling NMS. Use within 14 days of MAO inhibitor therapy is contraindicated.
Other serotonergic drugs (5-HT$_3$ antagonists, fentanyl, lithium, meperidine, tramadol, trazodone): May cause serotonin syndrome. Monitor patient closely.
Triptans (tryptophan): May cause serotonin syndrome or NMS-like reactions. Use together isn't recommended. If concomitant use can't be avoided, use cautiously and with increased monitoring at the start of therapy and with dosage increase.
Warfarin: May increase PT or INR. Monitor patient closely.
Drug-herb. *St. John's wort:* May cause serotonin syndrome. Monitor patient closely.
Drug-lifestyle. *Alcohol use:* May increase mental and psychomotor impairment. Avoid alcohol.

EFFECTS ON LAB TEST RESULTS
• May increase cholesterol and triglyceride levels.
• May decrease sodium level.
• May cause false-positive urine immunoassay screening tests for phencyclidine and amphetamine.

CONTRAINDICATIONS & CAUTIONS
• Contraindicated in patients hypersensitive to drug or within 14 days of stopping MAO inhibitor therapy. Don't start MAO inhibitor less than 7 days after stopping venlafaxine.
Boxed Warning Venlafaxine isn't approved for use in children. ∎
🔔 *Alert:* Concomitant use with serotonergic drugs, linezolid, or methylene blue can cause serotonin syndrome. Concomitant use of

these drugs and venlafaxine is recommended only for life-threatening or urgent conditions when the potential benefits outweigh the risks of toxicity.
• Use cautiously in patients with renal impairment, HTN, or diseases or conditions that could affect hemodynamic responses or metabolism, and in those with history of mania or seizures.
• Carefully evaluate patients for history of drug abuse and follow such patients closely, observing them for signs and symptoms of venlafaxine misuse or abuse (development of tolerance, dose incrementation, drug-seeking behavior).
• May trigger an angle-closure attack. Use cautiously in patients at risk for acute narrow-angle glaucoma.
• Hyponatremia can occur, which may be a result of SIADH. Older adults, patients who are volume-depleted, and those taking diuretics are at increased risk. Discontinue drug if patient develops symptomatic hyponatremia.
Dialyzable drug: Unlikely.
⚠ *Overdose S&S:* Altered level of consciousness, somnolence, paresthesia of all four limbs, tachycardia, bradycardia, mydriasis, seizures, vomiting, ECG changes, hypotension, liver necrosis, rhabdomyolysis, serotonin syndrome, vertigo, death.

PREGNANCY-LACTATION-REPRODUCTION
• There are no adequate studies during pregnancy. Use only if clearly needed and potential benefit justifies fetal risk.
🔔 *Alert:* Neonates exposed to drug during the late third trimester have developed complications (sometimes immediately upon delivery) that require respiratory support, tube feedings, and prolonged hospitalization.
• Drug may appear in human milk. Patient should discontinue breastfeeding or discontinue drug.

NURSING CONSIDERATIONS
Boxed Warning Drug may increase the risk of suicidality in children, adolescents, and young adults ages 18 to 24, especially during the first few months of treatment, especially those with major depressive disorder or other psychiatric disorder. ∎
Boxed Warning Closely monitor patients for signs and symptoms of clinical worsening and suicidality, especially at the beginning of therapy and with dosage adjustments.

Reactions in bold italics are *life-threatening*. Interactions may have a *rapid onset* or a *delayed onset*.

Signs and symptoms may include agitation, insomnia, anxiety, aggressiveness, or panic attacks. ∎

⊙ *Alert:* Sudden discontinuation or abrupt decrease in venlafaxine dose can lead to serotonin withdrawal (agitation, confusion, flulike symptoms, sensory disturbances, tremor). Reduce dosage gradually and watch for symptoms. Discontinuation may take several months in some patients.

⊙ *Alert:* If linezolid or methylene blue must be given, stop venlafaxine and monitor patient for serotonin toxicity for 2 weeks or until 24 hours after last dose of methylene blue or linezolid, whichever comes first. May resume serotonergic psychiatric drugs 24 hours after last dose of methylene blue or linezolid.

• Carefully monitor BP. Drug therapy may cause sustained, dose-dependent increases in BP.

• Monitor patient for hyponatremia (headache, difficulty concentrating, memory impairment, confusion, weakness, unsteadiness and, in severe cases, hallucinations, syncope, seizure, respiratory arrest, coma, death).

• Monitor weight, particularly in patients with depression who are underweight.

⊙ *Alert:* Monitor patient for signs and symptoms of serotonin syndrome, including restlessness, hallucinations, loss of coordination, tachycardia, rapid BP changes, increased body temperature, overactive reflexes, nausea, vomiting, and diarrhea. Serotonin syndrome may be more likely to occur when starting or increasing the dosage of triptan, SSRI, or SSNRI.

• SSNRIs may cause sexual dysfunction. Monitor patient for signs and symptoms and exclude other causes such as underlying psychiatric disorder. Inquire specifically about changes; patient may not report spontaneously.

PATIENT TEACHING

• Instruct patient in safe drug administration.

• Inform patient that if drug needs to be stopped, it should be tapered gradually by the prescriber and not stopped abruptly.

Boxed Warning Warn family members to closely monitor patient for signs or symptoms of worsening condition or suicidality. ∎

• Caution patient to avoid hazardous activities that require alertness and good coordination until effects of drug are known.

• Tell patient to avoid alcohol and to consult prescriber before taking other prescription or OTC drugs or supplements.

• Teach patient to recognize and immediately report signs and symptoms of serotonin toxicity (fever, mental status changes, muscle twitching, diaphoresis, shivering or shaking, diarrhea, loss of coordination).

• Advise patient to report pregnancy, plans to become pregnant, breastfeeding, or plans to breastfeed during therapy.

---

verapamil hydrochloride
ver-AP-a-mill

Calan SR, Isoptin SR✤, Verelan✐, Verelan PM

Therapeutic class: Antihypertensives
Pharmacologic class: Calcium channel blockers

AVAILABLE FORMS

Capsules (extended-release) ⓓ: 100 mg, 120 mg, 180 mg, 200 mg, 240 mg, 300 mg, 360 mg
Injection: 2.5 mg/mL
Tablets: 40 mg, 80 mg, 120 mg
Tablets (extended-release) ⓓ: 120 mg, 180 mg, 240 mg

INDICATIONS & DOSAGES

Adjust-a-dose (for all indications): In patients with severe liver dysfunction, give 30% of dose.

➤ **Vasospastic angina (Prinzmetal or variant angina); unstable angina; classic chronic, stable angina pectoris**
Adults: Initially, 80 to 120 mg (immediate-release) PO t.i.d. Increase dosage at daily or weekly intervals as needed. Some patients may require up to 480 mg daily. Don't exceed 480 mg/day.

Adjust-a-dose: In patients with renal or hepatic impairment, older adults, and patients with low weight, reduce initial dosage to 40 mg t.i.d.

➤ **To prevent paroxysmal supraventricular tachycardia**
Adults: 240 to 480 mg (immediate-release) PO daily, in three or four divided doses. Don't exceed 480 mg/day.

V

➤ **Atrial flutter or atrial fibrillation; supraventricular arrhythmias**
Adults: 0.075 to 0.15 mg/kg (5 to 10 mg) by IV push with ECG and BP monitoring. Repeat dose of 0.15 mg/kg (10 mg) in 30 minutes if inadequate response.
Children ages 1 to 15: Give 0.1 to 0.3 mg/kg as IV bolus; not to exceed 5 mg. Repeat dose in 30 minutes if inadequate response. Don't exceed 10 mg as a single dose.
Children younger than age 1: Give 0.1 to 0.2 mg/kg as IV bolus with continuous ECG monitoring. Repeat dose in 30 minutes if inadequate response.

➤ **Patients with chronic atrial fibrillation or flutter who are digitalized**
Adults: 240 to 320 mg (immediate-release) PO daily, in three or four divided doses.

➤ **HTN**
Adults: Initially, 80 mg immediate-release tablet PO t.i.d. May increase based on therapeutic effect to maximum of 480 mg/day. Or, initially, 240 mg extended-release tablet (Verelan) PO once daily in the morning. If response isn't adequate, may increase by 120 mg daily (maximum, 480 mg). If using Verelan PM, 200 mg PO daily at bedtime. May increase to 300 mg at bedtime if inadequate response. Maximum dose is 400 mg. If using Calan SR, give 180 mg PO in the morning. Evaluate weekly and approximately 24 hours after previous dose. May increase as follows: 240 mg each morning; 180 mg each morning plus 180 mg each evening, or 240 mg each morning plus 120 mg each evening; 240 mg every 12 hours.
Adjust-a-dose: In patients with renal or hepatic impairment, older adults, and patients with low weight, reduce initial dosage to 40 mg t.i.d. for immediate-release tablets, 120 mg once daily for Verelan or Calan SR, or 100 mg once daily for Verelan PM.

ADMINISTRATION
PO
• Pellet-filled capsules may be given by carefully opening the capsule and sprinkling the pellets on a spoonful of applesauce. This should be swallowed immediately without chewing, followed by a glass of cool water to ensure that all the pellets are swallowed.
• An oral suspension may be compounded by a pharmacist if needed.

• Give long-acting forms of the drug whole; don't crush or break tablet.
IV
▼ This form is contraindicated in patients receiving IV beta blockers and in those with ventricular tachycardia.
▼ Inject directly into a vein or into the tubing of a free-flowing, compatible solution, such as D_5W, half-NSS, NSS, Ringer solution, or lactated Ringer solution.
▼ Give doses over at least 2 minutes (3 minutes in older adults) to minimize risk of adverse reactions.
▼ Monitor ECG and BP continuously.
▼ **Incompatibilities:** Albumin, amphotericin B, hydralazine, solutions with a pH greater than 6, sulfamethoxazole–trimethoprim. Consult a drug incompatibility reference for more information.

ACTION
A calcium channel blocker that inhibits calcium ion influx across cardiac and smooth-muscle cells, thus decreasing myocardial contractility and oxygen demand; it also dilates coronary arteries and arterioles.

Route	Onset	Peak	Duration
PO	1–2 hr	1–2 hr	8–10 hr
PO (extended-release)	30 min	5–9 hr	24 hr
IV	Immediate	1–5 min	0.5–6 hr

Half-life: 2.8 to 12 hours (varies by product).

ADVERSE REACTIONS
CNS: dizziness, headache, fatigue, sleep disturbances, pain, lethargy. **CV:** transient hypotension, *HF, bradycardia, AV block, ventricular asystole, ventricular fibrillation,* edema, flushing, HTN, tachycardia. **EENT:** gingival hyperplasia. **GI:** constipation, nausea, diarrhea, dyspepsia. **Musculoskeletal:** myalgia. **Respiratory:** dyspnea. **Skin:** rash. **Other:** flulike syndrome, infection.

INTERACTIONS
Drug-drug. *Amiodarone:* May cause bradycardia and decrease cardiac output. Monitor patient closely.
Antihypertensives (ACE inhibitors, beta blockers, diuretics, vasodilators), quinidine: May cause hypotension. Monitor BP.
Barbiturates (phenobarbital): May increase verapamil clearance. Monitor response and adjust verapamil dose as needed.

Reactions in bold italics are *life-threatening*. Interactions may have a *rapid onset* or a *delayed onset*.

Beta blockers: May have additive effects on HR, AV conduction, or cardiac contractility. Use together cautiously.

Carbamazepine: May increase levels of carbamazepine. Monitor patient for toxicity and adjust dosage as needed.

Cyclosporine: May increase cyclosporine level. Monitor cyclosporine level.

Digoxin: May increase digoxin level and risk of toxicity. Monitor digoxin level and cardiac function closely and decrease dosages as needed.

Disopyramide: May cause HF. Avoid use 48 hours before or 24 hours after verapamil.

Dofetilide: May increase dofetilide level. Avoid using together.

Flecainide: May enhance negative inotropic effect and prolongation of AV conduction. Use together cautiously.

HMG-CoA reductase inhibitors that are substrates of CYP3A4 (atorvastatin, lovastatin, simvastatin): May elevate plasma concentrations of these drugs and risk of myopathy and rhabdomyolysis. If coadministration can't be avoided, limit dose of the HMG-CoA reductase inhibitor. Don't give doses greater than 10 mg daily of simvastatin or greater than 40 mg daily of lovastatin. Monitor drug levels closely and adjust dosage as needed.

Inhalation anesthetics (enflurane): May potentiate cardiac effects. Titrate doses carefully to avoid excessive CV depression.

Ivabradine: May increase ivabradine level and risk of bradycardia and conduction disturbances. Avoid use together.

Lithium: May decrease or increase lithium level. Monitor lithium level.

Macrolide antibiotics (clarithromycin, erythromycin): May increase macrolide and verapamil levels. Monitor cardiac function closely and adjust doses as needed.

Moderate CYP3A4 inducers (dabrafenib, modafinil, nafcillin): May decrease verapamil level. Use cautiously together.

Moderate and strong CYP3A4 inhibitors (ketoconazole, ritonavir): May increase verapamil level. Monitor therapy closely.

mTOR inhibitors (everolimus, sirolimus, tacrolimus): May increase levels of these drugs. Monitor drug levels closely and adjust dosage as needed.

Neuromuscular blockers: May potentiate the activity of these drugs. Monitor neuromuscular function, and adjust dosages of either drug as needed.

Rifampin: May decrease oral bioavailability of verapamil. Monitor patient for lack of effect.

Strong CYP3A4 inducers (dexamethasone, phenytoin): May decrease verapamil level. Monitor patient for verapamil effect; adjust dosage as needed.

Theophylline: May decrease clearance of theophylline. Monitor for signs of theophylline toxicity.

Drug-herb. *St. John's wort:* May decrease drug level and effect. Discourage use together.

Drug-food. *Grapefruit juice:* May increase drug level. Discourage use together.

Drug-lifestyle. *Alcohol use:* May increase serum concentration of alcohol. Discourage use together.

EFFECTS ON LAB TEST RESULTS
• May increase ALT, AST, ALP, and bilirubin levels.
• May cause false-positive urine detection of methadone.

CONTRAINDICATIONS & CAUTIONS
• Contraindicated in patients hypersensitive to drug and in those with severe left ventricular dysfunction, cardiogenic shock, second- or third-degree AV block, or sick sinus syndrome except in presence of functioning pacemaker, atrial flutter or fibrillation and an accessory bypass tract syndrome, severe HF (unless secondary to therapy), and severe hypotension.
• IV form is contraindicated in patients receiving IV beta blockers and in those with wide-complex ventricular tachycardia (QRS complex of 0.12 seconds or more).
• Use cautiously in older adults, children, and patients with increased ICP, hypertrophic cardiomyopathy, or hepatic or renal disease.
• Use cautiously in patients with Duchenne muscular dystrophy; drug may precipitate respiratory muscle failure.

Dialyzable drug: No.

⚠ **Overdose S&S:** Hypotension, bradycardia, arrhythmias, hyperglycemia, depressed mental status, noncardiogenic pulmonary edema, increasing AV block.

PREGNANCY-LACTATION-REPRODUCTION
• There are no adequate studies during pregnancy. Drug crosses the placental barrier. Use

only if clearly needed. Fetal monitoring is recommended.
• Drug appears in human milk. Some manufacturers recommend that patients stop breastfeeding.

NURSING CONSIDERATIONS
• Frequently monitor PR interval.
• Monitor BP at the start of therapy, during dosage adjustments, and routinely during therapy. Assist patient with walking because dizziness may occur.
• If signs and symptoms of HF occur, such as swelling of hands and feet and shortness of breath, notify prescriber.
• Monitor renal function test and LFT results during prolonged treatment.
• *Look alike–sound alike:* Don't confuse Verelan with Vivarin or Voltaren.

PATIENT TEACHING
• Tell patient to report all adverse reactions, especially palpitations, slow heartbeat, dizziness, dyspnea, or swelling.
• Instruct patient to take oral form of drug exactly as prescribed.
• Tell patient not to crush or chew extended-release forms.
• Caution patient against abruptly stopping drug.
• If patient continues nitrate therapy during oral verapamil dosage adjustment, urge continued adherence. SL nitroglycerin may be taken, as needed, for acute chest pain.
• Drug significantly inhibits alcohol elimination. Advise patient to avoid or severely limit alcohol use.

vericiguat
ver-i-SIG-ue-at

Verquvo

Therapeutic class: Pulmonary vasodilators
Pharmacologic class: Soluble guanylate cyclase stimulators

AVAILABLE FORMS
Tablets: 2.5 mg, 5 mg, 10 mg

INDICATIONS & DOSAGES
➤ **Reduces risk of CV death and HF rehospitalization after a hospitalization for HF or need for outpatient IV diuretics in patients with symptomatic chronic HF and ejection fraction less than 45%**
Adults: 2.5 mg PO once daily. Double the dose approximately every 2 weeks up to target maintenance dose of 10 mg once daily, as tolerated.

ADMINISTRATION
PO
• Give with food.
• May crush and mix with water immediately before giving.
• If dose is missed, give as soon as possible on the same day of missed dose; don't give two doses on the same day.
• Store tablets at 68° to 77° F (20° to 25° C).

ACTION
Directly stimulates soluble guanylate cyclase independently of and synergistically with nitric oxide, causing increased levels of intracellular cyclic guanosine monophosphate, leading to smooth muscle relaxation and vasodilation.

Route	Onset	Peak	Duration
PO	Unknown	4 hr (with food)	Unknown

Half-life: 30 hours.

ADVERSE REACTIONS
CV: hypotension. **Hematologic:** anemia.

INTERACTIONS
Drug-drug. *Other soluble guanylate cyclase stimulators (riociguat):* May increase risk of adverse effects. Contraindicated for use together.
PDE5 inhibitors (avanafil, sildenafil, vardenafil): May increase risk of hypotension. Avoid use together.

EFFECTS ON LAB TEST RESULTS
• May decrease RBC count.

CONTRAINDICATIONS & CAUTIONS
• Drug hasn't been studied in patients with eGFR less than 15 mL/minute/1.73 m^2 or severe hepatic impairment or in those who require dialysis.
• Safety and effectiveness in children haven't been established.
• Use cautiously in older adults.
Dialyzable drug: Unlikely.

PREGNANCY-LACTATION-REPRODUCTION

Boxed Warning Exclude pregnancy before starting therapy. ■

Boxed Warning Drug may cause fetal harm and is contraindicated in patients who are pregnant. ■

Boxed Warning Patients of childbearing potential must use effective forms of contraception during therapy and for 1 month after final dose. ■

• For patients exposed to drug during pregnancy, notify manufacturer (1-877-888-4231).
• It isn't known if drug appears in human milk or how drug affects milk production or infants who are breastfed. Patient shouldn't breastfeed during therapy.

NURSING CONSIDERATIONS

• Verify pregnancy status before starting drug.
• Monitor patient for hypotension.
• Monitor patient for anemia.

PATIENT TEACHING

• Instruct patient on proper self-administration.

Boxed Warning Advise patient to report pregnancy or plans to become pregnant during therapy. ■

Boxed Warning Tell patient of childbearing potential to use effective contraception during therapy and for 1 month after final dose. ■

• Inform patient not to breastfeed during therapy.

vibegron
vye-BEG-ron

Gemtesa

Therapeutic class: Bladder antispasmodics
Pharmacologic class: Beta-3 adrenergic agonists

AVAILABLE FORMS
Tablets: 75 mg

INDICATIONS & DOSAGES

➤ **Overactive bladder with symptoms of urge urinary incontinence, urgency, and urinary frequency**
Adults: 75 mg PO once daily.

ADMINISTRATION
PO
• Give without regard to food.

• Patient should swallow tablets whole with glass of water.
• May crush tablets and mix with approximately 15 mL of applesauce; give immediately and follow with a glass of water.
• Store tablets at 68° to 77° F (20° to 25° C).

ACTION
Relaxes detrusor smooth muscle and increases bladder capacity during bladder filling.

Route	Onset	Peak	Duration
PO	Unknown	1–3 hr	Unknown

Half-life: 30.8 hours.

ADVERSE REACTIONS
CNS: headache. **EENT:** dry mouth, nasopharyngitis. **GI:** constipation, diarrhea, nausea. **GU:** UTI, urine retention. **Respiratory:** bronchitis, URI. **Other:** hot flushes.

INTERACTIONS
Drug-drug. *Digoxin:* May increase serum digoxin level. Monitor digoxin level before and during therapy; adjust digoxin dosage as needed. Continue monitoring upon discontinuation of therapy and adjust digoxin dosage as needed.
Muscarinic antagonists (atropine, glycopyrrolate, ipratropium bromide, scopolamine): May increase risk of urine retention. Use cautiously together.

EFFECTS ON LAB TEST RESULTS
None reported.

CONTRAINDICATIONS & CAUTIONS
• Contraindicated in patients hypersensitive to drug or its components.
• Drug may increase risk of urine retention. Use cautiously in patients with bladder outlet obstruction.
• Avoid use in patients with eGFR less than 15 mL/minute/1.73 m^2 (with or without hemodialysis) and in those with severe hepatic impairment (Child-Pugh class C).
• Safety and effectiveness in children haven't been established.
Dialyzable drug: Unknown.

PREGNANCY-LACTATION-REPRODUCTION
• There are no adequate studies during pregnancy. Use only if benefit outweighs fetal risk.
• It isn't known if drug appears in human milk; drug was detected in animal milk

studies. Consider benefits and possible risk to the infant.

NURSING CONSIDERATIONS

• Monitor patient for urine retention. Discontinue drug if urine retention occurs.

• *Look alike–sound alike:* Don't confuse vibegron with vigabatrin or Vigadrone.

PATIENT TEACHING

• Inform patient that drug may cause urine retention and to report urinary hesitancy or urine retention.

• Teach patient proper drug administration and storage.

• Advise patient to report pregnancy, plans to become pregnant, or breastfeeding.

vigabatrin
veye-gah-BA-trin

Sabril, Vigadrone

Therapeutic class: Anticonvulsants
Pharmacologic class: GABA transaminase inhibitors

AVAILABLE FORMS
Powder for oral solution: 500 mg
Tablets: 500 mg

INDICATIONS & DOSAGES

Adjust-a-dose (for all indications): For patients with CrCl of 51 to 80 mL/minute, reduce dosage by 25%; for CrCl of 31 to 50 mL/minute, decrease dosage by 50%; for CrCl of 11 to 30 mL/minute, decrease dosage by 75%.

➤ **Refractory complex partial seizures in patients with inadequate response to several alternative treatments**

Adults and children age 17 and older and children weighing more than 60 kg: Initially, 500 mg PO b.i.d. May increase dosage weekly in 500-mg/day increments to maximum of 1,500 mg PO b.i.d.

Children ages 2 to 16 weighing 25 to 60 kg: Initially, 500 mg/day (250 mg b.i.d.) PO. Increase in weekly intervals to a maximum maintenance dose of 2,000 mg/day (1,000 mg b.i.d.) depending on response.

Children ages 2 to 16 weighing more than 20 to 25 kg: Initially, 500 mg/day (250 mg b.i.d.) PO. Increase in weekly intervals to a

maximum maintenance dose of 1,500 mg/day (750 mg b.i.d.) depending on response.

Children ages 2 to 16 weighing more than 15 to 20 kg: Initially, 450 mg/day (225 mg b.i.d.) PO. Increase in weekly intervals to a total maximum maintenance dose of 1,300 mg/day (650 mg b.i.d.) depending on response.

Children ages 2 to 16 weighing 10 to 15 kg: Initially, 350 mg/day (175 mg b.i.d.) PO. Increase in weekly intervals to a total maximum maintenance dose of 1,050 mg/day (525 mg b.i.d.) depending on response.

➤ **Infantile spasms**

Infants and children ages 1 month to 2 years: 50 mg/kg/day PO given in two divided doses. Titrate in 25- to 50-mg/kg/day increments every 3 days as needed. Maximum dose is 150 mg/kg/day (75 mg/kg b.i.d.).

ADMINISTRATION
PO

⚠ *Alert:* Hazardous drug; use safe handling and disposal precautions.

• Drug may be given with or without food.

• Empty entire contents of the appropriate number of packets (500 mg/packet) of powder into cup, and dissolve in 10 mL of cold or room-temperature water per packet. Use oral syringe supplied with the medication to measure the water and give the solution. The concentration of the final solution is 50 mg/mL. Use immediately after reconstitution and discard any unused portion.

• Discard solution if it isn't clear, colorless, and free of particles.

ACTION

Precise mechanism unknown. Thought to control seizures by inhibiting GABA transaminase, the enzyme responsible for metabolizing the inhibitory neurotransmitter GABA, thereby increasing GABA levels in the CNS.

Route	Onset	Peak	Duration
PO	Unknown	1–2.5 hr	Unknown

Half-life: 5.5 to 10.5 hours.

ADVERSE REACTIONS

CNS: abnormal behavior, abnormal coordination, abnormal dreams, abnormal thinking, anxiety, asthenia, attention disturbance, confusion, *seizures,* depression, dizziness, dysarthria, expressive language disorder, fatigue, drowsiness, fever, gait disorder, headache, hyperreflexia, hypoesthesia, hyporeflexia, ataxia, insomnia, irritability, lethargy, malaise, memory impairment, nervousness, paresthesia, peripheral neuropathy, postictal state, sedation, impaired consciousness, sensory disturbance, sensory loss, somnolence, *status epilepticus,* thirst, tremor, vertigo, dystonia, hypotonia, hypertonia. **CV:** chest pain, peripheral edema. **EENT:** asthenopia, blurred vision, diplopia, nystagmus, eye pain, strabismus, conjunctivitis, visual field defect, tinnitus, otitis media, sinus headache, nasal congestion, nasopharyngitis, pharyngolaryngeal pain, sinusitis, toothache. **GI:** abdominal distention, constipation, diarrhea, dyspepsia, nausea, stomach discomfort, abdominal pain, vomiting, thirst, gastroenteritis. **GU:** dysmenorrhea, erectile dysfunction, UTI. **Hematologic:** anemia. **Metabolic:** increased or decreased appetite, weight gain. **Musculoskeletal:** arthralgia, back pain, contusion, extremity pain, joint sprain, myalgia, muscle spasm, muscle strain, muscle twitching. **Respiratory:** bronchitis, cough, pulmonary congestion, URI, pneumonia, infectious croup. **Skin:** rash, wound secretion. **Other:** thirst, flulike syndrome, viral infection, candidiasis.

INTERACTIONS

Drug-drug. *Cannabidiol, cannabis:* May enhance CNS depressant effect of vigabatrin. Monitor therapy.
Clonazepam: May increase clonazepam level. Use together cautiously.
▪️**Boxed Warning** *Drugs associated with serious adverse ophthalmic effects , such as retinopathy (hydroxychloroquine) or glaucoma (corticosteroids, TCAs):* May increase risk of serious adverse ophthalmic effects. Avoid coadministration unless benefits clearly outweigh risks. ▪️
Fosphenytoin, phenytoin: May decrease phenytoin level, especially when drug is started or stopped. Monitor drug levels.
Drug-lifestyle. *Alcohol use:* May increase CNS depression. Patient should avoid alcohol.

EFFECTS ON LAB TEST RESULTS

• May decrease ALT and AST levels.
• May decrease Hb level, hematocrit, and RBC count.
• May increase amino acid levels in urine and lead to false-positive tests for genetic metabolic disorders.

CONTRAINDICATIONS & CAUTIONS

• Contraindicated in patients hypersensitive to drug or its components and as first-line therapy for complex partial seizures.
🜨 *Alert:* Use drug only when potential benefits outweigh risk of vision loss.
▪️**Boxed Warning** Drug may cause progressive and permanent bilateral concentric visual field constriction and may reduce visual acuity; the onset is unpredictable and can occur anytime during therapy. Risk of visual impairment increases with increasing dosage and cumulative exposure, but no dosage or exposure is known to be free of risk of vision loss, which may continue after drug is discontinued. Because of risk of permanent vision loss, drug is available only through the Vigabatrin REMS program. A visual exam should be performed before, every 3 months during, and 3 to 6 months after therapy. ▪️
▪️**Boxed Warning** Due to risk of vision loss, withdraw drug in patients who don't show substantial benefit within 3 months of initiation for refractory complex partial seizures and within 2 to 4 weeks of initiation in patients with infantile spasms, or sooner if treatment failure becomes obvious. Periodically reassess patient response to and continued need for drug. Use drug at lowest dosage with shortest exposure time as clinically necessary. ▪️
▪️**Boxed Warning** Don't use drug in patients who have or are at high risk for other types of irreversible vision loss unless benefits clearly outweigh risks. ▪️
• Drug may cause MRI abnormalities or neurotoxicity (intramyelinic edema). Drug may increase risk of peripheral neuropathy in adults.
• Use cautiously in patients with a history of depression, suicidality, or anemia.
Dialyzable drug: 40% to 60%.
⚠️ *Overdose S&S:* Unconsciousness, coma, drowsiness, vertigo, psychosis, apnea, respiratory depression, bradycardia, agitation, irritability, confusion, headache, hypotension, abnormal behavior, increased seizure activity, status epilepticus, speech disorder.

PREGNANCY-LACTATION-REPRODUCTION

• There are no adequate studies during pregnancy; animal studies suggest drug may cause fetal harm. Use only if potential benefit justifies fetal risk.

V

• Patients taking drug during pregnancy should enroll in the North American AED (Antiepileptic Drug) Pregnancy Registry (1-888-233-2334) or www.aedpregnancyregistry.org/.
• Drug appears in human milk. Patient should discontinue breastfeeding or discontinue drug.

NURSING CONSIDERATIONS

⚠ *Alert:* Closely monitor all patients taking or starting therapy with antiepileptics for changes in behavior indicating worsening suicidality or depression. Symptoms such as anxiety, agitation, hostility, mania, and hypomania may be precursors to emerging suicidality.
• Discontinue drug if patient fails to comply with therapy.
⚠ *Alert:* Don't withdraw drug suddenly. For adults, taper by decreasing daily dose by 1,000 mg/day weekly until discontinued. For children with complex partial seizures, taper daily dose by one third every week for 3 weeks. For infantile spasms, decrease daily dose at a rate of 25 to 50 mg/kg every 3 to 4 days.
• Monitor patient closely for such adverse effects as dizziness, which may lead to falls.
• Monitor patient closely for anemia, somnolence, fatigue, peripheral neuropathy, peripheral edema, and weight gain.
• Monitor ALT and AST levels; drug decreases levels, making these measurements unreliable for detecting early hepatic injury.

PATIENT TEACHING

• Instruct patient in safe drug administration and handling.
• Advise patient to read the manufacturer's medication guide before starting treatment and before each prescription refill.
• Warn patient that drug may cause dizziness and somnolence and to avoid driving or other hazardous activities until drug's effects are known.
Boxed Warning Inform patient that drug may cause vision loss, and explain the importance of regular eye exams and of the need for immediately reporting vision changes. Counsel patient that vision loss may be severe before it's detected. ∎
• Advise patient to call prescriber and not to stop drug suddenly if adverse reactions occur.
• Tell patient to report pregnancy or plans to become pregnant during therapy.

• Inform patient that drug appears in human milk and to avoid breastfeeding.

vilazodone hydrochloride
vil-AZ-oh-dohne

Viibryd◆

Therapeutic class: Antidepressants
Pharmacologic class: SSRIs–partial 5-HT$_{1A}$ receptor agonists

AVAILABLE FORMS
Tablets: 10 mg, 20 mg, 40 mg

INDICATIONS & DOSAGES
➤ **Major depressive disorder**
Adults: Initially, 10 mg PO daily for 7 days, then 20 mg PO daily. After 7 days, may increase to 40 mg PO daily. Recommended range, 20 to 40 mg.
Adjust-a-dose: Don't exceed 20 mg once daily when used in combination with a strong CYP3A4 inhibitor. Based on clinical response, consider increasing dosage twofold, up to a maximum 80 mg once daily, over 1 to 2 weeks in patients taking strong CYP3A4 inducers for more than 14 days.

ADMINISTRATION
PO
• Give drug with food.
• Give a missed dose as soon as possible. If it's almost time for the next dose, skip the missed dose and give the next dose at the regular time. Don't double dose.

ACTION
Binds to serotonin reuptake sites and 5-HT$_{1A}$ receptors; is a partial agonist at serotonergic 5-HT$_{1A}$ receptors.

Route	Onset	Peak	Duration
PO	Unknown	4–5 hr	Unknown

Half-life: 25 hours.

ADVERSE REACTIONS
CNS: dizziness, headache, somnolence, paresthesia, insomnia, abnormal dreams, restlessness, fatigue, sedation, tremor. **CV:** palpitations. **EENT:** dry mouth. **GI:** abdominal distention, abdominal pain, diarrhea, nausea, vomiting, dyspepsia, flatulence, gastroenteritis, increased appetite. **GU:** delayed

---

Reactions in bold italics are *life-threatening*. Interactions may have a *rapid onset* or a ***delayed onset***.

ejaculation, erectile dysfunction, sexual dysfunction, abnormal orgasm, decreased libido. **Metabolic:** weight gain. **Musculoskeletal:** arthralgia.

INTERACTIONS

Drug-drug. *Anticoagulants (apixaban, aspirin, heparin, NSAIDs, warfarin), antiplatelet agents:* May increase risk of bleeding. Monitor patient closely; adjust dosages of these drugs, or discontinue them.
CNS drugs: May cause additive effects. Use together cautiously.
Digoxin: May increase digoxin level. Monitor levels before and during use with vilazodone. Reduce digoxin dose as necessary.
MAO inhibitors, linezolid, methylene blue: May increase risk of serious or fatal adverse effects. Don't use concurrently with MAO inhibitor or within 14 days of starting or discontinuing an MAO inhibitor.
Serotonergics (buspirone, SSNRIs, SSRIs, tramadol, triptans): May cause serotonin syndrome. Use together with extreme caution.
Strong CYP3A4 inducers (carbamazepine, phenytoin, rifampin): May decrease vilazodone level. Monitor effectiveness; adjust vilazodone dosage as needed.
Strong CYP3A4 inhibitors (clarithromycin, itraconazole, voriconazole): May increase vilazodone level. Reduce vilazodone dosage to 20 mg daily.
Drug-herb. *Herbs with anticoagulant or antiplatelet properties (alfalfa, anise, bilberry):* May increase bleeding risk. Consider therapy modification.
St. John's wort: May increase risk of serotonin syndrome. Avoid use together.
Drug-lifestyle. *Alcohol use:* May increase bioavailability of vilazodone. Discourage use together.

EFFECTS ON LAB TEST RESULTS
• May decrease sodium level.

CONTRAINDICATIONS & CAUTIONS
🛈 *Alert:* Life-threatening serotonin syndrome (fever, mental status changes, muscle twitching, diaphoresis, shivering or shaking, diarrhea, loss of coordination) and NMS (hyperthermia, muscle rigidity, autonomic instability with possible rapid fluctuation of vital signs, mental status changes) have been reported with antidepressant use. Risk increases when antidepressants are used with other serotonergic drugs and with drugs that impair serotonin metabolism.
🛈 *Alert:* Concomitant use with methylene blue or linezolid can cause serotonin syndrome. Don't initiate drug in patients receiving linezolid or methylene blue.
• Contraindicated in patients hypersensitive to drug or its inactive components.
• Use cautiously in patients with history or family history of depression, hypomania, severe hepatic dysfunction, seizure disorder, or untreated angle-closure glaucoma.
Dialyzable drug: Unlikely.
⚠ *Overdose S&S:* Serotonin syndrome, lethargy, restlessness, hallucinations, disorientation.

PREGNANCY-LACTATION-REPRODUCTION
• Neonates born to patients who used drug in the third trimester can develop complications (including persistent pulmonary HTN of the newborn) upon delivery requiring prolonged hospitalization, respiratory support, and enteral feedings. Use drug during pregnancy only if potential benefits outweigh fetal risk.
• Patients taking drug during pregnancy should enroll in the North American AED (Antiepileptic Drug) Pregnancy Registry (1-888-233-2334 or www.aedpregnancyregistry.org/).
• Drug may appear in human milk. Use only when benefit outweighs risk to infant.

NURSING CONSIDERATIONS
• Evaluate patients for major depressive disorder.
Boxed Warning Drug may increase the risk of suicidality in children, adolescents, and young adults with major depressive disorder or other psychiatric disorders. Drug isn't approved for use in children. ∎
• Screen patients for risk of bipolar disorder. Vilazodone isn't approved for treatment of bipolar depression. Use of an antidepressant in patients with bipolar disorder may precipitate mixed or manic episodes.
🛈 *Alert:* If linezolid or methylene blue must be given concurrently with vilazodone (or other serotonergic drug), stop serotonergic drug and monitor patient for serotonin toxicity for 2 weeks (5 weeks if fluoxetine was taken) or until 24 hours after the last dose of methylene blue or linezolid, whichever comes first. May resume vilazodone

V

24 hours after last dose of methylene blue or linezolid.

• Evaluate patient for history of drug abuse, and watch closely for signs and symptoms of misuse or abuse (increased tolerance, drug-seeking behavior, requests for dosage increase).

• Closely monitor patient who had recently been taking MAO inhibitors for tremor, myoclonus, diaphoresis, nausea, vomiting, flushing, dizziness, hyperthermia with features that resemble NMS, seizures, rigidity, autonomic instability with possible rapid fluctuations of vital signs, and mental status changes that include extreme agitation progressing to delirium and coma.

• Monitor patient for NMS (hyperthermia, rigidity, autonomic instability with possible rapid fluctuations of vital signs, mental status changes).

• Monitor patients taking anticoagulants or antiplatelet agents for signs and symptoms of bleeding.

• When discontinuing vilazodone, avoid abrupt discontinuation. Gradually reduce dosage and monitor patient for adverse events. If withdrawal symptoms become intolerable, consider resuming the previous prescribed dosage and decreasing the dosage at a more gradual rate. Wait at least 14 days before starting an MAO inhibitor.

• Hyponatremia and SIADH, which may be life-threatening, have occurred as a result of treatment with other SSRIs and SSNRIs, especially in older adults and patients taking diuretics or who are otherwise volume-depleted. Discontinue vilazodone in patients with symptomatic hyponatremia and treat appropriately. Monitor patient for signs and symptoms of hyponatremia, such as headache, difficulty concentrating, memory impairment, confusion, weakness, unsteadiness, hallucinations, syncope, seizures, coma, and respiratory arrest.

• Monitor patients for acute-angle glaucoma. Many antidepressants, including vilazodone, may trigger an angle-closure attack in patients with anatomically narrow angles who don't have a patent iridectomy.

PATIENT TEACHING
Boxed Warning Advise families and caregivers to closely observe patient for increased suicidality. ∎

• Teach patient safe drug administration.

⚠ **Alert:** Teach patient to recognize and immediately report signs and symptoms of serotonin toxicity (fever, mental status changes, muscle twitching, diaphoresis, shivering or shaking, diarrhea, and loss of coordination) and NMS (hyperthermia, rigidity, autonomic instability with possible rapid fluctuations of vital signs, and mental status changes).

• Warn patient not to stop drug abruptly.

• Instruct patient to inform prescriber of all other medicines being taken to avoid dangerous interactions.

• Tell patient to immediately seek medical attention if fever, rigidity, rapid changes in pulse rate or BP, diaphoresis, or confusion occurs.

• Counsel patient to keep all appointments for monitoring blood work and for follow-up care.

• Advise patient to use caution when driving or operating hazardous equipment until effects of drug are known; drug may impair judgment, thinking, and motor skills.

• Caution patient and caregivers to watch for signs and symptoms of the onset of manic or hypomanic episodes.

• Warn patient to avoid alcohol during drug therapy.

• Advise patient to report pregnancy or plans to become pregnant or to breastfeed during therapy.

---

viloxazine
vye-LOX-a-zeen

Qelbree

Therapeutic class: ADHD drugs
Pharmacologic class: Selective norepinephrine reuptake inhibitors

AVAILABLE FORMS
Capsules (extended-release) ⒹⓃⒸ: 100 mg, 150 mg, 200 mg

INDICATIONS & DOSAGES
➤ **ADHD**
Children ages 12 to 17: Initially, 200 mg PO once daily. After 1 week, may titrate by 200-mg increments to maximum dose of 400 mg daily, depending on response and tolerability.
Children ages 6 to 11: Initially, 100 mg PO once daily. May titrate by 100-mg increments weekly to maximum dose of 400 mg daily, depending on response and tolerability.

Reactions in bold italics are *life-threatening*. Interactions may have a *rapid onset* or a *delayed onset*.

Adjust-a-dose: For severe renal impairment (eGFR less than 30 mL/minute/1.73 m²), starting dose is 100 mg once daily. May titrate weekly by 50- to 100-mg increments once daily to maximum dose of 200 mg once daily.

ADMINISTRATION
PO
- Give without regard for food.
- Give capsules whole; don't crush, cut, or allow patient to chew capsules.
- If patient can't swallow capsule whole, open capsule and sprinkle contents over a tsp of applesauce; have patient consume without chewing (within 2 hours). Don't store.
- Store capsules at 68° to 77° F (20° to 25° C).

ACTION
Exact mechanism unknown. Believed to inhibit reuptake of norepinephrine.

Route	Onset	Peak	Duration
PO	Unknown	5 hr	Unknown

Half-life: 7 hours.

ADVERSE REACTIONS
CNS: fatigue, fever, headache insomnia, irritability, lethargy, sedation, somnolence. **CV:** increased diastolic BP, tachycardia. **GI:** abdominal discomfort or pain, decreased appetite, nausea, vomiting. **Respiratory:** URI.

INTERACTIONS
Drug-drug. *CYP2D6 substrates (atomoxetine, desipramine, dextromethorphan, nortriptyline, metoprolol, perphenazine, risperidone, tolterodine, venlafaxine); CYP3A4 substrates (avanafil, buspirone, conivaptan, darifenacin, darunavir, ebastine, everolimus, ibrutinib, lomitapide, lovastatin, lurasidone, midazolam, naloxegol, nisoldipine, saquinavir, simvastatin, sirolimus, tipranavir, triazolam, vardenafil):* May increase substrate level and risk of adverse reactions. Monitor patient closely and adjust substrate dosage as clinically indicated.
MAO inhibitors (isocarboxazid, phenelzine, rasagiline, safinamide, selegiline, tranylcypromine): May increase risk of hypertensive crisis with concomitant use or within 14 days after discontinuing MAO inhibitor. Use during this time frame is contraindicated.
Moderately sensitive CYP1A2 substrates (clozapine, pirfenidone): May increase substrate level and risk of adverse reactions.

Avoid use together. If concomitant use is unavoidable, reduce substrate dosage.
Sensitive CYP1A2 substrates, CYP1A2 substrates with narrow therapeutic range (alosetron, duloxetine, ramelteon, tasimelteon, theophylline, tizanidine): May increase substrate level and risk of adverse reactions. Use together is contraindicated.

EFFECTS ON LAB TEST RESULTS
None reported.

CONTRAINDICATIONS & CAUTIONS
Boxed Warning Drug increases risk of suicidality. Monitor patient closely. ■
- Drug may induce mania or mixed episodes in patients with bipolar disorder. Screen patients for bipolar disorder before drug initiation.
- Use hasn't been studied in patients with hepatic impairment and isn't recommended.
- Use cautiously in patients with severe renal impairment.
- Safety and effectiveness in children younger than age 6 haven't been established.
Dialyzable drug: Unknown.
⚠ *Overdose S&S:* Drowsiness, impaired consciousness, diminished reflexes, increased HR.

PREGNANCY-LACTATION-REPRODUCTION
- Based on animal studies, drug may cause patient and fetal harm. Discontinue drug if pregnancy occurs.
- Enroll patients exposed to drug during pregnancy in the National Pregnancy Registry for Psychiatric Medications (1-866-961-2388 or www.womensmentalhealth.org/preg).
- It isn't known if drug appears in human milk or how drug affects milk production or infants who are breastfed. Weigh patient's clinical need and risk to the infant against benefits of breastfeeding.

NURSING CONSIDERATIONS
Boxed Warning Monitor patient for clinical worsening or emergence of suicidality, especially during drug initiation and dosage changes. If signs or symptoms occur, consider discontinuing drug. ■
- Assess patient for personal and family history of suicide, bipolar disorder, and depression before drug initiation.
- Assess HR and BP at baseline, after dosage increase, and periodically during therapy.

V

• Periodically assess need for drug and dosage adjustments in patient taking drug long term.

• Monitor patient for mania or hypomania and excessive fatigue or somnolence.

• *Look alike–sound alike:* Don't confuse viloxazine with vilazodone.

PATIENT TEACHING

Boxed Warning Caution patient or caregiver to immediately report suicidality or new behavioral signs or symptoms. ■

• Instruct patient and caregivers in proper drug administration and storage.

• Tell patient or caregiver to report signs and symptoms of mania and hypomania (extreme increase in activity and talking, racing thoughts, severe insomnia, reckless behavior, excessive happiness or irritability).

• Caution patient that drug may cause fatigue or somnolence. Warn patient not to perform hazardous tasks or those requiring mental alertness until effects of drug are known.

• Inform patient that changes in BP and HR will be monitored while on drug.

• Tell patient or caregiver that drug may affect body weight and weight will be monitored for changes.

• Instruct patient to report pregnancy or plans to become pregnant during therapy.

SAFETY ALERT!

vinBLAStine sulfate (VLB)
vin-BLAS-teen

Therapeutic class: Antineoplastics
Pharmacologic class: Vinca alkaloids

AVAILABLE FORMS
Injection: 1 mg/mL in 10-mL vials

INDICATIONS & DOSAGES

� *Alert:* Manufacturer's labeling may not reflect current clinical practice. Dosing and frequency may vary by treatment protocol or phase.

Adjust-a-dose (for all indications): For patients with serum bilirubin level above 3 mg/dL, give 50% of usual dose. After a dose produces a WBC count below 3,000/mm³, give maintenance doses of one increment less than this amount at weekly intervals.

➤ **Hodgkin lymphoma**
Adults: 3.7 mg/m² IV in combination with other chemotherapeutic drugs.
Children: 6 mg/m² IV in combination with other chemotherapeutic drugs.
Adjust-a-dose: Adjust dose based on WBC response. Frequency and duration of treatment vary based on concomitant drugs and hematologic response.

➤ **Non-Hodgkin lymphomas; Kaposi sarcoma**
Adults: 3.7 mg/m² IV in combination with other chemotherapeutic drugs.
Adjust-a-dose: Adjust dose based on WBC response. Frequency and duration of treatment vary based on concomitant drugs and hematologic response.

➤ **Letterer-Siwe disease (histiocytosis X)**
Children: 6.5 mg/m² IV as a single agent.

➤ **Testicular germ-cell carcinomas**
Adults: 3.7 mg/m² IV in combination with other chemotherapeutic drugs.
Children: 3 mg/m²/day IV on days 1 through 5 of each cycle in combination with other chemotherapeutic drugs.

➤ **Bladder cancer ◆**
Adults: 3 mg/m² IV on day 2 every 14 days in combination with other chemotherapeutic drugs.

ADMINISTRATION

IV

▼ Preparing and giving drug may be mutagenic, teratogenic, or carcinogenic.

Boxed Warning Drug is for IV use only; fatal if given by other routes. ■

☺ *Alert:* When drug is dispensed in other than the original container, it must be packaged in the overwrap provided and labeled, using the auxiliary sticker provided and must state "Do not remove covering until moment of injection. For intravenous use only. Fatal if given by other routes." A syringe containing a specific dose must be labeled, using the auxiliary sticker provided to state: "For intravenous use only. Fatal if given by other routes."

☺ *Alert:* The Institute for Safe Medication Practices strongly recommends dispensing vinblastine in a minibag (NOT in a syringe) to prevent inadvertent intrathecal use.

▼ If a minibag isn't possible, inject drug directly into tubing of running IV line over 1 minute.

Reactions in bold italics are *life-threatening*. Interactions may have a *rapid onset* or a *delayed onset*.

Boxed Warning Make sure catheter is properly positioned in vein. Drug is a vesicant; if extravasation occurs, stop infusion immediately and notify prescriber. Moderate heat applied to area of leakage and a local injection of hyaluronidase may help disperse drug. ■

▼ **Incompatibilities:** Cefepime, furosemide, pantoprazole.

ACTION

Arrests mitosis in metaphase, blocking cell division.

Route	Onset	Peak	Duration
IV	Unknown	Unknown	Unknown

Half-life: Initial phase, 3.7 minutes; second phase, 1.6 hours; terminal phase, 25 hours.

ADVERSE REACTIONS

CNS: loss of deep tendon reflexes, numbness, paresthesia, peripheral neuropathy and neuritis, *seizures, stroke,* depression, headache, malaise. **CV:** *MI,* HTN. **EENT:** pharyngitis, oral vesiculation. **GI:** anorexia, constipation, ileus, nausea, stomatitis, vomiting, abdominal pain, *bleeding ulcer,* diarrhea, *hemorrhagic enterocolitis.* **Hematologic:** anemia, *leukopenia, thrombocytopenia.* **Musculoskeletal:** muscle pain and weakness, bone pain, jaw pain. **Respiratory:** *acute bronchospasm,* shortness of breath. **Skin:** irritation, phlebitis, cellulitis, reversible alopecia, vesiculation and necrosis with extravasation. **Other:** pain at tumor site.

INTERACTIONS

Drug-drug. *Azole antifungals, erythromycin, other drugs that inhibit cytochrome P-450 pathway:* May increase vinblastine toxicity. Avoid combination if possible. Monitor patient closely for toxicity.
Mitomycin: May increase risk of bronchospasm and shortness of breath. Monitor patient's respiratory status.
Ototoxic drugs, such as platinum-containing antineoplastics: May cause temporary or permanent hearing impairment. Monitor hearing function.
Phenytoin: May decrease plasma phenytoin level. Monitor phenytoin level closely.
Vaccines (inactivated): May diminish therapeutic effect of vaccines. Complete all age-appropriate vaccinations at least 2 weeks before starting vinblastine. If patient is vaccinated during therapy, revaccinate at least 3 months after drug is stopped.
Vaccines (live): May enhance adverse or toxic effect of live-virus vaccines and diminish their therapeutic effect. Avoid use with vinblastine; don't vaccinate for at least 3 months after therapy ends.
Drug-herb. *St. John's wort:* May decrease vinblastine concentration. Avoid use together.

EFFECTS ON LAB TEST RESULTS

• May decrease Hb level and WBC and platelet counts.

CONTRAINDICATIONS & CAUTIONS

• Contraindicated in patients hypersensitive to drug and in those with severe leukopenia or bacterial infection or significant granulocytopenia unless it's a result of the disease being treated.
• Avoid use in older adults with cachexia or ulcerated skin due to increased leukopenic response.
• Use cautiously in patients with hepatic dysfunction, pulmonary dysfunction, or CV disease.
Dialyzable drug: No.
⚠ *Overdose S&S:* Exaggerated effects, neurotoxicity.

PREGNANCY-LACTATION-REPRODUCTION

• There are no adequate studies during pregnancy, but drug can cause fetal harm. If drug is used during pregnancy or if patient becomes pregnant during therapy, inform patient of potential fetal hazard. Patients of childbearing potential should avoid pregnancy during therapy.
• It isn't known if drug appears in human milk. Patient should discontinue breastfeeding or discontinue drug.

NURSING CONSIDERATIONS

Boxed Warning Drug should be administered by personnel experienced in vinblastine sulfate administration. ■
• To reduce nausea, give antiemetic before drug.
• Don't give drug into a limb with compromised circulation.
• Monitor infusion site closely to prevent extravasation.
🕑 *Alert:* After giving drug, monitor patient for life-threatening acute bronchospasm. If this occurs, notify prescriber immediately.

V

Reaction is most likely to occur in patients also receiving mitomycin.

• Monitor patient for stomatitis. If stomatitis occurs, stop drug and notify prescriber.

• Assess bowel activity. Give laxatives as indicated. Stool softeners may be used prophylactically.

• Don't repeat dosage more frequently than every 7 days or severe leukopenia will occur. Nadir occurs on days 5 to 10. WBC count recovers fairly rapidly, usually within another 7 to 14 days.

• Assess patient for numbness and tingling in hands and feet. Assess gait for early evidence of footdrop.

• Drug is less neurotoxic than vincristine.

• Stop drugs known to cause urine retention for first few days after therapy, particularly in older adults.

• *Look alike–sound alike:* Don't confuse vinblastine with vincristine or vinorelbine.

PATIENT TEACHING

• Tell patient to report evidence of infection (fever, sore throat, fatigue) and bleeding (easy bruising, nosebleeds, bleeding gums, melena). Tell patient to take temperature daily.

• Urge patient to report pain, swelling, burning, or any unusual feeling at injection site during infusion.

• Warn patient that hair loss may occur but that it's usually temporary.

• Caution patient to avoid pregnancy during therapy.

• Tell patient that pain may occur in jaw and in the organ with the tumor.

SAFETY ALERT!

vinCRIStine sulfate
vin-KRIS-teen

Therapeutic class: Antineoplastics
Pharmacologic class: Vinca alkaloids

AVAILABLE FORMS
Injection: 1 mg/mL in 1-mL, 2-mL preservative-free vials

INDICATIONS & DOSAGES
⚠ *Alert:* Manufacturer's labeling may not reflect current clinical practice. Dosage, frequency, and duration of treatment vary by treatment protocol or phase.

➤ **Acute lymphoblastic and other leukemias, Hodgkin lymphoma, malignant lymphoma, neuroblastoma, rhabdomyosarcoma, Wilms tumor**
Adults: 1.4 mg/m^2 IV weekly.
Children weighing more than 10 kg: 1.5 to 2 mg/m^2 IV weekly.
Children weighing 10 kg and less or with BSA less than 1 m^2: Initially, 0.05 mg/kg IV weekly. Titrate dosage as tolerated, up to 2 mg/dose.
Adjust-a-dose: For patients with direct bilirubin level above 3 mg/dL, reduce dosage by 50%.

ADMINISTRATION
IV
⚠ *Alert:* Preparing and giving drug may be mutagenic, teratogenic, or carcinogenic. Follow institutional policy to reduce risks.

▼ Inject directly into tube of running IV line of NSS or D$_5$W only, slowly over 1 minute.

⚠ *Alert:* To prevent inadvertent intrathecal administration, WHO and the Institute for Safe Medication Practices strongly recommend dispensing vincristine in a minibag (not in a syringe).

Boxed Warning Make sure catheter is positioned correctly in vein. Drug is a vesicant; if extravasation occurs, stop infusion immediately and notify prescriber. Local injection of hyaluronidase and application of moderate heat to area of leakage may help disperse drug. ■

Boxed Warning Administer by IV route only; fatal if given by other routes. ■

Boxed Warning Syringes containing this product should be labeled, using the auxiliary sticker provided, to state, "For intravenous use only. Fatal if given by other routes." Extemporaneously prepared syringes containing this product must be packaged in an overwrap that's labeled, "Do not remove covering until moment of injection. For intravenous use only. Fatal if given by other routes." ■

▼ If protocol requires a continuous infusion, use a central line. Give as a short 5- to 10-minute infusion in 25 to 50 mL of NSS or D$_5$W.

▼ All vials contain 1 mg/mL solution; refrigerate vials.

▼ **Incompatibilities:** Cefepime, furosemide, idarubicin, pantoprazole, phenytoin, sodium bicarbonate. Consult a drug incompatibility reference for more information.

Reactions in bold italics are *life-threatening*. Interactions may have a *rapid onset* or a *delayed onset*.

ACTION
Arrests mitosis in metaphase, blocking cell division.

Route	Onset	Peak	Duration
IV	Unknown	Unknown	Unknown

Half-life: Initial phase, 5 minutes; second phase, 2.25 hours; terminal phase, 6.5 days.

ADVERSE REACTIONS
CNS: loss of deep tendon reflexes, paresthesia, peripheral neuropathy, *coma, seizures,* ataxia, foot drop, cranial nerve palsies, fever, headache, sensory loss, neuritic pain, abnormal gait, dizziness, vertigo. **CV:** HTN, hypotension. **EENT:** blindness, diplopia, optic and extraocular neuropathy, photophobia, ptosis, visual disturbances, nystagmus, temporary or permanent deafness, vocal cord paralysis, hoarseness. **GI:** constipation, cramps, nausea, stomatitis, vomiting, *intestinal necrosis,* anorexia, diarrhea, dysphagia, ileus that mimics surgical paralytic ileus. **GU:** dysuria, polyuria, urine retention. **Hematologic:** *leukopenia, thrombocytopenia,* anemia. **Hepatic:** *hepatic veno-occlusive disease.* **Metabolic:** weight loss, dehydration, hyperuricemia. **Musculoskeletal:** cramps, jaw pain, myalgia, muscle weakness, muscle wasting. **Respiratory:** *acute bronchospasm,* dyspnea. **Skin:** phlebitis, cellulitis at injection site, rash, reversible alopecia, severe local reaction following extravasation. **Other:** hypersensitivity reactions.

INTERACTIONS
Drug-drug. *Fosphenytoin, phenytoin:* May reduce levels of these drugs. Monitor levels closely.
HIV protease inhibitors (atazanavir, ritonavir): May increase pharmacologic effects of vincristine. Monitor patient for profound neutropenia and severe neuropathy. Temporarily suspend HIV protease inhibitor or reduce vincristine dosage if significant hematologic or GI toxicity occurs.
Mitomycin: May increase frequency of bronchospasm and acute pulmonary reactions. Monitor patient's respiratory status.
Moderate CYP3A4 inhibitors (erythromycin, verapamil): May increase vincristine level. Use together cautiously.
Ototoxic drugs: May potentiate loss of hearing. Use together with caution.

P-gp inducers (rifampin, saquinavir), P-gp inhibitors (clarithromycin, cyclosporine, diltiazem): May alter vincristine level. Avoid use together.
Strong CYP3A4 inducers (phenobarbital, rifampin): May decrease vincristine level. Use together cautiously.
Strong CYP3A4 inhibitors (clarithromycin, ketoconazole): May increase vincristine level and risk of toxicities. Consider alternative therapy to inhibitor.
Triazole antifungals (itraconazole, posaconazole, voriconazole): Concomitant use may increase risk of neurotoxicity. Consider therapy modification.
Vaccines (inactivated): May diminish therapeutic effect of vaccines. Complete all age-appropriate vaccinations at least 2 weeks before starting vincristine. If patient is vaccinated during therapy, revaccinate at least 3 months after drug is stopped.
Vaccines (live): May enhance adverse or toxic effect of live-virus vaccines and diminish their therapeutic effect. Avoid use with vincristine; don't vaccinate for at least 3 months after drug is stopped.
Warfarin: May increase anticoagulant effects. Monitor INR and adjust warfarin dose as needed.
Drug-herb. *Echinacea, St. John's wort:* May decrease vincristine concentration. Avoid use together.

EFFECTS ON LAB TEST RESULTS
• May increase uric acid level.
• May decrease sodium level.
• May decrease Hb level and WBC and platelet counts.

CONTRAINDICATIONS & CAUTIONS
• Contraindicated in patients hypersensitive to drug and in those with demyelinating form of Charcot-Marie-Tooth syndrome.
• Don't give to patients who are receiving radiation therapy through ports that include the liver.
• Use cautiously in patients with hepatic dysfunction, neuromuscular disease, or infection.
Dialyzable drug: No.
⚠ **Overdose S&S:** Exaggerated effects, death.

PREGNANCY-LACTATION-REPRODUCTION
• There are no adequate studies during pregnancy, but drug may cause fetal harm. If used during pregnancy or if patient becomes

pregnant during therapy, inform patient of potential fetal hazard. Patients of childbearing potential should use effective contraception during therapy.
• It isn't known if drug appears in human milk. Patient should discontinue breastfeeding or discontinue drug.
• Drug may impair fertility.

NURSING CONSIDERATIONS
Boxed Warning Drug should be administered by personnel experienced in the administration of vincristine sulfate. ∎
• Watch for hyperuricemia, especially in patients with leukemia or lymphoma. Maintain hydration and give allopurinol to prevent uric acid nephropathy. Watch for toxicity.
• If SIADH (rare) develops, restrict fluids, if needed. Monitor fluid intake and output.
• Because of risk of neurotoxicity, don't give drug more often than once weekly. Children are more resistant to neurotoxicity than adults. Neurotoxicity is dose related and usually reversible.
• Older adults and patients with underlying neurologic disease may be more susceptible to neurotoxic effects.
• Monitor patient for depression of Achilles tendon reflex, numbness, tingling, footdrop or wristdrop, difficulty walking, ataxia, and slapping gait. Monitor patient's ability to walk on heels. Support patient while walking.
• Monitor bowel function. Constipation may be an early sign of neurotoxicity.
• Stop drugs known to cause urine retention, particularly in older adults, for first few days after therapy.
• *Look alike–sound alike:* Don't confuse vincristine with vincristine liposomal, vinblastine, or vinorelbine.

PATIENT TEACHING
• Advise patient to report all adverse reactions, especially pain or burning at injection site during or after administration.
• Instruct patient to report increased shortness of breath and evidence of infection (fever, sore throat, fatigue) and bleeding (easy bruising, nosebleeds, bleeding gums, melena). Tell patient to take temperature daily.
• Teach patient to follow a prophylactic bowel management plan and to report constipation.
• Warn patient that hair loss may occur, but explain that it's usually temporary.

• Caution patient not to breastfeed and to avoid becoming pregnant during therapy and to consult prescriber before becoming pregnant.

SAFETY ALERT!

vinorelbine tartrate
vin-oh-REL-been

Therapeutic class: Antineoplastics
Pharmacologic class: Semisynthetic vinca alkaloids

AVAILABLE FORMS
Injection: 10 mg/mL, 50 mg/5 mL

INDICATIONS & DOSAGES
🌜 *Alert:* Manufacturer's labeling may not reflect current clinical practice. Dosage, frequency, and duration of treatment vary by treatment protocol or phase.
Adjust-a-dose (for all indications): Refer to manufacturer's instructions for toxicity-related dosage adjustments.
➤ **As monotherapy for treatment of patients with metastatic NSCLC; in combination with cisplatin for first-line treatment of patients with locally advanced or metastatic NSCLC**
Adults: 30 mg/m^2 IV weekly as monotherapy. In combination treatment, 25 mg/m^2 IV weekly with cisplatin 100 mg/m^2 given every 4 weeks. Or, 30 mg/m^2 IV weekly in combination with cisplatin 120 mg/m^2 given on days 1 and 29, then every 6 weeks.
➤ **HER-2 positive advanced or metastatic breast cancer ◆**
Adults: 25 or 30 mg/m^2 IV every 7 days (as a single agent) until disease progression or unacceptable toxicity.

ADMINISTRATION
IV
🌜 *Alert:* Hazardous agent; use safe-handling and disposal precautions.
▼ Dilute to 0.5 to 2 mg/mL in an IV bag of D$_5$W, NSS, half-NSS, D$_5$W half-NSS, Ringer solution, or lactated Ringer solution.
▼ Give drug IV over 6 to 10 minutes into side port of a free-flowing IV line that is closest to IV bag; then flush with 75 to 125 mL or more of recommended solution for dilution.

Reactions in bold italics are *life-threatening*. Interactions may have a *rapid onset* or a **delayed onset**.

▼ The Institute for Safe Medication Practices strongly recommends dispensing vinca alkaloids in a minibag (not a syringe).

▼ Monitor site for irritation and infiltration because drug can cause localized tissue damage, necrosis, and thrombophlebitis.

⚠ Alert: Ensure proper IV catheter placement. If extravasation occurs, stop drug immediately and inject remaining dose into a different vein; notify prescriber.

▼ May store diluted drug for up to 24 hours at room temperature.

▼ **Incompatibilities:** None listed by manufacturer. Consult a drug incompatibility reference for more information.

ACTION

Exerts its primary antineoplastic effect by disrupting microtubule assembly, which in turn disrupts spindle formation and prevents mitosis.

Route	Onset	Peak	Duration
IV	Unknown	Unknown	Unknown

Half-life: About 27.5 to 43.6 hours.

ADVERSE REACTIONS

CNS: asthenia, fatigue, peripheral neuropathy, fever, taste alteration, neurotoxicity (paresthesia, hyperesthesia, hyporeflexia, weakness). **CV:** chest pain, localized phlebitis. **EENT:** ototoxicity. **GI:** anorexia, constipation, diarrhea, nausea, stomatitis, vomiting. **Hematologic:** anemia, *agranulocytosis, neutropenia, bone marrow suppression, granulocytopenia, thrombocytopenia, leukopenia.* **Hepatic:** hyperbilirubinemia, elevated AST level. **Musculoskeletal:** arthralgia, jaw pain, loss of deep tendon reflexes, myalgia. **Respiratory:** dyspnea, respiratory tract infection. **Skin:** alopecia, injection-site pain or reaction, rash. **Other:** infection, *sepsis.*

INTERACTIONS

Drug-drug. *Cisplatin:* May increase risk of bone marrow suppression when used with cisplatin. Monitor hematologic status closely.
CYP3A inhibitors (erythromycin, ketoconazole, ritonavir): May decrease metabolism of vinorelbine. Watch for increased adverse effects.
Macrolide antibiotics (clarithromycin, erythromycin): May increase vinorelbine level. Consider therapy modification.

Mitomycin: May increase risk of pulmonary reactions. Monitor respiratory status closely.
Paclitaxel: May increase risk of neuropathy. Monitor patient closely.
Posaconazole: May increase risk of neurotoxicity. Monitor patient closely.
Vaccines (inactivated): May diminish therapeutic effect of vaccines. Complete all age-appropriate vaccinations at least 2 weeks before starting vinorelbine. If patient is vaccinated during therapy, revaccinate at least 3 months after drug is stopped.
Vaccines, live-virus: May increase risk of live-virus vaccine–induced adverse reactions. Concurrent use isn't recommended.
Drug-herb. *Echinacea:* May diminish therapeutic effect of vinorelbine. Consider therapy modification.

EFFECTS ON LAB TEST RESULTS

• May increase creatinine and bilirubin levels and LFT values.
• May decrease Hb level and granulocyte, WBC, and platelet counts.

CONTRAINDICATIONS & CAUTIONS

• Use cautiously in patients whose bone marrow may have been compromised by previous exposure to radiation therapy or chemotherapy or whose bone marrow is still recovering from chemotherapy.

• Use cautiously in patients with hepatic impairment. Monitor liver function during treatment.

• Safety and effectiveness in children haven't been established.
Dialyzable drug: 0% to 24%.

⚠ Overdose S&S: Paralytic ileus, stomatitis, esophagitis, bone marrow aplasia, sepsis, paresis, death.

PREGNANCY-LACTATION-REPRODUCTION

• Drug can cause fetal harm when used during pregnancy. Patients of childbearing potential should use highly effective contraception during therapy and for 6 months after final dose.
• Drug may be hazardous to fetus if used during pregnancy. Inform patient of potential risk.
• Males with partners of childbearing potential should use highly effective contraception during therapy and for 3 months after final dose.

V

• It isn't known if drug appears in human milk. Patient should discontinue breastfeeding during treatment and for 9 days after final dose, or discontinue drug.

• Drug may impair male fertility.

NURSING CONSIDERATIONS

Boxed Warning Severe myelosuppression resulting in serious infection, septic shock, hospitalization, and death may occur. ∎

Boxed Warning Decrease dosage or withhold drug in accordance with recommended dosage modifications. Neutrophil count should be 1,000/mm³ or more before administration. ∎

• If neutrophil count falls below 1,000/mm³, withhold drug and notify prescriber. Neutrophil count nadir occurs between days 7 and 10.

• Monitor CBC before each dose. Don't give drug to patient with neutrophil count below 1,000 cells/mm³. Adjust dosage based on neutrophil count obtained on day of treatment.

• Patient may receive injections of G-CSF to promote cell growth and decrease risk of infection.

• Monitor liver enzyme levels in patients with hepatic impairment.

⚈ *Alert:* Drug is a vesicant. If extravasation occurs, stop infusion immediately, notify prescriber, and manage as directed.

⚈ *Alert:* Monitor deep tendon reflexes; loss may represent cumulative toxicity.

• Monitor patients closely for hypersensitivity and new or worsening signs and symptoms of neuropathy in those with prior history of or preexisting neuropathy.

• Severe acute bronchospasm, interstitial pneumonitis, and ARDS have been reported. Monitor patient for unexplained dyspnea or other signs and symptoms of pulmonary toxicity.

• Monitor patient for severe constipation and bowel obstruction. A prophylactic bowel regimen that includes adequate dietary fiber and fluid intake and routine use of stool softeners may be needed.

• As a guide to the effects of therapy, monitor patient's peripheral blood count and bone marrow.

• *Look alike–sound alike:* Don't confuse vinorelbine with vinblastine or vincristine.

PATIENT TEACHING

• Advise patient to report any pain or burning at site of injection.

• Instruct patient not to take other drugs, including OTC preparations, until approved by prescriber.

• Tell patient to report all adverse reactions, especially evidence of infection (fever, sore throat, fatigue) and bleeding (easy bruising, nosebleeds, bleeding gums, melena). Tell patient to take temperature daily.

• Advise patient to report increased or new shortness of breath, cough, or wheezing.

• Instruct patient to report constipation and to follow a prophylactic bowel management plan.

• Counsel patient of childbearing potential to use highly effective contraception during therapy and for 6 months after final dose and male patient with partner of childbearing potential to use highly effective contraception during therapy and for 3 months after final dose.

• Advise patient not to breastfeed during therapy.

SAFETY ALERT!

vismodegib
VIS-moe-DEG-ib

Erivedge

Therapeutic class: Antineoplastics
Pharmacologic class: Hedgehog pathway inhibitors

AVAILABLE FORMS
Capsules ⓄⓉⒸ: 150 mg

INDICATIONS & DOSAGES
➤ **Metastatic basal cell carcinoma; locally advanced basal cell carcinoma that has recurred following surgery or in patients who aren't candidates for surgery or radiation**
Adults: 150 mg PO once daily until disease progression or unacceptable toxicity.
Adjust-a-dose: Withhold drug for up to 8 weeks for intolerable adverse reactions until improvement or resolution. Treatment durations shorter than 8 weeks before interruptions haven't been studied. Permanently discontinue drug if patient experiences SCARs, including SJS, TEN, or DRESS syndrome.

ADMINISTRATION
PO
☙ *Alert:* Hazardous agent; use safe-handling and disposal precautions.
• May give with or without food.
• Patient should swallow capsule whole. Don't open, crush, or allow patient to chew capsules.
• If a dose is missed, omit the missed dose and resume dosing at the next scheduled time.
• Store capsules at room temperature.

ACTION
Inhibits Hedgehog signaling pathway by binding to and inhibiting Smoothened, a transmembrane protein involved in Hedgehog signal transmission. Inhibition of this protein slows pathway for tumor growth.

Route	Onset	Peak	Duration
PO	Unknown	2.4 days	Unknown

Half-life: 4 days with continued dosing; 12 days after one dose.

ADVERSE REACTIONS
CNS: fatigue, taste perversion, absence of taste. **GI:** nausea, diarrhea, vomiting, constipation, decreased appetite. **GU:** azotemia, amenorrhea. **Metabolic:** weight loss, *hyponatremia, hypokalemia.* **Musculoskeletal:** muscle spasms, arthralgia. **Skin:** alopecia.

INTERACTIONS
None reported.

EFFECTS ON LAB TEST RESULTS
• May increase CK, BUN, and creatinine levels.
• May decrease sodium and potassium levels.

CONTRAINDICATIONS & CAUTIONS
• Contraindicated in patients hypersensitive to drug.
• Premature fusion of the epiphyses has been reported in children taking drug. In some cases, fusion progressed after drug was discontinued. Drug isn't indicated for children.
• SCARs, including SJS, TEN, and DRESS syndrome, which could be life-threatening or fatal, have been reported.
Dialyzable drug: Unknown.

PREGNANCY-LACTATION-REPRODUCTION
Boxed Warning Contraindicated during pregnancy. Drug can cause embryo-fetal death or severe birth defects. ∎

Boxed Warning Verify pregnancy status within 7 days before start of therapy. Advise patient of fetal risk. ∎

Boxed Warning Patients of childbearing potential should use effective contraception during therapy and for 24 months after final dose; male patients should use condoms, even after a vasectomy, to avoid drug exposure to partners who are pregnant and to partners of childbearing potential during therapy and for 3 months after final dose. ∎

• Drug is present in semen but it isn't known if the amount in semen can cause embryofetal harm. Men shouldn't donate semen during therapy and for 3 months after therapy ends.
• Report exposure during pregnancy (directly or from seminal fluid) or within 7 months after treatment ends to Genentech at 1-888-835-2555.
• It isn't known if drug appears in human milk. Breastfeeding isn't recommended during therapy and for 24 months after final dose.
• Drug may cause amenorrhea, which may be irreversible.

NURSING CONSIDERATIONS
• Monitor patient for GI toxicities (decreased appetite, nausea, diarrhea, vomiting, abdominal pain, constipation).
• Monitor patient for skin alterations.
• *Look alike–sound alike:* Don't confuse vismodegib with vemurafenib or vandetanib.

PATIENT TEACHING
Boxed Warning Advise male and female patients of the risks to an embryo or fetus, the need for contraception during and after therapy, and the risk of drug exposure through semen. ∎

Boxed Warning Tell patient of childbearing potential to use highly effective contraception during therapy and for 24 months after final dose; advise male patient to use condoms, even after a vasectomy, to avoid drug exposure to partners who are pregnant and to partners of childbearing potential during therapy and for 3 months after final dose. ∎

• Instruct patient in proper drug administration.
• Warn patient to immediately report confirmed or suspected pregnancy after exposure to drug, or if patient has unprotected sex.
• Advise patient experiencing drug-induced amenorrhea that it's unknown if amenorrhea will be reversed after drug discontinuation.

V

• Caution patient not to donate blood or blood products while taking drug and for at least 24 months (or semen for 3 months) after last dose.

vorapaxar sulfate
VOR-a-PAX-ar

Zontivity

Therapeutic class: Antiplatelet drugs
Pharmacologic class: Platelet aggregation inhibitors

AVAILABLE FORMS
Tablets: 2.08 mg

INDICATIONS & DOSAGES
➤ **To reduce thrombotic CV events in patients with history of MI or peripheral arterial disease, in combination with aspirin or clopidogrel**
Adults: 1 tablet (2.08 mg) PO once daily.

ADMINISTRATION
PO
• May give with or without food.
• Store tablets in original package at room temperature. Keep the desiccant packet in the bottle to protect from moisture.

ACTION
Inhibits platelet aggregation. Drug is a reversible antagonist of the protease-activated receptor-1 expressed on platelets.

Route	Onset	Peak	Duration
PO	Unknown	1–2 hr	Unknown

Half-life: 5 to 13 days.

ADVERSE REACTIONS
CNS: depression, *intracranial bleeding.* **EENT:** retinopathy, retinal disorders, diplopia. **GI:** *GI bleeding.* **Hematologic:** *hemorrhage,* anemia, iron deficiency. **Skin:** rash, eruption, exanthemas.

INTERACTIONS
Drug-drug. *Drugs known to cause bleeding (anticoagulants, fibrinolytics, NSAIDs [long-term], SSNRIs, SSRIs, warfarin):* Increase risk of bleeding, including intracranial hemorrhage and fatal bleeding. Avoid use together.

Strong CYP3A inducers (carbamazepine, phenytoin, rifampin): May decrease vorapaxar level. Avoid use together.
Strong CYP3A inhibitors (boceprevir, clarithromycin, conivaptan, itraconazole, ketoconazole, nefazodone, nelfinavir, posaconazole, ritonavir, saquinavir, telaprevir, telithromycin): May increase vorapaxar level. Avoid use together.
Drug-herb. *Herbs with anticoagulant/antiplatelet properties (alfalfa, anise, bilberry):* May increase bleeding risk. Consider therapy modification.
St. John's wort: May decrease vorapaxar level. Avoid use together.

EFFECTS ON LAB TEST RESULTS
• May decrease RBC count.

CONTRAINDICATIONS & CAUTIONS
Boxed Warning Don't use in patients with history of intracranial hemorrhage, stroke, TIA, or active pathologic bleeding. Antiplatelet drugs, including vorapaxar, increase risk of bleeding, including intracranial hemorrhage and fatal bleeding. ■
• Drug has only been studied in combination with aspirin or clopidogrel.
• Use cautiously in patients with low body weight, reduced renal or hepatic function, or history of bleeding disorder; and in patients concomitantly using drugs known to increase bleeding.
• Use isn't recommended in patients with severe hepatic impairment.
• Older adults are at higher risk for bleeding. Consider patient's age before administering drug.
• Safety and effectiveness in children haven't been established.
Dialyzable drug: Unlikely.

PREGNANCY-LACTATION-REPRODUCTION
• Drug can cause serious adverse reactions, including maternal hemorrhage. Discontinue drug when pregnancy is detected and begin alternative therapy with a shorter duration of action.
• It isn't known if drug appears in human milk. Use during breastfeeding isn't recommended.

NURSING CONSIDERATIONS
🛑 **Alert:** Stopping drug briefly during an episode of acute bleeding won't be useful in managing bleeding, because of drug's long

---

*Reactions in bold italics are **life-threatening**. Interactions may have a *rapid onset* or a **delayed onset**.*

half-life. There's no known treatment to reverse the antiplatelet effect; drug will significantly inhibit platelet aggregation for 4 weeks after discontinuation.

• Discontinue drug if patient experiences a stroke, TIA, or intracranial hemorrhage.
• Monitor Hb level and hematocrit periodically. Monitor patient for bleeding.
• Evaluate patients with hypotension who have had recent coronary angiography, PCI, CABG, or other surgical procedure for possible bleeding.

PATIENT TEACHING

Boxed Warning Caution patient that drug increases risk of bleeding, including intracranial hemorrhage and fatal bleeding. ∎

• Advise patient to tell other providers about taking drug, especially before any surgery or dental procedure.
• Instruct patient to take drug exactly as prescribed in addition to aspirin or clopidogrel, and not to discontinue drug without first consulting prescriber.
• Teach patient to report bruising or severe prolonged or excessive unexplained bleeding (blood in stool, vomit, or urine and coughing up blood or blood clots).
• Advise patient to report all prescription and OTC medications, vitamins, herbs, and other dietary supplements being taken to prescriber and pharmacist so that they are aware of other treatment that may affect bleeding risk.
• Caution patient to immediately report pregnancy or plans to become pregnant.
• Tell patient that breastfeeding isn't recommended during therapy.

---

voriconazole 🔏
vor-ah-KON-ah-zole

Vfend

Therapeutic class: Antifungals
Pharmacologic class: Synthetic triazoles

AVAILABLE FORMS

Oral suspension: 200 mg/5 mL (40 mg/mL after reconstitution)
Powder for injection: 200 mg/vial
Tablets: 50 mg, 200 mg

INDICATIONS & DOSAGES

Adjust-a-dose (for all indications): For adults with mild or moderate hepatic impairment (Child-Pugh class A or B), decrease the maintenance dosage by 50%. In adults with a CrCl of less than 50 mL/minute, use PO form instead of IV form to prevent IV mixture component accumulation.

➤ **Esophageal candidiasis**
Adults, children ages 12 to 14 weighing 50 kg or more, and children age 15 and older regardless of body weight: 200 mg PO every 12 hours.
Adults weighing less than 40 kg: 100 or 150 mg PO every 12 hours.
Children ages 2 to younger than 12 and children ages 12 to 14 weighing less than 50 kg: Initially, 4 mg/kg IV every 12 hours. If patient can't tolerate 4-mg/kg IV dose, reduce dose by 1-mg/kg steps. If inadequate response and patient can tolerate initial IV dose, increase dose by 1-mg/kg steps. After at least 5 days of IV therapy and significant clinical improvement, consider an oral regimen of 9 mg/kg PO every 12 hours. If patient can't tolerate 9-mg/kg PO dose, reduce dose by 1-mg/kg or 50-mg steps. If inadequate response and patient can tolerate initial PO dose, increase dose by 1-mg/kg or 50-mg steps to a maximum of 350 mg PO every 12 hours.
Adjust-a-dose: For all patients, treat for at least 14 days and for at least 7 days after symptoms resolve.

➤ **Invasive aspergillosis; serious infections caused by *Fusarium* species and *Scedosporium apiospermum* in patients intolerant of or refractory to other therapy**
Adults, children ages 12 to 14 weighing 50 kg or more, and children age 15 and older regardless of body weight: Initially, 6 mg/kg IV every 12 hours for two doses; then maintenance dose of 4 mg/kg IV every 12 hours. If patient can't tolerate 4-mg/kg dose, decrease to 3 mg/kg. Continue IV therapy for at least 7 days. Switch to PO form as tolerated, using the maintenance dosages shown here.
Adults weighing 40 kg or more, children ages 12 to 14 weighing 50 kg or more, and children age 15 and older regardless of body weight: 200 mg PO every 12 hours. May increase to 300 mg PO every 12 hours, if needed. If patient can't tolerate the 300-mg dose, reduce dose in 50-mg decrements to a minimum of 200 mg every 12 hours.
Adults weighing less than 40 kg: 100 mg PO every 12 hours. May increase to 150 mg PO

V

every 12 hours, if needed. If patient can't tolerate the 150-mg dose, reduce dose to 100 mg every 12 hours.

Children ages 2 to younger than 12 and children ages 12 to 14 weighing less than 50 kg: Initially, 9 mg/kg IV every 12 hours for two doses; then maintenance dose of 8 mg/kg IV every 12 hours. If patient can't tolerate 8-mg/kg IV dose, reduce dose by 1-mg/kg steps. If inadequate response and patient can tolerate initial IV maintenance dose, increase dose by 1-mg/kg steps. Continue IV therapy for at least 7 days; then switch to 9 mg/kg PO every 12 hours. If patient can't tolerate 9-mg/kg PO dose, reduce dose by 1-mg/kg or 50-mg steps. If inadequate response and patient can tolerate initial PO maintenance dose, increase dose by 1-mg/kg or 50-mg steps to a maximum of 350 mg PO every 12 hours.

➤ **Candidemia in patients who are non-neutropenic;** *Candida* **infections of the kidney, abdomen, bladder wall, or wounds and disseminated skin infections**

Adults, children ages 12 to 14 weighing 50 kg or more, and children age 15 and older regardless of body weight: Initially, 6 mg/kg IV every 12 hours for two doses, then 3 to 4 mg/kg IV every 12 hours for maintenance, depending on severity of the infection. If patient can't tolerate 4-mg/kg dose, decrease to 3 mg/kg. Switch to PO form as tolerated, using the maintenance dosages shown here.

Adults weighing 40 kg or more, children ages 12 to 14 weighing 50 kg or more, and children age 15 and older regardless of body weight: 200 mg PO every 12 hours. May increase to 300 mg PO every 12 hours, if needed. If unable to tolerate the 300-mg dose, reduce dose in 50-mg decrements to a minimum of 200 mg every 12 hours.

Adults weighing less than 40 kg: 100 mg PO every 12 hours. May increase to 150 mg PO every 12 hours, if needed. If patient can't tolerate the 150-mg dose, reduce dose to 100 mg every 12 hours.

Children ages 2 to younger than 12 and children ages 12 to 14 weighing less than 50 kg: Initially, 9 mg/kg IV every 12 hours for two doses; then maintenance dose of 8 mg/kg IV every 12 hours. If patient can't tolerate 8-mg/kg IV dose, reduce dose by 1-mg/kg steps. If inadequate response and patient can tolerate initial IV maintenance dose, increase dose by 1-mg/kg steps. Continue IV therapy for at least 5 days; then switch to 9 mg/kg PO every 12 hours. If patient can't tolerate 9-mg/kg PO dose, reduce dose by 1-mg/kg or 50-mg steps. If inadequate response and patient can tolerate initial PO maintenance dose, increase dose by 1-mg/kg or 50-mg steps to a maximum of 350 mg PO every 12 hours.

Adjust-a-dose: Treat patients with candidemia for at least 14 days after symptoms resolve or after the last positive culture result, whichever is longer.

ADMINISTRATION

• Obtain specimens for fungal culture and other relevant lab studies (including histopathology) before starting therapy to isolate and identify causative organism(s). May start drug before study results are known. Adjust therapy when results become available if necessary.

🌙 *Alert:* Hazardous agent; use safe-handling and disposal precautions.

PO

• Give tablets or oral suspension at least 1 hour before or 1 hour after a meal or enteral tube feeding.

• For the oral suspension, use only the dispenser provided in the medication package.

• Don't mix oral suspension with other drugs or beverages.

• Shake suspension for 10 seconds before each use. Store at room temperature. Discard unused portion of suspension after 14 days.

IV

▼ In patients with CrCl less than 50 mL/minute, use IV form cautiously and closely monitor serum creatinine level. Change to PO form is recommended.

▼ Reconstitute powder with 19 mL of water for injection to obtain a volume of 20 mL of clear concentrate containing 10 mg/mL of drug. Discard vial if a vacuum doesn't pull the diluent into vial. Shake vial until powder completely dissolves. Use the reconstituted solution immediately.

▼ Further dilute the 10-mg/mL solution to 5 mg/mL or less. Follow manufacturer's instructions for diluting.

▼ Infuse over 1 to 3 hours at 5 mg/mL or less and a maximum hourly rate of 3 mg/kg/hour.

🌙 *Alert:* Don't administer as an IV bolus injection.

▼ Don't infuse concomitantly with any blood product or short-term infusion of concentrated electrolytes, even if the two infusions are running in separate IV lines (or cannulas).

Reactions in bold italics are *life-threatening*. Interactions may have a *rapid onset* or a ***delayed onset***.

▼ **Incompatibilities:** Blood products, electrolyte supplements, 4.2% sodium bicarbonate infusion. Consult a drug incompatibility reference for more information.

ACTION

Inhibits the cytochrome P-450–dependent synthesis of ergosterol, a vital component of fungal cell membranes.

Route	Onset	Peak	Duration
PO, IV	Immediate	1–2 hr	12 hr

Half-life: Variable depending on dose.

ADVERSE REACTIONS

CNS: fever, headache, hallucinations. **CV:** tachycardia, HTN, hypotension, peripheral edema. **EENT:** abnormal vision, photophobia, chromatopsia, epistaxis. **GI:** nausea, vomiting, abdominal pain, diarrhea, constipation, mucosal inflammation. **GU:** renal dysfunction, *acute kidney failure.* **Hematologic:** *thrombocytopenia.* **Hepatic:** abnormal LFT values, cholestatic jaundice. **Metabolic:** *hypokalemia.* **Respiratory:** cough, dyspnea, URI, hemoptysis. **Skin:** rash. **Other:** chills.

INTERACTIONS

Refer to prescribing information for additional drug interaction information.

Drug-drug. *Astemizole, cisapride, ivabradine, pimozide, quinidine, terfenadine:* May increase levels of these drugs, leading to torsades de pointes and prolonged QT interval. Use together is contraindicated.

Benzodiazepines, calcium channel blockers, methadone, NSAIDs, sulfonylureas, vinca alkaloids: May increase levels of these drugs. Adjust dosages of these drugs; monitor patient for adverse reactions.

Carbamazepine, long-acting barbiturates, rifabutin, rifampin, *ritonavir (high-dose therapy):* May decrease voriconazole level. Use together is contraindicated.

Cyclosporine, tacrolimus: May increase levels of these drugs. Adjust dosages; monitor levels.

Efavirenz: May significantly decrease voriconazole level while significantly increasing efavirenz level. Adjust dosage of both drugs. Use of voriconazole when efavirenz dosage is 400 mg or more/day is contraindicated. In adults also receiving efavirenz, increase voriconazole dosage to 400 mg PO every 12 hours and decrease efavirenz dosage to 300 mg PO every 24 hours. When treatment with voriconazole is stopped, restore initial efavirenz dosage.

Ergot alkaloids (ergotamine), tolvaptan: May increase levels of these drugs. Use together is contraindicated.

Fluconazole: May increase voriconazole level. Avoid use together. Monitor patient for adverse effects 24 hours after last fluconazole.

HIV protease inhibitors (amprenavir, nelfinavir, saquinavir), NNRTIs (delavirdine): May increase levels of both drugs. Monitor patient for adverse reactions and toxicity.

HMG-CoA reductase inhibitors (atorvastatin, fluvastatin, lovastatin, pravastatin, rosuvastatin, simvastatin): May increase levels and adverse effects, including rhabdomyolysis, of these drugs. Monitor patient closely and reduce dose of HMG-CoA reductase inhibitor as needed.

Letermovir: May decrease voriconazole level. Monitor effectiveness.

Lurasidone, sirolimus, tolvaptan: May significantly increase levels of these drugs. Use together is contraindicated.

Naloxegol: May increase naloxegol level and risk of opioid withdrawal symptoms. Use together is contraindicated.

Omeprazole: May increase omeprazole level. When initiating voriconazole therapy in patients already receiving omeprazole doses of 40 mg or greater, reduce omeprazole dose by half.

Opioids, long-acting (fentanyl, oxycodone): May increase levels of these drugs. Adjust doses of these drugs; monitor patient for adverse reactions.

Oral contraceptives containing ethinyl estradiol and norethindrone: May increase levels and adverse effects of these drugs. Monitor patient closely.

Phenytoin: May decrease voriconazole level and increase phenytoin level. Increase voriconazole maintenance dose; monitor phenytoin level. In adults also receiving phenytoin, increase maintenance dose of voriconazole to 5 mg/kg IV every 12 hours, or increase PO dose from 100 to 200 mg (in adults weighing 40 kg or less) or from 200 to 400 mg (in adults weighing more than 40 kg).

Ritonavir: May decrease voriconazole level. Use with ritonavir dosages of 400 mg b.i.d. is contraindicated. Avoid using with low-dose ritonavir (100 mg b.i.d.) unless benefits outweigh risks.

V

♣Canada   ◇OTC   ◆ Off-label use   ℰ Photoguide   ⊜ Do not crush   *Liquid contains alcohol   ▓ Genetic

Venetoclax: May increase risk of TLS during initiation and ramp-up phase of chronic lymphocytic leukemia or small lymphocytic lymphoma treatment. Use together is contraindicated.

Warfarin: May significantly prolong PT and increase INR. Monitor PT, INR, and bleeding.

Drug-herb. *St. John's wort:* May increase drug level. Use together is contraindicated.

Drug-lifestyle. *Sun exposure:* May cause photosensitivity. Advise patient to avoid excessive sunlight exposure.

EFFECTS ON LAB TEST RESULTS

• May increase CK, cholesterol, ALP, AST, ALT, bilirubin, creatinine, urine glucose, and urine albumin levels.
• May decrease albumin level.
• May increase or decrease glucose, calcium, magnesium, potassium, sodium, or phosphorus level.
• May decrease Hb level, hematocrit, and platelet, WBC, and RBC counts.

CONTRAINDICATIONS & CAUTIONS

• Contraindicated in patients hypersensitive to drug or its components.
🔲 Tablets are contraindicated in patients with rare hereditary galactose intolerance, Lapp lactase deficiency, or glucose-galactose malabsorption due to lactose content.
• May prolong QT interval. Rare cases of torsades de pointes, cardiac arrest, and sudden death have been reported. Use cautiously in patients with proarrhythmic conditions (congenital or acquired QT-interval prolongation, cardiomyopathy, sinus bradycardia, existing symptomatic arrhythmias) and in those taking concomitant drugs that can prolong QT interval.
• Use cautiously in patients hypersensitive to other azoles.
• Use cautiously in patients with risk factors for acute pancreatitis (recent chemotherapy, stem cell transplant).
• SCARs, including SJS, TEN, and DRESS syndrome, have been reported. Discontinue drug for exfoliative cutaneous reactions.
• IV administration is recommended in children ages 2 to 12 with malabsorption and very low body weight for age, because oral bioavailability may be limited.

Dialyzable drug: Yes.

⚠ *Overdose S&S:* Photophobia.

PREGNANCY-LACTATION-REPRODUCTION

• Drug can cause fetal harm. Use during pregnancy only if benefit clearly outweighs fetal risk. If used during pregnancy, inform patient of potential hazard to the fetus.
• Patient of childbearing potential should use effective contraception.
• It isn't known if drug appears in human milk. Patient should discontinue breastfeeding or discontinue drug.

NURSING CONSIDERATIONS

• Correct electrolyte disturbances before initiation of and during therapy.
• Obtain ECG for patients with concomitant medications or conditions that prolong the QT interval.
• Infusion reactions, including flushing, fever, diaphoresis, tachycardia, chest tightness, dyspnea, faintness, nausea, pruritus, and rash, may occur as soon as infusion starts. If reaction occurs, notify prescriber; infusion may need to be stopped.
• Monitor renal function and serum creatinine level closely.
• Monitor LFT results at start of and during therapy. Monitor patients who develop abnormal LFT results for more severe hepatic injury. If patient develops signs and symptoms of liver disease, drug may need to be stopped.
• Monitor patient for SCARs and photosensitivity skin reactions that could lead to melanoma or squamous cell carcinoma of the skin. Phototoxicity reactions occur more frequently in children.
• If drug is continued despite phototoxicity-related lesion, obtain regular dermatologic evaluations. Discontinue drug if patient develops a skin lesion consistent with squamous cell carcinoma or melanoma.
• Monitor patient for azole-induced adrenal insufficiency (fatigue, aches, weight loss, hypotension, loss of body hair, hyperpigmentation) and, in patients taking corticosteroids, Cushing syndrome (weight gain, round face, thinning skin, diaphoresis).
• If treatment lasts longer than 28 days, vision changes may occur.
• Skeletal fluorosis and periostitis have been reported with long-term therapy. Evaluate complaints of skeletal pain and discontinue drug for radiologic findings compatible with fluorosis or periostitis.
• *Look alike–sound alike:* Don't confuse voriconazole with fluconazole.

Reactions in bold italics are *life-threatening*. Interactions may have a *rapid onset* or a ***delayed onset***.

PATIENT TEACHING
• Teach patient safe drug administration and handling.
• Advise patient to avoid driving or operating machinery while taking drug, especially at night, because vision changes, including blurring, photophobia, and changes in color perception, may occur.
• Tell patient to avoid strong, direct sunlight and to use sun-protective measures.
• Advise patient to avoid becoming pregnant during therapy because of the risk of harm to the fetus.

---

vortioxetine hydrobromide ⌧
vor-tie-OX-e-teen

Trintellix

Therapeutic class: Antidepressants
Pharmacologic class: Multimodal antidepressants

AVAILABLE FORMS
Tablets: 5 mg, 10 mg, 20 mg

INDICATIONS & DOSAGES
➤ **Major depressive disorder**
Adults: 10 mg PO once daily. Increase as tolerated to targeted dose of 20 mg once daily.
Adjust-a-dose: If 10 mg once daily isn't tolerated, decrease dosage to 5 mg once daily. If discontinuing drug when patient is taking 15 or 20 mg daily, first decrease dosage to 10 mg daily for 1 week; then stop drug to avoid adverse reactions. Reduce dosage by 50% when giving with strong CYP2D6 inhibitor. Increase dosage by up to three times the original dose when giving with strong CYP inducer for more than 14 days.
⌧ For patients who are known CYP2D6 poor metabolizers, maximum recommended dose is 10 mg daily.

ADMINISTRATION
PO
• Give drug without regard to meals.
• Store tablets at room temperature.

ACTION
Antidepressant effect of vortioxetine isn't fully understood, but is thought to be related to its enhancement of serotonergic activity in the CNS through inhibition of the reuptake of serotonin (5-HT), as well as 5-HT$_3$ receptor antagonism and 5-HT$_{1A}$ receptor agonism.

Route	Onset	Peak	Duration
PO	2–4 wk	7–11 hr	Unknown

Half-life: 66 hours.

ADVERSE REACTIONS
CNS: dizziness, abnormal dreams. **EENT:** dry mouth. **GI:** nausea, diarrhea, constipation, vomiting, flatulence. **GU:** sexual dysfunction. **Skin:** pruritus.

INTERACTIONS
Drug-drug. *Aspirin, clopidogrel, heparin, NSAIDs, warfarin:* May increase risk of bleeding. Use together cautiously.
Diuretics: May increase risk of hyponatremia. Monitor patient carefully.
Linezolid, methylene blue: May increase risk of serotonin syndrome. Use together is contraindicated.
MAO inhibitors: May cause severe adverse effects from impaired serotonin metabolism. Concurrent use is contraindicated. Don't restart MAO inhibitor for at least 21 days after vortioxetine has been stopped. Start vortioxetine at least 14 days after MAO inhibitor has been stopped.
Serotonergics (buspirone, fentanyl, lithium, SSNRIs, SSRIs, TCAs, tramadol, triptans, tryptophan products): May increase risk of serotonin syndrome. Monitor patient carefully.
Strong CYP inducers (carbamazepine, phenytoin, rifampin): May decrease vortioxetine level if coadministered for more than 14 days. Consider increasing vortioxetine dosage with concurrent use, to maximum of three times original dose. Decrease vortioxetine dosage to original level within 14 days when strong CYP inducer is discontinued.
Strong CYP2D6 inhibitors (bupropion, fluoxetine, paroxetine, quinidine): May increase vortioxetine level. Decrease vortioxetine dosage by half when given together. Increase vortioxetine dosage to original level when CYP2D6 inhibitor is discontinued.
Drug-herb. *Herbs with anticoagulant/antiplatelet properties (alfalfa, anise, bilberry):* May increase bleeding risk. Consider therapy modification.
St. John's wort: May increase risk of serotonin syndrome. Don't use together.

V

Drug-lifestyle. *Alcohol use:* May increase psychomotor impairment. Patient should avoid alcohol.

EFFECTS ON LAB TEST RESULTS
• May decrease sodium level.

CONTRAINDICATIONS & CAUTIONS
• Contraindicated in patients hypersensitive to drug or its components.
• Use of MAO inhibitors to treat psychiatric disorders with vortioxetine or within 21 days of stopping vortioxetine is contraindicated because of an increased risk of serotonin syndrome.
Boxed Warning Drug isn't approved for use in children. ■
• Use cautiously in patients with a history or family history of bipolar disorder, mania, or hypomania.
• Use cautiously in patients taking diuretics or who are otherwise volume-depleted because of increased risk of hyponatremia.
• Drug may increase bleeding risk, particularly if used with aspirin, NSAIDs, warfarin, or other drugs or herbs that interfere with hemostasis.
• Drug may trigger an angle-closure attack in patients with anatomically narrow angles who don't have a patent iridectomy.
Dialyzable drug: Unknown.
⚠ *Overdose S&S:* Dizziness, diarrhea, abdominal discomfort, generalized pruritus, somnolence, flushing, nausea.

PREGNANCY-LACTATION-REPRODUCTION
• Drug's effects during pregnancy are unknown. Third-trimester use may increase risk of persistent pulmonary hypertension and withdrawal in newborns. Use only if potential benefits outweigh fetal risk.
• Encourage enrollment in the National Pregnancy Registry for Antidepressants (1-844-405-6185 or https://womensmentalhealth.org/clinical-and-research-programs/pregnancyregistry/antidepressants/).
• It isn't known if drug appears in human milk. Patient should discontinue breastfeeding or discontinue drug.

NURSING CONSIDERATIONS
Boxed Warning Drug increases risk of suicidality in children, adolescents, and young adults. ■

Boxed Warning Monitor patients for signs and symptoms of worsening depression, suicidality, or unusual changes in behavior, especially during initial treatment or with dosage changes, either increases or decreases. ■
• Screen patients for bipolar disorder before drug initiation. Drug isn't approved for use in bipolar depression.
• Monitor patients for signs and symptoms of hyponatremia and SIADH (headache, difficulty concentrating, memory impairment, confusion, weakness, unsteadiness, hallucination, syncope, seizure, coma, respiratory arrest, death). Discontinue drug if hyponatremia occurs.
• Monitor patients for signs and symptoms of serotonin syndrome, including mental status changes (agitation, hallucinations, delirium, coma), autonomic instability (tachycardia, labile blood pressure, dizziness, diaphoresis, flushing, hyperthermia), neuromuscular symptoms (tremor, rigidity, myoclonus, hyperreflexia, incoordination), seizures, or severe GI symptoms (nausea, vomiting, diarrhea). Discontinue drug immediately if signs and symptoms occur.
• Drug may cause withdrawal syndrome (dysphoric mood, irritability, agitation, dizziness, sensory disturbances, anxiety, confusion, headache, lethargy, emotional lability, insomnia, hypomania, tinnitus, and seizures). To discontinue therapy, reduce dosage of 15 mg once daily or more to 10 mg once daily for 1 week before full discontinuation to prevent withdrawal. If intolerable withdrawal signs and symptoms occur after dosage reduction or drug discontinuation, consider resuming previous dosage, then tapering more gradually.
• Serotonergic antidepressants may cause signs and symptoms of sexual dysfunction. Assess for sexual dysfunction before and during treatment.

PATIENT TEACHING
Boxed Warning Advise patient and caregivers to watch for signs and symptoms of suicidality, especially during dosage adjustment. ■
• Tell patient to report all adverse reactions to prescriber.
• Warn patient about signs and symptoms of serotonin syndrome or autonomic instability.
• Advise patient that nausea, xerostomia, dizziness, constipation, diarrhea, or sexual dysfunction may occur.

- Tell patient to immediately report behavioral changes, insomnia, or signs and symptoms of hyponatremia, hemorrhaging, or serotonin syndrome.
- Warn patient not to stop drug abruptly or without discussing with prescriber.
- Caution patient about operating machinery or doing tasks that require alertness while taking drug.

SAFETY ALERT!

warfarin sodium 🅰
WAR-far-in

Jantoven

Therapeutic class: Anticoagulants
Pharmacologic class: Vitamin K antagonists

AVAILABLE FORMS
Tablets: 1 mg, 2 mg, 2.5 mg, 3 mg, 4 mg, 5 mg, 6 mg, 7.5 mg, 10 mg

INDICATIONS & DOSAGES
➤ **Prophylaxis and treatment of venous thromboembolic disorders (DVT, PE) and embolic complications from atrial fibrillation or cardiac valve replacement; adjunct to reduce risk of systemic embolism after MI**
Adults: 2 to 5 mg PO daily for 2 to 4 days; then dosage based on daily PT and INR until stable in the therapeutic range. Usual maintenance dosage is 2 to 10 mg PO daily. Base dosages on INR target goals and other clinical factors. Individualize duration of treatment as clinically indicated.
🅰 *Adjust-a-dose:* Consider lower initiation and maintenance doses for older adults, patients who are debilitated, patients of Asian descent, and those with CYP2C9 and VKORC1 genotypes. Patients with CYP2C9 gene variant may require more time to achieve maximum INR effect. Monitor INR more frequently in patients with renal impairment.

ADMINISTRATION
PO
- Establish baseline coagulation parameters before therapy. PT and INR determinations are essential for proper control. Recommended INR ranges from 2 to 3 for most patients. Target INR in patients with tilting disk valves and bileaflet mechanical valves in mitral position or caged ball or caged disk valves ranges from 2.5 to 3.5.
- Give drug at same time daily.
- Give a missed dose as soon as possible on the same day; don't double dose to make up for a missed dose.

ACTION
Inhibits vitamin K–dependent activation of clotting factors II, VII, IX, and X, formed in the liver. Also inhibits anticoagulant proteins C and S.

Route	Onset	Peak	Duration
PO	Within 24 hr	4 hr	2–5 days

Half-life: 20 to 60 hours.

ADVERSE REACTIONS
CNS: taste perversion. **CV:** vasculitis. **GI:** abdominal pain, diarrhea, flatulence, bloating, nausea, vomiting. **Hematologic:** *hemorrhage.* **Hepatic:** *hepatitis,* elevated liver enzyme levels. **Respiratory:** tracheal or tracheobronchial calcification. **Skin:** alopecia, pruritus, rash, dermatitis. **Other:** chills, hypersensitivity or allergic reactions, including *anaphylactic reactions* and urticaria.

INTERACTIONS
🔵 *Alert:* Consult labeling of all concurrently used drugs to obtain further information about interactions with warfarin.
Drug-drug. *Acetaminophen:* May increase bleeding with long-term therapy (more than 2 weeks) at high doses (more than 2 g/day) of acetaminophen. Monitor therapy.
Allopurinol, **amiodarone**, **anabolic steroids**, *anticoagulants (argatroban, bivalirudin),* **azole antifungals**, *aspirin, beta blockers (atenolol, propranolol), cephalosporins, chloramphenicol, cimetidine, corticosteroids,* **danazol**, *diazoxide, diflunisal, disulfiram, erythromycin, ethacrynic acid, felbamate,* **fibric acids**, *fluoxymesterone, fluoroquinolones, furosemide, glucagon, HMG-CoA reductase inhibitors (lovastatin, simvastatin), heparin, isoniazid,* **lansoprazole**, *macrolide antibiotics (azithromycin, clarithromycin, erythromycin), meclofenamate, methimazole, methyldopa, methylphenidate,* **methyltestosterone**, **metronidazole**, *nalidixic acid, neomycin (oral),* **NSAIDs**, *omeprazole,* **oxandrolone**, *pentoxifylline, propafenone, propylthiouracil, quinidine, quinolones (ciprofloxacin,*

W

levofloxacin, ofloxacin), **salicylates,** *selective cyclo-oxygenase-2 inhibitors (celecoxib),* SSRIs, **sulfamethoxazole–trimethoprim, sulfonamides,** *tamoxifen, tetracyclines, thiazides, thrombolytics,* **thyroid drugs,** *ticlopidine, tramadol, vitamin E, valproic acid, zafirlukast:* May increase anticoagulant effect. Monitor patient carefully for bleeding. Reduce anticoagulant dosage as directed.
Aprepitant, ascorbic acid, **barbiturates,** *bosentan, carbamazepine, clozapine, corticotropin, cyclosporine, dicloxacillin, griseofulvin, haloperidol, meprobamate, mercaptopurine, nafcillin, oral contraceptives containing estrogen, protease inhibitors (ritonavir), raloxifene, ribavirin, rifampin, spironolactone, sucralfate, thiazide diuretics, trazodone, vitamin K:* May reduce PT and thereby decrease INR, which reduces the anticoagulant effect. Monitor PT and INR carefully. Increase warfarin dosage, as needed.
Cyclophosphamide, phenytoin, propylthiouracil, ranitidine: May affect PT and INR. Monitor PT and INR carefully.
Sulfonylureas (oral antidiabetics): May increase hypoglycemic response. Monitor glucose levels.
Drug-herb. *Coenzyme Q10, ginseng, St. John's wort:* May reduce action of warfarin. Modify therapy.
Green tea: May decrease anticoagulant effect caused by vitamin K content of green tea. Advise patient to minimize variable consumption of green tea.
Herbs with anticoagulant properties (dong quai, fenugreek, feverfew, garlic, ginger, **ginkgo,** *willow bark):* May increase risk of bleeding. Discourage use together.
Drug-food. **Cranberry juice:** May increase risk of severe bleeding. Discourage use together.
Foods, multivitamins, and other enteral products containing vitamin K: May impair anticoagulation. Tell patient to maintain consistent daily intake of foods containing vitamin K.
Drug-lifestyle. *Alcohol use:* May enhance anticoagulant effects. Tell patient to avoid large amounts of alcohol.

EFFECTS ON LAB TEST RESULTS
• May increase ALT and AST levels.
• May falsely decrease theophylline level.
• May increase INR and prolong PT and PTT.

CONTRAINDICATIONS & CAUTIONS
Boxed Warning Drugs, dietary changes, and other factors affect INR levels achieved with warfarin therapy. ■
• Contraindicated in patients hypersensitive to drug and in those with active ulceration or bleeding from the GI, GU, or respiratory tract; aneurysm; dissecting aorta; cerebrovascular hemorrhage; severe or malignant HTN; severe renal or hepatic disease; subacute bacterial endocarditis, pericarditis, or pericardial effusion; or blood dyscrasias or hemorrhagic tendencies.
• Contraindicated with recent or contemplated surgery involving large open areas, eye, brain, or spinal cord; recent prostatectomy; or major regional lumbar block anesthesia, spinal puncture, or diagnostic or therapeutic invasive procedures.
• Contraindicated in unsupervised patients with conditions that increase risk of nonadherence (senility, alcoholism, psychosis).
• Fatal and serious calciphylaxis (calcium uremic arteriolopathy) has been reported in patients with and without ESRD. If calciphylaxis is diagnosed, stop drug and treat calciphylaxis. Consider alternative anticoagulation.
• Avoid using in patients with a history of warfarin-induced necrosis; or in situations in which there are inadequate lab facilities for coagulation testing.
▓ Use cautiously in patients with infectious diseases or intestinal flora disturbance (sprue, antibiotic therapy), moderate to severe HTN, hepatic or renal disease, drainage tubes in any orifice, deficiency in protein C-mediated anticoagulant response, cataract surgery, polycythemia vera, vasculitis, or diabetes; with regional or lumbar block anesthesia; with heparin-induced thrombocytopenia; and in conditions that increase risk of hemorrhage.
• Acute kidney injury may occur in patients with altered glomerular integrity or with a history of kidney disease, possibly in relation to episodes of excessive anticoagulation and hematuria.
• Drug may increase release of atheromatous plaque emboli, most commonly affecting the kidneys, pancreas, spleen, and liver. Signs and symptoms depend on the site of embolization and may progress to necrosis and death.
Dializable drug: Unknown.

Reactions in bold italics are *life-threatening*. Interactions may have a *rapid onset* or a *delayed onset*.

⚠ *Overdose S&S:* Blood in stools or urine, excessive bruising, persistent oozing from superficial injuries, excessive menstrual bleeding, melena, petechiae.

PREGNANCY-LACTATION-REPRODUCTION
• Drug can cause fetal harm. Contraindicated during pregnancy except in patients with mechanical heart valves, who are at high risk for thromboembolism and for whom benefits of warfarin may outweigh fetal risks.
• Drug is contraindicated in patients experiencing threatened abortion, eclampsia, and preeclampsia.
• Verify pregnancy status before starting drug.
• Patients of childbearing potential should use effective contraception during therapy and for 1 month after final dose.
• Drug hasn't been detected in human milk. Use cautiously during breastfeeding. Monitor infants for bruising or bleeding.

NURSING CONSIDERATIONS
Boxed Warning Warfarin can cause major or fatal bleeding, which is more likely to occur during the starting period and with a higher dose. Regularly monitor INR in all patients. Consider more frequent INR monitoring in those at high risk for bleeding. ∎
• At the start of therapy, monitor INR daily until stabilized in the therapeutic range; then monitor every 1 to 4 weeks.
• Avoid IM injections when possible.
• Regularly inspect patient for bleeding gums, bruises on arms or legs, petechiae, nosebleeds, melena, hematuria, and hematemesis.
• Check for unexpected bleeding in infants who are breastfed by patients taking warfarin.
• Monitor patient for purple-toes syndrome due to microemboli, characterized by a dark purple or mottled color of the toes; may occur 3 to 10 weeks, or even later, after starting therapy.
🕙 *Alert:* Withhold drug and call prescriber at once in the event of fever or rash (signs of severe adverse reactions).
• No dosage adjustment is necessary for patients with renal failure. Monitor INR more frequently in patients with compromised renal function to maintain INR within therapeutic range.
• Effect can be neutralized by oral or parenteral vitamin K.

• Older adults, patients who are debilitated, and patients with renal or hepatic failure are especially sensitive to drug's effect.
• Make sure that patient isn't taking additional anticoagulants unless instructed by prescriber.
• *Look alike–sound alike:* Don't confuse Jantoven with Janumet or Januvia.

PATIENT TEACHING
• Stress importance of adhering to prescribed dosage and follow-up appointments for monitoring. Tell patient to carry a card that identifies patient's increased risk of bleeding.
Boxed Warning Tell patient and family about measures to prevent bleeding, to watch for signs of bleeding or abnormal bruising, and to call prescriber at once if they occur. ∎
• Warn patient to avoid OTC products containing aspirin, other salicylates, or drugs that may interact with warfarin unless ordered by prescriber.
🕙 *Alert:* Advise patient to consult prescriber before initiating any herbal therapy as many herbs have anticoagulant, antiplatelet, or fibrinolytic properties.
• Tell patient to consult prescriber before using miconazole vaginal cream or suppositories. Abnormal bleeding and bruising have occurred.
• Instruct patient to report heavier than usual menstruation. Dosage adjustment may be needed.
• Advise patient to use electric razor when shaving and to use a soft toothbrush.
• Caution patient to avoid activities or sports that may result in traumatic injury.
• Instruct patient to immediately report pain or discoloration of the skin, unusual symptom or pain (for example, sudden cool, painful, purple discoloration of toes), bruising, bleeding, blood in urine, bloody or black stools, headache, dizziness, or weakness.
• Tell patient to read food labels. Food, nutritional supplements, and multivitamins that contain vitamin K may impair anticoagulation.
• Inform patient that consuming foods high in vitamin K (such as green, leafy vegetables) can decrease anticoagulant effects. Tell patient to eat a balanced diet with consistent intake of vitamin K and to notify prescriber before making any dietary changes.
• Tell patient to inform all health care providers about taking warfarin and to inform

W

warfarin prescriber of new medication orders and upcoming surgeries or procedures.
• Advise patient to report serious illness, severe diarrhea, infections, or fever to prescriber.
• Caution patient of childbearing potential of the fetal risk and to report pregnancy or plans to become pregnant.

zafirlukast
zah-FUR-luh-kast

Accolate✑

Therapeutic class: Antiasthmatics
Pharmacologic class: Leukotriene receptor antagonists

AVAILABLE FORMS
Tablets: 10 mg, 20 mg

INDICATIONS & DOSAGES
➤ **Prevention and long-term treatment of asthma**
Adults and children age 12 and older: 20 mg PO b.i.d.
Children ages 5 to 11: 10 mg PO b.i.d.

ADMINISTRATION
PO
• Give drug 1 hour before or 2 hours after meals.
• Protect from light and moisture.

ACTION
Selectively competes for leukotriene receptor sites, blocking inflammatory action.

Route	Onset	Peak	Duration
PO	Rapid	2–3 hr	12 hr

Half-life: 10 hours.

ADVERSE REACTIONS
CNS: headache, asthenia, dizziness, pain, fever. **GI:** abdominal pain, diarrhea, dyspepsia, nausea, vomiting. **Musculoskeletal:** back pain, myalgia. **Other:** accidental injury, infection.

INTERACTIONS
Drug-drug. *Aspirin:* May increase zafirlukast level. Monitor patient for adverse effects.
Erythromycin, theophylline: May decrease zafirlukast level. Monitor patient for decreased effectiveness.

Lumacaftor: May increase or decrease serum concentration of CYP2C9 substrates (high risk with inhibitors or inducers). Monitor therapy.
Moderate and strong CYP2C9 inhibitors (fluconazole): May increase zafirlukast level. Use together cautiously.
Warfarin: May increase warfarin concentration, prolonging PT. Monitor PT and INR, and adjust anticoagulant dosage.
Drug-food. *Any food:* May reduce rate and extent of drug absorption. Advise patient to take drug 1 hour before or 2 hours after a meal.

EFFECTS ON LAB TEST RESULTS
• May increase ALT level.

CONTRAINDICATIONS & CAUTIONS
• Contraindicated in patients hypersensitive to drug and in those with hepatic impairment, including hepatic cirrhosis.
• Use cautiously in older adults.
• Safety and effectiveness in children younger than age 5 haven't been determined.
Dialyzable drug: Unknown.
⚠ **Overdose S&S:** Rash, upset stomach.

PREGNANCY-LACTATION-REPRODUCTION
• There are no adequate studies during pregnancy. Use during pregnancy only if clearly needed.
• Drug appears in human milk. Don't use during breastfeeding because of potential for tumorigenicity shown in animal studies.

NURSING CONSIDERATIONS
⟐ *Alert:* Reducing oral corticosteroid dose has been followed in rare cases by eosinophilia, vasculitic rash, worsening pulmonary symptoms, cardiac complications, or neuropathy, sometimes known as Churg-Strauss syndrome.
• Drug isn't indicated to reverse bronchospasm in acute asthma attacks, including status asthmaticus.
⟐ *Alert:* Drug may cause behavior and mood changes, including agitation, depression, insomnia, and suicidality. Monitor patient and consider discontinuing drug if neuropsychiatric symptoms develop.
⟐ *Alert:* Life-threatening hepatic failure has been noted in postmarketing reports. For suspected liver failure (right upper quadrant abdominal pain, nausea, fatigue, lethargy,

pruritus, jaundice, flulike symptoms, anorexia, enlarged liver), discontinue drug immediately.
• *Look alike–sound alike:* Don't confuse Accolate with Accupril or Accutane.

PATIENT TEACHING
• Instruct patient in safe drug administration and storage.
• Tell patient that drug is used for long-term treatment of asthma and to keep taking it even if symptoms resolve.
• Advise patient that drug isn't indicated for use in reversal of bronchospasm in acute asthma attacks, including status asthmaticus.
• Caution patient to continue taking other antiasthmatics, as prescribed.
• Warn patient that drug may cause behavior and mood changes (agitation, insomnia, depression, suicidality), and to report development of these symptoms to prescriber.
• Teach patient to report rare but serious signs and symptoms of hepatic dysfunction.

zaleplon
ZAL-e-plon

Therapeutic class: Hypnotics
Pharmacologic class: Pyrazolopyrimidines
Controlled substance schedule: IV

AVAILABLE FORMS
Capsules: 5 mg, 10 mg

INDICATIONS & DOSAGES
➤ **Short-term treatment of insomnia (up to 30 days)**
Adults: 10 mg PO daily at bedtime; may increase to 20 mg as needed. Reevaluate patient if drug is used for more than 2 to 3 weeks.
Adjust-a-dose: For older adults, low-weight adults, or patients who are debilitated, initially, 5 mg PO daily at bedtime; doses of more than 10 mg aren't recommended. For patients with mild to moderate hepatic impairment or those also taking cimetidine, 5 mg PO daily at bedtime.

ADMINISTRATION
PO
• Give drug immediately before bed or after patient has gone to bed and has experienced difficulty falling asleep.
• Don't give drug after a high-fat or heavy meal as onset may be delayed.

ACTION
A hypnotic with chemical structure unrelated to benzodiazepines that interacts with the GABA–benzodiazepine receptor complex in the CNS. Modulation of this complex is thought to be responsible for sedative, anxiolytic, muscle relaxant, and anticonvulsant effects of benzodiazepines.

Route	Onset	Peak	Duration
PO	Rapid	1 hr	Unknown

Half-life: 1 hour.

ADVERSE REACTIONS
CNS: amnesia, anxiety, asthenia, confusion, depersonalization, depression, difficulty concentrating, dizziness, drowsiness, fever, hallucinations, headache, hypertonia, hypoesthesia, malaise, migraine, nervousness, paresthesia, somnolence, tremor, vertigo, smell alteration, taste perversion. **CV:** chest pain, peripheral edema. **EENT:** abnormal vision, conjunctivitis, eye pain, ear pain, hyperacusis, epistaxis, dry mouth. **GI:** abdominal pain, anorexia, colitis, constipation, dyspepsia, nausea. **GU:** dysmenorrhea. **Musculoskeletal:** arthralgia, arthritis, back pain, myalgia. **Respiratory:** bronchitis. **Skin:** photosensitivity reactions, pruritus, rash.

INTERACTIONS
Drug-drug. *Carbamazepine, phenobarbital, phenytoin, rifampin, other CYP3A4 inducers:* May reduce zaleplon bioavailability and peak level. Consider using a different hypnotic.
Cimetidine: May increase zaleplon bioavailability and peak level. Use an initial zaleplon dose of 5 mg.
CNS depressants (imipramine, thioridazine): May cause additive CNS effects. Use together cautiously.
Opioid class warning: May cause slow or difficult breathing, sedation, and death. Avoid use together. If use together is necessary, limit dosage and duration of each drug to minimum necessary for desired effect.
Promethazine: May decrease zaleplon plasma level. Use together cautiously.
Drug-food. *Heavy meals, high-fat foods:* May prolong absorption, delaying peak drug level by about 2 hours; may delay sleep onset. Advise patient not to take with meals.
Drug-lifestyle. *Alcohol use:* May increase CNS effects. Discourage use together.

EFFECTS ON LAB TEST RESULTS
• May increase lipid levels.

CONTRAINDICATIONS & CAUTIONS
• Contraindicated in patients hypersensitive to drug or its components and in those with severe hepatic impairment.
• If hypersensitivity reactions occur, don't rechallenge patient.
• *Opioid class warning:* Opioids should only be prescribed with benzodiazepines or other CNS depressants to patients for whom alternative treatment options are inadequate.
Boxed Warning Drug may cause rare but serious injury, including death, due to complex sleep behaviors, such as sleepwalking, sleep driving, and engaging in other activities while not fully awake. These behaviors can occur even at the lowest recommended doses and after just one dose. Drug is contraindicated in patients with a history of complex sleep behavior while taking drug. ∎
• Avoid use in patients with sensitivity to tartrazine (FD&C Yellow No. 5), which is contained in capsules. Reactions may occur more frequently in patients with aspirin hypersensitivity.
• Use cautiously in older adults; in patients with depression or debilitation; in patients with history of drug dependence, benzodiazepine abuse, or benzodiazepine-like hypnotic abuse; and in patients with compromised respiratory function.
• Drug may cause changes in behavior and thinking, including out-of-character extroversion or aggressive behavior, loss of personal identity, confusion, strange behavior, agitation, hallucinations, worsening of depression, or suicidality.
Dialyzable drug: Unknown.
⚠ *Overdose S&S:* Drowsiness, confusion, lethargy, ataxia, hypotension, respiratory depression, coma, death.

PREGNANCY-LACTATION-REPRODUCTION
• There are no adequate studies during pregnancy. Use during pregnancy isn't recommended.
• Drug appears in human milk in a small amount, with highest amount occurring during a feeding at about 1 hour after administration. Use during breastfeeding isn't recommended.

NURSING CONSIDERATIONS
• Closely monitor patients who have compromised respiratory function caused by illness, older adults, and patients who are debilitated because they are more sensitive to respiratory depression.
• Start treatment only after carefully evaluating patient because sleep disturbances may be a symptom of an underlying physical or psychiatric disorder. Failure of drug to relieve insomnia after 7 to 10 days requires further evaluation.
• Adverse reactions are usually dose-related. Consult prescriber about dose reduction if adverse reactions occur.
• *Look alike–sound alike:* Don't confuse zaleplon with Zelapar, Zemplar, or zolpidem.

PATIENT TEACHING
• *Opioid class warning:* Caution patient or caregiver of patient taking an opioid with a benzodiazepine, CNS depressant, or alcohol to seek immediate medical attention for dizziness, light-headedness, extreme sleepiness, slowed or difficult breathing, or unresponsiveness.
Boxed Warning Warn patient of risk of injury or death related to complex sleep behaviors. Direct patient to stop drug and immediately report an episode of complex sleep behavior or if patient doesn't remember activities performed while taking drug. ∎
🕐 *Alert:* Warn patient that drug may cause allergic reactions. Advise patient to report these adverse effects.
• Advise patient that drug works rapidly and should only be taken immediately before bedtime or after going to bed when patient has had trouble falling asleep.
• Inform patient that risk of next-day psychomotor impairment increases if drug is taken with less than 7 to 8 hours sleep or is taken with other CNS depressants, including alcohol, or at higher than recommended dosage.
• Caution patient that drowsiness, dizziness, light-headedness, and coordination problems occur most often within 1 hour after taking drug.
• Advise patient to avoid alcohol use while taking drug and to notify prescriber before taking other prescription or OTC drugs.
• Tell patient not to take drug after a high-fat or heavy meal.

Reactions in bold italics are *life-threatening*. Interactions may have a *rapid onset* or a *delayed onset*.

• Advise patient to report sleep problems that continue despite use of drug.
• Notify patient that dependence can occur and that drug is recommended for short-term use only.
• Warn patient not to abruptly stop drug because of risk of withdrawal symptoms, including unpleasant feelings, stomach and muscle cramps, vomiting, diaphoresis, shakiness, and seizures.
• Notify patient that insomnia may recur for a few nights after stopping drug but should resolve on its own.
• Warn patient that drug may cause changes in behavior and thinking, including complex behaviors, out-of-character extroversion or aggressive behavior, loss of personal identity, confusion, strange behavior, agitation, hallucinations, worsening of depression, or suicidality. Tell patient to notify prescriber immediately if these symptoms occur as drug may need to be discontinued.
• Advise patient to consult prescriber before becoming pregnant or breastfeeding.

zidovudine
zid-oh-VEW-den

Retrovir♪

Therapeutic class: Antiretrovirals
Pharmacologic class: Nucleoside–nucleotide reverse transcriptase inhibitors

AVAILABLE FORMS
Capsules ⓓ: 100 mg
Injection: 10 mg/mL
Syrup: 50 mg/5 mL
Tablets ⓓ: 300 mg

INDICATIONS & DOSAGES
Adjust-a-dose (for all indications): In patients with significant anemia (Hb level less than 7.5 g/dL or more than 25% below baseline) or significant neutropenia (granulocyte count less than 750/mm³ or more than 50% below baseline), interrupt therapy until evidence proves marrow has recovered. In patients receiving hemodialysis or peritoneal dialysis, or with CrCl less than 15 mL/minute, give 100 mg PO or 1 mg/kg IV every 6 to 8 hours. For patients with mild to moderate hepatic dysfunction or liver cirrhosis, daily dose may need to be reduced.

➤ **HIV infection, with other antiretrovirals**
Adults: 300 mg PO b.i.d. with other antiretrovirals. If patient is unable to tolerate oral drug, give 1 mg/kg IV infused over 1 hour every 4 hours until PO form can be given.
Children ages 4 weeks to less than 18 years: Do not exceed the recommended adult dose. For patients weighing 30 kg or more, 300 mg PO b.i.d. or 200 mg PO t.i.d. For patients weighing 9 to less than 30 kg, 9 mg/kg PO b.i.d. or 6 mg/kg PO t.i.d. For patients weighing 4 to less than 9 kg, 12 mg/kg PO b.i.d. or 8 mg/kg PO t.i.d.
➤ **To prevent maternal-fetal transmission of HIV**
Patients who are pregnant and at more than 14 weeks' gestation: 100 mg PO five times daily until start of labor. Then, 2 mg/kg (total body weight) IV over 1 hour followed by a continuous IV infusion of 1 mg/kg/hour until umbilical cord is clamped.
Neonates: 2 mg/kg PO every 6 hours starting within 12 hours after birth and continuing until 6 weeks old. Or, give 1.5 mg/kg via IV infusion over 30 minutes every 6 hours.

ADMINISTRATION
⊘ *Alert:* Hazardous drug; use safe-handling and disposal precautions.
PO
• Give oral formulations without regard to meals.
• Use calibrated measuring device to accurately measure oral liquid dose.
• Don't keep capsules in places that may be damp or hot. Heat and moisture may cause the drug to break down.
• Give a missed dose as soon as possible unless it's close to the next scheduled dose.
IV
▼ Give by this route only until oral drug can be tolerated.
⊘ *Alert:* Vial stoppers contain natural rubber latex, which may cause allergic reactions in latex-sensitive individuals.
▼ Remove the calculated dose from the vial; add to D₅W to achieve a concentration no greater than 4 mg/mL.
▼ Infuse drug over 1 hour (adults) or 30 minutes (neonates) at a constant rate. Avoid rapid infusion or bolus injection.
▼ Don't give by IM injection.
▼ Protect undiluted vials from light.
▼ After dilution, solution remains stable for 24 hours at room temperature and for

Z

48 hours if refrigerated at 36° to 46° F (2° to 8° C). Administer diluted solution within 8 hours if stored at 77° F (25° C) or within 24 hours if refrigerated at 36° to 46° F.

▼ **Incompatibilities:** None listed by manufacturer. Consult a drug incompatibility reference for more information.

ACTION
NRTI that inhibits replication of HIV by blocking DNA synthesis.

Route	Onset	Peak	Duration
PO, IV	Unknown	30–90 min	Unknown

Half-life: 0.5 to 3 hours.

ADVERSE REACTIONS
CNS: asthenia, dizziness, fever, fatigue, headache, malaise, neuropathy, insomnia, paresthesia, somnolence, decreased reflexes, irritability. **CV:** lymphadenopathy, *HF,* ECG abnormality, left ventricular dilation, edema. **EENT:** ear symptoms, nasal discharge or congestion. **GI:** anorexia, nausea, vomiting, abdominal pain, cramps, constipation, diarrhea, dyspepsia, stomatitis. **GU:** hematuria. **Hematologic:** *agranulocytosis, neutropenia, severe bone marrow suppression, thrombocytopenia,* anemia. **Hepatic:** altered LFT values, hepatomegaly. **Metabolic:** increased lipase and amylase levels, weight loss. **Musculoskeletal:** arthralgia, myalgia, myopathy. **Respiratory:** cough, wheezing. **Skin:** rash. **Other:** chills, splenomegaly.

INTERACTIONS
Drug-drug. *Atovaquone, fluconazole, methadone, probenecid, trimethoprim, valproic acid:* May increase bioavailability of zidovudine. May need to adjust dosage.
Clarithromycin: May enhance myelosuppressive effect of zidovudine and decrease zidovudine serum concentration. Closely monitor response to zidovudine and consider staggering zidovudine and clarithromycin doses when possible to minimize potential for interaction. Consider therapy modification.
Doxorubicin, ribavirin, stavudine: May have antagonistic effects. Avoid using together.
Ganciclovir, interferon alfa, other bone marrow suppressive or cytotoxic drugs: May increase hematologic toxicity of zidovudine. Use together cautiously.
Orlistat: May decrease serum concentration of antiretrovirals. Monitor therapy.

EFFECTS ON LAB TEST RESULTS
• May increase lipase, amylase, bilirubin, ALT, AST, ALP, and LDH levels.
• May decrease Hb level and RBC, WBC, granulocyte, neutrophil, and platelet counts.

CONTRAINDICATIONS & CAUTIONS
• Contraindicated in patients who have had a potentially life-threatening hypersensitivity reaction to drug or its components.
• Potentially life-threatening hypersensitivity reactions, such as anaphylaxis and SJS, can occur.
Boxed Warning Use cautiously and with close monitoring in patients with advanced symptomatic HIV infection and in those with severe bone marrow depression. Use of this drug has been associated with hematologic toxicity, including neutropenia and severe anemia. ■
• Use cautiously in patients with hepatomegaly, hepatitis, or other risk factors for liver disease and in those with renal insufficiency. Monitor renal function tests and LFTs.
• Use cautiously in patients with granulocyte count less than 1,000 cells/mm³ or Hb level less than 9.5 g/dL.
Boxed Warning Prolonged use has been associated with myopathy. ■
Dialyzable drug: Unlikely.
⚠ *Overdose S&S:* Fatigue, headache, vomiting, hematologic disturbances.

PREGNANCY-LACTATION-REPRODUCTION
• U.S. Department of Health and Human Services Perinatal HIV Guidelines consider zidovudine in combination with lamivudine to be an alternative regimen for use during pregnancy in patients who are antiretroviral-naive.
• Administer zidovudine IV near delivery regardless of antepartum regimen or mode of delivery in patients with HIV RNA greater than 1,000 copies/mL or unknown HIV RNA status.
• Register patients exposed to zidovudine during pregnancy in the Antiretroviral Pregnancy Registry (1-800-258-4263).
• Drug appears in human milk. Because of potential for postnatal HIV-1 transmission, breastfeeding is contraindicated.
• In couples who want to conceive, the partner with HIV infection should attain maximum viral suppression before conception.

Reactions in bold italics are *life-threatening*. Interactions may have a *rapid onset* or a *delayed onset*.

NURSING CONSIDERATIONS

Boxed Warning Although rare, lactic acidosis without hypoxemia and severe hepatomegaly with steatosis may occur. Notify prescriber if patient develops unexplained tachypnea, dyspnea, or a decrease in bicarbonate level. Therapy may need to be suspended until lactic acidosis is ruled out. ■

• Frequently monitor blood studies to detect anemia or agranulocytosis or hepatic decompensation. Patients may need reduced dosage or temporary stop to therapy.

• Monitor patient for signs and symptoms of immune reconstitution syndrome (fever, pain, erythema, wound drainage, swollen lymph nodes, rash) and autoimmune disorders, which have been reported in patients treated with combination antiretroviral therapy.

• Monitor patient for signs of lipoatrophy (localized fatty tissue loss) during therapy. If feasible, switch to an alternative regimen if lipoatrophy is suspected.

• Drug may temporarily decrease morbidity and mortality in certain patients with AIDS.

• Health care providers caring for patients infected with HIV and their infants may call the National Perinatal HIV Hotline for clinical consultations (888-448-8765).

• *Look alike–sound alike:* Don't confuse Retrovir with ritonavir.

PATIENT TEACHING

• Teach patient safe drug administration and handling.

• Tell patient to take drug exactly as directed and not to share it with others.

• Remind patient to comply with the dosage schedule. Suggest ways to avoid missing doses, perhaps by using an alarm clock.

• Tell patient that dosages vary among patients and not to change dosing instructions unless directed to do so by prescriber.

• Warn patient not to take other drugs for AIDS unless prescriber has approved them.

• Advise patient that monotherapy isn't recommended and to discuss any questions with prescriber.

• Stress importance of complying with frequent lab testing because drug-related anemia may occur requiring blood transfusion.

• Advise patient who is pregnant and infected with HIV-1 that drug therapy only reduces the risk of HIV transmission to the newborn. Long-term risks to infants are unknown.

• Inform patient who is pregnant and considering use of zidovudine for prevention of HIV-1 transmission to the infant that transmission may still occur in some cases despite therapy.

• Advise patient who is pregnant and infected with HIV-1 not to breastfeed, to avoid postnatal transmission of HIV.

• Tell patient not to keep capsules in the kitchen, bathroom, or other places that may be damp or hot. Heat and moisture may cause the drug to break down and affect the intended results.

• Instruct patient to report loss of subcutaneous fat, most evident in face, limbs, and buttocks, which may be only partially reversible over months to years if therapy is changed to a non-zidovudine-containing regimen.

• Advise patient to report signs and symptoms of lactic acidosis (nausea, vomiting, shortness of breath, weakness).

• Warn patient that potentially life-threatening hypersensitivity reactions can occur and to immediately report any rash.

ziprasidone hydrochloride
zih-PRAZ-i-done

Geodon◆, Zeldox✤

ziprasidone mesylate
Geodon

Therapeutic class: Antipsychotics
Pharmacologic class: Benzisoxazole derivatives

AVAILABLE FORMS

Capsules 🄖 20 mg, 40 mg, 60 mg, 80 mg
IM injection: 20 mg/mL single-dose vials (after reconstitution)

INDICATIONS & DOSAGES

➤ **Symptomatic treatment of schizophrenia**
Adults: Initially, 20 mg PO b.i.d. with food. Dosages are highly individualized. Adjust dosage, if necessary, no more frequently than every 2 days; to allow for lowest possible doses, the interval should be several weeks to assess symptom response.

Effective dosage range is usually 20 to 100 mg b.i.d., but an increase to a dosage

Z

greater than 80 mg b.i.d. generally isn't recommended. Safety of dosages exceeding 100 mg b.i.d. hasn't been established.

➤ **Rapid control of acute agitation in patients with schizophrenia**

Adults: 10 to 20 mg IM as needed, up to a maximum dose of 40 mg daily. May give doses of 10 mg every 2 hours; may give doses of 20 mg every 4 hours to a maximum of 40 mg/day. If long-term therapy is indicated, replace with oral ziprasidone as soon as possible.

➤ **Acute bipolar I mania, including manic and mixed episodes, as monotherapy; maintenance treatment of bipolar I disorder as an adjunct to lithium or valproate**

Adults: 40 mg PO b.i.d. with food on day 1. Increase to 60 to 80 mg PO b.i.d. with food on day 2; then adjust dosage based on patient response from 40 to 80 mg b.i.d.

ADMINISTRATION
PO
• Always give with food.
• Patient must swallow capsules whole.

IM
• To prepare IM ziprasidone, add 1.2 mL of sterile water for injection to the vial and shake vigorously until drug is completely dissolved. Reconstituted solution contains 20 mg/mL ziprasidone.
• Don't mix injection with other medicinal products or solvents other than sterile water for injection.
• Inspect parenteral drug products for particulate matter and discoloration before administration. Discard unused portion of reconstituted solution.
• The effects of giving IM for more than 3 consecutive days are unknown. If long-term therapy is necessary, switch to PO as soon as possible.
• Store injection at controlled room temperature of 77° F (25° C); protect from light. After reconstituting, it may be stored away from light for up to 24 hours at 59° to 86° F (15° to 30° C) or up to 7 days refrigerated, 36° to 46° F (2° to 8° C).

ACTION
May inhibit dopamine and serotonin-2 receptors, causing reduction in schizophrenia symptoms.

Route	Onset	Peak	Duration
PO	Unknown	6–8 hr	12 hr
IM	Unknown	1 hr	Unknown

Half-life: PO, about 7 hours; IM, 2 to 5 hours.

ADVERSE REACTIONS
CNS: confusion, headache, somnolence, akathisia, dizziness, extrapyramidal symptoms (hypertonia, dystonia, dyskinesia, hypokinesia, tremor, paralysis, twitching), vertigo, abnormal gait, asthenia, hostility, tremor, fever, hypesthesia, ataxia, amnesia, delirium, akinesia, dysarthria, choreoathetosis, incoordination, neuropathy, anxiety, insomnia, hypertonia, agitation, cogwheel rigidity, paresthesia, personality disorder, psychosis, speech disorder, withdrawal syndrome. **CV:** *bradycardia,* orthostatic hypotension, tachycardia, chest pain, HTN, vasodilation. **EENT:** abnormal vision, rhinitis, dry mouth, facial edema, dysphagia, tongue edema, increased salivation, pharyngitis. **GI:** nausea, constipation, dyspepsia, diarrhea, anorexia, abdominal pain, *rectal hemorrhage,* vomiting, tooth disorder. **GU:** dysmenorrhea, priapism. **Metabolic:** hyperglycemia. **Musculoskeletal:** myalgia, flank pain, back pain. **Respiratory:** cough, dyspnea, infection. **Skin:** rash, injection-site pain, furunculosis, fungal dermatitis, diaphoresis, photosensitivity reaction. **Other:** accidental injury, flulike syndrome, chills.

INTERACTIONS
Drug-drug. *Antihypertensives:* May enhance hypotensive effects. Monitor BP.
Carbamazepine: May decrease ziprasidone level. May need to increase ziprasidone dose to achieve desired effect.
CYP3A4 inhibitors (itraconazole, ketoconazole): May increase ziprasidone level. Ziprasidone dosage reduction may be needed to achieve desired effect.
Drugs that decrease potassium or magnesium, such as diuretics: May increase risk of arrhythmias. Monitor potassium and magnesium levels if using these drugs together.
Opioid class warning: May cause slow or difficult breathing, sedation, and death. Avoid use together. If use together is necessary, limit dosage and duration of each drug to minimum necessary for desired effect.
QT interval–prolonging drugs such as antiarrhythmics (amiodarone, disopyramide,

---

Reactions in bold italics are *life-threatening*. Interactions may have a *rapid onset* or a **delayed onset**.

dofetilide, procainamide, quinidine, sotalol),
arsenic trioxide, dolasetron, droperidol,
mefloquine, pentamidine, phenothiazines,
pimozide, quinolones, tacrolimus: May increase risk of life-threatening arrhythmias.
Use together is contraindicated.

Serotonin modulators (nefazodone, tra-
zodone, vilazodone, vortioxetine): May increase risk of serotonin syndrome and NMS.
Monitor therapy.

Drug-lifestyle. *Alcohol use:* May increase
dizziness, drowsiness, confusion, and difficulty concentrating. Don't use together.

EFFECTS ON LAB TEST RESULTS
- May increase glucose and lipid levels.
- May decrease WBC count.

CONTRAINDICATIONS & CAUTIONS
- Contraindicated in patients hypersensitive
to drug and in those with recent MI or uncompensated HF.
- Contraindicated in patients with history of
prolonged QT interval or congenital long QT
syndrome and in those taking other drugs that
prolong QT interval.

Boxed Warning Older adults with
dementia-related psychosis treated with
antipsychotics are at increased risk for
death. Drug isn't approved for treatment of
dementia-related psychosis. ■

- *Opioid class warning:* Opioids should only
be prescribed with benzodiazepines or other
CNS depressants to patients for whom alternative treatment options are inadequate.
- **Alert:** Rarely drug is associated with
SCARs, including SJS and DRESS syndrome.
- Use cautiously in patients with history of
seizures, bradycardia, hypokalemia, or hypomagnesemia; in those with acute diarrhea;
and in those with conditions that may lower
the seizure threshold (such as Alzheimer dementia).
- Use cautiously in patients at risk for aspiration pneumonia.
- Use cautiously in patients at risk for falls,
including older adults and those with diseases
or conditions that may cause somnolence, orthostatic hypotension, or motor or sensory
instability and those taking medications that
may cause the same.
- Use cautiously in patients with known
CV disease (history of MI or ischemic heart
disease, HF, conduction abnormalities),

cerebrovascular disease, or conditions that
would predispose patient to hypotension (dehydration, hypovolemia, use of antihypertensives).
- Drug may elevate prolactin level and occurrence of galactorrhea, amenorrhea, gynecomastia, and erectile dysfunction.
- Don't use IM form in patients with
schizophrenia who are already taking oral
ziprasidone.
- Use cautiously in older adults and in patients with renal or hepatic impairment.

Dializable drug: No.

⚠ Overdose S&S: Sedation, slurred speech,
transitory HTN, anxiety, extrapyramidal
symptoms, somnolence, tremor.

PREGNANCY-LACTATION-REPRODUCTION
- There are no adequate studies during pregnancy. Use only if potential benefit justifies
fetal risk.
- **Alert:** Neonates exposed to antipsychotics
during the third trimester are at risk for developing extrapyramidal signs and symptoms
(repetitive movements of the face and body)
and withdrawal symptoms (agitation, abnormally increased or decreased muscle tone,
tremors, sleepiness, severe difficulty breathing, difficulty feeding) after delivery.
- Enroll patients exposed to drug during pregnancy in the National Pregnancy
Registry for Atypical Antipsychotics
(1-866-961-2388).
- It isn't known if drug or its metabolites
appear in human milk. Breastfeeding isn't
recommended.

NURSING CONSIDERATIONS
- **Alert:** Monitor patients and immediately
report signs and symptoms of DRESS syndrome (rash, fever, swollen glands) or other
SCARs. Discontinue drug for suspected
SCARs.
- **Alert:** Hyperglycemia may occur. Monitor
patients with diabetes regularly. Patients with
risk factors for diabetes should undergo fasting blood glucose testing at baseline and periodically. Monitor all patients for symptoms of
hyperglycemia, including excessive hunger or
thirst, frequent urination, and weakness. Hyperglycemia may be reversible when drug is
stopped.
- **Alert:** Monitor patient for symptoms of
metabolic syndrome (significant weight gain
and increased BMI, HTN, hyperglycemia,

hypercholesterolemia, and hypertriglyceridemia).

• Stop drug in patients with a QTc interval longer than 500 msec.

• Dizziness, palpitations, or syncope may be symptoms of a life-threatening arrhythmia such as torsades de pointes. Provide CV evaluation and monitoring in patients who experience these symptoms.

• Don't give to patients with electrolyte disturbances, such as hypokalemia or hypomagnesemia, because these increase the risk of arrhythmia. Assess serum electrolyte levels at baseline and periodically during therapy; correct abnormalities.

🕲 *Alert:* Patient taking an antipsychotic may develop life-threatening NMS (hyperpyrexia, muscle rigidity, altered mental status, and autonomic instability) or tardive dyskinesia. Assess abnormal involuntary movement before starting therapy, at dosage changes, and periodically thereafter, to monitor patient for tardive dyskinesia.

• Monitor patient for abnormal body temperature regulation, especially if patient is exercising strenuously, is exposed to extreme heat, is also receiving anticholinergics, or is at risk for dehydration.

• Assess fall risk when initiating treatment and recurrently for patients on long-term therapy, especially for older adults and patients with diseases or conditions or who are taking other drugs that could increase fall risk.

• Closely monitor patients at risk for suicide.

• Symptoms may not improve for 4 to 6 weeks.

• *Look alike–sound alike:* Don't confuse ziprasidone with trazodone, zafirlukast, zidovudine, zonisamide, or Zyprexa.

PATIENT TEACHING

• *Opioid class warning:* Caution patient or caregiver of patient taking an opioid with a benzodiazepine, CNS depressant, or alcohol to seek immediate medical attention for dizziness, light-headedness, extreme sleepiness, slowed or difficult breathing, or unresponsiveness.

• Teach patient safe drug administration.

• Tell patient to immediately report signs or symptoms of dizziness, fainting, irregular heartbeat, or relevant heart problems.

• Advise patient to report recent episodes of diarrhea, abnormal movements, sudden fever, muscle rigidity, or change in mental status.

🕲 *Alert:* Tell patient to immediately report rash (with or without blisters), fever, swollen lymph nodes, mouth ulcers, skin shedding, or targetlike spots in the skin.

• Advise patient to report pregnancy or plans to become pregnant.

• Tell patient that breastfeeding isn't recommended during therapy.

• Advise patient that drug can cause sleepiness and to use care when operating machinery or driving a motor vehicle.

• Inform patient that drug may cause somnolence, orthostatic hypotension, and motor and sensory instability, which may lead to falls and, consequently, fractures or other injuries.

• Advise patient that symptoms may not improve for 4 to 6 weeks.

zoledronic acid
zoh-leh-DROH-nik

Reclast

Therapeutic class: Antiosteoporotics
Pharmacologic class: Bisphosphonates

AVAILABLE FORMS
Injection as ready-to-infuse solution: 4 mg/100 mL, 5 mg/100 mL
Injection: 4 mg/5 mL vial

INDICATIONS & DOSAGES
➤ **Hypercalcemia caused by malignancy**
Adults: 4 mg by IV infusion over at least 15 minutes. If albumin-corrected calcium level doesn't return to normal, may repeat 4 mg. Let at least 7 days pass before retreatment to allow a full response to the first dose.
Adjust-a-dose: Assess serum creatinine level before each treatment or retreatment. Dosage adjustments aren't necessary for patients presenting with mild to moderate renal impairment before initiation of therapy (serum creatinine level less than 400 micromol/L or less than 4.5 mg/dL).
➤ **Multiple myeloma; bone metastases of solid tumors in conjunction with standard antineoplastics**
Adults: 4 mg IV infusion every 3 to 4 weeks. Treatment duration depends on type of cancer. Use for prostate cancer only after it has progressed after treatment with at least one course of hormonal therapy. Give patients an oral calcium supplement of 500 mg and a

multiple vitamin containing 400 international units of vitamin D daily.

Adjust-a-dose: For patients with CrCl of 50 to 60 mL/minute, give 3.5 mg. If 40 to 49 mL/minute, give 3.3 mg. If 30 to 39 mL/minute, give 3 mg. For patients with normal baseline creatinine level but an increase of 0.5 mg/dL and in those with abnormal baseline creatinine level who have an increase of 1 mg/dL, withhold drug. Resume treatment at the same dose as that before treatment interruption only when creatinine level has returned to within 10% of baseline value. If CrCl falls below 30 mL/minute, don't give drug.

➤ **Paget disease of bone (osteitis deformans)**
Adults: 5 mg by IV infusion. May repeat if relapse occurs. Patient also needs 1,500 mg elemental calcium in divided doses (750 mg b.i.d. or 500 mg t.i.d.) and 800 international units vitamin D daily, especially during the 2 weeks after dosing.

➤ **Treatment of osteoporosis in men; to reduce incidence of fractures in patients after menopause with osteoporosis; to treat and prevent glucocorticoid-induced osteoporosis in patients taking a daily dosage equivalent to 7.5 mg or greater of prednisone and who are expected to remain on glucocorticoids for at least 12 months**
Adults: 5 mg by IV infusion once a year.

➤ **Prevention of osteoporosis**
Adults who are postmenopausal: 5 mg by IV infusion once every 2 years.

➤ **Prevention of osteopenia secondary to androgen-deprivation therapy in prostate cancer ◆**
Adults: 4 mg IV every 3 months for 1 year or 4 mg every 12 months.

➤ **Prevention of osteopenia associated with aromatase inhibitor therapy in women with breast cancer ◆**
Adults: 4 mg IV every 6 months for 5 years.

ADMINISTRATION
IV
▼ Further dilute concentrate by withdrawing 5 mL to obtain 4 mg of drug and mix in 100 mL of NSS or D₅W. For ready-to-use bottles or bags, if reduced doses are needed for patients with renal impairment, withdraw appropriate volume of solution and label with final drug content and final volume. Refer to manufacturer's instructions.

▼ If drug isn't used immediately after reconstitution, refrigerate solution and give within 24 hours.

▼ If refrigerated, allow refrigerated solution to reach room temperature before administration.

▼ Infuse over not less than 15 minutes at a constant infusion rate to adequately hydrated patient. Give as a single IV solution through a separate infusion line.

▼ Flush IV line with 10 mL NSS after infusion.

▼ After opening, solution remains stable for 24 hours at 36° to 46° F (2° to 8° C).

▼ May store vials, bags, and bottles at room temperature.

▼ **Incompatibilities:** Solutions containing calcium (such as lactated Ringer solution) or other IV drugs.

ACTION

Inhibits bone resorption, probably by inhibiting osteoclast activity and osteoclastic resorption of mineralized bone and cartilage. Decreases calcium release induced by the stimulatory factors produced by tumors.

Route	Onset	Peak	Duration
IV	Unknown	Unknown	Unknown

Half-life: Triphasic with terminal half-life, 146 hours.

ADVERSE REACTIONS

CNS: headache, anxiety, somnolence, insomnia, confusion, agitation, depression, paresthesia, hypoesthesia, fatigue, weakness, dizziness, fever, asthenia, malaise, vertigo, lethargy. **CV:** hypotension, HTN, atrial fibrillation, leg edema, chest pain, palpitations. **EENT:** eye pain. **GI:** nausea, constipation, diarrhea, abdominal pain, vomiting, anorexia, dysphagia, decreased appetite, dyspepsia, abdominal distention, stomatitis. **GU:** *increased creatinine level,* UTI. **Hematologic:** anemia, *granulocytopenia, neutropenia, thrombocytopenia, pancytopenia.* **Metabolic:** dehydration, weight decrease, hypophosphatemia, *hypokalemia, hypomagnesemia.* **Musculoskeletal:** arthralgia, myalgia, back pain, osteonecrosis of the jaw, osteoarthritis, muscle spasms, bone pain, neck pain, shoulder pain, extremity pain. **Respiratory:** dyspnea, cough. **Skin:** alopecia, dermatitis, rash, pruritus, hyperhidrosis. **Other:** *progression of cancer,* rigors, infection, candidiasis, flulike symptoms.

INTERACTIONS
Drug-drug. *Aminoglycosides, calcitonin, loop diuretics:* May have additive effects that lower calcium level. Use together cautiously, and monitor calcium level.
Nephrotoxic drugs such as NSAIDs: Renal toxicity may be greater in patients with renal impairment. Use Reclast cautiously with other potentially nephrotoxic drugs. Monitor serum creatinine before each dose.

EFFECTS ON LAB TEST RESULTS
• May increase creatinine level.
• May decrease calcium, phosphorus, magnesium, and potassium levels.
• May decrease Hb level and hematocrit and RBC, WBC, and platelet counts.

CONTRAINDICATIONS & CAUTIONS
• Contraindicated in patients hypersensitive to drug, other bisphosphonates, or drug's ingredients. Reclast is contraindicated in patients with hypocalcemia, CrCl of less than 35 mL/minute, or evidence of acute renal impairment. Use in patients with severe renal impairment isn't recommended.
⏺ *Alert:* Reclast may increase risk of renal failure, especially in patients with underlying renal impairment, dehydration, and increased age. Screen patients before use and monitor them carefully.
⏺ *Alert:* There may be an increased risk of fractures of the thigh in patients treated with bisphosphonates.
• Patients must be adequately supplemented with calcium and vitamin D.
• Use cautiously in older adults and patients with aspirin-sensitive asthma because other bisphosphonates have been linked to bronchoconstriction in aspirin-sensitive patients with asthma.
• The optimal duration of Reclast use hasn't been determined. Consider patients at low risk for fracture for drug discontinuation after 3 to 5 years of use and reevaluate their risk of fracture periodically.
• Osteonecrosis of the neck and jaw has been reported with bisphosphonate use. Patient should receive preventive dental exams before starting and avoid invasive dental procedures.
Dialyzable drug: Unknown.
⚠ *Overdose S&S:* Hypocalcemia, hypophosphatemia, hypomagnesemia, renal impairment.

PREGNANCY-LACTATION-REPRODUCTION
• Drug shouldn't be used during pregnancy. Patients should avoid pregnancy during therapy. Discontinue drug when pregnancy is recognized.
• Drug may cause fetal harm if used during pregnancy or if patient becomes pregnant after completing therapy because drug binds to bone long term and may be released over weeks to years. Inform patient of potential fetal hazard.
• It isn't known if drug appears in human milk. Patient should discontinue breastfeeding or discontinue drug.

NURSING CONSIDERATIONS
• Hydrate patient adequately before giving; urine output should be about 2 L daily.
• Monitor calcium, phosphate, magnesium, and creatinine levels carefully. Monitor creatinine level before each dose. Correct decreased calcium, phosphorus, and magnesium levels using IV calcium gluconate, potassium and sodium phosphate, and magnesium sulfate.
• Monitor renal function closely. Patients with renal impairment may be at a greater risk for adverse reactions.
⏺ *Alert:* Patients, especially those who have cancer or poor oral hygiene or who are receiving chemotherapy or corticosteroids, should have a dental exam with appropriate preventive dentistry before therapy and avoid invasive dental procedures.
• Osteonecrosis of the jaw has been reported rarely in patients after menopause who have osteoporosis treated with bisphosphonates, including zoledronic acid. All patients should have a routine oral exam before treatment and should be monitored during therapy.
• Severe incapacitating bone, joint, and muscle pain may occur. Withhold future doses if severe symptoms occur. Symptoms may resolve partially or completely with drug stoppage.
• Adequately supplement patients with calcium and vitamin D.
• Administration of acetaminophen after administration may reduce the incidence of acute-phase reaction symptoms.

PATIENT TEACHING
• Review use and administration of drug with patient and family.

Reactions in bold italics are ***life-threatening***. Interactions may have a *rapid onset* or a ***delayed onset***.

• Instruct patient to report adverse effects promptly (such as fever, flulike symptoms, myalgia, arthralgia, headache, muscle cramps, numbness, tingling, difficulty swallowing, palpitations, jaw pain, thigh and bone pain, edema).

• Explain importance of periodic lab tests to monitor therapy and renal function.

• On day of treatment, instruct patient to drink at least two glasses of fluid such as water within a few hours before infusion. Advise patient of importance of calcium and vitamin D supplementation.

• Advise patient to report persistent pain or nonhealing sore of the mouth or jaw and to maintain good oral hygiene and receive routine dental checkups.

ZOLMitriptan
zohl-mah-TRIP-tan

Zomig

Therapeutic class: Antimigraine drugs
Pharmacologic class: Serotonin 5-HT₁ receptor agonists

AVAILABLE FORMS
Nasal spray: 2.5 mg, 5 mg
Tablets (immediate-release): 2.5 mg, 5 mg
Tablets (ODTs) ⓘ: 2.5 mg, 5 mg

INDICATIONS & DOSAGES
➤ **Acute migraine headaches**
Adults: Initially, 1.25 or 2.5 mg. Increase to 5 mg per dose, as needed. If using ODTs, initially, 2.5 mg PO. If headache returns after first dose, give a second dose no sooner than 2 hours after first dose. Maximum dosage is 10 mg in 24 hours.
Adjust-a-dose: In patients with moderate to severe hepatic impairment, give 1.25 mg. Limit total daily dose in patients with severe hepatic impairment to no more than 5 mg/day. In patients taking cimetidine, limit maximum single dose to 2.5 mg, not to exceed 5 mg in any 24-hour period.
Adults and children age 12 and older: Initially, 1 spray (2.5 mg) into nostril; may increase to maximum 5-mg single dose if needed. If headache returns after first dose, give a second dose no sooner than 2 hours after first dose. Maximum dose is 10 mg in 24 hours.

Adjust-a-dose: Nasal spray isn't recommended in patients with moderate or severe hepatic impairment. In patients taking cimetidine, limit maximum single dose to 2.5 mg, not to exceed 5 mg in any 24-hour period.

ADMINISTRATION
PO
• If patient needs a 1.25-mg dose, break a 2.5-mg immediate-release tablet in half.
• Give ODT immediately after opening.
• Don't break or crush ODT.
• Have patient dissolve ODT on the tongue and swallow with saliva, not fluid.
Intranasal
• Patient should gently blow nose before use.
• Remove cap and insert device into nostril while blocking the opposite nostril.
• Press plunger device while patient breathes gently in through the nose. Patient should then breathe gently through the mouth for 5 to 10 seconds.
• Don't test or prime spray before use; nasal sprayer contains only one dose.
• Discard after use.

ACTION
May act as an agonist at serotonin receptors on extracerebral intracranial blood vessels, which constricts the affected vessels, inhibits neuropeptide release, and reduces pain transmission in the trigeminal pathways.

Route	Onset	Peak	Duration
PO	Unknown	1.5–3 hr	Unknown
Intranasal	5 min	3 hr	Unknown

Half-life: 3 hours.

ADVERSE REACTIONS
CNS: dizziness, somnolence, vertigo, paresthesia, asthenia, pain, drowsiness, depersonalization, headache, dysgeusia, insomnia, hyperesthesia, warm or cold sensations. **CV:** palpitations; chest pain, pressure, tightness, or heaviness; facial edema. **EENT:** pain, tightness, or pressure in the neck, throat, or jaw; nasal irritation, dry mouth. **GI:** dyspepsia, dysphagia, nausea, abdominal pain, vomiting. **Musculoskeletal:** arthralgia, myalgia. **Skin:** diaphoresis. **Other:** chills, hypersensitivity reaction.

INTERACTIONS
Drug-drug. *Cimetidine:* May double half-life of zolmitriptan. Limit maximum single

Z

dose of zolmitriptan to 2.5 mg, not to exceed 5 mg in any 24-hour period. Monitor patient closely.

Ergot-containing drugs, other triptans: May exacerbate headaches and increase vasoconstricting effects. Avoid using within 24 hours of zolmitriptan.

MAO inhibitors: May increase zolmitriptan level. Avoid using within 2 weeks of MAO inhibitor.

Methylene blue: May enhance serotonergic effect and result in serotonin syndrome. Avoid combination.

SSRIs, tramadol: May cause additive serotonin effects, resulting in weakness, hyperreflexia, or incoordination. Monitor patient closely.

EFFECTS ON LAB TEST RESULTS
• None significant.

CONTRAINDICATIONS & CAUTIONS
• Contraindicated in patients hypersensitive to drug or its components and in patients with uncontrolled HTN, hemiplegic or basilar migraine, stroke, TIA history, PVD, ischemic bowel disease, Wolff-Parkinson-White syndrome or arrhythmias associated with other cardiac accessory conduction pathway disorders, ischemic heart disease (angina pectoris, history of MI or documented silent ischemia), symptoms of ischemic heart disease (coronary artery vasospasm, including Prinzmetal variant angina), or other significant heart disease.

• 5-HT$_1$ agonists may increase risk of serious cardiac, cerebrovascular, and other vasospastic adverse events (arrhythmias, MI, cerebral hemorrhage, subarachnoid hemorrhage, stroke, GI ischemia, splenic infarct).

• Use cautiously in patients with liver disease and in those who may be at risk for CAD (such as patients who are postmenopausal or men older than age 40) or with risk factors, such as HTN, hypercholesterolemia, obesity, diabetes, smoking, or family history.

• Partial vision loss and blindness, both transient and permanent, have been reported with 5-HT$_1$ agonists.

Dialyzable drug: Unknown.

⚠ *Overdose S&S:* Sedation.

PREGNANCY-LACTATION-REPRODUCTION
• Drug has caused fetal harm in animal studies, but there are no adequate studies during pregnancy. Use only if clearly needed and potential benefit justifies fetal risk.

• It isn't known if drug appears in human milk. Patient should discontinue breastfeeding or discontinue drug.

NURSING CONSIDERATIONS
• Drug isn't intended for preventing migraines or treating hemiplegic or basilar migraines.

• Safety of drug hasn't been established for cluster headaches or for treatment of an average of more than three headaches (oral formulation) or four headaches (intranasal formulation) in a 30-day period.

• A CV exam should be performed in patients who are triptan-naive and have multiple CV risk factors (increased age, diabetes, HTN, smoking, obesity, strong family history of CAD). Consider initiating therapy in a medically supervised setting with ECG monitoring. Patients with a negative CV exam should have periodic exams during therapy.

🜂 *Alert:* Combining drug with an SSRI or an SSNRI may cause serotonin syndrome. Signs and symptoms may include restlessness, hallucinations, loss of coordination, fast heartbeat, rapid changes in BP, increased body temperature, overactive reflexes, nausea, vomiting, and diarrhea. Serotonin syndrome may be more likely to occur when starting or increasing the dose of drug, SSRI, or SSNRI.

• Zomig ODT tablets contain phenylalanine, which can be harmful to patients with phenylketonuria.

• *Look alike–sound alike:* Don't confuse Zomig with Zoloft or Zonegran. Don't confuse zolmitriptan with rizatriptan, sumatriptan, or zolpidem.

PATIENT TEACHING
• Tell patient that drug is intended to relieve, not prevent, signs and symptoms of migraine. It isn't used to treat other types of headaches, and misuse of drug to treat more than 10 headaches per month may lead to worsening of headaches.

• Advise patient how to properly take drug and to take it as prescribed.

• Caution patient to immediately report pain or tightness in the chest or throat, heart throbbing, shortness of breath, slurred speech, rash, skin lumps, or swelling of the face, lips, or eyelids.

Reactions in bold italics are *life-threatening*. Interactions may have a *rapid onset* or a *delayed onset*.

- Tell patient to report pregnancy, plans to become pregnant, or breastfeeding before using drug.
- Warn patient that serotonin syndrome may occur if drug is used in combination with other drugs that increase serotonin level (SSRIs, SSNRIs).

SAFETY ALERT!

zolpidem tartrate ☒
ZOL-pih-dem

Ambien✍, Ambien CR, Edluar, Sublinox✤, Zolpimist

Therapeutic class: Hypnotics
Pharmacologic class: Imidazopyridines
Controlled substance schedule: IV

AVAILABLE FORMS
Oral spray: 5 mg/actuation
Tablets: 5 mg, 10 mg
Tablets (extended-release) ⓒ: 6.25 mg, 12.5 mg
Tablets (ODTs) ⓒ: 1.75 mg, 3.5 mg, 5 mg, 10 mg

INDICATIONS & DOSAGES
➤ **Short-term management of insomnia**
Adults: 5 or 10 mg (men) or 5 mg (women) immediate-release or 6.25 or 12.5 mg (men) or 6.25 mg (women) extended-release PO immediately before bedtime. Or, 5 or 10 mg (men) or 5 mg (women) SL tablet or spray once per night immediately before bedtime. At time of dose, at least 7 to 8 hours should remain before planned time of awakening. May increase to 10 mg as needed.
Adjust-a-dose: For older adults, patients who are debilitated, and patients with mild to moderate hepatic insufficiency, 5 mg PO or SL immediately before bedtime. Or, 6.25 mg of extended-release form. Maximum daily dose is 10 mg immediate-release and 12.5 mg extended-release.
➤ **Sleep maintenance in insomnia (SL tablets)**
Adults: 3.5 mg (men) or 1.75 mg (women) SL once per night as needed for middle-of-the-night awakening with at least 4 hours of bedtime remaining before planned waking.
Adjust-a-dose: For older adults, patients with hepatic impairment, or patients taking concomitant CNS depressant, 1.75 mg SL for women and men.

ADMINISTRATION
PO
- For rapid sleep onset, drug should not be taken with or immediately after meals.
- Don't crush, break, or divide extended-release tablets.
- Place SL tablet under tongue to disintegrate. Patient shouldn't swallow tablet whole or take with water.
- Prime oral spray pump with 5 sprays before first use or with 1 spray if pump hasn't been used for 14 days.
- Pump spray directly over tongue. Have patient press down fully to make sure full dose is delivered.

ACTION
Although drug interacts with one of three identified GABA–benzodiazepine receptor complexes, it isn't a benzodiazepine. It exhibits hypnotic activity and minimal muscle relaxant and anticonvulsant properties.

Route	Onset	Peak	Duration
PO	30 min	30–120 min	6–8 hr

Half-life: 1.5 to 8.5 hours.

ADVERSE REACTIONS
CNS: headache, amnesia, abnormal dreams, balance disorder, asthenia, attention disturbance, anxiety, fever, hallucination, disorientation, feeling intoxicated, ataxia, drowsiness, depression, dizziness, hypoesthesia, vertigo, confusion, disinhibition, lethargy, light-headedness, nervousness, sleep disorder, euphoria, mood swings, memory disorder, paresthesia. **CV:** palpitations, chest pain. **EENT:** diplopia, eye redness, abnormal vision, eye symptoms, tinnitus, pharyngitis, sinusitis, dry mouth, labyrinthitis, throat irritation. **GI:** abdominal pain, abdominal distress, abdominal tenderness, change in appetite, gastroenteritis, GERD, vomiting, constipation, diarrhea, hiccups, dyspepsia, nausea. **GU:** dysuria, UTI, menstrual disorder. **Musculoskeletal:** arthralgia, myalgia, back pain. **Respiratory:** respiratory tract infection, bronchitis, cough, dyspnea. **Skin:** rash, urticaria, bruising. **Other:** flulike syndrome, hypersensitivity reactions.

INTERACTIONS
Drug-drug. *Chlorpromazine, imipramine:* May cause additive effect of decreased alertness. Monitor patient closely.

Z

CNS depressants: May cause excessive CNS depression. Use together cautiously.

CYP3A4 inducers (rifampin): May decrease effects of zolpidem. Avoid use together.

CYP3A4 inhibitors (itraconazole, ketoconazole, verapamil): May increase zolpidem level. Use a low zolpidem dosage and monitor therapy.

Opioid class warning: May cause slow or difficult breathing, sedation, and death. Avoid use together. If use together is necessary, limit dosage and duration of each drug to minimum necessary for desired effect.

Drug-herb. *Calendula, chamomile, gotu kola, kava, valerian:* May increase risk of CNS depression. Avoid concomitant use.

St. John's wort: May decrease zolpidem level and effects. Avoid concomitant use.

Drug-food. *Grapefruit juice:* May decrease zolpidem metabolism. Avoid grapefruit juice.

Drug-lifestyle. *Alcohol use:* May cause excessive CNS depression. Discourage use together.

EFFECTS ON LAB TEST RESULTS
• May increase ALT, AST, and bilirubin levels.
• May decrease radioactive iodine uptake.

CONTRAINDICATIONS & CAUTIONS
• Contraindicated in patients hypersensitive to drug or its components.
• *Opioid class warning:* Opioids should only be prescribed with benzodiazepines or other CNS depressants to patients for whom alternative treatment options are inadequate.

Boxed Warning Drug may cause rare but serious injury, including death, due to complex sleep behaviors, such as sleepwalking, sleep driving, and engaging in other activities while not fully awake. These behaviors can occur even at the lowest recommended doses and after just one dose. Drug is contraindicated in patients with a history of complex sleep behavior while taking drug. ∎

• Avoid use in patients with severe hepatic impairment as it may contribute to encephalopathy.
• Use cautiously in patients with compromised respiratory status, mild or moderate hepatic impairment, myasthenia gravis, or a history of depression or worsening depression.
• *Alert:* Drug level may remain elevated the day after drug use, impairing mental alertness.

Risk increases if patient sleeps for less than 7 hours, takes drug with other CNS depressants including alcohol, or takes higher than recommended dose.

• *Alert:* Patients taking extended-release formulation shouldn't drive or engage in other activities that require complete mental alertness the day after taking drug because drug level can remain high enough to impair these activities.

• *Alert:* Drug can cause drowsiness and decreased level of consciousness, which may lead to falls and severe injuries, such as hip fractures and intracranial hemorrhage.

• Abnormal thinking and behavior changes have been reported in patients treated with zolpidem. Some of these changes included decreased inhibition (aggressiveness and extroversion that seemed out of character), bizarre behavior, agitation, and depersonalization. Visual and auditory hallucinations have been reported. Immediately evaluate signs or symptoms of new behaviors.

⚲ Women have a lower zolpidem clearance than men; lower initial doses are recommended in women.

Dialyzable drug: No.

⚠ *Overdose S&S:* Impaired consciousness, somnolence, coma, CV or respiratory compromise, death.

PREGNANCY-LACTATION-REPRODUCTION
• Drug crosses the placental barrier. Use during pregnancy only if potential benefit outweighs fetal risk.
• Monitor neonates exposed to zolpidem during pregnancy and labor for excess sedation, hypotonia, and respiratory depression and manage accordingly.
• Drug appears in human milk. Use cautiously during breastfeeding.
• Monitor infants exposed to zolpidem through human milk for excess sedation, hypotonia, and respiratory depression. Patient may consider expressing and discarding milk during treatment and for 23 hours after zolpidem administration to minimize infant's drug exposure.

NURSING CONSIDERATIONS
• *Alert:* Anaphylaxis and angioedema may occur as early as the first dose. Monitor patient closely. Discontinue drug and don't restart if these occur.

Reactions in bold italics are *life-threatening*. Interactions may have a *rapid onset* or a *delayed onset*.

• Use drug only for short-term management of insomnia, usually 7 to 10 days. Reevaluate patient if insomnia persists.
• Use the smallest effective dose in all patients.
• Take precautions to prevent hoarding by patients who are depressed, suicidal, or drug-dependent, or who have a history of drug abuse.
• Monitor patient for withdrawal signs and symptoms after rapid dosage reduction or abrupt drug discontinuation.
• *Look alike–sound alike:* Don't confuse Ambien with Abilify or Ativan. Don't confuse zolpidem with lorazepam, zaleplon, or zolmitriptan. ∎

PATIENT TEACHING
• *Opioid class warning:* Caution patient or caregiver of patient taking an opioid with a benzodiazepine, CNS depressant, or alcohol to seek immediate medical attention for dizziness, light-headedness, extreme sleepiness, slowed or difficult breathing, or unresponsiveness.

Boxed Warning Warn patient of risk of injury or death related to complex sleep behaviors, such as driving, eating, and making phone calls while asleep. Direct patient to stop drug and immediately report an episode of complex sleep behavior or if patient doesn't remember activities done while taking drug. ∎
• Instruct patient about how to properly take drug by prescribed formulation.
⊕ *Alert:* Warn patient that drug may cause allergic reactions, facial swelling, and respiratory depression. Advise patient to immediately report these adverse effects.
⊕ *Alert:* Tell patient that drug has the potential to cause next-day impairment, and that this risk increases if dosing instructions aren't carefully followed. Tell patient to wait for at least 8 hours after dosing before driving or engaging in other activities requiring full mental alertness. Inform patient that impairment can be present even if patient may feel fully awake.
⊕ *Alert:* Tell patient that drug can cause drowsiness and decreased level of consciousness, which may lead to falls and severe injuries.
• For rapid sleep onset, instruct patient not to take drug with or immediately after meals.
• Instruct patient to take drug immediately before going to bed; onset of action is rapid.

• Tell patient to avoid alcohol use while taking drug.
• Caution patient to avoid performing activities that require mental alertness or physical coordination during therapy.

---

zonisamide
zoh-NISS-a-mide

Zonegran, Zonisade

Therapeutic class: Anticonvulsants
Pharmacologic class: Sulfonamides

AVAILABLE FORMS
Capsules ⓓⓝⓖ: 25 mg, 50 mg, 100 mg
Oral suspension: 100 mg/5 mL

INDICATIONS & DOSAGES
➤ **Adjunctive therapy for partial seizures in patients with epilepsy**
Adults and children older than age 16: Initially, 100 mg PO daily for 2 weeks. Then, may increase dosage to 200 mg daily for at least 2 weeks. May increase dosage to 300 mg and then to 400 mg PO daily, with the dose stable for at least 2 weeks to achieve steady state at each level. Maximum recommended dose is 600 mg daily; however, there is no evidence of increased response with doses above 400 mg/day.
Adjust-a-dose: For patients with renal or hepatic impairment, titrate dosages more slowly and monitor patients more frequently.

ADMINISTRATION
PO
⊕ *Alert:* Hazardous drug; use safe-handling and disposal precautions.
• Give drug without regard for food.
• Don't crush or open capsule.
• May give solution once or twice daily.
• Shake solution well before giving.
• Measure and give solution using an accurate measuring device.
• Discard unused solution 30 days after opening the bottle.

ACTION
May stabilize neuronal membranes and suppress neuronal hypersynchronization at sodium and calcium channels, which prevents seizures.

Z

Route	Onset	Peak	Duration
PO (capsules)	Unknown	2–6 hr	Unknown
PO (solution)	Unknown	0.5–5 hr	Unknown

Half-life: 63 hours.

ADVERSE REACTIONS

CNS: dizziness, headache, somnolence, *seizures, status epilepticus,* abnormal gait, agitation or irritability, anxiety, asthenia, ataxia, confusion, depression, difficulties in concentration or memory, difficulties in verbal expression, fatigue, hyperesthesia, incoordination, insomnia, mental slowing, nervousness, paresthesia, schizophrenic or schizophreniform behavior, speech disorders, tremor, taste perversion. **EENT:** amblyopia, diplopia, nystagmus, tinnitus, pharyngitis, rhinitis, dry mouth. **GI:** anorexia, abdominal pain, constipation, diarrhea, dyspepsia, nausea, vomiting. **GU:** kidney stones. **Metabolic:** weight loss. **Respiratory:** cough. **Skin:** pruritus, rash, ecchymosis. **Other:** accidental injury, flulike syndrome.

INTERACTIONS

Drug-drug. *Other carbonic anhydrase inhibitors (acetazolamide, dichlorphenamide, topiramate):* May increase severity of metabolic acidosis; may increase risk of kidney stone formation. Monitor patient for development or worsening of metabolic acidosis.
Other CNS depressants: May cause CNS depression and other cognitive or neuropsychiatric adverse events. Use together cautiously.
Strong CYP3A4 inducers (carbamazepine, phenobarbital, phenytoin, valproate): May increase zonisamide clearance. Monitor patient closely.
Drug-herb. *Kava kava:* May enhance adverse or toxic effects of zonisamide. Monitor therapy.
Drug-lifestyle. *Alcohol use:* May cause CNS depression and other cognitive or neuropsychiatric adverse events. Use together cautiously.

EFFECTS ON LAB TEST RESULTS

• May increase chloride, ALP, BUN, and creatinine levels.
• May decrease serum bicarbonate, phosphorus, calcium, and albumin levels.

CONTRAINDICATIONS & CAUTIONS

• Contraindicated in patients hypersensitive to drug or to sulfonamides.

• Use cautiously in patients with renal and hepatic dysfunction or kidney stones. Avoid use in patients with eGFR less than 50 mL/minute.
• Use cautiously in patients with history of psychiatric symptoms.
• Use cautiously with other drugs that predispose patients to heat-related disorders, including but not limited to carbonic anhydrase inhibitors and drugs with anticholinergic activity.
• Drug may increase risk of SCARs.
• Safety and effectiveness in children younger than age 16 haven't been established; children are at increased risk for oligohidrosis and hyperthermia.
Dialyzable drug: Yes.
⚠ *Overdose S&S:* CNS symptoms, coma, bradycardia, hypotension, respiratory depression.

PREGNANCY-LACTATION-REPRODUCTION

• Drug may cause a variety of fetal abnormalities. Use in pregnancy only if potential benefit justifies fetal risk.
• Patients of childbearing potential should use effective contraception during therapy and for 1 month after final dose.
• Monitor neonates of patients treated with zonisamide during pregnancy for metabolic acidosis; transient metabolic acidosis may occur after birth.
• Encourage patients taking drug during pregnancy to enroll in the North American AED (Antiepileptic Drug) Pregnancy Registry (1-888-233-2334 or www.aedpregnancyregistry.org/).
• Drug appears in human milk. Patient should discontinue breastfeeding or discontinue drug.

NURSING CONSIDERATIONS

🛈 *Alert:* Monitor patient for signs and symptoms of hypersensitivity.
• Rarely, patients receiving sulfonamides have died because of severe reactions, such as SJS, fulminant hepatic necrosis, aplastic anemia, otherwise unexplained rashes, and agranulocytosis. If signs and symptoms of hypersensitivity or other serious reactions occur, stop drug immediately and notify prescriber.
🛈 *Alert:* Closely monitor all patients taking or starting AEDs for changes in behavior indicating worsening suicidality or depression. Symptoms such as anxiety, agitation,

---

Reactions in bold italics are *life-threatening*. Interactions may have a *rapid onset* or a *delayed onset*.

hostility, mania, and hypomania may be precursors to emerging suicidality.
• If patient develops acute renal failure or a significant sustained increase in creatinine or BUN level, stop drug and notify prescriber. Periodically monitor renal function.
• Drug can cause metabolic acidosis, especially in those with predisposing conditions or therapies. This risk is more frequent and severe in younger patients. Measure serum bicarbonate level before starting treatment and periodically during treatment, even in the absence of symptoms.
• Reduce dosage or stop drug gradually because abrupt discontinuation may increase seizures or cause status epilepticus.
• Achieving steady-state levels may take 2 weeks.
• Increase fluid intake and urine output to help prevent kidney stones, especially in patients with predisposing factors.
• Monitor patient for cognitive and neuropsychiatric adverse reactions, including psychomotor slowing, difficulty with concentration, speech or language problems (especially word-finding difficulties), somnolence or fatigue, depression, and psychosis.

PATIENT TEACHING
• Teach patient safe drug administration and handling.
• Advise patient to call prescriber immediately if rash develops or seizures worsen.
• Warn patient and family that drug may increase risk of suicidality and to be alert for new or worsening symptoms of depression, unusual changes in mood or behavior, or the emergence of suicidality. Tell them to report these signs or symptoms to prescriber immediately.
• Tell patient to immediately report sudden back or abdominal pain, pain when urinating, bloody or dark urine, fever, sore throat, mouth sores or easy bruising, decreased sweating, fever, depression, or speech or language problems.
• Advise patient to avoid dehydration and to maintain adequate fluid intake.
• Caution patient that drug can cause drowsiness and not to drive or operate dangerous machinery until drug's effects are known.
• Advise patient not to stop taking drug without prescriber's approval because abrupt withdrawal can cause seizures.

• Instruct patient of childbearing potential to report pregnancy, plans to become pregnant, or breastfeeding and to use contraception during therapy.

abrocitinib ⚠
a-broe-SYE-ti-nib

Cibinqo

Therapeutic class: Immunomodulators
Pharmacologic class: Janus kinase inhibitors

AVAILABLE FORMS
Tablets ⊡: 50 mg, 100 mg, 200 mg

INDICATIONS & DOSAGES
➤ **Refractory, moderate to severe atopic dermatitis not adequately controlled with other systemic drug products, including biologics, or when use of those therapies is inadvisable**
Adults: 100 mg PO once daily. May increase to 200 mg once daily if inadequate response after 12 weeks. Discontinue drug if inadequate response after 200-mg dose increase. Can use with or without topical corticosteroids.
🔲 *Adjust-a-dose:* For patients with moderate renal impairment (eGFR of 30 to 59 mL/minute) or patients who are known or suspected CYP2C19 poor metabolizers, reduce dosage to 50 mg once daily; if inadequate response after 12 weeks, may double the dose. Refer to manufacturer's instructions for toxicity-related dosage adjustments.

ADMINISTRATION
PO
• Give at same time each day without regard to food.
• Patient should swallow tablets whole with water. Don't allow patient to crush, split, or chew tablets.
• If a dose is missed, give as soon as possible. If missed dose is within 12 hours of the time before next dose, skip the missed dose and resume dosing at regular scheduled time.
• Store tablets at 68° to 77° F (20° to 25° C) in original container.

ACTION
Reversibly inhibits Janus kinase (JAK) by blocking the adenosine triphosphate binding site, possibly reducing inflammation.

Route	Onset	Peak	Duration
PO	Unknown	1 hr	Unknown

Half-life: 3 to 5 hours.

ADVERSE REACTIONS
CNS: dizziness, fatigue, headache. **CV:** HTN.
EENT: nasopharyngitis, oropharyngeal pain.
GI: abdominal discomfort, gastroenteritis, nausea, vomiting, upper abdominal pain. **GU:** UTI.
Hematologic: *thrombocytopenia.* **Metabolic:** increased CK level. **Skin:** acne, contact dermatitis, impetigo. **Other:** flulike symptoms, infections, herpes simplex, herpes zoster.

INTERACTIONS
Drug-drug. *Antiplatelet drugs (clopidogrel, prasugrel, ticagrelor [excluding low-dose aspirin]):* May increase risk of bleeding with thrombocytopenia. Avoid use together during first 3 months of therapy.
Moderate to strong CYP2C19 and CYP2C9 inhibitors (fluconazole): May increase abrocitinib level. Avoid use with drugs that are moderate to strong inhibitors of both CYP2C19 and CYP2C9.
Other JAK inhibitors, biologic immunomodulators, immunosuppressants: May enhance immunosuppressant effect. Avoid use together.
P-gp substrates (dabigatran, digoxin): May increase P-gp substrate level and risk of adverse reactions of substrate. Small increases may lead to serious or life-threatening toxicities. Monitor patient closely or titrate P-gp substrate dosage.
Strong CYP2C19 and CYP2C9 inducers (rifampin): May decrease abrocitinib level. Avoid use together.
Strong CYP2C19 inhibitors (fluvoxamine): May increase abrocitinib level. Reduce abrocitinib dosage.
Vaccines: May decrease therapeutic effect of inactivated vaccines and increase risk of infection from live vaccines. Give all immunizations, including herpes zoster, according to immunization guidelines before starting drug. Avoid live vaccines immediately before, during, and immediately after therapy.
Drug-lifestyle. *Smoking:* May increase risk of malignancies and CV events. Discourage smoking.
Sun exposure: May increase risk of skin cancer. Limit exposure to sunlight and UV light.

EFFECTS ON LAB TEST RESULTS
• May increase LDL, total cholesterol, HDL, and CK levels.
• May decrease Hb level, ANC, and platelet and lymphocyte counts.

CONTRAINDICATIONS & CAUTIONS
Boxed Warning Drug may increase risk of serious bacterial, fungal, viral, and opportunistic infections, leading to hospitalization or death. The most frequently reported serious infections were herpes simplex, herpes zoster, and pneumonia. Avoid use in patients with active, serious infection, including localized infections. Consider the risk and benefits of use in patients with chronic or recurrent infection. ∎
• Don't give to patients with active TB. Consider anti-TB treatment in patients with previously untreated latent TB, patients with a history of active TB if an adequate course of treatment can't be confirmed, and patients with a negative latent TB test but who have risk factors for TB infection.
Boxed Warning Patients age 50 and older with RA and at least one CV risk factor treated with a JAK inhibitor have an increased risk of major adverse CV events, including all-cause mortality. A higher rate of major adverse CV events (CV death, MI, stroke) and thrombosis (PE, venous,

arterial) have occurred with JAK inhibitors compared with TNF blockers in patients with RA. Patients who are current or past smokers are at additional risk. Discontinue drug in patients with MI, stroke, or signs or symptoms of thrombosis. Abrocitinib isn't approved for use in patients with RA. ■

Boxed Warning Lymphoma and other malignancies have been observed in patients treated with JAK inhibitors. Those receiving JAK inhibitors for RA have a higher rate of malignancies (excluding non-melanoma skin cancer) compared with TNF blockers. Patients who are current or past smokers are at increased risk. ■

Boxed Warning Serious and sometimes fatal thrombosis, including DVT, PE, and arterial thrombosis, have occurred in patients treated with JAK inhibitors. Consider risks and benefits. Use cautiously in patients at risk for thrombosis. ■

• Contraindicated in patients with active HBV or HCV infection.

• Avoid use in patients with severe (Child-Pugh class C) hepatic impairment.

• Use cautiously in patients with moderate renal impairment.

• Contraindicated in patients with severe renal impairment (eGFR of 15 to 29 mL/minute) or ESRD, platelet count less than 150,000/mm³, absolute lymphocyte count less than 500/mm³, ANC less than 1,000/mm³, or Hb level less than 8 g/dL.

▨ Use cautiously in older adults and patients who are CPY2C19 poor metabolizers.

• Safety and effectiveness in children haven't been established.

Dialyzable drug: Unknown.

PREGNANCY-LACTATION-REPRODUCTION

• There are no adequate studies during pregnancy. It isn't known if drug increases risk of major birth defects, miscarriage, or adverse maternal or fetal outcomes.

• Enroll patient exposed to drug during pregnancy in the pregnancy exposure registry (1-877-311-3770).

• It isn't known if drug appears in human milk or how drug affects milk production or infants who are breastfed. Patient shouldn't breastfeed during therapy and for 1 day after final dose.

• May impair fertility in patients of childbearing potential.

NURSING CONSIDERATIONS

Boxed Warning Monitor patient for infection during and after therapy. Stop drug if serious or opportunistic infection occurs. Initiate diagnostic testing and appropriate antimicrobial therapy. Weigh risks and benefits of restarting therapy. ■

Boxed Warning Test patient for latent TB before and during therapy. Treat TB before therapy. Monitor for active TB during therapy, even if patient initially tested negative for latent TB. ■

• Monitor patient for herpes zoster. If reactivation occurs, consider interrupting therapy until episode resolves.

• Screen and monitor patient for HBV infection reactivation before and during therapy. Monitor patient with inactive HBV infection for expression of HBV DNA during therapy. If HBV DNA is detected, consult liver specialist.

• Perform periodic skin exams in patient who is at increased risk for skin cancer.

• Monitor patient for serious CV events. Discontinue drug if MI or stroke occurs.

• Monitor patient for signs and symptoms of PE, DVT, and arterial thrombosis (edema; pain in one leg; sudden, unexplained chest pain; dyspnea). If signs or symptoms occur, stop drug, promptly evaluate, and treat as clinically indicated.

• Monitor patient for signs and symptoms of GI perforation (fever, abdominal pain, changes in bowel habits).

• Monitor CBC at baseline, 4 weeks after starting drug, 4 weeks after dosage increase, and as indicated for patients on long-term abrocitinib therapy who develop hematologic abnormalities.

• Monitor lipid levels 4 weeks after starting drug. Manage hyperlipidemia according to clinical guidelines.

• Ensure that patient is up to date with all immunizations, including herpes zoster, before starting drug.

• *Look alike-sound alike:* Don't confuse abrocitinib with axitinib, afatinib, alectinib, abciximab, abemaciclib, or acalabrutinib.

PATIENT TEACHING

• Instruct patient about safe drug administration and storage.

Boxed Warning Inform patient to immediately report signs or symptoms of infection (fever, diaphoresis, chills, shortness of breath, muscle aches, fatigue, weight loss, cough, hemoptysis, burning on urination, stomach pain, diarrhea, skin sores, or red, warm, painful skin). ■

Boxed Warning Tell patient about increased risk of certain cancers, such as skin cancer, and to obtain periodic skin exams during therapy. Advise patient to limit exposure to sunlight and UV light. ■

Boxed Warning Teach patient about increased risk of MI, stroke, DVT, and PE. Advise patient to seek immediate medical attention if experiencing chest or limb pain, extremity edema, dyspnea, numbness, difficulty walking or speaking, sudden headache, or confusion. ■

• Inform patient about immunizations required before therapy.

• Tell patient to immediately report sudden vision changes.

• Counsel patient to avoid receiving live-virus vaccines.

NEW DRUGS

NEW DRUGS

• Instruct patient of childbearing potential to report pregnancy or plans to become pregnant during therapy.
• Advise patient not to breastfeed during therapy and for 1 day after final dose.
• Advise patient of childbearing potential that drug may impair fertility.

SAFETY ALERT!

asciminib ⊠
as-KIM-i-nib

Scemblix

Therapeutic class: Antineoplastics
Pharmacologic class: Kinase inhibitors

AVAILABLE FORMS
Tablets ⊞: 20 mg, 40 mg

INDICATIONS & DOSAGES
Adjust-a-dose (for all indications): Refer to manufacturer's instructions for toxicity-related dosage adjustments.
➤ **Philadelphia chromosome–positive chronic myeloid leukemia in chronic phase previously treated with two or more tyrosine kinase inhibitors** ⊠
Adults: 80 mg PO once daily or 40 mg PO every 12 hours if clinical benefit is observed or until unacceptable toxicity occurs.
➤ **Philadelphia chromosome–positive chronic myeloid leukemia in chronic phase with the *T315I* mutation** ⊠
Adults: 200 mg PO every 12 hours.

ADMINISTRATION
PO
• Give at approximately same time each day or at 12-hour intervals.
• Avoid giving with food for at least 2 hours before and 1 hour after each dose.
• Don't allow patient to break, crush, or chew tablets or to swallow them whole.
• If a dose is missed by more than 12 hours on a once-daily regimen or by more than 6 hours on a twice-daily regimen, skip dose and take next dose as scheduled.
• Store tablets at 68° to 77° F (20° to 25° C).

ACTION
Inhibits the ABL1 kinase activity of the BCR-ABL1 fusion protein.

Route	Onset	Peak	Duration
PO	Unknown	2–3 hr	Unknown

Half-life: 5.5 to 9 hours.

ADVERSE REACTIONS
CNS: dizziness, fatigue, fever, headache, peripheral neuropathy. **CV:** arrhythmia, edema, HF, *hemorrhage*, HTN, palpitations, *prolonged QT interval.* **EENT:** blurred vision, dry eye. **GI:** abdominal pain, constipation, diarrhea, nausea, increased amylase and lipase levels, *pancreatitis,* vomiting. **GU:** increased creatinine level, UTI. **Hematologic:** anemia, *febrile neutropenia, lymphopenia, neutropenia, thrombocytopenia.* **Hepatic:** hyperbilirubinemia, increased ALT and AST levels. **Metabolic:** dyslipidemia, hypercholesterolemia, hypertriglyceridemia, hyperuricemia, *hypocalcemia, hypokalemia,* hypophosphatemia, hypothyroidism, increased CK level. **Musculoskeletal:** arthralgia, musculoskeletal pain. **Respiratory:** cough, dyspnea, pleural effusion, pneumonia, URI. **Skin:** hypersensitivity reaction, pruritus, rash.

INTERACTIONS
Drug-drug. *Certain P-gp substrates:* May increase substrate level. If concomitant use can't be avoided, closely monitor patient for substrate-related adverse reactions.
CYP2C9 substrates (warfarin): May increase risk of substrate-related adverse reactions. Avoid using together with asciminib 80 mg (total) daily; if concomitant use can't be avoided, reduce the substrate dose. Avoid using together with asciminib 200 mg b.i.d.; if concomitant use can't be avoided, consider alternative therapy with a non-CYP2C9 substrate.
CYP3A4 substrates (midazolam): May increase substrate level and risk of adverse reactions. Closely monitor patient treated with asciminib 80 mg daily with concomitant use of CYP3A4 substrates. Avoid using together with asciminib 200-mg b.i.d.
Itraconazole oral solution containing hydroxypropyl-β-cyclodextrin: May reduce asciminib level and effectiveness. Avoid use together.
Strong CYP3A4 inhibitors (clarithromycin): May increase asciminib level and risk of adverse reactions. Closely monitor patient treated with asciminib at 200 mg b.i.d.

EFFECTS ON LAB TEST RESULTS
• May increase amylase, AST, ALT, bilirubin, cholesterol, CK, creatinine, lipase, triglyceride, and uric acid levels.
• May decrease phosphate, corrected calcium, and potassium levels.
• May decrease Hb level and lymphocyte, neutrophil, and platelet counts.

CONTRAINDICATIONS & CAUTIONS
• Drug may increase risk of hypersensitivity reactions, HTN, pancreatic toxicity, severe thrombocytopenia, and neutropenia events.
• CV toxicity, including arrhythmias, prolonged QT interval, ischemic cardiac and CNS conditions, HF, and arterial, thrombotic, and embolic events, may occur. Patients with prior exposure to multiple tyrosine kinase inhibitors, preexisting cardiac conditions, or CV risk factors are at increased risk.

Reactions in bold italics are *life-threatening*. Interactions may have a *rapid onset* or a **delayed onset**.

- Safety and effectiveness in children haven't been established.
Dialyzable drug: No.

PREGNANCY-LACTATION-REPRODUCTION
- Drug can cause fetal harm. Advise patients who are pregnant of the risk.
- Patients of childbearing potential should use effective contraception during therapy and for 1 week after final dose.
- It isn't known if drug appears in human milk or how drug affects milk production or infants who are breastfed. Patient shouldn't breastfeed during therapy and for 1 week after final dose.
- Drug may impair fertility in patients of childbearing potential. Reversibility of the effect is unknown.

NURSING CONSIDERATIONS
- Verify pregnancy status in patients of childbearing potential before drug initiation.
- Monitor CBC every 2 weeks for the first 3 months and monthly thereafter, or as clinically indicated.
- Monitor patient for signs and symptoms of myelosuppression (fever, infection, easy bruising, bleeding).
- Monitor serum lipase and amylase levels monthly during therapy and as clinically indicated. Assess patient for pancreatitis when lipase elevation is accompanied by abdominal symptoms (nausea, vomiting, severe abdominal pain or discomfort).
- Monitor BP and manage HTN as clinically indicated.
- Monitor patient for signs and symptoms of hypersensitivity reaction (rash, edema, bronchospasm); initiate appropriate treatment as indicated.
- Monitor patient with CV risk factors for CV toxicity signs and symptoms. Initiate appropriate treatment as clinically indicated.

PATIENT TEACHING
- Advise patient about proper drug administration and storage.
- Inform patient of the need for routine blood testing during therapy.
- Warn patient about potential for low blood cell counts and to immediately report fever, and signs or symptoms of infection, bleeding, or easy bruising.
- Advise patient about the risk of pancreatitis and to contact prescriber if signs or symptoms occur.
- Inform patient about the risk of HTN. Advise patient to routinely monitor BP and report BP elevations or signs and symptoms of HTN (confusion, headache, dizziness, chest pain, shortness of breath).
- Tell patient to immediately stop drug and report signs or symptoms of hypersensitivity reaction (rash, edema, bronchospasm).

- Inform patient about the risk of CV toxicity, especially if the patient has CV risk factors. Tell patient to immediately contact prescriber or seek medical help if experiencing palpitations, edema, shortness of breath, chest pain, dizziness, weight gain, visual changes, numbness or weakness, trouble talking, severe stomach pain, or headache.
- Advise patient to report pregnancy or plans to become pregnant or to breastfeed.
- Advise patient of childbearing potential to use effective contraception during therapy and for 1 week after final dose.
- Warn patient not to breastfeed during therapy and for 1 week after final dose.
- Caution patient of childbearing potential that drug may impair fertility.

atogepant
a-TOE-je-pant

Qulipta

Therapeutic class: Antimigraine drugs
Pharmacologic class: Calcitonin gene-related peptide receptor antagonists

AVAILABLE FORMS
Tablets: 10 mg, 30 mg, 60 mg

INDICATIONS & DOSAGES
➤ **Prevention of episodic migraine headaches**
Adults: 1 tablet PO once daily.
Adjust-a-dose: If used concomitantly with a strong CYP3A4 inhibitor, give 10 mg PO once daily. If used concomitantly with a strong or moderate CYP3A4 inducer, give 30 or 60 mg PO once daily. If used concomitantly with an OATP inhibitor, give 10 or 30 mg PO once daily. In patients with CrCl less than 30 mL/minute, give 10 mg PO once daily.

ADMINISTRATION
PO
- Give without regard to food.
- If patient is receiving dialysis, give after treatment.
- Store tablets at 68° to 77° F (20° to 25° C).

ACTION
Antagonizes calcitonin gene-related peptide receptors.

Route	Onset	Peak	Duration
PO	Unknown	1–2 hr	Unknown

Half-life: 11 hours.

ADVERSE REACTIONS
CNS: fatigue, somnolence. **GI:** constipation, decreased appetite, nausea. **Hepatic:** elevated transaminase levels. **Metabolic:** weight loss.

NEW DRUGS

INTERACTIONS

Drug-drug. *OATP inhibitors (cyclosporine, rifampin):* May increase atogepant level. Adjust atogepant dosage.

Strong or moderate CYP3A4 inducers (carbamazepine, efavirenz, etravirine, phenytoin, rifampin): May decrease atogepant level. Adjust atogepant dosage.

Strong CYP3A4 inhibitors (clarithromycin, itraconazole, ketoconazole): May increase atogepant level. Adjust atogepant dosage.

Drug-herb. *St. John's wort:* May decrease atogepant level. Adjust atogepant dosage.

EFFECTS ON LAB TEST RESULTS

• May increase hepatic transaminase levels.

CONTRAINDICATIONS & CAUTIONS

• Avoid use in patients with severe hepatic impairment (Child-Pugh class C).
• Use cautiously in older adults. Initiate therapy at lowest dose.
• Safety and effectiveness in children haven't been established.

Dialyzable drug: Unknown.

PREGNANCY-LACTATION-REPRODUCTION

• Based on animal studies, drug may cause fetal harm. Advise patients who are pregnant of the fetal risk.
• Use during pregnancy only if clearly indicated and benefit outweighs fetal risk.
• It isn't known if drug appears in human milk or how drug affects milk production or infants who are breastfed. Before making the decision to breastfeed, consider patient's clinical need and risk to the infant.

NURSING CONSIDERATIONS

• Monitor LFT values when appropriate.

PATIENT TEACHING

• Instruct patient about proper drug administration and storage.
• Advise patient to report use of other prescription drugs, OTC drugs, or herbal products to prescriber.
• Inform patient that drug may interact with other drugs and that dosage modifications may be necessary.

---

avacopan
a-va-KOE-pan

Tavneos

Therapeutic class: Immunomodulators
Pharmacologic class: Complement inhibitors

AVAILABLE FORMS

Capsules 🔵: 10 mg

INDICATIONS & DOSAGES

➤ **Adjunctive treatment of severe active anti-neutrophil cytoplasmic autoantibody–associated vasculitis (granulomatosis with polyangiitis and microscopic polyangiitis), in combination with standard therapy, including glucocorticoids**

Adults: 30 mg PO b.i.d.

Adjust-a-dose: When used with a strong CYP3A4 inhibitor, reduce dosage to 30 mg PO once daily. If AST or ALT level is greater than $3 \times$ ULN, interrupt therapy. If AST or ALT level is greater than $5 \times$ ULN, or AST or ALT level is $3 \times$ ULN with bilirubin level elevation greater than $2 \times$ ULN, discontinue drug until avacopan-induced liver injury is ruled out.

ADMINISTRATION

PO
• Give with food.
• Don't allow patient to crush, open, or chew capsules.
• Don't make up a missed dose; give next dose at the scheduled time. Don't double the next dose.
• Store capsules at 68° to 77° F (20° to 25° C).

ACTION

Inhibits the interaction between C5aR and anaphylatoxin C5a to block C5a-mediated neutrophil activation and migration. Exact mechanism of therapeutic effect is unknown.

Route	Onset	Peak	Duration
PO	Unknown	2 hr	Unknown

Half-life: 97.6 hours (parent drug); 55.6 hours (active metabolite).

ADVERSE REACTIONS

CNS: dizziness, fatigue, headache, paresthesia. **CV:** HTN. **GI:** diarrhea, nausea, upper abdominal pain, vomiting. **GU:** elevated creatinine level. **Hepatic:** liver enzyme abnormalities. **Skin:** rash. **Other:** *angioedema*.

INTERACTIONS

Drug-drug. *CYP3A4 substrates (midazolam):* May increase risk of substrate-related adverse reactions. Monitor patient closely and consider dosage reduction of sensitive CYP3A4 substrates with a narrow therapeutic window.

Strong and moderate CYP3A4 inducers (rifampin): May decrease avacopan level. Avoid use together.

Strong CYP3A4 inhibitors (itraconazole): May increase avacopan level. Reduce avacopan dosage.

Drug-herb. *St. John's wort:* May decrease avacopan level. Avoid use together.

EFFECTS ON LAB TEST RESULTS

• May increase creatinine, AST, ALT, bilirubin, and CK levels.

CONTRAINDICATIONS & CAUTIONS

• Contraindicated in patients hypersensitive to drug or its components.

• Drug increases risk of serious and life-threatening events such as liver injury, transaminase elevations, and hepatobiliary events.

• Not recommended in patients with active, untreated or uncontrolled chronic liver disease (hepatitis B, hepatitis C, uncontrolled autoimmune hepatitis) or cirrhosis.

• Drug may cause reactivation of latent HBV infection and hypersensitivity reactions, including angioedema.

• Avoid use in patients with an active, serious infection.

• Use cautiously in patients with chronic or recurrent infection, TB exposure, history of serious or opportunistic infections, or underlying conditions that predispose them to infection. Also use cautiously in patients who have lived or traveled in areas of endemic TB or mycoses.

• Safety and effectiveness in children haven't been established.

Dialyzable drug: Unknown.

PREGNANCY-LACTATION-REPRODUCTION

• There are no studies during pregnancy. Use only if potential benefit justifies risk.

• It isn't known if drug appears in human milk or how it affects milk production or infants who are breastfed. Before making the decision to breastfeed, consider patient's clinical need and risk to the infant.

NURSING CONSIDERATIONS

• Before initiating drug, screen patient for HBV infection. If patient is HBsAg positive or HBsAg negative but anti-HBc positive, ensure patient is evaluated by a practitioner with expertise in management of HBV.

• Monitor LFT values and total bilirubin level at baseline, every 4 weeks for 6 months, then as clinically indicated.

• Monitor patient for serious hypersensitivity reactions, including angioedema. If angioedema occurs, discontinue drug immediately and provide supportive care. Don't reinitiate drug unless other causes have been determined.

• Monitor patient for clinical and laboratory signs of hepatitis or HBV reactivation during therapy and for 6 months after therapy ends. Immediately discontinue drug if reactivation occurs.

• Monitor patient for signs and symptoms of infection during therapy; treat promptly if infection occurs.

PATIENT TEACHING

• Instruct patient about proper medication administration and storage.

• Advise patient to stop drug and seek immediate medical attention if experiencing signs or symptoms

of angioedema (swelling of the face, extremities, eyes, lips, or tongue; difficulty swallowing or breathing).

• Tell patient to contact prescriber immediately for signs or symptoms of liver problems (yellowing of skin or eyes; dark brown or tea-colored urine; pain on upper right side of abdomen; abnormal bleeding or bruising).

• Inform patient that drug may increase risk of serious infection, including reactivation of HBV infection, and to immediately report signs or symptoms of infection to prescriber.

• Instruct patient to contact prescriber immediately if fever or signs and symptoms of infection develop.

---

cabotegravir
ka-boe-TEG-ra-vir

Apretude, Vocabria

Therapeutic class: Antiretrovirals
Pharmacologic class: HIV-1 integrase strand transfer inhibitors

AVAILABLE FORMS

Injection (extended-release): 600 mg/3 mL single-dose vial
Tablets: 30 mg

INDICATIONS & DOSAGES

➤ **Short-term treatment of HIV-1 infection in combination with rilpivirine in patients who are virologically suppressed (HIV-1 RNA less than 50 copies/mL) while on a stable antiretroviral regimen with no history of treatment failure and with no known or suspected resistance to either cabotegravir or rilpivirine**

Adults (lead-in therapy): 30 mg PO daily in combination with oral rilpivirine for at least 28 days as lead-in therapy to assess cabotegravir tolerability before starting cabotegravir and rilpivirine extended-release injections. Give final oral dose the same day as starting cabotegravir and rilpivirine injections.

Adults (bridging therapy): 30 mg PO daily in combination with oral rilpivirine for 2 months as bridging therapy for patients who plan to miss a scheduled injection by more than 7 days. Start first dose of bridging therapy 1 month after final cabotegravir and rilpivirine injection for patients on a monthly schedule, and about 2 months after last injection for patients on an every-2-month schedule. Continue oral dosing until injections are restarted.

➤ **Short-term preexposure prophylaxis (PrEP) to reduce risk of sexually acquired HIV-1 infection in patients at risk**

Adults and adolescents age 12 and older weighing at least 35 kg (lead-in therapy): 1 tablet PO daily for at least 28 days as lead-in therapy before starting cabotegravir extended-release injections. Give final

NEW DRUGS

oral dose on same day of or within 3 days after initiating cabotegravir injections.

Adults and adolescents age 12 and older weighing at least 35 kg (bridging therapy): 1 tablet PO daily to replace one every-2-month injection as bridging therapy for patients who plan to miss cabotegravir injection by more than 7 days. Start first dose of bridging therapy 2 months after final cabotegravir injection dose and continue until or within 3 days after injections are restarted. An alternative oral PrEP regimen is recommended when duration exceeds 2 months.

➤ **PrEP to reduce the risk of sexually acquired HIV-1 infection in patients at risk, with or without an oral lead-in with cabotegravir**

Adults and adolescents age 12 and older weighing at least 35 kg: Initially, 600 mg IM on the last day of or within 3 days after oral lead-in therapy (if used), followed by a second injection 1 month later. Continue with injections every 2 months thereafter.

ADMINISTRATION

Boxed Warning Don't initiate drug for PrEP unless negative infection status is confirmed. ▪

PO
- Give at same time each day with food.
- Give missed dose as soon as possible.
- Store tablets below 86° F (30° C).

IM
- Drug is provided in a kit with vial adapter, needle, and syringe.
- Allow vial to reach room temperature if stored in refrigerator.
- Inspect for particulate matter and discoloration. Discard if present.
- Shake vial vigorously until suspension appears uniform. Small air bubbles are expected and acceptable.
- Give as soon as possible. Suspension may remain in syringe for up to 2 hours. After 2 hours, discard drug and syringe. Don't refrigerate filled syringe.
- Inject into ventrogluteal area (preferred); dorsogluteal area (upper outer quadrant) is also acceptable.
- May need longer needle lengths sufficient to reach gluteus muscle for patients with BMI greater than 30 kg/m².
- May give injection up to 7 days before or after the date patient is to receive the injection.
- If patient plans to miss a scheduled every-2-month injection by more than 7 days, give oral cabotegravir bridge doses.
- If injection is missed or delayed more than 7 days and oral therapy hasn't been given, reassess patient to determine if resumption of injection dosing remains appropriate. Refer to manufacturer's instructions for recommendations on repeated missed injections and time since prior injection.
- Store suspension at 36° to 77° F (2° to 25° C). Don't freeze.

ACTION
Inhibits HIV integrase by binding to the integrase active site and blocking the strand transfer step of retroviral DNA integration.

Route	Onset	Peak	Duration
PO	Unknown	3 hr	Unknown
IM	Unknown	7 days	Unknown

Half-life: PO, 41 hours; IM, 5.6 to 11.5 weeks.

ADVERSE REACTIONS
CNS: abnormal dreams, asthenia, depressive disorders, dizziness, fatigue, fever, headache, mood swings, sleep disorder, somnolence. **GI:** abdominal pain, decreased appetite, diarrhea, flatulence, nausea, vomiting. **Hepatic:** *hepatotoxicity.* **Musculoskeletal:** back pain, myalgia. **Respiratory:** URI. **Other:** injection-site reactions, *suicidality.*

INTERACTIONS
Drug-drug. *Antacids containing aluminum, calcium carbonate, or magnesium:* May decrease oral cabotegravir level. Administer antacids at least 2 hours before or 4 hours after cabotegravir.

Methadone: May decrease methadone level. Monitor patient and adjust methadone dosage as needed.

Other antiretrovirals: Avoid use of other antiretrovirals with cabotegravir when used as monotherapy for PrEP or in combination with rilpivirine for treatment of HIV-1.

Rifabutin: May decrease cabotegravir level when given with extended-release injection. If used concomitantly, give the second injection of extended-release cabotegravir 2 weeks after initial dose, and give maintenance doses monthly while patient is receiving rifabutin.

Strong inducers of UGT1A1 or UGT1A9 (carbamazepine, oxcarbazepine, phenobarbital, phenytoin, rifampin, rifapentine): May significantly decrease cabotegravir level and cause loss of virologic response. Avoid use together.

EFFECTS ON LAB TEST RESULTS
- May increase AST, ALT, lipase, creatinine, fasting lipid, and CK levels.
- May decrease HDL level.

CONTRAINDICATIONS & CAUTIONS
- Contraindicated in patients hypersensitive to drug or its components.
- Contraindicated for PrEP in patients with unknown or positive HIV-1 status. Monotherapy with drug isn't a complete regimen for HIV-1 treatment.
- Time from initiation of HIV-1 PrEP to maximal protection is unknown.

Boxed Warning Risk of drug resistance may occur with use for HIV PrEP in patients with undiagnosed HIV-1 infection. Drug-resistant variants have been identified in patients with undiagnosed HIV-1 infections with use of cabotegravir injections. ▪

NEW DRUGS

- Serious or severe hypersensitivity reactions may occur with cabotegravir. Discontinue drug if hypersensitivity reactions occur.
- Drug may cause hepatotoxicity in patients with or without known preexisting hepatic disease or other risk factors. Use cautiously in patients with underlying hepatic disease or marked transaminase elevations before drug initiation.
- Residual extended-release formulation of drug may remain in circulation for 12 months or longer.
- Use cautiously in older adults and patients with severe or end-stage renal disease. Use in patients with severe hepatic impairment hasn't been studied.
- Safety and efficacy haven't been established with cabotegravir for treatment of HIV-1 infection in children, and for HIV-1 PrEP in children younger than age 12 or weighing less than 35 kg.
Dialyzable drug: Unlikely.

PREGNANCY-LACTATION-REPRODUCTION
- There are no studies during pregnancy. Cabotegravir injections aren't recommended for use in patients planning to become pregnant. Consider risks and benefits of therapy in patients of childbearing potential or who are pregnant.
- Enroll patients exposed to drug during pregnancy in the Antiretroviral Pregnancy Registry (1-800-258-4263).
- It isn't known if drug appears in human milk or how drug affects milk production or infants who are breastfed.
- Breastfeeding isn't recommended in patients who are HIV positive. For uninfected patients taking drug for PrEP, assess risks and benefits of therapy during breastfeeding. Extended-release formulation may appear in human milk 12 months or more after discontinuing drug.

NURSING CONSIDERATIONS
Boxed Warning Before starting drug (oral or IM) for PrEP and before each subsequent injection, test for HIV-1 infection using an FDA-approved or -cleared test for the diagnosis of acute primary HIV-1 infection. Patients who become infected with HIV-1 while receiving injections for PrEP must transition to a complete HIV-1 therapy regimen. ∎
- Evaluate patient for potential exposure events and signs and symptoms of acute HIV-1 infection. Test patient for HIV-1 infection if diagnosed with other sexually transmitted infections (STIs).
- Monitor patient for signs and symptoms of hypersensitivity reactions (severe rash or rash accompanied by fever; general malaise; fatigue; muscle or joint aches; blisters including oral blisters or lesions; conjunctivitis; facial edema; hepatitis; eosinophilia; angioedema; difficulty breathing); discontinue drug immediately if these occur.
- Monitor LFT values during therapy and as clinically indicated. Discontinue cabotegravir if hepatotoxicity is suspected.

- Monitor patient for depressive symptoms, and promptly evaluate for relation to cabotegravir.
- Refer to rilpivirine's prescribing information if rilpivirine is used with cabotegravir.

PATIENT TEACHING
- Inform patient taking cabotegravir for PrEP that it's part of an overall HIV-1 infection prevention strategy, including adherence to dosing schedule and safer sex practices, including condoms, to reduce the risk of STIs.
- Tell patient taking cabotegravir for PrEP that testing for HIV-1 is needed before therapy, before each injection, and if patient has been diagnosed with other STIs.
- Inform patient that drug isn't always effective in preventing HIV-1 infection.
- Advise patient to contact prescriber immediately if experiencing signs and symptoms of hypersensitivity reaction (severe rash, rash with fever, tiredness, muscle or joint aches, blisters, facial swelling, difficulty breathing, liver problems).
- Inform patient that LFT values will be monitored during therapy.
- Tell patient to promptly report depressive symptoms to prescriber.
- Advise patient to follow testing schedule, take drug as prescribed, and avoid missed doses as doing so increases the risk of acquiring HIV-1 infection and developing drug resistance.
- Advise patient of childbearing potential to report pregnancy or plans to become pregnant or breastfeed.

daridorexant
dar-i-doe-REX-ant

Quviviq

Therapeutic class: Hypnotics
Pharmacologic class: Orexin receptor antagonists
Controlled substance schedule: IV

AVAILABLE FORMS
Tablets: 25 mg, 50 mg

INDICATIONS & DOSAGES
➤ **Insomnia characterized by difficulties with sleep onset or sleep maintenance**
Adults: 25 to 50 mg PO nightly.
Adjust-a-dose: In patients with moderate hepatic impairment (Child Pugh score 7 to 9) or when drug is used concomitantly with moderate CYP3A4 inhibitor, maximum dose is 25 mg once nightly.

ADMINISTRATION
PO
- Give within 30 minutes of bedtime; ensure at least 7 hours remain before planned time of awakening.

NEW DRUGS

• May delay sleep onset if drug is given with or soon after a meal.
• Store tablets at 68° to 77° F (20° to 25°C).

ACTION
Blocks orexin receptors, suppressing the system responsible for promoting wakefulness.

Route	Onset	Peak	Duration
PO	Unknown	1–2 hr	Unknown

Half-life: 8 hours.

ADVERSE REACTIONS
CNS: fatigue, headache, somnolence. **GI:** nausea.

INTERACTIONS
Drug-drug. *CNS depressants (alprazolam, oxycodone):* May increase risk of CNS depression. Adjust daridorexant or CNS depressant dosage to limit additive effects.
Strong and moderate CYP3A4 inducers (efavirenz, phenytoin, rifampin): May decrease daridorexant level. Avoid use together.
Strong or moderate CYP3A4 inhibitors (clarithromycin, diltiazem, itraconazole): May increase daridorexant level and risk of adverse reactions. Avoid use with strong CYP3A4 inhibitors. Decrease daridorexant dosage to 25 mg once nightly with use of moderate CYP3A4 inhibitors.
Drug-food. *High-caloric, high-fat meals:* May delay sleep onset. Patient should avoid ingesting drug with or soon after a meal.
Drug-lifestyle. *Alcohol use:* May increase CNS depression. Discourage use together.

EFFECTS ON LAB TEST RESULTS
None reported.

CONTRAINDICATIONS & CAUTIONS
• Contraindicated in patients with narcolepsy.
• Use in patients with severe hepatic impairment isn't recommended.
• Use cautiously in patients with psychiatric disorders; drug may worsen depression or suicidality.
• Use cautiously in patients with a history of abuse of or addiction to alcohol or other substances.
• Use cautiously in patients with compromised respiratory function (obstructive sleep apnea, COPD).
• Use cautiously in older adults.
• Safety and effectiveness in children haven't been established.
• Drug can cause sleep paralysis, hallucinations, and cataplexy-like symptoms (periods of leg weakness lasting from seconds to a few minutes that may not be associated with an identified triggering event [laughter or surprise]).
Dialyzable drug: Unlikely.
⚠ Overdose S&S: Somnolence, muscle weakness, cataplexy-like symptoms, sleep paralysis, disturbance in attention, fatigue, headache, constipation.

PREGNANCY-LACTATION-REPRODUCTION
• There are no studies during pregnancy.
• Enroll patients exposed to drug during pregnancy in the pregnancy exposure registry (1-833-400-9611).
• It isn't known if drug appears in human milk or how drug affects milk production or infants who are breastfed. Drug was detected in animal milk studies.
• Before initiating breastfeeding, consider the patient's clinical need and risk to the infant. Monitor infant who is breastfed for excessive sedation.

NURSING CONSIDERATIONS
• Evaluate patient for comorbid diseases as the cause of insomnia before starting drug or if insomnia persists after 7 to 10 days of treatment.
• Monitor patient for sleep paralysis, hallucinations, cataplexy-like symptoms, and complex sleep behaviors (sleepwalking; sleep-driving; engaging in activities while not fully awake, including preparing and eating food, making phone calls, having sex). Discontinue drug if complex sleep behaviors occur.
• Monitor patient for worsening insomnia or the emergence of new cognitive or behavioral abnormalities and report these changes to prescriber. Abnormalities may be related to unrecognized underlying psychiatric or medical disorders and may become evident during therapy.
• Monitor respiratory status as clinically indicated.

PATIENT TEACHING
• Instruct patient about proper drug administration and storage.
• Tell patient and family to alert prescriber if adverse effects occur.
• **⊕ Alert:** Caution patient to immediately report suicidality or new behavioral signs or symptoms.
• Warn patient not to increase dose unless directed by prescriber.
• Tell patient about risk of decreased awareness and alertness. Warn patient to avoid performing activities that require mental alertness or physical coordination (such as driving or operating heavy machinery) until fully awake.
• Inform patient and family about the risk of sleep paralysis, hallucinations, and complex sleep behaviors.
• Tell patient to contact prescriber if insomnia worsens or hasn't improved within 7 to 10 days after starting drug.
• Warn patient to avoid alcohol while taking drug.
• Instruct patient of childbearing potential to report pregnancy or plans to become pregnant or to breastfeed.

Reactions in bold italics are *life-threatening*. Interactions may have a *rapid onset* or a **delayed onset**.

difelikefalin
dye-fel-i-KEF-a-lin

Korsuva

Therapeutic class: Miscellaneous CNS drugs
Pharmacologic class: Kappa opioid receptor agonists

AVAILABLE FORMS
Injection: 65 mcg/1.3 mL (50 mcg/mL)

INDICATIONS & DOSAGES
➤ **Moderate to severe pruritus associated with chronic kidney disease in patients on hemodialysis**
Adults: 0.5 mcg/kg IV bolus injection at end of each hemodialysis treatment.

ADMINISTRATION
IV

▼ Don't mix or dilute before administration.
▼ Inspect for particulate matter and discoloration; solution should be clear and colorless.
▼ Give as bolus injection into venous line of dialysis circuit at the end of hemodialysis treatment during or after rinse back. If given after rinse back, follow with 10 mL saline flush. If given during rinse back, additional saline flush isn't needed.
▼ Give dose within 60 minutes of syringe preparation.
▼ Store prepared syringes and vials at 68° to 77° F (20° to 25° C). Don't freeze.
▼ Discard unused drug.
▼ If patient misses a regularly scheduled hemodialysis treatment, don't give missed dose. Resume at end of next hemodialysis session.

ACTION
Exact mechanism is unknown.

Route	Onset	Peak	Duration
IV	Unknown	Unknown	Unknown

Half-life: 23 to 31 hours.

ADVERSE REACTIONS
CNS: dizziness, gait disturbances, headache, mental status change, somnolence. **GI:** diarrhea, nausea. **Metabolic:** *hyperkalemia*.

INTERACTIONS
Drug-drug. *CNS depressants, opioids, sedating antihistamines:* May increase risk of CNS adverse reactions. Use together cautiously.

EFFECTS ON LAB TEST RESULTS
• May increase potassium level.

CONTRAINDICATIONS & CAUTIONS
• Drug isn't recommended for patients with severe hepatic impairment or for those on peritoneal dialysis.
• Safety and effectiveness in children haven't been established.
Dialyzable drug: Yes.
⚠ **Overdose S&S:** Dizziness, somnolence, mental status changes, paresthesia, fatigue, hypertension, vomiting.

PREGNANCY-LACTATION-REPRODUCTION
• There are no studies during pregnancy. Use only if clearly needed.
• It isn't known if drug appears in human milk or how drug affects milk production or infants who are breastfed. Consider patient's clinical need and risks to infant.

NURSING CONSIDERATIONS
• Monitor patient for CNS adverse reactions, including dizziness, somnolence (especially in older adults), mental status changes, gait disturbances, and falls.

PATIENT TEACHING
• Warn patient about risk of CNS adverse effects.
• Tell patient not to drive or operate machinery until drug's effects are known.

ganaxolone 🧬
gan-AXE-oh-lone

Ztalmy

Therapeutic class: Anticonvulsants
Pharmacologic class: Neuroactive steroid GABA-A receptor modulators
Controlled substance schedule: V

AVAILABLE FORMS
Oral suspension: 50 mg/mL

INDICATIONS & DOSAGES
➤ **Seizures associated with cyclin-dependent kinase-like 5 deficiency disorder** 🧬
Patients age 2 and older weighing 29 kg or more:
Initially, 150 mg PO t.i.d. (450 mg daily). Titrate to 300 mg t.i.d., then 450 mg t.i.d. to maximum dose of 600 mg t.i.d. (1,800 mg daily) based on tolerability. Titrate no more frequently than every 7 days.
Patients age 2 and older weighing 28 kg or less:
Initially, 6 mg/kg PO t.i.d. (18 mg/kg/day). Titrate to 11 mg/kg t.i.d., then 16 mg/kg t.i.d. to maximum dose of 21 mg/kg t.i.d. (63 mg/kg/daily) based on tolerability.
Adjust-a-dose: When discontinuing drug, reduce dosage gradually to minimize risk of increased seizure frequency and status epilepticus. Monitor patients with hepatic impairment for adverse reactions; reduce dosage as needed.

ADMINISTRATION
PO
• Shake bottle for 1 minute, then wait 1 minute before measuring and giving drug.
• Use oral syringe(s) provided to measure dose. Don't use household spoon.
• Give with food.
• Store upright in original bottle at 59° to 86° F (15° to 30° C). Keep bottle tightly closed.
• Discard unused drug 30 days after opening or by the "Discard After" date on the bottle, whichever is sooner.

ACTION
Unknown. Thought to result from positive allosteric modulation of the GABA type A receptor in the CNS.

Route	Onset	Peak	Duration
PO	Unknown	2–3 hr	Unknown

Half-life: 34 hours.

ADVERSE REACTIONS
CNS: fever, *seizures*, somnolence, sedation. **EENT:** nasal congestion. **GI:** salivary hypersecretion. **Musculoskeletal:** gait disturbance. **Respiratory:** bronchitis, URI. **Other:** flulike syndrome, seasonal allergy.

INTERACTIONS
Drug-drug. *CNS depressants (antidepressants, opioids):* May cause somnolence and sedation. Use cautiously together.
Strong or moderate CYP450 inducers (antiepileptic drugs [carbamazepine, phenobarbital, phenytoin, primidone], rifampin): May decrease ganaxolone level. Avoid use together. If use together unavoidable, consider increasing ganaxolone dosage; don't exceed maximum daily dose. May need to increase ganaxolone dosage in patients on stable ganaxolone dose who are starting or increasing enzyme-inducing antiepileptic drug doses; don't exceed maximum daily dose.
Drug-lifestyle. *Alcohol use:* May increase somnolence and sedation. Discourage use together.

EFFECTS ON LAB TEST RESULTS
None reported.

CONTRAINDICATIONS & CAUTIONS
• Use cautiously in patients with hepatic impairment or depression.
🜂 *Alert:* Drug may increase risk of suicidality as soon as first week of treatment.
• Drug has potential for abuse. Don't abruptly discontinue antiepileptic drugs due to risk of seizures.
• Safety and effectiveness in children younger than age 2 haven't been established.
Dialyzable drug: Unknown.

PREGNANCY-LACTATION-REPRODUCTION
• There are no adequate studies during pregnancy.
• Enroll patient exposed to drug during pregnancy in the pregnancy exposure registry (1-888-233-2334 or https://www.aedpregnancyregistry.org/).
• Drug appears in human milk. It isn't known how drug affects milk production or infant who is breastfed. Use cautiously during breastfeeding.

NURSING CONSIDERATIONS
• Monitor patient for somnolence and sedation.
🜂 *Alert:* Avoid abruptly discontinuing drug.
🜂 *Alert:* Monitor patient for emergence or worsening of depression, suicidality, or unusual changes in mood or behavior.
• Monitor patient for potential drug abuse or dependence. Taper drug as recommended, unless symptoms warrant immediate discontinuation.
• Monitor patient with hepatic impairment for adverse reactions.
• *Look alike-sound alike:* Don't confuse ganaxolone with oxandrolone or gabapentin, or Ztalmy with Xtandi.

PATIENT TEACHING
• Instruct patient and caregiver about proper drug administration and storage.
• Tell patient that drug may cause somnolence. Caution patient not to drink alcohol, drive, or operate heavy machinery until drug's effects are known.
🜂 *Alert:* Instruct patient to avoid abrupt discontinuation of drug.
🜂 *Alert:* Warn patient and family that drug may increase risk of suicidality. Advise patient to report emergence or worsening of depression, suicidality, and unusual changes in mood or behavior.
• Advise patient about risk of abuse and dependence during therapy.
• Advise patient to report pregnancy or plans to become pregnant during therapy.

inclisiran ⌧
in-kli-SIR-an

Leqvio

Therapeutic class: Antilipemics
Pharmacologic class: Proprotein convertase subtilisin/kexin type 9 (PCSK9) mRNA inhibitors

AVAILABLE FORMS
Injection: 284 mg/1.5 mL (189 mg/mL) prefilled syringe

INDICATIONS & DOSAGES
➤ **Adjunct to diet and maximally tolerated statin therapy for the treatment of heterozygous familial hypercholesterolemia or clinical atherosclerotic CV**

NEW DRUGS

disease in patients who require additional lowering of LDL cholesterol ▧

Adults: 284 mg subcut for one dose. Repeat dose at 3 months, then every 6 months thereafter.

ADMINISTRATION
Subcutaneous
• Inspect solution before use. Solution is clear and colorless to pale yellow. Don't use if particulate matter or discoloration is present.
• Inject subcut into abdomen, upper arm, or thigh. Avoid areas of active skin disease or injury.
• If dose is missed by less than 3 months, give dose and maintain original dosing schedule. If missed dose is beyond 3 months, give dose and start a new schedule based on this date.
• Store at 59° to 86° F (15° to 30° C).

ACTION
Targets PCSK9 mRNA, which increases the breakdown of LDL receptors and results in lower LDL cholesterol levels in the blood.

Route	Onset	Peak	Duration
Subcut	Unknown	4 hr	Unknown

Half-life: 9 hours.

ADVERSE REACTIONS
GI: diarrhea. **GU:** UTI. **Musculoskeletal:** arthralgia, extremity pain. **Respiratory:** bronchitis, dyspnea. **Skin:** injection-site reactions (pain, erythema, rash).

INTERACTIONS
None.

EFFECTS ON LAB TEST RESULTS
None.

CONTRAINDICATIONS & CAUTIONS
• Use in patients with ESRD or severe hepatic impairment hasn't been studied.
• Drug's effect on CV morbidity and mortality hasn't been established.
• Safety and effectiveness in children haven't been established.
Dialyzable drug: Unknown.

PREGNANCY-LACTATION-REPRODUCTION
• There are no adequate studies during pregnancy. Drug may cause fetal harm.
• Discontinue drug if pregnancy occurs.
• It isn't known if drug appears in human milk or how drug affects milk production or infants who are breastfed. Before initiating breastfeeding, consider the patient's clinical need and risk to the infant.

NURSING CONSIDERATIONS
• Monitor LDL level periodically, beginning as early as 30 days after drug initiation.

PATIENT TEACHING
• Instruct patient of childbearing potential to report pregnancy or plans to become pregnant during therapy.
• Advise patient that injection-site reactions can occur.

maralixibat
mar-a-LIX-i-bat

Livmarli

Therapeutic class: Miscellaneous GI drugs
Pharmacologic class: Ileal bile acid transporter inhibitors

AVAILABLE FORMS
Oral solution: 9.5 mg/mL

INDICATIONS & DOSAGES
➤ **Cholestatic pruritus in patients with Alagille syndrome**
Adults and children age 1 and older: Initially, 190 mcg/kg PO once daily. After 1 week, increase dosage to 380 mcg/kg once daily as tolerated. Maximum dose is 28.5 mg (3 mL) daily in patients weighing 70 kg or more.
Adjust-a-dose: Decrease dosage or interrupt therapy for LFT abnormalities or GI adverse reactions. When LFT values return to baseline or stabilize at new baseline values, consider restarting at 190 mcg/kg and increase as tolerated. If LFT abnormalities or GI reactions recur, or signs and symptoms consistent with clinical hepatitis, portal HTN, or hepatic decompensation (variceal hemorrhage, ascites, hepatic encephalopathy) occur, discontinue therapy.

ADMINISTRATION
PO
• Give 30 minutes before first meal of the day.
• Use supplied measuring device (0.5 mL, 1 mL, or 3 mL) to measure and deliver dose.
• If a dose is missed, give as soon as possible within 12 hours of the regular time and resume normal schedule next day. If a dose is missed by more than 12 hours, skip dose and resume normal schedule next day.
• Store at 68° to 77° F (20° to 25° C).
• Discard drug if not used within 45 days after opening bottle.

ACTION
Reversible inhibitor of ileal bile acid transporter (IBAT) that decreases reabsorption of bile acids from the terminal ileum. The mechanism that improves pruritus is unknown, but it may involve inhibition of IBAT.

NEW DRUGS

Route	Onset	Peak	Duration
PO	Unknown	45 min	Unknown

Half-life: 1.6 hours.

ADVERSE REACTIONS

GI: abdominal pain, diarrhea, GI bleeding, nausea, vomiting. **Hepatic:** elevated LFT values. **Metabolic:** fat-soluble vitamin (FSV) deficiency. **Musculoskeletal:** fracture.

INTERACTIONS

Drug-drug. *Bile acid binding resins (cholestyramine, colesevelam, colestipol):* May bind maralixibat in the gut. Give binding resin 4 hours before or 4 hours after maralixibat.
OATP2B1 substrates (statins): May decrease absorption of OATP2B1 substrate. Monitor effect of the substrate.

EFFECTS ON LAB TEST RESULTS

• May increase ALT, AST, and bilirubin levels.
• May decrease FSV (A, D, E, and K) levels.
• May increase INR.

CONTRAINDICATIONS & CAUTIONS

• Safety and effectiveness in patients with clinically significant portal HTN or decompensated cirrhosis haven't been established.
• Safety and effectiveness in patients younger than age 1 or older than age 65 haven't been established.
Dialyzable drug: Unlikely.
⚠ *Overdose S&S:* From propylene glycol component of drug: CNS, CV, or respiratory effects; hyperosmolality.

PREGNANCY-LACTATION-REPRODUCTION

• Maternal use isn't expected to result in measurable fetal exposure because systemic absorption is low.
• It isn't known if drug appears in human milk or how drug affects milk production or infants who are breastfed. Use of drug at recommended dose isn't expected to result in infant exposure during breastfeeding.
• Increased maternal FSV supplementation during pregnancy and lactation may be necessary.

NURSING CONSIDERATIONS

• Obtain LFT values at baseline and monitor during therapy.
• Monitor patient for persistent diarrhea or diarrhea accompanied by bloody stool, vomiting, dehydration requiring treatment, and fever.
• If diarrhea or vomiting occurs, monitor patient for dehydration and treat promptly.
• Monitor serum FSV levels (vitamins A, D, E, K [measured using INR]) at baseline and during therapy. Observe patient for clinical manifestations of deficiency. Give FSV supplement if deficiency is diagnosed. Stop drug if deficiency persists or worsens despite supplementation.

PATIENT TEACHING

• Teach patient proper drug administration and storage.
• Instruct patient to contact prescriber if new-onset or worsening abdominal pain, vomiting, diarrhea, or dehydration occurs.
• Inform patient of need for blood tests to check liver function before and during therapy. Tell patient to report nausea, vomiting, yellowing of skin or whites of eyes, dark or brown urine, pain on right side of abdomen, or loss of appetite.
• Caution patient that drug may impair absorption of FSVs (A, D, E, and K). Explain need for lab testing before and periodically during therapy to monitor patient for development or worsening of FSV deficiency.

SAFETY ALERT!

maribavir ⬚
ma-RYE-ba-vir

Livtencity

Therapeutic class: Antivirals
Pharmacologic class: Kinase inhibitors

AVAILABLE FORMS

Tablets: 200 mg

INDICATIONS & DOSAGES

➤ **Posttransplant CMV infection or disease that's refractory to treatment with ganciclovir, valganciclovir, cidofovir, or foscarnet**
Adults and children age 12 and older weighing at least 35 kg: 400 mg PO b.i.d.
Adjust-a-dose: If drug is used concomitantly with carbamazepine, increase maribavir to 800 mg PO b.i.d. If used concomitantly with phenytoin or phenobarbital, increase maribavir to 1,200 mg PO b.i.d.

ADMINISTRATION

PO
• Give without regard for food.
• Store at 68° to 77° F (20° to 25° C).

ACTION

Inhibits protein kinase activity of CMV enzyme, which inhibits human CMV replication.

Route	Onset	Peak	Duration
PO	Unknown	1–3 hr	Unknown

Half-life: 4.32 hours in transplant patients.

ADVERSE REACTIONS

CNS: fatigue, taste disturbance. **GI:** diarrhea, nausea, vomiting. **GU:** *acute kidney injury.* **Hematologic:** anemia, *neutropenia.* **Other:** *recurrence of underlying CMV infection or disease.*

Reactions in bold italics are *life-threatening*. Interactions may have a *rapid onset* or a **delayed onset.**

INTERACTIONS

Drug-drug. *Carbamazepine, phenytoin, phenobarbital:* May decrease maribavir level. If taken concomitantly, increase maribavir dose.

Cyclosporine, everolimus, sirolimus, tacrolimus: May increase concentration of immunosuppressant. Monitor patient for increased drug level and adverse effects. Adjust immunosuppressant dosage as needed.

Digoxin: May increase digoxin level. Monitor digoxin level and adjust digoxin as needed.

Ganciclovir, valganciclovir: May decrease viral activity of these drugs. Avoid use together.

Rifabutin, rifampin: May decrease maribavir efficacy. Avoid use together.

Rosuvastatin: May increase statin concentration. Monitor patient closely for adverse effects, especially myopathy and rhabdomyolysis.

Strong CYP3A4 inducers (except carbamazepine, phenytoin, phenobarbital): May decrease maribavir level. Avoid use together.

Substrates of CYP3A, P-gp, and BCRP (cimetidine, fexofenadine, glyburide, midazolam): May increase substrate concentration. Avoid use together.

Drug-herb. *St. John's wort:* May decrease maribavir efficacy. Discourage use together.

EFFECTS ON LAB TEST RESULTS

- May increase creatinine level.
- May decrease Hb level and WBC and platelet counts.

CONTRAINDICATIONS & CAUTIONS

▨ Virologic failure due to resistance can occur during and after therapy, usually within 4 to 8 weeks after stopping drug.
- Safety and effectiveness in children younger than age 12 and weighing less than 35 kg haven't been established.

Dialyzable drug: Unlikely.

PREGNANCY-LACTATION-REPRODUCTION

- There are no adequate studies during pregnancy.
- It isn't known if drug appears in human milk or how drug affects milk production or infants who are breastfed. Before initiating breastfeeding, consider patient's clinical need and risk to the infant.

NURSING CONSIDERATIONS

- Monitor patient for drug interactions and drug levels per manufacturer's guidelines.
- Monitor patient for treatment failure. Assess CMV DNA levels and check for maribavir resistance if patient isn't responding to therapy or experiences relapse.

PATIENT TEACHING

- Instruct patient of childbearing potential to report pregnancy or plans to become pregnant during therapy.

- Instruct patient to inform prescriber if taking other prescription and OTC medications, herbs, and supplements, especially if taking medication for seizures.

---

mavacamten ▨
mav-a-KAM-ten

Camzyos

Therapeutic class: HF drugs
Pharmacologic class: Cardiac myosin inhibitors

AVAILABLE FORMS

Capsules: 2.5 mg, 5 mg, 10 mg, 15 mg

INDICATIONS & DOSAGES

➤ **Symptomatic NYHA Class II to III obstructive hypertrophic cardiomyopathy to improve functional capacity and symptoms**

Adults: Initially, 5 mg PO daily. Individualize dose based on patient's clinical status and echocardiographic assessment. Subsequent doses after titration may be 2.5, 5, 10, or 15 mg once daily. See manufacturer's instructions for initiation and maintenance dose algorithms based on LVEF and Valsalva left ventricular outflow tract assessments.

Adjust-a-dose: For patients on stable therapy with a weak CYP2C19 or moderate CYP3A4 inhibitor, start mavacamten at 5 mg PO once daily. For patients starting a weak CYP2C19 or moderate CYP3A4 inhibitor during therapy, reduce mavacamten dose by one level (15 mg to 10 mg; 10 mg to 5 mg; or 5 mg to 2.5 mg). Don't initiate concomitant weak CYP2C19 or moderate CYP3A4 inhibitors in patients on stable mavacamten 2.5 mg daily because a lower mavacamten dose isn't available.

ADMINISTRATION

PO
- Give without regard to food.
- Patient must swallow capsules whole; don't allow patient to break, open, or chew capsules.
- Give a missed dose as soon as possible that day; then give next dose at the usual time on the following day. Don't give two doses in the same day.
- Store at 38° to 77° F (20° to 25° C).

ACTION

Inhibits cardiac myosin, reduces dynamic left ventricular outflow tract obstruction, and improves cardiac filling pressures.

Route	Onset	Peak	Duration
PO	Unknown	1 hr	Unknown

Half-life: ▨ 6 days (normal CYP2C19 metabolizers) to 23 days (poor CYP2C19 metabolizers).

NEW DRUGS

ADVERSE REACTIONS
CNS: dizziness, syncope. **CV:** *HF,* reduced LVEF.

INTERACTIONS
Drug-drug. *Cimetidine:* May increase mavacamten level. Use together cautiously.

CYP2C8 (repaglinide), CYP2C9 (tolbutamide), CYP2C19 (omeprazole), CYP3A4 (midazolam, repaglinide) substrates: May reduce substrate levels. Monitor substrate levels.

Diltiazem with a beta blocker, disopyramide; ranolazine; verapamil with a beta blocker: Use with mavacamten hasn't been studied. Avoid use together.

Disopyramide with verapamil or diltiazem: May cause left ventricular dysfunction and HF in patients with obstructive hypertrophic cardiomyopathy. Avoid use together.

Hormonal contraceptives (ethinyl estradiol, progestin): May decrease ethinyl estradiol and progestin levels, leading to contraceptive failure or breakthrough bleeding. Patient should use contraceptive method unaffected by CYP450 enzyme induction (intrauterine system) or add nonhormonal contraceptives (condoms) during therapy and for 4 months after final dose.

Boxed Warning *Moderate to strong CYP2C19 or CYP3A4 inducers (rifampin):* May decrease mavacamten level and efficacy. Avoid use together. ■

Boxed Warning *Moderate to strong CYP2C19 inhibitors:* May increase mavacamten level and risk of HF. Avoid use together. ■

Negative inotropes (beta blockers, diltiazem, verapamil): May have additive effects. If concomitant use is unavoidable, monitor LVEF closely when initiating or increasing negative inotrope dosage until stable doses and clinical response are achieved.

Boxed Warning *Strong CYP3A4 inhibitors (ketoconazole):* May increase mavacamten level and risk of HF due to systolic dysfunction. Avoid use together. ■

Weak CYP2C19 inhibitors (esomeprazole, omeprazole), moderate CYP3A4 inhibitors (ciprofloxacin, cyclosporine): May increase mavacamten level. Adjust mavacamten dosage.

Drug-herb. *St. John's wort:* May decrease mavacamten level and effectiveness. Discourage use together.

Drug-food. *Grapefruit juice:* May increase mavacamten level and drug adverse effects. Discourage use together.

EFFECTS ON LAB TEST RESULTS
None reported.

CONTRAINDICATIONS & CAUTIONS
• Contraindicated in patients hypersensitive to drug or its components.

Boxed Warning Contraindicated with concomitant use of moderate to strong CYP2C19 inhibitors, strong CYP3A4 inhibitors, moderate to strong CYP2C19 inducers, or moderate to strong CYP3A4 inducers. ■

Boxed Warning Drug can cause HF due to systolic dysfunction. ■

Boxed Warning Echocardiogram assessments of LVEF are required before and during mavacamten use. ■

Boxed Warning Initiation in patients with LVEF less than 55% isn't recommended. Interrupt therapy if LVEF falls below 50% or if clinical status worsens. ■

• Consider interrupting therapy in patients with intercurrent illness because of possible exacerbation of cardiac symptoms.

• Safety and effectiveness in children haven't been established.

• Use cautiously in older adults.

Boxed Warning Because of the risk of systolic dysfunction and HF, drug is only available through the Camzyos REMS program. ■

Dialyzable drug: Unlikely.

⚠ **Overdose S&S:** Vasovagal reaction, hypotension, asystole, systolic dysfunction (dyspnea, edema, fatigue, dizziness, cough, wheezing).

PREGNANCY-LACTATION-REPRODUCTION
• Based on animal studies, drug may cause fetal harm.

• Patients of childbearing potential must use effective contraception during therapy and for 4 months after final dose.

• Patients using hormonal contraceptives should use additional or alternative contraceptive methods.

• Report pregnancies that occur during therapy to the Bristol Myers Squibb pregnancy outcomes study (1-800-721-5072 or www.bms.com).

• It isn't known if drug appears in human milk or how drug affects milk production or infants who are breastfed. Consider patient's clinical need and risk to the infant.

NURSING CONSIDERATIONS
• Verify pregnancy status before start of therapy.

• Daily dosing takes weeks to reach steady-state drug levels and therapeutic effects.

• Assess patient's clinical status and LVEF at baseline and at 4, 8, and 12 weeks during initiation phase, every 12 weeks during maintenance phase, and as clinically indicated. Adjust dosage according to manufacturer's algorithms.

• Schedule echocardiogram and clinical assessments 4 weeks after initiation of a CYP inhibitor; don't titrate up the mavacamten dose until 12 weeks after inhibitor initiation.

• Closely monitor patient for serious intercurrent illness (serious infection) or arrhythmia (atrial fibrillation or other uncontrolled tachyarrhythmia) due to risk of developing systolic dysfunction and HF.

• Monitor patient for new or worsening arrhythmia, dyspnea, chest pain, fatigue, palpitations, leg edema, or elevations in N-terminal pro B-type natriuretic peptide as these signs and symptoms

---

Reactions in bold italics are *life-threatening*. Interactions may have a *rapid onset* or a **delayed onset**.

may indicate HF and require prompt evaluation of cardiac function.

Consider pharmacogenomic evaluation to determine CYP2C19 poor metabolizers, as concentrations of drug may significantly increase.

PATIENT TEACHING

Alert: Advise patient of potential for drug interactions. Tell patient to report all prescription and OTC medications, herbal supplements, and vitamins taken before or during therapy.

• Tell patient that cardiac function assessment and echocardiography will be performed to monitor for HF. Tell patient to report signs or symptoms of HF immediately.

Boxed Warning Inform patient of the need to enroll in the drug's REMS program and the importance of adhering to monitoring requirements. ■

• Inform patient of childbearing potential to report known or suspected pregnancy.

• Advise patient of childbearing potential to use effective contraception during therapy and for 4 months after final dose.

• Counsel patient using hormonal contraceptive to use alternative or additional methods of contraception.

• Inform patient exposed to drug during pregnancy about the availability of a safety study that monitors pregnancy outcomes.

---

mitapivat
mye-ta-PIV-at

Pyrukynd

Therapeutic class: Hemolysis inhibitors
Pharmacologic class: Pyruvate kinase activators

AVAILABLE FORMS
Tablets : 5 mg, 20 mg, 50 mg

INDICATIONS & DOSAGES

➤ **Hemolytic anemia in patients with pyruvate kinase (PK) deficiency**

Adults: Initially, 5 mg PO b.i.d. for 4 weeks. If Hb level remains below normal range or patient required a transfusion within last 8 weeks, increase to 20 mg b.i.d. for 4 weeks. If Hb level remains below normal range or patient required a transfusion within last 8 weeks, increase to 50 mg b.i.d. If Hb level decreases during maintenance therapy of 5 or 20 mg b.i.d., consider titrating up to maximum of 50 mg b.i.d. Discontinue drug if no benefit is achieved by 24 weeks.

Adjust-a-dose: If using concomitantly with moderate CYP3A inhibitors, maximum mitapivat dose is 20 mg b.i.d. If using concomitantly with moderate CYP3A inducers, titrate mitapivat

beyond 50 mg b.i.d.; don't exceed maximum of 100 mg b.i.d.

For intolerability, Hb level above normal, or adverse reactions, reduce dosage to next lower dose level (20 mg b.i.d. or 5 mg b.i.d.). Taper dosage gradually to discontinue drug. If risk to patient is greater than risk of acute hemolysis due to sudden withdrawal of drug, stop drug without tapering.

ADMINISTRATION
PO
• Give without regard to food.
• Patient must swallow tablets whole. Don't allow patient to split, crush, dissolve, or chew tablets.
• If a dose is missed by less than 4 hours, give dose as soon as possible. If a dose is missed by more than 4 hours, skip missed dose and resume normal schedule.
• Store at 68° to 77° F (20° to 25° C). Store blister wallets in original carton until use.

ACTION
Binds to the PK tetramer and increases PK activity, which decreases hemolysis.

Route	Onset	Peak	Duration
PO	Unknown	30–60 min	Unknown

Half-life: 3 to 5 hours.

ADVERSE REACTIONS
CNS: paresthesia. **CV:** *arrhythmia,* flushing, hot flashes, HTN. **EENT:** dry mouth, oropharyngeal pain. **GI:** constipation, gastroenteritis. **Hematologic:** *acute hemolysis.* **Metabolic:** decreased estrone and estradiol levels (in males), increased testosterone level (in males), hypertriglyceridemia, increased urate level. **Musculoskeletal:** arthralgia, back pain, musculoskeletal pain. **Other:** breast discomfort.

INTERACTIONS
Drug-drug. *CYP2B6 substrates, CYP2C substrates, CYP3A substrates (hormonal contraceptives [ethinyl estradiol], midazolam), UGT1A1 substrates:* May decrease substrate level. Monitor patient for loss of therapeutic effect of substrates with narrow therapeutic index. Patient should use alternative nonhormonal contraceptive or add a barrier contraceptive.
Moderate CYP3A inducers (efavirenz): May decrease mitapivat level. Consider alternative therapy. If concomitant use is unavoidable, monitor Hb level and titrate mitapivat dosage.
Moderate CYP3A inhibitors (fluconazole): May increase mitapivat level and risk of adverse reactions. Monitor Hb level. Don't titrate mitapivat beyond 20 mg b.i.d.
P-gp substrates: May increase P-gp substrate level. Monitor patient for adverse reactions of P-gp substrates with narrow therapeutic index.

NEW DRUGS

🍁Canada ◆OTC ◇Off-label use *Photoguide ⓓDo not crush *Liquid contains alcohol Genetic

Strong CYP3A inducers (rifampin): May decrease mitapivat level. Avoid use together.

Strong CYP3A inhibitors (itraconazole): May increase mitapivat level and risk of adverse reactions. Avoid use together.

EFFECTS ON LAB TEST RESULTS
• May increase triglyceride and urate levels.
• May increase testosterone level in males.
• May decrease estrone and estradiol levels in males.
• May increase Hb level.

CONTRAINDICATIONS & CAUTIONS
• Avoid use in patients with moderate or severe hepatic impairment.
• Safety and effectiveness in children haven't been established.
Dialyzable drug: Unlikely.

PREGNANCY-LACTATION-REPRODUCTION
• There are no adequate studies during pregnancy. Use cautiously during pregnancy.
• Untreated PK deficiency during pregnancy may precipitate acute hemolysis, preterm labor, miscarriage, and severe anemia requiring frequent transfusion.
• Drug may reduce effectiveness of hormonal contraceptives.
• It isn't known if drug appears in human milk or how drug affects milk production or infants who are breastfed. Consider patient's clinical need and risk to the infant.

NURSING CONSIDERATIONS
• Avoid abrupt interruption or discontinuation of drug to avoid acute hemolysis. Taper dosage gradually and monitor patient for signs and symptoms of hemolysis (jaundice, scleral icterus, dark urine).
• Monitor Hb level periodically during therapy and before dosage increases.

PATIENT TEACHING
• Advise patient about safe drug administration.
⚠ *Alert:* Caution patient not to abruptly stop drug but to gradually taper dosage as instructed by prescriber. Tell patient to immediately report signs and symptoms of acute hemolysis (including jaundice, scleral icterus, dark urine, dizziness, confusion, fatigue, or shortness of breath).
• Tell patient to report all prescription and OTC medications and herbal products being taken.
• Inform patient taking hormonal contraceptives to use an alternative nonhormonal contraceptive method or to add a barrier method during therapy.

SAFETY ALERT!

mobocertinib ⬚
moe-boe-SER-ti-nib

Exkivity

Therapeutic class: Antineoplastics
Pharmacologic class: Kinase inhibitors

AVAILABLE FORMS
Capsules ⬚: 40 mg

INDICATIONS & DOSAGES
➤ **Locally advanced or metastatic NSCLC with *EGFR* exon 20 mutations, as detected by an FDA-approved test, with progression on or after platinum-based chemotherapy** ⬚
Adults: 160 mg PO daily until disease progression or unacceptable toxicity occurs.
Adjust-a-dose: See manufacturer's instructions for toxicity-related dosage adjustments. For patients unable to avoid taking a moderate CYP3A inhibitor, reduce mobocertinib dosage by approximately 50% and monitor QTc interval frequently. After moderate CYP3A inhibitor has been discontinued for 3 to 5 elimination half-lives, resume mobocertinib at dose taken before initiating CYP3A inhibitor.

ADMINISTRATION
PO
• Give at same time each day without regard to food.
• Patient must swallow capsule whole; don't allow patient to open, crush, or chew capsules.
• If a dose is missed by more than 6 hours, don't give missed dose; wait until next scheduled dose.
• If patient vomits after administration, don't give an additional dose but resume dosing at the next scheduled time.
• Store capsules at 68° to 77° F (20° to 25° C).

ACTION
Targets tumors by inhibiting cancer cell proliferation.

Route	Onset	Peak	Duration
PO	Unknown	4 hr	Unknown

Half-life: 18 hours.

ADVERSE REACTIONS
CNS: fatigue, fever, headache, peripheral neuropathy. **CV:** atrial fibrillation, edema, *HF*, HTN, *prolonged QT interval.* **EENT:** ocular toxicity. **GI:** abdominal pain, decreased appetite, diarrhea, dyspepsia, GERD, nausea, stomatitis, vomiting. **GU:** *acute kidney injury.* **Hematologic:** anemia, *leukocytopenia.* **Metabolic:** *hypokalemia; hypomagnesemia;* increased amylase, lipase, and creatinine levels; weight loss. **Musculoskeletal:** pain. **Respiratory:** cough, dyspnea, ILD, pleural

---

effusion, pneumonitis, rhinorrhea, URI. **Skin:** alopecia, dry skin, paronychia, pruritus, rash, palmar-plantar erythrodysesthesia.

INTERACTIONS

Drug-drug. *CYP3A substrates (midazolam):* May decrease substrate level. May increase substrate dosage if necessary.

Boxed Warning *Drugs that prolong the QTc interval (amiodarone, ciprofloxacin, haloperidol, lithium, methadone, procainamide, SSRIs, thioridazine, TCAs):* May significantly increase risk of QTc-interval prolongation. Avoid use together. If concomitant use can't be avoided, monitor QTc interval carefully. ■

Hormonal contraceptives: May decrease contraceptive level and cause therapeutic failure. Avoid use together.

Strong or moderate CYP3A inducers (efavirenz, rifampin): May decrease mobocertinib level and antitumor activity. Avoid use together.

Boxed Warning *Strong or moderate CYP3A inhibitors (itraconazole, ketoconazole):* May increase mobocertinib level. Avoid use together. If concomitant use can't be avoided, reduce mobocertinib dosage and monitor QTc interval more frequently with ECGs. Monitor patient for adverse reactions. ■

Drug-herb. *St. John's wort:* May decrease mobocertinib level. Discourage use together.

Drug-food. *Grapefruit, grapefruit juice:* May increase mobocertinib level. Discourage use together.

EFFECTS ON LAB TEST RESULTS

• May increase CK, amylase, lipase, ALP, ALT, and AST levels.
• May decrease albumin, magnesium, potassium, and sodium levels.
• May decrease Hb level and RBC, lymphocyte, platelet, and leukocyte counts.

CONTRAINDICATIONS & CAUTIONS

Boxed Warning Drug can cause life-threatening HR-corrected QTc-interval prolongation, including torsades de pointes, which can be fatal. Monitor QTc interval and electrolyte levels at baseline and periodically during therapy. Increase monitoring frequency in patients with risk factors for QTc-interval prolongation. ■

Boxed Warning Withhold drug, reduce dosage, or permanently discontinue drug based on severity of QTc-interval prolongation. ■

• Drug can increase risk of severe or life-threatening ILD or pneumonitis.
• Drug may increase risk of cardiac toxicity, including decreased ejection fractions, cardiomyopathy, and HF.
• Drug may cause diarrhea leading to dehydration or electrolyte imbalance, with or without renal impairment.

• Safety and effectiveness in children haven't been established.
• Use cautiously in older adults because of increased risk of adverse reactions.
• Recommended dosage for patients with severe renal or hepatic impairment hasn't been established. *Dialyzable drug:* Unlikely.

PREGNANCY-LACTATION-REPRODUCTION

• Drug may impair fertility.
• Drug can cause fetal harm. Advise patients who are pregnant of the risk.
• Patients of childbearing potential should use effective nonhormonal contraception during therapy and for 1 month after final dose. Males with partners of childbearing potential must use effective contraception during therapy and for 1 week after final dose.
• It isn't known if drug appears in human milk or how drug affects milk production or infants who are breastfed. Patient shouldn't breastfeed during therapy and for 1 week after final dose.

NURSING CONSIDERATIONS

• Verify the pregnancy status in patients of childbearing potential before drug initiation.
• Monitor cardiac function, including LVEF, at baseline and during therapy. Withhold drug, resume at reduced dosage, or permanently discontinue based on severity.
• Monitor electrolyte levels at baseline and during therapy.
• Monitor patient for diarrhea. Initiate antidiarrheal at first episode of diarrhea and increase fluid and electrolyte intake. Withhold drug, reduce dosage, or permanently discontinue drug based on severity.
• *Look alike-sound alike:* Don't confuse mobocertinib with ceritinib or osimertinib.

PATIENT TEACHING

• Instruct patient about proper drug administration and storage.
• Tell patient about risk of QTc-interval prolongation. Advise patient to report dizziness, lightheadedness, or syncope.
• Inform patient about risk of severe or fatal ILD or pneumonitis and to contact prescriber immediately if new or worsening cough, shortness of breath, or chest pain occurs.
• Advise patient to immediately report signs or symptoms of HF (palpitations, shortness of breath, chest pain, syncope).
• Tell patient to report diarrhea and to promptly start antidiarrheal (loperamide) and to increase oral fluid and electrolyte intake.
• Instruct patient of childbearing potential of the fetal risk and to report pregnancy or plans to become pregnant during therapy. Tell patient to use effective nonhormonal contraception during therapy and for 1 month after final dose.

NEW DRUGS

• Advise male with partner of childbearing potential to use effective contraception during therapy and for 1 week after final dose.
• Warn patient not to breastfeed during therapy and for 1 week after final dose.
• Inform (male and female) that drug may impair fertility.
• Counsel patient to inform prescriber of all drugs, vitamins, supplements, and OTC medications being taken. Tell patient to avoid grapefruit or grapefruit juice while taking drug.

---

oteseconazole
oh-tes-e-KON-a-zole

Vivjoa

Therapeutic class: Antifungals
Pharmacologic class: Azole antifungals

AVAILABLE FORMS
Capsules ⬤: 150 mg

INDICATIONS & DOSAGES
➤ **To reduce incidence of recurrent vulvovaginal candidiasis (RVVC) in patients with a history of RVVC who aren't of childbearing potential**
Adults: 600 mg PO as a single dose on day 1; followed by 450 mg as a single dose on day 2; then, on day 14, 150 mg every 7 days for 11 weeks (weeks 2 through 12). Or, if given in combination with fluconazole, give fluconazole 150 mg PO on days 1, 4, and 7; followed by oteseconazole 150 mg once daily on days 14 through 20; then, on day 28, oteseconazole 150 mg PO every 7 days for 11 weeks (weeks 4 through 14).

ADMINISTRATION
PO
• Give with food.
• Patient must swallow capsule whole. Don't allow patient to crush, open, dissolve, or chew capsule.
• Store at 68° to 77° F (20° to 25° C).

ACTION
Inhibits fungal cell membrane formation and integrity.

Route	Onset	Peak	Duration
PO	Unknown	5–10 hr	Unknown

Half-life: 138 days.

ADVERSE REACTIONS
CNS: headache. **GI:** dyspepsia, nausea. **GU:** dysuria; menorrhagia; metrorrhagia; vulvovaginal burning, discomfort, or pain. **Other:** hot flashes.

INTERACTIONS
Drug-drug. *BCRP substrates (rosuvastatin):* May increase level and adverse effects of substrate. Use lowest possible starting dose of substrate or consider reducing substrate dosage. Monitor patient for adverse effects.

EFFECTS ON LAB TEST RESULTS
• May increase CK level.

CONTRAINDICATIONS & CAUTIONS
• Contraindicated in patients hypersensitive to drug or its components.
• Safety and effectiveness in patients who are pre-menarchal haven't been established.
• Contraindicated in patients with moderate or severe hepatic impairment (Child-Pugh class B or C) or in patients with severe renal impairment or ESRD with or without dialysis.
• Use cautiously in older adults.
Dialyzable drug: Unlikely.

PREGNANCY-LACTATION-REPRODUCTION
• Based on animal studies, drug may cause fetal harm.
• Drug is contraindicated in patients of childbearing potential and during pregnancy.
• It isn't known if drug appears in human milk or how drug affects milk production. Patient shouldn't breastfeed during therapy.

NURSING CONSIDERATIONS
• If specimens for fungal culture are obtained before therapy, may start antifungal therapy before culture results are known. Adjust therapy once culture result is known.

PATIENT TEACHING
🔴 *Alert:* Explain that drug is contraindicated in patients of childbearing potential and during pregnancy and breastfeeding.
• Teach patient about safe drug administration.
• Ensure that patient fully understands the dosing schedule for oteseconazole or oteseconazole plus fluconazole.
• Advise patient to report all OTC and prescription medications, vitamins, or herbal supplements being taken.

---

tapinarof
ta-PIN-ar-of

Vtama

Therapeutic class: Aryl hydrocarbon receptor agonists
Pharmacologic class: Antipsoriatics

AVAILABLE FORMS
Cream: 1%

INDICATIONS & DOSAGES
➤ **Plaque psoriasis**
Adults: Apply a thin layer to psoriatic skin lesions once daily.

ADMINISTRATION
Topical
• Avoid applying to unaffected areas of skin.
• Not for oral, ophthalmic, or intravaginal use.
• Store at 38° to 77° F (20° to 25° C).

ACTION
Exact mechanism unknown.

Route	Onset	Peak	Duration
Topical	Unknown	Unknown	Unknown

Half-life: Unknown.

ADVERSE REACTIONS
CNS: headache. **EENT:** nasopharyngitis.
Skin: contact dermatitis, folliculitis, pruritus.
Other: flulike syndrome.

INTERACTIONS
None reported.

EFFECTS ON LAB TEST RESULTS
None reported.

CONTRAINDICATIONS & CAUTIONS
• Safety and effectiveness in children haven't been established.
Dialyzable drug: Unlikely.

PREGNANCY-LACTATION-REPRODUCTION
• There are no adequate studies during pregnancy. Use only if potential benefit justifies fetal risk.
• It isn't known if drug appears in human milk or how drug affects milk production or infants who are breastfed. Consider patient's clinical need and risk to the infant.

NURSING CONSIDERATIONS
• Monitor patient's skin for signs and symptoms of adverse skin reactions (itching, redness, burning, or peeling).

PATIENT TEACHING
• Instruct patient in safe application of drug.
• Remind patient or caregiver to wash hands after application unless treatment area is the hands.
• Advise patient to report pregnancy or plans to become pregnant or to breastfeed during therapy.

tirzepatide
tir-ZEP-a-tide

Mounjaro

Therapeutic class: Antidiabetics
Pharmacologic class: Glucose-dependent insulinotropic polypeptide receptor and glucagon-like peptide-1 receptor agonists

AVAILABLE FORMS
Injection: 2.5 mg/0.5 mL, 5 mg/0.5 mL, 7.5 mg/ 0.5 mL, 10 mg/0.5 mL, 12.5 mg/ mL, 15 mg/mL single-dose pens

INDICATIONS & DOSAGES
➤ **Adjunct to diet and exercise to improve glycemic control in adults with type 2 diabetes**
Adults: Initially, 2.5 mg subcut once weekly. After 4 weeks, increase to 5 mg subcut once weekly. If additional glycemic control is needed, increase in 2.5-mg increments after 4 weeks on current dose, up to maximum dose of 15 mg once weekly.

ADMINISTRATION
Subcutaneous
• Give drug at any time of day, without regard to food.
• Inspect solution before use. Solution should be clear and colorless to slightly yellow. Don't use if particulate matter or discoloration is present.
• Inject into abdomen, thigh, or upper arm.
• Rotate injection sites with each dose.
• Don't mix drug with insulin for injection. Give as separate injections in the same body region but not adjacent to each other.
• If a dose is missed, give dose as soon as possible within 4 days (96 hours) of the missed dose; then give next dose on regularly scheduled day and resume weekly schedule. If more than 4 days have passed, skip missed dose and give next dose on the regularly scheduled day and resume once weekly schedule.
• May change day of weekly administration if the time between two doses is at least 72 hours.
• Store at 36° to 46° F (2° to 8° C). May store pens unrefrigerated, below 86° F (30° C) for up to 21 days.

ACTION
Enhances insulin secretion and reduces glucagon levels.

Route	Onset	Peak	Duration
Subcut	Unknown	8–72 hr	Unknown

Half-life: About 5 days.

ADVERSE REACTIONS
CV: sinus tachycardia. **GI:** abdominal distention, abdominal pain, constipation, decreased appetite,

NEW DRUGS

diarrhea, dyspepsia, eructation, flatulence, GERD, nausea, vomiting. **Metabolic:** increased amylase and lipase levels. **Skin:** injection-site reaction. **Other:** hypersensitivity, anti-drug antibody development.

INTERACTIONS

Drug-drug. *Insulin, insulin secretagogues (sulfonylureas):* May increase risk of hypoglycemia. Monitor blood glucose level and reduce dosage of insulin or insulin secretagogues accordingly.
Oral contraceptives: May reduce contraceptive effectiveness due to delayed gastric emptying. Switch to nonoral contraceptive method, or add barrier contraceptive method for 4 weeks after starting tirzepatide and for 4 weeks after each dosage increase.
Oral medications: May affect absorption of concomitant oral medications. Use together cautiously.

EFFECTS ON LAB TEST RESULTS

• May increase amylase and lipase levels.
• May decrease blood glucose level.

CONTRAINDICATIONS & CAUTIONS

Boxed Warning Contraindicated in patients with a personal or family history of medullary thyroid carcinoma (MTC) and in patients with multiple endocrine neoplasia syndrome type 2. ■
Boxed Warning Thyroid C-cell adenomas and carcinomas occurred in animal studies. It isn't known if tirzepatide causes thyroid C-cell tumors, including MTC, in humans. ■
• Contraindicated in patients with known hypersensitivity to drug or its components.
• Monitor kidney function in patients with history of impaired kidney function who are reporting severe adverse GI reactions, especially if dehydration occurs.
• Drug is associated with GI adverse reactions, sometimes severe. Not recommended for use in patients with severe GI disease.
• Rapid improvement in glycemic control may be associated with temporary worsening of diabetic retinopathy. Monitor patient with history of diabetic retinopathy for disease progression.
• Safety and effectiveness in children haven't been established.
Dialyzable drug: Unlikely.

PREGNANCY-LACTATION-REPRODUCTION

• Based on animal studies, drug may cause fetal harm. Use only if potential benefit justifies fetal risk.
• It isn't known if drug appears in human milk or how drug affects milk production or infants who are breastfed. Use cautiously during breastfeeding.

NURSING CONSIDERATIONS

• Initiation dose isn't intended for glycemic control.
• Monitor patient for signs and symptoms of pancreatitis (persistent, severe abdominal pain, which may radiate to the back, and vomiting); discontinue drug if suspected.
• Concomitant use with an insulin secretagogue or insulin may increase risk of hypoglycemia, including severe hypoglycemia. Reduced dosage of insulin secretagogue or insulin may be necessary.
• Monitor patient for hypersensitivity reactions (rash, urticaria, wheezing); discontinue drug if suspected.
• Monitor patient for severe GI adverse reactions (nausea, vomiting, abdominal distention) and dehydration.
• Monitor kidney function in patients with impaired kidney function.
• Monitor patient for cholelithiasis (abdominal pain, nausea, vomiting, jaundice). If suspected, clinically evaluate.

PATIENT TEACHING

• Teach patient safe drug administration.
Boxed Warning Inform patient that drug causes thyroid C-cell tumors in rats and that the human relevance of tirzepatide-induced rodent thyroid C-cell tumors hasn't been determined. ■
• Counsel patient to report signs and symptoms of thyroid tumors (lump in neck, persistent hoarseness, dysphagia, dyspnea).
• Instruct patient to stop drug and report suspected pancreatitis.
• Caution patient about increased risk of hypoglycemia when drug is used with an insulin secretagogue (such as a sulfonylurea) or insulin.
• Educate patient on signs and symptoms of hypoglycemia (dizziness, sweating, confusion, drowsiness, headache, blurred vision, slurred speech, shakiness, jitteriness, tachycardia, anxiety, irritability, mood change, hunger, weakness).
• Advise patient to immediately report signs or symptoms of hypersensitivity and stop drug.
• Instruct patient to report severe or persistent GI symptoms (nausea, vomiting, diarrhea).
• Inform patient about risk of dehydration. Explain precautions to avoid fluid depletion.
• Educate patient on potential risk of worsening kidney function. Explain the signs and symptoms (fatigue and weakness, muscle cramps, urinating less, edema of legs, ankles, feet).
• Tell patient to report vision changes during therapy.
• Instruct patient to contact health care provider for clinical follow-up if gallbladder disease is suspected.
• Warn patient who is pregnant of fetal risk. Advise patient to report pregnancy or plans to become pregnant.
• Instruct patient that drug may reduce efficacy of oral contraceptives. Advise patient to switch to a nonoral contraceptive method or to add a barrier contraceptive for 4 weeks after initiation and 4 weeks after each dosage escalation.

vonoprazan–amoxicillin
von-OH-pra-zan/am-ox-i-SILL-in

Voquezna Dual Pak

Therapeutic class: Antacids–anti-infectives
Pharmacologic class: Potassium-
competitive acid blockers–antibacterials

AVAILABLE FORMS
Copackage containing:
Capsules: amoxicillin 500 mg
Tablets: vonoprazan 20 mg

INDICATIONS & DOSAGES
➤ **Helicobacter pylori infection**
Adults: Vonoprazan 20 mg PO b.i.d. plus amoxicillin 1,000 mg PO t.i.d. for 14 days.

ADMINISTRATION
PO
* Give without regard to food.
* If a dose is missed, give within 4 hours from scheduled dose. If more than 4 hours have elapsed, skip dose and give next dose at regularly scheduled time. Continue normal dosing schedule until medication is completed.
* Store at room temperature and protect from light.

ACTION
Vonoprazan is a proton pump inhibitor that blocks acid secretion. Amoxicillin inhibits bacterial cell-wall synthesis by binding to penicillin-binding proteins.

Route	Onset	Peak	Duration
PO (vonoprazan)	2–3 hr	2.5–3 hr	Unknown
PO (amoxicillin)	Unknown	1–2 hr	Unknown

Half-life: Vonoprazan, 7 hours; amoxicillin, 1 hour.

ADVERSE REACTIONS
CNS: dysgeusia, headache. **CV:** HTN. **EENT:** nasopharyngitis. **GI:** abdominal pain, diarrhea. **GU:** vulvovaginal candidiasis. **Other:** hypersensitivity reaction.

INTERACTIONS
Drug-drug. *Allopurinol:* May increase incidence of rash. Discontinue allopurinol at first sign of rash.
Atazanavir: May alter absorption of atazanavir. Avoid use together.
Clopidogrel: May reduce clopidogrel level and platelet inhibition. Carefully monitor efficacy of clopidogrel or use alternative antiplatelet therapy.
CYP2C19 substrates (cilostazol, citalopram): May increase substrate level. Monitor patient for adverse reactions.
CYP3A4 substrates (cyclosporine, tacrolimus): May increase substrate level and risk of adverse reactions of substrate. Monitor substrate level and watch for adverse effects.
Drugs dependent on gastric pH for absorption (antiretrovirals, dasatinib, erlotinib, iron salts, itraconazole, ketoconazole, mycophenolate mofetil, nilotinib): May decrease absorption and effectiveness of these drugs. If used concomitantly, refer to prescribing information for the individual drugs.
Nelfinavir: May alter nelfinavir absorption. Avoid use together.
Oral anticoagulants: May increase PT and INR. Monitor patient closely and adjust oral anticoagulant dosage as necessary.
Probenecid: May increase amoxicillin exposure and adverse reactions. Monitor patient for adverse reactions.
Rilpivirine: May alter rilpivirine absorption. Avoid use together.
Strong or moderate CYP3A inducers (efavirenz, rifampin): May decrease vonoprazan effectiveness. Avoid use together.

EFFECTS ON LAB TEST RESULTS
* May cause false-positive urine glucose test based on Benedict copper reduction reaction. Use test based on enzymatic glucose oxidase reactions when testing patients treated with drug.
* May cause false-positive serum chromogranin A (CgA) test for neuroendocrine tumors.

CONTRAINDICATIONS & CAUTIONS
* Contraindicated in patients hypersensitive to vonoprazan, amoxicillin, or other beta-lactams (penicillins or cephalosporins).
* Avoid use in patients with severe abnormal kidney function (eGFR less than 30 mL/minute) or moderate to severe hepatic impairment (Child-Pugh class B or C).
* Avoid use in patients with mononucleosis; drug may increase risk of erythematous rash.
* Serious and fatal hypersensitivity reactions, including anaphylaxis, have been reported. If hypersensitivity reactions occur, discontinue therapy and initiate immediate supportive care.
* SCARs have occurred. Discontinue at first sign or symptom of SCARs or other signs or symptoms of hypersensitivity and consider further evaluation.
* CDAD has been reported with use of acid-suppressing therapies and nearly all antibacterial agents.
* Safety and effectiveness in children haven't been established.
* Use cautiously in older adults.
Dialyzable drug: Vonoprazan, no. Amoxicillin, yes.
⚠ **Overdose S&S:** Amoxicillin: interstitial nephritis, crystalluria, reversible kidney impairment.

PREGNANCY-LACTATION-REPRODUCTION
* There are no adequate studies during pregnancy. Use with caution.

• It isn't known if drug appears in human milk or how drug affects infants who are breastfed or milk production. Patient who is breastfeeding should pump and discard milk during therapy and for 2 days after final dose, and feed infant stored human milk (collected before therapy) or formula.

• Enroll patient exposed to drug during pregnancy in the Phathom Pharmaceuticals pregnancy exposure registry (1-800-775-PHAT [7428]).

NURSING CONSIDERATIONS

• Monitor patient for hypersensitivity reactions. If reactions occur, discontinue drug and begin immediate supportive care.

• Monitor patient for SCARs. Discontinue drug at first sign or symptom and evaluate further.

• Monitor patient for diarrhea during and after therapy. If CDAD is confirmed, discontinue drug and manage patient as clinically indicated.

• If CgA testing is needed, assess CgA level 14 days after therapy ends and retest if CgA level is high.

• *Look alike–sound alike:* Don't confuse vonoprazan with voriconazole.

PATIENT TEACHING

• Teach patient safe drug administration.

• Advise patient to take drug as directed and complete full course of therapy, even if feeling better early in the course of therapy. Skipping doses or not completing full course may decrease effectiveness of treatment and increase the likelihood that bacteria will develop resistance.

• Counsel patient that treatment of *H. pylori* infection is important due to its association with stomach ulcers, atrophic gastritis, and increased risk of gastric cancer.

• Advise patient that hypersensitivity reactions can occur. Tell patient to immediately report a new rash, urticaria, drug eruptions, facial swelling, or difficulty breathing.

• Teach patient about risk of serious skin reactions. Tell patient to stop drug immediately and report signs or symptoms of rash, mucosal lesions, or other signs or symptoms of reaction.

• Advise patient of drug interactions and to report use of other medications, including natural substitutes and nutritional supplements.

• Inform patient that diarrhea may occur and that rarely, watery and bloody stools (with or without stomach cramps and fever) may develop as late as 2 or more months after the final dose. Tell patient experiencing watery and bloody stools to notify health care provider as soon as possible.

• Instruct patient who is breastfeeding to pump and discard milk during therapy and for 2 days after final dose.

vonoprazan–amoxicillin–clarithromycin ⚠

van-OH-pra-zan/am-ox-a-SILL-in/
klar-ITH-ro-my-sin

Voquezna Triple Pak

Therapeutic class: Antacids–anti-infectives
Pharmacologic class: Potassium-competitive acid blockers–antibacterials–antimicrobials

AVAILABLE FORMS
Copackage containing:
Capsules: amoxicillin 500 mg
Tablets: vonoprazan 20 mg and clarithromycin 500 mg

INDICATIONS & DOSAGES
➤ *Helicobacter pylori* **infection**
Adults: Vonoprazan 20 mg PO plus amoxicillin 1,000 mg PO plus clarithromycin 500 mg PO b.i.d. for 14 days.

ADMINISTRATION
PO
• Give without regard to food.
• Give doses in morning and evening approximately 12 hours apart.
• If a dose is missed, give within 4 hours from scheduled dose. If more than 4 hours has elapsed, skip dose and give next dose at regularly scheduled time. Continue normal dosing schedule until medication is completed.
• Store at room temperature and protect from light.

ACTION
Vonoprazan is a proton pump inhibitor that blocks acid secretion. Amoxicillin inhibits bacterial cell-wall synthesis by binding to penicillin-binding proteins. Clarithromycin binds to the 50S ribosomal subunit of susceptible bacteria, resulting in inhibition of protein synthesis.

Route	Onset	Peak	Duration
PO (vonoprazan)	2–3 hr	2.5–3 hr	Unknown
PO (amoxicillin)	Unknown	1–2 hr	Unknown
PO (clarithromycin)	Unknown	2–3 hr	Unknown

Half-life: Vonoprazan, 7 hours; amoxicillin, 1 hour; clarithromycin, 5 to 7 hours.

ADVERSE REACTIONS
CNS: dysgeusia, headache. **CV:** HTN. **EENT:** nasopharyngitis. **GI:** abdominal pain, diarrhea. **GU:** vulvovaginal candidiasis. **Other:** hypersensitivity reaction.

INTERACTIONS

Drug-drug. *Allopurinol:* May increase risk of rash. Discontinue allopurinol at first sign of rash.

Antiarrhythmics (amiodarone, dofetilide, procainamide, quinidine, sotalol): May increase risk of adverse reactions, including prolonged QT interval and cardiac arrhythmias. Avoid use together. If concomitant use can't be avoided, monitor patient for prolonged QTc interval.

Atazanavir, nelfinavir: May alter absorption of these drugs. Avoid use together.

Atorvastatin: May increase statin level. Avoid use together. If concomitant use can't be avoided, limit atorvastatin dosage to 20 mg daily.

Benzodiazepines (alprazolam, midazolam, triazolam): May increase benzodiazepine level. Closely monitor patient for increased or prolonged CNS effects and refer to benzodiazepine prescribing information for dosage recommendations.

Calcium channel blockers (amlodipine, diltiazem, nifedipine, verapamil): May increase calcium channel blocker level and risk of adverse reactions. Use together cautiously.

Clopidogrel: May reduce clopidogrel level and platelet inhibition. Carefully monitor clopidogrel level or use alternative antiplatelet therapy.

Colchicine: May increase colchicine level and risk of adverse reactions. Concomitant use is contraindicated in patients with abnormal kidney function or liver impairment. If used concomitantly in patients with normal kidney or liver function, monitor patient for colchicine toxicity.

CYP2C19 substrates (cilostazol, citalopram): May increase substrate level. Monitor patient for adverse reactions. Refer to prescribing information of substrate for dosage adjustments if used together.

CYP3A substrates (alfentanil, bromocriptine, cilostazol, cilostazol, methylprednisolone, phenobarbital, vinblastine): Clarithromycin may increase substrate level. Use together cautiously.

CYP3A4 substrates (cyclosporine, tacrolimus): May increase substrate level and risk of adverse reactions of substrate. Monitor substrate level and watch for adverse effects.

CYP450 substrates (hexobarbital, phenytoin, valproate): May increase substrate level and risk of adverse reactions. Use together cautiously.

Digoxin: Clarithromycin may increase digoxin level and risk of adverse reactions. Monitor digoxin level.

Disopyramide: May increase risk of adverse reactions, including cardiac arrhythmias and hypoglycemia. Avoid use together. If concomitant use can't be avoided, monitor patient for prolonged QTc interval and changes in blood glucose level.

Drugs dependent on gastric pH for absorption (antiretrovirals, dasatinib, erlotinib, iron salts, itraconazole, ketoconazole, mycophenolate mofetil, nilotinib): May decrease absorption and effectiveness of these drugs. If used concomitantly, refer to prescribing information for the individual drugs.

Ergot alkaloids (dihydroergotamine, ergotamine): May increase alkaloid level. Avoid use together.

Etravirine: Clarithromycin may increase risk of adverse reactions or reduce effectiveness of both agents. Avoid use together.

Fluvastatin: May increase fluvastatin level. Avoid use together. If concomitant use can't be avoided, give fluvastatin at lowest dose.

Hypoglycemic agents (insulin, nateglinide, pioglitazone, repaglinide, rosiglitazone): May increase hypoglycemic agent level and risk of hypoglycemia. Monitor glucose level.

Itraconazole: Clarithromycin may increase risk of adverse reaction of both agents. Monitor patient for adverse effects.

Lovastatin, simvastatin: May increase statin level. Avoid use together.

Maraviroc: Clarithromycin may increase maraviroc level. Use together cautiously. Refer to maraviroc prescribing information for appropriate dosing information.

Omeprazole: May increase clarithromycin level. Avoid use together.

Oral anticoagulants: May increase PT and INR. Monitor patient closely and adjust dosage of oral anticoagulants as necessary.

Phosphodiesterase inhibitors (sildenafil, tadalafil, vardenafil): Clarithromycin may increase inhibitor level and risk of adverse reactions. Avoid use together. If concomitant use can't be avoided, refer to inhibitor prescribing information for dosage adjustment.

Pimozide: May increase pimozide level, somnolence, risk of NMS, and risk of prolonged QT interval and arrhythmias. Avoid use together.

Pravastatin: May increase statin level. Avoid use together. If use together can't be avoided, limit pravastatin dosage to 40 mg daily.

Probenecid: May increase amoxicillin exposure and adverse reactions. Monitor patient for adverse reactions.

Quetiapine: May increase quetiapine level and risk of adverse reactions. Refer to quetiapine prescribing information for dosage reduction.

Rilpivirine-containing products: May alter rilpivirine absorption. Avoid use together.

Ritonavir: Clarithromycin may increase risk of adverse reactions or reduce effectiveness of both agents. Avoid use in patients with decreased kidney function.

Saquinavir: May increase risk of adverse reactions or reduce effectiveness of saquinavir and clarithromycin. Refer to saquinavir prescribing information for instructions on concomitant use.

Strong or moderate CYP3A inducers (efavirenz, rifampin): May decrease vonoprazan and clarithromycin effectiveness. Avoid use together.

Theophylline: Clarithromycin may increase theophylline level. Monitor serum theophylline level in patients receiving high theophylline doses or with baseline concentrations in the upper therapeutic range.

Tolterodine: May increase tolterodine level and risk of adverse reactions. Tolterodine 1 mg b.i.d. is recommended in patients deficient in CYP2D6 activity when concomitantly used with clarithromycin.

Zidovudine: May increase levels of zidovudine and clarithromycin. Separate drug administration by at least 2 hours.

Drug-herb. *St. John's wort:* May decrease clarithromycin level. Advise patient to use cautiously together.

EFFECTS ON LAB TEST RESULTS

• May increase liver enzyme levels.
• May cause false-positive urine glucose test based on Benedict copper reduction reaction. Use test based on enzymatic glucose oxidase reactions when testing patients treated with drug.
• May cause false-positive serum chromogranin A (CgA) test for neuroendocrine tumors.

CONTRAINDICATIONS & CAUTIONS

• Contraindicated in patients hypersensitive to vonoprazan, amoxicillin or other beta-lactams (penicillins or cephalosporins), or clarithromycin or other macrolide antibacterials.
• Contraindicated in patients with a history of cholestatic jaundice or hepatic dysfunction associated with clarithromycin.
• Serious and fatal reactions, including anaphylaxis, have been reported. If hypersensitivity reactions occur, discontinue therapy and initiate immediate supportive care.
• SCARs have occurred. Discontinue at first sign or symptom of SCAR or other signs and symptoms of hypersensitivity and consider further evaluation.
• CDAD has been reported with use of acid-suppressing therapies and nearly all antibacterial agents.
• Clarithromycin may increase risk of prolonged QT interval and arrhythmias, including torsades de pointes. Avoid use in patients with known prolonged QT interval or ventricular cardiac arrhythmia, proarrhythmic conditions such as uncorrected hypokalemia or hypomagnesemia, or significant bradycardia and in patients on drugs known to prolong QT interval.
• Avoid use in patients with mononucleosis; drug may increase risk of erythematous rash.
• Avoid use in patients with severe kidney impairment (eGFR less than 30 mL/minute) or moderate to severe hepatic impairment (Child-Pugh class B or C).
• Clarithromycin may exacerbate myasthenia gravis and prompt new onset of signs or symptoms of myasthenic syndrome.
• Safety and effectiveness in children haven't been established.
• Use cautiously in older adults.
Dialyzable drug: Vonoprazan, no; amoxicillin, yes; clarithromycin, no.

⚠ *Overdose S&S:* Amoxicillin: interstitial nephritis, crystalluria, reversible kidney impairment. Clarithromycin: GI symptoms.

PREGNANCY-LACTATION-REPRODUCTION

• There are no adequate studies during pregnancy for vonoprazan-associated risks. Clarithromycin may cause adverse fetal and pregnancy effects, including miscarriage. Use isn't recommended during pregnancy unless there are no appropriate alternative therapies.
• It isn't known if drug appears in human milk or how drug affects infants who are breastfed or milk production. Patient who is breastfeeding should pump and discard milk during therapy and for 2 days after final dose, and feed infant stored human milk (collected before therapy) or formula.
• Enroll patient exposed to drug during pregnancy in the Phathom Pharmaceuticals pregnancy exposure registry (1-800-775-PHAT [7428]).
• Based on animal studies, clarithromycin may impair fertility in males of reproductive potential.

NURSING CONSIDERATIONS

• Monitor patient with diabetes for hypoglycemia.
• Monitor patient for hypersensitivity reactions. If they occur, discontinue therapy and institute immediate supportive care.
• Monitor patient for SCARs. Discontinue drug at first sign or symptoms of SCARs and evaluate further.
• Monitor patient for diarrhea during and after therapy. If CDAD is confirmed, discontinue drug and manage patient as clinically indicated.
• If CgA testing is needed, assess CgA level 14 days after therapy ends and retest if CgA level is high.
• *Look alike–sound alike:* Don't confuse vonoprazan with voriconazole.

PATIENT TEACHING

• Teach patient safe drug administration.
• Advise patient to take drug as directed and complete full course of therapy, even if feeling better early in the course of therapy. Skipping doses or not completing full course may decrease effectiveness of treatment and increase the likelihood that bacteria will develop resistance.
• Counsel patient that treatment of *H. pylori* infection is important due to its association with stomach ulcers, atrophic gastritis, and increased risk of gastric cancer.
• Advise patient that hypersensitivity reactions can occur. Tell patient to immediately report a new rash, urticaria, drug eruptions, facial swelling, or difficulty breathing.
• Teach patient about risk of serious skin reactions. Tell patient to stop drug immediately and report signs or symptoms of rash, mucosal lesions, or other signs or symptoms of reaction.
• Warn patient that drug may interact with other medications. Advise patient to report use of other

NEW DRUGS

medications, including natural substitutes and nutritional supplements.

• Inform patient that diarrhea may occur with antibacterial use and that, rarely, watery and bloody stools (with or without stomach cramps and fever) may develop as late as 2 or more months after the final dose. If watery and bloody stools occur, tell patient to notify health care provider as soon as possible.

• Instruct patient who is breastfeeding to pump and discard milk during therapy and for 2 days after final dose.

• Advise male of reproductive potential that drug may impair fertility.

• Inform patient taking hypoglycemic agents about increased risk of hypoglycemia and to monitor glucose closely during therapy.

vosoritide
voe-SOR-i-tide

Voxzogo

Therapeutic class: Growth factors
Pharmacologic class: C-type natriuretic peptide analogues

AVAILABLE FORMS
Injection: 0.4 mg, 0.56 mg, 1.2 mg single-dose vial

INDICATIONS & DOSAGES
➤ **Increase of linear growth in patients with achondroplasia with open epiphyses**
Children age 5 and older: 0.24 to 0.8 mg subcut once daily, based on actual body weight. Refer to prescribing information for dosing table.
Adjust-a-dose: Adjust dose every 3 to 6 months, according to actual body weight. Permanently discontinue drug upon confirmation of closed epiphyses.

ADMINISTRATION
Subcutaneous
• Ensure that patient has adequate food intake and drinks approximately 240 to 300 mL (8 to 10 oz) of fluid 1 hour before drug administration.
• Give drug at same time each day.
• To reconstitute, let vial and prefilled diluent syringe containing sterile water for injection reach room temperature. Inject entire diluent volume into vial. Gently swirl vial until powder is completely dissolved; don't shake.
• Reconstituted solution should be a clear, colorless to yellow liquid. Discard if solution contains particulate matter or is cloudy or discolored.
• Concentration of drug in reconstituted 0.4-mg vial and 0.56-mg vial is 0.8 mg/mL; concentration of drug in reconstituted 1.2-mg vial is 2 mg/mL.
• May store prepared solution in vial at room temperature for a maximum of 3 hours.

• Withdraw dose from vial using supplied syringe.
• Give subcut injection into thigh, lower abdomen avoiding the 2 inches (5 cm) around the navel, buttock, or back of upper arm. Don't inject into same area on 2 consecutive days. Don't inject into skin that is red, swollen, or tender.
• Discard unused portion of drug remaining in vial. Don't mix with other medications.
• If a dose is missed beyond 12 hours of the scheduled dose, skip missed dose and continue with regular dosing schedule on the next day.
• Store vial and prefilled diluent syringe in refrigerator at 36° to 46° F (2° to 8° C); don't freeze. May store at room temperature at 68° to 77° F (20° to 25° C) out of direct sunlight for 90 days. Don't return drug to refrigerator after it's been at room temperature.

ACTION
Promotes bone growth by binding to natriuretic peptide receptor B and reduces fibroblast growth factor receptor 3 gene activity, a negative regulator of bone growth.

Route	Onset	Peak	Duration
Subcut	Unknown	15 min	Unknown

Half-life: 21 to 28 minutes.

ADVERSE REACTIONS
CNS: dizziness, fatigue. **CV:** hypotension. **EENT:** ear pain. **GI:** diarrhea, gastroenteritis, vomiting. **Musculoskeletal:** arthralgia. **Skin:** bruising, dry skin, discoloration or induration, hemorrhage, injection-site erythema, pain, pruritus, swelling, urticaria. **Other:** flulike symptoms, seasonal allergy.

INTERACTIONS
Drug-drug. *Antihypertensives:* May increase hypotensive effect. Use together cautiously.

EFFECTS ON LAB TEST RESULTS
• None reported.

CONTRAINDICATIONS & CAUTIONS
• Drug hasn't been studied in patients with significant cardiac or vascular disease.
• Drug isn't indicated for use in adults.
• Avoid use in patients with eGFR less than 60 mL/minute/1.73 m².
• Some dosage forms may contain polysorbate 80.
• Safety and effectiveness in children younger than age 5 haven't been established.
Dialyzable drug: No.

PREGNANCY-LACTATION-REPRODUCTION
• There are no adequate studies in pregnancy.
• It isn't known if drug appears in human milk or how drug affects milk production or infants who are breastfed. Before patient starts breastfeeding, consider the patient's clinical need and risk to the infant.
• There are no data on fertility.

NEW DRUGS

NURSING CONSIDERATIONS
• Monitor patient's weight, growth, and physical development every 3 to 6 months.
• Monitor patient for signs and symptoms of transient hypotension (dizziness, fatigue, nausea).
• Ensure patient is well hydrated and has had adequate food intake before giving drug.
• Caregiver can give drug after receiving proper training on preparation and administration by practitioner.

PATIENT TEACHING
• Instruct caregiver about proper drug administration and disposal of syringes and needles.
• Advise caregiver to reduce risk of hypotension by ensuring that the patient has adequate food intake and drinks 240 to 300 mL (8 to 10 oz) of fluid 1 hour before giving drug.

vutrisiran ☒
vue-tri-SIR-an

Amvuttra

Therapeutic class: Metabolic agents
Pharmacologic class: Anti-transthyretin (TTR) small interfering RNA (siRNA) agents

AVAILABLE FORMS
Injection: 25 mg/0.5 mL prefilled syringe

INDICATIONS & DOSAGES
➤ **Polyneuropathy of hereditary transthyretin-mediated amyloidosis** ☒
Adults: 25 mg subcut every 3 months.

ADMINISTRATION
Subcutaneous
• Drug should be given by a health care professional.
• Allow drug to reach room temperature for 30 minutes before use.
• Inspect solution for particulate matter and discoloration. Solution is clear, colorless to slightly yellow. Don't use if solution looks cloudy, discolored, or contains particulate matter.
• Check syringe for visible damage; ensure needle cap is attached to syringe.
• Inject into abdomen, thighs, or upper arms.
• Push plunger rod as far as it will go to inject drug completely and activate the needle shield.
• Give a missed dose as soon as possible. Resume dosing every 3 months thereafter.
• Store at 36° to 86° F (2° to 30° C) in original carton until ready for use. Don't freeze.

ACTION
Causes degradation of mutant and wild-type TTR mRNA, resulting in a reduction of serum TTR protein and TTR protein deposits in tissues.

Route	Onset	Peak	Duration
Subcut	Unknown	0.17–12 hr	Unknown

Half-life: 2.2 to 6.4 hours.

ADVERSE REACTIONS
CV: *AV block.* **Musculoskeletal:** arthralgia. **Respiratory:** dyspnea. **Skin:** injection-site reactions (bruising, erythema, pain, pruritus, warmth). **Other:** antidrug antibody development, vitamin A deficiency.

INTERACTIONS
None reported.

EFFECTS ON LAB TEST RESULTS
• May decrease vitamin A level.

CONTRAINDICATIONS & CAUTIONS
• Drug hasn't been studied in patients with kidney failure, ESRD, or moderate to severe hepatic impairment.
• Safety and effectiveness in children haven't been established.
Dialyzable drug: Unknown.

PREGNANCY-LACTATION-REPRODUCTION
• There are no adequate studies during pregnancy. Use only if benefit outweighs fetal risk.
• It isn't known if drug appears in human milk or how drug affects milk production or an infant who is breastfed. Use cautiously during breastfeeding.

NURSING CONSIDERATIONS
• Monitor patient for decreased vitamin A levels.
• Monitor patient for vision changes such as night blindness. Refer patient to an ophthalmologist as needed.
• Monitor patient for injection-site reactions.
• *Look alike-sound alike:* Don't confuse vutrisiran with patisiran.

PATIENT TEACHING
• Inform patient that therapy leads to decreased vitamin A levels.
• Instruct patient to take the recommended daily allowance of vitamin A.
• Advise patient to report vision changes, including night blindness.
• Counsel patient to report pregnancy or plans to become pregnant during treatment. Caution patient about fetal risk.

Appendices

Nursing process: Patient safety during drug therapy

Drug therapy is a complex process that can easily lead to adverse patient events. In 2007, the Institute of Medicine (IOM) released its report on the drug safety system, *The Future of Drug Safety: Promoting and Protecting the Health of the Public.* The IOM reported that approximately 400,000 preventable adverse drug events occurred each year in the United States. The IOM also estimated that preventable hospital medication errors occurred at a rate of 1/patient/day and contributed to 7,000 patient deaths/year. Although much progress has been made, problems with using medications safely remain. Medication errors are one of the top 10 most frequently reviewed sentinel events by The Joint Commission. Applying the nursing process (assessment, nursing diagnosis, planning, intervention, and evaluation) during drug therapy enables the nurse to systematically identify the drug therapy needs of each patient, thereby reducing the number of adverse events and providing safe patient care.

Nursing process step	Key points

Assessment	• Collect data—subjective and objective
	  ○ Current and prior health status
	  ○ Cultural considerations
	  ○ Lab values
	  ○ Allergies
	  ○ Physical assessment
	  ○ Medication history
	    ▪ Prescriptions and OTC drugs
	    ▪ Herbal supplements
	    ▪ Response to medications
	    ▪ Knowledge of medications
	    ▪ Medication adherence.

Nursing diagnosis or problem	• Identify all associated nursing diagnoses.
Planning	• Review patient allergies. • Review and reconcile prescribed medications. • Identify possible adverse effects of medications. • Identify potential interactions with other medications. • Determine route of administration. • Determine time of administration. • Develop patient teaching about medication administration.

Intervention	• Administer medication utilizing the "eight rights"
	  ○ Right patient
	  ○ Right drug
	  ○ Right dose
	  ○ Right time
	  ○ Right route
	  ○ Right reason
	  ○ Right response
	  ○ Right documentation.
	• Use technology such as bar coding to ensure safe and correct administration.
	• Teach patient about each medication at time of administration.

Evaluation	• Monitor patient's response to medication. • Monitor for possible adverse effects of medication. • Monitor for unexpected effects of medication. • Document medication administration.

Decision tree: Deciding about medication administration

Use this tool to help you determine whether or not to administer a medication. Be sure to consider all of the phases of medication administration in this document.

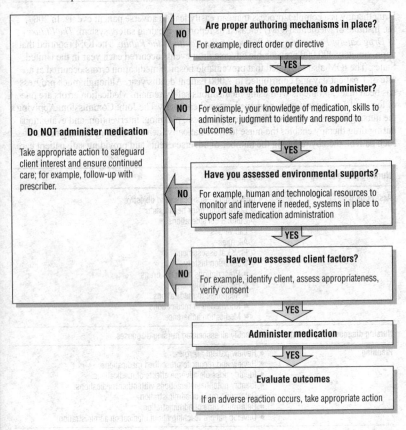

Do NOT administer medication

Take appropriate action to safeguard client interest and ensure continued care; for example, follow-up with prescriber.

Are proper authoring mechanisms in place?

For example, direct order or directive

NO / YES

Do you have the competence to administer?

For example, your knowledge of medication, skills to administer, judgment to identify and respond to outcomes

NO / YES

Have you assessed environmental supports?

For example, human and technological resources to monitor and intervene if needed, systems in place to support safe medication administration

NO / YES

Have you assessed client factors?

For example, identify client, assess appropriateness, verify consent

NO / YES

Administer medication

YES

Evaluate outcomes

If an adverse reaction occurs, take appropriate action

Adapted from College of Nurses of Ontario. (2019). *Practice Standard: Medication.* https://www.cno.org/globalassets/docs/prac/41007_medication.pdf

Avoiding common drug errors: Best practices and prevention

In addition to following your facility's administration policies, you can help prevent errors in drug administration by reviewing these common errors and ways to prevent them. The Joint Commission, the Institute for Safe Medication Practices (ISMP), and the FDA also maintain resources to help improve drug safety.

Topic	Error	Best practices and prevention
Drug orders		
Pharmacy computer system	The system may not detect all unsafe orders.	• Don't rely on the pharmacy computer system to detect all unsafe orders. • Before giving a drug, understand the correct indication, dosage, route, and potential adverse effects. • Consult the pharmacist if there is any question, and verify the information using an approved current drug reference.
Confusing drug names	Many drugs have names that look alike or sound alike and may easily be mistaken one for the other.	• Perform a medication reconciliation on admission, at each transition of care, and when the practitioner prescribes a new medication. Question any deviations from patient's routine. • Take your time and read the label carefully. • Consult the ISMP "List of Confused Drug Names" (www.ismp.org/recommendations/confused-drug-names-list). • Be aware of tall man lettering, which helps differentiate similar drug names.
Abbreviations	Using dangerous abbreviations can result in giving the wrong drug or wrong dose, by the wrong route, or at the wrong time.	• Don't abbreviate drug names. • Be aware of The Joint Commission's official "Do Not Use" list of drug abbreviations to avoid (see *Appendix 4: Abbreviations to avoid [The Joint Commission]*, page 1614). • Consult your facility's list of approved abbreviations and the ISMP's "List of Error-Prone Abbreviations, Symbols, and Dose Designations" (www.ismp.org/recommendations/error-prone-abbreviations-list).
Unclear order	A drug order with incomplete or unclear information can result in giving the wrong drug or wrong dose, by the wrong route, or at the wrong time.	• Ensure that each order specifies the correct drug name, concentration, dosage, route, and frequency of administration. • Clarify all incomplete or unclear orders with the prescriber. Utilize read-back and verify when taking phone and verbal orders.
Inadvertent overdose	A prescriber may write an order for a combination drug such as acetaminophen-opioid analgesic tablets without realizing the total acetaminophen dose could be toxic (don't exceed 4 g daily).	• Note the amount of acetaminophen in each combined formulation. • Warn patients not to take additional drugs that contain acetaminophen. • Verify any "as needed" pain or fever medication orders to check if they contain acetaminophen. Monitor patient's use of "as needed" drugs as prescribed.

(continued)

Topic	Error	Best practices and prevention
Anticoagulants	Lack of standardization for drug naming, labeling, and packaging can create confusion. Dosing regimens, assay methods, narrow therapeutic ranges, complex drug interactions, and drug monitoring methods create high potential for complications.	• Keep current with your facility's anticoagulant therapy protocol, the different dosing regimens, assay methods and their standardized range of normal values, drug interactions, monitoring methods, and reversal regimens for each anticoagulant given. • Don't confuse direct oral anticoagulants with one another because the drug names are similar, such as confusing rivaroxaban with edoxaban. • Use only unit-dose products if available. • Be especially aware of the correct doses and indications for neonates and children. • Teach patients to manage their therapy appropriately.

Drug preparation

Topic	Error	Best practices and prevention
Crushing drugs for oral or enteral administration	Crushing certain oral or enteral drugs may: • alter the drug's effects, causing overdose or other adverse reactions • result in skin irritation or other adverse reactions for the preparer • produce teratogenic effects when administered to patients who are pregnant (through exposure) • be hazardous if not done in an appropriate environment (e.g., chemotherapy and other hazardous drugs).	• Use a liquid formulation instead of crushing a drug whenever possible. • Before crushing a drug, always check with the pharmacist and established references, such as the ISMP's list of "Oral Dosage Forms That Should Not Be Crushed" (www.ismp.org/recommendations/do-not-crush).
Solution color change or particulate matter	Unusual appearance may indicate that: • the drug has been improperly stored or manufactured • the drug has expired • the wrong drug has been provided by the pharmacy • the wrong liquid was chosen out of patient's medication supply.	• Closely examine all solutions before giving them, and know what their appearance should be. • If you note a color change, contact the pharmacist who dispensed the solution and report it. • Don't give a drug until verifying that the drug has been correctly labeled and that it is safe to give. • Verify that you have chosen the correct solution from patient's supply if patient is on more than one liquid drug.
Incorrect drug storage	Incorrect storage may change a drug's physical properties or result in its being inadvertently administered.	• Follow your facility's policy for storing drugs. • Always store drugs in the appropriate container, in the appropriate place, at the appropriate temperature, for the appropriate duration.
Incomplete or incorrect drug labels	Incorrect or incomplete labeling can result in giving the wrong drug, formulation, or dose.	• Never give a drug whose label is incomplete or incorrect. Notify the pharmacy immediately and obtain the correctly labeled drug. • Properly label and verify all medications, medication containers, and other solutions on and off the sterile field.

Topic	Error	Best practices and prevention
Drug administration		
Using a parenteral syringe for oral or enteral drugs	Using a parenteral syringe with a luer-lock to prepare small amounts of oral or enteral drugs can result in misadministration because the drug could be accidentally injected into an IV line.	• Always use special oral syringes to give oral or enteral drugs. Their hubs won't support a needle and they don't have a luer-lock, so they can't be attached to IV lines. • Always properly label syringes (if they aren't thrown away immediately).
Infusion pump safety problems	Problems with infusion pumps (used to deliver controlled fluids, drugs, and nutrients) can cause fluid overload or administration of inaccurate doses.	• Make sure you know how to safely operate an infusion pump. Consult your facility's policy on proper usage. • Before beginning an infusion, always verify that the pump is working properly. Make sure all alarms are functional, and never bypass them. • Double-check all dosing to include the infusion rate. • Always double-check that the correct medication bag is hanging in the pump. • Consult ISMP's "Guidelines for Optimizing Safe Implementation and Use of Smart Infusion Pumps" for more information (www.ismp.org/guidelines/safe-implementation-and-use-smart-pumps).
Calculation errors	Dosage calculation errors can cause significant patient harm, especially with "high alert" medications, and in neonates and children.	• Be aware of medications that are considered high alert. Consult "ISMP List of High-Alert Medications in Acute Care Settings" (https://www.ismp.org/sites/default/files/attachments/2018-08/highAlert2018-Acute-Final.pdf) or "ISMP List of High-Alert Medications in Community/Ambulatory Healthcare" (https://www.ismp.org/sites/default/files/attachments/2017-11/highAlert-community.pdf). • Write out the mg/kg or mg/m^2 dose and the calculated dose as a safeguard. • Whenever a prescriber provides a calculation, double-check it and document that the dose was verified in the medical record. • Use only approved abbreviations, and be aware of the placement of decimal points.
OTC products and supplements (herbal supplements and vitamins)	Because OTC products, herbal supplements, and vitamins aren't subject to the same quality assurance standards as drugs, their labels may be misrepresented and their effects and interactions with drugs may not be well studied.	• Always assess and document all OTC drugs, herbal supplements, and vitamins patient is taking in patient's medical record. • Monitor patient carefully, and report unusual adverse reactions. • Consult an evidence-based drug reference for known drug-herb interactions. • Use extra care when combining herbal supplements with anticoagulants because bleeding times may increase.

Abbreviations to avoid (The Joint Commission)

The Joint Commission requires every health care facility to develop a list of approved abbreviations for staff use. Certain abbreviations should be avoided because they're easily misunderstood, especially when handwritten. The Joint Commission has identified a minimum list of dangerous abbreviations, acronyms, and symbols. This do-not-use list includes the following items.

Official "Do Not Use" List[1]		
Do not use	**Potential problem**	**Use instead**
U, u (unit)	Mistaken for "O" (zero), the number "4" (four), or "cc"	Write "unit"
IU (International Unit)	Mistaken for "IV" (intravenous) or the number "10" (ten)	Write "International Unit"
Q.D., QD, q.d., qd (daily)	Mistaken for each other	Write "daily"
Q.O.D., QOD, q.o.d, qod (every other day)	Period after the Q mistaken for "I" and the "O" mistaken for "I"	Write "every other day"
Trailing zero (X.0 mg)* Lack of leading zero (.X mg)	Decimal point is missed	Write "X mg" Write "0.X mg"
MS	Can mean morphine sulfate or magnesium sulfate	Write "morphine sulfate"
MSO_4 and $MgSO_4$	Confused for one another	Write "magnesium sulfate"

[1]Applies to all orders and all medication-related documentation that is handwritten (including free-text computer entry) or on preprinted forms.

*Exception: A "trailing zero" may be used only where required to demonstrate the level of precision of the value being reported, such as for laboratory results, imaging studies that report size of lesions, or catheter/tube size. It may not be used in medication orders or other medication-related documentation.

Do not use: Dangerous abbreviations, symbols, and dose designations (ISMP Canada)

The abbreviations, symbols, and dose designations found in this table have been reported as being frequently misinterpreted and involved in harmful medication errors. They should NEVER be used when communicating medication information.

Abbreviation	Intended meaning	Problem	Correction
U	unit	Mistaken for "0" (zero), "4" (four), or "cc"	Use "unit"
IU	international unit	Mistaken for "IV" (intravenous) or "10" (ten)	Use "unit"
Abbreviations for drug names		Misinterpreted because of similar abbreviations for multiple drugs; e.g., MS, MSO_4 (morphine sulphate), $MgSO_4$ (magnesium sulphate) may be confused for one another	Do not abbreviate drug names
QD QOD	every day every other day	QD and QOD have been mistaken for each other, or as "qid". The Q has also been misinterpreted as "2" (two).	Use "daily" and "every other day"
OD	every day	Mistaken for "right eye" (OD = oculus dexter)	Use "daily"
OS, OD, OU	left eye, right eye, both eyes	May be confused with one another	Use "left eye", "right eye", or "both eyes"
D/C	discharge	Interpreted as "discontinue whatever medications follow" (typically discharge medications)	Use "discharge"
cc	cubic centimetre	Mistaken for "u" (units)	Use "mL" or "millilitre"
µg	microgram	Mistaken for "mg" (milligram), resulting in one thousand-fold overdose	Use "mcg"

Symbol	Intended meaning	Potential problem	Correction
@	at	Mistaken for "2" (two) or "5"	Use "at"
>	greater than	Mistaken for "7" (seven) or the letter "L"	Use "greater than"/ "more than" or "less than"/"lower than"
<	less than	Confused with each other	

Dose designation	Intended meaning	Potential problem	Correction
Trailing zero	X.0 mg	Decimal point is overlooked, resulting in 10-fold dose error	Never use a zero by itself after a decimal point. Use "X mg"
Lack of leading zero	.X mg	Decimal point is overlooked, resulting in 10-fold dose error	Always use a zero before a decimal point. Use "0.X mg"

Adapted from ISMP's *List of Error-Prone Abbreviations, Symbols, and Dose Designations 2006*.
Available from: https://www.ismp-canada.org/download/ISMPCanadaListOfDangerousAbbreviations.pdf
Reprinted with permission from ISMP Canada, 2023.

Therapeutic drug monitoring guidelines

Lab value ranges may vary among labs. Be sure to compare test results with the normal values of the lab that performed the test.

Drug	Laboratory test monitored	Therapeutic ranges of test
ACE inhibitors (benazepril, captopril, enalapril, enalaprilat, fosinopril, lisinopril, moexipril, perindopril, quinapril, ramipril, trandolapril)	Creatinine BUN Potassium WBC with differential	Men: 0.9–1.3 mg/dL Women: 0.6–1.1 mg/dL 6–20 mg/dL 3.5–5.2 mEq/L *****
aminoglycoside antibiotics (amikacin, gentamicin, tobramycin)	Amikacin peak Amikacin trough Creatinine Gentamicin peak Tobramycin peak Gentamicin, tobramycin trough	20–30 mcg/mL 1–8 mcg/mL Men: 0.9–1.3 mg/dL Women: 0.6–1.1 mg/dL 6–10 mcg/mL 5–10 mcg/mL <2 mcg/mL
amphotericin B	BUN CBC with differential and platelets Creatinine Electrolytes (especially potassium and magnesium) Liver function	6–20 mg/dL ***** Men: 0.9–1.3 mg/dL Women: 0.6–1.1 mg/dL Potassium: 3.5–5.2 mEq/L Magnesium: 1.3–2.2 mEq/L Sodium: 135–147 mEq/L Chloride: 95–110 mEq/L *
antibiotics	Cultures and sensitivities WBC with differential	 *****
biguanides (metformin)	CBC Creatinine Fasting glucose HbA$_{1c}$ Vitamin B$_{12}$	***** Men: 0.9–1.3 mg/dL Women: 0.6–1.1 mg/dL ≤100 mg/dL 5%–7% of total Hb 190–900 ng/mL
carBAMazepine	BUN Carbamazepine CBC with differential Liver function Platelet count Sodium	6–20 mg/dL 4–12 mcg/mL ***** * 140–400 × 10^3/mm^3 136–145 mEq/L
corticosteroids (betamethasone, cortisone, dexamethasone, hydrocortisone, methylPREDNISolone, predniSONE, prednisoLONE, triamcinolone)	Electrolytes (especially potassium) Fasting glucose	Potassium: 3.5–5.2 mEq/L Magnesium: 1.8–2.6 mEq/L Sodium: 136–145 mEq/L Chloride: 96–106 mEq/L Calcium: 8.8–10.4 mg/dL ≤100 mg/dL

*****For those areas marked with asterisks, the following values can be used:
Hb: Women: 12–16 g/dL
    Men: 14–18 g/dL
Hematocrit: Women: 37%–48%
           Men: 42%–52%
RBCs: 4–5.5 × 10^3/mm^3
WBCs: 5–10 × 10^3/mm^3

Differential: Neutrophils: 45%–74%
        Bands: 0%–8%
        Lymphocytes: 16%–45%
        Monocytes: 4%–10%
        Eosinophils: 0%–7%
        Basophils: 0%–2%

Monitoring guidelines

Monitor WBC with differential before therapy, monthly during first 3 months, then periodically for first year. Monitor renal function and potassium level closely at start of therapy, after dosage changes, and periodically during therapy.

Check drug levels after third dose. Obtain blood for peak level 30 minutes after IV infusion ends or 60 minutes after IM injection. For trough levels, draw blood just before next dose. Dosage may need to be adjusted accordingly. Recheck after three doses. For extended-interval (once-daily) amikacin dosing, obtain a random amikacin level between 6 and 14 hours after start of amikacin infusion. Monitor creatinine and BUN levels and urine output for signs of decreasing renal function. Monitor urine for increased proteins, cells, and casts.

Monitor creatinine, BUN, and electrolyte levels at least daily at start of therapy, then as clinically indicated. Regularly monitor blood counts and LFT results during therapy.

Monitor WBC with differential weekly during therapy. Obtain specimen cultures and sensitivities to identify causative organism to determine best treatment.

Check renal function and hematologic values before starting therapy and at least annually thereafter. If patient has impaired renal function, don't use metformin because it may cause lactic acidosis. Monitor response to therapy by periodically evaluating fasting glucose and HbA_{1c} levels; a patient's home monitoring of glucose level helps monitor compliance and response. Monitor vitamin B_{12} level every 2 to 3 years.

Monitor blood counts and platelets before therapy; monitor closely during therapy. Check LFTs and BUN before and periodically during therapy.

Monitor electrolyte and glucose levels regularly during long-term therapy.

(continued)

---

*For those areas marked with one asterisk, the following values can be used:
ALT: 7–56 units/L
AST: 5–40 units/L
Alkaline phosphatase: 17–142 units/L
LDH: 140–280 units/L
GGT: <40 units/L
Total bilirubin: 0.2–1 mg/dL

Drug	Laboratory test monitored	Therapeutic ranges of test
digoxin	Creatinine	Men: 0.9–1.3 mg/dL
		Women: 0.6–1.1 mg/dL
	Digoxin	0.8–2 nanograms/mL
	Digoxin in HF	0.5–0.9 nanograms/mL
	Electrolytes	Potassium: 3.5–5.2 mEq/L
		Magnesium: 1.8–2.6 mEq/L
		Sodium: 136–145 mEq/L
		Chloride: 96–106 mEq/L
		Calcium: 8.8–10.4 mg/dL
epoetin alfa	CBC with differential	*****
	Hematocrit	Women: 36%–48%
		Men: 42%–52%
	Platelet count	$140–400 \times 10^3/mm^3$
	Serum ferritin	18–270 nanograms/mL
	Transferrin	250–425 mg/dL
gemfibrozil	CBC	*****
	Lipids	Total cholesterol: <200 mg/dL
		LDL: <130 mg/dL
		HDL: ≥35 mg/dL
		Triglycerides: <150 mg/dL
	Liver function	*
	Serum glucose	<100 mg/dL
	CK	26–174 units/L
heparin (unfractionated)	PTT	1.5–2 × control
	Hematocrit	*****
	Platelet count	$140–400 \times 10^3/mm^3$
HMG-CoA reductase inhibitors (atorvastatin, fluvastatin, lovastatin, pravastatin, rosuvastatin, simvastatin)	Lipids	Total cholesterol: <200 mg/dL
		LDL: <130 mg/dL
		HDL: ≥35 mg/dL
		Triglycerides: <150 mg/dL
	Liver function	*
insulin	Fasting glucose	≤100 mg/dL
	HbA$_{1c}$	<5%–7% of total Hb
isotretinoin	CBC with differential	*****
	Glucose	<100 mg/dL
	Liver function	*
	Lipids	Total cholesterol: <200 mg/dL
		LDL: <130 mg/dL
		HDL: ≥35 mg/dL
		Triglycerides: <150 mg/dL
	Platelet count	$140–400 \times 10^3/mm^3$
	Pregnancy test	Negative

*****For those areas marked with asterisks, the following values can be used:

Hb: Women: 12–16 g/dL
    Men: 14–18 g/dL
Hematocrit: Women: 37%–48%
    Men: 42%–52%
RBCs: $4–5.5 \times 10^3/mm^3$
WBCs: $5–10 \times 10^3/mm^3$

Differential: Neutrophils: 45%–74%
Bands: 0%–8%
Lymphocytes: 16%–45%
Monocytes: 4%–10%
Eosinophils: 0%–7%
Basophils: 0%–2%

Monitoring guidelines

Draw blood sample for digoxin level just before next dose or at least 6 hours after last dose. To monitor maintenance therapy, check drug level at least 1 week after initiation or change in therapy. Base therapy changes on clinical findings, not solely on drug level. Monitor electrolyte levels and renal function periodically during therapy.

After initiation or change in therapy, monitor hematocrit twice weekly for 2 to 6 weeks until stabilized in target range and a maintenance dose established. Monitor hematocrit regularly thereafter.

Therapy is usually withdrawn after 3 months if response is inadequate. Patient must be fasting to measure triglyceride levels. Periodically obtain blood counts and LFT values during first 12 months. Obtain CK for muscle pain or weakness.

When drug is given by continuous IV infusion, check PTT every 4 hours or according to facility policy in early stages of therapy, and daily thereafter. Check platelet counts and hematocrit, and test for occult blood in stools periodically during therapy.

Perform LFTs at baseline, 2 to 4 weeks after initiation or change in therapy (depending on drug), and periodically thereafter.

A patient's home monitoring of glucose level helps measure compliance and response. HbA$_{1c}$ level measures long-term control.

Use a serum or urine pregnancy test with a sensitivity of at least 25 milli-international units/mL. Perform one test before therapy and a second test during first 5 days of the menstrual cycle before therapy begins or at least 11 days after last unprotected sexual intercourse, whichever is later. Repeat pregnancy tests monthly during and 1 month after end of therapy. Obtain baseline LFTs and lipid levels; repeat every 1 to 2 weeks until response to treatment is established (usually 4 weeks).

(continued)

*For those areas marked with one asterisk, the following values can be used:
ALT: 7–56 units/L
AST: 5–40 units/L
Alkaline phosphatase: 17–142 units/L
LDH: 140–280 units/L
GGT: <40 units/L
Total bilirubin: 0.2–1 mg/dL

Drug	Laboratory test monitored	Therapeutic ranges of test
linezolid	Amylase CBC with differential Cultures and sensitivities Liver function Lipase Platelet count	25–125 international units/L ***** * 10–140 units/L $140–400 \times 10^3/mm^3$
lithium	BUN Creatinine CBC Electrolytes (especially calcium, potassium, and sodium) Fasting glucose Lithium Thyroid function tests	8–25 mg/dL Men: 0.9–1.3 mg/dL Women: 0.6–1.1 mg/dL ***** Calcium: 8.8–10.4 mg/dL Potassium: 3.5–5.2 mEq/L Magnesium: 1.8–2.6 mEq/L Sodium: 136–145 mEq/L Chloride: 96–106 mEq/L ≤100 mg/dL 0.6–1.2 mEq/L TSH: 0.45–4.5 microunits/mL T_3: 80–200 nanograms/dL T_4: 5.4–11.5 mcg/dL
methotrexate	CBC with differential Creatinine Liver function Methotrexate Platelet count	***** Men: 0.9–1.3 mg/dL Women: 0.6–1.1 mg/dL * Normal elimination: ~ 5 micromol/L 24 hours postdose ~ 0.5 micromol/L 48 hours postdose ~ <0.2 micromol/L 72 hours postdose $140–400 \times 10^3/mm^3$
NNRTIs (delavirdine, dora-virine, efavirenz, etravirine, nevirapine, rilpivirine)	Amylase CBC with differential and platelets Liver function Lipids Viral load	25–125 international units/L ***** * Total cholesterol: <200 mg/dL LDL: <130 mg/dL HDL: ≥35 mg/dL Triglycerides: <150 mg/dL
phenytoin	Albumin CBC Phenytoin	3.5–5.2 g/dL ***** 10–20 mcg/mL
procainamide	ANA titer CBC Liver function N-acetylprocainamide (NAPA) Procainamide	Negative ***** * 15–25 mcg/mL 3–10 mcg/mL

*****For those areas marked with asterisks, the following values can be used:

Hb: Women: 12–16 g/dL
   Men: 14–18 g/dL
Hematocrit: Women: 37%–48%
     Men: 42%–52%
RBCs: $4–5.5 \times 10^3/mm^3$
WBCs: $5–10 \times 10^3/mm^3$

Differential: Neutrophils: 45%–74%
   Bands: 0%–8%
   Lymphocytes: 16%–45%
   Monocytes: 4%–10%
   Eosinophils: 0%–7%
   Basophils: 0%–2%

Monitoring guidelines

Obtain baseline CBC with differential and platelet count weekly during therapy. Monitor LFTs and amylase and lipase levels during therapy.

Checking drug levels is crucial to safe use of drug. Consult prescribing information for optimal lithium therapeutic range for acute and maintenance treatment. Draw blood sample for level immediately before next dose. Monitor level twice weekly until stable. Once at steady state, check level weekly; when patient is on appropriate maintenance dose, check level every 2 or 3 months. Monitor CBC; creatinine, electrolyte, and fasting glucose levels; and thyroid function test results before therapy and periodically thereafter.

Monitor drug level according to dosing protocol. Monitor CBC with differential, platelet count, and LFT and renal function test results more frequently when therapy starts or changes, and when methotrexate levels may be elevated, such as when patient is dehydrated.

Obtain baseline LFTs and monitor closely during first 12 weeks of therapy. Continue to monitor regularly during therapy. Check CBC with differential and platelet count before and periodically during therapy. Monitor lipid levels periodically. Monitor amylase level during efavirenz and etravirine therapy.

Monitor drug level immediately before next dose and 7 to 10 days after therapy starts or changes. Obtain a CBC at baseline and monthly early in therapy. Watch for toxic effects at therapeutic levels. Adjust the measured level for hypoalbuminemia or renal impairment, which can increase free drug levels.

Measure drug level 6 to 12 hours after a continuous infusion is started or immediately before next oral dose. Combined procainamide and NAPA levels can be used as an index of toxicity when renal impairment exists. Obtain CBC, LFTs, and ANA titer periodically during longer-term therapy.

(continued)

*For those areas marked with one asterisk, the following values can be used:
ALT: 7–56 units/L
AST: 5–40 units/L
Alkaline phosphatase: 17–142 units/L
LDH: 140–280 units/L
GGT: <40 units/L
Total bilirubin: 0.2–1 mg/dL

Drug	Laboratory test monitored	Therapeutic ranges of test
quinidine	CBC	*****
	Creatinine	Men: 0.9–1.3 mg/dL
		Women: 0.6–1.1 mg/dL
	Electrolytes (especially potassium)	Potassium: 3.5–5.2 mEq/L
		Magnesium: 1.8–2.6 mEq/L
		Sodium: 136–145 mEq/L
		Chloride: 96–106 mEq/L
	Liver function	*
	Quinidine	2–6 mg/L
sulfonylureas	Fasting glucose	≤100 mg/dL
	HbA$_{1c}$	5%–7% of total Hb
	Creatinine	Men: 0.9–1.3 mg/dL
		Women: 0.6–1.1 mg/dL
theophylline	Theophylline	10–20 mcg/mL
thiazolidinediones (pioglitazone, rosiglitazone)	Fasting glucose	≤100 mg/dL
	HbA$_{1c}$	5%–7% of total Hb
	Liver function	*
thyroid hormones	Thyroid function tests	TSH: 0.45–5.4 microunits/mL
		T$_3$: 80–200 nanograms/dL
		T$_4$: 5.4–11.5 mcg/dL
valproate sodium, valproic acid, divalproex sodium	Ammonia	15–45 mcg/dL
	Amylase	25–125 international units/L
	BUN	8–25 mg/dL
	CBC with differential	*****
	Creatinine	Men: 0.9–1.3 mg/dL
		Women: 0.6–1.1 mg/dL
	Liver function	*
	Platelet count	140–400 × 10^3/mm^3
	PT	11–13 seconds
	Valproic acid	50–100 mcg/mL
vancomycin	Creatinine	Men: 0.9–1.3 mg/dL
		Women: 0.6–1.1 mg/dL
	Vancomycin	25–40 mcg/mL (peak)
		10–20 mcg/mL (trough)
warfarin	INR	For an acute MI, atrial fibrillation, treatment of pulmonary embolism, prevention of systemic embolism, tissue heart valves, valvular heart disease, or prophylaxis or treatment of venous thrombosis: 2–3 For mechanical prosthetic valves or recurrent systemic embolism: 2.5–3.5

*****For those areas marked with asterisks, the following values can be used:

Hb: Women: 12–16 g/dL
  Men: 14–18 g/dL
Hematocrit: Women: 37%–48%
       Men: 42%–52%
RBCs: 4–5.5 × 10^3/mm^3
WBCs: 5–10 × 10^3/mm^3

Differential: Neutrophils: 45%–74%
       Bands: 0%–8%
Lymphocytes: 16%–45%
Monocytes: 4%–10%
Eosinophils: 0%–7%
Basophils: 0%–2%

Monitoring guidelines

Obtain sample for level immediately before next oral dose and 30 to 35 hours after therapy starts or changes. Periodically obtain blood counts, LFT and renal function test results, and electrolyte levels.

Monitor response to therapy by periodically evaluating fasting glucose and HbA_{1c} levels. Patient should monitor glucose levels at home to help measure compliance and response.

Obtain sample for drug level right before next dose of sustained-release oral product and at least 2 days after therapy starts or changes.

Monitor response by evaluating fasting glucose and HbA_{1c} levels. Obtain baseline LFT results, and repeat tests periodically during therapy. Don't initiate therapy with pioglitazone or rosiglitazone if ALT level exceeds $2.5 \times$ ULN.

Monitor thyroid function test results every 2 to 3 weeks until appropriate maintenance dose is determined and every 6 to 12 months thereafter.

Monitor LFT results, ammonia level, coagulation test results, renal function test results, CBC, and platelet count at baseline and periodically during therapy. Closely monitor LFT results during first 6 months.

May check drug level with third dose administered, at the earliest. Draw peak level 1.5 to 2.5 hours after a 1-hour infusion or IV infusion is complete. Draw trough level within 1 hour of next dose administered. Renal function can be used to adjust dosing and intervals.

Check INR daily, beginning 3 days after therapy begins. Continue checking it until therapeutic goal is achieved, and monitor it periodically thereafter. Also check level 7 days after change in dose or start of a potentially interacting therapy.

*For those areas marked with one asterisk, the following values can be used:
ALT: 7–56 units/L
AST: 5–40 units/L
Alkaline phosphatase: 17–142 units/L
LDH: 140–280 units/L
GGT: <40 units/L
Total bilirubin: 0.2–1 mg/dL

Pregnancy risk categories: The FDA's Final Rule

In December 2014, the FDA published the *Content and Format of Labeling for Human Prescription Drug and Biological Products; Requirements for Pregnancy and Lactation Labeling*, referred to as the "Pregnancy and Lactation Labeling Rule," a final rule that set new standards for how information about using medications during pregnancy and breast-feeding is presented in the labels of biological products and prescription drugs. These standards went into effect June 30, 2015, for all newly approved drug and biological products.

The final rule recognizes that decisions for medication use during pregnancy and breastfeeding involve complex risk-benefit considerations and must be individualized because many patients who are pregnant or breastfeeding need medications to manage acute and chronic conditions. According to the final rule, the letter category system was often misinterpreted as a grading system and provided oversimplified information about a drug's risk. Consequently, the pregnancy risk categories (A, B, C, D, X) were replaced with three labeled subsections titled "Pregnancy," "Lactation," and "Females and Males of Reproductive Potential." These subsections provide more consistent, relevant explanations and information about a drug's risks and benefits in the real-world context of caring for patients. Information about active pregnancy exposure registries should be provided to patients when applicable. Patients who are pregnant or breastfeeding should always consult their health care professionals before taking any prescription or OTC medications or supplements.

Controlled substance schedules

Drugs regulated under the jurisdiction of the Controlled Substances Act of 1970 are divided into the following groups or schedules:
- Schedule I: High abuse potential, lack of accepted safety, and no accepted medical use. Examples include heroin and LSD.
- Schedule II/IIN: High abuse potential with severe dependence liability. Has an accepted medical use for treatment in the United States. Examples include opioids, amphetamines, and some barbiturates.
- Schedule III/IIIN: Less abuse potential than Schedule I or II drugs; abuse may cause moderate to low physical dependence or high psychological dependence. Has an accepted medical use for treatment in the United States. Examples include nonbarbiturate sedatives, nonamphetamine stimulants, anabolic steroids, and low doses of certain opioids.
- Schedule IV: Less abuse potential than Schedule III drugs and limited dependence liability. Has an accepted medical use for treatment in the United States. Examples include some sedatives, anxiolytics, and nonopioid analgesics.
- Schedule V: Less abuse potential with limited physical or psychological dependence compared to Schedule IV drugs. Has an accepted medical use for treatment in the United States. This category mainly includes low doses of opioids, such as codeine, used in antitussives or antidiarrheals. Under federal law, limited quantities of certain Schedule V drugs may be purchased without a prescription directly from a pharmacist if allowed under specific state statutes. Legal purchasing age is generally age 18 with valid identification. All such transactions and relevant personal information must be recorded by the dispensing pharmacist.

Canadian National Drug Schedules

The Canadian National Drug Schedules (NDS), issued by the National Association of Pharmacy Regulatory Authorities (NAPRA), is the regulatory model that defines the conditions of sale for all drug products sold in Canada. NAPRA assigns each drug product to one of four categories (Schedule I, II, III, or Unscheduled) depending on various factors, including the level of professional intervention required, public safety, and the drug's level of toxicity. The NDS is based on a cascading structure that allows regulators to use clinical judgment to determine market placement of the drug product: Schedule I products are considered the most highly regulated, and Unscheduled products have the least restrictions at point of sale.

Schedule	Description of regulatory drug categories
Schedule I drugs	• Drug requires a prescription by a licensed practitioner. • Ongoing drug monitoring and evaluation is required. • Appropriate drug use may cause dependency. • Serious drug reactions may occur at normal therapeutic dosages. • Narrow margin of safety exists between therapeutic and toxic dosages. • Serious drug interactions are known or may occur. • Drug's use may promote development of resistant strains of microorganisms. • Drug is new or the indication isn't appropriate for self-treatment and its safety in widespread use hasn't been established.
Schedule II drugs	• Drug isn't included in Schedule I and the initial need for the drug is identified or confirmed by a regulated health professional (i.e., pharmacist, physician). Prescription not required. • Drug should be administered in a health care setting or under the direction of a regulated health professional. • Drug must be readily available under exceptional circumstances when a prescription isn't practical. • Chronic therapy or subsequent retreatment requires monitoring by a pharmacist. • Drug requires intervention by a pharmacist to confirm that the patient has made an appropriate self-assessment, the condition is new to patient self-assessment, or the condition generally isn't appropriate for patient self-assessment. • Drug has significant potential for abuse or misuse. • Drug may cause serious adverse reactions not completely addressed in product label. • Safe use of drug requires a pharmacist to provide more detailed information and education than appear on the product label. • Drug may mask or delay signs and symptoms of a serious disease. • Drug is new or is in a new drug delivery system, for self-medication.
Schedule III drugs	• Drug isn't in Schedule I or II and is a new ingredient for self-medication, and advice from a pharmacist can support safe use. • Drug is used to treat a chronic or persistent condition, and advice from a pharmacist can support safe use. Prescription not required. • There is potential for abuse or misuse. • Drug may mask or delay signs and symptoms of a serious disease. • Advice from a pharmacist to explain, reinforce, or expand on product labeling information, or when product selection is likely to cause confusion, can promote safe use of drug. • Products may be located in the self-selection area of the pharmacy but must be under direct supervision of the pharmacist and clearly identified as the "professional services area" of the pharmacy.
Unscheduled drugs	• Drug can be sold from any retail outlet without professional supervision. • Acceptable and adequate label information is available for patients to make a safe drug choice. • Drug isn't included in Schedule I, II, or III.

Safe disposal of unused drugs: What patients need to know

Why is the safe disposal of unused drugs important?

It's reported that Americans fill more than 4.75 billion prescriptions annually, and many new drugs are approved each year. More drugs available and the saving of unused drugs create an increased potential for drug abuse, misuse, dependence, overdose, and accidental poisoning.

According to data from the 2020 National Survey on Drug Use and Health, 9.5 million Americans age 12 and older have misused opioids in the past year and among those people, 9.3 million misused prescription pain relievers. The Substance Abuse and Mental Health Services Administration reports that more than 50% of opioid abusers were first exposed by trying someone else's medication. Presently, steps are being taken to combat the growing epidemic of opioid abuse, dependence, and overdose in the United States: An FDA advisory committee will assess New Drug Applications for opioids that don't have abuse-deterrent formulations; the pharmaceutical industry is developing technologies to develop abuse-deterrent formulations; prescribers will have more training on long-acting and immediate-release opioid use and prescribing; immediate-release opioids will have stronger warnings similar to the warnings enacted for the long-acting formulations; and the FDA will require more postmarketing data to assess misuse and abuse of long-acting opioids. This ongoing assessment has resulted in naloxone, a life-saving drug, becoming more readily available to consumers and consumers' families (eg, OTC programs).

Other important drug safety considerations include unused drugs leading to harmful drug misuse and abuse, as well as accidental drug exposure and poisoning, particularly in children and pets. The U.S. Poison Control Center reported that in 2020, 76.9% of all reported poison exposures were unintentional. Pain medication was the most common substance linked to poison exposure in adults age 20 or older, followed by sedatives and sleeping

medications, antidepressants, and CV medications. According to Poison Control, analgesic drugs were the second most frequent cause of fatal poisonings in children between 2016 and 2020. The FDA has documented cases of accidental exposure to transdermal fentanyl pain patches. Most of these cases occurred in children younger than age 2, and 12 of these exposures resulted in death. Child-resistant containers are no guarantee that the container is child-proof; studies report that as many as 55% of accidental drug exposures in children were to drugs stored in child-resistant containers.

Now, more than ever, it's important for you as a health care provider to discuss the critical issue of safe disposal of prescribed drugs with all patients. Be sure to remind patients about the safe disposal of unused drugs at follow-up visits. Teaching patients to safely dispose of unused drugs helps protect household members and pets from accidental drug exposure and poisoning.

Patient-teaching points

Here are some important patient-teaching points about safe disposal of unused drugs:

• Tell patients that the FDA doesn't recommend the reuse or redistribution of an unused drug, because the safety and effectiveness of the drug can't be guaranteed once it's dispensed. Such factors as improper drug storage and possible drug tampering can alter the drug's safety and effectiveness. Federal law prohibits the redistribution of controlled substances.

• Counsel patients, caregivers, or family members to dispose of all unused drugs as soon as they are no longer needed.

• Advise patients to check for community drug take-back programs. These programs provide convenient disposal of drugs that can be harmful to others, such as psychotherapeutic drugs. Drug take-back programs have been designed by the U.S. Drug Enforcement Administration and are administered in conjunction with local law enforcement, usually twice a year. Patients can mail in their unused drugs or drop them off in person to local law enforcement personnel. Or, they can dispose of the drugs in a special receptacle (known as a "drop-box") located in local clinics or retail pharmacies. If drug take-back programs aren't locally available, advise patients to check with community resources or their pharmacist or prescriber to see if they may dispose of drugs themselves.

• Instruct patients that certain drugs considered harmful if ingested by others may be flushed down the sink or toilet; tell them to check the following resources to see if flushing is appropriate:

○ Medicines Recommended for Disposal by Flushing: https://www.fda.gov/drugs/safe-disposal-medicines/disposal-unused-medicines-what-you-should-know

○ DailyMed (official FDA drug label information and package inserts): https://dailymed.nlm.nih.gov/dailymed/. Search for the drug's name; then look for the following sections within the label:
  – Information for Patients and Caregivers
  – Patient Information
  – Patient Counseling Information
  – Safety and Handling Instructions
  – Medication Guide.

• Advise patients that nonharmful drugs may be disposed of by placing them intact (don't crush capsules or tablets) in a plastic bag or container filled with an undesirable substance, such as dirt, cat litter, or coffee grounds, and then placing the container in the household trash. Tell patients to make sure that children and pets can't access the trash receptacle.

• Warn patients to remove and destroy all labels from medication containers before recycling or disposing of them, to maintain privacy.

• Instruct patients to safely dispose of transdermal drug patches by folding them in half (sticky sides together) while avoiding contact with the sticky sides. Fentanyl patches should be immediately flushed down the toilet. Patches containing nitroglycerin or testosterone may be placed in the household trash.

Additional resources

Here are additional resources to find out more information about safe drug disposal of unused drugs:

• DEA Diversion Control Division–Drug Disposal Information: www.deadiversion.usdoj.gov/drug_disposal/index.html

• DEA Diversion Control Division–Controlled Substance Public Disposal Locations: https://apps.deadiversion.usdoj.gov/pubdispsearch/spring/main?execution=e1s1

• DEA Diversion Control Division–Registration call center: 1-800-882-9539

• FDA. Drug Disposal: Questions and Answers: www.fda.gov/drugs/disposal-unused-medicines-what-you-should-know/drug-disposal-questions-and-answers

• FDA. Don't Be Tempted to Use Expired Medicines: www.fda.gov/drugs/special-features/dont-be-tempted-use-expired-medicines

• FDA. Contact number: 1-888-INFO-FDA (1-888-463-6332).

Prescription drug abuse:
Identifying and treating toxicity

Prescription drugs have CNS effects that can be used or altered to achieve stimulant, euphoric, or mind-altering effects. Commonly used preparations (e.g., tablets and capsules) can be crushed, inhaled, or injected to produce quicker results. The table below lists commonly abused prescription drugs with examples of brand names, along with signs and symptoms of toxicity, potential adverse health effects, and treatment. Not all drugs have reversal agents that can be used to rapidly counteract adverse effects. General supportive care measures (respiratory and cardiac function support and IV fluids) are needed to improve clinical outcomes when prescription drugs are abused.

Substance	Toxicity signs & symptoms	Possible health effects	Toxicity care and treatment
Anesthetics			
cocaine • Medical uses: topical (ENT) anesthesia • Generic/brand names: cocaine • Routes: inhalation (nasal/oral), injection	↑HR, ↑BP, arrhythmias, chest pain, nosebleeds, vomiting, ↓appetite, dilated pupils, euphoria, insomnia, restlessness, anxiety, erratic behavior, paranoia, seizures	MI, stroke, cardiomyopathy, coma, ↑HIV risk from shared needles, ↓birth weight/premature delivery (if used during pregnancy), psychosis, hyperthermia, rhabdomyolysis	General supportive care; seizure control with IV benzodiazepines (e.g., diazepam, lorazepam). Dialysis and hemoperfusion are ineffective.
propofol • Medical uses: general anesthesia/sedation • Generic/brand names: propofol (Diprivan) • Routes: injection	Hyperthermia, ↓HR, ↓BP, ↑LFTs, nausea, vomiting, itching, wheezing, hypoxia, ↓consciousness, stupor, anxiety, confusion, delirium, seizures	MI, HF, metabolic acidosis, pancreatitis, liver damage, renal failure, respiratory depression, ↑HIV risk from shared needles	General supportive care; seizure control with IV benzodiazepines (e.g., diazepam, lorazepam). May consider hemofiltration for metabolic acidosis. Monitor urine output (urine may be rusty, tea-colored, green, or olive). Mechanical ventilation may be required.
ketamine • Medical uses: anesthesia, analgesia, sedation • Generic/brand names: ketamine (Ketalar) • Routes: injection, inhalation (nasal/oral)	↑HR, ↑BP, ↓respiratory rate, dysuria, diplopia, nystagmus, abnormal dreams, ↓consciousness, hallucinations, dysphoria, sedation, dizziness, palpitations, inability to speak, ↓coordination, seizures	Renal impairment, bladder dysfunction, respiratory depression, loss of memory, ↑HIV risk from shared needles	General supportive care; seizure control with IV benzodiazepines (e.g., diazepam, lorazepam). Treat dystonia with diphenhydramine.

Substance	Toxicity signs & symptoms	Possible health effects	Toxicity care and treatment
Opioid analgesics			
• Medical uses: pain treatment • Generic/brand names: codeine, fentanyl (Actiq, Fentora), hydrocodone bitartrate–acetaminophen (Lortab), hydromorphone hydrochloride (Dilaudid), meperidine (Demerol), methadone hydrochloride (Methadose), morphine sulfate (Duramorph, Infumorph, Mitigo, MS Contin), oxycodone hydrochloride (Oxaydo, OxyContin, Roxicodone, Xtampza ER), oxycodone hydrochloride–acetaminophen (Oxycet, Percocet), oxycodone–aspirin (Percodan), oxymorphone hydrochloride, tapentadol (Nucynta), tramadol hydrochloride (ConZip, Qdolo), tramadol hydrochloride–acetaminophen (Ultracet), tramadol hydrochloride–celecoxib (Seglentis) • Routes: oral, inhalation (nasal), injection, transdermal, buccal, sublingual	↓BP, ↓HR, ↓respiratory rate, nausea, vomiting, constipation, drowsiness, euphoria, ↓GI motility, sedation, seizures	Apnea, hypoxia, coma, CNS depression, respiratory depression, liver function abnormality/liver damage (associated with long-term acetaminophen use), death	General supportive care; seizure control with IV benzodiazepines (e.g., diazepam, lorazepam). Naloxone is the preferred reversal agent for opioids. Activated charcoal isn't recommended due to risk of CNS depression and aspiration. Mechanical ventilation may be required.
Stimulants			
Amphetamines • Medical uses: ADHD, narcolepsy • Generic/brand names: dextroamphetamine (Dexedrine), amphetamine–dextroamphetamine (Adderall XR, Dyanavel XR, Mydayis), lisdexamfetamine (Vyvanse) • Routes: oral, inhalation (nasal/oral), injection, transdermal	Hyperthermia, ↑HR, ↑BP, arrhythmias, palpitations, chest pain, diaphoresis, flushing, paranoia, agitation, abnormal behavior, dehydration, seizures	HF, MI, psychosis, renal/hepatic failure, serotonin syndrome, coma, ↑HIV risk from shared needles, rhabdomyolysis	General supportive care; seizure control with IV benzodiazepines (e.g., diazepam, lorazepam). Consider activated charcoal (most effective within 1 hour of toxic ingestion); dialysis and hemoperfusion are ineffective.
methylphenidate • Medical uses: ADHD, narcolepsy • Generic/brand names: methylphenidate (Aptensio XR, Cotempla XR, Daytrana, Jornay PM, Quillivant XR, Ritalin LA/SR) • Routes: oral, transdermal	Hyperthermia, ↑HR, ↑BP, arrhythmias, palpitations, chest pain, diaphoresis, flushing, nausea, headache, tremor, paranoia, agitation, abnormal behavior, euphoria, seizures, serotonin syndrome	HF, MI, pulmonary HTN, psychosis, renal failure, hepatic failure, coma, sudden death, rhabdomyolysis	General supportive care; seizure control with IV benzodiazepines (e.g., diazepam, lorazepam). Consider activated charcoal (most effective within 1 hour of toxic ingestion); dialysis and hemoperfusion are ineffective.
Sedatives			
Barbiturates • Medical uses: sedation, seizures, hypnotic • Generic/brand names: amobarbital (Amytal), butabarbital, pentobarbital (Nembutal), secobarbital • Routes: oral, injection	Hypothermia, ↓BP, ↓respiratory rate, ↓reflexes, drowsiness, slurred speech, nystagmus, confusion, ataxia	Respiratory failure, CV collapse, coma	General supportive care. Activated charcoal, urine alkalinization (not effective for short-acting barbiturates, which are primarily metabolized by the liver), hemoperfusion, hemofiltration, and dialysis have all been used with some success to increase elimination of barbiturates.

(continued)

Substance	Toxicity signs & symptoms	Possible health effects	Toxicity care and treatment
Sedatives (*continued*)			
Benzodiazepines • Medical uses: alcohol withdrawal, anxiety/panic disorder, insomnia, preoperative/moderate sedation, seizure disorder • Generic/brand names: alprazolam (Xanax), chlordiazepoxide, clobazam (Onfi, Sympazan) clonazepam (Klonopin), diazepam (Valium), lorazepam (Ativan, Valtoco), midazolam, oxazepam, quazepam (Doral), temazepam (Restoril), triazolam (Halcion) • Routes: oral, injection	Hypothermia, ↓BP, ↓respiratory rate, sedation, confusion, slurred speech, ataxia	Metabolic acidosis (from propylene glycol diluent used in Valium and Ativan injection preparations), respiratory failure, coma, rhabdomyolysis	General supportive care. Consider activated charcoal (most effective within 1 hour of toxic oral ingestion); hemodialysis and forced or enhanced diuresis are ineffective. Flumazenil is the reversal agent for benzodiazepines.
Sleep drugs • Medical uses: insomnia • Generic/brand names: eszopiclone (Lunesta), zaleplon, zolpidem (Ambien CR, Edluar, Zolpimist) • Routes: oral	↓BP, ↓respiratory rate, nausea, vomiting, abdominal pain, dizziness, confusion, ↓coordination, delusions, headache, sleep-eating, sleep-driving, slurred speech, somnolence	Respiratory depression, CV collapse, coma	General supportive care. Consider activated charcoal (most effective within 1 hour of toxic oral ingestion); hemodialysis is ineffective.
Miscellaneous drugs			
Cannabinoids • Medical uses: treatment of nausea, vomiting, appetite stimulant, epilepsy • Generic/brand names: cannabidiol (Epidiolex), dronabinol (Marinol, Syndros), nabilone • Routes: oral, inhalation (oral), injection (rare)	Lethargy, ↑HR, ataxia, muscle tremors, pulmonary irritation, sore throat, rhinitis, coughing, mydriasis, somnolence, euphoria, depersonalization, alteration of time sense, loss of social inhibition, mood alterations, memory impairment, cannabinoid hyperemesis syndrome	• Oral: significant altered mental status, hypotonia, coma • Injection (extract or oil): shock, DIC, rhabdomyolysis, acute renal failure, death	General supportive care; seizure control with IV benzodiazepines (e.g., diazepam, lorazepam). Absorption/elimination techniques (e.g., activated charcoal, hemodialysis, hemoperfusion, urine alkalinization) are ineffective.
Anabolic steroids • Medical uses: breast cancer, delayed puberty, hypogonadism • Generic/brand names: testosterone (Androderm, AndroGel, Aveed, Fortesta, Jatenzo, Kyzatrex, Tlando, Vogelxo), oxandrolone, oxymetholone • Routes: oral, injection, transdermal, intranasal	↑BP, acne, fluid retention, ↑lipid levels, jaundice, tendon rupture, breast enlargement (men), male-pattern baldness, changes in sex organs, infertility, libido changes, rage, aggression, mania, delusions, mood swings, insomnia, weight gain	Short stature, MI, hepatitis, hepatic tumors, hepatic failure, thrombosis, stroke, ↑HIV risk from shared needles	General supportive care. Absorption/elimination techniques (e.g., activated charcoal, hemodialysis, hemoperfusion, urine alkalinization) are ineffective. Benzodiazepines and antipsychotics may be considered for extreme aggression.

Serotonin syndrome: What you should know to protect your patient

Serotonin is a neurotransmitter involved in the conduction of nerve impulses. Serotonin syndrome, a drug reaction resulting from an increase in plasma serotonin levels, can range in severity from mild to life-threatening to fatal. It frequently occurs when drugs that affect serotonin levels are given together, causing serotonin levels to rise. Serotonin syndrome can occur within minutes or hours of drug administration and may cause ARDS, DIC, liver and renal failure, rhabdomyolysis, intractable myoclonus, and seizures. Identifying the symptoms and initiating prompt treatment can prevent a potentially fatal outcome. Some drugs commonly associated with serotonin syndrome include SSRIs (fluoxetine), SSNRIs (duloxetine), MAO inhibitors (phenelzine), methylene blue, opiates (methadone), antiemetics (ondansetron), antibiotics (linezolid), antiretrovirals (ritonavir), dextromethorphan, and herbal supplements (St. John's wort).

Key points	What you need to know or do
Risk factors	• Coadministration of medications that affect serotonin levels • Overdose of medications that affect serotonin levels
Signs and symptoms	• Agitation, restlessness, mental status changes, hallucinations • Headache, muscle pain • Loss of muscle coordination, muscle rigidity, seizures, muscle spasms, tremor • Fever, shivering, goose bumps, HTN, tachycardia, arrhythmia • Profound diaphoresis • Nausea, vomiting, diarrhea
Preventive measures	• Review medication history and drug therapy for potential interactions. • Identify patients at risk for serotonin syndrome. • Perform thorough baseline assessment.
Monitoring	• Monitor patient's condition closely. • Monitor temperature, HR (continuous cardiac monitoring), BP, fluid status, and urine output frequently. • Monitor oxygenation, mental status, and pain levels. • Monitor serum serotonin levels. • Monitor electrolyte and CK levels.
Treatment and interventions	• Discontinue drugs associated with serotonin syndrome. • Administer oxygen therapy, ventilation, and paralytics (succinylcholine chloride) as needed to maintain adequate ventilation. • Institute cooling measures (i.e., cooling baths, blankets) for fever. • Administer IV fluids to maintain hydration. • Administer medications to block serotonin production (antihistamines [cyproheptadine hydrochloride]), to control seizures and myoclonus (benzodiazepines [diazepam]), and to control HTN (nitroprusside), tachycardia (beta blockers [esmolol]), and pain (opioids if needed).

Tumor lysis syndrome: A life-threatening emergency

Tumor lysis syndrome is a potentially life-threatening oncologic emergency caused by a rapid and massive breakdown of tumor cells, usually within a week after chemotherapy, targeted therapy, or radiation administration. It can also occur spontaneously in rapidly growing neoplasms. The release of tumor cell debris into the bloodstream causes an array of metabolic disturbances, such as hyperkalemia, hyperphosphatemia, hyperuricemia, and hypocalcemia, which can lead to seizures, acute kidney injury, fluid overload, cardiac arrhythmias, cardiopulmonary arrest, and death. TLS is associated with treatment for hematologic cancers, including some leukemias and lymphomas, and with the use of such chemotherapeutic drugs as paclitaxel, fludarabine, etoposide, bortezomib, zoledronic acid, and hydroxyurea.

Key considerations	What you need to know or do
Risk factors	• Disease with high tumor-cell proliferation rate • Chemosensitivity of the malignancy, bulky tumor, or extensive metastasis; organ infiltration; bone marrow involvement • Pretreatment hyperuricemia, elevated LDH levels, renal impairment, nephrotoxic drugs
Signs and symptoms	• Lethargy, syncope, seizures, altered mental state • HF, arrhythmias, sudden death • Edema, weight gain, fluid overload • Renal failure, metabolic acidosis, decreased or absent urine output, urine sediment, flank pain, hematuria • Anorexia, nausea, vomiting, constipation, diarrhea • Muscle cramping, tetany • Hyperkalemia, hypocalcemia, hyperphosphatemia, hyperuricemia
Preventive measures	• Identify at-risk patients as soon as possible. • Obtain central venous access. • Obtain baseline ECG, vital signs, and hemodynamic status. • Administer IV hydration to improve renal perfusion and GFR. • Administer sodium bicarbonate for metabolic acidosis. • Administer pretreatment hypouricemics (allopurinol or rasburicase). • Avoid potassium-sparing diuretics. • Consider phosphate-binding agents for hyperphosphatemia.
Treatment and monitoring	• Monitor mental status. • Monitor respiratory status and oxygenation. Administer oxygen therapy as prescribed. • Institute continuous cardiac monitoring. • Closely monitor vital signs and fluid volume status (fluid intake, urine output, weight, edema). • Monitor serial electrolytes, acid-base balance, and BUN, creatinine, and uric acid levels every 4 to 6 hours or at a frequency determined by the prescriber. Monitor calcium, phosphate, and LDH levels. Correct abnormalities. • Monitor fluid volume and administer diuretics. • Renal replacement therapy or hemodialysis may be needed.

Severe cutaneous adverse reactions

Severe cutaneous adverse reactions (SCARs) are hypersensitivity reactions usually triggered by medications. SCARs include SJS, TEN, DRESS syndrome, and acute generalized exanthematous pustulosis (AGEP). These reactions may be life-threatening and can occur at any time during treatment and, in some cases, after treatment has stopped. Identifying the symptoms and initiating prompt treatment can prevent a potentially fatal outcome. Some drugs commonly associated with SCARs include anticonvulsants, sulfa-containing drugs, anti-infectives (antibiotics, antituberculotics, antivirals), NSAIDs, and uric acid-lowering agents (allopurinol).

SJS and TEN are essentially the same disorder differentiated by the extent of the reaction. SJS is the less severe, affecting up to 10% of the patient's BSA. The mortality rate for SJS and TEN increases in patients older than age 40, those in whom the reaction affects more than 10% of the BSA, and those with an HR over 120 beats/minute, the presence of malignancy, BUN level above 28 mg/dL, blood glucose level over 252 mg/dL, and blood bicarbonate level less than 20 mEq/L. Potential long-term complications of SJS and TEN include chronic eczema, pigment changes, alopecia, hyperhidrosis, impaired taste, difficulty urinating, dry eye syndrome, chronic conjunctivitis, and corneal erosions.

DRESS syndrome is the presence of three or more symptoms, including cutaneous reactions (rash, exfoliative dermatitis), eosinophilia, fever, lymphadenopathy, and one or more systemic complications (hepatitis, nephritis, pneumonitis, myocarditis, pericarditis). DRESS syndrome affects more than 50% of the patient's BSA. The mortality rate for DRESS syndrome increases with severe organ involvement, multiorgan failure, and viral reactivation of cytomegalovirus. Potential long-term complications of DRESS syndrome include permanent renal dysfunction, type 1 diabetes, thyroid disorders, and autoimmune diseases, including SLE.

AGEP generally develops rapidly after exposure, especially to an antibiotic or diltiazem. Spontaneous resolution often occurs with withdrawal of the causative agent. Long-term complications and death are rare.

Key points	What you need to know or do
Risk factors	• History of SCAR • Exposure to high-risk drugs • Family history of a SCAR • Certain genetic variations • HIV-positive status • Immunocompromise • Cancer (especially hematologic) • Viral infections

(continued)

Key points	What you need to know or do
Signs and symptoms	**SJS and TEN** • Flulike symptoms: fever, malaise • Blistering and peeling of face and chest • Spreading of blisters and erosion to other areas, including mucous membranes; sore throat, conjunctivitis, trouble swallowing and breathing, sores in the urinary tract or genitals • Skin pain • Dehydration • Secondary infection • Severe complications: pneumonia, sepsis, shock, multiple organ failure, death **DRESS syndrome** • Flulike symptoms: fever, malaise, lymphadenopathy • Maculopapular rash progressing to erythema • Other skin presentations: purpura, pustules, exfoliative dermatitis, targetlike lesions • Symmetrical distribution of lesions on trunk and extremities • Pruritus • Mucosal lesions and edema • Hematologic changes: eosinophilia, leukocytosis, neutrophilia, lymphocytosis, monocytosis, atypical lymphocytes • Liver injury: acute elevated liver enzyme levels • Kidney injury: proteinuria, acute interstitial nephritis, acute renal failure • Lung involvement: shortness of breath, dry cough, interstitial infiltrates and pleural effusions on x-ray • Heart involvement: hypotension, tachycardia, chest pain, ECG changes • Nervous system involvement: Bell's palsy, peripheral neuropathy, aseptic meningitis, cerebral vasculitis **AGEP** • Sudden onset of pustules and edematous erythema, especially at the major skin folds • Facial edema • Blisters • Mucosal lesions (rare, mild) • Fever • Leukocytosis • Major organ involvement in severe cases: liver, kidney, lung, and bone marrow abnormalities
Preventive measures	• Screen patient for prior allergic reactions. • Encourage patient to wear a medical alert necklace or bracelet. • Ensure that patient has an allergy alert bracelet in the hospital or other facility. • Advise patient to notify all providers and pharmacists of SCAR history. • Monitor patient receiving new medications. • Assess for genetic markers for specific drugs. • Teach patient to report symptoms.
Monitoring	• Monitor skin and mucous membranes closely. • Monitor fluid balance and electrolytes. • Monitor vital signs. • Monitor CBC. • Monitor nutritional status. • Monitor airway status.
Treatment and interventions	• Identification and immediate withdrawal of causative agent • Confirmation by histopathologic exam • Assessment and management of skin wounds • Management of fluid and nutrition status • Adequate pain control • Appropriate antibiotic therapy for secondary infections • Corticosteroids (systemic and topical) • Immunosuppression (cyclosporine, etanercept)

Anaphylaxis

Anaphylaxis, a potentially life-threatening allergic reaction, can occur within seconds or minutes of exposure to an allergen. Nonallergic mechanisms can also trigger anaphylaxis but are less common. The reaction causes the immune system to release chemical mediators, such as histamine, prostaglandin D2, and cytokines. Many of the mediators have overlapping and synergistic effects; for example, hypotension and bronchoconstriction may cause shock and respiratory distress. After an initial anaphylactic reaction, future reactions may be more severe.

Allergens can include food, insect bites, latex, and medications. Some drugs commonly associated with anaphylaxis include aspirin, NSAIDs, antibiotics, and IV contrast for imaging studies.

Identifying the symptoms and initiating prompt treatment can prevent a potentially fatal outcome.

Key points	What you need to know or do
Risk factors	• History of a mild anaphylactic reaction • Allergies • Asthma or COPD • Latex exposure • Heart disease • Mastocytosis or other mast cell disorders
Signs and symptoms	• Skin reactions, including hives, itching, flushing or pale skin, generalized urticaria, pruritus • Hypotension, tachycardia or bradycardia, weak pulse, arrhythmia, chest pain • Dizziness, syncope, collapse • Sneezing, rhinorrhea, hoarseness • Stridor, wheezing, dyspnea, persistent cough, cyanosis • Angioedema of eyes, lips, tongue, airway, hands, feet, genitals • Angioedema of the bowel wall presenting as abdominal pain, nausea, vomiting, or diarrhea • Respiratory arrest
Preventive measures	• Screen patient for prior allergic reactions. • Encourage patient to wear a medical alert necklace or bracelet. • Ensure that patient has an allergy alert bracelet in the hospital or other facility. • Advise patient to notify all providers and pharmacists of allergy. • Keep patient's medical record up to date. • Monitor patient receiving new medications closely. • Teach patient to report symptoms.
Monitoring	• Monitor patient's condition closely. • Monitor BP and cardiac rhythm continuously. • Monitor oxygenation by pulse oximetry. • Monitor fluid status and urine output frequently.
Treatment and interventions	• Administer IM epinephrine, and repeat every 5 to 15 minutes as needed. • Position patient supine or in Trendelenburg position, if necessary and tolerated. • Administer oxygen therapy. • Assist with ET intubation for imminent airway obstruction from angioedema. • Administer IV NSS by rapid bolus to treat hypotension, and repeat as needed. • Administer albuterol via nebulizer or metered-dose inhaler, and repeat as needed. • Administer H_1 antihistamine (diphenhydramine IV, cetirizine IV) for urticaria and itching only. • Administer H_2 antihistamine (famotidine IV). • Administer glucocorticoid (methylprednisolone). • For refractory symptoms, administer epinephrine by continuous infusion, add a second vasopressor, or administer glucagon to patients on beta blockers not responding to epinephrine.

Understanding biosimilar drugs

What are nonbiologic drug products and how are they approved?

Most drugs on the market are nonbiologic drugs that are made from chemicals with known structures that can be identically re-created. Brand-name nonbiologic drugs are first approved by the FDA through a New Drug Application approval process that requires evidence of safety and effectiveness of the drug, the quality of the product, and the accuracy of its labeling. Pharmaceutical companies file for patents or exclusive marketing rights with the FDA for each drug.

Once these patents expire, other pharmaceutical companies can manufacture the brand-name nonbiologic drug by making an identical (bioequivalent), less expensive, generic formulation (called an "innovator drug" by the FDA) of the same brand-name drug. Generic formulations are less expensive because the pharmaceutical companies file for an Abbreviated New Drug Application (ANDA) approval process, which doesn't require the pharmaceutical company to perform clinical trials and submit evidence of safety and effectiveness of the generic drug. The FDA's *Approved Drug Products with Therapeutic Equivalence Evaluations* (also known as the Orange Book) contains all of the FDA-approved drugs and identifies which drugs are therapeutically equivalent. If drugs are deemed therapeutically equivalent, a less costly drug may be able to be substituted for a higher-cost drug.

What are biological drug products?

In contrast to conventional drug products, which are pure chemical substances, biological drugs are made from living organisms (human or animal cells or tissues, proteins, microorganisms), and their manufacturing processes are more complex than those for conventional drugs and are also proprietary. Examples of biological products include vaccines, blood and blood products, and recombinant therapeutic proteins. Biological drugs work by targeting a certain biological structure, enzyme, pathway, or other mechanism; for example, they may change the way the immune system reacts to a virus or change cells and proteins involved in inflammation.

What are biosimilar drugs and how are they approved?

Just as nonbiologic drugs have brand-name and generic forms, biological drugs have brand-name and biosimilar forms. Unlike generic drugs, which are chemical replicas of the original brand-name drug, biosimilar drugs are similar to but not exact duplicates of the brand-name drug (biological reference product) because they are made from tissues and other nonchemical components. Each pharmaceutical company must demonstrate that its biosimilar drug is highly similar to a biological reference product that has already been FDA-approved. According to the FDA, biosimilar drugs must demonstrate that they have "no clinically meaningful differences in terms of safety and effectiveness from the reference product. Minor differences in clinically inactive components are allowed."

As with nonbiologic drugs, brand-name biological drugs are approved by the FDA through a Biologics License Application, which requires evidence of safety, purity, potency, and effectiveness of the biological drug.

An abbreviated licensure pathway for biological products is described in The Patient Protection and Affordable Care Act (Affordable Care Act) of 2010. Similar to the ANDA approval process, biological drugs have an abbreviated licensure pathway for biological products that are demonstrated to be "biosimilar" to or "interchangeable" with an FDA-licensed biological product. The Biologics Price Competition and Innovation Act (BPCI Act), part of the Affordable Care Act, provides this licensure pathway. According to the BPCI Act, an interchangeable biological drug may be substituted for the reference product by a pharmacist without the consultation or intervention of the prescriber.

Similar to the Orange Book for nonbiologic drugs, the FDA's *Lists of Licensed Biological Products with Reference Product Exclusivity and Biosimilarity or Interchangeability Evaluations* (also known as the Purple Book) states whether a biological product has been determined by the FDA to be biosimilar to or interchangeable with a biological reference product.

Why are biosimilar drugs important?

The FDA is expected to approve an increasing number of biosimilar drugs, as these drugs are expected to compete with each other in the medical marketplace and decrease consumer costs. The average sale price for biosimilar drugs can be as much as 50% less than the reference product. Some pharmaceutical companies have embraced the new technology of biosimilar drugs and have a pipeline of biosimilar drugs in the development or approval stage. Just like generics, biosimilar drugs can be made by more than one pharmaceutical company, thereby increasing competition and hopefully lowering overall health care costs.

What is important to know about biosimilar and biological reference drugs?

Biosimilarity is based on the product being highly similar to the biological reference product as determined by toxicity studies in animals and one or more clinical studies demonstrating the safety, purity, and potency of the product.

Biosimilar drugs:
• may be approved for the same or fewer indications as the biological reference drug. The number of approved indications may not exceed the number of approved indications for the reference drug.
• must have the same mechanism of action, route of administration, dosage forms, and strength as the reference drug.
• are expected to have no differences in safety and effectiveness compared to the reference drug.

How are biosimilar drug names determined?

Biological products and their biosimilar drugs share a nonproprietary name (also referred to as a "proper name"). Biosimilar drugs use the nonproprietary name plus a suffix composed of four lowercase letters, separated from the core name by a hyphen. These four letters are proposed by the manufacturer at the time of application or submission. Older suffixes may represent the name of the pharmaceutical company that holds the biosimilar drug's licensing agreement. On March 6, 2015, the FDA approved the very first biosimilar drug, filgrastim-sndz (Zarxio), licensed by the Sandoz Company. It's a biosimilar drug to the biological reference product filgrastim (Neupogen).

Additional information may be found at https://www.bbcic.org/resources/fda-guidance/Nonproprietary-Naming-Biological-Products.

Antacids: Indications and dosages

Refer to manufacturer's instructions for complete prescribing and safety information.

aluminum hydroxide
a-LOO-mi-num

Therapeutic class: Antacids
Pharmacologic class: Aluminum salts

AVAILABLE FORMS
Oral suspension: 320 mg/5 mL ◊

INDICATIONS & DOSAGES
➤ **Acid indigestion**
Adults: 640 mg PO five to six times daily after meals and at bedtime. Maximum dose, 3,840 mg/day.

aluminum hydroxide–magnesium carbonate
a-LOO-mi-num

Acid Gone ◊ , Gaviscon ◊

Therapeutic class: Antacids
Pharmacologic class: Aluminum salts

AVAILABLE FORMS
Oral suspension: 31.7 mg aluminum hydroxide/119.3 mg magnesium carbonate in 5 mL ◊ ; 254 mg aluminum hydroxide/237.5 mg magnesium carbonate in 5 mL ◊
Tablets (chewable): 160 mg aluminum hydroxide/105 mg magnesium carbonate ◊

INDICATIONS & DOSAGES
➤ **Acid indigestion, heartburn, sour stomach, GI upset**
Adults: 2 to 4 chewable tablets PO q.i.d.; maximum dose, 16 tablets/24 hours. Or, 10 to 20 mL (254 mg aluminum hydroxide/237.5 mg magnesium carbonate/5 mL) PO q.i.d.; maximum dose, 80 mL/24 hours.
Adults and children age 12 and older: 15 to 30 mL (31.7 mg aluminum hydroxide/119.3 mg magnesium carbonate/5 mL) PO q.i.d.; maximum dose, 120 mL/24 hours.

calcium carbonate
KAL-see-um

Alka-Seltzer Heartburn ◊ , Cal-Gest ◊ , Maalox ◊ , Maalox Children's ◊ , Titralac ◊ , Tums ◊

Therapeutic class: Antacids
Pharmacologic class: Calcium salts

AVAILABLE FORMS
Calcium carbonate contains 40% calcium; 20 mEq calcium per gram.
Oral suspension: 1,250 mg/5 mL ◊
Powder: 800 mg/2 g ◊
Tablets: 648 mg ◊ , 1,250 mg ◊ , 1,500 mg ◊
Tablets (chewable): 260 mg ◊ , 400 mg ◊ , 420 mg ◊ , 500 mg ◊ , 600 mg ◊ , 750 mg ◊ , 1,000 mg ◊ , 1,177 mg ◊ , 1,250 mg ◊

INDICATIONS & DOSAGES
➤ **Acid indigestion**
Adults: 1 to 4 tablets, 5 to 10 mL, or ½ teaspoon (1.3 g) PO when symptomatic. Maximum dose, 8,000 mg daily for up to 2 weeks.
Children age 12 and older: 500 to 3,000 mg when symptomatic. Maximum dose, 7,500 mg daily for up to 2 weeks.
Children ages 6 to 11, weighing at least 21.8 kg: 750 to 800 mg PO when symptomatic. Maximum dose, 2,400 mg daily for up to 2 weeks.
Children ages 2 to 5 weighing 10.9 to 21.3 kg: 375 to 400 mg PO when symptomatic. Maximum dose, 1,200 mg daily for up to 2 weeks.
➤ **Calcium supplement**
Adults: 500 mg to 4 g PO daily in one to three divided doses.

magnesium oxide
mag-NEE-see-um

Mag-200 ◊ , Mag-Ox 400 ◊ , Maox ◊ , Uro-Mag ◊

Therapeutic class: Antacids
Pharmacologic class: Magnesium salts

AVAILABLE FORMS
Capsules: 140 mg ◊
Tablets: 100 mg ◊ , 200 mg ◊ , 400 mg ◊ , 420 mg ◊ , 500 mg ◊

INDICATIONS & DOSAGES
➤ **Acid indigestion**
Adults: 1 tablet PO once daily or b.i.d. according to the package directions or as directed by prescriber. Maximum dosage, 2 tablets (800 mg)/day for up to 2 weeks.
➤ **Dietary supplement**
Adults: 1 to 2 tablets or 1 to 5 capsules PO daily or as directed by prescriber.

Antidiarrheals: Indications and dosages

Refer to manufacturer's instructions for complete prescribing and safety information.

bismuth subsalicylate
BIS-mith sub-sal-LIS-a-late

Bismatrol ◊, Kaopectate ◊,
Pepto-Bismol ◊, Pink Bismuth ◊,
Stomach Relief ◊

Therapeutic class: Antidiarrheals
Pharmacologic class: Adsorbents

AVAILABLE FORMS
Caplets ⊙: 262 mg ◊
Capsules ⊙: 262 mg ◊
Oral suspension: 262 mg/15 mL (regular strength) ◊,
525 mg/15 mL (maximum strength) ◊
Tablets (chewable): 262 mg ◊

INDICATIONS & DOSAGES
➤ **Diarrhea, gas, indigestion, heartburn, nausea; traveler's diarrhea**
Adults and children age 12 and older: 525 mg PO every 30 to 60 minutes or 1,050 mg PO every 60 minutes as needed for up to 2 days. Maximum, 4,200 mg/24 hours.

crofelemer
kro-FEL-e-mer

Mytesi

Therapeutic class: Antidiarrheals
Pharmacologic class: Antidiarrheals

AVAILABLE FORMS
Tablets (delayed-release) ⊙: 125 mg

INDICATIONS & DOSAGES
➤ **Noninfectious diarrhea in patients with HIV/ AIDS on antiretroviral therapy**
Adults: 125 mg PO b.i.d.

diphenoxylate hydrochloride– atropine sulfate
dye-fen-OKS-ul-ate/A-troe-peen

Lomotil*

Therapeutic class: Antidiarrheals
Pharmacologic class: Opioids
Controlled substance schedule: V

AVAILABLE FORMS
Liquid: 2.5 mg diphenoxylate and 0.025 mg atropine/5 mL*
Tablets: 2.5 mg diphenoxylate and 0.025 mg atropine

INDICATIONS & DOSAGES
➤ **Acute, nonspecific diarrhea**
Adults and children age 13 and older: Initially, 5 mg diphenoxylate PO q.i.d.; reduce dosage with initial control of symptoms. Maximum dosage, 20 mg/day.
Children ages 2 to 12: 0.3 to 0.4 mg/kg diphenoxylate liquid form PO daily in four divided doses. Maintenance, reduce dosage with initial control of symptoms; may reduce dosage by as much as 75%. Maximum, 10 mg/day. Don't use tablets in children younger than age 13.

loperamide hydrochloride
loe-PER-a-mide

Diamode ◊, Imodium A-D ◊

Therapeutic class: Antidiarrheals
Pharmacologic class: Piperidine derivatives

AVAILABLE FORMS
Capsules: 2 mg
Oral liquid: 1 mg/7.5 mL ◊
Tablets: 2 mg ◊

INDICATIONS & DOSAGES
Boxed Warning Don't exceed recommended dosages due to risk of torsades de pointes, cardiac arrest, and death. Use is contraindicated in children younger than age 2. ■
➤ **Acute, nonspecific diarrhea; reducing volume of discharge from ileostomies**
Adults and children older than age 12: Initially, give 4 mg PO; then 2 mg after each unformed stool. Maximum, 16 mg/day (prescription strength) or 8 mg/day (OTC) unless otherwise directed.
Children ages 9 to 11 weighing 27.1 to 43 kg: 2 mg PO; then 1 mg after each loose stool. Maximum, 6 mg daily.
Children ages 6 to 8 weighing 21 to 27 kg: 2 mg PO; then 1 mg after each loose stool. Maximum, 4 mg daily.
Children ages 2 to 5 weighing 13 to less than 21 kg (oral liquid only): 1 mg PO; then 1 mg after each loose stool. Maximum, 3 mg/day.
➤ **Chronic diarrhea associated with inflammatory bowel disease**
Adults: Initially, 4 mg PO; then 2 mg after each unformed stool until diarrhea subsides. Adjust dosage to individual response. Maximum, 16 mg/day (prescription strength).
➤ **Diarrhea, traveler's diarrhea (OTC)**
Adults and children age 12 and older: 4 mg PO followed by 2 mg after each subsequent loose stool for a maximum of 8 mg/24 hours.

telotristat ethyl
tel-OH-tri-stat

Xermelo

Therapeutic class: Antidiarrheals
Pharmacologic class: Tryptophan hydroxylase
inhibitors

AVAILABLE FORMS
Tablets: 250 mg

INDICATIONS & DOSAGES
➤ **Carcinoid syndrome diarrhea in combination
with somatostatin analogue (SSA) therapy in patients inadequately controlled by SSA therapy**
Adults: 250 mg PO t.i.d.

Laxatives: Indications and dosages

Refer to manufacturer's instructions for complete prescribing and safety information.

bisacodyl
bye-suh-KOH-dil

Bisacodyl EC ◇ , Biscolax ◇ , Carter's Little Pills ✽ ◇ , Codulax ✽ ◇ , Dulcolax ◇ , Ex-Lax Ultra ◇ , Feen-a-Mint ◇ , Fleet Bisacodyl ◇ , Silver Bullet ✽ ◇ , The Magic Bullet ◇ , Woman's Laxative ◇

Therapeutic class: Laxatives
Pharmacologic class: Diphenylmethane derivatives

AVAILABLE FORMS
Enema: 10 mg/30 mL ◇
Suppositories: 10 mg ◇
Tablets (delayed-release) **OTC**: 5 mg ◇

INDICATIONS & DOSAGES
➤ **Constipation; preparation for surgery or rectal or bowel exam**
Adults and children age 12 and older: 5 to 15 mg PO, PRN. Or, 10-mg suppository PR daily PRN. Or, 10-mg enema PR for evacuation before exam or surgery. May give enema as a single daily dose.
Children ages 6 to 11: 5 mg PO, PRN. Oral dose isn't recommended if child can't swallow tablet whole. Don't give enema in children younger than age 12.

calcium polycarbophil
FiberCon ◇ , Fiber-Lax ◇

Therapeutic class: Laxatives
Pharmacologic class: Hydrophilic drugs

AVAILABLE FORMS
Tablets: 625 mg ◇

INDICATIONS & DOSAGES
➤ **Constipation**
Adults and children older than age 12: 2 tablets (1,250 mg) PO once daily to q.i.d., PRN.

docusate calcium (dioctyl calcium sulfosuccinate)
DOK-yoo-sayt

Kao-Tin Capsule ◇ , Surfak ◇

docusate sodium (dioctyl sodium sulfosuccinate)
Colace ◇ , Correctol Extra Gentle ◇ , DocuSol Kids Enema ◇ , DOK ◇ , Dulcolax Stool Softener ◇ , Enemeez Mini ◇ , Pedia-Lax Liquid Stool Softener ◇ , Phillips Stool Softener ◇ , Selax ✽ ◇ , Silace ◇ , Surfak ◇

Therapeutic class: Laxatives
Pharmacologic class: Surfactants

AVAILABLE FORMS
docusate calcium
Capsules: 240 mg ◇
docusate sodium
Capsules: 100 mg ◇ , 200 mg ✽ ◇ , 240 mg ◇ , 250 mg ◇
Oral liquid: 50 mg/15 mL ◇ , 100 mg/10 mL ◇ , 150 mg/15 mL ◇
Rectal suspension: 100 mg/5 mL ◇ , 283 mg/5 mL ◇
Syrup: 60 mg/15 mL ◇
Tablets: 100 mg ◇

INDICATIONS & DOSAGES
➤ **Constipation (stool softener)**
Adults and children older than age 12: 50 to 360 mg docusate sodium PO daily in a single dose or in divided doses or 240 mg docusate calcium PO daily until bowel movements are normal. Or, give enema. Administer contents of 1 bottle PR once daily for up to 1 week.
Children ages 2 to 11: 50 to 150 mg docusate sodium PO daily as a single dose or in divided doses. Or, give 100 mg or 283 mg enema PR once daily for up to 1 week.

glycerin
GLI-ser-in

Avedana ◇ , Pedia-Lax ◇

Therapeutic class: Laxatives
Pharmacologic class: Trihydric alcohols

AVAILABLE FORMS
Enema: 5.4 g ◇
Liquid suppository: 2.8 g ◇
Suppositories: Adult and pediatric sizes (1 and 2 g) ◇

INDICATIONS & DOSAGES
➤ **Constipation**
Adults and children age 6 and older: 1 rectal suppository/day, or PR as enema, PRN.
Children ages 2 to younger than age 6: 1 rectal pediatric suppository/day.

lactitol
LAK-ti-tol

Pizensy

Therapeutic class: Laxatives
Pharmacologic class: Hyperosmolar agents

AVAILABLE FORMS
Powder for oral solution: 280 g, 560 g (multidose bottles); 10 g (single-dose packet)

INDICATIONS & DOSAGES
➤ **Chronic idiopathic constipation**
Adults: 20 g PO once daily, preferably with meals.
Adjust-a-dose: In patients with persistent loose stools, reduce to 10 g PO once daily.

lactulose
LAK-tyoo-lose

Constulose, Enulose, Generlac, Kristalose

Therapeutic class: Laxatives
Pharmacologic class: Disaccharides

AVAILABLE FORMS
Oral solution: 10 g/15 mL
Packets: 10 g, 20 g
Rectal solution: 10 g/15 mL, 20 g/30 mL

INDICATIONS & DOSAGES
➤ **Constipation**
Adults: 10 to 20 g PO daily, increased to 40 g, if needed.
➤ **To prevent and treat hepatic encephalopathy, including hepatic precoma and coma in patients with severe hepatic disease**
Adults: Initially, 20 to 30 g PO every 1 to 2 hours to produce two soft stools daily; then reduce frequency to t.i.d. or q.i.d. to produce two or three soft stools daily. Usual dose is 60 to 100 g daily in divided doses. Or, 200 g or 300 mL diluted with 700 mL of water or NSS and given as retention enema PR every 4 to 6 hours, as needed.
Older children and adolescents: Initially, 26.7 to 60 g/day (40 to 90 mL/day) PO in divided doses to produce two or three soft stools daily; then adjust dosage to maintain stool output.

Infants: Initially, 1.7 to 6.7 g/day (2.5 to 10 mL/day) PO in divided doses to produce two or three soft stools daily; then adjust dosage to maintain stool output.

linaclotide
LIN-a-KLOE-tide

Constella✢, Linzess

Therapeutic class: Laxatives
Pharmacologic class: Guanylate cyclase-C agonists

AVAILABLE FORMS
Capsules ⓞⓝⓒ: 72 mcg, 145 mcg, 290 mcg

INDICATIONS & DOSAGES
Boxed Warning Contraindicated in children younger than age 2 due to dehydration risk. Safety and effectiveness in children younger than age 18 haven't been established. ∎
➤ **IBS with constipation**
Adults: 290 mcg PO once daily on an empty stomach at least 30 minutes before first meal of the day.
➤ **Chronic idiopathic constipation**
Adults: 72 to 145 mcg PO once daily on an empty stomach at least 30 minutes before first meal of the day.

lubiprostone
loo-bee-PRAHS-tohn

Amitiza✐

Therapeutic class: Laxatives
Pharmacologic class: Chloride channel activators

AVAILABLE FORMS
Capsules ⓞⓝⓒ: 8 mcg, 24 mcg

INDICATIONS & DOSAGES
➤ **Chronic idiopathic constipation; opioid-induced constipation in patients with chronic, noncancer pain**
Adults: 24 mcg PO b.i.d. with food and water.
Adjust-a-dose: For patients with moderately impaired hepatic function (Child-Pugh class B), starting dose is 16 mcg b.i.d.; for those with severely impaired hepatic function (Child-Pugh class C), starting dose is 8 mcg b.i.d. May increase to full dose after appropriate interval if tolerated and an adequate response hasn't been obtained at initial dose. Monitor patient response.
➤ **IBS with constipation**
Women age 18 and older: 8 mcg PO b.i.d. with food and water.
Adjust-a-dose: For patients with severely impaired hepatic function (Child-Pugh class C), starting dose

is 8 mcg once daily. May increase to full dose after appropriate interval if tolerated and an adequate response hasn't been obtained at initial dose. Monitor patient response.

magnesium citrate (citrate of magnesia)
Citroma ◇, GoodSense Magnesium Citrate ◇

magnesium hydroxide (milk of magnesia)
Dulcolax ◇, Milk of Magnesia ◇, Milk of Magnesia-Concentrate ◇, Pedia-Lax Chewable Tablets ◇, Phillips' Milk of Magnesia ◇

magnesium sulfate ◇ (Epsom salts ◇)

Therapeutic class: Laxatives
Pharmacologic class: Magnesium salts

AVAILABLE FORMS
magnesium citrate
Oral solution: 1.75 g/30 mL ◇
Tablets: 100 mg ◇
magnesium hydroxide
Chewable tablets: 311 mg ◇, 400 mg ◇, 600 mg ◇
Oral suspension: 400 mg/5 mL ◇, 800 mg/5 mL ◇, 1,200 mg/15 mL ◇, 2,400 mg/10 mL ◇
magnesium sulfate
Granules: About 40 mEq magnesium/5 g ◇

INDICATIONS & DOSAGES
➤ **Constipation; to evacuate bowel before surgery**
Adults and children age 12 and older: 6.5 to 10 fluid oz (195 to 300 mL) magnesium citrate with 8 oz (240 mL) water PO in single or divided doses in 24 hours. Or, 2 to 4 tablets magnesium citrate PO daily at bedtime or in divided doses. Or, 8 chewable magnesium hydroxide tablets PO at bedtime or in divided doses. Or, 30 to 60 mL magnesium hydroxide liquid (400 mg/5 mL) PO as a single daily dose at bedtime or in divided doses. Or, 15 to 30 mL magnesium hydroxide liquid (800 mg/5 mL) PO as a single daily dose at bedtime or in divided doses. Or, 10 to 20 mL magnesium hydroxide (1,200 mg/5 mL) PO as a single daily dose at bedtime or in divided doses. Or, 10 to 20 g magnesium sulfate granules dissolved in 8 fluid oz water PO as a single dose; may repeat after 4 hours, PRN.
Children ages 6 to 11: 3 to 7 fluid oz magnesium citrate with 8 oz water PO in 24 hours as a single daily dose or in divided doses. Or, 2 to 6 chewable tablets magnesium hydroxide PO as a single daily dose or in divided doses. Or, 15 to 30 mL magnesium hydroxide liquid (400 mg/5 mL) as a single daily dose at bedtime or in divided doses. Or, 7.5 to 15 mL magnesium

hydroxide liquid (800 mg/5 mL) PO as a single daily dose at bedtime or in divided doses. Or, 5 to 10 mL magnesium hydroxide liquid (1,200 mg/5 mL) PO as a single daily dose at bedtime or in divided doses. Or, 5 to 10 g magnesium sulfate dissolved in 8 fluid oz water PO daily as a single dose; may repeat in 4 hours, PRN.
Children ages 3 to 5: One to three magnesium hydroxide chewable tablets PO as a single daily dose or in divided doses. Or, 5 to 15 mL magnesium hydroxide liquid (400 mg/5 mL) PO as a single daily dose or in two to four divided doses.

polyethylene glycol 3350 (PEG)
pol-ee-ETH-ih-leen

Clearlax✽◇, Comfilax✽◇, GaviLAX◇, GlycoLax◇, HealthyLax◇, Lax-A-Day✤◇, MiraLax◇, Pegalax✽◇, Relaxa✽◇, Restoralax✽

Therapeutic class: Laxatives
Pharmacologic class: Osmotic drugs

AVAILABLE FORMS
Powder: 17 g in single-dose packets

INDICATIONS & DOSAGES
➤ **Short-term (1 to 2 weeks) treatment of occasional constipation**
Adults and adolescents age 17 and older: 17 g (about 1 heaping tablespoon or one individual dose packet) powder PO dissolved in 120 to 240 mL beverage once daily.

polyethylene glycol–electrolyte solution (PEG-ES)
pol-ee-ETH-ih-leen

GaviLyte-C, GaviLyte-G, GoLYTELY, MoviPrep, Plenvu

Therapeutic class: Laxatives
Pharmacologic class: Osmotic laxatives

AVAILABLE FORMS
Oral solution: PEG 3350 (refer to individual manufacturer for strength and dosage of electrolytes)
Powder for oral solution: 4-L dose of solution contains PEG 3350 (refer to individual manufacturer for strength and dosage of electrolytes)

INDICATIONS & DOSAGES
➤ **Bowel preparation before GI exam**
Adults: 240 mL PO every 10 minutes until 4 L are consumed or rectal effluent is clear. Typically, give

4 hours before exam, allowing 3 hours for drinking and 1 hour for bowel evacuation. May give via NG tube: 20 to 30 mL/minute (1.2 to 1.8 L/hour) until 4 L is administered or rectal effluent is clear. Or, for MoviPrep or Plenvu, refer to package instructions for split-dose or full-dose regimen.
Children age 6 months and older: 25 mL/kg/hour PO or via NG tube until rectal effluent is clear and free of solid matter.

sodium phosphate monobasic monohydrate–sodium phosphate dibasic anhydrous
OsmoPrep

Therapeutic class: Laxatives
Pharmacologic class: Osmotic laxatives

AVAILABLE FORMS
Tablets: 1.5 g sodium phosphate (1.102 g sodium phosphate monobasic monohydrate and 0.398 g sodium phosphate dibasic anhydrous)

INDICATIONS & DOSAGES
Boxed Warning Acute phosphate nephropathy has been reported. Use the dose and dosing regimen as recommended (p.m./a.m. split dose). ▪

➤ **To cleanse bowel before colonoscopy**
Adults age 18 and older: 32 tablets taken in the following manner: The evening before the procedure, 4 tablets PO with 8 oz of clear liquid every 15 minutes for a total of 20 tablets (five doses); 3 to 5 hours before the procedure, 4 tablets PO with at least 8 oz of clear liquid every 15 minutes for a total of 12 tablets (three doses). A minimum of 7 days should elapse before repeating usage.

sodium phosphates
Fleet Enema◇, Fleet Enema Extra◇, Fleet For Children◇, Pedia-Lax◇

Therapeutic class: Laxatives
Pharmacologic class: Acid salts

AVAILABLE FORMS
Enema solution: 19 g monobasic sodium phosphate monohydrate and 7 g dibasic sodium phosphate heptahydrate in 118-mL, 133-mL, or 197-mL bottles◇
Enema solution (pediatric use): 9.5 g monobasic sodium phosphate monohydrate and 3.5 g dibasic sodium phosphate heptahydrate in 59-mL or 66-mL bottles◇

INDICATIONS & DOSAGES
➤ **Constipation**
Adults and children age 12 and older: 1 bottle PR as an enema once in 24 hours, PRN.
Children ages 5 to 11: 1 bottle enema for pediatric use PR as an enema once in 24 hours, PRN.
Children ages 2 to younger than 5: One-half bottle enema for pediatric use PR as an enema once in 24 hours, PRN.

sodium picosulfate–magnesium oxide–anhydrous citric acid
Clenpiq

Therapeutic class: Laxatives
Pharmacologic class: Peristaltic stimulants–osmotic agents

AVAILABLE FORMS
Oral solution: 10 mg sodium picosulfate, 3.5 g magnesium oxide, and 12 g anhydrous citric acid/160-mL bottle

INDICATIONS & DOSAGES
➤ **To cleanse colon in preparation for colonoscopy**
Adults and children age 9 and older: The split-dose method is preferred. Give first bottle during the evening before colonoscopy (5 p.m. to 9 p.m.) followed by at least five 8-oz (240 mL) drinks of clear liquids within 5 hours and before bed. Give second bottle next day, during the morning approximately 5 hours before colonoscopy. Follow dose with at least four 8-oz (240-mL) drinks of clear liquids before colonoscopy; continue with clear liquids within 5 hours and up to 2 hours before colonoscopy.

Vitamins and minerals: Indications and dosages

Refer to manufacturer's instructions for complete prescribing and safety information.

ferrous fumarate
FAIR-us

Ferretts ◇, Ferrimin 150 ◇, Ferrocite ◇

Therapeutic class: Iron supplements
Pharmacologic class: Hematinics

AVAILABLE FORMS
Each 100 mg of ferrous fumarate provides 33 mg of elemental iron.
Tablets ⓄⓉⒸ: 29 mg ◇, 150 mg ◇, 324 mg ◇, 325 mg ◇

INDICATIONS & DOSAGES
➤ **Iron deficiency**
Adults: 29 to 150 mg of elemental iron PO every other day between meals or as directed by prescriber. Daily dosing may decrease absorption.
Children: 3 to 6 mg/kg/day of elemental iron PO in one to three divided doses up to a maximum daily dose of 200 mg/day.

ferrous gluconate
FER-us

Ferate ◇, Fergon ◇, Ferrotabs ◇

Therapeutic class: Iron supplements
Pharmacologic class: Hematinics

AVAILABLE FORMS
Each 100 mg of ferrous gluconate provides 11.6 mg of elemental iron.
Tablets ⓄⓉⒸ: 240 mg ◇, 324 mg ◇

INDICATIONS & DOSAGES
➤ **Iron deficiency**
Adults: 29 to 150 mg of elemental iron PO every other day or as directed by prescriber. Daily dosing may decrease absorption.
Children: 3 to 6 mg/kg/day of elemental iron PO in one to three divided doses.

ferrous sulfate
FER-us

FeroSol ◇*, Fer-In-Sol ◇, Fe-Vit Iron ◇

ferrous sulfate (dried)
Feosol ◇, Feratab ◇, FeroSul ◇, Slow FE ◇, Slow Release Iron ◇

Therapeutic class: Iron supplements
Pharmacologic class: Hematinics

AVAILABLE FORMS
Each 100 mg of ferrous sulfate provides 20 mg of elemental iron or 30 mg of elemental iron in ferrous sulfate dried products.
Elixir: 220 mg/5 mL ◇*
Liquid: 75 mg/mL ◇, 300 mg/5 mL ◇
Tablets: 325 mg ◇
Tablets (extended-release) ⓄⓉⒸ: 142 mg ◇, 160 mg (dried) ◇, 324 mg ◇, 325 mg ◇

INDICATIONS & DOSAGES
➤ **Iron deficiency**
Adults, infants, and children: Refer to individual manufacturer's instructions for dosages or as directed by prescriber. Immediate-release products are usually given in divided doses daily. Extended-release formulations are given once daily. Lower daily doses may cause less GI adverse events in older adults. Daily dosing may decrease absorption.

vitamin A
Vitamin A Fish ◇

vitamin A palmitate
Aquasol A

AVAILABLE FORMS
Note: Each international unit is equivalent to 0.3 mcg retinol equivalent (RE).
Capsules: 7,500 international units ◇, 8,000 international units ◇, 10,000 international units ◇, 25,000 international units
Injection: 50,000 international units/mL in 2-mL vials
Tablets: 10,000 international units ◇, 15,000 international units ◇

INDICATIONS & DOSAGES
➤ **RDA**
Men and boys older than age 14: 900 mcg RE.
Women and girls older than age 14: 700 mcg RE.
Children ages 9 to 13: 600 mcg RE.
Children ages 4 to 8: 400 mcg RE.
Children ages 1 to 3: 300 mcg RE.
Infants ages 7 to 12 months: 500 mcg RE.

Neonates and infants younger than age 6 months: 400 mcg RE.
Women who are pregnant ages 14 to 18: 750 mcg RE.
Women who are pregnant ages 19 to 50: 770 mcg RE.
Women who are breastfeeding ages 14 to 18: 1,200 mcg RE.
Women who are breastfeeding ages 19 to 50: 1,300 mcg RE.

➤ **Severe vitamin A deficiency**
Adults and children older than age 8: 100,000 international units IM or PO for 3 days; then 50,000 international units PO or IM daily for 2 weeks. Follow with adequate dietary nutrition and RE vitamin A supplements.
Children ages 1 to 8: 17,500 to 35,000 international units IM daily for 10 days.
Infants: 7,500 to 15,000 international units IM daily for 10 days.

➤ **Maintenance dose to prevent recurrence of vitamin A deficiency**
Adults and children older than age 8: 10,000 to 20,000 international units PO daily for 2 months.
Children infants to age 8: Give 5,000 to 10,000 international units PO daily for 2 months; then adequate dietary nutrition and RE vitamin A supplements.

vitamin B$_{12}$ (cyanocobalamin)
Nascobal, Physicians EZ Use B-12, Vitamin Deficiency System-B12, Vibisone

hydroxocobalamin (vitamin B$_{12}$)
Cyanokit

AVAILABLE FORMS
cyanocobalamin
Injection*: 1,000 mcg/mL, 2,000 mcg/mL
Intranasal spray: 500 mcg/spray
Liquid (SL): 3,000 mcg ◇
Lozenges: 50 mcg ◇, 100 mcg ◇, 250 mcg ◇, 500 mcg ◇
Tablets: 100 mcg ◇, 250 mcg ◇, 500 mcg ◇, 1,000 mcg ◇
Tablets (extended-release): 1,000 mcg ◇
Tablets (SL): 2,500 mcg ◇
hydroxocobalamin
Injection: 1,000 mcg/mL, 5 g/vial

INDICATIONS & DOSAGES
➤ **RDA for cyanocobalamin**
Adults and children age 14 and older: 2.4 mcg.
Children ages 9 to 13: 1.8 mcg.
Children ages 4 to 8: 1.2 mcg.
Children ages 1 to 3: 0.9 mcg.
Infants ages 7 months to 1 year: 0.5 mcg.
Neonates and infants age 6 months and younger: 0.4 mcg.

Women who are pregnant: 2.6 mcg.
Women who are breastfeeding: 2.8 mcg.

➤ **Vitamin B$_{12}$ deficiency from inadequate diet, subtotal gastrectomy, or other condition, disorder, or disease, except malabsorption related to pernicious anemia or other GI disease**
Adults and children (cyanocobalamin): 100 mcg IM or deep subcut daily for 6 to 7 days. If improvement, give 100 mcg on alternate days for seven doses, then every 3 to 4 days for 2 to 3 weeks. Maintenance dose, 100 mcg IM or deep subcut monthly. For subsequent prophylaxis, advise adequate nutrition and daily RDA vitamin B$_{12}$ supplements.
Adults (hydroxocobalamin): 30 mcg IM daily for 5 to 10 days. Maintenance dose, 100 to 200 mcg IM monthly.
Children (hydroxocobalamin): 1 to 5 mg in single doses of 100 mcg IM over 2 or more weeks, depending on severity of deficiency. Maintenance dose is 30 to 50 mcg IM every 4 weeks. For subsequent prophylaxis, advise adequate nutrition and daily RDA vitamin B$_{12}$ supplements.

➤ **Pernicious anemia or vitamin B$_{12}$ malabsorption**
Adults: Initially, 100 mcg cyanocobalamin IM or deep subcut daily for 6 to 7 days. If response is observed, 100 mcg IM or deep subcut every other day for 7 doses, then 100 mcg every 3 to 4 days for 2 to 3 weeks; then 100 mcg IM or deep subcut once monthly.

➤ **Maintenance therapy for remission of pernicious anemia after IM vitamin B$_{12}$ therapy in patients without nervous system involvement; dietary deficiency, malabsorption disorders, and inadequate secretion of intrinsic factor**
Adults: Initially, 1 spray in one nostril once weekly (Nascobal). Give at least 1 hour before or after hot foods or liquids.

➤ **Schilling test flushing dose**
Adults and children: 1,000 mcg hydroxocobalamin IM as single dose.

➤ **Cyanide poisoning**
Adults: Initially, 5 g hydroxocobalamin IV over 15 minutes. Based on patient's condition, may repeat 5 g dose IV over 15 minutes to 2 hours.

coenzyme Q10
CoQ10 ◇, Mega CoQ10 ◇, Vitaline CoQ10 ◇

AVAILABLE FORMS
Capsules: 10 mg ◇, 30 mg ◇, 50 mg ◇, 60 mg ◇, 75 mg ◇, 100 mg ◇, 120 mg ◇, 125 mg ◇, 150 mg ◇, 200 mg ◇, 400 mg ◇
Capsules (extended-release): 100 mg ◇
Liquid (liposomal): 2.5 mg/drop ◇, 100 mg/mL ◇
Oral liquid: 6 mg/mL ◇
Syrup: 10 mg/mL ◇
Tablets: 50 mg ◇, 60 mg ◇, 100 mg ◇
Tablets (chewable): 30 mg ◇, 100 mg ◇
Wafers: 60 mg ◇, 100 mg ◇, 300 mg ◇, 400 mg ◇, 600 mg ◇

INDICATIONS & DOSAGES
➤ **Dietary supplement for conditions associated with coenzyme Q10 deficiency**

Adults: 10 to 300 mg/day PO in one dose or up to three divided doses. Higher doses (up to 3,000 mg/day) have been used.

---

folic acid (vitamin B$_9$)
FA-8 ◇

AVAILABLE FORMS
Injection: 10-mL vials (5 mg/mL)*
Capsules: 0.8 mg ◇, 5 mg ◇, 20 mg ◇
Tablets: 0.4 mg ◇, 0.8 mg ◇, 1 mg

INDICATIONS & DOSAGES
➤ **RDA**
Adults and children age 14 and older: 400 mcg.
Children ages 9 to 13: 300 mcg.
Children ages 4 to 8: 200 mcg.
Children ages 1 to 3: 150 mcg.
Infants ages 7 months to 1 year: 80 mcg.
Neonates and infants younger than age 6 months: 65 mcg.
Women who are pregnant: 600 mcg.
Women who are breastfeeding: 500 mcg.
➤ **Megaloblastic or macrocytic anemia from folic acid or other nutritional deficiency, hepatic disease, alcoholism, intestinal obstruction, or excessive hemolysis**
Adults and children: Initially, up to 1 mg PO, IM, IV, or subcut daily until anemia has resolved; then proper diet and RDA supplements are needed to prevent recurrence.
Maintenance dosing:
Adults and children age 4 and older: Up to 0.4 mg PO, IM, IV, or subcut daily.
Children younger than age 4: Up to 0.3 mg PO, IM, or subcut daily.
Infants: 0.1 mg PO, IM, IV, or subcut daily.
Women who are pregnant or breastfeeding: 0.8 mg PO, IM, IV, or subcut daily.

---

iron dextran
EYE-ern DEKS-tran

INFeD

Therapeutic class: Iron supplements
Pharmacologic class: Hematinics

AVAILABLE FORMS
1 mL iron dextran provides 50 mg elemental iron.
Injection: 50 mg elemental iron/mL in 2-mL single-dose vials

INDICATIONS & DOSAGES
➤ **Iron deficiency anemia**
Adults and children weighing more than 15 kg: IV or IM test dose is required. (See manufacturer's

instructions.) Total dose may be calculated using dosage table in manufacturer's instructions or by using the following formula:

$$\text{Dose (mL)} = 0.0442 \text{ (desired Hb}$$
$$- \text{observed Hb)} \times \text{LBW}$$
$$+ (0.26 \times \text{LBW})$$

Note: LBW = lean body weight in kg. For males, LBW = 50 kg + 2.3 kg for each inch of patient's height over 5 feet. For females, LBW = 45.5 kg + 2.3 kg for each inch of patient's height over 5 feet.
Children weighing 5 to 15 kg: Use dosage table in package insert or calculate dose as follows:

$$\text{Dose (mL)} = 0.0442 \text{ (desired Hb}$$
$$- \text{observed Hb)} \times \text{weight in kg}$$
$$+ (0.26 \times \text{weight in kg).}$$

IV
Adults and children: Inject 0.5-mL test dose over at least 30 seconds. If no reaction occurs in 1 hour, give remainder of therapeutic IV dose. Repeat therapeutic IV dose daily. Single daily dose shouldn't exceed 100 mL. Give slowly (50 mg [1 mL/minute]). Don't give drug in the first 4 months of life.
IM (by Z-track method)
Adults and children: Inject 0.5-mL test dose. If no reaction occurs in 1 hour, give remainder of dose. Daily dose ordinarily shouldn't exceed 0.5 mL (25 mg) for infants weighing less than 5 kg; 1 mL (50 mg) for those weighing less than 10 kg; and 2 mL (100 mg) for heavier children and adults. Don't give drug in the first 4 months of life.
➤ **Iron replacement for blood loss**
Adults and children older than age 4 months: Replacement iron (in mg) = [Blood loss (in mL) × hematocrit] ÷ 50 mg/mL.
Note: This formula is based on the approximation that 1 mL of normocytic, normochromic red cells contains 1 mg of elemental iron.

---

leucovorin calcium (citrovorum factor, folinic acid)

AVAILABLE FORMS
Injection: 50-mg, 100-mg, 200-mg, 350-mg, 500-mg vials for reconstitution (contains no preservatives)
Solution for injection: 100 mg/10-mL vials
Tablets: 5 mg, 10 mg, 15 mg, 25 mg

INDICATIONS & DOSAGES
➤ **Leucovorin rescue after high-dose methotrexate therapy**
Adults: 15 mg (approximately 10 mg/m^2) PO, IM, or IV every 6 hours for 10 doses starting 24 hours after start of methotrexate infusion. Continue treatment until methotrexate level is less than 5×10^{-8} M. See manufacturer's instructions for dosage adjustment guidelines for methotrexate toxicity.
➤ **Impaired methotrexate elimination or inadvertent overdose**

Adults: 10 mg/m^2 PO, IM, or IV every 6 hours until serum methotrexate level is less than 10^{-8} M. If 24-hour serum creatinine level increases 50% over baseline or if 24-hour methotrexate level is greater than 5×10^{-6} M or 48-hour level is greater than 9×10^{-7} M, increase dosage to 100 mg/m^2 IV every 3 hours until methotrexate level is less than 10^{-8} M.

➤ **Folic acid antagonist overdose (trimethoprim, pyrimethamine)**
Adults and children: 5 to 15 mg PO daily.

➤ **Folate-deficient megaloblastic anemia**
Adults and children: Up to 1 mg IM or IV daily.

➤ **Palliative treatment of advanced colorectal cancer**
Adults: 20 mg/m^2 IV daily followed by 5-FU 425 mg/m^2 IV. Or, 200 mg/m^2 IV daily for 5 days (over 3 minutes or longer) followed by 5-FU 370 mg/m^2 daily for 5 consecutive days. Repeat at 4-week intervals for two additional courses; then at intervals of 4 to 5 weeks, if tolerated. Give 5-FU and leucovorin separately to avoid precipitate formation.

niacin (nicotinic acid, vitamin B$_3$)
Endur-Acin ◇, Niacor, Niaspan, Slo-Niacin ◇

niacinamide ◇ (nicotinamide ◇)

AVAILABLE FORMS
niacin
Capsules (extended-release): 250 mg ◇, 500 mg
Tablets: 50 mg ◇, 100 mg ◇, 250 mg ◇, 500 mg
Tablets (extended-release): 250 mg ◇, 500 mg ◇, 750 mg ◇, 1,000 mg ◇
niacinamide
Tablets: 100 mg ◇, 500 mg ◇

INDICATIONS & DOSAGES
➤ **RDA**
Adult men and boys ages 14 to 18: 16 mg.
Adult women and girls ages 14 to 18: 14 mg.
Children ages 9 to 13: 12 mg.
Children ages 4 to 8: 8 mg.
Children ages 1 to 3: 6 mg.
Infants ages 7 months to 1 year: 4 mg.
Neonates and infants younger than age 6 months: 2 mg.
Women who are pregnant: 18 mg.
Women who are breastfeeding: 17 mg.

➤ **Niacin deficiency (except Niacor or Niaspan)**
Adults: Up to 100 mg PO daily.

➤ **Dyslipidemia when patient is unable to achieve desired response or is intolerant to other therapies**
Adults: 250 mg Niacor PO daily after evening meal. Increase at 4- to 7-day intervals up to 1 to 2 g PO daily in two or three divided doses. Maximum 6 g daily. Or, 500 mg Niaspan PO daily at bedtime with a low-fat snack. Increase at 4-week intervals by 500 mg daily to a maximum of 2 g daily.

paricalcitol
Zemplar

AVAILABLE FORMS
Capsules: 1 mcg, 2 mcg, 4 mcg
Injection: 2 mcg/mL, 5 mcg/mL

INDICATIONS & DOSAGES
➤ **To prevent or treat secondary hyperparathyroidism in patients with stage 3 or 4 chronic kidney disease**
Adults: Initial dose is based on baseline intact parathyroid hormone (iPTH) levels. If iPTH is less than or equal to 500 picograms (pg)/mL, give 1 mcg PO daily or 2 mcg PO three times weekly, no more often than every other day. If iPTH is greater than 500 pg/mL, give 2 mcg PO daily or 4 mcg PO three times weekly, no more often than every other day. Adjust dose at 2- to 4-week intervals, based on iPTH levels.
Children ages 10 to 16: Initially, 1 mcg PO three times weekly, no more frequently than every other day. As indicated, increase each dose every 4 weeks or decrease each dose at any time based on iPTH, serum calcium, and phosphorus levels.

➤ **To prevent or treat secondary hyperparathyroidism in patients with stage 5 chronic kidney disease on dialysis**
Adults: 0.04 to 0.1 mcg/kg (2.8 to 7 mcg) IV no more often than every other day during dialysis. May safely give doses as high as 0.24 mcg/kg. If satisfactory response isn't observed, increase dosage by 2 to 4 mcg at 2- to 4-week intervals. Or, calculate initial PO dose in mcg, based on baseline iPTH level divided by 80 and administered three times weekly, no more frequently than every other day. Initiate only after baseline serum calcium level has been adjusted to 9.5 mg/dL or less. Titrate as indicated by using most recent iPTH level divided by 80. Decrease dosage by 2 to 4 mcg if serum calcium level is elevated.
Children ages 10 to 16: Calculate initial PO dose in mcg, rounded down to the nearest whole number, based on baseline iPTH level divided by 120 and administered three times weekly, no more frequently than every other day. As indicated, increase each dose every 4 weeks or decrease each dose at any time to maintain iPTH within target range.

pyridoxine hydrochloride (vitamin B$_6$)
B-natal ◇

AVAILABLE FORMS
Capsules: 250 mg ◇
Injection: 100 mg/mL
Tablets: 25 mg ◇, 50 mg ◇, 100 mg ◇, 250 mg ◇, 500 mg ◇
Tablets (extended-release): 200 mg ◇

INDICATIONS & DOSAGES
➤ **RDA**

Adults ages 19 to 50: 1.3 mg.
Men age 51 and older: 1.7 mg.
Women age 51 and older: 1.5 mg.
Boys ages 14 to 18: 1.3 mg.
Girls ages 14 to 18: 1.2 mg.
Children ages 9 to 13: 1 mg.
Children ages 4 to 8: 0.6 mg.
Children ages 1 to 3: 0.5 mg.
Infants ages 7 months to 1 year: 0.3 mg (0.03 mg/kg).
Neonates and infants younger than age 6 months:
0.1 mg (0.01 mg/kg).
Women who are pregnant: 1.9 mg.
Women who are breastfeeding: 2 mg.
➤ **Dietary vitamin B₆ deficiency**
Adults: 10 to 20 mg IM or IV daily for 3 weeks; then
maintenance dose is 2 to 5 mg PO daily for several
weeks.

sodium fluoride
Fluoritab, Pharmaflur df,
Pharmaflur 1.1, Phos-Flur ◇

sodium fluoride, topical
ACT ◇, Denta5000 Plus, Fluoridex,
Gel-Kam, Gel-Tin ◇, Just For Kids ◇,
Listerine Total Care ◇, Prevident,
SF 5000 Plus

AVAILABLE FORMS
sodium fluoride
Lozenges: 1 mg
Solution: 0.125 mg/drop, 0.25 mg/drop, 0.2 mg/mL,
0.5 mg/mL
Tablets (chewable): 0.25 mg, 0.5 mg, 1 mg
sodium fluoride, topical
Cream: 1.1%
Gel: 0.4% ◇, 1.1%, 1.23%
Paste: 0.454% ◇, 1.1%
Rinse: 0.02% ◇, 0.04% ◇, 0.05%, 0.2%

INDICATIONS & DOSAGES
➤ **To prevent dental caries**
Adults and children older than age 6: 5 to 10 mL of
rinse once daily or b.i.d. (see product instructions) for
1 minute, or thin ribbon of gel applied to teeth with
toothbrush or mouth trays. Or, 1 lozenge PO once
daily (adults only).
*If fluoride ion level in drinking water is less than
0.3 parts/million (ppm)*
Children ages 6 to 16: 1 mg PO daily.
Children ages 3 to 5: 0.5 mg PO daily.
Infants and children ages 6 months to 2 years:
0.25 mg PO daily.
*If fluoride ion level in drinking water is 0.3 to
0.6 ppm*
Children ages 6 to 16: 0.5 mg PO daily.
Children ages 3 to 5: 0.25 mg PO daily.

thiamine hydrochloride (vitamin B₁)
Thiamiject ✦

AVAILABLE FORMS
Capsules: 50 mg ◇
Injection: 100 mg/mL
Tablets: 50 mg ◇, 100 mg ◇, 250 mg ◇

INDICATIONS & DOSAGES
➤ **RDA**

Adult men: 1.2 mg.
Adult women: 1.1 mg.
Boys ages 14 to 18: 1.2 mg.
Girls ages 14 to 18: 1 mg.
Children ages 9 to 13: 0.9 mg.
Children ages 4 to 8: 0.6 mg.
Children ages 1 to 3: 0.5 mg.
Infants ages 7 months to 1 year: 0.3 mg.
Neonates and infants younger than age 6 months:
0.2 mg.
Women who are pregnant: 1.4 mg.
Women who are breastfeeding: 1.4 mg.
➤ **Beriberi**
Adults: Depending on severity, 10 to 20 mg IM t.i.d.
for up to 2 weeks; then dietary correction and multi-
vitamin supplement containing 5 to 10 mg thiamine
daily for 1 month.
Children: 25 mg IV daily if infantile beriberi isn't
responsive to oral therapy.
➤ **Wet beriberi with myocardial failure**
Adults and children: 10 to 20 mg IV t.i.d. given slowly.
➤ **Thiamine deficiency**
Adults: Up to 100 mg/L IV by rapid infusion. Contin-
ue daily parenteral doses at RDA if GI disturbances
prevent adequate oral absorption. Or, 1 tablet or
capsule PO daily.
➤ **Neuritis of pregnancy in patients unable to take
adequate oral therapy due to vomiting**
Adults: 5 to 10 mg IM daily.
➤ **Wernicke encephalopathy** ◆
Adults: Initially, 100 mg IV; then 50 to 100 mg IM
daily until patient is consuming a regular balanced
diet.

vitamin C (ascorbic acid)
Ascor, C-Caps ◇, Halls Defense
Vitamin C Drops ◇, Nature's Way ◇

AVAILABLE FORMS
Capsules: 500 mg ◇
Capsules (timed-release): 500 mg ◇
Crystals: 1,000 mg/½ tsp
Injection: 500 mg/mL
Lozenges: 60 mg ◇
Oral solution: 100 mg/mL ◇, 500 mg/15 mL ◇
Powder: 60 mg/¼ tsp ◇, 1,000 mg/tsp ◇,
1,060 mg/¼ tsp ◇

Tablets: 250 mg ◊ , 500 mg ◊ , 1,000 mg ◊ , 1,500 mg ◊
Tablets (chewable): 100 mg ◊ , 250 mg ◊ , 400 mg ◊ ,
500 mg ◊
Tablets (timed-release): 500 mg ◊
Wafer: 500 mg ◊

INDICATIONS & DOSAGES
➤ RDA
Men age 19 and older: 90 mg.
Women age 19 and older: 75 mg.
Boys ages 14 to 18: 75 mg.
Girls ages 14 to 18: 65 mg.
Children ages 9 to 13: 45 mg.
Children ages 4 to 8: 25 mg.
Children ages 1 to 3: 15 mg.
Infants ages 7 months to 1 year: 50 mg.
Neonates and infants up to age 6 months: 40 mg.
Women who are pregnant: 85 mg.
Women who are breastfeeding: 120 mg.
Adult smokers: Add an extra 35 mg daily.
➤ Frank and subclinical scurvy
Adults: Depending on severity, 100 to 300 mg PO or
200 mg IV daily.
Children age 11 and older: 200 mg IV or IM daily.
Children ages 1 to younger than 11: 100 mg IV daily.
Infants ages 5 to younger than 12 months: 50 mg IV
daily.
➤ Extensive burns
Adults and children: 200 to 500 mg IV, daily for 7 to
10 days; 1 to 2 g daily for extensive burns.
➤ Postoperative wound healing
Adults and children: 300 to 500 mg IV once daily for
1 week to 10 days.

---

vitamin D cholecalciferol (vitamin D₃)
Bio-D-Mulsion ◊ , Decara, Dialyvite
Vitamin D3 Max ◊ , Kids First ◊ ,
VitaMelts ◊

ergocalciferol (vitamin D₂)
Calcidol ◊ , Drisdol

AVAILABLE FORMS
cholecalciferol
Capsules: 25 mcg (1,000 international units), 50 mcg
(2,000 international units), 125 mcg (5,000 international units), 250 mcg (10,000 international units),
625 mcg (25,000 international units), 1.25 mg
(50,000 international units)
Liquid: 400 international units/mL ◊ , 400 international units/0.03 mL ◊ , 2,000 international units/
0.03 mL ◊ , 5,000 international units/mL ◊
Tablets: 10 mcg (400 international units) ◊ , 20 mcg
(800 international units) ◊ , 25 mcg (1,000 international units) ◊ , 50 mcg (2,000 international units) ◊ ,
75 mcg (3,000 international units) ◊ , 125 mcg (5,000
international units) ◊ , 1,250 mcg (50,000 international units) ◊

Tablets (chewable): 10 mcg (400 international units) ◊ ,
25 mcg (1,000 international units) ◊ , 50 mcg (2,000
international units) ◊
ergocalciferol
Capsules: 1.25 mg (50,000 international units)
Oral liquid: 200 mcg (8,000 international units)/mL in
60-mL dropper bottle ◊
Tablets: 10 mcg (400 international units) ◊ , 50 mcg
(2,000 international units) ◊

INDICATIONS & DOSAGES
➤ RDA
Adults older than age 70: 20 mcg (international units).
Adults to age 70 and children age 1 and older: 15 mcg
(600 international units).
Children from birth to less than 12 months: 10 mcg
(400 international units).
Women who are pregnant or breastfeeding: 15 mcg
(600 international units).
➤ Rickets and other vitamin D deficiency diseases
Adults and children: Individualize cholecalciferol
dosage based on age and serum 25-hydroxyvitamin
D level. For vitamin D–resistant rickets, give 12,000
to 500,000 international units ergocalciferol PO daily.
After correction of deficiency, maintenance includes
adequate diet and RDA supplements.
➤ Hypoparathyroidism
Adults and children: 1.25 to 5 mg (50,000 to 200,000
international units) ergocalciferol PO daily with calcium supplement.

---

vitamin D analogue doxercalciferol
Hectorol

AVAILABLE FORMS
Capsules: 0.5 mcg, 1 mcg, 2.5 mcg
Injection: 2 mcg/mL in 1-mL, 2-mL vials

INDICATIONS & DOSAGES
➤ Secondary hyperparathyroidism in patients requiring dialysis for chronic kidney disease
Adults: Initially, 10 mcg PO three times weekly at
dialysis. Adjust dosage as needed to lower intact parathyroid hormone (iPTH) levels to 150 to 300 picograms (pg)/mL. Increase dose by 2.5 mcg at 8-week
intervals if iPTH level hasn't decreased by 50% and
fails to reach target range. Maximum dose is 20 mcg
PO three times weekly. If iPTH levels fall below
100 pg/mL, suspend drug for 1 week; then give dose
of at least 2.5 mcg less than last dose. Or, 4 mcg IV
bolus three times a week at the end of dialysis, no
more frequently than every other day. Adjust dose
as needed to lower iPTH levels to 150 to 300 pg/mL.
Dosage may be increased by 1 to 2 mcg at 8-week intervals if the iPTH level isn't decreased by 50% and
fails to reach target range. Maximum dose is 18 mcg
weekly. If iPTH levels go below 100 pg/mL, suspend
drug for 1 week, then resume at a dose that's at least
1 mcg PO lower than the last dose.

➤ **Secondary hyperparathyroidism in patients with stage 3 or 4 chronic kidney disease who are predialysis**

Adults: 1 mcg PO daily. Adjust dosage as needed to lower iPTH levels to 35 to 70 pg/mL for stage 3 or 70 to 110 pg/mL for stage 4. Increase dosage at 2-week intervals by 0.5 mcg if levels are above 70 pg/mL for stage 3 or above 110 pg/mL for stage 4. If level falls below 35 pg/mL for stage 3 or 70 pg/mL for stage 4, suspend treatment for 1 week, then give dose at least 0.5 mcg lower than last dose. Maximum dose, 3.5 mcg daily.

vitamin E (tocopherols)
E 1000 ◇, Natural Vitamin E ◇, SoluVita-E ◇

AVAILABLE FORMS
Capsules ⓄⓉⒸ: 100 international units ◇, 200 international units ◇, 400 international units ◇, 1,000 international units ◇
Liquid: 15 international units/0.3 mL ◇, 50 international units/mL ◇, 400 international units/15 mL ◇
Tablets: 100 international units ◇, 200 international units ◇, 400 international units ◇

INDICATIONS & DOSAGES
Note: RDAs for vitamin E have been converted to α-tocopherol equivalents (α-TE). One α-TE equals 1 mg of D-α tocopherol, or 1.49 international units.
➤ **RDA**
Adults and children ages 14 to 18: 15 mg.
Children ages 9 to 13: 11 mg.
Children ages 4 to 8: 7 mg.
Children ages 1 to 3: 6 mg.
Infants ages 7 months to 1 year: 5 mg.
Neonates and infants younger than age 6 months: 4 mg.
Women who are pregnant: 15 mg.
Women who are breastfeeding: 19 mg.
➤ **Dietary supplement**
Adults: Dosage of tablets and capsules varies by product and ranges from 100 to 1,000 mg/day. Or, 30 units (0.6 mL of the 15 units/0.3 mL drops) PO daily. Or, 100 units (0.25 mL of the 100 units/0.25 mL) PO daily.
Children (using the 15 units/0.3 mL drops): For children age 4 and older, give 30 units (0.6 mL) PO daily. For those ages 1 to 3, give 10 units (0.2 mL) PO daily. For those younger than age 1, give 5 units (0.1 mL) PO daily.

vitamin K analogue phytonadione (vitamin K₁)
K1-1000 ◇, Mephyton

AVAILABLE FORMS
Capsules: 1 mg ◇
Injection (emulsion): 1 mg/0.5 mL, 10 mg/mL
Tablets: 100 mcg ◇, 5 mg

INDICATIONS & DOSAGES
Boxed Warning Risk of severe and even fatal hypersensitivity reactions using IV or IM routes; restrict their use to situations in which the subcut route isn't feasible and the serious risk is justified. ▪
➤ **RDA**
Men age 19 and older: 120 mcg.
Women age 19 and older, including women who are pregnant or breastfeeding: 90 mcg.
Children ages 14 to 18: 75 mcg.
Children ages 9 to 13: 60 mcg.
Children ages 4 to 8: 55 mcg.
Children ages 1 to 3: 30 mcg.
Infants ages 7 months to 1 year: 2.5 mcg.
Neonates and infants younger than age 6 months: 2 mcg.
➤ **Hypoprothrombinemia caused by vitamin K malabsorption, drug therapy, or excessive vitamin A dosage**
Adults: Depending on severity, 2.5 to 25 mg PO or subcut; may repeat in 6 to 8 hours. May give IV at a rate of 1 mg/minute or more if unavoidable.
➤ **Hypoprothrombinemia caused by effect of oral anticoagulants**
Adults: 2.5 to 10 mg PO, IM, or subcut, based on PT and INR. May repeat in 12 to 48 hours. Or, 2.5 to 10 mg IV at a rate of no more than 1 mg/minute based on INR and severity of bleeding. May repeat after 6 to 12 hours as needed.
➤ **To prevent vitamin K–deficiency bleeding in neonates**
Neonates: 0.5 to 1 mg IM within 1 hour after birth.
➤ **To treat vitamin K–deficiency bleeding in neonates**
Neonates: 1 mg subcut or IM. Higher doses may be needed if mother has been receiving oral anticoagulants.

✦Canada   ◇ OTC   ♦ Off-label use   ⓄⓉⒸ Do not crush   *Liquid contains alcohol.

Additional OTC drugs: Indications and dosages

Refer to manufacturer's instructions for complete prescribing and safety information.

benzocaine
ben-ZOH-cane

Anacaine ◇, HurriCaine ◇, Ora-film ◇, Zilactin Baby ◇

Therapeutic class: Dermatologic agents
Pharmacologic class: Topical anesthetics

AVAILABLE FORMS
Gel: 7.5% ◇, 10% ◇, 20% ◇
Liquid: 10% ◇, 20% ◇
Lozenge: 15 mg ◇
Ointment: 5% ◇, 10% ◇, 20% ◇
Spray (external aerosol): 2% ◇, 5% ◇, 20% ◇
Spray (oral): 20% ◇

INDICATIONS & DOSAGES
Refer to individual manufacturer's instructions for use.
➤ **Sore throat**
Adults and children age 5 and older: Allow 1 lozenge to dissolve slowly in mouth. May repeat every 2 hours, PRN.
Adults and children age 2 and older: 1 spray to affected area or throat up to q.i.d., PRN.
➤ **Mouth and gum irritation**
Adults: 1 spray or thin layer of gel or ointment to the affected area up to q.i.d., PRN.
Children age 2 and older: Apply thin layer of gel, liquid, or ointment to affected area up to q.i.d., PRN.
➤ **Dermal irritation**
Adults and children age 2 and older: Apply ointment or spray to affected area up to q.i.d., PRN.
➤ **Hemorrhoids**
Adults: Apply ointment to affected area up to six times a day, PRN.

cetirizine hydrochloride
se-TEER-i-zeen

Reactine ❈ ◇, Zyrtec ◇, Zyrtec Children's Allergy ◇

Therapeutic class: Antihistamines
Pharmacologic class: Piperazine derivatives

AVAILABLE FORMS
Capsules: 10 mg ◇
Syrup: 5 mg/5 mL ◇
Tablets: 5 mg ◇, 10 mg ◇, 20 mg ❈ ◇
Tablets (chewable): 5 mg ◇, 10 mg ◇
Tablets (ODTs): 10 mg ◇

INDICATIONS & DOSAGES
Adjust-a-dose (for all indications): For adults and children age 6 and older receiving hemodialysis, those with hepatic impairment, those with CrCl less than 31 mL/minute, and patients age 65 and older, give 5 mg PO daily. Don't use in children younger than age 6 with renal or hepatic impairment.
➤ **Seasonal allergic rhinitis**
Adults and children age 6 and older: 5 to 10 mg PO once daily.
Children ages 2 to 5: 2.5 mg PO once daily. May increase to 2.5 mg b.i.d. or 5 mg daily. Maximum daily dose is 5 mg.
➤ **Perennial allergic rhinitis; chronic urticaria**
Adults and children age 6 and older: 5 to 10 mg PO once daily.
Children ages 1 to 5 years: 2.5 mg PO once daily; increase to maximum of 5 mg daily.
Children ages 12 to 23 months: 2.5 mg PO once daily or b.i.d.
Children ages 6 to 11 months: 2.5 mg PO once daily.

chlorpheniramine maleate
klor-fen-IR-a-meen

Allergy Relief ◇, Chlor-Trimeton ◇, Chlor-Trimeton Allergy ◇, Diabetic Tussin Allergy ◇, Pharbechlor ◇

Therapeutic class: Antihistamines
Pharmacologic class: Alkylamines

AVAILABLE FORMS
Liquid: 2 mg/mL ◇
Syrup: 2 mg/5 mL ◇ *
Tablets: 4 mg ◇
Tablets (extended-release) ⊙ⁿᶜ: 12 mg ◇

INDICATIONS & DOSAGES
➤ **Allergic rhinitis**
Adults and children age 12 and older: 4 mg PO every 4 to 6 hours, not to exceed 24 mg daily. Or, 12 mg extended-release PO every 12 hours, not to exceed 24 mg daily.
Children ages 6 to 12: 2 mg PO every 4 to 6 hours, not to exceed 12 mg daily.

cimetidine
sye-MET-i-deen

Tagamet HB ◇

cimetidine hydrochloride

Therapeutic class: Antiulcer drugs
Pharmacologic class: H₂-receptor
antagonists

AVAILABLE FORMS
Oral liquid: 300 mg/5 mL*
Tablets: 200 mg ◇, 300 mg, 400 mg, 800 mg

INDICATIONS & DOSAGES
Adjust-a-dose (for all indications): In patients
with renal impairment, decrease dosage to 300 mg PO
every 12 hours, increasing frequency to every 8 hours
with caution. A patient who is renally impaired and
also has liver dysfunction may require even further
dosage reduction. Schedule dose after hemodialysis.
➤ **Short-term treatment of duodenal ulcer; maintenance therapy**
Adults and children age 16 and older: 800 mg PO
at bedtime. Or, 400 mg PO b.i.d. and at bedtime or
300 mg PO q.i.d. (with meals and at bedtime). Or,
200 mg PO t.i.d. with a 400-mg bedtime dose. Treatment lasts 4 to 6 weeks unless endoscopy shows
healing.
   Alternatively, higher doses of 1,600 mg at bedtime
for 4 weeks may be beneficial for patients with
larger duodenal ulcers (larger than 1 cm defined
endoscopically) who are also heavy smokers (1 pack/
day or more) when it's important to ensure healing
within 4 weeks for this subpopulation.
   For maintenance therapy, 400 mg at bedtime.
➤ **Active benign gastric ulceration**
Adults: 800 mg PO at bedtime or 300 mg PO q.i.d.
(with meals and at bedtime) for up to 8 weeks.
➤ **Pathologic hypersecretory conditions, such as
Zollinger-Ellison syndrome, systemic mastocytosis,
and multiple endocrine adenomas**
Adults and children age 16 and older: 300 mg PO
q.i.d. with meals and at bedtime, adjusted to patient
needs. Maximum oral amount, 2,400 mg daily.
➤ **GERD with erosive esophagitis**
Adults: 800 mg PO b.i.d. or 400 mg PO q.i.d. before
meals and at bedtime for up to 12 weeks.
➤ **Heartburn (OTC only)**
Adults and children age 12 and older: 200 mg PO
with water as symptoms occur, or as directed, up to
b.i.d. For prevention, 200 mg PO right before or up to
30 minutes before eating food or drinking beverages
that cause heartburn. Maximum, 400 mg daily. Drug
shouldn't be taken daily for longer than 2 weeks.

dextromethorphan hydrobromide
dex-troe-meth-OR-fan

Balminil DM ✤ ◇, Buckley's Cough ◇,
Delsym ◇, ElixSure Cough ◇,
Hold ◇, Robitussin ◇, Robitussin
Children's Cough Long-Acting ◇,
Scot-Tussin Diabetes ◇, Triaminic
Long Acting Cough ◇ *

Therapeutic class: Antitussives
Pharmacologic class: Levorphanol
derivatives

AVAILABLE FORMS
Gelcaps: 15 mg ◇
Liquid (extended-release): 30 mg/5 mL ◇
Lozenges: 5 mg ◇
Solution: 3 mg/mL ✤ ◇, 7.5 mg/5 mL ◇, 10 mg/
5 mL ◇ *, 12.5 mg/5 mL ◇, 15 mg/5 mL ◇ *
Strips (orally disintegrating): 7.5 mg ◇ *
Syrup: 5 mg/5 mL ◇, 7.5 mg/5 mL ◇, 10 mg/5 mL ◇,
20 mg/15 mL ◇
Tablet: 15 mg ◇

INDICATIONS & DOSAGES
➤ **Cough suppressant**
Adults and children age 12 and older: 10 to 20 mg PO
every 4 hours, or 20 to 30 mg every 6 to 8 hours. Or,
60 mg extended-release liquid PO b.i.d. Maximum,
120 mg daily. Or 5 to 15 mg lozenges PO every
4 hours, up to 120 mg/day.
Children ages 6 to 11: 5 to 10 mg PO every 4 hours,
or 15 mg every 6 to 8 hours. Or, 30 mg extended-
release liquid PO b.i.d. Maximum, 60 mg daily.
Or 5 to 10 mg lozenges PO every 4 hours, up to
60 mg/day. Don't exceed four doses in 24 hours.
Children ages 4 to younger than 6: 2.5 to 5 mg PO
every 4 hours, or 7.5 mg every 6 to 8 hours. Or, 15 mg
extended-release liquid PO b.i.d. Maximum, 30 mg
daily.

fexofenadine hydrochloride
fecks-oh-FEN-a-deen

Allegra 12 Hour ✤ ◇, Allegra
24 Hour ◇, Allegra Allergy ◇,
Allegra Allergy Children's ◇

Therapeutic class: Antihistamines
Pharmacologic class: Piperidines

AVAILABLE FORMS
Oral suspension: 30 mg/5 mL ◇
Tablets: 60 mg ◇, 120 mg ✤ ◇, 180 mg ◇
Tablets (ODTs): 30 mg ◇

INDICATIONS & DOSAGES

Adjust-a-dose (for all indications): For patients with impaired renal function or need for dialysis, give adults and children age 12 and older 60 mg PO daily, and children ages 2 to 11 30 mg daily.

➤ **Seasonal allergies/hay fever**

Adults and children age 12 and older: 60 mg PO b.i.d., or 120 or 180 mg PO once daily.

Children ages 2 to 11: 30 mg PO every 12 hours. Maximum, 60 mg daily.

➤ **Chronic idiopathic urticaria** ♦

Adults and children age 12 and older: 60 mg PO b.i.d., or 180 mg PO once daily.

---

guaiFENesin (glyceryl guaiacolate)
gwye-FEN-e-sin

Altarussin ◇, Balminil DM✢◇, Diabetic Tussin ◇, Geri-Tussin ◇, Mucinex ◇, Mucosa ◇, Mucus Relief ◇, Refenesen 400 ◇, Robafen Mucus/Chest Congestion ◇, Tussin ◇

Therapeutic class: Expectorants
Pharmacologic class: Propanediol derivatives

AVAILABLE FORMS

Granules: 100 mg ◇
Liquid: 100 mg/5 mL ◇*, 200 mg/10 mL ◇, 300 mg/15 mL ◇, 400 mg/20 mL ◇
Syrup: 100 mg/5 mL ◇
Tablets: 200 mg ◇, 400 mg
Tablets (extended-release) ⓞ: 600 mg ◇, 1,200 mg ◇

INDICATIONS & DOSAGES

➤ **Expectorant**

Adults and children age 12 and older: 200 to 400 mg PO every 4 hours, or 600 to 1,200 mg (extended-release tablets) PO every 12 hours. Maximum, 2,400 mg daily.

Children ages 6 to 11: 100 to 200 mg PO every 4 hours. Maximum, 1,200 mg daily.

Children ages 4 to 5: 50 to 100 mg granules, syrup, or liquid every 4 hours as needed. Maximum, 600 mg daily.

---

loratadine
lor-AT-a-deen

Children's Claritin ◇, Children's Loratadine ◇, Claritin ◇, Claritin RediTabs ◇

Therapeutic class: Antihistamines
Pharmacologic class: Piperidines

AVAILABLE FORMS

Capsules: 10 mg ◇
Syrup: 5 mg/5 mL ◇
Tablets: 10 mg ◇
Tablets (chewable): 5 mg ◇
Tablets (ODTs): 5 mg ◇, 10 mg ◇

INDICATIONS & DOSAGES

Adjust-a-dose (for all indications): For adults with CrCl of 10 to 50 mL/minute, give 5 to 10 mg every 24 to 48 hours. For adults with CrCl less than 10 mL/minute, give dose every 48 hours.

➤ **Allergic rhinitis**

Adults and children age 6 and older: 10 mg PO daily. Or, 5 mg dispersible tablet b.i.d.

Children ages 2 to 5: 5 mg chewable tablets or syrup PO daily.

➤ **To relieve itching due to hives (urticaria)**

Adults and children age 6 and older: 10 mg PO daily.

---

meclizine hydrochloride (meclozine hydrochloride)
MEK-li-zeen

Antivert, Bonine ◇, Motion-Time ◇, Travel-Ease ◇

Therapeutic class: Antivertigo drugs
Pharmacologic class: Anticholinergics

AVAILABLE FORMS

Tablets: 12.5 mg ◇, 25 mg ◇, 50 mg
Tablets (chewable): 25 mg ◇

INDICATIONS & DOSAGES

➤ **Vertigo**

Adults and children age 12 and older: 25 to 100 mg PO daily in divided doses. Dosage varies with response.

➤ **Motion sickness**

Adults and children age 12 and older: 25 to 50 mg PO 1 hour before travel; then daily for duration of trip.

---

minoxidil (topical)
mi-NOX-i-dill

Men's Rogaine ◇, Minoxidil Extra Strength for Men ◇, Theroxidil ◇, Women's Rogaine ◇

Therapeutic class: Hair-growth stimulants
Pharmacologic class: Direct-acting vasodilators

AVAILABLE FORMS
Topical foam: 5% ◇
Topical solution: 2% ◇, 5% ◇

INDICATIONS & DOSAGES
➤ **Androgenetic alopecia**
Adults: 1 mL of solution to affected area b.i.d. or half a capful of foam applied to affected area b.i.d. (men) or daily (women). Maximum daily dose is 2 mL of solution.

oxymetazoline hydrochloride (intranasal)
ox-i-met-AZ-oh-leen

Afrin 12 Hour ◇, Dristan ◇, Duration 12 Hour Nasal Spray ◇

Therapeutic class: Decongestants
Pharmacologic class: Sympathomimetics

AVAILABLE FORMS
Nasal solution: 0.05% ◇

INDICATIONS & DOSAGES
➤ **Nasal congestion**
Adults and children age 6 and older: 2 to 3 sprays of 0.05% solution in each nostril b.i.d. Don't use for more than 3 days.

phenylephrine hydrochloride (intranasal)
fen-ill-EF-rin

4-Way Fast Acting ◇, 4-Way Menthol ◇, Nasal Four ◇, Neo-Synephrine Mild ◇, Neo-Synephrine Maximum ◇

Therapeutic class: Vasoconstrictors
Pharmacologic class: Adrenergics

AVAILABLE FORMS
Nasal solution: 0.25% ◇, 0.5% ◇, 1% ◇

INDICATIONS & DOSAGES
➤ **Nasal congestion**
Adults and children age 12 and older: 2 to 3 drops or 2 to 3 sprays of 0.25% to 1% solution in each nostril every 4 hours, PRN. Don't use for longer than 3 days.
Children ages 6 to 11: 2 to 3 drops or 2 to 3 sprays of 0.25% solution in each nostril every 4 hours, PRN. Don't use for longer than 3 days.
Children ages 2 to 5: 2 to 3 drops of 0.125% solution in each nostril every 4 hours, PRN. Don't use for longer than 3 days.

pseudoephedrine hydrochloride
soo-dow-e-FED-rin

Children's Sudafed ◇, Nexafed ◇, Sudafed ◇, SudoGest ◇, Zephrex-D ◇

Therapeutic class: Decongestants
Pharmacologic class: Adrenergics

AVAILABLE FORMS
Oral solution: 15 mg/5 mL ◇, 30 mg/5 mL ◇
Syrup: 15 mg/5 mL ◇, 30 mg/5 mL ◇
Tablets: 30 mg ◇, 60 mg ◇
Tablets (abuse-deterrent) ⓄⓃⒸ: 30 mg ◇
Tablets (extended-release) ⓄⓃⒸ: 120 mg ◇, 240 mg ◇

INDICATIONS & DOSAGES
⚠ *Alert:* Don't use drug with an MAO inhibitor or within 2 weeks of stopping an MAO inhibitor.
➤ **Nasal decongestant**
Adults and children age 12 and older: 60 mg PO every 4 to 6 hours; or 120 mg extended-release tablet PO every 12 hours; or 240 mg extended-release tablet PO once daily. Maximum dosage, 240 mg daily.
Children ages 6 to 11 (immediate-release products only): 30 mg PO every 4 to 6 hours. Maximum dosage, 120 mg daily.
Children ages 4 to 5 (immediate-release products only): 15 mg PO every 4 to 6 hours or 1 mg/kg/dose every 6 hours. Maximum dosage, 60 mg daily.

pyrethrins–piperonyl butoxide
pi-RETH-rinz/PI-per-oh-nel

LiceMD ◇, Lice Killing Shampoo ◇, RID ◇, VanaLice ◇

Therapeutic class: Pediculicides
Pharmacologic class: Pyrethrins

AVAILABLE FORMS
Gel: pyrethrins 0.3% and piperonyl butoxide 3.5%
Shampoo: pyrethrins 0.33% and piperonyl butoxide 4% ◇

INDICATIONS & DOSAGES

➤ *Pediculus humanus* infestations

Adults and children age 2 years and older: Apply to hair, scalp, or other infested areas until entirely wet. Allow to remain for 10 minutes but no longer. Wash thoroughly with warm water and soap or shampoo. Remove dead lice and eggs with fine-toothed comb. Repeat treatment in 7 to 10 days to kill newly hatched lice.

simethicone
sye-METH-ih-kone

Gas Relief ◇ , Gas-X ◇ , Gas-X Extra Strength ◇ , Gas-X Infant Drops ◇ , Infacol ✤ , Mylanta Gas Minis ◇ , Mylicon ◇ , Ovol ✤ , Pediacol ✤ ◇ , Phazyme ◇ , Simeped ◇

Therapeutic class: Antiflatulents
Pharmacologic class: Polydimethylsiloxanes

AVAILABLE FORMS

Capsules: 125 mg ◇ , 180 mg ◇ , 250 mg ◇
Drops: 40 mg/mL ✤ , 40 mg/0.6 mL ◇
Liquid: 20 mg/0.3 mL ◇
Strips (orally disintegrating): 40 mg ◇ , 62.5 mg ◇
Tablets (chewable): 80 mg ◇ , 125 mg ◇

INDICATIONS & DOSAGES

➤ GI gas retention

Adults and children older than age 12: 40 to 125 mg PO q.i.d. as needed after each meal and at bedtime; may give single doses of up to 160 to 500 mg after meals or at bedtime, up to 500 mg daily. For drops, 40 to 80 mg PO as needed after each meal and at bedtime, up to 500 mg daily.

Children ages 2 to 12 or weighing more than 11 kg: 40 mg PO q.i.d. as needed after meals and at bedtime, up to 480 mg daily.

Children younger than age 2 or weighing less than 11 kg: 20 mg PO q.i.d. as needed after meals and at bedtime, up to 240 mg daily.

terbinafine hydrochloride (topical)
ter-BIN-ah-fin

Lamisil ◇ , Lamisil AT ◇

Therapeutic class: Antifungals
Pharmacologic class: Allylamine derivatives

AVAILABLE FORMS

Cream: 1% ◇
Solution: 1% ◇
Spray: 1% ◇

INDICATIONS & DOSAGES

➤ Athlete's foot

Adults and children age 12 and older: For athlete's foot between the toes, apply b.i.d. (morning and night) for 1 week or as directed by prescriber. For athlete's foot on the bottom or sides of the foot, apply b.i.d. (morning and night) for 2 weeks or as directed by prescriber.

➤ Jock itch, ringworm

Adults and children age 12 and older: Apply once daily for 1 week or as directed by prescriber.

witch hazel
wich HA-zel

A.E.R. Witch Hazel ◇ , Preparation H Wipes ◇ , TN Dickinson's Witch Hazel ◇

Therapeutic class: Dermatologic agents
Pharmacologic class: Astringents

AVAILABLE FORMS

External pads: 20% ◇ , 50% ◇
External solution: 86% ◇

INDICATIONS & DOSAGES

➤ Anal or vaginal irritation

Adults and children age 12 and older: Apply to affected area up to six times daily or after each bowel movement.

➤ Minor skin irritation

Adults and children age 12 and older: Apply to affected area PRN.

✤Canada   ◇ OTC   ◆ Off-label use   ⓄⓉⒸDo not crush   *Liquid contains alcohol.

Common combination drugs: Indications and dosages

Refer to manufacturer's instructions for complete prescribing and safety information.

Analgesics

butalbital–acetaminophen–caffeine–codeine phosphate ⊠
Fioricet with Codeine
Controlled substance schedule: III

AVAILABLE FORMS
Capsules
50 mg butalbital, 300 mg acetaminophen, 40 mg caffeine, and 30 mg codeine phosphate

INDICATIONS & DOSAGES
Boxed Warning Acetaminophen has been associated with cases of acute liver failure and death. ▮

⊠ Boxed Warning Opioid use increases risk of addiction, abuse, and misuse. Opioids can cause fatal respiratory depression. Opioids can cause respiratory depression and death in children with ingestion of even one dose, particularly with ultra-rapid metabolizers. Opioids combined with benzodiazepines or CNS depressants can cause death. Use during pregnancy can cause neonatal opioid withdrawal syndrome. ▮

➤ **Tension headache**
Adults: 1 to 2 capsules PO every 4 hours PRN. Maximum dosage, 6 capsules in 24 hours.

butalbital–aspirin–caffeine–codeine phosphate ⊠
Ascomp with Codeine
Controlled substance schedule: III

AVAILABLE FORMS
Capsules
50 mg butalbital, 325 mg aspirin, 40 mg caffeine, and 30 mg codeine phosphate

INDICATIONS & DOSAGES
⊠ Boxed Warning Opioid use increases risk of addiction, abuse, and misuse. Opioids can cause fatal respiratory depression. Opioids can cause respiratory depression and death in children with ingestion of even one dose, particularly with ultra-rapid metabolizers. Opioids combined with benzodiazepines or CNS depressants can cause death. Use during pregnancy can cause neonatal opioid withdrawal syndrome. ▮

➤ **Tension headache**
Adults: 1 to 2 capsules PO every 4 hours PRN. Maximum dosage, 6 capsules in 24 hours.

hydrocodone bitartrate–ibuprofen
Controlled substance schedule: II

AVAILABLE FORMS
Tablets
5 mg hydrocodone bitartrate and 200 mg ibuprofen
7.5 mg hydrocodone bitartrate and 200 mg ibuprofen
10 mg hydrocodone bitartrate and 200 mg ibuprofen

INDICATIONS & DOSAGES
Boxed Warning Opioid use increases risk of addiction, abuse, and misuse. Opioids can cause fatal respiratory depression. Opioids can cause respiratory depression and death in children with ingestion of even one dose. Opioids combined with benzodiazepines or CNS depressants can cause death. Use during pregnancy can cause neonatal opioid withdrawal syndrome. ▮

➤ **Acute pain (short-term)**
Adults and children age 16 and older: 1 tablet PO every 4 to 6 hours, PRN. Maximum dosage, 5 tablets in 24 hours.

ibuprofen–famotidine
Duexis

AVAILABLE FORMS
Tablets ⓄⓃⒸ
800 mg ibuprofen and 26.6 mg famotidine

INDICATIONS & DOSAGES
Boxed Warning NSAIDs are contraindicated after CABG surgery and may cause an increased risk of serious CV thrombotic events, MI, stroke, and GI adverse reactions (bleeding, ulceration, and perforation), which can be fatal. ▮

➤ **RA and osteoarthritis**
Adults: 1 tablet PO t.i.d. Older adults may need reduced dosages. Use not recommended in patients with CrCl less than 50 mL/minute.

naproxen–esomeprazole
Vimovo

AVAILABLE FORMS
Tablets ⓄⓃⒸ
375 mg naproxen and 20 mg esomeprazole
500 mg naproxen and 20 mg esomeprazole

INDICATIONS & DOSAGES
Boxed Warning NSAIDs are contraindicated for use in CABG surgery and may cause an increased risk of serious CV thrombotic events, MI, stroke, and GI adverse reactions (bleeding, ulceration, and perforation), which can be fatal. ▮

➤ **Osteoarthritis, RA, or ankylosing spondylitis in patients at risk for gastric ulcer development**
Adults: 1 tablet PO b.i.d.

➤ **Juvenile idiopathic arthritis in patients at risk for gastric ulcer development**
Adults and adolescents age 12 and older weighing more than 50 kg: 1 tablet PO b.i.d.
Adolescents age 12 and older weighing 38 to less than 50 kg: 1 tablet (375 naproxen/20 mg esomeprazole) PO b.i.d.

oxyCODONE hydrochloride–aspirin
Controlled substance schedule: II

AVAILABLE FORMS
Tablets
4.8355 mg oxycodone hydrochloride and 325 mg aspirin

INDICATIONS & DOSAGES

Opioid use increases risk of addiction, abuse, and misuse. Opioids can cause fatal respiratory depression. Opioids can cause respiratory depression and death in children with ingestion of even one dose. Opioids combined with benzodiazepines or CNS depressants can cause death. Use during pregnancy can cause neonatal opioid withdrawal syndrome. ■

➤ **Moderate to moderately severe pain**
Adults: 1 tablet PO every 6 hours PRN. Maximum dosage, 12 tablets in 24 hours.

pentazocine–naloxone hydrochloride
Controlled substance schedule: IV

AVAILABLE FORMS
Tablets
50 mg pentazocine and 0.5 mg naloxone hydrochloride

INDICATIONS & DOSAGES
Boxed Warning Opioid use increases risk of addiction, abuse, and misuse. Opioids can cause fatal respiratory depression. Opioids can cause respiratory depression and death in children with ingestion of even one dose. Opioids combined with benzodiazepines or CNS depressants can cause death. Use during pregnancy can cause neonatal opioid withdrawal syndrome. ■

➤ **Moderate to severe pain**
Adults and children age 12 and older: 1 tablet PO every 3 to 4 hours. May increase to 2 tablets if necessary. Maximum dosage, 12 tablets in 24 hours.

tramadol hydrochloride–acetaminophen
Ultracet 🖉 ⚕
Controlled substance schedule: IV

AVAILABLE FORMS
Tablets
37.5 mg tramadol hydrochloride and 325 mg acetaminophen

INDICATIONS & DOSAGES
Boxed Warning Acetaminophen has been associated with acute liver failure and death. ■
Boxed Warning Opioid use increases risk of addiction, abuse, and misuse. Opioids can cause fatal respiratory depression. Opioids can cause respiratory depression and death in children with ingestion of even one dose. Opioids combined with benzodiazepines or CNS depressants can cause death. Use during pregnancy can cause neonatal opioid withdrawal syndrome. ■

➤ **Acute pain**
Adults: 2 tablets PO every 4 to 6 hours as needed for up to 5 days. Maximum dosage, 8 tablets in 24 hours.
Adjust-a-dose: Patients with CrCl less than 30 mL/minute shouldn't exceed 2 tablets every 12 hours.

Antiacne drugs

benzoyl peroxide–adapalene
Epiduo, Epiduo Forte
AVAILABLE FORMS
Topical gel
2.5% benzoyl peroxide and 0.1% adapalene
2.5% benzoyl peroxide and 0.3% adapalene

INDICATIONS & DOSAGES
➤ **Acne vulgaris**
Adults and children age 9 and older (Epiduo): Apply a thin film to affected areas of face or trunk once daily after washing.
Adults and children age 12 and older (Epiduo Forte): Apply a thin film to affected areas of face or trunk once daily after washing.

clindamycin phosphate–tretinoin
Veltin, Ziana
AVAILABLE FORMS
Topical gel
Clindamycin phosphate 1.2% and tretinoin 0.025%
INDICATIONS & DOSAGES
➤ **Acne vulgaris**
Adults and children age 12 and older: Apply pea-size amount to cover entire affected area once daily in the evening or at bedtime. Avoid eyes, lips, and mucous membranes.

Antidiabetics

alogliptin benzoate–metFORMIN hydrochloride
Kazano
AVAILABLE FORMS
Tablets
12.5 mg alogliptin benzoate and 500 mg metformin
12.5 mg alogliptin benzoate and 1,000 mg metformin
INDICATIONS & DOSAGES
Boxed Warning Metformin can cause serious and sometimes fatal lactic acidosis; prompt hemodialysis is recommended. ■

➤ **Adjunct to diet and exercise to improve glycemic control in patients with type 2 diabetes**
Adults: 1 tablet PO b.i.d. with food. Adjust dosage based on effectiveness and tolerability. Maximum daily dose, 25 mg alogliptin and 2,000 mg metformin.
Adjust-a-dose: Discontinue drug if eGFR falls below 30 mL/minute/1.73 m^2.

alogliptin benzoate–pioglitazone hydrochloride
Oseni
AVAILABLE FORMS
Tablets
12.5 mg alogliptin benzoate and 15 mg pioglitazone hydrochloride
12.5 mg alogliptin benzoate and 30 mg pioglitazone hydrochloride
12.5 mg alogliptin benzoate and 45 mg pioglitazone hydrochloride
25 mg alogliptin benzoate and 15 mg pioglitazone hydrochloride
25 mg alogliptin benzoate and 30 mg pioglitazone hydrochloride
25 mg alogliptin benzoate and 45 mg pioglitazone hydrochloride
INDICATIONS & DOSAGES
Boxed Warning Pioglitazone can cause or exacerbate HF. Drug isn't recommended in patients

with symptomatic HF and is contraindicated in patients with NYHA Class III or IV HF. ∎

➤ **Adjunct to diet and exercise to improve glycemic control in patients with type 2 diabetes**

Adults inadequately controlled on diet and exercise, inadequately controlled on metformin monotherapy, or who require additional glycemic control on alogliptin: Alogliptin 25 mg/pioglitazone 15 mg or alogliptin 25 mg/pioglitazone 30 mg PO once daily. May titrate to a maximum of alogliptin 25 mg/pioglitazone 45 mg once daily based on glycemic response as determined by HbA_{1c}.

Adults who require additional glycemic control on pioglitazone: Alogliptin 25 mg/pioglitazone 15 mg, alogliptin 25 mg/pioglitazone 30 mg, or alogliptin 25 mg/pioglitazone 45 mg PO once daily as appropriate based on current therapy. May titrate to a maximum of alogliptin 25 mg/pioglitazone 45 mg once daily based on glycemic response as determined by HbA_{1c}.

Adults switching from alogliptin administered with pioglitazone: Initiate at the dosage of alogliptin and pioglitazone based on current therapy. May titrate to a maximum of alogliptin 25 mg/pioglitazone 45 mg once daily based on glycemic response as determined by HbA_{1c}.

Adults with HF (NYHA Class I or II): Alogliptin 25 mg/pioglitazone 15 mg PO once daily. May titrate to a maximum of alogliptin 25 mg/pioglitazone 45 mg once daily based on glycemic response as determined by HbA_{1c}.

canagliflozin–metFORMIN hydrochloride
Invokamet, Invokamet XR
AVAILABLE FORMS
Tablets (immediate-release)
50 mg canagliflozin and 500 mg metformin
50 mg canagliflozin and 1,000 mg metformin
150 mg canagliflozin and 500 mg metformin
150 mg canagliflozin and 1,000 mg metformin
Tablets (extended-release) 🔵
50 mg canagliflozin and 500 mg extended-release metformin
50 mg canagliflozin and 1,000 mg extended-release metformin
150 mg canagliflozin and 500 mg extended-release metformin
150 mg canagliflozin and 1,000 mg extended-release metformin
INDICATIONS & DOSAGES
Boxed Warning Metformin can cause serious and sometimes fatal lactic acidosis; prompt hemodialysis is recommended. ∎

➤ **Adjunct to diet and exercise to improve glycemic control in patients with type 2 diabetes when treatment with both canagliflozin and metformin is appropriate; to reduce risk of major adverse CV events (CV death, nonfatal MI, nonfatal stroke), ESRD, doubling of serum creatinine level, and hospitalization for HF in patients with type 2 diabetes and diabetic nephropathy with albuminuria greater than 300 mg/day**

Adults not on canagliflozin or metformin: Initiate therapy with 50 mg canagliflozin and 500 mg metformin PO b.i.d. with meals. Or, 2 extended-release tablets, each containing 50 mg canagliflozin and 500 mg metformin, once daily with morning meal.

Adults already on metformin: 50 mg canagliflozin plus previously prescribed dose of metformin PO b.i.d. with meals. Or, extended-release tablets containing 100 mg canagliflozin plus previously prescribed dose of metformin PO once daily with morning meal.

Adults already on canagliflozin: 500 mg metformin plus previously prescribed dose of canagliflozin PO b.i.d. with meals. Or, extended-release tablets containing 1,000 mg metformin plus previously prescribed dose of canagliflozin PO once daily with morning meal.

Adults already on canagliflozin and metformin: Switch to the same total daily doses of each component PO b.i.d. with meals. Or, use extended-release product once daily with morning meal.

Adjust-a-dose: Increase dosage gradually if needed to reduce metformin's GI adverse effects. Don't exceed maximum daily dose of 2,000 mg of metformin and 300 mg of canagliflozin. Limit dose of the canagliflozin component to 50 mg b.i.d. in patients with moderate renal impairment with an eGFR of 45 to less than 60 mL/minute/1.73 m². Discontinue drug if eGFR falls below 45 mL/minute/1.73 m².

dapagliflozin–sAXagliptin
Qtern
AVAILABLE FORMS
Tablets 🔵
5 mg dapagliflozin and 5 mg saxagliptin
10 mg dapagliflozin and 5 mg saxagliptin
INDICATIONS & DOSAGES
➤ **Adjunct to diet and exercise to improve glycemic control in patients with type 2 diabetes who have inadequate control with dapagliflozin or who are already treated with dapagliflozin and saxagliptin**
Adults: 1 tablet daily in the morning.
Adults not on dapagliflozin: Initially, 5 mg dapagliflozin/5 mg saxagliptin PO once daily in the morning. May increase to 10 mg dapagliflozin/5 mg saxagliptin daily.

glipiZIDE–metFORMIN hydrochloride
AVAILABLE FORMS
Tablets
2.5 mg glipizide and 250 mg metformin hydrochloride
2.5 mg glipizide and 500 mg metformin hydrochloride
5 mg glipizide and 500 mg metformin hydrochloride
INDICATIONS & DOSAGES
Boxed Warning Metformin can cause serious and sometimes fatal lactic acidosis; prompt hemodialysis is recommended. ∎

Adjust-a-dose (for all indications): Discontinue drug if eGFR falls below 30 mL/minute/1.73 m².

➤ **As initial adjunctive therapy to diet and exercise to improve glycemic control in patients with type 2 diabetes**

Adults: Initially, glipizide 2.5 mg/metformin 250 mg once a day with a meal. In patients with fasting plasma glucose level of 280 to 320 mg/dL, consider initiating therapy with glipizide 2.5 mg/metformin 500 mg b.i.d. May increase dosage every 2 weeks per glycemic response to maximum daily dose of 10 mg glipizide with 2,000 mg metformin in divided doses.

➤ **Second-line therapy when diet, exercise, and initial treatment with a sulfonylurea or metformin don't achieve glycemic control**

Adults: Initially, 2.5 mg glipizide/500 mg metformin or 5 mg glipizide/500 mg metformin PO b.i.d. Increase dosage in increments of no more than glipizide 5 mg/metformin 500 mg up to a maximum daily dose of glipizide 20 mg/metformin 2,000 mg.

glyBURIDE–metFORMIN hydrochloride

AVAILABLE FORMS
Tablets
1.25 mg glyburide and 250 mg metformin hydrochloride
2.5 mg glyburide and 500 mg metformin hydrochloride
5 mg glyburide and 500 mg metformin hydrochloride

INDICATIONS & DOSAGES
Boxed Warning Metformin can cause serious and sometimes fatal lactic acidosis; prompt hemodialysis is recommended. ∎

➤ **Adjunctive therapy to diet and exercise to improve glycemic control in patients with type 2 diabetes**

Adults: Initially, glyburide 1.25 mg/metformin 250 mg PO daily or b.i.d. with meals.

Adults inadequately controlled on metformin, glyburide, or another sulfonyluric monotherapy: Glyburide 2.5 mg/metformin 500 mg or glyburide 5 mg/metformin 500 mg PO b.i.d. with meals.

Adults currently on metformin and glyburide or other sulfonyluric: Switch to same total daily doses.

Adjust-a-dose: Gradually increase dosage according to glycemic control and tolerability up to maximum dosage of glyburide 20 mg and metformin 2,000 mg daily. Discontinue drug if eGFR falls below 30 mL/minute/1.73 m².

linagliptin–metFORMIN hydrochloride

Jentadueto, Jentadueto XR

AVAILABLE FORMS
Tablets
2.5 mg linagliptin and 500 mg metformin hydrochloride
2.5 mg linagliptin and 850 mg metformin hydrochloride
2.5 mg linagliptin and 1,000 mg metformin hydrochloride

Tablets (extended-release) ⊙
2.5 mg linagliptin and 1,000 mg extended-release metformin hydrochloride
5 mg linagliptin and 1,000 mg extended-release metformin hydrochloride

INDICATIONS & DOSAGES
Boxed Warning Metformin can cause serious and sometimes fatal lactic acidosis; prompt hemodialysis is recommended. ∎

➤ **Adjunct to diet and exercise to improve glycemic control in adults with type 2 diabetes when treatment with both linagliptin and metformin is appropriate**

Adults already on metformin: 2.5 mg linagliptin PO b.i.d. or 5 mg linagliptin extended-release PO once daily plus current dose of metformin already being taken.

Adults not on metformin: 2.5 mg linagliptin/500 mg metformin PO b.i.d. or 5 mg linagliptin/1,000 mg metformin extended-release PO once daily.

Adjust-a-dose: Gradually titrate dosage to achieve glycemic control. Maximum dose, 2.5 mg linagliptin and 1,000 mg metformin b.i.d. Discontinue drug if eGFR falls below 30 mL/minute/1.73 m².

pioglitazone hydrochloride–metFORMIN hydrochloride

ActoPlus Met

AVAILABLE FORMS
Tablets
15 mg pioglitazone and 500 mg metformin hydrochloride
15 mg pioglitazone and 850 mg metformin hydrochloride

INDICATIONS & DOSAGES
Boxed Warning Pioglitazone can cause or exacerbate HF. Drug isn't recommended in patients with symptomatic HF and is contraindicated in patients with NYHA Class III or IV HF. Metformin can cause serious and sometimes fatal lactic acidosis; prompt hemodialysis is recommended. ∎

➤ **Adjunct to diet and exercise to improve glycemic control in patients with type 2 diabetes**

Adults already on metformin: 15 mg pioglitazone/500 mg metformin or 15 mg pioglitazone/850 mg metformin PO once daily or b.i.d. with food based on current metformin dosage.

Adults already on pioglitazone: 15 mg pioglitazone/500 mg metformin PO b.i.d. or 15 mg pioglitazone/850 mg metformin PO once daily.

Adults with HF (NYHA Class I or II): 15 mg pioglitazone/500 mg metformin or 15 mg pioglitazone/850 mg metformin PO once daily.

Adults already on metformin and pioglitazone: Switch to the same total daily doses of each component.

Adjust-a-dose: Gradually titrate dosage to achieve glycemic control. Maximum dosage, 45 mg pioglitazone and 2,550 mg metformin per day. Discontinue drug if eGFR falls below 30 mL/minute/1.73 m².

sitagliptin phosphate–metFORMIN hydrochloride

Janumet, Janumet XR

AVAILABLE FORMS
Tablets
50 mg sitagliptin phosphate and 500 mg metformin hydrochloride
50 mg sitagliptin phosphate and 850 mg metformin hydrochloride ♣

50 mg sitagliptin phosphate and 1,000 mg metformin hydrochloride

Tablets (extended-release) ⓘ
50 mg sitagliptin phosphate and 500 mg extended-release metformin hydrochloride
50 mg sitagliptin phosphate and 1,000 mg extended-release metformin hydrochloride
100 mg sitagliptin phosphate and 1,000 mg extended-release metformin hydrochloride

INDICATIONS & DOSAGES

Boxed Warning Metformin can cause serious and sometimes fatal lactic acidosis; prompt hemodialysis is recommended. ∎

➤ **Adjunct to diet and exercise to improve glycemic control in patients with type 2 diabetes when treatment with both sitagliptin and metformin is appropriate**

Adults already on metformin (immediate-release):
50 mg sitagliptin PO b.i.d. plus the dose of metformin already being taken. If necessary for patients taking 850 mg metformin PO b.i.d., recommended starting dosage is 50 mg sitagliptin/1,000 mg metformin PO b.i.d.

Adults already on metformin (extended-release):
100 mg/day sitagliptin plus previously prescribed dose of metformin. For patients taking 850 mg immediate-release metformin PO b.i.d. or 1,000 mg metformin PO b.i.d., recommended starting dosage is 100 mg sitagliptin/2,000 mg extended-release metformin PO once daily.

Adults not on metformin: 50 mg sitagliptin/500 mg metformin PO b.i.d. or 100 mg sitagliptin/1,000 mg extended-release metformin PO once daily.

Adjust-a-dose: Gradually titrate dosage to achieve glycemic control. Maximum dosage, 100 mg sitagliptin and 2,000 mg metformin. Discontinue drug if eGFR falls below 30 mL/minute/1.73 m².

Antigout drugs

probenecid–colchicine
AVAILABLE FORMS
Tablets
500 mg probenecid and 0.5 mg colchicine
INDICATIONS & DOSAGES
➤ **Chronic gouty arthritis**
Adults: 1 tablet PO daily for 1 week; then 1 tablet PO b.i.d. If necessary, increase daily dosage by 1 tablet every 4 weeks within tolerance (usually not above 4 tablets daily) if symptoms aren't controlled or 24-hour uric acid excretion isn't above 700 mg.
Adjust-a-dose: Probenecid may not be effective if eGFR falls below 30 mL/minute/1.73 m².

Antihypertensives

aliskiren hemifumarate–hydroCHLOROthiazide
Tekturna HCT
AVAILABLE FORMS
Tablets
150 mg aliskiren hemifumarate and 12.5 mg hydrochlorothiazide

150 mg aliskiren hemifumarate and 25 mg hydrochlorothiazide
300 mg aliskiren hemifumarate and 12.5 mg hydrochlorothiazide
300 mg aliskiren hemifumarate and 25 mg hydrochlorothiazide
INDICATIONS & DOSAGES
Boxed Warning Renin inhibitors can cause fetal harm; when pregnancy is detected, discontinue drug as soon as possible. ∎
➤ **HTN**
Adults: Initially, 150 mg aliskiren/12.5 mg hydrochlorothiazide PO daily. Titrate up as needed after 2 to 4 weeks to a maximum of 300 mg aliskiren/25 mg hydrochlorothiazide daily. Or substitute at same dosage for individual components.

amLODIPine besylate–benazepril hydrochloride
Lotrel
AVAILABLE FORMS
Capsules
2.5 mg amlodipine besylate and 10 mg benazepril hydrochloride
5 mg amlodipine besylate and 10 mg benazepril hydrochloride
5 mg amlodipine besylate and 20 mg benazepril hydrochloride
5 mg amlodipine besylate and 40 mg benazepril hydrochloride
10 mg amlodipine besylate and 20 mg benazepril hydrochloride
10 mg amlodipine besylate and 40 mg benazepril hydrochloride
INDICATIONS & DOSAGES
Boxed Warning Drugs that act directly on the renin-angiotensin system can cause fetal harm; when pregnancy is detected, discontinue drug as soon as possible. ∎
➤ **HTN**
Adults: Initially, 2.5 mg amlodipine/10 mg benazepril PO daily in morning. Titrate dosage based on BP response. Maximum dosage, 10 mg amlodipine and 40 mg benazepril. Or substitute at same dosage for individual components.
Adjust-a-dose: Consider lower initial doses for older adults and patients with hepatic impairment. Drug isn't recommended in patients with CrCl of 30 mL/minute or less.

amLODIPine besylate–hydroCHLOROthiazide–olmesartan medoxomil
Tribenzor
AVAILABLE FORMS
Tablets
5 mg amlodipine besylate, 12.5 mg hydrochlorothiazide, and 20 mg olmesartan medoxomil
5 mg amlodipine besylate, 12.5 mg hydrochlorothiazide, and 40 mg olmesartan medoxomil
5 mg amlodipine besylate, 25 mg hydrochlorothiazide, and 40 mg olmesartan medoxomil

10 mg amlodipine besylate, 12.5 mg hydrochlorothiazide, and 40 mg olmesartan medoxomil

10 mg amlodipine besylate, 25 mg hydrochlorothiazide, and 40 mg olmesartan medoxomil

INDICATIONS & DOSAGES

Boxed Warning Drugs that act directly on the renin-angiotensin system can cause fetal harm; when pregnancy is detected, discontinue drug as soon as possible. ∎

➤ **HTN**

Adults: Adjust dosage of individual products; then switch to appropriate combination product. One tablet PO daily. May increase dosage after 2 weeks. Maximum recommended dose, 10 mg amlodipine/25 mg hydrochlorothiazide/40 mg olmesartan.

Adjust-a-dose: Drug isn't recommended in patients with CrCl of 30 mL/minute or less.

amLODIPine besylate–olmesartan medoxomil

Azor

AVAILABLE FORMS

Tablets

5 mg amlodipine besylate and 20 mg olmesartan medoxomil

5 mg amlodipine besylate and 40 mg olmesartan medoxomil

10 mg amlodipine besylate and 20 mg olmesartan medoxomil

10 mg amlodipine besylate and 40 mg olmesartan medoxomil

INDICATIONS & DOSAGES

Boxed Warning Drugs that act directly on the renin-angiotensin system can cause fetal harm; when pregnancy is detected, discontinue drug as soon as possible. ∎

➤ **HTN**

Adults: Initially, 5 mg amlodipine/20 mg olmesartan PO once daily. Titrate as needed every 1 to 2 weeks up to maximum of 10 mg amlodipine/40 mg olmesartan once daily.

amLODIPine besylate–telmisartan

AVAILABLE FORMS

Tablets

5 mg amlodipine besylate and 40 mg telmisartan

5 mg amlodipine besylate and 80 mg telmisartan

10 mg amlodipine besylate and 40 mg telmisartan

10 mg amlodipine besylate and 80 mg telmisartan

INDICATIONS & DOSAGES

Boxed Warning Drugs that act directly on the renin-angiotensin system can cause fetal harm; when pregnancy is detected, discontinue drug as soon as possible. ∎

➤ **HTN**

Adults: 1 tablet PO daily. Substitute for its individually titrated components or initiate therapy with 5 mg amlodipine/40 mg telmisartan or 5 mg amlodipine/80 mg telmisartan. May increase dosage after at least 2 weeks. Maximum dosage is 10 mg amlodipine/80 mg telmisartan.

amLODIPine besylate–valsartan

Exforge

AVAILABLE FORMS

Tablets

5 mg amlodipine besylate and 160 mg valsartan

5 mg amlodipine besylate and 320 mg valsartan

10 mg amlodipine besylate and 160 mg valsartan

10 mg amlodipine besylate and 320 mg valsartan

INDICATIONS & DOSAGES

Boxed Warning Drugs that act directly on the renin-angiotensin system can cause fetal harm; when pregnancy is detected, discontinue drug as soon as possible. ∎

➤ **HTN**

Adults: Substitute for its individually titrated components or initiate therapy with 5 mg amlodipine/160 mg valsartan PO once daily if patient isn't volume depleted. Increase after 1 to 2 weeks to desired effect or a maximum of 10 mg amlodipine/320 mg valsartan daily.

amLODIPine besylate–valsartan–hydroCHLOROthiazide

Exforge HCT

AVAILABLE FORMS

Tablets

5 mg amlodipine besylate, 160 mg valsartan, and 12.5 mg hydrochlorothiazide

10 mg amlodipine besylate, 160 mg valsartan, and 12.5 mg hydrochlorothiazide

5 mg amlodipine besylate, 160 mg valsartan, and 25 mg hydrochlorothiazide

10 mg amlodipine besylate, 160 mg valsartan, and 25 mg hydrochlorothiazide

10 mg amlodipine besylate, 320 mg valsartan, and 25 mg hydrochlorothiazide

INDICATIONS & DOSAGES

Boxed Warning Drugs that act directly on the renin-angiotensin system can cause fetal harm; when pregnancy is detected, discontinue drug as soon as possible. ∎

➤ **HTN**

Adults: 1 tablet PO once daily as a substitute for the individually titrated components. Or, initiate in patients not adequately controlled on any two of the following antihypertensive classes: calcium channel blockers, ARBs, and diuretics. May increase dosage after 2 weeks. Maximum recommended dosage, 10 mg amlodipine/320 mg valsartan/25 mg hydrochlorothiazide.

Adjust-a-dose: In older adults and patients with hepatic impairment, use lower doses and titrate cautiously.

atenolol–chlorthalidone

Tenoretic

AVAILABLE FORMS

Tablets

50 mg atenolol and 25 mg chlorthalidone

100 mg atenolol and 25 mg chlorthalidone

INDICATIONS & DOSAGES

➤ **HTN**

Adults: Initially, 50 mg atenolol/25 mg chlorthalidone PO daily in the morning. May increase to 100 mg atenolol/25 mg chlorthalidone if needed.

Adjust-a-dose: If CrCl is 15 to 35 mL/minute/1.73 m², maximum dose is 50 mg atenolol/25 mg chlorthalidone daily. If CrCl is less than 15 mL/minute/1.73 m², maximum dose is 50 mg atenolol/25 mg chlorthalidone every other day.

---

benazepril hydrochloride–hydroCHLOROthiazide

Lotensin HCT

AVAILABLE FORMS

Tablets

5 mg benazepril and 6.25 mg hydrochlorothiazide
10 mg benazepril and 12.5 mg hydrochlorothiazide
20 mg benazepril and 12.5 mg hydrochlorothiazide
20 mg benazepril and 25 mg hydrochlorothiazide

INDICATIONS & DOSAGES

Boxed Warning Drugs that act directly on the renin-angiotensin system can cause fetal harm; when pregnancy is detected, discontinue drug as soon as possible. ■

➤ **HTN**

Adults: 1 tablet PO daily in the morning. Initially, 10 mg benazepril and 12.5 mg hydrochlorothiazide in patients not adequately controlled on individual component as monotherapy. Or substitute for individually titrated components. Wait 2 to 3 weeks before increasing hydrochlorothiazide dose. Maximum dose is 20 mg benazepril and 25 mg hydrochlorothiazide daily.

Adjust-a-dose: Drug isn't recommended in patients with CrCl of 30 mL/minute/1.73 m² or less.

---

bisoprolol fumarate–hydroCHLOROthiazide

Ziac

AVAILABLE FORMS

Tablets

2.5 mg bisoprolol fumarate and 6.25 mg hydrochlorothiazide
5 mg bisoprolol fumarate and 6.25 mg hydrochlorothiazide
10 mg bisoprolol fumarate and 6.25 mg hydrochlorothiazide

INDICATIONS & DOSAGES

➤ **HTN**

Adults: Initially, 2.5 mg bisoprolol/6.25 mg hydrochlorothiazide PO daily. Increase dosage in 14-day intervals; optimal antihypertensive effect may require 2 to 3 weeks. Or, substitute for previously titrated individual components. Maximum dosage, 20 mg bisoprolol and 12.5 mg hydrochlorothiazide daily.

Adjust-a-dose: Use caution when titrating drug in patients with renal or hepatic impairment.

---

candesartan cilexetil–hydroCHLOROthiazide

Atacand HCT

AVAILABLE FORMS

Tablets

16 mg candesartan cilexetil and 12.5 mg hydrochlorothiazide
32 mg candesartan cilexetil and 12.5 mg hydrochlorothiazide
32 mg candesartan cilexetil and 25 mg hydrochlorothiazide

INDICATIONS & DOSAGES

Boxed Warning Drugs that act directly on the renin-angiotensin system can cause fetal harm; when pregnancy is detected, discontinue drug as soon as possible. ■

➤ **HTN**

Adults: Initially, 16 mg candesartan/12.5 mg hydrochlorothiazide PO daily in one or two divided doses in patients who aren't controlled on monotherapy with individual product or who are volume-depleted. Titrate dosage to clinical effect. Maximum effect can be expected within 4 weeks of drug initiation or dosage change. Or, substitute for previously titrated individual components.

---

enalapril maleate–hydroCHLOROthiazide

Vaseretic

AVAILABLE FORMS

Tablets

5 mg enalapril maleate and 12.5 mg hydrochlorothiazide
10 mg enalapril maleate and 25 mg hydrochlorothiazide

INDICATIONS & DOSAGES

Boxed Warning Drugs that act directly on the renin-angiotensin system can cause fetal harm; when pregnancy is detected, discontinue drug as soon as possible. ■

➤ **HTN**

Adults: Initially, 5 mg enalapril maleate/12.5 mg hydrochlorothiazide or 10 mg enalapril/25 mg hydrochlorothiazide PO daily in patients not adequately controlled with either enalapril or hydrochlorothiazide monotherapy. Increase dosage based on response after 2 to 3 weeks. Or, substitute for previously titrated individual components. Maximum dosage, 20 mg enalapril and 50 mg hydrochlorothiazide daily.

---

fosinopril–hydroCHLOROthiazide

AVAILABLE FORMS

Tablets

10 mg fosinopril sodium and 12.5 mg hydrochlorothiazide
20 mg fosinopril sodium and 12.5 mg hydrochlorothiazide

INDICATIONS & DOSAGES

Boxed Warning Drugs that act directly on the renin-angiotensin system can cause fetal harm; when pregnancy is detected, discontinue drug as soon as possible. ■

➤ **HTN**

Adults: 1 tablet PO per day in the morning in patients not adequately controlled on either fosinopril or hydrochlorothiazide monotherapy. Titrate based on clinical effect. Or, substitute for previously titrated individual components.

---

irbesartan–hydroCHLOROthiazide
Avalide
AVAILABLE FORMS
Tablets
150 mg irbesartan and 12.5 mg hydrochlorothiazide
300 mg irbesartan and 12.5 mg hydrochlorothiazide
INDICATIONS & DOSAGES
Boxed Warning Drugs that act directly on the renin-angiotensin system can cause fetal harm; when pregnancy is detected, discontinue drug as soon as possible. ▪
➤ HTN
Adults: Initially, 150 mg irbesartan/12.5 mg hydrochlorothiazide PO daily in patients not adequately controlled on either irbesartan or hydrochlorothiazide monotherapy or as initial therapy. Titrate based on clinical effect; dosage can be increased after 1 to 2 weeks. Or, substitute for previously titrated individual components. Maximum daily dose, 300 mg irbesartan and 25 mg hydrochlorothiazide.

losartan potassium–hydroCHLOROthiazide
Hyzaar
AVAILABLE FORMS
Tablets
50 mg losartan potassium and 12.5 mg hydrochlorothiazide
100 mg losartan potassium and 12.5 mg hydrochlorothiazide
100 mg losartan potassium and 25 mg hydrochlorothiazide
INDICATIONS & DOSAGES
Boxed Warning Drugs that act directly on the renin-angiotensin system can cause fetal harm; when pregnancy is detected, discontinue drug as soon as possible. ▪
➤ HTN; risk reduction for stroke in patients with HTN and left ventricular hypertrophy
Adults: 1 tablet PO daily as a substitute for individual titrated components or in patients not adequately controlled with monotherapy with either of the component products. May use as initial therapy in severe HTN when benefits outweigh risk. Titrate after 3 weeks. Maximum dose: Losartan 100 mg/hydrochlorothiazide 25 mg once daily.

metoprolol tartrate–hydroCHLOROthiazide
AVAILABLE FORMS
Tablets
50 mg metoprolol tartrate and 25 mg hydrochlorothiazide
100 mg metoprolol tartrate and 25 mg hydrochlorothiazide
100 mg metoprolol tartrate and 50 mg hydrochlorothiazide
INDICATIONS & DOSAGES
➤ HTN
Adults: Adjust dosage using individual products; then switch to appropriate combination product. Usual dosage is 100 to 200 mg metoprolol/25 to 50 mg hydrochlorothiazide PO once daily or 50 to 100 mg

metoprolol/12.5 to 25 mg hydrochlorothiazide PO b.i.d.

moexipril hydrochloride–hydroCHLOROthiazide
AVAILABLE FORMS
Tablets
7.5 mg moexipril hydrochloride and 12.5 mg hydrochlorothiazide
15 mg moexipril hydrochloride and 12.5 mg hydrochlorothiazide
15 mg moexipril hydrochloride and 25 mg hydrochlorothiazide
INDICATIONS & DOSAGES
Boxed Warning Drugs that act directly on the renin-angiotensin system can cause fetal harm; when pregnancy is detected, discontinue drug as soon as possible. ▪
➤ HTN
Adults: Initially, 7.5 mg moexipril/12.5 mg hydrochlorothiazide, or 15 mg moexipril/12.5 mg hydrochlorothiazide, or 15 mg moexipril/25 mg hydrochlorothiazide PO once daily in patients not adequately controlled on moexipril or hydrochlorothiazide monotherapy. Or, substitute for previously titrated individual components. Adjust dosage based on clinical response.

olmesartan medoxomil–hydroCHLOROthiazide
Benicar HCT 🖉
AVAILABLE FORMS
Tablets
20 mg olmesartan medoxomil and 12.5 mg hydrochlorothiazide
40 mg olmesartan medoxomil and 12.5 mg hydrochlorothiazide
40 mg olmesartan medoxomil and 25 mg hydrochlorothiazide
INDICATIONS & DOSAGES
Boxed Warning Drugs that act directly on the renin-angiotensin system can cause fetal harm; when pregnancy is detected, discontinue drug as soon as possible. ▪
➤ HTN
Adults: Initially in patients not controlled on olmesartan monotherapy, 40 mg olmesartan/12.5 mg hydrochlorothiazide PO daily. Initially in patients not controlled on hydrochlorothiazide monotherapy, 20 mg olmesartan/12.5 mg hydrochlorothiazide PO daily. May titrate dosage at 2- to 4-week intervals. Or, substitute for previously titrated individual components. Maximum dosage, 40 mg olmesartan/25 mg hydrochlorothiazide.

quinapril hydrochloride–hydroCHLOROthiazide
Accuretic
AVAILABLE FORMS
Tablets
10 mg quinapril hydrochloride and 12.5 mg hydrochlorothiazide

20 mg quinapril hydrochloride and 12.5 mg hydrochlorothiazide

20 mg quinapril hydrochloride and 25 mg hydrochlorothiazide

INDICATIONS & DOSAGES

Boxed Warning Drugs that act directly on the renin-angiotensin system can cause fetal harm; when pregnancy is detected, discontinue drug as soon as possible. ■

➤ **HTN**

Adults: Initially, 10 mg quinapril/12.5 mg hydrochlorothiazide or 20 mg quinapril/12.5 mg hydrochlorothiazide PO daily in patients not adequately controlled on quinapril monotherapy or who are controlled on 25 mg hydrochlorothiazide daily but experience significant potassium loss. May titrate dosage at 2- to 3-week intervals. Or, substitute for previously titrated individual components.

Adjust-a-dose: Discontinue drug if eGFR falls below 30 mL/minute/1.73 m² or serum creatinine level is more than 3 mg/dL.

telmisartan–hydroCHLOROthiazide
Micardis HCT

AVAILABLE FORMS

Tablets

40 mg telmisartan and 12.5 mg hydrochlorothiazide

80 mg telmisartan and 12.5 mg hydrochlorothiazide

80 mg telmisartan and 25 mg hydrochlorothiazide

INDICATIONS & DOSAGES

Boxed Warning Drugs that act directly on the renin-angiotensin system can cause fetal harm; when pregnancy is detected, discontinue drug as soon as possible. ■

➤ **HTN**

Adult: Initially, 80 mg telmisartan/12.5 mg hydrochlorothiazide PO per day in patients without adequate control with monotherapy on either of the component drugs or who are controlled on 25 mg hydrochlorothiazide daily but experience significant potassium loss. May adjust up to 160 mg telmisartan and 25 mg hydrochlorothiazide, based on patient's response after 2 to 4 weeks of therapy. Or, substitute for previously titrated individual components. Not for use as initial therapy.

Adjust-a-dose: In patients with mild to moderate hepatic impairment or biliary obstructive disorders, begin therapy with 40 mg telmisartan/12.5 mg hydrochlorothiazide PO once daily. Don't use in patients with severe hepatic impairment. Drug isn't recommended in patients with CrCl of 30 mL/minute/ 1.73 m² or less.

trandolapril–verapamil hydrochloride

AVAILABLE FORMS

Tablets (extended-release)

1 mg trandolapril and 240 mg verapamil hydrochloride

2 mg trandolapril and 180 mg verapamil hydrochloride

2 mg trandolapril and 240 mg verapamil hydrochloride

4 mg trandolapril and 240 mg verapamil hydrochloride

INDICATIONS & DOSAGES

Boxed Warning Drugs that act directly on the renin-angiotensin system can cause fetal harm; when pregnancy is detected, discontinue drug as soon as possible. ■

➤ **HTN**

Adults: 1 tablet PO per day with food. Adjust dosage using the individual products; then switch to appropriate combination product.

Adjust-a-dose: In patients with hepatic or renal impairment (CrCl of less than 30 mL/minute), lower doses are recommended.

valsartan–hydroCHLOROthiazide
Diovan HCT *◆*

AVAILABLE FORMS

Tablets

80 mg valsartan and 12.5 mg hydrochlorothiazide

160 mg valsartan and 12.5 mg hydrochlorothiazide

160 mg valsartan and 25 mg hydrochlorothiazide

320 mg valsartan and 12.5 mg hydrochlorothiazide

320 mg valsartan and 25 mg hydrochlorothiazide

INDICATIONS & DOSAGES

Boxed Warning Drugs that act directly on the renin-angiotensin system can cause fetal harm; when pregnancy is detected, discontinue drug as soon as possible. ■

➤ **HTN**

Adults: Initially, 160 mg valsartan/12.5 mg hydrochlorothiazide PO daily. Titrate to desired effect after 1 to 2 weeks. Or, substitute for previously titrated individual components. Maximum dose, 320 mg valsartan/25 mg hydrochlorothiazide.

Antilipemics

ezetimibe–simvastatin
Vytorin *◆* ▨

AVAILABLE FORMS

Tablets

10 mg ezetimibe with 10, 20, 40, or 80 mg simvastatin

INDICATIONS & DOSAGES

➤ **Homozygous familial hypercholesterolemia, primary hyperlipidemia or mixed hyperlipidemia** ▨

Adults: 1 tablet PO daily in the evening in combination with a cholesterol-lowering diet and exercise. May adjust dosage of simvastatin in combination based on patient response.

Only use 10 mg ezetimibe/80 mg simvastatin in patients who have been taking drug long-term without evidence of muscle toxicity. In patients unable to achieve their LDL cholesterol goal using 10 mg ezetimibe/40 mg simvastatin, don't titrate to the 10 mg ezetimibe/80 mg simvastatin dose; use an alternative therapy.

If giving drug with a bile acid sequestrant, give drug at least 2 hours before or 4 hours after the bile acid sequestrant.

Adjust-a-dose: For patients with moderate to severe renal impairment (GFR less than 60 mL/minute), give 10 mg ezetimibe/20 mg simvastatin once daily in the evening. Refer to manufacturer's instructions for dosage adjustments when used with concomitant drugs.

Use with niacin doses of 1,000 mg or more isn't recommended when treating patients who are Chinese because of an increased risk of myopathy.▓

Antimigraine drugs

ergotamine tartrate–caffeine
Cafergot, Migergot
AVAILABLE FORMS
Tablets
1 mg ergotamine tartrate and 100 mg caffeine
Suppositories
2 mg ergotamine tartrate and 100 mg caffeine
INDICATIONS & DOSAGES
Boxed Warning Use with potent CYP3A4 inhibitors, including protease inhibitors and macrolide antibiotics, can cause serious vasospasm and is contraindicated. ■
➤ **Prevention and treatment of vascular headache**
Adults: 2 tablets PO at first sign of attack. Follow with 1 tablet every 30 minutes, if needed. Maximum dose is 6 tablets per attack. Don't exceed 10 tablets per week. Or, 1 suppository PR at first sign of attack; follow with second dose after 1 hour, if needed. Maximum dose is 2 suppositories per attack. Don't exceed 5 suppositories per week.

SUMAtriptan succinate–naproxen sodium
Treximet
AVAILABLE FORMS
Tablets
85 mg sumatriptan succinate and 500 mg naproxen sodium
INDICATIONS & DOSAGES
Boxed Warning NSAIDs may cause an increased risk of serious and sometimes fatal CV thrombotic events, MI, stroke, and GI adverse reactions. Contraindicated after CABG surgery. ■
➤ **Migraine headache**
Adults: One 85 mg sumatriptan/500 mg naproxen tablet PO at first sign of migraine. May follow with a second dose 2 hours later. Maximum dosage, 2 tablets in 24 hours. Limit use to 5 migraine headaches in 30-day period.

Antiplatelet drugs

dipyridamole–aspirin
AVAILABLE FORMS
Capsules ⓞⓣⓒ
200 mg dipyridamole and 25 mg aspirin
INDICATIONS & DOSAGES
➤ **To reduce stroke risk**
Adults: 1 capsule PO b.i.d. in morning and evening. Not interchangeable with the individual components of aspirin and dipyridamole tablets.

Antiretrovirals

abacavir sulfate–lamiVUDine
Epzicom ▓
AVAILABLE FORMS
Tablets
600 mg abacavir and 300 mg lamivudine

INDICATIONS & DOSAGES
▓ **Boxed Warning** Contraindicated in patients with prior hypersensitivity reaction to abacavir and in patients who are positive for HLA-B*5701; screen for the HLA-B*5701 allele before starting drug. Never restart drug in patients who have had a hypersensitivity reaction to abacavir; severe signs and symptoms, including death, can occur within hours. Severe acute exacerbations of HBV infection have been reported in patients infected with both HBV and HIV who have discontinued lamivudine. Monitor patients closely for at least several months after stopping drug. ■
➤ **HIV infection**
Adults and children weighing 25 kg or more:
1 tablet PO daily in combination with other antiretrovirals.
Adjust-a-dose: Use isn't recommended in patients with CrCl less than 50 mL/minute or moderate to severe hepatic impairment.

abacavir sulfate–lamiVUDine–zidovudine
Trizivir ▓
AVAILABLE FORMS
Tablets
300 mg abacavir sulfate, 150 mg lamivudine, and 300 mg zidovudine
INDICATIONS & DOSAGES
▓ **Boxed Warning** Contraindicated in patients with prior hypersensitivity reaction to abacavir and in patients positive for HLA-B*5701; screen for the HLA-B*5701 allele before starting drug. Never restart drug in patients who have had a hypersensitivity reaction to abacavir; severe signs and symptoms, including death, can occur within hours. Hematologic toxicity, myopathy, lactic acidosis, and severe hepatomegaly with steatosis, including fatal cases, have been reported. Severe acute exacerbations of HBV infection have been reported in patients infected with both HBV and HIV who have discontinued lamivudine. Monitor patients closely for at least several months after stopping drug. ■
➤ **HIV infection**
Adults and children weighing 40 kg or more: 1 tablet PO b.i.d., alone or with other antiretrovirals.
Adjust-a-dose: Use isn't recommended in patients with CrCl less than 50 mL/minute or mild hepatic impairment. Use is contraindicated in moderate to severe hepatic impairment.

bictegravir–emtricitabine–tenofovir alafenamide
Biktarvy
AVAILABLE FORMS
Tablets
30 mg bictegravir, 120 mg emtricitabine, and 15 mg tenofovir alafenamide
50 mg bictegravir, 200 mg emtricitabine, and 25 mg tenofovir alafenamide

INDICATIONS & DOSAGES

Boxed Warning Severe, acute reactivations of HBV infection have been reported in patients infected with both HIV and HBV who have discontinued emtricitabine or tenofovir. Close monitoring over several months is recommended. If appropriate, initiate anti–hepatitis B therapy. ■

➤ **HIV-1 infection in adults and children weighing at least 25 kg who have no antiretroviral treatment history or to replace current antiretroviral regimen in patients who are virologically suppressed (HIV-1 RNA less than 50 copies/mL) on a stable antiretroviral regimen for at least 3 months with no history of treatment failure and no known substitutions associated with resistance to the individual components**

Adults and children weighing at least 25 kg: 1 tablet of 50 mg bictegravir, 200 mg emtricitabine, and 25 mg tenofovir alafenamide PO daily.

Children weighing 14 to less than 25 kg: 1 tablet of 30 mg bictegravir, 120 mg emtricitabine, and 15 mg tenofovir alafenamide PO daily.

efavirenz–emtricitabine–tenofovir disoproxil fumarate

Atripla

AVAILABLE FORMS

Tablets

600 mg efavirenz, 200 mg emtricitabine, and 300 mg tenofovir disoproxil fumarate

INDICATIONS & DOSAGES

Boxed Warning Severe, acute reactivations of HBV infection have been reported in patients infected with both HIV and HBV who have discontinued emtricitabine or tenofovir. Close monitoring over several months is recommended. If appropriate, initiate anti–hepatitis B therapy. ■

➤ **HIV infection**

Adults and children weighing at least 40 kg: 1 tablet PO daily on empty stomach. Dosing at bedtime may improve tolerability of nervous system symptoms.

Adjust-a-dose: If given with rifampin in patients weighing 50 kg or more, give additional 200 mg of efavirenz per day. Use isn't recommended in patients with CrCl less than 50 mL/minute or moderate to severe hepatic impairment.

emtricitabine–rilpivirine–tenofovir disoproxil fumarate

Complera

AVAILABLE FORMS

Tablets

200 mg emtricitabine, 25 mg rilpivirine, and 300 mg tenofovir disoproxil fumarate

INDICATIONS & DOSAGES

Boxed Warning Severe, acute reactivations of HBV infection have been reported in patients infected with both HIV and HBV who have discontinued emtricitabine or tenofovir. Close monitoring over several months is recommended. If appropriate, initiate anti–hepatitis B therapy. ■

➤ **HIV infection**

Adults and children weighing 35 kg or more: 1 tablet PO once daily with food.

Adjust-a-dose: Use isn't recommended in patients with CrCl less than 50 mL/minute.

emtricitabine–tenofovir disoproxil fumarate

Truvada

AVAILABLE FORMS

Tablets

100 mg emtricitabine and 150 mg tenofovir disoproxil fumarate

133 mg emtricitabine and 200 mg tenofovir disoproxil fumarate

167 mg emtricitabine and 250 mg tenofovir disoproxil fumarate

200 mg emtricitabine and 300 mg tenofovir disoproxil fumarate

INDICATIONS & DOSAGES

Boxed Warning For preexposure prophylaxis, confirm that patient is HIV-negative immediately before initiating and periodically (at least every 3 months) during use to decrease risk of drug resistance. Severe acute exacerbations of HBV infection have been reported in HBV-infected patients who have discontinued drug. Monitor patients closely for at least several months after stopping drug. ■

➤ **Preexposure prophylaxis (adults and adolescents) and treatment of HIV infection in combination with other retrovirals**

Adults and adolescents (preexposure prophylaxis and treatment) and children (treatment) weighing 35 kg or more: 200 mg emtricitabine/300 mg tenofovir disoproxil fumarate PO daily.

Children weighing 28 to less than 35 kg: 167 mg emtricitabine/250 mg tenofovir disoproxil fumarate PO daily.

Children weighing 22 to less than 28 kg: 133 mg emtricitabine/200 mg tenofovir disoproxil fumarate PO daily.

Children weighing 17 to less than 22 kg: 100 mg emtricitabine/150 mg tenofovir disoproxil fumarate PO daily.

Adjust-a-dose: For adults with CrCl of 30 to 49 mL/minute, give dose every 48 hours; withhold drug for CrCl of less than 30 mL/minute. There are no dosage recommendations for children with renal impairment. Not recommended for preexposure prophylaxis in individuals with estimated CrCl below 60 mL/minute.

lamiVUDine–zidovudine

Combivir *⚭*

AVAILABLE FORMS

Tablets

150 mg lamivudine and 300 mg zidovudine

INDICATIONS & DOSAGES

Boxed Warning Hematologic toxicity, myopathy, lactic acidosis, severe hepatomegaly (including fatal cases), and exacerbations of HBV infection have been reported. ■

➤ **HIV infection**

Adults and children weighing 30 kg or more: 1 tablet PO b.i.d.

Adjust-a-dose: Use isn't recommended in patients with CrCl less than 50 mL/minute or hepatic impairment.

Antiulcer drugs

bismuth subcitrate potassium–metroNIDAZOLE–tetracycline hydrochloride
Pylera

AVAILABLE FORMS
Capsules
140 mg bismuth subcitrate potassium, 125 mg metronidazole, and 125 mg tetracycline hydrochloride

INDICATIONS & DOSAGES

Boxed Warning Metronidazole has been shown to be carcinogenic in mice and rats. It's unknown if it's carcinogenic in humans. ∎

➤ **Eradication of *Helicobacter pylori* infection; active duodenal ulcers associated with *H. pylori* infection**

Adults: Give each dose (which includes all 3 capsules) PO q.i.d. after meals and at bedtime for 10 days with omeprazole 20 mg PO b.i.d. (after the morning and evening meals) for 10 days.

lansoprazole–amoxicillin–clarithromycin

AVAILABLE FORMS
Daily administration pack
Two 30-mg lansoprazole capsules, four 500-mg amoxicillin capsules, and two 500-mg clarithromycin tablets

INDICATIONS & DOSAGES

➤ **Eradication of *Helicobacter pylori* infection**

Adults: 30 mg lansoprazole, 1 g amoxicillin, and 500 mg clarithromycin PO b.i.d. before eating (morning and evening) for 10 to 14 days.

⚠ *Alert:* Clarithromycin may increase risk of death, especially in patients with heart disease. Avoid use in patients at high risk, and weigh risks and benefits of therapy in all patients. In patients with heart disease, consider the use of alternative antibiotics.

Benign prostatic hyperplasia drug

dutasteride–tamsulosin hydrochloride
Jalyn

AVAILABLE FORMS
Capsules ⓄⓃⒸ
0.5 mg dutasteride and 0.4 mg tamsulosin hydrochloride

INDICATIONS & DOSAGES

➤ **Symptomatic BPH**

Adult men: 1 capsule PO daily 30 minutes after same meal each day.

Contraceptives

segesterone acetate–ethinyl estradiol
Annovera

AVAILABLE FORMS
Vaginal ring
103 mg segesterone acetate and 17.4 mg ethinyl estradiol delivering an average of 0.15 mg segesterone acetate and 0.013 mg ethinyl estradiol daily

INDICATIONS & DOSAGES

Boxed Warning Cigarette smoking increases risk of serious CV events from combination hormonal contraceptives; use should be avoided in individuals older than age 35 who smoke. ∎

➤ **Contraception**

Patients of childbearing potential: 1 vaginal ring inserted into the vagina and left in place continuously for 21 days, followed by a 7-day vaginal ring–free interval. One vaginal ring provides 13 cycles of contraception for approximately 1 year.

Diuretics

aMILoride hydrochloride–hydroCHLOROthiazide

AVAILABLE FORMS
Tablets
5 mg amiloride hydrochloride and 50 mg hydrochlorothiazide

INDICATIONS & DOSAGES

Boxed Warning May cause potentially fatal hyperkalemia; monitor serum potassium levels carefully. ∎

➤ **HF or HTN**

Adults: 1 to 2 tablets PO per day as a single daily dose or in divided dose with food.

spironolactone–hydroCHLOROthiazide
Aldactazide

AVAILABLE FORMS
Tablets
25 mg spironolactone and 25 mg hydrochlorothiazide
50 mg spironolactone and 50 mg hydrochlorothiazide

INDICATIONS & DOSAGES

Adjust-a-dose (all indications): In older adults, initiate with lowest available dose. Avoid spironolactone doses of more than 25 mg/day in older adults with HF or renal impairment.

➤ **Edema**

Adults: 25 to 200 mg spironolactone/25 to 200 mg hydrochlorothiazide PO in single or divided doses daily.

➤ **HTN**

Adults: 50 to 100 mg spironolactone/50 to 100 mg hydrochlorothiazide PO in single or divided doses daily.

Heart failure drugs

isosorbide dinitrate–hydrALAZINE hydrochloride ⊠
BiDil

AVAILABLE FORMS
Tablets
20 mg isosorbide dinitrate and 37.5 mg hydralazine

INDICATIONS & DOSAGES

➤ **Adjunct to standard HF therapy in patients who self-identify as Black** ⊠

Adults: 1 to 2 tablets PO t.i.d. Maximum, 2 tablets PO t.i.d.

Menopause drugs

conjugated estrogens–bazedoxifene acetate

Duavee

AVAILABLE FORMS
Tablets
0.45 mg conjugated estrogens and 20 mg bazedoxifene acetate

INDICATIONS & DOSAGES
Boxed Warning May increase risk of endometrial cancer. Product isn't for use for preventing CV disease or dementia. Product shouldn't be used with additional estrogens; use at lowest effective doses, for shortest duration, consistent with treatment goals and risks for the individual patient. ■
➤ **Vasomotor symptoms associated with menopause; postmenopausal osteoporosis prevention**
Adults: 1 tablet PO once daily.

conjugated estrogens/conjugated estrogens–medroxyPROGESTERone acetate

Premphase

AVAILABLE FORMS
Tablets
0.625 mg conjugated estrogens; 0.625 mg conjugated estrogens and 5 mg medroxyprogesterone acetate

INDICATIONS & DOSAGES
Boxed Warning Product may increase risk of endometrial and breast cancer and CV disease. Product isn't for use for preventing dementia or CV disease. Use at lowest effective doses, for the shortest duration, consistent with treatment goals and risks for the individual patient. ■
➤ **Moderate to severe symptoms (vasomotor, vulvar, and vaginal atrophy) of menopause; to prevent osteoporosis**
Patients with intact uterus: 1 tablet PO per day. Use estrogen (maroon tablet) alone on days 1 to 14 and estrogen–medroxyprogesterone acetate (light blue tablet) on days 15 to 28.

conjugated estrogens–medroxyPROGESTERone acetate

Prempro

AVAILABLE FORMS
Tablets
0.3 mg conjugated estrogens and 1.5 mg medroxyprogesterone
0.45 mg conjugated estrogens and 1.5 mg medroxyprogesterone
0.625 mg conjugated estrogens and 2.5 mg medroxyprogesterone
0.625 mg conjugated estrogens and 5 mg medroxyprogesterone

INDICATIONS & DOSAGES
Boxed Warning Product may increase risk of endometrial and breast cancer and CV disease. Product isn't for use for preventing dementia. Use at lowest effective doses, for the shortest duration, consistent with treatment goals and risks for the individual patient. ■
➤ **Symptoms of menopause (vasomotor, vulvar, and vaginal atrophy); to prevent osteoporosis**
Patients with intact uterus: 1 tablet PO per day.

Miscellaneous cardiac drugs

amLODIPine besylate–atorvastatin calcium ▓

Caduet

AVAILABLE FORMS
Tablets
2.5 mg amlodipine besylate with 10 mg, 20 mg, or 40 mg atorvastatin calcium
5 mg amlodipine besylate with 10 mg, 20 mg, 40 mg, or 80 mg atorvastatin calcium
10 mg amlodipine besylate with 10 mg, 20 mg, 40 mg, or 80 mg atorvastatin calcium

INDICATIONS & DOSAGES
Adjust-a-dose (all indications): For small or fragile patients, older adults, or patients with hepatic insufficiency, initially, 2.5 mg amlodipine once daily. Atorvastatin is contraindicated in patients with active liver disease or unexplained LFT elevations. Refer to manufacturer's instructions for dosage adjustments when used with concomitant drugs.
➤ **HTN, CAD (amlodipine); prevention of CV disease, hyperlipidemia (atorvastatin)**
Adults: Determine the most effective dose for each component; then select the most appropriate combination product. When titrating amlodipine, wait 7 to 14 days between titration steps. When titrating atorvastatin, adjust dosage at intervals of 4 weeks or more. Maximum dose, amlodipine 10 mg and atorvastatin 80 mg daily.

aspirin–omeprazole

Yosprala

AVAILABLE FORMS
Tablets (delayed-release) ⊙
81 mg delayed-release aspirin and 40 mg immediate-release omeprazole
325 mg delayed-release aspirin and 40 mg immediate-release omeprazole

INDICATIONS & DOSAGES
➤ **To reduce risk of aspirin-associated gastric ulcers in patients who require aspirin for the secondary prevention of CV and cerebrovascular events**
Adults: 1 tablet PO once daily 60 minutes before a meal.

Opioid agonists

buprenorphine hydrochloride–naloxone hydrochloride

Suboxone, Zubsolv
Controlled substance schedule: III

AVAILABLE FORMS
SL tablets
2 mg buprenorphine and 0.5 mg naloxone
8 mg buprenorphine and 2 mg naloxone
SL tablets (Zubsolv)
0.7 mg buprenorphine and 0.18 mg naloxone
1.4 mg buprenorphine and 0.36 mg naloxone

2.9 mg buprenorphine and 0.71 mg naloxone
5.7 mg buprenorphine and 1.4 mg naloxone
8.6 mg buprenorphine and 2.1 mg naloxone
11.4 mg buprenorphine and 2.9 mg naloxone
SL film (Suboxone)
2 mg buprenorphine and 0.5 mg naloxone
4 mg buprenorphine and 1 mg naloxone
8 mg buprenorphine and 2 mg naloxone
12 mg buprenorphine and 3 mg naloxone
INDICATIONS & DOSAGES
➤ **Induction of opioid dependence treatment**
Refer to manufacturer's instructions for specific product.
➤ **Opioid dependence**
Adults: Maintenance dose is based on buprenorphine. Refer to manufacturer's instructions for specific product.

Psychotherapeutics

chlordiazePOXIDE–amitriptyline
Controlled substance schedule: IV
AVAILABLE FORMS
Tablets
5 mg chlordiazepoxide and 12.5 mg amitriptyline
10 mg chlordiazepoxide and 25 mg amitriptyline
INDICATIONS & DOSAGES
Boxed Warning Not approved for use in children because of increased suicide risk. Monitor patients on antidepressants for appearance or worsening of suicidal thoughts and behaviors. Benzodiazepine use with opioids can cause sedation and fatal respiratory depression. Use of product increases risk of addiction, abuse, and misuse. ■
➤ **Severe depression**
Adults: 10 mg chlordiazepoxide/25 mg amitriptyline PO t.i.d. to up to six times daily. For patients who don't tolerate higher doses, 5 mg chlordiazepoxide/ 12.5 mg amitriptyline PO t.i.d. to q.i.d. Reduce dosage after initial response.
Adjust-a-dose: Older adults may need lower dosages.

OLANZapine–FLUoxetine hydrochloride
Symbyax
AVAILABLE FORMS
Capsules
3 mg olanzapine and 25 mg fluoxetine
6 mg olanzapine and 25 mg fluoxetine
6 mg olanzapine and 50 mg fluoxetine
12 mg olanzapine and 25 mg fluoxetine
12 mg olanzapine and 50 mg fluoxetine
INDICATIONS & DOSAGES
Boxed Warning Drug increases risk of suicidality. Not approved for use in children younger than age 10 because of suicide risk or in patients with dementia-related psychosis because of increased risk of death. ■
➤ **Bipolar I disorder or depression**
Adults: 1 capsule PO daily in the evening. Initially, 6 mg olanzapine/25 mg fluoxetine capsule, adjusted according to effectiveness and tolerability.

Children age 10 and older with bipolar depression:
Initially, 3 mg olanzapine/25 mg fluoxetine PO daily in the evening, adjusted according to effectiveness and tolerability.

perphenazine–amitriptyline hydrochloride
AVAILABLE FORMS
Tablets
2 mg perphenazine and 10 mg amitriptyline hydrochloride
2 mg perphenazine and 25 mg amitriptyline hydrochloride
4 mg perphenazine and 10 mg amitriptyline hydrochloride
4 mg perphenazine and 25 mg amitriptyline hydrochloride
4 mg perphenazine and 50 mg amitriptyline hydrochloride
INDICATIONS & DOSAGES
Boxed Warning Drug increases risk of suicidality. Not approved for use in children because of suicide risk or in patients with dementia-related psychosis because of increased risk of death. ■
➤ **Anxiety, agitation, or depression**
Adults: 2 to 4 mg perphenazine/10 to 25 mg amitriptyline PO t.i.d. to q.i.d. or 4 mg perphenazine/50 mg amitriptyline PO b.i.d. Reduce dosage after initial response. In severely ill patients with schizophrenia, give initial dose of 2 tablets (4 mg perphenazine/ 25 mg amitriptyline) PO t.i.d.; if needed, a fourth dose may be added at bedtime.

Respiratory tract drugs

budesonide–formoterol fumarate dihydrate
Symbicort
AVAILABLE FORMS
Aerosol inhalation
80 mcg budesonide and 4.5 mcg formoterol fumarate dihydrate per actuation
160 mcg budesonide and 4.5 mcg formoterol fumarate dihydrate per actuation
INDICATIONS & DOSAGES
➤ **Asthma, COPD**
Adults and children age 12 and older: Initially, 2 inhalations b.i.d. approximately 12 hours apart. For COPD, use only 160 mcg budesonide and 4.5 mcg formoterol fumarate dihydrate.
Children ages 6 to younger than 12: 2 inhalations of 80 mcg budesonide and 4.5 mcg formoterol fumarate dihydrate b.i.d.

chlorpheniramine polistirex–HYDROcodone polistirex
Controlled substance schedule: II
AVAILABLE FORMS
Oral solution (extended-release)
8 mg chlorpheniramine polistirex and 10 mg hydrocodone polistirex (equivalent to 10 mg hydrocodone bitartrate)/5 mL

INDICATIONS & DOSAGES

Boxed Warning *Opioid class warning:* Opioids combined with benzodiazepines or CNS depressants can cause death. Serious, life-threatening, or fatal respiratory depression may occur. Drug exposes users to risks of addiction, abuse, and misuse, which can lead to overdose and death. Dosing errors can result in accidental overdose and death. Avoid use in patients taking CYP3A4 inhibitors or inducers. Accidental ingestion, especially by children, can result in a fatal overdose. Prolonged use during pregnancy can result in neonatal opioid withdrawal syndrome. ■

➤ **Cough and upper respiratory signs and symptoms associated with allergy or cold**

Adults: 8 mg chlorpheniramine polistirex/10 mg hydrocodone polistirex PO every 12 hours. Maximum dose, 16 mg chlorpheniramine polistirex and 20 mg hydrocodone polistirex in 24 hours.

---

ipratropium bromide–albuterol sulfate

Combivent Respimat

AVAILABLE FORMS

Metered-dose inhaler

20 mcg ipratropium bromide and 100 mcg albuterol sulfate

Nebulizer solution

0.5 mg ipratropium bromide and 2.5 mg albuterol sulfate/3 mL

INDICATIONS & DOSAGES

➤ **COPD in patients who require more than a single bronchodilator**

Adults: 1 inhalation q.i.d. May give additional doses as needed up to maximum of 6 total inhalations in 24 hours. Or, 1 nebulization every 6 hours. May give up to 6 nebulizations (18 mL) in 24 hours.

---

loratadine–pseudoephedrine sulfate

Alavert Allergy/Sinus ◇, Claritin-D ◇, Claritin-D 24 Hour ◇

AVAILABLE FORMS

Tablets (extended-release) ⓓⓃⓒ

5 mg loratadine and 120 mg pseudoephedrine
10 mg loratadine and 240 mg pseudoephedrine

INDICATIONS & DOSAGES

➤ **Cold; allergy symptoms**

Adults and children age 12 and older: 5 mg loratadine/120 mg pseudoephedrine PO b.i.d., or 10 mg loratadine/240 mg pseudoephedrine PO daily. Maximum dosage, 10 mg loratadine/240 mg pseudoephedrine per day.

---

mometasone furoate–formoterol fumarate dihydrate

Dulera

AVAILABLE FORMS

Oral inhalation

50 mcg mometasone furoate and 5 mcg formoterol fumarate dihydrate
100 mcg mometasone furoate and 5 mcg formoterol fumarate dihydrate
200 mcg mometasone furoate and 5 mcg formoterol fumarate dihydrate

INDICATIONS & DOSAGES

➤ **Asthma**

Adults and children older than age 12: 2 inhalations b.i.d. Base starting dose on prior therapy with inhaled corticosteroids.

Children ages 5 to younger than 12: Using a 50-mcg mometasone furoate/5 mcg formoterol fumarate dihydrate inhaler, 2 inhalations b.i.d. (morning and evening). Maximum dosage, 200 mcg mometasone furoate/20 mcg formoterol fumarate dihydrate per day.

Adjust-a-dose: Titrate to the lowest effective dose after 2 to 3 months when asthma becomes well controlled.

Antidotes: Indications and dosages

Refer to manufacturer's instructions for complete prescribing and safety information.

activated charcoal

Actidose-Aqua, Actidose with Sorbitol, Char-Flo with Sorbitol, EZ Char, Insta-Char Aqueous, Insta-Char in Sorbitol

Therapeutic class: Antidotes
Pharmacologic class: Adsorbents

AVAILABLE FORMS

Liquid: 15 g* ◇, 25 g* ◇, 50 g* ◇
Oral suspension: 25 g ◇
Powder for reconstitution: 25 g ◇

INDICATIONS & DOSAGES

➤ Poisoning
Adjust-a-dose (all indications): Product and dosing should be used as directed by prescriber, including a poison control center. Dosing may vary depending on poison ingested, age, weight, and formulation used.
Adults and children age 12 and older weighing more than 32 kg: 50 to 100 g PO (aqueous base) or 50 g PO (sorbitol base). Or, 25 to 100 g powder PO mixed with water, then 12.5 g every hour or 25 g every other hour.
Children ages 1 to 12 weighing 16 to 32 kg: 25 g PO (sorbitol base). Or, 25 to 50 g or 0.5 to 1 g/kg powder PO mixed with water, then 1 to 2 g/kg every 2 to 4 hours.
Children younger than age 1 (aqueous only): 1 g/kg. May repeat every 4 to 6 hours if necessary.
Adults and children (EZ Char): For patients weighing 22 kg or more, give entire amount of reconstituted liquid (25 g); for those weighing 11 to less than 22 kg, give 60 to 120 mL (4 to 8 tablespoons) of reconstituted liquid; for those weighing 5.5 to less than 11 kg, give 30 to 60 mL (2 to 4 tablespoons) of reconstituted liquid; for those weighing 2.7 to less than 5.5 kg, give 15 to 30 mL (1 to 2 tablespoons) of reconstituted liquid. Repeat dose immediately, if necessary.

amifostine
am-i-FOS-steen

Ethyol

Therapeutic class: Cytoprotective drugs
Pharmacologic class: Organic thiophosphates

AVAILABLE FORMS

Injection: 500 mg in single-use vials

INDICATIONS & DOSAGES

Adjust-a-dose (all indications): Refer to manufacturer's instructions for interrupting therapy if hypotension occurs.

➤ **Reduction of cumulative renal toxicity associated with repeated administration of cisplatin in patients with advanced ovarian cancer**
Adults: 910 mg/m^2 once daily as a 15-minute IV infusion, starting 30 minutes before chemotherapy. Premedication with antiemetics, including dexamethasone 20 mg IV and a serotonin 5-HT$_3$ receptor antagonist, are recommended.
➤ **Moderate to severe xerostomia in patients undergoing postoperative radiation treatment for head and neck cancer, when the radiation port includes a substantial portion of the parotid glands**
Adults: 200 mg/m^2 once daily as a 3-minute IV infusion, starting 15 to 30 minutes before standard fraction radiation therapy. Premedication with oral 5-HT$_3$ receptor antagonists, alone or in combination with other antiemetics, is recommended.

deferasirox
de-FER-a-sir-ox

Exjade, Jadenu, Jadenu Sprinkle

Therapeutic class: Chelating agents
Pharmacologic class: Heavy metal antagonists

AVAILABLE FORMS

Sprinkles: 90 mg, 180 mg, 360 mg
Tablets: 90 mg, 180 mg, 360 mg
Tablets for oral suspension ⬛ : 125 mg, 250 mg, 500 mg

INDICATIONS & DOSAGES

Boxed Warning Drug can cause fatal renal failure, hepatic failure, and GI hemorrhage. Monitor patient carefully. Contraindicated in adults and children with eGFR less than 40 mL/minute/1.73 m^2; avoid use in patients with severe (Child-Pugh class C) hepatic impairment. Evaluate baseline renal function before starting drug or increasing dosage in all patients. Measure serum transaminase and bilirubin levels in all patients before initiating treatment, every 2 weeks during first month, and at least monthly thereafter. Monitor patients and discontinue deferasirox for suspected GI ulceration or hemorrhage. ∎
Adjust-a-dose (for all indications): When converting therapy from Exjade to Jadenu, the dose of Jadenu should be approximately 30% lower (rounded to the nearest whole tablet) than the current dose of Exjade.

Contraindicated in patients with platelet count less than 50,000/mm^3. Discontinue drug if eGFR is less than 40 mL/minute/1.73 m^2.

Start older adults at low end of dosing range.

Avoid use in patients with severe (Child-Pugh class C) hepatic impairment. Reduce starting dose by 50% in patients with moderate (Child-Pugh class B)

hepatic impairment. Closely monitor all patients with mild (Child-Pugh class A) or moderate hepatic impairment for effectiveness and adverse reactions. Reduce starting dose by 50% in patients with eGFR of 40 to 60 mL/minute/1.73 m². Use cautiously in children with eGFR between 40 and 60 mL/minute/1.73 m². If treatment is needed, use the minimum effective dose and monitor renal function frequently.

For unavoidable use with a bile acid sequestrant or UDP-glucuronosyltransferase (UGT) inducer, increase deferasirox dosage by 50% and monitor ferritin level.

➤ **Chronic iron overload caused by blood transfusions (transfusional hemosiderosis)**

Adults and children age 2 and older with eGFR greater than 60 mL/minute/1.73 m²: Exjade oral suspension: Initially, 20 mg/kg PO daily on an empty stomach 30 minutes before eating. Monitor serum ferritin level monthly, and adjust dose every 3 to 6 months by 5 or 10 mg/kg based on ferritin trends. Don't exceed 40 mg/kg daily. Interrupt therapy and continue monthly monitoring if serum ferritin level drops below 500 mcg/L.

Jadenu: Initially, 14 mg/kg PO once daily on an empty stomach or with a light meal. Monitor serum ferritin level monthly, and adjust dose every 3 to 6 months by increments of 3.5 or 7 mg/kg, based on serum ferritin trends. Don't exceed 28 mg/kg. If serum ferritin level falls below 1,000 mcg/L at two consecutive visits, consider dosage reduction, especially if dose is greater than 17.5 mg/kg/day. Interrupt therapy if serum ferritin level drops below 500 mcg/L and continue monthly monitoring.

Adjust-a-dose: Interrupt therapy for children with acute illnesses that can cause volume depletion and monitor more frequently. Resume therapy as appropriate.

For adults: If serum creatinine level increases by 33% or more above the average baseline measurement, repeat serum creatinine within 1 week and, if still elevated by 33% or more, reduce Exjade dose by 10 mg/kg or Jadenu dose by 7 mg/kg.

For children ages 2 to 17: Reduce Exjade dose by 10 mg/kg/day or Jadenu dose by 7 mg/kg if eGFR decreases by greater than 33% below the average baseline measurement and repeat eGFR within 1 week.

➤ **Chronic iron overload in patients with non-transfusion-dependent thalassemia syndromes and with a liver iron (Fe) concentration (LIC) of at least 5 mg Fe per gram of dry weight (dw) and a serum ferritin level greater than 300 mcg/L**

Adults and children age 10 and older with eGFR greater than 60 mL/minute/1.73 m²: Exjade oral suspension: Initially, 10 mg/kg PO once daily 30 minutes before food. If baseline LIC is greater than 15 mg Fe/g dw, may increase to 20 mg/kg/day after 4 weeks. Interrupt treatment when serum ferritin level is less than 300 mcg/L, and obtain LIC to determine if LIC is less than 3 mg Fe/g dw. If LIC remains greater than 7 mg Fe/g dw after 6 months of therapy, increase dosage to maximum of 20 mg/kg/day. If LIC is 3 to 7 mg Fe/g

dw after 6 months, continue treatment at maximum of 10 mg/kg/day. If LIC is less than 3 mg Fe/g dw, stop treatment. Continue to monitor LIC, and restart treatment when LIC rises again to more than 5 mg Fe/g dw.

Jadenu: Initially, 7 mg/kg PO once daily on an empty stomach or with a light meal. If baseline LIC is greater than 15 mg Fe/g dw, may increase to 14 mg/kg/day after 4 weeks. Interrupt treatment when serum ferritin level is less than 300 mcg/L, and obtain LIC to determine if LIC is less than 3 mg Fe/g dw. If LIC remains greater than 7 mg Fe/g dw after 6 months of therapy, increase dosage to maximum of 14 mg/kg/day. If LIC is 3 to 7 mg Fe/g dw after 6 months, continue treatment at maximum of 7 mg/kg/day. If LIC is less than 3 mg Fe/g dw, stop treatment. Continue to monitor LIC and restart treatment when LIC rises again to more than 5 mg Fe/g dw.

Adjust-a-dose: Increase monitoring frequency and consider dose interruption for children who have acute illness that can cause volume depletion.

For adults: If serum creatinine level increases by 33% or more above the average baseline measurement, repeat serum creatinine within 1 week and, if still elevated by 33% or more, interrupt Exjade therapy if dose is 5 mg/kg, or reduce by 50% if dose is 10 or 20 mg/kg; interrupt Jadenu therapy if dose is 3.5 mg/kg, or reduce by 50% if dose is 7 or 14 mg/kg.

For children ages 10 to 17: Reduce Exjade dose by 5 mg/kg/day or Jadenu dose by 3.5 mg/kg if eGFR decreases by greater than 33% below the average baseline measurement and repeat eGFR within 1 week.

deferiprone
de-FER-i-prone

Ferriprox

Therapeutic class: Chelating drugs
Pharmacologic class: Heavy metal antagonists

AVAILABLE FORMS
Solution: 100 mg/mL
Tablets: 500 mg, 1 g

INDICATIONS & DOSAGES
Boxed Warning Drug can cause agranulocytosis that can lead to serious infections and death. Measure ANC before therapy and weekly during therapy. Interrupt therapy for neutropenia or infection. Advise patients to immediately report signs or symptoms of infection. ■

Adjust-a-dose (for all indications): To minimize GI upset when initiating therapy, may start at 45 mg/kg/day and increase weekly by 15 mg/kg/day. If serum ferritin level falls consistently below 500 mcg/L, consider temporary therapy interruption. For ANC less than 1,500/mm³, interrupt therapy immediately and monitor until recovery; don't rechallenge unless potential benefit outweighs risk. For ANC less than

500/mm³, consider hospitalization and other clinically appropriate management; don't resume unless potential benefits outweigh risks.

➤ **Transfusional iron overload due to thalassemia syndromes, sickle cell disease, or other anemias**
Adults and children age 8 and older: Initially, 25 mg/kg tablets or oral solution PO t.i.d., or 25 mg/kg tablets PO b.i.d., for a total of 75 mg/kg/day. May titrate to maximum dosage of 99 mg/kg/day based on patient response and therapeutic goals. Round dose to nearest 500 mg (one-half 1-g tablet), 250 mg (one-half 500-mg tablet) or 2.5 mL of oral solution.
Children age 3 and older: Initially, 25 mg/kg oral solution PO t.i.d., for a total of 75 mg/kg/day. May titrate to maximum dosage of 99 mg/kg/day based on patient response and therapeutic goals. Round dose to nearest 2.5 mL of oral solution.

digoxin immune Fab (ovine)
di-JOX-in

DigiFab

Therapeutic class: Antidotes
Pharmacologic class: Antibody fragments

AVAILABLE FORMS
Injection: 40-mg vial

INDICATIONS & DOSAGES
➤ **Life-threatening digoxin toxicity**
Adults and children: Base dosage on ingested amount or level of digoxin. When calculating amount of antidote, round up to the nearest whole number. Each vial of digoxin immune Fab binds to about 0.5 mg of digoxin. For digoxin tablets, calculate number of antidote vials as follows: multiply ingested amount by 0.8; then divide answer by 0.5. For example, if patient takes 25 tablets of 0.25 mg digoxin, the ingested amount is 6.25 mg. Multiply 6.25 mg by 0.8 and divide answer by 0.5 to obtain 10 vials of antidote. If digoxin level is known, determine the number of antidote vials as follows: multiply the digoxin level in nanograms per milliliter by patient's weight in kilograms; then divide by 100.
➤ **Acute toxicity or if estimated ingested amount or digoxin level is unknown**
Adults and children: Consider giving 10 vials of digoxin immune Fab and observing patient's response. Follow with another 10 vials if indicated. Dosage should be effective in most life-threatening cases in adults and children but may cause volume overload in young children.
➤ **Toxicity during prolonged therapy if digoxin level is unknown**
Adults and children: 6 vials of antidote in patients weighing 20 kg or more, or 1 vial of antidote in patients weighing less than 20 kg.

dimercaprol
dye-mer-KAP-role

BAL in Oil

Therapeutic class: Chelating drugs
Pharmacologic class: Heavy metal antagonists

AVAILABLE FORMS
Injection: 100 mg/mL

INDICATIONS & DOSAGES
➤ **Severe arsenic or gold poisoning**
Adults and children: 3 mg/kg deep IM every 4 hours for 2 days; then q.i.d. on third day; then b.i.d. for 10 days.
➤ **Mild arsenic or gold poisoning**
Adults and children: 2.5 mg/kg deep IM q.i.d. for 2 days; then b.i.d. on third day; then once daily for 10 days.
➤ **Mercury poisoning**
Adults and children: Initially, 5 mg/kg deep IM; then 2.5 mg/kg daily or b.i.d. for 10 days.
➤ **Acute lead encephalopathy**
Adults and children: 4 mg/kg given alone by deep IM; then every 4 hours with edetate calcium disodium administered at a separate site for 2 to 7 days. For less severe poisoning, reduce dose to 3 mg/kg after first dose.

doxapram hydrochloride
DOKS-a-pram

Dopram

Therapeutic class: CNS stimulants
Pharmacologic class: Analeptics

AVAILABLE FORMS
Injection: 20 mg/mL*

INDICATIONS & DOSAGES
➤ **Postanesthesia respiratory stimulation**
Adults: 0.5 to 1 mg/kg as a single IV injection (not to exceed 1.5 mg/kg) or as multiple injections every 5 minutes, total not to exceed 2 mg/kg or 3 g daily. Or, 250 mg in 250 mL of NSS, D_5W, or $D_{10}W$ infused at initial rate of 5 mg/minute IV until satisfactory response is achieved. Maintain at 1 to 3 mg/minute. Don't exceed total dose for infusion of 4 mg/kg or 3 g daily.
➤ **Drug-induced CNS depression**
Adults: For injection, priming dose of 1 to 2 mg/kg IV, repeated in 5 minutes and again every 1 to 2 hours until patient awakens (and if relapse occurs). Maximum daily dose is 3 g.

For intermittent infusion, priming dose of 1 to 2 mg/kg IV, repeated in 5 minutes and again in 1 to 2 hours, if needed. If response occurs, give IV infusion (1 mg/mL) at 1 to 3 mg/minute until patient awakens.

Don't infuse for longer than 2 hours or give more than 3 g/day. May resume IV infusion after rest period of 30 minutes to 2 hours, if needed.

➤ **COPD related to acute hypercapnia**

Adults: 1 to 2 mg/minute by IV infusion using 2 mg/mL solution. Maximum, 3 mg/minute. Don't infuse for longer than 2 hours. Discontinue infusion if blood gas levels deteriorate.

edetate calcium disodium
ED-e-tate

Calcium Disodium Versenate

Therapeutic class: Chelating drugs
Pharmacologic class: Heavy metal antagonists

AVAILABLE FORMS
Injection: 200 mg/mL

INDICATIONS & DOSAGES
Boxed Warning Toxic effects of drug can be fatal. Use with extreme caution in patients with lead encephalopathy and cerebral edema. Never exceed the recommended daily dosage and avoid rapid IV infusion. ∎

➤ **Acute lead encephalopathy or lead level greater than 70 mcg/dL**

Adults and children: Use in conjunction with dimercaprol. Consult published protocols and specialized references for dosage recommendations.

➤ **Lead poisoning without encephalopathy or asymptomatic with lead level less than 70 mcg/dL but greater than 20 mcg/dL**

Adults and children: 1 g/m^2/day IV infused over 8 to 12 hours once daily or 1 g/m^2 IM daily in divided doses spaced 8 to 12 hours apart for 5 days. Or, for adults with lead nephropathy, give as follows: If serum creatinine level is 2 to 3 mg/dL, give 500 mg/m^2 every 24 hours for 5 days; if serum creatinine level is 3 to 4 mg/dL, give 500 mg/m^2 every 48 hours for three doses; if serum creatinine level is more than 4 mg/dL, give 500 mg/m^2 once weekly. These regimens may be repeated at 1-month intervals.

glucarpidase
gloo-KAR-pid-ase

Voraxaze

Therapeutic class: Antidotes
Pharmacologic class: Recombinant bacterial enzymes

AVAILABLE FORMS
Powder for injection: 1,000 units/vial

INDICATIONS & DOSAGES
➤ **Methotrexate toxicity (more than 1 micromole/L) in patients with impaired renal function**

Adults and children age 1 month and older: 50 units/kg as a single IV injection over 5 minutes.

lanthanum carbonate
LAN-thah-num

Fosrenol

Therapeutic class: Antihyperphosphatemics
Pharmacologic class: Non-calcium, non-aluminum phosphate binders

AVAILABLE FORMS
Oral powder: 750 mg, 1 g
Tablets (chewable): 500 mg, 750 mg, 1 g

INDICATIONS & DOSAGES
➤ **Reduction of serum phosphate level in patients with ESRD**

Adults: Initially, 500 mg PO t.i.d. with meals. Adjust every 2 to 3 weeks by 750 mg daily until reaching desired phosphate level. Reducing phosphate level to less than 6 mg/dL usually requires 1,500 to 3,000 mg daily. Maximum daily dose is 4,500 mg.

◑ *Alert:* Drug has the potential to bind other orally administered drugs. Consider separating the administration of other oral medications by at least 2 hours.

mesna
MES-na

Mesnex

Therapeutic class: Cytoprotective drugs
Pharmacologic class: Antidotes

AVAILABLE FORMS
Injection: 100 mg/mL*
Tablets: 400 mg

INDICATIONS & DOSAGES
➤ **Prophylaxis of ifosfamide-induced hemorrhagic cystitis**

Adults (IV only regimen): Total daily mesna dose is 60% of ifosfamide dose. Give 20% of ifosfamide dose weight by weight (w/w) IV bolus injection at the time of ifosfamide administration, then at 4 and 8 hours after ifosfamide dose. For example, if ifosfamide dose is 1.2 g/m^2, the mesna dose is 240 mg/m^2 given at the same time as ifosfamide and then 4 hours and 8 hours after ifosfamide. Dosing schedule is repeated each day ifosfamide is given.

Adults (IV and PO dosing regimen): Total daily mesna dose is 100% of ifosfamide dose. Give 20% of ifosfamide dose (w/w) IV bolus injection at the same time ifosfamide is given. Then give 40% of ifosfamide dose (w/w) as PO tablets at 2 hours and 6 hours after ifosfamide dose. Dosing schedule is repeated each day ifosfamide is given. This ratio of IV and oral dosing hasn't been established as effective for daily ifosfamide doses higher than 2 g/m^2.

Adjust-a-dose: If ifosfamide dosage is increased or decreased, the mesna dosage should also be modified to maintain the mesna-to-ifosfamide ratio.

➤ **Prevention of cyclophosphamide-induced hemorrhagic cystitis (with high-dose cyclophosphamide)**

Adults younger than age 40: 2,100 mg/m^2/day continuous IV infusion (mesna dose is equivalent to the cyclophosphamide dose) for 2 days with cyclophosphamide infusion during cycles 1, 2, 3, and 6.

naloxegol oxalate
nal-OX-ee-gol

Movantik

Therapeutic class: Antidotes
Pharmacologic class: Opioid antagonists

AVAILABLE FORMS
Tablets: 12.5 mg, 25 mg

INDICATIONS & DOSAGES
➤ **Opioid-induced constipation in patients with chronic noncancer pain, including patients with chronic pain related to prior cancer or its treatment who don't require frequent opioid dosage escalation**

Adults: 25 mg PO once daily in the morning at least 1 hour before or 2 hours after the first meal of the day. If 25 mg isn't tolerated, reduce to 12.5 mg once daily.
Adjust-a-dose: For CrCl less than 60 mL/minute, decrease starting dose to 12.5; if tolerated, may increase to 25 mg if needed. If use with a moderate CYP3A4 inhibitor is necessary, decrease dosage to 12.5 mg daily.

phentolamine mesylate
fen-TOLE-a-meen

OraVerse

Therapeutic class: Antidotes
Pharmacologic class: Alpha blockers

AVAILABLE FORMS
Injection: 0.4 mg/1.7 mL, 5 mg/mL

INDICATIONS & DOSAGES
➤ **Prevention of dermal necrosis from norepinephrine extravasation (excluding OraVerse)**
Adults: Add 10 mg of phentolamine to each liter of solution containing norepinephrine; the pressor effect of norepinephrine is unaffected.
➤ **Dermal necrosis and sloughing after IV extravasation of norepinephrine or dopamine (excluding OraVerse)**
Adults: Infiltrate area with 5 to 10 mg phentolamine in 10 mL of NSS within 12 hours of extravasation.
➤ **Reversal of soft-tissue anesthesia (OraVerse only)**

Adults and children age 6 and older weighing more than 30 kg: Dosage depends on amount of anesthetic used. Refer to manufacturer's instructions.
➤ **Diagnosis of pheochromocytoma, to control or prevent HTN before or during pheochromocytomectomy (excluding OraVerse)**
Adults: IV or IM diagnostic dose is 5 mg with close monitoring of BP. Give 5 mg IV or IM 1 to 2 hours before surgical removal of tumor. During surgery, patient may need an additional 5 mg IV.
Children: IV diagnostic dose is 1 mg, and IM diagnostic dose is 3 mg with close monitoring of BP. Give 1 mg IV or IM 1 to 2 hours before surgical removal of tumor. During surgery, patient may need an additional 1 mg IV.

pralidoxime chloride (2-PAM chloride, 2-pyridine-aldoxime methochloride)
pra-li-DOKS-eem

Protopam Chloride

Therapeutic class: Antidotes
Pharmacologic class: Quaternary ammonium oximes

AVAILABLE FORMS
Injection: 1 g/20 mL in 20-mL vial
Injection (for IM use): 300 mg/mL

INDICATIONS & DOSAGES
➤ **Antidote for organophosphate poisoning in combination with atropine**
Adults: 1 to 2 g in 100 mL of NSS by IV infusion over 15 to 30 minutes. If not practical or if pulmonary edema is present, give dose of 1 g in 20 mL of sterile water by slow IV push over at least 5 minutes. Repeat in 1 hour if muscle weakness persists. May give additional doses cautiously. May use IM or subcut injection if IV isn't feasible.

For IM dosing: *For mild symptoms,* give 600 mg (2 mL) IM. Wait 15 minutes; if symptoms persist, give a second dose. May give a third dose after an additional 15 minutes. If at any time after the first dose patient develops severe symptoms, give two additional 600-mg doses in rapid succession for a total cumulative dose of 1,800 mg. *For severe symptoms,* give three 600-mg doses (three doses of 2 mL each) in rapid succession. If symptoms persist after the complete 1,800-mg regimen (three injections of 600 mg each), may repeat the series beginning approximately 1 hour after the last injection.
Children age 16 and younger (IV dosing): Give loading dose of 20 to 50 mg/kg (maximum 2 g) IV over 15 to 30 minutes, followed by 10 to 20 mg/kg/hour by continuous IV infusion. Or, give initial dose of 20 to 50 mg/kg IV over 15 to 30 minutes, then give second dose of 20 to 50 mg/kg IV in 1 hour if muscle weakness persists. May repeat dose every 10 to 12 hours PRN. Maximum is 2 g/dose. Or, if pulmonary edema

is present or it isn't practical to give intermittent or continuous IV infusions, give dose of 20 to 50 mg/kg as 50-mg/mL solution in water by IV push slowly over 5 minutes. If muscle weakness persists, may give additional doses every 10 to 12 hours.

Children age 16 and younger with mild symptoms who weigh 40 kg or more (IM dosing): Give 600 mg IM. If symptoms persist after 15 minutes, give second dose of 600 mg IM. If symptoms persist 15 minutes after second dose, give third dose of 600 mg IM. Maximum combined dose for three injections is 1,800 mg. If patient develops severe symptoms at any time after first dose, administer second and third doses in rapid succession. For severe symptoms, give all three doses of 600 mg IM each in rapid succession for total combined dose of 1,800 mg.

Children age 16 and younger with mild symptoms who weigh less than 40 kg (IM dosing): Give 15 mg/kg IM in anterolateral thigh. If symptoms persist after 15 minutes, give second dose of 15 mg/kg IM. If symptoms persist after second dose, give third dose of 15 mg/kg IM. If patient develops severe symptoms at any time after first dose, give second and third doses in rapid succession. For severe symptoms, give all three doses of 15 mg/kg IM each in rapid succession. Maximum combined dose for three injections is 45 mg/kg.

➤ **Control of overdosage by anticholinesterase drugs used in the treatment of myasthenia gravis**
Adults: 1 to 2 g IV; then 250 mg IV every 5 minutes PRN.

---

protamine sulfate
PROE-ta-meen

Therapeutic class: Antidotes
Pharmacologic class: Heparin antagonists

AVAILABLE FORMS
Injection: 10 mg/mL

INDICATIONS & DOSAGES
Boxed Warning Drug can cause severe hypotension, CV collapse, noncardiogenic pulmonary edema, catastrophic pulmonary vasoconstriction, and pulmonary HTN. Keep vasopressors and resuscitation equipment immediately available. Don't give when bleeding occurs without prior heparin use. ■

➤ **Heparin overdose**
Adults: Dosage should be guided by blood coagulation studies. 1 mg of protamine sulfate neutralizes not less than 100 USP heparin units. Give by slow IV injection over 10 minutes in doses not to exceed 50 mg.

---

rasburicase ▨
ras-BUR-ih-kase

Elitek

Therapeutic class: Replacement enzymes
Pharmacologic class: Recombinant urate-oxidases

AVAILABLE FORMS
Injection: 1.5 mg, 7.5 mg in single-dose vials with diluent

INDICATIONS & DOSAGES
Boxed Warning Drug can cause serious and fatal hypersensitivity reactions. Don't give to patients with G6PD deficiency due to risk of hemolysis; screen those at higher risk before starting therapy. Drug can cause methemoglobinemia. Immediately and permanently discontinue drug if a serious hypersensitivity reaction, hemolysis, or methemoglobinemia occurs. Drug degrades uric acid in blood samples left at room temperature. Collect sample in prechilled tubes containing heparin, and immediately immerse and maintain sample in an ice water bath. Assay sample within 4 hours of collection. ■

➤ **Initial management of plasma uric acid levels in patients with leukemia, lymphoma, and solid tumor malignancies who are receiving chemotherapy that's expected to result in tumor lysis and subsequent elevation of plasma uric acid level**
Adults and children: 0.2 mg/kg IV infusion over 30 minutes daily for up to 5 days. Drug is only indicated for a single course of treatment.

---

sodium polystyrene sulfonate
pol-ee-STYE-reen

Kayexalate ♣, SPS

Therapeutic class: Potassium-removing resins
Pharmacologic class: Cation-exchange resins

AVAILABLE FORMS
Powder: 3.5 g/tsp in 1-lb jar
Suspension: 15 g/60 mL*

INDICATIONS & DOSAGES
➤ **Hyperkalemia**
Adults: 15 g PO daily to q.i.d. in water or syrup (3 to 4 mL/g of resin). Or, mix powder with appropriate medium (aqueous suspension or diet appropriate for renal failure) and instill through NG tube. Or, 30 to 50 g as a suspension or in 100 mL of an aqueous vehicle every 6 hours as warm emulsion (at body temperature) deep into sigmoid colon (20 cm). Following retention period, irrigate colon to remove resin.
Children: 1 g/kg/dose PO or by NG tube every 6 hours.

Infants and small children: 1 mEq potassium/g of resin PO or by NG tube daily to q.i.d. May be given rectally in 10% dextrose in water if unable to give orally. Following retention period, irrigate colon to remove resin.

Neonates: 0.5 to 1 g/kg as rectal suspension. Use minimum effective dosage. Following retention, irrigate colon to remove resin.

---

succimer
SUX-i-mer

Chemet

Therapeutic class: Chelating drugs
Pharmacologic class: Heavy metal chelators

AVAILABLE FORMS
Capsules: 100 mg

INDICATIONS & DOSAGES
➤ **Lead poisoning in children with lead levels greater than 45 mcg/dL**
Children age 12 months and older: Initially, 10 mg/kg or 350 mg/m^2 PO every 8 hours for 5 days. Then reduce to 10 mg/kg or 350 mg/m^2 PO every 12 hours for additional 14 days. Maximum, 500 mg/dose.

---

sugammadex sodium
su-GAM-ma-dex

Bridion

Therapeutic class: Antidotes
Pharmacologic class: Modified gamma cyclodextrins

AVAILABLE FORMS
Injection: 200 mg/2 mL, 500 mg/5 mL in single-dose vials

INDICATIONS & DOSAGES
➤ **Reversal of neuromuscular blockade induced by rocuronium bromide and vecuronium bromide in patients undergoing surgery**
Adults and children age 2 and older (routine reversal of rocuronium- and vecuronium-induced neuromuscular blockade): Base doses and timing of drug administration on monitoring for twitch responses and extent of spontaneous recovery that has occurred. Give 4 mg/kg IV bolus over 10 seconds if recovery of the twitch response has reached one to two posttetanic counts (PTC) and there are no twitch responses to train-of-four (TOF) stimulation. Give 2 mg/kg IV over 10 seconds if spontaneous recovery has reached the reappearance of the second twitch (T$_2$) in response to TOF stimulation.
Adults (immediate reversal of rocuronium-induced neuromuscular blockade): If there is a clinical need to reverse neuromuscular blockade (approximately 3 minutes) after administration of a single 1.2-mg/kg

dose of rocuronium, give sugammadex 16 mg/kg IV over 10 seconds. Immediate reversal of rocuronium-only induced neuromuscular blockade hasn't been studied in children.

Selected ophthalmic drugs: Indications and dosages

Refer to manufacturer's instructions for complete prescribing and safety information.

aflibercept
a-FLIB-er-sept

Eylea

Therapeutic class: Vascular endothelial growth factor inhibitors
Pharmacologic class: Antiangiogenetic drugs

AVAILABLE FORMS
Intravitreal injection: 2 mg in 0.05-mL single-use vial and prefilled syringe

INDICATIONS & DOSAGES
➤ **Neovascular (wet) age-related macular degeneration**
Adults: 2 mg (0.05 mL) intravitreal injection every 4 weeks for first 12 weeks; then 2 mg (0.05 mL) once every 8 weeks. Some patients may need every-4-week dosing after first 12 weeks.
➤ **Macular edema following retinal vein occlusion**
Adults: 2 mg (0.05 mL) intravitreal injection once every 4 weeks.
➤ **Diabetic macular edema and diabetic retinopathy**
Adults: 2 mg (0.05 mL) intravitreal injection every 4 weeks for first 5 injections; then 2 mg (0.05 mL) every 8 weeks. Some patients may need every-4-week dosing after first five injections.

alcaftadine
al-CAFF-tuh-deen

Lastacaft ◇

Therapeutic class: Antihistamines
Pharmacologic class: Histamine$_1$-receptor antagonists

AVAILABLE FORMS
Ophthalmic solution: 0.25% (2.5 mg/mL) ◇

INDICATIONS & DOSAGES
➤ **Itching associated with allergic conjunctivitis**
Adults and children age 2 and older: Instill 1 drop in each eye once daily.

bepotastine besilate
beh-POT-uh-steen

Bepreve

Therapeutic class: Antihistamines (ophthalmic)
Pharmacologic class: Histamine$_1$-receptor antagonists

AVAILABLE FORMS
Ophthalmic solution: 1.5%

INDICATIONS & DOSAGES
➤ **Itching associated with allergic conjunctivitis**
Adults and children age 2 and older: Instill 1 drop into affected eye(s) b.i.d.

besifloxacin hydrochloride
beh-sih-FLOX-ah-sin

Besivance

Therapeutic class: Antibiotics
Pharmacologic class: Fluoroquinolones

AVAILABLE FORMS
Ophthalmic suspension: 0.6%

INDICATIONS & DOSAGES
➤ **Conjunctivitis caused by CDC coryneform group G, *Aerococcus viridans, Corynebacterium pseudodiphtheriticum, C. striatum, Haemophilus influenzae, Moraxella catarrhalis, M. lacunata, Pseudomonas aeruginosa, Staphylococcus aureus, S. epidermidis, S. hominis, S. lugdunensis, S. warneri, Streptococcus mitis* group, *S. oralis, S. pneumoniae,* or *S. salivarius***
Adults and children age 1 and older: Instill 1 drop into affected eye t.i.d., 4 to 12 hours apart, for 7 days.

bimatoprost
by-MAT-oh-prost

Durysta, Latisse, Lumigan, Vistitan ✦

Therapeutic class: Antiglaucoma drugs
Pharmacologic class: Prostaglandin analogues

AVAILABLE FORMS
Intraocular implant: 10 mcg
Ophthalmic solution: 0.01%, 0.03%
Topical ophthalmic solution: 0.03%

INDICATIONS & DOSAGES

➤ **Increased IOP in patients with open-angle glaucoma or ocular HTN**

Adults and adolescents age 16 and older: Instill 1 drop ophthalmic solution in conjunctival sac of affected eye(s) once daily in the evening.

Adults: Insert 1 implant in anterior chamber of affected eye. Don't exceed 1 implant per eye.

➤ **Hypotrichosis of the eyelashes (Latisse)**

Adults and children age 5 and older: Apply 1 drop topical ophthalmic solution nightly directly to skin of upper eyelid margin at base of eyelashes with single-use applicator, using a second applicator for a second eye (if needed).

---

brinzolamide–brimonidine tartrate

brin-ZOL-ah-mide/brih-MOE-neh-deen

Simbrinza

Therapeutic class: Antiglaucoma drugs
Pharmacologic class: Carbonic anhydrase inhibitors–alpha$_2$ adrenergic receptor agonists

AVAILABLE FORMS

Ophthalmic suspension: brinzolamide 1% and brimonidine 0.2%

INDICATIONS & DOSAGES

➤ **Reduction of IOP in patients with open-angle glaucoma or ocular HTN**

Adults and children age 2 and older: Instill 1 drop into affected eye(s) t.i.d.

Adjust-a-dose: Use not recommended if eGFR falls below 30 mL/minute/1.73 m^2.

---

brolucizumab-dbll

broe-lue-SIZ-ue-mab

Beovu

Therapeutic class: Immunomodulators
Pharmacologic class: Vascular endothelial growth factor inhibitors

AVAILABLE FORMS

Solution for intravitreal injection: 6 mg/0.05 mL in single-use vial or prefilled syringe

INDICATIONS & DOSAGES

➤ **Neovascular (wet) age-related macular degeneration**

Adults: 6 mg intravitreal injection monthly (every 25 to 31 days) for three doses; then every 8 to 12 weeks thereafter.

✳ *NEW INDICATION:* **Diabetic macular edema**

Adults: 6 mg intravitreal injection every 6 weeks (every 39 to 45 days) for five doses; then every 8 to 12 weeks thereafter.

---

bromfenac sodium

BROM-fen-ak

BromSite, Prolensa

Therapeutic class: Anti-inflammatory drugs (ophthalmic)
Pharmacologic class: NSAIDs

AVAILABLE FORMS

Ophthalmic solution: 0.07%, 0.075%, 0.09%

INDICATIONS & DOSAGES

➤ **Inflammation and pain after cataract surgery**

Adults: For 0.07% solution and 0.09% solution, instill 1 drop in affected eye(s) once daily beginning 1 day before surgery, continued on the day of surgery and for the first 14 days after surgery. For 0.075% solution, instill 1 drop in affected eye(s) b.i.d. (morning and evening) beginning 1 day before surgery, continued on the day of surgery and for the first 14 days after surgery.

---

carteolol hydrochloride

KAR-tee-oh-lol

Therapeutic class: Antiglaucoma drugs
Pharmacologic class: Nonselective beta blockers

AVAILABLE FORMS

Ophthalmic solution: 1%

INDICATIONS & DOSAGES

➤ **Chronic open-angle glaucoma, intraocular HTN**

Adults: Instill 1 drop in each affected eye b.i.d.

---

cenegermin-bkbj

sen-EH-jer-min bkbj

Oxervate

Therapeutic class: Growth factors
Pharmacologic class: Human nerve growth factors

AVAILABLE FORMS

Ophthalmic solution: 0.002% (20 mcg/mL) multidose vial

INDICATIONS & DOSAGES

➤ **Neurotrophic keratitis**

Adults and children age 2 and older: Instill 1 drop into affected eye(s) every 2 hours six times a day for 8 weeks.

---

ciprofloxacin hydrochloride (ophthalmic)

si-proe-FLOX-a-sin

Ciloxan

Therapeutic class: Antibiotics
Pharmacologic class: Fluoroquinolones

AVAILABLE FORMS
Ophthalmic ointment: 0.3%
Ophthalmic solution: 0.3%

INDICATIONS & DOSAGES
➤ **Corneal ulcers caused by *Pseudomonas aeruginosa*, *Staphylococcus aureus*, *S. epidermidis*, *Streptococcus pneumoniae*, or possibly *Serratia marcescens* or *Streptococcus* viridans group**
Adults and children older than age 1: Instill 2 drops in affected eye every 15 minutes for first 6 hours; then 2 drops every 30 minutes for remainder of first day. On the second day, instill 2 drops hourly. On days 3 to 14, instill 2 drops every 4 hours. Treatment may be continued after day 14 if reepithelialization hasn't occurred.
➤ **Bacterial conjunctivitis caused by *Haemophilus influenzae*, *Staphylococcus aureus*, *S. epidermidis*, *Streptococcus pneumoniae* or *S. viridans* group**
Adults and children older than age 1: Instill 1 or 2 drops into conjunctival sac of affected eye every 2 hours while awake for first 2 days. Then, 1 or 2 drops every 4 hours while awake for next 5 days.
Adults and children older than age 2: Instill ½-inch (1.27-cm) ribbon of ointment into conjunctival sac t.i.d. for the first 2 days, then ½-inch ribbon b.i.d. for next 5 days.

cycloSPORINE (ophthalmic emulsion)

cy-cloh-SPORE-inn

Cequa, Restasis, Verkazia

Therapeutic class: Immunomodulators
Pharmacologic class: Calcineurin inhibitors

AVAILABLE FORMS
Ophthalmic emulsion: 0.05%, 0.1%
Ophthalmic solution: 0.09%

INDICATIONS & DOSAGES
➤ **To increase tear production in patients whose tear production is presumed to be suppressed due to ocular inflammation associated with keratoconjunctivitis sicca**
Adults: Instill 1 drop of 0.05% emulsion or 0.09% solution in each eye b.i.d. approximately 12 hours apart.

➤ **Vernal keratoconjunctivitis**
Adults and children age 4 and older: Instill 1 drop of 0.1% emulsion in each affected eye q.i.d. (morning, noon, afternoon, and evening).

dexamethasone (ophthalmic)

dex-a-METH-a-sone

Dextenza, Dexycu, Maxidex, Ozurdex

dexamethasone sodium phosphate

Therapeutic class: Anti-inflammatory drugs (ophthalmic)
Pharmacologic class: Corticosteroids

AVAILABLE FORMS
dexamethasone (ophthalmic)
Insert (ophthalmic): 0.4 mg
Intraocular implant: 0.7 mg
Intraocular suspension: 9%
Ophthalmic suspension: 0.1%
dexamethasone sodium phosphate
Ophthalmic solution: 0.1%

INDICATIONS & DOSAGES
➤ **Uveitis; iridocyclitis; inflammatory conditions of eyelids, conjunctiva, cornea, and anterior segment of globe; corneal injury from chemical or thermal burns or penetration of foreign bodies; allergic conjunctivitis; suppression of graft rejection after keratoplasty; acne rosacea**
Adults and children: Initially, instill 1 or 2 drops of solution into conjunctival sac every hour during the day and every 2 hours during the night. Decrease to 1 drop every 4 hours when favorable response is noted. As condition improves, taper to 1 drop t.i.d. or q.i.d. to control symptoms. Treatment may extend from a few days to several weeks. Or, instill 1 or 2 drops of suspension in the conjunctival sac up to six times daily. In severe disease, drops may be used hourly, being tapered to discontinuation as inflammation subsides.
➤ **Macular edema; posterior-segment uveitis; diabetic macular edema**
Adults: Inject 1 implant (0.7 mg) intravitreally into each affected eye.
➤ **Ocular postoperative inflammation**
Adults: Inject 0.005 mL (517 mcg) of 9% suspension into posterior chamber at the end of ocular surgery or place single 0.4-mg insert into the lower lacrimal canaliculus.
✷ *NEW INDICATION:* **Ocular itching associated with allergic conjunctivitis**
Adults: Place single 0.4-mg insert into the lower lacrimal canaliculus.

difluprednate
die-FLU-pred-nate

Durezol

Therapeutic class: Anti-inflammatory drugs (ophthalmic)
Pharmacologic class: Corticosteroids

AVAILABLE FORMS
Ophthalmic emulsion: 0.05%

INDICATIONS & DOSAGES
➤ **Inflammation and pain associated with ocular surgery**
Adults and children: Instill 1 drop into the conjunctival sac of the affected eye q.i.d. beginning 24 hours after surgery for 2 weeks, then decrease to b.i.d. for 1 week, and then taper according to response.
➤ **Endogenous anterior uveitis**
Adults: Instill 1 drop into the conjunctival sac of the affected eye q.i.d. for 14 days, then taper as clinically indicated.

dorzolamide hydrochloride
dor-ZOLE-ah-mide

Trusopt

Therapeutic class: Antiglaucoma drugs
Pharmacologic class: Carbonic anhydrase inhibitors–sulfonamides

AVAILABLE FORMS
Ophthalmic solution: 2%

INDICATIONS & DOSAGES
➤ **Increased IOP in patients with ocular HTN or open-angle glaucoma**
Adults and children: Instill 1 drop into conjunctival sac of affected eye(s) t.i.d.

epinastine hydrochloride
ep-ih-NAS-teen

Therapeutic class: Antihistamines
Pharmacologic class: H$_1$-receptor antagonists–mast cell stabilizers

AVAILABLE FORMS
Ophthalmic solution: 0.05%

INDICATIONS & DOSAGES
➤ **To prevent pruritus from allergic conjunctivitis**
Adults and children age 2 and older: Instill 1 drop into each eye b.i.d. Continue treatment as long as allergen is present, even if symptoms resolve.

fluorometholone
flur-oh-METH-oh-lone

FML, FML Forte

fluorometholone acetate
Flarex

Therapeutic class: Anti-inflammatory drugs (ophthalmic)
Pharmacologic class: Corticosteroids

AVAILABLE FORMS
fluorometholone
Ophthalmic ointment: 0.1%
Ophthalmic suspension: 0.1%, 0.25%
fluorometholone acetate
Ophthalmic suspension: 0.1%

INDICATIONS & DOSAGES
➤ **Inflammatory and allergic conditions of cornea, conjunctiva, sclera, or anterior uvea**
Adults and children older than age 2 (acetate form not for use in children of any age): Instill 1 drop b.i.d. to q.i.d. or ½-inch ribbon of ointment once daily to t.i.d. For first 24 to 48 hours, may increase dosing frequency to every 4 hours. For fluorometholone acetate, instill 1 to 2 drops q.i.d.; may give 2 drops every 2 hours during initial 24 to 48 hours of treatment.

gatifloxacin
ga-ti-FLOKS-a-sin

Zymar✦, Zymaxid

Therapeutic class: Antibiotics
Pharmacologic class: Fluoroquinolones

AVAILABLE FORMS
Solution: 0.3%✦, 0.5%

INDICATIONS & DOSAGES
➤ **Bacterial conjunctivitis caused by *Staphylococcus aureus*, *S. epidermidis*, *Streptococcus pneumoniae*, or *Haemophilus influenzae***
Adults and children age 1 and older: Instill 1 drop of Zymar into affected eye every 2 hours while patient is awake, up to eight times daily for 2 days. Then instill 1 drop up to q.i.d. while patient is awake on days 3 to 7.
➤ **Bacterial conjunctivitis caused by *Streptococcus mitis* group, *S. aureus*, *S. epidermidis*, *S. oralis*, *S. pneumoniae*, or *Haemophilus influenzae***
Adults and children age 1 and older: Instill 1 drop Zymaxid into affected eye every 2 hours while patient is awake, up to eight times on day 1. Then instill 1 drop b.i.d. to q.i.d. while patient is awake on days 2 to 7.

gentamicin sulfate (ophthalmic)
jen-ta-MYE-sin

Gentak

Therapeutic class: Antibiotics
Pharmacologic class: Aminoglycosides

AVAILABLE FORMS
Ophthalmic ointment: 0.3%
Ophthalmic solution: 0.3%

INDICATIONS & DOSAGES
➤ **External ocular infections (conjunctivitis, keratoconjunctivitis, corneal ulcers, blepharitis, blepharoconjunctivitis, acute meibomianitis, and dacryocystitis) caused by susceptible organisms (*Staphylococcus aureus*, *S. epidermidis*, *Streptococcus pyogenes*, *S. pneumoniae*, *Klebsiella aerogenes*, *K. pneumoniae*, *Escherichia coli*, *Haemophilus influenzae*, *Neisseria gonorrhoeae*, *Pseudomonas aeruginosa*, *Serratia marcescens*)**
Adults and children age 1 month and older: Instill 1 to 2 drops in affected eye every 4 hours. In severe infections, up to 2 drops every hour. Or, apply ointment (approximately ½-inch [1.25 cm] ribbon) to lower conjunctival sac b.i.d. or t.i.d.

ketorolac tromethamine (ophthalmic)
KEE-toe-role-ak

Acular, Acular LS, Acuvail

Therapeutic class: Anti-inflammatory drugs (ophthalmic)
Pharmacologic class: NSAIDs

AVAILABLE FORMS
Ophthalmic solution: 0.4%, 0.45%, 0.5%

INDICATIONS & DOSAGES
➤ **Relief from ocular itching caused by seasonal allergic conjunctivitis (Acular)**
Adults and children age 2 and older: Instill 1 drop of 0.5% solution into conjunctival sac in each eye q.i.d.
➤ **Relief of postoperative inflammation after cataract extraction (Acular)**
Adults and children age 2 and older: Instill 1 drop of 0.5% solution to affected eye q.i.d. beginning 24 hours after cataract surgery and continuing through first 2 weeks of postoperative period.
➤ **To reduce ocular pain, burning, and stinging after corneal refractive surgery (Acular LS)**
Adults and children age 3 and older: Instill 1 drop 0.4% solution q.i.d. to affected eye, as needed, for up to 4 days after surgery.

➤ **To reduce pain and inflammation after cataract surgery (Acuvail)**
Adults: Instill 1 drop 0.45% solution b.i.d. to affected eye beginning 1 day before surgery, continuing on day of surgery, and through first 2 weeks after surgery.

ketotifen fumarate
kee-toe-TYE-fen

Alaway ◇, Zaditor ◇

Therapeutic class: Antihistamines (ophthalmic)
Pharmacologic class: H₁-receptor antagonists–mast cell stabilizers

AVAILABLE FORMS
Ophthalmic solution: 0.025%

INDICATIONS & DOSAGES
➤ **To temporarily prevent eye itching from allergic conjunctivitis or temporarily relieve itchy eyes due to pollen, ragweed, grass, animal hair, and dander**
Adults and children age 3 and older: Instill 1 drop in each affected eye every 8 to 12 hours but not more than b.i.d.

latanoprost
lah-TAN-oh-prost

Xalatan, Xelpros

Therapeutic class: Antiglaucoma drugs
Pharmacologic class: Prostaglandin analogues

AVAILABLE FORMS
Ophthalmic solution: 0.005% (50 mcg/mL)

INDICATIONS & DOSAGES
➤ **Increased IOP in patients with ocular HTN or open-angle glaucoma**
Adults: Instill 1 drop in each affected eye once daily in the evening.

levobunolol hydrochloride
LEE-voe-BYOO-no-lahl

Betagan

Therapeutic class: Antiglaucoma drugs
Pharmacologic class: Nonselective beta blockers

AVAILABLE FORMS
Ophthalmic solution: 0.5%

INDICATIONS & DOSAGES
➤ **Chronic open-angle glaucoma, ocular HTN**
Adults: Instill 1 or 2 drops 0.5% solution once daily.
May give 1 drop of 0.5% solution b.i.d. with more
severe or uncontrolled glaucoma.

lifitegrast
LIF-i-teg-rast

Xiidra

Therapeutic class: Anti-inflammatory drugs
(ophthalmic)
Pharmacologic class: Lymphocyte
function-associated antigen-1 antagonists

AVAILABLE FORMS
Ophthalmic solution: 5%

INDICATIONS & DOSAGES
➤ **Dry eye disease**
Adults: Instill 1 drop into each eye b.i.d., approximately
12 hours apart.

naphazoline hydrochloride
naf-AZ-oh-leen

Clear Eyes Redness Relief ◊

Therapeutic class: Vasoconstrictors
Pharmacologic class: Alpha-1 agonists

AVAILABLE FORMS
Ophthalmic solution: 0.0125% ◊ , 0.03%

INDICATIONS & DOSAGES
➤ **Eye redness, irritation, or itching**
Adults: Instill 1 or 2 drops into the conjunctival sac of
affected eye(s) up to q.i.d.

netarsudil
ne-TAR-soo-dil

Rhopressa

Therapeutic class: Antiglaucoma drugs
Pharmacologic class: Rho kinase inhibitors

AVAILABLE FORMS
Ophthalmic solution: 0.02%

INDICATIONS & DOSAGES
➤ **To reduce elevated IOP in patients with
open-angle glaucoma or ocular HTN**
Adults: Instill 1 drop into affected eye(s) once daily in
the evening.

netarsudil–latanoprost
ne-TAR-soo-dil/la-TAN-oh-prost

Rocklatan

Therapeutic class: Antiglaucoma drugs
Pharmacologic class: Rho kinase
inhibitors–prostaglandin F2 alpha
analogues

AVAILABLE FORMS
Ophthalmic solution: netarsudil 0.2 mg/mL (0.02%)/
latanoprost 0.05 mg/mL (0.005%)

INDICATIONS & DOSAGES
➤ **To reduce elevated IOP in patients with
open-angle glaucoma or ocular HTN**
Adults: Instill 1 drop into affected eye(s) once daily in
the evening.

ofloxacin (ophthalmic)
oh-FLOX-a-sin

Ocuflox

Therapeutic class: Antibiotics
Pharmacologic class: Fluoroquinolones

AVAILABLE FORMS
Ophthalmic solution: 0.3%

INDICATIONS & DOSAGES
➤ **Conjunctivitis caused by *Staphylococcus aureus,
S. epidermidis, Streptococcus pneumoniae, Entero-
bacter cloacae, Haemophilus influenzae, Proteus
mirabilis,* or *Pseudomonas aeruginosa***
Adults and children older than age 1: Instill 1 or
2 drops in conjunctival sac every 2 to 4 hours daily
while patient is awake, for first 2 days; then 1 or
2 drops q.i.d. on days 3 through 7.
➤ **Bacterial corneal ulcer caused by *Staphylococcus
aureus, S. epidermidis, Streptococcus pneumoniae,
Pseudomonas aeruginosa, Serratia marcescens,* or
*Propionibacterium acnes***
Adults and children older than age 1: Instill 1 or
2 drops every 30 minutes while patient is awake and
1 or 2 drops every 4 to 6 hours after patient goes to
bed on days 1 and 2. On day 3, instill 1 or 2 drops
hourly while patient is awake; continue for 4 to 6 days.
Then, instill 1 or 2 drops q.i.d. for an additional 3 days
or until cured.

phenylephrine hydrochloride (ophthalmic)
fen-ill-EF-rin

Mydfrin ✤

Therapeutic class: Mydriatics
Pharmacologic class: Sympathomimetic amines–adrenergics

AVAILABLE FORMS
Ophthalmic solution: 2.5%, 10%

INDICATIONS & DOSAGES
➤ **Mydriasis**
Adults and children age 1 and older: Instill 1 drop of 2.5% or 10% solution every 3 to 5 minutes, up to 3 drops per eye. May repeat dose.
Children younger than age 1: Instill 1 drop of 2.5% solution every 3 to 5 minutes, up to 3 drops per eye.

pilocarpine hydrochloride (ophthalmic)
pie-low-KAR-peen

Isopto Carpine, Vuity

Therapeutic class: Miotics
Pharmacologic class: Direct-acting parasympathomimetics

AVAILABLE FORMS
Ophthalmic solution: 1%, 1.25%, 2%, 4%

INDICATIONS & DOSAGES
➤ **Primary open-angle glaucoma or ocular HTN**
Adults and children age 2 and older: Instill 1 drop daily up to q.i.d.; adjust concentration and frequency to control IOP. Start pilocarpine-naive patients on the 1% concentration.
Children younger than age 2: Instill 1 drop of 1% solution in eye t.i.d.
➤ **Management of acute angle-closure glaucoma**
Adults and children age 2 and older: Instill 1 drop of 1% or 2% solution in affected eye up to three times in a 30-minute period.
Children younger than age 2: Instill 1 drop of 1% solution in eye t.i.d.
➤ **Prevention of postoperative elevated IOP associated with laser surgery**
Adults and children age 2 and older: Instill 1 drop of 1%, 2%, or 4% solution in affected eye 15 to 60 minutes before surgery. May instill 2 drops, spaced at least 5 minutes apart.
➤ **Induction of miosis**
Adults and children age 2 and older: Instill 1 drop of 1%, 2%, or 4% solution in the eye. May give 2 drops, spaced at least 5 minutes apart.

➤ **Induction of miosis before goniotomy or trabeculotomy**
Children: Instill 1 drop of 1% or 2% solution in eye 15 to 60 minutes before surgery.
✴ *NEW INDICATION:* **Presbyopia (Vuity)**
Adults: Instill 1 drop of 1.25% solution in each eye once daily.

sulfacetamide sodium 10%
sul-fah-SEE-tah-mide

Therapeutic class: Antibiotics
Pharmacologic class: Sulfonamides

AVAILABLE FORMS
Ophthalmic ointment: 10%
Ophthalmic solution: 10%

INDICATIONS & DOSAGES
➤ **Conjunctivitis and other superficial ocular infections due to susceptible microorganisms**
Adults and children age 2 months and older: Instill 1 or 2 drops into lower conjunctival sac every 2 to 3 hours. Increase interval as condition responds. Or, apply ½-inch ribbon of 10% ointment into conjunctival sac every 3 to 4 hours and at bedtime. Ointment may be used at night along with drops during the day. Usual duration of treatment is 7 to 10 days.
➤ **Trachoma**
Adults and children age 2 months and older: Instill 2 drops into lower conjunctival sac every 2 hours with systemic sulfonamide therapy.

tafluprost
TA-floo-prost

Zioptan

Therapeutic class: Antiglaucoma drugs
Pharmacologic class: Prostaglandin analogues

AVAILABLE FORMS
Ophthalmic solution: 0.0015%

INDICATIONS & DOSAGES
➤ **Increased IOP in patients with open-angle glaucoma or ocular HTN**
Adults: Instill 1 drop in conjunctival sac of affected eye once daily in the evening.

tetrahydrozoline hydrochloride (ophthalmic)
tet-rah-hi-DRAZ-oh-leen

Visine Red Eye Comfort ◇

Therapeutic class: Vasoconstrictors
Pharmacologic class: Sympathomimetics

AVAILABLE FORMS
Ophthalmic solution: 0.05% ◇

INDICATIONS & DOSAGES
➤ **Conjunctival congestion, irritation, and allergic conditions**
Adults (all products) and children age 6 and older (Visine products): Instill 1 or 2 drops in affected eye up to q.i.d., or as directed by prescriber.

timolol maleate
tye-MOE-lol

Betimol, Istalol, Timoptic

Therapeutic class: Antiglaucoma drugs
Pharmacologic class: Nonselective beta blockers

AVAILABLE FORMS
Ophthalmic gel-forming solution: 0.25%, 0.5%
Ophthalmic solution: 0.25%, 0.5%
Ophthalmic solution (preservative-free): 0.25%, 0.5%

INDICATIONS & DOSAGES
➤ **To reduce IOP in ocular HTN or open-angle glaucoma**
Adults: Initially, instill 1 drop of 0.25% solution in each affected eye b.i.d.; maintenance dosage is 1 drop once daily. If no response, instill 1 drop of 0.5% solution in each affected eye b.i.d. If IOP is controlled, reduce dosage to 1 drop daily. Or, instill 1 drop of gel-forming solution (0.25% or 0.5%) in each affected eye once daily. Or, for Istalol, initially instill 1 drop 0.5% solution in each affected eye once daily in the morning. If response is unsatisfactory, concomitant therapy may be considered.
Children age 2 and older: Initially, instill 1 drop of 0.25% Timoptic or timolol generic solution in each affected eye b.i.d. If no response, increase to 1 drop of 0.5% solution in each affected eye b.i.d. If IOP is controlled, reduce dosage to 1 drop daily.

travoprost
TRA-voe-prost

Izba✦, Travatan Z

Therapeutic class: Antiglaucoma drugs
Pharmacologic class: Prostaglandin analogues

AVAILABLE FORMS
Ophthalmic solution: 0.003%✦, 0.004%

INDICATIONS & DOSAGES
➤ **To reduce IOP in patients with open-angle glaucoma or ocular HTN**
Adults and children age 16 and older: Instill 1 drop in each affected eye once daily in the evening.
Adults (Izba): Instill 1 drop in each affected eye once daily in the evening.

voretigene neparvovec-rzyl ☒
vor-RET-i-jeen ne-PAR-voe-vek

Luxturna

Therapeutic class: Ophthalmic gene therapies
Pharmacologic class: Adeno-associated virus gene therapies

AVAILABLE FORMS
Injection: 0.5 mL single-use vial with two vials of diluent

INDICATIONS & DOSAGES
➤ **Confirmed biallelic *RPE65* mutation–associated retinal dystrophy ☒**
Adults younger than age 65 and children age 1 and older: Subretinal injection of 0.3 mL (1.5×10^{11} vector genomes [vg]) to each eye on separate days within a close interval, but no fewer than 6 days apart.

Selected biologicals and blood derivatives: Indications and dosages

albumin 5%
al-BYOO-min

Albuked-5, Albuminex 5%, AlbuRx 5%, Albutein 5%, Flexbumin 5%, Plasbumin-5

albumin 25%
Albuked-25, Albuminex 25%, Albutein 25%, Flexbumin 25%, Human Albumin Grifols 25%, Kedbumin 25%, Plasbumin-25

Therapeutic class: Plasma volume expanders
Pharmacologic class: Blood derivatives

AVAILABLE FORMS
albumin 5%
Injection: 50 mg/mL in 50-mL, 100-mL, 250-mL, 500-mL vials
albumin 25%
Injection: 250 mg/mL in 20-mL, 50-mL, 100-mL vials

INDICATIONS & DOSAGES
➤ **Hypovolemic shock**
Adults: Initially, 12.5 to 25 g (250 to 500 mL) of 5% solution by IV infusion, repeated every 15 to 30 minutes, as needed. As plasma volume approaches normal, rate of infusion of 5% solution shouldn't exceed 2 to 4 mL/minute. Dosage of 25% solution varies with patient's condition and response. As plasma volume approaches normal, rate of infusion of 25% solution shouldn't exceed 1 mL/minute.
Older children and adolescents: Initially, 12.5 to 25 g IV (250 to 500 mL) of albumin 5%; repeat in 30-minute intervals as needed.
Infants and younger children: Initially, 0.5 to 1 g/kg/dose IV (10 to 20 mL/kg/dose of albumin 5%); repeat at 30-minute intervals as needed.
➤ **ARDS**
Adults: 25 g of 25% solution by IV infusion over 30 minutes; may repeat at 8-hour intervals for 3 days if necessary. Titrate to fluid loss and normalization of serum total protein.
➤ **Burns**
Adults: 25% solution infused no faster than 2 to 3 mL/minute (for Flexbumin, 1 mL/minute) to maintain plasma albumin concentration at approximately 2.5 ± 0.5 g/100 mL with a plasma oncotic pressure of 20 mm Hg (equal to a total plasma protein concentration of 5.2 g/100 mL). The duration of therapy is determined by the loss of protein from burned areas and in the urine.
➤ **Hypoproteinemia**
Adults: 200 to 300 mL of 25% albumin. Dosage varies with patient's condition and response. Usual daily dose is 50 to 75 g. Rate of infusion shouldn't exceed 2 to 3 mL/minute.
Children: Usual daily dosage is 25 g of 25% albumin. Rate of infusion shouldn't exceed 2 mL/minute.
➤ **Prevention of central volume depletion after paracentesis due to cirrhotic ascites**
Adults: 5 to 10 g of 25% solution IV infusion for every 1 L of ascitic fluid removed or 50 g total for paracentesis volumes of 5 L or more.
➤ **Ovarian hyperstimulation syndrome**
Adults: 50 to 100 g of 25% solution IV infusion over 4 hours; may repeat at 4- to 12-hour intervals as necessary.
➤ **Acute nephrosis**
Adults: 100 mL of 25% albumin daily for 7 to 10 days in combination with a loop diuretic.
➤ **Hemolytic disease of the newborn**
Children: 1 g/kg body weight of 25% albumin IV before or during exchange transfusion.

antihemophilic factor (AHF, factor VIII)

Advate, Adynovate, Afstyla, Eloctate, Esperoct, Hemofil M, Jivi, Koate, Kogenate FS, Kovaltry, Novoeight, Nuwiq, Obizur, Recombinate, Xyntha

Therapeutic class: Clotting factors
Pharmacologic class: Plasma proteins

AVAILABLE FORMS
Injection: Vials, with diluent; units specified on label

INDICATIONS & DOSAGES
➤ **Factor VIII deficiency, hemophilia A**
Drug provides hemostasis in factor VIII deficiency, hemophilia A. Specific dosage depends on patient's weight, severity of hemorrhage, and presence of inhibitors. Mild bleeding episodes require a circulating factor VIII level 20% to 40% of normal; moderate to major bleeding episodes and minor surgery, a level 30% to 60% of normal; severe bleeding or major surgery, a level 60% to 100% of normal depending on product used. Refer to specific brand for actual dosage.

anti-inhibitor coagulant complex (human)
Feiba, Feiba NF✚

Therapeutic class: Clotting factors
Pharmacologic class: Plasma proteins

AVAILABLE FORMS
Injection: Number of units of factor VIII correctional activity indicated on label of vial

INDICATIONS & DOSAGES
Boxed Warning   Thrombotic and thromboembolic events have been reported during postmarketing surveillance. ∎

➤ **To prevent or control hemorrhagic episodes in patients with hemophilia A and B with inhibitors**
Adults and children age 31 days and older: For joint hemorrhage, 50 to 100 units/kg IV every 12 hours until pain and acute disabilities improve. For mucous membrane hemorrhage, 50 to 100 units/kg IV every 6 hours for at least 1 day or until bleeding resolves. For soft-tissue hemorrhage, 100 units/kg IV every 12 hours until bleeding resolves. For other severe hemorrhage, 100 units/kg IV every 6 to 12 hours until bleeding resolves. For all indications, don't exceed a single dose of 100 units/kg body weight or a daily dose of 200 units/kg body weight.

➤ **Management of perioperative bleeding in patients with hemophilia A and B with inhibitors**
Adults and children age 31 days and older: 50 to 100 units/kg IV immediately before surgery as a one-time dose; then 50 to 100 units/kg IV every 6 to 12 hours postoperatively until bleeding resolves and healing is achieved. Don't exceed a single dose of 100 units/kg body weight or a daily dose of 200 units/kg body weight.

➤ **Routine prophylaxis to prevent or reduce frequency of bleeding episodes in patients with hemophilia A and B with inhibitors**
Adults and children age 31 days and older: 85 units/kg IV every other day.

beractant
ber-AKT-ant

Survanta

Therapeutic class: Lung surfactants
Pharmacologic class: Bovine lung extracts

AVAILABLE FORMS
Suspension for intratracheal instillation: 25 mg/mL

INDICATIONS & DOSAGES
➤ **To prevent respiratory distress syndrome (RDS), also known as hyaline membrane disease, in premature neonates weighing 1,250 g or less at birth or having symptoms consistent with surfactant deficiency**
Neonates: 4 mL/kg intratracheally. Divide each dose into four quarter-doses and give each quarter-dose over 2 to 3 seconds with infant in a different position to ensure even distribution of drug; between quarter-doses, manually ventilate infant for at least 30 seconds or until stable. Give drug as soon as possible, preferably within 15 minutes of birth. Repeat in 6 hours if respiratory distress continues. Don't exceed four doses in 48 hours.

➤ **Rescue treatment of RDS in premature infants**
Neonates: 4 mL/kg intratracheally. Divide each dose into four quarter-doses and give each quarter-dose over 2 to 3 seconds with infant in a different position to ensure even distribution of drug; between quarter-doses, manually ventilate for at least 30 seconds or until stable. Give dose as soon as RDS is confirmed by X-ray, preferably within 8 hours of birth. Repeat in 6 hours if respiratory distress continues. Don't exceed four doses in 48 hours.

calfactant
kal-FAK-tant

Infasurf

Therapeutic class: Lung surfactants
Pharmacologic class: Bovine lung extracts

AVAILABLE FORMS
Intratracheal suspension: 35 mg phospholipids and 0.7 mg proteins/mL in 3-mL, 6-mL vials

INDICATIONS & DOSAGES
➤ **To prevent respiratory distress syndrome (RDS) in premature infants younger than 29 weeks' gestational age at high risk for RDS; to treat infants younger than age 72 hours who develop RDS (confirmed by clinical and radiologic findings) and need an endotracheal tube**
Neonates: 3 mL/kg of body weight at birth intratracheally, given in two aliquots of 1.5 mL/kg each, every 12 hours for a total of up to three doses.

caplacizumab-yhdp
kap-la-SIZ-ue-mab

Cablivi

Therapeutic class: Immunomodulators
Pharmacologic class: Anti–von Willebrand factors

AVAILABLE FORMS
Injection: 11 mg single-dose vial

INDICATIONS & DOSAGES
➤ **Acquired thrombotic thrombocytopenic purpura (aTTP), in combination with plasma exchange and immunosuppressive therapy**
Adults: On day 1 of plasma exchange therapy, give 11 mg IV bolus at least 15 minutes before plasma exchange, followed by 11 mg subcut after completion of plasma exchange. On subsequent days during daily plasma exchange, give 11 mg subcut once daily following plasma exchange. Continue 11 mg subcut once daily for 30 days following the last daily plasma exchange. After initial treatment course, if signs and symptoms of persistent underlying disease such as suppressed ADAMTS13 activity levels remain, may extend treatment for a maximum of 28 days. Discontinue drug if patient experiences more than two recurrences of aTTP during therapy.

coagulation factor Xa (recombinant), inactivated-zhzo
Andexxa

Therapeutic class: Antidotes
Pharmacologic class: Factor Xa proteins

AVAILABLE FORMS
Injection: 200-mg vials

INDICATIONS & DOSAGES
Boxed Warning Use of drug has been associated with thromboembolic and ischemic events, including MI, stroke, cardiac arrest, and sudden death. Monitor patient for thromboembolic events and initiate anticoagulation when appropriate. ∎
➤ **Reversal of anticoagulation in patients treated with rivaroxaban or apixaban in life-threatening or uncontrolled bleeding**
Adults: Base dosing on the specific factor Xa inhibitor, dose of factor Xa inhibitor, and time since patient's last dose of factor Xa inhibitor. If last dose of rivaroxaban was 10 mg or less taken less than 8 hours or an unknown time ago; last dose of apixaban was 5 mg or less taken less than 8 hours or an unknown time ago; or either rivaroxaban or apixaban at any dose was taken 8 hours or more ago, give initial bolus dose of 400 mg IV at a target rate of 30 mg/minute followed 2 minutes later with an IV infusion of 4 mg/minute for up to 120 minutes.

If last dose of rivaroxaban was greater than 10 mg or the last dose is unknown and was taken less than 8 hours or an unknown time ago; or last dose of apixaban was greater than 5 mg or the last dose is unknown, give initial bolus dose of 800 mg IV at a target rate of 30 mg/minute followed 2 minutes later with an IV infusion of 8 mg/minute for up to 120 minutes.

emicizumab-kxwh
em-i-SIZ-ue-mab

Hemlibra

Therapeutic class: Antibodies
Pharmacologic class: Monoclonal IgG4 antibodies

AVAILABLE FORMS
Injection: 30 mg/mL, 60 mg/0.4 mL, 105 mg/0.7 mL, 150 mg/mL single-dose vials

INDICATIONS & DOSAGES
Boxed Warning Thrombotic events have been reported after average cumulative amount of more than 100 units/kg was given within 24 hours of activated prothrombin complex concentrate (aPCC). Discontinue aPCC or suspend emicizumab dose if symptoms occur. ▨
➤ **Routine prophylaxis to prevent or reduce frequency of bleeding episodes in patients with hemophilia A (congenital factor VIII deficiency) with or without factor VIII inhibitors** ▨
Adults and children: 3 mg/kg subcut once weekly for 4 weeks; then 1.5 mg/kg once weekly or 3 mg/kg subcut once every 2 weeks or 6 mg subcut once every 4 weeks.

factor IX complex
Profilnine, Profilnine SD

factor IX (human)
AlphaNine SD, Immunine VH ✤

factor IX (recombinant)
Alprolix, BeneFIX, Ixinity, Rixubis

factor IX (recombinant [glycopegylated])
Rebinyn

Therapeutic class: Clotting factors
Pharmacologic class: Plasma proteins

AVAILABLE FORMS
Injection: Vials, with diluent; international units specified on label

INDICATIONS & DOSAGES
➤ **Factor IX deficiency (also called hemophilia B or Christmas disease)**
Adults and children: Dosage is highly individualized, depending on degree of deficiency, level of factor IX desired, patient's weight and condition, and severity of bleeding. Infusion rates vary with product and patient comfort. Refer to manufacturer's instructions for each product to calculate dosage.

hepatitis B immune globulin (human)

hep-ah-TYE-tis

HepaGam B, HyperHEP B, Nabi-HB

Therapeutic class: Prophylaxis drugs
Pharmacologic class: Immune serums

AVAILABLE FORMS

Injection: 1-mL, 5-mL vials; 0.5-mL neonatal single-dose syringe; 1-mL single-dose syringe

INDICATIONS & DOSAGES

➤ **Postexposure HBV prophylaxis**
Adults and children: 0.06 mL/kg (usual dose is 3 to 5 mL) IM as soon as possible (within 24 hours if possible) but within 7 days after exposure (within 14 days if sexual exposure). Repeat dose 28 days after exposure if patient doesn't elect to receive or doesn't respond to the hepatitis B vaccine.
Infants younger than age 12 months if primary caregiver has acute HBV infection: 0.5 mL IM.
Neonates born to HBsAg-positive patients: 0.5 mL IM within 12 hours of birth. Active vaccination with hepatitis B vaccine may begin at the same time.
➤ **To prevent recurrence of HBV infection after liver transplantation in patients who are HBsAg-positive (HepaGam B only)**
Adults: 20,000 international units IV at rate of 2 mL/minute. Give first dose simultaneously with the grafting of the transplanted liver (anhepatic phase); then give daily on days 1 through 7, every 2 weeks from day 14 through 12 weeks, and monthly from month 4 onward.
Adjust-a-dose: Adjust dose in patients who don't reach anti-HBs levels of 500 international units/L within the first week after transplantation. In patients with surgical bleeding or abdominal fluid drainage of more than 500 mL, or those undergoing plasmapheresis, give 10,000 international units IV every 6 hours until target level is reached.

luspatercept-aamt

lus-PAT-er-sept

Reblozyl

Therapeutic class: Hematopoietics
Pharmacologic class: Erythroid maturation agents

AVAILABLE FORMS

Injection: 25 mg, 75 mg single-use vials

INDICATIONS & DOSAGES

Adjust-a-dose (for all indications): Review Hb and transfusion record before each dose; follow manufacturer's instructions for dosage modifications if insufficient response to treatment or rapid rise in Hb, or for predose Hb of 11.5 g/dL or greater. For grade 3 or 4 hypersensitivity reactions, discontinue treatment. For other grade 3 or 4 adverse reactions, interrupt treatment until adverse reaction resolves to no higher than grade 1; then restart treatment at next lower dose. Discontinue treatment if dose delay continues for longer than 12 consecutive weeks.
➤ **Anemia in patients with beta-thalassemia who require regular RBC transfusions**
Adults: 1 mg/kg subcut once every 3 weeks. Titrate dose by response to maximum dose of 1.25 mg/kg.
➤ **Anemia in patients who fail an erythropoiesis-stimulating agent and require two or more RBC transfusions over 8 weeks with very low- to intermediate-risk myelodysplastic syndrome with ring sideroblasts or with myelodysplastic or myeloproliferative neoplasm with ring sideroblasts and thrombocytosis**
Adults: 1 mg/kg subcut once every 3 weeks. Titrate dose by response to maximum dose of 1.75 mg/kg.

lusutrombopag

loo-soo-TROM-boe-pag

Mulpleta

Therapeutic class: Hematopoietics
Pharmacologic class: Thrombopoietin receptor agonists

AVAILABLE FORMS

Tablets: 3 mg

INDICATIONS & DOSAGES

➤ **Thrombocytopenia in patients with chronic liver disease scheduled to undergo a procedure**
Adults: 3 mg PO once daily for 7 days, beginning 8 to 14 days before procedure. Procedure should occur 2 to 8 days after final dose.

lymphocyte immune globulin (antithymocyte globulin [equine], ATG, LIG)

Atgam

Therapeutic class: Immunosuppressants
Pharmacologic class: Immunoglobulins

AVAILABLE FORMS

Injection: 50 mg of equine IgG/mL in 5-mL ampules

INDICATIONS & DOSAGES

Boxed Warning Drug can cause anaphylaxis. Only use drug in facilities with adequate laboratory and supportive medical resources. ■

➤ **Acute renal allograft rejection**
Adults and children: 10 to 15 mg/kg IV daily for 14 days. Additional alternate-day therapy to total of 21 doses can be given. Start therapy when rejection is diagnosed.
➤ **Aplastic anemia**
Adults and children: 10 to 20 mg/kg IV daily for 8 to 14 days. Additional alternate-day therapy to total of 21 doses can be given.

plasma protein fraction
Plasmanate

Therapeutic class: Plasma volume expanders
Pharmacologic class: Plasma proteins

AVAILABLE FORMS
Injection: 5% (50 mg/mL) solution in 50-mL, 250-mL, 500-mL vials

INDICATIONS & DOSAGES
➤ **Shock**
Adults: Dosage varies with patient's condition and response. Typical minimum effective dose is 250 to 500 mL. Adjust rate according to clinical response.

SAFETY ALERT!

protein C concentrate ▨
Ceprotin

Therapeutic class: Anticoagulants
Pharmacologic class: Protein C replacements

AVAILABLE FORMS
Injection: 500 international units/vial, 1,000 international units/vial

INDICATIONS & DOSAGES
Adjust-a-dose (for all indications): Adjust dose based on severity of protein C deficiency, plasma level of protein C, and patient's age and condition.
➤ **Venous thrombosis and purpura fulminans in patients with severe congenital protein C deficiency** ▨
Adults, neonates, and children: Initially for acute episodes and short-term prophylaxis, 100 to 120 international units/kg IV; then, 60 to 80 international units/kg IV every 6 hours for subsequent three doses to maintain peak protein C activity of 100%. Maintenance dose of 45 to 60 international units/kg IV every 6 to 12 hours to maintain trough protein C activity levels above 25%.
➤ **Long-term prevention of venous thrombosis and purpura fulminans**
Adults, neonates, and children: 45 to 60 international units/kg IV every 12 hours to maintain trough protein C activity levels above 25%.

rabies immune globulin (human)
HyperRAB, Imogam Rabies-HT, Kedrab

Therapeutic class: Antibodies
Pharmacologic class: Immunoglobulins

AVAILABLE FORMS
Injection: 150 international units/mL in 2-mL, 10-mL vials; 300 international units/mL in 1-mL, 3-mL, 5-mL vials

INDICATIONS & DOSAGES
➤ **Rabies exposure**
Adults and children: 20 international units/kg IM at time of first dose of rabies vaccine. If anatomically feasible, up to the full dose is used to infiltrate wound area; remainder is given IM in a different site.

Rh₀(D) immune globulin intramuscular (human) (IGIM)
HyperRHO S/D Full Dose, HyperRHO S/D Mini-Dose, MICRhoGAM, RhoGAM

Rh₀(D) immune globulin intravenous (human) (IGIV)
Rhophylac, WinRho SDF

Therapeutic class: Immune globulins
Pharmacologic class: Immunoglobulins

AVAILABLE FORMS
IGIM
Injection: 50-mcg syringe (250 international units, microdose), 300-mcg syringe (1,500 international units, standard dose)
IGIV
Injection: 120-mcg (600 international units), 300-mcg (1,500 international units), 500-mcg (2,500 international units), 1,000-mcg (5,000 international units), 3,000-mcg (15,000 international units) vials; 300-mcg (1,500 international units) syringe

INDICATIONS & DOSAGES
Boxed Warning Intravascular hemolysis leading to compromising anemia, multisystem organ failure, and death have been reported in patients treated for ITP with IGIV. ∎
➤ **Rh exposure after abortion, miscarriage, ectopic pregnancy, or childbirth**
Adults: Transfusion unit or blood bank determines fetal RBC volume entering patient's blood; 300 mcg IGIM is given IM if fetal RBC volume is less than 15 mL. More than one dose may be needed if severe

feto-maternal hemorrhage occurs; must be given within 72 hours after delivery or miscarriage.

➤ **To prevent Rh antibody formation after abortion or miscarriage**
Adults: Consult transfusion unit or blood bank. Up to and including 12 weeks' gestation, one IGIM microdose vial (50 mcg) IM will suppress immune reaction to 2.5 mL $Rh_0(D)$-positive RBCs. At 13 weeks' gestation and later, use one IGIM standard dose (300 mcg). Ideally, give within 3 hours, but may be given up to 72 hours after abortion or miscarriage.

➤ **Rh exposure after abortion, amniocentesis after 34 weeks' gestation, or other manipulations past 34 weeks' gestation with increased risk of Rh isoimmunization**
Adults: 120 mcg IGIV, given IV or IM within 72 hours of delivery, miscarriage, or manipulation.

➤ **To suppress Rh isoimmunization during pregnancy**
Adults: 300 mcg IV or IM at 28 weeks' gestation. If given early in pregnancy, give additional doses at 12-week intervals to maintain adequate levels of passively acquired anti-Rh antibodies. Then, within 72 hours of delivery, give 120 mcg WinRho or 300 mcg HyperRHO, RhoGAM, or Rhophylac IM or IV. If 72 hours have elapsed, give drug as soon as possible, up to 28 days.

➤ **Incompatible blood transfusion**
Adults: Total dose depends on volume of RBCs or whole blood infused. Consult blood bank or transfusion unit at once; must be given within 72 hours. Give 600 mcg WinRho IV every 8 hours or 1,200 mcg IM every 12 hours until total dose has been given.

➤ **Chronic ITP in patients who are $Rh_0(D)$ antigen-positive; ITP secondary to HIV; acute ITP in children**
Adults and children: Initially, 50 mcg/kg IV as single dose or divided into two doses on separate days. If Hb level is less than 10 g/dL, reduce first dose to 25 to 40 mcg/kg. Then, give 25 to 60 mcg/kg IV as needed to elevate platelet count with specific individually determined dosage.

romiplostim
roh-mih-PLOH-stim

Nplate

Therapeutic class: Hematopoietics
Pharmacologic class: Thrombopoietin receptor agonists

AVAILABLE FORMS
Injection: 125-mcg, 250-mcg, 500-mcg single-use vials

INDICATIONS & DOSAGES
➤ **ITP in patients who have had an insufficient response to corticosteroids, immunoglobulins, or splenectomy**

Adults; children age 1 and older with ITP for at least 6 months: Initially, 1 mcg/kg subcut once weekly. Adjust dosage in increments of 1 mcg/kg/week to maintain platelet count of 50×10^9/L or higher, as needed, to reduce the risk of bleeding. Maximum dose, 10 mcg/kg weekly. Refer to manufacturer's instructions for dosage adjustments for platelet counts. Discontinue if platelet count doesn't increase after 4 weeks at maximum dose.

➤ **To increase survival in patients (including term neonates) acutely exposed to myelosuppressive doses of radiation**
Adults and children: 10 mcg/kg subcut as soon as possible after suspected or confirmed exposure to radiation level greater than 2 gray (Gy).

tetanus immune globulin (human)
HyperTET S/D

Therapeutic class: Prophylaxis drugs
Pharmacologic class: Immunoglobulins

AVAILABLE FORMS
Injection: 250-unit vial or syringe

INDICATIONS & DOSAGES
➤ **Postexposure prevention of tetanus after injury in patients whose immunization is incomplete or unknown**
Adults and children age 7 and older: 250 units deep IM injection.
Children younger than age 7: 250 units deep IM injection is recommended; may also give 4 units/kg.

Vaccines and toxoids: Indications and dosages

Refer to manufacturer's instructions for complete prescribing and safety information.

anthrax vaccine, adsorbed
BioThrax

Pharmacologic class: Vaccines

AVAILABLE FORMS
Injection: 0.5 mL/dose in 5-mL multidose vial

INDICATIONS & DOSAGES
➤ **Preexposure prophylaxis of disease caused by *Bacillus anthracis* in persons at high risk of exposure**
Adults ages 18 through 65: 0.5 mL IM at day 0, month 1, and month 6, followed by booster doses at 12 and 18 months. Yearly booster injections of 0.5 mL IM are recommended for those who remain at risk. Or, 0.5 mL subcut at 0, 2, and 4 weeks and 6 months, with booster doses at 12 and 18 months and at 1-year intervals thereafter.
➤ **Postexposure prophylaxis of disease following suspected or confirmed *B. anthracis* exposure, in conjunction with recommended antibacterial drugs**
Adults ages 18 through 65: 0.5 mL subcut 0, 2, and 4 weeks after exposure. Administer with concomitant antibiotic therapy.

cholera vaccine, live
Vaxchora

Pharmacologic class: Vaccines

AVAILABLE FORMS
Suspension: 100-mL package

INDICATIONS & DOSAGES
➤ **Active immunization against disease caused by *Vibrio cholerae***
Adults age 18 through 64 and children age 6 and older: One dose in 100 mL reconstituted buffer solution PO 10 days before potential exposure.
Children ages 2 to younger than 6: One dose in 50 mL reconstituted buffer solution PO 10 days before potential exposure.

COVID-19 vaccine
Emergency use authorization: Janssen vaccine, Novavax
Pharmacologic class: Vaccines

AVAILABLE FORMS
Injection: Multidose vials with 5 (Janssen) or 10 (Novavax) doses

INDICATIONS & DOSAGES
➤ **To prevent coronavirus disease 2019 (COVID-19)**
Adults age 18 and older (Janssen): 0.5 mL IM as a single dose. May give a single 0.5-mL booster dose at least 2 months after primary vaccination.
Adults and children age 12 and older (Novavax): 0.5 mL IM as a series of two doses (0.5 mL each) 3 weeks apart.
➤ **Booster dose after completion of primary vaccination with another authorized or approved COVID-19 vaccine (Janssen only)**
Eligible patients: May give 0.5 mL IM as a single dose to the eligible population at the dosing interval authorized for a booster dose of the vaccine used for primary vaccination.

COVID-19 vaccine, mRNA
Comirnaty, Spikevax

Emergency use authorization: Moderna or Pfizer bivalent (original and omicron) vaccines
Pharmacologic class: Vaccines

AVAILABLE FORMS
ⓘ *Alert:* Read labels carefully. Vials are age specific.
Injection: 0.2 mL, 0.3 mL dose (Comirnaty/Pfizer); 0.25 mL, 0.5 mL dose (Spikevax/Moderna)

INDICATIONS & DOSAGES
➤ **To prevent coronavirus disease 2019 (COVID-19) caused by severe acute respiratory syndrome coronavirus (SARS-CoV-2) (Comirnaty)**
Adults and adolescents age 12 and older: 0.3 mL IM as a series of two doses, 3 weeks apart.
Children ages 5 to younger than 12 (EUA): 0.2 mL IM as a series of two doses, 3 weeks apart.
Children ages 6 months through 4 years (EUA): 0.2 mL IM as an initial series of two doses, 3 weeks apart, followed by a third dose at least 8 weeks after the second dose.
Adjust-a-dose: Under an EUA, may give a third dose at least 28 days after the second dose to patients age 5 and older who have undergone solid organ transplantation or who are diagnosed with conditions considered to have an equivalent level of immuno-compromise.
➤ **To prevent COVID-19 caused by SARS-CoV-2 (Spikevax)**
Adults age 18 and older: 0.5 mL IM as a series of two doses, 4 weeks apart.
Adjust-a-dose: May give a third dose at least 1 month after second dose to patients who have under-gone solid organ transplantation or who are diagnosed with conditions considered to have an equivalent level of immunocompromise.

Children age 12 to younger than 18 years (EUA):
0.5 mL IM as a series of two doses, 4 weeks apart.
May give a third dose at least 28 days after the second
dose to patients who are immunocompromised.
Children age 6 to younger than 12 years (EUA):
0.5 mL IM as a series of two doses, 4 weeks apart.
May give a third dose at least 28 days after the second
dose to patients who are immunocompromised.
*Children age 6 months to younger than 6 years
(EUA):* 0.25 mL IM as a series of two doses, 4 weeks
apart. May give a third dose at least 28 days after the
second dose to patients who are immunocompromised.
➤ **Booster dose after completion of primary
vaccination with another authorized or approved
COVID-19 vaccine (EUA for Comirnaty and
Spikevax vaccines)**
Eligible patients: May give 0.3 mL (Comirnaty) or
0.25 mL (Spikevax) IM as a single dose to the eligible population at the dosing interval authorized for a
booster dose of the vaccine used for primary vaccination.
✱ *NEW INDICATION:* **Booster after completion
of primary vaccination or most recent booster
with any authorized or approved monovalent
COVID-19 vaccine (EUA for bivalent vaccines)**
Eligible patients: May give single booster dose of
0.3 mL (Pfizer) or 0.5 mL (Moderna) at least 2 months
after completion of primary vaccination or most recent
booster.

diphtheria and tetanus toxoids and acellular pertussis vaccine adsorbed (DTaP)
Daptacel, Infanrix

tetanus toxoid and reduced diphtheria toxoid and acellular pertussis vaccine adsorbed (Tdap)
Adacel, Boostrix

Pharmacologic class: Vaccines/toxoids

AVAILABLE FORMS
DTaP
Daptacel
Injection: 15 limit flocculation (Lf) units diphtheria
toxoid, 5 Lf units tetanus toxoid, and 10 mcg pertussis
toxoid adsorbed per 0.5 mL
Infanrix
Injection: 25 Lf units diphtheria toxoid, 10 Lf units
tetanus toxoid, and 25 mcg inactivated pertussis toxins
adsorbed per 0.5 mL
Tdap
Adacel
Injection: 5 Lf units tetanus toxoid, 2 Lf units diph-
theria toxoid, and 2.5 mcg detoxified pertussis toxins
adsorbed per 0.5 mL

Boostrix (preservative-free)
Injection: 5 Lf units tetanus toxoid, 2.5 Lf units diphtheria toxoid, and 8 mcg inactivated pertussis toxins
adsorbed per 0.5 mL

INDICATIONS & DOSAGES
➤ **Primary immunization (Daptacel, Infanrix)**
*Children ages 6 weeks to 6 years (before 7th birth-
day):* 0.5 mL IM at 2, 4, 6, and 15 to 20 months and
a fifth dose at age 4 to 6 years. May give first dose as
early as 6 weeks; then every 4 to 8 weeks for Infanrix
or every 6 to 8 weeks for Daptacel.
➤ **Booster immunization; tetanus prophylaxis for
wound management**
Adults and children ages 10 to 64 (Adacel): 0.5 mL
IM as a single dose at least 5 years after the last DTaP
or Td vaccination.
Adults and children age 10 and older (Boostrix):
0.5 mL IM as a single dose at least 5 years after the
last DTaP or Td vaccination.
✱ *NEW INDICATION:* **Immunization during third
trimester to prevent pertussis in infants younger
than age 2 months**
Patients during third trimester: 0.5 mg IM as a single
dose.

diphtheria and tetanus toxoids, acellular pertussis adsorbed, hepatitis B (recombinant), and inactivated poliovirus vaccine combined
Pediarix

Pharmacologic class: Vaccines/toxoids

AVAILABLE FORMS
Injection: 0.5-mL single-dose prefilled syringe; each
0.5 mL contains 25 Lf units diphtheria toxoid, 10 Lf
units tetanus toxoid, acellular pertussis antigens,
10 mcg HBsAg, and inactivated poliovirus types 1,
2, and 3

INDICATIONS & DOSAGES
➤ **Active immunization**
Children ages 6 weeks to younger than 7 years:
Primary series is three 0.5-mL doses IM at 6- to
8-week intervals (preferably 8), usually starting at
age 2 months; may start at age 6 weeks.

diphtheria and tetanus toxoids, acellular pertussis adsorbed, and inactivated poliovirus combination vaccine (DtaP/IPV)
Kinrix, Quadracel

Pharmacologic class: Vaccines/toxoids

AVAILABLE FORMS
Injection (Kinrix: preservative-free): 25 Lf units diphtheria toxoid, 10 Lf units tetanus toxoid, 25 mcg inactivated pertussis toxin (PT), and inactivated poliovirus types 1, 2, and 3 per 0.5 mL
Injection (Quadracel): 15 Lf units diphtheria toxoid, 5 Lf units tetanus toxoid, 20 mcg detoxified PT, and inactivated poliovirus types 1, 2, and 3 per 0.5 mL

INDICATIONS & DOSAGES
➤ **Active immunization against diphtheria, tetanus, pertussis, and poliomyelitis as the fifth dose in the DTaP vaccine series and the fourth dose in the IPV series (Kinrix), or as the fifth dose in the DTaP vaccine series and as a fourth or fifth dose in the IPV series (Quadracel)**
Children ages 4 through 6: 0.5 mL IM, preferably in the deltoid muscle of the upper arm as a single dose. Refer to manufacturer's instructions for use with prior specific vaccine products.

diphtheria and tetanus toxoids, acellular pertussis adsorbed, inactivated poliovirus, and *Haemophilus influenzae* type b conjugate vaccine combined
Pentacel

Pharmacologic class: Vaccines/toxoids

AVAILABLE FORMS
Injection: 15 Lf units diphtheria toxoid, 5 Lf units tetanus toxoid, 20 mcg inactivated pertussis toxin, inactivated poliovirus types 1, 2, and 3, and 10 mcg *H. influenzae* type b covalently bound to 24 mcg tetanus toxoid per 0.5 mL

INDICATIONS & DOSAGES
➤ **Active immunization against diphtheria, tetanus, pertussis, poliomyelitis, and invasive disease caused by *H. influenzae* type b**
Children ages 6 weeks to 4 years (before 5th birthday): 0.5 mL IM as a four-dose series at ages 2, 4, 6, and 15 through 18 months. The first dose may be given as early as age 6 weeks.

Haemophilus b conjugate vaccine, meningococcal protein conjugate (PRP-OMP)
PedvaxHIB

Haemophilus b conjugate, tetanus toxoid conjugate (PRP-T)
ActHIB, Hiberix

Pharmacologic class: Vaccines

AVAILABLE FORMS
Hib conjugate vaccine, meningococcal protein conjugate
Injection: 7.5 mcg of Hib PRP and 125 mcg *N. meningitides* OMPC per 0.5 mL
Hib conjugate vaccine, tetanus toxoid conjugate
Injection: 10 mcg Hib capsular polysaccharide and 24 mcg tetanus toxoid (ActHIB) or 10 mcg Hib capsular polysaccharide and 25 mcg tetanus toxoid (Hiberix)

INDICATIONS & DOSAGES
➤ **Active immunization for the prevention of invasive disease caused by Hib (PedvaxHIB)**
Infants, including preterm infants: 0.5 mL IM at age 2 months; repeat at age 4 months. May give first dose as early as age 6 weeks. Give booster dose at age 12 to 15 months when primary two-dose regimen is completed before 12 months. When first dose is given between 11 and 14 months, omit the booster after primary two-dose regimen.
Previously unvaccinated children ages 15 months to 6 years: 0.5 mL IM. Booster dose isn't needed.
➤ **Active immunization for the prevention of invasive disease caused by Hib (ActHIB, Hiberix)**
Children ages 2 months through 5 years (before 6th birthday) (ActHIB): 0.5 mL IM at age 2 months. Repeat at ages 4 and 6 months. Give booster dose at ages 15 to 18 months.
Children ages 6 weeks to 4 years (before 5th birthday) (Hiberix): 0.5 mL IM at age 2 months. Repeat at ages 4 and 6 months. Give booster dose at ages 15 to 18 months. May give first dose as early as age 6 weeks.

hepatitis A vaccine, inactivated
Havrix, Vaqta

Pharmacologic class: Vaccines

AVAILABLE FORMS
Havrix
Injection: 0.5 mL, 1 mL prefilled syringes
Vaqta
Injection: 0.5 mL vials or prefilled syringes

INDICATIONS & DOSAGES

➤ **Active immunization against hepatitis A virus**

Adults: 1 mL Havrix or 1 mL Vaqta IM as single dose. For booster dose, give 1 mL Havrix 6 to 12 months after first dose or 1 mL Vaqta IM 6 to 18 months after first dose. Booster is recommended for prolonged immunity.

Children ages 12 months to 18 years: 0.5 mL Havrix or 0.5 mL Vaqta IM as single dose. Then, give booster dose of 0.5 mL Havrix 6 to 12 months after first dose or 0.5 mL Vaqta IM 6 to 18 months after first dose. Booster is recommended for prolonged immunity.

hepatitis B vaccine, recombinant
Engerix-B, PreHevbrio, Recombivax HB, Recombivax HB Dialysis Formulation

Pharmacologic class: Vaccines

AVAILABLE FORMS
Engerix-B
Injection: 0.5 mL, 1 mL prefilled syringes; 1 mL single-dose vials
PreHevbrio
Injection: 1 mL single-dose vials
Recombivax HB
Injection: 0.5 mcg HBsAg/0.5 mL, 10 mcg HBsAg/mL single-dose vials and prefilled syringes
Recombivax HB, adult dialysis formulation
Injection: 40 mcg HBsAg/mL single-dose vials

INDICATIONS & DOSAGES

➤ **Immunization against infection from all known subtypes of HBV**

Adults age 20 and older (Engerix-B); adults age 18 and older (PreHevbrio): Initially, 1 mL IM; then second dose of 1 mL IM after 30 days. A third dose of 1 mL IM is given 6 months after first dose.

Adults undergoing dialysis (Engerix-B): Initially, 2 mL IM; then second dose of 2 mL IM after 30 days. Third dose of 2 mL IM is given 2 months after first dose. Fourth dose of 2 mL IM is given 6 months after first dose. Assess need for booster doses with antibody testing annually. Give 2 mL booster when antibody level declines below 10 milli-international units/mL.

Neonates and children up to age 19: Initially, 0.5 mL IM; then second dose of 0.5 mL IM 30 days later. Give third dose of 0.5 mL IM 6 months after first dose.

Adjust-a-dose (Engerix-B): See manufacturer's instructions for alternative dosage and administration schedules.

➤ **Recombivax HB**

Adults age 20 and older: Initially, 1 mL IM; then second dose of 1 mL IM after 30 days. Give third dose of 1 mL IM 6 months after first dose.

Adjust-a-dose: For adults who are predialysis or undergoing dialysis, initially, 1 mL of 40 mcg IM dialysis formulation; then second dose of 40 mcg IM in 30 days, and final dose of 40 mcg IM 6 months after first dose. A booster or revaccination may be indicated if anti-HBs titer is below 10 mIU/mL 1 to 2 months after third dose and annually thereafter.

Infants, children, and adolescents age 19 or younger: Initially, 0.5 mL IM; then second dose of 0.5 mL IM after 30 days. Give third dose of 0.5 mL IM 6 months after first dose. Or, in adolescents ages 11 to 15, give 1 mL IM; then second dose of 1 mL 4 to 6 months later.

human papillomavirus recombinant vaccine, 9-valent
Gardasil 9

Pharmacologic class: Virus antigens

AVAILABLE FORMS
Injection: 0.5 mL single-dose vial, prefilled syringe

INDICATIONS & DOSAGES

➤ **To prevent cervical, vulvar, vaginal, and anal cancer caused by human papillomavirus (HPV) types 16, 18, 31, 33, 45, 52, and 58; genital warts caused by HPV types 6 and 11; cervical adenocarcinoma in situ, and cervical, vulval, vaginal, and anal intraepithelial neoplasias caused by HPV types 6, 11, 16, 18, 31, 33, 45, 52, and 58**

Women and girls ages 15 to 45: Three separate IM injections of 0.5 mL each. Give second injection 2 months after first; then give third injection 6 months after the first.

Girls ages 9 to 14: Two-dose regimen of 0.5 mL IM injection at 0 and 6 to 12 months. (If second dose is administered earlier than 5 months after first dose, administer a third dose at least 4 months after second dose.) Or, three-dose regimen of 0.5 mL IM injection at 0, 2, and 6 months.

➤ **To prevent genital warts caused by HPV types 6 and 11; anal, oropharyngeal, and other head and neck cancers caused by HPV types 6, 18, 31, 33, 45, 52, and 58; anal intraepithelial neoplasia caused by HPV types 6, 11, 16, 18, 31, 33, 45, 52, and 58**

Men and boys ages 15 to 45: Three separate IM injections of 0.5 mL each. Give second injection 2 months after first; then give third injection 6 months after first.

Boys ages 9 to 14: Two-dose regimen of 0.5 mL IM injection at 0 and 6 to 12 months. (If second dose is administered earlier than 5 months after first dose, administer a third dose at least 4 months after second dose.) Or, three-dose regimen of 0.5 mL IM injection at 0, 2, and 6 months.

influenza virus vaccine, inactivated

Afluria Quadrivalent, Fluad Quadrivalent, Fluarix Quadrivalent, Flucelvax Quadrivalent, FluLaval Quadrivalent, Fluzone High-Dose Quadrivalent, Fluzone Quadrivalent

influenza virus vaccine, live

FluMist Quadrivalent

Pharmacologic class: Vaccines

AVAILABLE FORMS
Injection: 0.5-mL, 0.7 mL prefilled syringes; 0.5 mL single-dose vials; 5 mL multidose vials
Intranasal: 0.2 mL prefilled sprayer

INDICATIONS & DOSAGES
➤ **Active immunization to prevent disease caused by influenza A and B viruses**
Patients age 9 and older: 0.5 mL IM as a single dose (Afluria Quadrivalent, Fluarix Quadrivalent, Flucelvax Quadrivalent, FluLaval Quadrivalent, Fluzone Quadrivalent).
Children ages 3 to 8: 0.5 mL IM as a single dose (FluLaval Quadrivalent, Fluzone Quadrivalent). May need to repeat dose based on previous vaccination status.
Children ages 3 to 8: 0.5 mL (Afluria Quadrivalent, Fluzone Quadrivalent) IM as one dose if previously vaccinated; may need to be repeated per immunization guidelines. Give two doses of 0.5 mL at least 4 weeks apart if patient hasn't been previously vaccinated or vaccination history is unknown.
Children ages 6 to 35 months: 0.25 mL or 0.5 mL IM as a single dose (Afluria Quadrivalent, Fluzone Quadrivalent) if previously vaccinated. Give two doses of 0.25 mL or 0.5 mL at least 4 weeks apart if patient hasn't been previously vaccinated or vaccination history is unknown.
Children age 6 months to younger than 9 years: 0.5 mL (Fluarix Quadrivalent, Flucelvax Quadrivalent, FluLaval Quadrivalent) IM as a single dose. May need to repeat dose based on previous vaccination status.
Older adults (age 65 and older) (Fluad Quadrivalent, Fluzone High-Dose Quadrivalent): 0.5 mL IM as a single dose or 0.7 mL IM high-dose as a single dose.
Patients ages 9 to younger than 50: 0.2 mL FluMist intranasally (0.1 mL per nostril) once per season.
Children ages 2 to younger than 9: 0.2 mL FluMist intranasally (0.1 mL per nostril). May need to repeat dose based on previous vaccination status.

Japanese encephalitis virus vaccine

Ixiaro

Pharmacologic class: Vaccines

AVAILABLE FORMS
Injection: 0.5 mL single-dose syringe

INDICATIONS & DOSAGES
➤ **To prevent disease caused by Japanese encephalitis virus**
Adults and children age 3 and older: Two doses of 0.5 mL IM 28 days apart. Complete immunization at least 1 week before exposure. If primary series of two doses was completed more than a year previously, may give a booster dose if ongoing exposure or reexposure is expected.
Children ages 2 months to younger than 3 years: Two doses of 0.25 mL IM 28 days apart.

measles, mumps, and rubella virus vaccine, live

M-M-R II, Priorix

Pharmacologic class: Vaccines

AVAILABLE FORMS
Injection: 0.5 mL single-dose vial

INDICATIONS & DOSAGES
➤ **Routine immunization**
Adults: 0.5 mL subcut. May need to repeat dose based on immunosuppression status and vaccination history.
Children age 12 months and older: 0.5 mL subcut. A two-dose schedule is recommended, with first dose given between ages 12 and 15 months (between ages 6 and 12 months in high-risk areas) and second dose given at ages 4 to 6.
➤ **Postexposure prophylaxis for measles**
Adults and children age 12 months and older: 0.5 mL subcut within 72 hours of exposure.

measles, mumps, rubella, and varicella (MMRV) virus vaccine, live, attenuated

ProQuad

Pharmacologic class: Vaccines

AVAILABLE FORMS
Injection: 0.5 mL single-dose vial

INDICATIONS & DOSAGES
➤ **Routine immunization**
Children ages 12 months to 12 years: 0.5 mL subcut. The first dose is usually given between ages 12 and 15 months but may be given any time through age 12. A second dose, if needed, is usually given between ages 4 and 6. At least 1 month should elapse between a dose of a measles-containing vaccine and a dose of MMRV vaccine. If a second dose of a varicella-containing vaccine is required, at least 3 months should elapse between administration of the two doses.

meningococcal (groups A, C, Y, and W-135) conjugate vaccine (MCV4)
Menactra, MenQuadfi, Menveo

meningococcal (group B) vaccine
Bexsero, Trumenba

Pharmacologic class: Vaccines

AVAILABLE FORMS
Injection: 0.5 mL single-dose vials and prefilled syringes

INDICATIONS & DOSAGES
➤ **Active immunization for the prevention of invasive meningococcal disease caused by** *Neisseria meningitidis* **serogroups A, C, Y, and W-135**
Menactra
Adults and children ages 2 to 55: 0.5 mL IM as a single dose, preferably in the deltoid muscle.
Adults and children ages 15 to 55 who are at continued risk for meningococcal disease: 0.5 mL IM as a booster at least 4 years after prior dose.
Children ages 9 months to 23 months: 0.5 mL IM given as a two-dose series 3 months apart.
MenQuadfi
Adults and children older than age 2: 0.5 mL IM as a single dose. Patients age 15 and older at continued risk may receive a single booster at least 4 years after prior dose.
Menveo
Patients ages 2 to 55: 0.5 mL IM as a single dose, preferably into deltoid muscle. For patients ages 15 to 55 at continued high risk for meningococcal disease, a second dose may be given at least 4 years after a prior dose of meningococcal conjugate vaccine.
Children age 2 to younger than 11: 0.5 mL IM as a single dose. For children age 2 to younger than 6 at continued high risk, a second dose may be given 2 months after the first dose.
Children ages 7 to 23 months: 0.5 mL IM given as a two-dose series with second dose in the second year of life and at least 3 months after first dose.
Infants age 2 months to 12 months: 0.5 mL IM given as a four-dose series at 2, 4, 6, and 12 months.

➤ **Active immunization for the prevention of invasive meningococcal disease caused by** *N. meningitidis* **serogroup B**
Adults through age 25 and children age 10 and older: 0.5 mL/dose (Bexsero) IM as a two-dose series at least 1 month apart. Or, 0.5 mL/dose (Trumenba) IM at 0 and 6 months (two-dose schedule), or at 0 month and then a second dose at either 1 or 2 months and then a third dose at 6 months (three-dose schedule).

palivizumab
Synagis

Pharmacologic class: Monoclonal antibodies

AVAILABLE FORMS
Injection: 50 mg, 100 mg vials

INDICATIONS & DOSAGES
➤ **Prevention of serious lower respiratory tract disease caused by RSV**
High-risk infants age 24 months and younger: 15 mg/kg IM monthly throughout RSV season. Give first dose before commencement of RSV season. Children undergoing cardiopulmonary bypass should receive an additional dose as soon as possible after the procedure, then monthly as scheduled.

pneumococcal vaccine, polyvalent

23-valent conjugate vaccine
Pneumovax 23

20-valent conjugate vaccine
Prevnar 20

15-valent conjugate vaccine
Vaxneuvance

13-valent conjugate vaccine
Prevnar 13

Pharmacologic class: Vaccines

AVAILABLE FORMS
Pneumovax 23
Injection: 25 mcg each of 23 *Streptococcus pneumoniae* polysaccharide isolates per 0.5 mL in single-dose vials or prefilled syringes
Prevnar 20
Injection: 2.2 mcg each of 20 *S. pneumoniae* serotypes per 0.5 mL in single-dose prefilled syringes
Vaxneuvance
Injection: 2.0 mcg of 15 *S. pneumoniae* serotypes per 0.5 mL in single-dose prefilled syringes
Prevnar 13
Injection: 2.2 mcg each of 13 *S. pneumoniae* serotypes per 0.5 mL in single-dose prefilled syringes

INDICATIONS & DOSAGES
➤ **Pneumococcal immunization**
Adults age 50 and older; adults and children age 2 and older at high risk: 0.5 mL Pneumovax IM or sub-cut. Patients at high risk may be reimmunized following Advisory Committee on Immunization Practices guidelines.
➤ **Immunization against invasive disease caused by *S. pneumoniae* serotypes**
Prevnar 13
Children ages 6 to younger than 18): 0.5 mL IM as a single dose.
Infants ages 6 weeks to younger than 6 years: 0.5 mL IM for a total of four doses at ages 2, 4, 6, and 12 to 15 months. See manufacturer's instructions for catch-up schedule.
Vaxneuvance
Children age 6 weeks and older: 0.5 mL IM for a total of four doses at ages 2, 4, 6, and 12 to 15 months. See manufacturer's instructions for catch-up schedule.
➤ **Otitis media caused by susceptible *S. pneumoniae* serotypes (Prevnar 13)**
Infants ages 6 weeks to younger than 6 years: 0.5 mL IM for a total of four doses at ages 2, 4, 6, and 12 to 15 months. See manufacturer's instructions for catch-up schedule.
➤ **Immunization against *S. pneumoniae* (Prevnar 13, Prevnar 20, Vaxneuvance)**
Adults age 18 and older: 0.5 mL IM as a single dose.

poliovirus vaccine, inactivated (IPV)
IPOL

Pharmacologic class: Vaccines

AVAILABLE FORMS
Injection: 5 mL multidose vials

INDICATIONS & DOSAGES
➤ **Poliovirus immunization, inactivated**
Unvaccinated adults: 0.5 mL subcut or IM; give second dose 4 to 8 weeks later. Give third dose 6 to 12 months later.
Vaccinated adults: 0.5 mL subcut or IM booster may be given to patients at increased risk of exposure.
Children: 0.5 mL subcut or IM at ages 2 months and 4 months. Give third dose at ages 6 to 18 months. Give a booster dose of 0.5 mL subcut at ages 4 to 6.

rabies vaccine
Imovax Rabies, RabAvert

Pharmacologic class: Vaccines

AVAILABLE FORMS
Injection: 2.5 international units rabies antigen/mL, in single-dose vial with diluent

INDICATIONS & DOSAGES
➤ **Postexposure antirabies immunization**
Adults and children: Five 1-mL doses IM. Give first dose as soon as possible after exposure in conjunction with rabies immune globulin; give additional doses on days 3, 7, 14, and 28 after first dose. If no antibody response occurs after this primary series, booster dose is recommended.
➤ **Postexposure antirabies immunization in people who are previously immunized**
Adults and children: 1 mL IM immediately and 1 mL IM 3 days later.
➤ **Preexposure preventive immunization for persons in high-risk groups**
Adults and children: Three 1-mL injections IM. Give first dose on day 0 (first day of therapy), second dose on day 7, and third dose on day 21 or 28. Assess rabies antibodies every 2 years in patients at continued high risk. Give booster dose if titer is less than complete neutralization at 1:5 serum dilutions by RFFIT. Booster can be given in absence of titer test.

rotavirus, live
Rotarix, RotaTeq

Pharmacologic class: Vaccines

AVAILABLE FORMS
Lyophilized powder for oral suspension: single-dose vial with 1 mL liquid diluent in prefilled oral applicator
Oral suspension: 2 mL single-dose tubes

INDICATIONS & DOSAGES
➤ **Prevention of rotavirus gastroenteritis**
RotaTeq
Children ages 6 to 32 weeks: Give first dose of 2 mL PO at 6 to 12 weeks. Give second and third doses at 4- to 10-week intervals. The three-dose series should be completed by age 32 weeks.
Rotarix
Infants ages 6 to 24 weeks: Give first dose of 1 mL PO at age 6 weeks. Give another 1-mL dose PO after at least 4 weeks. The two-dose series should be completed by age 24 weeks.

smallpox and monkeypox vaccine
Jynneos

Pharmacologic class: Vaccines

AVAILABLE FORMS
Injection: 0.5 mL single-dose vials

INDICATIONS & DOSAGES
➤ **Prevention of smallpox and monkeypox in high-risk patients**
Adults: 0.5 mL subcut for two doses 4 weeks apart.

tetanus and diphtheria toxoid, adsorbed (Td)
TdVax, Tenivac

Pharmacologic class: Vaccines

AVAILABLE FORMS
Injection: 0.5 mL single-dose vials or syringes

INDICATIONS & DOSAGES
➤ **Primary immunization to prevent tetanus and diphtheria**
Adults and children age 7 and older: 0.5 mL IM 4 to 8 weeks apart for two doses; then give third dose 6 to 12 months (TdVax) or 6 to 8 months (Tenivac) after second.
➤ **Booster dose to prevent tetanus and diphtheria**
Adults and children age 7 and older: 0.5 mL IM at age 11 to 12 years, then at 10-year intervals.
➤ **Postexposure prevention of tetanus**
Adults and children age 7 and older: For a clean, minor wound, give emergency booster dose if more than 10 years have elapsed since last dose. For all other wounds, give booster dose if more than 5 years have elapsed since last dose.

tick-borne encephalitis vaccine
Ticovac

Pharmacologic class: Vaccines

AVAILABLE FORMS
Injection: 1.2 mcg inactivated virus/0.25 mL, 2.4 mcg inactivated virus/0.5 mL suspension in single-dose prefilled syringes

INDICATIONS & DOSAGES
➤ **Active immunization to prevent tick-borne encephalitis**
Adults and adolescents age 16 and older: 0.5 mL IM as a series of three doses at day 0, 14 days to 3 months after first vaccination, and 5 to 12 months after second vaccination. May give booster (fourth dose) at least 3 years after completing primary series if ongoing exposure or reexposure to tick-borne encephalitis virus.
Children ages 1 to 15: 0.25 mL IM as a series of three doses at day 0, 1 to 3 months after first vaccination, and 5 to 12 months after second vaccination. May give booster (fourth dose) at least 3 years after completing primary series if ongoing exposure or reexposure to tick-borne encephalitis virus.

varicella virus vaccine
Varivax

Pharmacologic class: Vaccines

AVAILABLE FORMS
Injection: 0.5 mL single-dose vials

INDICATIONS & DOSAGES
➤ **To prevent varicella zoster (chickenpox) infections**
Adults and children age 13 and older: 0.5 mL subcut; then, second 0.5-mL dose 4 to 8 weeks later.
Children ages 1 to 12: 0.5 mL subcut at 12 to 15 months; then, second 0.5-mL dose at 4 to 6 years. If a second dose is given, allow a minimum interval of 3 months between a dose of varicella-containing vaccine and Varivax.

zoster vaccine recombinant, adjuvanted
Shingrix

Pharmacologic class: Vaccines

AVAILABLE FORMS
Injection: 0.5-mL vials

INDICATIONS & DOSAGES
➤ **Prevention of herpes zoster (shingles)**
Adults age 50 and older: 0.5 mL IM as a two-dose series, with first dose given at month 0 and second dose given anytime between 2 and 6 months later.
Adults age 18 and older who are or will be immunodeficient or immunosuppressed by known disease or therapy: 0.5 mL IM as a two-dose series, with first dose given at month 0 and second dose given 1 to 2 months later.

Less commonly used drugs: Indications and dosages

Refer to manufacturer's instructions for complete prescribing and safety information.

SAFETY ALERT!

acalabrutinib
a-KAL-a-broo-ti-nib

Calquence

Therapeutic class: Antineoplastics
Pharmacologic class: Kinase inhibitors

AVAILABLE FORMS
Capsules 🔵: 100 mg

INDICATIONS & DOSAGES
Adjust-a-dose (for all indications): Refer to manufacturer's instructions for toxicity-related dosage adjustments. Avoid concomitant use with CYP3A inhibitors, but if a CYP3A inhibitor is necessary and will be used short term (up to 7 days), interrupt acalabrutinib therapy. If patient is taking acalabrutinib with a moderate CYP3A inhibitor, reduce acalabrutinib dosage to 100 mg once daily. Avoid concomitant use with strong CYP3A inducers, but if use together can't be avoided, increase acalabrutinib dosage to 200 mg b.i.d.

➤ **Mantle cell lymphoma in patients who have received at least one prior therapy**
Adults: 100 mg PO approximately every 12 hours until disease progression or unacceptable toxicity occurs.
➤ **Chronic lymphocytic leukemia (CLL) or small lymphocytic lymphoma (SLL)**
Adults: 100 mg PO approximately every 12 hours; continue until disease progression or unacceptable toxicity occurs. Or, with obinutuzumab for patients with previously untreated CLL or SLL, 100 mg PO approximately every 12 hours until disease progression or unacceptable toxicity occurs, beginning with cycle 1 (each cycle is 28 days). Start obinutuzumab at cycle 2 for six cycles. Refer to obinutuzumab prescribing information for recommended dosing. Give acalabrutinib before obinutuzumab when given on same day.

SAFETY ALERT!

acarbose
a-KAR-boz

Glucobay✥

Therapeutic class: Antidiabetics
Pharmacologic class: Alpha-glucosidase inhibitors

AVAILABLE FORMS
Tablets: 25 mg, 50 mg, 100 mg

INDICATIONS & DOSAGES
➤ **Adjunct to diet and exercise to improve glycemic control in patients with non-insulin-dependent type 2 diabetes**

Adults: Dosages individualized. Initially, 25 mg PO t.i.d. with first bite of each main meal. Adjust dosage every 4 to 8 weeks, based on 1-hour postprandial glucose level or HbA$_{1c}$ levels and tolerance. Maintenance dosage is 50 to 100 mg PO t.i.d. For patients who weigh less than 60 kg, don't exceed 50 mg PO t.i.d. For patients who weigh more than 60 kg, don't exceed 100 mg PO t.i.d.

aclidinium bromide
a-cli-DIN-ee-um

Tudorza Pressair

Therapeutic class: Miscellaneous respiratory drugs
Pharmacologic class: Anticholinergics

AVAILABLE FORMS
Dry powder inhaler: 400 mcg/actuation

INDICATIONS & DOSAGES
➤ **Maintenance treatment of COPD**
Adults: 400 mcg (1 inhalation) b.i.d.

afamelanotide
a-fa-me-LAN-oh-tide

Scenesse

Therapeutic class: Dermatologic agents
Pharmacologic class: Alpha-melanocyte stimulating hormone analogues

AVAILABLE FORMS
Implant: 16 mg

INDICATIONS & DOSAGES
➤ **To increase pain-free light exposure in patients with a history of phototoxic reactions from erythropoietic protoporphyria**
Adults: 16 mg subcut every 2 months above the anterior suprailiac crest.

SAFETY ALERT!

afatinib dimaleate
a-FA-ti-nib

Gilotrif

Therapeutic class: Antineoplastics
Pharmacologic class: Tyrosine kinase inhibitors

AVAILABLE FORMS
Tablets: 20 mg, 30 mg, 40 mg

INDICATIONS & DOSAGES
➤ **Metastatic, squamous NSCLC that has progressed after platinum-based chemotherapy; first-line treatment of patients with metastatic NSCLC whose tumors have epidermal growth factor receptor exon 19 deletions or exon 21 (*L858R*) substitution mutations**

Adults: 40 mg PO once daily on an empty stomach until disease progression or intolerability occurs.
Adjust-a-dose: For patients with preexisting renal impairment (eGFR of 15 to 29 mL/minute/1.73 m²), give 30 mg PO once daily. For patients who require long-term therapy with a P-gp inducer, increase afatinib daily dose by 10 mg as tolerated. Resume the previous dose 2 to 3 days after discontinuation of the P-gp inducer.

For patients who require therapy with a P-gp inhibitor, reduce afatinib daily dose by 10 mg if concomitant therapy isn't tolerated. Resume previous dose after discontinuation of the P-gp inhibitor as tolerated. Refer to manufacturer's instructions for toxicity-related dosage adjustments.

alfuzosin hydrochloride
al-foo-ZOE-sin

Uroxatral🔎

Therapeutic class: BPH drugs
Pharmacologic class: Alpha₁ blockers

AVAILABLE FORMS
Tablets (extended-release): 10 mg

INDICATIONS & DOSAGES
➤ **BPH**
Adults: 10 mg PO once daily.

alirocumab ▨
AL-i-rok-ue-mab

Praluent

Therapeutic class: Antilipemics
Pharmacologic class: Proprotein convertase subtilisin/kexin type 9 antibody inhibitors

AVAILABLE FORMS
Injection: 75 mg/mL, 150 mg/mL in single-dose prefilled pens

INDICATIONS & DOSAGES
➤ **Adjunct to diet, alone or in combination with other LDL cholesterol (LDL-C)–lowering therapies, to treat primary hyperlipidemia, including heterozygous familial hypercholesterolemia (HeFH); to reduce risk of MI, stroke, and unstable angina requiring hospitalization in patients with established CV disease who require additional lowering of LDL-C levels ▨**
Adults: 75 mg subcut every 2 weeks or 300 mg subcut every 4 weeks. If LDL-C response is inadequate (within 4 to 8 weeks), may increase dosage to maximum of 150 mg every 2 weeks. Recommended dosage in patients with HeFH undergoing LDL apheresis is 150 mg subcut every 2 weeks, without regard to the timing of apheresis.
➤ **Adjunct to other LDL-C–lowering therapies in patients with homozygous familial hypercholesterolemia to reduce LDL-C levels ▨**
Adults: 150 mg subcut every 2 weeks.

alosetron hydrochloride
a-LOE-se-tron

Lotronex

Therapeutic class: Anti-IBS drugs
Pharmacologic class: Selective 5-HT₃ receptor antagonists

AVAILABLE FORMS
Tablets: 0.5 mg, 1 mg

INDICATIONS & DOSAGES
Boxed Warning Drug is only appropriate for adult females with severe diarrhea-predominant IBS who haven't responded to conventional therapy. Infrequent but serious GI adverse reactions have been reported and resulted in hospitalization and, rarely, blood transfusion, surgery, and death. ■
➤ **Severe diarrhea-predominant IBS**
Adult females: 0.5 mg PO b.i.d. If, after 4 weeks, drug is well tolerated but doesn't adequately control IBS symptoms, increase to 1 mg b.i.d. (maximum dose, 2 mg/day). After 4 weeks at this dosage, if symptoms aren't controlled, stop drug.

SAFETY ALERT!

alprostadil (injection)
al-PROS-ta-dill

Prostin VR Pediatric

Therapeutic class: Prostaglandins
Pharmacologic class: Prostaglandins

AVAILABLE FORMS
Injection: 500 mcg/mL

INDICATIONS & DOSAGES
Boxed Warning Apnea may occur, especially in neonates weighing less than 2 kg at birth and during first hour of infusion. ■
➤ **Palliative therapy for temporary maintenance of patency of ductus arteriosus until surgery can be performed**
Neonates: 0.05 to 0.1 mcg/kg/minute by IV infusion. When therapeutic response is achieved, reduce infusion rate to lowest dose that will maintain response. Maximum dose is 0.4 mcg/kg/minute. Or, give drug through umbilical artery catheter placed at ductal opening.

alprostadil (intracavernosal injection; urogenital suppository)
al-PROSS-ta-dil

Caverject, Caverject Impulse, Edex, Muse

Therapeutic class: Erectile dysfunction drugs
Pharmacologic class: Prostaglandins

AVAILABLE FORMS
Intracavernosal injection: 20 mcg/vial, 40 mcg/vial
Intracavernosal injection (injection device): 10 mcg/cartridge, 20 mcg/cartridge, 40 mcg/cartridge
Intracavernosal injection (syringe): 10 mcg/syringe, 20 mcg/syringe

Urethral suppository: 125 mcg, 250 mcg, 500 mcg, 1,000 mcg

INDICATIONS & DOSAGES

➤ **Erectile dysfunction of vasculogenic, psychogenic, or mixed causes**

Injection

Adults: Dosages highly individualized; initially, inject 2.5 mcg intracavernosally. If partial response occurs, give second dose of 2.5 mcg; increase by 5 to 10 mcg until patient achieves erection suitable for intercourse lasting no longer than 1 hour. If no response to first dose, increase second dose to 7.5 mcg within 1 hour; then increase by 5 to 10 mcg until patient achieves suitable erection. After initial doses, patient must remain in prescriber's office until complete detumescence occurs. Don't repeat for at least 24 hours. For Edex, give 1 to 40 mcg by intracavernosal injection over 5 to 10 seconds. Use the lowest effective dose no more than three times per week with at least 24 hours between doses.

Urethral suppository

Adults: Initially, 125 to 250 mcg, under supervision of prescriber. Adjust dosage as needed until response is sufficient for sexual intercourse. Maximum of two administrations in 24 hours; maximum dose is 1,000 mcg.

➤ **Erectile dysfunction of neurogenic cause (spinal cord injury)**

Adults: Dosages highly individualized; initially, inject 1.25 mcg intracavernosally. If partial response occurs, give second dose of 1.25 mcg. Increase in increments of 2.5 mcg, to dose of 5 mcg; then increase in increments of 5 mcg until patient achieves erection suitable for intercourse lasting no longer than 1 hour. If no response to first dose, give next higher dose within 1 hour. After initial doses, patient must remain in prescriber's office until complete detumescence occurs. Don't repeat procedure for at least 24 hours. For Edex, give 1 to 40 mcg by intracavernosal injection over 5 to 10 seconds. Use the lowest effective dose no more than three times per week with at least 24 hours between doses.

alvimopan
al-VIM-oh-pan

Entereg

Therapeutic class: Bowel restorative drugs
Pharmacologic class: Peripherally acting mu-opioid receptor antagonists

AVAILABLE FORMS
Capsules: 12 mg

INDICATIONS & DOSAGES
Boxed Warning Due to risk of MI, drug is for short-term use in hospitalized patients. Only available through a REMS program. ∎

➤ **Management of postoperative ileus to accelerate recovery after partial large- or small-bowel resection surgery with primary anastomosis**

Adults: 12 mg PO 30 minutes to 5 hours before surgery, followed by 12 mg PO b.i.d. beginning first day after surgery for up to 7 days or maximum of 15 in-hospital doses (180 mg).

amifampridine
AM-i-fam-pri-deen

Firdapse

Therapeutic class: Cholinergic agonists
Pharmacologic class: Potassium channel blockers

AVAILABLE FORMS
Tablets: 10 mg

INDICATIONS & DOSAGES
➤ **Lambert-Eaton myasthenic syndrome**

Adults and children ages 6 to younger than 17 weighing 45 kg or more: 15 to 30 mg/day PO in three to four divided doses. May increase by 5 mg daily every 3 or 4 days. Maximum single dose is 20 mg; maximum daily dose is 80 mg.

Children ages 6 to younger than 17 weighing less than 45 kg: 5 to 15 mg/day PO in three to four divided doses. May increase by 2.5 daily every 3 to 4 days. Maximum single dose, 10 mg; maximum daily dose, 40 mg.

Adjust-a-dose: In patients with renal impairment (CrCl of 15 to 90 mL/minute) or any degree of hepatic impairment, or in known N-acetyltransferase poor metabolizers, starting dose is the lowest recommended initial daily dosage in divided doses.

amikacin liposome inhalation suspension
am-i-KAY-sin

Arikayce

Therapeutic class: Antibacterials
Pharmacologic class: Aminoglycosides

AVAILABLE FORMS
Inhalation: 590 mg/8.4 mL unit-dose vial

INDICATIONS & DOSAGES
Boxed Warning Increased risk of respiratory reactions, including hypersensitivity pneumonitis, hemoptysis, bronchospasm, or exacerbation of pulmonary disease. ∎

➤ **MAC lung disease as part of a combination antibacterial drug regimen in patients who don't achieve negative sputum cultures after a minimum of 6 consecutive months of a multidrug background regimen therapy and who have limited or no alternative treatment options**

Adults: 590 mg/8.4 mL oral inhalation once daily using the Lamira Nebulizer System over 14 to 20 minutes.

amisulpride
am-ee-SUL-pride

Barhemsys

Therapeutic class: Antiemetics
Pharmacologic class: Dopamine antagonists

AVAILABLE FORMS
Injection: 5 mg/2 mL, 10 mg/4 mL

INDICATIONS & DOSAGES
➤ **Prevention of postoperative nausea and vomiting, either alone or in combination with antiemetic of a different class**
Adults: 5 mg IV as a single dose over 1 to 2 minutes at time of anesthesia induction.
➤ **Postoperative nausea and vomiting in patients who have received antiemetic prophylaxis with agent of a different class or haven't received prophylaxis**
Adults: 10 mg IV as a single dose infused over 1 to 2 minutes in the event of nausea or vomiting after surgical procedure.

anakinra
ann-ACK-in-rah

Kineret

Therapeutic class: Immunomodulators
Pharmacologic class: Interleukin-1 receptor antagonists

AVAILABLE FORMS
Injection: 100 mg/0.67 mL in a prefilled glass syringe

INDICATIONS & DOSAGES
Adjust-a-dose (for all indications): In severe renal insufficiency or ESRD (CrCl less than 30 mL/minute), consider every-other-day dosing.
➤ **Neonatal-onset multisystem inflammatory disease**
Adults and children: Initially, 1 to 2 mg/kg subcut once daily. May increase in 0.5- to 1-mg/kg increments to maximum dose of 8 mg/kg daily. Maintenance dose is 3 to 4 mg/kg daily. May divide total daily dose into two equal doses.
➤ **To reduce signs and symptoms and slow progression of structural damage in moderately to severely active RA after one or more failures with DMARDs, alone or combined with DMARDs other than TNF blockers**
Adults: 100 mg subcut daily at the same time each day.
➤ **Interleukin-1 receptor antagonist deficiency**
Adults and children: Initially, 1 to 2 mg/kg subcut once daily. May increase in 0.5- to 1-mg/kg increments to maximum dose of 8 mg/kg daily.

angiotensin II
an-jee-oh-TEN-sin

Giapreza

Therapeutic class: Vasoconstrictors
Pharmacologic class: Angiotensin II analogues

AVAILABLE FORMS
Injection: 2.5 mg/mL in 1-mL single-dose vials

INDICATIONS & DOSAGES
➤ **To increase BP in patients with septic or other distributive shock**
Adults: Initially, 20 nanograms/kg/minute IV infusion. May titrate by up to 15 nanograms/kg/minute every 5 minutes as needed to achieve or maintain target BP. Don't exceed 80 nanograms/kg/minute during first 3 hours of treatment. Doses as low as 1.25 nanograms/kg/minute may be effective. Maintenance doses shouldn't exceed 40 nanograms/kg/minute. Once shock has sufficiently improved, wean patient by down-titrating every 5 to 15 minutes by increments of up to 15 nanograms/kg/minute.

anidulafungin
ah-nid-doo-la-FUN-jin

Eraxis

Therapeutic class: Antifungals
Pharmacologic class: Echinocandins

AVAILABLE FORMS
Powder for injection: 50 mg/vial, 100 mg/vial

INDICATIONS & DOSAGES
➤ **Candidemia and other *Candida* infections (intra-abdominal abscess, peritonitis)**
Adults: A single 200-mg loading dose by IV infusion at no more than 1.1 mg/minute on day 1; then 100 mg daily for at least 14 days after last positive culture result.
Children age 1 month and older: A single 3-mg/kg loading dose (not to exceed 200 mg) by IV infusion at no more than 1.1 mg/minute on day 1; then 1.5 mg/kg (not to exceed 100 mg) daily for at least 14 days after last positive culture result.
➤ **Esophageal candidiasis**
Adults: A single 100-mg loading dose by IV infusion at no more than 1.1 mg/minute on day 1; then 50 mg daily for at least 14 days and for at least 7 days after symptoms resolve.

apomorphine hydrochloride
ah-poe-MORE-feen

Apokyn, Kynmobi

Therapeutic class: Antiparkinsonian drugs
Pharmacologic class: Nonergot-derivative dopamine agonists

AVAILABLE FORMS
SL film ⓄⓊⓉ: 10 mg, 15 mg, 20 mg, 25 mg, 30 mg
Solution for injection*: 10 mg/mL (contains benzyl alcohol)

INDICATIONS & DOSAGES
➤ **Intermittent hypomobility, "off" episodes caused by advanced Parkinson disease (given with an antiemetic)**
Adults: Initially, give a 1-mg or 2-mg subcut test dose when patient is in an "off" episode. Measure supine and standing BP before first dose and every 20 minutes for at least the first hour. If patient tolerates and responds to drug, start with the same dose as needed as outpatient. Titrate dosage in 1-mg increments every few days to effect and tolerance. Don't exceed 6 mg. Separate doses by at least 2 hours.

If patient tolerates test dose but doesn't respond adequately or doesn't tolerate test dose, refer to manufacturer's instructions for further medically supervised dosing.

Or, initially, give 10 mg SL during an "off" state achieved by patient withholding the regular morning dose of carbidopa–levodopa and any other adjunctive Parkinson disease medications from midnight the night before. If patient tolerates 10 mg and responds adequately, continue 10 mg PRN up to five times daily. If 10 mg was tolerated but response was insufficient, resume usual Parkinson disease medications and up-titrate SL apomorphine in increments of 5 mg. Maximum single dose is 30 mg. Separate doses by at least 2 hours.

Treatment with concomitant antiemetic is recommended starting 3 days before drug initiation and continued as necessary to control nausea and vomiting, generally up to 2 months.
Adjust-a-dose: In patients with mild to moderate renal impairment, give test and starting doses of 1 mg subcut.

arformoterol tartrate
arr-fohr-MOH-tur-ahl

Brovana

Therapeutic class: Bronchodilators
Pharmacologic class: Long-acting selective beta₂ agonists

AVAILABLE FORMS
Solution for inhalation: 15 mcg/2 mL vials

INDICATIONS & DOSAGES
➤ **Maintenance treatment of bronchoconstriction in patients with COPD**
Adults: 15 mcg inhaled via nebulizer every 12 hours. Maximum dose is 30 mcg daily.

armodafinil
ar-moe-DAF-i-nil

Nuvigil

Therapeutic class: Stimulants
Pharmacologic class: CNS stimulants
Controlled substance schedule: IV

AVAILABLE FORMS
Tablets: 50 mg, 150 mg, 200 mg, 250 mg

INDICATIONS & DOSAGES
➤ **To improve wakefulness in patients with excessive sleepiness caused by narcolepsy, obstructive sleep apnea (OSA), or shift-work sleep disorder**
Adults: 150 to 250 mg PO daily in morning. For OSA, doses exceeding 150 mg daily may not be more effective. For shift-work sleep disorder, 150 mg PO daily, 1 hour before start of shift.
Adjust-a-dose: Reduce dosage in patients with severe hepatic impairment. Consider lower doses in older adults.

artemether–lumefantrine
art-TEM-mah-ther/loo-meh-FAN-treen

Coartem

Therapeutic class: Antimalarials
Pharmacologic class: Schizontocides

AVAILABLE FORMS
Tablets: artemether 20 mg and lumefantrine 120 mg

INDICATIONS & DOSAGES
➤ **Uncomplicated malaria caused by *Plasmodium falciparum***
Adults and children weighing 35 kg or more: Initially, 4 tablets PO, followed by 4 tablets in 8 hours, then 4 tablets b.i.d. for the next 2 days. Total course is 24 tablets.
Children weighing 25 to less than 35 kg: Initially, 3 tablets PO, followed by 3 tablets in 8 hours, then 3 tablets b.i.d. for the next 2 days. Total course is 18 tablets.
Children weighing 15 to less than 25 kg: Initially, 2 tablets PO, followed by 2 tablets in 8 hours, then 2 tablets b.i.d. for the next 2 days. Total course is 12 tablets.
Children weighing 5 to less than 15 kg: Initially, 1 tablet PO, followed by 1 tablet in 8 hours, then 1 tablet b.i.d. for the next 2 days. Total course is 6 tablets.

SAFETY ALERT!

atezolizumab
a-te-zoe-LIZ-ue-mab

Tecentriq

Therapeutic class: Antineoplastics
Pharmacologic class: Monoclonal antibodies

AVAILABLE FORMS
Injection: 840 mg/14 mL, 1,200 mg/20 mL single-dose vial

INDICATIONS & DOSAGES
Adjust-a-dose (for all indications): Dosage reductions aren't recommended for toxicities; drug is either withheld or permanently discontinued. Refer to manufacturer's instructions for toxicity-related dosage modifications.
➤ **Locally advanced or metastatic urothelial carcinoma in patients who are not eligible for cisplatin-containing chemotherapy and whose tumors express PD-L1 (PD-L1 stained tumor-infiltrating immune cells covering 5% or more of the tumor**

area), or aren't eligible for platinum-containing chemotherapy regardless of PD-L1 status ▧

Adults: 840-mg IV infusion every 2 weeks, 1,200-mg IV infusion every 3 weeks, or 1,680-mg IV infusion every 4 weeks until disease progression or unacceptable toxicity occurs.

➤ **First-line treatment of extensive-stage small cell lung cancer, in combination with carboplatin and etoposide**

Adults: 840-mg IV infusion every 2 weeks, 1,200-mg IV infusion every 3 weeks, or 1,680-mg IV infusion every 4 weeks. If using with carboplatin and etoposide, give before chemotherapy when given on same day.

Adjust-a-dose: Dosage reductions aren't recommended for toxicities; drug is either withheld or permanently discontinued. Refer to manufacturer's instructions for toxicity-related treatment. Refer to prescribing information for chemotherapy agents for dosing information.

➤ **First-line treatment for metastatic nonsquamous NSCLC in patients with no *EGFR* or *ALK* genomic tumor aberrations, in combination with paclitaxel protein-bound particles and carboplatin or in combination with bevacizumab, paclitaxel, and carboplatin** ▧

Adults: 840-mg IV infusion every 2 weeks, 1,200-mg IV infusion every 3 weeks, or 1,680-mg IV infusion every 4 weeks. Infuse before chemotherapy and bevacizumab when given on same day.

Adjust-a-dose: Refer to manufacturer's instructions for toxicity-related treatment. Refer to prescribing information for the chemotherapy agents or bevacizumab for dosing information. After completion of four to six cycles of chemotherapy, and if bevacizumab is discontinued, atezolizumab may be continued. Recommended atezolizumab dosage is 840 mg every 2 weeks, 1,200 mg every 3 weeks, or 1,680 mg every 4 weeks via IV infusion until disease progression or unacceptable toxicity occurs.

➤ **Metastatic NSCLC in patients whose tumors have high PD-L1 expression, with no *EGFR* or *ALK* genomic tumor aberrations, or have disease progression during or after platinum-containing chemotherapy (Patients with NSCLC and *EGFR* or *ALK* genomic tumor aberrations should have disease progression on FDA-approved therapy for these aberrations before starting drug.)** ▧

Adults: 840-mg IV infusion every 2 weeks, 1,200-mg IV infusion every 3 weeks, or 1,680-mg IV infusion every 4 weeks until disease progression or unacceptable toxicity occurs. Give first infusion over 60 minutes; if tolerated, may give all subsequent infusions over 30 minutes.

✳ *NEW INDICATION:* **Adjuvant treatment after resection and platinum-based chemotherapy for patients with stage II to IIIA NSCLC whose tumors express PD-L1**

Adults: 840-mg IV infusion every 2 weeks, 1,200-mg every 3 weeks, or 1,680-mg IV infusion every 4 weeks until disease progression or unacceptable toxicity occurs, or up to 1 year.

➤ **Unresectable or metastatic hepatocellular carcinoma in combination with bevacizumab in patients who haven't received prior systemic therapy**

Adults: 840-mg IV infusion every 2 weeks, 1,200-mg IV infusion every 3 weeks, or 1,680-mg IV infusion every 4 weeks. Give 15 mg/kg bevacizumab after atezolizumab on same day every 3 weeks until disease progression or unacceptable toxicity occurs. If bevacizumab is discontinued, give atezolizumab 840-mg IV infusion every 2 weeks, 1,200-mg IV infusion every 3 weeks, or 1,680-mg IV infusion every 4 weeks. Give first infusion over 60 minutes; if tolerated, may give all subsequent infusions over 30 minutes. Refer to manufacturer's instructions for bevacizumab prescribing information.

➤ ***BRAF* V600 mutation-positive unresectable or metastatic melanoma in combination with cobimetinib and vemurafenib** ▧

Adults: After completion of 28-day cycle of cobimetinib and vemurafenib, give atezolizumab 840-mg IV infusion every 2 weeks, 1,200-mg IV infusion every 3 weeks, or 1,680-mg IV infusion every 4 weeks with cobimetinib 60 mg PO once daily (21 days on/7 days off) and vemurafenib 720 mg PO b.i.d. until disease progression or unacceptable toxicity occurs. Give first infusion over 60 minutes; if tolerated, give all subsequent infusions over 30 minutes. Refer to manufacturer's instructions for cobimetinib and vemurafenib prescribing information.

SAFETY ALERT!

atracurium besylate
at-truh-KYOO-ree-um

Therapeutic class: Skeletal muscle relaxants
Pharmacologic class: Nondepolarizing neuromuscular blockers

AVAILABLE FORMS
Injection: 10 mg/mL

INDICATIONS & DOSAGES

➤ **Adjunct to general anesthesia to facilitate ET intubation and relax skeletal muscles during surgery or mechanical ventilation**

Adults and children age 2 and older: 0.4 to 0.5 mg/kg by IV bolus. Give maintenance dose of 0.08 to 0.1 mg/kg within 20 to 45 minutes during prolonged surgery and every 15 to 25 minutes in patients receiving balanced anesthesia. For prolonged procedures, use a constant infusion at 9 to 10 mcg/kg/minute initially; then reduce to 5 to 9 mcg/kg/minute. For infusion in the ICU, an infusion rate of 11 to 13 mcg/kg/minute should provide adequate neuromuscular blockade.

Children ages 1 month to 2 years: First dose, 0.3 to 0.4 mg/kg IV for those under halothane anesthesia. Frequent maintenance doses may be needed.

Adjust-a-dose: In adults, adolescents, children, or infants with significant CV disease or history suggesting a greater risk of histamine release (anaphylactic reaction, asthma), give initial dose of 0.3 to 0.4 mg/kg slowly or in divided doses over 1 minute. In adults receiving enflurane or isoflurane at the same time, reduce initial atracurium dose by 33% (0.25 to 0.35 mg/kg). In adults receiving atracurium following succinylcholine, initial dose is 0.3 to 0.4 mg/kg.

avanafil
a-VAN-a-fill

Stendra

Therapeutic class: Erectile dysfunction drugs
Pharmacologic class: PDE5 inhibitors

AVAILABLE FORMS
Tablets: 50 mg, 100 mg, 200 mg

INDICATIONS & DOSAGES
➤ **Erectile dysfunction**
Adults: 100 mg PO daily as needed 15 minutes before sexual activity. May increase to a maximum of 200 mg daily 15 minutes before sexual activity or decrease to 50 mg daily 30 minutes before sexual activity. Use lowest effective dosage. Maximum, one dose daily.
Adjust-a-dose: In patients taking moderate CYP3A4 inhibitors, maximum dosage is 50 mg PO daily. Don't use in patients taking strong CYP3A4 inhibitors. In patients taking a stable dose of alpha blocker, initially give 50 mg PO daily; adjust as needed and tolerated.

SAFETY ALERT!

avapritinib 🗲
a-va-PRI-ti-nib

Ayvakit

Therapeutic class: Antineoplastics
Pharmacologic class: Tyrosine kinase inhibitors

AVAILABLE FORMS
Tablets: 25 mg, 50 mg, 100 mg, 200 mg, 300 mg

INDICATIONS & DOSAGES
Adjust-a-dose (for all indications): Reduce starting dose to 100 mg once daily for metastatic GI stromal tumor (GIST) or 50 mg for advanced systemic mastocytosis (AdvSM) when giving with moderate CYP3A inhibitor. Refer to manufacturer's instructions for toxicity-related dosage adjustments. Permanently discontinue if patient with GIST can't tolerate 100 mg once daily or if patient with AdvSM can't tolerate 25 mg once daily. There are no dosage recommendations for patients with severe renal impairment, ESRD, or severe hepatic impairment.
➤ **Unresectable or metastatic GIST in patients with *PDGFRA* exon 18 and *PDGFRA* D842V mutations 🗲**
Adults: 300 mg PO once daily. Continue therapy until disease progression or unacceptable toxicity occurs.
➤ **AdvSM**
Adults: 200 mg PO once daily. Continue therapy until disease progression or unacceptable toxicity occurs.

SAFETY ALERT!

avatrombopag maleate
a-va-TROM-boe-PAG

Doptelet

Therapeutic class: Hematopoietics
Pharmacologic class: Thrombopoietin receptor agonists

AVAILABLE FORMS
Tablets: 20 mg

INDICATIONS & DOSAGES
➤ **Thrombocytopenia in patients with chronic liver disease scheduled to undergo a procedure**
Adults: Begin dosing 10 to 13 days before scheduled procedure. For platelet count of 40×10^9/L to less than 50×10^9/L, give 40 mg PO once daily for 5 consecutive days. For platelet count less than 40×10^9/L, give 60 mg PO once daily for 5 consecutive days. Patient should undergo procedure within 5 to 8 days after final dose.
➤ **Chronic immune thrombocytopenia in patients who have had an insufficient response to a previous treatment**
Adults: 20 mg PO once daily. Adjust dosage or frequency of dosing to maintain platelet count of 50×10^9/L or greater. Maximum dosage is 40 mg/day.

SAFETY ALERT!

azaCITIDine
ay-za-SYE-ti deen

Onureg, Vidaza

Therapeutic class: Antineoplastics
Pharmacologic class: Pyrimidine nucleoside analogues

AVAILABLE FORMS
Powder for injection: 100-mg vials
Tablets: 200 mg, 300 mg

INDICATIONS & DOSAGES
Adjust-a-dose (for all indications): Refer to manufacturer's instructions for toxicity-related dosage adjustments.
➤ **Myelodysplastic syndrome, including refractory anemia, refractory anemia with ringed sideroblasts (if patient has neutropenia or thrombocytopenia, or needs transfusions), refractory anemia with excess blasts, refractory anemia with excess blasts in transformation, or chronic myelomonocytic leukemia**
Adults: Initially, 75 mg/m² subcut or IV daily for 7 days; repeat cycle every 4 weeks. May increase to 100 mg/m² if no response after two treatment cycles and nausea and vomiting are the only toxic reactions. Minimum of four treatment cycles are recommended. Continue treatment as long as patient continues to benefit.
➤ **Continued treatment of adults with acute myeloid leukemia who achieved first complete remission or complete remission with incomplete blood**

count recovery following intensive induction chemotherapy and who aren't able to complete intensive curative therapy

Adults: 300 mg PO once daily on days 1 through 14 of each 28-day cycle. Continue until disease progression or unacceptable toxicity occurs. Give an antiemetic before each dose for at least the first two cycles.

✳ **NEW INDICATION: Newly diagnosed juvenile myelomonocytic leukemia (JMML)**

Children age 1 year and older weighing 10 kg or more: 75 mg/m² IV infusion daily for 7 days in a 28-day cycle. Treat for minimum of three cycles and maximum of six cycles.

Children age 1 month to younger than 1 year or weighing less than 10 kg: 2.5 mg/kg IV infusion daily for 7 days in a 28-day cycle. Treat for minimum of three cycles and maximum of six cycles.

Adjust-a-dose: Can consider treatment delays up to 14 days for nonhematologic toxicities. Hematologic toxicity will be difficult to differentiate from natural course of JMML; dosage reduction for hematologic toxicity isn't recommended during first three cycles. Discontinue therapy if neutrophil count is less than 0.5×10^9/L at end of cycle 3 or on day 1 of cycles 5 or 6.

➤ **Acute myeloid leukemia ♦**

Adults: 75 mg/m²/day subcut or IV for 7 days every 4 weeks for at least six cycles. May continue treatment as long as patient continues to benefit or until disease progression or unacceptable toxicity occurs.

---

azelaic acid
aze-eh-LAY-ik

Azelex, Finacea

Therapeutic class: Antiacne drugs
Pharmacologic class: Dicarboxylic acids

AVAILABLE FORMS
Cream: 20%
Foam: 15%
Gel: 15%

INDICATIONS & DOSAGES
➤ **Mild to moderate inflammatory acne vulgaris**
Adults and children age 12 and older: Apply thin film of cream (Azelex) and gently but thoroughly massage into affected areas b.i.d., in morning and evening. Can reduce to once daily if persistent skin irritation occurs.
➤ **Mild to moderate rosacea**
Adults: Apply thin film of foam or gel (Finacea) and gently but thoroughly massage into affected areas b.i.d., in morning and evening. Reassess if no improvement in 12 weeks.

---

azilsartan kamedoxomil
ay-zil-SAR-tan

Edarbi

Therapeutic class: Antihypertensives
Pharmacologic class: ARBs

AVAILABLE FORMS
Tablets: 40 mg, 80 mg

INDICATIONS & DOSAGES
Boxed Warning Drugs that act directly on the renin-angiotensin system can cause fetal harm; when pregnancy is detected, discontinue drug as soon as possible. ∎
➤ **HTN (alone or in combination with other antihypertensives)**
Adults: 80 mg PO once daily.
Adjust-a-dose: For patients treated with high doses of diuretics, consider initiating therapy at 40 mg PO daily.

SAFETY ALERT!

bedaquiline fumarate
bed-AK-wi-leen

Sirturo

Therapeutic class: Antituberculotics
Pharmacologic class: Diarylquinolines

AVAILABLE FORMS
Tablets: 20 mg, 100 mg

INDICATIONS & DOSAGES
Boxed Warning Due to increased risk of death, drug should be reserved for use when an effective treatment regimen can't otherwise be provided. QT-interval prolongation can occur; avoid concomitant drugs that prolong QT interval. ∎
➤ **Pulmonary multidrug-resistant TB as part of combination therapy**
Adults and children age 5 and older weighing at least 30 kg: Weeks 1 and 2, 400 mg PO once daily. Weeks 3 to 24, 200 mg PO three times a week (48 hours between doses) for a total of 600 mg/week.
Children age 5 and older weighing 15 to less than 30 kg: Weeks 1 and 2, 200 mg PO once daily. Weeks 3 to 24, 100 mg PO three times a week (48 hours between doses) for a total of 300 mg/week.
Adjust-a-dose: In first 2 weeks, if a dose is missed, don't make it up but continue the dosing schedule. From 3 weeks on, if a dose is missed, have patient take dose as soon as possible, then resume the three-times-a-week schedule.

SAFETY ALERT!

belinostat ▨
be-LIN-oh-stat

Beleodaq

Therapeutic class: Antineoplastics
Pharmacologic class: Histone deacetylase inhibitors

AVAILABLE FORMS
Injection: 500-mg single-use vial

INDICATIONS & DOSAGES
➤ **Relapsed or refractory peripheral T-cell lymphoma**
Adults: 1,000 mg/m² IV infusion over 30 minutes once daily on days 1 through 5 of a 21-day cycle. Repeat cycles until disease progression or unacceptable toxicity occurs.

Adjust-a-dose: For patients homozygous for the *UGT1A1*28* allele, reduce starting dose to 750 mg/m^2 because drug clearance may be decreased. (This may affect 20% of Blacks, 10% of Whites, and 2% of Asians.) ▨

For patients who are obese, use patient's actual body weight for calculating BSA or weight-based dosing.

Refer to manufacturer's instructions for toxicity-related dosage adjustments.

belumosudil
bel-ue-MOE-soo-dil

Rezurock

Therapeutic class: Immunomodulators
Pharmacologic class: Kinase inhibitors

AVAILABLE FORMS
Tablets ⓓ: 200 mg

INDICATIONS & DOSAGES
➤ **Chronic GVHD after failure of at least two prior lines of systemic therapy**
Adults and children age 12 and older: 200 mg PO daily until progression of chronic GVHD requires new systemic therapy.
Adjust-a-dose: Refer to manufacturer's instructions for toxicity-related dosage adjustments. If drug is used concomitantly with strong CYP3A inducers or PPIs, increase dosage to 200 mg b.i.d.

bempedoic acid ▨
bem-pe-DOE-ik

Nexletol

Therapeutic class: Antilipemics
Pharmacologic class: Adenosine triphosphate-citrate lyase inhibitors

AVAILABLE FORMS
Tablets: 180 mg

INDICATIONS & DOSAGES
➤ **Heterozygous familial hypercholesterolemia or established atherosclerotic CV disease as an adjunct to diet and maximally tolerated statin therapy in patients who require additional lowering of LDL cholesterol** ▨
Adults: 180 mg PO once daily.

SAFETY ALERT!

bendamustine hydrochloride
ben-dah-MOO-steen

Belrapzo, Bendeka, Treanda

Therapeutic class: Antineoplastics
Pharmacologic class: Mechlorethamine derivatives

AVAILABLE FORMS
Injection solution: 100 mg/4 mL in vials
Lyophilized powder for injection: 25 mg, 100 mg in single-use vials

INDICATIONS & DOSAGES
Adjust-a-dose (for all indications): Refer to manufacturer's instructions for dosage adjustments for hematologic and nonhematologic toxicities.
◑ **Alert:** Available formulations have different concentrations; don't mix or combine. See manufacturer's instructions for preparation.
➤ **Chronic lymphocytic leukemia**
Adults: 100 mg/m^2 IV on days 1 and 2 of a 28-day cycle, given for up to six cycles.
➤ **Indolent B-cell non-Hodgkin lymphoma that has progressed during or within 6 months of treatment with rituximab or a rituximab-containing regimen**
Adults: 120 mg/m^2 IV on days 1 and 2 of a 21-day cycle, given for up to eight cycles.

benzonatate
ben-ZOE-na-tate

Therapeutic class: Antitussives
Pharmacologic class: Local anesthetics

AVAILABLE FORMS
Capsules ⓓ: 100 mg, 150 mg, 200 mg

INDICATIONS & DOSAGES
➤ **Symptomatic relief of cough**
Adults and children older than age 10: 100 to 200 mg PO t.i.d. PRN; up to 600 mg daily.

berotralstat ▨
ber-oh-TRAL-stat

Orladeyo

Therapeutic class: Miscellaneous hematologic drugs
Pharmacologic class: Plasma kallikrein inhibitors

AVAILABLE FORMS
Capsules: 110 mg, 150 mg

INDICATIONS & DOSAGES
➤ **Prophylaxis to prevent attacks of hereditary angioedema** ▨
Adults and children age 12 and older: 150 mg PO once daily.
Adjust-a-dose: For patients with moderate or severe hepatic impairment (Child-Pugh class B or C), concomitant use with P-gp or BCRP inhibitors, or persistent GI reactions, decrease dose to 110 mg PO once daily.

betaxolol hydrochloride
beh-TAX-oh-lol

Betoptic S

Therapeutic class: Antiglaucoma drugs–antihypertensives
Pharmacologic class: Beta blockers

AVAILABLE FORMS
Ophthalmic solution: 0.5%
Ophthalmic suspension: 0.25%
Tablets: 10 mg, 20 mg

INDICATIONS & DOSAGES

➤ **Chronic open-angle glaucoma, ocular HTN (ophthalmic only)**

Adults: Instill 1 or 2 drops of solution or 1 drop of suspension in affected eye(s) b.i.d.

➤ **HTN**

Adults: 10 mg PO once daily. May increase dose to 20 mg if desired response isn't achieved after 7 to 14 days.

Adjust-a-dose: To prevent bradycardia, reduce starting dose to 5 mg in older adults. In patients with severe renal impairment and those on dialysis, reduce initial dose to 5 mg daily. May increase dosage by 5 mg/day every 2 weeks to a maximum dose of 20 mg/day. Taper dosage over 2 weeks before discontinuing drug.

SAFETY ALERT!

bexarotene

bex-AR-oh-teen

Targretin

Therapeutic class: Antineoplastics
Pharmacologic class: Retinoids

AVAILABLE FORMS

Capsules: 75 mg
Topical gel: 1%

INDICATIONS & DOSAGES

Boxed Warning Oral drugs in the retinoid class are associated with birth defects in humans; don't give during pregnancy. ∎

Adjust-a-dose (for all indications): Refer to manufacturer's instructions for toxicity-related dosage adjustments.

➤ **Cutaneous manifestations of cutaneous T-cell lymphoma (CTCL) in patients refractory to at least one prior systemic therapy**

Adults: Initially, 300 mg/m² PO once daily. If no tumor response after 8 weeks and if initial dose of 300 mg/m²/day is well tolerated, may increase dosage to 400 mg/m²/day with careful monitoring. Continue until disease progression or unacceptable toxicity occurs.

➤ **Cutaneous lesions in patients with CTCL (Stage IA and IB) with refractory or persistent disease after receiving other therapies or in those who haven't tolerated other therapies**

Adults: Apply sufficient gel to cover lesion with a generous coating. Initially apply once every other day for first week. Increase application frequency at weekly intervals to once daily, then b.i.d., then t.i.d., and finally q.i.d. according to individual lesion tolerance; continue as long as patient derives benefits. Most patients can tolerate a dosing frequency of two to four times per day.

bezlotoxumab

BEZ-loe-tox-ue-mab

Zinplava

Therapeutic class: Toxin binders
Pharmacologic class: Monoclonal antibodies

AVAILABLE FORMS

Injection: 1,000 mg/40 mL (25 mg/mL) in single-dose vials

INDICATIONS & DOSAGES

➤ **To reduce recurrence of *Clostridioides difficile* infection (CDI) in patients receiving antibacterial treatment for CDI and who are at high risk for CDI recurrence**

Adults: 10 mg/kg by IV infusion over 60 minutes as a one-time dose during antibacterial treatment for CDI.

SAFETY ALERT!

bicalutamide

bye-ka-LOO-ta-mide

Casodex

Therapeutic class: Antineoplastics
Pharmacologic class: Androgen receptor inhibitors

AVAILABLE FORMS

Tablets: 50 mg

INDICATIONS & DOSAGES

➤ **Metastatic prostate cancer in combination with a luteinizing hormone-releasing hormone analogue**

Adult males: 50 mg PO once daily.

blinatumomab ▨

blin-a-TOOM-oh-mab

Blincyto

Therapeutic class: Antineoplastics
Pharmacologic class: Monoclonal antibodies

AVAILABLE FORMS

Injection: 35-mcg single-use vial

INDICATIONS & DOSAGES

Boxed Warning Drug can cause fatal cytokine release syndrome and neurologic toxicities. ∎

⊙ *Alert:* Strictly follow instructions for preparation (including admixing) and administration to minimize medication errors.

Adjust-a-dose (for all indications): If the interruption after an adverse event is no longer than 7 days, continue the same cycle to a total of 28 days of infusion inclusive of days before and after the interruption in that cycle. If an interruption due to an adverse event is longer than 7 days, start a new cycle. Refer to manufacturer's instructions for toxicity-related dosage adjustments.

➤ **Relapsed or refractory B-cell precursor acute lymphoblastic leukemia (ALL) ▨**

Adults and children: A treatment course consists of up to two induction cycles followed by three additional consolidation cycles and up to four additional cycles of continued therapy. A single cycle of treatment induction or consolidation consists of 28 days of continuous IV infusion followed by a 14-day treatment-free interval (total 42 days). A single cycle of continued therapy consists of 28 days of continuous IV infusion followed by a 56-day treatment-free interval (total 84 days).

For patients weighing 45 kg or more, for cycle 1, initially give 9 mcg/day by continuous IV infusion on days 1 through 7, then 28 mcg/day by continuous IV infusion on days 8 through 28, followed by a 14-day treatment-free interval (total 42 days). For subsequent induction and consolidation cycles, give 28 mcg/day on days 1 through 28, each cycle followed by a 14-day treatment-free interval (total 42 days). For each cycle of continued therapy, give 28 mcg/day, followed by a 56-day treatment-free interval (total 84 days).

For patients weighing 22 to less than 45 kg, the dose is calculated using patient's BSA. For cycle 1, initially give 5 mcg/m^2/day (not to exceed 9 mcg/day) by continuous IV infusion on days 1 through 7, then 15 mcg/m^2/day (not to exceed 28 mcg/day) by continuous IV infusion on days 8 through 28, followed by a 14-day treatment-free interval (total 42 days). For subsequent induction and consolidation cycles, give 15 mcg/m^2/day (not to exceed 28 mcg/day) on days 1 through 28, each cycle followed by a 14-day treatment-free interval (total 42 days). For each cycle of continued therapy, give 15 mcg/m^2/day (not to exceed 28 mcg/day), followed by a 56-day treatment-free interval (total 84 days). Drug isn't recommended for use in patients weighing less than 22 kg.

➤ **B-cell precursor ALL in first or second complete remission with minimal residual disease greater than or equal to 0.1%**
Adults and children: A treatment course consists of one induction cycle followed by up to three additional cycles for consolidation.

For patients weighing 45 kg or more, the dose for a single cycle of treatment induction or consolidation is 28 mcg/day continuous IV infusion for 28 days, followed by a 14-day treatment-free interval (total 42 days). For patients weighing 22 to less than 45 kg, the dose for a single cycle of treatment induction or consolidation, calculated using patient's BSA, is 15 mcg/m^2/day (not to exceed 28 mcg/day) continuous IV infusion for 28 days, followed by a 14-day treatment-free interval (total 42 days). Drug isn't recommended for use in patients weighing less than 22 kg.

bosutinib ▨
boe-SUE-ti-nib

Bosulif

Therapeutic class: Antineoplastics
Pharmacologic class: Kinase inhibitors

AVAILABLE FORMS
Tablets: ⓄⓉⒸ 100 mg, 400 mg, 500 mg

INDICATIONS & DOSAGES
Adjust-a-dose (for all indications): If CrCl is 30 to 50 mL/minute at start of therapy, give 400 mg once daily for resistant therapy and 300 mg once daily for newly diagnosed chronic phase; if CrCl is less than 30 mL/minute, give 300 mg once daily for resistant therapy and 200 mg once daily for newly diagnosed chronic phase. For preexisting hepatic impairment (Child-Pugh class A, B, or C) at start of therapy, give

200 mg once daily. Refer to manufacturer's instructions for dosage adjustments based on hematologic and nonhematologic toxicities.
➤ **Chronic, accelerated, or blast-phase Philadelphia chromosome–positive (Ph+) chronic myelogenous leukemia (CML) with resistance or intolerance to prior therapy** ▨
Adults: 500 mg PO once daily with food. Consider dosage escalation to 600 mg once daily in patients who don't reach complete hematologic response by week 8 or a complete cytogenetic response by week 12, who didn't have grade 3 or higher adverse reactions, and who are currently taking 500 mg daily.
➤ **Newly diagnosed chronic phase Ph+ CML** ▨
Adults: 400 mg PO once daily with food until disease progression or unacceptable toxicity occurs. Consider dosage escalation by 100-mg increments to a maximum of 600 mg once daily in patients who don't achieve or maintain a hematologic, cytogenetic, or molecular response and who don't have grade 3 or higher adverse reactions at the recommended starting dosage.

bremelanotide
bre-me-LAN-oh-tide

Vyleesi

Therapeutic class: Miscellaneous CNS drugs
Pharmacologic class: Melanocortin receptor agonists

AVAILABLE FORMS
Injection: 1.75 mg/0.3 mL single-dose autoinjector

INDICATIONS & DOSAGES
➤ **Acquired, generalized hypoactive sexual desire disorder in women who are premenopausal**
Adults: 1.75 mg subcut at least 45 minutes before anticipated sexual activity, not to exceed one dose in 24 hours or eight doses in a month. Discontinue drug if patient doesn't report symptom improvement after 8 weeks of treatment.

brexanolone
brex-AN-oh-lone

Zulresso

Therapeutic class: Antidepressants
Pharmacologic class: GABA$_A$ receptor modulators
Controlled substance schedule: IV

AVAILABLE FORMS
Injection: 100 mg/20 mL single-dose vial

INDICATIONS & DOSAGES
Boxed Warning Drug can cause excessive sedation or sudden loss of consciousness. Monitoring is recommended. ▮
➤ **Postpartum depression**
Patients age 15 and older: Give as a continuous IV infusion over a total of 60 hours, titrating dosage as follows: 0 to 4 hours, 30 mcg/kg/hour; 4 to 24 hours, increase infusion rate to 60 mcg/kg/hour; 24 to

52 hours, increase infusion rate to 90 mcg/kg/hour or consider a dosage of 60 mcg/kg/hour if higher infusion rate isn't tolerated; 52 to 56 hours, decrease infusion rate to 60 mcg/kg/hour; 56 to 60 hours, decrease infusion rate to 30 mcg/kg/hour.

Adjust-a-dose: For excessive sedation, stop infusion until symptoms resolve and resume at the same or lower infusion rate.

SAFETY ALERT!

brigatinib ⚕

bri-GA-ti-nib

Alunbrig

Therapeutic class: Antineoplastics
Pharmacologic class: Tyrosine kinase inhibitors

AVAILABLE FORMS

Tablets: 30 mg, 90 mg, 180 mg

INDICATIONS & DOSAGES

➤ **Anaplastic lymphoma kinase–positive metastatic NSCLC** ⚕

Adults: 90 mg PO once daily for 7 days. If tolerated, increase dosage to 180 mg once daily. Continue until disease progression or unacceptable toxicity occurs. If drug is interrupted for 14 days or more for reasons other than toxicity, resume treatment at 90 mg once daily for 7 days before escalating dosage to the previously tolerated dose.

Adjust-a-dose: If concomitant use of a strong CYP3A inhibitor is unavoidable, reduce brigatinib once-daily dose by approximately 50%; if concomitant use of a moderate CYP3A inhibitor is unavoidable, reduce brigatinib once-daily dose by 40%. After a strong or moderate CYP3A inhibitor is discontinued, resume the brigatinib dose that was tolerated before initiating the strong CYP3A inhibitor.

If concomitant use of a moderate CYP3A inducer is unavoidable, increase brigatinib once-daily dose in 30-mg increments after 7 days of treatment with the current brigatinib dose as tolerated, up to a maximum of twice the brigatinib dose that was tolerated before initiating the moderate CYP3A inducer. After discontinuing a moderate CYP3A inducer, resume the brigatinib dose that was tolerated before initiation of the moderate CYP3A inducer.

If CrCl is 15 to 29 mL/minute, reduce dose by about 50%. For severe hepatic impairment (Child-Pugh class C), reduce dose by about 40%.

Refer to manufacturer's instructions for toxicity-related dosage adjustments and drug discontinuation.

brivaracetam

briv-a-RA-se-tam

Briviact

Therapeutic class: Anticonvulsants
Pharmacologic class: Anticonvulsants
Controlled substance schedule: V

AVAILABLE FORMS

Tablets ⊘: 10 mg, 25 mg, 50 mg, 75 mg, 100 mg
Injection: 50 mg/5 mL single-dose vial
Oral solution: 10 mg/mL

INDICATIONS & DOSAGES

➤ **Adjunctive therapy or monotherapy for partial-onset seizures in patients with epilepsy**

Adults and children age 16 and older: Initially, 50 mg PO or IV b.i.d. Titrate dosage to individual patient tolerability and therapeutic response to a minimum dose of 25 mg b.i.d. and a maximum dose of 100 mg b.i.d.

Children age 4 and older weighing 50 kg or more: 25 to 50 mg PO b.i.d. Adjust dosage based on clinical response and tolerability. Minimum dose, 25 mg b.i.d.; maximum dose, 100 mg b.i.d.

Children age 4 and older weighing 20 to less than 50 kg: 0.5 to 1 mg/kg PO b.i.d. Adjust dosage based on clinical response and tolerability. Minimum dose, 0.5 mg/kg b.i.d.; maximum dose, 2 mg/kg b.i.d.

Children age 4 and older weighing 11 to less than 20 kg: 0.5 to 1.25 mg/kg PO b.i.d. Adjust dosage based on clinical response and tolerability. Minimum dose, 0.5 mg/kg b.i.d.; maximum dose, 2.5 mg/kg b.i.d.

Children age 1 month and older weighing 20 to less than 50 kg: 0.5 to 1 mg/kg PO b.i.d. Adjust dosage based on clinical response and tolerability. Minimum dose, 0.5 mg/kg b.i.d.; maximum dose, 2 mg/kg b.i.d.

Children age 1 month and older weighing 11 to less than 20 kg: 0.5 to 1.25 mg/kg PO b.i.d. Adjust dosage based on clinical response and tolerability. Minimum dose, 0.5 mg/kg b.i.d.; maximum dose, 2.5 mg/kg b.i.d.

Children age 1 month and older weighing less than 11 kg: 0.75 to 1.5 mg/kg PO b.i.d. Adjust dosage based on clinical response and tolerability. Minimum dose, 0.75 mg/kg b.i.d.; maximum dose, 3 mg/kg b.i.d.

Adjust-a-dose: Refer to manufacturer's instructions for dosage adjustments in adults and children with hepatic impairment. In patients also taking rifampin, increase brivaracetam dosage by up to 100% (double the dose).

bromocriptine mesylate

broe-moe-KRIP-teen

Cycloset, Parlodel

Therapeutic class: Antiparkinsonian drugs
Pharmacologic class: Dopamine receptor agonists

AVAILABLE FORMS

Capsules: 5 mg
Tablets: 0.8 mg (Cycloset), 2.5 mg (Parlodel)

INDICATIONS & DOSAGES

➤ **Parkinson disease (except Cycloset)**

Adults: 1.25 mg PO b.i.d. with meals. Increase dosage by 2.5 mg/day every 14 to 28 days to lowest dosage producing an optimal therapeutic response. Maximum, 100 mg daily.

➤ **Hyperprolactinemia-associated disorders, including amenorrhea with or without galactorrhea, hypogonadism, or infertility (except Cycloset)**

Adults and adolescents age 16 and older: 1.25 to 2.5 mg PO daily, increased by 2.5 mg daily at 2- to 7-day intervals until desired effect occurs. Usual therapeutic daily dose is 2.5 to 15 mg.

Children ages 11 to 15: 1.25 to 2,5 mg PO daily. May increase as tolerated until therapeutic response is achieved. Range, 2.5 to 10 mg daily in children with prolactin-secreting pituitary adenomas.

➤ **Acromegaly (except Cycloset)**

Adults: 1.25 to 2.5 mg PO with bedtime snack for 3 days. May add another 1.25 to 2.5 mg every 3 to 7 days as tolerated until therapeutic benefit occurs. Maximum, 100 mg daily. Usual therapeutic dose is 20 to 30 mg daily.

➤ **Type 2 diabetes (Cycloset only)**

Adults: Initially, 0.8 mg PO daily within 2 hours after waking in the morning. May increase by 0.8 mg weekly until maximum tolerated dosage of 1.6 to 4.8 mg daily is achieved.

Adjust-a-dose: Dosage shouldn't exceed 1.6 mg once daily during concomitant use of a moderate CYP3A4 inhibitor. Avoid use with strong CYP3A4 inhibitors.

SAFETY ALERT!

busulfan
byoo-SUL-fan

Busulfex, Myleran

Therapeutic class: Antineoplastics
Pharmacologic class: Alkyl sulfonates

AVAILABLE FORMS
Injection: 6 mg/mL
Tablets ⓄⓃⓄ: 2 mg

INDICATIONS & DOSAGES
Boxed Warning Injection causes severe and prolonged myelosuppression at recommended dosage. Hematopoietic progenitor cell transplantation is required to prevent potentially fatal complications. Oral form can induce severe bone marrow hypoplasia. Should only be prescribed by experienced health care professionals. ▪

➤ **Hematopoietic stem-cell conditioning regimen for chronic myelocytic leukemia, in combination with cyclophosphamide**

Adults: 0.8 mg/kg (ideal or actual body weight, whichever is lower) IV over 2 hours every 6 hours for 4 days (a total of 16 doses) beginning 7 days before transplant. Give cyclophosphamide 60 mg/kg IV over 1 hour daily for 2 days beginning no sooner than 6 hours after 16th dose of IV busulfan.

➤ **Palliative treatment of chronic myelogenous (myeloid, myelocytic, granulocytic) leukemia**

Adults: 4 to 8 mg (60 mcg/kg or 1.8 mg/m^2) PO daily until WBC count falls to 15,000/mm^3. Stop drug until WBC count rises to approximately 50,000/mm^3; then resume dosage as before. When remission is shorter than 3 months, may give maintenance therapy of 1 to 3 mg PO daily.

C1 esterase inhibitor subcutaneous (human) 🕱
ES-ter-ase

Berinert, Cinryze, Haegarda

Therapeutic class: Miscellaneous hematologic drugs
Pharmacologic class: Serine protease inhibitors

AVAILABLE FORMS
Injection: 500 international units (Berinert, Cinryze); 2,000 international units, 3,000 international units (Haegarda) in single-use vials packaged with sterile water for injection

INDICATIONS & DOSAGES
➤ **Routine prophylaxis to prevent hereditary angioedema (HAE) attack (except Berinert)** 🕱

Adults and adolescents age 12 and older: 60 international units/kg Haegarda subcut twice weekly (every 3 or 4 days). Or, 1,000 international units Cinryze IV at a rate of 1 mL/minute (10 minutes) every 3 or 4 days. May consider doses up to 2,000 international units (not exceeding 80 units/kg) IV based on individual patient response.

Children age 6 to 11: 60 international units/kg Haegarda subcut twice weekly (every 3 or 4 days). Or, 500 international units Cinryze IV at a rate of 1 mL/minute (5 minutes) every 3 or 4 days. May consider doses up to 1,000 international units IV based on individual patient response.

➤ **Treatment of HAE attack (Berinert only)** 🕱

Adults and children age 6 and older: 20 international units/kg by slow IV injection at a rate of approximately 4 mL/minute.

SAFETY ALERT!

cabazitaxel
ka-baz-ih-TAX-el

Jevtana

Therapeutic class: Antineoplastics
Pharmacologic class: Taxoids

AVAILABLE FORMS
Injection: 60 mg/1.5 mL

INDICATIONS & DOSAGES
Boxed Warning Drug is associated with severe hypersensitivity and neutropenic deaths. Monitor patient and blood cell counts closely and provide appropriate therapy. Contraindicated for use in patients with history of severe hypersensitivity reaction to drug or drugs formulated with polysorbate 80. ▪

➤ **In combination with prednisone for metastatic castration-resistant prostate cancer previously treated with docetaxel-containing treatment regimen**

Adults: 20 mg/m^2 IV over 1 hour every 3 weeks. A dose of 25 mg/m^2 can be used in select patients at the discretion of the treating health care provider. Give oral prednisone 10 mg daily throughout cabazitaxel therapy. Premedicate at least 30 minutes before each dose of cabazitaxel with the following IV medications to reduce risk or severity of hypersensitivity: antihistamine (5 mg dexchlorpheniramine, or 25 mg diphenhydramine or equivalent antihistamine), corticosteroid (8 mg dexamethasone or equivalent steroid), and H₂ antagonist. Antiemetic prophylaxis is recommended and can be given PO or IV as needed.

Adjust-a-dose: Refer to manufacturer's instructions for toxicity-related dosage adjustments, hepatic impairment, and use with strong CYP3A inhibitors.

canakinumab ⚕
kan-ah-KIN-yoo-mab

Ilaris

Therapeutic class: Anti-autoimmune agents
Pharmacologic class: Monoclonal antibodies

AVAILABLE FORMS
Injection: 150 mg in single-use vials

INDICATIONS & DOSAGES
➤ **Cryopyrin-associated periodic syndromes (familial cold autoinflammatory syndrome and Muckle-Wells syndrome)** ⚕
Adults and children age 4 and older weighing more than 40 kg: 150 mg subcut every 8 weeks.
Adults and children age 4 and older weighing 15 to 40 kg: 2 mg/kg subcut every 8 weeks; may increase dosage to 3 mg/kg in children weighing 15 to 40 kg who have an inadequate response.
➤ **Still disease (adult-onset and active systemic juvenile idiopathic arthritis)** ⚕
Children age 2 and older weighing at least 7.5 kg: 4 mg/kg subcut every 4 weeks. Maximum dose is 300 mg.
➤ **TNF receptor-associated periodic syndrome; hyperimmunoglobulin D syndrome/mevalonate kinase deficiency; familial Mediterranean fever** ⚕
Adults and children age 2 and older weighing more than 40 kg: Initially, 150 mg subcut every 4 weeks; may increase to 300 mg every 4 weeks if clinical response is inadequate.
Adults and children age 2 and older weighing 15 to 40 kg: Initially, 2 mg/kg subcut every 4 weeks; may increase dosage to 4 mg/kg every 4 weeks if clinical response isn't adequate.

cannabidiol
kan-a-bi-DYE-ol

Epidiolex

Therapeutic class: Anticonvulsants
Pharmacologic class: Cannabinoids
Controlled substance schedule: V

AVAILABLE FORMS
Oral solution: 100 mg/mL

INDICATIONS & DOSAGES
➤ **Seizures associated with Lennox-Gastaut syndrome, Dravet syndrome, or tuberous sclerosis complex (TSC)**

Adults and children age 1 and older: Initially, 2.5 mg/kg PO b.i.d. After 1 week, increase to a maintenance dosage of 5 mg/kg PO b.i.d. If necessary, may further increase dose, as tolerated, in weekly increments of 2.5 mg/kg b.i.d. to a maximum maintenance dosage of 10 mg/kg b.i.d. for Lennox-Gastaut syndrome and Dravet syndrome, or 12.5 mg/kg b.i.d. for TSC. For patients in whom a more rapid titration is warranted, may increase dosage no more frequently than every other day.

Adjust-a-dose: For moderate hepatic impairment (Child-Pugh class B), initiate therapy at 1.25 mg/kg PO b.i.d. Increase to maintenance dose of 5 mg/kg or 6.25 mg/kg for tuberous sclerosis complex (TSC) PO b.i.d. For severe hepatic impairment (Child-Pugh class C), initiate therapy at 0.5 mg/kg PO b.i.d. Increase to maintenance dose of 2.5 mg/kg PO b.i.d. Discontinue drug in patients with transaminase elevations greater than $3 \times$ ULN and bilirubin levels greater than $2 \times$ ULN, and in those with sustained transaminase elevations greater than $5 \times$ ULN.

SAFETY ALERT!

capmatinib ⚕
kap-MA-ti-nib

Tabrecta

Therapeutic class: Antineoplastics
Pharmacologic class: Kinase inhibitors

AVAILABLE FORMS
Tablets ⊙: 150 mg, 200 mg

INDICATIONS & DOSAGES
➤ **Metastatic NSCLC in patients whose tumors have a mutation that leads to mesenchymal-epithelial transition exon 14 skipping as detected by an FDA-approved test** ⚕
Adults: 400 mg PO b.i.d.

Adjust-a-dose: If adverse reactions occur, lower dosage to 300 mg PO b.i.d. for first dosage reduction, and 200 mg PO b.i.d. for a second dosage reduction. Permanently discontinue drug in patients unable to tolerate 200 mg PO b.i.d. See manufacturer's instructions for specific dosage reductions due to severity of adverse reactions.

carboprost tromethamine
KAR-boe-prost

Hemabate

Therapeutic class: Oxytocics
Pharmacologic class: Prostaglandins

AVAILABLE FORMS
Injection: 250 mcg/mL

INDICATIONS & DOSAGES
Boxed Warning Strictly adhere to recommended dosages and only use in a hospital that can provide immediate intensive and acute surgical care. ∎
➤ **To terminate pregnancy between weeks 13 and 20 of gestation**
Adults: Initially, 250 mcg deep IM; optionally, a 100-mcg IM test dose may be given. Give subsequent

doses of 250 mcg at intervals of 1.5 to 3.5 hours, depending on uterine response. Dosage may be increased in increments of 500 mcg if contractility is inadequate after several 250-mcg doses. Total dose shouldn't exceed 12 mg or continuous administration for more than 2 days.

➤ **Refractory postpartum hemorrhage**
Adults: 250 mcg by deep IM injection. Repeat doses every 15 to 90 minutes as needed. Maximum total dose is 2 mg (eight doses).

SAFETY ALERT!

carfilzomib
car-FIL-zoe-mib

Kyprolis

Therapeutic class: Antineoplastics
Pharmacologic class: Proteasome inhibitors

AVAILABLE FORMS
Powder for injection: 10 mg, 30 mg, 60 mg in single-use vials

INDICATIONS & DOSAGES
◑ *Alert:* See manufacturer's instructions for administration precautions.

➤ **Relapsed or refractory multiple myeloma**
Adults: Calculate dosage using patient's actual BSA at baseline. In patients with BSA greater than 2.2 m², calculate dosage based on BSA of 2.2 m². For monotherapy, 20 mg/m² IV over 10 minutes on 2 consecutive days each week for 3 weeks (days 1, 2, 8, 9, 15, and 16), followed by 12-day rest period (days 17 to 28). If tolerated, may increase to 27 mg/m² in cycle 1 days 8, 9, 15, and 16 and to 27 mg/m² for subsequent cycles. From cycle 13 on, omit day 8 and 9 doses.

Or, 20 mg/m² IV over 30 minutes on 2 consecutive days each week for 3 weeks (days 1, 2, 8, 9, 15, 16), followed by 12-day rest period (days 17 to 28). If tolerated, may increase to 56 mg/m² in cycle 1 days 8, 9, 15, and 16 and to 56 mg/m² for subsequent cycles. From cycle 13 on, omit day 8 and 9 doses. Treatment may continue until disease progression or unacceptable toxicity occurs.

For the combination regimens, refer to manufacturer's instructions

Adjust-a-dose: Refer to manufacturer's instructions for dosage adjustments based on toxicities.

carisoprodol
kar-eye-soe-PROE-dol

Soma✔

Therapeutic class: Skeletal muscle relaxants
Pharmacologic class: Carbamate derivatives
Controlled substance schedule: IV

AVAILABLE FORMS
Tablets: 250 mg, 350 mg

INDICATIONS & DOSAGES
➤ **Relief of discomfort associated with acute, painful musculoskeletal conditions**

Adults: 250 to 350 mg PO t.i.d. and at bedtime for a maximum of 2 to 3 weeks.

cefiderocol
sef-i-DER-oh-kol

Fetroja

Therapeutic class: Antibiotics
Pharmacologic class: Cephalosporins

AVAILABLE FORMS
Injection: 1-g vials

INDICATIONS & DOSAGES
Adjust-a-dose (for all indications): If CrCl is 120 mL/minute or greater, give 2-g IV infusion every 6 hours; if CrCl is 30 to 59 mL/minute, give 1.5-g IV infusion every 8 hours; if CrCl is 15 to 29 mL/minute, give 1-g IV infusion every 8 hours; if CrCl is less than 15 mL/minute, give 0.75-g IV infusion every 12 hours. Refer to manufacturer's instructions for patients receiving continuous renal replacement therapy.

➤ **Complicated UTI caused by *Escherichia coli, Klebsiella pneumoniae, Proteus mirabilis, Pseudomonas aeruginosa,* and *Enterobacter cloacae* complex in patients with limited or no other treatment options**
Adults: 2-g IV infusion every 8 hours given over 3 hours. Recommended duration is 7 to 14 days.

➤ **Hospital-acquired bacterial pneumonia and ventilator-associated bacterial pneumonia caused by *Acinetobacter baumannii* complex, *E. coli, E. cloacae* complex, *K. pneumoniae, P. aeruginosa,* and *Serratia marcescens***
Adults: 2-g IV infusion every 8 hours given over 3 hours. Recommended duration is 7 to 14 days.

cefOXitin sodium
se-FOKS-i-tin

Therapeutic class: Antibiotics
Pharmacologic class: Second-generation cephalosporins

AVAILABLE FORMS
Infusion: 1 g, 2 g

INDICATIONS & DOSAGES
Adjust-a-dose (for all indications): For adults with renal insufficiency, give loading dose of 1 to 2 g. For adults with CrCl of 30 to 50 mL/minute, give 1 to 2 g every 8 to 12 hours; if CrCl is 10 to 29 mL/minute, 1 to 2 g every 12 to 24 hours; if CrCl is 5 to 9 mL/minute, 0.5 to 1 g every 12 to 24 hours; and if CrCl is less than 5 mL/minute, 0.5 to 1 g every 24 to 48 hours. For patients receiving hemodialysis, give a loading dose of 1 to 2 g after each hemodialysis session; then give the maintenance dose based on creatinine level. For patients receiving continuous ambulatory peritoneal dialysis, give 1 g every 24 hours.

➤ **Serious infection of the respiratory or GU tracts; gynecologic, skin, soft-tissue, bone, or joint infection; bloodstream or intra-abdominal infection caused by susceptible organisms (such** as *Escherichia coli* and other coliform bacteria, penicillinase- and non–penicillinase-producing *Staphylococcus aureus, Staphylococcus epidermidis,* streptococci, *Klebsiella, Haemophilus influenzae, Neisseria gonorrhoeae, Clostridium* species, *Peptococcus niger, Peptostreptococcus* species, and *Bacteroides,* including *B. fragilis*)

Adults: 1 to 2 g IV every 6 to 8 hours for uncomplicated infections. May use up to 12 g daily in life-threatening infections.

Children older than age 3 months: 80 to 160 mg/kg daily IV in four to six equally divided doses. Maximum daily dose, 12 g.

➤ **Perioperative prophylaxis**

Adults: 2 g IV 30 to 60 minutes before initial surgical incision; then 2 g IV every 6 hours for up to 24 hours. For patients undergoing cesarean section, give 2 g IV as soon as the umbilical cord is clamped; may give additional 2-g doses 4 and 8 hours after initial dose.

Children age 3 months and older: 30 to 40 mg/kg IV 30 to 60 minutes before initial surgical incision; then 30 to 40 mg/kg every 6 hours for up to 24 hours.

ceftaroline fosamil
sef-TAR-oh-leen

Teflaro

Therapeutic class: Antibiotics
Pharmacologic class: Fifth-generation cephalosporins

AVAILABLE FORMS
Injection: 400 mg, 600 mg in single-use vials

INDICATIONS & DOSAGES
➤ **Acute bacterial skin and skin-structure infections caused by susceptible isolates of *Staphylococcus aureus, Streptococcus pyogenes, Streptococcus agalactiae, Escherichia coli, Klebsiella pneumoniae,* or *Klebsiella oxytoca;* community-acquired bacterial pneumonia (CABP) caused by susceptible isolates of *Streptococcus pneumoniae, S. aureus, Haemophilus influenzae, K. pneumoniae, K. oxytoca,* or *E. coli***

Adults: 600 mg IV over 5 to 60 minutes every 12 hours. For skin and skin-structure infections, continue treatment for 5 to 14 days; for CABP, continue treatment for 5 to 7 days.

Children older than age 2 and younger than 18 weighing more than 33 kg: 400 mg IV every 8 hours or 600 mg IV every 12 hours for 5 to 14 days.

Children older than age 2 and younger than 18 weighing 33 kg or less: 12 mg/kg IV every 8 hours for 5 to 14 days.

Children age 2 months to younger than 2 years: 8 mg/kg IV every 8 hours for 5 to 14 days.

Adjust-a-dose: For adults with CrCl of 31 to 50 mL/minute, give 400 mg IV every 12 hours. If CrCl is 15 to 30 mL/minute, give 300 mg IV every 12 hours. For patients with ESRD, including those on hemodialysis, give 200 mg IV every 12 hours. Administer after dialysis treatment.

➤ **Acute bacterial skin and skin-structure infections caused by susceptible isolates of *Staphylococcus aureus, Streptococcus pyogenes, Streptococcus agalactiae, Escherichia coli, Klebsiella pneumoniae,* or *Klebsiella oxytoca***

Infants with gestational age of at least 34 weeks and postnatal age of at least 12 days to less than 2 months: 6 mg/kg IV infusion over 30 to 60 minutes every 8 hours for 5 to 14 days.

cenobamate
sen-oh-BAM-ate

Xcopri

Therapeutic class: Anticonvulsants
Pharmacologic class: Anticonvulsants
Controlled substance schedule: V

AVAILABLE FORMS
Tablets ⊕*:* 12.5 mg, 25 mg, 50 mg, 100 mg, 150 mg, 200 mg

INDICATIONS & DOSAGES
➤ **Partial-onset seizures**

Adults: Initially, 12.5 mg PO once daily on weeks 1 and 2; then 25 mg once daily weeks 3 and 4; 50 mg once daily weeks 5 and 6; 100 mg once daily weeks 7 and 8; and 150 mg once daily weeks 9 and 10. Maintenance dose of 200 mg once daily at week 11. If necessary, may increase dosage above 200 mg by increments of 50 mg once daily every 2 weeks to a maximum of 400 mg.

Adjust-a-dose: In patients with mild to moderate hepatic impairment (Child-Pugh class A or B), maximum dose is 200 mg once daily. Consider dosage reduction in patients with mild to severe renal impairment. If phenytoin is used concomitantly, gradually decrease phenytoin dosage by up to 50% as cenobamate is being increased. Avoid abrupt withdrawal; gradually reduce dosage over at least 2 weeks if discontinuing drug.

SAFETY ALERT!

ceritinib ⊠
se-RI-ti-nib

Zykadia

Therapeutic class: Antineoplastics
Pharmacologic class: Kinase inhibitors

AVAILABLE FORMS
Tablets: 150 mg

INDICATIONS & DOSAGES
➤ **Anaplastic lymphoma kinase-positive metastatic NSCLC ⊠**

Adults: 450 mg PO once daily with food until disease progression or unacceptable toxicity occurs.

Adjust-a-dose: Refer to manufacturer's instructions for toxicity-related dosage adjustments and discontinuation.

🍁Canada   ◇OTC   ◆Off-label use   🖉Photoguide   ⊕Do not crush   *Liquid contains alcohol   ⊠Genetic

cetrorelix acetate
set-roe-REL-iks

Cetrotide

Therapeutic class: Infertility drugs
Pharmacologic class: Gonadotropin-releasing hormone antagonists

AVAILABLE FORMS
Powder for injection: 0.25 mg

INDICATIONS & DOSAGES
➤ **To inhibit premature luteinizing hormone surges in patients undergoing controlled ovarian stimulation**

Adults: Ovarian stimulation therapy with gonadotropins is started on cycle day 2 or 3. Give cetrorelix acetate 0.25 mg subcut on stimulation day 5 (morning or evening) or day 6 (morning), and continue once daily until day of hCG administration.

cevimeline hydrochloride
seh-vih-MEH-leen

Evoxac

Therapeutic class: Cholinergic agonists
Pharmacologic class: Cholinergic agonists

AVAILABLE FORMS
Capsules: 30 mg

INDICATIONS & DOSAGES
➤ **Dry mouth in patients with Sjögren syndrome**
Adults: 30 mg PO t.i.d.

SAFETY ALERT!

chlorambucil
klor-AM-byoo-sill

Leukeran

Therapeutic class: Antineoplastics
Pharmacologic class: Nitrogen mustards

AVAILABLE FORMS
Tablets: 2 mg

INDICATIONS & DOSAGES
Boxed Warning Drug can severely suppress bone marrow function; is a carcinogen, and probably mutagenic and teratogenic; and produces human infertility. ∎

➤ **Chronic lymphocytic leukemia; malignant lymphomas, including lymphosarcoma, giant follicular lymphoma, and Hodgkin lymphoma**
Adults: For initiation of therapy or for short courses of treatment, 0.1 to 0.2 mg/kg PO daily for 3 to 6 weeks (usually 4 to 10 mg daily). Maintenance dosage shouldn't exceed 0.1 mg/kg/day and may be as low as 0.03 mg/kg/day. Adjust dosage according to patient response; reduce when WBC count falls abruptly. For intermittent dosing schedule, give initial single dose of 0.4 mg/kg. Then give doses at biweekly or monthly intervals, increasing by 0.1-mg/kg increments until lymphocytosis is controlled or toxicity occurs.

Adjust-a-dose: Reduce first dose if given within 4 weeks after a full course of radiation therapy or myelosuppressive drugs, or if pretreatment WBC or platelet count is depressed from bone marrow disease.

chloramphenicol sodium succinate
klor-am-FEN-i-kole

Therapeutic class: Antibiotics
Pharmacologic class: Dichloroacetic acid derivatives

AVAILABLE FORMS
Injection: 1-g vials

INDICATIONS & DOSAGES
Boxed Warning Drug is associated with serious and fatal blood dyscrasias. Use alternative therapies when possible. Patient should be hospitalized during therapy to closely monitor blood lab levels. ∎
➤ ***Haemophilus influenzae* meningitis, acute *Salmonella typhi* infection, and meningitis, bacteremia, or other severe infections caused by sensitive *Salmonella* species, rickettsia, lymphogranuloma, psittacosis, or various sensitive gram-negative organisms**
Adults: 50 mg/kg IV daily, divided every 6 hours. Increased dosage, up to 100 mg/kg daily, may be needed.
Full-term infants older than age 2 weeks with normal metabolic processes and children: Up to 50 mg/kg IV daily, divided every 6 hours. May use up to 100 mg/kg/day in four divided doses for bacteremia or meningitis; reduce to 50 mg/kg/day as soon as possible.
Neonates age 2 weeks and younger: 25 mg/kg IV daily divided every 6 hours.
Preterm infants, and children and infants with suspected immature metabolic processes: 25 mg/kg IV once daily.
Adjust-a-dose: For patients with renal or hepatic impairment, excessive blood levels may result from administration of the recommended dosage. Determine drug blood concentration at appropriate intervals and adjust dosage accordingly.

SAFETY ALERT!

chlordiazePOXIDE hydrochloride
klor-dye-az-e-POX-ide

Therapeutic class: Anxiolytics
Pharmacologic class: Benzodiazepines
Controlled substance schedule: IV

AVAILABLE FORMS
Capsules: 5 mg, 10 mg, 25 mg

INDICATIONS & DOSAGES
Boxed Warning Benzodiazepine use exposes patient to risks of abuse, misuse, and addiction, which can lead to overdose or death. Benzodiazepine use with opioids can cause sedation and fatal respiratory depression. ∎

✦Canada ◇OTC ◆Off-label use ✐Photoguide ⓓⓝⓒDo not crush *Liquid contains alcohol ▨Genetic

Boxed Warning Abrupt discontinuation or rapid dosage reduction of benzodiazepines after continued use may precipitate acute and life-threatening withdrawal reactions. To reduce risk, gradually taper drug to discontinue or reduce dosage. ■

Adjust-a-dose (for all indications): In older adults or patients who are debilitated, give 5 mg PO b.i.d. to q.i.d. Use smallest effective dose, to prevent oversedation or ataxia.

➤ **Mild to moderate anxiety**
Adults: 5 to 10 mg PO t.i.d. or q.i.d.
Children older than age 6: 5 mg PO b.i.d. to q.i.d. Maximum, 10 mg PO b.i.d. or t.i.d.

➤ **Severe anxiety**
Adults: 20 to 25 mg PO t.i.d. or q.i.d.

➤ **Withdrawal symptoms of acute alcoholism**
Adults: 50 to 100 mg PO. Repeat as needed, up to 300 mg daily.

➤ **Preoperative apprehension and anxiety**
Adults: 5 to 10 mg PO t.i.d. or q.i.d. on days before surgery.

chlorproMAZINE hydrochloride
klor-PROE-ma-zeen

Therapeutic class: Antipsychotics
Pharmacologic class: Phenothiazines

AVAILABLE FORMS
Injection: 25 mg/mL
Oral solution: 30 mg/mL, 100 mg/mL
Tablets: 10 mg, 25 mg, 50 mg, 100 mg, 200 mg

INDICATIONS & DOSAGES
Boxed Warning Older adults with dementia-related psychosis treated with antipsychotics are at an increased risk of death. Drug isn't approved to treat these patients. ■

➤ **Psychosis, mania**
Adults and children older than age 12: For patients with acute disease who are hospitalized, 25 mg IM; may give an additional 25 to 50 mg IM in 1 hour if needed. Increase over several days to 400 mg every 4 to 6 hours for severe cases. Switch to oral therapy as soon as possible. Or, 25 mg PO t.i.d. initially; then gradually increase to 500 mg (400 mg in patients less acutely disturbed) daily in divided doses. For outpatients, 30 to 75 mg daily in two to four divided doses. Increase dosage by 20 to 50 mg twice weekly until symptoms are controlled.

➤ **Nausea and vomiting**
Adults and children older than age 12: 10 to 25 mg PO every 4 to 6 hours PRN. Or, 25 mg IM initially. If no hypotension occurs, may give 25 to 50 mg IM every 3 to 4 hours PRN, until vomiting stops. Or, during surgery, may give 12.5 mg IM, repeated in 30 minutes if needed, or fractional 2-mg doses IV at 2-minute intervals to maximum dose of 25 mg.
Children ages 6 months to 12 years: 0.55 mg/kg PO every 4 to 6 hours or IM every 6 to 8 hours PRN. Maximum IM dose in children younger than age 5 or weighing less than 23 kg is 40 mg. Maximum IM

dose in children ages 5 to 12 or weighing 23 to 45 kg is 75 mg.

➤ **Acute intermittent porphyria, intractable hiccups**
Adults and children older than age 12: 25 to 50 mg PO t.i.d. or q.i.d. If hiccups persist for 2 to 3 days on oral therapy, give 25 to 50 mg IM. If hiccups still persist, give 25 to 50 mg diluted in 500 to 1,000 mL of NSS and infused slowly with patient in supine position. For porphyria, give 25 mg IM t.i.d. or q.i.d. until patient can take oral therapy.

➤ **Tetanus**
Adults and children older than age 12: 25 to 50 mg IV or IM t.i.d. or q.i.d.
Children ages 6 months to 12 years: 0.55 mg/kg IM or IV every 6 to 8 hours. Maximum parenteral dosage in children weighing less than 23 kg is 40 mg daily; for children weighing 23 to 45 kg, may give 75 mg, except in severe cases. If giving IV, dilute to 1 mg/mL with NSS and administer at a rate of 0.5 mg/minute.

➤ **Behavioral disorders, hyperactivity**
Children ages 6 months to 12 years: For outpatients, 0.55 mg/kg PO every 4 to 6 hours or IM every 6 to 8 hours, as needed. For patients who are hospitalized, start with low oral doses and increase gradually. In severe behavioral disorders, 50 to 100 mg PO daily or, in older children, 200 mg/day or more PO may be necessary. There is little evidence that improvement in patients who are severely disturbed and intellectually disabled is enhanced by doses beyond 500 mg/day. In patients age 5 or younger or weighing less than 23 kg who are hospitalized, don't exceed 40 mg/day IM. In children ages 5 to 12 weighing 23 to 45 kg, don't exceed 75 mg/day IM, except in unmanageable cases.

➤ **Preoperative sedation, anxiety**
Adults and children older than age 12: Preoperatively, 25 to 50 mg PO 2 to 3 hours before surgery or 12.5 to 25 mg IM 1 to 2 hours before surgery.
Children ages 6 months to 12 years: Preoperatively, 0.55 mg/kg PO 2 to 3 hours before surgery or IM 1 to 2 hours before surgery.
Older adults: Lower dosages are sufficient; dosage increments should be more gradual than in younger adults.

chlorthalidone
klor-THAL-i-done

Thalitone

Therapeutic class: Antihypertensives
Pharmacologic class: Thiazide diuretics

AVAILABLE FORMS
Tablets: 15 mg, 25 mg, 50 mg

INDICATIONS & DOSAGES
➤ **Edema**
Adults: 50 to 100 mg PO daily, or 100 mg PO on alternating days (maximum, 200 mg/day).

➤ **HTN**
Adults: 15 to 25 mg PO daily.

cholestyramine
koe-LESS-tir-a-meen

Prevalite, Questran, Questran Light

Therapeutic class: Antilipemics
Pharmacologic class: Bile acid sequestrants

AVAILABLE FORMS
Powder for oral suspension: 4-g single-dose packets; multidose cans with each level scoop equivalent to 4 g of cholestyramine resin

INDICATIONS & DOSAGES
➤ **Primary hyperlipidemia or pruritus caused by partial bile obstruction; adjunct for reduction of increased cholesterol level in patients with primary hypercholesterolemia**
Adults: 4 g PO once daily or b.i.d. Maintenance dose is 8 to 16 g daily divided into two doses. Maximum daily dose is 24 g.
Children: 240 mg/kg/day PO in two to three divided doses, not to exceed 8 g/day.

SAFETY ALERT!

cidofovir
sye-DOE-fo-veer

Therapeutic class: Antivirals
Pharmacologic class: Nucleosides–nucleotides

AVAILABLE FORMS
Injection: 75 mg/mL

INDICATIONS & DOSAGES
Boxed Warning Cidofovir is indicated only for the treatment of CMV retinitis in patients with AIDS. ∎
➤ **CMV retinitis in patients with AIDS**
Adults: Initially, 5 mg/kg IV infused over 1 hour once weekly for 2 consecutive weeks; then maintenance dose of 5 mg/kg IV infused over 1 hour once every 2 weeks. Give probenecid and prehydration with IV NSS simultaneously to reduce risk of nephrotoxicity.
Adjust-a-dose: For patients with creatinine level of 0.3 to 0.4 mg/dL above baseline, reduce dosage to 3 mg/kg at same rate and frequency. If creatinine level reaches 0.5 mg/dL or more above baseline, or patient develops 3+ or higher proteinuria, stop drug.

Don't start drug if serum creatinine level is more than 1.5 mg/dL, CrCl is 55 mL/minute or less, or urine protein level is 100 mg/dL or more (at least 2+ proteinuria).

ciprofloxacin hydrochloride (otic)
si-proe-FLOX-a-sin

Cetraxal, Otiprio

Therapeutic class: Antibiotics
Pharmacologic class: Fluoroquinolones

AVAILABLE FORMS
Otic solution: 0.2% (5 mg in 0.25-mL single-use container)

Suspension, intratympanic: 6% (60 mg/1-mL single-use vial)

INDICATIONS & DOSAGES
➤ **Acute otitis externa caused by susceptible isolates of *Pseudomonas aeruginosa* or *Staphylococcus aureus***
Adults and children age 1 and older: Instill 0.5 mg (0.25 mL) of 0.2% solution (contents of one single-dose container) into affected ear b.i.d. for 7 days.
Adults and children age 6 months and older: Instill 12 mg (0.2 mL) of 6% suspension into affected ear as a single dose.
➤ **Bilateral otitis media with effusion at time of tympanostomy tube placement**
Children age 6 months and older: 0.1 mL (6 mg) of 6% suspension into each affected ear after suctioning of middle ear effusion.

SAFETY ALERT!

cladribine
KLA-dri-been

Mavenclad

Therapeutic class: Immunomodulators
Pharmacologic class: Purine antimetabolites

AVAILABLE FORMS
Tablets ⓒ: 10 mg

INDICATIONS & DOSAGES
Boxed Warning Drug can cause fetal harm; use is contraindicated in adults of reproductive potential who don't plan to use effective contraception. Drug can increase risk of malignancy; use is contraindicated in patients with current malignancy. ∎
➤ **Relapsing forms of MS, including relapsing-remitting disease and active secondary progressive disease, in patients who have had inadequate response to, or are unable to tolerate, other MS therapies**
Adults weighing 40 kg or more: 3.5 mg/kg PO over 2 years, administered as 1.75 mg/kg each year. Divide the 1.75-mg/kg dose over two cycles, each lasting 4 to 5 consecutive days. Don't administer more than 2 tablets (20 mg) daily. For first year of treatment, start first cycle at any time. Administer second cycle 23 to 27 days after last dose of first cycle. For second year of treatment, start first cycle at least 43 weeks after last dose of first year's second cycle. Administer second cycle 23 to 27 days after last dose of second year's first cycle. Following 2 years of treatment, don't administer additional doses of drug during the next 2 years.
Adjust-a-dose: Lymphocytes must be within normal limits before start of treatment. Lymphocyte count must be at least 800 cells/mm³ before start of second treatment course. If needed, delay second treatment course for up to 6 months to allow lymphocyte recovery to at least 800 cells/mm³. If this recovery takes more than 6 months, discontinue treatment.

cloBAZam ⚥
KLOE-ba-zam

Onfi, Sympazan

Therapeutic class: Anticonvulsants
Pharmacologic class: Benzodiazepines
Controlled substance schedule: IV

AVAILABLE FORMS
Oral film: 5 mg, 10 mg, 20 mg
Oral suspension: 2.5 mg/mL
Tablets: 10 mg, 20 mg

INDICATIONS & DOSAGES
Boxed Warning Benzodiazepine use exposes patient to risks of abuse, misuse, and addiction, which can lead to overdose or death. Benzodiazepine use with opioids can cause sedation and fatal respiratory depression. ■
Boxed Warning Abrupt discontinuation or rapid dosage reduction of benzodiazepines after continued use may precipitate acute and life-threatening withdrawal reactions. To reduce risk, gradually taper drug to discontinue or reduce dosage. ■
➤ **Adjunctive treatment of seizures associated with Lennox-Gastaut syndrome**
Adults and children age 2 and older weighing more than 30 kg: Initially, 5 mg PO b.i.d. for 6 days. On day 7, increase to 10 mg PO b.i.d.; on day 14, titrate to 20 mg PO b.i.d. as tolerated. Dosage escalation shouldn't proceed more rapidly than weekly. Maximum dose is 40 mg/day.
Adults and children age 2 and older weighing 30 kg or less: Initially, 5 mg PO once daily for 6 days. On day 7, increase to 5 mg PO b.i.d.; on day 14, titrate to 10 mg PO b.i.d. as tolerated. Dosage escalation shouldn't proceed more rapidly than weekly. Maximum dose is 20 mg/day.
⚥ *Adjust-a-dose:* For older adults, patients with mild to moderate hepatic impairment (Child-Pugh score of 5 to 9), and those who are poor CYP2C19 metabolizers, initially 5 mg PO daily for 1 week; then titrate according to weight but at half the recommended dose as tolerated. If necessary, may start an additional titration to maximum dosage (20 or 40 mg/day depending on weight) on day 21.

clomiPHENE citrate
KLOE-mi-feen

Therapeutic class: Ovulation stimulants
Pharmacologic class: Chlorotrianisene derivatives

AVAILABLE FORMS
Tablets: 50 mg

INDICATIONS & DOSAGES
➤ **Ovulatory dysfunction**
Adults: 50 mg PO daily for 5 days, starting on day 5 of menstrual cycle (first day of menstrual flow is day 1) if bleeding occurs, or at any time if patient hasn't had recent uterine bleeding. If ovulation doesn't occur, may increase dosage to 100 mg PO daily for 5 days

as soon as 30 days after first course. Repeat until conception occurs or until three courses of therapy are completed.

clomiPRAMINE hydrochloride
kloe-MI-pra-meen

Anafranil

Therapeutic class: Antidepressants
Pharmacologic class: TCAs

AVAILABLE FORMS
Capsules: 25 mg, 50 mg, 75 mg

INDICATIONS & DOSAGES
Boxed Warning Drug increases risk of suicidality in children, adolescents, and young adults. ■
➤ **OCD**
Adults: Initially, 25 mg PO daily with meals, gradually increased to 100 mg/day in divided doses during first 2 weeks. Thereafter, increase every 2 to 3 weeks to maximum dose of 250 mg/day in divided doses with meals, as needed. After adjustment, may give total daily dose at bedtime.
Children age 10 and older and adolescents: Initially, 25 mg PO daily with meals, gradually increased over first 2 weeks to maximum of 3 mg/kg daily or 100 mg PO daily in divided doses, whichever is smaller. Maximum daily dose is 3 mg/kg or 200 mg, whichever is smaller; give at bedtime after adjustment.
Adjust-a-dose: Reassess and adjust dosage periodically to maintain patient on lowest effective dosage.

SAFETY ALERT!

cobimetinib fumarate ⚥
koe-bi-ME-ti-nib

Cotellic

Therapeutic class: Antineoplastics
Pharmacologic class: Kinase inhibitors

AVAILABLE FORMS
Tablets ⓓⓒ: 20 mg

INDICATIONS & DOSAGES
➤ **Unresectable or metastatic melanoma with a *BRAF* V600E or V600K mutation in combination with vemurafenib** ⚥
Adults: 60 mg PO once daily for first 21 days of each 28-day treatment cycle until disease progression or unacceptable toxicity occurs.
Adjust-a-dose: Refer to manufacturer's instructions for toxicity-related dosage adjustments.

colesevelam hydrochloride ⚥
koe-leh-SEVE-eh-lam

Welchol🗸

Therapeutic class: Antilipemics
Pharmacologic class: Bile acid sequestrants

AVAILABLE FORMS
Powder for oral suspension: 3.75-g packets
Tablets: 625 mg

🍁Canada ◇OTC ◆Off-label use 🗸Photoguide ⓓⓒDo not crush *Liquid contains alcohol ⚥Genetic

INDICATIONS & DOSAGES

➤ Adjunct to diet and exercise to reduce elevated LDL cholesterol (LDL-C) in patients with primary hyperlipidemia; to reduce LDL-C in children who are postmenarchal with heterozygous familial hypercholesterolemia and unable to reach LDL-C target levels despite adequate trial of diet and lifestyle modification ▨

Adults: 3 tablets (1,875 mg) PO b.i.d. or 6 tablets (3,750 mg) PO once daily. Or, one 3.75-g packet PO once daily.

Children ages 10 to 17: One 3.75-g packet PO once daily.

➤ Adjunct to diet and exercise to improve glycemic control in type 2 diabetes

Adults: 3 tablets (1,875 mg) PO b.i.d. or 6 tablets (3,750 mg) PO once daily. Or, one 3.75-g packet PO once daily.

BIOSIMILAR DRUG

collagenase *Clostridium histolyticum*
kuh-LAJ-eh-nase klos-TRID-ee-um hiss-toe-LIH-teh-kum

Xiaflex

collagenase *Clostridium histolyticum*-aaes
QWO

Therapeutic class: Anticollagen drugs
Pharmacologic class: Enzymes

AVAILABLE FORMS
Powder for injection: 0.9 mg, 1.84 mg single-use vials

INDICATIONS & DOSAGES

Boxed Warning Xiaflex is associated with penile fracture and other related penile injuries, which may require surgery. ∎

➤ Dupuytren contracture with palpable cord (Xiaflex)

Adults: 0.58 mg injected into palpable cord with contracture of metacarpophalangeal joint or proximal interphalangeal joint. May repeat up to three times per cord at 4-week intervals.

➤ Peyronie disease with palpable plaque and curvature deformity of at least 30 degrees at start of therapy (Xiaflex)

Adults: Initially, 0.58 mg injected into the target plaque once; then repeat injection 1 to 3 days later. May repeat up to four treatment cycles of two injections at approximately 6-week intervals. Discontinue treatment if curvature deformity is less than 15 degrees after any cycle.

➤ Moderate to severe cellulite in the buttocks (QWO)

Women: 0.84 mg subcut per treatment area; may repeat every 21 days for a total of three treatment visits. Maximum, 12 injections (3.6 mL) in a single buttock.

conivaptan hydrochloride
kah-nih-VAP-tan

Vaprisol

Therapeutic class: Vasopressin antagonists
Pharmacologic class: Arginine vasopressin receptor antagonists

AVAILABLE FORMS
Injection (premixed): 20 mg/100 mL D_5W

INDICATIONS & DOSAGES

➤ Euvolemic hyponatremia (as from SIADH, hypothyroidism, adrenal insufficiency, pulmonary disorders) and hypervolemic hyponatremia in patients who are hospitalized

Adults: Loading dose of 20 mg IV over 30 minutes followed by continuous infusion of 20 mg IV over 24 hours for 2 to 4 days. If sodium level isn't rising at desired rate, increase to maximum dose of 40 mg over 24 hours by continuous infusion. Total duration of infusion shouldn't exceed 4 days.

Adjust-a-dose: If sodium level rises more than 12 mEq/L in 24 hours, stop infusion. If hyponatremia persists or recurs and patient has had no adverse neurologic effects from the rapid rise in sodium level, restart infusion at a reduced dose. If patient develops hypotension or hypovolemia, stop infusion. Monitor vital signs and volume status often. If hyponatremia persists once patient is no longer hypotensive and volume returns to normal, restart infusion at a reduced dose. In patients with hepatic impairment (Child-Pugh class B or C), give a loading dose of 10 mg over 30 minutes followed by a continuous infusion of 10 mg over 24 hours for 2 to 4 days. If serum sodium level isn't rising at desired rate, may titrate dosage upward to 20 mg over 24 hours. Don't use if CrCl is less than 30 mL/minute.

SAFETY ALERT!

copanlisib dihydrochloride
ko-PAN-li-sib

Aliqopa

Therapeutic class: Antineoplastics
Pharmacologic class: Kinase inhibitors

AVAILABLE FORMS
Injection (lyophilized, preservative-free): 60-mg single-dose vials

INDICATIONS & DOSAGES

➤ Relapsed follicular lymphoma in patients who have received at least two prior systemic therapies

Adults: 60 mg IV infusion over 1 hour on days 1, 8, and 15 of a 28-day treatment cycle on an intermittent schedule (3 weeks on and 1 week off). Continue until disease progression or unacceptable toxicity occurs.

Adjust-a-dose: Reduce dosage to 45 mg in patients with moderate hepatic impairment (Child-Pugh class B) or to 30 mg in patients with severe hepatic impairment (Child-Pugh class C). If concomitant use of a strong CYP3A inhibitor is unavoidable, reduce copanlisib dosage to 45 mg. Refer to manufacturer's

---

instructions for toxicity-related dosage adjustments and drug discontinuation.

crizanlizumab-tmca
kriz-an-LIZ-ue-mab

Adakveo

Therapeutic class: Immunomodulators
Pharmacologic class: Monoclonal antibodies

AVAILABLE FORMS
Injection: 100 mg/10 mL single-dose vials

INDICATIONS & DOSAGES
➤ **To reduce frequency of vaso-occlusive crises in patients with sickle cell disease**
Adults and children age 16 and older: 5 mg/kg IV infusion over 30 minutes at week 0, week 2, then every 4 weeks thereafter. Give with or without hydroxyurea.

SAFETY ALERT!

crizotinib ▨
kriz-OH-ti-nib

Xalkori

Therapeutic class: Antineoplastics
Pharmacologic class: Tyrosine kinase inhibitors

AVAILABLE FORMS
Capsules: 200 mg, 250 mg

INDICATIONS & DOSAGES
Adjust-a-dose (for all indications): Refer to manufacturer's instructions for toxicity-related dosage adjustments.
➤ **Metastatic NSCLC that's anaplastic lymphoma kinase (ALK)- or ROS1-positive ▨**
Adults: 250 mg PO b.i.d. until disease progression or intolerance occurs.
Adjust-a-dose: For patients with CrCl less than 30 mL/minute (not requiring dialysis), give 250 mg once daily. For patients with preexisting moderate hepatic impairment, give 200 mg b.i.d. For patients with preexisting severe hepatic impairment, give 250 mg once daily. For unavoidable use with strong CYP3A inhibitors, decrease crizotinib dose to 250 mg once daily.
➤ **Relapsed or refractory systemic anaplastic large cell lymphoma that's ALK-positive ▨**
Children age 1 and older and young adults: 280 mg/m² PO b.i.d. until disease progression or unacceptable toxicity occurs.
Adjust-a-dose: Refer to manufacturer's instructions for dosage adjustment for renal or hepatic impairment, or unavoidable use with CYP3A inhibitor.
✷ *NEW INDICATION:* **Unresectable, recurrent or refractory ALK-positive inflammatory myofibroblastic tumor ▨**
Adults: 250 mg PO b.i.d. until disease progression or unacceptable toxicity occurs.
Children age 1 and older: 280 mg/m² PO b.i.d. until disease progression or unacceptable toxicity occurs.

Adjust-a-dose: Refer to manufacturer's instructions for dosage adjustment for renal or hepatic impairment, or unavoidable use with CYP3A inhibitor.

crotamiton
kroe-TAM-ih-tuhn

Crotan

Therapeutic class: Scabicides–pediculicides
Pharmacologic class: Scabicides

AVAILABLE FORMS
Lotion: 10%

INDICATIONS & DOSAGES
➤ **Parasitic infestation (scabies)**
Adults: Wash entire body with soap and water. Then thoroughly massage lotion into skin from the chin down to the toes (with special attention to skinfolds, creases, interdigital spaces, and genital area). Put lotion under fingernails after trimming the nails short. Apply second coat in 24 hours. Change clothing and bed linen the next morning. Wait another 48 hours after last application; then wash off.
➤ **Itching**
Adults: Apply locally, massaging gently into affected area until completely absorbed; repeat PRN.

SAFETY ALERT!

dacomitinib ▨
dak-oh-MI-ti-nib

Vizimpro

Therapeutic class: Antineoplastics
Pharmacologic class: Epidermal growth factor receptor inhibitors

AVAILABLE FORMS
Tablets: 15 mg, 30 mg, 45 mg

INDICATIONS & DOSAGES
➤ **First-line treatment of patients with metastatic NSCLC with epidermal growth factor receptor (*EGFR*) exon 19 deletion or exon 21 L858R substitution mutations ▨**
Adults: 45 mg PO once daily until disease progression or unacceptable toxicity occurs.
Adjust-a-dose: Refer to manufacturer's instructions for toxicity-related dosage adjustments.

dalfampridine
dal-FAM-prih-deen

Ampyra

Therapeutic class: MS drugs
Pharmacologic class: Potassium channel blockers

AVAILABLE FORMS
Tablets (extended-release) ⊕ : 10 mg

INDICATIONS & DOSAGES
➤ **To improve walking in patients with MS**
Adults: 10 mg PO every 12 hours (maximum, 20 mg daily).

✳Canada   ◇OTC   ◆Off-label use   ✐Photoguide   ⊕Do not crush   *Liquid contains alcohol   ▨Genetic

dantrolene sodium
DAN-troe-leen

Dantrium, Dantrium IV, Revonto, Ryanodex

Therapeutic class: Skeletal muscle relaxants
Pharmacologic class: Hydantoin derivatives

AVAILABLE FORMS
Capsules: 25 mg, 50 mg, 100 mg
Injection: 20 mg/vial, 250 mg/vial

INDICATIONS & DOSAGES
Boxed Warning Drug can cause hepatotoxicity; only use for indicated conditions and at lowest effective dose. Stop drug if benefits aren't evident within 45 days. ▪

➤ **Spasticity and sequelae from severe chronic disorders, such as MS, cerebral palsy, spinal cord injury, and stroke**
Adults and children age 5 and older weighing 50 kg or more: Initially, 25 mg PO daily; then 25 mg t.i.d., 50 mg t.i.d., and finally, 100 mg t.i.d. Maintain each dosage level for 7 days to determine response. May increase t.i.d. to q.i.d. if necessary. Maximum, 400 mg daily.
Children age 5 and older weighing less than 50 kg: Initially, 0.5 mg/kg PO daily; then 0.5 mg/kg t.i.d., 1 mg/kg t.i.d., and finally, 2 mg/kg t.i.d. Maintain each dosage level for 7 days to determine response. May increase t.i.d. to q.i.d. if necessary. Maximum, 100 mg q.i.d.
Adjust-a-dose: If no further benefit is observed at the next higher dose, decrease dosage to the previous lower dose.
➤ **To manage malignant hyperthermic crisis**
Adults and children: Initially, 1 mg/kg IV push. Repeat, as needed, up to cumulative dose of 10 mg/kg. Or, follow Malignant Hyperthermia Association of the United States (MHAUS) recommendations.
➤ **To prevent or attenuate malignant hyperthermic crisis in susceptible patients who need surgery**
Adults and children age 5 and older: 4 to 8 mg/kg PO daily in three or four divided doses for 1 or 2 days before procedure. Give final dose 3 or 4 hours before procedure. Or, 2.5 mg/kg IV about 1.25 hours before anesthesia; infuse Dantrium or Revonto over 1 hour, or Ryanodex over at least 1 minute. Or, follow MHAUS recommendations.
➤ **To prevent recurrence of malignant hyperthermic crisis**
Adults and children age 5 and older: 4 to 8 mg/kg PO daily in four divided doses for up to 3 days after hyperthermic crisis. Or, follow MHAUS recommendations.

darunavir ethanolate ▨
dar-OO-na-veer

Prezista

Therapeutic class: Antiretrovirals
Pharmacologic class: Protease inhibitors

AVAILABLE FORMS
Oral suspension: 100 mg/mL
Tablets ⊙ₒ: 75 mg, 150 mg, 600 mg, 800 mg

INDICATIONS & DOSAGES
➤ **HIV infection, with ritonavir and other antiretrovirals** ▨
Adults who are treatment-experienced with at least one darunavir resistance–associated substitution or when genotypic testing isn't feasible (testing is recommended): 600 mg PO b.i.d., given with 100 mg ritonavir PO b.i.d.
Adults who are treatment-naive or treatment-experienced with no darunavir resistance–associated substitutions: 800 mg PO once daily, given with ritonavir 100 mg PO once daily.
Patients who are pregnant: 600 mg PO b.i.d., given with ritonavir 100 mg or cobicistat 150 mg PO b.i.d. May consider 800 mg PO once daily, given with ritonavir 100 mg PO once daily only in certain patients who are pregnant and are already on a stable 800-mg dose with ritonavir 100-mg once-daily regimen before pregnancy, are virologically suppressed (HIV-1 RNA less than 50 copies/mL), and in whom a change to twice-daily darunavir 600 mg with ritonavir 100 mg may compromise tolerability or adherence.
Children ages 3 to younger than 18 who are treatment-naive or treatment-experienced with no darunavir resistance–associated substitutions: 35 mg/kg PO once daily with ritonavir 7 mg/kg PO once daily. Don't exceed recommended dosage for adults who are treatment-experienced. Refer to manufacturer's prescribing information for weight-based dosage table.
Children ages 3 to younger than 18 who are treatment-experienced with at least one darunavir resistance–associated substitution: 20 mg/kg PO b.i.d. with ritonavir 3 mg/kg PO b.i.d. Don't exceed recommended dosage for adults who are treatment-experienced. Refer to manufacturer's prescribing information for weight-based dosage table.

SAFETY ALERT!

dasatinib ▨
duh-SAH-tin-nib

Sprycel

Therapeutic class: Antineoplastics
Pharmacologic class: Protein–tyrosine kinase inhibitors

AVAILABLE FORMS
Tablets ⊙ₒ: 20 mg, 50 mg, 70 mg, 80 mg, 100 mg, 140 mg

INDICATIONS & DOSAGES
Adjust-a-dose (for all indications): If patient has hematologic toxicity, such as neutropenia or thrombocytopenia, consider reducing dose or interrupting or stopping therapy. If patient has severe, nonhematologic toxicity, withhold dose until condition resolves; then resume at previous or reduced dose as appropriate. Refer to manufacturer's instructions for toxicity-related dosage adjustments.
➤ **Chronic, accelerated, or myeloid or lymphoid blast phase Philadelphia chromosome–positive (Ph+) chronic myeloid leukemia (CML) with resistance or intolerance to earlier treatment, including**

♣ Canada   ◇ OTC   ◆ Off-label use   ✐ Photoguide   ⊙ₒ Do not crush   *Liquid contains alcohol   ▨ Genetic

imatinib; Ph+ acute lymphoblastic leukemia with resistance or intolerance to prior therapy ▨
Adults: 140 mg PO once daily. If patient tolerates this dose but fails to respond to treatment, increase to 180 mg PO once daily. Continue until disease progresses or intolerable adverse effects occur.
➤ **Newly diagnosed Ph+ chronic-phase CML; children with Ph+ CML in chronic phase** ▨
Adults: 100 mg PO daily. May increase to 140 mg daily.
Children weighing 45 kg or more: 100 mg PO once daily. May increase to 120 mg daily.
Children weighing 30 to less than 45 kg: 70 mg PO once daily. May increase to 90 mg daily.
Children weighing 20 to less than 30 kg: 60 mg PO once daily. May increase to 70 mg daily.
Children weighing 10 to less than 20 kg: 40 mg PO once daily. May increase to 50 mg daily.
Adjust-a-dose: Recalculate pediatric dose every 3 months, or more often if necessary, based on changes in body weight. Continue until disease progresses or intolerable adverse effects occur.
➤ **Newly diagnosed Ph+ acute lymphoblastic leukemia in combination with chemotherapy** ▨
Children age 1 and older weighing 45 kg or more: 100 mg PO once daily.
Children age 1 and older weighing 30 to less than 45 kg: 70 mg PO once daily.
Children age 1 and older weighing 20 to less than 30 kg: 60 mg PO once daily.
Children age 1 and older weighing 10 to less than 20 kg: 40 mg PO once daily.
Adjust-a-dose: Recalculate pediatric dose every 3 months, or more often if necessary, based on changes in body weight. Continue treatment for up to 2 years.

SAFETY ALERT!

DAUNOrubicin hydrochloride
daw-nah-ROO-buh-sin

Therapeutic class: Antineoplastics
Pharmacologic class: Anthracycline glycoside antibiotics

AVAILABLE FORMS
Injection: 5 mg/mL

INDICATIONS & DOSAGES
Boxed Warning Inject into a rapidly flowing IV infusion; never give by IM or subcut route as severe local tissue necrosis may result. Drug may cause severe myelosuppression or myocardial toxicity in the form of potentially fatal HF, during therapy or months to years afterward. Reduce dosage for renal or hepatic impairment. Should only be used by health care professional experienced in leukemia chemotherapy. ∎
Adjust-a-dose (for all indications): For patients with impaired hepatic and renal function, reduce dosage as follows: If bilirubin level is 1.2 to 3 mg/dL, give three-fourths normal dose; if bilirubin or creatinine level exceeds 3 mg/dL, give half normal dose. Dosages vary. Check treatment protocol with prescriber.

➤ **To induce remission in acute nonlymphocytic (myelogenous, monocytic, erythroid) leukemia**
Adults age 60 and older: 30 mg/m^2/day IV on days 1, 2, and 3 of first course and on days 1 and 2 of subsequent courses in combination with cytarabine infusions. Maximum lifetime cumulative dose is 550 mg/m^2; in patients who received mediastinal radiation, maximum lifetime cumulative dose is 400 mg/m^2.
Adults younger than age 60: 45 mg/m^2/day IV on days 1, 2, and 3 of first course and on days 1 and 2 of subsequent courses in combination with cytarabine infusions. Maximum lifetime cumulative dose is 550 mg/m^2; in patients who received mediastinal radiation, maximum lifetime cumulative dose is 400 mg/m^2.
➤ **To induce remission in acute lymphocytic leukemia (with combination therapy)**
Adults: 45 mg/m^2/day IV on days 1, 2, and 3 of first course. Maximum lifetime cumulative dose is 550 mg/m^2; in patients who received mediastinal radiation, maximum lifetime cumulative dose is 400 mg/m^2.
Children age 2 and older: 25 mg/m^2 IV on day 1 every week for up to 6 weeks, if needed. Maximum lifetime cumulative dose is 300 mg/m^2.
Children younger than age 2 or with BSA less than 0.5 m^2: 1 mg/kg/dose for 1 to 3 days (dose based on body weight, not BSA). Administration frequency is specific to each combination chemotherapy regimen. Maximum lifetime cumulative dose is 10 mg/kg.

daunorubicin liposome–cytarabine liposome
daw-nah-ROO-buh-sin/sye-TARE-a-been

Vyxeos

Therapeutic class: Antineoplastics
Pharmacologic class: Anthracycline topoisomerase inhibitors–nucleoside metabolic inhibitors

AVAILABLE FORMS
Injection (liposomes as a lyophilized cake): 44 mg daunorubicin/100 mg cytarabine in single-dose vials

INDICATIONS & DOSAGES
Boxed Warning Verify drug name and dosage before preparation and administration to avoid dosing errors. ∎
➤ **Newly diagnosed, therapy-related acute myeloid leukemia (t-AML) or AML with myelodysplasia-related changes (AML-MRC)**
Adults and children age 1 and older: A full course of therapy consists of one to two induction cycles followed by up to two consolidation cycles.
    For initial induction cycle, 44 mg/m^2 daunorubicin and 100 mg/m^2 cytarabine IV infusion on days 1, 3, and 5. For patients who fail to achieve a response with first induction cycle, give a second induction cycle of 44 mg/m^2 daunorubicin and 100 mg/m^2 cytarabine IV infusion on days 1 and 3. May give second induction cycle 2 to 5 weeks after first induction cycle if no unacceptable toxicity occurred with previous cycle.

Give first consolidation cycle 5 to 8 weeks after start of the last induction. Recommended dose for each consolidation cycle is 29 mg/m^2 daunorubicin and 65 mg/m^2 cytarabine IV infusion on days 1 and 3. Give second consolidation cycle 5 to 8 weeks after start of first consolidation cycle in patients without disease progression or unacceptable toxicity.
Adjust-a-dose: Refer to manufacturer's instructions for toxicity-related dosage adjustments.

defibrotide sodium
dee-FIB-roe-tide

Defitelio

Therapeutic class: Thrombolytics
Pharmacologic class: Thrombolytics

AVAILABLE FORMS
Injection: 200 mg/2.5 mL (80 mg/mL)

INDICATIONS & DOSAGES
➤ **Hepatic veno-occlusive disease (VOD), also known as sinusoidal obstruction syndrome, with renal or pulmonary dysfunction after hematopoietic stem-cell transplantation**
Adults and children: 6.25 mg/kg IV given as a 2-hour infusion every 6 hours. Administer for a minimum of 21 days; if after 21 days signs and symptoms of hepatic VOD haven't resolved, continue until resolution of VOD or to a maximum of 60 days.
Adjust-a-dose: Refer to manufacturer's instructions for toxicity-related dosage interruption and discontinuation.

deflazacort
de-FLAZE-a-kort

Emflaza

Therapeutic class: Muscular dystrophy drugs
Pharmacologic class: Corticosteroids

AVAILABLE FORMS
Oral suspension*: 22.75 mg/mL
Tablets: 6 mg, 18 mg, 30 mg, 36 mg

INDICATIONS & DOSAGES
➤ **Duchenne muscular dystrophy**
Adults and children age 2 and older: 0.9 mg/kg PO once daily.
Adjust-a-dose: Round dose up to nearest 0.1 mL when using oral suspension. Round dose up to nearest possible dose based on available tablet strengths. Decrease dosage to one-third of recommended dosage when used with moderate or strong CYP3A4 inhibitors.

deoxycholic acid
dee-OX-i-koe-lik

Kybella

Therapeutic class: Lipolytic agents
Pharmacologic class: Lipolytics

AVAILABLE FORMS
Injection: 10 mg/mL in 2-mL single-use vials*

INDICATIONS & DOSAGES
➤ **Improvement in appearance of moderate to severe convexity or fullness associated with submental fat**
Adults: Inject subcut into the submental region using an area-adjusted dose of 2 mg/cm^2. A single treatment consists of a maximum of 50 injections (up to a total of 10 mL), 0.2 mL each, spaced 1 cm apart. A maximum of six single treatments may be administered at intervals no less than 1 month apart. Tailor the number of injections and the number of treatments to patient's submental fat distribution and treatment goals.

desipramine hydrochloride
des-IP-ra-meen

Norpramin

Therapeutic class: Antidepressants
Pharmacologic class: TCAs

AVAILABLE FORMS
Tablets: 10 mg, 25 mg, 50 mg, 75 mg, 100 mg, 150 mg

INDICATIONS & DOSAGES
Boxed Warning Antidepressants increase risk of suicidality in children, adolescents, and young adults with depression and other psychiatric disorders. Drug isn't approved for use in children. ∎
➤ **Depression**
Adults: Initially, 25 to 50 mg PO once daily or in divided doses; increase based on tolerance and clinical response. Usual dosage, 100 to 200 mg daily in single dose or divided doses; maximum, 300 mg daily.
Adolescents and older adults: 25 to 100 mg PO once daily or in divided doses; increase gradually to maximum of 150 mg daily, if needed.

desloratadine
dess-lor-AT-a-deen

Clarinex✿

Therapeutic class: Antihistamines
Pharmacologic class: Piperidines

AVAILABLE FORMS
Oral solution: 0.5 mg/mL
Tablets: 5 mg
Tablets (ODTs): 2.5 mg, 5 mg

INDICATIONS & DOSAGES
➤ **Seasonal allergic rhinitis (patients age 2 and older); perennial allergic rhinitis or chronic idiopathic urticaria (patients age 6 months and older)**
Adults and children age 12 and older: 5 mg tablets or solution PO once daily.
Children ages 6 to 11: 2.5 mg ODT or solution PO once daily.
Children ages 12 months to 5 years: 1.25 mg solution PO once daily.
Infants ages 6 to 11 months: 1 mg solution PO once daily.
Adjust-a-dose: In adults with hepatic or renal impairment, start dosage at 5 mg PO every other day.

✚Canada ◇OTC ◆Off-label use ✐Photoguide ⬤Do not crush *Liquid contains alcohol ▨Genetic

deutetrabenazine ⓖ
doo-tet-ra-BEN-a-zeen

Austedo

Therapeutic class: Antichorea drugs
Pharmacologic class: Vesicular monoamine transporter 2 inhibitors

AVAILABLE FORMS
Tablets ⓓⓝⓒ: 6 mg, 9 mg, 12 mg

INDICATIONS & DOSAGES
Boxed Warning Drug can increase risk of depression and suicidality in patients with Huntington disease. Contraindicated for use in patients who are suicidal or those with untreated or inadequately treated depression. ∎

➤ **Chorea associated with Huntington disease or tardive dyskinesia**
Adults: Initially, 6 mg PO b.i.d. with food in patients not being switched from tetrabenazine. Titrate up at weekly intervals by 6 mg/day to a tolerated dose that reduces chorea, up to a maximum of 48 mg/day. If total daily dose is 12 mg or more, give in two divided doses. Can discontinue drug without tapering. To resume after treatment interruption of more than 1 week, retitrate dosage. To resume after treatment interruption of less than 1 week, resume at previous dosage without titration.

If switching from tetrabenazine to deutetrabenazine, stop tetrabenazine and initiate deutetrabenazine the next day. Refer to manufacturer's prescribing information for deutetrabenazine dosage based on last tetrabenazine dose.

✐ *Adjust-a-dose:* In patients currently receiving strong CYP2D6 inhibitors or for those who are known poor CYP2D6 metabolizers, don't exceed 36 mg/day (or 18 mg as a single dose).

dexlansoprazole
deks-lan-SOE-pra-zole

Dexilant✐

Therapeutic class: Antiulcer drugs
Pharmacologic class: PPIs

AVAILABLE FORMS
Capsules: 30 mg, 60 mg

INDICATIONS & DOSAGES
➤ **Healing of erosive esophagitis**
Adults and children age 12 and older: Initially, 60-mg capsule PO once daily for up to 8 weeks.
Adjust-a-dose: For patients with moderate hepatic impairment (Child-Pugh class B), maximum dose is 30-mg capsule PO daily for up to 8 weeks.

➤ **Maintenance of healed erosive esophagitis; heartburn relief**
Adults and children age 12 and older: One 30-mg capsule PO daily for up to 6 months in adults and 16 weeks in patients ages 12 to 17.

➤ **Symptomatic nonerosive GERD**
Adults and children age 12 and older: One 30-mg capsule PO daily for 4 weeks.

dexmedetomidine hydrochloride
deks-MED-e-toe-mi-deen

Igalmi, Precedex

Therapeutic class: Sedatives
Pharmacologic class: Alpha₂-adrenergic agonists

AVAILABLE FORMS
Injection (concentrate): 100 mcg/mL in 2-mL and 10-mL single-use vials
Injection (ready-to-use): 4 mcg/mL in 20-mL single-use vials and 50-mL, 100-mL, and 250-mL single-use bottles
SL film ⓓⓝⓒ: 120 mcg, 180 mcg

INDICATIONS & DOSAGES
Adjust-a-dose (for all indications): In patients with impaired hepatic function (Child-Pugh class A, B, or C) and in those older than age 65, consider reducing dosage.

➤ **ICU sedation**
Adults: Loading infusion of 1 mcg/kg IV over 10 minutes, then maintenance infusion of 0.2 to 0.7 mcg/kg/hour adjusted to achieve desired level of sedation. Infusion not to exceed 24 hours.
Adjust-a-dose: For conversion from alternative sedative therapy, a loading infusion may not be needed.

➤ **Procedural sedation**
Adults: Loading infusion of 1 mcg/kg IV over 10 minutes. Then give maintenance infusion, generally initiated at 0.6 mcg/kg/hour and adjusted to achieve desired clinical effect; dosages range from 0.2 to 1 mcg/kg/hour.
Adjust-a-dose: For less invasive procedures such as ophthalmic surgery, a loading infusion of 0.5 mcg/kg IV given over 10 minutes may be suitable. In patients older than age 65, give a loading infusion of 0.5 mcg/kg IV over 10 minutes.

➤ **Awake fiber-optic intubation**
Adults: Initial loading infusion of 1 mcg/kg IV over 10 minutes, then maintenance infusion of 0.7 mcg/kg/hour until endotracheal tube is secured.

✳ *NEW INDICATION:* **Acute treatment of agitation associated with schizophrenia or bipolar I or II disorder**
Adults: 120 mcg SL or buccally for mild or moderate agitation; if agitation persists, may give up to two additional 60-mcg doses at least 2 hours apart. Or, 180 mcg SL or buccally for severe agitation; if agitation persists, may give up to two additional 90-mcg doses at least 2 hours apart.
Adults age 65 or older: 120 mcg SL or buccally for mild, moderate, or severe agitation; if agitation persists, may give up to two additional 60-mcg doses at least 2 hours apart.
Adjust-a-dose: For patients with mild or moderate hepatic impairment, give 90 mcg for mild or moderate agitation or 120 mcg for severe agitation. For severe hepatic impairment, give 60 mcg for mild or moderate agitation, or 90 mcg for severe agitation. If agitation

---

persists in patients with hepatic impairment, may give up to two additional 60-mcg doses at least 2 hours apart. If systolic BP (SBP) is less than 90 mm Hg, diastolic BP (DBP) is less than 60 mm Hg, HR is less than 60 beats per minute, or postural decrease in SBP is more than 20 mm Hg or DBP is more than 10 mm Hg after prior dose, don't repeat dose.

dimenhyDRINATE
dye-men-HYE-dri-nate

Dramamine ◇, Driminate ◇, Gravol ✚◇, Travel Tabs ✚◇

Therapeutic class: Antivertigo drugs
Pharmacologic class: Anticholinergics

AVAILABLE FORMS
Caplets (long-acting): 100 mg✚◇
Capsules: 50 mg✚◇
Injection: 50 mg/mL
Oral solution: 15 mg/5 mL✚◇
Suppositories: 25 mg✚◇, 50 mg✚◇, 100 mg✚◇
Tablets: 15 mg✚◇, 50 mg◇
Tablets (chewable): 15 mg✚◇, 50 mg◇

INDICATIONS & DOSAGES
➤ **To prevent and treat motion sickness**
Adults and children age 12 and older: 50 to 100 mg PO every 4 to 6 hours; 50 mg IM every 4 hours PRN; 50 mg IV diluted in 10 mL NSS for injection, injected over 2 minutes every 4 hours PRN. May give 100 mg IV every 4 hours PRN when drowsiness isn't objectionable or is even desirable. Maximum, 400 mg daily. For prevention, use drug at least 30 minutes before motion exposure.
Children ages 6 to 11: 25 to 50 mg PO every 6 to 8 hours, not to exceed 150 mg in 24 hours. Or, 1.25 mg/kg or 37.5 mg/m² IM q.i.d.
Children age 8 and older: 25 to 50 mg PR b.i.d. to t.i.d. PRN. For prevention, use drug at least 30 minutes and preferably 1 to 2 hours before traveling.
Children ages 2 to 5: 12.5 to 25 mg PO every 6 to 8 hours, not to exceed 75 mg in 24 hours. Or, 1.25 mg/kg or 37.5 mg/m² IM q.i.d. Maximum, 300 mg daily.

dimethyl fumarate
dye-METH-il

Tecfidera

Therapeutic class: Immunomodulators
Pharmacologic class: Nuclear factor–like 2 pathway activators

AVAILABLE FORMS
Capsules (delayed-release) ⓓⓝⓒ: 120 mg, 240 mg

INDICATIONS & DOSAGES
➤ **Relapsing MS**
Adults: Initially, 120 mg PO b.i.d. for 7 days; then increase to maintenance dosage of 240 mg b.i.d.
Adjust-a-dose: Consider temporary dosage reduction to 120 mg b.i.d. for patient who can't tolerate maintenance dose. Resume recommended dose of 240 mg

b.i.d. within 4 weeks; then consider discontinuing drug if patient is unable to tolerate return to maintenance dose.

Consider interrupting or discontinuing therapy in patients with lymphocyte count of less than 500/mm³ persisting for more than 6 months. Consider withholding drug in patients with serious infections until resolution. Individualize decisions about restarting therapy based on clinical circumstances.

dinoprostone
dye-noe-PROST-ohn

Cervidil, Prepidil

Therapeutic class: Oxytocics
Pharmacologic class: Prostaglandins

AVAILABLE FORMS
Endocervical gel: 0.5 mg/application (2.5-mL syringe)
Vaginal insert: 10 mg

INDICATIONS & DOSAGES
➤ **To ripen an unfavorable cervix at or near term in patients who are pregnant**
Adults: Apply 0.5 mg endocervical gel intravaginally; if cervix remains unfavorable after 6 hours, repeat dose. Don't exceed 1.5 mg (three applications) within 24 hours. After obtaining desired response, wait 6 to 12 hours before giving IV oxytocin. Or, place 10-mg vaginal insert transversely in posterior vaginal fornix immediately after removing insert from foil. Take insert out when active labor begins or after 12 hours have passed, whichever occurs first. After insert removal, wait at least 30 minutes before giving oxytocin.

SAFETY ALERT!

dinutuximab
din-ue-TUX-i-mab

Unituxin

Therapeutic class: Antineoplastics
Pharmacologic class: GD2-binding monoclonal antibodies

AVAILABLE FORMS
Injection: 17.5 mg/5 mL (3.5 mg/mL) in single-use vials

INDICATIONS & DOSAGES
Boxed Warning Life-threatening infusion reactions can occur. Give required prehydration and premedication before each infusion and monitor patient for infusion reaction during and for at least 4 hours after infusion. Interrupt drug for infusion reaction and permanently discontinue for anaphylaxis. Drug causes severe neuropathic pain and requires IV opioids before, during, and after infusion. Discontinue drug for severe unresponsive pain and severe sensory or motor neuropathy. ■
➤ **High-risk neuroblastoma, in combination with granulocyte-macrophage colony-stimulating factor, interleukin-2, and 13-*cis*-retinoic acid, in patients who achieved at least a partial response to prior first-line multiagent, multimodality therapy**

Children: 17.5 mg/m^2/day IV over 10 to 20 hours for 4 consecutive days for up to five cycles. Cycles 1, 3, and 5 are 24 days in duration, and drug is administered on days 4, 5, 6, and 7. Cycles 2 and 4 are 32 days in duration, and drug is administered on days 8, 9, 10, and 11.

Adjust-a-dose: Refer to manufacturer's instructions for toxicity-related dosage adjustments and drug discontinuation.

disulfiram
dye-SUL-fi-ram

Therapeutic class: Alcohol deterrents
Pharmacologic class: Aldehyde dehydrogenase inhibitors

AVAILABLE FORMS
Tablets: 250 mg, 500 mg

INDICATIONS & DOSAGES
Boxed Warning Never give drug to a patient who is intoxicated or without patient's full knowledge. ∎
➤ **Alcohol use disorder, moderate to severe**
Adults: 250 to 500 mg PO as single dose in morning for 1 to 2 weeks (or in evening if drowsiness occurs) after patient has abstained from alcohol for at least 12 hours. Maintenance dosage is 125 to 500 mg PO daily (average 250 mg) until permanent self-control is established. Treatment may continue for months or years.

dolutegravir sodium
doe-loo-TEG-ra-vir

Tivicay, Tivicay PD

Therapeutic class: Antiretrovirals
Pharmacologic class: Integrase strand transfer inhibitors

AVAILABLE FORMS
Tablets: 10 mg, 25 mg, 50 mg
Tablets for oral suspension: 5 mg

INDICATIONS & DOSAGES
⚠ *Alert:* Tivicay tablets and tablets for oral suspension can't be interchanged on a milligram-per-milligram basis. Children weighing 3 to 14 kg should only receive oral suspension. ∎
➤ **HIV-1 infection in adults who are treatment-naive or treatment-experienced and in children who are treatment-naive or treatment-experienced and are integrase strand transfer inhibitor (INSTI)–naive, in combination with other antiretrovirals**
Tivicay
Adults and children weighing 20 kg or more: 50 mg PO once daily.
Children weighing 14 to less than 20 kg: 40 mg PO once daily.
Tivicay PD
Children weighing 20 kg or more: 30 mg once daily.
Children weighing 14 to less than 20 kg: 25 mg once daily.

Children age 4 weeks and older weighing 10 to less than 14 kg: 20 mg once daily.
Children age 4 weeks and older weighing 6 to less than 10 kg: 15 mg once daily.
Children age 4 weeks and older weighing 3 to less than 6 kg: 5 mg once daily.
Adjust-a-dose: If administered with the potent UGT1A/CYP3A inducers carbamazepine, efavirenz, fosamprenavir/ritonavir, tipranavir/ritonavir, or rifampin, for adults give dolutegravir 50 mg b.i.d. For children, increase the weight-based dose of dolutegravir to b.i.d.
➤ **HIV-1 infection in patients who are INSTI-experienced with certain INSTI-associated resistance substitutions or clinically suspected INSTI resistance, or in patients who are treatment-naive or treatment-experienced INSTI-naive when administered with certain UGT1A or CYP3A inducers**
Adults: 50 mg PO b.i.d.
➤ **HIV-1 infection with rilpivirine as a complete regimen to replace the current antiretroviral regimen in patients who are virologically suppressed (HIV-1 RNA less than 50 copies/mL) on a stable antiretroviral regimen for at least 6 months with no history of treatment failure or known substitutions associated with resistance to either antiretroviral**
Adults: 50 mg PO once daily with rilpivirine PO once daily.

dolutegravir–lamivudine
doe-loo-TEG-ra-vir/la-MI-vyoo-deen

Dovato

Therapeutic class: Antiretrovirals
Pharmacologic class: Integrase strand transfer inhibitors–nucleoside analogues/reverse transcriptase inhibitors

AVAILABLE FORMS
Tablets: 50 mg dolutegravir/300 mg lamivudine

INDICATIONS & DOSAGES
Boxed Warning Screen all patients for coinfection with HBV to prevent emergence from lamivudine-resistant HBV variants and potential exacerbation of HBV infection when lamivudine is discontinued. Additional anti-HBV therapy may be necessary. ∎
➤ **HIV-1 infection in patients with no antiretroviral treatment history; HIV-1 infection as replacement for a current stable antiretroviral regimen in patients who are virologically suppressed (HIV-1 RNA less than 50 copies/mL) with no history of treatment failure and no known substitutions associated with resistance to the individual components**
Adults: 1 tablet PO once daily.
Adjust-a-dose: If administered with carbamazepine or rifampin, give 1 tablet PO once daily followed by an additional dolutegravir 50-mg tablet approximately 12 hours from the combination product dose. If a dosage reduction of lamivudine is needed for patients with CrCl of less than 50 mL/minute, use individual components of this product.

---

droxidopa

droks-eye-DOE-pa

Northera

Therapeutic class: Vasopressors
Pharmacologic class: Norepinephrine precursors

AVAILABLE FORMS
Capsules: 100 mg, 200 mg, 300 mg

INDICATIONS & DOSAGES

Boxed Warning Increased risk of supine HTN; monitor supine BP before and during treatment and more frequently with dosage increases. Elevating head of the bed lessens risk. Reduce dosage or discontinue drug if supine HTN can't be managed with head elevation. ∎

➤ **Symptomatic neurogenic orthostatic hypotension caused by primary autonomic failure (Parkinson disease, multiple system atrophy, and pure autonomic failure), dopamine beta-hydroxylase deficiency, nondiabetic autonomic neuropathy**
Adults: Initially, 100 mg PO t.i.d. in morning, at midday, and in late afternoon at least 3 hours before bedtime. Titrate to symptomatic response in increments of 100 mg t.i.d. every 24 to 48 hours. Maximum dose is 600 mg t.i.d.

dupilumab

doo-PIL-ue-mab

Dupixent

Therapeutic class: Immunomodulators
Pharmacologic class: Monoclonal antibodies

AVAILABLE FORMS
Injection: 100 mg/0.67 mL, 200 mg/1.14 mL, 300 mg/2 mL in single-dose prefilled syringes

INDICATIONS & DOSAGES

➤ **Moderate to severe atopic dermatitis not adequately controlled with topical therapy or when other therapies aren't advisable**
Adults and children ages 6 to 17 weighing 60 kg or more: Initially, 600 mg subcut given as two 300-mg injections in different sites followed by 300 mg subcut every other week.
Children ages 6 to 17 weighing 30 to less than 60 kg: Initially, 400 mg subcut given as two 200-mg injections in different sites followed by 200 mg subcut every other week.
Children ages 6 to 17 weighing 15 to less than 30 kg: Initially, 600 mg subcut given as two 300-mg injections in different sites, followed by 300 mg subcut every 4 weeks.
Children ages 6 months to 5 years weighing 15 to less than 30 kg: 300 mg subcut every 4 weeks.
Children ages 6 months to 5 years weighing 5 to less than 15 kg: 200 mg subcut every 4 weeks.

➤ **Add-on maintenance treatment for inadequately controlled chronic rhinosinusitis with nasal polyposis**
Adults: 300 mg subcut every other week.

➤ **Add-on maintenance treatment in patients with moderate to severe asthma with an eosinophilic phenotype or with oral corticosteroid–dependent asthma**
Adults and children age 12 and older: Initially, 400 mg subcut (two 200-mg injections) followed by 200 mg every other week. Or, initially 600 mg subcut (two 300-mg injections) followed by 300 mg every other week. Or, for patients requiring concomitant oral corticosteroids or with comorbid moderate to severe atopic dermatitis for which drug is indicated, initially 600 mg subcut followed by 300 mg every other week.
Children ages 6 to 11 weighing 30 kg or more: 200 mg subcut every other week.
Children ages 6 to 11 weighing 15 to less than 30 kg: 100 mg subcut every other week or 300 mg every 4 weeks.

✳ **NEW INDICATION: Eosinophilic esophagitis**
Adults and children age 12 and older weighing at least 40 kg: 300 mg subcut once a week.

✳ **NEW INDICATION: Prurigo nodularis**
Adults: Initially, 600 mg subcut given as two 300-mg injections in different sites followed by 300 mg subcut every other week.

SAFETY ALERT!

durvalumab

dur-VAL-ue-mab

Imfinzi

Therapeutic class: Antineoplastics
Pharmacologic class: Monoclonal antibodies

AVAILABLE FORMS
Injection: 500 mg/10 mL, 120 mg/2.4 mL single-dose vials

INDICATIONS & DOSAGES

Adjust-a-dose (for all indications): Refer to manufacturer's instructions for toxicity-related withholding or drug discontinuation.

➤ **Unresectable, stage III NSCLC in patients whose disease hasn't progressed after concurrent platinum-based chemotherapy and radiation therapy**
Adults weighing 30 kg or more: 10 mg/kg IV infusion every 2 weeks or 1,500 mg every 4 weeks until disease progression, unacceptable toxicity, or a maximum of 12 months.
Adults weighing less than 30 kg: 10 mg/kg IV infusion every 2 weeks until disease progression, unacceptable toxicity, or a maximum of 12 months.

➤ **First-line treatment of extensive-stage small-cell lung cancer, in combination with etoposide and either carboplatin or cisplatin**
Adults weighing 30 kg or more: 1,500 mg IV infusion before chemotherapy (on the same day) every 3 weeks for four cycles, followed by 1,500 mg every 4 weeks as a single agent, until disease progression or unacceptable toxicity occurs.
Adults weighing less than 30 kg: 20 mg/kg IV infusion before chemotherapy (on the same day) every 3 weeks (21 days) for four cycles, followed by 10 mg/kg every

2 weeks as a single agent until disease progression or unacceptable toxicity occurs.

✳ *NEW INDICATION:* **Metastatic or locally advanced biliary tract cancer, in combination with gemcitabine and cisplatin**

Adults weighing 30 kg or more: 1,500-mg IV infusion every 3 weeks (21 days) for up to eight cycles in combination with chemotherapy, followed by 1,500 mg every 4 weeks as a single agent until disease progression or unacceptable toxicity occurs.

Adults weighing less than 30 kg: 20 mg/kg IV infusion every 3 weeks (21 days) for up to eight cycles in combination with chemotherapy, followed by 20 mg/kg every 2 weeks as a single agent until disease progression or unacceptable toxicity occurs.

---

ecallantide ▨
ee-KAL-lan-tide

Kalbitor

Therapeutic class: Protein inhibitors
Pharmacologic class: Human plasma kallikrein inhibitors

AVAILABLE FORMS
Injection: 10 mg/mL vials

INDICATIONS & DOSAGES
Boxed Warning Anaphylaxis has been reported after administration. ∎
➤ **Acute attacks of hereditary angioedema ▨**
Adults and adolescents age 12 and older: 30 mg subcut given as three 10-mg injections; give additional 30-mg dose within 24 hours if attack persists.

---

econazole nitrate
ee-KOE-na-zole

Ecoza, Zolpak

Therapeutic class: Antifungals
Pharmacologic class: Imidazole derivatives

AVAILABLE FORMS
Cream: 1%
Foam: 1%

INDICATIONS & DOSAGES
➤ **Tinea corporis, tinea cruris, tinea pedis, tinea versicolor**
Adults and children: Rub cream into affected areas daily for at least 2 weeks (1 month for tinea pedis).
Adults and children age 12 and older (tinea pedis only): Apply foam to affected areas daily for 4 weeks.
➤ **Cutaneous candidiasis**
Adults and children: Rub cream into affected areas b.i.d. (morning and evening) for 2 weeks.

SAFETY ALERT!

eculizumab
eck-u-LIZ-uh-mob

Soliris

Therapeutic class: Hemolysis inhibitors
Pharmacologic class: Monoclonal IgG antibodies

AVAILABLE FORMS
Injection: 10 mg/mL in 300-mg single-use vials

INDICATIONS & DOSAGES
Boxed Warning Life-threatening and fatal meningococcal infections have occurred. Meningococcal vaccine is required at least 2 weeks before administration of eculizumab unless risks of delaying treatment outweigh risks of infection. Access is restricted through a REMS program and prescribers must be enrolled. ∎
➤ **Hemolysis in patients with paroxysmal nocturnal hemoglobinuria**
Adults: 600 mg IV every 7 days for 4 weeks, 900 mg 7 days later, then 900 mg every 14 days thereafter.
➤ **Atypical hemolytic-uremic syndrome**
Adults and children weighing 40 kg or more: 900 mg IV weekly for 4 weeks, then 1,200 mg at week 5, then 1,200 mg every 2 weeks.
Children age 2 months and older weighing 30 to 39 kg: 600 mg IV weekly for 2 weeks, then 900 mg at week 3, then 900 mg every 2 weeks.
Children age 2 months and older weighing 20 to 29 kg: 600 mg IV weekly for 2 weeks, then 600 mg at week 3, then 600 mg every 2 weeks.
Children age 2 months and older weighing 10 to 19 kg: 600 mg IV weekly for one dose, then 300 mg at week 2, then 300 mg every 2 weeks.
Children age 2 months and older weighing 5 to 9 kg: 300 mg IV weekly for one dose, then 300 mg at week 2, then 300 mg every 3 weeks.
Adjust-a-dose: Give a supplemental dose within 60 minutes after each plasmapheresis or plasma exchange session. If most recent dose was 300 mg, give 300-mg supplemental dose. If most recent dose was 600 mg or more, give 600-mg supplemental dose. For patients receiving fresh frozen plasma, if most recent dose was 300 mg or more, give 300-mg supplemental dose 1 hour before each unit of fresh frozen plasma.
➤ **Refractory generalized myasthenia gravis in patients who are anti-acetylcholine receptor antibody-positive; neuromyelitis optica spectrum disorder in patients who are anti-aquaporin-4 antibody positive**
Adults: 900 mg IV weekly for 4 weeks; then 1,200 mg at week 5; then 1,200 mg every 2 weeks.
Adjust-a-dose: Give a supplemental dose within 60 minutes after each plasmapheresis or plasma exchange session. If most recent dose was 300 mg, give 300-mg supplemental dose. If most recent dose was 600 mg or more, give 600-mg supplemental dose. For patients receiving fresh frozen plasma, if most recent dose was 300 mg or more, give 300-mg supplemental dose 1 hour before each unit of fresh frozen plasma.

---

edaravone

ed-a-RAV-one

Radicava

Therapeutic class: Miscellaneous CNS drugs
Pharmacologic class: Free radical scavengers

AVAILABLE FORMS
Injection: 30 mg/100 mL premixed bags
Suspension: 105 mg/5 mL

INDICATIONS & DOSAGES
➤ **ALS**
Adults: For initial treatment cycle, give 60 mg IV infusion over 60 minutes daily for 14 days, followed by a 14-day drug-free period. Or, for initial treatment cycle, 105 mg PO or NG for 14 days, followed by a 14-day drug-free period. For all subsequent treatment cycles, give 60 mg IV infusion daily, or 105 mg PO or NG, for 10 out of 14 days, followed by a 14-day drug-free period. Give PO or NG in the morning after overnight fasting.
Adjust-a-dose: May switch patient from 60 mg IV to 105 mg PO solution daily.

efinaconazole

ef-in-a-KON-a-zole

Jublia

Therapeutic class: Antifungals
Pharmacologic class: Azole antifungals

AVAILABLE FORMS
Topical solution: 10%

INDICATIONS & DOSAGES
➤ **Toenail onychomycosis due to *Trichophyton rubrum* or *Trichophyton mentagrophytes***
Adults and children age 6 and older: Apply solution to affected toenails using the brush applicator once daily for 48 weeks.

elapegademase-lvlr 🧬

EL-a-peg-ad-e-mase

Revcovi

Therapeutic class: Replacement enzymes
Pharmacologic class: Recombinant adenosine deaminase enzymes

AVAILABLE FORMS
Injection: 2.4 mg/1.5 mL (1.6 mg/mL) single-dose vial

INDICATIONS & DOSAGES
➤ **Adenosine deaminase (ADA) severe combined immune deficiency** 🧬
Adults and children who are pegademase bovine–naive: Initially, 0.2 mg/kg (based on ideal body weight or actual weight, whichever is greater) IM twice a week for at least 12 to 24 weeks until immune reconstitution is achieved. Then, may adjust dosage to maintain trough ADA activity greater than 30 mmol/hour/L,

trough deoxyadenosine nucleotide (dAXP) levels less than 0.02 mmol/L, or adequate immune reconstitution based on clinical assessment.
Adults and children transitioning from pegademase bovine to elapegademase-lvlr: If weekly pegademase bovine dose is unknown or is 30 units/kg or lower, begin elapegademase-lvlr at 0.2 mg/kg IM once weekly. If weekly pegademase bovine dose is greater than 30 units/kg, calculate an equivalent weekly elapegademase-lvlr dose (mg/kg) by dividing the pegademase bovine dose (units/kg) by 150. May increase dosage by increments of 0.033 mg/kg weekly if trough ADA activity is under 30 mmol/hr/L, trough dAXP levels are greater than 0.02 mmol/L, and/or immune reconstitution is inadequate based on clinical assessment. The total weekly dose may be divided into multiple IM administrations during a week.

elexacaftor–tezacaftor–ivacaftor and ivacaftor 🧬

el-ex-a-KAF-tor/tez-a-KAF-tor/eye-va-KAF-tor

Trikafta

Therapeutic class: Metabolic agents
Pharmacologic class: Cystic fibrosis transmembrane conductance regulator (CFTR) facilitators (elexacaftor and tezacaftor)–CFTR potentiators (ivacaftor)

AVAILABLE FORMS
Tablets 🍬: 50 mg elexacaftor, 25 mg tezacaftor, 37.5 mg ivacaftor (fixed-dose combination) copackaged with 75 mg ivacaftor; 100 mg elexacaftor, 50 mg tezacaftor, 75 mg ivacaftor (fixed-dose combination) copackaged with 150 mg ivacaftor

INDICATIONS & DOSAGES
➤ **Cystic fibrosis in patients who have at least one F508del mutation in the *CFTR* gene**
Adults and children age 12 and older: 2 tablets (each containing 100 mg elexacaftor, 50 mg tezacaftor, and 75 mg ivacaftor) PO in the morning, followed by one 150-mg ivacaftor tablet in the evening about 12 hours later.
Children ages 6 to younger than 12 weighing 30 kg or more: 2 tablets (each containing 100 mg elexacaftor, 50 mg tezacaftor, and 75 mg ivacaftor) PO in the morning, followed by one 150-mg ivacaftor tablet in the evening about 12 hours later.
Children ages 6 to younger than 12 weighing less than 30 kg: 2 tablets (each containing 50 mg elexacaftor, 25 mg tezacaftor, and 37.5 mg ivacaftor) PO in the morning, followed by one 75-mg ivacaftor tablet in the evening about 12 hours later.
Adjust-a-dose: For patients with moderate hepatic impairment (Child-Pugh class B), 2 tablets (each containing elexacaftor, tezacaftor, and ivacaftor) PO in the morning on day 1, alternating with 1 tablet in the morning on day 2. Patient shouldn't take an evening dose of ivacaftor. For patients currently receiving moderate and strong CYP3A inhibitors, refer to manufacturer's instructions for dosage adjustments.

🍁Canada   ◇OTC   ◆Off-label use   ✐Photoguide   🍬Do not crush   *Liquid contains alcohol   🧬Genetic

eltrombopag ☒

ell-trom-BOW-pag

Promacta, Revolade✦

Therapeutic class: Hematopoietics
Pharmacologic class: Thrombopoietin
receptor agonists

AVAILABLE FORMS

Powder for oral suspension: 12.5-mg, 25-mg packets
Tablets ⓞⓝⓒ: 12.5 mg, 25 mg, 50 mg, 75 mg

INDICATIONS & DOSAGES

Boxed Warning Drug increases risk of hepatotoxicity. In patients with HCV infection, use with interferon and ribavirin may increase risk of hepatic decompensation. Consult prescribing information for specific monitoring guidelines. ■

➤ **Thrombocytopenia associated with chronic ITP when response to corticosteroids, immunoglobulins, or splenectomy is inadequate**

Adults and children age 6 and older: Initially, 50 mg PO once daily.
Children ages 1 to 5: Initially, 25 mg PO once daily.
☒ *Adjust-a-dose:* Adjust dosage as necessary to achieve and maintain platelet count at 50×10^9/L or greater; maximum dosage is 75 mg daily. For patients older than age 6 and of East Asian descent or those with mild, moderate, or severe hepatic impairment, reduce dosage to 25 mg once daily. For patients older than age 6 of East Asian descent and any hepatic impairment, reduce dosage to 12.5 mg once daily. Refer to manufacturer's instructions for dosage adjustments based on hematologic parameters.

➤ **Thrombocytopenia in patients with chronic HCV infection to allow use of interferon-based therapy**

Adults: Initially, 25 mg PO once daily. Increase by 25-mg increments every 2 weeks as necessary to achieve target platelet count required to initiate antiviral therapy. Maximum dose is 100 mg daily.
Adjust-a-dose: During antiviral therapy, adjust dosage to avoid peginterferon dose reduction. Refer to manufacturer's instructions for dosage adjustments based on hematologic parameters. Discontinue drug when antiviral treatment is stopped.

➤ **Severe aplastic anemia when response to immunosuppressive therapy is insufficient**

Adults: Initially, 50 mg PO once daily. Adjust dosage as necessary in 50-mg increments every 2 weeks to achieve target platelet count of 50×10^9/L or greater. Maximum dosage is 150 mg daily.
☒ *Adjust-a-dose:* In patients of East Asian descent or those with mild, moderate, or severe hepatic impairment, reduce initial dosage to 25 mg once daily. Refer to manufacturer's instructions for dosage adjustments based on hematologic parameters.

If no hematologic response has occurred after 16 weeks of therapy, or new cytogenetic abnormalities are observed, discontinue drug.
➤ **First-line treatment of severe aplastic anemia, in combination with standard immunosuppressive therapy**

Adults and children age 12 and older: 150 mg PO once daily for 6 months.
Children ages 6 to 11: 75 mg PO once daily for 6 months.
Children ages 2 to 5: 2.5 mg/kg PO once daily for 6 months.
☒ *Adjust-a-dose:* In patients of East Asian descent or those with mild, moderate, or severe hepatic impairment (Child-Pugh class A, B, C), reduce initial dosage by 50%. Don't initiate if baseline ALT or AST level is more than $6 \times$ ULN. Refer to manufacturer's instructions for toxicity-related dosage adjustments.

emapalumab-lzsg

em-a-PAL-ue-mab

Gamifant

Therapeutic class: Immunomodulators
Pharmacologic class: Monoclonal antibodies

AVAILABLE FORMS

Injection: 10 mg/2 mL, 50 mg/10 mL, 100 mg/20 mL single-dose vials

INDICATIONS & DOSAGES

➤ **Primary hemophagocytic lymphohistiocytosis (HLH) in patients with refractory, recurrent, or progressive disease or intolerance to conventional HLH therapy**

Adults and children: 1 mg/kg IV infusion over 1 hour twice weekly (every 3 to 4 days) until hematopoietic stem cell transplantation or unacceptable toxicity.
Adjust-a-dose: If unsatisfactory improvement in clinical condition, may increase dose to 3 mg/kg on day 3; to 6 mg/kg from day 6 onwards; to 10 mg/kg on day 9 onwards. See manufacturer's information for specific criteria for dosage increases. After clinical condition is stabilized, decrease dosage to previous level to maintain clinical response.

SAFETY ALERT!

enasidenib ☒

en-a-SID-e-nib

Idhifa

Therapeutic class: Antineoplastics
Pharmacologic class: Isocitrate
dehydrogenase-2 inhibitors

AVAILABLE FORMS

Tablets: 50 mg, 100 mg

INDICATIONS & DOSAGES

Boxed Warning Drug may cause differentiation syndrome (including fever, dyspnea, acute respiratory distress, pulmonary infiltrates, pleural or pericardial effusions, rapid weight gain or peripheral edema, lymphadenopathy, bone pain, and hepatic, renal, or multiorgan dysfunction), which can be fatal if not treated. If differentiation syndrome is suspected, initiate corticosteroid therapy and hemodynamic monitoring until symptom resolution. ■

✦Canada   ◇ OTC   ◆ Off-label use   ✐ Photoguide   ⓞⓝⓒ Do not crush   *Liquid contains alcohol   ☒ Genetic

➤ **Relapsed or refractory acute myeloid leukemia in patients with an isocitrate dehydrogenase-2 mutation** ✂

Adults: 100 mg PO once daily until disease progression or unacceptable toxicity. For patients without disease progression or unacceptable toxicity, treat for at least 6 months to allow time for clinical response.

Adjust-a-dose: Refer to manufacturer's instructions for toxicity-related dosage adjustments.

---

entacapone

en-TA-ka-pone

Comtan

Therapeutic class: Antiparkinsonian drugs
Pharmacologic class: Catechol-O-methyltransferase inhibitors

AVAILABLE FORMS
Tablets ⊙: 200 mg

INDICATIONS & DOSAGES
➤ **Adjunct to levodopa–carbidopa for treatment of idiopathic Parkinson disease in patients with signs and symptoms of end-of-dose wearing-off**
Adults: 200 mg PO with each dose of levodopa–carbidopa, up to eight times daily. Maximum, 1,600 mg daily. May need to reduce daily levodopa dose or extend the interval between levodopa doses to optimize patient's response.

SAFETY ALERT!

---

entrectinib ✂

en-TREK-ti-nib

Rozlytrek

Therapeutic class: Antineoplastics
Pharmacologic class: Kinase inhibitors

AVAILABLE FORMS
Capsules: 100 mg, 200 mg

INDICATIONS & DOSAGES
Adjust-a-dose (for all indications): For adults and children age 12 and older with BSA greater than 1.50 m^2, decrease entrectinib dosage to 200 mg PO once daily if given with a moderate CYP3A inhibitor or to 100 mg PO once daily if given with a strong CYP3A inhibitor. After discontinuation of the CYP3A inhibitor for three to five elimination half-lives, resume entrectinib dosage given before initiating the CYP3A inhibitor. Refer to manufacturer's instructions for toxicity-related dosage adjustments.

➤ **ROS1-positive metastatic NSCLC** ✂
Adults: 600 mg PO once daily until disease progression or unacceptable toxicity.

➤ **Solid tumors that have a neurotrophic tyrosine receptor kinase gene fusion without a known acquired resistance mutation, that are metastatic or when surgical resection is likely to result in severe morbidity, and that have progressed after treatment or have no satisfactory alternative** ✂

Adults and children age 12 and older with BSA greater than 1.50 m^2: 600 mg PO once daily until disease progression or unacceptable toxicity.
Children age 12 and older with BSA of 1.11 to 1.50 m^2: 500 mg PO once daily until disease progression or unacceptable toxicity.
Children age 12 and older with BSA of 0.91 to 1.10 m^2: 400 mg PO once daily until disease progression or unacceptable toxicity.
Adjust-a-dose: Avoid use with moderate or strong CYP3A4 inhibitors in children with BSA less than 1.5 m^2.

SAFETY ALERT!

---

enzalutamide

en-za-LOO-ta-mide

Xtandi

Therapeutic class: Antineoplastics
Pharmacologic class: Androgen receptor inhibitors

AVAILABLE FORMS
Capsules ⊙: 40 mg
Tablets ⊙: 40 mg, 80 mg

INDICATIONS & DOSAGES
Adjust-a-dose (for all indications): If use with strong CYP3A4 inducers is unavoidable, increase dosage to 240 mg once daily. If use with strong CYP2C8 inhibitors is unavoidable, reduce dosage to 80 mg once daily. Refer to manufacturer's instructions for toxicity-related dosage adjustments.
➤ **Castration-resistant prostate cancer; metastatic castration-sensitive prostate cancer**
Adults: 160 mg PO once daily after a bilateral orchiectomy or with a GnRH analogue. Continue until disease progression or unacceptable toxicity.

---

eravacycline

er-a-va-SYE-kleen

Xerava

Therapeutic class: Antibiotics
Pharmacologic class: Tetracyclines

AVAILABLE FORMS
Injection: 50-mg, 100-mg single-dose vial

INDICATIONS & DOSAGES
➤ **Complicated intra-abdominal infections caused by susceptible microorganisms (*Escherichia coli, Klebsiella pneumoniae, Citrobacter freundii, Enterobacter cloacae, Klebsiella oxytoca, Enterococcus faecalis, Enterococcus faecium, Staphylococcus aureus, Streptococcus anginosus* group, *Clostridium perfringens, Bacteroides* species, and *Parabacteroides distasonis*)**
Adults: 1 mg/kg IV over 60 minutes every 12 hours for 4 to 14 days as determined by the severity and location of the infection and clinical response.
Adjust-a-dose: For patients with severe hepatic impairment (Child-Pugh class C), give 1 mg/kg IV every 12 hours on day 1 followed by 1 mg/kg IV every 24 hours starting on day 2 for 4 to 14 days. If drug is

---

used with a strong CYP3A inducer, give 1.5 mg/kg IV every 12 hours for 4 to 14 days.

SAFETY ALERT!

erdafitinib ▨
er-da-FI-ti-nib

Balversa

Therapeutic class: Antineoplastics
Pharmacologic class: Kinase inhibitors

AVAILABLE FORMS
Tablets: 3 mg, 4 mg, 5 mg

INDICATIONS & DOSAGES
➤ **Locally advanced or metastatic urothelial carcinoma with susceptible *FGFR3* or *FGFR2* genetic alterations and that has progressed during or following at least one line of prior platinum-containing chemotherapy, including within 12 months of neoadjuvant or adjuvant platinum-containing chemotherapy** ▨
Adults: 8 mg PO once daily. May increase to 9 mg once daily if serum phosphate level is less than 5.5 mg/dL and there are no ocular disorders or grade 2 or greater adverse reactions 14 to 21 days after start of treatment. Continue treatment until disease progression or unacceptable toxicity occurs.
Adjust-a-dose: Refer to manufacturer's instructions for toxicity-related dosage adjustments.

eslicarbazepine acetate
es-li-kar-BAZ-e-peen

Aptiom

Therapeutic class: Anticonvulsants
Pharmacologic class: Carboxamide derivatives

AVAILABLE FORMS
Tablets: 200 mg, 400 mg, 600 mg, 800 mg

INDICATIONS & DOSAGES
➤ **Partial-onset seizures**
Adults: Initially, 400 mg PO once daily; may initiate treatment at 800 mg daily if need for additional seizure reduction outweighs an increased risk of adverse reactions. May increase in weekly increments of 400 to 600 mg once daily to a recommended maintenance dose of 800 to 1,600 mg once daily.

For monotherapy, consider the 800-mg once-daily maintenance dose in patients unable to tolerate 1,200-mg daily dose. For adjunctive therapy, consider the 1,600-mg daily dose in patients who didn't achieve a satisfactory response with a 1,200-mg daily dose.
Children ages 4 to 17: Dosage is based on body weight; increase based on clinical response and tolerability, but no more frequently than once per week.

For patients weighing more than 38 kg, initially 400 mg PO once daily; titrate in 400-mg increments to 800 to 1,200 mg PO once daily. For those weighing 32 to 38 kg, initially 300 mg PO once daily; titrate in 300-mg increments to 600 to 900 mg PO once daily. For those weighing 22 to 31 kg, initially 300 mg PO once daily;

titrate in 300-mg increments to 500 to 800 mg PO once daily. For those weighing 11 to 21 kg, initially 200 mg PO once daily; titrate in 200-mg increments to 400 to 600 mg PO once daily.
Adjust-a-dose: For patients with moderate to severe renal impairment (CrCl of less than 50 mL/minute), the initial, titration, and maintenance doses should generally be reduced by 50%. Maintenance doses may be adjusted according to clinical response. Consider adjusting dosages of both eslicarbazepine and carbamazepine if given concurrently. Consider increasing eslicarbazepine dosage if given with enzyme-inducing AEDs, such as phenobarbital, primidone, or phenytoin.

etelcalcetide
e-tel-KAL-se-tide

Parsabiv

Therapeutic class: Hyperparathyroidism drugs
Pharmacologic class: Calcimimetics

AVAILABLE FORMS
Injection: 2.5 mg/0.5 mL, 5 mg/mL, 10 mg/2 mL in single-dose vials

INDICATIONS & DOSAGES
➤ **Secondary hyperparathyroidism in patients with chronic kidney disease on hemodialysis**
Adults: Initially, 5 mg IV bolus injection three times per week at end of hemodialysis treatment; maintenance dosage is individualized and determined by titration based on parathyroid hormone (PTH) level and corrected serum calcium response. Dosage range is 2.5 to 15 mg three times weekly. Increase dosage in 2.5- or 5-mg increments based on PTH level in patients with corrected serum calcium level within the normal range and PTH level above recommended target range. Increase dosage no more frequently than every 4 weeks.
Adjust-a-dose: If PTH level is below target range, decrease dosage or temporarily discontinue drug. In patients with corrected serum calcium level below lower limit of normal (LLN), but at or above 7.5 mg/dL without symptoms of hypocalcemia, consider decreasing dosage or temporarily discontinuing drug or use concomitant therapies to increase corrected serum calcium level.

If drug is stopped, reinitiate at a lower dose when PTH level is within target range and hypocalcemia has been corrected. If corrected serum calcium level falls below LLN or signs or symptoms of hypocalcemia develop, start or increase calcium supplementation (calcium, calcium-containing phosphate binders, or vitamin D sterols or increases in dialysate calcium concentration). Etelcalcetide dosage reduction or discontinuation may be necessary.

If corrected serum calcium level falls below 7.5 mg/dL or patient reports signs and symptoms of hypocalcemia, stop drug and treat hypocalcemia; when corrected serum calcium level is within normal limits, signs and symptoms of hypocalcemia have resolved, and predisposing factors for hypocalcemia have been addressed, reinitiate at a dose 5 mg lower than last administered dose. If last administered dose was 2.5 or 5 mg, reinitiate at 2.5-mg dose.

etodolac
ee-toe-DOE-lak

Therapeutic class: Anti-inflammatory drugs
Pharmacologic class: NSAIDs

AVAILABLE FORMS
Capsules: 200 mg, 300 mg
Tablets: 400 mg, 500 mg
Tablets (extended-release): 400 mg, 500 mg, 600 mg

INDICATIONS & DOSAGES
Boxed Warning NSAIDs may cause an increased risk of serious and sometimes fatal CV thrombotic events, MI, stroke, and GI adverse reactions. Contraindicated after CABG surgery. ■
➤ **Acute pain**
Adults: 200 to 400 mg (immediate-release) PO every 6 to 8 hours, not to exceed 1,000 mg daily.
➤ **Short- and long-term management of osteoarthritis and RA**
Adults: 600 to 1,000 mg (immediate-release) PO daily, divided into two or three doses. Maximum daily dose is 1,000 mg. For extended-release tablets, 400 to 1,000 mg PO daily.
➤ **Juvenile RA**
Children ages 6 to 16 weighing more than 60 kg: 1,000 mg (extended-release) PO once daily.
Children ages 6 to 16 weighing 46 to 60 kg: 800 mg (extended-release) PO once daily.
Children ages 6 to 16 weighing 31 to 45 kg: 600 mg (extended-release) PO once daily.
Children ages 6 to 16 weighing 20 to 30 kg: 400 mg (extended-release) PO once daily.

evolocumab
e-voe-LOK-ue-mab

Repatha

Therapeutic class: Antilipemics
Pharmacologic class: Proprotein convertase subtilisin kexin type 9 antibody inhibitors

AVAILABLE FORMS
Injection: 140 mg/mL solution in single-dose prefilled syringe or autoinjector
Injection (Pushtronex system): 420 mg/3.5 mL

INDICATIONS & DOSAGES
➤ **Adjunct to diet, alone or in combination with other low-density lipoprotein cholesterol (LDL-C)–lowering therapies, in patients with primary hyperlipidemia, including heterozygous familial hypercholesterolemia (HeFH), who require additional lowering of LDL-C**
Adults: 140 mg subcut every 2 weeks or 420 mg subcut once monthly. When switching dosage regimens, give first dose of new regimen on next scheduled date of prior regimen.

➤ **Adjunct to diet and other LDL-C lowering therapies in children with HeFH who require additional lowering of LDL-C**
Children age 10 and older: 140 mg subcut every 2 weeks or 420 mg subcut once monthly. When switching dosage regimens, give first dose of new regimen on next scheduled date of prior regimen.
➤ **Adjunct to other LDL-C lowering therapies (statins, ezetimibe, LDL apheresis) in patients with homozygous familial hypercholesterolemia in patients who require additional lowering of LDL-C**
Adults and children age 10 and older: 420 mg subcut once monthly. May increase to 420 mg every 2 weeks if clinically meaningful response isn't achieved in 12 weeks. Patients on lipid apheresis may begin treatment with 420 mg every 2 weeks to correspond with their apheresis schedule, given after apheresis session.
➤ **To reduce risk of MI, stroke, and coronary revascularization in patients with established CV disease**
Adults: 140 mg subcut every 2 weeks or 420 mg subcut once monthly. When switching dosage regimens, give first dose of new regimen on next scheduled date of prior regimen.

SAFETY ALERT!

exemestane
ex-e-MES-tane

Aromasin

Therapeutic class: Antineoplastics
Pharmacologic class: Aromatase inhibitors

AVAILABLE FORMS
Tablets: 25 mg

INDICATIONS & DOSAGES
Adjust-a-dose (for all indications): In patients also taking strong CYP3A4 inducers, increase daily dose to 50 mg.
➤ **Advanced breast cancer in patients who are postmenopausal whose disease has progressed after treatment with tamoxifen**
Adults: 25 mg PO once daily after a meal.
➤ **Early-stage estrogen receptor–positive breast cancer in patients who are postmenopausal who have taken tamoxifen for 2 to 3 years**
Adults: 25 mg PO once daily after a meal to complete a 5-year course, unless cancer recurs or is found in the other breast.
➤ **First-line adjuvant treatment of estrogen receptor–positive early breast cancer in patients who are postmenopausal ♦**
Adults: 25 mg PO once daily after a meal for 5 years.
➤ **Adjuvant therapy for hormone receptor-positive high-risk disease, in combination with ovarian function suppression ♦**
Patients who are premenopausal: 25 mg PO once daily after a meal after completion of chemotherapy or 6 to 8 weeks after ovarian functions suppression begins.

➤ **To reduce risk of breast cancer** ◆
Patients who are postmenopausal age 35 and older: 25 mg PO once daily after a meal for 5 years.

SAFETY ALERT!

fedratinib
fed-RA-ti-nib

Inrebic

Therapeutic class: Antineoplastics
Pharmacologic class: Kinase inhibitors

AVAILABLE FORMS
Capsules: 100 mg

INDICATIONS & DOSAGES
Boxed Warning Serious and fatal encephalopathy, including Wernicke, can occur. Assess thiamine levels in all patients before and periodically during treatment, and as clinically indicated. Don't start fedratinib in patients with thiamine deficiency. If encephalopathy is suspected, immediately discontinue fedratinib and initiate parenteral thiamine. ∎
➤ **Intermediate-2 or high-risk primary or secondary (post–polycythemia vera or post–essential thrombocythemia) myelofibrosis**
Adults: 400 mg PO once daily if baseline platelet count is 50×10^9/L or greater.
Adjust-a-dose: In patients with severe renal impairment (CrCl of 15 to 29 mL/minute), decrease dose to 200 mg once daily. If administering with strong CYP3A4 inhibitors, reduce dose to 200 mg PO once daily. When administration with a strong CYP3A4 inhibitor is discontinued, increase fedratinib dose to 300 mg once daily during first 2 weeks after discontinuation; then increase to 400 mg once daily as tolerated. Refer to manufacturer's instructions for toxicity-related dosage adjustments.

ferumoxytol
fer-yoo-MOX-i-tol

Feraheme

Therapeutic class: Iron salts
Pharmacologic class: Iron supplements

AVAILABLE FORMS
Injection: 510 mg elemental iron per 17 mL (30 mg/mL) single-dose vial

INDICATIONS & DOSAGES
Boxed Warning Fatal and serious hypersensitivity reactions, including anaphylaxis, can occur even if drug was previously tolerated. Give as an IV infusion over at least 15 minutes and only when personnel and therapies are immediately available to treat hypersensitivity reactions. ∎
➤ **Iron deficiency anemia (IDA) in patients intolerant of or who have had an unsatisfactory response to oral iron, or who have chronic kidney disease**
Adults: 510 mg IV infusion over at least 15 minutes. Repeat in 3 to 8 days. If IDA persists or recurs 1 month after the second infusion, may repeat the two-dose treatment course.

fesoterodine fumarate
fes-oh-TER-oh-deen

Toviaz

Therapeutic class: Antispasmodics
Pharmacologic class: Muscarinic receptor antagonists

AVAILABLE FORMS
Tablets (extended-release) ⊚*:* 4 mg, 8 mg

INDICATIONS & DOSAGES
➤ **Urge incontinence, urinary urgency, and urinary frequency from overactive bladder**
Adults: 4 mg PO once daily; increase to 8 mg once daily if needed.
Adjust-a-dose: Don't exceed 4 mg daily in patients with CrCl of less than 30 mL/minute and in those taking potent CYP3A4 inhibitors.
✳ *NEW INDICATION:* **Neurogenic detrusor overactivity**
Children age 6 and older weighing more than 35 kg: 4 mg PO once daily for 1 week; then increase to 8 mg once daily.
Children age 6 and older weighing more than 25 and up to 35 kg: 4 mg PO once daily. May increase to 8 mg once daily if needed.
Adjust-a-dose: If child weighs more than 25 and up to 35 kg, drug isn't recommended if eGFR is 29 mL/minute/1.73 m². If child weighs 35 kg or more and eGFR is 29 mL/minute/1.73 m², recommended dose is 4 mg daily; drug isn't recommended if eGFR is less than 15 mL/minute/1.73 m². If coadministering strong CYP3A4 inhibitors in child weighing more than 35 kg, maximum dose is 4 mg daily; coadministration isn't recommended in child weighing more than 25 and up to 35 kg.

fish oil triglycerides emulsion
fish oyl try-GLYC-e-rides

Omegaven

Therapeutic class: Nutritional supplements
Pharmacologic class: Essential fatty acid supplements

AVAILABLE FORMS
Injection: 5 g/50 mL, 10 g/100 mL single-dose bottles

INDICATIONS & DOSAGES
➤ **Source of calories and fatty acids in patients with parenteral nutrition–associated cholestasis**
Children: Recommended and maximum dosage is 1 g/kg/day by IV infusion. Initial rate of infusion shouldn't exceed 0.05 mL/minute for first 15 to 30 minutes of infusion; if tolerated, gradually increase until reaching the required rate after 30 minutes. Maximum infusion rate shouldn't exceed 1.5 mL/kg/hour.
Adjust-a-dose: If triglyceride levels are greater than 250 mg/dL in neonates and infants or greater than 400 mg/dL in older children, consider stopping drug for 4 hours and obtain a repeat serum triglyceride level. Resume therapy based on new result as

indicated. If triglyceride levels remain elevated, consider a reduced dose of 0.5 to 0.75 g/kg/day with an incremental increase to 1 g/kg/day.

flibanserin
flib-AN-ser-in

Addyi

Therapeutic class: Miscellaneous sexual dysfunction aids
Pharmacologic class: Serotonin agonist/antagonist agents

AVAILABLE FORMS
Tablets: 100 mg

INDICATIONS & DOSAGES
Boxed Warning Drug interacts with alcohol. Drug is contraindicated for use with strong or moderate CYP3A4 inhibitors and in patients with hepatic impairment. ■

➤ **Acquired, generalized hypoactive sexual desire disorder in patients who are premenopausal**
Adults: 100 mg PO once daily at bedtime. If no improvement after 8 weeks, discontinue drug.

SAFETY ALERT!

fludarabine phosphate
floo-DARE-a-been

Therapeutic class: Antineoplastics
Pharmacologic class: Purine antagonists

AVAILABLE FORMS
Powder for injection: 50 mg
Solution for injection: 50 mg/2 mL

INDICATIONS & DOSAGES
Boxed Warning Drug may cause severe bone marrow suppression, neurotoxicity, and autoimmune disorders, such as hemolytic anemia, thrombocytopenia, and acquired hemophilia. Use in combination with pentostatin for the treatment of refractory chronic lymphocytic leukemia (CLL) isn't recommended due to high risk of fatal pulmonary toxicity. Drug should only be given under the supervision of a health care provider experienced with antineoplastic therapy. ■

➤ **B-cell CLL in patients with no or inadequate response to at least one standard alkylating drug regimen**
Adults: 25 mg/m² IV over 30 minutes daily for 5 consecutive days. Repeat cycle every 28 days. The optimal duration of treatment hasn't been established, but it's recommended to give three additional cycles after maximal response is obtained.
Adjust-a-dose: In patients with CrCl of 30 to 70 mL/minute, reduce dose by 20%. If CrCl is less than 30 mL/minute, don't give drug.

➤ **Newly diagnosed pediatric acute myeloid leukemia as part of a multiagent chemotherapy regimen, in combination with cytarabine and idarubicin during consolidation phase of treatment ◆**

Children: 10.5 mg/m² IV over 15 minutes as a single dose, followed by a continuous IV infusion of 30.5 mg/m²/day for 48 hours during consolidation phase of treatment.

➤ **Allogeneic hematopoietic stem cell transplantation in older adults as a myeloablative conditioning regimen, in combination with busulfan ◆**
Adults: 40 mg/m²/day IV for 4 days (in combination with busulfan) beginning 6 days before transplantation.

fludrocortisone acetate
floo-droe-KOR-ti-sone

Therapeutic class: Mineralocorticoids
Pharmacologic class: Mineralocorticoids

AVAILABLE FORMS
Tablets: 0.1 mg

INDICATIONS & DOSAGES
➤ **Salt-losing adrenogenital syndrome (congenital adrenal hyperplasia)**
Adults: 0.1 to 0.2 mg PO daily.

➤ **Addison disease (adrenocortical insufficiency)**
Adults: 0.1 mg PO daily. Usual dosage range is 0.1 mg three times weekly to 0.2 mg daily. Decrease dosage to 0.05 mg daily if transient HTN develops.

flunisolide (intranasal)
floo-NISS-oh-lide

Therapeutic class: Corticosteroids
Pharmacologic class: Corticosteroids

AVAILABLE FORMS
Nasal spray: 25 mcg/spray

INDICATIONS & DOSAGES
➤ **Symptoms of seasonal or perennial allergic rhinitis**
Adults and children age 15 and older: Starting dose is 2 sprays in each nostril b.i.d. If needed, may increase dosage to 2 sprays in each nostril t.i.d. Maximum total daily dose is 8 sprays in each nostril per day.
Children ages 6 to 14: Starting dose is 1 spray in each nostril t.i.d. or 2 sprays in each nostril b.i.d. Maximum total daily dose is 4 sprays in each nostril per day.

fluPHENAZine decanoate
floo-FEN-a-zeen

fluPHENAZine hydrochloride
Therapeutic class: Antipsychotics
Pharmacologic class: Phenothiazines

AVAILABLE FORMS
fluphenazine decanoate
Depot injection: 25 mg/mL*
fluphenazine hydrochloride
Elixir: 2.5 mg/5 mL*
IM injection: 2.5 mg/mL
Oral concentrate: 5 mg/mL*
Tablets: 1 mg, 2.5 mg, 5 mg, 10 mg

INDICATIONS & DOSAGES
Boxed Warning Drug isn't indicated for use in older adults with dementia-related psychosis because of increased risk of death. ■
➤ **Psychotic disorders**
Adults: Initially, 2.5 to 10 mg fluphenazine hydrochloride PO daily in divided doses every 6 to 8 hours; may increase cautiously to 20 mg/day. Maintenance dose is 1 to 5 mg PO daily. IM doses are one-third to one-half of PO doses. Usual initial IM dose is 1.25 mg. Give more than 10 mg daily with caution.

Or, 12.5 to 25 mg of fluphenazine decanoate IM or subcut every 3 to 4 weeks (response may last up to 6 weeks in some patients); maintenance dose is 25 to 100 mg, as needed.
Older adults: 1 to 2.5 mg fluphenazine hydrochloride PO daily.

fosamprenavir calcium
foss-am-PREN-ah-ver

Lexiva

Therapeutic class: Antiretrovirals
Pharmacologic class: Protease inhibitors

AVAILABLE FORMS
Oral suspension: 50 mg/mL
Tablets: 700 mg

INDICATIONS & DOSAGES
Adjust-a-dose (for all indications excluding adults):
There are no dosing recommendations for children with hepatic impairment. Dosage for children shouldn't exceed recommended adult dosage of 700 mg fosamprenavir with ritonavir 100 mg b.i.d. Drug isn't approved for once-daily dosing in children.
➤ **HIV infection, with other antiretrovirals**
Adults: In patients not previously treated, 1,400 mg PO b.i.d. (without ritonavir). Or, 1,400 mg PO once daily with ritonavir 100 to 200 mg PO once daily. Or, 700 mg PO b.i.d. with ritonavir 100 mg PO b.i.d. In patients previously treated with a protease inhibitor, 700 mg PO b.i.d. plus ritonavir 100 mg PO b.i.d.
Adjust-a-dose: If patient has mild hepatic impairment (Child-Pugh score of 5 to 6), reduce dosage to 700 mg PO b.i.d. without ritonavir (in patients who are therapy-naive) or 700 mg b.i.d. plus ritonavir 100 mg once daily (in patients who are therapy-naive or protease inhibitor–experienced). If patient has moderate hepatic impairment (Child-Pugh score of 7 to 9), reduce dosage to 700 mg b.i.d. (in patients who are therapy-naive) without ritonavir or 450 mg b.i.d. plus ritonavir 100 mg once daily (in patients who are therapy-naive or protease inhibitor–experienced). If patient has severe hepatic impairment (Child-Pugh score of 10 to 15), reduce dosage to 350 mg b.i.d. without ritonavir (in patients who are therapy-naive) or 300 mg b.i.d. plus ritonavir 100 mg once daily (in patients who are therapy-naive or protease inhibitor–experienced).
➤ **HIV infection with other antiretrovirals for protease inhibitor–naive children age 4 weeks and older**

Children ages 4 weeks to 18 years weighing 20 kg or more: 18 mg/kg PO with ritonavir 3 mg/kg b.i.d.
Children ages 4 weeks to 18 years weighing 15 to less than 20 kg: 23 mg/kg PO with ritonavir 3 mg/kg b.i.d.
Children ages 4 weeks to 18 years weighing 11 to less than 15 kg: 30 mg/kg PO with ritonavir 3 mg/kg b.i.d.
Children ages 4 weeks to 18 years weighing less than 11 kg: 45 mg/kg PO with ritonavir 7 mg/kg b.i.d.
➤ **HIV infection with other antiretrovirals for protease inhibitor–experienced children age 6 months and older**
Children ages 6 months to 18 years weighing 20 kg or more: 18 mg/kg PO with ritonavir 3 mg/kg b.i.d.
Children ages 6 months to 18 years weighing 15 to less than 20 kg: 23 mg/kg PO with ritonavir 3 mg/kg b.i.d.
Children ages 6 months to 18 years weighing 11 to less than 15 kg: 30 mg/kg PO with ritonavir 3 mg/kg b.i.d.
Children ages 6 months to 18 years weighing less than 11 kg: 45 mg/kg PO with ritonavir 7 mg/kg b.i.d.
➤ **HIV infection without ritonavir in protease inhibitor–naive children**
Children age 2 years and older: 30 mg/kg PO b.i.d. For patients weighing at least 47 kg, may use the adult regimen of fosamprenavir 1,400 mg b.i.d. Maximum dose is 1,400 mg b.i.d.

fostamatinib disodium hexahydrate
FOS-tam-A-ti-nib

Tavalisse

Therapeutic class: Immunomodulators
Pharmacologic class: Spleen tyrosine kinase inhibitors

AVAILABLE FORMS
Tablets: 100 mg, 150 mg

INDICATIONS & DOSAGES
➤ **Thrombocytopenia in patients with chronic ITP who have had an insufficient response to previous treatment**
Adults: Initially, 100 mg PO b.i.d. If platelet count hasn't increased to at least 50×10^9/L after 4 weeks, increase dosage to 150 mg b.i.d. Use lowest dosage possible to achieve and maintain platelet count of at least 50×10^9/L as necessary to reduce the risk of bleeding. Discontinue fostamatinib after 12 weeks if platelet count hasn't increased to a level adequate to avoid clinically important bleeding.
Adjust-a-dose: Refer to manufacturer's instructions for toxicity-related dosage adjustments.

fostemsavir
fos-TEM-sa-vir

Rukobia

Therapeutic class: Antiretrovirals
Pharmacologic class: HIV-1 gp120 attachment inhibitors

AVAILABLE FORMS

Tablets (extended-release) ⓓⓝⓒ: 600 mg

INDICATIONS & DOSAGES

➤ **HIV-1 infection, in combination with other antiretrovirals, in patients with multidrug-resistant HIV-1 infection who are heavily treatment-experienced but failing their current antiretroviral regimen due to resistance, intolerance, or safety considerations**

Adults: 600 mg PO b.i.d.

---

fremanezumab-vfrm

FRE-ma-nez-ue-mab

Ajovy

Therapeutic class: Antimigraine drugs
Pharmacologic class: Calcitonin gene-related peptide antagonists

AVAILABLE FORMS

Injection: 225 mg/1.5 mL single-dose prefilled syringe or autoinjector

INDICATIONS & DOSAGES

➤ **Prevention of migraine headache**

Adults: 225 mg subcut once a month or 675 mg (three consecutive injections of 225 mg each) subcut every 3 months (quarterly).

---

galantamine hydrobromide

gah-LAN-tah-meen

Razadyne ER

Therapeutic class: Anti-Alzheimer drugs
Pharmacologic class: Cholinesterase inhibitors

AVAILABLE FORMS

Capsules (extended-release): 8 mg, 16 mg, 24 mg
Oral solution: 4 mg/mL
Tablets: 4 mg, 8 mg, 12 mg

INDICATIONS & DOSAGES

➤ **Mild to moderate Alzheimer dementia**

Adults: Initially, 4 mg immediate-release tablets or solution PO b.i.d., preferably with morning and evening meals. If dose is well tolerated after minimum of 4 weeks of therapy, increase dosage to 8 mg b.i.d. A further increase to 12 mg b.i.d. may be attempted, but only after at least 4 weeks of therapy at the previous dosage. Dosage range is 16 to 24 mg daily in two divided doses.

Or, 8 mg extended-release capsule PO once daily in the morning with food. Increase to 16 mg PO once daily after a minimum of 4 weeks. May further increase to 24 mg once daily after a minimum of 4 weeks, based on patient response and tolerability. Dosage range is 16 to 24 mg daily.

Adjust-a-dose: For patients with moderate hepatic impairment (Child-Pugh score of 7 to 9) or moderate renal impairment (CrCl of 9 to 59 mL/minute), dosage usually shouldn't exceed 16 mg daily. Drug isn't recommended for patients with severe hepatic impairment or CrCl less than 9 mL/minute.

---

galcanezumab-gnlm

GAL-ka-nez-ue-mab

Emgality

Therapeutic class: Antimigraine drugs
Pharmacologic class: Monoclonal antibodies

AVAILABLE FORMS

Injection: 100 mg/mL single-dose prefilled syringe; 120 mg/mL in single-dose autoinjector or prefilled syringe

INDICATIONS & DOSAGES

➤ **Prevention of migraine headache**

Adults: Initially, 240 mg subcut (administered as two consecutive injections of 120 mg each) once as a loading dose, followed by 120 mg subcut once monthly.

➤ **Episodic cluster headache**

Adults: Initially, 300 mg subcut (three consecutive injections of 100 mg) once at onset of the cluster period, then monthly until end of the cluster period.

SAFETY ALERT!

gilteritinib ✂

GIL-te-ri-ti-nib

Xospata

Therapeutic class: Antineoplastics
Pharmacologic class: Kinase inhibitors

AVAILABLE FORMS

Tablets: 40 mg

INDICATIONS & DOSAGES

Boxed Warning Drug can cause differentiation syndrome (fever, dyspnea, hypoxia, pulmonary infiltrates, pleural or pericardial effusions, rapid weight gain or peripheral edema, hypotension, or renal dysfunction), which can be fatal or life-threatening if not treated. If differentiation syndrome is suspected, initiate corticosteroid therapy and hemodynamic monitoring. ▮

➤ **Relapsed or refractory acute myeloid leukemia with an *FLT3* mutation** ✂

Adults: 120 mg PO once daily for a minimum of 6 months.

Adjust-a-dose: See manufacturer's instructions for toxicity-related dosage adjustments, including for QT-interval prolongation.

---

givosiran

giv-oh-SIR-an

Givlaari

Therapeutic class: Endocrine-metabolic agents
Pharmacologic class: Aminolevulinate synthase 1–directed small interfering RNAs

AVAILABLE FORMS

Injection: 189 mg/mL single-dose vial

INDICATIONS & DOSAGES
➤ **Acute hepatic porphyria**
Adults: 2.5 mg/kg subcut once monthly.
Adjust-a-dose: For patients with severe or significant transaminase elevations who subsequently improve after dose interruption, reduce dosage to 1.25 mg/kg once monthly. For those who resume dosing at 1.25 mg/kg once monthly without recurrence of severe or significant transaminase elevations, increase dose to 2.5 mg/kg once monthly.

SAFETY ALERT!

glasdegib
glas-DEG-ib

Daurismo

Therapeutic class: Antineoplastics
Pharmacologic class: Hedgehog pathway inhibitors

AVAILABLE FORMS
Tablets: 25 mg, 100 mg

INDICATIONS & DOSAGES
Boxed Warning Drug can cause severe birth defects and fetal death. ∎
➤ **Newly diagnosed acute myeloid leukemia, in combination with low-dose cytarabine, in patients who are age 75 and older or who have comorbidities that preclude the use of intensive induction chemotherapy**
Adults: 100 mg PO once daily on days 1 to 28, in combination with cytarabine 20 mg subcut b.i.d. on days 1 to 10 of each 28-day cycle. Treat for a minimum of six cycles to allow time for clinical response or until unacceptable toxicity or loss of disease control.
Adjust-a-dose: Refer to glasdegib manufacturer's instructions for toxicity-related dosage adjustments. Refer to cytarabine manufacturer's instructions for dosing and toxicity-related information.

glucagon
GLOO-ka-gon

GlucaGen Diagnostic Kit, GlucaGen HypoKit, Gvoke HypoPen, Gvoke PFS

Therapeutic class: Diagnostic agents
Pharmacologic class: Antihypoglycemics

AVAILABLE FORMS
Powder for injection: 1-mg (1-unit) vials
Solution: 0.5 mg/0.1 mL, 1 mg/0.2 mL prefilled syringe or autoinjector; 1 mg/0.2 mL vial

INDICATIONS & DOSAGES
➤ **Hypoglycemia**
Glucagon
Adults and children weighing more than 20 kg or older than age 6: 1 mg (1 unit) IV, IM, or subcut. May repeat in 15 minutes, if needed. IV glucose must be given if patient fails to respond.
Children weighing 20 kg or less: 0.5 mg (0.5 unit) or 20 to 30 mcg/kg IV, IM, or subcut; maximum dose,

1 mg. May repeat in 15 minutes, if needed. IV glucose must be given if patient fails to respond.
GlucaGen
Adults and children weighing more than 25 kg or age 6 or older or when weight is unknown: 1 mg (1 mL) IV, IM, or subcut.
Children weighing less than 25 kg or younger than age 6 when weight is unknown: 0.5 mg (0.5 mL) IV, IM, or subcut.
Gvoke (subcut only)
Adults and children age 2 and older weighing 45 kg or more: 1 mg subcut into lower abdomen, outer thigh, or outer upper arm. May repeat in 15 minutes if no response.
Children age 2 to younger than 12 weighing less than 45 kg: 0.5 mg subcut into lower abdomen, outer thigh, or outer upper arm. May repeat in 15 minutes if no response.
➤ **Diagnostic aid for radiologic exam of the GI tract**
Adults: 0.2 to 2 mg IV or 1 mg IM before radiologic exam. Refer to manufacturer's instruction for dosage by anatomic area.

SAFETY ALERT!

goserelin acetate
GOE-se-rel-in

Zoladex

Therapeutic class: Antineoplastics
Pharmacologic class: Gonadotropin-releasing hormone analogues

AVAILABLE FORMS
Implants: 3.6 mg, 10.8 mg

INDICATIONS & DOSAGES
➤ **Endometriosis, including pain relief and lesion reduction**
Adults: 3.6 mg subcut every 28 days into the anterior abdominal wall below the navel. Maximum length of therapy is 6 months.
➤ **Endometrial thinning before endometrial ablation**
Adults: 3.6 mg subcut into the anterior abdominal wall below the navel. Give one or two implants, 4 weeks apart. When one depot is given, surgery should be performed at 4 weeks; when two depots are given, surgery should be performed within 2 to 4 weeks after second depot.
➤ **Palliative treatment of advanced breast cancer in patients who are premenopausal and perimenopausal**
Adults: 3.6 mg subcut every 28 days into anterior abdominal wall below navel.
➤ **Palliative treatment of advanced prostate cancer**
Men: 3.6 mg subcut every 28 days or 10.8 mg subcut every 12 weeks into anterior abdominal wall below navel.
➤ **Stage B2-C prostate cancer in combination with radiotherapy and flutamide**

✤Canada   ◇ OTC   ◆ Off-label use   ✐Photoguide   ⓓⓞDo not crush   *Liquid contains alcohol   ✂Genetic

Men: Start 8 weeks before initiating radiotherapy and continue during radiation therapy. Give 3.6 mg subcut into anterior abdominal wall below navel 8 weeks before radiotherapy, followed in 28 days by 10.8 mg subcut. Or, give four injections of 3.6 mg at 28-day intervals, two injections preceding and two during radiotherapy.

guanFACINE hydrochloride
GWAHN-fa-seen

Intuniv

Therapeutic class: Antihypertensives
Pharmacologic class: Centrally acting antiadrenergics

AVAILABLE FORMS
Tablets: 1 mg, 2 mg
Tablets (extended-release) ⒪: 1 mg, 2 mg, 3 mg, 4 mg

INDICATIONS & DOSAGES
➤ **HTN**

Adults and children age 12 and older: Initially, 1 mg immediate-release tablet PO once daily at bedtime. If response isn't adequate after 3 to 4 weeks, may increase dosage to 2 mg daily.

➤ **ADHD**

Children ages 6 to 17: Extended-release form only. Initially, 1 mg PO once daily in a.m. or p.m. at approximately same time each day. Adjust dosage in increments of 1 mg/week as needed. Target dosage range is 0.05 to 0.12 mg/kg PO once daily. Adjust dosage up to 0.12 mg/kg once daily if well tolerated and necessary. Doses above 4 mg/day haven't been evaluated in children ages 6 to 12 or above 7 mg/day in adolescents ages 13 to 17.

Adjust-a-dose: Refer to manufacturer's instructions for dosage adjustment for use with CYP3A4 inhibitors or inducers.

HYDROXYprogesterone caproate
hye-drox-ee-proh-JESS-te-rone

Makena

Therapeutic class: Hormones
Pharmacologic class: Progestins

AVAILABLE FORMS
Injection: 250 mg/mL in single-dose and multidose vials; 275 mg/1.1 mL autoinjector

INDICATIONS & DOSAGES
➤ **To reduce risk of preterm birth in patients with singleton pregnancy and history of singleton spontaneous preterm birth**

Adolescents and patients who are pregnant age 16 and older: 250 mg IM in gluteus maximus (if using vial) or 275 mg subcut in back of either upper arm (if using autoinjector) once weekly starting between 16 weeks, 0 days and 20 weeks, 6 days of gestation and continuing until week 37 (through 36 weeks, 6 days) of gestation or delivery, whichever occurs first.

ibalizumab-uiyk
eye-ba-LIZ-ue-mab

Trogarzo

Therapeutic class: Antiretrovirals
Pharmacologic class: CD4-directed postattachment HIV-1 inhibitors

AVAILABLE FORMS
Injection: 200 mg/1.33 mL (150 mg/mL) single-dose vials

INDICATIONS & DOSAGES
➤ **HIV-1 infection, in combination with other antiretrovirals, in patients with multidrug-resistant HIV-1 infection who are heavily treatment-experienced and failing their current antiretroviral regimen**

Adults: 2,000 mg IV infusion loading dose followed by 800 mg IV infusion maintenance doses every 2 weeks.

icosapent ethyl
eye-KOE-sa-pent

Vascepa

Therapeutic class: Antilipemics
Pharmacologic class: Ethyl esters

AVAILABLE FORMS
Capsules ⒪: 500 mg, 1 g

INDICATIONS & DOSAGES
➤ **Adjunct to diet to reduce triglyceride levels 500 mg/dL or more**

Adults: 2 g PO b.i.d. with food.

➤ **Adjunct to maximally tolerated statin therapy to reduce risk of MI, stroke, coronary revascularization, and unstable angina requiring hospitalization in patients with elevated triglyceride levels (150 mg/dL or more) and established CV disease, or in patients with diabetes and two or more additional risk factors for CV disease**

Adults: 2 g PO b.i.d. with food.

SAFETY ALERT!

IDArubicin hydrochloride
eye-da-ROO-bi-sin

Idamycin PFS

Therapeutic class: Antineoplastics
Pharmacologic class: Semisynthetic anthracyclines

AVAILABLE FORMS
Injection: 1 mg/mL in 5-, 10-, and 20-mL single-dose vials

INDICATIONS & DOSAGES
Dosages vary. Check treatment protocol with prescriber.

Boxed Warning Reduce dosage in patients with hepatic or renal impairment. Don't give idarubicin if bilirubin level exceeds 5 mg/dL. Severe local tissue necrosis can occur with extravasation. Give slowly into a freely flowing IV infusion. Drug can cause myocardial toxicity leading to HF, and severe myelo-suppression. Drug should be given under supervision of a physician experienced in leukemia chemothera-py in a facility with appropriate lab and supportive resources. ■

➤ **Acute myeloid leukemia with other approved antileukemic drugs**
Adults: 12 mg/m^2 daily for 3 days by slow IV injec-tion (over 10 to 15 minutes) with 100 mg/m^2 daily of cytarabine for 7 days by continuous IV infusion. Or, cytarabine may be given as 25-mg/m^2 bolus; then 200 mg/m^2 daily for 5 days by continuous IV infusion. May give a second course, if needed.
Adjust-a-dose: If patient experiences severe mucositis, delay second course of therapy until recovery is com-plete; reduce dosage by 25%. Consider dosage reduction if bilirubin or creatinine level is above normal range. ♦
➤ **Acute myeloid leukemia (newly diagnosed)** ♦
Infants, children, adolescents: Per clinical trial CCG-2961, for induction and consolidation, 5 mg/m^2/dose IV daily for 4 days on days 0 to 3 in combination with cytarabine, etoposide, thioguanine, and dexametha-sone. Or, for consolidation only, 12 mg/m^2/dose IV daily for 3 days on days 0 to 2 in combination with fludarabine and cytarabine.

SAFETY ALERT!

ifosfamide
eye-FOSS-fa-mide

Ifex

Therapeutic class: Antineoplastics
Pharmacologic class: Nitrogen mustards

AVAILABLE FORMS
IV solution: 1 g/20 mL
Powder for injection: 1-g, 3-g vials

INDICATIONS & DOSAGES
➤ **Germ cell testicular cancer as third-line chemo-therapy in combination with certain other antineo-plastics and mesna**
Adults: 1.2 g/m^2 IV daily for 5 consecutive days. Re-peat treatment every 3 weeks or after patient recovers from hematologic toxicity. Don't repeat doses until WBC count exceeds 2,000/mm^3 and platelet count ex-ceeds 50,000/mm^3.
➤ **Ewing sarcoma** ♦
Adults: 1,800 mg/m^2/day IV for 5 days (VAC/IE regimen; in combination with mesna and etoposide); alternate with VAC (vincristine, doxorubicin, and cyclophosphamide) every 3 weeks for a total of 17 courses.
   Or, 3,000 mg/m^2/day IV on days 1, 2, 22, 23, 43, and 44 for four courses (VAIA regimen; in combi-nation with vincristine, doxorubicin, dactinomycin, and mesna).
   Or, 2,000 mg/m^2/day IV for 3 days every 3 weeks for 14 courses (in combination with vincristine, doxo-rubicin, dactinomycin, and mesna).

   Or, 3,000 mg/m^2/day IV over 1 to 3 hours for 3 days every 3 weeks for six courses (VIDE regimen; in combination with vincristine, doxorubicin, etopo-side, and mesna).
   Or, 1,800 mg/m^2/day IV over 1 hour for 5 days ev-ery 3 weeks for 12 cycles (IE regimen; in combination with etoposide and mesna).
   Or, 1,800 mg/m^2/day IV for 5 days every 3 weeks for up to 12 cycles (ICE regimen; in combination with carboplatin and etoposide [and mesna]).
Children: 1,800 mg/m^2/day IV for 5 days (IE regi-men; in combination with mesna and etoposide); alter-nate with VAC (vincristine, doxorubicin, and cyclo-phosphamide) every 3 weeks for a total of 17 courses.
   Or, 1,800 mg/m^2/day IV for 5 days every 3 to 4 weeks for two courses (ICE regimen; in combina-tion with carboplatin and etoposide [and mesna]), fol-lowed by CAV (cyclophosphamide, doxorubicin, and vincristine).
   Or, 3,000 mg/m^2/day IV on days 1, 2, 22, 23, 43, and 44 for four courses (VAIA regimen; in combi-nation with vincristine, doxorubicin, dactinomycin, and mesna).
   Or, 2,000 mg/m^2/day IV for 3 days every 3 weeks for 14 courses (in combination with vincristine, doxo-rubicin, dactinomycin, and mesna).
   Or, 3,000 mg/m^2/day IV over 1 to 3 hours for 3 days every 3 weeks for 6 courses (VIDE regimen; in combination with vincristine, doxorubicin, etoposide, and mesna).
   Or, 1,800 mg/m^2/day IV over 1 hour for 5 days ev-ery 3 weeks for 12 cycles (IE regimen; in combination with etoposide and mesna).
   Or, 1,800 mg/m^2/day IV for 5 days every 3 weeks for up to 12 cycles (ICE regimen; in combination with carboplatin and etoposide [and mesna]).
➤ **Soft tissue sarcoma** ♦
Adults: 3,000 mg/m^2/day IV over 4 hours for 3 days every 3 weeks for at least two cycles or until disease progression.
   Or, 1,500 mg/m^2/day IV for 4 days every 3 weeks until disease progression or unacceptable toxicity (EIA regimen; in combination with etoposide, doxoru-bicin, and regional hyperthermia).
   Or, 2,000 mg/m^2/day IV continuous infusion for 3 days every 3 weeks (MAID regimen; in combina-tion with mesna, doxorubicin, and dacarbazine).
   Or, 2,500 mg/m^2/day IV continuous infusion for 3 days every 3 weeks (in combination with mesna, doxorubicin, and dacarbazine); reduce ifosfamide to 1,500 mg/m^2/day if prior pelvic irradiation.
   Or, 1,800 mg/m^2/day IV over 1 hour for 5 days every 3 weeks for five cycles (in combination with mesna and epirubicin).
   Or, 1,500 mg/m^2/day IV over 2 hours for 4 days every 3 weeks for four to six cycles (AIM regimens; in combination with mesna and doxorubicin).
   Or, 2,000 to 3,000 mg/m^2/day IV over 3 hours for 3 days (in combination with mesna and doxorubicin).

---

imipenem–cilastatin sodium–relebactam

im-i-PEN-em/sye-la-STAT-in/rel-e-BAK-tam

Recarbrio

Therapeutic class: Anti-infectives
Pharmacologic class: Penem antibacterials–renal dehydropeptidase inhibitors–beta-lactamase inhibitors

AVAILABLE FORMS

Injection: 1.25-g (imipenem 500 mg, cilastatin 500 mg, relebactam 250 mg) vial

INDICATIONS & DOSAGES

Adjust-a-dose (for all indications): For CrCl of 60 to 89 mL/minute, give 1 g IV every 6 hours (imipenem 400 mg, cilastatin 400 mg, relebactam 200 mg); for CrCl of 30 to 59 mL/minute, give 750 mg IV every 6 hours (imipenem 300 mg, cilastatin 300 mg, relebactam 150 mg); for CrCl of 15 to 29 mL/minute, give 500 mg IV every 6 hours (imipenem 200 mg, cilastatin 200 g, relebactam 100 mg); for CrCl less than 15 mL/minute, don't administer unless hemodialysis is instituted within 48 hours. For patients with ESRD on hemodialysis, give 500 mg IV every 6 hours. Give after hemodialysis and at intervals timed from the end of that hemodialysis session.

➤ **Complicated UTIs, including pyelonephritis, caused by susceptible gram-negative microorganisms (*Enterobacter cloacae, Escherichia coli, Klebsiella aerogenes, Klebsiella pneumoniae,* and *Pseudomonas aeruginosa*) in patients with limited or no alternative treatment options**

Adults: 1.25 g by IV infusion over 30 minutes every 6 hours. Recommended duration of treatment is 4 to 14 days guided by the severity and location of the infection, and clinical response.

➤ **Complicated intra-abdominal infections caused by susceptible gram-negative microorganisms (*Bacteroides caccae, Bacteroides fragilis, Bacteroides ovatus, Bacteroides thetaiotaomicron, Bacteroides uniformis, Bacteroides vulgatus, Bifidobacterium stercoris, Citrobacter freundii, E. cloacae, E. coli, Fusobacterium nucleatum, K. aerogenes, Klebsiella oxytoca, K. pneumoniae, Parabacteroides distasonis,* and *P. aeruginosa*) in patients with limited or no alternative treatment options**

Adults: 1.25 g by IV infusion over 30 minutes every 6 hours. Recommended duration of treatment is 4 to 14 days guided by the severity and location of the infection, and clinical response.

➤ **Hospital-acquired pneumonia and ventilator-associated pneumonia caused by susceptible gram-negative organisms (*Acinetobacter calcoaceticus-baumannii* complex, *E. cloacae, E. coli, Haemophilus influenzae, K. aerogenes, K. oxytoca, K. pneumoniae, P. aeruginosa,* and *Serratia marcescens*)**

Adults: 1.25 g by IV infusion over 30 minutes every 6 hours. Recommended duration of treatment is 4 to 14 days guided by the severity and location of the infection, and clinical response.

imiquimod

ih-mih-KWI-mahd

Aldara, Vyloma✚, Zyclara

Therapeutic class: Immunosuppressants (topical)
Pharmacologic class: Immune response modifiers

AVAILABLE FORMS

Cream: 2.5%, 3.75% in 30-mL pump bottles (one dose is one full actuation); 3.75% % in single-use packets

INDICATIONS & DOSAGES

➤ **External genital and perianal warts**

Adults and adolescents age 12 and older: Apply thin layer of 3.75% cream once daily before sleep; leave on for 8 hours. Continue up to 8 weeks. Or, apply thin layer of 5% cream three times per week before sleep; leave on for 6 to 10 hours. Continue for up to 16 weeks.

➤ **Typical, nonhyperkeratotic, nonhypertrophic actinic keratoses on the face or scalp in immunocompetent adults**

Adults: Wash area with mild soap and water, and allow to dry for at least 10 minutes. Apply 5% cream to face or scalp, but not both concurrently, twice weekly at bedtime; wash off after about 8 hours. Treat for 16 weeks. Or, apply 2.5% or 3.75% cream once daily at bedtime for two 2-week cycles. Separate cycles by a 2-week no-treatment period.

➤ **Superficial basal cell carcinoma**

Adults: Wash area with mild soap and water, and allow to dry thoroughly. Apply a thin layer of 5% cream to the biopsy-confirmed area, including 1 cm of skin surrounding tumor, five times a week at bedtime; wash off after about 8 hours. Treat for 6 weeks.

indapamide

in-DAP-a-mide

Therapeutic class: Diuretics/antihypertensives
Pharmacologic class: Thiazide-like diuretics

AVAILABLE FORMS

Tablets: 1.25 mg, 2.5 mg

INDICATIONS & DOSAGES

➤ **Edema of HF**

Adults: Initially, 2.5 mg PO daily in the morning, increased to 5 mg daily after 1 week, if needed.

➤ **HTN**

Adults: Initially, 1.25 mg PO daily in the morning, increased to 2.5 mg daily after 4 weeks, if needed. Increased to 5 mg daily after 4 more weeks, if needed. If response is inadequate, a second antihypertensive, given at 50% of the usual starting dose, may be needed.

---

inotersen ⚥

in-oh-TER-sen

Tegsedi

Therapeutic class: Endocrine-metabolic agents
Pharmacologic class: Antisense oligonucleotides

AVAILABLE FORMS

Injection: 284 mg/1.5 mL single-dose, prefilled syringe

INDICATIONS & DOSAGES

Boxed Warning Drug can cause glomerulonephritis that may require immunosuppressive therapy and may result in dialysis-dependent renal failure. Testing before and monitoring during treatment is required. ∎

Boxed Warning Drug can cause sudden and unpredictable thrombocytopenia that can be life-threatening and is contraindicated with platelet count less than 100×10^9/L. Testing before and monitoring during treatment is required. ∎

➤ **Polyneuropathy of hereditary transthyretin–mediated amyloidosis** ⚥

Adults: 284 mg subcut once weekly on the same day every week.

Adjust-a-dose: Refer to manufacturer's instructions for monitoring and dosage adjustments based on platelet counts.

SAFETY ALERT!

inotuzumab ozogamicin

in-oh-TOOZ-ue-mab

Besponsa

Therapeutic class: Antineoplastics
Pharmacologic class: Antibody–drug conjugates

AVAILABLE FORMS

Injection (lyophilized): 0.9 mg lyophilized powder in single-dose vials

INDICATIONS & DOSAGES

Boxed Warning Hepatotoxicity, including fatal and life-threatening hepatic veno-occlusive disease (VOD), has occurred. Permanently discontinue drug if VOD occurs. A higher posthematopoietic stem cell transplant (HSCT) nonrelapse mortality rate occurred in patients receiving inotuzumab. ∎

➤ **Relapsed or refractory B-cell precursor acute lymphoblastic leukemia**

Adults: Premedicate with a corticosteroid, antipyretic, and antihistamine. For cycle 1, total dose is 1.8 mg/m² given as three divided doses on days 1, 8, and 15 of a 21-day treatment cycle. On day 1, give 0.8 mg/m² IV infusion; on days 8 and 15, give 0.5 mg/m² IV infusion. Cycle 1 is 3 weeks in duration, but may be extended to 4 weeks if patient achieves a complete remission (CR) or CR with incomplete hematologic recovery (Cri), or to allow recovery from toxicity.

For subsequent cycles in patients who achieve a CR or CRi, total dose per cycle is 1.5 mg/m² given as three divided doses on days 1, 8, and 15 of a 28-day treatment cycle. On days 1, 8, and 15, give 0.5 mg/m² IV infusion. Subsequent cycles are 4 weeks in duration.

For subsequent cycles in patients who don't achieve a CR or CRi, total dose per cycle is 1.8 mg/m² given as three divided doses on days 1, 8, and 15 of a 28-day treatment cycle. On day 1, give 0.8 mg/m² IV infusion; on days 8 and 15, give 0.5 mg/m² IV infusion. Subsequent cycles are 4 weeks in duration, but discontinue drug in patients who don't achieve CR or CRi within three cycles.

For patients proceeding to HSCT, recommended treatment duration is two cycles. May consider a third cycle for those who don't achieve a CR or CRi and minimal residual disease negativity after two cycles.

For patients not proceeding to HSCT, may give additional cycles of treatment, up to a maximum of six cycles.

Adjust-a-dose: Refer to manufacturer's instructions for toxicity-related dosage adjustments and drug discontinuation.

SAFETY ALERT!

interferon gamma-1b

in-ter-FEER-on

Actimmune

Therapeutic class: Immune response modifiers
Pharmacologic class: Biological response modifiers

AVAILABLE FORMS

Injection: 100 mcg (2 million international units) in 0.5-mL vials

INDICATIONS & DOSAGES

➤ **Chronic granulomatous disease in adults and children age 1 year and older; severe malignant osteopetrosis in adults and children age 1 month and older**

Adults and children with BSA greater than 0.5 m²: Give 50 mcg/m² (1 million international units/m²) subcut three times weekly, preferably at bedtime.
Adults and children with a BSA of 0.5 m² or less: 1.5 mcg/kg subcut three times weekly.

Adjust-a-dose: If patient has severe reaction, decrease dosage by 50% or stop drug until reaction subsides.

SAFETY ALERT!

irinotecan liposome ⚥

eye-rye-no-TEE-kan

Onivyde

Therapeutic class: Antineoplastics
Pharmacologic class: DNA topoisomerase inhibitors

AVAILABLE FORMS

Injection: 43 mg/10 mL in single-use vials

✦Canada   ◇OTC   ◆Off-label use   ⊘Photoguide   ⊛Do not crush   *Liquid contains alcohol   ⚥Genetic

INDICATIONS & DOSAGES

Boxed Warning Drug may cause severe diarrhea. Contraindicated in patients with bowel obstruction. Withhold drug and initiate loperamide for late-onset diarrhea of any severity. Administer IV or subcut atropine 0.25 to 1 mg (unless clinically contraindicated) for early-onset diarrhea of any severity. Drug may cause fatal neutropenic sepsis and severe or life-threatening neutropenic fever. Withhold drug for ANC below 1,500/mm³ or neutropenic fever. Monitor CBC periodically during treatment. ■

➤ **Metastatic adenocarcinoma of the pancreas after disease progression after gemcitabine-based therapy, in combination with 5-FU and leucovorin** ▨

Adults: 70 mg/m² IV infusion over 90 minutes every 2 weeks. Premedicate with a corticosteroid and an antiemetic 30 minutes before infusion.

Adjust-a-dose: Refer to manufacturer's instructions for patients known to be homozygous for the UGT1A1*28 allele and for toxicity-related dosage adjustments and discontinuation.

---

isavuconazonium sulfate
eye-sa-vue-koe-na-ZOE-nee-um

Cresemba

Therapeutic class: Antifungals
Pharmacologic class: Triazole antifungals

AVAILABLE FORMS

Capsules: 186 mg (equal to isavuconazole 100 mg)
Injection: 372 mg (equal to isavuconazole 200 mg)/vial

INDICATIONS & DOSAGES

➤ **Invasive aspergillosis; invasive mucormycosis fungal infection**

Adults: Give loading doses of 372 mg IV or PO every 8 hours for six doses (48 hours); then give maintenance dose of 372 mg IV or PO once daily. Initiate maintenance dose 12 to 24 hours after last loading dose. Switching between IV and PO formulations of isavuconazonium sulfate is acceptable for maintenance dosing. It isn't necessary to restart dosing with a loading dose when switching between formulations.

---

isoproterenol hydrochloride
eye-soe-proe-TER-e-nole

Isuprel

Therapeutic class: Bronchodilators, inotropes
Pharmacologic class: Nonselective beta-adrenergic agonists

AVAILABLE FORMS

Injection: 0.2 mg/mL in 1-mL, 5-mL ampules or vials

INDICATIONS & DOSAGES

➤ **Bronchospasm during anesthesia**

Adults: Dilute 1 mL (0.2 mg) with 9 mL of NSS or D₅W. Give 0.01 to 0.02 mg IV and repeat as necessary.

➤ **Heart block, Adams-Stokes attacks except when caused by ventricular tachycardia or fibrillation; cardiac arrest until electric shock or pacemaker therapy is available**

Adults: Initially, 0.02 to 0.06 mg IV bolus or via infusion at 5 mcg/minute IV; then 0.01 to 0.2 mg IV bolus. Or, initially, 0.2 mg IM or subcut; then 0.02 to 1 mg IM or 0.15 to 0.2 mg subcut as needed. Or, initially 0.02 mg intracardiac.

➤ **Shock**

Adults: 0.5 to 5 mcg/minute (0.25 to 2.5 mg) by continuous IV infusion. Usual concentration is 1 mg in 500 mL D₅W. Titrate infusion rate according to HR, central venous pressure, BP, and urine flow.

---

istradefylline
iz-TRA-de-FYE-leen

Nourianz

Therapeutic class: Antiparkinsonian drugs
Pharmacologic class: Adenosine receptor antagonists

AVAILABLE FORMS

Tablets: 20 mg, 40 mg

INDICATIONS & DOSAGES

➤ **Adjunct to levodopa–carbidopa in patients with Parkinson disease experiencing "off" episodes**

Adults: 20 mg PO once daily. May increase to a maximum of 40 mg PO once daily based on individual need and tolerability.

Adjust-a-dose: For patients with moderate hepatic impairment (Child-Pugh class B) or concomitant use of strong CYP3A4 inhibitors, maximum recommended dosage is 20 mg PO once daily. For patients who use tobacco in amounts of 20 or more cigarettes per day (or the equivalent of another tobacco product), recommended dosage is 40 mg PO once daily.

SAFETY ALERT!

---

ivosidenib ▨
EYE-voe-SID-e-nib

Tibsovo

Therapeutic class: Antineoplastics
Pharmacologic class: Isocitrate dehydrogenase-1 inhibitors

AVAILABLE FORMS

Tablets ⊕ 250 mg

INDICATIONS & DOSAGES

Boxed Warning Can cause differentiation syndrome (fever, dyspnea, hypoxia, pulmonary infiltrates, pleural or pericardial effusions, rapid weight gain or peripheral edema, hypotension, and hepatic, renal, or multiorgan dysfunction), which can be fatal if not treated. If differentiation syndrome is suspected, initiate corticosteroid therapy and hemodynamic monitoring until symptom resolution. ■

Adjust-a-dose (for all indications): Refer to manufacturer's instructions for toxicity-related dosage adjustments.

♣Canada ◇OTC ◆Off-label use ✐Photoguide ⊕Do not crush *Liquid contains alcohol ▨Genetic

➤ **Relapsed or refractory acute myeloid leukemia (AML) with a susceptible *IDH1* mutation** 🔬
Adults: 500 mg PO daily. Treat for a minimum of 6 months to allow time for clinical response or until disease progression or unacceptable toxicity.
➤ **Newly diagnosed AML with a susceptible *IDH1* mutation in patients age 75 and older or who have comorbidities that preclude use of intensive induction chemotherapy, in combination with azacitidine** 🔬
Adults age 75 and older: 500 mg PO daily with azacitidine 75 mg/m² subcut or IV once daily on days 1 to 7 (on days 1 to 5 and 8 to 9) of each 28-day cycle until disease progression or unacceptable toxicity occurs. Treat for a minimum of 6 months to allow time for clinical response. Refer to azacitidine manufacturer's instructions for additional dosing information.
➤ **Locally advanced or metastatic cholangiocarcinoma with *IDH1* mutation in patients who have been previously treated** 🔬
Adults: 500 mg PO daily until disease progression or unacceptable toxicity occurs.

SAFETY ALERT!

ixabepilone
ecks-ah-BEH-pill-own

Ixempra Kit

Therapeutic class: Antineoplastics
Pharmacologic class: Microtubule inhibitors

AVAILABLE FORMS
Injection: 15-mg, 45-mg vials

INDICATIONS & DOSAGES
Boxed Warning Drug is contraindicated in patients with AST or ALT level greater than 2.5 × ULN or bilirubin level 1 × ULN when used with capecitabine due to increased toxicity and neutropenia-related death. ∎
➤ **With capecitabine for metastatic or locally advanced breast cancer, after failure of anthracycline and a taxane, or in patients whose cancer is taxane-resistant and for whom further anthracycline therapy is contraindicated; or alone for metastatic or locally advanced breast cancer, after failure of anthracycline, taxanes, and capecitabine**
Adults: 40 mg/m² IV over 3 hours every 3 weeks. Doses for patients with BSA greater than 2.2 m² should be calculated based on 2.2 m². Premedicate with an H₁-receptor antagonist, such as diphenhydramine 50 mg PO (or equivalent), and an H₂-receptor antagonist 1 hour before ixabepilone infusion. For patients who experienced a prior hypersensitivity reaction, premedicate with corticosteroids (such as dexamethasone 20 mg IV 30 minutes before infusion or PO 60 minutes before infusion) in addition to the H₁- and H₂-receptor antagonists.
Adjust-a-dose: Refer to manufacturer's instructions for monotherapy and combination therapy dosage adjustments for toxicities and hepatic failure.

ketoprofen
kee-toe-PROE-fen

Therapeutic class: Anti-inflammatory drugs
Pharmacologic class: NSAIDs

AVAILABLE FORMS
Capsules: 25 mg, 50 mg, 75 mg
Capsules (extended-release): 200 mg

INDICATIONS & DOSAGES
Boxed Warning NSAIDs may increase risk of serious CV thrombotic events, MI, stroke, and GI adverse reactions. Contraindicated for use in CABG surgery. ∎
Adjust-a-dose (for all indications): For patients age 75 and older, reduce dosage. For patients with mildly impaired renal function, maximum daily dose is 150 mg. For patients with GFR of less than 25 mL/minute/1.73 m², ESRD, or impaired liver function and serum albumin level less than 3.5 g/dL, maximum daily dose is 100 mg.
➤ **RA, osteoarthritis**
Adults: 75 mg PO t.i.d. or 50 mg PO q.i.d., or 200 mg as an extended-release capsule once daily. Maximum dose is 300 mg daily, or 200 mg daily for extended-release capsules.
➤ **Mild to moderate pain, dysmenorrhea**
Adults: 25 to 50 mg PO every 6 to 8 hours PRN. Maximum dose is 300 mg daily.
➤ **Ankylosing spondylitis ♦**
Adults: 100 mg PO b.i.d.

lanadelumab-flyo
LAN-a-del-ue-mab

Takhzyro

Therapeutic class: Prophylaxis drugs
Pharmacologic class: Monoclonal antibodies

AVAILABLE FORMS
Injection: 300 mg/2 mL single-dose vial or prefilled syringe

INDICATIONS & DOSAGES
➤ **Prevention of hereditary angioedema attacks**
Adults and children age 12 and older: Initially, 300 mg subcut every 2 weeks. If patient is attack-free for more than 6 months, may consider decreasing dosing to 300 mg subcut every 4 weeks.

SAFETY ALERT!

lapatinib 🔬
lah-PAH-tih-nihb

Tykerb

Therapeutic class: Antineoplastics
Pharmacologic class: Kinase inhibitors

AVAILABLE FORMS
Tablets: 250 mg

INDICATIONS & DOSAGES
Boxed Warning Severe and fatal hepatotoxicity has been observed. ∎

✚Canada   ◇OTC   ♦Off-label use   ✐Photoguide   ⊜Do not crush   *Liquid contains alcohol   🔬Genetic

Adjust-a-dose (for all indications): Refer to manufacturer's instructions for toxicity-related dosage adjustments and use with strong CYP34A4 inhibitors and CYP3A4 inducers.

➤ **Advanced or metastatic breast cancer with capecitabine when tumors overexpress HER2 and patient has had prior therapy, including an anthracycline, a taxane, and trastuzumab** ▧

Adults: 1,250 mg (5 tablets) PO once daily as a single dose on days 1 through 21, with 2,000 mg/m²/day capecitabine given PO in two doses 12 hours apart on days 1 to 14. Repeat 21-day cycle. Continue until disease progression or unacceptable toxicity occurs.

➤ **HER2-positive, hormone receptor–positive metastatic breast cancer in patients who are postmenopausal** ▧

Adults: 1,500 mg PO once daily in combination with letrozole 2.5 mg PO once daily.

SAFETY ALERT!

larotrectinib ▧
lar-oh-TREK-ti-nib

Vitrakvi

Therapeutic class: Antineoplastics
Pharmacologic class: Kinase inhibitors

AVAILABLE FORMS
Capsules: 25 mg, 100 mg
Oral solution: 20 mg/mL

INDICATIONS & DOSAGES
➤ **Solid tumors that have a neurotrophic receptor tyrosine kinase gene fusion without a known acquired resistance mutation, are metastatic or where surgical resection is likely to result in severe morbidity, and have no satisfactory alternative treatments or have progressed after treatment** ▧

Adults and children age 1 month and older with BSA of at least 1 m²: 100 mg PO b.i.d., until disease progression or unacceptable toxicity.

Children age 1 month and older with BSA less than 1 m²: 100 mg/m² PO b.i.d., until disease progression or unacceptable toxicity.

Adjust-a-dose: For moderate (Child-Pugh class B) to severe (Child-Pugh class C) hepatic impairment, reduce the starting dose by 50%. If administration with a strong CYP3A4 inhibitor is unavoidable, reduce larotrectinib dose by 50%. If administration with a strong CYP3A4 inducer is unavoidable, double larotrectinib dose. If CYP3A4 drug is discontinued, allow 3 to 5 elimination half-lives before resuming prior larotrectinib dose. Refer to manufacturer's instructions for toxicity-related dosage adjustment.

lasmiditan
las-MID-i-tan

Reyvow

Therapeutic class: Antimigraine drugs
Pharmacologic class: Serotonin receptor agonists
Controlled substance schedule: V

AVAILABLE FORMS
Tablets ⊚*:* 50 mg, 100 mg

INDICATIONS & DOSAGES
➤ **Acute treatment of migraine with or without aura**
Adults: 50 mg, 100 mg, or 200 mg PO, as needed. Maximum daily dose is one dose in 24 hours.

lefamulin
lef-a-MUE-lin

Xenleta

Therapeutic class: Antibacterials
Pharmacologic class: Pleuromutilin anti-infectives

AVAILABLE FORMS
Injection: 150 mg/15 mL vial
Tablets ⊚*:* 600 mg

INDICATIONS & DOSAGES
➤ **Community-acquired bacterial pneumonia caused by susceptible strains of *Streptococcus pneumoniae*, *Staphylococcus aureus* (methicillin-susceptible isolates), *Haemophilus influenzae*, *Legionella pneumophila*, *Mycoplasma pneumoniae*, and *Chlamydophila pneumoniae***
Adults: 150 mg IV infusion over 60 minutes every 12 hours for 5 to 7 days, or 600 mg PO every 12 hours for 5 days. May switch from IV form to oral form to complete treatment course.

Adjust-a-dose: For patients with severe hepatic impairment (Child-Pugh class C), reduce IV dose to 150 mg infused every 24 hours. Tablets aren't recommended for moderate (Child-Pugh class B) or severe hepatic impairment.

lenvatinib mesylate
len-VA-ti-nib

Lenvima

Therapeutic class: Antineoplastics
Pharmacologic class: Kinase inhibitors

AVAILABLE FORMS
Capsules: 4 mg, 10 mg

INDICATIONS & DOSAGES
Adjust-a-dose (for all indications): See manufacturer's instructions for toxicity-related dosage adjustments and management.

➤ **Locally recurrent or metastatic, progressive, radioactive iodine-refractory differentiated thyroid cancer**
Adults: 24 mg PO daily until disease progression or unacceptable toxicity occurs.

Adjust-a-dose: For preexisting severe renal impairment (CrCl less than 30 mL/minute) or severe hepatic impairment (Child-Pugh class C), decrease dosage to 14 mg PO daily.

➤ **Advanced renal cell carcinoma after one prior antiangiogenic therapy, in combination with everolimus**

♣Canada   ◇OTC   ◆Off-label use   ✐Photoguide   ⊚Do not crush   *Liquid contains alcohol   ▧Genetic

Adults: 18 mg PO once daily with everolimus 5 mg PO once daily until disease progression or unacceptable toxicity occurs. Refer to everolimus prescribing information for recommended dosage information.
Adjust-a-dose: For preexisting severe renal impairment (CrCl less than 30 mL/minute) or severe hepatic impairment (Child-Pugh class C), decrease lenvatinib dosage to 10 mg PO daily.
➤ **Advance renal cell carcinoma as first-line treatment, in combination with pembrolizumab**
Adults: 20 mg PO once daily with pembrolizumab 200 mg IV infusion over 30 minutes every 3 weeks. Continue until disease progression or unacceptable toxicity occurs or for up to 2 years. Refer to pembrolizumab prescribing information for recommended dosage information.
Adjust-a-dose: For preexisting severe renal impairment (CrCl less than 30 mL/minute) or severe hepatic impairment (Child-Pugh class C), decrease lenvatinib dosage to 10 mg PO daily.
➤ **Unresectable hepatocellular carcinoma, first-line treatment**
Adults weighing 60 kg or more: 12 mg PO once daily until disease progression or unacceptable toxicity occurs.
Adults weighing less than 60 kg: 8 mg PO once daily until disease progression or unacceptable toxicity occurs.
➤ **Advanced endometrial carcinoma microsatellite instability-high or mismatch repair-deficient in patients who have disease progression after prior systemic therapy and aren't candidates for curative surgery or radiation, in combination with pembrolizumab**
Adults: 20 mg PO once daily with pembrolizumab 200 mg IV infusion every 3 weeks until disease progression or unacceptable toxicity. Refer to pembrolizumab prescribing information for recommended dosage information.
Adjust-a-dose: For preexisting severe renal impairment (CrCl less than 30 mL/minute) or severe hepatic impairment (Child-Pugh class C), decrease lenvatinib dosage to 10 mg PO daily.

letermovir
let-ER-moe-vir

Prevymis

Therapeutic class: Antivirals
Pharmacologic class: CMV DNA terminase complex inhibitors

AVAILABLE FORMS
Injection: 240 mg/12 mL, 480 mg/24 mL single-use vials
Tablets (ⓓⓝⓒ): 240 mg, 480 mg

INDICATIONS & DOSAGES
➤ **Prophylaxis of CMV infection and disease in CMV-seropositive recipients [R+] of an allogeneic hematopoietic stem cell transplant**

Adults: 480 mg PO or 480-mg IV infusion over 1 hour once daily beginning between day 0 and day 28 post-transplant and continuing through day 100 posttransplant.
Adjust-a-dose: If drug is administered with cyclosporine, decrease dose to 240 mg PO or IV once daily. If cyclosporine is initiated after start of letermovir, decrease next dose of letermovir to 240 mg once daily. If cyclosporine is discontinued after start of letermovir, increase next dose of letermovir to 480 mg once daily. If cyclosporine dosing is interrupted due to high cyclosporine level, no letermovir dosage adjustment is needed.

levomilnacipran hydrochloride
lee-voe-mil-NAY-sih-pran

Fetzima

Therapeutic class: Antidepressants
Pharmacologic class: SSNRIs

AVAILABLE FORMS
Capsules (extended-release) (ⓓⓝⓒ): 20 mg, 40 mg, 80 mg, 120 mg

INDICATIONS & DOSAGES
Boxed Warning Antidepressants increase risk of suicidality in children, adolescents, and young adults. Drug isn't approved for use in children. ∎
➤ **Major depressive disorder**
Adults: Initially, 20 mg PO once daily for 2 days; then increase to 40 mg once daily. May increase in increments of 40 mg at intervals of 2 or more days. Maximum dosage is 120 mg once daily.
Adjust-a-dose: For patients with CrCl of 30 to 59 mL/minute, maximum maintenance dosage is 80 mg once daily. If CrCl is 15 to 29 mL/minute, maximum maintenance dosage is 40 mg once daily. Don't use for patients with ESRD.

L-glutamine
ell-GLOO-ta-meen

Endari

Therapeutic class: Miscellaneous hematologic drugs
Pharmacologic class: Amino acids

AVAILABLE FORMS
Oral powder: 5 g per packet

INDICATIONS & DOSAGES
➤ **To reduce acute complications of sickle cell disease**
Adults and children age 5 and older weighing more than 65 kg: 15 g (3 packets) PO b.i.d.
Adults and children age 5 and older weighing 30 to 65 kg: 10 g (2 packets) PO b.i.d.
Children age 5 and older weighing less than 30 kg: 5 g (1 packet) PO b.i.d.

---

lidocaine (intradermal, ophthalmic, topical)
LYE-doe-kane

Lidocaine, Lidoderm

lidocaine hydrochloride
Akten, AneCream ◇, AneCream 5, Glydo, Lidodan✣◇, LidoPatch ◇, Maxilene✣◇, RectiCare ◇, Solarcaine ◇, Xolido ◇, Xylocaine, Zingo

Therapeutic class: Analgesics
Pharmacologic class: Local anesthetics

AVAILABLE FORMS
Cream: 2%◇, 3%, 3.88%, 4%◇, 4.12%, 5%◇, 10%
Gel: 2%◇, 2.8%, 3%◇, 4%◇, 5%◇
Jelly: 2%
Lotion: 1%◇, 2.75%, 3%, 3.5%, 4%
Ointment: 4%◇, 5%
Ophthalmic gel: 3.5%
Patch: 1.8%, 3.5%, 4%◇, 5%
Powder for injection: 0.5-mg single-use intradermal injection system
Topical solution: 2%, 4%
Topical spray: 0.5%
Viscous oral solution: 2%, 4%

INDICATIONS & DOSAGES
Boxed Warning Postmarketing cases of seizures, cardiopulmonary arrest, and death in patients younger than age 3 have been reported with use of lidocaine 2% viscous solution when it wasn't administered in strict adherence to the dosing and administration recommendations. Lidocaine 2% viscous solution isn't approved for teething pain. ∎

Adjust-a-dose (for all indications): Decrease dosage as needed based on patient's age, weight, and physical condition.

➤ **Urethra anesthesia and treatment of painful urethritis**
Male adults and children: Slowly instill 15 mL (300 mg lidocaine) 2% jelly into urethra using an easy syringelike action, until patient has a feeling of tension or until about 15 mL is instilled. Apply penile clamp for 5 to 10 minutes at the corona; then, if needed, an additional 15 mL may be instilled as needed for adequate anesthesia. Before catheterization, 5 to 10 mL (100 to 200 mg) is usually adequate. Maximum dose for adults is 600 g in any 12-hour period. Maximum dose for children is 4.5 mg/kg.
Women and children: Slowly instill 3 to 5 mL (60 to 100 mg) of 2% jelly into urethra. A small amount of jelly may be applied to cotton swab and deposited into the urethral opening before instillation. Allow several minutes for anesthetic effect to occur. Maximum dose for adults is 600 g in any 12-hour period. Maximum dose for children is 4.5 mg/kg.

➤ **Anesthetic lubricant for ET intubation**
Adults and children: Apply moderate amount of 2% jelly to external surface of ET tube shortly before use. Maximum adult dose is 30 mL (600 mg) in any 12-hour period. Maximum dose in children is

4.5 mg/kg. Or, apply up to 5 g per single application, approximately 6 inches, of 5% ointment to external surface of ET tube shortly before use. Maximum adult dose of 5% ointment is 20 g (equivalent to lidocaine base 1,000 mg) per day. Maximum dose in children is 4.5 mg/kg.

➤ **Topical anesthesia of accessible mucous membranes of oral and nasal cavities and proximal portions of digestive tract**
Adults: 15 mL 2% oral topical viscous solution to affected areas not more frequently than every 3 hours. Maximum dose, 4.5 mg/kg, not to exceed 300 mg/dose.
Adults and children age 10 and older: Apply 1 to 5 mL (40 to 200 mg) 4% oral topical solution to affected area as a spray, applied with cotton applicators or packs, as when instilled into a cavity. Maximum dose is 4.5 mg/kg, not to exceed 300 mg/dose.
Children younger than age 10 who have a normal lean body mass and normal body development: Apply 4% oral topical solution to affected area as a spray, applied with cotton applicators or packs, as when instilled into a cavity. May determine dose by applying one of the standard pediatric drug formulas. Maximum dose is 4.5 mg/kg.

➤ **Oropharynx anesthetic**
Adults and children (used in dentistry): Apply 5% ointment to previously dried oral mucosa. For use in adults with the insertion of new dentures, apply to all denture surfaces with mucosal contact. Maximum dose for adults is 5 g/single application (equivalent to lidocaine base 250 mg or 6 inches of ointment) or 20 g of ointment (equivalent to 1,000 g lidocaine base) per day. Patient should consult a dentist at least every 48 hours throughout denture-fitting period. Maximum dose for children is 5 g/single application (equivalent to 250 mg lidocaine base or approximately 6 inches of ointment) or 4.5 mg/kg lidocaine base.
Adults: 15 mL 2% solution swished in the mouth and spit out or gargled and swallowed no more frequently than every 3 hours. Maximum dose for adults is 4.5 mg/kg/dose (or 300 mg/dose); eight doses per 24 hours.
Children age 3 and older: Don't exceed 4.5 mg/kg/dose (or 300 mg/dose) swished in the mouth and spit out no more frequently than every 3 hours (four doses in 12 hours).
Children younger than age 3: 1.2 mL 2% solution applied to immediate area with a cotton-tipped applicator no more frequently than every 3 hours. Maximum is four doses in 12 hours and 1.2 mL/dose.

➤ **Skin discomfort (irritation, itching, pain)**
⊙ *Alert:* For children weighing less than 10 kg, a single application should be applied over an area no greater than 100 cm². For children weighing between 10 and 20 kg, a single application should be applied over an area no greater than 600 cm².
Adults and children (5% ointment): Apply ointment topically for adequate control of symptoms. Maximum dose for adults is 5 g/single application (equivalent to lidocaine base 250 mg or approximately 6 inches of ointment) or 20 g of ointment (equivalent

to lidocaine base 1,000 mg)/day. Maximum dose for children is 5 g/single application (equivalent to lidocaine base 250 mg or approximately 6 inches of ointment), or 4.5 mg/kg lidocaine base.
Adults and children age 2 and older (cream, gel, spray): Apply 4% cream or 4% gel or spray to affected areas t.i.d. to q.i.d. Or apply 2% gel to affected areas t.i.d. as needed.

➤ **Local analgesia for venipuncture (Zingo)**
Adults and children age 3 and older: Apply one intradermal lidocaine (0.5 mg) device to site planned for venipuncture 1 to 3 minutes before needle insertion.

➤ **Anorectal discomfort**
Adults and children age 12 and older: Apply 5% cream or 5% gel up to six times a day.

➤ **Postherpetic neuralgia**
Adults: Apply 5% patch to most painful area for up to 12 hours in any 24-hour period. Maximum dose is 3 patches in a single application.

➤ **Ocular surface anesthesia (Akten)**
Adults and children: Apply 2 drops to ocular surface in area of planned procedure. Reapply as needed to maintain anesthetic effect.

---

lindane
LIN-dayn

Therapeutic class: Scabicides–pediculicides
Pharmacologic class: Ectoparasiticides–ovicides

AVAILABLE FORMS
Shampoo: 1%

INDICATIONS & DOSAGES
Boxed Warning Only use in patients who can't tolerate or have failed first-line treatment with safer medications. Drug can cause seizures and death. Use with caution in infants, children, older adults, individuals with other skin conditions, and those who weigh less than 50 kg; they may be at risk for serious neurotoxicity. Use is contraindicated in premature infants and patients with known uncontrolled seizure disorders. ∎

➤ **Head lice (*Pediculosis capitis*), crab lice (*Pthirus pubis*)**
Adults and children age 10 and older: Apply shampoo undiluted to dry hair and work into lather for 4 minutes; small amounts of water may increase lathering. Give special attention to the fine hairs along the neck. Apply 30 mL of shampoo for short hair, 45 mL for medium-length hair, or 60 mL for long hair. Allow shampoo to remain in place for 4 minutes only. Then, add small quantities of water to form a good lather. Rinse thoroughly and rub dry briskly with towel. Comb with a fine-tooth comb and remove nits with a nit comb or tweezers. Don't retreat.
Older adults: May need to reduce dosage because of increased skin absorption.

---

liothyronine sodium (T₃)
lye-oh-THYE-roe-neen

Cytomel, Triostat

Therapeutic class: Thyroid hormone replacements
Pharmacologic class: Thyroid hormones

AVAILABLE FORMS
Injection: 10 mcg/mL in 1-mL vials*
Tablets: 5 mcg, 25 mcg, 50 mcg

INDICATIONS & DOSAGES
Boxed Warning Drugs with thyroid hormone activity, alone or with other therapeutic agents, shouldn't be used for treatment of obesity or for weight loss. Dosage beyond daily hormonal requirements may produce serious or even life-threatening toxicity. ∎

➤ **Congenital hypothyroidism**
Children: Initially, 5 mcg PO daily; increase by 5 mcg every 3 to 4 days until desired response is achieved. For maintenance: Infants may require only 20 mcg daily; children ages 1 to 3 may require 50 mcg daily; and children older than age 3 may require full adult dosage.

➤ **Myxedema coma, premyxedema coma**
Adults: Initially, 10 to 20 mcg IV for patients with CV disease; 25 to 50 mcg IV for patients who don't have CV disease. Adjust dosage based on patient's condition and response. Switch patient to oral therapy as soon as possible.

➤ **Thyroid hormone replacement**
Adults: Initially, 25 mcg PO daily; increase by up to 25 mcg every 1 to 2 weeks until satisfactory response occurs. Usual maintenance dosage, 25 to 75 mcg daily.
Children: 5 mcg daily; increase by 5 mcg daily every 3 to 4 days until desired response.
Adjust-a-dose: For older adults and patients with CV disease, give 5 mcg once daily; may increase by 5 mcg/day every 2 weeks.

➤ **TSH suppression in patients with well-differentiated thyroid cancer**
Adults: Adjust PO dosage based on desired therapeutic range.

➤ **T₃ suppression test to differentiate hyperthyroidism from euthyroidism**
Adults: 75 to 100 mcg PO daily for 7 days; radioactive iodine uptake is determined before and after hormone administration.

---

lomitapide mesylate ⊠
lom-i-TA-pide

Juxtapid

Therapeutic class: Antilipemics
Pharmacologic class: Microsomal triglyceride transfer protein inhibitors

AVAILABLE FORMS
Capsules: 5 mg, 10 mg, 20 mg, 30 mg

✚Canada   ◇OTC   ◆Off-label use   ✐Photoguide   ⓓⓝⓒDo not crush   *Liquid contains alcohol   ⊠Genetic

INDICATIONS & DOSAGES

➤ As an adjunct to low-fat diet and other lipid-lowering treatments, including LDL apheresis where available, to reduce LDL, total cholesterol, apolipoprotein B, and non-HDL cholesterol levels in patients with homozygous familial hypercholesterolemia ⬚

Adults: 5 mg PO once daily. May increase to 10 mg daily after at least 2 weeks; may increase at least 4 weeks later to 20 mg, then at least 4 weeks later to 40 mg, then at least 4 weeks later to 60 mg. Measure ALT, AST, ALP, and total bilirubin levels with any dosage increase. Maximum daily dosage is 60 mg.

Adjust-a-dose: In patients with ESRD receiving dialysis and in patients with mild hepatic impairment (Child-Pugh class A), don't exceed 40 mg PO daily. Maximum dose is 30 mg daily with concomitant weak CYP3A4 inhibitors and 40 mg daily with concomitant oral contraceptives. Refer to manufacturer's instructions for drug-interaction and toxicity-related dosage adjustments.

SAFETY ALERT!

lomustine (CCNU)
loe-MUS-teen

Gleostine

Therapeutic class: Antineoplastics
Pharmacologic class: Nitrosoureas

AVAILABLE FORMS
Capsules: 10 mg, 40 mg, 100 mg

INDICATIONS & DOSAGES

Boxed Warning Drug can cause severe and fatal myelosuppression. Monitor blood cell counts weekly for at least 6 weeks after a dose. Ensure that patient is prescribed and takes only a single dose every 6 weeks. Fatal toxicity occurs with overdose. ∎

➤ Brain tumor, Hodgkin lymphoma

Adults and children: 130 mg/m² PO as single dose every 6 weeks. Round doses to nearest 10 mg. Don't give repeat doses until WBC exceeds 4,000/mm³ and platelet count is greater than 100,000/mm³.

Adjust-a-dose: Reduce dosage to 100 mg/m² once every 6 weeks in patients with compromised bone marrow function. Refer to manufacturer's instructions for dosage adjustments for hematologic toxicity or when used with other myelosuppressive drugs.

SAFETY ALERT!

lorlatinib ⬚
lor-LA-ti-nib

Lorbrena

Therapeutic class: Antineoplastics
Pharmacologic class: Tyrosine kinase inhibitors

AVAILABLE FORMS
Tablets: 25 mg, 100 mg

INDICATIONS & DOSAGES

➤ Anaplastic lymphoma kinase (ALK)-positive metastatic NSCLC ⬚

Adults: 100 mg PO once daily until disease progression or unacceptable toxicity.

Adjust-a-dose: If CrCl is 15 to less than 30 mL/minute, reduce dosage to 75 mg once daily. Refer to manufacturer's instructions for toxicity-related dosage adjustments. If use with CYP3A inhibitors is unavoidable, reduce lorlatinib starting dose to 75 mg once daily. In patients who have had a lorlatinib dosage reduction to 75 mg once daily due to adverse reactions and who begin a strong CYP3A inhibitor, reduce lorlatinib dose to 50 mg once daily. If the strong CYP3A inhibitor is discontinued, increase the lorlatinib dose (after three plasma half-lives of the strong CYP3A inhibitor) to the dose that was used before initiation of the strong CYP3A inhibitor. If concomitant use with moderate CYP3A inducers is unavoidable, increase the lorlatinib dose to 125 mg once daily. Avoid use with strong CYP3A inducers.

luliconazole
loo-li-KON-a-zole

Luzu

Therapeutic class: Antifungals
Pharmacologic class: Azole antifungals

AVAILABLE FORMS
Cream: 1%

INDICATIONS & DOSAGES

➤ Interdigital tinea pedis (athlete's foot) caused by *Trichophyton rubrum* or *Epidermophyton floccosum*

Adults: Apply thin layer to affected area and approximately 1 inch (2.5 cm) of surrounding area once daily for 2 weeks.

➤ Tinea cruris (jock itch) and tinea corporis (ringworm) caused by *T. rubrum* or *E. floccosum*

Adults: Apply thin layer to affected area and approximately 1 inch (2.5 cm) of surrounding area once daily for 1 week.

lumacaftor–ivacaftor ⬚
LOO-ma-kaf-tor/EYE-va-kaf-tor

Orkambi

Therapeutic class: Metabolic agents
Pharmacologic class: Cystic fibrosis transmembrane conductance regulator (CFTR) potentiators

AVAILABLE FORMS
Granules: lumacaftor 75 mg/ivacaftor 94 mg, 100 mg lumacaftor/125 mg ivacaftor, 150 mg lumacaftor/188 mg ivacaftor
Tablets: 100 mg lumacaftor/125 mg ivacaftor, 200 mg lumacaftor/125 mg ivacaftor

INDICATIONS & DOSAGES

➤ Cystic fibrosis in patients who are homozygous for the F508del mutation in the *CFTR* gene ⬚

Adults and children age 12 and older: 400 mg lumacaftor/250 mg ivacaftor PO every 12 hours with fat-containing food.

Children ages 6 to 11: 200 mg lumacaftor/250 mg ivacaftor PO every 12 hours with fat-containing food.
Children ages 2 to 5 weighing 14 kg or more: 150 mg lumacaftor/188 mg ivacaftor packet of granules every 12 hours with fat-containing food.
Children ages 2 to 5 weighing less than 14 kg: 100 mg lumacaftor/125 mg ivacaftor packet of granules PO every 12 hours with fat-containing food.
Children ages 1 to 2 weighing 14 kg or more: lumacaftor 150 mg/ivacaftor 188 mg packet of granules PO every 12 hours with fat-containing food.
Children ages 1 to 2 weighing 9 to less than 14 kg: lumacaftor 100 mg/ivacaftor 125 mg packet of granules PO every 12 hours with fat-containing food.
Children ages 1 to 2 weighing 7 to less than 9 kg: lumacaftor 75 mg/ivacaftor 94 mg packet of granules PO every 12 hours with fat-containing food.
Adjust-a-dose: Refer to manufacturer's instructions for hepatic impairment, drug-interaction, and toxicity-related dosage adjustments.

lumasiran
loo-ma-SIR-an

Oxlumo

Therapeutic class: Metabolic agents
Pharmacologic class: Hydroxyacid oxidase 1-directed small interfering RNA

AVAILABLE FORMS
Injection: 94.5 mg/0.5 mL single-dose vials

INDICATIONS & DOSAGES
➤ **Primary hyperoxaluria type 1 to lower urinary oxalate levels**
Adults and children weighing 20 kg or more: 3 mg/kg subcut once monthly for 3 months; then 3 mg/kg subcut once every 3 months.
Children weighing 10 to less than 20 kg: 6 mg/kg subcut once monthly for 3 months; then 6 mg/kg subcut once every 3 months.
Children weighing less than 10 kg: 6 mg/kg subcut once monthly for 3 months; then 3 mg/kg subcut once monthly.

lumateperone
loo-ma-TE-per-one

Caplyta

Therapeutic class: Antipsychotics
Pharmacologic class: Central serotonin and dopamine receptor antagonists

AVAILABLE FORMS
Capsules: 5 mg, 21 mg, 42 mg

INDICATIONS & DOSAGES
Boxed Warning Antidepressants increase risk of suicidality in children, adolescents, and young adults. Drug isn't approved for use in children. ■
Boxed Warning Older adults with dementia-related psychosis treated with antipsychotics are at increased risk for death; drug isn't approved for treatment of dementia-related psychosis. ■

Adjust-a-dose (all indications): For patients with moderate or severe hepatic impairment (Child-Pugh class B or C) or if administered with moderate CYP3A4 inhibitor, decrease lumateperone dosage to 21 mg once daily. If administered with strong CYP3A4 inhibitor, decrease lumateperone dosage to 10.5 mg once daily.
➤ **Schizophrenia**
Adults: 42 mg PO once daily.
✳ **NEW INDICATION: Depressive episodes associated with bipolar I or II disorder (bipolar depression) as monotherapy or as adjunctive therapy with lithium or valproate**
Adults: 42 mg PO once daily.

SAFETY ALERT!

lurbinectedin
loor-bin-EK-te-din

Zepzelca

Therapeutic class: Antineoplastics
Pharmacologic class: Alkylating agents

AVAILABLE FORMS
Injection: 4-mg single-dose vial

INDICATIONS & DOSAGES
➤ **Metastatic small-cell lung cancer with disease progression on or after platinum-based chemotherapy**
Adults: 3.2 mg/m^2 IV infusion over 60 minutes every 21 days until disease progression or unacceptable toxicity occurs.
Adjust-a-dose: Refer to manufacturer's instructions for toxicity-related dosage adjustments.

mecasermin ▨
meh-KAH-sur-men

Increlex

Therapeutic class: Growth factors
Pharmacologic class: Human insulin growth factors

AVAILABLE FORMS
Injection: 10 mg/mL

INDICATIONS & DOSAGES
➤ **Growth failure in children with severe primary insulin growth factor-1 deficiency or children with growth hormone gene deletion who have developed neutralizing antibodies to growth hormone** ▨
Children age 2 and older: Initially, 0.04 to 0.08 mg/kg subcut b.i.d. If well tolerated for at least 1 week, may increase by 0.04 mg/kg per dose, to the maximum dose of 0.12 mg/kg b.i.d.

meloxicam
mel-OX-i-kam

Anjeso, Mobic✿, Vivlodex

Therapeutic class: Antirheumatics
Pharmacologic class: NSAIDs

AVAILABLE FORMS

Capsules: 5 mg, 10 mg
Injection: 30 mg/mL single-dose vial
Oral suspension: 7.5 mg/5 mL
Tablets: 7.5 mg, 15 mg

INDICATIONS & DOSAGES

Boxed Warning NSAIDs may increase risk of serious CV thrombotic events, MI, stroke, and GI adverse reactions. Contraindicated for use in CABG surgery. ■

Adjust-a-dose (for all indications): Use of PO forms isn't recommended in patients with CrCl of less than 20 mL/minute as drug hasn't been studied in this population. Use of IV form isn't recommended in patients with eGFR less than 60 mL/minute/1.73m². If patient is receiving hemodialysis, give no more than 7.5-mg tablet or oral suspension, or 5-mg capsule once daily.

➤ **To relieve signs and symptoms of osteoarthritis or RA**
Adults: 7.5 mg PO once daily. May increase as needed to maximum dosage of 15 mg daily. For osteoarthritis only, give 5 mg Vivlodex PO once daily. May increase to 10 mg in patients who require additional analgesia. Use lowest effective dose for shortest duration consistent with individual patient treatment goals.

➤ **To relieve signs and symptoms of pauciarticular or polyarticular course juvenile RA**
Children weighing 60 kg or more: 7.5 mg PO daily.
Children age 2 and older: 0.125 mg/kg oral suspension PO once daily, up to maximum of 7.5 mg.

➤ **Moderate to severe pain, alone or in combination with non-NSAID analgesics**
Adults: 30 mg IV bolus over 15 seconds once daily. Use for shortest duration consistent with individual patient treatment goals.

---

menotropins

men-oh-TROE-pins

Menopur

Therapeutic class: Ovulation stimulants
Pharmacologic class: Gonadotropins

AVAILABLE FORMS

Injection: 75 international units of luteinizing hormone and 75 international units of FSH activity per vial

INDICATIONS & DOSAGES

➤ **Assisted reproductive technologies**
Adults: Initially, 225 units subcut into lower abdomen daily starting on cycle day 2 or 3. Menopur may be used in combination with urofollitropin, but total initial dose of both shouldn't exceed 225 units (150 international units of menotropins and 75 international units of urofollitropin or 75 international units of menotropins and 150 international units of urofollitropin). Adjust dosage after 5 days, based on ovarian response as determined by ultrasound evaluation of follicular growth and serum estradiol levels. Don't make additional adjustments more frequently than

every 2 days and not to exceed 150 units per adjustment. Maximum daily dosage is 450 units. Use for maximum of 20 days.

---

mepolizumab

me-poe-LIZ-ue-mab

Nucala

Therapeutic class: Miscellaneous respiratory drugs
Pharmacologic class: Monoclonal antibodies

AVAILABLE FORMS

Injection: 40 mg/0.4 mL, 100 mg/mL single-dose pre-filled syringe; 100 mg/mL single-dose autoinjector; 100-mg single-dose vials

INDICATIONS & DOSAGES

➤ **Add-on maintenance treatment of severe asthma in patients with an eosinophilic phenotype**
Adults and children age 12 and older: 100 mg subcut every 4 weeks into upper arm, thigh, or abdomen.
Children age 6 to 11: 40 mg subcut every 4 weeks into upper arm, thigh, or abdomen.

➤ **Eosinophilic granulomatosis with polyangiitis**
Adults: 300 mg given as three separate 100-mg subcut injections into the upper arm, thigh, or abdomen once every 4 weeks.

➤ **Hypereosinophilic syndrome persisting for 6 months or more without an identifiable nonhematologic secondary cause**
Adults and children age 12 and older: 300 mg given as three separate 100-mg subcut injections into upper arm, thigh, or abdomen once every 4 weeks.

➤ **Maintenance treatment of chronic rhinosinusitis with nasal polyps in patients with inadequate response to nasal corticosteroids**
Adults: 100 mg subcut once every 4 weeks in to upper arm, thigh, or abdomen.

---

methylergonovine maleate

meth-il-er-goe-NOE-veen

Methergine

Therapeutic class: Oxytocics
Pharmacologic class: Ergot alkaloids

AVAILABLE FORMS

Injection: 0.2 mg/mL in 1-mL vials
Tablets: 0.2 mg

INDICATIONS & DOSAGES

➤ **To prevent and treat postpartum hemorrhage caused by uterine atony or subinvolution; for control of uterine hemorrhage in second stage of labor**
Adults: 0.2 mg IM after delivery of the anterior shoulder, after delivery of the placenta, or during the puerperium. May repeat every 2 to 4 hours as needed. During life-threatening emergencies, 0.2 mg IV over at least 1 minute while monitoring BP and uterine contractions. During puerperium, 0.2 mg PO every 6 to 8 hours for up to 7 days. Decrease dosage if severe cramping occurs.

---

midostaurin ⚇
mi-doe-STOR-in

Rydapt

Therapeutic class: Antineoplastics
Pharmacologic class: Tyrosine kinase inhibitors

AVAILABLE FORMS
Capsules: 25 mg

INDICATIONS & DOSAGES
Adjust-a-dose (for all indications): Refer to manufacturer's instructions for toxicity-related adjustments.
➤ **Newly diagnosed acute myeloid leukemia in patients with *FLT3* mutation in combination with daunorubicin and cytarabine** ⚇
Adults: 50 mg PO b.i.d. with food on days 8 to 21 of each induction cycle (in combination with daunorubicin and cytarabine) and on days 8 to 21 of each consolidation cycle (in combination with high-dose cytarabine).
➤ **Aggressive systemic mastocytosis, systemic mastocytosis with associated hematologic neoplasm, or mast cell leukemia**
Adults: 100 mg PO b.i.d. with food until disease progression or unacceptable toxicity occurs.

migalastat hydrochloride ⚇
mi-GAL-a-stat

Galafold

Therapeutic class: Metabolic agents
Pharmacologic class: Pharmacological chaperones

AVAILABLE FORMS
Capsules ⓓ*:* 123 mg

INDICATIONS & DOSAGES
➤ **Confirmed Fabry disease with an amenable galactosidase alpha gene variant** ⚇
Adults: 123 mg PO once every other day, at the same time of day.

miSOPROStol
mye-soe-PROST-ole

Cytotec

Therapeutic class: Antiulcer drugs
Pharmacologic class: Prostaglandin E₁ analogues

AVAILABLE FORMS
Tablets: 100 mcg, 200 mcg

INDICATIONS & DOSAGES
Boxed Warning Drug can cause abortion, premature birth, birth defects, and uterine rupture and is contraindicated during pregnancy. Advise patients of the risk; warn them not to give drug to others. ∎

➤ **Prevention of NSAID-induced gastric ulcer**
Adults: 200 mcg PO q.i.d. with food; if not tolerated, decrease to 100 mcg PO q.i.d. Give dosage for duration of NSAID therapy.

moexipril hydrochloride
moe-EX-eh-pril

Therapeutic class: Antihypertensives
Pharmacologic class: ACE inhibitors

AVAILABLE FORMS
Tablets: 7.5 mg, 15 mg

INDICATIONS & DOSAGES
Boxed Warning Drugs that act directly on the renin-angiotensin system can cause fetal harm; when pregnancy is detected, discontinue as soon as possible. ∎
➤ **HTN, alone or in combination with thiazide diuretics**
Adults: Initially, 7.5 mg PO once daily as monotherapy, given 1 hour before a meal. Or initially, 3.75 mg if diuretic therapy can't be discontinued. Increase dosage incrementally according to BP response. Recommended dosage range is 7.5 to 30 mg daily in one or two divided doses.
Adjust-a-dose: For patients currently being treated with a diuretic, if possible stop diuretic 2 to 3 days before therapy is initiated to reduce likelihood of hypotension. If BP isn't adequately controlled with moexipril alone, may reinstitute diuretic therapy. For patients with CrCl of 40 mL/minute/1.73 m² or less, cautiously give initial dose of 3.75 mg once daily. May titrate dosage upward to a maximum daily dosage of 15 mg.

mogamulizumab-kpkc ⚇
moe-GAM-ue-LIZ-ue-mab

Poteligeo

Therapeutic class: Antineoplastics
Pharmacologic class: Monoclonal antibodies

AVAILABLE FORMS
Injection: 4 mg/mL in 5-mL single-use vial

INDICATIONS & DOSAGES
➤ **Relapsed or refractory mycosis fungoides or Sézary syndrome after at least one prior systemic therapy**
Adults: Initially, 1 mg/kg IV infusion over at least 60 minutes on days 1, 8, 15, and 22 of the first 28-day cycle; then on days 1 and 15 of each subsequent 28-day cycle until disease progression or unacceptable toxicity occurs.
Adjust-a-dose: Refer to manufacturer's instructions for toxicity-related dosage adjustments.

---

moxetumomab pasudotox-tdfk
MOX-e-toom-oh-mab pa-SOO-doe-tox

Lumoxiti

Therapeutic class: Antineoplastics
Pharmacologic class: Anti-CD22s

AVAILABLE FORMS
Injection (lyophilized cake or powder): 1 mg/mL single-dose vial

INDICATIONS & DOSAGES
Boxed Warning Drug can cause capillary leak syndrome and hemolytic-uremic syndrome. Monitor patient closely and delay or discontinue drug as recommended. ■

➤ **Relapsed or refractory hairy cell leukemia who received at least two prior systemic therapies, including treatment with a purine nucleoside analogue**

Adults: 0.04 mg/kg IV infusion over 30 minutes on days 1, 3, and 5 of each 28-day cycle. Continue treatment for a maximum of six cycles, unless disease progression or unacceptable toxicity occurs.

Adjust-a-dose: Refer to manufacturer's information for toxicity-related dosage adjustments.

nafarelin acetate ⬚
nah-FAR-eh-lin

Synarel

Therapeutic class: Endocrine-metabolic agents
Pharmacologic class: Gonadotropin-releasing hormone analogues

AVAILABLE FORMS
Nasal spray: 2 mg/mL (200 mcg/spray)

INDICATIONS & DOSAGES
➤ **Central precocious puberty ⬚**

Children age 8 years or younger (female), or age 9 or younger (male): 2 sprays (400 mcg) into each nostril in the morning and evening for a total of 8 sprays (1,600 mcg) per day. If necessary, may increase dosage to a total of 9 sprays (1,800 mcg) per day, administered as 3 sprays (600 mcg) into alternating nostrils t.i.d. Continue treatment until resumption of puberty is desired.

➤ **Endometriosis**

Adults: Begin treatment between days 2 and 4 of menstrual cycle. Administer 1 spray (200 mcg) into one nostril in the morning and 1 spray (200 mcg) into the other nostril in the evening for a total of 2 sprays (400 mcg) per day. If persistent regular menstruation continues after 2 months of treatment, increase dose to 1 spray (200 mcg) into each nostril in the morning and 1 spray (200 mcg) into each nostril in the evening for a total of 4 sprays (800 mcg) per day. Recommended duration of treatment is 6 months.

nefazodone hydrochloride
ne-FAZ-oh-done

Therapeutic class: Antidepressants
Pharmacologic class: Antidepressants

AVAILABLE FORMS
Tablets: 50 mg, 100 mg, 150 mg, 200 mg, 250 mg

INDICATIONS & DOSAGES
Boxed Warning Antidepressants increase risk of suicidality in children, adolescents, and young adults. Drug isn't approved for use in children. Life-threatening hepatic failure has been reported; discontinue drug if clinical signs or symptoms suggest liver failure or hepatocellular injury. ■

➤ **Depression**

Adults: Initially, 100 mg/day PO b.i.d. Increase dosage in increments of 100 to 200 mg/day in two divided doses at intervals of no less than 1 week. Effective dosage range is 300 to 600 mg/day.

Adjust-a-dose: In older adults or patients who are debilitated, especially women, initially 50 mg PO b.i.d. Don't start drug until 14 days after administration of an MAO inhibitor.

SAFETY ALERT!

nelarabine
neh-LAR-uh-been

Arranon, Atriance⬥

Therapeutic class: Antineoplastics
Pharmacologic class: DNA demethylation agents; prodrugs of cytotoxic deoxyguanosine

AVAILABLE FORMS
Injection: 5 mg/mL in 50-mL vials

INDICATIONS & DOSAGES
Boxed Warning Severe neurologic adverse reactions have been reported, including altered mental states, CNS effects (including seizures), and peripheral neuropathy, ranging from numbness and paresthesia to motor weakness and paralysis. ■

➤ **Relapsed or refractory T-cell acute lymphoblastic leukemia and T-cell lymphoblastic lymphoma after treatment with at least two chemotherapy regimens**

Adults: 1,500 mg/m² IV over 2 hours on days 1, 3, and 5. Repeat every 21 days.

Children age 1 year and older: 650 mg/m² IV over 1 hour daily for 5 consecutive days. Repeat every 21 days.

Adjust-a-dose: Continue therapy until transplant, disease progression, or unacceptable toxicity occurs or until patient no longer benefits from therapy. Refer to manufacturer's information for toxicity-related dosage adjustments.

---

niMODipine
nye-MOE-dih-peen

Nymalize

Therapeutic class: Vasodilators
Pharmacologic class: Calcium channel blockers

AVAILABLE FORMS
Capsules ⓓⓝⓒ: 30 mg
Oral solution: 6 mg/mL in 5-mL and 10-mL prefilled syringe; 60 mg/10 mL in 237-mL bottle

INDICATIONS & DOSAGES
Boxed Warning Don't administer parenterally; may cause life-threatening reactions and death. ■
➤ **To improve neurologic deficits after subarachnoid hemorrhage from ruptured intracranial berry aneurysm**
Adults: 60 mg PO every 4 hours, given 1 hour before or 2 hours after a meal, for 21 days. Begin therapy within 96 hours after subarachnoid hemorrhage.
Adjust-a-dose: For patients with hepatic failure or cirrhosis, 30 mg PO every 4 hours for 21 days.

nintedanib esylate
nin-TED-a-nib

Ofev

Therapeutic class: Miscellaneous respiratory drugs
Pharmacologic class: Tyrosine kinase inhibitors

AVAILABLE FORMS
Capsules ⓓⓝⓒ: 100 mg, 150 mg

INDICATIONS & DOSAGES
➤ **Idiopathic pulmonary fibrosis; chronic fibrosing ILD with a progressive phenotype; to slow rate of decline in pulmonary function in patients with systemic sclerosis-associated ILD**
Adults: 150 mg PO b.i.d. approximately 12 hours apart with food.
Adjust-a-dose: In patients with mild hepatic impairment (Child-Pugh class A), give 100 mg b.i.d. approximately 12 hours apart with food. Refer to manufacturer's instructions for toxicity-related dosage adjustments.

nisoldipine
nye-SOHL-di-peen

Sular

Therapeutic class: Antihypertensives
Pharmacologic class: Calcium channel blockers

AVAILABLE FORMS
Tablets (extended-release) ⓓⓝⓒ: 8.5 mg, 17 mg, 20 mg, 25.5 mg, 30 mg, 34 mg, 40 mg

INDICATIONS & DOSAGES
➤ **HTN**
Adults: Dosage must be adjusted to each patient's needs. Initially, 17 mg PO once daily, 1 hour before or 2 hours after a meal, increased by 8.5 mg/week or at longer intervals, as needed. Usual maintenance dose is 17 to 34 mg daily. Doses of more than 34 mg daily aren't recommended. Or, initially, 20 mg PO once daily, 1 hour before or 2 hours after a meal, increased by 10 mg/week or at longer intervals, as needed. Usual maintenance dose is 20 to 40 mg daily. Doses of more than 60 mg daily aren't recommended.
Patients older than age 65: Initially, 8.5 to 10 mg PO once daily; adjust dosage as for other adults.
Adjust-a-dose: For patients with hepatic impairment, initially 8.5 to 10 mg PO once daily; adjust dosage as for other adults.

nitazoxanide
nye-te-ZOCKS-a-nide

Alinia

Therapeutic class: Antiprotozoals
Pharmacologic class: Antiprotozoals

AVAILABLE FORMS
Oral suspension: 100 mg/5 mL
Tablets: 500 mg

INDICATIONS & DOSAGES
➤ **Diarrhea caused by *Cryptosporidium parvum* or *Giardia lamblia***
Adults and children age 12 and older: 500 mg PO with food every 12 hours for 3 days.
Children ages 4 to 11: 200 mg (10 mL) PO with food every 12 hours for 3 days.
Children ages 1 to 3: 100 mg (5 mL) PO with food every 12 hours for 3 days.

nusinersen sodium
neu-si-NER-sen

Spinraza

Therapeutic class: Miscellaneous CNS drugs
Pharmacologic class: Antisense oligonucleotides

AVAILABLE FORMS
Injection: 12 mg/5 mL single-use vials

INDICATIONS & DOSAGES
➤ **Spinal muscular atrophy**
Adults and children: Initially, 12 mg (5 mL) intrathecally once every 14 days for three doses; then 12 mg intrathecally once 30 days after third dose. Administer a maintenance dose of 12 mg intrathecally once every 4 months thereafter.

✦Canada   ◇OTC   ◆Off-label use   ✐Photoguide   ⓓⓝⓒ Do not crush   *Liquid contains alcohol   ▓Genetic

obeticholic acid
oh-BET-i-kol-ik

Ocaliva

Therapeutic class: Miscellaneous GI drugs
Pharmacologic class: Farnesoid X receptor agonists

AVAILABLE FORMS
Tablets: 5 mg, 10 mg

INDICATIONS & DOSAGES
Boxed Warning Hepatic decompensation and failure, in some cases fatal, have been reported in patients with primary biliary cholangitis with cirrhosis. Permanently discontinue in patients with clinical evidence of hepatic decompensation, compensated cirrhosis with evidence of portal HTN, or clinically significant hepatic adverse reactions. ∎

➤ **Primary biliary cholangitis in combination with ursodeoxycholic acid (UDCA) in patients with an inadequate response to UDCA, or as monotherapy in patients unable to tolerate UDCA**
Adults: 5 mg PO once daily in patients without cirrhosis or with compensated cirrhosis without portal HTN who haven't achieved an adequate biochemical response to an appropriate dosage of UDCA for at least 1 year or are intolerant to UDCA. If an adequate reduction in alkaline phosphatase or total bilirubin level hasn't been achieved after 3 months and patient is tolerating drug, increase to maximum dosage of 10 mg once daily.

obiltoxaximab
oh-bil-tox-AX-i-mab

Anthim

Therapeutic class: Antibodies
Pharmacologic class: Monoclonal antibodies

AVAILABLE FORMS
Injection: 600 mg/6 mL single-dose vials

INDICATIONS & DOSAGES
Boxed Warning Because of risk of hypersensitivity and anaphylaxis, administer drug in a setting monitored by trained personnel and equipped to manage anaphylaxis. ∎

➤ **Inhalational anthrax due to *Bacillus anthracis* in combination with appropriate antibacterial drugs; prophylaxis of inhalational anthrax due to *B. anthracis* when alternative therapies aren't available or aren't appropriate**
Adults and children weighing more than 40 kg: 16 mg/kg/dose IV over 90 minutes as a single dose.
Adults weighing 40 kg or less, and children weighing more than 15 to 40 kg: 24 mg/kg/dose IV over 90 minutes as a single dose.
Children weighing 15 kg or less: 32 mg/kg/dose IV over 90 minutes as a single dose.

odevixibat ⊠
oh-de-VIX-i-bat

Bylvay

Therapeutic class: Miscellaneous GI drugs
Pharmacologic class: Bile acid transporter inhibitors

AVAILABLE FORMS
Capsules ⊙ɴᴇ: 400 mcg, 1,200 mcg
Oral pellets: 200 mcg, 600 mcg

INDICATIONS & DOSAGES
➤ **Pruritus in patients with progressive familial intrahepatic cholestasis** ⊠
Adults and children age 3 months and older: 40 mcg/kg PO daily with morning meal. If no improvement after 3 months, increase dosage in 40-mcg/kg increments up to 120 mcg/kg PO daily. Maximum total daily dose is 6 mg.
Adjust-a-dose: Interrupt therapy if new-onset LFT abnormalities or signs and symptoms of clinical hepatitis are observed. Once LFT values return to baseline or stabilize at new baseline, restart drug at 40 mcg/kg/day and increase dosage as tolerated. Consider permanently stopping drug if LFT abnormalities recur. Interrupt therapy if persistent diarrhea occurs. Restart drug at 40 mcg/kg/day when diarrhea resolves and increase dosage as tolerated. Stop drug if diarrhea persists and no alternative etiology is identified.

ofloxacin (otic)
of-FLOKS-a-sin

Therapeutic class: Antibiotics
Pharmacologic class: Fluoroquinolones

AVAILABLE FORMS
Otic solution: 0.3%

INDICATIONS & DOSAGES
➤ **Chronic suppurative otitis media with perforated tympanic membrane**
Adults and children age 12 and older: 10 drops instilled into the affected ear b.i.d. for 14 days.
➤ **Otitis externa**
Adults and children age 13 and older: 10 drops instilled into the affected ear once daily for 7 days.
Children ages 6 months to younger than 13 years: 5 drops into the affected ear once daily for 7 days.
➤ **Acute otitis media in children with tympanostomy tubes**
Children ages 1 to 12: 5 drops instilled into the affected ear b.i.d. for 10 days.

SAFETY ALERT!

olaparib ⊠
oh-LAP-a-rib

Lynparza

Therapeutic class: Antineoplastics
Pharmacologic class: Poly ADP-ribose polymerase inhibitors

AVAILABLE FORMS
Tablets (omc): 100 mg, 150 mg

INDICATIONS & DOSAGES
Adjust-a-dose (for all indications): For patients with moderate renal impairment (CrCl of 31 to 50 mL/minute), reduce dosage to 200 mg PO b.i.d. Refer to manufacturer's instructions for toxicity-related dosage adjustments and drug's use with CYP3A inhibitors.

➤ **Maintenance treatment of recurrent epithelial ovarian, fallopian tube, or primary peritoneal cancer in patients who are in a complete or partial response to platinum-based chemotherapy**
Adults: 300 mg PO b.i.d. Continue treatment until disease progression or unacceptable toxicity occurs.

➤ **First-line maintenance treatment (in combination with bevacizumab) of advanced epithelial ovarian, fallopian tube, or primary peritoneal cancer in adults who are in complete or partial response to first-line, platinum-based chemotherapy and whose cancer is associated with homologous recombination deficiency–positive status, defined by either a deleterious or suspected deleterious *BRCA*-mutation or genomic instability** ▧
Adults: 300 mg PO b.i.d., continued until disease progression or unacceptable toxicity occurs, or up to 2 years in patients with complete response. Give in combination with bevacizumab 15 mg/kg IV infusion every 3 weeks for a total of 15 months, including chemotherapy and maintenance doses.

✳ *NEW INDICATION:* **Maintenance treatment of deleterious or suspected deleterious germline or somatic *BRCA*-mutated advanced epithelial ovarian, fallopian tube, or primary peritoneal cancer in patients who are in complete or partial response to first-line platinum-based chemotherapy** ▧
Adults: 300 mg PO b.i.d. continued until disease progression or unacceptable toxicity occurs, or up to 2 years in patients with complete response. Patient may continue beyond 2 years if continued treatment is beneficial.

➤ **Deleterious or suspected deleterious germline *BRCA*-mutated (*gBRCAm*), HER2-negative metastatic breast cancer in patients previously treated with chemotherapy in the neoadjuvant, adjuvant, or metastatic setting** ▧
Adults: 300 mg PO b.i.d. for a total daily dose of 600 mg until disease progression or unacceptable toxicity occurs.

➤ **Adjuvant treatment of deleterious or suspected deleterious *gBRCAm* HER2-negative, high risk early breast cancer** ▧
Adults: 300 mg PO b.i.d. for 1 year, or until disease recurrence or unacceptable toxicity occurs.

➤ **First-line maintenance treatment of deleterious or suspected deleterious *gBRCAm* metastatic pancreatic adenocarcinoma in adults whose disease hasn't progressed on at least 16 weeks of a first-line, platinum-based chemotherapy regimen** ▧
Adults: 300 mg PO b.i.d. until disease progression or unacceptable toxicity.

➤ **Deleterious or suspected deleterious germline or somatic homologous recombination repair gene-mutated metastatic castration-resistant prostate cancer in adults who have progressed after prior enzalutamide or abiraterone treatment** ▧
Adults: 300 mg PO b.i.d. until disease progression or unacceptable toxicity. Patients should also receive a GnRH analogue or have had bilateral orchiectomy.

olopatadine hydrochloride
oh-loh-PAT-ah-dine

Pataday, Patanase

Therapeutic class: Antihistamines
Pharmacologic class: H₁-receptor antagonists

AVAILABLE FORMS
Nasal spray: 665 mcg/spray
Ophthalmic solution: 0.1%◇, 0.2%◇, 0.7%◇

INDICATIONS & DOSAGES
➤ **Seasonal allergic rhinitis (nasal)**
Adults and children age 12 and older: 2 sprays into each nostril b.i.d.
Children ages 6 to 11: 1 spray into each nostril b.i.d.
➤ **Allergic conjunctivitis**
Adults and children age 3 and older: 1 drop (0.1%) in each affected eye b.i.d. at an interval of 6 to 8 hours.
Adults and children age 2 and older: 1 drop (0.2%, 0.7%) in each affected eye once a day.

olsalazine sodium
ol-SAL-uh-zeen

Dipentum

Therapeutic class: Anti-inflammatory drugs
Pharmacologic class: Salicylates

AVAILABLE FORMS
Capsules: 250 mg

INDICATIONS & DOSAGES
➤ **Maintenance of remission of ulcerative colitis in patients intolerant of sulfasalazine**
Adults: 500 mg PO b.i.d.

ombitasvir–paritaprevir–ritonavir and dasabuvir
om-BIT-as-vir/par-i-TA-pre-vir/ri-TOE-na-vir/da-SA-bue-vir

Viekira Pak

Therapeutic class: Antivirals
Pharmacologic class: Antivirals

AVAILABLE FORMS
Copackaged 28-day supply:
Tablets: 12.5 mg ombitasvir/75 mg paritaprevir/50 mg ritonavir
Tablets: dasabuvir 250 mg

INDICATIONS & DOSAGES

➤ **Chronic HCV genotype 1 infection, including patients with compensated cirrhosis, with or without ribavirin**

Adults: For Viekira Pak, give 2 ombitasvir–paritaprevir–ritonavir tablets PO once daily (in morning) and 1 dasabuvir tablet PO b.i.d. (morning and evening), with a meal.

Adjust-a-dose: For patients with HCV genotype 1a infection or unknown genotype without cirrhosis, give Viekira Pak plus ribavirin for 12 weeks. For patients with genotype 1a infection or unknown genotype with compensated cirrhosis, give Viekira Pak plus ribavirin for 24 weeks. For patients with genotype 1b infection with or without compensated cirrhosis, give Viekira Pak for 12 weeks. For patients with liver transplant and normal hepatic function and mild fibrosis, regardless of genotype 1 subtype, give Viekira Pak plus ribavirin for 24 weeks. For ALT level greater than $10 \times$ ULN, consider discontinuing antiviral therapy. If ALT level is elevated and associated with liver inflammation, increasing bilirubin or ALP level or INR, discontinue treatment.

Use in patients with Child-Pugh class B or C is contraindicated.

onasemnogene abeparvovec-xioi ✂
on-a-SEM-noe-jeen a-be-PAR-voe-vek

Zolgensma

Therapeutic class: CNS agents
Pharmacologic class: Gene therapies

AVAILABLE FORMS
Injection: 2.0×10^{13} vector genomes (vg)/mL in vials of 5.5 mL or 8.3 mL in a kit of two to nine vials

INDICATIONS & DOSAGES
Boxed Warning Drug can cause serious acute liver injury and acute liver failure. Assess liver function before infusion and monitor patient for at least 3 months post infusion. Give corticosteroids to all patients before and after drug infusion. ■

➤ **Spinal muscular atrophy with bi-allelic mutations in the survival motor neuron 1 gene** ✂
Children younger than age 2: 1.1×10^{14} vg/kg body weight as a single IV infusion over 60 minutes.

orlistat
ORE-lah-stat

Alli ◇, Xenical

Therapeutic class: Antiobesity drugs
Pharmacologic class: Lipase inhibitors

AVAILABLE FORMS
Capsules: 60 mg ◇, 120 mg

INDICATIONS & DOSAGES
➤ **To manage obesity, including weight loss and weight maintenance with a reduced-calorie diet; to reduce risk of weight gain after previous weight loss**

Adults and children ages 12 and older: 120 mg PO t.i.d. with or up to 1 hour after each main meal containing fat.

➤ **Weight loss (OTC formulation)**
Adults age 18 and older: One 60-mg capsule PO with each meal containing fat. Dosage shouldn't exceed 3 capsules a day.

oxacillin sodium
oks-a-SIL-in

Therapeutic class: Antibiotics
Pharmacologic class: Penicillins

AVAILABLE FORMS
Injection: 1-g, 2-g, 10-g vials; 1 g/50 mL, 2 g/50 mL premixed solution

INDICATIONS & DOSAGES
➤ **Infections caused by penicillinase-producing staphylococci that have demonstrated susceptibility to the drug; empirical therapy in suspected cases of resistant staphylococcal infections**

Adults: For mild to moderate infections, 250 to 500 mg IV or IM every 4 to 6 hours. For severe infections, 1 g IV or IM every 4 to 6 hours.

Infants and children weighing less than 40 kg: For mild to moderate infections, 50 mg/kg/day IV or IM in equally divided doses every 6 hours. For severe infections, 100 mg/kg/day IV or IM in equally divided doses every 4 to 6 hours.

Premature infants and neonates: 25 mg/kg/day IV or IM.

Adjust-a-dose: Duration of therapy depends on type and severity of the infection and overall condition of patient. In severe infections, continue drug for at least 14 days. Continue drug for at least 48 hours after patient is afebrile and asymptomatic and cultures are negative. Treatment of endocarditis and osteomyelitis may require a longer duration of therapy. Consider dosage reduction in patients with known or suspected renal impairment.

ozanimod
oh-ZAN-i-mod

Zeposia

Therapeutic class: MS drugs
Pharmacologic class: Sphingosine 1-phosphate receptor modulators

AVAILABLE FORMS
Capsules ⓓ: 0.23 mg, 0.46 mg, 0.92 mg

INDICATIONS & DOSAGES
➤ **Relapsing forms of MS, including clinically isolated syndrome, relapsing-remitting disease, and active secondary progressive disease; moderate to severe active ulcerative colitis**

Adults: Initially, 0.23 mg PO once daily on days 1 to 4, then 0.46 mg PO once daily on days 5 to 7, then maintenance dose of 0.92 mg PO once daily.

ozenoxacin
oz-en-OX-a-sin

Xepi

Therapeutic class: Antibiotics
Pharmacologic class: Quinolone antibiotics

AVAILABLE FORMS
Cream: 1%

INDICATIONS & DOSAGES
➤ **Impetigo due to *Staphylococcus aureus* or *Streptococcus pyogenes***
Adults and children age 2 months and older: Apply a thin layer topically to affected areas b.i.d. for 5 days.

SAFETY ALERT!

panitumumab ⚇
pan-eh-TOO-moo-mab

Vectibix

Therapeutic class: Antineoplastics
Pharmacologic class: Monoclonal antibodies

AVAILABLE FORMS
Solution for infusion: 20 mg/mL

INDICATIONS & DOSAGES
Boxed Warning Dermatologic toxicities occur in 90% of patients receiving monotherapy, and are severe in 15%. ∎

➤ **Wild-type RAS (defined as wild-type in both KRAS and NRAS) metastatic colorectal cancer as first-line therapy in combination with FOLFOX (5-FU, leucovorin, oxaliplatin); as monotherapy following disease progression during or after fluoropyrimidine-, oxaliplatin-, and irinotecan-containing regimens**
Adults: 6 mg/kg IV infusion over 60 minutes every 14 days as a single agent or in combination with FOLFOX. For doses greater than 1,000 mg, infuse over 90 minutes.
Adjust-a-dose: For patients with mild or moderate (grade 1 or 2) infusion reactions, reduce infusion rate by 50%. For patients with severe infusion reactions, stop drug permanently. Refer to manufacturer's instructions for toxicity-related dosage adjustments and drug discontinuation.

parathyroid hormone
par-a-THYE-roid

Natpara

Therapeutic class: Hormone replacements
Pharmacologic class: Parathyroid hormone analogues

AVAILABLE FORMS
Injection: 25 mcg, 50 mcg, 75 mcg, 100 mcg multi-dose cartridges

INDICATIONS & DOSAGES
Boxed Warning May increase risk of osteosarcoma. Reserve use for patients for whom the potential benefits outweigh this risk. ∎

➤ **Adjunct to calcium and vitamin D to control hypocalcemia in patients with hypoparathyroidism who can't be well controlled on calcium supplements and active forms of vitamin D alone**
Adults: Initially, 50 mcg subcut once daily in the thigh. Titrate maintenance dose to lowest dose that achieves a total albumin-corrected serum calcium level within the lower half of the normal total serum calcium range (between 8 and 9 mg/dL) without the need for active forms of vitamin D and with calcium supplementation sufficient to meet daily requirements. Maximum dose is 100 mcg daily.
Adjust-a-dose: If albumin-corrected serum calcium level can't be maintained above 8 mg/dL without an active form of vitamin D or oral calcium supplementation, may increase Natpara dosage in increments of 25 mcg every 4 weeks to a maximum daily dose of 100 mcg. If total serum calcium level is repeatedly above 9 mg/dL after active form of vitamin D has been discontinued and calcium supplement has been decreased to a dosage sufficient to meet daily requirements, may decrease Natpara dosage to 25 mcg/day.

patiromer sorbitex calcium
pa-TIR-oh-mer

Veltassa

Therapeutic class: Potassium-removing resins
Pharmacologic class: Cation exchange polymers

AVAILABLE FORMS
Oral powder: 8.4-g, 16.8-g, 25.2-g packets

INDICATIONS & DOSAGES
➤ **Nonemergency treatment of hyperkalemia**
Adults: Initially, 8.4 g PO once daily. Monitor serum potassium level and adjust dosage based on potassium level at intervals of 1 week or longer, in increments of 8.4 g, to reach desired potassium concentration. Maximum dosage is 25.2 g once daily.

patisiran ⚇
PAT-i-sir-an

Onpattro

Therapeutic class: Metabolic agents
Pharmacologic class: Anti-transthyretin small interfering RNA agents

AVAILABLE FORMS
Injection: 2 mg/mL in 5-mL single-dose vials

INDICATIONS & DOSAGES
➤ **Polyneuropathy of hereditary transthyretin-mediated amyloidosis ⚇**
Adults weighing 100 kg or more: 30 mg IV infusion over 80 minutes once every 3 weeks. Premedicate with a corticosteroid, acetaminophen, an H_1 blocker, and an H_2 blocker at least 60 minutes before administration.
Adults weighing less than 100 kg: 0.3 mg/kg IV infusion over 80 minutes once every 3 weeks. Premedicate

with a corticosteroid, acetaminophen, an H_1 blocker, and an H_2 blocker at least 60 minutes before administration.

SAFETY ALERT!

PAZOPanib
paz-OH-pa-nib

Votrient

Therapeutic class: Antineoplastics
Pharmacologic class: Multi-tyrosine kinase inhibitors

AVAILABLE FORMS
Tablets ⓒ: 200 mg

INDICATIONS & DOSAGES
Boxed Warning Severe and fatal hepatotoxicity has been observed in clinical trials. ■
➤ **Advanced renal cell carcinoma; advanced soft-tissue sarcoma in patients who have received prior chemotherapy**
Adults: 800 mg PO daily at least 1 hour before or 2 hours after a meal. Continue until disease progression or unacceptable toxicity occurs.
Adjust-a-dose: For patients with moderate hepatic impairment, 200 mg PO daily. Drug isn't recommended for patients with severe hepatic impairment. When coadministration of strong CYP3A4 inhibitors is necessary, decrease pazopanib dosage to 400 mg PO daily. Refer to manufacturer's instructions for toxicity-related dosage adjustments.

pegcetacoplan
peg-set-a-KOE-plan

Empaveli

Therapeutic class: Immunomodulators
Pharmacologic class: Complement inhibitors

AVAILABLE FORMS
Injection: 1,080 mg/20 mL (54 mg/mL) single-dose vial

INDICATIONS & DOSAGES
➤ **Paroxysmal nocturnal hemoglobinuria**
Adults: 1,080 mg subcut infusion twice weekly.
Adjust-a-dose: For LDH level greater than $2 \times$ ULN, give 1,080 mg subcut infusion every 3 days. Monitor LDH level twice weekly for at least 4 weeks after dosage increase. To reduce risk of hemolysis with abrupt treatment discontinuation when switching from eculizumab, initiate pegcetacoplan while continuing eculizumab at its current dose; after 4 weeks, discontinue eculizumab and continue pegcetacoplan. When switching from ravulizumab, initiate pegcetacoplan no more than 4 weeks after last dose of ravulizumab.

peginterferon beta-1a
peg-in-ter-FEER-on

Plegridy, Plegridy Starter Pack (subcut), Plegridy Titration Kit (IM)

Therapeutic class: Antivirals
Pharmacologic class: Biological response modifiers

AVAILABLE FORMS
Injection (IM): 125 mcg/0.5 mL in prefilled syringe
Injection (subcut): 63 mcg/0.5 mL, 94 mcg/0.5 mL, 125 mcg/0.5 mL in prefilled pen-injector or prefilled syringe

INDICATIONS & DOSAGES
➤ **Relapsing forms of MS**
Adults: On day 1, 63 mcg subcut or IM. On day 15, 94 mcg subcut or IM. On day 29 and every 14 days thereafter, 125 mcg subcut or IM.

pegloticase ☒
peg-LOE-ti-kase

Krystexxa

Therapeutic class: Antigout agents
Pharmacologic class: Uric acid–specific enzymes

AVAILABLE FORMS
Injection: 8 mg/mL in 2-mL single-use vial

INDICATIONS & DOSAGES
Boxed Warning Drug can cause G6PD deficiency–associated hemolysis and methemoglobinemia. Screen patients at risk for G6PD deficiency before initiation. Due to risk of hypersensitivity and anaphylaxis, administer drug in a setting monitored by trained personnel and equipped to manage anaphylaxis, and premedicate with antihistamines and corticosteroids. Assess uric acid level before infusions and discontinue treatment if level increases above 6 mg/dL. ■
➤ **Chronic gout in patients refractory to conventional therapy**
Adults: 8 mg by IV infusion over no less than 120 minutes every 2 weeks.

pegvaliase-pqpz
peg-VAL-i-ase pqpz

Palynziq

Therapeutic class: Phenylalanine reducers
Pharmacologic class: Phenylalanine-metabolizing enzymes

AVAILABLE FORMS
Injection: 2.5 mg/0.5 mL, 10 mg/0.5 mL, 20 mg/mL in single-dose prefilled syringes

INDICATIONS & DOSAGES
Boxed Warning Due to risk of hypersensitivity and anaphylaxis, administer initial dose in a setting monitored by trained personnel and equipped to

manage anaphylaxis. Instruct patient and patient's observer (if applicable) to recognize signs and symptoms of anaphylaxis if self-administering, and confirm their competency. ∎

➤ **To reduce blood phenylalanine concentrations in patients with phenylketonuria who have uncontrolled blood phenylalanine concentrations greater than 600 micromol/L on existing management**
Adults: Initially, 2.5 mg subcut once weekly for 4 weeks. Then titrate dosage in step-wise fashion over at least 5 weeks to achieve a dosage of 20 mg subcut once daily as follows: 2.5 mg subcut twice weekly for 1 week, then 10 mg subcut once weekly for 1 week, then 10 mg subcut twice weekly for 1 week, then 10 mg subcut four times per week for 1 week, then 10 mg subcut once daily for 1 week, then maintenance dose of 20 mg subcut once daily for at least 24 weeks.

Consider a dosage increase to 40 mg subcut once daily in patients who have been maintained continuously on 20 mg once daily for at least 24 weeks and who haven't achieved a blood phenylalanine concentration of 600 micromol/L or less. Consider increasing to a maximum of 60 mg subcut once daily in patients who haven't achieved a response with 40 mg once daily continuous treatment for at least 16 weeks. Use lowest effective and tolerated dosage.
Adjust-a-dose: For patients with blood phenylalanine concentrations less than 30 micromol/L, may reduce dosage with or without dietary protein and phenylalanine intake modification to maintain phenylalanine level above 30 micromol/L. Discontinue drug in patients who haven't achieved a response after 16 weeks of continuous treatment with 60 mg subcut once daily.

---

pentoxifylline
pen-tox-IH-fi-leen

Therapeutic class: Hemorrheologic drugs
Pharmacologic class: Xanthine derivatives

AVAILABLE FORMS
Tablets (extended-release) ⓒ: 400 mg

INDICATIONS & DOSAGES
➤ **Intermittent claudication from chronic occlusive vascular disease**
Adults: 400 mg PO t.i.d. with meals for at least 8 weeks.
Adjust-a-dose: For CrCl less than 30 mL/minute, reduce dosage to 400 mg once daily.

May decrease to 400 mg b.i.d. if GI and CNS adverse effects occur. If adverse effects persist, discontinue drug.

---

perampanel
per-AMP-an-ell

Fycompa

Therapeutic class: Anticonvulsants
Pharmacologic class: Noncompetitive AMPA receptor antagonists
Controlled substance schedule: III

AVAILABLE FORMS
Oral suspension: 0.5 mg/mL
Tablets: 2 mg, 4 mg, 6 mg, 8 mg, 10 mg, 12 mg

INDICATIONS & DOSAGES
Boxed Warning   Serious or life-threatening psychiatric and behavioral adverse reactions have been reported in patients with and without prior psychiatric history. ∎

Adjust-a-dose (for all indications): In older adults, don't increase dosage more frequently than every 2 weeks. In patients with mild hepatic impairment, increase daily dose by 2 mg no more frequently than every 2 weeks; maximum is 6 mg once daily. In patients with moderate hepatic impairment, increase daily dose by 2 mg no more frequently than every 2 weeks; maximum is 4 mg once daily. Refer to manufacturer's instructions for use with CYP3A4 inducers.

➤ **Monotherapy or adjunctive therapy for partial-onset seizures with or without secondarily generalized seizures in patients with epilepsy**
Adults and children age 4 and older: Initially, 2 mg PO once daily at bedtime. Increase dosage in increments of 2 mg once daily based on clinical response and tolerability and not more frequently than at weekly intervals. Recommended maintenance dose is 8 to 12 mg once daily at bedtime, although some patients may respond to 4 mg once daily.

➤ **Adjunctive therapy in treatment of primary generalized tonic-clonic seizures in patients with epilepsy**
Adults and children age 12 and older: Initially, 2 mg PO once daily at bedtime. Increase dosage in increments of 2 mg once daily based on clinical response and tolerability and not more frequently than at weekly intervals. Recommended maintenance dose in monotherapy or adjunctive therapy is 8 mg once daily at bedtime, although if needed, may increase dosage to 12 mg once daily.

---

peramivir
per-AM-i-vir

Rapivab

Therapeutic class: Antivirals
Pharmacologic class: Neuraminidase inhibitors

AVAILABLE FORMS
Injection: 200 mg/20 mL (10 mg/mL) vials

INDICATIONS & DOSAGES
➤ **Acute uncomplicated influenza in patients who have been symptomatic for no more than 2 days**
Adults and adolescents age 13 and older: 600 mg IV infusion over 15 to 30 minutes as a single dose.
Adjust-a-dose: For patients with CrCl of 30 to 49 mL/minute, dose is 200 mg; for patients with CrCl of 10 to 29 mL/minute, dose is 100 mg. For patients with ESRD requiring dialysis, give after dialysis at a dose adjusted for renal function.
Children ages 6 months to 12 years: 12 mg/kg (up to 600 mg) IV infusion over 15 to 30 minutes as a single dose.

✚Canada   ◇ OTC   ◆ Off-label use   ✐Photoguide   ⓒDo not crush   *Liquid contains alcohol   ▓Genetic

Adjust-a-dose: For patients with CrCl of 30 to 49 mL/minute, dose is 4 mg/kg; for patients with CrCl of 10 to 29 mL/minute, dose is 2 mg/kg. For patients with ESRD requiring dialysis, give after dialysis at a dose adjusted for renal function.

No data are available to support a recommended dosage adjustment for patients age 6 months to younger than 2 years with CrCl less than 50 mL/minute.

perindopril erbumine
pur-IN-doh-pril

Coversyl ♣

Therapeutic class: Antihypertensives
Pharmacologic class: ACE inhibitors

AVAILABLE FORMS
Tablets: 2 mg, 4 mg, 8 mg

INDICATIONS & DOSAGES
Boxed Warning Drugs that act directly on the renin-angiotensin system can cause fetal harm; when pregnancy is detected, discontinue drug as soon as possible. ∎

Adjust-a-dose (for all indications): For patients with CrCl of 30 mL/minute or greater, initially 2 mg PO daily. Maximum daily maintenance dose is 8 mg. Not recommended for patients with CrCl of less than 30 mL/minute. For patients taking diuretics, consider reducing the diuretic dose before initiating drug. If diuretic therapy can't be altered, monitor patient closely for at least 2 hours after initiating perindopril and until BP has stabilized for another hour. Adjust dosage based on patient's BP response.

➤ **To reduce the risk of CV death or nonfatal MI in patients with stable CAD**
Adults age 70 or younger: 4 mg PO once daily for 2 weeks; then, increase as tolerated to 8 mg once daily.
Adults older than age 70: Initially, 2 mg PO once daily for the first week; then, 4 mg once daily for the second week and 8 mg once daily after that, if tolerated.

➤ **Essential HTN**
Adults: Initially, 4 mg PO once daily. Increase dosage until BP is controlled or to maximum of 16 mg/day; usual maintenance dosage is 4 to 8 mg once daily; may be given in two divided doses.
Adults older than age 65: Initially, 4 mg PO daily as one dose or in two divided doses. May increase dosage by more than 8 mg/day with careful BP monitoring.

permethrin
per-METH-rin

Kwellada-P ♣ ◇ , Nix ◇

Therapeutic class: Scabicides–pediculicides
Pharmacologic class: Pyrethroids

AVAILABLE FORMS
Cream: 5%
Crème rinse: 1% ◇
Lotion: 1% ♣ , 5% ♣

INDICATIONS & DOSAGES
➤ **Infestation with *Pediculus humanus capitis* (head louse) and its nits (lotion)**
Adults and children age 2 months and older: Use after hair has been washed with conditioner-free shampoo, rinsed with water, and towel dried. Apply a sufficient amount (25 to 50 mL) of 1% formulation to saturate hair and scalp. Allow drug to remain on hair for 10 minutes before rinsing off with warm water. Remove remaining nits with comb. Usually only one application is needed. May repeat 7 days after first treatment if lice or nits are still present.

➤ **Infestation with *Sarcoptes scabiei* (5% cream or lotion)**
Adults and children age 2 months and older: Thoroughly massage into the skin from the head to the soles of feet. Treat infants on hairline, neck, scalp, temple, and forehead. Wash cream off after 8 to 14 hours. Usually one application is needed. May retreat if living mites are observed 14 days after first treatment.

perphenazine
per-FEN-uh-zeen

Therapeutic class: Antipsychotics
Pharmacologic class: Phenothiazines

AVAILABLE FORMS
Tablets: 2 mg, 4 mg, 8 mg, 16 mg

INDICATIONS & DOSAGES
Boxed Warning Older adults with dementia-related psychosis treated with antipsychotics are at an increased risk for death. Drug isn't approved to treat these patients. ∎

➤ **Schizophrenia in patients who are nonhospitalized**
Adults and children older than age 12: Initially, 4 to 8 mg PO t.i.d.; reduce as soon as possible to minimum effective dose.

➤ **Schizophrenia in patients who are hospitalized**
Adults and children older than age 12: Initially, 8 to 16 mg PO b.i.d., t.i.d., or q.i.d.; increase to 64 mg daily, as needed.

➤ **Severe nausea and vomiting**
Adults: 8 to 16 mg PO daily in divided doses to maximum of 24 mg. Reduce dosage as soon as possible to minimum effective dose.

SAFETY ALERT!

pexidartinib hydrochloride
pex-i-DAR-ti-nib

Turalio

Therapeutic class: Antineoplastics
Pharmacologic class: Kinase inhibitors

AVAILABLE FORMS
Capsules: 200 mg

INDICATIONS & DOSAGES
Boxed Warning Drug can cause serious and potentially fatal liver injury. ∎

➤ **Symptomatic tenosynovial giant cell tumor associated with severe morbidity or functional limitations and not amenable to improvement with surgery**

Adults: 400 mg PO b.i.d. until disease progression or unacceptable toxicity.

Adjust-a-dose: For patients with mild to severe renal impairment (CrCl of 15 to 89 mL/minute), give 200 mg PO in the morning and 400 mg PO in the evening. For patients with moderate hepatic impairment (total bilirubin level greater than 1.5 and up to 3 × ULN), give 200 mg b.i.d. For patients taking concurrent strong CYP3A inhibitors or UGT inhibitors, if planned daily dose was 600 or 800 mg/day, reduce to 200 mg PO b.i.d. If planned dose was 400 mg/day, reduce to 200 mg PO daily. Refer to manufacturer's instructions for toxicity-related dosage adjustments.

---

pimavanserin tartrate
pim-a-VAN-ser-in

Nuplazid

Therapeutic class: Antipsychotics
Pharmacologic class: 5-HT receptor inverse agonist and antagonists

AVAILABLE FORMS
Capsules: 34 mg
Tablets: 10 mg

INDICATIONS & DOSAGES
Boxed Warning Older adults with dementia-related psychosis treated with antipsychotics are at an increased risk for death. Drug isn't approved to treat these patients. ∎
➤ **Hallucinations and delusions associated with Parkinson disease psychosis**
Adults: 34 mg PO once daily.
Adjust-a-dose: If drug is used with strong CYP3A4 inhibitors, reduce pimavanserin dosage to 10 mg once daily.

---

pirfenidone
pir-FEN-i-done

Esbriet

Therapeutic class: Miscellaneous respiratory drugs
Pharmacologic class: Antifibrotics

AVAILABLE FORMS
Capsules ⬤: 267 mg
Tablets: 267 mg, 534 mg, 801 mg

INDICATIONS & DOSAGES
➤ **Idiopathic pulmonary fibrosis**
Adults: Initially, 267 mg PO t.i.d. days 1 to 7 of therapy; then increase to 534 mg PO t.i.d. for 7 more days (days 8 to 14); then increase to 801 mg PO t.i.d. starting on day 15 of therapy. Maintenance dosage is 801 mg PO t.i.d. Maximum dose is 2,403 mg/day.
Adjust-a-dose: If treatment is interrupted for 14 or more consecutive days, restart drug with 2-week titration period. Refer to manufacturer's instructions for

toxicity-related dosage adjustments and use with CYP1A2 inhibitors.

---

pitolisant hydrochloride ☒
pi-TOL-i-sant

Wakix

Therapeutic class: CNS stimulants
Pharmacologic class: Histamine-3 receptor antagonist/inverse agonists

AVAILABLE FORMS
Tablets: 4.45 mg, 17.8 mg

INDICATIONS & DOSAGES
➤ **Excessive daytime sleepiness or cataplexy in patients with narcolepsy**
Adults: Dosage range is 17.8 to 35.6 mg PO once daily in the morning upon wakening. Titrate dosage as follows: Week 1: Initiate with 8.9 mg (two 4.45-mg tablets) PO once daily. Week 2: Increase to 17.8 mg (one 17.8-mg tablet) PO once daily. Week 3: May increase to the maximum recommended dosage of 35.6 mg (two 17.8-mg tablets) PO once daily based on tolerability.
☒ *Adjust-a-dose:* For patients with moderate hepatic impairment, initiate at 8.9 mg PO once daily and increase after 14 days to a maximum dosage of 17.8 mg PO once daily. For patients with moderate to severe renal impairment or patients known to be poor CYP2D6 metabolizers, initiate at 8.9 mg PO once daily and increase after 7 days to a maximum dosage of 17.8 mg PO once daily.

---

plerixafor
pleh-RIX-uh-for

Mozobil

Therapeutic class: Hematopoietics
Pharmacologic class: CXCR4 chemokine receptor inhibitors

AVAILABLE FORMS
Injection: 24 mg/1.2 mL in single-use vials

INDICATIONS & DOSAGES
➤ **To mobilize hematopoietic stem cells for collection and subsequent autologous transplantation in patients with non-Hodgkin lymphoma and multiple myeloma**
Adults: Initiate plerixafor treatment once daily, 0.24 mg/kg (actual body weight) subcut; or for patients weighing 83 kg or less, give 20 mg fixed dose subcut, approximately 11 hours before initiation of each apheresis, after patient has received G-CSF 10 mcg/kg once daily in the morning for 4 days. Repeat plerixafor dose for up to 4 consecutive evenings and administer G-CSF 10 mcg/kg on each day before apheresis. Don't exceed 40 mg/day.
Adjust-a-dose: For patients with CrCl of 50 mL/minute or less, give 0.16 mg/kg once daily (not to exceed 27 mg/day), or for patients weighing 83 kg or less, give fixed dose of 13 mg.

⬧Canada ◇ OTC ◆ Off-label use ✔Photoguide ⬤Do not crush *Liquid contains alcohol ☒Genetic

potassium iodide
po-TASS-ee-um

Iosat ◇, ThyroSafe ◇

Therapeutic class: Antihyperthyroid drugs
Pharmacologic class: Salts of stable iodine

AVAILABLE FORMS
Oral solution: 65 mg/mL
Tablets: 65 mg, 130 mg

INDICATIONS & DOSAGES
➤ **Radiation protectant for thyroid gland**
Adults and children ages 12 to 18 weighing at least 68 kg: 130 mg PO every 24 hours for 10 to 14 days as directed by public health authorities. Start no later than 3 to 4 hours after exposure. Avoid repeat dosing in patients who are pregnant or breastfeeding.
Children ages 3 to 12 or children ages 12 to 18 weighing less than 68 kg: 65 mg PO every 24 hours as directed by public health authorities. Start no later than 3 to 4 hours after exposure.
Children older than 1 month to 3 years: 32.5 mg PO every 24 hours as directed by public health authorities. Start no later than 3 to 4 hours after exposure.
Neonates from birth to 1 month: 16.25 mg PO every 24 hours as directed by public health authorities. Start no later than 3 to 4 hours after exposure. Avoid repeat dosing, if possible.

prabotulinumtoxinA-xvfs
pra-bot-ue-LYE-num-TOX-in-A

Jeuveau

Therapeutic class: Neuromuscular transmission blockers
Pharmacologic class: Acetylcholine release inhibitors

AVAILABLE FORMS
Injection: 100 units/single-dose vial

INDICATIONS & DOSAGES
Boxed Warning All botulinum toxin products can spread beyond intended injection area to produce symptoms lasting hours to weeks post injection. Drug isn't approved for treatment of spasticity. ■
➤ **Temporary improvement in the appearance of moderate to severe glabellar lines associated with corrugator or procerus muscle activity**
Adults: Inject 0.1 mL (4 units) IM into each of the five sites for a total dose of 20 units. See prescribing information for diagram and complete administration instructions. Retreatment may occur no less than 3 months from prior dose. Consider cumulative dose if other botulinum toxin agents have been used to treat other conditions.

PRALAtrexate
pral-ah-TREX-ate

Folotyn

Therapeutic class: Antineoplastics
Pharmacologic class: Folate analogue metabolic inhibitors

AVAILABLE FORMS
Injection: 20 mg/mL, 40 mg/2 mL in single-use vials

INDICATIONS & DOSAGES
➤ **Relapsed or refractory peripheral T-cell lymphoma**
Adults: 30 mg/m^2 IV push over 3 to 5 minutes weekly for 6 weeks in 7-week cycles until disease progresses or unacceptable toxicity develops. Initiate supplementation with folic acid and vitamin B_{12} before treatment.
Adjust-a-dose: Refer to manufacturer's instructions for dosage adjustments for adverse reactions.

pralsetinib ▨
pral-SE-ti-nib

Gavreto

Therapeutic class: Antineoplastics
Pharmacologic class: Kinase inhibitors

AVAILABLE FORMS
Capsules: 100 mg

INDICATIONS & DOSAGES
Adjust-a-dose (for all indications): Refer to manufacturer's instructions for toxicity-related dosage adjustments. For patients taking a combined P-gp and strong CYP3A inhibitor with pralsetinib 300 mg or 400 mg once daily, decrease pralsetinib dosage to 200 mg once daily; for patients taking a combined P-gp and strong CYP3A inhibitor with pralsetinib 200 mg once daily, decrease pralsetinib dosage to 100 mg once daily. Permanently discontinue pralsetinib in patients unable to tolerate 100 mg once daily.
    For patients taking pralsetinib with a strong CYP3A inducer, increase pralsetinib starting dose to double current dose beginning on day 7 of coadministration. After inducer has been discontinued for 14 days, resume pralsetinib at dose taken before initiation of the strong CYP3A inducer.
➤ **Metastatic *RET* fusion-positive NSCLC as detected by an FDA-approved test** ▨
Adults: 400 mg PO once daily. Continue until disease progression or unacceptable toxicity occurs.
➤ **Advanced or metastatic *RET*-mutant medullary thyroid cancer in patients who require systemic therapy** ▨
Adults and children age 12 and older: 400 mg PO once daily. Continue until disease progression or unacceptable toxicity occurs.
➤ **Advanced or metastatic *RET* fusion-positive thyroid cancer in patients who require systemic**

therapy and are radioactive iodine–refractory (if radioactive iodine is appropriate) ▨
Adults and children age 12 and older: 400 mg PO once daily. Continue until disease progression or unacceptable toxicity occurs.

prasterone
PRAS-ter-one

Intrarosa

Therapeutic class: Hormone replacements
Pharmacologic class: Synthetic steroids

AVAILABLE FORMS
Vaginal insert: 6.5 mg

INDICATIONS & DOSAGES
➤ **Moderate to severe dyspareunia, a symptom of vulvar and vaginal atrophy, due to menopause**
Adults: 1 vaginal insert intravaginally once daily at bedtime.

pretomanid
pre-TOE-ma-nid

Therapeutic class: Antituberculotics
Pharmacologic class: Nitroimidazoles

AVAILABLE FORMS
Tablets: 200 mg

INDICATIONS & DOSAGES
➤ **Pulmonary extensively drug-resistant, treatment-intolerant, or nonresponsive multidrug-resistant TB, in combination with bedaquiline and linezolid**
Adults: 200 mg PO once daily for 26 weeks. Give in combination with bedaquiline 400 mg PO once daily for 2 weeks followed by 200 mg 3 × per week, with at least 48 hours between doses, for 24 weeks for a total of 26 weeks and linezolid 1,200 mg daily PO for up to 26 weeks. May extend dosing of combination regimen beyond 26 weeks if necessary. Give regimen by directly observed therapy.
Adjust-a-dose: If aminotransferase elevations are accompanied by total bilirubin elevation greater than 2 × ULN, or are greater than 8 × ULN, or are greater than 5 × ULN and persist beyond 2 weeks, interrupt treatment with the entire regimen. If myelosuppression, peripheral neuropathy, or optic neuropathy due to linezolid occurs, decrease linezolid dosage to 600 mg daily and, if necessary, further reduce dosage to 300 mg daily or interrupt dosing.

primaquine phosphate
PRIM-a-kwin

Therapeutic class: Antimalarials
Pharmacologic class: Aminoquinolines

AVAILABLE FORMS
Tablets: 26.3 mg (equivalent to 15-mg base)

INDICATIONS & DOSAGES
➤ **To prevent relapse of *Plasmodium vivax* malaria**
Adults: 1 tablet (15 mg base) PO daily for 14 days. Give concurrently with chloroquine.

primidone
PRI-mi-done

Mysoline

Therapeutic class: Anticonvulsants
Pharmacologic class: Barbiturate analogues

AVAILABLE FORMS
Tablets: 50 mg, 250 mg

INDICATIONS & DOSAGES
➤ **Grand mal, psychomotor, and focal epileptic seizures**
Adults and children age 8 and older: Initially, 100 to 125 mg PO at bedtime on days 1 to 3; then 100 to 125 mg PO b.i.d. on days 4 to 6; then 100 to 125 mg PO t.i.d. on days 7 to 9, followed by maintenance dose of 250 mg PO t.i.d. May increase maintenance dose to 250 mg q.i.d., if needed. May increase dosage to maximum of 2 g daily in divided doses. See manufacturer's instructions for beginning therapy in patients already receiving other anticonvulsants.
Children younger than age 8: Initially, 50 mg PO at bedtime for 3 days; then 50 mg PO b.i.d. for days 4 to 6; then 100 mg PO b.i.d. for days 7 to 9, followed by maintenance dose of 125 to 250 mg PO t.i.d. or 10 to 25 mg/kg daily in divided doses.

probenecid
proe-BEN-e-sid

Therapeutic class: Uricosurics
Pharmacologic class: Sulfonamide derivatives

AVAILABLE FORMS
Tablets: 500 mg

INDICATIONS & DOSAGES
➤ **Adjunct to penicillin therapy**
Adults and children age 15 and older weighing more than 50 kg: 500 mg PO q.i.d.
Children ages 2 to 14 or weighing 50 kg or less: Initially, 25 mg/kg or 0.7 g/m² PO; then 40 mg/kg/day or 1.2 g/m² in four divided doses daily.
➤ **Hyperuricemia of gout, gouty arthritis**
Adults: 250 mg PO b.i.d. for first week; then 500 mg b.i.d. Review maintenance dose every 6 months and reduce daily dosage by increments of 500 mg, if indicated.

prucalopride succinate
proo-KAL-oh-pride

Motegrity

Therapeutic class: GI drugs
Pharmacologic class: Selective serotonin-4 (5-HT₄) receptor agonists

AVAILABLE FORMS
Tablets: 1 mg, 2 mg

INDICATIONS & DOSAGES
➤ **Chronic idiopathic constipation**
Adults: 2 mg PO once daily.
Adjust-a-dose: For severe renal impairment (CrCl less than 30 mL/minute), decrease dose to 1 mg PO once daily.

pyrazinamide
peer-a-ZIN-a-mide

Therapeutic class: Antituberculotics
Pharmacologic class: Nicotinamide analogues

AVAILABLE FORMS
Tablets: 500 mg

INDICATIONS & DOSAGES
➤ **Initial treatment of active TB with other anti-tuberculotics or after treatment failure with other primary drugs in any form of active TB**
Adults and children: 15 to 30 mg/kg PO once daily. Don't exceed 3 g/day. Or, 50 to 70 mg/kg lean body weight PO twice weekly. This dosage may exceed the recommended 3-g/day maximum dose, but an increased incidence of adverse reactions hasn't been reported. Administer pyrazinamide for first 2 months of a 6-month or longer treatment regimen for drug-susceptible TB. Treat known or suspected drug-resistant infections with individualized regimens, which may frequently include pyrazinamide.

Patients with HIV infection may need longer courses of therapy. Refer to the CDC (www.CDC.gov) for current treatment recommendations and complete drug regimens.
Adjust-a-dose: For older adults, use doses at the low end of the dosing range.

SAFETY ALERT!

quiNIDine gluconate
KWIN-i-deen

quiNIDine sulfate
Therapeutic class: Antiarrhythmics
Pharmacologic class: Cinchona alkaloids

AVAILABLE FORMS
quinidine gluconate (62% quinidine base)
Tablets (extended-release) ⓪: 324 mg
quinidine sulfate (83% quinidine base)
Tablets: 200 mg, 300 mg

INDICATIONS & DOSAGES
Boxed Warning Therapy for non-life-threatening arrhythmias may result in increased mortality; risk is probably greatest in patients with structural heart disease. ∎
Adjust-a-dose (for all indications): In patients with hepatic impairment or HF, reduce dosage.

Discontinue drug if QRS complex widens to 130% of pretreatment duration, QTc interval widens to 130% of pretreatment duration and is longer than 500 msec,

P waves disappear, or patient develops significant tachycardia, symptomatic bradycardia, or hypotension.
➤ **Atrial flutter or fibrillation (pharmacologic conversion)**
Adults: 400 mg quinidine sulfate PO every 6 hours. If no cardioversion after four or five doses, may increase cautiously to desired effect. Or, quinidine gluconate 648 mg (two 324-mg tablets) PO every 8 hours if no cardioversion after three or four doses, may increase cautiously to desired effect.
➤ **Paroxysmal atrial fibrillation or flutter; maintenance of sinus rhythm**
Adults: For quinidine gluconate, initially 324 mg (extended-release) every 8 to 12 hours. May increase dosage cautiously to desired effect to usual dosage range of 324 to 648 mg every 8 hours. For quinidine sulfate, initially 200 mg (immediate-release) every 6 hours. May increase dosage cautiously to desired effect.
➤ **Ventricular arrhythmias**
Note: Dosing regimens for suppression of life-threatening ventricular arrhythmias haven't been adequately studied. For patients with structural heart disease or other risk factors for toxicity, initiate or adjust dosage in a setting where continuous monitoring and resuscitation are available. Monitor patients for 2 to 3 days once the appropriate dosage has been achieved.
Adults: For quinidine gluconate, 324 mg (extended-release) every 8 to 12 hours. May increase dosage cautiously up to 648 mg every 8 to 12 hours. For quinidine sulfate, initially 200 mg (immediate-release) every 6 hours. May increase dosage cautiously up to 600 mg every 6 to 12 hours.

quinupristin–dalfopristin
QUIN-uh-pris-tin/DALF-oh-pris-tin

Synercid

Therapeutic class: Antibiotics
Pharmacologic class: Streptogramins

AVAILABLE FORMS
Injection: 500-mg vials (150 mg quinupristin and 350 mg dalfopristin)

INDICATIONS & DOSAGES
➤ **Complicated skin and skin-structure infections caused by methicillin-susceptible *Staphylococcus aureus* or *Streptococcus pyogenes***
Adults and adolescents age 16 and older: 7.5 mg/kg IV over 1 hour every 12 hours for at least 7 days.

SAFETY ALERT!

radioactive iodine (sodium iodide, ¹³¹I)
Hicon

Sodium Iodide ¹³¹I Therapeutic

Therapeutic class: Radiopharmaceuticals
Pharmacologic class: Antithyroid drugs

AVAILABLE FORMS
All radioactivity concentrations are determined at time of calibration.

Capsules: Radioactivity range, 100 mCi/capsule
Concentrated solution for preparation of capsules or oral solution: 250 mCi/0.25mL, 500 mCi/0.5 mL, 1,000 mCi/mL vials

INDICATIONS & DOSAGES
➤ **Hyperthyroidism**
Adults: Usual dosage is 4 to 10 mCi PO. Dosage is based on estimated weight of thyroid gland and thyroid uptake.
➤ **Thyroid cancer**
Adults: Initially, 30 to 100 mCi PO, with subsequent doses of 100 to 200 mCi for metastases. Dosage is based on estimated malignant thyroid tissue and metastatic tissue as determined by total body scan. Repeat treatment according to clinical status.

---

ravulizumab-cwvz
rav-ue-LIZ-ue-mab

Ultomiris

Therapeutic class: Immunomodulators
Pharmacologic class: Complement inhibitors

AVAILABLE FORMS
Injection: 300 mg/30 mL (10 mg/mL), 300 mg/3 mL (100 mg/mL), 1,100 mg/11 mL (100 mg/mL) single-dose vials

INDICATIONS & DOSAGES
Boxed Warning   Risk of life-threatening meningococcal infections and sepsis. ■
Adjust-a-dose (for all indications): Supplemental dosing is required for patients weighing 40 kg or more receiving concomitant plasma exchange (PE), plasmapheresis (PP), or intravenous immunoglobulin (IVIg). Additional dose is given within 4 hours after PE, PP, or IVIg and is based on weight, current dose, and concomitant treatment. Refer to manufacturer's instructions for ravulizumab-cwvz dosing.
➤ **Paroxysmal nocturnal hemoglobinuria; inhibition of complement-mediated thrombotic microangiopathy in patients with atypical hemolytic-uremic syndrome**
Adults and children age 1 month and older weighing 100 kg or more: 3,000 mg IV infusion loading dose, followed in 2 weeks by maintenance dose of 3,600 mg IV infusion once every 8 weeks.
Adults and children age 1 month and older weighing 60 to less than 100 kg: 2,700 mg IV infusion loading dose, followed in 2 weeks by maintenance dose of 3,300 mg IV infusion once every 8 weeks.
Adults and children age 1 month and older weighing 40 to less than 60 kg: 2,400 mg IV infusion loading dose, followed in 2 weeks by maintenance dose of 3,000 mg IV infusion once every 8 weeks.
Children age 1 month and older weighing 30 to less than 40 kg: 1,200-mg IV loading dose, followed in 2 weeks by maintenance dose of 2,700-mg IV infusion once every 8 weeks.
Children age 1 month and older weighing 20 to less than 30 kg: 900-mg IV infusion loading dose, followed in 2 weeks by maintenance dose of 2,100-mg IV infusion once every 8 weeks.

Children age 1 month and older weighing 10 to less than 20 kg: 600-mg IV infusion loading dose, followed in 2 weeks by maintenance dose of 600-mg IV infusion once every 4 weeks.
Children age 1 month and older weighing 5 to less than 10 kg: 600-mg IV infusion loading dose, followed in 2 weeks by maintenance dose of 300-mg IV infusion once every 4 weeks.
Patients switching from eculizumab to ravulizumab: Administer a ravulizumab loading dose 2 weeks after last eculizumab infusion; then follow maintenance dosing according to patient's weight.
✳ *NEW INDICATION:* **Generalized myasthenia gravis in patients who are anti-acetylcholine receptor antibody-positive**
Adults weighing 100 kg or more: 3,000 mg IV infusion loading dose, followed in 2 weeks by maintenance dose of 3,600 mg IV infusion once every 8 weeks.
Adults weighing 60 to less than 100 kg: 2,700 mg IV infusion loading dose, followed in 2 weeks by maintenance dose of 3,300 mg IV infusion once every 8 weeks.
Adults weighing 40 to less than 60 kg: 2,400 mg IV infusion loading dose, followed in 2 weeks by maintenance dose of 3,000 mg IV infusion once every 8 weeks.
Patients switching from eculizumab to ravulizumab: Administer a ravulizumab loading dose 2 weeks after last eculizumab infusion or 1 week after last eculizumab induction infusion; then follow maintenance dosing according to patient's weight.

SAFETY ALERT!

regorafenib ▨
re-goe-RAF-e-nib

Stivarga

Therapeutic class: Antineoplastics
Pharmacologic class: Kinase inhibitors

AVAILABLE FORMS
Tablets: 40 mg

INDICATIONS & DOSAGES
Boxed Warning   May cause severe or fatal hepatotoxicity. Monitor closely. ■
Adjust-a-dose (for all indications): Refer to manufacturer's instructions for toxicity-related dosage adjustments and discontinuation.
➤ **Metastatic colorectal cancer previously treated with fluoropyrimidine-, oxaliplatin-, and irinotecan-based chemotherapy, an anti–vascular endothelial growth factor therapy and, if *KRAS* wild type, an anti–epidermal growth factor receptor therapy** ▨
Adults: 160 mg PO once a day for first 21 days of each 28-day cycle. Continue therapy until disease progression or unacceptable toxicity occurs.
➤ **Locally advanced, unresectable, or metastatic GI stromal tumor previously treated with imatinib mesylate and sunitinib malate**

Adults: 160 mg PO once daily for first 21 days of each 28-day cycle. Continue therapy until disease progression or unacceptable toxicity occurs.

➤ **Hepatocellular carcinoma in patients previously treated with sorafenib**

Adults: 160 mg PO once daily for first 21 days of each 28-day cycle. Continue treatment until progression or unacceptable toxicity occurs.

retapamulin
re-te-PAM-ue-lin

Altabax

Therapeutic class: Antibiotics
Pharmacologic class: Pleuromutilins

AVAILABLE FORMS
Topical ointment: 1%

INDICATIONS & DOSAGES
➤ **Impetigo due to** *Staphylococcus aureus* **(meth-icillin-susceptible isolates only) or** *Streptococcus pyogenes*

Adults and children age 9 months and older: Apply a thin layer to affected area (up to 100 cm² in total BSA in adults or 2% total BSA in children) b.i.d. for 5 days.

SAFETY ALERT!

reteplase (recombinant)
RET-ah-place

Retavase Half-Kit, Retavase Kit

Therapeutic class: Thrombolytics
Pharmacologic class: Tissue plasminogen activators

AVAILABLE FORMS
Injection: 10 units/vial, in a kit with components for reconstitution of one or two single-use vials

INDICATIONS & DOSAGES
➤ **Acute ST-elevation MI (STEMI)**

Adults: Give bolus injection of 10 units as soon as possible after onset of STEMI. If complications, such as serious bleeding or anaphylactoid reaction, don't occur after first bolus, give second bolus 30 minutes after start of first. Give each bolus IV over 2 minutes.

revefenacin
REV-e-fen-a-sin

Yupelri

Therapeutic class: Bronchodilators
Pharmacologic class: Anticholinergics

AVAILABLE FORMS
Solution for inhalation: 175 mcg/3 mL unit-dose vial

INDICATIONS & DOSAGES
➤ **Maintenance treatment of COPD**

Adults: 175 mcg oral inhalation via nebulizer once daily.

rifabutin
rif-ah-BYOO-tin

Mycobutin

Therapeutic class: Antituberculotics
Pharmacologic class: Semisynthetic ansamycins

AVAILABLE FORMS
Capsules: 150 mg

INDICATIONS & DOSAGES
➤ **To prevent disseminated** *Mycobacterium avium* **complex in patients with advanced HIV infection**

Adults: 300 mg PO daily as a single dose or in two divided doses. May give with food or give 150 mg b.i.d. to minimize GI distress.

Adjust-a-dose: For patients with CrCl of less than 30 mL/minute, reduce rifabutin dosage by 50%.

rifamycin
rif-a-MYE-sin

Aemcolo

Therapeutic class: Antibiotics
Pharmacologic class: Ansamycins

AVAILABLE FORMS
Tablets (delayed-release): 194 mg

INDICATIONS & DOSAGES
➤ **Travelers' diarrhea caused by noninvasive strains of** *Escherichia coli*

Adults: 388 mg PO b.i.d. for 3 days.

riluzole
RIL-yoo-zole

Exservan, Rilutek, Tiglutik

Therapeutic class: Neuroprotectors
Pharmacologic class: Benzothiazoles

AVAILABLE FORMS
Film: 50 mg
Tablets: 50 mg
Suspension (oral): 50 mg/10 mL

INDICATIONS & DOSAGES
➤ **Amyotrophic lateral sclerosis**

Adults: 50 mg PO every 12 hours, taken on empty stomach 1 hour before or 2 hours after a meal.

rimegepant
ri-ME-je-pant

Nurtec ODT

Therapeutic class: Antimigraine drugs
Pharmacologic class: Calcitonin gene-related peptide receptor antagonists

AVAILABLE FORMS
Tablets (ODTs): 75 mg

INDICATIONS & DOSAGES

➤ **Acute migraine with or without aura**
Adults: 75 mg PO as a single dose. Maximum dose, 75 mg in 24 hours.
➤ **Prevention of episodic migraine**
Adults: 75 mg PO every other day.

riociguat
RYE-oh-sig-ue-at

Adempas

Therapeutic class: Vasodilators
Pharmacologic class: Soluble guanylate cyclase stimulators

AVAILABLE FORMS
Tablets: 0.5 mg, 1 mg, 1.5 mg, 2 mg, 2.5 mg

INDICATIONS & DOSAGES
Boxed Warning Drug may cause fetal harm. Exclude pregnancy before treatment; patient should avoid pregnancy for 1 month after treatment. For females, Adempas is available only through the Adempas REMS Program. ▮
➤ **Chronic thromboembolic pulmonary HTN (CTEPH) (WHO Group 4), after surgical treatment, or inoperable CTEPH, to improve exercise capacity and WHO functional class; pulmonary artery HTN (WHO Group 1) to improve exercise capacity and WHO functional class and to delay clinical worsening**
Adults: Initially, 1 mg PO t.i.d. Increase dosage by 0.5 mg t.i.d. if systolic BP remains greater than 95 mm Hg and patient has no signs or symptoms of hypotension. Dosage increases should occur no less than 2 weeks apart. Titrate to highest tolerated dosage; maximum dose is 2.5 mg PO t.i.d.
Adjust-a-dose: Patients unable to tolerate initial 1-mg dosage due to hypotension may start at 0.5 mg PO t.i.d. Decrease dosage by 0.5 mg PO t.i.d. in patients experiencing hypotension. Patients who smoke may need dosages titrated higher than 2.5 mg PO t.i.d. Patients who quit smoking during treatment may need a dosage decrease. Consider a starting dose of 0.5 mg PO t.i.d. for patients taking strong CYP and P-gp/BCRP inhibitors.

SAFETY ALERT!

ripretinib
rip-RE-ti-nib

Qinlock

Therapeutic class: Antineoplastics
Pharmacologic class: Tyrosine kinase inhibitors

AVAILABLE FORMS
Tablets ⬤: 50 mg

INDICATIONS & DOSAGES
➤ **Advanced GI stromal tumor in patients who have received prior treatment with three or more kinase inhibitors, including imatinib**
Adults: 150 mg PO once daily until disease progression or unacceptable toxicity occurs.

Adjust-a-dose: For patients unable to avoid taking with a moderate CYP3A inducer, increase ripretinib dosage to 150 mg b.i.d. during coadministration. Resume once-daily ripretinib dosing 14 days after moderate CYP3A inducer is discontinued. Refer to manufacturer's instructions for toxicity-related dosage adjustments. Permanently discontinue drug if patient can't tolerate 100-mg dose.

risankizumab-rzaa
ris-an-KIZ-ue-mab

Skyrizi

Therapeutic class: Immunomodulators
Pharmacologic class: Interleukin-23 receptor antagonists

AVAILABLE FORMS
Injection (IV): 600 mg/10 mL single-dose vial
Injection (subcut): 75 mg/0.83 mL prefilled syringe; 150 mg/mL prefilled syringe or pen; 360 mg/2.4 mL prefilled cartridge

INDICATIONS & DOSAGES
➤ **Moderate to severe plaque psoriasis in patients who are candidates for systemic therapy or phototherapy**
Adults: 150 mg (two 75-mg injections) subcut at weeks 0 and 4 and every 12 weeks thereafter.
➤ **Active psoriatic arthritis**
Adults: 150 mg (two 75-mg injections) subcut at weeks 0 and 4 and every 12 weeks thereafter.
➤ **Moderately to severely active Crohn disease**
Adults: 600 mg IV infusion over at least 1 hour at weeks 0, 4, and 8; then 360 mg subcut at week 12 and every 8 weeks thereafter.

risdiplam ⬝
ris-DIP-lam

Evrysdi

Therapeutic class: Miscellaneous CNS drugs
Pharmacologic class: Survival of motor neuron 2–directed RNA splicing modifiers

AVAILABLE FORMS
Oral solution: 0.75 mg/mL (60-mg bottles)

INDICATIONS & DOSAGES
➤ **Spinal muscular atrophy** ⬝
Adults and children age 2 and older weighing 20 kg or more: 5 mg PO daily.
Children age 2 and older weighing less than 20 kg: 0.25 mg/kg PO daily.
Children age 2 months to younger than 2 years: 0.2 mg/kg PO daily.

---

romiDEPsin
roh-mih-DEP-sin

Istodax

Therapeutic class: Antineoplastics
Pharmacologic class: Histone deacetylase
inhibitors

AVAILABLE FORMS
Injection: 27.5 mg/5.5 mL, 10 mg/2 mL vials
Injection (powder for solution): 10-mg vial

INDICATIONS & DOSAGES
➤ **Cutaneous T-cell lymphoma and peripheral T-cell lymphoma in patients who have received at least one prior systemic therapy**
Adults: 14 mg/m^2 by IV infusion over 4 hours on days 1, 8, and 15 of 28-day cycle. Repeat every 28 days if effective and well tolerated.
Adjust-a-dose: Refer to manufacturer's instructions for toxicity-related dosage adjustments and discontinuation.

romosozumab-aqqg
roe-moe-SOZ-ue-mab

Evenity

Therapeutic class: Antiosteoporotics
Pharmacologic class: Sclerostin inhibitors

AVAILABLE FORMS
Injection: 105 mg/1.17 mL single-use prefilled syringe

INDICATIONS & DOSAGES
Boxed Warning Drug can increase risk of MI, stroke, and CV death. ∎
➤ **Osteoporosis in patients after menopause at high risk for fracture; or in patients who have failed or are intolerant of other osteoporosis therapy**
Adults: 210 mg (two syringes) subcut once every month for 12 months.

rufinamide
roo-FIN-ah-mide

Banzel

Therapeutic class: Anticonvulsants
Pharmacologic class: Triazole derivatives

AVAILABLE FORMS
Suspension: 40 mg/mL
Tablets: 200 mg, 400 mg

INDICATIONS & DOSAGES
➤ **Adjunct treatment of seizures associated with Lennox-Gastaut syndrome**
Adults and children age 17 and older: Initially, 400 to 800 mg PO daily in two equally divided doses. Increase dosage by 400 to 800 mg/day every 2 days to 3,200 mg PO daily in divided doses.
Children ages 1 to less than 17: Initially, 10 mg/kg/day PO in two equally divided doses. Increase dosage by 10 mg/kg every other day to 45 mg/kg/day or 3,200 mg (whichever is less) PO daily in divided doses.

Adjust-a-dose: Dialysis clears drug by 30%; dosage adjustment may be necessary. For patients taking valproate, start rufinamide at dosages less than 400 mg/day (adults) or less than 10 mg/kg/day (children).

ruxolitinib phosphate
rux-oh-LI-ti-nib

Jakafi

Therapeutic class: Antineoplastics
Pharmacologic class: Janus-associated kinase inhibitors

AVAILABLE FORMS
Tablets: 5 mg, 10 mg, 15 mg, 20 mg, 25 mg

INDICATIONS & DOSAGES
Adjust-a-dose (for all indications): Refer to manufacturer's instructions for toxicity-related dosage adjustments, dosage modifications for renal or hepatic impairment, or use with strong CYP3A4 inhibitors or fluconazole.
➤ **Intermediate or high-risk myelofibrosis, including primary myelofibrosis, post–polycythemia vera myelofibrosis, and post–essential thrombocythemia myelofibrosis**
Adults: Initially, 20 mg PO b.i.d. if platelet count is greater than 200×10^9/L, 15 mg PO b.i.d. if platelet count is 100 to 200×10^9/L, or 5 mg PO b.i.d. if platelet count is 50 to less than 100×10^9/L. May increase in 5-mg increments b.i.d. to a maximum of 25 mg b.i.d. Don't increase during the first 4 weeks of therapy and not more frequently than every 2 weeks.

Consider dosage increases in patients who meet all of the following conditions: failure to achieve either a 50% reduction from pretreatment baseline in palpable spleen length or a 35% reduction in spleen volume as measured by CT scan or MRI; platelet count greater than 125×10^9/L at 4 weeks and never below 100×10^9/L; and ANC greater than 0.75×10^9/L.

Long-term maintenance at a 5-mg b.i.d. dosage hasn't shown response; limit continued use at this dosage to patients in whom benefits outweigh risks.

Discontinue drug after 6 months if there is no spleen reduction or symptom improvement. If drug needs to be stopped for any reason except thrombocytopenia, taper gradually by 5 mg b.i.d. each week.
➤ **Polycythemia vera in patients with an inadequate response to or who are intolerant of hydroxyurea**
Adults: Initially, 10 mg PO b.i.d. If response is inadequate and platelet count is 140×10^9 or greater, Hb level is 12 g/dL or greater, and ANC is 1.5×10^9/L or greater, may increase dose by 5 mg b.i.d. to a maximum of 25 mg b.i.d. (Maximum is 50 mg/day.) Doses shouldn't be increased during first 4 weeks of therapy and not more frequently than every 2 weeks. Inadequate response is defined as one of the following: continued need for phlebotomy, WBC count higher than ULN, platelet count greater than ULN, or palpable spleen that's reduced by less than 25% from baseline.

> **Steroid-refractory acute GVHD**

Adults and children age 12 and older: Initially 5 mg PO b.i.d. May increase to 10 mg b.i.d. after at least 3 days of treatment if ANC and platelet counts aren't decreased by 50% or more from first day of dosing.

Adjust-a-dose: After 6 months of treatment in patients who have discontinued corticosteroids, taper drug by one dose level every 8 weeks (10 mg b.i.d. to 5 mg b.i.d. to 5 mg once daily). Consider retreatment if acute GVHD recurs during or after taper.

> **Chronic GVHD after failure of one or two lines of systemic therapy**

Adults and children age 12 and older: 10 mg PO b.i.d.

Adjust-a-dose: After 6 months of treatment in patients who have discontinued corticosteroids, taper drug by one dose level every 8 weeks (10 mg b.i.d. to 5 mg b.i.d. to 5 mg once daily). Consider retreatment if GVHD recurs during or after taper.

---

sarecycline
sar-e-SYE-kleen

Seysara

Therapeutic class: Antibiotics
Pharmacologic class: Tetracyclines

AVAILABLE FORMS
Tablets: 60 mg, 100 mg, 150 mg

INDICATIONS & DOSAGES
> **Inflammatory lesions of nonnodular moderate to severe acne vulgaris**

Adults and children age 9 and older weighing 85 to 136 kg: 150 mg PO once daily.

Adults and children age 9 and older weighing 55 to 84 kg: 100 mg PO once daily.

Adults and children age 9 and older weighing 33 to 54 kg: 60 mg PO once daily.

---

secnidazole
sek-NID-a-zole

Solosec

Therapeutic class: Antibiotics
Pharmacologic class: Nitroimidazoles

AVAILABLE FORMS
Oral granules: 2 g/packet

INDICATIONS & DOSAGES
> **Bacterial vaginosis**

Patients age 12 and older: One single dose of 2 g PO.

> **Trichomoniasis**

Adults and children age 12 and older: One single dose of 2 g PO. Treat sexual partners at same dose at same time.

---

secukinumab
sek-ue-KIN-ue-mab

Cosentyx

Therapeutic class: Immunomodulators
Pharmacologic class: Human IgG1 monoclonal antibodies

AVAILABLE FORMS
Injection: 75 mg/0.5 mL prefilled syringe, 150 mg/mL autoinjector or prefilled syringe
Injection (lyophilized powder): 150 mg in single-use vials

INDICATIONS & DOSAGES
> **Moderate to severe plaque psoriasis in patients who are candidates for systemic therapy or phototherapy; psoriatic arthritis in patients with coexistent moderate to severe plaque psoriasis**

Adults: 300 mg as two subcut injections of 150 mg each on weeks 0, 1, 2, 3, and 4; then 300 mg every 4 weeks thereafter. If clinically indicated, a 150-mg dose may be acceptable for some patients with plaque psoriasis.

> **Moderate to severe plaque psoriasis in patients who are candidates for systemic therapy or phototherapy**

Children age 6 and older weighing 50 kg or more: 150 mg subcut at weeks 0, 1, 2, 3, and 4; then 150 mg every 4 weeks thereafter.

Children age 6 and older weighing less than 50 kg: 75 mg subcut at weeks 0, 1, 2, 3, and 4; then 75 mg every 4 weeks thereafter.

> **Active psoriatic arthritis**

Adults: To use with a loading dose, give 150 mg subcut once weekly at weeks 0, 1, 2, 3, and 4; then 150 mg subcut every 4 weeks. To use without a loading dose, give 150 mg subcut every 4 weeks. May consider increasing dosage to 300 mg subcut every 4 weeks.

Children age 2 and older weighing 50 kg or more: 150 mg subcut at weeks 0, 1, 2, 3, and 4; then 150 mg every 4 weeks thereafter.

Children age 2 and older weighing 15 to less than 50 kg: 75 mg subcut at weeks 0, 1, 2, 3, and 4; then 75 mg every 4 weeks thereafter.

> **Active ankylosing spondylitis; active nonradiographic axial spondyloarthritis with objective signs of inflammation**

Adults: To use with a loading dose, give 150 mg subcut once weekly at weeks 0, 1, 2, 3, and 4; then 150 mg subcut every 4 weeks. To use without a loading dose, give 150 mg subcut every 4 weeks. For active psoriatic arthritis, may consider increasing dosage to 300 mg subcut every 4 weeks.

✳ *NEW INDICATION:* **Enthesitis-related arthritis**

Adults and children age 4 and older weighing 50 kg or more: 150 mg subcut at weeks 0, 1, 2, 3, and 4; then 150 mg every 4 weeks thereafter.

Adults and children age 4 and older weighing 15 to less than 50 kg: 75 mg subcut at weeks 0, 1, 2, 3, and 4; then 75 mg every 4 weeks thereafter.

---

selexipag
se-LEX-i-pag

Uptravi

Therapeutic class: Vasodilators
Pharmacologic class: Prostacyclin receptor agonists

AVAILABLE FORMS
Injection (lyophilized powder): 1,800-mg vial
Tablets (extended-release) ⓒⓇⓊ: 200 mcg, 400 mcg, 600 mcg, 800 mcg, 1,000 mcg, 1,200 mcg, 1,400 mcg, 1,600 mcg

INDICATIONS & DOSAGES
➤ **PAH (WHO Group I) to delay disease progression and reduce risk of hospitalization**
Adults: Initially, 200 mcg PO b.i.d. Increase dosage by increments of 200 mcg b.i.d. at weekly intervals to the highest tolerated dose. If dose isn't tolerated, decrease dosage to the previous tolerated dose. Maximum dose is 1,600 mcg b.i.d. If patient can't take oral form, may temporarily give by IV infusion at patient's current dose of tablets over 80 minutes b.i.d. Refer to manufacturer's instructions for IV dosing table.
Adjust-a-dose: For patients with moderate hepatic impairment (Child-Pugh class B), initiate therapy at 200 mcg once daily and increase by 200-mcg increments once daily at weekly intervals, as tolerated. Avoid use in patients with severe hepatic impairment (Child-Pugh class C). If administered with moderate CYP2C8 inhibitor, reduce dosing to once daily.

selinexor
sel-i-NEX-or

Xpovio

Therapeutic class: Antineoplastics
Pharmacologic class: Nuclear export inhibitors

AVAILABLE FORMS
Tablets: 20 mg, 40 mg, 50 mg, 60 mg

INDICATIONS & DOSAGES
Adjust-a-dose (for all indications): Follow manufacturer's instructions for toxicity-related dosage adjustments.
➤ **Relapsed or refractory multiple myeloma in combination with dexamethasone in patients who have received at least four prior therapies and whose disease is refractory to at least two proteasome inhibitors, at least two immunomodulatory agents, and an anti-CD38 monoclonal antibody**
Adults: 80 mg PO with dexamethasone 20 mg PO on days 1 and 3 of each week until disease progression or unacceptable toxicity.
➤ **Relapsed or refractory diffuse large B-cell lymphoma after at least two lines of systemic therapy**
Adults: 60 mg PO on days 1 and 3 of each week until disease progression or unacceptable toxicity occurs.
➤ **Multiple myeloma, in combination with bortezomib and dexamethasone, in patients who have received at least one prior therapy**
Adults: 100 mg once weekly in combination with bortezomib and dexamethasone. Refer to manufacturer's instructions for bortezomib and dexamethasone for additional dosing information.

selumetinib
sel-ue-ME-ti-nib

Koselugo

Therapeutic class: Antineoplastics
Pharmacologic class: Kinase inhibitors

AVAILABLE FORMS
Capsules ⓒⓇⓊ: 10 mg, 25 mg

INDICATIONS & DOSAGES
➤ **Neurofibromatosis type 1 with symptomatic, inoperable plexiform neurofibromas**
Children age 2 and older: 25 mg/m^2 PO b.i.d. until disease progression or unacceptable toxicity.
Adjust-a-dose: For patients with moderate hepatic impairment (Child-Pugh class B), reduce dose to 20 mg/m^2 b.i.d. If patient is taking selumetinib with strong or moderate CYP3A4 inhibitor or fluconazole, and current dose is 25 mg/m^2 b.i.d., reduce to 20 mg/m^2 b.i.d.; if current dose is 20 mg/m^2 b.i.d., reduce to 15 mg/m^2 b.i.d. After discontinuing strong or moderate CYP3A4 inhibitor or fluconazole, wait for three elimination half-lives; then resume selumetinib at dose taken before initiation of the inhibitor or fluconazole. Refer to manufacturer's instructions for toxicity-related dosage adjustments.

sertaconazole nitrate
sir-tah-KAHN-uh-zole

Ertaczo

Therapeutic class: Antifungals
Pharmacologic class: Imidazoles

AVAILABLE FORMS
Topical cream: 2%

INDICATIONS & DOSAGES
➤ **Interdigital tinea pedis caused by *Trichophyton rubrum*, *Trichophyton mentagrophytes*, or *Epidermophyton floccosum* in patients who are immunocompetent**
Adults and children age 12 and older: Apply cream b.i.d. to affected areas between toes and healthy surrounding areas for 4 weeks.

silver sulfadiazine
sul-fa-DYE-a-zeen

Flamazine ✤, Silvadene, SSD, Thermazene

Therapeutic class: Antibacterials (topical)
Pharmacologic class: Broad-spectrum sulfonamides

AVAILABLE FORMS
Cream: 1%

INDICATIONS & DOSAGES
➤ **To prevent or treat wound infection in second- and third-degree burns**
Adults: Apply one-sixteenth-inch thickness of cream to clean, debrided wound daily or b.i.d. Burn areas

should be covered with cream at all times. Reapply to areas from which it has been removed by patient activity.

siponimod 🧬
si-PON-i-mod

Mayzent

Therapeutic class: MS drugs
Pharmacologic class: Sphingosine
1-phosphate receptor modulators

AVAILABLE FORMS
Tablets ⊙: 0.25 mg, 1 mg, 2 mg

INDICATIONS & DOSAGES
➤ **Relapsing forms of MS with CYP2C9 genotype *1/*1, *1/*2, or *2/*2** 🧬
Adults: Start drug with a 5-day titration to help reduce cardiac effects. Initially, on days 1 and 2, give 0.25 mg PO once daily; on day 3, give 0.5 mg PO once daily; on day 4, give 0.75 mg PO once daily; on day 5, give 1.25 mg PO once daily; on day 6, begin maintenance dosage of 2 mg PO once daily.
➤ **Relapsing forms of MS with CYP2C9 genotype *1/*3 or *2/*3** 🧬
Adults: Start drug with a 4-day titration to help reduce cardiac effects. Initially, on days 1 and 2, give 0.25 mg PO once daily; on day 3, give 0.5 mg PO once daily; on day 4, give 0.75 mg PO once daily; on day 5, begin maintenance dosage of 1 mg PO once daily.

sodium bicarbonate
Therapeutic class: Antacids
Pharmacologic class: Alkalinizers

AVAILABLE FORMS
Injection: 4.2% (0.5 mEq/1 mL), 7.5% (0.9 mEq/1 mL), 8.4% (1 mEq/1 mL)
Powder: 2,616 mg/½ tsp ◇
Tablets: 325 mg ◇, 650 mg ◇

INDICATIONS & DOSAGES
➤ **Metabolic acidosis**
Adults and children: Dosage depends on blood carbon dioxide content, pH, and patient's condition; usually, 2 to 5 mEq/kg IV infused over 4- to 8-hour period. Base subsequent doses on patient's acid-base status.
➤ **Urinary alkalinization**
Adults: Initially, 4,000 mg PO; then 1,000 to 2,000 mg PO every 4 hours; dosage based on urine pH.
Children: 84 to 840 mg/kg PO daily in four divided doses. Titrate based on urine pH.
➤ **Antacid**
Adults younger than age 60: 650 to 2,600 mg PO up to every 4 hours with a glass of water. Maximum, 15,600 mg/day.
Adults age 60 and older: 650 to 1,300 mg PO up to every 4 hours with a glass of water. Maximum, 7,800 mg/day.
Adults and children older than age 12: ½ tsp (2,616 mg) oral powder in 120 mL water PO every 2 hours up to six doses daily for patients younger than age 60, or three doses daily for patients older than age 60.

➤ **Cardiac arrest**
Adults and children age 2 and older: Administer according to results of arterial blood pH, partial pressure of arterial carbon dioxide, and calculated base deficit. Initially, 44.6 to 100 mEq of bicarbonate IV. Then redetermine serum pH and bicarbonate concentration. May give 44.6 to 50 mEq every 5 to 10 minutes if necessary.
Children younger than age 2: 1 to 2 mEq/kg IV slowly followed by 1 mEq/kg every 10 minutes of arrest. Don't give more than 8 mEq/kg IV total; a 4.2% solution may be preferred.
➤ **Prevention of contrast media nephrotoxicity ◆**
Adults: 154 mEq/L in dextrose 5% infusion as an IV bolus of 3 mL/kg/hour for 1 hour immediately before contrast administration, followed by an infusion of 1 mL/kg/hour for 6 hours after the procedure.

SAFETY ALERT!

sonidegib phosphate
soe-ni-DEG-ib

Odomzo

Therapeutic class: Antineoplastics
Pharmacologic class: Hedgehog pathway inhibitors

AVAILABLE FORMS
Capsules: 200 mg

INDICATIONS & DOSAGES
Boxed Warning Drug can cause birth defects or embryo-fetal death if used during pregnancy. Females must use contraception during therapy and for 20 months after last dose. Males must use condoms and shouldn't donate sperm during therapy and for at least 8 months after last dose. ∎
➤ **Locally advanced basal cell carcinoma that has recurred after surgery or radiation therapy, or in patients who aren't candidates for surgery or radiation therapy**
Adults: 200 mg PO once daily at least 1 hour before or 2 hours after a meal. Administer until disease progression or unacceptable toxicity occurs.
Adjust-a-dose: Refer to manufacturer's instructions for toxicity-related dosage adjustments and discontinuation.

SAFETY ALERT!

SORAfenib tosylate
sohr-uh-FEN-ib

NexAVAR

Therapeutic class: Antineoplastics
Pharmacologic class: Multi-kinase inhibitors

AVAILABLE FORMS
Tablets: 200 mg

INDICATIONS & DOSAGES
➤ **Advanced renal cell carcinoma; unresectable hepatocellular carcinoma; locally advanced or metastatic, progressive, differentiated thyroid carcinoma refractory to radioactive iodine treatment**

🍁Canada   ◇OTC   ◆Off-label use   🖉Photoguide   ⊙Do not crush   *Liquid contains alcohol   🧬Genetic

Adults: 400 mg PO b.i.d. at least 1 hour before or 2 hours after eating. Continue until disease progresses or unacceptable toxicity occurs.

Adjust-a-dose: Refer to manufacturer's instructions for dosage adjustments for dermatologic and other toxicities.

spinosad
SPIN-oh-sad

Natroba

Therapeutic class: Scabicides–pediculicides
Pharmacologic class: Topical actinomycete bacterium derivatives

AVAILABLE FORMS
Topical solution: 0.9%*

INDICATIONS & DOSAGES
➤ **Head lice infestation**
Adults and children age 6 months and older: Apply only amount needed to adequately cover scalp and hair, up to 120 mL. Leave on for 10 minutes (start timing after scalp and hair have been completely covered); then thoroughly rinse off with warm water. If live lice are seen 7 days after first treatment, apply a second treatment.

➤ **Scabies infestation**
Adults and children age 4 and older: Apply to skin to completely cover body from neck to soles of feet. For patients with balding scalp, also apply to scalp, hairline, temples, and forehead. Allow skin to dry for 10 minutes before patient dresses. Leave on skin for 6 hours before patient showers or bathes.

stiripentol
stir-i-PEN-tol

Diacomit

Therapeutic class: Anticonvulsants
Pharmacologic class: Anticonvulsants

AVAILABLE FORMS
Capsules: 250 mg, 500 mg
Powder for oral suspension: 250 mg, 500 mg

INDICATIONS & DOSAGES
➤ **Seizures associated with Dravet syndrome in patients taking clobazam**
Adults: 50 mg/kg/day PO in two or three divided doses with a meal.
Children age 1 year and older weighing 10 kg or more: 25 mg/kg PO b.i.d. or 16.67 mg/kg PO t.i.d.
Children age 1 year and older weighing 7 to less than 10 kg: 25 mg/kg PO b.i.d.
Children ages 6 months to younger than 1 year weighing 7 kg or more: 25 mg/kg PO b.i.d.
Adjust-a-dose: If exact dosage can't be achieved with the available strengths, round to the nearest dosage, which is usually within 50 to 150 mg of the recommended 50 mg/kg/day. Maximum dose, 3,000 mg/day. If somnolence occurs, consider reducing clobazam dosage by 25%. If somnolence persists, consider decreasing clobazam dosage by an additional 25%.

Consider adjusting the dosage of other concomitant anticonvulsants with sedating properties.

tacrolimus 🗶
tack-ROW-lim-us

Advagraf♣, Astagraf XL, Envarsus XR, Prograf

Therapeutic class: Immunosuppressants
Pharmacologic class: Calcineurin inhibitors

AVAILABLE FORMS
Capsules ⓘ: 0.5 mg, 1 mg, 5 mg
Capsules (extended-release) ⓘ: 0.5 mg, 1 mg, 3 mg♣, 5 mg
Granules for oral suspension: 0.2 mg, 1 mg unit-dose packets
Injection: 5 mg/mL*
Tablets (extended-release) ⓘ: 0.75 mg, 1 mg, 4 mg

INDICATIONS & DOSAGES
Boxed Warning Drug increases risk of serious infections and malignancies. Increased mortality reported in women with transplants using Astagraf XL. Astagraf XL isn't approved for use in transplantation. ∎

🗶 *Adjust-a-dose (for all indications):* Give lowest recommended oral and IV dosages to older adults and patients with renal or hepatic impairment. Patients who are Black with renal transplants may need higher dosages than patients who are White to attain comparable trough concentrations.

⚠ *Alert:* Individualizing dosing regimen is necessary for optimal therapy. Frequently monitor trough concentrations in the early transplant period to ensure adequate drug exposure. Extended-release capsules aren't interchangeable or substitutable with other tacrolimus extended-release or immediate-release products.

➤ **To prevent organ rejection in allogenic liver, kidney, heart, or lung transplant (with other immunosuppressants)**
Adults: For patients who can't take drug PO, 0.03 to 0.05 mg/kg/day (liver or kidney), 0.01 mg/kg/day (heart), or 0.01 to 0.03 mg/kg/day (lung) IV as continuous infusion at least 6 hours after liver, heart, or lung transplant or within 24 hours of kidney transplant if renal function has recovered. Switch to oral therapy as soon as possible, with first dose 8 to 12 hours after stopping IV infusion. For renal transplant, give oral dose within 24 hours of transplantation after renal function has recovered. Initial immediate-release oral dosages: For liver transplant, 0.1 to 0.15 mg/kg PO daily in two divided doses every 12 hours; for kidney transplant, 0.2 mg/kg PO daily (in combination with azathioprine) or 0.1 mg/kg PO daily (in combination with mycophenolate mofetil [MMF] and interleukin-2 receptor agonist) in two divided doses every 12 hours; for heart or lung transplant, 0.075 mg/kg PO daily in two divided doses every 12 hours (in combination with azathioprine or MMF). Adjust dosages based on patient response. Adjunct therapy with adrenal corticosteroids is recommended early posttransplant.

♣Canada   ◇ OTC   ◆ Off-label use   ⏥Photoguide   ⓘ Do not crush   *Liquid contains alcohol   🗶 Genetic

For Astagraf XL extended-release (ER) form (renal transplant only): When using with basiliximab induction, MMF, and corticosteroids, administer initial dose of 0.15 to 0.2 mg/kg PO once daily before or within 48 hours of completion of transplant procedure, but may delay until renal function has recovered. When using in combination with corticosteroids and MMF without basiliximab induction, give 0.1 mg/kg PO once daily (preoperative within 12 hours before reperfusion); 0.2 mg/kg PO once daily (postoperative at least 4 hours after preoperative dose and within 12 hours of reperfusion).

To convert from immediate-release form to Astagraf XL, initiate ER treatment in a 1:1 ratio (mg:mg) using previously established total daily dose of immediate-release form. Give once daily. To convert from immediate-release form to Envarsus XR, initiate ER treatment with a once-daily dose that's 80% of the total daily dose of the immediate-release product.
Children (liver transplant only): 0.03 to 0.05 mg/kg IV daily as continuous infusion.
Children (liver, kidney, or heart transplant): For kidney transplant, 0.3 mg/kg/day immediate-release capsules or oral suspension, divided in two doses, administered every 12 hours or, within 24 hours of reperfusion, give 0.3 mg/kg Astagraf XL PO once daily in combination with basiliximab induction, MMF, and corticosteroids; for liver transplant, 0.15 to 0.2 mg/kg/day immediate-release capsules or 0.2 mg/kg/day oral suspension, divided in two doses, administered every 12 hours; for heart or lung transplant, 0.3 mg/kg/day immediate-release capsules or oral suspension or 0.1 mg/kg/day if cell-depleting induction treatment is administered, divided in two doses, administered every 12 hours. Children in general need higher tacrolimus doses compared to adults: The higher dose requirements may decrease as the child grows older. Patients with cystic fibrosis may require higher doses.
➤ **To prevent organ rejection in patients with de novo kidney transplant, in combination with other immunosuppressants (Envarsus XR)**
Adults: Initially, 0.14 mg/kg/day PO. Titrate dosage based on clinical assessments of rejection and tolerability and to achieve tacrolimus whole blood trough concentration range of 6 to 11 ng/mL during the first month, then 4 to 11 ng/mL during all subsequent months.

tafamidis ▧
ta-FAM-id-is

Vyndamax

tafamidis meglumine
Vyndaqel

Therapeutic class: Endocrine-metabolic agents
Pharmacologic class: Transthyretin stabilizers

AVAILABLE FORMS
tafamidis
Capsules: 61 mg

tafamidis meglumine
Capsules: 20 mg

INDICATIONS & DOSAGES
➤ **Cardiomyopathy of wild-type or hereditary transthyretin-mediated amyloidosis to reduce CV mortality and CV-related hospitalization** ▧
Adults: 80 mg tafamidis meglumine (four 20-mg capsules) PO once daily, or 61 mg tafamidis PO once daily.

tafenoquine succinate ▧
ta-FEN-Oh-kwin

Arakoda, Krintafel

Therapeutic class: Antimalarials
Pharmacologic class: Aminoquinolines

AVAILABLE FORMS
Tablets (OTC): 100 mg, 150 mg

INDICATIONS & DOSAGES
➤ **Prevention of relapse of *Plasmodium vivax* malaria in patients who have tested negative for G6PD deficiency and who are receiving chloroquine therapy for acute *P. vivax* infection (Krintafel)** ▧
Adults and children age 16 and older: Single dose of 300 mg PO given as two 150-mg tablets taken together. Coadminister on first or second day of chloroquine therapy for acute *P. vivax* malaria.
➤ **Malaria prophylaxis in patients who have tested negative for G6PD deficiency (Arakoda)** ▧
Adults: 200 mg PO once daily for 3 days before travel to a malarious area; then while patient is in malarious area, 200 mg once weekly beginning 7 days after the last dose of the loading regimen. After patient leaves the malarious area, 200 mg PO as a single dose 7 days after the last dose of maintenance regimen.

SAFETY ALERT!

tagraxofusp-erzs
tag-RAX-oh-fusp

Elzonris

Therapeutic class: Antineoplastics
Pharmacologic class: Anti-CD123 agents

AVAILABLE FORMS
Injection: 1,000 mcg/1 mL single-dose vial

INDICATIONS & DOSAGES
Boxed Warning Drug can cause capillary leak syndrome, which can be life-threatening or fatal. ■
➤ **Blastic plasmacytoid dendritic cell neoplasm**
Adults and children age 2 and older: 12 mcg/kg IV infusion once daily on days 1 to 5 of a 21-day cycle. May extend dosing period for dose delays up to day 10. Premedicate with an H_1-antagonist, an H_2-antagonist, a corticosteroid, and acetaminophen before each transfusion. Continue treatment until disease progression or unacceptable toxicity occurs.
Adjust-a-dose: Refer to manufacturer's instructions for toxicity-related dosage adjustments.

SAFETY ALERT!

tapentadol hydrochloride
tah-PEN-tah-dol

Nucynta✐, Nucynta ER✐, Nucynta IR✥

Therapeutic class: Opioid analgesics
Pharmacologic class: Centrally acting synthetic opioid analgesics
Controlled substance schedule: II

AVAILABLE FORMS
Tablets: 50 mg, 75 mg, 100 mg
Tablets (extended-release) ⓒ: 50 mg, 100 mg, 150 mg, 200 mg, 250 mg

INDICATIONS & DOSAGES
Boxed Warning Opioid use increases risk of addiction, abuse, and misuse. Opioids can cause fatal respiratory depression. Opioids can cause respiratory depression and death in children with ingestion of even one dose. Opioids combined with benzodiazepines or CNS depressants, including alcohol, can cause death. Use during pregnancy can cause neonatal opioid withdrawal. ∎

Adjust-a-dose (for all indications): Use lowest effective dosage for shortest duration consistent with individual patient treatment goals. Don't stop drug abruptly; withdraw slowly and individualize gradual taper plan to prevent signs and symptoms of withdrawal.

➤ **Acute pain severe enough to require an opioid analgesic and for which alternative treatments are inadequate (immediate-release only)**
Adults: 50 to 100 mg PO every 4 to 6 hours, as needed, for pain. On day 1, may give second dose in 1 hour if first dose is ineffective. Adjust subsequent dosing to maintain adequate pain control. Maximum daily dose, 700 mg on day 1; 600 mg on subsequent days.
Adjust-a-dose: For patients with moderate hepatic impairment (Child-Pugh class B), initially give 50 mg PO every 8 hours. Maximum, three doses (150 mg) in 24 hours; the interval between doses should be no less than 8 hours.

➤ **Severe chronic pain when continuous, around-the-clock opioid analgesia is needed for an extended period (extended-release); neuropathic pain associated with diabetic peripheral neuropathy (extended-release)**
Adults: Initially, 50 mg PO b.i.d. (approximately every 12 hours). Titrate with dosage increases of 50 mg no more than b.i.d. every 3 days. Therapeutic range is 100 to 250 mg PO b.i.d. Maximum daily dose is 500 mg.
Adjust-a-dose: For patients with moderate hepatic impairment (Child-Pugh class B), initially 50 mg (extended-release) PO once every 24 hours. Maximum dose is 100 mg (extended-release) once daily. Monitor patient closely for respiratory and CNS depression, particularly during initiation and titration.

tavaborole
tah-vah-BOR-ole

Kerydin

Therapeutic class: Antifungals
Pharmacologic class: Antifungals

AVAILABLE FORMS
Topical solution: 5%

INDICATIONS & DOSAGES
➤ **Onychomycosis of toenails due to *Trichophyton rubrum* or *Trichophyton mentagrophytes***
Adults: Apply once daily for 48 weeks to entire surface of affected toenail and under the tip of affected toenail.

tecovirimat
tek-oh-VIR-i-mat

Tpoxx

Therapeutic class: Antivirals
Pharmacologic class: Antivirals

AVAILABLE FORMS
Capsules: 200 mg
Injection: 200 mg/20 mL

INDICATIONS & DOSAGES
Adjust-a-dose (for all indications): Don't use with CrCl less than 30 mL/minute.
➤ **Human smallpox disease caused by variola virus**
PO
Adults and children weighing 120 kg or more: 600 mg PO every 8 hours for 14 days.
Adults and children weighing 40 to less than 120 kg: 600 mg PO every 12 hours for 14 days.
Adults and children weighing 25 to less than 40 kg: 400 mg PO every 12 hours for 14 days.
Adults and children weighing 13 to less than 25 kg: 200 mg PO every 12 hours for 14 days.
IV
Adults and children weighing 120 kg or more: 300 mg IV infusion over 6 hours every 12 hours for up to 14 days.
Adults and children weighing 35 to less than 120 kg: 200 mg IV infusion over 6 hours every 12 hours for up to 14 days.
Adults and children weighing 3 to less than 35 kg: 6 mg/kg IV infusion over 6 hours every 12 hours for up to 14 days.

tedizolid phosphate
ted-eye-ZOE-lid

Sivextro

Therapeutic class: Antibiotics
Pharmacologic class: Oxazolidinones

AVAILABLE FORMS
Injection: 200 mg/vial
Tablets: 200 mg

INDICATIONS & DOSAGES

➤ Acute bacterial skin and skin-structure infections caused by susceptible gram-positive isolates (*Staphylococcus aureus* [including MRSA and methicillin-susceptible strains], *Streptococcus pyogenes*, *Streptococcus agalactiae*, *Streptococcus anginosus* group [including *S. anginosus*, *Streptococcus intermedius*, and *Streptococcus constellatus*], and *Enterococcus faecalis*)
Adults and children age 12 and older: 200 mg PO or IV once daily for 6 days.

tegaserod maleate
teg-a-SER-od

Zelnorm

Therapeutic class: Anti-IBS drugs
Pharmacologic class: Serotonin-4 (5-HT$_4$) receptor agonists

AVAILABLE FORMS
Tablets: 6 mg

INDICATIONS & DOSAGES
➤ IBS with constipation
Women younger than age 65: 6 mg PO b.i.d. 30 minutes before meals. Discontinue in patients with inadequate response after 4 to 6 weeks of treatment.

SAFETY ALERT!

temozolomide
teh-moh-ZOH-loh-mide

Temodal ✦, Temodar

Therapeutic class: Antineoplastics
Pharmacologic class: Alkylating drugs

AVAILABLE FORMS
Capsules ⓓⓃⓒ: 5 mg, 20 mg, 100 mg, 140 mg, 180 mg, 250 mg
Injection: 100 mg/vial

INDICATIONS & DOSAGES
Adjust-a-dose (for all indications): Refer to manufacturer's instructions for toxicity-related dosage adjustments.
➤ Newly diagnosed glioblastoma in combination with radiation therapy
Adults: Initially, 75 mg/m^2 IV infusion or PO once daily for 42 days (up to 49 days if no toxicity). Maintenance dose is 150 mg/m^2 IV infusion or PO once daily on days 1 to 5 of a 28-day cycle for six cycles; may increase dose to 200 mg/m^2 for cycles two to six if CTCAE is grade 2 or less, ANC is 1.5×10^9/L or more, and platelet count is 100×10^9/L or more. If dose was increased in cycle two, maintain dose at 200 mg/m^2 for days 1 to 5 of subsequent cycles, unless toxicity occurs. If dose wasn't increased in cycle two, don't increase in subsequent cycles.
➤ Refractory anaplastic astrocytoma
Adults: Initially, 150 mg/m^2 IV infusion or PO once daily for 5 days of a 28-day treatment cycle. May increase dose to 200 mg/m^2 for 5 days of a 28-day

treatment cycle, if nadir and day 1 of next cycle ANC is 1.5×10^9/L or more and platelet count is 100×10^9/L or more. Continue until disease progression or unacceptable toxicity.

SAFETY ALERT!

temsirolimus
tem-sir-OH-li-mus

Torisel

Therapeutic class: Antineoplastics
Pharmacologic class: Kinase inhibitors

AVAILABLE FORMS
IV solution: 25 mg/mL

INDICATIONS & DOSAGES
➤ Advanced renal cell carcinoma
Adults: 25 mg IV over 30 to 60 minutes once weekly until disease progresses or unacceptable toxicity occurs. Give diphenhydramine 25 to 50 mg IV 30 minutes before each dose.
Adjust-a-dose: Reduce dosage to 15 mg once weekly in patients with bilirubin level more than 1 to $1.5 \times$ ULN or AST level more than ULN with normal bilirubin level. Refer to manufacturer's instructions for toxicity-related dosage adjustments.
  If use with a strong CYP3A4 inhibitor is necessary, consider a dosage reduction to 12.5 mg once weekly. If use with a strong CYP3A4 inducer is necessary, increase dosage to 50 mg once weekly.

tenapanor hydrochloride
ten-A-pa-nor

Ibsrela

Therapeutic class: Miscellaneous GI drugs
Pharmacologic class: Sodium/hydrogen exchanger 3 inhibitors

AVAILABLE FORMS
Tablets: 50 mg

INDICATIONS & DOSAGES
Boxed Warning Due to risk of dehydration, drug is contraindicated in children younger than age 6. Avoid use in children ages 6 to younger than 12. Safety and effectiveness in patients younger than age 18 haven't been established. ∎
➤ IBS with constipation
Adults: 50 mg PO b.i.d.

SAFETY ALERT!

tepotinib ✗
tep-OH-ti-nib

Tepmetko

Therapeutic class: Antineoplastics
Pharmacologic class: Kinase inhibitors

AVAILABLE FORMS
Tablets ⓓⓃⓒ: 225 mg

INDICATIONS & DOSAGES
➤ **Metastatic NSCLC harboring mesenchymal-epithelial transition (*MET*) exon 14 skipping alterations** ▨
Adults: 450 mg PO daily until disease progression or unacceptable toxicity occurs.
Adjust-a-dose: Refer to manufacturer's instructions for toxicity-related dosage adjustments. Permanently discontinue drug if patient can't tolerate 225 mg PO once daily.

terbutaline sulfate
ter-BYOO-ta-leen

Therapeutic class: Bronchodilators
Pharmacologic class: Beta$_2$ agonists

AVAILABLE FORMS
Injection: 1 mg/mL
Tablets: 2.5 mg, 5 mg

INDICATIONS & DOSAGES
Boxed Warning Drug hasn't been approved and shouldn't be used for tocolysis. Serious adverse reactions may occur.■
➤ **Prevention and reversal of bronchospasm in patients with asthma and reversible bronchospasm associated with bronchitis and emphysema**
Adults and children age 12 and older: 0.25 mg subcut. If needed, repeat in 15 to 30 minutes. Maximum, 0.5 mg in 4 hours. If patient fails to respond to second dose, consider other measures.
Adults and adolescents older than age 15: 2.5 to 5 mg PO t.i.d. every 6 hours while awake. Maximum, 15 mg daily.
Children ages 12 to 15: 2.5 mg PO t.i.d. every 6 hours while awake. Maximum, 7.5 mg daily.

SAFETY ALERT!

teriflunomide
ter-i-FLOO-noe-mide

Aubagio

Therapeutic class: Immunomodulators
Pharmacologic class: Pyrimidine synthesis inhibitors

AVAILABLE FORMS
Tablets: 7 mg, 14 mg

INDICATIONS & DOSAGES
Boxed Warning Severe and fatal liver injury can occur. May cause major birth defects. Contraindicated during pregnancy. ■
➤ **Relapsing forms of MS**
Adults: 7 or 14 mg PO once daily.

tezacaftor–ivacaftor and ivacaftor ▨
tez-a-KAF-tor/eye-va-KAF-tor

Symdeko

Therapeutic class: Metabolic agents
Pharmacologic class: Cystic fibrosis transmembrane conductance regulator (CFTR) facilitators (tezacaftor); CFTR potentiators (ivacaftor)

AVAILABLE FORMS
Tablets: 50 mg tezacaftor/75 mg ivacaftor fixed-dose combination tablets copackaged with ivacaftor 75-mg tablets;100 mg tezacaftor/150 mg ivacaftor fixed-dose combination tablets copackaged with ivacaftor 150-mg tablets

INDICATIONS & DOSAGES
➤ **Cystic fibrosis in patients homozygous for the F508del mutation or who have at least one mutation in the *CFTR* gene that's responsive to tezacaftor–ivacaftor based on in vitro data or clinical evidence** ▨
Adults, children age 12 and older, and children age 6 to younger than 12 weighing 30 kg or more: 100 mg tezacaftor/150 mg ivacaftor (1 combination tablet) PO in the morning and 150 mg ivacaftor (1 tablet) PO in the evening, approximately 12 hours apart.
Children age 6 to younger than 12 weighing less than 30 kg: 50 mg tezacaftor/75 mg ivacaftor (1 combination tablet) PO in the morning and 75 mg ivacaftor (1 tablet) PO in the evening, approximately 12 hours apart.
Adjust-a-dose: For patients with moderate or severe hepatic impairment (Child-Pugh class B or C), omit the ivacaftor evening dose. For patients with Child-Pugh class C hepatic failure, consider giving the morning ivacaftor dose less frequently. For patients also taking CYP3A inhibitors, refer to manufacturer's instructions for dosage adjustments.

theophylline
thee-OFF-i-lin

Elixophyllin*, Theo ER♣, Theo-24

Therapeutic class: Bronchodilators
Pharmacologic class: Xanthine derivatives

AVAILABLE FORMS
Capsules (extended-release) ⓓ*:* 100 mg, 200 mg, 300 mg, 400 mg
Infusion: 400 mg/500 mL
Syrup: 80 mg/15 mL*
Tablets (extended-release) ⓓ*:* 100 mg, 200 mg, 300 mg, 400 mg, 450 mg, 600 mg

INDICATIONS & DOSAGES
🕚 *Alert:* Don't use extended-release preparations to treat acute bronchospasm.
➤ **Parenteral theophylline (preferred route) for acute bronchospasm in patients not currently receiving theophylline**

Loading dose: 4.6 mg/kg ideal body weight IV over 30 minutes; then maintenance infusion.
Nonsmoking adults younger than age 60 and children older than age 16: 0.4 mg/kg/hour IV (maximum 900 mg daily).
Nonsmoking children ages 12 to 16: 0.5 mg/kg/hour IV (maximum 900 mg daily).
Children ages 12 to 16 who smoke and children ages 9 to 12: 0.7 mg/kg/hour IV.
Children 1 to 9: 0.8 mg/kg/hour IV.
Infants ages 6 weeks to 1 year: Calculate mg/kg/hour IV dosage as follows: 0.008 × (age in weeks) + 0.21.
Neonates older than 24 days: 1.5 mg/kg IV every 12 hours to achieve target theophylline concentration of 7.5 mcg/mL.
Neonates 24 days old and younger: 1 mg/kg IV every 12 hours to achieve a target theophylline concentration of 7.5 mcg/mL.
Adjust-a-dose: For adults older than age 60, give 0.3 mg/kg/hour IV, up to a maximum of 17 mg/hour. For adults with HF, cor pulmonale, liver disease, sepsis with multiorgan failure, or shock, give 0.2 mg/kg/hour IV, up to a maximum infusion rate of 17 mg/hour unless serum theophylline concentrations are monitored at 24-hour intervals. Maximum daily dose is 400 mg.
➤ **Oral theophylline for acute bronchospasm in patients not currently receiving theophylline**
Adults age 60 and younger, children ages 16 and older, and children ages 1 to 15 weighing 45 kg or more: 5 mg/kg PO, then 300 mg (immediate-release syrup) PO daily in divided doses every 6 to 8 hours for 3 days. If tolerated, increase to 400 mg PO daily in divided doses every 6 to 8 hours. If necessary, dosage may be increased after 3 days to 600 mg PO daily in divided doses every 6 to 8 hours.
Children ages 1 to 15 weighing less than 45 kg: 5 mg/kg PO, then 12 to 14 mg/kg immediate-release (maximum 300 mg) PO daily in divided doses every 4 to 6 hours for 3 days. If tolerated, increase to 16 mg/kg (maximum 400 mg) PO daily in divided doses every 4 to 6 hours. After 3 days, if necessary, increase to 20 mg/kg (maximum 600 mg) PO daily in divided doses every 4 to 6 hours.
Adjust-a-dose: For children ages 1 to 15 with risk factors for reduced theophylline clearance or for whom serum concentrations can't be monitored, give 5 mg/kg PO, then 12 to 14 mg/kg (maximum 300 mg) PO daily in divided doses every 4 to 6 hours for 3 days. If tolerated, increase to 16 mg/kg (maximum 400 mg) PO daily in divided doses every 4 to 6 hours. For children age 16 and older and adults with risk factors for reduced theophylline clearance or for whom serum concentrations can't be monitored, give 5 mg/kg PO, then 300 mg PO daily in divided doses every 6 to 8 hours for 3 days. If tolerated, increase to 400 mg PO daily in divided doses every 6 to 8 hours.
➤ **Chronic bronchospasm using extended-release preparations**
Adults age 60 or younger, children age 16 and older, and children ages 6 to 15 weighing more than 45 kg: 300 mg PO daily in divided doses every 8 to 12 hours or 300 to 400 mg (24-hour extended-release capsule)

PO daily for 3 days. If tolerated, increase to 400 mg PO in divided doses every 8 to 12 hours or 400 to 600 mg (24-hour extended-release capsule) PO daily. After 3 more days, if necessary, increase dose to 600 mg PO daily in divided doses every 8 to 12 hours. Titrate dosages greater than 600 mg according to serum blood levels.
Children ages 6 to 15 weighing less than 45 kg: 12 to 14 mg/kg (maximum 300 mg extended-release tablet) daily in divided doses every 8 to 12 hours for 3 days. If tolerated, increase to 16 mg/kg (maximum 400 mg extended-release tablet) daily in divided doses every 8 to 12 hours. After 3 more days, if necessary, increase to 20 mg/kg (maximum 600 mg extended-release tablet) daily in divided doses every 8 to 12 hours.
Adjust-a-dose: For children ages 6 to 15 with risk factors for reduced theophylline clearance or for whom serum concentrations can't be monitored, give 12 to 14 mg/kg (maximum 300 mg) daily in divided doses for 3 days. If tolerated, increase to a maximum of 16 mg/kg (maximum 400 mg) PO daily in divided doses every 8 to 12 hours. For children age 16 and older and adults age 60 or younger or for whom serum concentrations can't be monitored, give 300 mg PO daily in divided doses every 8 to 12 hours. After 3 days, if necessary, increase to maximum of 400 mg PO daily in divided doses every 8 to 12 hours. For adults older than age 60, the recommended maximum daily dose is 400 mg PO per day in divided doses every 8 to 12 hours unless symptoms continue and peak serum concentration is less than 10 mcg/mL. Administer dosages greater than 400 mg PO daily cautiously. See manufacturer's instructions for dosage adjustment guided by theophylline concentration.

thioridazine hydrochloride
thye-oh-RYE-da-zeen

Therapeutic class: Antipsychotics
Pharmacologic class: Phenothiazines

AVAILABLE FORMS
Tablets: 10 mg, 25 mg, 50 mg, 100 mg

INDICATIONS & DOSAGES
Boxed Warning May prolong QTc interval. Risk of life-threatening ventricular arrhythmias. Older adults with dementia-related psychosis treated with antipsychotics are at increased risk of death. Drug isn't approved to treat patients with dementia-related psychosis. ∎
➤ **Schizophrenia in patients who don't respond to treatment with at least two other antipsychotics**
Adults: Initially, 50 to 100 mg PO t.i.d.; increase gradually to 800 mg daily in divided doses, as needed. Daily maintenance doses range from 200 to 800 mg divided into two to four doses.
Children: Initially, 0.5 mg/kg PO daily in two to four divided doses. Increase gradually to optimal therapeutic effect; maximum dose is 3 mg/kg daily.

♣Canada   ◇OTC   ◆Off-label use   ✐Photoguide   ⊜Do not crush   *Liquid contains alcohol   ▓Genetic

tigecycline
tye-gah-SYE-klin

Tygacil

Therapeutic class: Antibiotics
Pharmacologic class: Glycylcycline
antibacterials

AVAILABLE FORMS
Lyophilized powder: 50-mg vial

INDICATIONS & DOSAGES
Boxed Warning Compared to other drugs used to
treat serious infections, tigecycline has an increased
mortality risk. Use only in situations in which alternative treatments aren't suitable. ■
Adjust-a-dose (for all indications): For adults
with severe hepatic impairment (Child-Pugh class C),
give initial dose of 100 mg IV; then 25 mg IV every
12 hours.
➤ **Community-acquired bacterial pneumonia**
Adults: Initially, 100 mg IV; then 50 mg IV every
12 hours for 7 to 14 days. Infuse drug over 30 to
60 minutes.
Children ages 12 to 17: 50 mg IV every 12 hours for
7 to 14 days.
Children ages 8 to 11: 1.2 mg/kg IV every 12 hours
for 7 to 14 days. Maximum dose, 50 mg every
12 hours.
➤ **Complicated skin or skin-structure infection;
complicated intra-abdominal infection**
Adults: Initially 100 mg IV; then 50 mg every
12 hours for 5 to 14 days. Infuse drug over 30 to
60 minutes.
Children ages 12 to 17: 50 mg IV every 12 hours for
5 to 14 days.
Children ages 8 to 11: 1.2 mg/kg IV every 12 hours
for 5 to 14 days. Maximum dose, 50 mg every
12 hours.

tildrakizumab-asmn
til-dra-KIZ-ue-mab

Ilumya

Therapeutic class: Antipsoriatics
Pharmacologic class: Interleukin-23
antagonists

AVAILABLE FORMS
Injection: 100 mg/mL single-dose prefilled syringes

INDICATIONS & DOSAGES
➤ **Moderate to severe plaque psoriasis in patients
who are candidates for systemic therapy or phototherapy**
Adults: 100 mg subcut at weeks 0, 4, and every
12 weeks thereafter.

tinidazole
teh-NID-ah-zol

Therapeutic class: Antiprotozoals
Pharmacologic class: Antiprotozoals

AVAILABLE FORMS
Tablets: 250 mg, 500 mg

INDICATIONS & DOSAGES
Boxed Warning Use tinidazole only for the conditions for which it's indicated. Avoid long-term use. ■
Adjust-a-dose (for all indications): For patients
receiving hemodialysis, give an additional dose equal
to half the recommended dose after the hemodialysis
session.
➤ **Bacterial vaginosis in patients who aren't preg-
nant**
Adults: 2 g PO once daily for 2 days, or 1 g PO once
daily for 5 days.
➤ **Trichomoniasis caused by *Trichomonas vag-
inalis***
Adults: 2 g PO as a single dose. Sexual partners
should be treated at the same time with the same dose.
➤ **Giardiasis caused by *Giardia lamblia (Giardia
duodenalis)***
Adults: 2 g PO as a single dose.
Children age 3 and older: Give 50 mg/kg (up to 2 g)
PO as a single dose.
➤ **Intestinal amebiasis caused by *Entamoeba his-
tolytica***
Adults: 2 g PO daily for 3 days.
Children age 3 and older: Give 50 mg/kg (up to 2 g)
PO daily for 3 days.
➤ **Amebic liver abscess (amebiasis)**
Adults: 2 g PO daily for 3 to 5 days.
Children age 3 and older: Give 50 mg/kg (up to 2 g)
PO daily for 3 to 5 days.

SAFETY ALERT!

tirofiban hydrochloride
tye-row-FYE-ban

Aggrastat

Therapeutic class: Antiplatelet drugs
Pharmacologic class: Glycoprotein IIb/IIIa
receptor antagonists

AVAILABLE FORMS
Injection (premixed bag): 50 mcg/mL in 100 mL,
250 mL
Injection (vials): 50 mcg/mL in 100 mL, 250 mcg/mL
in 15 mL (bolus)

INDICATIONS & DOSAGES
➤ **In patients with non-ST elevation ACS to
reduce rate of thrombotic CV events (combined
endpoint of death, MI, or refractory ischemia or
repeat cardiac procedure)**
Adults: IV loading dose of 25 mcg/kg administered
within 5 minutes, followed by 0.15 mcg/kg/minute for
up to 18 hours.
Adjust-a-dose: If CrCl is 60 mL/minute or less, use
an IV loading dose of 25 mcg/kg administered within
5 minutes, followed by 0.075 mcg/kg/minute for up
to 18 hours.

tisagenlecleucel
tiss-a-GEN-lek-LOO-sel

Kymriah

Therapeutic class: Antineoplastics
Pharmacologic class: CD19-directed
genetically modified autologous T-cell
immunotherapies

AVAILABLE FORMS
IV infusion: Patient-specific; single-dose 10- to 50-mL infusion bag containing chimeric antigen receptor (CAR)–positive viable T cells

INDICATIONS & DOSAGES
Boxed Warning Don't give drug to patients with active infection or inflammatory disorders. Fatal or life-threatening cytokine release syndrome (CRS) and neurologic toxicities have occurred. Only available through a restricted program called Kymriah REMS. ■

Adjust-a-dose (for all indications): Refer to manufacturer's instructions for specific lymphodepleting chemotherapy and for management of severe toxicities, including CRS.

➤ **B-cell precursor acute lymphoblastic leukemia that's refractory or in second or later relapse**
Patients younger than age 25 weighing more than 50 kg: 0.1 to 2.5×10^8 total CAR-positive viable T cells IV infusion 2 to 14 days after completion of lymphodepleting chemotherapy. Don't determine dose based on body weight.
Patients younger than age 25 weighing 50 kg or less: 0.2 to 5.0×10^6 CAR-positive viable T cells/kg body weight IV infusion 2 to 14 days after completion of lymphodepleting chemotherapy.

➤ **Relapsed or refractory large B-cell lymphoma after two or more lines of systemic therapy, including diffuse large B-cell lymphoma (DLBCL) not otherwise specified, high-grade B-cell lymphoma, and DLBCL arising from follicular lymphoma**
Adults: 0.6 to 6.0×10^8 CAR-positive viable T cells IV infusion 2 to 11 days after completion of lymphodepleting chemotherapy. May omit lymphodepleting chemotherapy if patient's WBC count is 1×10^9/L or less within 1 week before tisagenlecleucel infusion.

✷ *NEW INDICATION:* **Relapsed or refractory follicular lymphoma after two or more lines of systemic therapy**
Adults: 0.6 to 6.0×10^8 CAR-positive viable T cells IV infusion 2 to 6 days after completion of lymphodepleting chemotherapy.
Adjust-a-dose: May omit lymphodepleting chemotherapy if patient's WBC count is less than 1×10^9/L within 1 week before tisagenlecleucel infusion.

tivozanib
tye-VOE-za-nib

Fotivda

Therapeutic class: Antineoplastics
Pharmacologic class: Kinase inhibitors

AVAILABLE FORMS
Capsules ⓞⓝⓒ: 0.89 mg, 1.34 mg

INDICATIONS & DOSAGES
➤ **Relapsed or refractory advanced renal cell carcinoma after two or more prior systemic therapies**
Adults: 1.34 mg PO once daily for 21 days followed by 7 days off for a 28-day cycle. Continue until disease progression or unacceptable toxicity occurs.
Adjust-a-dose: In patients with moderate hepatic impairment (total bilirubin level greater than 1.5 to $3 \times$ ULN with any AST level), decrease dose to 0.89 mg. Refer to manufacturer's instructions for toxicity-related dosage adjustments.

tolcapone
TOLE-ka-pone

Tasmar

Therapeutic class: Antiparkinsonian drugs
Pharmacologic class: Catechol-O-methyltransferase inhibitors

AVAILABLE FORMS
Tablets: 100 mg

INDICATIONS & DOSAGES
Boxed Warning Risk of liver injury. Stop drug if patient shows no benefit within 3 weeks. ■

➤ **Adjunct to levodopa–carbidopa for signs and symptoms of idiopathic Parkinson disease in patients who have symptom fluctuation or haven't responded to other adjunctive treatment**
Adults: Initially, 100 mg PO t.i.d. with levodopa–carbidopa. May increase dosage to 200 mg PO t.i.d. if clinical benefit is justified, as this dosage is associated with increased frequency of ALT elevation. Levodopa dosage may need to be reduced by about 30% to minimize risk of dyskinesias, especially when levodopa dose is over 600 mg daily.

toremifene citrate
tore-EM-ah-feen

Fareston

Therapeutic class: Antineoplastics
Pharmacologic class: Nonsteroidal antiestrogens

AVAILABLE FORMS
Tablets: 60 mg

INDICATIONS & DOSAGES
Boxed Warning May prolong QTc interval and risk of fatal ventricular arrhythmias. ■

➤ **Metastatic breast cancer in patients who are postmenopausal with estrogen receptor–positive or estrogen receptor–unknown tumors**
Adults: 60 mg PO once daily. Continue until disease progresses.

trandolapril ▓
tran-DOE-la-pril

Therapeutic class: Antihypertensives
Pharmacologic class: ACE inhibitors

AVAILABLE FORMS
Tablets: 1 mg, 2 mg, 4 mg

INDICATIONS & DOSAGES
Boxed Warning   Drugs that act directly on the re-nin-angiotensin system can cause fetal harm; when pregnancy is detected, discontinue drug as soon as possible. ∎
Adjust-a-dose (for all indications): If CrCl is below 30 mL/minute or patient has hepatic cirrhosis, first dose is 0.5 mg daily.
➤ **HTN** ▓
Adults: For patients not taking a diuretic, initially 2 mg PO for a patient who is Black and 1 mg PO for all other patients, once daily. If control isn't adequate, increase dosage at intervals of at least 1 week. Maintenance doses for most patients: 2 to 4 mg daily. Some patients taking once-daily doses of 4 mg may need b.i.d. doses. For patients also taking a diuretic, initially, 0.5 mg PO once daily. Subsequent dosage adjustment is based on BP response.
➤ **HF or left ventricular dysfunction after MI**
Adults: Initially, 1 mg PO daily, adjusted to 4 mg PO daily. If patient can't tolerate 4 mg, continue at highest tolerated dose.

treprostinil
tra-PROS-tin-ill

Remodulin, Tyvaso

treprostinil diolamine
Orenitram

Therapeutic class: Antihypertensives
Pharmacologic class: Vasodilators

AVAILABLE FORMS
Injection: 1 mg/mL, 2.5 mg/mL, 5 mg/mL, 10 mg/mL in 20-mL vials
Powder for inhalation: 16 mcg, 32 mcg, 48 mcg, 64 mcg single-dose cartridges
Solution for inhalation: 1.74 mg/2.9 mL ampule
Tablets (extended-release): 0.125 mg, 0.25 mg, 1 mg, 2.5 mg, 5 mg

INDICATIONS & DOSAGES
➤ **To reduce symptoms caused by exercise in patients with NYHA Class II to IV PAH**
Adults: Initially, 1.25 nanograms/kg/minute by continuous subcut infusion. If patient doesn't tolerate initial dose, reduce infusion rate to 0.625 nanogram/kg/minute. Increase by 1.25 nanograms/kg/minute each week for the first 4 weeks and then by no more than

2.5 nanograms/kg/minute each week for the remaining duration of infusion. Experience with treprostinil dosages exceeding 40 nanograms/kg/minute is limited. May be given IV through a central venous catheter if subcut route isn't tolerated.
Adjust-a-dose: For patients with mild or moderate hepatic insufficiency, initially, 0.625 nanogram/kg ideal body weight/minute, and increase cautiously.
➤ **To decrease rate of clinical deterioration in patients with NYHA Class II to IV PAH requiring transition from Flolan (epoprostenol sodium)**
Adults: Start treprostinil subcut or IV infusion at 10% of the current IV epoprostenol dose; increase dose as the epoprostenol dose is reduced. Decrease epoprostenol dose in 20% increments and increase treprostinil in 20% increments, always maintaining a total dose of 110% of epoprostenol starting dose. Once epoprostenol is at 20% of starting dose and treprostinil is at 90%, decrease epoprostenol to 5% and increase treprostinil to 110%. Finally, stop epoprostenol and maintain treprostinil dose at 110% of epoprostenol starting dose plus an additional 5% to 10% as needed. Change rate based on individual patient response. Treat worsening of PAH symptoms with increases in treprostinil dose. Treat adverse effects associated with prostacyclin and prostacyclin analogues with decreases in epoprostenol dose.
➤ **PAH in patients with WHO Group I signs and symptoms to improve exercise capacity**
Adults: 0.25 mg PO every 12 hours or 0.125 mg PO every 8 hours. May increase in increments of 0.25 or 0.5 mg every 12 hours or 0.125 mg every 8 hours every 3 to 4 days as tolerated to achieve optimal clinical response. If incremental increases aren't tolerated, consider slower titration. Maximum dose is determined by tolerability. If patient is taking strong CYP2C8 inhibitors, initiate at 0.125 mg PO every 12 hours; increase in increments of 0.125 mg every 12 hours every 3 to 4 days.

For solution inhalation: Initially, 18 mcg (3 inhalations) q.i.d. every 4 hours while patient is awake; if 3 inhalations aren't tolerated, reduce to 1 or 2 inhalations, then increase to 3 inhalations as tolerated. For maintenance, increase each dose by 3 inhalations at approximately 1- to 2-week intervals; target and maximum dose is 54 mcg (9 inhalations) q.i.d.

For powder inhalation: Initially, 16 mcg (1 inhalation) q.i.d. May increase by 16 mcg per treatment every 1 to 2 weeks as tolerated. Target maintenance dose is 48 to 64 mcg per session.

To transition from subcut or IV to PO administration, refer to manufacturer's instructions.
Adjust-a-dose: If intolerable adverse effects occur, decrease PO dose in 0.25-mg increments. To discontinue therapy, reduce dose in steps of 0.5 to 1 mg/day; avoid discontinuing drug abruptly. If patient is unable to continue oral treatment, consider a temporary infusion of subcut or IV treprostinil. For patients with mild hepatic impairment, initiate drug at 0.125 mg PO every 12 hours and increase in increments of 0.125 mg every 12 hours every 3 to 4 days.

If patient is taking strong CYP2C8 inhibitors, initiate at 0.125 mg PO every 12 hours; increase in increments of 0.125 mg every 12 hours every 3 to 4 days.

➤ **PAH associated with ILD in patients (WHO Group 3) to improve exercise ability**

Adults: For solution inhalation: Initially, 3 breaths (18 mcg) per treatment session q.i.d., approximately 4 hours apart. Increase by 3 breaths in 1- to 2-week intervals, as tolerated, to target maintenance dose of 9 breaths (54 mcg) q.i.d. If 3 breaths aren't tolerated initially, decrease to 1 or 2 breaths and increase as tolerated.

For powder inhalation: Initially, 16 mcg (1 inhalation) q.i.d. May increase by 16 mcg per treatment every 1 to 2 weeks as tolerated. Target maintenance dose is 48 to 64 mcg per session.

---

triclabendazole
tri-kla-BEN-da-zole

Egaten

Therapeutic class: Anthelmintics
Pharmacologic class: Anthelmintics

AVAILABLE FORMS
Tablets: 250 mg

INDICATIONS & DOSAGES
➤ **Fascioliasis**
Adults and children age 6 and older: 10 mg/kg PO every 12 hours for two doses.

---

trifarotene
trye-FAR-oh-teen

Aklief

Therapeutic class: Antiacne drugs
Pharmacologic class: Retinoids

AVAILABLE FORMS
Cream: 0.005%

INDICATIONS & DOSAGES
➤ **Acne vulgaris**
Adults and children age 9 and older: Apply a thin layer to affected areas of face or trunk once daily in the evening on clean and dry skin.

SAFETY ALERT!

---

trifluridine–tipiracil hydrochloride
trye-FLURE-i-deen/tye-PIR-a-sil

Lonsurf

Therapeutic class: Antineoplastics
Pharmacologic class: Pyrimidine analogues

AVAILABLE FORMS
Tablets: 15 mg trifluridine/6.14 mg tipiracil, 20 mg trifluridine/8.19 mg tipiracil

INDICATIONS & DOSAGES
Adjust-a-dose (for all indications): Refer to manufacturer's instructions for dosage adjustments for hematologic and nonhematologic toxicities.

➤ **Metastatic colorectal cancer in patients previously treated with fluoropyrimidine-, oxaliplatin-, and irinotecan-based chemotherapy, an antivascular endothelial growth factor biological therapy and, if RAS wild-type, an anti-epidermal growth factor receptor therapy**

Adults: 35 mg/m² (based on the trifluridine component) PO b.i.d. with food up to a maximum of 80 mg/dose (based on trifluridine component) on days 1 through 5 and days 8 through 12 of a 28-day cycle. Round doses to nearest 5-mg increment. Continue until disease progression or unacceptable toxicity occurs.

➤ **Metastatic gastric or gastroesophageal junction adenocarcinoma previously treated with at least two lines of chemotherapy that included a fluoropyrimidine, a platinum, either a taxane or irinotecan and, if appropriate, HER2/neu-targeted therapy**

Adults: 35 mg/m² (based on trifluridine component) PO b.i.d. with food up to a maximum of 80 mg/dose (based on trifluridine component) on days 1 through 5 and days 8 through 12 of a 28-day cycle. Round doses to nearest 5-mg increment. Continue until disease progression or unacceptable toxicity occurs.

SAFETY ALERT!

---

trilaciclib
trye-la-SYE-klib

Cosela

Therapeutic class: Antineoplastics
Pharmacologic class: Kinase inhibitors

AVAILABLE FORMS
Injection: 300 mg single-dose vial

INDICATIONS & DOSAGES
➤ **To decrease incidence of chemotherapy-induced myelosuppression when administered before platinum/etoposide-containing regimen or topotecan-containing regimen for extensive-stage small cell lung cancer**

Adults: 240 mg/m² IV infusion over 30 minutes completed within 4 hours before start of chemotherapy on each day of chemotherapy. If given on sequential days, interval between trilaciclib doses shouldn't be greater than 28 hours.
Adjust-a-dose: Refer to manufacturer's instructions for toxicity-related dosage adjustments.

---

trimethobenzamide hydrochloride
trye-meth-oh-BEN-za-mide

Tigan

Therapeutic class: Antiemetics
Pharmacologic class: Anticholinergics

AVAILABLE FORMS
Capsules: 300 mg
Injection: 100 mg/mL

INDICATIONS & DOSAGES
➤ **Postoperative nausea and vomiting; nausea associated with gastroenteritis**
Adults: 300 mg PO or 200 mg IM t.i.d. or q.i.d.

Adjust-a-dose: Dosage reduction or increased dosing interval is recommended in older adults and patients with renal impairment (CrCl of 70 mL/minute/1.73 m²).

triptorelin pamoate
trip-toe-REL-in

Trelstar Mixject, Triptodur

Therapeutic class: Hormone analogues
Pharmacologic class: Gonadotropin releasing hormone agonists

AVAILABLE FORMS
Injectable suspension (Trelstar Mixject): 3.75 mg, 11.25 mg, 22.5 mg in Mixject single-dose delivery systems
Injectable suspension (extended-release) (Triptodur): 22.5 mg single-dose vials packaged with 2 mL of diluent sterile water for injection

INDICATIONS & DOSAGES
➤ **Palliative treatment of advanced prostate cancer (Trelstar Mixject only)**
Adults: 3.75 mg IM once every 4 weeks, or 11.25 mg IM once every 12 weeks, or 22.5 mg IM once every 24 weeks. Because of different release characteristics, dosing schedule depends on the product selected.
➤ **Central precocious puberty (Triptodur only)**
Children age 2 and older: 22.5 mg IM once every 24 weeks. Treatment should be discontinued at the appropriate age of onset of puberty at the discretion of the physician.

SAFETY ALERT!

tucatinib ⚉
too-KA-ti-nib

Tukysa

Therapeutic class: Antineoplastics
Pharmacologic class: Tyrosine kinase inhibitors

AVAILABLE FORMS
Tablets ⏺: 50 mg, 150 mg

INDICATIONS & DOSAGES
➤ **In combination with trastuzumab and capecitabine in patients with advanced unresectable or metastatic HER2-positive breast cancer, including those with brain metastases, who have received one or more prior anti-HER2-based regimens in the metastatic setting ⚉**
Adults: 300 mg PO b.i.d. approximately 12 hours apart until disease progression or unacceptable toxicity. Refer to prescribing information for trastuzumab and capecitabine for additional information.
Adjust-a-dose: For patients with severe hepatic impairment (Child-Pugh class C), reduce dosage to 200 mg b.i.d. Concomitant use of strong CYP2C8 inhibitors isn't recommended; if use can't be avoided, reduce tucatinib dosage to 100 mg b.i.d. Refer to prescribing information for toxicity-related dosage adjustments.

ubrogepant
ue-BROE-je-pant

Ubrelvy

Therapeutic class: Antimigraine drugs
Pharmacologic class: Calcitonin gene-related peptide antagonists

AVAILABLE FORMS
Tablets: 50 mg, 100 mg

INDICATIONS & DOSAGES
➤ **Acute treatment of migraine with or without aura**
Adults: 50 or 100 mg PO, as needed. May repeat once at least 2 hours after initial dose, if needed. Maximum dose, 200 mg a day.
Adjust-a-dose: For patients with severe hepatic or severe renal impairment, give 50 mg; if needed, may give a second 50-mg dose at least 2 hours after initial dose. For patients receiving moderate and weak CYP3A inhibitors, moderate and weak CYP3A4 inducers, BCRP or P-gp only inhibitors, refer to manufacturer's instructions for dosage adjustments.

upadacitinib
ue-pad-a-SYE-ti-nib

Rinvoq

Therapeutic class: Antirheumatics
Pharmacologic class: Janus kinase inhibitors

AVAILABLE FORMS
Tablets (extended release): 15 mg

INDICATIONS & DOSAGES
Boxed Warning Drug increases risk of TB and invasive fungal, bacterial, viral, and opportunistic infections. Prescreen patients for latent TB. Drug increases risk of CV events, all-cause mortality, malignancies, and thrombotic events, some resulting in death. ■
➤ **Moderate to severe active RA in patients who have had an inadequate response or intolerance to methotrexate**
Adults: 15 mg PO once daily. Drug may be used as monotherapy or in combination with methotrexate or other nonbiologic DMARDs.
Adjust-a-dose: If serious infection develops, interrupt drug until the infection is controlled. Interrupt therapy if ANC is less than 1,000 cells/mm³ or absolute lymphocyte count (ALC) is less than 500 cells/mm³ or Hb level is less than 8 g/dL. May restart drug once ANC, ALC, or Hb level returns to above this value. If hepatic transaminase levels rise and drug-induced liver injury is suspected, interrupt treatment.
✳ *NEW INDICATION:* **Psoriatic arthritis in patients with inadequate response or intolerance to one or more TNF blockers**
Adults: 15 mg PO once daily.
Adjust-a-dose: If serious infection develops, interrupt drug until infection is controlled. Interrupt therapy if ANC is less than 1,000 cells/mm³, absolute

lymphocyte count (ALC) is less than 500 cells/mm³, or Hb level is less than 8 g/dL. Restart drug once ANC, ALC, or Hb level returns to above these values. If hepatic transaminase levels rise and drug-induced liver injury is suspected, interrupt therapy.

✱ ***NEW INDICATION:*** **Refractory, moderate to severe atopic dermatitis not adequately controlled with other systemic drugs, including biologicals, or when use of those therapies is inadvisable**

Adults and children age 12 and older weighing at least 40 kg: Initially, 15 mg PO once daily. May increase to 30 mg once daily. If adequate response isn't achieved with 30-mg dose, stop therapy. Use lowest effective dose needed to maintain response.

Adjust-a-dose: In older adults or patients with severe renal impairment (CrCl less than 30 mL/minute), give 15 mg once daily. If used concomitantly with strong CYP3A4 inhibitors, give 15 mg once daily. Not recommended for patients with severe hepatic impairment.

✱ ***NEW INDICATION:*** **Moderate to severe ulcerative colitis after inadequate response or intolerance to one or more TNF blockers**

Adults: 45 mg PO once daily for 8 weeks, followed by maintenance dose of 15 mg once daily. May increase maintenance dose to 30 mg once daily for patients with refractory, severe, or extensive disease. If patient response to 30-mg dose is inadequate, discontinue drug. Use lowest effective dose needed to maintain response.

Adjust-a-dose: If patient has severe renal impairment (eGFR of 15 to 29 m/L/minute/1.73m²) or mild to moderate hepatic impairment (Child-Pugh class A or B) or is taking a strong CYP3A4 inhibitor, give induction dose, 30 mg once daily for 8 weeks; then maintenance dose, 15 mg once daily.

✱ ***NEW INDICATION:*** **Ankylosing spondylitis after an inadequate response or intolerance to one or more TNF blockers**

Adults: 15 mg PO once daily.

Adjust-a-dose: If serious infection develops, interrupt therapy until infection is controlled. Interrupt therapy if ANC is less than 1,000 cells/mm³, ALC is less than 500 cells/mm³, or Hb level is less than 8 g/dL. May restart drug once ANC, ALC, or Hb level returns to above these values. If hepatic transaminase levels rise and drug-induced liver injury i suspected, interrupt therapy.

uridine triacetate ⧖

URE-i-deen

Vistogard, Xuriden

Therapeutic class: Replacement enzymes
Pharmacologic class: Uridine replacements

AVAILABLE FORMS

Oral granules (DNC): 2-g, 10-g single-use packets

INDICATIONS & DOSAGES

➤ **Hereditary orotic aciduria (Xuriden)** ⧖

Adults and children: 60 mg/kg PO daily; may increase to 120 mg/kg daily for insufficient efficacy. Maximum dose is 8 g/day. See manufacturer's instructions for weight-based dosing tables.

➤ **Fluoropyrimidine overdose (emergency treatment of 5-FU or capecitabine overdose; or early-onset severe or life-threatening cardiac or CNS toxicity; or early-onset, unusually severe adverse reactions [e.g., GI toxicity or neutropenia] within 96 hours after end of 5-FU or capecitabine administration) (Vistogard)**

Adults: 10 g PO every 6 hours for a total of 20 doses beginning as soon as possible after overdose or early-onset toxicity within 96 hours after end of 5-FU or capecitabine administration. Maximum, 10 g/dose.

Children: 6.2 g/m² PO not to exceed 10 g/dose every 6 hours for 20 doses beginning as soon as possible after overdose or early-onset toxicity within 96 hours after end of 5-FU or capecitabine administration. Refer to manufacturer's information for weight-based dosing tables.

valbenazine ⧖

val-BEN-a-zeen

Ingrezza

Therapeutic class: Neuromuscular transmission blockers
Pharmacologic class: Vesicular monoamine transporter 2 inhibitors

AVAILABLE FORMS

Capsules: 40 mg, 60 mg, 80 mg

INDICATIONS & DOSAGES

➤ **Tardive dyskinesia**

Adults: Initially, 40 mg PO once daily for 1 week, then 80 mg once daily; for some patients, 40 or 60 mg once daily may be appropriate.

⧖ ***Adjust-a-dose:*** For moderate to severe hepatic impairment (Child-Pugh score 7 to 15) or when drug is administered with a strong CYP3A4 inhibitor, give 40 mg once daily. If drug is administered with a strong CYP2D6 inhibitor, or for patients who are known poor metabolizers of CYP2D6, consider a dosage reduction.

valGANciclovir hydrochloride

val-gan-SYE-kloe-veer

Valcyte

Therapeutic class: Antivirals
Pharmacologic class: Nucleosides—nucleotides

AVAILABLE FORMS

Oral solution: 50 mg/mL

Tablets (DNC): 450 mg

INDICATIONS & DOSAGES

Boxed Warning Drug can cause severe bone marrow suppression and suppression of fertility in both males and females. Animal data suggest fetal harm and potential carcinogenic effects in humans. ■

Adjust-a-dose (for all indications): For adults with CrCl of 40 to 59 mL/minute, induction dosage is 450 mg b.i.d.; maintenance dosage is 450 mg daily. If CrCl is 25 to 39 mL/minute, induction dosage is 450 mg daily; maintenance dosage is 450 mg every

2 days. If CrCl is 10 to 24 mL/minute, induction dosage is 450 mg every 2 days; maintenance dosage is 450 mg twice weekly. Drug isn't recommended for patients with CrCl of less than 10 mL/minute.

➤ **To prevent CMV disease in heart, kidney, and kidney-pancreas transplantation in patients at high risk (donor CMV-seropositive or recipient CMV-seronegative)**

Adults: For patients with a heart or kidney-pancreas transplant, 900 mg PO once daily starting within 10 days of transplantation until 100 days post-transplantation. For patients with a kidney transplant, 900 mg PO daily starting within 10 days of transplantation until 200 days post-transplantation.

➤ **To prevent CMV disease in children with kidney transplant who are at high risk**

Children age 4 months to 16 years: Give dose once daily starting within 10 days of transplantation until 200 days post-transplantation of kidney, based on BSA and CrCl (modified Schwartz formula):

$$\text{Dose (mg)} = 7 \times \text{BSA} \times \text{CrCl}$$

Adjust-a-dose: For children, maximum calculated CrCl (modified Schwartz formula) to be used is 150 mL/minute/1.73 m², even if the calculated value is greater. The maximum pediatric dose is 900 mg, even if the calculated dose is greater.

➤ **To prevent CMV disease in children with heart transplant who are at high risk**

Children ages 1 month to 16 years: Give dose once daily starting within 10 days of transplantation until 100 days posttransplantation of heart, based on BSA and CrCl (modified Schwartz formula):

$$\text{Dose (mg)} = 7 \times \text{BSA} \times \text{CrCl}$$

Maximum dose is 900 mg once daily.

➤ **CMV retinitis in patients with AIDS**

Adults: For active disease, give 900 mg PO b.i.d. for 21 days; maintenance dose is 900 mg PO daily. For inactive disease, give 900 mg PO once daily.

SAFETY ALERT!

vandetanib
van-DET-a-nib

Caprelsa

Therapeutic class: Antineoplastics
Pharmacologic class: Kinase inhibitors

AVAILABLE FORMS
Tablets: 100 mg, 300 mg

INDICATIONS & DOSAGES
Boxed Warning May prolong QTc interval and increase risk of fatal ventricular arrhythmias. ∎

➤ **Symptomatic or progressive medullary thyroid cancer in patients with unresectable locally advanced or metastatic disease**

Adults: 300 mg PO daily until disease progression or unacceptable toxicity occurs.

Adjust-a-dose: In patients with moderate renal impairment (CrCl of 30 to less than 50 mL/minute), initiate therapy at 200 mg PO daily. Refer to manufacturer's instructions for toxicity-related dosage adjustment.

vedolizumab
ve-doe-LIZ-ue-mab

Entyvio

Therapeutic class: Immune response modifiers
Pharmacologic class: Humanized IgG1 monoclonal antibodies

AVAILABLE FORMS
Injection: 300 mg single-use vials

INDICATIONS & DOSAGES
➤ **Moderate to severe Crohn disease or ulcerative colitis**

Adults: 300 mg IV infusion over 30 minutes, administered at weeks 0, 2, and 6, then every 8 weeks thereafter. Discontinue use if no evidence of therapeutic benefit by week 14.

SAFETY ALERT!

vemurafenib ▨
vem-ue-RAF-e-nib

Zelboraf

Therapeutic class: Antineoplastics
Pharmacologic class: Kinase inhibitors

AVAILABLE FORMS
Tablets ⓜ: 240 mg

INDICATIONS & DOSAGES
➤ **Unresectable or metastatic melanoma with *BRAF* V600E mutation; Erdheim-Chester disease with *BRAF* V600 mutation** ▨

Adults: 960 mg PO every 12 hours. Continue until disease progression or unacceptable toxicity occurs.

Adjust-a-dose: Avoid concomitant use of strong CYP3A4 inducers. If use together is unavoidable, increase vemurafenib dosage by 240 mg (1 tablet) as tolerated. After discontinuation of a strong CYP3A4 inducer for 2 weeks, resume prior vemurafenib dosage. Refer to manufacturer's instructions for toxicity-related dosage adjustments.

SAFETY ALERT!

voclosporin
vok-loe-SPOR-in

Lupkynis

Therapeutic class: Immunomodulators
Pharmacologic class: Calcineurin inhibitors

AVAILABLE FORMS
Capsules ⓜ: 7.9 mg

INDICATIONS & DOSAGES
➤ **Active lupus nephritis in combination with a background immunosuppressive therapy regimen**

Adults: 23.7 mg PO b.i.d. in combination with mycophenolate mofetil and corticosteroids.

Adjust-a-dose: If eGFR is less than 60 mL/minute/1.73 m² and reduced from baseline by more than 20% and less than 30%, reduce dosage by 7.9 mg b.i.d.; if eGFR is still reduced from baseline by more than 20% within 2 weeks, reduce dosage again by 7.9 mg b.i.d. If eGFR is less than 60 mL/minute/1.73 m² and reduced from baseline by 30% or more, discontinue drug. Consider restarting at 7.9 mg b.i.d. only if eGFR has returned to 80% or more of baseline within 2 weeks.

If a dosage decrease due to eGFR was made, consider increasing dosage by 7.9 mg b.i.d. for each eGFR measurement that is 80% or more of baseline; don't exceed starting dose. Avoid use in patients with baseline eGFR less than 45 mL/minute/1.73 m² unless benefit exceeds risk.

If used in patients with severe renal impairment at baseline, give 15.8 mg b.i.d. For patients with mild and moderate hepatic impairment (Child-Pugh class A and B), give 15.8 mg b.i.d. If concomitantly used with moderate CYP3A4 inhibitors, give 15.8 mg in the morning and 7.9 mg in the evening.

voxelotor
vox-EL-oh-tor

Oxbryta

Therapeutic class: Miscellaneous hematologic drugs
Pharmacologic class: Hemoglobin S polymerization inhibitors

AVAILABLE FORMS
Tablets ⓓ: 500 mg
Tablets for suspension: 300 mg

INDICATIONS & DOSAGES
➤ **Sickle cell disease**
Adults and children age 12 and older: 1,500 mg PO once daily, with or without hydroxyurea.
Children age 4 to younger than 12 weighing 40 kg or more: 1,500 mg PO once daily, with or without hydroxyurea.
Children age 4 to younger than 12 weighing 20 to less than 40 kg: 900 mg PO once daily, with or without hydroxyurea.
Children age 4 to younger than 12 weighing 10 to less than 20 kg: 600 mg PO once daily, with or without hydroxyurea.
Adjust-a-dose: For adults and children age 12 and older with severe hepatic impairment (Child-Pugh class C), reduce dosage to 1,000 mg PO once daily. For adults and children age 12 and older currently receiving a strong CYP3A4 inhibitor or fluconazole, decrease dosage to 1,000 mg PO once daily. For adults and children age 12 and older currently receiving a strong or moderate CYP3A4 inducer, increase dosage to 2,500 mg PO once daily.

For children age 4 to younger than 12 with severe hepatic impairment (Child-Pugh class C), reduce dosage based on body weight: If 40 kg or more, give 1,000 mg (two 500-mg tablets) or 900 mg (three 300-mg tablets for oral suspension) daily; if 20 to less than 40 kg, give 600 mg daily; if 10 to less than 20 kg, give 300 mg daily.

For children age 4 to younger than 12 currently receiving a strong or moderate CYP3A4 inducer, see manufacturer's instructions for dosage adjustment based on weight.

zanamivir
zan-AM-ah-veer

Relenza Diskhaler

Therapeutic class: Antiretrovirals
Pharmacologic class: Selective neuraminidase inhibitors

AVAILABLE FORMS
Powder for inhalation: 5 mg/blister

INDICATIONS & DOSAGES
➤ **Uncomplicated acute illness caused by influenza virus A and B in patients who have had symptoms for no longer than 2 days**
Adults and children age 7 and older: 2 oral inhalations (one 5-mg blister per inhalation for total dose of 10 mg) b.i.d. using the dry-powder inhalation device for 5 days. Give two doses on first day of treatment, allowing at least 2 hours to elapse between doses. Give subsequent doses about 12 hours apart (in the morning and evening) at about the same time each day. Some guidelines suggest that longer treatment duration may be considered in patients who remain severely ill after 5 days.
➤ **Prevention of influenza in a household setting**
Adults and children age 5 and older: 2 oral inhalations (one 5-mg blister per inhalation for total dose of 10 mg) once daily for 10 days.
➤ **Prevention of influenza in a community setting**
Adults and adolescents ages 12 to 16: 2 oral inhalations (one 5-mg blister per inhalation for total dose of 10 mg) once daily for 28 days.

SAFETY ALERT!

zanubrutinib
zan-ue-BROO-ti-nib

Brukinsa

Therapeutic class: Antineoplastic agents
Pharmacologic class: Tyrosine kinase inhibitors

AVAILABLE FORMS
Capsules ⓓ: 80 mg

INDICATIONS & DOSAGES
➤ **Mantle cell lymphoma in patients who have received at least one prior therapy; Waldenström macroglobulinemia; marginal zone lymphoma**
Adults: 160 mg PO b.i.d. or 320 mg PO once daily. Continue treatment until disease progression or unacceptable toxicity occurs.
Adjust-a-dose: For patients with severe hepatic impairment (Child-Pugh class C), reduce dosage to 80 mg PO b.i.d. If given with strong CYP3A inhibitor, decrease dosage to 80 mg PO once daily. If given with moderate CYP3A inhibitor, decrease dosage to 80 mg PO b.i.d. After discontinuation of a CYP3A inhibitor, resume previous zanubrutinib dosage. Refer to manufacturer's instructions for toxicity-related dosage adjustments.

♣Canada   ◇ OTC   ♦ Off-label use   ✐ Photoguide   ⓓDo not crush   *Liquid contains alcohol   ▒ Genetic

SAFETY ALERT!

ziv-aflibercept
ziv-a-FLIB-er-sept

Zaltrap

Therapeutic class: Antineoplastics
Pharmacologic class: Vascular endothelial growth factor inhibitors

AVAILABLE FORMS
Injection: 100 mg/4 mL, 200 mg/8 mL in single-use vials

INDICATIONS & DOSAGES
➤ **Metastatic colorectal cancer that is resistant or has progressed after an oxaliplatin-containing regimen in combination with FOLFIRI regimen**
Adults: 4 mg/kg IV infusion over 1 hour every 2 weeks until disease progression or unacceptable toxicity occurs. Give before any component of FOLFIRI regimen on day of treatment. Continue until disease progression or unacceptable toxicity occurs.
Adjust-a-dose: Refer to manufacturer's instructions for toxicity-related dosage adjustments.

Index

Boldface refers to full color photographs.

Boldface refers to full color photographs.

Boldface refers to full color photographs.

Boldface refers to full color photographs.